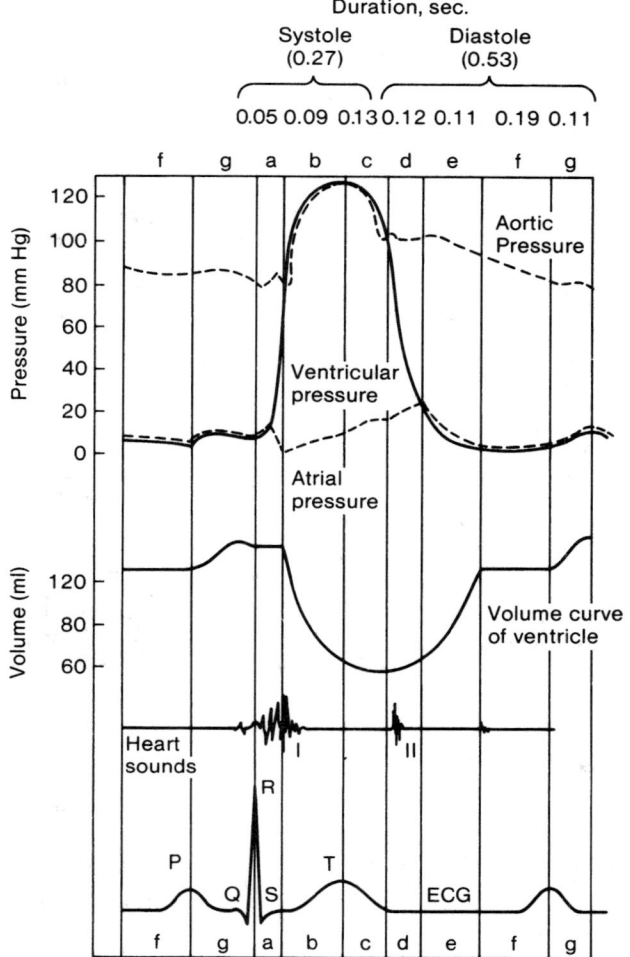

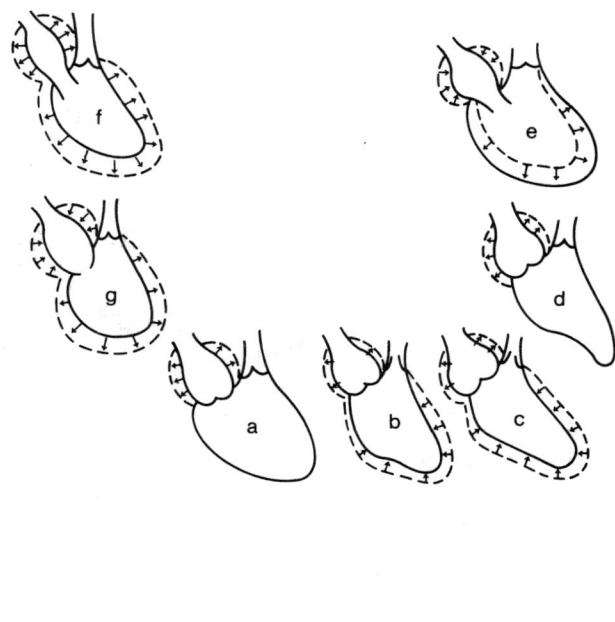

The cardiac cycle, illustrating the changes in aortic, left ventricular, and left atrial pressures, and in left ventricular volume, in relation to the phono-cardiogram and the electrocardiogram. The duration of each phase at a heart rate of approximately 75 beats/min is indicated at the top of the figure. a, isovolumetric ventricular contraction; b, rapid ventricular ejection; c, slow ventricular ejection; d, isovolumetric relaxation; e, rapid ventricular filling; f, diastasis; g, atrial contraction; I, first heart sound; II, second heart sound. Insets: Changes in the configuration of the left atrium, mitral valve, left ventricle, and aortic valve during various phases of the cycle. (Adapted from Wiggens. [1952]. *Circulatory dynamics*. New York: Grune & Stratton.)

Cardiac Nursing

5TH EDITION

HA, FAAN
Ith Systems
nic Services
of Nursing
Washington
Washington

RN, FAAN
Professor
cal Nursing
l of Nursing
idemiology
of Medicine
in Francisco
, California

RN, FAHA
ite Professor
alth Systems
l of Nursing
Washington
Washington

RN, CCNS
Commander
h Squadron
edical Wing
1 AFB, Texas

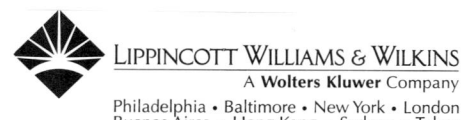

LIPPINCOTT WILLIAMS & WILKINS
A **Wolters Kluwer** Company
Philadelphia • Baltimore • New York • London
Buenos Aires • Hong Kong • Sydney • Tokyo

Acquisitions Editor: Patricia Casey
Editorial Assistant: Dana Irwin
Senior Production Editor: Tom Gibbons
Director of Nursing Production: Helen Ewan
Managing Editor/Production: Erika Kors
Design Coordinator: Brett MacNaughton
Cover Designer: Deborah Lynam
Interior Designer: Joan Wendt
Senior Manufacturing Manager: William Alberti
Indexer: Ann Cassar
Compositor: TechBooks
Printer: Courier-Westford

5th Edition

9 8 7 6 5 4 3 2 1

Library of Congress Cataloging-in-Publication Data
Cardiac nursing / [edited by] Susan L. Woods . . . [et al.]. — 5th ed.
    p. ; cm.
    Includes bibliographical references and index.
    ISBN 0-7817-4718-X (hardcover : alk. paper)
        1. Heart—Diseases—Nursing.   I. Woods, Susan L.
    [DNLM: 1. Heart Diseases—nursing. 2. Heart Diseases—prevention & control—Nurses' Instruction.
WY 152.5 C2672 2005]
    RC674.C3 2005
    616.1′20231—dc22
                                                                        2004010830

LWW.com

Dedication

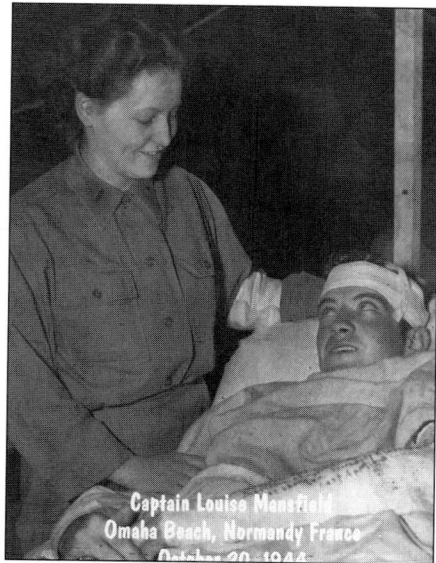

Captain Louise Mansfield
Omaha Beach, Normandy France

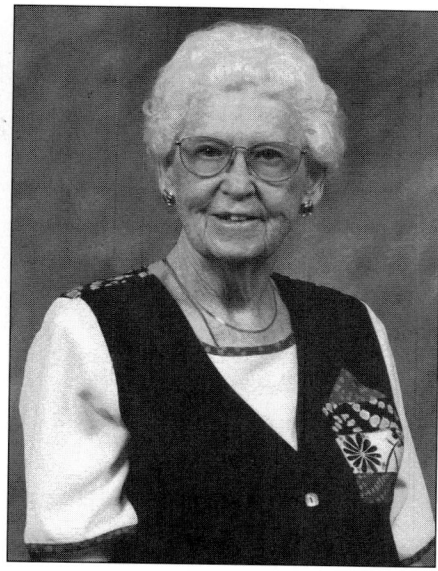

The photo on the left of Susie caring for a wounded soldier at Normandy was used on the cover of the *American Journal of Nursing*, 45(5), May 1945. The more recent photo on the right is how many of us remember her.

This fifth edition of *Cardiac Nursing* is dedicated to the memory of Louise "Susie" Wasson Mansfield, R.N., M.A., Professor of Nursing, Emeritus, University of Washington. Susie played a major role in the professional careers of the editors: Sue, Sandy, and Erika, and indirectly in the career of Liz. Additionally, she influenced the careers of many of our contributors throughout the five editions. Susie inspired, guided, and supported us in the first edition of *Cardiac Nursing*, published in 1982. The second edition was dedicated to her.

Susie was an extraordinary mentor, teacher, researcher, nurse, and friend. As our way of honoring Susie, we want to tell you something about her life. Susie was born February 19, 1916 in Blountsville, Indiana, and died on October 19, 2003 in Seattle, Washington. In 1937 she graduated from Samaritan Hospital School of Nursing, Nampa, Idaho, with her diploma in nursing. She obtained a Bachelor of Science in Education cum laude in 1947 from Ohio State University. She received her Master of Arts degree from Columbia University Teachers College, New York, New York, with a major in nursing education, in 1951. She continued post-master's study at Columbia during 1951, but rather than completing her doctorate, she married Glen Mansfield and raised five children. From 1959 to 1962 she studied physiology and related fields at the University of Washington.

Susie was a staff nurse and head nurse at Harborview Hospital, Seattle, Washington, from 1938 to 1942, when she joined the U.S. Army Nurse Corps and remained on active duty until 1946. During World War II, she was stationed with the 50th General Field Hospital at Normandy Beach, landing with the fifth wave of infantry. Additionally, she served at a field hospital in Glasgow, Scotland. She cared for many of the D-Day casualties as they were processed on their way back home. She retired from the U.S. Army Reserves as a Major in 1965. She entered academia as an instructor of surgical nursing at University of Oregon Medical School, Department of Nursing, Portland, Oregon. In 1951, she joined the faculty at the University of Washington School of Nursing, Seattle, where she retired as Emeritus Professor in 1979.

Susie devoted her life to the profession of nursing and made a vital contribution to the field of cardiovascular nursing. She set a standard of excellence for nursing practice, education, and research. She shared her knowledge in the classroom as a professor at the University of Washington, School of Nursing. Susie was a past chairperson of the American Heart Association Council on Cardiovascular Nursing and editor of its scientific publication, *Cardiovascular Nursing*, and she pioneered the introduction of nursing research presentations at the Annual Scientific Sessions of the American Heart Association. She was honored for her vast contributions with the American Heart Association's Gold Heart Award, bestowed to only the most outstanding and deserving volunteers. From 1977 to 1979, Susie led a U.S.P.H.S. grant, "Controlled study of earlier cardiac rehabilitation," with cardiologist Robert A. Bruce at a time when persons following acute myocardial infarction were kept at strict bedrest for extended periods. Her legacy continues to inspire cardiovascular nurses and teachers around the world.

Susie and Glen Mansfield were married for 45 years. Her sincere caring for others sets an example for us all. The Louise "Susie" Mansfield Endowed Scholarship at the University of Washington School of Nursing has been established for the education of future cardiovascular graduate nursing students. Her presence is missed.

Contributors

Bradley E. Aouizerat, BS, PhD
Assistant Professor
Department of Physiological Nursing
School of Nursing
University of California San Francisco
San Francisco, California

Gaylene Altman, MN, PhD, RN
Assistant Professor
Department of Biobehavioral Nursing and Health Systems
School of Nursing
University of Washington
Seattle, Washington

Kathy Berra, MSN, NP, FAAN
Clinical Trial Director
Stanford Center for Research in Disease Prevention
Stanford Medical School
Palo Alto, California

Susan Jean Blancher, MN, ARNP
Electrophysiology Nurse Practitioner
Cardiology Department
Virginia Mason Medical Center
Seattle, Washington

Eleanor F. Bond, BSN, MA, PhD, FAAN
Professor
Department of Biobehavioral Nursing and Health Systems
School of Nursing
University of Washington
Seattle, Washington

Lora E. Burke, PhD, MPH, RN
Associate Professor of Nursing and Epidemiology
University of Pittsburgh
Health and Community Systems
Pittsburgh, Pennsylvania

Robert L. Burr, MSEE, PhD
Research Associate Professor
Department of Biobehavioral Nursing and Health Systems
School of Nursing
University of Washington
Seattle, Washington

Mary M. Canobbio, MN, RN, FAAN
Lecturer,
School of Nursing
University of California, Los Angeles
Administrative Coordinator for Research, Clinical Program and
  Fund Development
Ahmanson-UCLA Adult Congenital Heart Disease Center
Los Angeles, California

Meghan A. Cartwright, MA, RD
Research Associate
Health and Community Systems
School of Nursing
University of Pittsburgh
Pittsburgh, Pennsylvania

Ruth F. Craven, EdD, RN, BC, FAAN
Professor
Department of Biobehavioral Nursing and Health Systems
Associate Dean
Educational Outreach and Community Relations
School of Nursing
University of Washington
Seattle, Washington

Susanna Garner Cunningham, BScN, MA, PhD
Professor
Department of Biobehavioral Nursing and Health Systems
School of Nursing
University of Washington
Seattle, Washington

Michaelene Hargrove Deelstra, MSN, ARNP
Cardiology/Acute Care Nurse Practitioner
Summit Cardiology/Swedish Physician Division
Clinical Instructor
Department of Biobehavioral Nursing and Health Systems
School of Nursing
University of Washington
Seattle, Washington

Sherri Del Bene, MN, RN, CNAA, BC
Director, Patient Care Services
University of Washington Medical Center
Clinical Instructor
Department of Biobehavioral Nursing and Health Systems
School of Nursing
University of Washington
Seattle, Washington

Sandra B. Dunbar, RN, DSN, FAAN
Charles Howard Candler Professor
Nell Hodgson Woodruff School of Nursing

Emory University
Atlanta, Georgia

Joan M. Fair, RN, ANP, PhD
Research Project Director
Stanford Research Prevention Center
School of Medicine
Stanford University
Stanford, California

Linda Felver, PhD, RN
Associate Professor
School of Nursing
Oregon Health & Science University
Portland, Oregon

Polly Gardner, MN, ARNP, ACNP
Cardiology Nurse Practitioner
Overlake Internal Medicine, Cardiology
Bellevue, Washington
Clinical Instructor
Department of Biobehavioral Nursing and Health Systems
School of Nursing
University of Washington
Seattle, Washington

Donna Gerity, MN, RN
Clinical Nurse Specialist
Minor & James Medical Cardiology Department
Staff Nurse
Electrophysiology Lab
Swedish Medical Center
Seattle, Washington

Margaret Hall, MD
Cardiologist
Summit Cardiology
Seattle, Washington

Margaret Hanrahan, MN, ARNP
Nurse Practitioner, Cardiology
Harborview Medical Center
Seattle, Washington

Margaret Heitkemper, PhD, RN, FAAN
Professor and Chair
Department of Biobehavioral Nursing and Health Systems
School of Nursing
Corbally Professor for Public Service
University of Washington
Seattle, Washington

Jon Huseby, MD
Internal Medicine, Pulmonary and Critical Care Medicine
Polyclinic
Swedish Hospital Providence Campus

Clinical Professor of Pulmonary and Critical Care Medicine
School of Medicine
University of Washington
Seattle, Washington

Carol Jacobson, MN, RN
Swedish Medical Center
Clinical Instructor
Department of Biobehavioral Nursing and Health Systems
School of Nursing
University of Washington
Director
Quality Education Services
Seattle, Washington

Debra Laurent, MN, ARNP, ACNP
Cardiology Acute Care Nurse Practitioner
Seattle Heart Clinic
Swedish Heart Institute
Clinical Assistant Professor
Department of Biobehavioral Nursing and Health Systems
School of Nursing
University of Washington
Seattle, Washington

Denise LeDoux, MN, ARNP, ACNP
Teaching Associate
Cardiac Surgery
Department of Surgery
University of Washington
Doctoral Student
School of Nursing
University of Washington
Seattle, Washington

Barbara S. Levine, PhD, CRNP
Nurse Practitioner
Cardiovascular Healthcare Consultants, P.C.
Paoli, Pennsylvania

Helen Luikart, MS, RN
Clinical Research Coordinator/Transplant Coordinator
Division of Cardiovascular Medicine
Stanford University Medical Center
Stanford, California

Simone K. Madan, PhD
Assistant Clinical Professor
Department of Medicine
University of California San Francisco
San Francisco, California

Kirsten Martin, MS, RN
Nursing Faculty
Los Medanos College
Pittsburg, California

Diana E. McMillan, PhD, RN
Assistant Professor
Faculty of Nursing
University of Manitoba
Winnipeg, Manitoba, Canada

Lt. Col. Margaret M. McNeill, BSN, MS, CCRN, CAN, CCNS
Chief Nurse/Deputy Commander
Air Force Center for Sustainment of Trauma and Readiness Skills
Shock Trauma Center
University of Maryland Medical System
Baltimore, Maryland

Nancy Houston Miller, BSN, RN
Associate Director
Stanford Cardiac Rehabilitation Program
Stanford University
Palo Alto, California

Nancy Munro, MN, CCRN, ACNP
Cardiovascular/Thoracic Services
INOVA Alexandria Hospital
Alexandria, Virginia
Clinical Instructor, ACNP Program
University of Maryland School of Nursing
Baltimore, Maryland

Jonathan Myers, PhD
Health Research Scientist
Cardiology Division
Palo Alto VA Health Care System
Clinical Associate Professor of Medicine
Stanford University
Palo Alto, California

Katherine M. Newton, PhD, RN
Associate Investigator
Center for Health Studies
Group Health Cooperative
Affiliate Assistant Professor
Department of Biobehavioral Nursing and Health Systems
School of Nursing
Department of Epidemiology
School of Public Health
University of Washington
Seattle, Washington

Martha Nolte, MD
Medical Director
University of California San Francisco
Diabetes Teaching Center
San Francisco, California

Kathy P. Parker, PhD, RN, FAAN
Edith F. Honeycutt Professor
Nell Hodgson Woodruff School of Nursing
Emory University
Atlanta, Georgia

Therese A. Polakoski, MS, HFI

Susan L. Reed, MN, ARNP, CCRN
Cardiology Nurse Practitioner
Seattle Heart Clinic
Seattle, Washington

Joseph O. Schmelz, PhD, RN, CIP
Research Administrator
Wilford Hall Medical Center
Lackland AFB
San Antonio, Texas

Julie A. Shinn, MA, RN, CCRN, FAAN
Cardiovascular Clinical Nurse Specialist
Patient Care Services
Stanford University Medical Center
Stanford, California
Clinical Associate Professor
University of California, San Francisco
School of Nursing
San Francisco, California

Laurie Soine, MN, ARNP, ACNP
Nurse Practitioner, Nuclear Cardiology
Teaching Associate
Department of Radiology
University of Washington Medical Center
Clinical Instructor
Department of Biobehavioral Nursing and Health Systems
School of Nursing
University of Washington
Seattle, Washington

Dorothy L. Tschirpke, BSN, RN

Anne T. Falsone Vaughan, MSN, RN
Clinical Instructor
Medical Surgical and Critical Care Nursing
Bellarmine University
Louisville, Kentucky

Margaret I. Wallhagen, PhD, RN, CS, GNP
Associate Professor
Department of Physiological Nursing
University of California San Francisco
School of Nursing
San Francisco, California

Reviewers

About the Editors

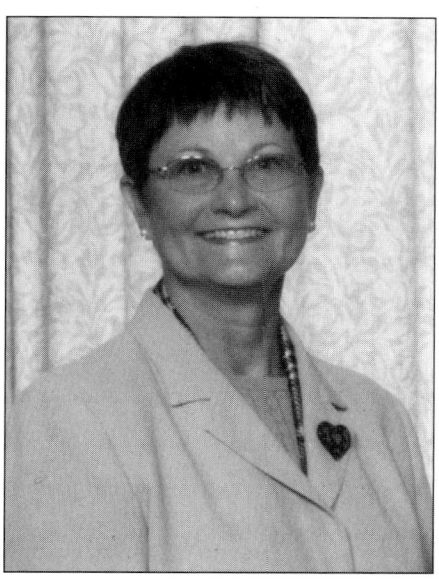

Susan L. Woods, PhD, RN, FAHA, FAAN

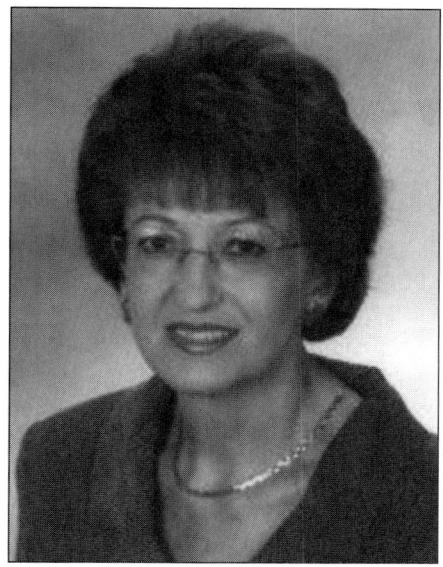

Erika Sivarajan Froelicher, RN, MA, MPH, PhD, FAAN

Susan has been on the faculty at the University of Washington School of Nursing since 1975, where she has taught both undergraduate and graduate courses. She is currently Professor of Biobehavioral Nursing and Health Systems and the Associate Dean for Academic Services in the School of Nursing. Her clinical and research focus is in all aspects of cardiac nursing, particularly in measurement of cardiovascular variables and chronobiology. Susan was a founding board member of the Commission on Collegiate Nursing Education (CCNE) and is a current member of the CCNE Accreditation Review Committee. She has been the recipient of the Distinguished Research Award from the American Association of Critical Care Nursing and the Katherine Lembright Award from the American Heart Association Council on Cardiovascular Nursing. Susan has also received the Alumni All-Around Award from Oregon Health Science University, where she obtained a PhD in Nursing. She is a fellow in the American Academy of Nursing and the American Heart Association. Susan has two children, Jaime Rose Navetta and Jennifer Mary Woods, and is married to Jim Woods. She enjoys traveling, gardening, swimming, and collecting shells.

Erika has advanced degrees in nursing, public health, and epidemiology. During more than 30 years of nursing and public health experience, she has been an emergency room nurse, a psychiatric nurse, a center director, a researcher, an epidemiologist, and a university professor. As a consultant, she has advised hospitals, businesses, and foundations in the areas of nursing and cardiac care. Currently, she serves on the editorial board of *Heart and Lung, Human Kinetics, Cardiovascular Nursing,* and *European Journal for Cardiovascular Nursing* and is both a Founding and Associate Editor for *Journal of Cardiovascular and Pulmonary Rehabilitation* as well as having reviewed for many other medical and nursing journals.

Erika has presented papers and given invited lectures on coronary disease prevention and rehabilitation to more than 100 national and international groups. Her articles and abstracts have appeared in such publications as *New England Journal of Medicine, Circulation, Heart and Lung, American Journal of Nursing, Advanced Journal for Nursing Scholarship, Patient Education and Counseling,* and *Circulation.* As coauthor, she has published books on critical care nursing and cardiac care.

She has dedicated herself to research and teaching in nursing and medicine internationally in Asia, Europe, South America, Canada, Australia, and Africa through consultation, collaborative research and guest faculty as visiting professor in Hong Kong, University of Basel Switzerland, University of Natal South Africa, and the University of Vienna, among others.

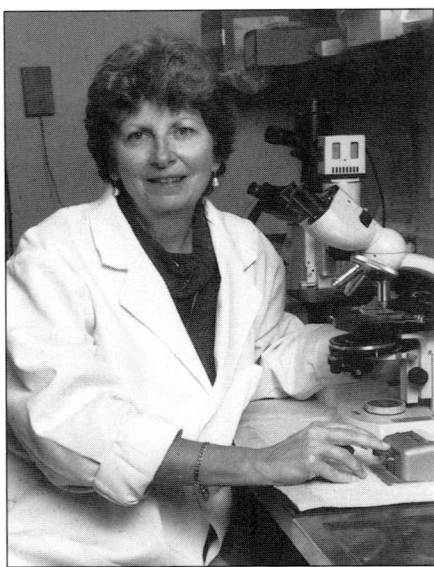

Sandra Adams (Underhill) Motzer, PhD, RN, FAHA

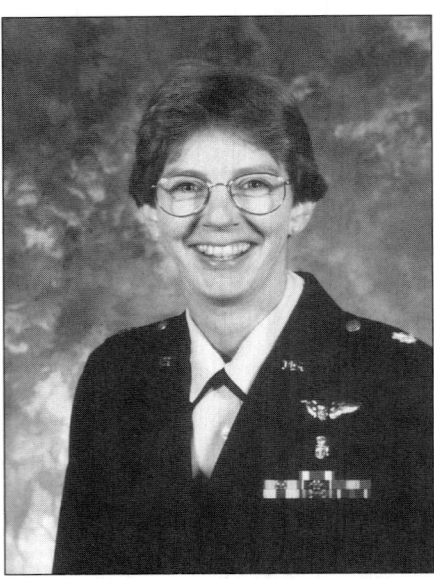

Elizabeth J. Bridges, Col. (s) USAF NC, PhD, RN, CCNS

Sandy is a diploma graduate from Washington Hospital Center School of Nursing, Washington, DC. She earned her BSN and MN at the University of Washington and her PhD at Oregon Health Sciences University, Portland. She completed a post-doctoral fellowship at the University of Washington. Sandy was a founding co-editor of the journal *Progress in Cardiovascular Nursing* and is a charter Fellow of the American Heart Association's Council on Cardiovascular Nursing as well as the American Heart Association (FAHA). She is a past president of the Puget Sound Chapter of the American Association of Critical Care Nurses and is active in Sigma Theta Tau at the international and local levels. Sandy has taught cardiovascular nursing for many years at all academic levels and in the community. Currently she directs the master's-level medical-surgical nurse educator and clinical nurse specialist tracks at the University of Washington School of Nursing. She teaches graduate-level courses in advanced pathophysiology, practice teaching, and, for the clinical nurse specialist and nurse educator students, clinical specialization and role development. Her funded research involves the effects of chronic health disturbances on immune function across the menstrual cycle and the effects of exercise on sleep in persons with heart failure. Sandy and her husband Tim enjoy hiking, beach walking, and traveling.

Elizabeth has been a critical care nurse in the United States Air Force for 21 years. For the past 5 years she has served as the Deputy Commander of the 59th Clinical Research Squadron and Senior Nurse Researcher at the 59th Medical Wing at Lackland AFB, Texas. In September of 2004, she will be joining the faculty at the University of Washington as an Assistant Professor of Biobehavioral Nursing and Health Systems. Her clinical research focuses on the integration of hemodynamic monitoring into the care of critically ill patients and the care of critically ill patients in military, unique, and austere environments. Specifically, she is studying hemodynamic monitoring at altitude, aspects of thermal stress and the maintenance of body temperature in critically ill patients under field conditions and long-distance aeromedical transport, factors that affect the efficacy of CPR under field conditions, and interventions to prevent decubitus ulcer formation during long-distance aeromedical transport. Elizabeth is a primary instructor for the United States Air Force Critical Care Air Transport Team program, the Critical Care Nursing program director at the Defense Institute for Medical Operations, and a course director for the international course Trauma Systems and Disaster Response. This latter course works with host nations around the world to assist them in the development of their trauma and disaster response systems and to build international health care bridges.

Preface to the 5th Edition

Cardiac Nursing continues to be *the* reference book for nurses caring for patients who have or are at risk for developing cardiac disease. *Cardiac Nursing,* Fifth Edition, provides the basic and advanced nurse with the most comprehensive evidence-based practice information. We believe that bedside nurses, clinical nurse specialists, nurse practitioners, nurse educators, and nurse researchers all will benefit from the content in this edition.

New to This Edition

Dr. Elizabeth J. Bridges has been added as an editor to the fifth edition. She has participated as a contributor to the past two editions and has written several chapters in this edition as well. Global perspectives of cardiovascular disease have been included in all chapters where appropriate, which enhances the usefulness and generalizability of the content. There have been many changes in the care of cardiac patients since the fourth edition. Thus, all chapters have been updated to reflect the most current evidence-based practice guidelines. To make more explicit the evidence base of the references and to facilitate students' linking the evidence with the researchers, the referencing format has been revised so that authors' names and dates of publication are now in text. Seven new chapters have been added: Genetics, Inflammation, Atherosclerosis, Heart Rate Variability, Congenital Heart Disease, Complementary and Alternative Medicine, and Disease Management Models. Additionally, two chapters from the fourth edition each receive their own full chapter status—Echocardiography (Chapter 16) and Nuclear and Other Scans (Chapter 17)—and the Myocardial Ischemia and Infarction chapter is now Pathophysiology of Acute Coronary Syndrome (Chapter 25), Acute Coronary Syndromes (Chapter 26), Inflammation (Chapter 6), and Atherosclerosis (Chapter 7).

Content and Organization

The emphasis on health promotion, health maintenance, and disease management has been maintained throughout the text. By adding, reorganizing and revising chapters and content, the fifth edition will help all cardiac nurses provide care more confidently and effectively within the changing health care and economic environment across all practice settings. There are five parts in this edition:

PART ONE: ANATOMY AND PHYSIOLOGY. Includes chapters on anatomy and physiology, systemic and pulmonary circulation and gas transport, and the regulation of cardiac output and blood pressure.

PART TWO: PHYSIOLOGIC AND PATHOPHYSIOLOGIC RESPONSES. Includes chapters on genetics; inflammation; atherosclerosis; hematopoiesis, coagulation, and bleeding; fluid and electrolyte balances and imbalances; acid-base balances and imbalances; sleep; and aging.

PART THREE: ASSESSMENT OF HEART DISEASE. Includes chapters on history taking and physical examination; laboratory tests; radiologic examination of the chest; echocardiography; nuclear and other scans; electrocardiography; arrhythmias and conduction disturbances; cardiac electrophysiologic procedures; exercise testing; cardiac catheterization; hemodynamic monitoring; and heart rate variability.

PART FOUR: PATHOPHYSIOLOGY AND MANAGEMENT OF HEART DISEASE. Includes chapters on the pathophysiology of acute coronary syndrome; acute coronary syndrome; interventional cardiology techniques; heart failure; cardiac surgery; shock; sudden cardiac death and cardiac arrest; pacemakers and implantable defibrillators; acquired valvular heart disease; pericardial, myocardial and endocardial disease; and congenital heart disease.

PART FIVE: HEALTH PROMOTION AND DISEASE PREVENTION. Includes chapters on the assessment and management of coronary heart disease risk factors and disease prevention; psychosocial interventions; smoking cessation and relapse prevention; hypertension; hyperlipidemia; activity and exercise; obesity; diabetes; adherence; complementary and alternative medicine; and disease management models.

The Tradition of Excellence

The fifth edition continues our tradition of excellence in nursing care found in the previous four editions by having over 90% of the chapters written by cardiac nursing experts. The "red book" maintains our nursing philosophy by organizing the content within the framework of the nursing process, and includes numerous nursing care plans. Where possible, the rationale and evidence for treatments and interventions are included.

We sincerely appreciate all the comments we received about the previous editions. We hope you find that the fifth edition lives up to our standard of excellence of the past four editions, and that it becomes your primary reference source for cardiac nursing.

Susan L. Woods, PhD, RN, FAAN, FAHA
Erika S. Sivarajan Froelicher, PhD, RN, FAAN, FAHA
Sandra Adams (Underhill) Motzer, PhD, RN, FAHA
Elizabeth J. Bridges, Col. (s) USAF NC, PhD, RN, CCNS

Table of Contents

PART I
Anatomy and Physiology **1**

1   Cardiac Anatomy and Physiology   3
ELEANOR F. BOND

General Anatomic Description   3
Cardiac Structures   6
Cardiac Tissue   9
Coronary Circulation   12
Cardiac Innervation   16
Myocardial Cell Structure   16
Myocardial Cell Electrical Characteristics   17
Cardiac Action Potential   22
Sarcolemmal Ionic Currents   26
Factors Modifying Electrophysiologic Function   28
Propagation of the Cardiac Impulse   29
Mechanical Characteristics of Cardiac Cells   32
Mechanical Properties of the Myocardium   35
Myocardial Metabolism   41
Physiology of the Coronary Circulation   41
The Cardiac Cycle   43

2   Systemic Circulation   49
ELIZABETH J. BRIDGES

Structural Characteristics of the Vasculature and
    Lymphatics   49
Local Regulation   53
Neurohumoral Stimulation   58
Calcium   60
Volume and Flow Distribution   61
The Arterial System   63
The Venous System   64
Microcirculatory Exchange   65
The Lymphatic System   67

**3   Pulmonary Circulation
      and Gas Transport   71**
JOSEPH O. SCHMELZ
POLLY E. GARDNER

Structural/Anatomic   71
Physiology   72
Gas Transport   75

Oxygen Delivery, Consumption, Extraction and
    Cardiac Output   77
Oxygen Consumption-Delivery Relationship   78
Monitoring Oxygenation   78

**4   Regulation of Cardiac
      Output and Blood Pressure   81**
ELIZABETH J. BRIDGES

Afferent Input and Receptor   81
Central Nervous System Regulation   83
Autonomic Nervous System Regulation   84
Systemic Hormones   89
Heart Rate   92
Intrinsic Cardiac Control   93
Extrinsic Control: Pericardial Limitation   94
Long-Term Control of Blood Pressure   94
Local Regulation of Systemic Microvascular Beds   96
Venous System   98
Models of Cardiac Performance   99
Additional Effects of Respiration   102
Overall Control   102

PART II
Physiologic and Pathologic Responses **109**

5   Genetics   111
BRADLEY AOUIZERAT

DNA   111
DNA and Human Diversity   113
Genetic Variation   113
Gene Testing   114
The Human Genome Project   114
Pharmacogenomics   114
Biochemical Basis of Genetic Disease   115
Overview: Heart Disease   115
The Genetics of Cardiovascular Disease   116
Evidence for a Genetic Basis of Coronary
    Artery Disease   118
Diagnosis and Risk Assessment: Application of
    Genetic Susceptibility Information in the
    Prevention of Coronary Artery Disease   120
Ethical Considerations   121
Summary   121

6 Inflammation   **127**

BRADLEY AOUIZERAT

Introduction   127
Overview of the Pathophysiology of
   Cardiovascular Disease   128
Brain Natriuretic Peptide   129
Circulating Adhesion Molecules   129
Fibrinogen   130
High Sensitivity C-Reactive Protein   130
Homocysteine   131
Interleukin 6   132
Serum Amyloid A   133
Tumor Necrosis Factor Alpha   133
von Willebrand Factor   134
Conclusion   134

7 Atherosclerosis   **139**

BRADLEY AOUIZERAT

American Heart Association Lesion
   Classification System   139
Cells and Extracellular Matrix of Lesions   143
Vascular Surface Defects and Hematoma   145
Lesion Types and Morphology: Correlation
   with Clinical Syndromes   146
Conclusion   146

**8 Hematopoiesis, Coagulation,
   and Bleeding**   **150**

NANCY MUNRO

Hematopoietic Cells   150
Hemostasis   154
Coagulation–Inflammation Link   157
Bleeding Disorders   158
Clotting Disorders   162

**9 Fluid and Electrolyte Balance
   and Imbalance**   **173**

LINDA FELVER

Principles of Fluid Balance   173
Extracellular Fluid Volume Balance   175
Osmolality Balance   176
Principles of Electrolyte Balance   177
Electrolyte Imbalances   179
Summary   186

**10 Acid-Base Balance and
   Imbalances**   **189**

LINDA FELVER

Principles of Acid-Base Balance   189
Acid-Base Imbalances   191
Summary   195

11 Sleep   **197**

KATHY P. PARKER
SANDRA B. DUNBAR

Normal Sleep   197
The Regulation of Sleeping and Waking   202
Physiology During Sleep   202
Impaired Sleep, Sleep Disorders, and Excessive
   Daytime Sleepiness   204
Sleep in Patients with Cardiovascular Disease   205
Cardiac Events in Sleep   208
Sleep-Related Disordered Breathing   209
Sleep-Related Adverse Outcomes in Patients
   with Cardiovascular Disease   210
Nursing Management   211
The Health Care Providers' Sleep   213
Summary   213

**12 Physiologic Adaptations
   with Aging**   **220**

BARBARA S. LEVINE
RUTH F. CRAVEN

General Physiologic Changes   221
Cardiovascular Changes   222
Respiratory Changes   223
Renal Changes   224
Hepatic Changes   225
Effects of Aging on Pharmacokinetics   225
Summary   225

PART III
Assessment of Heart Disease   ***227***

**13 History Taking and Physical
   Examination**   **229**

BARBARA S. LEVINE

Cardiovascular History   229
Physical Assessment   234

14 Laboratory Tests Using Blood   **265**

SUSAN L. REED

Blood Specimen Collection   265
Cardiac Markers   269
Blood Lipids   276
Additional Laboratory Tests Associated with
   Cardiac Disease   278
Hematologic Studies   281
Blood Cultures   283
Coagulation Studies   283
Arterial Blood Gases   286
Blood Chemistries   286

Selected Chemistries   288
Serum Concentration of Selected Drugs   291

15 Radiologic Examination of the Chest   296

JON S. HUSEBY
DENISE LEDOUX

How X-Rays Work   296
Interpretation of Chest Radiographs   297
Chest Film Findings in Acute Care Determining
Line, Tube, and Catheter Placement   297
Chest Film Findings in Cardiovascular Disease   297

16 Echocardiography   307

MARGARET L. HALL

Technical Aspects   308
Special Techniques   309
Echocardiography of Cardiac Structures
in Health and Disease   312
Newer Techniques   317
Conclusion   318

17 Nuclear and Other Imaging Studies   319

LAURIE SOINE
MARGARET HANRAHAN

Nuclear Studies of the heart   319

18 Electrocardiography   326

CAROL JACOBSON

Electrical Conduction Through the Heart   326
Basic Electrocardiography   328
The 12-Lead Electrocardiogram   330
Axis Determination   336
Intraventricular Conduction Abnormalities   337
Ischemia, Injury, and Infarction   342
Atrial and Ventricular Enlargement   349
Electrolyte Imbalances   353
Wellens Syndrome   356
Brugada Syndrome   357

19 Arrhythmias and Conduction Disturbances   361

CAROL JACOBSON

Mechanisms of Arrhythmias   361
Basic Arrhythmias and Conduction Disturbances   365
Complex Arrhythmias and Conduction
Disturbances   391

20 Cardiac Electrophysiology Procedures   425

SUSAN BLANCHER

Diagnostic Electrophysiology Studies   425
Interventional Electrophysiology and Catheter
Ablation   430
Nursing Care of the Patient Undergoing
Electrophysiology Procedures   436

21 Exercise Testing   439

JONATHAN MYERS

Indications and Objectives   439
Safety and Personnel   439
Pretest Considerations   440
Exercise Test Selection   442
Interpretation of Exercise Test Responses   445
Test Termination   450
Recovery Period   452
Assessing Test Accuracy   452
Ancillary Methods for the Detection of
Coronary Artery Disease   453
Gas Exchange Techniques   454
Prognosis   455
Exercise Testing in Special Populations   455
Summary   456

22 Cardiac Catheterization   459

MICHAELENE HARGROVE DEELSTRA
CAROL JACOBSON

Indications   459
Contraindications   460
Patient Preparation   461
Procedure   463
The Nurse in the Cardiac Catheterization
Laboratory   472
Interpretation of Data   474

23 Hemodynamic Monitoring   478

ELIZABETH J. BRIDGES

Technical Aspects of Invasive Pressure Monitoring   478
Direct Arterial Pressure Monitoring   483
Central Venous Pressure Monitoring   488
Pulmonary Artery Pressure Monitoring   489
Functional Hemodynamic Indices   500
Cardiac Output Measurement   503
Ventricular Function Curves   505
Continuous Cardiac Output   506
Less Invasive Methods for Cardiac Output
Monitoring   507
Oxygen Supply and Demand   512

24 Heart Rate Variability   **527**

DIANA MCMILLAN
ROBERT BURR

Mechanisms of Heart Rate Variability 527
Heart Rate Variability Measurement 527
HRV Patterns in Common Cardiovascular Conditions 530
Factors Influencing Heart Rate Variability 532
Impact of Interventions on HRV 535
Summary 536

PART **IV**
*Pathophysiology and Management
of Heart Disease*   **539**

**25 Pathophysiology of Acute
Coronary Syndrome**   **541**

POLLY GARDNER
GAYLENE ALTMAN

Introduction 541
Mechanisms That Regulate Coronary Blood Flow 542
Causes of Myocardial Ischemia and Infarction 542
Risk Factors for Coronary Artery Disease 543
Incidence of Myocardial Ischemia 543
Incidence of Myocardial Infarction 545
Implications for Nurses 547

26 Acute Coronary Syndromes   **550**

SHERRI DEL BENE
ANNE VAUGHAN

Angina Pectoris 550
Myocardial Infarction 556

**27 Interventional Cardiology
Techniques**   **585**

MICHAELENE HARGROVE DEELSTRA

Percutaneous Coronary Interventions 585
Percutaneous Coronary Procedures 587
Complications Associated with PCI 592
Late Complications of PCI 594
Adjunctive Modalities 595
Anticoagulation Options for PCI 596
Noncoronary Devices 596
Nursing Management 597

28 Heart Failure   **601**

DEBRA LAURENT

Etiologies and Definitions 601
Pathophysiology and Pathogenesis 603
Clinical Manifestations 610

Classification 612
Medical Management 613
Nursing Management 621

29 Cardiac Surgery   **628**

DENISE LEDOUX
HELEN LUIKART

Evolving Trends in Cardiac Surgery 628
Preoperative Assessment and Preparation 628
Surgical Techniques 629
Cardiac Surgery Procedures for Coronary Artery
    Revascularization 631
Cardiac Surgery Procedures for Acquired
    Structural Heart Disease 634
Cardiac Transplantation 642

30 Acute Heart Failure and Shock   **659**

DEBRA LAURENT
JULIE A. SHINN

Database for Nursing Management 659
Nursing Management Plan for the Patient
    in Shock 674

**31 Sudden Cardiac Death and
Cardiac Arrest**   **689**

DONNA GERITY

Definition of Sudden Death 689
Pathophysiology and Cause of Sudden Cardiac Arrest 689
Management of Sudden Cardiac Arrest 691
Survivors of Cardiac Arrest 704
Summary 707

**32 Pacemakers and Implantable
Defibrillators**   **709**

CAROL JACOBSON
DONNA GERITY

Pacemakers 709
Implantable Cardioverter Defibrillators 738
Conclusion 754

33 Acquired Valvular Heart Disease   **756**

DENISE LEDOUX

Database for Nursing Management 756

**34 Pericardial, Myocardial, and
Endocardial Disease**   **776**

MARGARET M. MCNEILL

Pericardial Disease 776
Cardiomyopathies 782
Endocardial Disease 787

35 Congenital Heart Disease   794
MARY M. CANOBBIO

Incidence and Prevalence   794
Congenital Heart Defects   794
Normal Pulmonary Blood Flow-Impairment or
    Obstruction to Ventricular Outflow   794
Left-to-Right Shunts with Increased
    Pulmonary Blood Flow   798
Cyanotic Right-to-Left Shunts with Decreased
    Pulmonary Blood Flow   800
Cyanotic Congenital Heart Defects with Increased
    Pulmonary Blood Flow   801
Medical Management Plan   803

PART V
*Health Promotion and
Disease Prevention   807*

**36 Coronary Heart Disease
Risk Factors   809**
KATHERINE M. NEWTON
ERIKA SIVARAJAN FROELICHER

Demographic Characteristics   810
Family History of Cardiovascular Disease   810
Cigarette Smoking   811
Hypertension   812
Serum Lipids and Lipoproteins   812
Physical Activity   813
Diabetes Mellitus   815
Body Weight   817
Reproductive Hormones   818
Folate and Homocysteine   819
Antioxidants   820
Conclusions   820

**37 Psychosocial Risk Factors: Assessment
and Management Interventions   825**
SIMONE K. MADAN
ERIKA SIVARAJAN FROELICHER

Psychosocial Risk Factors and CHD   825
Mechanisms for Psychosocial Risk Factors
    and CHD   828
Assessment of Psychosocial Risk Factors   829
Management Interventions for Psychosocial
    Risk Factors   830
Pharmacological Interventions   834
Summary   835

**38 Smoking Cessation: A Systematic
Approach to Managing Patients
with Coronary Heart Disease   838**
KIRSTEN MARTIN
ERIKA SIVARAJAN FROELICHER

Harmful Effects of Smoking   839
Benefits of Smoking Cessation   840
Theoretical Framework for Smoking Cessation   840
Smoking Cessation Interventions in the Coronary
    Heart Disease Population   840
General Trends in Smoking Cessation Interventions   841
Treating Tobacco Use and Dependence: Clinical
    Practice Guideline   841
Special Areas on Which to Focus   849
Summary   852

39 Hypertension   856
SUSANNA CUNNINGHAM

Database for Management   856
Management of High BP   867

**40 Lipid Management and Coronary
Heart Disease   897**
JOAN M. FAIR
KATHLEEN A. BERRA

Blood Lipids: Structure and Functions   897
Lipid Metabolism and Transport   898
Reverse Cholesterol Transport   899
Low-Density Lipoprotein Variants   900
Cholesterol and Endothelial Function   900
Dyslipidemic Disorders   901
Hypercholesterolemia   901
The Management of High Blood Cholesterol   902
Evaluation of the Patient with Elevated Cholesterol   905
Lipoprotein Measurement   905
Dietary Management of Hyperlipidemia   905
Weight Control and Lipid Management   908
Alcohol and Lipoproteins   909
Physical Activity and Lipoproteins   909
Hormones and Lipoproteins   909
Pharmacologic Management of
    Hyperlipidemia   910

41 Exercise and Activity   916
JONATHAN MYERS

Role of Exercise in Cardiovascular Health   916
Cardiac Rehabilitation   921
Closing Comment   933

**42 Obesity: An Overview of
Assessment and Treatment   937**

LORA E. BURKE
MEGHAN A. CARTWRIGHT

Identification and Assessment of the
Overweight or Obese Patient   938
Clinical Evaluation   939
Treatment of Overweight and Obesity   941
Components of the Treatment   942
Summary   945

43 Diabetes Mellitus   948

MARGARET I. WALLHAGEN
MARTHA S. NOLTE

Definition and Diagnosis   948
Prevalence and Consequences of Diabetes   948
Pathophysiology of Diabetes Mellitus   949
Complications of Diabetes Mellitus   951
Pathophysiology of Complications   952
Nursing Management of Diabetes   953
Health Screening and Monitoring   958
Summary   958

**44 Adherence to Cardiovascular
Treatment Regimens   961**

LORA E. BURKE
DOROTHY TSCHIRPKE
THERESE A. POLAKOSKI

Significance of Nonadherence   961
Methods of Measurement   962
Determinants of Adherence   965
Models of Behavior Change   966
Adherence-Enhancing Strategies   966
Educational Strategies to Improve Adherence   969
Questionnaires Relevant to Adherence-Enhancing
Interventions   969

Building a Therapeutic Relationship with
the Patient   970
Summary   971

**45 Complementary and Alternative
Medicine in Cardiac and Vascular
Disease   974**

ELEANOR F. BOND
MARGARET M. HEITKEMPER

CAM Definitions and Characteristics   974
CAM Domains   974
Prevalence of CAM   975
Alternative Medical Systems   975
Mind–Body Interventions for Cardiovascular
Disease   976
Biologically Based Treatments   978
Manipulative and Body-Based Methods and Energy
Therapies   982
Legal Aspects of CAM   982
Integration of CAM into Nursing Assessment
and Clinical Management   982
Summary   983

**46 Disease Management Models
for Cardiovascular Care   986**

NANCY HOUSTON MILLER
ERIKA SIVARAJAN FROELICHER

Disease Management: Definition and Models   987
Various Models of Disease Management in
Cardiovascular Care   987
Components of Disease Management Systems   988
Training and Job Qualifications for Disease
Management   992
The Unresolved Issues for Disease Management   992

Index   997

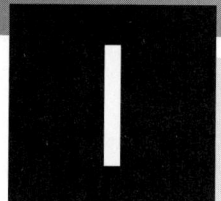

PART

I

Anatomy and Physiology

Cardiac Anatomy and Physiology

ELEANOR F. BOND*

An understanding of cardiac anatomy is helpful for understanding cardiac physiology and the functional consequences of disease. This chapter describes normal human adult cardiac anatomy, cellular structure, and ultrastructure. The chapter also discusses the electrical, mechanical, and metabolic activities that underlie cardiac pump performance. The coronary circulation is described and discussed in the context of its linkage to changing demands of cardiac tissue for nutrient delivery and waste removal. Finally, integrated cardiac performance is discussed.

GENERAL ANATOMIC DESCRIPTION

The heart is a hollow muscular organ encased and cushioned in its own serous membrane, the pericardium. It lies in the middle mediastinal compartment of the thorax between the two pleural cavities. Two thirds of the heart extends to the left of the body's midline (Fig. 1-1).

The heart consists of four muscular chambers, two atria and two ventricles, and associated structures. The right heart (right atrium and ventricle) receives blood from the body and pumps it into the low-pressure pulmonary arterial system. The left heart (left atrium and ventricle) receives oxygenated blood from the lungs and pumps it into the high-pressure systemic arterial system. Interatrial and interventricular septa separate the right and left atria and ventricles from each other.

The long axis of the heart is directed obliquely, leftward, downward, and forward. Any factor that changes the shape of the thorax changes the position of the heart and modifies the directional axis. Respiratory alterations in the diaphragm and the rib cage constantly cause small changes the cardiac axis. Thus, with a deep inspiration, the heart descends and becomes more vertical. Factors that may cause long-term axis variations in healthy people include age, weight, pregnancy, body shape, and shape of the thorax. A tall, thin person usually has a more vertical heart, whereas a short, obese person usually has a more

horizontal heart. Pathologic conditions of the heart, lungs, abdominal organs, and other structures influence the direction of the cardiac axis.

The surfaces of the heart are used to reference its position in relation to other structures and to describe the location of damage, as in a myocardial infarction. The right ventricle and parts of the right atrium and the left ventricle form the anterior (or sternocostal) cardiac surface (Figs. 1-1 and 1-2). The right atrium and ventricle lie anteriorly and to the right of the left atrium and ventricle in the frontal plane. Thus, when viewed from the front of the body, the heart appears to be lying sideways, directed forward and leftward, with the right heart foremost.

The small portion of the lower left ventricle that extends anteriorly forms a blunt tip composed of the apical part of the interventricular septum and the left ventricular free wall. Because of the forward tilt of the heart, movement of this apex portion of the left ventricle during cardiac contraction usually forms the *point of maximal impulse,* which can be observed in healthy people in the fifth intercostal space at the left midclavicular line, 7 to 9 cm from midline. The sternum, costal cartilages of the third to sixth ribs, part of the lungs, and, in children, the thymus, overlie the anterior cardiac surface.

The left atrium and a small section of the right atrium and ventricle comprise the base of the heart, which is directed backward and forms the posterior surface of the heart (Fig. 1-3). The thoracic aorta, esophagus, and vertebrae are posterior to the heart. The inferior or diaphragmatic surface of the heart, comprising chiefly the left ventricle, lies almost horizontally on the upper surface of the diaphragm (Fig. 1-4). The right ventricle forms a portion of the inferior cardiac surface.

The right atrium forms the lateral right heart border and, therefore, the right atrium and right lung lie close together. The entire right margin of the heart extends laterally from the superior vena cava along the right atrium and then toward the diaphragm to the cardiac apex. The lateral wall of the left ventricle and a small part of the left atrium form most of the left heart border. This portion of the left ventricle is next to the left lung and sometimes is referred to as the *pulmonary surface.*

The coronary (or atrioventricular [AV]) sulcus (groove) is the external landmark denoting the separation of the atria from the ventricles. The AV sulcus encircles the heart obliquely and

*The material in this chapter was originally coauthored with Carol Jean Halpenny.

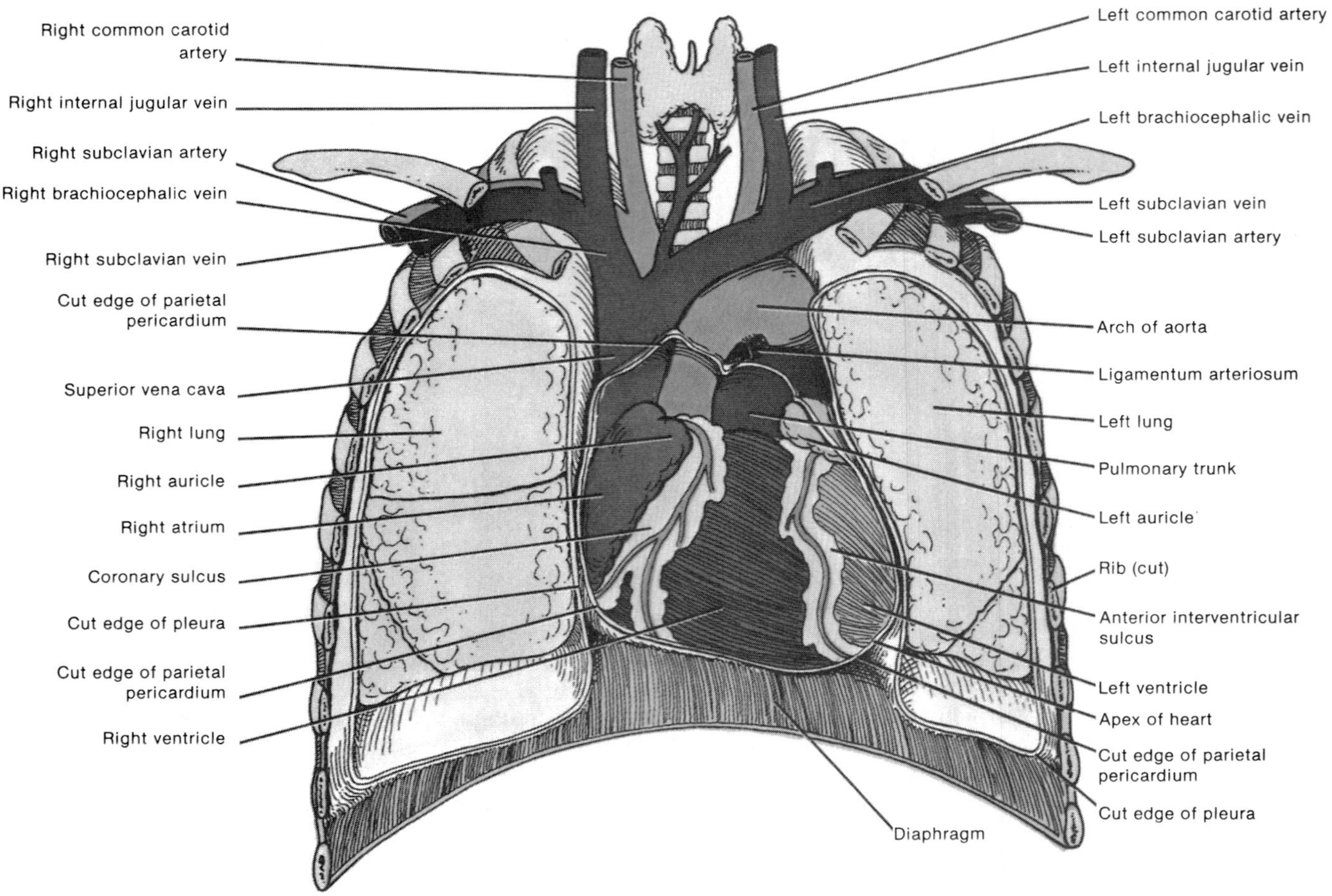

Right common carotid artery

Right internal jugular vein

Right subclavian artery

Right brachiocephalic vein

Right subclavian vein

Cut edge of parietal pericardium

Superior vena cava

Right lung

Right auricle

Right atrium

Coronary sulcus

Cut edge of pleura

Cut edge of parietal pericardium

Right ventricle

Left common carotid artery

Left internal jugular vein

Left brachiocephalic vein

Left subclavian vein

Left subclavian artery

Arch of aorta

Ligamentum arteriosum

Left lung

Pulmonary trunk

Left auricle

Rib (cut)

Anterior interventricular sulcus

Left ventricle

Apex of heart

Cut edge of parietal pericardium

Cut edge of pleura

Diaphragm

■ **Figure 1–1.** Anterior view of the heart, illustrating the position of the heart and associated structures in the thoracic cavity. (From Tortora, G.J. [1986]. *Principles of human anatomy* [4th ed., p. 302]. New York: Harper & Row.)

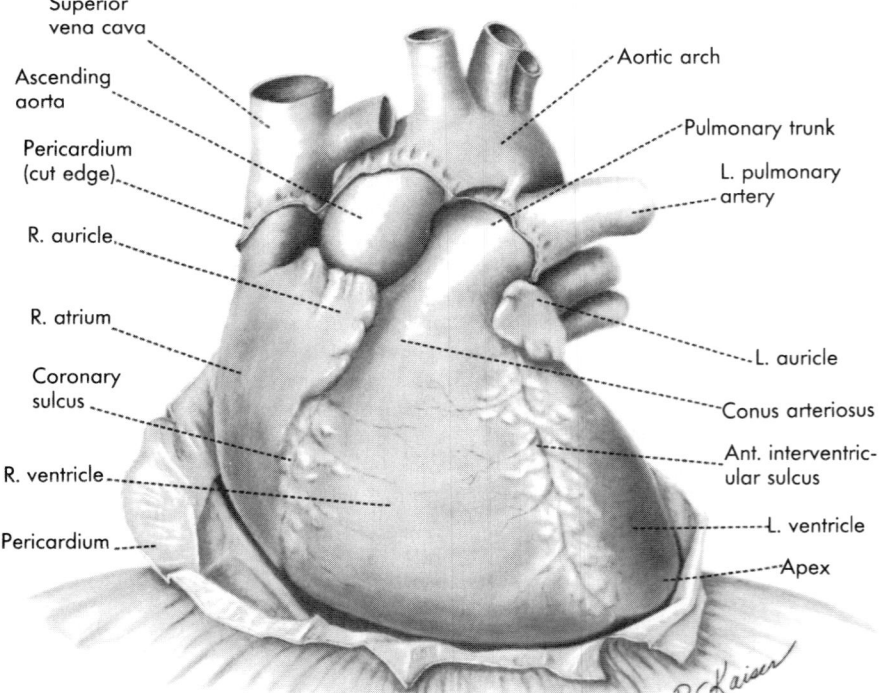

■ **Figure 1–2.** Anterior view of the heart, illustrating the cardiac structures. The pericardial sac has been cut open and reflected toward the diaphragm. (From Hollinshead, W.H., & Rosse, C. [1985]. *Textbook of anatomy* [4th ed. p. 523]. Philadelphia: Harper & Row.)

Superior vena cava

Ascending aorta

Pericardium (cut edge)

R. auricle

R. atrium

Coronary sulcus

R. ventricle

Pericardium

Aortic arch

Pulmonary trunk

L. pulmonary artery

L. auricle

Conus arteriosus

Ant. interventricular sulcus

L. ventricle

Apex

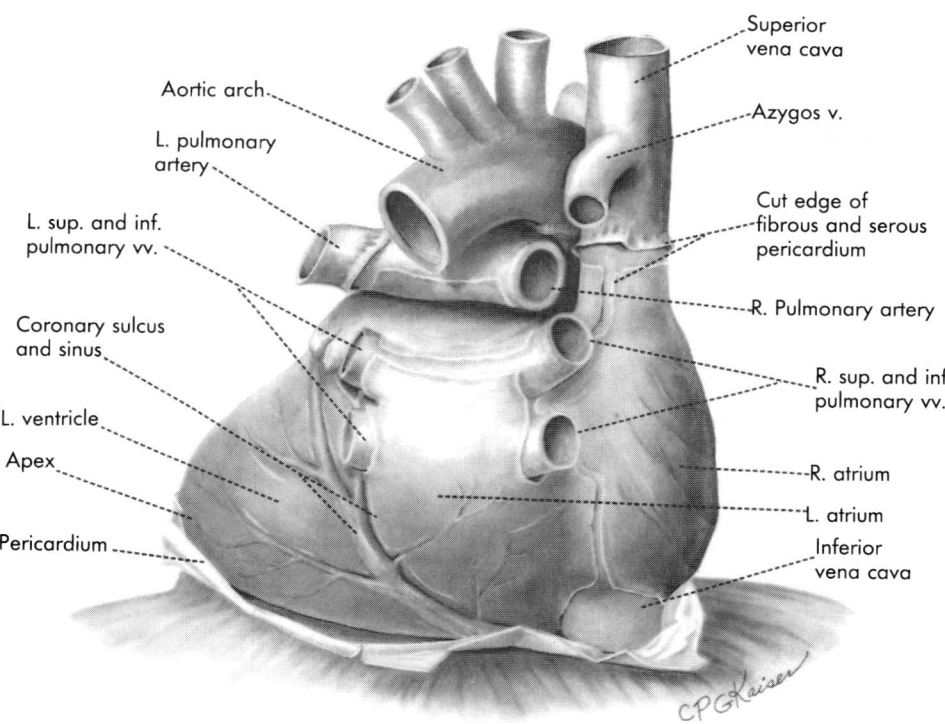

Figure 1–3. Posterior view of the heart, (From Hollinshead, W.H., & Rosse, C. [1985]. *Textbook of anatomy* [4th ed., p. 523]. Philadelphia: Harper & Row.)

contains coronary blood vessels, cardiac nerves, and epicardial fat. The aorta and pulmonary artery interrupt the AV sulcus anteriorly. The anterior and posterior interventricular sulci separate the right and left ventricles on the external heart surface. The crux of the heart is the point on the external posterior heart surface where the posterior interventricular sulcus intersects the coronary (AV) sulcus externally and where the interatrial septum joins the interventricular septum internally.

The average adult heart is approximately 12 cm long from its base at the beginning root of the aorta to the left ventricular apex, 8 to 9 cm wide transversely at the widest part, and 6-cm-thick anteroposteriorly. Tables have been derived to indicate normal ranges of heart size for various body weights and heights (Ungerleider & Clark, 1939).

The adult male heart comprises approximately 0.43% of body weight, 280 to 350 g, with an average weight of 300 g

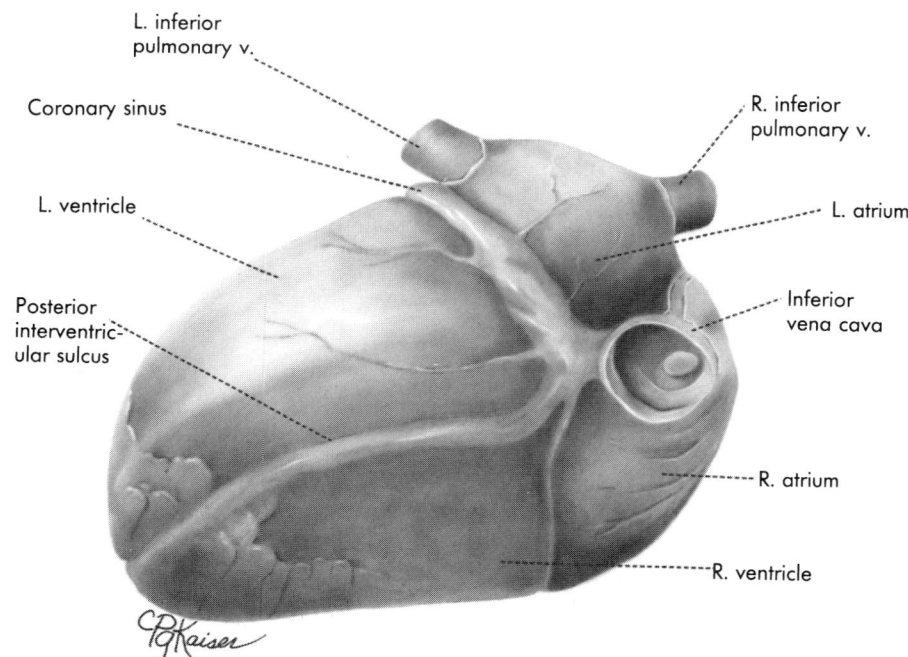

Figure 1–4. Inferior or diaphragmatic heart surface, with the pericardial sac reflected. (From Hollinshead, W.H., & Rosse, C. [1985]. *Textbook of anatomy* [4th ed., p. 524]. Philadelphia: Harper & Row.)

(Reiner et al., 1959; Smith & Smith, 1928). The adult female heart comprises approximately 0.40% of body weight, 230 to 300 g, with an average weight of 250 g (Reiner et al., 1959; Smith & Smith, 1928). Age, body build, frequency of physical exercise, and heart disease influence heart size and weight.

CARDIAC STRUCTURES

Fibrous Skeleton

Four adjacent, dense, fibrous connective tissue rings, the annuli fibrosi, surround the cardiac valves and provide an internal supporting structure for the heart. The annuli are attached together and connected by a central fibrous core (Fig. 1-5). Each annulus and valve has a slightly different orientation, but the entire connective tissue structure, termed the *fibrous skeleton,* is oriented obliquely within the mediastinum.

The fibrous skeleton divides the atria from the ventricles. It provides the attachment site for some of the atrial and ventricular cardiac muscle fibers. A portion of the fibrous skeleton extends downward between the right atrium and left ventricle, forming the upper or membranous part of the interventricular septum.

Chambers

The wall thickness of each of the four cardiac chambers reflects the amount of force generated by that chamber. The two thin-walled atria serve functionally as reservoirs and conduits for blood that is being funneled into the ventricles; they add a small amount of force to the moving blood. The left ventricle, which adds the greatest amount of energy to the flowing blood, is two to three times as thick as the right ventricle. The approximate normal wall thicknesses of the chambers are as follows: right atrium, 2 mm; right ventricle, 3 to 5 mm; left atrium, 3 mm; and left ventricle, 13 to 15 mm.

The interatrial septum between right and left atria extends obliquely forward from right to left. The interatrial septum includes the fossa ovalis, a remnant of a fetal structure, the foramen ovale. The lower portion of the interatrial septum is formed by the lower medial right atrial wall on one side and the aortic outflow tract of the left ventricular wall on the other side. The lower muscular portion of the interventricular septum extends downward from the upper membranous part of the interventricular septum. The clinical significance of these structures has recently received increased attention. A pooled analysis of autopsy studies has demonstrated that the prevalence of patent foramen ovale in adults is approximately 26% (Windecker & Meier, 2002). This is clinically significant, providing a potential conduit for a shunt from the right atrium to the left atrium and possibly accounting for increased risk of stroke (Overell et al., 2000) and migraine headache (Milhaud et al., 2001).

In considering the internal surfaces of the cardiac chambers, it is helpful to remember that blood flows more smoothly and with less turbulence across walls that are smooth than across ridged walls. Blood pools more frequently in appendages or other areas out of the direct blood flow path.

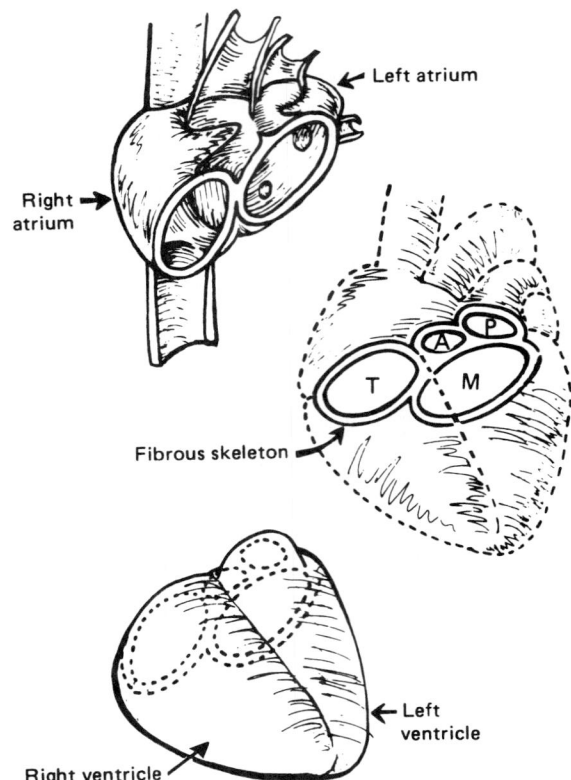

■ **Figure 1–5.** Schematic view of the fibrous skeleton, illustrating the attachment of the cardiac valves and chambers. The four annuli and their extensions lie in different planes, so it is impossible to depict them accurately on a plane surface. T, tricuspid valve; M, mitral valve; A, aortic valve; P, pulmonic valve. (Adapted from Rushmer, R.F. [1976]. *Cardiovascular dynamics* [p. 77]. Philadelphia: WB Saunders.)

Right Heart

The posterior and septal walls of the right atrium are smooth, whereas the lateral wall and the right atrial appendage (auricle) have parallel muscular ridges, termed *pectinate muscles.* The right auricle extends over the aortic root externally.

The inferior wall of the right atrium and part of the superior wall of the right ventricle are formed by the tricuspid valve (Fig. 1-6). The anterior and inferior walls of the right ventricle are lined by muscle bundles, the trabeculae carneae, which form a rough-walled inflow tract for blood. One muscle group, the septomarginal trabecula or moderator band, extends from the lower interventricular septum to the anterior right ventricular papillary muscle.

Another thick muscle bundle, the christa supraventricularis, extends from the septal wall to the anterolateral wall of the right ventricle. The christa supraventricularis helps to divide the right ventricle into an inflow and outflow tract. The smooth-walled outflow tract, called the *conus arteriosus,* or *infundibulum,* extends to the pulmonary artery.

The concave free wall of the right ventricle is attached to the slightly convex septal wall. The internal right ventricular cavity is crescent or triangle shaped. The right ventricle also forms a crescent laterally around the left ventricle. Right ventricular contraction causes the right ventricular free wall to move

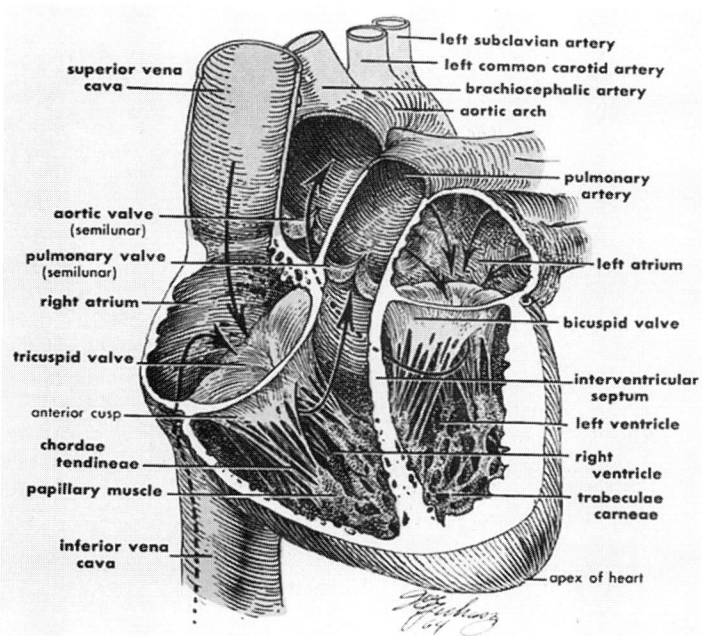

■ **Figure 1–6.** Schematic illustration of cardiac structures. (From Crouch, J.E. [1985]. *Functional human anatomy* [4th ed., p. 403]. Philadelphia: Lea & Febiger.)

toward the interventricular septum. This bellows-like action is effective in ejecting large and variable volumes into a low-pressure system (Fig. 1-7).

Venous blood enters the right atrium from the upper and lower posterior part of the atrium through the superior and inferior venae cavae. Most of the venous drainage from the heart enters the right atrium through the coronary sinus, which is located between the entrance of the inferior vena cava into the right atrium and the orifice of the tricuspid valve. Blood flows medially and anteriorly from the right atrium through the tricuspid orifice into the right ventricle.

Blood enters the right ventricle in an almost horizontal but slightly leftward, anterior, and inferior direction. It is ejected superiorly and posteriorly through the pulmonary valve (Fig. 1-8).

Left Heart

The left atrium is a cuboid structure that lies between the aortic root and the esophagus. The left atrial appendage, or auricle, extends along the border of the pulmonary artery. The walls of the left atrium are smooth except for pectinate muscle bundles in the atrial appendage.

The left ventricle's cone or oval shape is caused by the generally concave left ventricular free wall and interventricular septum. The mitral valve and its attachments form the left ventricular inflow tract. The outflow tract is formed by the anterior surface of the anterior mitral valve cusp, the septum, and the aortic vestibule. The lower muscular interventricular septum and free walls of the left ventricle are deeply ridged with trabeculae carneae muscle bundles, so most of the interior surface of the ventricle is rough. The upper membranous septum and aortic vestibule region have smooth walls. The interventricular septum is functionally and anatomically a more integral part of the left ventricle than the right ventricle. The septum is triangular, with its base at the aortic area. The upper

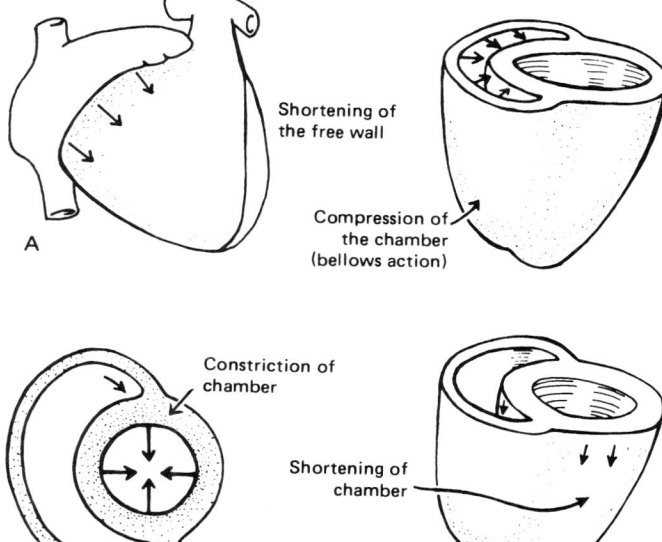

■ **Figure 1–7.** Right and left ventricular contraction. (*A*) Right ventricular contraction. Right ventricular ejection of blood is accomplished primarily by shortening and movement of the free wall toward the interventricular septum. Note the crescent shape of the right ventricle. (*B*) Blood is ejected from the left ventricle primarily by a reduction in the diameter of the chamber. There is some ventricular shortening. (Adapted from Rushmer, R. [1976]. *Cardiovascular dynamics* [p. 92]. Philadelphia: WB Saunders.)

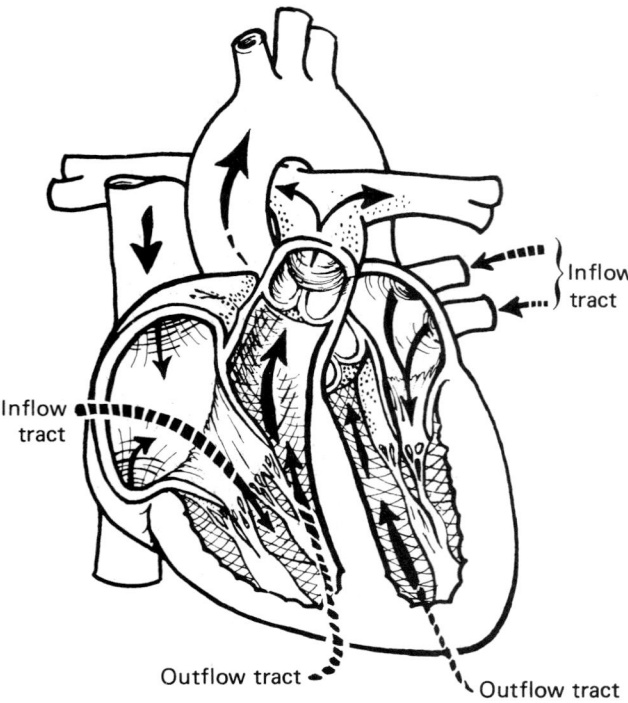

■ **Figure 1–8.** Blood flow through cardiac chambers and valves.

septum separates the right atrium from the left ventricle and is often called the *AV septum.*

Blood is ejected from the left ventricle mainly by circumferential contraction of the muscular wall, that is, by decreasing the diameter of the cylinder (see Fig. 1-7). There is some longitudinal shortening. The ventricular cavity has a small surface area in relation to the volume contained, but high pressure can be developed because of the amount of ventricular muscle, the shape of the cavity, and the way the muscles contract.

Four pulmonary veins return blood from the lungs to openings in the posterolateral wall of the left atrium. Blood is directed obliquely forward out of the left atrium and enters the left ventricle in an anterior, leftward, inferior direction. Blood flows out of the ventricle from the apex toward the aorta in a superior and rightward direction (see Fig. 1-8).

Thus, blood flows from posterior orifices into both ventricles in a leftward direction and is ejected superiorly toward the center of the heart. The right ventricular outflow tract is more tubular; the left ventricular outflow tract more conical (see Fig. 1-8).

Valves

Atrioventricular Valves

The AV tricuspid and bicuspid (mitral) valve complexes are composed of six components that function as a unit: the atria, the valve rings or annuli fibrosi of the fibrous skeleton, the valve cusps or leaflets, the chordae tendineae, the papillary muscles, and the ventricular walls (see Fig. 1-6). The mitral and tricuspid valve cusps are composed of fibrous connective tissue covered by endothelium. They attach to the fibrous skeleton valve rings. Fibrous cords called *chordae tendineae* connect the free valve margins and ventricular surfaces of the valve cusps to papillary muscles and ventricular walls. The papillary muscles are trabeculae carneae muscle bundles oriented parallel to the ventricular walls, extending from the walls to the chordae tendineae (see Fig. 1-6). The chordae tendineae provide many cross-connections from one papillary muscle to the valve cusps or from trabeculae carneae in the ventricular wall directly to valves.

In the adult, the tricuspid orifice is larger (approximately 11 cm in circumference, or capable of admitting three fingers) than the mitral orifice (approximately 9 cm in circumference, or capable of admitting two fingers). The combined surface area of the AV valve cusps is larger than the surface area of the valvular orifice because the cusps resemble curtain-like, billowing flaps.

Most commonly, there are three tricuspid valve cusps: the large anterior, the septal, and the posterior (inferior); There are usually two principal right ventricular papillary muscles, the anterior and the posterior (inferior), and a smaller set of accessory papillary muscles attached to the ventricular septum.

The arrangement of the two triangular bicuspid valve cusps has been compared with a bishop's hat, or miter; hence the structure is called the "mitral" valve. The smaller, less mobile posterior cusp is situated posterolaterally, behind, and to the left of the aortic opening. The larger, more mobile anterior cusp extends from the anterior papillary muscle to the ventricular septum.

The left ventricle most commonly has two major papillary muscles: the posterior papillary muscle attached to the diaphragmatic ventricular wall and the anterior papillary muscle attached to the sternocostal ventricular wall. Thus, the posteromedial papillary muscle extends to the posterolateral valve leaflet, and the anterolateral papillary muscle extends to the anteromedial valve leaflet. Chordae tendineae from each papillary muscle go to both mitral cusps.

During diastole, the AV valves open passively when pressure in the atria exceeds that in the ventricles. The papillary muscles are relaxed. The valve cusps part and project into the ventricle, forming a funnel and thus promoting blood flow into the ventricles (see Fig. 1-8). Toward the end of diastole, the deceleration of blood flowing into the ventricles, the movement of blood in a circular motion behind the cusps, and the increasing pressures in the ventricle compared with lessening pressures in the atria, help to close each valve. During systole, the free edges of the valve cusps are prevented from being everted into the atria by contraction of the papillary muscles and tension in the chordae tendineae. Thus, blood is prevented from flowing backward into the atria despite the high systolic ventricular pressures.

Semilunar Valves

The two semilunar (pulmonary [or pulmonic] and aortic) valves are each composed of three cup-shaped cusps of approximately equal size that attach at their base to the fibrous skeleton. The valve cusps are convex from below, with thickened nodules at the center of the free margins.

The cusps are composed of fibrous connective tissue lined with endothelium. The endothelial lining on the nonventricular side of the valves closely resembles and merges with that of the intima of the arteries beyond the valves. The aortic cusps are thicker than the pulmonic; both are thicker than the AV cusps.

The pulmonary valve orifice is approximately 8.5 cm in circumference. The pulmonic valve cusps are termed *right anterior* (right), *left anterior* (anterior), and *posterior* (left). The aortic valve is approximately 7.5 cm in circumference. The sinuses of Valsalva are pouch-like structures immediately behind each semilunar cusp. The coronary arteries branch from the aorta from two of the pouches or sinuses of Valsalva. The aortic cusps are designated by the name of the nearby coronary artery: right coronary (right or anterior) aortic cusp, left coronary (left or left posterior) aortic cusp, and noncoronary (posterior or right posterior) aortic cusp.

The two semilunar valves are approximately at right angles to each other in the closed position. The pulmonic valve is anterior and superior to the other three cardiac valves. When closed, the semilunar valve cusps contact each other at the nodules and along crescentic arcs, called *lunulae,* below the free margins. During systole, the cusps are thrust upward as blood flows from an area of greater pressure in the ventricle to an area of lesser pressure in the aorta or the pulmonary artery. The effect of the deceleration of blood in the aorta during late systole on small circular currents of blood in the sinuses of Valsalva helps passively to close the semilunar valve cusps. Backflow into the ventricles during diastole is prevented because of the cusps' fibrous strength, their close approximation, and their shape.

CARDIAC TISSUE

The heart wall is composed mainly of a muscular layer, the myocardium. The epicardium and the pericardium cover the external surface. Internally, the endocardium covers the surface.

Epicardium and Pericardium

The epicardium is a layer of mesothelial cells that forms the visceral or heart layer of the serous pericardium. Branches of the coronary blood and lymph vessels, nerves, and fat are enclosed in the epicardium and the superficial layers of the myocardium.

The epicardium completely encloses the external surface of the heart and extends several centimeters along each great vessel, encircling the aorta and pulmonary artery together. It merges with the tunica adventitia of the great vessels, at which point it doubles back on itself as the parietal pericardium. This continuous membrane thus forms the pericardial sac and encloses a potential space, the pericardial cavity (see Fig. 1-1). The serous parietal pericardium lines the inner surface of the thicker, tougher fibrous pericardial membrane. The pericardial membrane extends beyond the serous pericardium and is attached by ligaments and loose connections to the sternum, diaphragm, and structures in the posterior mediastinum.

The pericardial cavity is usually filled with 10 to 30 mL of thin, clear serous fluid. The main function of the pericardium and its fluid is to lubricate the moving surfaces of the heart. The pericardium also helps to retard ventricular dilation, helps to hold the heart in position, and forms a barrier to the spread of infections and neoplasia.

Pathophysiological conditions such as cardiac bleeding or an exudate-producing pericarditis may lead to a sudden or large accumulation of fluid within the pericardial sac. This may impede ventricular filling (see Chapter 34). From 50 to 300 mL of pericardial fluid may be accumulated without serious ventricular impairment. When greater volumes accumulate, ventricular filling is impaired, which is a condition known as cardiac tamponade. If this happens slowly, the ventricles may be able to maintain an adequate cardiac output by contracting more vigorously. The pericardium is histologically similar to pleural and peritoneal serous membranes, so inflammation of all three membranes may occur with certain systemic conditions such as rheumatoid arthritis.

Myocardium

The myocardial layer is composed of cardiac muscle cells interspersed with connective tissue and small blood vessels. Some atrial and ventricular myocardial fibers are anchored to the fibrous skeleton (see Fig. 1-5). The thin-walled atria are composed of two major muscle systems: one that surrounds both the atria, and another that is arranged at right angles to the first and that is separate for each atrium.

Each ventricle is a single muscle mass of nested figure eights of individual muscle fiber path spirals anchored to the fibrous skeleton (Robb et al., 1942; Streeter et al., 1969). Ventricular muscle fibers spiral downward on the epicardial ventricular wall, pass through the wall, spiral up on the endocardial surface, cross the upper part of the ventricle, and go back down through the wall (Fig. 1-9). This vortex arrangement allows for the circumferential generation of tension throughout the ventricular wall and thus is functionally efficient for ventricular contraction. Some fiber paths spiral around both ventricles. The fibers form a fan-like arrangement of interconnecting muscle fibers when dissected horizontally through the ventricular wall (Streeter et al., 1969). The orientation of these fibers gradually rotates through the thickness of the wall (Fig. 1-10).

The myocardial tissue consists of several functionally specialized cell types:

Working myocardial cells generate the contractile force of the heart. These cells have a markedly striated appearance because of the orderly arrays of the abundant contractile

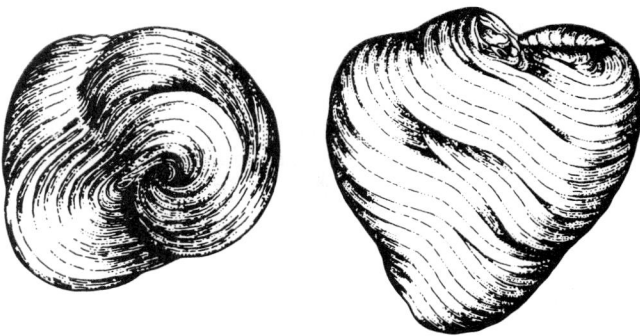

■ **Figure 1–9.** Schematic view of spiral arrangement of ventricular muscle fibers. (From Katz, A. [1977]. *Physiology of the heart* [p. 4]. New York: Raven Press.)

Endocardium

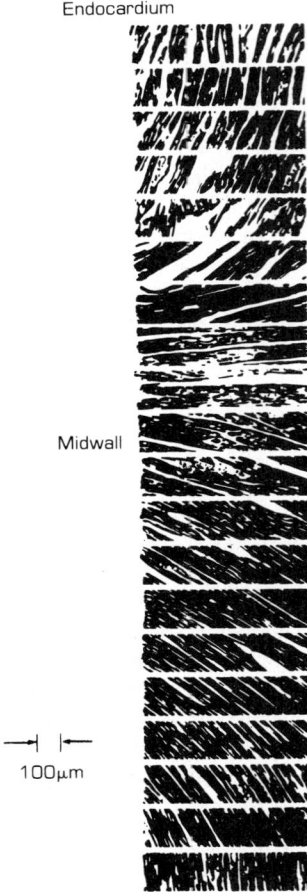

Midwall

100μm

Epicardium

■ **Figure 1–10.** Changing ventricular muscle fiber angles at different depths. Reconstructed from a series of microphotographs. (From Streeter, D.D. Jr, Spotnitz, H.M., & Patel, D.P. et al. [1969]. Fiber orientation in the canine left ventricle during diastole and systole. *Circulation Research,* 24, 342. By permission of the American Heart Association, Inc.)

protein filaments. Working myocardial cells comprise the bulk of the walls of both atrial and both ventricular chambers.

Nodal cells are specialized for pacemaker function. They are found in clusters in the sinus node and AV node. These cells contain few contractile filaments, little sarcoplasmic reticulum (SR), and no transverse tubules. They are the smallest myocardial cells.

Purkinje cells are specialized for rapid conduction of electrical impulses, especially through the thick ventricular wall. The large size, elongated shape, and sparse contractile protein composition reflect this specialization. These cells are found in the common His bundle and in the left and right bundle branches as well as in a diffuse network throughout the ventricles. Purkinje cell cytoplasm is rich in glycogen granules, thus making these cells more resistant to damage during anoxia. A secondary function of the Purkinje cells is to serve as a potential pacemaker locus. In the absence of an overriding impulse from the sinus node, Purkinje cells initiate electrical impulses.

In areas of contact between diverse cell types, there is usually an area of gradual transition in which the cells are intermediate in appearance.

Endocardium

The endocardium is composed of a layer of endothelial cells and a few layers of collagen and elastic fibers. The endocardium is in continuation with the tunica intima of the blood vessels.

Conduction Tissues

In the normal sequence of events, the specialized nodal myocardial cells depolarize spontaneously, generating electrical impulses that are conducted to the larger mass of working myocardial cells (Fig. 1-11). The sequential contraction of the atria and ventricles as coordinated units depends on the anatomic arrangement of the specialized cardiac conducting tissue. Small cardiac nerves, arteries, and veins lie close to the specialized conducting cells, providing neurohumoral modulation of cardiac impulse generation and conduction.

Keith and Flack first described the sinus node in 1907. It lies close to the epicardial surface of the heart, above the tricuspid valve, near the anterior entrance of the superior vena cava into the right atrium. The sinus node is also referred to as the *sinoatrial node.* It is approximately 10 to 15 mm long, 3 to 5 mm wide, and 1 mm thick. Small nodal cells are surrounded by and interspersed with connective tissue. They merge with the larger working atrial muscle cells.

Bachmann (1916) originally described an interatrial myocardial bundle conducting impulses from the right atrium to the left atrium. James (1963) presented evidence for three *internodal conduction pathways* from the sinus node to the AV node. It is unclear whether the pathways are ever of functional significance (Scher & Spach, 1979; Spach & Barr, 1976). It is generally believed that the cardiac impulse spreads from the sinus node to the AV node via cell-to-cell conduction through the atrial working myocardial cells (Fawcett, 1986).

Tarawa (1906) initially described the AV node in 1906. It is located subendocardially on the right atrial side of the central fibrous body, in the lower interatrial septal wall. The AV node is close to the septal leaflet of the tricuspid valve and anterior to the coronary sinus. A group of fibers connects the AV node to working myocardial cells in the left atrium (Fabiato, 1983). The AV node is approximately 7 mm long, 3 mm wide, and 1 mm thick (Titus et al., 1963). Nodal fibers are interspersed with normal working myocardial fibers; it is difficult to precisely identify the AV node boundaries. There are several zones of specialized conducting tissue in the AV junction area: the compact AV node, a transition zone containing small nodal and larger working atrial myocardial cells, the penetrating AV bundle, and the branching AV bundle (Anderson et al., 1975a; Hecht et al., 1973).

Fibers from the AV node converge into a shaft termed the *bundle of His* (also called the *penetrating AV bundle* or *common bundle*). It is approximately 10 mm long and 2 mm in diameter (Titus et al., 1963). The bundle of His passes from the lower right atrial wall anteriorly and laterally through the central fibrous body, which is part of the fibrous skeleton.

As first noted by His in 1893, the His bundle provides the only cellular connection between the atria and ventricles. The His bundle is of pivotal functional importance. Cardiac impulse transmission is slowed at this site, providing time for

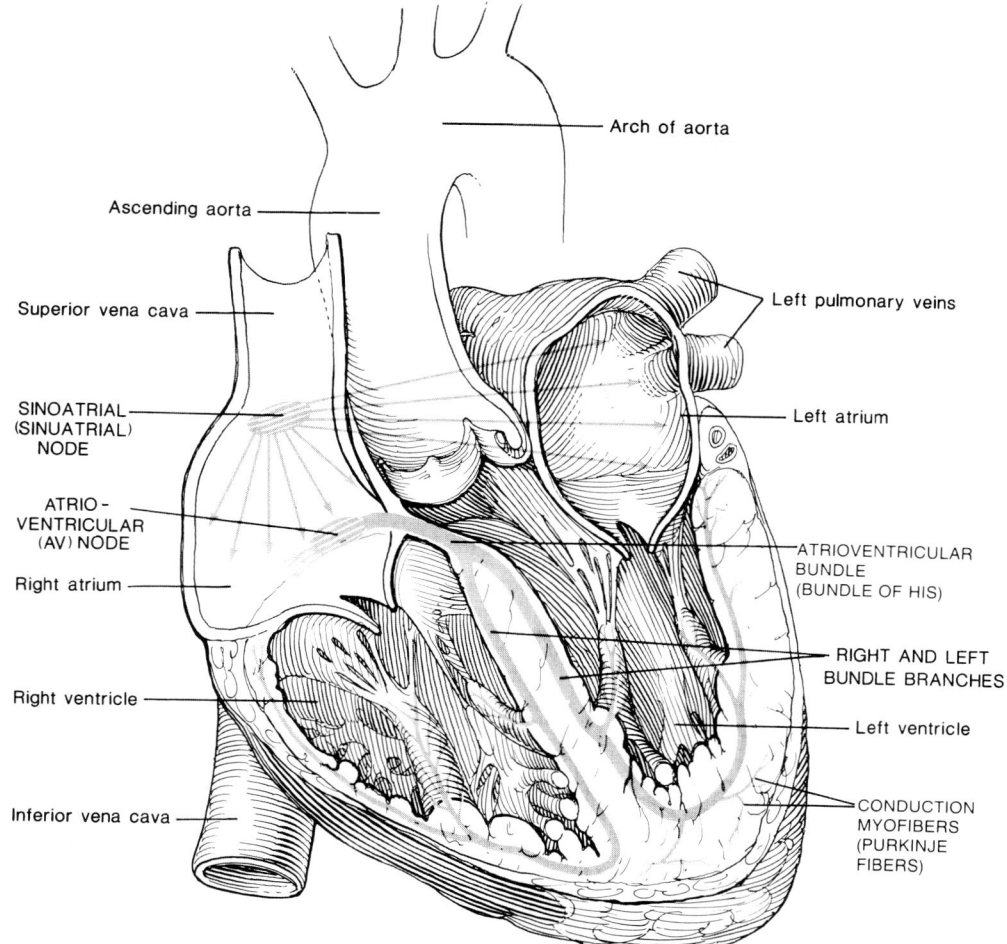

Arch of aorta

Ascending aorta

Superior vena cava

Left pulmonary veins

SINOATRIAL
(SINUATRIAL)
NODE

Left atrium

ATRIO-
VENTRICULAR
(AV) NODE

ATRIOVENTRICULAR
BUNDLE
(BUNDLE OF HIS)

Right atrium

RIGHT AND LEFT
BUNDLE BRANCHES

Right ventricle

Left ventricle

Inferior vena cava

CONDUCTION
MYOFIBERS
(PURKINJE
FIBERS)

■ **Figure 1–11.** Schematic illustration of the human cardiac conducting system. (From Tortora, G.J. [1986]. *Principles of human anatomy* [4th ed., p. 311]. New York: Harper & Row.)

atrial contraction to dispel blood from the atria into the ventricles. This boosts the ventricular volume and increases the cardiac output during subsequent ventricular contraction. At the membranous septal region of the heart, the right atrium and left ventricle are opposite each other across the septum, with the right ventricle in close proximity. Three of the four cardiac valves are nearby (Hudson, 1967) (Fig. 1-12). Thus, pathological problems of the fibrous skeleton or of the tricuspid, mitral, or aortic valves may affect functioning of one or more of the other valves or may affect cardiac impulse conduction. Dysfunction of the AV conducting tissue may affect the coordinated functioning of the atria and ventricles.

Abnormal accessory pathways, termed *Kent bundles*, occasionally join the atria and ventricles through connections outside the main AV node and His bundle (Kent, 1893, 1914). Tracts from the His bundle to upper interventricular septum (termed *paraspecific fibers of Mahaim*) sometimes occur and are also abnormal (Mahaim, 1947; Mahaim & Winston, 1941). AV conduction is accelerated when impulses bypass the delay-producing AV junction and travel instead through these abnormal connections. When accelerated AV conduction occurs, cardiac output often decreases because there is inadequate time

for atrial contraction to boost ventricular filling (Anderson et al., 1975b).

The His bundle begins branching in the region of the crest of the muscular septum (see Fig. 1-11). The right bundle branch typically continues as a direct extension of the His bundle. The right bundle branch is a well-defined, single, slender group of fibers approximately 45 to 50 mm long and 1 mm thick. It initially courses downward along the right side of the interventricular septum, continues through the moderator band of muscular tissue near the right ventricular apex, and then continues to the base of the anterior papillary muscle. If a small segment of the bundle is damaged, the entire distal distribution is affected because of the right bundle's thinness, length, and relative lack of arborization.

The left bundle branch arises almost perpendicularly from the His bundle as the common left bundle branch. This common left bundle, approximately 10 mm long and 4 to 10 mm wide, then divides into two discrete divisions, the left anterior bundle branch and the left posterior bundle branch. The left anterior bundle branch, or left anterior fascicle, is approximately 25 mm long and 3 mm thick. It usually arises directly from the common left bundle after the origin of the posterior

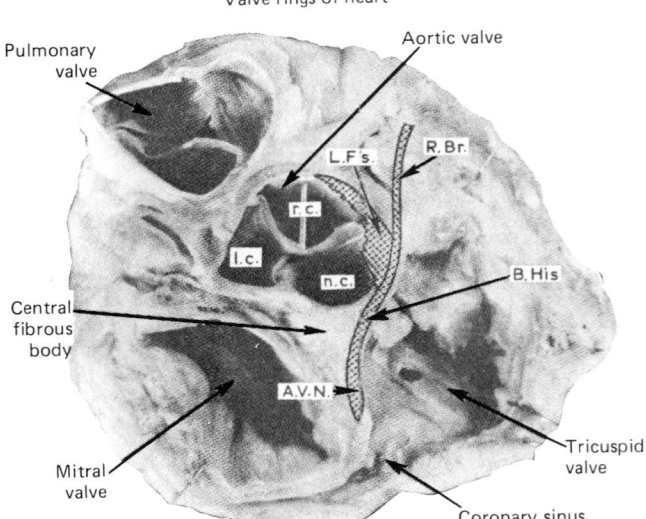

Valve rings of heart

Pulmonary valve

Aortic valve

L.F's   R. Br.

r.c.

l.c.

n.c.

B. His

Central fibrous body

A.V.N.

Mitral valve

Tricuspid valve

Coronary sinus

■ **Figure 1–12.** Schematic illustration of the relation of the atrioventricular conducting system to cardiac valves. Viewed from above. Note the proximity of the atrioventricular node (A.V.N.) to the aortic, mitral, and tricuspid valves and the proximity of the valves to each other. L.F., left ventricular conducting fiber; R. Br., right bundle branch; B. His, bundle of His; r.c., l.c., and n.c., right, left, and noncoronary cusps of the aortic valve. (From Hudson, R.E.B. [1967]. Surgical pathology of the conducting system of the heart. *British Heart Journal*, 29, 652, 1967.)

fascicle and close to the origin of the right bundle. It ramifies to the anterior septum and courses over the left ventricular anterior (superior) wall to the anterior papillary muscle, crossing the aortic outflow tract. Anterior and septal myocardial infarctions and aortic valve dysfunction often affect the left anterior bundle branch.

The large, thick, left posterior bundle branch, or left posterior fascicle, arises either from the first portion of the common left bundle or from the His bundle directly. The left posterior fascicle goes inferiorly and posteriorly across the left ventricular inflow tract to the base of the posterior papillary muscle, and then spreads diffusely through the posterior inferior left ventricular free wall. It is approximately 20 mm long and 6 mm thick. This fascicle is often the least vulnerable segment of the ventricular conducting system because of its diffuseness, its location in a relatively protected nonturbulent portion of the ventricle, and its dual blood supply (Table 1-1).

Three, rather than two, major divisions of the left bundle branch are sometimes found, with a group of fibers ramifying from the left posterior fascicle and terminating in the lower septum and apical ventricular wall (Hecht et al., 1973). This trifascicular configuration of the bundles explains some conduction defects involving partial bundle-branch block. Sometimes instead of three discrete bundles the common left bundle fans out diffusely along the septum and the free ventricular wall (Massing & James, 1976) (see Fig. 1-12).

Purkinje fibers, first described in 1845, form a complex network of conducting tissue ramifications that provide a continuation of the bundle branches in each ventricle (Purkinje, 1845). They course down toward the ventricular apex and then

up toward the fibrous rings at the ventricular bases. They spread over the subendocardial ventricular surfaces and then spread from the endocardium through the myocardium, thus spreading from inside outward, providing extensive contacts with working myocardial cells, and coupling myocardial excitation with muscular contraction.

■ CORONARY CIRCULATION

The heart is continuously active. Like all tissues, it must receive oxygen and metabolic substrates and have carbon dioxide and other wastes removed to maintain aerobic metabolism and contractile activity. However, unlike other tissues, it must generate the force to power its own perfusion. The heart requires large perfusion volumes.

Coronary Arteries

The major coronary arteries in humans are the right coronary artery and the left coronary artery, sometimes called the *left main coronary artery.* These arteries branch from the aorta in the region of the sinus of Valsalva (Figs. 1-13 and 1-14). They extend over the epicardial surface of the heart and branch several times. The branches usually emerge at a right angle from the parent artery (James, 1961). The arteries plunge inward through the myocardial wall and undergo further branching. The epicardial branches exit first. The more distal branches supply the endocardial (internal) myocardium. The arteries continue branching and eventually become arterioles, then capillaries. Partially because the blood supply originates more distally, the endocardium is more vulnerable to compromised blood supply than is the epicardial (outer) myocardium.

There is much individual variation in the pattern of coronary artery branching. In general, the right coronary artery supplies the right atrium and ventricle. The left coronary artery supplies much of the left atrium and ventricle. The following discussion describes the most common arterial pattern. Table 1-1 lists the major cardiac structures, their usual arterial supply, and some common variations (e.g., either the right or the left coronary artery may supply the AV node).

Individual anatomic variation should be considered in analyzing individual patient data. For example, angiographic visualization of the left circumflex artery might show severe stenosis. Although it is not likely that AV node and His bundle perfusion would be affected (because the right coronary artery typically perfuses these structures), in approximately 10% of cases the structures would be at risk. Thus, angiographic information is validated with clinical data. Also, apparently attenuated or narrowed vessels may be normal anatomic variants.

Vessel Dominance

Dominance (or *preponderance*), a term commonly used in describing coronary vasculature, refers to the distribution of the terminal portion of the arteries. The artery that reaches and

Table 1–1 ■ AREA SUPPLIED BY COMMON ARTERIES*

Structure	Usual Arterial Supply	Common Variants
Right atrium	Sinus node artery, branch of RCA (55%)	Sinus node artery, branch of L circumflex (45%)
Left atrium	Major L circumflex†	Sinus node artery, branch of L circumflex (45%)
Right ventricle		
Anterior	Major RCA	
	Minor LAD	
Posterior	Major RCA; posterior descending branch of RCA	Posterior descending may branch from L circumflex (10%)
	Minor LAD (ascending portion)	LAD terminates at apex (40%)
Left ventricle		
Posterior (diaphragmatic)	Major L circumflex, posterior descending branch of RCA	Posterior descending may branch from L circumflex (10%)
	Minor LAD (ascending portion)	LAD terminates at apex (40%)
Anterior	L coronary artery; L circumflex and LAD	
Apex	Major LAD	
Intraventricular septum	Major septal branches of LAD	Minor posterior descending may branch from L circumflex,
	Minor posterior descending branch of RCA and AV nodal branch of RCA	AV nodal may branch from L circumflex
Left ventricular papillary muscles		
Anterior	Diagonal branch of LAD; other branches of LAD, other branches of L circumflex	Diagonal may branch from circumflex
Posterior	RCA and L circumflex	RCA and LAD
Sinus node	Nodal artery from RCA (55%)	Nodal artery from L circumflex (45%)
AV node	RCA (90%)	L circumflex (10%)
Bundle of His	RCA (90%)	L circumflex (10%)
Right bundle	Major LAD septal branches	
	Minor AV nodal artery	
Left anterior bundle	Major LAD septal branches	
	Minor AV nodal artery	
Left posterior bundle	LAD septal branches and AV nodal artery	

* Percentages in parentheses denote frequency of occurrence in autopsy studies.
† Major and minor refer to degree of predominance of an artery in perfusing a structure.
RCA, right coronary artery; LAD, left anterior descending artery; L, left; LV, left ventricle; AV, atrioventricular.
Data from James, T.N. (1961). *Anatomy of the coronary arteries.* New York: Paul B. Hoeber; James, T.N. (1978). Anatomy of the coronary arteries and veins. In J.W. Hurst (Ed.), *The heart* (4th ed., pp 32–47). New York: McGraw-Hill.

crosses the *crux* (where the right and left AV grooves cross the posterior interatrial and interventricular grooves) is said to be *dominant.* In approximately 85% of cases, the right coronary artery crosses the crux and is dominant. The term can be confusing because in most human hearts, the left coronary artery is of wider caliber and perfuses the largest proportion of myocardium. Thus, the dominant artery usually does not perfuse the largest percentage of myocardial mass. The dominant artery supplies the posterior diaphragmatic interventricular septum and diaphragmatic surface of the left ventricle.

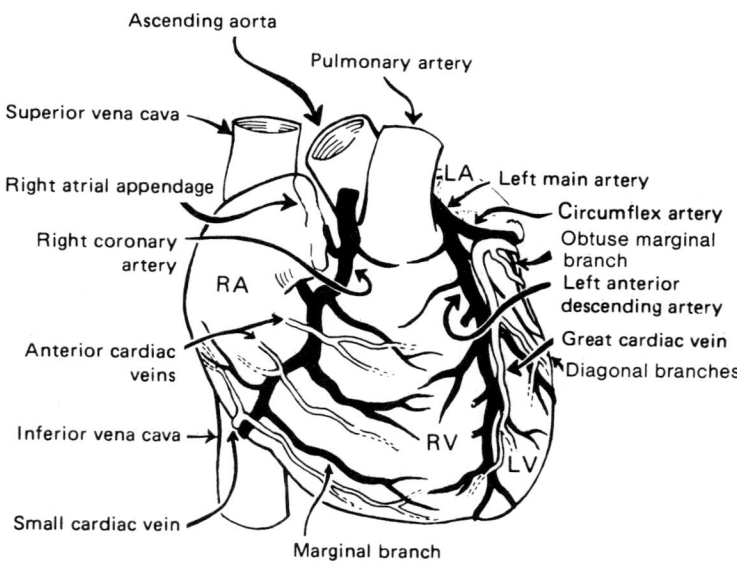

■ Figure 1–13. Principal arteries and veins on the anterior surface of the heart. Part of the right atrial appendage has been resected. The left coronary artery arises from the left coronary aortic sinus behind the pulmonary trunk. RA, right atrium; RV, right ventricle; LA, left atrium; LV, left ventricle. (Adapted from Walmsley R., & Watson, H. [1978]. *Clinical anatomy of the heart* [p. 203]. New York: Churchill Livingston.)

■ **Figure 1–14.** Principal arteries and veins on the infero-posterior surfaces of the heart. This schematic drawing illustrates the heart tilted upward at a nonphysiological angle; normally, little of the inferior cardiac surface is visible posteriorly. The right coronary artery is shown to cross the crux and to supply the atrioventricular node. The artery to the sinus node in this figure arises from the right coronary artery. RA, right atrium; RV, right ventricle; LA, left atrium; LV, left ventricle. (Adapted from Walmsley, R., & Watson, H. [1978]. *Clinical anatomy of the heart* [p. 205]. New York: Churchill Livingston.)

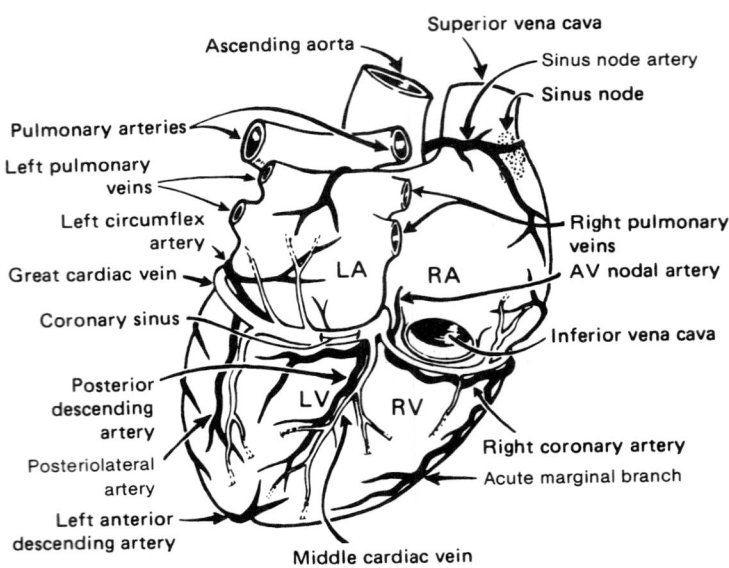

Right Coronary Artery

The right coronary artery supplies the right atrium, right ventricle, and a portion of the posterior and inferior surfaces of the left ventricle. It supplies the AV node and bundle of His in 90% of hearts, and the sinus node in 55% of hearts (James, 1961). It originates behind the right aortic cusp and passes behind the pulmonary artery, coursing in the right AV groove laterally to the right margin of the heart and then posteriorly. The major branches of the right coronary artery, in order of origin, are as follows:

1. Conus branch
2. Sinus node artery
3. Right ventricular branches
4. Right atrial branch
5. Acute marginal branch
6. AV nodal branch
7. Posterior descending branch
8. Left ventricular branch
9. Left atrial branch

The *conus branch* is small and exits within the first 2 cm of the right coronary artery in 60% of cases. It sometimes originates as a separate vessel with an ostium within a millimeter of the right coronary artery (Kelly & Gensini, 1975). The branch proceeds centrally to the left of the pulmonic valve. It supplies the upper part of the right ventricle, near the outflow tract at the level of the pulmonic valve. When the conus branch anastomoses with a right ventricular branch of the left anterior descending artery, the resulting structure is called the *circle of Vieussens,* an important collateral link between left and right coronary arteries.

The sinus node artery arises from the right coronary artery in 55% of cases (Kelly & Gensini, 1975). It proceeds in the opposite direction from the conus branch, coursing cranially and to the right, encircling the superior vena cava. It usually has two branches: one supplies the sinus node and parts of the right atrium, and the other branches to the left atrium.

The right coronary artery courses along the AV groove, giving rise next to one or more *right ventricular branches* that vary in length and distribute to the right ventricular wall. The *right atrial branch* proceeds cranially toward the right heart border and perfuses the right atrium.

The *acute marginal branch* is a fairly large branch of the right coronary artery. It originates at the acute margin of the heart near the right atrial artery and courses in the opposite direction, toward the apex. It perfuses the inferior and diaphragmatic surfaces of the right ventricle and occasionally the posterior apical portion of the interventricular septum.

The *AV nodal branch* is slender and straight. It originates at the crux and is directed inward toward the center of the heart. It perfuses the AV node and the lower portion of the interatrial septum.

The *posterior descending branch* is an important branch of the right coronary artery. It supplies the posterosuperior portion of the interventricular septum. It exits at the crux and courses in the posterior interventricular sulcus.

The *left ventricular branch* originates just beyond the crux. It runs centrally in the angle formed by the left posterior AV groove and the posterior interventricular sulcus. It perfuses the diaphragmatic aspect of the left ventricle.

A *left atrial branch* may course along the posterior left AV groove and perfuse the left atrium.

Left Coronary Artery

The left main coronary artery arises from the aorta in the ostium behind the left cusp of the aortic valve. This artery passes between the left atrial appendage and the pulmonary artery and then typically divides into two major branches: the *left anterior descending artery* and the *left circumflex artery.*

Left Anterior Descending Artery. The left anterior descending artery supplies portions of the left and right ventricular myocardium and much of the interventricular septum. The left anterior descending artery appears to be a continuation of the left main coronary artery. It passes to the left of the pulmonic valve region, courses in the anterior interventricular sulcus to the apex, then courses around the apex to terminate in the inferior portion of the posterior interventricular sulcus. Occasionally, the posterior descending branch of the right coronary artery extends around the apex from the posterior surface; the left anterior descending artery ends short of the apex. The major branches of the left anterior descending artery, in the order in which they branch, are the following:

1. First diagonal branch
2. First septal branch
3. Right ventricular branch
4. Minor septal branches
5. Second diagonal branch
6. Apical branches

The *first diagonal branch* is usually a large artery. It originates close to the bifurcation of the left main coronary artery and passes diagonally over the free wall of the left ventricle. It perfuses the high lateral portion of the left ventricular free wall. Several smaller diagonal branches may exit from the left side of the left anterior descending artery and run parallel to the first diagonal branch. The one referred to as the *second diagonal branch* takes its origin approximately two thirds of the way from the origin to the termination of the left anterior descending artery. This second diagonal branch perfuses the lower lateral portion of the free wall to the apex.

A variable number of septal branches occur. The *first septal branch* is the first to exit the left anterior descending artery. The others are referred to as *minor septal branches*. The septal branches exit at a 90-degree angle and course in the septum from the front to the back and caudally. Together, the septal branches perfuse two thirds of the upper portion of the septum and most of the inferior portion of the septum. The remaining superoposterior section of the septum is supplied by branches from the posterior descending artery, which usually derives from the right coronary artery.

One or more *right ventricular branches* may exist. One runs toward the conus branch of the right coronary artery and may anastomose into the circle of Vieussens.

The final branches are the *apical branches.* These perfuse the anterior and diaphragmatic aspects of the left ventricular free wall and apex.

Circumflex Artery. The *circumflex artery* supplies blood to parts of the left atrium and left ventricle. In 45% of cases, it supplies the major perfusion of the sinus node; in 10% of cases, it supplies the AV node (Kelly & Gensini, 1975). The circumflex artery exits from the left main coronary artery at a near-right angle and courses posteriorly in the AV groove toward, but usually not reaching, the crux. If the circumflex reaches the crux, it gives rise to the posterior descending artery. In the 15% of cases in which this occurs, the left coronary artery supplies the entire septum and possibly the AV node (Kelly & Gensini, 1975). The branches of the circumflex artery, in order of origin, are as follows:

1. Atrial circumflex branch
2. Sinus node artery
3. Obtuse marginal branches
4. Posterolateral branches

The *atrial circumflex branch* is usually small in caliber but may be as wide as the remaining portion of the circumflex. It runs along the left AV groove and perfuses the left atrial wall.

In 45% of cases, the *sinus node artery* originates from the initial portion of the circumflex; it runs cranially and dorsally, to the base of the superior vena cava in the region of the sinus node (Kelly & Gensini, 1975). This artery perfuses portions of the left and right atria as well as the sinus node.

From one to four *obtuse marginal branches* may be seen. These vary greatly in size. They run along the ventricular wall laterally and posteriorly, toward the apex, along the obtuse margin of the heart. The marginal branches supply the obtuse margin of the heart and the adjacent posterior wall of the left ventricle above the diaphragmatic surface.

The *posterolateral branches* arise from the circumflex artery in 80% of cases (Kelly & Gensini, 1975). These branches originate in the terminal portion of the circumflex artery and course caudally and to the left on the posterior left ventricular wall, supplying the posterior and diaphragmatic wall of the left ventricle.

The *posterior descending* and AV nodal arteries occasionally arise from the circumflex. When they do, the entire septum is supplied by branches of the left coronary artery.

Coronary Capillaries

Blood passes from arteries into arterioles, then into capillaries, where exchange of oxygen and other materials takes place. The heart has a dense capillary network with approximately 3,300 capillaries/mm^2, or approximately 1 capillary per muscle fiber (Wearn, 1940). Blood flow through coronary capillaries is regulated according to myocardial metabolic needs (see later).

When myocardial cells hypertrophy, the cell radius increases. The capillary network, however, does not appear to proliferate (Armour & Hopkins, 1984). The same capillaries must perfuse a larger mass of tissue. The distance over which materials must diffuse is increased. Thus, with hypertrophy, the coronary circulation perfuses a larger tissue mass. At the same time, efficiency of exchange may be diminished.

Coronary Veins

Most of the venous drainage of the heart is through epicardial veins. The large veins course close to the coronary arteries. Two veins sometimes accompany an artery (James, 1961). The major veins feed into the great cardiac vein, which runs alongside the circumflex artery, becomes the coronary sinus, and then empties into the right atrium (see Fig. 1-14). An incompetent (incompletely shut) semilunar valve, called the valve of Vieussens, marks the junction between the great cardiac vein and the coronary sinus. A similar structure, the thebesian valve, is also incompetent and is found at the entry of the coronary sinus into the right atrium. Venous blood from the right ventricular muscle is drained primarily by two to four anterior cardiac veins that empty directly into the right atrium, bypassing the coronary sinus (see Fig. 1-13).

Some veins, known as *thebesian veins,* empty directly into the ventricles (Fig. 1-15). They are more common on the right

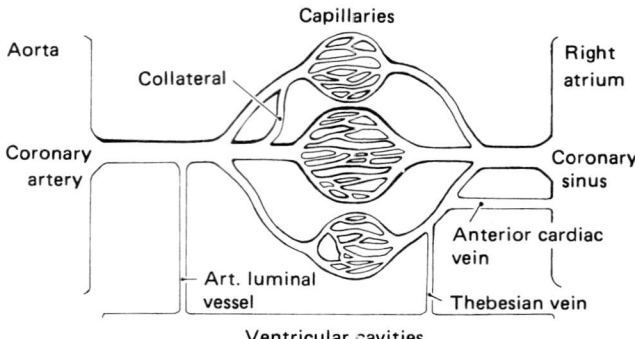

■ **Figure 1–15.** Schematic model of coronary circulation. As in other circulatory beds, the coronary circulation includes arteries, capillaries, and veins. Some veins drain directly into the ventricles. Collateral channels may link arterial vessels. Art, arterial. (Adapted from Ruch, T.C. & Patton, H.D. [1974]. *Physiology and biophysics* [20th ed., Vol. 2, p. 249]. Philadelphia: WB Saunders.)

side of the heart, where the pressure gradient is favorable for such flow. Only a small amount of venous blood is returned directly to the left ventricle. When blood is returned to the left ventricle, it constitutes a component of physiologic shunt, or unoxygenated blood entering the systemic circulation. Many collateral channels are found in the venous drainage system.

Lymph Drainage

Cardiac contraction promotes lymphatic drainage in the myocardium through an abundant system of lymphatic vessels, most of which eventually converge into the principal left anterior lymphatic. Lymph from this vessel empties into the pretracheal lymph node and then proceeds by way of two channels to the cardiac lymph node, the right lymphatic duct, and then into the superior vena cava (Miller, 1982).

The importance of a normally functioning lymphatic system in maintaining an appropriate environment for cardiac cell function is frequently overlooked. Although complete cardiac lymph obstruction is rarely observed, experimental acute and chronic lymphatic impairment causes cellular myocardial and endocardial changes, particularly when occurring in conjunction with venous congestion (Miller, 1982). Experimentally induced myocardial infarction in animals with chronically impaired lymphatic drainage causes more extensive cellular necrosis, an increased and prolonged inflammatory response, and a greater amount of fibrosis than infarction in animals without lymphatic obstruction (Miller, 1982).

CARDIAC INNERVATION

Sensory nerve fibers from ventricular walls, the pericardium, coronary blood vessels, and other tissues transmit impulses by way of the cardiac nerves to the central nervous system. Motor nerve fibers to the heart are autonomic. Sympathetic stimulation accelerates firing of the sinus node, enhances conduction through the AV node, and increases the force of cardiac contraction. Parasympathetic stimulation slows the heart rate, slows conduction through the AV node, and may decrease ventricular contractile force.

Sympathetic preganglionic cardiac nerves arise from the first four or five thoracic spinal cord segments. The nerves synapse with long postganglionic fibers in the superior, middle, and cervicothoracic or stellate ganglia adjacent to the spinal cord. Most postganglionic sympathetic nerves to the heart travel through the superior, middle, and inferior cardiac nerves. However, several cardiac nerves with variable origins have been identified (Armour & Hopkins, 1984; Randall, 1984). Parasympathetic preganglionic cardiac nerves arise from the right and left vagus nerves and synapse with postganglionic nerves close to their target cardiac cells.

Both vagal and sympathetic cardiac nerves converge in the cardiac plexus. The cardiac plexus is situated superior to the bifurcation of the pulmonary artery, behind the aortic arch, and anterior to the trachea at the level of tracheal bifurcation. From the cardiac plexus, the cardiac nerves course in two coronary plexuses along with the right and left coronary blood vessels.

Sympathetic fibers are richly distributed throughout the heart. Right sympathetic ganglia fibers most commonly innervate the sinus node, the right atrium, the anterior ventricular walls, and to some extent the AV node. Most commonly, left sympathetic ganglia fibers extensively innervate the AV junctional area and the posterior and inferior left ventricle (Randall, 1984).

A dense supply of vagal fibers innervates the sinus node, AV node, and ventricular conducting system. Consequently, many parasympathetic ganglia are found in the region of the sinus and AV nodes. Vagal fibers also innervate both atria and, to a lesser extent, both ventricles (Randall, 1984). Right vagal fibers have more effect on the sinus node; left vagal fibers have more effect on the AV node and ventricular conduction system. However, there is overlap. The clinical importance of vagal stimulation for ventricular function continues to be debated.

Although neurotransmitters from cardiac nerves are important modulators of cardiac activity, the success of cardiac transplantation illustrates the capacity of the heart to function without nervous innervation.

MYOCARDIAL CELL STRUCTURE

Myocardial cells are long, narrow, and often branched. A limiting membrane, the sarcolemma, surrounds each cell. Specialized surface membrane structures include the intercalated disc, nexus, and transverse tubules (T-tubules). Major intracellular components are contractile protein filaments (called myofibrils), mitochondria, SR, and nucleus. There is a small amount of cytoplasm, called *sarcoplasm* (Fig. 1-16).

The *sarcolemma* is a thin phospholipid bilayer separating the intracellular and extracellular spaces. Across the barrier of the sarcolemma are marked differences in ionic composition and electrical charge. Proteins embedded in the sarcolemma serve multiple functions. Embedded receptors bind substances present in the extracellular space. That binding in turn activates or inhibits cell electrical, contractile, metabolic, or other functions. Embedded ion channels regulate membrane ion permeability

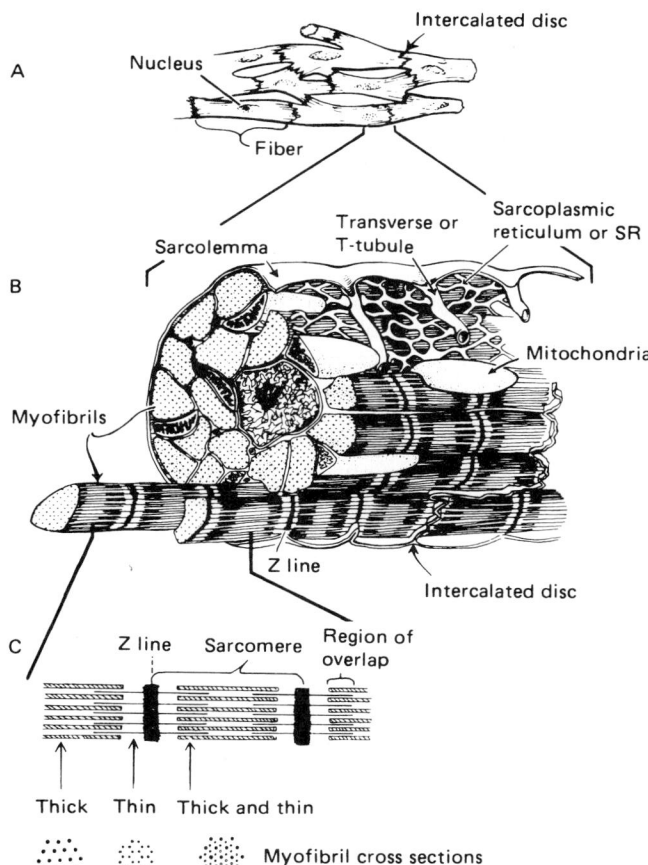

A

B

C

Thick Thin Thick and thin

Myofibril cross sections

■ **Figure 1–16.** The microscopic structure of working myocardial cells. (*A*) Working myocardial cells as seen under the light microscope. Note the branching network of fibers and intercalated discs. (*B*) Schematic illustration of the internal structure of the working myocardial cell. Note the striated appearance of the myofibrils, the intimate association of the sarcoplasmic reticulum with the myofibrils, the presence of T-tubules, and the large number of mitochondria. (*C*) Structure of the sarcomere, illustrating alignment of thick and thin filaments. Cross-sections taken at three different positions along the sarcomere illustrate a region with only thick filaments, a region with only thin filaments, and a region of overlap where the thick and the thin filaments interdigitate. (Adapted from Braunwald, E., Ross, J., & Sonnenblick, E. [1976]. *Mechanisms of contraction of the normal and failing heart* [2nd ed., p. 3]. Boston: Little, Brown.)

and electrical function. Various carrier proteins facilitate the uptake of metabolic substrates such as glucose. Some sarcolemma proteins add structural stability.

Structurally, each myocardial cell is distinct. The *intercalated disc* forms a mechanical and electrical junction between adjacent cells. A specialized type of cell-to-cell connection, the *nexus* (sometimes called the *gap junction*), is present in the intercalated disc. The nexus is the site of direct exchange of small molecules. The nexus also provides a low-resistance electrical path between cells, thus facilitating rapid impulse conduction. Physiologic conditions alter the permeability of the nexus. For example, two substances that vary with physiologic state are adenosine triphosphate (ATP) and cyclic adenosine monophosphate (cAMP) -dependent protein kinases. Both

alter nexus permeability (De Mello, 1990; Sperelakis, 1979). Because of these junctions, the heart functions as a syncytium of coordinated cells, although anatomically the cells are discrete units.

Another specialized membrane structure, the *T-tubule system*, is an extensive labyrinthine network of membrane-lined tubes systematically tunneling inward throughout each cell. It is formed by invaginations of the sarcolemma, continuous with the surface membrane. The T-tubule lumen contains extracellular fluid. The T-tubular network carries electrical excitation to the central portions of myocardial cells, thus allowing near-simultaneous activation of deep and superficial parts of cells.

Myofibrils are long, rod-like structures that extend the length of the cell. They contain the contractile proteins, which convert the chemical energy of ATP into mechanical energy and heat. Muscle contraction involves the generation of force, shortening by the myofibrils, or both. The highly organized alignment of the contractile proteins in myofilaments gives the myocardial cell its striated (striped) appearance.

Mitochondria are small, rod-shaped membranous structures located within the cell. Breakdown of substrates and synthesis of high-energy compounds occurs in the mitochondria. The relative abundance of mitochondria in cardiac muscle cells reflects the high level of biochemical activity required to support continuous contractile activity.

The *sarcoplasmic reticulum* is an extensive, self-contained internal membrane system. Both the T-tubules and SR contribute to linking of electrical depolarization of the membrane to the mechanical activity of the contractile protein filaments. This functional coordination is called excitation—contraction coupling. The SR is the major storage depot for calcium ion, releasing then taking up calcium ion with each contraction of the heart.

The *nucleus* contains the genetic material of the cell; it is the site where new proteins are synthesized.

MYOCARDIAL CELL ELECTRICAL CHARACTERISTICS

An electrical charge exists across the myocardial sarcolemma. The charge is called a *potential difference* and is measured in millivolts (mV). During the interim between excitations, the intracellular space of the cell is negative compared with the extracellular space. This potential difference is called the *membrane resting potential*. During excitation, the potential difference changes: the inside of the cell becomes less negative, or slightly positive compared with the extracellular space. This type of potential difference change is called *depolarization*. After depolarization, the membrane potential difference again becomes negative, returning the membrane electrical charge to the resting potential value. This type of potential difference change is called *repolarization*. The normal depolarization—repolarization cycle is known as the *action potential*. The electrical excitation of the action potential is the signal that evokes contraction. Until the cell repolarizes sufficiently, there can be no action potential. If the potential difference becomes more negative than the usual resting potential, the membrane is said to be *hyperpolarized*. The more hyperpolarized the membrane, the more current is required to evoke an action potential.

Some myocardial cells have *automaticity*, that is, an intrinsic ability to depolarize spontaneously and initiate an action potential. The action potential generated in such a cell is then propagated throughout cardiac tissue. Depolarization of one cardiac cell initiates depolarization of adjacent cells and ultimately leads to cell contraction.

It is estimated that there are approximately 19 billion cells in the adult heart; these cells must depolarize in an orderly sequence if the heart is to undergo a coordinated contraction that is able to add force to moving blood. Impulses generated in ectopic sites in the heart are less likely to depolarize in an orderly sequence and less likely to contract in an orderly fashion that effectively pumps blood.

Basis for Myocardial Excitation: Characteristics of Biologic Membranes

Intracellular and extracellular spaces are separated by a thin insulating membrane, the sarcolemma. These spaces have very different ionic compositions. The intracellular space contains high concentrations of potassium ion (positively charged) and protein (negatively charged) and has low concentration of sodium ion (positively charged). The extracellular space consists of high concentrations of sodium ion and chloride ion (negatively charged); extracellular potassium ion concentration is low.

For each ion, concentration differences across the sarcolemma are determined by the sarcolemma's permeability to that ion and the strength of the forces moving the ion from one to the other side of the membrane. Electrical and concentration differences are maintained by a number of active and passive processes. Typical concentration differences are outlined in Table 1-2.

The sarcolemma is composed of phospholipid molecules. Each molecule consists of a charged hydrophilic (water-attracting) globular head and a noncharged hydrophobic (water-repelling) tail. The molecules organize into thin sheets, with the heads oriented in a consistent direction. Two sheets are aligned tail-to-tail to form a double layer (bilayer). The tails form the core of the sheet, and the heads are directed outward in both directions. The result is a 7- to 9-nm, high-resistance, insulated barrier to ionic movement.

Proteins are embedded within the phospholipid bilayer and may comprise more than half the mass of the membrane. The proteins act as receptors, channels, pumps, or structural stabilizers. They may be inserted into the intracellular or extracellular side of the bilayer or span its full thickness. Some of the proteins contain a water-filled pore that spans the membrane connecting the intracellular and extracellular spaces, forming a channel through which ions can pass. Membrane channels open and close in response to a stimulus (electrical, mechanical, or chemical), allowing passage of specific ions when open. The opening and closing properties of a channel are called its *gating* characteristics. The ability of a channel to selectively allow passage of certain ions while restricting other ions is called its *selectivity* property. Many ion channels are named after the ion for which they have selectivity. Some common types are sodium channels, potassium channels, and calcium channels (Fig. 1-17).

Mechanisms of Ion Distribution Across the Myocardial Membrane

Ions are distributed across the membrane according to the membrane permeability to the ion and the electrical and diffusion forces on the ion. For each ion that can penetrate the membrane, there is a continual movement toward equilibrium. When equilibrium is reached, forces driving ion movement are balanced, and there is no additional net change in the ion distribution. The Nernst equation, discussed later, is useful in understanding the relationship between electrical and diffusional forces driving ion movement. It is useful to remember that the permeability properties of the living membrane change continually.

Table 1–2 ■ APPROXIMATE INTRACELLULAR AND EXTRACELLULAR ION CONCENTRATIONS AND ACTIVITIES IN CARDIAC MUSCLE*

Ion[†]	Extracellular Concentration[‡]	Intracellular Concentration[§11]	Ratio of Extracellular to Intracellular Concentration	E_1	Intracellular Activity[#]
Na$^+$	145 mM	15 mM	9.7	+60 mV	7.0 mM
K$^+$	4 mM	150 mM	0.027	−94 mV	125 mM
Cl$^−$	120 mM	5 mM	24	−83 mV	15 mM
Ca^{2+}	2 mM	10^{-4} M	2×10^4	+129 mV	8×10^{-6} mM

*Values given are approximations and vary according to the cardiac tissue, species, and method used for measurement.

[†]Na$^+$, sodium; K$^+$, potassium; Cl$^−$, chloride; Ca^{2+}, calcium.

[‡]mM, millimolar.

[11]Most of the intracellular calcium is bound to proteins or sequestered in intracellular organelles; thus, total intracellular calcium content approximates 1 to 2 mm. During contraction, measurable intracellular calcium concentration approximates 10^{-5} mm.

[§]E_1, equilibrium potential; mV, millivolt. [#]Median values from summarized data; these values should be considered as subject to revision. Concentrations and equilibrium potentials from Sperelakis, N. (1979). Origin of the cardiac resting potential. In R.M. Berne (Ed.), *Handbook of physiology, Section 2: The cardiovascular system, vol 1, the heart* (p. 193.) Bethesda: American Physiological Society. Activities are approximations from Lee, C.O. (1981). Ionic activities in cardiac muscle cells and application of ion-sensitive microelectrodes, *American Journal of Physiology*, 10, H461, H464; and Fozzard, H.A., Wasserstrom, J.A. (1985). Voltage dependence of intracellular sodium and control of contraction. In P.P. Zipes, & J. Jalife. *Cardiac electrophysiology and arrhythmias* (p. 52.) Orlando: Grune & Stratton.

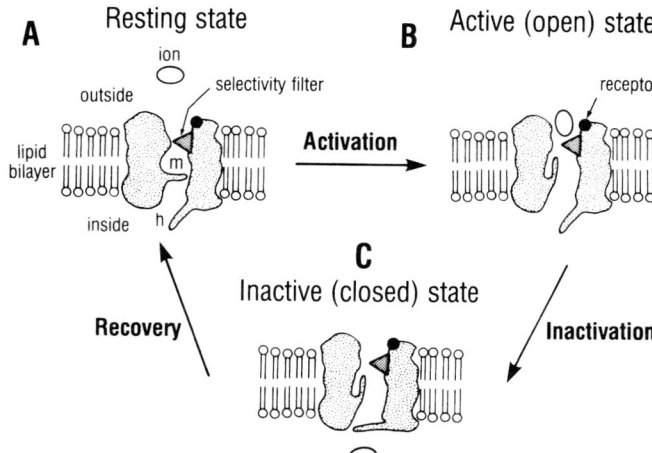

A Resting state   **B** Active (open) state

C Inactive (closed) state

■ **Figure 1–17.** Schematic illustration of the three hypothetical states of voltage-dependent ion channels in cardiac cell membranes, such as those for sodium. In the resting state (*A*), the activation (m) gate is closed and the inactivation (h) gate is open; ions are prevented from crossing the membrane through the channel. Depolarization to threshold activates the channel to the active state (*B*), opening the activation gate and allowing ions to traverse the channel. Closure of the inactivation gate terminates the ion flux and inactivates the channel (*C*). Repolarization reactivates the channel to the resting, ready-to-be-activated state. Selectivity filters in the channel may determine the ion type or types admitted through the channel. (◄, selectivity filter.) (Adapted from Sperelakis, N. [1984]. Hormonal and neurotransmitter regulation of Ca^{++} influx through voltage-dependent slow channels in cardiac muscle membrane. *Membrane Biochemistry,* 5, 134.)

Diffusional Force

Particles in solution move, or diffuse, from an area of higher concentration to an area of lower concentration. In the case of uncharged, soluble molecules, diffusion proceeds until there is a uniform distribution of the molecules within the solution. The solution is then said to be in equilibrium. At equilibrium, there is still particle movement within the solution, but no net change in overall distribution of particles. Charged particles also diffuse. The diffusion of charged particles is influenced not only by the concentration gradient but also by the electrical field.

Electrical Force And Current

Like charges repel, opposite charges attract. Positively charged particles tend to flow toward negatively charged particles and regions; similarly, negatively charged particles are attracted to positive ions and regions. The electrical (or electromotive) force difference between regions is called the *potential difference* and is expressed in volts (1 mV = 0.001 V). The net flow of charges is called *current* (measured in amperes). *Resistance* is the opposition to the flow of current, measured in ohms. Ohm's law (electromotive force = current × resistance) describes the relation among current, voltage, and resistance.

When charged particles have different concentrations in the solutions separated by a cell membrane, and some of the particles are able to permeate the membrane and others are not, an electrical force is established. This force influences the distribution of all other charged particles. The potential difference

across biologic membranes is described by comparing the interior of the cell with the external solution. In the typical quiescent or resting myocardial cell, the potential difference is −70 to −90 mV; that is, the cell interior is negative with respect to the exterior (Fig. 1-18). When positively charged ions move from the extracellular fluid to the intracellular fluid, the current is said to be *inward*. With inward current, the cell interior becomes less negative, that is, it depolarizes. When positively charged ions flow into the extracellular space from the interior of the cell, the current is said to be *outward;* the cell repolarizes. Movement of negatively charged ions in one direction is electrically equivalent to an opposite-directed movement of positively charged ions. Thus, the inward movement of an anion such as chloride is called an outward current. This, too, causes repolarization.

Nernst Equation Calculation of Equilibrium Potential for Specific Ions. The Nernst equation is used to calculate the *equilibrium potential* for a particular ion. If the potential difference across the membrane were the same as that calculated by the Nernst equation as the equilibrium potential for a particular ion, then the electrical force would counterbalance the concentration difference of that specific ion. If the membrane were permeable to the ion, there would be no net ion movement. An understanding of the equilibrium potential is basic to an understanding of the electrical characteristics of biologic membranes.

Potassium is an important and useful example for discussion of the Nernst equation. Potassium, a positive ion, has a much higher concentration inside the myocardial cell than in the extracellular space. To balance the force of the concentration difference, the inside of the myocardial cell would need to be approximately −94 mV compared with outside of the membrane. That charge, −94 mV, is known as the potassium equilibrium potential or the potassium Nernst potential for the cell. The resting myocardial membrane is permeable to potassium. The large concentration gradient is maintained because the actual voltage across the membrane between activation cycles, approximately −90 mV (inside negative), is nearly sufficient to

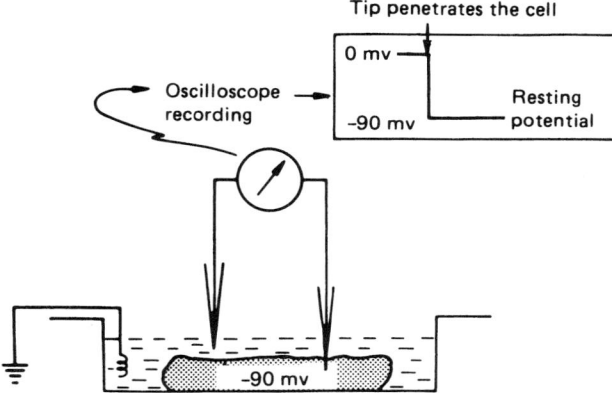

Tip penetrates the cell

0 mv

Oscilloscope recording

Resting potential

−90 mv

−90 mv

■ **Figure 1–18.** Schematic illustration of how intracellular electrical changes are recorded. When the tip of one microelectrode penetrates a cell, the oscilloscope trace shifts from the reference 0 potential and records the intracellular negative resting potential. (Adapted from Vassale, M. [1976]. *Cardiac physiology for the clinician* [p. 2]. New York: Academic Press.)

hold the potassium inside the cell. The slow outward trickle of potassium is corrected by a membrane pump that moves potassium back into the cell (and moves sodium out of the cell). If the resting potential were −94 mV, there would be no net potassium ion movement.

The following illustrates the Nernst equation calculation of the equilibrium potential for potassium ion:

$$E_K = \frac{RT}{FZ_K} \mathrm{Ln} \frac{[K^+]_o}{[K^+]_i}$$

Where E_K = equilibrium potential for K^+
R = gas constant
T = absolute temperature
F = the Faraday (number of coulombs per mole of charge)
Z_K = the valence of K^+ (+1)
$[K^+]_O$ = K^+ concentration outside the cell (e.g., 4mM)
$[K^+]_i$ = K^+ concentration inside the cell (e.g., 155mM)

Converting from the natural log to the base 10 log and replacing the constants measured at 37°C with numeric values, the equation becomes approximately as follows:

$$E_K = 61 \log_{10} \frac{[K^+]_o}{[K^+]_i}$$

$$E_K = 61 \log_{10} \frac{4}{155} = -97 \mathrm{mV}$$

According to the Nernst equation, the higher the potassium ion concentration in the external solution, the more depolarized is the *potassium equilibrium potential*. If the resting membrane were highly permeable to potassium, then the higher the external potassium concentration, the more depolarized would be the *resting potential*. If one were to perform such an experiment, placing an intact muscle cell in a dish bathed in solutions with varying potassium concentrations, one would observe that this is the case. As the potassium concentration in the external solution is raised, the membrane becomes more depolarized. When the concentration of potassium ion in the extracellular fluid becomes equal to the concentration in the intracellular fluid, the membrane potential is 0 mV.

In cardiac surgery, when it is important to have a heart without electrical and mechanical activity, the organ is sometimes perfused with the cool cardioplegic solution. The perfusate typically contains 15 to 35 mM potassium. As would be predicted from the Nernst equation, the cell membranes depolarize. The depolarized cells no longer experience an action potential, resulting in a motionless surgical field.

Each ion has a different equilibrium potential that depends on the relative concentration on the two sides of the membrane (see Table 1-2). In each case, the equilibrium potential is calculated using the Nernst equation. For example, given typical sodium ion concentrations as in Table 1-2, the equilibrium potential for sodium is approximately +60 mV. This means that if the membrane were permeable to sodium, then the membrane potential would have to be +60 mV to halt net inward sodium current. At typical resting potentials of +90 mV, a large electromotive force favors inward sodium current. The sodium concentration is markedly higher in the extracellular space than it is in the intracellular area. Thus, diffusion forces also favor inward sodium current. At rest, however, there is minimal net movement of sodium ion because the sodium channels are closed. When the channels open during activation, the diffusional and electrical forces combine to produce a large, but transient, inward current carried by sodium ion. The result is rapid depolarization.

The chloride ion concentration is higher in the extracellular space than in the intracellular space. Thus, diffusional force favors inward movement of chloride ion. However, the resting membrane potential is at approximately the chloride ion equilibrium potential. Thus, the negative potential opposes the net inward movement of chloride. The resting muscle membrane is permeant to chloride, but there is scant net chloride movement.

The sarcoplasmic calcium ion concentration is extremely low. Calcium ion is actively removed from the sarcoplasm. It is taken up into the SR and pumped outward into the extracellular space. The extracellular calcium ion concentration is in the millimolar range, approximately 100,000-times higher than the intracellular concentration. Thus, a powerful concentration gradient would move calcium ion inward if a path were available. A powerful electrical force also favors inward movement. The calcium ion equilibrium potential calculated from the Nernst equation is more positive than +100 mV. However, the resting membrane is not permeant to calcium ion. As with the sodium ion, the opening of a channel for calcium ion movement evokes a large inward current. This happens during activation. The presence of intracellular calcium ion signals metabolic and contractile changes.

Calculation of the Membrane Resting Potential. At high external potassium concentrations, the Nernst equation for potassium ion predicts resting membrane potential with good accuracy. In and below the physiologic range of external potassium ion concentrations, the membrane potential is slightly less negative than would be predicted based on potassium ion concentrations. This is because at very low external potassium concentrations, the membrane is slightly permeable to sodium ion. Because concentration and electrical gradients for sodium ion both favor inward movement of sodium ion, a slight sodium permeability results in a trickling inward of sodium ions (an inward current). The membrane depolarizes slightly, becoming several millivolts more positive than the potassium equilibrium potential. The ratio of potassium and sodium permeabilities determines the extent to which the resting membrane potential deviates from the potassium equilibrium potential. Equations have been developed to predict resting membrane potential based on permeabilities and concentrations of the permeating ions. These computations assume that the membrane is in a steady state and that there are no active ion pumps producing current.

Typically, cardiac muscle cells have a resting membrane potential of approximately −90 mV between excitations. Excitation and propagation of excitation depend on the resting membrane potential. The more negative the resting membrane potential, the more current is required to initiate excitation, but the speed and amplitude of depolarizing excitation are greater. The less negative the resting membrane potential, the less current required to initiate excitation; the speed and amplitude of depolarization are less. If the resting potential is depolarized a substantial amount, then the cell can be impossible to activate. The resting membrane potential is altered by changes in the ionic milieu on either side of the membrane and by hormones or drugs that alter the relative permeabilities of potassium or sodium ion. Factors that alter the action of the sodium-potassium pump alter the resting membrane potential. These include insulin and epinephrine (hyperpolarizing influences) and digoxin-like drugs (depolarizing influence).

Ionic Activity. Although electrochemical gradients are most frequently explained in terms of chemical concentration gradients, it is actually each ion's chemical activity that affects most cellular functions. Ionic activity reflects interactions between ions as well as the ion concentration. An ion's activity is equal to its concentration times its activity coefficient. It is possible to make reasonably accurate measurements of ionic activities within cells. However, most descriptions of ion movements are based on ion concentration.

Ion Movement Across the Myocardial Cell Membrane

Passive Ion Movement. Ions traverse the sarcolemma passively through membrane-bound, water-filled pores called *channels*. When the channel is open, any ions that are able to pass through the channel move according to the concentration and electrical gradient, as constrained by the channel dimensions. When the channel is closed, ions do not penetrate. The opening and closing properties of an ion channel are referred to as its *gating* characteristics. The signal to open may be a change in the electrical field (voltage-gated channel) or a change in the chemical milieu (receptor-gated channel). Changes in the internal or external milieu may modify the gating of a channel. Further, there may be time-dependent effects. For example, a small depolarization opens the sodium channel, and then it closes after a few milliseconds.

An important channel characteristic is its ability to allow passage of some ions while excluding others. This is called *selective permeability*. A theoretical model of an ionic channel is given in Figure 1-17.

In Nobel prize–winning work, Hodgkin and Huxley (1952) characterized the sodium current of the squid giant axon. The sodium channel is one of the most common in excitable cells and is well characterized. At rest, there is a negative resting membrane potential, perhaps -90 mV. Sodium ion concentration is high in the extracellular space, low inside the cell. Electrical and diffusion gradients favor inward sodium ion movement, but there is no path for movement. The sodium channel is closed at the resting membrane potential. With a small electrical signal, the channel opens. The opening of the sodium channel in response to a small depolarizing current is sometimes described as opening of the *activation gate*. When the activation gate opens, the sodium channel is then open. Because the sodium channel is selectively permeable to sodium ion, sodium ions flow through the channel according to the electrical and concentration gradients. Both those forces favor the inward movement of sodium-an inward current. An intense current flows. After a few milliseconds, however, another gate (sometimes called the *inactivation gate* or *h gate*) closes, halting the current. The h gate remains closed until the membrane is restored to a negative voltage. At that time, the inactivation gate opens (but no current flows because the activation gate is closed). With the closing of either gate, current is halted. To summarize, the sodium channel is conceptualized as having

two gates. At resting membrane potential, the channel is closed because the activation gate is closed. Depolarization opens that gate but, after a brief lag, the inactivation gate closes, again closing the channel. Repolarization opens the inactivation gate but closes the activation gate.

Scores of channels have been described, each with characteristic gating and selectivity profiles. The mixing of a selection of channel populations can produce a rich repertoire of biologic operating characteristics in various membranes. The membrane of vertebrate cardiac muscle is especially complex, with a diverse mix of channels. The result is a dynamic, responsive membrane that can be finely tuned to varying operating conditions. Some of the other major channels of the vertebrate heart are described later in this chapter.

Active Ion Transport. Any movement of ion against its electrochemical gradient is said to be *active movement* or *active transport*. To move any ion against its electrochemical gradient, energy must be used. The energy may be stored in ATP. In some cases, the energy stored in one ion's electrochemical gradient can be expended to power the movement of another ion against its electrochemical gradient. The former ion is said to be moving "downhill" or in the direction of a lower energy state. The ion that is moved against the gradient is said to be transported "uphill."

Sodium-Potassium-Adenosine Triphosphatase Pump. A slight trickling inward of sodium ions from the extracellular fluid occurs while the cell is at resting potential. In addition, with each activation, many cells experience a large transient inward sodium current. If these concentration shifts were not corrected, there would eventually be a loss of the sodium ion concentration gradient. This does not happen because the cardiac muscle membrane (as well as many other types of membranes) has a pump that moves sodium ion out of the cell in exchange for an inward movement of potassium ions. In this case, both ions are moving against a concentration gradient. The pump is powered by the energy stored in ATP; hence, the pump is known as the *sodium-potassium pump* or *sodium-potassium-ATPase*. This pump helps to reestablish the resting concentrations of intracellular sodium and potassium after cardiac depolarization. The ratio of sodium ions pumped out to potassium ions pumped in is usually 3:2. This ratio of 3:2 results in a net outward movement of charge and hyperpolarization of the resting membrane. A primary regulator of this pump is the intracellular sodium concentration. Other factors influencing pump activity include extracellular sodium concentration, and intracellular and extracellular potassium concentration. Digoxin-like drugs block the sodium-potassium pump (Glynn, 1993). Epinephrine and insulin both stimulate the sodium-potassium pump, causing uptake of potassium into cells. Clinicians capitalize on this feature when they administer insulin and glucose to the hyperkalemic patient. Epinephrine and insulin can be associated with hypokalemia.

Sodium-Calcium Exchange. Another important cardiac membrane pump is the sodium-calcium pump. Calcium ion moves across the sarcolemma into the cell to activate contraction. It must be removed. Although there is some harvesting of calcium ion into the intracellular sequestering sites such as SR, the inward movement and storage cannot go on unopposed. Calcium ion is moved back into the extracellular space by means of an exchange pump. The energy stored in the sodium gradient powers the movement of calcium ion. In other words, sodium ion is moved downhill to pump calcium ion uphill (Langer, 1982). Usually, this exchange mechanism transports three sodium ions into the cell for one calcium ion transported out of the cell. In this situation, the pump is electrogenic, but the direction or ratios of transmembrane ion exchanges may be reversed or changed. When the concentration of intracellular sodium ion is increased (e.g., when the use of digoxin-like drugs has partially blocked the sodium-potassium-ATPase pump), there is less energy stored in the sodium gradient. This exchange mechanism does not promote as great a sodium influx and calcium efflux. There is then more calcium ion stored in the SR and more calcium ion released during activation, with net positive inotropic effects.

Calcium Atpase Pumps. The cardiac SR actively pumps calcium ion uphill into its core in a process that hydrolyzes ATP as an energy source. An active calcium pump in the cardiac sarcolemma also extrudes calcium ion from the cell. The latter may be more important in vascular tissue than in cardiac muscle.

CARDIAC ACTION POTENTIAL

Each type of cardiac cell (e.g., working myocardial cells, nodal cells, Purkinje cells) has characteristic action potential features. In general, there are two types of action potentials, sometimes called *fast-* and *slow-response* cells. Fast-response cells, such as Purkinje cells and the working myocardial cells of the atrium and ventricle, have a rapid depolarization, then a period of sustained depolarization called the *plateau phase.* Conduction to the adjacent cells is rapid. During the interim between action potentials, the resting potential is fairly constant. Slow-response cells, such as the sinus and AV node cells, spontaneously depolarize slowly during the action potential, and have a shorter, nonprominent plateau phase that merges into a slower repolarization period. The latter conduct more slowly (Fig. 1-19). Differences in the ionic currents account for differences in the shape of the action potential.

In the following sections, the action potential of a fast-response cell (working myocardial cell) is characterized, and then

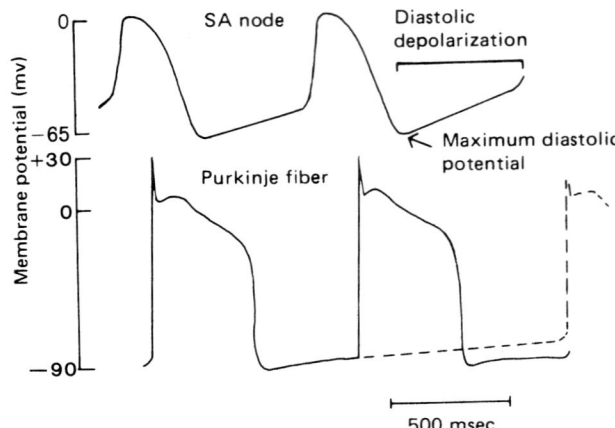

■ **Figure 1–19.** Action potentials of sinus node cells and Purkinje cells. Purkinje cell action potentials are usually elicited by propagated impulses. If Purkinje cells are not discharged by impulses from the sinus node or elsewhere, the Purkinje diastolic depolarization progresses enough to attain threshold. (Adapted from Vassale, M. [1976]. *Cardiac physiology for the clinician* [p. 35]. New York: Academic Press.)

the typical slow-responding cell is described. Finally, distinctive features of the other cell types are noted. Table 1-3 summarizes the electrophysiological properties of the various tissue types.

Action Potential of Working Myocardial Cells

During the interim between contractions, the working myocardial cell has a resting membrane potential of approximately −90 mV. Excitation of the cell begins with a small depolarization to threshold potential, which is usually approximately −70 mV. This small depolarization evokes a large depolarization, the cardiac action potential upstroke. The

Table 1–3 ■ CARDIAC ACTION POTENTIAL PROPERTIES*

	Fast-Conducting Tissue			**Slow-Conducting Tissue**	
	Purkinje	Atrial Muscle	Ventricular Muscle	Sinus Node	Atrioventricular Node
Resting potential	−90 to −95 mV	−80 to −90 mV	−80 to −90 mV	−50 to −60 mV	−60 to −70 mV
Activation threshold	−70 to −60 mV			−40 to −30 mV	
Action potential					
Rate of phase 0 (V_{max})	500 to 800 V/s	100 to 200 V/s	100 to 200 V/s	1 to 10 V/s	5 to 15 V/s
Amplitude	120 mV	110 to 120 mV	110 to 120 mV	60 to 70 mV	70 to 80 mV
Overshoot	30 mV	30 mV	30 mV	0 to 10 mV	5 to 15 mV
Duration	300 to 500 ms	100 to 300 ms	200 to 300 ms	100 to 300 ms	100 to 300 ms
Diastolic depolarization		Not prominent		Prominent	
(major ion)					
Depolarizing current		Na^+		Ca^{2+}	
Channel blocked by	Tetrodotoxin, type I antiarrhythmics, or sustained depolarization at -40 mV			Mn^{2+}, La^{3+}, verapamil, nifedipine, other inorganic substances, type IV antiarrhythmics	
Effect of adrenergic stimulation	Not pronounced			Pronounced	

* Values are approximations and vary with methods and specific tissue used.
Adapted from Bigger, J.T. (1984). Electrophysiology for the clinician. *European Heart Journal,* 5(Suppl. B), 2; Opie, L. (1984). *The heart* (p. 44) Orlando: Grune & Stratton; Sperelakis, N. (1979). Origin of the cardiac resting potential. In R.E. Berne (Ed.), *Handbook of physiology, sec 2, the cardiovascular system, vol 1, the heart,* (p. 190). Bethesda, MD: American Physiological Society; Zipes, D.P. (1984). Genesis of cardiac arrhythmias. In E. Braunwald (Ed.), *Heart disease,* (2nd ed., p. 615) Philadelphia. WB Saunders.

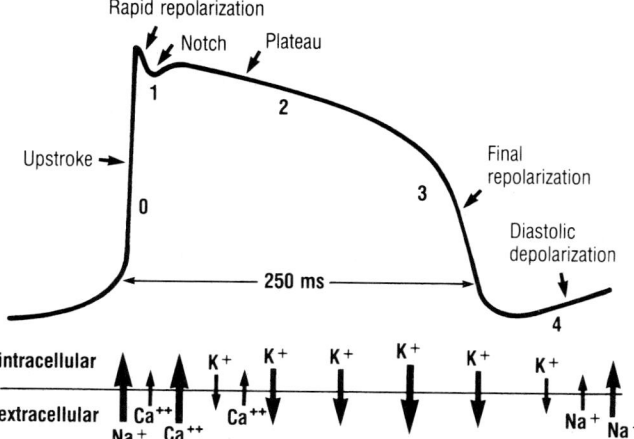

■ **Figure 1–20.** Schematic illustration of major ionic movements during a Purkinje cell action potential, with the cell depicted as exhibiting spontaneous depolarization. Arrows indicate approximate times when the indicated ion movement influences membrane potential. Pumps, exchanges, and leaks are not illustrated. Under normal physiologic conditions, Purkinje cells do not exhibit spontaneous depolarization. (Adapted from Ten Eick, R.E., Baumgarten, C.M., & Sunger, D.H. [1981]. Ventricular dysrhythmia: Membrane basis of currents, channels, gates and cables. *Progress in Cardiovascular Disease*, 24, 159; Fozzard, H.A., & Gibbons, W.R. [1973]. Action potential and contraction of heart muscle. *American Journal of Cardiology*, 31, 183.)

action potential propagates the full length of the cell membrane and communicates to adjacent cells by means of current flow across the low-resistance path of the nexus. These cells are called *fast myocytes* because the initial depolarization rate is rapid.

The five phases of the cardiac action potential are summarized, and then described in detail (Fig. 1-20). Briefly, phase 0 is the initial period of rapid depolarization, the action potential upstroke. The membrane potential changes from resting potential (approximately −90 mV) to a value positive to 0 mV (e.g., +30 mV). After this brief (<1 to 2 milliseconds) phase, there is a period of sustained depolarization called the *plateau phase*. Conduction to adjacent cells is rapid. During the interim between action potentials, the resting potential is fairly constant. Slow-response cells, such as the sinus and AV node cells, spontaneously depolarize between action potentials, depolarize slowly during the action potential, and have a shorter, nonprominent plateau phase that there are three repolarizing phases. In phase 1, there is a small, early, rapid repolarization. Phase 2 is the so-called plateau phase. There is some minor additional depolarization and a prolonged slow repolarization. In phase 3, repolarization becomes rapid, returning the membrane to resting potential. Phase 4 describes the interval between action potentials. During phase 4, the membrane is in the repolarized state preceding another depolarization. The cardiac action potential may take hundreds of milliseconds. The duration and amplitude of each phase depends on the opening and closing of a variety of ion channel gates. This in turn depends on the ionic and neurohormonal milieu.

Phase 0: Action Potential Upstroke

The working myocardial cell action potential is initiated by an inward current flowing primarily by way of the low-resistance

nexus. This small current depolarizes the cell to threshold (approximately −70 mV; Fig. 1-21). Once threshold voltage is reached, the sodium channel activation gate opens, thus opening the sodium channel. There follows a large inward current carried by sodium ions. The depolarizing current opens more sodium channels, producing the propagating, regenerating, swift depolarization of the action potential upstroke. The peak voltages attained are +30 to +40 mV, approaching but not attaining the sodium equilibrium potential (which is approximately +65 mV). Depolarization closes the inactivation gate. The channel closes, halting the current, stopping depolarization.

The maximal velocity of phase 0 depolarization is sometimes called V_{max} (to be distinguished from the contractile variable, the maximal velocity of shortening, also called V_{max}).

The speed of impulse conduction through the myocardium depends on the V_{max} for the individual cells. V_{max} reflects sodium channel activity. Factors that alter the resting potential or the sodium gradient alter V_{max}. Such factors include ionic milieu and certain drugs, including many antiarrhythmic drugs. Class I antiarrhythmic agents (lidocaine, quinidine, procainamide, others) block the fast sodium channel, slowing the rate of phase 0 depolarization.

The more negative the resting membrane potential, the faster is V_{max} and the greater is the amplitude of the depolarization. Hyperpolarization opens the inactivation gate. When depolarization opens the activation gate, the sodium channel is open, and the current is intense. Conversely, a less negative membrane voltage before threshold is associated with a slower V_{max} caused by failure adequately to remove inactivation (i.e., failure to open the inactivation gate). Hyperkalemia causes such depolarization; the condition is associated with arrhythmias.

Phase 1: Early Repolarization

The rapid upstroke ceases when sodium channels close spontaneously after a few milliseconds (caused by inactivation). Another transient current is activated, the transient outward current. This outward current is carried primarily by potassium ion and results in the slight repolarization of the cell to approximately +10 mV. Some chloride ions flow inward. This,

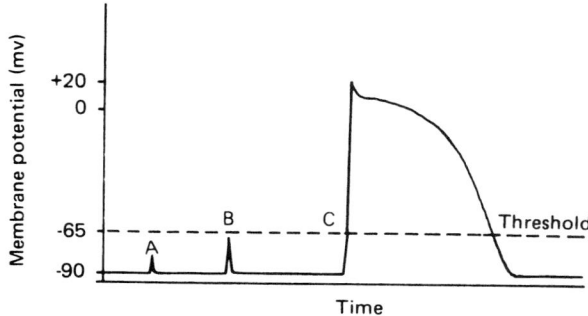

■ **Figure 1–21.** Schematic illustration of the initiation of an action potential when the membrane potential is depolarized to threshold. Small depolarizing stimuli (*A* and *B*) that fail to reach threshold (dashed line) are unable to initiate an action potential. When depolarization reaches threshold (*C*), a regenerative action potential is produced. Once the latter begins, further depolarization becomes independent of the initial stimulus. (From Katz, A.M. [1977]. *Physiology of the heart* [p. 236]. New York: Raven Press.)

too, is an "outward" current because of the negative charge on the chloride ion. When the voltage is positive, both the concentration gradient and the electrical force (inside positive the positive potassium ion) favor outflow of potassium ion from the cell. This is an outward current. Similarly, with chloride ion, when the membrane potential is positive, the electrical gradient amplifies the concentration gradient, both favoring the inward movement of the negatively charged chloride ion. The inward movement of negative ions is electrically indistinguishable from an outward movement of positive ions; both are called *outward current.*

Phase 1 ends with the closure of the current-bearing channels. A "notch" appears on the action potential profile. The voltage of the notch region has important effects on subsequent gating of other channels and can affect the shape of the remainder of the action potential.

Phase 2: Action Potential Plateau

During the plateau, little net current flows. Inward (depolarizing) and outward (repolarizing) currents are nearly balanced; thus, there is little change in membrane voltage. Inward currents are carried by sodium and calcium ions. Calcium ion in turn evokes additional calcium ion release from internal stores, and contraction ensues. Outward currents are carried by potassium ions. Over time, the calcium channels slowly inactivate; the repolarizing outward potassium current predominates; the membrane slowly repolarizes. The phase ends when the calcium channels are closed.

During the plateau phase, sodium currents may travel through a few fast sodium channels that failed to inactivate. At least two types of calcium channels are active. Both types of calcium channels open with depolarization, and then close spontaneously after a certain period of time. β-adrenergic agonists potentiate calcium currents, thus increasing the amplitude and duration of the plateau. The increase in calcium ion in turn has a positive inotropic effect on contraction. Calcium channel blockers, acidosis, and ATP depletion diminish calcium currents, diminish the plateau, and diminish the force generated during contraction (called negative inotropes).

The counterbalancing outward current is carried by potassium ion through multiple channel types. One type of potassium channel that is important in disease is the ATP-sensitive potassium current. This potassium channel is activated or opened when the ATP concentration falls, such as during ischemia. This in turn greatly shortens the duration of the plateau and hastens the onset of rapid repolarization phase. Shortened depolarization diminishes the calcium current and thus the contractile force (another negative inotropic influence).

The plateau phase distinguishes cardiac muscle from skeletal muscle or nerve tissue. The plateau provides for greater inward calcium currents in cardiac muscle. Because the tissue is refractory to stimulation for the duration of phase 2 and much of phase 3, cardiac muscle cannot experience tetany.

Phase 3: Late Rapid Repolarization

The calcium currents that sustained the plateau eventually stop. The calcium channels close, and repolarization proceeds unopposed, with outward movement of potassium ions. As the membrane voltage becomes increasingly negative, sodium channel inactivation is removed. The sodium channel can once again be excited or activated (as soon as a small depolarization opens the activation gate).

Phase 4: Interim Between Action Potentials

During rapid repolarization (phase 3), the membrane potential is restored to the resting potential. Phase 4 is the interim between the end of rapid repolarization and the start of the next action potential. During this phase, the membrane is permeable to potassium ion. The membrane voltage is close to the potassium equilibrium potential. The type of potassium channel open during this phase is called the *inward rectifier* (so called because it allows inward current more readily than outward current). Because the membrane potential is slightly more positive than the potassium equilibrium potential, potassium trickles outward.

Action Potential of Sinus Node-Type Cells

Sinus node-type cells are called *slow myocytes* because phase 0 depolarization is slower than in fast myocytes. Phase 1 is absent, and phase 2 is abbreviated. Phase 3 is similar to that in fast myocytes, although slow myocytes repolarize to a less negative voltage than fast myocytes. Maximal negative voltage at the start of phase 4 is approximately -60 mV. During phase 4, there is spontaneous depolarization (see Fig. 1-19).

Phase 0 depolarization in slow myocytes is carried primarily by calcium ion rather than sodium ion. There is a less abrupt transition in the rate of depolarization before and after reaching threshold in sinus node cells.

Phase 1 is absent. There is no notch, and there is no large transient outward potassium current.

Phase 2 is present but abbreviated. Slow repolarization begins after the maximal positive voltage is reached. As in other cells, potassium efflux evokes repolarization in slow myocytes.

Phase 3, rapid repolarization, is similar to that in fast myocytes. The rate of repolarization is slower and the maximal diastolic potential attained is less negative than in fast-response cells.

During phase 4, the slow-response cells continually depolarize toward threshold. Because phase 4 coincides with the diastolic phase of the cardiac cycle, the membrane potential during phase 4 is frequently termed the *diastolic potential change* in automatic cells. The voltage at the start of phase 4 is the most negative voltage attained in these cells and is termed *maximal diastolic potential.*

Phase 4 spontaneous depolarization is caused by the following sequence of currents: a nonselective channel opens, allowing inward sodium current; outward potassium current declines after some depolarization; transient (T)-type calcium channels open, allowing inward calcium current; and long-lasting (L)-type calcium channels open, allowing the full action potential depolarization.

Cells in the sinus node spontaneously depolarize to threshold more rapidly than do other automatic cardiac cells. Thus, the slope of phase 4 is steeper in sinus node cells than in other

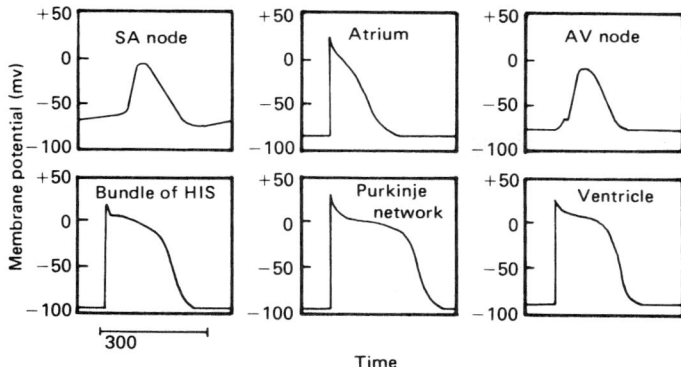

■ **Figure 1–22.** Characteristic action potentials in different regions of the heart. See text for description. (From Katz, A.M. [1977]. *Physiology of the heart* [p. 251]. New York: Raven Press.)

automatic cells. The ion current changes that account for the diastolic depolarization include a decrease in a stabilizing potassium current, an increase in a sodium current, some ongoing leakage of sodium ions, and eventually opening of the T-type calcium channels (Irisawa & Noma, 1984; Maylie & Morad, 1984).

Ionic currents flowing in slow-type myocytes are modulated by autonomic innervation. Adrenergic stimulation increases the potassium current, causing the cell to repolarize to a more negative potential, and the action potential to proceed more swiftly. Acetylcholine, the parasympathetic mediator, slows the pacemaker currents.

Action Potential of Purkinje-Type Cells

The action potential of the Purkinje cell is similar to that of the working myocardial cell, although somewhat prolonged in duration of the plateau. Hypoxia and acidosis in ischemic Purkinje cells may produce conditions in which the fast sodium channel is not opened. Phase 0 depolarization is then due to slow channel activation, carried primarily by calcium ion.

Action Potential of Atrial Cells

Atrial working myocardial cells undergo rapid depolarization. These cells have essentially no plateau period, but repolarization is slower than in Purkinje cells (Fig. 1-22). The total action potential duration of atrial cells is shorter than that of Purkinje cells. Atrial muscle cells do not spontaneously depolarize under physiologic conditions. Spontaneous depolarization can occur under nonphysiological conditions.

Cells in the Atrioventricular Node

In general, spontaneously depolarizing cells of the AV node are similar to sinus node cells in the rate of phase 0 depolarization and of maximal repolarization voltage (see Fig. 1-22).

Figure 1-23 illustrates the different electrophysiological characteristics of cells termed *atrionodal, nodal,* and *nodal-His;* these action potentials have been identified as originating from the upper, middle, and lower junctional areas, respectively

(Noma & Shibasaki, 1985). Other investigators contend that the electrophysiological properties of atrionodal, nodal, and nodal—His cells are not correlated with definite anatomic areas (Hecht et al., 1973).

Cells in the Bundle of His

The electrophysiological characteristics of His bundle cells closely resemble those of Purkinje cells in the distal conducting system. The duration of the His bundle action potential, however, is slightly less than that of cells in the Purkinje network. The most rapid period of depolarization and the longest period of repolarization occur in Purkinje cells at the distal end of the conducting system (see Fig. 1-22).

Refractory Periods

The period after depolarization, during which it is difficult or impossible to re-excite the cell, is termed the *refractory period* (Fig. 1-24). Refractoriness reflects the effects on depolarization of time and voltage requirements for the activation, inactivation, and recovery of ion channels.

During the *effective refractory period,* no action potential can be initiated by an external electrical stimulus. The duration of this period depends on the time it takes to remove inactivation from the sodium and calcium channels. The effective refractory period extends from phase 0 through the middle of phase 3.

During the *relative refractory period,* only a stimulus greater than normal can initiate an action potential. The relative refractory period occurs during the latter part of repolarization (late phase 3).

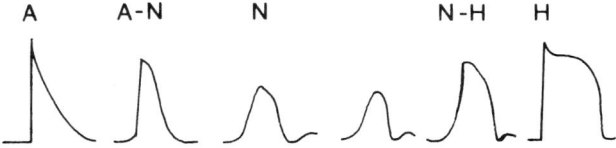

■ **Figure 1–23.** Schematic illustration of action potentials from atrial (A), atrionodal (A-N), nodal (N), nodal-His (N-H), and His bundle (H) cells. See text for discussion. (From Myerburg, R., & Lazzara, R. [1973]. Electrophysiologic basis of cardiac arrhythmias and conduction disturbances. *Cardiovascular Clinics,* 5, 9.)

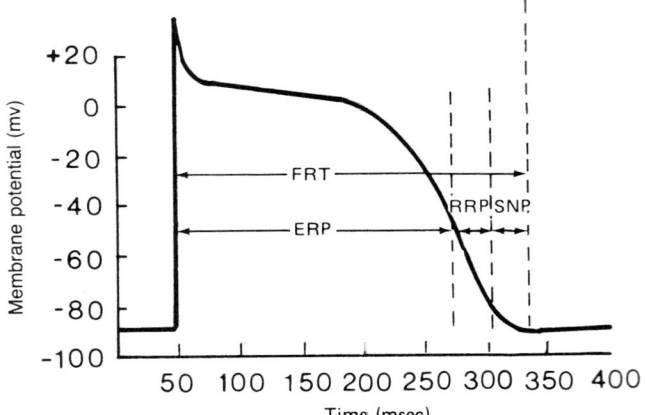

■ **Figure 1–24.** Excitability during the cardiac action potential. The effective refractory period (ERP), during which electrical stimuli of any strength are unable to initiate a propagated action potential, is followed by the relative refractory period (RRP), during which only stimuli greater than those that normally reach threshold can cause a propagated action potential. This is followed by the supernormal period (SNP), during which stimuli slightly less than those that normally reach threshold can cause a propagated action potential. The action potentials generated during the RRP and SNP usually propagate slowly. Full recovery time (FRT) is the interval after depolarization, after which threshold returns to normal and stimulation produces a normally propagated action potential. (Adapted from Katz, A.M. [1977]. *Physiology of the heart* [p. 248]. New York: Raven Press.)

The entire period between depolarization and complete repolarization is termed the *full recovery time.* Under normal conditions, cardiac cells are not depolarized until they have had time to recover fully from the previous depolarization. Usually, cells with long refractory periods have long action potential durations. The upper limits of normal heart rate responses and the time allowed for ventricular filling depend on normal cardiac electrical refractoriness.

Under certain conditions, a stimulus can initiate an action potential during the last part of phase 3 and the beginning of phase 4. Cardiac arrhythmias may occur during this period, especially when pathophysiological situations, such as ischemia, promote abnormal refractory periods (see Chapter 19).

■ SARCOLEMMAL IONIC CURRENTS

The currents that combine to orchestrate the action potential can be studied independently. Neurohormonal and ionic milieu, pharmacologic agents, and pathologic processes variably influence each current. Powerful techniques using the patch clamp and molecular biology have extended our understanding of the individual channels and hold the promise of increasing our understanding of important issues such as the generation of arrhythmias in disease states. New treatments are being developed. Some of the major channels are discussed individually (Table 1-4).

Table 1–4 ■ CARDIAC IONIC CURRENTS

Current*	Charge Carrier	Activation Mechanism	Function
Inward Currents			
I_{Na}	Na^+	Voltage	AP upstroke
I_{Ca} (I_{Si}, I_{Caf}, I_{Cas})	Ca^{2+}	Voltage	AP plateau
			E-C coupling
			AP upstroke
			Sinus pacemaker
$I_f(I_h)$	Na^+ and K^+	Voltage	Spontaneous depolarization
$I_{ti}(I_t, I_{Na,K})$	Na^+ and K^+	?$[(Ca^{2+}]_i$	After-depolarization
Outward Currents			
$I_K(I_x, I_{x1}, I_{x2})$	K^+ (Na^+)	Voltage	Repolarization
I_{to}	K^+	Voltage, ?$[Ca^{2+}]$	Early repolarization
I_{K1}	K^+	Voltage	Resting potential
			Repolarization
			?Plateau potential
I_{KCa}	K^+	$[Ca^{2+}]_i$	Repolarization
I_{KAch}	K^+	ACh, ? voltage	Inhibition
Pump/Exchange Currents			
I_p	Na^+, K^+	$[K^+], [Na^+]$	Na^+-K^+-ATPase pump
$I_{Na, Ca}$	Na^+, Ca^{2+}	$[Ca^{2+}], [Na^+]$	Na^+-Ca^{2+} exchange
Background Currents			
I_{bNa}	Na^+	?	Inward leakage
I_{bCa}	Ca^{2+}	?	? Inward leakage
? I_{bCl}	Cl^-	?	?

* Currents identified in multicellular preparations are labeled I and currents identified in single-cell preparations are labeled i. Some of these currents are speculative (see text).
Ach, acetylcholine; AP, action potential; E-C, excitation-contraction; [ ], concentration of ion indicated.
Adapted from Brown, H.F. (1982). Electrophysiology of the sinoatrial node. *Physiology Review,* 62, 506; Nobel, D. (1981). The surprising heart. *Journal of Physiology,* 353, 43; Opie, L. (1984). *The heart,* (p. 47). Orlando: Grune & Stratton; and Reuter, H. (1984). Ion channels in cardiac cell membranes. *Annual Review of Physiology,* 46, 474.

Inward Currents

The inward currents are carried by sodium or calcium ions moving into the cell. For each ion, there are several different types of channels, each with its own gating characteristics.

Fast Inward Current I_{NA}

The fast sodium current is activated to cause rapid depolarization in phase 0 of fast-response cells. It was discussed in some detail previously. Briefly, the sodium channel opens with depolarization to threshold (-70 to -60 mV) but quickly closes because of inactivation. Repolarization is necessary to remove the inactivation (Hodgkin & Huxley, 1952). The fast sodium current is blocked by the puffer fish poison tetrodotoxin. Many antiarrhythmic agents, particularly class I agents, alter this current.

Calcium Currents

The two major types of calcium channels are termed L (long-lasting) and T (transient). The L current activates with depolarizations beyond -40 mV and then slowly inactivates. The T current activates at -70 mV and rapidly decays. Both channels probably contribute to the plateau of the cardiac action potential. The T channels contribute to phase 0 spontaneous depolarization in pacemaker cells and the L channels contribute to the action potential in these cells. These currents may be potentiated by β-adrenergic (catecholamine) stimulation and diminished by acetylcholine and acidosis (Sperelakis, 1984) (see later discussion). The current is blocked by inorganic compounds such as lanthanum, cobalt, nickel, and manganese. Organic charged tertiary amines, such as verapamil, block the slow channel at the inner membrane. The block depends on membrane potential and the rate of stimulation. Organic dihydropyridines, such as nifedipine, also block the channel.

Pacemaker Current

Pacemaking results from the combining of at least four currents. There is a time-dependent inactivation of the potassium current, and thus a loss of outward current (which would tend to hyperpolarize). This alone does not produce depolarization: channels that carry ions with an equilibrium potential positive to the membrane potential also must open. The currents involved are I_h, I_{Ca}, and background sodium current. I_h channels open at negative (hyperpolarized) potentials (hence the designation "h"), close at positive potentials, and allow passage of both sodium (hence a depolarizing influence) and potassium. Gating is slow. Similarly, a sodium leak current occurs and is a depolarizing influence. Calcium channels are activated with depolarization. With increasing depolarization, the calcium T channels open, carrying inward depolarizing calcium current (I_{Ca}) (DiFrancesco, 1981).

Transient Diastolic Inward Current I_{ti}

The transient diastolic inward current is a nonselective current that carries both sodium and potassium and may be activated by intracellular calcium. It is not normally active but may be involved in initiating delayed depolarizations and triggering arrhythmias in Purkinje and ventricular muscle cells, particularly when extracellular potassium concentration is low.

Other inward currents have been identified. Sodium and calcium "leak" currents and the sodium-calcium exchange mechanisms can generate small inward currents.

Outward Currents

A cell can experience outward current in two primary ways: (1) potassium can flow out of the cell; or (2) chloride can flow inward. Both tend to repolarize the membrane that had been depolarized. Both tend to stabilize the resting membrane potential. There are many types of potassium currents in cardiac muscle.

Outward Rectifying Current I_K

The outward rectifying current causes repolarization after an action potential. It opens slowly after depolarization, so it is also called the *delayed rectifying current*. It carries potassium, and it closes with repolarization. It also may be labeled I_x, and has been subdivided into I_{x1} early rapid component and I_{x2} late slower component.

Background Outward Current I_{K1}

This potassium current flows through channels that close with depolarization and open with repolarization. Thus, when the cell is depolarized during the plateau phase, the channel is closed. Were the channel open, potassium would flow outward, resulting in a repolarization. This would abort the plateau and halt the calcium current, which activates contraction. Hence, it is efficient that this channel is closed during depolarization. It is open with repolarization and serves to stabilize the membrane potential close to the potassium equilibrium potential. It is sometimes called the *inward rectifier* because it is highly permeant to inward potassium currents but less permeant to outward currents. When the membrane is depolarized and potassium can flow outward, the channel closes. It is sensitive to the extracellular potassium concentration.

Transient Outward Current I_{to}

This potassium current is linked with early (phase 1) rapid repolarization. It opens when a cell is depolarized after a period of hyperpolarization, and it closes quickly.

Other Potassium Currents

A nonvoltage-dependent potassium current that is activated by an increase in the intracellular calcium concentration, I_{Kca}, may participate in the maintenance of the plateau and in repolarization. This current may be the same as or similar to the transient outward current (I_{to}).

Of potential importance in the diseased heart is the ATP-dependent potassium channel. This channel opens when the ATP concentration falls to 10% to 20% of normal (Noma & Shibasaki, 1985). The action potential becomes abbreviated during ischemia. This channel may account for such a phenomenon. It would open when the ATP level dropped, shorten the action potential duration, and result in less contraction when the substrate needed for contraction was unavailable (Nichols et al., 1991).

Acetylcholine activates potassium channels whose outward currents decrease during depolarization. Although this phenomenon may be related to potentiation of the background outward potassium current (I_{K1}), there is evidence for a separate voltage-responsive potassium current, I_{KACh}, whose channels are regulated by muscarinic cholinergic receptors.

Other outward currents have been identified. The sodium-potassium-ATPase pump usually generates a small outward current, I_p.

FACTORS MODIFYING ELECTROPHYSIOLOGIC FUNCTION

Factors that alter cardiac cell depolarization and repolarization do so by affecting the rates of voltage changes, the magnitudes of voltage changes, or the timing of the phases of the cardiac action potential. Such changes affect cardiac impulse generation, impulse conduction, or both, and reflect the effects of environmental alterations on transcellular ionic fluxes.

Impulse generation, or *automaticity,* is influenced by a cardiac cell's maximal diastolic repolarization, threshold level, and rate of spontaneous depolarization to threshold (slope of phase 4). If maximal diastolic repolarization becomes more negative, if threshold becomes less negative, or if the slope of phase 4 becomes less steep, the rate at which the entire cell is spontaneously depolarized can become slower; opposite effects can lead to a more rapid rate of spontaneous depolarization (see Chapter 19).

Cardiac impulse conduction velocity is influenced by the rate of depolarization (slope of phase 0), the magnitude of depolarization (amplitude of phase 0), the distance from resting potential to threshold level, the action potential and refractory period durations, and the resistance to current flow. If the rate or amplitude of phase 0 is decreased, the difference between resting potential and threshold is increased, the action potential or refractory periods are lengthened, or the resistance to current flow is increased, the rate of conduction can slow. For example, Purkinje cells have faster conduction velocities than nodal cells because the Purkinje cells have rapid sodium channels that create fast and large depolarization.

The responsiveness of cardiac cells is described by the relation between the membrane potential before rapid depolarization and the maximal velocity of conduction during rapid depolarization. Cardiac cell excitability is described by the current required to alter the membrane potential from resting to threshold (Singer et al., 1981). Although once threshold is reached, the cell completely depolarizes, the amplitude of the action potential can be decreased if the distance between the resting potential and the threshold potential is less than usual. Stimuli that are insufficient to depolarize a cell to threshold are not effective in initiating action potentials, but such stimuli can have an effect on ionic movements, and in pathophysiological situations, these stimuli may influence cardiac arrhythmia generation and conduction (see Chapter 19).

Cardiac impulse generation, conduction, or both can be altered by the effects on cardiac cells of changes in the ratio of extracellular to intracellular ionic concentrations, acid—base changes, sympathetic and parasympathetic stimulation, myocardial stretch, cooling, ischemia, and heart rate changes. These factors often affect different cardiac cells in different ways; the following section discusses general selected examples of some of these alterations. (The effects of alterations in extracellular ionic concentrations on cardiac electrical and mechanical functions are discussed in Chapters 9 and 10.)

Adrenergic and Cholinergic Effects

Catecholamines

This broad class of biologically active compounds includes many natural hormones and neurotransmitters (epinephrine, norepinephrine, dopamine) as well as pharmacological agents. These compounds have metabolic, endocrine, central nervous system and other actions. In the heart they are generally excitatory, increasing the strength and or the frequency of contraction. In the blood vessels, these substances can evoke constriction or dilation. There are several receptor subtypes producing complex and sometimes conflicting effects on cardiac cell action potentials. Generally, catecholamines increase the magnitude and rate of diastolic depolarization in both Purkinje and sinus nodal cells. Repolarization becomes faster, and the action potential duration is shortened. The increased rate of sinus node spontaneous depolarization (slope of phase 4) appears to be the most important mechanism by which adrenergic effects increase heart rate (Fig. 1-25). Catecholamines increase the amplitude and rate of rise of phase 0 in junctional cells, which increases conduction velocity through the AV node. Catecholamines also increase myocardial contractility. Most of catecholamine effects on the cardiac action potential are caused by β-adrenergic receptors.

Acetylcholine

The cholinergic effects of parasympathetic (vagal) nerve stimulation are more pronounced on the sinus node, the AV node, and atrial muscle than on ventricular muscle where the receptors are the most common. Acetylcholine slows the rate of diastolic depolarization (slope of phase 4) in sinus node cells; thus, the maximal diastolic potential becomes more negative with vagal stimulation. The heart rate is slowed (Fig. 1-26). The sinus node action potential duration and refractory period are both shortened. There is a decreased rate of rise and amplitude of phase 0 in AV nodal cells in response to acetylcholine, leading to slowed AV conduction. The AV refractory period may also be prolonged. Atrial contractile strength is decreased. Cholinergic cardiac receptor stimulation inhibits cardiac catecholamine effects by inhibiting the β-adrenergic effects of cAMP and inhibiting prejunctional norepinephrine release.

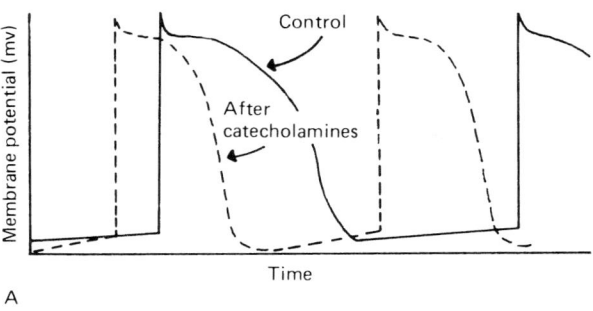
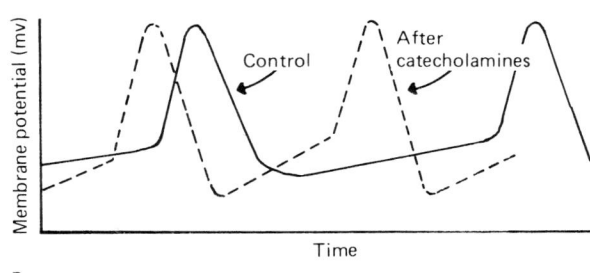

■ **Figure 1–25.** Schematic illustration of the general electrophysiologic effects of catecholamines on (*A*) Purkinje cells and (*B*) sinus node cells. (From Katz, A.M. [1977]. *Physiology of the heart* [pp. 366, 367]. New York: Raven Press.)

Effects of Acidosis and Alkalosis

Acidosis slows repolarization and prolongs the action potential duration in Purkinje fibers. Cardiac calcium channels are blocked by acidosis, resulting in a cardiac action potential with a slower rate of rise, amplitude, and duration (Overell et al., 2000). Acidosis induces decreased contractility by decreasing calcium ion influx and decreasing the sensitivity of the myofibrils to calcium ion (Donaldson et al., 1981).

Alkalosis can shorten the action potential duration. Purkinje automaticity is increased owing to an increased rate of diastolic depolarization (Singer et al., 1981).

Other Effects

The action potential duration is related to the length of the preceding diastolic interval. When heart rate increases (thus the interval between successive cardiac impulses decreases), then repolarization is usually faster, also. The action potential is shorter in duration. At slower heart rates, the action potential duration lengthens.

In experimental situations, the effects of *warming the heart* are somewhat similar to adrenergic effects (e.g., diastolic depolarization is increased in automatic fibers). *Cooling the heart* depresses spontaneous depolarization in automatic cells. Repolarization is delayed, and conduction is decreased. Arrhythmias may occur during cooling, which is clinically relevant for the cardiac surgical patient who has been subjected to hypothermia (see Chapter 29) and for the patient experiencing hypothermia caused by exposure.

Stretching cardiac fibers increases the rate of diastolic depolarization and makes the maximal diastolic potential less negative in automatic fibers. Myocardial fiber stretch may cause arrhythmias during heart failure. The effects of *hypoxemia* and *ischemia* on the action potential are discussed in Chapter 25.

▋ PROPAGATION OF THE CARDIAC IMPULSE

The spread of the cardiac impulse through the heart depends several factors, including the following: (1) the anatomic characteristics of the conducting system; (2) structural characteristics of cells (e.g., cardiac cell type and diameter, arrangement of low-resistance intercalated discs, and contiguity to other cells capable of conducting current); and (3) electrophysiological state of the cell membrane (i.e., resting potential, ionic concentrations and conductance, threshold membrane potential, rate and magnitude of depolarization, rate and magnitude of repolarization, duration of the action potential, and the refractory period). As in a battery, there is energy stored across the cell membrane. When one segment of the membrane depolarizes, positive charge enters the cell, and an electrical circuit is established along the cell (Overell et al., 2000).

In general, current flows more easily inside the cell and to adjacent cells across the intercalated discs at tight junctions than laterally across adjacent, highly resistant areas of cell membranes. If the current is sufficient to depolarize adjacent cells, a wave of depolarization is propagated and spreads

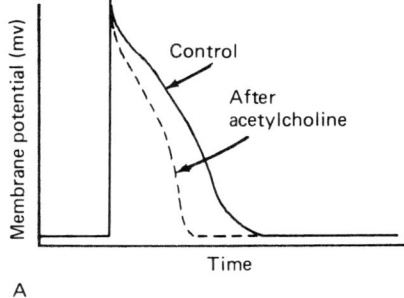
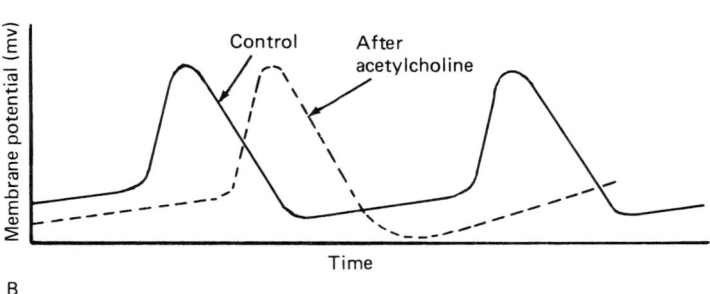

■ **Figure 1–26.** Schematic illustration of the general electrophysiologic effects of acetylcholine (vagal stimulation) on (*A*) atrial muscle cells and (*B*) sinus node cells. (From Katz, A.M. [1977]. *Physiology of the heart* [pp. 362, 363]. New York: Raven Press.)

Table 1–5 ■ NORMAL CARDIAC ACTIVATION SEQUENCE

Normal Sequence of Activation	Conduction Velocity (m/s)	Time for Impulse to Traverse Structure (s)	Rate of Automatic Discharge (per minute)
Sinoatrial node	—	} ~0.15	60–100
Atrial myocardium	0.8–1 m/s		None
AV node	0.02–0.05		See text
AV bundle	1.2–2	} ~0.08	40–55
Bundle branches	1.5–2		
Purkinje network	2–4	} ~0.08	25–40
Ventricular myocardium	0.3–1		None

AV, atrioventricular; m, meters; s, second; ~, approximately.
Adapted from Katz, A.M. (1977). *Physiology of the heart* (p. 259). New York: Raven Press.

rapidly from cell to cell. Thus, the cardiac tissue behaves essentially as a syncytium, although propagation may be somewhat discontinuous (Spach & Lootsey, 1983).

As the impulse spreads through the heart, it depolarizes tissue that has recovered and is excitable, but it cannot depolarize tissue that is still refractory. Because the cardiac impulse spreads rapidly through the atria, slowly through the AV junction, and then rapidly through the ventricles, both atria contract almost synchronously, the ventricles have time to receive blood from the contracting atria, and then both ventricles contract almost synchronously.

Atrial Conduction

Sinus node cells normally have the fastest rate of spontaneous depolarization and thus set the pace of cardiac excitation. The sinus node normally initiates the electrical impulse that is then conducted to other areas of the myocardium, depolarizing other cells of the conducting system before those cells have time to depolarize spontaneously to threshold. The electrical impulse appears to spread outward in relatively concentric circles from the sinus node through the atria, moving in approximately 0.1 seconds from the upper right atrium to the posterior left atrium. Conduction velocity (speed with which the impulse spreads) through the atria is approximately 0.8 to 1 m/s (Table 1-5). Conduction velocities are not equal through the atria; conduction is more rapid by way of the Bachman bundle into the left atrium than in other areas of the interatrial septum. Although there are specialized conduction pathways in the atrium as in the ventricle, the functional significance of the atrial fibers is less clear. Generally, the impulse travels radially within the atria. Atrial repolarization appears to spread in the same direction as depolarization.

Junctional Conduction

The cardiac impulse is not conducted through the connective tissue of the cardiac skeleton, so cardiac muscle tissue in the AV junction provides the only pathway for electrical conduction from the atria to the ventricles. Conduction velocity through the AV node is approximately 0.05 m/s, although in some areas it has been found to be as slow as 0.02 m/s.

The rate of impulse conduction through the AV junction is influenced by the atrial site at which the impulse enters the junctional area (Maylie & Morad, 1984). An initial normal slowing of conduction through the AV junction with a later increase in the speed of conduction is correlated with electrophysiological differences in atrionodal, nodal, and nodal-His cells (Paes de Carvalho & de Almeida, 1960) (see Fig. 1-23). Other mechanisms have been postulated for the slowing of conduction through the junction, including the small size of the junctional conducting cells and the amounts of connective tissue interspersed among conducting cells.

The property of a propagating impulse becoming successively weaker is termed *decremental conduction*. The extent to which this occurs in the AV junction under normal circumstances continues to be debated. Extreme decremental conduction leads to AV blocks (see Chapter 19).

The slowing of the cardiac impulse at the AV junction prevents the atria and ventricles from contracting at the same time and protects the ventricles from the abnormally fast heart rates that can be generated in the atria under abnormal situations. Pre-excitation syndromes can be explained on the basis of accessory junctional pathways (Anderson et al., 1975b) (see Chapter 19).

Ventricular Conduction

The excitation impulse travels quickly through the His-Purkinje system. The His-Purkinje cells have the most rapid conduction velocities in the heart, approximately 1.5 to 2 m/s in the His bundle and 2 to 4 m/s in the Purkinje system (Singer et al., 1981). The cardiac impulse next spreads in a rapid (approximately 0.08 seconds), sequential manner from the common. His bundle through the bundle branches, then through the extensive ramifications of the Purkinje fiber system, and finally through ventricular muscle. Ventricular activation occurs in three general phases: septal depolarization, apex depolarization, and basal depolarization (Fig. 1-27).

The depolarization wave moves through the interventricular septum from left to right. The middle left septal area and the anterior and posterior left paraseptal areas are depolarized within the first 0 to 10 milliseconds (Durrer et al., 1970).

Most of the left and right ventricular cavities are depolarized within 20 to 40 milliseconds (Durrer et al., 1970). Activation spreads from the endocardium toward the epicardium.

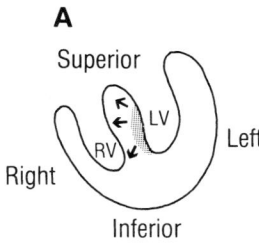

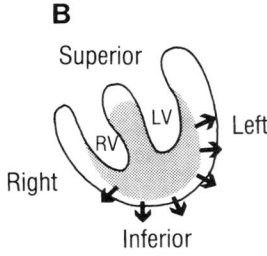

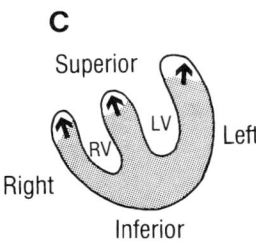

■ **Figure 1–27.** Schematic illustration of the sequence of ventricular depolarization. See text for description. RV, right ventricle; LV, left ventricle. (Adapted from Katz. A.M. [1977]. *Physiology of the heart* [pp. 275, 276]. New York: Raven Press.)

Although the impulse travels more rapidly through left ventricular tissue, the right ventricular wall is thinner. Thus, the full thickness of the right ventricle is generally depolarized prior to the left. The first epicardial depolarization is usually in the lower right ventricular wall because of its thinness.

Purkinje fibers are sparsely distributed in the basal (upper) sections of the ventricles and septum, particularly in the right ventricle and the septum. The basal and posterior portions of both ventricles and the basal interventricular septum are the last areas to be activated, at approximately 80 milliseconds (Durrer et al., 1970).

Although Purkinje fibers conduct the cardiac impulse more rapidly than other cardiac cells, Purkinje cells in the distal terminations of the conducting system have longer action potential durations and refractory periods than do ventricular muscle fibers (see previous). Because conduction is slower in cells with longer action potential durations and refractory periods, the conduction velocity of the cardiac impulse is slowed at the point where Purkinje fibers connect with ventricular muscle cells. In theory, the distal Purkinje fibers then function like a gate, the length of the refractory period in distal Purkinje fibers normally controlling the rate at which ventricular muscle fibers depolarize (Weidmann, 1982). Excitation–contraction coupling and the rate of cardiac contraction may be controlled by this gating

mechanism. The clinical importance of this gating mechanism is not clear (Lazzara et al., 1976).

Ventricular repolarization proceeds in general from the epicardium to the endocardium and spreads from the ventricular bases to the apices (Cohen, 1985). Thus, ventricular repolarization proceeds in a direction that is opposite to the direction of depolarization; thus the QRS and T waves are generally oriented in the same direction under normal circumstances. All portions of the ventricle recover at approximately the same time. However, ventricular repolarization is not homogeneous; under pathophysiological conditions, this may help create situations that promote ventricular arrhythmias (see Chapter 19).

Excitation–Contraction Coupling

Electrical excitation (i.e., depolarization of the myocardial cell membrane during the action potential) causes cardiac muscle contraction. The linking of electrical activity to mechanical activity is called *excitation–contraction coupling*. As identified by Ringer more than 100 years ago, an increase in the cytosolic calcium concentration is necessary to trigger this process (Ringer, 1883). Electrical excitation results in increases in intracellular calcium ion concentration. Intracellular calcium ion in turn is the key that initiates contractile protein interaction during contraction. The removal of calcium ion turns the process off and results in relaxation of the contractile apparatus. Thus, calcium ion is the link between electrical excitation and mechanical contraction. Calcium ion flows inward across the cell membrane during the action potential. Intracellular calcium ion stimulates release of calcium ion from internal stores such as the sarcoplasmic reticulum (SR). Removal of calcium ion from the myoplasm evokes relaxation. The mechanisms by which ionic fluxes across the sarcolemma evoke contraction and relaxation are illustrated in Figure 1-28.

Calcium influx across the sarcolemma in response to cardiac membrane depolarization triggers the release of calcium by the SR (Fabiato, 1983). The terminal cisternae of the SR press closely on the T-tubule. Electron-dense bridges or "feet" are visible with electron microscopy spanning the distance between the two membrane systems (Franzini-Armstrong, 1970). These structures, the so-called *ryanodine receptors* (because of binding properties), communicate the signal for SR calcium ion release.

The primary cardiac contractile proteins are actin, myosin, troponin, and tropomyosin. In cardiac cells, tropomysin inhibits interaction between action and myosin. When calcium ion binds with troponin following electrical excitation, this alters tropomyosin in such a way that the resting inhibition by tropomyosin ceases. Myosin interacts with actin, binding and forming crossbridges.

Calcium exerts several of its internal effects through combining with an intracellular protein called *calmodulin*. In cardiac myocardial cells, the calcium-calmodulin complex promotes calcium ion binding to troponin and thus promotes contraction. Calcium–calmodulin also may stimulate the calcium pumps on the SR and the sarcolemma and may stimulate sodium–calcium exchange; all these actions help remove calcium ion from the cytosol. Calcium-calmodulin influences the synthesis and breakdown of cAMP and may help promote

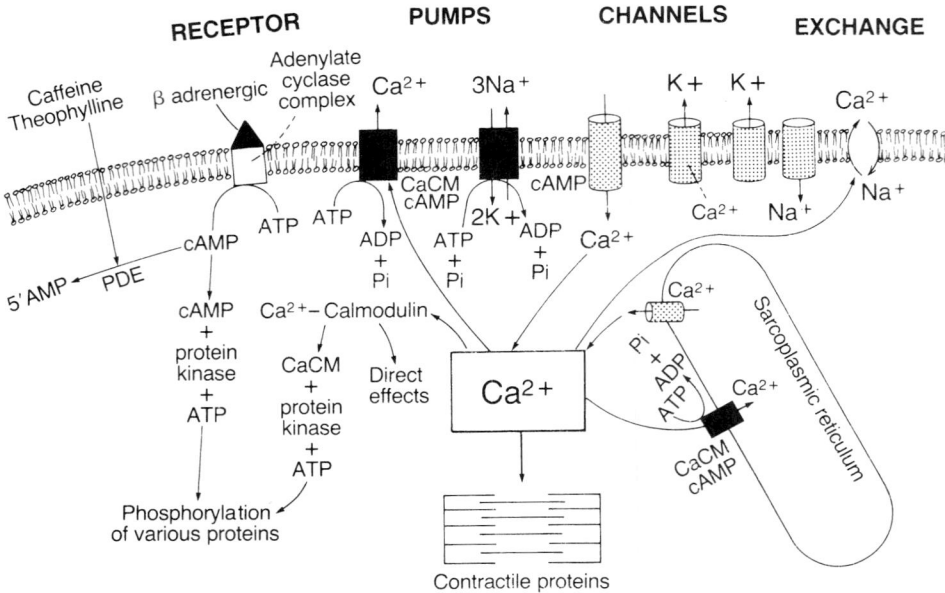

■ **Figure 1–28.** Schematic illustration of cardiac membrane transport processes and excitation-contraction coupling. CaCM, calcium calmodulin; cAMP, cyclic adenosine monophosphate; ADP, adenosine monophosphate; ATP, adenosine triphosphate; PDE, phosphodiesterase. (Adapted from Shamoo, A.E., & Ambudkar, I.S. [1984]. Regulation of calcium transport in cardiac cells. *Canadian Journal of Physiology and Pharmacology, 62,*13; Sperelakis, N. [1984]. Hormonal and neurotransmitter regulation of Ca^{++} influx through voltage-dependent slow channels in cardiac membrane. *Membrane Biochemistry,* 5(2), 153; and Tibbits, G.F., unpublished diagram.)

sarcolemmal calcium influx. Calcium may exert several other effects, either directly or by combining with other intracellular proteins, and thus may modulate myocardial cell contraction and relaxation through several different mechanisms.

Stimulation of (β-adrenergic receptors on the cardiac cell membrane influences transmembrane calcium fluxes and cardiac contraction through the intracellular production of cAMP from ATP, which in turn initiates several series of reactions involving intracellular protein phosphorylation (transfer of high-energy phosphates) by protein kinases. The metabolic actions of cAMP help to provide energy substrates for cardiac muscle contraction and relaxation. Phosphorylation of a sarcolemmal calcium channel membrane protein by cAMP creates a conformation or pore diameter change that places the calcium channel in a functional state available for voltage activation (Sperelakis, 1979). cAMP may also facilitate the SR release of calcium. Both actions promote an increased cytosolic calcium concentration and thus promote muscle contraction.

Phospholamban is an SR membrane protein that activates the SR calcium pump. Phosphorylation of phospholamban by cAMP, and by calmodulin at a different site, stimulates the calcium pump, increases SR calcium uptake, and promotes relaxation. cAMP phosphorylation of troponin influences the interaction between troponin and calcium, which also promotes relaxation.

Although uptake of calcium ion into the SR promotes relaxation, mechanisms that increase the amount of calcium ion in the SR promote increased calcium ion availability for tension generation during subsequent contractions. Thus, the increased rate and strength of contraction produced by β adrenergic stimulation and other combined chronotropic-inotropic mechanisms appear to be matched by mechanisms that enhance the rate of cardiac relaxation (Sperelakis, 1979).

Calcium, through its role as a regulator of contraction and its possible role as an initiator of contraction, is the major link

between excitation and contraction. The intracellular calcium concentration is directly and indirectly influenced by the amount of calcium transported in and out of the cell across the sarcolemma (Sperelakis, 1979). Calcium sarcolemmal fluxes are affected by the membrane potential and by sodium and potassium concentrations and transcellular fluxes. Conversely, potassium flux through the calcium-regulated potassium channel and sodium flux during sodium-calcium exchange are affected by the intracellular concentration of calcium.

MECHANICAL CHARACTERISTICS OF CARDIAC CELLS

Overview of Contraction

As seen in Figure 1-16, the myofibril is composed of a series of repeating units, called *sarcomeres*. Sarcomeres are the basic functional and structural units of the myofibril. Dark-staining Z lines mark the ends of the sarcomere. Attached to the Z line are the thin filaments. The center of the sarcomere is composed of the dark-appearing thick filaments. Interdigitating thin and thick filaments overlap to a variable extent. The amount of overlap is altered during shortening, when thick and thin filament proteins interact, and the filaments slide past one another.

The individual thick and thin filaments do not themselves change in length; the sarcomere (and the muscle as a whole) shortens. If shortening of the sarcomere (or the muscle cell) is prevented, the interaction of thick and thin filaments is manifested as tension or force generation. Such a contraction is termed *isometric.* When a stimulated muscle is allowed to shorten, tension is not increased, and the contraction is said to be *isotonic* (Figs. 1-29 and 1-30). In the heart, early systolic

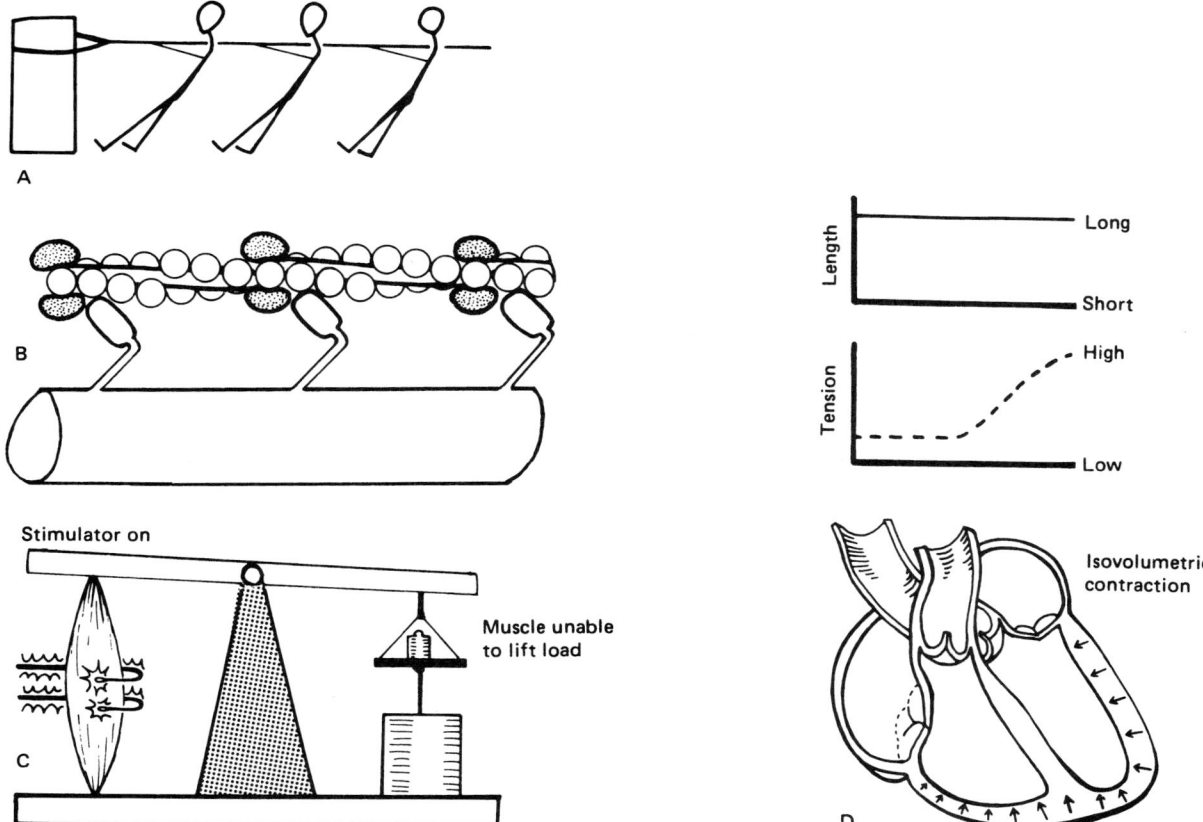

■ **Figure 1–29.** Isometric contraction. (*A*) In an isometric contraction, force is generated while muscles are held at a constant length. Schematically, this is analogous to the stick men pulling a load they cannot dislodge: A large force is generated, but no movement takes place. (*B*) At the molecular level, myosin heads attach to actin and pull, but filaments do not slide significantly past one another. (*C*) An experimental preparation producing isometric contraction consists of a muscle mounted on a lever with a very large load as counterweight. The muscle generates a force when stimulated, but the load is so great that the muscle cannot lift it. (*D*) In the heart, ventricular contraction is primarily isometric before the opening of the semilunar valves: Tension increases but no major shortening takes place. (*A* and *B* adapted from Katz, A.M. [1977]. *Physiology of the heart* [p. 118]. New York: Raven Press.)

contraction is primarily isometric: tension increases and muscle length remains fairly constant. Later in systole, the contraction is primarily isotonic: the heart muscle shortens, and the blood is expelled into the aorta. Little additional tension is developed.

Molecular Basis for Contraction

The *thick filaments* are composed primarily of the protein myosin. Myosin is large, consisting of six subunits: two heavy chains and four light chains per molecule. The two heavy chain subunits are coiled to form a long, rod-like tail at one end. At the opposite end of the long myosin heavy chain, a head protrudes from each subunit. Groups of myosin tails are arranged to form the rigid backbone of the thick filament. The heads are the site of ATP breakdown and interaction with the thin filaments. Heads project outward in a spiral along the length of the thick filament. At the center of the filament, the molecules reverse direction, leaving a bare region from which no heads protrude. The small light chains are nestled in the angle between head and tail, two per heavy chain. Both heavy and light chains are members of multigene families and exist in

several forms, called *isoforms*. Variation in isoform composition may modify the rate or intensity of myosin chemical activity. This in turn may modify the contractile properties of the tissue. Age, mechanical loading, or metabolic or hormonal state may modify isoform composition.

The *thin filaments* are composed primarily of bead-shaped molecules of the protein actin arranged in an intercoiled, double-stranded chain. Two other proteins, troponin and tropomyosin, are located on the thin filaments at periodic intervals (Fig. 1-31). Actin interacts with the thick-filament protein, myosin, resulting in the transduction of the chemical energy of ATP into mechanical energy. Troponin and tropomyosin are called *regulatory proteins* because they modify the interaction of actin and myosin.

Myosin is an enzyme that breaks down the high-energy ATP molecule. During the resting state, the products of ATP breakdown remain bound to the myosin head. When myosin interacts with actin, the rate of ATP turnover is greatly increased. The chemical energy released from ATP is converted to the mechanical energy of contraction and heat.

According to the *cross-bridge theory*, a bond or crossbridge forms during muscle contraction, linking thick and thin

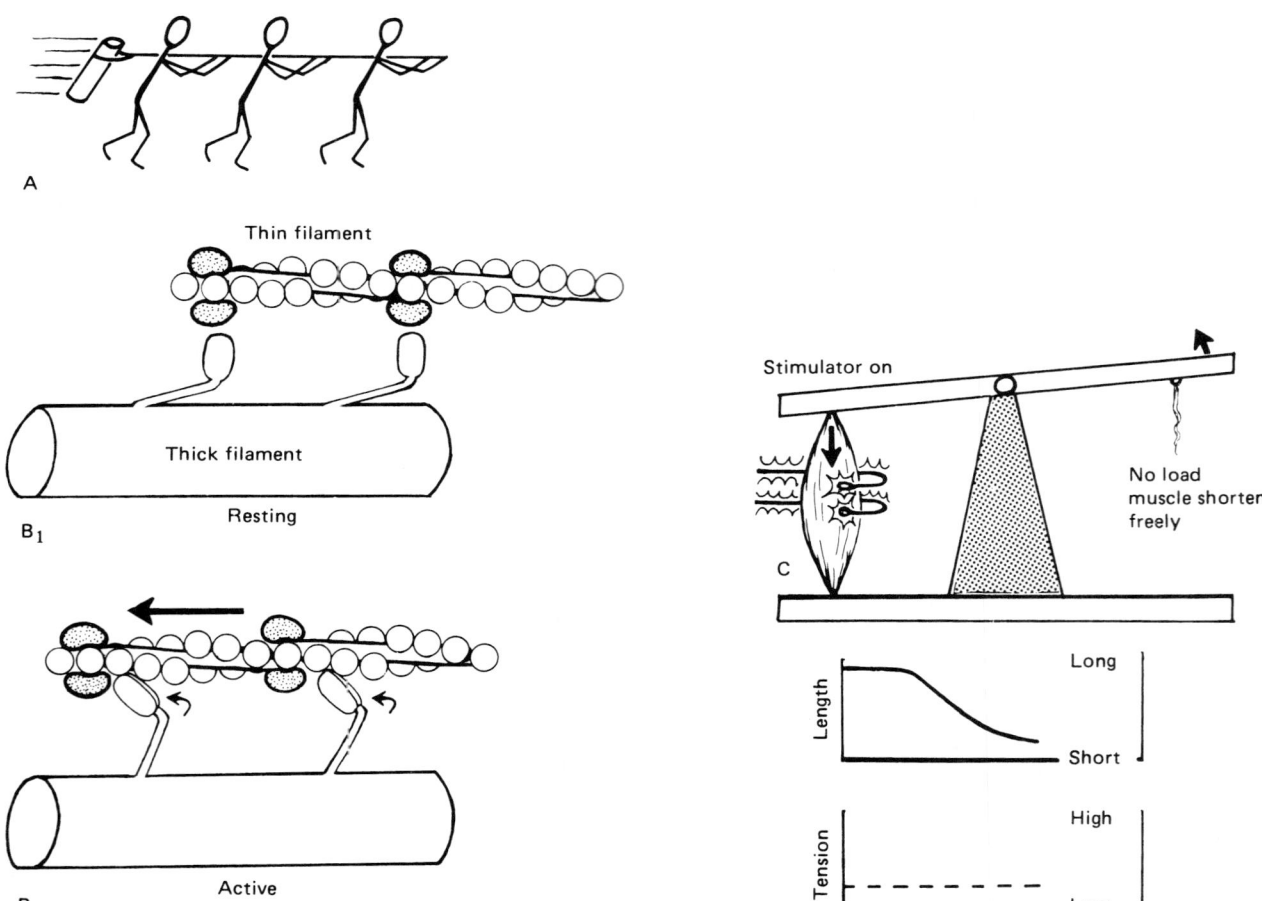

■ **Figure 1–30.** Isotonic contraction. (*A*) In an isotonic contraction, muscles shorten freely, and little tension is developed. Schematically, this is analogous to the stick men running with a very small load. Little force is generated, but movement takes place. (*B*) At the molecular level, myosin heads attach briefly to actin and pull the thin filament, then release in a cyclic fashion. The sarcomere shortens. (*C*) An experimental preparation producing isotonic contraction consists of a muscle mounted on a lever without significant counterload. The stimulated muscle shortens freely, not increasing its tension. (*A* and *B* adapted from Katz, A.M. [1977]. *Physiology of the heart* [pp. 87, 112]. New York: Raven Press.)

filaments. The protuberant myosin head contains an actin-binding site and forms the cross-bridge. This crossbridge is capable of binding, flexing, releasing, and binding again, thus pulling the thin filament toward the center of the sarcomere in an isotonic contraction. If the muscle is held at a fixed length and is unable to shorten (an isometric contraction), tension is generated by the pulling of the cross-bridge.

When the muscle is relaxed during diastole, the interaction of myosin and actin is inhibited by tropomyosin and troponin. Electrical signals across the cell membrane trigger the release of calcium ion into the sarcoplasm from within the SR and from extracellular fluid by way of the sarcolemma and T-tubule membranes. This increase in intracellular calcium ion concentration is in turn a trigger for contraction. Calcium ion binds troponin; tropomyosin rotates in a manner such that resting inhibition to cross-bridge formation is removed, and cross-bridges form (see Fig. 1-31).

At relaxation, calcium ion concentration is very low in the sarcoplasm. When calcium ion concentration rises, contraction occurs. The sarcoplasmic calcium ion concentration determines

the forcefulness of contraction. Figure 1-32 illustrates the relation: the higher the sarcoplasmic calcium ion concentration, the greater is the tension or pull the heart muscle can generate until a saturating concentration is attained.

Molecular Basis for Relaxation

Contraction ceases when calcium ion is removed from the sarcoplasm. Troponin releases its bound calcium ion; tropomyosin returns to the position in which actin and myosin interaction was blocked. The cell relaxes again (see Fig. 1-31).

Removal of calcium ion is essential in this sequence. Two mechanisms are important in this process. The SR pumps calcium ion into its core. This is an active process and requires chemical energy from ATP breakdown. Also, calcium ion is pumped outward across the sarcolemma. This, too, is an active process because calcium ion must be moved against electrical and concentration gradients. Rather than using ATP directly, this process uses the energy stored in the sodium ion gradient.

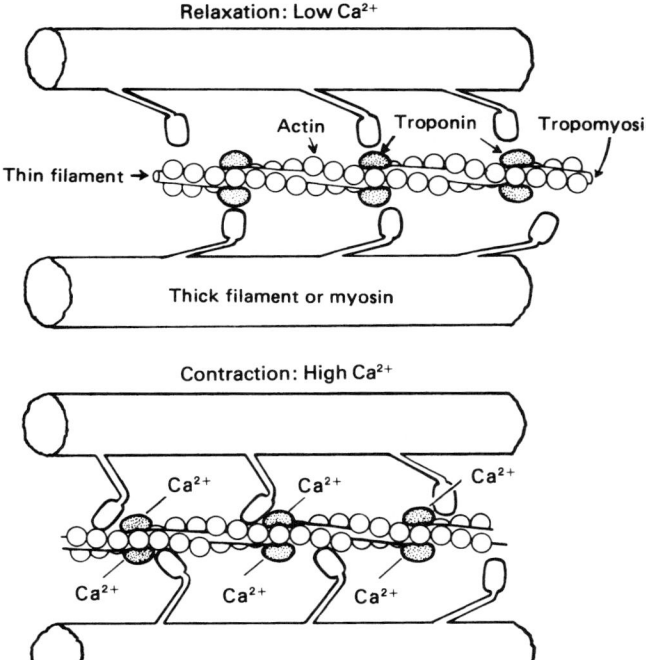

Figure 1–31. Molecular interactions during relaxation and contraction proposed by the cross-bridge theory of muscle contraction. During relaxation, when calcium ion (Ca^{2+}), concentration is low, no cross-bridges form. When intracellular Ca^{2+} concentration rises as it does after the action potential, troponin combines with Ca^{2+}, and the tropomyosin-troponin system changes in such a way as to allow attachment and pulling by crossbridges. Adapted from Alpert, N.R. & Hamrell, B.B. [1976]. Cardiac hypertrophy: A compensatory and anticompensatory response to stress. In M. Vassalle [Ed.], *Cardiac physiology for the clinician* [p. 196]. New York: Academic Press.)

In conjunction with sodium ion moving inward down its concentration gradient, calcium ion is forced outward. The sodium ion gradient, in turn, is maintained by the sodium-potassium pump, which is powered by ATP.

The ATP required for the removal of calcium ion from the cell and for the cycling of cross-bridges may be depleted, for

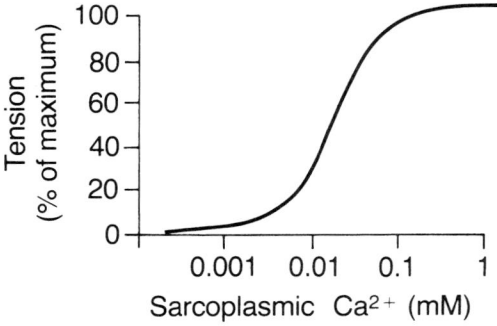

Figure 1–32. The calcium ion (Ca^{2+}) concentration versus tension relation. The higher the sarcoplasmic Ca^{2+} concentration, the more tension the heart muscle is able to generate until a maximum level is attained. Note the range of intracellular Ca^{2+} concentrations is significantly lower than the 1- to 2-mM concentration in the extracellular space.

example, in myocardial ischemia. When this happens, cross-bridges form and are not broken; the muscle is stiff.

Modulation of Sarcoplasmic Calcium Ion Concentration

Interventions that alter the sarcoplasmic calcium ion concentration alter the force generated in a contraction. For example, β-adrenergic drugs such as epinephrine may increase inward calcium current through calcium channels opened during the action potential, increasing sarcoplasmic calcium ion concentration and, thus, force of contraction. Certain antiarrhythmic drugs such as procainamide are associated with decreased calcium ion release from the SR and, thus, decreased systolic tension generation and blood pressure (Hunter et al., 1982).

Digitalis-like drugs increase the force of contraction. A prominent theory postulates that this effect is mediated by changes in the sarcoplasmic calcium ion concentration. Digitalis-like drugs partially block the sodium—potassium pump. As the transmembrane sodium ion gradient decreases, less calcium ion is pumped out across the sarcolemma. The intracellular calcium ion stores and calcium ion level during contraction increase. The end result is augmented contractile strength.

MECHANICAL PROPERTIES OF THE MYOCARDIUM

The heart is a pump. Its function is to add energy to the flowing blood, thus propelling it through the systemic and pulmonary circulations. The performance of the heart as a pump can be described in terms of the cardiac output (CO). CO is the volume of blood pumped by one ventricle in 1 minute. It is equal to the stroke volume (SV), or volume of blood pumped with each beat, times the number of cardiac contractions (heart rate, HR) in 1 minute: (CO = SV × HR). Typical normal values in a 70-kg man at rest (HR: 68 beats/min; SV: 80 mL) produce a cardiac output of 5,440 mL/min or 5.4 L/min.

Stroke volume is determined by the degree of ventricular filling during diastole, or preload, the force against which the ventricle must pump, or afterload, the contractile state of the myocardium, and by the heart rate. In the remainder of this section, these factors are discussed in more detail, and the manner in which they interact to influence the mechanical function of the heart is described.

Preload and Afterload

Preload

Preload is the distending force that stretches the ventricular muscle immediately before electrical excitation and contraction. Figure 1-33 further defines preload and illustrates the role of preload in the contraction of a simple muscle preparation and in the heart. Left ventricular end-diastolic pressure is the left ventricular preload. In the absence of pathologic mitral valve changes, left atrial pressure is an indicator of left ventricular

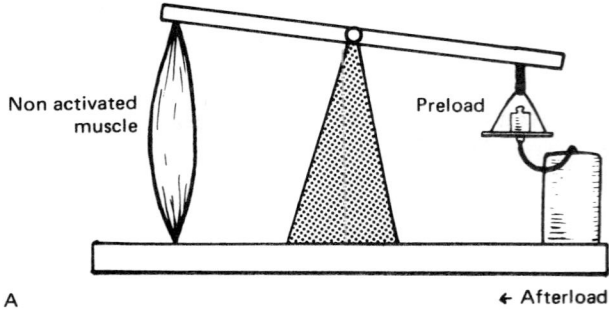

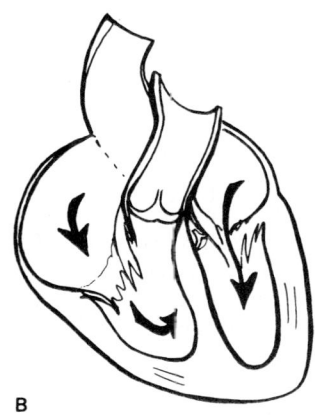

Preload = load stretching the
resting ventricle to its end-
diastolic volume

■ **Figure 1–33.** Preload. (*A*) In the isolated muscle preparation, preload is the load stretching the resting muscle. Thus, preload determines the resting length of the muscles. (*B*) In the heart, the ventricular preload is determined by the volume of blood stretching the resting ventricles.

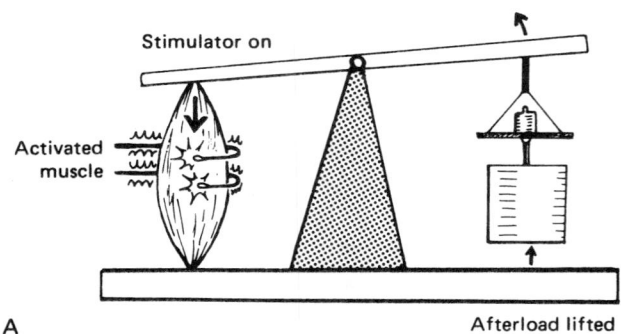

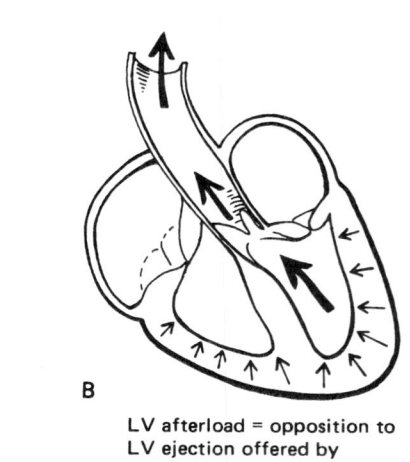

LV afterload = opposition to
LV ejection offered by
aortic pressure

■ **Figure 1–34.** Afterload. (*A*) In the isolated muscle preparation, afterload is the force opposing shortening. The muscle must generate enough tension to lift the afterload before it can shorten. (*B*) In the heart, the afterload is the force opposing ventricular ejection.

preload. In order to make clinical judgments about left ventricular preload, clinicians measure the pulmonary artery pressures and the pulmonary capillary end diastolic pressure. If there is no pulmonary hypertension as well as no mitral valve pathology, then these pressures are useful indices of left ventricular preload. Central venous pressure, in the absence of tricuspid valve disease, is an index of right ventricular preload (see Chapter 23).

Afterload

A related term often used to describe cardiac mechanical function is *afterload.* This is the force that opposes ventricular ejection (i.e., the forces that the muscle must overcome to move the blood during contraction). Figure 1-34 illustrates the role of afterload in a simple muscle preparation and in the heart.

Left ventricular afterload is determined by the *volume and mass of blood* ejected by the ventricle, by the *resistance to blood flow* (determined mainly by the cross-sectional area of the small arterioles, known as resistance vessels), by the *aortic impedance* (amount of pressure change for a given volume of blood ejected into the aorta; this depends on the elasticity of the aorta and branching arteries), and intrathoracic pressures. The arterial systolic pressure is a good clinical indicator of the afterload of

the left ventricle; pulmonary systolic pressure indicates right ventricular afterload. Total systemic vascular resistance (SVR) and total pulmonary vascular resistance (PVR) are used to indicate left and right ventricular afterload, respectively.

Preload Role: Length-Tension Relationship

Early in this century, Starling observed that within limits, an increase in left ventricular volume at the end of diastole results in the generation of increased active pressure and increased volume pumped during the ensuing contraction. Beyond a certain volume, this mechanism is no longer operational; increased end-diastolic volume results instead in decreased pressure developing and a decreased volume of blood being ejected (Patterson et al., 1914). This property is known as *Starling's law of the heart* or the *length-tension relation of cardiac muscle* (or sometimes, the *Frank-Starling law of the heart*). It is commonly illustrated in a graph (Fig. 1-35). Although the left ventricular *volume* at the end of diastole is factor that determines the subsequent force of contraction, clinician's measure pressures increments, not volume. However, the volume and the pressure are related, as discussed later (see section on Compliance).

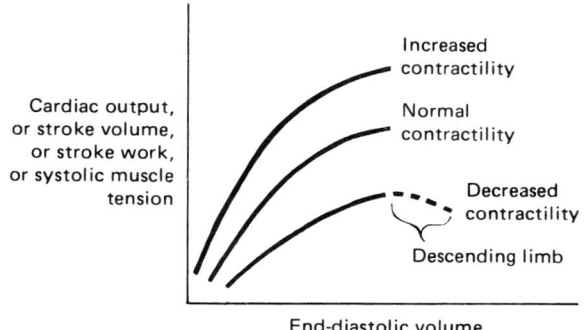

■ Figure 1–35. The length-tension relation of the heart. End-diastolic volume determines the end-diastolic length of the ventricular muscle fibers and is proportional to tension generated during systole as well as to cardiac output, stroke volume, and stroke work. A change in cardiac contractility causes the heart to perform on a different length-tension curve.

The length-tension mechanism is a functional one; it is thought to help maintain overall matching between left and right ventricular output. For instance, if a person reclines after being in a standing position (or elevates the legs when in a reclining position), the volume of blood returning to the heart transiently increases. The right ventricle is stretched and increases its force of contraction, pumping a larger stroke volume to the lungs and generating higher pressures. Pulmonary vascular pressures rise. This raises the left ventricular filling pressure or preload. Left ventricular filling volume increases. The left ventricle generates increased active pressure and pumps a larger stroke volume, and arterial vascular pressures rise (see Chapter 4). This intrinsic ability of the heart to match increased cardiac volume return is useful in case of the cardiac transplant patient, providing a mechanism to increase cardiac output, particularly early in exercise.

Some forms of therapy are designed to take advantage of the length—tension characteristics of the heart. Examples of this are leg raising and intravascular volume expansion in the patient with shock. These therapies increase central blood volume and improve cardiac contractile force; they are easily and rapidly accessible. They are, however, associated with an increase in myocardial oxygen consumption and should be used carefully in the patient at risk for myocardial ischemia. These patients should be monitored for ECG signs of myocardial and for symptoms such as chest pain when interventions may result in increased preload.

It is often clinically useful to graph an indicator of cardiac length (such as pulmonary artery wedge pressure) against an indicator of the tension generated (such as cardiac output). These length-tension diagrams characterize the mechanical functioning of the heart and can be used to judge the impact of therapies (see Fig. 1-35). Positive inotropic factors, that is, factors that increase the contractility of the heart, such as sympathetic stimulation, alter the length-tension relation, so that a higher tension is generated at the same left ventricular end-diastolic volume. In the failing heart, the same stretch generates much less tension and cardiac output does not substantially increase with volume. The heart is said to be refractory to inotropic stimulation; it may be said that the Starling curve is reduced.

The cross-bridge theory of muscle contraction partly accounts for the length-tension relation of cardiac muscle (Fig. 1-36). Tension generated by muscle is proportional to the number of cross-bridges formed. At short lengths, thin filaments overlap one another and interfere with crossbridge formation. Maximal tension development occurs in the range of muscle lengths at which the myosin crossbridge regions maximally overlap the thin filaments without the thin filaments overlapping one another. If the muscle is stretched still further, then the region of cross-bridge overlap is diminished and less tension is developed (Gordon et al., 1966).

Other factors also contribute to the shape of the Starling curve. For example, when the heart is stretched, more cells may be brought into parallel with the axis of shortening and may be able to contribute more effectively to the total development of force within the ventricle. Calcium ion, which grades the force of contraction, may enter the sarcoplasm in larger quantities for longer periods of time. Contractile filaments may be more sensitive to calcium ion at longer sarcomere lengths.

Compliance. Starling's law of the heart relates end-diastolic length, rather than end-diastolic pressure, to the strength of

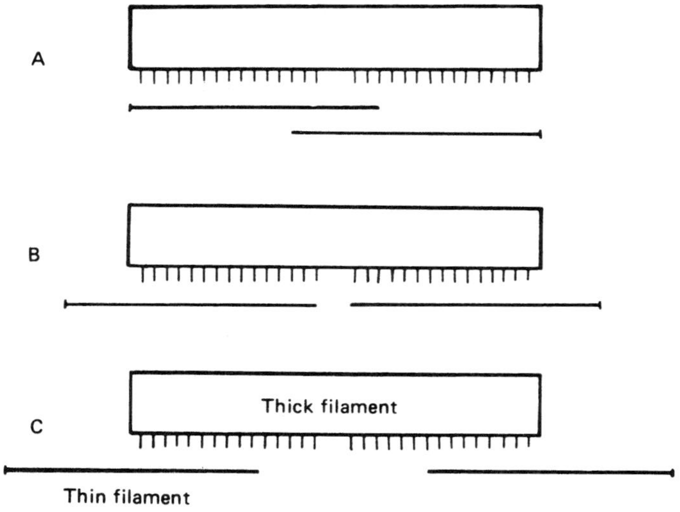

■ Figure 1–36. Schematic view of variations in overlap between the thick and thin filaments that account for the length-tension relation of cardiac muscle. (*A*) Sarcomere on ascending limb of length-tension curve. The thin filaments begin overlapping, interfering with attachment by cross-bridges. (*B*) Sarcomere with maximal effective overlap of thin and thick filaments and hence at the peak of the length-tension curve. (*C*) Sarcomere stretched beyond maximal overlap and hence on the descending limb of the length-tension curve. As the actin chains are pulled farther out, fewer actin sites are available for crossbridge attachment. (*A* and *B* adapted from Katz, A.M. [1977]. *Physiology of the heart* [pp. 129, 130]. New York: Raven Press.)

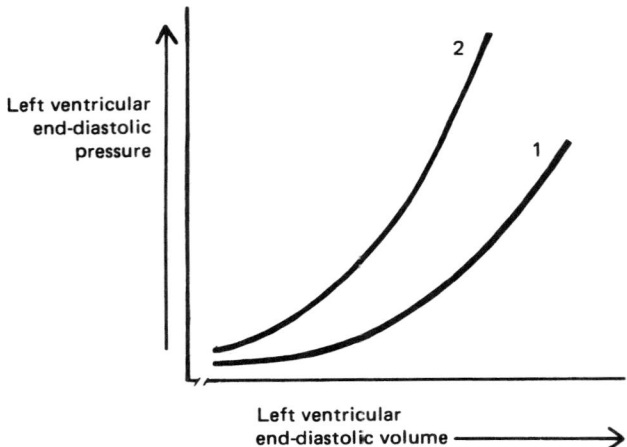

■ **Figure 1–37.** The stiffness of the left ventricle. Stiffness is the slope of the pressure-volume relation. Curve 1 represents normal stiffness; curve 2 represents an increase in stiffness such as that which might occur after a myocardial infarction. In both cases, increases in volume result in increased pressure and an increased increment in pressure for a given increment in volume. Compliance is the inverse of stiffness. (Adapted from Forrester, J.S., & Diamond, G.A. [1973]. Clinical application of left ventricular pressures. In E. Corday, & H.J.C. Swan [Eds.], *Myocardial infarction: New perspectives in diagnosis and management* [pp. 143–148]. Baltimore: Williams & Wilkins.)

contraction. End-diastolic length and pressure are, however, related. *Compliance* is the term used to describe that relation. Compliance (*C*) is the change in volume (ΔV) that results for a given change in pressure (ΔP):

$$C = \Delta V / \Delta P$$

Stiffness (*S*) is the inverse of compliance ($S = \Delta P / \Delta V$). Increased stiffness is the same as decreased compliance.

Compliance of the heart is determined by inherent properties of the cardiac muscle tissue, by cardiac chamber geometry, and by the state of the pericardium. The myocardial tissue is stiffer with hypoxia, ischemia, and scarring, such as after a myocardial infarction (Lewis & Gotsman, 1980) (curve 2 in Fig. 1-37). Infiltrative myocardial diseases such as amyloidosis increase muscle stiffness. Geometry changes that result in increased stiffness include hypertrophy. When operating at a more distended volume, the heart is invariably stiffer: it requires larger increments in filling pressure to achieve a given increment in volume (see Fig. 1-37). Pericardial conditions that increase cardiac stiffness include pericarditis and tamponade. The ability of the cardiac muscle to relax, expand, and stretch in response to a volume is called "lusitropy."

Implications for Patient Care. It is important to consider left ventricular compliance in patient care. In monitoring preload, the nurse commonly measures indices of left ventricular end-diastolic *pressure*. Yet, therapeutic goals are related to achieving an end-diastolic *volume* change that will take advantage of the length-tension relation of the heart to maintain or increase cardiac output. The pressure change is important, too, because elevated left ventricular filling pressures result in pulmonary congestion and edema.

For example, the first few days after a myocardial infarction are usually characterized by an increase in myocardial stiffness (Hood et al., 1970) (see Fig. 1-37). The same end-diastolic volume may be accompanied by such a markedly increased end diastolic pressure that signs of left ventricular failure such as crackles appear (see Chapter 13). In this case, inotropic agents (which increase the force of contraction) would be of little or no benefit. Unloading therapies, however, that may decrease the end-diastolic volume can eliminate the damaging elevation in end-diastolic pressures. Furthermore, lowered ventricular pressures throughout diastole may improve coronary arterial filling. Better perfusion can improve tissue oxygenation and further diminish stiffness.

Afterload Role: Force-Velocity Relationship

The heart's ability to contract is influenced by the amount of pressure above the preload it must actively generate. With a smaller afterload, the heart is able to contract more rapidly. Against very large afterload, contraction is much slower. This is often referred to as the *force-velocity of shortening relation*, or simply the *force-velocity relation* (Fig. 1-38). Changes in the initial muscle length or changes in contractility can alter the force-velocity relation.

An intuitive understanding of the force-velocity relation can be gained by reviewing the stick-figure cartoons in Figure 1-38. The lighter the load, the faster A, B, and C run; the heavier the

■ **Figure 1–38.** Approximation of the force-velocity of shortening relation of cardiac muscle. Velocity of shortening is maximal with extremely light afterload. Shortening is impossible with large afterloads. (Adapted from Katz, A.M. [1977]. *Physiology of the heart* [pp. 87, 126]. New York: Raven Press.)

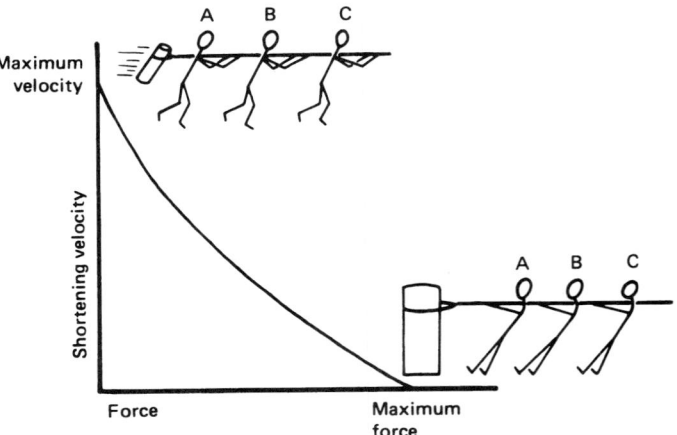

load, the slower they can move. If the load they are trying to pull is sufficiently heavy, they are unable to move it at all.

At the molecular level, the rate of cycling of crossbridges may be equated to the speed of shortening. Generation of tension may be equated to attachment and pulling by the crossbridges. The amount of tension the muscle can generate is determined by the number of cross-bridges the muscle is able to form. This is determined in part by the preload, or the amount of diastolic stretch placed on the muscle. Once a critical amount of force equivalent to the afterload, or force opposing ejection, is generated, the muscle shortens. The speed of that shortening may be equated with the speed of cycling of cross-bridges and is determined in part by the afterload.

Effect of Afterload on the Volume Ejected by the Ventricle. In addition to influencing the speed of shortening, afterload is related to extent of shortening. Increases in SVR, at a constant end-diastolic pressure, result in decreased volume pumped by the left ventricle. When pumping against decreased aortic pressure, the left ventricle pumps a larger volume.

Implications for Patient Care. It is important to consider the force-velocity relation in myocardial performance. Vasopressors that increase the SVR increase the afterload. Because of the inverse nature of the force—velocity relation, the development of greater force is accompanied by a slower velocity of shortening. There may be a concomitant decrease in stroke volume and cardiac output. Further, there is an increase in the oxygen requirements of the cardiac tissue when afterload is increased.

Conversely, therapies that decrease the afterload are associated with faster and more extensive shortening and a larger volume pumped. The cardiac output increases. Increases in cardiac output achieved in this manner have the unique advantage of decreasing myocardial oxygen consumption. Reduction of afterload, however, is associated with decreased coronary perfusion pressure. Signs of myocardial ischemia may develop in patients with partially obstructed coronary arteries.

Contractility of Cardiac Muscle

Contractility describes the heart's ability to contract: it describes the ability of the heart muscle to shorten, develop tension, or both. Altered contractility is a change in the ability of the heart to contract independent of variations induced by altering either preload or afterload (see Fig. 1-35; Fig. 1-39). In Figure 1-35, the curves other than "normal" represent alterations in contractility.

Contractility is a property intrinsic to the muscle. Its physiological basis is not yet understood. Although contractility is difficult to define or measure, it is a property of critical importance because abnormalities in contractility are a major problem in the failing heart. Many therapies are designed to enhance contractility.

Contractility is not equivalent to cardiac performance, which can be influenced by valvular function and circulating blood volume as well as by myocardial contractility. Factors that affect the contractility of the heart are called *inotropic agents*. Positive inotropic agents increase contractility. These include sympathetic stimulation, excess thyroid hormone, epinephrine, norepinephrine, dopamine, dobutamine, isoproterenol infusion, and calcium salt infusion. Digitalis-like drugs have positive inotropic action. Negative inotropic agents decrease contractility; these include

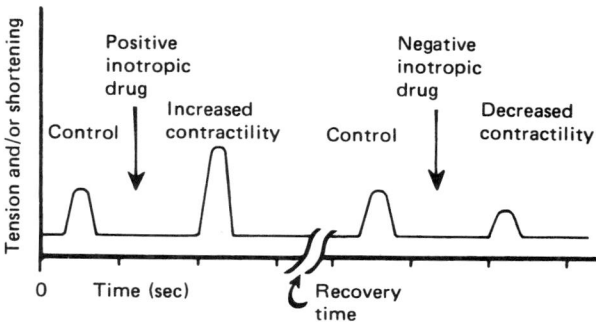

■ Figure 1–39. Positive and negative inotropic effects on tension development or myocardial shortening. An increase in myocardial contractility enhances the amount of tension developed, the rate of shortening, or both, without an increase in initial cardiac muscle length. A decrease in myocardial contractility reduces the amount of tension developed, the rate of shortening, or both, without a decrease in initial cardiac muscle length. (Adapted from Katz, A.M. [1977]. *Physiology of the heart* [p. 166]. New York: Raven Press.)

myocardial hypoxia, ischemia, acidosis, barbiturates, alcohol, procainamide and quinidine, propranolol, and possibly lidocaine.

Therapies that increase contractility increase myocardial oxygen consumption. Agents such as catecholamines increase both contractility and afterload and result in substantial increase in myocardial oxygen consumption.

Treppe

Heart rate is the fourth major determinant of the force of contraction. Alteration in the force of contraction with heart rate is called the *Treppe* or *staircase phenomenon*. In an experimental preparation with the preload held constant, the faster the rate of stimulation, the stronger is the force of contraction. Conversely, in the same preparation, slower rates of stimulation result in less forceful contraction. In the intact organism, as heart rate increases, there is decreased time for filling. The Treppe phenomenon provides some compensation for the decrement (Fig. 1-40).

Treppe is an intrinsic property of the heart muscle, independent of hormones or innervation. It is present in the transplanted heart. The physiological basis for Treppe may be rate-driven variations in sarcoplasmic calcium ion concentration.

Two other types of rate-related alterations occur in force of contraction. A pause augments the force of the ensuing beat. This is called *rest potentiation*. After an extra beat, the force of the ensuing contraction is increased. This effect is called *postextrasystolic potentiation*.

The manner in which variations in cardiac rate or rhythm induce changes in cardiac output in the intact heart is complex. Rate-related variations in force of contraction and filling interact; the amount pumped depends on that complex interaction.

Cardiac Reserve

The interaction of the mechanical properties of the heart can be illustrated by considering the reserve capacity of the heart. *Cardiac reserve* refers to the ability of the heart to increase its

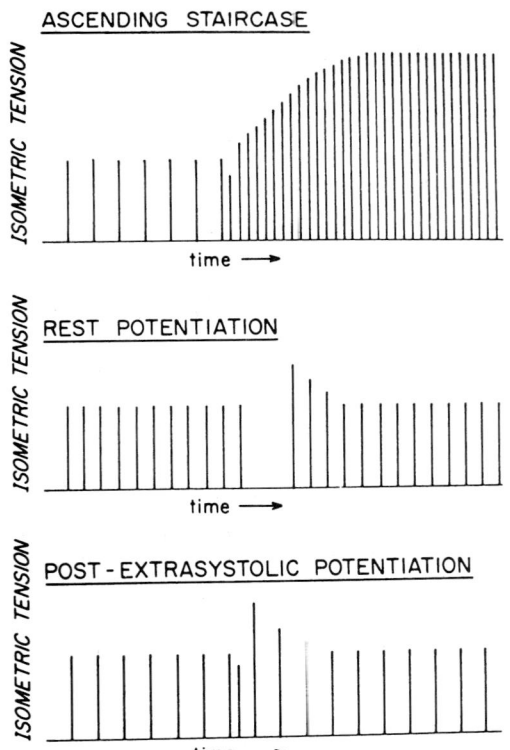

■ Figure 1–40. Changes in isometric force generated in cardiac muscle when the stimulation frequency is altered. (From Feigl, E.O. [1974]. *Physiology and biophysics* [20th ed., vol. 2, p. 37]. Philadelphia: WB Saunders.)

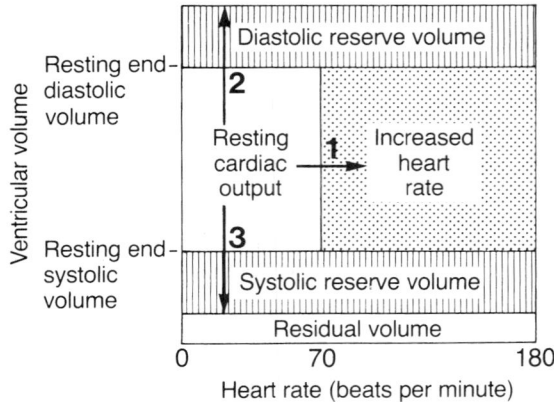

■ Figure 1–41. Cardiac reserve describes the ability of the heart to increase its output. Increases in heart rate increase the cardiac output (arrow 1). Stroke volume increases also increase the cardiac output. This can be accomplished by an increase in preload (diastolic reserve, arrow 2) or by contracting to a smaller end-systolic volume (systolic reserve, arrow 3). (From Rushmer, R.F. [1976]. *Cardiovascular dynamics* [p. 274]. Philadelphia: WB Saunders.)

output. In the healthy person, the reserve capacity is used to meet demands for increased blood flow, such as during exercise. Normal cardiac output is 5.5 L/min in a healthy, 70-kg man. Use of cardiac reserve typically increases cardiac output with activity to 18 L/min. Heart disease often limits the total possible output and the patient may have to rely on reserve capacity simply to maintain a normal cardiac output at rest. The two components of cardiac reserve are increases in heart rate and stroke volume (Fig. 1-41).

Increases in heart rate increase the cardiac output. As the heart beats more rapidly, there is less time for filling. The rate-related increase in force of contraction partially compensates for the lower end-diastolic filling. At rates higher than approximately 180 beats/min; however, diastole is so shortened that diastolic filling is reduced. Stroke volume is then diminished, as predicted by the Starling relation. Furthermore, the coronary arteries are perfused during diastole, and fast heart rates diminish coronary blood flow. This may result in ischemia, which in turn diminishes myocardial compliance and contractility. The stiff ventricle requires greater filling pressures to expand it to the same diastolic volume and may well operate at a smaller volume, further diminishing stroke volume, again as defined by the Starling relation. Beyond a certain point, increasing the heart rate so decreases the volume pumped per beat that cardiac output decreases.

During diastole, the heart can fill to a larger volume than usual, thereby increasing its stroke volume as defined by the Starling relation. This is sometimes called the *diastolic cardiac reserve.* Increases in diastolic volume are accompanied by increases in end-diastolic pressure. Left ventricular end-diastolic pressures beyond approximately 20 to 25 mm Hg typically result in pulmonary congestion and edema. The more dilated the ventricle, the more oxygen it requires (discussed later); this may be a limiting problem in the patient with coronary artery disease.

The heart is capable of ejecting a larger portion of its volume than it normally does; that is, it can contract to a smaller end-systolic volume. This is sometimes called the *systolic reserve;* it comes into play when the afterload is decreased (force—velocity relation) or contractility is increased. Increases in the velocity of contraction or contractility also make extra demands on the heart in terms of oxygen requirements and may be intolerable for the patient with coronary artery disease.

Factors involved in mechanical performance interact continuously. For example, an increase in afterload may result in a decrease in the stroke volume ejected. This in turn results in a larger volume of blood in the heart at end systole. The addition of an unchanged amount of blood during the subsequent diastole increases the end diastolic volume. The ensuing contraction is more forceful, and stroke volume is increased owing to the Starling effect.

In hemorrhage, the filling pressure may diminish; the stroke volume decreases as predicted by the Starling relation. However, the afterload may also decrease. This tends to raise the stroke volume. Adrenergic outflow also contributes to increased stroke volume. The cardiac output may increase despite lowered filling pressures.

This section has discussed means by which the heart can increase its output. Just as a budget deficit can be corrected either by increasing income or by carefully managing spending, the cardiovascular system can meet demands for increased perfusion both by increasing output and by more efficiently using its present output. It can, for instance, shift blood flow to more active regions and extract more oxygen from the blood (see Chapter 4).

Assessment of the Patient's Pump Performance

Assessment of the patient includes the evaluation of numerous indices of overall pump performance, as follows:

- Urine output, mental status, skin color, and temperature are indices of the adequacy of cardiac output to various organs and tissues
- Cardiac output may be measured directly
- Left ventricular preload is estimated from the pulmonary artery wedge pressure
- SVR (index of left ventricular afterload) is calculated
- Blood pressure is the product of cardiac output and SVR

These observations measure end products of many complexly interacting variables that together compose the reserve capacity of the cardiovascular system. In making these assessments, the nurse not only should ask whether blood flow and pressure are adequate but also should probe more deeply:

- How much of the patient's reserve capacity must be used to maintain the current level of functioning?
- Is the patient already tachycardic, with a dilated left ventricle?
- Is the patient's heart already receiving a high level of endogenous catecholaminergic outflow?
- How much of the patient's reserve capacity is left? Of that left, how much can be used in planning the patient's care?
- What is the cost of the patient's current functional state in terms of myocardial oxygen consumption?

MYOCARDIAL METABOLISM

The chemical energy of ATP powers myocardial contraction, ion pumping, and many other activities. ATP is broken down (hydrolyzed) into adenosine diphosphate and inorganic phosphate. With hydrolysis, chemical energy is transformed into mechanical energy and heat. Because the heart is continuously active, ATP must be continuously available. The usual intramyocardial cellular concentrations of ATP (estimated at 5 mM) are sufficient to power contraction mechanical activity for only a few beats.

Creatine phosphate is a backup source of high-energy phosphate to replenish the ATP supply. However, energy stores in ATP and creatine phosphate together supply enough energy only for several minutes of activity. Thus, the heart depends on ongoing ATP synthesis. This occurs in a series of efficient, but complex, enzyme-dependent reactions. The bulk of myocardial ATP is synthesized in an aerobic environment. The presence of large amounts of mitochondria, the sites of aerobic synthesis of ATP in the myocardial cell, attest to the need for oxygen as an energy substrate. The myocyte contains more mitochondria than any other type of muscle cell.

Free fatty acids are the preferred myocardial fuel, particularly when the patient is in the fasting state. *Glucose* or its storage form, glycogen, can serve as an additional substrate for energy metabolism. Whereas glucose contributes only 15% to myocardial ATP synthesis in the fasting patient, its role

increases to nearly 50% in the postprandial state. *Amino acids* play a minor role in energy metabolism of the heart. In starvation, however, amino acid intermediates are metabolized to maintain energy stores.

PHYSIOLOGY OF THE CORONARY CIRCULATION

Under normal conditions at rest, the heart extracts a large amount of oxygen from the blood that perfuses the heart: the difference in oxygen content between the coronary arterial and coronary sinus blood is approximately 11.4 mL O_2/100 mL blood (Regan et al., 1963). The total oxygen content of arterial blood is normally approximately 20 mL O_2/100 mL blood, so this represents extraction of more than 50% of the arterial oxygen content.

It is difficult to extract much more oxygen than this, yet the oxygen requirement of the heart may increase many fold. This additional oxygen can be supplied only by increasing the coronary blood flow. Coronary blood flow increases proportionately to myocardial metabolism and oxygen consumption.

Determinants of Myocardial Oxygen Consumption

Some oxygen is used in the "housekeeping" activities of the heart cells. This refers to those activities that are independent of contraction and includes such functions as maintenance of the proper ionic environment and repair or replacement of intracellular proteins. The amount of oxygen used in these functions is relatively small and stable.

Each contraction of the heart involves movements of ions across the cell membranes. By removing calcium ion from the fluid bathing the heart cells, the heart can be excited without actively developing tension. The oxygen requirement electrical depolarization and repolarization is small (Klocke et al., 1966), accounted for by the cycling of pumps that maintain sodium and potassium ion concentrations.

In addition to these two fairly constant and low requirements for oxygen, factors related to activity and the state of the heart that determine how much oxygen the heart needs. These constitute the major determinants of myocardial oxygen consumption ($M\dot{V}O_2$) and include intramyocardial tension, heart rate, shortening, and contractile state.

Intramyocardial Tension

The *law of Laplace* is used to calculate intramyocardial tension. This law states

$$T \approx \frac{P \times R}{Th}$$

where T = intramyocardial wall tension, P = internal pressure within the ventricular cavity, R = radius of the ventricular cavity, Th = thickness of the ventricular wall, and $\approx$ signifies "proportional to." An increase in the afterload of the left ventricle causes the left ventricle to develop more pressure during the systolic period, thereby increasing intramyocardial tension and oxygen consumption. An increase in the preload or filling pressures of the left ventricle increases tension because both internal pressure and the radius of the ventricular cavity are increased and the thickness is decreased. Again, $M\dot{V}O_2$ is increased.

Heart Rate

Increased heart rate (at the same preload and afterload) increases the $M\dot{V}O_2$. Each beat represents the generation of tension by the myocardium.

Shortening

In an *isotonic twitch,* there is a component of the oxygen consumption that is proportional to the amount of shortening by a muscle. That is, there is a metabolic cost that is related to shortening. This is sometimes called the *Fenn effect* and is a characteristic of cardiac as well as of skeletal muscle. In cardiac muscle, a contraction with a large amount of shortening is one that expels a large stroke volume.

Contractile State

Contractility correlates with the amount of oxygen consumed by the heart. Positive inotropic factors increase the $M\dot{V}O_2$. Negative inotropic agents diminish $M\dot{V}O_2$.

Pressure Versus Volume Work

Work done by the heart is proportional to the pressure generated times the volume pumped (stroke work = [mean arterial pressure − left atrial pressure] × stroke volume). Pressure generated is a component of the intramyocardial tension as described by the Laplace relation and thus contributes to the overall $M\dot{V}O_2$. The size of the stroke volume is related to the amount of myocardial shortening, and thus it too contributes to the $M\dot{V}O_2$. Although equal amounts of work can be obtained by altering pressure or volume, the cost in terms of $M\dot{V}O_2$ is much greater for high-pressure work than for high-volume work. Thus, cardiac work is poorly correlated with $M\dot{V}O_2$.

Indices of Myocardial Oxygen Consumption

No single indicator of the oxygen requirements of the myocardium is available. Ideally, such an indicator would take into account all major determinants of the $M\dot{V}O_2$. The pressure—rate product and the tension—time index are two commonly used methods of estimation that have been validated (Robb et al., 1942). Each takes into account one of the major determinants of the $M\dot{V}O_2$, the heart rate. Another major determinant, tension, is also considered in these indices. What is actually measured, however, is pressure. For pressure to be an indicator of tension, the other factors in the Laplace equation, that is, radius of the ventricular cavity and thickness of the ventricular wall must be constant.

The pressure—rate product is calculated by multiplying the heart rate by either systolic or mean arterial pressure and dividing by 100.

The tension-time index more appropriately may be called the pressure-time index. It is calculated by multiplying the area under the left ventricular pressure curve by the heart rate.

Myocardial Oxygen Supply

Control of Coronary Blood Flow

Flow of blood in the coronary circulation is, as in all vascular beds, proportional to the perfusion pressure and inversely proportional to the resistance of the bed. Resistance in the coronary bed is altered by compression on it during systole and by metabolic, neural, and hormonal factors. Coronary artery disease can impose significant resistance.

The pressure difference that drives cardiac perfusion is the gradient between aortic pressure and the pressure in the right atrium, into which most of the coronary perfusion ultimately returns. The coronary circulation, however, is autoregulated. This means that changes in the perfusion pressure over a range of pressures (approximately 60 to 180 mm Hg) make little difference in the amount of blood flowing to the heart if the other factors influencing perfusion are held constant.

Because the heart develops its own perfusion pressure, a fall in aortic pressure can reduce coronary perfusion, which in turn may further decrease cardiac function and pressure development. A cycle of deterioration may result.

During systole, the tension in the myocardial wall is high. This compresses the coronary arteries and prevents perfusion. Thus, the heart has the unique property of receiving most of its blood flow during diastole (Fig. 1-42). Rapid heart rates decrease the time spent in diastole and may impinge on coronary perfusion.

Intramyocardial tension tends to be highest in the subendocardial regions of the left ventricle. Thus, $M\dot{V}O_2$ is probably highest in this region; yet systolic compression is also greatest here. This in part explains why this area has an increased incidence of infarction. In transmural infarctions (i.e., ones that

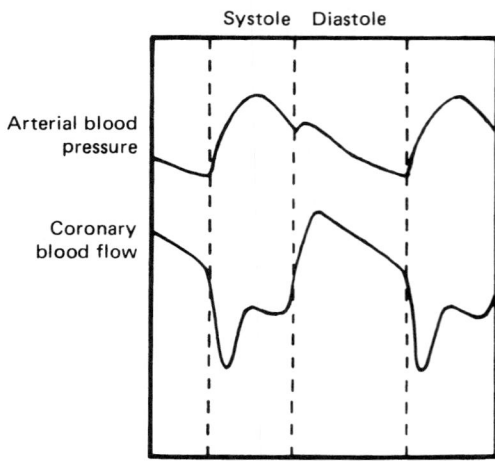

■ **Figure 1–42.** Effect of systolic compression on coronary blood flow. Note the decrease in flow during systole and the increase during diastole. (From Folkow, B., & Neil, E. [1971]. *Circulation* [p. 421]. Oxford: Oxford University Press.)

involve the full thickness of the left ventricular wall), the area of involvement is typically greater on the subendocardial surface than on the subepicardial surface (see Chapter 20??[1]). A factor that also contributes to this pattern of involvement in infarction is the pattern of coronary artery distribution. Because arteries enter the myocardium on the epicardial surface and plunge inward through the wall, the most easily compromised distal segments of the coronary arteries perfuse the endocardium.

The coronary arteries are innervated by α-sympathetic and parasympathetic fibers. The direct effects of neural outflow are the same in the coronary bed as in other systemic beds. α-Adrenergic stimulation (or norepinephrine) constricts arteries, and parasympathetic (vagal) stimulation dilates them. Pharmacologic doses of the β-adrenergic drug isoproterenol dilate the coronary artery bed. Often, however, the direct effect of neural outflow on the coronary bed is masked because the autonomic nervous system also affects myocardial metabolism and contractility, and the effect of these latter factors predominates.

Local metabolic conditions are the predominant determinants of coronary perfusion. Increased metabolism or hypoxia leads to vasodilation and increased myocardial blood flow. The mechanism that mediates this effect is unknown. One hypothesis suggests that adenosine is released from myocardial tissue in proportion to the amount of oxygen being consumed, and that perfusion correlates with the amount of adenosine released (Ahmed et al., 1972).

With atherosclerosis, significant resistance can develop in the coronary arteries. Lesions that occupy more than two thirds of the vessel's cross-sectional area may impinge significantly on flow at rest. Such lesions can prevent the increases in flow necessary when myocardial oxygen demand increases.

Collateral Circulation

Collateral arteries are interarterial vessels that can connect two branches of a single coronary artery or connect branches of the right coronary artery with branches of the left. In the human heart, collaterals are found through the full thickness of the myocardium, with the highest density near the endocardial surface. Although they are present at birth, collaterals do not become functionally significant unless the myocardium experiences hypoxic or ischemic insult. Before transformation, the collateral arteries are very narrow. They are devoid of smooth muscle and therefore are unable to respond to pharmacologic or metabolic vasoactive substances. After being stimulated to develop, the collateral tracts increase in diameter and develop a smooth muscle layer until; ultimately, the vessels are histologically similar to arterioles. When fully developed, these vessels are able to vasodilate when nitrates are administered and may autoregulate (Cohen, 1985). The time course from ischemic insult until significant enlargement is seen may be as short as 9 days (Siepser et al., 1972).

Three conditions are correlated with collateral development: coronary artery disease, chronic myocardial hypoxia, and myocardial hypertrophy. In coronary artery disease, the collateral diameter increases in proportion to the severity of coronary artery narrowing. Functionally significant increases in collateral structure are seen with a 75% or greater reduction in the luminal diameter of a major vessel. Chronic hypoxic myocardium is seen in patients with anemia, cyanotic heart disease, and chronic obstructive pulmonary disease (Zimmerman, 1952). There is also an increase in collateral diameter in hypertrophied hearts (Barmeyer, 1971). Attempts to stimulate development of collaterals with exercise programs have not been successful (Cohen, 1985). Collaterals frequently disappear after successful aortocoronary bypass grafting (Levin et al., 1981).

Blood flow through collateral vessels may contribute significantly to myocardial perfusion. Patients with similar coronary occlusions have smaller areas of infarction when collateral development has occurred. Patients with abundant and well-developed collaterals sometimes have a totally occluded coronary artery but no evidence of infarction. Blood flow through collateral vessels may be insufficient to meet increased demand, such as during exercise, and is insufficient to prevent necrosis in most cases.

Clinical Implications

It is important to analyze the effect of altered clinical states on the myocardial oxygen need. It is useful to consider the Laplace relation when evaluating oxygen demand in clinical states. For example, *hypertrophy of ventricular muscle* results in an increase in the thickness of the ventricular wall. This is advantageous in that wall tension is lower for the same left ventricular cavity size (same end-diastolic volume); hence, oxygen consumption is decreased. However, development of hypertrophy is a two-edged sword. At the same time that wall tension is decreased, the mass of tissue requiring oxygen is increased; the net result may well be a greater demand by the heart for oxygen. Furthermore, because hypertrophy tends to increase the size of the muscle cells without increasing the tissue capillarity, diffusional distances are increased. The supply of oxygen to the interior of the fiber may be significantly impaired.

With *cardiac dilation,* the radius of the left ventricle is increased. A larger end-diastolic volume is associated with higher end-diastolic pressure and increased pressure generation during systole, according to the Starling law. The Laplace relation predicts that both factors lead to increased intramyocardial wall tension. The stretching out of the heart wall is associated with decreased wall thickness, further increasing intramyocardial wall tension. The increase in oxygen demand can be significant.

THE CARDIAC CYCLE

Every ventricular contraction that propels blood to the body or the lungs is the result of the sequential activation of the cardiac chambers through the coordinated functioning of the electrical and mechanical factors. This section describes the changing cardiac pressures and volumes that coincide with the time sequence of cardiac events. An understanding of normal or abnormal cardiac functioning depends on familiarity with the cardiac cycle, which is represented graphically in Figure 1-43.

For the sake of simplicity, the description of events that occur during the cardiac cycle begins with events in the left

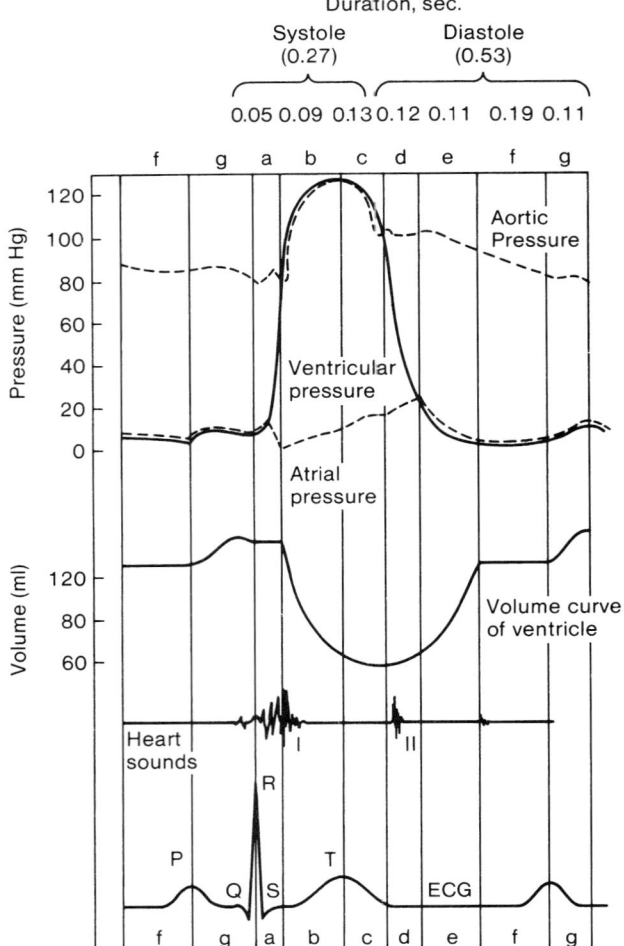

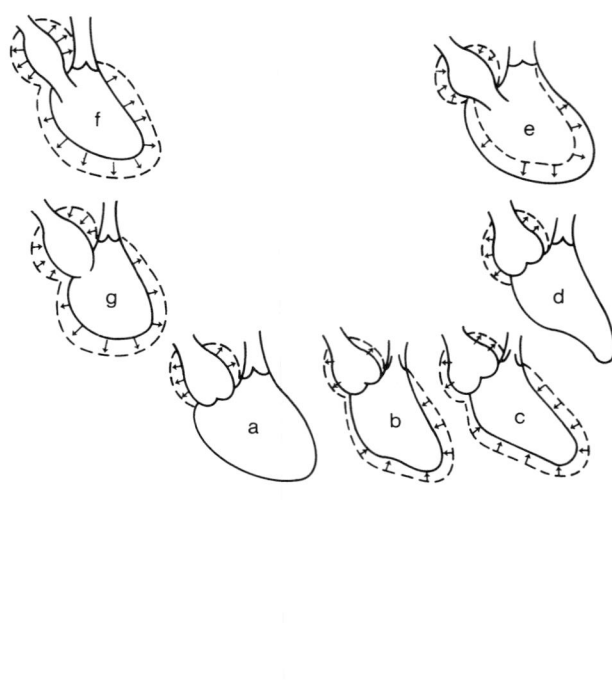

■ **Figure 1–43.** The cardiac cycle, illustrating the changes in aortic, left ventricular, and left atrial pressures, and in left ventricular volume, in relation to the phonocardiogram and the electrocardiogram. The duration of each phase at a heart rate of approximately 75 beats/min is indicated at the top of the figure. a, isovolumetric ventricular contraction; b, rapid ventricular ejection; c, slow ventricular ejection; d, protodiastole and isovolumetric relaxation; e, rapid ventricular filling; f, diastasis; g, atrial contraction; I, first heart sound; II, second heart sound. Insets: Changes in the configuration of the left atrium, mitral valve, left ventricle, and aortic valve during various phases of the cycle. (Adapted from Wiggens. [1952]. *Circulatory dynamics.* New York: Grune & Stratton.)

heart. Figure 1-43 should be referred to frequently to obtain an understanding of what is occurring concurrently with respect to electrical activity; atrial, ventricular, and aortic pressures; atrial and ventricular volumes; valvular activity; and heart sounds.

Some general points about pressures and timing should be remembered during the following discussion. Blood flows from a chamber with a greater pressure to a chamber with a lower pressure. When valves are open between two chambers, pressures in both chambers change until they are approximately equal. When valves between two chambers are closed, the pressures in the chambers change relatively independently of each other.

Ventricular systole and diastole divide the cardiac cycle into two major phases. The cardiac cycle can be further subdivided into several separate periods during systole and diastole. Because the cardiac cycle is continuous, the description of these periods can begin at any point.

Left Ventricular Cardiac Events

Ventricular Systole

Isovolumic Ventricular Contraction (Period a, Fig. 1-43). Ventricular contraction follows ventricular depolarization (reflected by the ECG QRS wave). Ventricular pressure increases rapidly. At the onset of this period, pressures in the atrium and ventricle are approximately equal, but atrial pressure decreases with atrial muscle relaxation. Closure of the mitral valve buffers the atria from the high ventricular pressures.

The mitral valve closes when the ventricle contracts. Pressure in the ventricle becomes higher than in the atrium. The aortic valve remains closed until left ventricular pressure becomes greater than aortic pressure. Bulging of the cardiac valves due to abrupt ventricular pressure increases may cause slight increases in atrial and aortic pressures recorded during this period.

During the brief time when both mitral and aortic valves are closed, there are no actual changes in ventricular volume because no blood is flowing into or out of the ventricle. The ventricle changes shape during this period. The apparent increase in ventricular volume recorded on the ventricular volume curve in Figure 1-43 occurs when ventricular volume is calculated from the ventricular circumference.

Besides being called the *isovolumic* or *isovolumetric period*, this time has been termed the *isometric phase* of ventricular contraction because tension is increasing rapidly, whereas the muscle fibers do not shorten much until they overcome the afterload of aortic pressure. Muscle contraction is not completely isometric, however, because the ventricles change dimensions.

Rapid Ventricular Ejection (Period b, Fig. 1-43). Ventricular muscle contraction continues, and the aortic valve opens as long as left ventricular pressure exceeds aortic pressure. The aorta and left ventricle are essentially a common cavity at this time. Ventricular pressure continues to rise rapidly during the initial part of this period, and then rises less rapidly during the latter part of the period to approximately the systolic pressure (120 mm Hg in the figure).

Ventricular volume decreases rapidly during ventricular ejection; two thirds or more of the stroke volume is ejected during this approximately 0.09-second period (Table 1-6). Aortic flow reaches peak velocity during the early part of the rapid ejection period before the point of maximal ventricular pressure. Aortic pressure may actually slightly exceed ventricular pressure during the latter period of rapid ventricular ejection, but blood continues to flow into the aorta because of the forward momentum of the blood. Much of the stroke volume is accommodated in the elastic proximal aorta.

The left atrium is relaxed at this time. Atrial pressure slowly begins to increase as blood from the lungs accumulates in the atrium. Ventricular repolarization begins.

Reduced Ventricular Ejection (Period c, Fig. 1-43). Ventricular and aortic pressures begin to decrease approximately 0.13 seconds before the end of ventricular contraction. During this time, ventricular muscle fibers are no longer contracting as forcefully as during the previous period. The fibers have reached a shorter length. Ventricular volume continues to fall, although at a slower rate than during rapid ejection, and blood continues to flow into the aorta. This period of reduced ventricular ejection comprises approximately the latter two thirds of the total ejection period (see Table 1-6).

Atrial pressure and volume continue to increase. Ventricular repolarization is usually complete by this time, as indicated by the end of the T wave.

Ventricular Diastole

Protodiastole (Initial Part of Period d, Fig. 1-43). As ventricular muscle relaxation begins, there is a brief period before ventricular pressure becomes lower than aortic pressure when no blood is being ejected from the ventricle. Blood flow momentarily reverses. This backflow at a time when ventricular pressure is becoming less than aortic pressure facilitates the closure of the aortic valve. The second heart sound occurs. During this time, a slight transient decrease in atrial pressure may occur, reflecting the effect of ventricular relaxation.

Table 1–6 ■ DURATION OF CARDIAC CYCLE PERIODS*

Cycle Phase	Duration (in seconds)
Isometric contraction	0.05
Maximal ejection	0.09
Reduced ejection	0.13
Total systole	0.27
Protodiastole	0.04
Isometric relaxation	0.08
Rapid inflow	0.11
Diastasis	0.19
Atrial systole	0.11
Total diastole	0.53

*Numbers shown are for heart rate of approximately 75 beats/min.
From Scher, A.M. (1974). Mechanical events of the cardiac cycle. In T.C. Ruch, H.D. Patton (Eds.), *Physiology and biophysics* (20th ed., Vol. II, pp. 102–116) Philadelphia: WB Saunders.

Isovolumic Ventricular Relaxation (Latter Part of Period d, Fig. 1-43). Ventricular pressure decreases rapidly as the ventricle relaxes. There is no change in ventricular volume during this period when all the cardiac valves are closed. After closure of the aortic valve, aortic pressure increases by a few millimeters of mercury, and the incisura or dicrotic notch is inscribed on the aortic pressure tracing. Atrial pressure continues to increase as the atrium continues to receive pulmonary venous blood.

Rapid Ventricular Filling (Period e, Fig. 1-43). The AV (mitral) valve opens when atrial pressure exceeds ventricular pressure. The ventricle fills rapidly with blood that has been accumulating in the atrium, but ventricular pressure continues to decrease during this period because ventricular relaxation continues. Most of the blood that was sequestered in the atrium during systole is emptied into the ventricle by the time the ventricle reaches maximal diastolic size. Atrial pressure decreases as the atria empty but remains slightly greater than ventricular pressure throughout this period.

Late Diastole (Diastasis; Period f, Fig. 1-43). The mitral valve remains open, and pressures in the atrium and ventricle equilibrate in the time after rapid ventricular filling and before the beginning of atrial contraction. Blood from the lungs continues to enter the left ventricle passively, so ventricular volume and pressure slowly increase. Coronary artery blood flow usually is maximal during late diastole. The beginning of atrial depolarization is indicated by the upstroke of the ECG P wave.

Atrial Contraction (Period g, Fig. 1-43). Atrial muscle contraction follows atrial depolarization and results in an increase in left atrial pressure. Ventricular volume and pressure are increased slightly as the atrium forces most of its remaining blood into the ventricles.

Between 15% and 25% of the end-diastolic ventricular volume consists of blood that has been ejected from the atrium during atrial contraction. The contribution of atrial contraction to total ventricular volume depends on venous return and heart rate; it is greater at faster heart rates. This atrial contribution to ventricular volume may be lost when the atria and ventricles are electrically and mechanically dissociated, such as during atrial fibrillation or complete heart block (see Chapter 19). Aortic pressure continues to decrease as blood in the aorta flows into the periphery.

Toward the end of this period, the ventricles begin to depolarize. Diastole ends with the onset of ventricular contraction. The cardiac cycle is repeated.

Right Ventricular Cardiac Cycle

The sequence of events in the right ventricle during the cardiac cycle is exactly the same as in the left ventricle, but the timing of events in the two ventricles is slightly different. Right ventricular and pulmonary artery pressures are much lower than left ventricular and aortic pressures and right atrial pressures are usually slightly less than left atrial pressures.

Several factors lead to differences in the timing of events between the right and left heart. Contraction of the left ventricle begins before contraction of the right ventricle. Left ventricular isovolumetric contraction and relaxation last longer than right ventricular isovolumetric contraction and relaxation, presumably because the left ventricle must develop more contractile force to overcome higher systemic pressures. Right ventricular ejection begins before, lasts longer than, and ends after left ventricular ejection, possibly because pressures in the pulmonary artery are lower than in the aorta. Thus, right ventricular filling and ejection periods are longer than left ventricular periods, but the durations of left and right ventricular electromechanical systole are almost equal.

Cardiac Valvular Events and Normal Heart Sounds

Valvular Events

The differences in timing of right and left ventricular events lead to differences in timing of right and left valvular events. The AV valves close at the onset of ventricular systole. The mitral valve normally closes before the tricuspid valve because left ventricular contraction begins before right ventricular contraction.

The aortic and pulmonic valves open when ventricular pressures exceed arterial pressures. The pulmonic valve opens before the aortic valve. Right ventricular isovolumetric contraction is shorter than left ventricular isovolumetric contraction.

The aortic and pulmonic valves close when ventricular pressures fall below arterial pressures. The aortic valve closes before the pulmonic valve. The right ventricular ejection period is longer than the left.

The AV valves open during diastole when ventricular pressures are lower than atrial pressures. The tricuspid valve opens before the mitral valve because of the more rapid isovolumetric right ventricular relaxation.

Normal Heart Sounds

The specific mechanisms responsible for heart sounds continue to be disputed. Sudden accelerations and decelerations of blood, turbulent blood flow, and the movements of valves, heart walls, and blood vessels may all contribute to the production of vibrations and sounds audible at the body surface.

First Heart Sound. Closure of the mitral valve and oscillations in the movement of blood in the ventricles are associated with vibrations of the entire valvular apparatus and of atrial and ventricular walls. This creates the early components of the first heart sound. Later components of the first heart sound may be due to the acceleration of blood ejected into the aorta.

Second Heart Sound. The second heart sound actually begins before semilunar valve closure. The mechanisms responsible for the second heart sound include arterial blood flow decelerations caused by ventricular relaxation, blood vessel wall vibrations, and semilunar valvular vibrations.

The closure of the pulmonic valve after the aortic valve leads to a two-component sound, which is accentuated during inspiration (see Chapter 13). During inspiration, the time between closure of the aortic and pulmonic valves is increased, probably because a decrease in pulmonary vascular impedance leads to a longer right ventricular ejection time.

Clinical Applications of Cardiac Events

Systolic Events

The stroke volume is the volume ejected by the ventricle in a single contraction. Stroke volume multiplied by the number of cardiac cycles per minute (heart rate) equals the cardiac output. A typical volume ejected by the ventricle is 60 to 130 mL/m^2 body surface area (BSA)/second, illustrated by the ventricular volume downstroke of Figure 1-43. The stroke volume is the difference between the ventricular end-diastolic and end-systolic volume. The stroke volume is approximately 24 to 36 mL/beat per meters squared.

The *ejection fraction* is the percentage of total ventricular volume ejected during each contraction (i.e., the stroke volume divided by end-diastolic volume). The ejection fraction is a frequently used index of ventricular function; normally, it is greater than 55% and usually is approximately 65%.

The maximal rate of left ventricular force development and rise of left ventricular pressure over time (peak *dP/dt*) occurs during isovolumic ventricular contraction. Peak *dP/dt* is sometimes used as a clinical measure of ventricular contractility.

Specific phases of the left ventricular systolic time intervals, such as the pre-ejection period, left ventricular ejection time, total electromechanical systole (Q-S), and the preejection period, left ventricular ejection time ratio are derived from simultaneous noninvasive ECG, phonocardiogram, and carotid artery pulse tracing recordings. The value of systolic time interval measurements in the diagnosis and prognosis of ventricular dysfunction due to ischemic heart disease continues to be debated (Ahmed et al., 1972; Mangschau et al., 1984). The tension—time index is also used to assess ventricular function. These intervals vary with heart rate.

Diastolic Events

Diastole comprises a greater portion of the cardiac cycle (approximately 65%) than does systole (approximately 35%) at normal heart rates (see Table 1-6). At faster heart rates, both systole and diastole are shortened, diastole proportionally more so than systole. For example, at a heart rate of 180 beats/min, diastole comprises approximately 40% and systole approximately 60% of the cardiac cycle. At fast heart rates, diastolic filling is increasingly important in terms of the decreased amount of time available for ventricular and coronary artery filling, which may lead to impaired myocardial functioning.

The jugular venous and the carotid arterial pulses normally reflect right and left heart events, respectively. All cardiovascular assessment and treatment plans intimately depend on an appreciation of the cardiac cycle.

REFERENCES

Ahmed, S., Levinson, G., Schwart, C., & Ettinger, P. (1972). Systolic time intervals as measures of the contractile state of the left ventricular myocardium in man. *Circulation, 46*(3), 559–571.

Anderson, R., Becker, A., Brechenmacher, C., Davies, M., & Rossi, L. (1975a). The human atrioventricular junctional area. A morphological study of the A-V node and bundle. *European Journal of Cardiology, 3*(1), 11–25.

Anderson, R., Becker, A., Brechenmacher, C., Davies, M., & Rossi, L. (1975b). Ventricular preexcitation: A proposed nomenclature for its substrates. *European Journal of Cardiology, 3*(1), 27–36.

Armour, J., & Hopkins, D. (1984). Anatomy of the efferent autonomic nerves and ganglia innervating the heart. In W. Randall (Ed.), *Nervous control of cardiovascular function* (pp. 20–45). New York: Oxford University Press.

Bachman, G. (1916). The inter-auricular time interval. *American Journal of Physiology, 41*, 309–320.

Barmeyer, J. (1971). Postmortem measurement of intracoronary anastomotic flow in normal and diseased heart. A quantitative study. *Vascular Surgery, 5*, 239–248.

Cohen, M. (1985). *Coronary collaterals: Clinical and experimental observation.* Mt. Kisco, New York: Futura.

De Mello, N. (1990). Effect of isoproterenol and 3-isobutyl-1-methylxanthine on junctional conductance in heart cell pairs. *Biochim Biophys Acta, 1012*(3), 291–298.

DiFrancesco, D. (1981). A new interpretation of the pacemaker current in calf Purkinje fibres. *Journal of Physiology (London), 314*, 359–376.

Donaldson, S., Bond, E., & Seeger, L. (1981). Intracellular pH vs MgATP^{+2} concentration as determinants of Ca^{+2} activated force generation of disrupted rabbit cardiac cells. *Cardiovascular Research, 15*, 268–275.

Durrer, D., van Dama, R., Freud, G., Janse, M., Meijler, F., & Arzbaecher, R. (1970). Total excitation of the isolated human heart. *Circulation, 41*(6), 899–912.

Fabiato, A. (1983). Calcium-induced release of calcium from the cardiac sarcoplasmic reticulum. *American Journal of Physiology, 245*, C1–C14.

Fawcett, D. (1986). *A textbook of histology* (11th ed.). Philadelphia: W.B. Saunders.

Franzini-Armstrong, C. (1970). Studies of the triad: Structure of the junction in frog twitch fibers. *Journal of Cell Biology, 47*, 488–499.

Glynn, I. (1993). Annual review prize lecture: All hands to the sodium pump. *Journal of Physiology (Lond), 462*, 1–30.

Gordon, A., Huxley, A., & Julian, F. (1966). The variation of isometric tension with sarcomere length in vertebrate muscle fibres. *Journal of Physiology (Lond), 184*, 170–192.

Hecht, H., Kossmann, C., Childers, R., Langendorf, R., Lev, M., Rosen, K., et al. (1973). Atrioventricular and intraventricular conduction: revised nomenclature and concepts. *American Journal of Cardiology, 31*(2), 232–244.

His, W.J. (1893). Die Thatigkeit des embryonalen Herzens unde deren Bedeutung fur die Lehre von der Herzbewegun beim Erwachsenen. *Arbeiten aus der Med Klin zu Leipzig, 1*, 14–50.

Hodgkin, A., & Huxley, A. (1952). Currents carried by sodium and potassium ions through the membrane of the giant axon of *Logilo. Journal of Physiology (London), 116*, 449–472.

Hood, W.J., Bianco, J., Kumar, R., & Whiting, R. (1970). Experimental myocardial infarction. IV. Reduction of left ventricular compliance in the healing phase. *Journal of Clinical Investigation, 49*, 1316–1323.

Hudson, R. (1967). Surgical pathology of the conducting system of the heart. *British Heart Journal, 29*, 646–670.

Hunter, D., Haworth, R., & Berkoff, H. (1982). Cellular calcium turnover in perfused rat heart. *Circulation Research, 51*, 363–370.

Irisawa, H., & Noma, A. (1984). Pacemaker currents in mammalian nodal cells. *Journal of Molecular and Cellular Cardiology, 16*, 777–781.

James, T. (1961). *Anatomy of the Coronary Arteries.* New York: Paul B Hoeber.

James, T. (1963). The connecting pathways between the sinus node and AV node and between the right and left atrium in the human heart. *American Heart Journal, 66*, 498–508.

Keith, A., & Flack, M. (1907). The form and nature of the muscular connections between the primary divisions of the vertebrate heart. *Journal of Anatomy and Physiology, 41*, 172–189.

Kelly, A., & Gensini, G. (1975). Coronary arteriography and left heart studies. *Heart and Lung, 4*, 85–98.

Kent, A. (1893). Researches on the structure and function of the mammalian heart. *Journal of Physiology (Lond), 14*, 233–254.

Kent, A. (1914). The right lateral auriculo-ventricular junction of the heart. *Journal of Physiology (Lond), 48*, 22–24.

Klocke, F., Braunwald, E., & Ross, J.J. (1966). Oxygen cost of electrical activation of the heart. *Circulation Research, 18*, 357–365.

Langer, G. (1982). Sodium-calcium exchange in the heart. *Annual Review of Physiology, 44*, 435–449.

Lazzara, R., el-Sherif, N., Befeler, F., & Scherlag, B. (1976). Regional refractoriness within the ventricular conduction system. An evaluation of the "gate" hypothesis. *Circulation Research, 39*(2), 254–262.

Levin, D., Beckmann, C., Sos, T., & Sniderman, K. (1981). The effect of coronary artery bypass on collateral circulation. *Radiology, 141*(2), 317–322.

Lewis, B., & Gotsman, M. (1980). Current concepts of left ventricular relaxation and compliance. *American Heart Journal, 99*, 101–112.

Mahaim, I. (1947). Kent's fibers and the A-V paraspecific conduciton through the upper connections of the bundle of His-Tarawa. *American Heart Journal, 33*, 651–653.

Mahaim, I., & Winston, T. (1941). Recherches d'anotomie comparee et de pathologie experimentale sur les connexions hautes du faisceau de His-Tarawa. *Cardiologia, 5*, 189–260.

Mangschau, A., Karlsen, R., Lippestad, C., & Nerdrum, H. (1984). Systolic time intervals and ejection fraction in assessing left ventricular performance following acute myocardial infarction. *Acta Medica Scandinavica, 215*(4), 341–347.

Massing, G., & James, T. (1976). Anatomical configuration of the His bundle and bundle branches in the human heart. *Circulation, 53*, 609–621.

Maylie, J., & Morad, M. (1984). Ionic currents responsible for the generation of pacemaker current in the rabbit sino-atrial node. *Journal of Physiology, 363*, 463–480.

Milhaud, D., Bogousslavsky, J., van Melle, G., & Liot, P. (2001). Ischemic stroke and active migraine. *Neurology, 57*(10), 1805–1811.

Miller, A. (1982). *Lymphatics of the heart.* New York: Raven Press.

Nichols, C., Ripoli, C., & Ledere, W. (1991). ATP-sensitive potassium channel modulation of the guinea pig ventricular action potential and contraction. *Circulation Research, 68*, 280–287.

Noma, A., & Shibasaki, T. (1985). Membrane current through adenosinetriphosphate-regulated potassium channels in guinea pig ventricular cells. *Journal of Physiology (London), 363*, 463–480.

Overell, J., Bone, I., & Lees, K. (2000). Interatrial septal abnormalities and stroke: a meta-analysis of case-control studies. *Neurology, 55*, 1172–1179.

Paes de Carvalho, A., & de Almeida, D. (1960). Spread activity through atrioventricular node. *Circulation Research, 8*, 801–809.

Patterson, S., Per, H., & Starling, E. (1914). The regulation of the heart beat. *Journal of Physiology (Lond), 48*, 465–513.

Purkinje, J. (1845). Mikroskopisch-neurologische beobachtungen. *Arch Anat Physiol Wiss Med, 12*, 281.

Randall, W. (1984). Selective autonomic innervation of the heart. In W. Randall (Ed.), *Nervous control of cardiovascular function* (pp. 46–67). New York: Oxford University Press.

Regan, T., Frank, M., Lehan, P., Galante, J., & Hellems, H. (1963). Myocardial blood flow and oxygen uptake during acute red cell volume increments. *Circulation Research, 13*, 172–181.

Reiner, L., Massolene, A., Rodriguez, F., & Freudenthal, R. (1959). The weight of the human heart. I. Normal cases. *Archives of Pathology, 68*(1), 58–73.

Ringer, S. (1883). A further contribution regarding the influence of the different constituents of the blood on the contraction of the heart. *Journal of Physiology (Lond), 4*, 29–42.

Robb, J., Robb, J., & Robb, R. (1942). The normal heart. *Heart Journal, 23*, 455–467.

Scher, A., & Spach, M. (1979). Cardiac depolarization and repolarization and the electrocardiogram. In R. Berne (Ed.), *Handbook of physiology. Section 2. The cardiovascular system, vol. 1, the heart* (pp. 357-392). Bethesda, MD: American Physiological Society.

Siepser, S., Kaltman, A., Mills, N., Pughkem, T., & Fox, A. (1972). Coronary collateral flow after traumatic fistula between right coronary artery and right atrium. *New England Journal Medicine,* 287(15), 754–756.

Singer, D., Baumgarten, C., & Ten Eick, R. (1981). Cellular electrophysiology of ventricular and other dysrhythmias. Studies on diseased and ischemic heart. *Progress in Cardiovascular Disease,* 24, 97–156.

Smith, H., & Smith, H. (1928). The relation of the weight of the heart to the weight of the body and the weight of the heart to age. *American Heart Journal,* 4, 79–93.

Spach, M., & Barr, R. (1976). Cardiac anatomy from an electrophysiological viewpoint. In C. Nelson, & D. Geselvitz (Eds.), *The theoretical basis of electrocardiology* (pp. 3–20). Oxford: Clarendon, Press.

Spach, M., & Lootsey, J. (1983). The nature of electrical propagation in cardiac muscle. *American Journal of Physiology,* 244, H3–H22.

Sperelakis, N. (1979). Propagation mechanisms of the heart. *Annual Review of Physiology,* 41, 441–457.

Sperelakis, N. (1984). Hormonal and neurotransmitter regulation of Ca^{2+} influx through voltage-dependent slow channels in cardiac muscle cell membrane. *Membrane Biochemistry,* 5, 131–166.

Streeter, D.J., Spotnitz, H., Patel, D., Ross, J.J., & Sonnenblick, E. (1969). Fiber orientation in the canine left ventricle during systole and diastole. *Circulation Research,* 24(3), 339–347.

Tarawa, S. (1906). *Das Reisleitungs system des Saugetierherzens [Monograph].* Jena, Germany: G. Fischer.

Titus, J., Daugherty, G., & Edwards, J. (1963). Anatomy of the normal human atrioventricular junctional area: A morphological study of the AV node and bundle. *American Journal of Anatomy,* 113, 407–415.

Ungerleider, H., & Clark, C. (1939). A study of the transverse diameter of the heart silhouette with prediction based on the teleoroentgenogram. *American Heart Journal,* 17, 92–102.

Wearn, J. (1940). Morphological and functional alterations of the coronary circulation. *Harvey Lectures,* 35, 243–270.

Weidmann, S. (1982). Cardiac cellular physiology and its contribution to electrocardiography. *Japanese Heart Journal,* 23 (Suppl), 12–16.

Windecker, S., & Meier, B. (2002). Patent foramen ovale and atrial septal aneurysm: when and how should they be treated. *American College of Cardiolgy Current Journal Review,* 11, 97–101.

Zimmerman, H. (1952). The coronary circulation in patients with severe emphysema, cor pulmonale, cyanotic congenital heart disease, and severe anemia. *Diseases of the Chest,* 22, 269–273.

2

Systemic Circulation

ELIZABETH J. BRIDGES*

The structural and functional characteristics of the systemic circulation determine the continuous adjustments in flow, pressure, and resistance that occur in each vascular bed and that are vital determinants of tissue function. Blood flow and nutrient exchange in various vascular beds are affected by the structural and metabolic characteristics of the vascular bed, the physical factors that affect flow and the exchange of materials across the blood vessel wall, the local factors originating from the metabolically active cells and vascular endothelium that regulate flow to individual vascular beds, and local and systemic neuroendocrine regulation. The combined regulation of cardiac output, blood pressure, and systemic vascular resistance (SVR) determines tissue blood flow and, ultimately, the survival of each organ system and the body as a whole. This chapter describes the basic anatomy and physiology of the systemic circulation; Chapter 4 describes the overall regulation of cardiac output and blood pressure.

STRUCTURAL CHARACTERISTICS OF THE VASCULATURE AND LYMPHATICS

Blood vessels are usually classified in the following manner: aorta, large arteries; main arterial branch, small arteries, arterioles; terminal arterioles, capillaries, postcapillary venules; venules, small veins, main venule branch, large veins, and the vena cava (Rhodin, 1980; Rothe, 1983; Wiedeman, 1963). These classifications are based on structural characteristics such as diameter, wall thickness, and the presence of muscle (Fig. 2-1). Although vessel sizes are given in Figure 2-1, blood vessel diameter is not an appropriate criterion to use for classification, because differences in vessel size reflect the state of vessel contraction as well as differences between organ systems and species (Rhodin, 1980, 1981).

The views expressed in this chapter are those of the author and do not reflect the official policy of the Department of Defense or other departments of the United States Government.

*The author wishes to acknowledge Dr. B. Zane Atkins, Major USAF MC for his review of this chapter.

With the exception of the capillaries, the systemic vasculature is composed of three layers: the tunica intima or internal layer, which consists of the endothelium and the basal membrane; the tunica media, which consists of smooth muscle and a matrix of collagen, elastin, and glycoproteins; and the tunica adventitia, which consists of connective tissue (Ross & Glomset, 1976) (Fig. 2-2). In the larger arteries and veins, the tunica adventitia also contains blood vessels that supply the vessel wall (vasa vasorum) (Opie, 1998; Rhodin, 1980). The vascular endothelium has gained importance as a primary mediator of vascular function and is discussed in detail.

Arteries

Arteries with large diameters, in which the media contains smooth muscle and elastin, are called *elastic arteries* (Rhodin, 1980). Because of the considerable amount of elastin, these large conducting arteries are able to distend to twice their unloaded length. The ability of the capacitive arteries to distend is important in cushioning pulsatile flow, such that the blood flow to the organs/tissue is almost a constant flow. During systole, the aorta and proximal large vessels store approximately 50% to 60% of the stroke volume. During diastole, the distended vessels recoil and move the remaining blood to the periphery. This phenomenon is referred to as a "Windkessel function," which is the transformation of pulsatile flow in the central arteries to constant flow in the periphery (Belz, 1995; London & Guerin, 1999). As the arteries approach the periphery, they become smaller in diameter, and there is a relative decrease in elastin and a relative increase in smooth muscle in the tunica media (Mulvany, 1996; Mulvany & Aalkjær, 1990). These peripheral arteries are referred to as *muscular arteries*.

The small arteries (prearteriolar vessels with a diameter less than 500 mm) receive nervous stimulation primarily from noradrenergic stimuli, with the nerve terminals located in the adventitia. Unlike the larger arteries, in which sympathetic neural constriction is activated by α_1 and postsynaptic α_2 receptors, the small arteries are noradrenergically constricted mainly by the postsynaptic α_2 receptors (Faber, 1988; Mulvany, 1996; Mulvany & Aalkjær, 1990). The small arteries are also

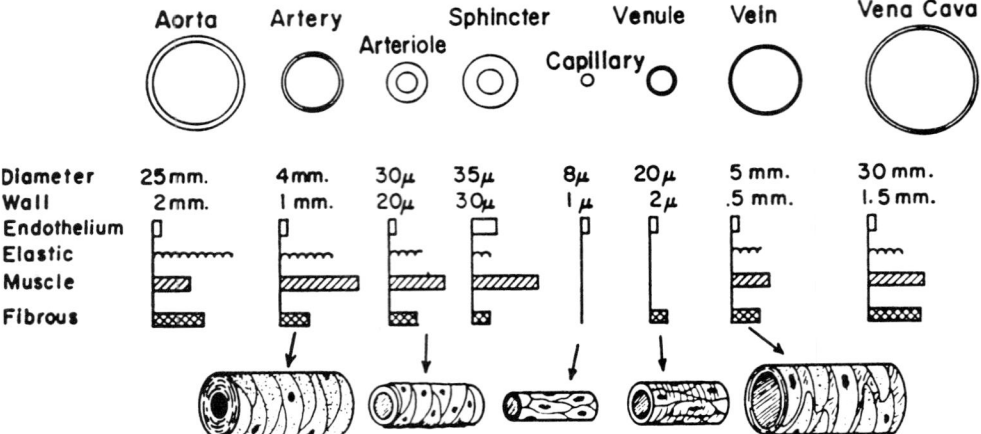

■ Figure 2–1. Schematic drawing of the major structural characteristics of the principal segments of blood vessels. The relative amounts of elastic tissue and fibrous tissues are largest in the aorta and least in small branches of the arterial tree. Small vessels have more prominent smooth muscle in the media. Capillaries consist only of endothelial cells. The walls of the veins are much like the arterial walls, but are thinner in relation to their caliber. (Rushmer, R.F. [1976]. *Cardiovascular dynamics* [4th ed., p. 135]. Philadelphia: WB Saunders.)

sensitive to endothelium-derived relaxing and contracting factors, which are described later.

Microvascular Bed

The term *microcirculation* denotes the vascular and lymphatic microcirculation. The vascular microcirculation consists of: (1) large and small arterioles (*precapillary resistance vessels*); (2) terminal arterioles, which in many tissues serve as so-called precapillary sphincters; and (3) other precapillary structures such as capillaries; and (4) nonmuscular venules, known collectively as the exchange vessels, and muscular venules (postcapillary resistance vessels). The term *lymphatic microvasculature* refers specifically to the terminal lymphatic vessels (Renkin, 1984; Rhodin, 1981).

Arterioles

As the vessel diameter decreases from the small arteries to the arterioles, the number of smooth muscle layers decreases from approximately six layers in the 300-μm vessels to a single layer of irregularly dispersed smooth muscle in the 30- to 50-μm vessels (Mulvany & Aalkjeær, 1990). At this point, the vessels are referred to as *arterioles*. The smallest arteriolar branches (8 to 20 μm in diameter) are called the *terminal arterioles* (Renkin, 1989). In some cases, smooth muscle extends beyond the intersection of the terminal arterioles with the nonmuscular capillaries into structures known as *precapillary sphincters* (Renkin, 1984). The terminal arterioles and precapillary sphincters control the distribution of blood supply to the exchange vessels (Berg & Sarelius, 1995; Sarelius et al., 2000).

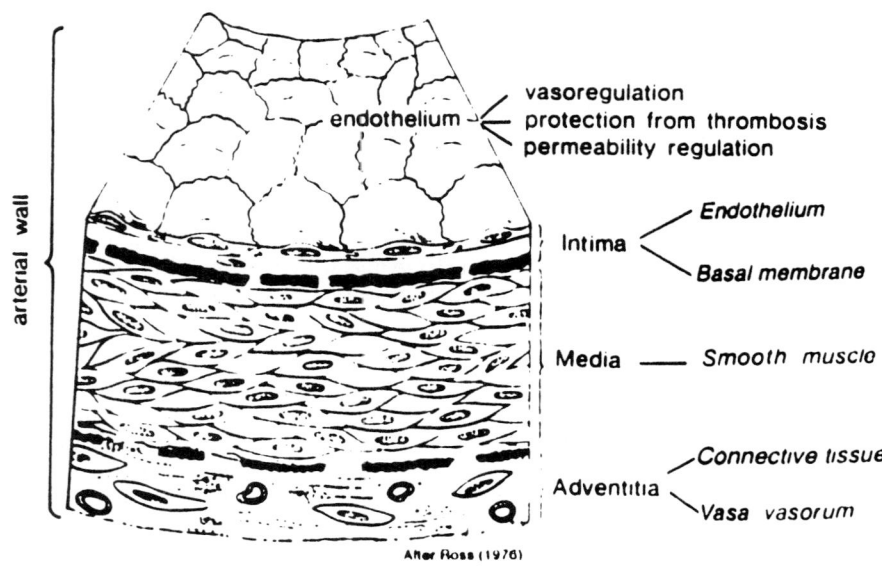

■ Figure 2–2. Histologic structure of the normal muscular artery demonstrating the different roles of the endothelium, smooth muscle, and fibrous tissue. (Adapted from Ross, R. M., & Glomset, J. [1998]. The pathogenesis of atherosclerosis. *New England Journal of Medicine, 295,* 369–377. In Opie, L. H. [1998]. *The heart: Physiology from cell to circulation,* p. 234. Philadelphia: Lippincott-Raven.)

Capillaries

Capillaries branch from terminal arteriolar segments. The capillary wall consists of endothelial cells and basal lamina; there is no tunica media or adventitia. Capillary diameter is 4 to 8 mm, which is just large enough to allow the deformable red blood cells to pass through (Renkin, 1984; Simionescu & Simionescu, 1984). Not all exchange vessels in an area are simultaneously open. During periods of increased metabolism, capillary recruitment increases the number of open and perfused exchange vessels, thereby decreasing the distances for diffusion between exchange blood vessels and cells, as well as increasing the total surface area for exchange between the capillaries and cells (Renkin, 1989).

In microvascular beds located in the ears, fingers, and toes in humans and many other mammals, there are arteriovenous vascular channels that bypass the exchange vessels and allow blood to flow directly from arterioles to venules (Renkin, 1989; Rhodin, 1980). These arteriovenous anastomoses, which are richly innervated by the sympathetic nervous system, are important in local temperature control in these areas and even of the whole body in some conditions (Charkoudian, 2003; Johnson, 1989).

Exchange Vessel Endothelium

The endothelium of exchange vessels in various organs contains at least four different structures that determine the rate of filtration and bulk transport of water and solutes and the exchange of larger molecules. The structure of the membrane (continuous, fenestrated, discontinuous, or tight junction) varies depending on the location of the vascular bed (Renkin, 1977, 1989; Simionescu & Simionescu, 1984). All four types of endothelium have a continuous basement membrane, with the exception of the discontinuous endothelium.

Continuous endothelium is found in skin; skeletal, smooth, and cardiac muscle; and the lungs. There are several mechanisms by which substances pass through continuous endothelium. Water and solutes pass through intercellular junctions (40Å to 1Å) driven predominantly by a pressure gradient (ΔP) driving fluid out of the vessels. This outward flow is partly counterbalanced by forces drawing water back into the vessels. Lipid-soluble substances (CO_2, O_2) pass directly through the cell by diffusion; cytoplasmic vesicles transport solutes and water back and forth through the endothelium; and vesicles intermittently fuse to create channels in the cell. The junctions between the cells are responsible for the high permeability of the membrane to "ultrafiltrate," or protein-free fluid, and for the rapid diffusion of small ions. The continuous endothelium is relatively impermeable to plasma proteins and large molecules.

Fenestrated vascular endothelium is located in the gastrointestinal mucosa, glands, renal glomerular capillaries, and peritubular capillaries. The endothelium has openings (fenestrae) that expose the basement membrane (renal glomerular capillaries) or are covered by a thin diaphragm (gastrointestinal mucosa, renal peritubular capillaries). The fenestrated endothelium has a higher permeability to water and small solute molecules than continuous endothelium, whereas its permeability to plasma proteins is low, similar to continuous endothelium (Renkin, 1989).

Discontinuous endothelium is located in the hepatic cells, bone marrow, and splenic sinusoids. Discontinuous endothelium contains gaps in the endothelium and basement membrane and is permeable to proteins and other large molecules.

Tight-junction endothelium is located in the central nervous system and retina. It is the least permeable. The endothelial cells are connected by tight junctions that effectively restrict passage of all substances. Water- and lipid-soluble molecules pass directly through the endothelium, whereas ions and lipid-insoluble substances, such as glucose and amino acids, are transported by membrane carriers (Wolburg & Lippoldt, 2002).

Venules

Venous capillaries extend to the postcapillary venules (nonmuscular, 7 to 50 μm) and collecting venules. Along with the capillaries, the nonmuscular venules act as exchange vessels. Smooth muscle reappears in venules that are approximately 30 to 50 μm in diameter. These venules, which receive adrenergic innervation, are referred to as the muscular venules, postcapillary resistance vessels, or capacitance vessels (Renkin, 1984, 1989; Rhodin, 1980; Rothe, 1983; Simionescu & Simionescu, 1984). As discussed later in the section on microcirculation, postcapillary resistance tends to be far less than precapillary resistance and has almost no effect on overall systemic vascular resistance. The veins contain approximately 70% of total blood volume, with approximately 25% of this volume in the venules (Rothe, 1983).

Veins

In general, veins have a larger diameter and thinner, more compliant walls than arteries at equivalent branches of the vascular tree (Rothe, 1983) (see Fig. 2-1). However, the thickness of the venous walls is variable, and in tall animals like humans and giraffes, the thickness depends on the location of the vein in the body. For example, the veins in the legs and feet, which withstand the high hydrostatic pressure associated with standing, are thick-walled, whereas the veins near or above the level of the heart are thin-walled (Conrad, 1971; Rowell, 1986). The veins contain all three vascular layers found in the arteries; however, these layers are often indistinct (Rhodin, 1980). Superficial veins form a rich anastomosis with deeper veins via vessels that perforate the muscles. These perforating veins allow venous return from cold skin to be diverted to warm muscle, providing a thermal short circuit, and they are particularly important for function of the muscle pump, which is described in Chapter 4.

Venous Valves

With the exception of the intrathoracic and intracerebral veins, the medium-sized veins contain valves that are oriented in the direction of blood flow, thus preventing retrograde blood flow into the muscle (Rothe, 1983). The presence of competent valves, in conjunction with the muscle pump in the lower extremities, is crucial to the ability to stand erect and in maintaining a reasonably low capillary pressure, because the valves interrupt the hydrostatic column that extends from the right atrium to the feet after each leg muscle contraction (Raju et al., 1993). After humans with normal valvular function stand up, the valves in dependent veins initially interrupt the hydrostatic column. However, over a period of approximately 2 to 3 minutes, as the veins fill with blood, the valves can no longer interrupt the hydrostatic column as volume continues to accumulate. At this time, there is a displacement of approximately 600 mL of blood from the central circulation into the legs and pelvic organs (Rowell, 1993). In conditions in which blood flow is high, the hydrostatic effects associated with the loss of valvular function occur within 2 to 3 seconds. If the hydrostatic effects are not overcome by the muscle pump in the lower extremities, then arterial hypotension and syncope result. This phenomenon is readily seen in the soldier who faints while standing motionless at attention.

Venoconstriction

In contrast to the arteries, not all veins constrict when exposed to norepinephrine. For example, the postcapillary venules ranging from 0.007 to 2 mm in diameter do not have smooth muscle and therefore cannot constrict (Rowell, 1986). Most larger venules and small veins (including veins in the skeletal muscle) contain some smooth muscle (Rothe, 1983), but they are sparsely innervated and are not considered sites of vasoconstriction. The lack of venoconstriction in the skeletal muscle is important because the leg veins do not constrict in orthostasis. The splanchnic organs (liver, gastrointestinal tract, pancreas, and spleen) are the exception because they are richly innervated by sympathetic noradrenergic fibers and are capable

of venoconstriction. In addition, the veins in the skin respond to thermoregulatory reflexes. In humans, significant venoconstriction occurs only in the splanchnic circulation; in response to thermoregulatory reflexes, the veins in the skin constrict and dilate (Hainsworth, 1986; Rowell, 1986; Rowell et al., 1996).

Lymphatics

The lymphatics are a system of thin-walled vessels that collect and conduct lymph from the microvasculature to the central circulation. Lymph consists primarily of ultrafiltrate and proteins that have been filtered from exchange vessels. The initial lymphatic vessels (also known as terminal lymphatics or lymph capillaries), which consist of endothelialized tubes, originate in large, blind-terminal bulbs located in the connective tissue of most organ systems (Renkin, 1989; Schmid-Schonbein, 1990). The lymphatic capillaries empty into collecting lymphatics, which in turn empty into transporting lymphatic vessels (Fig. 2-3). The central lymphatic vessels empty into the left and right lymphatic ducts, which empty into the subclavian veins.

A very small and transient pressure gradient between the interstitium and the terminal lymphatics promotes fluid movement into the lymphatics (Aukland & Reed, 1993; Schmid-Schonbein, 1990). Beginning at the level of the collecting capillaries, there are bicuspid valves, and the larger lymphatics contain smooth muscle that spontaneously contracts in a rhythmic manner (Trzewik et al., 2001; Van Helden & Zhao, 2000). The primary mechanism underlying lymphatic flow is the intrinsic contraction of the lymphangions, which are the functional unit of lymphatic vessels, consisting of the valve and

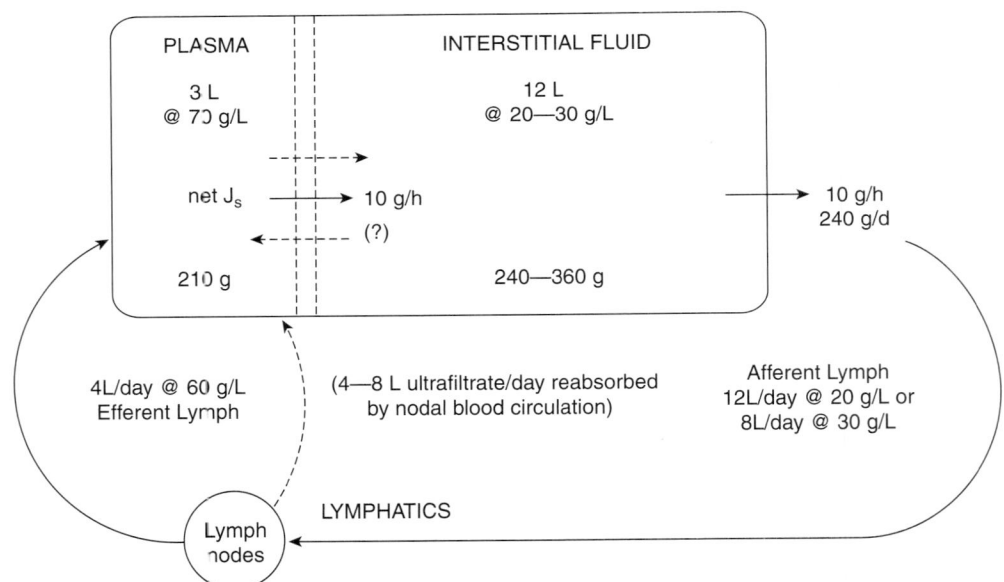

■ **Figure 2–3.** Steady-state distribution and circulation of fluid (ultrafiltrate) and plasma proteins in a normal human (weight, 65 kg). The double dashed line between plasma and interstitial fluid represents exchange vessel endothelium. The weights at the bottoms of the boxes represent the total content of each. (Renkin, E. M. [1986]. Some consequences of capillary permeability to macromolecules: Starling's hypothesis reconsidered. *American Journal of Physiology, 250,* H706–H710.)

portion of the vessel surrounding the valve. The intrinsic contraction remains active during rest, anesthesia, and immobilization (Olszewski, 2002). Lymphatic flow is also facilitated by lymph formation, skeletal muscle contractions (e.g., walking, foot flexing), respiration, fluctuations of central venous pressure, gastrointestinal peristalsis, and arterial pulsations (Gashev, 2002).

Vascular Smooth Muscle

Vascular smooth muscle contains the contractile filaments, actin and myosin; however, unlike striated smooth muscle (cardiac), the filaments are not organized in any fashion (Small & Gimona, 1998). Although the sarcoplasmic reticulum is not as prominent in vascular smooth muscle as in cardiac muscle, it serves as the primary intracellular source of calcium (Somlyo & Somlyo, 2002). Additionally, the amount of myosin in smooth muscle is approximately one-fifth that found in striated muscle. Despite this lower amount of myosin, smooth muscle develops higher force per cross-sectional area than striated muscle. Vascular smooth muscle also usually contracts more slowly than striated muscle, and it maintains tonic contractions with lower energy (adenosine triphosphate [ATP]) expenditure (Murphy, 1994).

Smooth muscle is characterized as "phasic" and "tonic." Phasic vascular smooth muscle, which is capable of high shortening velocities, is located in the portal veins. Tonic vascular smooth muscle is located in most of the small arteries and arterioles and has a slower shortening velocity, but it is capable of maintaining sustained vascular tone (Horowitz et al., 1996). As in cardiac and skeletal muscle, contraction of vascular smooth muscle is related to the formation and release of cross-bridges by the cyclic attachment and detachment of the heads of the contractile protein myosin with actin (see Chapter 1). Tonic contractions allow for the maintenance of a basal vascular tone, which is crucial for the maintenance of arterial blood pressure. These tonic contractions are the result of a "latch bridge," which is a slowing in the crossbridge cycling rate. The exact mechanism of the latch bridge has yet to be elucidated (Hai & Murphy, 1988; Sweeney, 1998).

LOCAL REGULATION

In addition to the systemic factors that affect vascular resistance, there are local factors that control resistance. These factors include autacoids, endothelium-derived vasoactive substances, local metabolic factors that match blood flow (oxygen transport) to metabolism, autoregulation (see Chapter 4), and local heating and cooling (as described in the section on venoconstriction).

Autacoids

The autacoids (vasoactive substances) include histamine, serotonin, prostaglandin, and bradykinin. These factors most often compete with adrenergic (vasoconstrictive) effects and exert a

Table 2–1 ■ FUNCTIONS OF THE VASCULAR ENDOTHELIUM RELATED TO VASOMOTOR FUNCTION

Action	Factors Responsible
Release of vasodilatory agents	Nitric oxide Prostacyclin Endothelium-derived hyperpolarizing factor
Release of vasoconstrictor agents	Endothelin-1 Angiotensin/angiotensin II Prostaglandin H2 Thromboxane A2 Superoxide anions
Antiaggregatory effects	Nitric oxide Prostacyclin Thromboresistant endothelium

local vasodilatory effect, which can improve tissue perfusion. The autacoids are not involved in systemic regulation of blood pressure or total peripheral resistance; however, as described later, they initiate or modify the vascular response to other stimuli.

Endothelium-Derived Vasoactive Substances

The vascular endothelium, which is a single layer of squamous cells in the tunica intima, modulates vascular tone by secreting dilator and constrictor substances (Mombouli & Vanhoutte, 1999). In addition, the endothelium affects platelet adhesion and aggregation and the regulation of vascular smooth muscle proliferation (Heydrick, 2000; Loscalzo, 2001; Sarkar & Webb, 1998). The proposed functions of the vascular endothelium (Table 2-1) require an intact endothelium (Furchott & Zawadzki, 1980). The endothelium-produced vasodilator substances include endothelium-derived relaxing factors (EDRF), prostaglandins, and endothelium-derived hyperpolarizing factor (Fig. 2-4). A discussion of each of these factors follows, and a summary of the stimuli that cause the release of each of the factors is presented in Table 2-2.

Endothelium-Derived Relaxing Factors

The seminal observation that endothelium is a key mediator of vascular reactivity was made in 1980 (Furchott & Zawadzki, 1980). The ability of the artery to relax was attributed to the elusive substance, EDRF, which was later identified as nitric oxide (NO) (Ignarro, 1989; Ignarro et al., 1987). Although other relaxing factors such as prostacyclin (prostaglandin I_2 [PGI_2]) and endothelial-derived hyperpolarizing factor (EDHF) are also produced, the major EDRF is NO.

Nitric Oxide. Nitric oxide is a gas with an extremely short half-life (seconds) that diffuses into vascular smooth muscle cells and causes vasodilation (Luscher, 1991; Moncada et al., 1991; Palmer et al., 1987). Nitric oxide's existence is elaborated by the enzyme nitric oxide synthase, which exists in three

Table 2–2

Factors	Stimuli
Vasodilating Factors	
Nitric oxide Endothelium-derived relaxing factor Prostacyclin Endothelium-derived hyperpolarizing factor	Acetylcholine, histamine, arginine vasopressin, epinephrine, norepinephrine, bradykinin, adenosine diphosphate, serotonin (from aggregating platelets), thrombin (from coagulation cascade)
Vasoconstricting Factors	
Endothelium-derived contracting factor	Physical stimuli (mechanical stretch), arachidonic acid (endothelial injury and platelet aggregation), serotonin, adenosine diphosphate
Endothelin-1	Thrombin, interleukin-1, epinephrine, angiotensin II, arginine vasopressin
Prostanoids	Endothelin-1, endothelial membrane damage
Superoxide anions	Physical stress (e.g., shear stress, postischemic reperfusion), chemical endothelial stimulants (bradykinin, cytokines)

ENDOTHELIUM-DEPENDENT RESPONSES
(not present in all blood vessels)

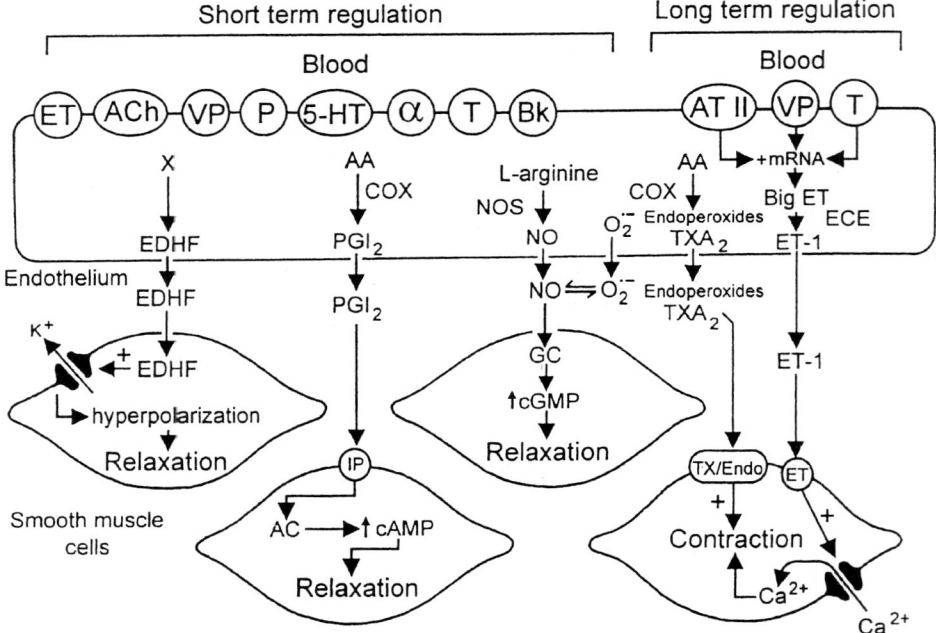

■ **Figure 2–4.** Activation of endothelial receptors can stimulate NO synthase (NOS, with the production of nitric oxide [NO]), and cyclooxygenase (COX), which produces prostacyclin (PGI$_2$) from arachidonic acid (AA) and can lead to the release of endothelium-derived hyperpolarizing factor (EDHF). NO causes relaxation by activating the formation of cyclic GMP (cGMP) from guanosine triphosphate (GTP) by soluble guanylate cyclase (GC). Prostacyclin (PGI$_2$) causes relaxation by activating adenylate cyclase (AC) leading to the formation of cyclic AMP (cAMP). EDHF causes hyperpolarization and relaxation by opening K$^+$ channels. Any increase in cytosolic calcium (including that induced by calcium ionophore A23187) causes the release of relaxing factors. In certain blood vessels, contracting substances can be released from the endothelial cells, which include superoxide anions (O$_2^-$), thromboxane A$_2$ (TXA$_2$), endoperoxides and possibly endothelin-1 (ET$_1$). Thromboxane A$_2$ and endoperoxides activate specific receptors (TX/Endo) on the vascular smooth muscle, as does ET$_1$. Such activation causes an increase in intracellular Ca^{2+} leading to contraction. The production of ET$_1$ (catalyzed by endothelin converting enzyme [ECE]) can be augmented by angiotensin II (ATII), vasopressin (VP) or thrombin (T). The neurohumoral mediators that cause the release of endothelium-derived relaxing factors (and sometimes contracting factors) through activation of specific endothelial receptors (circles) include acetylcholine (ACh), adenosine diphosphate (P), bradykinin (BK), endothelin (ET), adrenaline (α), serotonin (5HT), thrombin (T) and vasopressin (VP). (From Vanhoutte, P.M. [1999]. How to assess endothelial function in human blood vessels. *Journal of Hypertension, 17,* 1047–1058.)

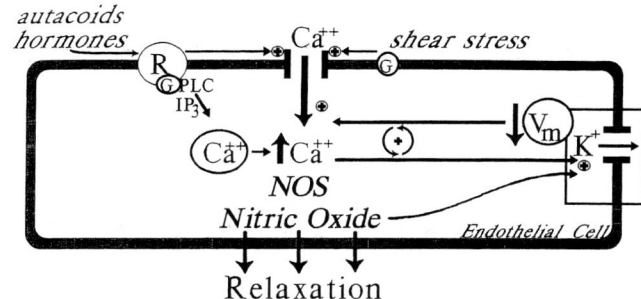

■ Figure 2–5. Scheme demonstrating the release of NO from endothelial cells. Hormones and autocoids acting at endothelial membrane receptors (R) or shear stress cause G-protein (G) mediated increases in calcium (Ca^{2+}) influx and phospholipase C (PLC)-mediated hydrolysis of phosphatidyl inositol biphosphate yielding inositol triphosphate (IP_3), which releases calcium from intracellular stores. The resulting increase in calcium activates NOS to produce NO. The endothelial cell membrane potential (Vm) is hyperpolarized possibly due to activation of calcium-dependent potassium channels, either by the rise in calcium or by NO acting in an autocrine manner. The resulting hyperpolarization accentuates calcium influx due to the increased electrochemical gradient for calcium, and thereby through positive-feedback potentiates the release of NO. (Revised from Cohen, R.A., & Vanhoutte, P.M. [1995]. Endothelium-dependent hyperpolarization: Beyond nitric oxide and cyclic GMP. *Circulation, 92*(11), 3337–3349.)

forms: constitutive or endothelial (cNOS or eNOS), inducible (iNOS), and bnos, which is found in the central nervous system.

Shear stress is a primary factor involved in the release of NO (Fig. 2-5). Although the exact mechanism of action is unknown, shear stress appears to activate potassium-channels in the cell membrane. This activation causes cellular hyperpolarization, which allows calcium to flow into the cell (Cohen, 2000; Cohen & Vanhoutte, 1995). The increased intracellular calcium activates the endothelial enzyme, nitric oxide synthase (eNOS), which catalyzes the conversion of L-arginine to NO. After forming in the endothelial cells, NO diffuses extraluminally into the smooth muscle cells, where it stimulates the release of guanylyl cyclase (GC) and causes cellular hyperpolarization, which ultimately results in vasodilation (Fig. 2-6). Nitric oxide also has secondary vasodilatory effects through the inhibition of the release of the vasoconstrictor endothelin-1 (ET_1), although this beneficial effect decreases with age (Alonso & Radomski, 2003; Heydrick, 2000; Vanhoutte, 2000).

In addition to shear stress, autocoids and hormones increase the release of NO from the endothelium (see Fig. 2-5). These substances (see Table 2-2) cause the release of inositol triphosphate (IP_3), which leads to an increase in intracellular calcium and subsequently stimulates the release of NO. Additionally, NO decreases sympathetic vasoconstriction by inhibiting the release of norepinephrine at the supraspinal, spinal, and synaptic levels (Iida, 1999). Clinically, nitrovasodilators (e.g., nitroglycerin and sodium nitroprusside) cause vasodilation by the donation of NO or NO-like compound (Ignarro et al., 2002; McHugh & Cheek, 1998). Of note, nitroglycerin-induced coronary artery vasodilation does not require the presence of an intact endothelium. In addition, ACE inhibitors, calcium channel blockers, statins, and phosphodiesterase inhibitors

indirectly stimulate NO release or enhance its bioavailability (Ignarro et al., 2002).

Nitric oxide also inhibits platelet activation, aggregation, and adhesion (Loscalzo, 2001); smooth muscle proliferation (Sarkar & Webb, 1998); and endothelial cell apoptosis (Heydrick, 2000) (Fig. 2-7). Of importance, the protective effect of NO against platelet aggregation and vasoconstriction decreases naturally with age and is also diminished with disease processes (e.g., hypertension, diabetes, postmyocardial infarction reperfusion injuries) and altered defense mechanisms (Guzik et al., 2002; Kojda & Harrison, 1999; Landmesser et al., 2000). The loss of the protective endothelium, decreased NO production, and increased NO degradation may foster increased platelet aggregation and vascular proliferation, which are keys to the development of atherosclerosis (Behrendt & Ganz, 2002; Kojda & Harrison, 1999; Sarkar & Webb, 1998). Conversely, increased NO synthesis by inducible NOS (iNOS) may be responsible for the hypotension, decreased vascular tone, and vascular hyporeactivity observed in hemorrhagic and septic shock (Murray et al., 2000).

Prostacyclin. Prostacyclin is a vasodilator prostaglandin that is released by stimulation of endothelial-specific receptors (Naruko et al., 1996). Prostacyclin receptor stimulation, which acts through adenylate cyclase, increases cAMP formation (Fig. 2-8). Increased cAMP stimulates potassium-induced cellular hyperpolarization and also increases calcium extrusion from the cell. Prostacyclin also increases NO release and, concomitantly,

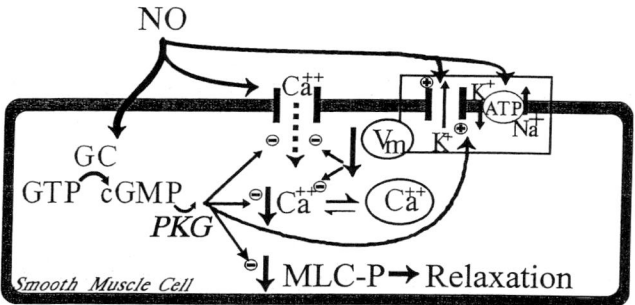

■ Figure 2–6. Scheme showing the mechanisms by which vascular smooth muscle cells respond to NO. NO stimulates guanylyl cyclase (GC), which converts guanosine triphosphate (GTP) to cyclic guanosine monophosphate (cGMP). The cyclic nucleotide through protein kinase G (PKG) phosphorylates proteins, which favor reuptake of calcium, increases calcium extrusion from the cell, and inhibits calcium influx, all leading to a decrease in intracellular free calcium and relaxation. Cyclic GMP may also hyperpolarize the smooth muscle cells by activating potassium channels. NO may also have direct calcium inhibitory effects, as well as direct hyperpolarizing actions via activation of potassium channels or the Na^+/K^+ ATPase. The resulting hyperpolarization decreases smooth muscle cell calcium levels by inhibiting influx through voltage-dependent calcium channels and favoring the reuptake of calcium into intracellular stores and extrusion of calcium from the cell, resulting in a decrease in intracellular free calcium levels. The decrease in myosin light-chain kinase phosphorylation (MLC-P) by the calcium-dependent myosin light-chain kinase relaxes the smooth muscle cell. (Revised from Cohen, R.A., & Vanhoutte, P.M. [1995]. Endothelium-dependent hyperpolarization: Beyond nitric oxide and cyclic GMP. *Circulation, 92*(11), 3337–3349.)

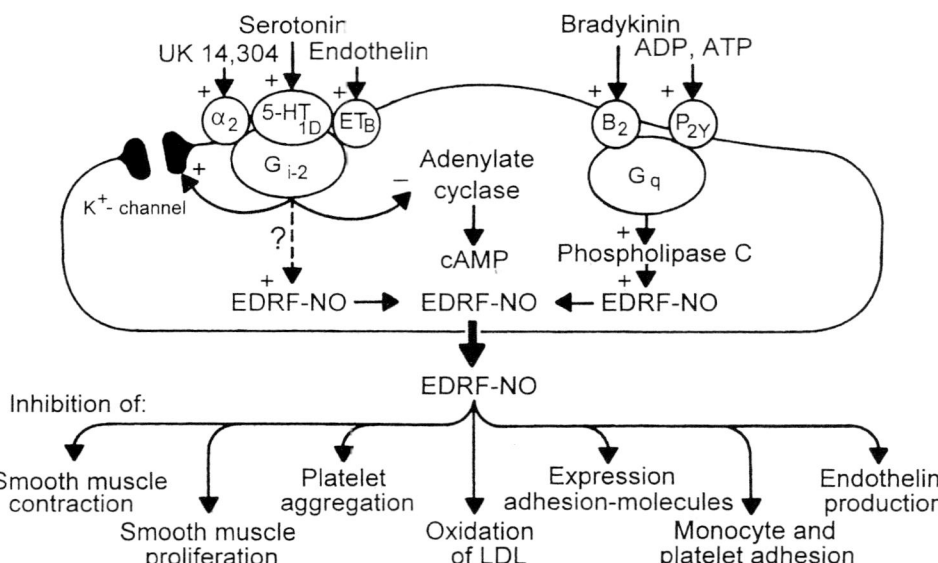

■ **Figure 2–7.** Postulated signal transduction processes in a normal endothelial cell. Activation of the cell causes the release of EDRF-NO, which has important protective effects in the vascular wall. α, alpha-adrenergic, T-HT, serotonin receptor; ET, endothelin receptors; B, bradykinin receptor; P, purinoreceptor; G, coupling proteins; cAMP, cyclic adenosine monophosphate; NO, nitric oxide; LDL, low density lipoproteins; + activation; − inhibition. (Modified from Vanhoutte, P.M. [1999]. Endothelial dysfunction and vascular disease. In J.A. Panza, & R.O. Cannon (Eds.), *Endothelium, nitric oxide and atherosclerosis.* New York: Futura Publishing.)

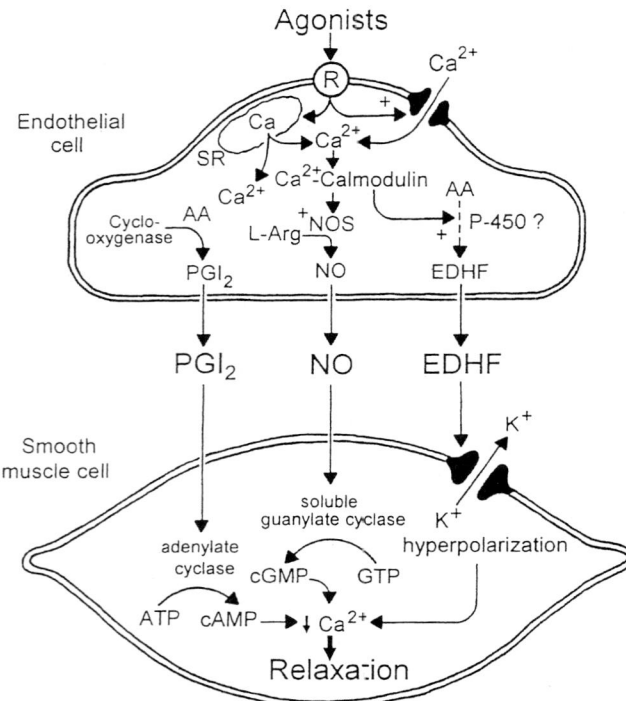

■ **Figure 2–8.** Schematic summarizing the release of relaxing factors from endothelial cells and their effect on vascular smooth muscle cells. Ach, acetylcholine; A23187, calcium ionophore A21837; BK, bradykinin; B2, bradykinin B2 receptor; cAMP, cyclic adenosine monophosphate; cGMP, cyclic guanosine monophosphate; EDHF, endothelium-derived hyperpolarizing factor; EET, epoxyeicosatrienoic acid; K⁺; potassium channel; M1, M3, muscarinic M1 or M3 receptor subtypes; NOS, nitric oxide synthase; PGI₂, prostacyclin; P450, cytochrome P450 monooxygenase; TBA, tetrabutylammonium; TEA, tetraethylammonium. The *broken line* indicates the action of an inhibitor or an antagonist. (From Mombouli, J. V., & Vanhoutte, P. M. [1999]. Endothelial dysfunction: From physiology to therapy. *Journal of Molecular Cell Cardiology, 31,* 61–74.)

NO prolongs the effect of prostacyclin by inhibiting its breakdown (Mombouli & Vanhoutte, 1999).

Endothelium-Derived Hyperpolarizing Factors. Vasodilation may also be mediated by non-NO/non-prostanoid EDHF (Busse et al., 2002). Shear stress and agonist-receptor stimulation, mediated by factors such as bradykinin and acetylcholine, cause an increase in intracellular calcium. In addition to activating NO, the increased calcium also stimulates the release of EDHF (Cohen & Vanhoutte, 1995; Takamura et al., 1999). The putative EDHF (the exact substance remains unknown) is thought to be formed by the action of the calcium-calmodulin complex and the enzyme cytochrome p450 monooxygenase (cytochrome P-450) on an arachidonic acid (epoxyeicosatrienoic acid). The EDHF acts by either opening potassium channels or hyperpolarizing the cell via electrical coupling between the endothelial and vascular smooth muscle cells (Busse et al., 2002; Feletou & Vanhoutte, 1999, 2000; Triggle & Ding, 2002). Cellular hyperpolarization augments calcium movement into the cell and, through a positive feedback mechanism, further increases calcium influx. The hyperpolarization of the endothelial cells then spreads to the smooth muscle cells through a yet to be described mechanism. The vasodilatory role of EDHF increases in vessels of smaller diameter (i.e., resistance arteries) in contrast to larger vessels (Shimokawa et al., 1996; Urakami-Harasawa et al., 1997). In diseases such as diabetes and hypertension, there is a decrease in EDHF-mediated hyperpolarization, which may contribute to the pathologic changes associated with these diseases (Puddu et al., 2000; Taddei et al., 1995). However, this pathological process may be offset by ACE inhibitors and exercise (Griffin et al., 2001; Minami et al., 2002; Roks, 2002).

Endothelium-Derived Contracting Factors

The EDCF include endothelin-1 (ET₁), the vasoconstrictor prostanoids, prostaglandin H2 (PGH2), and the precursor of thromboxane A2 (TXA$_2$); superoxide anions (O$_2^-$); and components of the renin-angiotensin-aldosterone system (RAAS). These substances are released in response to vasoconstrictive stimuli (Vanhoutte, 1997, 1999) (see Fig. 2-4). Vasoconstriction also occurs as a result of a decrease in endothelial production of NO.

Endothelin-1. Endothelin-1 is an amino acid peptide that binds to vascular smooth muscle membrane receptors (ET$_A$ and ET$_B$). Under normal resting conditions, the circulating plasma level of ET$_1$ is very low and it acts locally, in a paracrine fashion, to cause vasodilation through the endothelial synthesis of NO, PGI$_2$, and EDHF (Vanhoutte, 1997, 1999). Conversely, at increased levels, ET$_1$ directly stimulates the vascular smooth muscle (primarily via ET$_A$ receptors) and is the most potent vasoconstrictor known (Yanigisawa et al., 1988). The production of ET$_1$ can be augmented by angiotensin II (ATII), vasopressin, oxygen free radicals, thrombin, and platelet-derived transforming growth factor (Kaddoura & Poole-Wilson, 1996; Luscher et al., 1996). Endothelin-1, along with other contractile agonists (norepinephrine and angiotensin II), causes vasoconstriction by stimulating phospholipase-C, which leads to the formation of inositol triphosphate (IP$_3$) and the subsequent increase in intracellular calcium (Schiffrin & Touyz, 1998). This latter action is inhibited by NO (Vanhoutte, 2000) (Fig. 2-9).

The effects of ET$_1$ are important clinically for at least two reasons. First, in pathological conditions such as congestive heart failure, increased ET$_1$ levels are associated with increased morbidity and mortality and may play an important role in the disease process (Duchman et al., 2000). For example, ET$_1$ stimulates the RAAS, which enhances the conversion of angiotensin I to angiotensin II, causing a synergistic augmentation of vasoconstriction and sodium retention. In addition, the plasma level of ET$_1$ is inversely related to exercise capacity (Krum et al., 1995) and antagonism of ET$_1$ receptors has been shown to improve cardiac function in decompensated heart failure (Duchman et al., 2000). Second, ET$_1$ may play an important role in cardiovascular disease because of its role in cellular proliferation and apoptosis, which contributes to the progression of atherosclerosis, restenosis after angioplasty, and cell loss in heart failure (Best & Lerman, 2000). Endothelin (particularly through ET$_B$ receptors) activates macrophages, which leads to the oxidation of LDL cholesterol and subsequently increases NO degradation and enhances atherosclerosis (Lavallee et al., 2001).

Prostanoids. In response to ET$_1$ and endothelial membrane damage by diseases such as diabetes, hypertension, and hypercholesterolemia, the vascular smooth muscle is exposed to vasoconstrictive substances such as serotonin (5HT), which is released from aggregating platelets, and the vasoconstrictor prostanoids, PGH2 and TXA$_2$, whose production is accelerated by the effect of superoxide anions on arachidonic acid (Vanhoutte, 1999). Prostaglandin H2 and TXA$_2$, which interfere with the normal vasodilatory, antithrombotic, and homeostatic functions of the endothelium, act directly on the vascular smooth muscle, causing adherence and aggregation of platelets as well as vasoconstriction (Lüscher & Vanhoutte, 1990; Mombouli & Vanhoutte, 1999; Vanhoutte & Boulanger, 1995; Vanhoutte & Mombouli, 1996).

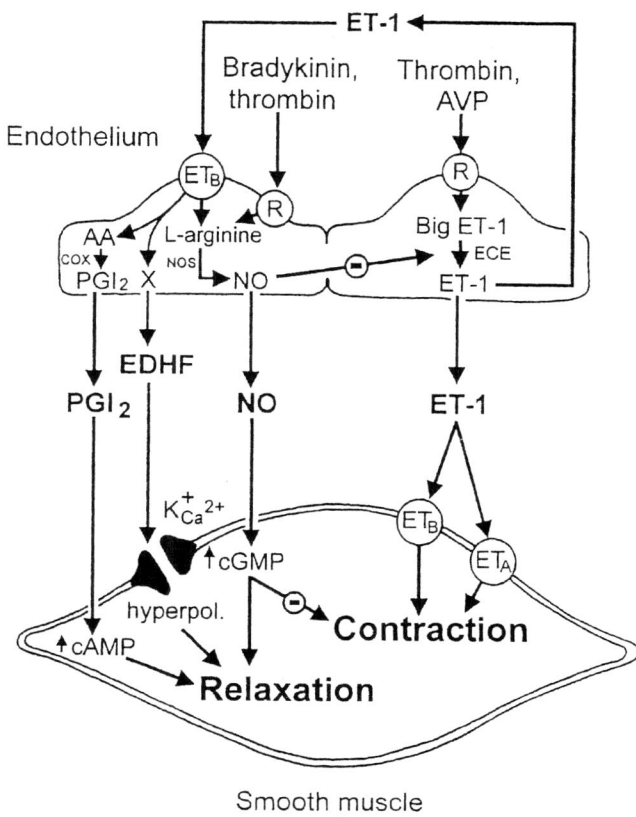

■ **Figure 2–9.** Interaction between endothelin-1 and endothelial-derived relaxing factors. AA, arachidonic acid; cAMP, cyclic AMP; cGMP, cyclic GMP; COX, cyclooxygenase; ECE, endothelin converting enzyme; EDHF, endothelium-derived hyperpolarizing factor; ET, endothelin, endothelin receptor; hyperpol, hyperpolarization; K$_{Ca}^+$$^{2+}$, calcium-dependent potassium channel; NO, nitric oxide; NOS, nitric oxide synthase; PGI$_2$, prostacyclin; R, receptor; X unknown precursor. (From Vanhoutte, P.M. [1999]. Endothelial dysfunction and vascular disease. In J.A. Panza & R.O. Cannon [Eds.], *Endothelium, nitric oxide and atherosclerosis.* New York: Futura Publishing.)

Thromboxane A$_2$ is catalyzed from arachidonic acid by prostaglandin H synthase (PGHS-1), also known as cyclooxygenase-1 (COX-1) (Davidge, 2001). TXA$_2$ causes platelet activation, vasoconstriction, and smooth muscle proliferation, and it is thought to play an important role in the pathogenesis of myocardial infarction (Bing, 2001; Jneid et al., 2003). The reason for the administration of PGHS-1 or COX-1 antagonists (e.g., NSAIDs, aspirin) in cardiovascular disease is to inhibit platelet production of TXA$_2$, because it has been shown to reduce cardiovascular morbidity and mortality. Additionally TXA$_2$ antagonists used in conjunction with glycoprotein IIb/IIIa receptor-blocking antibodies (e.g., C7E3 Fab, abciximab) enhance thrombolysis and decrease the incidence of coronary reocclusion (Coller, 1997; Zusman, 1992). A negative side effect of the COX-1 antagonists is that they are toxic to the gastric mucosa. Use of selective PGHS-2 or COX-2 inhibitors, which are not toxic to the gastrointestinal tract, may be beneficial (FitzGerald et al., 2001). Despite this beneficial effect, the COX-2 inhibitors do not inhibit thromboxane,

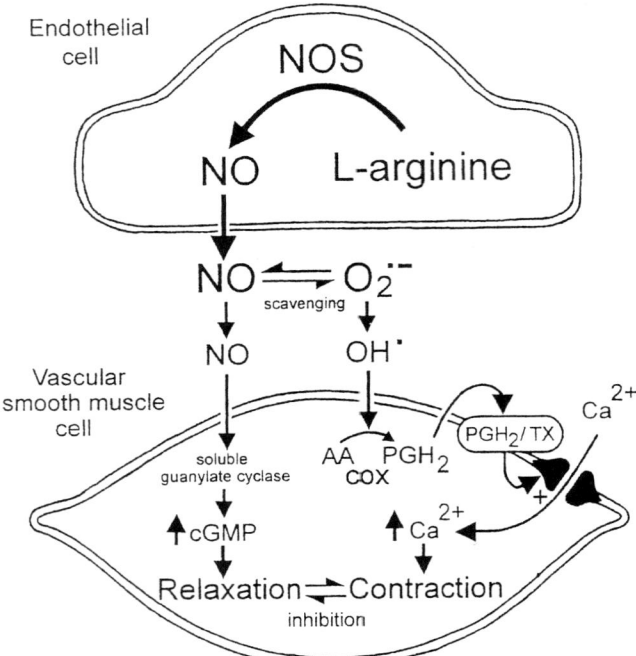

■ **Figure 2–10.** Interactions between nitric oxide (NO) and superoxide anions (O_2^-). Superoxide anions cause contraction of vascular smooth muscle by scavenging endothelium-derived NO and by activating the production of vasoconstrictor prostaglandins in the vascular smooth muscle cells, presumably after transformation of hydroxyl radicals (OH^-). AA, arachidonic acid; COX, cyclooxygenase; cGMP, cyclic GMP; NOS, nitric oxide synthase; PGH_2, endoperoxides; TX, thromboxane. (From Vanhoutte, P. M. [1999]. Endothelial dysfunction and vascular disease. In J. A. Panza & R. O. Cannon (Eds.), *Endothelium, nitric oxide and atherosclerosis.* New York: Futura Publishing.)

whereas they may inhibit vascular prostacyclin, which has vasodilatory effects and inhibits platelet aggregation. Research is ongoing to determine if COX-2 inhibitors increase the risk of cardiovascular disease caused by the creation of a prothrombotic state (FitzGerald, 2002; Konstam & Weir, 2002).

Superoxide Anions. In response to physical stresses, such as shear stress, postischemic reperfusion, and chemical endothelial stimulants (bradykinin, cytokines, angiotensin II), the endothelium produces reactive oxygen species (e.g., superoxide anions and oxidized LDL cholesterol). These ROS inactivate NO (Fig. 2-10), increase the production of the vasoconstrictors PGH2 and TXA_2, and, in conjunction with impaired NO release, decrease NO-mediated vasorelaxation (Harrison et al., 2003; Landmesser et al., 2000). In contrast, superoxide dismutase (an enzyme system that breaks down the free radicals into nontoxic substances and inhibits the breakdown of NO by superoxide anions) inhibits pathologic ET_1 production and augments

endothelial relaxation (Hornig et al., 2001; Kojda & Harrison, 1999). Clinically, ACE inhibitors, which prevent angiotensin-II from inducing oxidative stress, may improve NO availability (Behrendt & Ganz, 2002; Dzau et al., 2002; Hornig et al., 2001). Of note, a recent meta-analysis failed to find any beneficial effects from vitamin E (an antioxidant) in the reduction of cardiovascular mortality or death (Vivekananthan et al., 2003).

Local Metabolic Control of Blood Flow

Local metabolic factors that control arteriolar resistance play a role in matching blood flow (oxygen transport) to metabolism. These factors may accumulate in low-flow conditions and cause vasodilation by inhibition of basal tone (Fig. 2-11). The increased flow that occurs as a result of the vasodilation is referred to as *reactive hyperemia*. Metabolic factors that have been shown to interact and contribute to reactive hyperemia include adenosine and adenosine triphosphate (ATP), nitric oxide, prostaglandins, and potassium (Marshall, 2002; Ralevic, 2002; Ray et al., 2002). Other metabolic factors include hydrogen, phosphate, carbon dioxide, lactic acid, intermediates of the Krebs cycle, vasoactive peptides, osmolarity, and a local decrease in oxygen (Hudlicka, 1985; Rowell, 1993; Sheperd, 1983; Sparks, 1980; Vanhoutte, 1988). Many of these factors (i.e., potassium, osmolarity, PO_2) appear to play a role in the initiation of exercise-induced hyperemia, but other factors are responsible for sustained vasodilation. An increase in flow-dependent shear stress on the endothelium has also been shown to cause vasodilation in skeletal muscle and venules. This vasodilation is mediated in part by the release of NO and prostaglandin (Koller & Bagi, 2002; Koller et al., 1998; Koller & Kaley, 1998).

■ NEUROHUMORAL STIMULATION

In addition to stimulation by endothelium-derived vasodilating and vasoconstricting factors, neurohumoral factors bind with receptors on vascular smooth muscle. The effects of this stimulation vary throughout the vascular system.

Adrenergic Stimulation

α-Adrenergic Stimulation

The α-adrenergic receptors are generally categorized as α_1 and α_2 receptors (Flavahan et al., 1987). Molecular cloning techniques have lead to a further division of the α-receptor subtypes. The α_1-adrenergic receptors, which are now characterized as subtypes α_{1A}, α_{1B}, and α_{1D}, are located in arteries, arterioles, and cutaneous and visceral veins. The α_{1A} receptors are responsible for vessel contraction. The α_{1B} receptors are thought to contribute to the

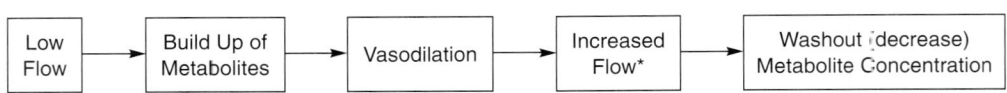

*Increased flow called reactive hyperemia.

■ **Figure 2–11.** Mechanism of local metabolic control of resistance. (Courtesy of Loring B. Rowell, University of Washington, Seattle, WA, 1998.)

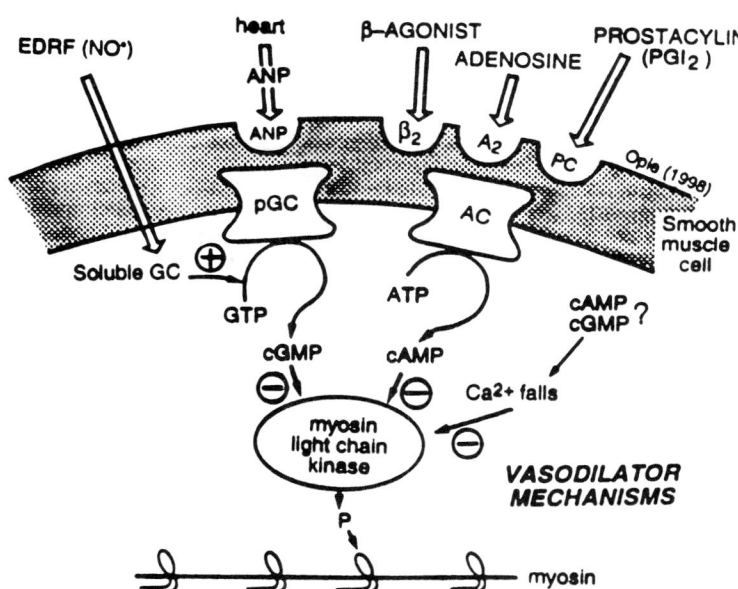

■ **Figure 2–12.** Vasodilatory mechanisms. Most act by formation of cyclic nucleotides, cyclic guanosine monophosphate (cGMP) and cyclic adenosine monophosphate (cAMP), both of which are vasodilatory, possibly through inhibition of myosin light-chain kinase. GMP is the messenger for guanylate cyclase (GC), which in turn is stimulated by atrial natriuretic polypeptide (ANP) or by EDRF (i.e., nitric oxide). Vasodilatory cAMP is formed by stimulation of adenylate cyclase (AC) in response to β_2-stimulation or by adenosine (A) stimulation through A_2-receptors, or by prostacyclin (PO; PGI_2) receptor. ATP, adenosine triphosphate; pGC, prostacyclin C (G kinase). (Opie, L.H. [1998]. *The heart: Physiology from cell to circulation* [3rd ed., p. 240]. Philadelphia: Lippincott-Raven.)

maintenance of basal vascular tone and arterial blood pressure in conscious animals and are sensitive to exogenous agonists. Finally, the α_{1D} receptors also play a role in vascular contraction, although they have a lesser effect than the α_{1B} receptors (Civantos Calzada & Aleixandre de Artinano, 2001).

The α_2 receptors, which have presynaptic and postsynaptic functions, are characterized as $\alpha_{2A/D}$, α_{2B}, and α_{2C}. The $\alpha_{2A/D}$ and α_{2B} receptors are present in large arteries but are located with greater density on the terminal arterioles, which act as precapillary sphincters to control the number of open capillaries and total capillary blood flow. The $\alpha_{2A/D}$ receptors play the primary role in vasoconstriction (Kable et al., 2000). The α_{2B} receptors also play a role in vasoconstriction and may contribute to the onset of hypertension. The α_{2C} receptors are responsible for venoconstriction (Civantos Calzada & Aleixandre de Artinano, 2001; Leech & Faber, 1996).

Whereas stimulation of the presynaptic α_2 receptors inhibits norepinephrine, stimulation of the postsynaptic α_2 receptors located on the vascular smooth muscle causes norepinephrine release and subsequent vasoconstriction (Sperelakis & Ohya, 1990; Sperelakis et al., 1992). However, the α_2-mediated vasoconstriction is attenuated by the α_2 presynaptic inhibition of norepinephrine release. In addition, in contrast to α_1 receptor stimulation, the effect of norepinephrine on α_2 in terminal arterioles is inhibited by metabolites, thus fostering metabolic vasodilation even when vasoconstrictor tone to blood vessels in the skeletal muscle is high.

β-Adrenergic Stimulation

In the heart, β_1 receptors predominate (60%—80%), although there are also a smaller number of β_2 receptors (20%—30%), with the latter receptors playing a role in coronary vasodilation (del Monte et al., 1993; Feigl, 1998). There is also a small number (<1%) of β_3 adrenergic receptors in cardiomyocytes (Gauthier et al., 1996). The β_3 receptors, which mediate negative inotropy via a NO-dependent pathway (Gauthier et al.,

1998; Varghese et al., 2000), become important during heart failure when they are up-regulated and may contribute to functional degradation of the failing heart (Moniotte et al., 2001).

In vascular smooth muscle, the β-adrenergic receptors are predominantly of the β_2-subtype. Stimulation of these receptors causes relaxation (Lands et al., 1967) via activation of cyclic adenosine monophosphate (cAMP), which in turn activates a protein kinase that phosphorylates the myosin light-chain kinase (MLCK) enzyme (Fig. 2-12). Phosphorylation inactivates MLCK and as a result, the MLCK is unable to participate in the phosphorylation of the myosin and the promotion of the active myosin kinase-calmodulin-calcium complex. Failure to form the calmodulin-calcium complex inhibits cross-bridge formation. β_2-adrenergic stimulation also decreases intracellular calcium by hyperpolarization of the vascular smooth muscle, which decreases the influx of calcium into the cell, increases cAMP-mediated extrusion of calcium from the cell, and promotes calcium uptake by the sarcoplasmic reticulum (Sperelakis et al., 1994). There are also a small number of β_3 receptors in the vascular smooth muscle, which are thought to be responsible for vasodilation in the skin and fat, although this finding remains to be demonstrated in humans (Berlan et al., 1994; Berlan et al., 1995; Trochu et al., 1997).

Intracellular Signals for Vasodilation and Vasoconstriction

The two major messengers for vasodilation are the intracellular nucleotides cyclic adenosine monophosphate (cAMP, described previously) and cyclic guanosine monophosphate (cGMP). The primary messenger for vasoconstriction is inositol triphosphate (IP_3).

Cyclic GMP

Nitric oxide, atrial natriuretic peptides, and nitrovasodilators (e.g., nitroglycerin and nitroprusside) activate guanylate cyclase

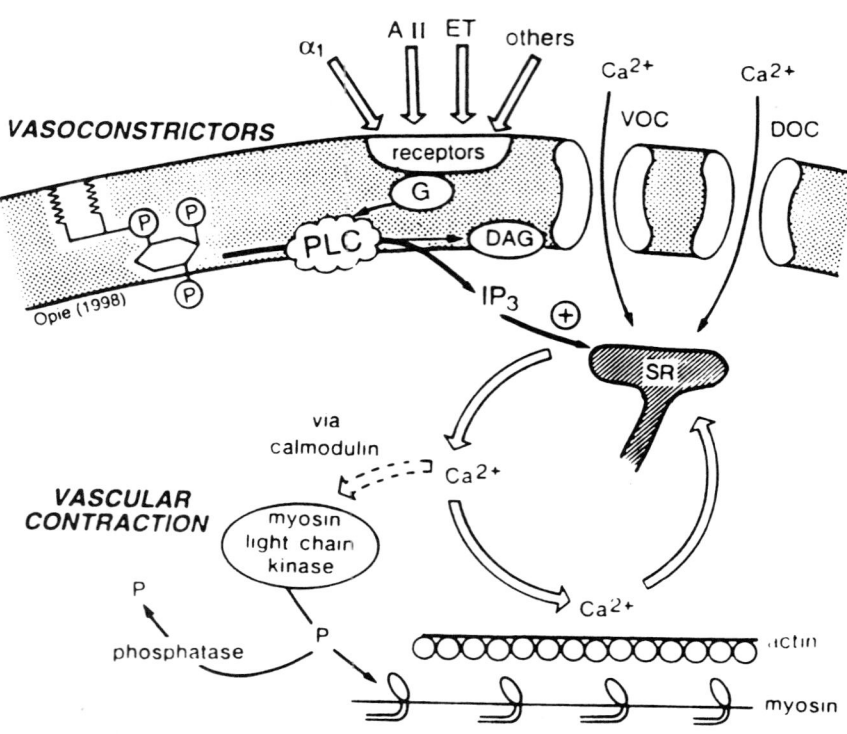

■ **Figure 2–13.** Vasoconstrictory mechanisms. Several act by releasing calcium from the sarcoplasmic reticulum (SR). For example, stimulation of vascular receptors by endothelin (ET), angiotensin II (AII), or norepinephrine (NE) leads to increased activity of phospholipase C (PLC), which splits phosphatidyl inositol into two messengers: IP₃ (inositol triphosphate) and 1,2-DAG (1, 2-diaclyglycerol). IP₃ promotes the release of calcium from the SR. Membrane-bound DAG activates protein kinase C. Vasoconstriction also occurs in response to enhanced activity of the calcium channels. (From Opie, L.H. [1998]. *The heart: Physiology from cell to circulation* [3rd ed., p. 239]. Philadelphia: Lippincott-Raven.)

(GC), which generates cGMP from guanosine triphosphate (GTP). The cGMP activates the cGMP-dependent kinase known as phosphokinase G (PKG), which is proposed to decrease intracellular calcium and subsequently vasorelaxation by: (1) increasing the uptake or extrusion of calcium by the cytoplasm; (2) inhibiting calcium release from the sarcoplasmic reticulum; (3) regulating the levels of IP₃; (4) inhibiting calcium-activated potassium channels; and (5) decreasing contractile protein sensitivity to calcium (Cohen et al., 1999; Heydrick, 2000; Komalavilas & Lincoln, 2000). Phosphokinase G also directly inhibits MLCK, thus inhibiting contraction. Additionally, cGMP hyperpolarizes the cell, which further decreases intracellular calcium (Cohen, 2000).

Inositol Triphosphate (IP₃)

In response to vasoconstrictor stimuli (e.g., norepinephrine, angiotensin II [AII], and endothelin), the enzyme phospholipase C (PLC) located in the cell wall splits phosphatidyl inositol into IP₃ and diacylglycerol (DAG) (Fig. 2-13). Inositol triphosphate is the primary messenger for vasoconstriction and acts on a special calcium-receptor channel on the sarcoplasmic reticulum to release calcium. Conversely, cGMP inhibits the accumulation of IP₃, which leads to a decrease in cytosolic calcium levels and vasorelaxation (Komalavilas & Lincoln, 2000).

▓ CALCIUM

The major endpoint of extrinsic neurohormonal factors and local regulation of vascular tone involves a cascade of messengers that influence calcium movement in and out of the cell or sarcoplasmic reticulum, thus influencing the contractile process (Berridge, 1993; Berridge, 1997). Knowledge of the role of calcium is important because the modulation of calcium flux is the focus of pharmacologic control of vascular resistance.

As with cardiac and skeletal muscle, the changes in intracellular calcium are responsible for vascular smooth muscle contraction and relaxation. However, unlike skeletal and cardiac muscle in which calcium reverses the inhibitory effect of troponin on the actin-myosin interaction, vascular smooth muscle cross-bridge formation and muscle contraction result from the indirect activation of myosin by calcium (Horowitz et al., 1996; Somlyo & Somlyo, 1994).

Sources of Calcium

The increased intracellular calcium comes from an influx of calcium across the sarcolemma and from the sarcoplasmic reticulum (Somlyo & Somlyo, 1994). The calcium influx across the sarcolemma is through voltage-gated ion channels, which are altered by the activation of the IP₃-regulated channels or ryanodine receptors. These receptors display calcium-induced calcium release (Berridge, 2002; Berridge et al., 1999; Bootman et al., 2002).

Calcium Signaling

The increased intracellular calcium binds with calmodulin, a small protein found in the cytosol of vascular smooth muscle (Fig. 2-14). The calcium-calmodulin complex activates the enzyme myosin light-chain kinase, which in turn phosphorylates

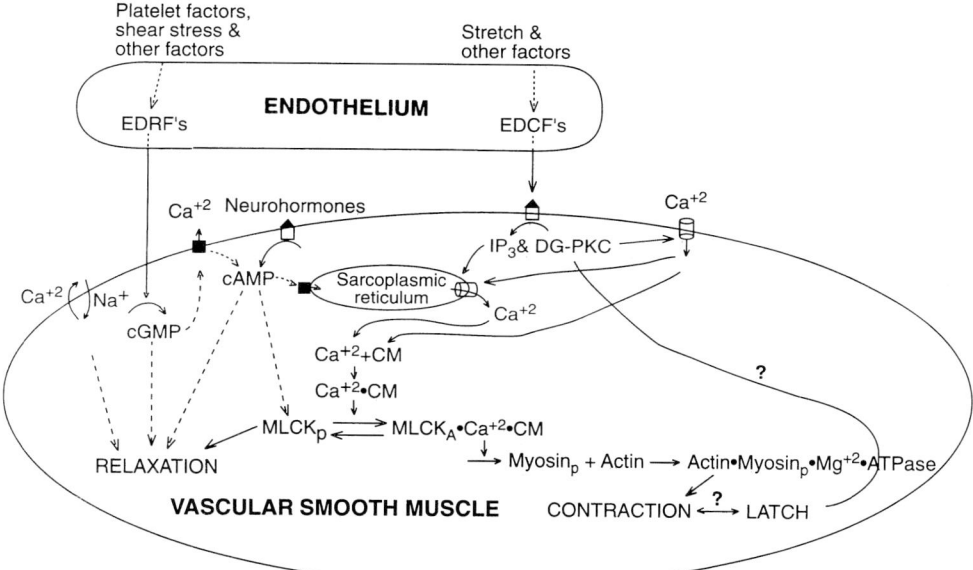

■ **Figure 2–14.** Hypothetical simplified illustration of interactions between endothelial and vascular smooth muscle cells. Physical forces or circulating factors from nerves, platelets, or other sources trigger the endothelial cell to produce endothelium-derived relaxing (EDRFs) and contracting factors (EDCFs), which diffuse into vascular smooth muscle or stimulate membrane receptors (⌂). Calcium enters the cell through voltage-operated channels (▯) and may be released from intracellular stores such as sarcoplasmic reticulum (SR). Calcium (Ca^{+2}) interacts with calmodulin (CM), and together they activate myosin light-chain kinase (MLCK), which in turn phosphorylates (P) myosin so it can react with actin and cause vascular smooth muscle contraction. EDCFs activate inositol triphosphate (IP_3), which may promote the release of calcium from SR, and diacylglycerol (DG), which activates protein kinase C (PKC). PKC may influence the contractile proteins or promote the latch state. Cyclic guanosine monophosphate (cGMP), initiated by EDRFs, or cyclic adenosine monophosphate (cAMP), initiated by adrenergic and other vascular smooth muscle cell membrane receptor stimuli, may promote calcium cellular extrusion or uptake by the SR through activating membrane pumps (▪).

the light protein chains of the myosin head. The phosphorylation activates the myosin (increases the ATPase activity) such that the myosin can interact with actin. The process of phosphorylation is considered the primary mechanism of smooth muscle contraction. Conversely, a decrease in the cytoplasmic calcium concentration inactivates the MLCK and permits dephosphorylation of myosin by the enzyme myosin light-chain phosphatase. The dephosphorylation facilitates the detachment of myosin from actin, resulting in relaxation (Somlyo & Somlyo, 1994).

The cytoplasmic calcium concentration is decreased through uptake of calcium into the sarcoplasmic reticulum and transport out of the cell across the plasma membrane by Ca^{2+}-ATPase exchanger or a probable Na^+/Ca^{2+} exchanger (Marin et al., 1999; Somlyo & Somlyo, 2002). Additionally, calcium is decreased by closure of the membrane calcium channels through hyperpolarization (Patterson et al., 2002) or pharmacologically with calcium channel blockers.

VOLUME AND FLOW DISTRIBUTION

Resistance

The pressure decrease from the aorta to the small arteries is relatively small, approximately 25 mm Hg (Fig. 2-15) (Sheperd & Vanhoutte, 1979). As much as 50% of the peripheral resistance

appears to occur proximal to vessels with diameters of 100 mm. This finding indicates the primary sites for peripheral vascular resistance are the small arteries and the arterioles, although the exact location of the resistance vessels remains equivocal (Christensen & Mulvany, 2001; Mulvany & Aalkjeær, 1990; Renkin, 1989).

Alterations in the diameter of the terminal arterioles or precapillary blood vessels control capillary and venous pressures, microvascular blood flow and exchange, and postcapillary venous volume (Duling, 1981; Duling & Klitzman, 1980). Although the radius of the capillaries is considerably smaller than the radius of the arterioles, the resistance is lower because of the increase in cross-sectional area.

Volume Distribution

At rest, the systemic veins contain as much as 60% to 80% of the total blood volume, with 25% to 50% of this volume in the small veins (<1 mm in diameter). One-fourth of the total blood volume is in the capacious splanchnic circulation. Although the cross-sectional area is largest at the end of the capillaries, the largest volume of blood, as demonstrated in Fig. 2-16, is in the venules because of the combination of cross-sectional area and the length of the venules (Scher, 1989). The remainder of the blood is distributed in the aorta and systemic arteries (10%), the capillaries (5%), and the pulmonary bed and heart (15% to 25%) (Rothe, 1983; Zweifach & Lipowsky, 1984).

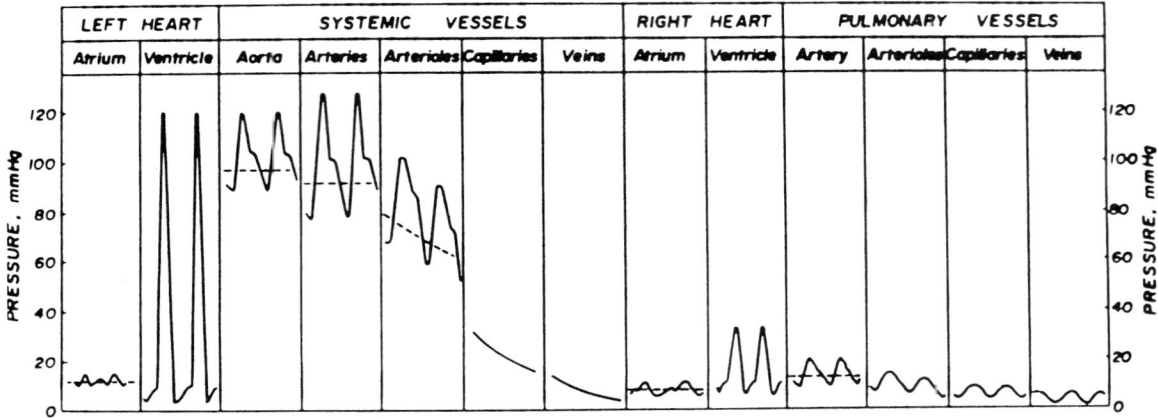

■ **Figure 2–15.** Pressure changes in the human cardiovascular system. In the left atrium, the pressure is low but pulsatile because of the rhythmic contractions of the atrial muscle. The main generator of pressure is the muscle of the left ventricle; in the latter cavity, the pressure alternates with each cardiac cycle from near 0 (diastole) to approximately 120 mm Hg (systole). When the pressure in the ventricle exceeds that in the aorta, the aortic semilunar valve opens, the ventricle and aorta become a common chamber, and the pressure in both rises in unison. The rise in aortic pressure causes an expansion of the aorta and the large arteries because of their elasticity and because blood enters the arterial trees faster than it leaves it through the small-bore arterioles. When the ventricle starts to relax, the aortic valve closes. As the ventricle continues to relax, the pressure within it drops quickly to near 0, but the pressure in the aorta falls slowly throughout ventricular diastole as the distended arterial tree recoils and blood continues to flow to the capillaries through the arterioles. The major loss of pressure occurs at the arterioles because of the high resistance to flow that they offer. The pressure in the capillaries and veins decreases further to approximately 0 in the great veins entering the right atrium; the flow in the systemic capillaries and veins is relatively nonpulsatile. The right side of the heart generates a pressure pattern similar to that in the systemic circulation, but the systolic pressure in the pulmonary artery is approximately six times less than that of the aorta, and the flow in the pulmonary capillaries is pulsatile. Mean pressures are indicated by dotted lines. In large arteries, the mean pressure is lower than in the aorta, although the systolic pressure is higher because of reflection of the pulse waves. (From Shepherd, J.T., & Vanhoutte, P.M. [1979]. *The human cardiovascular system: Facts and concepts* [p. 78.] New York: Raven Press.)

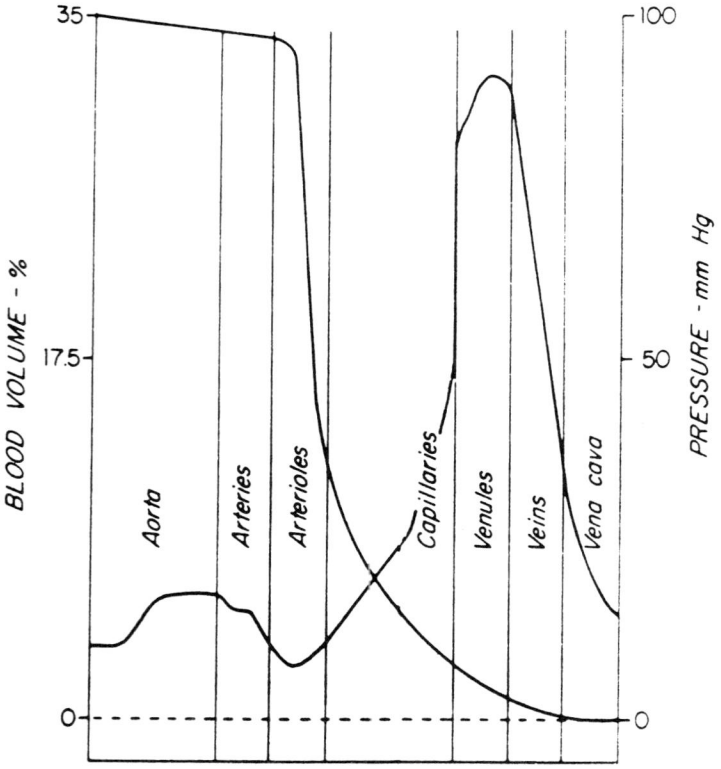

■ **Figure 2–16.** Changes in estimated blood volume (%) and blood pressure in consecutive segments of the systemic blood vessels. Note that the volume is predominantly in the venules. The pressure is high in the aorta and arteries, falls rapidly in the arterioles, and then falls more slowly from the capillaries to the vena cava. (From Scher, A.M. [1989]. The veins and venous return. In H.D. Patton, A. Fuchs, B. Hille et al. [Eds.], *Textbook of physiology, Vol. 2* [21st ed., p. 880.]. Philadelphia: WB Saunders.)

Blood Flow

Definition of Flow

Blood flow ($\dot{Q}$) is expressed in terms of volume of blood per unit of time (volume/time). For example, the cardiac output, which is defined as the liters of blood pumped out of the left ventricle into the systemic circulation each minute, is usually expressed as liters per minute.

Determinants of Flow

Nonturbulent flow ($\dot{Q}$) in a segment of an isogravitational blood vessel (i.e., a blood vessel on the same horizontal level) is determined by the pressure difference (ΔP) between the inflow and outflow ends of that segment divided by the resistance (R) to flow provided by that segment. The relationship that demonstrates that flow will change as the result of a change in pressure or the change in resistance across a vascular bed is expressed in the following equation:

$$\dot{Q} = \Delta P/R$$

Substituting physiological values into this equation gives:

$$CO = MAP - RAP/SVR$$

where MAP − RAP is the difference between the mean arterial pressure (MAP; as an indicator of aortic or upstream pressure) and right atrial pressure (RAP; downstream pressure) divided by the SVR.

Pressure. Blood pressure is the force exerted by the blood in a blood vessel. Clinically, pressure is expressed as millimeters of mercury, torr, or centimeters of H_2O. The relationship between these various measures is:

$$1 \text{ mm Hg} = 1 \text{ torr} = 1.36 \text{ cm } H_2O$$

Pressure in blood vessels has three components: (1) static pressure, which is related to the fullness of the vascular system at zero flow; (2) hydrostatic pressure, which is equal to the height of the column of liquid (h) multiplied by the density of the liquid (p) multiplied by the gravitational force (g), hydrostatic pressure = pgh; and (3) dynamic pressure, which is the pressure generated by the heart and is equal to flow multiplied by resistance (pressure = flow × resistance). The static pressure and the hydrostatic pressure are added to the dynamic pressure to give blood pressure. The hydrostatic pressure, and particularly the effect of the height of the fluid column, is especially important in the upright position, because the fluid column between the heart and the feet may add an additional 100 mm Hg of hydrostatic pressure to the dynamic pressure (100 mm Hg). In the systemic circulation, blood flows from the aorta, where the MAP is 100 mm Hg, to the right atrium (mean pressure = 0 to 6 mm Hg).

Resistance. Based on an analogy to Ohm's law, resistance (R) is equal to a pressure gradient (ΔP) divided by blood flow ($\dot{Q}$):

$$R = \Delta P/\dot{Q}$$

According to Poiseuille's law for laminar nonpulsatile flow of a substance with uniform viscosity, vascular resistance is proportional to a constant ($8/\pi$), the viscosity of the blood (η), and the length of the vessel (L). It is inversely proportional to the fourth power of the radius (r^4):

$$R = \frac{8L\eta}{\pi r^4}$$

Thus the resistance to flow depends on only the dimension length (L) and radius (r) of the vessel and the viscosity (η) of the fluid. The radius of the blood vessel is the primary factor determining resistance in the vascular system. For example, if all other factors are held constant, decreasing the vessel radius by 50% increases resistance 16-fold, because resistance is inversely proportional to the fourth power of the radius. An increase in blood viscosity causes resistance to increase, although this increased viscosity is seldom an acute event (Badeer, 2001). However, an increase in the hematocrit (e.g., polycythemia caused by high altitude) can increase blood viscosity, causing resistance to increase (Hlastala & Berger, 2001). A limitation of Poiseuille's law is that it is based on rigid tubes and predicts a linear relationship between pressure and flow. However, because of the elastic properties of blood vessels, the relationship between pressure and flow is nonlinear (Boulpaep, 2003). Depending on the starting pressure and the vasoconstrictive state of the vessel, an initial increase in pressure may distend the vessel but have limited effect on flow.

The SVR is calculated by the following equation:

$$SVR = (MAP - RAP/CO) \times 80$$

In this equation, 80 is a conversion factor for adjusting mm Hg·L^{-1} × min^{-1} to dyne/sec/cm^{-5}. The normal SVR ranges from 800 to 1,200 dynes/sec/cm^{-5}.

Pulmonary vascular resistance is calculated:

$$PVR = [PAM - PAWP/CO] \times 80$$

where PAM is mean pulmonary artery pressure and PAWP is pulmonary artery wedge pressure. In the pulmonary circulation, the entire cardiac output flows from the pulmonary artery (pressure ranges from 7 to 18 mm Hg) to the left atrium (pressure ranges from 2 to 12 mm Hg, mean = 8 mm Hg), with a change in pressure of only approximately 10 mm Hg. The total pulmonary vascular resistance (PVR) is approximately 10% of the SVR. The PVR ranges from 20 to 120 dynes/sec/cm^{-5}, with an average of 100 dynes/sec/cm^{-5} (see Chapter 3). Changes in the PVR, however, may occur with changes in gravity, body position, lung volume, alveolar and intrapleural pressures, intravascular pressures, and right ventricular output, without any change in pulmonary vascular tone (Hlastala & Berger, 2001; Levitzky, 1995). Thus, changes in PVR as an indicator of pulmonary vascular tone must be interpreted with caution.

THE ARTERIAL SYSTEM

Arterial Pressure

Systolic and diastolic blood pressures describe the high and low values of pressure fluctuations around the mean of the arterial pressure wave (Gallagher & O'Rourke, 1993). The MAP in the ascending aorta depends on the cardiac output and SVR:

$$MAP = CO \times SVR$$

whereas arterial distensibility and left ventricular stroke volume determine the amplitude and contour of the pressure wave (Gallagher & O'Rourke, 1993). The peak systolic pressure is determined by the volume and velocity of left ventricular ejection (i.e., the larger the SV, the larger the pulse pressure at any given distensibility), peripheral arterial resistance, the distensibility of the arterial wall, the viscosity of blood, and the end-diastolic volume in the arterial blood (O'Rourke, 1990a). During diastole, arterial pressure decreases until the next ventricular contraction, so the minimal diastolic pressure is determined by factors that affect the magnitude and rate of the diastolic pressure drop. Factors that affect diastolic blood pressure include blood viscosity, arterial distensibility, peripheral resistance, and the length of the cardiac cycle (O'Rourke, 1990b).

During systole, the elastic walls of the aorta and large arteries stretch as more blood enters than runs off into the periphery. Thus, a portion of the stroke volume is stored in the relatively distensible aorta during systole. During diastole, there is passive elastic recoil of the arterial walls, causing continued, but decreasing, ejection of blood out of the aorta and into the peripheral arteries (Fig. 2-17). The elastic recoil transforms pulsatile flow into more continuous flow in the smaller vessels and

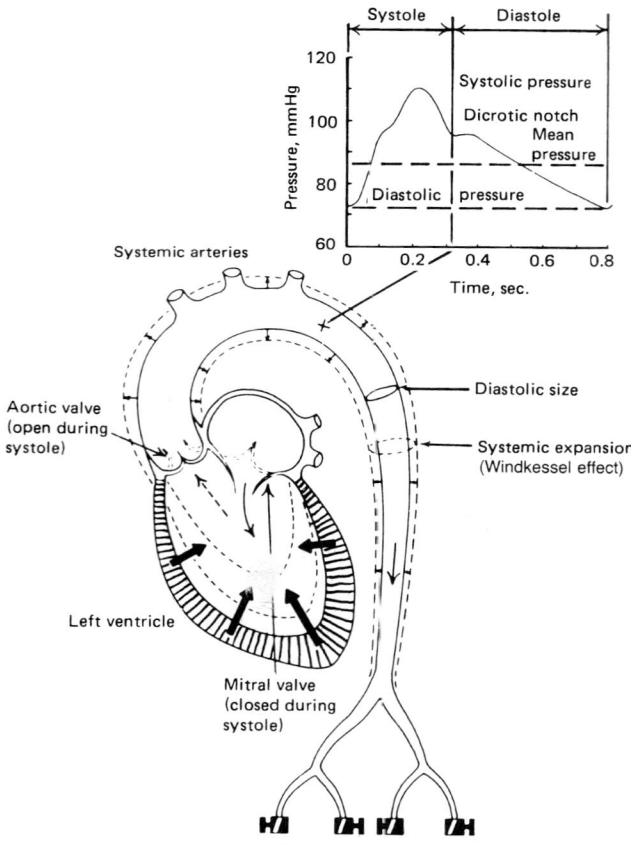

■ **Figure 2–17.** Schematic illustration of changes in aortic pressure during the cardiac cycle and the dampening role of the aorta and large arteries on the pulsatile flow from the heart during systole (sometimes termed the Windkessel effect). (From Shepherd, J.T., & Vanhoutte, P.M. [1979]. *The human cardiovascular system: Facts and concepts* [p. 78]. New York: Raven Press.)

explains why the blood pressure does not drop to zero during periods of no flow (e.g., diastole) (Mohrman & Heller, 2003).

Pulse pressure is the difference between the systolic and diastolic pressures. The aortic pulse pressure is directly proportional to left ventricular stroke volume and inversely related to arterial compliance, with changes in SV responsible for most acute changes.

$$\text{Pulse pressure} \cong \text{Stroke volume/arterial compliance}$$

A normal pulse pressure at the brachial artery is approximately 40 mm Hg. A higher pulse pressure may reflect where the pressure is measured in the body (increased pulse pressure in the periphery). Ejection velocity also affects the pulse pressure, whereas the SVR does not affect the pulse pressure as it affects both systolic and diastolic pressures.

THE VENOUS SYSTEM

The venous system transports blood back to the heart from the microcirculation of each organ system and plays a crucial role in the maintenance of thoracic intravascular volume. The veins also serve as a low-pressure reservoir with the capacity to contain a large and variable volume of blood (similar to a giant capacitor sitting next to the right ventricle). The veins are innervated by α-adrenergic fibers but not β-adrenergic fibers. Only the splanchnic and cutaneous veins receive extensive innervation. The veins constrict in response to α-adrenergic stimuli and dilate as the result of withdrawal of the α-adrenergic stimuli or in response to increased transmural pressure (i.e., passive vasodilation). There are no active vasodilatory mechanisms in the veins (Rowell, 1986).

Venous Pressure and Resistance

In the supine position, the pressure generated by the heart in the large arteries is approximately 100 mm Hg. However, as demonstrated in Fig. 2-15, the pressure decreases across the arterioles and capillaries, with a resultant pressure in the small veins of only 15 to 20 mm Hg. The right atrial pressure is approximately 0 to 5 mm Hg (depending on position, the state of hydration, and cardiac output). Thus, the pressure driving blood flow from the left side of the heart to the capillaries is approximately 80 mm Hg, whereas the driving pressure from the postcapillary vessels to the right atrium is only 15 to 20 mm Hg (difference between the postcapillary vessels and the right atrium). Interestingly, in the upright position, despite the addition of hydrostatic pressure (determined by the height of a continuous column of blood between any given point and the heart), this gradient is unchanged.

Skeletal muscle contractions in the extremities (the muscle pump) and respiration (respiratory pump) play an essential role in propelling venous blood from the veins to the right atrium (see Chapter 4). In addition, the venous valves prevent backward flow into the muscle. Valvular function is particularly important during standing and exercise (Criado et al., 1995; Hosoi et al., 2002; Raju et al., 1993). The valves also promote the one-way flow of blood through perforating veins that lie between the superficial and deep veins.

Venous Compliance

When empty, the thin walls of the veins are flattened and the vessels are elliptical. As the veins fill with blood, they passively change to a circular shape. Because of this passive accommodation to an increase in volume, the veins are capable of receiving large volumes of fluid with only small increases in transmural pressure; that is, they are compliant. Because of their ability to serve as a volume reservoir, the veins are referred to as capacitance vessels. At increased pressures, the veins become distended and less compliant; thus, any given pressure change is associated with a smaller change in volume (Rowell, 1986). Because of the compliant nature of the veins, the venous system plays an important role in altering thoracic intravascular volume (Hainsworth, 1986).

MICROCIRCULATORY EXCHANGE

Flow Through the Microvascular Circulation

Blood flow ($\dot{Q}$) through the microcirculation (or any organ) is directly related to the difference in pressure between the arterial end of the vascular segment (P_A) and venous pressure (P_v) and is inversely related to vascular resistance (R_T) (Levick, 1991; Renkin, 1984, 1989):

$$\text{Flow} = (P_A - P_V)/R_T$$

In the absence of changes in arterial pressure (P_A), changes in local vascular resistance and intravascular pressure are caused by vasodilation and vasoconstriction of the arterioles. Any alteration in the tone of the muscular venules contributes little to the change in resistance.

Microvascular Transport Mechanisms

Solutes and water passively move across the endothelium as the result of two processes, diffusion and ultrafiltration. Diffusion is the result of the random kinetic motion of ions and molecules. Diffusion results in the net transport of substances along a concentration gradient from high to low concentration. Ultrafiltration is the combined movement of fluid and solutes in a unilateral direction through a membrane, except that the movement of the solutes is restricted by the membrane. The driving force for ultrafiltration is the difference between hydrostatic pressure and oncotic pressure across the membrane. Ultrafiltration is the primary mechanism for controlling plasma and interstitial fluid volume (Renkin, 1989).

Diffusion

Concentration gradients, created by the production or consumption of specific substances, are the primary driving forces for diffusion (with the exception of the tight-junction capillaries, which are affected by electrical gradients). Because diffusion in or out of a blood vessel creates a concentration gradient along the vessel, diffusion exchange is strongly influenced by blood flow, particularly for those substances that rapidly diffuse through the membrane wall (Crone & Levitt, 1984; Renkin, 1984). The rate of diffusion of a solute across the capillary wall (J_s) is proportional to the concentration gradient, that is, the difference between the concentration in the plasma (C_p) and interstitial concentration (C_i), the permeability (P_s) of the endothelium to the solute, and the surface area (A) available for exchange.

$$J_s = P_s A (C_p - C_i)$$

For substances that diffuse rapidly through the capillary endothelium (e.g., O_2, CO_2), the transport of the solute depends on the concentration gradient and blood flow (through the delivery or removal of the substance). The rate of diffusion (J_s) is described as *flow-limited*.

$$J_s = (C_a - C_i)\dot{Q}$$

where C_a is the concentration of the substance in the arterial blood, C_i is the concentration of the substance in the interstitium, and $\dot{Q}$ is the rate of blood flow. Flow-limited diffusion has potentially important implications for oxygen delivery in the setting of decreased oxygen delivery (e.g., cardiogenic shock or during severe exercise when flow rates are so high that diffusion is limited). However, most substances have intermediate endothelial permeability, and the rate of diffusion depends on endothelial permeability and flow (Renkin, 1989).

Most solutes, including small lipophilic and hydrophilic molecules and macromolecules, move through membranes of exchange vessels by diffusion. The route of diffusion depends on the type of membrane (continuous, fenestrated, discontinuous, and tight-junction) and the characteristics of the substance (e.g., lipid soluble, ionic, large macromolecule). Water diffuses through the endothelium primarily through intercellular clefts (Curry, 1984; Michel, 1984, 1988). Lipid-soluble substances, such as O_2, CO_2, and anesthetic gases, which pass easily through the lipid bilayer of the microvascular wall, diffuse relatively rapidly through the endothelium. Small hydrophilic solutes, such as ions and simple sugars, pass primarily through fenestrae, junctions between cells, or intracellular clefts (Curry, 1984; Michel, 1996; Simionescu & Simionescu, 1984). The primary mode of macromolecular transport is through vesicles or possibly large pores (Michel, 1996). The transport or movement of the macromolecules into the interstitium contributes to interstitial oncotic pressure.

Ultrafiltration

Starling's hypothesis of microvascular fluid exchange is described by the following equation (Landis, 1927; Levick, 1991; Michel, 1997; Renkin, 1986; Starling, 1896):

$$J_v/A = L_p ([P_c - P_i] - \sigma[\pi_c = \pi_i])$$

J_v/A = fluid filtration across the capillary wall per unit area
L_p = hydraulic permeability of the capillary wall
P_c = global value for capillary pressure
P_i = global value for interstitial pressure
σ = osmotic reflection coefficient

π_c = global value for capillary oncotic pressure
π_i = global value for interstitial oncotic pressure

In Starling's initial conceptualization of ultrafiltration, it was thought that at the arterial end of the capillary, the net forces favored the movement of fluid out of the vessel (filtration). Somewhere in the middle of the vessel, an equilibrium point was reached at which there was neither a gain nor a loss of fluid. Finally, on the venous end of the exchange vessel, the net forces favored reabsorption. Although the validity of Starling's equation has been repeatedly confirmed, the conceptualization of upstream filtration and downstream reabsorption has been questioned (Levick, 1997; Michel, 1997). In general, the forces opposing filtration (see later) do not exceed capillary pressure, and filtration occurs along the entire length of the exchange vessel (Levick, 1991, 1997). The net filtration is necessary to wash out the proteins that are continuously diffusing out of the vessels into the interstitium (Aukland & Reed, 1993; Levick, 1997) The ultrafiltrate and proteins that cross the vessel wall into the interstitial fluid are subsequently removed by the lymphatic system (Levick, 1991).

The primary direction of ultrafiltration is out of the vessel (filtration versus reabsorption), with the rate of fluid movement across a short segment of exchange vessel (J_v/A) having a curvilinear relationship to the net pressure difference (i.e., limited fluid movement at low P_c) across the vessel wall (Michel, 1997). In Starling's initial conceptualization, the net pressure difference reflected the algebraic sum of four pressures: intravascular (capillary) pressure (P_c), interstitial fluid pressure (P_i), plasma oncotic pressure (π_c), and interstitial oncotic pressure (π_i). The true pressure opposing filtration (P_o) is not simply plasma oncotic pressure, but rather oncotic plasma pressure minus interstitial oncotic pressure plus interstitial hydrostatic pressure and the reflection coefficient:

$$P_o = \sigma\,(\pi_p - \pi_i) + P_i$$

However, recent studies indicate that the effective oncotic force that opposes fluid filtration across the microvessel wall is the local oncotic pressure difference across the endothelial surface glycocalyx (the structure that covers the entire capillary endothelium and is the primary filter for proteins) and not the global difference between the oncotic pressure in the plasma and tissue (Hu & Weinbaum, 1999; Michel, 1997). Models of this new conceptualization suggest that the oncotic pressure opposing filtration is greater than estimated from blood-tissue protein concentration differences, and transcapillary fluid flux is smaller than predicted from the original Starling equation. Therefore, in the aforementioned Starling equation, the pressures P_i and π_i are the local hydrostatic pressure behind the glycocalyx and oncotic pressure on the tissue side of the matrix layer, respectively, and not the values from the tissue space (Hu & Weinbaum, 1999).

Capillary pressure (P_c) is the primary force behind filtration. Mean capillary pressure (P_c) is determined by the arterial and venous pressures and the ratio of postcapillary resistance (R_v) to precapillary resistance (R_a), as described by the following equation (Pappenheimer & Soto-Rivera, 1948):

$$P_c = \frac{(P_v + P_a) \times (R_v/R_a)}{1 + (R_v/R_a)}$$

where P_v is venous pressure, P_a is arterial pressure, R_v is postcapillary midpoint resistance, and R_a is precapillary midpoint resistance (where $R_v + R_a = R_{Total}$). An increase in either P_a or P_v results in an increase in P_c, unless counteracted by a decrease in the R_v/R_a ratio. The lower the R_v/R_a ratio (i.e., increased precapillary resistance or decreased postcapillary resistance), the lower the capillary pressure. It is the adjustment in R_v/R_a ratio, primarily through regulation of precapillary resistance (R_a) in the skeletal muscle and skin, that constitutes the primary effector mechanism for the central nervous system-mediated control of plasma volume (Aukland & Nicolaysen, 1981; Groebe, 1996; Mellander, 1978). However, the centrally mediated decrease in mean capillary pressure occurs only to the extent allowed by local autoregulatory adjustments.

In response to hypovolemic hypotension, compensatory precapillary vasoconstriction (increased R_a) decreases the mean P_c, and the net pressure in the downstream (venous) segment of the exchange vessel favors transient reabsorption (Fig. 2-18).

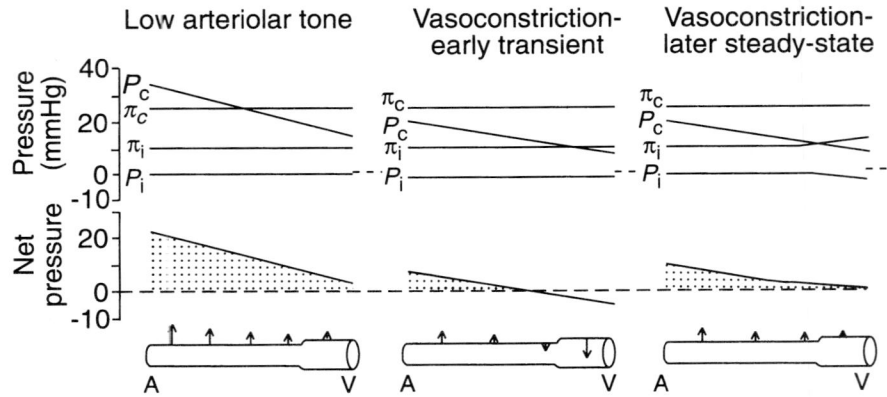

■ **Figure 2–18.** (*Top*) Axial gradient of four Starling pressures. (*Middle*) Net pressure. (*Bottom*) Direction of fluid flux. (*Left*) Control values. (*Middle*) Precapillary constriction lowers capillary pressure, resulting in transient fluid absorption. (*Right*) Final steady state (filtration) after interstitial fluid pressure and oncotic pressure have readjusted. P_c, capillary hydrostatic pressure; P_i, tissue hydrostatic pressure, π_c, capillary oncotic pressure; π_i, tissue oncotic pressure; A, arterial end of capillary; V, venular end of capillary. (From Levick, J.R. [1991]. Capillary filtration-absorption balance reconsidered in light of dynamic extravascular factors. *Experimental Physiology, 76,* 846.)

This autotransfusion is the result of a change in the ratio of the postcapillary to precapillary resistance on mean capillary pressure (Lanne & Lundvall, 1992). Of note, this response is decreased in older individuals, which may impair their response to orthostasis or hemorrhage (Olsen et al., 2000).

In addition to the hydrostatic and oncotic forces, two other factors affect fluid movement across the exchange vessel: the hydraulic conductivity of the wall (L_p) and the reflection coefficient (σ). Hydraulic conductivity is a measure of the permeability of the exchange vessel to fluid, with the highest L_p values for fenestrated endothelia and lowest for tight-junction endothelia (Renkin, 1989). Hydraulic conductivity is difficult to measure and is estimated by the capillary filtration coefficient. The capillary filtration coefficient, which is equal to the product of hydraulic conductivity and the available area (L_pA), is expressed as milliliters of net filtrate formed in 100 g of tissue per minute for each milliliter increase in mean capillary filtration pressure ($ml \times min^{-1} mm\,Hg^{-1} \times 100\,g^{-1}$). The capillary filtration coefficient is a useful indicator of capillary permeability (Aukland & Reed, 1993). A decrease in the capillary filtration coefficient, for example by a decrease in the area available for exchange, reduces the rate of net capillary filtration for any given net filtration pressure. The second factor, the reflection coefficient (σ), represents the osmotic pressure exerted by a difference in the concentration gradient of a substance across a membrane (oncotic effect of the concentration gradient) and is affected by the ratio of the solute size to pore size. The greater the ratio, the greater the reflection coefficient (Levick, 1991).

The reflection coefficient is close to 1 for tight-junction endothelium, which is completely impermeable to protein. In normal systemic exchange vessels in the skin and skeletal muscle, with continuous or fenestrated endothelium, the reflection coefficient ranges from 0.8 to 0.95 for albumin and total protein (Aukland & Reed, 1993; Levick, 1997), which indicates that these vessels are not completely impermeable to proteins (Levick, 1991; Michel, 1988; Renkin, 1989). In the lungs, the reflection coefficients are, in general, lower for albumin (0.5 to 0.6) and protein (0.5 to 0.7) (Aukland & Reed, 1993). In cases of injury to the endothelium, the reflection coefficient is markedly reduced, allowing increased movement of large molecules (e.g., protein) out of the exchange vessels.

THE LYMPHATIC SYSTEM

Removal of fluid and plasma proteins from the interstitium by the terminal lymphatics is essential in the maintenance of an equilibrium in microvascular-interstitial exchange (Levick, 1991). Depending on the protein concentration in the lymph, 8 to 12 L/d of lymph, which reflects net filtration caused by movement of fluid out of the vascular bed, is removed from the interstitium by the lymphatic system (Levick, 1991; Renkin, 1986) (see Fig. 2-3). Approximately 4 to 8 L of the ultrafiltrate is directly reabsorbed from the lymphatic vessels back into the blood vessels, and the remaining 4 L of efferent lymph, which includes all of the filtered protein, is delivered back to the central circulation (Aukland & Reed, 1993; Renkin, 1986). These findings are relatively new and indicate that lymph flow

is two-times greater than previously thought. This high level of lymphatic flow supports the idea that filtration (return of lymph to the systemic vasculature) occurs along the entire length of lymphatic bed and not just in the central circulation.

REFERENCES

Alonso, D., & Radomski, M. W. (2003). The nitric oxide-endothelin-1 connection. *Heart Failure Review*, 8(1), 107–115.
Aukland, K., & Nicolaysen, G. (1981). Interstitial fluid volume: local regulatory mechanisms. *Physiological Reviews*, 61, 556–643.
Aukland, K., & Reed, R. (1993). Interstitial-lymphatic mechanisms in the control of extracellular fluid volume. *Physiological Reviews*, 73(1), 1–78.
Badeer, H. (2001). Hemodynamics for medical patients. *Advances in Physiological Education*, 25(1–4), 44–52.
Behrendt, D., & Ganz, P. (2002). Endothelial function. From vascular biology to clinical applications. *American Journal Cardiology*, 90(10C), 40L–48L.
Belz, G. G. (1995). Elastic properties and Windkessel function of the human aorta. *Cardiovascular Drugs and Therapy*, 9(1), 73–83.
Berg, B. R., & Sarelius, I. H. (1995). Functional capillary organization in striated muscle. *American Journal of Physiology*, 268(3 Pt 2), H1215–1222.
Berlan, M., Galitzky, J., Bousquet-Melou, A., Lafontan, M., & Montastruc, J. L. (1994). Beta-3 adrenoreceptor-mediated increase in cutaneous blood flow in dog. *Journal Pharmacology and Experimental Therapeutics*, 268(3), 1444–1451.
Berlan, M., Galitzky, J., & Montastruc, J. L. (1995). Beta 3-adrenoceptors in the cardiovascular system. *Fundamental and Clinical Pharmacology*, 9(3), 234–239.
Berridge, M. (1993). Inositol triphosphate and calcium signalling. *Nature*, 361, 315–325.
Berridge, M. (1997). Elementary and global aspects of calcium signalling. *Journal of Experimental Biology*, 200, 315–319.
Berridge, M. (2002). The endoplasmic reticulum: a multifunctional signalling organelle. *Cell Calcium*, 32(5–6), 235–249.
Berridge, M., Lipp, P., & Bootman, M. (1999). Calcium signalling. *Current Biology*, 9(5), R157–159.
Best, P. J., & Lerman, A. (2000). Endothelin in cardiovascular disease: from atherosclerosis to heart failure. *Journal of Cardiovascular Pharmacology*, 35(4 Suppl 2), S61–63.
Bing, R. J. (2001). Myocardial ischemia and infarction: growth of ideas. *Cardiovascular Research*, 51(1), 13–20.
Bootman, M. D., Berridge, M. J., & Roderick, H. L. (2002). Calcium signalling: more messengers, more channels, more complexity. *Current Biology*, 12(16), R563–565.
Boulpaep, E. (2003). Arteries and veins. In W. Boron & E. Boulpaep (Eds.), *Medical physiology: A cellular and molecular approach* (pp. 447–462). Philadelphia: Saunders.
Busse, R., Edwards, G., Feletou, M., Fleming, I., Vanhoutte, P. M., & Weston, A. H. (2002). EDHF: bringing the concepts together. *Trends in Pharmacological Sciences*, 23(8), 374–380.
Charkoudian, N. (2003). Skin blood flow in adult human thermoregulation: How it works, when it does not, and why. *Mayo Clinics Proceeding*, 78(5), 603–612.
Christensen, K. L., & Mulvany, M. J. (2001). Location of resistance arteries. *Journal of Vascular Research*, 38(1), 1–12.
Civantos Calzada, B., & Aleixandre de Artinano, A. (2001). Alpha-adrenoceptor subtypes. *Pharmacological Research*, 44(3), 195–208.
Cohen, R. (2000). Role of nitric oxide in vasomotor regulation. In J. Loscalzo, & J. Vita (Eds.), *Contemporary cardiology: Nitric oxide and the cardiovascular system* (Vol. 4, pp. 105–122). Totowa, NJ: Humana Press.
Cohen, R., & Vanhoutte, P. (1995). Endothelium-dependent hyperpolarization. Beyond nitric oxide and cyclic GMP. *Circulation*, 92(11), 3337–3349.
Cohen, R., Weisbrod, R., Gericke, M., Yaghoubi, M., Bierl, C., & Bolotina, V. (1999). Mechanism of nitric oxide-induced vasodilatation: refilling of intracellular stores by sarcoplasmic reticulum Ca2+ ATPase and inhibition of store-operated Ca2+ influx. *Circulation Research*, 84(2), 210–219.
Coller, B. (1997). GPIIb/IIIa antagonists: pathophysiologic and therapeutic insights from studies of c7E3Fab. *Thrombosis and Haemostasis*, 78(1), 730–735.
Conrad, M. (1971). *Functional anatomy of the circulation of the lower extremities*. Chicago: Year Book.

Criado, E., Daniel, P., Marston, W., Mansfield, D., & Keagy, B. (1995). Physiologic variations in lower extremity venous valvular function. *Annals of Vascular Surgery*, 9(1), 102–108.

Crone, E., & Levitt, D. (1984). Capillary permeability to small solutes. In E. Renkin & C. Michel (Eds.), *Handbook of physiology* (Sec. 2, Vol. IV. *Microcirculation*, pp. 411–466). Bethesda: American Physiological Society.

Curry, R. (1984). Mechanics and thermodynamics of transcapillary exchange. In E. Renkin & C. Michel (Eds.), *Handbook of physiology* (Sec. 2, Vol. IV. *Microcirculation*, pp. 309–374). Bethesda, MD: American Physiological Society.

Davidge, S. T. (2001). Prostaglandin H synthase and vascular function. *Circulation Research*, 89(8), 650–660.

del Monte, F., Kaumann, A., & Poole-Wilson, P. (1993). Coexistence of functioning beta-1 and beta-2 adrenoreceptors in single myocytes from human ventricle. *Circulation*, 88, 854–863.

Duchman, S. M., Thohan, V., Kalra, D., & Torre-Amione, G. (2000). Endothelin-1: A new target of therapeutic intervention for the treatment of heart failure. *Current Opinion in Cardiology*, 15(3), 136–140.

Duling, B. (1981). Coordination of microcirculatory function with oxygen demand in skeletal muscle. In A. Kovach, J. Hamar, & L. Szabo (Eds.), *Advances in physiology: Cardiovascular physiology: Microcirculation and capillary exchange* (Vol. 7, pp. 1–16). Budapest: Akademiai Kaido.

Duling, B. R., & Klitzman, B. (1980). Local control of microvascular function: role in tissue oxygen supply. *Annual Review of Physiology*, 42, 373–382.

Dzau, V. J., Bernstein, K., Celermajer, D., Cohen, J., Dahlof, B., Deanfield, J., et al. (2002). Pathophysiologic and therapeutic importance of tissue ACE: a consensus report. *Cardiovascular Drugs and Therapy*, 16(2), 149–160.

Faber, J. (1988). In situ analysis of alpha-adrenoreceptors on arteriolar and venular smooth muscle in rat skeletal muscle microcirculation. *Circulation Research*, 62(1), 37–50.

Feigl, E. O. (1998). Neural control of coronary blood flow. *Journal of Vascular Research*, 35(2), 85–92.

Feletou, M., & Vanhoutte, P. M. (1999). The third pathway: endothelium-dependent hyperpolarization. *Journal Physiology and Pharmacology*, 50(4), 525–534.

Feletou, M., & Vanhoutte, P. M. (2000). Endothelium-dependent hyperpolarization of vascular smooth muscle cells. *Acta Pharmacologica Sinica*, 21(1), 1–18.

FitzGerald, G. A. (2002). Cardiovascular pharmacology of nonselective nonsteroidal anti-inflammatory drugs and coxibs: clinical considerations. *American Journal Cardiology*, 89(6A), 26D–32D.

FitzGerald, G. A., Cheng, Y., & Austin, S. (2001). COX-2 inhibitors and the cardiovascular system. *Clinical Experience in Rheumatology*, 19(6 (Suppl 5), S31–36.

Flavahan, N., Cooke, J., Shepherd, J., & Vanhoutte, P. (1987). Human postjunctional alpha-1 and alpha-2 adrenoreceptors: differential distribution in arteries and limbs. *Journal Pharmacology and Experimental Therapeutics*, 241(2), 361–365.

Furchott, R., & Zawadzki, J. (1980). The obligatory role of endothelial cells in the relaxation of arterial smooth muscle by acetylcholine. *Nature*, 288, 373–376.

Gallagher, D., & O'Rourke, M. (1993). What is the arterial pressure? In M. O'Rourke, M. Safar, & V. Dzau (Eds.), *Arterial vasodilation: Mechanisms and therapy* (pp. 134–148). Philadelphia: Lea & Febiger.

Gashev, A. A. (2002). Physiologic aspects of lymphatic contractile function: current perspectives. *Annals of the New York Academy of Sciences*, 979, 178–187; discussion 188–196.

Gauthier, C., Leblais, V., Kobzik, L., Trochu, J., Khandoudi, N., Bril, A., et al. (1998). The negative inotropic effect of B3-Adrenoreceptor stimulation is mediated by activation of nitric oxide synthase pathway in human ventricle. *Journal Clinical Investigation*, 102, 1377–1384.

Gauthier, C., Tavernier, G., Charpentier, F., Langin, D., & Le Marec, H. (1996). Functional beta3-adrenoreceptor in the human heart. *Journal Clinical Investigation*, 98(2), 556–562.

Griffin, K. L., Woodman, C. R., Price, E. M., Laughlin, M. H., & Parker, J. L. (2001). Endothelium-mediated relaxation of porcine collateral-dependent arterioles is improved by exercise training. *Circulation*, 104(12), 1393–1398.

Groebe, K. (1996). Precapillary servo control of blood pressure and postcapillary adjustment of flow to tissue metabolic status. A new paradigm for local perfusion regulation. *Circulation*, 94(8), 1876–1885.

Guzik, T. J., Mussa, S., Gastaldi, D., et al. (2002). Mechanisms of increased vascular superoxide production in human diabetes mellitus: role of NAD(P)H oxidase and endothelial nitric oxide synthase. *Circulation*, 105(14), 1656–1662.

Hai, C., & Murphy, R. (1988). Cross-bridges phosphorylation and regulation of latch state in smooth muscle. *American Journal Physiology*, 254, C99–C106.

Hainsworth, R. (1986). Vascular capacitance: its control and importance. *Reviews of Physiology Biochemistry and Pharmacology*, 105, 101–173.

Harrison, D., Griendling, K. K., Landmesser, U., Hornig, B., & Drexler, H. (2003). Role of oxidative stress in atherosclerosis. *American Journal of Cardiology*, 91(3A), 7A–11A.

Heydrick, s. (2000). Cellular signal transduction and nitric oxide. In J. Loscalzo & J. Vita (Eds.), *Contemporary cardiology: Nitric oxide and the cardiovascular system* (Vol. 4, pp. 33–49). Totowa, NJ: Humana Press.

Hlastala, M., & Berger, A. (2001). *Physiology of respiration*. New York: Oxford University Press.

Hornig, B., Landmesser, U., Kohler, C., Ahlersmann, D., Spiekermann, S., Christoph, A., et al. (2001). Comparative effect of ace inhibition and angiotensin II type 1 receptor antagonism on bioavailability of nitric oxide in patients with coronary artery disease: role of superoxide dismutase. *Circulation*, 103(6), 799–805.

Horowitz, A., Menice, C., Laporte, R., & Morgan, K. (1996). Mechanisms of smooth muscle contraction. *Physiological Reviews*, 76(4), 967–1003.

Hosoi, Y., Zukowski, A., Kakkos, S., & Nicolaides, A. N. (2002). Ambulatory venous pressure measurements: new parameters derived from a mathematic hemodynamic model. *Journal of Vascular Surgery*, 36(1), 137–142.

Hu, X., & Weinbaum, S. (1999). A new view of Starling's Hypothesis at the microstructural level. *Microvascular Research*, 58(3), 281–304.

Hudlicka, O. (1985). Regulation of muscle blood flow. *Clinical Physiology*, 5(3), 201–229.

Ignarro, L. J. (1989). Biological actions and properties of endothelium-derived nitric oxide formed and released from artery and vein. *Circulation Research*, 65(1), 1–21.

Ignarro, L. J., Buga, G. M., Wood, K. S., Byrns, R. E., & Chaudhuri, G. (1987). Endothelium-derived relaxing factor produced and released from artery and vein is nitric oxide. *Proceedings of the National Academy of Sciences of the United States of America*, 84(24), 9265–9269.

Ignarro, L. J., Napoli, C., & Loscalzo, J. (2002). Nitric oxide donors and cardiovascular agents modulating the bioactivity of nitric oxide: an overview. *Circulation Research*, 90(1), 21–28.

Iida, N. (1999). Nitric oxide mediates sympathetic vasoconstriction at supraspinal, spinal, and synaptic levels. *American Journal of Physiology*, 276(3), H918–H925.

Jneid, H., Bhatt, D., Corti, R., Badimon, J., Fuster, V., & Francis, G. (2003). Aspirin and clopedigrol in acute coronary syndromes: therapeutic insights from the CURE study. *Archives of Internal Medicine*, 163(10), 1145–1153.

Johnson, J. (1989). Circulation to the skin. In H. Patton, A. Fuchs, B. Hille, A. Scher, & R. Steiner (Eds.), *Textbook of physiology* (21st ed., Vol. 2, pp. 898–910). Philadelphia: W.B. Saunders.

Kable, J., Murrin, L., & Bylund, D. B. (2000). In vivo gene modification elucidates subtype-specific functions of alpha (2)-adrenergic receptors. *Journal of Pharmacology and Experimental Therapeutics*, 293(1), 1–7.

Kaddoura, S., & Poole-Wilson, P. (1996). Endothelin-1 in heart failure: A new therapeutic target? *Lancet*, 348(9025), 418–419.

Kojda, G., & Harrison, D. (1999). Interactions between NO and reactive oxygen species: Pathophysiological importance in atherosclerosis, hypertension, diabetes and heart failure. *Cardiovascular Research*, 43(3), 562–571.

Koller, A., & Bagi, Z. (2002). On the role of mechanosensitive mechanisms eliciting reactive hyperemia. *American Journal of Physiology*, 283(6), H2250–2259.

Koller, A., Dornyei, G., & Kaley, G. (1998). Flow-induced responses in skeletal muscle venules: modulation by nitric oxide and prostaglandins. *American Journal of Physiology*, 275(3 Pt 2), H831–836.

Koller, A., & Kaley, G. (1998). Shear stress-induced dilation of arterioles. *American Journal of Physiology*, 274(1 Pt 2), H382–383.

Komalavilas, P., & Lincoln, T. (2000). Regulation of intracellular $Ca+2$ by cyclic GMP-dependent protein kinase in vascular smooth muscle. In P. J. Kadowitz & D. McNamara (Eds.), *Nitric oxide and the regulation of peripheral circulation* (pp. 15–32). Boston: Birkhauser.

Konstam, M. A., & Weir, M. R. (2002). Current perspective on the cardiovascular effects of coxibs. *Cleveland Clinic Journal of Medicine*, 69 Suppl 1, SI47–52.

Krum, H., Goldsmith, R., Wilshire-Clement, M., Miller, M., & Packer, M. (1995). Role of endothelin in the exercise intolerance of chronic heart failure. *American Journal Cardiology*, 75, 1282–1283.

Landis, E. (1927). Micro-injection studies of capillary permeability II. *American Journal of Physiology*, 82(2), 217–238.

Landmesser, U., Merten, R., Spiekermann, S., Buttner, K., Drexler, H., & Hornig, B. (2000). Vascular extracellular superoxide dismutase activity in patients with coronary artery disease: relation to endothelium-dependent vasodilation. *Circulation*, 101(19), 2264–2270.

Lands, A. M., Arnold, A., McAuliff, J. P., Luduena, F. P., & Brown, T. G., Jr. (1967). Differentiation of receptor systems activated by sympathomimetic amines. *Nature*, 214(88), 597–598.

Lanne, T., & Lundvall, J. (1992). Mechanisms in man for rapid refill of the circulatory system in hypovolaemia. *Acta Physiologica Scandinavia*, 146(3), 299–306.

Lavallee, M., Takamura, M., Parent, R., & Thorin, E. (2001). Crosstalk between endothelin and nitric oxide in the control of vascular tone. *Heart Failure Review*, 6(4), 265–276.

Leech, C. J., & Faber, J. E. (1996). Different alpha-adrenoceptor subtypes mediate constriction of arterioles and venules. *American Journal of Physiology*, 270(2 Pt 2), H710–722.

Levick, J. (1991). Capillary filtration-absorption balance reconsidered in light of dynamic extravascular factors. *Experimental Physiology*, 76(6), 825–857.

Levick, J. (1997). Fluid exchange across the endothelium. *International Journal of Microcirculation: Clinical and Experimental*, 17(5), 241–247.

Levitzky, M. (1995). *Pulmonary physiology* (4th ed.). New York: McGraw-Hill.

London, G. M., & Guerin, A. P. (1999). Influence of arterial pulse and reflected waves on blood pressure and cardiac function. *American Heart Journal*, 138(3 Pt 2), 220–224.

Loscalzo, J. (2001). Nitric oxide insufficiency, platelet activation, and arterial thrombosis. *Circulation Research*, 88(8), 756–762.

Luscher, T., Oemar, B., Boulanger, B., & Hahn, A. (1996). Molecular and cellular biology of endothelin and its receptors. In K. Lindpainter & D. Ganten (Eds.), *Molecular reviews* (pp. 96–104). London: Chapman & Hall.

Lüscher, T., & Vanhoutte, P. (1990). *The endothelium: Modulation of cardiovascular function*. Boca Raton, FL: CRC Inc.

Luscher, T. F. (1991). Endothelium-derived nitric oxide: the endogenous nitrovasodilator in the human cardiovascular system. *European Heart Journal*, 12 Suppl E, 2–11.

Marin, J., Encabo, A., Briones, A., Garcia-Cohen, E., & Alonso, M. (1999). Mechanisms involved in the cellular calcium homeostasis in vascular smooth muscle: calcium pumps. *Life Sciences*, 64(5), 279–303.

Marshall, J. M. (2002). Roles of adenosine in skeletal muscle during systemic hypoxia. *Clinical and Experimental Pharmacology and Physiology*, 29(9), 843–849.

McHugh, J., & Cheek, D. J. (1998). Nitric oxide and regulation of vascular tone: pharmacological and physiological considerations. *American Journal of Critical Care*, 7(2), 131–140; quiz 141–132.

Mellander, S. (1978). On the control of capillary fluid transfer by precapillary and postcapillary vascular adjustment. *Microvascular Research*, 15, 319–330.

Michel, C. (1984). Fluid movements through capillary walls. In E. Renkin & C. Michel (Eds.), *Handbook of physiology* (Sec. 2, Vol. IV. *Microcirculation*, pp. 375–409). Bethesda, MD: American Physiological Society.

Michel, C. (1988). Capillary permeability and how it may change. *Journal of Physiology*, 404, 1–29.

Michel, C. (1996). Transport of macromolecules through microvascular walls. *Cardiovascular Research*, 32(4), 644–653.

Michel, C. (1997). Starling: the formulation of his hypothesis of microvascular fluid exchange and its significance after 100 years. *Experimental Physiology*, 82(1), 1–30.

Minami, A., Ishimura, N., Harada, N., Sakamoto, S., Niwa, Y., & Nakaya, Y. (2002). Exercise training improves acetylcholine-induced endothelium-dependent hyperpolarization in type 2 diabetic rats, Otsuka Long-Evans Tokushima fatty rats. *Atherosclerosis*, 162(1), 85–92.

Mohrman, D., & Heller, J. M. (2003). *Cardiovascular physiology* (5th ed.). New York: Lange Medical Books/McGraw-Hill.

Mombouli, J. V., & Vanhoutte, P. M. (1999). Endothelial dysfunction: from physiology to therapy. *Journal of Molecular and Cellular Cardiology*, 31(1), 61–74.

Moncada, S., Palmer, R., & Higgs, E. (1991). Nitric oxide: Physiology, pathophysiology, and pharmacology. *Pharmacological Reviews*, 43(2), 109–142.

Moniotte, S., Kobzik, L., Feron, O., Trochu, J., Gauthier, C., & Ballingand, J. (2001). Upregulation of beta(3)-adrenoreceptors and altered contractile response to inotropic amines in human failing myocardium. *Circulation*, 103(12), 1649–1655.

Mulvany, M. (1996). The Seventh Heymans Memorial Lecture Ghent, February 18, 1995. Physiological aspects of small arteries. *Archives Internationales de Pharmacodynamie et de Therapie*, 331(1), 1–31.

Mulvany, M., & Aalkjeær, C. (1990). Structure and function of small arteries. *Physiological Reviews*, 70(4), 922–961.

Murphy, R. (1994). What is special about smooth muscle? The significance of covalent crossbridge regulation. *FASEB*, 8, 311–318.

Murray, P. T., Wylam, M. E., & Umans, J. G. (2000). Nitric oxide and septic vascular dysfunction. *Anesthesia Analgesia*, 90(1), 89–101.

Naruko, T., Ueda, M., van der Wal, A. C., van der Loos, C. M., Itoh, H., Nakao, K., et al. (1996). C-type natriuretic peptide in human coronary atherosclerotic lesions. *Circulation*, 94(12), 3103–3108.

Olsen, H., Vernersson, E., & Lanne, T. (2000). Cardiovascular response to acute hypovolemia in relation to age. Implications for orthostasis and hemorrhage. *American Journal of Physiology*, 278(1), H222–232.

Olszewski, W. L. (2002). Contractility patterns of normal and pathological changed human lymphatics. *Annals of the New York Academy of Sciences*, 979, 52–63; discussion 76–59.

Opie, L. (1998). *The heart: Physiology from cell to circulation*. Philadelphia: Lippincott-Raven.

O'Rourke, M. (1990a). The measurement of systemic blood pressure: normal and abnormal pulsations of the arteries and veins. In J. Hurst & R. Schlant (Eds.), *The heart arteries and veins* (7th ed., pp. 149–162). New York: McGraw-Hill.

O'Rourke, M. (1990b). What is blood pressure? *American Journal of Hypertension*, 3(10), 803–810.

Palmer, R., Ferrige, A., & Moncada, S. (1987). Nitric oxide release accounts for the biological activity of endothelium-derived relaxing factor. *Nature*, 327, 524–526.

Pappenheimer, J., & Soto-Rivera, A. (1948). Effective osmotic pressure of the plasma proteins and other quantities associated with capillary circulation in the hindlimbs of cats and dogs. *American Journal of Physiology*, 152(3), 471–491.

Patterson, A., Henrie-Olsen, J., & Brenner, R. (2002). Vasoregulation at the molecular level: a role for the beta1 subunit of the calcium-activated potassium (BK) channel. *Trends in Cardiovascular Medicine*, 12(2), 78–82.

Puddu, P., Puddu, G. M., Zaca, F., & Muscari, A. (2000). Endothelial dysfunction in hypertension. *Acta Cardiologica*, 55(4), 221–232.

Raju, S., Fredericks, R., Lishman, P., Neglen, P., & Morano, J. (1993). Observations on the calf venous pump mechanism: Determinants of postexercise pressure. *Journal of Vascular Surgery*, 17(3), 459–469.

Ralevic, V. (2002). Hypoxic vasodilatation: is an adenosine-prostaglandins-NO signalling cascade involved? *Journal of Physiology*, 544(Pt 1), 2.

Ray, C. J., Abbas, M. R., Coney, A. M., & Marshall, J. M. (2002). Interactions of adenosine, prostaglandins and nitric oxide in hypoxia-induced vasodilatation: in vivo and in vitro studies. *Journal of Physiology*, 544(Pt 1), 195–209.

Renkin, E. (1977). Multiple pathways of capillary permeability. *Circulation Research*, 41, 735–743.

Renkin, E. (1984). Control of microcirculation and blood-tissue exchange. In E. Renkin & C. Michel (Eds.), *Handbook of physiology* (Vol. IV, Part 2, pp. 627–687). Bethesda: American Physiological Society.

Renkin, E. (1986). Some consequences of capillary permeability to macromolecules: Starling's hypothesis reconsidered. *American Journal of Physiology*, 250, H706–H710.

Renkin, E. (1989). Microcirculation and exchange. In H. Patton, A. Fuches, B. Hille, A. Scher, & R. Steiner (Eds.), *Textbook of physiology* (21st ed., Vol. 2, pp. 860–878). Philadelphia: WB Saunders.

Rhodin, J. (1980). Architecture of the vessel wall. In H. Sparks (Ed.), *Handbook of physiology* (Sec. 2, Vol. 2, pp. 1–31). Bethesda, MD: American Physiological Society.

Rhodin, J. (1981). Anatomy of the microcirculation. In J. Ditzel (Ed.), *Microcirculation* (pp. 11–17). New York: Academic Press.

Roks, A. J. (2002). Improvement of endothelium-derived hyperpolarizing factor function by renin-angiotensin system inhibition: paving the way towards prevention of age-related endothelial dysfunction. *Journal of Hypertension*, 20(3), 363–365.

Ross, R., & Glomset, J. (1976). The pathogenesis of atherosclerosis. *New England Journal of Medicine*, 295(7), 369–377.

Rothe, C. (1983). Venous system: physiology of the capacitance vessels. In F. Abboud (Ed.), *Handbook of physiology. The cardiovascular system. Peripheral circulation and organ blood flow* (Sec. 2, Vol. III, Part 1, pp. 397–452). Bethesda, MD: American Physiological Society.

Rowell, L. (1986). *Human circulation: Regulation during physical stress*. New York: Oxford University Press.

Rowell, L. (1993). *Human cardiovascular control*. New York: Oxford University Press.

Rowell, L. B., O'Leary, D. S., & Kellogg, D. L. J. (1996). Integration of cardiovascular control systems in dynamic exercise. In J. Sheperd (Ed.), *Handbook of physiology, exercise: Regulation and integration of multiple systems* (Sec. 12, pp. 770–838). Bethesda MD: Oxford University Press.

Sarelius, I. H., Cohen, K. D., & Murrant, C. L. (2000). Role for capillaries in coupling blood flow with metabolism. *Clinical and Experimental Pharmacology and Physiology*, 27(10), 826–829.

Sarkar, R., & Webb, R. C. (1998). Does nitric oxide regulate smooth muscle cell proliferation? A critical appraisal. *Journal of Vascular Research*, 35(3), 135–142.

Scher, A. (1989). The veins and venous return. In H. Patton, A. Fuchs, & B. Hille (Eds.), *Textbook of physiology* (21st ed., Vol. 2, pp. 879–886). Philadelphia: WB Saunders.

Schiffrin, E. L., & Touyz, R. M. (1998). Vascular biology of endothelin. *Journal of Cardiovascular Pharmacology*, 32 Suppl 3, S2–13.

Schmid-Schonbein, G. (1990). Microlymphatics and lymph flow. *Physiological Reviews*, 70(4), 987–1028.

Sheperd, J. (1983). Circulation to skeletal muscle. In J. Sheperd, F. M. Abboud, & J. P. Geiger (Eds.), *Handbook of physiology: The cardiovascular system: Peripheral circulation and organ blood flow* (Sec. 2, Vol. III [Part I], pp. 319–370). Bethesda, MD: American Physiological Society.

Sheperd, J., & Vanhoutte, P. (1979). *The human cardiovascular system: Facts and concepts*. New York: Raven Press.

Shimokawa, H., Yasutake, H., Fujii, K., Owada, M. K., Nakaike, R., Fukumoto, Y., et al. (1996). The importance of the hyperpolarizing mechanism increases as the vessel size decreases in endothelium-dependent relaxations in rat mesenteric circulation. *Journal of Cardiovascular Pharmacology*, 28(5), 703–711.

Simionescu, M., & Simionescu, N. (1984). Ultrastructure of the microvascular wall: Functional correlations. In E. Renkin, & C. Michel (Eds.), *Handbook of physiology: Microcirculation* (Sec. 2, Vol. IV, pp. 41–101). Bethesda, MD: American Physiological Society.

Small, J., & Gimona, M. (1998). The cytoskeleton of the vertebrate smooth muscle cell. *Acta Physiologica Scandinavia*, 164(4), 341–348.

Somlyo, A., & Somlyo, A. (1994). Signal transduction and regulation in smooth muscle. *Nature*, 372(17), 231–236.

Somlyo, A., & Somlyo, A. (2002). The sarcoplasmic reticulum: then and now. *Novartis Foundation Symposium*, 246, 258–268; discussion 268–271, 272–256.

Sparks, H. (1980). Effect of local metabolic factors on vascular smooth muscle. In D. Bohr, A. Somlyo, & H. Sparks (Eds.), *Handbook of physiology: The cardiovascular system: Vascular smooth muscle* (Sec. 2, Vol. II, pp. 475–513). Bethesda, MD: American Physiological Society.

Sperelakis, N., & Ohya, Y. (1990). Cyclic nucleotide regulation of Ca^{2+} slow channels and neurotransmitter release in vascular muscle. *Progress in Clinical and Biological Research*, 5(327), 277–298.

Sperelakis, N., Tohse, N., & Ohya, Y. (1992). Regulation of calcium slow channels in cardiac muscle and vascular smooth muscle cells. *Advances in Experimental Medicine Biology*, 311, 163–187.

Sperelakis, N., Tohse, N., Ohya, Y., & Masuda, H. (1994). Cyclic GMP regulation of calcium slow channels in cardiac muscle and vascular smooth muscle cells. *Advances in Pharmacology*, 26, 217–252.

Starling, E. (1896). On the absorption of fluids from the connective tissue spaces. *Journal of Physiology (Lond)*, 19, 312–316.

Sweeney, H. (1998). Regulation and tuning of smooth muscle myosin. *American Journal of Respiratory and Critical Care Medicine*, 158, S95–S99.

Taddei, S., Virdis, A., Mattei, P., Ghiadoni, L., Gennari, A., Fasolo, C. B., et al. (1995). Aging and endothelial function in normotensive subjects and patients with essential hypertension. *Circulation*, 91(7), 1981–1987.

Takamura, Y., Shimokawa, H., Zhao, H., Igarashi, H., Egashira, K., & Takeshita, A. (1999). Important role of endothelium-derived hyperpolarizing factor in shear stress—induced endothelium-dependent relaxations in the rat mesenteric artery. *Journal of Cardiovascular Pharmacology*, 34(3), 381–387.

Triggle, C. R., & Ding, H. (2002). Endothelium-derived hyperpolarizing factor: is there a novel chemical mediator? *Clinical and Experimental Pharmacology and Physiology*, 29(3), 153–160.

Trochu, J., Le Marec, H., Beverelli, F., Berdeaux, A., & Gauthier, C. (1997). Vasorelaxation induced by beta3-adrenoreceptor stimulation is mainly mediated by endothelium-derivated NO. *Circulation*, 96(8S), 676–I (abstract).

Trzewik, J., Mallipattu, S. K., Artmann, G. M., Delano, F. A., & Schmid-Schonbein, G. W. (2001). Evidence for a second valve system in lymphatics: endothelial microvalves. *FASEB Journal*, 15(10), 1711–1717.

Urakami-Harasawa, L., Shimokawa, H., Nakashima, M., Egashira, K., & Takeshita, A. (1997). Importance of endothelium-derived hyperpolarizing factor in human arteries. *Journal of Clinical Investigation*, 100(11), 2793–2799.

Van Helden, D. F., & Zhao, J. (2000). Lymphatic vasomotion. *Clinical and Experimental Pharmacology and Physiology*, 27(12), 1014–1018.

Vanhoutte, P., & Boulanger, C. (1995). Endothelium-dependent responses in hypertension. *Hypertension Research*, 18(2), 87–98.

Vanhoutte, P., & Mombouli, J. (1996). Vascular endothelium: vasoactive mediators. *Progress in Cardiovascular Disease*, 39(3), 229–238.

Vanhoutte, P. M. (1988). *Vasodilatation: Vascular smooth muscle, peptides, autonomic nerves, and endothelium*. New York: Raven Press.

Vanhoutte, P. M. (1997). Endothelial dysfunction and atherosclerosis. *European Heart Journal*, 18 Suppl E, E19–29.

Vanhoutte, P. M. (1999). How to assess endothelial function in human blood vessels. *Journal of Hypertension*, 17(8), 1047–1058.

Vanhoutte, P. M. (2000). Say NO to ET. *Journal of the Autonomic Nervous System*, 81(1–3), 271–277.

Varghese, P., Harrison, R., Lofthouse, R., Georgeakopolous, D., Berkowitz, D., & Hare, J. (2000). B3-adrenoreceptor deficiency blocks nitric oxide-dependent inhibition of myocardial contractility. *Journal of Clinical Investigation*, 106(5), 697–703.

Vivekananthan, D., Penn, M., Sapp, S., Hsu, A., & Topol, E. (2003). Use of antioxidant vitamins for the prevention of cardiovascular disease: meta-analysis of randomised trials. *Lancet*, 361(9374), 2017–2023.

Wiedeman, M. (1963). Dimensions of blood vessels from distributing artery to collecting vein. *Circulation Research*, 12, 375–378.

Wolburg, H., & Lippoldt, A. (2002). Tight junctions of the blood-brain barrier: development, composition and regulation. *Vasculare Pharmacology*, 38(6), 323–337.

Yanigisawa, M., Kurihara, H., & Kimura, S. (1988). A novel potent vasoconstrictor peptide produced by vascular endothelial cells. *Nature*, 332, 411–415.

Zusman, R. (1992). Eicosanoids: Prostaglandins, thromboxane, and prostacyclin. In H. Fozzard, E. Haber, R. Jennings, A. Katz, & E. Morgan (Eds.), *The heart and cardiovascular system* (Vol. 2, pp. 1797–1815). New York: Raven Press.

Zweifach, B., & Lipowsky, H. (1984). Pressure-flow relations in blood and lymph microcirculation. In E. Renkin, & C. Michel (Eds.), *Handbook of physiology* (Sec. 2, Vol. IV. *Microcirculation*, pp. 251–307). Bethesda, MD: American Physiological Society.

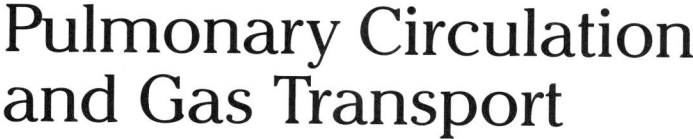

3

Pulmonary Circulation and Gas Transport

JOSEPH O. SCHMELZ • POLLY E. GARDNER

The pulmonary circulation removes oxygen from the atmosphere, transfers the oxygen to the blood via the alveoli, and exchanges carbon dioxide. Once oxygen has diffused from the alveoli to the pulmonary blood, the systemic circulation transports oxygen and nutrients from the gastrointestinal tract to the various tissues of the body. The systemic circulation also transports electrolytes, hormones, cells, and immune substances and carries waste products to the excretory organs for disposal.

Each tissue controls its internal environment depending on its specific needs. The amount of oxygen released into the tissues and the amount of carbon dioxide released from the tissues are regulated by tissue activity. Oxygen delivery or transport to a particular tissue depends on the amount of oxygen inspired during ventilation, the adequacy of pulmonary gas exchange, perfusion of blood flow to the tissues, and the capacity of the blood to carry oxygen (Guyton & Hall, 2001). The blood flow to a particular vascular bed depends on the cardiac output and the tone of the vascular bed. Thus, the chief aim of both circuits is to maintain a balance between oxygen consumption and delivery for the various tissues of the body.

This chapter completes the discussion of blood flow started in Chapter 2, Systemic Circulation, by addressing the anatomy and physiology of the pulmonary circulation, pulmonary gas exchange, and the transport of oxygen and carbon dioxide. See Table 3-1 for a summary of abbreviations in this chapter.

STRUCTURAL/ANATOMIC

Gross Anatomy

Pulmonary Circulation

The primary function of the pulmonary circulation is to expose the blood to alveolar air so that oxygen can be taken up by the blood and so carbon dioxide can be excreted. The pulmonary circulation is in series with the systemic circulation and receives the same cardiac output, approximately 5 to 6 L/min at rest for an adult weighing 70 kg. The pulmonary circulation has only 10% the capacity of the systemic circulation, yet it must accommodate the same ejected volume. No other single organ receives the entire output of one ventricle.

Although pulmonary blood flow is equal to that of the systemic system, its vascular resistance is seven to eight times lower than systemic resistance. Consequently, the pulmonary circulation has high blood flow and acts as a reservoir for the right ventricle. The pulmonary vascular bed is regulated by passive factors, such as lung volume, and active factors, such as alveolar gas. These mechanisms alter pulmonary vascular resistance.

Pulmonary blood volume decreases or is diverted to the systemic circulation in conditions such as generalized systemic vasodilation, the standing position, positive end-expiratory pressure, or circulatory shock. Conditions that increase pulmonary blood volume include generalized systemic vasoconstriction, (Berne & Levy, 2000) the supine position, mitral stenosis, and left heart failure.

Pulmonary Vessels

The pulmonary circulation originates from the base of the right ventricle, extends 5 cm, and divides into the right and left pulmonary arteries. As the pulmonary artery rises, the right pulmonary artery is positioned posterior to the aorta and superior vena cava and anterior to the right mainstem bronchus. The left pulmonary artery extends over the left main bronchus and divides into lobar branches. The pulmonary arteries and segmental and lobar branches are composed of elastic arteries to maintain low vascular resistance. These arteries contain smooth muscle with the capability of vasoconstriction and vasodilatation.

The muscular arteries have internal and external elastic laminae with a layer of smooth muscle cells. The acinour and supernumerary arteries (precapillary arteries) are muscular. Increases in pulmonary vascular resistance come from the precapillary arteries.

Arterioles are vessels with a thin intima and a single elastic lamina. These vessels make up the accessory branches of the respiratory tree and end at the alveolar capillary network.

Table 3–1 ▪ ABBREVIATIONS

V_T	Tidal volume
V_E	Expired volume
V_D	Dead space volume
V_A	Alveolar volume
P_A	Alveolar pressure
Pa	Arterial pressure
Pv	Venous pressure
$P_{A_{O2}}$	Alveolar partial pressure of oxygen
$P_{A_{CO2}}$	Alveolar partial pressure of carbon dioxide
Pa_{O2}	Arterial partial pressure of oxygen
Pa_{CO2}	Arterial partial pressure of carbon dioxide
$P\bar{v}_{O2}$	Mixed venous partial pressure of oxygen
P_{CO2}	Partial pressure of carbon dioxide
P_{O2}	Partial pressure of oxygen
$F_{I_{O2}}$	Fraction of inspired oxygen
$P_{I_{O2}}$	Pressure of inspired oxygen
P_{50}	Partial pressure of oxygen at which Hgb is 50% saturated
Sa_{O2}	Arterial blood saturation
Ca_{O2}	Oxygen content of arterial blood
Cv_{O2}	Oxygen content of mixed venous blood
$C(a\text{-}v)_{O2}$	Difference between arterial and venous oxygen content
$S\bar{v}_{O2}$	Mixed venous oxygen saturation
O_2ER	Oxygen extraction ratio
Sp_{O2}	Pulse oximetry oxygen saturation
$\dot{V}/\dot{Q}$	Ventilation perfusion ratio
$\dot{V}_{O2}$	Oxygen consumption
$\dot{D}_{O2}$	Oxygen delivery
$\dot{Q}_{O2}$	Oxygen transport
WOB	Work of breathing
Hgb	Hemoglobin

Muscles of Respiration

The inspiratory and expiratory muscles determine the rate of inspiratory and expiratory airflow and generate negative and positive intrathoracic pressures. The primary muscles of inspiration include the diaphragm and the parasternal inter-cartilaginous, external intercostal, and scalenus muscles. The sternocleidomastoid muscles serve as accessory muscles of inspiration. During inspiration, the diaphragm and parasternal and external intercostals contract, producing deflation of the rib cage. Abdominal muscles contribute to expiration under conditions of increased ventilatory demand such as exercise or hypercapnia.

Cellular/Hormonal

The entire pulmonary vascular bed is lined with endothelium. The endothelium serves a number of functions, including modulating vascular smooth muscle tone, releasing relaxing and contracting mediators, and activating or deactivating circulating mediators. Endothelial cells act to maintain vascular tone by releasing various relaxing and constricting factors in response to physical and hormonal stimuli. The primary endothelium relaxing factors released by the endothelial cells are nitric oxide and prostacyclin. The constricting factors include endothelin, superoxide anion, thromboxane, and prostaglandin H2.

A number of circulating factors effect vasomotor tone. Vasoconstriction is induced by $\alpha1$ and $\alpha2$ receptors, whereas $\beta2$ receptors mediate vasodilation. Serotonin and histamine mediate vasoconstriction in the pulmonary circulation. Angiotensin II is a potent pulmonary vasoconstrictor. Other vasodilator peptides include bradykinin, calcitonin, and substance P.

Angiotensin-converting enzyme, released by the pulmonary endothelium, is responsible for the conversion of angiotensin I to angiotensin II. This enzyme also deactivates the peptide bradykinin. In addition, the endothelium contains adhesion molecules that migrate to areas of inflammation when activated by local chemoattractants.

Other Non-Gas Exchange Functions

In addition to gas exchange, the lungs metabolize several substances and produce hormones and cytokines. Lung capillary endothelial cells produce, remove, modify, and inactivate many bioactive substances. For example, bradykinin, prostaglandins, and serotonin are inactivated in the lungs. During passage through the lungs, these substances can be partially or completely removed from the blood. The lungs can also add substances to the blood, such as histamine, bradykinin, and prostaglandins. Angiotensin I is activated in the pulmonary circulation to angiotensin II (West, 2000). The lungs can serve as a filter, trapping and dissolving small clots produced in the systemic circulation (West & Wagner, 2000).

▪ PHYSIOLOGY

Respiration is a process consisting of four major events: (1) pulmonary ventilation, which is the bulk movement of air between the atmosphere and the alveoli in the lungs; (2) diffusion of gases (oxygen and carbon dioxide) across the respiratory membrane between the alveoli and blood; (3) transport of gases to and from the cells of the body; and (4) other non-gas exchange functions (e.g., hormonal activity) (Guyton & Hall, 2001). Maintenance of adequate tissue oxygenation depends on complex mechanisms, including transport of oxygen, microvascular control (systemic and local), and intact metabolic cellular function. Figure 3-1 illustrates the processes by which oxygen is transported from the atmosphere to the mitochondria.

Ventilation is the process of the exchange of air between the atmosphere (external environment) and alveoli. It involves the distribution of air into the pulmonary structures of the tracheobronchial tree to the alveoli of the lung (Fauci et al., 1998). Air flow in the conducting airways (first 17 airway generations) is along a pressure gradient. Air moves from higher outside pressure (atmospheric) to lower airway pressure (sub-atmospheric). As air enters the alveolar region of the lung, the movement of gases becomes less dependent on the pressure gradient and diffusion becomes increasingly important (West, 2000; Roca et al., 2000).

Diffusion is the process of movement of gases from an area of high partial pressure to an area of low partial pressure. Toward

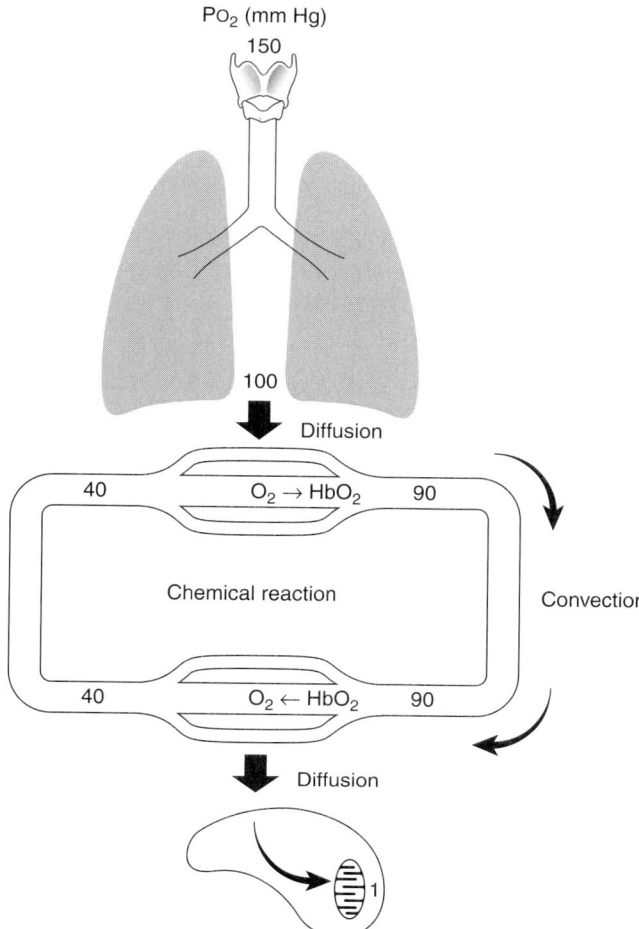

PO$_2$ (mm Hg)

150

100

Diffusion

40   O$_2 \rightarrow$ HbO$_2$ 90

Chemical reaction

Convection

40   O$_2 \leftarrow$ HbO$_2$ 90

Diffusion

1

■ **Figure 3–1.** The processes when oxygen is transported from atmosphere to the mitochondria. (From Dantzker, D. R., & Scharf, S. M. [1998.] *Cardiopulmonary critical care* [3rd ed., p. 175.]. Philadelphia: WB Saunders.)

the end of the airways, at the alveoli, diffusion is the driving force behind the movement of oxygen and carbon dioxide across the alveolar membrane into the pulmonary capillaries.

Perfusion is the process of transporting gases to and from the cells of the body. This event includes mixed venous blood flow to the pulmonary capillaries where gases are exchanged between the alveoli and blood, and blood flow to the systemic capillaries where gases are exchanged between the blood and the surrounding body fluids.

Other lung functions that affect respiration but do not involve gas exchange include hormonal activity (discussed earlier) and the work of breathing (WOB). WOB is the metabolic demand of breathing. It includes the energy needed to move the lung and chest wall and results in a demand for oxygen.

Dead Space

Ventilation must keep pace with the constant demand to replenish oxygen and eliminate carbon dioxide exchanged in the alveoli. Dead space is the volume of inspired air that does

not participate in gas exchange (Muller, 2002). The volume of gas in a normal breath is measured as the tidal volume (V$_T$). This volume is multiplied by the number of breaths per minute to calculate minute volume (V$_E$). Minute volume represents the total volume of air moved through the airways to and from the alveoli. A portion of this volume will reach the alveoli where gas exchange can occur (alveolar volume), while the remainder will stay in the conducting airways and will not contribute to gas exchange (anatomic dead space) (V$_T$ = V$_D$ + V$_A$). In disease states, some lung regions may continue to receive ventilation but will not get normal blood flow. The result is wasted ventilation, adding to dead space volume (physiologic dead space) (Weinberger, 2004).

West Zones

Because the alveolar air spaces surround collapsible capillaries, intrapleural and alveolar pressures affect pulmonary capillary pressures. Pulmonary blood flow reflects this influence during respiration in the upright and lateral recumbent positions. Inspiration and expiration induce fluctuating intrathoracic pressures that influence the pulmonary vessels. Pulmonary capillaries are also affected by alveolar pressure to a certain degree. However, the capillary-alveolar membrane is thin and compliant enough to approximate pulmonary capillary pressure to alveolar pressure. With a change from supine to standing position, a hydrostatic pressure difference of 20 cm H$_2$O is created between the apex and base of the lung.

West (West & Wagner, 2000; West, 2003) described the hydrostatic effect of body position on pulmonary capillary flow by dividing the lung into three regions (Fig. 3-2). Zone 1 is represented above the heart in an upright body position, where pulmonary alveolar pressure (PA) may exceed pulmonary arterial pressure (Pa) and pulmonary venous pressure (Pv) (PA > Pa > Pv). In a normal physiologic state,

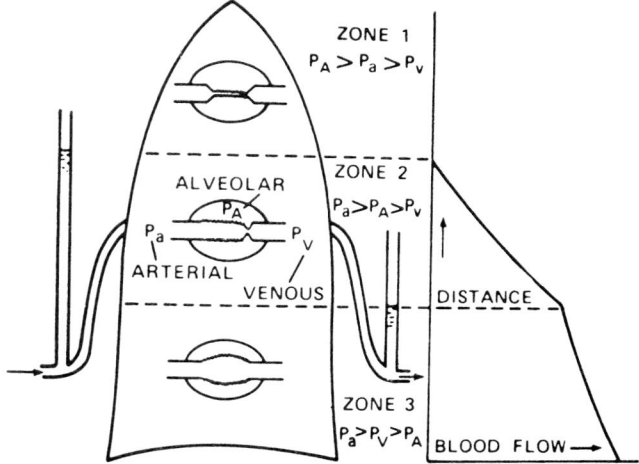

ZONE 1
P$_A$ > P$_a$ > P$_v$

ALVEOLAR
P$_A$

ZONE 2
P$_a$ > P$_A$ > P$_v$

P$_a$ P$_v$

ARTERIAL

VENOUS   DISTANCE

ZONE 3
P$_a$ > P$_v$ > P$_A$ BLOOD FLOW

■ **Figure 3–2.** Model to explain the zones of the lungs. PA, alveolar pressure; Pa, pulmonary arterial pressure; Pv, pulmonary venous pressure. (From West, J. B. [1979]. *Respiratory physiology: The essentials* [2nd ed., p. 43.]. Baltimore: Williams & Wilkins.)

pulmonary arterial pressure is sufficient to maintain blood flow to the top of the lung. Thus, this zone does not usually develop. However, in conditions that reduce arterial pressure (e.g., hemorrhage) or increase alveolar pressure (e.g., positive end-expiratory pressure), a zone 1 region may be created. In this state, the apex of the lung is ventilated yet unperfused, creating alveolar dead space that is ineffective for gas exchange.

The region of zone 2 is represented at the level of the left atrium of the heart, where pulmonary arterial pressure increases because of the hydrostatic effect. At this point, Pa exceeds PA, which continues to exceed venous pressures (Pa > PA > Pv). Although Pa exceeds PA, alveolar pressure is still higher than the pressure of the left atrium.

The region of zone 3, below the left atrium, is where both Pa and left atrial pressures exceed PA (Pa > Pv > PA). Blood flow, determined by the difference between arterial and venous pressures, is increased markedly in this region of the lung because of capillary distention. A zone 3 region creates a continuous column of fluid between the pulmonary artery and the left atrium. Reliable pulmonary artery pressure measurements can be obtained when the tip of the pulmonary artery catheter is located in zone 3.

This model of blood flow distribution is adequate for understanding the range of ventilation and perfusion relationships throughout the lung as a whole. New high-resolution imaging technology has found that within a given isogravitational plane, there is greater heterogeneity than explained by the West zones, and that gravity plays less of a role in the distribution of blood flow than previously thought (Glenny, 1998).

Diffusion

Each gas in a mixture of gases behaves as if it alone occupies the total volume and exerts a partial pressure independent of the other gases present. Diffusion is the process of movement of molecules. In conditions in which a gas has an area of high concentration and an area of low concentration, the net diffusion of gas will be from the area of high to low. In addition to the difference in pressure, the solubility of the gas in the body fluid (primarily water), the cross-sectional area of the exchange surface (alveolar–pulmonary capillary interface), and the distance the gas must travel are among the factors that affect the net diffusion in fluids. Carbon dioxide is approximately 20-times more soluble in water than in oxygen. Some pathologic conditions (e.g., pulmonary edema) can affect cross-sectional area and distance (Guyton & Hall, 2001).

Ventilation-Perfusion Matching

Pulmonary precapillary vasomotor and bronchiolar responses serve to match pulmonary capillary perfusion to alveolar ventilation. Unlike in the systemic circulation where hypoxemia, decreased pH, or increased amounts of carbon dioxide cause local vasodilation, any of these conditions in the pulmonary circulation may cause arteriolar vasoconstriction. In well-ventilated regions, there is little vasoconstriction in response to deoxygenated blood. In poorly ventilated areas where the amount of alveolar oxygen is less than normal, such as when a bronchus is obstructed, vasoconstriction occurs and blood is shunted to other lung areas.

Hypoxic vasoconstriction serves a useful role in diverting blood flow to areas of the lung with more abundant oxygen, thus improving gas exchange. Hypoxic vasoconstriction occurs in conditions such as high altitude or in patients with chronic obstructive pulmonary disease. When blood flow to a certain lung area is reduced, there is a subsequent decrease in the alveolar carbon dioxide concentration. The bronchial smooth muscle responds to the decreased alveolar carbon dioxide levels by constricting, thus shifting ventilation away from a poorly perfused area (West & Wagner, 2000).

Constriction of the pulmonary vessels can be induced by pharmacologic agents such as norepinephrine, serotonin, histamine, and prostaglandins (Guyton & Hall, 2001). Pharmacologic agents that induce vasodilation of the pulmonary vessels include isoproterenol, beta adrenergic type 2 agents, nitroprusside, nitroglycerine, prostacyclin, and acetylcholine.

Ventilation and perfusion must occur in equal proportion in the various regions of the lung to achieve adequate gas exchange. Gas exchange determines the levels of alveolar oxygen partial pressure (PA_{O2}) and carbon dioxide partial pressure (PA_{CO2}). An adequate alveolar PO_2 depends on a balance of two factors: the rate of removal of oxygen by the pulmonary arterial blood and the rate of replenishment of oxygen by alveolar ventilation. An adequate PA_{CO2} depends on the rate of removal of carbon dioxide by alveolar ventilation. A key concept used to understand pulmonary gas exchange is the ventilation-perfusion ratio ($\dot{V}/\dot{Q}$). The concentration of gases (i.e., oxygen, carbon dioxide, nitrogen) in the various regions of the lung is determined by the ratio of the rate of ventilation to the rate of perfusion (blood flow). Obstruction to ventilation or perfusion leads to alteration in this ratio and, consequently, the composition of gases. Inequality in ventilation-perfusion hinders the lungs' ability to replenish oxygen and remove carbon dioxide.

Impairment of gas exchange can result in a decrease in Pa_{O2} and an increase in tissue PCO_2. Clinically, these conditions can result in hypoxemia.

Causes of Arterial Hypoxemia

The sources of arterial hypoxemia can be categorized as follows:

- Decreased partial pressure of inspired oxygen
- Decreased percentage of inspired oxygen (decreased fraction of inspired oxygen, FI_{O2})
- Diffusion limitation
- Hypoventilation
- $\dot{V}/\dot{Q}$ Mismatch
- Shunt

Decreases in the atmospheric pressure related to higher altitude result in a proportional decrease in the partial pressure of inspired oxygen (PI_{O2}). These conditions are common to high-altitude locations and air travel; however, they are rarely encountered in the clinical setting. Decreased percentage of inspired oxygen (FI_{O_2}) occurs in situations in which other gases may displace oxygen and lower the overall percentage of oxygen below 21% (e.g., diagnostic testing). Diffusion limitation can potentially cause abnormal diffusion of oxygen across the alveolar-capillary membrane. Diffusion limitation can be caused by increases in the thickness of the diffusion pathway and/or decreased transit time through the pulmonary circulation. Hypoventilation can result in a decrease in alveolar PO_2 caused by insufficient gas exchange between the external environment and the alveoli. Hypoventilation can result from trauma to the chest wall, paralysis of the respiratory muscles, and medications such as morphine sulfate and barbiturates, which depress the respiratory center (Dantzker & Scharf, 1998; West & Wagner, 2000; Sibbald, 2002).

Matching ventilation of the alveoli with perfusion of the pulmonary capillary bed is a delicate balance. $\dot{V}/\dot{Q}$ matching is a dynamic process with different distributions occurring simultaneously within the regions of the lungs. In disease, there is a myriad of $\dot{V}/\dot{Q}$ relationships exemplified by regions receiving excessive ventilation (dead space), normal ventilation and perfusion (ideal), and excessive perfusion (shunt).

Shunt refers to the condition when blood passes into the systemic circulation without passing through a ventilated region of the lung. Under normal conditions, there exists a small physiological shunt because of the difference in PO_2 between alveolar gas and end-capillary blood. Physiologically, mixed venous blood from the pulmonary arterial bed mixes with capillary blood from pulmonary venous beds, thereby lowering the end-capillary PO_2. This difference can become larger in conditions such as ventricular septal defect, in which greater amounts of venous blood are added to arterial blood across the defect, resulting in a lower Pa_{O_2}.

An important clinical characteristic of a shunt is that the hypoxemia cannot be completely resolved by placing the patient on an inspired oxygen fraction (FI_{O_2}) of 100%. Because the shunt blood bypasses the ventilated regions of the lung, it is not exposed to the higher alveolar PO_2. In patients with shunt, the arterial PCO_2 may be low, normal, or high, depending on the capacity to increase respiratory drive in response to hypoxemia.

GAS TRANSPORT

Gas Exchange

In the lungs, oxygen and carbon dioxide equilibrate across the alveolar-capillary membranes by simple passive diffusion, moving from an area of greater partial pressure to a region of lesser partial pressure. The partial pressure of oxygen in pulmonary arterial blood (venous blood from the body) is approximately 40 mm Hg, whereas pulmonary alveolar partial pressure of oxygen is approximately 100 mm Hg; thus, oxygen diffuses into the blood. The partial pressure of systemic arterial oxygen is slightly less than 100 mm Hg because of the admixture of oxygenated and deoxygenated blood. Blood from pulmonary veins is mixed with some deoxygenated blood from bronchial veins, and in the left heart it is mixed with deoxygenated blood

from thebesian veins draining cardiac muscle tissue (physiological shunt).

Carbon dioxide is removed in the pulmonary capillaries. The partial pressure of carbon dioxide in pulmonary arterial blood (systemic venous blood) is 46 mm Hg and that of blood leaving the lung (which becomes systemic arterial blood) is 40 mm Hg. The release of carbon dioxide is aided by the conversion of hemoglobin to oxyhemoglobin.

Oxygen reaching the tissues must dissociate from hemoglobin and pass out of the red blood cells and move to the mitochondria. Just as in the lungs, once the oxygen molecule leaves the cell, passive diffusion becomes the driving force in the movement of oxygen. Unlike the relatively short distances encountered in the lung, the oxygen diffusion from the blood to the mitochondria in the target cell is much greater. The partial pressure of oxygen at the arterial end of the capillary, approximately 90 mm Hg, quickly drops to approximately 30 mm Hg in the tissues and to approximately 1 to 3 mm Hg in the mitochondria (Dantzker & Scharf, 1998; Roca, et al., 2000). Factors other than diffusion that influence oxygen delivery include the rate of oxygen delivery, the position of the P_{50} (right or left shift), and the rate of cellular oxygen consumption (Leach & Treacher, 2002). Oxygen carriers, such as myoglobin, within the target cells offset the diffusion limitation (Walley, 2002).

Transport of carbon dioxide in the blood begins with the diffusion of carbon dioxide out of the tissue cells. The PCO_2 of the tissues (50 mm Hg) is greater than the $PaCO_2$ in systemic capillaries (46 mm Hg). Thus, carbon dioxide diffuses from the tissues into the blood. The PCO_2 in the tissues is proportional to the amount of energy expended. Once carbon dioxide has diffused into the capillaries, a series of chemical reactions can occur. Carbon dioxide is carried in the blood by three mechanisms. Approximately 6% is carried in the dissolved state, 20% to 25% combines with hemoglobin, and most of it combines with hydrogen to form bicarbonate. In the normal physiological state, an average of 4 mL of carbon dioxide is transported from the tissues to the lungs in each 100 mL of blood. The amount of carbon dioxide carried in the blood can greatly alter the acid-base balance and must be carefully monitored in the critically ill patient (Berry & Pinard, 2002). The diffusion of carbon dioxide into the blood is determined by two factors, the PCO_2 of the tissues and the oxygen content of the blood; both factors are in turn determined by the environment of the tissues. Thus, the physiochemical state that results from this exchange of gases is controlled by the metabolic demands of the tissues.

Gas Transport

Hemoglobin

In the red blood cell, the hemoglobin (Hgb) molecule acts as an oxygen-binding site responsible for carrying 97% of the oxygen in the blood. Hemoglobin is a protein of four subunits of porphyrin and iron. The molecule is composed of two alpha and two beta polypeptide chains, each with an iron-containing heme molecule capable of binding oxygen. Theoretically, 1 g of hemoglobin is capable of transporting 1.39 mL of oxygen. However, some of the heme sites are in an alternate form (methemoglobin) that is not capable of combining with oxygen. The maximum amount of oxygen that can be transported is approximately 1.34 to 1.36 milliliters per gram of hemoglobin (some authors suggest this number may be lower, approximately 1.31; Lumb, 2000). Hemoglobin has a unique chemical structure that accounts for the differences in the speed at which oxygen binds with hemoglobin (affinity). Oxygen affinity increases as more hemoglobin is saturated with oxygen, so that the affinity of the last heme unit is greater than the first unit. This relationship explains the non-linear curve represented in the oxyhemoglobin dissociation (or equilibrium) curve (Hlastala & Berger, 2001).

Partial Pressure of Oxygen

Alveolar oxygen diffuses into the pulmonary capillaries. The amount of oxygen transferred depends on the mechanics of the ventilation-perfusion relationship of the lungs and the amount of inspired oxygen. The majority (97%) of the oxygen transported by the blood is bound to hemoglobin (Hgb).

The remaining 3% of the oxygen transported by the blood (0.3 mL/dL) comprises oxygen dissolved in plasma. The Pa_{O_2}, a measurement of oxygen tension, is simply a reflection of the patient's plasma oxygenation. The Pa_{O_2} is an excellent indication of the patient's capacity for bonding oxygen to hemoglobin and the ability of oxygen to be released into the interstitial tissues. The body's plasma may carry a small percentage of the arterial oxygen, but measurement of its oxygen tension is an indirect method for determining the patient's oxygen-hemoglobin affinity (Roca, et al., 2000)

Arterial Oxygen Saturation

As the partial pressure of oxygen in the pulmonary capillaries increases, oxygen binds with hemoglobin to form oxyhemoglobin in the manner described. After leaving the pulmonary circulation, arterial blood can be sampled to measure the partial pressure of oxygen Pa_{O_2}. Because oxygen binds with hemoglobin in a predictable manner, the saturation of hemoglobin in the arterial blood (Sa_{O_2}) can be calculated (or measured directly by co-oximetry). The quantity of oxyhemoglobin, reflecting the amount of hemoglobin bound to oxygen, is measured as oxygen saturation. Saturation can be expressed as a percentage when multiplied by 100.

Oxyhemoglobin Dissociation Curve

The essential relationship between Pa_{O_2} and Sa_{O_2} is graphically illustrated by the oxyhemoglobin dissociation curve (Fig. 3-3), originally described by Hufner in 1890. The sigmoid, or S, shape of this curve reflects the optimal conditions that facilitate oxygen loading in the lungs and oxygen release to the tissues. To describe these processes in relation to the curve, it is often divided into two segments: the association segment and the dissociation segment.

The upper portion of the curve, or the association segment, represents oxygen uptake, where large decreases in Pa_{O_2} elicit only small decreases in Sa_{O_2}. For example, in the association segment, a 40% reduction in the Pa_{O_2} (mm Hg) from 100 to

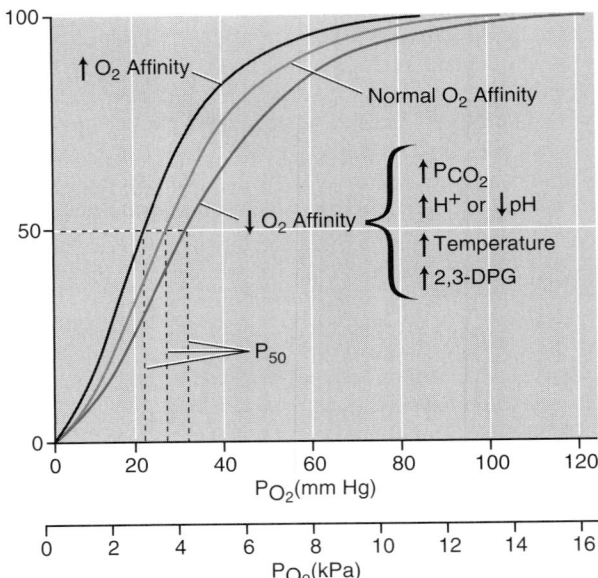

■ Figure 3–3. Changes in O_2 affinity of the O_2 saturation curve. Three curves are shown with progressively decreasing O_2 affinity indicated by increasing P_{50}. (From Hlastala, M. P., & Berger, A. J. [2001]. *Physiology of respiration* [2nd ed., p. 99]. New York: Oxford University Press.)

60 only results in a 7% drop in oxygen saturation. The association segment also represents the body's protective mechanism to ensure that, even with a substantial decrease in Pa_{O_2}, adequate arterial oxygen content is available for transport to the cells. The lower portion of the curve, or the dissociation segment, reflects the release of oxygen to the tissues. Here, small changes in Pa_{O_2} result in large changes in Sa_{O_2}, protecting the tissues by releasing large amounts of oxygen with minimal changes in oxygen tension. Unlike in the association segment, a 40% reduction in the Pa_{O_2} results in a 20% drop in oxygen saturation.

Changes in oxyhemoglobin affinity affect the oxyhemoglobin dissociation curve and need to be considered in tissue oxygen assessment (Berry & Pinard, 2002). Increased affinity, caused by hypothermia, alkalosis, or decreased levels of 2,3-diphosphoglycerate (2,3,-DPG), decreases oxyhemoglobin affinity, shifting the curve to the right and thus allowing more oxygen to be released. In this way, tissue oxygenation is enhanced in the presence of decreased saturation and increased demand.

Change in the Pa_{CO_2} can also cause shifts in the hemoglobin dissociation curve; this is termed the *Bohr effect* (Bohr et al., 1978). As blood perfuses through the lungs, carbon dioxide diffuses from the blood to the alveoli. As a result of this movement of carbon dioxide, the Pa_{CO_2} is reduced, and there is a subsequent increase in pH. The hemoglobin dissociation curve shifts to the left, thus increasing the binding of hemoglobin to oxygen and allowing greater oxygen transport to the tissues (Berne & Levy, 2000; Guyton & Hall, 2001). At the tissue level, however, carbon dioxide displaces oxygen from the hemoglobin. The hemoglobin dissociation curve shifts to the right at the tissue level, facilitating higher oxygen delivery to the tissues (opposite to what occurs in the lungs). Shifts in the oxygen-hemoglobin dissociation curve have greater affects on events in the tissues than in the lungs because the relationships in the lungs are described in the flat upper position of the curve.

A frequently used index of right and left shifts of the dissociation curve is the P_{50}, which is the Pa_{O_2} at which hemoglobin is 50% saturated. A higher than normal P_{50} value indicates a lower than normal affinity for oxygen. Under normal conditions (37°C, pH 7.40, PCO_2 40 mm Hg, and normal hemoglobin), the P_{50} is 27 mm Hg.

Blood Oxygen Content

Blood oxygen content reflects the amount of oxygen dissolved in plasma ($0.0031 \times PO_2$) and the amount bound to hemoglobin (Hgb) ($1.36 \times$ hemoglobin $\times Sa_{O_2}$), where 1.36 is the maximum amount of oxygen carried by 1 gram of hemoglobin. This expression is depicted in the following equation (Roca, et al., 2000):

$$(Hgb \times 1.36 \times Sa_{O_2}) + (0.0031 \times Pa_{O_2})$$
$$97\% \qquad\qquad 3\%$$

Assuming a normal hemoglobin of 15 grams, arterial Pa_{O_2} equal to 100 mm Hg, and 98% saturation, the arterial oxygen content (Ca_{O_2}) is 20 mL/dL. The equation can also be used to determine venous oxygen content (Cv_{O_2}). Assuming no change in the hemoglobin and a venous Pa_{O_2} of 40 mm Hg and 75% saturation, the venous oxygen content is 15 mL/dL.

The delivery of adequate oxygen for normal cellular function depends not only on the total amount of oxygen in the arterial blood (arterial oxygen content) but also on the ability of the heart to provide adequate blood flow (cardiac output).

▪ OXYGEN DELIVERY, CONSUMPTION, EXTRACTION AND CARDIAC OUTPUT

Oxygen Delivery

Oxygen delivery ($\dot{D}O_2$) is the supply of oxygen to the body and is defined as the transport of oxygen to the tissues per minute. Oxygen delivery is determined by the combined processes of ventilation and diffusion (pulmonary function), hemoglobin binding capacity, convective movement of blood (cardiac function), microvascular distribution, and delivery of oxygen to the mitochondria (passive diffusion) (Roca, et al., 2000).

Measurement of Oxygen Delivery

Measurement of oxygen delivery ($\dot{D}O_2$) or transport ($\dot{Q}O_2$) is calculated by multiplying total arterial oxygen content by cardiac output (CO):

$$\dot{D}O_2 = CO \times Ca_{O_2} \times 10$$

where $Ca_{O_2} = (Hgb \times 1.36 \times Sa_{O_2}) + (0.0031 \times Pa_{O_2})$

$$= CO \times Hgb \times Sa_{O_2} \times 13.6$$

In patients with cardiac output of 5 L/min and a Ca_{O_2} of 20 mL/dL, arterial oxygen delivery ($\dot{D}O_2$) is 1,000 mL of oxygen/min.

Delivery of oxygen to support aerobic metabolism can be limited anywhere along the route from the environment through the alveolar-pulmonary interface, the systemic circulation, and the capillary-tissue junction to the mitochondria. Hypoxia is the shortage of oxygen at the tissue level. Hypoxia can be classified as: (1) **hypoxic hypoxia,** caused by a decreased PO_2; (2) **anemic hypoxia,** insufficient hemoglobin carrying capacity and normal PO_2; (3) **ischemic (stagnant) hypoxia,** caused by a lack of blood flow to the tissue; and (4) **histotoxic (cytopathic) hypoxia,** normal oxygen delivery; however, the cell is unable to process the oxygen and produce adenosine triphosphate (ATP) (Fink, 2002; Dantzker & Scharf, 1998).

Oxygen Consumption

Oxygen consumption ($\dot{V}O_2$) is the body's demand for oxygen and is defined as the amount of oxygen consumed at the tissue level per minute. Oxygen consumption can be calculated by determining the difference between the quantity of oxygen carried by the arterial system to the tissues (Ca_{O_2}) and the quantity remaining in the blood returning in the venous system to the lungs (Cv_{O_2}) (Leach & Treacher, 2002):

$$\dot{V}O_2 = (CO \times Ca_{O_2} \times 10) - (CO \times Cv_{O_2} \times 10)$$
$$\dot{V}O_2 = Ca_{O_2} - Cv_{O_2}$$

By combining the factors, the preceding can be simplified to the following equation:

$$\dot{V}O_2 = CO \times Hgb \times 13.6 \times (Sa_{O_2} - S\bar{v}O_2)$$

This equation is a restatement of the Fick equation, placing $\dot{V}O_2$ on the left instead of cardiac output. This formula identifies all components of oxygen supply and demand. In a patient with normal values in a relatively steady state, normal $\dot{V}O_2$ is between 200 and 250 mL/min (or estimates of 3.5 mL/kg), as shown in the following equation (Roca et al., 2000):

$$\dot{V}O_2 = 5\ L/min \times 15\ g/dL \times 13.6 \times (0.98 - 0.75)$$
$$\dot{V}O_2 = 234\ mL/min$$

Oxygen consumption is affected by several factors. Blood flow depends on the cardiac output and on the degree of constriction of the vascular bed in the tissue (vasoregulatory mechanisms). Low hemoglobin, such as in anemia, reduces the amount of available oxygen to be delivered to the tissues. Reduced Pa_{O_2} can affect the driving force needed to load the oxygen molecule on the hemoglobin. Decreased Sa_{O_2} affects the affinity between oxygen and hemoglobin, enhancing the release of oxygen to the tissues. The metabolic rate of the tissues also affects the affinity of oxygen to be released.

Oxygen Extraction Ratio

The percentage of oxygen extracted by the tissues is a useful indicator of the balance between oxygen delivery and consumption.

Oxygen extraction represents the difference between arterial and venous oxygen contents (normal 5 mL/dL or 25%) and is known as the $C(a-v)_{O_2}$ difference or oxygen extraction ratio (O_2ER). This ratio increases in pathological conditions characterized by an imbalance between oxygen delivery and $\dot{V}O_2$. O_2ER is increased by factors such as decreased cardiac output, increased oxygen consumption (e.g., shivering), anemia, and decreased arterial oxygenation. O_2ER is decreased in conditions where $\dot{V}O_2$ is relatively low in proportion to oxygen delivery, such as in sepsis, hypothermia, high-flow states, peripheral shunting, or inability of tissue to use oxygen (Des Jardins, 2002; Leach & Treacher, 2002).

Cardiac Output

Cardiac output is a main determinant of oxygen delivery. Reduction in blood flow decreases the supply of oxygen to the cells, thereby initiating a series of compensatory mechanisms to increase oxygen transport and extraction. Careful monitoring of the determinants of cardiac output—heart rate, preload, afterload, and contractility—is necessary to optimize oxygen delivery. Arterial oxygen content and cardiac output are combined in the oxygen delivery ($\dot{D}O_2$) equation to measure the amount of oxygen delivered to the tissues in a given unit of time.

OXYGEN CONSUMPTION-DELIVERY RELATIONSHIP

Three main compensatory mechanisms are needed to balance delivery and consumption to maintain aerobic metabolism. These mechanisms are:

1. Cardiac output: As oxygen demand and consumption increase, cardiac output increases to maintain adequate oxygen delivery.
2. Vasoregulatory mechanisms (systemic vascular resistance): The cardiac output and systemic vascular resistance actually work in conjunction with each other. Peripheral tissue beds shunt blood (vasoconstrict) to organs of greater demand (Snyder, 1987).
3. Oxygen delivery–extraction (mixed venous oxygen saturation, $S\bar{v}O_2$): Diminished oxygen delivery results in an increased oxygen extraction, reducing the amount of oxygen in venous blood returning to the heart (Jesurum, 2001).

The balance between oxygen supply and demand can be challenged by a number of factors. An increase $\dot{V}O_2$ is a threat to the oxygen supply-demand balance (Leach & Treacher, 2002). For the most part, the body consumes the oxygen it demands as long as there is adequate oxygen delivery. Once oxygen demand increases, the body's compensatory mechanisms must work to maintain oxygen delivery. If $\dot{V}O_2$ increases in a healthy person, cardiac output increases to maintain the balance between oxygen delivery and demand. If additional oxygen is required, then extraction of available oxygen increases, causing a decrease in $S\bar{v}O_2$.

A decrease in hemoglobin is another threat. As discussed previously, hemoglobin carries approximately 97% of the oxygen to the tissues. Except in certain situations, such as large volume replacements, hemoglobin is a very slowly changing value. However, frank hemorrhage or hidden intra-abdominal bleeding would result in a rapid decrease in hemoglobin. In the healthy person with mild anemia or a reduced level of hemoglobin, cardiac output usually increases as a compensatory measure to increase the delivery of oxygen.

As with other threats to the oxygen supply-demand balance, increasing oxygen extraction is a second compensatory mechanism that increases the delivery of oxygen. Failure of the ventilatory process is also a threat. In most instances, even in patients with severe pulmonary disease, the Sa_{O_2} remains above 90% and poses little threat to the oxygen supply-demand balance. If the Sa_{O_2} decreases to an unacceptable range, the body responds by increasing cardiac output (Roca et al., 2000). An increase in oxygen extraction results if increases in cardiac output fail to meet oxygen demand. A decrease in cardiac output is perhaps the most serious threat to the patient because an inadequate cardiac output eliminates one of the most important compensatory mechanisms.

MONITORING OXYGENATION

Arterial Blood Gas

Arterial blood gas (ABG) testing is routinely performed in clinical practice as a measure of gas exchange. Three measurements are typically obtained: arterial PO_2, PCO_2 and pH. The normal range for PO_2 is between 80 and 100 mm Hg. The normal value decreases with age. Factors that affect the oxygen dissociation curve (temperature, PCO_2, and pH) should be considered whenever reviewing a blood gas report. Reduced PO_2 results from reduced inspired PO_2, hypoventilation, diffusion impairment, shunt, and ventilation–perfusion inequality. Arterial PCO_2 is normally between 36 and 44 mm Hg, and unlike PO_2 is rarely affected by age. Increases in arterial PCO_2 are caused by hypoventilation and ventilation–perfusion inequality. Arterial pH is a measure of hydrogen ion concentration in the blood. Normal pH ranges between 7.35 and 7.45. Values lower than 7.35 indicate a higher hydrogen ion concentration (acidosis), whereas pH values higher than 7.45 signify a lower concentration of hydrogen (alkalosis). Pulmonary and metabolic factors interact in determining the pH value (West, 2003; Weinberger, 2004)

Traditional ABG testing involves intermittent sampling of arterial blood. Recent advances in technology have lead to the development of continuous monitoring devices that use either indwelling electrochemical sensors or optical sensors. Continuous ABG monitoring may decrease response time to changes in critically ill patients, which may translate into improved clinical outcomes.

Pulse Oximetry

Pulse oximetry (Sp_{O_2}) is a noninvasive clinical tool that determines the percentage of hemoglobin saturation by measuring the absorbency of two wavelengths of light detected in a vascular bed. Pulse oximetry demonstrates higher accuracy at saturations of 90% or more. At saturations less than 80% it may be less reliable. Sp_{O_2} measurement is also influenced by jaundice, shock states, and reduced body temperature. Sp_{O_2} monitors are not capable of detecting carbon monoxide or methemoglobinemia elevated levels of carboxyhemoglobin, severe hypoxic states. In addition, the presence of nail polish on the patient's finger may invalidate the Sa_{O_2} measurement. The earlobe and bridge of the nose are alternative sites to the finger (Caples & Hubmayr, 2003).

Transcutaneous Monitoring

Transcutaneous monitoring of P_{O_2} and P_{CO_2} offers an alternative, noninvasive method of oxygen monitoring. These monitors work by warming the skin to induce local vasodilation and detecting diffusion of oxygen and carbon dioxide from the skin. Unlike pulse oximetry that monitors oxygen saturation of hemoglobin, transcutaneous oxygen monitors approximate P_{O_2}. However, reliance on local skin warming and perfusion limits the use of these devices (Caples & Hubmayr, 2003).

Continuous S$\bar{v}$O$_2$ Interpretation

Mixed venous oxygen saturation is an index measured in the pulmonary arterial bed that is influenced by and dependent on the interaction between oxygen delivery and consumption (White, 1987a; White, 1987b). Monitoring and trending the S$\bar{v}$O$_2$ provides critical information on the adequacy of the balance between oxygen delivery and consumption (Jesurum, 2001).

Continuous S$\bar{v}$O$_2$ generally reflects the total body's adequacy of tissue oxygenation. The S$\bar{v}$O$_2$ parameter is considered a "global" indicator of the whole body's oxygen supply–demand balance. One of the limitations of this indicator is that it is unable to specify which tissue bed or organ is suffering from an imbalance in delivery and consumption (Snyder, 1987).

Sampling from various venous sites in the body would give very different results. Each organ system uses oxygen in differing amounts and therefore returns blood with various S$\bar{v}$O$_2$ levels. For instance, the coronary circulation has the greatest need for oxygen and P$\bar{v}$O$_2$ values are lowest at 30 mm Hg (57% saturation). However, the integumentary system has a lower demand for oxygen, often returning venous blood values of 75 mm Hg (95% saturation). The S$\bar{v}$O$_2$ can be measured by the conventional method of sending a pulmonary arterial sample to the laboratory for interpretation or by means of a pulmonary artery catheter with a fiberoptic photometric lumen, which allows continuous monitoring of S$\bar{v}$O$_2$.

Regional Measures of Oxygenation

A method to monitor regional or tissue oxygenation is still being sought by clinicians (Dantzker, 2001). Currently, gastric

tonometry and infrared spectroscopy are the only technologies available that have clinical applications (Leach & Treacher, 2002). Gastric tonometry has been tested in the stomach and intestine. The tonometer balloon provides an indirect measure of changes in tissue CO_2 (an index of tissue hydrogen ion concentration (pHi). Increases in regional CO_2 are assumed to be related to cellular hypoxia. Sublingual measures of pHi have also been explored.

Other methods of monitoring tissue oxygenation are under evaluation. Spectophometic analysis of hemoglobin saturation in the microvascular is one method being evaluated for future clinical use. Spectophotometry uses optical density measures similar to pulse oximetry. Functional MRI is another method currently being explored to measure changes in capillary oxygenation. This method combined with flow-sensitive MRI may be effective in quantifying changes in flow with changes in oxygen metabolism. P_{O_2} microelectrodes that can be either implanted transcutaneously or applied to the surface are another method used to target oxygenation to a specific target organ. The intrusive nature of these electrodes limits the validity of their results and usefulness in clinical practice. Finally, metabolic activity (i.e., hypoxia) measurement using PET imaging has been used to determine areas of hypoxia in tumors. (Lewis & Welch, 2001). In general, many of these measurements are difficult to conduct in the clinical setting, require specialized equipment and procedures, and are not widely available (Leach & Treacher, 2002).

REFERENCES

Berne, R. M., & Levy, M. N. (2000). *Principles of physiology* (3rd ed., pp. 323–341). St Louis: Mosby.

Berry, B. E., & Pinard, A. E. (2002). Assessing tissue oxygenation. *Critical Care Nurse, 22*(3), 22–42.

Bohr, D. F., Greenberg S., & Bonaccorsi A. (1978). Mechanisms of action of vasoactive agents. In G. Kaley & B. Altura (Eds.), *Micro-circulation* (Vol. II, pp. 311–348). Baltimore: University Park Press.

Boron, W. F. (2003). *Mechanics of Respiration*. In W. Boron & E. Boulpaep (Eds.), *Medical physiology* (pp. 607–632). Philadelphia: Saunders.

Caples, S. M., & Hubmayr, R. D. (2003). Respiratory monitoring tools in the intensive care unit. *Current Opinions in Critical Care, 9*, 230–235.

Dantzker, D. R. (2001). Monitoring issue oxygenation: The quest continues [editorial]. *Chest, 120*(3), 701–702.

Dantzker, D. R., & Scharf, S.M. (1998). *Cardiopulmonary critical care* (3rd ed., pp. 29–42; 173–221). Philadelphia: WB Saunders.

Des Jardins, T. (2002). *Cardiopulmonary anatomy and physiology: Essentials for respiratory care* (4th ed., pp. 11–53). Albany: Delmar.

Fauci, A. S., Braunwald, E., Isselbacher, K. J. et al. (1998). *Harrison's principles of internal medicine* (14th ed.). New York: McGraw-Hill.

Fink, M. P. (2002). Cytopathic hypoxia: mitochondrial dysfunction as a potential mechanism contributing to organ failure in sepsis. In W. Sibbald, K. Messmer, & M. Fink (Eds.), *Tissue oxygenation in acute medicine* (pp. 128–137). Berlin: Springer-Verlag.

Gleeny, R. W. (1998). Blood flow distribution in the lung. *Chest, 114*, 8S–16S.

Guyton, A. C., & Hall, J. E. (2001). *Human physiology and mechanisms of disease* (6th ed., pp. 324–336). Philadelphia: WB Saunders.

Hlastala, M. P., & Berger, A. J. (2001). *Physiology of respiration* (2nd ed., pp. 97–133). New York: Oxford University Press.

Jesurum, J. (2001). SvO2 Monitoring. *Critical Care Nurse, 21*(1), 79–83.

Leach, R. M., & Treacher, D. F. (2002). The pulmonary physician in critical care 2: Oxygen delivery and consumption in the critically ill. *Thorax, 57*, 170–177.

Levitzky, M. G. (2002). *Pulmonary physiology* (6th ed., pp. 113–129). New York: McGraw-Hill.

Lewis, J. S., & Welch, M. J. (2001). PET imaging of hypoxia. *Quarterly Journal of Nuclear Medicine, 45*(2), 183–188.

Lumb, A. B. (2000). *Nunn's applied respiratory physiology* (5th ed., pp.163–199). Oxford: Butterworth Heinemann.

Muller, B. F. (2002). Mechanics of respiration. In E. Bittar (Ed.), *Pulmonary biology in health and disease* (pp. 166–167). New York: Springer.

Pinsky, M. R. (2002). Role of cardiorespiratory system in delivering oxygen. In W. Sibbald, K. Messmer, & M. Fink (Eds.), *Tissue oxygenation in acute medicine* (pp. 3–13). Berlin: Springer-Verlag.

Roca, J., Rodriguez-Roisin, R., & Wagner, P.D. (2000). Pulmonary and peripheral gas exchange and their interactions. In J. Roca , & R. Rodriguez-Roisin (Eds.), *Pulmonary and peripheral gas exchange in health and disease* (pp. 1–27). New York: Marcel Dekker.

Snyder, J. V. (1987). Assessment of systemic oxygen transport. In J. Snyder & M. Pinsky (Eds.), *Oxygen transport in the critically ill* (pp 179–198). Chicago: Year Book.

Walley, K. R. (2002). Hypoxic hypoxia. In W. Sibbald, K. Messmer, & M. Fink (Eds.), *Tissue oxygenation in acute medicine* (pp. 3–13). Berlin: Springer-Verlag.

Weinberger, S. E. (2004). *Principles of pulmonary medicine* (4th ed., pp. 1–19). Philadelphia: WB Saunders.

West, J. B. (2003). *Pulmonary pathophysiology: The essentials* (6th ed., pp. 17–36). Philadelphia: Lippincott Williams & Wilkins.

West, J. B., & Wagner, P. D. (2000). Ventilation, blood flow, and gas exchange. In J. Murray & J. Nadel (Eds.), *Textbook of respiratory medicine* (3rd ed., pp. 55–89). Philadelphia: WB Saunders.

White, K. M. (1987a). Continuous monitoring of mixed venous oxygen saturation (SvO2): A new assessment tool in critical care nursing: Part I. *Cardiovascular Nursing,* 23(1), 1–6.

White, K. M. (1987b). Continuous monitoring of mixed venous oxygen saturation (SvO2): A new assessment tool in critical care nursing: Part II. *Cardiovascular Nursing,* 23(2), 1–7.

4

Regulation of Cardiac Output and Blood Pressure

ELIZABETH J. BRIDGES*

This chapter reviews the neurohumoral control of the cardiovascular system as it relates to the rapid and more long-term control of cardiac output and blood pressure and the local control of blood flow (autoregulatory, metabolic, autacoid). Several models of cardiac function are presented, including the relationship between cardiac output and central venous pressure, the Krogh model of the effect of distribution of blood volume on cardiac output, and the arterial baroreflex responses to decreased and increased blood pressure.

AFFERENT INPUT AND RECEPTOR

Arterial Baroreceptors

The arterial baroreceptors are responsible for the reflex control of blood pressure. These baroreceptors are undifferentiated nerve fibers located in the adventitia of the carotid sinus (at the bifurcation of the carotid artery) and the aortic arch (between the arch of the aorta and the bifurcation of the subclavian artery; Fig. 4-1). The receptors are mechanoreceptors that respond to distortion or a change in transmural pressure or stretch (ds/dt) of the vascular bed in which they are located. For example, the carotid baroreceptors are sensitive to external compression or massage, both of which unload them (decrease transmural pressure). Although baroreceptors are often referred to as "pressoreceptors," they in fact do not sense pressure directly, but instead only indirectly through change in stretch.

The baroreceptors respond to two types of input: static input (i.e., mean arterial pressure) and phasic input (i.e., pulsatile changes). Therefore, the baroreceptors are responsive to mean arterial pressure, pulse pressure, and the number of pulses per minute (e.g., heart rate) (Scher, 1989). The static response has a threshold effect, that is, below a certain threshold of mean arterial pressure (20 to 50 mm Hg), the receptor stops firing. Above this

threshold there is an increase in rate of receptor firing in proportion to the increase in mean pressure, until a plateau of the output is reached at saturation. The phasic response increases when the rate of change of pressure rises (increasing pressure) and decreases when the rate of change in pressure decreases. A discussion of the central nervous system regulation is presented below.

Cardiopulmonary Receptors

Cardiopulmonary or low-pressure baroreceptors are located in the atria, ventricles, and pulmonary arteries and veins, with the cardiac baroreceptors providing the primary afferent input for the vagal cardioreflex (McMahon et al., 2000a, 2000b; Minisi, 1998). The properties of the cardiopulmonary baroreceptors are similar to those of the arterial baroreceptors, that is, a decrease in transmural pressure in the chamber or vessel results in a decrease in the firing rate of receptors, and vice versa.

Input to the central nervous system from the ventricular receptors, which are sensitive to mechanical and chemical stimuli, is through nonmyelinated vagal afferents (C fibers) (Hainsworth, 1995a). In response to an increase in ventricular pressure, the mechanoreceptors were previously thought to stimulate a depressor response (decreased heart rate/vasodilation). While the depressor reflex is observed as a decreased heart rate, recent studies suggest that this reflex plays a minimal role in the alteration in vascular tone in contrast to the vascular response induced by increases in carotid or coronary arterial pressure. The ventricular mechanoreceptors appear to play a role only in protection from gross overdistention, possibly during myocardial ischemia (Wright et al., 2000; Wright et al., 2001).

Bezold-Jarisch Reflex

The Bezold-Jarisch reflex, which is the most commonly used model to explain the triggering of vasovagal syncope, is manifested as a triad of symptoms (bradycardia, apnea, and hypotension) (Fenton et al., 2000). This reflex is mediated through cardiopulmonary vagal afferents with receptors located in the inferoposterior wall of the left ventricle (Aviado & Guevara Aviado, 2001). Stimulation of these mechanoreceptors and

The views expressed in this chapter are those of the author and do not reflect the official policy of the Department of Defense or other departments of the United States Government.

*The author thanks Dr. B. Zane Atkins for his review of this chapter.

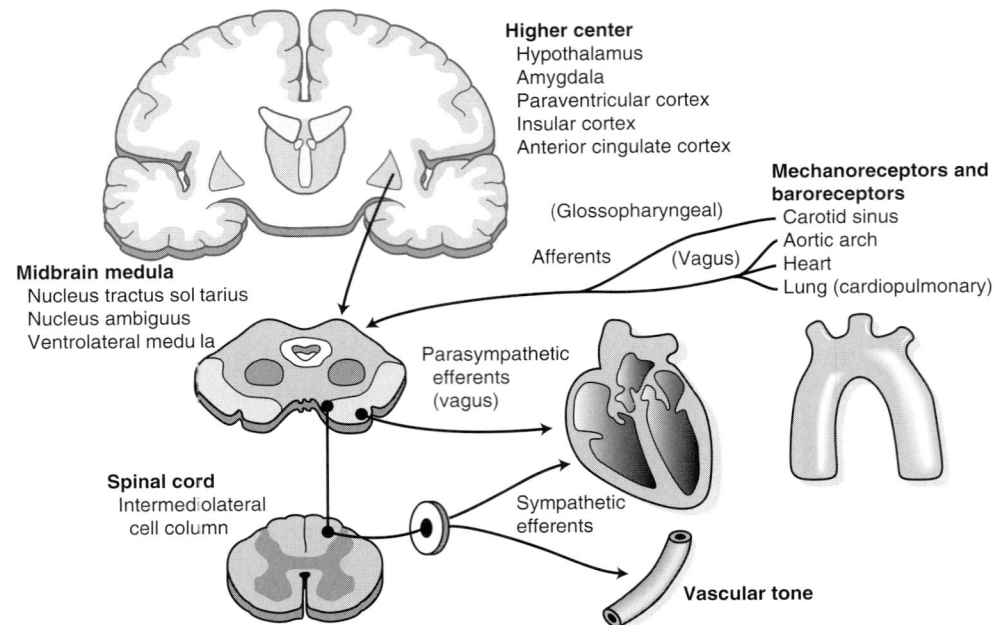

Higher center
Hypothalamus
Amygdala
Paraventricular cortex
Insular cortex
Anterior cingulate cortex

Mechanoreceptors and baroreceptors
(Glossopharyngeal)   Carotid sinus
                     Aortic arch
Afferents   Heart
         (Vagus)   Lung (cardiopulmonary)

Midbrain medula
Nucleus tractus sol tarius
Nucleus ambiguus
Ventrolateral medu la

Parasympathetic
efferents
(vagus)

Spinal cord
Intermediolateral
cell column

Sympathetic
efferents

Vascular tone

■ **Figure 4–1.** Autonomic nervous system regulation of cardiovascular hemodynamic responses. The baroreceptors (mechanoreceptors), which are located in the carotid sinus, the aortic arch and in the heart and lungs, send afferent impulses to the nucleus tractus solitarius. The vagal fibers to the heart arise from the vagal nucleus in the brainstem. This nucleus is governed by the nucleus tractus solitarius, which is the main receiving station for afferent information from the peripheral mechanoreceptors and chemoreceptors. The medullary centers also receive input from higher brain centers. The vagal nerve alters hear: rate through its effect on the sinoatrial (SA) and atrioventricular (AV) nodes. Sympathetic fibers innervate the SA and AV nodes and the ventricular myocardium, and affect heart rate and contractility. In addition, the sympathetic fibers innervate the vasculature, and thus alter vascular tone. (From Fenton, A.M., et al. [2000]. Vasovagal syncope. *Annals of Internal Medicine, 133,* 714–725.)

chemoreceptors leads to an inhibitory or depressor reflex causing a vagally mediated decrease in heart rate and withdrawal of sympathetic stimulation to the peripheral vasculature with subsequent vasodilation. Stimulation of this reflex may occur with pathological conditions, such as myocardial infarction (MI), administration of thrombolytic therapy, hemorrhage, aortic stenosis or syncope. It is important to note that vasovagal syncope may also occur in patients with transplanted (denervated) hearts; thus, factors other than those traditionally attributed to the Bezold-Jarish reflex must be considered (Fenton et al., 2000). Examples of other causative factors that inhibit sympathetic nervous system activation may include the release of endogenous opioids or nitric oxide, an abnormal serotonergic response, or impaired cerebral autoregulation with paradoxical cerebral vasoconstriction (Grubb & Karas, 1998; Morillo et al., 1997; Rea & Thames, 1993; van Lieshout et al., 1997). Figure 4-2 characterizes the numerous putative causes of vasovagal syncope. During an acute inferoposterior MI (particularly because of right coronary artery occlusion) and at the time of reperfusion of these infarctions, the transient bradycardia observed is thought to be a manifestation of the depressor effect of vagal receptors located in the inferoposterior wall of the left ventricle (Serrano et al., 1999). During ischemia, these receptors, which are mechanosensitive or chemosensitive, may be distorted by bulging of the ventricular wall during systole (Thoren, 1972) or by the presence of reactive oxygen species, serotonin, bradykinin, thromboxane A$_2$, or adenosine (Longhurst et al., 2001; Thames et al., 1996; Wacker et al., 2003). During thrombolytic therapy, the occur-

rence of vagally mediated bradycardia may be an indicator of reperfusion and sustained vessel patency, particularly with an inferior MI (Chiladakis et al., 2003). These receptors are also thought to mediate the reflex bradycardia and hypotension that occur during coronary angiography, particularly during injection of contrast material into the arteries that supply the inferoposterior surface of the left ventricle (e.g., circumflex, right coronary artery) (Perez-Gomez & Garcia-Aguada, 1977).

In severe aortic stenosis, some patients experience exertional syncope and even sudden death. The probable mechanism of the syncope is an exercise-induced increase in left ventricular pressure, which is extreme because of high aortic valve resistance, despite a decrease in aortic blood pressure. This high left ventricular pressure stimulates the ventricular baroreceptors and is manifested by a Bezold-Jarisch response (Mark et al., 1973; Mark & Mancia, 1983; Minisi & Thames, 1991; Omran et al., 1996). This abnormal cardiovascular response may also play a role in triggering sudden death (Lim et al., 2002). Once these patients undergo surgical correction of the stenosis, however, the normal sympathetic vasoconstrictor response to exercise is restored. Finally, in cases of severe hemorrhage or during head-up tilt (particularly in patients receiving a concurrent infusion of isoproterenol), the ventricular depressor reflex was thought to be initiated by the acute distortion of the ventricular mechanoreceptors by a forceful ventricular contraction on a relatively empty ventricle or simply forceful contraction alone (Lee et al., 1996; Morillo et al., 1997; Sander-Jensen, 1991). However, this abnormal response may also reflect a decrease in baroreceptor sensitivity causing a decrease in peripheral vasoconstriction

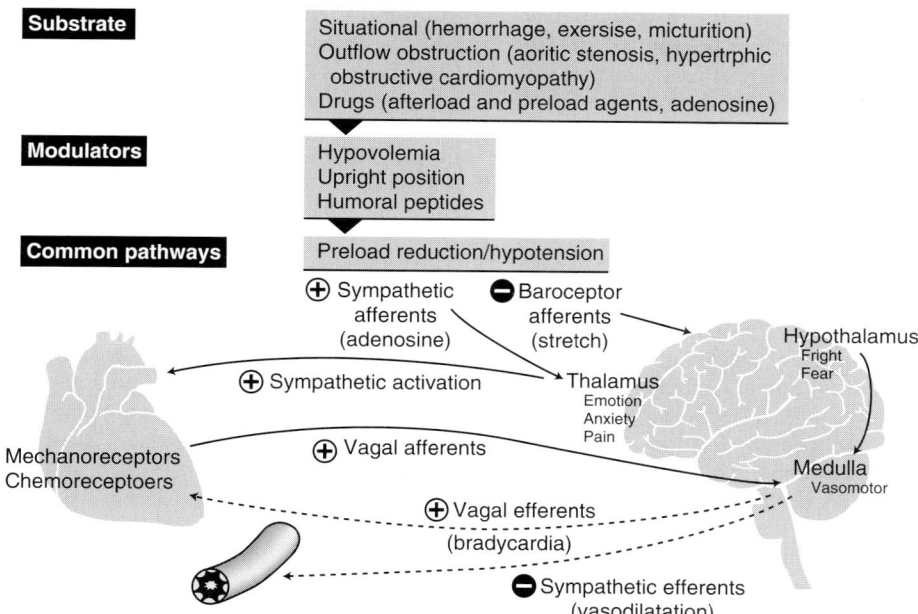

■ **Figure 4–2.** The Bezold-Jarisch reflex indicates that the neurocardiogenic reflex is initiated by cardiac mechanoreceptor activation. This information is transmitted by the vagal afferents to the cardiovascular respiratory center in the medulla. The negative feedback response is transmitted by an activation of the vagal efferents and an inhibition of the sympathetic efferents. Inputs to the medulla may originate from extracardiac locations as well as directly from the higher central nervous system. (From Fenton, A.M., et al. [2000]. Vasovagal syncope. *Annals of Internal Medicine, 133,* 714–725.)

(Flevari et al., 2002) or an altered hormonal response. In individuals in whom syncope develops, there is a plateau in norepinephrine levels and no change or a paradoxical increase in epinephrine (leading to β-adrenergic mediated vasodilation) compared with individuals who are not syncopal (Evans et al., 2001; Rowell & Blackmon, 1989). Another causative factor may be the abnormal activation of the serotonergic system, which leads to withdrawal of sympathetic support (Grubb & Karas, 1998; Theodorakis et al., 2003; Theodorakis et al., 1997).

Chemoreceptors

Peripheral chemoreceptors located in the carotid and aortic bodies are sensitive to decreased arterial Pa_{O2} or an increase in Pa_{CO2} or $[H^+]$, whereas central chemoreceptors, which are located in the medulla are sensitive to increased Pa_{CO2} (Hlastala & Berger, 2001). Stimulation of these receptors leads to hyperventilation and sympathetic activation, which causes vasoconstriction in most vascular beds, except the brain and heart. While an increase in blood pressure is an outcome of the chemoreflex, an increase in baroreceptor stimulation (i.e., increased arterial blood pressure) inhibits the chemoreflex response. Conversely, the chemoreflexes potentiate the baroreflex mediated vasoconstriction in response to decreased arterial blood pressure (Kara et al., 2003). In hypertension and sleep apnea, the peripheral chemoreflex response to hypoxemia is enhanced, with a resultant increase in sympathetic activation. Of clinical importance, there is a strong relationship between hypertension and sleep apnea (i.e., individuals with sleep apnea have a high prevalence of hypertension) (Peppard et al., 2000).

In heart failure, both the peripheral and central chemoreflex responses may be enhanced, as manifested by increased sympathetic activation (Narkiewicz & Somers, 2003). This enhanced response may contribute to genesis of sleep apnea in these patients, which is associated with a poorer prognosis (Javaheri, 2003; Lanfranchi et al., 1999).

CENTRAL NERVOUS SYSTEM REGULATION

The *nucleus tractus solitarius* is an ovoid area located in the medulla that receives efferent input from cardiovascular, respiratory, and gastrointestinal sites (see Fig. 4-1). The *nucleus tractus solitarius* serves as the first relay station for reflexes (e.g., baroreceptor reflex) that control circulation and respiration. From the *nucleus tractus solitarius,* there are multiple projections to areas such as: (1) the ventrolateral medulla, which is responsible for sympathetic efferent activity; (2) the *nucleus ambiguus* or "cardioinhibitory center" of the medulla, which is the location of the cell bodies of the vagal parasympathetic nerves; and (3) the median preoptic nuclei, which affect the release of vasopressin. The output from the medulla depends on the perturbation of the system (i.e., an increase or decrease in blood pressure). The complete baroreflex response is discussed later. From the central nervous system, the efferent arm of the rapid control of blood pressure operates through the autonomic nervous system.

From the carotid sinus, afferent input to the nucleus tractus solitarius in the medulla is through the carotid sinus nerve (nerve of Hering), which joins the ninth cranial nerve (glossopharyngeal). The sensory input from the aortic arch is through the 10th cranial nerve (vagus). Through synaptic connections to areas located in cental and rostral ventrolateral medulla and *nucleus ambiguus,* sympathetic and parasympathetic output, respectively, is modified by afferent feedback from the baroreceptors (Schreihofer & Guyenet, 2002). Of particular importance, output from the lateral ventrolateral medulla, which is directly projected to spinal sympathetic outflow via the bulbospinal (or medullispinal) tract, is responsible for maintaining tonic sympathetic activity, and thus resting arterial blood pressure (Dampney et al., 2002; Pilowsky & Goodchild, 2002). In addition, baroreceptor signals are transmitted to the forebrain. The forebrain plays a role in the release of vasopressin in response to a sustained decrease in blood pressure and influences the sympathoexcitatory vasomotor neurons in the medulla (Dampney, 1994; Verberne & Owens, 1998). The excitation or inhibition of the sympathetic and parasympathetic systems depends on the direction of the change in arterial pressure. For example, an increase in blood pressure elicits acute parasympathetic activation and sympathetic inhibition, which decreases the heart rate, cardiac contractility, vascular resistance, and venous return. Conversely, a decrease in blood pressure results in increased sympathetic activation and parasympathetic withdrawal.

AUTONOMIC NERVOUS SYSTEM REGULATION

The autonomic nervous system, which is one branch of the peripheral nervous system, is responsible for coordination of body functions that ensure homeostasis. The autonomic nervous system is further divided into two major components: the sympathetic nervous system and the parasympathetic nervous system (Fig. 4-3).

Sympathetic Nervous System

Efferent projections from the hypothalamus and medulla terminate in the intermediolateral cells located in the gray matter of the thoracic and lumbar (thoracolumbar) sections of the spinal column (specifically, T-1 to L-2). Hence, the sympathetic nervous system is often referred to as the thoracolumbar division of the autonomic nervous system. The neuronal cell bodies, which are located in the spinal column, are generally the origin of short preganglionic efferent fibers that innervate postsynaptic sympathetic neurons located in three general groupings of ganglia (a group of nerve cell bodies). The paravertebral ganglia are located in a bilateral chain-like structure adjacent to the spinal column. This chain extends from the superior cervical ganglia, located at the level of the bifurcation of the carotid artery, to ganglia located in the sacral region. The prevertebral ganglia, which lays midline and anterior to the aorta and vertebral column, include the celiac, aorticorenal, and superior and inferior mesenteric ganglia. The third group of ganglia comprises the previsceral or terminal ganglia, which are located close to the target organs of the sympathetic nervous system. The previsceral ganglia have long preganglionic

fibers and short postganglionic fibers. In contrast, the paravertebral and prevertebral ganglia give rise to long postganglionic fibers, which extend to the target organs of the sympathetic nervous system (e.g., heart, lungs, vascular smooth muscle, liver, kidneys, bladder, and reproductive organs; see Fig. 4-3). Of particular importance to the control of blood pressure are the sympathetic receptors located in the heart, vasculature, kidneys, and renal medulla.

Adrenoreceptors

At the target organs, the postganglionic fibers terminate at the neuroeffector junction and are separated from the adrenergic receptors (adrenoreceptors) by only a small junctional gap or cleft. The adrenoreceptors have been classified into two general groups: α-adrenergic receptors and β-adrenergic receptors. The receptor groups are further divided into general subtypes, β_1, β_2, and β_3 and α_1 and α_2 (Table 4-1) (Bylund et al., 1994; Lands et al., 1967). Based on molecular cloning techniques, the α-receptors are further subdivided, with the α_1 subclassified as (α_{1A}, α_{1B}, α_{1D}) (Guimaraes & Moura, 2001). The α_1 receptors on the vasculature may be further subclassified as α_{1H}, α_{1L}, and α_{1N} (Tsuru et al., 2002), although additional research needs to be conducted to determine if these latter receptor subtypes are distinct entities or conformational states of the α_{1A} receptor (Guimaraes & Moura, 2001). The α_2 receptor has also been subclassified (α_{2A}, α_{2B}, and α_{2C}) (Hein et al., 1999).

The effects of dopamine are mediated by two families of receptors (D_1 and D_2) (Amenta et al., 2001). The D1 receptors (D_1 and D_5 receptor subtypes) couple with G proteins to activate adenyl cyclase and the D_2 receptors (D_2, D_3, and D_4 receptor subtypes) inhibit adenyl cyclase release and activate potassium channels (Emilien et al., 1999; Missale et al., 1998). Dopamine is a precursor of norepinephrine. In the heart, dopamine exerts its indirect inotropic and chronotropic effects through the release of norepinephrine. Stimulation of postjunctional D_1 receptors in the renal, mesenteric, and splenic arteries produces vasodilation and natriuresis. Stimulation of prejunctional D_2 receptors in blood vessels inhibits norepinephrine release causing vasodilation. Additionally, in the kidneys stimulation of the D_2 receptor inhibits norepinephrine release and plays a synergistic role in modulating natriuresis via inhibition of aldosterone secretion (Jose et al., 1998). Exogenous administration of low-dose dopamine (<4 μg/kg per minute) causes vasodilation of the renal and splanchnic vascular beds and increases sodium excretion. However, low-dose dopamine has not been found to be renoprotective (Kellum & Decker, 2001; Marik, 2002). Intermediate doses of exogenous dopamine (2–10 μg/kg per minute) stimulate β1-adrenergic receptors in the heart and increases contractility. Higher doses (>10 μg/kg per minute) stimulate α-adrenergic receptors in the peripheral vasculature and cause vasoconstriction.

Heart. In the heart, β_1 receptors predominate (60%—80%), although there is also a smaller number of β_2 receptors (20%—30%), with the latter receptors playing a role in coronary vasodilation (del Monte et al., 1993; Feigl, 1998). Stimulation of the β_1 and β_2 receptors in the heart increases: (1) the rate of discharge of the sinoatrial node; (2) conduction across the atrioventricular node; and (3) speed of contraction in the atria and

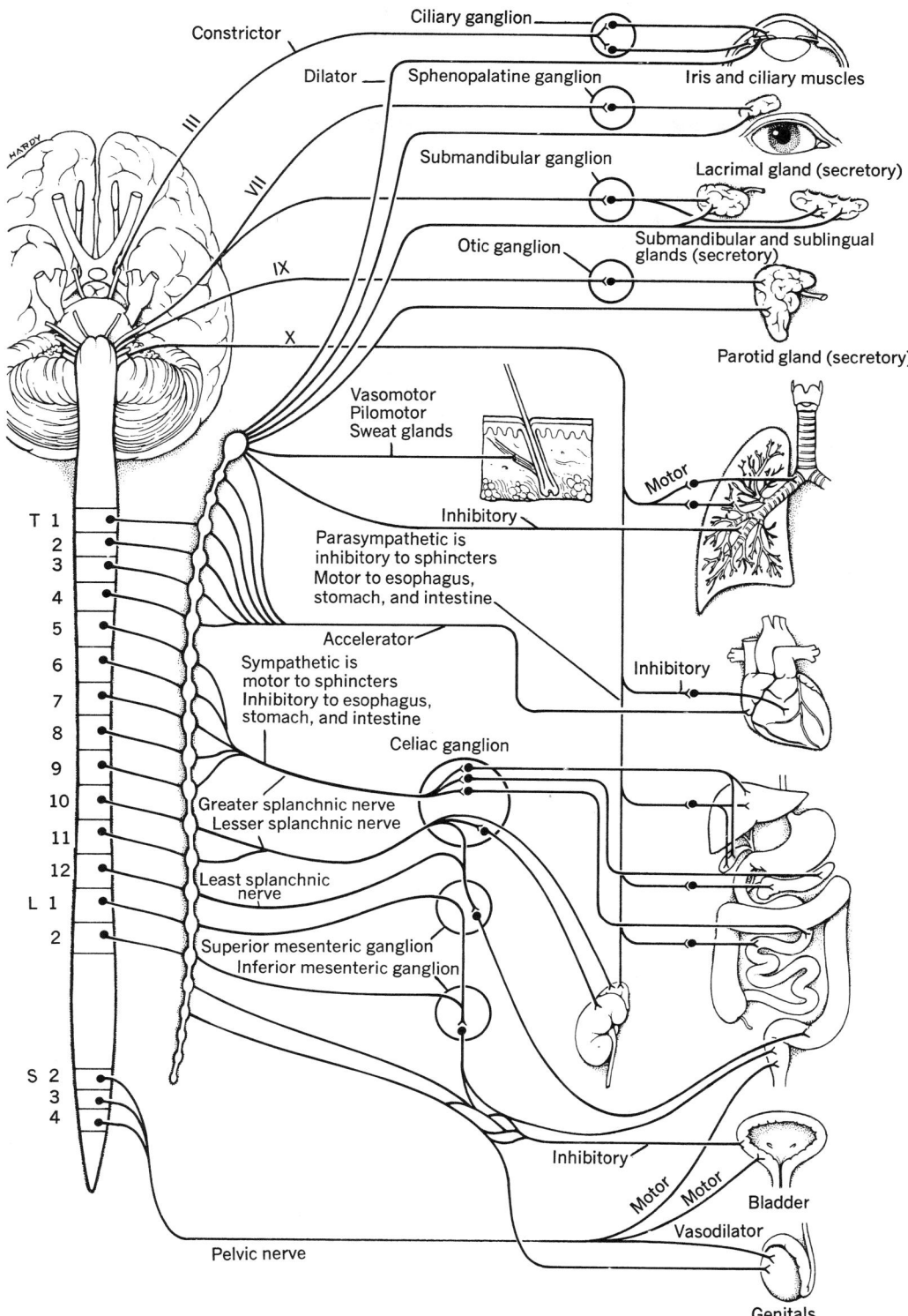

■ **Figure 4–3.** The autonomic nervous system. Parasymphathetic (craniosacral) divisions send long preganglionic fibers that synapse with a second nerve in ganglia located close to or within the organs that are then innervated by short postganglionic fibers. The sympathetic (thoracolumbar) division sends relatively short preganglionic fibers to the chains of paravertebral ganglia and to certain outlying ganglia. The second cell then sends relatively long postganglionic fibers to the organs they innervate. (From Rodman, M.J. & Smith, D.W. [1985]. *Pharmacology and drug therapy in nursing* [3rd ed., p. 302]. Philadelphia: JB Lippincott.)

Table 4–1 ■ CARDIOVASCULAR EFFECTS OF AUTONOMIC NERVOUS SYSTEM INNERVATION

Organ	Site	Effects	
		Sympathetic Stimulation	Parasympathetic Stimulation
Heart	Sinoatrial/atrioventricular nodes, His-Purkinje system	+ Chronotrope (β_1, β_2)	− Chronotrope
	Myocardium	+ Inotrope (β_1, β_2, presynaptic α_{2A}, presynaptic α_{2C})	− Inotrope (minor)
	Coronary arteries	Vasoconstriction (α_{1D}, α_2) Vasodilation (β_2)	Dilation
Systemic vasculature	Skeletal muscle	Vasodilation ($\beta_1 < \beta_2$, β_3, presynaptic α_2) Vasoconstriction (postsynaptic α_2)	—
	Splanchnic bed	Vasoconstriction (α, postsynaptic α_2)	—
	Renal	Vasoconstriction (α_1)	—
	Cutaneous veins	Vasoconstriction (postjunctional α_1, α_2)	Vasodilation

ventricles (chronotropic effect). In addition, β_1 stimulation increases cardiac contractility (inotropic effect). There is also a small number (<1%) of β_3 adrenergic receptors in cardiomyocytes (Gauthier et al., 1996). The β_3 receptors, which mediate negative inotropy via a nitric oxide-dependent pathway (Gauthier et al., 1998; Varghese et al., 2000), become important during heart failure when they are up-regulated and may contribute to functional degradation of the failing heart (Moniotte et al., 2001). In the murine model, there is also a putative β_4 receptor in the heart that has inotropic effects, although this receptor has not yet been identified in humans (Guimaraes & Moura, 2001; Kaumann, 1997; Kaumann et al., 1998). There are small number (approximately 14%) of α_1 receptors located in the atria and ventricles (Bristow et al., 1988). Stimulation of the α_1 receptors creates a modest inotropic response (Franchini & Cowley, 1996).

Vasculature. Sympathetic stimulation of the arterial tree extends to the level of the terminal arterioles and is also present on capacitance vessels, primarily in the splanchnic bed. The primary transmitter of the vascular smooth muscle sympathetic neuroeffector junction is norepinephrine. Binding of norepinephrine to the vascular smooth muscle α_1 receptor initiates vasoconstriction. The distribution of the α_1 subtypes varies depending on the vascular bed. For example, α_{1A} adrenoreceptors predominate in coronary, splanchnic, renal, and pulmonary vessels, whereas central arteries and veins express all three α_1 receptor subtypes (Rudner et al., 1999). Stimulation of presynaptic α_2 receptors inhibits norepinephrine release and decreases vasoconstriction, a process called *passive vasodilation*. Conversely, stimulation of the postsynaptic α_2 receptors, which are located on large arterioles and perhaps most importantly on the terminal arterioles, causes vasoconstriction (Faber, 1988; Leech & Faber, 1996; Ohyanagi et al., 1991). This vasoconstriction determines the number of open capillaries, and thus capillary blood flow. The α_2-mediated vasoconstriction of the terminal arterioles can be inhibited by metabolic vasodilators (e.g., oxygen, potassium), particularly in the skeletal muscles. Additionally, there are smooth muscle β_2 receptors. Stimulation of the noncardiac β_2 receptors results in relaxation of smooth muscle, with subsequent bronchodilation and peripheral vasodilation.

Cutaneous Vasculature

Control of the cutaneous circulation arises from both thermoregulatory and nonthermoregulatory reflexes. The cutaneous circulation has an extensive distribution of both α_1 and α_2 adrenoreceptors, but virtually no β adrenoreceptors (Borbujo et al., 1989). The glabrous skin (e.g., palms/soles) is innervated only by vasoconstrictive nerves. In contrast, nonglabrous skin receives both vasoconstrictive and vasodilator innervation (Johnson & Proppe, 1996). The sympathetic vasoconstrictor nerves release norepinephrine and may also release vasoconstrictive co-transmitters (neuropeptide Y or adenosine triphosphate), although this latter mechanism remains to be elucidated in humans (Charkoudian, 2003).

In a thermoneutral environment, the cutaneous resistance vessels in the acral regions (e.g., ears) are tonically constricted, whereas the nonacral regions (limbs, head, trunk) have minimal constriction (Pergola et al., 1994; Rowell, 1993). Vasodilation in the acral regions is primarily caused by withdrawal of vasoconstrictive tone (passive vasodilation), whereas vasodilation in nonacral regions is the result of an active process, which is sympathetically (but not adrenergically) mediated (Roddie, 1983; Rowell et al., 1996). Within a "neutral zone," thermoregulation is controlled entirely by changes in cutaneous vasomotor tone (Savage & Brengelmann, 1996). An active increase in adrenergic tone causes vasoconstriction in response to hypothermia. Conversely, a decrease in adrenergic stimulation causes passive vasodilation and is responsible for 10% to 20% of vasodilation in response to hyperthermia (Charkoudian, 2003; Johnson & Proppe, 1996; Rowell, 1983). Cholinergic nerves, which innervate the sweat glands, release a yet to be described co-transmitter that may be functionally linked to the large and important active cutaneous vasodilation seen in heat stress (Kellogg et al., 1995; Roddie, 1983; Rowell et al., 1996). Additionally, under conditions of hyperthermia, nitric oxide appears to be necessary for the vasodilatory response (Kellogg et al., 1998; Shibasaki et al., 2002). The cutaneous veins constrict in response to local cold and are reflexly constricted in response a decrease in skin or core body temperature (Joyner & Dietz, 2003).

Nonthermoregulatory control of the cutaneous circulation via the arterial and cardiopulmonary baroreflexes plays a role in blood pressure control. For example, under normothermic conditions, "unloading" of the baroreflex causes cutaneous vasoconstriction. Because of the normally low cutaneous blood flow during normothermia, this vasoconstriction contributes little to blood pressure maintenance. However, under conditions of hyperthermia and during exercise, when there is significant blood flow to the cutaneous vasculature, baroreflex-mediated vasoconstrictive may offset thermoregulatory vasodilation and play an important role in maintenance of blood pressure (Johnson & Proppe, 1996; Rowell et al., 1996). Of note, the baroreflex sensitivity is not impaired by whole-body heating as previously thought; however, heat stress may decrease peripheral vasoconstrictor responsiveness, which contributes to an increased susceptibility to orthostatic intolerance (Crandall et al., 2003).

Neurotransmitters

The sympathetic postganglionic fibers that innervate the arterial tree are in general noradrenergic (i.e., release norepinephrine). The only exceptions are the postganglionic fibers that innervate the sweat glands (sudomotor neurons), which have acetylcholine as their neurotransmitter and the extrapyramidal system, which has dopamine as the primary neurotransmitter (Hoffman & Taylor, 2001). Norepinephrine is synthesized from tyrosine and is stored in sympathetic nerve terminals. In response to neuronal stimulation, the "packets" or quanta of norepinephrine are extruded from the axon vesicles by exocytosis. The vesicular release of norepinephrine is enhanced by angiotensin II and cold, whereas the prejunctional effects of potassium, decreased PO_2, heat, autacoids (adenosine, bradykinin, serotonin, prostaglandins), nitric oxide, and acetylcholine inhibit its release (Vanhoutte & Leusen, 1981) (Fig. 4-4). The neurotransmitters diffuse over varying small distances, depending on the width of the junctional cleft, to receptors located on effector organs. Norepinephrine, as discussed later, is also considered a systemic hormone because of its spillover into the interstitial space.

Parasympathetic Nervous System

The second branch of the autonomic nervous system is the parasympathetic nervous system. The primary parasympathetic outflow is through four cranial nerves (III, VII, IX, and X). Of importance to blood pressure and cardiac output control, cardiac vagal (cranial nerve X) motorneurons are located in the nucleus ambiguus and dorsal vagal nucleus of the medulla (Spyer, 2000). In addition, there are cell bodies located in the spinal cord gray matter at S-2 through S-4. Hence, the parasympathetic nervous system is referred to as the *craniosacral* branch of the autonomic nervous system. In contrast to the sympathetic nervous system, the preganglionic fibers of the parasympathetic nervous system are long fibers, synapsing on ganglia that are close to or directly attached to the effector organ. The postsynaptic fibers are relatively short, in contrast to the fibers of the sympathetic nervous system.

Receptors

In the parasympathetic nervous system, the nerve fibers are cholinergic, which means they liberate acetylcholine. Despite a common neurotransmitter (acetylcholine), stimulation of various receptors in the parasympathetic nervous system causes different effects. The reason for the variable response is that there are two general types of cholinergic receptors: nicotinic and muscarinic.

Preganglionic cholinergic receptors, which are found in the sympathetic and parasympathetic nervous systems, are nicotinic. The nicotinic receptors are located on autonomic ganglia and skeletal muscle endplates. Stimulation of the nicotinic receptors is excitatory and short-term (milliseconds). These receptors are blocked by curare. In clinical practice, blockade of the nicotinic receptors with various neuromuscular blocking agents (e.g., succinylcholine, pancuronium) causes musculoskeletal paralysis (blockade at the skeletal muscle endplate) and may potentially cause hypotension because of blockade at the autonomic ganglia (Hoffman & Taylor, 2001).

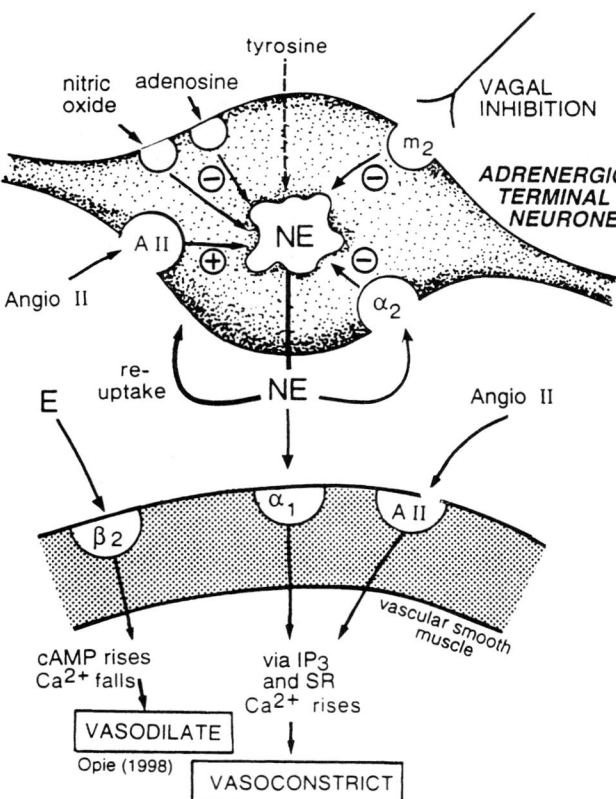

■ **Figure 4–4.** Arteriolar constriction and dilation. Norepinephrine (NE), released from the storage granules of the terminal neurons into the synaptic cleft, has predominantly vasoconstrictive effects acting through postsynaptic α_1 receptors. In addition, presynaptic α_2 receptors are stimulated to allow feedback inhibition of its release to modulate any excess release of NE. Parasympathetic cholinergic stimulation releases acetylcholine (Ach), which stimulates the muscarinic (m_2) receptors to inhibit the release of NE and thereby indirectly cause vasodilation. Circulating epinephrine (E) stimulates vasodilatory α_2 receptors. Angiotensin II (Angio II), formed ultimately in response to renin released from the kidneys, is also powerfully vasoconstrictive, acting both by enhancement of NE release and directly on arteriolar receptors. cAMP, cyclic adenosine monophosphate; SR, sarcoplasmic reticulum; IP_3, inositol triphosphate, AII, angiotensin II. (From Opie, L.H. [1998]. *The heart: Physiology from cell to circulation* [3rd ed., p. 28.]. Philadelphia: Lippincott-Raven.)

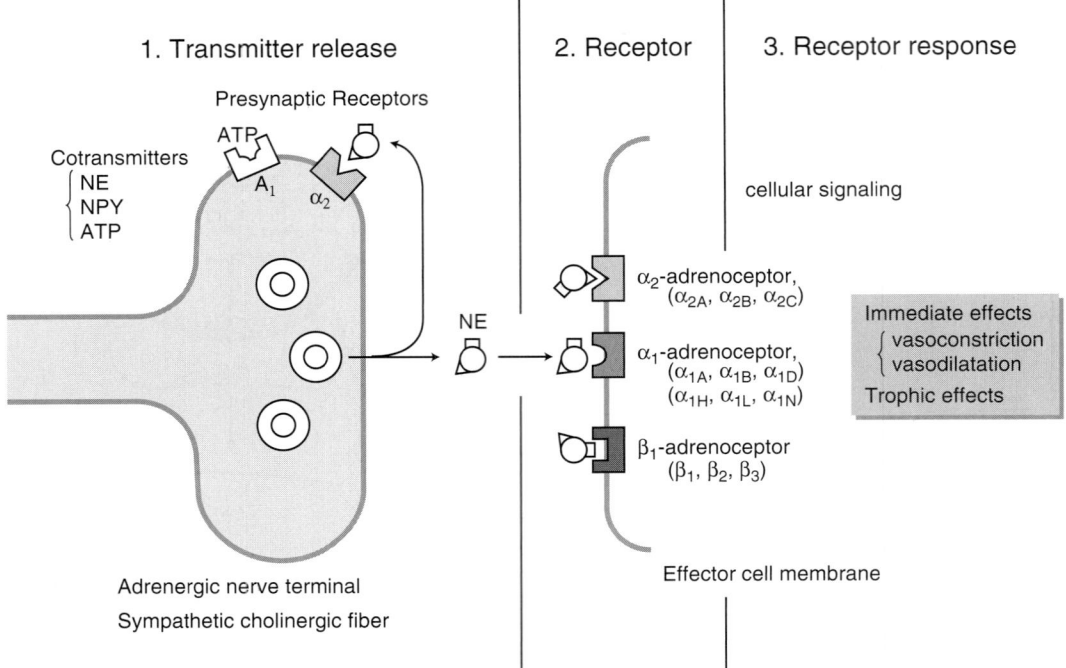

■ **Figure 4–5.** Diagram of the sympathetic nerve and adrenergic neuroeffector mechanism. 1. Transmitter release from the sympathetic terminal. Sympathetic nerve may contain three cotransmitters, i.e., norepinephrine (NE), neuropeptide Y (NPY) and ATP. Release of main transmitter NE may be presynaptically modulated by α_2-adrenoreceptor, A_1 adenosine receptor, etc. 2. Adrenoreceptors on the effector cell membrane. There are α- and β-adrenoreceptors and subtypes $\alpha_1(\alpha_{1A}, \alpha_{1B}, $ and $\alpha_{1D}; \alpha_{1H}, \alpha_{1L}$ and $\alpha_{1N}), \alpha_2 (\alpha_{2A}, \alpha_{2B}$ and $\alpha_{2C})$, and β_1, β_2 and β_3. There may be regional differences in the population of adrenoreceptors. 3. Effector responses. Sympathetic nerves have both immediate effects—contraction and dilation, differing from vessel to vessel—as well as long term trophic effect on blood vessels. (From Tsuru, H. et al. [2002]. Role of perivascular sympathetic nerves and regional differences in the features in sympathetic innervation of the vascular system. *Japanese Journal of Pharmacology,* 88[1], 9–13.)

The primary postganglionic receptor in the heart, smooth muscle, and glandular tissue is muscarinic, with its actions mediated by coupling with G-protein receptors. These receptors are stimulated by muscarine and can be antagonized by atropine and scopolamine. There are subtypes of the muscarinic receptors that result in varied responses. For example, stimulation of muscarinic subtype 1 (M_1) receptors is responsible for the release of norepinephrine from the sympathetic neurons. Conversely, stimulation of muscarinic subtype 2 (M_2) receptors, which are specifically associated with vagal nerve endings in the heart, has direct and indirect negative inotropic and chronotropic effects. The direct effects are secondary to occupation of the ß-adrenergic receptors and inhibition of norepinephrine release, and the indirect effects occur through inhibition of the adrenergic second messenger cAMP (Brodde & Michel, 1999; Brown & Taylor, 2001). Of clinical importance, the negative chronotropic and inotropic effects associated with the M_2 receptor are blocked by atropine.

Co-transmitters

At the preganglionic synapse, the primary neurotransmitter for the sympathetic and parasympathetic nervous systems is acetylcholine. At the neuroeffector junction in the sympathetic nervous system, the primary neurotransmitters are norepinephrine and its precursor, dopamine, whereas the primary neurotransmitter of the postganglionic fibers of the parasympathetic nervous system is acetylcholine. However, other neurotransmitters that augment or modify the effects of the primary neurotransmitter are co-released, and are referred to as *co-transmitters* (Fig. 4-5) (Burnstock, 1995). The most prominent co-transmitter in the sympathetic nervous system ganglia is neuropeptide Y (NPY), and a lesser effect is observed from adenosine triphosphate (ATP) (Tsuru et al., 2002). Vasoactive intestinal peptide (VIP) is the prominent co-transmitter in the parasympathetic nervous system ganglia and nonadrenergic, noncholinergic nerves (Burnstock, 1986).

Neuropeptide Y

Neuropeptide Y (NPY) is an amino acid peptide released with norepinephrine from sympathetic nerve terminals. Neuropeptide Y has direct pressor effects and also exerts a prejunctional modulation of the release of other neurotransmitters. For example, neuropeptide Y inhibits the release of acetylcholine from vagal nerve endings, thus attenuating the effects of the parasympathetic system on heart rate, atrioventricular conduction, and atrial contractility (Franchini & Cowley, 1996). In addition, NPY potentiates the postjunctional contractile effects of norepinephrine. In the mesentery, 30% of the sympathetic nervous system induced vasoconstriction depends on NPY (Han et al., 1998; Westfall et al., 1998), although the role of NPY varies depending on the vascular bed.

VIP

Vasoactive intestinal peptide (VIP) is present in the peripheral and central circulation, where it acts as a nonadrenergic, noncholinergic neurotransmitter or neuromodulator. Endogenous VIP is a potent vasodilator. It is released in response to vagal stimulation in the heart, where it produces coronary vasodilation as well as positive inotropic (particularly in the right atria and ventricle) and chronotropic effects (Feliciano & Henning, 1998; Henning & Sawmiller, 2001). VIP-induced peripheral vasodilation is caused by increased calcium-extrusion or sequestration induced by VIP or natriuretic protein-C receptor stimulation. This peripheral vasodilation enhances the VIP-mediated inotropic effects (Colston & Freeman, 1992; Lundberg, 1996).

■ SYSTEMIC HORMONES

In addition to the rapid control of arterial pressure by the autonomic nervous system, hormones such as epinephrine and arginine vasopressin directly and indirectly affect the baroreceptor reflex and play an important role in the rapid control of blood pressure. Three interrelated systems (natriuretic peptide system, renin-angiotensin-aldosterone system [RAAS] and the kallikrein-kinin system [KKS]) also contribute to the regulation of the arterial blood pressure and fluid volume (Fig. 4-6). Finally, a spillover of norepinephrine into the systemic circulation also affects blood pressure and cardiac output.

Epinephrine

In response to physical or emotional stressors (mental stress, exercise, hyperthermia, hypoglycemia), epinephrine is secreted into the plasma by the adrenal medulla, causing the plasma level of epinephrine to increase. Epinephrine stimulates β_1 receptors in the heart and has positive chronotropic and inotropic effects. The net effect of this cardiac stimulation is an increase in cardiac output. Epinephrine also acts on the vasculature and stimulates the β_2 receptors in the skeletal muscles and splanchnic arterioles, which causes vasodilation in these two large regions and potentially large decrements in the systemic vascular resistance (see Fig. 4-3). In the skin and kidneys, epinephrine stimulates the α-adrenergic receptors and causes vasoconstriction (Opie, 1998; Rowell, 1986).

Exogenously administered epinephrine has dose-specific effects. Low-dose epinephrine (0.005 to 0.02 µg/kg per minute in adults) stimulates the β adrenoreceptors and causes vasodilation and increased heart rate and contractility. Increased doses (>0.2 µg/kg per minute) stimulate the α-adrenoreceptors and increases vascular resistance and blood pressure (Hoffman, 2001). Knowledge of these dose-specific effects is important, and although epinephrine is often administered for its vasoconstrictive effects, it may cause vasodilation if a large-enough dose is not administered.

Arginine Vasopressin

Arginine vasopressin (AVP), or antidiuretic hormone (ADH), is a neurotransmitter synthesized in the hypothalamus and released

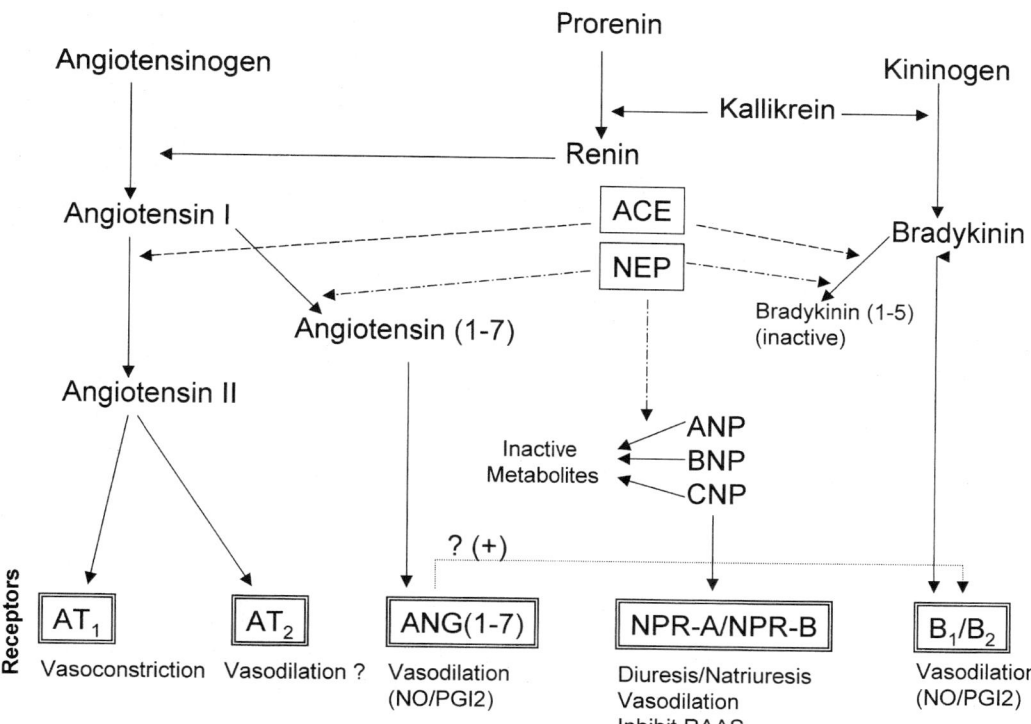

■ **Figure 4–6.** Interaction of the renin-angiotensin-aldosterone system (RAAS), kallikrein-kinin system (KKS), and natriuretic peptides (Burnett, 1999; Schmaier, 2002, 2003; Tschope et al., 2002).

from the neurohypophysis of the pituitary gland (posterior pituitary gland). Vasopressin is primarily released in response to changes in plasma osmolality; however, AVP may also be released in response to a decrease in blood volume or blood pressure. As the osmolality increases, AVP secretion increases. In humans, the primary effect of AVP is its antidiuretic effect, which is caused by stimulation of water absorption at the distal and collecting tubules of the kidney (Giebisch & Windhager, 2003; Knepper - et al., 2000). The change in water absorption affects plasma osmolality. Vasopressin is exquisitely sensitive to changes in osmolality; for example, a 5- to 10-mOsm increase in osmolality causes an increase in plasma AVP (Bie, 1980; Ramsay et al., 1988). The close relation between osmolality and AVP maintains plasma osmolality within 3% of normal in most conditions.

The sensitivity of the baroreceptor system is less than that of the osmoreceptors, as demonstrated by the large (5% to 10%) iso-osmotic change in plasma volume required before vasopressin secretion is altered. However, during hemorrhage (plasma volume decreased by >5% to 10%), plasma levels of vasopressin are increased, in some cases 100-fold (Shen et al., 1991) (Fig. 4-7). In this case, vasopressin acts in a manner similar to renin and norepinephrine, causing vasoconstriction and playing a supporting role to the sympathetic nervous system in the maintenance of blood pressure (Jackson, 2001b). The mechanism for the hemorrhage-induced change in vasopressin secretion was previously thought to be the Henry-Gauer (cardiorenal) reflex. Current evidence suggests that the arterial baroreceptors, and not the cardiac receptors, are the primary reflex controllers of the plasma volume-mediated release of this hormone (Rowell, 1993; Thrasher et al., 2000; Thrasher & Keil, 1998). In the case of hemorrhage, the change in intrathoracic volume alters the arterial systolic blood pressure, which decreases arterial baroreceptor stimulation, and leads to increased vasopressin secretion (Thrasher & Keil, 2000).

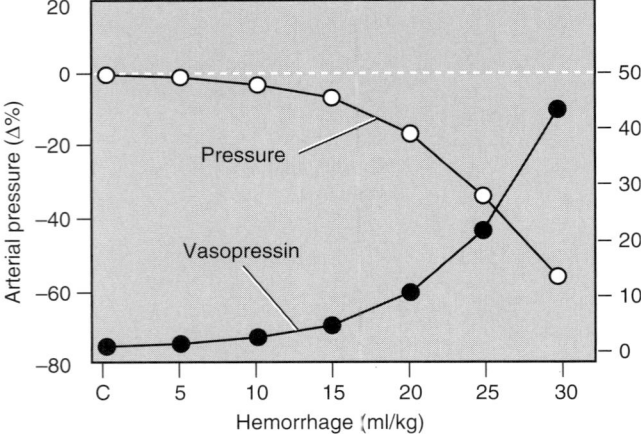

■ **Figure 4–7.** Mean percentage changes in arterial blood pressure and in plasma vasopressin concentration in response to blood loss (0.5 ml/kg/min) in a group of 12 dogs; the maximal volume of blood withdrawn was 30 ml/kg. (Redrawn from Shen, Y.-T., Cowley, A.W., J., & Vatner, S.F. [2001]. Relative roles of cardiac and arterial baroreceptors in vasopressin regulation during hemorrhage in conscious dogs. *Circulation Research, 68,* 1422. From Berne, R.M., & Levy, M.N. [2001]. *Cardiovascular physiology* [8th ed.]. St. Louis: Mosby.)

Natriuretic Peptides

There are three natriuretic peptides (A, B, and C) that contribute to the regulation of blood pressure and electrolyte and volume homeostasis (Levin et al., 1998; Rubattu & Volpe, 2001). Atrial natriuretic peptide (ANP) and brain natriuretic peptide (B-type natriuretic peptide [BNP]) are released from granules in the atria and ventricles in response to increased stretch (increased preload and afterload) (Ruskoaho et al., 1997) and hormonal stimuli (e.g., angiotensin II, glucocorticoids, endothelin I, catecholamines) (Rubattu & Volpe, 2001). Brain natriuretic peptide was first discovered in the brain but is found in a greater concentration in the ventricles; hence, the term B-type natriuretic peptide or BNP is a more appropriate term. The actions of BNP are similar to ANP. C-type natriuretic peptide is widely distributed in the brain, kidneys, lungs, heart, and endothelial cells, and is released in response to shear stress. The natriuretic peptides are metabolized by three mechanisms: (1) binding with natriuretic peptide receptor-C (NPR-C); (2) metabolism by neutral endopeptidase (NEP), which is located in the renal tubules, lung, intestine, seminal vesicles, and neutrophils; and (3) renal clearance.

The cardiac natriuretic peptides, which bind with natriuretic peptide receptor A (NPR-A), cause diuresis and natriuresis, which decreases cardiac preload and subsequently decreases the blood pressure (Dhingra et al., 2002). Preload reduction may occur because of shifting of fluid from the intravascular to the extravascular space (increased vascular endothelial permeability) and possibly increased capillary hydrostatic pressure along with natriuresis (Levin et al., 1998). Additionally, ANP and BNP decrease sympathetic tone to the peripheral vasculature both centrally and peripherally, inhibit the renin-angiotensin-aldosterone system by inhibiting angiotensin II-stimulated sodium and water transport in the proximal tubules, improve ventricular relaxation, and lower the activation threshold for the vagal afferents, which suppresses the reflex tachycardia and vasoconstriction associated with the decrease in preload and cardiac output (Burnett, 1999; Rubattu & Volpe, 2001) (Fig. 4-8). Clinically, the short-term administration of intravenous B-type natriuretic peptide nesiritide (Natrecor) has been shown to improve hemodynamic function and decrease symptoms of acute decompensated heart failure compared with standard therapy (Colucci et al., 2000; Keating & Goa, 2003; Mills et al., 1999).

Atrial natriuretic protein has an acute hypotensive effect mediated by a decrease in cardiac output and may also play a role in long-term reduction of blood pressure (Melo et al., 2000). The long-term blood pressure effect reflects a decrease in vascular resistance and is mediated indirectly by prejunctional attenuation of sympathetic tone to resistance vessels (Melo et al., 1999). In the presence of heart failure, the role of ANP and BNP in blood pressure control remains unclear (Cowley, 1992). In severe heart failure, increased levels of ANP may offset the detrimental effects of increased angiotensin-aldosterone and the sympathetic nervous system. However, in early heart failure, impaired release of ANP may contribute to sodium retention and disease progression (Rubattu & Volpe, 2001).

C-type natriuretic peptide binds to natriuretic peptide receptor-B (NPR-B), leading to the generation of intracellular guanosine 3'5'-monophosphate (cGMP). CNP is a selective

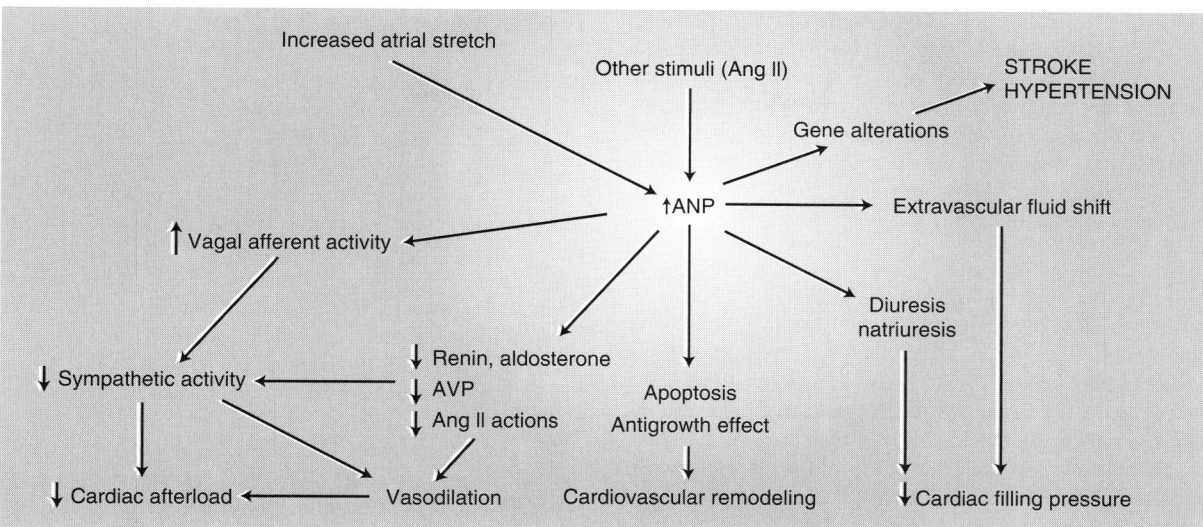

■ **Figure 4–8.** Schematic representation of the regulation and function of atrial natriuretic peptide (ANP). Along with the classical circulatory effects, the new emerging functional properties of the atrial natriuretic peptides are shown. AVP, vasopressin; ANG II, angiotensin II. (From Rubattu, S., & Volpe, M. [2001]. The atrial natriuretic peptide: A changing view. *Journal of Hypertension, 19,* 1925.)

endothelium-independent vasodilator (effects greater on pre-contracted veins than arteries). This vascular effect decreases venous return and subsequently decreases cardiac filling pressures, cardiac output, and arterial blood pressure. Unlike ANP and BNP, CNP has minimal renal actions (Stingo et al., 1992). CNP is a potent coronary vasodilator (Chen & Burnett, 1998) and also has an anti-mitogenic effect on vascular smooth muscle, which may be protective against atheroma development and restenosis (Naruko et al., 1996).

Renin-Angiotensin-Aldosterone System

The renin-angiotensin-aldosterone system (RAAS) plays an important role in the long-term control of arterial blood pressure, regional blood flow, and sodium balance. The RAAS acts in a cascade fashion, initiated by the stimulation of renin release from the kidney. Renin is stored in and released from the juxtaglomerular cells near the renal afferent arterioles. Renin release is stimulated by three mechanisms. First, renin release occurs in response to increased sympathetic nervous system stimulation of the afferent and efferent arterioles in the renal glomeruli. The ß-adrenergic receptors in the cells of the juxtaglomerular apparatus are sensitive to neurally released and systemic catecholamines. Note, this neurally mediated response can be blocked by ß-adrenergic blockers (e.g., propranolol). Second, renin release is stimulated by decreased renal perfusion pressure, distending the afferent arterioles (intrarenal baroreceptor pathway). Below a mean arterial pressure of 80 to 90 mm Hg, renin secretion is a steep and linear function of renal perfusion pressure. Finally, decreased sodium chloride concentration in the macula densa, which is located in the early distal tubule, stimulates the juxtaglomerular apparatus to secrete renin (Jackson, 2001a). Increased blood pressure decreases renin release by activating the baroreceptors caus-

ing a decrease in sympathetic tone, increasing pressure in the renal arterioles, and decreasing sodium chloride reabsorption in the proximal tubule, causing increased sodium chloride to reach the macula densa.

Angiotensin II is released through the proteolytic effects of renin on the plasma protein, angiotensinogen, which is synthesized and released into the plasma from the liver. Renin converts angiotensinogen to angiotensin I. Angiotensin I, which is inactive, is converted to angiotensin II by an angiotensin converting enzyme (ACE) located in the plasma and vascular endothelium throughout the body (Jackson, 2001a). Pharmacologically, ACE inhibitors exert their effect at this level of the renin-angiotensin system (Dzau et al., 2001).

Angiotensin II has two primary actions: vasoconstriction and stimulation of aldosterone release. Angiotensin II causes vasoconstriction of the arterioles through a direct effect on the vascular smooth muscle (Jackson, 2001a). Angiotensin II indirectly affects vascular tone by stimulating the formation of superoxide anions, which inhibit NO-mediated vasodilation, and by inducing endothelin-1 formation to cause further vasoconstriction (Griendling et al., 1997; Harrison et al., 2003; Harrison, 1997; Mombouli & Vanhoutte, 1999). The renal and splanchnic circulations are particularly sensitive to angiotensin II. Angiotensin II increases vascular resistance and stimulates the heart indirectly through its potentiating actions on the sympathetic nervous system. These effects include: (1) accelerating the synthesis and release of norepinephrine; (2) delaying neuronal reuptake of norepinephrine; (3) directly stimulating the sympathetic ganglia; and (4) facilitating the response to sympathetic activity and vasoconstrictor drugs (Rowell, 1993).

Angiotensin II also has a long-term effect on blood pressure through stimulation of aldosterone synthesis and secretion, which increases blood volume. Aldosterone, a mineralocorticoid synthesized and secreted by the adrenal cortex, increases sodium reabsorption in the loop of Henle and decreases sodium excretion, which together lead to retention of water and expansion of blood volume. The change in blood volume is a slow process, which is important in the long-term control of blood pressure. Angiotensin II may also play a role in a sustained increase in sympathetic vasomotor or cardiac sympathetic activity by modification of sympathetic nervous system activity perhaps by action at the level of the paraventricular nucleus (Brooks & Osborn, 1995; Dampney et al., 2002). This latter mechanism may contribute to long-term control of sympathetic activity.

Kallikrein-Kinin System

The kallikrein-kinin system (KKS) plays a role in blood pressure control and may have a protective cardiovascular effect. Kinins (e.g., bradykinin and kallidin), which are produced by the action of the enzyme kallikrein on kininogens, bind with B_1 and B_2 receptors. Binding of kinins with the B_1-receptor causes the release of NO and prostacyclin (PGI_2) from endothelial cells and subsequent vasodilation. The B_2 receptors appear to play a role in pathological conditions such as pain, inflammation and hypertension. Stimulation of the B_2 receptor causes the release of NO and PGI_2 and may be cardioprotective via vasodilation and anti-ischemic and anti-proliferative effects (Sharma & Sharma, 2002). A deficient KKS may play a role in the pathogenesis of hypertension through altered sodium excretion (Sharma & Sharma, 2002).

Interaction Between the KKS, RAAS, and Natriuretic Hormones

The KKS, RAAS, and the natriuretic hormones interact via the actions of angiotensin-converting enzyme (ACE) and NEP (see Fig 4-6). ACE stimulates the conversion of angiotensin I to angiotensin II and degrades kinins (Burnett, 1999; Schmaier, 2002, 2003). NEP, which is the principle enzyme responsible for degrading the natriuretic peptides, also stimulates the formation of angiotensin (1–7) from angiotensin I. Angiotensin (1–7) has vasodilatory and antiproliferative effects that inhibit ACE and also counteract the actions of angiotensin II (Tschope et al., 2002). Angiotensin (1–7) also enhances the effects of bradykinin through yet to be identified mechanisms. Kallikrein, which is the enzyme involved in the formation of bradykinin, may also stimulate the conversion of prorenin to renin (Schmaier, 2003). Renin subsequently causes the conversion of angiotensinogen to angiotensin I. Exploitation of the physiological interactions between these three systems may be useful in the treatment of heart failure and hypertension (Burnett, 1999). For example, ACE inhibition exerts its antihypertensive effects by decreasing angiotensin II, increasing angiotensin (1–7) levels and potentiating the effects of bradykinin by increasing its level and through direct effect on the B_2-receptor (Tschope et al., 2002). Omapatrilat, which inhibits ACE and NEP activity, decreased the risk of death and hospitalization in chronic heart failure compared to ACE inhibition alone (enalapril and lisinopril) (Packer et al., 2002; Rouleau et al., 2000) and may decrease vascular tone and blood pressure in hypertension (Mitchell et al., 2002; Waeber, 2000).

Norepinephrine Spillover

Approximately 80% of the norepinephrine secreted at the neuroeffector junction is either taken-up by sympathetic neurons (neuronal reuptake) or broken-down by the enzymes monoamine oxidase or catechol-O-methyl transferase. The remaining 20% may spill into the systemic circulation. The spillover is usually proportional to the increase in sympathetic nervous system activation; thus, the plasma norepinephrine level can be used as an approximate indicator of SNS activity (Esler, 1993). Direct measurement of sympathetic nerve traffic via microneurography and spectral analysis are alternative methods to measures SNS activity (Grassi & Esler, 1999). Factors such as the nerve-firing rate, blood flow, neuronal uptake of norepinephrine, capillary permeability, and width of the junctional cleft can also affect the level of plasma norepinephrine. The width of the junctional cleft is particularly important in the pulmonary vasculature, where spillover is predominantly the result of the wide junctional clefts and not of a high rate of sympathetic nervous system activation or norepinephrine release (Bevan, 1977, 1979; Bevan & Su, 1974).

■ HEART RATE

Control of Heart Rate

The intrinsic heart rate at rest, without any neurohumoral influence, is approximately 100 to 120 beats per minute. The heart rate in the intact, resting person reflects a balance between the tonically active sympathetic and parasympathetic nervous systems, with the parasympathetic nervous system predominating (Hainsworth, 1995b; Levy & Martin, 1979; Spyer, 2000). The predominance of the parasympathetic nervous system is manifested by a resting heart rate that is lower than the intrinsic rate. Parasympathetic predominance may also be demonstrated by abolishing the vagal influence with the administration of atropine.

Vagal stimulation of the sinoatrial and atrioventricular nodes leads to a rapid (within one to two beats) decrease in heart rate. When vagal stimulation is discontinued, the heart rate increases rapidly. The rapid response to vagal stimulation and the presence of a large amount of cholinesterase (the enzyme that degrades the acetylcholine that is released from the parasympathetic fibers) allows the vagus nerve to exert beat-to-beat control of heart rate. Conversely, the heart rate response to sympathetic stimulation is gradual in onset, and once the sympathetic stimulation is terminated, the heart rate slowly decreases (Levy & Martin, 1979; Levy, 1997).

As discussed later, there is an inverse relation between heart rate and arterial blood pressure. The inverse changes in heart rate are in response to baroreceptor stimulation, with the response most pronounced over a mean arterial pressure of 70 to 160 mm Hg. The alterations in heart rate are achieved by a reciprocal relationship between sympathetic and parasympathetic cardiac stimulation.

Changes in heart rate also occur as a result of chemosensor reflexes (Pa_{O_2}) mediated by the carotid chemoreceptors. For example, a relatively slight excitation of the chemoreceptors leads to stimulation of the vagal center in the medulla and a decrease in heart rate. This response, which is seldom seen clinically, is considered the primary reflex effect of chemosensor stimulation (Mohrman & Heller, 1997). With increased levels of stimulation (e.g., a marked decrease in Pa_{O_2}), a secondary reflex is initiated that leads to depression of the primary chemoreceptor reflex and an increase in heart rate. This reflex is caused by pulmonary hyperventilation, which leads to hypocapnia and activation of pulmonary stretch receptors. The chemosensor reflex plays only a minimal role in the control of heart rate because the primary and secondary reflexes tend to offset one another.

Resting Sinus Arrhythmia

There is a direct relation between heart rate and respiration (Hainsworth, 1995b). During inspiration the heart rate increases, then it decreases during expiration. This respiratory-induced cyclical variation in heart rate is referred to as a *sinus arrhythmia*. The sinus arrhythmia also may occur in the absence of ventilatory movement, indicating a central control mechanism (Anrep et al., 1936). Sinus arrhythmia is thought to reflect vagal cardiac nerve activity. Of interest, respiratory activity phasically alters vagal motorneuron responsiveness, with decreased vagal output during inspiration compared to expiration (Eckberg, 2000). An in-depth discussion of this subject is presented in Chapter 24.

Heart Rate and Cardiac Output

The relationship between heart rate and cardiac output is defined by the equation: cardiac output = stroke volume × heart rate. The effect of heart rate on cardiac output can vary over a wide range because of changes in stroke volume. As is discussed in the section on models of cardiac performance, a small increase in heart rate causes an increase in cardiac output and a decrease in stroke volume. The decrease in stroke volume is due to the effect of increased cardiac output on the peripheral volume, and a subsequent decrease in central venous pressure (Janicki et al., 1996; Sheriff, Zhou et al., 1993). In this case, the increase in heart rate is not the direct cause of the decrease in stroke volume. It is not until the heart rate exceeds 150 beats/min that the cardiac output is decreased secondary to inadequate diastolic filling time, which decreases stroke volume. Conversely, below a heart rate of 50 beats/min, the stroke volume is relatively fixed, and a further decrease in heart rate causes a decrease in cardiac output (Bevegård et al., 1967; Hainsworth, 1995b; Miller et al., 1962; Rushmer, 1959).

INTRINSIC CARDIAC CONTROL

In addition to cardiac control through the autonomic nervous system and systemic hormones, cardiac output is modified by the intrinsic factors: preload, afterload, and contractility. The following discussion focuses on how these factors affect cardiac output.

Preload

At the level of the muscle fiber, preload is defined as the force acting to stretch the ventricular fibers at end-diastole. Preload

is related to cardiac output by the Frank-Starling law of the heart (length-tension relationship), which states that an increase in myocardial muscle fiber length is associated with an increase in the force of contraction (Sonnenblick, 1962; Starling, 1918), and the subsequent increase in stroke volume and cardiac output (Sarnoff, 1955; Weber et al., 1974). In the case of preload/afterload dependent changes in contractile function, the mechanism of increased contractile force is known as length-dependent activation, whereby the myofilaments increase their sensitivity to cytosolic calcium as the sarcomere length increases to maximum (Hancock et al., 1993; Opie, 1998). This mechanism is contrary to traditional descriptions of Starling's law of the heart, which had maximal cardiac function occurring at an "optimal sarcomere length" (Lakatta, 1987). According to this conceptualization, an increase in sarcomere length was thought to give rise to optimal overlap of actin and myosin. This conceptualization has been challenged because the cardiac sarcomere normally operates at 80% to 85% of optimal length with only 10% of maximal force developed.

Afterload

In muscle fiber experiments, preload is the tension in the muscle before contraction and afterload is the additional tension that develops in the muscle during contraction before shortening occurs (Brady, 1991; Sonnenblick, 1962). At the level of the ventricle, afterload is defined as ventricular wall tension during the shortening phase of contraction and reflects the sum of the forces against which the ventricle must act to eject blood (Janicki et al., 1996). However, given the heterogeneous direction of myocardial fibers and the torsion or twisting of the ventricle during systole, a single measure of ventricular wall tension is inadequate to define afterload. In the intact system in vivo, afterload is defined as the pressure in the aorta during systole (Hedges, 1983). The aortic blood pressure is essentially equal to left ventricular pressure during the ejection phase of systole; thus, these values are interchangeable. The key factors that affect aortic blood pressure during ejection are arterial compliance, arterial resistance, and the reflection of pulse waves from the periphery.

As described by the force-velocity relation, for any given preload there is an inverse relation between afterload and muscle shortening, and thus stroke volume (Covell & Ross, 2002). Although this relationship is observed in the isolated muscle fiber, it is not clinically apparent in people with normal cardiac function (Janicki et al., 1996). However, in people with a chronically depressed inotropic state (e.g., heart failure, cardiomyopathy), a steady state with altered ventricular dimensions (hypertrophy, dilatation) and maximal use of the length-tension relation occurs. Therefore, in these people in the face of an increase in afterload, the reserve provided by the length-tension relationship is exhausted and stroke volume decreases acutely (Ross, 1976). These findings help to explain the use of afterload-reducing agents in patients with heart failure.

In clinical practice, systemic vascular resistance, which is often considered *the* indicator of afterload, is used interchangeably with afterload. This conceptualization is incorrect because afterload can change independently of vascular resistance. For example, in a patient who has experienced a severe hemorrhage, despite the fact that the systemic vascular resistance is increased (often to extreme), afterload is actually decreased. Recalling the original definition of afterload as the additional tension that develops in the muscle during contraction before shortening occurs helps to clarify this area of confusion. The tension or stress that develops in the ventricular wall according to the Laplace relation is:

$$T = \frac{PR}{2h}$$

where T is average circumferential wall stress (force/cross-sectional area), P is intraventricular pressure, R is the radius of curvature of the wall, and h is wall thickness. In hemorrhage, the radius of the ventricle is decreased, and if the compensatory actions of increased heart rate and systemic vasoconstriction are inadequate to maintain pressure, the intraventricular pressure also decreases. Thus, despite an increase in systemic vascular resistance, ventricular afterload decreases.

Contractility

Contractility refers to the intrinsic properties of cardiac myocytes that reflect the activation, formation, and cycling of cross-bridges between actin and myosin filaments. In the intact heart, a change in contractility is defined as an alteration in cardiac performance that is independent of preload and afterload. An increase in contractility results in greater magnitude and velocity of shortening and augmented stroke volume (Opie, 1997; Sonnenblick, 1962). Contractility, which reflects the availability of calcium to the myofilament and sensitivity of the myofilament to calcium, can be increased by an increase in circulating epinephrine and norepinephrine released from cardiac sympathetic nerves, and by a decrease in the interval between beats (increasing heart rate), a phenomenon known as the treppe (staircase) effect (Covell & Ross, 2002). There is also an important relationship between heart rate and β-adrenergic stimulation and myocardial contractility, with the effects of β-adrenergic stimulation expressed only when there is a concomitant increase in heart rate (Ross et al., 1995; Ross, 2000). This relationship has been exemplified by the progressive increase in contractility (measured by dP/dt) with incremental doses of dobutamine (Kambayashi et al., 1992). This latter relationship is now considered the fourth intrinsic factor influencing myocardial contractility, along with length-dependent activation, basal force frequency effect, and direct positive inotropic effect of myocardial β-adrenergic receptor stimulation (Covell & Ross, 2002). Clinically, loss of the force-frequency relationship during heart block and downregulation of β-adrenergic stimulation during heart failure contributes to impaired cardiac function.

EXTRINSIC CONTROL: PERICARDIAL LIMITATION

Under normal resting conditions, the pericardium has little or no effect on cardiac filling; however, during acute increases in cardiac volume, the pericardium affects ventricular interaction and plays a role in the compensatory increase or decrease in stroke volume between the two ventricles (Kroeker et al., 2003). Additionally, in the face of increased filling pressures, the pericardium restricts cardiac filling, which is important in preventing excessive dilation during acute increases in cardiac volume (Spodick, 1997). In chronic cardiac dilation, however, there is growth of new pericardial tissue or slippage of the collagen fibers, and the pericardium actually enlarges in size and mass. As a result of this pericardial distortion, there is no increase in pericardial constraint in chronic cardiac dilation (Horne et al., 2000; Kardon et al., 2000).

After pericardiectomy there is an increase in the maximal cardiac output, O_2 consumption, and left ventricular end-diastolic segment length (Hammond et al., 1992). The increase in cardiac output is caused by an increase in stroke volume, which is caused by an increase in end-diastolic volume and myocardial fiber length, as described by the Frank-Starling law of the heart (De Hert et al., 2001). However, the effects of pericardiectomy on stroke volume and cardiac output are apparent only during exercise (Stray-Gundersen et al., 1986).

In cases in which the pericardium has been opened and reapproximated, pericardial constraint increases because of development of adhesions between the pericardium and the heart (Hunter et al., 1992). The increased constraint is manifested as an increase in intraventricular pressure for any given volume, which reflects an increase in juxtacardiac pressure (Rao et al., 1999). Consideration of the increased juxtacardiac pressure is important in the interpretation of hemodynamic data (increased pressure for any given volume) in postcardiac surgery patients who have had pericardial reapproximation.

LONG-TERM CONTROL OF BLOOD PRESSURE

Although the sympathetic nervous system, through the sinoaortic baroreceptor reflex, plays a primary role in the rapid (minutes to hours) regulation of blood pressure, this reflex appears to be less important than neuroendocrine factors in the long-term control of arterial pressure. The probable method for the long-term control of arterial pressure is the much slower-acting fluid volume regulation, with the hypothesized mechanism being renal pressure diuresis-natriuresis (Cowley, 1992; Granger et al., 2002; Osborn, 1997).

While blood volume is not directly linked to arterial pressure, long-term arterial blood pressure control is based on the idea that arterial pressure is maintained at a level required by the kidneys to excrete a volume of urine approximately equivalent to the daily fluid intake (minus extrarenal fluid losses). The kidneys sense a change in blood volume through the arterial pressure (Brooks & Osborn, 1995; Cowley, 1992). That arterial pressure and not fluid volume is sensed is demonstrated in disease processes associated with a combination of increased extracellular volume and decreased arterial pressure (e.g., heart failure, cirrhosis with ascites). In these cases, the kidneys retain fluid despite expanded fluid volume.

Based on this hypothesis, an increase in renal perfusion pressure causes a decrease in sodium reabsorption and an increase in sodium and water excretion, although the exact mechanism remains unknown (Granger et al., 2002). As long as sodium and water intake remained stable, the enhanced sodium excretion will decrease extracellular volume and blood volume, and arterial pressure will decrease. According to this mechanism, an increase in systemic vascular resistance and subsequent increase in renal perfusion pressure would not cause a long-term increase in arterial pressure, unless renal function was impaired (Cowley, 1992).

Renal Excretion of Sodium Chloride and Water

Despite the putative primacy of the renal diuresis-natriuresis mechanism in the long-term control of blood pressure, a hypothesis receiving some support is that arginine vasopressin and angiotensin II provide long-term feedback to the central nervous system. In addition, neural and hormonal factors modulate the renal diuresis-natriuresis response. For example, a decrease in sodium intake stimulates renin activity, which leads to the generation of angiotensin II. An increase in angiotensin II decreases renal blood flow and the glomerular filtration rate, which indicates a shift of the pressure-natriuresis response (i.e., increased response to decreased sodium). Thus, angiotensin II appears to have an important role in the long-term modulation of renal function and the control of blood pressure (Cowley, 1992).

Basal Tone

All arterioles exhibit a basal level of vasoconstriction or tone. Basal tone, which is the intrinsic level of vascular tone, is independent of neural or humoral influences and serves as the baseline around which neural or humorally mediated vasoconstriction or vasodilation occurs (Fig. 4-9). Basal tone varies among organs; it is lowest in the kidneys and highest in the skeletal muscles, heart, and brain (Mellander, 1989). The maintenance of arteriolar tone through tonic rhythmic vasoconstriction is essential for the maintenance of blood pressure. For example, it is estimated that if this basal myogenic tone were eliminated, a minimal cardiac output of 60 to 75 L/min would be required to maintain a normal blood pressure (Mellander, 1989; Rowell, 1986). In contrast, if the sympathetic input associated with resting tone were withdrawn, the blood pressure would decrease only from 100 to 86 mm Hg. This small decrease in blood pressure occurs because the vascular bed with the highest resting tone (skeletal muscle) normally receives only 15% of the cardiac output.

Nitric oxide affects basal arteriolar tone and blood pressure, with a greater effect in larger (>200 μm) than in smaller resistance vessels (<200 μm) (Vallance et al., 1990). Nitric oxide also affects large-artery distensibility (Joannides et al., 1995; Wilkinson et al., 2002). The reduction or absence of

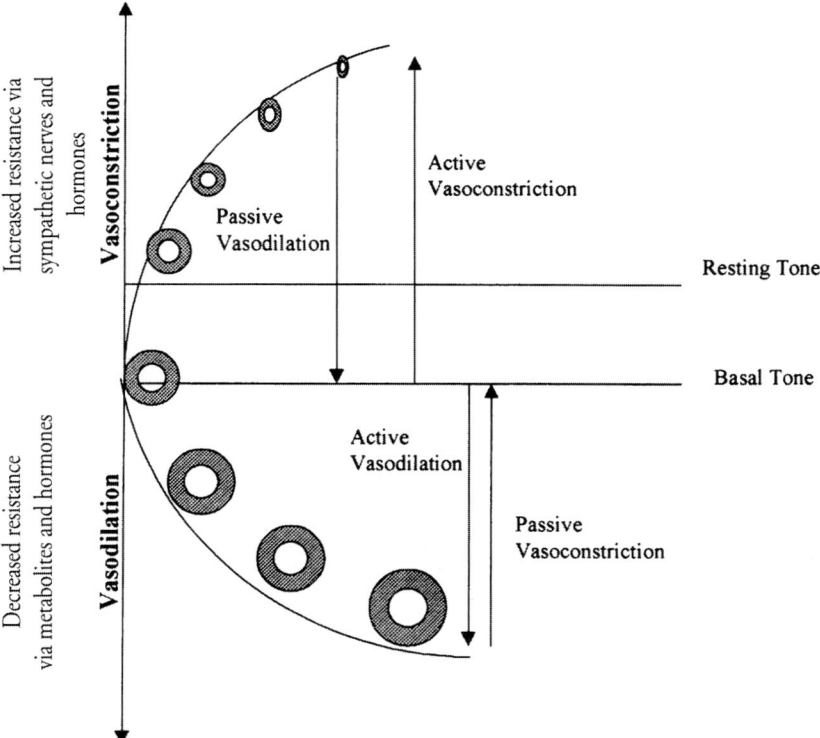

■ **Figure 4–9.** Schematic of active and passive changes in vascular resistance. The vascular bed is tonically constricted (basal tone) as a result of neurohumoral and local factors (autoregulation). In addition, some vascular beds have a higher level of tone (resting tone) indicating sympathetic nervous system (SNS) stimulation. Passive vasodilation is the passive release of SNS stimulation, dilating the vessel toward basal tone. Passive vasoconstriction is the release of active vasodilatory stimuli. Active vasodilation is vascular dilation below basal tone and active vasoconstriction is constriction above basal tone. (Courtesy of Loring B. Rowell, University of Washington, Seattle, WA.)

tonic NO release causes increased mean arterial blood pressure and may be a cause of pathological conditions characterized by increased blood pressure (Sorrentino & Pinto, 1997; Wilkinson et al., 2002).

As demonstrated in Figure 4-9, active and passive vasomotion occurs around the basal and resting tone of the vascular bed. Four terms define this vasomotion (Celander, 1954; Rowell, 1986):

1. *Active vasoconstriction,* which is mediated by sympathetic stimulation, is the increase in vascular resistance above the basal level.
2. *Passive vasodilation,* in contrast to active vasoconstriction, is the reduction in vascular resistance back to the basal level caused by the withdrawal of the sympathetic stimulation associated with active vasoconstriction. In some vascular beds, resistance may be increased above basal tone by tonic sympathetic stimulation. This increase in vascular tone is referred to as *resting tone.* Passive vasodilation is most easily seen in vascular beds with increased resting tone (e.g., acral regions).
3. If a vascular bed has high basal tone, *active vasodilation,* which is a decrease in vascular resistance below the level maintained by basal tone, may occur (i.e., vasodilation beyond that which exists after all neural and hormonal influences are removed). In this case, the vasodilation is not merely the result of withdrawal of sympathetic tone, because this action causes passive vasodilation.
4. *Passive vasoconstriction* is caused by withdrawal of the stimulation causing active vasodilation.

The skeletal muscle arterioles have a high basal tone and therefore are capable of a wide range of vasoconstriction and vasodilation, because there is an increased level of basal tone to be modulated. In contrast, the renal vasculature has a low basal and resting tone that can be markedly increased through sympathetic stimulation, but has little capability to undergo active vasodilation because there is so little basal tone to inhibit.

LOCAL REGULATION OF SYSTEMIC MICROVASCULAR BEDS

Arteriolar resistance vessels are partially constricted under normal circumstances by a tonic rhythmic myogenic tone, and this level of tone is modulated by neurogenic or other factors that cause active vasoconstriction or vasodilation. In the intact organism, blood flow and vascular hydrostatic pressure in the microvasculature of each organ system are controlled by complex interrelations among the effects of physical factors, locally released substances, circulating hormones, and above all by neurotransmitters secreted in response to central activation of the sympathetic nervous system. The relative predominance of local versus centrally mediated control of the microvascular bed varies among vascular beds, and it also varies among resistance, precapillary, and postcapillary blood vessels within a given vascular bed.

The large and medium-sized arterioles, which are the predominant sites of vascular resistance, are primarily under the control of the sympathetic nervous system and centrally mediated neurohumoral factors (e.g., angiotensin II). These vascular segments are influential in the control of arterial blood pressure and, by virtue of their position, they control the total amount of blood entering a specific vascular area; therefore, the distribution of blood flow between the different vascular beds. The terminal arterioles or precapillary vascular segments control the number of open capillaries and are under sympathetic nervous system and local control (Johanson, 1980). Local control mechanisms (autoregulation) that affect the terminal arterioles may have a substantial influence on exchange vessel pressures and flows and on the vascular tissue exchange of fluid and solutes.

Autoregulation

Autoregulation, which appears to occur in all organs except the lung, is the intrinsic tendency of an organ or vascular bed to maintain constant blood flow through alteration in its arteriolar tone, despite changes in arterial pressure. Autoregulation can occur in some organs over a range of perfusion pressure of 60 to 80 mm Hg to an upper limit of 150 mm Hg (Fig. 4-10), and is independent of neural and hormonal control. There are three hypotheses to explain autoregulation: the myogenic, metabolic, and tissue pressure hypotheses (Johnson, 1986; Renkin, 1984). It appears that none of these mechanisms works in isolation and, as described later, the tissue pressure hypothesis may apply only in pathological conditions. In addition, under certain conditions (e.g., a marked decrease in arterial perfusion with hypoxemia and decreased transmural pressure), metabolic and myogenic control promote vasodilation in an additive manner (Borgström et al., 1984; Renkin, 1984). Conversely, with increased venous pressure, the myogenic and metabolic control systems may compete. In this case (low-flow, high venous pressure), metabolically induced vasodilatation usually predominates over the myogenic response to increased vascular distention, which should stimulate vasoconstriction (Johnson, 1980; Lombard & Duling, 1977; Renkin, 1984).

Myogenic Hypothesis

The myogenic hypothesis refers to the acute reaction of a blood vessel to a change in intraluminal pressure, that is a pressure-induced stretch in vascular smooth muscle results in vasoconstriction and subsequently decreases the flow (Johansson, 1989; Renkin, 1984; Schubert & Mulvany, 1999). Conversely, when the intraluminal pressure is decreased, the stimulus for the myogenic response is decreased, the vessel dilates, and blood flow is returned toward control levels (Johnson, 1980). Much is unknown about the myogenic response. For example, exactly what is sensed to stimulate the myogenic response (e.g., change in pressure, stretch of the vascular smooth muscle, or change in wall tension) remains unclear. Possible mechanisms for sensing the myogenic stimulus include depolarization of the vascular smooth muscle, activation of mechanosensitive ion channels, modulation of carrier-mediated ion exchangers, transmission of the alteration in the cytoskeleton and extracellular matrix via surface receptors (e.g., integrins), and activation of membrane-bound enzymes (Davis & Hill, 1999). Endothelial-derived nitric oxide or, in the absence of the

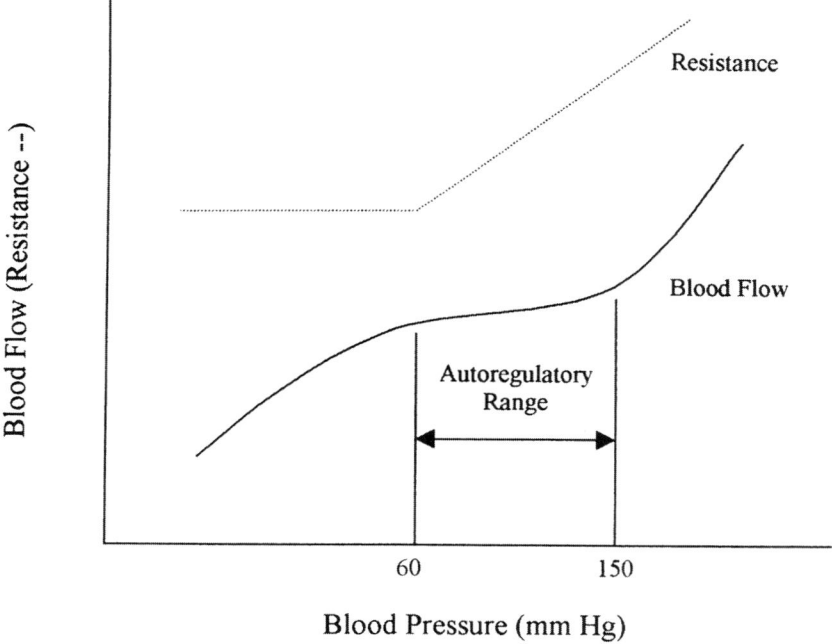

■ **Figure 4–10.** A schematic representation of autoregulation. The blood flow is relatively constant between an arterial pressure of 60 and 150 mm Hg because of an active increase in resistance. Below a mean pressure of 60 mm Hg and above 150 mm Hg, the flow is directly related to pressure.

endothelium, an EDHF-like substance may provide modulation of myogenic tone in small arteries via a negative feedback mechanism (Schubert & Mulvany, 1999; Scotland et al., 2001). While it is uncertain how the myogenic signal is coupled to the contractile response, it appears to involve increased intracellular calcium, which contributes to contraction through calcium-calmodulin-myosin light-chain kinase phosphorylation of myosin, with the subsequent interaction of actin and myosin. Additional calcium regulatory mechanisms include alterations in intracellular calcium, calcium-induced changes in ion channels, and alteration in calcium sensitivity (Hill et al., 2001).

There are two arguments against the myogenic hypothesis. First, the myogenic response senses local pressure rather than flow to control flow (Price, 1991; Rowell, 1986). Autoregulation is related to the control of flow, not the control of pressure; thus, although the myogenic response may play some role in the local control of blood flow, its role in the central control of blood flow remains to be demonstrated. Second, to increase resistance and maintain a constant flow, the caliber of the arteriole must be smaller than it was before the vessel was stretched by the increased pressure. If this vasoconstriction does not occur, flow rises (Rowell, 1986). The myogenic response appears to play a greater role in autoregulation when both the arterial and venous pressures change equally (i.e., during postural changes). This latter action may be related to the release of NO in response to changes in flow and pressure (Davis & Hill, 1999).

Metabolic Hypothesis

The metabolic hypothesis is considered a special case of metabolic control of blood flow and is based on the idea that the concentration of a large number of metabolites and metabolic substrates (e.g., potassium, hydrogen, O_2, CO_2, adenosine) in the interstitial space controls vascular tone. In this case, the vascular smooth muscle acts as a chemosensor. According to this hypothesis, a decrease in blood flow leads to an increase in the local concentration of a metabolite and causes vasodilation and increased blood flow (Feigl, 1989; Renkin, 1984; Rowell, 1986). Recent research suggests that a metabolite (possibly a byproduct of arachidonic acid) is released from the venous system that vasodilates the adjacent arteriole. The exact stimulus is unknown, but it may be related to a hypoxia-induced release of ATP from red blood cells leading to the release of arachidonic acid (Hester & Hammer, 2002). The metabolic hypothesis has been suggested as a mechanism for autoregulation in organs or tissues where the primary function of blood supply is to support local metabolism. In this case, there is a close relation between blood flow and metabolic needs. However, in organ systems with high blood flow (e.g., kidney, skin), where blood flow occurs in excess of metabolic needs, there is a limited relationship between blood flow and metabolism (Rowell, 1986), and the metabolic hypothesis as a factor in the autoregulatory control of blood flow has not been supported.

An important point is that metabolic autoregulation is not the same as metabolically induced active and reactive hyperemia (increased blood flow), which occur in response to increased metabolic demand (e.g., intestinal vasculature during digestion or cardiac and skeletal muscle during activity) or interruption of blood flow to a vascular bed, respectively (Renkin, 1984). Active hyperemia is the adaptive increase in blood flow in response to changes in the local metabolic rate caused by variation in the functional activity of the surrounding cells (Renkin, 1984). In response to this change in functional status, the vascular resistance decreases almost immediately. In addition, there is an increase in the number of perfused capillaries (capillary recruitment) in response to metabolic stimulation. The magnitude of the reactive hyperemia response depends on the duration of the vascular obstruction and the metabolic rate of the given vascular bed. Unlike "pure" metabolic autoregulation, this response is a combination of three components: (1) passive changes in vessel diameter caused by a change in transmural pressure; (2) a myogenic response to the change in transmural pressure; and (3) a metabolic component (Johnson, 1980; Lombard & Duling, 1977; Renkin, 1984).

Tissue Pressure Hypothesis

The tissue pressure hypothesis states that an increase in external pressure (e.g., interstitial pressure) decreases transmural pressure (pressure inside minus pressure outside the vessel), which passively decreases the vessel diameter and decreases flow (Renkin, 1984). The effect of external compression on blood flow normally occurs during ventricular systole, when the coronary arteries are compressed. Clinically, the effect of transmural compression is more likely to be observed in organs constrained in a rigid container (e.g., brain, where increased cerebrospinal fluid pressure may compress cerebral vessels) or a stiff capsule (e.g., kidney) (Renkin, 1984; Rowell, 1986). In the lung, vascular compression caused by increased external (alveolar) pressure, such as with the application of high levels of positive end-expiratory pressure, may also affect blood flow.

Under physiological conditions, tissue pressure probably does not play a major role in the control of blood flow, but it may be particularly important under pathological conditions such as edema, hemorrhage into the interstitial space, or cellular swelling caused by injury or hypoxemia (compartment syndrome) (Renkin, 1984). In the latter cases, external compression may decrease blood flow below a physiologically safe level.

VENOUS SYSTEM

The primary functions of the venous system are to return blood from the capillaries to the heart and to serve as a reservoir that counterbalances the transient imbalance between cardiac output and venous return. However, because of its capacious nature, the venous system serves not only as a reservoir, storing approximately 70% of the total blood volume (approximately 33% of total blood volume is stored in the splanchnic bed—liver, stomach, spleen, and intestines), but also as a buffer against changes in cardiac output and blood pressure (Pang, 2001). The venous system can play both an active (venoconstriction) and, more importantly, a passive role in the maintenance of thoracic blood volume.

Neurohumoral Stimulation

The only neural control of veins is through the α-adrenergic fibers of the sympathetic nervous system (Rothe, 1983). Release of norepinephrine from α-adrenergic fibers causes constriction in the splanchnic and cutaneous veins, whereas withdrawal of

sympathetic stimulation results in passive vasodilation. The cutaneous veins are densely innervated with α-adrenergic receptors, predominantly postsynaptic α₂-receptors (Flavahan et al., 1985). There is limited β-adrenergic stimulation in the cutaneous veins, and the veins of the skeletal muscle and the small venules have virtually no innervation. Epinephrine is the primary humoral factor that affects the veins, with actions on cutaneous vessels and, more importantly, splanchnic vessels. Given the preponderance of α-adrenergic receptors on the veins, epinephrine stimulation causes venoconstriction.

Passive Versus Active Effects

As noted, neurohumoral stimulation primarily affects the most capacious volume reservoirs (splanchnic and cutaneous venous bed). The question is whether translocation of blood from the venous system is primarily the consequence of active venoconstriction or of the passive effects that stem from the substantial changes in venous transmural pressure caused by arteriolar vasoconstriction or vasodilation.

Changes in upstream arteriolar tone alter downstream venous transmural pressure and the volume of blood that flows through the venous system. For example, arteriolar vasodilation increases blood flow into the highly capacious postcapillary venous beds, and the increase in their transmural venular pressure passively expands their volume. Given that total blood volume is constant, an increase in blood volume in the peripheral venous system means a decrease in the volume of the central veins that fill the heart. Conversely, vasoconstriction decreases flow into the postcapillary venous system, venous transmural pressure decreases, and the elastic recoil of the veins passively expels their volume toward the central thoracic veins (Rothe & Gaddis, 1990).

The magnitude of passive change in venous transmural pressure depends on where the changes occur along the venous volume-pressure curve. For example, as demonstrated in Figure 4-11, at a low venous transmural pressure, the pressure-volume curve is steep. A small change in distending pressure causes a large change in volume, that is, arteriolar vasodilation, which increases venous blood flow and venous transmural pressure, which causes a larger increase in venous volume expansion when the veins are not initially distended compared with the volume expansion that would occur if the veins were fully distended with decreased compliance. Conversely, passive vasoconstriction translocates a larger volume of blood to the central circulation when venular volume is normal or increased, in contrast to a situation such as hemorrhage, in which the volume is already diminished (e.g., no further volume to move into the central circulation).

The passive effects of an alteration in blood flow on venous volume are exemplified in a study that evaluated the effect of a pacing-induced increase or decrease in cardiac output on central venous pressure (Sheriff, Zhou et al., 1993). A decrease in cardiac output, which resulted in a 17-mm Hg decrease in arterial pressure, was associated with a 3.9-mm Hg increase in central venous pressure. The increase in central venous pressure reflects the decrease in venous flow and transmural pressure associated with the decrease in cardiac output and the resultant passive recoil of the veins and the translocation of their blood centrally. The relation between venous volume and cardiac output is

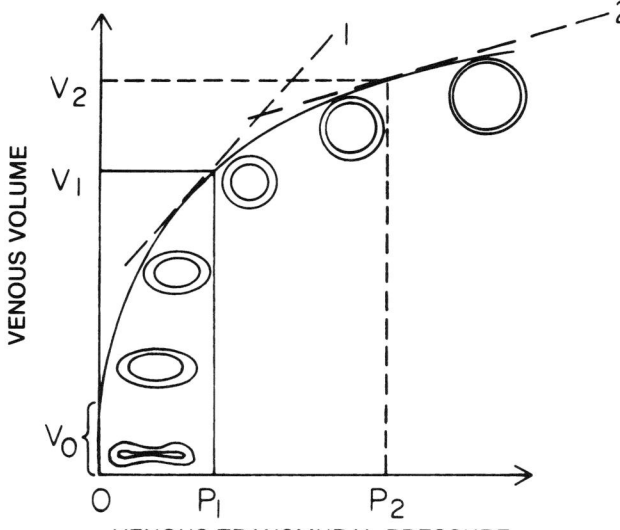

■ **Figure 4–11.** Typical volume-pressure curve of an isolated vein. Dashed lines (1 and 2) show the compliance ($\Delta V/\Delta P$) at two venous transmural pressures, P_1 and P_2. Note that compliance varies with pressure, being greatest at the lower pressures (line 1) and decreasing as the pressure increases (line 2). V_0 is the unstressed volume, which is the volume contained at 0 transmural pressure. The change in volume from V_2 to V_1 is the passive effect of changing pressures from P_2 to P_1. Note how changing cross-sectional geometry contributes to passive emptying. (From Rowell, L.B. [1986]. *Human circulation: Regulation during physical stress* [p. 46]. New York: Oxford University Press.)

addressed further in the sections on the relation between cardiac output and central venous pressure, and the Krogh model.

The dominance of passive venous volume mobility can be altered in conditions such as hemorrhage, in which active venoconstriction of the richly innervated splanchnic veins can also play a role in the translocation of blood back to the central circulation (Hainsworth, 1986; Rowell, 1986). In addition, vasoconstriction continues to exert its effects on venous volume, as previously described. In a study that examined the effects of a 27% decrease in cardiac output, with and without the presence of reflexes, active constriction of the splanchnic veins accounted for 21% of the translocated blood volume, whereas passive vasodilation accounted for the remaining 79% (Rothe & Gaddis, 1990). Thus, when active and passive effects are combined, the passive effects of decreased blood flow on venous volume mobility exceed the effect of simultaneous active venoconstriction (Rothe & Gaddis, 1990; Rowell, 1993).

▉ MODELS OF CARDIAC PERFORMANCE

Relation Between Cardiac Output and Central Venous Pressure

In the 1950s, Guyton and colleagues (Guyton, 1955; Guyton et al., 1959; Guyton et al., 1957) developed a model in which central venous pressure was presumed to affect cardiac output

in a retrograde fashion. However, a more useful conceptualization is a model of the anterograde relationship between cardiac output and central venous pressure, that is, cardiac output affects central venous pressure (Rowell, 1993; Brengelmann, 2003). Guyton and colleagues (Guyton et al., 1962) addressed this anterograde relationship. They stated:

> The normal [i.e., at rest] circulatory system operates near this limit [i.e., collapse of central veins due to increased cardiac output] so that an increase in efficacy of the heart as a pump cannot by itself increase cardiac output more than a few percent, unless some simultaneous effect takes place in the peripheral circulatory system at the same time to translocate blood from the peripheral vessels to the heart.

The concept put forward in this statement provides answers to two questions raised by Guyton's statement. First, why, at rest, does an increase in cardiac output decrease the central venous pressure? Conversely, why does a decrease in cardiac output increase the central venous pressure? Second, is it possible to correct the problem and maintain end-diastolic volume?

Why Does an Increase in Cardiac Output Decrease Central Venous Pressure?

In experiments, an increase in cardiac output secondary to an increase in heart rate was limited by a decrease in central venous pressure (Bevegård et al., 1967). This inverse relationship between cardiac output and central venous pressure is demonstrated in Figure 4-12. The resistive and

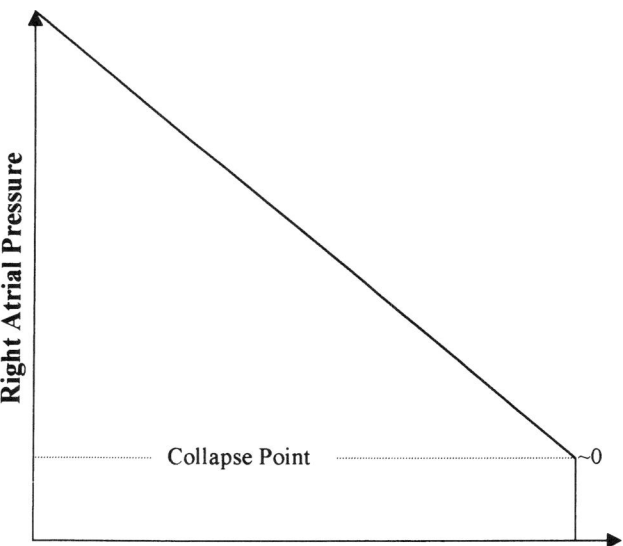

■ **Figure 4–12.** Schematic demonstrating the effect of raising or lowering cardiac output on right atrial pressures, which is caused in turn by the effect of blood flow on peripheral vascular volume. (Modified from Rowell, L.B. [1993]. *Human cardiovascular control* [p. 45]. New York: Oxford University Press.)

capacitive properties of the arteries and veins help to explain this relationship (Janicki et al., 1996; Rowell, 1986). Of particular importance is the highly capacious nature of the postcapillary venules and small veins in most vascular beds. In response to increased blood flow (increased cardiac output), transmural pressure in the veins rises, and thus their volume rises as well. The consequent shift in blood volume from the central to the peripheral veins lowers the central venous pressure (Janicki et al., 1996; Rowell et al., 1996; Sheriff, Zhou et al., 1993). If cardiac output continues to increase, the central venous pressure approaches 0 mm Hg, and eventually the central venous vasculature collapses, making it impossible to increase cardiac output further (Janicki et al., 1996). This constitutes an autolimitation on our ability to increase cardiac output when there is no extra cardiac force available to match increased venous return with cardiac output.

In contrast to the effects of increased cardiac output on central venous pressure, a decrease in cardiac output causes peripheral venous transmural pressure to decrease. The decrease in transmural pressure allows the venous beds to collapse passively and expel their blood volume into the central circulation, thus raising end-diastolic volume, central venous pressure, and stroke volume.

Krogh Model. The ideas expressed about the inverse relationship between cardiac output and central venous pressure bring to life the importance of a simple and highly insightful model of the circulation proposed by Krogh in 1912 that helps us to understand the importance of the distribution of cardiac output on end-diastolic volume and stroke volume (Krogh, 1912). The Krogh model (Fig. 4-13) divides the circulation into two circuits, one compliant and the other noncompliant. In humans, the two compliant vascular beds are the splanchnic region (liver, gastrointestinal tract, pancreas) and the skin, whereas the remaining vascular beds are noncompliant (Rothe, 1983; Rowell, 1993). Cardiac filling pressures depend on the ratio of flow through the noncompliant versus compliant vascular beds. For example, if, with all else constant, flow is increased to the splanchnic region relative to the skeletal muscle, cardiac filling pressures would be expected to decrease as a consequence of the distention and increased volume in the compliant splanchnic veins, whereas the volume in the noncompliant veins in the muscle would not be expected to change. This relationship can be visualized as running fluid through a piece of highly compliant tubing, such as a Penrose drain, versus running the same flow and volume through a rigid pipe. The volume in the compliant tubing increases, whereas the volume in the rigid tubing remains constant.

A clinical demonstration of the Krogh model can be achieved by administering a vasoconstricting α-adrenergic agent to a patient who is vasodilated. Vasoconstriction of blood vessels leading into compliant vascular beds (e.g., splanchnic) results in the passive collapse of the bed, with translocation of blood into the central circulation and a subsequent increase in blood return to the heart. However, as observed in clinical practice, a decrease in blood flow to the splanchnic region is not risk-free; for example, decreased gastrointestinal tract perfusion and ischemic bowel can occur if the decrease in flow is too great.

The Krogh model is also useful for understanding the potentially negative consequences of recreational hyperthermia (i.e., hot tub or sauna) on coronary blood flow and cardiac output in a person with coronary artery disease. Normally, resting skin blood flow is approximately 200 to 500 mL/min. With hyperthermia, the highly compliant cutaneous vascular bed dilates, with up to 60% of the cardiac output directed to the skin to facilitate heat dissipation (Johnson & Proppe, 1996; Rowell et al., 1996). Generally, the redistribution of blood volume does not compromise oxygen delivery to vital organs. However, in individuals with compromised coronary circulation, there is a potential for a decrease in blood volume available to the heart and a subsequent decrease in cardiac output and coronary artery perfusion. In addition, the vasodilation accelerates the rate of increase in body core temperature because of the increased cutaneous volume exposed to the hot water or air (Rowell, 1986, 1993).

The effects of environmental thermal stress plus exercise can also precipitate problems. In this case, the ability to increase cardiac output is limited by the decrease in central

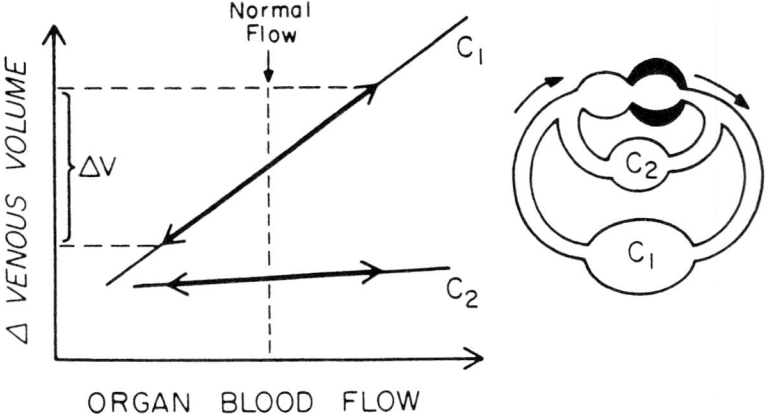

■ **Figure 4–13.** (*Right*) The Krogh model divides the circulation between two circuits, one compliant (C_1) and the other noncompliant (C_2). (*Left*) The relation between the change in organ venous volume and blood flow through a compliant organ (C_1) and a noncompliant organ (C_2). The volume of blood available to the heart is determined by the distribution of blood flow between such circuits. For example, in hyperthermia there is increased blood volume in the compliant vascular beds of the skin, and the amount of blood available to the heart is decreased. (From Rowell, L.B. [1986]. *Human circulation: Regulation during physical stress* [p. 60]. New York: Oxford University Press.)

venous pressure and stroke volume, which is caused by vasodilation of the cutaneous vascular bed and the subsequent large increase in venous volume. The body compensates (according to the Krogh model) by marked vasoconstriction in the visceral organs (including the kidneys), which can lead to ischemia and injury of these organs as well as a severe overload on the heart (Rowell, 1986). This finding has important implications for exercise programs that are a part of cardiac rehabilitation and highlights the need for control of ambient temperature to maximize the benefits of exercise (Rowell, 1986, 1993).

How is it Possible to Correct the Problem and Maintain End-Diastolic Volume?

The second question is, "How is it possible to correct the problem of increased peripheral blood volume to maintain end-diastolic volume when cardiac output increases?" For example, in response to the stress of standing, blood volume is transferred to the periphery, and a reflex increase in heart rate and cardiac output is initiated to maintain blood pressure. The increase in cardiac output is maintained for only a few beats, as the left ventricular reservoir (the pulmonary veins) is rapidly depleted. As discussed, the beneficial effect of increasing cardiac output is ultimately limited by the flow-induced "relative sequestration or pooling" of blood in the periphery. Any further increase in heart rate or cardiac output is met by a decrease in central venous pressure, and thus in a circular manner the cardiac output decreases (Bevegård et al., 1967; Lancon et al., 1994; Schaefer et al., 1988). Therefore, as Guyton (1962) stated, for cardiac output to be maintained it is imperative that a "simultaneous effect takes place in the peripheral circulatory system at the same time to translocate blood from the peripheral vessels to the heart." Two factors that aid in the translocation of blood from the peripheral vessels to the central circulation are the muscle pump and the respiratory pump.

Muscle Pump. During passive upright posture or tilt, blood volume in the dependent (below heart level) veins increases by 500 to 700 mL, and then it slowly increases further because of filtration and slow venous expansion (i.e., creep). Although the increase in peripheral blood volume may be temporarily offset by the presence of intact venous valves, the central venous pressure, stroke volume, and cardiac output fall progressively to a point where the arterial blood pressure begins to fall, eventually resulting in fainting. However, the key to surviving the stress of passive upright posture is the contraction of skeletal muscles in the legs (Gauer & Thron, 1965).

When the skeletal muscles in the leg relax, they do so rapidly. The sudden release of muscular compression pulls the collapsed veins open and creates negative transmural pressure (assuming the valves are competent) (Laughlin & Schrage, 1999). This negative pressure occurs because the veins, which are tethered to the muscle, are pulled open as the muscle recoils and create an arteriovenous pressure gradient that facilitates movement of blood into the venous beds (Rowell et al., 1996). During muscle contraction, the muscle pump generates a gradient for flow between the venous beds and the right

atrium and can expel blood against the 100 mm Hg venous hydrostatic pressure that develops during quiet standing. The muscle pump, with a pumping capability *equal to that of the left ventricle,* is so important that it is often referred to as the "second heart" (Rowell et al., 1996; Sheriff, Rowell et al., 1993; Sheriff & Van Bibber, 1998). Without the muscle pump, we would be unable to maintain an upright position or exercise (Laughlin & Schrage, 1999; Notarius & Magder, 1996; Sheriff, Zhou et al., 1993).

Respiratory Pump. The second, but less important, mechanism that promotes blood return to the heart is the respiratory pump. The respiratory pump augments the effect of the muscle pump on venous blood flow by 1.5 to 2.3 times compared to arrested ventilation (Osada et al., 2002). The pressure difference promoting flow from the venules to the right atrium is affected by changes in intrathoracic and intra-abdominal pressures (Brecher, 1956). During inspiration, the diaphragm descends and intrathoracic pressure decreases and intra-abdominal pressure increases. These pressure changes create a gradient for blood flow from the point where the vena cava enters the thoracic cavity to the right atrium and thereby increases venous return to the heart. During expiration, the diaphragm relaxes and intrathoracic pressure increases, whereas intra-abdominal pressure decreases. The increased intrathoracic pressure impedes thoracic venous flow; however, there is an increase in blood flow from the lower extremities. During mechanical ventilation, the relation between the respiratory cycle and venous return is reversed (Michard & Teboul, 2000).

Normally, the changes in venous return are not readily apparent because the liver serves as a sump to smooth out the fluctuations in venous return (Moreno et al., 1967). The liver is able to do this because it is a highly compliant vascular bed. During inspiration, the diaphragm compresses the hepatic veins and essentially stops venous outflow. However, arterial inflow continues, and the liver swells with blood. During expiration, the diaphragm ascends and the compression of the hepatic veins is released. The liver discharges the increased blood volume to the right atrium, which smoothes the expected respiratory oscillations.

An increase in respiratory oscillations may be observed in patients with a noncompliant liver, such as those with hepatic engorgement secondary to right heart failure or hepatic cirrhosis. In these cases, the respiration-induced fluctuations are more apparent because the liver cannot serve as a sump for blood (Moreno & Burchell, 1982). Pericardial constriction, restrictive cardiomyopathy, and right ventricular infarction are other clinical conditions to consider when a respiration-induced increase in right atrial pressure (Kussmaul's sign) is observed (Spodick, 1997). In these cases, the paradoxical increase in right atrial pressure is caused by the inspiration-induced increase of venous return into the nondistensible right atrium or ventricle (Spodick, 1975). Clinically, evaluation of respiratory-induced changes in right atrial pressure provide insight into whether stroke volume will increase in response to volume loading (Magder et al., 1992; Magder et al., 2001; Michard & Teboul, 2000). This latter concept, which is based on a respiratory-induced change in stroke volume and cardiac output, is further discussed in Chapter 23.

ADDITIONAL EFFECTS OF RESPIRATION

In addition to the effects of the respiratory pump on returning blood to the heart, the normal rhythmic changes in intrathoracic pressure also directly affect stroke volume, cardiac output, and blood pressure (see Chapter 23). Extreme changes in intrathoracic pressure (Valsalva maneuver) also have potentially serious consequences for patients with cardiovascular disease.

Valsalva Maneuver

The Valsalva maneuver, which is a deep breath followed by straining to expire against a closed glottis, causes an abnormal increase in intrathoracic pressures. The hemodynamic response to the sudden increase in intrathoracic pressure associated with the Valsalva maneuver can be subdivided into four phases (Hamilton et al., 1936; Hamilton et al., 1944; Levin, 1966) (Fig. 4-14). During the initial phase (phase 1: strain phase), which is produced by forcefully exhaling against a closed glottis, there is a transient increase in arterial systolic and diastolic pressures due to aortic compression caused by increased intrathoracic pressure, and a marked decrease in venous return subsequent to compression of the vena cava and a decrease in pulse pressure. During the remainder of the strain phase (phase 2), there is a progressive decrease in blood pressure and cardiac output due to a decrease in venous return and left ventricular filling and stroke volume subsequent to compression of the vena cava. The decrease in cardiac output and arterial pulse pressure, which increases baroreflex-mediated sympathetic activity, is manifested as a compensatory increase in heart rate and

peripheral resistance (Smith et al., 1996). On release of the strain (phase 3), there is an abrupt decrease in arterial pressure (release of aortic compression) and a rapid rise in venous return (decreased caval compression with restoration of the inferior vena cava to right atrial pressure gradient) without a change in heart rate (Aebischer et al., 1995). Finally, during phase 4 (overshoot), when the increased venous return reaches the left ventricle, there is a progressive increase in left ventricular stroke volume, blood pressure, and pulse pressure above baseline caused by an increase in cardiac output, secondary to the increased venous return into the vasoconstricted systemic vasculature (Brooker et al., 1974; Hamilton et al., 1936; Smith et al., 1996). The overshoot of blood pressure, pulse pressure, and cardiac output stimulates vagal activity, leading to reflex bradycardia (Smith et al., 1996).

In the clinical setting, the effects of the Valsalva maneuver may be observed when a patient strains during defecation or vomiting (McGuire et al., 1950). It is the reflex bradycardia and the sequelae of the Valsalva maneuver (cardiac arrhythmias, sudden cardiac arrest, cerebral and subarachnoid hemorrhage, rupture of a dissecting aortic aneurysm) that are observed clinically (Metzger & Therrien, 1990). Patients who may be at increased risk for an adverse response to the Valsalva maneuver include those with cardiac disease (e.g., heart failure) and older individuals, because the response to the maneuver has been shown to decrease with age (Levin, 1966; Sharpey-Schafer, 1955; Storm et al., 1989). Interventions to protect this high-risk group from the sequelae of the Valsalva maneuver (e.g., positioning, and avoiding straining during a bowel movement or vomiting) need to be performed.

OVERALL CONTROL

Baroreflex Control of Blood Pressure

The arterial baroreflex is considered the primary mechanism of control for the short-term or rapid control of arterial blood pressure. Neurohumoral factors (predominantly the control of sodium excretion) are responsible for long-term or slower blood pressure control.

Arterial Baroreceptor Response to Decreased Arterial Pressure

A decrease in blood pressure may be the result of loss of blood (hemorrhage) or a shift in blood away from the heart (standing up). In response to a decrease in arterial pressure, the baroreceptor firing rate decreases, and the firing rate through the sinus node and vagal afferents is reduced. The clinical manifestations of this response are relatively slow in contrast to the almost instantaneous response to an increase in blood pressure (Fig. 4-15) (Toska & Walloe, 2002; Wieling et al., 1998). The response to a decrease in arterial pressure is described as follows (Fig. 4-16):

Increased Sympathetic Nervous System Activity. The primary result is an increase in total vascular resistance. This

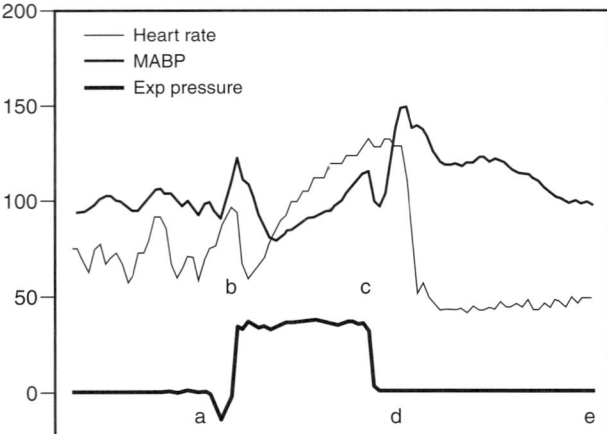

■ **Figure 4–14.** The normal hemodynamic response to a Valsalva maneuver. Phase 1: a–b; phase 2: b–c; phase 3: c–d; phase 4: d–e. MABP, mean arterial blood pressure; Exp pressure, expiratory pressure. (From Freeman, R. [1997]. Noninvasive evaluation of heart rate variability. In P.A. Low [Ed.], *Clinical autonomic disorders* [2nd ed., p. 302]. Philadelphia: Lippincott-Raven.)

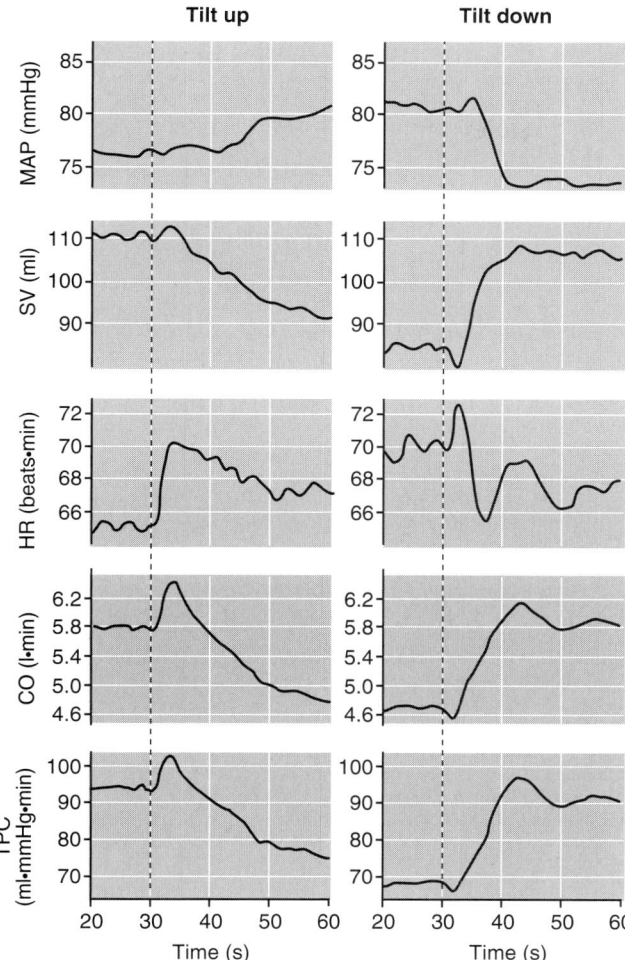

■ **Figure 4–15.** Average response to 30° head up tilt (HUT) and tilt back to supine position in seven subjects (41 experiments). (From Toska, K., & Walløe, L. [2002]. Dynamic time course of hemodynamic responses after passive head up tilt and tilt back to supine position. *Journal of Applied Physiology, 92,* 1674.)

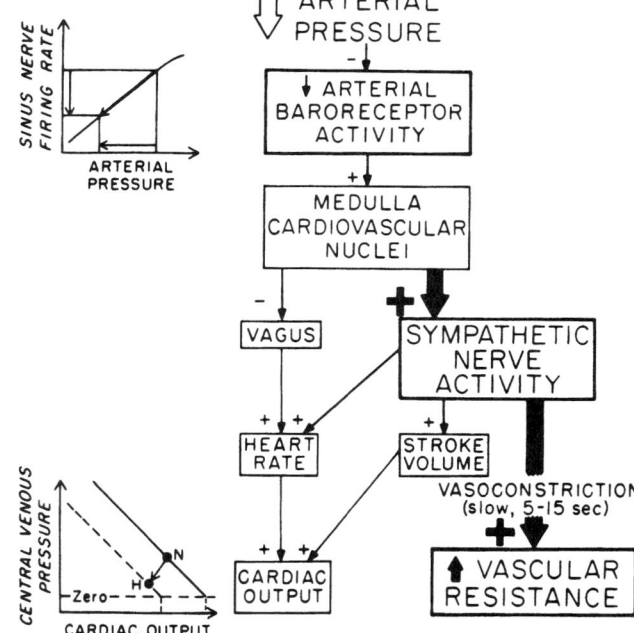

■ **Figure 4–16.** Summary of how the arterial baroreflex restores blood pressure back toward normal during arterial hypotension. Correction is by relatively slow (5 to 15 seconds) vasoconstriction. Increased heart rate has little or no effect if cardiac filling pressure is low and cardiac output cannot be increased, for reasons illustrated in the small graph next to "cardiac output" (central venous pressure vs. cardiac output). When normal (N) cardiac output increases, central venous pressure falls. When both cardiac output and central venous pressure are low during hemorrhage (H), cardiac output cannot rise much without collapsing central veins as central venous pressure goes to 0. (From Rowell, L.B. [1993]. *Human cardiovascular control* [p. 57]. New York: Oxford University Press.)

Arterial Baroreceptor Response to Increased Arterial Pressure

An acute increase in blood pressure results in increased stimulation of the sinoaortic baroreceptors. The increased baroreceptor firing rate increases sinus and vagal afferent input into the nucleus tractus solitarius of the medulla. In response to the increased baroreceptor input, the following occur (Fig. 4-17):

1. A rapid (within one beat) decrease in heart rate, secondary to a sudden increase in vagal tone
2. A secondary decrease in stroke volume due to the negative inotropic effects of the increased vagal tone (minor effect)
3. A sympathetic nervous system-mediated decrease in vascular tone (minor effect)

The net result is a decrease in heart rate, with a subsequent decrease in cardiac output and blood pressure. The most important point is that the response, which occurs within one beat, is mediated by a vagally-induced decrease in heart rate and cardiac output (Toska et al., 1994). The rapid response is extremely important in the protection of the cerebral vessels (Heistad & Kontos, 1983). Passive vasodilation due to a decrease in sympathetic tone occurs only in the skeletal muscles, and thus does not contribute greatly to the sudden lowering of arterial blood pressure (Rowell, 1993).

response is relatively slow (5 to 15 seconds). A small increase in stroke volume secondary to ß1 stimulation and increased contractility also occurs. The increase in vascular resistance is the primary mechanism for restoring blood pressure, because an increase in heart rate is relatively ineffective in raising cardiac output. As previously described, if the cardiac output increases without an increase in peripheral vascular tone, then the central venous pressure decreases. The sympathetic nervous system-mediated vasoconstriction decreases blood flow to the splanchnic region, thereby causing a passive release of 300 to 500 mL of blood from its capacious veins into the central circulation (Rothe & Gaddis, 1990; Rowell, 1977; Scott-Douglas et al., 2002).

Decreased Vagal Activity Resulting in an Increase in Heart Rate. The increase in heart rate is not a primary compensatory response to a decrease in blood pressure. As described by the cardiac output-central venous pressure relation, an increase in heart rate-induced central venous pressure is of limited efficacy in increasing the cardiac output.

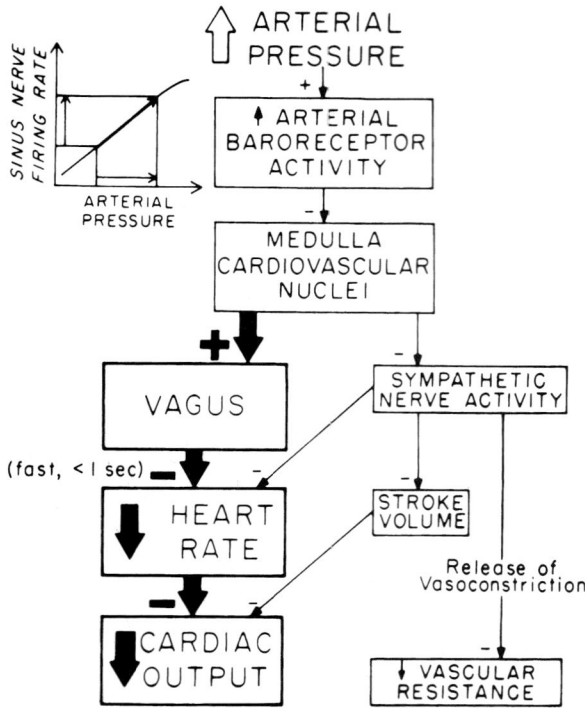

■ **Figure 4–17.** Summary of how the arterial baroreflex restores blood pressure back toward normal after sudden hypertension. Correction is rapid and achieved by immediate vagal activation and reduced heart rate and cardiac output. Release of tonic vasoconstriction is slow and has a minimal effect because only skeletal muscle has significant tonic vasoconstriction to be withdrawn in resting humans. (From Rowell, L.B. [1993]. *Human cardiovascular control,* [p. 58.]. New York: Oxford University Press.)

REFERENCES

Aebischer, N., Malhotra, R., Coonors, L., Kappenberger, L., & Parisi, A. (1995). Ventricular interdependence during Valsalva maneuver as seen by two-dimensional echocardiography: new insights about an old method. *Journal of the American Society of Echocardiography,* 8(4), 536–542.

Amenta, F., Ricci, A., Rossodivita, I., Avola, R., & Tayebati, S. K. (2001). The dopaminergic system in hypertension. *Clinical and Experimental Hypertension,* 23(1–2), 15–24.

Anrep, G., Pascual, W., & Rossler, R. (1936). Respiratory variations in heart rate. II. The central mechanism of the respiratory arrhythmia and the inter-relations between the central and reflex mechanisms. *Proceedings of the Royal Society of London. Series B: Biological Sciences,* 119, 218–230.

Aviado, D. M., & Guevara Aviado, D. (2001). The Bezold-Jarisch reflex. A historical perspective of cardiopulmonary reflexes. *Annals of the New York Academy of Sciences,* 940, 48–58.

Bevan, J. A. (1977). Some functional consequences of variation in adrenergic synaptic cleft width and in nerve density and distribution. *Federation Proceedings,* 36(10), 2439–2443.

Bevan, J. A. (1979). Some bases of differences in vascular response to sympathetic activity. *Circulation Research,* 45(2), 161–171.

Bevan, J. A., & Su, C. (1974). Variation of intra- and perisynaptic adrenergic transmitter concentrations with width of synaptic cleft in vascular tissue. *Journal of Pharmacology and Experimental Therapeutics,* 190(1), 30–38.

Bevegård, S., Jonsson, B., Karlof, I., Lagergren, H., & Sowton, E. (1967). Effect of changes in ventricular rate on cardiac output and central pressures at rest and during exercise in patients with artificial pacemakers. *Cardiovascular Research,* 1, 21–33.

Bie, P. (1980). Osmoreceptors, vasopressin, and control of renal water excretion. *Physiological Reviews,* 60(4), 961–1048.

Borbujo, J., Garcia-Villalon, A., Valle, J., Gomez, B., & Diequez, G. (1989). Postjunctional alpha-1 and alpha-2 adrenoreceptors in human skin arteries.

An in vitro study. *Journal of Pharmacology and Experimental Therapeutics,* 249(1), 284–287.

Borgström, P., Grände, P., & Mellander, S. (1984). An evaluation of the metabolic interaction with myogenic reactivity during blood flow autoregulation. *Acta Physiologica Scandinavia,* 122, 275–284.

Brady, A. (1991). Mechanical properties of isolated cardiac myocytes. *Physiological Reviews,* 71(2), 413–428.

Brecher, G. (1956). *Venous return.* New York: Grune & Stratton.

Brengelmann, G. (2003). A critical analysis of the view that right atrial pressure determines venous return. *Journal of Applied Physiology,* 94(3), 849–859.

Bristow, M., Monobe, W., Pasmussen, R., Hershberger, R., & Hoffman, B. (1988). Alpha-1 adrenergic receptors in the nonfailing and failing human heart. *Journal Pharmacology and Experimental Therapeutics,* 247(3), 1039–1045.

Brodde, O. E., & Michel, M. C. (1999). Adrenergic and muscarinic receptors in the human heart. *Pharmacological Reviews,* 51(4), 651–690.

Brooker, J., Alderman, E., & Harrison, D. (1974). Alterations in left ventricular volumes induced by Valsalva manouvre. *British Heart Journal,* 36, 713–718.

Brooks, V., & Osborn, J. (1995). Hormonal-sympathetic interactions in long-term regulation of arterial pressure: an hypothesis. *American Journal Physiology,* 268(37), R1343–R1358.

Brown, J., & Taylor, P. (2001). Muscarinic receptor agonists and antagonists. In J. Hardman & L. Limbird (Eds.), *Goodman & Gillman's the pharmacological basis of therapeutics* (10th ed., pp. 155–173). New York: McGraw-Hill.

Burnett, J. C., Jr. (1999). Vasopeptidase inhibition: a new concept in blood pressure management. *Journal of Hypertension (Supplement),* 17(1), S37–43.

Burnstock, G. (1986). Purines and cotransmitters in adrenergic and cholinergic neurones. *Progress in Brain Research,* 68, 193–203.

Burnstock, G. (1995). Noradrenaline and ATP: cotransmitters and neuromodulators. *Journal Physiology and Pharmacology,* 46(4), 365–384.

Bylund, D. B., Eikenberg, D. C., Hieble, J. P., Langer, S. Z., Lefkowitz, R. J., Minneman, K. P., et al. (1994). International Union of Pharmacology nomenclature of adrenoceptors. *Pharmacological Reviews,* 46(2), 121–136.

Celander, O. (1954). The range of control exercised by sympathicoadrenal system. *Acta Physiologica Scandinavia,* 32 (Suppl 116), 1–132.

Charkoudian, N. (2003). Skin blood flow in adult human thermoregulation: How it works, when it does not, and why. *Mayo Clinics Proceeding,* 78(5), 603–612.

Chen, H. H., & Burnett, J. C., Jr. (1998). C-type natriuretic peptide: the endothelial component of the natriuretic peptide system. *Journal of Cardiovascular Pharmacology,* 32 Suppl 3, S22–28.

Chiladakis, J. A., Patsouras, N., & Manolis, A. S. (2003). The Bezold-Jarisch reflex in acute inferior myocardial infarction: clinical and sympathovagal spectral correlates. *Clinical Cardiology,* 26(7), 323–328.

Colston, J. T., & Freeman, G. L. (1992). Beneficial influence of vasoactive intestinal peptide on ventriculovascular coupling in closed-chest dogs. *American Journal Physiology,* 263(4 Pt 2), H1300–1305.

Colucci, W. S., Elkayam, U., Horton, D. P., Abraham, W. T., Bourge, R. C., Johnson, A. D., et al. (2000). Intravenous nesiritide, a natriuretic peptide, in the treatment of decompensated congestive heart failure. Nesiritide Study Group. *New England Journal of Medicine,* 343(4), 246–253.

Covell, J., & Ross, J. (2002). Systolic and diastolic function (mechanics) of the intact heart. In E. Page, H. Fozzard, & R. Solaro (Eds.), *Handbook of physiology: Section 2. The cardiovascular system* (Vol. 2., The heart, pp. 741–784). Bethesda, MD: American Physiological Society.

Cowley, A. J. (1992). Long-term control of arterial blood pressure. *Physiological Reviews,* 72(1), 231–300.

Crandall, C. G., Cui, J., & Wilson, T. E. (2003). Effects of heat stress on baroreflex function in humans. *Acta Physiologica Scandinavia,* 177(3), 321–328.

Dampney, R. A. (1994). Functional organization of central pathways regulating the cardiovascular system. *Physiological Reviews,* 74(2), 323–364.

Dampney, R. A., Coleman, M. J., Fontes, M. A., et al. (2002). Central mechanisms underlying short- and long-term regulation of the cardiovascular system. *Clinical and Experimental Pharmacology and Physiology,* 29(4), 261–268.

Davis, M., & Hill, M. (1999). Signaling mechanisms underlying the vascular myogenic response. *Physiological Reviews,* 79(2), 387–423.

De Hert, S. G., ten Broecke, P. W., Rodrigus, I. E., Mertens, E., Stockman, B. A., & Vermeyen, K. M. (2001). The effects of the pericardium on length-dependent regulation of left ventricular function in coronary artery surgery patients. *Journal of Cardiothoracic Vascular Anesthesiology,* 15(3), 300–305.

del Monte, F., Kaumann, A., & Poole-Wilson, P. (1993). Coexistence of functioning beta-1 and beta-2 adrenoreceptors in single myocytes from human ventricle. *Circulation,* 88, 854–863.

Dhingra, H., Roongsritong, C., & Kurtzman, N. A. (2002). Brain natriuretic peptide: role in cardiovascular and volume homeostasis. *Seminars in Nephrology*, 22(5), 423–437.

Dzau, V. J., Bernstein, K., Celermajer, D., Cohen, J., Dahlof, B., Deanfield, J., et al. (2001). The relevance of tissue angiotensin-converting enzyme: manifestations in mechanistic and endpoint data. *American Journal of Cardiology*, 88(9 Suppl), 1L–20L.

Eckberg, D. L. (2000). Physiological basis for human autonomic rhythms. *Annals of Medicine*, 32(5), 341–349.

Emilien, G., Maloteaux, J. M., Geurts, M., Hoogenberg, K., & Cragg, S. (1999). Dopamine receptors—physiological understanding to therapeutic intervention potential. *Pharmacology and Therapeutics*, 84(2), 133–156.

Esler, M. (1993). Clinical application of noradrenaline spillover methodology: delineation of regional human sympathetic nervous responses. *Pharmacology Toxicology*, 73(5), 243–253.

Evans, J. M., Leonelli, F. M., Ziegler, M. G., McIntosh, C. M., Patwardhan, A. R., Ertl, A. C., et al. (2001). Epinephrine, vasodilation and hemoconcentration in syncopal, healthy men and women. *Autonomic Neuroscience*, 93(1–2), 79–90.

Faber, J. (1988). In situ analysis of alpha-adrenoreceptors on arteriolar and venular smooth muscle in rat skeletal muscle microcirculation. *Circulation Research*, 62(1), 37–50.

Feigl, E. (1989). The arterial system. In H. Patton, A. Fuchs, B. Hille, A. Scher, & R. Steiner (Eds.), *Textbook of physiology* (21st ed., Vol. 2, pp. 849–859). Philadelphia: WB Saunders.

Feigl, E. O. (1998). Neural control of coronary blood flow. *Journal of Vascular Research*, 35(2), 85–92.

Feliciano, L., & Henning, R. J. (1998). Vagal nerve stimulation during muscarinic and beta-adrenergic blockade causes significant coronary artery dilation. *Journal of the Autonomic Nervous System*, 68(1–2), 78–88.

Fenton, A. M., Hammill, S. C., Rea, R. F., Low, P. A., & Shen, W. K. (2000). Vasovagal syncope. *Annals of Internal Medicine*, 133(9), 714–725.

Flavahan, N., Linblad, L., Verbeuren, T., Shepherd, J., & Vanhoutte, P. (1985). Cooling and alpha-1 and alpha-2 adrenergic response in cutaneous veins: role of receptor reserve. *American Journal of Physiology*, 249, H950–H955.

Flevari, P. P., Livanis, E. G., Theodorakis, G. N., Mesiskli, T., Zarvalis, E., & Kremastinos, D. T. (2002). Baroreflexes in vasovagal syncope: two types of abnormal response. *Pacing and Clinical Electrophysiology*, 25(9), 1315–1323.

Franchini, K., & Cowley, A. J. (1996). Autonomic control of cardiac function. In D. Robertson, P. Low, & R. Polinsky (Eds.), *Primer on the autonomic nervous system* (pp. 42–48). San Diego: Academic Press.

Gauer, O., & Thron, H. (1965). Postural changes in the circulation. In W. Hamilton, & P. Dow (Eds.), *Handbook of physiology: Circulation* (Sec. 2, Vol. III, pp. 2409–2439). Bethesda: American Physiological Society.

Gauthier, C., Leblais, V., Kobzik, L., Trochu, J., Khandoudi, N., Bril, A., et al. (1998). The negative inotropic effect of B3-Adrenoreceptor stimulation is mediated by activation of nitric oxide synthase pathway in human ventricle. *Journal of Clinical Investigation*, 102, 1377–1384.

Gauthier, C., Tavernier, G., Charpentier, F., Langin, D., & Le Marec, H. (1996). Functional beta3-adrenoreceptor in the human heart. *Journal of Clinical Investigation*, 98(2), 556–562.

Giebisch, G., & Windhager, E. (2003). Urine concentration and dilution. In W. Boron, & E. Boulpaep (Eds.), *Medical physiology* (pp. 828–844). Philadelphia: WB Saunders.

Granger, J. P., Alexander, B. T., & Llinas, M. (2002). Mechanisms of pressure natriuresis. *Current Hypertension Report*, 4(2), 152–159.

Grassi, G., & Esler, M. (1999). How to assess sympathetic activity in humans. *Journal of Hypertension*, 17(6), 719–734.

Griendling, K. K., Ushio-Fukai, M., Lassegue, B., & Alexander, R. W. (1997). Angiotensin II signaling in vascular smooth muscle. New concepts. *Hypertension*, 29(1 Pt 2), 366–373.

Grubb, B. P., & Karas, B. J. (1998). The potential role of serotonin in the pathogenesis of neurocardiogenic syncope and related autonomic disturbances. *Journal of Interventional Cardiac Electrophysiology*, 2(4), 325–332.

Guimaraes, S., & Moura, D. (2001). Vascular adrenoceptors: an update. *Pharmacological Reviews*, 53(2), 319–356.

Guyton, A. (1955). Determination of cardiac output by equating venous return curves with cardiac response curves. *Physiological Reviews*, 35, 123–129.

Guyton, A., Abernathy, B., Langston, J., Kaufmann, B., & Fairchild, H. (1959). Relative importance of venous and arterial resistances in controlling venous return and cardiac output. *American Journal of Physiology*, 196(5), 1008–1014.

Guyton, A., Douglas, B., Langston, J., & Richardson, T. (1962). Instaneous increase in mean circulatory pressure and cardiac output at onset of muscular activity. *Circulation Research*, 11, 431–444.

Guyton, A., Lindsey, A., Abernathy, B., & Richardson, T. (1957). Venous return at various right atrial pressures and the normal venous return curve. *American Journal of Physiology*, 189(3), 609–615.

Hainsworth, R. (1986). Vascular capacitance: its control and importance. *Reviews of Physiology Biochemistry and Pharmacology*, 105, 101–173.

Hainsworth, R. (1995a). Cardiovascular reflexes from ventricular and coronary receptors. *Advances in Experimental Medicine and Biology*, 381, 157–174.

Hainsworth, R. (1995b). The control and physiological importance of heart rate. In M. Malik, & A. Camms (Eds.), *Heart rate variability* (pp. 3–19). Armonk, NY: Futura Publishing.

Hamilton, W., Woodbury, R., & Harper, H. (1936). Physiologic relationships between intrathoracic, intraspinal, and arterial pressures. *JAMA*, 107(11), 853–856.

Hamilton, W., Woodbury, R., & Harper, H. (1944). Arterial, cerebrospinal and venous pressures in man during cough and strain. *American Journal of Physiology*, 141, 42–50.

Hammond, H., White, F., Bhargava, V., & Shabetai, R. (1992). Heart size and maximal cardiac output are limited by the pericardium. *American Journal of Physiology*, 263, H1675–H1681.

Han, S., Yang, C. L., Chen, X., Naes, L., Cox, B. F., & Westfall, T. (1998). Direct evidence for the role of neuropeptide Y in sympathetic nerve stimulation-induced vasoconstriction. *American Journal of Physiology*, 274(1 Pt 2), H290–294.

Hancock, W. O., Martyn, D. A., & Huntsman, L. L. (1993). Ca2+ and segment length dependence of isometric force kinetics in intact ferret cardiac muscle. *Circulation Research*, 73(4), 603–611.

Harrison, D., Griendling, K. K., Landmesser, U., Hornig, B., & Drexler, H. (2003). Role of oxidative stress in atherosclerosis. *American Journal of Cardiology*, 91(3A), 7A–11A.

Harrison, D. G. (1997). Endothelial function and oxidant stress. *Clinical Cardiology*, 20(11 Suppl 2), II-11-17.

Hedges, J. R. (1983). Preload and afterload revisited. *Journal of Emergency Nursing*, 9(5), 262–267.

Hein, L., Altman, J. D., & Kobilka, B. K. (1999). Two functionally distinct alpha2-adrenergic receptors regulate sympathetic neurotransmission. *Nature*, 402(6758), 181–184.

Heistad, D., & Kontos, H. (1983). Cerebral circulation. In J. Shepherd, F. Abboud, & S. Geiger (Eds.), *Handbook of Physiology. The cardiovascular system: Peripheral circulation and organ blood flow* (Part 2, Vol. III, pp. 137–182). Bethesda: American Physiological Society.

Henning, R. J., & Sawmiller, D. R. (2001). Vasoactive intestinal peptide: cardiovascular effects. *Cardiovascular Research*, 49(1), 27–37.

Hester, R. L., & Hammer, L. W. (2002). Venular-arteriolar communication in the regulation of blood flow. *American Journal of Physiology*, 282(5), R1280–1285.

Hill, M. A., Zou, H., Potocnik, S. J., Meininger, G. A., & Davis, M. J. (2001). Invited review: arteriolar smooth muscle mechanotransduction: Ca(2+) signaling pathways underlying myogenic reactivity. *Journal of Applied Physiology*, 91(2), 973–983.

Hlastala, M., & Berger, A. (2001). *Physiology of respiration*. New York: Oxford University Press.

Hoffman, B. (2001). Catecholamines, sympathomimetic drugs, and adrenergic receptor agonists. In J. Hardman, & L. Limbird (Eds.), *Goodman & Gillman's the pharmacological basis of therapeutics* (10th ed., pp. 215–268). New York: McGraw-Hill.

Hoffman, B., & Taylor, P. (2001). Neurotransmission. The autonomic and somatic nervous systems. In J. Hardman, & L. Limbird (Eds.), *Goodman & Gilman's the pharmacological basis of therapeutics* (10th ed., pp. 115–153). New York: McGraw Hill.

Horne, S. G., Belenkie, I., Tyberg, J. V., & Smith, E. R. (2000). Pericardial pressure in experimental chronic heart failure. *Canadian Journal Cardiology*, 16(5), 607–613.

Hunter, S., Smith, G. H., & Angelini, G. D. (1992). Adverse hemodynamic effects of pericardial closure soon after open heart operation. *Annals of Thoracic Surgery*, 53(3), 425–429.

Jackson, E. (2001a). Renin and angiotensin. In J. Hardman & L. Limbird (Eds.), *Goodman & Gillman's the pharmacological basis of therapeutics* (pp. 809–841). New York: McGraw-Hill.

Jackson, E. (2001b). Vasopressin and other agents affecting renal water conservation. In J. Hardman & L. Limbird (Eds.), *Goodman & Gillman's the pharmacological basis of therapeutics* (10th ed., pp. 789–808). New York: McGraw Hill.

Janicki, J., Sheriff, D., Robotham, J., & Wise, R. (1996). Cardiac output during exercise: Contributions of the cardiac, circulatory, and respiratory systems. In L. Rowell, & J. Sheperd (Eds.), *Handbook of physiology. Exercise: Regulation and integration of multiple systems* (Sec. 12, pp. 649–704). Bethesda, MD: Oxford University Press.

Javaheri, S. (2003). Heart failure and sleep apnea: emphasis on practical therapeutic options. *Clinics in Chest Medicine*, 24(2), 207–222.

Joannides, R., Richard, V., Haefeli, W., Linder, L., Luscher, T., & Thuillez, C. (1995). Role of basal and stimulated release of nitric oxide in the regulation of radial artery caliber in humans. *Hypertension*, 26(2), 327–331.

Johanson, B. (1980). Myogenic responses of vascular smooth muscle. In N. Stevens (Ed.), *Smooth muscle contraction* (pp. 457–472). New York: Marcel Dekker.

Johansson, B. (1989). Myogenic tone and reactivity: definitions based on muscle physiology. *Journal of Hypertension*, 7 (Suppl 4), S5–S8.

Johnson, J., & Proppe, D. (1996). Cardiovascular adjustments to heat stress. In M. Fregly, & C. Blatteis (Eds.), *Handbook of physiology: Section 4, environmental physiology* (Vol. 1, pp. 215–243). New York: Oxford University Press.

Johnson, P. (1980). The myogenic response. In D. Bohr, A. Somlyo, & H. Sparks (Eds.), *Handbook of physiology* (Sec. 2, Vol. II, *Vascular smooth muscle*, pp. 409–442). Bethesda: American Physiological Society.

Johnson, P. (1986). Autoregulation of blood flow. *Circulation Research*, 59, 483–495.

Jose, P. A., Eisner, G. M., & Felder, R. A. (1998). Renal dopamine receptors in health and hypertension. *Pharmacology and Therapeutics*, 80(2), 149–182.

Joyner, M. J., & Dietz, N. M. (2003). Sympathetic vasodilation in human muscle. *Acta Physiologica Scandinavia*, 177(3), 329–336.

Kambayashi, M., Miura, T., Oh, B. H., Rockman, H. A., Murata, K., & Ross, J., Jr. (1992). Enhancement of the force-frequency effect on myocardial contractility by adrenergic stimulation in conscious dogs. *Circulation*, 86(2), 572–580.

Kara, T., Narkiewicz, K., & Somers, V. K. (2003). Chemoreflexes—physiology and clinical implications. *Acta Physiologica Scandinavia*, 177(3), 377–384.

Kardon, D. E., Borczuk, A. C., & Factor, S. M. (2000). Mechanism of pericardial expansion with cardiac enlargement. *Cardiovascular Pathology*, 9(1), 9–15.

Kaumann, A. J. (1997). Four beta-adrenoceptor subtypes in the mammalian heart. *Trends in Pharmacological Sciences*, 18(3), 70–76.

Kaumann, A. J., Preitner, F., Sarsero, D., Molenaar, P., Revelli, J. P., & Giacobino, J. P. (1998). (-)-CGP 12177 causes cardiostimulation and binds to cardiac putative beta 4-adrenoceptors in both wild-type and beta 3-adrenoceptor knockout mice. *Molecular Pharmacology*, 53(4), 670–675.

Keating, G. M., & Goa, K. L. (2003). Nesiritide: a review of its use in acute decompensated heart failure. *Drugs*, 63(1), 47–70.

Kellogg, D. L., Jr., Crandall, C. G., Liu, Y., Charkoudian, N., & Johnson, J. M. (1998). Nitric oxide and cutaneous active vasodilation during heat stress in humans. *Journal of Applied Physiology*, 85(3), 824–829.

Kellogg, D. L., Jr., Pergola, P. E., Piest, K. L., Kosiba, W. A., Crandall, C. G., Grossmann, M., et al. (1995). Cutaneous active vasodilation in humans is mediated by cholinergic nerve cotransmission. *Circulation Research*, 77(6), 1222–1228.

Kellum, J., & Decker, J. (2001). Use of dopamine in acute renal failure: a meta-analysis. *Critical Care Medicine*, 29(8), 1526–1531.

Knepper, M., Valtin, H., & Sands, J. (2000). Renal action of vasopressin. In J. Fray, & H. Goodman (Eds.), *Handbook of physiology. Section 7, The endocrine system* (pp. 496–529). Washington: American Physiological Society.

Kroeker, C. A., Shrive, N. G., Belenkie, I., & Tyberg, J. V. (2003). Pericardium modulates left and right ventricular stroke volumes to compensate for sudden changes in atrial volume. *American Journal of Physiology*, 284(6), H2247–2254.

Krogh, A. (1912). The regulation of the supply of blood to the right heart. *Skandinavisches Archiv fur Physiologie*, 27, 227–248.

Lakatta, E. G. (1987). Starling's law of the heart is explained by an intimate interaction of muscle length and myofilament calcium activation. *Journal of the American College of Cardiology*, 10(5), 1157–1164.

Lancon, J., Pillet, M., Gabrielle, F., Fayollle, J., & Tatou, E. (1994). Effects of atrial pacing on right ventricular contractility after coronary artery surgery. *Journal of Cardiothoracic and Vascular Anesthesia*, 8(5), 536–540.

Lands, A. M., Arnold, A., McAuliff, J. P., Luduena, F. P., & Brown, T. G., Jr. (1967). Differentiation of receptor systems activated by sympathomimetic amines. *Nature*, 214(88), 597–598.

Lanfranchi, P. A., Braghiroli, A., Bosimini, E., Mazzuero, G., Colombo, R., Donner, C. F., et al. (1999). Prognostic value of nocturnal Cheyne-Stokes respiration in chronic heart failure. *Circulation*, 99(11), 1435–1440.

Laughlin, M. H., & Schrage, W. G. (1999). Effects of muscle contraction on skeletal muscle blood flow: When is there a muscle pump? *Medicine and Science in Sports*, 31(7), 1027–1035.

Lee, T. M., Chen, M. F., Su, S. F., Chao, C. L., Liau, C. S., & Lee, Y. T. (1996). Excessive myocardial contraction in vasovagal syncope demonstrated by echocardiography during head-up tilt test. *Clinical Cardiology*, 19(2), 137–140.

Leech, C. J., & Faber, J. E. (1996). Different alpha-adrenoceptor subtypes mediate constriction of arterioles and venules. *American Journal of Physiology*, 270(2 Pt 2), H710–722.

Levin, A. (1966). A simple test of cardiac function based upon the heart rate changes induced by the Valsalva Maneuver. *American Journal of Cardiology*, 18, 90–99.

Levin, E. R., Gardner, D. G., & Samson, W. K. (1998). Natriuretic peptides. *New England Journal of Medicine*, 339(5), 321–328.

Levy, M., & Martin, P. (1979). Neural control of the heart. In R. Berne (Ed.), *Handbook of physiology* (Sec. 2, Vol. 1, pp. 581–620). Bethesda, MD: American Physiological Society.

Levy, M. N. (1997). Neural control of cardiac function. *Baillieres Clinical Neurology*, 6(2), 227–244.

Lim, P. O., Morris-Thurgood, J. A., & Frenneaux, M. P. (2002). Vascular mechanisms of sudden death in hypertrophic cardiomyopathy, including blood pressure responses to exercise. *Cardiology Review*, 10(1), 15–23.

Lombard, J., & Duling, B. (1977). Relative importance of tissue oxygenation and vascular smooth muscle hypoxia in determining arteriolar response to occlusion in the hamster cheek pouch. *Circulation Research*, 41, 365–373.

Longhurst, J. C., Tjen, A. L. S. C., & Fu, L. W. (2001). Cardiac sympathetic afferent activation provoked by myocardial ischemia and reperfusion. Mechanisms and reflexes. *Annals of the New York Academy of Sciences*, 940, 74–95.

Lundberg, J. M. (1996). Pharmacology of cotransmission in the autonomic nervous system: integrative aspects on amines, neuropeptides, adenosine triphosphate, amino acids and nitric oxide. *Pharmacological Reviews*, 48(1), 113–178.

Magder, S., Georgiadis, G., & Cheong, T. (1992). Respiratory variation in right atrial pressure predict the response to fluid challenge. *Journal of Critical Care*, 7(2), 76–85.

Magder, S., Lagonidis, D., & Erice, F. (2001). The use of respiratory variations in right atrial pressure to predict the cardiac output response to PEEP. *Journal of Critical Care*, 16(3), 108–114.

Marik, P. E. (2002). Low-dose dopamine: a systematic review. *Intensive Care Medicine*, 28(7), 877–883.

Mark, A., Abboud, F., Schmid, P., Heistad, D., & Johannsen, U. (1973). Reflex vascular response to left ventricular outflow obstruction and activation of ventricular baroreceptors in dogs. *Journal of Clinical Investigation*, 52, 1147–1153.

Mark, A., & Mancia, G. (1983). Cardiopulmonary baroreflexes in humans. In J. Sheperd, & F. Abboud (Eds.), *Handbook of physiology. Section 2. The cardiovascular system* (Vol. III., Part 2, pp. 795–813). Bethesda, MD: American Physiological Society.

McGuire, J., Green, R., Hauenstein, V., Courter, S., Braunstein, J., Plessinger, V., et al. (1950). Bed pan deaths. *American Practitioner*, 1(1), 23–28.

McMahon, N. C., Drinkhill, M. J., Myers, D. S., & Hainsworth, R. (2000a). Absence of reflex vascular responses from the intrapulmonary circulation in anaesthetised dogs. *Experimental Physiology*, 85(4), 421–430.

McMahon, N. C., Drinkhill, M. J., Myers, D. S., & Hainsworth, R. (2000b). Reflex responses from the main pulmonary artery and bifurcation in anaesthetised dogs. *Experimental Physiology*, 85(4), 411–420.

Mellander, S. (1989). Functional aspects of myogenic vascular control. *Journal of Hypertension*, 7 (suppl 4), S21–S30.

Melo, L. G., Steinhelper, M. E., Pang, S. C., Tse, Y., & Ackermann, U. (2000). ANP in regulation of arterial pressure and fluid-electrolyte balance: lessons from genetic mouse models. *Physiological Genomics*, 3(1), 45–58.

Melo, L. G., Veress, A. T., Ackermann, U., Steinhelper, M. E., Pang, S. C., Tse, Y., et al. (1999). Chronic regulation of arterial blood pressure in ANP transgenic and knockout mice: role of cardiovascular sympathetic tone. *Cardiovascular Research*, 43(2), 437–444.

Metzger, B., & Therrien, B. (1990). Effect of position on cardiovascular response during the Valsalva Maneuver. *Nursing Research*, 39(4), 198–202.

Michard, F., & Teboul, J. L. (2000). Using heart-lung interactions to assess fluid responsiveness during mechanical ventilation. *Critical Care*, 4(5), 282–289.

Miller, D., Gleason, W., & Whalen, R. (1962). Effect of ventricular rate in the cardiac output in the dog with chronic heart block. *Circulation Research*, 10, 658–663.

Mills, R. M., LeJemtel, T. H., Horton, D. P., Liang, C., Lang, R., Silver, M. A., et al. (1999). Sustained hemodynamic effects of an infusion of nesiritide (human b-type natriuretic peptide) in heart failure: a randomized, double-blind, placebo-controlled clinical trial. Natrecor Study Group. *Journal of the American College of Cardiology*, 34(1), 155–162.

Minisi, A., & Thames, M. (1991). Reflexes from ventricular receptors with vagal afferents. In I. Zucker, & J. Gilmore (Eds.), *Reflex control of circulation* (pp. 359–405). Boca Raton, FL: CRC Press.

Minisi, A. J. (1998). Vagal cardiopulmonary reflexes after total cardiac deafferentation. *Circulation*, 98(23), 2615–2620.

Missale, C., Nash, S. R., Robinson, S. W., Jaber, M., & Caron, M. G. (1998). Dopamine receptors: from structure to function. *Physiological Reviews*, 78(1), 189–225.

Mitchell, G. F., Izzo, J. L., Jr., Lacourciere, Y., Ouellet, J. P., Neutel, J., Qian, C., et al. (2002). Omapatrilat reduces pulse pressure and proximal aortic stiffness in patients with systolic hypertension: results of the conduit hemodynamics of omapatrilat international research study. *Circulation*, 105(25), 2955–2961.

Mohrman, D., & Heller, L. (1997). *Cardiovascular physiology* (4th ed.). New York: McGraw-Hill.

Mombouli, J. V., & Vanhoutte, P. M. (1999). Endothelial dysfunction: from physiology to therapy. *Journal of Molecular and Cellular Cardiology*, 31(1), 61–74.

Moniotte, S., Kobzik, L., Feron, O., Trochu, J., Gauthier, C., & Ballingand, J. (2001). Upregulation of beta(3)-adrenoreceptors and altered contractile response to inotropic amines in human failing myocardium. *Circulation*, 103(12), 1649–1655.

Moreno, A., & Burchell, A. (1982). Respiratory regulation of splanchnic and systemic venous return in normal subjects and in patients with hepatic cirrhosis. *Surgery, Gynecology and Obstetrics*, 154, 257–267.

Moreno, A., Burchell, A., van der Woude, R., & Burke, J. (1967). Respiratory regulation of splanchnic and venous return. *American Journal of Physiology*, 213, 455–465.

Morillo, C. A., Ellenbogen, K. A., & Fernando Pava, L. (1997). Pathophysiologic basis for vasodepressor syncope. *Cardiology Clinics*, 15(2), 233–249.

Narkiewicz, K., & Somers, V. K. (2003). Sympathetic nerve activity in obstructive sleep apnoea. *Acta Physiologica Scandinavia*, 177(3), 385–390.

Naruko, T., Ueda, M., van der Wal, A. C., van der Loos, C. M., Itoh, H., Nakao, K., et al. (1996). C-type natriuretic peptide in human coronary atherosclerotic lesions. *Circulation*, 94(12), 3103–3108.

Notarius, C. F., & Magder, S. (1996). Central venous pressure during exercise: role of muscle pump. *Canadian Journal of Physiology and Pharmacology*, 74(6), 647–651.

Ohyanagi, M., Faber, J., & Nishigaki, K. (1991). Differential activation of alpha 1- and alpha 2-adrenoceptors on microvascular smooth muscle during sympathetic nerve stimulation. *Circulation Research*, 68(1), 232–244.

Omran, H., Fehske, W., Rabahieh, R., Hagendorff, A., Pizzulli, L., Zirbes, M., et al. (1996). Valvular aortic stenosis: risk of syncope. *Journal of Heart Valve Disease*, 5(1), 31–34.

Opie, L. (1997). Mechanisms of cardiac contraction and relaxation. In E. Braunwald (Ed.), *Heart disease: A textbook of cardiovascular medicine* (Vol. 1, pp. 360–393). Philadelphia: WB Saunders.

Opie, L. (1998). *The heart: Physiology from cell to circulation*. Philadelphia: Lippincott-Raven.

Osada, T., Katsumura, T., Hamaoka, T., Murase, N., Naka, M., & Shimomitsu, T. (2002). Quantitative effects of respiration on venous return during single knee extension-flexion. *International Journal of Sports Medicine*, 23(3), 183–190.

Osborn, J. W. (1997). The sympathetic nervous system and long-term regulation of arterial pressure: what are the critical questions? *Clinical and Experimental Pharmacology and Physiology*, 24(1), 68–71.

Packer, M., Califf, R. M., Konstam, M. A., Krum, H., McMurray, J. J., Rouleau, J. L., et al. (2002). Comparison of omapatrilat and enalapril in patients with chronic heart failure: the Omapatrilat Versus Enalapril Randomized Trial of Utility in Reducing Events (OVERTURE). *Circulation*, 106(8), 920–926.

Pang, C. C. (2001). Autonomic control of the venous system in health and disease: effects of drugs. *Pharmacology and Therapeutics*, 90(2–3), 179–230.

Peppard, P. E., Young, T., Palta, M., & Skatrud, J. (2000). Prospective study of the association between sleep-disordered breathing and hypertension. *New England Journal of Medicine*, 342(19), 1378–1384.

Perez-Gomez, F., & Garcia-Aguada, A. (1977). Origin of ventricular reflexes caused by coronary arteriography. *British Heart Journal*, 39, 967–973.

Pergola, P. E., Kellogg, D. L., Jr., Johnson, J. M., & Kosiba, W. A. (1994). Reflex control of active cutaneous vasodilation by skin temperature in humans. *American Journal of Physiology*, 266(5 Pt 2), H1979–1984.

Pilowsky, P. M., & Goodchild, A. K. (2002). Baroreceptor reflex pathways and neurotransmitters: 10 years on. *Journal of Hypertension*, 20(9), 1675–1688.

Price, J. (1991). Influence of pressure and flow on constriction of blood vessels. *Journal of the Florida Medical Association*, 78(12), 825–827.

Ramsay, D. J., Thrasher, T. N., & Bie, P. (1988). Endocrine components of body fluid homeostasis. *Comparative Biochemistry and Physiology*, 90(4), 777–780.

Rao, V., Komeda, M., Weisel, R. D., Cohen, G., Borger, M. A., & David, T. E. (1999). Should the pericardium be closed routinely after heart operations? *Annals of Thoracic Surgery*, 67(2), 484–488.

Rea, R. F., & Thames, M. D. (1993). Neural control mechanisms and vasovagal syncope. *Journal of Cardiovascular Electrophysiology*, 4(5), 587–595.

Renkin, E. (1984). Control of microcirculation and blood-tissue exchange. In E. Renkin & C. Michel (Eds.), *Handbook of physiology* (Vol. IV (Part 2), pp. 627–687). Bethesda: American Physiological Society.

Roddie, I. (1983). Circulation to skin and adipose tissue. In J. Shepherd & F. M. Abboud (Eds.), *Handbook of physiology: The cardiovascular system, peripheral circulation and organ blood flow* (pp. 285–317). Bethesda, MD: American Physiological Society.

Ross, J., Jr., Miura, T., Kambayashi, M., Eising, G. P., & Ryu, K. H. (1995). Adrenergic control of the force-frequency relation. *Circulation*, 92(8), 2327–2332.

Ross, J. J. (2000). Adrenergic regulation of the force-frequency effect. In G. Hasenfuss, & H. Just (Eds.), *Heart rate as a determinant of cardiac function: Basic mechanism and clinical significance* (pp. 155–165). Darmstadt: Springer.

Ross, J. R. (1976). Afterload mismatch and preload reserve: A conceptual framework for the analysis of ventricular function. *Progress in Cardiovascular Disease*, 18(4).

Rothe, C. (1983). Venous system: Physiology of the capacitance vessels. In J. Shepherd, & F. Abboud (Eds.), *Handbook of Physiology: The cardiovascular system, peripheral circulation and organ blood flow* (Sec. 2, Vol. III, Part 1, pp. 397–452). Bethesda, MD: American Physiological Society.

Rothe, C., & Gaddis, M. (1990). Autoregulation of cardiac output by passive elastic characteristics of the vascular capacitance system. *Circulation*, 81(1), 360–368.

Rouleau, J. L., Pfeffer, M. A., Stewart, D. J., Isaac, D., Sestier, F., Kerut, E. K., et al. (2000). Comparison of vasopeptidase inhibitor, omapatrilat, and lisinopril on exercise tolerance and morbidity in patients with heart failure: IMPRESS randomised trial. *Lancet*, 356(9230), 615–620.

Rowell, L. (1983). Cardiovascular adjustments to thermal stress. In J. Shepherd, & F. M. Abboud (Eds.), *Handbook of physiology: Section 2: The cardiovascular system* (Vol. 3, Part 2, pp. 967–1023). Bethesda, MD: American Physiological Society.

Rowell, L. (1986). *Human circulation: Regulation during physical stress*. New York: Oxford University Press.

Rowell, L. (1993). *Human cardiovascular control*. New York: Oxford University Press.

Rowell, L., & Blackmon, J. (1989). Hypotension induced by central hypovolaemia and hypoxaemia. *Clinical Physiology*, 9, 269–277.

Rowell, L., O'Leary, D., & Kellogg, D. (1996). Integration of cardiovascular control systems in dynamic exercise. In L. Rowell, & J. Sheperd (Eds.), *Handbook of physiology: Exercise: Regulation and integration of multiple systems* (Vol. Section 12, pp. 770–838). Bethesda: Oxford University Press.

Rowell, L. B. (1977). Reflex control of the cutaneous vasculature. *Journal of Investigative Dermatology*, 69(1), 154–166.

Rubattu, S., & Volpe, M. (2001). The atrial natriuretic peptide: a changing view. *Journal of Hypertension*, 19(11), 1923–1931.

Rudner, X. L., Berkowitz, D. E., Booth, J. V., Funk, B. L., Cozart, K. L., D'Amico, E. B., et al. (1999). Subtype specific regulation of human vascular alpha(1)-adrenergic receptors by vessel bed and age. *Circulation*, 100(23), 2336–2343.

Rushmer, R. (1959). Constance of stroke volume in ventricular responses to exertion. *American Journal of Physiology*, 196, 745–750.

Ruskoaho, H., Leskinen, H., Magga, J., Taskinen, P., Mantymaa, P., Vuolteenaho, O., et al. (1997). Mechanisms of mechanical load-induced atrial natriuretic peptide secretion: role of endothelin, nitric oxide, and angiotensin II. *Journal of Molecular Medicine*, 75(11–12), 876–885.

Sander-Jensen, K. (1991). Heart and endocrine changes during central hypovolemia in man. *Danish Medical Bulletin*, 38(6), 443–457.

Sarnoff, S. J. (1955). Myocardial contractility as described by ventricular function curves; observations on Starling's Law of the Heart. *Physiological Reviews*, 35, 107–122.

Savage, M. V., & Brengelmann, G. L. (1996). Control of skin blood flow in the neutral zone of human body temperature regulation. *Journal of Applied Physiology*, 80(4), 1249–1257.

Schaefer, S., Taylor, A., Lee, H., Niggemann, E., Levine, B., Popma, J., et al. (1988). Effect of increasing heart rate on left ventricular performance in patients with normal cardiac function. *American Journal of Cardiology*, 16, 617–620.

Scher, A. (1989). Cardiovascular control. In H. Patton, A. Fuchs, B. Hille, A. Scher, & R. Steiner (Eds.), *Textbook of physiology. Circulation, respiration, body fluids, metabolism, and endocrinology* (21st ed., Vol. 2, pp. 972–990). Philadelphia: WB Saunders.

Schmaier, A. H. (2002). The plasma kallikrein-kinin system counterbalances the renin-angiotensin system. *Journal of Clinical Investigation*, 109(8), 1007–1009.

Schmaier, A. H. (2003). The kallikrein-kinin and the renin-angiotensin systems have a multilayered interaction. *American Journal of Physiology*, 285(1), R1–13.

Schreihofer, A. M., & Guyenet, P. G. (2002). The baroreflex and beyond: control of sympathetic vasomotor tone by GABAergic neurons in the ventrolateral medulla. *Clinical and Experimental Pharmacology and Physiology*, 29(5–6), 514–521.

Schubert, R., & Mulvany, M. J. (1999). The myogenic response: Established facts and attractive hypotheses. *Clinical Science*, 96(4), 313–326.

Scotland, R., Chauhan, S., Vallance, P., & Ahluwalia, A. (2001). An endothelium-derived hyperpolarizing factor-like factor moderates myogenic constriction of mesenteric resistance arteries in the absence of endothelial nitric oxide synthase-derived nitric oxide. *Hypertension*, 38(4), 833–839.

Scott-Douglas, N. W., Robinson, V. J., Smiseth, O. A., Wright, C. I., Manyari, D. E., Smith, E. R., et al. (2002). Effects of acute volume loading and hemorrhage on intestinal vascular capacitance: a mechanism whereby capacitance modulates cardiac output. *Canadian Journal of Cardiology*, 18(5), 515–522.

Serrano, C. V., Jr., Bortolotto, L. A., Cesar, L. A., Solimene, M. C., Mansur, A. P., Nicolau, J. C., et al. (1999). Sinus bradycardia as a predictor of right coronary artery occlusion in patients with inferior myocardial infarction. *International Journal of Cardiology*, 68(1), 75–82.

Sharma, J. N., & Sharma, J. (2002). Cardiovascular properties of the kallikrein-kinin system. *Current Medical Research and Opinion*, 18(1), 10–17.

Sharpey-Schafer, E. (1955). Effects of Valsalva's Manoeuvre on the normal and failing circulation. *British Medical Journal*, 1, 693–695.

Shen, Y. T., Cowley, A. W., Jr., & Vatner, S. F. (1991). Relative roles of cardiac and arterial baroreceptors in vasopressin regulation during hemorrhage in conscious dogs. *Circulation Research*, 68(5), 1422–1436.

Sheriff, D., Rowell, L., & Scher, A. (1993). Is the rapid rise in vascular conductance at onset of dynamic exercise due to the muscle pump? *American Journal of Physiology*, 265, H1227–H1234.

Sheriff, D., & Van Bibber, R. (1998). Flow-generating capability of the isolated skeletal muscle pump. *American Journal of Physiology*, 274(5 Pt 2), H1502–1508.

Sheriff, D., Zhou, X., Scher, A., & Rowell. L. (1993). Dependence of cardiac filling pressure on cardiac output during rest and dynamic exercise in dogs. *American Journal of Physiology*, 265(1 Pt 2), H316–322.

Shibasaki, M., Wilson, T. E., Cui, J., & Crandall, C. G. (2002). Acetylcholine released from cholinergic nerves contributes to cutaneous vasodilation during heat stress. *Journal of Applied Physiology*, 93(6), 1947–1951.

Smith, M., Beightol, L., Fritsch-Yelle, J., Ellenboge, K., Porter, T., & Eckberg, D. (1996). Valvalva's maneuver revisited a quantitative method yielding insights into human autonomic control. *American Journal of Physiology*, 271(3 (Part 2)), Hi1240–1249.

Sonnenblick, E. H. (1962). Force-velocity relations in mammalian heart muscle. *American Journal of Physiology*, 202(5), 931–939.

Sorrentino, R., & Pinto, A. (1997). The increase in blood pressure induced by inhibition of nitric oxide synthase in anesthetized Wistar rats is inversely related to basal blood pressure value. *Journal of Cardiovascular Pharmacology*, 29(5), 599–604.

Spodick, D. (1975). Kussmaul's sign. *New England Journal of Medicine*, 293, 1047–1048.

Spodick, D. (1997). *The pericardium: A comprehensive textbook*. New York: Marcel Dekker, Inc.

Spyer, M. (2000). Vagal preganglionic neurons innervating the heart. In E. Page, H. Fozzard, & R. Solaro (Eds.), *Handbook of physiology, Section 2: The cardiovascular system, Vol. I: The heart* (pp. 213–239). Bethesda, MD: American Physiological Society.

Starling, E. (1918). *The Linacre lecture on the law of the heart, given at Cambridge, 1915*. London: Longmans, Green.

Stingo, A. J., Clavell, A. L., Aarhus, L. L., & Burnett, J. C., Jr. (1992). Cardiovascular and renal actions of C-type natriuretic peptide. *American Journal of Physiology*, 262(1 Pt 2), H308–312.

Storm, D., Metzger, B., & Therrien, B. (1989). Effects of age on autonomic cardiovascular responsiveness in healthy men and women. *Nursing Research*, 38, 326–330.

Stray-Gundersen, J., Musch, T., Haidet, G., Swain, D., Ordway, G., & Mitchell, J. (1986). The effect of pericardiectomy on maximal oxygen consumption and maximal cardiac output in untrained dogs. *Circulation Research*, 58(4), 523–530.

Thames, M. D., Dibner-Dunlap, M. E., Minisi, A. J., & Kinugawa, T. (1996). Reflexes mediated by cardiac sympathetic afferents during myocardial ischaemia: role of adenosine. *Clinical Experimental Pharmacology and Physiology*, 23(8), 709–714.

Theodorakis, G. N., Livanis, E. G., Leftheriotis, D., Flevari, P., Markianos, M., & Kremastinos, D. T. (2003). Head-up tilt test with clomipramine challenge in vasovagal syndrome—a new tilt testing protocol. *European Heart Journal*, 24(7), 658–663.

Theodorakis, G. N., Markianos, M., Livanis, E. G., Zarvalis, E., Flevari, P., & Kremastinos, D. T. (1997). Hormonal responses during tilt-table test in neurally mediated syncope. *American Journal of Cardiology*, 79(12), 1692–1695.

Thoren, P. (1972). Left ventricular receptors activated by severe asphyxia and by coronary artery occlusion. *Acta Physiologica Scandinavia*, 85, 455.

Thrasher, T. N., Chen, H. G., & Keil, L. C. (2000). Arterial baroreceptors control plasma vasopressin responses to graded hypotension in conscious dogs. *American Journal of Physiology*, 278(2), R469–475.

Thrasher, T. N., & Keil, L. C. (1998). Arterial baroreceptors control blood pressure and vasopressin responses to hemorrhage in conscious dogs. *American Journal of Physiology*, 275(6 Pt 2), R1843–1857.

Thrasher, T. N., & Keil, L. C. (2000). Systolic pressure predicts plasma vasopressin responses to hemorrhage and vena caval constriction in dogs. *American Journal of Physiology*, 279(3), R1035–1042.

Toska, K., Eriksen, M., & Walloe, L. (1994). Short-term cardiovascular responses to a step decrease in peripheral conductance in humans. *American Journal of Physiology*, 266(1 Pt 2), H199–211.

Toska, K., & Walloe, L. (2002). Dynamic time course of hemodynamic responses after passive head-up tilt and tilt back to supine position. *Journal of Applied Physiology*, 92(4), 1671–1676.

Tschope, C., Schultheiss, H. P., & Walther, T. (2002). Multiple interactions between the renin-angiotensin and the kallikrein-kinin systems: role of ACE inhibition and AT1 receptor blockade. *Journal of Cardiovascular Pharmacology*, 39(4), 478–487.

Tsuru, H., Tanimitsu, N., & Hirai, T. (2002). Role of perivascular sympathetic nerves and regional differences in the features of sympathetic innervation of the vascular system. *Japanese Journal of Pharmacology*, 88(1), 9–13.

Vallance, P., Collier, J., & Moncada, S. (1990). Effects of endothelium-derived nitric oxide on peripheral arteriolar tone in man. *Lancet*, 189(2), 997–1000.

van Lieshout, J. J., Wieling, W., & Karemaker, J. M. (1997). Neural circulatory control in vasovagal syncope. *Pacing and Clinical Electrophysiology*, 20(3 Pt 2), 753–763.

Vanhoutte, P., & Leusen, I. (1981). *Vasodilatation*. New York: Raven Press.

Varghese, P., Harrison, R., Lofthouse, R., Georgeakopolous, D., Berkowitz, D., & Hare, J. (2000). B3-adrenoreceptor deficiency blocks nitric oxide-dependent inhibition of myocardial contractility. *Journal of Clinical Investigation*, 106(5), 697–703.

Verberne, A. J., & Owens, N. C. (1998). Cortical modulation of the cardiovascular system. *Progress in Neurobiology*, 54(2), 149–168.

Wacker, M. J., Wilhelm, H. L., Gomez, S. E., Floor, E., & Orr, J. A. (2003). Role of serotonin in thromboxane A2-induced coronary chemoreflex. *American Journal of Physiology*, 284(3), H867–875.

Waeber, B. (2000). Vasopeptidase inhibition: A new approach to the management of cardiovascular disease. *Journal of Clinical Hypertension*, 2(2), 87–93.

Weber, K., Janicki, J., Reeves, R., Hefner, L., & Reeves, J. (1974). Determinants of stroke volume in the isolated canine heart. *Journal of Applied Physiology*, 37(5), 742–747.

Westfall, T. C., McCullough, L. A., Vickery, L., Naes, L., Yang, C. L., Han, S. P., et al. (1998). Effects of neuropeptide Y at sympathetic neuroeffector junctions. *Advances in Pharmacology*, 42, 106–110.

Wieling, W., Van Lieshout, J. J., & Ten Harkel, A. D. (1998). Dynamics of circulatory adjustments to head-up tilt and tilt-back in healthy and sympathetically denervated subjects. *Clinical Science*, 94(4), 347–352.

Wilkinson, I., Qasem, A., McEniery, C., Webb, D., Avolio, A., & Cockcroft, J. R. (2002). Nitric oxide regulates local arterial distensibility in vivo. *Circulation*, 105, 213–217.

Wright, C., Drinkhill, M. J., & Hainsworth, R. (2000). Reflex effects of independent stimulation of coronary and left ventricular mechanoreceptors in anaesthetised dogs. *Journal of Physiology*, 528 Pt 2, 349–358.

Wright, C. I., Drinkhill, M. J., & Hainsworth, R. (2001). Responses to stimulation of coronary and carotid baroreceptors and the coronary chemoreflex at different ventricular distending pressures in anaesthetised dogs. *Experimental Physiology*, 86(3), 381–390.

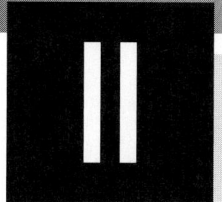
Physiologic and Pathologic Responses

5

Genetics

BRADLEY AOUIZERAT

A little more than 50 years ago, Watson and colleagues discovered the secret of life when they published the chemical structure of DNA (Watson, 2000). The double helix structure made immediately obvious how this molecular archive of life could encode information in the copious quantities necessary to program a living cell. This discovery set into motion a revolution that has continued to unfold to this day, much of it guided by this original discovery.

Research is a slow process, often with years between each sensation, and even today the DNA revolution remains largely behind laboratory doors, in the form of scientists' ever-increasing understanding of the mechanisms of life. But a few powerful inventions—forensic DNA examination, DNA-based drug discovery, and specific disease susceptibility mutation screening—have enjoyed a significant active contribution to society (see Display 5-1 for definitions).

DNA underlies almost every aspect of human health. Obtaining a detailed picture of how genes and other DNA sequences function together and interact with environmental factors ultimately will lead to the discovery of pathways involved in normal processes and in disease pathogenesis. Such knowledge will have a profound impact on the way disorders are diagnosed, treated, and prevented, and will bring about revolutionary changes in clinical and public health practice. Some of these transformative developments are described herein.

How do scientists study and find these genetic mutations? They have available to them a variety of tools and technologies to compare a DNA sequence isolated from a healthy person to the same region of DNA extracted from an afflicted person. Advanced computer technologies, combined with the explosion of genetic data currently being generated from the various whole-genome sequencing projects, enable scientists to use these molecular genetic tools to more accurately diagnose disease and to design new therapeutic interventions. This chapter reviews some common principles that geneticists—scientists who study the inheritance pattern of specific traits—can use to inform clinical practice.

DNA

Molecular genetics is the study of the different word, maybe the units, which pass information from generation to generation. These molecules, our genes, are long sequences of deoxyribonucleic acid, or DNA. Just four chemical building blocks or bases, deoxyguanine (G), deoxyadenine (A), deoxy1thymine (T), and deoxycytosine (C), are placed in a unique order (or unique combinations) to code for all of the heritable units in all living organisms (Fig. 5-1).

DNA is the chemical responsible for preserving, copying, and transmitting information within cells. DNA, located in the nucleus of every cell, harbors the instructions that provide almost all of the information necessary for a living organism to grow and function. The DNA molecule resembles a twisted ladder, usually described as a double helix. The rungs are repeating units called nucleotides, which are the quantum building blocks of DNA. Nucleotides are composed of one sugar—phosphate molecule (the linear strands or outer rails of the DNA ladder) and one base (Fig. 5-2). DNA in eukaryotic cells consists of two nucleotide strands joined by weak chemical bonds between the two bases, forming base pairs. Therefore, a base pair constitutes a "rung" on the ladder of the DNA. The four bases organize in two fundamental pairs, A with T and C with G. One rail of a DNA ladder is a single strand of DNA that is denoted by a sequence of nucleotides (e.g., ACGTGCTGACCTGACGTAGGGCATA), which has complementary bases on the opposite rail, forming complementary nucleotide strands. Within the regions of DNA that express information, these strings of nucleotides are organized into three unit "words" termed *codons*. These codons are organized into groups, called *exons*. Ultimately, these exons form sentences, or *genes*. Genes encode all of the necessary information to produce a messenger molecule composed of ribonucleic acids (RNA), which are composed of four other nucleotides: guanine (G), adenine (A), cytosine (C), and uracil (U). The DNA sentences are *transcribed* into RNA messages, which are single-stranded complementary copies of DNA. Once processed, these messages leave the nucleus and enter another cellular compartment where they are threaded into cellular machinery, which *translates* the information into its final state, the *protein*. Proteins are required for the structure, function, and regulation of the body's cells, tissues, and organs. This process, DNA transcribed into RNA, which can then be translated into proteins, represents the central dogma of molecular biology. It is worth noting that a small subset of the genes expresses RNA without being translated into proteins. These other forms of RNA play crucial roles in the biology of the cell.

DEFINITIONS

Amino acids. The building block for proteins. Humans use 20 amino acids.

Chromosome. An arrangement of tightly packed and coiled DNA and protein. Diploid cells such as the human body cells have 23 sets of chromosomes; haploid cells such as gametes — sperm or ova—have only a single set of chromosomes.

DNA. Deoxyribonucleic acid, the double helix, which codes for the proteins and other elements necessary to construct an organism.

Exon. Regions of DNA that are expressed, coding for RNA and/or protein.

Gamete. A sex cell, such as egg or sperm, capable of joining with an opposite gamete (egg plus sperm) to make a zygote.

Gene. A gene is a segment of DNA or RNA that performs a specific function; usually, it is a segment of DNA that codes for some molecular product, often a protein. Aside from the nucleotides that code for the protein, a gene also consists of segments that determine the type, quantity and timing of protein expression. Genes can produce different combinations of proteins under different stimuli.

Genome. The sum total of genetic material in an individual organism.

Genotype. A relative term that can refer to a particular nucleotide position, or even an entire segment of DNA. A genotype has two components, one from the same position on each chromosome.

Intron. In most eukaryotic cells, introns are segments of DNA that are a component of gene structure but do not generally code for proteins. Introns are processed out of transcribed messenger RNA (mRNA) before it is excised by ribosomes.

Mutation. An alteration in a gene or segment of DNA; mutations are largely accidental and unproductive. On rare occasions mutations can be dangerous and even more rarely they are beneficial. Mutations can lead to variation in the phenotype of an organism.

Phenotype. The physical structure and/or composition of an organism, or group of organisms. Genotypes expressed and developed within an environment determines phenotype.

Protein. Genes often code for proteins, which help form and regulate all organisms. Proteins are molecular machines composed of strings of twenty different types of amino acids. Proteins can in turn form complexes, which interact to perform more complex actions and functions.

Ribosomes. Ribosomes are complexes of RNA and protein, which use the information encoded in mRNA to assemble specific proteins out of amino acids.

RNA. Ribonucleic acid; an intermediate, complementary copy of DNA. Messenger RNA (mRNA) is used by ribosomes as templates of constructed proteins.

Sex chromosomes. In humans, the X and Y chromosomes. Two X chromosomes produce a female, while and X and a Y chromosome results in a male. Other species have different types of sex chromosomes.

Synteny. Segments of chromosomes, which contain the same sequence of genes, which are shared between different organisms.

Humans have approximately 3 billion base pairs of DNA in most of our cells. This complete set of genes is called a genome. The exact sequence of the bases is different for everyone, which makes each of us unique. DNA is an exquisitely small yet extremely long molecule that lacks the tensile strength to remain unprotected during cell division. Accordingly, DNA molecules are packaged into tightly coiled units called *chromosomes,* found in the nucleus of every cell. Chromosomes consist of the double helix of DNA wrapped around proteins, called histones. DNA in the human genome is arranged into 24 distinct

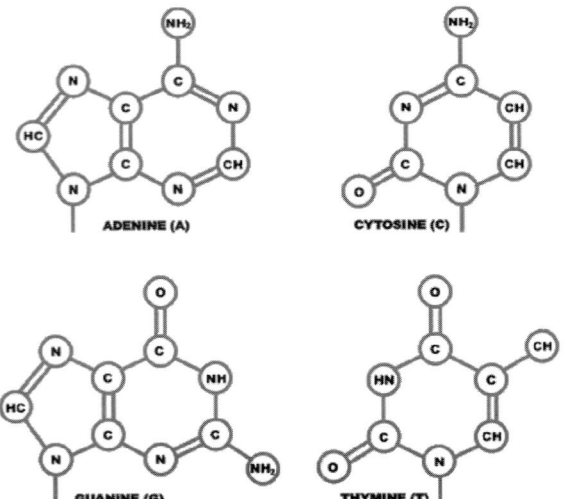

■ **Figure 5–1.** The four DNA bases. Each DNA is made up of the sugar 2'-deoxyribose linked to a phosphate group and one of the four bases depicted above.

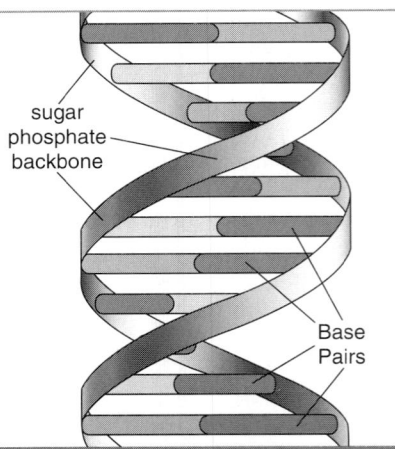

■ **Figure 5–2.** The DNA molecule consists of two anti-parallel, complementary strands of nucleotides that pair A+T or G+C.

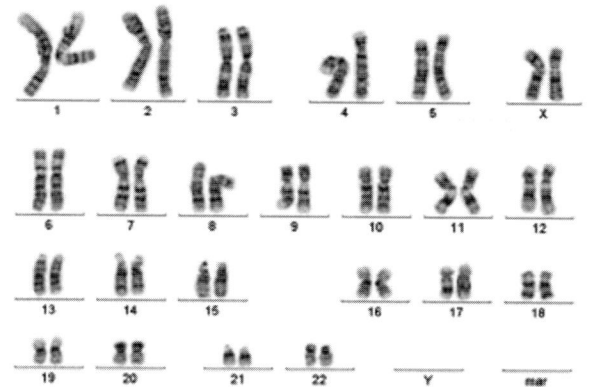

■ **Figure 5–3.** An example of the human genome condensed into the 22 chromosome pairs (autosomes) and the 2 sex chromosomes.

chromosomes, physically separate molecules that range in length from about 50 million to 250 million base pairs. In addition, there are two sex chromosomes that determine gender; two copies of the "X" chromosome result in female gender, while one copy each of the "X" and "Y" chromosomes determines male gender (Fig. 5-3). A few types of major chromosomal abnormalities, including missing or extra chromosome copies or gross chromosomal breaks that rejoin at another chromosome location (translocations), can be detected by microscopic examination. Most changes in DNA, however, are far subtler and require a much closer analysis of the DNA molecule.

Genes

Each chromosome contains many genes, the basic physical and functional units of heredity in living cells. Genes constitute approximately 2% of the human genome; the remainder consists of noncoding regions, whose functions may include providing chromosomal structural integrity and regulating where, when, and in what quantity proteins are made. Genes consist of a length of DNA that encodes instructions for making a specific RNA or protein. Through these molecular products, our genes influence almost everything about us, including how we grow, process foods, reproduce, respond to environmental influences including infections and medicines, and perhaps most importantly our susceptibility and response to disease.

On cell division, DNA becomes tightly packed into a complex structure called chromatin, which is arranged into chromosomes in each cell nucleus. With a few exceptions, such as red blood cells, platelets, and specialized immune cells and platelets, the DNA in each cell of the human body is complete and identical. The human genome—the complete collection of genetic instructions—is estimated to be composed of approximately 35,000 genes. Genes are defined as the segments of DNA that contain the code for all proteins. Proteins are molecular machines that can perform a vast array of diverse and complex functions. DNA is the template that guides the synthesis of those machines through the direction of DNA's intermediate, messenger ribonucleic acid (mRNA), which

leaves the nucleus to be processed in the cytoplasm. Ribosomes (a complex of protein and RNA) then use the mRNA to translate the original DNA instructions and synthesize proteins. Some genes perform other functions, such as making the RNA constituents of ribosomes.

When DNA is transcribed to RNA, many lengths of nucleotides do not code for proteins. These segments of RNA are called *introns* and are processed out of the RNA segments. The segments that remain (termed *exons*) are spliced together, forming the mature *messenger RNA;* these abridged versions of our genes code for proteins. In some cases, a length of newly transcribed RNA can be processed in different iterations; the sequence of exons used can be spliced together in different combinations to make a variety of different proteins. Thus, a single gene can produce or express a diverse series of protein products, depending on the cell type, timing, and ambient activating conditions. This explains in part how identical embryonic cells differentiate to become a variety of different tissues. Similarly, cardiac cells synthesize proteins required for that organ's structure and function, whereas liver cells make proteins important in the metabolic functions of that organ.

DNA AND HUMAN DIVERSITY

Although we all look quite different from one another, we are surprisingly alike at the genetic level. The DNA of most people is 99.9% identical. Only approximately 3 million base pairs are responsible for the differences among us, which is only one tenth of 1% of our genome. Yet these DNA base sequence variations influence most of our physical differences and many other characteristics, also. Gene sequence variations occur in our genes and a subset of the variations results in different forms of the same gene and are called alleles. People can have two identical or two different alleles for a particular gene.

Genes determine hereditary traits such as eye color or hair color. They do this by providing precise instructions for how every activity in every cell of our body should be performed. For example, a gene may guide a liver cell to remove excess cholesterol from our bloodstream. How does a gene do this? It will instruct the cell to make a particular protein and this protein then performs the actual task. In the case of excess blood cholesterol, it is the receptor proteins on the outside of a liver cell that bind to and remove cholesterol from the blood. The cholesterol molecules can then be transported into the cell, where they are further processed by other proteins.

GENETIC VARIATION

A *mutation,* more neutrally referred to as a genetic variation, is a change in the DNA sequence of a gene (e.g., an "A" is altered into a C, G, or T) or even a gross alteration in the chromosomes. Polymorphisms (*poly* meaning many, and *morph* meaning forms) are arbitrarily defined as common differences in the sequence of DNA, occurring in at least 1% of the population. Mutations are less common differences, which occur in less than 1% of the population. Most DNA variation is functionally neutral (neither beneficial nor harmful), but harmful sequence changes sometimes do occur. Changes within genes can result in proteins that do not work normally or do not work at all, which can contribute to disease or affect how an individual responds to a medicine. Mutations may be passed down from parent to child (in the sperm or egg cells), may occur around the time of conception, or may be acquired during a person's lifetime. Mutations can arise spontaneously during normal cell functions, such as when a cell divides or in response to environmental factors such as toxins, radiation, hormones, and even diet.

Many diseases are caused by mutations or changes in the DNA sequence of a gene. When the information coded by a gene changes, the resulting protein may not function properly or may not even be made at all. In either case, the cells containing that genetic change may no longer perform as expected. For example, it is now known that mutations in the gene that codes for the cholesterol receptor protein are associated with a disease called familial hypercholesterolemia. The cells of most individuals with this disease exhibit reduced receptor function and, as a result, cannot remove a sufficient amount of low-density lipoprotein (LDL), which carries cholesterol from their bloodstream. Such an affected person may then have dangerously high levels of cholesterol, a known risk factor for development of atherosclerosis, putting him or her at increased risk for cardiovascular disease such as heart attack and stroke.

Genetic variations are differences in DNA sequence among individuals that may underlie differences in health. Genetic variations occurring in more than 1% of a population would be considered useful polymorphisms for population genetic analyses. Polymorphism types include single nucleotide polymorphisms (SNPs), small-scale insertions/deletions, and repetitive elements (satellite DNA). Satellite DNA is common throughout the genome. These groups of variations are segments of DNA that are repeated in tandem and can be used to differentiate individuals with differing numbers of repeats. The most common variations found in genes are SNPs, which can change the protein product, alter the temporal or spatial expression of a gene, or silence its expression altogether. A comprehensive and complex system of repair genes encodes enzymes that correct nearly all DNA errors. As our bodies change in response to age, illness, and other factors, our DNA repair systems may become less efficient and uncorrected mutations can accumulate, resulting in diseases such as cancer.

GENE TESTING

DNA-based tests are among the first commercial medical applications of the new genetic discoveries. Gene tests can be used to diagnose disease, confirm, and more precisely define a clinical diagnosis, provide prognostic information about the course of a disease, or confirm the existence of a disease in asymptomatic individuals.

Currently, several hundred genetic tests are in clinical use, with a large expansion in available tests expected as a result of the Human Genome Project. Most current tests detect mutations associated with rare genetic disorders that follow Mendelian inheritance patterns. These include cystic fibrosis, sickle cell anemia, and Huntington disease. Recently, tests have been developed to detect mutations for a few more complex conditions such as breast, ovarian, and colon cancers. Although they have limitations, these tests sometimes are used to make risk estimates in asymptomatic individuals with a family history of the disorder. One potential benefit to using such gene tests is that they may provide information to help health care providers and patients manage the disease more effectively.

THE HUMAN GENOME PROJECT

The Human Genome Project (HGP) traces its roots to an initiative in the United States Department of Energy (DOE), which since 1947 has supported the development of new energy resources and technologies and acquiring a deeper understanding of potential health and environmental risks posed by their production and use. In 1986, the DOE announced the Human Genome Initiative, the result of which would provide a reference human genome sequence. Soon thereafter, the DOE joined with the National Institutes of Health (NIH) to develop a plan for a joint HGP that officially began in 1990. During the early years of the HGP, the Wellcome Trust in the United Kingdom joined the effort as a major partner. Important contributions also came from other collaborators around the world, including researchers in Japan, France, Germany, and China. The ultimate goal of the HGP was to generate a high-quality reference DNA sequence for the human genome and to identify all human genes. Other important goals included sequencing the genomes of model organisms to complement our exploration of human DNA, enhancing computational resources to support future research and commercial applications, exploring gene function through mouse— human comparisons, studying human variation, and training future scientists in genomics.

In June 2000, scientists announced the completion of the first working draft of the entire human genome (Lander et al., 2001; Venter et al., 2001). The high-quality reference sequence was completed 2 years ahead of schedule in April 2003, marking the end of the HGP. Available to researchers worldwide, the human genome reference sequence provides an unprecedented biological resource that will accelerate research and discovery, which are expected to seed a myriad of practical applications. The draft sequence has already aided locating genes associated with human disease. Hundreds of other genome sequence projects on microbes, plants, and animals have been completed since the initiation of the HGP, which have enabled detailed comparisons among organisms.

PHARMACOGENOMICS

It is estimated that more than 100,000 people die each year from adverse responses to medications. Another 2.2 million individuals experience serious reactions, while others fail to respond at all. Researchers are beginning to correlate DNA variants with individual responses to medical treatments, permitting identification of particular subgroups of patients, and develop drugs customized for those populations. The discipline that blends pharmacology with genomic capabilities is called *pharmacogenomics.*

DNA variants in genes involved in drug metabolism are the focus of much current research in this area. Enzymes encoded by these genes are responsible for metabolizing most drugs used today, including many for treating cardiovascular diseases. Enzyme function affects patient responses to both the drug and its dose response. Future advances will enable rapid testing to determine the patient's genotype and guide treatment with the most effective drugs, in addition to drastically reducing adverse reactions.

Genomic data and technologies also are expected to make drug development faster, cheaper, and more effective. New drugs aimed at specific sites in the body and at particular biochemical events leading to disease will cause fewer side effects than many current medicines. Ideally, the new genomic drugs could be administered earlier in the disease process. As knowledge becomes available to select patients most likely to benefit from a potential drug, pharmacogenomics will speed the design of clinical trials to bring the drugs into clinical use sooner.

BIOCHEMICAL BASIS OF GENETIC DISEASE

Our genetic constitution, the way in which our individual genome interacts with the environment, can impact our health in many ways. An individual can inherit genetic diseases, caused by abnormal groups of genes passed down from one generation to the next. Such heritable disorders are in three general classes. The first class is single mutant genes of large effect, which can be readily identified given detailed family history review coupled with appropriate genetic testing (e.g., familial hypercholesterolemia). This class of genetic disorders is commonly referred to as mendelian disorders, named after the founder of the modern principles of genetics, Gregor Mendel (Mendel, 1965). The more common class of heritable disorders are those of multifactorial inheritance, caused by the complex interplay of several genes and environmental factors (e.g., diabetes, hypertension, and atherosclerosis). The last class is chromosomal aberrations, abnormalities of either chromosomal structure or number. Such gross alterations to the genome can result from a cellular "accident" or from a parent who carries a chromosomal aberration (e.g., trisomy 21 or Down syndrome).

Altered gene function can manifest at the molecular level in several ways. Genetic alterations can result in enzyme defects, which result in the synthesis of a defective enzyme with reduced activity or reduce quantity. This can lead to substrate accumulation, a metabolic block with a decreased amount of end product, or the failure to inactivate a tissue damaging substrate. Another mechanism of disease is malfunctions in receptors and transport systems. For example, in familial hypercholesterolemia, a reduced function of LDL receptor leads to an inability to transport LDL into the cell, which causes elevated levels of plasma cholesterol and accelerates atherosclerosis.

As the science of genetics has matured, research has shifted focus from rare, single gene disorders to common, multifactorial chronic diseases. Chronic disease affects more than 90 million Americans, accounting for 70% of all deaths and 60% of the nation's medical costs. As research progresses, genetics offers the opportunity to target health promotion and disease prevention programs better and the possibility to conserve health care program resources. However, the contribution of genetics to chronic disease is complex, reflecting the interaction of many genes with the environment and with one another.

OVERVIEW: HEART DISEASE

Cardiovascular Disease

According to the Centers for Disease Control and Prevention, cardiovascular disease, principally heart disease and stroke, is the leading cause of death among men and women in all racial and ethnic groups. Cardiovascular disease affects approximately 58 million Americans and costs the nation $274 billion each year, including health expenditures and lost productivity. Research has begun to uncover a number of potential genetic susceptibility genes for heart disease and stroke and their risk factors (e.g., obesity and high blood pressure).

Heart disease has become a major focus of genetic research. In the past decade, the number of publications on genetic contributions to heart disease has risen exponentially. Genetic mutations have been associated with various risk factors for heart disease, including lipid metabolism and transport, hypertension, and elevated plasma homocysteine levels. It is believed that while traditional risk factors including environmental influences explain approximately 50% of cardiovascular disease, genetics may help explain the remaining disease burden.

Stroke

Studies also have indicated a genetic predisposition to ischemic and hemorrhagic stroke. Although single gene disorders explain a small fraction of strokes, the genetic contribution to stroke most likely will be multifactorial and complex. Recent family studies, including the Framingham Heart Study, have highlighted a significant genetic component to stroke. Twin and family studies provide evidence that genetic factors contribute to the risk of stroke and that their role may be at least as important in stroke as in coronary heart disease. Genetic variation of cystathionine B synthase or methylenetetrahydrofolate reductase (Kelly et al., 2002) result in markedly elevated plasma homocysteine levels and homocystinuria (Wald et al., 2002). Homocysteine is a sulfur-containing amino acid derivative formed during methionine metabolism. Homocystinemia has been demonstrated to increase the risk of coronary artery disease, peripheral artery disease, stroke, and venous thrombosis; and it is a risk factor for premature vascular disease (Engman, 1998). The angiotensin-1 converting enzyme (ACE) gene is known to be a polymorphism, which in some but not all studies is a risk factor for myocardial infarction. Similar studies in stroke patients also show inconsistent results, but most of these studies have been underpowered to detect a small contribution to stroke risk from the ACE gene. Recent meta-analysis shows that the polymorphism, acting recessively, is a modest but independent risk factor for ischemic stroke onset (Sharma, 1998); i.e., apolipoprotein E ε_4 allele has been associated with increased risk of coronary heart disease and is also a major genetic susceptibility locus for Alzheimer disease. Some studies have shown an association between apoE ε polymorphism and ischemic stroke or outcome after stroke. Carriers of the rare ε_4 are more frequent among patients with ischemic cerebrovascular disease compared with control subjects. A recent meta-analysis provides evidence for a role for the apoE genotype in the pathogenesis of some cases of ischemic cerebrovascular disease (McCarron et al., 1999).

Atherosclerosis

Atherosclerosis is a progressive disease characterized by the accumulation of lipids and fibrous elements in the large arteries (see Chapter 7). The early lesions of atherosclerosis consist of subendothelial accumulations of cholesterol-engorged macrophages called foam cells. Lesions can usually be found in the aorta in the first decade of life, the coronary arteries in the second decade, and the cerebral arteries in the third or fourth decades. Because of differences in blood flow dynamics, there are preferred sites of lesion formation within the arteries. Plaques can become increasingly complex, involving calcification, ulceration, and hemorrhage from small vessels within the lesion. Although advanced lesions may encroach and block blood flow, the critical clinical complication is an acute occlusion caused by thrombus formation, resulting in angina, myocardial infarction or stroke.

Sudden Cardiac Death

Although coronary artery disease accounts for the majority of sudden death in cases of cardiac arrest cases, a small proportion (<5%) are attributable to sudden arrhythmia death syndrome. A prolonged QT interval is a common thread among the various phenotypes associated with this phenomenon. A number of drugs are known to cause QT prolongation, as well as disorders of potassium, calcium, and magnesium homeostasis, myocarditis, and endocrine and nutritional disorders. Recently, attention has focused on a group of inherited gene mutations in cardiac ion channels that cause long QT syndrome with an increased risk for sudden death. The age of onset for long QT-related death is the early 30s, with men disproportionately affected. Most cardiac events are precipitated by intense exercise or emotional stress, but they also can occur during sleep. Unfortunately, not all persons with long QT syndrome have previous symptoms or identifiable ECG abnormalities and may present with sudden death. Anti-arrhythmic agents and implantable defibrillators are used for the treatment of long QT syndrome, although identification of the specific gene variants underlying this syndrome will almost certainly better direct prophylactic therapy (Meyer et al., 2003).

THE GENETICS OF CARDIOVASCULAR DISEASE

Epidemiological studies over the past 50 years have identified many risk factors for atherosclerosis (Table 5-1). Dyslipidemia appears to be of primary importance, because raised levels of

Table 5–1 ■ GENETIC AND ENVIRONMENTAL FACTORS ASSOCIATED WITH ATHEROSCLEROSIS AND CORONARY HEART DISEASE.

Trait	Epidemiologic Studies	Population Genetic Studies	Animal Models of Disease	Clinical Trials	Reference
Factors with a strong genetic component					
↑ LDL/VLDL	•	•	•	•	Assmann et al., 1999
↓ HDL cholesterol	•	•	•		Gordon & Rifkind, 1989
↑ Lipoprotein(a)	•		•		Kronenberg et al., 1999
↑ Blood pressure	•			•	Assmann et al., 1999; Glassman, 1998
↑ Homocysteine	•	•			Gerhard & Duell, 1999
↑ Triglycerides	•	•		•	Fruchart & Duriez, 2002
Family history	•	•			Goldbourt & Neufeld, 1986
Diabetes and obesity	•	•	•		Assmann et al., 1999
↑ Hemostatic factors		•			Assmann et al., 1999
Depression and other behavioral traits		•			Glassman, 1998
Gender (male)	•	•			Shepard et al., 2003
Systemic inflammation	•	•		•	Kugiyama et al., 1999
Metabolic syndrome	•	•			Lusis, 1998
Environmental factors					
High-fat diet	•	•	•		Assmann et al., 1999
Smoking	•			•	Assmann et al., 1999
↓ Antioxidant levels	•		•	•	Steinberg, 1999
Lack of exercise	•	•			Assmann et al., 1999
Infectious agents	•	•	•		Hu et al., 1999

Adapted from Lusis, 2000.

atherogenic lipoproteins are a prerequisite for most forms of atherosclerosis. With the exception of gender and the level of lipoprotein(a), each of the genetic risk factors involves multiple genes. An added level of complexity involves the interactions between risk factors that are often not simply additive. For example, the effects of hypertension on coronary artery disease (CAD) are considerably amplified if cholesterol levels are high (Lusis, 1998).

The importance of genetics and environment in human CAD has been examined in many family and twin studies (Goldbourt & Neufeld, 1986). The heritability (the portion attributed to genetic factors) of atherosclerosis has been high in most population studies, often in excess of 50%. It is also evident that the environment explains much of the variation in disease incidence between populations. Thus, the common forms of CAD result from the combination of unfavorable genetic and environmental factors and our increased lifespan (Lusis, 1998).

Generally, the manifestation of CAD is caused by the interaction of several genetic and environmental factors, with those patients with the greatest number of risk factors, including genetic and environmental, facing the highest risk at earlier ages. Several biochemical processes are involved in atherosclerosis formation, progression, and culmination as acute coronary syndromes. Lipid and apolipoprotein metabolism, inflammatory response, endothelial function, platelet function, thrombosis, fibrinolysis, homocysteine metabolism, insulin sensitivity, and blood pressure regulation have been demonstrated to influence disease pathophysiology (Lefkowitz & Willerson, 2001; Rauch et al., 2001; Weissberg, 2000). Each of these biochemical processes involves the complex interplay of enzymes, receptors, and ligands encoded by our genes, the expressions of which are also influenced by environmental factors. Genetic variations can modulate the function of these constituents, resulting in altered susceptibility to the development and progression of CAD (Scheuner, 2001). Several well-established environmental risk factors that predispose to CAD have also been identified (Table 5-2).

The treatment and prevention of CAD has improved greatly in the past decades; however, it remains the leading cause of death and premature disability in the United States (Association, 2000).

Table 5–2 ■ GENETIC CHANGES RELEVANT TO HEART DISEASE.

Trait	Mendelian Characteristics
↑ LDL/VLDL levels	Familial hypercholesterolemia → LDL receptor gene defects resulting in a dominant disorder resulting very high LDL-cholesterol levels and early CAD (Lusis, 1998) Familial defective apoB-100 →Dominant disorder caused by apoB mutations that affect binding to LDL receptor (Lusis, 1998); less severe than FH
↓ HDL cholesterol levels	ApoAI deficiency (apoAI) (Lusis, 1998); In the homozygous state, null mutations of apoAI result in the virtual absence of HDL and early CAD Tangier disease (ABC1 transporter) (Orso et al., 2000; Young & Fielding, 1999). This recessive disorder results in the inability of cells to export cholesterol and phospholipids, resulting in very low levels of HDL
Coagulation	Various genetic disorders of genetic hemostasis (Lusis, 1998): unlike rare disorders of lipid metabolism where atherosclerotic disease is a primary manifestation, disorders of hemostasis usually present either as increased risk of bleeding or as thrombosis (usually venous), with no outstanding effect on atherogenesis
Elevated homocysteine	Homocystinuria (cystathionine β-synthetase): recessive metabolic disorder resulting in very high levels of homocysteine and severe occlusive vascular disease (Gerhard & Duell, 1999)
Diabetes, type 2	MODY1 (hepatocyte nuclear factor 4a), MODY2 (glucokinase), and MODY3 (hepatocyte nuclear factor 1a) (Lusis, 1998): MODY1, 2, and 3 are characterized by the development of non-insulin-dependent diabetes mellitus in young adults
Hypertension	Glucorticoid-remediable aldosteronism: a dominant disorder with early-onset hypertension and stroke (hybrid gene from crossover of 11-b-hydroxylase and aldosterone synthase) (Luft, 1998) Liddle syndrome (epithelial sodium: dominant disorder with hypertension and metabolic alkalosis channel) (Luft, 1998) Mineralocorticoid receptor (Geller et al., 2000): early-onset hypertension associated with pregnancy

Common genetic variations contributing to heart disease and its risk factors

LDL/VLDL	ApoE (Lusis, 1998): three common missense alleles explain ~5% of variance in cholesterol levels
HDL levels	Hepatic lipase (Cohen et al., 1994): promoter polymorphism ApoAI-CIII-AIV cluster (Cohen et al., 1994): multiple polymorphisms Cholesteryl ester transfer: common null mutations (Japanese); protein (Lusis, 1998) missense polymorphisms Lipoprotein lipase (Wittrup et al., 1999): missense polymorphisms
Lipoprotein(a)	Apolipoprotein(a) (Kronenberg et al., 1999): many alleles explain >90% variance
Homocysteine	Methylene tetrahydrofolate: missense polymorphism reductase (Lusis, 1998)
Coagulation	Fibrinogen B (Lusis, 1998): promoter polymorphism Plasminogen activator: promoter polymorphism inhibitor type 1 (Lusis, 1998) Factor VIII (Lusis, 1998): missense polymorphism
Blood pressure	Angiotensinogen (Luft, 1998): missense and promoter polymorphisms β2-adrenergic receptor (Luft, 1998): missense polymorphism Alpha-adducin (Luft, 1998): missense polymorphism
CAD	Angiotensin-converting insertion–deletion polymorphism enzyme (Samani et al., 1996) Serum paraoxonase (Hegele, 1999; Shih et al., 1999): missense polymorphism affecting enzymatic activity Hemachromatosis: missense polymorphism associated gene (Tuomainen et al., 1999) Endothelial nitric oxide: missense polymorphism synthase (Hingorani et al., 1999) Factor XIII (Franco et al., 2000): missense polymorphism

Only genes exhibiting evidence of linkage or association in two or more studies are cited. Adapted from Lusis, 2000.

The cumulative risk for CAD by age 70 is 30% and 15% in males and females, respectively, and increasing to 48% and 30% by the age of 90 years (Lloyd-Jones et al., 1999). Moreover, it is now clear that disability and mortality from CAD at young ages is particularly devastating to families and has a substantial impact on our economy. Understanding the genetic basis of CAD is expected to improve disease management by providing improved diagnosis, targeted therapies, and prognosis.

Genetic Aspects/Dissection of Atherosclerosis

Although the common forms of atherosclerosis are multifactorial, studies of rare, mendelian forms have contributed vital insights into disease pathogenesis (see Table 5-2). Studies of familial hypercholesterolemia helped unravel the pathways that regulate plasma cholesterol metabolism, knowledge of which was important for the development of cholesterol-lowering interventions. In contrast to the mendelian disorders, dissecting the genetic contribution of common, complex forms of CAD has proven more difficult. Studies of candidate genes have suggested a number of genes influencing the traits relevant to atherosclerosis, but our understanding remains incomplete (see Table 5-2). Large-scale sequencing is now underway to identify polymorphisms for many other candidate genes for hypertension, diabetes, and other traits relevant to atherosclerosis (Cargill et al., 1999). In an attempt to identify further atherosclerosis genes, whole-genome scans (a method of fingerprinting the entire genome in attempts to identify genes shared in affected individuals more often than with their relatives) for loci associated with diabetes, hyperlipidemia, low high-density lipoprotein (HDL) levels, and hypertension have been performed (Krushkal et al., 1999), but few loci with significant evidence of linkage have been found, emphasizing the complexity of these traits.

As a result of the genome projects and large-scale sequencing, hundreds of thousands of gene variations are being identified and a catalogued. Given the rapid development of DNA chip technology, it will soon be possible to genotype large numbers of such polymorphisms in many thousands of individuals. However, appropriate methods to analyze such data are currently unavailable (Risch, 2000).

▪ EVIDENCE FOR A GENETIC BASIS OF CORONARY ARTERY DISEASE

Significant amounts of research support a genetic basis for coronary heart disease and its risk factors. The methods of investigation include family and twin studies, animal models, and gene association studies. Although, historically, single gene mutation was the first to be described as a class, only rarely is susceptibility to atherosclerosis the result of a single gene mutation. The most familiar single gene mutation is familial hypercholesterolemia, which is caused by disruptive mutations of the LDL receptor or apolipoprotein B (Day et al., 1997; Hobbs et al., 1992; Tybjaerg-Hansen et al., 1998).

Twin Studies

Twins have been useful in studying the genetic contribution to many common diseases. A higher concordance of a trait is found in monozygotic twins who share all of their genes compared with dizygotic twins who share only half suggests a genetic component. Several large twin registries, including the Danish Twin Registry, which includes approximately 8,000 unselected twin pairs, observed a significant difference in concordance of CAD deaths in monozygotic twins compared with dizygotic twins in men and women (Allen et al., 1967; Berg, 1984; Cederlof et al., 1967; de Faire et al., 1975; Marenberg et al., 1994; Mosteller, 1993; Reed et al., 1991). A common observation was the delayed age of onset of CAD in women versus men.

Familial Aggregation

A genetic epidemiologic study analyzing data regarding 19 traditional risk factors from cases with myocardial infarction before age 55 compared with matched controls (Nora et al., 1980) suggested the highest odds ratio was associated with a family history of a first-degree relative with CAD before age 55. The risk increased 7.1-fold if the CAD was diagnosed before age 55. These risks were substantially greater than those associated with elevated cholesterol, smoking, or inactivity. Population studies have shown on average a 2- to 3-fold increase in CAD risk in first-degree relatives of cases (Geller et al., 2000; Rissanen, 1979; Rose, 1964; Slack, 1966; Thomas & Cohen, 1955), and prospective studies have shown a 1.5- to 2-fold increase in CAD risk associated with a positive family history (Barrett-Connor & Khaw, 1984; Colditz et al., 1991; Colditz et al., 1986; Hopkins et al., 1988; Phillips et al., 1988; Schildkraut et al., 1989; Sholtz et al., 1975). The observation of aggregation of CAD-associated risk factors (e.g., dyslipidemia, hypertension, obesity, and diabetes) in families with CAD further suggests a genetic basis for these conditions and explains, in part, the familial aggregation of CAD (Adlersberg, 1949; Becker et al., 1988; Berg et al., 1979; Blumenthal et al., 1975; Hamby, 1981; Rissanen & Nikkila, 1977; Rosengren et al., 1990; Thomas & Cohen, 1955).

Angiography studies have confirmed that family history of CAD is an independent risk factor for angiographically evident CAD (Anderson et al., 1979; Hamby, 1981; Sharp et al., 1992). Many studies of familial aggregation of CAD have indicated that the age of onset of a case is inversely proportional to the risk to relatives and that the risk of disease is typically several times greater in relatives of females with CAD compared with males with CAD (Rissanen, 1979; Slack, 1966). The heritability for CAD is estimated at approximately 56%, suggesting more than half of premature CAD (diagnosed before age 55) is caused by the contribution of genes. Moreover, in families with CAD onset before age 46, heritability was estimated at 90% to 100%, whereas within families of the oldest cases the heritability ranged from 15 to 30% (Rissanen, 1979).

Animal Models

In the past two decades, understanding of the molecular mechanisms in atherogenesis has been revolutionized by studies in genetically engineered animal models (Smithies & Maeda, 1995). These models include studies in rabbits, pigs, nonhuman primates, and rodents. Mice deficient in apolipoprotein E (apo E) or the LDL receptor have advanced lesions and are the models most used in genetic and physiological studies (Tamminen et al., 1999). These have permitted in vivo testing of hypotheses. Caveats to such studies are the limits imposed by species differences compared with humans.

Excellent animal models exist for the study of heart disease and the associated conditions of diabetes, dyslipidemia, hypertension, and obesity. Use of animals eliminates problems caused by genetic heterogeneity (mixed population backgrounds) and environmental influences. Given a controlled environment, trait differences between animal strains are best explained by genetic factors. Gene associations in animal models can result in the identification of candidate genes for study in human families, because conserved chromosomal segments exist between model animals and humans (synteny) (Mehrabian, 1992).

The use of animal models is a potentially powerful way of identifying genes that contribute to common forms of atherosclerosis. Many animal models have common variations in many traits relevant to atherosclerosis, and orthologous genes (those having an evolutionary counterpart in other species) frequently contribute to a trait in rodents and humans (Stoll et al., 2000). Mapping and identification of genes contributing to complex traits is easier in animals than in humans. During this decade, it is likely that genome scan approaches and that large-scale gene expression studies in animal models of disease will become widely used in atherosclerosis research.

Gene Associations

Many polymorphisms have been associated with atherosclerosis (Lusis, 2000; Villa-Colinayo et al., 2000) (Table 5-3). Because of methodological constraints, these genes were historically identified as a result of their participation in biochemical pathways implicated in the development and progression of atherosclerosis. There are also numerous studies that have found gene associations with related disorders that are indirectly implicated in the development and progression of CAD, diabetes (Altshuler et al., 2000; Hart et al., 1999; Horikawa et al., 2000; Reis et al., 2000; Stone et al., 1996; Vinik & Bell, 1988), hypertension (Frossard et al., 1999; Geller et al., 2000; Krushkal et al., 1998; Williams et al., 1994), and obesity (Heinonen et al., 1999; Large et al., 1997; Mitchell et al., 1998; Nagase et al., 1997; Ristow et al., 1998; Sina et al., 1999; Walder et al., 1998). Recent investigations using genome scan approaches, which are unbiased screens of the entire genome that can implicate novel genes, have identified additional genetic loci associated with CAD, hypertension, and diabetes, which might provide additional insight to genetic factors contributing to atherosclerosis (Aouizerat et al., 1999; Bray et al., 2000; Ghosh et al., 2000; Hein et al., 1995; Krushkal et al., 1999; Pajukanta

et al., 2000; Vionnet et al., 2000; Watanabe et al., 2000). Genetic factors have been identified that accelerate progression and clinical coronary events by influencing the response to risk factor modification such as diet, alcohol, and use of postmenopausal hormone replacement therapy (Girelli et al., 2000; Kuivenhoven et al., 1998; Psaty et al., 2001). For example, the risk of myocardial infarction is lower in men with an alcohol dehydrogenase variation that is associated with a slower rate of ethanol metabolism, and a significant interaction between this genetic variation and alcohol intake was found (Hines et al., 2001). Those who were homozygous for the susceptibility allele and drank at least one drink per day had the greatest reduction in risk for myocardial infarction and the highest HDL cholesterol levels. Genetic variation also plays a role in response to diet (McCombs et al., 1994; Ordovas, 1999; Tall et al., 1997). A recent study found that 40% of the inter-individual variation in LDL cholesterol levels in response to a low-saturated-fat diet is a familial trait (Denke et al., 2000).

Table 5–3 ■ CANDIDATE GENES IMPLICATED IN RISK FOR HEART DISEASE IN HUMANS.

Candidate Genes

Lipid Metabolism
Apoliproprotein (a) (LPA) (Berg et al., 1979; Kraft et al., 1996)
Apolipoprotein B (Tybjaerg-Hansen et al., 1998)
Apolipoprotein E (Hixson, 1991; Moore et al., 1997; Wang et al., 1995; Wilson et al., 1996)
Cholesterol ester transfer protein (Gudnason et al., 1997; Kuivenhoven et al., 1998)
LDL receptor (Day et al., 1997; Hobbs et al., 1992)
Lipoprotein lipase (Jukema et al., 1996)
Paraoxonase (Sanghera et al., 1998)

Blood Pressure Regulation
Angiotensinogen (Gardemann et al., 1999; Wang & Staessen, 2000; Winkelmann et al., 1999)
Angiotensin II receptor, type 1 (Tiret et al., 1994; Wang & Staessen, 2000)
Angiotensin converting enzyme inhibitor (Cambien et al., 1992; Keavney et al., 2000; Tiret et al., 1994; Wang & Staessen, 2000)

Thrombosis
Factor II (Prothrombin) (Psaty et al., 2001)
Factor V (Factor V Leiden) (Le et al., 2000; Rosendaal et al., 1997)
Factor VII (Di Castelnuovo et al., 2000; Feng et al., 2000; Girelli et al., 2000; Green et al., 1993)

Fibrinolysis
Fibrinogen (Green et al., 1993; Humphries et al., 1997; Tybjaerg-Hansen et al., 1997; Yu et al., 1996)
Plasminogen activator inhibitor-1b (Pastinen et al., 1998)
Platelet function Glycoprotein IIIa (Hooper et al., 1999; Ridker et al., 1997; Weiss et al., 1996)

Endothelial Function/Inflammatory Response
Endothelial leukocyte adhesion molecule-1 (E-selectin) (Wenzel et al., 1994)
Endothelial cell nitric oxide synthase (Hooper et al., 1999)

Homocysteine Metabolism
Cystathionine beta synthase (Boers, Fowler et al., 1985; Boers, Smals et al., 1985; Franken et al., 1996)
Methylene tetrahydrofolate reductase (Christensen et al., 1997; Frosst et al., 1995; Kang et al., 1993)

Adapted from Lusis, 2000.

Although genetic association studies have generated a veritable tidal wave of attractive candidate genes, an important caveat to such studies exists. While these studies may provide strong and exciting correlations between particular genetic variations and disease, they must be replicated and generalized to the population (by their study in large epidemiologic studies) before their clinical usefulness can be accepted and realized.

DIAGNOSIS AND RISK ASSESSMENT: APPLICATION OF GENETIC SUSCEPTIBILITY INFORMATION IN THE PREVENTION OF CORONARY ARTERY DISEASE

Coronary artery disease is a heterogeneous disorder; logically, no universal path of prevention exists for all patients (Mirvis & Chang, 1997). In the future, knowledge of a patient's genetic risk factors will identify important biologic differences that could improve disease prevention and management through targeted interventions. Failure to recognize these differences may deny appropriate access to care for those patients who may benefit from alternative prevention and management strategies.

Cardiovascular disease is heterogeneous in manifestation, and the most appropriate therapy will depend on the particular subtype of disease. Therefore, one application of screening would be to distinguish different forms of the disease so that pharmacological intervention can be more effectively targeted. Classification is already used clinically because patients are grouped according to the variety of risk factors they display, but genetic testing will greatly expand the subdivisions of the disease.

Because heart disease and stroke are diseases of adulthood, knowledge of susceptibility to disease could be available years before clinical disease develops, permitting earlier intervention. Testing for elevated LDL cholesterol and decreased HDL cholesterol and blood pressure have long been advocated as a way of identifying individuals at increased risk, and other factors have emerged more recently as risk indicators (see Table 5-1). Once the genes contributing to common forms of the disease have been identified, along with their underlying genetic lesions, genetic tests will add greatly to our ability to assess risk.

Cholesterol lowering is a central tenet of primary and secondary prevention of CAD (Blankenhorn et al., 1993; Blankenhorn et al., 1987; Brown et al., 1990; Downs et al., 1998; Effect of simvastatin, 1994; Jukema et al., 1995; Randomised trial of cholesterol, 1994; Summary of the Second Report, 1993). However, despite effective lipid lowering, CAD will develop in a substantial proportion of individuals, or those with CAD will have progression of their disease (Kreisberg, 1996). Moreover, elevated plasma cholesterol is not a sensitive predictor of individuals with the greatest genetic susceptibility to CAD (Genest et al., 1992). Elevated levels of lipoprotein(a) [Lp(a)], a pro-inflammatory subpopulation of LDL particles modified by the apolipoprotein (a) protein, is not currently detected with routine cholesterol screening, and only 3% of patients with hyper-Lp(a) had elevated LDL cholesterol values. Epidemiological studies have shown that plasma HDL cholesterol is inversely related to CAD and that there is an inverse relationship between HDL cholesterol and triglyceride levels. Also, hypertriglyceridemia is an independent risk factor for CAD (Fruchart & Duriez, 2002). Fibrates reduce death from CAD and nonfatal myocardial infarction in secondary prevention of CAD in men with low levels of HDL cholesterol. During fibrate treatment, HDL cholesterol levels predicted the magnitude of reduction in risk for CAD events. Supplementation with the cofactors involved in homocysteine metabolism, vitamins B6, B12, and folate are effective in reducing homocysteine levels, particularly if there is a vitamin deficiency (Brattstrom et al., 1990; Brattstrom et al., 1988; Ubbink, 1997), although the long-term effect of cofactor supplementation on reducing cardiovascular events is still undergoing study. However, data are lacking regarding the efficacy of these agents on reducing cardiovascular events in individuals who have modified novel genetic risk factors contributing to unfavorable homocysteine and lipoprotein(a) levels. Despite this lack of evidence, knowledge of genetic susceptibility to CAD has value in providing risk information and can guide decision-making regarding lifestyle modification and participation in disease prevention and management strategies.

Early detection strategies for CAD are generally not recommended for the general population, because many lack adequate sensitivity and specificity whereas others are too invasive and costly. However, use of early detection strategies such as electron beam CT may ultimately prove to be more cost-effective for genetically susceptible persons at high risk. There is consistent evidence that coronary calcification correlates highly with the presence and degree of obstructive and nonobstructive plaque (Bielak et al., 2000; Budoff et al., 1996; Nallamothu et al., 2001; Rumberger et al., 1995; Schmermund et al., 1998), nonfatal infarction, and need for subsequent coronary revascularization in asymptomatic individuals (Arad et al., 1996; Raggi et al., 2000; Secci et al., 1997) and patients undergoing coronary angiography (Detrano et al., 1996). Once CAD is identified in high-risk individuals with a genetic susceptibility, more aggressive risk factor modification, for example pharmacological intervention and procedures such as angioplasty or revascularization, can be considered.

Genetic susceptibility to disease can be assessed by direct DNA-based testing, direct measurement of biochemical traits, physical and pathologic characteristics, and personal and family history collection. Physical examination findings can be instrumental in identifying a genetic risk for CAD (e.g., tendon xanthomas and xanthelasma seen in hereditary lipid disorders). However, many hereditary syndromes are rare and account for only a small percentage of cardiovascular disease. Conversely, DNA markers associated with common forms of disease are generally prevalent and of low magnitude, and thus in isolation are not highly predictive of CAD risk. Moreover, modeling the cumulative risk of the multiple low-magnitude genetic risk factors is still evolving and their application to clinical risk assessment is currently premature. Therefore, the systematic collection of family history information currently appears to be the most appropriate screening approach for identification of individuals with a genetic susceptibility to CAD (see Tables 5-1 and 5-2).

In addition to identifying individuals with increased cardiovascular risk, the family history can also identify qualitative characteristics of CAD risk, which are important when planning disease prevention and management strategies (Scheuner et al., 1997). Familial aggregation of CAD, dyslipidemia, hypertension, stroke, and type 2 diabetes suggests insulin resistance (commonly referred to as the metabolic syndrome) (Reaven, 1988). Altered hemostasis may be suspected in a family that features multiple affected relatives with early onset of CAD and stroke or other thromboembolic events. Recognition of these qualitative features may have important implications for recommending appropriate diagnostic tests as well as individualized surveillance and prevention strategies.

Family history reports of CAD, diabetes, and hypertension are generally accurate, with sensitivity of a case report for CAD ranging from 67% to 85% (Bensen et al., 1999; Kahn et al., 1990; Kee et al., 1993). Specificity values for family history reports of these conditions approach 90% (Bensen et al., 1999). A positive family history can generally be used with a high degree of confidence for the identification of individuals who may be at increased risk for CAD. Nonetheless, when possible, verification of family history by review of medical records and death certificates is preferable, although not always feasible. Studies of family history validity indicate some under-reporting of disease in relatives; thus, a negative report should not be used as an indicator of a minimum or decreased disease risk (less than the general population risk).

An important goal of genetic evaluation for CAD is the development of individualized preventive strategies based on genetic risk assessment and the personal medical history and lifestyle. Patient participation in the process is vital to the success of the prevention plan. Genetic counseling is an integral component of the genetic evaluation, helping to identify a patient's motivations and understanding of the genetic risk assessment and perceived barriers and benefits to learning of a genetic risk (Fraser, 1974). This communication process ensures the opportunity to provide an informed consent, including discussion of the potential benefits, risks, and limitations regarding genetic risk assessment and testing (ASHG Report, 1996; Geller et al., 1997; McKinnon et al., 1997; Statement on use of DNA testing for presymptomatic identification of cancer risk, 1994).

Generally, individuals are motivated to participate in genetic risk assessment with the hope that it will clarify the most appropriate plan for disease management and prevention and for the benefit that such genetic information may have for family members. Several studies have shown that family history can influence compliance with lipid screening and other preventive interventions (Tamragouri et al., 1986). Common barriers to obtaining genetic risk information for common disease include fear of discrimination in the workplace and by insurers, cost, and uncertainty about the value of interventions (Croyle et al., 1997; Hudson et al., 1995; Lerman et al., 1996; Rothenberg et al., 1997). The evidence regarding genetic discrimination of otherwise healthy individuals is minimal, although uncertain (Billings et al., 1992; Geller et al., 1996). Yet because of the fear of potential discrimination, individuals may choose to forego genetic risk assessment that may deprive a patient of beneficial surveillance or therapeutic measures to reduce disease risk. The past 15 years has seen escalating interest regarding the use of genetic information by health insurers (Reilly, 1998). In 1996, the Health Insurance Portability and Accountability Act (HIPAA) became the first federal law to limit the use of genetic data by health insurers. It forbids, among other features, health insurers from using genetic predisposition to disease as a "preexisting" condition that could delay or limit coverage.

ETHICAL CONSIDERATIONS

Sharing information about the risk of future disease can have significant emotional and psychological effects, also. The lack of sufficient privacy and legal protections could lead to discrimination in employment and insurance or other misuse of personal genetic information. Additionally, because genetic tests identify information about individuals and their families, test results can impact family dynamics. Results also can pose risks for population groups if they lead to group stigmatization. Families or individuals who have genetic disorders or who are at risk for them often seek help from medical geneticists and genetic counselors. These professionals can diagnose and explain disorders, review available options for testing, preventive strategies, and treatment, and provide emotional support. Other issues related to genetic tests include their effective introduction into clinical practice, the regulation of laboratory genetic testing quality assurance, the availability of testing, and the education of health care providers and patients about correct interpretation and attendant risks.

SUMMARY

Coronary artery disease management and prevention can improve with genetic risk assessment. Our genetic profile contributes to susceptibility, development, and progression of cardiovascular diseases and our response to risk factor modification and lifestyle choices. Identification of genetically susceptible individuals through the family history and biochemical and DNA testing is possible, and many inherited cardiovascular risk factors are modifiable. Early detection of CAD may be appropriate for genetically susceptible individuals to guide decision-making about risk factor modification. However, data are lacking regarding the efficacy of this approach in preventing clinical events. Research is necessary to investigate the outcome of genetic risk assessment in the management of CAD. Despite the current paucity of evidence, knowledge of genetic CAD susceptibility likely has value in providing risk information and guiding subsequent clinical decision-making. Genetics will play an important role in health promotion and prevention and treatment strategies for chronic diseases such as cardiovascular disease. There is a need for informing the public about the significance of genetic discovery and health status. Translational research that takes the discovery of disease susceptibility genes and creates opportunities for better-targeted prevention and treatment strategies is imperative to decrease the effect of cardiovascular morbidity and mortality.

REFERENCES

Adlersberg, D., Parets, A. D., & Boas, E. P. (1949). Genetics of atherosclerosis. Studies of families with xanthoma and unselected patients with coronary artery disease under the age of fifty years. *Journal of the American Medical Association, 141*, 246.

Allen, G., Harvald, B., & Shields, J. (1967). Measures of twin concordance. *Acta Genet Stat Med, 17*(6), 475–481.

Altshuler, D., Hirschhorn, J. N., Klannemark, M., Lindgren, C. M., Vohl, M. C., Nemesh, J., et al. (2000). The common PPARgamma Pro12Ala polymorphism is associated with decreased risk of type 2 diabetes. *Natural Genetics, 26*(1), 76–80.

American Heart Association. (2000). *Heart and Stroke Statistical Update*, from www.americanheart.org

Anderson, A. J., Loeffler, R. F., Barboriak, J. J., & Rimm, A. A. (1979). Occlusive coronary artery disease and parental history of myocardial infarction. *Preventive Medicine, 8*(3), 419–428.

Aouizerat, B. E., Allayee, H., Cantor, R. M., Davis, R. C., Lanning, C. D., Wen, P. Z., et al. (1999). A genome scan for familial combined hyperlipidemia reveals evidence of linkage with a locus on chromosome 11. *American Journal of Human Genetics, 65*(2), 397–412.

Arad, Y., Spadaro, L. A., Goodman, K., Lledo-Perez, A., Sherman, S., Lerner, G., et al. (1996). Predictive value of electron beam computed tomography of the coronary arteries. 19-month follow-up of 1173 asymptomatic subjects. *Circulation, 93*(11), 1951–1953.

ASHG report. Statement on informed consent for genetic research. The American Society of Human Genetics. (1996). *American Journal of Human Genetics, 59*(2), 471–474.

Assmann, G., Cullen, P., Jossa, F., Lewis, B., & Mancini, M. (1999). Coronary heart disease: reducing the risk: the scientific background to primary and secondary prevention of coronary heart disease. A worldwide view. International Task Force for the Prevention of Coronary Heart Disease. *Arterioscler Thromb Vasc Biol, 19*(8), 1819–1824.

Barrett-Connor, E., & Khaw, K. (1984). Family history of heart attack as an independent predictor of death due to cardiovascular disease. *Circulation, 69*(6), 1065–1069.

Becker, D. M., Becker, L. C., Pearson, T. A., Fintel, D. J., Levine, D. M., & Kwiterovich, P. O. (1988). Risk factors in siblings of people with premature coronary heart disease. *Journal of the American College of Cardiology, 12*(5), 1273–1280.

Bensen, J. T., Liese, A. D., Rushing, J. T., Province, M., Folsom, A. R., Rich, S.S., et al. (1999). Accuracy of proband reported family history: the NHLBI Family Heart Study (FHS). *Genet Epidemiol, 17*(2), 141–150.

Berg, K. (1984). Twin studies of coronary heart disease and its risk factors. *Acta Genet Med Gemellol (Roma), 33*(3), 349–361.

Berg, K., Dahlen, G., & Borresen, A.L. (1979). Lp(a) phenotypes, other lipoprotein parameters, and a family history of coronary heart disease in middle-aged males. *Clinical Genetics, 16*(5), 347–352.

Bielak, L. F., Rumberger, J. A., Sheedy, P F., 2nd, Schwartz, R. S., & Peyser, P. A. (2000). Probabilistic model for prediction of angiographically defined obstructive coronary artery disease using electron beam computed tomography calcium score strata. *Circulation, 102*(4), 380–385.

Billings, P. R., Kohn, M. A., de Cuevas, M., Beckwith, J., Alper, J. S., & Natowicz, M. R. (1992). Discrimination as a consequence of genetic testing. *American Journal of Human Genetics, 50*(3), 476–482.

Blankenhorn, D. H., Azen, S. P., Kramsch, D. M., Mack, W. J., Cashin-Hemphill, L., Hodis, H. N., et al. (1993). Coronary angiographic changes with lovastatin therapy. The Monitored Atherosclerosis Regression Study (MARS). The MARS Research Group. *Annals of Internal Medicine, 119*(10), 969–976.

Blankenhorn, D. H., Nessim, S. A., Johnson, R. L., Sanmarco, M. E., Azen, S. P., & Cashin-Hemphill, L. (1987). Beneficial effects of combined colestipol-niacin therapy on coronary atherosclerosis and coronary venous bypass grafts. *JAMA, 257*(23), 3233–3240.

Blumenthal, S., Jesse, M. J., Hennekens, C. H., Klein, B. E., Ferrer, P. L., & Gourley, J. E. (1975). Risk factors for coronary artery disease in children of affected families. *Journal of Pediatrics, 87*(6 PT 2), 1187–1192.

Boers, G. H., Fowler, B., Smals, A. G., Trijbels, F. J., Leermakers, A. I., Kleijer, W. J., et al. (1985). Improved identification of heterozygotes for homocystinuria due to cystathionine synthase deficiency by the combination of methionine loading and enzyme determination in cultured fibroblasts. *Human Genetics, 69*(2), 164–169.

Boers, G. H., Smals, A. G., Trijbels, F J., Fowler, B., Bakkeren, J. A., Schoonderwaldt, H. C., et al. (1985). Heterozygosity for homocystinuria in premature peripheral and cerebral occlusive arterial disease. *New England Journal of Medicine, 313*(12), 709–715.

Brattstrom, L. E., Israelsson, B., Jeppsson, J. O., & Hultberg, B. L. (1988). Folic acid—an innocuous means to reduce plasma homocysteine. *Scandinavian Journal of Clinical Laboratory Investigation, 48*(3), 215–221.

Brattstrom, L., Israelsson, B., Norrving, B., Bergqvist, D., Thorne, J., Hultberg, B., et al. (1990). Impaired homocysteine metabolism in early-onset cerebral and peripheral occlusive arterial disease. Effects of pyridoxine and folic acid treatment. *Atherosclerosis, 81*(1), 51–60.

Bray, M. S., Krushkal, J., Li, L., Ferrell, R., Kardia, S., Sing, C. F., et al. (2000). Positional genomic analysis identifies the beta(2)-adrenergic receptor gene as a susceptibility locus for human hypertension. *Circulation, 101*(25), 2877–2882.

Brown, G., Albers, J. J., Fisher, L. D., Schaefer, S. M., Lin, J. T., Kaplan, C., et al. (1990). Regression of coronary artery disease as a result of intensive lipid-lowering therapy in men with high levels of apolipoprotein B. *New England Journal of Medicine, 323*(19), 1289–1298.

Budoff, M. J., Georgiou, D., Brody, A., Agatston, A. S., Kennedy, J., Wolfkiel, C., et al. (1996). Ultrafast computed tomography as a diagnostic modality in the detection of coronary artery disease: a multicenter study. *Circulation, 93*(5), 898–904.

Cambien, F., Poirier, O., Lecerf, L., Evans, A., Cambou, J. P., Arveiler, D., et al. (1992). Deletion polymorphism in the gene for angiotensin-converting enzyme is a potent risk factor for myocardial infarction. *Nature, 359*(6396), 641–644.

Cargill, M., Altshuler, D., Ireland, J., Sklar, P., Ardlie, K., Patil, N., et al. (1999). Characterization of single-nucleotide polymorphisms in coding regions of human genes. *Natural Genetics, 22*(3), 231–238.

Cederlof, R., Friberg, L., & Jonsson, E. (1967). Hereditary factors and "angina pectoris". A study on 5,877 twin-pairs with the aid of mailed questionnaires. *Archives of Environmental Health, 14*(3), 397–400.

Christensen, B., Frosst, P., Lussier-Cacan, S., Selhub, J., Goyette, P., Rosenblatt, D. S., et al. (1997). Correlation of a common mutation in the methylenetetrahydrofolate reductase gene with plasma homocysteine in patients with premature coronary artery disease. *Arterioscler Thromb Vasc Biol, 17*(3), 569–573.

Cohen, J. C., Wang, Z., Grundy, S. M., Stoesz, M. R., & Guerra, R. (1994). Variation at the hepatic lipase and apolipoprotein AI/CIII/AIV loci is a major cause of genetically determined variation in plasma HDL cholesterol levels. *Journal of Clinical Investigation, 94*(6), 2377–2384.

Colditz, G. A., Rimm, E. B., Giovannucci, E., Stampfer, M. J., Rosner, B., & Willett, W. C. (1991). A prospective study of parental history of myocardial infarction and coronary artery disease in men. *American Journal of Cardiology, 67*(11), 933–938.

Colditz, G. A., Stampfer, M. J., Willett, W. C., Rosner, B., Speizer, F. E., & Hennekens, C. H. (1986). A prospective study of parental history of myocardial infarction and coronary heart disease in women. *American Journal of Epidemiology, 123*(1), 48–58.

Croyle, R. T., Smith, K. R., Botkin, J. R., Baty, B., & Nash, J. (1997). Psychological responses to BRCA1 mutation testing: preliminary findings. *Health Psychology, 16*(1), 63–72.

Day, I. N., Whittall, R. A., O'Dell, S. D., Haddad, L., Bolla, M. K., Gudnason, V., et al. (1997). Spectrum of LDL receptor gene mutations in heterozygous familial hypercholesterolemia. *Human Mutatation, 10*(2), 116–127.

de Faire, U., Friberg, L., & Lundman, T. (1975). Concordance for mortality with special reference to ischaemic heart disease and cerebrovascular disease. A study on the Swedish Twin Registry. *Preventive Medicine, 4*(4), 509–517.

Denke, M. A., Adams-Huet, B., & Nguyen, A.T. (2000). Individual cholesterol variation in response to a margarine- or butter-based diet: A study in families. *JAMA, 284*(21), 2740–2747.

Detrano, R., Hsiai, T., Wang, S., Puentes, G., Fallavollita, J., Shields, P., et al. (1996). Prognostic value of coronary calcification and angiographic stenoses in patients undergoing coronary angiography. *Journal of the American College of Cardiology, 27*(2), 285–290.

Di Castelnuovo, A., D'Orazio, A., Amore, C., Falanga, A., Donati, M. B., & Iacoviello, L. (2000). The decanucleotide insertion/deletion polymorphism in the promoter region of the coagulation factor VII gene and the risk of familial myocardial infarction. *Thrombosis Research, 98*(1), 9–17.

Downs, J. R., Clearfield, M., Weis, S., Whitney, E., Shapiro, D. R., Beere, P. A., et al. (1998). Primary prevention of acute coronary events with lovastatin in men and women with average cholesterol levels: results of AFCAPS/TexCAPS. Air Force/Texas Coronary Atherosclerosis Prevention Study. *JAMA, 279*(20), 1615–1622.

Effect of simvastatin on coronary atheroma: the Multicentre Anti-Atheroma Study (MAAS). (1994). *Lancet, 344*(8923), 633–638.

Engman, M. (1998). Homocysteinemia: new information about an old risk factor for vascular disease. *Journal of Insur Medicine, 30*(4), 231–236.

Feng, D., Tofler, G. H., Larson, M. G., O'Donnell, C. J., Lipinska, I., Schmitz, C., et al. (2000). Factor VII gene polymorphism, factor VII levels, and prevalent cardiovascular disease: the Framingham Heart Study. *Arterioscler Thromb Vasc Biol, 20*(2), 593–600.

Franco, R. F., Pazin-Filho, A., Tavella, M. H., Simoes, M. V., Marin-Neto, J. A., & Zago, M. A. (2000). Factor XIII val34leu and the risk of myocardial infarction. *Haematologica, 85*(1), 67–71.

Franken, D. G., Boers, G. H., Blom, H. J., Cruysberg, J. R., Trijbels, F. J., & Hamel, B. C. (1996). Prevalence of familial mild hyperhomocysteinemia. *Atherosclerosis, 125*(1), 71–80.

Fraser, F. C. (1974). Genetic counseling. *American Journal of Human Genetics, 26*(5), 636–661.

Frossard, P. M., Lestringant, G. G., Malloy, M. J., & Kane, J. P. (1999). Human renin gene BglI dimorphism associated with hypertension in two independent populations. *Clinical Genetics, 56*(6), 428–433.

Frosst, P., Blom, H. J., Milos, R., Goyette, P., Sheppard, C. A., Matthews, R. G., et al. (1995). A candidate genetic risk factor for vascular disease: a common mutation in methylenetetrahydrofolate reductase. *Natural Genetics, 10*(1), 111–113.

Fruchart, J. C., & Duriez, P. (2002). HDL and triglyceride as therapeutic targets. *Current Opinion in Lipidology, 13*(6), 605–616.

Gardemann, A., Stricker, J., Humme, J., Nguyen, Q. D., Katz, N., Philipp, M., et al. (1999). Angiotensinogen T174M and M235T gene polymorphisms are associated with the extent of coronary atherosclerosis. *Atherosclerosis, 145*(2), 309–314.

Geller, D. S., Farhi, A., Pinkerton, N., Fradley, M., Moritz, M., Spitzer, A., et al. (2000). Activating mineralocorticoid receptor mutation in hypertension exacerbated by pregnancy. *Science, 289*(5476), 119–123.

Geller, G., Botkin, J. R., Green, M. J., Press, N., Biesecker, B. B., Wilfond, B., et al. (1997). Genetic testing for susceptibility to adult-onset cancer. The process and content of informed consent. *JAMA, 277*(18), 1467–1474.

Geller, L. N., Alper, J. S., Billings, P. R., Barash, C. I., Beckwith, J., & Natowicz, M.R. (1996). Individual, family, and societal dimensions of genetic discrimination: a case study analysis. *Science Eng Ethics, 2*(1), 71–88.

Genest, J. J., Jr., Martin-Munley, S. S., McNamara, J. R., Ordovas, J. M., Jenner, J., Myers, R. H., et al. (1992). Familial lipoprotein disorders in patients with premature coronary artery disease. *Circulation, 85*(6), 2025–2033.

Gerhard, G. T., & Duell, P. B. (1999). Homocysteine and atherosclerosis. *Current Opinions in Lipidology, 10*(5), 417–428.

Ghosh, S., Watanabe, R. M., Valle, T. T., Hauser, E. R., Magnuson, V. L., Langefeld, C. D., et al. (2000). The Finland-United States investigation of non-insulin-dependent diabetes mellitus genetics (FUSION) study. I. An autosomal genome scan for genes that predispose to type 2 diabetes. *American Journal of Human Genetics, 67*(5), 1174–1185.

Girelli, D., Russo, C., Ferraresi, P., Olivieri, O., Pinotti, M., Friso, S., et al. (2000). Polymorphisms in the factor VII gene and the risk of myocardial infarction in patients with coronary artery disease. *New England Journal of Medicine, 343*(11), 774–780.

Glassman, A. H., & Shapiro, P. A. (1998). Depression and the course of coronary artery disease. *American Journal of Psychiatry, 155*, 4–11.

Goldbourt, U., & Neufeld, H.N. (1986). Genetic aspects of arteriosclerosis. *Arteriosclerosis, 6*(4), 357–377.

Gordon, D. J., & Rifkind, B. M. (1989). High-density lipoprotein—the clinical implications of recent studies. *New England Journal of Medicine, 321*(19), 1311–1316.

Green, F., Hamsten, A., Blomback, M., & Humphries, S. (1993). The role of beta-fibrinogen genotype in determining plasma fibrinogen levels in young survivors of myocardial infarction and healthy controls from Sweden. *Thromb Haemost, 70*(6), 915–920.

Gudnason, V., Thormar, K., & Humphries, S. E. (1997). Interaction of the cholesteryl ester transfer protein I405V polymorphism with alcohol consumption in smoking and non-smoking healthy men, and the effect on plasma HDL cholesterol and apoAI concentration. *Clinical Genetics, 51*(1), 15–21.

Hamby, R. I. (1981). Hereditary aspects of coronary artery disease. *American Heart Journal, 101*(5), 639–649.

Hart, L. M., Stolk, R. P., Dekker, J. M., Nijpels, G., Grobbee, D. E., Heine, R.J., et al. (1999). Prevalence of variants in candidate genes for type 2 diabetes mellitus in The Netherlands: the Rotterdam study and the Hoorn study. *Journal of Clinical Endocrinology and Metabolism, 84*(3), 1002–1006.

Hegele, R. A. (1999). Paraoxonase genes and disease. *Annals of Medicine, 31*(3), 217–224.

Hein, L., Barsh, G. S., Pratt, R. E., Dzau, V. J., & Kobilka, B. K. (1995). Behavioural and cardiovascular effects of disrupting the angiotensin II type-2 receptor in mice. *Nature, 377*(6551), 744–747.

Heinonen, P., Koulu, M., Pesonen, U., Karvonen, M. K., Rissanen, A., Laakso, M., et al. (1999). Identification of a three-amino acid deletion in the alpha2B-adrenergic receptor that is associated with reduced basal metabolic rate in obese subjects. *Journal of Clinical Endocrinology and Metabolism, 84*(7), 2429–2433.

Hines, L. M., Stampfer, M. J., Ma, J., Gaziano, J. M., Ridker, P. M., Hankinson, S. E., et al. (2001). Genetic variation in alcohol dehydrogenase and the beneficial effect of moderate alcohol consumption on myocardial infarction. *New England Journal of Medicine, 344*(8), 549–555.

Hingorani, A. D., Liang, C. F., Fatibene, J., Lyon, A., Monteith, S., Parsons, A., et al. (1999). A common variant of the endothelial nitric oxide synthase (Glu298—>Asp) is a major risk factor for coronary artery disease in the UK. *Circulation, 100*(14), 1515–1520.

Hixson, J. E. (1991). Apolipoprotein E polymorphisms affect atherosclerosis in young males. Pathobiological Determinants of Atherosclerosis in Youth (PDAY) Research Group. *Arterioscler Thromb, 11*(5), 1237–1244.

Hobbs, H. H., Brown, M. S., & Goldstein, J. L. (1992). Molecular genetics of the LDL receptor gene in familial hypercholesterolemia. *Human Mutation, 1*(6), 445–466.

Hooper, W. C., Lally, C., Austin, H., Benson, J., Dilley, A., Wenger, N. K., et al. (1999). The relationship between polymorphisms in the endothelial cell nitric oxide synthase gene and the platelet GPIIIa gene with myocardial infarction and venous thromboembolism in African Americans. *Chest, 116*(4), 880–886.

Hopkins, P. N., Williams, R. R., Kuida, H., Stults, B. M., Hunt, S. C., Barlow, G. K., et al. (1988). Family history as an independent risk factor for incident coronary artery disease in a high-risk cohort in Utah. *American Journal of Cardiology, 62*(10 Pt 1), 703–707.

Horikawa, Y., Oda, N., Cox, N. J., Li, X., Orho-Melander, M., Hara, M., et al. (2000). Genetic variation in the gene encoding calpain-10 is associated with type 2 diabetes mellitus. *Natural Genetics, 26*(2), 163–175.

Hu, H., Pierce, G. N., & Zhong, G. (1999). The atherogenic effects of chlamydia are dependent on serum cholesterol and specific to Chlamydia pneumoniae. *Journal of Clinical Investigation, 103*(5), 747–753.

Hudson, K. L., Rothenberg, K. H., Andrews, L. B., Kahn, M. J., & Collins, F. S. (1995). Genetic discrimination and health insurance: an urgent need for reform. *Science, 270*(5235), 391–393.

Humphries, S. E., Panahloo, A., Montgomery, H. E., Green, F., & Yudkin, J. (1997). Gene-environment interaction in the determination of levels of haemostatic variables involved in thrombosis and fibrinolysis. *Thromb Haemost, 78*(1), 457–461.

Jukema, J. W., Bruschke, A. V., van Boven, A. J., Reiber, J. H., Bal, E. T., Zwinderman, A. H., et al. (1995). Effects of lipid lowering by pravastatin on progression and regression of coronary artery disease in symptomatic men with normal to moderately elevated serum cholesterol levels. The Regression Growth Evaluation Statin Study (REGRESS). *Circulation, 91*(10), 2528–2540.

Jukema, J. W., van Boven, A. J., Groenemeijer, B., Zwinderman, A. H., Reiber, J. H., Bruschke, A. V., et al. (1996). The Asp9 Asn mutation in the lipoprotein lipase gene is associated with increased progression of coronary atherosclerosis. REGRESS Study Group, Interuniversity Cardiology Institute, Utrecht, The Netherlands. Regression Growth Evaluation Statin Study. *Circulation, 94*(8), 1913–1918.

Kahn, L. B., Marshall, J. A., Baxter, J., Shetterly, S. M., & Hamman, R. F. (1990). Accuracy of reported family history of diabetes mellitus. Results from San Luis Valley Diabetes Study. *Diabetes Care, 13*(7), 796–798.

Kang, S. S., Passen, E. L., Ruggie, N., Wong, P. W., & Sora, H. (1993). Thermolabile defect of methylenetetrahydrofolate reductase in coronary artery disease. *Circulation, 88*(4 Pt 1), 1463–1469.

Keavney, B., McKenzie, C., Parish, S., Palmer, A., Clark, S., Youngman, L., et al. (2000). Large-scale test of hypothesised associations between the angiotensin-converting-enzyme insertion/deletion polymorphism and myocardial infarction in about 5000 cases and 6000 controls. International Studies of Infarct Survival (ISIS) Collaborators. *Lancet, 355*(9202), 434–442.

Kee, F., Tiret, L., Robo, J.Y., Nicaud, V., McCrum, E., Evans, A., et al. (1993). Reliability of reported family history of myocardial infarction. *British Medical Journal, 307*(6918), 1528–1530.

Kelly, P.J., Rosand, J., Kistler, J.P., Shih, V.E., Silveira, S., Plomaritoglou, A., et al. (2002). Homocysteine, MTHFR 677C—>T polymorphism, and risk of ischemic stroke: results of a meta-analysis. *Neurology, 59*(4), 529–536.

Kraft, H. G., Lingenhel, A., Kochl, S., Hoppichler, F., Kronenberg, F., Abe, A., et al. (1996). Apolipoprotein(a) kringle IV repeat number predicts risk for coronary heart disease. *Arterioscler Thromb Vasc Biol,* 16(6), 713–719.

Kreisberg, R. A. (1996). Cholesterol-lowering and coronary atherosclerosis: good news and bad news. *American Journal of Medicine,* 101(5), 455–458.

Kronenberg, F., Kronenberg, M. F., Kiechl, S., Trenkwalder, E., Santer, P., Oberhollenzer, F., et al. (1999). Role of lipoprotein(a) and apolipoprotein(a) phenotype in atherogenesis: prospective results from the Bruneck study. *Circulation,* 100(11), 1154–1160.

Krushkal, J., Ferrell, R., Mockrin, S. C., Turner, S. T., Sing, C. F., & Boerwinkle, E. (1999). Genome-wide linkage analyses of systolic blood pressure using highly discordant siblings. *Circulation,* 99(11), 1407–1410.

Krushkal, J., Xiong, M., Ferrell, R., Sing, C. F., Turner, S. T., & Boerwinkle, E. (1998). Linkage and association of adrenergic and dopamine receptor genes in the distal portion of the long arm of chromosome 5 with systolic blood pressure variation. *Human Molecular Genetics,* 7(9), 1379–1383.

Kugiyama, K., Ota, Y., Takazoe, K., Moriyama, Y., Kawano, H., Miyao, Y., et al. (1999). Circulating levels of secretory type II phospholipase A(2) predict coronary events in patients with coronary artery disease. *Circulation,* 100(12), 1280–1284.

Kuivenhoven, J. A., Jukema, J. W., Zwinderman, A. H., de Knijff, P., McPherson, R., Bruschke, A.V., et al. (1998). The role of a common variant of the cholesteryl ester transfer protein gene in the progression of coronary atherosclerosis. The Regression Growth Evaluation Statin Study Group. *New England Journal of Medicine,* 338(2), 86–93.

Lander, E. S., Linton, L. M., Birren, B., Nusbaum, C., Zody, M. C., Baldwin, J., et al. (2001). Initial sequencing and analysis of the human genome. *Nature,* 409(6822), 860–921.

Large, V., Hellstrom, L., Reynisdottir, S., Lonnqvist, F., Eriksson, P., Lannfelt, L., et al. (1997). Human beta-2 adrenoceptor gene polymorphisms are highly frequent in obesity and associate with altered adipocyte beta-2 adrenoceptor function. *Journal of Clinical Investigation,* 100(12), 3005–3013.

Le, W., Yu, J. D., Lu, L., Tao, R., You, B., Cai, X., et al. (2000). Association of the R485K polymorphism of the factor V gene with poor response to activated protein C and increased risk of coronary artery disease in the Chinese population. *Clinical Genetics,* 57(4), 296–303.

Lefkowitz, R. J., & Willerson, J. T. (2001). Prospects for cardiovascular research. *JAMA,* 285(5), 581–587.

Lerman, C., Narod, S., Schulman, K., Hughes, C., Gomez-Caminero, A., Bonney, G., et al. (1996). BRCA1 testing in families with hereditary breast-ovarian cancer. A prospective study of patient decision making and outcomes. *JAMA,* 275(24), 1885–1892.

Lloyd-Jones, D. M., Larson, M. G., Beiser, A., & Levy, D. (1999). Lifetime risk of developing coronary heart disease. *Lancet,* 353(9147), 89–92.

Luft, F. C. (1998). Molecular genetics of human hypertension. *Journal of Hypertension,* 16(12 Pt 2), 1871–1878.

Lusis, A. J. (2000). Atherosclerosis. *Nature,* 407(6801), 233–241.

Lusis, A. J., Weinreb, A., & Drake, T. A. (1998). *Textbook of cardiovascular medicine.* Philadelphia: Lippincott-Raven.

Marenberg, M. E., Risch, N., Berkman, L. F., Floderus, B., de Faire, U. (1994). Genetic susceptibility to death from coronary heart disease in a study of twins. *New England Journal of Medicine,* 330(15), 1041–1046.

McCarron, M. O., Delong, D., & Alberts, M. J. (1999). APOE genotype as a risk factor for ischemic cerebrovascular disease: a meta-analysis. *Neurology,* 53(6), 1308–1311.

McCombs, R.J., Marcadis, D.E., Ellis, J., & Weinberg, R.B. (1994). Attenuated hypercholesterolemic response to a high-cholesterol diet in subjects heterozygous for the apolipoprotein A-IV-2 allele. *New England Journal of Medicine,* 331(11), 706–710.

McKinnon, W. C., Baty, B. J., Bennett, R. L., Magee, M., Neufeld-Kaiser, W. A., Peters, K. F., et al. (1997). Predisposition genetic testing for late-onset disorders in adults. A position paper of the National Society of Genetic Counselors. *JAMA,* 278(15), 1217–1220.

Mehrabian, M., Lusis, A. J. (1992). *Molecular genetics of coronary artery disease. Candidate genes and processes in atherosclerosis.* New York: Karger.

Mendel, G. (1965). *Experiments in plant hybridisation.* London: Oliver and Boyd.

Meyer, J. S., Mehdirad, A., Salem, B. I., Kulikowska, A., & Kulikowski, P. (2003). Sudden arrhythmia death syndrome: importance of the long QT syndrome. *American Family Physician,* 68(3), 483–488.

Mirvis, D. M., & Chang, C. F. (1997). Managed care, managing uncertainty. *Archives of Internal Medicine,* 157(4), 385–388.

Mitchell, B. D., Blangero, J., Comuzzie, A. G., Almasy, L. A., Shuldiner, A. R., Silver, K., et al. (1998). A paired sibling analysis of the beta-3 adrenergic receptor and obesity in Mexican Americans. *Journal of Clinical Investigation,* 101(3), 584–587.

Moore, J. H., Reilly, S. L., Ferrell, R. E., & Sing, C. F. (1997). The role of the apolipoprotein E polymorphism in the prediction of coronary artery disease age of onset. *Clinical Genetics,* 51(1), 22–25.

Mosteller, M. (1993). A genetic analysis of cardiovascular disease risk factor clustering in adult female twins. *Genetics and Epidemiology,* 10(6), 569–574.

Nagase, T., Aoki, A., Yamamoto, M., Yasuda, H., Kado, S., Nishikawa, M., et al. (1997). Lack of association between the Trp64 Arg mutation in the beta 3-adrenergic receptor gene and obesity in Japanese men: a longitudinal analysis. *Journal of Clinical Endocrinology and Metabolism,* 82(4), 1284–1287.

Nallamothu, B. K., Saint, S., Bielak, L. F., Sonnad, S. S., Peyser, P. A., Rubenfire, M., et al. (2001). Electron-beam computed tomography in the diagnosis of coronary artery disease: a meta-analysis. *Archives of Internal Medicine,* 161(6), 833–838.

Nora, J. J., Lortscher, R. H., Spangler, R. D., Nora, A. H., & Kimberling, W. J. (1980). Genetic—epidemiologic study of early-onset ischemic heart disease. *Circulation,* 61(3), 503–508.

Ordovas, J.M. (1999). The genetics of serum lipid responsiveness to dietary interventions. *Proc Nutr Soc,* 58(1), 171–187.

Orso, E., Broccardo, C., Kaminski, W. E., Bottcher, A., Liebisch, G., Drobnik, W., et al. (2000). Transport of lipids from golgi to plasma membrane is defective in tangier disease patients and Abc1-deficient mice. *Natural Genetics,* 24(2), 192–196.

Pajukanta, P., Cargill, M., Viitanen, L., Nuotio, I., Kareinen, A., Perola, M., et al. (2000). Two loci on chromosomes 2 and X for premature coronary heart disease identified in early- and late-settlement populations of Finland. *American Journal of Human Genetics,* 67(6), 1481–1493.

Pastinen, T., Perola, M., Niini, P., Terwilliger, J., Salomaa, V., Vartiainen, E., et al. (1998). Array-based multiplex analysis of candidate genes reveals two independent and additive genetic risk factors for myocardial infarction in the Finnish population. *Human Molecular Genetics,* 7(9), 1453–1462.

Phillips, A. N., Shaper, A. G., Pocock, S. J., & Walker, M. (1988). Parental death from heart disease and the risk of heart attack. *European Heart Journal,* 9(3), 243–251.

Psaty, B. M., Smith, N. L., Lemaitre, R. N., Vos, H. L., Heckbert, S. R., LaCroix, A. Z., et al. (2001). Hormone replacement therapy, prothrombotic mutations, and the risk of incident nonfatal myocardial infarction in postmenopausal women. *JAMA,* 285(7), 906–913.

Raggi, P., Callister, T. Q., Cooil, B., He, Z.X., Lippolis, N. J., Russo, D. J., et al. (2000). Identification of patients at increased risk of first unheralded acute myocardial infarction by electron-beam computed tomography. *Circulation,* 101(8), 850–855.

Randomised trial of cholesterol lowering in 4444 patients with coronary heart disease: the Scandinavian Simvastatin Survival Study (4S). (1994). *Lancet,* 344(8934), 1383–1389.

Rauch, U., Osende, J. I., Fuster, V., Badimon, J. J., Fayad, Z., & Chesebro, J. H. (2001). Thrombus formation on atherosclerotic plaques: pathogenesis and clinical consequences. *Annals of Internal Medicine,* 134(3), 224–238.

Reaven, G. M. (1988). Banting lecture 1988. Role of insulin resistance in human disease. *Diabetes,* 37(12), 1595–1607.

Reed, T., Quiroga, J., Selby, J. V., Carmelli, D., Christian, J. C., Fabsitz, R. R., et al. (1991). Concordance of ischemic heart disease in the NHLBI twin study after 14-18 years of follow-up. *Journal of Clinical Epidemiology,* 44(8), 797–805.

Reilly, P. R. (1998). Genetic risk assessment and insurance. *Genetics Testing,* 2(1), 1–2.

Reis, A. F., Ye, W. Z., Dubois-Laforgue, D., Bellanne-Chantelot, C., Timsit, J., & Velho, G. (2000). Association of a variant in exon 31 of the sulfonylurea receptor 1 (SUR1) gene with type 2 diabetes mellitus in French Caucasians. *Human Genetics,* 107(2), 138–144.

Ridker, P. M., Hennekens, C. H., Schmitz, C., Stampfer, M. J., & Lindpaintner, K. (1997). PIA1/A2 polymorphism of platelet glycoprotein IIIa and risks of myocardial infarction, stroke, and venous thrombosis. *Lancet,* 349(9049), 385–388.

Risch, N. J. (2000). Searching for genetic determinants in the new millennium. *Nature,* 405(6788), 847–856.

Rissanen, A. M. (1979). Familial occurrence of coronary heart disease: effect of age at diagnosis. *American Journal of Cardiology,* 44(1), 60–66.

Rissanen, A. M., & Nikkila, E. A. (1977). Coronary artery disease and its risk factors in families of young men with angina pectoris and in controls. *British Heart Journal,* 39(8), 875–883.

Ristow, M., Muller-Wieland, D., Pfeiffer, A., Krone, W., & Kahn, C. R. (1998). Obesity associated with a mutation in a genetic regulator of adipocyte differentiation. *New England Journal of Medicine,* 339(14), 953–959.

Rose, G. (1964). Familial patterns in ischaemic heart disease. *British Journal of Preventive Society Medicine,* 18, 75–80.

Rosendaal, F. R., Siscovick, D. S., Schwartz, S. M., Beverly, R. K., Psaty, B. M., Longstreth, W. T., Jr., et al. (1997). Factor V Leiden (resistance to activated protein C) increases the risk of myocardial infarction in young women. *Blood,* 89(8), 2817–2821.

Rosengren, A., Wilhelmsen, L., Eriksson, E., Risberg, B.,& Wedel, H. (1990). Lipoprotein (a) and coronary heart disease: a prospective case-control study in a general population sample of middle aged men. *British Medical Journal,* 301(6763), 1248–1251.

Rothenberg, K., Fuller, B., Rothstein, M., Duster, T., Ellis Kahn, M. J., Cunningham, R., et al. (1997). Genetic information and the workplace: legislative approaches and policy changes. *Science,* 275(5307), 1755–1757.

Rumberger, J. A., Simons, D. B., Fitzpatrick, L. A., Sheedy, P. F., & Schwartz, R. S. (1995). Coronary artery calcium area by electron-beam computed tomography and coronary atherosclerotic plaque area. A histopathologic correlative study. *Circulation,* 92(8), 2157–2162.

Samani, N. J., Thompson, J. R., O'Toole, L., Channer, K., & Woods, K. L. (1996). A meta-analysis of the association of the deletion allele of the angiotensin-converting enzyme gene with myocardial infarction. *Circulation,* 94(4), 708–712.

Sanghera, D. K., Aston, C. E., Saha, N., & Kamboh, M. I. (1998). DNA polymorphisms in two paraoxonase genes (PON1 and PON2) are associated with the risk of coronary heart disease. *American Journal of Human Genetics,* 62(1), 36–44.

Scheuner, M. T. (2001). Genetic predisposition to coronary artery disease. *Current Opinion in Cardiology,* 16(4), 251–260.

Scheuner, M. T., Wang, S. J., Raffel, L. J., Larabell, S. K., & Rotter, J. I. (1997). Family history: a comprehensive genetic risk assessment method for the chronic conditions of adulthood. *American Journal of Medical Genetics,* 71(3), 315–324.

Schildkraut, J. M., Myers, R. H., Cupples, L. A., Kiely, D. K., & Kannel, W.B. (1989). Coronary risk associated with age and sex of parental heart disease in the Framingham Study. *American Journal of Cardiology,* 64(10), 555–559.

Schmermund, A., Baumgart, D., Adamzik, M., Ge, J., Gronemeyer, D., Seibel, R., et al. (1998). Comparison of electron-beam computed tomography and intracoronary ultrasound in detecting calcified and noncalcified plaques in patients with acute coronary syndromes and no or minimal to moderate angiographic coronary artery disease. *American Journal of Cardiology,* 81(2), 141–146.

Secci, A., Wong, N., Tang, W., Wang, S., Doherty, T., & Detrano, R. (1997). Electron beam computed tomographic coronary calcium as a predictor of coronary events: comparison of two protocols. *Circulation,* 96(4), 1122–1129.

Sharma, P. (1998). Meta-analysis of the ACE gene in ischaemic stroke. *Journal of Neurology, Neurosurgery and Psychiatry,* 64(2), 227–230.

Sharp, S. D., Williams, R. R., Hunt, S. C., & Schumacher, M. C. (1992). Coronary risk factors and the severity of angiographic coronary artery disease in members of high-risk pedigrees. *American Heart Journal,* 123(2), 279–285.

Shepard, D. R., Jneid, H., & Thacker, H. L. (2003). Gender, hyperlipidemia, and coronary artery disease. *Comprehensive Therapy,* 29(1), 7–17.

Shih, P. T., Brennan, M. L., Vora, D. K., Territo, M. C., Strahl, D., Elices, M. J., et al. (1999). Blocking very late antigen-4 integrin decreases leukocyte entry and fatty streak formation in mice fed an atherogenic diet. *Circulation Research,* 84(3), 345–351.

Sholtz, R. I., Rosenman, R. H., & Brand, R. J. (1975). The relationship of reported parental history to the incidence of coronary heart disease in the Western Collaborative Group Study. *American Journal of Epidemiology,* 102(4), 350–356.

Sina, M., Hinney, A., Ziegler, A., Neupert, T., Mayer, H., Siegfried, W., et al. (1999). Phenotypes in three pedigrees with autosomal dominant obesity caused by haploinsufficiency mutations in the melanocortin-4 receptor gene. *American Journal of Human Genetics,* 65(6), 1501–1507.

Slack, J., & Evans, K. A. (1966). The increased risk of death from ischaemic heart disease in first-degree relatives of 121 men and 96 women with ischaemic heart disease. *Journal of Medical Genetics,* 3, 239–257.

Smithies, O., & Maeda, N. (1995). Gene targeting approaches to complex genetic diseases: atherosclerosis and essential hypertension. *Proceedings of the National Academy of Sciences, U S A,* 92(12), 5266–5272.

Statement on use of DNA testing for presymptomatic identification of cancer risk. National Advisory Council for Human Genome Research. (1994). *JAMA,* 271(10), 785.

Steinberg, D. W., J. L. (1999). *Molecular basis of cardiovascular disease.* Philadelphia: Saunders.

Stoll, M., Kwitek-Black, A. E., Cowley, A. W., Jr., Harris, E. L., Harrap, S. B., Krieger, J. E., et al. (2000). New target regions for human hypertension via comparative genomics. *Genome Research,* 10(4), 473–482.

Stone, L. M., Kahn, S. E., Fujimoto, W. Y., Deeb, S. S., & Porte, D., Jr. (1996). A variation at position -30 of the beta-cell glucokinase gene promoter is associated with reduced beta-cell function in middle-aged Japanese-American men. *Diabetes,* 45(4), 422–428.

Summary of the second report of the National Cholesterol Education Program (NCEP) Expert Panel on Detection, Evaluation, and Treatment of High Blood Cholesterol in Adults (Adult Treatment Panel II). (1993). *JAMA,* 269(23), 3015–3023.

Tall, A., Welch, C., Applebaum-Bowden, D., & Wassef, M. (1997). Interaction of diet and genes in atherogenesis. Report of an NHLBI working group. *Arterioscler Thromb Vasc Biol,* 17(11), 3326–3331.

Tamminen, M., Mottino, G., Qiao, J. H., Breslow, J. L., & Frank, J. S. (1999). Ultrastructure of early lipid accumulation in ApoE-deficient mice. *Arterioscler Thromb Vasc Biol,* 19(4), 847–853.

Tamragouri, R. N., Martin, R. W., Cleavenger, R. L., & Sieber, W. K., Jr. (1986). Cardiovascular risk factors and health knowledge among freshman college students with a family history of cardiovascular disease. *Journal of the American College of Health,* 34(6), 267–270.

Thomas, C. B., & Cohen, B. H. (1955). The familial occurrence of hypertension and coronary artery disease, with observations concerning obesity and diabetes. *Annals of Internal Medicine,* 42(1), 90–127.

Tiret, L., Bonnardeaux, A., Poirier, O., Ricard, S., Marques-Vidal, P., Evans, A., et al. (1994). Synergistic effects of angiotensin-converting enzyme and angiotensin-II type 1 receptor gene polymorphisms on risk of myocardial infarction. *Lancet,* 344(8927), 910–913.

Tuomainen, T. P., Kontula, K., Nyyssonen, K., Lakka, T. A., Helio, T., & Salonen, J. T. (1999). Increased risk of acute myocardial infarction in carriers of the hemochromatosis gene Cys282Tyr mutation : a prospective cohort study in men in eastern Finland. *Circulation,* 100(12), 1274–1279.

Tybjaerg-Hansen, A., Agerholm-Larsen, B., Humphries, S. E., Abildgaard, S., Schnohr, P., & Nordestgaard, B.G. (1997). A common mutation (G-455—> A) in the beta-fibrinogen promoter is an independent predictor of plasma fibrinogen, but not of ischemic heart disease. A study of 9,127 individuals based on the Copenhagen City Heart Study. *Journal of Clinical Investigation,* 99(12), 3034–3039.

Tybjaerg-Hansen, A., Steffensen, R., Meinertz, H., Schnohr, P., & Nordestgaard, B. G. (1998). Association of mutations in the apolipoprotein B gene with hypercholesterolemia and the risk of ischemic heart disease. *New England Journal of Medicine,* 338(22), 1577–1584.

Ubbink, J. B. (1997). The role of vitamins in the pathogenesis and treatment of hyperhomocyst(e)inaemia. *Journal of Inherited Metabolic Disorders,* 20(2), 316–325.

Venter, J. C., Adams, M. D., Myers, E. W., Li, P. W., Mural, R. J., Sutton, G. G., et al. (2001). The sequence of the human genome. *Science,* 291(5507), 1304–1351.

Villa-Colinayo, V., Shi, W., Araujo, J., & Lusis, A. J. (2000). Genetics of atherosclerosis: the search for genes acting at the level of the vessel wall. *Curentr Atherosclerosis Report,* 2(5), 380–389.

Vinik, A., & Bell, G. (1988). Mutant insulin syndromes. *Hormone and Metabolism Research,* 20(1), 1–10.

Vionnet, N., Hani El, H., Dupont, S., Gallina, S., Francke, S., Dotte, S., et al. (2000). Genomewide search for type 2 diabetes-susceptibility genes in French whites: evidence for a novel susceptibility locus for early-onset diabetes on chromosome 3q27-qter and independent replication of a type 2-diabetes locus on chromosome 1q21-q24. *American Journal of Human Genetics,* 67(6), 1470–1480.

Wald, D.S., Law, M., & Morris, J.K. (2002). Homocysteine and cardiovascular disease: evidence on causality from a meta-analysis. *British Medical Journal,* 325(7374), 1202.

Walder, K., Norman, R. A., Hanson, R. L., Schrauwen, P., Neverova, M., Jenkinson, C. P., et al. (1998). Association between uncoupling protein polymorphisms (UCP2-UCP3) and energy metabolism/obesity in Pima indians. *Human Molecular Genetics,* 7(9), 1431–1435.

Wang, J. G., & Staessen, J. A. (2000). Genetic polymorphisms in the renin-angiotensin system: relevance for susceptibility to cardiovascular disease. *European Journal of Pharmacology,* 410(2-3), 289–302.

Wang, X. L., McCredie, R. M., & Wilcken, D. E. (1995). Polymorphisms of the apolipoprotein E gene and severity of coronary artery disease defined by angiography. *Arterioscler Thromb Vasc Biol,* 15(8), 1030–1034.

Watanabe, R. M., Ghosh, S., Langefeld, C. D., Valle, T. T., Hauser, E. R., Magnuson, V. L., et al. (2000). The Finland-United States investigation of non-insulin-dependent diabetes mellitus genetics (FUSION) study. II. An autosomal genome scan for diabetes-related quantitative-trait loci. *American Journal of Human Genetics,* 67(5), 1186–1200.

Watson, J. (2000). The double helix revisited. The man who launched the Human Genome Project celebrates its success. *Time,* 156(1), 30.

Weiss, E. J., Bray, P. F., Tayback, M., Schulman, S. P., Kickler, T. S., Becker, L. C., et al. (1996). A polymorphism of a platelet glycoprotein receptor as an inherited risk factor for coronary thrombosis. *New England Journal of Medicine,* 334(17), 1090–1094.

Weissberg, P. L. (2000). Atherogenesis: current understanding of the causes of atheroma. *Heart,* 83(2), 247–252.

Wenzel, K., Felix, S., Kleber, F. X., Brachold, R., Menke, T., Schattke, S., et al. (1994). E-selectin polymorphism and atherosclerosis: an association study. *Human Molecular Genetics,* 3(11), 1935–1937.

Williams, R. R., Hunt, S. C., Hopkins, P N., Wu, L. L., & Lalouel, J. M. (1994). Evidence for single gene contributions to hypertension and lipid disturbances: definition, genetics, and clinical significance. *Clinical Genetics,* 46(1 Spec No), 80–87.

Wilson, P. W., Schaefer, E. J., Larson, M. G., & Ordovas, J. M. (1996). Apolipoprotein E alleles and risk of coronary disease. A meta-analysis. *Arterioscler Thromb Vasc Biol,* 16(10), 1250–1255.

Winkelmann, B. R., Russ, A. P., Nauck, M., Klein, B., Bohm, B. O., Maier, V., et al. (1999). Angiotensinogen M235T polymorphism is associated with plasma angiotensinogen and cardiovascular disease. *American Heart Journal,* 137(4 Pt 1), 698–705.

Wittrup, H. H., Tybjaerg-Hansen, A., & Nordestgaard, B.G. (1999). Lipoprotein lipase mutations, plasma lipids and lipoproteins, and risk of ischemic heart disease. A meta-analysis. *Circulation,* 99(22), 2901–2907.

Young, S. G., & Fielding, C. J. (1999). The ABCs of cholesterol efflux. *Natural Genetics,* 22(4), 316–318.

Yu, Q., Safavi, F., Roberts, R., & Marian, A. J. (1996). A variant of beta fibrinogen is a genetic risk factor for coronary artery disease and myocardial infarction. *Journal of Investigative Medicine,* 44(4), 154–159.

WEB RESOURCES

International Societies of Nurses in Genetics:
http://www.globalreferrals.com/isong.html
National Center for Biotechnology Information:
http://www.ncbi.nlm.nih.gov
Department of Energy/Human Genome Project Information:
http://www.ornl.gov/TechResources/Human_Genome/publicat/primer/index.html
The International Atherosclerosis Society:
http://www.athero.org/
The American Heart Association:
http://www.americanheart.org

6

INFLAMMATION

BRADLEY AOUIZERAT

It is now abundantly clear that cardiovascular disease is the result of the interaction of multiple physiological processes. Myriad population studies, animal models of disease, and biochemical studies have demonstrated the participation and interaction of lipid metabolism, endothelial function, carbohydrate metabolism, thrombogenesis, oxidative stress, and inflammation in the occurrence of cardiovascular disease (Fig. 6-1). Inflammation is the process by which the body responds to injury. Whereas the pathophysiological importance of myocardial inflammation was recognized more than three centuries ago (Lower, 1669), formal recognition that inflammatory mediators were activated in the setting of heart failure occurred little more than one decade ago (Levine et al., 1990). Laboratory evidence and findings from clinical and population studies suggest that inflammation plays an important role in all stages of atherosclerosis (Libby et al., 2002). The demonstration of the presence of inflammatory cytokines in patients with heart failure immediately sparked interest in the role that these molecules play in regulating cardiac structure and function, particularly with respect to their potential role in the progression of heart failure.

The goal of understanding the role of inflammatory mediators in heart failure derives from the observation that many aspects of the syndrome of heart failure can be explained in large part by the biological effects of proinflammatory cytokines. When expressed in the circulation at sufficiently high concentrations, cytokines are potent enough to recapitulate many facets of heart failure, including progressive left ventricular (LV) dysfunction and remodeling, pulmonary edema, and cardiomyopathy (Bozkurt, 1998; Kubota, 1997; Thaik, 1995). Growing experimental evidence suggests that heart failure progresses in part as a result of the deleterious effects of cytokines in the heart and peripheral circulation, thus exacerbating heart failure (Seta, 1996). What is also clear is that the sustained expression (in clinical terms), caused by high-level production of inflammatory mediators inducing maladaptive effects in the heart or cardiovascular system as a whole.

Appreciation of the pathophysiological consequences of sustained expression of proinflammatory mediators in preclinical and clinical heart failure models has led to a series of multicenter clinical trials in patients with moderate to advanced heart failure. The often contradictory outcomes of these clinical trials underscore the complex participation of proinflamma-

tory mediators in the initiation and progression of cardiovascular disease (Alexander, 1994). To that end, this chapter will summarize the tremendous growth of knowledge that has recently occurred in the field of cardiovascular disease, combining what we have learned from basic research and clinical trials, as well as the potential directions of future research endeavors in this area.

INTRODUCTION

Biomarkers for disease can be defined as biological agents, whose concentration or presence informs an altered risk for development of a particular disease or the development of a disease, reflecting the extent of such disease. Some biomarkers have causal roles in disease development, such that modifications lead to reduction in risk. Two time-proven examples are the decreased risk inherent to reduction in plasma cholesterol level and the cessation of smoking. Yet other factors that are not involved in the mechanism of disease can still serve as useful indicators of disease risk or response to treatment (e.g., interleukin 6). Epidemiological research in large cohort studies over the past three decades (e.g. the Framingham Heart Study and the Multiple Risk Factor Intervention Trial) has resulted in the elucidation of several risk factors for cardiovascular disease (CVD) (Kannel, 1997; Kannel et al., 1976). Such studies have established the following risk factors for CVD: age, male gender, hypertension, diabetes mellitus, dyslipidemia, and smoking. Strong evidence also exists to implicate lack of physical activity, obesity, and alcohol intake. While recognition and control of these risk factors have engendered a substantial reduction in CVD-related morbidity and mortality, more than 35% of CVD occurs among those without any known risk factors (Koenig, 2001). This observation motivates a large part of the medical research community to identify novel markers of disease, including inflammatory markers of CVD. For the purposes of clarity and focus, this chapter will exclude other important risk markers such as psychosocial determinants, and those based on mechanical quantification of existing atherosclerotic burden. This chapter will assess the role of inflammatory markers in terms of causality, predictive ability, and potential clinical applicability (modified from Bradford-Hill, 1965). It is critical

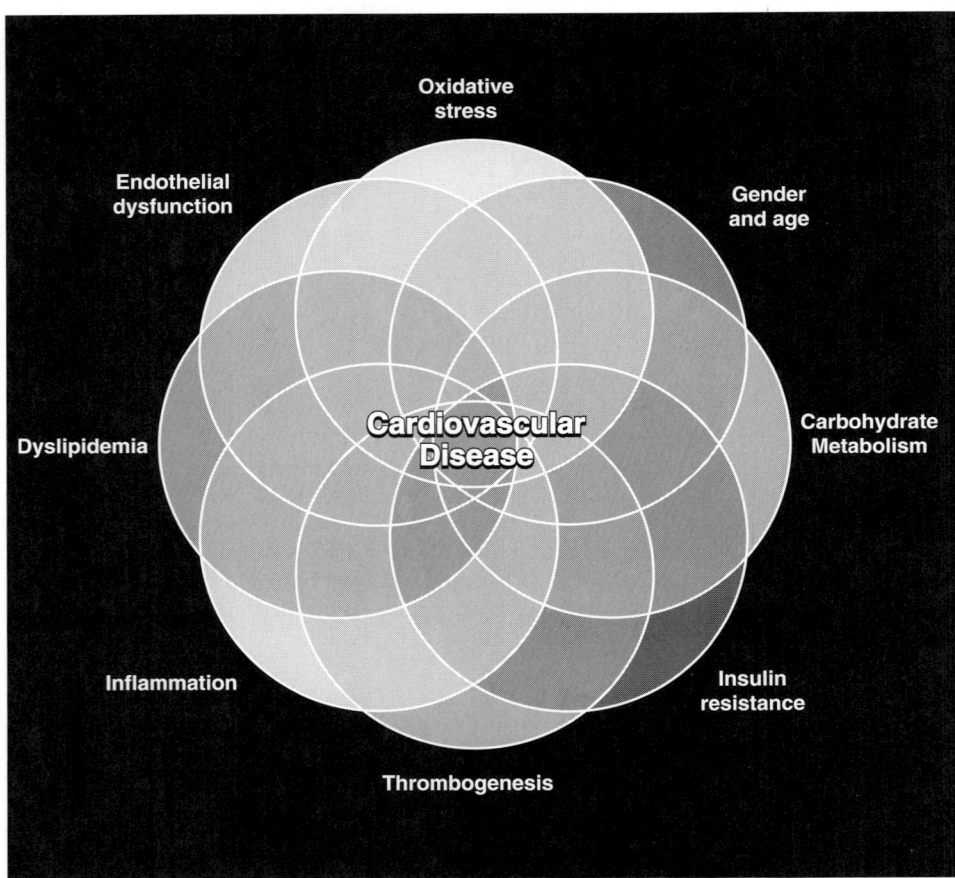

■ **Figure 6–1.** Myriad population studies, animal models of disease, and biochemical studies have demonstrated the participation and complex interaction of lipid metabolism, endothelial function, carbohydrate metabolism, thrombogenesis, oxidative stress, and inflammation in the occurrence of cardiovascular disease.

to note that these serve as potential markers, because, at present, there remains insufficient evidence to support incorporation of any of these risk markers into routine clinical practice.

OVERVIEW OF THE PATHOPHYSIOLOGY OF CARDIOVASCULAR DISEASE

Atherosclerosis is a manifestation of CVD (reviewed in Chapter 7). Briefly, atherosclerosis is a disease of the large arteries and is caused by the accumulation of plaques within the arterial wall. Over time, these plaques become progressively more rigid and the affected arteries may eventually stenose. Plaque rupture with subsequent local thrombosis usually results in acute arterial occlusion and thromboembolism. Atherosclerosis is initiated by endothelial activation and/or damage, which stimulates release of inflammatory mediators (Boring et al., 1998; Gu et al., 1998; Mach et al., 1999); this also encourages arterial smooth muscle cell proliferation. These inflammatory mediators recruit monocytes and lymphocytes, which cross the endothelial barrier and accumulate in the intima, mounting or sustaining a local inflammatory response. Monocytes differentiate into macrophages and express scavenger receptors. The macrophages consume lipoproteins, which accumulate in this subendothelial space, eventually becoming lipid-laden foam cells, which lose the ability to re-enter the circulation. These foam cells coalesce, forming fatty streaks. Fibrogenic mediators are released from activated leukocytes and the endothelium in an attempt to remodel the lesion by promoting the replication of smooth muscle cells, which in turn secrete enzymes that degrade elastin and collagen in response to inflammatory stimuli. The degradation of the arterial extracellular matrix permits the penetration of smooth muscle cells through the elastic laminae and collagenous matrix resulting in the production of a dense extracellular matrix referred to as the growing plaque (Ross, 1993). Over time, the plaque acquires a fibrous cap and may calcify. Eventually, inflammatory mediators contribute further to the disease process by inhibiting collagen synthesis and provoke secretion of collagenases by foam cells, resulting in plaque instability. This process thins the fibrous cap, rendering it weak and susceptible to rupture when potent procoagulant tissue factors expressed within the atheroma then trigger localized thrombogenesis, acute vascular occlusion, and clinical symptoms (Gu et al., 1998).

As described, inflammation is a key feature of all stages of atherothrombogenesis. This paradigm shift has prompted the search for inflammatory, as well as hemostatic, markers, which may reflect current risk or predict future CVD. Their identification is also tantalizing in their potential to serve as targets for new therapeutic interventions, or provide more appropriate targeting of established therapies.

BRAIN NATRIURETIC PEPTIDE

The heart is an endocrine organ. Natriuretic peptides are neurohormones produced by the heart, which participate in an important counter-regulatory system to balance the effects of sympathetic neurohormones. Brain natriuretic peptide (BNP) is a cardiac neurohormone secreted from the ventricles of the heart in response to ventricular volume expansion and pressure overload (Tateyama et al., 1990). BNP is a diuretic, a natriuretic, and a vasorelaxant (MacGregor et al., 1999). Secreted in a precursor form (ProBNP), it is cleaved into two fragments: physiologically active BNP and a biologically inactive fragment (NTproBNP) (Hunt et al., 1997). NTproBNP has a longer biological half-life than BNP, is more stable in serum and plasma, and is a more specific marker of cardiac activity than BNP.

Epidemiologic studies indicate that BNP and NTproBNP are useful prognostic indicators after the onset of heart failure (Dries & Stevenson, 2000; McDonagh et al., 2001), transmural myocardial infarction (MI), (Richards et al., 1998; Richards et al., 1999) and non-ST segment elevation acute coronary syndromes (de Lemos et al., 2001). In addition, they appear to be sensitive diagnostic markers of myocardial diseases: hypertrophy and ventricular dysfunction (Dries & Stevenson, 2000; McDonagh et al., 1998). Therapy that modifies NTproBNP has been shown to not only reduce total cardiovascular events but also delay time to first event (Troughton et al., 2000). Of particular interest is the mounting evidence that these biomarkers are effective prognostic indicators of mortality in the general population (McDonagh et al., 2001; Wallen et al., 1997).

BNP and NTproBNP are easily and reliably measured by radioimmunoassay. The level of BNP is increased in patients with myocardial infarction, ventricular hypertrophy, cardiomyopathy, and chronic obstructive pulmonary disease. Exploring the use of BNP to predict primary risk of CVD is of great importance given the preliminary data on the prediction of risk of all-cause mortality.

CIRCULATING ADHESION MOLECULES

When inflammatory markers come into contact with endothelial cell membranes, they produce a series of proteins termed adhesion molecules. Activation of endothelial cells and platelets is an important mediator of atherothrombosis (Cherian et al., 2003). Adhesion molecules are specific proteins that regulate the different steps of leukocyte migration from the blood stream into the vessel wall (Jang et al., 1994; Luscinskas & Gimbrone, 1996; Springer, 1995). Markers of endothelial cell and platelet activation such as soluble adhesion molecules can be measured in plasma. Soluble forms of adhesion molecules occur on enzymatic cleavage of membrane-bound molecules, which serve as markers of endothelial cell activation and inflammation (Blann & McCollum, 1994). Intracellular adhesion molecule I (ICAM-I), vascular adhesion molecule I (VCAM-I), and E-selectin are three such proteins that are expressed in response to inflammatory markers such as interleukin 1 (IL-1), tumor necrosis factor alpha (TNF-α), and interferon gamma (IFN-γ) (Fukumoto et al., 1997; Pober et al., 1986). Leukocyte migration is a definitive early event in atherogenesis, and expression of these adhesion molecules can be detected in atherosclerotic plaques (Cybulsky et al., 2001; Davies et al., 1993; Li et al., 1993). Elevated levels of the soluble forms of E-selectin, ICAM-1, and VCAM-1 are found in the plasma of patients with stable angina and acute coronary syndromes (Haught et al., 1996).

Recent evidence indicates that circulating adhesion molecules can remain elevated as much as 6 months after unstable angina (Mulvihill et al., 2000). The clinical relevance of prolonged elevation of circulating adhesion molecules is unclear. Recent evidence points to the usefulness of these factors as biomarkers of disease independent of other risk factors, in which high levels may predict future vascular events (Libby, 2000). Soluble (s) VCAM-1, sICAM-1, and sE-selectin are currently measured by commercial enzyme-linked immunoabsorbent assay (ELISA); these assays are sensitive (being able to detect less than one 1/100 of the physiological concentration of each adhesion molecule) and 100% specific (no cross-reaction with other serum components occurs).

Recent data from the Atherosclerosis Risk in Communities studies revealed a five-fold increased risk of coronary heart disease (CHD) and a two-fold increased risk of carotid atherosclerosis between the extreme quartiles of plasma ICAM-1 levels (Hwang et al., 1997). Analysis of ICAM-1 levels in the Physicians' Health Study (PHS) revealed a 1.6-fold increase risk of MI in men with ICAM-1 concentrations in the highest quartile compared with those in the lowest quartile (Ridker, Hennekens et al., 1998). Evidence from the ARIC study indicates that E-selectin is more closely associated with carotid disease (Hwang et al., 1997). The fact that no association was demonstrated for VCAM-1 levels in the ARIC cohort (Hwang et al., 1997) is potentially caused by the fact that VCAM-1 production is limited to vascular wall components, whereas ICAM-1 is also expressed by fibroblasts and hemopoietic cells. This implies that ICAM-1 acts as a more general marker of inflammation. In the secondary preventive setting, all three biomarkers appear to be significantly and independently related to future death from cardiovascular causes in patients with confirmed coronary artery disease (Blankenberg et al., 2001). This study also indicated that VCAM-1 levels increased the predictive value of classic risk factors. Taken together, these data suggest that ICAM-1 has predictive usefulness for CVD in healthy people, whereas VCAM-1 is an appropriate biomarker in individuals with established atherosclerotic disease. In a recent population genetic study, several soluble adhesion molecules (soluble P-selectin, soluble intercellular adhesion molecule-1, and soluble vascular cell adhesion molecule-1) were found to be lower in individuals of West African origin (a population with lower risk for coronary heart disease) compared with European individuals (Miller et al., 2003).

Circulating adhesion molecules are currently measured by commercially available ELISA, a method that is resource-intensive. Moreover, measurement of these adhesion molecules by ELISA is limited to specialized laboratories. Although preliminary evidence supports a role for circulating adhesion molecules as predictors of CVD risk, additional research is necessary before widespread clinical use.

FIBRINOGEN

Fibrinogen is an acute phase reactant synthesized in the liver and is the substrate of the enzyme thrombin and the precursor to fibrin. Fibrinogen binds platelet glycoproteins, which facilitates platelet aggregation, and plays a central role in the coagulation cascade (Lefkovits et al., 1995; Lefkovits & Topol, 1995). These properties make fibrinogen an important determinant of thrombogenesis and plasma viscosity, and thus a potentially useful candidate biomarker of CVD risk. While its association with the development of CVD is well established (Ernst & Resch, 1993; Meade et al., 1986), evidence of causality has not been demonstrated. Fibrinogen modulates atherothrombosis, in part by binding low-density lipoproteins (LDL) and homing in on lesions and inducing proliferation of vascular smooth muscle (Eber & Schumacher, 1993; Smith, 1986). Fibrinogen is involved in the initial stages of plaque formation, where its integration into the artery wall leads to its conversion to fibrin and fibrinogen degradation products. It also binds to HDL, which sequesters more fibrinogen (Ernst & Resch, 1993). Moreover, fibrinogen and fibrinogen degradation products stimulate smooth muscle cell proliferation and migration (Smith et al., 1990; Thompson & Smith, 1989) and may mediate the adhesion of macrophages into the subendothelial space and further migration into the intima (Miyao et al., 1993).

A host of epidemiological evidence is consistent with a positive correlation between plasma fibrinogen levels and risk of CVD (Danesh et al., 1998; Folsom, Aleksic et al., 2001; Kannel et al., 1987; Lee et al., 1993; Ma et al., 1999; Maresca et al., 1999; Meade et al., 1986; Sato et al., 2000; Tracy et al., 1999; Tracy et al., 1995). Taken together, there exists an approximate doubling in risk for CHD between individuals from the extreme quartiles for plasma fibrinogen. Plasma fibrinogen levels have been variably correlated with incidence of ischemic stroke (Folsom et al., 1999; Kannel et al., 1987; Smith et al., 1997). The observation that fibrinogen levels increase along with many other well-established risk factors for CVD begs the possibility that associations may be caused by confounding factors. Fibrinogen levels positively co-vary with age, plasma total cholesterol, LDL cholesterol and plasma triglycerides, obesity, smoking, hypertension, diabetes mellitus, and socioeconomic factors (Genest & Cohn, 1995; Muldoon et al., 1995). Fibrinogen is a routinely measured blood parameter that is simple, reliable, and reproducible (Di Minno & Mancini, 1990; Sweetnam et al., 1998). While no specific treatment currently exists that can affect plasma fibrinogen levels directly, diffuse modulation of the coagulation cascade is routinely performed for other therapeutic or preventive purposes.

HIGH SENSITIVITY C-REACTIVE PROTEIN

C-reactive protein (CRP) is a small protein complex produced by the liver in response to inflammatory stimuli (Libby et al., 2002; Pepys, 1995). The synthesis of CRP is stimulated by cytokines, primarily IL-6 released from inflamed tissue. Levels of CRP can increase up to 1,000-fold during acute inflammation. It is not clear yet whether it is locally expressed (secreted) or absorbed from the blood stream. Initially, assays were designed to detect and measure large elevations in CRP, because such elevations are readily observed in inflammatory diseases such as rheumatoid arthritis. Recently, appreciation of the presence of minor elevation in CRP levels in individuals without gross inflammation has lead to the development of a high-sensitivity test, which permits detection of minor fluctuations of CRP not detectable by conventional assays. Several large epidemiological studies have supported a role for elevated high-sensitivity (hs) CRP predicting future CVD.

The Physicians' Health Study (PHS) consists of a cohort of nearly 15,000 middle-aged to elderly men followed-up prospectively. Enrolled subjects were initially free of disease. When subjects with baseline levels of hsCRP in the lowest quartile were compared with individuals in the highest quartile, they exhibited a two-fold increase in the risk of subsequent stroke or peripheral vascular disease and a three-fold increase in the risk of MI (Ridker, 1998; Ridker et al., 1997; Ridker, Cushman et al., 1998). These findings have already been consistently supported by six other large population studies: the Air Force/Texas Coronary Atherosclerosis Prevention Study (AFCAPS/TexCAPS) (Ridker et al., 2001), smokers from the Multiple Risk Factor Intervention Trial (MRFIT) study (Kuller et al., 1996), elderly patients from the Cardiovascular Health Study (CHS) (Tracy, 1999; Tracy et al., 1997), postmenopausal women in the Women's Health Study (WHS) (Ridker, Buring et al., 1998), the Augsburg cohort of the Monitoring Trends and Determinants in Cardiovascular Disease (MONICA) Study (Koenig et al., 1999), and the Helinski Heart Study (Roivainen et al., 2000).

High-sensitivity CRP was the strongest independent risk factor for future MI in the PHS and the WHS studies, even considering traditional risk factors or equivalent levels of homocysteine (Kuller et al., 1996; Ridker, 1998; Ridker, Buring et al., 1998; Ridker et al., 1997; Ridker, Hennekens et al., 2000). Modeling of risk factors indicated that an absolute risk assessment incorporating the ratio of total cholesterol to high-density lipoprotein (HDL) cholesterol and hsCRP resulted in the most accurate estimation of overall cardiovascular risk (Fig. 6-2). Moreover, in studies of patients suffering acute coronary syndromes, elevated hsCRP levels were associated with poorer outcomes (Biasucci, Liuzzo, Buffon et al., 1999; de Winter et al., 1999; Liuzzo et al., 1994), suggesting prognostic usefulness in secondary preventive settings.

Although no specific treatment currently exists for the modulation of the determinants of elevated CRP, the predictive value of hsCRP measurement in conjunction with other established risk factors appears to more accurately quantify CVD risk. Preliminary studies support the usefulness of incorporating hsCRP in more accurate and informed primary and secondary preventive strategies. Males with the highest baseline hsCRP levels were found to experience the greatest risk reduction after the use of aspirin in the PHS study (Ridker et al., 1997; Ridker et al., 2001), whereas added benefit of pravastatin treatment was observed in individuals with elevated hsCRP in the Cholesterol and Recurrent Events (CARE) trial (Sacks et al., 1996). In the AFCAPS/TexCAPS, treatment with lovastatin was also associated with reduction in hsCRP levels (Ridker et al., 2001).

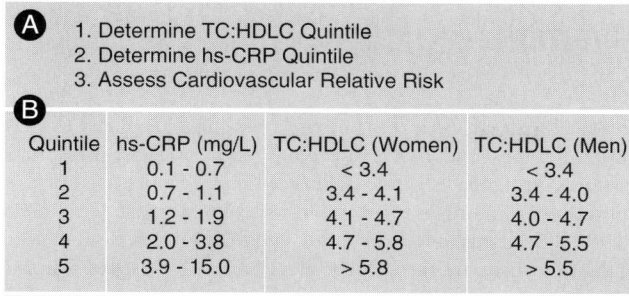

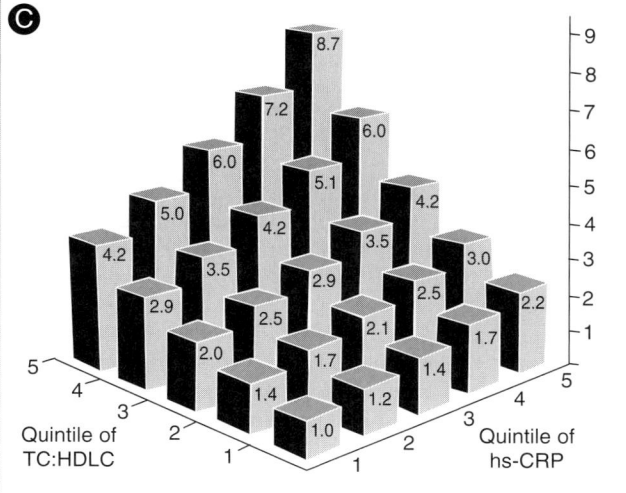

■ Figure 6–2. Proposed cardiovascular risk assessment tool using hs-CRP and lipid screening. (*A*) Steps in risk assessment. (*B*), hs-CRP and total cholesterol (TC): HDL-C quintiles used for the risk assessment. (*C*) Three-dimensional column plot showing relative risk for future cardiovascular events based on quintile of hs-CRP and quintile of TC:HDL-C ratio. The distribution of hs-CRP was derived form ongoing population-based surveys. The lipid cutoffs and risk estimates for incident cardiovascular disease were derived from studies by Ridker and co-workers (Ridker, 1998; Ridker, Buring et al., 1998; Ridker, Cushman et al., 1998). (From Rifai, N. & Ridker, P.M. [2001]. Proposed cardiovascular risk assessment algorithm using high-sensitivity C-reactive protein and lipid screening. *Clinical Chemistry,* 47, 28–30.)

In addition to its role as a biomarker of vascular inflammation, emerging data indicate CRP participates in the atherothrombogenic process, although its precise role is unclear. Natural enzymatic cleavage of CRP results in the production of small peptides, which exhibit a potent effect on immune activity (Heuertz et al., 1993; Robey et al., 1987; Tilg et al., 1993). CRP may further promote thrombosis by activation and co-localization of complement and stimulation of monocytes resulting in synthesis of procoagulant tissue factor (de Winter et al., 1999). In the ARIC studies (Folsom et al., 2002), hsCRP related poorly with subclinical atherosclerosis as measured by carotid intimal media thickness after adjustment for conventional risk factors, suggesting that CRP may be more associated with thrombosis than atherosclerosis. Thus CRP, through its derivative peptides, may contribute to the formation of atheroma and eventual plaque rupture.

At the present time, hsCRP represents the most promising of all new risk biomarkers of CVD. The American Heart Association (AHA) and the Centers for Disease Control and Prevention recently published a joint scientific statement about using inflammatory markers in clinical and public health practice (Pearson et al., 2003) after systematically reviewing the evidence of association between inflammatory markers (mainly CRP) and coronary heart disease and stroke. CRP levels show a consistent dose-dependent and independent association with cardiovascular risk, and it can be measured reliably and relatively cheaply (Folsom, Pankow et al., 2001). These preliminary studies suggest that hsCRP may be able to predict response to aspirin and lipid-lowering therapy, although more data are required to confirm if interventions can be reliably targeted to and guided by hsCRP levels. However, limitations in the use of this biomarker exist, namely its lack of specificity and the uncertainty surrounding its etiological roles (Yu & Rifai, 2000).

HOMOCYSTEINE

Homocysteine (Hcy) is a sulphur-containing amino acid that is closely related to the essential amino acid methionine and to cysteine (http://www.homocysteine.net). Hcy is formed during the metabolism of methionine in the methionine cycle and is metabolized through two pathways: re-methylation or trans-sulphuration. The re-methylation of homocysteine is performed by the enzyme methionine synthase, which requires vitamin B_{12} and methyltetrahydrofolate. In the liver and kidneys, an alternative pathway for the re-methylation of homocysteine exists, but most tissues are entirely dependent on the former mechanism of homocysteine recycling. The remaining homocysteine is converted in the trans-sulphuration pathway to cysteine in two reactions requiring vitamin B_6. Cysteine is a precursor to glutathione, the major cellular reduction/oxidation (redox) buffer, which in turn regulates various aspects of cellular function. The trans-sulphuration pathway also directs Hcy to degradation and its ultimate removal as sulphate through the kidneys.

Homocysteine exists in several forms; the combined measurement is termed total homocysteine (tHcy). Plasma tHcy increases throughout life, being low in childhood and increasing during puberty, with the relative increase being greater in males. It is at this time that population differences start to emerge. On menopause, the gender-related differences in tHcy diminish, but concentrations remain lower in women than in men. The higher tHcy concentrations seen in the elderly may be caused by many factors such as malabsorption, insufficient dietary supply, reduced metabolic activity, reduced kidney function, and other physiological age-related changes. In addition, many drugs affect tHcy levels either by reducing the absorption of co-factors or by increasing their catabolism. Certain diseases also influence homocysteine metabolism. Nutritional and other lifestyle factors are important determinants of tHcy and may explain part of the observed variation between different populations (Display 6-1).

A role for homocysteine levels in the risk of CVD was first suggested by detection of an association between hyperhomocystinemia and premature vascular disease in individuals with inherited homocystinuria (Folsom et al., 1999; McCully,

DISPLAY   6-1

PHYSIOLOGIC DETERMINANTS OF TOTAL HOMOCYSTEINE LEVELS

Age
CVD
Diabetes
Drugs
Gender
Genetics
Lifestyle
Proliferative disease
Renal Failure
Sex steroid hormones
Thyroid disease
Vitamin status

Italicized physiologic determinants represent interactive determinants that modulate total homocysteine, which in turn modulates disease progression.

1969). Subsequent studies exploring the potential of modest changes in plasma Hcy levels correlating with risk of CVD yielded mixed results (Boushey et al., 1995; Christen et al., 2000). Results have not been consistent but seem to support a continuous positive relationship with risk, in addition to a potential threshold effect. A preliminary meta-analysis revealed a positive association with CVD risk in which every 5 mmol/L increase in Hcy increased the risk of incident coronary disease by 60% in men and 80% in women (Boushey et al., 1995). However, this report was not corroborated in a subsequent study (Christen et al., 2000). Several hypotheses may prove to account for the association of Hcy with risk of CVD. They include the ability of Hcy to stimulate the endothelium directly, thereby increasing proliferation of smooth muscle cells (Tsai et al., 1994) and the tendency toward thrombosis (Boushey et al., 1995). The correlation of Hcy with renal dysfunction, smoking, fibrinogen levels, and plasma CRP levels suggests the potential for confounding (El-Khairy et al., 1999).

That folic acid and vitamins B_6 and B_{12} participate in Hcy metabolism provides a ready target for intervention; several studies have demonstrated dose-dependent reductions in Hcy after supplementation of folic acid, vitamin B_6, and vitamin B_{12} (Eikelboom et al., 1999; Lowering blood homocysteine. . ., 1998). Measurement of Hcy is inexpensive and reliable (Shipchandler & Moore, 1995; Zighetti et al., 2002). Because dietary intervention and supplementation could alter CVD risk by lowering plasma Hcy, it makes Hcy an attractive biomarker. The AHA has not yet defined hyperhomocystinemia (high plasma homocysteine levels) as a major risk factor for CVD and does not yet recommend widespread use of folic acid and B vitamin supplements to reduce the risk of heart disease and stroke (http://www.american-heart.org). Randomized clinical trials incorporating clinical outcomes are ongoing and are expected to provide definitive evidence as to the usefulness of using and modulating plasma Hcy (Ford et al., 2002).

INTERLEUKIN 6

Interleukin 6 (IL-6) is a pleiotropic cytokine produced by several cell types and is a central mediator of the acute-phase response. It regulates humoral and cellular responses and plays a central role in inflammation and tissue injury (Van Snick, 1990). The effects of IL-6 are mediated through the interaction of IL-6 with its receptor complex, IL-6R. IL-6 is the primary determinant of CRP release from the liver and is produced in response to several factors, including IL-1, IFN-γ, and TNF (Baumann & Gauldie, 1990). This cytokine is the only known biomarker that can induce the synthesis of all acute phase proteins. In addition to its role in inflammatory processes, experimental evidence suggests that IL-6 possesses procoagulant activity (Mestries et al., 1994). IL-6 is synthesized in the endothelial and smooth muscle cells from normal and aneurysmal arteries (Loppnow & Libby, 1989a; Loppnow & Libby, 1989b). Large quantities of IL-6 have been identified in human atherosclerotic plaques (Rus et al., 1996). Approximately one third of circulating IL-6 is synthesized from adipose tissue, which suggests that IL-6 and obesity may be interrelated (Herity, 2000; Mohamed-Ali et al., 1997); this is particularly relevant given that obesity is a risk factor for CVD. Some cytokines have been demonstrated to inhibit insulin signaling (Hotamisligil et al., 1994), induce hypertriglyceridemia (Hardardottir et al., 1994), and cause endothelial activation (van der Poll et al., 1992). Recent epidemiological studies suggest that chronic inflammatory states are associated with insulin resistance and endothelial dysfunction (Yudkin et al., 2000).

Whereas the epidemiological evidence demonstrating an association between IL-6 and CVD independent of CRP is mixed and limited, it remains suggestive. After adjustment for CRP and other cardiovascular risk factors, men segregated in the highest quartile of baseline IL-6 levels from the PHS cohort exhibited greater than twice the risk of first MI than did those in the lowest quartile (Ridker, Rifai et al., 2000). Complimentary results were observed in women with CVD participating in the Women's Health and Ageing Study. Similarly, after adjustment for CRP and other cardiovascular risk factors, women found in the highest tertile of the cohort's IL-6 levels displayed a three-fold increased risk of death compared with members of the lowest tertile (Volpato et al., 2001). In contrast, the associated risk of mortality and IL-6 and CRP in the elderly was found to be similar for those with and without CVD, although their effects were not assayed independently (Harris et al., 1999). In a population-based cross-sectional study, electrocardiogram abnormalities were found to be associated independently with elevated IL-6 (Mendall et al., 1997). This biomarker appears to be predictive of future heart disease (Harris et al., 1999) and is elevated in patients with unstable angina (Biasucci et al., 1996). Patients displaying persistent IL-6 elevation tend to experience a worse in-hospital outcome after admission with unstable angina (Biasucci, Liuzzo, Fantuzzi et al., 1999; Biasucci, Liuzzo, Grillo et al., 1999).

The current method of IL-6 measurement is by ELISA, which is expensive and tends to make large-scale testing problematic (Harris et al., 1999). A complicating factor is the circadian variation of IL-6, which is only partially corrected by limiting the timing of blood sampling. Like CRP, IL-6 is a systemic bio-marker not specific to CVD, which means routine cardiovascular risk evaluation cannot be based on isolated consideration of IL-6 levels. Taken with the lack of a specific treatment for elevated IL-6 levels, more data are required before the clinical use of this promising biomarker.

SERUM AMYLOID A

Serum amyloid A (SAA) proteins, a family of inflammatory apolipoproteins, are major acute-phase reactants that are produced in response to various insults (Malle et al., 1993). Their concentrations can increase up to 1,000-fold during inflammation (Benditt, 1962; Gabay & Kushner, 1999). They bind HDL with high affinity after their synthesis and participate in modifying cholesterol transport during inflammatory conditions (Banka et al., 1995; Malle & De Beer, 1996). SAA is synthesized primarily in the liver (Gabay & Kushner, 1999) and, to a lesser extent, in extrahepatic tissues (Urieli-Shoval et al., 1998) and has been identified in human atherosclerotic plaque (Yamada et al., 1996).

The exact role of SAA in atherogenesis has not been fully defined. It is complicated by its role in the metabolism of HDL, in which evidence suggests it may act as a signal for redirecting HDL to sites of tissue destruction and cholesterol accumulation (Kisilevsky & Subrahmanyan, 1992). In addition, SAA might influence HDL-mediated cholesterol efflux by displacing apolipoprotein A-I from HDL (Coetzee et al., 1986) and by modulating the activity of lecithin cholesterol acyltransferase (Steinmetz et al., 1989). SAA may contribute further to atherogenesis by participating in the remodeling of atherosclerotic plaque by inducing the secretion of collagenase from smooth muscle cells (Brinckerhoff et al., 1989; Migita et al., 1998). This in turn affects thrombus formation by inhibiting platelet aggregation and adhesion at the endothelial cell surface (Shainkin-Kestenbaum et al., 1996; Syversen et al., 1994; Zimlichman et al., 1990) and increasing the oxidation of LDL. This causes adhesion and chemotactic recruitment of inflammatory cells to the sites of inflammation in atherosclerotic coronary arteries (Shainkin-Kestenbaum et al., 1996; Syversen et al., 1994; Zimlichman et al., 1990). SAA concentrations parallel those of C-reactive protein; some studies suggest SAA is a more sensitive marker of inflammatory disease (Malle & De Beer, 1996). At present, assays for SAA are not widely available. Concentrations of SAA are increased in patients with coronary heart disease and seem to have a useful prognostic utility with acute coronary syndromes (Cushman et al., 1999; Haverkate et al., 1997; Morrow et al., 1998; Ridker, Hennekens et al., 2000). Further epidemiological studies testing the diagnostic and/or prognostic usefulness of SAA are required.

TUMOR NECROSIS FACTOR ALPHA

Tumor necrosis factor *alpha* (TNF-α) was originally identified as an anti-tumor agent. TNF-α is now well-established as a cytokine with a variety of biological functions (Bemelmans et al.,

1996). While TNF-α exhibits potent cytostatic (having an inhibitory action on cell growth or cell division) and cytotoxic effects on select tumor cell-types, it is now more generally recognized as a primary proinflammatory cytokine with a potent negative inotropic effect (affecting the contraction of muscle, especially heart muscle) (Levine et al., 1990). It is a circulating protein with two known cell surface target receptors, TNF receptor I (p55) and TNF receptor II (p75) (Tartaglia & Goeddel, 1992; Tartaglia et al., 1991). With the exception of erythrocytes, the TNF receptors have been identified on all examined cell types (Tartaglia & Goeddel, 1992; Tartaglia et al., 1991), which emphasizes the more ubiquitous role of TNF-α as a proinflammatory cytokine. Both p55 and p75 can be cleaved, releasing soluble proteins capable of binding TNF-α. These soluble receptors compete with the cellular forms and can inhibit the effects of TNF-α and thus titrate the effective concentration of TNF-α locally and systemically (Hale et al., 1995).

TNF-α is a multifunctional circulating cytokine produced in a variety of cell types including T-lymphocytes, natural killer cells, smooth muscle cells, endothelial cells, and some tumor cells, but the largest sources of TNF-α are monocytes and macrophages (Bemelmans et al., 1996). After modified LDL promotes the differentiation of monocytes into macrophages, the macrophages release a variety of chemicals, including TNF α and IL-1, and activate endothelial cells to express adhesion molecules that bind monocytes, making them available for recruitment into the subendothelial space (Nathan, 1987).

TNF-α is involved with several cardiovascular processes and is elevated in advanced heart failure. High levels of TNF-α can produce left ventricular dysfunction, pulmonary edema, and cardiomyopathy. Taken together with the fact that it has also been detected in human atherosclerotic plaques (Barath et al., 1990), TNF-α was expected to have a major role in the pathogenesis of CAD. Elevated levels of TNF-α have been observed after acute myocardial infarction (Maury & Teppo, 1989), and the concentration of the soluble TNF receptors (p55 and p75) also increases rapidly after acute MI (Pannitteri et al., 1997). Presumably, the increase in these soluble receptors represents a protective mechanism against TNF-α release. Similar to IL-6, TNF-α participates in the regulation of the synthesis of other acute-phase proteins that are risk factors for atherosclerosis (e.g., fibrinogen and factor VIII) (Baumann & Gauldie, 1994). TNF-α also modulates insulin sensitivity, which produces changes in lipid (Feingold & Grunfeld, 1992) and glucose parameters associated with cardiovascular risk (Hotamisligil et al., 1995; Hotamisligil et al., 1993).

There exists a wealth of preclinical data and early clinical studies that have suggested a role for TNF antagonism in heart failure (Deswal, 2001; Mann, 2002; Torre-Amione et al., 1996). Plasma TNF-α was measured in patients after MI enrolled in the CARE trial with levels measured again 9 months after initial infarct. The excess risk of recurrent coronary events after myocardial infarction was predominantly seen among individuals with the highest level of TNF-α; those with levels in excess of the 95th percentile of the control distribution had an approximately three-fold increase in risk. Risk estimates were independent of other risk factors and were similar to subgroup analysis limited to cardiovascular death or to recurrent nonfatal myocardial infarction (Ridker, 2000). Given the strong data suggesting a role for TNF antagonism in heart failure, the negative results of the clinical trials have been disappointing (Mann et al., 2002;

Packer, 2002). However, analysis of the aggregate clinical trial data provides some hint as to why these studies have been negative. Neither the trials with etanercept nor the trial with infliximab was neutral in terms of effect (Homeister, 1994; Klein, 1995; Torre-Amione, 1996). In both trials, a dose-dependent and time-dependent progression of heart failure and/or worsening outcomes was observed, with two explanations worthy of consideration. The first is that the agents that were used had intrinsic toxicity, and the second is that TNF antagonism has problematic effects in the setting of heart failure. There exists a strong possibility that the attempts to mitigate the atherogenic effect of TNF-α were premature, and that the results of these intervention trials will help to direct further study of the biochemical and pathophysiologic mechanisms of TNF action.

VON WILLEBRAND FACTOR

Factor VIII is one of the plasma proteins important for coagulation. It is a complex of two components, each with a different genetic control and biochemical function: (1) factor VIIIc, a coagulation protein; and (2) factor VIIIvW, a platelet adhesion protein (also known as von Willebrand factor). von Willebrand factor (vWF) is a large protein complex necessary for normal platelet adhesion and acts as a bridge between a receptor on the platelet surface and the exposed basement membrane or subendothelial collagen. Factor VIIIc forms a complex with vWF in plasma, with the latter acting as a carrier protein. von Willebrand factor, a glycoprotein synthesized in endothelial cells and megakaryocytes, promotes thrombus formation by mediating platelet adhesion and aggregation (Ruggeri, 1997). It is released from endothelial cells and platelets after endothelial damage and is a marker of endothelial dysfunction, which in turn is an indicator of early atherogenesis (Ruggeri, 1992).

Several epidemiological studies have established an independent positive association between vWF and CHD (Folsom, 2001; Meade et al., 1994; Rumley et al., 1999). One compelling report provided evidence of increased risk of re-infarction and mortality in survivors of MI with elevated levels of vWF (Jansson et al., 1991). Initial reports of increased risk of stroke (Folsom, 2001) failed to be corroborated in other population studies (Folsom, 2001; Smith et al., 1997; Thogersen et al., 1998).

While measurement of vWF is not standardized, the different assays used by investigators conducting the relevant epidemiological studies have reported comparable and reproducible results. In any case, a commercially available and reliable ELISA has recently been released (Murdock et al., 1997). von Willebrand factor is a sensitive marker of many adaptive conditions, including the acute phase of an inflammatory response, and preliminary evidence supports a role for vWF in the risk of CHD and potentially of stroke.

CONCLUSION

It is now generally recognized that inflammation plays a crucial role in the development of atherothrombosis. In defining the value of any novel risk marker, the evidence of its usefulness must be evaluated not only in terms of causality but also in terms of potential clinical usefulness and additive predictive capacity. In addition, the clinical usefulness of measuring such markers must be accurate, precise, reliable, reproducible, and cost-effective. Therefore, further well-designed prospective evaluation of each of these markers is needed before their use in routine clinical practice. Many of the biomarkers discussed display an encouraging potential for the prediction of risk for different acute coronary syndromes and may correlate with severity and future risk for CVD. As our understanding of the pathophysiology of CVD improves, so will the potential to identify biomarkers of disease. Many such markers have been studied (in-depth reviews are available) (Magliano et al., 2003; Mann, 2002; Saadeddin et al., 2002), with many new candidates on the horizon (MCP-1, IL-1, IL-8, P selectin, L selectin, IL-18). Thus far, the search for such biomarkers has focused on inflammatory and hemostatic markers, with growing interest in neurohormonal factors. Given the burden of CVD, identification of novel risk markers is important in that their measurement may improve risk estimation and lead to more effective and efficient targeting of existing preventive and therapeutic strategies, or ultimately, they may represent new therapeutic opportunities.

REFERENCES

Alexander, R. W. (1994). Inflammation and coronary artery disease. *New England Journal of Medicine*, 331(7), 468–469.

Banka, C. L., Yuan, T., de Beer, M. C., Kindy, M., Curtiss, L. K., & de Beer, F. C. (1995). Serum amyloid A (SAA): influence on HDL-mediated cellular cholesterol efflux. *Journal of Lipid Research*, 36(5), 1058–1065.

Barath, P., Fishbein, M. C., Cao, J., Berenson, J., Helfant, R. H., & Forrester, J. S. (1990). Detection and localization of tumor necrosis factor in human atheroma. *American Journal of Cardiology*, 65(5), 297–302.

Baumann, H., & Gauldie, J. (1990). Regulation of hepatic acute phase plasma protein genes by hepatocyte stimulating factors and other mediators of inflammation. *Molecular and Biological Medicine*, 7(2), 147–159.

Baumann, H., & Gauldie, J. (1994). The acute phase response. *Immunology Today*, 15(2), 74–80.

Bemelmans, M. H., van Tits, L. J., & Buurman, W. A. (1996). Tumor necrosis factor: function, release and clearance. *Critical Reviews in Immunology*, 16(1), 1–11.

Benditt, E. P., Lagunoff, D., Eriksen, N., & seri, O.A. (1962). Amyloid: extraction and preliminary characterization of some proteins. *Archives of Pathology and Laboratory Medicine*, 74, 323–330.

Biasucci, L. M., Liuzzo, G., Buffon, A., & Maseri, A. (1999). The variable role of inflammation in acute coronary syndromes and in restenosis. *Seminars in Interventional Cardiology*, 4(3), 105–110.

Biasucci, L. M., Liuzzo, G., Fantuzzi, G., Caligiuri, G., Rebuzzi, A. G., Ginnetti, F., Dinarello, C. A., & Maseri, A. (1999). Increasing levels of interleukin (IL)-1Ra and IL-6 during the first 2 days of hospitalization in unstable angina are associated with increased risk of in-hospital coronary events. *Circulation*, 99(16), 2079–2084.

Biasucci, L. M., Liuzzo, G., Grillo, R. L., Caligiuri, G., Rebuzzi, A. G., Buffon, A., Summaria, F., Ginnetti, F., Fadda, G., & Maseri, A. (1999). Elevated levels of C-reactive protein at discharge in patients with unstable angina predict recurrent instability. *Circulation*, 99(7), 855–860.

Biasucci, L. M., Vitelli, A., Liuzzo, G., Altamura, S., Caligiuri, G., Monaco, C., Rebuzzi, A. G., Ciliberto, G., & Maseri, A. (1996). Elevated levels of interleukin-6 in unstable angina. *Circulation*, 94(5), 874–877.

Blankenberg, S., Rupprecht, H. J., Bickel, C., Peetz, D., Hafner, G., Tiret, L., & Meyer, J. (2001). Circulating cell adhesion molecules and death in patients with coronary artery disease. *Circulation*, 104(12), 1336–1342.

Blann, A. D., & McCollum, C. N. (1994). Circulating endothelial cell/leukocyte adhesion molecules in atherosclerosis. *Thromb Haemost*, 72(1), 151–154.

Boring, L., Gosling, J., Cleary, M., & Charo, I. F. (1998). Decreased lesion formation in CCR2-/- mice reveals a role for chemokines in the initiation of atherosclerosis. *Nature, 394*(6696), 894–897.

Boushey, C. J., Beresford, S. A., Omenn, G. S., & Motulsky, A. G. (1995). A quantitative assessment of plasma homocysteine as a risk factor for vascular disease. Probable benefits of increasing folic acid intakes. *JAMA, 274*(13), 1049–1057.

Bozkurt, B., Kribbs, S., Clubb, F. J. Jr., Michael, L. H., Didenko, V. V., Hornsby, P. J., Seta, Y., Oral, H., Spinale, F. G., & Mann, D. L. (1998). Pathophysiologically relevant concentrations of tumor necrosis factor promote progressive left ventricular dysfunction and remodeling in rats. *Circulation, 97*, 1382–1391.

Bradford-Hill, A. (1965). The environment and disease: Association or causation? President's address. *Proceedings of the Royal Society of Medicine, 58*, 295.

Brinckerhoff, C. E., Mitchell, T. I., Karmilowicz, M. J., Kluve-Beckerman, B., & Benson, M. D. (1989). Autocrine induction of collagenase by serum amyloid A-like and beta 2-microglobulin-like proteins. *Science, 243*(4891), 655–657.

Cherian, P., Hankey, G. J., Eikelboom, J. W., Thom, J., Baker, R. I., McQuillan, A., Staton, J., & Yi, Q. (2003). Endothelial and platelet activation in acute ischemic stroke and its etiological subtypes. *Stroke, 34*(9), 2132–2137.

Christen, W. G., Ajani, U. A., Glynn, R. J., & Hennekens, C. H. (2000). Blood levels of homocysteine and increased risks of cardiovascular disease: causal or casual? *Archives of Internal Medicine, 160*(4), 422–434.

Coetzee, G. A., Strachan, A. F., van der Westhuyzen, D. R., Hoppe, H. C., Jeenah, M. S., & de Beer, F. C. (1986). Serum amyloid A-containing human high density lipoprotein 3. Density, size, and apolipoprotein composition. *Journal of Biology and Chemistry, 261*(21), 9644–9651.

Cushman, M., Lemaitre, R. N., Kuller, L. H., Psaty, B. M., Macy, E. M., Sharrett, A. R., & Tracy, R. P. (1999). Fibrinolytic activation markers predict myocardial infarction in the elderly. The Cardiovascular Health Study. *Arterioscler Thromb Vasc Biol, 19*(3), 493–498.

Cybulsky, M. I., Iiyama, K., Li, H., Zhu, S., Chen, M., Iiyama, M., Davis, V., Gutierrez-Ramos, J. C., Connelly, P. W., & Milstone, D. S. (2001). A major role for VCAM-1, but not ICAM-1, in early atherosclerosis. *Journal of Clinical Investigation, 107*(10), 1255–1262.

Danesh, J., Collins, R., Appleby, P., & Peto, R. (1998). Association of fibrinogen, C-reactive protein, albumin, or leukocyte count with coronary heart disease: meta-analyses of prospective studies. *JAMA, 279*(18), 1477–1482.

Davies, M. J., Gordon, J. L., Gearing, A. J., Pigott, R., Woolf, N., Katz, D., & Kyriakopoulos, A. (1993). The expression of the adhesion molecules ICAM-1, VCAM-1, PECAM, and E-selectin in human atherosclerosis. *Journal of Pathology, 171*(3), 223–229.

de Lemos, J. A., Morrow, D. A., Bentley, J. H., Omland, T., Sabatine, M. S., McCabe, C. H., Hall, C., Cannon, C. P., & Braunwald, E. (2001). The prognostic value of B-type natriuretic peptide in patients with acute coronary syndromes. *New England Journal of Medicine, 345*(14), 1014–1021.

de Winter, R. J., Bholasingh, R., Lijmer, J. G., Koster, R. W., Gorgels, J. P., Schouten, Y., Hoek, F. J., & Sanders, G. T. (1999). Independent prognostic value of C-reactive protein and troponin I in patients with unstable angina or non-Q-wave myocardial infarction. *Cardiovascular Research, 42*(1), 240–245.

Deswal, A., Petersen, N. J., Feldman, A. M., Young, J. B., White, B. G., & Mann, D. L. (2001). Cytokines and cytokine receptors in advanced heart failure: an analysis of the cytokine database from the Vesnarinone Trial (VEST). *Circulation, 103*, 2055–2059.

Di Minno, G., & Mancini, M. (1990). Measuring plasma fibrinogen to predict stroke and myocardial infarction. *Arteriosclerosis, 10*(1), 1–7.

Dries, D. L., & Stevenson, L. W. (2000). Brain natriuretic peptide as bridge to therapy for heart failure. *Lancet, 355*(9210), 1112–1113.

Eber, B., & Schumacher, M. (1993). Fibrinogen: its role in the hemostatic regulation in atherosclerosis. *Semin Thromb Hemost, 19*(2), 104–107.

Eikelboom, J. W., Lonn, E., Genest, J., Jr., Hankey, G., & Yusuf, S. (1999). Homocyst(e)ine and cardiovascular disease: a critical review of the epidemiologic evidence. *Annals of Internal Medicine, 131*(5), 363–375.

El-Khairy, L., Ueland, P. M., Nygard, O., Refsum, H., & Vollset, S. E. (1999). Lifestyle and cardiovascular disease risk factors as determinants of total cysteine in plasma: the Hordaland Homocysteine Study. *American Journal of Clinical Nutrition, 70*(6), 1016–1024.

Ernst, E., & Resch, K. L. (1993). Fibrinogen as a cardiovascular risk factor: a meta-analysis and review of the literature. *Annals of Internal Medicine, 118*(12), 956–963.

Feingold, K. R., & Grunfeld, C. (1992). Role of cytokines in inducing hyperlipidemia. *Diabetes, 41*(Suppl. 2), 97–101.

Folsom, A. R. (2001). Hemostatic risk factors for atherothrombotic disease: an epidemiologic view. *Thromb Haemost, 86*(1), 366–373.

Folsom, A. R., Aleksic, N., Ahn, C., Boerwinkle, E., & Wu, K. K. (2001). Beta-fibrinogen gene -455G/A polymorphism and coronary heart disease incidence: the Atherosclerosis Risk in Communities (ARIC) Study. *Annals of Epidemiology, 11*(3), 166–170.

Folsom, A. R., Aleksic, N., Catellier, D., Juneja, H. S., & Wu, K. K. (2002). C-reactive protein and incident coronary heart disease in the Atherosclerosis Risk In Communities (ARIC) study. *American Heart Journal, 144*(2), 233–238.

Folsom, A. R., Pankow, J. S., Tracy, R. P., Arnett, D. K., Peacock, J. M., Hong, Y., Djousse, L., & Eckfeldt, J. H. (2001). Association of C-reactive protein with prevalent atherosclerotic disease. *American Journal of Cardiology, 88*(2), 112–117.

Folsom, A. R., Rosamond, W. D., Shahar, E., Cooper, L. S., Aleksic, N., Nieto, F. J., Rasmussen, M. L., & Wu, K. K. (1999). Prospective study of markers of hemostatic function with risk of ischemic stroke. The Atherosclerosis Risk in Communities (ARIC) Study Investigators. *Circulation, 100*(7), 736–742.

Ford, E. S., Smith, S. J., Stroup, D. F., Steinberg, K. K., Mueller, P. W., & Thacker, S. B. (2002). Homocyst(e)ine and cardiovascular disease: a systematic review of the evidence with special emphasis on case-control studies and nested case-control studies. *International Journal of Epidemiology, 31*(1), 59–70.

Fukumoto, Y., Shimokawa, H., Ito, A., Kadokami, T., Yonemitsu, Y., Aikawa, M., Owada, M. K., Egashira, K., Sueishi, K., Nagai, R., Yazaki, Y., & Takeshita, A. (1997). Inflammatory cytokines cause coronary arteriosclerosis-like changes and alterations in the smooth-muscle phenotypes in pigs. *Journal of Cardiovascular Pharmacology, 29*(2), 222–231.

Gabay, C., & Kushner, I. (1999). Acute-phase proteins and other systemic responses to inflammation. *New England Journal of Medicine, 340*(6), 448–454.

Genest, J., Jr., & Cohn, J. S. (1995). Clustering of cardiovascular risk factors: targeting high-risk individuals. *American Journal of Cardiology, 76*(2), 8A–20A.

Gu, L., Okada, Y., Clinton, S. K., Gerard, C., Sukhova, G. K., Libby, P., & Rollins, B. J. (1998). Absence of monocyte chemoattractant protein-1 reduces atherosclerosis in low density lipoprotein receptor-deficient mice. *Molecular Cell, 2*(2), 275–281.

Hale, K. K., Smith, C. G., Baker, S. L., Vanderslice, R. W., Squires, C. H., Gleason, T. M., Tucker, K. K., Kohno, T., & Russell, D. A. (1995). Multifunctional regulation of the biological effects of TNF-alpha by the soluble type I and type II TNF receptors. *Cytokine, 7*(1), 26–38.

Hardardottir, I., Moser, A. H., Memon, R., Grunfeld, C., & Feingold, K. R. (1994). Effects of TNF, IL-1, and the combination of both cytokines on cholesterol metabolism in Syrian hamsters. *Lymphokine Cytokine Research, 13*(3), 161–166.

Harris, T. B., Ferrucci, L., Tracy, R. P., Corti, M. C., Wacholder, S., Ettinger, W. H., Jr., Heimovitz, H., Cohen, H. J., & Wallace, R. (1999). Associations of elevated interleukin-6 and C-reactive protein levels with mortality in the elderly. *American Journal of Medicine, 106*(5), 506–512.

Haught, W. H., Mansour, M., Rothlein, R., Kishimoto, T. K., Mainolfi, E. A., Hendricks, J. B., Hendricks, C., & Mehta, J. L. (1996). Alterations in circulating intercellular adhesion molecule-1 and L-selectin: further evidence for chronic inflammation in ischemic heart disease. *American Heart Journal, 132*(1 Pt 1), 1–8.

Haverkate, F., Thompson, S. G., Pyke, S. D., Gallimore, J. R., & Pepys, M. B. (1997). Production of C-reactive protein and risk of coronary events in stable and unstable angina. European Concerted Action on Thrombosis and Disabilities Angina Pectoris Study Group. *Lancet, 349*(9050), 462–466.

Herity, N. A. (2000). Interleukin 6: a message from the heart. *Heart, 84*(1), 9–10.

Heuertz, R. M., Piquette, C. A., & Webster, R. O. (1993). Rabbits with elevated serum C-reactive protein exhibit diminished neutrophil infiltration and vascular permeability in C5a-induced alveolitis. *American Journal of Pathology, 142*(1), 319–328.

Homeister, J. W., & Lucchesi, B. R. (1994). Complement activation and inhibition in myocardial ischemia and reperfusion injury. *Annual Review of Pharmacology and Toxicology, 34*, 17–40.

Hotamisligil, G. S., Arner, P., Caro, J. F., Atkinson, R. L., & Spiegelman, B. M. (1995). Increased adipose tissue expression of tumor necrosis factor-alpha in human obesity and insulin resistance. *Journal of Clinical Investigation, 95*(5), 2409–2415.

Hotamisligil, G. S., Murray, D. L., Choy, L. N., & Spiegelman, B. M. (1994). Tumor necrosis factor alpha inhibits signaling from the insulin receptor. *Proceedings of the National Academy of Sciences of the USA, 91*(11), 4854–4858.

Hotamisligil, G. S., Shargill, N. S., & Spiegelman, B. M. (1993). Adipose expression of tumor necrosis factor-alpha: direct role in obesity-linked insulin resistance. *Science, 259*(5091), 87–91. http://www.americanheart.org.

Retrieved, from the World Wide Web:[AQ1] http://www.homocysteine.net.
Retrieved, from the World Wide Web: Hunt, P. J., Richards, A. M., Nicholls, M. G., Yandle, T. G., Doughty, R. N., & Espiner, E. A. (1997). Immunoreactive amino-terminal pro-brain natriuretic peptide (NT-PROBNP): a new marker of cardiac impairment. *Clinical Endocrinology (Oxford)*, 47(3), 287–296.

Hwang, S. J., Ballantyne, C. M., Sharrett, A. R., Smith, L. C., Davis, C. E., Gotto, A. M., Jr., & Boerwinkle, E. (1997). Circulating adhesion molecules VCAM-1, ICAM-1, and E-selectin in carotid atherosclerosis and incident coronary heart disease cases: the Atherosclerosis Risk In Communities (ARIC) study. *Circulation*, 96(12), 4219–4225.

Jang, Y., Lincoff, A. M., Plow, E. F., & Topol, E. J. (1994). Cell adhesion molecules in coronary artery disease. *Journal of the American College of Cardiology*, 24(7), 1591–1601.

Jansson, J. H., Nilsson, T. K., & Johnson, O. (1991). von Willebrand factor in plasma: a novel risk factor for recurrent myocardial infarction and death. *British Heart Journal*, 66(5), 351–355.

Kannel, W. B. (1997). Cardiovascular risk factors in the elderly. *Coronary Artery Disease*, 8(8-9), 565–575.

Kannel, W. B., D'Agostino, R. B., & Belanger, A. J. (1987). Fibrinogen, cigarette smoking, and risk of cardiovascular disease: insights from the Framingham Study. *American Heart Journal*, 113(4), 1006–1010.

Kannel, W. B., McGee, D., & Gordon, T. (1976). A general cardiovascular risk profile: the Framingham Study. *American Journal of Cardiology*, 38(1), 46–51.

Kisilevsky, R., & Subrahmanyan, L. (1992). Serum amyloid A changes high density lipoprotein's cellular affinity. A clue to serum amyloid A's principal function. *Laboratory Investigation*, 66(6), 778–785.

Klein, B., & Brailly, H. (1995). Cytokine-binding proteins: stimulating antagonists. *Immunology Today*, 16, 216–220.

Koenig, W. (2001). Inflammation and coronary heart disease: an overview. *Cardiology Review*, 9(1), 31–35.

Koenig, W., Sund, M., Frohlich, M., Fischer, H. G., Lowel, H., Doring, A., Hutchinson, W. L., & Pepys, M. B. (1999). C-Reactive protein, a sensitive marker of inflammation, predicts future risk of coronary heart disease in initially healthy middle-aged men: results from the MONICA (Monitoring Trends and Determinants in Cardiovascular Disease) Augsburg Cohort Study, 1984 to 1992. *Circulation*, 99(2), 237–242.

Kubota, T., McTiernan, C.F., Frye, C.S., Slawson, S.E., Lemster, B.H., Koretsky, A.P., Demetris, A.J., & Feldman, A.M. (1997). Dilated cardiomyopathy in transgenic mice with cardiac specific overexpression of tumor necrosis factor-alpha. *Circulation Research*, 81, 627–635.

Kuller, L. H., Tracy, R. P., Shaten, J., & Meilahn, E. N. (1996). Relation of C-reactive protein and coronary heart disease in the MRFIT nested case-control study. Multiple Risk Factor Intervention Trial. *American Journal of Epidemiology*, 144(6), 537–547.

Lee, A. J., Lowe, G. D., Woodward, M., & Tunstall-Pedoe, H. (1993). Fibrinogen in relation to personal history of prevalent hypertension, diabetes, stroke, intermittent claudication, coronary heart disease, and family history: the Scottish Heart Health Study. *British Heart Journal*, 69(4), 338–342.

Lefkovits, J., Plow, E. F., & Topol, E. J. (1995). Platelet glycoprotein IIb/IIIa receptors in cardiovascular medicine. *New England Journal of Medicine*, 332(23), 1553–1559.

Lefkovits, J., & Topol, E. J. (1995). Platelet glycoprotein IIb/IIIa receptor inhibitors in ischemic heart disease. *Current Opinion in Cardiology*, 10(4), 420–426.

Levine, B., Kalman, J., Mayer, L., Fillit, H. M., & Packer, M. (1990). Elevated circulating levels of tumor necrosis factor in severe chronic heart failure. *New England Journal of Medicine*, 323(4), 236–241.

Li, H., Cybulsky, M. I., Gimbrone, M. A., Jr., & Libby, P. (1993). Inducible expression of vascular cell adhesion molecule-1 by vascular smooth muscle cells in vitro and within rabbit atheroma. *American Journal of Pathology*, 143(6), 1551–1559.

Libby, P. (2000). Changing concepts of atherogenesis. *Journal of Internal Medicine*, 247(3), 349–358.

Libby, P., Ridker, P. M., & Maseri, A. (2002). Inflammation and atherosclerosis. *Circulation*, 105(9), 1135–1143.

Liuzzo, G., Biasucci, L. M., Gallimore, J. R., Grillo, R. L., Rebuzzi, A. G., Pepys, M. B., & Maseri, A. (1994). The prognostic value of C-reactive protein and serum amyloid a protein in severe unstable angina. *New England Journal of Medicine*, 331(7), 417–424.

Loppnow, H., & Libby, P. (1989a). Adult human vascular endothelial cells express the IL6 gene differentially in response to LPS or IL1. *Cellular Immunology*, 122(2), 493–503.

Loppnow, H., & Libby, P. (1989b). Comparative analysis of cytokine induction in human vascular endothelial and smooth muscle cells. *Lymphokine Research*, 8(3), 293–299.

Lower, R. (1669). *Tractatus de Corde: De Motu & Colore Sagnuinus & Chyli in Eum Tranfitu* (1st ed.). London, UK: Jacobi Alleftry.

Lowering blood homocysteine with folic acid based supplements: meta-analysis of randomised trials. Homocysteine Lowering Trialists' Collaboration. (1998). *British Medical Journal*, 316(7135), 894–898.

Luscinskas, F. W., & Gimbrone, M. A., Jr. (1996). Endothelial-dependent mechanisms in chronic inflammatory leukocyte recruitment. *Annual Review of Medicine*, 47, 413–421.

Ma, J., Hennekens, C. H., Ridker, P. M., & Stampfer, M. J. (1999). A prospective study of fibrinogen and risk of myocardial infarction in the Physicians' Health Study. *Journal of the American College of Cardiology*, 33(5), 1347–1352.

MacGregor, A. S., Price, J. F., Hau, C. M., Lee, A. J., Carson, M. N., & Fowkes, F. G. (1999). Role of systolic blood pressure and plasma triglycerides in diabetic peripheral arterial disease. The Edinburgh Artery Study. *Diabetes Care*, 22(3), 453–458.

Mach, F., Sauty, A., Iarossi, A. S., Sukhova, G. K., Neote, K., Libby, P., & Luster, A. D. (1999). Differential expression of three T lymphocyte-activating CXC chemokines by human atheroma-associated cells. *Journal of Clinical Investigation*, 104(8), 1041–1050.

Magliano, D. J., Liew, D., Ashton, E. L., Sundararajan, V., & McNeil, J. J. (2003). Novel biomedical risk markers for cardiovascular disease. *Journal of Cardiovascular Risk*, 10(1), 41–55.

Malle, E., & De Beer, F. C. (1996). Human serum amyloid A (SAA) protein: a prominent acute-phase reactant for clinical practice. *European Journal of Clinical Investigation*, 26(6), 427–435.

Malle, E., Steinmetz, A., & Raynes, J. G. (1993). Serum amyloid A (SAA): an acute phase protein and apolipoprotein. *Atherosclerosis*, 102(2), 131–146.

Mann, D. L. (2002). Inflammatory mediators and the failing heart: past, present, and the foreseeable future. *Circulation Research*, 91(11), 988–998.

Mann, D. L., Swedberg, K., Packer, M., Fleming, T., Djian, J., Warren, M. S., & McMurray, J. J. (2002, September 25th). Effects of cytokine antagonism with etanercept on morbidity and mortality in patients with chronic heart failure: results of the RENAISSANCE, RECOVERY and RENEWAL trials. Paper presented at the Annual Meeting of the Heart Failure Society of America, Boca Raton, Fla.

Maresca, G., Di Blasio, A., Marchioli, R., & Di Minno, G. (1999). Measuring plasma fibrinogen to predict stroke and myocardial infarction: an update. *Arterioscler Thromb Vasc Biol*, 19(6), 1368–1377.

Maury, C. P., & Teppo, A. M. (1989). Circulating tumour necrosis factor-alpha (cachectin) in myocardial infarction. *Journal of Internal Medicine*, 225(5), 333–336.

McCully, K. S. (1969). Vascular pathology of homocysteinemia: implications for the pathogenesis of arteriosclerosis. *American Journal of Pathology*, 56(1), 111–128.

McDonagh, T. A., Cunningham, A. D., Morrison, C. E., McMurray, J. J., Ford, I., Morton, J. J., & Dargie, H. J. (2001). Left ventricular dysfunction, natriuretic peptides, and mortality in an urban population. *Heart*, 86(1), 21–26.

McDonagh, T. A., Robb, S. D., Murdoch, D. R., Morton, J. J., Ford, I., Morrison, C. E., Tunstall-Pedoe, H., McMurray, J. J., & Dargie, H. J. (1998). Biochemical detection of left-ventricular systolic dysfunction. *Lancet*, 351(9095), 9–13.

Meade, T. W., Cooper, J. A., Stirling, Y., Howarth, D. J., Ruddock, V., & Miller, G. J. (1994). Factor VIII, ABO blood group and the incidence of ischaemic heart disease. *British Journal of Haematology*, 88(3), 601–607.

Meade, T. W., Mellows, S., Brozovic, M., Miller, G. J., Chakrabarti, R. R., North, W. R., Haines, A. P., Stirling, Y., Imeson, J. D., & Thompson, S. G. (1986). Haemostatic function and ischaemic heart disease: principal results of the Northwick Park Heart Study. *Lancet*, 2(8506), 533–537.

Mendall, M. A., Patel, P., Asante, M., Ballam, L., Morris, J., Strachan, D. P., Camm, A. J., & Northfield, T. C. (1997). Relation of serum cytokine concentrations to cardiovascular risk factors and coronary heart disease. *Heart*, 78(3), 273–277.

Mestries, J. C., Kruithof, E. K., Gascon, M. P., Herodin, F., Agay, D., & Ythier, A. (1994). In vivo modulation of coagulation and fibrinolysis by recombinant glycosylated human interleukin-6 in baboons. *European Cytokine Network*, 5(3), 275–281.

Migita, K., Kawabe, Y., Tominaga, M., Origuchi, T., Aoyagi, T., & Eguchi, K. (1998). Serum amyloid A protein induces production of matrix metalloproteinases by human synovial fibroblasts. *Laboratory Investigation*, 78(5), 535–539.

Miller, M. A., Sagnella, G. A., Kerry, S. M., Strazzullo, P., Cook, D. G., & Cappuccio, F. P. (2003). Ethnic differences in circulating soluble adhesion molecules: the Wandsworth Heart and Stroke Study. *Clinical Science (London),* 104(6), 591–598.

Miyao, Y., Yasue, H., Ogawa, H., Misumi, I., Masuda, T., Sakamoto, T., & Morita, E. (1993). Elevated plasma interleukin-6 levels in patients with acute myocardial infarction. *American Heart Journal,* 126(6), 1299–1304.

Mohamed-Ali, V., Goodrick, S., Rawesh, A., Katz, D. R., Miles, J. M., Yudkin, J. S., Klein, S., & Coppack, S. W. (1997). Subcutaneous adipose tissue releases interleukin-6, but not tumor necrosis factor-alpha, in vivo. *Journal of Clinical Endocrinology and Metabolism,* 82(12), 4196–4200.

Morrow, D. A., Rifai, N., Antman, E. M., Weiner, D. L., McCabe, C. H., Cannon, C. P., & Braunwald, E. (1998). C-reactive protein is a potent predictor of mortality independently of and in combination with troponin T in acute coronary syndromes: a TIMI 11A substudy. Thrombolysis in Myocardial Infarction. *Journal of the American College of Cardiology,* 31(7), 1460–1465.

Muldoon, M. F., Herbert, T. B., Patterson, S. M., Kameneva, M., Raible, R., & Manuck, S. B. (1995). Effects of acute psychological stress on serum lipid levels, hemoconcentration, and blood viscosity. *Archives of Internal Medicine,* 155(6), 615–620.

Mulvihill, N. T., Foley, J. B., Murphy, R., Crean, P., & Walsh, M. (2000). Evidence of prolonged inflammation in unstable angina and non-Q wave myocardial infarction. *Journal of the American College of Cardiology,* 36(4), 1210–1216.

Murdock, P. J., Woodhams, B. J., Matthews, K. B., Pasi, K. J., & Goodall, A. H. (1997). von Willebrand factor activity detected in a monoclonal antibody-based ELISA: an alternative to the ristocetin cofactor platelet agglutination assay for diagnostic use. *Thromb Haemost,* 78(4), 1272–1277.

Nathan, C. F. (1987). Secretory products of macrophages. *Journal of Clinical Investigation,* 79, 319–326.

Packer, M., Chung, E., Batra, S., Lo, K. H., Kereiakes, D. J., & Willerson, J. T. (2002). Randomized placebo-controlled dose-ranging trial of infliximab, a monoclonal antibody to tumor necrosis factor-alpha, in moderate to severe heart failure. Paper presented at the Annual Meeting of the Heart Failure Society of America, Boca Raton, Fla.

Pannitteri, G., Marino, B., Campa, P. P., Martucci, R., Testa, U., & Peschle, C. (1997). Interleukins 6 and 8 as mediators of acute phase response in acute myocardial infarction. *American Journal of Cardiology,* 80(5), 622–625.

Pearson, T. A., Mensah, G. A., Alexander, R. W., Anderson, J. L., Cannon, R. O., 3rd, Criqui, M., Fadl, Y. Y., Fortmann, S. P., Hong, Y., Myers, G. L., Rifai, N., Smith, S. C., Jr., Taubert, K., Tracy, R. P., & Vinicor, F. (2003). Markers of inflammation and cardiovascular disease: application to clinical and public health practice: A statement for healthcare professionals from the Centers for Disease Control and Prevention and the American Heart Association. *Circulation,* 107(3), 499–511.

Pepys, M. B. (1995). The acute phase response and C-reactive protein. In *Oxford textbook of medicine (Vol. 2).* Oxford, UK: Oxford University Press.

Pober, J. S., Bevilacqua, M. P., Mendrick, D. L., Lapierre, L. A., Fiers, W., & Gimbrone, M. A., Jr. (1986). Two distinct monokines, interleukin 1 and tumor necrosis factor, each independently induce biosynthesis and transient expression of the same antigen on the surface of cultured human vascular endothelial cells. *Journal of Immunology,* 136(5), 1680–1687.

Richards, A. M., Nicholls, M. G., Yandle, T. G., Frampton, C., Espiner, E. A., Turner, J. G., Buttimore, R. C., Lainchbury, J. G., Elliott, J. M., Ikram, H., Crozier, I. G., & Smyth, D. W. (1998). Plasma N-terminal pro-brain natriuretic peptide and adrenomedullin: new neurohormonal predictors of left ventricular function and prognosis after myocardial infarction. *Circulation,* 97(19), 1921–1929.

Richards, A. M., Nicholls, M. G., Yandle, T. G., Ikram, H., Espiner, E. A., Turner, J. G., Buttimore, R. C., Lainchbury, J. G., Elliott, J. M., Frampton, C., Crozier, I. G., & Smyth, D. W. (1999). Neuroendocrine prediction of left ventricular function and heart failure after acute myocardial infarction. The Christchurch Cardioendocrine Research Group. *Heart,* 81(2), 114–120.

Ridker, P. M. (1998). C-reactive protein and risks of future myocardial infarction and thrombotic stroke. *European Heart Journal,* 19(1), 1–3.

Ridker, P. M., Buring, J. E., Shih, J., Matias, M., & Hennekens, C. H. (1998). Prospective study of C-reactive protein and the risk of future cardiovascular events among apparently healthy women. *Circulation,* 98(8), 731–733.

Ridker, P. M., Cushman, M., Stampfer, M. J., Tracy, R. P., & Hennekens, C. H. (1997). Inflammation, aspirin, and the risk of cardiovascular disease in apparently healthy men. *New England Journal of Medicine,* 336(14), 973–979.

Ridker, P. M., Cushman, M., Stampfer, M. J., Tracy, R. P., & Hennekens, C. H. (1998). Plasma concentration of C-reactive protein and risk of developing peripheral vascular disease. *Circulation,* 97(5), 425–428.

Ridker, P. M., Hennekens, C. H., Buring, J. E., & Rifai, N. (2000). C-reactive protein and other markers of inflammation in the prediction of cardiovascular disease in women. *New England Journal of Medicine,* 342(12), 836–843.

Ridker, P. M., Hennekens, C. H., Roitman-Johnson, B., Stampfer, M. J., & Allen, J. (1998). Plasma concentration of soluble intercellular adhesion molecule 1 and risks of future myocardial infarction in apparently healthy men. *Lancet,* 351(9096), 88–92.

Ridker, P. M., Rifai, N., Clearfield, M., Downs, J. R., Weis, S. E., Miles, J. S., & Gotto, A. M., Jr. (2001). Measurement of C-reactive protein for the targeting of statin therapy in the primary prevention of acute coronary events. *New England Journal of Medicine,* 344(26), 1959–1965.

Ridker, P. M., Rifai, N., Stampfer, M. J., & Hennekens, C. H. (2000). Plasma concentration of interleukin-6 and the risk of future myocardial infarction among apparently healthy men. *Circulation,* 101(15), 1767–1772.

Ridker, P. M., Rifai, N., Pfeffer, M., Sacks, F., Lepage, S., & Braunwald, E. (2000). Elevation of tumor necrosis factor-a and increased risk of recurrent coronary events after myocardial infarction. *Circulation,* 101, 2149–2153.

Rifai, N., & Ridker, P. M. (2001). Proposed cardiovascular risk assessment algorithm using high-sensitivity C-reactive protein and lipid screening. *Clinical Chemistry,* 47(1), 28–30.

Robey, F. A., Ohura, K., Futaki, S., Fujii, N., Yajima, H., Goldman, N., Jones, K. D., & Wahl, S. (1987). Proteolysis of human C-reactive protein produces peptides with potent immunomodulating activity. *Journal of Biology and Chemistry,* 262(15), 7053–7057.

Roivainen, M., Viik-Kajander, M., Palosuo, T., Toivanen, P., Leinonen, M., Saikku, P., Tenkanen, L., Manninen, V., Hovi, T., & Manttari, M. (2000). Infections, inflammation, and the risk of coronary heart disease. *Circulation,* 101(3), 252–257.

Ross, R. (1993). The pathogenesis of atherosclerosis: a perspective for the 1990s. *Nature,* 362(6423), 801–809.

Ruggeri, Z. M. (1992). von Willebrand factor as a target for antithrombotic intervention. *Circulation,* 86(6 Suppl), III26–29.

Ruggeri, Z. M. (1997). von Willebrand factor. *Journal of Clinical Investigation,* 99(4), 559–564.

Rumley, A., Lowe, G. D., Sweetnam, P. M., Yarnell, J. W., & Ford, R. P. (1999). Factor VIII, von Willebrand factor and the risk of major ischaemic heart disease in the Caerphilly Heart Study. *British Journal of Haematology,* 105(1), 110–116.

Rus, H. G., Vlaicu, R., & Niculescu, F. (1996). Interleukin-6 and interleukin-8 protein and gene expression in human arterial atherosclerotic wall. *Atherosclerosis,* 127(2), 263–271.

Saadeddin, S. M., Habbab, M. A., & Ferns, G. A. (2002). Markers of inflammation and coronary artery disease. *Medical Science Monitoring,* 8(1), RA5–12.

Sacks, F. M., Pfeffer, M. A., Moye, L. A., Rouleau, J. L., Rutherford, J. D., Cole, T. G., Brown, L., Warnica, J. W., Arnold, J. M., Wun, C. C., Davis, B. R., & Braunwald, E. (1996). The effect of pravastatin on coronary events after myocardial infarction in patients with average cholesterol levels. Cholesterol and Recurrent Events Trial investigators. *New England Journal of Medicine,* 335(14), 1001–1009.

Sato, S., Nakamura, M., Iida, M., Naito, Y., Kitamura, A., Okamura, T., Nakagawa, Y., Imano, H., Kiyama, M., Iso, H., Shimamoto, T., & Komachi, Y. (2000). Plasma fibrinogen and coronary heart disease in urban Japanese. *American Journal of Epidemiology,* 152(5), 420–423.

Seta, Y., Shan, K., Bozkurt, B., Oral, H., & Mann, D.L. (1996). Basic mechanisms in heart failure: the cytokine hypothesis. *Journal of Cardiac Failure,* 2, 243–249.

Shainkin-Kestenbaum, R., Zimlichman, S., Lis, M., Preciado-Patt, L., Fridkin, M., & Berenheim, J. (1996). Modulation of prostaglandin I2 production from bovine aortic endothelial cells by serum amyloid A and its N-terminal tetradecapeptide. *Biomedical Peptides, Proteins and Nucleic Acids,* 2(4), 101–106.

Shipchandler, M. T., & Moore, E. G. (1995). Rapid, fully automated measurement of plasma homocyst(e)ine with the Abbott IMx analyzer. *Clinical Chemistry,* 41(7), 991–994.

Smith, E. B. (1986). Fibrinogen, fibrin and fibrin degradation products in relation to atherosclerosis. *Clinical Haematology,* 15(2), 355–370.

Smith, E. B., Keen, G. A., Grant, A., & Stirk, C. (1990). Fate of fibrinogen in human arterial intima. *Arteriosclerosis,* 10(2), 263–275.

Smith, F. B., Lee, A. J., Fowkes, F. G., Price, J. F., Rumley, A., & Lowe, G. D. (1997). Hemostatic factors as predictors of ischemic heart disease and stroke in the Edinburgh Artery Study. *Arterioscler Thromb Vasc Biol,* 17(11), 3321–3325.

Springer, T. A. (1995). Traffic signals on endothelium for lymphocyte recirculation and leukocyte emigration. *Annual Review of Physiology,* 57, 827–872.

Steinmetz, A., Hocke, G., Saile, R., Puchois, P., & Fruchart, J. C. (1989). Influence of serum amyloid A on cholesterol esterification in human plasma. *Biochim Biophys Acta,* 1006(2), 173–178.

Sweetnam, P. M., Yarnell, J. W., Lowe, G. D., Baker, I. A., O'Brien, J. R., Rumley, A., Etherington, M. D., Whitehead, P. J., & Elwood, P. C. (1998). The relative power of heat-precipitation nephelometric and clottable (Clauss) fibrinogen in the prediction of ischaemic heart disease: the Caerphilly and Speedwell studies. *British Journal of Haematology,* 100(3), 582–588.

Syversen, P. V., Saeter, U., Cunha-Ribeiro, L., Orvim, U., Sletten, K., Husby, G., & Sakariassen, K. S. (1994). The effect of serum amyloid protein A fragment-SAA25-76 on blood platelet aggregation. *Thrombosis Research,* 76(3), 299–305.

Tartaglia, L. A., & Goeddel, D. V. (1992). Two TNF receptors. *Immunology Today,* 13(5), 151–153.

Tartaglia, L. A., Weber, R. F., Figari, I. S., Reynolds, C., Palladino, M. A., Jr., & Goeddel, D. V. (1991). The two different receptors for tumor necrosis factor mediate distinct cellular responses. *Proceedings of the National Academy of Sciences of the USA,* 88(20), 9292–9296.

Tateyama, H., Hino, J., Kangawa, K., Ogihara, T., & Matsuo, H. (1990). Characterization of immunoreactive brain natriuretic peptide in human cardiac atrium. *Biochem Biophys Res Commun,* 166(3), 1080–1087.

Thaik, C. M., Calderone, A., Takahashi, N., & Colucci, W.S. (1995). Interleukin-1 modulates the growth and phenotype of neonatal rat cardiac myocytes. *Journal of Clinical Investigation,* 96, 1093–1099.

Thogersen, A. M., Jansson, J. H., Boman, K., Nilsson, T. K., Weinehall, L., Huhtasaari, F., & Hallmans, G. (1998). High plasminogen activator inhibitor and tissue plasminogen activator levels in plasma precede a first acute myocardial infarction in both men and women: evidence for the fibrinolytic system as an independent primary risk factor. *Circulation,* 98(21), 2241–2247.

Thompson, W. D., & Smith, E. B. (1989). Atherosclerosis and the coagulation system. *Journal of Pathology,* 159(2), 97–106.

Tilg, H., Vannier, E., Vachino, G., Dinarello, C. A., & Mier, J. W. (1993). Antiinflammatory properties of hepatic acute phase proteins: preferential induction of interleukin 1 (IL-1) receptor antagonist over IL-1 beta synthesis by human peripheral blood mononuclear cells. *Journal of Experimental Medicine,* 178(5), 1629–1636.

Torre-Amione, G., Kapadia, S., Benedict, C. R., Oral, H., Young, J. B., & Mann, D. L. (1996). Proinflammatory cytokine levels in patients with depressed left ventricular ejection fraction: a report from the Studies of Left Ventricular Dysfunction (SOLVD). *Journal of the American College of Cardiology,* 27, 1201–1206.

Torre-Amione, G., Kapadia, S., Lee, J., Durand, J. B., Bies, R. D., Young, J. B., & Mann, D. L. (1996). Tumor necrosis factor-alpha and tumor necrosis factor receptors in the failing human heart. *Circulation,* 93, 704–711.

Tracy, R. P. (1999). Inflammation markers and coronary heart disease. *Current Opinion in Lipidology,* 10(5), 435–441.

Tracy, R. P., Arnold, A. M., Ettinger, W., Fried, L., Meilahn, E., & Savage, P. (1999). The relationship of fibrinogen and factors VII and VIII to incident cardiovascular disease and death in the elderly: results from the cardiovascular health study. *Arterioscler Thromb Vasc Biol,* 19(7), 1776–1783.

Tracy, R. P., Bovill, E. G., Yanez, D., Psaty, B. M., Fried, L. P., Heiss, G., Lee, M., Polak, J. F., & Savage, P. J. (1995). Fibrinogen and factor VIII, but not factor VII, are associated with measures of subclinical cardiovascular disease in the elderly. Results from The Cardiovascular Health Study. *Arterioscler Thromb Vasc Biol,* 15(9), 1269–1279.

Tracy, R. P., Lemaitre, R. N., Psaty, B. M., Ives, D. G., Evans, R. W., Cushman, M., Meilahn, E. N., & Kuller, L. H. (1997). Relationship of C-reactive protein to risk of cardiovascular disease in the elderly. Results from the Cardiovascular Health Study and the Rural Health Promotion Project. *Arterioscler Thromb Vasc Biol,* 17(6), 1121–1127.

Troughton, R. W., Frampton, C. M., Yandle, T. G., Espiner, E. A., Nicholls, M. G., & Richards, A. M. (2000). Treatment of heart failure guided by plasma aminoterminal brain natriuretic peptide (N-BNP) concentrations. *Lancet,* 355(9210), 1126–1130.

Tsai, J. C., Perrella, M. A., Yoshizumi, M., Hsieh, C. M., Haber, E., Schlegel, R., & Lee, M. E. (1994). Promotion of vascular smooth muscle cell growth by homocysteine: a link to atherosclerosis. *Proceedings of the National Academy of Sciences of the USA,* 91(14), 6369–6373.

Urieli-Shoval, S., Cohen, P., Eisenberg, S., & Matzner, Y. (1998). Widespread expression of serum amyloid A in histologically normal human tissues. Predominant localization to the epithelium. *Journal of Histochemistry and Cytochemistry,* 46(12), 1377–1384.

van der Poll, T., van Deventer, S. J., Pasterkamp, G., van Mourik, J. A., Buller, H. R., & ten Cate, J. W. (1992). Tumor necrosis factor induces von Willebrand factor release in healthy humans. *Thromb Haemost,* 67(6), 623–626.

Van Snick, J. (1990). Interleukin-6: an overview. *Annual Review of Immunology,* 8, 253–278.

Volpato, S., Guralnik, J. M., Ferrucci, L., Balfour, J., Chaves, P., Fried, L. P., & Harris, T. B. (2001). Cardiovascular disease, interleukin-6, and risk of mortality in older women: the women's health and aging study. *Circulation,* 103(7), 947–953.

Wallen, T., Landahl, S., Hedner, T., Nakao, K., & Saito, Y. (1997). Brain natriuretic peptide predicts mortality in the elderly. *Heart,* 77(3), 264–267.

Yamada, T., Kakihara, T., Kamishima, T., Fukuda, T., & Kawai, T. (1996). Both acute phase and constitutive serum amyloid A are present in atherosclerotic lesions. *Pathology International,* 46(10), 797–800.

Yu, H., & Rifai, N. (2000). High-sensitivity C-reactive protein and atherosclerosis: from theory to therapy. *Clinical Biochemistry,* 33(8), 601–610.

Yudkin, J. S., Kumari, M., Humphries, S. E., & Mohamed-Ali, V. (2000). Inflammation, obesity, stress and coronary heart disease: is interleukin-6 the link? *Atherosclerosis,* 148(2), 209–214.

Zighetti, M. L., Chantarangkul, V., Tripodi, A., Mannucci, P. M., & Cattaneo, M. (2002). Determination of total homocysteine in plasma: comparison of the Abbott IMx immunoassay with high performance liquid chromatography. *Haematologica,* 87(1), 89–94.

Zimlichman, S., Danon, A., Nathan, I., Mozes, G., & Shainkin-Kestenbaum, R. (1990). Serum amyloid A, an acute phase protein, inhibits platelet activation. *Journal of Laboratory Clinical Medicine,* 116(2), 180–186.

7

Atherosclerosis

BRADLEY AOUIZERAT

Atherosclerosis is a thickening or hardening of arteries. It is a progressive disease that evolves from deposits of lipids, cellular debris, calcium, and fibrin (a clotting agent) that accumulate in the lining of large arteries, all of which intiates and is compounded by a progressive inflammatory component. The later stages of these lesions are termed plaques. While atherosclerosis is primarily a disease of the large arteries, medium-size vessels can also be affected, with significant inter-individual variation in the sites and rate of plaque formation. Plaques can enlarge to partially or completely impede blood flow through an artery. Some plaques may hemorrhage within the plaque or rupture, initiating thrombus formation (blood clot) at the site with possible embolic consequences. Occlusion of arterial blood flow can lead to angina, myocardial infarction, or stroke.

Deposition of lipids, platelets, cellular debris, and calcium stimulate cells in the locale of the damaged artery wall to produce still other substances that contribute further to the atherosclerotic process. This results in recruitment of immune cells into the lesion as well as proliferation of arterial smooth muscle cells in an attempt to "heal" the lesion. As a result, the innermost layer of the artery, the intima, thickens, enlarges, and eventually encroaches on the vessel lumen, progressively restricting the flow of blood (and thus oxygen) to the vascular bed. Critical reductions in the supply of oxygen to the heart can result in angina or myocardial infarction or ischemic stroke in the brain, often exacerbated by arterial thrombus formation.

Atherosclerosis is a slow progressive disease that may start in childhood. In some persons, this condition may progress rapidly to cause symptoms in their third decade, whereas in others it does not become clinically significant until the fifth or sixth decades. In industrialized nations, it accounts for more than 50% of all cause adult mortality. Epidemiological studies have identified many important genetic and environmental risk factors associated with atherosclerosis (Table 7-1). However, the underlying complexity of the disease has made precise delineation of the cellular and molecular mechanisms involved difficult. Over the past decade, new investigative tools have contributed to a clearer picture of the molecular mechanisms underlying the development of atherosclerotic plaque. It is clear that atherosclerosis is not simply an inevitable consequence of ageing.

AMERICAN HEART ASSOCIATION LESION CLASSIFICATION SYSTEM

More than a decade ago, the American Heart Association (AHA) endeavored to provide an organized system for the categorization of lesions based on histological and morphological data (Stary et al., 1992). This system has helped standardize research in atherosclerosis though modifications have recently been proposed (Stary, 2000).

Coronary artery lesions can be grouped into seven major types (I-VII) (Stary, 1990, 1992, 1994; Stary et al., 1992; Stary et al., 1994). Consistent morphologic data would seem to indicate that each lesion type is relatively stable and will not progress to the next lesion type without additional factors or pressures. While the advanced lesions (type IV-VII) can manifest clinically, the early lesions (type I-III) are clinically silent and can be organized temporally. Types I and II are generally found in children, whereas type III tends to occur later and bridges early and advanced lesions. Perhaps the most important observation is that the clinically silent lesion types (I through III) have been shown capable of regression in animal models. Advanced lesions are generally disorganized and lead to thickening and eventual compromise of the vessel wall. Lipid-laden macrophages (termed "foam cells") are the predominant cellular components of type I lesions. In type II and III lesions, intimal smooth muscle cells dominate, with minimal involvement of lymphocytes, plasma cells, and mast cells in the pathological processes. This group of inflammatory cells becomes quite active in advanced (type IV and V) lesions. Figures 7-1 and 7-2 summarize the essential characteristics and temporal occurrence of atherosclerotic lesions.

Type I Lesions

Type I lesions, often termed the "initial lesion," are the earliest detectable lesion type. The lesion can only be observed microscopically and histochemically (by staining for lipid deposits) in the intima. Type I lesions are most often observed in infants and children (Stary, 1987), although they are readily identifiable in adults with little atherosclerosis or in areas of the vasculature not prone to arteriosclerosis. These lesions occur in regions of

Table 7–1 ■ CARDIOVASCULAR RISK FACTORS

Cardiovascular Risk Factors

Non-modifiable Risk Factors

Age   Male Gender

Modifiable Risk Factors

Alcohol intake	Hypertension	Overweight and obesity
Diabetes	Lack of exercise	Positive family history
Hypercholesterolemia	Left ventricular hypertrophy	Smoking

Emerging Risk Factors

C-reactive protein	Hypertriglyceridemia	Renin
Fibrinogen	Hyper-Lp(a)	Uricemia
Hyperhomocysteinuria	Microalbuminuria	

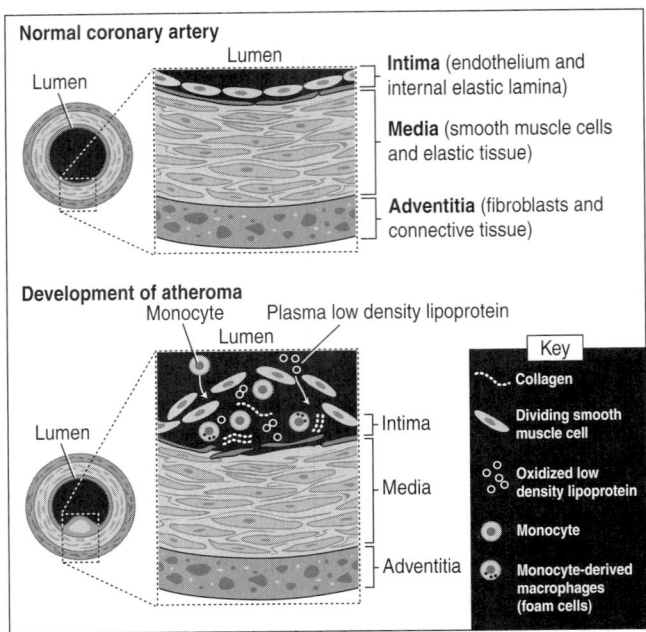

■ **Figure 7–2.** Schematic representation of normal coronary artery wall (*top*) and development of atheroma (*bottom*). (Modified from Grech, E.D. [2003]. ABC of interventional cardiology: percutaneous coronary intervention. II: the procedure. *BMJ,* 326[7399], 1137–1140.)

the intima that display adaptive intimal thickening caused by the hemodynamic force of blood flow. These regions eventually evolve into type II and type III lesions. Although more common to early adulthood, the occurrence of type III lesions has been reported as early as the first year of life (Stary, 1987, 1989). The accumulation of intimal foam cells is a consequence and a marker of pathological accumulation of atherogenic lipoproteins.

Type II Lesions

Type II lesions, also known as fatty streaks that are visible on gross inspection, are yellow spots or streaks on arterial intima. Visualization of fatty streaks can be enhanced by Sudan red staining (Guzman et al., 1968). Microscopic evaluation of the intima may provide further information, even when fatty streaks are not grossly apparent. The transmigration of macrophages into the subendothelial space and their subsequent transformation into foam cells produces an adaptive intimal thickening, which may obscure the fatty streak, potentially leading to an underestimate of the extent of these lesions. Recruitment of macrophages to the

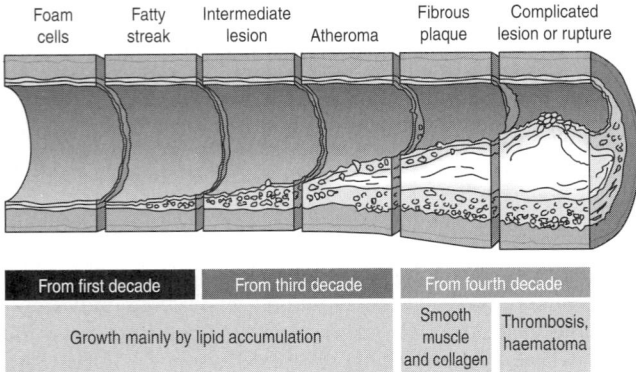

■ **Figure 7–1.** Progression of atheromatous plaque from initial lesion to complex and ruptured plaque. (Modified from Grech, E.D. [2003]. ABC of interventional cardiology: percutaneous coronary intervention. II: the procedure. *BMJ,* 326[7399], 1137–1140.)

intima marks one of the defining events in the initiation of the atherosclerotic lesion (see Chapter 6). Specific adhesion molecules expressed on the surface of vascular endothelial cells mediate leucocyte adhesion: the selectins and members of the immunoglobulin superfamily such as vascular cell adhesion molecule-1. Once adherent, the macrophages enter the artery wall in part because of the chemoattractant properties of another chemokine, macrophage chemoattractant protein-1. Modified lipoproteins contain oxidized phospholipids that induce the expression of adhesion molecules and cytokines implicated in early atherogenesis (Libby, 2000).

Progression of atheroma involves accumulation of smooth muscle cells that elaborate extracellular matrix macromolecules. Microscopic examination of type II lesions reveals that the foam cells are more organized, stratifying into layers, and that smooth muscle cells also begin to show signs of intracellular lipid accumulation. The properties of these lesions results in continued recruitment of macrophage and evidence suggests that T-lymphocytes and mast cells (components of the immune system) begin to invade the lesion (Katsuda et al., 1992; Munro et al., 1987; Stary, 1990). At this stage, the preponderance of the lipid in type II lesions resides in cells, with the majority found in foam cells. A limited amount of extracellular lipid (droplets) can also be detected.

While the ability to reproduce this lesion type in experimental models has yielded much information, the mechanisms of its progression to frank atherosclerosis remains unclear. However, some distinctions can be made. Consistent co-localization of type II lesions to specific portions of the arterial tree is characteristic (Cornhill et al., 1990). Additionally, subgroups of type II lesions can be described dependent on their location and the lipoprotein profile of the individual. Type IIa lesions represent the subset of lesions that may potentially progress to type III lesions over time or with increases in atherogenic (triglyceride- and cholesterol-enriched) lipoproteins. This smaller subgroup of type II lesions occurs in predictable locations in the arterial tree (proximal to bifurcations), where adaptive intimal thickenings occur, and are also termed progression-prone or advanced lesion-prone. Type IIb (progression-resistant or advanced lesion-resistant) lesions consist of the larger subset of type II lesions that are less likely to progress and are located in regions with relatively normal intima with little subendothelial smooth muscle cell invasion or proliferation. Type IIb lesions *do* have the potential to progress, particularly in persons with high plasma levels of atherogenic lipoproteins. Type IIb lesions are further distinguished from IIa by the presence of smooth muscle cells that produce intercellular matrix in the region of adaptive thickening. In type IIb lesions, macrophages without lipid are found mostly near the endothelial surface; foam cells are found deeper within the intima; and the extracellular lipid accumulates even deeper within the adaptive thickening.

The fate of a type II lesion, to become progression-prone or progression-resistant, is dependent not only on the relative atherogenicity of one's plasma lipoprotein profile but also on the direct mechanical forces that act on the vessel wall. The flow of blood through the vasculature causes nonuniform distributions of mechanical force, particularly immediately distal to vessel bifurcations. Lesion-prone regions experience greater shear stress, which increases the opportunity for blood-borne components (e.g. lipids) and the vessel wall to interact, facilitating greater transendothelial diffusion (Glagov et al., 1988). Clearly, individuals with greater plasma concentrations of atherogenic lipoproteins will provide the opportunity for accelerated influx and early accumulation of lipid in the lesion-prone areas. In individuals with very high plasma levels of atherogenic lipoproteins, such as those with familial hypercholesterolemia, type II lesions rapidly evolve into advanced lesions, even in arterial locations outside the progression-prone zones. It is noteworthy that by middle age, the development of advanced lesions outside the progression-prone areas occurs even in the absence of high plasma cholesterol (i.e., even in individuals free of premature risk factors). Several *in vivo* and *in vitro* methods have been used to map and quantify visible type II lesions. These include planimetry (Bernard et al., 1997; Okura et al., 1997), point-counting (Hansen, 1978; Rissanen, 1975), polar mapping (Goris et al., 1987; Parson et al., 1982), and computer-assisted angiographic methods (Cornhill et al., 1990). These methods are based on Sudan red dye-mediated visualization of lipid deposits within longitudinally bisected arteries.

Prevalence and Location of Type II Lesions

Ninety-nine percent of children (aged 2 to 15 years) have type II lesions in the aorta. Type II lesions generally increase in extent throughout the length of the aorta around puberty (Stary, 1989; Weingand et al., 1986). While fatty streaks develop in larger arteries in infancy, type II lesions emerge in the coronary arteries around puberty (Hansen et al., 1995; Stary, 1989; Strong & McGill, 1969) and are only rarely identified before the age of 9,

given no known predisposing risk factors (Eggen & Solberg, 1968; Hansen et al., 1995; Stary, 1989). In one report, 65% of children aged 12 to 14 years were found to have type I or type II lesions and 8% had advanced lesions (Hansen et al., 1995; Stary, 1989). While the factors affecting this rapid increase in type II lesions are unknown, elevated cholesterol levels and blood pressure have been identified as potential risk factors even at this age (Ellefson et al., 1978; Lauer et al., 1985; Newman et al., 1986; Tell et al., 1985; Viikari et al., 1985).

Type III Lesions

Type III lesions are also known as intermediate or transitional lesions or preatheroma. Type III lesions contain more free cholesterol, fatty acid, sphingomyelin, lysolecithin, and triglyceride than type II lesions (Katsuda et al., 1992; Small, 1988). Fatty acid composition differs between type II and more advanced lesions and may be explained by the overall increase in lipids and the change from intracellular to predominantly extracellular storage. Type III lesions contain extracellular lipid deposits (droplets and particles) among the layers of smooth muscle cells that tend to occur adjacent to areas of adaptive intimal thickening. These dispersed droplets accumulate beneath the macrophage/foam cell layer, replace cellular matrix proteoglycans and fibers, and also divide smooth muscle cells. This lipid-variegation destabilizes the integrity of intimal smooth muscle cells and is characteristic of type III lesions.

Type IV Lesions

This lesion, referred to as atheroma is the first "advanced" lesion of atherosclerosis, characterized histologically by a lipid core, intimal disorganization, and arterial deformity, which predispose this lesion type to sudden progression that may precipitate clinical symptoms. Macrophages within the lesions are primed for immune and/or inflammatory responses, expressing major histocompatibility complex receptors and, a variety of cytokines and growth regulatory molecules. These lesions possess a large, well-defined intimal pool of extracellular lipid known as the lipid core. The type IV lesion is also known as an atheroma. The continued growth of these extracellular lipid pools is a result of continued transmigration from the plasma, encouraged by the areas of decreased local blood flow (called eddies) at lesion-prone sites. Initially, these lesions co-localize with adaptive intimal thickenings. Lipid cores thicken the artery wall and are clearly visible when the luminal surface of the lesion is examined, although thickening usually occurs at the external boundry and contributes little to narrowing of the vessel lumen at this stage (Glagov et al., 1988).

This lesion type is characterized by displacement of the intimal smooth muscle cells and the intercellular matrix of the deep intima by accumulating pools of extracellular lipid. The dispersed cells appear attenuated and elongated with thickening of the basement membranes. Calcium particles are often found within the lipid cores and even within the organelles of some of the smooth muscle cells. In addition, capillaries may be readily identified around the lipid core and are most common at the lateral margins and facing the lumen. Macrophages, smooth muscle cells, and even mast cells and lymphocytes, populate the region between the lipid core and the endothelial surface. Coalescence of the lipid core leads to a subsequent increase in fibrous tissue (mainly collagen), which will in turn alter the intima above the lipid core. When the fibrous tissue enrichment of the intima covering the lipid core occurs, the lesion is classified as type V. In either conventional histological sections, or by examination by the unaided eye, the upper intimal layer of a type IV lesion is indistinguishable from the fibrotic cover (also known as the fibrous cap) of a type V lesion. This explains why type IV and type V lesions are both referred to as fibrous plaques.

Although this lesion class only minimally contributes to luminal narrowing, type IV lesions have important clinical significance. Enrichment of the region between the lipid core and the lesion surface with proteoglycans, foam cells, and dispersed smooth muscle cells with decreased collagen content renders the lesion susceptible to fissures or ulceration. Ominously, localization and accumulation of macrophages in the periphery of advanced lesions, particularly type IV, makes them vulnerable to sudden rupture.

Type V Lesions

This next stage in lesion progression is referred to as a fibroatheroma, because of the intimal accumulation of abundant fibrous connective tissue adjacent to a lipid core. When a type V lesion has both a lipid core and calcification within the lesion, it is referred to as a type Vb lesion. Type Vc lesions are devoid of a lipid core and contain minimal lipid deposition. Type V lesions tend to cause a more noticeable narrowing of arteries than type IV lesions and are particularly clinically relevant given their susceptibility to fissure, hemorrhage, and rupture with hematoma and/or thrombus formation.

Population studies of advanced lesion histology reveal that reparative smooth muscle cells infiltrate regions of the intima in which lipid cores disturb or disrupt the cell and intercellular matrix structure. This fibrous tissue often accounts for more of the thickness of the lesion than its underlying lipid core. The new tissue is composed of both collagen and smooth muscle cells. These new smooth muscle cells are distinct from their older counterparts in that they are enriched in rough-surfaced endoplasmic reticulum. Previous thrombi appear to result in thicker lesions and surrounding tissue as they are incorporated into the growing lesion. Type V lesions also contain large, numerous, and newly formed vessel capillaries at the periphery of the lipid core. The media adjacent to the intima of type V lesions are characterized by depletion and disorganization of smooth muscle cells. The surrounding media and adjacent adventitia are enriched in lymphocytes, macrophages, and macrophage foam cells.

Type Va lesions can form larger compound lesions, composed of irregular intercalating lipid cores separated by thick layers of fibrous connective tissue (variably termed multilayered fibroatheroma). Both hemodynamic and tensile forces may contribute to the formation of such compound lesions; as lesions impinge on the circulation, alterations in blood flow promote asymmetric vascular narrowing and a redistribution of the regions of predisposition to lesion formation (Glagov et al.,

1988). An alternate explanation may be the serial rupture of the lesion surface, hematoma formation, and thrombosis followed by fibrious organization.

Though type Vb lesions are primarily differentiated by calcification, they tend to possess greater fibrous connective tissue compared to earlier lesion types. Mineral deposits may eventually replace a lesion's core (an accumulation of dead cells and extracellular lipid). Such calcified lesions are variably also termed a type VII lesion (Stary, 1992, 1994).

The type Vc lesions, being fibrotic and largely devoid of lipid core, often occur in the arteries in the lower extremities (Ross et al., 1984) and have been referred to as a type VIII lesion by some investigators (Stary, 1992, 1994). These lesions may form by one of several mechanisms, including thrombus organization, extension of the fibrous component of an adjacent fibroatheroma, or resorption of lipid cores. Although fibrotic lesions rarely possess a lipid core, a positive stain for lipids is not uncommon in this lesion type. It is noteworthy that wall shear stress caused by increased hydrostatic pressure is common in the lower extremities and could conceivably provide another mechanism for this lesion formation.

Type VI Lesions

Lesion types V and VI may undergo disruption of the lesion surface or develop hematoma, hemorrhage, or thrombotic deposits. They account for the majority of atherosclerotic morbidity and mortality. Any one of these complications is sufficient to re-categorize type IV or V lesions as type VI lesions; they are also referred to as complicated lesions. Moreover, the particular complicating event permits subdividion of type VI lesions into three subtypes according to (a) disruption; (b) hemorrhage; or (c) thrombosis, although practically, lesions are often complex and rarely conform perfectly to the lesion classification criteria. Indeed, instances of surface disruptions, hematoma, and thrombosis superimposed on other lesions types or even on intima without a noticeable lesion are not uncommon. The composition of blood, the integrity of the intima, the sensitivity of the inflammatory response, and the dynamic range of shear and tensile forces to which the lesion or intima is exposed varies greatly between persons. While physiological and biochemical studies aimed at characterizing both the determinants and mechanisms resulting in the spectrum of lesion types is ongoing, continued innovation in clinical imaging of lesions has contributed much to the more accurate identification of lesion types and their associated clinical syndromes.

In the past, clinical assessment of atherosclerotic lesions was confined to advanced, gross vascular abnormalities, including aneurysms and vascular stenoses. But the integration of newer and emerging technologies has permitted more accurate depiction of lesion morphology, which in turn informs more specific interventions (Table 7-2). Targeting of treatment has been honed further by the growing understanding of the pathophysiology of lesion progression and associated clinical events. This has permitted clinicians to move beyond simple diagnosis to proactive prevention of complicated lesions through detection of earlier lesions and more accurate lesion characterization.

Table 7–2 ■ NEW TECHNOLOGIES PERMITTING EARLIER DETECTION AND ESTIMATION OF LESION VOLUME ARE LISTED

Method	Features Detected
B-mode ultrasonography and Doppler flow	Permits measurement of the severity of stenosis in peripheral arteries
Intravascular ultrasound	Produces cross-sectional images of the vascular wall, revealing lesion composition and lumen contour
Magnetic resonance angiography	A noninvasive alternative to angiography, permitting study of major vessels (the aorta and carotid arteries and coronary arteries)
Angioscopy	Direct vascular vascularization detects specific morphological features such as thrombus
Ultrafast computed tomography	A noninvasive method detecting coronary artery calcium

While angiography is the definitive method for evaluation of the vascular lumen, it cannot detail the vascular wall. The sensitivity of coronary angiography for early detection of atherosclerosis may be increased by these methods. Emerging methodologies that may allow noninvasive monitoring of atherosclerosis include magnetic resonance spectroscopy, labeled antiplatelet monoclonal antibody imaging, and radiolabeling of low-density lipoproteins and monocytes.

CELLS AND EXTRACELLULAR MATRIX OF LESIONS

A host of changes exist in the cellular compartment and extracellular matrix composition of lesions. Interaction of the apolipoprotein B on LDL with cell surface glycosaminoglycans appears to be a mechanism for trapping LDL in the arterial intima. Moreover, production of glycosaminoglycans increases during the early stages of atherosclerosis, which contribute to more avid cellular lipoprotein recruitment (Stevens et al., 1976; Tammi et al., 1978; Wagner & Salisbury, 1978). Dermatan sulfate proteoglycans are another surface moiety hypothesized to increase the rate of progression of atherosclerosis (Wagner & Salisbury, 1978). This class of molecules also binds plasma LDL under physiological conditions with increased affinity in comparison with other molecules of this class (Iverius, 1972). In vitro studies of smooth muscle cells exposed to conditioned media from cultured macrophages provides evidence for a role for macrophages in modulating the type and amount of proteoglycans found in the developing lesion (Edwards et al., 1990). Macrophage accumulation in type II lesions leads to the production of enzymes capable of degrading proteoglycans within the lesion locale. Enzymatic digestion of the chondroitin sulfate proteoglycan, versican, leads to progression of the lesion because of its role in maintaining the viscoelasticity and the integrity of the vessel wall against the passage of plasma materials.

Although there are significant decreases in elastin content in advanced atherosclerotic lesions, few changes are reported in initial and fatty streak lesions. A variety of elastases attack elastic fibers, and the possibility exists for macrophages (Banda & Werb, 1981) and smooth muscle cells (Robert et al., 1984) to produce such proteases. This results in a decrease in structural

intergrity. Moreover, degradation of elastic fibers may have significant consequences in early lesions, because elastin-derived peptides are extremely chemotactic for macrophages.

Smooth Muscle Cells

Alterations in the functional properties and amount of smooth muscle cells are a central feature of atherogenesis. Changes result from stimuli, including lipid accumulation, disruption of intimal structure, damage to intimal cells and matrix, and deposits of platelets and fibrinogen. These stimuli activate resident cells to produce mitogenic factors, spurring smooth muscle cell proliferation, and ultimately contributing to lesion progression.

Macrophages

Whereas macrophages are generally located proximal to the lumen, foam cells are trapped within the intima. However, this distribution becomes less obvious in complicated lesions or regions in which the intima is relatively thin. When a lipid core is present, macrophage foam cells are usually most evident along the luminal aspect and at the lateral margins of the core. Macrophage foam cells are more numerous and found closer to the surface of the lesion boarder, largely because of a lack of intimal thickening at the lesion periphery. Foam cells eventually die as the lesion develops, contributing to the growth of what is more appropriately termed a "necrotic" core, being composed of extracellular lipid and necrotizing cells. Unfortunately, there are currently no appropriate biomarkers for defining this type of cellular injury.

An accumulating body of evidence indicates that in addition to lipid accumulation, macrophages contribute to atherogenesis by secretion of a range of factors modulating the formation and modeling of advanced lesions, including monocyte chemotactic protein-1 (MCP-1) and tumor necrosis factor (TNF) (Barath et al., 1990). Lesions laden with monocytes and macrophage foam cells (Davies et al., 1993; Falk, 1992) are more prone to rupture because of the release of proteolytic enzymes (e.g., collagenase and elastase) by the macrophages. It is not clear yet if macrophages secrete these enzymes throughout lesion formation or only as they die. The capacity of macrophages to express cytokines and growth regulatory molecules was reviewed earlier (Stary et al., 1994).

Lymphocytes

Monoclonal antibodies against CD antigens reveal the presence of T (CD4+ T helper and CD8+ T killer) and B lymphocytes in advanced lesions (Jonasson et al., 1986). It is yet unclear to what extent these immune cells participate in the atherogenic process. Macrophage foam cell-derived oxidized lipids constitute a significant but variable component of the core of advanced lesions (Ball et al., 1995; Mitchinson et al., 1985; Rosenfeld & Ross, 1990). Autoantibodies that recognize oxidized LDL have been isolated from human sera (Palinski et al., 1989), and the titers of these antibodies may potentially be diagnostic of advanced atherosclerosis (Salonen et al., 1992). In addition, viral and bacterial (e.g. chlamydia) antigens have been found in advanced human lesions using molecular and immunocytochemical techniques (Kuo et al., 1993).

Lipid and Lipoprotein in the Extracellular Matrix

While the transfer of lipoproteins from the plasma into the intima is a physiological process, the concentrations of these particles are particularly elevated in advanced lesions (Stary et al., 1994). Definitive identification of the types and amounts of extracellular lipid are difficult and depend largely on methods of tissue preparation and study. More extracellular lipid is observed in lesion types III, IV, Va, and VI. In addition, extracellular lipid accumulates and pools, forming "lipid cores," in lesion types IV, Va, and VI. Lesions contain many lipid-laden cells that die or can be found in various stages of disintegration, evidence that much of the extracellular lipid is derived from cells and lipoproteins originally internalized by cells (Ball et al., 1995; Mitchinson et al., 1985). In addition, intracytoplasmic lipid can also be expelled from intact cells into the extracellular space (Schmitz & Muller, 1991). Extracellular lipid is also derived in part by direct coalescence of plasma-derived lipoproteins (Guyton & Klemp, 1989, 1994).

Fibrinogen

The degree and extent to which fibrinogen accumulates in advanced lesions or parts of advanced lesions varies. Immunohistochemical techniques show that the cores of advanced lesions stain for fibrinogen more than any other part of advanced lesions, except superimposed thrombi. It must be recalled that immunohistochemical staining alone cannot distinguish thrombus-associated fibrinogen from physiological infiltration of fibrinogen from the plasma. However, it is generally accepted that intensely fibrinogen-positive bands found in the majority of advanced lesions constitute evidence of incorporated past thrombi (Bini et al., 1989). Fibrinogen contributes directly and indirectly (by promoting smooth muscle cell growth) to the volume of most advanced lesions.

Proteoglycans

Proteoglycans are a class of glycosylated proteins that have covalently linked sulfated glycosaminoglycans, (i.e., chondroitin sulfate, dermatan sulfate, heparan sulfate, heparin). The protein component of proteoglycans is a core protein that is modified by the addition of a complex set of sugar groups. Glycosaminoglycans are sulfated polysaccharides made of repeating disaccharides (40 to 100 repeats, on average). These complex groups endow proteoglycans with unique properties. In contrast to arterial glycosaminoglycans, little is known about qualitative changes in specific proteoglycan molecules in atherosclerotic lesions. Large extracellular proteoglycans, mainly chondroitin sulfate-containing molecules,

function in arterial permeability, ion exchange, transport, and deposition of plasma materials such as LDL. Extracellular heparin sulfate proteoglycans possessing particular oligosaccharide or carbohydrate sequences have different functional properties. Functions attributed to specific oligosaccharides include antiproliferative effects on arterial smooth muscle cells (Schmidt et al., 1992), fibroblast growth factor binding (Turnbull et al., 1992; Tyrrell et al., 1993), lipoprotein lipase binding (Parthasarathy et al., 1994), and antithrombin III binding (Rosenberg et al., 1979). While hypotheses regarding the concentrations, composition, and function of various proteogyclans are currently being evaluated, the lack of clinical studies to inform the clinical relevance of such hypotheses makes discussion of these molecules premature in this venue.

Collagen

Second only to lipids, collagen is the major extracellular component of type V lesions. The increased collagen of atherosclerotic lesions is produced by intimal smooth muscle cells. The major collagen type of advanced lesions is the fibrillar collagen type I. Type I collagen is particularly prevalent in the fibrous cap and in vascularized regions of advanced lesions (Rekhter et al., 1993). A significant and consistent change in the minor collagen types of advanced atherosclerotic lesions includes type V collagen, which increases with advancing fibrosis (Morton & Barnes, 1982; Murata et al., 1986; Ooshima, 1981) and plays a role in cell migration (Stenn et al., 1979); and type IV collagen, which is associated with the basement membranes of smooth muscle cells. The exact stimulus for collagen accumulation in atherosclerosis is unknown, although redistribution of mechanical stress has been shown to produce changes in matrix production.

Elastin

The relative concentration and localization of elastin fibers varies with the location and type of lesion. De novo synthesis of subendothelial, medial, and adventitial elastin is common in type V lesions, along with collagen. Whereas the smooth muscle cells of advanced lesions produce elastin, integration of the protein into a functional elastic fiber may be impaired.

Split or frayed elastic fibers tend to associate closely with lipid and calcium deposits. Lipid bound to elastic fibers may change elasticity of tissue by modifying the functionality of the elastin fibers and increase their susceptibility to proteolytic degradation (Chaudiere et al., 1980; Guantieri et al., 1983). Both calcium and magnesium may increase the degradation of elastin (Bernier et al., 1981), the degradation products of which have been reported to produce chemotactic derivatives, which recruit macrophages (Senior et al., 1980).

Calcium

Mineralization of atherosclerotic lesions is a well-substantiated phenomenon. Accumulation of calcium in the arterial wall in the course of the atherogenic process is considered to be a manifestation of advanced atherosclerosis. Unfortunately, very little is known about the factors controlling the quantity of calcium in the lesions. Vesicles in the extracellular matrix of advanced lesions may serve as sites for calcification (Kim, 1976). Mineral deposits in atherosclerosis may also be associated with elastic fibers (Urry, 1971).

VASCULAR SURFACE DEFECTS AND HEMATOMA

As lesions progress, disruptions of the lesion surface may present as fissures or even ulcerations and are highly variable in their severity and scope. Fissures of the lesion surface vary in length and depth and most likely reseal, leading to lesion progression by incorporating hematoma and thrombus (Davies & Thomas, 1985; Falk, 1992). Ulcerations can range from minor focal loss of a microscopic portion of the endothelial cell layer to deep ulcerations that can expose lipid cores and release lipid and other components that activate the coagulation cascade. Atheromatous lesions (types IV and Va) are particularly prone to intimal disruptions and ultimately thrombosis (Davies & Thomas, 1985; Falk, 1989, 1992; Richardson et al., 1989). This susceptibility is caused in part by the presence of activated inflammatory cells within the lesions (Tracy et al., 1985; van der Wal et al., 1994), the release of proteolytic enzymes by macrophages within the lesions (Davies et al., 1993; Henney et al., 1991; Steinberg & Witztum, 1990), coronary spasm (Nobuyoshi et al., 1991), structural weakness related to lesion composition (Richardson et al., 1989), the release of toxic factors from cell death (necrosis), and shear stress (Glagov et al., 1988; Ku et al., 1985). In addition to intimal hematoma caused by tearing of the lesion surface, some hemorrhage may begin internally from disruption of newly formed vessels within the lesion (Barger et al., 1984).

Thrombosis

Advanced atherosclerotic lesions containing thrombi or their remnants become common by the fourth decade of life, ranging in size from microscopic to grossly visible deposits, with some consisting of stratified layers of lesions of different ages (Bini et al., 1989). Incorporation of recurrent hematomas and thrombi over time (months to years) results in the progressive narrowing of the arterial lumen. Thrombus remnants contain increasing numbers of smooth muscle cells derived by ingrowth from the intima. These smooth muscle cells synthesize collagen, providing the stratum for overgrowth of endothelial cells at the lumen. Ultimately, thrombi may continue to enlarge, with the potential to rapidly occlude the lumen of a medium-sized artery (within days or even hours).

Several mechanisms can influence the location, frequency, concentration, and size of thrombi. Shear stress participates in lesion progression, with thrombotic occlusions being common at vessel bifurcations and locations of arterial angulation (Taeymans et al., 1992). Increased levels of low-density lipoproteins (demonstrated to impair platelet function) (Aviram & Brook, 1987; Brook & Aviram, 1988), nutrition (Betteridge, 1987), contents of cigarette smoke (Miller, 1992), and elevated lipoprotein (a) levels (Loscalzo, 1990; Scanu, 1991), have been associated with greater risk for clinical coronary artery disease. Taken together, systemic factors play a significant role in modulating the development of thrombi.

Atherosclerotic Aneurysms

A common sequela of advanced lesions (types IV, V, and VI) is the developement of distensions in the entire vascular wall. These outward bulges or aneurysms are most commonly associated with type VI lesions when the intimal surface is eroded. Both old and new mural thrombi permeate atherosclerotic aneurysms, and the thrombi become layered in older aneurysms. Whereas the thrombi can form large masses that can fill an aneurysm, the underlying lumen remains generally well-preserved and approximates the dimensions of the original vessel. The evolution of atherosclerotic aneurysms is preceded by a series of changes in the locale of the lesion. Matrix fibers are continuously degraded and resynthesized (Dobrin et al., 1984), causing a progressive decay of matrix architecture that results in dilation and potentially rupture (Langille & O'Donnell, 1986). Susceptibility to atherosclerotic aneurysm is modulated by secondary risk factors resulting in increased hemodynamic and/or tensile stress (e.g. hypertension) and by genetic variation. The search for genetic factors predisposing to atherosclerotic aneurysm development is ongoing.

Severity of Stenosis

The severity of lesion stenosis modulates the degree of impaired blood flow. The degree of stenosis is estimated by the ratio of the maximum diameter of a stenosed artery in comparison to an adjacent normal arterial diameter. Coronary artery blood flow begins to decrease to a clinically significant degree with 50% stenosis and blood flow decreases rapidly when stenosis exceeds 70% (Gould & Lipscomb, 1974), and the determination of stenosis is of particular clinical benefit above and below these cut-offs. However, this physiological marker (decrease in blood flow) is technically difficult to measure accurately and fails to account for other factors that can influence the clinical impact of stenosis on a patient (e.g., rate of lesion growth and lesion length and/or geometry) (Goldstein et al., 1987). Percent diameter stenosis assumes that the arterial lumen measured is approximately circular in cross-section; however, stenosis of coronary arteries will often result in an elliptical, D-shaped, slit-like, or crescent-shaped lumen (Glagov et al., 1987; Nissen et al., 1991; Thomas et al., 1986; Zarins et al., 1988). Thus, whereas percent stenosis measured on any *single* view can misrepresent the cross-sectional area, the accuracy of this measure is greatly increased by the use of two or more views, a fact commonly used in the angiographic evaluation of arterial anatomy (Brown et al., 1977; Zarins et al., 1988).

Another caveat to this methodology is that the selection of a "normal" reference segment is not always obvious given that adjacent coronary arteries may look normal but are seldom free of disease (Glagov et al., 1987; Zarins et al., 1988). Nevertheless, percent stenosis measured by a variety of means provides a powerful tool with significant clinical usefulness in the evaluation of coronary disease (Arnett et al., 1979; Blankenhorn & Curry, 1982; Markis et al., 1976).

LESION TYPES AND MORPHOLOGY: CORRELATION WITH CLINICAL SYNDROMES

In addition to the severity of stenosis, atherosclerotic lesions can be characterized by key aspects of their morphology. Comparison of postmortem coronary angiograms with histological sections has defined the pathological significance of key morphological descriptors (Levin & Fallon, 1982). These include lesion length, texture of lumen outline, abrupt or tapered lesion shoulders, and defects caused by thrombus, presence of calcification, and lesion eccentricity or ectasia. The composition of atherosclerotic lesions correlates with the clinical status of the patient; in some patients, these measures are better predictors of clinical outcome than severity of stenosis (O'Holleran et al., 1987).

Acute or Unstable Ischemic Coronary Syndromes

Lesion disruption followed by intraluminal thrombus is central to the pathogenesis of unstable syndromes of coronary heart disease. The severity of lesion disruption influences the characteristics of the subsequent clinical state. If lesion disruption and thrombosis are limited, then the result is usually asymptomatic lesion growth. A deeper disruption (e.g., fissuring) can result in a transient thrombotic occlusion that may last only minutes and can reccur (Falk, 1989, 1992). This can result in unstable angina (Fuster et al., 1988). If disruption is very deep or ulceration exposes the lipid core, which contains highly reactive tissue factors and other elements, then a persistant thrombotic occlusion (lasting a few hours or longer) may culminate in acute myocardial infarction (Fuster et al., 1988; Davies et al., 1991; Nakagawa et al., 1988). Angiographic studies have repeatedly confirmed these events and subsequent clinical manifestations (Ambrose et al., 1986; Levin & Fallon, 1982; Little et al., 1988).

Chronic Stable Angina and Silent Occlusion

The clinical angiographic morphology associated with chronic stable angina resembles that of uncomplicated lesions (Levin & Fallon, 1982), tending toward a smooth outline and tapered shoulders, appearing symmetric with a broad neck (Ambrose et al., 1985; Ellis et al., 1989). Lesions tend to be fibrotic and stable (Kragel et al., 1991). Interestingly, although severe stenoses tend to progress to total thrombotic occlusion more often than less severe lesions, they are less likely to lead to infarct (Fuster et al., 1979), potentially because of the presence of collateral vessels that have had time to develop. In contrast to unstable lesions, the residual thrombus is usually found on the downstream side of the stenosis.

Aortic and Peripheral Atherosclerosis

Aortic atherosclerosis typically manifests in the abdominal aorta between the level of the renal arteries and the iliac bifurcation. Because of its size, sudden obstruction of the aorta is relatively uncommon, whereas atherosclerotic disease in the iliac and femoral arteries is often severe. Advanced lesions (i.e., type VI) can result in distal emboli, stenosis, and acute vessel occlusion. In addition, atrophy of the media associated with large eroded lesions can culminate in aneurysm formation.

Cerebrovascular Atherosclerosis

Similar to coronary atherosclerosis, luminal surface disruption predisposes to lesion instability and manifests most often at the carotid bifurcation. Lesion rupture can result in distal emboli and/or occlusion. This can result in transient or more permanent cerebral symptoms. Severe stenosis at the proximal internal carotid and in intracerebral branches can result in obstruction and cerebral ischemia.

CONCLUSION

Atherosclerosis accounts for more than 50% of all-cause adult mortality in Westernized countries. It is a slow progressive disease that may start in childhood but does not become significant until the fifth or sixth decades of life in the absence of predisposing risk factors (see Table 7-1). Atherosclerosis is a progressive disease that evolves from deposits of lipids, cellular debris, calcium and fibrin, and inflammation. It is a disease that affects the large arteries and medium-size vessels and displays significant inter-individual variation in the sites and in the rate of plaque formation. Plaques can enlarge to partially or completely impede blood flow through an artery, and occlusion of arterial blood flow (and thus oxygen supply) and the local inflammatory sequelae caused by plaque rupture and thrombosis can lead to angina, myocardial infarction, or stroke. Morphological, immunohistochemical, and epidemiological data have supported the construction of a lesion classification system, which has helped clinical decision-making and research into the underlying pathophysiology and potential therapeutic intervention (Table 7-3).

Table 7–3 ▪ TERMS USED TO DESIGNATE DIFFERENT TYPES OF HUMAN ATHEROSCLEROTIC LESIONS IN PATHOLOGY

Terms for Atherosclerotic Lesions in Histological Classification		Other Terms for the Same Lesions Often Based on Appearance With the Unaided Eye	
Type lesion I	Initial lesion	Fatty dot or streak	Early lesions
Type lesion IIa	Progression-prone type II lesion		
IIb	Progression-resistant type II		
Type lesion III	Intermediate lesion (preatheroma)		
Type lesion IV	Atheroma	Atheromatous plaque, fibrolipid plaque, fibrous plaque	
Type lesion Va	Fibroatheroma (type V lesion)		Advanced lesions, raised lesions
Vb	Calcific lesion (type VII lesion)	Calcified plaque	
Vc	Fibrotic lesion (type VIII lesion)	Fibrous plaque	
Type lesion VI	Lesion with surface defect, and/or hematoma–hemorrhage, and/or thrombotic deposit	Complicated lesion, complicated plaque	

Reproduced from Stary et al. (1995). A report from the Committee on Vascular Lesions of the Council on Arteriosclerosis, American Heart Association. *Arterioscler Thromb Vasc Biol*, 15, 1512–1531.

REFERENCES

Ambrose, J. A., Winters, S. L., Arora, R. R., Eng, A., Riccio, A., Gorlin, R., & Fuster, V. (1986). Angiographic evolution of coronary artery morphology in unstable angina. *Journal of the American College of Cardiology*, 7(3), 472–478.

Ambrose, J. A., Winters, S. L., Stern, A., Eng, A., Teichholz, L. E., Gorlin, R., & Fuster, V. (1985). Angiographic morphology and the pathogenesis of unstable angina pectoris. *Journal of the American College of Cardiology*, 5(3), 609–616.

Arnett, E. N., Isner, J. M., Redwood, D. R., Kent, K. M., Baker, W. P., Ackerstein, H., & Roberts, W. C. (1979). Coronary artery narrowing in coronary heart disease: comparison of cineangiographic and necropsy findings. *Annals of Intern Medicine*, 91(3), 350–356.

Aviram, M., & Brook, J. G. (1987). Platelet activation by plasma lipoproteins. *Progress in Cardiovascular Disease*, 30(1), 61–72.

Ball, R. Y., Stowers, E. C., Burton, J. H., Cary, N. R., Skepper, J. N., & Mitchinson, M. J. (1995). Evidence that the death of macrophage foam cells contributes to the lipid core of atheroma. *Atherosclerosis*, 114(1), 45–54.

Banda, M. J., & Werb, Z. (1981). Mouse macrophage elastase. Purification and characterization as a metalloproteinase. *Biochemical Journal*, 193(2), 589–605.

Barath, P., Fishbein, M. C., Cao, J., Berenson, J., Helfant, R. H., & Forrester, J. S. (1990). Detection and localization of tumor necrosis factor in human atheroma. *American Journal of Cardiology*, 65(5), 297–302.

Barger, A. C., Beeuwkes, R., 3rd, Lainey, L. L., & Silverman, K. J. (1984). Hypothesis: vasa vasorum and neovascularization of human coronary arteries. A possible role in the pathophysiology of atherosclerosis. *New England Journal of Medicine*, 310(3), 175–177.

Bernard, Y., Meneveau, N., Vuillemenot, A., Magnin, D., Anguenot, T., Schiele, F., & Bassand, J. P. (1997). Planimetry of aortic valve area using multiplane transoesophageal echocardiography is not a reliable method for assessing severity of aortic stenosis. *Heart*, 78(1), 68–73.

Bernier, F., Bakala, H., & Wallach, J. (1981). Effect of Mg2+ and Ca2+ on enzymatic elastolysis of insoluble elastin determined by a conductimetric method. *Connective Tissue Research*, 8(2), 71–75.

Betteridge, J. (1987). Nutrition and platelet function in atherogenesis. *Proceedings of the Nutrition Society*, 46(3), 345–359.

Bini, A., Fenoglio, J. J., Jr., Mesa-Tejada, R., Kudryk, B., & Kaplan, K. L. (1989). Identification and distribution of fibrinogen, fibrin, and fibrin(ogen) degradation products in atherosclerosis. Use of monoclonal antibodies. *Arteriosclerosis*, 9(1), 109–121.

Blankenhorn, D. H., & Curry, P. J. (1982). The accuracy of arteriography and ultrasound imaging for atherosclerosis measurement. A review. *Archives of Pathological Laboratory Medicine*, 106(10), 483–489.

Brook, J. G., & Aviram, M. (1988). Platelet lipoprotein interactions. *Semin Thromb Hemost*, 14(3), 258–265.

Brown, B. G., Bolson, E., Frimer, M., & Dodge, H. T. (1977). Quantitative coronary arteriography: estimation of dimensions, hemodynamic resistance, and atheroma mass of coronary artery lesions using the arteriogram and digital computation. *Circulation*, 55(2), 329–337.

Chaudiere, J., Derouette, J. C., Mendy, F., Jacotot, B., & Robert, L. (1980). In vitro preparation of elastin—triglyceride complexes. Fatty acid uptake and modification of the susceptibility to elastase action. *Atherosclerosis*, 36(2), 183–194.

Cornhill, J. F., Herderick, E. E., & Stary, H. C. (1990). Topography of human aortic sudanophilic lesions. *Monographs in Atherosclerosis*, 15, 13–19.

Davies, M. J., Richardson, P. D., Woolf, N., Katz, D. R., & Mann, J. (1993). Risk of thrombosis in human atherosclerotic plaques: role of extracellular lipid, macrophage, and smooth muscle cell content. *British Heart Journal*, 69(5), 377–381.

Davies, M. J., & Thomas, A. C. (1985). Plaque fissuring—the cause of acute myocardial infarction, sudden ischaemic death, and crescendo angina. *British Heart Journal*, 53(4), 363–373.

Davies, S. W., Marchant, B., Lyons, J. P., Timmis, A. D., Rothman, M. T., Layton, C. A., & Balcon, R. (1991). Irregular coronary lesion morphology after thrombolysis predicts early clinical instability. *Journal of the American College of Cardiology*, 18(3), 669–674.

Dobrin, P. B., Baker, W. H., & Gley, W. C. (1984). Elastolytic and collagenolytic studies of arteries. Implications for the mechanical properties of aneurysms. *Archives of Surgery*, 119(4), 405–409.

Edwards, I. J., Wagner, W. D., & Owens, R. T. (1990). Macrophage secretory products selectively stimulate dermatan sulfate proteoglycan production in cultured arterial smooth muscle cells. *American Journal of Pathology*, 136(3), 609–621.

Eggen, D. A., & Solberg, L. A. (1968). Variation of atherosclerosis with age. *Laboratory Investigation*, 18(5), 571–579.

Ellefson, R. D., Elveback, L. R., Hodgson, P. A., & Weidman, W. H. (1978). Cholesterol and triglycerides in serum lipoproteins of young persons in Rochester, Minnesota. *Mayo Clinic Proceedings*, 53(5), 307–320.

Ellis, S., Alderman, E. L., Cain, K., Wright, A., Bourassa, M., & Fisher, L. (1989). Morphology of left anterior descending coronary territory lesions as a predictor of anterior myocardial infarction: a CASS Registry Study. *Journal of the American College of Cardiology*, 13(7), 1481–1491.

Falk, E. (1989). Morphologic features of unstable atherothrombotic plaques underlying acute coronary syndromes. *American Journal of Cardiology*, 63(10), 114E–120E.

Falk, E. (1992). Why do plaques rupture? *Circulation*, 86(6 Suppl), III30–42.

Fuster, V., Badimon, L., Cohen, M., Ambrose, J. A., Badimon, J. J., & Chesebro, J. (1988). Insights into the pathogenesis of acute ischemic syndromes. *Circulation*, 77(8), 1213–1220.

Fuster, V., Frye, R. L., Kennedy, M. A., Connolly, D. C., & Mankin, H. T. (1979). The role of collateral circulation in the various coronary syndromes. *Circulation*, 59(6), 1137–1144.

Glagov, S., Weisenberg, E., Zarins, C. K., Stankunavicius, R., & Kolettis, G. J. (1987). Compensatory enlargement of human atherosclerotic coronary arteries. *New England Journal of Medicine*, 316(22), 1371–1375.

Glagov, S., Zarins, C., Giddens, D. P., & Ku, D. N. (1988). Hemodynamics and atherosclerosis. Insights and perspectives gained from studies of human arteries. *Archives of Pathological Laboratory Medicine*, 112(10), 1018–1031.

Goldstein, R. A., Kirkeeide, R. L., Demer, L. L., Merhige, M., Nishikawa, A., Smalling, R. W., Mullani, N. A., & Gould, K. L. (1987). Relation between geometric dimensions of coronary artery stenoses and myocardial perfusion reserve in man. *Journal of Clinical Investigation*, 79(5), 1473–1478.

Goris, M. L., Boudier, S., & Briandet, P. A. (1987). Two-dimensional mapping of three-dimensional SPECT data: a preliminary step to the quantitation of thallium myocardial perfusion single photon emission tomography. *American Journal of Physiological Imaging*, 2(4), 176–180.

Gould, K. L., & Lipscomb, K. (1974). Effects of coronary stenoses on coronary flow reserve and resistance. *American Journal of Cardiology*, 34(1), 48–55.

Grech, E. D. (2003). ABC of interventional cardiology: percutaneous coronary intervention. II: the procedure. *BMJ*, 326(7399), 1137–1140.

Guantieri, V., Tamburro, A. M., & Gordini, D. D. (1983). Interactions of human and bovine elastins with lipids: their proteolysis by elastase. *Connective Tissue Research*, 12(1), 79–83.

Guyton, J. R., & Klemp, K. F. (1989). The lipid-rich core region of human atherosclerotic fibrous plaques. Prevalence of small lipid droplets and vesicles by electron microscopy. *American Journal of Pathology*, 134(3), 705–717.

Guyton, J. R., & Klemp, K. F. (1994). Development of the atherosclerotic core region. Chemical and ultrastructural analysis of microdissected atherosclerotic lesions from human aorta. *Arterioscler Thromb*, 14(8), 1305–1314.

Guzman, M. A., McMahan, C. A., McGill, H. C., Jr., Strong, J. P., Tejada, C., Restrepo, C., Eggen, D. A., Robertson, W. B., & Solberg, L. A. (1968). Selected methodologic aspects of the International Atherosclerosis Project. *Laboratory Investigation*, 18(5), 479–497.

Hansen, B. F. (1978). Heart autopsy in ischemic heart disease. An autopsy protocol. *Acta Pathol Microbiol Scand [A]*, 86(3), 241–244.

Hansen, M. E., Valentine, R. J., McIntire, D. D., Myers, S. I., Chervu, A., & Clagett, G. P. (1995). Age-related differences in the distribution of peripheral atherosclerosis: when is atherosclerosis truly premature? *Surgery*, 118(5), 834–839.

Henney, A. M., Wakeley, P. R., Davies, M. J., Foster, K., Hembry, R., Murphy, G., & Humphries, S. (1991). Localization of stromelysin gene expression in atherosclerotic plaques by in situ hybridization. *Proceedings of the National Academy of Sciences of the USA*, 88(18), 8154–8158.

Iverius, P. H. (1972). The interaction between human plasma lipoproteins and connective tissue glycosaminoglycans. *Journal of Biology and Chemistry*, 247(8), 2607–2613.

Jonasson, L., Holm, J., Skalli, O., Bondjers, G., & Hansson, G. K. (1986). Regional accumulations of T cells, macrophages, and smooth muscle cells in the human atherosclerotic plaque. *Arteriosclerosis*, 6(2), 131–138.

Katsuda, S., Boyd, H. C., Fligner, C., Ross, R., & Gown, A. M. (1992). Human atherosclerosis. III. Immunocytochemical analysis of the cell composition of lesions of young adults. *American Journal of Pathology*, 140(4), 907–914.

Kim, K. M. (1976). Calcification of matrix vesicles in human aortic valve and aortic media. *Fed Proc*, 35(2), 156–162.

Kragel, A. H., Gertz, S. D., & Roberts, W. C. (1991). Morphologic comparison of frequency and types of acute lesions in the major epicardial coronary arteries in unstable angina pectoris, sudden coronary death and acute myocardial infarction. *Journal of the American College of Cardiology*, 18(3), 801–808.

Ku, D. N., Giddens, D. P., Zarins, C. K., & Glagov, S. (1985). Pulsatile flow and atherosclerosis in the human carotid bifurcation. Positive correlation between plaque location and low oscillating shear stress. *Arteriosclerosis*, 5(3), 293–302.

Kuo, C. C., Shor, A., Campbell, L. A., Fukushi, H., Patton, D. L., & Grayston, J. T. (1993). Demonstration of Chlamydia pneumoniae in atherosclerotic lesions of coronary arteries. *Journal of Infectious Disease*, 167(4), 841–849.

Langille, B. L., & O'Donnell, F. (1986). Reductions in arterial diameter produced by chronic decreases in blood flow are endothelium-dependent. *Science*, 231(4736), 405–407.

Lauer, R. M., Burns, T. L., & Clarke, W. R. (1985). Assessing children's blood pressure—considerations of age and body size: the Muscatine Study. *Pediatrics*, 75(6), 1081–1090.

Levin, D. C., & Fallon, J. T. (1982). Significance of the angiographic morphology of localized coronary stenoses: histopathologic correlations. *Circulation*, 66(2), 316–320.

Libby, P. (2000). Changing concepts of atherogenesis. *Journal of Internal Medicine*, 247(3), 349–358.

Little, W. C., Constantinescu, M., Applegate, R. J., Kutcher, M. A., Burrows, M. T., Kahl, F. R., & Santamore, W. P. (1988). Can coronary angiography predict the site of a subsequent myocardial infarction in patients with mild-to-moderate coronary artery disease? *Circulation*, 78(5 Pt 1), 1157–1166.

Loscalzo, J. (1990). Lipoprotein(a). A unique risk factor for atherothrombotic disease. *Arteriosclerosis*, 10(5), 672–679.

Markis, J. E., Joffe, C. D., Cohn, P. F., Feen, D. J., Herman, M. V., Gorlin, R. (1976). Clinical significance of coronary arterial ectasia. *American Journal of Cardiology*, 37(2), 217–222.

Miller, G. J. (1992). Hemostasis and cardiovascular risk. The British and European experience. *Archives of Pathology and Laboratory Medicine*, 116(12), 1318–1321.

Mitchinson, M. J., Hothersall, D. C., Brooks, P. N., & De Burbure, C. Y. (1985). The distribution of ceroid in human atherosclerosis. *Journal of Pathology*, 145(2), 177–183.

Morton, L. F., & Barnes, M. J. (1982). Collagen polymorphism in the normal and diseased blood vessel wall. Investigation of collagens types I, III and V. *Atherosclerosis*, 42(1), 41–51.

Munro, J. M., van der Walt, J. D., Munro, C. S., Chalmers, J. A., & Cox, E. L. (1987). An immunohistochemical analysis of human aortic fatty streaks. *Human Pathology*, 18(4), 375–380.

Murata, K., Motayama, T., & Kotake, C. (1986). Collagen types in various layers of the human aorta and their changes with the atherosclerotic process. *Atherosclerosis*, 60(3), 251–262.

Nakagawa, S., Hanada, Y., Koiwaya, Y., & Tanaka, K. (1988). Angiographic features in the infarct-related artery after intracoronary urokinase followed by prolonged anticoagulation. Role of ruptured atheromatous plaque and adherent thrombus in acute myocardial infarction in vivo. *Circulation*, 78(6), 1335–1344.

Newman, W. P., 3rd, Freedman, D. S., Voors, A. W., Gard, P. D., Srinivasan, S. R., Cresanta, J. L., Williamson, G. D., Webber, L. S., & Berenson, G. S. (1986). Relation of serum lipoprotein levels and systolic blood pressure to early atherosclerosis. The Bogalusa Heart Study. *New England Journal of Medicine*, 314(3), 138–144.

Nissen, S. E., Gurley, J. C., Grines, C. L., Booth, D. C., McClure, R., Berk, M., Fischer, C., & DeMaria, A. N. (1991). Intravascular ultrasound assessment of lumen size and wall morphology in normal subjects and patients with coronary artery disease. *Circulation*, 84(3), 1087–1099.

Nobuyoshi, M., Tanaka, M., Nosaka, H., Kimura, T., Yokoi, H., Hamasaki, N., Kim, K., Shindo, T., & Kimura, K. (1991). Progression of coronary atherosclerosis: is coronary spasm related to progression? *Journal of the American College of Cardiology*, 18(4), 904–910.

O'Holleran, L. W., Kennelly, M. M., McClurken, M., & Johnson, J. M. (1987). Natural history of asymptomatic carotid plaque. Five year follow-up study. *American Journal of Surgery*, 154(6), 659–662.

Okura, H., Yoshida, K., Hozumi, T., Akasaka, T., & Yoshikawa, J. (1997). Planimetry and transthoracic two-dimensional echocardiography in noninvasive assessment of aortic valve area in patients with valvular aortic stenosis. *Journal of the American College of Cardiology*, 30(3), 753–759.

Ooshima, A. (1981). Collagen alpha B chain: increased proportion in human atherosclerosis. *Science*, 213(4508), 666–668.

Palinski, W., Rosenfeld, M. E., Yla-Herttuala, S., Gurtner, G. C., Socher, S. S., Butler, S. W., Parthasarathy, S., Carew, T. E., Steinberg, D., & Witztum, J. L. (1989). Low density lipoprotein undergoes oxidative modification in vivo. *Proceedings of the National Academy of Sciences of the USA*, 86(4), 1372–1376.

Parson, I., Mendler, P., & Downar, E. (1982). On-line cardiac mapping: an analog approach using video and multiplexing techniques. *American Journal of Physiology*, 242(4), H526–535.

Parthasarathy, N., Goldberg, I. J., Sivaram, P., Mulloy, B., Flory, D. M., & Wagner, W. D. (1994). Oligosaccharide sequences of endothelial cell surface heparan sulfate proteoglycan with affinity for lipoprotein lipase. *Journal of Biology and Chemistry*, 269(35), 22391–22396.

Rekhter, M. D., Zhang, K., Narayanan, A. S., Phan, S., Schork, M. A., & Gordon, D. (1993). Type I collagen gene expression in human atherosclerosis. Localization to specific plaque regions. *American Journal of Pathology*, 143(6), 1634–1648.

Richardson, P. D., Davies, M. J., & Born, G. V. (1989). Influence of plaque configuration and stress distribution on fissuring of coronary atherosclerotic plaques. *Lancet*, 2(8669), 941–944.

Rissanen, V. (1975). Coronary atherosclerosis in cases of coronary death as compared with that occurring in the populatiom. A study of a medico-legal autopsy series of coronary deaths and violent deaths. *Annals of Clinical Research*, 7(6), 412–425.

Robert, L., Jacob, M. P., Frances, C., Godeau, G., & Hornebeck, W. (1984). Interaction between elastin and elastases and its role in the aging of the arterial wall, skin and other connective tissues. A review. *Mechanisms of Ageing and Development*, 28(2–3), 155–166.

Rosenberg, R. D., Jordan, R. E., Favreau, L. V., & Lam, L. H. (1979). Highly active heparin species with multiple binding sites for antithrombin. *Biochem Biophys Res Commun*, 86(4), 1319–1324.

Rosenfeld, M. E., & Ross, R. (1990). Macrophage and smooth muscle cell proliferation in atherosclerotic lesions of WHHL and comparably hypercholesterolemic fat-fed rabbits. *Arteriosclerosis*, 10(5), 680–687.

Ross, R., Wight, T. N., Strandness, E., & Thiele, B. (1984). Human atherosclerosis. I. Cell constitution and characteristics of advanced lesions of the superficial femoral artery. *American Journal of Pathology*, 114(1), 79–93.

Salonen, J. T., Yla-Herttuala, S., Yamamoto, R., Butler, S., Korpela, H., Salonen, R., Nyyssonen, K., Palinski, W., & Witztum, J. L. (1992). Autoantibody against oxidised LDL and progression of carotid atherosclerosis. *Lancet*, 339(8798), 883–887.

Scanu, A. M. (1991). Lp(a) as a marker for coronary heart disease risk. *Clinical Cardiology*, 14(2 Suppl 1), I35–39.

Schmidt, A., Yoshida, K., & Buddecke, E. (1992). The antiproliferative activity of arterial heparan sulfate resides in domains enriched with 2-O-sulfated uronic acid residues. *Journal of Biology and Chemistry*, 267(27), 19242–19247.

Schmitz, G., & Muller, G. (1991). Structure and function of lamellar bodies, lipid-protein complexes involved in storage and secretion of cellular lipids. *Journal of Lipid Research*, 32(10), 1539–1570.

Senior, R. M., Griffin, G. L., & Mecham, R. P. (1980). Chemotactic activity of elastin-derived peptides. *Journal of Clinical Investigation*, 66(4), 859–862.

Small, D. M. (1988). George Lyman Duff memorial lecture. Progression and regression of atherosclerotic lesions. Insights from lipid physical biochemistry. *Arteriosclerosis*, 8(2), 103–129.

Stary, H. C. (1987). Macrophages, macrophage foam cells, and eccentric intimal thickening in the coronary arteries of young children. *Atherosclerosis*, 64(2–3), 91–108.

Stary, H. C. (1989). Evolution and progression of atherosclerotic lesions in coronary arteries of children and young adults. *Arteriosclerosis*, 9(1 Suppl), I19–32.

Stary, H. C. (1990). The sequence of cell and matrix changes in atherosclerotic lesions of coronary arteries in the first forty years of life. *European Heart Journal*, 11 Suppl E, 3–19.

Stary, H. C. (1992). Composition and classification of human atherosclerotic lesions. *Virchows Arch A Pathol Anat Histopathol*, 421(4), 277–290.

Stary, H. C. (1994). Changes in components and structure of atherosclerotic lesions developing from childhood to middle age in coronary arteries. *Basic Research in Cardiology*, 89 Suppl 1, 17–32.

Stary, H. C. (2000). Natural history and histological classification of atherosclerotic lesions: an update. *Arterioscler Thromb Vasc Biol*, 20(5), 1177–1178.

Stary, H. C., Blankenhorn, D. H., Chandler, A. B., Glagov, S., Insull, W., Jr., Richardson, M., Rosenfeld, M. E., Schaffer, S. A., Schwartz, C. J., Wagner, W. D., et al. (1992). A definition of the intima of human arteries and of its atherosclerosis-prone regions. A report from the Committee on Vascular Lesions of the Council on Arteriosclerosis, American Heart Association. *Circulation*, 85(1), 391–405.

Stary, H. C., Chandler, A. B., Glagov, S., Guyton, J. R., Insull, W., Jr., Rosenfeld, M. E., Schaffer, S. A., Schwartz, C. J., Wagner, W. D., & Wissler, R. W. (1994). A definition of initial, fatty streak, and intermediate lesions of atherosclerosis. A report from the Committee on Vascular Lesions of the Council on Arteriosclerosis, American Heart Association. *Circulation*, 89(5), 2462–2478.

Steinberg, D., & Witztum, J. L. (1990). Lipoproteins and atherogenesis. Current concepts. *JAMA*, 264(23), 3047–3052.

Stenn, K. S., Madri, J. A., & Roll, F. J. (1979). Migrating epidermis produces AB2 collagen and requires continual collagen synthesis for movement. *Nature*, 277(5693), 229–232.

Stevens, R. L., Colombo, M., Gonzales, J. J., Hollander, W., & Schmid, K. (1976). The glycosaminoglycans of the human artery and their changes in atherosclerosis. *Journal of Clinical Investigation*, 58(2), 470–481.

Strong, J. P., & McGill, H. C., Jr. (1969). The pediatric aspects of atherosclerosis. *Journal of Atheroscler Research*, 9(3), 251–265.

Taeymans, Y., Theroux, P., Lesperance, J., & Waters, D. (1992). Quantitative angiographic morphology of the coronary artery lesions at risk of thrombotic occlusion. *Circulation*, 85(1), 78–85.

Tammi, M., Seppala, P. O., Lehtonen, A., & Mottonen, M. (1978). Connective tissue components in normal and atherosclerotic human coronary arteries. *Atherosclerosis*, 29(2), 191–194.

Tell, G. S., Mittelmark, M. B., & Vellar, O. D. (1985). Cholesterol, high density lipoprotein cholesterol and triglycerides during puberty: the Oslo Youth Study. *American Journal of Epidemiology*, 122(5), 750–761.

Thomas, A. C., Davies, M. J., Dilly, S., Dilly, N., & Franc, F. (1986). Potential errors in the estimation of coronary arterial stenosis from clinical arteriography with reference to the shape of the coronary arterial lumen. *British Heart Journal*, 55(2), 129–139.

Tracy, R. E., Devaney, K., & Kissling, G. (1985). Characteristics of the plaque under a coronary thrombus. *Virchows Arch A Pathol Anat Histopathol*, 405(4), 411–427.

Turnbull, J. E., Fernig, D. G., Ke, Y., Wilkinson, M. C., & Gallagher, J. T. (1992). Identification of the basic fibroblast growth factor binding sequence in fibroblast heparan sulfate. *Journal of Biology and Chemistry*, 267(15), 10337–10341.

Tyrrell, D. J., Ishihara, M., Rao, N., Horne, A., Kiefer, M. C., Stauber, G. B., Lam, L. H., & Stack, R. J. (1993). Structure and biological activities of a heparin-derived hexasaccharide with high affinity for basic fibroblast growth factor. *Journal of Biology and Chemistry*, 268(7), 4684–4689.

Urry, D. W. (1971). Neutral sites for calcium ion binding to elastin and collagen: a charge neutralization theory for calcification and its relationship to atherosclerosis. *Proceedings of the National Academy of Sciences of the USA*, 68(4), 810–814.

van der Wal, A. C., Becker, A. E., van der Loos, C. M., & Das, P. K. (1994). Site of intimal rupture or erosion of thrombosed coronary atherosclerotic plaques is characterized by an inflammatory process irrespective of the dominant plaque morphology. *Circulation*, 89(1), 36–44.

Viikari, J., Akerblom, H. K., Nikkari, T., Seppanen, A., Uhari, M., Pesonen, E., Dahl, M., Lahde, P. L., Pietikainen, M., & Suoninen, P. (1985). Atherosclerosis precursors in Finnish children and adolescents. IV. Serum lipids in newborns, children and adolescents. *Acta Paediatr Scand Suppl*, 318, 103–109.

Wagner, W. D., & Salisbury, B. G. (1978). Aortic total glycosaminoglycan and dermatan sulfate changes in atherosclerotic rhesus monkeys. *Laboratory Investigation*, 39(4), 322–328.

Weingand, K. W., Clarkson, T. B., Adams, M. R., & Bostrom, A. D. (1986). Effects of age and/or puberty on coronary artery atherosclerosis in cynomolgus monkeys. *Atherosclerosis*, 62(2), 137–144.

Zarins, C. K., Weisenberg, E., Kolettis, G., Stankunavicius, R., & Glagov, S. (1988). Differential enlargement of artery segments in response to enlarging atherosclerotic plaques. *Journal of Vascular Surgery*, 7(3), 386–394.

Hematopoiesis, Coagulation, and Bleeding

NANCY MUNRO

The physiological functions of blood include nutrition, oxygenation, respiration, and excretion. These functions are accomplished by the various components of blood. Approximately 55% of blood volume is composed of plasma, which is a transport medium for ions, proteins, hormones, and end products of cellular metabolism. The most important ions carried in the plasma are sodium, potassium, chloride, hydrogen, magnesium, and calcium. Examples of proteins transported in the plasma are immunoglobulins and the coagulation proteins. Formed elements or cells including red blood cells (RBC; erythrocytes), white blood cells (WBC; leukocytes), and platelets (thrombocytes) constitute the other 45% of blood volume. Erythrocytes transport uoxygen to the tissues and carbon dioxide to the lungs for excretion. Leukocytes protect against infection and play a major role in the inflammatory process. Thrombocytes, along with coagulation proteins, protect against blood loss through the formation of blood clots (Owen & Webster, 1998).

Because these functions are vital, a significant blood loss has devastating consequences for all body tissues. Protection against such blood losses and potential exsanguination from injuries is achieved by a complex series of events leading to hemostasis. The endothelium of the vasculature plays a vital role in the coagulation process and is now considered an organ by the Margaux III Conference on Critical Illness: The Endothelium: An Under-recognized Organ in Critical Illness (Dhainaut et al., 2002). The endothelial cell participates by releasing mediators that effect coagulation and the role of the vessel's participation in hemostasis. This system is balanced by the equally complex mechanism of fibrinolysis, which dissolves clots. Normal blood flow through the vasculature is dependent in part on the balance of these two systems, hemostasis and fibrinolysis. Recent research has also revealed that there is a link between coagulation and the inflammatory process that has caused the scientific community to re-examine the process of atherosclerosis (Libby, 2002). Knowledge of these normal processes is important as a basis for understanding the many alterations that may occur as a result of disease states or drug administration

HEMATOPOIETIC CELLS

Hematopoiesis, or the production of blood cells, occurs primarily in the bone marrow. The liver, spleen, lymph nodes, and thymus are involved in hematopoiesis during embryonic life, but after birth extramedullary (outside the bone marrow) hematopoiesis occurs only during abnormal circumstances. If it occurs at all after birth, extramedullary hematopoiesis occurs mainly in the liver and spleen. The pluripotent hematopoietic stem cell resides mainly in the bone marrow and in small numbers in the peripheral blood. It is the source of all the types of blood cells: red blood cells (RBC), white blood cells (WBC), and platelets.

The stem cell is an immature (undifferentiated) cell that has the capacity to reproduce itself and to mature (differentiate) into any of the different types of blood cells. As the stem cell divides and matures, it differentiates into one of two committed cell lines: lymphoid or myeloid. The committed lymphoid cells eventually mature into T or B lymphocytes. The committed myeloid stem cell develops into what is called a colony-forming unit granulocyte, erythrocyte, macrophage, megakaryocyte (CFU-GEMM) (Shoemaker et al., 2000). This colony-forming unit, in turn, has the potential to develop along discrete cell lines: the erythroid line (leading to the formation of RBC), the granulocyte-monocyte line (leading to the formation of the phagocytic WBC), the megakaryocyte line (leading to the formation of platelets), the eosinophil line, and the basophil line. As the various types of blood cells mature, they are released into the peripheral circulation. Figure 8-1 shows a model for hematopoietic cell differentiation and the growth factors involved at the various stages of differentiation. Colony-stimulating factors (CSF) are cell-derived glycoproteins that are released by various cells including endothelial cells and will influence the development and function of the stem cell at various stages of maturation. Table 8-1 lists most of the known hematopoietic growth factors and the type of cell they are thought to stimulate.

Red Blood Cells

The major role of the RBC is respiration, which is the exchange of gases. The mature RBC is a biconcave disc filled with hemoglobin but does not have a nucleus. The lack of a nucleus allows the RBC to change shape and facilitates movement through small capillary beds. Heme, the iron-containing pigment, is the actual oxygen-transporting portion of the hemoglobin molecule. Oxygen diffuses from the alveoli into the alveolar capillaries and binds to each of 4 to 5 sites on the heme portion of hemoglobin. One gram of hemoglobin can carry 1.34 to 1.36 milliliters of oxygen. The remarkable oxygen-binding capacities of the RBC are influenced by three factors that affect the oxyhemoglobin dissociation curve: pH, temperature, and the amount of 2,3 diphosphogylcerate (2,3 DPG) (see Chapter 3). Tissue metabolism produces carbon dioxide as a waste product that is also transported from the tissues by the RBC. Carbon dioxide diffuses into the RBC and combines with water to form carbonic acid that further dissociates to the hydrogen and bicarbonate ions. The bicarbonate ion is inactivated when combined with hydrogen ions to again form water and carbon dioxide that is eliminated at the alveoli.

All tissues of the body require a constant supply of oxygen to survive. The RBC binds oxygen at the alveolar level and transports it to the tissues that will use oxygen, depending on multiple factors. The correct number of RBC is crucial. If the number of RBC is too low (anemia), the oxygen-carrying

Table 8–1 ■ HEMATOPOIETIC GROWTH FACTORS AND SOME OF THEIR CHARACTERISTICS

Factor*	Cells Stimulated
M-CSF	Monocytes
GM-CSF	All granulocytes, megakaryocytes, erythrocytes, and stem cells
G-CSF	Granulocytes, macrophages, endothelial cells
IL-3	Granulocytes, erythroid cells, multipotential progenitors
IL-4	B cells, T cells
IL-5	B cells, CFU-Eo
IL-6	B cells, T cells, CFU-GEMM, CFU-GM, BFU-E, macrophages, neural cells, hepatocytes
IL-7	B cells
IL-8	T cells, neutrophils
IL-9	BFU-E, CFU-GEMM
IL-11	B, T cells, CFU-GEMM, macrophages
Erythropoietin	CFU-E, BFU-E
c-kit ligand	Primitive progenitors ("stem cell factor")

*CSF, colony-stimulating factor; GM, granulocyte-macrophage; IL, interleukin; CFU, colony-forming unit; Eo, eosinophil; BFU, burst-forming unit; E, erythrocyte; GEMM, granulocytes, erythrocytes, macrophages, megakaryocytes.
Adapted from Rothstein, G. (1993). Origin and development of the blood and blood-forming tissues. In Lee, G.R., Bithell, T.C., Foerster, J., et al. (Eds.), *Wintrobe's clinical hematology* (9th ed., p. 53). Philadelphia: Lea & Febiger.

capacity is compromised. Too many RBC (polycythemia) increase the viscosity of the blood and thus slow the flow to the tissues. The rate of bone marrow stem cell differentiation into

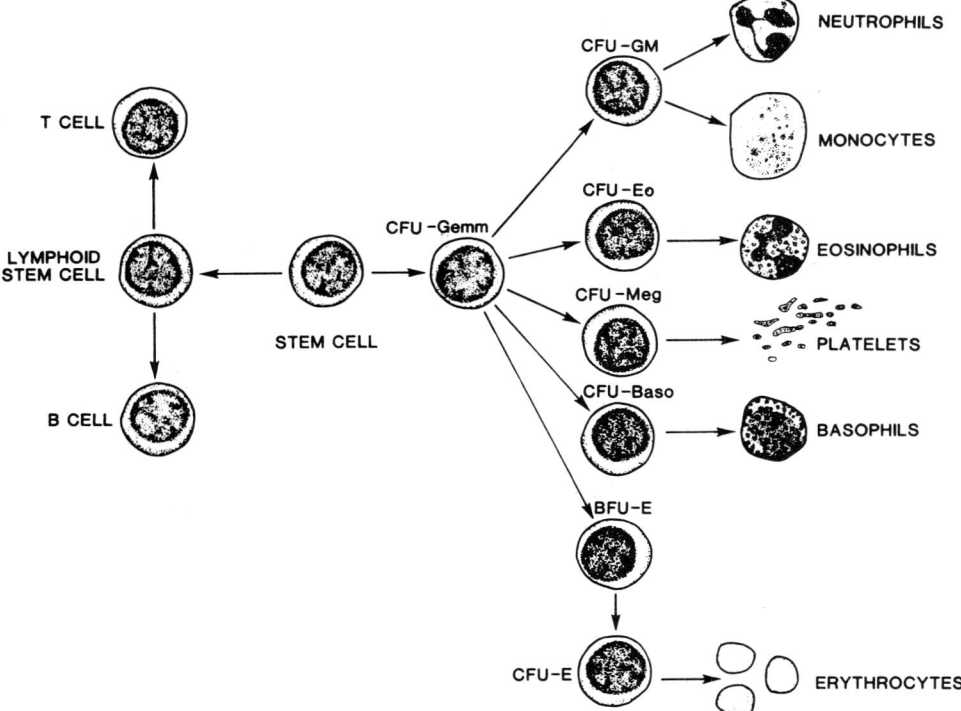

■ **Figure 8–1.** Diagram of hematopoiesis. The various progenitors are schematically represented. CFU-GEMM, multipotential progenitor for granulocytes, erythrocytes, macrophages, megakaryocytes; CFU-GM, progenitor for neutrophils and monocytes; CFU-Eo, progenitor for eosinophils; CFU-Meg, progenitor for megakaryocytes; CFU-Baso, progenitor for basophils; BFU-E, most primitive, committed progenitor for erythroid line; GFU-E more mature progenitor for erythroid line. (From Rothstein, G. [1993] Origin and development of the blood and blood forming tissues. In G. R. Lee, T. C. Bithel, J. Foerster, et al. [Eds.], *Wintrobe's clinical hematology* [9th ed., p. 51.]. Philadelphia: Lea & Febiger.)

erythrocytes is primarily controlled by erythropoietin. Most of this hormone is produced by the kidney. The creation of RBC is influenced by the oxygen content of the blood as sensed by the kidneys. Production also requires necessary substrates including vitamin B_{12}, vitamin B_6, folic acid, and iron. The vitamins and folic acid are obtained from dietary sources, as is iron. However, most iron is gained through the recycling of the RBC in the spleen. RBC production is increased at times of blood loss, at high altitude, and in pulmonary diseases that affect the transport of oxygen from the lungs to the blood. It takes approximately 3 to 5 days for RBC to mature in the marrow and be released into the peripheral circulation. RBCs live approximately 120 days, at which time they are recycled by the spleen.

White Blood Cells

White blood cells can be divided into two major categories: phagocytes and lymphocytes. The primary role of phagocytes is to locate and kill invading microorganisms or foreign antigens. The primary role of lymphocytes is to initiate and direct the immune response including the manufacture of antibodies. White blood cells travel throughout the body and will migrate into different tissues depending on chemical mediators that signal the cells. Phagocytes perform their role primarily out in the tissues, where they travel toward the site of an inflammation (chemotaxis) and kill microbes by engulfing them (phagocytosis). Many substances, including complement fragments and bacterial products, stimulate this chemotactic migration. Phagocytosis is an active process that uses energy derived from anaerobic glycolysis. Phagocytic cells are divided into two subgroups: granulocytes (granular substances within the cell after staining) and monocytes. The granulocytes include neutrophils ("polys"), basophils, and eosinophils. Neutrophils compose 60% to 70% of all WBC. Neutrophil maturation in the marrow takes 7 to 10 days. Their main function is to find and kill bacteria, especially resident microorganisms such as staphylococci and Gram-negative enteric flora (Jerius, 1998). They also play an important role in acute inflammatory processes. Neutrophils are one of the first phagocytic cells to appear at the site of an acute inflammation. During severe inflammatory reactions, neutrophils can actually cause damage to surrounding tissues by releasing proteolytic enzymes and oxygen-free radicals. Once in the bloodstream, some of the neutrophils freely circulate while others linger along the blood vessel wall, which is called margination. Substances emanating from an injury or from an organism make the blood vessel wall sticky, so that the marginated neutrophils adhere to the vessel walls. The neutrophil releases substances that allow the endothelial cells to separate and permit the neutrophil to crawl into the connective tissue (diapedesis). The neutrophil migrates to the area of injury through chemotaxis. The migration of neutrophils to the tissues takes place rapidly, within 12 hours on entering the bloodstream. Once in the bloodstream, the neutrophil must be able to differentiate cells or substances that are foreign. Opsonization is a process in which molecules in the plasma coat the microorganism, making it more recognizable to the neutrophil.

Esosinophils and basophils are WBC that have specific functions that are also important in the defense of the body. Eosinophils develop in the marrow along the same maturation process as neutrophils. They make up only approximately 4% of a normal WBC count. Eosinophils have been postulated to play a defensive role against parasites and allergic reactions. Basophils account for only 0.5% to 1% of the total WBC count. The role of the basophil is not well clarified, but these cells are known to play a part in immediate hypersensitivity reactions. Basophils release histamine when stimulated, which in turn results in the signs and symptoms of allergic reaction such as rhinitis, bronchospasm, urticaria, angioedema, and anaphylaxis. The relationship between basophils and mast cells, similar cells that reside in tissues, is not clearly understood.

Agranular leukocytes are WBC without granular substances within the cells after staining. Monocytes and lymphocytes are agranular leukocytes. Monocytes constitute 4% to 8% of the total WBC count. Within 24 to 36 hours of entering the circulation, they migrate into the tissues where they undergo further maturation and are called macrophages. Hepatic Kupffer cells, alveolar macrophages, and peritoneal macrophages are examples of tissue macrophages. Once lodged in their target organ, macrophages can live for up to 60 days. In the bloodstream, monocytes have similar functions to the neutrophil. However, in addition, monocytes and macrophages play a crucial role in recognizing foreign invaders and presenting foreign antigens to lymphocytes, thus stimulating the immune response. They are important in killing bacteria, protozoa, cells infected with viruses, and tumor cells. In addition to their phagocytic activity, macrophages secrete biologically active products, including cytokines that modulate the immune response.

Lymphocytes are essential components of the immune system. They recognize and are instrumental in the elimination of foreign proteins, pathogens, and tumor cells. Lymphocytes control the intensity and specificity of the immune response. There are two general types of lymphocytes, T lymphocytes (or T cells), which provide cell-mediated and B lymphocytes (B cells), which produce the antibodies of humoral immunity. Stem cell differentiation for the production of lymphocytes occurs in the bone marrow. During fetal life, lymphocytes that will become T cells migrate to the thymus gland and mature into T cells ready to participate in cell-mediated immune reactions. It is in the thymus that T cells learn to differentiate self from nonself. There are four separate subsets of T cells: helper T cells, suppressor T cells, cytotoxic T cells, and memory T cells. Cell-mediated activities are of great importance in delayed hypersensitivity reactions; graft rejection; graft-versus-host disease; and in defense against fungal, protozoal, and most viral infections. Another important function of T cells is to regulate immune activities through the secretion of lymphokines.

B lymphocytes mature into cells that respond to stimulation from foreign proteins by differentiating into memory cells and plasma cells. The plasma cells produce specific antibodies that inactivate or destroy foreign proteins and pathogens. These antibodies are particularly effective against bacterial infections, especially encapsulated bacteria, such as pneumococci, streptococci, meningococci, and hemophilus influenzae, as well as certain viruses. The helper cells of the T cells stimulate B cells to produce antibodies. Another subset of T cells, the suppressor cells help slow the production of antibodies and prevent uncontrolled immune reactions. Memory B and T cells impart immunologic memory. These cells respond to repeated exposures

Table 8–2 ■ WHITE BLOOD CELLS

Name	Function
White blood cell (WBC) or leukocyte	Combat pathogens and other foreign substances that enter the body
Granular Leukocytes	
Neutrophils	Phagocytosis or the destruction of bacteria with lysozyme, defensins and strong oxidants
Eosinophils	Combat the effects of histamine in allergic reactions, phagocytize antigen-antibody complexes
Basophils	Liberate heparin, histamine and serotonin in allergic reactions that intensify the overall inflammatory response
Agranular Leukocytes	
Lymphocytes (T cells, B cells, natural killer cells)	Mediate immune responses including antigen–antibody reactions
Monocytes	Phagocytosis after transforming into macrophages

Adapted from Tortora, G. & Grabowski, S. (2003). *Principles of anatomy and physiology.* New York: John Wiley & Sons, Inc.

to specific antigens with greater efficiency than during the first exposure. This memory provides the rationale for vaccinations. Natural killer cells, another subset of lymphocytes, kill tumor cells and cells infected by viruses. They play an important role in tumor surveillance. The activities of phagocytes and immune cells overlap in numerous mutually beneficial ways. For example, immune cells often participate in chronic inflammatory reactions. Conversely, engulfment of foreign protein by macrophages is a preparatory step leading to antibody production. Table 8-2 summarizes the WBC and their function.

Because blood cells have a limited lifespan, they need to be replaced constantly. Usually, the number of cells produced is fairly constant, but depending on environmental stimuli such as bleeding, infection, or inflammation various cells may be needed in larger than normal quantities at times. Thus, each of these cell lines is regulated by cytokines that influence the rate of growth and differentiation of the stem cells in the marrow. Cytokines are proteins that are made by cells of the immune system and regulate the immune response. Some examples of cytokines are granulocyte-macrophage colony-stimulating factor (GM-CSF), which stimulates the growth of granulocytes and macrophages, and interleukin-3 (IL-3), which stimulates the stem cell. Cytokines also stimulate the function of mature immune cells.

Platelets

Platelets are small cell fragments that are produced by the disintegration of megakaryocytes in the bone marrow, producing several thousand platelets that are released into the circulation. They are tiny, disc-shaped fragments that are capable of changing shape and have a high metabolic rate. It takes approximately 5 days for a stem cell to differentiate along the megakaryocyte line and produce platelets. Under normal circumstances, platelets circulate in the bloodstream for approximately 10 days. The production of platelets is regulated by thrombopoietin, which is a humoral hormone-like substance. Platelets are also called

thrombocytes, which means *clot cell.* They play a major role in hemostasis by adhering to a damaged blood vessel wall and aggregating together to form a mechanical barrier to the flow of blood thereby preventing blood loss. Platelets will then release various mediators to attract other cells and components to the site so that fibrin formation can start. There are three storage granules in the platelets: alpha granules, dense bodies, and lysomes. Alpha granules contain and release fibrinogen. Dense bodies release adenine nucleotides, serotonin, and platelet factor 4 (PF-4). Lysomes contain degradative acid hydrolases (Owen & Webster, 1998). Platelets are sequestered in the spleen and are released as needed to combat bleeding. Their function is vital to the coagulation process, so much so that many cardiac interventions are now aimed at disabling platelet function.

Coagulation Factors

The major component of blood, plasma, contains many particles including proteins (clotting factors) that are involved in coagulation. To standardize the identification of these proteins, an international committee assigned a nomenclature for these proteins using Roman numerals listed in order of their discovery. However, the order does not refer to the sequence of reactions in the coagulation cascade. A lowercase "a" is also used to indicate the activated form of a clotting factor. Table 8-3 lists these clotting factors. The liver plays a significant role in maintaining adequate amounts of these clotting factors, because it is the primary site of protein synthesis. Tissue thromboplastin, or tissue factor (III), is an exception that can be found in most body tissues, especially around vessels and organs. Antihemophilic factor (VIII) is a factor that is synthesized in the endothelial cells. It is also important to recognize that there are multiple enzymes and mediators that play key roles in the activation of these clotting factors. The environment must be optimal for this intricate cascade to function properly. All these proteins

Table 8–3 ■ BLOOD COAGULATION PROTEINS

Number	Name(s)
I	Fibrinogen
II	Prothrombin
III	Tissue factor (thromboplastin)
IV	Calcium ions
V	Proaccelerin, labile factor, or accelerator globulin (AcG)
VII	Serum prothrombin conversion accelerator (SPCA), stable factor, or proconvertin
VIII	Antihemophilic factor (AHF), antihemophilic factor A, or antimophilic globulin (AHG)
IX	Christmas factor, plasma thromboplastin component (PTC), or anthemophilic factor B
X	Stuart factor, Prower factor, or thrombokinase
XI	Plasma thromboplastin antecedent (PTA) or antihemophilic factor C
XII	Hageman factor, glass factor, contact factor, or antihemophilic factor D
XIII	Fibrin-stabilizing factor (FSF)

Adapted from Tortora, G. & Grabowski, S. (2003). *Principles of anatomy and physiology.* New York: John Wiley & Sons, Inc.

require a very specific chemical environment to function and are dependent on proper pH and temperature for the reactions to occur. Synthesis of factors II, VII, IX, and X requires vitamin K to be present, and these are known as vitamin K-dependent factors. It is also important to recognize that calcium is also a coagulation factor whose role can be underestimated. To balance the coagulation process, there are also a number of proteins and systems that will inhibit coagulation including antithrombin III, proteins C and S, as well as components of the fibrinolytic cascade. The interaction of all these proteins in a chemical sequence will produce a clot to repair blood vessels and then dissolve the clot so that normal flow can be restored.

HEMOSTASIS

The normal hemostatic system is designed to protect against bleeding from injured blood vessels. Hemostasis is usually accomplished by a sequence of interrelated processes involving blood vessels and endothelial activity, platelets, and coagulation proteins. This complex system is highly regulated to ensure that clotting occurs only at a site of injury and only as long as the integrity of the vessel is compromised. The process of hemostasis consists of several components: (1) blood vessel spasm; (2) formation of a platelet plug; (3) contact between damaged blood vessel, blood platelet, and coagulation proteins; (4) development of a blood clot around the injury; and (5) fibrinolytic removal of excess hemostatic material to reestablish vascular integrity (Turgeon, 1999). Coagulation proteins comprise the coagulation cascade, which consists of three components: the intrinsic pathway (vascular trauma), the extrinsic pathway (tissue trauma), and the common pathway leading to fibrin formation. The clotting processes are balanced by the complex mechanism of fibrinolysis, which breaks-down clots and maintains or re-establishes blood flow once the vessel damage has healed. The balance between these two mechanisms and their activators and inhibitors is vital. An imbalance in one direction leads to excessive bleeding, whereas an imbalance in the other direction leads to excessive clotting. The following sections present the normal sequence of coagulation and fibrinolysis, as well as selected coagulation disorders most commonly associated with the patient experiencing cardiovascular disease.

Vascular Spasm

The sympathetic nervous system is automatically stimulated when a blood vessel is injured. Epinephrine and norepinephrine are released causing contraction of the vascular smooth muscle and vasoconstriction. Endothelin I, which is a peptide produced by the endothelial cell, angiotensin II, and vasoconstrictor prostaglandins are additional agents that contribute to vasoconstriction (Turgeon, 1999). The stenosis of smaller vessels, i.e., venules and arterioles, may be sufficient to decrease blood flow and close disrupted capillaries. Larger vessels may require longer periods of more intense vasoconstriction to assist with hemostasis but may ultimately require surgical intervention.

Role of the Endothelium in Hemostasis

The endothelial cell was once thought to be inert and have no specific role in maintaining vascular integrity. Research over the years has proven this hypothesis to be incorrect. The endothelial cell is a vital component of normal homeostasis. In normal conditions, the endothelium surface is intact and there is minimal interaction with platelets or the coagulation proteins. The function of the endothelium is to promote blood flow. The endothelial cell inhibits blood coagulation by: (1) expressing thrombomodulin, a clotting enzyme that binds thrombin; (2) changing the specificity of thrombomodulin from fibrin to protein C, which blocks the ability to convert fibrinogen to fibrin; (3) using proteoglycans on their surfaces to bind and potentiate the coagulation inhibitors antithrombin III and tissue factor pathway inhibitor (TFPI); (4) releasing small amounts of plasminogen activator tissue-type plasminogen activator (tPA); (5) inhibiting platelet aggregation by producing prostacyclin and nitric oxide (NO), which vasodilates the microcirculation; and (6) inhibiting adherence of peripheral blood cells (Hack & Zeerleder, 2001). These interactions maintain the anticoagulant properties of the endothelium by keeping platelets inactive and inhibiting key coagulation proteins such as tissue factor and thrombin.

However, once the endothelial surface is disrupted by various factors including physical injury or circulating mediators, it will develop procoagulant properties. When the endothelium is stimulated by inflammatory cytokines such as interleukin (IL) ILα, ILβ, or tumor necrosis factor (TNF) α, it is referred to as activated endothelium. Once the subendothelial connective tissue is exposed and activated, it will lose thrombomodulin and heparin sulfate and begin to synthesize tissue factor (factor III). Factor III interacts with factor VII to start the extrinsic pathway. Therefore, protein C is not activated and the action of clotting inhibitor systems will be lost. This activation of the cascade will further incite the endothelial cell to produce more inflammatory mediators (cytokines and chemokines) that will start the expression of adhesion molecules. Leukocytes will adhere to the endothelial cell and become activated by the production of leukocyte agonists such as platelet activating factor (PAF) (Hack & Zeerleder, 2001). Platelets are now attracted to the site and augment the coagulation process.

Platelet Phase

The platelet phase refers to the formation of a soft mass of aggregated platelets that provides a temporary patch over the injured vessel. Almost immediately after vascular injury, platelets begin to adhere to the exposed subendothelial basement membrane and collagen fibers. Adherent platelets release adenosine diphosphate (ADP), which causes platelets to change from their normal disc shape into a spherical form with pseudopods that attach along the surface and allow platelets to clump together (Turgeon, 1999). During activation, the platelets become sticky when bridges formed by fibrinogen in the presence of calcium cause platelets to adhere to each other, increasing the size of the platelet plug. ADP and collagen also trigger formation of arachidonic acid from phospholipids in the platelet membrane. This acid leads to the formation of thromboxane A_2, a substance that induces further platelet aggregation. Thromboxane A_2 causes conformational changes in glycoprotein IIb/IIIa, a receptor on the platelet surface, which exposes fibrinogen binding sites. Fibrinogen builds bridges to adjacent platelets, a process called platelet adhesion, which advances platelet aggregation. When these aggregates are reinforced with fibrin, they are referred to as a thrombus (Turgeon, 1999). Ultimately, aggregated platelets plug the injured vessel.

Coagulation Cascade

The final phase of hemostasis is the formation of a fibrin blood clot. The coagulation process is most commonly viewed as a series of enzymatic reactions in which clotting factors are sequentially activated. This process is known as the coagulation cascade. The clotting factors are all present in the circulating blood in their inactive form until a stimulus for clot formation occurs. Twelve different substances have been officially designated as clotting factors (see Table 8-3). As studied in the laboratory, the coagulation process can be initiated by two different pathways: the extrinsic pathway and the intrinsic pathway. Although differentiating between them is helpful for understanding pathologic mechanisms, medication actions, and coagulation tests, these two pathways are functionally inseparable in vivo. The extrinsic pathway, whose major mediators are rapidly inactivated, is the primary initiator of the clotting cascade. The intrinsic pathway, whose major mediators are more slowly degraded, is thought to be important for maintenance and amplification of the clotting cascade. Both extrinsic and intrinsic mechanisms eventually lead to the activation of factor X, with the remaining steps of the coagulation sequence being identical and referred to as the common pathway. The sequence of the coagulation process is shown in Figure 8-2.

Extrinsic Pathway

The extrinsic pathway is initiated by the combination of tissue factor with factor VIIa and ionized calcium, which together convert factor X to its activated form, factor Xa. The function of the extrinsic pathway is tested in the laboratory by the prothrombin time (PT). Tissue factor, also called tissue thromboplastin (formerly factor III), is a membrane glycoprotein that is particularly prevalent in tissues, where it plays a vital role in the prevention of hemorrhage. Tissue factor is exposed to and binds to factor VII, which is activated to factor VIIa. Factor VIIa is a potent enzyme that activates factor X to Xa. The reactions from this step on are referred to as the common pathway. Calcium plays a significant role in each step leading to the formation of thrombin (Turgeon, 1999).

Intrinsic Pathway

Because the intrinsic pathway is initiated by a separate set of factors that is not degraded by rapid-acting inhibitors, the process may proceed more slowly and the results may last longer and be more pronounced than those initiated by the extrinsic pathway. The function of the intrinsic pathway is commonly analyzed by the partial thromboplastin time (PTT). Intrinsic activation is initiated when blood is exposed to a negatively charged surface, such as the site of blood vessel injury. The negative charge, along with

collagen and endotoxin, attracts factor XII, which binds to the surface and autoactivates to factor XIIa. Factor XIIa converts prekallikrein to kallikrein, which in turn converts circulating factor XII to its activated form, XIIa. Both the activated form of factor XII and kallikrein catalyze the activation of factor XI into XIa. Factor XIa, together with ionized calcium, cleaves factor IX at two sites to produce factor IXa. Factor IXa, together with factor VIII, phospholipid, and ionized calcium convert factor X to its activated form, factor Xa. As discussed previously, factor X can also be activated through the extrinsic pathway. From here, the coagulation process proceeds along the common pathway, regardless of whether initiation was extrinsic or intrinsic (Turgeon, 1999).

Common Pathway and Fibrin Formation

The final common sequence involves the combination of factors Xa and V, phospholipid, and ionized calcium into a complex that converts prothrombin to thrombin. The thrombin formed subsequently cleaves the long molecule fibrinogen to fibrin. The fibrin monomer is able to polymerize spontaneously to form a loose web of fibers that is capable of stopping the bleeding in small and medium-sized arteries and veins. The fibrin clot is eventually stabilized and thickened by the action of factor XIII, which is activated by the presence of ionized calcium and thrombin. Fibrin forms a loose covering over the injured area and reinforces the platelet plug. After a short period of time, the clot begins to retract. This process is thought to be a reaction of the platelets, which send out cytoplasmic processes that attach to the fibrin and pull the fibers closer (Turgeon, 1999). Plasminogen and other components of the fibrinolytic mechanism are incorporated into the fibrin clot as it solidifies.

Fibrinolysis

The removal of clots when the site of vessel injury has healed is as important as the formation of the clot itself. Fibrinolysis is the physiological process that removes insoluble fibrin deposits by enzymatic digestion of the stabilized fibrin polymers (Turgeon, 1999). The process of fibrinolysis reestablishes blood flow. Plasmin dissolves clots by digesting fibrin and fibrinogen using hydrolysis. Plasminogen is a glycoprotein and an inactive form of plasmin, which is synthesized by the liver. It is activated to plasmin by the activity of proteolytic enzymes, the kinases that cleave a bond on the plasminogen molecule. Activators of plasminogen are found in various tissues, blood, and urine. The best-known endogenous activators are tissue plasminogen activator (tPA) and urokinase, which is a urinary activator of plasminogen. Some exogenous plasminogen activators are related to types of bacteria such as streptokinase and staphylokinase (Turgeon, 1999). Drugs have been developed to mimic the activity of these kinases to dissolve clots. Fragments of the fibrin clot, known as fibrin degradation products (FDP), are released into the circulation as the clot is broken down. FDP are potent inhibitors of coagulation. They act by binding to thrombin, thus inhibiting its action, and by interfering with the binding of fibrin threads to form the fibrin clot. Except in some abnormal situations, FDP are present in such small numbers that their anticoagulant effect is not clinically

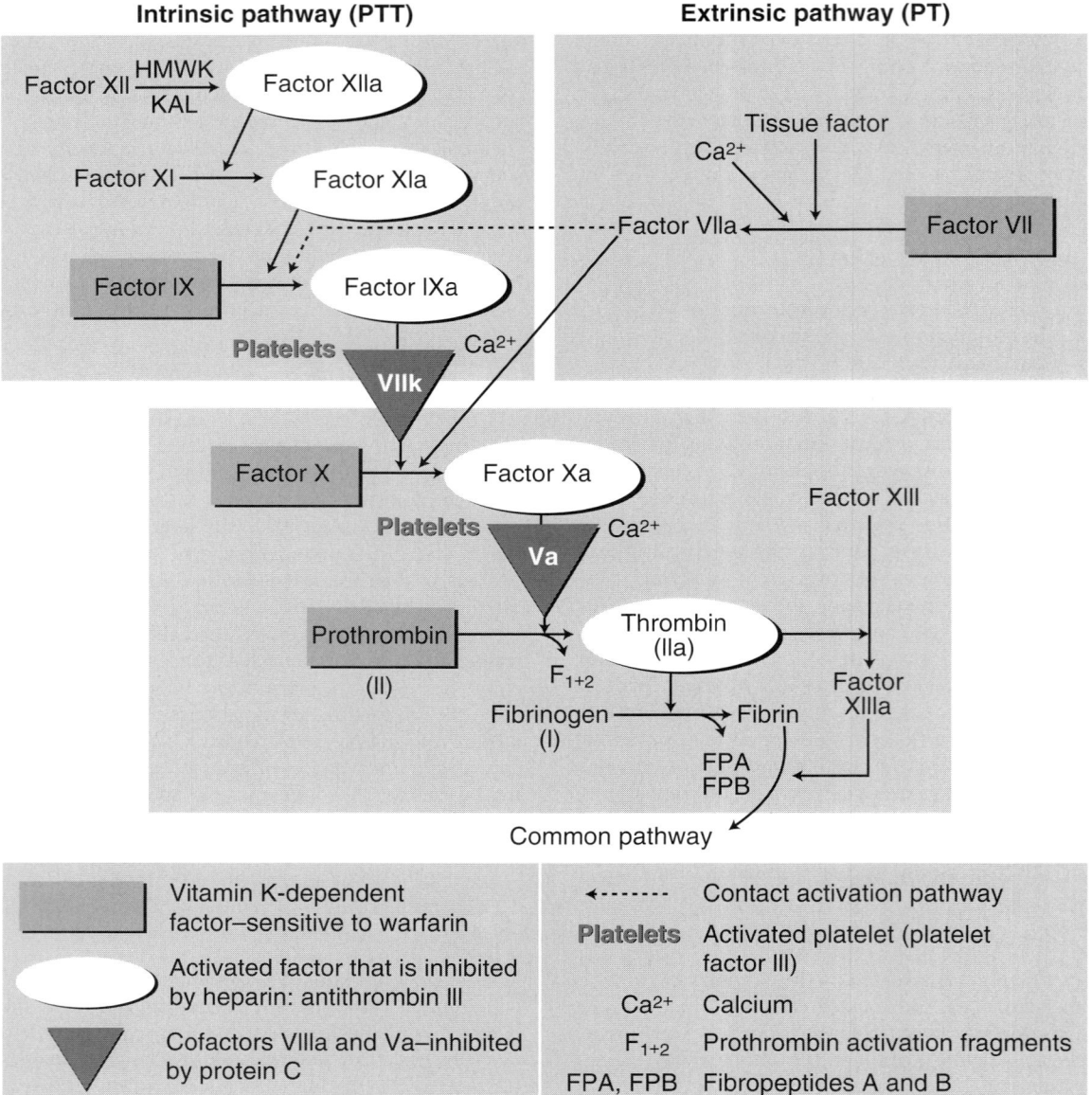

Intrinsic pathway (PTT)

Extrinsic pathway (PT)

Vitamin K-dependent
factor–sensitive to warfarin

Activated factor that is inhibited
by heparin: antithrombin III

Cofactors VIIIa and Va–inhibited
by protein C

Contact activation pathway

Platelets Activated platelet (platelet factor III)

Ca^{2+} Calcium

F_{1+2} Prothrombin activation fragments

FPA, FPB Fibropeptides A and B

■ **Figure 8–2.** The intrinsic, extrinsic and common coagulation pathways. Lower-case "a" denotes an activated factor. The protime (PT) measures the function of the extrinsic and common pathways; the partial thromboplastin time (PTT or aPTT) measures the activity of the intrinsic and common pathways. HMWK = High molecular weight kininogen; KAL = kallikrein. (Reproduced with permission from Dipiro, J. T., Talbert. R. L., Yee, G. C., et al. [1997]. *Pharmacotherapy: A pathophysiologic approach* [3rd ed.]. Stamford, CT: Appleton & Lange.)

important. Plasminogen is then converted back to plasmin and neutralized by a number of antiplasmin and inhibitor systems. All these reactions that occur in the coagulation cascade and fibrinolytic system are time dependent and can be monitored using laboratory testing as listed in Table 8-4.

Natural Anticoagulant Systems

Coagulation is regulated by three major mechanisms: the elimination of activated clotting factors, the protease inhibitors (inhibitors of coagulation), and the destruction of the fibrin clot.

There must be a balance between coagulation and anticoagulation processes in the body to maintain homeostasis. The natural anticoagulant systems include antithrombin III (AT-III), heparin cofactor II, and protein C and its cofactor, protein S.

Antithrombin III is an alpha-2 globulin glycoprotein, which is considered the major inhibitor of coagulation. It slowly inactivates thrombin as well as factors Xa, IXa, XIa, and XIIa. In the presence of heparin, antithrombin III-thrombin binding is increased significantly. This is thought to be the main mechanism for heparin's anticoagulation ability and its interaction with antithrombin III and tissue factor pathway inhibitor.

Table 8–4 ■ COAGULATION LABORATORY TESTS

Test	Normal Value	Coagulation Correlation	Clinical Significance
Activated partial thromboplastin time (aPTT)	<35 seconds	Generation of thrombin and fibrin to via intrinsic and common pathway	**Increased** with heparin or thrombin inhibitortherapy
Prothrombin time (PT)	10–13 seconds	Generation of thrombin and fibrin via extrinsic and common pathway	**Increased** with liver disease, extrinsic factor deficiencies, or oral anticoagulants.
International normalized ratio (INR)	Therapy goal dependent	Standardized values used to correct for different thromboplastin reagents inused PT calculations.	See American College of Chest (ACCP) Guidelines
Thrombin time (TT)	<20 seconds	Rate of thrombin induced cleavage of fibrinogen to fibrin	**Increased** with low fibrinogen levels, DIC, liver disease, increased FDP
Fibrinogen	200–400 mg/dL	Deficiencies in fibrinogen and alterations in conversion of fibrinogen to fibrin	**Increased** with inflammatory rsponse **Decreased** with liver disease or consumption of fibrinogen with intravascular clotting
Fibrin degradation products (FDP)	<8–10 μg/mL	Generation of fibrin fragments upon degeneration	**Increased** in fibrinolysis, DIC
Platelet count	150,000–400,000/mm^3	Amount of circulating platelets; does not reflect functional ability	**Increased** in myeloproliferative disorders, inflammation, post splenectomy **Decreased** in consumptive states, DIC, drug reactions, platelet disorders
Bleeding time (BT)	2–9 minutes, depending on reagent	Determines platelet adhesion and aggregation	**Increased** with platelet abnormalities, aspirin, severe liver disease
Protein C	4–5μg/mL	Determines activity of natural anticoagulation systems	**Increased** in inflammation **Decreased** in consumptive disorders
D-dimer assay	<400 ng/mL	Determines the level of endogenous thrombolysis; plasmin activity on fibrin	**Increased** with excessive endogenous thrombolysis
Activated clotting time (ACT)	46–70 seconds or 1.5–2.5-times control	Alternative test that can be performed at the bedside to determine heparin's anticoagulation level	**Increased** with heparin therapy **Decreased** with protamine administration

Modified from Kinney, M., et al. (1998). *AACN clinical reference for critical care nursing.* St. Louis: C.V. Mosby.

Heparin cofactor II is a heparin-dependent thrombin inhibitor whose activity is also accelerated by the presence of heparin. This cofactor not only inhibits thrombin but also thrombin induced platelet aggregation and release (Turgeon, 1999).

Protein C and protein S are major natural anticoagulants in the body and have a powerful role in anticoagulation. Deficiency in either of these proteins can lead to the development of thrombus. Protein C is a vitamin K-dependent protein, which is synthesized in the liver and circulates as a zymogen, an inactive precursor form in the blood. Activation occurs faster when thrombin, in the presence of thrombomodulin, assists with proteolytic cleavage that converts protein C to its active enzymatic form, activated protein C (APC). Protein S must also be present to help APC proteolytically cleave factors Va and VIIIa, which will decrease the conversion of prothrombin to thrombin, and acts as a regulatory feedback loop to balance coagulation. The dual role of thrombin in both coagulation and anticoagulation is exemplified here. Protein C also has a function in promoting fibrinolysis by neutralizing the inhibitors of tPA that allow the conversion of plasminogen to plasmin. Inactivation of APC is a slower process with a plasma protease inhibitor that has a short half-life intimating that other unidentified direct cell mechanisms (Turgeon, 1999). The properties of protein C have been applied clinically

with the development of Drotrecogin C (Xigris). Drotrecogin C is a recombinant intravenous form of protein C that is now being trialed in the septic patient population to try to decrease the occurrence of multisystem organ dysfunction secondary to microemboli formation in organs in severe sepsis. Activated protein C has a major role as an agent that suppresses inflammation and prevents microvascular coagulation. These properties were first discovered by Taylor et al. (1987) when it was discovered that protein C prevented coagulopathic and lethal effects of *Escherichia coli* infusion in baboons. Although the major side effect of APC is bleeding, recent studies have shown the efficacy and safety of APC for severe sepsis (Bernard et al., 2001).

COAGULATION—INFLAMMATION LINK

The role of the inflammatory process has become a major focus of study in many areas of medicine, especially inflammation's role in the atherosclerosis process. The study of the relationship between coagulation and inflammation is focused on the integrity of the endothelium and the recruitment of leukocytes

(Libby et al., 2002). Normally, the endothelium does not encourage the binding of white blood cells to the wall. However, with elevated levels of low-density lipoproteins (LDL), the excess LDL molecules will begin to infiltrate the endothelial wall and experience oxidation and glycation (Libby, 2002). These chemical changes will cause the endothelial cell to express an adhesion molecule, vascular cell adhesion molecule I (VCAM-I) that will bind various types of leukocytes, especially monocytes and T lymphocytes. This process occurs especially at arterial branch points where the endothelial cells are exposed to abnormal laminar flow. This abnormal laminar flow decreases the endothelial cells protective ability to secrete nitric oxide and to limit the expression of VCAM-I (Libby et al., 2002).

Once the monocyte is attached to the endothelial wall, it releases monocyte chemoattractant protein-1 (MCP-1), which will help the migration of the monocyte into the intima. With the assistance of macrophage colony-stimulating factor (M-CSF), the monocyte starts to ingest the excess lipids and transform itself into a macrophage foam cell. The macrophage foam cells are the trigger for activating the coagulation system. They release proteolytic enzymes that degrade the collagen fibers that compose the fibrous cap, so that it weakens and can rupture. The macrophage foam cell also produces tissue factor (Factor III) and once the plaque cap ruptures and exposes the tissue factor to the circulating blood, coagulation will ensue (Libby et al., 2002). The T cells also release cytokines such as tumor necrosis factor (TNF-β), which stimulates the macrophages, endothelial cells, and the smooth muscles. Peptide growth factors are released that promote the replication of smooth muscle cells into an extracellular matrix, which is characteristic of an atherosclerotic lesion (Libby et al., 2002).

However, this link between coagulation and inflammation may not only be limited to the atherosclerosis process. Hypertension may also be linked to inflammation because angiotensin II not only may be a vasoconstrictor but also may cause intimal inflammation by stimulating the smooth muscle and endothelial cells to express proinflammatory cytokines such as interleukin 6 (IL6) and monocyte chemoattractant protein-1 (MCP-1) (Krazhofer et al., 1999). Hyperglycemia associated with diabetes can lead to the formation of advance glycation end products (AGE) that may augment the secretion of proinflammatory cytokines (Schmidt et al., 1999). Even chronic extravascular infections such as gingivitis, prostatitis, bronchitis, etc., can augment extravascular production of inflammatory cytokines that can accelerate the evolution of atherosclerotic lesions (Libby et al., 2002). This new scientific insight into the role of inflammation in the development of atherosclerosis has led to using new markers to determine the degree of inflammation. Findings of a relationship between increased C-reactive protein levels and unfavorable cardiovascular outcomes have led to new therapeutic considerations for acute coronary syndrome (Libby et al., 2002).

◼ BLEEDING DISORDERS

Bleeding can occur when the intricate relationship between the various elements of the hemostatic system is disturbed. Bleeding defects in the hemostatic system can be categorized into three areas: vascular issues, platelet dysfunction, or coagulation dysfunction. Vascular issues generally cause endothelial damage by an autoimmune process (allergy induced), endotoxins from infections, or abnormal vascular structure. Platelet dysfunction can present as thrombocytopenia (low platelet count) or thrombocytosis (high platelet count). Thrombocytopenia can result from decreased production, decreased distribution, or increased destruction of platelets. Thrombocytosis can result from either a primary or a secondary cause. Coagulation dysfunction can be either congenital or acquired deficiencies in the factors (Display 8-1). In each case, bleeding is the primary manifestation. The bleeding may be minor, such as petechiae and easy bruising of the skin, or major, with massive hemorrhage.

The focus of cardiac interventions today emphasizes maintaining blood flow with percutaneous interventions (vascular injury) and anticoagulation to prevent thrombus formation. This intentional disruption of the coagulation system can potentially lead to bleeding disorders or even shock with excessive blood loss from percutaneous interventions and/or thrombolysis. Shock can lead to hypoperfusion and decreased oxygen delivery, which can trigger the intrinsic and extrinsic pathways simultaneously. Disseminated intravascular coagulation (DIC) is a complication of shock. Although DIC is actually a disorder of coagulation, it is discussed as a bleeding disorder because its major manifestation is bleeding.

Disseminated Intravascular Coagulation

Disseminated intravascular coagulation (DIC) is a pathological syndrome resulting in the indiscriminate formation of fibrin clots throughout all or most of the microvasculature. Paradoxically, diffuse bleeding occurs as a result of the consumption of clotting factors and is usually the hallmark sign of the syndrome. It is a disorder in which the coagulation cascade has been "pathologically activated" either by the extrinsic pathway releasing tissue factor or by the intrinsic pathway with endothelial injury (Owen & Webster, 1998). It is considered a complication of many different diseases and is known as a consumptive coagulopathy or defibrination syndrome (Turgeon, 1999). Successful treatment of DIC must include treatment of the primary cause of the disorder as well as the hematologic consequences. (See Display 8-2 for diseases associated with disseminated intravascular coagulation.)

Etiology

Inappropriate coagulation results from the presence of thromboplastic substances in the bloodstream. These thromboplastic substances stimulate clotting despite the lack of actual bleeding. Tissue thromboplastin (tissue factor) is released into the circulation by damaged cells in massive burns, injuries, and systemic infections. DIC is a common complication of serious infections, especially Gram-negative sepsis. The fetus, placenta, and amniotic fluid contain thromboplastic substances that are released into the maternal circulation during obstetric complications such as abruptio placentae and amniotic fluid embolism. Certain malignant tumors release small amounts of thromboplastic substances

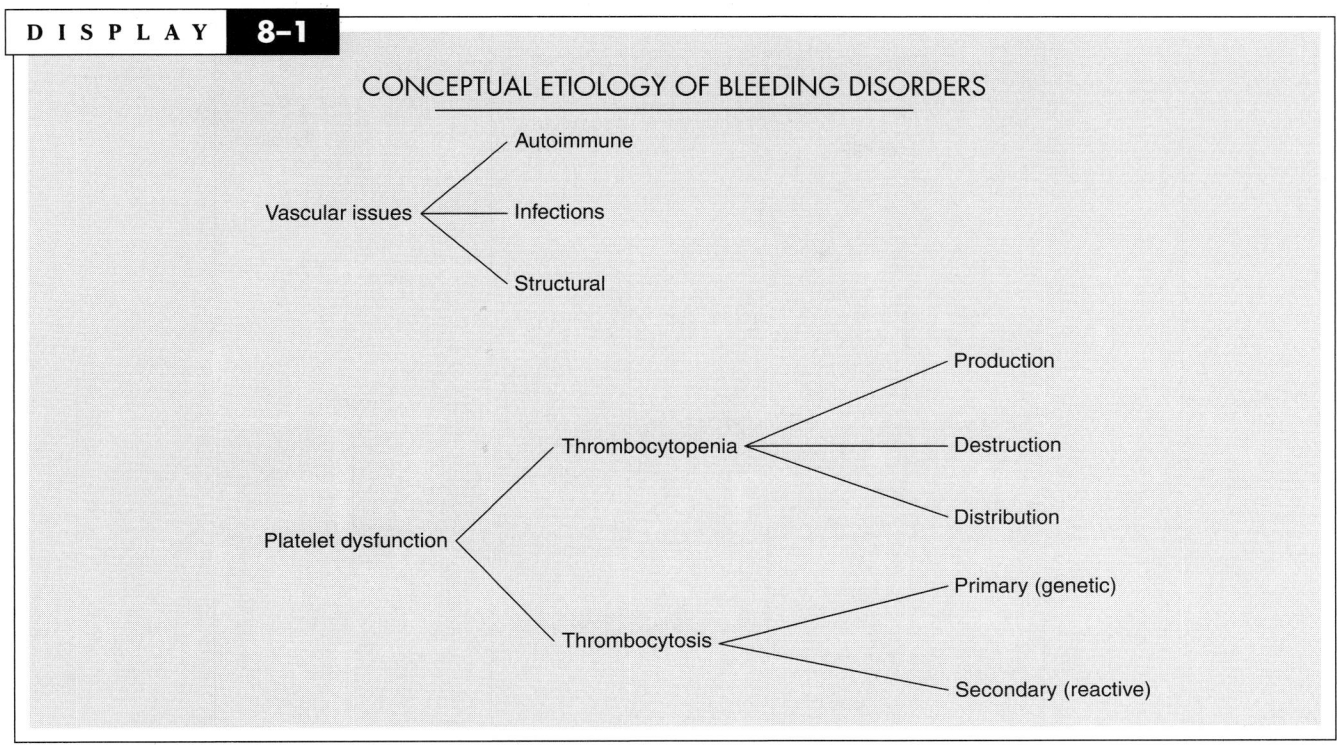

CONCEPTUAL ETIOLOGY OF BLEEDING DISORDERS

into the circulation. Chemotherapy or radiation treatment can cause tumor cells to die and release massive amounts of thromboplastin into the circulation (Owen & Webster, 1998). In the patient with cardiovascular disease, DIC is most likely to develop as a result of cardiogenic, septic, or hemorrhagic shock; acidosis; or extracorporeal circulation, which can all lead to cellular death and thromboplastin release. Figure 8-2 provides a conceptual model of the cause of DIC.

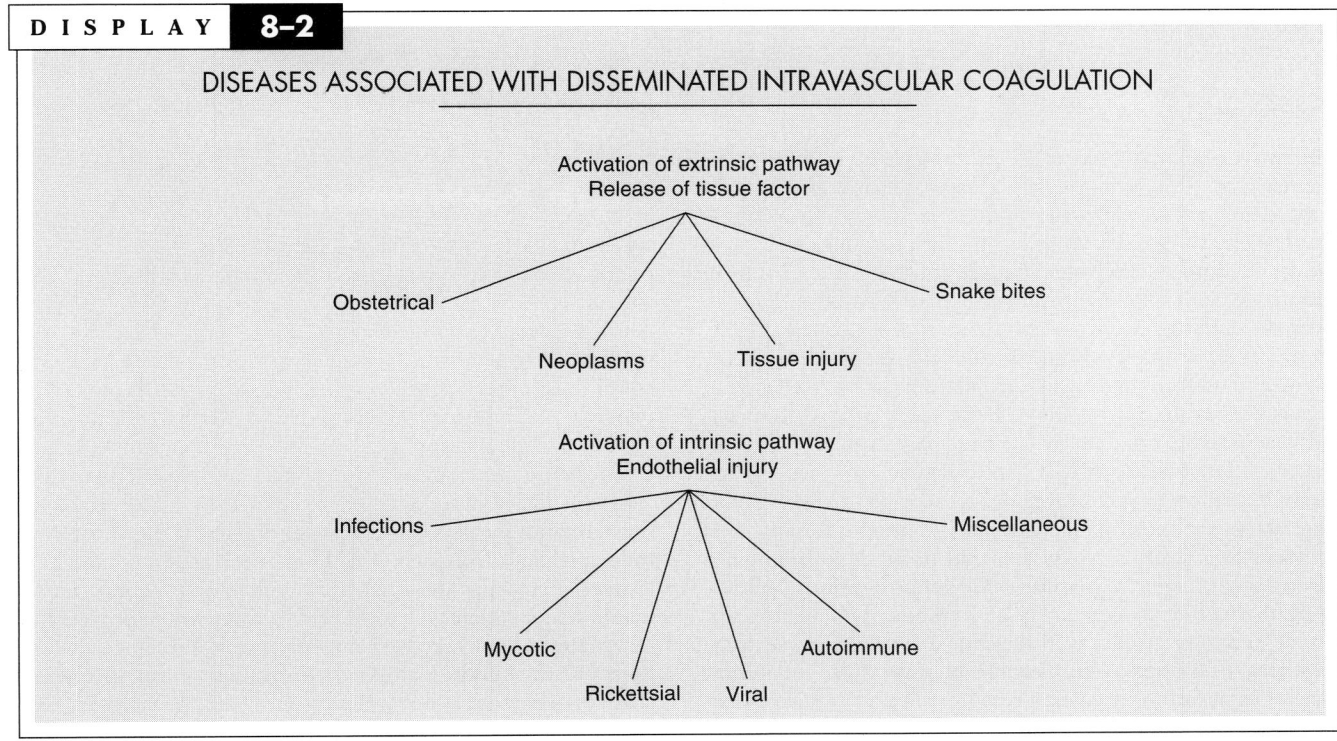

DISEASES ASSOCIATED WITH DISSEMINATED INTRAVASCULAR COAGULATION

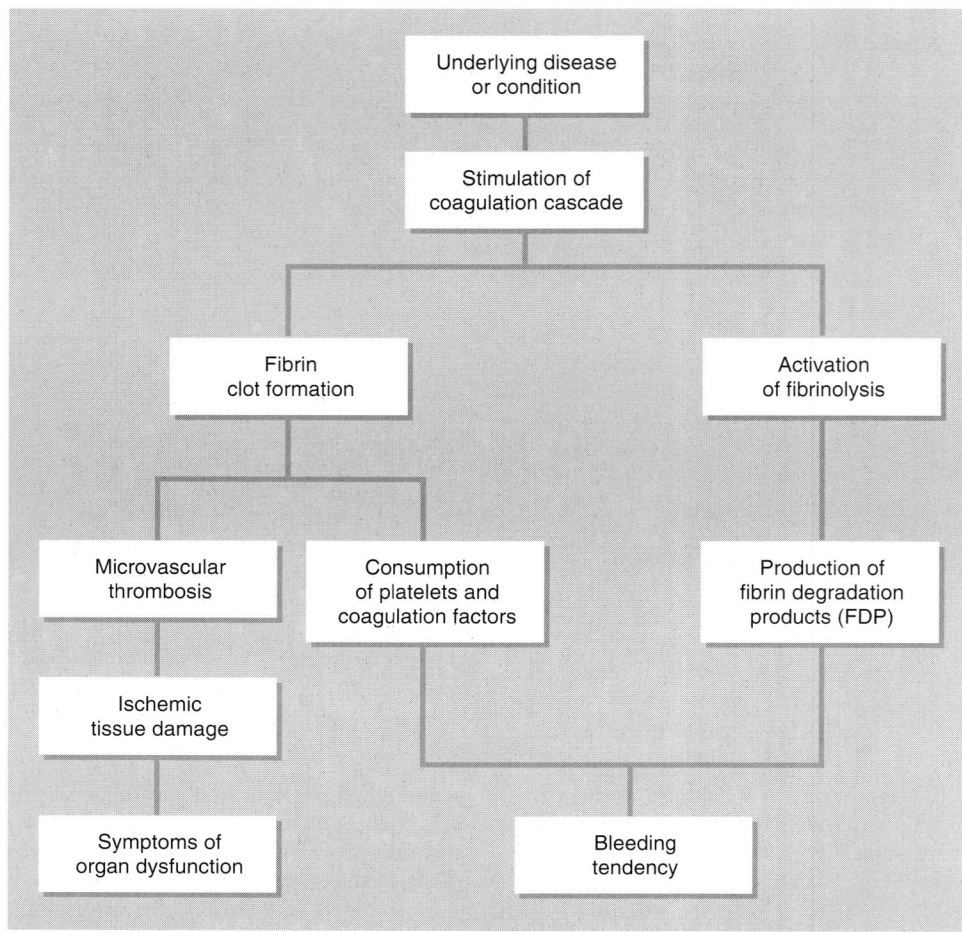

■ **Figure 8–3.** Pathophysiology of DIC. (From Kinney, M., Dunbar S. Brooks-Brun, J., et al. [1998]. *AACN's clinical reference for critical care nursing.* St. Louis: CV Mosby.)

Pathophysiology

The two major consequences of DIC are bleeding and organ ischemia (Fig. 8-3). Endothelial damage and/or tissue damage initiate the pathways and activation of the coagulation factors that leads to the formation of thrombin. Thrombin influences the coagulation system by: (1) cleaving fibrinogen to fibrin; (2) activating factor XIII; (3) stimulating platelets resulting in decreased circulating numbers; and (4) activating protein C (Turgeon, 1999). Widespread intravascular clotting resulting in the deposition of fibrin in the microcirculation leads to ischemia in organs such as the kidney, lungs, brain, skin, and gastrointestinal system. RBC are damaged as they pass through the fibrin strands. These damaged RBC are called schistocytes. As the disseminated clotting continues, circulating platelets and clotting factors are consumed and bleeding ensues. Fibrinolysis is activated as a result of the widespread fibrin deposition, converting plasminogen to plasmin, which destroys fibrin and fibrinogen, yielding abnormally large amounts of circulating fibrin degradation products (Turgeon, 1999). In these large numbers, FDPs aggravate bleeding because they: (1) inhibit platelet aggregation by coating receptor sites, (2) act as anticoagulants by competing with thrombin; and (3) impair fibrin

polymerization (Turgeon, 1999). Consumption of the factors is so rapid that repletion cannot be maintained.

Clinical Manifestations

Disseminated intravascular coagulation can occur in a chronic or acute form. The chronic form is subtler and easily goes unrecognized. The acute form tends to be more severe and sudden in onset. The astute clinician should have a high index of suspicion when patients experience any of the aforementioned conditions, observing for subtle signs of DIC. All organ systems are susceptible to the intravascular clotting that can occur. Classically, skin disruptions such as petechiae, purpura, and ecchymosis are very common. Continual bleeding and/or oozing from any skin disruption such as venipunctures or vascular access sites are another familiar sign. Neurological signs and symptoms can range from decreased level of consciousness and restlessness to seizures or coma. Respiratory dysfunction can be manifested by increased work of breathing with long expiratory times, use of accessory muscles, tachypnea, and adventitious breath sounds. Cardiac decompensation can encompass changes in rhythm and blood pressure as the sympathetic nervous system attempts compensation. The clinical presentation can range from hypertension to hypoperfusion. Hemodynamic indices may be decreased with hypovolemia or pulmonary artery pressures may be increased in the presence of a pulmonary embolism. Hypovolemic shock may result if blood loss is severe. Potential spaces for bleeding, especially the retroperitoneal space and thighs, need to be closely observed when femoral vascular access devices are in place or are removed. Acute abdominal signs such as distention, tenderness, pain, and decreased or absent bowel sounds may indicate major gastrointestinal dysfunction. Urine output may be decreased and signs of renal failure, such as an increase in creatinine, may occur. It is important to remember that the primary disorder that led to DIC must also be treated to correct DIC.

Medical Management

The diagnosis of DIC should be suspected whenever abnormal bleeding occurs in association with any of the primary disorders described previously. Multiple coagulation test abnormalities are found in DIC. These include prolonged PT, PTT, and thrombin time; decreased fibrinogen and platelet counts; and decreased levels of factors II, V, VIII, and X indicate the consumption of clotting factors. The elevation of FDP and the D-dimer levels confirm fibrinolysis. D-dimer levels indicate the level of activity of plasmin on fibrin, i.e., thrombolysis. Schistocytes may also be present. The presence of clotting and fibrinolysis with a suspicious clinical presentation can assist the practitioner in making the diagnosis of DIC. The prognosis of DIC varies markedly depending on the underlying cause and the amount of intravascular clotting. DIC may cease spontaneously, it may respond to prompt and aggressive treatment, or it may lead to organ ischemia, bleeding, and potentially death. Disseminated intravascular coagulation always occurs as the result of some other underlying abnormality, and thus the treatment of DIC is directed toward improvement of the underlying disorder. For example, infection requires the use of antibiotics. General supportive measures, such as fluid and blood replacement, mechanical ventilation, and vasoactive drugs to maintain tissue perfusion are essential. Transfusions of platelets, fresh-frozen plasma, red blood cells, and cryoprecipitate will be needed to attempt to replace consumed coagulation factors. The use of heparin, a potent anticoagulant that inactivates the intravascular clotting and thus inhibits consumption of the coagulation factors, is very controversial and probably inappropriate in the face of active bleeding.

Nursing Interventions

Perceptive nursing skill can be the pivotal factor in the patient with DIC. Early recognition of the subtle signs could avert further decompensation. If the patient displays any sign of restlessness or agitation, physiological factors such as hypoxemia should be the first consideration. Monitoring oxygenation using pulse oximetry will give some estimate of oxygenation that can be confirmed with an arterial blood gas. If gas exchange is adequate and restlessness and agitation persist, neurological causes must be considered and sedation should be avoided unless indicated. The patient's heart rate, rhythm, and blood pressure should be continually monitored for any changes. If manual or noninvasive blood pressure monitoring is being used, rotation of the cuff should be implemented because ecchymotic areas under the cuff can develop. Hemodynamic monitoring may be used and variations in indices may indicate cardiac failure, hypovolemia, or pulmonary complications such as pulmonary embolism. Monitoring urine output for at least 0.5 mL/kg per hour should be routine practice. Removal of large catheters used for percutaneous interventions should always be performed with care. Achieving and maintaining hemostasis is dependent on technique. Manual pressure should be applied slightly above the insertion site of the vessel and minimal padding should be used to control bleeding. This technique will allow visualization of the site for continual monitoring and lessen the chance of hematoma formation. Once adequate hemostasis is achieved, other devices can be applied to assure adequate clot formation at the puncture site. Proper technique in hemostasis control is especially important for patients with a coagulopathy.

If hemorrhage is present, the priority should be volume resuscitation. Blood products should be replaced depending on estimated blood loss and laboratory values. Aggressive fluid resuscitation should be performed through short, large-bore venous access using pressure bags if the patient is hypotensive to assure fast intravascular volume repletion (FCCS, 1998). While infusing blood products, the nurse should observe for allergic reactions (Tables 8-5 and 8-6). Continual bleeding may require massive blood product replacement, which can cause a "washout" effect of most of the functioning coagulation proteins, and paradoxically cause further coagulopathy (FCCS, 1998). It is also important to keep accurate records as to the number of various blood products received. Red blood cell loss needs to be replaced, but it is important to realize that a transfusion is not a benign intervention. Critically ill patients may

Table 8–5 ■ AGENTS USED TO PROMOTE COAGULATION BLOOD PRODUCTS

Product	Standard Volume	Administration	Factor Replaced
Platelets (random donor)	Usually 8–10 donors/unit at 50–70 mL/unit	Rapid administration increases possible allergic reaction	
Platelets (single donor)	One donor/200–300 mL	Rapid administration possible allergic reaction	
Packed red blood cells (RBC)	250–350 mL/unit	Rapid administration; blood type mismatch	
Fresh frozen plasma (FFP)	200–250 mL/unit	Rapid administration	II, V, VII, IX, X, XI, XII
Cryoprecipitate	Usually 8–10 donors/unit at 10–20 mL/unit	Rapid administration increases possible allergic reaction	I

Modified from Kinney, M. et al. (1998). *AACN clinical reference for critical care nursing.* St. Louis: C.V. Mosby.

TABLE 8–6 ■ DRUGS USED TO PROMOTE COAGULATION

Drug	Dose	Side Effects	Mechanism
Protamine	1 mg for every 100 units of IV heparin	Hypotension; possible anaphylaxis if exposed to NPH	Binds heparin to neutralize anticoagulant effect
Desarginine vasopressin (DDAVP)	0.3 μg/kg IV at 12–24-hour interval	Mild flushing, headache, mild to moderate abdominal pain	Temporarily improves platelet function in patient with renal or liver disease; mechanism not clear

Hardman, J. & Limbard, L. (2000). *Goodman and Gilman's the pharmacological basis of therapeutics.* New York: McGraw-Hill Company.

be at risk for immunosuppressive and microcirculatory complications with red cell transfusions (Hebert et al., 1999). A restrictive transfusion strategy (transfuse for a hemoglobin <7.0 g/dL) has been shown to be as effective as a liberal strategy (transfuse for a hemoglobin <10 g/dL) with a decrease in mortality (Hebert et al., 1999). The only two groups of patients that may require the more liberal transfusion strategy are patients with an acute myocardial infarction or unstable angina (Hebert et al., 1999). Observation for bleeding should include monitoring of all vascular accesses as well as the area around the site. Vigilant surveys by the nurse of the skin surface and digits are necessary to observe for petechiae, ecchymosis, and other skin disruptions that may provide early warning signs of impending DIC (see Display 8-3 for nursing interventions with bleeding disorders).

■ CLOTTING DISORDERS

Excessive or inappropriate coagulation is also of great clinical significance. Venous thrombosis involves the interacting conditions of stasis, vascular damage, and hypercoagulability. Its the most common life-threatening complication, pulmonary embolism, is a major cause of mortality in hospitalized patients. Recognition of patients likely to have any of these conditions is a nursing responsibility.

Clot Formation

A thrombus is a clot or solid mass formed by blood components. Thrombosis refers to the formation or presence of blood clots in a vessel. A thrombus that breaks loose and travels in the blood vessel is termed an embolus, hence the term thromboembolism. The potential outcome from either thrombosis or embolism is ischemia, leading to infarction with cellular and tissue necrosis. A thrombus develops when the normal process of hemostasis is inappropriately activated. Three factors (vessel injury, stasis, and hypercoagulability) can predispose a patient to thrombosis. These three factors are commonly known as Virchow's triad (Shoemaker et al., 2001) (Fig. 8-4).

DISPLAY 8-3

NURSING INTERVENTIONS WITH BLEEDING DISORDERS

Non-Emergent Interventions

1. Close observation of skin, mucus membranes, wounds, and intravascular access sites, especially femoral areas.
2. Assess for decreased tissue perfusion.
   a) Cerebral: Decreased level of consciousness, restlessness, agitation, apprehension
   b) Myocardial: Chest pain, EKG changes, respiratory distress
   c) Renal: Decreased urine output, rising BUN and creatinine
3. Test all body secretions for occult blood.
4. Measure and record blood loss.
5. Prevent injury.
   a) Soft toothbrush/swab for oral care
   b) Use electric razor
   c) No IM/SQ injections
   d) Minimize blood drawing and venipunctures
   e) Avoid invasive procedures (ie, NG tubes, rectal tubes, etc.)
6. Support patient and family.
   a) Provide calm environment
   b) Explain all procedures
   c) Provide frequent progress reports
   d) Allow flexible visiting hours
   e) Encourage proper sleep patterns

Emergent Interventions

1. Aggressive volume resuscitation through short, large-bore catheters; use warming devices for temperature <36°
2. Controlling bleeding at access sites using manual pressure applied slightly above site and minimal dressing to observe site closely
3. Accurate hemodynamic monitoring (see Chapter 23)
4. Supportive ventilator care

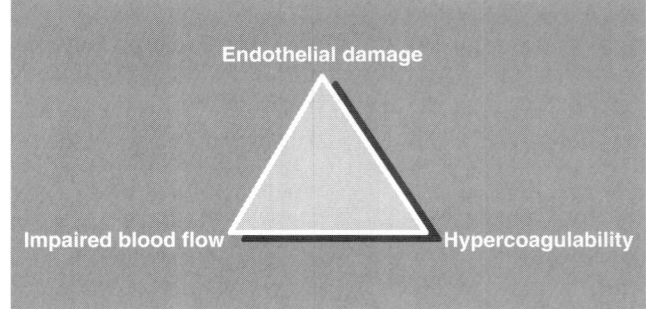

■ **Figure 8–4.** Virchow's triad.

First, the vessel involved must have suffered some type of injury, particularly damage to the endothelial layer. Vessel injury may be the result of sustained pressure on the vessel or surrounding tissue, as might occur from prolonged immobility of an extremity or pressure points caused by crossed legs, elastic-topped knee socks, or a bed where the knee gatch is raised too high. Vessel wall injury can also result from direct trauma by surgery or, more commonly, by intravenous (IV) or arterial catheters. Underlying vascular disease also creates vessel wall abnormalities. Chemical irritation may result from intravenous solutions and drugs. Anything that exposes collagen fibers in the vessel wall of arteries and veins may cause rapid platelet adhesion, aggregation, and thrombus formation. In addition, injury to vessels activates an inflammatory response that can be seen histologically and, in most cases, is seen most vividly in the lower extremities. When an extremity is immobile for any period of time, the pumping action is lost, resulting in venous stasis. For example, during the postoperative period there is a decrease in total limb blood flow because of immobility. Stasis may also result from reduced cardiac output caused by heart failure or shock. Alteration in blood flow leading to arterial thrombosis may be caused by turbulent flow at points of arterial bifurcation or stenosis, or with aneurysms. Fortunately, the rapid blood flow in arteries tends to discourage thrombus formation. Reduced blood flow in the atria occurs with atrial fibrillation, leading to thrombus formation. When the patient's cardiac rhythm converts to a regular sinus rhythm, these thrombi can be expelled into the lungs or systemic circulation (Shoemaker et al., 2001).

The final predisposing factor of Virchow's triad is hypercoagulability of the blood. Changes in blood leading to hypercoagulability may occur during pregnancy or in women using oral contraceptive drugs, which can cause elevated levels of coagulation factors. Changes in blood constituents may also occur in polycythemia, in severe anemia, or with circulating endotoxins from systemic infections. Deficiencies in antithrombin III and decreased hepatic function may be thrombogenic in patients with liver disease and in premature infants. The type of thrombus formed usually differs between arteries and veins. Arterial thrombi usually begin at the site of endothelial injury or turbulence. A venous thrombus is almost always occlusive. In the slower-moving blood of the veins, the thrombus frequently creates a long cast in the lumen of the vessel. No matter what type of clot is present, embolic disorders are a clinical challenge in which tissue perfusion will be compromised and intervention is needed.

Deep Vein Thrombosis

The clinical problems associated with venous thromboembolism (VTE) include deep vein thrombosis (DVT) and pulmonary embolism (PE). One of the most common and potentially life-threatening problems confronting health care professionals is the diagnosis, prophylaxis, and treatment of DVT and PE in both medical and surgical patients. The major risk associated with DVT is that it can lead to PE, which is responsible for 150,000 to 200,000 deaths per year in the United States (Hull et al., 2001). Venous thrombosis in the lower extremity can involve superficial leg veins, the deep veins of the calf (calf vein thrombosis), and the more proximal veins, in-

cluding the popliteal veins, the superficial femoral, common femoral, and iliac veins. In superficial vein thrombosis, sometimes called thrombophlebitis, the thrombosis is the result of inflammation in the venous wall of the superficial venous system and is benign and self-limiting.

Etiology

The risk factors associated with venous thromboembolism can be divided into two categories: primary and secondary hypercoaguable states. Virchow's triad (see Fig. 8-4) theory can be applied to some of these risk factors (Table 8-7).

Pathophysiology

Thrombi can form because the balance that is maintained in normal homeostasis has been disrupted. Coagulation is enhanced or fibrinolysis is impaired, which can lead to a hypercoaguable state. Primary inherited disorders that cause a hypercoaguable state are usually deficiencies in factors that inhibit coagulation, so there is less counterbalance to the coagulation process. The three main deficiencies are antithrombin III, protein C, and protein S (Turgeon, 1999). Secondary hypercoaguable states may result from endothelial activation by cytokines that will lead to loss of normal vessel wall anticoagulant surface functions with conversion to proinflammatory thrombogenic functions (Turgeon, 1999). Vascular endothelial damage can expose circulating blood components to subendothelial structures that initiate thrombosis. This process can also lead to vasoconstriction, which causes stasis and makes it easier for platelets to detach from flowing blood. The accumulation of platelets can furnish phospholipid for the intrinsic pathway, promoting thrombin formation by absorbing activated factor X to their surface (Turgeon, 1999). Platelets can also undergo alterations in their surface area that can lead to spontaneous aggregation or increased adhesiveness (Turgeon, 1999). Increased blood viscosity may also predispose thrombosis. Patients with increased levels of fibrinogen can induce erythrocyte aggregation, increasing viscosity and decreasing blood flow (Turgeon, 1999).

Table 8–7 ■ RISK FACTORS PREDISPOSING TO VENOUS THROMBOEMBOLISM

Primary Hypercoaguable States
Protein C deficiency
Protein S deficiency
Antithrombin III deficiency
Dysfibrinogenemia
Heparin-induced thrombocytopenia

Secondary Hypercoaguable States
Surgical and nonsurgical trauma
Previous venous thromboembolism
Immobilization (paralysis, extended bedrest or sitting)
Age > 40 years
Obesity
Heart disease
Malignant disease
Estrogens (pregnancy, oral contraceptives)

Modified from Turgeon, M. (1999). *Clinical hematology: Theory and procedures.* Philadelphia: Lippincott Williams & Wilkins.

Clinical Manifestations

The classic signs and symptoms of pain, edema, warmth, erythema, and tenderness of the leg are common with DVT but can also be caused by nonthrombotic events. There can also be a palpable cord, discoloration, cyanosis, venous distention, and prominence of the superficial veins (Hull et al., 2001). The size of the thrombus, the location of the affected vein, and the adequacy of collateral channels are some of the factors that cause the variability of the clinical presentation (Fahey, 2000). In the past, a positive Homans' sign, which is pain occurring in the affected calf with forceful dorsiflexion of the foot, was thought to be diagnostic for a DVT. However, a positive Homans' sign is not specific for thrombotic disease and could indicate minor muscle injury or other lower leg disorder (Fahey, 2000). Therefore, caution must be used when interpreting Homans' sign because any inflammation near the calf muscles may also elicit similar pain. Asymmetry between two extremities may also be present, with the affected limb being slightly larger because of the congestion and edema associated with the inflammatory process. These signs and symptoms in combination with the presence of the associated risk factors should assist in the diagnostic process. The clinical manifestations of DVT are sometimes elusive and should always be confirmed by objective diagnostic tests.

Medical Management

Objective testing and a careful history and physical examination should be obtained if a DVT is suspected. The patient's history and physical examination are important components of the diagnostic process, because they may reveal an alternative cause of the patient's symptoms. Diagnostic studies for DVT include B-mode or duplex ultrasonography, venography, and impedence plethysmography. Some form of ultrasound, either compression or color duplex, is usually the most common test used for diagnosing DVT because it is more specific and sensitive. Venography is used but is technically difficult to perform and requires experience to execute the test accurately. Impedence plethysmography is also used but is not sensitive to calf vein thrombosis (Hull et al., 2001). Once the diagnosis of DVT is confirmed, anticoagulation will be initiated immediately. Prevention is also an important priority to deter further decompensation of the patient's condition. Both these interventions will be discussed and more radical interventions, such as venous filters, will be discussed in the treatment of pulmonary embolism.

Anticoagulation

The main goal of therapy for VTE, of any origin, is anticoagulation to prevent further formation of thrombi. Depending on the severity of the embolism, anticoagulation can be used conservatively or aggressively if thrombolytic therapy is needed to lyse a life-threatening clot. The Sixth American College of Chest Physicians (ACCP) Consensus Conference on Antithrombotic Therapy (2001) recommends these drugs to be used for anticoagulation with VTE: the heparins, oral anticoagulants, and thrombolytic agents. The most common and one of the oldest drugs used for anticoagulation is heparin. Heparin is a glycosaminoglycan that binds to and activates antithrom-

bin III and reduces the formation of thrombin and fibrin. The best method of administering heparin is according to a weight-based protocol, which starts with a bolus loading dose of 5,000 units or 75 units/kg intravenously (IV) followed by a heparin IV drip at 18 units/kg per hour. The dose is then regulated by aPTT results that are sampled initially every 6 hours, with the aPTT goal of 1.5- to 2-times the normal aPTT. The use of a heparin weight-based protocol has been found to be more efficient in achieving an aPTT above the lower limit of the therapeutic range in 24 hours (Raskob et al., 2001). The goal for anticoagulation is that the dose of unfractionated heparin should be sufficient to prolong the aPTT to a range that corresponds to a plasma heparin level of 0.2 to 0.4 IU/mL by protamine sulfate or 0.3 to 0.6 IU/mL by an amidolytic anti-Xa assay (Hirsch, et al., 2001). Another group of drugs in the same class are the low-molecular-weight heparins (LMWH), which have a reduced ability to catalyze the inhibition of thrombin while retaining the ability to inhibit the activity of factor Xa. The advantage to the LMW heparins is that they do not bind to most plasma proteins, which contribute to a more predictable anticoagulant dose, and there is no need for laboratory monitoring. Enoxaparin (Lovenox) is the more common LMWH used currently and it can be administered either once or twice per day subcutaneously (SQ). If prescribed once daily, the dose is 1.5 mg/kg and if prescribed twice daily (BID), the dose is 1.0 mg/kg. Another LMWH is Dalteparin (Fragmin) (Raskob et al., 2001). There are other LMWH agents such as tinzaparin, nadroparin, and reviparin that are used less commonly.

The next drug category used for anticoagulation for VTE is oral anticoagulants. Warfarin (Coumadin) is the primary drug used. There are other oral agents available, such as dicumarol, which are not used as much because of erratic absorption and gastrointestinal side effects (Hardman et al., 2001). The major action of oral anticoagulants is that they are antagonists of vitamin K. The starting dose is usually 5 mg orally (po) and is then adjusted according to prothrombin time (PT) and international normalized ratio (INR). When prescribing warfarin, it is important to remember that the effect of the dose administered today will not be reflected in the PT/INR until approximately 3 days after that dose is administered. The anticoagulation treatment for VTE is initially heparin, which is administered for 5 days. Oral anticoagulant therapy overlaps with heparin therapy for at least 4 to 5 days until the INR goal of 2.0 to 3.0 is achieved (ACCP, 2001). Once the target for INR is reached and the level remains stable, the heparin can be discontinued and the warfarin dose adjusted further until stable and then followed-up by intermittent INR sampling. Oral anticoagulation is continued for at least 3 months up to as long as 6 months, depending on the reason for the development of VTE (ACCP, 2001).

When a DVT dislodges and becomes a life-threatening pulmonary embolism, thrombolytic agents can be used. Thrombolytic agents can be used in patients with hemodynamically unstable pulmonary embolism or massive iliofemoral thrombosis, and in those who are also at low risk for bleeding (ACCP, 2001). These agents are used as fibrinolytic therapy, which are designed to facilitate thrombolysis and decrease the ischemic damage produced by thrombotic events (Loscalzo, 2001). The drugs used for this purpose are known as plasminogen activators that bind to or induce a conformational change in plasminogen, proteolytically cleaving plasminogen to plasmin,

Table 8–8 ■ DRUGS USED TO PROMOTE ANTICOAGULATION

Drug Category	Mechanism	Dose
Heparin, unfractionated	Binds to and activates antithrombin III and reduces the formation of thrombin and fibrin	Load: 5,000 u or 75 u/kg followed by initial infusion 18 u/kg/min; adjust according weight based protocol using aPTT (goal is usuallytwice the normal aPTT value ~70 seconds)
Heparin, low-molecular-weight	Similar to heparin but reduced ability to catalyze the inhibition of thrombin with retained ability to inhibit activity of factor Xa	1.5 mg/kg if dosed QD 1.0 mg/kg if dosed BID; these doses are for enoxaparin (lovenox)
Oral anticoagulants, coumadin	Antagonist of vitamin K	Dosed according to PT/INR (goal is related to reason for anticoagulation; usual INR goal is 2.0–3.0)
Plasminogen activator, streptokinase	Induce a conformational change in plasminogen byproteolytically cleaving plasminogen to plasmin, enhancing fibrinolysis; no fibrin specificity	250,000 u IV load followed byinfusion 100,000 IU/h for 24 h
Plasminogen activator, urokinase	Same as streptokinase	2,000 IU IV load followed by infusion 2000 IU/h for 24–48 h
Plasminogen activator, t-PA	Same as streptokinase but has relative fibrin specificity	100 mg over 2 h
Thrombin inhibitors, argatroban	Directly inhibits thrombin formation enhancing fibrinolysis	1–2 mcg/kg/min infusion not to exceed 10 mcg/kg/min
Thrombin inhibitors, lepirudin	Same as argatroban	0.4 mg/kg loading dose followed by 0.15 mg/kg/h infusion

Adapted from Raskob, G., et al. (2001). In *Williams' hematology* (6th ed.). New York: McGraw-Hill Publishing.

thereby enhancing the fibrinolytic system (Loscalzio, 2001). Steptokinase is the oldest plasminogen activator approved for use with DVTs and is administered intravenously with a loading dose of 250,000 IU, followed by a 100,000 IU/h infusion for 24 hours. A limiting factor in the use of streptokinase is that patients can have an allergic reaction to the drug if they have had a recent streptococcal infection that can generate antibodies. Urokinase is another plasminogen activator that is administered intravenously with a loading dose of 2,000 IU followed by an infusion at 2,000 IU/kg per hour for 24 to 48 hours (Loscalzio, 2001). The disadvantage of both these drugs is that they lack fibrin specificity and will induce a systemic lytic effect (Hardman et al., 2001). Tissue plasminogen activator (t-PA) is also approved for use in the treatment of these patients. It is also administered intravenously and for DVT, the dose is 100 mg over the course of 2 hours (Loscalzio, 2001). Unlike the other two drugs, t-PA does have relative fibrin specificity, which may not be as important as once thought, but the lytic state produced by t-PA is less pronounced than streptokinase or urokinase (Loscalzio, 2001). There is no laboratory test that correlates with clinical efficacy of fibrinolytic therapy. However, a fibrinogen level less than 100 mg/dL has been associated with an increased hemorrhagic risk (Loscalzio, 2001). Table 8-8 summarizes the anticoagulants used for treating DVT.

The obvious side effect of any type of anticoagulation is bleeding. If the INR goal of 2.0 to 3.0 is attained, the risk of bleeding is minimal (Dalen, 2002). Careful consideration must be given to the patient's situation before starting anticoagulation, especially with the use of fibrinolytic therapy. Absolute contraindications for fibrinolytic therapy include active internal bleeding, hemorrhagic stroke, nonhemorrhagic stroke within the past year, intracranial neoplasm, and suspected aortic dissection. Relative contraindications can include prolonged cardiopulmonary resuscitation, severe hypertension, trauma within the past 4 weeks, surgery within the past 3

weeks, a history of bleeding diathesis, pregnancy, and active peptic ulcer disease (Loscalzio, 2001). The use of thrombolytic agents in the treatment of venous thromboembolism should be individualized and careful consideration must be given to the risks and benefits of this type of intervention (ACCP, 2001).

Bleeding associated with anticoagulant therapy can be treated with various reversal agents such as protamine sulfate for heparin and vitamin K for coumadin. Treatment is also directed at correction of coagulopathies, as indicated by abnormal coagulation studies (e.g., PT/PTT). Use of blood products such as fresh-frozen plasma, cryoprecipitate, and platelets may be able to stop or decrease bleeding. Repletion of blood loss may also be necessary. Locating the major site of bleeding is very important but can be a challenging task, especially if the site is more occult in nature. Surgical intervention may be required, and this type of high-risk patient will need to be optimized before surgery.

Prophylaxis

Although treatment for DVT has become more delineated over the years, the key intervention with DVT and possible pulmonary embolism is prevention. The most common and oldest intervention is the use of low-dose unfractionated subcutaneous heparin of 5,000 units every 8 to 12 hours. Low-molecular-weight heparin has also been shown to be effective in preventing VTE, especially in surgical patients, even with patients undergoing hip and knee surgery (Dalen, 2002). Other medications are not as effective when used for prophylaxis. Oral anticoagulants are not used because of the higher rate of bleeding. Aspirin is also considered ineffective for VTE prophylaxis (Dalen, 2002, ACCP 2001). External pneumatic compression is a non-pharmacologic intervention that has proven valuable in many types of surgical patients including hip procedures. Elastic stockings are also used and found to be useful in nonorthopedic, moderate-risk surgical patient (Dalen, 2002).

Table 8–9 ■ ACCP DVT RISK CATEGORIES

Risk Category	Prophylaxis
Low Risk	
General surgery patients undergoing minor procedures <40 years old Have no additional risk factors	No specific prophylaxis except early ambulation
Moderate Risk	
Minor surgery but other thrombosis risk factors Non-major surgery between ages 40–60 years old Major surgery <40 years old	Low-dose unfractionated heparin Low-molecular-weight heparin Elastic (graduated compression) stockings or Intermittent pneumatic compression
High Risk	
Non-major surgery. >60 years old or with additional risk factors Major surgery >40 years old or with additional risk factors	Low-dose unfractionated heparin Low-molecular-weight heparin or Intermittent pneumatic compression

There are many more recommendations for specific surgeries such as urologic, hip replacement, gynecologic, orthopedic, hip fracture, trauma and neurosurgery.

Adapted from Geerts, W., et al. (2001). Prevention of venous thromboembolism. *Chest,* 119 (1 Suppl.), 132s–175s.

These prophylactic measures are stratified for use depending on the risk for DVT (Table 8-9).

Nursing Interventions

The primary approach to nursing management of the patient at risk for DVT includes identifying the risk category for a patient and implementing preventive strategies. Such strategies include active or passive leg exercises and early ambulation to increase muscle activity, thereby improving venous blood flow. Frequent turning, coughing, and deep breathing help to improve venous return. Other measures to promote venous return are pneumatic compression stockings, graduated compression stockings, elevating the foot of the bed 6 to 8 inches, and not raising the knee gatch to avoid excessive popliteal pressure. A thorough history of the patient's risk factors along with the vigilant physical assessment of extremities for any evidence of inflammation, such as redness, swelling, asymmetry, and tenderness, are critical. If any signs and symptoms are observed, objective diagnostic testing should be pursued. Bleeding is the most common complication of anticoagulant and fibrinolytic therapy. The patient must be observed for subtle signs of bleeding. Careful monitoring of all puncture sites is mandatory, especially femoral interventional sites, with special attention to the abdomen and flank areas where large amounts of blood can sequester before the patient becomes symptomatic. Gastrointestinal bleeding is also another mechanism for blood loss. Assessing for symptoms of abdominal discomfort as well as guiac testing of excretions of patients on anticoagulation should be routine nursing interventions. Patient education regarding PT monitoring, anticoagulant medications and their side effects and interactions with other drugs should be reviewed. Leg elevation while sitting should be emphasized and the importance of physical activity when discharged should be emphasized. Risk factors such as obesity, smoking, and estrogen therapy should be identified and interventions designed to assist the patient to modify them as appropriate (Fahey, 1999). Be-

cause embolization is always a threat, special attention to the assessment of cardiopulmonary indicators is paramount. Pulmonary embolism may present with sudden onset of dyspnea, chest pain, and tachypnea, accompanied by other symptoms that will be discussed in the next section.

Pulmonary Embolism

Although diagnostic and therapeutic modalities have improved over the years, pulmonary embolism (PE) remains a challenging clinical entity. The incidence of symptomatic PE is estimated to occur in more than 600,000 patients annually in the United States and contributes to 50,000 to 200,000 deaths (Wood, 2002). Two thirds of patients with fatal cases will die within 1 hour of presentation (Wood, 2002). The mortality rate for hospitalized patients with PE has remained at approximately 15% over the past 40 years (Wood, 2002). Similar information has been gleaned from the International Cooperative Pulmonary Embolism Registry (ICOPER), which is a collaborative study developed to gather worldwide data about PE. The overall 3-month mortality rate for all PE patients in the ICOPER was 17.4% (Goldhaber et al., 1999). An interesting finding of the ICOPER is that postoperative prophylaxis is not instituted in more than half the patients in that database. Concern regarding lack of prophylaxis was echoed in the ACCP Consensus Conference (2001), who recommended that every hospital develop a formal strategy that addresses the prevention of thromboembolic complications with a written thromboprophylaxis policy, especially for high-risk groups.

Pulmonary embolism may be the result of either arterial or venous thrombi. Common sources of PE include deep venous thrombi from the lower legs, right atrial thrombi, septic foci (often related to intravenous drug abuse or infected vascular access sites), and tumors. Other sources of emboli are amniotic fluid, fat, air, bone marrow, and other foreign bodies. These latter sources have a pathophysiology that is different from the usual venous source and occur less frequently. Many factors predispose patients to PE and are similar to those risk factors for development of DVT discussed earlier. One unique factor that predisposes patients to PE is an inherited predisposition to hypercoagulability caused by a resistance to activated protein C. This inherited predisposition manifests itself as a gene mutation known as factor V Leiden in the factor V gene. Factor V Leiden is the most common of all the other inherited hypercoaguable states (Goldhaber, 2001).

Pathophysiology

A PE is a mechanical complete or partial obstruction to blood flow from the right to left heart. The physiological response of the patient is dependent on the degree of obstruction and the underlying cardiopulmonary function (Wood, 2002). A patient with good cardiopulmonary function and a complete obstruction may have the same outcome as a patient with poor cardiopulmonary function and a partial obstruction. Cardiac failure with a massive PE is caused by increased wall stress and ischemia that comprises the right ventricular (RV) function quickly and eventually impacts left ventricular (LV) function (Wood, 2002). With obstruction of blood flow out of the right side of the heart, an increased afterload develops. Additional factors that increase afterload are neural reflexes, the release of humoral factors, mediators that are released by platelets (platelet activating factor and serotonin) and systemic arterial hypoxemia (Wood, 2002). The cardiac output (CO) is initially maintained by increased catecholamine release resulting in an increased heart rate and contractility (Wood, 2002). The RV will attempt to contract against the resistance presented by the embolism but will eventually decompensate leading to an increase in RV volume. This increased RV preload leads to increased wall stress and compromised RV coronary blood flow and ischemia. Increased RV volume will also cause a septal shift that will decrease LV distensibility and decrease LV preload. This alteration in preload will lead to a decrease in CO and mean arterial pressure (MAP). RV coronary perfusion pressure (CPP) is dependent on the gradient between the MAP and the RV subendocardial pressure (Wood, 2002). The decrease in MAP will aggravate the compromised RV oxygen supply. Further RV ischemia will perpetuate decreased RV performance and the cycle will continue until complete decompensation occurs. This pathophysiological cycle is summarized in Figure 8-5.

The emboli itself can lead to a local aggregation of platelets and the release of vasoactive substances, which increase vasoconstriction. Gas exchange abnormalities are related to the size and type of embolic material, the extent of the occlusion and the underlying cardiopulmonary status and length of time since embolization (Wood, 2002). With PE, there is initial adequate ventilation coupled with inadequate perfusion (i.e., alveolar deadspace). The persistent obstruction and associated vasoconstriction can lead to bronchoconstriction, which produce shunting, another ventilation-perfusion (VQ) imbalance.

Any sustained VQ mismatch results in arterial hypoxemia. The hemodynamic and gas exchange consequences of a massive PE can lead to a dramatic clinical presentation.

Clinical Manifestations

Pulmonary embolism may occur with a sudden, abrupt onset, or have an insidious onset that mimics other cardiopulmonary disorders. Dyspnea is the most common symptom associated with PE and tachypnea is the most frequent sign (Goldhaber, 2001). Other signs such as pleuritic pain, cough or hemoptysis can be present and may indicate a small PE located near the pleura (Goldhaber, 2001). Classic cardiac signs such as tachycardia, low-grade fever, and neck vein distention can also be observed on presentation but may also be the function of age, the size of the PE and the underlying cardiopulmonary status. Younger patients may not have any of these signs whereas older patients may present with several or all of these signs (Goldhaber, 2001). There may also be vague complaints of chest discomfort, which can also be associated with acute coronary ischemic syndromes.

The presentation of a patient with a massive PE can be very similar to the signs and symptoms mentioned above. The only difference is that the signs and symptoms are a more extreme and exaggerated response to the embolic event. The classic clinical presentation of a massive PE can include syncope, cyanosis, tachycardia (heart rate >120 beats/min), tachypnea (respiratory rate >30 breaths/min), and hepatomegaly (Wood, 2002). Because symptoms of a massive PE can be so vague, it is

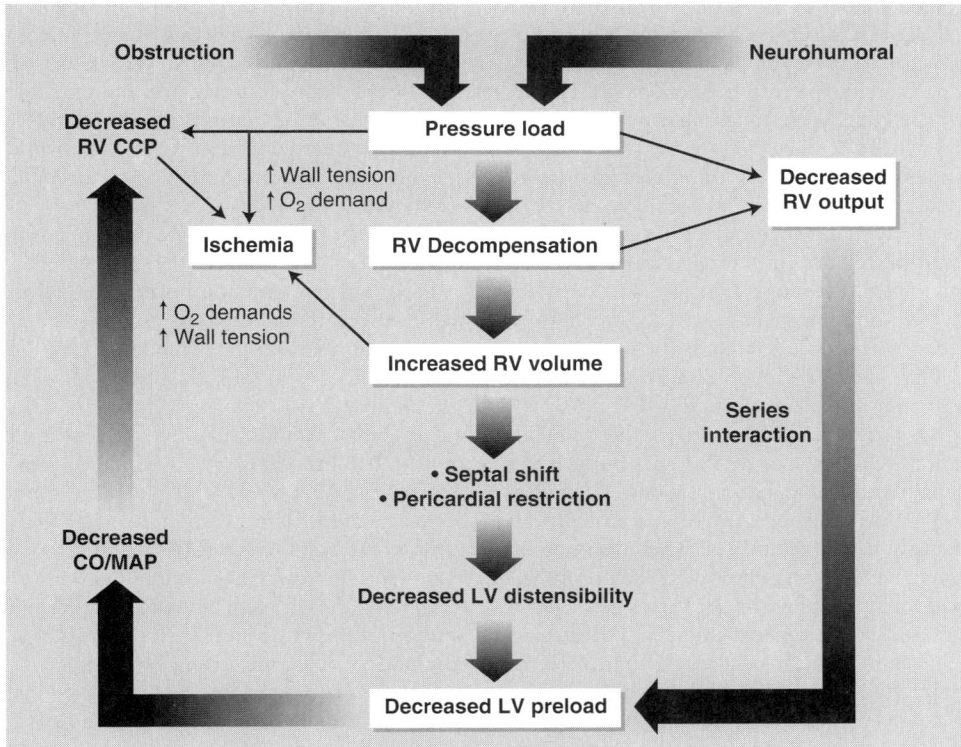

■ **Figure 8–5.** Pathophysiology of PE. (From Wood, K. [2002]. Major pulmonary embolism. Review of pathophysiologic approach to the golden hour of hemodynamically significant pulmonary embolism. *Chest, 121* [3], 877–905.)

important to gather data about patients and continually consider what their risk factors are for having a pulmonary embolism.

Medical Management

The diagnosis of PE is challenging, because PE can mimic other cardiorespiratory or musculoskeletal disorders such as myocardial infarction, pneumonia, congestive heart failure, asthma, or costochondritis. The diagnosis of PE should always be confirmed by objective tests. However, there are few tests that are specific for PE. Because the protective mechanism of fibrinolysis is triggered with the formation of a clot, tests reflecting fibrinolysis have been helpful in making the diagnosis of PE. The quantitative plasma D-dimer enzyme-linked immunosorbent assay (ELISA) level is elevated (>500 ng/mL) in more than 90% of patients with PE (Goldhaber, 2001). Arterial blood gas (ABG) values are not valuable in the diagnosis of PE, which is contrary to classic teaching (PIOPED, 1990). The expected hypoxemia associated with PE was not found to be consistently present in patients with documented PE. The ECG may be abnormal with an S wave in lead I, a Q wave in lead III, and inverted T wave in lead III; however, these changes are usually seen in patients with a massive PE. A normal chest radiograph in a dyspneic patient could suggest a possible PE (Goldhaber, 2001). However, a more definitive diagnosis can be made by means of a noninvasive lung ventilation/perfusion (VQ) scan. In PE, a defect is evident in the perfusion portion of the scan in conjunction with a normal ventilation scan. An abnormal VQ scan suggests PE. If the VQ scan is normal, the likelihood of PE is low. This test needs to be carefully evaluated since pre-existing cardiopulmonary disease can distort the interpretation and both the ventilation and perfusion portion of the test should be performed. The V/Q scan can be used in conjunction with a chest radiograph by performing the perfusion portion and matching it with the radiograph. If there is a perfusion defect when the chest radiograph is normal, then a PE is suspected (ACCP, 1998).

If the VQ scan is nondiagnostic, a pulmonary angiogram should be performed and is considered the gold standard. A definitive diagnosis of PE is best made by pulmonary angiography because a well-performed pulmonary angiogram excludes the diagnosis of PE. Although the time and costs involved with the invasive pulmonary angiography preclude its routine use in the diagnosis of PE, it remains the most reliable clinical study available. Recent radiological advances now include the spiral chest computed tomography (CT), which is a newer test used in diagnosing PE. The strength of the spiral CT is its ability to detect emboli in the central arteries but it is not as sensitive for finding peripheral emboli in the pulmonary vasculature (ACCP, 1998) Both tests require a significant contrast dye load and this fact should be considered when deciding on the test. Acetylcysteine (Mucomyst) can be given before and after the test to decrease the possibility of decreasing renal function (Tepel et al., 2000). Contrast-agent-induced reduction in renal function may be caused by direct toxic effects on the tubular epithelial cells by the formation of reactive oxygen species or reduced antioxidant activity (Tepel et al., 2000). Decreased renal function from contrast dye load may also be caused by an alteration in renal hemodynamics. Acetylcysteine, which has been recommended as prophylaxis for dye-induced renal dysfunction, has been shown to have renal vasodilatory effects as well as antioxidant benefits (Tepel et al., 2000).

Once PE is diagnosed, anticoagulation is the first intervention. The previous section on anticoagulation for DVT discusses the usual approach for treatment. If the patient is severely compromised and experiencing cardiopulmonary failure due to a PE, thrombolytic therapy is indicated. Caval interruption or inferior vena cava filter can also be used to treat a PE. This intervention helps prevent passage of emboli to the lung and is used in cases where anticoagulation may not be appropriate. There are two types of filters: bird's nest filter, which is placed infrarenally, and the Greenfield filter, which is placed suprarenally (Goldhaber, 2001). In rare instances, pulmonary embolectomy may be performed in conjunction with cardiopulmonary bypass. Mortality rates with this procedure can exceed 50% and should be performed only in institutions that can quickly mobilize a cardiac surgery team (Wood, 2002). With prompt identification and treatment, prognosis is good for patients with PE. Successful treatment results in little long-term morbidity. Sequelae such as pulmonary hypertension and cor pulmonale may be seen in patients with underlying cardiopulmonary disease or those with massive emboli.

Nursing Interventions

Because PE can be a life-threatening event, the emphasis of nursing management is on prevention. As discussed previously, prevention of thrombus formation and early detection of PE is essential. Fifty percent of those patients who die of PE do so within the first hour. Any patient experiencing a sudden onset of dyspnea, tachypnea, and possible chest pain must be evaluated for the possibility of PE. Assessing the character of the patient's chest pain is important because most patients describe their pain as pleuritic. A 12-lead ECG and an ABG also provide useful data. Explaining all procedures and tests helps reassure patients during a time of discomfort and anxiety about the sudden change of their condition. Once the diagnosis of PE has been established, continued nursing management of the patient's cardiopulmonary function is essential.

Because profound arterial hypoxemia can accompany PE, the primary goal is to normalize gas exchange. By normalizing the exchange of gases and minimizing the VQ mismatch, other systemic effects of impaired gas exchange can also be ameliorated. Interventions to support respiratory function by patient positioning and the use of supplemental oxygen may help decrease the degree of hypoxemia accompanying PE. Supplemental oxygen may be administered by face mask or, if necessary, by endotracheal intubation and mechanical ventilation. Positioning the patient with the head of the bed elevated allows for better chest expansion with respiration. Coaching of the patient to promote the best respiratory pattern can be very important and maintaining a calm environment and approach to the patient can make the difference in the patient's course. The administration of prescribed analgesics and sedatives may help relieve the patient's discomfort and anxiety. By reducing discomfort and anxiety, respiratory rate may also decrease, thus reducing the additional vasoconstriction and bronchoconstriction caused by lower $PaCO_2$ levels. Anticoagulants and thrombolytic agents, as described earlier, are usually ordered by the physician. These agents help decrease the recurrence of emboli and may help lyse the embolus, thus restoring normal blood flow through the pulmonary vasculature.

Frequent assessment of cardiopulmonary function is also important. Vital signs, particularly respiratory rate, heart rate, and blood pressure should be assessed and documented hourly and as needed. Normal vital signs may indicate improved gas exchange. ABG analysis offers a quantitative assessment of gas exchange. Because of the prolonged duration of anticoagulant therapy, patients require extensive teaching about the administration and follow-up schedules of oral anticoagulants, a medication identification card or band, potential hazards associated with therapy, and the signs and symptoms of bleeding and recurrent VTE. Dietary restrictions and foods that contain large amounts of vitamin K should be reviewed. This is a disease with long-term implications that can be successfully managed with patient participation and education.

Heparin-Induced Thrombocytopenia

Anticoagulation is a key intervention in treating cardiovascular disease. The primary agent that has been used for years is heparin and with an increased use of heparin, a new syndrome has been identified. Heparin-induced thrombocytopenia (HIT) is a challenging immunohematologic issue that was originally described in the early 1960s. Key elements of the syndrome were discovered in the mid 1970s, and the antigen target of the HIT antibody was identified in 1992 (Warkentin, 1999). However, knowledge about this disease is still in the developmental stages. With more patients being exposed to heparin or related drugs, the occurrence of HIT is increasing. One issue with the disease is that it is difficult to diagnose and unpredictable in incidence but can have some devastating outcomes. Unlike other clotting disorders, HIT is the result of an immunohematologic reaction.

HIT is a drug-induced immunoglobulin-mediated thrombocytopenic disorder that is frequently complicated by life- and limb-threatening thrombotic complications (Warkentin et al., 1998). HIT is a potentially devastating thrombotic disorder that can generate heparin dependent antibodies 5 to 8 days after initiation of heparin or sooner if there has been previous exposure to heparin. The recognition of this syndrome has been an issue because it can be difficult to recognize and there can be various reasons for thrombocytopenia. There are two types of HIT. Type I HIT is associated with a mild decrease in platelet count within 4 days of exposure that will recover despite the continued use of heparin (Warkentin et al., 1998). This condition is usually associated with large dosing of heparin such as after thrombolytic therapy or intraoperative interventions with cardiac surgery. The decrease in platelets may be the result of a direct activating effect on platelets by heparin and there has been no diagnostic test for this event. Another name for this type I HIT is non-immune heparin-associated thrombocytopenia, because there is no generation of an immunoglobulin (Warkentin et al., 1998). Type II HIT is the clinicopathologic syndrome that is diagnosed by two criteria: (1) one or more clinical events, primarily thrombocytopenia and possibly thrombosis; and (2) laboratory evidence for a heparin-dependent immunoglobulin (Warkentin et al., 1998).

Unlike other platelet disorders, HIT is associated with thrombosis, not bleeding.

Etiology

The cause of HIT is the exposure to heparin leading to the development of immunoglobulin, IgG that becomes detectable 5 days or more after exposure to heparin. It has also been discovered that there is a 100% cross reactivity with low-molecular-weight heparin and heparinoids and HIT IgG, which is different that immunogenicity. In the latter case, there is still a possibility of developing HIT even though it is less likely (Kelton & Warkentin, 1998). Of the patients exposed to heparin, heparin-dependent antibodies develop in up to 50% (Warkentin et al., 1995), and HIT develops in approximately 3% (Warkentin & Kelton, 1990). Thromboembolic complications occur in approximately 50% of HIT patients (Brieger et al., 1998). Although HIT can develop in any patient who has exposure to heparin, there are certain patient populations that seem to have a higher incidence. These populations include the orthopedic and the cardiac surgery patient.

Pathophysiology

The development of the pathogenic IgG is the key to this disorder (Fig. 8-6). The heparin binds with platelet factor 4 (PF4)

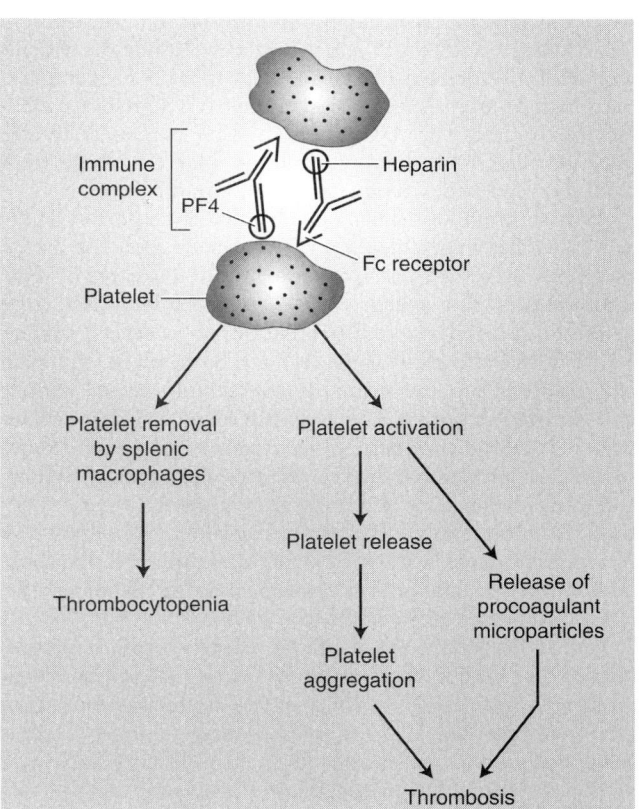

■ **Figure 8–6.** Pathophysiology of HIT. (From Chong, B. [1995]. Heparin-induced thrombocytopenia. *British Journal of Haematology,* 89(3), 431–439.)

that leads to the development of a highly reactive antigenic complex. Pathogenic IgG is formed and activates the platelets (Warkentin et al., 1998). The major target antigen is a macromolecular complex comprising heparin or other high-sulfated oligosaccharides and PF4, which binds to the platelet surface (Warkentin et al., 1998). Thrombocytopenia develops as the reticuloendothelial system consumes activated platelets, platelet microaggregates, and IgG-coated platelets (Chong, 1995). This activation results in the generation of procoagulant platelet-derived microparticles and also the activation of the endothelium with the recognition of the HIT antibodies and a thrombotic state is created (Warkentin et al., 1998). Arterial and venous thrombus can form, which can lead to devastating outcomes.

Clinical Presentation

The initial presentation of HIT is thrombocytopenia during or after heparin therapy. The platelet count will either decrease to less than 50% of baseline or decrease to a count of less than 100,000/μL (Warkentin, 1999). With type I HIT, thrombocytopenia will be the only symptom that will gradually recover. Type II HIT is more destructive and can have multisystem involvement because the thrombus can form in any vessel of any organ. However, there is a pattern emerging with the more common thrombus formation. Venous thrombotic complications include deep vein thrombosis (DVT), pulmonary embolism, and venous gangrene, which are precipitated by warfarin (Coumadin). Deep vein thrombosis is the most common clinical feature and occurs in approximately 50% of the patients with HIT (Warkentin, 1999). Arterial thrombotic complications include arterial occlusion of a limb vessel, myocardial infarction, or stroke (arterial and venous). Skin necrosis at heparin injection sites is another presentation that can range from painful erythematous papules to dermal necrosis.

Arterial thrombosis usually involves the distal portion of the aorta, and the symptoms can vary in degree depending on the thrombus size. The classic presentation for acute arterial thrombosis is known as the "6 Ps": pallor, pulselessness, pain, paresthesias, paralysis, and poikilothermy (coolness) (Fahey, 1999). Either the arms or the legs can be involved. The pain and paralysis are the result of nerve and skeletal muscle ischemia that can occur as early as 4 to 6 hours after the occlusion. Beyond this time period, the situation can progress to potential compartment syndrome with severe pain, tense swelling, and muscle tenderness of the affected extremity (Fahey, 1999). In HIT, limb amputation is not uncommon. Embolization of thrombus from the heart or proximal aorta can occur that could lead to microvascular ischemic events involving the mesenteric, renal, or spinal arteries (Warkentin, 1999).

Venous limb gangrene is a more recently recognized complication of HIT that can be caused with warfarin anticoagulation. A typical DVT can progress to venous limb gangrene despite an INR that is greater than 4.0. This coagulation abnormality is thought to reflect an imbalance of the anticoagulant/procoagulant components of the cascade, which may be caused by a rapidly acquired protein C insufficiency (Warkentin, 1999). Prevention and early interventions are the goals of all interventions. Table 8-10 summarizes the complications of HIT.

Table 8–10 ■ COMMON COMPLICATIONS OF HIT

Venous Thrombosis
Deep vein thrombosis
Coumarin-induced venous limb gangrene
Pulmonary embolism
Cerebral venous thrombosis
Adrenal vein thrombosis leading to infarction

Arterial Thrombosis
Lower limb artery thrombosis
Cerebrovascular accident
Myocardial infarction
Other

Skin Lesions (at heparin injection sites)
Skin necrosis
Erythematous plaques

Acute Systemic Reaction (after heparin bolus)

Hypofibrinogenemia (secondary to decompensated DIC)

Modified from Warkentin, T. (2002). Platelet count monitoring and laboratory testing for HIT: Recommendations of the College of American Pathologists. *Archives of Pathology Laboratory Medicine*, 126, 1415–1423.

Medical Management

Medical management is challenged with making the diagnosis of HIT. The diagnosis of HIT is based on the patient's exposure to heparin, which can extend to 100 days before the event (Warkentin, 2002). The diagnostic process continues with the assessment of the platelet count. Thrombocytopenia after heparin exposure is the hallmark signal to indicate HIT but other reasons for a decrease in platelets also need to be considered. However, if heparin exposure is documented and the platelet count decrease to 50% of baseline or less than 100,000/μL, then the presumptive diagnosis is HIT. Any source of heparin or heparinoids must be discontinued. Even the smallest amounts of heparin such as heparin-coated catheters or heparin flush solutions must be eliminated. The next step is to order a heparin-associated platelet antibody (HAPA) test, which is based on enzyme-linked immunosorbent assay (ELISA) (Warkentin, 1999). The College of American Pathologists recommend that HIT antibody testing be performed on patients in whom there is clinical suspicion of HIT based on temporal occurrence of thrombocytopenia or the occurrence of new thrombosis during or soon after heparin therapy (Warkentin, 2002). The presence of antibodies may not always confirm the diagnosis of HIT. HIT antibodies develop into clinical HIT in only a minority of patients (Warkentin, 1999). This is the reason why Warkentin has described HIT as a "clinicopathologic syndrome." Once thrombocytopenia associated with heparin administration is suspected, a search for new thrombosis should begin. Thrombosis can occur throughout the body, but there are selected complications (Table 8-10) that have greater frequency. The occurrence of thrombosis with HIT can be catastrophic. Limb amputation is not uncommon, and death as a result of end organ damage is approximately 30% (Brieger et al., 1998). Supportive care of these complications will then be the focus for the clinician.

The major decision will be starting anticoagulation using thrombin inhibitors such as argatroban or lepirudin (see Table 8-7). These drugs have been developed for use when heparin is contraindicated. Research is ongoing to determine what drug is most effective in treating thrombosis formed in HIT but there is not definitive answer at present. Argatroban is a thrombin inhibitor that is approved for the treatment of HIT and is administered intravenously. The dose of argatroban is 1 to 2 mcg/kg per minute not to exceed a rate of 10 mcg/kg per minute or an aPTT more than 100 seconds (GlaxoSmithKline, 2001). Lepirudin is a recombinant hirudin that has also been approved for use with HIT and is administered intravenously. Hirudin is the most potent natural thrombin inhibitor that is found in the salivary gland of the medicinal leech and lepirudin is a derivative of hirudin using recombinant DNA therapy. The loading dose of lepirudin is 0.4 mg/kg followed by an infusion of 0.15 mg/kg per hour. A baseline aPTT should be obtained before the start of therapy. Infusion doses of both these drugs are maintained to achieve an aPTT 1.5- to 2.5-times the normal value, similar to the goal of heparin therapy. The aPTT is usually sampled every 6 hours, but with lepirudin, the first aPTT should be drawn in 4 hours and then at least once per day (Raskob et al., 2001). Low-molecular-weight heparin (LMWH) and danaparoid, a heparinoid, were initially used to treat HIT but have been contraindicated since cross-reactivity has been discovered (Kelton and Warkentin, 1998). Argatroban and lepirudin are continued until an oral anticoagulant can be safely initiated and therapeutic anticoagulation goals are achieved (see anticoagulation section).

Nursing Interventions

This clinicopathological syndrome requires the most astute observational and correlation skills of a nurse. A high index of suspicion is needed especially with postoperative orthopedic, cardiac, and vascular surgical patients who are receiving prophylactic doses of unfractionated heparin for at least 5 days (Warkentin, 2002). A thorough history of the patient's possible exposure to heparin, including 100 days before the event, must be obtained (Warkentin, 2002). Platelet count should be measured promptly in these patient populations and monitored closely. Recommendations from the College of American Pathologists include the following: (1) monitoring is crucial between days 4 to 10+ after starting heparin, when the highest platelet count from day 4 onward represents "baseline"; (2) for a patient recently exposed to heparin (within the past 100 days), a repeat platelet count obtained within 24 hours after re-initiation of heparin is recommended to identify patients with rapid-onset HIT caused by already-circulating HIT antibodies; (3) a platelet count should be measured promptly and compared with recent values in a patient in whom thrombosis develops during or soon after heparin therapy; and (4) a platelet count decrease of 50% or more from baseline can indicate HIT, even if the platelet count nadir remains above 150×10^9/L (Warkentin, 2002, p. 1421).

A decreasing platelet count should cause suspicion and the search for possible thrombosis formation should begin.

Vigilant physical assessment of extremities for any evidence of embolic events such as erythema, asymmetrical edema of the extremities, and/or tenderness is critical. The "6 Ps" should provide guidelines for monitoring limb perfusion. Early observation of limb compromise may allow appropriate vascular intervention, which could avert amputation. Further evaluation and observation of all body systems, especially neurological, pulmonary, and cardiac, may reveal early signs and symptoms

of embolic events. If the patient displays any sign of restlessness or agitation, physiological factors such as hypoxemia should be the first consideration. Monitoring oxygenation using pulse oximetry will give some estimate of oxygenation that can be confirmed with an arterial blood gas. If gas exchange is adequate and restlessness and agitation persist, neurological causes must be considered and sedation should be avoided unless indicated. Respiratory distress with tachypnea, dyspnea on exertion, prolonged expiratory time as well as restlessness, and agitation could be indications of pulmonary emboli. The patient's heart rate, rhythm, and blood pressure should be continually monitored for any changes. Hemodynamic monitoring may be used and variations in indices may indicate cardiac failure, myocardial infarction, or pulmonary complications such as pulmonary embolism depending on the situation and the primary disorder. Gastrointestinal dysfunction can present with a wide range of signs and symptoms from nausea and vomiting to acute abdominal pain. Assessment of the abdomen should never be omitted and given special attention if HIT is suspected. Any abdominal discomfort should be carefully considered and monitored for any progression. Monitoring urine output for at least 0.5 mL/kg per hour should be routine practice. The BUN and creatinine trends should also be closely reviewed. If these organ systems are severely compromised, multisystem organ dysfunction may be the end result, with poor outcomes. HIT can be a devastating syndrome.

REFERENCES

ACCP Consensus Committee on Pulmonary Embolism. (1998). Opinions regarding the diagnosis and management of venous thromboembolic disease. *Chest,* 113(2), 499–505.

Bernard, G. R., Vincent, J. L., Laterre, P. F., et al.(2001). Recombinant human protein C worldwide evaluation in severe sepsis (PROWESS) study group. Efficacy and safety of recombinant human activated protein C for severe sepsis. *New England Journal of Medicine,* 344(10), 699–709.

Beutler, E., Coller, B., Lichtman, M., et al. (2001). *'s hematology* (6th ed.). New York: McGraw-Hill Medical Publishing Division.

Braunwald, E., Fauci, A., Kasper, D., et al. (2001). *Harrison's principles of internal medicine* (15th ed.). New York: McGraw-Hill Medical Publishing Division.

Brieger, D., Mak, K., Hottke-Marchant, K., & Topol, E. J. (1998). Heparin-induced thrombocytopenia. *Journal of American College of Cardiology,* 31(7), 1449–1459.

Chong, B. (1995). Heparin-induced thrombocytopenia. *British Journal of Haematology,* 89(3), 431–439.

Dalen, J. (2002).Pulmonary embolism: What have we learned since Virchow? Treatment and prevention *Chest,* 122(5), 1801–1817.

Dhainaut, J., Abraham, E. & Opol, S. (2002). Introduction to the Third Margaux Conference on Critical Illness: The Endothelium: An under-recognized organ of critical illness. *Critical Care Medicine,* 30(5), 179–180.

Dipiro, J. T., Talbert, R. N., Yee, G. C., et al. (1997). *Pharmacotherapy: A pathophysiologic approach* (3rd ed.). Stamford, CT: Appleton & Lange.

Fahey, V. (1999). *Vascular nursing* (3rd ed.). Philadelphia: WB Saunders.

Geerts, W., Heit, J., Clagett, G., et al. (2001). Prevention of venous thromboembolism. *Chest,* 119(1 Suppl.), 132s–175s.

Goldhaber, S., Vasani, L., & DeRosa, M. (1999). Acute pulmonary embolism: Clinical outcomes in the International Cooperative Pulmonary Embolism registry (ICOPER). *Lancet,* 353(9162), 1386–1389.

Goldhaber, S. (2001). Pulmonary thromboembolism. In *Harrison's principles of internal medicine* (15th ed.). New York: McGraw-Hill Medical Publishing Division.

Hack, C. & Zeerleder, S. (2001). The endothelium in sepsis: Source of and target for inflammation. *Critical Care Medicine,* 29(7), S21–26.

Hardman, J. & Limbird, L. (2000).*Goodman and Gillman's the pharmacological basis of therapeutics* (10th ed.). New York: McGraw-Hill Medical Publishing Division.

Hebert, P., Wells, G., Blajchman, M., et al., and the Transfusion Requirements in Critical Care Investigators for the Canadian Critical Care Trials Group. (1999). A multicenter, randomized, controlled clinical trial of transfusion requirements in critical care. *New England Journal of Medicine*, 340(6), 409–417.

Hirsh, J., Dalen, J., & Guyatt, G. (2000). The sixth ACCP guidelines for antithrombotic therapy for prevention and treatment of thrombosis. American College of Chest Physicians. *Chest*, 119(1 Suppl.), 132s–175s.

Hull, R., Pineo, G., & Raskob, G. (2000). Diagnosis and treatment of venous thromboembolism. In *Textbook on critical care medicine* (4th ed.). Philadelphia: WB Saunders.

Jerius, H., Beall, A., Woodrum, D. et al. (1998). Thrombin-induced vasospasm: Cellular signaling mechanisms. *Surgery*, 1, 46–50.

Kelton, J. & Warkentin, T. (1998). Heparin-induced thrombocytopenia: Diagnosis, natural history and treatment options. *Postgraduate Medicine*, 103(2), 169–177.

Kinney, M., Dunbar, S., Brooks-Brun, J., et al. (1998). *AACN's clinical reference for critical care nursing*. St. Louis: CV Mosby.

Libby, P. (2002). Atherosclerosis: The new view. *Scientific American*, 286(5), 46–55.

Libby, P., Redker, P. & Maseri, A. (2002). Inflammation and atherosclerosis. *Circulation*, 105(9), 1135–1143.

Owen, D. & Webster, J. (1998). Hematology: Clinical physiology. In *AACN clinical reference for critical care nursing*. St Louis: CV Mosby.

Shoemaker, W., Ayres, S., Grenvik, A., & Holbrook, P. (2000). *Textbook on critical care medicine* (4th ed.). Philadelphia: WB Saunders.

Society of Critical Care Medicine (1998). *Fundamental critical care support (FCCS)*. Chicago: Society of Critical Care Medicine.

Taylor, F. B., Chang, A., Esmon, C. T., et al. (1987). Protein C prevents coagulopathic and lethal effects of *Escherichia coli* infusion in the baboon. *Journal of Clinical Investigation*, 79(3), 918–925.

Tepel, M., Van der Giet, M., Schwarzfeld, C., et al. (2000). Prevention of radiographic-contrast-agent-induced reductions in renal function by acetylcysteine. *New England Journal of Medicine*, 343(3), 180–184.

Tortora, G. & Grabowski, S. (2003). *Principles of anatomy and physiology*. New York: John Wiley & Sons, Inc.

Turgeon, M. (1999). *Clinical hematology: Theory and procedures*. Philadelphia: Lippincott Williams & Wilkins.

Warkentin, T. (1999). Heparin-induced thrombocytopenia: A clinicopathologic syndrome. *Thrombosis and Haemostasis*, 82(2), 439–447.

Warkentin, T. (2002). Platelet count monitoring and laboratory testing for heparin-induced thrombocytopenia: Recommendation of the College of American Pathologists. *Archives of Pathology Laboratory Medicine*, 126(11), 1415–1423.

Warkentin, T., Chong, B., & Greinacher, A. (1998). Heparin-induced thrombocytopenia: Towards concensus. *Thrombosis and Haemostasis*, 79(1), 1–7.

Warkentin, T. & Kelton, J. (1990). Heparin and platelets. *Hematology Oncology Clinics of North America*, 4(1), 243–264.

Wood, K. (2002). Major pulmonary embolism. *Chest*, 121(3), 877–905.

WEBSITES

www.accp.org
www.argatroban.com
www.guidelines.gov
www.xigris.com

9

Fluid and Electrolyte Balance and Imbalances

LINDA FELVER

PRINCIPLES OF FLUID BALANCE

The fluid in the body serves many vital functions. In addition to being the milieu in which cellular chemistry occurs, it provides the transport medium for oxygen and other nutrients to reach the cells and for carbon dioxide and other metabolic waste products to be removed from the body. Technically, *fluid* is water plus the substances dissolved in it.

The amount of water in the body decreases as a person ages. The body ranges from 70% water by weight (newborn infant) to 60% (young or middle-aged adult) to 45% (elderly woman). Women have less water by weight than men because a higher percentage of their weight is fat. Similarly, water is a lower percentage of body weight in obese people. One liter of water weighs 1 kg (2.2 lb). Thus, a standard 70-kg (154-lb) middle-aged man (60% water) has 42 L of body water (70 kg × 0.60 = 42 kg; 42 kg = 42 L) (Felver, 2000).

Body Fluid Compartments

The fluid in the body lies in several compartments. The *extracellular fluid* consists primarily of vascular and interstitial fluid. Some extracellular fluid is located in bone and dense connective tissue; this fluid is not considered accessible for dynamic exchange. *Intracellular fluid*, as the name indicates, lies in the cells. *Transcellular fluid* is fluid that is secreted by epithelial cells. Examples of transcellular fluid are cerebrospinal fluid, saliva, and intestinal secretions. Many of the transcellular fluids are reabsorbed by the body after they have been secreted.

More water is located inside the cells than outside of them. Clinically, approximately two thirds of body water in adults is considered intracellular and one-third extracellular. Thus, the 70-kg man who has 42 L of body water can be considered to have approximately 28 L of water inside the cells and 14 L of extracellular water. This extracellular water is approximately one-third vascular and two-thirds interstitial. For clinical purposes, the 70-kg man can be considered to have approximately 4.5 L of water in the vascular compartment and approximately 9.5 L in the interstitial compartment.

Osmolality

The relative proportion of water to particles in body fluid is measured as osmolality. Osmolality can be considered to be the degree of concentration. Technically, osmolality is defined as the number of moles of particles per kilogram of water. The normal range of osmolality of the blood is 280 to 300 mOsm/kg (lower in normal pregnancy) (Blackburn, 2003). Fluids that have osmolality within this normal range are called *isotonic*. Extracellular and intracellular fluids have the same osmolality. If the osmolality of the extracellular fluid is increased or decreased, then the osmolality of the intracellular fluid changes rapidly until intracellular and extracellular fluids again have the same osmolality. This process is discussed later in the section on Fluid Distribution.

Although the osmolality of intracellular and extracellular fluids is the same, the ion composition of the two fluids differs. Thus, they have the same particle concentration, but the specific kinds of particles are different in the two fluids. Intracellular fluid has a higher concentration of protein and potassium, magnesium, and phosphate ions; extracellular fluid has a higher concentration of sodium, calcium, chloride, and bicarbonate ions (Rose & Post, 2001). Transcellular fluids are usually hypotonic; their ion composition varies widely depending on their physiologic function.

Processes Involved in Fluid Balance

Fluid balance is the net result of fluid intake, fluid distribution, fluid excretion, and fluid loss by abnormal routes. Fluid balance is maintained when fluid excretion and fluid loss through any abnormal routes are matched by fluid intake and when the fluid is distributed normally into its compartments (Felver, 2000).

Fluid Intake

The major determinant of fluid intake in a healthy adult is habit. Thirst, another important determinant of fluid intake, can be caused by several physiologic mechanisms. These include dryness of the oral mucous membranes, increase in osmolality of the body fluids (osmoreceptor-mediated thirst), decrease in extracellular fluid volume (ECV) (baroreceptor-mediated thirst), and increased renin secretion (angiotensin-mediated thirst). Osmoreceptor-mediated thirst is the most common cause of thirst in healthy adults. This mechanism becomes less effective with aging. Thus, elderly adults often have a greater need for water before they become thirsty. Cultural factors have an important influence on fluid intake. For example, intake of certain herbal teas may be considered necessary by some patients when they become ill. In clinical settings, health care professionals often regulate the fluid intake. Routes of fluid intake include oral, rectal, intravenous, and intraosseous, as well as through tubes into body cavities. Oral fluid intake includes liquids and the water contained in food, as well as water made by cellular metabolism of ingested nutrients.

Fluid Distribution

Two types of fluid distribution operate in the body. First, fluid is distributed between the vascular and interstitial spaces, the two subcompartments of the extracellular compartment. Second, fluid is distributed between the extracellular and intracellular compartments. Different processes regulate these two types of fluid distribution.

Fluid distribution between the vascular and interstitial spaces is regulated by filtration. Filtration is the net result of four opposing forces. Two of these forces tend to move fluid out of the capillaries, whereas the other two tend to move fluid into the capillaries. Which direction the fluid moves in any one location depends on which forces are stronger. The two forces that tend to move fluid out of capillaries are the blood hydrostatic pressure (outward force against the capillary walls) and the interstitial fluid osmotic pressure (inward pulling force caused by particles in interstitial fluid). The two forces that tend to move fluid into capillaries are the blood osmotic pressure (inward pulling force caused by particles in blood) and the interstitial fluid hydrostatic pressure.

Usually, the blood hydrostatic pressure is highest at the arterial end of a capillary, and there is filtration from the capillary into the interstitial fluid. This flow of fluid out of the capillaries is useful in carrying oxygen, glucose, amino acids, and other nutrients to the cells that are surrounded by interstitial fluid. Most proteins are too large to cross into the interstitial fluid and remain in the capillary. At the venous end of a capillary, the blood hydrostatic pressure is usually lower and the blood osmotic pressure higher because fluid has left the capillary but the proteins have remained. These changes cause a net flow of fluid from the interstitial space back into the venous end of a capillary. The flow of fluid back into the capillaries is physiologically useful in carrying carbon dioxide, metabolic acids, and other waste products into the blood for further metabolism or excretion.

Changes in any of the four forces that determine the direction of filtration at the capillaries can cause abnormal distribution between the vascular and interstitial compartments. The most common abnormal distribution is edema, which is expansion of the interstitial space. Edema can be caused by increased blood hydrostatic pressure (e.g., venous congestion), increased interstitial fluid osmotic pressure (e.g., proteins in interstitial fluid), decreased blood osmotic pressure (e.g., hypoproteinemia), or blockage of the lymphatic system, which normally removes excess fluid from the interstitial space and returns it to the vascular compartment.

The second type of fluid distribution occurs between the extracellular and intracellular compartments. This process is regulated by osmosis. Cell membranes are freely permeable to water, but the passage of ions and other particles depends on membrane transport processes. Osmotic pressure is an inward-pulling force caused by particles in a fluid. Both the extracellular and intracellular fluids exert osmotic pressure. Because the osmolality of the two compartments is normally the same, the osmotic pressures are the same. Therefore, the force pulling water into the cells is balanced by the force pulling water into the interstitial space, and the normal fluid distribution is maintained. If the osmolality of the extracellular fluid changes, however, then osmosis occurs, altering the fluid distribution until the osmolality in the extracellular and intracellular compartments is again the same. For example, if the extracellular fluid becomes more concentrated (increased osmolality), then the osmotic pressure of the extracellular fluid becomes higher than the osmotic pressure of the intracellular fluid. Water leaves the intracellular compartment until the intracellular fluid becomes as concentrated as the extracellular fluid. This process decreases the amount of water that is distributed into the intracellular compartment. Similarly, if the extracellular fluid becomes more dilute (decreased osmolality), then the osmotic pressure of the extracellular fluid becomes lower than the osmotic pressure of the intracellular fluid. Water moves by osmosis into the intracellular compartment until the intracellular fluid becomes as dilute as the extracellular fluid. This process increases the amount of water that is distributed into the intracellular compartment.

In summary, fluid distribution between the vascular and interstitial compartments depends on filtration, the net result of four forces that act on fluid at the capillary level. Fluid distribution between the extracellular and intracellular compartments depends on osmosis, the movement of water across cell membranes to equilibrate particle concentrations.

Fluid Excretion

The normal routes of fluid excretion are respiratory tract, urine, feces, and skin (insensible perspiration and sweat). In a standard adult, approximately 400 mL of water is excreted daily through the respiratory tract, even if the person is fluid-depleted. This amount increases during fever. The urine volume of a healthy adult varies according to the fluid intake, the needs of the body, and the hormonal status. It averages 1,500 mL. Major hormones that regulate urinary excretion of fluid are summarized in Table 9-1. Diuretics, ethanol, and caffeine increase urine volume. Fecal excretion of water averages 200 mL per day in healthy adults who have a normal fluid balance and a fully functioning bowel. Diarrhea causes a dramatic increase in fecal excretion of water. Insensible perspiration is fluid excretion through the skin that is not visible. It averages 500 mL per day in a healthy adult. Insensible perspiration occurs even if the person is fluid depleted. It increases during fever. Sweat is visible fluid excretion through the skin. The volume of sweat varies greatly depending primarily on thermoregulatory needs.

Fluid Loss by Abnormal Routes

Examples of abnormal routes of fluid loss are emesis, drains, suction, paracentesis, and hemorrhage. Third-spacing (e.g., ascites) can be considered abnormal fluid loss, even though the

Table 9–1 ■ HORMONES THAT REGULATE RENAL FLUID EXCRETION

Hormone	Physiologic Source	Major Physiologic Actions	Stimuli That Increase Hormone Secretion	Stimuli That Decrease Hormone Secretion
Aldosterone	Adrenal cortex (zona glomerulosa)	Kidneys retain more saline (expands extracellular fluid volume) Kidneys excrete more potassium and hydrogen ions	Angiotensin II (from the renin-angiotensin system; kidneys release more renin during hypovolemia and other causes of decreased blood flow through the renal artery and by stimulation of renal sympathetic nerves)	Decreased angiotensin II Hypokalemia
Natriuretic peptides	*A-type natriuretic peptide:* atrial myocardium *B-type natriuretic peptide:* ventricular myocardium *C-type natriuretic peptide:* endothelial cells	Natriuresis (kidneys excrete more saline, which reduces extracellular fluid volume) Vasodilation (suppresses endothelin; arterioles dilate, which reduces peripheral vascular resistance and lowers blood pressure) Suppression of renin-angiotensin system	*A-type natriuretic peptide:* atrial dilation (stretch) *B-type natriuretic peptide:* increased ventricular end-diastolic pressure and volume *C-type natriuretic peptide:* vascular shear stress	*A-type natriuretic peptide:* lack of atrial dilation (decreased stretch) *B-type natriuretic peptide:* normal or decreased ventricular end-diastolic pressure and volume *C-type natriuretic peptide:* reduced vascular shear stress
Antidiuretic hormone (ADH)	Synthesized in preoptic and paraventricular nuclei of hypothalamus Secreted from posterior pituitary gland	Kidneys retain more water (dilutes body fluids, decreasing osmolality)	Increased osmolality of body fluids Hypovolemia Physiologic and psychological stressors; surgery/anesthesia; trauma; pain; nausea	Decreased osmolality of body fluids Hypervolemia Ethanol

fluid remains in the body, because the fluid is not freely available to the normal fluid compartments.

Summary of Fluid Balance

In summary, the processes of fluid intake, fluid distribution, fluid excretion, and fluid loss by abnormal routes must act together to maintain fluid balance. A change in one of these processes must be matched by a change in another to maintain fluid balance. For example, if an increased urine output is matched by an increased fluid intake, then fluid balance can be maintained. If changes in one or more of these processes are not matched by changes in the others, however, then a fluid imbalance occurs. Fluid imbalances may be characterized by altered *volume* of fluid (ECV imbalances), altered *concentration* of fluid (osmolality imbalances), or a combination of the two.

■ EXTRACELLULAR FLUID VOLUME BALANCE

The ECV is the net result of fluid intake, fluid distribution, fluid excretion, and fluid loss by abnormal routes. A normal ECV is maintained when fluid excretion and any fluid loss are balanced by fluid intake and when the fluid distribution is normal. The body's responsiveness to administration of a fluid load has a circadian rhythm (i.e., varies in a cyclic manner over 24 hours). The kidneys can excrete an excess fluid load more efficiently if it is administered during the time that the person is normally active than if it is administered during a person's customary sleeping time.

The blood volume is an important determinant of the work of the heart and provides the medium for oxygen delivery to

tissues. Therefore, ECV imbalances can interfere with cardiac function and tissue oxygenation.

Extracellular Fluid Volume Deficit

Extracellular fluid volume deficit is caused by removal of sodium-containing fluid from the vascular and interstitial spaces. Usually, the fluid is removed from the body; however, in some cases, fluid is sequestered in the peritoneal cavity, the intestinal lumen, or some other "third space." ECV deficits occur when intake of sodium-containing fluid does not keep pace with increased fluid excretion or loss of fluid through abnormal routes. Clinical causes of ECV deficit are presented in Table 9-2. ECV deficit may develop in patients with cardiac disease who use diuretics if the dosage is excessive.

Table 9–2 ■ CAUSES OF EXTRACELLULAR FLUID VOLUME DEFICIT

Category	Clinical Examples
Excessive removal of gastrointestinal fluid	Diarrhea Emesis GI fistula drainage Nasogastric or intestinal tube suctioning or drainage
Excessive renal excretion of saline	Adrenal insufficiency Diuresis due to bed rest Excessive use of diuretics
Excessive removal of sodium-containing fluid by other routes	Hemorrhage Third-space accumulation Burns Excessive diaphoresis

The clinical manifestations of ECV deficit include sudden weight loss (unless there is third-spacing), decreased skin turgor, dryness of opposing mucous membranes, hard dry stools, longitudinal furrows in the tongue, absence of tears and sweat, and soft sunken eyeballs. Although weight loss occurs immediately, most of these signs appear only after substantial fluid depletion. Cardiovascular manifestations are among the early signs; these are discussed next.

Many of the clinical manifestations of ECV deficit are evident in the cardiovascular system. Decreased volume in the vascular compartment causes postural blood pressure drop, increased small vein filling time, flat neck veins when supine (or neck veins that collapse during inspiration), and decreased central venous pressure.

A postural blood pressure drop is present if the following criteria are met in an adult: (1) blood pressure is measured with the patient supine and then standing or sitting with the legs dependent (not horizontal); (2) systolic blood pressure decreases more than 15 mm Hg; (3) diastolic blood pressure decreases 10 mm Hg or more; and (4) heart rate increases. The increase in heart rate indicates that autonomic reflexes are functioning and rules out autonomic insufficiency, which may cause the upright blood pressure to decrease when the ECV is normal. Postural blood pressure drop is not a reliable assessment for ECV deficit in patients who have transplanted hearts. The heart rate may not increase in these patients when their blood pressure drops from ECV deficit.

Small vein filling time is assessed by placing a patient's hand or foot below the level of the heart, occluding a small vein, milking it flat by stroking toward the heart, and then releasing it. If the vein takes longer than 3 to 5 seconds to refill, then the patient probably has an ECV deficit (unless occlusive arterial disease is present).

The decreased preload of ECV deficit leads to decreased cardiac output, with resulting dizziness, syncope, and oliguria. If ECV deficit becomes severe, tachycardia, pallor caused by cutaneous vasoconstriction, and other manifestations of hypovolemic shock occur (see Chapter 30).

Extracellular Fluid Volume Excess

Excess ECV is an overload of fluid in the vascular and interstitial compartments. It is common in patients with heart failure because their decreased cardiac output activates the renin-angiotensin-aldosterone system (Struthers, 2002). Aldosterone causes renal retention of sodium and water, which expands the extracellular volume. In patients who have hypertension caused by elevated renin, ECV excess also develops. Other causes of ECV excess are listed in Table 9-3. Clinical manifestations of ECV excess include sudden weight gain, peripheral edema, and the cardiovascular effects described next.

Increased vascular volume is manifested by bounding pulse, distended neck veins when upright, and elevated central venous pressure. The crackles, dyspnea, and orthopnea of pulmonary edema may be present. A sudden overload of isotonic fluid increases cardiac work and may cause heart failure, especially in an older adult or an infant.

Table 9–3 ■ CAUSES OF EXTRACELLULAR FLUID VOLUME EXCESS

Category	Clinical Examples
Excessive infusion of isotonic, sodium-containing solutions Renal retention of saline	Excessive normal saline (0.9% NaCl) Excessive Ringer's or lactated Ringer's Endocrine: Excessive aldosterone (CHF, cirrhosis, hyperaldosteronism); excessive glucocorticoids (Cushing syndrome, pharmacologic doses of glococorticoids) Renal: Oliguric renal failure

■ OSMOLALITY BALANCE

The osmolality of body fluids is determined by the relative proportion of particles and water. The serum sodium concentration usually parallels the osmolality of the blood. When the serum sodium concentration is abnormally low, the osmolality is decreased; in other words, the blood is relatively too dilute. Conversely, when the serum sodium concentration is elevated, the osmolality is increased; in that case, the blood is relatively too concentrated. Antidiuretic hormone (see Table 9-1) is the major regulator of osmolality (Robertson, 2001).

Hyponatremia

Hyponatremia is a relative excess of water that causes a decreased serum sodium concentration. It is caused by a gain of water relative to salt or a loss of salt relative to water (Table 9-4). Antidiuretic hormone increases the reabsorption of water by the renal tubules and thus dilutes the body fluids. In patients who have had cardiac surgery, hyponatremia

Table 9–4 ■ CAUSES OF HYPONATREMIA

Category	Clinical Examples
Gain of water relative to salt	Endocrine: Excessive ADH (ectopic production; stimulation by surgery/anesthesia, stressors, pain, nausea) Iatrogenic: Excessive infusion of D5W, tap water enemas, or water ingestion (after poisoning or before ultrasound examination); absorption of water from hypotonic irrigation solution Other: Near-drowning in fresh water; excessive ingestion of low-sodium fluid such as water (psychogenic polydipsia) or beer (beer potomania)
Loss of salt relative to water	Gastrointestinal: Replacement of water but not salt after emesis, diarrhea, or nasogastric suction; removal of sodium with hypotonic irrigation Renal: Diuretics, especially thiazides; salt-wasting renal diseases Other: Replacement of water but not salt after excessive diaphoresis

may occur in the first few days after surgery if excess free water is administered because the stressors of surgery, anesthesia, pain, and nausea increase the secretion of antidiuretic hormone (Felver, 2000). Hyponatremia is common in patients with severe congestive heart failure because their decreased cardiac output triggers release of ADH. Although ACE inhibitors have the potential to cause hyponatremia, these drugs are sometimes used to reverse hyponatremia in patients who have severe CHF because they restore perfusion and decrease the baroreceptor stimulus to ADH release (Rose & Post, 2001).

Medications used by patients with cardiac disease that may cause hyponatremia include thiazide diuretics and ACE inhibitors (Al-Salman & Pursell, 2001; Rose & Post, 2001; USP, 2003). Hyponatremia from thiazide diuretics occurs more frequently in women than men, especially in older women (Chapman et al., 2002).

The hypo-osmolality of hyponatremia causes water to enter cells by osmosis. The clinical manifestations of hyponatremia are primarily nonspecific markers of cerebral dysfunction: malaise, confusion, lethargy, seizures, and coma. The extent of these manifestations depends on the speed with which hyponatremia develops as well as its severity (Gross et al., 2001). Hyponatremia does not have significant clinical effects on cardiac electrophysiology or function.

Hypernatremia

Hypernatremia is a relative deficit of water that causes an increased serum sodium concentration. It is caused by a loss of water relative to salt or a gain of salt relative to water (Table 9-5). The hyperosmolality of hypernatremia causes water to leave cells by osmosis. The clinical manifestations are similar to those of hyponatremia: malaise, confusion, lethargy, seizures, and coma (Rose & Post, 2001). Thirst (except in some older adults) and oliguria (except in hypernatremia caused by decreased antidiuretic hormone) may also occur. As with hyponatremia, the extent of these manifestations depends on the speed with which hypernatremia develops as well as its severity (DePetris et al., 2001). Hypernatremia

Table 9–5 ■ CAUSES OF HYPERNATREMIA

Category	Clinical Examples
Loss of water relative to salt	Endocrine: Lack of ADH (diabetes insipidus) Renal: Osmotic diuresis; renal concentrating disorders Other: Inadequate water replacement after diarrhea or excessive diaphoresis
Gain of salt relative to water	Decreased intake of water: Inability to respond to thirst (coma, aphasia, paralysis, confusion); lack of access to water; difficulty swallowing fluids (advanced Parkinsonism); prolonged nausea Increased intake of salt: Excessive hypertonic NaCl or $NaHCO_3$; near-drowning in salt water; tube feedings without adequate water intake

also does not have significant clinical effects on cardiac electrophysiology or function.

Mixed Extracellular Fluid Volume and Osmolality Imbalances

Extracellular fluid volume and osmolality imbalances may occur at the same time in the same person. For example, in a person who has severe gastroenteritis without proper fluid replacement, concurrent ECV deficit and hypernatremia (clinical dehydration) will develop. The fluid lost in the emesis and diarrhea, plus the usual daily fluid excretion (urine, feces, respiratory, insensible through skin), is hypotonic sodium-containing fluid (analogous to isotonic saline that has extra water added). The signs and symptoms of such mixed fluid imbalances are a combination of the clinical manifestations of the two separate imbalances. In the example of clinical dehydration, the patient has the sudden weight loss, manifestations of decreased vascular volume, and signs of decreased interstitial volume that result from ECV deficit plus the thirst and nonspecific signs of cerebral dysfunction that result from hypernatremia (Rose & Post, 2001).

▓ PRINCIPLES OF ELECTROLYTE BALANCE

Electrolyte balance is the net result of several concurrent dynamic processes. These processes are electrolyte intake, absorption, distribution, excretion, and loss through abnormal routes (Felver, 2000) (Table 9-6). Electrolyte intake in healthy people is primarily by the oral route; other routes of electrolyte intake include the intravenous and rectal routes, and also through tubes into various body cavities. Electrolytes that are taken into the gastrointestinal tract must be absorbed into the blood. Although some electrolytes (e.g., potassium) are absorbed readily by mechanisms based on gradients, the absorption of other electrolytes (e.g., calcium and magnesium) is more complex and can be impaired by many factors.

Electrolytes are distributed into all body fluids, but their concentrations in the different body fluid compartments vary greatly. Substantial amounts of most electrolytes are located in pools outside the extracellular fluid. For example, the major pool of potassium is inside cells; the major pool of calcium is in the bones.

Electrolyte excretion occurs through the normal routes of urine, feces, and sweat. Any removal of electrolytes through other routes can be considered loss of electrolytes through an abnormal route. Examples of these abnormal routes are emesis, nasogastric suction, fistula drainage, and hemorrhage.

To maintain normal balance of any specific electrolyte, electrolyte intake and absorption must equal electrolyte excretion and electrolyte loss through abnormal routes, and the electrolyte must be distributed properly within the body. Alterations in any of these processes can cause an electrolyte imbalance (Felver, 2000).

Table 9–6 ■ ELECTROLYTE HOMEOSTASIS

Electrolyte	Sources of Intake	Absorption	Electrolyte Pool	Distribution	Excretion
Potassium (K$^+$)	*Foods:* Almonds Apricots Bananas Cantaloupe Coffee (instant) Dates Molasses Oranges Peaches Potatoes Prunes Raisins Strawberries *Intravenous:* Packed red blood cells or whole blood; penicillin G	Based on gradient between lumen and blood concentrations	Inside cells	*Cause shift into cells:* β-adrenergic agonists Insulin Alkalosis *Cause shift out of cells:* Acidosis caused by mineral acids Lack of insulin Cell death	*Urinary:* Increased by in- creased flow, glucocorticoids Aldosterone causes K$^+$ excretion *Fecal:* Increased with diarrhea *Sweat*
Calcium (Ca^{2+})	*Foods:* Beet greens Broccoli Dairy products Farina Kale Milk chocolate Oranges Salmon (canned) Sardines Tofu	Most efficient in duodenum; increased by vitamin D Decreased by phosphates, phytates, oxalates, increased intestinal pH, undigested fat, diarrhea, glucocorticoids	Physiologically unavailable when bound in blood to proteins and small organic anions Bones	*Cause more binding in blood:* Alkalosis Citrate in blood products Protein plasma expanders Increased free fatty acids *Cause shift into bones:* Lack of parathyroid hormone *Cause shift from bones:* Parathyroid hormone High-protein diet Glucocorticoids Immobility	*Urinary:* Decreased by parathyroid hormone Increased by saline diuresis, high protein diet *Fecal:* Increased with undigested fat *Sweat*
Magnesium (Mg^{2+})	*Foods:* Cocoa Chocolate Dried beans and peas Green leafy vegetables Hard water Nuts Peanut butter Sea salt Whole grains	Most efficient in terminal ileum Decreased by phosphates, phytate, undigested fat, alcohol, diarrhea Increased by lactose	Physiologically unavailable when bound in blood to proteins and small organic anions Bones Inside cells	*Cause more binding in blood:* Citrate in blood products Increased free fatty acids *Cause shift from bones:* Parathyroid hormone *Cause shift into cells:* Epinephrine Insulin	*Urinary:* Increased with extracellular fluid volume expansion, rising blood alcohol, high- protein diet, acidosis *Fecal:* Increased with undigested fat, increased aldosterone *Sweat*
Phosphate (P$_i$)	*Foods:* Eggs Meat Milk Processed foods Almost all foods have some phosphates	Decreased by aluminum and magnesium antacids, diarrhea	Inside cells Bones	*Cause shift into cells:* Epinephrine Insulin Increased cellular metabolism *Cause shift out of cells:* Ketoacidosis Cell death *Cause shift out of bones:* Parathyroid hormone Immobility	*Urinary:* Increased by parathyroid hormone, extracellular fluid volume expansion *Fecal* *Sweat*

From Felver, L. (1995). Fluid and electrolyte balance and imbalances. In S.L. Woods, E.S. Froelicher, C.J. Halpenny et al. (Eds.), *Cardiac nursing* (3rd ed., p. 126). Philadelphia: JB Lippincott.

ELECTROLYTE IMBALANCES

Plasma electrolyte imbalances may have profound effects on cardiovascular function. Because cardiac function depends on ion currents across myocardial cell membranes, action potential generation, impulse conduction, and myocardial contraction are all vulnerable to alterations in electrolyte status. In addition to their effects on the myocardium itself, some electrolyte imbalances have vascular effects.

Potassium Balance

Potassium balance is the net result of potassium intake and absorption, distribution, excretion, and abnormal losses. These components are summarized in Table 9-6. Although the plasma potassium concentration describes the status of potassium in the extracellular fluid, it does not necessarily reflect the amount of potassium inside the cells. The plasma potassium concentration has a circadian rhythm, rising during the hours a person is usually active and reaching its trough when a person is usually asleep. A classic study demonstrated that the kidneys handle an intravenous potassium load much less efficiently during the hours a person is customarily asleep, which has implications for potassium administration to ICU patients (Moore-Ede et al., 1978).

The potassium concentration of the extracellular fluid has a major influence on the function of the myocardium. Specifically, the resting membrane potential of cardiac cells is proportional to the ratio of potassium concentrations in the extracellular and intracellular fluids. The potassium concentration within cardiac cells is approximately 140 mEq/L; the normal potassium concentration of the extracellular fluid is 3.5 to 5 mEq/L. A small change in the extracellular concentration of potassium has a large effect on the extracellular-to-intracellular concentration ratio because the initial extracellular value is relatively small. A similar change in the intracellular potassium concentration has a lesser effect because the initial intracellular value is so large.

Hypokalemia

Hypokalemia, a decrease in the plasma potassium concentration, is caused by decreased potassium intake, shift of potassium ions from the extracellular fluid into the cells, increased excretion of potassium, loss of potassium through an abnormal route, or any combination of these factors (Felver, 2000). Some specific etiologic factors in these categories are listed in Table 9-7. Hypokalemia is common in patients with heart failure because of their increased secretion of aldosterone and their diuretic therapy (Laragh & Sealey, 2001).

Catecholamines and beta agonist drugs cause potassium ions to shift into cells by a β_2-adrenergic mechanism. This effect can produce hypokalemia (Hahn & Lofgren, 2000; Wong et al., 2001). Plasma catecholamines increase rapidly during myocardial infarction (MI) and hypokalemia is common during acute coronary syndromes (Foo et al., 2003). This hypokalemic effect is not as strong in persons who have diabetic autonomic neuropathy (Foo et al, 2003). Transient

Table 9-7 ■ CAUSES OF HYPOKALEMIA

Category	Clinical Examples
Decreased potassium intake	NPO orders
	Anorexia
	Fad diets
	Fasting
	Prolonged intravenous therapy without K^+
Potassium shift into cells	Alkalosis
	Excessive beta-adrenergic stimulation (epinephrine, beta agonists)
	Hypothermia (accidental or induced)
	Excessive insulin
	Rapid correction of acidosis during hemodialysis
	Familial periodic paralysis
Increased potassium excretion	Diarrhea (includes laxative overuse)
	Hyperaldosteronism (increases renal excretion of potassium)
	Chronic excessive ingestion of black licorice (contains aldosterone-like compounds)
	Excessive glucocorticoids (Cushing's syndrome; glucocorticoid therapy)
	Hypomagnesemia (causes renal potassium wasting)
	Diuretic therapy with loop or thiazide diuretics
	Polyuria
	High-dose penicillin therapy (nonreabsorbable anion effect in kidney)
Potassium loss by abnormal route	Emesis
	Nasogastric suction
	Drainage from gastrointestinal fistula
	Dialysis

hypokalemia associated with catecholamine release during a MI may cause further impairment of an already compromised myocardium (see Chapter 25).

The increased potassium excretion caused by many types of diuretics is well known (Chapman et al., 2002; USP, 2003). Hypokalemia caused by diuretic therapy occurs most frequently within 2 to 8 weeks, although it may arise after more than 1 year (Blanning & Westfall, 2001). The necessity of monitoring the plasma potassium concentration in patients using diuretics, especially older adults, is clear (Zuccala et al., 2000). Patients with hypokalemia have significantly more ventricular arrhythmias after MI than do normokalemic patients. The hypokalemic effect of catecholamines is stronger in patients who are using thiazide diuretics than it is in those who are not using diuretics.

Because of the cardiac effects of hypokalemia (discussed later), the National Council on Potassium in Clinical Practice has established guidelines for potassium replacement (Cohn et al., 2000). For patients with hypertension, the guideline is to maintain a serum potassium concentration of at least 4.0 mEq/L. Potassium replacement should be considered routinely in patients with CHF, even with a serum potassium level of 4.0 mEq/L. Potassium levels of at least 4.0 mEq/L are necessary in patients who have cardiac arrhythmias. The guidelines also emphasize the necessity of routine monitoring of serum potassium in patients who have CHF or cardiac arrhythmias.

The clinical manifestations of hypokalemia include diminished bowel sounds, abdominal distention, constipation, polyuria, skeletal muscle weakness, flaccid paralysis, cardiac arrhythmias, and postural hypotension. Cardiac and vascular effects of hypokalemia are discussed next.

Cardiac Effects of Hypokalemia. The cardiac effects of hypokalemia include changes in cell membrane resting potential. When the extracellular potassium concentration decreases, the extracellular/intracellular potassium concentration ratio decreases. This change in ratio causes cardiac muscle cells to hyperpolarize (i.e., the resting membrane potential becomes more negative). In hyperpolarized cells, the distance between resting potential and action potential is increased; hyperpolarized cells are less responsive to stimuli than are normal cells. The hyperpolarizing effect of hypokalemia on cardiac cells does not occur at all levels of hypokalemia. At low plasma potassium concentrations, a *hypopolarizing* effect may be seen. This is probably caused by decreased potassium conductance (analogous to decreased potassium permeability) of the cell membrane. The specific alteration of cardiac cell membrane resting potential thus depends on the degree of hypokalemia. In any case, the normal resting potential is altered, which contributes to the development of arrhythmias.

In addition to its effect on cell membrane resting potential, hypokalemia increases the rate of cardiac cell diastolic depolarization. Diastolic depolarization is the normal mechanism that initiates the depolarization of pacemaker cells (see Chapter 19). Under usual circumstances, diastolic depolarization is fastest in the sinus node cells; consequently, the sinus node serves as the predominant pacemaker. During hypokalemia, however, the rate of diastolic depolarization increases in other myocardial cells, especially in diseased myocardium. Ectopic beats may arise, even from hyperpolarized cells.

Other effects of hypokalemia on the myocardium also predispose to arrhythmias. Hypokalemia decreases conduction velocity, especially in the atrioventricular node. Hypokalemia prolongs the action potential by decreasing the rate of repolarization, at least in part by decreasing cardiac cell membrane permeability to potassium efflux. It increases the dispersion of ventricular repolarization, which may contribute to cardiac arrhythmias (Yelamanchi et al., 2001). The absolute refractory period is shorter than normal; the relative refractory period is prolonged. These changes in the refractory period predispose to the development of extrasystoles and reentrant arrhythmias (see Chapter 19).

The cardiac alterations of hypokalemia may cause many types of arrhythmias. Hypokalemia-induced arrhythmias include supraventricular premature depolarizations and tachycardias, atrial flutter, ventricular ectopic beats and ventricular tachycardia, torsade de pointes, and ventricular fibrillation (Araki et al., 2003; Boccalandro et al., 2003; Demir et al., 2000; Glauser, 2001; Kusano et al., 2001; Slovis & Jenkins, 2002). Hypokalemia potentiates digitalis toxicity and may reduce the effectiveness of disopyramide (USP, 2003). Animal studies indicate that down-regulation of gap junction proteins in diabetic cardiomyopathy increases the vulnerability to ventricular fibrillation in hypokalemia (Okruhlicova et al., 2002).

As might be expected from the previous discussion, electrocardiographic (ECG) changes are seen in patients with hypokalemia (see Chapter 19). A characteristic change is the development of U waves (Webster et al., 2002). Other ECG changes include flattened T waves, ST segment depression, and prolonged PR interval (Hahn & Lofgren, 2000; Webster

et al., 2002). A prolonged QT interval may also occur in hypokalemia; the QRS complex may widen (Demir et al., 2000; Marinella & Burdette, 2000; Slovis & Jenkins, 2002; Yelamanchi et al., 2001).

Long-standing hypokalemia is associated with selective myocardial cell necrosis. As discussed in Chapter 31, selective myocardial cell necrosis is associated with sudden cardiac death.

Vascular Effects of Hypokalemia. In addition to the multiple cardiac effects discussed previously, hypokalemia has vascular effects. Postural hypotension often occurs in hypokalemia (Rose and Post, 2001), most likely caused by impaired smooth muscle function.

Classic studies indicate that chronic potassium depletion in humans impairs vasodilation during strenuous exercise (Knochel & Schlein, 1972). The resulting impaired muscle blood flow decreases oxygen delivery and contributes to the rhabdomyolysis that occurs with whole-body potassium depletion (Lane & Phillips, 2003; Ozgur & Kursat, 2002; Prat et al., 2001).

Hyperkalemia

Hyperkalemia, an increased plasma potassium concentration, results from increased potassium intake, shift of potassium ions from the cells to the extracellular fluid, decreased potassium excretion, or any combination of these factors (Felver, 2000). Examples of specific etiologic factors in each of these categories are listed in Table 9-8. Hyperkalemia may occur during hemorrhagic or hypovolemic shock and during cardiopulmonary resuscitation.

Some medications that are commonly administered to patients with cardiac disease may cause hyperkalemia. *Angiotensin-converting enzyme (ACE) inhibitors,* such as captopril and enalapril, and *angiotensin II receptor blockers,* such as losartan, decrease the release of aldosterone. Aldosterone normally

Table 9–8 ■ CAUSES OF HYPERKALEMIA

Category	Clinical Examples
Increased potassium intake	Excessive intravenous potassium
	Insufficiently mixed KCl in flexible plastic intravenous bag
	Massive transfusion of blood stored longer than 3 days (K^+ leaves red blood cells)
	Large doses of intravenous potassium penicillin G (contains 1.6 mEq K^+/million units)
	Large oral intake only if decreased renal excretion
Potassium shift out of cells	Acidosis due to mineral acids (not organic acids like ketoacids)
	Insulin deficiency
	Massive cell death (crushing injuries, burns, cytotoxic drugs)
	Large digitalis overdose
	Familial periodic paralysis
Decreased potassium excretion	Oliguria
	Extracellular fluid volume depletion
	Oliguric renal failure
	Decreased aldosterone from any cause (Addison's disease, chronic heparin administration, lead poisoning, ACE inhibitors, angiotensin II receptor antagonists)
	Potassium-sparing diuretics

facilitates renal excretion of potassium. When these drugs decrease the availability of aldosterone, hyperkalemia may occur (USP, 2003). Severe hyperkalemia from ACE inhibitors occurs more commonly in people older than age 70 years. *Potassium-sparing diuretics,* such as triamterene, spironolactone, and amiloride, may cause hyperkalemia, especially if given with potassium supplementation or ACE inhibitors (Blaustein et al., 2002; USP, 2003). *Beta-adrenergic blockers* (those with β_2 action) promote the development of hyperkalemia by blocking catecholamine-induced potassium entry into cells. Hemodialysis patients and persons who have undergone renal transplantation have increased risk of hyperkalemia from beta-blockers (McCauley et al., 2002; Nowicki & Miszczak-Kuban, 2002; Nowicki et al., 2002). The hyperkalemic effect of beta-blockade is especially pronounced during exercise, which has relevance to treadmill stress testing (Lucia et al., 2002). Administration of *unfractionated heparin,* even in low-dose therapy, decreases the synthesis of aldosterone; hyperkalemia is likely to occur in heparinized persons who have even mild renal insufficiency (Day et al., 2002; Rose & Post, 2001). Low-molecular-weight heparin does not seem to have this effect (Abdel-Raheem et al., 2002). A massive overdose of *digitalis* causes hyperkalemia by allowing intracellular potassium to leak into the extracellular fluid (USP, 2003).

Another cardiovascular-related source of hyperkalemia is massive blood transfusion (Downes & Sarode, 2001). While blood is stored, potassium ions leak from the erythrocytes into the plasma. The longer the storage time, the greater the potassium load contained in a unit of blood (Knichwit et al., 2002). A classic study indicates that if the blood has been in storage for more than 3 days, rewarming the blood before administration causes only minimal return of potassium to the cells (Eurenius & Smith, 1973). Patients receiving more than 10 units of stored blood within a few hours are considered at high risk for severe hyperkalemia; however, fatal hyperkalemia has occurred with transfusion of fewer units.

Hyperkalemia may be manifested clinically by intestinal cramping and diarrhea, skeletal muscle weakness, flaccid paralysis, cardiac arrhythmias, and cardiac arrest. The cardiac effects of hyperkalemia are potentially fatal; they are discussed in the next section.

Cardiac Effects of Hyperkalemia. Hyperkalemia alters myocardial cell function in several ways. When the plasma potassium concentration increases, the extracellular/intracellular potassium concentration ratio increases. Consequently, the resting membrane potential of cardiac cells becomes partially depolarized (hypopolarized). Initially, the partial depolarization of resting cardiac cells increases their excitability because the resting potential is close to threshold potential (see Chapter 19). As the extracellular potassium concentration increases, however, the cardiac cells depolarize to the extent that they cannot repolarize. Cells in this state are nonexcitable; no further contractile activity occurs. The ability of hyperkalemia to cause asystolic cardiac arrest is exploited by using potassium as a cardioplegic agent during cardiac surgery (Li et al., 2002).

Other effects of hyperkalemia include decreased duration of the action potential at all heart rates and increased rate of repolarization, the latter due to increased permeability of the cardiac cell membrane to potassium efflux (Yelamanchi et al., 2001). Hyperkalemia lengthens the effective refractory period of atrial muscle and slows diastolic depolarization of pacemaker cells, two antiarrhythmic effects. Cardiac cells vary in their sensitivity to the effects of hyperkalemia. Atrial cells are more sensitive than ventricular cells; the conduction system is the least affected by hyperkalemia.

As the plasma potassium increases, the rate of rise of the action potential decreases. Slow upstroke velocity decreases cell-to-cell conduction velocity (see Chapter 19). Hyperkalemia decreases conduction velocity at all levels of the conduction system: atrial, atrioventricular nodal, and intraventricular (Gennari, 2002). In severe hyperkalemia, intraventricular conduction may be completely inhibited. Bundle-branch block or, less frequently, complete heart block may occur (Webster et al., 2002).

Although some of the cellular effects of hyperkalemia are anti-arrhythmogenic, cardiac arrhythmias do occur in hyperkalemia. The differential effects of hyperkalemia on different cell types cause slow and nonhomogeneous conduction to cells with variable degrees of excitability. When intra-atrial conduction is decreased, sinus node impulses may be delayed in exit or may fail to propagate. This situation gives rise to Wenckebach (type I) or Mobitz (type II) sinoatrial block (see Chapter 19). Reentrant ventricular arrhythmias may arise. Ventricular tachycardia may terminate in ventricular fibrillation (Webster et al., 2002). Asystolic cardiac arrest is also a potentially fatal event (Slovis & Jenkins, 2002). Hyperkalemia may cause heart block with digitalis and serious arrhythmias with concurrent use of disopyramide (USP, 2003).

The characteristic ECG changes of hyperkalemia arise from the electrophysiologic changes previously described. The T waves become peaked (tented) with a narrow base and symmetric shape (Somers et al., 2002). The QRS complex widens; ST depression may occur. Hyperkalemia also causes decreased amplitude and prolongation of P waves and PR prolongation. As the plasma potassium concentration increases to high levels, the P waves disappear. A sine-wave pattern appears in severe, often terminal, hyperkalemia (Slovis & Jenkins, 2002; Webster et al., 2002).

The ECG changes of hyperkalemia are not well correlated with plasma potassium levels (Webster et al., 2002). Although the ECG is usually abnormal with severe hyperkalemia (serum potassium greater than 8 mEq/L), minimal ECG changes have been observed in patients with serum potassium concentrations greater than 9 mEq/L. The rate of increase of the plasma potassium concentration may contribute more to the ECG changes in hyperkalemia than does the absolute plasma potassium level. Hemodialysis patients may not exhibit the characteristic peaked T wave or other ECG signs when they are severely hyperkalemic. This may be caused in part by concurrent hypercalcemia, which can flatten the T wave (Aslam et al., 2002). The ECG changes of hyperkalemia are also blunted during hypothermia (Mattu et al., 2002). Occasionally, the ECG in hyperkalemia mimics MI; the ECG will normalize after treatment of the hyperkalemia (Webster et al., 2002).

During myocardial ischemia, potassium concentration increases quickly in the extracellular spaces of the myocardium. The clinical effect of these localized areas of high potassium concentration is not yet understood. During exercise, elevated catecholamines counteract the negative cardiac effects of hyperkalemia in normal hearts; this protective effect is diminished in ischemic hearts.

Hyperkalemia also has an indirect cardiac effect in that it stimulates aldosterone secretion. Through its saline-retaining action on the kidneys, aldosterone expands the ECV, which may have a detrimental effect on patients in heart failure.

Vascular Effects of Hyperkalemia. Hyperkalemia reduces the smooth muscle relaxation normally mediated by endothelium-derived hyperpolarizing factor (EDHF) (Long et al., 2002). In high concentrations, potassium ions cause contraction of smooth muscle of coronary arteries (Krassoi et al., 2003).

Calcium Balance

Calcium balance is the net result of calcium intake and absorption, distribution, excretion, and abnormal losses. These components are summarized in Table 9-6. Calcium in the plasma exists in three forms: protein bound, complexed, and ionized (free). The calcium that is bound to plasma proteins and complexed with small anions (e.g., citrate) is physiologically inactive. Only the ionized calcium is physiologically active. The commonly used laboratory measure for extracellular calcium is the total calcium concentration (bound, complexed, and ionized), although ionized calcium measurements are available clinically in many locations.

Calcium ions play crucial roles in the automaticity of the sinus and atrioventricular nodes, in the plateau phase of the Purkinje and ventricular cell action potentials, in excitation-contraction coupling, and in cardiac and vascular muscle contraction (see Chapters 1 and 19). Not unexpectedly, one of the cardiac effects of an abnormal extracellular calcium concentration is altered duration of the plateau phase. Extracellular fluid calcium imbalances are less likely to cause cardiac arrhythmias than are potassium imbalances, but arrhythmias associated with hypercalcemia have been fatal. In addition to their cardiac effects, acute calcium imbalances also affect the vasculature.

Hypocalcemia

Hypocalcemia may be defined as a decreased extracellular *total* calcium concentration or as a decreased extracellular *ionized* calcium concentration. The first definition refers to the commonly measured total calcium value. The second definition of hypocalcemia, however, is used in this chapter because decreases in ionized calcium concentration cause physiologic effects even if the total plasma concentration is within normal limits.

Hypocalcemia results from decreased calcium intake or absorption, decreased physiologic availability of calcium, increased calcium excretion, loss of calcium by an abnormal route, or any combination of these factors (Felver, 2000). Table 9-9 lists specific causative factors for hypocalcemia. Several of these specific factors may cause hypocalcemia in patients with cardiac disease. The preservative used in storage of blood contains citrate, which complexes with calcium ions. Large or rapid transfusions of citrated blood cause hypocalcemia by decreasing the physiologic availability of calcium in the blood (Downes & Sarode, 2001; Zixin et al., 2001). The hypocalcemic effect of blood transfusions is greater in critically ill patients (Carlstedt & Lind, 2001). Similarly, rapid administra-

Table 9–9 ▪ CAUSES OF HYPOCALCEMIA

Category	Clinical Examples
Decreased calcium intake or absorption	Diet deficient in calcium
	Diet deficient in vitamin D
	Malabsorption syndromes
	Chronic diarrhea (including laxative overuse)
	Steatorrhea
	Pancreatitis
Shift of calcium into physiologically unavailable form or into bones	Alkalosis
	Massive blood transfusion (citrate binds Ca^{2+})
	Rapid infusion of albumin
	Pancreatitis
	Lack of PTH (hypoparathyroidism; surgical removal of parathyroid gland during thyroid surgery)
	Hypomagnesemia
	Hyperphosphatemia (overuse of phosphate-containing laxatives or enemas; excessive oral or IV phosphate intake; tumor lysis syndrome)
	Acute fluoride poisoning
Increased calcium excretion	Gastrointestinal: Pancreatitis
	Renal: Chronic renal insufficiency
Loss of calcium by abnormal route	Wound exudate

tion of proteinaceous plasma expanders such as albumin also decreases the physiologic availability of plasma calcium and may cause symptomatic hypocalcemia.

Hypocalcemia increases neuromuscular excitability. The clinical manifestations of hypocalcemia may include digital and perioral paresthesias, positive Chvostek's sign, positive Trousseau's sign, muscle twitching and cramping, grimacing, hyperactive reflexes, tetany, carpopedal spasm, laryngospasm, seizures, cardiac arrhythmias, cardiac arrest, and hypotension (with acute hypocalcemia).

Cardiac Effects of Hypocalcemia. Hypocalcemia prolongs the plateau phase, thereby increasing the duration of the cardiac action potential. In addition, hypocalcemia slows atrioventricular and intraventricular conduction to a moderate degree (Al-Wahab & Munyard, 2001).

These hypocalcemia-related changes in the myocardium usually are not great enough to give rise to significant cardiac arrhythmias in clinical settings, although they may occasionally predispose to ventricular arrhythmias, including torsade de pointes (RuDusky, 2001). Hypocalcemia does cause characteristic alterations in the ECG. Hypocalcemia prolongs the ST segment (Keegan et al., 2002). This finding is not unexpected because hypocalcemia prolongs the plateau phase of the action potential. The prolongation of the ST segment causes a prolonged QT interval (Nishra et al., 2001; Peterson, 2001; Slovis & Jenkins, 2002). The degree of prolongation of the QT interval is not a reliable indicator of the degree of hypocalcemia or of the decrease in ionized calcium concentration, but it is influenced by the rate of decrease of the ionized calcium (Zivin et al., 2001). Concurrent hypomagnesemia magnifies the ECG effects of hypocalcemia. ECG changes in patients with hypocalcemia and hypomagnesemia may mimic myocardial infarction (Lehmann et al., 2000).

Hypocalcemia impairs myocardial contractility and thus may cause heart failure (Gulati et al., 2001; Kashyap & Kashyap,

2001). Patients who already have heart failure may decompensate if they become hypocalcemic. Hypocalcemia-associated heart failure may be unresponsive to digitalis until the hypocalcemia is corrected (USP, 2003). Although the role of calcium ions in the regulation of myocardial contraction is clear (see Chapter 19), the mechanism by which hypocalcemia interferes with this process is not fully understood. Because most of the calcium ions that initiate myocardial contraction come from the sarcoplasmic reticulum rather than directly from the extracellular fluid, the depressive effect of hypocalcemia on myocardial contractility is probably most important in patients who have pre-existing down-regulation of beta-adrenergic receptors (Lehmann et al., 2000). In a normal heart, hypocalcemia reduces stroke work at any particular left ventricular end-diastolic pressure. This impairment is even greater in an ischemic heart. A classic study showed that patients who are administered albumin for resuscitation during hypovolemic shock may also exhibit impaired myocardial contractility when the ionized calcium binds to the albumin and becomes physiologically unavailable (Kovalik et al., 1981).

Vascular Effects of Hypocalcemia. Calcium ions play several important roles in contraction of vascular smooth muscle. They are involved in the action potential, in the regulation of cell membrane permeability, and in excitation-contraction coupling. In smooth muscle, as well as in cardiac muscle, contraction is initiated by an increase in cytoplasmic calcium. Most of the calcium ions that initiate the contraction come from the sarcoplasmic reticulum rather than from the extracellular fluid. Any short-term effects of hypocalcemia on the vasculature are more likely to arise from alterations in cell membrane permeability than from alteration in the contractile mechanisms. Acute (but not chronic) hypocalcemia causes hypotension. The mechanisms involved are not completely understood but likely include decreased peripheral vascular resistance and impaired cardiac function.

Hypercalcemia

Hypercalcemia is caused by increased intake or absorption of calcium, shift of calcium from the bones into the extracellular fluid, decreased calcium excretion, or any combination of these factors (Felver, 2000). Specific causative factors are listed under these categories in Table 9-10. Note that thiazide diuretics, often administered to patients with cardiac disease, decrease the urinary excretion of calcium (Sato et al., 2002;

Table 9–10 ■ CAUSES OF HYPERCALCEMIA

Category	Clinical Examples
Increased calcium intake or absorption	Milk-alkali syndrome
	Excessive vitamin D
Shift of calcium out of bone	Hyperparathyroidism
	Prolonged immobility
	Bone tumors
	Multiple myeloma
	Cancers that produce parathyroid hormone-related factor and other bone-resorbing factors
Decreased calcium excretion	Thiazide diuretics
	Familial hypocalciuric hypercalcemia

USP, 2003). Another type of diuretic should be substituted if hypercalcemia develops.

The clinical manifestations of hypercalcemia include anorexia, nausea, vomiting, constipation, abdominal pain, polyuria, renal calculi, skeletal muscle weakness, diminished reflexes, confusion, lethargy, possible personality change, frank psychosis, cardiac arrhythmias, and hypertension (with acute hypercalcemia).

Cardiac Effects of Hypercalcemia. Hypercalcemia shortens the plateau phase of the cardiac action potential, thereby decreasing the duration of the action potential. In addition, it increases the rate of diastolic depolarization of sinus node cells and may increase the initial rate of increase and amplitude of the action potential. It may also delay atrioventricular conduction.

Cardiac arrhythmias that have been reported to arise from hypercalcemia include various types of heart block, paroxysmal atrial fibrillation, and severe bradycardia (Wolf et al., 2000). Hypercalcemia potentiates digitalis toxicity (Slovis & Jenkins, 2002). Patients using digitalis may acquire heart block if they become hypercalcemic (USP, 2003). Sudden death has occurred in severe hypercalcemia, possibly caused by ventricular fibrillation.

The ECG in hypercalcemia reflects the short plateau phase in a shortened ST segment. The QT interval is decreased as a result (Slovis & Jenkins, 2002). The length of the QT interval is a clinically unreliable index of the extent of hypercalcemia. Hypercalcemia has been accompanied by lengthening of the QRS complex and diffuse flattening of T waves (Ashizawa et al., 2003).

Vascular Effects of Hypercalcemia. In persons who have intact parathyroid glands, acute hypercalcemia causes vasoconstriction and raises systolic blood pressure by impairing the vasodilatory function of the endothelium (Nilsson et al., 2001). Increased intracellular calcium in vascular smooth muscle also causes increased vascular resistance. In many people with essential hypertension, increased intracellular calcium occurs with normal plasma calcium levels. Parathyroid hormone and parathyroid hormone-related factor are implicated in transepithelial calcium transport and likely play a role in the hypertensive mechanism.

Magnesium Balance

Magnesium balance is the net result of magnesium intake and absorption, distribution, excretion, and abnormal losses. These components are summarized in Table 9-6. Similar to calcium, magnesium in the plasma exists in three forms: protein-bound, complexed, and ionized (free). Only the ionized magnesium is physiologically active; however, the only widely available clinical laboratory measure for magnesium is the total serum magnesium concentration (bound, complexed, and ionized).

Magnesium, like potassium, is primarily an intracellular ion. For this reason, plasma levels of magnesium do not necessarily reflect the intracellular magnesium content. Total-body magnesium depletion may be present even when the plasma magnesium is normal. Intracellular magnesium is a cofactor for many enzymes, including Na^+-K^+ adenosine triphosphatase (ATPase). Changes in magnesium balance, especially hypomagnesemia, cause alterations in ion transport across membranes. Because the function of cardiac and smooth muscle depends on ion fluxes, magnesium imbalances have myocardial and vascular effects.

Table 9–11 ■ CAUSES OF HYPOMAGNESEMIA

Category	Clinical Examples
Decreased magnesium intake or absorption	Prolonged IV therapy without Mg^{2+}
	Chronic malnutrition
	Chronic diarrhea
	Steatorrhea
	Pancreatitis
	Malabsorption syndromes
	Chronic alcoholism
	Ileal resection
Increased magnesium excretion	Gastrointestinal: Steatorrhea
	Renal: Diabetic ketoacidosis; diuretic therapy; increased aldosterone (CHF, cirrhosis, hyperaldosteronism); chronic alcoholism; renal damage from drugs (amphotericin B, aminoglycosides)
Magnesium loss by abnormal route	Emesis
	Nasogastric suctioning
	Drainage from GI fistula

Hypomagnesemia and Total-Body Magnesium Depletion

Hypomagnesemia and total-body magnesium depletion are caused by decreased magnesium intake or absorption, decreased physiologic availability of magnesium, increased magnesium excretion, loss of magnesium by an abnormal route, or any combination of these factors (Felver, 2000). Specific causative factors for hypomagnesemia are listed in Table 9-11. Hypomagnesemia and total-body magnesium depletion are common in chronic alcoholism; therefore, patients with alcoholic cardiomyopathy need assessment for hypomagnesemia.

Diuretics (except for spironolactone, triamterene, and amiloride) and digitalis cause increased renal excretion of magnesium and can lead to hypomagnesemia. Patients with heart failure are at high risk for hypomagnesemia or total-body magnesium depletion (Cohen et al., 2003). In addition to diuretic and digitalis therapy, they often have congestion of the splanchnic vessels, which decreases magnesium absorption. Also, the secondary hyperaldosteronism and elevated catecholamines of heart failure increase urinary excretion of magnesium. Hypomagnesemic patients who have congestive heart failure have more arrhythmias than normomagnesemia patients (Oladapo & Falese, 2000). Patients with acute MI often have ionized hypomagnesemia (Elming et al., 2000). Hypomagnesemia may be a causative factor for MI as well as a result of pathophysiologic changes immediately after MI.

Hypomagnesemia causes increased neuromuscular excitability. The signs and symptoms of hypomagnesemia include hyperactive reflexes, positive Chvostek's sign, positive Trousseau's sign, leg and foot cramps, muscle twitching, grimacing, tremors, dysphagia, nystagmus, ataxia, tetany, seizures, extreme confusion, cardiac arrhythmias, and hypertension.

Cardiac Effects of Hypomagnesemia and Total-Body Magnesium Depletion. Magnesium is a cofactor for Na^+-K^+ ATPase, the enzyme that plays a major role in the regulation of intracellular potassium concentration in the myocardium. When magnesium is deficient, the decreased intracellular

magnesium leads to decreased activity of this enzyme. As a result, the intracellular potassium ion concentration decreases and intracellular sodium concentration increases in myocardial cells. Decreased activity of Na^+-K^+ ATPase interferes with the reentry of potassium ions into depolarized cells and promotes diastolic leak of potassium from cells that are already depolarized. In addition, hypomagnesemia causes increased membrane permeability to potassium, an effect that also tends to decrease intracellular potassium concentration in the myocardium.

In hypomagnesemia, the sinus node has an increased spontaneous firing rate, and there is a rate-dependent decrease in the duration of the cardiac action potential. The absolute refractory period is shortened, and the relative refractory period is lengthened. Hypomagnesemia thus predisposes to arrhythmias, especially tachyarrhythmias. The imbalance is associated with supraventricular tachycardia, supraventricular ectopy, ventricular ectopic beats, ventricular tachycardia, ventricular fibrillation, and torsade de pointes (Klevay & Milne, 2002; Mela et al., 2002; Onagawa et al., 2003). Whether these arrhythmias are caused directly by the hypomagnesemia itself or by hypomagnesemia-induced changes in potassium transport across myocardial membranes is uncertain. What is clear, however, is that both hypomagnesemia and total-body magnesium depletion lead to cardiac arrhythmias that can be corrected only by the administration of magnesium. Clinical studies demonstrate that correction of ionized hypomagnesemia during coronary artery bypass surgery (CABG) leads to fewer postoperative episodes of ventricular tachycardia (Wilkes et al., 2002). Administration of magnesium reduces postoperative arrhythmias in CABG patients and in children having surgery for congenital heart defects, regardless of whether they are initially hypomagnesemic (Dorman et al., 2000; Speziale et al., 2000). In patients who are not hypomagnesemic, magnesium has been used pharmacologically to treat arrhythmias, including atrial fibrillation, ventricular tachycardia, and torsade de pointes, and to reduce arrhythmias in acute MI and in heart failure (Ceremuzynski et al., 2000; Kaye & O'Sullivan, 2002).

A classic study demonstrated that heart muscle magnesium content decreases after acute MI (Speich et al., 1980). This post-MI magnesium decrease may be caused by leakage of magnesium from necrotic cells and interference with ion transport in hypoxic cells. Another mechanism for the cardiac muscle magnesium decrease after MI may be the action of catecholamines. It is likely that localized decreases of myocardial magnesium after acute MI predispose to the development of cardiac arrhythmias. Animal studies show decreased tolerance to ischemic stress with chronic magnesium deficiency (Kramer et al., 2003).

Hypomagnesemia potentiates digitalis toxicity (USP, 2003). Hypomagnesemia-related digitalis toxicity arises in part from the intracellular potassium deficiency caused by the magnesium imbalance. Digitalis toxicity arrhythmias have been observed in patients with therapeutic digitalis levels and either decreased serum magnesium levels or normal serum levels with total-body magnesium depletion.

The ECG changes in hypomagnesemia are not easily characterized; rather, they are somewhat nonspecific. Prolongation of the QT interval is frequently observed in hypomagnesemia

(Onagawa et al., 2003). This ECG change probably occurs because of altered potassium transport caused by hypomagnesemia. Other ECG changes that have been seen with hypomagnesemia, such as ST segment depression, prolonged PR interval, wide QRS complex, and T-wave abnormalities, may be caused by multiple electrolyte imbalances that occur in conjunction with hypomagnesemia, or by the hypomagnesemia itself.

Vascular Effects of Hypomagnesemia and Total-Body Magnesium Depletion. Hypomagnesemia has important effects on vascular smooth muscle. A decrease in the extracellular magnesium concentration causes arteriolar vasoconstriction, in part by increasing the intracellular calcium concentration in vascular smooth muscle. The resulting increased peripheral vascular resistance causes the hypertension that often accompanies acute or chronic hypomagnesemia. In addition to this direct vasoconstrictive effect, hypomagnesemia also decreases the vasodilation response to acetylcholine (Touyz et al., 2002). Low levels of dietary magnesium and low serum magnesium are associated with increased prevalence of hypertension (Fox et al., 2003).

The vascular actions of hypomagnesemia promote the occurrence of vasospasm (Fox et al., 2001). The coronary arteries are extremely sensitive to the effects of hypomagnesemia. Coronary artery spasm may cause acute myocardial ischemia in clinical hypomagnesemia (Ortega-Carnicier et al., 2001). Sudden-death ischemic heart disease, associated with a reduced dietary intake of magnesium, may be the result of coronary vasospasm. Plasma free fatty acids bind ionized magnesium, rendering it physiologically inactive. An increase in plasma free fatty acids thus causes a decrease in the amount of ionized magnesium. In patients who have total-body magnesium depletion, it is possible that epinephrine-induced increases in plasma free fatty acids are a triggering factor for coronary vasospasm (and subsequent sudden death).

Total-body magnesium depletion (with or without hypomagnesemia) appears to play an important role in the development of atherosclerosis and ischemic heart disease. Animal studies show hypertension, endothelial dysfunction, and vascular remodeling with chronic magnesium deficiency (Touyz et al., 2002). Animal studies demonstrate plasma elevation of pro-inflammatory cytokines and neuropeptides that stimulate free radical formation (Kramer et al., 2003). Thus, magnesium deficiency can cause changes that are part of the atherosclerotic process.

In summary, the vascular effects of hypomagnesemia include vasoconstriction, increased peripheral resistance, hypertension, impaired vasodilation, and a tendency to vasospasm. Current evidence relates total-body magnesium depletion, with or without hypomagnesemia, to congestive heart failure, ischemic heart disease, and essential hypertension.

Hypermagnesemia

Hypermagnesemia is caused by increased magnesium intake or absorption, increased physiologic availability of magnesium, decreased magnesium excretion, or any combination of these factors (Felver, 2000). Specific causative factors for hypermagnesemia are listed in Table 9-12. Older adults who use magnesium-containing antacids and laxatives are at especially high risk for development of hypermagnesemia, in part because they

Table 9–12 ■ CAUSES OF HYPERMAGNESEMIA

Category	Clinical Examples
Increased magnesium intake or absorption	Excessive use of Mg^{2+}-containing laxatives, antacids, or urologic irrigation solutions
	Excessive intravenous infusion of Mg^{2+}
	Aspiration of sea water
Decreased magnesium excretion	Oliguric renal failure
	Adrenal insufficiency

may have unrecognized renal insufficiency (Schelling, 2000; Zaman & Abreo, 2003).

The cardiac effects (bradycardia, arrhythmias, cardiac arrest) and vascular effects (flushing, hypotension) of hypermagnesemia are discussed next. In addition to these effects, hypermagnesemia may cause a subjective sensation of warmth, diaphoresis, drowsiness, lethargy, coma, diminished deep tendon reflexes, flaccid skeletal muscle paralysis, and respiratory depression.

Cardiac Effects of Hypermagnesemia. A plasma excess of magnesium interferes with cardiac conduction throughout the heart. AV block or complete heart block may occur at high plasma levels of magnesium (Harker & Majcher, 2000; Zaman & Abreo, 2003). Hypermagnesemia inhibits myocardial contraction and depresses membrane excitability, although intracellular contractile mechanisms remain intact (USP, 2003).

Hypermagnesemia suppresses the SA node and causes sympathetic nervous system blockade (Schelling, 2000). Both of these factors contribute to clinically significant supraventricular bradycardia. Cardiac arrest in asystole may be fatal in severe hypermagnesemia. ECG changes associated with hypermagnesemia include prolonged PR interval and increased duration of the QRS complex (Birrer et al., 2002; Zaman & Abreo, 2003). These changes are somewhat variable and do not present a classic, easily recognizable picture.

Vascular Effects of Hypermagnesemia. Hypermagnesemia reduces peripheral vascular resistance by inhibiting calcium movement into vascular smooth muscle cells, inhibiting calcium release from intracellular storage, and depressing contractile responses to vasoactive substances such as epinephrine and angiotensin II (USP, 2003). The peripheral vasodilation caused by these mechanisms leads to hypotension (Birrer et al., 2002). Vasodilation of cutaneous vessels in hypermagnesemia causes flushing.

Phosphate Balance

Phosphate balance is the net result of phosphate intake and absorption, distribution, excretion, and abnormal losses. These components are summarized in Table 9-6.

The normal range of serum phosphate concentration is 2.5 to 4.5 mg/dL. Mild or moderate hypophosphatemia (1.0 to 2.4 mg/dL) may be asymptomatic. Severe hypophosphatemia, with a serum phosphate less than 1 mg/dL, usually has dramatic clinical manifestations.

Severe Hypophosphatemia

Hypophosphatemia is caused by decreased intake or absorption of phosphate, shift of phosphate into cells, or increased phosphate excretion (Felver, 2000). Specific causative factors included in these categories are presented in Table 9–13.

Of importance to patients with cardiac disease is the decrease in plasma phosphate concentration that occurs with intravenous glucose administration. Glucose infusion by itself does not usually cause severe hypophosphatemia; however, if glucose infusion is combined with other factors, such as diuretics that increase phosphate excretion, severe hypophosphatemia may result. Insulin, as well as glucose, promotes the movement of phosphate into cells. Catecholamines and β-adrenergic agonist drugs also shift phosphate into cells and predispose to hypophosphatemia (Subramanian & Khardori, 2000).

Hypophosphatemia is common in chronic alcoholism (Miller & Slovis, 2000; Shiber & Mattu, 2002). Patients with newly diagnosed alcoholic cardiomyopathy need to have their phosphate levels checked. If they undergo alcohol withdrawal, then they will likely be hyperventilating and respiratory alkalosis will develop, which also causes hypophosphatemia; therefore, their phosphate levels will need continued monitoring.

The signs and symptoms of severe hypophosphatemia include anorexia, nausea, malaise, diminished reflexes, paresthesias, muscle aching, muscle weakness, rhabdomyolysis, severe debility, acute respiratory failure, hemolysis (possible hemolytic anemia), confusion, stupor, seizures, coma, and impaired cardiac function. These effects of hypophosphatemia are caused primarily by decreased intracellular ATP and by decreased 2,3-diphosphoglycerate (2,3-DPG) in the red blood cells. Decreased erythrocyte 2,3-DPG causes tissue hypoxia by increasing hemoglobin-oxygen affinity, which reduces oxygen release. Administration of phosphate to hypophosphatemic patients increases erythrocyte 2,3-DPG, which decreases hemoglobin-oxygen affinity and allows greater tissue oxygenation (Miller & Slovis, 2000).

Cardiac Effects of Severe Hypophosphatemia. Severe hypophosphatemia impairs myocardial function by decreasing cardiac contractility. This cardiac impairment may progress to acute congestive failure or congestive cardiomyopathy (Claudius et al., 2002; Miller & Slovis, 2000). The decreased cardiac performance of hypophosphatemia is reversed by the intravenous administration of phosphate (Claudius, Sachs, & Shamji, 2002; Subramanian & Khardori, 2000).

The role of severe hypophosphatemia in cardiac arrhythmias is not well understood. Arrhythmias do occur in these patients. However, many patients who have severe hypophosphatemia also have hypokalemia or hypocalcemia or multiple electrolyte imbalances, so it may be difficult to isolate the effect of the decreased phosphate.

Vascular Effects of Severe Hypophosphatemia. Clinically, any vascular effects of severe hypophosphatemia are difficult to separate from the cardiac effects. Mean arterial pressure in hypophosphatemic patients increases after phosphate repletion (Claudius et al., 2002). It is possible that this effect is caused by a vascular as well as a myocardial action; however, clearly the cardiac effect predominates in most situations.

SUMMARY

Fluid balance is determined by the interplay of fluid intake, distribution, excretion, and fluid loss through abnormal routes. The two types of fluid imbalances are ECV imbalances and osmolality imbalances. ECV imbalances are increases or decreases in the amount of fluid in the vascular and interstitial compartments. Osmolality imbalances are alterations in the concentration of body fluids and result in movement of water into or out of cells caused by osmosis. Extracellular volume and osmolality imbalances may occur concurrently or separately in patients with cardiac disease.

A normal plasma electrolyte concentration is necessary for optimal cardiovascular function. Because electrolytes play important roles in the generation of action potentials and the contraction of cardiac and smooth muscle, electrolyte imbalances exert cardiac and vascular effects. The effects of a specific electrolyte imbalance depend on the specific role of that electrolyte in normal cardiovascular function.

People who do not have cardiovascular disease may acquire an electrolyte imbalance that subsequently causes cardiovascular impairment. In addition, patients who have pre-existing cardiovascular disease have specific risk factors for electrolyte imbalances. If imbalances develop in these patients, then the cardiovascular effects of the electrolyte imbalances may cause severe disturbance to an already compromised cardiovascular system. Successful nursing management of these patients involves careful assessment of risk factors, elimination of those risk factors when possible, surveillance for the manifestations of fluid and electrolyte imbalances, and nursing interventions to protect and support function during the correction of fluid and electrolyte imbalances (Felver, 2000).

Table 9–13 ■ CAUSES OF HYPOPHOSPHATEMIA

Category	Clinical Examples
Decreased phosphate intake or absorption	Prolonged or excessive antacid use
	Starvation
	Malabsorption syndromes
	Chronic diarrhea
	Chronic alcoholism
Shift of phosphate into cells	Total parenteral nutrition
	Rapid cell proliferation (refeeding after starvation or malnutrition; leukemic blast crisis)
	Respiratory alkalosis (hyperventilation)
	Insulin
	Epinephrine, beta-adrenergic agonists
	Infusion of IV glucose, fructose, or lactate
Increased phosphate excretion	Diabetic ketoacidosis
	Alcohol withdrawal
	Diuretic phase after severe burns
	Infusion of IV bicarbonate
	Renal tubular acidosis
	Diuretic therapy
	Glucocorticoid therapy
Phosphate loss by abnormal route	Emesis
	Hemodialysis

REFERENCES

Abdel-Raheem, M., Potti, A., Tadros, S., Koka, V., Hanekom, D., Fraiman, G., & Danielson, B. D. (2002). Effect of low-molecular-weight heparin on potassium homeostasis. *Pathophysiology of Haemostasis & Thrombosis, 32,* 107–110.

Al-Salman, J., & Pursell, R. (2001). Hyponatremic encephalopathy induced by thiazides. *Western Journal of Medicine, 175,* 87.

Al-Wahab, S., & Munyard, P. (2001). Functional atrioventricular block in a preterm infant. *Archives of Diseases of Childhood,* 85, F220–F221.

Araki, T., Konno, T. Itoh, H., Ino, H., & Shimizu, M. (2003). Brugada syndrome with ventricular tachycardia and fibrillation related to hypokalemia. *Circulation Journal, 67,* 93–95.

Ashizawa, N., Arakawa, S., Koide, Y., Toda, G., Seto, S., & Yano, K. (2003). Hypercalcemia due to vitamin D intoxication with clinical features mimicking acute myocardial infarction. *Internal Medicine, 42,* 340–344.

Aslam, S., Friedman, E. A., & Ifudu, O. (2002). Electrocardiography is unreliable in detecting potentially lethal hyperkalaemia in haemodialysis patients. *Nephrology Dialysis Transplantation,* 17, 1639–1642.

Birrer, R. B., Shallash, A. J., & Totten, V. (2002). Hypermagnesemia-induced fatality following epsom salt gargles. *Journal of Emergency Medicine, 22,* 2002, 185–188.

Blackburn, S. T. (2003). *Maternal, fetal, and neonatal physiology* (2nd ed.). Philadelphia: WB Saunders.

Blanning, A., & Westfall, J. M. (2001). How soon should serum potassium levels be monitored for patients started on diuretics? *Journal of Family Practice,* 50, 207–208.

Blaustein, D., Babu, K., Reddy, A., Schwenk, M., & Avram, M. (2002). Estimation of glomerular filtration rate to prevent life-threatening hyperkalemia due to combined therapy with spironolactone and angiotensin-converting enzyme inhibition or angiotensin receptor blockade. *American Journal of Cardiology, 90,* 662–663.

Boccalandro, C., Lopez-Penabad, L., Boccalandro, F., & Lavis, V. (2003). Ventricular fibrillation in a young Asian man. *Lancet, 361,* 1432.

Carlstedt, F., & Lind, L (2001). Hypocalcemic syndromes. *Critical Care Clinics, 17,* 139–153.

Ceremuzynski, L., Gebalska, J., Wolk, R., & Makowska, E. (2000). Hypomagnesemia in heart failure with ventricular arrhythmias. Beneficial effects of magnesium supplementation. *Journal of Internal Medicine, 247,* 78–86.

Chapman, M., Hanrahan, R., McEwen, J., & Marley, J.E. (2003). Hyponatremia and hypokalemia due to indapamide. *Medical Journal of Australia,* 176, 219–222.

Claudius, I., Sachs, C., & Shamji, T. (2002). Hypophosphatemia-induced heart failure. *American Journal of Emergency Medicine, 20,* 369–370.

Cohen, N., Almoznino-Sarafian, D., Zaidenstein, R., et al. (2003). Serum magnesium aberrations in furosemide (frusemide) treated patients with congestive heart failure: pathophysiological correlates and prognostic evaluation. *Heart, 89,* 411–416.

Day, J., Chaudhry, A., Hunt, I., & Taylor, K. (2002). Heparin-induced hyperkalemia after cardiac surgery. *Annals of Thoracic Surgery,* 74,1698–1700.

Demir, A.D., Soylu, M., Tikiz, H., Tezcan, U.K., Balbay, Y., & Kutuk, E. (2000). Polymorphic ventricular tachycardia due to renal artery stenosis—a case report. *Angiology, 51,* 1039–1043.

De Petris, L., Luchetti, A., & Emma, F. (2001). Cell volume regulation and transport mechanisms across the blood-brain barrier: implications for the management of hypernatraemic states. *European Journal of Pediatrics,* 160(2), 71–77.

Dorman, B. H., Sade, R.M., Burnette, J. S., Wiles, H. B., Pinosky, M, L., Reeves, S. T., et al. (2000). Magnesium supplementation in the prevention of arrhythmias in pediatric patients undergoing surgery for congenital heart defects. *American Heart Journal,* 139, 522–558.

Downes, K., & Sarode, R. (2001). Massive blood transfusion. *Indian Journal of Pediatrics, 68,* 145–149.

Elming, H., Seibaek, M., Ottesen, M. M., Torp-Pedersen, C., Holm, E., Thode, J., et al. (2000). Serum-ionised magnesium in patients with acute myocardial infarction. Relation to cardiac arrhythmias, left ventricular function and mortality. *Magnesium Research,* 13, 285–292.

Eurenius, S., & Smith, R. M. (1973). The effect of warming on the serum potassium content of stored blood. *Anesthesiology,* 38, 482–484.

Felver, L. (2000). Fluid and electrolyte homeostasis and imbalances. In L. Copstead & J. Banasik (Eds.), *Perspectives on pathophysiology* (2nd ed., pp. 538–545). Philadelphia: W.B. Saunders.

Foo K., Sekhri N., Deaner A., Knight C., Suliman A., Ranjadayalan K., & Timmis A.D. (2003). Effect of diabetes on serum potassium concentrations in acute coronary syndromes. *Heart (British Cardiac Society),* 89, 31–35.

Fox, C. H., Mahoney, M. C., Ramsoomair, D., & Carter, C. A. (2003). Magnesium deficiency in African-Americans: does it contribute to increased cardiovascular risk factors? *Journal of the National Medical Association,* 95, 257–262.

Fox, C., Ramsoomair, D., & Carter, C. (2001). Magnesium: its proven and potential clinical significance. *Southern Medical Journal,* 94, 1195–1201.

Gennari, F. J. (2002). Disorders of potassium homeostasis: hypokalemia and hyperkalemia. *Critical Care Clinics,* 18, 273–288.

Glauser, J. (2001). Cardiac arrhythmias, respiratory failure, and profound hypokalemia in a trauma patient. *Cleveland Clinic Journal of Medicine, 68,* 401, 405–410, 413.

Greenberg, A. (2000). Diuretic complications. *American Journal of the Medical Sciences, 319,* 10–24.

Gross, P., Reimann, D., Henschkowski, J., & Damian, M. (2001). Treatment of severe hyponatremia: conventional and novel aspects. *Journal of the American Society of Nephrology,* 12 (Suppl. 17), S10–S14.

Gulati, G., Bajpai, A., Juneja, R., Kabra, M., Bagga, A., & Kalra, V. (2001). Hypocalcemic heart failure masquerading as dilated cardiomyopathy. *Indian Journal of Pediatrics, 68,* 287–290.

Hahn, R. G., & Lofgren, A. (2000). Epinephrine, potassium and the electrocardiogram during regional anaesthesia. *European Journal of Anaesthesiology,* 17, 132–137.

Harker, H. E., & Majcher, T. A. (2000). Hypermagnesemia in a pediatric patient. *Anesthesia and Analgesia,* 91, 1160–1162.

Jeegan, M. T., Bondy, L.R., Blackshear, J. L., & Lanier, W. L. (2002). Hypocalcemia-like electrocardiographic changes after administration of intravenous fosphenytoin. *Mayo Clinic Proceedings,* 77, 584–586.

Kashyap, A. S., & Kashyap, S. (2001). Heart failure, a thick tongue, and an abnormal cranial computed tomogram. *Postgraduate Medical Journal,* 77, 535, 545–546.

Kaye, P., & O'Sullivan, I. (2002). The role of magnesium in the emergency department. *Emergency Medicine Journal,* 19, 288–291.

Klevay, L. M., & Milne, D. B. (2002). Low dietary magnesium increases supraventricular ectopy. *American Journal of Clinical Nutrition,* 75, 550–554.

Knichwit, G., Zahl, M., Van Aken, H., Semjonow, A., & Booke, M. (2002). Intraoperative washing of long-stored packed red blood cells by using an autotransfusion device prevents hyperkalemia. *Anesthesia and Analgesia,* 95, 324–325.

Knochel, J, & Schlein, E. (1972). On the mechanism of rhabdomyolysis in potassium depletion. *Journal of Clinical Investigation,* 51, 1750–1758.

Kovalik, S. G., Ledgerwood, A. M., Lucas, C. E., et al. (1981). The cardiac effect of altered calcium homeostasis after albumin resuscitation. *Journal of Trauma,* 21, 275–279.

Kramer, J. H., Mak, I. T., Phillips, T. M., & Weglicki, W. B. (2003). Dietary magnesium intake influences circulating pro-inflammatory neuropeptide levels and loss of myocardial tolerance to postischemic stress. *Experimental Biology & Medicine,* 228, 665–673.

Krassoi, I., Pataricza, J., & Papp, J. G. (2003). Thiorphan enhances bradykinin-induced vascular relaxation in hypoxic/hyperkalaemic porcine coronary artery. *Journal of Pharmacy & Pharmacology,* 55, 339–345.

Kusano, K. F., Hata, Y., Yumoto, A., Emori, T., Sato, T., & Ohe, T. (2001). Torsade de pointes with a normal QT interval associated with hypokalemia: a case report. *Japanese Circulation Journal,* 65, 757–760.

Lane, R., & Phillips, M. (2003). Rhabdomyolysis. *BMJ,* 27(7407), 115–116.

Laragh, J. H., & Sealey, J. E. (2001). K(+) depletion and the progression of hypertensive disease or heart failure. The pathogenic role of diuretic-induced aldosterone secretion. *Hypertension,* 37, 806–810.

Lehmann, G., Deisenhofer, I., Ndrepepa, G., & Schmitt, C. (2000). ECG changes in a 25-year-old woman with hypocalcemia due to hypoparathyroidism: hypocalcemia mimicking acute myocardial infarction. *Chest,* 118, 260–262.

Li, H. Y., Wu, S., He, G. W., & Wong, T. M. (2002). Aprikalim reduces the Na+-Ca2+ exchange outward current enhanced by hyperkalemia in rat ventricular myocytes. *Annals of Thoracic Surgery,* 73, 1253–1259.

Long, C., Li, W., Lin, D. M., & Yang, J. G. (2002). Effect of potassium-channel openers on the release of endothelium-derived hyperpolarizing factor in porcine coronary arteries stored in cold hyperkalemic solution. *Journal of Extra-Corporeal Technology,* 34, 125–129.

Lucia, A., Hoyos, J., Santalla, A., et al. (2002). Lactic acidosis, potassium, and the heart rate deflection point in professional road cyclists. *British Journal of Sports Medicine,* 36, 113–117.

McCauley, J., Murray, J., Jordan, M., et al. (2002). Labetalol-induced hyperkalemia in renal transplant recipients. *American Journal of Nephrology, 22,* 347–351.

Marinella, M. A., & Burdette, S. D. (2000). Hypokalemia-induced QT interval prolongation. *Journal of Emergency Medicine, 4,* 375–376.

Mattu, A., Brady, W. J., & Perron, A. D. (2002). Electrocardiographic manifestations of hypothermia. *American Journal of Emergency Medicine, 20,* 314–326.

Mela, T., Galvin, J. M., & McGovern, B. A. (2002). Magnesium deficiency during lactation as a precipitant of ventricular tachyarrhythmias. *Pacing & Clinical Electrophysiology, 25,* 231–233.

Miller, D. W., & Slovis, C. M. (2000). Hypophosphatemia in the emergency department therapeutics. *American Journal of Emergency Medicine, 18,* 457–461.

Moore-Ede, M. C., Meguid, M., Fitzpatrick, G., et al. (1978). Circadian variation in response to potassium infusion. *Clinical Pharmacology and Therapeutics, 23,* 218–227.

Nilsson, I. L., Rastad, J., Johansson, K., & Lind, L. (2001). Endothelial vasodilatory function and blood pressure response to local and systemic hypercalcemia. *Surgery, 130,* 986–990.

Nishra, A., Wong, L., & Jonklaas, J. (2001). Prolonged, symptomatic hypocalcemia with pamidronate administration and subclinical hypoparathyroidism. *Endocrine Journal, 14,* 159–164.

Nowicki, M., & Miszczak-Kuban, J. (2002). Nonselective beta-adrenergic blockade augments fasting hyperkalemia in hemodialysis patients. *Nephron, 91,* 222–227.

Nowicki, M., Szewczyk-Seifert, G., Klimek, D., & Kokot, F. (2002). Carvedilol does not modulate moderate exercise-induced hyperkalemia in hemodialysis patients. *Clinical Nephrology, 57,* 352–358.

Oladapo, O. O., & Falase, A. O. (2000). Congestive heart failure and ventricular arrhythmias in relation to serum magnesium. *African Journal of Medicine & Medical Sciences, 29,* 265–268.

Okruhlicova, L., et al. (2002). Gap junction remodelling is involved in the susceptibility of diabetic rats to hypokalemia-induced ventricular fibrillation. *Acta Histochemica, 104,* 387–391.

Onagawa, T., Ohkuchi A., Ohki, R., et al. (2003). Woman with postpartum ventricular tachycardia and hypomagnesemia. *Journal of Obstetrics & Gynaecology Research, 29,* 92–95.

Ortega-Carnicier, J., de la Nieta, D. S., & Alcazar, R. (2001). Acute myocardial injury caused presumably by coronary spasm after magnesium fluorosilicate ingestion. *Journal of Electrocardiography, 34,* 335–337.

Ozgur, B., & Kursat, S. (2002). Hypokalemic rhabdomyolysis aggravated by diuretics complicating Conn's syndrome without acute renal failure. *Clinical Nephrology, 57,* 89–91.

Peterson, B. L (2001). A 6-month-old infant with prolonged QTc interval. *Journal of Pediatric Health Care, 15,* 263-263; 275–276.

Prat, G., Petrognani, R., Diatta, B., Dufau, J. P., & Theobald, X. (2001). Hypokalemia causing rhabdomyolysis and precordialgia. *Intensive Care Medicine, 27,* 1096.

Robertson, G. L. (2001). Antidiuretic hormone: normal and disordered function. *Endocrinology and Metabolism Clinics of North America, 30,* 671–694.

Rose, B. D., & Post, T. (2001). *Clinical physiology of acid-base and electrolyte disorders* (5th ed.). New York: McGraw-Hill.

RuDusky, B. M.. (2001). ECG abnormalities associated with hypocalcemia. *Chest, 119,* 668–669.

Sato, K., Hasegawa, Y., Nakae, J., Nanao, K., Takahashi, I., Tajima, T., Shinohara, N., & Fujieda, K. (2002). Hydrochlorothiazide effectively reduces urinary calcium excretion in two Japanese patients with gain-of-function mutations of the calcium-sensing receptor gene. *Journal of Clinical Endocrinology and Metabolism, 87,* 3068–3073.

Schelling, J. R. (2000). Fatal hypermagnesemia. *Clinical Nephrology, 53,* 61–65.

Shiber, J. R., & Mattu, A. (2002). Serum phosphate abnormalities in the emergency department. *Journal of Emergency Medicine, 23,* 395–400.

Somers, M. P., Brady, W. J., Perron, A. D., & Mattu, A. (2002). The prominant T wave: electrocardiographic differential diagnosis. *American Journal of Emergency Medicine, 20,* 243–251.

Speich, M., Bousquet, B., & Nicolas, G. (1980). Concentrations of magnesium, calcium, potassium, and sodium in human heart muscle after acute myocardial infarction. *Clinical Chemistry, 2,* 1662–1665.

Speziale, G., Ruvolo, G., Fattouch, K., Macrina, F., Tonelli, E., Donnetti, M., et al. (2000). Arrhythmia prophylaxis after coronary artery bypass grafting: regimens of magnesium sulfate administration. *Thoracic and Cardiovascular Surgeon, 48,* 22–26.

Struthers, A. D. (2002). Aldosterone: cardiovascular assault. *American Heart Journal, 144*(5 Suppl), S2–S7.

Subramanian, R., & Khardori, R. (2000). Severe hypophosphatemia: pathophysiologic implications, clinical presentations, and treatment. *Medicine, 79,* 1–8.

Touyz, R. M., Pu, Q., He, G., et al. (2002). Effects of low dietary magnesium intake on development of hypertension in stroke-prone spontaneously hypertensive rats: role of reactive oxygen species. *Journal of Hypertension, 20,* 2221–2232.

United States Pharmacopeial Convention (USP), Inc. (2003). *USP dispensing information - Volume I: Drug information for the health care professional* (23rd ed.). Greenwood Village, CO: Thomson MICROMEDEX.

Webster, A., Brady, W., & Morris, F. (2002). Recognising signs of danger: ECG changes resulting from an abnormal serum potassium concentration, *Emergency Medicine, 19,* 74–77.

Wilkes, N. J,., Mallett, S. V., Peachey, T., Di Salvo, C., & Walesby, R. (2002). Correction of ionized plasma magnesium during cardiopulmonary bypass reduces the risk of postoperative cardiac arrhythmia. *Anesthesia and Analgesia, 95,* 828–834.

Wolf, M. E., Ranade, V., Molnar, J., Somberg, J., & Mosnaim, A. D. (2000). Hypercalcemia, arrhythmia, and mood stabilizers. *Journal of Clinical Psychopharmacology, 20,* 260–264.

Wong, K., Chak, W., Cheung, C., Choi, K., & Li, C. (2001). Hypokalemic metabolic alkalosis attributed to cough mixture abuse. *American Journal of Kidney Diseases [Online], 38,* 390–394.

Yelamanchi, V. P., Molnar, J., Ranade, V., Somberg, J.C. (2001). Influence of electrolyte abnormalities on interlead variability of ventricular repolarization times in 12-lead electrocardiography. *American Journal of Therapeutics, 8,* 117–122.

Zaman, F., & Abreo, K. (2003). Severe hypermagnesemia as a result of laxative use in renal insufficiency. *Southern Medical Journal, 96,* 102–103.

Zivin, J. R., Gooley, T., Zager, R. A., & Ryan, M. J. (2001). Hypocalcemia: a pervasive metabolic abnormality in the critically ill. *American Journal of Kidney Diseases, 37,* 689–698.

Zuccala, G., Pedone, C., Cocchi, A., Pahor, M., Carosella, L., Carbonin, P., Bernabei, R. (2000). Older age and in-hospital development of hypokalemia from loop diuretics: results from a multicenter survey. *Journals of Gerontology, 55,* M232-M238.

Acid-Base Balance and Imbalances

LINDA FELVER

PRINCIPLES OF ACID-BASE BALANCE

The degree of acidity of the body fluids plays an important role in physiology. It influences the structure and function of many enzymes and also modifies the affinity between oxygen and hemoglobin. Deviations of acid-base balance from normal can affect cellular function and tissue oxygenation. In the extreme, they can be fatal.

Terminology Review

An *acid* is a substance that donates hydrogen ions (H^+) in solution. A *base* is a substance that accepts hydrogen ions. The more hydrogen ions a solution contains, the more acidic it is. The actual number of hydrogen ions in extracellular fluid is small and unwieldy to write (0.00004 mmol/L) (Guyton & Hall, 2000). Therefore, the degree of acidity of body fluids is reported as the pH. The pH is the negative logarithm of the hydrogen ion concentration. It ranges from 1 (very acidic) to 14 (very alkaline). A pH of 7 is neutral. The blood is normally slightly alkaline. The normal pH range of the blood is 7.35 to 7.45. If the pH of the blood falls below the normal range (i.e., becomes more acidic), a patient has *acidemia*. The process that tends to decrease the pH is called *acidosis*. Similarly, if the pH of the blood rises above the normal range (i.e., becomes more alkaline), a patient has *alkalemia*. The process that tends to increase the pH is called *alkalosis*.

Processes Involved in Acid-Base Balance

Normal cellular metabolism continually produces acids, which can cause dangerous acidemia without the closely regulated processes by which the body maintains pH within the normal range. After acid production, the processes of acid buffering and acid excretion work to maintain or reestablish a normal pH.

Acid Production

Cellular metabolism produces two types of acids: carbonic acid and metabolic acids. Carbonic acid (H_2CO_3) is produced as carbon dioxide (CO_2); the enzyme carbonic anhydrase combines the CO_2 with water (H_2O) to produce carbonic acid. In a standard adult, approximately 15,000 mmol of carbonic acid are generated per day from metabolism of carbohydrates and fats (Rose & Post, 2000).

Metabolic acids are produced primarily from the metabolism of phosphate-containing compounds and amino acids that contain sulfur. These metabolic acids include sulfuric and phosphoric acids. Metabolic acids are handled differently by the body than carbonic acid. For this reason, they are sometimes called *noncarbonic acids*.

Cellular metabolism also produces small amounts of base (bicarbonate ions; HCO_3^-) as a result of oxidation of small organic anions such as citrate. Much more metabolic acid is produced than base. In a standard adult, a net 50 to 100 mEq of hydrogen ions is generated per day from metabolism (Rose & Post, 2000).

Acid Buffering

Buffers in the body act to minimize changes in pH because of gain of acid or base. They neutralize acids by taking up excess hydrogen ions and neutralize bases by releasing hydrogen ions. Buffers are located in all body fluids; however, the most important roles are played by the buffers in the extracellular fluid, intracellular fluid, bone, and urine. Different body fluids contain different buffers, which meet specific needs (Table 10-1).

The major extracellular buffer is the carbonic acid-bicarbonate-carbon dioxide buffer system (commonly termed the *bicarbonate buffer system*). Carbonic acid is a weak acid, which means that it dissociates partially when in solution so that it is in equilibrium with bicarbonate and hydrogen ions. The carbonic acid concentration can be altered by variations in alveolar ventilation (variations in CO_2 excretion). The chemical equation for the bicarbonate buffer system is written as follows:

$$CO_2 + H_2O \rightleftharpoons H_2CO_3 \rightleftharpoons H^+ + HCO_3^-$$

carbon　　water　　carbonic　　hydrogen　　bicarbonate
dioxide　　　　　　acid　　　　ion　　　　ion

Table 10–1 ■ THE MAJOR BUFFERS

Extracellular Fluid	Intracellular Fluid	Bone	Urine
Bicarbonate	Proteins	Carbonates	Inorganic phosphates
Inorganic phosphates	Organic and inorganic phosphates	Phosphates	
Plasma proteins	Hemoglobin (in erythrocytes)		

To maintain the pH of the blood within the normal range, there must be 20 bicarbonate ions for every carbonic acid molecule. The Henderson-Hasselbalch equation, a mathematical description of the pH of a buffered solution, shows how this 20:1 ratio is necessary:

$$pH = pKa + \log \frac{[A^-]}{[HA]} \quad \text{(general equation)}$$

$$pH = 6.1 + \log \frac{[HCO_3^-]}{[H_2CO_3]} \quad \begin{array}{l}\text{(substituting values for} \\ \text{bicarbonate buffer system)}\end{array}$$

$$pH = 6.1 + \log \frac{20}{1}$$

$$pH = 6.1 + 1.3$$

$$pH = 7.4$$

A buffer system cannot buffer its own acid. Thus, the bicarbonate buffer system cannot buffer carbonic acid. The carbonic acid that is produced by cells (as CO_2 and H_2O) is buffered primarily by intracellular buffers. The bicarbonate buffer system is a major buffer for metabolic acids. Table 10-2 summarizes the role of buffers with respect to acid or base loads.

Acid Excretion

Even though the buffers minimize pH changes as acid is produced, they have a limited capacity. Therefore, acid excretion mechanisms are necessary to maintain acid-base balance. The body has two acid excretion methods: the lungs excrete carbonic acid and the kidneys excrete metabolic acids.

Role of the Lungs. The lungs excrete carbonic acid in the form of carbon dioxide and water. They cannot excrete metabolic acids. When alveolar ventilation increases (increased rate and depth of ventilation), more carbonic acid is excreted. Conversely, when alveolar ventilation decreases, less carbonic acid is excreted. Because carbonic acid is essentially carbon dioxide

and water, the body actually senses and regulates the partial pressure of carbon dioxide ($PaCO_2$).

If carbonic acid begins to accumulate (increased $PaCO_2$), chemoreceptors in the medulla and carotid and aortic bodies are stimulated by the increased $PaCO_2$ and decreased pH (Guyton & Hall, 2000). The resulting increase in alveolar ventilation causes the excretion of the excess carbonic acid. Similarly, if too little carbonic acid is present (decreased $PaCO_2$), the chemoreceptors are less stimulated, and alveolar ventilation decreases somewhat to retain carbonic acid in the body. Hypoxia, sensed by the carotid chemoreceptors, stimulates alveolar ventilation and may override the suppression of ventilation from decreased $PaCO_2$. In a healthy person, alveolar ventilation changes rapidly in response to changes in $PaCO_2$, and thus carbonic acid is excreted at a rate effective in maintaining acid-base balance.

Role of the Kidneys. The kidneys excrete metabolic acids. They cannot excrete carbonic acid. The renal epithelial cells that line the proximal tubules secrete hydrogen ions into the renal tubular fluid and reabsorb bicarbonate ions in the process. Bicarbonate is the major extracellular buffer of metabolic acids. Therefore, the bicarbonate ion concentration indicates how much metabolic acid is present. A decreased serum bicarbonate concentration indicates increased amounts of metabolic acid. When the proximal tubular cells secrete hydrogen ions that are eventually excreted in the urine, they replenish the bicarbonate ions that were used in buffering. Hydrogen ions are also secreted into the renal tubular fluid by cells that line the distal tubules and collecting ducts. The distal tubular cells can also secrete bicarbonate into the tubular fluid or reabsorb it into the blood.

If the urine were to become too acidic, it could damage the cells that line the urinary tract. Fortunately, the urine does not become dangerously acidic because the hydrogen ions in the renal tubules are buffered by the urine buffers or combine chemically with ammonia. Ammonia (NH_3) is produced by renal tubular cells and then diffuses into the tubular fluid (Guyton and Hall, 2000). Hydrogen ions combine with ammonia in the tubular fluid to produce ammonium ions (NH_4^+). Because ammonium ions are charged particles, they cannot cross the cell membranes to enter the blood; thus, they are "trapped" in the renal tubular fluid and excreted in the urine. An increase of acid in the body (decreased pH) causes the production of more ammonia, which facilitates renal excretion of acid. This process begins within 2 hours but takes several days to be maximally effective (Rose & Post, 2000).

Thus, the kidneys have several mechanisms that result in the excretion of metabolic acids that are produced by cellular metabolism. These mechanisms can be adjusted to excrete

Table 10–2 ■ ROLE OF BUFFERS WITH RESPECT TO AN ACID OR BASE LOAD

Buffer	Role with Carbonic Acid Load	Role with Metabolic Acid Load	Role with Base (Bicarbonate) Load
Extracellular bicarbonate	Not effective	Major role (immediate action)	Not effective
Other extracellular buffers	Minor role (immediate action)	Minor role (immediate action)	Minor role (immediate action)
Intracellular buffers	Major role (10–30 minutes)	Important role (2–4 hours)	Important role (hours)
Bone buffers	Probably not important	Important role (2–4 hours)	Important role (hours)

Table 10–3 ■ SUMMARY OF PHYSIOLOGIC RESPONSES THAT MAINTAIN ACID-BASE BALANCE

Physiological Mechanism	Response to Decreased pH (too much acid in blood)	Response to Increased pH (too much bicarbonate in blood)
Buffers	Accept hydrogen ions	Release hydrogen ions
Respiratory system	Excretes carbonic acid by increasing rate and depth of respiration	Retains carbonic acid in the body by decreasing rate and depth of respiration
Kidneys	Excrete more metabolic acid by increasing secretion of H^+ into renal tubular fluid, increasing reabsorption of bicarbonate, and increasing production of NH_3	Excrete less metabolic acid by decreasing secretion of H^+ into renal tubular fluid, decreasing reabsorption of bicarbonate, and decreasing production of NH_3

more acid or less acid, thereby maintaining the bicarbonate ion concentration within normal limits. Changes in renal function with normal aging cause older adults to excrete acid loads more slowly than younger adults.

Summary of Acid-Base Balance

Cellular metabolism produces carbonic acid and metabolic acids. These acids must be excreted to maintain normal acid-base balance. Buffers in all body fluids act to minimize changes in pH due to an acid load or a bicarbonate (base) load. Carbonic acid is excreted by the lungs; increases or decreases in alveolar ventilation regulate the amount of carbonic acid excretion. The $PaCO_2$ is the clinical indicator of carbonic acid. Metabolic acids are excreted by the kidneys, which can excrete more or less acid as needed. The plasma bicarbonate ion concentration is the clinical indicator of the amount of metabolic acid. Table 10-3 summarizes the physiologic responses that maintain acid-base balance.

ACID-BASE IMBALANCES

Acid-base imbalances occur when the capacity of the buffers to modulate pH changes is exceeded. Two terms are important in understanding the physiologic responses to acid-base imbalances. *Correction* of the imbalance occurs when the original problem is fixed so that the pH, $PaCO_2$, and plasma bicarbonate ion concentration can return to normal. *Compensation* for an acid-base imbalance restores the pH toward normal but does not correct the problem that originally caused the imbalance. In many cases, an acid-base imbalance persists long enough that compensatory physiologic processes occur. A partially compensated acid-base imbalance is characterized by abnormal pH, $PaCO_2$, and plasma bicarbonate ion concentration. However, the pH is not as abnormal as it was before the partial compensation. When an acid-base imbalance is fully compensated, the pH is in the normal range, but the $PaCO_2$ and plasma bicarbonate ion concentration are both abnormal. By moving the pH toward normal, compensation for an acid-base imbalance helps to protect cells from death.

Acidosis

A patient who has acidosis has processes that tend to decrease the pH of the blood below normal by creating a relative excess of acid. The resulting acidemia may persist or may be lessened by the body's compensatory response. A pH below 6.9 is usually fatal. Acidosis is classified as respiratory or metabolic, depending on what type of acid is initially in relative excess.

Respiratory Acidosis

Respiratory acidosis occurs when too much carbonic acid accumulates in the blood. Clinically, the increase of carbonic acid is measured as an increased $PaCO_2$. Carbonic acid is normally excreted by the lungs. Thus, any factor that decreases respiration or ventilation can cause respiratory acidosis (Table 10-4). Patients in whom cor pulmonale develops because of chronic lung disease commonly have chronic respiratory acidosis.

Carbon dioxide diffuses readily through membranes. Thus, the pH of cerebrospinal fluid (CSF) decreases when respiratory acidosis occurs. As excess CO_2 enters the brain cells, intracellular acidosis alters enzyme activity and central nervous system (CNS) depression results. The clinical manifestations of respiratory acidosis are CNS depression (disorientation, lethargy, somnolence), headache, blurred vision, tachycardia, and cardiac arrhythmias.

Respiratory acidosis can be corrected only by restoring lung function because the lungs are the only route of excretion of carbonic acid. If the kidneys compensate by excreting more than the usual amount of metabolic acids, then the pH moves back toward normal, even though the blood chemistry remains abnormal. Excretion of more metabolic acids raises the bicarbonate ion concentration because fewer bicarbonate ions are used in buffering. Thus, renal compensation for respiratory acidosis restores the 20:1 ratio of bicarbonate to carbonic acid, even though the absolute values of both are elevated. Restoring the 20:1 ratio normalizes the pH. Renal compensation for respiratory acidosis takes 3 to 5 days to be fully effective. A compensated respiratory acidosis is characterized by an elevated $PaCO_2$ (the sign of the primary problem), an elevated bicarbonate ion concentration (the sign of the renal compensation), and a pH that is decreased (partially compensated) or normal (fully compensated).

In respiratory acidosis, excess CO_2 diffuses into cardiac cells. Although intracellular buffering of carbonic acid may protect intracellular pH in cardiac cells more effectively than in many other types of cells, the intracellular pH in cardiac cells does decrease (Kupriyanov et al., 2002). Respiratory acidosis depresses cardiac contractility (Kalinin, 2002). The negative effects of decreased myocardial cell contractility in respiratory acidosis are partially offset by increased sympathetic neural discharge and

Table 10–4 ■ CAUSES OF RESPIRATORY ACIDOSIS

Category	Clinical Examples
Decreased gaseous exchange (problem in the airways or alveoli of lungs)	Decreased alveolar ventilation for any reason
	Acute airway obstruction by foreign body
	Severe asthma
	Sleep apnea (obstructive type)
	Chronic obstructive pulmonary disease (COPD) type A (emphysema) in end-stage
	Chronic obstructive pulmonary disease (COPD) type B (chronic bronchitis)
	Atelectasis
	Pneumonia
	Adult respiratory distress syndrome (ARDS)
	Pulmonary edema
	Hypoventilation with mechanical ventilator
Impaired neuromuscular function of chest (problem in the chest muscles or nerves)	Chest injury
	Surgical incision in chest or upper abdomen (pain limits chest expansion)
	Respiratory muscle fatigue
	Severe hypokalemia
	Poliomyelitis
	Guillain-Barré syndrome
	Myasthenia gravis
	Kyphoscoliosis
	Pickwickian syndrome (obesity limits chest expansion)
Suppression of respiratory neurons in brainstem (medulla) (problem in the brainstem)	Opioids
	Barbiturates
	Anesthetics
	Sleep apnea (central type)

increased catecholamine levels (Mizukoshi et al., 2001). Tachycardia and cardiac arrhythmias in patients with respiratory acidosis may be caused by the increased circulating catecholamines.

Respiratory acidosis also affects blood vessels, altering both peripheral vascular resistance and distribution of blood flow. Peripheral vascular resistance decreases, owing to peripheral vasodilation (Kazmaier et al., 1998). Coronary vasodilation also occurs (Phillis et al., 2000). The peripheral vasculature becomes less sensitive to alpha- and beta-adrenergic stimulation. Decreased peripheral vascular resistance and decreased cardiac contractility cause hypotension. The hypotension may be diminished by constriction in splanchnic and peripheral venous beds (the venous capacitance beds). This response increases central arterial blood volume.

The decreased pH in the CSF causes cerebral vasodilation, increasing cerebral blood flow (Najarian et al., 2000). This is the cause of the headache that is experienced by many patients with respiratory acidosis. Increased cerebral blood flow from cerebral vasodilation may also raise CSF pressure and cause papilledema. In contrast to its effect on other vascular beds, respiratory acidosis causes vasoconstriction in the pulmonary vasculature (Mizuno et al., 2002). The resulting increase in pulmonary vascular resistance may worsen the clinical status of patients with preexisting right heart failure.

In summary, the major cardiovascular effects of respiratory acidosis are tachycardia, cardiac arrhythmias, decreased cardiac contractility, decreased peripheral vascular resistance, increased pulmonary vascular resistance, and shift of blood flow from the venous capacitance beds into the central and cerebral arterial beds.

Metabolic Acidosis

Metabolic acidosis is caused by relatively too much metabolic acid. It can be due to a gain of acid or a loss of base. Acid can be gained from intake of acids or substances that are converted to acid in the body, from an increased rate of normal metabolism, from production of unusual acids due to altered metabolic processes, or from factors that decrease renal excretion of acid. Bicarbonate ions (base) can be lost in the urine or through the gastrointestinal tract. Table 10-5 lists clinical conditions that cause metabolic acidosis by each of these mechanisms. Cardiogenic shock causes metabolic acidosis by accumulation of lactic acid from anaerobic metabolism and through failure of the decreased circulation to deliver metabolic acids to the kidneys for excretion. No matter what its cause, metabolic acidosis is characterized by a decreased plasma bicarbonate ion concentration. The bicarbonate is either depleted by being used to buffer excess metabolic acids or is lost directly from the body.

Metabolic acidosis can be corrected physiologically only by the kidneys, which are the sole excretory route for metabolic acids. Renal correction of metabolic acidosis may take several days. Meanwhile, respiratory compensation occurs within hours. The respiratory compensation for metabolic acidosis is hyperventilation. By increasing the excretion of carbonic acid, hyperventilation makes the blood less acid. This makes the blood chemistry more abnormal (decreased $PaCO_2$) but tends to restore the 20:1 ratio of bicarbonate to carbonic acid and move the pH toward the normal range, thus helping to preserve

Table 10–5 ■ CAUSES OF METABOLIC ACIDOSIS

Category	Clinical Examples
Acid accumulation by ingestion or infusion of acid or acid precursors	Aspirin (acetylsalicylic acid)
	Boric acid
	Ammonium chloride (releases H^+)
	Methanol (converts to formic acid)
	Antifreeze (ethylene glycol converts to oxalic acid)
	Paraldehyde (converts to acetic and chloroacetic acids)
	Elemental sulfur (converts to sulfuric acid)
Acid accumulation by increased production of normal metabolic acids	Hyperthyroidism
	Hypermetabolic state after burns, trauma, or sepsis
	Lactic acidosis
	Shock
Acid accumulation by utilization of abnormal or incomplete metabolic pathways	Alcoholic ketoacidosis
	Diabetic ketoacidosis
	Starvation ketoacidosis
Acid accumulation by impaired acid exceration	Prolonged oliguria from any cause
	Oliguric renal failure
	Severe hypovolemia
	Shock
	Renal tubular acidosis (type 1)
	Hypoaldosteronism
Loss of bicarbonate	Severe diarrhea
	Intestinal decompression
	Fistula drainage from pancreas or intestine
	Vomiting of intestinal contents
	Ureterosigmoidostomy
	Renal tubular acidosis (type 2)

Table 10–6 ▪ VASCULAR EFFECTS OF ACID-BASE IMBALANCES

Vascular Bed	Respiratory Acidosis	Metabolic Acidosis	Respiratory Alkalosis	Metabolic Alkalosis
Peripheral	Vasodilation	Vasodilation	Vasoconstriction (debatable)	Vasoconstriction (likely)
Coronary	Vasodilation	Vasodilation	Vasoconstriction	Vasoconstriction
Cerebral	Vasodilation	Vasodilation	Vasoconstriction	Vasoconstriction
Pulmonary	Vasoconstriction	Vasoconstriction	Vasodilation	Vasodilation

cellular function. Compensated metabolic acidosis is characterized by a decreased $PaCO_2$ (the sign of the respiratory compensation), a decreased bicarbonate ion concentration (the sign of the primary problem), and a pH that is decreased (partially compensated) or normal (fully compensated).

The clinical manifestations of metabolic acidosis include headache, abdominal pain, cardiac arrhythmias, and CNS depression (confusion, drowsiness, lethargy, stupor, coma). The CNS depression arises from decreased pH of the CSF and resultant intracellular acidosis of brain cells. The exact cause of the abdominal pain is not clearly understood. Patients are tachypneic from the compensatory hyperventilation.

Metabolic acidosis depresses cardiac contractility by causing intracellular acidosis, which alters delivery of calcium ions to the myofilaments and inhibits myofilament responsiveness to calcium (Kalinin, 2002; Takahashi, 2001). Cardiac arrhythmias may be related to an increase in circulating catecholamine levels caused by metabolic acidosis or other concurrent pathophysiological processes. A catecholamine increase helps preserve cardiac output during mild metabolic acidosis. However, in more severe metabolic acidosis the decreased myocardial contractility predominates. Coronary artery occlusion causes myocardial acidosis, so that these cardiac effects occur in patients with myocardial infarction without the systemic effects of metabolic acidosis.

Increased circulating catecholamines also protect the arterial blood pressure from the peripheral vasodilation caused by acidosis. This peripheral vasodilation is caused by increased release of nitric oxide by the vascular endothelium (Hattori, 2002). The vascular bed becomes hyporesponsive to vasopressors. Coronary vasodilation and pulmonary vasoconstriction occur (Kitakaze et al., 2001; Mizuno et al., 2002). Mild cerebral vasodilation is probably responsible for the headache experienced by some patients (Horiuchi et al., 2002; Najarian et al., 2000). Constriction of the venous capacitance vessels increases central blood volume. The vascular effects of acid-base imbalances are summarized in Table 10-6. A syndrome characterized by hypotension, acidosis, and vasodilation (HAV syndrome), in which the cardiac and vascular effects of metabolic acidosis likely play a role (Chemmalakuzhy et al., 2001), sometimes develops in patients who have undergone heart transplantation.

Alkalosis

A patient who has alkalosis has processes that tend to increase the pH of the blood above normal by creating a relative excess of base (a relative deficit of acid). The resulting alkalemia may persist or may be modulated by a compensatory response. A pH above 7.8 is usually fatal. Alkalosis is classified as respiratory or metabolic, depending on what type of acid is initially in relative deficit.

Respiratory Alkalosis

Respiratory alkalosis occurs when there is too little carbonic acid in the blood. Clinically, the decreased carbonic acid is measured as a decreased $PaCO_2$. Any factor that causes hyperventilation can cause excretion of too much carbonic acid, leading to respiratory alkalosis (Table 10-7).

Note that hypoxia, as from pulmonary embolism or severe anemia, causes appropriate hyperventilation with resultant respiratory alkalosis. In such cases, the cause of the hypoxia should be the primary focus of treatment rather than the respiratory alkalosis.

Patients who have respiratory alkalosis may evidence light-headedness, diaphoresis, paresthesias (digital and circumoral), muscle cramps, carpal and pedal spasms, tetany, syncope, and cardiac arrhythmias. Most of these manifestations are the result of increased neuromuscular excitability. The CSF becomes alkalotic. Chvostek and Trousseau signs (nonspecific signs of increased neuromuscular excitability) are positive in many of these patients.

Respiratory alkalosis can be corrected only by the lungs. If any compensation occurs, it is performed by the kidneys, which increase the urinary excretion of bicarbonate ions to restore the 20:1 ratio of bicarbonate ion to carbonic acid. Renal compensation for a respiratory acid-base imbalance requires several days. Most cases of respiratory alkalosis have a short duration; therefore, the disorder is often uncompensated or

Table 10–7 ▪ CAUSES OF RESPIRATORY ALKALOSIS

Category	Clinical Examples
Hyperventilation due to hypoxemia	Pulmonary disease that causes decreased PaO_2 Pulmonary embolism High altitude
Hyperventilation due to situational factors	Anxiety or fear Pain Prolonged crying and gasping Hyperventilation with mechanical ventilator
Hyperventilation due to stimulation of respiratory neurons in brainstem (medulla)	High fever Encephalitis Meningitis Salicylates (overdose) Gram-negative sepsis

partially compensated. Compensated respiratory alkalosis is characterized by a decreased $PaCO_2$ (the sign of the primary problem), a decreased bicarbonate ion concentration (the sign of the renal compensation), and a pH that is increased (partially compensated) or normal (fully compensated).

Respiratory alkalosis causes increased pH inside myocardial cells and increases cardiac contractility by increasing the calcium sensitivity of myofibrils (Hunjan et al., 1998). The imbalance increases sympathetic nervous system activity and circulating catecholamine levels. Cardiac arrhythmias may result. Although respiratory alkalosis may cause peripheral vasodilation, which decreases peripheral vascular resistance, it is likely to cause peripheral vasoconstriction and increased peripheral vascular resistance (Jundi et al., 2000; Kazmaier et al., 1998). Respiratory alkalosis also causes coronary vasoconstriction and cerebral vasoconstriction (Zuccarello et al., 2000). This latter effect reduces intracranial pressure and cerebral blood flow and may be the reason for the light-headedness and syncope experienced by some patients with respiratory alkalosis. In contrast to its effect on other blood vessels, respiratory alkalosis causes pulmonary vasodilation (Mizuno et al., 2002). This effect is reduced in conditions with chronically increased pulmonary blood flow, such as some congenital heart defects (Cornfield, 2002).

Metabolic Alkalosis

Metabolic alkalosis is caused by relatively too little metabolic acid. It can be due to a loss of acid or a gain of base. Acid can be lost through the gastrointestinal tract or in the urine. Acid may also be shifted into cells and thus "lost" from the blood. Base (bicarbonate ions) may be gained from intake of bicarbonate or of substances that are converted to bicarbonate in the body. Patients receiving the combination of loop diuretics and thiazide diuretics for treatment of severe congestive heart failure may develop "contraction alkalosis," metabolic alkalosis associated with extracellular volume contraction (Rose & Post, 2000). In a patient with hypovolemic shock from hemorrhage, a metabolic alkalosis may develop if eight or more units of packed red cells or other forms of blood are infused in a short time because the liver metabolizes the citrate in the blood into bicarbonate. Additional causes of metabolic alkalosis are listed in Table 10-8.

The initial clinical manifestations of metabolic alkalosis are often milder than those of respiratory alkalosis because bicarbonate ions cross membranes (and thus alter CSF and intracellular pH) less rapidly than does carbon dioxide. These clinical manifestations may include light-headedness, paresthesias, muscle cramps, carpal and pedal spasms, and cardiac arrhythmias. An initial CNS excitation is followed by the CNS depression of severe metabolic alkalosis: confusion, lethargy, and coma. The plasma bicarbonate ion concentration is elevated.

Correction of metabolic alkalosis must be accomplished by the kidneys because they are the excretory organs for bicarbonate ions. Compensation for the disorder, therefore, is the role of the lungs. Because the bicarbonate ion concentration is increased in metabolic alkalosis, the 20:1 ratio of bicarbonate ion to carbonic acid that creates a normal pH can be restored by increasing the amount of carbonic acid in the blood. Thus, the respiratory compensation for metabolic alkalosis is decreased

Table 10–8 ■ CAUSES OF METABOLIC ALKALOSIS

Category	Clinical Examples
Decrease of acid	Emesis
	Gastric suction
	Hyperaldosteronism (increases renal excretion of acid)
	Chronic excessive ingestion of black licorice (contains aldosterone-like compounds)
	Glucocorticoid excess
	Diuretic therapy
	Hypokalemia (acid moves into cells)
Increase of base (bicarbonate ions)	Excess ingestion of baking soda or bicarbonate antacids
	Excess infusion of $NaHCO_3$
	Excess administration of lactate or acetate (convert to bicarbonate)
	Massive blood transfusion (citrate converts to bicarbonate
	Extracellular fluid volume deficit (contraction alkalosis)

rate and depth of respiration. This compensatory hypoventilation retains carbonic acid (carbon dioxide and water) in the body, which tends to normalize the pH. Compensatory hypoventilation, however, is limited by the body's need for oxygen, so full compensation for metabolic alkalosis is not common. Compensated metabolic alkalosis is characterized by an increased $PaCO_2$ (the sign of the respiratory compensation), an increased bicarbonate ion concentration (the sign of the primary problem), and a pH that is somewhat increased (partially compensated).

Metabolic alkalosis causes increased cardiac contractility by increasing calcium sensitivity, although intracellular pH does not increase in myocardial cells as it does in respiratory alkalosis (Hunjan et al., 1998). Cardiac arrhythmias may occur. Vascular effects are likely to include peripheral vasoconstriction. Other vascular effects of metabolic alkalosis are coronary vasoconstriction, pulmonary vasodilation, and cerebral vasoconstriction with resulting decreased cerebral blood flow and light-headedness (Mizuno et al., 2002; Zuccarello et al., 2000).

Principles of Interpreting Arterial Blood Gas Reports

Arterial blood gases are used to assess a patient's acid-base status. The material presented earlier in this chapter provides the basis for understanding and interpreting acid-base aspects of arterial blood gases. The principles are summarized in this section. The PaO_2, a measure of oxygenation, is not discussed here.

The first laboratory value to consider is the pH. If it is below the normal range (less than 7.35 or the reported laboratory normal), then the patient has acidosis. If it is above the normal range (greater than 7.45 or the reported laboratory normal), then the patient has alkalosis. If the pH is within the normal range, there may be no acid-base imbalance, or the patient may have a fully compensated imbalance. For purposes of interpretation, then, if the pH is less than 7.40, the patient is tentatively

Table 10–9 ▪ MIXED ACID-BASE IMBALANCES

Concurrent Primary Acid-Base Imbalances	Effect on pH	Clinical Examples	Blood Gas Values
Respiratory acidosis plus metabolic alkalosis	Opposing effect on pH	Person with type B COPD (chronic bronchitis) develops repeated emesis	pH possibly near normal $PaCO_2$ increased HCO_3^- increased
Respiratory alkalosis plus metabolic acidosis	Opposing effect on pH	Person with encephalitis develops circulatory shock	pH possibly near normal $PaCO_2$ decreased HCO_3^- decreased
Metabolic acidosis plus metabolic alkalosis	Opposing effect on pH	Person with chronic renal failure develops repeated emesis	Vary, depending on severity and duration of imbalances
Respiratory acidosis and metabolic acidosis	Same effect on pH	Person with type B COPD (chronic bronchitis) develops prolonged diarrhea	pH greatly decreased $PaCO_2$ increased HCO_3^- decreased
Two different types of metabolic acidosis	Same effect on pH	Person with diabetic ketoacidosis becomes dehydrated and develops lactic acidosis from poor tissue perfusion	pH greatly decreased $PaCO_2$ likely decreased (compensation) HCO_3^- greatly decreased
Metabolic alkalosis and respiratory alkalosis	Same effect on pH	Person who received massive blood transfusion hyperventilates from pain and fear	pH greatly increased $PaCO_2$ decreased HCO_3^- increased

considered to have acidosis; if the pH is greater than 7.40, the patient is tentatively considered to have alkalosis.

The next value to consider is the $PaCO_2$. If the $PaCO_2$ is above the normal range, then the patient has respiratory acidosis. This respiratory acidosis may be the primary problem, or it may be compensatory. On the other hand, if the $PaCO_2$ is below the normal range, then the patient has respiratory alkalosis. This respiratory alkalosis may be the primary problem or it may be compensatory. If the $PaCO_2$ is within the normal range, then the patient does not have a respiratory acid-base disorder.

A basic understanding of acid-base imbalances facilitates differentiating between primary and compensatory respiratory imbalances. If the patient has *primary respiratory acidosis,* then the pH would be expected to be below 7.40. A *compensatory respiratory acidosis* would occur in response to a metabolic alkalosis, so the pH would be above 7.40.

The third laboratory value to consider is the bicarbonate ion concentration. If it is above the normal range, the patient has metabolic alkalosis, which may be the primary problem or may be compensatory. If the bicarbonate ion concentration is below the normal range, then the patient has primary or compensatory metabolic acidosis. A bicarbonate ion concentration within the normal range indicates no metabolic acid-base disorder. The differentiation between primary and compensatory imbalances is made by considering the pH. A patient who has a *primary metabolic acidosis* would be expected to have a pH below 7.40. A *compensatory metabolic acidosis* would be a response to a primary respiratory alkalosis, so the pH would be above 7.40. Following similar logic, with a *primary metabolic alkalosis,* the pH would be above 7.40; with a *compensatory metabolic alkalosis,* the pH would be below that value.

Once the three values have been examined, the final step in interpreting arterial blood gas values is to compare the interpretation with the patient's history and condition to verify that it makes sense. The principles of laboratory value interpretation presented in this section apply to patients who have only one primary acid-base imbalance. Mixed acid-base imbalances (more than one concurrent primary imbalance) are presented in the next section.

Mixed Acid-Base Imbalances

Occasionally, a patient may have more than one primary acid-base imbalance at the same time. In this circumstance, coexisting primary acidosis and alkalosis may somewhat neutralize each other so that the pH is near normal while the $PaCO_2$ and bicarbonate ion concentration are grossly abnormal. Alternatively, two primary disorders that cause the same pH alteration (e.g., types of coexisting alkalosis) can create a pH that rapidly approaches the fatal limit. Examples of mixed acid-base imbalances are presented in Table 10-9.

SUMMARY

This chapter describes the mechanisms by which the body maintains acid-base balance and explains acid-base imbalances. Respiratory acid-base imbalances are disorders of too much or too little carbonic acid (carbon dioxide and water). Their laboratory marker is an altered $PaCO_2$. The body compensates for an ongoing respiratory acid-base disorder by excreting more or fewer metabolic acids in the urine to normalize the pH.

Metabolic acid-base imbalances are disorders of too many or too few metabolic acids. Their laboratory marker is an altered bicarbonate ion concentration. The body compensates for metabolic acid-base disorders by adjusting alveolar ventilation to excrete more or less carbonic acid to normalize the pH. In addition to their other effects, acid-base imbalances alter cardiac contractility and may cause cardiac arrhythmias. They influence the degree of vasoconstriction in various vascular beds. Thus, an understanding of acid-base balance and imbalances is important in the care of cardiac patients.

REFERENCES

Chemmalakuzhy, J., Costanzo, M.R., Meyer, P., Piccione, W., Kao, W., Winkel, E., Saltzberg, M., Heroux, A., & Parrillo, J. (2001). Hypotension, acidosis, and vasodilatation syndrome post-heart transplant: prognostic variables and outcomes. *Journal of Heart and Lung Transplantation, 20,* 1075–1083.

Cornfield, D., Resnik, E., Herron, J., Reinhartz, O., & Fineman, J. (2002). Pulmonary vascular K+ channel expression and vasoreactivity in a model of congenital heart disease. *American Journal of Physiology, 283,* L1210–L1219.

Guyton, A. C., & Hall, J. E. (2000). *Textbook of medical physiology* (10th ed.). Philadelphia: W.B. Saunders.

Hattori, K., Tsuchida, S., Tsukahara, H., Mayumi, M., Tanaka, T., Zhang, L., Taniguchi, T., & Muramatsu, I. (2002). Augmentation of NO-mediated vasodilation in metabolic acidosis. *Life Sciences, 71,* 1439–1447.

Horiuchi, T., Dietrich, H., Hongo, K., Goto, T., & Dacey, R. (2002). Role of endothelial nitric oxide and smooth muscle potassium channels in cerebral arteriolar dilation in response to acidosis. *Stroke, 33,* 844–849.

Hunjan, S., Mason, R. P., Mehta, V. D, Kulkarni, P. V., Aravind, S., Arora, V., & Antich, P. P. (1998). Simultaneous intracellular and extracellular pH measurement in the heart by 19F NMR of 6-fluoropyridoxol. *Magnetic Resonance in Medicine, 39,* 551–556.

Jundi, K., Barrington, K. J., Henderson, C., Allen, R. G., & Finer, N. N. (2000). The hemodynamic effects of prolonged respiratory alkalosis in anesthetized newborn piglets. *Intensive Care Medicine, 26,* 449–456.

Kalinin, A., & Gessler, H. (2002). Oxygen consumption and force development in turtle and trout cardiac muscle during acidosis and high extracellular potassium. *Journal of Comparative Physiology B, Biochemical, Systemic, and Environmental Physiology, 172,* 145–151.

Kazmaier, S., Weyland, A., Buhre, W., Stephan, H., Rieke, H., Filoda, K., & Sonntag, H. (1998). Effects of respiratory alkalosis and acidosis on myocardial blood flow and metabolism in patients with coronary artery disease. *Anesthesiology, 89,* 831–837.

Kitakaze, M., Node, K., Takashima, S., Asanuma, H., Akasura, M., Sanada, S., Shinokazi, Y., Mori, H., Sato, H., Kuzuya, T., & Hori, M. (2001). Role of cellular acidosis in production of nitric oxide in canine ischemic myocardium. *Journal of Molecular and Cellular Cardiology, 33,* 1727–1737.

Kupriyanov, V. V., Xiang, B., Sun, J., Jilkina, O., & Deslauriers, R. (2002). Effects of regional hypoxia and acidosis on Rb(+) uptake and energetics in isolated pig hearts: (87)Rb MRI and (31)P MR spectroscopic study. *Biochimica et Biophysica Acta, Molecular Basis of Disease, 1586,* 57–70.

Mizukoshi, Y., Shibata, K., & Yoshida, M. (2001). Left ventricular contractility is reduced by hypercapnic acidosis and thoracolumbar epidural anesthesia in rabbits. *Canadian Journal of Anaesthesia, 48,* 557–562.

Mizuno, S., Demura, Y., Ameshima, S., Okamura, S., Miyamori, I., & Ishizaki, T. (2002). Alkalosis stimulates endothelial nitric oxide synthase in cultured human pulmonary arterial endothelial cells. *American Journal of Physiology, 283,* L113–L119.

Najarian, T., Marrache, A. M., Dumont, I., Hardy, P., Beauchamp, M. H., Hou, X., Peri, K., Gobeil, F., Jr., Varma, D.R., & Chemtob, S. (2000). Prolonged hypercapnia-evoked cerebral hyperemia via K+ channel- and prostaglandin E2-dependent endothelial nitric oxide synthase induction. *Circulation Research, 87,* 1149–1156.

Phillis, J. W., Song, D., & O'Regan, M.H. (2000). Mechanisms involved in coronary artery dilatation during respiratory acidosis in the isolated perfused rat heart. *Basic Research in Cardiology, 95,* 93–97.

Rose, B. D., & Post, T. (2000). *Clinical physiology of acid-base and electrolyte disorders* (5th ed.). New York: McGraw-Hill.

Takahashi, R., Shimazaki, Y., & Endoh, M. (2001). Decrease in Ca(2+)-sensitizing effect of UD-CG 212 Cl, a metabolite of pimobendan, under acidotic condition in canine ventricular myocardium. *Journal of Pharmacology and Experimental Therapeutics, 298,* 1060–1066.

Zuccarello, M., Lee, B., & Rapoport, R. M. (2000). Hypocapnic constriction in rabbit basilar artery in vitro: triggering by serotonin and dependence on endothelin-1 and alkalosis. *European Journal of Pharmacology, 407,* 191–195.

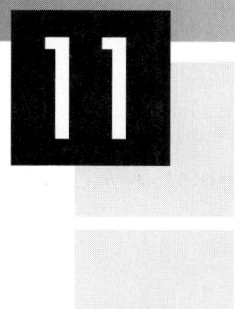

SLEEP

KATHY P. PARKER • SANDRA B. DUNBAR

The physiological changes that accompany normal sleep may have adverse effects on patients with cardiovascular disease (Redeker, 2002). Because this group also has a high prevalence of sleep abnormalities, these changes may be particularly problematic (Krieger & Redeker, 2002; Parker & Dunbar, 2002; Redeker & Hedges, 2002a; Richards, Anderson, Chesson, & Nagel, 2002). Thus, achieving a more complete understanding of the effects of sleep and sleep-related problems experienced by these patients is absolutely imperative if optimizing health outcomes is the goal (Weaver, 2001). Clinicians and researchers alike face numerous challenges in this regard, especially when considering the complex clinical presentation and treatment needs typical of these patients. To assist nurses in helping patients with cardiovascular disease achieve adequate, restful, and restorative sleep, this chapter reviews normal sleep and sleepiness, changes in cardiopulmonary and other system functions during sleep, sleep problems commonly seen in patients with cardiovascular disease, and appropriate nursing management.

NORMAL SLEEP

Sleep and Sleepiness

The human need for sleep has been recognized throughout the centuries, and few physiological phenomena have received as much attention from scholars, scientists, poets, and other literary figures (Thorpy, 1991). Before the 20th century, sleep was thought to be a simple, passive phenomenon—a state often described as existing between waking and death (Thorpy, 1991). Today, although much remains to be fully understood about the topic, the modern study of sleep has revealed some of its secrets. It is now known that sleep is an active process regulated by a multiplicity of behavioral, neuroendocrine, and central nervous system factors (Aldrich, 1999; Carskadon & Dement, 2000). It is also becoming increasingly well recognized that insufficient and/or poor-quality nocturnal sleep and daytime sleepiness adversely affect important clinical outcomes (Newman et al., 2000; Nugent et al., 2001; Whitney et al., 1998). Numerous primary sleep disorders (84 of them) (ASDA, 1997) have been either recognized or proposed, and the field of sleep medi-

cine has now become a bona fide, empirically based subspecialty (Aldrich, 1999).

The modern textbook definition describes sleep as "a reversible behavioral state of perceptual disengagement from and unresponsiveness to the environment" (Carskadon & Dement, 2000). Sleep is further defined according to behavioral and physiological criteria. Behavioral criteria include quiescence, closed eyes, decreased response to external stimuli, recumbent position, and reversible unconsciousness (Carskadon & Dement, 2000; Chokroverty, 1999; Tobler, 1995). The physiological criteria are based on polysomnographic recordings that include electroencephalography (EEG), electro-oculography (EOG), and electromyography (EMG) (Rechtschaffen & Kales, 1968) (Figs. 11-1 and 11-2).

Daytime sleepiness refers to the tendency or propensity to fall asleep during the day. In normal individuals, sleepiness typically has a biphasic circadian rhythm (Richardson, Carskadon, Orav, & Dement, 1982; Roehrs, Carskadon, Dement, & Roth, 2000), with an increased sleep tendency in the mid afternoon and, as is well known to nightshift workers, in the early morning hours (Kecklund & Akerstedt, 1995) (Fig.11-3). In fact, a continuum between being very alert and very sleepy (often referred to as *arousal state*) provides a background for all waking endeavors and is a far more important dimension of human function than commonly recognized. Many adults are chronically sleepy in the daytime because of insufficient or disrupted nighttime sleep. The problem may initially go unnoticed when masked by stimulating factors such as movement, excitement, high motivation, or hunger. However, daytime sleepiness can be unmasked by situational factors such as boredom, a warm dark room, or a prolonged dull task (Roehrs et al., 2000). Although poor nocturnal sleep can cause sleepiness, abnormal daytime sleep can also adversely affect nocturnal sleep. Thus, a complete assessment includes an examination of nocturnal and daytime sleep/wake patterns.

Measurement of Sleep and Sleepiness

There are three primary ways in which sleep and sleepiness are measured: subjectively, behaviorally, and objectively. In sleep and health, these measures are often, but not always, congruent;

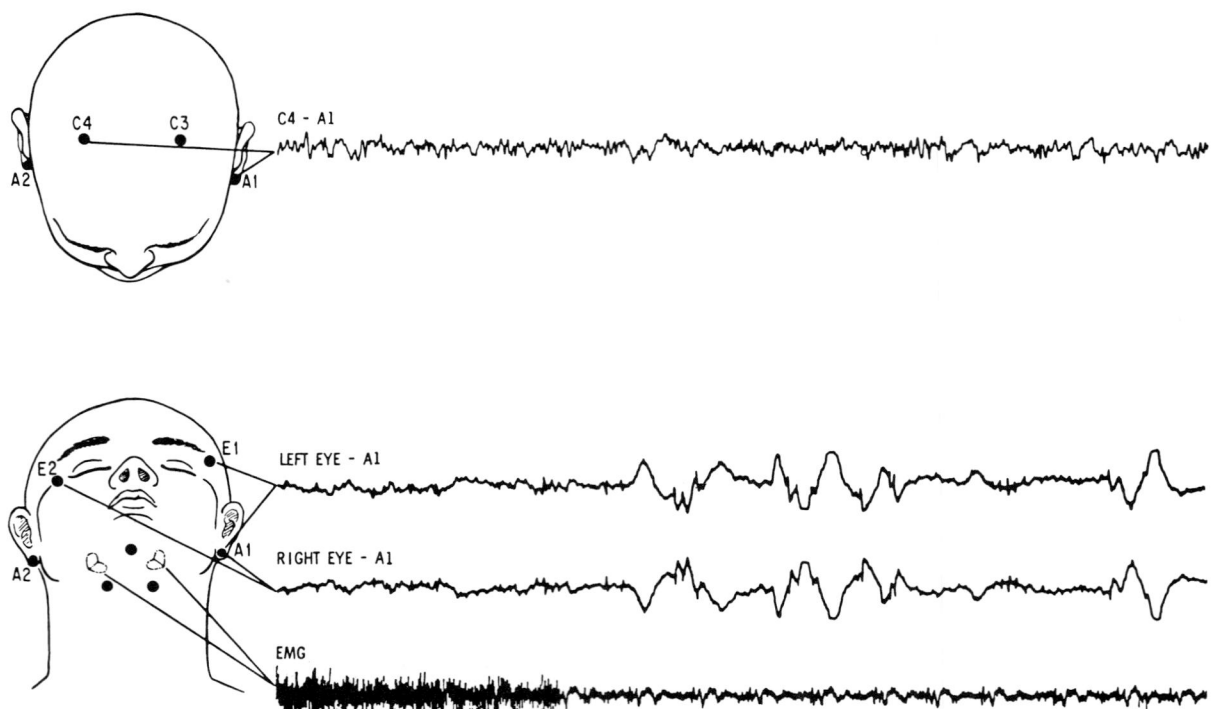

■ **Figure 11–1.** Placement of electrodes for (*top*) electroencephalogram and (*bottom*) electro-oculogram and electromyogram in polygraphic sleep recordings. (From Rechtschaffen, A., & Kales, A. [Eds.][1968]. *A manual of standardized terminology, techniques and scoring system for sleep stages of human subjects* [p. 15]. Los Angeles, CA: Brain Information Service/Brain Research Institute, University of California, 1968.)

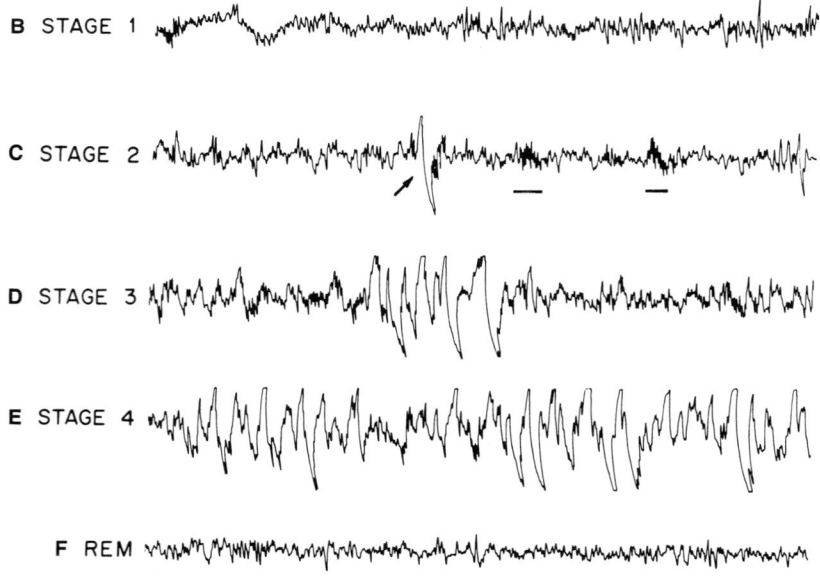

■ **Figure 11–2.** Electroencephalogram patterns in wakefulness and sleep in a young adult. (*A*) Rhythmic α-wave activity at 8 to 10 Hz in relaxed wakefulness with the eyes closed. (*B*) Mixed-frequency, relatively low-amplitude waves in non-rapid-eyemovement stage 1, with a vertex sharp wave toward the end of the tracing. (*C*) K complex (*arrow*) and sleep spindles (*underscored*) begin in stage 2. (*D, E*) Progressively greater percentages of slow, high-amplitude waves in stages 3 and 4. (*F*) Mixed-frequency, relatively low-amplitude waves in rapid-eye-movement sleep, similar to the pattern in stage 1. (From Dement, W., Richardson, G., Prinz, P. et al. [1985]. Changes of sleep and wakefulness with age. In C.E. Finch, & E.L. Schneider [Eds.], *Handbook of the biology of aging,* [2nd ed., p. 694]. New York: Van Nostrand Reinhold.)

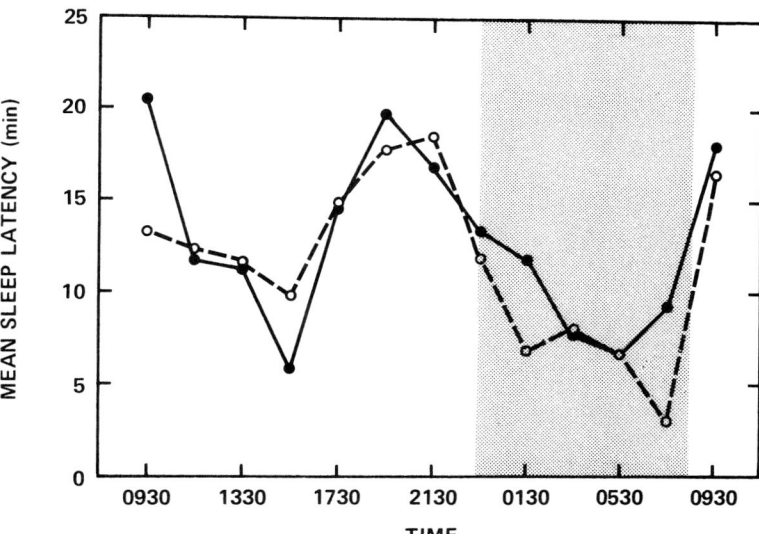

■ **Figure 11–3.** Mean sleep latency in minutes in young adults (*open circles*) and old adults (*solid circles*) at different times of day. The shaded area represents the nighttime sleep period. A biphasic rhythm exists with maximal sleepiness in the mid-afternoon and early morning, as indicated by shorter latencies. (From Richardson, G.S., Carskadon, M.A., Orav, E.F., et al. [1982]. Circadian variation of sleep tendency in elderly and young adult subjects. *Sleep,* 5 [Suppl. 2], S87.)

however, they become much less well associated when impaired sleep or other health problems are present (Baker, Maloney, & Driver, 1999; D'Hoore & D'Hoore, 1990; Griefahn, Schuemer-Kohrs, Schuemer, Moehler, & Mehnert, 2000; McCall, Turpin, Reboussin, Edinger, & Haponik, 1995; Rotenberg, Indursky, Kayumov, Sirota, & Melamed, 2000; Tsuchiyama, Nagayama, Kudo, Kojima, & Yamada, 2003; Yagi et al., 1998).

Subjective Measurement

Subjective measures of sleep can be particularly useful for screening, triage, and assessing the effects of treatment (Cohen, 1997). Types of information typically obtained include an individual's assessment of sleep latency (time from lights out to the onset of sleep), number of awakenings, depth and length of sleep, refreshing quality of sleep, satisfaction with sleep, and soundness of sleep (Shaver & Giblin, 1989). This information can be collected through the use of sleep questionnaires, i.e., the Pittsburgh Sleep Quality Index (Buysse, Reynolds, Monk, Berman, & Kupfer, 1989; Buysse et al., 1991), St. Mary's Hospital Sleep Questionnaire (Ellis et al., 1981), Sleep Disorders Questionnaire (Douglass et al., 1994), sleep diaries, visual analogue scales (Leed's Sleep Evaluation Questionnaire (Parrott & Hindmarch, 1980), and interviews (Shaver & Giblin, 1989).

Daytime sleepiness can also be measured using subjective assessments such as the Epworth Sleepiness Scale (ESS), an instrument that has been widely used in the clinical and research settings (Johns, 1991, 1992, 2000; Roehrs et al., 2000). Test scores greater than 10 or 11 have been reported in patients with sleep disorders that cause excessive daytime sleepiness (EDS); the average score for control subjects is 6 (possible range of scores is 0 to 24; higher score = greater subjective sleepiness) (Johns, 1991, 2000). Although the results of studies examining the relationship between ESS scores and sleep apnea severity, for example, have been equivocal (Chervin & Aldrich, 1999; Johns, 1993), improvement

in scores after treatment of apnea with continuous positive airway pressure (CPAP) has been described (Monasterio et al., 2001; Sin, Mayers, Man, & Pawluk, 2002). Thus, the instrument may be sensitive to and particularly helpful in evaluating clinical responses to interventions designed to improve sleep (Table 11-1).

Table 11–1 ■ EPWORTH SLEEPINESS SCALE

Name: _____

Today's date: _____ Your age: _____

Your sex (male = M; female = F): _____

How likely are you to doze off or fall asleep in the following situations, in contrast to feeling just tired? This refers to your usual way of life in recent times. Even if you have not done some of these things recently, try to work out how they would have affected you. Use the following scale to choose the *most appropriate number* for each situation:

0 = would *never* doze
1 = *slight* chance of dozing
2 = *moderate* chance of dozing
3 = *high* chance of dozing

Situation	Chance of Dozing
Sitting and reading	_____
Watching TV	_____
Sitting, inactive in a public place (theater or meeting)	_____
As a passenger in a car for an hour without a break	_____
Lying down to rest in the afternoon when circumstances permit	_____
Sitting and talking to someone	_____
Sitting quietly after a lunch without alcohol	_____
In a care, while stopped for a few minutes in traffic	_____

Johns, M. W. (1991). A new method for measuring daytime sleepiness: the Epworth sleepiness scale. *Sleep,* 14(6), 540–545.

Behavioral Assessment

Assessment of behaviors related to sleep and sleepiness are an important part of a thorough assessment. In fact, observation is considered the "gold standard" for sleep monitoring in infants. Typically, individuals who are sleepy or sleep-deprived manifest characteristic behaviors including yawning, eye rubbing, head nodding, ptosis of the eyelids, irritability, and slowed movement. Other observable waking behaviors that can be noted include automatic behavior, unintentional sleep episodes, cataplexy (a stereotypical feature of narcolepsy in which there is a sudden decrement in muscle tone and loss of deep tendon reflexes leading to muscle weakness, paralysis, and/or postural collapse), and sleep drunkenness (ASDA, 1997). Although lying quietly in a horizontal position is typical, movements and position changes can occur and are a normal part of sleep behavior (Gardner & Grossman, 1975; Johnson, Swan, & Weigand, 1930; Kleitman, Cooperman, & Mullin, 1933). Abnormal sleep-related behaviors include bizarre postures, restless sleep, jerking of the extremities, seizure activity, and dream enactment. Video recordings of these behaviors during polysomnography (PSG) are often made to assist in the assessment and diagnosis of sleep problems. Observations of patients' nocturnal behaviors by health care providers, bed partners, or parents often play an important role in the diagnosis and treatment of sleep disorders (Cohen, 1997).

Objective Measurement

The structure and timing of sleep stages and cycles can be studied objectively using polysomnography (PSG), a procedure involving the simultaneous recording of the EEG, the EMG, and the EOG. At the usual recording speed of 1 centimeter per second, a standard 30-centimeter page represents a 30-second period, or *epoch*. Each epoch is assigned a single sleep-stage score based primarily on changes in EEG frequency (in cycles/second, or hertz [Hz]) and amplitude (in microvolts [μV]), with confirmation by the EOG and EMG patterns (Rechtschaffen & Kales, 1968). In addition to sleep-staging signals, polysomnography often includes the measurement of other physiological parameters, such as respiratory movements of the chest and abdomen, airflow at the nose and mouth, arterial oxygen saturation, electrocardiogram (ECG), and leg movements (anterior tibialis EMG).

Daytime sleepiness (daytime sleep propensity or tendency) can be quantified using the Multiple Sleep Latency Test (MSLT) (ASDA, 1986). Beginning 1.5 to 2 hours at the end of a nocturnal polysomnographic recording, four to five 20-minute nap opportunities are typically given in 2-hour intervals. The sleep latency of any given nap opportunity is defined as the time from lights out to the first 30-second epoch scored as sleep. The average sleep latency across all naps is calculated and expressed as the mean sleep latency. The range of possible mean sleep latency scores on the MSLT is 0 to 20 minutes, with a low score indicating greater sleepiness. An MSLT score less than 5 minutes indicates pathological sleepiness and is a level at which patients often experience marked impairment of social and/or occupational functioning and at which they are generally advised against driving or operating heavy equipment (Richardson et al., 1978; Thorpy, 1992). Scores between 5 and 10 minutes are considered to be in the "diagnostic gray zone," whereas scores greater than 10 are considered normal.

An alternative method sometimes used to objectively measure sleep/wake patterns, actigraphy, relies on monitoring periods of activity and rest (Ancoli-Israel et al., 2003). Using a battery-operated wristwatch-size microprocessor that senses movement with a piezoelectric beam, continuous motion data can be obtained for long periods. Computer algorithms allow for analysis of activity and nonactivity, as well as (Pollak, Tryon, Nagaraja, & Dzwonczyk, 2001) scoring of sleep and wakefulness. While actigraphy cannot determine sleep stages, information on total sleep time, percent of time spent awake, number of awakenings, time between awakenings, and sleep onset latency can be obtained. Actigraphy data correlate well with PSG data, particularly when sleep is normal (Ancoli-Israel et al., 2003; Jean-Louis et al., 1996). Correlations decrease when sleep is disturbed or activity is limited (Pollak et al., 2001; Sadeh & Acebo, 2002; Sadeh, Hauri, Kripke, & Lavie, 1995).

Stages of Sleep

Typical EEG patterns during wakefulness and sleep are shown in Figure 11-2. During relaxed wakefulness with the eyes open, the EEG consists predominantly of mixed frequency (cycle per second; Hz), low-voltage activity (low amplitude), or *desynchronized* brain-wave activity. Rapid eye movements and blinks may occur, and muscle tone is usually at its highest level. With eyes closed, alpha waves are often noted (8 to 12 Hz) (Carskadon, 2000).

Sleep onset is heralded by a general slowing of the EEG activity and the emergence of theta waves (4 to 7 Hz) during more than 50% of the epoch. Sleep then progresses through several stages of nonrapid eye movement (NREM) and rapid eye movement (REM) sleep and cycles (a NREM/REM cycle) that are well described and form characteristic patterns in individuals and groups (Carskadon & Dement, 2000). NREM sleep is divided somewhat arbitrarily into four stages based on the EEG pattern. Sleep depth increases from stage 1 to 4 in that the sleeper becomes more difficult to awaken.

In stages 1 and 2, or light sleep, the EEG consists of relatively low-amplitude waves with a predominant frequency of 2 to 7 Hz. High, narrow, vertex, sharp waves may appear late in stage 1. Stage 2 is identified by two sporadic waveforms that stand out from the background EEG: sleep spindles and K complexes. Sleep spindles are waxing–waning bursts of waves in the 12 to 14 Hz range (Carskadon, 2000; Rechtschaffen & Kales, 1968). They originate in the thalamus and are thought to reflect impulses that inhibit the relay of sensory information to the cerebral cortex (Chase, 2000). K complexes consist of a sharp negative wave (upward deflection by EEG recording convention) followed by a slower positive wave (downward deflection). They occur spontaneously and in response to mild external stimuli, such as sounds. Stages 3 and 4, also called slow-wave or deep sleep, are differentiated by the percentage of slow (0.5 to 2 Hz), high-amplitude (>75 μV) EEG waves (referred to as *synchronized* brain-wave activity). They account for 20% to 50% of the epoch in stage 3 and more than 50% in stage 4. The eyes are relatively quiet during NREM sleep, except for slow rolling movements that usually occur at the beginning of stage 1 and disappear in stage 2. Muscle tone is moderately reduced from the waking level (Carskadon, 2000).

There are two types of REM sleep. Similar to waking, *tonic REM sleep* is characterized by desynchronized brain activity—a mixed frequency, relatively low-amplitude EEG. However, in REM sleep there is also a complete loss of postural muscle tone caused by hyperpolarization of brainstem and spinal motoneurons (Siegel, 2000). The sleeper has an active brain in a paralyzed body, with only the diaphragm and extraocular muscles retaining substantial tone. Some suggest that the purpose of this physiological phenomenon is to prevent the enactment of dreams. REM behavior disorder, in which there is loss of this normally occurring paralysis, is typified by abnormal movements, behaviors, and dream enactment during REM sleep. *Phasic REM sleep* occurs intermittently and is characterized by bursts of REMs (for which the stage is named), muscle twitches in the face and distal extremities (potent motor excitation briefly overrides the paralysis), and fluctuations in blood pressure, heart rate, and breathing (Lee, 2003; Parmeggaiani, 2000).

Approximately 80% of people awakened from REM sleep and 40% awakened from NREM sleep report having dreams. In NREM sleep, the mental activity tends to have a dull, sketchy quality without much basis in reality. In contrast, dreams recalled from REM sleep are usually vivid, well-formed, story-like narratives. Dreams include more visual imagery and emotional tone as the night progresses in relation to longer REM periods and greater intensity of phasic events (Carskadon & Dement, 2000). Penile and clitoral erections also often occur during REM sleep.

The Sleep Cycle

Most people have their major sleep period at night, organized in a rhythmic sequence of sleep stages (Fig. 11-4). After a short period of relaxed wakefulness, a young adult enters stage 1 sleep, followed by a descent into stage 2 for 10 to 25 minutes, a few minutes of stage 3, and approximately 20 to 40 minutes of stage 4. The sleeper then goes through stages 3 and 2 and has a brief REM period approximately 90 minutes after sleep onset (the period from sleep onset to the first REM period is referred to as REM latency). The cycle begins again and repeats another four to six times during the night. Slow-wave sleep occupies less of the second cycle and may then disappear, whereas REM periods lengthen across the night. Therefore, most slow wave sleep occurs in the first third of the night, and most REM sleep occurs in the last third. If an awakening occurs, then the sleep cycle typically starts again with stage 1 sleep. Frequent disruptions of sleep prevent the normal progression into slow-wave and REM sleep and increase stage 1 and 2 sleep (Carskadon & Dement, 2000).

Adults typically change their body position 40 to 50 times during a normal sleep period; the characteristics and number of movements that occur are relatively stable personal traits (Johnson et al., 1930; Kleitman et al., 1933; Moses, Lubin, Naitoh, & Johnson, 1972). Major body shifts often occur at changes from stage 4 to lighter NREM stages or from REM to NREM sleep. A sudden muscle contraction involving all or part of the body (hypnic jerk or hypnic myoclonus) often accompanied by intense visual imagery occasionally occurs at sleep onset and is normal; however, the frequency of the events may increase with stress or irregular sleep schedules (ASDA, 1997).

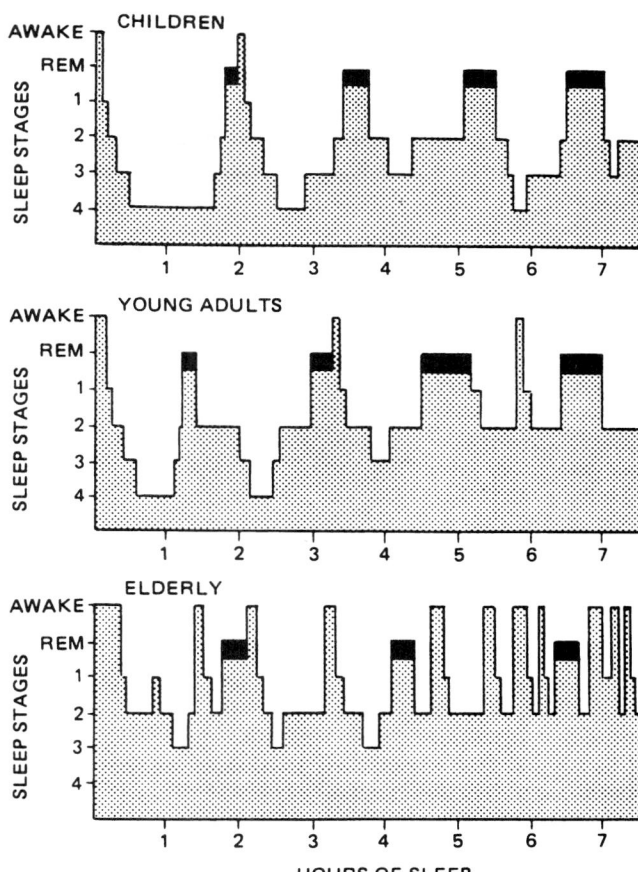

■ **Figure 11–4.** Normal sleep cycles in children, young adults, and the elderly. Rapid-eye-movement (REM) sleep (*darkened area*) occurs cyclically throughout the night at intervals of approximately 90 minutes in all age groups and shows little variation in the different age groups, whereas stage 4 non-REM (NREM) sleep decreases with age. In addition, the elderly have frequent awakenings and a marked increase in total wake time. (From Kales, A., & Kales, J.D. [1974]. Sleep disorder. *New England Journal of Medicine, 290,* 488.)

Sleep in Aging

With increasing age, particularly in men, sleep becomes lighter and more fragmented (see Fig. 11-4). In contrast to young adults, older people usually spend more time in bed but less time asleep (reduced sleep efficiency) and are more easily awakened from sleep. The time needed to fall asleep (sleep latency) shows little change with aging, but more nighttime awakenings, brief arousals, and stage changes occur (Bliwise, 2000). There is a striking reduction in slow-wave sleep (stages 3 and 4) and an increase in stage 1 sleep, with little change in the percentages of stage 2 and REM sleep (Carskadon & Dement, 2000). Bedtime and wake-up time come earlier (circadian phase advance), the daytime sleep tendency may be increased, daytime napping is more common, and tolerance for changes in the sleep–wake schedule is reduced. Sleep apnea (discussed later) and periodic leg movements (involuntary repetitive jerks) are more common in older adults and can contribute to sleep disruption (Ancoli-Israel, 2000; Ancoli-Israel et al., 1991; Ancoli-Israel, et al.,

2002; Cohen-Zion et al., 2001). Other factors may include poor sleep habits, a reduced activity level, psychological concerns, physical illness, and medications (Bliwise, 2000). Not surprisingly, older people often are dissatisfied with their sleep and use sleeping pills more often than other age groups (Wysowski & Baum, 1991). In elders, increased sleep latency and reduced sleep efficiency have been linked to greater mortality (Dew et al., 2003).

The Function of Sleep

The function of sleep remains a topic surrounded by controversy. Some have postulated that it is important for mental and physical restoration (Adam & Oswald, 1984) and energy conservation (Zepelin & Rechtschaffen, 1974). Others propose that the primary function of sleep is the maintenance of synaptic and neuronal network function (Kavanau, 1997, 2000; Krueger & Obal, 2002; Zepelin & Rechtschaffen, 1974). Sleep deprivation studies have shown that total and partial sleep loss impair well-being and functioning, with mood being the most strongly affected, followed by cognitive and motor performance (Dinges et al., 1997). Most agree that although the exact function of sleep remains to be discovered, it fulfills a vital need, one that is essential to human health and well being (Lee, 2003).

Sleep appears to play an important role in thermoregulatory (McGinty & Szymusiak, 1990; Szymusiak & McGinty, 1990) and immune processes (Benca et al., 1989; Dinges, Douglas, Hamarman, Zaugg, & Kapoor, 1995). Special areas in the hypothalamus and basal forebrain integrate temperature and sleep control through a network of complex interactive processes. For example, an increase in brain temperature before sleep onset increases sleep depth while deep sleep increases heat loss by stimulating vasodilatation and reduction of the metabolic rate. Peripheral signals coming from skin thermosensors going to these brain regions can also have a significant affect on sleep/wake state (Van Someren, 2000). In fact, the vasodilatation of blood vessels in the feet in response to local warmth was recently shown to be an independent predictor of sleep onset (Krauchi, et al., 1999; Krauchi & Wirz-Justice, 2001). Many immune factors such as interleukin-1, interleukin-2, and tumor necrosis factor (TNF)-α have been shown to promote deep sleep, possibly because of the associated increased heat production (Krueger & Obal, 2002). Thus, the interaction of sleep, thermoregulation, and immunological responses may explain why patients become sleepy when having fevers and infections. Sleep deprivation has also been associated with reduction in the activity of natural killer (NK) cells in response to a bacterial or viral load, also suggesting a direct link between sleep and immune function (Irwin et al., 1996; Krueger, et al., 1999).

■ THE REGULATION OF SLEEPING AND WAKING

According to the Two-Process Model of Sleep Regulation (Borbely & Acherman, 2000), the major mechanisms controlling sleep and waking across time are: (a) a homeostatic process determined by previous sleep and waking; and (b) a circadian

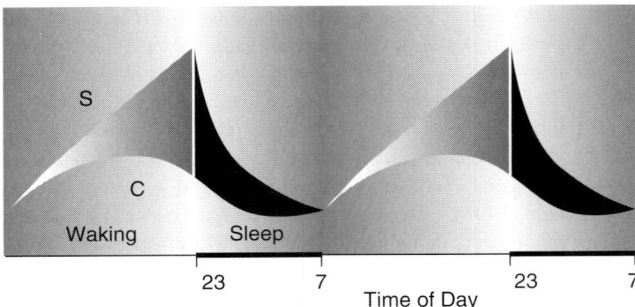

■ **Figure 11–5.** The two-process model of sleep regulation. Two primary processes regulate sleep: a homeostatic process determined by prior sleep and waking, and a circadian process that designates periods of high and low sleep propensity.

process that designates periods of high and low sleep propensity. The homeostatic process reflects the physiological need for sleep, which builds across the day and dissipates throughout the night (Fig.11-5). A key indicator of this process is EEG slow wave activity, which is high during the beginning of a sleep episode but decreases as the night progresses. The circadian process, a sinusoidal rhythm of approximately 24 hours, is controlled by a biologic oscillator (suprachiasmatic nucleus). This process regulates sleep propensity and its effects are greatest in the early morning hours. The rhythm of core body temperature is a key indicator of the circadian process. The timing and duration of sleep are determined by the combined action of homeostatic and circadian processes via their influence on thermoregulatory and neuronal/neurohormonal systems (Borbely & Acherman, 2000; Van Someren, 2000). Factors that either oppose or enhance these processes can have significant effects on the timing, duration, and structure of sleep as well as daytime alertness.

■ PHYSIOLOGY DURING SLEEP

The physiological basis of nursing care has rested almost entirely on studies of responses during wakefulness. However, NREM sleep, REM sleep, and wakefulness are very different physiological states associated with state-dependent changes in the function of most body systems. In healthy individuals, these changes are well tolerated; but in patients with cardiovascular disease, the sleep state may make them vulnerable to serious, sometimes fatal, complications.

Cardiovascular Function in Sleep

Cardiovascular control during sleep is primarily determined by variation in autonomic nervous system activity, which causes changes in blood pressure and heart rate, major determinants of myocardial oxygen demand (Khatri & Freis, 1967; Verrier, 2002). Increased parasympathetic tone and, to a lesser extent, decreased sympathetic tone, lead to a reduction in heart rate and cardiac output in NREM sleep. Vasodilatation causes a reduction in systemic vascular resistance and a 5% to 15% decrease in blood pressure. In contrast, pulmonary artery pressure increases slightly (Coccagna, et al., 1972; Lugaresi et al., 1978). Baroreceptor gain is heightened and contributes to the reduction and stability of blood pressure. Brief surges in blood pressure and heart rate occur with K complexes, arousals, and large body movements (Blasi et al., 2003; Catcheside, et al., 2002; Lugaresi et al., 1978; Tank et al., 2003). An age-related reduction in this response has been demonstrated in middle aged subjects in comparison to younger subjects, possibly reflecting a decline in parasympathetic functions that occurs with increasing age (Gosselin, et al., 2002). Sharp increases in heart rate and blood pressure occur with morning awakening and beginning the day's activities (Floras et al., 1978; Mulcahy et al., 1993) as well as after other periods of sleep, such as afternoon naps (Mulcahy et al., 1993).

Rapid eye movement sleep brings an increase in cardiovascular demands. Although blood pressure and heart rate have average levels near those observed in light NREM sleep or quiet wakefulness, their variability increases markedly during phasic REM sleep, with wide, erratic fluctuations (Coccagna & Lugaresi, 1978; Monti, et al., 2002; Murali, Svatikova, & Somers, 2003; Somers, Dyken, Mark, & Abboud, 1993). These changes are related to bursts of increased sympathetic activity and to reduced vagal input to the heart (Monti et al., 2002). Cardiac efferent vagal tone and baroreceptor regulation are generally suppressed during REM sleep (Verrier, 2002).

Respiratory Function in Sleep

Sleep alters breathing patterns, ventilation, and arterial blood gas values. Periodic breathing, a cyclic waxing and waning of tidal volume, sometimes with brief apnea, is common at sleep onset in association with fluctuations between wakefulness and light sleep. Breathing is remarkably regular, however, in stable stage 2 and slow-wave sleep. The pattern becomes faster and more erratic during phasic REM sleep (Krieger, 2000; Simon et al., 2002).

Minute ventilation falls, mainly because of reduced tidal volume, with an average decrease of approximately 13% in stage 2 and 15% in stage 4 compared with quiet wakefulness. This hypoventilation leads to small changes in arterial blood gases, including a mild hypercapnia (increases of 2 to 7 mm Hg in carbon dioxide tension), decreases of 0.01 to 0.06 units in pH, and a mild hypoxemia (decreases of 3 to 10 mm Hg in oxygen tension and 2% or less in oxygen saturation) (Krieger, 2000). Data regarding REM sleep are somewhat contradictory but suggest that minute ventilation, tidal volume, and respiratory frequency are similar to those in NREM sleep, with similar or somewhat greater changes in blood gas values (Krieger, 2000; Simon et al., 2002).

Other factors that contribute to hypoventilation in NREM sleep include reduced central drive to breathe caused by loss of the wakefulness stimulus and increased upper airway resistance to airflow due to reduced pharyngeal muscle tone (Krieger, 2000; Simon et al., 2002). Tone in the intercostal muscles and diaphragm, however, is maintained. In REM sleep, tone is lost in both the intercostal and upper airway muscles, reducing the rib cage contribution to breathing and increasing upper airway resistance; however, the diaphragm is relatively spared from REM-related paralysis. Phasic REM sleep also includes dysrhythmic changes in the stimulation of brainstem respiratory neurons, resulting in an erratic breathing pattern (Krieger, 2000; Simon et al., 2002).

The arterial blood gas changes stimulate an adaptive increase in ventilation, although the response is less effective in sleep than in wakefulness. In men, the ventilatory responses to both hypercapnia and hypoxemia decrease by approximately half from wakefulness to NREM sleep, with a further reduction in REM sleep. Women respond similarly to hypercapnia but somewhat differently to hypoxemia. Women have a lower ventilatory response than men when awake and little change in NREM sleep, but a similar fall in REM sleep (Berthon-Jones & Sullivan, 1984; Davis, Loh, Nodal, & Charnock, 1978; Douglas, 2000). Previous sleep deprivation impairs the ventilatory responses during wakefulness (Cooper & Phillips, 1982; Schiffman, et al., 1983; White et al., 1983).

Arousal from sleep is a second adaptive response to blood gas changes because the change stimulates ventilation and permits voluntary action to cope with the situation, such as moving a pillow that interferes with breathing. Hypercapnia is a relatively effective arousal stimulus, awakening most healthy subjects before carbon dioxide tension rises 15 mm Hg; concurrent hypoxemia enhances the response. Hypoxemia alone, however, is a poor arousal stimulus; study subjects often fail to awaken despite an oxygen saturation as low as 70% (Krieger, 2000; Simon et al., 2002).

Adaptive responses that protect the airways are less effective during sleep. Respiratory secretions are cleared less readily because of diminished mucociliary clearance (Bateman, Pavia, & Clarke, 1978), and the tendency to aspirate increases (Huxley, et al., 1978). In addition, sleep suppresses the cough reflex to irritating substances in the airways in both REM and NREM sleep (Douglas, 2000; Power et al., 1984).

Thermoregulation in Sleep

Body temperature is regulated at a lower set point in NREM sleep than in wakefulness. In combination with reduced motor activity, this results in a decrease in temperature at sleep onset (Barrett et al., 1993; Van Someren, 2000). The normal temperature regulating mechanisms are markedly inhibited during REM sleep; during this stage of sleep, body temperature is influenced more by the environment than the hypothalamus (Skinner, 2002). Body temperature also has an independent circadian rhythm that typically peaks in the late afternoon and reaches a minimum in the early morning hours of sleep (Skinner, 2002).

Sleep length depends on the phase of the circadian temperature rhythm at bedtime because the rising phase triggers awakening from sleep. A sleep period that begins when body temperature is low—for example, going to bed at 3:00 AM—is relatively short because temperature soon rises. In contrast, a sleep period that begins when temperature is high is relatively long because a rise in temperature does not occur for some time (Czeisler & Khalsa, 2000; Czeisler et al., 1980; Skinner, 2002). The body temperature rhythm shifts a little earlier (phase advance) with aging, which may partly explain why many older people have an earlier wake-up time than younger adults (Czeisler et al., 1992).

Cerebral Blood Flow, Intracranial Pressure, and Cerebral Metabolism in Sleep

Brain blood flow increases in sleep in comparison to waking. A small to moderate increase in brain blood flow occurs in NREM sleep, an observation likely related to the mild hypercapnia associated with reduced ventilation. The marked increase in brain blood flow in REM sleep, however, cannot be explained by hypercapnia alone (Douglas, 2000; Simon et al., 2002). Brain imaging techniques show that metabolic activity in the brain in NREM sleep is approximately one-fourth to one-third lower than in quiet wakefulness, whereas in REM sleep it is similar to the waking level. Areas with higher metabolic activity in REM sleep include the left side of the brain (right side when awake), limbic system (involved in emotions), and visual association areas (Madsen et al., 1991). Poor performance on tasks after sleep deprivation is associated with reduced metabolic activity in the frontal lobes, thalamus, and midbrain, which may be associated with the state of reduced alertness (Wu et al., 1991). Intracranial pressure appears to increase at sleep onset and during light sleep, decrease variably during slow-wave sleep, and rise significantly during REM sleep, perhaps reflecting changes in brain blood flow.

Renal Function in Sleep

Urine flow is reduced and more concentrated during sleep with a decreased excretion of sodium, chloride, potassium, and calcium. The mechanisms involved in these changes in urine flow and electrolyte excretion are complex and include changes in renal blood flow, glomerular filtration, hormone secretion (vasopressin, aldosterone, prolactin, parathormone), and sympathetic neural stimulation (Buxton, Spiegel, & Van Cauter, 2002; Cianci et al., 1991; Van Cauter, 2000). Because nighttime potassium excretion is reduced, potassium infusions given at that time may lead to higher serum levels than daytime infusions (Moore-Ede et al., 1978).

From infancy to old age, males have penile erections (nocturnal penile tumescence) during REM sleep. Total tumescence time is greatest just before and during puberty and then may gradually decline. Sleep-related erectile activity can be monitored to aid in differentiating physical and psychological components of impotence (Ware & Hirshkowitz, 2000).

Endocrine Function in Sleep

Endocrine hormone secretion is influenced by sleep. For example, growth hormone secretion is highly sleep-dependent and most secretion occurs during the first few hours after sleep onset during slow-wave sleep. If sleep is advanced or delayed, growth hormone secretion shifts accordingly. In contrast, thyroid hormone and cortisol secretions have independent circadian rhythms. Thyroid hormone secretion increases in the late evening; cortisol concentration increases in the latter half of the night and peaks toward the end of the normal sleep period or soon after awakening (Van Cauter, 2000).

The hormone melatonin, secreted by the pineal gland, induces sleepiness and is under study as a therapeutic agent. Melatonin has a marked circadian rhythm that is closely linked to the light–dark cycle and to the sleep–wake, temperature, and cortisol rhythms. A late evening surge in melatonin begins at darkness, approximately 2 hours before bedtime, and is considered a marker of the body's circadian timing system. Secretion peaks at approximately 3:00 AM, then is suppressed by daylight to levels that are barely detectable. Bright light exposure suppresses melatonin secretion and can be used to help reset a person's circadian clock (Lewy, 1999; Lewy & Sack, 1989; Nathan, et al., 1997; Owen & Arendt, 1992).

IMPAIRED SLEEP, SLEEP DISORDERS, AND EXCESSIVE DAYTIME SLEEPINESS

Impaired sleep can be generally categorized as either sleep deprivation (resulting from inadequate sleep) or sleep disruption (resulting from fragmented sleep during the night) (Lee, 2003) (Fig. 11-6). Sleep deprivation frequently occurs in association with particular lifestyles or stages of development. Sleep disruption is often seen in health-related conditions. Both sleep deprivation and sleep disruption result in sleep loss (Lee, 2003). Important information has been obtained through sleep deprivation studies that have shown that sleep loss has numerous adverse effects including fatigue, anxiety, increase illness, increased sensitivity to pain, decreased immune response, restlessness, disorientation, decreased alertness/attention during the day, and decreased sense of well-being (Adam & Oswald, 1984; Anderson et al., 2003; Dinges et al., 1997; Hong & Dimsdale, 2003; Miller, 2003; Nicassio, et al., 2002). It is interesting to note that Kripke et el. recently demonstrated an increased risk of mortality associated with chronic nocturnal sleep periods less than or equal to 6 hours (Kripke, 2003). In a 10-year follow-up from NHANES I, Qureshi et al. also found an increase in stroke in persons who reported greater than 8 hours or less than 6 hours per night (Qureshi et al., 1997).

Sleep disorders, specific diagnostic entities, include a wide array of problems characterized by insomnia (difficulty initiating or maintaining sleep or early morning awakening), excessive daytime sleepiness, and/or abnormal movements, behaviors, or sensations during sleep (Table 11-2) (ASDA, 1997). There are three primary groups of sleep disorders outlined in the International Classification of Sleep Disorders (ASDA, 1997). *Dyssomnias* are those disorders that produce difficulty initiating or maintaining sleep or excessive sleepiness. Dyssomnias may be related to intrinsic factors (idiopathic insomnia, obstructive sleep apnea, periodic limb movements), extrinsic factors (medications, environmental conditions), or circadian rhythm factors (shift work, irregular sleep–wake pattern, and advanced or delayed sleep phase). *Parasomnias* include abnormal behaviors, movements, or sensations during sleep, such as nightmares, sleep walking, sleep terrors, rapid eye movement (REM) behavioral disorder, and bruxism. The third category, *sleep disorders associated with mental, neurologic, or other medical disorders,* includes sleep abnormalities associated with conditions such as Parkinson

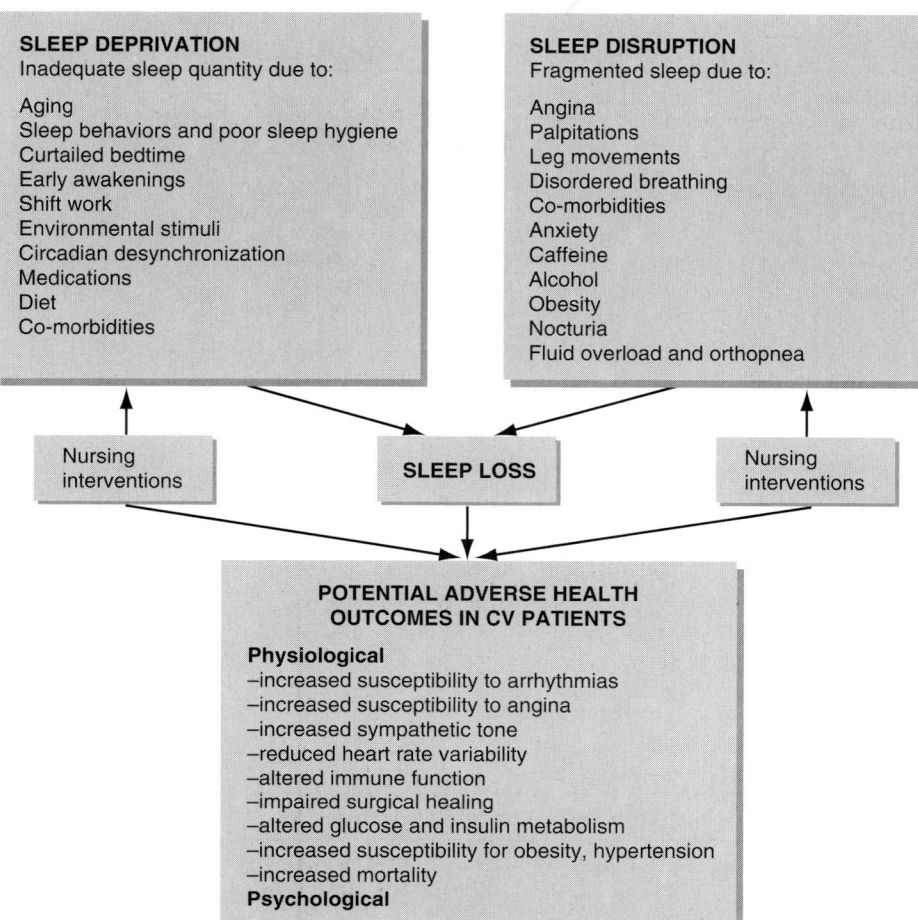

■ **Figure 11–6.** Conceptual model of impaired sleep in cardiovascular patients). (Adapted from Lee, K. A. [2003]. Impaired sleep. In V. Carrieri-Kolilman et. al [Eds.], *Pathophysiological phenomena in nursing: Human responses to illness* [pp. 363–385]. St. Louis: Saunders.)

disease, sleep-related epilepsy, mood disorders, nocturnal cardiac ischemia, sleep-related gastroesophageal reflux, and chronic obstructive pulmonary disease. A final category of *proposed sleep disorders,* for which there is insufficient information available to confirm the unequivocal existence of the disorders (i.e., short sleeper, long sleep, and sleep choking syndrome), is also included in the taxonomy.

Excessive daytime sleepiness (EDS), the inability to maintain the alert awake state, is the most common consequence of sleep disorders and/or insufficient or poor sleep and is the most prevalent symptom of patients seen in sleep disorders centers in the United States (D'Alessandro et al., 1995). However, because of its often vague and nonspecific clinical presentation, the condition is frequently unrecognized by health care providers in other clinical settings (ASDA, 1997; El-Ad & Korczyn, 1998). Patients themselves may have very little insight into the nature and severity of the problem and the negative effects that EDS has on their lives. For in its milder forms, EDS may cause only minor, barely perceived decrements in social and occupational functioning (ASDA, 1997). When severe, however, it can be debilitating, causing a broad range of neuropsychological deficits affecting daytime functioning and quality of life. EDS can even be life threatening because of associated alterations in alertness and reactivity (Connor et al., 2001; Lloberes et al., 2000; Lyznicki et al., 1998a, 1998b). Increased napping has

also been associated with increased mortality in the elderly (Bursztyn et al., 1999; Bursztyn et al., 2002).

SLEEP IN PATIENTS WITH CARDIOVASCULAR DISEASE

Sleep in Coronary Heart Disease

Although more than 13 million Americans are estimated to have coronary heart disease (AHA, 2003), research about their sleep patterns remains relatively limited. Several recent large studies, such as the Sleep Heart Health Study, have begun to link sleep symptoms and sleep-disordered breathing with cardiovascular disease (Newman et al., 2001; Shahar et al., 2001). Assessing these relationships is often complicated by variations in age, sex, type and severity of cardiovascular impairment, and medications. However, the existing research conveys consistent themes suggesting that sleep disorders increase cardiovascular risk and that patients with coronary heart disease often have disturbed sleep.

Impaired cardiac function from multiple causes can produce symptoms such as chest pain and dyspnea that interfere with sleep. Even when patients with a variety of diseases are

Table 11–2 ■ INTERNATIONAL CLASSIFICATION OF SLEEP DISORDERS (ASDA, 1997)

Dyssomnias

Intrinsic Sleep Disorders	*Extrinsic Sleep Disorders*	*Circadian Rhythm Sleep Disorders*
Psychophysiologic insomnia	Inadequate sleep hygiene	Time zone change (jet-lag) syndrome
Sleep state misperception	Environmental sleep disorder	Shift-work sleep disorder
Idiopathic insomnia	Altitude insomnia	Irregular sleep-wake pattern
Narcolepsy	Adjustment sleep disorder	Delayed sleep phase syndrome
Recurrent hypersomnia	Insufficient sleep syndrome	Advanced sleep phase syndrome
Idiopathic hypersomnia	Limit-setting sleep disorder	Non-24-hour sleep-wake disorder
Obstructive sleep apnea syndrome	Sleep-onset association disorder	
Central sleep apnea syndrome	Food allergy insomnia	
Central alveolar hypoventilation syndrome	Nocturnal eating (drinking) syndrome	
Periodic limb movement disorder	Hypnotic-dependent sleep	
Restless legs syndrome	Stimulant-dependent sleep disorder	
	Alcohol-dependent sleep disorder	
	Toxin-induced sleep disorder	

Parasomnias

Arousal Disorders	*Parasomnias Usually Associated With REM Sleep*	*Other Parasomnias*
Confusional arousals	Nightmares	Sleep bruxism
Sleepwalking	Sleep paralysis	Sleep enuresis
Sleep terrors	Impaired sleep-related penile erections	Sleep-related abnormal swallowing syndrome
Sleep-Wake Transition Disorders	Sleep related painful erections	Nocturnal paroxysmal dystonia
Rhythmic movement disorder	REM sleep-related sinus arrest	Sudden unexplained nocturnal death syndrome
Sleep starts	REM sleep behavior disorder	Primary snoring
Sleeptalking		Infant sleep apnea
Nocturnal leg cramps		Congenital central hypoventilation syndrome
		Sudden infant death syndrome
		Benign neonatal sleep myoclonus

Sleep Disorders Associated With Medical or Psychiatric Disorders

Associated With Mental Disorders	*Associated With Neurological Disorders*	*Associated With Other Medical Disorders*
Psychoses	Cerebral degenerative disorders	Sleeping sickness
Mood disorders	Dementia	Nocturnal cardiac ischemia
Anxiety disorders	Parkinsonism	Chronic obstructive pulmonary disease
Panic disorder	Fatal familial insomnia	Sleep-related asthma
Alcoholism	Sleep-related epilepsy	Sleep-related gastroesophageal reflux
	Electrical status epilepticus of sleep	Peptic ulcer disease
	Sleep-related headaches	Fibromyalgia

Proposed Sleep Disorders

Short sleeper		Terrifying hypnagogic hallucinations
Long sleeper	Menstrual-associated sleep disorder	
Subwakefulness syndrome	Pregnancy-associated sleep disorder	Sleep-related neurogenic tachypnea
Fragmentary myoclonus		
Sleep hyperhidrosis	Sleep choking syndrome	Sleep-related laryngospasm

ASDA.(1997). *The international classification of sleep disorders.* Rochester, MN: American Sleep Disorders Association.

considered, cardiovascular symptoms are a major factor associated with symptoms of reduced total sleep and increased nighttime wakefulness (Johns et al., 1970). The psychological impact of heart disease also has a major impact on sleep. A myocardial infarction (MI), for example, not only affects physical health and comfort but also influences social relationships, living patterns, work options and income, and sense of personal vulnerability. Fears of death, reinfarction, or inability to resume former living patterns are common (Alonzo, 1999; Alonzo & Reynolds, 1998). It is not surprising that anxiety and depression, typically accompanied by poor sleep, are common after an MI; many patients report troublesome

insomnia that lasts for months and sometimes years (Littrell & Schumann, 1989; Schleifer et al., 1989; Stern et al., 1977; Stern et al., 1976; Wishnie et al., 1971).

Sleep apnea may increase the risk of coronary heart disease via pathways mediated by hypertension and the metabolic consequences of increased oxidative stress, C-reactive protein, and insulin resistance. Patients with sleep apnea may also be obese and have a greater prevalence of other underlying cardiovascular risk factors suggesting a bidirectional relationship (Newman et al., 2001; Shamsuzzaman et al., 2002). Poor sleep appears to be a precursor to MI as symptoms of insomnia, habitual short sleep, waking up exhausted, daytime sleepiness, and frequent napping are common in the preceding months. A common link with the period of depression and elevated inflammatory markers that often precedes MI is a possible explanation for these symptoms (Carney et al., 2002; Miller et al., 2002). Some describe these clusters of symptoms as "vital exhaustion," a state characterized by unusual fatigue and lack of energy, increased irritability, and depressive symptoms, including demoralization (Appels et al., 2000; McSweeney & Crane, 2000). Such precursor or prodromal symptoms have been particularly noted in women before acute MI (McSweeney & Crane, 2000).

Sleep in the Coronary Care Unit

Specialized coronary care units (CCUs) convincingly reduce hospital deaths after MI, but they can be far from optimal environments for sleep. The setting is unfamiliar and perhaps frightening to patients, the schedule and bedtime routine differ from those at home, noise and lighting may never be completely suppressed, interruptions for patient care procedures are frequent, and personnel may lack awareness that patients have a problem sleeping (Freedman et al., 1999). In addition, some medications may result in the appearance of "sleep" when in fact the patient is merely experiencing the sedating side effect of the medication and is not truly asleep or perceiving that sleep occurred.

In polysomnographic studies, CCU patients typically have a pattern of light, fragmented sleep with reduced slow-wave and REM sleep, frequent stage changes, and considerable nighttime wakefulness (Richards & Bairnsfather, 1988a). Although total sleep time is not necessarily reduced, the normal circadian sleep–wake rhythm is disrupted, with sleep occurring off and on during the 24 hours. Sleep is more disturbed as illness severity increases, with MI compared with angina, and during hemodynamic monitoring (Dohno et al., 1977). Sleep patterns usually improve over time, probably in relation to such factors as improved health status, fewer interruptions for care, and increased familiarity with the CCU environment (Simpson et al., 1996).

Sleep After Cardiac Surgery

Sleep disruption after surgery is related to the magnitude of procedure and associated postoperative care. Patients who undergo cardiac surgery experience dramatic sleep pattern disturbances. Severe sleep deprivation is common in the early postoperative period, with only a few hours of fragmented sleep each 24 hours and virtual absence of slow-wave and REM sleep (Redeker & Hedges, 2002b; Simpson et al., 1996). One small study comparing preoperative and postoperative polysomnographic recordings in six men who underwent coronary artery bypass grafting (CABG) surgery revealed a significant decrease in mean sleep time, mean percentage stage 3–4 sleep, and mean REM sleep with reduced sleep time correlated with behavioral and mental changes (Edell-Gustafsson et al., 1997). Cardiac surgical patients report sleep disturbances and distress at uninterrupted sleep because of nursing care (Doering et al., 2002). Contributing environmental and clinical factors to postoperative sleep problems include persistent interruptions and activity, high noise and lighting levels, anxiety, pain, and medications (Doering et al., 2002; Edell-Gustafsson et al., 1999; Simpson et al., 1996). Additionally, cardiac surgery patients may be elderly and have pre-existing sleep disorders (Redeker, 2002). Sleep deprivation often is implicated as a risk factor for the postoperative delirium that develops in some cardiac surgical patients.

Although sleep patterns gradually improve after cardiac surgery, slow-wave and REM sleep may be suppressed for several weeks after the patient returns home, with many patients reporting continuing sleep disturbances (King & Parrinello, 1988). An initial contributing factor for some patients with heart valve replacements is noise generated by the mechanical valve prosthesis, including audible high-frequency closing clicks and low-frequency sounds conducted by body tissues that the patient becomes accustomed to over time (Moritz et al., 1992). Although very few interventions have been tested for their effects on promoting sleep after cardiac surgery, attention to reducing noxious environmental stimuli is an obvious approach. Examples are found in studies reporting positive effects of structured quiet time, guidelines to reduce noise, and providing patients with earplugs while in intensive care units (Olson et al., 2001; Walder et al., 2000; Wallace et al., 1999). Other interventions such as white noise and music therapy suggest promising directions (Williamson, 1992; Zimmerman et al., 1996). Because sleep disruptions after cardiac surgery are multifactorial and include environmental, treatment-related, and intrinsic factors, a comprehensive approach to management of these problems is essential.

Sleep in Heart Failure

Sleep problems, fatigue, and daytime sleepiness are extremely prevalent in patients with heart failure. As with other cardiac patients, precipitating factors include increased age, co-morbidities, and medications, especially diuretics and beta-blocking agents, and mood disturbances such as anxiety and depression (Parker & Dunbar, 2002). Cheyne-Stokes respiration (CSR) is a form of sleep-disordered breathing documented in 40% to 50% of heart failure patients with left ventricular ejection fraction less than 40% (Quaranta et al., 1997). Patients with CSR have fragmented sleep with frequent arousals and nocturnal oxygen desaturations resulting in poor sleep efficiency. Sleep-disordered breathing and central sleep apnea (CSA) increase arrhythmia risk and mortality in persons with heart failure or left ventricular dysfunction (Javaheri et al., 1998; Lanfranchi et al., 1999; Lanfranchi et al., 2003). Heart failure patients may have a high prevalence of periodic limb movements (PLM) leading to recurrent arousals from sleep and symptoms of insomnia and daytime sleepiness (Hanly & Zuberi-Khokhar, 1996).

Although sleep problems, increased fatigue, and daytime sleepiness are common in heart failure patients, few studies have fully explored these symptoms. Heart failure patients perceive that sleep is affected by demands of daily activities and cardiac symptoms (Brostrom et al., 2001). Subjective sleep symptoms have also been linked to increased BMI, increased extracellular fluid volume, depression, and lower perceived quality of life (Dunbar et al., 2001; Hanly & Zuberi-Khokhar, 1995).

Sleep in Hypertension

Age and sleep-disrupting medications are important contributors to sleep disturbances in patients with hypertension. In some patients with hypertension, faulty baroreceptor activation can lead to higher nocturnal arterial blood pressure, and these patients may be referred to as "nondippers," reflecting the loss of usual decline in blood pressure during the nocturnal period. Increased microarousals, reduced length and depth of nonrapid eye movement sleep, and shortened rapid eye movement latency have been documented in this population (George, 2000). In patients with mild to moderate hypertension, sleep deprivation increased sympathetic nervous activity during the night and after morning, leading to increased blood pressure and heart rate, thereby increasing risk for target organ damage and acute cardiovascular events (Lusardi et al., 1999).

Sleep in Chronic Obstructive Pulmonary Disease

During REM sleep, patients with COPD can have repeated episodes of hypoventilation, with large decreases in oxygen saturation and a mild hypercapnia, as REM-related changes in breathing interact with disease-related alterations in pulmonary function. For example, REM sleep and COPD are associated with reduced ventilation and with diminished ventilatory and arousal responses to arterial blood gas changes. In addition, patients with COPD increasingly depend on the intercostal and accessory muscles of breathing, yet their activity is inhibited during REM sleep (Douglas, 1992: Douglas, 2000b). Alcohol consumed before sleep may worsen nocturnal hypoxemia and increase ventricular ectopic frequency in patients with COPD and should be discouraged particularly before bedtime (Douglas, 2000a). Hypnotic agents are not recommended for hypercapnic patients and have varied results in normocapnic patients with COPD, thus caution is warranted (Douglas, 2000a).

Cardiovascular consequences of sleep-related hypoxemia in COPD included marked elevations in pulmonary artery pressure, daytime pulmonary hypertension, increased frequency of PVCs, and an increase in myocardial oxygen demand to a level much like that in maximal exercise at the time when the arterial oxygen supply is low (Mohsenin, 2002). Not surprisingly, patients with COPD often sleep badly, with light sleep that is fragmented by arousals. Use of low-flow nocturnal oxygen to relieve nocturnal hypoxemia reduces cardiovascular complications, probably improves sleep, and may prolong survival (Douglas, 2000a; Mohsenin, 2002).

◼ CARDIAC EVENTS IN SLEEP

Angina

Anginal chest pain results from myocardial ischemia, an imbalance between coronary blood flow and myocardial requirements (see Chapter 25). In its classic form, angina is precipitated by physical exertion or other situations that increase myocardial oxygen demand. Blood pressure and heart rate characteristically increase before appearance of ischemic changes in the ECG in daytime and sleep-related anginal episodes (see Chapter 18).

Classic (effort) angina and the full spectrum of cardiac ischemic syndromes including unstable angina, non-Q—wave myocardial infarction, and variant angina occur more often in the morning hours and early after awakening than at night (Cannon et al., 1997; Onaka et al., 1998; Willich, 1999). Sleep is generally a time of reduced myocardial demand because of decreased blood pressure and heart rate. However, in persons with stable coronary artery disease and normal left ventricular function, REM-induced surges in heart rate can increase metabolic demands in the context of stenotic blood flow, thereby setting up a cascade of events that can lead to plaque disruption and arrhythmias (Verrier, 2002). Patients with known daytime ischemia report relatively few nighttime anginal episodes and usually have reduced or unchanged ECG evidence of ischemia. Circadian rhythms in levels of plasma endothelin-1 are likely linked with these differences in ischemic thresholds (Li et al., 2002). When greater ischemic changes occur at night, they are often asymptomatic (silent ischemia), and nocturnal chest pain is more likely to occur in older and sicker patients and those with other symptoms of cardiac impairment, such as congestive failure. (Peters et al., 2002; Verrier, 2002).

Variant (Prinzmetal) angina is a less common form of ischemic chest pain. It is caused by coronary artery spasm and is characterized by angina at rest and ST segment elevation. Variant angina has a clear circadian rhythm, with episodes clustering in the early morning hours of sleep. At one time, increased sympathetic activity during REM sleep was believed to be the mechanism for nocturnal coronary spasm; however, more contemporary understandings have emerged from research documenting circadian alterations in endothelial function and reduced nocturnal vagal nerve and cardiac parasympathetic activity (Burger et al., 1999; Kawano et al., 2002; Mori, 1994).

Arrhythmias

Sinus bradycardia and sinus arrhythmia are the most frequent changes in heart rhythm during sleep in healthy people, consistent with the dominance of parasympathetic activity. Bradycardia during sleep is more common in men than in women, and the difference between daytime and nighttime heart rates decreases with age. Although heart rate usually is lowest in slow-wave sleep, little information is available about sleep stage relationships with bradyarrhythmias. Bradycardia dependent changes in atrial repolarization predisposing to intra-atrial re-entry have been suggested to lead to vagally mediated atrial fibrillation during sleep in susceptible patients (Coccagna et al., 1997; Gillis, 2000).

Premature ventricular contractions (PVCs) are common after MI and, when frequent or complex, carry a higher mortality risk. Sleep usually suppresses arrhythmogenesis and the frequency of PVCs in healthy people (Friedman, 1997; Gillis, 2000). Nighttime PVCs have no consistent relation to sleep stage in that some experience greater numbers during the wake sleep transition and others during REM (Gillis, 2000). PVC frequency, however, also may be independently related to heart rate and is increased by factors such as hypoxemia, increased circulating catecholamines, and loss of vagal activity during the night. Hypoxemia is especially important in patients with sleep apnea and chronic obstructive pulmonary disease (COPD), in whom PVCs are clearly more common during sleep than wakefulness (see following discussion).

The influence of sleep on ventricular arrhythmias and sudden cardiac death is gaining attention in the clinical and scientific communities because of the nonuniform distributions of these events across the day. Sleep-state—dependent fluctuations in autonomic nervous system activity may in fact trigger the onset of major cardiovascular events such as sudden cardiac death and ventricular tachyarrhythmias in susceptible individuals (Lavery et al., 1997). Genetic influences may play a role in that it has been recently observed that cardiac events are rare in persons with long QT syndrome in subgroup LQT1 but frequent in subgroup LQT3 (Stramba-Badiale et al., 2000). These subgroups are characterized by different genetic mutations.

SLEEP-RELATED DISORDERED BREATHING

Sleep-related changes in breathing and oxygenation have important cardiovascular consequences. This section focuses on the cardiovascular impact of sleep in obstructive sleep apnea, central sleep apnea, and snoring.

Obstructive Sleep Apnea

Patients with sleep apnea repeatedly stop breathing during sleep for periods of 10 seconds or longer (AASM, 1999; ASDA, 1997) (Fig. 11-7). Apnea can be obstructive (a collapsed upper airway blocks airflow despite effort to breathe), central (no respiratory effort), or mixed (central, then obstructive component). A predominance of obstructive apnea is the most common pattern and can lead to repetitive episodes of hypoxemia that are terminated by brief arousals. Typical patients are middle-aged men who are overweight, snore loudly during sleep, and experience daytime sleepiness that interferes with normal activities; women with sleep apnea are usually postmenopausal (ASDA, 1997; Bassiri & Guilleminault, 2000; Collop & Kaye, 2002; Guilleminault et al., 1988). Sleep apnea is likely to be worsened by sleep deprivation (Guilleminault & Rosekind, 1981; White et al., 1983), alcohol ingestion (Block, et al., 1986; Issa & Sullivan, 1982; Scrima et al., 1982), and sedative or hypnotic use (Dolly & Block, 1982).

Obstructive sleep apnea has significant cardiovascular consequences. Systemic and pulmonary arterial pressures increase in a stepwise fashion with repeated apnea. Daytime systemic hypertension occurs in 40% to 60% of patients and, conversely, approximately 20% to 30% of hypertensive patients have sleep apnea (Carlson et al., 1994; Shepard, 1992). Whether the hypertension is caused directly by sleep apnea or a related common factor, such as obesity, is unclear (Hoffstein et al., 1991; Millman et al., 1991; Rauscher et al., 1992). Several recent studies suggest that obstructive sleep apnea has an independent effect on blood pressure levels (Bixler et al., 2000; Peppard et al.,

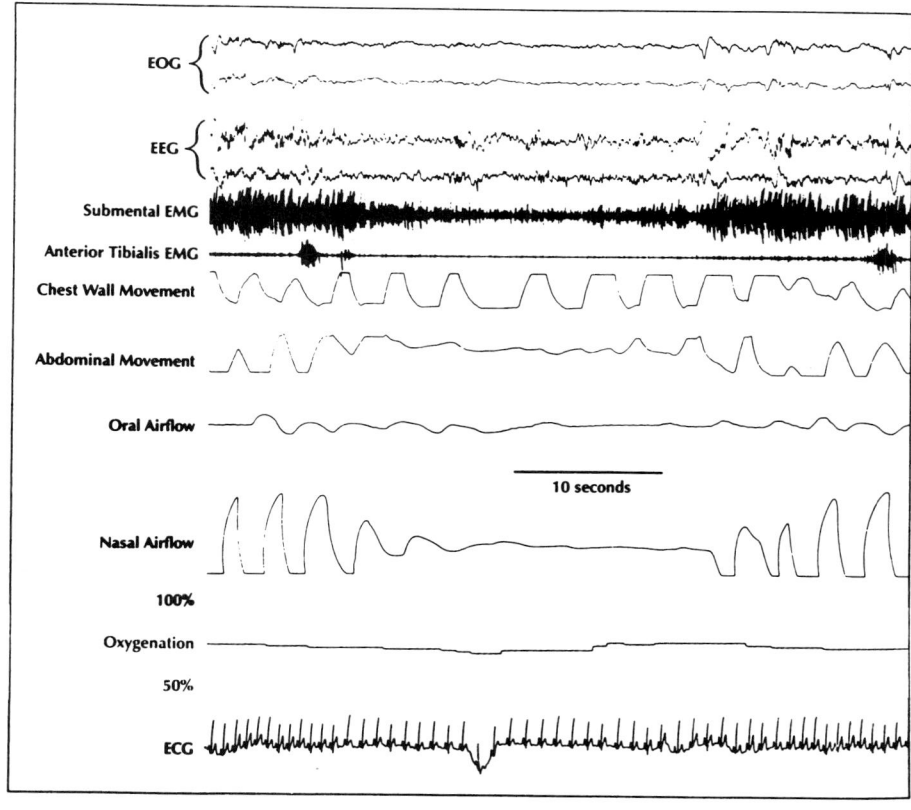

■ **Figure 11–7.** Recording of multiple physiologic signals in a formal polysomnographic sleep evaluation. In this example, the patient has an obstructive apnea with cessation of oral and nasal airflow despite effort to breathe. The interrupted breathing is accompanied by a decrease in oxygen saturation and slowing of the heart rate and is followed by an arousal. ECG, electrocardiogram; EEG, electroencephalogram; EMG, electromyogram: EOG, electro-oculogram. (From White, D. [1992]. Obstructive sleep apnea. *Hospital Practice,* 27[5A], 68.)

2000; Worsnop et al., 1998). The Wisconsin sleep cohort study prospectively evaluated the clinical course of hypertension in patients with obstructive sleep apnea and found that blood pressure increased linearly with apnea severity (Hla et al., 1994; Young et al., 1997). The Sleep Heart Health Study, the largest prospective performed to date, found that although some of the association was related to body mass index, there was a significant relationship between apnea severity and hypertension (Nieto et al., 2000).

Cardiac arrhythmias are relatively common and include PVCs, atrioventricular block, and bradycardia. Apneas are often associated with a progressive sinus bradycardia, sometimes with a prolonged sinus pause, followed by an abrupt increase in heart rate when breathing resumes (Hoffstein & Mateika, 1994; Liston et al., 1994). A fall and subsequent rise in cardiac output parallels the heart rate changes (Weiss et al., 1996).

To minimize possible complications, early diagnosis and treatment are critical (Achermann & Borbely, 1990; He et al., 1988; Redline & Strohl, 1998; Young et al., 1993). The treatment of choice for obstructive sleep apnea is nasally applied continuous positive airway pressure (CPAP). A soft, firmly fitting nasal mask is held in place by straps and attached to a bedside blower that provides continuous pressure (usually 5 to 15 cm H_2O) to prevent collapse of the upper airway. Recent improvements in CPAP devices include gradual onset of pressure and separate control of inspiratory and expiratory pressures (Littner et al., 2002). Conservative treatment strategies include weight loss, learning to sleep in a side-lying position (as by putting a ball in a pouch on the pajama back), and avoidance of alcohol and sedatives. Pharmacological approaches with purported respiratory stimulants (e.g., acetazolamide, methylprogesterone, and protriptyline) have had variable effectiveness. Occasionally, surgery is performed to enlarge the upper airway (uvulopalatopharyngoplasty) or to bypass it (tracheostomy) when other measures do not alleviate the apnea (AASM, 1995, 1996). If the patient has been receiving antihypertensive medication, the dosage may need to be reduced when the sleep apnea is effectively managed.

Central Sleep Apnea

Patients with severe congestive heart failure often have a pattern of periodic (Cheyne-Stokes; Cheyne, 1818; Stokes, 1854) breathing during light sleep in which periods of central apnea alternate with hyperpnea. This breathing pattern causes recurrent episodes of hypoxemia that can further impair the failing heart. Frequent arousals during the hyperpneic phase that disrupt sleep can impair daytime alertness (Hanly & Zuberi-Khokhar, 1995; Staniforth, et al., 2001; Staniforth, Kinnear, et al., 1998; Yamashiro & Kryger, 1993). One mechanism for the abnormal breathing pattern is prolonged circulation time that delays the ventilatory responses to blood gas changes. The resulting hypoxemia sets up a vicious cycle whereby increased ventilation improves oxygenation but lowers carbon dioxide tension below the apneic threshold; the resulting apnea then leads to hypoxemia, which perpetuates the cycle. In addition, cardiac enlargement and pulmonary congestion reduce gas stores in the lungs, which allows wider swings in blood gas values with changes in ventilation (Wuyam, Pepin, et al., 2000; Yamashiro & Kryger, 1993). Effective treatment of the heart

failure (Javaheri, 2000) and low-flow oxygen therapy during sleep help to correct the hypoxemia and stabilize the breathing pattern (Krachman et al., 1999; Resta et al., 1999; Staniforth et al., 1998). Use of nasal CPAP has also been shown to decrease the severity of central apneas in patients with heart failure (Krachman et al., 1999; Sin et al., 2000).

Snoring and Upper Airway Resistance

Epidemiologic studies indicate that habitual snoring is associated with a greater prevalence of coronary heart disease (D'Alessandro et al., 1990; Koskenvuo et al., 1987; Koskenvuo et al., 1985; Koskenvuo et al., 1994), hypertension (Gislason et al., 1987), and stroke (Koskenvuo et al., 1987; Palomaki, 1991; Palomaki et al., 1992). Snoring is more common and becomes habitual earlier in men than in women. Snoring is a primarily inspiratory (but may also be expiratory) noise during sleep caused by partial upper airway obstruction and vibration of the soft tissues. Snoring intensifies as NREM sleep deepens and diminishes in REM sleep. Heavy snoring is associated with reduced ventilation, obstructive apnea during light sleep and especially REM sleep, transient falls in arterial oxygen, and elevated systemic and pulmonary arterial pressures. Factors that worsen snoring include obesity, supine position, sleep deprivation, use of alcohol or sedatives, and smoking (Hoffstein, 2000). Upper airway resistance syndrome (UARS) is a condition marked by frequent arousals from sleep related to an increase in respiratory effort needed to overcome resistance to air flow resulted in disturbed sleep and EDS (Guilleminault et al., 1992). Snoring may or may not be a symptom of UARS. Treatment options for these conditions include CPAP, posterior pharyngeal airway surgery, or a dental appliance (used to move the lower jaw and tongue forward, thus increasing the posterior pharyngeal airway space) (AASM, 1995).

SLEEP-RELATED ADVERSE OUTCOMES IN PATIENTS WITH CARDIOVASCULAR DISEASE

In the physiological domain, sleep loss results in changes in body temperature regulation, autonomic function, metabolic regulation involving glucose tolerance and insulin production, thyroid secretion, cortisol secretion and circadian rhythm, and immunocompetence (Speigel, Leproult & Cauter, 1999). The accumulation of these changes is significant as documented in the Cardiovascular Health Study findings of increased daytime sleepiness being associated with increased risk of mortality or incident cardiovascular disease of acute myocardial infarction and HF (Newman, 2000).

Additional consequences of sleep loss are cognitive and behavioral changes in the form of mood disturbances, problems with impaired short-term memory, and excessive daytime sleepiness. In the Sleep Heart Health Study (SHHS), an assessment of more than 5,000 adults, sleep difficulties were associated with impaired quality of life and vitality (Baldwin, 2001).

In the social realm, sleep loss can lead to impaired interactions with family and co-workers and reduced productivity and efficiency in work related tasks. Significant relationships are found between sleep loss and increased risk for accidents as well as increased overall health care use (Kapur, 2002). Figure 11-6 presents a conceptual model of impaired sleep related to the cardiovascular patient.

NURSING MANAGEMENT

Assessment

A sleep assessment (Table 11-3) is a systematic collection of data that includes information about a patient's usual sleep patterns, sleep effectiveness, bedtime routines, and sleep environment. Because sleep-related breathing disorders predominate in the same group at highest risk for cardiovascular disease, the patient (or bed partner) should be asked about two cardinal symptoms of sleep apnea: snoring and daytime sleepiness. The patient's physical appearance provides additional data. A variety of factors related to the patient's underlying pathophysiological disorder, treatments, environment, personal habits or concerns, and maturational status can contribute to sleep problems, and these should be explored. If the patient can be observed during sleep, then a variety of physi-

ological variables can be monitored. Objective data from a PSG sleep study may be available for occasional patients; but for most, a sleep history and direct observation are the primary assessment methods. When disturbed sleep is a significant ongoing problem, a sleep diary is an excellent way to document frequency and severity of symptoms and their effect on daily activities, evaluate progress of treatment, and promote self-management.

Sleep clinicians often use the acronym "BEARS" as a format to organize available subjective, behavioral, and objective information in performing a sleep history (Lee, 2003; see the web site of the American Academy of Sleep Medicine: www.aasmnet.org):

B   Bedtime problems
E   Excessive daytime sleepiness
A   Awakenings during the night
R   Regularity and duration of sleep
S   Sleep-disordered breathings

Precipitating Factors

A careful sleep assessment will elucidate demographic and physiological, psychological, behavioral, and environmental factors that contribute to sleep disorders in cardiac patient. The incidence of cardiovascular disease increases with the *aging* of the population and, as noted earlier, sleep difficulties frequently

Table 11–3 ▪ SLEEP ASSESSMENT

Pathophysiology and Symptoms	**Physiological Alterations in Sleep**
Insomnia	Heart rate/rhythm
Excessive daytime sleepiness	Hemodynamic monitoring
Fatigue	Respiratory pattern
Depression	Respiratory pauses
Pain	Snoring
Dyspnea	
Nausea	**Sleep Patterns**
Mobility restriction	Bedtime/wake time
Restless legs	Time to fall asleep
Others	Mid-sleep awakenings
	Time of final awakening
Treatment	Total sleep time
Medications	Movement during sleep
Monitoring devices	Number and duration of naps
Other treatments	
Surgical recovery	**Sleep Effectiveness**
	Refreshing quality of sleep
Environment	Subjective sleep quality
Bed/Bedding	Daytime alertness
Lighting	Excessive daytime sleepiness
Sound	Ability to perform daytime activities
Temperature	
Interruption by caregivers	**Bedtime Routines**
Bed partner	Bedtime rituals
	Use of sleep medication
Personal Behaviors and Concerns	Use of other sleep aids
Sleep-wake schedule changes	Sleep positions
Worry about illness	
Concerns about family/work	***Physical Observations***
Depression	Yawning
	Dozing
Maturational Status	Decreased attention span
Age	Irritability
Menopausal status	Obesity

accompany aging. *Medications* used to treat cardiac disorders may increase the risk for sleep problems. Diuretic drugs inappropriately timed may lead to nocturia. Beta-blocking agents can lead to insomnia, nightmares, hallucinations at night, and decreased REM sleep. Beta antagonists with alpha$_1$-blocking activity are associated with fatigue, somnolence, and insomnia. Antiarrhythmia drug regimens that include amiodarone or diltiazem are associated with abnormal dreams. Centrally acting antihypertensive drugs such as clonidine or reserpine can cause sedation, drowsiness, nightmares, and insomnia. The presence of *co-morbidities* is another important contributor to sleep difficulties including COPD, arthritis, fibromyalgia, chronic pain, and glucose and metabolic abnormalities. *Psychological states* of anxiety and depression also have a significant negative influence on sleep. Environmental noise and excessive light are major disrupters of sleep in the hospital and critical care setting.

Nursing Diagnosis

A nursing diagnosis of impaired sleep is made when patients experience or are at risk of experiencing a change in the quantity or quality of sleep that causes discomfort or interferes with daily life. The typical presenting complaint is either insomnia (difficulty falling asleep or staying asleep) or excessive sleepiness. The diagnostic statement should include the related factors that contribute to the problem to provide specificity and suggest direction for intervention. The statement may also include the signs and symptoms that indicate sleep is disturbed. For example, a patient with a recent MI may have a nursing diagnosis of "impaired sleep related to intermittent chest pain, anxiety, and disruptions of care as evidenced by difficulty falling asleep and frequent nighttime awakenings." A patient with COPD complicated by heart failure may have a diagnosis of "impaired sleep related to recurrent nighttime hypoxemia evidenced by frequent nighttime awakenings and excessive daytime sleepiness."

Nursing Goals

The general nursing management plan focuses on promoting adequate, restful sleep for patients with cardiovascular disorders. This can be accomplished first by preventing or reducing the factors that are disturbing the patient's sleep or have the potential to do so. A second goal is to provide bedtime routines, comfort measures, and a setting conducive to sleep. A third goal is to detect alterations in physiological function that are caused by or may accentuate the underlying health problem. A fourth goal is to assist patients to learn behavioral patterns that enhance the quality of their sleep (Lee, 2003; Parker, 1995).

Interventions

Sleep Hygiene

Sleep hygiene refers to practices of daily living that promote good sleep (Zarcone, 2000). These behaviors reinforce the time and place for sleep and control factors that interfere with sleep. Sleep hygiene is an effective, low-technology approach that fits with common sense and principles of sleep regulation. It is the

foundation for intervention when sleep is disturbed and is an important component of patient teaching for health maintenance (Lee, 2003).

To reinforce the time for sleep, patients should be advised to go to bed and get up at approximately the same times each day, perform a regular bedtime routine, and limit napping. Exposure to outdoor morning light helps to maintain the setting of the circadian timing system. To the extent possible in hospital settings, patients should have the opportunity to sleep during accustomed hours and to maintain familiar routines. Increased napping commonly occurs during illness and may be particularly important during recovery from cardiac surgery or other cardiac events (Redeker & Hedges, 2002a; Simpson et al., 1996), but the effect on nighttime sleep and physical recovery in cardiovascular patients has not been studied.

The place for sleep should be physically comfortable and psychologically conducive to sleep. To keep the bed associated with sleep, it should be reserved for that purpose rather than serving as a hub for other activities. When lying in bed does not lead to sleep, the patient should be advised to get up, engage in quiet activity until drowsy, and then return to bed. Trying too hard to sleep is counterproductive; it is better to engage in some distraction and let sleep come naturally. The psychological associations that are established when patients must spend considerable waking time in bed have not been studied.

Strenuous physical activity, worry, and anxiety lead to physiological arousal that interferes with sleep. Moderate exercise usually is perceived as more beneficial to sleep when performed early in the day rather than late in the evening (Young-McCaughan et al., 2003). If patients tend to dwell on their concerns after going to bed, setting aside planned "worry time" an hour or two before bedtime may be helpful. Consumption of stimulants such as caffeine-containing beverages should be restricted to the early part of the day (Walsh et al., 1990); nicotine in tobacco products is also a mild stimulant that interferes with falling sleep (Phillips & Danner, 1995). Although alcohol in moderate doses helps some people fall asleep, their subsequent sleep will likely be fragmented by brief, frequent arousals, and their total sleep time will be reduced (Roehrs & Roth, 2001; Wessendorf & Teschler, 2002). Massage and other relaxation measures have been shown to be beneficial in reducing anxiety and inducing sleep in critically ill patients (Richards & Bairnsfather, 1988b).

Environmental Management

Nurses have considerable control over the hospital patient's physical environment, particularly lighting and sound levels. Most people prefer a darkened, quiet room for sleep. The level of noise tends to be particularly high in intensive care units, and a major source of that noise is the staff (Simpson et al., 1996; Topf, et al., 1996; Topf & Thompson, 2001). Noise can be reduced by conscious effort to avoid unnecessary or loud conversation, close doors to patients' rooms, use equipment quietly, turn off unnecessary equipment or alarms, consider sound level when deciding on equipment purchases, and give attention to acoustic features when participating in design of hospital units (Dracup, 1988). Some patients may find that soothing background sounds, such as provided by audiotapes of ocean surf or patter of rain, or music aid their sleep (Williamson, 1992).

A major challenge to nurses working in hospital settings, especially intensive care units, is limiting disruptions of patients' sleep while still providing the care necessary in cardiovascular disorders and surgery. Nursing care should be planned to protect, or at least minimally disrupt, the hours patients spend in sleep. Most patients' daily life schedules include the major sleep period at night, and routine procedures should be avoided during that time. Research is needed to determine the success of these sleep opportunities and possible adverse effects of grouping patient care procedures.

Nurses have the opportunity to lead the multidisciplinary team in understanding the patient's need for sleep and in identifying untimely disruptions. Skills of diplomacy, coordination, and priority setting are needed to get important procedures accomplished without fragmenting either the patient's sleep or the health care provider's routine. Sophisticated monitoring equipment permits assessment of many physiological parameters without disturbing the patient. Necessary interruptions should, when possible, occur at times when otherwise unavoidable activities occur.

Drawing morning blood specimens for laboratory tests is routine in many hospital settings, and in intensive care units, personal care also may occur at times when patients would otherwise be asleep. Although this helps to distribute workload across the 24 hours and to prepare patients and their laboratory data for the day shift and morning physicians' rounds, it shortens the total sleep period and particularly interferes with REM sleep. Health care providers should reevaluate these traditional practices.

Comfort and Relaxation

Patients with pain, dyspnea, or simply wrinkled bedding can find it difficult to sleep or even rest at ease. Analgesics should be administered when indicated to alleviate pain. Careful positioning and dry, wrinkle-free beds enhance patient comfort. Enabling patients to perform their desired bedtime rituals may facilitate sleep onset. Assisting them to a side lying position may have a beneficial effect on sleep and may facilitate optimal breathing. Various kinds of relaxation techniques may be used to produce a calm inner state through reduction of arousal.

Medications

In general, sleep hygiene and other nonpharmacologic strategies should be used before sleep-promoting medications are considered in managing sleep problems (Chesson et al., 1999). However, with acute or short-term insomnia, the use of medications may be indicated. Benzodiazepines or benzodiazepine-like medications are generally the hypnotics of choice. Short-acting agents such as zaleplon, triazolam, or zolpidem are preferred to avoid a daytime carryover effect. If daytime sedation is desired, longer-acting agents such as flurazepam, temazepam, or estazolam can be used. When hypnotics are abruptly discontinued, sleep is likely to worsen (rebound insomnia), an effect that can be reduced by tapering the dose. Patients with sleep apnea or heavy snoring are not good candidates for hypnotic medications because they may worsen hypoxemia and the related sleep disturbance. Long-term use of hypnotics has been associated with increased risk of mortality (Kripke et al., 1998).

Outcome Criteria

Ideally, patients should be able to fall asleep easily at bedtime and sustain sleep for an adequate period. They should awaken feeling rested and refreshed and remain alert during normal daily activities. They should be able to describe and perform practices of daily living that promote good sleep quality and daytime alertness.

THE HEALTH CARE PROVIDERS' SLEEP

Hospital nurses, physicians, and others who work the night shift or rotating schedules often experience irregular sleep–wake schedules and inferior sleep, causing reduced alertness and general fatigue. This is accentuated by the pronounced circadian alertness–sleepiness rhythm, with maximal sleepiness and lowest performance at approximately 4:00 to 5:00 AM, at the low point of the body temperature rhythm (Akerstedt, 2003). Mental tasks that require sustained visual attention, such as monitoring an ECG oscilloscope or driving home from work, are more affected than are physical tasks (Daly & Wilson, 1983; Gold et al., 1992). Suggested coping strategies include staying on a night schedule on nonwork days (often socially unattractive), using rotation schedules that move forward around the clock rather than backward, and taking a nap before going to work (Akerstedt, 1998, 2003; Sharkey, et al., 2001). Use of melatonin in the evening to help reset the circadian timing system or bright light therapy to suppress natural melatonin secretion from the pineal gland also appear to be promising strategies (Sharkey et al., 2001).

SUMMARY

Patients with cardiovascular disease often have disturbed sleep, especially in intensive cardiac care settings, and may be at risk for physiological changes during sleep that adversely affect their health status. Despite the widely held belief that sleep promotes well being, hospital practices are rarely designed to encourage optimal sleep. Research is needed to clarify the role of nighttime sleep and daytime naps in recovery from cardiovascular disease and surgery (e.g., what are optimal sleep patterns?) and to identify nursing interventions that prevent sleep deprivation, minimize adverse sleep-related physiological changes, and promote good sleep.

REFERENCES

AASM. (1995). Practice parameters for the treatment of snoring and obstructive sleep apnea with oral appliances. American Sleep Disorders Association. *Sleep,* 18(6), 511–513.
AASM. (1996). Practice parameters for the treatment of obstructive sleep apnea in adults: the efficacy of surgical modifications of the upper airway. Report of the American Sleep Disorders Association. *Sleep,* 19(2), 152–155.
AASM. (1999). Sleep-related breathing disorders in adults: recommendations for syndrome definition and measurement techniques in clinical research. The Report of an American Academy of Sleep Medicine Task Force. *Sleep,* 22(5), 667–689.

Achermann, P., & Borbely, A. A. (1990). Simulation of human sleep: ultradian dynamics of electroencephalographic slow-wave activity. *Journal of Biological Rhythms*, 5(2), 141–157.

Adam, K., & Oswald, I. (1984). Sleep helps healing. *British Medical Journal (Clinical Research Edition)*, 289(6456), 1400–1401.

AHA. (2003). *Heart and stroke facts*. Dallas, TX: American Heart Association.

Akerstedt, T. (1998). Is there an optimal sleep-wake pattern in shift work? *Scandinavian Journal of Work Environmental Health*, 24(Suppl. 3), 18–27.

Akerstedt, T. (2003). Shift work and disturbed sleep/wakefulness. *Occupational Medicine (London)*, 53(2), 89–94.

Aldrich, M. S. (1999). Normal human sleep. In M. S. Aldrich (Ed.), *Sleep medicine* (pp. 3–26). New York: Oxford.

Alonzo, A. A. (1999). Acute myocardial infarction and posttraumatic stress disorder: the consequences of cumulative adversity. *Journal of Cardiovascular Nursing*, 13(3), 33–45.

Alonzo, A. A., & Reynolds, N. R. (1998). The structure of emotions during acute myocardial infarction: a model of coping. *Social Science & Medicine*, 46(9), 1099–1110.

Ancoli-Israel, S. (2000). Insomnia in the elderly: a review for the primary care practitioner. *Sleep*, 23(Suppl. 1), S23–S30; discussion S36–S28.

Ancoli-Israel, S., Cole, R., Alessi, C., Chambers, M., Moorcroft, W., & Pollak, C. P. (2003). The role of actigraphy in the study of sleep and circadian rhythms. *Sleep*, 26(3), 342–392.

Ancoli-Israel, S., Kripke, D. F., Klauber, M. R., Mason, W. J., Fell, R., & Kaplan, O. (1991). Sleep-disordered breathing in community-dwelling elderly. *Sleep*, 14(6), 486–495.

Ancoli-Israel, S., Martin, J. L., Kripke, D. F., Marler, M., & Klauber, M. R. (2002). Effect of light treatment on sleep and circadian rhythms in demented nursing home patients. *Journal of the American Geriatrics Society*, 50(2), 282–289.

Anderson, K. O., Getto, C. J., Mendoza, T. R., Palmer, S. N., Wang, X. S., Reyes-Gibby, C. C., & Cleeland, C. S. (2003). Fatigue and sleep disturbance in patients with cancer, patients with clinical depression, and community-dwelling adults. *Journal of Pain Symptom Management*, 25(4), 307–318.

Appels, A., Kop, W. J., & Schouten, E. (2000). The nature of the depressive symptomatology preceding myocardial infarction. *Behavioral Medicine*, 26(2), 86–89.

ASDA. (1986). Guidelines for the Multiple Sleep Latency Test (MSLT): A standard measure of sleepiness. *Sleep*, 9(4), 519–524.

ASDA. (1997). *The international classification of sleep disorders*. Rochester, MN: American Sleep Disorders Association.

Baker, F. C., Maloney, S., & Driver, H. S. (1999). A comparison of subjective estimates of sleep with objective polysomnographic data in healthy men and women. *Journal of Psychosomatic Research*, 47(4), 335–341.

Barrett, J., Lack, L., & Morris, M. (1993). The sleep-evoked decrease of body temperature. *Sleep*, 16(2), 93–99.

Bassiri, A. G., & Guilleminault, C. (2000). Clinical features and evaluation of obstructive sleep apnea-hypopnea syndrome. In M. H. Kryger, T. Roth & W. C. Dement (Eds.), *Principles and practice of sleep medicine* (3rd ed., pp. 869–878). Philadelphia: W.B. Saunders Company.

Bateman, J. R., Pavia, D., & Clarke, S. W. (1978). The retention of lung secretions during the night in normal subjects. *Clinical Science Molecular Medicine (Suppl.)*, 55(6), 523–527.

Benca, R. M., Kushida, C. A., Everson, C. A., Kalski, R., Bergmann, B. M., & Rechtschaffen, A. (1989). Sleep deprivation in the rat: VII. Immune function. *Sleep*, 12(1), 47–52.

Berthon-Jones, M., & Sullivan, C. E. (1984). Ventilation and arousal responses to hypercapnia in normal sleeping humans. *Journal of Applied Physiology*, 57(1), 59–67.

Bixler, E. O., Vgontzas, A. N., Lin, H. M., Ten Have, T., Leiby, B. E., Vela-Bueno, A., & Kales, A. (2000). Association of hypertension and sleep-disordered breathing. *Archives of Internal Medicine*, 160(15), 2289–2295.

Blasi, A., Jo, J., Valladares, E., Morgan, B. J., Skatrud, J. B., & Khoo, M. C. (2003). Cardiovascular variability after arousal from sleep: time-varying spectral analysis. *Journal of Applied Physiology*, 95(4), 1394–1404.

Bliwise, D. L. (2000). Normal aging. In M. H. Kryger, T. Roth & W. C. Dement (Eds.), *Principles and practice of sleep medicine* (third ed., pp. 26–42). Philadelphia: W.B. Saunders.

Block, A. J., Hellard, D. W., & Slayton, P. C. (1986). Effect of alcohol ingestion on breathing and oxygenation during sleep. Analysis of the influence of age and sex. *American Journal of Medicine*, 80(4), 595–600.

Borbely, A. A., & Acherman, P. (2000). Sleep homeostasis and models of sleep regulation. In M. H. Kryger, T. Roth & W. C. Dement (Eds.), *Principles and practice of sleep medicine* (3rd ed., pp. 377–390). Philadelphia: W.B. Saunders.

Brostrom, A., Stromberg, A., Dahlstrom, U., & Fridlund, B. (2001). Patients with congestive heart failure and their conceptions of their sleep situation. *Journal of Advanced Nursing*, 34(4), 520–529.

Burger, A. J., Charlamb, M., & Sherman, H. B. (1999). Circadian patterns of heart rate variability in normals, chronic stable angina and diabetes mellitus. *International Journal of Cardiology*, 71(1), 41–48.

Bursztyn, M., Ginsberg, G., Hammerman-Rozenberg, R., & Stessman, J. (1999). The siesta in the elderly: risk factor for mortality? *Archives of Internal Medicine*, 159(14), 1582–1586.

Bursztyn, M., Ginsberg, G., & Stessman, J. (2002). The siesta and mortality in the elderly: effect of rest without sleep and daytime sleep duration. *Sleep*, 25(2), 187–191.

Buxton, O. M., Spiegel, K., & Van Cauter, E. (2002). Modulation of endocrine function and metabolism by sleep and sleep loss. In T. L. Lee-Chiong, M. J. Sateia, & M. A. Carskadon (Eds.), *Sleep medicine* (pp. 59–69). Philadelphia: Hanley & Belfus.

Buysse, D. J., Reynolds, C. F., Monk, T. H., Berman, S. R., & Kupfer, D. J. (1989). The Pittsburgh Sleep Quality Index: a new instrument for psychiatric practice and research. *Psychiatry Research*, 28(2), 193–213.

Buysse, D. J., Reynolds, C. F., Monk, T. H., Hoch, C. C., Yeager, A. L., & Kupfer, D. J. (1991). Quantification of subjective sleep quality in healthy elderly men and women using the Pittsburgh Sleep Quality Index (PSQI) [published erratum appears in Sleep 1992 Feb;15(1):83]. *Sleep*, 14(4), 331–338.

Cannon, C. P., McCabe, C. H., Stone, P. H., Schactman, M., Thompson, B., Theroux, P., Gibson, R. S., Feldman, T., Kleiman, N. S., Tofler, G. H., Muller, J. E., Chaitman, B. R., & Braunwald, E. (1997). Circadian variation in the onset of unstable angina and non-Q-wave acute myocardial infarction (the TIMI III Registry and TIMI IIIB). *American Journal of Cardiology*, 79(3), 253–258.

Carlson, J. T., Hedner, J. A., Ejnell, H., & Peterson, L. E. (1994). High prevalence of hypertension in sleep apnea patients independent of obesity. *American Journal of Respiratory Critical Care Medicine*, 150(1), 72–77.

Carney, R. M., Freedland, K. E., Miller, G. E., & Jaffe, A. S. (2002). Depression as a risk factor for cardiac mortality and morbidity: a review of potential mechanisms. *Journal of Psychosomatic Research*, 53(4), 897–902.

Carskadon, M., & Dement, W. C. (2000). Normal human sleep: An overview. In M. H. Kryger, T. Roth & W. C. Dement (Eds.), *Principles and practice of sleep medicine* (3rd ed., pp. 15–25). Philadelphia: W.B. Saunders Company.

Carskadon, M. A., & Dement, W. C. (2000). Normal human sleep: an overview. In M. H. Kruger, T. Roth & W. C. Dement (Eds.), *Principles and practice of sleep medicine* (3rd ed., pp. 15–25). Philadelphia: W.B. Saunders Company.

Carskadon, M. A., Rechtschaffen, A. (2000). Monitoring and staging of human sleep. In M. H. Kryger, Roth, T., & Dement, W.C. (Eds.), *Principles and practice of sleep medicine* (3rd ed., pp. 1197–1216). Philadelphia: W.B. Saunders Company.

Catcheside, P. G., Chiong, S. C., Mercer, J., Saunders, N. A., & McEvoy, R. D. (2002). Noninvasive cardiovascular markers of acoustically induced arousal from non-rapid-eye-movement sleep. *Sleep*, 25(7), 797–804.

Chase, M. H. (2000). Sleep mechanisms. In M. H. Kryger, Roth, T. & W. C. Dement (Eds.), *Principles and practice of sleep medicine* (pp. 93–168). Philadelphia: W.B. Saunders Company.

Chervin, R. D., & Aldrich, M. S. (1999). The Epworth Sleepiness Scale may not reflect objective measures of sleepiness or sleep apnea. *Neurology*, 52(1), 125–131.

Chesson, A. L., Jr., Anderson, W. M., Littner, M., Davila, D., Hartse, K., Johnson, S., Wise, M., & Rafecas, J. (1999). Practice parameters for the nonpharmacologic treatment of chronic insomnia. An American Academy of Sleep Medicine report. Standards of Practice Committee of the American Academy of Sleep Medicine. *Sleep*, 22(8), 1128–1133.

Cheyne, J. (1818). A case of apoplexy in which the fleshy part of the heart was converted into fat. *Dublin Hospital Reports*, 2, 216–222.

Chokroverty, S. (1999). An overview of sleep. In S. Chokroverty (Ed.), *Sleep disorders medicine* (2nd ed., pp. 7–20). Boston: Butterworth Heinemann.

Cianci, T., Zoccoli, G., Lenzi, P., & Franzini, C. (1991). Loss of integrative control of peripheral circulation during desynchronized sleep. *American Journal of Physiology*, 261(2 Pt 2), R373–377.

Coccagna, G., Capucci, A., Bauleo, S., Boriani, G., & Santarelli, A. (1997). Paroxysmal atrial fibrillation in sleep. *Sleep*, 20(6), 396–398.

Coccagna, G., & Lugaresi, E. (1978). Arterial blood gases and pulmonary and systemic arterial pressure during sleep in chronic obstructive pulmonary disease. *Sleep*, 1(2), 117–124.

Coccagna, G., Mantovani, M., Brignani, F., Parchi, C., & Lugaresi, E. (1972). Continuous recording of the pulmonary and systemic arterial pressure during sleep in syndromes of hypersomnia with periodic breathing. *Bulletin Physiopathology Respiration*, 8(5), 1159–1172.

Cohen-Zion, M., Stepnowsky, C., Marler, Shochat, T., Kripke, D. F., & Ancoli-Israel, S. (2001). Changes in cognitive function associated with sleep disordered breathing in older people. *Journal of the American Geriatrics Society*, 49(12), 1622–1627.

Collop, N. A., & Kaye, D. K. (2002). Snoring and sleep-disordered breathing. In T. L. Lee-Chiong, M. J. Sateia, & M. A. Carskadon (Eds.), *Sleep medicine* (pp. 349–356). Philadelphia: Hanley & Belfus.

Connor, J., Norton, R., Ameratunga, S., Robinson, E., Wigmore, B., & Jackson, R. (2001). Prevalence of driver sleepiness in a random population-based sample of car driving. *Sleep*, 24(6), 688–694.

Cooper, K. R., & Phillips, B. A. (1982). Effect of short-term sleep loss on breathing. *Journal of Applied Physiology*, 53(4), 855–858.

Czeisler, C. A., Dumont, M., Duffy, J. F., Steinberg, J. D., Richardson, G. S., Brown, E. N., Sanchez, R., Rios, C. D., & Ronda, J. M. (1992). Association of sleep-wake habits in older people with changes in output of circadian pacemaker. *Lancet*, 340(8825), 933–936.

Czeisler, C. A., & Khalsa, S. B. S. (2000). The human circadian timing system and sleep-wake regulation. In M. H. Kryger, T. Roth, & W. C. Dement (Eds.), *Principles and practice of sleep medicine* (3rd ed., pp. 353–375). Philadelphia: W.B. Saunders Company.

Czeisler, C. A., Weitzman, E., Moore-Ede, M. C., Zimmerman, J. C., & Knauer, R. S. (1980). Human sleep: its duration and organization depend on its circadian phase. *Science*, 210(4475), 1264–1267.

D'Alessandro, R., Magelli, C., Gamberini, G., Bacchelli, S., Cristina, E., Magnani, B., & Lugaresi, E. (1990). Snoring every night as a risk factor for myocardial infarction: a case-control study. *BMJ*, 300(6739), 1557–1558.

D'Alessandro, R., Rinaldi, R., Cristina, E., Gamberini, G., & Lugaresi, E. (1995). Prevalence of excessive daytime sleepiness—an open epidemiological problem. *Sleep*, 18(5), 389–391.

Daly, B. J., & Wilson, C. A. (1983). The effect of fatigue on the vigilance of nurses monitoring electrocardiograms. *Heart Lung*, 12(4), 384–388.

Davis, J. N., Loh, L., Nodal, J., & Charnock, M. (1978). Effects of sleep on the pattern of CO2 stimulated breathing in males and females. *Advances in Experimental Medicine Biology*, 99, 79–83.

Dew, M. A., Hoch, C. C., Buysse, D. J., Monk, T. H., Begley, A. E., Houck, P. R., Hall, M., Kupfer, D. J., & Reynolds, C. F., 3rd. (2003). Healthy older adults' sleep predicts all-cause mortality at 4 to 19 years of follow-up. *Psychosomatic Medicine*, 65(1), 63–73.

D'Hoore, W., & D'Hoore, K. (1990). [Analysis of the relations between polysomnographic data and subjective evaluation of sleep in a group of normal subjects]. *Encephale*, 16(5), 383–388.

Dinges, D. F., Douglas, S. D., Hamarman, S., Zaugg, L., & Kapoor, S. (1995). Sleep deprivation and human immune function. *Advances in Neuroimmunology*, 5(2), 97–110.

Dinges, D. F., Pack, F., Williams, K., Gillen, K. A., Powell, J. W., Ott, G. E., Aptowicz, C., & Pack, A. I. (1997). Cumulative sleepiness, mood disturbance, and psychomotor vigilance performance decrements during a week of sleep restricted to 4–5 hours per night. *Sleep*, 20(4), 267–267.

Doering, L. V., McGuire, A. W., & Rourke, D. (2002). Recovering from cardiac surgery: what patients want you to know. *American Journal of Critical Care*, 11(4), 333–343.

Dohno, S., Lynch, J. J., Paskewitz, D. A., Gimbel, K. S., & Thomas, S. A. (1977). Sleep-waking changes in cardiac arrhythmia in a coronary care patient. *Psychosomatic Medicine*, 39(1), 39–43.

Dolly, F. R., & Block, A. J. (1982). Effect of flurazepam on sleep-disordered breathing and nocturnal oxygen desaturation in asymptomatic subjects. *American Journal of Medicine*, 73(2), 239–243.

Douglas, N. (1992). Nocturnal hypoxemia in patients with chronic obstructive pulmonary disease. *Clinics in Chest Medicine*, 13, 523–532.

Douglas, N. J. (2000a). Chronic obstructive pulmonary disease. In M. Kryger, R. T & W. C. Dement (Eds.), *Principles and practices of sleep medicine* (3 ed., pp. 965–975). Philadelphia: W. B. Saunders.

Douglas, N. J. (2000b). Respiratory physiology: control of ventilation. In M. H. Kryger, T. Roth & W. Dement (Eds.), *Principles and practice of sleep medicine* (3rd ed., pp. 221–228). Philadelphia: W.B. Saunders Company.

Douglass, A. B., Bornstein, R., Nino-Murcia, G., Keenan, S., Miles, L., Zarcone, V. P., Jr., Guilleminault, C., & Dement, W. C. (1994). The Sleep Disorders Questionnaire. I: Creation and multivariate structure of SDQ. *Sleep*, 17(2), 160–167.

Dracup, K. (1988). Are critical care units hazardous to health? *Applied Nursing Research*, 1(1), 14–21.

Dunbar, S. B., Clark, P. C., & Deaton, C., Parker, K.P., De, A.K. (2001). Correlates of sleep and daytime sleepiness in persons with heart failure. *Journal of Heart Failure*, 7(Suppl. 2)(5), 77 [abstract].

Edell-Gustafsson, U. M., Hetta, J. E., & Aren, C. B. (1999). Sleep and quality of life assessment in patients undergoing coronary artery bypass grafting. *Journal of Advanced Nursing*, 29(5), 1213–1220.

Edell-Gustafsson, U. M., Hetta, J. E., Aren, C. B., & Hamrin, E. K. F. (1997). Measurement of sleep and quality of life before and after coronary artery bypass grafting: a pilot study. *International Journal of Nursing Practice*, 3(4), 239–246.

El-Ad, B., & Korczyn, A. D. (1998). Disorders of excessive daytime sleepiness—an update. *Journal of Neurological Science*, 153(2), 192–202.

Ellis, B. W., Johns, M. W., Lancaster, R., Raptopoulos, P., Angelopoulos, N., & Priest, R. G. (1981). The St. Mary's Hospital sleep questionnaire: a study of reliability. *Sleep*, 4(1), 93–97.

Floras, J. S., Jones, J. V., Johnston, J. A., Brooks, D. E., Hassan, M. O., & Sleight, P. (1978). Arousal and the circadian rhythm of blood pressure. *Clinical Science Molecular Medicine* (Suppl.), 4, 395s–397s.

Freedman, N. S., Kotzer, N., & Schwab, R. J. (1999). Patient perception of sleep quality and etiology of sleep disruption in the intensive care unit. *American Journal of Respiratory & Critical Care Medicine*, 159(4 Pt 1), 1155–1162.

Friedman, E. H. (1997). Neurobiology of sleep suppression of ventricular arrhythmias.[comment]. *European Heart Journal*, 18(2), 349–350.

Gardner, J., & Grossman, W. (1975). Normal motor patterns in sleep in man. In *Advances in sleep research* (pp. 67–107). New York: Spectrum Publications.

George, C. F. P. (2000). Hypertension, ischemic heart disease, and stroke. In M. Kryger, R. T & W. C. Dement (Eds.), *Principles and practices of sleep medicine* (3rd ed., pp. 1030–1039). Philadelphia: W. B. Saunders.

Gillis, A. M. (2000). Cardiac arrhythmias. In M. Kryger, R. T & W. C. Dement (Eds.), *Principles and practice of sleep medicine* (3rd ed.). Philadelphia: W.B. Saunders.

Gislason, T., Aberg, H., & Taube, A. (1987). Snoring and systemic hypertension—an epidemiological study. *Acta Medica Scandinavia*, 222(5), 415–421.

Gold, D. R., Rogacz, S., Bock, N., Tosteson, T. D., Baum, T. M., Speizer, F. E., & Czeisler, C. A. (1992). Rotating shift work, sleep, and accidents related to sleepiness in hospital nurses. *American Journal of Public Health*, 82(7), 1011–1014.

Gosselin, N., Michaud, M., Carrier, J., Lavigne, G., & Montplaisir, J. (2002). Age difference in heart rate changes associated with micro-arousals in humans. *Clinical Neurophysiology*, 113(9), 1517–1521.

Griefahn, B., Schuemer-Kohrs, A., Schuemer, R., Moehler, U., & Mehnert, P. (2000). Physiological, subjective, and behavioural responses during sleep to noise from rail and road traffic. *Noise and Health*, 3(9), 59–71.

Guilleminault, C., Quera-Salva, M. A., Partinen, M., & Jamieson, A. (1988). Women and the obstructive sleep apnea syndrome. *Chest*, 93(1), 104–109.

Guilleminault, C., & Rosekind, M. (1981). The arousal threshold: sleep deprivation, sleep fragmentation, and obstructive sleep apnea syndrome. *Bulletin of European Physiopathology and Respiration*, 17(3), 341–349.

Guilleminault, C., Stoohs, R., Clerk, A., Simmons, J., & Labanowski, M. (1992). From obstructive sleep apnea syndrome to upper airway resistance syndrome: consistency of daytime sleepiness. *Sleep*, 15(6 Suppl.), S13–16.

Hanly, P., & Zuberi-Khokhar, N. (1995). Daytime sleepiness in patients with congestive heart failure and Cheyne- Stokes respiration. *Chest*, 107(4), 952–958.

Hanly, P. J., & Zuberi-Khokhar, N. (1996). Periodic limb movements during sleep in patients with congestive heart failure. *Chest*, 109(6), 1497–1502.

He, J., Kryger, M. H., Zorick, F. J., Conway, W., & Roth, T. (1988). Mortality and apnea index in obstructive sleep apnea. Experience in 385 male patients. *Chest*, 94(1), 9–14.

Hla, K. M., Young, T. B., Bidwell, T., Palta, M., Skatrud, J. B., & Dempsey, J. (1994). Sleep apnea and hypertension. A population-based study. *Annals of Internal Medicine*, 120(5), 382–388.

Hoffstein, V. (2000). Snoring. In M. H. Kryger, T. Roth & W. C. Dement (Eds.), *Principles and practice of sleep medicine* (3rd ed., pp. 813–826). Philadelphia: W.B. Saunders.

Hoffstein, V., Chan, C. K., & Slutsky, A. S. (1991). Sleep apnea and systemic hypertension: a causal association review. *American Journal of Medicine*, 91(2), 190–196.

Hoffstein, V., & Mateika, S. (1994). Cardiac arrhythmias, snoring, and sleep apnea. *Chest*, 106(2), 466–471.

Hong, S., & Dimsdale, J. E. (2003). Physical activity and perception of energy and fatigue in obstructive sleep apnea. *Medical Science Sports Exercise,* 35(7), 1088–1092.

Huxley, E. J., Viroslav, J., Gray, W. R., & Pierce, A. K. (1978). Pharyngeal aspiration in normal adults and patients with depressed consciousness. *American Journal of Medicine,* 64(4), 564–568.

Irwin, M., McClintick, J., Costlow, C., Fortner, M., White, J., & Gillin, J. C. (1996). Partial night sleep deprivation reduces natural killer and cellular immune responses in humans. *FASEB Journal,* 10(5), 643–653.

Issa, F. G., & Sullivan, C. E. (1982). Alcohol, snoring and sleep apnea. *Journal of Neurological and Neurosurgical Psychiatry,* 45(4), 353–359.

Javaheri, S. (2000). Treatment of central sleep apnea in heart failure. *Sleep,* 23 Suppl 4, S224–227.

Javaheri, S., Parker, T. J., Liming, J. D., Corbett, W. S., Nishiyama, H., Wexler, L., & Roselle, G. A. (1998). Sleep apnea in 81 ambulatory male patients with stable heart failure. Types and their prevalences, consequences, and presentations. *Circulation,* 97(21), 2154–2159.

Jean-Louis, G., von Gizycki, H., Zizi, F., Fookson, J., Spielman, A., Nunes, J., Fullilove, R., & Taub, H. (1996). Determination of sleep and wakefulness with the actigraph data analysis software (ADAS). *Sleep,* 19(9), 739–743.

Johns, M. W. (1991). A new method for measuring daytime sleepiness: the Epworth sleepiness scale. *Sleep,* 14(6), 540–545.

Johns, M. W. (1992). Reliability and factor analysis of the Epworth Sleepiness Scale. *Sleep,* 15(4), 376–381.

Johns, M. W. (1993). Daytime sleepiness, snoring, and obstructive sleep apnea. The Epworth Sleepiness Scale. *Chest,* 103(1), 30–36.

Johns, M. W. (2000). Sensitivity and specificity of the multiple sleep latency test (MSLT), the maintenance of wakefulness test and the Epworth sleepiness scale: failure of the MSLT as a gold standard. *Journal of Sleep Research,* 9(1), 5–11.

Johns, M. W., Egan, P., Gay, T. J., & Masterton, J. P. (1970). Sleep habits and symptoms in male medical and surgical patients. *British Medical Journal,* 2(708), 509–512.

Johnson, H., Swan, T., & Weigand, G. (1930). In what positions do healthy people sleep? *JAMA,* 94, 2058–2062.

Kavanau, J. L. (1997). Memory, sleep and the evolution of mechanisms of synaptic efficacy maintenance. *Neuroscience,* 79(1), 7–44.

Kavanau, J. L. (2000). Sleep, memory maintenance, and mental disorders. *Journal of Neuropsychiatry and Clinical Neuroscience,* 12(2), 199–208.

Kawano, H., Motoyama, T., Yasue, H., Hirai, N., Waly, H. M., Kugiyama, K., & Ogawa, H. (2002). Endothelial function fluctuates with diurnal variation in the frequency of ischemic episodes in patients with variant angina. *Journal of the American College of Cardiology,* 40(2), 266–270.

Kecklund, G., & Akerstedt, T. (1995). Effects of timing of shifts on sleepiness and sleep duration. *Journal of Sleep Research,* 4(S2), 47–50.

Khatri, I. M., & Freis, E. D. (1967). Hemodynamic changes during sleep. *Journal of Applied Physiology,* 22(5), 867–873.

King, K., & Parrinello, K. (1988). Patient perceptions of recovery from coronary artery bypass grafting after discharge from the hospital. *Heart Lung,* 17, 708–715.

Kleitman, N., Cooperman, N., & Mullin, F. (1933). Studies on the physiology of sleep IX. Motility and body temperature during sleep. *American Journal of Physiology,* 105, 574–584.

Koskenvuo, M., Kaprio, J., Heikkila, K., Sarna, S., Telakivi, T., & Partinen, M. (1987). Snoring as a risk factor for ischaemic heart disease and stroke in men. *British Medical Journal (Clinical Research Edition),* 294(6572), 643.

Koskenvuo, M., Kaprio, J., Partinen, M., Langinvainio, H., Sarna, S., & Heikkila, K. (1985). Snoring as a risk factor for hypertension and angina pectoris. *Lancet,* 1(8434), 893–896.

Koskenvuo, M., Partinen, M., Kaprio, J., Vuorinen, H., Telakivi, T., Kajaste, S., Salmi, T., & Heikkila, K. (1994). Snoring and cardiovascular risk factors. *Annals of Medicine,* 26(5), 371–376.

Krachman, S. L., D'Alonzo, G. E., & Berger, T. J., & Eisen, H. J. (1999). Comparison of oxygen therapy with nasal continuous positive airway pressure on Cheyne-Stokes respiration during sleep in congestive heart failure. *Chest,* 116(6), 1550–1557.

Krauchi, K., Cajochen, C., Werth, E., & Wirz-Justice, A. (1999). Warm feet promote the rapid onset of sleep. *Nature,* 401(6748), 36–37.

Krauchi, K., & Wirz-Justice, A. (2001). Circadian clues to sleep onset mechanisms. *Neuropsychopharmacology,* 25(5 Suppl.), S92–96.

Krieger, A. C., & Redeker, N. S. (2002). Obstructive sleep apnea syndrome: its relationship with hypertension. *Journal of Cardiovascular Nursing,* 17(1), 1–11.

Krieger, J. (2000). Respiratory physiology: Breathing in normal subjects. In W. C. Dement (Ed.), *Principles and practice of sleep medicine* (3rd ed., pp. 229–241). Philadelphia: W.B. Saunders Company.

Kripke, D. F. (2003). Sleep and mortality. *Psychosomatic Medicine,* 65(1), 74.

Kripke, D. F., Klauber, M. R., Wingard, D. L., Fell, R. L., Assmus, J. D., & Garfinkel, L. (1998). Mortality hazard associated with prescription hypnotics. *Biological Psychiatry,* 43(9), 687–693.

Krueger, J. M., Fang, J., & Floyd, R. A. (1999). Relationship between sleep and immune function. In F. W. Turek & P. C. Zee (Eds.), *Regulation of sleep and circadian rhythms* (Vol. 133, pp. 427–464). New York: Marcel Dekker, Inc.

Krueger, J. M., & Obal, F. J. (2002). Function of sleep. In M. A. Carskadon (Ed.), *Sleep medicine* (pp. 23–30). Philadelphia: Hanley & Belfus, Inc.

Lanfranchi, P. A., Braghiroli, A., Bosimini, E., Mazzuero, G., Colombo, R., Donner, C. F., & Giannuzzi, P. (1999). Prognostic value of nocturnal Cheyne-Stokes respiration in chronic heart failure. *Circulation,* 99(11), 1435–1440.

Lanfranchi, P. A., Somers, V. K., Braghiroli, A., Corra, U., Eleuteri, E., & Giannuzzi, P. (2003). Central sleep apnea in left ventricular dysfunction: prevalence and implications for arrhythmic risk. *Circulation,* 107(5), 727–732.

Lashley, F. R. (2004). Measuring sleep. In M. Frank-Stromborg & S. J. Olsen (Eds.), *Instruments for clinical health-care research* (pp. 293–314). Boston: Jones and Bartlett Publishers.

Lavery, C. E., Mittleman, M. A., Cohen, M. C., Muller, J. E., & Verrier, R. L. (1997). Nonuniform nighttime distribution of acute cardiac events: a possible effect of sleep states. *Circulation,* 96(10), 3321–3327.

Lee, K. A. (2003). Impaired sleep. In V. Carrieri-Kohlman, A. M. Lindsey & C. M. West (Eds.), *Pathophysiological phenomena in nursing: Human responses to illness* (pp. 363–385). St. Louis: Saunders.

Lewy, A. J. (1999). The dim light melatonin onset, melatonin assays and biological rhythm research in humans. *Biological Signals Reception,* 8(1–2), 79–83.

Lewy, A. J., & Sack, R. L. (1989). The dim light melatonin onset as a marker for circadian phase position. *Chronobiology International,* 6(1), 93–102.

Li, J. J., Huang, C. X., Fang, C. H., Chen, F., Jiang, H., Tang, Q. Z., & Li, G. S. (2002). Circadian variation in ischemic threshold in patients with stable angina: relation to plasma endothelin-1. *Angiology,* 53(4), 409–413.

Liston, R., Deegan, P. C., McCreery, C., & McNicholas, W. T. (1994). Role of respiratory sleep disorders in the pathogenesis of nocturnal angina and arrhythmias. *Postgraduate Medicine Journal,* 70(822), 275–280.

Littner, M., Hirshkowitz, M., Davila, D., Anderson, W. M., Kushida, C. A., Woodson, B. T., Johnson, S. F., & Merrill, S. W. (2002). Practice parameters for the use of auto-titrating continuous positive airway pressure devices for titrating pressures and treating adult patients with obstructive sleep apnea syndrome. An American Academy of Sleep Medicine report. *Sleep,* 25(2), 143–147.

Littrell, K., & Schumann, L. L. (1989). Promoting sleep for the patient with a myocardial infarction. *Critical Care Nurse,* 9(3), 44–49.

Lloberes, P., Levy, G., Descals, C., Sampol, G., Roca, A., Sagales, T., & de la Calzada, M. D. (2000). Self-reported sleepiness while driving as a risk factor for traffic accidents in patients with obstructive sleep apnoea syndrome and in non-apnoeic snorers. *Respiratory Medicine,* 94(10), 971–976.

Lugaresi, E., Coccagna, G., Cirignotta, F., Farneti, P., Gallassi, R., Di Donato, G., & Verucchi, P. (1978). Breathing during sleep in man in normal and pathological conditions. *Advances in Experimental Medicine and Biology,* 99, 35–45.

Lusardi, P., Zoppi, A., Preti, P., Pesce, R. M., Piazza, E., & Fogari, R. (1999). Effects of insufficient sleep on blood pressure in hypertensive patients: a 24-h study. *American Journal of Hypertension,* 12(1 Pt 1), 63–68.

Lyznicki, J. M., Doege, T. C., Davis, R. M., & Williams, M. A. (1998a). Sleepiness, driving, and motor vehicle crashes. Council on Scientific Affairs, American Medical Association. *JAMA,* 279(23), 1908–1913.

Lyznicki, J. M., Doege, T. C., Davis, R. M., & Williams, M. A. (1998b). Sleepiness, driving, and motor vehicle crashes. Council on Scientific Affairs, American Medical Association [see comments]. *JAMA,* 279(23), 1908–1913.

Madsen, P. L., Holm, S., Vorstrup, S., Friberg, L., Lassen, N. A., & Wildschiodtz, G. (1991). Human regional cerebral blood flow during rapid-eye-movement sleep. *Journal of Cerebral Blood Flow Metabolism,* 11(3), 502–507.

McCall, W. V., Turpin, E., Reboussin, D., Edinger, J. D., & Haponik, E. F. (1995). Subjective estimates of sleep differ from polysomnographic measurements in obstructive sleep apnea patients. *Sleep,* 18(8), 646–650.

McGinty, D., & Szymusiak, R. (1990). Keeping cool: a hypothesis about the mechanisms and functions of slow-wave sleep. *Trends in Neuroscience*, 13(12), 480–487.

McSweeney, J. C., & Crane, P. B. (2000). Challenging the rules: women's prodromal and acute symptoms of myocardial infarction. *Research in Nursing & Health*, 23(2), 135–146.

Miller, A. H. (2003). Cytokines and sickness behavior: implications for cancer care and control. *Brain Behavioral Immunology*, 17(Suppl. 1), S132–134.

Miller, G. E., Stetler, C. A., Carney, R. M., Freedland, K. E., & Banks, W. A. (2002). Clinical depression and inflammatory risk markers for coronary heart disease. *American Journal of Cardiology*, 90(12), 1279–1283.

Millman, R. P., Redline, S., Carlisle, C. C., Assaf, A. R., & Levinson, P. D. (1991). Daytime hypertension in obstructive sleep apnea. Prevalence and contributing risk factors. *Chest*, 99(4), 861–866.

Mohsenin, V. (2002). Breathing and sleep in chronic obstructive pulmonary disease and asthma. In M. A. Carskadon (Ed.), *Sleep medicine*. Philadelphia: Hanley & Belfus, Inc.

Monasterio, C., Vidal, S., Duran, J., Ferrer, M., Carmona, C., Barbe, F., Mayos, M., Gonzalez-Mangado, N., Juncadella, M., Navarro, A., Barreira, R., Capote, F., Mayoralas, L. R., Peces-Barba, G., Alonso, J., & Montserrat, J. M. (2001). Effectiveness of continuous positive airway pressure in mild sleep apnea-hypopnea syndrome. *American Journal of Respiratory Critical Care Medicine*, 164(6), 939–943.

Monti, A., Medigue, C., Nedelcoux, H., & Escourrou, P. (2002). Autonomic control of the cardiovascular system during sleep in normal subjects. *European Journal of Applied Physiology*, 87(2), 174–181.

Moore-Ede, M. C., Meguid, M. M., Fitzpatrick, G. F., Boyden, C. M., & Ball, M. R. (1978). Circadian variation in response to potassium infusion. *Clinics in Pharmacological Therapeutics*, 23(2), 218–227.

Mori, H. (1994). The relationship between the circadian variation of total vascular tone and autonomic nervous activity in patients with vasospastic angina. *Nippon Rinsho - Japanese Journal of Clinical Medicine*, 52(Suppl., Pt. 2), 235–240.

Moritz, A., Steinseifer, U., et al. (1992). Closing sounds and related complaints after heart valve replacement with St Jude Medical, Duromedics Edwards, Bjårk-Shiley Monostrut, and Carbomedics prostheses. *British Heart Journal*, 67, 460–465.

Moses, J., Lubin, A., Naitoh, P., & Johnson, L. C. (1972). Reliability of sleep measures. *Psychophysiology*, 9(1), 78–82.

Mulcahy, D., Wright, C., Sparrow, J., Cunningham, D., Curcher, D., Purcell, H., & Fox, K. (1993). Heart rate and blood pressure consequences of an afternoon SIESTA (Snooze-Induced Excitation of Sympathetic Triggered Activity). *American Journal of Cardiology*, 71(7), 611–614.

Murali, N. S., Svatikova, A., & Somers, V. K. (2003). Cardiovascular physiology and sleep. *Frontiers of Bioscience*, 8, s636–652.

Nathan, P. J., Burrows, G. D., & Norman, T. R. (1997). The effect of dim light on suppression of nocturnal melatonin in healthy women and men. *Journal of Neural Transmission*, 104(6–7), 643–648.

Newman, A. B., Nieto, F. J., Guidry, U., Lind, B. K., Redline, S., Pickering, T. G., Quan, S. F., & Sleep Heart Health Study Research, G. (2001). Relation of sleep-disordered breathing to cardiovascular disease risk factors: the Sleep Heart Health Study. *American Journal of Epidemiology*, 154(1), 50–59.

Newman, A. B., Spiekerman, C. F., Enright, P., Lefkowitz, D., Manolio, T., Reynolds, C. F., & Robbins, J. (2000). Daytime sleepiness predicts mortality and cardiovascular disease in older adults. The Cardiovascular Health Study Research Group. *Journal of the American Geriatrics Society*, 48(2), 115–123.

Nicassio, P. M., Moxham, E. G., Schuman, C. E., & Gevirtz, R. N. (2002). The contribution of pain, reported sleep quality, and depressive symptoms to fatigue in fibromyalgia. *Pain*, 100(3), 271–279.

Nieto, F. J., Young, T. B., Lind, B. K., Shahar, E., Samet, J. M., Redline, S., D'Agostino, R. B., Newman, A. B., Lebowitz, M. D., & Pickering, T. G. (2000). Association of sleep-disordered breathing, sleep apnea, and hypertension in a large community-based study. Sleep Heart Health Study. *JAMA*, 283(14), 1829–1836.

Nugent, A. M., Gleadhill, I., McCrum, E., Patterson, C. C., Evans, A., & MacMahon, J. (2001). Sleep complaints and risk factors for excessive daytime sleepiness in adult males in Northern Ireland. *Journal of Sleep Research*, 10(1), 69–74.

Olson, D. M., Borel, C. O., Laskowitz, D. T., Moore, D. T., & McConnell, E. S. (2001). Quiet time: a nursing intervention to promote sleep in neurocritical care units. *American Journal of Critical Care*, 10(2), 74–78.

Onaka, H., Hirota, Y., Shimada, S., Mishima, T., Shimoyama, H., Sakai, Y., & Kawamura, K. (1998). Circadian variation of myocardial ischemia in patients with unstable angina pectoris secondary to fixed and/or spastic coronary narrowing. *American Journal of Cardiology*, 81(5), 629–632.

Owen, J., & Arendt, J. (1992). Melatonin suppression in human subjects by bright and dim light in antarctica: time and season-dependent effects. *Neuroscience Letters, 137*(2), 181–184.

Palomaki, H. (1991). Snoring and the risk of ischemic brain infarction. *Stroke*, 22(8), 1021–1025.

Palomaki, H., Partinen, M., Erkinjuntti, T., & Kaste, M. (1992). Snoring, sleep apnea syndrome, and stroke. *Neurology*, 42(7 Suppl 6), 75–81; discussion 82.

Parker, K. P. (1995). Promoting sleep and rest in critically ill patients. *Critical Care Nursing Clinics of North Ameerica*, 7(2), 337–349.

Parker, K. P., & Dunbar, S. B. (2002). Sleep and heart failure. *Journal of Cardiovascular Nursing*, 17(1), 30–41.

Parmeggaiani, P. L. (2000). Physiological regulation in sleep. In M. H. Kryger, T. Roth & W. Dement (Eds.), *Principles and practice of sleep medicine* (3rd ed., pp. 169–178). Philadelphia: W.B. Saunders.

Parrott, A. C., & Hindmarch, I. (1980). The Leeds Sleep Evaluation Questionnaire in psychopharmacological investigations—a review. *Psychopharmacology (Berlin)*, 71(2), 173–179.

Peppard, P. E., Young, T., Palta, M., & Skatrud, J. (2000). Prospective study of the association between sleep-disordered breathing and hypertension. *New England Journal of Medicine*, 342(19), 1378–1384.

Peters, R. W., Zoble, R. G., & Brooks, M. M. (2002). Onset of acute myocardial infarction during sleep. *Clinical Cardiology*, 25(5), 237–241.

Phillips, B. A., & Danner, F. J. (1995). Cigarette smoking and sleep disturbance. *Archives of Internal Medicine*, 155(7), 734–737.

Pollak, C. P., Tryon, W. W., Nagaraja, H., & Dzwonczyk, R. (2001). How accurately does wrist actigraphy identify the states of sleep and wakefulness? *Sleep*, 24(8), 957–965.

Power, J. T., Stewart, I. C., Connaughton, J. J., Brash, H. M., Shapiro, C. M., Flenley, D. C., & Douglas, N. J. (1984). Nocturnal cough in patients with chronic bronchitis and emphysema. *American Review of Respiratory Disease*, 130(6), 999–1001.

Quaranta, A. J., D'Alonzo, G. E., & Krachman, S. L. (1997). Cheyne-Stokes respiration during sleep in congestive heart failure. *Chest*, 111(2), 467–473.

Qureshi, A. I., Giles, W. H., Croft, J. B., & Bliwise, D. L. (1997). Habitual sleep patterns and risk for stroke and coronary heart disease: a 10-year follow-up from NHANES I. *Neurology*, 48(4), 904–911.

Rauscher, H., Popp, W., & Zwick, H. (1992). Systemic hypertension in snorers with and without sleep apnea. *Chest*, 102(2), 367–371.

Rechtschaffen, A., & Kales, A. (1968). *A manual of standard terminology: techniques and scoring system for sleep stages in human subjects*. (Institute of Health Publication No. 204). Washington, D.C.: U.S. Government Printing Office.

Redeker, N. S. (2002). Why is sleep relevant to cardiovascular disease. *Journal of Cardiovascular Nursing*, 17(1), v–xi.

Redeker, N. S., & Hedges, C. (2002a). Sleep during hospitalization and recovery after cardiac surgery. *Journal of Cardiovascular Nursing*, 17(1), 56–68; quiz 82–53.

Redeker, N. S., & Hedges, C. (2002b). Sleep during hospitalization and recovery after cardiac surgery. *Journal of Cardiovascular Nursing*, 17(1), 56–68.

Redline, S., & Strohl, K. P. (1998). Recognition and consequences of obstructive sleep apnea hypopnea syndrome. *Clinics in Chest Medicine*, 19(1), 1–19.

Resta, O., Foschino-Barbaro, M. P., Bonfitto, P. G., Talamo, S., Nocerino, M. C., Stefa no, A., & Biasco, G. (1999). Nocturnal oxygen desaturation in patients with congestive heart failure. *Boll Soc Ital Biol Sper*, 75(5–6), 31–38.

Richards, K. C., Anderson, W. M., Chesson, A. L., Jr., & Nagel, C. L. (2002). Sleep-related breathing disorders in patients who are critically ill. *Journal of Cardiovascular Nursing*, 17(1), 42–55.

Richards, K. C., & Bairnsfather, L. (1988a). A description of night sleep patterns in the critical care unit. *Heart & Lung: Journal of Acute & Critical Care*, 17(1), 35–42.

Richards, K. C., & Bairnsfather, L. (1988b). A description of night sleep patterns in the critical care unit. *Heart Lung*, 17(1), 35–42.

Richardson, G. S., Carskadon, M. A., Flagg, W., Van den Hoed, J., Dement, W. C., & Mitler, M. M. (1978). Excessive daytime sleepiness in man: multiple sleep latency measurement in narcoleptic and control subjects. *Electroencephalographic Clinics in Neurophysiology*, 45(5), 621–627.

Richardson, G. S., Carskadon, M. A., Orav, E. J., & Dement, W. C. (1982). Circadian variation of sleep tendency in elderly and young adult subjects. *Sleep*, 5(Suppl. 2), S82–94.

Roehrs, T., Carskadon, M. A., Dement, W. C., & Roth, T. (2000). Daytime sleepiness and alertness. In M. H. Kryger, T. Roth & W. C. Dement (Eds.), *Principles and practice of sleep medicine* (3rd ed., pp. 43–52). Philadelphia: W.B. Saunders Company.

Roehrs, T., & Roth, T. (2001). Sleep, sleepiness, sleep disorders and alcohol use and abuse. *Sleep Medicine Review*, 5(4), 287–297.

Rotenberg, V. S., Indursky, P., Kayumov, L., Sirota, P., & Melamed, Y. (2000). The relationship between subjective sleep estimation and objective sleep variables in depressed patients. *International Journal of Psychophysiology*, 37(3), 291–297.

Sadeh, A., & Acebo, C. (2002). The role of actigraphy in sleep medicine. *Sleep Medicine Review*, 6(2), 113–124.

Sadeh, A., Hauri, P. J., Kripke, D. F., & Lavie, P. (1995). The role of actigraphy in the evaluation of sleep disorders. *Sleep*, 18(4), 288–302.

Schiffman, P. L., Trontell, M. C., Mazar, M. F., & Edelman, N. H. (1983). Sleep deprivation decreases ventilatory response to CO2 but not load compensation. *Chest*, 84(6), 695–698.

Schleifer, S. J., Macari-Hinson, M. M., Coyle, D. A., Slater, W. R., Kahn, M., Gorlin, R., & Zucker, H. D. (1989). The nature and course of depression following myocardial infarction. *Archives of Internal Medicine*, 149(8), 1785–1789.

Scrima, L., Broudy, M., Nay, K. N., & Cohn, M. A. (1982). Increased severity of obstructive sleep apnea after bedtime alcohol ingestion: diagnostic potential and proposed mechanism of action. *Sleep*, 5(4), 318–328.

Shahar, E., Whitney, C. W., Redline, S., Lee, E. T., Newman, A. B., Javier Nieto, F., O'Connor, G. T., Boland, L. L., Schwartz, J. E., & Samet, J. M. (2001). Sleep-disordered breathing and cardiovascular disease: cross-sectional results of the Sleep Heart Health Study.[comment]. *American Journal of Respiratory & Critical Care Medicine*, 163(1), 19–25.

Shamsuzzaman, A. S., Winnicki, M., Lanfranchi, P., Wolk, R., Kara, T., Accurso, V., & Somers, V. K. (2002). Elevated C-reactive protein in patients with obstructive sleep apnea. *Circulation*, 105(21), 2462–2464.

Sharkey, K. M., Fogg, L. F., & Eastman, C. I. (2001). Effects of melatonin administration on daytime sleep after simulated night shift work. *Journal of Sleep Research*, 10(3), 181–192.

Shaver, J. L., & Giblin, E. C. (1989). Sleep. *Annual Review of Nursing Research*, 7, 71–93.

Shepard, J. W., Jr. (1992). Hypertension, cardiac arrhythmias, myocardial infarction, and stroke in relation to obstructive sleep apnea. *Clinical Chest Medicine*, 13(3), 437–458.

Siegel, J. M. (2000). Brain mechanisms generating REM sleep. In M. H. Kryger, T. Roth & W. Dement (Eds.), *Principles and practice of sleep medicine* (3rd ed., pp. 112–133). Philadelphia: W.B. Saunders.

Simon, P. M., Landry, S. H., & Leiter, J. C. (2002). Respiratory control during sleep. In M. A. Carskadon et al. (Eds.), *Sleep medicine* (pp. 41–51). Philadelphia: Hanley & Belfus.

Simpson, T., Lee, E. R., & Cameron, C. (1996). Relationships among sleep dimensions and factors that impair sleep after cardiac surgery. *Research in Nursing & Health*, 19(3), 213–223.

Sin, D. D., Logan, A. G., Fitzgerald, F. S., Liu, P. P., & Bradley, T. D. (2000). Effects of continuous positive airway pressure on cardiovascular outcomes in heart failure patients with and without Cheyne-Stokes respiration. *Circulation*, 102(1), 61–66.

Sin, D. D., Mayers, I., Man, G. C., & Pawluk, L. (2002). Long-term compliance rates to continuous positive airway pressure in obstructive sleep apnea: a population-based study. *Chest*, 121(2), 430–435.

Skinner, R. D. (2002). Temperature regulation during sleep. In T. L. Lee-Chiong, M. J. Sateia & M. A. Carskadon (Eds.), *Sleep medicine* (pp. 71–75). Philadelphia: Hanley & Belfus.

Somers, V. K., Dyken, M. E., Mark, A. L., & Abboud, F. M. (1993). Sympathetic-nerve activity during sleep in normal subjects. *New England Journal of Medicine*, 328(5), 303–307.

Staniforth, A. D., Kinnear, W. J., & Cowley, A. J. (2001). Cognitive impairment in heart failure with Cheyne-Stokes respiration. *Heart*, 85(1), 18–22.

Staniforth, A. D., Kinnear, W. J., Starling, R., & Cowley, A. J. (1998). Nocturnal desaturation in patients with stable heart failure. *Heart*, 79(4), 394–399.

Staniforth, A. D., Kinnear, W. J., Starling, R., Hetmanski, D. J., & Cowley, A. J. (1998). Effect of oxygen on sleep quality, cognitive function and sympathetic activity in patients with chronic heart failure and Cheyne-Stokes respiration. *European Heart Journal*, 19(6), 922–928.

Stern, M. J., Pascale, L., & Ackerman, A. (1977). Life adjustment postmyocardial infarction: determining predictive variables. *Archives of Internal Medicine*, 137(12), 1680–1685.

Stern, M. J., Pascale, L., & McLoone, J. B. (1976). Psychosocial adaptation following an acute myocardial infarction. *Journal of Chronic Diseases*, 29(8), 513–526.

Stokes, W. (1854). *The disease of the heart and aorta*. Dublin: Hodges & Smith.

Stramba-Badiale, M., Priori, S. G., Napolitano, C., Locati, E. H., Vinolas, X., Haverkamp, W., Schulze-Bahr, E., Goulene, K., & Schwartz, P. J. (2000). Gene-specific differences in the circadian variation of ventricular repolarization in the long QT syndrome: a key to sudden death during sleep?[comment]. *Italian Heart Journal: Official Journal of the Italian Federation of Cardiology*, 1(5), 323–328.

Szymusiak, R., & McGinty, D. (1990). Control of slow wave sleep by thermoregulatory mechanisms. *Progress in Clinical Biological Research*, 345, 53-64; discussion 65–56.

Tank, J., Diedrich, A., Hale, N., Niaz, F. E., Furlan, R., Robertson, R. M., & Mosqueda-Garcia, R. (2003). Relationship between blood pressure, sleep K-complexes, and muscle sympathetic nerve activity in humans. *American Journal of Physiology Regul Integr Comp Physiol*, 285(1), R208–214.

Thorpy, M. J. (1991). History of sleep and man. In M. J. Thorpy & J. Yager (Eds.), *The encyclopedia of sleep and sleep disorders* (pp. ix-xxxiii). New York: Oxford.

Thorpy, M. J. (1992). The clinical use of the Multiple Sleep Latency Test. The Standards of Practice Committee of the American Sleep Disorders Association. *Sleep*, 15(3), 268–276.

Tobler, I. (1995). Is sleep fundamentally different between mammalian species? *Behavioral Brain Research*, 69(1-2), 35–41.

Topf, M., Bookman, M., & Arand, D. (1996). Effects of critical care unit noise on the subjective quality of sleep. *Journal of Advanced Nursing*, 24(3), 545–551.

Topf, M., & Thompson, S. (2001). Interactive relationships between hospital patients' noise-induced stress and other stress with sleep. *Heart Lung*, 30(4), 237–243.

Tsuchiyama, K., Nagayama, H., Kudo, K., Kojima, K., & Yamada, K. (2003). Discrepancy between subjective and objective sleep in patients with depression. *Psychiatry Clinics in Neuroscience*, 57(3), 259–264.

Van Cauter, E. (2000). Endocrine physiology. In M. H. Kryger, T. Roth & W. C. Dement (Eds.), *Principles and practice of sleep medicine* (3rd ed., pp. 266-278). Philadelphia: W.B. Saunders Company.

Van Someren, E. J. (2000). More than a marker: interaction between the circadian regulation of temperature and sleep, age-related changes, and treatment possibilities. *Chronobiology International*, 17(3), 313–354.

Verrier, R. L. (2002). Cardiac physiology during sleep. In M. A. Carskadon et al. (Eds.), *Sleep medicine* (pp. 53–57). Philadelphia: Hanley & Belfus.

Verrier, R. L. (2002). Cardiovascular disorders and sleep. In M. A. Carskadon et al. (Eds.), *Sleep medicine* (pp. 447–454). Philadelphia: Hanley & Belfus, Inc.

Walder, B., Francioli, D., Meyer, J. J., Lancon, M., & Romand, J. A. (2000). Effects of guidelines implementation in a surgical intensive care unit to control nighttime light and noise levels.[comment]. *Critical Care Medicine*, 28(7), 2242–2247.

Wallace, C. J., Robins, J., Alvord, L. S., & Walker, J. M. (1999). The effect of earplugs on sleep measures during exposure to simulated intensive care unit noise. *American Journal of Critical Care*, 8(4), 210–219.

Walsh, J. K., Muehlbach, M. J., Humm, T. M., Dickins, Q. S., Sugerman, J. L., & Schweitzer, P. K. (1990). Effect of caffeine on physiological sleep tendency and ability to sustain wakefulness at night. *Psychopharmacology (Berl)*, 101(2), 271–273.

Ware, J. C., & Hirshkowitz, M. (2000). Assessment of sleep-related erections. In M. H. Kryger, T. Roth & W. C. Dement (Eds.), *Principles and practice of sleep medicine* (pp. 1231–1238). Philadelphia: W.B. Saunders.

Weaver, T. E. (2001). Outcome measurement in sleep medicine practice and research. Part 1: assessment of symptoms, subjective and objective daytime sleepiness, health-related quality of life and functional status. *Sleep Medicine Review*, 5(2), 103–128.

Weiss, J. W., Remsburg, S., Garpestad, E., Ringler, J., Sparrow, D., & Parker, J. A. (1996). Hemodynamic consequences of obstructive sleep apnea. *Sleep*, 19(5), 388–397.

Wessendorf, T. E., & Teschler, H. (2002). Sleep disorders and alcohol. *Sleep Medicine Review*, 6(1), 71.

White, D. P., Douglas, N. J., Pickett, C. K., Zwillich, C. W., & Weil, J. V. (1983). Sleep deprivation and the control of ventilation. *American Review of Respiratory Diseases*, 128(6), 984–986.

Whitney, C. W., Enright, P. L., Newman, A. B., Bonekat, W., Foley, D., & Quan, S. F. (1998). Correlates of daytime sleepiness in 4578 elderly persons: the Cardiovascular Health Study. *Sleep*, 21(1), 27–36.

Williamson, J. W. (1992). The effects of ocean sounds on sleep after coronary artery bypass graft surgery. *American Journal of Critical Care,* 1(1), 91–97.

Willich, S. N. (1999). European survey on circadian variation of angina pectoris (ESCVA): design and preliminary results. *Journal of Cardiovascular Pharmacology,* 34(Suppl 2), S9-13; discussion S29–31.

Wishnie, H. A., Hackett, T. P., & Cssem, N. H. (1971). Psychological hazards of convalescence following myocardial inarction. *JAMA,* 215(8), 1292–1296.

Worsnop, C. J., Naughton, M. T., Barter, C. E., Morgan, T. O., Anderson, A. I., & Pierce, R. J. (1998). The prevalence of obstructive sleep apnea in hypertensives. *American Journal of Respiratory Critical Care Medicine,* 157(1), 111–115.

Wu, J. C., Gillin, J. C., Buchsbaum, M. S., Hershey, T., Hazlett, E., Sicotte, N., & Bunney, W. E., Jr. (1991). The effect of sleep deprivation on cerebral glucose metabolic rate in normal humans assessed with positron emission tomography. *Sleep,* 14(2), 155–162.

Wuyam, B., Pepin, J. L., Tremel, F., & Levy, P. (2000). Pathophysiology of central sleep apnea syndrome. *Sleep,* 23(Suppl. 4), S213–219.

Wysowski, D. K., & Baum, C. (1991). Outpatient use of prescription sedative-hypnotic drugs in the United States, 1970 through 1989. *Archives of Internal Medicine,* 151(9), 1779–1783.

Yagi, T., Noda, A., Itoh, R., Yamada, H., Nakashima, N., Yokota, M., & Koike, Y. (1998). [The relationship between subjective sleepiness and polysomnographic findings in sleep apnea syndrome]. *Rinsho Byori,* 46(11), 1168–1172.

Yamashiro, Y., & Kryger, M. H. (1993). Review: sleep in heart failure. *Sleep,* 16(6), 513–523.

Young, T., Palta, M., Dempsey, J., Skatrud, J., Weber, S., & Badr, S. (1993). The occurrence of sleep-disordered breathing among middle-aged adults. *New England Journal of Medicine,* 328(17), 1230–1235.

Young, T., Peppard, P., Palta, M., Hla, K. M., Finn, L., Morgan, B., & Skatrud, J. (1997). Population-based study of sleep-disordered breathing as a risk factor for hypertension. *Archives of Internal Medicine,* 157(15), 1746–1752.

Young-McCaughan, S., Mays, M. Z., Arzola, S. M., Yoder, L. H., Dramiga, S. A., Leclerc, K. M., Caton, J. R., Sheffler, R. L., & Nowlin, M. U. (2003). Research and commentary: Change in exercise tolerance, activity and sleep patterns, and quality of life in patients with cancer participating in a structured exercise program. *Oncology Nursing Forum,* 30(3), 441-454; discussion 441–454.

Zarcone, V. P. (2000). Sleep hygiene. In W. C. Dement (Ed.), *Principles and practice of sleep medicine* (3rd ed., pp. 657–661). Philadelphia: W.B. Saunders Company.

Zepelin, H., & Rechtschaffen, A. (1974). Mammalian sleep, longevity, and energy metabolism. *Brain Behavioral Evolution,* 10(6), 425–470.

Zimmerman, L., Nieveen, J., Barnason, S., & Schmaderer, M. (1996). The effects of music interventions on postoperative pain and sleep in coronary artery bypass graft (CABG) patients. *Scholarly Inquiry for Nursing Practice,* 10(2), 153-170; discussion 171–174.

12

Physiologic Adaptations With Aging

BARBARA S. LEVINE • RUTH F. CRAVEN

Aging is a normal developmental process during which physiological and psychosocial changes occur. Wide variation in the aging process exists among individuals as a result of varied environmental exposures, social relationships, genetic endowment, and health status. Whereas maximum lifespan (the age reached by the longest-lived survivors) for humans is 114 to 120 years, the average human lifespan is approximately 75 years. Developmental changes and adaptations continue throughout aging until death.

The lifespan is divided into phases, with the commonly used periods for these phases being infancy (birth to 1 year), early childhood (1 to 6 years), late childhood (7 to 10 years), adolescence (11 to 18 years), young adulthood (19 to 35 years), early middle age (36 to 49 years), late middle age (50 to 64 years), young—old (65 to 74 years), old (75 to 85 years), and old–old (86 years and older). The group of people who are aged 85 years or older is the most rapidly growing segment of the older population (Fig. 12-1). People in this age group typically have a noticeable decline in functional ability and have one or more chronic disorders.

Aging is a multifactorial process with genetic and environmental components. Each system in an organism, each tissue in a system, and each cell type in a tissue appear to have its own trajectory of aging (Cristofalo et al., 1994). Theories of the biologic aspects of aging have been developed and studied (Kane et al., 1999). The theories can be divided into three groups: organ theories, physiological theories, and genome-based theories. The organ theories examine age changes in the body brought about by the possible initiation from a "master" organ system, such as the immune or neurological system. The physiologic theories analyze cell functioning as related to waste product accumulation or molecular changes. The genome-based theories attribute age changes to the individual's genetic endowment and suggest that a predetermined series of events programmed into cells or random mutations or cell errors are responsible for the process of aging. Probably no one theory can totally explain the aging process, but some or all of these theories may be involved in the complete explanation.

The nurse needs to be aware of several concepts in addressing the health care needs of older adults:

1. Age-related changes are gradual and individual, and different systems age at different rates within an individual. There is more intra-individual variability among older people than there is among younger people.
2. Complex functions that require multisystem coordination show the most obvious decline and require the greatest compensation and support.
3. Vulnerability to disease increases with age.
4. Stressful situations (physiologic or psychosocial) produce a more pronounced reaction in the elderly and require a longer period of time for readjustment (Berry & Davignon, 1991).

Although Americans are living longer, they are not necessarily healthier. With increasing age, they are at increased risk for illness. Chronic illnesses, such as arthritis, cardiac and vascular problems, and diabetes, are the major health problems of older people (Fig. 12-2). Because of the lifestyle changes in young and middle-aged adults, particularly in the areas of diet and exercise, in the near future, older adults may be sufficiently healthier that definitions and expectations of the aging process may need to be revised. At present, however, heart disease and stroke are the first and third leading cause of death of older adults (Fig. 12-3).

When older people become ill, there is frequently an atypical presentation, such as missing or altered symptoms. Confusion is often one of the earliest indications of a change in health status. Restlessness, confusion, or altered mentation often occur in the presence of illness and should not be confused with dementia, providing that dementia was not present before the illness. Acute onset or unexplained deterioration of health should be carefully evaluated and not accepted as a normal concomitant of aging.

The older person who is ill has many adjustments and adaptations to make. The social supports (family and friends) available to that person may be fewer or less able to be supportive because of their own debilities, such as a spouse who is also ill or an adult child who has other responsibilities.

Apprehension, worry, and fear of becoming dependent and helpless may add to the emotional burden of the current illness. Of those older adults between 80 and 84 years of age, 30% require assistance with daily activities, and of those adults who are 85 years and older, 50% require assistance.

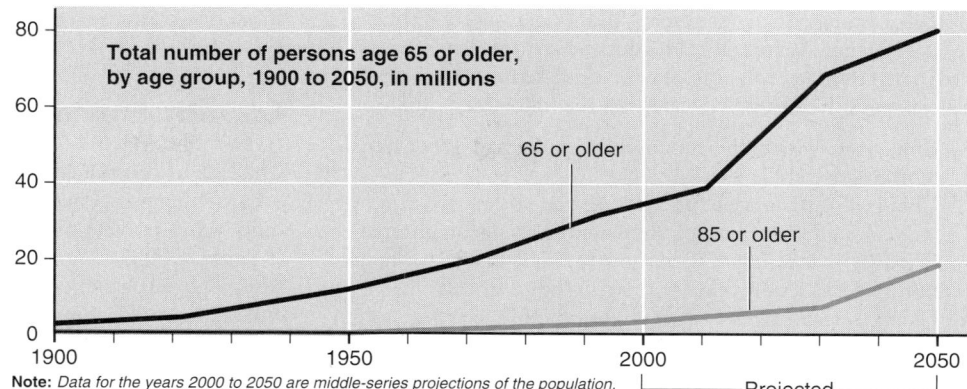

■ **Figure 12–1.** Projected growth in population (65 years and older), by age group, in millions, 1900–2050. (From Federal Interagency Forum on Aging-Related Statistics. [2000]. *Older Americans 2000: Key indicators of well-being.* Federal Interagency Forum on Aging-Related Statistics, Washington, DC: U.S. Government Printing Office.)

Note: *Data for the years 2000 to 2050 are middle-series projections of the population.*
Reference population: *These data refer to the resident population.*
Source: *U.S. Census Bureau, Decennial Census Data and Population Projections*

- In 2000, there are an estimated 35 million people age 65 or older in the United States, accounting for almost 13% of the total population. The number of older Americans has increased more than ten-fold since 1900, when there were 3 million people age 65 or older (4% of the total population). Despite the growth of the older population, the United States is a relatively young country when compared with other developed nations. In many industrialized countries, older persons account for 15% or more of the total population.

- In 2011, the "baby boom" generation will begin to turn 65, and by 2030, it is projected that one in five people will be age 65 or older. The size of the older population is projected to double over the next 30 years, growing to 70 million by 2030.

- As in most countries of the world, there are more older women than older men in the United States, and the proportion of the population that is female increases with age. In 2000, women are estimated to account for 58% of the population age 65 and older and 70% of the population age 85 and older.

- The population age 85 and older is currently the fastest growing segment of the older population. In 2000, an estimated 2% of the population is age 85 and older. By 2050, the percentage in this age group is projected to increase to almost 5% of the U.S. population. The size of this age group is especially important for the future of our health care system, because these individuals tend to be in poorer health and require more services than the younger old.

Older patients require careful, thorough nursing management during an acute illness and afterward. Discharge planning that begins with the admission process and includes consideration of living arrangements, care providers, and support services is especially important for older patients, who are often adversely affected by the shorter hospitalizations and fewer home nursing care visits that accompany managed care.

GENERAL PHYSIOLOGIC CHANGES

Aging is an integral part of the continuum that begins at conception and ends at death. As contrasted with the developmental growth and maturation of childhood and adolescence, aging is characterized by a decline in function and by changes that are decremental in nature. The inability to maintain homeostasis

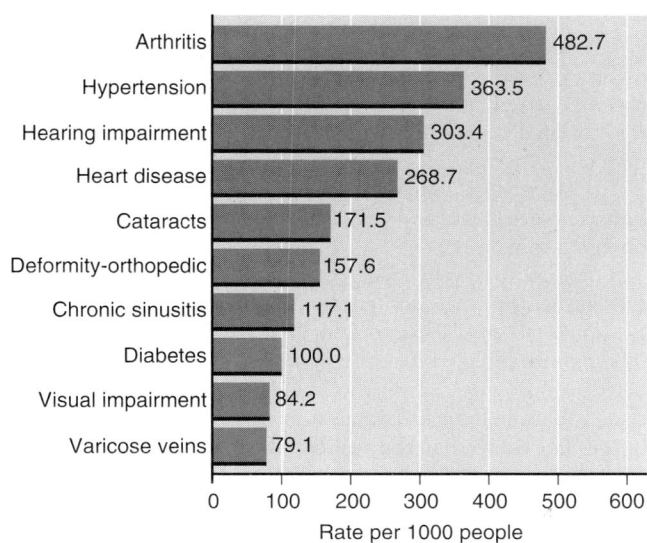

■ **Figure 12–2.** The top 10 chronic conditions for people older than 65 years of age, 1996. (From Adams, P. F., Hendershot, G. E. & Marano, M. A. [1999]. Current estimates from the National Health Interview Survey, 1996. National Center for Health Statistics, *Vital Health Statistics,* 10 [200], 1–148).

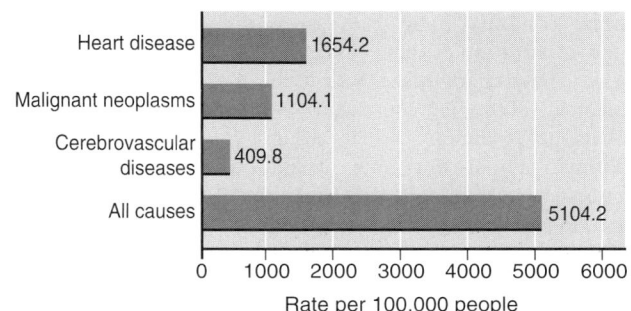

■ **Figure 12–3.** The top causes of death among older people, 65 or older. (From Arias, E. & Smith B. L. [2003]. Deaths: Preliminary data for 2001. *National Vital Statistics Reports,* 51 [5], p. 27.)

in a broad range of environments and with a variety of physiologic challenges is central to the decline in function.

Changes related to aging may be classified or categorized in several ways. Kenny (1985) suggests the following scheme:

1. Change in which the function is totally lost (e.g., female reproductive ability)
2. Changes in or loss of function related to loss of structure (e.g., altered kidney function related to loss of nephrons)
3. Changes in efficiency without structural loss (e.g., reduction in conduction velocity in aging nerve fibers)
4. Changes resulting from interruptions in a control system (e.g., the increase in gonadotropins in women with the reduction in feedback control of sex hormones)
5. Rarely, increased function (e.g., secretion of antidiuretic hormone in response to osmotic challenge)

In reviewing the age-related changes in selected systems, the changes in structure and function of each system are discussed along with the clinical implications of the changes.

CARDIOVASCULAR CHANGES

One of the challenges in discussing aging changes in any system is that of separating changes that can be attributed only to age from changes related to disease. This is particularly true in the cardiovascular system. This discussion attempts to identify what is known about changes in cardiovascular structure and function that result from aging changes and, subsequently, increase vulnerability to disease.

Cardiac Structural Changes

Although there are some differences in findings, it is now agreed that there is myocardial hypertrophy from aging alone. Cross-sectional studies of normotensive subjects without cardiovascular disease indicate that left ventricular wall thickness increases progressively with age in men and women (Lakatta & Levy, 2003b). The total number of left ventricular (LV) myocytes decreases with advancing age (Lakatta, 2000). Some myocytes are lost because of apoptosis and are replaced by fibrous tissue. Age-related increases in the amount of collagen and changes in collagen structure (increased cross-linkages) occur within the myocardium (Lakatta & Levy, 2003b). Surviving myocytes increase in size, producing age-related hypertrophy. A modest increase in LV cavitary size may occur and the cardiac silhouette may be enlarged slightly on the chest x-ray. These changes are within the clinically normal range (Lakatta, 2000).

Changes in the myocardial cells include the accumulation of lipofuscin (a lipid-containing material), which is thought to be a consequence of biologic aging; deposits of amyloid; and an increase in myocardial collagen and connective tissues (Kane et al., 1999; Taffet & Lakatta, 2003). The effects of these changes on function are unclear but may contribute to increased ventricular stiffness associated with aging and with hypertension.

Aging changes in the valves are characterized by increases in fibrosis, collagen degeneration, lipid accumulation, and calcification. Calcifications of the aortic valve ring can contribute to stenosis and valvular incompetence in aging (Taffet & Lakatta, 2003).

Cardiac Functional Changes

Changes in ventricular filling (preload) and diastolic function occur with aging. There is progressive slowing of the early diastolic filling rate coupled with augmented late diastolic filling (Lakatta, 2003). Augmentation of late diastolic filling results from vigorous atrial contraction and is accompanied by atrial enlargement. Despite these changes in filling, end-diastolic volume in the sitting or supine position is not usually reduced in women and is slightly increased in men (Lakatta, 2003). The change in end diastolic volume from rest to exercise increases with age (Fleg et al., 1995). This refutes the widely held belief that LV filling is impaired in the healthy, older heart.

Clinical implications of age-related changes in ventricular filling include greater dependence on atrial contraction, which is lost with atrial fibrillation, and greater sensitivity to hypovolemia. The importance of adequate intravascular volume increases further with tachycardia, which limits filling time.

There is no change in resting systolic function, heart rate, or cardiac output during healthy aging (Lakatta, 2003). Maximum heart rate during dynamic exercise decreases with age (maximum heart rate = 220 − age). This age-related decrease in maximum heart rate explains the age-related decrease in maximum cardiac output in healthy people. Maximum cardiac output reserve is approximately 3.5-fold in younger and 2.5-fold in older people (Lakatta, 2003).

Electrical System

Controversy and conflicting evidence exists about the effects of aging on the cardiac electrical system. In the absence of disease or extreme stress on the cardiac function, the electrical system is adequate for normal conductivity. Limited data support a marked age-associated increase in the prevalence and complexity of ventricular ectopy at rest and during exercise (Lakatta, 2003). In the Baltimore Longitudinal Study on Aging, isolated ventricular ectopy occurred at rest in 8.6% of men older than age 60 years compared with 0.5% in men aged 20 to 40 years (Fleg & Kennedy, 1982). The relationship between older age and greater ventricular ectopy was not observed in women.

There appears to be a decrease in the number of pacemaker cells in the sinus node and greater irregularity in their shape. By age 75 years, only 10% of original nodal cells remain, although this is compatible with normal pacemaker activity. The number of conducting cells in the atrioventricular (AV) node and the left bundle branch decreases in people older than 70 years of age. The decrease in the number of cells in the bundle of His begins after age 40, and after age 50 years in the right bundle. Some studies have noted increases in fat and collagen in the AV node and bundle (Klausner & Schwartz, 1985). Idiopathic bundle-branch fibrosis is a common cause of chronic atrioventricular block in people older than 65 years of age. The atrial and AV nodal refractory periods increase with age. It is not clear whether these changes are caused by altered catecholamine or vagal stimulation with age.

The normal electrocardiogram shows little change with age. There may be small increases in the PR, QRS, and QT intervals, along with a small decrease in the amplitude of the QRS complex. When challenged by disease or adverse circumstances, the age-dependent changes in the electrical system increase the potential for conduction difficulties.

Vascular System

Structural Changes

With advancing age, a series of structural changes take place in the vascular system. Central arterial vessel diameter tends to increase and the intimal and medial layers tend to thicken (Bilato & Crow, 1996). In the arterial intima, the endothelial cells become irregular in size and shape with an increase in connective tissue. Calcification and lipid deposition also occur. Some scientists argue that intimal media (IM) thickening is an early stage of atherosclerosis. IM thickness predicts the co-existence of silent coronary artery disease in screened subjects (Nagai et al., 1998). However, IM thickening may be an intrinsic age-related change that provides a foundation for the subsequent development of atherosclerosis (Lakatta & Levy, 2003a). Similar controversy surrounds age-associated endothelial dysfunction, systemic arterial stiffening, and arterial pulse-pressure widening. Whether age-related changes or early atherosclerosis, combinations of these processes occur to varying degrees in older people. Age-associated vascular changes interact with traditional cardiovascular risk factors to produce clinical atherosclerosis.

Functional Changes

Age-associated increase in IM thickness is accompanied by increased arterial stiffness. Arterial stiffness increases the pulse-wave velocity (PWV), transmitting the pulse wave faster than the actual movement of blood. When the pulse wave reaches branch points in the arterial tree, the wave is reflected back toward the heart. At distal locations, the reflected waves augment systolic pressure and reduce diastolic pressure (Rooke, 2000). Data from epidemiological studies indicate that increased PWV is seen with age and also in the context of atherosclerosis and diabetes (Dart & Kingwell, 2001; Gimbrone, 2001).

Elevation of the blood pressure is not a normal age change; however, it is a change that frequently occurs with the process of aging. Isolated systolic hypertension, in particular, is a distinct pathologic process and accounts for more than 50% of cases of hypertension. It is defined as a systolic pressure greater than 140 mm Hg and diastolic pressure below 90 mm Hg and is probably the result of arterial stiffening and loss of arterial compliance that occur with aging (Chobanian et al., 2003). Treatment of systolic hypertension follows the same principles as treatment of hypertension in general (see Chapter 39).

Autonomic Nervous System Modulation

Optimal cardiovascular function requires communications between the cardiovascular system and autonomic nervous system (ANS). Under stress the sympathetic component of the ANS prevails, producing arterial vasoconstriction while increasing heart rate and contractility. At rest the parasympathetic nervous system prevails, slowing down the heart rate. The extent of parasympathetic tone is small in older people. Heart rate variability, a reflection of balance between the sympathetic and parasympathetic nervous systems, declines steadily with aging (Lakatta & Levy, 2003b). The decline in heart rate variability is related to decreased parasympathetic activity, because it is the low frequency component that is reduced (Tappet & Lakatta, 2003). Decreased heart rate variability has been associated with poor outcomes in people with cardiovascular disease.

The aging cardiovascular system demonstrates decreased response to beta-adrenoreceptor stimulation (Rooke, 2000). Decreased responsiveness is not caused by a reduced number of beta-receptors, but to a decrease in affinity of beta-agonists for the receptors and reduced efficacy of postreceptor intercellular coupling responsible for muscle contraction (Lakatta, 1993). Stimulation of beta$_1$-receptors in the ventricles increases heart rate and contractility. Increased end-diastolic volume also increases cardiac contractility (Frank-Starling mechanism). If the ventricular response to beta$_1$-receptor stimulation is reduced in the aging heart, the ventricles are more dependent on adequate filling. Consequently, the aging heart is less tolerant of hypovolemia. Decreased beta-receptor responsiveness in the vasculature produces less vasodilation and higher resting blood pressure.

RESPIRATORY CHANGES

In the absence of disease, the changes that occur in the lungs from maturity through the aging process are so gradual that the lungs are capable of providing normal gas exchange throughout life. However, the lungs are continuously exposed to the external environment and to various internal assaults; hence, it is difficult to separate changes caused solely by aging from those related to injury or disease processes.

Structural Changes

The aging lung undergoes gradual, subtle changes. Host defense mechanisms of airway clearance and immune system function respond less vigorously with age. Studies of bronchoalveolar lavage show more neutrophils and fewer macrophages in fluid from older (70 to 80 years) than from younger subjects (19 to 34 years) (Thompson et al., 1992). The activity of the cilia is decreased, producing less ciliary clearance. Decreased cough reflex related to decreased cilia activity together with decreased immune system function increase susceptibility to lower respiratory infection, mechanical irritation, and, possibly, tumor formation.

There is an age-related increase in the ratio of elastin-to-collagen in the lung parenchyma that may contribute to increased lung compliance, reduced expiratory airway diameter, or airflow limitation (Zeleznik, 2003). Increased calcification of the thoracic joints (spine, ribs, and sternum) and reduced intercostal muscle strength produce a decrease in chest wall compliance with aging and an increased anteroposterior diameter of the chest. The resulting reduced mobility of the thorax leads to increased residual air volume and to a breathing pattern that is augmented by the increased use of diaphragmatic and abdominal muscles in breathing.

Functional Changes

The typical changes in lung function with age include decreased lung recoil, increased closing volume, altered lung volumes, and decreased maximum expiratory flow volume (Krumpe et al., 1985). Non-emphysematous enlargement of the alveoli is accepted as a normal change of aging. The effect of this change is decreased efficiency of gas-diffusing capacity and increased residual volume.

During expiration, airways in the dependent lung regions close and no longer participate in respiration. With aging, the lung volume at which these airways close (closing volume) may exceed the functional residual capacity, leading to closure of distal airways before the end of a normal breath (McClaren et al., 1995). Loss of lung recoil and the effects of gravity on the dependent areas of the lungs allow the airways to close at a higher lung volume and lead to nonuniformity of ventilation (Fig. 12-4).

After adjustment for height, total lung capacity does not change with age (McClaran et al., 1995). There is an increase, however, in residual volume for reasons previously discussed and in the ratio of residual volume-to-total lung capacity. When increased closing capacity closes terminal airways, these airways no longer actively participate in ventilation, resulting in reduced maximal expiratory flow (V_{max}) and in decreased expiratory volume measured in the first second of forced expiration (FEV_1).

As a result of changes in airway closure, diffusing capacity, lung volumes, and lung structure, a lower arterial oxygen tension

is seen in older adults. The arterial oxygen (PaO_2) decreases and alveolar—arterial oxygen difference (A-aO_2) widens, whereas arterial carbon dioxide ($PaCO_2$) and pH remain unchanged.

In summary, although the lung undergoes some structural and functional changes, the nondiseased respiratory system continues to be capable of supporting daily function throughout life. The effect of changes in the respiratory system may become evident under situations of high physiologic demand.

RENAL CHANGES

The kidney is an organ with complex functions that are intimately related with other organ systems, such as the cardiovascular, endocrine, and neurological systems. In discussing the aging kidney, changes are discussed as they relate to intrinsic changes in the kidney as well as those adaptive changes that result from the effects of other systems.

Structural Changes

The volume and weight of the kidney reach maximum in the third decade of life, start to decline during the fourth decade, and continue to decline throughout the remainder of the lifespan. Most of the decline in volume and weight is in the cortex, with a steady decline in the number of nephrons. Renal arteries undergo age-related thickening, producing a decline in renal blood flow and an increase in vascular resistance with age.

Functional Changes

Average renal blood flow decreases approximately 10% per decade, and the majority of older adults lose approximately 10% of glomerular filtration rate (GFR) per decade after the fourth decade. The reduced renal blood flow and decreased number of nephrons contribute to the reduction of GFR. Because of the decrease in muscle mass with aging, increased serum creatinine does not correspond with reduced GFR. Creatinine clearance, not serum creatinine, should be the criterion for assessing renal function in older people. The Cockcroft-Gault equation predicts creatinine clearance from serum creatinine. For men: creatinine clearance = (140 − age) (weight in kg) ÷ (72 × serum creatinine measured in mg/dL). The results are adjusted for women by multiplying by 0.85.

The clinical importance of this formula is apparent when determinations about kidney function and appropriate drug dosage need to be made. The steady decline in renal function impairs the ability of the kidney to excrete a salt or water load and reduces the renal clearance of those medications normally removed by the kidney (Wiggins, 2003).

The aging kidney's tendency to lose salt is related to nephron loss, with increased osmotic load per nephron leading to mild osmotic diuresis and the age-related changes in the renin-aldosterone system. Lower levels of renin (decreased by 30% to 50% in older adults) are related to 30% to 50% reductions in plasma concentration of aldosterone. When this is combined with the decreased GFR, older people are at risk for expansion

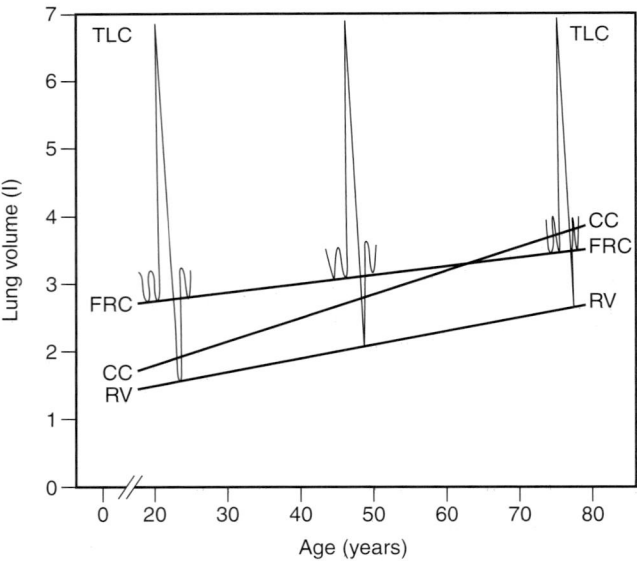

■ **Figure 12–4.** Changes in lung volumes with age. CC, closing capacity; FRC, functional residual capacity; RV, residual volume; TLC, total lung capacity. (Peterson, D. D., & Fishman, A. P. [1982]. The lungs in later life. In A. P. Fishman [Ed.], *Update: Pulmonary diseases and disorders* [pp. 123–136]. New York: McGraw-Hill.)

of extracellular fluid volume when faced with an acute salt load (from diet, drugs, or intravenous fluids).

The limited ability of the kidney to regulate salt balance is compounded by changes in water regulation. The aging kidney exhibits a modest age-related impairment in the ability to dilute urine and excrete a water load. Inability to dilute urine maximally is related to decreased GFR and an inability to suppress antidiuretic hormone. The ability to concentrate urine declines moderately also, with the usual value (specific gravity) of 1.032 decreasing to 1.024 at age 80 years (Miller, 2003). Therefore, the older person has more difficulty retaining fluid when it is necessary, as in situations of decreased circulating fluid volume (e.g., dehydration), and in excreting fluid, as in situations of excess circulating fluid volume (e.g., congestive heart failure).

Although baseline homeostasis of fluids and electrolytes is maintained with normal aging, there is a progressive loss of renal reserve. Vitamin D hydroxylation in the kidney is reduced and may contribute to a decreased intestinal absorption of calcium. Decreased renal reserve manifests in older patients' vulnerability to renal failure during acute illness. There are many functions of the kidney (e.g., erythropoietin production, hormone metabolism) that have yet to be thoroughly studied. Of those changes that have been described, the clinical effects on drugs and their excretion and on fluid balance are of primary importance.

HEPATIC CHANGES

Structural Changes

The proportion of liver to body weight remains constant through middle age and decreases gradually after age 70 years (Mezey, 2003). Liver histology in older adults shows more lipofuscin pigment and giant hepatocytes than in younger individuals. In healthy subjects, liver size, blood flow, and perfusion decrease by 30% to 40% between the third and tenth decade (Hall, 2003).

Functional Changes

There is no change in level of serum bilirubin, aminotransferases, or alkaline phosphatase with aging. Age-related change in liver function is small and, with the exception of some enzymes involved in drug metabolism, is not clinically significant. There is a decrease in the hepatic clearance of drugs, particularly those that have a low-extraction ratio and whose elimination is dependent on the cytochrome P450 system.

EFFECTS OF AGING ON PHARMACOKINETICS

Drug Absorption

Little is known about absorption of oral drugs from the intestines, but it seems to be mildly decreased or unchanged with age. Absorption appears to be the pharmacokinetic parameter least affected by advancing age.

Drug Distribution

Decreased serum albumin concentration is linked to decreased binding capacity of drugs. Drugs that are bound are inactive in terms of therapeutic effect. Unbound, or free, drug is free to exert therapeutic effects. This is one reason why a smaller dosage of drug may exert the same therapeutic effect in an older person as a standard dosage in a younger person.

With aging, lean body mass decreases by approximately 10% and body fat increases by the same amount. This, along with decreased total body water, may also contribute to the retention of fat-soluble drugs, so that they exert effects over a longer period of time because of depot action.

Drug Metabolism and Excretion

The effects of aging on drug metabolism depend on the pathway of metabolism in the liver. There is evidence that first-phase metabolism decreases with age (Kane et al., 1999). The liver microsomal drug oxidation/reduction system (P450 system) is responsible for the metabolism of many drugs. Although drug-metabolizing enzymes in the cytochrome P450 system do not decrease with age, hepatic clearance of drugs metabolized by this system is often reduced in older people. This is likely caused by the multiple drug and environmental factors that affect the cytochrome P450 system.

The other route of drug excretion is the kidney. As was previously described, changes in renal plasma flow and GFR may lead to decreased excretion of active drug with consequent prolonged half-lives of drugs and sustained or increased levels of free drug in the serum.

As a result of these changes in absorption, distribution, metabolism, and excretion, greater care must be exercised with drug administration to older patients. Administering drugs in smaller doses and less frequently may accomplish an adequate therapeutic effect. If adverse reactions or side effects occur, it may be more prudent to discontinue a suspected drug rather than add another drug to counteract the effects. Older people are vulnerable to adverse effects from drugs for many reasons (e.g., age changes, chronic conditions, polypharmacy). Consequently, clinical professionals must exercise caution and responsibility when drugs and older adults are concerned.

SUMMARY

In summary, cardiovascular function declines progressively with age, and because of the inter-relatedness of the major systems, it is affected by and affects the other systems as well. Respiratory, renal, and hepatic functions are independent and interconnected with cardiovascular function so that normal age-related changes in any or all of these systems exacerbate changes in other systems. One significant area in which this interconnectedness is exemplified is in drug therapy. The ongoing question and dilemma for the health care provider is differentiating between decline in function that occurs with age and problems resulting from specific cardiovascular diseases.

REFERENCES

Adams, P. F., Hendershot, G. E. & Marano, M. A. (1999). Current estimates from the National Health Interview Survey, 1996. National Center for Health Statistics. *Vital Health Statistics,* 10 (200).

Berry, A. L. & Davignon, D. (1991). Changes with aging. In M. Patrick et al. (Eds.), *Medical-surgical nursing* (2nd ed., pp. 55–70). Philadelphia: Lippincott.

Bilato, C. & Crow, M. T. (1996). Atherosclerosis and vascular biology of aging. *Aging,* 8, 221–234.

Chobanian, A. V., Bakris, G. L., Black, H. R. et al. (2003). The seventh report of the Joint National Committee on Prevention, Detection, Evaluation, and Treatment of High Blood Pressure: The JNC 7 Report. *JAMA,* 289, 2560–2572.

Cristofalo, V. J., Gerhard, G. S., & Pignolo, R. J. (1994). Molecular biology of aging. *Surgical Clinics of North Ameerica,* 74, 1–21.

Dart, A. M., & Kingwell, B. A. (2001). Pulse pressure: a review of mechanisms and clinical relevance. *Journal of the American College of Cardiology,* 37, 975–984.

Federal Interagency Forum on Aging-Related Statistics (2000). *Older Americans 2000: Key indicators of well-being.* Federal Interagency Forum on Aging-Related Statistics, Washington, DC: U.S. Government Printing Office.

Fleg, J. L., O'Connor, R. C., & Gerstenblith, G., et al. (1995). Impact of age on the cardiovascular response to dynamic upright exercise in healthy men and women. *Journal of Applied Physiology,* 78, 890–900.

Fleg, J. L., & Kennedy, H. L. (1982). Cardiac arrhythmias in a healthy elderly population: detection by 24-hour ambulatory electrocardiography. *Chest,* 81, 302–307.

Gimbrone, M. A. (1999). Vascular endothelium, hemodynamic forces, and atherogenesis. *American Journal of Pathology,* 155, 1–5.

Hall, K. E. (2003). Effect of aging on gastrointestinal function. In W. R. Hazzard, J. P. Blass, & J. B. Halter, et al. (Eds.), *Principles of geriatric medicine & gerontology* (5th ed., pp. 593–600). New York: McGraw-Hill.

Kane, R. L., Ouslander, J. G., & Abrass, I. B. (1999). *Essentials of clinical geriatrics* (4th ed.). New York: McGraw-Hill.

Kenny, R. A. (1985). Physiology of aging. *Clinics in Geriatric Medicine,* 1, 37–60.

Klausner, S. & Schwartz, A. (1985). The aging heart. *Clinics in Geriatric Medicine,* 1, 119–142.

Krumpe, P., Knudson, R., & Parsons, G., et al. (1985). The aging respiratory system. *Clinics in Geriatric Medicine,* 1, 143–176.

Lakatta, E. G. (2000). Cardiovascular aging in health. *Clinics in Geriatric Medicine,* 16, 419–444.

Lakatta, E. G. (2003). Arterial and cardiac aging: Major shareholders in cardiovascular disease enterprises. Part III: Cellular and molecular clues to heart and arterial aging. *Circulation,* 107, 490–497.

Lakatta, E. G., & Levy, D. (2003a). Arterial and cardiac aging: Major shareholders in cardiovascular disease enterprises. Part I: Aging arteries: A "set up" for vascular disease. *Circulation,* 107, 139–146.

Lakatta, E. G., & Levy, D. (2003b). Arterial and cardiac aging: Major shareholders in cardiovascular disease enterprises. Part II: The aging heart in health: Links to heart disease. *Circulation,* 107, 346–354.

McClaran, S. R., Babcock, M. A., & Pegelow, D. F., et al. (1995). Longitudinal effects of aging on lung function at rest and exercise in healthy active fit elderly adults. *Journal of Applied Physiology,* 78, 1957–1968.

Miller, M. (2003). Disorders of fluid balance. In W. R. Hazzard, J. P. Blass, & J. B. Halter, et al. (Eds.), *Principles of geriatric medicine & gerontology* (5th ed., pp. 581–592). New York: McGraw-Hill.

Nagai, J., Metter, E. J., & Earley, C. J., et al (1998). Increased carotid artery intimal-medial thickness in asymptomatic older subjects with exercise-induced myocardial ischemia. *Circulation,* 98, 1504–1509.

Peterson, D. D., & Fishman, A. P. (1982). The lungs in later life. In A. P. Fishman (Ed.), *Update: Pulmonary diseases and disorders* (pp. 123–136). New York: McGraw-Hill.

Rooke, G. A. (2000). Autonomic and cardiovascular function in the geriatric patient. *Anesthesiology Clinics of North America,* 18, 31–46.

Taffet, G. E., & Lakatta, E. G. (2003). Aging of the cardiovascular system. In W. R. Hazzard, J. P. Blass, J. B. Halter, J. G. Ouslander, & M. E. Tinetti (Eds.), *Principles of geriatric medicine & gerontology* (5th ed., pp. 403–421). New York: McGraw-Hill.

Thompson, A. B., Scholer, S. G., & Daughton, D. M., et al. (1992). Altered epithelial lining fluid parameters in old normal individuals. *Journal of Gerontology,* 47, 171–176.

Wiggins, J. (2003). Changes in renal function. In W. R. Hazzard, J. P. Blass, & J. B. Halter, et al. (Eds.), *Principles of geriatric medicine & gerontology* (5th ed., pp. 543–549). New York: McGraw-Hill.

Zeleznik, J. (2003). Normative aging of the respiratory system. *Clinics in Geriatric Medicine,* 19, 1–18.

Assessment of Heart Disease

13

History Taking and Physical Examination

BARBARA S. LEVINE

Assessment data, which are obtained from the patient's history, physical examination, and diagnostic tests, are used to formulate clinical diagnoses, establish patient goals, plan care, and evaluate patient outcomes. A complete history and physical examination includes the same content areas, whether elicited by nurses or physicians. A complete history and physical examination is impractical in most clinical situations. The inclusion of appropriate content areas is determined by the patient's clinical condition and the purpose and context of the clinical encounter. Specific content areas may be investigated in greater detail by clinicians from different disciplines, and the data may be used in different ways. Nurses must be able to incorporate historical data into the nursing assessment so the interdependent nursing and medical responsibilities are completed in the correct priority sequence. Conversely, physicians need to be aware of the data elicited by nurses so the complete database is the foundation for the total plan of care.

The provision of culturally appropriate care requires understanding of and sensitivity to differences in health beliefs and practices that reflect cultures or subcultures. The challenge is to be sensitive to cultural influences that may affect the clinical encounter without stereotyping the patient based on limited knowledge of the culture of origin. Three overarching concepts that are influenced by culture and affect the clinical encounter are perception of illness or explanatory model, patterns of kinship and decision making, and comfort with touch (Abbott et al., 2002).

This chapter focuses on history taking and physical examination of the patient with heart disease. Emphasis is placed on those sections of the health history and physical examination that are affected by heart disease. General assessment techniques, with their rationale, are described. Competence in obtaining a history and in performing a physical examination cannot be achieved simply by reading the material presented. It is vitally important to become actively involved in clinical assessment, ideally with a qualified preceptor. Many hours of practice are required before the beginning student becomes skilled in assessment techniques.

CARDIOVASCULAR HISTORY

Cardiac patients who are acutely ill require a different initial history than do cardiac patients with stable or chronic conditions. A patient experiencing a myocardial infarction requires immediate, and possibly life-saving, medical and nursing interventions (e.g., relief of chest discomfort and treatment of arrhythmia) rather than an extensive interview. For this patient, asking a few, well-chosen questions regarding chest discomfort using the patient's descriptors is important. In addition, associated symptoms (such as shortness of breath or palpitations), drug allergies and reactions, current medications, history of cardiac and other major illnesses, and smoking history should be determined while assessing vital signs (heart rate and rhythm and blood pressure) and starting an intravenous line. As the patient's condition stabilizes, a more extensive history should be obtained. Cardiac patients who are not acutely ill benefit from a more detailed history and physical examination.

A comprehensive history includes the following areas:

- Identifying information
- Chief complaint or presenting problem
- History of the present illness
- Past history
- Review of systems
- Family history
- Personal and social history
- Perceived health status
- Functional patterns

The responsibility for obtaining particular portions of the health history varies with practice model and setting. In traditional, hospital-based practice models, the first six areas of the history are usually obtained by a physician, some data related to personal and social history are obtained by a physician and some by a nurse, and data related to perceived health status and functional patterns are obtained by a nurse. In collaborative practice models, all data may be obtained by an advanced-practice nurse, or responsibility for all areas of data collection

229

Table 13-1 ■ DIFFERENTIAL DIAGNOSIS OF EPISODIC CHEST PAIN RESEMBLING ANGINA PECTORIS

Diagnosis	Duration	Quality	Provocation	Relief	Location	Comment
Effort angina	5–15 min	Visceral (pressure)	During effort or motion	Rest, nitroglycerin	Substernal radiates	First episode vivid
Rest angina	5–15 min	Visceral (pressure)	Spontaneous	Nitroglycerin	Substernal radiates	Often nocturnal
Mitral prolapse	Minutes to hours	Superficial (rarely visceral)	Spontaneous (no pattern)	Time	Left anterior	No pattern, variable character
Esophageal reflux	10–60 min	Visceral	Recumbency, lack of food	Food, antacid	Substernal epigastric	Rarely radiates
Esophageal spasm	50–60 min	Visceral	Spontaneous, cold liquids, exercise	Nitroglycerin	Substernal radiates	Mimics angina
Peptic ulcer	Hours	Visceral (burning)	Lack of food, "acid" foods	Food, antacids	Epigastric substernal	
Biliary disease	Hours	Visceral (wax and wane)	Spontaneous, food	Time, analgesia	Epigastric radiates	Colic
Cervical disc	Variable (gradually subsides)	Superficial	Head and neck movement, palpation	Time, analgesia	Arm, neck	Not relieved by rest
Hyperventilation	2–3 min	Visceral	Emotion tachypnea	Stimulus removal	Substernal	Facial paresthesia
Musculoskeletal	Variable	Superficial	Movement, palpation	Time, analgesia	Multiple	Tenderness
Pulmonary	30 minutes+	Visceral (pressure)	Often spontaneous	Rest, time, bronchodilator	Substernal	Dyspneic

From Christie, L. G. Jr., & Conti, C. R. (1981). Systematic approach to the evaluation of angina-like chest pain. *American Heart Journal, 102,* 899.

may be shared by the physician, advanced-practice nurse, nurse, and other members of the health care team. The cardiac nurse uses the data to make informed clinical judgments, to monitor change over time, to identify patient and family learning needs, and to coordinate care across settings.

Health History

The health history is the patient's story of his or her diseases, symptoms, illness experiences, and responses to actual and potential health problems. Because concepts of health and healing are rooted in culture, it is essential to elicit information about the person's beliefs about the causes, symptoms, and treatment of illness. Empathy, openness, and interest communicated by the clinician will enable patients to share their perspectives and beliefs.

The history-taking process may be the first phase in establishing a therapeutic relationship. The history is a precise, concise, chronologic description of the patient's current health status. The patient is the primary source of historical data; however, questioning of family members or close friends may provide essential information about symptoms and the impact of heart disease on family members. For example, the bed partner is more likely than the patient to provide a history of periodic respiration or sleep apnea. Review of records from previous encounters is a valuable secondary source of historical data.

The primary symptoms of heart disease include chest discomfort, dyspnea, syncope, palpitations, edema, cough, hemoptysis, and excess fatigue. Heart disease develops slowly, and the patient may have a long period of asymptomatic disease and may present initially with acute collapse. To describe the health history, a sample symptom, chest discomfort, is used throughout. Guidelines are useful in differentiating chest discomfort due to

serious, life-threatening conditions from those conditions that are less serious or would be treated in a different manner (Goldman, 1998). Table 13-1 summarizes conditions associated with chest discomfort.

Identifying Information

The patient's name, the name by which he or she prefers to be called, his or her age and birth date, and date and time of the interview are all recorded under identification of the patient. Country of origin, religious or cultural group, education, and socioeconomic level constitute optional information that may be included. It is assumed that all data in the history are obtained from the patient; when this is not the case, secondary data sources (e.g., family member, clinical records) should be identified. The use of an interpreter should also be recorded.

Chief Complaint or Presenting Problem

The chief complaint or presenting problem is the reason the person has sought health care and represents his or her priority for treatment. It should be recorded within quotation marks exactly as stated. The chief complaint also should indicate duration, such as "chest discomfort for 2 hours."

An asymptomatic patient may present because of a community screening activity (e.g., "high blood cholesterol discovered on finger-stick last month") or because of a positive diagnostic result (e.g., "positive perfusion scan last week").

A patient may have more than one chief complaint. Some complaints are closely related and may be listed together, such as "chest discomfort and weakness for 2 hours." If complaints are unrelated, they should be listed separately in the order of importance to the patient. In general, "the greater the number of symptoms, the less the significance of each" (Marriott, 1993).

There are four important points to remember when evaluating chest discomfort (Underhill, 1984):

1. For a patient who has a history of or who is at risk for development of coronary heart disease, always assume that the chest discomfort is secondary to ischemia until proven otherwise. This practice is important because unrelieved myocardial ischemia is immediately life threatening and can extend infarct size, resulting in serious complications such as lethal arrhythmia or cardiogenic shock. Chest discomfort related to other conditions, such as pulmonary emboli, usually is not as immediately life threatening.

2. There may be little correlation between the severity of the chest discomfort and the gravity of its cause. That is, pain is a subjective experience and depends, in part, on a lifetime of learned reactions to it. A stoic person may not admit to having much discomfort and yet may be having a large myocardial infarction. Another person may express extreme pain and yet may be experiencing stable angina rather than an acute myocardial infarction. Stress can increase pain. Taking into account the patient's usual response to pain (often obtained from a family member) may help the nurse interpret the patient's pain response better. In addition, older adults or people with diabetes may have altered sensory perception and little or no discomfort in the presence of severe disease (Chatterjee, 1991b). When present, positive objective signs, such as ST segment shifts on the electrocardiogram (ECG), are clear indicators of the significance of the subjective symptom. It is important to realize that the absence of electrocardiographic criteria for ischemia or infarction does not eliminate the clinical significance of the chest pain.

3. There is a poor correlation between the location of chest discomfort and its source because of the concept of "referred pain," which is pain originating in one location but being interpreted by the patient as occurring in another location. Commonly, cardiac discomfort is perceived as being in the arm, jaw, neck, or epigastric area rather than in the chest.

4. The patient may have more than one clinical problem occurring simultaneously, particularly if he or she has delayed seeking medical assistance.

History of The Present Illness

For the symptomatic patient, obtaining the history of the present illness starts with a more detailed discussion of the chief complaint. Begin with an open-ended question, such as "Tell me more about your chest discomfort." There is a wide range in patients' abilities to express thoughts accurately, chronologically, and succinctly. Some patients need guidance more than others. Listen to the patient. It is best to let patients tell their stories in a comfortable manner. However, patients who appear to be rambling need to be redirected by clarifying or leading questions. The information that must be obtained when describing any symptom is the time and manner of onset, frequency and duration, location, quality, quantity, setting, associated symptoms, alleviating or aggravating factors, pertinent negative responses, impact of the symptom on usual or desired activities, and the meaning attributed to the symptom by the patient.

The *time of onset* should be recorded, when possible, with both the date and time (e.g., "9 PM on December 22nd." When the patient presents with chest discomfort, it is essential to know how long the discomfort has been present and if it has been present continuously since onset. The *manner of onset* is the way in which the symptom began. For example, discomfort may begin suddenly and reach maximum intensity immediately, or there may be a growing awareness of the discomfort over time. *Frequency and duration* should be stated specifically rather than generally (e.g., "once a week," "once a day," or "more than three times a day"). Likewise, patients should be assisted to express the duration of the discomfort, as in "2 minutes," "15 minutes," or "1 hour." For patients with a history of angina, it is also important to determine if there has been any change in frequency or duration of chest discomfort, which suggests worsening of the underlying disease.

Ask the patient to describe the exact *location* of the symptom by pointing to it. Cardiac pain is diffuse, and the patient often rubs a hand over the sternum and precordium. Chest pain that can be precisely located with a fingertip is usually related to chest wall abnormalities (Braunwald, 2001). If the pain radiates, the patient should trace its path with a fingertip. The *quality* of a symptom refers to its unique characteristics, such as color, appearance, and texture. Chest discomfort is so subjective that its quality is particularly difficult to describe. Thus, whenever possible, it is important to use the patient's own words (in quotation marks). *Angina* means tightening, and the discomfort associated with angina may be described as "pressing," "squeezing," "tightening," "strangling," or "constricting" (Braunwald, 2001). The patient's response to the symptom also should be recorded (e.g., "It makes me stop what I'm doing and sit down," or "I can continue my activities without stopping").

Quantity refers to the size, extent, or amount of the symptom. The quantity of the chest discomfort is described in terms of its severity. Again, quantity is extremely subjective and might be rated best on a 10-point scale, ranging from "barely noticeable" (1) to "the worst pain ever" (10). The severity of pain should be recorded as a fraction (e.g., 2/10 or 10/10).

Ask patients to describe the *setting* and if they were alone or with someone when the symptom occurred. If the symptom has occurred before, ascertain if the setting, circumstances, or the presence of another person is consistent during symptom onset. This information may be useful later in counseling or helping a patient gain insight into the development of his or her symptoms. Chest discomfort that is reliably associated with activity (e.g., walking up hill) is a specific indicator of cardiac ischemia.

The patient should be asked to describe any *associated symptoms* that always accompany the chief complaint. For example, palpitations and dizziness might always precede the chest discomfort. If the patient mentions associated symptoms, these should be described in the same manner as the chief complaint (i.e., quality, quantity, onset, duration). It is important to note whether these associated symptoms occur consistently with the chief complaint or occur independently at other times.

Alleviating factors, such as resting, changing position, or taking medication, should be noted. Change in the time it takes for alleviating factors to be effective should be identified. For example, if, in the past, the chest discomfort resolved with 5 minutes of rest and now requires 10 minutes, worsening or a new pathologic process is suggested. *Aggravating factors,* such as eating, exercising, or being in a cold climate, also must be recorded. These factors can provide helpful diagnostic information. To complete the present illness history, it is also important to record any *pertinent negative responses* to the interviewer's questions, such as "The chest discomfort is not made worse by strenuous exercise." The patient should be specifically asked about palpitations, dizziness, syncope, dyspnea, orthopnea, and paroxysmal nocturnal dyspnea, if these symptoms have not already been described.

Impact of the symptom on usual or desired activities should be explored. Some people with recurrent chest discomfort reduce their activity over time to try and prevent chest discomfort. It is essential that clinicians understand how the symptom or disease has affected the patient's activity and perceived quality of life.

Throughout the interview, the nurse observes the patient carefully and may begin to understand the meaning the illness has for the patient. The personal meaning of the illness can amplify or reduce the symptom experience and course of action. When interviewing members of a culture not one's own, ask "Can you tell me what caused your illness?" and about the use of home remedies, foods, or traditional healers (Staff Development Workgroup, 1999).

The results of diagnostic or laboratory testing specifically related to heart disease are included in the *history of present illness.* Prior cardiac events (e.g., coronary artery bypass surgery or myocardial infarction) are included also.

Cardiovascular risk factors and current activity may be added in a separate paragraph to the conventional content of the history of present illness. Risk factors for coronary heart disease are discussed in Chapter 36.

Sample questions that may be used in assessing the patient with acute or recurrent chest discomfort are listed below. Similar questions may be generated to assess patients with other symptoms. However, it is important to phrase the questions according to the appropriateness of the situation and logically to pursue areas where further clarification is necessary.

- When exactly do you get the discomfort? Are you having discomfort now?
- What were you doing when the chest discomfort occurred?
- Exactly how often does the chest discomfort occur?
- How many minutes does it usually last?
- Can you point to the exact location where it starts?
- Does the discomfort move anywhere else?
- If so, can you trace its path with your fingertip?
- What words would you use to describe how the discomfort feels?
- What do you do when you have the chest discomfort?
- Quantify your discomfort on a 1-to-10 scale.
- Where were you when the discomfort occurred?
- If the chest discomfort has occurred before, have you always been in the same place?
- Were you alone at the time or with someone?
- Did you notice any other symptoms that occurred at the same time?
- If yes, does this other symptom ever occur by itself?
- What can you do to make the chest discomfort better?
- What can you do to make it worse?
- Are you taking any medication, herbs, or foods to improve your chest discomfort?

- If yes, what is the medication, herb, or food?
- Does any medication you are taking affect your chest discomfort?
- If yes, what is the medication?
- What time of day do you prefer to take your medication?
- What activities have you given up because of your chest discomfort?
- What do you think this chest discomfort means?
- Do you know anyone else who has had this kind of discomfort?

Past History

The past history includes past illnesses and interventions not directly related to the present illness. For a patient with chest discomfort, the history of a previous myocardial infarction, coronary artery bypass surgery, or cholecystectomy belongs in the *history of present illness,* whereas a remote appendectomy does not. Major elements of the *past history* include childhood and adult illnesses, accidents and injuries, current health status, current medications, allergies, and health maintenance. Always ask about major illnesses such as chronic obstructive airway disease, diabetes mellitus, bleeding disorders, and acquired immuno deficiency syndrome (AIDS).

Allergic reactions (e.g., to drugs, food, environmental agents, or animals) also should be noted. Always ask if the patient has an allergy to penicillin or to commonly used emergency drugs, such as lidocaine hydrochloride and morphine sulfate. Allergy to shellfish suggests iodine sensitivity and is important because agents used in cardiac diagnostic tests may contain iodine. Both the allergen and the reaction should always be noted, because some patients confuse an allergic reaction with a drug's side effect.

Medication history includes all prescription and over-the-counter drugs and home remedies. Over-the-counter preparations that increase heart rate or afterload may precipitate or worsen symptoms. If the patient has brought medications with him or her, these should be reviewed by the nurse and then sent home or to the appropriate area for safekeeping.

Family History

The major purpose of the family history is to assess risk factors affecting the patient's current or future health. Notations regarding the age and health status of each first-degree family member are made: living and well, deceased, and the possible or confirmed diagnosis now or at death. Family occurrences of diabetes, kidney disease, tuberculosis, cancer, arthritis, asthma, allergies, mental illness, alcoholism, and drug addiction are included. A family history of coronary heart disease, myocardial infarction, or sudden death would be included in the history of present illness for a patient presenting with chest discomfort.

Personal and Social History

The personal and social history includes important and relevant information about the patient as a person. A person's response to illness is determined in part by his or her cultural background, socioeconomic standing, education, and beliefs about the illness. Major elements include health habits, home situation, and supports and resources. Occupational history may be included here or in the past history. *Health habits* include alcohol, drug, or tobacco use; nutrition; sleep; and physical activity. Use of alcohol and the amount per time period (day, week, year) should be recorded. The use of recreational drugs, especially cocaine, should also be assessed. The cigarette smoking history should be recorded as the number of pack-years (packs per day multiplied by the number of years) the patient has smoked. Other tobacco use, such as pipe or cigar smoking or chewing tobacco, should be recorded. Special diets, such as low-sodium or low-fat diets, should be identified, and the patient's usual eating pattern should be described. The usual number of hours the patient sleeps and circumstances that impair or facilitate sleep should be assessed.

Current Living Circumstances. These include marital status, number of children, occupation, financial resources, and hobbies.

Perceived Health and Coping Challenges. The patient's perception of his or her current health status as either good or bad is helpful in assessing how he or she views its effect on daily living. For example, a 42-year-old man with an old anterior myocardial infarction is seen in the clinic. His chief complaint is extreme fatigue that prevents him from working a full 8-hour day at the office. Initial investigation focuses on ruling out any new process affecting the adequacy of cardiac output, such as a left ventricular aneurysm. Nonpathophysiologic causes for fatigue must be considered also, such as fear of overstressing his heart and sudden death, changes in the work situation, family difficulties, or depression.

Being aware of patients' goals in terms of health and lifestyle is important in determining whether their expectations are realistic. "What do you see yourself doing 3 months from now?" is a good way to ask the patient to define the goal. Another approach is ascertaining what changes the patient would be willing to make in life if the goal could not be achieved.

Assessing the patient's and family's expectations of health care has implications for teaching. For example, is the patient with unstable angina pectoris who has been admitted after "cardiac catheterization" able to explain what the test was and why it resulted in admission? Communication among the health care team members is essential before planning any teaching.

Resources and Support System. It is important to consider the patient's strengths and support system when planning care across the continuum: environmental resources, such as the proximity to the hospital; personal-social support, such as a spouse to provide home care; and economic support, such as adequate insurance, are all examples. Needed resources that are not readily available also must be considered. Knowledge of the patient's health benefits and financial status assists the health care team in designing an affordable therapeutic regimen (e.g., the avoidance of expensive combination or sustained-release medications when other drugs and dosage forms that are as effective and less costly are available).

Review of Systems

To ensure that all important areas have been considered, a systematic review of all body systems is conducted. Lists of major symptoms associated with each body system are included in health assessment textbooks (Bickley & Szilagyi, 2003; Seidel

et al., 2003). Some clinicians prefer to conduct the review of systems simultaneously with the physical examination. For the patient with chest discomfort, the review of the cardiac, pulmonary, and gastrointestinal systems is logically included in the history of present illness.

Functional Patterns

Clinical information related to function is collected in the following areas (Gordon, 1994):

- Health perception–health management
- Nutrition–metabolism
- Elimination
- Activity–exercise
- Cognitive–perceptual
- Sleep–rest
- Self-perception–self-concept
- Roles and relationships
- Sexuality
- Coping–stress
- Values–beliefs

Information collected within these functional patterns does not duplicate information collected within other areas of the health history. The sequence of data gathered in the functional assessment is determined by the patient's clinical condition and the purpose of the encounter. Relevant data obtained earlier in the history should not be repeated.

For the acutely ill cardiac patient who is admitted to the hospital, areas that affect the hospital experience are assessed first. As the patient is able, all functional patterns are assessed. To facilitate the gathering of subjective information for the functional assessment, examples of questions, using the sample symptom of chest discomfort, are listed below. Functional assessment is an ongoing process that evaluates the effect of intervention on patient outcome.

Health Perception–Health Management. Collect the following information:

- What concerns do you have about your health or hospitalization?
- What things are important to you while you are hospitalized? How can we make this experience as easy as possible for you?
- What do you think caused this illness (symptom)?
- Compared with others your age, how would you rate your general health?
- What things do you believe are important to maintain your health?

Nutrition–Metabolism. Collect the following information:

- What do you like to eat (including cultural or ethnic favorites)?
- How are your foods prepared (canned or commercially prepared foods versus fresh foods)?
- Do you usually eat in a restaurant, fast-food outlet, or at home?
- Who shops for groceries?
- Who prepares the meals?
- Are you on a special diet?

Elimination. Collect the following information:

- Is the amount that you urinate normal for you?
- Do you ever get up at night to use the bathroom? If so, how many times?
- If there was a change in elimination pattern, when did you notice it?
- Do you sometimes lose urine or find that you cannot quite make it to the bathroom?
- Do you take a diuretic? If so, when do you take it?
- What is your usual frequency of bowel movements? When was your last movement?
- Are there things you do to maintain that pattern?

Activity–Exercise. Collect the following information:

- Have you noticed a change in your usual or desired activity level?
- Do you have sufficient energy for your desired activities?
- What is the most strenuous activity you perform on a regular basis? How often and how long?
- What leisure or recreational activities do you enjoy? Are you currently able to participate in these activities?
- Are you satisfied with your current level of activity?

Cognitive–Perceptual. Collect the following information:

- Do you have any difficulty with seeing or hearing? Glasses or hearing aid?
- Do you think as fast as you used to? As clearly?
- In general, what is the easiest way for you to learn new material? Any learning difficulties?
- Do you understand why you are in the hospital?
- What does your diagnosis mean to you?
- What is your understanding of the treatment plan?
- Do you understand the risk factors for heart disease and how to modify them?
- Do you understand how long you will be in the hospital and when you can return to your usual activities of daily living?

Sleep–Rest. Collect the following information:

- How many hours do you usually sleep? What hours?
- Do you have difficulty falling asleep or staying asleep? Has this been a change for you or have you always had this difficulty?
- Do you follow a specific bedtime routine or ritual?

Self-Perception–Self-Concept. Collect the following information:

- How would you describe yourself? Your personality? Your approach to life?
- Most of the time, do you feel good about yourself?
- Have you noticed changes in yourself or your body? Do these changes concern you?

Roles and Relationships. Collect the following information:

- Do you live alone? With whom do you live?
- Do you have a close friend or confidant?
- How do you and those close to you feel about your illness?
- Do you often feel lonely? Do you feel part of the neighborhood in which you live?

Sexuality. Collect the following information:

- Have you experienced any changes in your sexuality? Problems in sexual relationships?
- For women: are you still menstruating? Are you taking hormone replacements?

Coping–Stress. Collect the following information:

- Do you feel tense or anxious much of the time? What helps? Do you use medicines for this?
- When you feel stressed, who is most helpful to you?
- When you have big problems in your life, how do you handle them? Does that usually work for you?

Values–Beliefs. Collect the following information:

- Are you generally satisfied with your life?
- Is religion important to you?
- Do you hold religious or other beliefs that you wish to observe here?

Functional and Therapeutic Classification

After the history is completed, it may be possible to categorize the patient according to the New York Heart Association's Functional and Therapeutic Classification (Table 13-2) (NYHA, 1964). This classification may be helpful in assessing symptom severity and monitoring effects of treatment over time. The patient's functional classification may improve as recovery from an acute event, such as myocardial infarction, occurs or as intervention is optimized. Conversely, it may decline with worsening or additional disease.

■ PHYSICAL ASSESSMENT

Assessment of physical findings confirms or expands data obtained in the health history. Baseline information is obtained at the initial encounter, and frequency of subsequent assessments is based on the clinical encounter. Change in the data over time documents progression of, or recovery from, acute disease; new disease; the effectiveness of current interventions; and the patient's current functional status. The type, degree, and rate of change assist the nurse in identifying or predicting immediate or long-term problems, formulating nursing diagnoses, planning care, and establishing individual patient outcome criteria.

In the acutely ill cardiac patient, segments of the physical examination are performed every 2 to 4 hours or more frequently if indicated. Although some data may be available from monitoring devices, physical examination assists in evaluating the accuracy of those data. As the acutely ill patient improves, assessments are routinely done once per shift or more frequently if indicated. If a rapid change in patient condition occurs, the initial assessment is problem focused and the complete assessment is done at a later time. Because nurses spend 24 hours per day with the hospitalized patient, they are in the best position to identify any changes that occur. It is to

Table 13–2 ■ FUNCTIONAL AND THERAPEUTIC CLASSIFICATION OF PATIENTS WITH DISEASES OF THE HEART

Functional Classification		Therapeutic Classification	
Class I	Patients with cardiac disease but without resulting limitations of physical activity. Ordinary physical activity does not cause undue fatigue, palpitation, dyspnea, or anginal pain.	Class A	Patients with cardiac disease whose physical activity need not be restricted in any way.
Class II	Patients with cardiac disease resulting in slight limitation of physical activity. They are comfortable at rest. Ordinary physical activity results in fatigue, palpitation, dyspnea, or anginal pain	Class B	Patients with cardiac disease whose ordinary physical activity need not be restricted, but who should be advised against servere or competitive efforts.
Class III	Patients with cardiac disease resulting in marked limitation of physical activity. They are comfortable at rest. Less than ordinary physical activity causes fatigue, palpitation, dyspnea, or anginal pain.	Class C	Patients with cardiac disease whose ordinary physical activity should be moderately restricted and whose more strenuous efforts should be discontinued.
Class IV	Patients with cardiac disease resulting in inability to carry on any physical activity without discomfort. Symptoms of cardiac insufficiency or of the anginal syndrome may be present even at rest. If any physical activity is undertaken, discomfort is increased.	Class D	Patients with cardiac disease whose ordinary physical activity should be markedly restricted.
		Class E	Patients with cardiac disease who should be at complete rest, confined to bed or chair.

From New York Heart Association Criteria Committee (1964). *Diseases of the heart and blood vessels: Nomenclature and criteria for diagnosis* (6th ed.) Boston, Little, Brown.

the patient's benefit for changes to be detected early, before serious complications develop. Any changes observed in the examination should be documented in the patient's record and reported to the physician. To collect, correlate, and interpret the data accurately, a thorough understanding of the cardiac cycle (see Chapter 1) is essential. A cardiac physical assessment should include an evaluation of:

■ The heart as a pump—reduced pulse pressure, cardiac enlargement, and presence of murmurs and gallop rhythms
■ Filling volumes and pressures—the degree of jugular venous pressure and the presence or absence of crackles, peripheral edema, and postural changes in blood pressure
■ Cardiac output—heart rate, blood pressure, pulse pressure, systemic vascular resistance, urine output, and central nervous system manifestations
■ Compensatory mechanisms—increased filling volumes, peripheral vasoconstriction, and elevated heart rate

The order and techniques of examination proceed logically. The precise order may vary with the setting and the condition of the patient. With practice, the focused cardiovascular examination can be done in approximately 10 minutes:

■ General appearance
■ Head
■ Arterial pulse
■ Jugular venous pressure
■ Blood pressure
■ Peripheral vasculature
■ Heart
■ Lungs
■ Abdomen

General Appearance

Observe the general appearance of the patient while the history is being obtained (Braunwald & Perloff, 2001). The patient's appearance and responses provide cues to the cardiovascular

status. Note general build, skin color, presence of shortness of breath, and distention of neck veins. Assess the patient's level of distress. If he or she is in pain, the patient's response to it may assist in the differential diagnosis. For example, moving about is a characteristic response to the pain of myocardial infarction, whereas sitting quietly is more characteristic of angina, and leaning forward is more characteristic of pericarditis (Chatterjee, 1991b). Some abnormalities of the arterial pulses may be observed unobtrusively. For example, patients with severe aortic insufficiency may have bounding pulses that cause the head to bob. Note appropriateness of weight; malnutrition and cachexia are associated with chronic, severe heart failure (Braunwald & Perloff, 2001). Skeletal manifestations of Marfan's syndrome, tall stature and arachnodactyly, may be observed. Level of consciousness should be described. Appropriateness of thought content, reflecting the adequacy of cerebral perfusion, is particularly important to evaluate. Family members who are most familiar with the patient can be of help in alerting the examiner to subtle behavior changes. The nurse also should be aware of the patient's anxiety level, not only to attempt to put the patient more at ease, but to realize its effects on the cardiovascular system.

Height and Weight

Height and weight are best measured using a standing platform scale with a height attachment. Weak, immobile, or critically ill patients may require a bed or chair scale for weighing, and it may be necessary to rely on the patient's self-reported height. Weight is an indicator of nutritional and fluid status; excessive weight indicates increased cardiovascular risk.

Body mass index (BMI) describes relative weight for height. BMI is calculated as weight in kilograms (kg) divided by the square of the height in meters (m²). In adults, obesity is defined as a BMI of 30 kg/m² or more; overweight is a BMI of 25 kg/m² or more (U. S. Department of Health and Human Services, 2000).

Larger BMI and abdominal fat distribution are associated with increased cardiovascular risk. (Poirer & Despres, 2003). In overweight people, waist circumference of 102 cm (40 inches) in men or 88 cm (35 inches) in women indicates increased risk.

Head

The examination of the head includes assessment of facial characteristics, color, temperature, and eyes. Advanced practice nurses may examine the fundi and retinal vasculature.

Facial Characteristics

Examination of the facial characteristics may aid in the recognition of disorders affecting the cardiovascular system (Braunwald & Perloff, 2001). *Coronary heart disease* is suggested by the presence of an earlobe crease in a person younger than 45 years of age. *Rheumatic heart disease* with severe mitral stenosis is associated with a malar flush, cyanotic lips, and slight jaundice from hepatic congestion. With severe aortic regurgitation, head bobbing with each heartbeat (de Musset's sign) may be present. Infective endocarditis is associated with a "café au lait" complexion. *Constrictive pericarditis* and *tricuspid valve disease* tend to cause facial edema. *Pheochromocytoma* is associated with episodic facial flushing, as well as severe hypertension and tachyarrhythmia.

Systemic conditions may affect or reflect cardiovascular function or treatment. (Braunwald & Perloff, 2001; O'Rourke, Silverman & Schlant, 1994). *Systemic lupus erythematosus* may present with a butterfly rash on the face and may suggest inflammatory heart disease. A systemic lupus erythematosus-like syndrome frequently occurs with procainamide administration but disappears after discontinuation of the drug. *Myxedema* is characterized by dry, sparse hair; loss of lateral eyebrows; a dull, expressionless face; and periorbital puffiness. Because a myocardial effect of hypothyroidism is reduced cardiac output, heart failure may develop in these patients. *Cushing's syndrome* is characterized by moon facies, hirsutism, acne, and centripetal obesity with thin extremities. High blood pressure frequently occurs with Cushing's syndrome.

Color

Cyanosis is the bluish discoloration seen through the skin and mucous membranes when the concentration of reduced hemoglobin exceeds 5 g/100 mL of blood. *Peripheral cyanosis* implies reduced blood flow to the periphery. Because more time is available for the tissues to extract oxygen from the hemoglobin molecule, the arteriovenous oxygen difference widens. Cyanosis of the nose, lips, and earlobes is considered peripheral. Peripheral cyanosis may occur physiologically with the vasoconstriction associated with anxiety or a cold environment, or pathologically in conditions that reduce blood flow to the periphery, such as cardiogenic shock.

Central cyanosis, as observed in the buccal mucosa, implies serious heart or lung disease and is accompanied by peripheral cyanosis. In severe heart disease, a right-to-left shunt exists in which blood passes through the lungs without being fully oxygenated, as happens in severe heart failure with interstitial pulmonary edema. In severe lung disease, changes produced by chronic obstructive airway disease or fibrosis impede oxygenation. *Pallor* can denote anemia (with concomitant decreased oxygen-carrying capacity) or an increased systemic vascular resistance. *Jaundice* can be associated with hepatic engorgement from right ventricular failure.

Temperature

Temperature reflects the balance of heat production and dissipation in the body. Normal oral temperature is considered to be 37°C (98.6°F). However, there is a diurnal pattern of temperature fluctuation, with temperatures as low as 35.8°C (96.4°F) orally in the early morning to as high as 37.3°C (99.1°F) orally in the late afternoon or evening. Oral temperatures average 0.5°C (1.0°F) lower than rectal temperatures, but this difference is quite variable (Bickley & Szilagyi, 2003). Normal body temperature may be less than 37°C in older adults because of reduced heat production (lower metabolic activity, less muscle mass and activity) and conservation (less insulation; Kenney, 1997).

In hospitalized patients, body temperature usually is measured on admission and then every 4 hours or more often if indicated. After cardiac surgery, temperature is measured every 15 to 30 minutes until rewarming is complete, and every 1 to 4 hours until normothermia is achieved. Measure the temperature orally unless the patient is unconscious or unable to close his or her mouth. Body temperatures also may be measured rectally, by means of a pulmonary artery catheter equipped with a thermistor, by means of a thermistor-equipped urinary bladder catheter, or with a device that measures temperature in the insulated auditory meatus close to the tympanic membrane. Pulmonary artery, urinary bladder, tympanic, and rectal temperatures are all considered to be core temperatures; however, they actually measure somewhat different things, and simultaneous measurements may not agree, especially during hypothermia. Pulmonary artery temperature measures the mean blood temperature that results from core thermogenesis and peripheral heat loss or gain. Because urine is a filtrate of blood, urinary bladder temperature also reflects mean blood temperature, but may be falsely low in the setting of low-output renal failure. During hypothermia after cardiac surgery, rectal temperatures reflect peripheral, rather than core, temperatures (Ponte, 1998).

Eyes

The eyes are examined for vision and appearance. A funduscopic examination may be performed.

Vision. Vision is assessed to determine if defects exist that may affect activities of daily living. The examination is as simple as having the patient read a name tag or identify an object.

Appearance. *Corneal arcus,* a thin, grayish-white circle around the iris, may occur normally with aging (Fig. 13-1*A*). When seen in white people younger than age 40 years, corneal arcus suggests hyperlipidemia. *Xanthelasmas* are slightly raised, yellowish plaques of cholesterol in the skin that appear along the nasal side of one or both eyelids (see Fig. 13-1*B*). They are

A Corneal Arcus

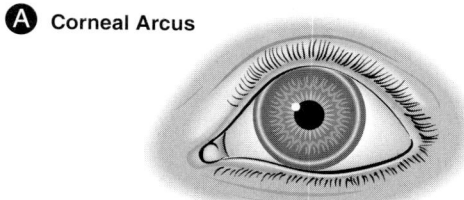

A corneal arcus is a thin grayish white arc or circle not quite at the edge of the cornea. It accompanies normal aging but may also be seen in younger people, especially African Americans. In young people, a corneal arcus suggests the possibility of hyperlipoproteinemia but does not prove it. Some surveys have revealed no relationship.

B Xanthelasmas

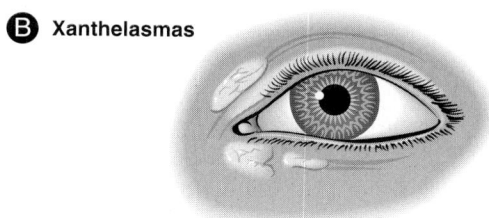

Slightly raised, yellowish, well circumscribed plaques in the skin, xanthelasmas appear along the nasal portions of one or both eyelids. They may accompany lipid disorders (e.g., hyphercholesterolemia), but may also occur independently.

■ **Figure 13–1.** Eye changes suggestive of hyperlipoproteinemia. (*A*) Corneal arcus. (*B*) Xanthelasmas.

associated with hyperlipidemia but also may occur normally. *Ophthalmitis* and *petechial* and *subconjunctival hemorrhages* of the upper and lower eyelids are seen with bacterial endocarditis.

Fundi. Examination of the ocular fundi provides the only opportunity for direct visualization of blood vessels. Vascular changes from high blood pressure and diabetes mellitus can be detected in the arteries and small veins of the retina. In general health care, funduscopic examination is conducted without pharmacologic dilation of the pupils. Physiologic dilation may be maximized by darkening the room and asking the patient to gaze off in the distance. Photographs printed in books are taken through a maximally dilated pupil with a special camera. The view through the ophthalmoscope is only a small portion of the retina. It is necessary to direct the ophthalmoscope in varying directions, following blood vessels and observing the retinal structures and background.

The *funduscopic examination technique* is as follows (Bickley & Szilagyi, 2003):

■ Darken the room.
■ Turn on the ophthalmoscope light; select the large round beam of white light.
■ Adjust the lens disc to 0 diopter. Keep your index finger on the lens disc throughout the examination.
■ Use your right hand and right eye to examine the patient's right eye; use your left hand and left eye to examine the patient's left eye.
■ Place your opposite thumb over the patient's eyebrow to gain proprioceptive guidance as you move closer to the patient.

■ Ask the patient to look straight ahead and to fix his or her gaze on a distant point.
■ Brace the ophthalmoscope firmly against your face, with your eye directly behind the sight hole.
■ Position yourself 15 inches away from the patient and 15 degrees lateral to his or her line of vision. Shine the light beam on the patient's pupil and note the *red reflex.* Absence of a *red reflex* suggests a lens opacity, such as a cataract.
■ With both of your eyes open and keeping the light beam focused on the red reflex, move horizontally at a 15-degree angle slowly toward the patient. When you are approximately 1.5 to 2 inches (3 to 5 cm) from the patient, the optic disc or blood vessels should come into view (Fig. 13-2). Rotate lenses with your index finger until fundic structures are as clearly visible as possible.
■ To overcome corneal reflection (light reflected back into the examiner's eye), direct the light beam toward the edge of the pupil rather than through its center.
■ Examine the *optic disc,* a yellowish-orange to creamy pink oval or round structure. If you do not see the disc, follow a blood vessel centrally (by noting the angles of vessel branching and the progressive enlargement of vessel size toward the disc) until it is visible. Assess disc border clarity (nasal margin may be normally somewhat blurred) and color.
■ Identify the *retinal arteries* and *veins* using the differential criteria of color, size, and light reflex (or reflection; Fig. 13-3*A*). Arteries and veins appear to originate from the *physiologic cup,* a small, white depression in the optic disc. Arteries are light red, are two thirds to four fifths the diameter of veins, and have a bright light reflex. Veins are dark red, are larger than arteries, and have an inconspicuous or absent light reflex. Follow the vessels peripherally in all directions, noting the character of the arteriovenous crossings. To examine the extreme periphery, instruct the patient to look up, down, temporally, and nasally.
■ Assess the retina for any *lesions,* noting size, shape, color, and distribution. *Optic disc edema* (swollen optic disc with blurred margins) is present in patients with increased intracranial pressure, retinal venous outflow obstruction, inflammation, or ischemia (Bickley & Szilagyi, 2003; Fig. 13-4). *Beading* (abnormal constriction) of a retinal vein is common in diabetic retinopathy. With high blood pressure, thickening of the walls and narrowing of the lumen of retinal arteries develop.

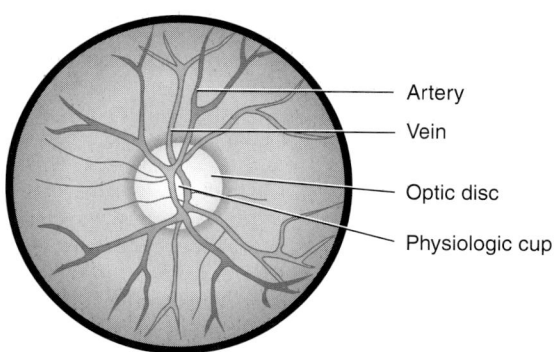

Artery
Vein
Optic disc
Physiologic cup

■ **Figure 13–2.** Funduscopic examination of retinal structures.

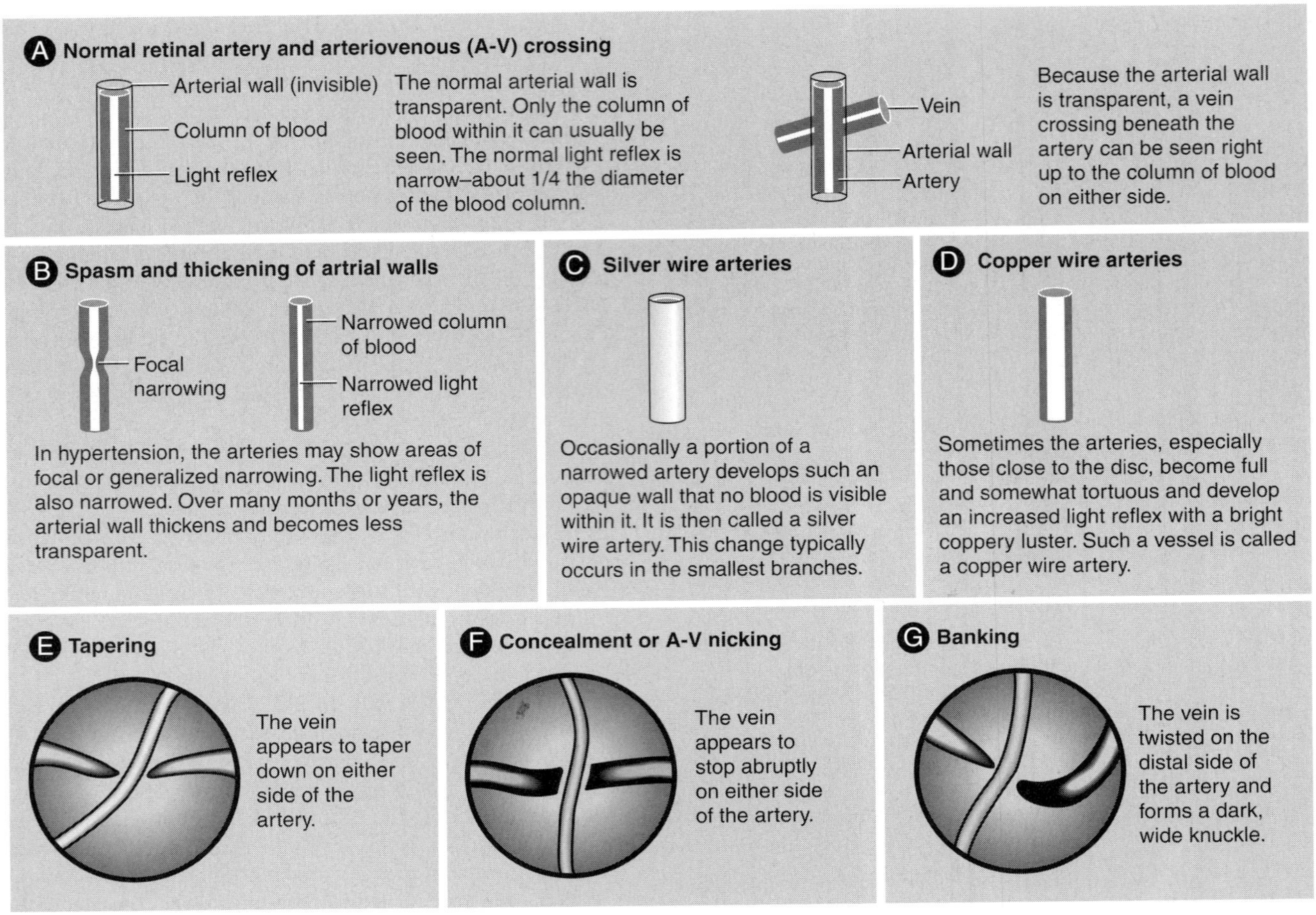

A **Normal retinal artery and arteriovenous (A-V) crossing**

Arterial wall (invisible)
Column of blood
Light reflex

The normal arterial wall is transparent. Only the column of blood within it can usually be seen. The normal light reflex is narrow–about 1/4 the diameter of the blood column.

Vein
Arterial wall
Artery

Because the arterial wall is transparent, a vein crossing beneath the artery can be seen right up to the column of blood on either side.

B **Spasm and thickening of artrial walls**

Focal narrowing
Narrowed column of blood
Narrowed light reflex

In hypertension, the arteries may show areas of focal or generalized narrowing. The light reflex is also narrowed. Over many months or years, the arterial wall thickens and becomes less transparent.

C **Silver wire arteries**

Occasionally a portion of a narrowed artery develops such an opaque wall that no blood is visible within it. It is then called a silver wire artery. This change typically occurs in the smallest branches.

D **Copper wire arteries**

Sometimes the arteries, especially those close to the disc, become full and somewhat tortuous and develop an increased light reflex with a bright coppery luster. Such a vessel is called a copper wire artery.

E **Tapering**

The vein appears to taper down on either side of the artery.

F **Concealment or A-V nicking**

The vein appears to stop abruptly on either side of the artery.

G **Banking**

The vein is twisted on the distal side of the artery and forms a dark, wide knuckle.

■ **Figure 13–3.** Vascular changes associated with high blood pressure. (*A*) Normal. (*B*) Spasm and thickening of arteriolar walls. (*C*) Silver wire arterioles. (*D*) Copper wire arterioles. (*E*) Venous tapering. (*F*) Arteriovenous nicking. (*G*) Venous banking.

These changes are observed as *focal narrowing,* a *narrowed column of blood,* and a *narrowed light reflex* (see Fig. 13-3*B*). If opacity is such that no blood column is visible, the artery appears as a *silver wire artery* (see Fig. 13-3*C*). With increased filling and tortuosity, arteries closest to the optic disc manifest an increased light reflex and are known as *copper wire arteries* (see Fig. 13-3*D*). Arteriovenous crossings also are affected by thickening of the artery walls, demonstrated by *tapering* of the vein on either side of the artery (see Fig. 10-3*E*), *arteriovenous nicking* (abrupt cessation of the vein on either side of the artery; see Fig. 13-3*F*), or *banking* of the vein (venous twisting distal to the artery, forming a dark, wide buckle; see Fig. 13-3*G;* Bickley & Szilagyi, 2003; Frank, 2003).

Red spots in the retina may be due to hemorrhage or microaneurysms, which can be associated with hypertension, diabetes, or a number of other conditions (Anderson, 1994; Bickley & Szilagyi, 2003). *Roth's spots,* hemorrhages with white centers, occur with subacute bacterial endocarditis and leukemia (Anderson, 1994; Bickley & Szilagyi, 2003) *Cotton wool patches* are white or gray and have large irregular shapes and fuzzy borders (Fig. 13-5*A*). They occur with hypertension and are seen frequently in patients

with AIDS. *Hard exudates* are small, creamy white or yellow lesions with well-defined borders (see Fig. 13-5*B*). They occur frequently in clusters and are indicative of diabetes, hypertension, and other conditions (Bickley & Szilagyi, 2003). Abnormalities of the fundi are difficult to see, require much practice, and may require eye drops to dilate the pupil.

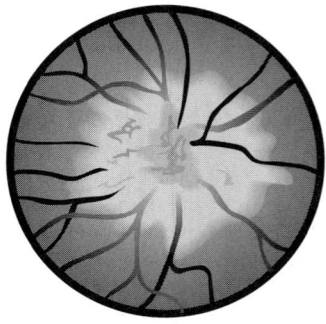

■ **Figure 13–4.** Papilledema. The optic disc is swollen, its margins are blurred, and the physiologic cup is not visible.

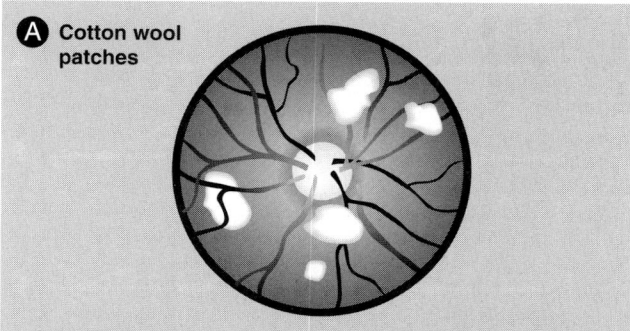

A Cotton wool patches

Cotton wool patches are white or grayish, ovoid lesions with irregular (thus "soft") borders. They are moderate in size but usually smaller than the disc. They result from infarcted nerve fibers and are seen with hypertension and many other conditions.

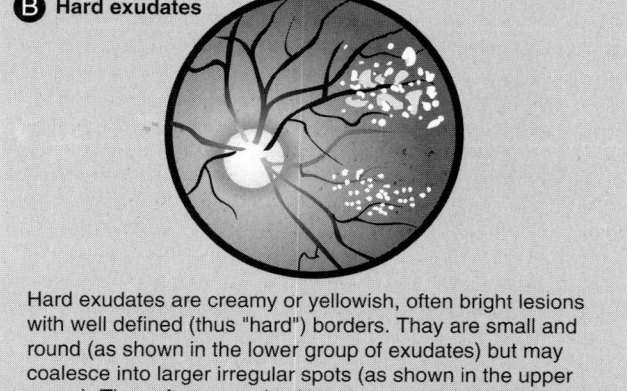

B Hard exudates

Hard exudates are creamy or yellowish, often bright lesions with well defined (thus "hard") borders. Thay are small and round (as shown in the lower group of exudates) but may coalesce into larger irregular spots (as shown in the upper group). They often occur in clusters or in circular, linear, or star-shaped patterns. Causes include diabetes and hypertension.

■ **Figure 13–5.** Light-colored spots in the retina. (*A*) Cotton wool patches. (*B*) Hard exudates.

Arterial Pulse

Information about pulse rate, rhythm, amplitude and contour, and obstruction to blood flow is obtained from palpation of the arterial pulse. Pulses should be evaluated at baseline, before and after vascular procedures that might impair blood flow, and with the onset of any symptom associated with reduced peripheral flow or ischemia. On initial examination, both carotid, both radial, both femoral, both tibial, and both dorsal pulses should be assessed.

Pulse Rate and Rhythm

Pulse rate and rhythm commonly are assessed in the radial artery. However, in certain clinical situations, such as shock (with very low-amplitude or absent peripheral pulses) or during cardiac arrest (when information about central blood flow is essential), pulses should be assessed in the more centrally located carotid artery.

Pulse Rate. The pulse rate at rest usually is between 60 and 100 (average of approximately 70) pulsations per minute. A lower resting heart rate is common in athletes. Conditions or activities such as exercise, fever, and stress increase the pulse rate. Hypothermia, certain drugs, and heart blocks, for example, decrease the pulse rate. Each pulse wave is indicative of a cardiac contraction. However, each cardiac contraction does not necessarily result in a peripheral pulse. In patients with heart disease, pulse rate may be slower than heart rate because not all cardiac contractions are perfused peripherally. Extremely fast heart rates, such as atrial fibrillation with an uncontrolled ventricular response or premature supraventricular or ventricular contractions, have shortened diastolic filling times, resulting in reduced stroke volume and, therefore, diminished or absent pulses. For this reason, pulse rate should not be recorded from the heart rate display on the cardiac monitor or counted from an electrocardiographic strip.

Using the pads of the index and middle fingers, compress the artery until maximum pulsation is detected. Count the rate. If regular, count for 15 seconds and multiply by 4; if irregular, count for a full minute, noting the variations in rhythm and volume.

In all cardiac patients and in any patient with an irregular heart rate, simultaneously auscultate the apical rate and palpate the peripheral rate (*apical–radial rate*); record both rates. It is important that the apical–radial rates be counted during the *same* minute. If the apical–radial difference is very large, if the rate is very fast, or if the examiner is not yet skilled, it may be helpful to have two people count for the same minute.

Pulse Rhythm. Pulse rhythm is normally regular. Physiologic variation can occur with respiration. During inspiration, blood flow to the right heart is increased, right ventricular output is enhanced, and pulmonary venous capacitance is increased. Consequently, blood flow to the left heart is reduced, causing a drop in left ventricular stroke volume. Cardiac output is maintained by a compensatory increase in heart rate (mediated by the baroreceptors). During expiration, the large amount of blood residing in the pulmonary vascular bed during inspiration reaches the left heart. Left ventricular contractility is enhanced by means of the Frank-Starling mechanism, increasing left ventricular stroke volume. Because an increased heart rate is no longer needed to maintain cardiac output, the heart rate returns to baseline. This physiologically irregular rhythm is termed *sinus arrhythmia*. It is common in people younger than 40 years of age. Other irregular rhythms are not normal. The irregularity should be described as regularly irregular (e.g., every other pulse wave is early) or irregularly irregular (e.g., atrial fibrillation). Occasional, early pulsations that are perceived as transient skips or breaks in an otherwise regular rhythm are common and are not necessarily abnormal.

Pulse Amplitude and Contour

Pulses are described in a variety of ways. The simplest classification is absent, present, and bounding. A 0-to-4 scale is often used, and pulses are graded as follows: absent (0), diminished (1+), normal (2+), moderately increased (3+), and markedly increased (4+; O'Rourke et al., 1994). This scale is fairly subjective, and, although an individual tends to be internally consistent over time, different people may grade the same pulse differently. There are also other scales in which the numbers are defined differently.

The amplitude of an arterial pulse is a function of the pulse pressure, which is related to stroke volume, elasticity of the arterial tree, and velocity of left ventricular ejection. Increased stroke volume, as occurs with exercise or excitement, results in increased amplitude and a bounding arterial pulse.

Small, weak pulses (Fig. 13-6*B*) have a diminished pulse pressure, which is indicative of a reduced stroke volume and ejection fraction and of increased systemic vascular resistance.

Large, bounding pulses result from an increased pulse pressure (see Fig. 13-6*C*). Increased pulse pressure is caused by increased stroke volume and ejection velocity and by diminished peripheral vasoconstriction. *Corrigan's pulse* is a bounding pulse visible in the carotid artery. It occurs with aortic regurgitation.

The amplitude of a pulse contributes to its contour, but contour refers to the rate of rise and the shape of the arterial pulse. Because of the distortion that occurs when the pulse wave is transmitted peripherally, pulse contour is best assessed in the carotid arteries. The *normal pulse contour* has a rapid and smooth upstroke. The dicrotic notch is not palpable (see Fig. 13-6*A*), although the dicrotic wave (see Fig. 13-6*I*) may be palpable in heart failure and in febrile states (O'Rourke et al., 1994). Usually it is palpable only in the peripheral arteries.

Pulsus bisferiens (see Fig. 13-6*D*) is characterized by a rapid upstroke and double systolic peak. This pulse may be present in idiopathic hypertrophic subaortic stenosis, aortic stenosis with regurgitation, and pure aortic insufficiency.

Pulsus alternans (see Fig. 13-6*E*) is a regular rhythm in which strong pulse waves alternate with weak ones. It is an ominous sign when it occurs at normal heart rates and suggests serious heart disease. The difference in amplitude may be slight and difficult to palpate. The presence of pulsus alternans can be confirmed with a sphygmomanometer. The cuff is inflated above systolic pressure and slowly released until the first heart sound is audible. Cuff pressure is held at this point, and the pulse is palpated to determine if every pulse is audible.

Bigeminal pulses (see Fig. 13-6*F*), which should not be confused with pulsus alternans, are caused by a bigeminal, premature ectopic rhythm. Note that every other pulse wave is not only diminished but is early.

Pulsus paradoxus (see Fig. 13-6*G*) is the reduction in strength of the arterial pulse that can be felt during abnormal inspiratory decline of left ventricular filling. However, it is more apparent and can be quantified if sphygmomanometry is used. (Refer to the discussion of the determination of paradoxical blood pressure below.)

Pulsus parvus et tardus (see Fig. 13-6*H*) is found in severe aortic stenosis. It resembles the double systolic beat in pulsus bisferiens, but its upstroke is more gradual and the pulse pressure is smaller. Usually it is palpable only in the carotid artery.

Carotid Pulse. The carotid artery is best for assessing pulse-wave amplitude and contour. Observe the neck for pulsations. Carotid pulsations are visible bilaterally just medial to the sternocleidomastoid muscle. Place your fingertips along the medial border of the sternocleidomastoid muscle in the lower half of the neck. Press posteriorly to feel the artery. Palpate well below the upper border of the thyroid cartilage to

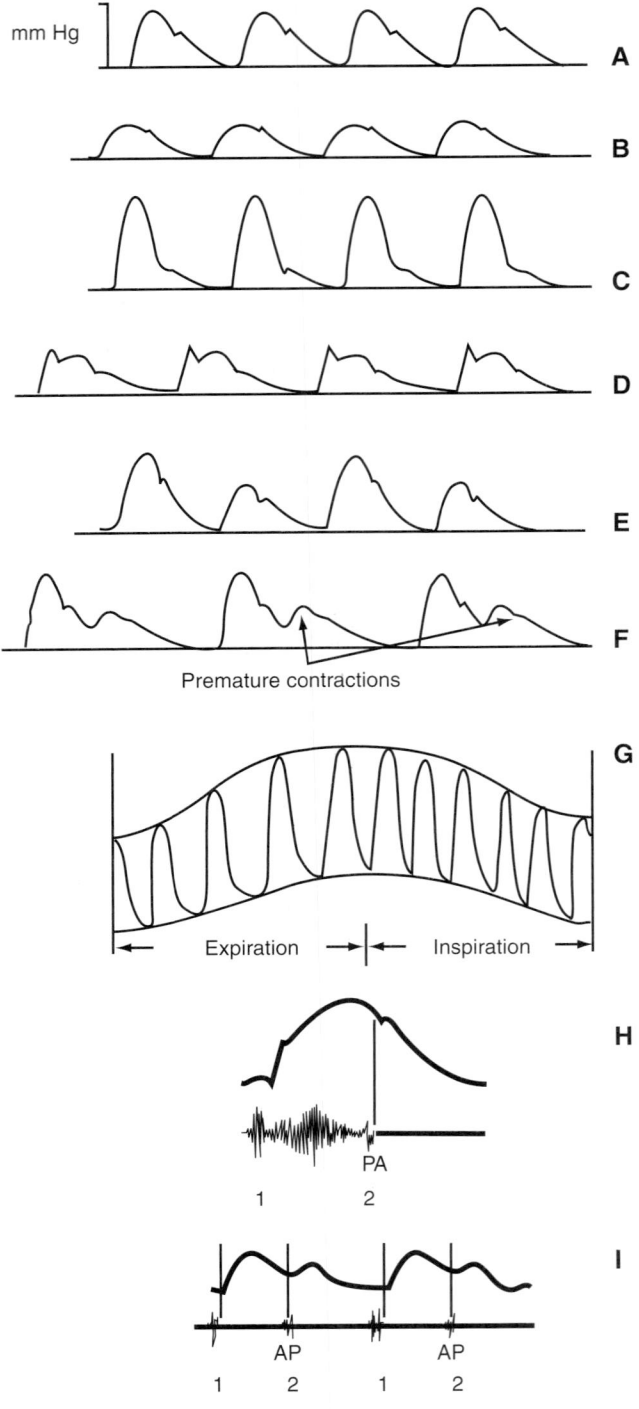

■ **Figure 13–6.** Normal and abnormal pulses. (*A*) Normal. (*B*) Small and weak. (*C*) Large and bounding. (*D*) Bisferiens. (*E*) Pulsus alternans. (*F*) Bigeminal. (*G*) Pulsus paradoxus. (*H*) Parvus et tardus. (*I*) Dicrotic.

avoid compressing the carotid sinus, which might result in a reflex drop in heart rate or blood pressure. Compare one side with the other, but do not palpate both sides simultaneously because brain blood flow might be interrupted. Using the side with the strongest pulsations, assess the amplitude and contour of the pulse wave and determine whether it occurs in early systole or has a delayed upstroke.

Peripheral Circulation. In the legs, assess femoral, popliteal, dorsalis pedis, and posterior tibial pulses (Fig. 13-7). The popliteal pulse is not directly palpable; only the transmitted pulsations can be detected. Pedal pulses should be assessed in a dependent position before determining that they are absent (O'Rourke et al., 1994). In the arms, assess brachial, radial, and ulnar pulses. When assessing peripheral circulation, always compare one side with the other. An *Allen test* should be performed before radial arterial cannulation to evaluate radial and ulnar arterial patency. Simultaneously compress the radial and ulnar arteries and ask the patient to make a fist. The hand blanches. Ask the patient to open his or her fist. Release the pressure from the ulnar artery while maintaining pressure on the radial artery. The hand color returns to normal if the ulnar artery is patent. Repeat the process releasing pressure from the radial artery. If dual circulation to the hand is not present, do not attempt radial arterial puncture or cannulation.

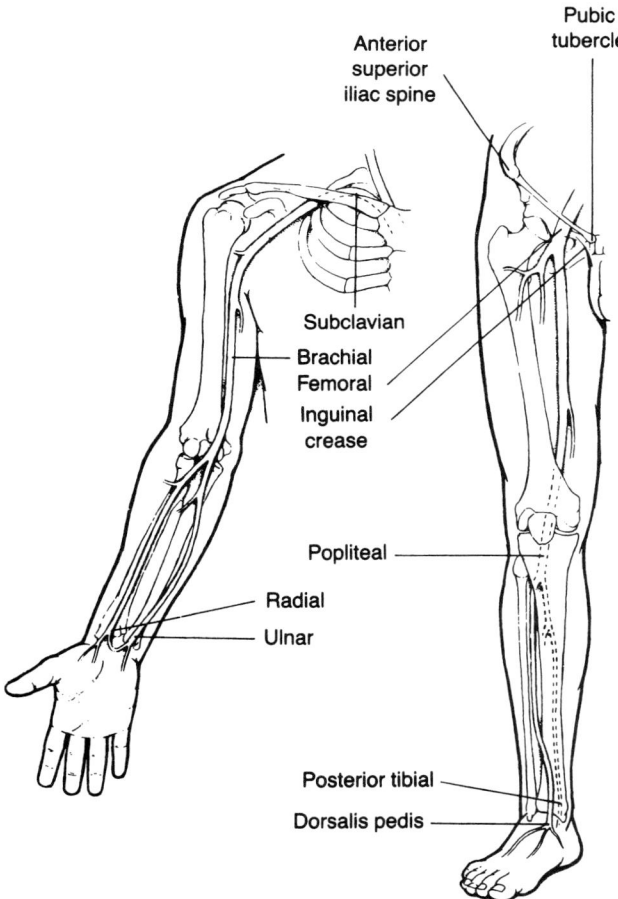

■ **Figure 13–7.** Peripheral arteries and their landmarks. (From Boozer, M. & Craven, R. F. [1986]. Assessment of vascular function. In M. L. Patrick, S. L. Woods, R. F. Craven, et al. [Eds.], *Medical-surgical nursing: Pathophysiological concepts* [p. 595]. Philadelphia: Lippincott.)

In shock states associated with reduced cardiac output and elevated systemic vascular resistance, or with arterial insufficiency, pulses may not be palpable in the periphery. In this case, *Doppler ultrasound* should be used to evaluate arterial flow. Using light pressure so that the artery is not occluded, place the Doppler probe (with conducting gel) over the general area of the artery to be assessed. Move the probe until the arterial signal is audible. Mark the location of the pulse with indelible ink.

Bruits

Bruits are arterial sounds, similar to cardiac murmurs, that occur with turbulence of blood flow. Bruits in the carotid arteries may indicate a partial obstruction to cerebral blood flow, whereas bruits in the femoral arteries suggest partial obstruction to blood flow to the legs. When listening for carotid bruits, instruct the patient to exhale and then hold his or her breath during the examination to prevent bruits from being obscured by respiratory sounds. Auscultate for bruits with the diaphragm of the stethoscope over the carotid, renal, iliac, and femoral arteries.

Jugular Venous Pulse

Inspection of the jugular venous pulse can reveal important information about right heart hemodynamics. The level of the jugular venous pressure reflects the right atrial pressure and, in most instances, reflects the right ventricular diastolic pressure (filling pressure). The pattern of the jugular venous pulse can reveal abnormalities of conduction and abnormal function of the tricuspid valve (Braunwald & Perloff, 2001). Assess the right side of the neck because right heart hemodynamics are transmitted more directly to the right, rather than to the left, jugular vein. It is important to inspect the skin for evidence of previous cannulation of the vessel that may result in thrombosis and affect the accuracy of pressure measurement. Oblique light may assist in visualizing the jugular veins.

Jugular Venous Pressure

Jugular venous pressure reflects filling volume and pressure on the right side of the heart. Jugular veins act like manometers; blood in the jugular veins assumes the level that corresponds to the right atrial (central venous) pressure. The normal jugular venous pressure is less than 9 cm H_2O (Bickley & Szilagyi, 2003). The right internal jugular vein provides the most accurate reflection of right heart hemodynamics because it is in an almost straight line with the innominate vein and the superior vena cava (Bickley & Szilagyi, 2003). It lies deep to the sternocleidomastoid muscle; however, the pulsations are usually transmitted to the skin. The top level of skin pulsation is recorded as the jugular venous pressure. If the right internal jugular vein is not visible, the right external jugular vein may be used to measure jugular venous pressure, although it is more subject to thrombosis or compression, and the presence of venous valves may make the data less reliable (McGee,

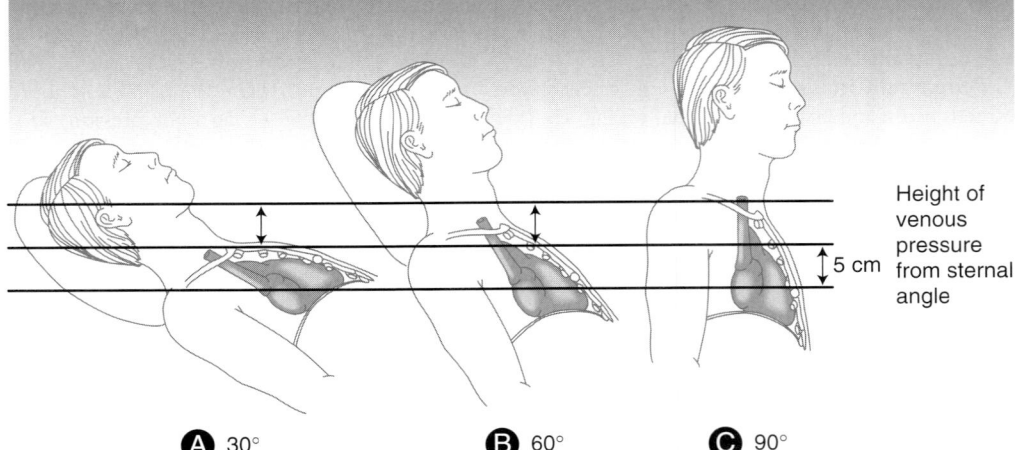

■ **Figure 13–8.** Assessment of jugular venous pressure.

Ⓐ 30°   Ⓑ 60°   Ⓒ 90°

Height of venous pressure from sternal angle

5 cm

1998). To measure the jugular venous pressure, follow these steps (Fig. 13-8):

■ Begin with the patient supine; the head and trunk should be in a straight line without significant flexion of the neck.
■ Position the patient's backrest so that the jugular meniscus can be seen in the lower half of the neck. Elevating the backrest 15 to 30 degrees above horizontal is usually sufficient.
■ Visualize the right internal jugular vein and identify the level of peak excursion. If the external jugular vein is used, identify the level at which it appears collapsed.
■ Place a ruler vertically on the sternal angle (angle of Lewis). Position a straight edge (e.g., tongue blade) horizontally at the highest point of the jugular vein so that it intersects the ruler at a right angle, and measure the vertical distance above the sternal angle.

If the top of the neck veins is more than 3 cm above the sternal angle, venous pressure is abnormally elevated. Elevated venous pressure reflects right ventricular failure (and is a late finding in left ventricular failure), reduced right ventricular compliance, pericardial disease, hypervolemia, tricuspid valve stenosis, and obstruction of the superior vena cava (O'Rourke et al., 1994). During inspiration, the jugular venous pressure normally declines, although the amplitude of the a wave may increase (Braunwald & Perloff, 2001). With the patient in the horizontal position, if the neck veins collapse on deep inspiration (intrathoracic pressure of -5 cm H_2O), the central venous pressure is less than 5 cm H_2O.

Abdominojugular reflux occurs in right ventricular failure. It can be demonstrated by pressing the periumbilical area firmly for 30 to 60 seconds and observing the jugular venous pressure. If there is a rise in the jugular venous pressure by 1 cm or more that is sustained throughout pressure application, abdominojugular reflux is present (Marriott, 1993). *Kussmaul's sign* is a paradoxical elevation of jugular venous pressure during inspiration and may occur in patients with chronic constrictive pericarditis, heart failure, or tricuspid stenosis.

Patterns of the Venous Pulse

Before evaluating the venous pulse, it is important to discriminate between venous and carotid pulsations. Venous pulse waves are observed more readily than they are palpated. The descents are often more easily seen than the peaks and are inward movements (Marriott, 1993). The carotid pulsation is a brisk, outward movement. Palpation of the jugular vein obliterates the pulsations except in extreme venous hypertension (O'Rourke et al., 1994). Palpation of the carotid does not obliterate the observable pulsation in the neck.

Right atrial systole increases right atrial pressure and causes venous distention and the resulting a wave (Fig. 13-9). Atrial emptying and relaxation, and descent of the atrial floor during ventricular systole, results in the x descent. The c wave occurs simultaneously with the carotid arterial pulse, interrupting the x descent. The c wave may be related to tricuspid valve closure and bulging into the right atrium, or it may be an artifact from the adjacent carotid pulse. The v wave reflects the rise in right atrial pressure from atrial filling during ventricular contraction while the tricuspid valve is closed. The y descent results from reduction in right atrial volume and pressure when the tricuspid valve opens (O'Rourke et al., 1994).

Timing of the venous pulse can be appreciated by auscultating the heart or palpating the carotid artery on the opposite side of the neck. The a wave occurs just before the first heart sound or carotid pulse and has a sharp rise followed by the rapid x descent. The v wave occurs immediately after the arterial pulse and has a slower, undulating pattern. The y descent is

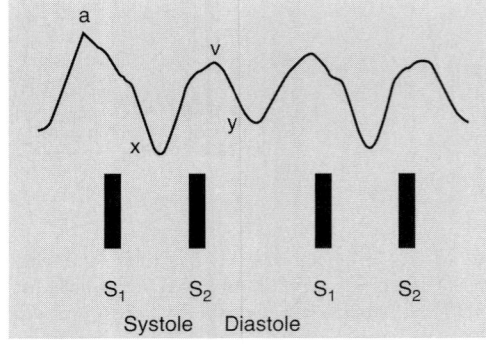

■ **Figure 13–9.** Patterns of the venous pulse.

less steep than the *x* descent. Consistently large a waves are seen in tricuspid stenosis, pulmonary hypertension, and right ventricular failure. *Cannon a waves* are seen in patients with atrioventricular dissociation as the right atrium contracts against the closed tricuspid valve (Marriott, 1993). The a wave is absent in atrial fibrillation because of the absence of coordinated atrial contraction. Elevated v waves and rapid *y* descents suggest tricuspid regurgitation or increased intravascular volume. Blunting of the *y* descent suggests impaired atrial emptying in early ventricular diastole, such as occurs in tricuspid stenosis, pericardial disease, or cardiac tamponade.

Blood Pressure

Systemic arterial blood pressure can be measured indirectly or directly. Indirect measurement of blood pressure is most common and is described in this section. Direct measurement of blood pressure, an invasive technique requiring placement of an arterial catheter, may be necessary in certain conditions, such as clinical shock. Direct measurement of blood pressure is discussed in Chapter 23.

Blood pressure should be measured at each health encounter. The auscultatory method of measurement with a properly calibrated and validated instrument should be used. Patients should be seated quietly in a chair, with feet on the floor and arm supported for at least 5 minutes before measurement (Chobanian et al., 2003).

Evaluate the patient's current blood pressure. If it differs greatly from the usual, immediate intervention may be required. Normal blood pressure in people 18 years of age or older is defined as less than 120/80 mm Hg, and prehypertension is defined as systolic pressure of 120 to 139 mm Hg or diastolic pressure of 80 to 90 mm Hg. Patients with prehypertension are at increased risk for progression to hypertension (Chobanian et al., 2003). Hypertension is defined as systolic blood pressure of 140 mm Hg or greater, diastolic blood pressure of 90 mm Hg or greater, or taking antihypertensive medication (Chobanian et al., 2003). (See Chapter 39 for treatment of hypertension.) In western societies, blood pressure tends to increase with increasing age. This is not biologic, and there is clear evidence that lowering blood pressure in older adults reduces the risk of stroke, cardiac disease, and all-cause mortality (Insuna et al., 1994). The higher the blood pressure, the greater the increase in the heart's work and oxygen consumption. Blood pressures less than 90/60 mm Hg may decrease blood and oxygen delivery to an already compromised myocardium. Taking into account symptoms of myocardial ischemia and adequacy of cerebral and peripheral perfusion may enable the examiner to judge more accurately the clinical significance of blood pressure changes in the cardiac patient.

Sphygmomanometer

Blood pressure is measured indirectly using a sphygmomanometer (inflatable bladder inside a pressure cuff, a manometer, and an inflation system) and stethoscope. Stethoscopes are described later in this chapter.

Table 13–3 ■ ACCEPTABLE BLADDER DIMENSIONS (IN CM) FOR ARMS OF DIFFERENT SIZES*

Cuff	Bladder Width (cm)	Bladder Length (cm)	Arm Circumference Range at Midpoint (cm)
Newborn	3	6	≤6
Infant	5	15	6–15[†]
Child	8	21	16–21[†]
Small adult	10	24	22–26
Adult	13	30	27–34
Large adult	16	38	35–44
Adult thigh	20	42	45–52

*There is some overlapping of the recommended range for arm circumferences to limit the number of cuffs; it is recommended that the larger cuff be used when available.
[†]To approximate the bladder width : arm circumference ratio of 0.40 more closely in infants and children, additional cuffs are available.
From Perloff, D., Grim, C., Flack, J., et al. (2001). *Human blood pressure determination by sphygmomanometry.* Dallas, TX: American Heart Association.

Bladder and Cuff. The inflatable bladder fits inside a nondistensible covering, termed the *cuff.* Size and placement of the bladder (rather than the cuff) are crucial in obtaining accurate blood pressure measurements. The bladder width should be 40% of the circumference of the limb (usually the arm) to be used. Bladders that are too narrow for the size of the limb reflect a falsely elevated blood pressure, whereas bladders that are too wide reflect an erroneously low blood pressure. Bladder length, which also affects accuracy of measurement, should be approximately twice that of width, or 80% of the limb circumference. Inflatable bladders and cuffs are available in various sizes. Table 13-3 summarizes recommended bladder dimensions for blood pressure cuffs. It is important to remember that cuff size is determined by patient size, not patient age (Grim & Grim, 2003).

Manometers. There are two types of manometers: mercury and aneroid. *Mercury manometers,* which are the most reliable, can be mounted either on a portable stand or on the wall above the bed or table. A reservoir of mercury (Hg) is attached to the bottom of the manometer, which is calibrated in millimeters (mm). In response to pressure exerted on the bulb, mercury rises vertically in the manometer. As pressure is released from the bag, the column of mercury falls, and blood pressure can be measured in millimeters of mercury. It is important that the meniscus of the mercury be at eye level when the blood pressure is measured. The blood pressure reading should be taken at the top of the meniscus. If the wall mounting is too high or the portable stand too low, errors in blood pressure determinations will be made.

In response to efforts by the Environmental Protection Agency to reduce potential mercury spills and exposure, many clinical facilities are using aneroid gauges or electronic monitoring devices. To date, mercury manometers remain the gold standard. Accurate measurement of blood pressure with nonmercury instruments requires sufficient standards of validation and stringent programs of calibration (Jones et al., 2001).

Aneroid manometers have round gauges calibrated in millimeters of mercury, or torr (1 torr = 1 mm Hg), and affixed to the blood pressure cuff. Advantages of the aneroid manometer are that it is easily seen, is conveniently portable, and, with the cuff, composes one unit. Unfortunately, the calibration of the dial frequently

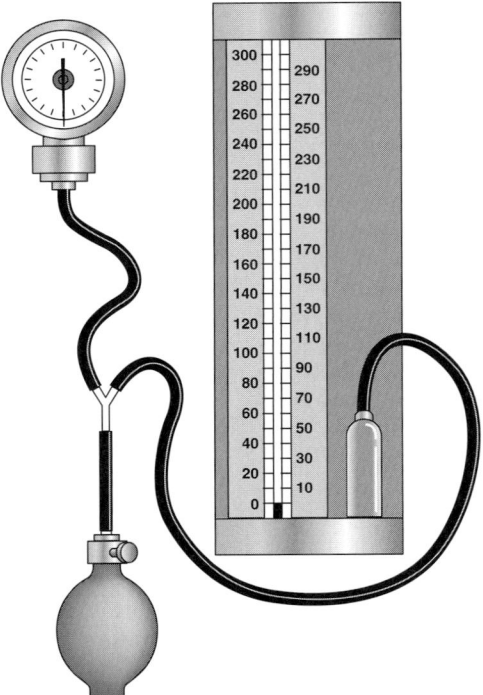

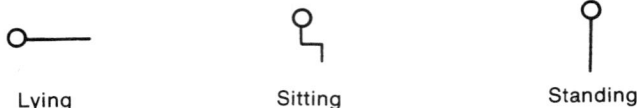

■ **Figure 13–11.** Symbols used to record a patient's position during blood pressure determination.

■ **Figure 13–10.** Calibration of an aneroid manometer. Disconnect the cuffs from both the aneroid and reference manometers. Attach a bulb to a Y connector and the Y connector to the tubes to each of the manometers. Inflate the bulb and observe the pressure at several points over the entire range on both manometers. The pressures should be equal on both manometers.

becomes inaccurate. It is important before each use to check that the indicator needle is pointing to the zero mark on the dial. If the needle is either below or above this mark, the blood pressure reading will be incorrect and the scale may no longer be linear.

Calibration of an aneroid manometer is performed using a mercury manometer as the reference manometer (Fig. 13-10; Grim & Grim, 2003). The mercury manometer must be functioning correctly to obtain reliable results). Aneroid manometers should be recalibrated by qualified personnel at least yearly or whenever the needle does not point to zero.

The inflation system of aneroid manometers consists of the bulb, exhaust valve, and tubing. The bladder should be able to be inflated and deflated gradually or rapidly. Check frequently for pressure leaks greater than 1 mm Hg per second and for smooth, efficient functioning of the apparatus.

Electronic devices can be used for measuring blood pressure, but the accuracy of these devices and stringent programs of calibration are necessary. Electronic devices are more sensitive to artifact such as patient movement or muscle contraction than are mercury and aneroid devices. Electronic devices do not require use of a stethoscope and may be used by patients for self-monitoring of blood pressure.

Technique

On initial examination, blood pressure should be recorded in both arms and, in infants, in one leg as well. Subsequently, the arm with the higher blood pressure should be used. Indicate whether the blood pressure was taken on the right arm or left arm. Avoid possible development of lymphedema after mastectomy by always taking the patient's blood pressures on the arm *opposite* the affected side. Avoid taking blood pressure on an arm with an arteriovenous shunt or fistula, as well as those with subclavian stenosis (Perloff et al., 1993).

Differences in blood pressure between the arms or between the arms and the legs have important diagnostic implications. In patients with occlusive arterial disease of the subclavian artery, the blood pressure is lower in the affected arm. In patients with coarctation of the aorta or dissecting aortic aneurysm, depending on the location of the lesion, the blood pressure may be higher in one arm than the other, or in both arms (proximal) compared with the legs (distal).

Bladder and Cuff Position. The deflated cuff is placed snugly around the arm, with the bladder covering the inner aspect of the arm and the brachial artery. The lower margin of the cuff should be 2.5 cm above the antecubital space.

Arm Position. As long as the patient's arm is at heart level, the blood pressure can be determined with the patient in any position. Errors up to 10 mm Hg, both systolic and diastolic, can be made if the arm is not at the correct level. Falsely elevated pressures are obtained if the arm is lower than the heart; falsely low pressures are measured if the arm is higher than the heart. The arm must be supported during pressure determination.

Patient Position. The patient's position during blood pressure measurement always should be recorded. Use the symbols or drawings shown in Figure 13-11.

Palpation. After the cuff is in place, the brachial artery is palpated continuously. Once the brachial or radial pulse is obtained, the cuff is inflated rapidly. The pressure at which the pulse disappears should be noted, but the cuff inflation should continue for another 30 mm Hg before the actual measurement of the blood pressure begins. For example, if the brachial pulse disappears when the cuff pressure is 110 mm Hg, the cuff should be pumped to 140 mm Hg before starting. The cuff should not be inflated further than necessary, because high cuff pressures are uncomfortable, create undue anxiety in the patient, and tend to raise the patient's blood pressure. The pressure in the cuff should be reduced gradually by 2 to 3 mm Hg per second. The point at which the brachial pulse is first detected on expiration is the systolic blood pressure. Diastolic blood pressure cannot be determined accurately by palpation. Once measurement is made, the cuff should be deflated rapidly. If possible, allow a minimum of 1 to 2 minutes before the blood pressure is measured again to release venous blood.

Systolic blood pressure is measured by palpation in patients whose blood pressures cannot be heard (e.g., patients in shock). It is also useful when checking blood pressures frequently (e.g., every 1 to 2 minutes). Palpated blood pressures are charted using "P" as diastolic pressure (e.g., 90/P).

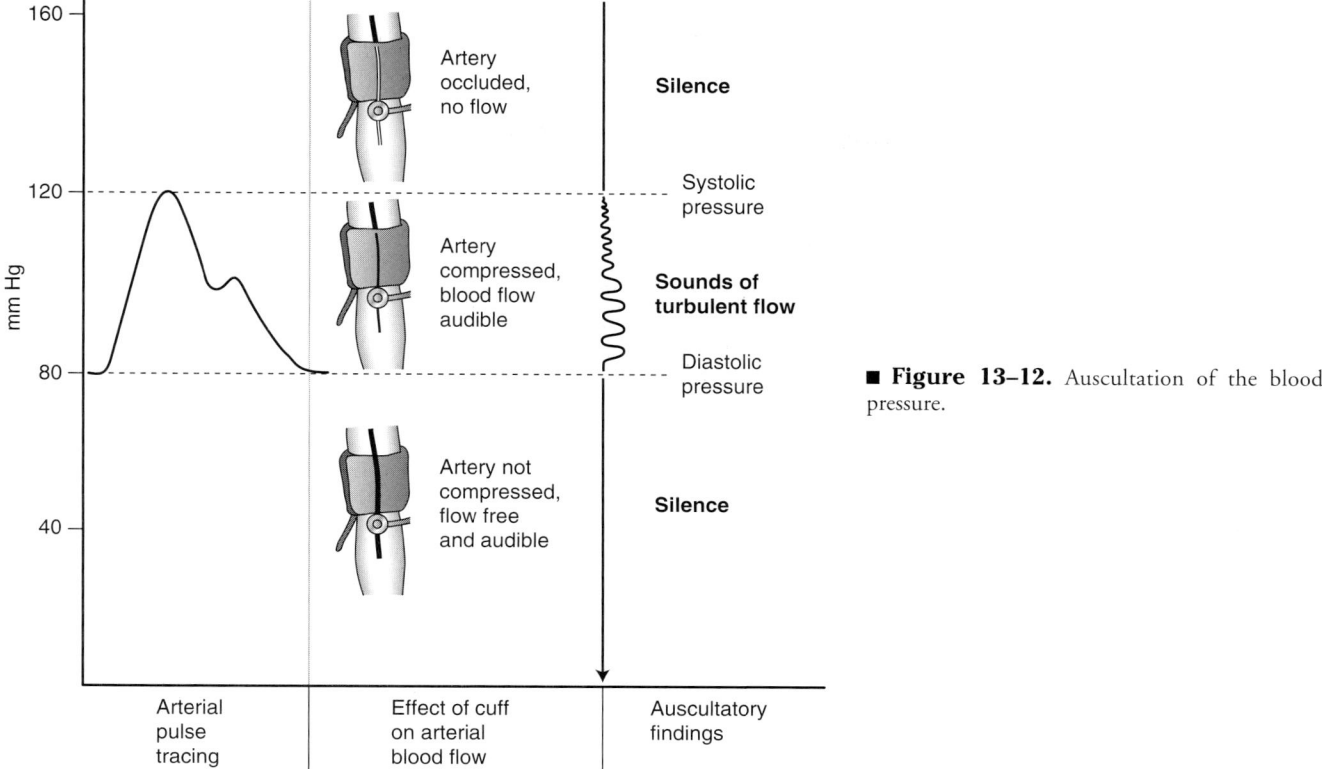

■ **Figure 13–12.** Auscultation of the blood pressure.

Auscultation. Preparation of the patient and use of the blood pressure equipment are identical in the auscultatory method. After the brachial pulse has been located, the stethoscope is applied over the artery using light pressure. Heavy pressure might partially occlude the artery, creating turbulence in the blood flow, prolonging phase IV (see below), and falsely lowering the diastolic blood pressure. Care must be taken to avoid causing extraneous noise, such as from the stethoscope touching the cuff or any other material.

Korotkoff sounds are the sounds created by turbulence of blood flow within the vessel caused by constriction of the blood pressure cuff (Fig. 13-12). The five Korotkoff sounds are summarized in Table 13-4.

Systolic blood pressure is the highest point at which initial tapping (phase I) is heard in two consecutive beats (to ascertain that the sound is not extraneous) during expiration. Systolic blood pressure is higher in the expiratory phase compared to the inspiratory phase of the respiratory cycle (see section on Measurement of Paradoxical Blood Pressure, below). Systolic blood pressure should be read to the nearest 2 mm Hg mark on the manometer.

Diastolic blood pressure is equated with disappearance of Korotkoff sounds (phase V) in adults. Phase V most closely approximates intra-arterial diastolic pressure. Muffling of sounds (phase IV) usually occurs at pressures 5 to 10 mm Hg higher than intra-arterial diastolic pressures and, therefore, is not a good indicator of diastolic blood pressure in adults. However, muffling, rather than disappearance of sounds, is a better index of intra-arterial diastolic pressure in children and in adults with hyperkinetic states. Hyperkinetic conditions, including hyperthyroidism, aortic insufficiency, and exercise, increase the rate of blood flow, resulting in disappearance of

sounds (absence of turbulence) far below intra-arterial diastolic pressure. In children and adults with hyperkinetic states, sounds can be detected below muffling for much longer than normal (Grim & Grim, 2003). As with systolic blood pressure, read diastolic pressure to the nearest 2 mm Hg mark on the

Table 13–4 ■ PHASES OF THE KOROTKOFF SOUNDS*

Phase 1
  The pressure level at which the first faint, consistent tapping sounds are heard. The sounds gradually increase in intensity as the cuff is deflated. The first of at least two of these sounds is defined as the *systolic pressure*.
Phase 2
  The time during cuff deflation when a murmur of swishing sounds is heard.
Phase 3
  The period during which sounds are crisper and increase in intensity.
Phase 4
  The time when a distinct, abrupt, muffling of sound (usually of a soft blowing quality) is heard. This is defined as the *diastolic pressure* in anyone in whom sounds continue to zero.
Phase 5
  The pressure level when the last regular blood pressure sound is heard and after which all sound disappears. This is defined as the *diastolic pressure* unless sounds are heard to zero.

* To avoid error, the observer must be prepared to recognize two normal Korotkoff sound variations associated with blood pressure (BP) readings. The auscultatory gap is a period of silence occurring during Korotkoff phases 1 and 2. This disappearance of sound is temporary and is usually short, but the gap can occur over a period of 40 mm Hg. It seems to be associated with higher BP readings. An absent Korotkoff phase 5 occurs when sounds are heard to zero. When this is the case, phase 4 should be recorded along with phase 5. In this case, phase 4 is the best reference for diastolic pressure.
Grim, C. M., & Grim, C. E. (2003). Blood pressure measurement. In J. L. Izzo, & H. R. Black (Eds.), *Hypertension primer* (3rd ed.). Dallas, TX: American Heart Association.

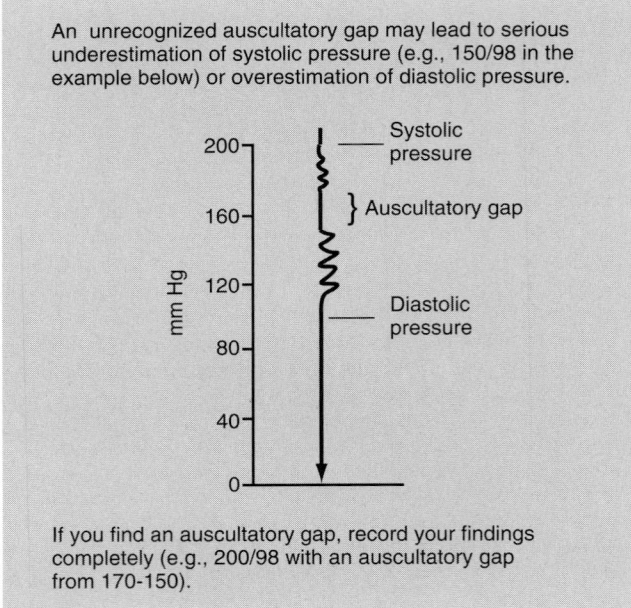

An unrecognized auscultatory gap may lead to serious underestimation of systolic pressure (e.g., 150/98 in the example below) or overestimation of diastolic pressure.

If you find an auscultatory gap, record your findings completely (e.g., 200/98 with an auscultatory gap from 170-150).

■ **Figure 13–13.** Auscultatory gap.

manometer. If there is a difference of 10 mm Hg or more between disappearance and muffling of sounds, record both diastolic pressures (e.g., 140/56/20 mm Hg; Grim & Grim, 2003).

In some patients, Korotkoff sounds may be soft and could result in falsely low blood pressure values. To augment the loudness of Korotkoff sounds, increase brachial flow by having the patient open and clench a fist; quickly inflate cuff to a value 30 mm above the palpable systolic blood pressure.

Auscultatory gap is a temporary disappearance of sound that occurs during the latter part of phase I and phase II (Fig. 13-13).

It is particularly common in patients with high blood pressure (Perloff et al., 1993), venous distention, or reduced velocity of arterial flow (e.g., severe aortic stenosis; O'Rourke et al., 1994). The auscultatory gap can be as wide as 40 mm Hg. Serious errors in blood pressure measurement can be made if the cuff is not inflated high enough to exceed true systolic pressure. Systolic blood pressure would be underestimated if the second appearance of the Korotkoff sounds were recorded as phase I. Diastolic blood pressure would be overestimated if the first muffling of sounds was considered to be phase IV. The auscultatory gap can be avoided if a preliminary palpable blood pressure is obtained before auscultation.

Measurement of Pulse Pressure

Pulse pressure is the difference between the systolic and diastolic blood pressures, expressed in millimeters of mercury. For example, if the blood pressure is 120/80 mm Hg, the pulse pressure is 40 mm Hg (Fig. 13-14). Pulse pressure reflects stroke volume, ejection velocity, and systemic vascular resistance. Use pulse pressure as a noninvasive indicator of the patient's ability to maintain cardiac output.

Pulse pressure is increased in many situations. A widened pulse pressure is seen in sinus bradycardia, complete heart block, aortic regurgitation, anxiety, exercise, and catecholamine infusion, which are examples of situations characterized by increased stroke volume. Examples of conditions that increase pulse pressure by reducing systemic vascular resistance are fever, hot environment, and exercise. Conditions such as atherosclerosis, aging, and high blood pressure widen the pulse pressure because of decreased distensibility of the aorta, arteries, and arterioles. A narrowed pulse pressure also can be caused by many factors: reduced ejection velocity in heart failure, shock, and hypovolemia; mechanical obstruction to systolic outflow in aortic stenosis, mitral stenosis, and mitral

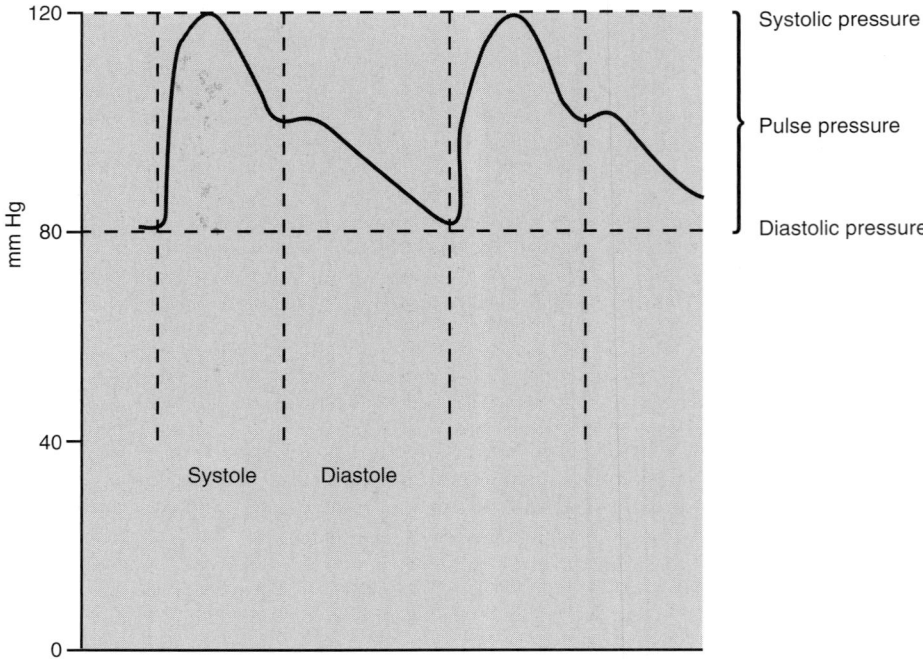

■ **Figure 13–14.** Measurement of pulse pressure.

insufficiency; peripheral vasoconstriction in shock and with certain drugs; and artifactually from an auscultatory gap (Braunwald & Perloff, 2001; O'Rourke et al., 1994). If the pulse pressure in the cardiac patient falls below 30 mm Hg, further assessment of the patient's cardiovascular status may be indicated.

Measurement of Postural Blood Pressure

Postural (orthostatic) hypotension occurs when the blood pressure drops after an upright posture is assumed. It usually is accompanied by dizziness, lightheadedness, or syncope. Although there are many causes of postural hypotension, the three most commonly seen in the cardiac patient are (1) intravascular volume depletion, which often results from aggressive diuretic therapy, inadequate intake, or intravascular to extravascular fluid shift; (2) inadequate vasoconstrictor mechanisms, which may be a primary pathologic process but also result from immobility; and (3) autonomic insufficiency, which is often related to the sympathetic blocking drugs used in the cardiac patient. Postural changes in blood pressure, along with the appropriate history, can help the clinician differentiate between them (Calkins & Zipes, 2001; Robertson, 2003). Postural changes in blood pressure and pulse should be measured in patients who are older than age 65 years, diabetic, receiving antihypertensive therapy, or who complain of dizziness or syncope. Important points to remember are the following:

- Position the patient supine and as flat as symptoms permit for 10 minutes before the initial measurement of blood pressure and heart rate.
- Always check supine measurements before upright measurements.
- Always record both heart rate and blood pressure at each postural change.
- Do not remove the blood pressure cuff between position changes, but do check to see that it remains placed correctly.
- Safety considerations may require assessment of blood pressure and pulse with the patient seated with legs in the dependent position before standing. Measurement of blood pressure and pulse in this position is not sufficient to rule out orthostasis (Calkins & Zipes, 2001).
- Have the patient assume a standing position. Measure the blood pressure and pulse immediately and after 2 minutes. If orthostasis is strongly suspected and not apparent after 2 minutes, continue to monitor blood pressure and pulse every 2 minutes for 10 minutes. If the purpose of collecting the data is to assess the risk of falling, another approach is to ask the patient to get out of bed as he or she normally does and evaluate the change in pulse rate and blood pressure and associated symptoms at the patient's rate of position change.
- Be alert for any signs or symptoms of patient distress, including dizziness, weakness, blurring of vision, and syncope. When the patient returns to a recumbent position, these symptoms should reverse and the blood pressure and pulse return to normal.
- Record any signs or symptoms that accompany the postural change.

Normal postural responses are a transient increased heart rate of 5 to 20 beats per minute (to offset reduced stroke volume and to maintain cardiac output), a drop in systolic pressure of less than 10 mm Hg, and an increase in diastolic pressure of approximately 5 mm Hg. *Orthostasis* is defined as a drop in systolic pressure of 20 mm Hg or greater or a drop in diastolic pressure of at least 10 mm Hg within 3 minutes of standing (Calkins & Zipes, 2001), although any drop in diastolic pressure may be cause for concern. The change from lying to sitting position is not sufficient to make a diagnosis of orthostasis; it may be used as a screening test because decreased blood pressure, increased pulse, or symptoms in the sitting position presage similar events in the erect position. Often, the change in blood pressure does not meet the criteria for orthostasis, but it is accompanied by a significant change in heart rate or associated symptoms, or both. These circumstances identify people at risk and should prompt further investigation by the cardiac nurse of the patient's present volume status and vasodilatory or cardioinhibitory drug regimen.

The presence of intravascular volume depletion (such as with diuretic therapy) should be suspected when, in response to sitting or standing, the heart rate increases and the systolic pressure decreases by 15 mm Hg and the diastolic blood pressure drops by 10 mm Hg (Calkins & Zipes, 2001). It is difficult to differentiate intravascular volume loss from inadequate vasoconstrictor mechanisms solely by changes in vital signs accompanying postural changes. With intravascular volume depletion, reflexes to maintain cardiac output (increased heart rate and peripheral vasoconstriction) function correctly, but, because of reduced intravascular fluid volume, these reflexes are not adequate to maintain systemic arterial pressure and the blood pressure falls. With inadequate vasoconstrictor mechanisms, the heart rate responds appropriately also, but blood pressure drops because of diminished peripheral vasoconstriction. Differentiation, therefore, depends in part on the patient's history. However, intravascular depletion and inadequate vasoconstrictor mechanisms are not mutually exclusive. The following is an example of a postural blood pressure recording showing either saline depletion or inadequate vasoconstrictor mechanisms:

Blood Pressure	Heart Rate	Patient Position
120/70 mm Hg	70 bpm	
100/55 mm Hg	90 bpm	
98/52 mm Hg	94 bpm	
150/90 mm Hg	60 bpm	
100/60 mm Hg	60 bpm	

Measurement of Paradoxical Blood Pressure

Paradoxical blood pressure is an exaggerated decrease in the systolic blood pressure during inspiration. The mechanism is complex and controversial. Normally, during inspiration, blood flow into the right heart is increased, right ventricular output is enhanced, and pulmonary venous capacitance is increased. Consequently, less blood reaches the left ventricle, which reduces left ventricular stroke volume and arterial pressure (Parati, Izzo & Gavish, 2003).

During cardiac tamponade, effects of respiration on both right and left ventricular filling appear to be greater than normal,

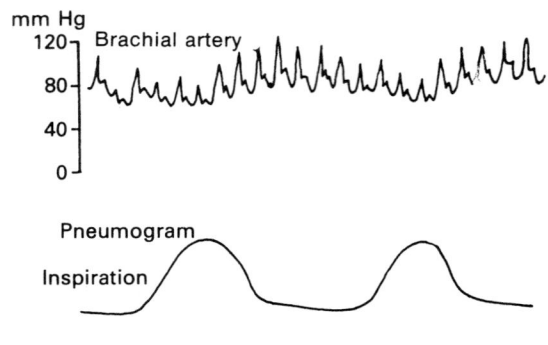

CARDIAC TAMPONADE

■ **Figure 13–15.** Paradoxical blood pressure in cardiac tamponade. The paradox is greater than 20 mm Hg. (Adapted from Fowler, N. O. [1972]. *Examination of the heart, part 2: Inspection and palpation of arterial and venous pulses* [p. 33]. New York: American Heart Association. By permission of the American Heart Association, Inc.)

causing a reduction of 10 mm Hg or more in systolic pressure during normal inspiration (Spodick, 2001; Fig. 13-15). In addition, echocardiography has demonstrated a shift of the intraventricular septum to the left, further impairing left ventricular filling and stroke volume. With high intrapericardial pressures, the thin-walled right ventricle may collapse during diastole, further impairing venous return and cardiac output (Spodick, 2001). Chronic obstructive airway disease, constrictive pericarditis, pulmonary emboli, restrictive cardiomyopathy, and cardiogenic shock have also been associated with an abnormal inspiratory decline of blood pressure. Echocardiographic studies of patients with emphysema demonstrate both an augmented inspiratory filling of the right ventricle and an exaggerated inspiratory decline of left ventricular filling (Chatterjee, 1991a).

The patient should breathe normally and must not exaggerate respiratory effort during an examination for a paradoxical blood pressure. As before, the nurse should inflate and gradually deflate the cuff until the first systolic sound is heard on expiration and continue slowly releasing the cuff pressure until sounds are heard both on inspiration and expiration. The difference between the two is termed the *paradox,* and it normally is less than 10 mm Hg (Spodick, 2001). For example, if the first systolic sound occurs at 140 mm Hg during expiration and Korotkoff sounds begin appearing with both inspiration and expiration at 120 mm Hg, the paradox is 20 mm Hg. Paradoxical blood pressures should be determined as a baseline in all patients on the cardiac care unit and routinely in all patients with pericarditis or with heart catheters, such as a temporary pacing wire.

Blood Pressure Measurement Under Special Conditions

Arrhythmia. With very irregular rhythms, accurate assessment of blood pressure is difficult because of the beat-to-beat variation in both stroke volume and blood pressure. Systolic blood pressure is related directly to the stroke volume and duration of the preceding cycle. Pulse pressure is related inversely to pulse cycle duration. A short cycle (reduced ventricular filling time) increases the diastolic blood pressure of that cycle and

reduces systolic blood pressure during the next cycle. A long pulse cycle (increased ventricular filling time) causes a decreased diastolic blood pressure in that cycle but an increased systolic blood pressure in the next cycle (Marriott, 1993).

Any arrhythmia that alters stroke volume and cardiac output can be detected during blood pressure measurement. Always record the presence of an irregular cardiac rhythm along with the blood pressure.

Premature ectopic beats (either ventricular or supraventricular) have a short cycle followed by a long cycle (post extrasystolic beat). If they occur only occasionally, they have minimal effects on blood pressure. In *bigeminal rhythms,* as the blood pressure cuff is deflated, Korotkoff sounds of the alternate strong beats are heard first and are half as fast as the heart rate. Further reduction in cuff pressure enables the listener to hear the alternating weaker sounds produced by the ectopic impulses as well.

Pulsus alternans, indicative of severe organic heart disease and left heart failure, also is manifested by alternating strong and weak pulses but with a regular cadence. Pulsus alternans can occur with ectopic bigeminal rhythms that are interpolated rather than premature, but, in this instance, it does not necessarily indicate severe organic heart disease.

Because pulse cycle length changes constantly in *atrial fibrillation,* both systolic and diastolic blood pressures must be approximated (Perloff et al., 1993). For systolic blood pressure, average a series of readings (three to five) of phase I pressures. For diastolic blood pressure, average the pressure readings obtained in phases IV and V.

Atrioventricular dissociation can be detected during auscultation of blood pressure. Examples of rhythms with atrioventricular dissociation include *ventricular tachycardia, high-grade* or *complete atrioventricular block,* and *asynchronous ventricular pacing.* In atrioventricular dissociation, an occasional, well-timed atrial contraction contributes to diastolic ventricular filling. This "atrial kick" augments the stroke volume for that beat. As the cuff bladder is deflated, phase I sounds periodically are increased.

Clinical Shock. In shock states associated with reduced cardiac output and elevated systemic vascular resistance, Korotkoff sounds may not be generated in the periphery. Direct measurement of blood pressure may be required to manage these critically ill patients. When indirect cuff measurements are compared with direct (femoral arterial) pressure measurements, direct pressures are higher than auscultated pressures. In hypotensive states, when direct measurement of blood pressure is not feasible, *Doppler ultrasound* may provide a more reliable indirect measurement of systolic blood pressure than the auscultatory method. Place the Doppler probe (with conducting gel) over the patient's artery. As in auscultatory measurement, inflate the cuff and listen for the arterial signal as the bladder is deflated. Cuff widths of 50% of the arm circumference have been recommended for the Doppler technique (Perloff et al., 1993).

Obesity. Cuff size and bladder size frequently are too small for use in the obese patient. If a proper-sized cuff cannot be used, apply a standard cuff to the forearm 13 cm from the elbow and auscultate the radial artery to obtain the blood pressure measurement.

Thigh Blood Pressure Measurement. Blood pressures are measured in the thigh if the arms cannot be used or to confirm or rule out certain conditions that alter circulation, such as coarctation of the aorta or dissecting aortic aneurysm.

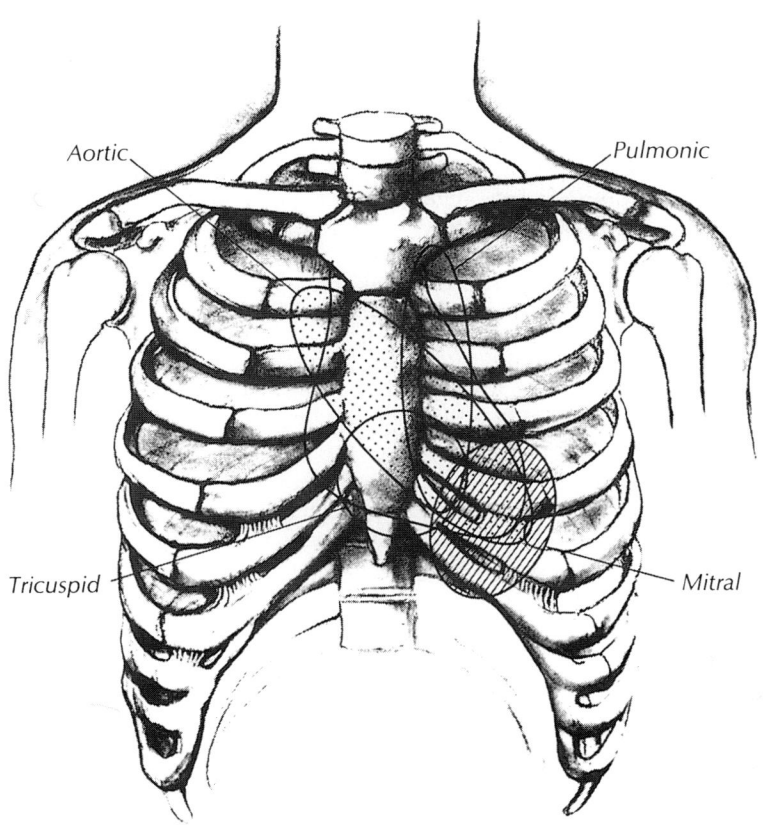

■ **Figure 13–17.** Areas to be assessed in the precordial examination. (Drawn from Leatham, A. [1979]. *An introduction to the examination of the cardiovascular system* [2nd ed., p. 20]. Oxford: Oxford University Press.)

Aortic

Pulmonic

Tricuspid

Mitral

When visible, the normal *apex impulse* can be seen within the fifth ICS at or just medial to the MCL. It is an early systolic pulsation with a rapid upstroke and downstroke. A late systolic retraction, 1 to 2 cm long, in the fourth or fifth ICS may also be normally seen and is produced by ventricular emptying. The apex impulse cannot be seen in every patient. It is easily detected in thin patients, whereas it may not be visible in those who are obese or have large breasts or barrel chests. An apex impulse that is below the fifth ICS, lateral to the MCL, or seen in more than one ICS represents left ventricular enlargement.

Slight movement over the sternum or the epigastrium can be normal in thin people and in those with fever or anemia who may have hyperdynamic heartbeats. A *sternal rise* that is sustained after systole begins usually indicates right ventricular enlargement. Pulsations in other areas are abnormal. For example, pulsation over the second right ICS may represent an aortic aneurysm, and pulsation over the second left ICS can represent increased filling pressure or flow in the pulmonary artery.

Paradoxical movement of the left anterior precordium is suggestive of a left ventricular aneurysm. With paradoxical movement, as the apex contracts, the aneurysmic area bulges. This ectopic impulse usually is seen above the apex impulse. The visibility of abnormal pulsations can be enhanced by balancing a tongue depressor on the chest over the pulsation.

Palpation

Movement that was not visible on inspection may be detected by palpation. All areas should be palpated using either the ball of the palm (at the base of the fingers) or the fingertips. In gen-

eral, the palm surface is more sensitive to *thrills* (vibrations), whereas fingertips are more sensitive to *pulsations*. Thrills indicate turbulence of blood flow and are associated with murmurs. Impulses are described in terms of *location, size, amplitude, duration,* and *time in the cardiac cycle* (systole or diastole). To facilitate measurement of the horizontal location in centimeters from the MCL, or the size of the impulse, it is helpful for the examiner to measure his or her hand and use it as a "ruler." For example, the distance from the tip of the finger to the first joint, the second joint, and the third joint can be used.

Assess the apex impulse for location, size, amplitude, and duration. The apex impulse is, by definition, the furthest point leftward and downward at which a cardiac pulsation can be seen or felt (Marriott, 1993). The normal apex impulse is felt as a light tap, extending over 3 cm or less. The apex impulse is felt immediately after the first heart sound and lasts halfway through systole. An impulse that is diffuse (felt over two ICSs), increased in amplitude, or laterally or inferiorly displaced suggests increased volume load and left ventricular dilatation, such as occurs in mitral insufficiency or left ventricular failure. An impulse that is sustained, enlarged, and, sometimes, laterally displaced suggests obstruction to outflow with increased ventricular pressure load and concentric hypertrophy of the muscle, such as occurs in aortic stenosis or systemic hypertension (Braunwald & Perloff, 2001). If the apex impulse cannot be felt with the patient lying supine, examine the patient in the left lateral position, which brings the apex of the heart against the chest wall; the quality of the apex beat still can be determined even though its size and position may be slightly altered. A diastolic outward pulsation indicates impaired ventricular filling and corresponds to an S_3 (early to mid-diastole) or S_4 (late diastole) heard on auscultation.

Next, palpate the right ventricular area. The presence of a pulsation suggests right ventricular enlargement. Palpation of the epigastrium, by placing the palmar surface of the hand over the area and sliding the fingers toward the xiphoid, can also detect right ventricular enlargement. Pulsations beating down on the fingertips indicate right ventricular movement. Pulsations pushing upward against the hand originate in the aorta. An increased aortic pulse could indicate abdominal aortic aneurysm or aortic regurgitation. Hepatic pulsations may be felt in the epigastrium but also over the right upper abdomen. The liver may pulsate with tricuspid valve disease, severe right ventricular failure, or pulmonary hypertension (Marriott, 1993). A thrill at the lower left sternal border suggests tricuspid valve disease.

Then, palpate the third left ICS and the second left and right ICSs. Systolic pulsations in the second left or right ICS suggest increased pressure or enlargement of the pulmonary artery or the aorta, respectively; thrills suggest pulmonary or aortic valve abnormalities.

Auscultation

Stethoscope. A good-quality stethoscope is required for cardiac auscultation. Although the human ear is able to hear sounds ranging in frequency from 20 cycles per second, or Hertz (Hz), to 20,000 Hz, it is most sensitive to 1,000 to 5,000 Hz. The frequency of most heart sounds is less than 1,000 Hz. The stethoscope must transmit these low-frequency sounds to the ear.

The parts of the stethoscope are the ear pieces, tubing, and chest pieces. The ear pieces should fit comfortably into the ear canal and be snug enough so that extraneous sound cannot enter. They also must be kept free of ear wax. Double tubing with a small internal diameter (3 mm) should extend from the ear pieces to the chest pieces. In addition, the tubing should be reasonably short (25 to 30 cm) so the sound is not diluted and should be thick to minimize room noise (Tilkian & Conover, 2001).

There are two basic types of chest pieces, the diaphragm and the bell. The *diaphragm,* which brings out higher frequencies and filters out the lower ones, is useful for listening to the first and second heart sounds (S_1 and S_2), high-frequency murmurs, and lung sounds. The diaphragm should be pressed firmly against the chest wall. The *bell* filters out high-frequency sounds and accentuates the low-frequency ones. Diastolic filling sounds and the low-frequency murmurs of mitral and tricuspid stenosis are heard best with the bell (Tilkian & Conover, 2001). The bell should rest lightly on the chest; if firm pressure is applied, the skin becomes taut and acts like a diaphragm. When auscultating heart sounds, the nurse stands on the patient's right side so that, as he or she places the bell of the stethoscope on the patient's chest, the chest piece is balanced. Because the bell does not have to be held in place, the possibilities of creating extraneous sounds and filtering out low frequencies are reduced.

As part of a cardiac examination, all areas identified in Figure 13-17 should be auscultated except the epigastrium. The listener's goals when auscultating the precordium are to identify normal heart sounds, the heart rate, and rhythm; extra diastolic and systolic sounds; murmurs; and pericardial friction rubs.

Technique. The stethoscope is placed directly on the chest wall; adequate auscultation of the heart and lungs through clothing is impossible. The room should be quiet; the patient and examiner should be comfortable. Cardiac auscultation should be performed with the patient in three positions: supine, lying partially on the left side, and sitting up, leaning forward. The examiner can begin listening either at the cardiac apex or at the base. Beginning at the apex allows the examiner to focus initially on the first heart sound, clearly identify systole and diastole, and think through the cardiac cycle while listening at each site. The apex is the location of the apex impulse identified by palpation. Remember that left ventricular enlargement shifts the apex from the normal location. The timing of extra sounds in the cardiac cycle, the location in which they are best heard, and the quality of the sound are used to differentiate one from another.

It is important to proceed in a systematic manner. Inching the stethoscope up and down the chest wall is a useful technique and allows the examiner to focus on specific events in the cardiac cycle (Table 13-5). At each location, listen sequentially to four events: S_1, systole (interval between S_1 and S_2), S_2, and diastole (interval between S_2 and S_1). For example, begin at the apical area with the diaphragm of the stethoscope and focus on S_1 and S_2. Normally, S_1 is louder than or equal to S_2 at the apex. Listen carefully during systole and during diastole for clicks, murmurs, or other extra sounds. Inch the stethoscope toward the sternum to the right ventricular area and listen for a split S_1. Continue to move the stethoscope up the left sternal border to the second left ICS and note the change in relative intensity of the heart sounds. Normally, S_2 is louder than S_1 at the base. Continue to listen for splitting of the second heart sound and, if present, determine whether it is physiologic or abnormal. Move the stethoscope to the second right ICS and listen for an ejection sound in early systole after S_1. Listen with the bell along the lower sternal border for right ventricular S_3 and S_4. Move the bell to the apical area and listen for left ventricular S_3 and S_4. An opening sound of the mitral valve (high frequency) can be distinguished from an S_3 by pressing firmly with the bell to stretch the skin. Stretching the skin causes it to act as a diaphragm and filters out low-frequency sounds.

Normal Heart Sounds. Normal heart sounds consist of the first and second heart sounds, S_1 and S_2. Both are of relatively high frequency and can, therefore, be heard clearly with the diaphragm of the stethoscope. Systole is normally shorter than

Table 13–5 ■ AUSCULTATORY TECHNIQUE

Location	Chest Piece	Sounds
Apex	Diaphragm	S_1 intensity; opening sounds; murmurs from aortic and mitral valve
	Bell	Left S_3, S_4; murmurs
Left sternal border	Diaphragm	S_2 intensity; split S_1; murmurs from tricuspid and pulmonic valves and from atrial septal defects
	Bell	Right S_3, S_4
Base	Diaphragm	Split S_2; ejection sounds; murmurs from aortic valve
	Bell	Murmurs from aortic valve or dilated aorta

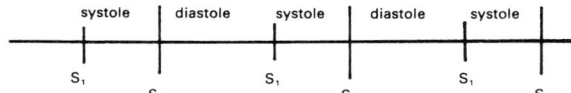

■ **Figure 13–18.** Normal heart sounds.

diastole; with slow heart rates (less than 100 beats/min), the two sounds are easily distinguished by the cadence of the rhythm (Fig. 13-18). However, in more rapid rhythms, diastole shortens so that systole and diastole are of equal duration or, as the rate increases further, diastole becomes shorter than systole. To identify systole and diastole properly in this instance, the examiner should palpate the carotid artery while listening to the heart; the carotid upstroke immediately follows S_1.

Phonocardiograms or echocardiograms can be used to validate the auscultatory findings. In a phonocardiogram, heart sounds, ECG, and carotid pulse tracings are recorded simultaneously. Phonocardiograms are most often used for research or teaching. Echocardiograms are used clinically to demonstrate abnormalities of valve structure and cardiac function (Armstrong & Feigenbaum, 2001).

The *first heart sound* is due primarily to closure of the mitral and tricuspid valves and is, therefore, heard loudest at the apex of the heart. Phonetically, if the heart sounds are "lub-dup," S_1 is the "lub." Mitral and tricuspid closure usually is heard as a single sound.

The intensity of the S_1 depends on leaflet mobility, position of the atrioventricular valves at the onset of systole, and the rate of ventricular upstroke. A loud S_1 is noted clinically in mitral stenosis when the cusps are mobile; with a short PR interval (0.08 to 0.13 second) because the leaflets are wide open when systolic contraction begins; in tachycardia, hyperthyroidism, or exercise because of an increased rate of pressure rise in the ventricle; and in the presence of a mechanical prosthetic mitral valve. Most commonly, a soft S_1 is due to poor conduction of sound through the chest wall, but other causes include a fixed or immobile valve; a long PR interval (0.20 to 0.26 second) or a slow heart rate, which allows the atrioventricular valves to float back into position before the onset of ventricular systole; low flow at the end of diastole; and β-adrenergic or calcium channel blockers that reduce the rate of rise of ventricular pressure. The intensity of S_1 varies from beat to beat in atrial fibrillation because diastolic filling time is not constant. In a regular rhythm with a variable S_1 intensity, complete heart block should be suspected (Ronan, 1992a). Variation in the intensity of S_1 can be evaluated by listening carefully to the relative intensity of S_1 and S_2 at the apex and the base. For example, when the intensity of S_1 is increased, it may be equal to or louder than S_2 at the base (Ronan, 1992a). When assessing variation in S_1, it is helpful to have the patient hold his or her breath because respiratory movements may cause variation in the intensity of heart sounds.

Splitting of the first heart sound occurs when tricuspid closure is delayed and is best heard at the lower left sternal border. Pathologic splitting of S_1 results from right bundle-branch block, tricuspid stenosis, and atrial septal defect (Ronan, 1992a). Splitting of S_1 helps to differentiate supraventricular from ventricular tachycardia. In supraventricular rhythms, S_1 is normal; in ventricular rhythms it is split (Marriott, 1993).

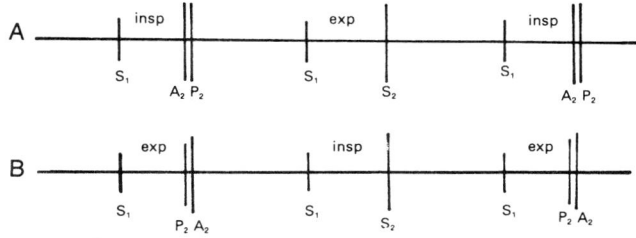

■ **Figure 13–19.** Splitting of the S_2. (*A*) Physiologic splitting. During inspiration (*insp*), the P_2 sound is delayed. (*B*) Paradoxical splitting. During expiration (*exp*), A_2 is delayed.

Unfortunately, when supraventricular rhythms are conducted aberrantly, S_1 is split.

The *second heart sound* results primarily from closure of the aortic and pulmonic valves and is loudest at the base of the heart. Phonetically, the "dup" of the "lub-dup" is the S_2. The intensity of S_2 is determined by the pressure in the receiving vessels, the mobility of the valve leaflets, the degree of apposition of the leaflets, and the size of the aortic root. Intensity is increased with systemic or pulmonary hypertension, ascending aortic aneurysm, and in the presence of a mechanical prosthetic aortic valve. Intensity may be diminished in heart failure, myocardial infarction, pulmonary embolism, clinical shock, and stenosis of the aortic or pulmonic valve (Ronan, 1992a).

Physiologic (normal) *splitting* of S_2 occurs during inspiration. During inspiration, an increased amount of blood is returned to the right side of the heart and a decreased amount of blood is returned to the left side of the heart due to trapping in the expanded lung. Pulmonic valve closure (P_2) is delayed because of the extra time needed for the increased blood volume to pass through the pulmonic valve, and aortic valve closure (A_2) occurs slightly early because of the relatively smaller amount of blood ejected from the left ventricle. In addition, the time of closure of P_2 is affected by the "hang out" interval, which is inversely related to pulmonary vascular impedance. During inspiration, the pulmonary vascular impedance decreases and P_2 is delayed; on expiration the opposite occurs (Ronan, 1992a). If the two components are fairly close together, it is difficult to appreciate two distinct and separate sounds. A physiologic split S_2 may seem muffled or sound like a short drum roll on inspiration compared with expiration. On expiration, the split sounds merge (Fig. 13-19*A*). Normal splitting should be evaluated during quiet respiration and may be better heard with the patient sitting (Marriott, 1993). In pathologic splitting of S_2 (wide or fixed splits), the second sound is split during both inspiration and expiration, although there may be some respiratory variation in the amount of the split.

Paradoxical (abnormal) *splitting* of S_2 also can occur. Paradoxical splitting is due to any mechanism that causes late aortic valve closure (A_2), such as electrical delay (left bundle-branch block, right ventricular pacing, or right ventricular ectopy), mechanical obstruction (aortic stenosis or systolic hypertension), or impaired left ventricular contractile function (left ventricular failure or left ventricular ischemia; see Fig. 13-19*B*). Because P_2 is soft and A_2 is comparably loud and easily transmitted, a split S_2 is heard best in the second left ICS (pulmonary outflow tract). In paradoxical splitting, the second component (aortic closure) is louder than the first component (pulmonic closure).

Normally, A_2 is louder than P_2, even in the pulmonic area, and P_2 is not well heard, if at all, in other areas of the precordium. In pulmonary hypertension, the intensity of P_2 increases so that A_2 less than or equal to P_2. The loud P_2 can be heard in other areas of the precordium, particularly the lower left sternal border and the cardiac apex (Bickley & Szilagyi, 2003).

Extra Diastolic Sounds. Extra diastolic sounds consist of diastolic filling sounds and opening snaps. *Diastolic filling sounds* (S_3 and S_4) occur as blood enters a noncompliant ventricle during the two phases of rapid ventricular filling; the end of the early rapid filling phase, as active ventricular relaxation ceases (S_3); and, with atrial contraction, the active, rapid filling phase (S_4). Three theories have been proposed to explain the generation of the third and fourth heart sounds: the mitral valve theory, the chest wall theory, and the ventricular wall vibration theory. The last is the most widely accepted theory. Sound is produced within the ventricle by the abrupt decrease in wall motion (S_3) or with rapid filling of a noncompliant ventricle that causes a rapid deceleration of blood flow (Ronan, 1992b). Diastolic filling sounds can arise from either or both ventricles. The cadence suggests the sound of a galloping horse, and these sounds are sometimes called diastolic gallops.

A *physiologic S_3* can be heard in healthy children or young adults but usually disappears by 40 years of age. Its disappearance with advancing age has been attributed to decreased ventricular wall compliance with reduced early ventricular filling (Marriott, 1993). An S_3 in people older than age 40 years is usually pathologic and signals impaired systolic function (Ronan, 1992b). It is one of the first clinical findings associated with cardiac decompensation, such as left ventricular heart failure (left ventricular S_3), primary pulmonary hypertension and cor pulmonale (right ventricular S_3), or insufficiency of the mitral, aortic, or tricuspid valves. An S_3 follows the S_2 in a "lub-dup-*ta*" cadence (Fig. 13-20). Using the bell of the stethoscope, listen for a left ventricular S_3 over the apex of the heart; for a right ventricular S_3, listen over the lower left sternal border. By having the patient in the left lateral position, the apex is brought forward against the chest wall, making the left ventricular S_3 louder and, therefore, easier to hear.

The S_4 occurs after atrial contraction as the blood is ejected into a noncompliant ventricle, producing a rapid elevation of ventricular pressure, and signals diastolic dysfunction. Although it is the fourth heart sound, because the S_4 occurs at the end of

ventricular diastole, it is heard immediately before S_1 and sounds like "*ta*-lub-dup" (Fig. 13-21). The S_4 is heard in most patients who have had a myocardial infarction, in a large number of patients experiencing angina pectoris, and in patients with coronary heart disease. It is also heard in patients with left ventricular hypertrophy due to hypertension, hypertrophic cardiomyopathy, or aortic stenosis. It is common in the elderly because of the decreased compliance of the ventricle that occurs with age and the prevalence of hypertension and aortic stenosis in this population. An S_4 does not necessarily imply cardiac failure in people with ventricular hypertrophy. Because atrial contraction is necessary to produce an S_4, it is not heard in patients with atrial fibrillation. As with the S_3, listen for an S_4 using the bell of the stethoscope. A left ventricular S_4 is heard best at the apex, with the patient lying in the left lateral position; right ventricular S_4 is loudest over the lower left sternal border. Inching the stethoscope from the apex to the lower left sternal border can be helpful in differentiating right- and left-sided sounds. Left-sided sounds fade and right-sided sounds get louder as the stethoscope approaches the sternum.

A *quadruple rhythm* may be heard in patients with severe cardiac failure and both systolic and diastolic dysfunction. If the heart rate is slow enough, four distinct heart sounds (S_1, S_2, and both S_3 and S_4) can be heard (Fig. 13-22). However, if a patient is ill enough to have a quadruple rhythm, tachycardia also usually is present. In this case, a *summation gallop* is heard, in which the S_3 and S_4 gallops fuse in mid-diastole to one loud diastolic sound. The summation gallop resembles the sound of a galloping horse (Fig. 13-23).

It stands to reason that in a noncompliant ventricle there should be more resistance to active ventricular filling than to passive ventricular filling; therefore, an S_4 gallop should be generated more easily than an S_3 gallop. Therefore, one would expect all patients with normal sinus rhythm who have an S_3 gallop to have an S_4 gallop as well. However, patients with normal sinus rhythm frequently have only an S_3. The cause for this finding is unknown, although one possibility may be an absence of actual mechanical atrial contraction in spite of electrical atrial activity.

Opening snaps are associated with the opening of a stenotic mitral valve. Opening sounds are not heard with normal valves. The sound is heard in very early diastole, medial to the cardiac apex. The sound can be loud and transmitted throughout the precordium (Fig. 13-24). Unlike an S_3, an opening snap has a high-pitched, snapping quality and is heard best with the diaphragm of the stethoscope (Tilkian & Conover, 2001).

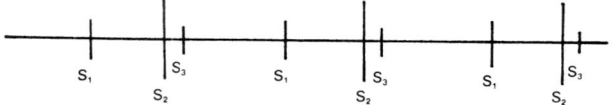

■ **Figure 13–20.** An S_3 gallop immediately follows the S_2.

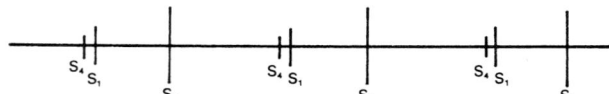

■ **Figure 13–21.** An S_4 gallop immediately precedes the S_1.

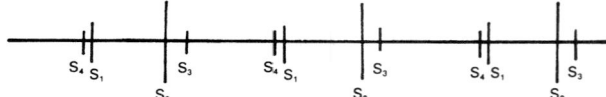

■ **Figure 13–22.** Quadruple rhythm.

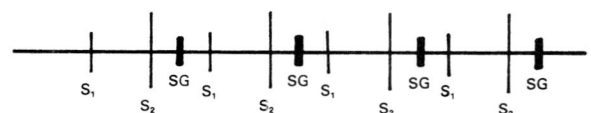

■ **Figure 13–23.** Summation gallop.

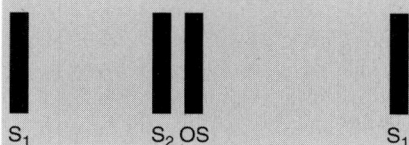

■ **Figure 13–24.** Opening snap (OS).

Extra Systolic Sounds. Extra systolic sounds consist of early systolic ejection sounds and systolic clicks. *Early ejection sounds* (Fig. 13-25) coincide with the opening of the aortic and pulmonic valves. They are heard shortly after S_1 and are high-pitched and clicking in quality. An *aortic ejection sound* is heard at the base or apex and accompanies a dilated aorta or aortic stenosis. *Pulmonic ejection sounds* are heard loudest in the second or third left ICSs and occur with pulmonary artery dilatation, pulmonary hypertension, and pulmonary stenosis (Tilkian & Conover, 2001). *Mid- to late systolic clicks* are associated with mitral valve prolapse; they occur from tensing of the leaflet or chordae when the limit of excursion is reached, and frequently they are followed by a murmur (Fig. 13-26).

Murmurs. Heart murmurs are sounds produced in the heart or great vessels by turbulent blood flow. Turbulent blood flow can be produced by (Tilkian & Conover, 2001):

- Increased rate of flow across a normal valve (exercise, pregnancy, anemia)
- Flow across a partial obstruction (valvular stenosis, pulmonary or systemic hypertension)
- Flow across an irregularity without obstruction (bicuspid aortic valve, thickening of aortic cusps with aging)
- Flow into a dilated vessel (dilation of the aortic root)
- Backward flow across an incompetent valve or through a ventricular septal defect

Murmurs are classified according to systolic or diastolic *timing* (Fig. 13-27); *intensity* (Table 13-6); *location* (where the murmur is heard loudest); *radiation,* such as to the back, neck, or axilla; *configuration* (Fig. 13-28); *quality,* such as harsh, rough, rumbling, blowing, squeaking, or musical; and *duration* (see Fig. 13-27; Braunwald & Perloff, 2001; Tilkian & Conover, 2001). Murmurs may be organic (due to intrinsic cardiovascular disease), functional (produced by circulatory

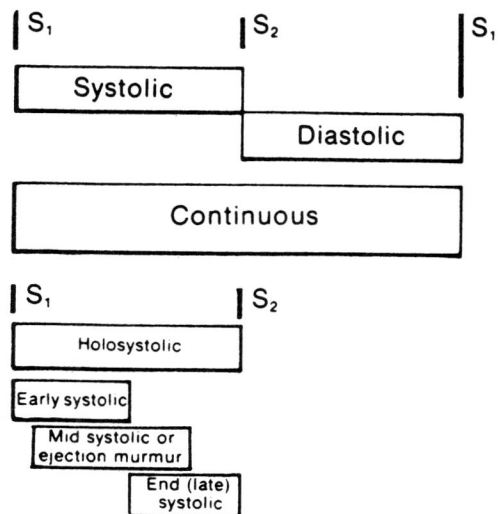

■ **Figure 13–27.** Classification of murmurs by timing. (From Tilkian, A. & Conover, M. [1993]. *Understanding heart sounds and murmurs* [3rd ed., p. 99]. Philadelphia: Saunders.)

disturbances such as anemia, pregnancy), or innocent (occur in the absence of disease; Marriott, 1993).

In adults, the most common systolic murmurs are produced by semilunar valve stenosis (ejection murmurs), atrioventricular valve insufficiency (regurgitant or holosystolic murmurs), and ventricular septal defect (early systolic murmurs) secondary to myocardial infarction. In older adults, the murmur of aortic sclerosis (thickening of aortic valve leaflets) is common. The most common diastolic murmurs are produced by the reverse set of circumstances: insufficiency of semilunar valves (early regurgitant murmurs) and stenosis of the atrioventricular valves (mid- to late diastolic rumbles). The loudness of the murmur may not correlate with the severity of the valvular lesion (e.g., a patient with a grade V to VI murmur in whom cardiogenic shock develops actually may have reduced intensity of the murmur because of diminished cardiac blood flow). Refer to Chapter 33 for descriptions of the murmurs of aortic and mitral stenosis and regurgitation.

Recognizing an innocent murmur is an important and difficult skill. The innocent murmur can often be diagnosed by its

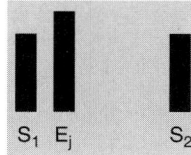

■ **Figure 13–25.** Early systolic ejection sound.

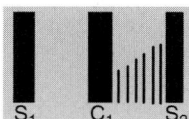

■ **Figure 13–26.** Mid to late systolic click.

Table 13–6 ■ GRADATIONS OF MURMURS

Grade	Description
Grade 1	Very faint, heard only after listener has "tuned in"; may not be heard in all positions
Grade 2	Quiet, but heard immediately after placing the stethoscope on the chest
Grade 3	Moderately loud
Grade 4	Loud, with palpable thrill
Grade 5	Very loud, with thrill. May be heard when the stethoscope is partly off the chest
Grade 6	Very loud, with thrill. May be heard with stethoscope entirely off the chest

Bickley, L. S. & Szilagyi, P.G. (2003). *Bates' guide to physical examination and history taking* (8th ed.). Philadelphia: Lippincott Williams & Wilkins.

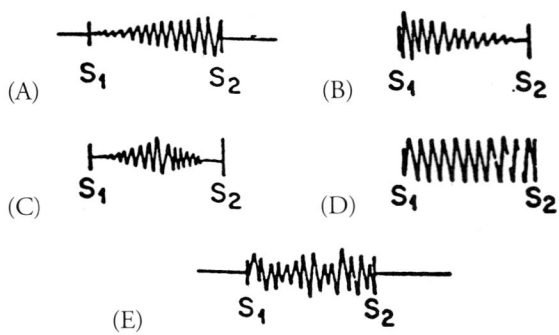

■ **Figure 13–28.** Configuration of murmurs. (*A*) Crescendo. (*B*) Decrescendo. (*C*) Crescendo-decrescendo (diamond). (*D*) Plateau (even). (*E*) Variable (uneven). (From Perloff, J. K. [1990]. *Physical examination of the heart and circulation* [p. 208]. Philadelphia: W. B. Saunders.)

clinical features and the absence of other clinical abnormalities. Clinical features of innocent murmurs include the following: always systolic, soft, short, modified by change in posture, normal S_2, and most common at left sternal border (Marriott, 1993). Echocardiography may be needed to confirm its innocence, and follow-up is essential. The precordial "whoop" or "honk" may be an innocent finding in patients without organic heart disease or may represent an exaggerated phase of an organic murmur (Marriott, 1993; Tilkian & Conover, 2001).

In the cardiac care unit, nurses are most often concerned with changes in murmurs rather than in their diagnosis. However, it is important accurately to diagnose the onset of murmurs of papillary muscle dysfunction and aortic insufficiency.

Normally, papillary muscle contraction allows for complete closure of the atrioventricular valves. However, when the papillary muscles are ischemic (most often in the left ventricle), they are unable to contract properly, preventing the chordae tendineae from being held tautly and, in turn, from holding the mitral valve leaflets closed during left ventricular contraction. Blood is, therefore, allowed to flow backward through the mitral valve (mitral regurgitation) during systole. The murmur of mitral regurgitation secondary to papillary muscle dysfunction is systolic (occurring in early to mid-systole) and usually soft, high pitched, and crescendo–decrescendo in configuration. In the presence of heart failure or angina, the murmur may become holosystolic.

A new murmur of *papillary muscle dysfunction* in the patient with acute myocardial infarction must be recognized immediately because interventions must be instituted to relieve the papillary muscle ischemia and prevent progression to papillary muscle infarction. Should the papillary muscles infarct, they also may rupture; there is a high mortality rate associated with papillary muscle rupture because of the development of sudden and profound heart failure.

In the setting of acute aortic dissection, coronary artery bypass grafting with a friable aorta, or aortic valve replacement, *new-onset aortic insufficiency* indicates retrograde dissection of the aorta, or valve dehiscence. The murmur of aortic insufficiency is an early diastolic, decrescendo murmur, heard at the second right or third left ICS that radiates toward the apex. In acute aortic insufficiency, the intensity of S_1 is frequently diminished because of the increase in ventricular volume, and

P_2 may be accentuated because of the rapid rise in pulmonary vascular pressure (Tilkian & Conover, 2001). Acute left ventricular failure may result from volume overload alone or, in the case of continued retrograde dissection, from myocardial infarction secondary to dissection of the coronary arteries.

Pericardial Friction Rubs. Pericardial friction rubs are characteristic of pericarditis, which occurs in more than 15% of patients with acute myocardial infarction. A pericardial friction rub develops in approximately 7% of patients with myocardial infarction, commonly by the fourth day after myocardial infarction. Rubs may be transient, lasting only several hours. The rub occurs with heart movement; each movement creates its own short, scratchy sound (Fig. 13-29). Pericardial friction rubs are classified as three-component (atrial systole, ventricular systole, and ventricular diastole), two-component (ventricular systole and diastole), or one component (ventricular systole) rubs. One-component rubs may be difficult to differentiate from a murmur. Rubs are best heard either with the patient sitting upright and leaning forward with the breath expelled (most appropriate for the patient with an acute myocardial infarction) or with the patient on his or her hands and knees in bed or on the examination table (useful in a nonacute situation). A peri-

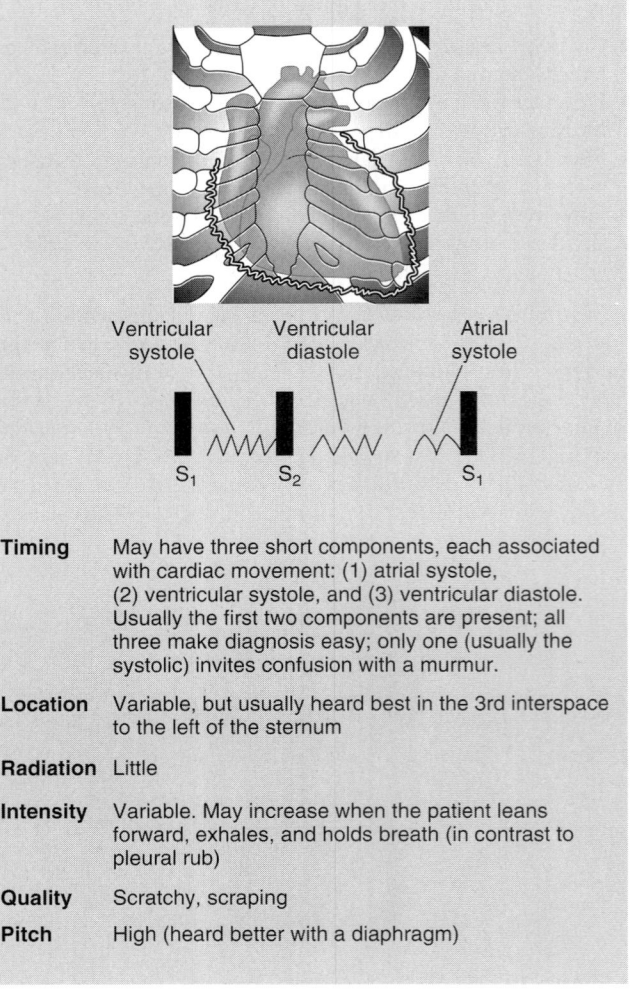

Timing	May have three short components, each associated with cardiac movement: (1) atrial systole, (2) ventricular systole, and (3) ventricular diastole. Usually the first two components are present; all three make diagnosis easy; only one (usually the systolic) invites confusion with a murmur.
Location	Variable, but usually heard best in the 3rd interspace to the left of the sternum
Radiation	Little
Intensity	Variable. May increase when the patient leans forward, exhales, and holds breath (in contrast to pleural rub)
Quality	Scratchy, scraping
Pitch	High (heard better with a diaphragm)

■ **Figure 13–29.** Pericardial friction rub.

cardial friction rub can be heard with or without a pericardial effusion. Pericardial friction rubs can be differentiated from pleural friction rubs by having the patient hold his or her breath.

Pericardial friction rubs are common in postoperative cardiac patients. Also, a respirophasic squeak may be heard that is related to mediastinal or pleural tubes. Air in the mediastinum produces a crunching sound (Hamman's sign) during auscultation of the precordium.

Dynamic Auscultation. Dynamic auscultation can be used to aid in the interpretation of heart sounds and murmurs. A variety of physiologic or pharmacologic maneuvers can be used to alter circulatory dynamics: respiration, postural changes, the Valsalva maneuver, postextrasystolic beats, isometric exercise, and vasoactive agents (Bickley & Szilagyi, 2003). Table 13-7 summarizes the auscultatory effects of these maneuvers.

Respiration affects blood flow. *Inspiration* increases venous return to the right heart, increasing right ventricular diastolic pressure, stroke volume, and ejection time. Pulmonary vascular impedance is reduced, with increases in pulmonary vascular capacitance. With a normal respiratory rate, blood return to the left ventricle is reduced, resulting in decreased left ventricular diastolic pressure, stroke volume, and ejection time. Transmission of the augmented right ventricular volume to the left ventricle is delayed by three to four cardiac cycles in the pulmonary vasculature. All of the auscultatory events generated by the right heart are augmented during inspiration (Tilkian & Conover, 2001). The use of the Müller maneuver (sustained inspiratory effort against a closed glottis) further augments the auscultatory effects of inspiration. *Expiration* increases venous return to the left heart, increasing left ventricular diastolic pressure, stroke volume, and ejection time (Braunwald & Perloff, 2001).

The *Valsalva maneuver* (forced expiration against a closed glottis) has variable effects associated with each of its four phases. In *phase I,* the *initial* phase, intrathoracic pressure increases, causing a transient elevation in left ventricular output. In *phase II,* the *straining* phase, venous return is decreased;

Table 13–7 ■ AUSCULTATORY EFFECTS OF PHYSIOLOGIC AND PHARMACOLOGIC MANEUVERS

Maneuver	Effect	Maneuver	Effect
Inspiration	Physiologically splits S_2	Valsalva maneuver	
	Attenuates left ventricular S_3 and S_4, mitral opening snap, and pulmonic ejection sound	Phase II	Attenuates S_3 and S_4 Narrows A_2–P_2 interval
	Accentuates right ventricular S_3 and S_4, tricuspid opening snap, and right heart murmurs	Phase III Phase IV	Widens A_2–P_2 interval Returns to baseline or transiently accentuates S_3 and S_4
	Hastens and accentuates click-murmur of mitral valve prolapse	Postextrasystolic beats	Augments murmurs of aortic and pulmonic stenosis, tricuspid and aortic regurgitation, and hypertrophic obstructive cardiomyopathy
Expiration	Paradoxically splits S_2		Delays click, murmur of mitral valve prolapse
	Accentuates left ventricular S_3 and S_4, mitral opening snap, and left heart murmurs		
	Attenuates right ventricular S_3 and S_4, and tricuspid opening snap	Isometric exercise	Accentuates left ventricular S_3 and S_4 and murmurs of aortic regurgitation, rheumatic mitral regurgitation, ventricular septal defect, mitral stenosis
Lying down	Widens split S_2 in all respiratory phases		Attenuates murmur of aortic stenosis
	Augments first right, then left, ventricular S_3 and S_4		Delays click, murmur of mitral valve prolapse
	Augments most systolic murmurs		
	Diminishes systolic murmur of hypertrophic obstructive cardiomyopathy	Amyl nitrate	Augments opening snaps; S_3; and murmurs of aortic, pulmonic, mitral, and tricuspid stenosis, and tricuspid regurgitation
	Delays and attenuates click, murmur of mitral valve prolapse		Diminishes murmurs of mitral and aortic regurgitation, ventricular septal defect, and Austin Flint
Sudden standing	Narrows split S_2 in all respiratory phases		Hastens click, murmur of mitral valve prolapse
	Diminishes first right, then left, ventricular S_3 and S_4		
	Diminishes most systolic murmurs		
	Accentuates systolic murmur of hypertrophic obstructive cardiomyopathy	Methoxamine and phenylephrine	Accentuates murmurs of aortic and mitral regurgitation, and ventricular septal defect
	Hastens and accentuates click, murmur of mitral valve prolapse		Diminishes murmurs of hypertrophic obstructive cardiomyopathy and aortic stenosis
Squatting	Augments right and left ventricular S_3 and S_4, and most murmurs		Delays click, murmur of mitral valve prolapse
	Delays click and murmur of mitral valve prolapse		

Adapted from Braunwald, E. (1984). The physical examination. In E. Braunwald(Ed.). *Heart disease A textbook of cardiovascular medicine,* (2nd ed., pp. 35–38). Philadelphia: WB Saunders.

first right, then left ventricular filling is reduced; stroke volume, mean arterial pressure, and pulse pressure are reduced; and heart rate is increased. In *phase III,* the *release* phase, venous return is increased, with subsequent increases in right, then left, ventricular filling. In *phase IV,* the *overshoot* phase, right ventricular filling and stroke volume return to baseline or may be elevated briefly. The return to baseline of left ventricular hemodynamics is delayed for six to eight beats and also may be elevated briefly (Braunwald & Perloff, 2001; Tilkian & Conover, 2001). During phase II, all murmurs diminish except those of hypertrophic cardiomyopathy and mitral valve prolapse. The Valsalva maneuver should not be held for more than 10 seconds because it reduces cardiac output.

Postural change from sitting or standing to lying down increases venous return first to the right and then to the left ventricle. Recumbence and passive leg raising cause most auscultatory cardiac events to increase except the murmurs of idiopathic hypertrophic subaortic stenosis and mitral valve prolapse. Sudden standing has the opposite effect; it reduces venous return and causes most murmurs, except hypertrophic cardiomyopathy and mitral valve prolapse, to decrease. Squatting simultaneously increases venous return and systemic vascular resistance (Braunwald & Perloff, 2001).

Postextrasystolic beats, if followed by a pause, increase ventricular filling and cardiac contractility. Similar hemodynamic changes occur with diastolic pauses in atrial fibrillation and sinus arrhythmia (Braunwald & Perloff, 2001).

Isometric exercise increases systemic vascular resistance, arterial pressure, heart rate, cardiac output, left ventricular filling pressure, and heart size. Using a calibrated handgrip device, the patient sustains the handgrip for 20 to 30 seconds. The handgrip enhances S_3 and S_4 and aortic regurgitant murmurs. Avoid isometric exercise in patients with myocardial ischemia or ventricular arrhythmia. The patient should not perform the Valsalva maneuver simultaneously with isometric exercise.

Pharmacologic agents used in dynamic auscultation are amyl nitrate, methoxamine, and phenylephrine (Braunwald & Perloff, 2001). Inhalation of *amyl nitrate* for 10 to 15 seconds causes marked vasodilatation, reducing systemic arterial pressure and producing a reflex tachycardia, followed by an increase in stroke volume and venous return. *Methoxamine* and *phenylephrine* increase systemic vascular resistance. Both cause a reflex drop in heart rate and decrease contractility and cardiac output. Methoxamine, 3 to 5 mg intravenously, results in blood pressure changes of 20 to 40 mm Hg, lasting 10 to 20 minutes. Phenylephrine, 0.5 mg intravenously, elevates blood pressure 30 mm Hg for 3 to 5 minutes.

Lungs

The respiratory assessment described in this chapter is elementary and is designed to assist the cardiac nurse in identifying respiratory manifestations seen in patients with heart disease. The room should be quiet and the patient's chest exposed. Proceed in a systematic manner: inspect, palpate, percuss, and auscultate. Always compare one side with the other; always place the stethoscope in direct contact with the chest wall. Begin with examination of the posterior chest, if possible, with the patient sitting upright and arms folded across the chest.

Follow with assessment of the anterior chest with the patient lying down. Only the upper and lower lobes of the lung are accessible by posterior chest examination; to assess the right middle lobe, the lateral and anterior chest must be examined (Bickley & Szilagyi, 2003; Fig. 13-30).

Inspection

Respiratory Rate, Depth, Rhythm, and Effort. Normally, the respiratory rate is less than 16 breaths per minute and the rhythm is regular (Fig. 13-31*A*). *Tachypnea,* rapid, shallow breathing, may be noted in patients who have heart failure, pain, or anxiety (see Fig. 13-31*B*). *Bradypnea,* slow breathing, can be noted during sleep or after administration of respiratory depressant agents, such as morphine sulfate or anesthesia (see Fig. 13-31*C*). *Cheyne-Stokes respirations,* characterized by periods of alternating deep breathing and apnea, occur in patients with severe left ventricular failure (see Fig. 13-31*D*). Of particular concern is the duration of the apneic period. Use of accessory muscles of respiration, an upright, forward-leaning position, and pursed-lip breathing are visible signs of increased respiratory effort. Retraction of the ICSs is seen in severe asthma or upper airway obstruction (Bickley & Szilagyi, 2003). A prolonged expiratory phase is associated with early airway obstruction.

Cough and Sputum. A dry, hacking *cough* from irritation of small airways is common in patients with pulmonary congestion from heart failure or patients taking angiotensin-converting enzyme inhibitors. *Pink, frothy sputum* is indicative of pulmonary edema. Although an occasional cough may be normal, sputum production is always abnormal.

Chest Configuration. With *normal* chest configuration, the anteroposterior to lateral diameter ratio ranges from 1 : 2 to 5 : 7 (Fig. 13-32*A*). With a *barrel chest,* associated with pulmonary emphysema and aging, the anteroposterior to lateral diameter ratio increases to 1 : 1 or more (see Fig. 13-32*B*). *Kyphoscoliosis,* an abnormal spinal curvature, may prevent the patient from fully expanding his or her lungs (see Fig. 13-32*C*).

Posterior Chest

Palpation. Palpation is performed to identify areas of tenderness, respiratory excursion, and any observed abnormality and to elicit tactile fremitus. To assess *respiratory excursion,* the examiner places his or her thumbs slightly to either side of the spine and parallel to the 10th ribs (Fig. 13-33). As the patient inhales deeply, the examiner evaluates the depth and symmetry of the patient's breath by the movement of his or her thumbs.

Fremitus is the palpable vibration transmitted to the chest wall through the bronchopulmonary system when the patient speaks. The patient is asked to repeat the word "ninety-nine," and the nurse uses the ball of his or her hand to palpate and compare areas over the posterior chest. Fremitus is decreased with air or fluid in the pleural space and by an obstructed bronchus; it is increased by lung consolidation. To estimate the level of the diaphragm bilaterally, the examiner places the ulnar surface of his or her hand parallel to its expected level and progressively moves the hand downward until fremitus is no longer felt. Posteriorly, the diaphragm is located between the 10th and 12th (with deep inspiration) ribs. An abnormally high diaphragm suggests a pleural effusion or atelectasis.

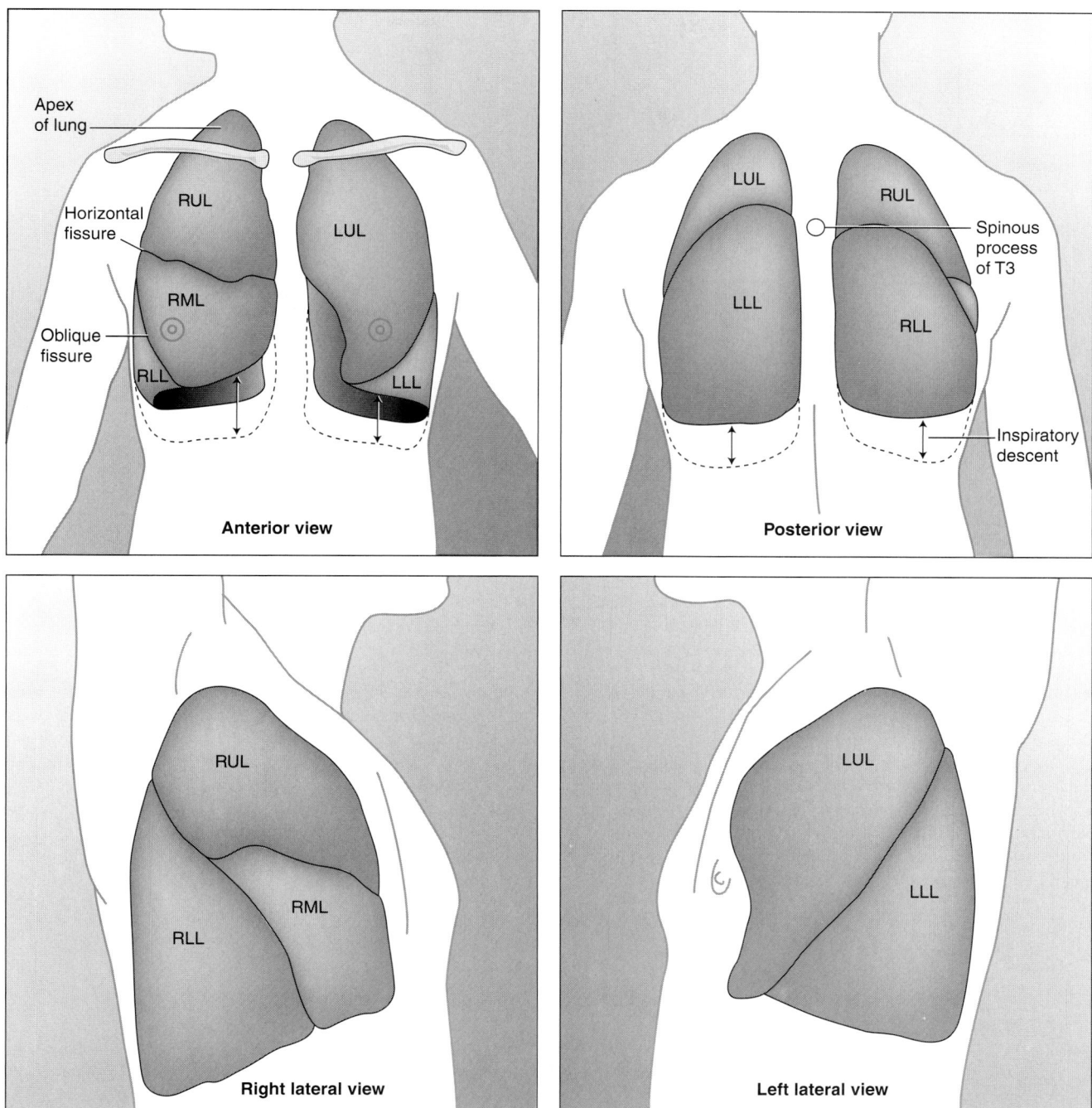

Anterior view

- Apex of lung
- Horizontal fissure
- Oblique fissure
- RUL
- LUL
- RML
- RLL
- LLL

Posterior view

- LUL
- RUL
- Spinous process of T3
- LLL
- RLL
- Inspiratory descent

Right lateral view

- RUL
- RML
- RLL

Left lateral view

- LUL
- LLL

■ **Figure 13–30.** Lobar localization.

Percussion. Percussion causes vibrations in the underlying tissues, resulting in sounds that indicate if the tissues are solid or filled with fluid or air (Table 13-8). The technique of percussion involves the examiner placing the passive finger firmly over the area to be percussed and striking the distal interphalangeal joint of the middle finger of that hand with the middle finger of the opposite hand (Fig. 13-34). Percuss across both shoulders and then at 5-cm intervals down the back (Fig. 13-35), making side-to-side comparisons. Normal lung tissue (air-filled) produces *resonance. Dullness* replaces resonance when fluid or solid tissue replaces air-filled tissue. In patients with emphysema and air trapping, *hyper-resonance* replaces resonance. *Diaphragmatic excursion* can be ascertained by percussion of the border between resonance (lung tissue) and dullness (muscle) in expiration and inspiration. Normal excursion is 5 to 6 cm.

Auscultation. Airflow, obstruction, and the condition of the lungs and pleural space can be assessed with auscultation. Use the diaphragm of the stethoscope pressed firmly on the skin in the sequence illustrated in Figure 13-36. Ask the patient to breathe slowly and deeply through his or her mouth

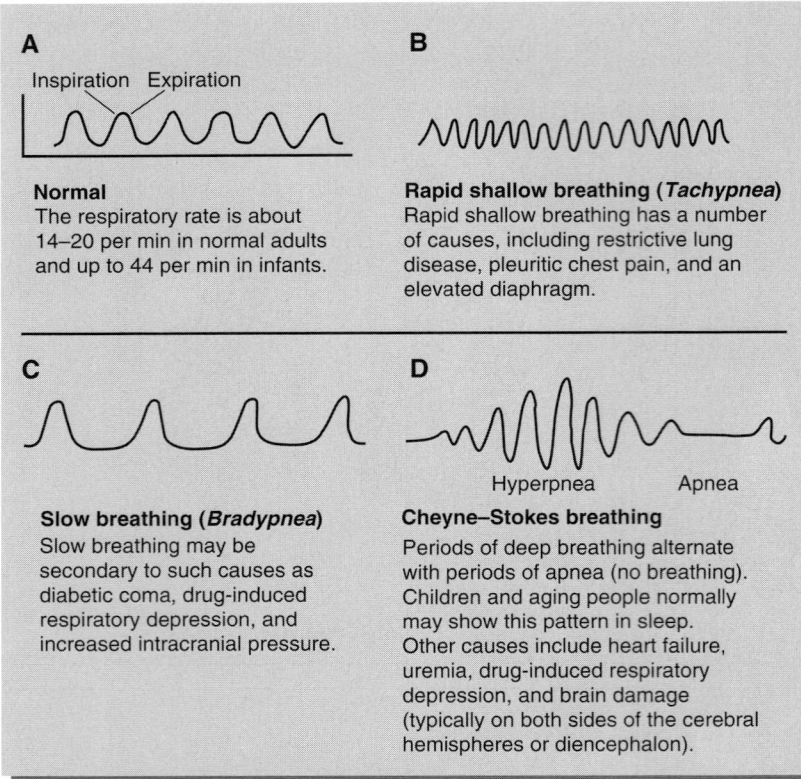

A

Inspiration Expiration

Normal
The respiratory rate is about 14–20 per min in normal adults and up to 44 per min in infants.

B

Rapid shallow breathing (*Tachypnea*)
Rapid shallow breathing has a number of causes, including restrictive lung disease, pleuritic chest pain, and an elevated diaphragm.

C

Slow breathing (*Bradypnea*)
Slow breathing may be secondary to such causes as diabetic coma, drug-induced respiratory depression, and increased intracranial pressure.

D

Hyperpnea   Apnea

Cheyne–Stokes breathing
Periods of deep breathing alternate with periods of apnea (no breathing). Children and aging people normally may show this pattern in sleep. Other causes include heart failure, uremia, drug-induced respiratory depression, and brain damage (typically on both sides of the cerebral hemispheres or diencephalon).

■ **Figure 13–31.** Respiratory rate and rhythm. (*A*) Normal. (*B*) Tachypnea. (*C*) Bradypnea. (*D*) Cheyne-Stokes.

because nose breathing changes the pitch of the sounds. Listen through one full breath in each location for pitch, intensity, and duration of inspiration and expiration.

Normal breath sounds (vesicular) are heard in peripheral lung tissue away from large airways. They are soft, low-pitched, blowing sounds. The inspiratory–expiratory time ratio is 5 : 2. Normal breath sounds are diminished at the bases. The sounds are decreased in obese patients and with shallow breathing or pleural effusion, and they are increased with exercise.

Bronchovesicular sounds are heard normally in the areas around the mainstem bronchi (below the clavicles and between the scapulae). They have moderate pitch and intensity, with an inspiratory-expiratory time ratio of 1 : 1. These sounds are abnormal if heard in the lung periphery.

Bronchial sounds, heard normally over the bronchial areas, are loud and high pitched. Expiratory time is greater than inspiratory time. If heard in the lung periphery, bronchial sounds are abnormal.

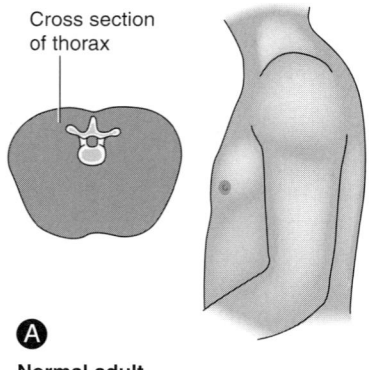

Cross section of thorax

A

Normal adult
The thorax in the normal adult is wider than it is deep. Its lateral diameter is larger than its anteroposterior diameter.

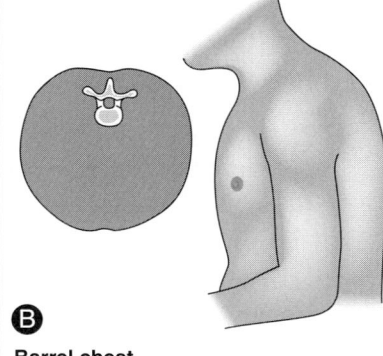

B

Barrel chest
A barrel chest has an increased anteroposterior diameter. This shape is normal during infancy, and often accompanies normal aging and chronic obstructive pulmonary disease.

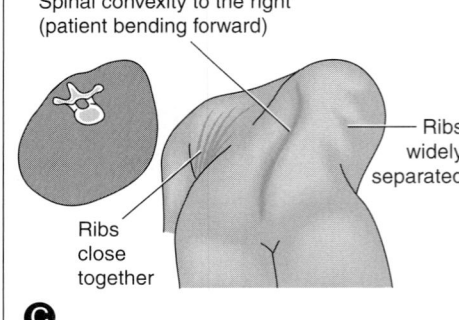

Spinal convexity to the right (patient bending forward)

Ribs widely separated

Ribs close together

C

Thoracic kyphoscoliosis
In thoracic kyphoscoliosis, abnormal spinal curvatures and vertebral rotation deform the chest. Distortion of the underlying lungs may make interpretation of lung findings very difficult.

■ **Figure 13–32.** Chest wall configurations. (*A*) Normal. (*B*) Barrel chest. (*C*) Kyphoscoliosis.

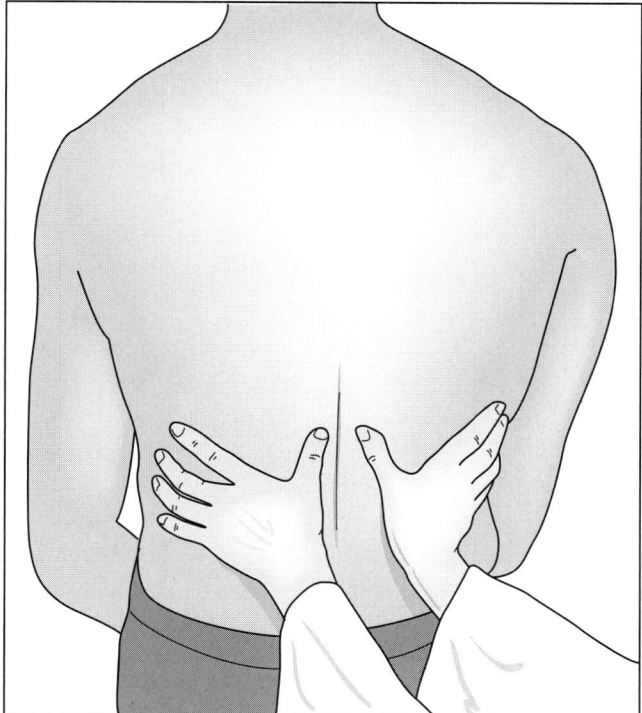

■ **Figure 13–33.** Assessment of respiratory excursion.

Adventitious breath sounds are superimposed over normal breath sounds. There are two categories of adventitious sounds: discontinuous (crackles) and continuous (wheezes and pleural friction rubs). When adventitious breath sounds are heard, note loudness, pitch, duration, number, timing (phase of respiratory cycle), location on the chest wall, and persistence from breath to breath. Have the patient cough, and note any change in adventitious sounds.

Crackles are discrete, discontinuous sounds that are similar to the sound generated by rubbing hairs together in front of the ears (Fig. 13-36A). Crackles are attributed to fluid in the alveoli or to explosive reopening of alveoli. Heart failure or atelectasis associated with bed rest, splinting from ischemic or incisional pain, or the effects of pain medication and sedatives often result in development of crackles. Typically, crackles are noted first at the bases (because of gravity's effect on fluid accumulation and decreased ventilation of basilar tissue), but may progress to all portions of the lung fields.

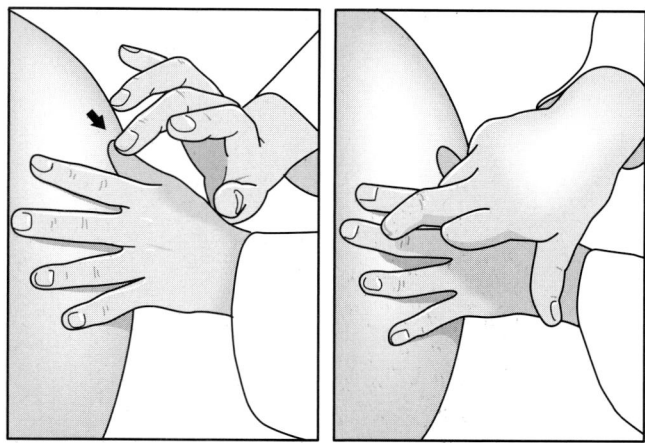

■ **Figure 13–34.** The technique of percussion.

Wheezes are continuous, musical sounds from rapid air movement through constricted airways. They are heard most often on expiration but can be heard during both inspiration and expiration (see Fig. 13-36B). Although wheezes are characteristic of obstructive lung disease, they can be caused by interstitial pulmonary edema compressing small airways. β-adrenergic blocking agents, such as propranolol, may precipitate airway narrowing, especially in patients with underlying pulmonary disease. A fixed wheeze is characteristic of an endobronchial mass or tumor.

Transmitted voice sounds may be louder and clearer than normal (bronchophony, whispered pectoriloquy) when heard through the chest wall. The quality of voice sounds may have a nasal or bleating character (egophony). Transmitted voice sounds suggest consolidation of lung tissue.

Pleural friction rubs result from inflamed pleura rubbing together. A pleural friction rub, characteristic of pleuritis, is a coarse, grating sound that can be heard on inspiration and expiration (see Fig. 13-36C).

Anterior Chest

Palpation. Tenderness of the pectoral muscles or costal cartilage suggests a musculoskeletal origin of chest pain. Respiratory excursion is assessed in the same manner as on the posterior chest, except that the examiner's thumbs are placed along each costal margin. Assess vocal or tactile fremitus. Fremitus normally is diminished over the precordium.

Table 13–8 ■ PERCUSSION NOTES AND THEIR CHARACTERISTICS

	Relative Intensity	Relative Pitch	Relative Duration	Example of Location
Flatness	Soft	High	Short	Thigh
Dullness	Medium	Medium	Medium	Liver
Resonance	Loud	Low	Long	Normal lung
Hyperresonance	Very loud	Lower	Longer	None normally
Tympany	Loud	High*	*	Gastric air bubble or puffed-out cheek

* Distinguished mainly by its musical timbre.
Bickley, L. S., & Szilagyi, P. G. (2003). *Bates' guide to physical examination and history taking* (8th ed.). Philadelphia: Lippincott Williams & Wilkins.

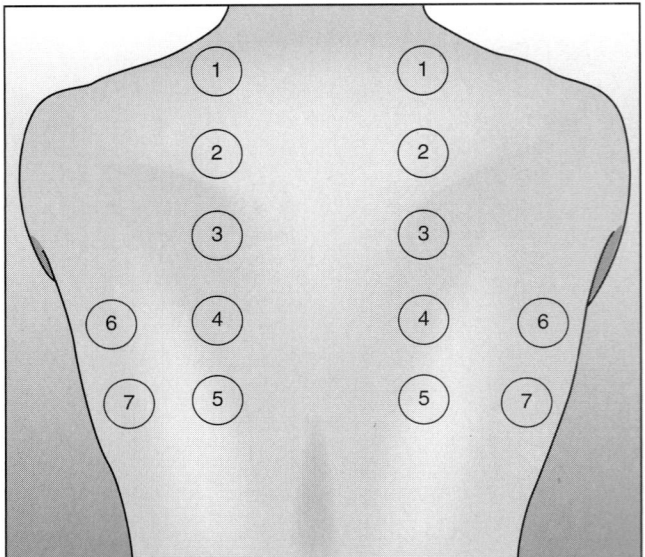

■ **Figure 13–35.** Sequence of posterior percussion and auscultation.

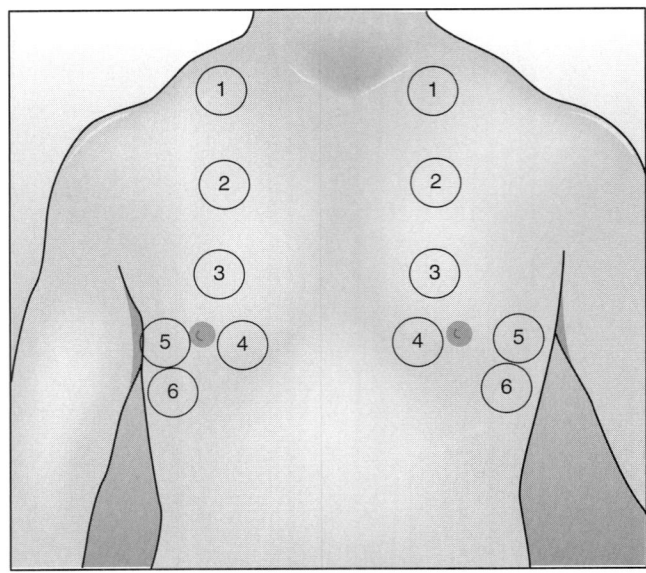

■ **Figure 13–37.** Sequence of anterior percussion and auscultation.

Percussion. The pattern for percussion of the anterior chest is diagrammed in Figure 13-37. Gently displace a female patient's breast before percussion. The heart produces dullness between the third and fifth ICSs. Note and mark the upper border of liver dullness.

Auscultation. Listen for breath sounds over the patient's anterior and lateral chest. Place the stethoscope in the sequence illustrated in Figure 13-37. If indicated, assess for transmitted voice sounds.

Abdomen

The abdominal examination presented here has a narrow focus. Purposes include evaluation of bowel tones, determination of liver size, assessment of bladder distention, and auscultation for bruits. After anesthesia, resumption of bowel tones must be confirmed before initiating a diet. Liver engorgement occurs because of decreased venous return secondary to right ventricular failure. Urine output is an important indicator of cardiac output. In a patient who is unable to void (e.g., secondary to

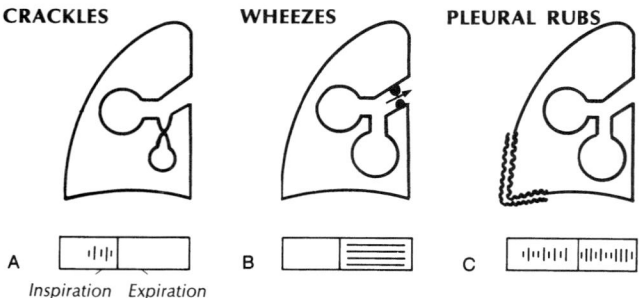

■ **Figure 13–36.** Adventitious breath sounds. (*A*) Crackles. (*B*) Wheezes. (*C*) Pleural friction rubs. (From Bates, B. [1987]. *A guide to physical examination* [4th ed., pp. 248–249]. Philadelphia: Lippincott.)

strict bed rest or after atropine sulfate administration) or who has not voided despite adequate fluid intake, always assess for bladder distention before initiating other measures.

Inspection

Observe the abdomen for symmetry and visible peristalsis. Note the presence of abdominal distention. Abdominally localized obesity (waist circumference >35 inches for women or >40 inches for men) is associated with coronary artery disease and with adult-onset diabetes mellitus.

Ausculation

Auscultate the abdomen after observation because palpation and percussion can either increase or diminish bowel sounds. Gently place the diaphragm of the stethoscope on the abdomen. Listen over all quadrants. Normal bowel sounds consist of clicks and gurgles, at a frequency of 5 to 34 per minute. It is necessary to listen for 2 minutes or more to determine that bowel sounds are absent. Borborygmi (prolonged gurgles of hyperperistalsis) also may be heard. Bowel sounds are increased with diarrhea and early intestinal obstruction, and they are decreased or absent with paralytic ileus and peritonitis (Bickley & Szilagyi, 2003). Listen for bruits over the renal, ischial, and femoral arteries.

Percussion

Determination of Liver Size. Percussion of the liver (Fig. 13-38) should start in the right MCL, at or below the umbilicus, and proceed upward from an area of tympany (intestine) to an area of dullness (liver). Identify the lower edge of the liver in the MCL. Next, percuss downward at the MCL from resonance (lung) to dullness (liver). Measure the distance from the upper to the lower liver edge at the MCL; the normal

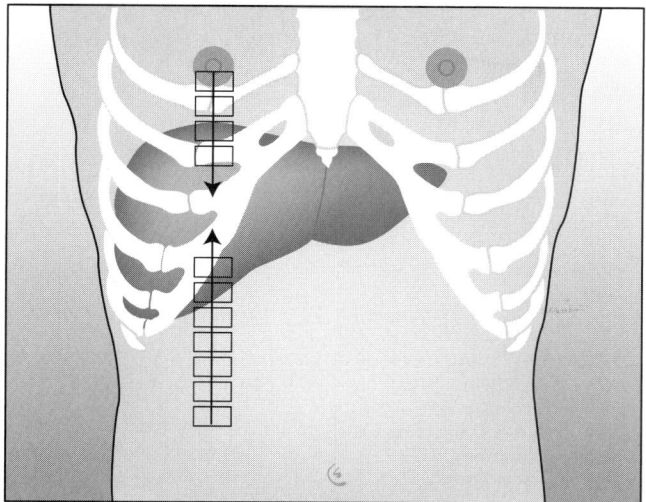

■ **Figure 13–38.** Percussion of the liver.

liver span is 6 to 12 cm (Fig. 13-39). A right pleural effusion or lung consolidation (dullness) may obscure the upper border. Gas in the colon (tympany) may obscure the lower edge.

Assessment of Bladder Distention. Percuss downward from the umbilicus to the symphysis pubis. Suprapubic dullness may indicate a distended urinary bladder. If percussion does not confirm suspicions of a distended urinary bladder, palpate gently above the symphysis pubis. If ascites is present, neither abdominal percussion nor palpation may reveal bladder distention.

Palpation

Determination of Liver Size. Deep palpation is necessary to feel the liver. It is imperative that the patient is relaxed. Place the left hand under the patient's 11th and 12th ribs for support. The liver is easier to palpate if the examiner pushes up with this hand. Place the right hand on the abdomen below the

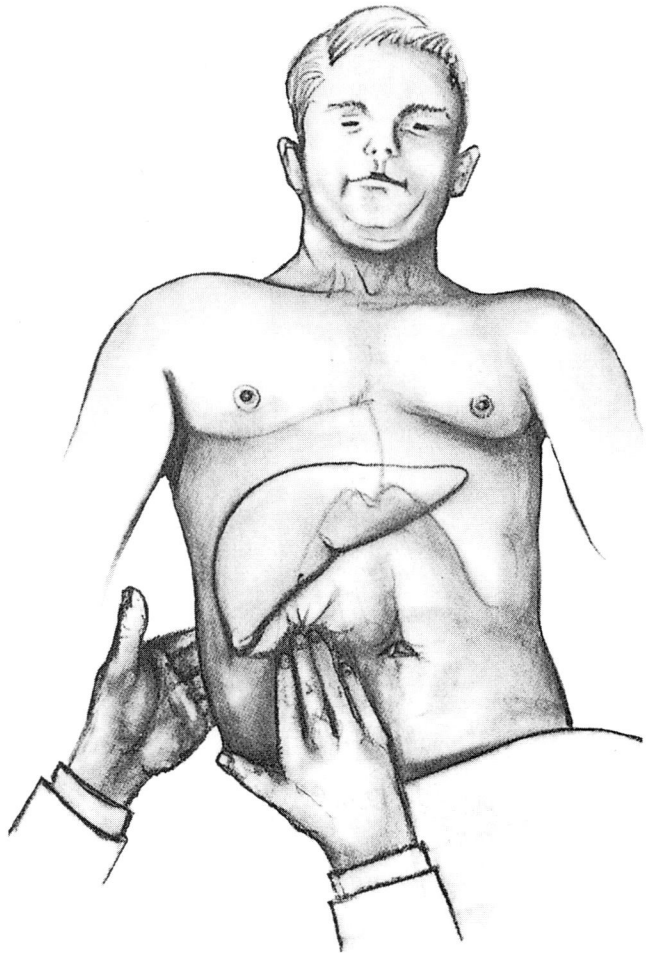

■ **Figure 13–40.** Palpation of the liver. (From Bates, B. [1987]. *A guide to physical examination* [4th ed.]. Philadelphia: Lippincott.)

lower edge of dullness, with the fingers pointing toward the right costal margin. As the patient takes a deep abdominal breath and then exhales, gently but firmly push in and up with the fingers (Fig. 13-40). With each exhalation, move the hand further toward the liver. The liver edge should come down to meet the fingers. Normally, it feels firm with a smooth edge. It should not be tender. With venous engorgement from right heart failure, the liver is enlarged, firm, tender, and smooth.

REFERENCES

Abbott, P. D., Short, E., Dodson, S., Garcia, C., Perkins, J., & Wyant, S. (2002). Improving your cultural awareness with Culture Clues. *The Nurse Practitioner*, 27(2), 44–51.

Anderson, W. B. (1994). Examination of the retina. In R. C. Schlant & R. W. Alexander (Eds.), *Hurst's the heart arteries and veins* (8th ed., pp. 315–320). New York: McGraw-Hill.

Armstrong, W. F., & Feigenbaum, H. (2001). Echocardiography. In E. Braunwald, D. P. Zipes & P. Libby (Eds.), *Heart disease: A textbook of cardiovascular medicine* (6th ed., pp. 160–236). Philadelphia: W. B. Saunders.

Bates, B. (1991). *A guide to physical examination*, (5th ed., p. 208). Philadelphia: J. B. Lippincott.

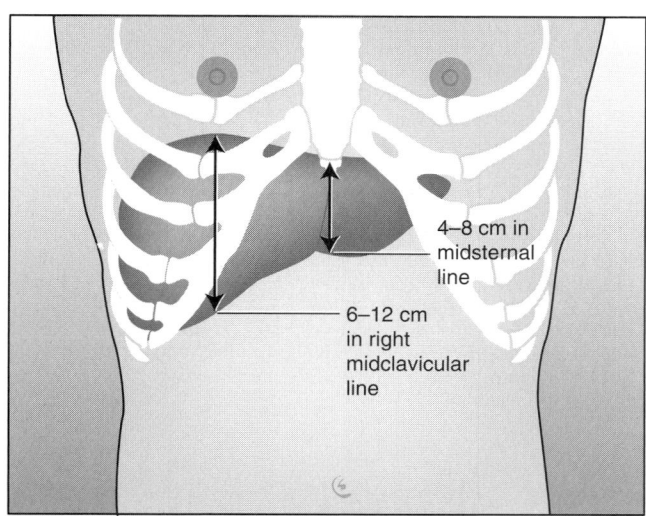

■ **Figure 13–39.** Measurement of liver span.

4–8 cm in midsternal line

6–12 cm in right midclavicular line

Bates, B. (1987). *A guide to physical examination*, (4th ed., p. 301). Philadelphia: J. B. Lippincott.

Bates, B. (1983). *A guide to physical examination*, (3rd ed., p. 79). Philadelphia: J. B. Lippincott.

Bickley, L. S., & Szilagyi, P. G. (2003). *Bates' guide to physical examination and history taking* (8th ed.). Philadelphia: Lippincott Williams & Wilkins.

Boozer, M., & Craven, R. F. (1986). Assessment of vascular function. In M. L. Patrick, S. L. Woods, R. F. Craven, et al. (Eds.), *Medical surgical nursing: Pathophysiological concepts* (pp. 593–599). Philadelphia: J. B. Lippincott.

Braunwald, E. (2001). The history. In E. Braunwald, D. P. Zipes & P. Libby (Eds.), *Heart disease: A textbook of cardiovascular medicine* (6th ed., pp. 27–44). Philadelphia: W. B. Saunders.

Braunwald, E. (1984). The physical examination. In E. Braunwald (Ed.), *Heart disease: A textbook of cardiovascular medicine* (2nd ed., pp. 35–38). Philadelphia: W. B. Saunders.

Braunwald, E., & Perloff, J. K. (2001). Physical examination of the heart and circulation. In E. Braunwald, D. P. Zipes & P. Libby (Eds.), *Heart disease: A textbook of cardiovascular medicine* (6th ed., pp. 45–81). Philadelphia: W. B. Saunders.

Calkins, H., & Zipes, D. P. (2001). Hypotension and syncope. In E. Braunwald, D. P. Zipes, & P. Libby (Eds.), *Heart disease: A textbook of cardiovascular medicine* (6th ed., pp. 932–940). Philadelphia: W. B. Saunders.

Charan, N. B., & Carvalho, P. (1992). Cardinal symptoms and signs in respiratory disease. In D. J. Pierson & R. M. Kacmarek (Eds.), *Foundations of respiratory care* (pp. 672–674). New York: Churchill Livingston.

Chatterjee, K. (1991a). Bedside evaluation of the heart: The physical examination. In W. Parmley & K. Chatterjee (Eds.), *Cardiology* (2nd ed., vol. 1, pp. 3.11–3.53). Philadelphia: J. B. Lippincott.

Chatterjee, K. (1991b). The history. In W. Parmley & K. Chatterjee (Eds.), *Cardiology* (2nd ed., vol. 1, pp. 3.2–3.10). Philadelphia: J. B. Lippincott.

Chobanian, A. V., Bakris, G. L., Black, H. R., et al. (2003). The seventh report of the Joint National Committee on Prevention, Detection, Evaluation, and Treatment of High Blood Pressure. *Journal of the American Medical Association, 289* (DOI 10.1001/jama.289.19.2560).

Christie, L. G., Jr., & Conti, C. R. (1981). Systematic approach to the evaluation of angina-like chest pain. *American Heart Journal, 102,* 897–912.

Creager, M. A., & Dzau, V. J. (1994). Vascular diseases of the extremities. In K. J. Isselbacher, E. Braunwald, J. D. Wilson, et al. (Eds.), *Harrison's principles of internal medicine* (13th ed., pp. 1135–1143). New York: McGraw-Hill.

Cunningham, S. L. (1986). Hypertension. In M. L. Patrick, S. L. Woods, R. F. Craven, et al. (Eds.), *Medical-surgical nursing: Pathophysiological concepts* (pp. 603–621). Philadelphia: J. B. Lippincott.

Fowler, N. O. (1972). *Examination of the heart. Part 2: Inspection and palpation of arterial and venous pulses* (p. 33). New York: American Heart Association.

Frank, R. N. (2003). The eye in hypertension. In J. L. Izzo & H. R. Black (Eds.), *Hypertension primer* (3rd ed., pp. 117–120). From the Council on High Blood Pressure Research, American Heart Association. Philadelphia: Lippincott Williams & Wilkins.

Franklin, S. S., & Izzo, J. L, (2003). Aging, hypertension, and arterial stiffness. In J. L. Izzo & H. R. Black (Eds.), *Hypertension primer* (3rd ed., pp. 170–175). From the Council on High Blood Pressure Research, American Heart Association. Philadelphia: Lippincott Williams & Wilkins.

Frohlich, E. D., Grim, C., Labarthe, D. R., et al. (Eds.) (1987). *Recommendations for human blood pressure determination by sphygmomanometers* (p. 10). Dallas: American Heart Association.

Goldhaber, S. Z. (2001). Pulmonary embolism. In E. Braunwald, D. P. Zipes & P. Libby (Eds.), *Heart disease: A textbook of cardiovascular medicine* (6th ed., pp. 1886–1907). Philadelphia: W. B. Saunders.

Goldman, L. (1998). *Primary cardiology.* Philadelphia: W. B. Saunders.

Gordon, M. (1994). *Nursing diagnosis process and application* (2nd ed.). New York: McGraw-Hill.

Grim, C. M., & Grim, C. E. (2003). Blood pressure measurement. In J. L. Izzo & H. R. Black (Eds.), *Hypertension primer,* (3rd ed., pp. 321–324). From the Council on High Blood Pressure Research, American Heart Association. Philadelphia: Lippincott Williams & Wilkins.

Hansen-Flaschen, J., & Nordberg, J. (1987). Clubbing and hypertrophic osteoarthropathy. *Clinics in Chest Medicine, 8,* 291.

Hurst, J. W., & Schlant, R. C. (1978). Examination of the arteries and their pulsation. In J. W. Hurst, R. B. Logue, R. C. Schlant, et al. (Eds.), *The heart* (4th ed., pp. 186–187). New York: McGraw-Hill.

Insuna, J. T., Sacks, H. S., Lau, T. S., et al. (1994). Drug treatment of hypertension in the elderly: A meta-analysis. *Annals of Internal Medicine, 121,* 355–362.

Jones, D. W., Frolich, E. D., Grim, C. M., et al. (2001). Mercury sphygmomanometers should not be abandoned: An advisory statement from the Council for High Blood Pressure Research, American Heart Association. *Hypertension, 37,* 185–186.

Kenney, W. L. (1997). Thermoregulation at rest and during exercise in healthy older adults. *Exercise and Sport Science Review, 25,* 41–76.

Leatham, A. (1979). *An introduction to the examination of the cardiovascular system* (2nd ed., p. 20). Oxford: Oxford University Press.

Marriott, H. J. L. (1993). *Bedside cardiac diagnosis.* Philadelphia: J. B. Lippincott.

McGee, S. R. (1998). Physical examination of venous pressure: A critical review. *American Heart Journal, 136,* 10–18.

New York Heart Association Criteria Committee. (1964). *Diseases of the heart and blood vessels: Nomenclature and criteria for diagnosis* (6th ed.). Boston: Little, Brown.

O'Rourke, R. A., Silverman, M. E., & Schlant, R. C. (1994). General examination of the patient. In R. C. Schlant & R. W. Alexander (Eds.), *Hurst's the heart, arteries, and veins* (8th ed., pp. 217–251). New York: McGraw-Hill.

Parati, G., Izzo, J. L., & Gavish, B. (2003). Respiration and blood pressure. In J. L. Izzo & H. R. Black (Eds.), *Hypertension primer* (3rd ed., pp. 117–120). From the Council on High Blood Pressure Research, American Heart Association. Philadelphia: Lippincott Williams & Wilkins.

Perloff, D., Grim, C., Flack, J., et al. (2001). Human blood pressure determination by sphygmomanometry. *Circulation, 88,* 2460–2470.

Perloff, J. K. (1990). *Physical examination of the heart and circulation* (p. 208). Philadelphia: W. B. Saunders.

Poirer, P., & Despres, J. P. (2003). Waist circumference, visceral obesity, and cardiovascular risk. *Journal of Cardiopulmonary Rehabilitation, 23*(3), 161–169.

Ponte, J. (1998). Warming the core after cardiac surgery. *Journal of Cardiothoracic Vascular Anesthesia, 12*(4), 496.

Robertson, D. (2003). Treatment of orthostatic disorders and baroreflex failure. In J. L. Izzo & H. R. Black (Eds.), *Hypertension primer* (3rd ed., pp. 479–482). From the Council on High Blood Pressure Research, American Heart Association. Philadelphia: Lippincott Williams & Wilkins.

Ronan, J. (1992a). Cardiac auscultation: The first and second heart sounds. *Heart Disease and Stroke, 1,* 113–116.

Ronan, J. (1992b). Cardiac auscultation: The third and fourth heart sounds. *Heart Disease and Stroke, 1,* 267–270.

Runge, M. S., & Harker, L. A. (1994). Thrombus formation and dissolution. In R. C. Schlant & R. W. Alexander (Eds.), *Hurst's the heart, arteries, and veins* (8th ed., pp. 173–183). New York: McGraw-Hill.

Seidel, H. M., Ball, J. W., Davis, J. E., et al. (2003). *Mosby's guide to physical examination* (5th ed.). St. Louis: Mosby.

Spodick, D. H. (2001). Pericardial diseases. In E. Braunwald, D. P. Zipes & P. Libby (Eds.), *Heart disease: A textbook of cardiovascular medicine* (6th ed., pp. 1823–1876). Philadelphia: W. B. Saunders.

Staff Development Workgroup. (1999). Culture Clues™: Communicating with your Latino patient. [On-line]. Available: http//depts.washin gton.edu/pfes/cultureclues.html.

Tilkian, A., & Conover, M. (2001). *Understanding heart sounds and murmurs with an introduction to lung sounds* (4th ed.). Philadelphia: W. B. Saunders.

Tilkian, A., & Conover, M. (1993). *Understanding heart sounds and murmurs with an introduction to lung sounds* (3rd ed.). Philadelphia: W. B. Saunders.

Underhill, S. L. (1984). Assessment of cardiovascular function. In L. S. Brunner & D. S. Suddarth (Eds.), *Textbook of medical-surgical nursing* (5th ed., pp. 457–563). Philadelphia: J. B. Lippincott.

U. S. Department of Health and Human Services. (2000). *Healthy people 2010: Understanding and improving health* (2nd ed., pp. 28–29). Washington, DC: U. S. Government Printing Office.

LABORATORY TESTS USING BLOOD

SUSAN L. REED

Diagnosis, treatment, and management of patients require a multimodal, multidisciplinary approach. Along with an in-depth history and physical, the clinician frequently depends on test results to complete the assessment picture. One of the most frequently used testing modalities is laboratory testing of blood specimens. Laboratory analysis composes approximately 43% of the data used by health care workers to make clinical decisions (Giuliano & Grant, 2002). A host of variables can affect interpretation of blood specimen results. Accurate interpretation starts with proper specimen collection. The nurse has a key role in maximizing the conditions under which specimens are collected (Kee, 1999; McFarland & Grant, 1994), thereby controlling for as many variables as possible.

BLOOD SPECIMEN COLLECTION

Collection of blood specimens is a process that involves three phases: patient preparation, collection of the blood sample, and interpretation of results. The nurse plays an important role during this process.

Patient Preparation

Adequate preparation of patients and their families involves education. Frequently, proper specimen collection and interpretation requires compliance with instructions about food or fluid restrictions, administering or withholding medications, and meeting criteria for proper timing of the blood sample (McFarland & Grant, 1994). When the blood sample is taken, patients should receive an explanation about what tests are being performed, why they have been ordered, and when results will be available. If the sample is being obtained by venipuncture, arterial puncture, or vascular port access, preparation of the patient includes a reminder about pain during the procedure and the importance of complying with instructions to maintain a certain body position.

Universal Precautions

All blood is considered a source of potential infection. Universal precautions, as well as organizational policies and procedures, should be followed when collecting and transporting specimens. Universal precautions include the use of gloves during phlebotomy (or at any time there is risk of exposure to blood or body fluids), complete avoidance of recapping needles, proper disposal of sharps, and proper handwashing. When there is the potential that blood or body fluids will splash, protective clothing and eyewear should be worn. Spills should be cleaned with an Environmental Protection Agency (EPA)–approved germicide or a 1:100 solution of household bleach, and soiled linen should be bagged at the location where it was used. Last, institutional policies should be followed with regard to isolation or transport of patients who have highly transmittable organisms and to disposal of infective waste (McFarland & Grant, 1994; Pagana & Pagana, 1998).

Blood Sample Collection

General guidelines for blood sample collection have been developed that help to ensure patient and clinician safety and maximize interpretation of results. The clinician should consider the policies and procedures of his or her organization with regard to blood specimen collection, as well as the standards for professional, national, and international organizations.

Control of variability can be enhanced by use of proper technique during collection and processing of the specimen. The practice of having patients clench and unclench fists in preparation for specimen collection from arms should be avoided. This maneuver causes an increase in the metabolic activity of muscle tissue, thereby affecting certain laboratory results. With just 1 minute of fist clenching, plasma potassium can increase by as much as 1.0 to 1.5 mmol/L. The possibility for hemolysis is enhanced by repeatedly clenching the fist during specimen withdrawal (Henry et al., 1974).

The use of a tourniquet produces changes as well. Once a tourniquet is placed on the arm, veins dilate because of their inability to drain. Under these conditions, return of fluid and electrolytes to the vein is decreased or prohibited, resulting in a hemoconcentrated specimen (Kee, 1999). In addition, despite decreased circulation of fresh blood to the tissues, cells continue their metabolic processes, leading to an increased concentration in metabolic waste products, such as lactate. In this more acidic environment, potassium leaks out of cells (Dufour, 1998). In general, the tourniquet should not be left on more than 1 or 2 minutes. Cellular injury and hemolysis can be caused by the prolonged use of a tourniquet, described as 3 minutes or longer (Statland et al., 1974). Longer use may be unavoidable during a difficult venipuncture. In such cases, information about a difficult venipuncture should be noted on the laboratory slip to assist with interpretation of results (McFarland & Grant, 1994).

Blood specimens can be contaminated in several ways. During collection, contamination may occur from intravenous (IV) fluids. Blood draws should not be performed on the same arm as an infusion. If the infusion arm cannot be avoided, a tourniquet may be placed between the IV site and the phlebotomy site. Slowing the IV to a keep-open rate (if not contraindicated) for 3 to 5 minutes before the draw may help to reduce contamination of the blood sample (McFarland & Grant, 1994). In any event, it should be noted on the laboratory slip that the sample was obtained under these conditions.

Contamination may also be introduced by improper use of blood tubes. Most specimen collection tubes contain some form of anticoagulant. If blood has been mistakenly collected in one tube containing anticoagulant, it should never be poured into a different tube. Also, blood entering one tube should never be allowed to contaminate remaining blood that will be introduced into another tube.

Another source of contamination is introduced when routine samples are drawn from arterial lines, vascular catheters, or ports. The use of an indwelling intravascular catheter allows access to the patient's blood supply without further invasive procedure. Comfort for the patient, ease, and speed of periodic specimen collection are some of the benefits of using an intravascular line for blood sampling. Intravascular catheters may be kept patent by continuous or intermittent infusion, or by instilling saline or heparin solutions. Sometimes, solutions delivered through the catheter may contain medications. The infusate or any additives may dilute blood constituents. This dilution would have the effect of lowering the concentration of the desired sample.

The diameter and length of the catheter are important determinants when considering this hemodilution. Several studies have been successful in establishing accuracy for specific laboratory tests after a minimal blood discard volume. Research has explored the use of central venous, intra-arterial, and pulmonary artery catheters, including both the RA port and vascular infusion port (VIP). Certain precisely controlled studies have quantified a discard volume for specific blood tests. Research has demonstrated that a 1- to 6-mL discard volume is sufficient for most intravascular catheters (Burns et al., 1985; Carlson, 2001; Coombs et al., 1984; Gregersen et al., 1983; Gregersen et al., 1987; Krueger et al., 1980; Russo et al., 1984; Statland et al., 1974; Wallace et al., 1986). At the very minimum, the initial discard needs to equal the dead space of the device or tubing. The institution's policy and procedure manual should be consulted for recommended withdrawal and dis-

card from vascular devices. Additional sources, such as professional nursing society standards, may assist in making decisions about recommended discard volumes.

Whether sampling from a pulmonary artery catheter, central venous line, arterial catheter, or other intravascular catheter, attention should be paid to the feasibility of interruption of the system. The pulmonary artery catheter presents particular problems. Both the RA port and VIP are useful for the administration of drugs and fluids. Although the RA port allows access to the central circulation, use of this port for thermodilution cardiac output calculations makes it difficult to infuse drugs or fluids (a large amount of the infusate might be delivered during delivery of the cardiac output injectate). Consequently, the VIP is chosen for fluid and drug infusion. In this situation, the use of the RA port may be preferable for blood withdrawal. If vasoactive drugs are not infusing through the VIP, it may also be used for blood sampling. The proximal opening into the RA is upstream of any drugs or fluid infusing through the RA port; therefore, the possibility of contamination of the blood sample by infusates is minimized. Typically, the distal port of the pulmonary artery catheter is only used for blood sampling when measuring a mixed venous blood gas from the pulmonary artery where venous blood mixes after circulating through the superior and inferior vena cavae, coronary sinuses, and the chambers in the right side of the heart.

Many institutions have shifted to the use of saline alone in lieu of heparin solution in IV lines and pressure tubing; however, questions persist about appropriate discard from vascular catheters (instilled with heparin) when drawing blood for coagulation studies. Inconsistent results may increase the cost to the patient through repeated testing, wasted blood, or erroneous treatment decisions (Cannon et al., 1985; Krueger et al., 1980). Various studies indicate that accurate results for activated partial thromboplastin time (aPTT) can be obtained if a minimal amount is withdrawn and discarded before filling blood specimen tubes. However, recommendations differ with respect to how much should be withdrawn and discarded (Heap et al., 1997; Laxson & Titler, 1994; Lew et al., 1991; Templin et al., 1993). Reliable results have been established for the PTT drawn from a heparinized catheter (Gregersen et al., 1987). However, sampling for thrombin time and PT has been shown to produce inaccurate results, particularly when a heparinized catheter is used (Baranowski, 1993; Gregersen et al., 1987; Snyder et al., 1986). Heparin adhering to a catheter can alter the test results (Costentino, 1987; "Intravenous Nursing Standards of Practice," 1990). Again, the nurse may refer to policy and procedure manuals or professional organization standards for guidance. In any event, coordination in obtaining multiple blood specimens decreases the amount of blood that is eventually discarded and the number of times that the sterile system is invaded, thus reducing risk of introducing infection.

Early investigations of sepsis associated with intravascular monitoring equipment discouraged frequent blood sampling from the system (Spaccavento & Hawley, 1982). These reports identified stopcocks and pressure transducers as the most frequent reservoirs for endemic contamination (Walrath et al., 1979; Weinstein et al., 1976). The incidence of local infection and bacteremia has been reduced by the use of disposable transducers and the percutaneous sheath systems used to introduce pulmonary artery catheters (Wiedemann et al., 1984).

The withdrawal of blood from an intravascular catheter should be considered a sterile procedure. Once removed, caps used to cover stopcock openings should always be replaced with a sterile cap. The person performing the procedure should be gloved. Syringes, used once, should be discarded.

Types of Specimens

When blood is withdrawn from the body, it eventually clots. The fluid that separates from the clot is called *serum*. Plasma, from unclotted blood, contains fibrinogen, which is eventually converted to fibrin. Most blood tests are performed on serum and therefore require use of a tube that allows blood to clot. Red-top tubes contain no additives; they are used for chemistries, drug monitoring, radioimmunoassays, serology, and blood typing. Lavender-top tubes, which contain ethylenediaminetetraacetic acid (EDTA), are usually used for hematology and certain other chemistries. Green-top tubes contain heparin as the anticoagulant and can be used for chemistries, arterial blood gases, hormone levels, and some immune function studies. Blue-top tubes, used for coagulation studies, contain citrate. Sodium fluoride, found in gray-top tubes, prevents glycolysis and may be used to test blood glucose in its in vivo state (Kee, 1999).

When multiple blood samples are drawn at the same collection time, the preferred order is as follows: tubes with no preservative (red top); tubes with mild anticoagulants (green, gray, blue, or black top); and tubes with EDTA (lavender top) should be collected last. Blood for coagulation studies should never be drawn first, because tissue injury can initiate the clotting process and result in falsely low levels of coagulation factors (Dufour, 1998). Specimens in tubes with additives should be rotated gently to mix the anticoagulant with the blood. They should never be shaken (Kee, 1999).

Hemolysis refers to the lysis of red blood cells. When extracellular fluid (plasma) is used for analysis, inaccurate results are produced if the specimen is hemolyzed. Hemolysis may occur in vivo, as in hemolytic disease states such as transfusion reactions. Hemolysis may also occur in some infections and with the use of some drugs (Dufour, 1998). A deficiency of the enzyme glucose-6-phosphate dehydrogenase, responsible for generating chemicals needed for maintenance of normal red cell fragility, contributes to hemolysis.

Hemolysis may also occur as a result of improper specimen collection technique or specimen transport. Hemolysis is the cause for specimen rejection in most non-emergent situations (Jacobs & DeMott, 2001). Specimens may be hemolyzed if they are collected from a poorly flowing venipuncture. Greater hemolysis occurs with the use of a large-bore needle than with a small-bore needle (Calam, 1977; Dufour, 1998), although Kennedy and colleagues (1996) found a greater incidence of hemolysis in emergency room patients who had blood samples drawn from small-gauge peripheral IV catheters compared to blood samples drawn from venipuncture using a Vacutainer or peripheral IV catheters with large-gauge needles. Failure to dry alcohol from the venipuncture site also results in hemolysis (Statland & Winkel, 1979). Blood should never be forcibly withdrawn from the venipuncture, nor should it be forcibly entered into the collection tube by pushing on the syringe barrel to fill faster (Dufour, 1998).

Specimens should be handled carefully when placed in collection tubes and when transported to the laboratory; rough handling may lead to hemolysis. Hemolysis increases the laboratory values of potassium, magnesium, calcium, phosphorus, lactate dehydrogenase (LDH), bilirubin, aspartate aminotransferase (AST), alanine aminotransferase (ALT), and creatine kinase (CK) (Jacobs & DeMott, 2001; Wallach, 1992). Hemolysis invalidates the results of most coagulation tests and can mask hemolyzing antibodies in the antibody screen and crossmatch (Jacobs & DeMott, 2001). If unexpected elevated laboratory values are reported, then the blood should be redrawn if hemolysis is suspected.

Proper specimen collection includes accurate identification of the patient and accurate labeling of the specimen at the site of collection (McFarland & Grant, 1994). It also includes rapid transport to the laboratory, because cells remain viable after collection and continue their metabolic processes. Specimens that are left to stand unprocessed often yield inaccurate results (Dufour, 1998).

Interpretation of Results

Inherent physiologic variability exists based on patient age, gender, ethnicity, and health status (such as pregnancy or post-MI). These physiologic differences affect interpretation of results. Physiologic changes associated with the aging process bring concomitant changes in some expected laboratory results. Because men usually have more muscle mass than women, gender differences are seen in substances related to muscle function or metabolism, such as creatinine. According to Dufour (1998) numerous studies have documented significant differences among European, African, and Asian populations in testing for cholesterol, enzymes, and hormones. Various physiologic states, such as pregnancy, stress, obesity, and endurance exercise, also introduce situational changes in expected results (Dufour, 1998; Jacobs & DeMott, 2001).

Cyclic variability produces daily, monthly, or yearly patterns in physiologic states. These cycles are often taken into consideration in the collection or interpretation of laboratory results (Jacobs & DeMott, 2001). As a result, most routine specimens, at least in the hospital setting, are drawn in the early morning to control for any circadian variability.

Blood tests are sometimes affected by the ingestion of food or fluids. Not only are results affected by the absorption of dietary components into the blood after a meal, but hormonal and metabolic changes also occur. Partial control for the variability introduced by food or fluid ingestion can be achieved either by drawing early morning, pre-meal specimens, or by having the patient fast for 8 to 12 hours. The latter is especially important in lipid testing (National Cholesterol Education Program, 2001).

Sometimes, differences based on position are negligible. In other cases, they are significant. Patient position during (and before) sampling can affect results. In the upright position, there may be a shift in extracellular fluid volume into the tissues. With the resulting increased concentration of proteins and protein-bound substances in the vascular space, samples for proteins, enzymes, Hct, Hb, calcium, iron, hormones, and several drugs may show an average 5% to 8% increase. Redistribution of extracellular fluid volume and electrolytes within the vascular space does not stabilize until a patient has assumed the sitting position for at least 15 minutes (from a standing position) (Dufour, 1998), and in some cases 20 to 30 minutes (Kee, 1999). In some settings, such as the hospital, it is not difficult to stabilize the patient's position and thus reduce variability (McFarland & Grant, 1994). In other settings, such as ambulatory care, significant variability is introduced if the patient is not made to sit for at least 15 minutes before the blood draw. Because control over sitting time is not usually feasible or practical, care should be taken in the interpretation of results. Exercising immediately before blood sample collection frequently produces significantly erroneous results, especially with enzyme evaluation. Forearm exercises before blood withdrawal may lead to hemolysis (Kee, 1999; Romano & Yourn, 1977).

The timing of blood sampling should include consideration of the effect of medications on the interpretation of results. Medications affect results of many specimens drawn for chemistry, hematology, coagulation, hormonal, and enzyme studies. Knowledge of the effect of the drug assists in proper timing or subsequent interpretation of the results. Consideration should also be given to the effects of other influences, including over-the-counter medications, caffeine, nicotine, ethanol (Dufour, 1998), home remedies, and herbal therapies.

In therapeutic drug monitoring, blood drug levels are monitored to evaluate the effects of drug therapy, make decisions regarding dosage, prevent toxicity, and monitor patient adherence. Timing of the blood sample usually depends on the half-life of the drug; samples drawn at projected peak level assist in monitoring for toxicity, whereas levels drawn at trough help to verify the minimum satisfactory therapeutic level for that patient (Chernecky & Berger, 1997; Tilkian et al., 1995; Treseler, 1988). Regardless of the purpose of the blood sample, drugs that may affect interpretation of results should be noted on the laboratory slip. For therapeutic drug monitoring, it is important to note the date and time of the last dose (McFarland & Grant, 1994).

Different laboratories use different equipment and methods by which to test specimens. Specific reference ranges are usually reported alongside the patient's results on the laboratory report. In an effort to establish a standard for communicating laboratory results, the World Health Organization has recommended that the medical and scientific community throughout the world adopt the use of the International System of Units (ISU) (Kee, 1999). An international unit is defined as the number of moles of substrate converted per second under defined conditions (Treseler, 1995). Thus, many laboratories may report results in different ways, depending on their accepted standard of practice (Kratz & Lewandrowski, 1998). Most laboratories also report critical (or panic) values. These values should be reported promptly to the provider so that results may be evaluated (and decisions made) in light of patient condition.

Most reference ranges have been established for venous blood samples. Because arterial blood has higher concentrations of glucose and oxygen and lower concentrations of waste products (i.e., ammonia, potassium, and lactate), an arterial source (instead of venous) should be noted on the laboratory slip. Capillary samples yield results that are closer to arterial blood than venous.

Critical evaluation of laboratory results should take into account how the reference or "normal" values were determined. Patients that have been seen for a long time by the same provider, or those who have been seen within the same health care organization, sometimes establish their own reference range. Reference ranges for a specific disease are sometimes established through large-scale clinical trials.

In most circumstances, each laboratory establishes its own reference values by testing a group that is easy to recruit. It is possible, however, that this technique may not reflect the usual values or range of values of the group that the organization serves. When samples are taken from volunteers, such as those who agree to give a blood sample for reference testing in exchange for a free cholesterol screening, bias may be introduced because those who are likely to volunteer may be those who have or suspect they have illness already. When reference samples are taken from patients who are undergoing routine physical examinations or elective surgery, results may reflect a mix of the surrounding population. Again, these reference values need to be considered in light of who was included or excluded from testing. Usually, those who drink alcohol, smoke, or take certain medications are excluded from reference range testing. However, this exclusion is likely to establish a narrow range of "normal" values, thereby increasing the number of people in the served population who fall outside the established range. Additional care should be taken in interpreting results if the laboratory reports only one set of reference values (Dufour, 1998).

Clinicians who are aware of how reference ranges are obtained are in a better position to interpret laboratory results accurately for their patients. In all situations, interpretation of results should be performed in light of all factors that introduce variability, and in light of the clinical condition, remembering that "normal" values do not necessarily indicate absence of disease, just as "abnormal" values do not necessarily establish a pathologic state (Dufour, 1998).

Sensitivity and Specificity of Laboratory Tests

Clinicians should use measures of test performance to judge the quality of a diagnostic test for a particular disease. The ability of a laboratory test to identify a particular disease is quantified by two measurements: sensitivity and specificity (Nicoll et al., 2001; Oxley et al., 2001).

Sensitivity is the frequency of a positive (abnormal) test result among all patients with a particular disease or the likelihood that a diseased patient has a positive test. If all patients with a given disease have a positive test, then the test sensitivity is 100%. Sensitivity is calculated by testing a population of patients who have been found to have a particular disease by some "gold standard" method (a procedure that defines the true disease state of the patient) (Nicoll et al., 2001; Oxley et al., 2001).

Specificity is the frequency of a negative (normal) test among all persons who do not have the disease or the likelihood that a healthy patient has a negative test. If all patients who do not have a particular disease have a negative test, then the test specificity is 100%. A test with a high specificity is helpful to confirm a diagnosis, because a highly specific test will have few results that are falsely positive. Specificity is calculated by testing a population of patients who have been found to have a particular disease by some gold standard method (Nicoll et al., 2001; Oxley et al., 2001).

Point-of-Care Testing

Point-of-care testing (POCT), also known as bedside testing or alternative site testing, is the laboratory testing of blood that is performed outside of a central laboratory (Jacobs & DeMott, 2001). The goal of POCT is to reduce the time it takes to diagnose and treat (decision cycle time). Because laboratory analysis of blood comprises approximately 43% of the data used by health care workers to make clinical decisions (Giuliano & Grant, 2002), POCT provides a decrease in the number of steps required to obtain a blood sample, process the sample, and receive the data, and therefore reduces decision cycle time. POCT is ideal in intensive care units, emergency departments, cardiac catheterization laboratories, and surgical suites where the need for rapid turnaround time of laboratory data is desired. Additional benefits of POCT include improved patient management, increased patient satisfaction, improved job satisfaction of nurses and physicians, decreased operating room time, decreased mortality and morbidity, and less blood sample volume (Jacobs & DeMott, 2001).

Glucose monitoring has been available for years as POCT to guide dosage of insulin administration. Hospitals have also used portable activated coagulation time (ACT) monitors to guide anticoagulation and heparin administration during interventional cardiology procedures and during cardiovascular surgery. In addition to glucose and ACT, POCT assays that are available for care of cardiac patients include Hct, Hb, ABGs, electrolytes, BUN, creatinine, ethanol, drugs of abuse, troponin-I, troponin-T, myoglobin, CK-MB, and B-type natriuretic peptide (BNP) (Jacobs & DeMott, 2001).

To ensure accuracy of data, a POCT system requires that there be up-front training of non-laboratory personnel on how to use new equipment, continued proficiency testing of staff, and assurance that electronic quality control requirements are met. It is important that POCT systems are linked to hospital or laboratory systems by radiofrequency and infrared to ensure that information handling, storage, and billing are performed properly.

Possible limitations of using a POCT system include its use by personnel with limited training in laboratory technology and the lack of understanding of quality control. POCT is considered to be more expensive than traditional laboratory analysis because the cost of cartridges is more expensive. Cost analysis needs to include the decreased labor by nursing and laboratory personnel plus the ability to make rapid decisions about acutely ill patients that may alter their course of illness (Giuliano & Grant, 2002).

Administration of a POCT system includes designating someone to be responsible for the POCT service, which would include: knowing who is performing POCT and which test they are performing, maintaining quality control documentation, selecting appropriate equipment, troubleshooting all

aspects of POCT, coordinating training, and serving as a liaison between nursing and other services (Jacobs & DeMott, 2001).

An example of a POCT study that demonstrates decreased decision cycle time is from Ng and colleagues (2001). These researchers used POCT of CK-MB, troponin-I, and myoglobin to study its use in the triaging of patients with chest pain. The researchers showed that POCT of cardiac markers allowed for correct diagnosis of MI in all patients in the study within 90 minutes of presentation; 90% of patients who had negative cardiac markers and a negative ECG were discharged within 90 minutes of presentation (Ng et al., 2001).

CARDIAC MARKERS

The internal environment of the healthy person is in a state of balance with respect to water, electrolytes, energy storage and use, and metabolic end products. Stability is maintained through homeostatic mechanisms that regulate the activities of cells and organs. During periods of critical illness, a disruption in cell membrane stability may cause chemical substances that are responsible for intracellular homeostatic mechanisms to appear in the blood. Frequent evaluation of blood results is a means by which the status of the internal environment and the extent and nature of tissue damage can be monitored.

Certain intracellular enzymes and proteins are rarely found in measurable amounts in the blood of healthy people. However, after an event leading to cellular injury, these substances may leak into the blood. In irreversible cellular damage, smaller intracellular components are released earlier than larger ones, accounting for differences in timing in the appearance of these substances in the blood after damage has occurred (Dufour, 1998). Because of the importance of the timing of the appearance (and disappearance) of enzymes and proteins in the blood, it is crucial that ordered tests are drawn on time. It is equally important that the date and time of the blood draw are noted on the laboratory slip so that the temporal sequence of the rise and fall can be established by those interpreting the results (Kee, 1998; Pagana & Pagana, 1998).

Initial diagnosis of MI, reinfarction, or other types of myocardial damage is made through evaluation of clinical signs and symptoms, 12-lead ECG, myocardial proteins (troponins), myoglobin, and enzymes (CK and its isoenzymes, isoforms, and mass activity).

Myocardial Proteins

Troponins

Troponins are protein complexes that regulate the calcium-dependent interaction of myosin with actin in the muscle contractile apparatus of striated muscle. They are found in both cardiac and skeletal muscle. Three isotypes have been identified: troponin-I (cTnI), troponin-T (cTnT), and troponin-C (cTnC) (Pagana & Pagana, 1998). Isotypes T and I are both found in the myocardium. Troponin-T binds the troponin complex to tropomyosin, and troponin-I inhibits the muscle

Table 14–1 ■ COMPARISON OF SENSITIVITY AND SPECIFICITY OF VARIOUS TESTS FOR MYOCARDIAL INFARCTION

Test	Sensitivity (%)	Specificity (%)
Electrocardiogram*	63–84	100
AST increased*	89–97	48–88
CK increased[†]	69–99	68–84
CK-MB increased[†]	79–80	96
LDH increased*	87	88
Myoglobin[†]	92	94
Troponin-I[†]	90–100	83–96
Troponin-T[†]	93	85

AST, Aspartate aminotransferase; CK, creatine kinase; LDH, lactate dehydrogenase.
　Range of values provided because different studies used various methods, periods after onset of symptoms, serial tests, benchmarks for establishing the diagnosis, and so forth. Refers to levels in serum.
* From Wallach, J. (1992). *Interpretation of diagnostic tests: A synopsis of laboratory medicine*, [5th ed.]. Boston: Little, Brown.
[†] Balk, E. M., et al. (2001). Accuracy of biomarkers to diagnose acute cardiac ischemia in the emergency department: A meta-analysis. *Annals of Emergency Medicine, 37*, 478–494.

Table 14–2 ■ TIMING OF APPEARANCE AND DISAPPEARANCE OF COMMONLY USED CARDIAC MARKERS AND ENZYMES IN RELATION TO ONSET OF CARDIAC SYMPTOMS

Marker or enzyme	Starts to rise (hours)	Peaks (hours)	Returns to normal (days)
AST	8	24–48	4
Total CK	4–6	24	3–4
CK-MB	4	18	2
LDH	24	72	8–9
Myoglobin	2–4	8–12	1–2
Troponin-I	4–6	10–24	4
Troponin-T	4–6	10–24	10

From Pagana, K. D. & Pagana, T. J. (2002). *Mosby's manual of diagnostic and laboratory tests* (p. 192). St. Louis: Mosby.

contraction in the absence of calcium and troponin-C (Sarko & Pollack, 2002). Troponin-C lacks cardiac specificity; therefore, it is the least studied of the troponins and has no assay available in the clinical setting. The normal range for troponin-I is 0 to 0.2 ng/mL, and the normal range for troponin-T is 0 to 0.03 ng/mL. Both are elevated in MI (Dufour, 1998). A troponin-I level greater than 1.5 ng/mL is consistent with acute MI (Kratz & Lewandrowski, 1998).

For patients with suspected acute coronary syndrome, troponin-I is the laboratory marker of choice because it is found exclusively in the myocardium. Because of its specificity and sensitivity for detecting myocardial injury, it has become the most important addition to clinical laboratory testing for assessment of myocardial injury (Jacobs & DeMott, 2001). In a meta-analysis by Balk and colleagues (2001), serial testing of troponin-I had 90% to 100% sensitivity and 83% to 96% specificity for detecting acute MI. Troponin-T had similar results showing 93% sensitivity and 85% specificity (Balk et al., 2001). See Table 14-1.

Troponin-I is typically not elevated in patients with either acute or chronic severe skeletal muscle injury, despite elevation in CK-MB (Adams et al., 1993); therefore, it is useful in detecting acute myocardial infarction after noncardiac surgery (Jacobs & DeMott, 2001). The troponins are enormously useful markers in the early diagnosis of MI because they are either low or undetectable in healthy people, but in the event of an MI, they are detectable as early as 3 to 4 hours after injury (Chernecky & Berger, 1997; Dufour, 1998; Pagana & Pagana, 2002). Because most troponin is so tightly bound to muscle, it is released slowly and may remain detectable for 1 to 2 weeks after MI (Adams et al., 1993; Dufour, 1998). This late-phase presence of troponins represents death of the contractile apparatus (Mangano, 1994). Troponin-I levels remain elevated after acute MI for 7 to 10 days or longer, and troponin-T levels remain elevated for up to 10 to 14 days. Because troponins remain elevated longer than CK-MB and are more specific than LDH, they are now the preferred test for patients who seek medical attention more than 24 to 48 hours after myocar-

dial injury. If reinfarction is suspected, troponin is not helpful because it may still be elevated from the first event (Pagana & Pagana, 2002). See Table 14-2 and Figure 14-1.

Between 15% to 48% of patients with unstable angina have an elevated troponin level with normal CK-MB. On coronary angiography, these patients frequently have active, unstable plaques, whereas patients without elevated troponin levels have stable plaques. These patients were considered to have minor myocardial damage. Patients with detectable levels of troponin have a higher in-hospital chance of having an adverse cardiac event. The risk is correlated with level of troponin: the higher the troponin, the worse the outcome (Sarko & Pollack, 2002).

Troponin-I levels may also be used to estimate the size of MI approximately 4 weeks after the initial event. Late elevations of troponin levels are inversely related to left ventricular ejection

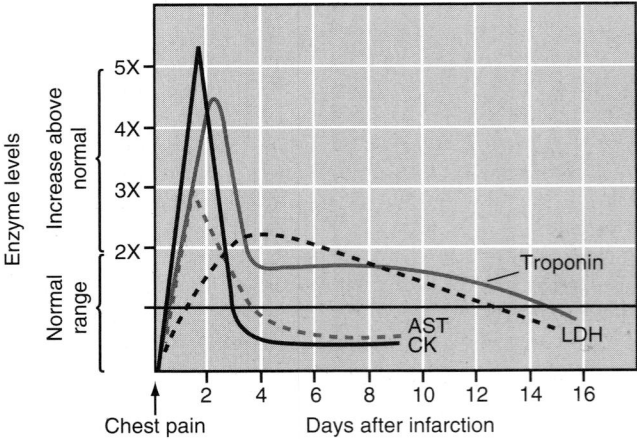

■ **Figure 14–1.** Patterns and timing of elevation for aspartate aminotransferase (AST), creatine kinase (CK), lactate dehydrogenase (LDH), and troponin. (Adapted and reproduced with permission from Ravel, R. [1984]. *Clinical laboratory medicine: Clinical application of laboratory data* [4th ed.]. Chicago: Year Book Medical Publishers, Inc., and Pagana, K. D., & Pagana, T. J. [2002]. *Mosby's manual of diagnostic and laboratory tests* [2nd ed.]. St. Louis: Mosby.)

fraction. Degradation of the myocardial contractile apparatus causes the abnormal troponin levels in this late period (Pagana & Pagana, 2002).

After coronary angiography, rapid peak or "washout" of troponin-I is seen, indicating reperfusion of the ischemic muscle tissue. This elevation is considered a favorable prognostic indicator (Pagana & Pagana, 2002; Sarko & Pollack, 2002).

Given the high rate of false-positive and false-negative CK-MB results in diagnosing blunt cardiac trauma (Miller, 1996), troponin-I has emerged as an accurate test for confirming presence of myocardial damage during cardiac contusion (Adams et al., 1996; Velmahos et al., 2003). Unlike CK-MB or troponin-T, troponin-I elevations are not found in the blood of marathon runners or patients with muscle disease (acute or chronic) unless there has been injury to the myocardium (Mangano, 1994). Troponin-I is not elevated in patients with renal insufficiency or failure (Birdi et al., 1997).

Troponin-T is not tested as often as troponin-I because it may be elevated in muscle damage (including rhabdomyolysis, polymyositis, and dermatomyositis) (Jacobs and DeMott, 2001; Sarko & Pollack, 2002) and may be falsely elevated in renal failure and dialysis patients (Chernecky & Berger, 1997; Dufour, 1998). It has been suggested that troponin-T concentrations may be of use in diagnosing perioperative MI after CABG. Troponin-T may also be a strong predictor of significant complication after MI, helping to identify those who require bypass surgery. In addition, release of troponin-T in donor hearts correlates with the need for inotropic support after cardiac transplantation, and may be of some use in evaluating high-risk donor hearts (Birdi et al., 1997). It has not been found useful as a predictor of cardiac allograft rejection (Wang et al., 1996). See Table 14-3.

Testing for troponins is typically performed at the time of the initial workup for suspected acute coronary syndrome, 6 to 12 hours later, followed by daily testing for 3 to 5 days or until the troponin level has peaked. Testing for troponins requires a 5-mL specimen in a red-top tube (Pagana & Pagana, 2002).

Myoglobin

Myoglobin is a low-molecular-weight oxygen-binding protein. Found in the myocardium and skeletal muscle, it is similar to hemoglobin (Hb) (Birdi et al., 1997). Myoglobin is released into the circulation after damage to the heart or skeletal muscle. In a meta-analysis by Balk and colleagues (2001), serial myoglobin has a sensitivity of 92% with a specificity of 94% for detecting acute MI (Balk et al., 2001). See Table 14-1. False-positive rates range anywhere from 0% to 22% because of its release from other muscle tissues (Pagana & Pagana, 1998; Tilkian et al., 1995). After MI, levels increase in 2 to 4 hours, peak in 8 to 12 hours, and return to normal (undetectable) as early as 12 hours but more typically after 24 to 30 hours. Because of the rapid increase in myoglobin levels after myocardial injury, it is useful as a basis for making decisions about thrombolytic therapy or emergency angioplasty within 6 hours of MI (Pagana & Pagana, 1998; Sobel & Jaffe, 1993). See Table 14-2.

Elevated myoglobin levels are seen after MI, reinfarction, skeletal muscle injury, trauma, severe burns, electrical shock,

Table 14–3 ■ NONCARDIAC DISORDERS RESULTING IN ELEVATION OF CREATINE KINASE-MB, LACTATE DEHYDROGENASE, AND TROPONINS

Elevated Creatine Kinase-MB
Muscular dystrophies
Hypothermia, hyperthermia
Hypothyroidism
Acute cholecystitis
Duchenne muscular dystrophy
Alcohol overdose
Delirium tremens
Polymyositis
Carcinomas (e.g., prostate, breast)
Dermatomyositis
Viral myositis
Extreme exercise
Peripartum period
Severe skeletal muscle trauma (rhabdomyolysis caused by crush injury or viral infection)
Reye syndrome
Poisoning

Elevated Lactate Dehydrogenase
Pulmonary embolism
Acute renal infarction
Hemolytic anemia
Pernicious anemia
Hemolysis associated with prosthetic heart valves
Pregnancy

Elevated Troponin-I
Hematologic malignancies
Subarachnoid hemorrhage
Cerebrovascular accident
Endocrine disease
Septic, intubated medical patients

Elevated Troponin-T
Polymyositis
Dermatomyositis
Renal failure/dialysis patients

polymyositis, alcoholic myopathy, delirium tremens, metabolic disorders (e.g., myxedema), malignant hyperthermia, systemic lupus erythematosus, muscular dystrophy, rhabdomyolysis, and seizures (Kee, 1999; Pagana & Pagana, 1998). Very high levels of myoglobin are toxic to the kidneys, and careful monitoring of renal function is warranted (Pagana & Pagana, 1998; Treseler, 1988). False-positive results occur in renal failure, when myoglobin is not excreted (McFarland & Grant, 1994). Myoglobin levels are usually evaluated along with serial determinations of troponin, CK and its isoenzymes, serial ECGs, and assessment of patient signs and symptoms. Tests for myoglobin require 5 mL of venous blood in a red-top tube (Kee, 1999).

Cardiac Enzymes

Enzymes are protein substances that catalyze chemical reactions in cells but do not themselves enter into the reaction. Substrates in the cells bind to the enzymes and form products. After the reaction, the enzyme molecule is free to undergo the same reaction with other substrate molecules. Specific enzymes are responsible for nearly every chemical reaction in the body.

Table 14–4 ■ DISTRIBUTION OF TOTAL CREATINE KINASE AND CREATINE KINASE ISOENZYMES IN HUMAN TISSUE

Tissue	Total CK	CK-MM (%)	CK-BB (%)	CK-MB (%)
Normal serum	Trace	97–100	0	0–3
Skeletal muscle	1894–3281	99–100	<1	<1
Heart	356–402	76–78	0–2	22
Bladder	162	2	92	6
Bowel	125–160	3–4	96	0–1
Brain	157	0	100	0
Lung	8.7–14	16–35	64–84	0–1

CK, creatine kinase. Expressed in units per liter (U/L) Expressed as percentage of total CK. Data from Galen, R. S. (1977). Myocardial infarction: A clinician's guide to the isoenzymes. *Resident and Staff Physician,* 23, 67–75; Lott, J. A. & Stang, J. M. (1980). Serum enzymes and isoenzymes in the diagnosis and differential diagnosis of myocardial ischemia and necrosis. *Clinical Chemistry,* 26, 1241–1250; and Tsung, S. M. (1976). Creatine kinase isoenzyme patterns in human tissue obtained at surgery. *Clinical Chemistry,* 22, 173–175.

Some enzymes are present in almost all cells; others are specific to cells of certain organs.

Creatine Kinase

Creatine kinase is an enzyme specific to cells of the brain, myocardium, and skeletal muscle, but it also is found in minimal amounts in other tissues such as smooth muscle. In these organ systems, the function of CK is primarily that of energy production, where it serves as a catalyst in the phosphorylation of adenosine diphosphate (ADP) to creatine and adenosine triphosphate (ATP). In this manner, CK is responsible for the transfer of an energy-rich bond to ADP. This reaction provides a rapid means of forming ATP for contractile activity in muscle as well as for energy requirements in nonmuscle tissue. The reaction is reversible, and ATP can phosphorylate creatine to form creatine phosphate and ADP during periods of rest (McFarland & Grant, 1988, 1994; Treseler, 1988).

In an acute MI, inadequate oxygen delivery to the myocardium causes cell injury. An acidic environment promotes the activity of lysosomal enzymes, which are responsible for cell membrane damage or destruction. CK is among the cellular enzymes that diffuse from the damaged cell into the blood. It is released after irreversible injury (Treseler, 1988). The appearance of CK in the blood indicates cardiac, cerebral, or skeletal muscle necrosis or injury and follows a predictable rise and fall over a specified time (see Fig. 14-1). Its presence may also indicate a neurologic pathologic process (Pagana & Pagana, 1998).

The average peak CK level after MI is approximately 1,200 units per liter of blood (U/L). The MB fraction averages 11%, with a relative index of 6% (Dufour, 1998). Total CK increases are seen in acute MI (Kee, 1999; McFarland & Grant, 1994; Pagana & Pagana, 1998), unstable angina (Kee, 1998; Pagana & Pagana, 1998; Treseler, 1988), shock, malignant hyperthermia, myopathies, myocarditis (Kee, 1999; Pagana & Pagana, 1998), cardiac aneurysm surgery, cardiac defibrillation (Kee, 1998; Pagana & Pagana, 1998), and sustained ventricular arrhythmias (Kee, 1998; Pagana & Pagana, 1998). Less frequent causes are electrical cardioversion, cardiac catheterization, and stroke (McFarland & Grant, 1994). Rises in total CK are also seen with major surgery, vigorous exercise, and alcoholic myopathy, and after IM injections (Kee, 1999; McFarland & Grant, 1994). Just one IM injection 24 to 48 hours before measurement may increase CK by more than 1,000 U/L

(Dufour, 1998; Kee, 1998; McFarland & Grant, 1994; Pagana & Pagana, 1998). CK levels as high as 5,000 to 10,000 U/L can be seen after cardiopulmonary resuscitation (Dufour, 1998). It is thought that CK-MB levels rise only slightly after cardiac pacemaker implantation and therefore should not interfere with attempts to evaluate such patients for MI (Gram-Hansen et al., 1990).

Specimens for CK are collected on admission, 8 to 12 hours later, and then every day for 3 days (Kee, 1998; Pagana & Pagana, 1998). CK and CK isoenzyme results should be evaluated along with troponin, myoglobin, ECG results, and clinical signs and symptoms. Laboratory slips should be marked with the date and time of any IM injections administered to the patient in the previous 24 to 48 hours. Caution should be exercised in interpretation of CKs drawn in the emergency department. Only 25% to 40% of patients who are having an MI have an abnormal CK at that point. An initial normal CK level should *never* be used to make a decision about discharge from the emergency department, or to withhold thrombolytic therapy (Dufour, 1998; Sobel & Jaffe, 1993).

The importance of monitoring the concentration of serum CK is related to its specificity in the organ in which it functions. Slightly different molecular forms (isoenzymes or *isozymes*) of CK have different tissues of origin (Table 14-4). The three CK isoenzymes are combinations of the protein subunits, M and B, named for their primary sites of isolation, the muscle (M) and brain (B) (Galen, 1981). CK-MM is the predominant muscle isoenzyme, found in cardiac and skeletal muscle. It also can be detected in normal serum. The myocardium is primarily responsible for the CK-MB form. CK-BB is present in the brain, lung, stomach, prostate, and smooth muscle of the gastrointestinal tract and bladder (Galen, 1981; Tsung, 1976). Diagnostic precision depends on laboratory analysis of CK isoenzymes and may well be imperative in critically ill patients with multiple organ system involvement.

Because of the wide range in baseline values among "healthy" people and various enzyme assay techniques, there are no uniform reference values for CK and CK isoenzymes (Dufour, 1998). Consequently, the practice of reporting the isoenzyme as a percentage of the total CK, as well as in U/L, has been encouraged (Lott & Stang, 1980). A nationwide survey of the analyses for CK and its isoenzymes revealed that 99% of 300 participating laboratories reported CK isoenzyme results in U/L, and 69% of the laboratories also reported isoenzymes as a percentage of the total CK activity (Boone et al., 1984). The reference values reported by laboratories may vary, suggesting possible regional variations in normal serum levels for CK and its isoenzymes.

Age, gender, race, physical activity, lean body mass, medications, and other unidentified factors are known to affect total CK. A patient's baseline CK level is related to his or her overall muscle mass (Pagana & Pagana, 1998). Adults have lower values than children. Serum CK declines with age; the older adults have very low values, sometimes making the diagnosis of MI difficult. CK values measured in women are lower than those of men; whites have lower values than blacks. Chronic exercise raises serum CK levels; however, there is a training effect, and well-trained athletes have smaller increases in CK after physical exertion (Lott & Stang, 1989). Medications that may increase CK include anticoagulants, aspirin, furosemide, captopril, lidocaine, propranolol, and morphine (Pagana & Pagana, 1998).

Creatine Kinase-BB. The brain fraction CK-BB (CK-1) is seen infrequently in serum. Its rare appearance has been associated with Reye syndrome, brain trauma, cerebral contusions, and cerebrovascular accidents (Hans et al., 1983; McFarland & Grant, 1994; Nordby and Urdal, 1985; Phillips et al., 1980; Ruzak-Skocir, 1991; Skogseid et al., 1992). The presence of CK-BB in association with cancer has been reported (Coolen et al., 1979). Other causes of serum CK-BB activity include malignant hyperpyrexia, bowel infarctions, renal failure, and central nervous system surgery (Fried et al., 1991; Galen, 1981). More recently, however, serum CK-BB has been reported after cardiac arrest (Longstreth et al., 1981; Longstreth et al., 1984; Massey & Goe, 1984). The presence of CK-BB after cardiac arrest has implications in the care of postarrest survivors. Investigators have been able to show that the maximum cerebrospinal fluid CK-BB concentration is related to neurologic outcome, Glasgow Coma Scale scores, the presence of intracranial pressure plateau waves, and histologic brain damage on death (Bakay & Ward, 1983; Hans et al., 1983; Kjekshus et al., 1980; Longstreth et al., 1984; Wallach, 1992). Studies have attempted to correlate serum CK-BB levels with neurologic outcome (Longstreth et al., 1981; Massey & Goe, 1984). Some researchers have suggested that a more favorable outcome is associated with a return to normal of serum CK-BB within 36 hours of a cerebral injury. Longstreth and coworkers (1981) suggested that persistence or reappearance of serum CK-BB more than 6 hours after cardiac arrest was associated with poor outcome (Longstreth et al., 1981). In a study by Massey and Goe (1984), no relationship was shown (Massey & Goe, 1984).

Creatine Kinase-MM. Creatine kinase–MM constitutes almost all CK in healthy people. Skeletal muscle injury or severe muscle exertion is the most frequent source of high-serum CK-MM (CK-3) levels. Specific examples include myopathy, vigorous exercise, multiple IM injections, electroconvulsive therapy, cardioversion, surgery (Pagana & Pagana, 1998), muscular dystrophy, convulsions, and delirium tremens. Elevations in CK-MM fractions have also been noted in conditions producing less obvious effects on muscle, such as hypokalemia and hypothyroidism. Alcohol has a direct toxic effect on muscle, and elevations of CK-MM can be detected in alcoholic patients (Ravel, 1984).

Some controversy continues as to whether skeletal muscle also contains CK-MB. One investigator reported that type I muscle fibers contain CK-MM, and that type II muscle fibers contain both CK-MM and CK-MB (Ravel, 1984). However, tissue studies performed by Tsung (1976) determined that CK-MB in skeletal muscle is responsible for less than 1% of the total CK activity in skeletal muscle, and that CK-MM is the primary muscle isoenzyme.

The analysis of blood for CK-MM can be a useful tool for differential diagnosis in complex situations. The normal range of CK-MM in the blood is 94% to 100% (Kee, 1999). Isoforms MM1 and MM3 are the most useful for evaluation of cardiac disease. A ratio of MM3:MM1 greater than 1 is suggestive of acute myocardial injury. The presence of CK-MM, rather than CK-MB, in the serum of patients who experienced electric countershock accounted for a total CK elevation in 30 patients studied by Ehsani and coworkers (Ehsani et al., 1976). This finding supported the belief that myocardial injury in such situations was minimal and that CK-MB was likely to appear in the serum only after abnormally vigorous and repetitive countershock. It is now accepted that total CK elevation after electric countershock, formerly thought to be of myocardial origin, is of skeletal muscle origin (CK-MM).

Exercise stress testing may negligibly elevate the total serum CK (Lott & Stang, 1980). A study of the sera of 62 subjects after performance of stress exercise to a symptom-tolerated maximum revealed that CK elevations, if present, were of the CK-MM fraction and were associated with the amount of work performed (Steele et al., 1978). Of marathon participants, 14% to 100% have elevated CK-MB (Lott & Stang, 1989).

A study of 210 patients after cardiac catheterization demonstrated that an increase in the serum activity of total CK activity was also of the CK-MM fraction. This issue was first examined by Roberts and coworkers (1975), who showed similar results in 42 patients. After balloon angioplasty of the coronary arteries, subtle myocardial injury may be reflected by increased CK-MB (Lott & Stang, 1989). If CK-MB is seen after cardiac catheterization without balloon angioplasty, injury to the myocardium should be considered (Lott & Stang, 1980).

At one time, it was thought that victims of primary cardiac arrest had experienced an MI, based on the case history and total CK elevation. In 1975, Cobb and coworkers (1975) reported that the CK elevation was not of myocardial origin (CK-MB) but was probably caused by cardiopulmonary resuscitation (CK-MM). This information has become an important determinant in the implication of several other cardiovascular diseases or processes that are now known to lead to primary cardiac arrest.

Creatine Kinase-MB. Since 1975, CK-MB (CK-2) isoenzyme analysis has been an accepted means for diagnosis of an acute MI. Roberts and associates (1975) examined tissue extracts obtained during surgery and demonstrated that the myocardium was the only tissue containing sufficient CK-MB to account for serum increases. The same studies revealed sera of 300 hospitalized patients had elevated CK-MB levels after MI (0.089 IU/mL), but low levels after cardiac catheterization and noncardiac surgery (0.004 IU/mL) (Roberts et al., 1975). This study was followed by others that determined that CK-MB isoenzyme activity was most specific in differentiating an MI from other myocardial events and could be defined by a predictable rise and fall over a period of 3 days (Smith et al., 1976).

When CK-MB is released from myocardial tissue, it has a biologic half-life in blood of hours to days (see Fig. 14-1). Total CK and CK-MB increase within 4 to 6 hours after an acute MI. Peak levels are seen within 12 to 24 hours and are more than six-times their normal value. If no additional myocyte necrosis occurs, levels return to normal within 3 to 4 days (Kee, 1998) (see Table 14- 2). Elevated CK-MB levels have also been reported after myocardial damage from unstable angina (Treseler, 1988), in cardiac surgery or coronary angioplasty, after defibrillation, in vigorous exercise, and after IM injections, trauma, and surgery (McFarland & Grant, 1994). Early and abnormally high increases in CK are sometimes seen after reperfusion by PTCA or thrombolytic agents (Prinkey, 1992). By 6 to 8 hours postangioplasty, 20% of patients have a mild increase in CK-MB. Elevations are occasionally seen in pericarditis, myocarditis, viral myositis, and sustained tachyarrhythmias (Tilkian et al., 1995). An increase in CK-MB may occur after cardioversion, but only with the use of 400 joules or more. The time course for increase is different for that of MI, with the mild increase of CK-MB peaking within 4 hours of cardioversion.

Although not very specific, CK-MB increases are seen after blunt cardiac trauma, as happens in steering-wheel injuries. However, they are so nonspecific that much doubt has been shed on the usefulness of CK and CK-MB levels in ruling out myocardial contusion. These tests may be abandoned in favor of the high specificity of troponin-I (Adams et al., 1996; Gunnar et al., 1991; Healey et al., 1990; Paone et al., 1993). Noncardiac increases in CK-MB are seen with trauma, skeletal muscle disease, Reye syndrome, hypothyroidism, labor, and in the peripartum period (Gersh, 1996).

Since 1975, studies have attempted to quantify the increase in CK-MB with such factors as ejection fraction and infarct size. Dyskinesis and akinesis have been associated with a higher CK level than hypokinesis in 21 patients studied by Hori and coworkers. They also found that the ejection fraction in patients with anterior wall MI was lower than that in those with inferior wall MI with the same CK-MB values (Hori et al., 1979). However, neither the ejection fraction values nor the clinical importance of the values was discussed.

Elevated CK-MB levels occur after PTCA and intracoronary thrombolysis. Normally there is no elevation of CK-MB with PTCA unless the procedure is performed early in an evolving MI in an effort to limit the infarct size. Monitoring of CK-MB after elective PTCA, however, has been suggested as important in ruling out myocardial damage. After successful elective PTCA, an elevation of CK-MB of 2% to 21% was found in 20% of 128 patients studied by Oh and colleagues (Oh et al., 1985). A mild myocardial necrosis was suspected in these patients. Length of hospital stay was twice that of patients without an elevated CK-MB, although it is not clear if the patients were kept in the hospital because of the elevated CK-MB or for other reasons. A high CK-MB is anticipated after fibrinolytic therapy, which takes place during the first few hours of symptoms suggestive of an acute MI. Early high CK-MB activity is considered to indicate successful reperfusion of the coronary artery. This "washout" of CK-MB, indicating revascularization, can be differentiated from the elevated CK-MB occurring after

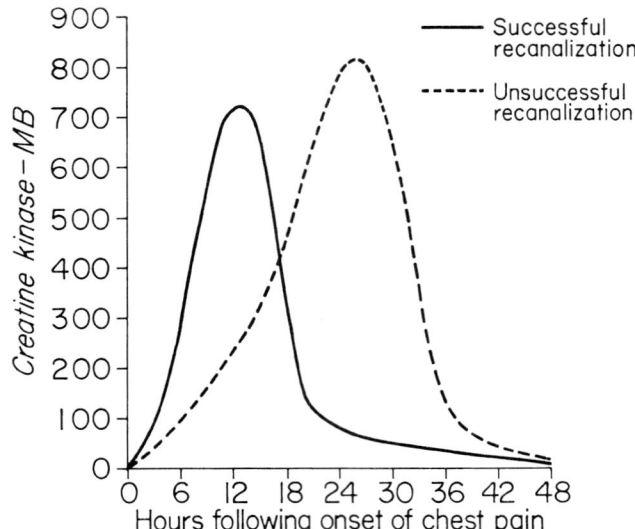

■ **Figure 14–2.** The pattern of total creatine kinase-MB (CK-MB) activity after successful emergency percutaneous transluminal coronary angioplasty (PTCA) or thrombolytic therapy (*solid line*) and unsuccessful PTCA or thrombolytic therapy (*dashed line*). Successful recanalization results in a "washout" of CK-MB (units/liter) at approximately 13 hours after onset of symptoms; an appearance of CK-MB at 22 to 30 hours indicates unsuccessful recanalization. (From Goe, M. R. [1987]. Creatine kinase enzyme determination: Implications for cardiovascular nursing. *Progress in Cardiovascular Nursing, 2, 48.*)

myocardial injury by its peak at approximately 12 to 14 hours after symptom onset (Mathey et al., 1981) (Fig. 14-2).

Other clinical situations may lead to a rise in serum CK-MB and are associated with myocardial cell injury or selected necrosis. Creatine kinase may be elevated with heart failure (without MI) and is usually attributed to circulatory failure secondary to heart failure or myocardial injury. In the presence of CHD, tachyarrhythmias compromise diastolic filling time and may lead to focal cell injury. The CK-MB in this situation is abnormal. Dysrhythmias without CHD do not lead to the release of CK-MB (Lott, 1984; Lott & Stang, 1980).

Just as the ECG may show changes with brain injury, such as subdural hematoma, CK-MB levels may also be elevated. Although the exact mechanism is not known, it is believed that a selected myocardial cell necrosis accompanies some head injuries. Subendocardial hemorrhage has been shown at autopsy of patients with CK-MB elevations after head injury (Kee, 1999). Finally, the appearance of CK-MM and CK-MB after extreme hypothermia reflects severe skeletal and cardiac muscle damage (Lott & Stang, 1980).

The patient in the critical care unit may have been admitted to rule out MI, for recovery after surgery, or after cardiovascular surgery. In addition, patients admitted with other diagnoses, including primary cardiac arrest, metabolic disorders, trauma, or respiratory disorders, can be found in these units. Each of these patients is at risk for myocardial injury and presents a complex diagnostic picture if acute MI develops. Assays of CK-MB or troponins are helpful in making a differential diagnosis. Serum CK-MB greater than 5% of the total CK indicates myocardial injury. Comparison of total CK to CK-MB

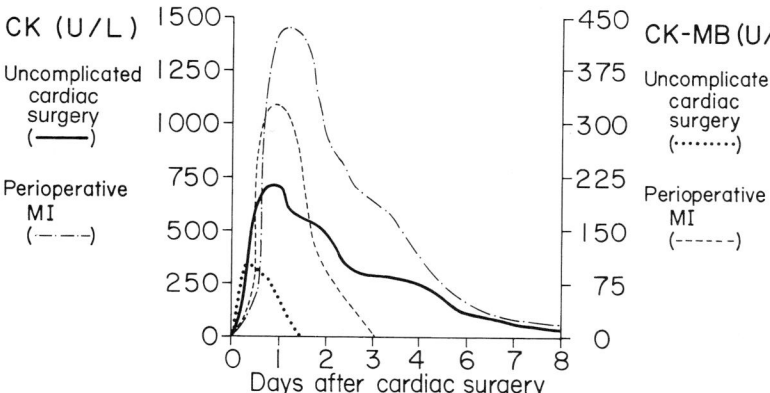

■ **Figure 14–3.** The pattern of total creatine kinase (CK) and creatine kinase-MB (CK-MB) activity after uncomplicated cardiac surgery (*dark lines*) and cardiac surgery with perioperative myocardial infarction (MI; *lighter lines*). After surgery, peak CK activity occurs at 22 hours and returns to normal after 5 days. The CK-MB activity appears approximately 4 hours after surgery and disappears within 48 hours. With an acute MI, CK-MB activity is considerably higher, occuring at approximately 21 to 24 hours after the onset of symptoms (the same time as total CK). (From Goe, M. R. [1987]. Creatine kinase enzyme determination: Implications for cardiovascular nursing. *Progress in Cardiovascular Nursing,* 2, 47.)

can be diagnostic, with a relative index greater than 2.5 highly suggestive of an acute MI (Pagana & Pagana, 1998).

CK-MB can be an accurate indicator of myocardial damage. In a meta-analysis by Balk and colleagues (2001), serial measurements of CK-MB were shown to have a sensitivity of 79% to 80% and a specificity of 96% for detecting MI (see Table 14-1) (Balk et al., 2001). CK-MB can also be found in other cardiac and noncardiac disorders (see Table 14-3), which can usually be distinguished clinically from an MI and present no diagnostic problem.

Creatine Kinase Activity After Cardiac Surgery. Until recently, the enzymatic criteria for diagnosis of a perioperative MI during CABG surgery remained a problem because of the myocardial cellular injury produced during surgery (Galen, 1981). Elevations in CK-MB have been associated with aortic cross-clamp time and duration of extracorporeal circulation (Tsung, 1976). At one time, it was thought that only a total CK level of 1200 U/L or greater could be diagnostic of perioperative infarct (Bolooki, 1973). However, studies have revealed that a small peak of CK-MB, having a shorter peak time and a rapid disappearance, was present after CABG surgery, whereas a peak CK-MB occurred later and lasted longer after an acute MI (Farah et al., 1984; Graeber, 1985; Koch-Weser, 1972). A peak activity seen 4 to 7 hours after CABG surgery reflects reversible myocardial ischemia, whereas a peak of more than 50 U/L occurring at 21 hours may indicate MI (Farah et al., 1984). Because perioperative MI has an influence on surgical prognosis, it has been suggested that multiple determinants of CK-MB be performed beyond 48 hours after cardiac surgery to rule out the occurrence of perioperative MI. Mass concentration of CK-MB and determination of the CK-MB time–activity curve are also sensitive diagnostic aids (Gulbis et al., 1990). With multiple determinations, the finding of a delayed peak or reappearance of CK-MB would be indicative of myocardial cell necrosis, a meaningful event in terms of length of hospitalization, treatment decisions, and rehabilitation. Figure 14-3 illustrates the typical patterns after CABG surgery and an acute MI.

The techniques used during valve replacement and atriotomy cause a postoperative elevation of CK-MB that is greater than that in patients who have had CABG surgery (Ganong, 1987; Jarvinen et al., 1983). This pattern of CK-MB activity led one group of investigators to suggest that the appearance of mean CK-MB levels of 93 to 103 U/L at 18 hours after aortic or mitral valve replacement precluded the diagnosis of perioperative MI (percentage of total CK was not discussed) (Jarvinen et al., 1983). However, it has been suggested that the diagnosis of perioperative MI is possible if two determinations of CK-MB are made between 18 and 30 hours after surgery, by which time CK-MB activity from other tissues (skeletal muscle or atrial myocardium) has disappeared. Sensitivity and specificity for MI were said to approach 99% if the two CK-MB determinations taken between 18 and 30 hours were 5% or more of the total CK (Graeber, 1985). Autotransfusion of shed mediastinal blood may complicate the assessment of perioperative MI after cardiac surgery. Reinfusion of autotransfused blood after internal mammary artery dissection is associated with high levels of total CK (MB fraction is normal) and LDH. Care should be taken when interpreting serial enzyme results in such a situation (Nguyen et al., 1996).

It is clear that whenever the question of myocardial damage arises, the analysis of CK isoenzymes is of diagnostic value. Identification of the isoenzyme responsible for total CK elevation in complex clinical situations could eliminate or confirm cardiac disease as a consideration in further treatment.

Creatine Kinase-MB Mass Concentration. Analysis of CK isoenzyme types depends on assessing functional "activity." An alternate approach has been developed that directly measures the mass concentration of CK (mg/L). Techniques to measure mass concentration allow CK to be determined more quickly. Rapid determination is of value in the emergency room when treatment decisions are being made, when coronary patency is evaluated after thrombolysis (Christenson et al., 1990), after cardiac surgery when perioperative MI is evaluated (Gulbis et al., 1990), and to select high-risk patients with unstable angina (Markenvard et al., 1992). Collinson and coworkers (1992) looked at 73 patients who had a diagnostic increase in CK; they measured CK-MB concentration and determined the slope in the rise of CK. They reported that 100% sensitivity and specificity for MI was shown within 4 hours of admission (Collinson et al., 1992).

Creatine Kinase Isoforms. Serum isoforms similar to CK-MM and CK-MB are part of the normal clearance process for CK and are present in all human sera. After release from injured myocardium, isoforms of CK-MM and CK-MB are converted in the circulation into three CK-MM isoforms and two CK-MB isoforms (Roberts et al., 1994). Studies have now shown that CK-MM isoform patterns provide a means of assessing the time of necrosis (Kanemitsu & Okigake, 1992). Similar results have been demonstrated for isoforms of CK-MB. Normally, MB-1 and MB-2 isoforms are found in a 1:1 ratio. However, when infarction occurs, the total CK-MB level may be normal, but a change in the ratio of MB-2 to MB-1 of 1.5 or greater is diagnostic of MI (Roberts et al., 1994). These isoforms have appeared in sera early after MI (1 to 4 hours), whereas total CK and CK-MB are still within normal limits (Kanemitsu & Okigake, 1992). The significance of these findings is that isoforms have become potential early indicators of MI capable of facilitating rapid diagnosis and intervention (Apple, 1989; Kanemitsu & Okigake, 1992; Schofer et al., 1992; Wu, 1989).

Laboratory Measurement of Creatine Kinase. Serum CK sampling is among the most common laboratory assays. It is particularly useful in the cardiac care unit, where the presence of CK isoenzymes has many important and life-threatening implications. The determination of an accurate serum CK level depends on several variables in measurement and procedural techniques. Table 14-5 describes typical serum CK values found in patients with MI and in healthy people.

The collection of blood for CK interpretation presents some problems in methodology. Dilution of the CK specimen with either distilled water or saline may lead to changes in enzyme kinetic activity (an indicator of enzyme concentration) when certain assay techniques are used (Henry et al., 1974). The test requires 1 to 3 mL of blood. CK must be collected in a timely manner because the half-life of the isoenzyme in the body may be as short as 2 to 5 hours. Any delay in collection of blood for CK-BB activity should be particularly avoided. The CK-BB isoenzyme is unstable in blood already collected, and serum should be frozen as soon as possible after the blood is drawn to minimize inactivation in the tube. Methods to reactivate this isoenzyme in serum may make this test less sensitive to time delay (Abbott & Lott, 1984; Longstreth et al., 1984). A baseline CK-MB, drawn during the first 4 hours after a suspected MI, may be of value in identifying atypical, chronically elevated CK (the immunoglobulin complex of CK-BB or CK of mitochondrial, rather than cytoplasmic, origin) when certain assay techniques are used (Massey & Butts, 1983).

Serum should be separated from the erythrocytes immediately after clotting is completed. Assays for CK-MB or CK-BB require that the serum be frozen until assayed. Results are reported in units per liter. However, measurement of CK-MM is not sensitive to storage. Isoenzyme results are also described as a percentage of the total CK. The assay is performed at either 30°C (room temperature) or 37°C (Baer & Dito, 1981). The assay temperature should be reported with the results.

Slight hemolysis can be tolerated for CK assay because red blood cells do not contain CK. However, specimens with a visible degree of hemolysis may contain adenylate kinase, which may falsely increase CK-MB results (Ravel, 1984). Assay mixtures for total CK used by many clinical laboratories now contain specific inhibitors of adenylate kinase, preventing falsely elevated total CK results.

Creatine kinase isoenzymes can be analyzed using several techniques, which accounts for the wide diversity in normal ranges (reference intervals) as well as diagnostic values. Because

Table 14–5 ■ REFERENCE VALUES FOR CREATINE KINASE AND CREATINE KINASE-MB*

Population	Total CK (U/L)	CK-MB (U/L)	CK-MB (%)
Ranges reported as normal	95–100	0–5	0–5
Healthy laboratory controls	42–123	0–1.4	0–2
Hospitalized patients	217–1140	0–8	0–1.1
Acute myocardial infarction patients	144–4125	6.8–336	4–19

CK, creatine kinase.
* UL = international units per liter of blood.
% = CK-MB/Total CK × 100
Results are usually reported in units per liter or percentage at either 30°C or 37°C.
From Boone, D. J. et al. (1984). "Results of a nationwide survey of analyses for creatine kinase and creatine kinase isoenzymes," *Clinical Chemistry,* 30, 33–37; and Varat, M. A. & Mercer, D. W. (1975). Cardiac specific creatine phosphokinase isoenzyme in the diagnosis of acute myocardial infarction. *Circulation,* 51, 855–859.

immunoassay is simple, relatively speedy, and precise, it is the most widely used technique for measuring CK. Electrophoresis is less sensitive and less accurate (Jacobs & DeMott, 2001). Immunoinhibition is not widely used because false-positive results are relatively common (Dufour, 1998). The range of reference values for upper limits of normal for the CK isoenzymes is given in Table 14-6.

BLOOD LIPIDS

An accumulation of lipids within the arterial wall is considered a part of the process of atherogenesis (Ross, 1999). Alteration of blood lipid levels has been identified as a CHD risk factor (Kannel, 1978). Certain lipoproteinemias have been identified as contributing to total plasma cholesterol levels. Plasma normally contains insoluble lipid elements: free fatty acids; exogenous triglycerides; endogenous triglycerides, which are manufactured in the liver; cholesterol; and phospholipids. To be transported, each is attached to a protein. Distinguishing lipoprotein abnormalities is useful because therapy is based on an understanding of the origin of the problem (see Chapter 40).

Blood Lipid Laboratory Measurement

Elevated lipid levels are considered a risk factor for cardiovascular disease. Cholesterol and the protein components of HDL, LDL, and triglycerides are evaluated by electrophoresis when hyperlipoproteinemia is suspected. In most people, the cholesterol values remain constant over 24 hours; a nonfasting blood sample for measurement of total blood cholesterol is acceptable. However, a nonfasting sample for HDL, LDL, and triglyceride levels is of less value (Cooper et al., 1992; Pagana & Pagana, 2002). National Cholesterol Education Program

Table 14–6 ■ NORMAL REFERENCE RANGES FOR LABORATORY BLOOD TESTS*

Blood Test	Reference Range
Hematologic Studies	
Red blood cell count	
Males	$4.6–6.2 \times 10^6$
Females	$4.2–5.4 \times 10^6$
Hematocrit	
Males	40%–50%
Females	38%–47%
Hemoglobin	
Males	13.5–18.0 g/100 mL
Females	12.0–16.0 g/100 mL
Corpuscle indices	
Mean corpuscular volume	82–98 fL
Mean corpuscular hemoglobin	27–31 pg
Mean corpuscular hemoglobin concentration	32%–36%
White blood cell count	
Total	4,500–11,000/mm³
Differential (in number of cells/mm³ blood)	
Total leukocytes	5,000–10,000 (100%)
Total neutrophils	3,000–7,000 (60%–70%)
Lymphocytes	1,500–3,000 (20%–30%)
Monocytes	375–500 (2%–6%)
Eosinophils	50–400 (1%–4%)
Basophils	0–50 (0.1%)
Sedimentation rate	0–30 mm/hr
Coagulation Studies	
Platelet count	250,000–500,000/mm³
Prothrombin time	12–15 sec
Partial thromboplastin time	60–70 sec
Activated partial thromboplastin time	35–45 sec
Activated coagulation time	75–105 sec
Fibrinogen level	160–300 mg/dL
Thrombin time	11.3–18.5 sec
Blood Chemistries	
Serum electrolytes	
Sodium	135–145 mEq/L
Potassium	3.3–4.9 mEq/L
Chloride	97–110 mEq/L
Carbon dioxide	22–31 mEq/L
Blood gases	
pH	7.35–7.45
$PaCO_2$	35–45 mm Hg
PaO_2	80–105 mm Hg
Bicarbonate	22–29 mEq/L
Base excess, deficit	0 ± 2.3 mEq/L
SaO_2	98%
SvO_2	60%–80%

Blood Test	Reference Range
Blood Chemistries–(cont.)	
Alkaline phosphatase	35–125 IU/L
Alanine aminotransferase-ALT	0–40 IU/L
Aspartate aminotransferase-AST	5–40 IU/L
Bilirubin	
Total	0.2–1.3 mg/dL
Direct	0–0.4 mg/dL
Calcium	
Total	8.9–10.3 mg/dL
Free (ionized)	4.6–5.1 mg/dL
Creatinine	
Males	0.9–1.4 mg/dL
Females	0.8–1.3 mg/dL
Glucose (fasting)	65–110 mg/dL
Hb A1c (varies with laboratory method used)	
Nondiabetic adult	2.2%–4.8%
Good diabetic control	2.5%–5.9%
Fair diabetic control	6%–8%
Poor diabetic control	>8%
LDH	20–200 IU/L
Magnesium	1.3–2.2 mEq/L
Phosphorus	2.5–4.5 mg/dL
Protein (total)	6.5–8.5 g/dL
Urea nitrogen	8–26 mg/dL
Uric acid	
Males	4.0–8.5 mg/dL
Females	2.8–7.5 mg/dL
Serum Enzymes	
CK-MM	95%–100%
CK-MB	0%–5%
CK-BB	0%
Myocardial Proteins	
Troponin-I	0–0.2 ng/mL
Troponin-T	0–0.03 ng/mL
Myoglobin	
Males	20–90 ng/mL
Females	10–75 ng/mL
hs-CRP	
Low	<1.0 mg/L
Average	1.0–3.0 mg/L
High	>3.0 mg/L
Homocysteine	
Optimal	<12 μmol/L
Borderline	12–15 μmol/L
High risk for cardiovascular disease	>15μmol/L
BNP (B-type natriuretic peptide)	
Most diagnostic of heart failure	>100 pg/mL

*Examples: regional laboratory techniques and methods may result in variations.

(NCEP), 2001 guidelines on cholesterol *screening* recommend everyone older than age 20 have a fasting lipoprotein profile (total cholesterol, LDL, HDL, and triglycerides) every 5 years (National Cholesterol Education Program, 2001). Table 14-7 lists lipid profile reference values. Lipoprotein electrophoresis is necessary to evaluate serum for hyperlipoproteinemia. LDL is difficult to isolate and measure. Therefore, if LDL is not measured in a screening lipoprotein test, it may be calculated using the Friedewald formula (see Table 14-8). The Friedewald formula is inaccurate if the triglycerides are greater than 400 mg/dL (Baron, 2001; Pagana & Pagana, 2002).

Very-low-density lipoprotein (VLDL) is also measured in people with known elevated lipid levels. VLDL is the predominant carrier of blood triglycerides. Excess levels of VLDL is considered a risk factor for atherosclerotic disease. VLDL is typically expressed as a percentage of total cholesterol (Pagana & Pagana, 2002).

Investigators have now broken-down lipoproteins into some of their components. Research continues on which components of the lipid profile contribute more to atherosclerotic disease (Pagana & Pagana, 2002). The protein component of lipoproteins is composed of polypeptides known as apolipoproteins.

Table 14–7 ■ LIPID PROFILE REFERENCE RANGES

Lipid Profile

Total blood cholesterol*

Desirable	<200 mg/dL
Borderline high	200–239 mg/dL
High	≥240 mg/dL

HDL-cholesterol*

Low, A major risk factor for CHD	<40 mg/dL
Better	40–59 mg/dL
High, Considered protective against heart disease	≥60 mg/dL

LDL-cholesterol*

Optimal	<100 mg/dL
Near or above optimal	100–129 mg/dL
Borderline high	130–159 mg/dL
High	160–189 mg/dL
Very high	>190 mg/dL

LDL cholesterol treatment goals*

No CHD or DM with 1 or no risk factors	<160 mg/dL
No CHD or DM with 2 or more risk factors	<130 mg/dL
CHD or DM patients	<100 mg/dL

Triglyceride*

Normal	<150 mg/dL
Borderline high	150–199 mg/dL
High	200–499 g/dL
Very high	≥500 mg/dL

Apolipoprotein A-I[†]

Males	Normal 75–160 mg/dL
Females	Normal 80–175 mg/dL

Apolipoprotein B-100[†]

Males	Normal 50–125 mg/dL
Females	Normal 45–12 mg/dL

CHD, coronary heart disease; DM, diabetes mellitus.
* From National Cholesterol Education Program (2001). Executive summary of The Third Report of The National Cholesterol Education Program (NCEP) Expert Panel on Detection, Evaluation, and Treatment of High Blood Cholesterol in Adults (Adult Treatment Panel III). *JAMA, 285,* 2486–2497.
† From Pagana, K. D. & Pagana, T. J. (2002). *Mosby's manual of diagnostic and laboratory tests* (pp. 106–107). St. Louis: Mosby.

Table 14–8 ■ COMPUTATION FORMULAS

Computation of LDL Cholesterol
Friedewald Formula *
LDL cholesterol = Total cholesterol − HDL cholesterol − (Triglycerides divided by 5)

Computation of Ionized Calcium
Serum calcium can be presumed to be normal if:
(4.5 − albumin level) = (0.8) + laboratory value for total calcium = 8.8 to 11.0 mEq/L

1. Obtain total calcium level (normal = 8.8–10.5 mEq/L). If it is less than normal (e.g., ,8.8 mEq/L), follow the steps below.
2. Obtain serum albumin level (normal = 4.5 g/dL).
3. If serum albumin level is decreased, subtract the decreased level from normal value for albumin (e.g., albumin level is measured at 3.0; 4.5 [normal] − 3.0 [measured] = 1.5).
4. For every 1.0 decrease in albumin, add 0.8 to calcium level (e.g., 1.5 × 0.8 = 1.2).
5. Add the calculated figure to the total calcium level (e.g., 7.8 + 1.2 = 9 mEq/L, calcium is within normal range).
6. One-half of this level (9/2) is 4.5, within the normal range for ionized calcium (normal ionized calcium = 4.5–5.0).

Computation of Anion Gap
Anion gap = [sodium (140) + potassium (4.0)] 2 − [bicarbonate (24) + chloride (110)] = 10–12 mEq/L

Computation of Serum Osmolality
Two times the serum sodium + serum glucose (Glu) divided by 18 + blood urea nitrogen (BUN) divided by 1.8 = serum osmolality ([2 × Sodium] + [Glucose/18] + [BUN/1.8]) = 280 − 300 mOsm/kg (e.g., (2 × 122) + (198/2) + (18/1.8) = 265 mOsm (water or intracellular fluid excess); (2 × 155) + (108/2) + (5.4/1.8) = 318 mOsm [water or intracellular fluid deficit])

*Formula valid for estimating LDL cholestrol if the triglyceride level is <400 mg/dL.

studied as a possible risk factor for CHD and Alzheimer disease (Jacobs & DeMott, 2001; Pagana & Pagana, 2002). Additional measurements of apolipoproteins may be included in the lipoprotein assay in assessing the risk of CHD but are typically reserved for patients with known CHD, suspected familial hypercholesterolemia, or other rare lipid metabolism disorders (Baron, 2001; Genest et al., 1992; Schaefer & Levy, 1985). Because lipids may be abnormal if drawn while the patient is having an acute MI or is otherwise undergoing considerable acute stress, it is recommended that lipid studies be performed at another time (Jacobs and DeMott, 2001). It is recommended that lipid profile tests should be performed after a 12- to 14-hour fast and after a stable diet for 2 to 3 weeks before testing (Jacobs & DeMott, 2001). A number of factors are known to influence LDL and HDL levels (Table 14-9).

■ ADDITIONAL LABORATORY TESTS ASSOCIATED WITH CARDIAC DISEASE

Nearly half of all patients with known CHD have no established coronary risk factors (i.e., hypertension, hypercholesterolemia, cigarette smoking, diabetes mellitus, marked obesity, and physical inactivity) (Braunwald, 1997). Atherosclerosis is now considered an inflammatory disease, with cytokines and other bioactive molecules involved in most steps of the atherogenesis process (Kuller et al., 1996; Ross, 1999) (see Chapters 6 and 7).

The major apolipoprotein of HDL is apolipoprotein A (apo-A), which has 2 major forms: apolipoprotein A-I (apo A-I) (75%) and apolipoprotein-II (20%). Apo A-I testing is primarily used for patients who have low HDL levels (Jacobs & DeMott, 2001). Many researchers believe apo A-I may be a better marker of atherogenic risk than HDL, but this conclusion remains controversial (Jacobs and DeMott, 2001; Pagana & Pagana, 2002).

LDL and VLDL both contain the protein component known as apolipoprotein B (apo B). Apo B exists in 2 forms: apo B-100 and apo B-48. Apo B-100 participates in the delivery and deposition of cholesterol to the tissues and has an affinity for the LDL receptor. Elevated Apo B-100 has been described as a good predictor of and a risk factor for CHD (Jacobs & DeMott, 2001; Pagana & Pagana, 2002; Schaefer & Levy, 1985; Wallach, 1992). A low ratio of apo A-I to apo B-100 may be a highly accurate predictor of CHD (Genest et al., 1992; Pagana & Pagana, 2002; Wallach, 1992). Lp(a), "lipoprotein little a," contains both apo B-100 and apo-A. Lp(a) and is being studied as a risk factor for CHD (Jacobs & DeMott, 2001). Apolipoprotein E (apo E) is another protein component involved in cholesterol transport. Apo E has 3 alleles: E2, E3, and E4. Apo E4 is being

Table 14–9 ■ FACTORS THAT INFLUENCE LOW-DENSITY LIPOPROTEIN (LDL) AND HIGH-DENSITY LIPOPROTEIN (HDL) LEVELS

LDL Levels	HDL Levels
Increased with:	*Increased with:*
Diets high in cholesterol	Not smoking
Diets high in saturated fat	Lean body mass
Alcohol	Estrogen
Strict vegetarian diet	Vigorous exercise
Hypothyroidism	Diet low in sucrose and starch
Obesity	Increased clearance of very-low-density lipoprotein (triglyceride)
Obstructive liver disease	Alcohol
Nephrotic syndrome	
Thiazide diuretics	*Decreased with:*
β-Adrenergic blocking agents	Cigarette smoking
Progestin and anabolic steroids	Obesity
	Progesterone
Decreased with:	Male gender
Low-cholesterol diet	Sedentary lifestyle
Low-fat diet	Hypertriglyceridemia
Alcohol restriction	Hepatocellular disease
Regular strenuous exercise	Non-insulin-dependent diabetes mellitus
	Hypoproteinemia
	Strict vegetarian diet
	Hypertriglyceridemia
	Anabolic steroids
	Starvation
	β-Adrenergic blocking agents
	Infectious illness

Other Cardiovascular Risk Factor Laboratory Tests

With the knowledge that atherosclerosis is an inflammatory disease, researchers are studying different markers to determine if there are other independent risk factors for the disease and if these markers can be used to identify individuals at high risk for CHD who may not have traditional risk factors. Markers being studied include, but are not limited to, adhesion molecules, C-reactive protein, cytokines, fibrinogen, homocysteine, lipoprotein-associated phospholipase A_2, serum amyloid A, tissue-type plasminogen activator, and WBC count. Homocysteine is being researched extensively and is in use as a possible risk factor for CHD. C-reactive protein is showing promise from a clinical chemistry perspective and research perspective as a risk factor for CHD (Pearson et al., 2003).

C-reactive Protein

C-reactive protein (CRP) is an acute-phase reactant protein that is produced primarily by the liver during the acute inflammatory process. CRP is a nonspecific but sensitive indicator of inflammation, bacterial infection, or acute injury. CRP is a more sensitive indicator of inflammation and responds more rapidly to inflammation than erythrocyte sedimentation rate (ESR). CRP was discovered approximately 70 years ago and has been used for decades to monitor the effectiveness of treatment for patients with systemic lupus erythematosus, rheumatoid arthritis, and other immune-related conditions (Jacobs & DeMott, 2001; Macy et al., 1997; Pagana & Pagana, 2002). Patients with acute MI, sepsis, or who have undergone surgery have elevated CRP levels (Jacobs & DeMott, 2001).

Interest in CRP changed since 1996 because of studies that link elevated CRP levels to increased CHD risk (see Figure 14-4). CRP has been studied to determine its usefulness in detecting a low-level acute-phase response caused by chronic atherosclerotic disease (Macy et al., 1997). In 1997, Ridker and colleagues (1997) established that men in the Physician's Health

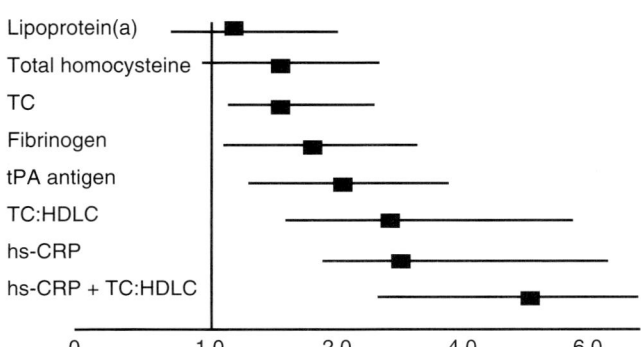

■ **Figure 14–4.** Relative risk for future myocardial infarction among apparently healthy middle-aged men in the Physician's Health Study according to baseline levels of lipoprotein(a), total plasma homocysteine, total cholesterol (TC), fibrinogen, tissue-type plasminogen activator (tPA) antigen, the ratio of total cholesterol to high-density lipoprotein cholesterol (TC: HDLC), and high-sensitivity C-reactive protein (hs-CRP). (From Ridker, P. M. [1999]. Evaluating novel cardiovascular risk factors: Can we better predict heart attacks? *Annals of Internal Medicine, 130,* 933–937.)

Study who had the highest CRP levels had three-times greater risk of MI and two-times greater risk of ischemic stroke than the men who had the lowest CRP levels. Other studies have continued to demonstrate a link between elevated CRP levels and increased risk of CHD in healthy middle-aged men (Koenig et al., 1999), healthy but high-risk men (Kuller et al., 1996), women from the Women's Health Study (Ridker et al., 2000), and the elderly (Tracy et al., 1997). CRP levels have also been shown to be elevated in overweight and obese young adults and older adults (Visser et al., 1999). Ridker and colleagues (2002) demonstrated that CRP was a stronger predictor of cardiovascular events than LDL level in 15,745 women participants in the Women's Health Study.

Increased body mass index, insulin resistance, hypertension, an intrauterine device (IUD), cigarette smoking, chronic infections (e.g., gingivitis, bronchitis), or chronic inflammation (e.g., rheumatoid arthritis) can increase CRP levels (Pearson et al., 2003). Drugs that may cause an increase in CRP include exogenous hormones. Increased activity, weight loss, and moderate alcohol consumption decrease CRP levels. Drugs that decrease CRP levels include fibrates, HMG-CoA reductase inhibitors (statins), nicotinic acid (niacin), nonsteroidal anti-inflammatory agents, salicylates, and steroids (Pagana & Pagana, 2002; Pearson et al., 2003). Many laboratories offer a routine CRP level or a high-sensitivity CRP (hs-CRP) level (see Table 14-6 for reference range). To evaluate CRP as a risk factor for CHD, the hs-CRP is monitored. As more information is available about CRP as a risk factor for CHD, reference values may change. To classify an individual's risk for atherosclerotic disease, it is recommended that two separate "fasting" hs-CRP measurements be evaluated. At this point, it is not recommended that all individuals be screened for CRP (Pearson et al., 2003).

Homocysteine

Homocysteine (Hcy) is an intermediate amino acid formed during protein catabolism by the conversion of methionine to cysteine. Vitamins B_6, folic acid, B_{12}, and riboflavin are all required for this metabolism. Epidemiologic studies first showed an association of high levels of Hcy with an increased incidence of atherosclerotic disease (Lily, 2001). Elevated Hcy is believed to be a part of the process of atherosclerosis by participating in endothelial damage, promoting LDL deposition, decreasing the availability of nitrous oxide, and promoting vascular smooth muscle growth. Research remains controversial that elevated Hcy levels may be an independent risk factor for CHD and carotid and peripheral vascular atherosclerosis (Ridker, 1999). A meta-analysis of observational studies performed by the Homocysteine Studies Collaboration (2002) found Hcy to be only a modest independent predictor of ischemic heart disease and stroke in healthy populations. A meta-analysis on cohort studies showed that elevated Hcy moderately increases the risk of a first cardiovascular event, regardless of age and follow-up duration (Bautista et al., 2002). Cleophas and colleagues (2000) in their meta-analysis found that elevated Hcy levels may not be as harmful to the heart as first thought, but may indicate an unhealthy lifestyle. Preliminary research suggests treatment of high Hcy levels with B_6, B_{12}, and folic acid improves Hcy and may alter CHD (Chambers et al., 2000; de Bree et al., 2003; Doshi et al., 2002; Schnyder et al., 2001; Title et al., 2000; Wald et al., 2001).

Elevated Hcy levels can be genetic or acquired. Hyperhomocystinemia can be caused by a genetic defect in Hcy metabolism. Children with this disease have very premature and accelerated atherosclerosis during childhood. Hcy testing should be performed when there is a strong familial predisposition for atherosclerotic disease or with a progressive or an early onset of atherosclerotic disease is suspected (Pagana & Pagana, 2002).

Elevated Hcy levels may also be acquired from a dietary deficiency of vitamins B_6, B_{12}, or folate. Obtaining Hcy levels in the elderly, alcoholics, or drug abusers may be helpful in the diagnosis of nutritional deficiencies. Individuals with megaloblastic anemia may have elevated Hcy levels before anemia and macrocytosis are evident (Jacobs & DeMott, 2001; Pagana & Pagana, 2002).

Patients with decreased renal function and hypothyroidism have increased Hcy levels. Men tend to have higher levels of Hcy than premenopausal women. Smoking is associated with higher levels of Hcy. Drugs that may increase Hcy levels include carbamazepine, corticosteroids, cyclosporine, methotrexate, nitrous oxide, theophylline, and phenytoin. Drugs that may decrease Hcy levels include folic acid, oral contraceptives, and tamoxifen (Pagana & Pagana, 2002). A fasting blood sample is recommended when testing Hcy levels. Meat contains elevated levels of Hcy and may alter results (Jacobs & DeMott, 2001; Pagana & Pagana, 2002). See Table 14-6 for reference range.

Lipoprotein-Associated Phospholipase A₂

Lipoprotein-associated phospholipase A_2, also known as platelet-activating factor acetylhydrolase or Lp-PLA_2, is presently being studied as an inflammatory marker of cardiovascular risk. Lp-PLA_2 is an enzyme regulated by inflammatory cytokines and is found predominately on LDL cholesterol. Lp-PLA_2 may contribute directly to atherogenesis, by hydrolyzing oxidized phospholipids into pro-atherogenic fragments and by generating lysolecithin, which has proinflammatory properties (Rader, 2000). Recent studies by Caslake and coinvestigators (2000) and Packard and researchers (2000) showed a strong correlation between Lp-PLA_2 levels and risk of CHD in men. By contrast, results from the Women's Health Study showed Lp-PLA_2 was not a strong predictor of future cardiovascular risk in females (Blake et al., 2001). Further research is needed to assess Lp-PLA_2 ability to predict cardiovascular risk and establish plasma levels.

Cardiac Natriuretic Peptide Markers

The natriuretic peptide system is part of the neurohormonal system that participates in cardiovascular homeostasis (Grantham & Burnett, 1997). Investigators have identified three natriuretic peptides. Type A and type B originate in the cardiac myocyte and type C originates in the endothelial and renal epithelial cells. A-type natriuretic peptide (ANP) originates in the atrium and is released into the bloodstream when the atrium is stretched beyond normal capacity. B-type natriuretic peptide (BNP) (also known as brain natriuretic peptide because it was first identified in small amounts in the brain) is produced and stored in the ventricles of the heart and is released when ventricular diastolic pressure rises (Maisel et al., 2002). Researchers believe that ANP is released as an acute response to increased volume in the heart, whereas BNP acts as a backup hormone only activated after prolonged volume overload (Grantham & Burnett, 1997). Both hormones act in a similar manner to increase the loss of water and sodium through the kidneys. Renin and aldosterone are suppressed by the hormones. Glomerular filtration rate is increased by renal vasculature dilation. ANP and BNP have diuretic and antihypertensive effects. BNP concentrations are elevated in heart failure and correlate well with measured left heart pressures.

Although ANP and BNP both have laboratory assays available, BNP has emerged as the laboratory marker of choice for evaluating dyspnea and heart failure because it is synthesized and secreted by the left ventricle. BNP concentrations have been correlated with the New York Heart Association Functional Classification of severity of heart failure, as well as prognosis in heart failure (Berger et al., 2002; Grantham & Burnett, 1997; Maisel et al., 2002; Wieczorek et al., 2002).

BNP testing is available as a rapid point-of-care test or can be performed in a centralized laboratory. McCullough and colleagues (2002) determined that BNP concentrations greater than 100 pg/mL had 90% sensitivity, 73% specificity, and a 90% negative predictive value for diagnosing heart failure. Wieczorek and researchers (2002) found similar results with a BNP assay of greater than 100 pg/mL having 82% sensitivity and 99% specificity for distinguishing control patients from those patients who had heart failure. Typically, BNP concentrations are being used in emergency departments to help differentiate heart failure from other causes of dyspnea. Research indicates BNP is a valuable tool to help clinicians diagnose heart failure (Berger et al., 2002; Maisel et al., 2002; McCullough et al., 2002; Sabatine et al., 2002; Wieczorek et al., 2002). Because BNP concentrations decrease as ventricular pressures are lowered, BNP might also be useful in the in-hospital management of patients with heart failure but is not approved for that use at this time. Along with hemodynamic monitoring, BNP might help clinicians in titrating therapy for heart failure (Wieczorek et al., 2002). See Table 14-6 for reference range.

HEMATOLOGIC STUDIES

Cells in the circulating blood are responsible for oxygen and carbon dioxide transport and the body's immune response. Erythrocytes (red blood cells), leukocytes (white blood cells), and platelets are formed in the bone marrow and are suspended in the plasma (see Chapter 8). Blood is also the transport system for electrolytes, products of metabolism, hormones, and plasma proteins. The blood volume in a normal adult is approximately 8% of the body weight (Ganong, 1987). An appreciation of the roles of erythrocytes, leukocytes, and other hematologic parameters is an important prerequisite to understanding deviations from normal. This approach is helpful in planning care based on an assessment of the demands of daily living. Each of the aspects of a hematologic study has meaning for patients in terms of their ability to withstand the effects of a cardiac event.

Complete Blood Cell Count

A complete blood cell count (CBC) is important for evaluating the oxygen-carrying capacity of the blood and the response of the body to invasion by foreign cells such as bacteria. Because excessive bleeding, bone marrow disease, hemolytic disorders, some drugs, and infections can alter the number of leukocytes, erythrocytes, or platelets in the blood, the CBC of the patient with cardiac disease is closely monitored. A baseline study can be compared with subsequent studies to evaluate bleeding, the effects of treatment, or the presence of infection (see Table 14-6).

Red Blood Cell Count

Red blood cells (RBCs; erythrocytes) are formed in the bone marrow and constitute the majority of peripheral cells. They contain Hb and are responsible for transporting oxygen to the tissues (and carbon dioxide from tissues). The average lifespan of an RBC is 120 days, after which it is removed from the blood by the liver, spleen, or bone marrow.

When the RBC count is more than 10% below the expected normal value, the patient is said to be anemic. Conditions under which there are a decreased number of RBCs include cirrhosis, hemorrhage, presence of prosthetic valves, renal disease, chronic illnesses, and various malignancies of the bone marrow (Chernecky & Berger, 1997; Pagana & Pagana, 1998). Anemia from any cause must be looked for in the patient with cardiac disease because it may precipitate angina, aggravate heart failure, or contribute to a diagnosis of subacute bacterial endocarditis (Tilkian et al., 1987). An Hb reduced to 5 g/dL manifests clinically as cyanosis.

An RBC increase is seen in congenital heart disease, severe chronic obstructive pulmonary disease, and polycythemia vera. It is falsely high in extracellular fluid deficit (volume contraction) and falsely low with extracellular fluid excess (Pagana & Pagana, 1998). The production of RBCs is inhibited by a rise in circulating RBC levels and stimulated by anemia and hypoxemia. The RBC count represents the number of RBCs in 1 μL of whole blood.

Hematocrit. The Hct is the volume of packed RBCs found in 100 mL of blood. As an indirect measure of the RBC count, Hct increases and decreases with the RBC count. Normal ranges for Hct differ by sex and age group (Pagana & Pagana, 1998). Physical training is known to decrease the Hct level. Findings suggest that physical training may be of value in lowering blood viscosity in patients after MI (Suzuki et al., 1992).

Hemoglobin. The RBCs contain a complex protein compound called *hemoglobin* (Hb). Hb is the oxygen-carrying protein of the RBC and is an important component of the acid–base buffer system. Insufficient amounts of Hb place a strain on the cardiovascular system and may cause MI, angina, congestive heart failure (CHF), or stroke. There is a diurnal variation in Hb, which varies by as much as 1 g/dL between its peak at 8 AM and its nadir at 8 PM (Pagana & Pagana, 1998).

Corpuscular Indices. With the RBC count, the quantity of Hb, and the Hct, the characteristics of individual RBCs can be described in terms of cell size (mean corpuscular volume [MCV]), amount of Hb present in a single cell (mean corpuscular Hb [MCH]), and the proportion of each cell occupied by

Hb (mean corpuscular Hb concentration [MCHC]). The indices are calculated by these formulas (Widmann, 1983):

MCV = Hematocrit (as %) × 10 ÷ RBC count (millions per mm³)

MCH = Hemoglobin (as g/100 mL) × 10 ÷ RBC count

MCHC = Hemoglobin ÷ Hematocrit

White Blood Cell Count

The WBCs, or leukocytes, work to defend against foreign matter and cells in the body. There are five types of WBCs: neutrophils, eosinophils, basophils, monocytes, and lymphocytes. Neutrophils, the most numerous circulating WBCs, are responsible for phagocytosis and are stimulated by acute bacterial infections or trauma. When their production is significantly increased, immature forms (bands) are released in the blood. Eosinophils are able to phagocytize antigen–antibody complexes and are increased during allergic and parasitic conditions. Basophils (mast cells) are increased during the healing phase of infection or inflammation. Monocytes are capable of fighting bacteria in a way similar to neutrophils, as well as removing debris and microorganisms from the blood. Lymphocytes play a role in chronic or viral infections. T lymphocytes, which mature in the thymus, are responsible for cellular-type immune reactions. B lymphocytes, which mature in the bone marrow, play a major role in humoral immunity (antibody production) (Kee, 1998, 1999; Pagana & Pagana, 1998).

Elevated WBC counts in the patient with cardiac disease may be caused by MI, bacterial endocarditis, or Dressler syndrome. After MI, the elevation may be a result of the body's normal response to stress. On approximately the fourth day after an acute MI, WBCs may be elevated. Leukocytosis occurs as the infarcted site is invaded by leukocytes and macrophages that engulf and phagocytose necrotic tissue.

Although an elevated temperature after MI may be expected, an elevated WBC count should always suggest the possibility of concomitant infection. A urinary or respiratory tract infection or an infection secondary to an invasive procedure is a possibility during an extended illness. In this case, the presence of band cells (immature neutrophils), coupled with leukocytosis, suggests the bone marrow is putting out more cells in response to stress or infection. An elevated WBC count has also been associated with CHD. WBC counts were obtained from participants in the Framingham, Massachusetts offspring study. An increase in WBC count in men was related to the development of cardiovascular disease (Kannel et al., 1992).

Drugs that may cause an increase in WBCs include aspirin, procainamide, allopurinol, heparin, digoxin, and epinephrine. WBCs have a diurnal variation, with counts generally lower in the morning than in the afternoon (Kee, 1999).

White Cell Differential. The differential count is a descriptive list of the types of WBCs. The differential for each of the five leukocyte types is usually expressed as a percentage of the total leukocyte count; the total should add up to 100 (see Table 14-6).

Cell Morphology

Occasionally, a CBC includes a description of any abnormal cell types. Immature RBCs (reticulocytes) may be noted. The presence of these cells is a clue that there may be increased demands on RBC production or that cell function may be impaired. Normoblasts appear in blood after severe stress, such as massive hemorrhage or hemolysis, or cardiac arrest. Megaloblasts can be seen in a severe vitamin B$_{12}$ or folate deficiency. Fragmented RBCs may suggest disseminated intravascular coagulopathy (DIC) (Abbey, 1983) and are also seen in people with prosthetic valves. Microcytes may indicate a nutritional iron-deficiency anemia. Target cells are seen in liver disease. The appearance of nucleated RBCs and immature WBCs (myelocytes) may indicate severely depressed bone marrow activity, requiring measures to protect the patient from infection. If the neutrophil count is less than 1,000 cells/mm³, then there is a slight risk of infection; if the count is less than 500 cells/mm³, then infection is frequent (Finch, 1983).

Erythrocyte Sedimentation Rate

The erythrocyte sedimentation rate (ESR) measures the speed at which anticoagulated erythrocytes settle in a long, narrow tube. The speed depends on the size of the clumps into which the cells aggregate in the presence of blood fibrinogen. The ESR is a nonspecific indicator of inflammatory disease. It may be elevated in MI and bacterial endocarditis; it is usually low in heart failure (Kee, 1999; McFarland & Grant, 1994). Although many factors affect the ESR and it is considered a test with neither disease nor organ specificity, it is a useful test in differentiating the pain of pericarditis and Dressler syndrome from anginal pain. The degree of increase of the ESR does not correlate with severity or prognosis (Wallach, 1992).

Complete Blood Count After Cardiac Surgery

The Hb and Hct levels are monitored after cardiac surgery to evaluate blood loss. Immediately after cardiac surgery, there are rapid shifts in extracellular fluid volume status because of the hemodilutional effects of cardiopulmonary bypass and the rewarming that follows induced hypothermia. This fluid shift may be reflected in a reduced Hb or Hct level. Frequent monitoring of the WBC count helps identify any leukocytosis and infection. Cardiopulmonary bypass results in a period of reduced phagocytic activity that renders the patient more at risk for infection (Silva et al., 1974).

Laboratory Measurement of Complete Blood Cell Values

The RBC and WBC counts are performed by an automated counter that directly measures all parameters, including Hct, corpuscular indices, and platelets. The precision of the Hct analysis is ±2 points. Consequently, a change in measurement by as much as 4 points may not indicate a change in the true Hct.

Activity and change in position may increase Hct and Hb levels; Hb may be higher by 8% in the morning than in the evening (Dacie & Lewis, 1984). A minimum of 2 mL of blood is required for assay. The usual precautions should be taken to avoid hemolysis and ensure accuracy. The specimen should be rapidly transported to the laboratory to avoid changes in distribution of the cells within the plasma. Red blood cell tests can be performed using capillary blood, but massage of the fingertip or earlobe can lead to cell destruction and alter the sample. If difficulty is encountered in locating a vein, then the tourniquet should be removed long enough to allow restoration of circulation to avoid a hemoconcentrated sample (Treseler, 1988). In one study, application of a tourniquet for 3 minutes led to an increase of 3.9 points in Hct; hemolysis was avoided when the tourniquet was applied for less than 1 minute (Masouredes, 1990). A blood smear should also be examined if there is an abnormality in one or more of the CBC parameters to evaluate the size, shape, and color of the RBCs, WBCs, and platelets.

BLOOD CULTURES

Blood cultures are indicated when a fever of unknown origin is present. Blood cultures aid in identifying specific bacterial organisms in the blood (bacteremia), and when combined with antibiotic sensitivity tests can provide information to clinicians about which antibiotic works best against that particular species of bacteria. Policies differ with regard to the number and timing of cultures considered adequate for diagnosis; the policy and procedure of the institution should be followed. Regardless of the number of cultures recommended and the timing between them, collection of blood cultures requires meticulous technique to protect the specimen from contamination. Sampling should be performed while the temperature is still elevated and before treatment with antibiotics. Blood cultures may be obtained from a central intravenous catheter, but only if it is to determine if the bacterial contamination is from the intravenous line (Garza & Becan-McBride, 2002). The blood is drawn and placed into specialized culture media. The blood samples are cultured in the laboratory at 37°C. Preliminary results should be available within 24 hours, but final results may not be available for a week or more.

COAGULATION STUDIES

Drug-induced anticoagulation is a routine procedure in the cardiac care unit and requires close monitoring of blood coagulation mechanisms. Anticoagulation is used after thrombolytic therapy, during cardiac surgery, to prevent formation of venous thrombus associated with prolonged bed rest and hemostasis, to prevent formation of intracardiac thrombus, and in treatment for established thrombus and embolus (see Chapter 8 for a discussion of coagulation).

The prevention and treatment of blood coagulation are complex and involve a number of hemostatic functions that play roles in the body's homeostasis. Therapy involves interference with this homeostatic mechanism. An understanding of the laboratory tests used to evaluate the effectiveness of treatment is vital to prevent undesired outcomes of anticoagulation therapy. The normal ranges for the coagulation factors and the methods used depend on the laboratory. Typical reference ranges, however, are listed in Table 14-6.

Platelet Count

Platelets are elements of the blood that promote coagulation and are produced by the bone marrow. They contribute to blood clotting by clumping or sticking to rough surfaces and injured sites (Kee, 1999). The average life span of a platelet is 7 to 9 days.

Platelet counts are useful for monitoring the course of a disease or treatment. Thrombocytopenia (low platelet count) is a common cause of abnormal bleeding (Abbey, 1983). There is a serious risk of hemorrhage when the platelet count is less than $50,000/mm^3$ (Adams et al., 1996), and a spontaneous bleed may occur when platelets are less than $20,000/mm$ (Adams et al., 1996). Bleeding caused by thrombocytopenia is characterized by petechiae, bleeding from the gums or tongue, or epistaxis (Weiss, 1977). Thrombocytopenia may occur by several mechanisms: reduced platelet production, sequestration of platelets, accelerated platelet destruction, loss from hemorrhage, and dilution from massive blood transfusions that contain few platelets.

Specific conditions that may cause a decrease in platelets include hemorrhage, hypersplenism, leukemia, prosthetic heart valves, heparin-induced thrombocytopenia (HITS), disseminated intravascular coagulation (DIC), systemic lupus erythematosus, hemolytic anemia, and infection. Other situations may give rise to thrombocytopenia, including idiopathic thrombocytopenic purpura, systemic lupus erythematosus, chronic lymphocytic leukemia, and lymphoma (Abbey, 1983). Medications that decrease the platelet count include acetaminophen, aspirin, chemotherapy, histamine blocking agents, heparin, hydralazine, quinidine, and thiazide diuretics (Pagana & Pagana, 1998). Nonsteroidal anti-inflammatory drugs may cause a decrease in platelet aggregation (Gutierrez, 1999a). The concurrent use of heparin with antiplatelet agents increases the risk of bleeding. After a large number of blood transfusions (14 units or more), and occasionally after extracorporeal circulation, the platelet count is low (Masouredes, 1990).

Aspirin has been incorporated into the treatment plan after MI to prevent hypercoagulability caused by platelet aggregation. Antiplatelet agents (clopidogrel and ticlopidine) help prevent platelet aggregation by inhibiting fibrinogen binding and platelet–platelet interaction. Antiplatelet agents have been incorporated into many treatment plans to prevent arterial thrombus including after MI, PTCA/stent placement, cardiovascular surgery, and other vascular surgeries. Patients receiving antiplatelet drugs may have a normal platelet count but have increased bleeding because of the drug. The drug alters the platelets for the life of platelets; therefore, increased bleeding may be seen for 7 to 14 days after discontinuation of treatment (Gutierrez, 1999a). Glycoprotein IIb/IIIa receptor inhibitors are also used to decrease platelet aggregation in acute MI and after PTCA/stent placement patients. Patients who receive glycoprotein IIb/IIIa agents should be monitored for signs of bleeding and thrombocytopenia.

Increased amounts of platelets may be seen in malignant disorders, polycythemia vera, postsplenectomy syndrome, and rheumatoid arthritis (Pagana & Pagana, 1998). Platelet counts may also be increased in those who live at high altitudes or exercise strenuously.

Prothrombin Time

The prothrombin time (PT) is used to evaluate the extrinsic system and common pathway in the clotting mechanism. Specifically, it measures the activity of prothrombin, fibrinogen, and factors V, VII, and X. Prothrombin is synthesized by the liver. PT may be prolonged in heart failure, vitamin K deficiency, liver disease, bile duct obstruction, DIC, massive blood transfusion, salicylate intoxication, and alcohol use (Kee, 1998, 1999; Pagana & Pagana, 1998). Severe liver damage may prolong PT. Drugs that may prolong PT include some antibiotics, allopurinol, cimetidine, warfarin, heparin, quinidine, and aspirin (Kee, 1999). Decreased PT is seen in thrombophlebitis, MI, and pulmonary embolus. Medications that may decrease PT include digitalis preparations, diuretics, diphenhydramine, and metaproterenol (Kee, 1999).

The PT is used mainly for monitoring patients on warfarin (Coumadin). Warfarin inhibits vitamin K-dependent synthesis of clotting factors II, VII, IX, and X. Therapeutic prothrombin times are considered to be 1.5- to 2-times normal, or a 15% to 50% change in the normal value. If the PT is allowed to prolong greater than 2.5-times the control value, then there is a risk of bleeding (Kee, 1998).

The international normalized ratio (INR) has now been adopted for reporting PT. The INR is calculated from the observed PT ratio. The INR is equivalent to the PT ratio that would have been obtained if the patient's PT had been compared to a PT value obtained using the International Reference Preparation, a standard human brain thromboplastin prepared by the World Health Organization. With the INR, standardized PT results are available for physicians in different parts of the country and the world. These standardized results are independent of the reagents used and adjust for the type of instrument used (Ansell, 2001; Gutierrez, 1999a). The therapeutic INR in most situations ranges from 2.0 to 3.5. However, different ranges have been established for deep vein thrombosis prophylaxis (1.5 to 2.0), deep vein thrombosis (2.0 to 3.0), prevention of embolus in atrial fibrillation (2.0 to 3.0), pulmonary embolism (3.0 to 4.0), and prosthetic valve prophylaxis (2.5 to 3.5). The INR should not be used to initiate warfarin therapy; it should be used only once the patient is thought to be on a stable dose (Kee, 1999; Pagana & Pagana, 1998; Severson et al., 1997).

Partial Thromboplastin Time and Activated Partial Thromboplastin Time

The partial thromboplastin time (PTT) and activated partial thromboplastin time (aPTT) measure the intrinsic coagulation system and are used in assessing patients receiving unfractionated heparin. With low-molecular-weight heparin, neither PTT nor aPTT changes, so laboratory monitoring is not required (Huang & Shimamura, 1998; Turpie, 1998). The PTT measures deficiencies in all factors except factors VII and XIII, whereas the

aPTT measures all coagulation factors except platelet factor III, factor XIII, and factor VII (Abbey, 1983). The aPTT is measured by adding test reagents to PTT to shorten clotting time. When clotting time is shortened, minor clotting defects can be detected (Kee, 1999; Pagana & Pagana, 1998).

The therapeutic range for PTT and aPTT is maintained at 1.5- to 2.5-times the patient's baseline value. The PTT and aPTT is usually drawn 30 to 60 minutes before the patient's next dose of heparin. For PTT and aPTT results less than 50 seconds, an increase in the heparin dose should be considered. Conversely, a decrease in dose should be considered for PTT and aPTT values greater than 100 seconds (Pagana & Pagana, 1998).

The PTT and aPTT are prolonged in heparin administration, congenital clotting factor deficiencies, cirrhosis of the liver, vitamin K deficiency, and DIC. Antihistamines, ascorbic acid, chlorpromazine, and salicylates may also cause an increase.

Activated Coagulation Time

The activated coagulation time (ACT) is used during cardiac surgery and cardiac catheterization to monitor heparinization. The time it takes whole blood to clot reflects the activity of the intrinsic clotting mechanism (Treseler, 1988). During extracorporeal heparin therapy, the ACT is kept at four- to six-times the baseline value.

Tests to measure ACT are simple and easy to use at the bedside. The use of ACT rather than aPTT to monitor heparin therapy in patients with unstable angina or acute MI may result in much steadier levels of anticoagulation and prevent ischemic recurrences (Melandri et al., 1993).

Fibrinogen Level

Fibrinogen is a plasma protein synthesized by the liver (Kee, 1998). This test measures the conversion of fibrinogen to fibrin by thrombin (Treseler, 1988). Fibrinogen levels are elevated in acute infections, collagen disease, inflammatory diseases, and hepatitis. Decreased levels are seen in severe liver disease, DIC, leukemia, and obstetric complications. Thrombolytic therapy may also affect fibrinogen levels. Intracoronary and intravenous (IV) streptokinase therapies lower fibrinogen levels to less than 100 mg/dL. Urokinase therapy, however, minimally decreases fibrinogen, whereas tissue plasminogen activator therapy does not reduce fibrinogen (Sipperly, 1985). Low fibrinogen levels (<100 mg/dL) may occur as a result of cardiac surgery, DIC, or other fibrinolytic disorders (Abbey, 1983). The most common use of the test is in differentiating these clinical conditions from liver disease, in which the fibrinogen level is rarely less than 100 mg/dL.

Thrombin Time

The time required for a thrombin solution to clot plasma is measured with the thrombin time (Abbey, 1983). Thrombin is the factor that directly converts fibrinogen to fibrin, and the formation of thrombin is the common pathway for both the intrinsic and extrinsic coagulation systems. The thrombin time moderates the thrombin–fibrinogen reaction and adequate formation of a fibrin clot (Treseler, 1988). Thrombin time is elevated by liver disorders, systemic lupus erythematosus, uremia, and DIC. The thrombin time may be used after fibrinolytic enzyme therapy (streptokinase) to assess the extent of hypofibrinogenemia. The thrombin time is prolonged after streptokinase therapy if antibody has not combined with the streptokinase antigen. In the rare event that thrombin time is not elevated after streptokinase infusion, the patient is presumed to have a large amount of streptococcal antibody, which renders streptokinase therapy ineffective. The thrombin time is prolonged with the use of urokinase and heparin and is too sensitive to heparin to monitor heparin therapy. Heparin contamination of specimens is common. The PTT, PT, and thrombin time should be measured concurrently because the thrombin time is too nonspecific to be used alone to assess anticoagulation therapy.

Protein C and Protein S

Protein C, with cofactor protein S, is a natural anticoagulant protein whose function is to degrade activated factor V and VIII. Deficiency in either protein C or S can lead to a hypercoagulable state that may cause venous thrombosis. For protein C to be activated, it needs to interact with the thrombin–thrombomodulin complex on the surface of endothelial cells. Protein C is vitamin K-dependent and indirectly promotes fibrinolysis. Hereditary protein C deficiency accounts for approximately 3% to 9 % of patients with venous thrombosis. Hereditary protein S deficiency accounts for 2% to 7% of patients with venous thrombosis (Jacobs & DeMott, 2001).

Acquired conditions that cause protein C or protein S deficiency include liver disease, vitamin K deficiency or warfarin use, consumption of protein C or protein S from thrombosis, DIC, or surgery. Protein S deficiency may also be acquired by use of estrogen, including oral contraceptives or estrogen replacement therapy, or pregnancy. Protein S may also be decreased in nephrotic syndrome, HIV infection, or varicella infection. A rapid decrease in protein C or protein S can be caused by initiating warfarin therapy without first reducing other coagulation factors with heparin. This rapid decrease in protein C or protein S can cause hypercoagulability and cause warfarin-induced skin necrosis. Warfarin-induced skin necrosis causes thrombosis of skin vessels that can lead to infarction and necrosis. Treatment requires discontinuation of warfarin and vitamin K administration (Jacobs & DeMott, 2001).

Warfarin should be discontinued for at least 10 days before testing for protein C or protein S. Reference range for protein C or protein S is reported as a percentage of the amount expected in normal plasma. The reference range is approximately 70% to 140% (Jacobs & DeMott, 2001).

Coagulation Studies After Cardiac Surgery

The nature of cardiac surgery calls for close attention to coagulation factors. Prolonged extracorporeal circulation, heparinization during surgery, and coagulopathies can contribute to bleeding after surgery. Tests commonly performed immediately after surgery are platelet count, fibrinogen level, PT, and PTT (Markmann & Wallace, 1985). After valve replacement or revascularization, commonly administered medications include heparin therapy, oral anticoagulant therapy, and antiplatelet agents (low-dose salicylates, clopidogrel, and ticlopidine). Heparin is administered either through infusion or subcutaneously during the early postoperative period; the PTT is considered the best index of unfractionated heparin activity. Low-molecular-weight heparin is also commonly administered subcutaneously in the postoperative period instead of unfractionated heparin, because it does not require PTT monitoring. The PT is monitored for patients receiving warfarin during and after hospital discharge because the risk for bleeding accompanies long-term anticoagulation therapy (Ansell, 2001; Gutierrez, 1999a).

Laboratory Measurement of Coagulation Studies

Blood specimens for coagulation studies should be placed in collection tubes prepared specifically for this purpose. The laboratory should be contacted for specifics such as type of collection tube and amount of blood required. For most studies, an exact amount of blood is required: exactly 1 mL for ACT and exactly 4.5 mL for thrombin, PT, and PTT, protein C, and protein S. Care must be taken after the specimen is withdrawn to prevent bleeding from a venipuncture site; pressure should be maintained over the site for a minimum of 3 to 5 minutes (Calam, 1977). Rapid transportation of the specimen to the laboratory is essential because analysis should be performed immediately.

A number of factors may contribute to the variability of coagulation studies. The timing of the determination of the test is critical, and the maximum effect of the anticoagulant must be considered. Results of coagulation studies require careful assessment because they are influenced by diet, medications (including over-the-counter medications), alcohol consumption, and physical activity. Circadian variations in the response of the coagulation may influence therapeutic response to anticoagulants (Becker & Corrao, 1989). Other unknown factors affect laboratory coagulation studies. Consequently, dose adjustments of anticoagulants should be followed-up by repeated testing.

Nursing Considerations After Hematologic Studies

Abnormal bleeding, anemias, the inflammatory response, and infection indicate several nursing diagnoses, including decreased cardiac output, fluid volume deficit, altered tissue perfusion, and impaired tissue integrity. The cardiac nurse should be aware of any actual or potential problems related to hematologic abnormalities. Knowledge of normal values, as well as those factors that alter function of the cells or homeostatic mechanisms, is required for recognition of deviations from normal. Attention to the results is important; communication to the physician, if necessary, should be based on an understanding of the ramifications of an altered value. Intervention should be based on a physiologic conceptualization of the mechanisms involved in altered hematologic values. Attention to the hematologic values alone, however, should never become the focus of nursing intervention. The ability of the patient to tolerate the condition should be assessed from a daily living status that incorporates resources as well as the demands of the illness (Carnevali, 1983).

ARTERIAL BLOOD GASES

Arterial blood gases are frequently assessed in the patient with cardiac disease. Tissue oxygenation, carbon dioxide removal, and acid–base status are analyzed through the assay of arterial blood gases. Arterial blood gas results guide treatment decisions in ventilated patients and critically ill, nonventilated patients. They are also drawn to establish a preoperative baseline (Pagana & Pagana, 1998). A complete discussion of these parameters can be found in Chapter 10. Knowledge of the normal blood gas values and the meaning of deviation from normal are essential to treatment decisions.

The arterial oxygen saturation (SaO_2) and the mixed venous oxygen saturation (SvO_2) reflect the relationship between oxygen supply and demand and the extent of overall tissue use of O_2. Continuous monitoring of SaO_2 (oxygen supply) can be achieved through pulse oximetry; laboratory analysis, however, is useful in distinguishing the SaO_2 at PaO_2 levels above 65 mm Hg (Luce et al., 1984). A fiberoptic pulmonary artery catheter is capable of evaluating SvO_2 levels continuously. This information is useful in determining the ideal mode of respiratory intervention, the effect of nursing care on tissue O_2 demands, physiologic alterations requiring increased supply of O_2, and the reflection of physiologic changes on cardiac output (White, 1985). Calibration of the SvO_2 catheter oximeter should be performed every 24 hours by laboratory co-oximeter saturation analysis. Table 14-6 provides normal values for SaO_2 and SvO_2.

BLOOD CHEMISTRIES

The body's homeostatic mechanisms are responsible for a stable internal environment. The chemical regulation of cellular and plasma metabolites is among the most precise mechanisms in the body. During periods of critical illness, these mechanisms may be inadequate or dramatically altered. The functional alterations that result from altered values are sometimes life threatening. An awareness of the factors affecting blood chemistry homeostasis, as well as the consequences of elevated or decreased levels, aids the nurse in making appropriate patient care decisions.

Some blood chemistry tests are performed routinely on admission to the hospital to establish the patient's baseline. Other tests are performed frequently during the day and may indicate the need for intervention in the form of altered therapy and treatment modalities. "Normal" or reference values may differ between laboratories or among populations. Typical reference ranges for selected blood chemistry values can be found in Table 14-6.

Serum Electrolytes

Sodium. Sodium is the major cation in the extracellular space. It has several major functions: maintenance of osmotic pressure, regulation of acid–base balance (by combining with chloride or bicarbonate ions), and transmission of nerve impulses by the sodium pump (Chernecky & Berger, 1997; Pagana & Pagana, 1998; Treseler, 1988). Sodium balance is regulated by aldosterone, atrial natriuretic hormone, and antidiuretic hormone (ADH). Aldosterone causes sodium conservation (and water retention) by stimulating the kidneys to reabsorb sodium. Aldosterone is secreted in response to low extracellular sodium levels, an increase in intracellular potassium, low blood volume or cardiac output, and physical or emotional stress (McFarland & Grant, 1994; Pagana & Pagana, 1998). When serum sodium levels are too high, atrial natriuretic hormone is secreted from the atrium and acts as an antagonist to renin and aldosterone (Kee, 1999). ADH, secreted by the posterior pituitary gland, controls serum sodium by regulation of the amount of intracellular fluid reabsorbed at the distal tubules (McFarland & Grant, 1994; Pagana & Pagana, 1998).

Potassium. Potassium is the major intracellular cation, in concentrations of approximately 150 mEq/L. It is regulated in a very strict range in the extracellular fluid. Potassium plays a crucial role in initiating and sustaining cardiac and skeletal muscle contraction. It is also important for acid–base balance and maintenance of oncotic pressure.

Maintenance of potassium within the normal range is crucial in the care of a patient with cardiac disease. Failure to do so results in dangerous sequelae for the patient. In general, potassium levels in patients with cardiac disease are maintained above 4.0 mEq/L. Special care should be taken in patients with cardiac disease receiving potassium-sparing diuretics or angiotensin-converting enzyme inhibitors, especially in light of decreased renal blood flow. Potassium levels are falsely elevated by analysis of hemolyzed specimens. Prolonged use of a tourniquet, having the patient clench and unclench a fist before blood draw, or delayed processing of the specimen all may cause hemolysis (Rose, 1984; Wallach, 1992).

Chloride. Chloride is the major extracellular anion. It helps to maintain electrical neutrality and acts as an acid–base buffer. The rise and fall of chloride levels follows sodium and bicarbonate shifts. When carbon dioxide increases, chloride shifts to the intracellular space as bicarbonate goes extracellular. Along with sodium, chloride also helps to maintain osmotic pressure. Found primarily in hydrochloric acid in stomach secretions, chloride also provides the acid medium for digestion and enzyme activation (Kee, 1999; McFarland & Grant, 1994; Pagana & Pagana, 1998).

Calcium. Calcium is found mainly in the bones and teeth, with only approximately 10% found in the blood (McFarland & Grant, 1994). Calcium is essential for the formation of bones and for blood coagulation. Calcium ions affect neuromuscular excitability and cellular and capillary permeability (Widmann, 1983). It is essential for nerve transmission and cardiac and skeletal muscle contraction. Calcium also contributes to anion–cation balance. Calcium can be found ionized (free) in the serum or bound to serum albumin. The ionized calcium, which is approximately one-half the total calcium, is the fraction important to cardiac and neuromuscular excitability (Pagana & Pagana, 1998). In acidosis, more calcium appears in the ionized form; in alkalotic environments, most of the calcium remains protein-bound (Kee, 1999).

Calcium levels in the blood follow a diurnal variation, with the lowest values occurring in the early morning and highest values occurring during the mid-evening (Chernecky & Berger, 1997). Ionized calcium is difficult to measure, so total calcium is reported in most hospitals. In some situations, the measured calcium level may be low, but by estimating the amount bound to protein, the ionized calcium may be found to be normal. The formula for the computation of ionized calcium is shown in Table 14-8. Decreased serum sodium (<120 mEq/L) increases protein-bound calcium and consequently increases the total calcium; the opposite is true of increased serum sodium (Wallach, 1992).

Magnesium. Magnesium is essential for more than 300 enzymatic activities involving lipid, carbohydrate, and protein metabolism. It is the second most predominant intracellular cation (Ryan et al., 1999). Most of the body's magnesium is stored in the bones in an insoluble state; one-third is bound to protein and approximately 1% is found in the serum. Because of its importance in phosphorylation of ATP, magnesium is seen as a critical component of almost all metabolic processes (Pagana & Pagana, 1998). Its importance in the care of patients with cardiac disease stems from its role in neuromuscular regulation.

Ventricular arrhythmias after MI have been associated with magnesium deficiency. Routine prophylactic use of magnesium sulfate for patients with myocardial infarction is no longer recommended by the American Heart Association. Magnesium sulfate 1 to 2 grams IV should be considered in ventricular fibrillation or ventricular tachycardia for patients with alcoholism or malnutrition with suspected low levels of magnesium (hypomagnesemia). It is recommended that magnesium sulfate should be administered to patients with ventricular fibrillation or ventricular tachycardia with a torsades de pointes pattern, although there are no randomized controlled trials that have shown its efficacy (American Heart Association, 2001).

Hypomagnesemia may precipitate cardiac arrhythmias, including atrial fibrillation, because of enhanced myocardium excitability. Hypomagnesemia is very common after cardiovascular surgery and has been found to be an independent risk factor for atrial fibrillation after cardiac surgery (Zaman et al., 1997), most likely caused by hemodilution, elevated epinephrine levels, increased loss through the urine, or the use of diuretics (Solomon et al., 2000). Atrial fibrillation is a common complication after cardiovascular surgery, occurring in approximately 20% to 40% of cases. The effectiveness of supplemental magnesium sulfate administration in preventing atrial fibrillation after cardiovascular surgery is controversial. Research on the administration of magnesium sulfate before and/or after cardiovascular surgery has shown mixed results. Neither Solomon and colleagues (2000) nor Kaplan and coinvestigators (2003) found that magnesium sulfate and propranolol administration reduced the incidence of atrial fibrillation

after CABG surgery. By contrast, Toraman and colleagues (2001) found a significant decrease in the incidence of atrial fibrillation with the use magnesium sulfate and Forlani and coinvestigators (2002) found an even greater decrease in the incidence of atrial fibrillation when magnesium sulfate was used in combination with sotalol. Therefore, research seems to indicate that use of magnesium sulfate alone may not decrease the incidence of atrial fibrillation after CABG surgery, but the use of beta-blockers and magnesium sulfate may be effective.

Hypermagnesemia results in decreased neuromuscular conduction, and consequent slowing of conduction in the heart. Magnesium levels should be monitored carefully in patients using digitalis preparations. Low magnesium levels are known to enhance the effect of digitalis, leading to toxicity (Kee, 1998, 1999; McFarland & Grant, 1994; Pagana & Pagana, 1998; Tilkian et al., 1995).

Carbon Dioxide. Measurement of carbon dioxide assists the clinician in evaluation of electrolyte status and acid–base balance. Because approximately 80% of carbon dioxide is found as bicarbonate, it is a good reflection of the bicarbonate level. The carbon dioxide level should not be confused with the PCO_2 obtained from blood gas readings.

Anion Gap. The anion gap measures the normal balance between positive and negative electrolytes in the serum. It describes the relationship between serum sodium (a cation) and bicarbonate and chloride (anions). A normal anion gap is 12 mEq/L. A value greater than 12 mEq/L is considered abnormal. This test is useful in determining whether an acid–base imbalance is caused by an increase in organic acid (increased lactic acid or ketoacids, or ingestion of acid such as salicylic acid). In this case, the anion gap increases. With mineral acid problems (decreased bicarbonate or increased hydrochloric acid), the anion gap is normal. A formula for computation of the anion gap is given in Table 14-8.

Serum Osmolality

Serum osmolality reflects the osmotic property of the blood. It is an important parameter in determining whether water excess or deficit exists. Either of these problems can present in the cardiac care unit, where fluid management is often a problem. The most dramatic alterations in osmolality can be seen with inappropriate ADH secretion or failure of ADH secretion in conditions characterized by low blood volume (see Chapter 9). Normal serum osmolality is 280 to 300 mOsm/kg. The osmolality can be measured in the laboratory or calculated with a simple formula (see Table 14-8.)

Serum Electrolytes After Cardiac Surgery

Fluid volume shifts and changes in electrolytes and serum osmolality are common after cardiac surgery. The examination of serum electrolytes at least every 3 to 4 hours during the first 24 hours after surgery has been recommended. Potassium changes may be rapid, sodium may be increased, total calcium and magnesium may be decreased, and total circulating volume may be increased. The hemodilutional effects of cardiopulmonary bypass are responsible for these changes as well as changes in renal function that, in turn, may affect fluid volume and electrolyte status (Markmann & Wallace, 1985). During and after cardiac surgery, changes in plasma potassium concentration may develop (Lim et al., 1983; Schwartz & Geer, 1985). There appears to be a decrease in potassium during hypothermia and an increase during rewarming, which has been attributed to washout of ischemic areas or to a direct effect of temperature on the transmembrane distribution of potassium (Lim et al., 1983). Sodium, chloride, calcium, and magnesium have not shown changes. However, serum sodium does decrease after surgery if large amounts of glucose-containing fluids have been infused. In this situation, glucose is metabolized slowly and draws fluid from the cells by its osmotic effect. Consequently, the sodium is diluted (Miyazawa et al., 1985).

Errors in measurement can be costly to the patient in terms of safety, health status, and cost-effective practice. Because changes in potassium are closely watched and treatment is initiated when the level falls within a very narrow range, the chances for error are great. It has been suggested that potassium replacement during rewarming be handled cautiously (Lim et al., 1983).

SELECTED CHEMISTRIES

Alkaline Phosphatase

Alkaline phosphatase is an enzyme released in liver and bone disease. An increased serum level suggests an abnormality in the liver or bones but can be associated with chronic therapeutic use of anticonvulsant drugs such as phenobarbital or phenytoin (Wallach, 1992). In addition, lipid-lowering agents such as bile acid resins, HMG-CoA reductase inhibitors (statins), and nicotinic acid can alter alkaline phosphatase and other liver tests. Alkaline phosphatase along with other liver enzymes (i.e., alanine aminotransferase [ALT], aspartate aminotransferase [AST]) is typically measured before initiation of lipid-lowering therapy, every 4 to 6 weeks at the start of therapy, every 6 to 12 weeks for the first year of therapy, and then every 6 months throughout treatment (Gutierrez, 1999b).

Alanine Aminotransferase

Alanine aminotransferase (ALT), formerly known as serum glutamic-pyruvic transaminase (SGPT) is found predominately in liver tissue but is also present in kidney, heart, and skeletal muscle tissue. This hepatocellular enzyme is released into the bloodstream when there is injury or disease affecting liver parenchyma, making ALT a specific and sensitive laboratory test. In hepatocellular disease other than viral hepatitis, the ALT-to-AST ratio is less than 1. In viral hepatitis, the ratio is greater than 1 (Pagana & Pagana, 2002).

ALT may be elevated with hepatitis, hepatic necrosis, hepatic ischemia, cholestasis, hepatic tumor, hepatotoxic drugs, obstructive jaundice, severe burns, myositis, pancreatitis, infectious mononucleosis, and shock (Pagana & Pagana, 2002). Drugs that may increase ALT levels include acetaminophen, allopurinol, ampillicin, cephalosporins, chlordiazepoxide, chlorpropamide, clofibrate, codeine, nicotinic acid, nonsteroidal antiinflammatory drugs, oral contraceptives, phenytoin, procainamide, propranolol, salicylates, and verapamil (Gutierrez, 1999b; Pagana & Pagana, 2002). The reference range for normal ALT is listed in Table 14-6.

Aspartate Aminotransferase

Aspartate aminotransferase (AST), formerly known as serum glutamic-oxaloacetic transaminase (SGOT or GOT), is located in the cell cytoplasm and in the mitochondria, where it catalyzes amino acid activity (Halsted, 1976). This enzyme, although not specific to myocardial tissue, was the first to be used extensively to confirm an MI (LaDue et al., 1954). The enzyme is widely distributed, with high concentrations in the liver, skeletal muscle, kidney, red blood cells, and myocardium (Halsted, 1976). It is found in lesser amounts in the lungs, pancreas, and brain (Kee, 1998; McFarland & Grant, 1994; Treseler, 1988). The presence of AST in so many organ systems reduces its specificity for MI (Lott and Stang, 1989). With its reduced specificity and newer, more specific and sensitive tests, AST is no longer used to diagnosis MI. AST is now used to evaluate, diagnose, and monitor hepatocellular diseases.

AST may be elevated with cardiac surgery, cardiac catheterization and angioplasty (Pagana & Pagana, 1998), severe angina, acute pulmonary embolus (Kee, 1998), renal infarction (Chernecky & Berger, 1997), acute pancreatitis, musculoskeletal diseases, trauma, and strenuous exercise. In alcoholic hepatitis, AST is usually elevated but rarely greater than 300 u/L, but AST is almost invariably twice as high as ALT (Koff, 2001). Drugs that may increase AST levels include antihypertensives, digitalis preparations, salicylates, verapamil (Kee, 1998; Pagana & Pagana, 1998), theophylline (McFarland & Grant, 1994), and lipid-lowering agents such as bile acid resins, HMG-CoA reductase inhibitors (statins), and nicotinic acid (niacin) (Gutierrez, 1999b). False elevations are seen in pyridoxine deficiency (beriberi, pregnancy), uremia, or diabetic ketoacidosis. Levels are slightly increased in the elderly (Kee, 1999). In chronic conditions, such as severe longstanding liver disease, the elevation is usually persistent (Pagana & Pagana, 1998). The reference range for normal AST is listed in Table 14-6.

Bilirubin

Bilirubin is a product of Hb breakdown and is removed from the body by the liver. Elevated direct bilirubin is the result of obstructive jaundice caused by extrahepatic (stones or tumor) or intrahepatic (damaged liver cells) conditions. Increases in indirect bilirubin occur with hepatocellular dysfunction or an increase in RBC destruction (e.g., transfusion reaction or hemolytic anemia). Care should be taken not to hemolyze the sample. The sample should also be protected from bright light, because bilirubin levels are reduced after 1 hour of such exposure (Chernecky & Berger, 1997; Kee, 1998, 1999; Pagana & Pagana, 1998).

Catecholamines

Epinephrine and norepinephrine are elevated in pheochromocytoma, a tumor of the adrenal medulla. Pheochromocytoma is a cause of high blood pressure.

Creatinine

Creatinine is a waste product formed during muscle protein metabolism. Serum creatinine is a reflection of the excretory function of the kidney. It is evaluated in conjunction with blood urea nitrogen (BUN), but is a more sensitive indicator of renal function. People with large muscle mass have higher serum creatinine levels than do those with less muscle, such as the elderly, amputees, and patients with muscle disease (Kee, 1998, 1999; McFarland & Grant, 1994; Pagana & Pagana, 1998; Treseler, 1988).

Glucose

Glucose is elevated whenever endogenous epinephrine is mobilized, such as in chronic renal failure, acute pancreatitis, acute MI, CHF, extensive surgery, and infections. Mild hyperglycemia can be expected whenever the patient is under stress. Diabetes mellitus is frequently the cause of marked hyperglycemia. MI may precipitate diabetes in a person with latent diabetes (Wallach, 1992). Ideally, blood specimens for glucose determination should be drawn when the patient is fasting (see Chapter 43).

Glycated Hemoglobin or HbA₁c

Glycated hemoglobin (GHb), also referred to as glycohemoglobin, glycosylated hemoglobin, HbA1c, or HbA_1, are terms used to describe a series of stable minor Hb components formed slowly and nonenzymatically from Hb and glucose (American Diabetes Association, 2003b). The rate at which glycated hemoglobin is formed is proportional to the concentration of blood glucose (Rohlfing et al., 2002). Because RBCs survive an average of 120 days, the measurement of glycated hemoglobin provides an index of a person's average blood glucose concentration during a 2- to 3-month period (Pagana & Pagana, 2002).

Glycated hemoglobin comprises a chemically heterogeneous group of substances formed by the reaction between sugars and hemoglobin. In adults, approximately 98% of the Hb in the RBC is hemoglobin A. Approximately 7% of hemoglobin A consists of a type called HbA1 that can combine strongly with glucose in a process called "glycosylation." Once glycosylation occurs, it is not easily reversible. HbA1c is one of three components of HbA_1 and combines most strongly with glucose (Pagana & Pagana, 2002). HbA1c is a specific form of glycated hemoglobin that has become the most accurate laboratory blood test in assessing long-term glycemic control in diabetic subjects (Jacobs & DeMott, 2001).

Multiple laboratory methods are used to measure the many components of GHb. Some assays measure all GHb components in a sample, whereas other assays measure only one or two components. International efforts are being made to standardize the measurement of GHb, and now most assays measure HbA1c or are calibrated to produce a result equivalent to that measurement (Jacobs & DeMott, 2001). The American Diabetes Association (2003) recommends that laboratories use only methods certified as traceable to the Diabetes Control and Complications Trial (DCCT) reference method. Regardless of the assay method type and specific analyte qualified, all results should be reported as "% HbA1c" or "% HbA1c equivalents."

The advantage of testing HbA1c over plasma glucose testing for long-term diabetes mellitus management is that the sample can be drawn at any time because it is not affected by short-term variations (e.g., food intake, exercise, stress, hypoglycemic agents). HbA1c testing is beneficial for evaluating the success and patient compliance of diabetic treatment, determining the duration of hyperglycemia in patients with newly diagnosed diabetes mellitus, individualizing diabetic control regimens, evaluating the diabetic glucose levels that change significantly day to day, and, in the hospital, differentiating short-term hyperglycemia in patients who do not have diabetes mellitus (e.g., recent stress from illness or MI) from those who do have diabetes mellitus (in which the glucose has been persistently elevated) (Pagana & Pagana, 2002). In nondiabetic patients, increased levels of HbA1c may be seen with Cushing syndrome, pheochromocytoma, corticosteroid therapy, and acromegaly; HbA1c levels may be decreased in patients with hemolytic anemias, chronic blood loss, and chronic renal failure (Pagana & Pagana, 2002).

Prospective, randomized, clinical trials such as the DCCT and the U.K. Prospective Diabetes Study (UKPDS) have shown that treatment regimens that reduced average HbA1c to approximately 7% (approximately 1% above the upper limits of normal) was associated with fewer long-term microvascular complications including rates of retinopathy, nephropathy, and neuropathy (The Diabetes Control and Complications Trial Research Group, 1993; UK Prospective Diabetes Study Group, 1998). However, in these trials, intensive control was found to increase the risk of severe hypoglycemia and weight gain. The reference range for HbA_{1c} is listed in Table 14-6.

Rohlfing and researchers (2002) analyzed data from the DCCT to determine the relationship between HbA1c and plasma glucose levels in patients with type 1 diabetes mellitus. Approximate levels of plasma glucose and corresponding HbA1c levels are shown in Table 14-10. Guidelines from the American Diabetes Association (2003a) recommend that HbA1c testing be performed at least two times per year in patients who are meeting treatment goals (and who have stable glycemic control) and quarterly in patients whose therapy has changed or who are not meeting glycemic goals (see Chapter 43).

Glycated Serum Protein (GSP)

In situations in which the HbA1c test cannot be measured or may not be useful (e.g., hemolytic anemias), GSP may be of value in the assessment of diabetic control. Human serum albumin has a turnover rate much shorter than erythrocytes (half life 14–20 days vs. a lifespan of 120 days); therefore, the degree of glycation of serum proteins (mostly albumin) provides

Table 14–10 ■ CORRESPONDENCE BETWEEN HBA1C LEVEL AND MEAN PLASMA GLUCOSE LEVELS

HbA1c %	Mean Plasma Glucose	
	mg/dL	mmol/L
6	135	7.5
7	170	9.5
8	205	11.5
9	240	13.5
10	275	15.5
11	310	17.5
12	345	19.5

From Rohlfing, C. L. et al. (2002). Defining the relationship between plasma glucose and HbA1c: Analysis of glucose profiles and HbA1c in the diabetes control and complications trial. *Diabetes Care, 25*, 276.

an index of glycemic control over a shorter period of time (1–2 weeks) than HbA1c. Measurements of total GSP correlate well with HbA1c. Values for GSP vary with changes in the synthesis or clearance of serum proteins that can occur with acute systemic illness or with liver disease. GSP assays must be performed on a monthly basis to gather the same information as measured by the HbA1c test. Unlike the HbA1c test, GSP has not yet been shown to be related to the risk of the development or progression of chronic complications of diabetes mellitus (American Diabetes Association, 2003b).

Lactate Dehydrogenase

Lactate dehydrogenase is an enzyme that catalyzes the reversible conversion of lactate to pyruvate, providing ATP for energy during periods of anaerobic metabolism (Ravel, 1984; Treseler, 1988). LDH is present in nearly all metabolizing cells and is released during tissue injury (McFarland & Grant, 1994). LDH is widely distributed in the body. It can be found in skeletal muscle, red blood cells, kidney, liver, pancreas, lungs, and brain (Galen, 1981; Pagana & Pagana, 1998; Ravel, 1984). Because of its presence in multiple organs throughout the body, evaluation of LDH is used to help establish many diagnoses. LDH has become obsolete in its use as a diagnostic aid in MI because of the more specific and sensitive troponin markers. Drugs that may cause an elevated LDH include clofibrate, codeine, meperidine, morphine, procainamide (McFarland & Grant, 1994), and lipid-lowering agents such as HMG-CoA reductase inhibitors (statins) and nicotinic acid (Gutierrez, 1999b).

Five main fractions (isoenzymes) of LDH are available for assay. LDH-1 is found in the heart, kidney, and red blood cells and is the fraction observed after MI. Lactate dehydrogenase isoenzymes are best analyzed by electrophoresis. The quality of the enzyme samples and the handling in the laboratory determines whether valid results are obtained. Because of the amount of LDH in red blood cells, hemolyzed specimens may not be used for analysis (Dufour, 1998; Kee, 1999; McFarland & Grant, 1994). A minimum of 2 mL of blood is required for assay (Halsted, 1976). The serum can be stored at room temperature for up to 48 hours if it cannot be analyzed for LDH immediately. However, if LDH isoenzyme analysis is desired, the sample should be stored at 25°C and analyzed within 24 hours. The normal reference range for LDH is listed in Table 14-6.

Protein

Total protein measurement includes albumin (53%) and globulin (15% α, 12% β, and 20% γ). These protein components can be quantified with the use of protein electrophoresis. Albumin (4 to 5.5 g/dL) contributes to the balance of osmotic pressure between blood and tissues. Globulins (2 to 3 g/dL) influence osmotic pressure and include the immunoglobulins (antibodies). Because albumin is produced in the liver, a low serum albumin level is seen in liver disease. Low-serum albumin also reflects poor nutritional status, and the finding should prompt a complete nutritional assessment. The half-life of albumin is 18 days. If albumin is reduced, then edema results, because albumin accounts for 90% of the serum colloid osmotic pressure. Albumin is reduced in heart failure because of hypervolemic dilution (Wallach, 1992). The α- and β-globulins tend to decrease with abnormal liver function. The γ-globulins, the body's antibodies, increase with chronic disease (Widmann, 1983).

Urea Nitrogen

Urea nitrogen is the end product of protein metabolism. It is produced by the liver and excreted by the kidney. Increases in BUN are referred to as *azotemia*. Prerenal azotemia occurs whenever a disease or condition affects urea nitrogen before the kidneys are actually damaged or diseased. Postrenal azotemia is the result of any condition that affects BUN after it has cleared the kidney, such as in ureteral and urethral obstruction. BUN levels in the elderly may be slightly higher because the number of nephrons tends to decrease in the aging process. The BUN may be higher in hospitalized patients because of their increased catabolic state (Chernecky & Berger, 1997; Kee, 1998; McFarland & Grant, 1994; Pagana & Pagana, 1998; Treseler, 1988).

Uric Acid

Uric acid is the end product of purine metabolism and is increased in gout. Severe renal disease results in a high level of serum uric acid because excretion is reduced. Large doses of salicylates may interfere with accurate test results (Widmann, 1983).

Selected Chemistries After Cardiac Surgery

Blood test results related to renal function are of particular importance after cardiac surgery. Anesthesia and the length of time associated with cardiopulmonary circulatory bypass present potential hazards to the surgical patient. The anesthetic agent may produce hypotension and subsequent reduced renal perfusion and injury to the glomeruli. Cardiopulmonary bypass may damage cellular elements, which must be cleared from the system. Observation of the renal system parameters (BUN and creatinine) gives clues to kidney function.

Laboratory Blood Chemistry Analysis

The sampling of serum for chemistry measurement requires 1 mL of blood for most tests. If a multichannel, random-access analyzer is used for a defined battery of tests, 2.5 mL of serum is required. Hemolysis should be avoided for most tests. Delays before analysis lead to prolonged contact of cells with serum and should be avoided for most samples because some products can shift from the cells into the serum. Preservatives may allow for increased stability of samples for some laboratory values, which can increase the storage time up to 48 hours. Once the laboratory work is completed, the results should be communicated rapidly to a health team member if intervention is indicated.

Nursing Considerations After Blood Chemistry Measurement

Variations in blood chemistry can substantiate nursing diagnoses of intracellular fluid volume excess or deficit, altered (decreased) cardiac output related to extracellular volume deficit or electromechanical conduction disturbances, impaired gas exchange, impaired physical mobility, altered patterns of urinary elimination, activity intolerance, and altered tissue perfusion.

■ SERUM CONCENTRATION OF SELECTED DRUGS

Serum levels of cardiac drugs are frequently obtained to determine the effectiveness of drug therapy. Usual ranges of therapeutic and toxic serum concentrations of selected drugs are given in Table 14–11.

The serum concentrations must always be interpreted in the context of all the clinical data. For example, digitalis intoxication can occur within the usual range of therapeutic serum concentrations if the patient has hypokalemia, hypercalcemia, hypomagnesemia, acid–base imbalances, increased adrenergic tone, hypothyroidism, hypoxemia, or myocardial ischemia (Koch-Weser, 1972).

Digitoxin, phenytoin, and quinidine are chiefly bound to serum albumin. Bound fractions have no pharmacologic effect. The determination of a drug in the serum is usually the total amount bound and unbound. Usually, the amount of unbound drug is a fairly constant percentage of the total. In situations in which there is less albumin or when the drug-binding ability of the albumin is decreased (such as in uremia), or in which other drugs that are highly bound to protein are also given, the amount of drug bound is less. Thus, serious toxicity can result even within the normal therapeutic range because of an increase in nonprotein-bound drug (Aronson et al., 1992b; Koch-Weser, 1972).

Serum concentrations of drugs can be altered by many mechanisms. A number of factors are known to alter digoxin concentration when the dosage is kept constant, including altered absorption, impaired renal excretion, drug interaction, and impaired metabolism (Aronson et al., 1992a). Theophylline

Table 14–11 ■ THERAPEUTIC REFERENCE RANGES AND TOXIC LEVELS OF COMMON DRUGS

Drug	Therapeutic Range	Toxic Level
Amiodarone	1.0–3.4 μg/mL	
Bretylium	0.8–2.4 μg/mL	
Digitoxin	15 ng/mL	>40 ng/mL
Digoxin	0.5–2.0 μg/mL	>4.0 ng/mL
Diltiazem	100–200 ng/mL	
Disopyramide	1.5–5.0 μg/mL	>9.0 μg/mL
Encainide	10.0–135 μg/mL	
Flecainide	0.2–1.0 μg/mL	
Lidocaine	1.5–5.0 μg/mL	>6.0 μg/mL
Lorcainide	200–500 ng/mL	
Metoprolol	120–200 ng/mL	
Mexiletine	0.5–2.0 μg/mL	>3.0 μg/mL
N-Acetylprocainamide (NAPA)	2.0–22.0 μg/mL	
Nifedipine	50–100 ng/mL	
Phenytoin	10–20 μg/mL	>18 μg/mL
Procainamide	4.0–8.0 μg/mL	>10 μg/mL
Propafenone	64–1044 ng/mL	
Propranolol	30–50 ng/mL	
Quinidine	2.5–5.0 μg/mL	>6.0 μg/mL
Theophylline	10–20 μg/mL	>20 μg/mL
Tocainide	4.0–10.0 μg/mL	>10 μg/mL
Verapamil	50–400 ng/mL	

From Taylor, W. J. & Caviness, M. H. D. (1986). *A textbook for the clinical application of therapeutic drug monitoring.* Irving, TX: Abbott Laboratories; Tilkian, S. M. et al. (1987). *Clinical implications of laboratory tests* (4th ed.). St. Louis: CV Mosby; and Woodley, M. & Whelan, A. (1992). *Manual of medical therapeutics* (27th ed., pp. 517–523). Boston: Little, Brown.

concentration is increased in neonates, in the elderly, with obesity, with high-carbohydrate diets, and with some comorbid conditions. Theophylline concentration is reduced in children, with a low-carbohydrate diet, with eating charcoal-cooked meats, and with some drugs (Aronson et al., 1992c). There is as much as a 50-fold difference in plasma concentration of phenytoin among patients using the same dosage; altered metabolism and altered protein-binding account for the large individual variation in the disposition of phenytoin (Aronson et al., 1992b).

The blood specimen to determine serum concentration of a drug usually is drawn 1 to 2 hours after an oral drug is administered because absorption and distribution are usually complete by this time (Koch-Weser, 1972). However, peak and trough times are frequently defined for individual drugs; these times should be considered in the timing of specimens for therapeutic drug level monitoring.

REFERENCES

Abbey, E. E. (1983). Bleeding disorders. In J. W. Campbell, & M. Frisse (Eds.), *Manual of medical therapeutics* (24th ed., pp. 285–288). Boston: Little, Brown.

Abbott, L. B., & Lott, J. A. (1984). Reactivation of serum creatine kinase isoenzyme BB inpatients with malignancies. *Clinical Chemistry,* 30, 1861–1863.

Adams, J. E., 3rd, Bodor, G. S., Dávila-Román, V. G., Delmez, J. A., Apple, F. S., Ladenson, J. H., & Jaffe, A. S. (1993). Cardiac troponin I: A marker with high specificity for cardiac injury. *Circulation,* 88, 101–106.

Adams, J. E., 3rd, Dávila-Román, V. G., Bessey, P. Q., Blake, D. P., Ladenson, J. H., & Jaffe, A. S. (1996). Improved detection of cardiac contusion with cardiac troponin I. *American Heart Journal,* 131, 308–312.

American Diabetes Association. (2003a). Standards of medical care for patients with diabetes mellitus. *Diabetes Care, 26*(90001), 33S–50.

American Diabetes Association. (2003b). Tests of glycemia in diabetes. *Diabetes Care, 26*(90001), 106S–108.

American Heart Association. (2001). *ACLS provider manual.* Dallas, TX: Author.

Ansell, J. E. (2001). Hemorrhagic and thrombotic disorders. In J. Noble (Ed.), *Textbook of primary care medicine* (3rd ed., pp. 1044–1052). St. Louis: Mosby.

Apple, F. S. (1989). Diagnostic use of CK-MM and CK-MB isoforms for detecting myocardial infarction. *Clinical Chemistry and Laboratory Medicine, 9,* 643–655.

Aronson, J. K., Hardman, M., & Reynolds, D. J. M. (1992a). ABC of monitoring drug therapy: Digoxin. *BMJ, 305,* 1149–1152.

Aronson, J. K., Hardman, M., & Reynolds, D. J. M. (1992b). ABC of monitoring drug therapy: Phenytoin. *BMJ, 305,* 1215–1218.

Aronson, J. K., Hardman, M., & Reynolds, D. J. M. (1992c). ABC of monitoring drug therapy: Theophylline. *BMJ, 305,* 1355–1358.

Baer, D. M., & Dito, W. R. (1981). Interpretations in therapeutic drug monitoring (pp. 90). Chicago, ASCP.

Bakay, R. A. E., & Ward, A. A. (1983). Enzymatic changes in serum and cerebrospinal fluid in neurological injury. *Journal of Neurosurgery, 58,* 27–37.

Balk, E. M., Ioannidis, J. P. A., Salem, D., Chew, P. W., & Lau, J. (2001). Accuracy of biomarkers to diagnose acute cardiac ischemia in the emergency department: A meta-analysis. *Annals of Emergency Medicine, 37,* 478–494.

Baranowski, L. (1993). Central venous access devices: Current technologies, uses, and management strategies. *Journal of Intravenous Nursing, 16,* 167–191.

Baron, R. B. (2001). Lipid abnormalities. In L. M. Tierney, S. J. McPhee, & M. A. Papadakis (Eds.), *Current: Medical diagnosis & treatment 2001* (40th ed., pp. 1208–1221). New York: Lange Medical Books/McGraw-Hill.

Bautista, L. E., Arenas, I. A., Penuela, A., & Martinez, L. X. (2002). Total plasma homocysteine level and risk of cardiovascular disease: A meta-analysis of prospective cohort studies. *Journal of Clinical Epidemiology, 55*(9), 882–887.

Becker, R. C., & Corrao, J. M. (1989). Circadian variations in cardiovascular disease. *Cleveland Clinic Journal of Medicine, 56,* 676–679.

Berger, R., Huelsman, M., Strecker, K., Bojic, A., Moser, P., Stanek, B., & Pacher, R. (2002). B-type natriuretic peptide predicts sudden death in patients with chronic heart failure. *Circulation, 105,* 2392–2397.

Birdi, I., Angelini, G. D., & Bryan, A. J. (1997). Biochemical markers of myocardial injury during cardiac operations. *The Annals of Thoracic Surgery, 63,* 879–874.

Blake, G. J., Dada, N., Fox, J. C., Manson, J. E., & Ridker, P. M. (2001). A prospective evaluation of lipoprotein-associated phospholipase A(2) levels and the risk of future cardiovascular events in women. *Journal of the American College of Cardiology, 38*(5), 1302–1306.

Bolooki, H. (1973). The significance of serum enzyme studies in patients undergoing direct coronary artery surgery. *Journal of Thoracic and Cardiovascular Surgery, 65,* 863.

Boone, D. J., Duncan, P. H., MacNeil, M. L., Smith, B. F., Houston, B., & Hearn, T. L. (1984). Results of a nationwide survey of analyses for creatine kinase and creatine kinase isoenzymes. *Clinical Chemistry, 33–37.*

Braunwald, E. (1997). Shattuck Lecture- Cardiovascular medicine at the turn of the millennium: Triumphs, concerns, and opportunities. *New England Journal of Medicine, 337,* 1360–1369.

Burns, P. K., Gregersen, R. A., & Underhill, S. L. (1985). Adequate discard volume determinations to obtain accurate coagulation studies from heparinized arterial lines [abstract]. *Circulation, 72,* II–96.

Calam, R. R. (1977). Reviewing the importance of specimen collection. *Journal of American Medical Technologists, 39,* 297–301.

Cannon, K., Mitchell, K. A., & Fabian, T. C. (1985). Prospective randomized evaluation of two methods of drawing coagulation studies from heparinized arterial lines. *Heart & Lung, 14,* 392–395.

Carlson, G. (2001). The value of point-of-care testing when instituting an insulin drip protocol. *Critical Care Nurse Quarterly, 24*(1), 49–53.

Carnevali, D. (1983). *Nursing care planning: Diagnosis and management* (3rd ed.). Philadelphia: JB Lippincott.

Caslake, M. J., Packard, C. J., Suckling, K. E., Holmes, S. D., Chamberlain, P., & Macphee, C. H. (2000). Lipoprotein-associated phospholipase A(2), platelet-activating factor acetylhydrolase: A potential new risk factor for coronary artery disease. *Atherosclerosis, 150*(2), 413–419.

Chambers, J. C., Ueland, P. M., Obeid, O. A., Wrigley, J., Refsum, H., & Kooner, J. S. (2000). Improved vascular endothelial function after oral B vitamins: An effect mediated through reduced concentrations of free plasma homocysteine. *Circulation, 102*(20), 2479–2483.

Chernecky, C. C., & Berger, B. J. (1997). *Laboratory tests and diagnostic procedures* (2nd ed.). Philadelphia: WB Saunders.

Christenson, R. H., Clemmensen, P., Ohman, E. M., Toffaletti, J., Silverman, L. M., Grande, P., Vollmer, R. T., & Wagner, G. S. (1990). Relative increase in creatine kinase MB isoenzyme during reperfusion after myocardial infarction is method dependent. *Clinical Chemistry, 36,* 1444–1449.

Cleophas, T. J., Hornstra, N., van Hoogstraten, B., & van der Meulen, J. (2000). Homocysteine, a risk factor for coronary artery disease or not? A meta-analysis. *The American Journal of Cardiology, 86*(9), 1005–1009.

Collinson, P. O., Rosalki, S. B., Kuwana, T., Garratt, H. M., Ramhamadamy, E. M., Baird, I. M., & Greenwood, T. W. (1992). Early diagnosis of acute myocardial infarction by CK-MB mass measurements. *Annals of Clinical Biochemistry, 29,* 43–47.

Coolen, R. B., Pragay, D. A., Nosanchuk, J. S., & Belding, R. (1979). Elevation of brain-type creatine kinase in serum from patients with carcinoma. *Cancer, 44,* 1414–1418.

Coombs, D. L., Russo, L. E., & Underhill, S. L., et al. (1984). Withdrawal of blood specimens from radial artery catheters for serum sodium and hematocrit studies (Abstract). *Circulation, 70,* II288.

Cooper, G. R., Myers, G. L., Smith, S. J., & Schlant, R. C. (1992). Blood lipid measurements: Variations and practical utility. *JAMA, 267,* 1652–1660.

Costentino, F. (1987). Central venous catheters. In A. Plumer (Ed.), *Principles and practices of intravenous therapy* (pp. 323–369). Boston: Little, Brown.

Dacie, J. V., & Lewis, S. M. (1984). *Practical hematology* (6th ed., pp. 7–12). Edinburgh: Churchill Livingstone.

de Bree, A., Verschuren, W. M., Blom, H. J., Nadeau, M., Trijbels, F. J., & Kromhout, D. (2003). Coronary heart disease mortality, plasma homocysteine, and B-vitamins: a prospective study. *Atherosclerosis, 166*(2), 369–377.

Doshi, S. N., McDowell, I. F., Moat, S. J., Payne, N., Durrant, H. J., Lewis, M. J., & Goodfellow, J. (2002). Folic acid improves endothelial function in coronary artery disease via mechanisms largely independent of homocysteine lowering. *Circulation, 105*(1), 22–26.

Dufour, D. R. (1998). *Clinical use of laboratory data: A practical guide.* Baltimore: Williams & Wilkins.

Ehsani, A., Ewy, G. A., & Sobel, B. E. (1976). Effects of electrical countershock on serum creatine phosphokinase (CPK) isoenzyme activity. *American Journal of Cardiology, 37,* 12–18.

Farah, S. Y., Moss, D. W., Ribeiro, P., Oakley, C. M., & Sapsford, R. N. (1984). Interpretation of changes in the activity of creatine kinase MB isoenzyme in serum after coronary artery bypass grafting. *Clinica Chimica Acta, 141,* 219–225.

Finch, S. C. (1983). Neutropenia. In W. J. Williams, B. Buetler, & A. J. Erslev, et al. (Eds.), *Hematology* (3rd ed., pp. 773–793). New York: McGraw-Hill.

Forlani, S., De Paulis, R., de Notaris, S., Nardi, P., Tomai, F., Proietti, I., Ghini, A. S., & Chiariello, L. (2002). Combination of sotalol and magnesium prevents atrial fibrillation after coronary artery bypass grafting. *Annals of Thoracic Surgery, 74*(3), 720–725.

Fried, M. W., Murthy, U. K., Hassig, S. R., Woo, J., & Oates, R. P. (1991). Creatine kinase isoenzymes in the diagnosis of intestinal infarction. *Digestive Diseases and Sciences, 36,* 1589–1593.

Galen, R. S. (1977). Myocardial infarction: A clinician's guide to the isoenzymes. *Resident and Staff Physician, 23,* 67–75.

Galen, R. S. (1981). Isoenzymes in cardiac and noncardiac disorders. In R. S. Galen & L. Brennan (Eds.), *Laboratory diagnosis and patient monitoring: Clinical chemistry* (pp. 113–136). Oradell, NJ: Medical Economics.

Ganong, W. F. (1987). Circulating body fluids. In W. F. Ganong (Ed.), *Review of medical physiology* (13th ed., pp. 429–449). Los Altos, CA: Lange Medical.

Garza, D., & Becan-McBride, K. (2002). *Phlebotomy handbook: Blood collection essentials* (6th ed.). Upper Saddle River, NJ: Prentice-Hall/Pearson.

Genest, J., JR., McNamara, J. R., Ordovas, J. M., Jenner, J. L., Silberman, S. R., Anderson, K. M., Wilson, P. W., Salem, D. N., & Schaefer, E. J. (1992). Lipoprotein cholesterol, apolipoprotein A-1 and B and lipoprotein (a) abnormalities in men with premature coronary artery disease. *Journal of the American College of Cardiology, 19,* 792–802.

Gersh, B. J. (1996). Acute myocardial infarction. In E. Giuliani, B J. Gersh, & M. D. McGoon, et al. (Eds.), *Mayo clinic practice of cardiology* (3rd ed.). St. Louis: Mosby.

Giuliano, K. K., & Grant, M. E. (2002). Blood analysis at the point of care: Issues in application for use in critically ill patients. *AACN Clinical Issues, 13*(2), 204–219.

Goe, M. R. (1987). Creatine kinase enzyme determination: Implications for cardiovascular nursing. *Progress in Cardiovascular Nursing, 2*(2), 48.

Graeber, G. M. (1985). Creatine kinase (CK): Its use in the evaluation of perioperative MI. *Surgical Clinics of North America*, 65, 539–551.

Gram-Hansen, P., Nielsen, F. E., & Kalusen, I. C. (1990). Creatine kinase-MB activity after implantation of a cardiac pacemaker. *American Journal of Cardiology*, 66, 862–863.

Grantham, J. A., & Burnett, J. C. (1997). BNP: Increasing importance in the pathophysiology and diagnosis of congestive heart failure. *Circulation*, 96, 388–390.

Gregersen, R. A., Underhill, S. L., & Detter, J. C. (1983). Withdrawal of blood specimens from heparinized radial artery catheters for coagulation studies [abstract]. *Circulation*, 68, III–23.

Gregersen, R. A., Underhill, S. L., Detter, J. C., Schmer, G., & Lax, K. (1987). Accurate coagulation studies from heparinized radial artery catheters. *Heart & Lung*, 16, 686–693.

Gulbis, B., Unger, P., Lenaers, A., Desment, J. M., & Ooms, H. A. (1990). Mass concentration of creatine kinase MB isoenzyme and lactate dehydrogenase isoenzyme 1 in diagnosis of perioperative myocardial infarction after coronary bypass surgery. *Clinical Chemistry*, 36, 1784–1788.

Gunnar, W. P., Martin, M., Smith, R. F., Manglano, R., Resnick, D. J., Lopez, V., & Barrett, J. A. (1991). The utility of cardiac evaluation in the hemodynamically stable patient with suspected myocardial contusion. *American Surgeon*, 57, 373–377.

Gutierrez, K. (1999a). Anticoagulant and antiplatelet drugs. In K. Gutierrez (Ed.), *Pharmacotherapeutics: Clinical decision-making in nursing* (pp. 774–789). Philadelphia: W. B. Saunders.

Gutierrez, K. (1999b). Antilipemic drugs. In K. Gutierrez (Ed.), *Pharmacotherapeutics: Clinical decision-making in nursing* (pp. 754–772). Philadelphia: W. B. Saunders.

Halsted, J. A. (1976). Diagnostic procedures and tests. In J. A. Halsted (Ed.), *The laboratory in clinical medicine* (pp. 530–535). Philadelphia: WB Saunders.

Hans, P., Born, J. D., Chapelle, J. P., & Milbouw, G. (1983). Creatine kinase isoenzymes in severe head injury. *Journal of Neurosurgery*, 58, 689–692.

Healey, M. A., Brown, R., & Fleiszer, D. (1990). Blunt cardiac injury: Is this diagnosis necessary? *Journal of Trauma*, 30, 137–146.

Heap, M. J., Ridley, S. A., Hodson, K., & Martos, F. J. (1997). Are coagulation studies on blood sampled from arterial lines valid? *Anaesthesia*, 52, 640–645.

Henry, R. J., Cannon, D. C., & Winkelman, J. W. (1974). Enzymes. In R. J. Henry, D. C. Cannon, & W. J. W. (Eds.), *Clinical chemistry: Principles and techniques* (pp. 818–904). Hagerstown, MD: Harper & Row.

Homocysteine Studies Collaboration. (2002). Homocysteine and risk of ischemic heart disease and stroke. *JAMA*, 16, 2015–2022.

Hori, M., Inoue, M., Fukui, S., Shimazu, T., Mishima, M., Ohgitani, N., Minamino, T., & Abe, H. (1979). Correlation of infarct size estimated from the total CK released in patients with acute myocardial infarction. *British Heart Journal*, 41, 433–440.

Huang, J. N., & Shimamura, A. (1998). Low-molecular-weight heparins. *Hematology/Oncology Clinics of North America*, 12, 1251–1281.

Intravenous Nursing Standards of Practice. (1990). *Journal of Intravenous Nursing*, 13(Suppl), S1–S98.

Jacobs, D. S., & DeMott, W. R. (2001). *Laboratory test handbook* (5th ed.). Hudson, OH: Lexi-Comp/NC.

Jarvinen, A., Mattila, T., & Kyosola, K. (1983). Serum CK-MB isoenzyme after aortic and mitral valve replacements. *Annals of Clinical Research*, 15, 189–193.

Kanemitsu, F., & Okigake, T. (1992). Creatine kinase MB isoforms for early diagnosis and monitoring of acute myocardial infarction. *Clinica Chimica Acta*, 206, 191–199.

Kannel, W. B. (1978). Recent findings of the Framingham Study. *Resident and Staff Physician*, 24, 56–71.

Kannel, W. B., Anderson, K., & Wilson, P. F. (1992). White blood cell count and cardiovascular disease: Insights from the Framingham Study. *JAMA*, 267, 1253–1256.

Kaplan, M., Kut, M. S., Icer, U. A., & Demirtas, M. M. (2003). Intravenous magnesium sulfate prophylaxis for atrial fibrillation after coronary artery bypass surgery. *Journal of Thoracic and Cardiovascular Surgery*, 125(2), 344–352.

Kee, J. L. (1998). *Handbook of laboratory diagnostic tests with nursing implications* (3rd ed.). Stamford, CT: Appleton & Lange.

Kee, J. L. (1999). *Laboratory and diagnostic tests with nursing implications* (5th ed.). Stamford, CT: Appleton & Lange.

Kennedy, C., Angermuller, S., King, R., Noviello, S., Walker, J., Warden, J., & Vang, S. (1996). A comparison of hemolysis rates using intravenous catheters versus venipuncture tubes for obtaining blood samples. *Journal of Emergency Nursing*, 22(6), 566–569.

Kjekshus, J. K., Vaagenes, P., & Hetland, O. (1980). Assessment of cerebral injury with spinal fluid creatine kinase (CSF-CK) in patients after cardiac resuscitation. *Scandinavian Journal of Clinical and Laboratory Investigation*, 40, 437–444.

Koch-Weser, J. (1972). Serum drug concentrations as therapeutic guides. *New England Journal of Medicine*, 287, 227–231.

Koenig, W., Sund, M., Frohlich, M., Fischer, H. G., Lowel, H., Doring, A., Hutchinson, W. L., & Pepys, M. B. (1999). C-Reactive protein, a sensitive marker of inflammation, predicts future risk of coronary heart disease in initially healthy middle-aged men: results from the MONICA (Monitoring Trends and Determinants in Cardiovascular Disease) Augsburg Cohort Study, 1984 to 1992. *Circulation*, 99(2), 237–242.

Koff, R. S. (2001). *Liver disease*. In J. Noble (Ed.), *Textbook of primary care medicine* (3rd ed., pp. 928–943). St. Louis: Mosby.

Kratz, A. K., & Lewandrowski, K. B. (1998). Normal reference laboratory values. *New England Journal of Medicine*, 339, 1063–1072.

Krueger, K. E., Carrico, C. J., Detter, J. C., Raisys, V. A., & Underhill, S. L. (1980). The reliability of laboratory data from blood samples collected through pulmonary artery catheters. *Archives of Pathology and Laboratory Medicine*, 105, 343–344.

Kuller, L. H., Tracy, R. P., Shaten, J., & Meilahn, E. N. (1996). Relation of C-reactive protein and coronary heart disease in the MRFIT nested case-control study. *American Journal of Epidemiology*, 144, 537–547.

LaDue, J. S., Wroblewski, F., & Karmen, A. (1954). Serum glutamic oxaloacetic transaminase activity in human acute transmural myocardial infarction. *Science*, 120, 497–499.

Laxson, C. J., & Titler, M. G. (1994). Drawing coagulation studies from arterial lines: An integrative literature review. *American Journal of Critical Care*, 3, 16–22.

Lew, J. K. L., Hutchinson, R., & Lin, E. S. (1991). Intra-arterial blood sampling for clotting studies: Effects of heparin contamination. *Anaesthesia*, 46, 719–721.

Lily, L. S. (2001). Ischemic heart disease. In J. Noble (Ed.), *Textbook of primary care medicine* (3rd ed., pp. 545–570). St. Louis: Mosby.

Lim, M., Linton, A. F., & Band, D. M. (1983). Rise in plasma potassium during rewarming in open-heart surgery. *Lancet*, 1, 241–242.

Longstreth, W. T., Clayson, K. J., & Sumi, S. M. (1981). Cerebrospinal fluid and serum creatine kinase BB activity after out-of-hospital cardiac arrest. *Neurology*, 31, 455–458.

Longstreth, W. T., Jr, Clayson, K. J., Chandler, W. L., & Sumi, S. M. (1984). Cerebrospinal fluid creatine kinase activity and neurologic recovery after cardiac arrest. *Neurology*, 34, 834–837.

Lott, J. A. (1984). Serum enzyme determinations in the diagnosis of acute myocardial infarction: An update. *Human Pathology*, 15, 706–716.

Lott, J. A., & Stang, J. M. (1980). Serum enzymes and isoenzymes in the diagnosis and differential diagnosis of myocardial ischemia and necrosis. *Clinical Chemistry*, 26, 1241–1250.

Lott, J. A., & Stang, J. M. (1989). Differential diagnosis of patients with abnormal serum creatine kinase isoenzymes. *Clinical Chemistry and Laboratory Medicine*, 9, 627–642.

Luce, J. M., Tyler, M. L., & Pierson, D. J. (1984). *Intensive respiratory care*. Philadelphia: WB Saunders.

Macy, E. M., Hayes, T. E., & Tracy, R. P. (1997). Variability in the measurement of C-reactive protein in healthy subjects: Implications for reference intervals and epidemiological applications. *Clinical Chemistry*, 43, 52–58.

Maisel, A. S., Krishnaswamy, P., Nowak, R. M., McCord, J., Hollander, J. E., Duc, P., Omland, T., Storrow, A. B., Abraham, W. T., Wu, A. H. B., Clopton, P., Steg, P. G., Westheim, A., Knudsen, C. W., Perez, A., Kazanegra, R., Herrmaan, H. C., & McCullough, P. A. (2002). Rapid measurement of B-type natriuretic peptide in the emergency diagnosis of heart failure. *New England Journal of Medicine*, 347(3), 161–167.

Mangano, D. T. (1994). Beyond CK-MB: Biochemical markers for perioperative myocardial infarction. *Anesthesiology*, 81, 1317–1320.

Markenvard, J., Dellborg, M., Jagenberg, R., & Swedberg, K. (1992). The predictive value of CK-MB mass concentration in unstable angina pectoris: Preliminary report. *Journal of Internal Medicine*, 231, 433–436.

Markmann, P. J., & Wallace, P. (1985). Nursing care in the intensive care unit. In K. M. McCauley, A. N. Brest, & D. C. McGoon (Eds.), *McGoon's cardiac surgery: An interprofessional approach to patient care* (pp. 319–354). Philadelphia: FA Davis.

Masouredes, S. P. (1990). Preservation and clinical use of erythrocytes and whole blood. In W. J. Williams, E. Buetler, & A. J. Erslev, et al. (Eds.), *Hematology* (4th ed., pp. 1628–1646). New York: McGraw-Hill.

Massey, T. H., & Butts, W. C. (1983). Development and clinical evaluation of a microcentrifugal analyzer method for determining creatine kinase MB isoenzyme. *Clinical Chemistry,* 29, 533–538.

Massey, T. H., & Goe, M. R. (1984). Transient creatine kinase-BB activity in serum or plasma after cardiac or respiratory arrest. *Clinical Chemistry,* 30, 50–55.

Mathey, D. G., Kuck, K. H., Tilsner, V., Krebber, H. J., & Bleifeld, W. (1981). Non surgical coronary recanalization in acute transmural myocardial infarction. *Circulation,* 63, 481–497.

McCullough, P. A., Nowak, R. M., McCord, J., Hollander, J. E., Herrmaan, H. C., Steg, P. G., Duc, P., Westheim, A., Omland, T., Knudsen, C. W., Storrow, A. B., Abraham, W. T., Lamba, S., Wu, A. H. B., Perez, A., Clopton, P., Krishnaswamy, P., Kazanegra, R., & Maisel, A. S. (2002). B-type natriuretic peptide and clinical judgment in emergency diagnosis of heart failure. *Circulation,* 106, 416–422.

McFarland, M. B., & Grant, M. M. (1988). *Nursing implications of laboratory tests.* New York: Wiley Medical.

McFarland, M. B., & Grant, M. M. (1994). *Nursing implications of laboratory tests* (3rd ed.). Albany, NY: Delmar.

Melandri, G., Branzi, A., Traini, A. M., Semprini, F., Cervi, V., & Magnani, B. (1993). On the value of the activated clotting time for monitoring heparin therapy in acute coronary syndromes. *American Journal of Cardiology,* 71, 469–470.

Miller, F. A. (1996). Cardiac trauma. In E. Giuliani, B. J. Gersh, & M. D. McGoon, et al. (Eds.), *Mayo clinic practice of cardiology* (3rd ed.). St. Louis: Mosby.

Miyazawa, K., Fukuyama, H., Yamaguchi, I., Kobayashi, M., Washio, M., & Oda, J. (1985). Serial determinations of serum enzymes following aorta-coronary bypass surgery and acute myocardial infarction. *Japan Heart Journal,* 26, 45–52.

National Cholesterol Education Program (2001). Executive Summary of The Third Report of The National Cholesterol Education Program (NCEP) Expert Panel on Detection, Evaluation, and Treatment of High Blood Cholesterol in Adults (Adult Treatment Panel III). *JAMA,* 285(19), 2486–2497.

Ng, S. M., Krishnaswamy, P., Morissey, R., Clopton, P., Fitzgerald, R., & Maisel, A. S. (2001). Coronary artery disease/Accelerated pathway for chest pain evaluation. *American Journal of Cardiology,* 88, 611–617.

Nguyen, D. M., Gilfix, B. M., Dennis, F., Blank, D., Latter, D. A., Ergina, P. L., Morin, J. E., & de Varennes, B. (1996). Impact of transfusion of mediastinal shed blood on serum levels of cardiac enzymes. *Annals of Thoracic Surgery,* 62, 109–114.

Nicoll, C. D., Pignone, M., & Detmer, W. M. (2001). Diagnostic testing & medical decision making. In L. M. J. Tierney, S. J. McPhee, & M. A. Papadakis (Eds.), *Current medical diagnosis & treatment 2001* (40th ed., pp. 1617–1627). New York: Lange Medical Books/McGraw-Hill.

Nordby, H. K., & Urdal, P. (1985). Creatine kinase BB in blood as index or prognosis and effect of treatment after severe head injury. *Acta Neurochirurgica,* 76, 131–136.

Oh, J. K., Shub, C., Ilstrup, D. M., & Reeder, G. S. (1985). Creatine kinase release after successful percutaneous transluminal coronary angioplasty. *American Heart Journal,* 109, 1225–1231.

Oxley, D. K., Garg, U., & Olsowka, E. S. (2001). Maximizing the information from laboratory tests-The Ulysses syndrome: Tests in search of disease. In D. S. Jacobs, & W. R. DeMott (Eds.), *Laboratory test handbook* (5th ed., pp. 15–23). Hudson, OH: Lexi-Comp/NC.

Pagana, K. D., & Pagana, T. J. (1998). *Mosby's manual of diagnostic and laboratory tests.* St. Louis: Mosby.

Pagana, K. D., & Pagana, T. J. (2002). *Mosby's manual of diagnostic and laboratory tests* (2nd ed.). St. Louis: Mosby.

Paone, R. F., Peacock, J. B., & Smith, D. L. T. (1993). Diagnosis of myocardial contusion. *Southern Medical Journal,* 86, 867–870.

Pearson, T. A., Mensah, G. A., Alexander, R. W., Anderson, J. L., Cannon, R. O., III., Criqui, M., Fadl, Y. Y., Fortmann, S. P., Hong, Y., Myers, G. L., Rifai, N., Smith, S. C., Jr., Taubert, K., Tracy, R. P., & Vinicor, F. (2003). Markers of inflammation and cardiovascular disease: Application to clinical and public health practice. *Circulation,* 107, 499–511.

Phillips, J. P., Jones, H. M., Hitchcock, R., Adama, N., & Thompson, R. J. (1980). Radioimmunoassay of serum creatine kinase BB as index of brain damage after head injury. *BMJ,* 281, 777–779.

Prinkey, L. A. (1992). Diagnostic testing. In C. E. Guzzetta, & B. M. Dossey (Eds.), *Cardiovascular nursing: Holistic practice* (pp. 128–130). St. Louis: Mosby.

Rader, D. J. (2000). Inflammatory markers of coronary risk. *New England Journal of Medicine,* 343(16), 1179–1182.

Ravel, R. (1984). Cardiac, pulmonary, and miscellaneous diagnostic procedures. In R. Ravel (Ed.), *Clinical laboratory medicine: Clinical application of laboratory data* (4th ed., pp. 227–441). Chicago: Year Book.

Ridker, P. M. (1999). Evaluating novel cardiovascular risk factors: Can we better predict heart attacks? *Annals of Internal Medicine,* 130, 933–937.

Ridker, P. M., Cushman, M., Stampfer, M. J., Tracy, R. P., & Hennekens, C. H. (1997). Inflammation, aspirin, and the risk of cardiovascular disease in apparently healthy men. *New England Journal of Medicine,* 336, 973–979.

Ridker, P. M., Hennekens, C. H., Buring, J. E., & Rifai, N. (2000). C-reactive protein and other markers of inflammation in the prediction of cardiovascular disease in women. *New England Journal of Medicine,* 342(12), 836–843.

Ridker, P. M., Rifai, N., Rose, L., Buring, J. E., & Cook, N. R. (2002). Comparison of C-reactive protein and low-density lipoprotein cholesterol levels in the prediction of first cardiovascular events. *New England Journal of Medicine,* 347(20), 1557–1565.

Roberts, R., Gowda, K. S., Ludbrook, P. A., & Sobel, B. E. (1975). Specificity of elevated serum MB creatine phosphokinase activity in the diagnosis of acute myocardial infarction. *American Journal of Cardiology,* 36, 433–437.

Roberts, R., Morris, D., & Pratt, C. M., et al. (1994). Pathophysiology, recognition and treatment of acute myocardial infarction and its complications. In R. C. Schlant, & R. W. Alexander (Eds.), *Hurst's the heart: Arteries and veins* (8th ed., pp. 1117–1122). New York: McGraw-Hill.

Rohlfing, C. L., Wiedmeyer, H.-M., Little, R. R., England, J. D., Tennill, A., & Goldstein, D. E. (2002). Defining the relationship between plasma glucose and HbA1c: Analysis of glucose profiles and HbA1c in the Diabetes Control and Complications Trial. *Diabetes Care,* 25(2), 275–278.

Romano, A. T., & Yourn, G. W. (1977). Mild forearm exercise during exercise and its effect on potassium determinations. *Clinical Chemistry,* 23, 303–304.

Rose, B. D. (1984). *Clinical physiology of acid-base and electrolyte disorders* (2nd ed., pp. 275–276). New York: McGraw-Hill.

Ross, R. (1999). Atherosclerosis- An inflammatory disease. *New England Journal of Medicine,* 340, 115126.

Russo, L. E., Coombs, D. L., & Underhill, S. L., et al. (1984). Reliable measurements of serum potassium and glucose from radial artery lines (Abstract). *Heart & Lung,* 13, 310.

Ruzak-Skocir, B. (1991). Cerebrospinal fluid CK enzyme and CK isoenzymes in the outcome prognosis of cerebrovascular disease. *Neurologia/Croatica,* 40, 247–256.

Ryan, T. J., Antman, E. M., Brooks, N. H., Califf, R. M., Hillis, L. D., Hiratzka, L. F., Rapaport, E., Riegel, B., Russell, R. O., Smith, E. E., III., & Weaver, W. D. (1999). ACC/AHA guidelines for the management of patients with acute myocardial infarction: 1999 update: a report of the American College of Cardiology/American Heart Association Task Force on Practice Guidelines (Committee on Management of Acute Myocardial Infarction). Available: www.acc.org [2003, April 5].

Sabatine, M. S., Morrow, D. A., de Lemos, J. A., Gibson, C. M., Murphy, S. A., Rifai, N., McCabe, C. E. M. A., Cannon, C. P., & Braunwald, E. (2002). Multimarker approach to risk stratification in non-ST elevation acute coronary syndromes. *Circulation,* 105, 1760–1763.

Sarko, J., & Pollack, C. V., Jr. (2002). Cardiac troponins. *Journal of Emergency Medicine,* 23(1), 57–65.

Schaefer, E. R., & Levy, R. L. (1985). Pathogenesis and management of lipoprotein disorders. *New England Journal of Medicine,* 312, 1300–1310.

Schnyder, G., Roffi, M., Pin, R., Flammer, Y., Lange, H., Eberli, F. R., Meier, B., Turi, Z. G., & Hess, O. M. (2001). Decreased rate of coronary restenosis after lowering of plasma homocysteine levels. *New England Journal of Medicine,* 345(22), 1593–1600.

Schofer, J., Ress-Grigolo, G., Voigt, K. D., & Mathey, D. G. (1992). Early detection of coronary artery patency after thrombolysis by determination of the MM creatine kinase isoforms in patients with acute myocardial infarction. *American Heart Journal,* 123, 846–853.

Schwartz, A. J., & Geer, R. T. (1985). Cardiac anesthesia. In K. M. McCauley & A. N. Brest, & D. C. McGoon (Eds.), *McGoon's cardiac surgery: An interprofessional approach to care* (pp. 289–315). Philadelphia: FA Davis.

Severson, A. L., Baldwin, L. R., & DeLoughery, T. G. (1997). International normalized ratio in anticoagulant therapy: Understanding the issues. *American Journal of Critical Care, 6,* 88–94.

Silva, J., Hoekesma, H., & FeKety, F. R. (1974). Transient defects in phagocytic functions during cardiopulmonary bypass. *Journal of Thoracic and Cardiovascular Surgery, 67,* 175–183.

Sipperly, M. E. (1985). Thrombolytic therapy update. *Critical Care Nurse, 5*(6), 30–34.

Skogseid, I. M., Nordby, H. K., Urdal, P., Paus, E., & Lilleaas, F. (1992). Increased serum creatine kinase BB and neuron specific enolase following head injury indicates brain damage. *Acta Neurochirurgica, 115,* 106–111.

Smith, A. F., Radford, D., Wong, C. P., & Oliver, M. F. (1976). Creatine kinase MB isoenzyme studies in diagnosis of myocardial infarction. *British Heart Journal, 38,* 225–232.

Snyder, M., Gregersen, R., & Underhill, S. L., et al. (1986). Partial thromboplastin and thrombin time blood specimens collection through pulmonary artery catheters (Abstract). *Heart & Lung, 15,* 315.

Sobel, B. E., & Jaffe, A. S. (1993). The value and limitations of cardiac enzymes in the recognition of acute myocardial infarction. *Heart Disease and Stroke, 2*(1), 26–32.

Solomon, A. J., Berger, A. K., Trivedi, K. K., Hannan, R. L., & Katz, N. M. (2000). The combination of propranolol and magnesium does not prevent postoperative atrial fibrillation. *Annals of Thoracic Surgery, 69,* 126–129.

Spaccavento, L. J., & Hawley, H. (1982). Infections associated with intraarterial lines. *Heart & Lung, 11,* 118–122.

Statland, B. E., Bokelund, H., & Winkel, P. (1974). Factors contributing to intra-individual variations of serum constituents: Effects of posture and tourniquet application on variation of serum constituents in healthy subjects. *Clinical Chemistry, 20,* 1513–1519.

Statland, B. E., & Winkel, P. (1979). Sources of variation in laboratory measurements. In J. B. Henry (Ed.), *Clinical diagnosis and management by laboratory methods* (pp. 3–28). Philadelphia: WB Saunders.

Steele, B. W., Gobel, F. L., Nelson, R. R., & Yasmineh, W. G. (1978). Creatine kinase isoenzyme activity following cardiac catheterization and exercise stress testing. *Chest, 73,* 489–496.

Suzuki, T., Yamauchi, K., Yamada, Y., Furumichi, T., Furui, H., Tsuzuki, J., Hayashi, H., Sotobata, I., & Saito, H. (1992). Blood coagulability and fibrolytic activity before and after physical training during the recovery phase of acute myocardial infarction. *Clinical Cardiology, 15,* 358–364.

Taylor, W. J., & Caviness, M. H. D. (1986). *A textbook for the clinical application of therapeutic drug monitoring.* Irving, TX: Abbott Laboratories.

Templin, K., Shively, M., & Riley, J. (1993). Accuracy of drawing coagulation samples from heparinized arterial lines. *American Journal of Critical Care, 2,* 88–95.

The Diabetes Control and Complications Trial Research Group. (1993). The effect of intensive treatment of diabetes on the development and progression of long-term complications in insulin-dependent diabetes mellitus. *New England Journal of Medicine, 329*(14), 977–986.

Tilkian, S. M., Conover, M. B., & Tilkian, A. (1987). *Clinical implications of laboratory tests* (4th ed.). St. Louis: CV Mosby.

Tilkian, S. M., Conover, M. B., & Tilkian, A. G. (1995). *Clinical and nursing implications of laboratory tests* (5th ed.). St. Louis: Mosby.

Title, L. M., Cummings, P. M., Giddens, K., Genest, J. J., Jr., & Nassar, B. A. (2000). Effect of folic acid and antioxidant vitamins on endothelial dysfunction in patients with coronary artery disease. *Journal of the American College of Cardiology, 36*(3), 758–765.

Toraman, F., Karabulut, E. H., Alhan, H. C., Dagdelen, S., & Tarcan, S. (2001). Magnesium infusion dramatically decreases the incidence of atrial fibrillation after coronary artery bypass grafting. *Annals of Thoracic Surgery, 72*(4), 1256-1261; discussion 1261–1252.

Tracy, R. P., Lemaitre, R. N., Psaty, B. M., Ives, D. G., Evans, R. G., Cushman, M., Meilahn, E. N., & Kuller, L. H. (1997). Relationship of C-reactive protein to risk of cardiovascular disease in the elderly. *Arteriosclerosis, Thrombosis, and Vascular Biology, 17,* 1121–1127.

Treseler, K. M. (1988). *Clinical laboratory tests: Significance and implications for nursing* (2nd ed.). Englewood Cliffs, NJ: Prentice-Hall.

Treseler, K. M. (1995). *Clinical laboratory and diagnostic tests: Significance and nursing implications* (3rd ed.). Norwalk, CT: Appleton & Lange.

Tsung, S. M. (1976). Creatine kinase isoenzyme patterns in human tissue obtained at surgery. *Clinical Chemistry, 22,* 173–175.

Turpie, A. G. G. (1998). Antithrombotic therapy in coronary ischaemia: The expanding role of low-molecular-weight heparin. *Haemostasis, 28*(Suppl 3), 35–42.

UK Prospective Diabetes Study (UKPDS) Group. (1998). Intensive blood-glucose control with sulphonylureas or insulin compared with conventional treatment and risk of complications in patients with type 2 diabetes (UKPDS 33). *Lancet, 352*(9131), 837–853.

Varat, M. A., & Mercer, D. W. (1975). Cardiac specific creatine phosphokinase isoenzyme in the diagnosis of acute myocardial infarction. *Circulation, 51,* 855–859.

Velmahos, G. C., Karaiskakis, M., Salim, A., Toutouzas, K. G., Murray, J., Asensio, J., & Demetriades, D. (2003). Normal electrocardiography and serum troponin I levels preclude the presence of clinically significant blunt cardiac injury. *Journal of Trauma, 54*(1), 45–50; discussion 50–41.

Visser, M., Bouter, L. M., McQuillan, G. M., Wener, M. H., & Harris, T. B. (1999). Elevated C-reactive protein levels in overweight and obese adults. *JAMA, 282,* 2131–2135.

Wald, D. S., Bishop, L., Wald, N. J., Law, M., Hennessy, E., Weir, D., McPartlin, J., & Scott, J. (2001). Randomized trial of folic acid supplementation and serum homocysteine levels. *Archives of Internal Medicine, 161*(5), 695–700.

Wallace, H. H., Carlson, K. K., & Snyder, M. L., et al. (1986). Obtaining reliable plasma glucose and potassium values from intraarterial catheters [abstract]. *Heart & Lung, 15,* 317.

Wallach, J. (1992). *Interpretation of diagnostic tests: A synopsis of laboratory medicine* (5th ed.). Boston: Little, Brown.

Walrath, J. M., Abbott, N. K., Caplan, E., & Scanlan, E. (1979). Stopcocks: Bacterial contamination in invasive monitoring systems. *Heart & Lung, 8,* 100–104.

Wang, C. W., Steinhubl, S. R., Castellani, W. J., Van Lente, F., Miller, D. P., James, K. B., & Young, J. B. (1996). Inability of serum myocyte death markers to predict acute cardiac allograft rejection. *Transplantation, 62,* 1938–1941.

Weinstein, R. A., Emori, T. G., Anderson, R. L., & Stamm, W. E. (1976). Pressure transducers as a source of bacteremia after open heart surgery. *Chest, 69,* 338–344.

Weiss, H. J. (1977). Platelet physiology and abnormalities of platelet function. *New England Journal of Medicine, 293,* 531–540.

White, K. M. (1985). Completing the hemodynamic picture: SvO_2. *Heart & Lung, 14,* 272–280.

Widmann, F. K. (1983). *Goodale's clinical interpretation of laboratory tests* (9th ed.). Philadelphia: FA Davis.

Wieczorek, S. J., Wu, A. H., Christenson, R., Krishnaswamy, P., Gottlieb, S., Rosano, T., Hager, D., Gardetto, N., Chiu, A., Bailly, K. R., & Maisel, A. (2002). A rapid B-type natriuretic peptide assay accurately diagnoses left ventricular dysfunction and heart failure: A multicenter evaluation. *American Heart Journal, 144,* 834–839.

Wiedemann, H. P., Matthay, M. A., & Matthay, R. A. (1984). Cardiovascularpulmonary monitoring in the intensive care unit, part 2. *Chest, 85,* 656–668.

Woodley, M., & Whelan, A. (1992). *Manual of medical therapeutics* (27th ed., pp. 517–523). Boston: Little, Brown.

Wu, A. H. (1989). Creatine kinase isoforms in ischemic heart disease. *Clinical Chemistry, 35,* 7–13.

Zaman, A. G., Alamgir, F., Richens, T., Williams, R., Rothman, M. T., & Mills, P. G. (1997). The role of signal averaged P wave duration and serum magnesium as a combined predictor of atrial fibrillation after elective coronary artery bypass surgery. *Heart, 77*(6), 527–531.

Radiologic Examination of the Chest

JON S. HUSEBY • DENISE LEDOUX

The chest radiography is one of the most common diagnostic tools used in the evaluation of cardiovascular disease and the critically ill. Although a variety of other imaging modalities are available, chest radiography remains fundamental because of its ready availability in most settings, relative inexpensive cost, and the ability to interpret films by a wide variety of health care providers.

The cardiac care nurse may be the first health care professional to see the chest radiograph of a patient in acute distress. Valuable time may be saved if the nurse is able to recognize the presence of an abnormality. Knowledge of chest radiograph interpretation and the disease processes that an abnormal film indicates can help in the nurse's understanding of disease pathophysiology, thereby allowing for better patient care; dual reading of radiographs significantly increases diagnostic accuracy and decreases the incidence of missed abnormalities. This chapter is divided into four sections:

1. How x-rays work
2. Interpretation of chest radiographs
3. Chest film findings in acute care determining line placement
4. Chest film findings in cardiovascular disease and acute care

HOW X-RAYS WORK

X-rays are radiant energy, like light, except that these waves are shorter and can pass through opaque objects. They are produced by bombarding a tungsten target with an electron beam and are channeled so that a narrow but diverging beam is emitted from the tube. When an x-ray exposure is taken, the tube is usually aimed so that the rays pass through the subject to the x-ray film in either a posterior to anterior (posteroanterior) or anterior to posterior (anteroposterior) direction (Figs. 15-1 and 15-2). Because the x-rays are diverging and subject to reflection (scatter), structures more distant from the film are magnified and less distinctly outlined. In general, chest radiographs are taken in the posteroanterior direction because

this places the heart, an anterior structure, closer to the film, resulting in less magnification and allowing the cardiac outline to be seen clearly.

Anteroposterior chest radiographs are often taken in cardiac care units (CCU) because it is difficult to put the x-ray tube behind the patient. The x-ray film is therefore placed behind the patient. Because the heart is relatively far away from the x-ray film, its outline is somewhat less distinct and the heart size is magnified. Moreover, the distance between the tube and the patient in CCU is shorter than usual to cut-down x-ray scatter. This also results in greater magnification.

The degree of darkness of the x-ray film depends on how much x-ray energy traverses the patient and exposes the film. This depends on the density of the material through which the x-ray beam passes. The chest has four major types of tissue densities through which rays must pass: bone, water, fat, and air. Because bone is the densest of these, fewer and less energetic x-rays pass through this substance. Thus, the shadow on the x-ray film cast by bone is light. (An x-ray picture is like a photographic negative, with white color indicating lack of exposure and black color indicating intense exposure.) The lung, which is largely air, is least dense; therefore, it appears black on a chest radiograph. Soft tissues and blood are largely water, with similar densities, between those of bone and air. Fat is usually visibly less dense than other soft tissues. Thus, a chest radiograph is actually a shadowgraph.

The reason a structure can be outlined is that the shadow of one density contrasts with that of an adjacent density. If two structures are of equal density and adjacent to each other, then a single combined shadow results. If two structures of similar density are in different planes or are separated by a structure of a different density, then the two structures are seen on x-ray film as separate. This property of the x-ray shadowgraph is helpful in determining where a certain density lies. For example, if a density on a posteroanterior chest radiograph is inseparable from and therefore adjacent to the descending thoracic aorta, then the observer knows that this abnormal density is in the posterior chest; if the

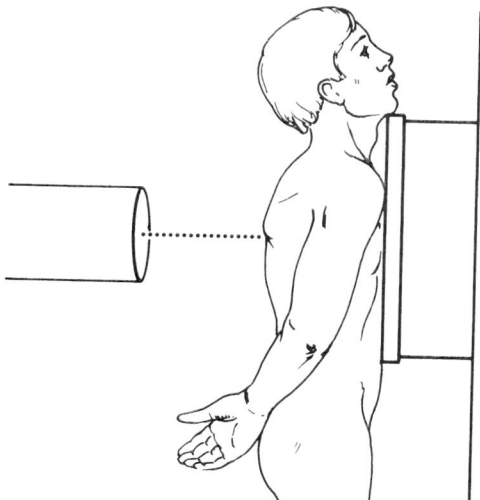

■ **Figure 15–1.** Positioning a patient for a posteroanterior (PA) frontal chest radiograph. The x-ray tube is behind the patient, and the x-ray film is close to his anterior chest.

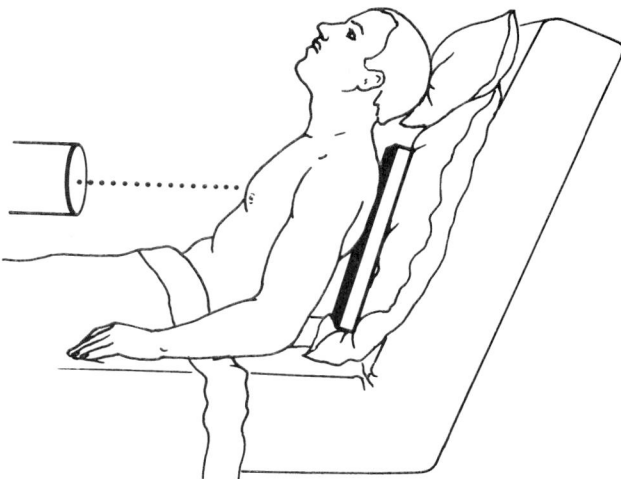

■ **Figure 15–2.** Typical cardiac care unit (CCU) patient positioned for an anteroposterior (AP) chest radiograph. Note that, as often occurs in the CCU, the patient's chest is not perfectly perpendicular to the x-ray tube. This placement is called a lordotic position and causes the heart to appear large and indistinct.

density is inseparable from the right heart border, then the density is in an anterior position, because the heart is an anterior structure.

INTERPRETATION OF CHEST RADIOGRAPHS

The chest radiograph is read as though the reader were looking at the patient. Traditionally, the x-ray film is placed on a view box or light box that allows the radiograph to be backlit so it can be viewed and interpreted. More recently, digital imaging technology is used increasingly in radiology allowing for rapid viewing of films on monitors rather than light boxes. Computerized radiographs can be viewed immediately on monitors on the CCU and stored images allow the provider to readily compare current films with previous images (Connolly, 2001). To ensure that all anatomic structures are seen, radiographs are read according to a certain pattern. This method is called the directed search method. It is common practice to look at soft tissues, bones, and diaphragms first, then at the lungs from apex to base, and finally at the outline of the heart and the aorta. Most structures in the chest, except the heart, are bilateral. Thus, if an abnormality is found on one side of the chest, the other side should be observed to ensure that this "abnormality" is not also present. Even if an obvious abnormality is present, a directed search should be completed so that additional disease is not missed. Figure 15-3*A* is a normal posteroanterior chest radiograph, and Figure 15-3*B* indicates what structures the shadows represent. Figure 15-4*A* shows the location of various lung lobes on a frontal projection and Figure 15-4*B*, a lateral film, shows the location of these lobes when the chest is viewed from the side.

CHEST FILM FINDINGS IN ACUTE CARE DETERMINING LINE, TUBE, AND CATHETER PLACEMENT

Bedside radiographs are used not only to assess for cardiopulmonary abnormalities, but also to evaluate placement of lines, tubes, and devices used in acute care. In addition to providing valuable information regarding the patient's cardiopulmonary status, the chest radiograph allows for early recognition of complications related to line placement as well as to evaluate therapeutic result after interventions such as drainage of a pleural effusion by chest tube placement. Table 15-1 lists invasive lines, tubes, and devices commonly used in acute cardiovascular care and describes radiologic findings. Figures 15-5 through 15-13 demonstrate radiologic appearance of a variety of invasive lines and devices.

CHEST FILM FINDINGS IN CARDIOVASCULAR DISEASE

The chest radiograph provides useful data that aid in the complete assessment of the patient in the CCU. While the patient with an uncomplicated acute coronary syndrome may present with a normal CXR, early chest radiography is essential as part of the diagnostic evaluation of aortic dissection, valvular heart disease, congestive heart failure, and pericardial effusion. Table 15-2 lists common cardiovascular clinical diagnoses and their associated radiologic findings. Figures 15-14 through 15-24 illustrate a variety of radiologic findings associated with cardiovascular pathophysiology. Early diagnosis of complications and improperly placed invasive lines improves patient care, and knowledge of the radiographic findings in disease processes augments the nurse's understanding of cardiopulmonary pathophysiology.

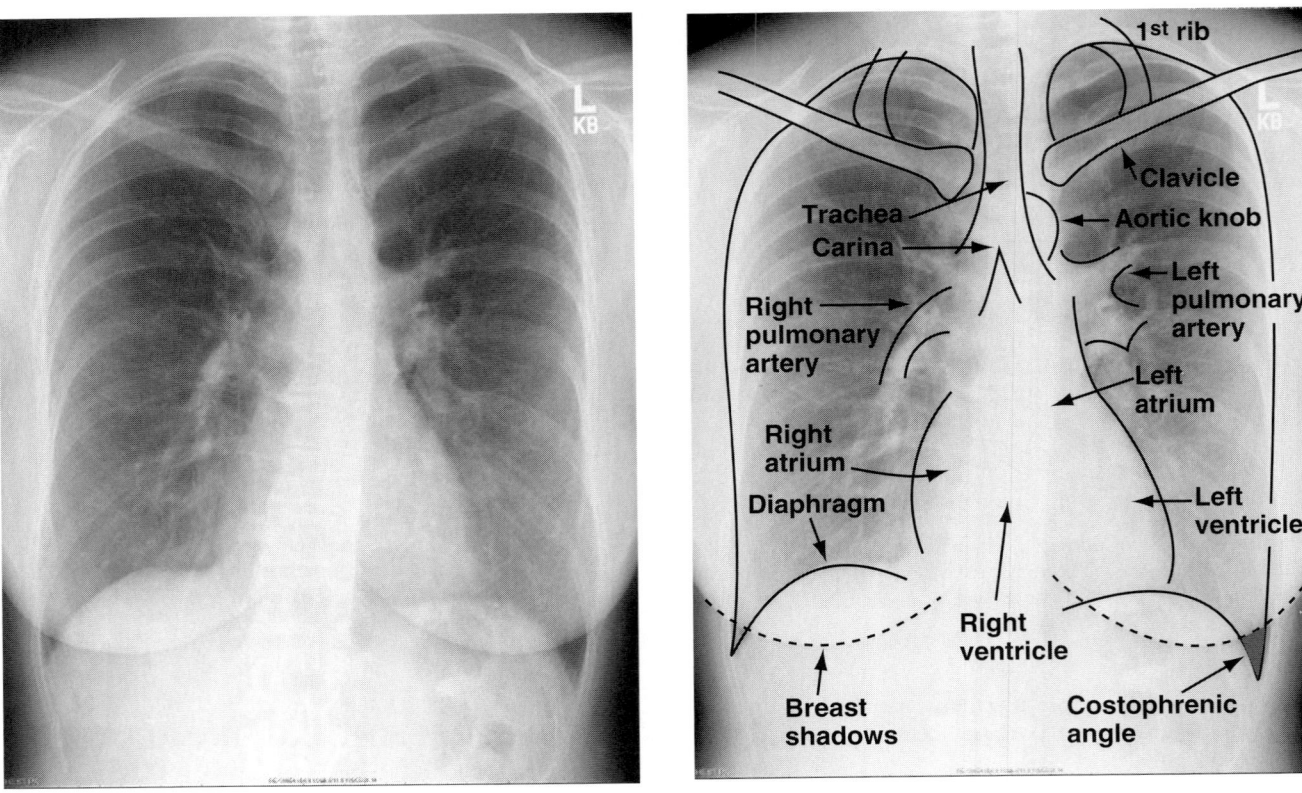

■ **Figure 15–3.** *(A)* Normal posteroanterior chest radiograph. *(B)* Outline of structures visible on normal posteroanterior chest radiograph.

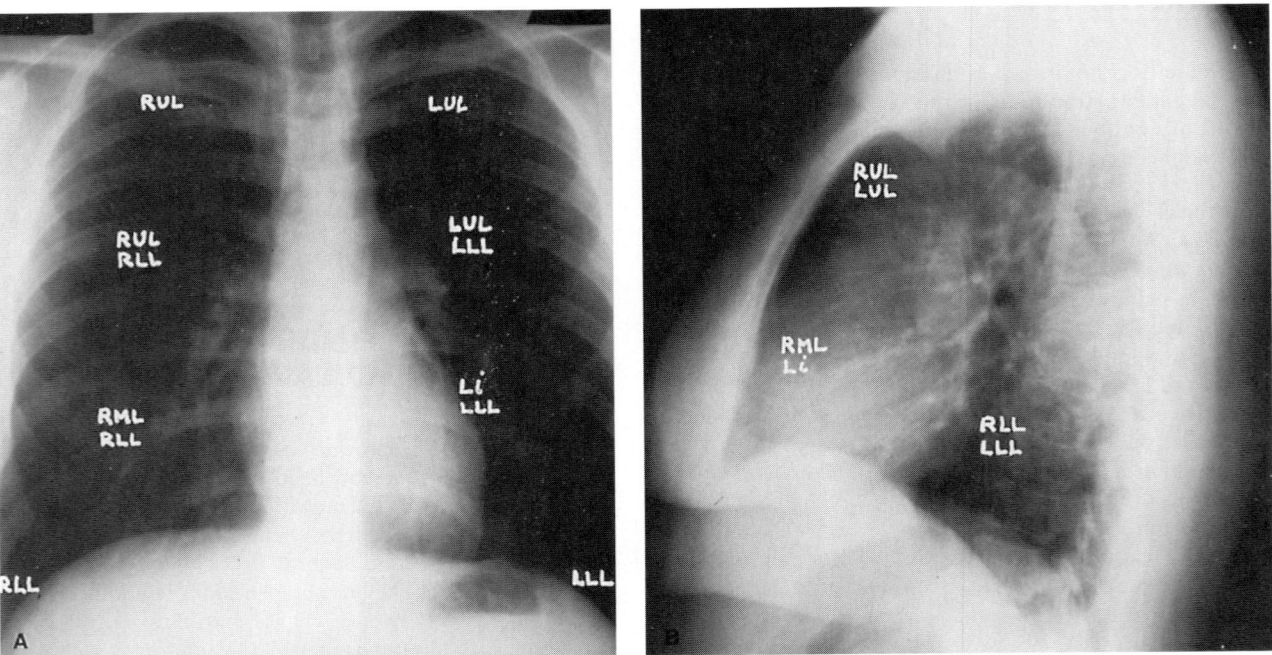

■ **Figure 15–4.** *(A)* Location of the lung lobes on the frontal chest radiograph. Because some lobes are anterior and some posterior, an abnormality in a certain area on a frontal chest radiograph can be in one of two lobes. Obtaining a lateral film or noticing whether an anterior or posterior structure is obliterated by an abnormal density can help with localization. RUL, right upper lobe; RLL, right lower lobe; LLL, left lower lobe; RML, right middle lobe; LUL, left upper lobe; Li, lingula. *(B)* Location of lung lobes on a lateral radiograph. Abnormalities of the right middle lobe and lingula would go undetected with posterior chest auscultation.

Table 15–1 ■ RADIOLOGIC APPEARANCE OF INVASIVE LINES AND DEVICES IN CARDIOVASCULAR CARE

Invasive Line or Device	Description of Radiologic Appearance for Correct Position
Central venous pressure catheter (CVP) or peripheral inserted central catheter (PICC)	Ideal position is in the superior vena cava. The CVP line tip should always be above the level of the right atrium or the catheter tip may slip into the right atrium or ventricle and produce arrhythmias, or rarely, cardiac perforation. Central lines can be misplaced into the subclavian artery or misdirected up into the internal jugular vein. You should trace the central line from its point of vascular entry to the tip to insure appropriate placement.
Pulmonary artery catheter (PAC)	The PAC tip should been within the main right or left pulmonary arteries and should extend no more than 2–4 cm beyond the vertebral midline. If the catheter tip is beyond this point there is increased risk of pulmonary artery occlusion, infarction, and rupture. The course of the PAC should be traced from its entry point to insure there is no looping in the ventricle. If the catheter tip is in the right ventricle, ventricular tachycardia may result from endocardial irritation.
Endotracheal tube (ETT)	The ETT should be visible as a radiopaque line within the trachea. The distal tip of the ETT should be a minimum of 4 cm above the main carina to avoid accidental right or left mainstem intubation. The ETT distal tip should be no higher than the level of the clavicles to avoid accidental extubation. Position of the head effects the location of the ETT tip. Flexion of the head towards the chest pulls the ETT up the trachea, while extension pushes the tube tip further into the trachea.
Chest tube (CT)	Chest tubes are used to drain air or fluid from the pleural cavity. Chest tubes inserted for pneumothorax are inserted towards the apex where gas or air collects and CTs inserted to drain fluid are inserted toward dependent areas around the base of the lungs. All of the islets that promote drainage (positioned along the proximal portion of the CT) need to be projected within the chest wall.
Intraaortic balloon pump (IABP)	The tip of the IABP should be located in the distal aortic arch, just below the aortic knob and distal to the left subclavian artery. The oblong radiopaque IABP tip has the appearance of a large grain of rice.
Transvenous pacer (TVP)	Pacemaker leads extend from their point of entry in the right or left brachiocephalic veins into the right atrium (atrial lead) and the trabeculae of the right ventricle (ventricular lead). If the pacer is malfunctioning, the CXR may show fractured or misplaced leads.
Feeding tube (FT)	The entire FT is radiopaque. One should be able to trace the FT through the esophagus, stomach, and into the duodenum.
Tracheostomy tube	Midline within the trachea with the tip several cm above the main carina.

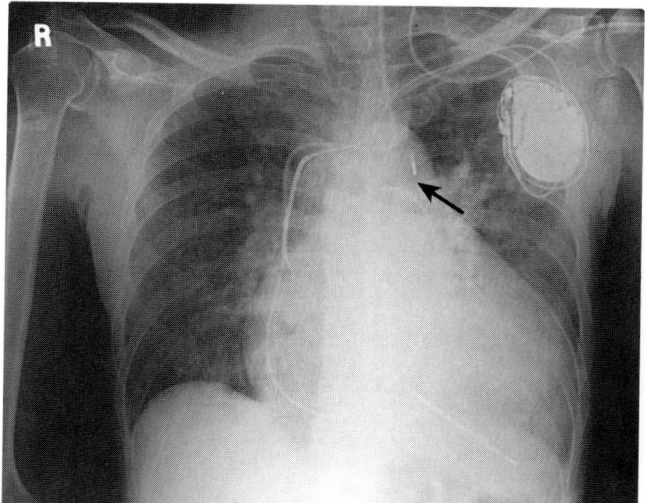

■ **Figure 15–5.** Correct IABP placement in aortic knob. The *small arrow* denotes the IABP tip just distal to the left subclavian artery. The patient has end-stage heart failure and is awaiting cardiac transplant. Note that the patient has significant cardiomegaly and also has an implantable defibrillator/pacer and lead in the right ventricle, in addition to a pulmonary artery catheter entering the left internal jugular with the tip visible in the main pulmonary artery.

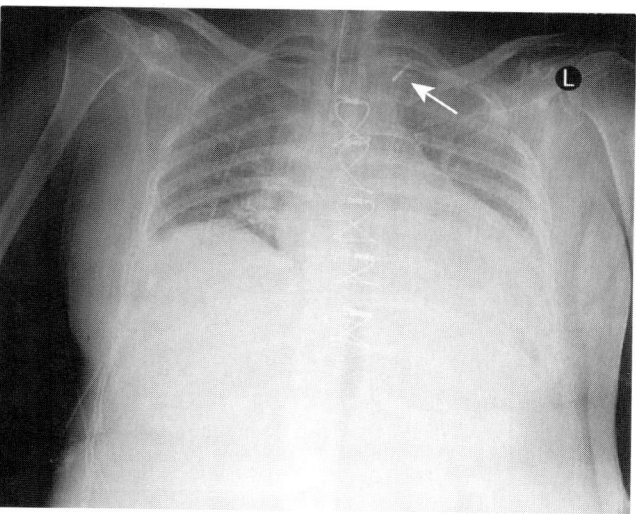

■ **Figure 15–6.** IABP placed too high into left subclavian artery. This IABP was emergently inserted at the bedside for a cardiac transplant patient in acute rejection and cardiogenic shock. The tip is above the aortic knob into the left subclavian artery. On exam, the patient had no left radial or brachial pulse until the IABP was pulled back 4 cm.

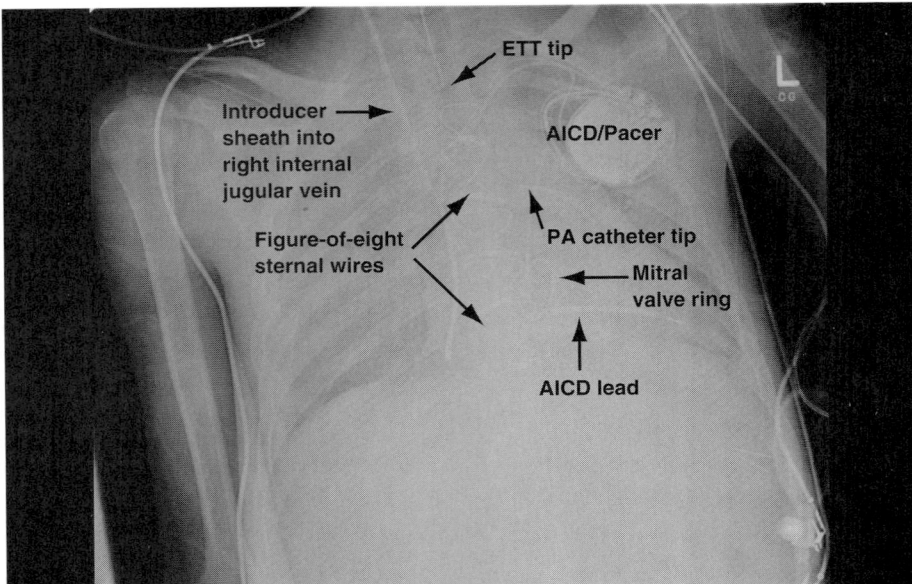

■ **Figure 15–7.** Line placement after cardiac surgery. This is a 17-year-old patient immediately postoperative after a mitral valve repair. Note the tip of the ETT at the level of the clavicles, in addition to his multiple other invasive lives including PA catheter and AICD. The ovoid object in the heart is his radiopaque mitral valve annuloplasty ring.

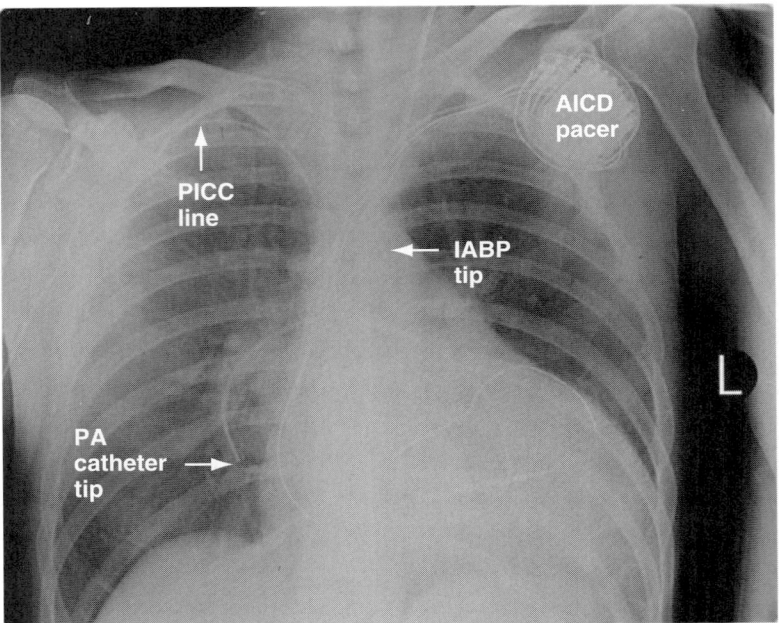

■ **Figure 15–8.** The PA catheter tip is out too far. The tip of the pulmonary artery catheter lies several cm beyond the hilum and is at risk for spontaneous wedge and pulmonary infarction. Patient also has an AICD, PICC line, and IABP.

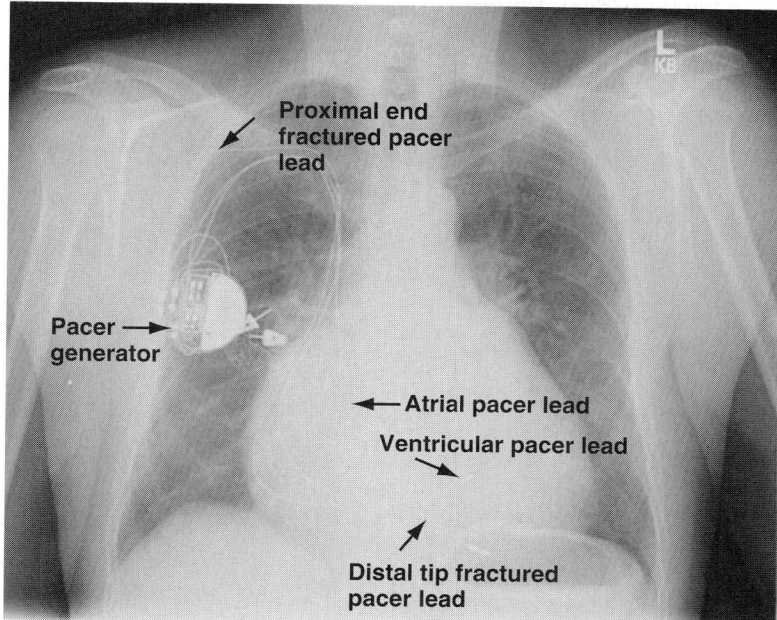

■ **Figure 15–9.** Pacemaker in-patient with cardiomegaly. Patient is a 27-year-old male with congenital heart disease. He had a previous pacer, but his original leads fractured and a new device and leads were placed. New leads can be seen in both the right atrium and right ventricle. A second ventricular lead can be seen in the right ventricle; if you trace this lead back, you will find it is fractured at the proximal end.

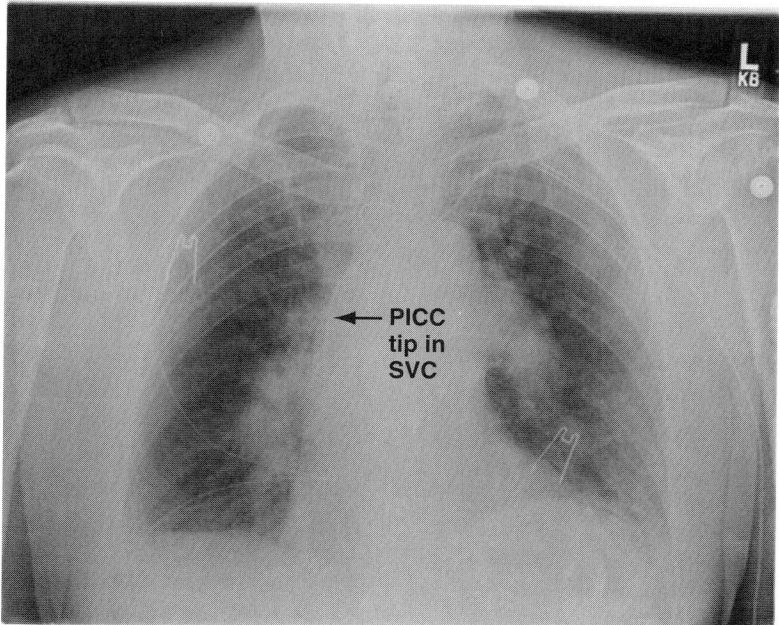

■ **Figure 15–10.** PICC line placement. Patient is a 56-year-old male with history of severe pulmonary hypertension secondary to chronic thromboembolic disease. Patient was postoperative after a pulmonary thromboendarterectomy. The tip of the PICC inserted into his left antecubital vein is correctly positioned in the superior vena cava. Note that, in addition to bilateral pleural effusions (see blunted costal phrenic angles), this individual also has very large pulmonary arteries extending from his hilum.

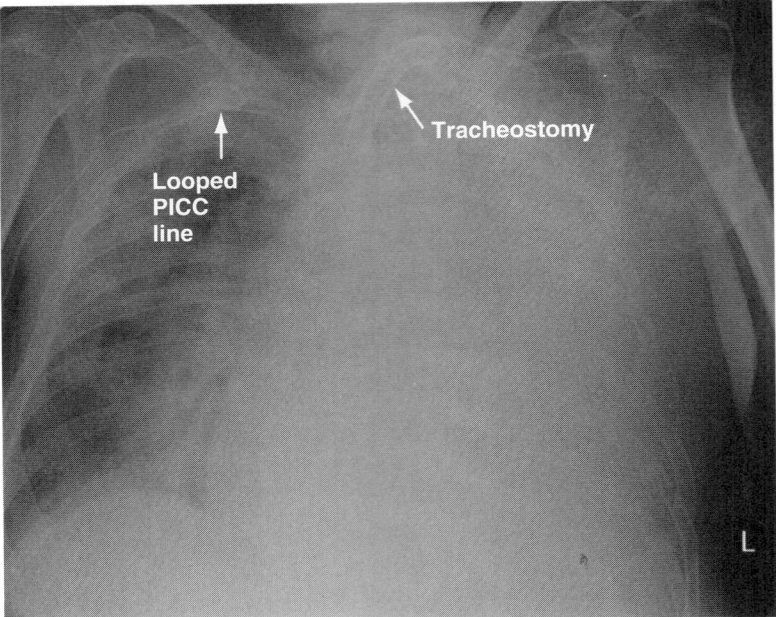

■ **Figure 15–11.** The PICC is looped in the right subclavian vein. Patient is a 55-year-old male who had multiple complications after emergent repair of a ruptured descending aortic aneurysm. Note that he also has a massive left hemothorax and tracheostomy tube in correct position.

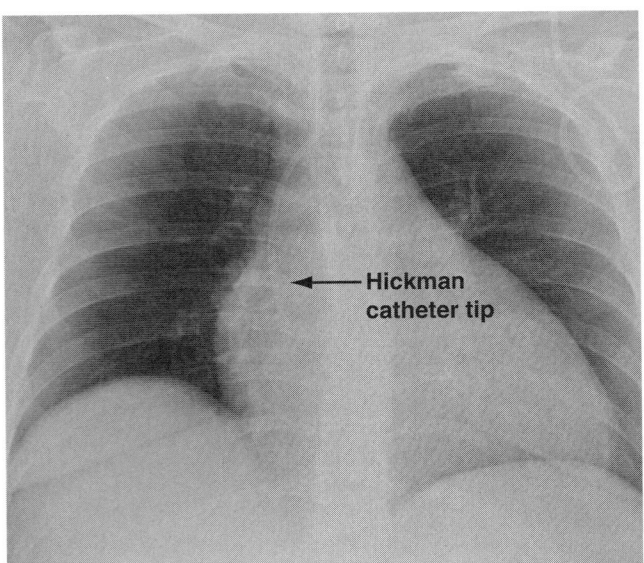

■ **Figure 15–12.** Hickman central line placement. Tunneled central line with correct position into the superior vena cava.

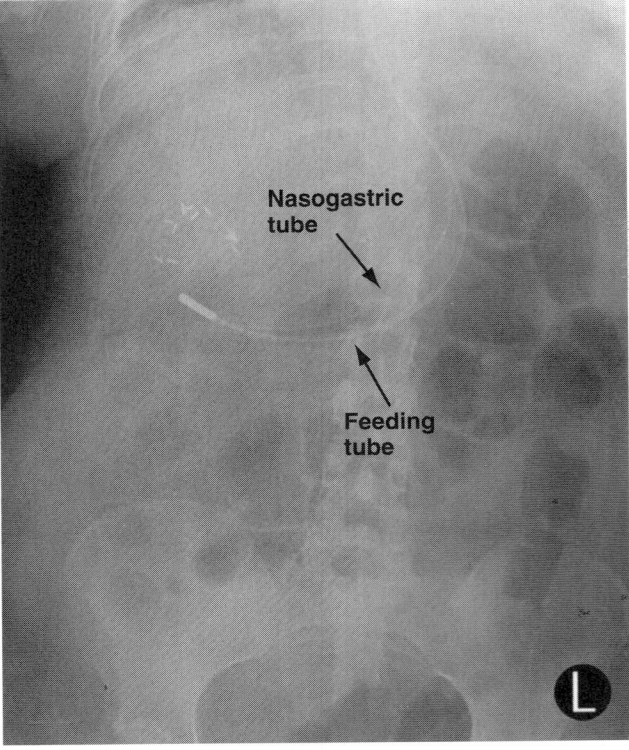

■ **Figure 15–13.** Feeding tube placement. Abdominal radiograph showing both the feeding tube and the nasogastric tube in the duodenum.

Table 15–2 ■ COMMON CLINICAL PRESENTATIONS IN ACUTE CARE AND RADIOLOGIC FINDINGS

Clinical Diagnosis	Radiologic Findings
Pericardial effusion	Enlarged cardiac silhouette with a "water bottle" appearance.
	May look very similar to cardiomegaly.
	Diagnosis of pericardial effusion should be verified with echocardiography.
Congestive heart failure (CHF)	In chronic CHF the heart is usually enlarged; in acute heart failure the heart may be of normal size.
	May have cephalization of blood vessels (increased size and number of blood vessels near the lung apices).
	May have interstitial fluid that begins at the lung bases and extends upwards.
	Frank pulmonary edema and pleural effusions may develop.
Aortic aneurysm	Ascending and/or descending aorta are enlarged.
	Widened mediastinum.
	New pleural effusion if leak or rupture.
Pneumothorax	Frontal, full upright CXR shows the visceral pleura as a thin white line.
	There is a hyperlucent area where there are no bronchovascular or lung markings.
	Pneumothorax is more difficult to see in supine film.
Pleural effusion	Fluid moves to dependent areas of pleural space and is best seen on upright or decubitus (side lying) CXR views.
	At least 200 to 300 cc must be present in the pleural space to cause costophrenic blunting.
	By doing decubitus views (side lying), one may determine if the effusion is free flowing and amenable to thoracentesis.
Pneumonia	Alveolar or interstitial pattern of white opacity.
	May be localized to a single lobe or be more diffuse.
	Air bronchograms are frequently present in lobar pneumonia.
Acute respiratory distress syndrome (ARDS)	Diffuse bilateral patchy infiltrates, "ground glass" appearance.
	May be confused with CHF.

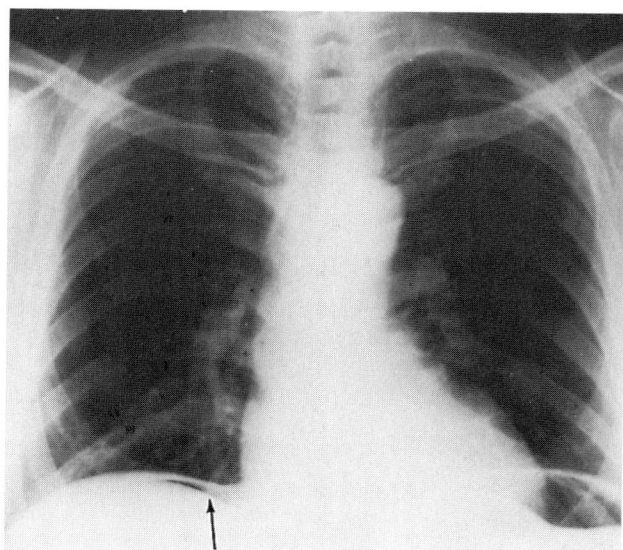

■ **Figure 15–14.** Free air under the diaphragm (*arrow*). This patient had epigastric pain and diaphoresis. The admission radiograph showed free air under the diaphragm consistent with a perforated viscus. At operation, a perforated peptic ulcer was found. The patient must be upright for the air to be seen under the diaphragm.

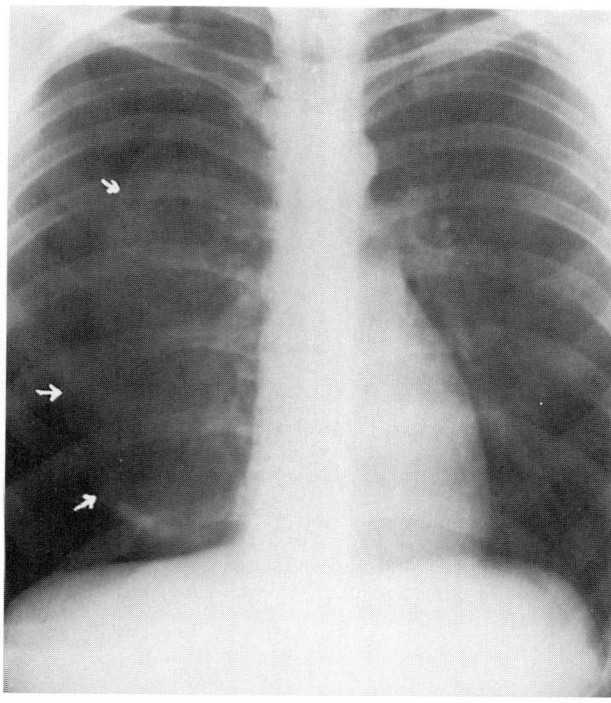

■ **Figure 15–15.** Pneumothorax. The patient may have acute chest pain and shortness of breath. Physical findings include absent or reduced breath sounds on the side of the pneumothorax and tympany or a hollow sound on chest percussion, with possibly a shift of the trachea to the side away from the pneumothorax. The *arrows* indicate the outer border of the right lung. The remainder of the right chest cavity is filled with air in the pleural space.

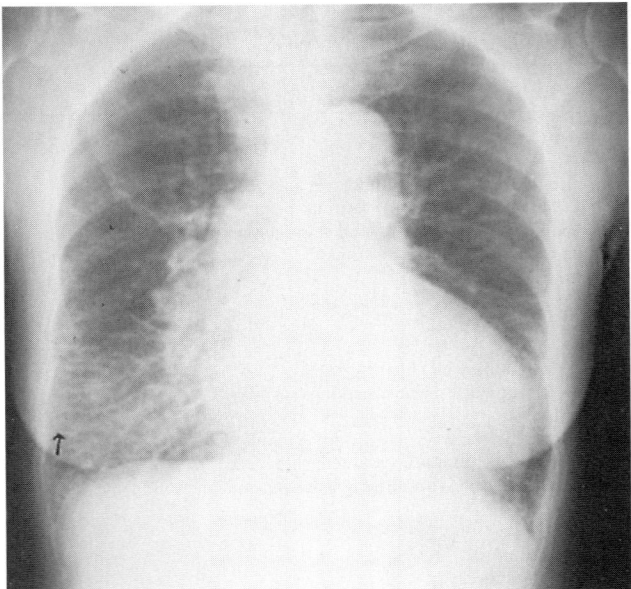

■ **Figure 15–16.** Cardiogenic pulmonary edema with cardiomegaly. In this radiograph, Kerley B lines are seen (*arrow*). These represent dilated pulmonary lymph vessels, which facilitate pulmonary edema removal from the alveolar spaces.

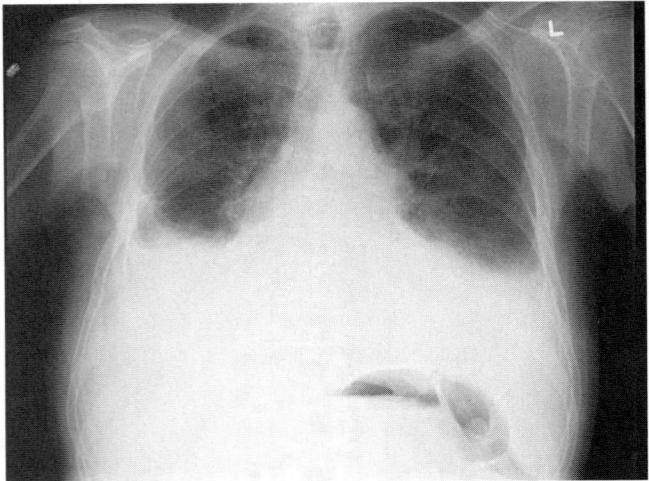

■ **Figure 15–17.** Congestive heart failure with bilateral pleural effusions. This 88-year-old man with severe aortic stenosis was admitted with severe shortness of breath and worsening heart failure.

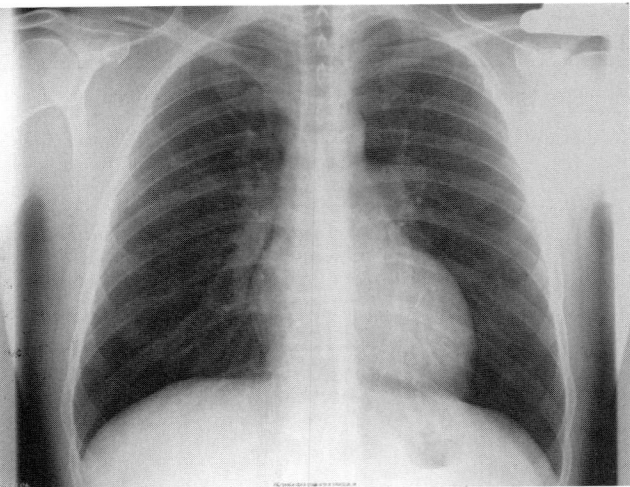

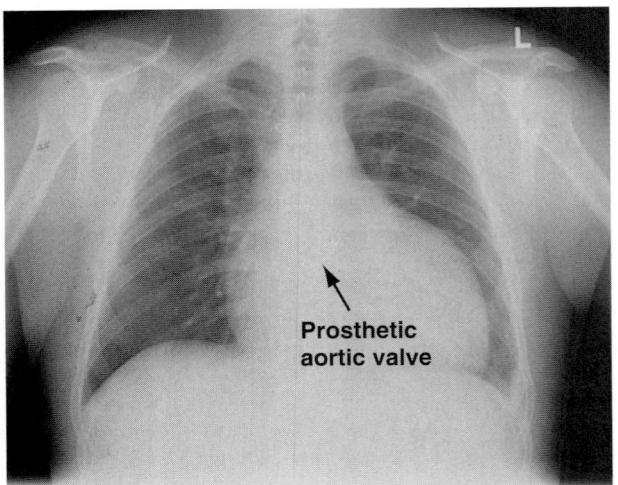

■ **Figure 15–18.** (*A*) Preoperative patient with aortic regurgitation. (*B*) Same patient 3 weeks after aortic valve replacement. Patient now has a large pericardial effusion creating tamponade physiology.

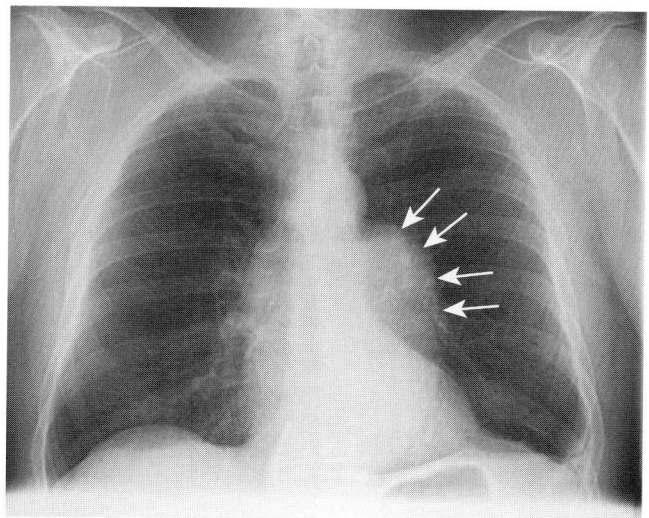

■ Figure 15–19. Descending thoracic aortic aneurysm. "Bulging" of the descending aorta noted by *arrows* in a 57-year-old male with history of blunt trauma to chest as well as hypertension.

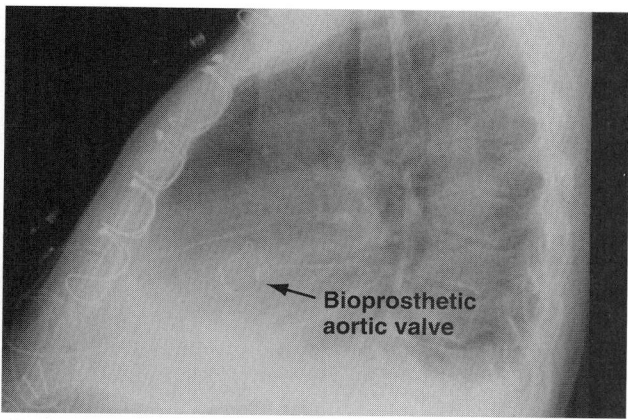

■ Figure 15–21. Radiologic appearance of stented bioprosthetic aortic valve replacement in lateral CXR view. Stents point toward blood flow.

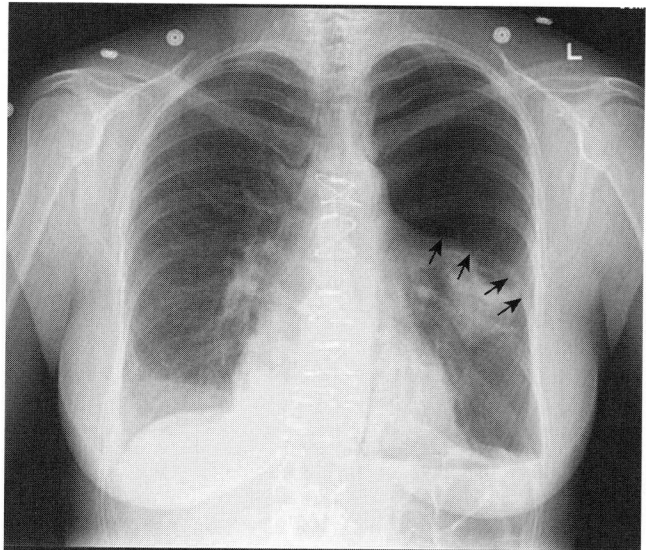

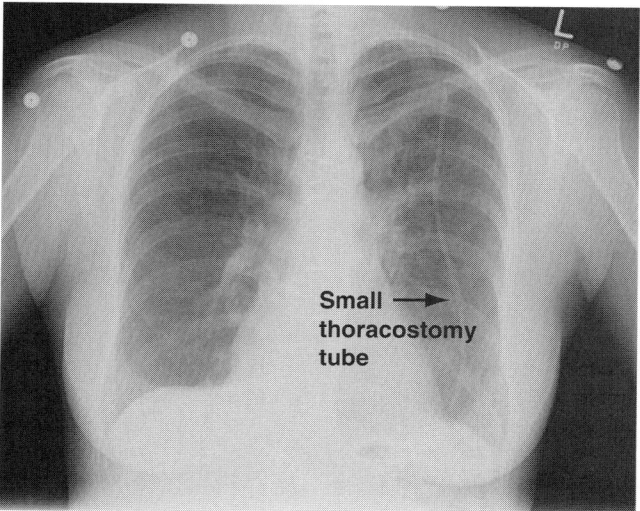

■ Figure 15–20. *(A)* Large left pneumothorax after surgical repair of a patent foramen ovale. *(B)* Re-expansion of left lung after placement of small thoracostomy tube in interventional radiology department.

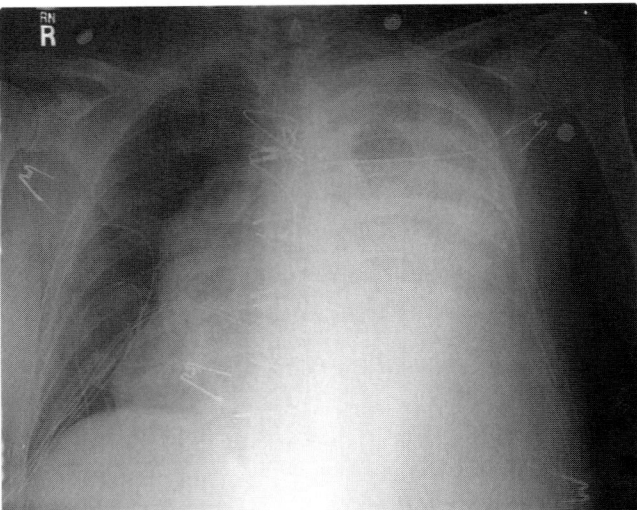

■ **Figure 15–22.** Massive left pleural effusion with mediastinal shift. This 62-year-old man had massive left pleural effusion causing severe orthopnea and shortness of breath. Patient underwent thoracentesis three times in a 24-hour period to drain a total of 3500 cc of serosanguineous fluid.

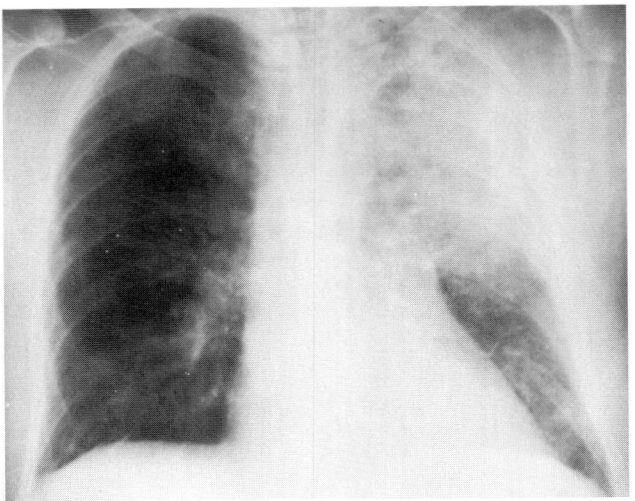

■ **Figure 15–24.** Left upper lobe pneumonia. Signs of consolidation (bronchial breathing, crackles, and dullness to percussion) are heard over the left upper chest. In pneumonia, egophony is heard over areas of consolidated lung. The patient is instructed to say the letter "e," and the lung is auscultated to demonstrate this finding. Normally the "e" sound is heard, but consolidated lung changes the "e" to an "a" that sounds like the "bleating of a goat." This sign is also known as "an e-to-a change."

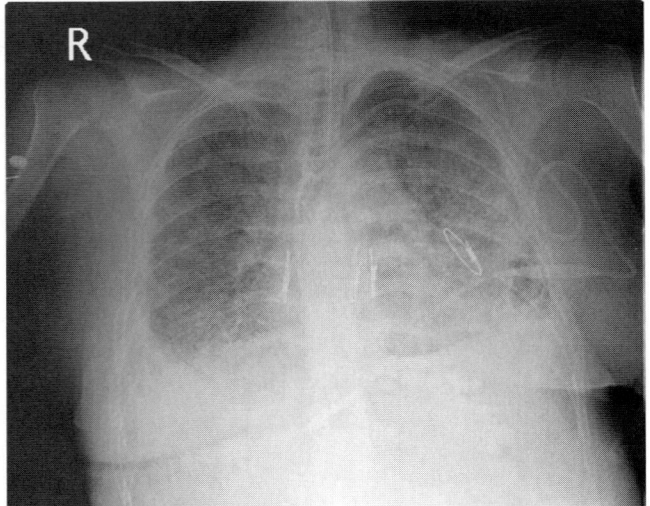

■ **Figure 15–23.** Acute respiratory distress syndrome. Diffuse bilateral opacities in patient postoperatively after bilateral lung transplantation.

REFERENCES

Blumenthal, N. P., & Miller, W. T. (1997). Radiographic pulmonary infiltrates. *AACN Clinical Issues*, 8(3), 411–424.

Brady, T. J., Grist, T. M., Westra, S. J., et al. (2003). Valvular. In *Pocket radiologist: Cardiac top 100 diagnoses* (pp. 53–75). Salt Lake City, UT: Amirsys.

Chapman, S., & Nakielny, R. (2003). *Aids to radiological differential diagnosis* (pp. 195–210). Edinburgh, Scotland: Saunders.

Connolly, M. A. (2001). Black, white, and shades of gray: common abnormalities in chest radiographs. *AACN Clinical Issues*, 12(2), 259–269.

Dettenmeier, P. A.(1995). *Radiographic assessment for nurses* (pp. 1–106). St. Louis, MO: Mosby.

Evans, T. J. (1992). AANA journal course: Update for nurse anesthetists—fundamentals of chest radiography: techniques and interpretation for the anesthetist. *Journal of AANA*, 60(1), 45–60.

Fraser, R. G., Pare, J. A. P., Pare, P. D., et al. (1988). *Diagnosis of diseases of the chest* (pp. 1–295). Philadelphia:WB Saunders.

George, R. B., Light, R. W., Matthay, M. A., et al. (1995). *Chest medicine: Essentials of pulmonary and critical care medicine* (pp. 81–92). Baltimore: Williams & Wilkins.

Groskin, S. A. (1998). Tubes, lines, and catheters. In D. S. Katz, K. R. Math & S. A. Groskin, *Radiology secrets* (pp. 39–45). Philadelphia: Hanley & Belfus.

Lillington, G. A. (1987). *A diagnostic approach to chest diseases* (pp. 23–27). Baltimore: Williams & Wilkins.

Stern, E. J. & White, C. S. (2003). Tube and line positions. In *Chest radiology companion* (pp. 17–32). Philadelphia: Lippincott Williams & Wilkins.

Echocardiography

MARGARET L. HALL

Many of the advances in diagnostic cardiology over the last half of the twentieth century were directed toward identifying anatomic and physiologic "noninvasive" tests, which can be performed with minimal risk and discomfort to the patient and maximum diagnostic accuracy and reproducibility. Development of many of our newer diagnostic modalities has evolved hand-in-hand with the arrival and evolution of the computer era, which has revolutionized data acquisition and manipulation. These rapid advances continue, providing ever-improving image resolution among other benefits. Echocardiography is one discipline in which these advances have not only improved diagnostic accuracy, but have actually contributed to the improved understanding of disease states. Currently, the diagnostic transthoracic echocardiogram is second only to the electrocardiogram in the frequency of its use in cardiac diagnosis.

Trained sonographers in multiple settings including the outpatient clinic, the hospital ward, the intensive care unit, and the emergency room routinely perform transthoracic echocardiograms and Doppler ultrasound examinations. Transesophageal echocardiograms are performed both in specially equipped and staffed diagnostic laboratories as well as in the operating room. In some hospitals, emergency room physicians (Mandavia et al., 2001) and anesthesiologists have been trained to perform and interpret echocardiograms in certain clinical situations. The American College of Cardiology and American Heart Association in collaboration with the American Society of Echocardiography, the Society of Cardiovascular Anesthesiologists and the Society of Pediatric Echocardiography have collaborated to develop competency standards for these examinations (Quinones et al., 2003). In this chapter we will explore some of the technical aspects of transthoracic echocardiography (TTE), diagnostic Doppler ultrasound and transesophageal echocardiography (TEE). In the second part of the chapter we will explore the echocardiographic and Doppler ultrasound findings in normal and pathologic conditions. Finally, we will touch upon newer and experimental techniques based on variations of echocardiographic technology.

The cardiac nurse can participate in the successful completion of these examinations by having an understanding of what the examination can add to understanding of the patient's condition and by educating the patient regarding the test procedure. This is relatively straightforward for the transthoracic echocardiogram. This test requires patient cooperation for body positioning and breathing; the pressure of the transducer against the chest or abdomen may be mildly uncomfortable for some individuals. Patient instruction for transesophageal echocardiography is much more complicated. In addition to stable positioning the patient needs to be oriented to the effects of conscious sedation, if used, and to the procedure of endoscope placement, similar to diagnostic upper gastrointestinal endoscopy. Achieving nursing goals in this setting rests on an understanding of the patient's condition, the specific clinical questions that may be answered by the test, and the general principles of the examination.

The importance of the sonographer in the successful acquisition of a diagnostic study cannot be overestimated. These individuals must possess sophisticated knowledge of cardiac anatomy, physiology and pathology. They must master the technical skills required to obtain diagnostic images and must demonstrate high degrees of technical skill to obtain a clinically accurate study. They must understand the physics and mechanics that govern examination equipment and techniques (Ehler et al., 2001). The sonographer's ability to vary the testing routine intelligently based on preliminary findings is so important that some centers perform echocardiography with a physician in attendance solely to guide the information collection. Other centers devote long training and mentoring periods for sonographers so that they may perform examinations independently which are then reviewed and interpreted by physicians at a later time. Whenever possible, it is helpful for nurses to view the echocardiograms on their patients. These studies provide a wonderful opportunity to study cardiac anatomy and physiology in disease states and can greatly enhance the nurse's understanding of the patient's condition (Fig. 16-1).

In contrast to transthoracic echocardiograms, transesophageal echocardiograms are typically performed by physicians who introduce the endoscope into the esophagus and manipulate it to obtain the various echocardiographic views. Most frequently this is a cardiologist in the diagnostic laboratory and a cardiac anesthesiologist in the operating room. The sonographer manages the machine settings during image acquisition. The trained nurse assists with topical anesthesia, administration of conscious sedation and intravenous contrast agents, monitoring vital signs during the procedure and post-sedation patient recovery.

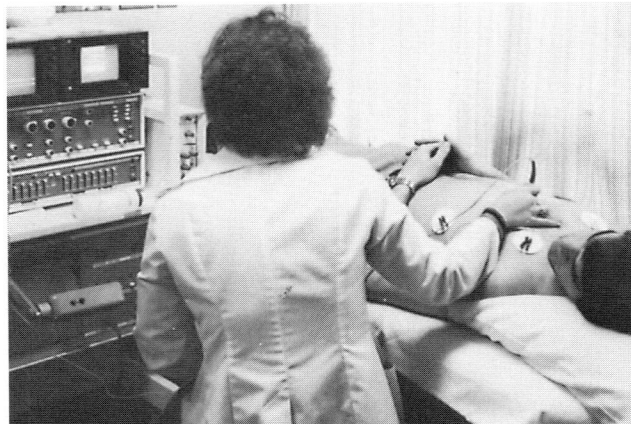

■ **Figure 16–1.** Position of patient and examiner for echocardio-gram. Portable machinery permits the examination at bedside with no loss in quality. (From Chang, S. [1976]. *M-mode echocardiographic techniques and pattern recognition.* Philadelphia: Lea & Febiger.)

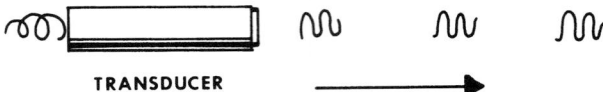

■ **Figure 16–2.** Transducer emits short bursts of sound.

TECHNICAL ASPECTS

Transthoracic Echocardiography

The study of ultrasound, the designation given to sound waves of frequencies higher than the human ear can detect, began nearly a century ago. The development of sonar (from so*u*nd *na*vigation *ranging) probably represents the first wide-spread use of pulsed ultrasound for remote object detection and localization. Today, ultrasound technology is used extensively for diagnosis in other parts of the body and in fetal evaluation and is therefore frequently familiar to patients and their families.

Echocardiography and Doppler imaging operate much like SONAR, and this analogy is often useful in explaining the test to patients. The ultrasound transducer serves both as a sender and a detector of sound waves. These high-frequency (2.5 to 5 MHz) waves are generated by the application of changing voltage to a substance called a *piezoelectric crystal.* This crystal deforms slightly under the influence of the electrical current, and a sound wave is generated. The waves are generated in short bursts (e.g., 1 microsecond), after which the transducer operates as a receiver for the remainder of 1 millisecond, then another short burst of sound is generated and received (Fig. 16-2). These sound waves cannot be heard or felt by the patient and produce no known damaging effect on tissues (Feigenbaum, 1994).

The speed of sound through any medium is determined by the density of the medium. Denser media transmit sound faster than less dense media. Whenever the ultrasound wave strikes a change in tissue density (such as that between blood and muscle or between soft tissue and bone), a portion of the wave is reflected back to the transducer. The density differences within the body are relatively minor. This means that the speed of the sound wave can be assumed to be nearly constant, and therefore the time between sound emission and sound detection can be used to calculate the distance between

the transducer and the reflected tissue interface. The intensity of returning sound is greatest when the tissue interface is perpendicular to the sound beam and least when parallel to the sound beam.

When the ultrasound signal returns to the crystal, it once again deforms it and thereby generates a voltage. The voltage is processed by the computer to supply images in several ways.

The transducer sound beam is like a flashlight beam shined into a darkened room. Changes in the angulation of the transducer demonstrate different structures or parts of structures. If the objects in the room are stationary, then moving the flashlight through several degrees of arc illuminates each of the objects in the room.

For moving structures like the heart, such a system would result in an unclear sound signal because, over a period of time, the distance from transducer to tissue density interface would change continuously. This problem was first solved by the development of what is called *M-mode* (*M* for *motion*) *echocardiography.* A schematic representation of an M-mode scan is shown in Figure 16-3. In this figure, the transducer is slowly rotated on the chest wall, as shown in Figure 16-4. The contours in the M-mode tracing are caused by cardiac motion relative to the transducer and thus bear little resemblance to our usual visual image of the heart. On an M-mode scan, time is on the horizontal axis, and the distance from the tissue density interface to the transducer is on the vertical axis.

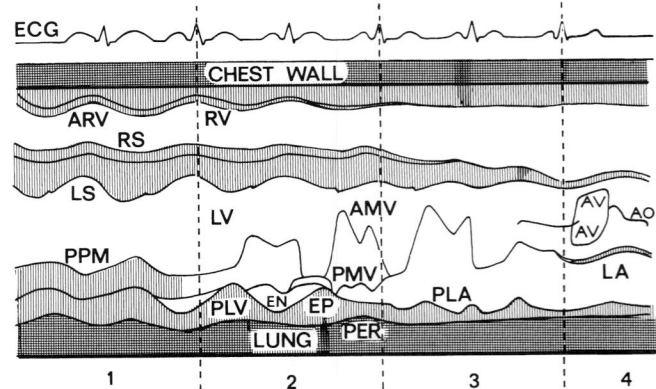

■ **Figure 16–3.** Schematic representation of an echocardiogram from the four-transducer positions, illustrated in Figure 16-4. ARV, anterior right ventricular wall; RS, right side of interventricular septum; LS, left side of ventricular septum; PPM, posterior papillary muscle; RV, right ventricle; LV, left ventricle; PLV, posterior left ventricular wall; EN, endocardium; EP, epicardium; PER, pericardium; AMV, anterior mitral valve leaflet; PMV, posterior mitral valve leaflet; PLA, posterior left atrial wall; AV, aortic valve cusps; AO, aorta; LA, left atrium. (Adapted from Feigenbaum, H. [1972]. Clinical application of echocardiography. *Progress in Cardiovascular Disease, 14,* 531.)

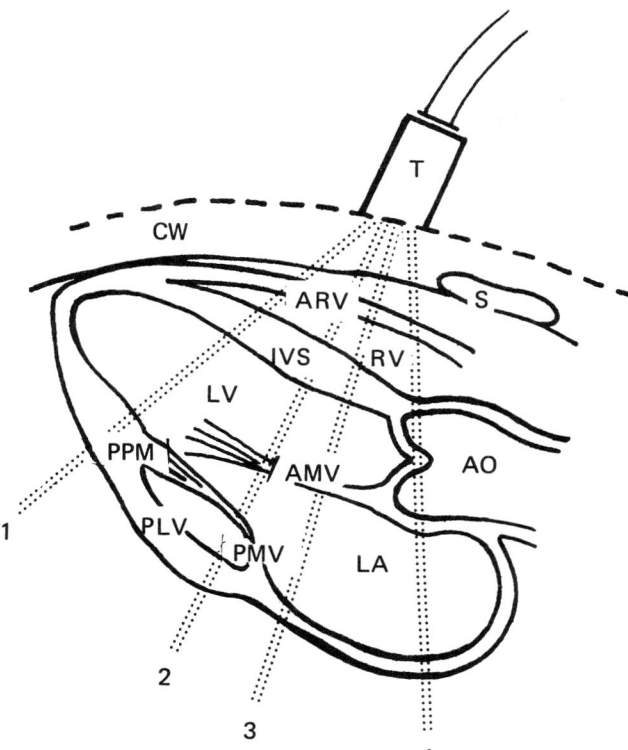

■ **Figure 16–4.** Schematic representation of the course of the ultrasonic beam to achieve the echo represented in Figure 16-3. CW, chest wall; T, transducer; S, sternum. Other abbreviations are defined in the legend to Figure 16-3. (Adapted from Feigenbaum, H. [1972]. Clinical application of echocardiography. *Progress in Cardiovascular Disease*, 14, 531.)

Two-dimensional (2-D) echocardiography is a further refinement on this technique. In 2-D echocardiography, the transducer sender-detector rotates automatically and rapidly through several degrees of arc. The resulting image is displayed on a video screen and recorded on videotape. It represents a tomographic "slice" of cardiac structures, thereby more closely resembling recognizable cardiac anatomy. Incorrect positioning or beam angulation, however, can significantly alter the appearance in 2-D echocardiography and obscure diagnostic information. Just as the body can be examined from several different views, so the cardiac anatomy can be viewed from several acoustic "windows." Because sound waves are diffused by air (lung) and totally reflected by bone (ribs), only a few surface locations on the chest and abdomen can be used for examination of the heart. The most common of these are shown in Figures 16-5 through 16-10, with the usual images they produce. Many modifications of these views are routinely used by experienced sonographers. Echocardiographic measurements are frequently obtained on-line from the M-mode images because the resolution is usually better than that on the corresponding 2-D study. The exact methods of measuring the dimensions or motion of each structure are standardized by convention. Because of anatomic variation, all such measurements cannot be obtained in all patients, so some parameters may be evaluated qualitatively rather than quantitatively by the experienced interpreter.

Doppler Echocardiography

The *Doppler principle* states that the frequency of sound emitted or reflected from the moving object is changed in a predictable way by the motion of the object. When the object moves toward the detector, the frequency increases; when the object moves away from the detector, the frequency decreases. This principle is best illustrated by the change in pitch (sound frequency) detected as a whistling train approaches and then recedes. In clinical Doppler, sound waves are reflected off moving red blood cells. The Doppler frequency shift is in the audible range and can be displayed as an audible signal or as a visual image graphed with frequency on the vertical axis and time on the horizontal axis (Fig. 16-11). The Doppler waveform can be recorded with the same transducer used for 2-D and M-mode echocardiography. It can be focused to "listen" at a certain point in the 2-D image so as to "hear" blood flow velocity at that point. This process is known as *pulsed Doppler*. Alternatively, the transducer may "listen" for all the velocities generated along the line of the sound beam. This is known as *continuous wave Doppler*. Technical aspects govern the choice between these two modes. Doppler shift is greatest when flow is exactly parallel to the sound beam (in contrast to M-mode or 2-D echocardiography). The magnitude of the frequency change is related to the velocity of blood flow in the sampled area. The pressure *difference,* but not the absolute pressure as blood flows from one area to another (e.g., across a valve orifice, through a conduit) can be approximated by the formula $P = 4V^2$, where P is the peak pressure gradient across the orifice and V is the velocity (in meters per second) of the sampled red blood cells. The timing of the waveform (systolic versus diastolic) is determined from the superimposed ECG. By convention, flow toward the transducer is indicated as a positive waveform and flow away from the transducer as a negative waveform. Thus, Doppler can record the location, timing, direction, and magnitude of blood flow velocity.

The 2-D equivalent of the visual or audible Doppler signal is *color flow Doppler*. This technique transforms sectors of recorded flow signals into different colors that are then superimposed on the real-time 2-D image. By convention, red is used for signals moving toward the transducer and blue is used for signals moving away from the transducer. The intensity of the color indicates velocity, with faster signals appearing lighter and slower signals appearing darker. Turbulence is indicated by a mosaic color pattern or by color mixture (e.g., green, yellow). Because an entire sector is imaged, color Doppler is much less tedious than pulsed Doppler mapping and is useful as a screening tool for valvular regurgitation. Good quality scans give a sense of the pattern of blood flow within the chamber through the cardiac cycle.

SPECIAL TECHNIQUES

Stress Echocardiography

The two techniques of exercise (bicycle or treadmill) testing and echocardiography can be used together to increase the diagnostic accuracy of standard exercise testing. In this technique,

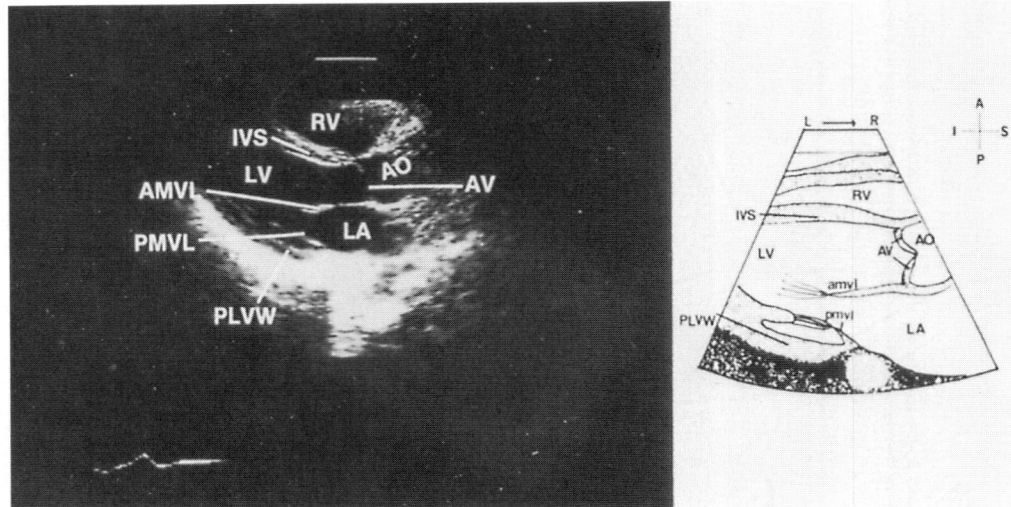

■ **Figure 16–5.** Parasternal long-axis view of the left ventricle. Still frame (*left*) with schematic drawing (*right*) of the long-axis left ventricular view. The aorta (AO) and aortic valve (AV) are seen at the right of the screen, and the left ventricle (LV) is at the left. The interventricular septum (IVS) is relatively horizontal and continuous with the anterior wall of the aorta. The right ventricle (RV) is anterior, and the posterior left ventricular wall (PLVW) and the left atrium (LA) are posterior. The anterior mitral valve leaflet (AMVL) and the posterior mitral valve leaflet (PMVL) are seen in the center of the picture. (From Levine, R.B., Brown, S.A., Janko, C. et al. [1984]. *Two-dimensional and Doppler echocardiographic technique* [p. 8]. Seattle, WA: University of Washington.)

four standard echocardiographic views (parasternal long axis, parasternal short axis, apical four chamber, apical two chamber) are obtained with ECG gating before exercise testing and displayed on a single screen image as a "cine loop" or single recurring cardiac cycle. Stress testing is performed in the standard fashion, and the four views are obtained rapidly during the first 90 seconds of recovery. The images can then be shuffled or reformatted with computer-assisted techniques to juxtapose the pre-exercise and post exercise images from each view.

The normal response to exercise is an increase in contractility. Areas of hypoperfusion appear normal on the rest images and become relatively hypokinetic with exercise. Areas of infarction show hypokinesis or akinesis at rest and with exercise. In stress echocardiography, it is extremely important to obtain all the images within the shortest possible period of time after exercise. Patients must be carefully coached to assist the sonographer by breathing properly during this image acquisition sequence.

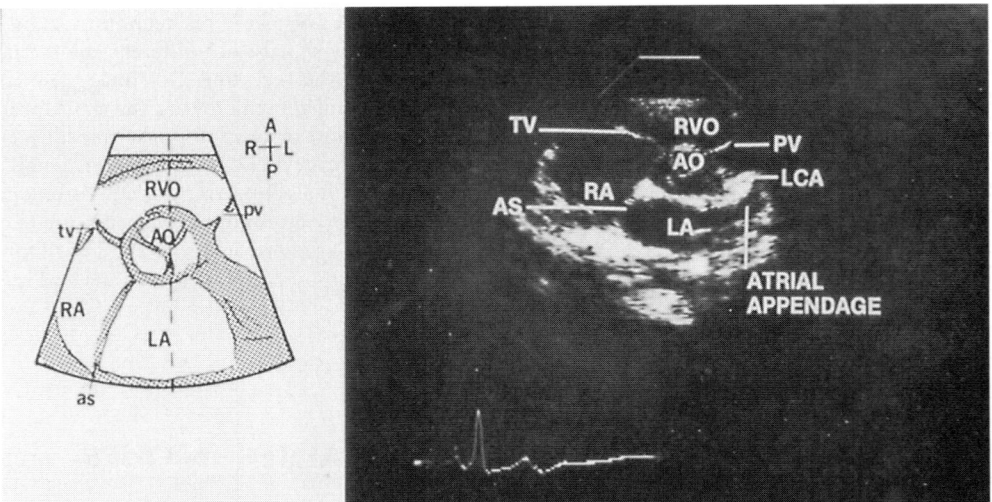

■ **Figure 16–6.** Parasternal short-axis view at level of great vessels. Still frame (*right*) with schematic drawing (*left*) of the short-axis great vessels view. The right ventricular outflow tract (RVO) is seen anteriorly, and the aorta (AO) with the three aortic valve leaflets is noted in the center of the picture. The left atrium (LA) is beneath the aorta, with the interatrial septum (AS) usually identifiable. The tricuspid valve (TV) is noted to the left of the screen, and the pulmonic valve (PV) is frequently seen to the right. LCA, left coronary artery. (From Levine, R.B., Brown, S.A., Janko, C. et al. [1984]. *Two-dimensional and Doppler echocardiographic technique* [p. 21]. Seattle, WA: University of Washington.)

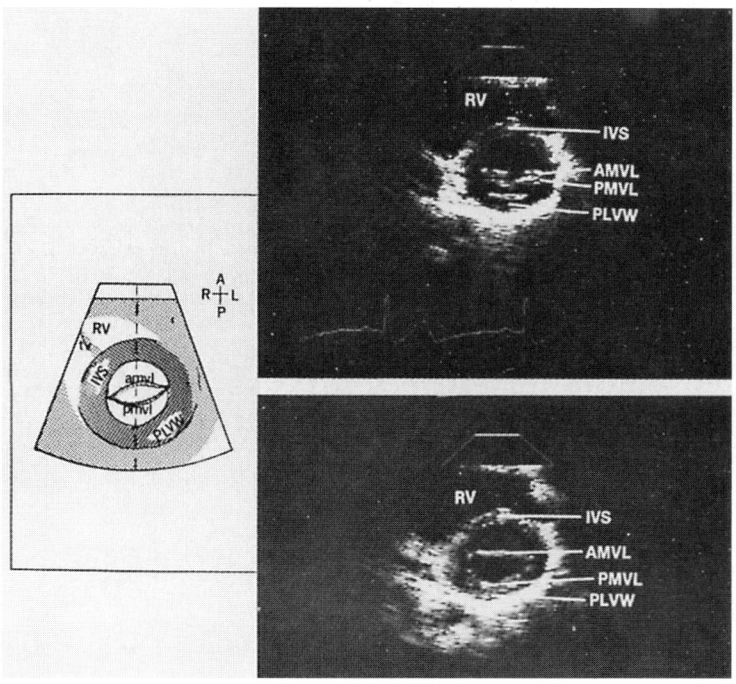

■ **Figure 16–7.** Parasternal short-axis view at level of mitral valve. Still frames (*right*) with schematic drawing (*left*) of the short-axis mitral valve view. The anterior and posterior mitral valve leaflets (AMVL and PMVL) are seen with the left ventricle posterior to the right ventricle (RV). The left ventricular walls, interventricular septum (IVS), and posterior wall (PLVW) are identified. The still frame on the top shows the mitral valve leaflets closed in systole. The still frame on the bottom shows the mitral valve leaflets open in diastole. (From Levine, R.B., Brown, S.A., Janko, C. et al. [1984]. *Two-dimensional and Doppler echocardiographic technique* [p. 15]. Seattle, WA: University of Washington.)

In patients who are unable to perform exercise, progressively increasing doses of dobutamine can be infused, beginning at 5–10 μg/kg/min and increasing to as much as 40 μg/kg/min in stepwise fashion. The same echocardiographic views are serially recorded. Atropine can be used in small doses for heart rate augmentation in patients who fail to achieve an adequate heart rate response with dobutamine alone. Cardiac response to dobutamine closely approximates that which would be expected from exercise. Exercise echocardiography and dobutamine stress echocardiography are extremely sensitive for two and three-vessel disease and somewhat more sensitive than standard exercise testing for single-vessel disease. Dipyridamole stress testing for individuals who cannot exercise and cannot tolerate dobutamine has been shown to have lesser sensitivity but greater specificity compared with exercise (de Albuquerque & Picano, 2001).

Transesophageal Echocardiography

A piezoelectric crystal can be mounted on an endoscope, replacing the fiberoptics used by the gastroenterologist to view the upper gastrointestinal tract. Echocardiographic images are obtained from within the esophagus or stomach and are often of much higher quality than transthoracic images because of elimination of acoustic impedance from ribs, sternum, and air-filled lungs. Obviously, this procedure is somewhat more invasive than standard transthoracic echocardiography. The complications relate primarily to the esophageal intubation and include trauma to the oropharynx, esophagus, or stomach; hypoxemia; aspiration; and rare vagal reaction. It is essential to have one practitioner, often a cardiac or gastroenterology nurse, devoted to monitoring the patient. Most complications can be prevented by careful manipulation of

the scope by experienced operators, meticulous attention to airway management, appropriate sedation of the patient, and continuous oxygen and ECG monitoring.

Technique

The oropharynx is anesthetized, and the patient is given sufficient sedation to be relaxed but not asleep because patient cooperation to swallow the endoscope is necessary. The operator may prefer the sitting or the left lateral decubitus position for scope introduction. The scope is advanced to the stomach, where flexion of the tip allows imaging of the heart through the stomach wall and diaphragm. The endoscope is then slowly withdrawn and views of cardiac structures are obtained at several levels in the esophagus in various 2-D planes. The imaging crystal of the endoscope can be rotated posteriorly on withdrawal to survey the descending thoracic aorta. The entire procedure usually takes approximately 15 to 20 minutes.

Indications

Transesophageal echocardiography is indicated when views obtained from transthoracic windows are of inadequate diagnostic quality. It is also indicated for several specific conditions in which the transesophageal approach has been shown to be more sensitive or to provide information that would not be shown on a transesophageal study. These include bacterial endocarditis, aortic dissection, regurgitation through or around a prosthetic mitral or tricuspid valve, LA thrombus (particularly involving the LA appendage), intracardiac source of embolus in stroke or systemic embolization, interatrial septal defect, and in some forms of congenital heart disease.

Transesophageal echocardiography is used for continuous monitoring of myocardial function during cardiac surgery and

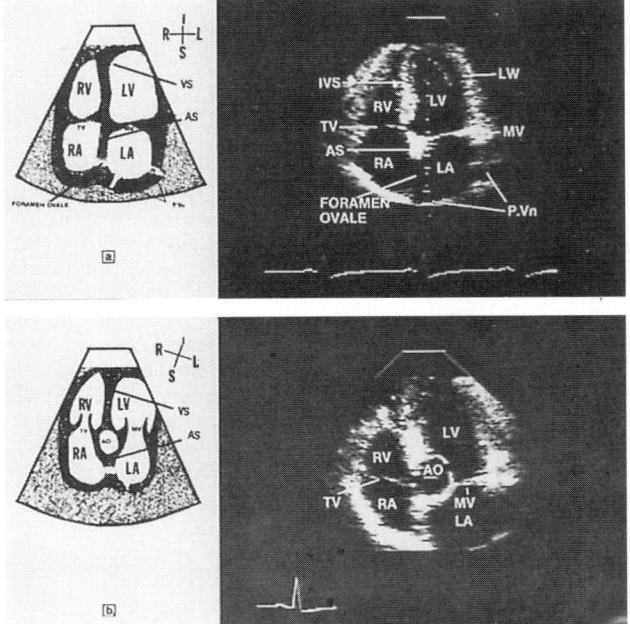

■ **Figure 16–8.** Apical four-chamber view. Still frames (*right*) with schematic drawings (*left*) of the apical views. The upper panel shows the four-chamber view. The left ventricle (LV) and left atrium (LA) appear on the right of the screen, with the mitral valve (MV) between the two. The right ventricle (RV) and right atrium (RA) are on the left, with the tricuspid valve (TV) between them. The interventricular septum (IVS) is seen at the top center of the screen, extending inferiorly and continuous with the interatrial septum (AS). Note the clear space at the level of the foramen ovale and the pulmonary veins (P.Vn) entering the left atrium. AO, aorta; LW, left ventricular wall. (From Levine, R.B., Brown, S.A., Janko, C. et al. [1984]. *Two-dimensional and Doppler echocardiographic technique* [p. 27]. Seattle, WA: University of Washington.)

noncardiac surgery in patients with heart disease. During cardiac surgery, transesophageal echocardiography is routinely used to confirm the adequacy and competence of mitral valve repair before the chest is closed. In coronary artery bypass surgery, the left ventricle can be surveyed before and after revascularization for segmental wall function. During noncardiac surgery in patients with known CHD, transesophageal echocardiography can be used to survey for wall motion abnormalities that may indicate the presence of myocardial ischemia.

ECHOCARDIOGRAPHY OF CARDIAC STRUCTURES IN HEALTH AND DISEASE

Left Ventricle

In high-quality echocardiograms, the distance from the transducer to the endocardial and epicardial surfaces of both the posterior LV wall and the interventricular septum can be measured. The thickness measured in diastole correlates well with actual anatomic wall thickness, and, when increased, is diagnostic

of LV hypertrophy. The distance between the posterior wall and septum in the parasternal long-axis view is the LV intracavitary dimension. This dimension increases with LV dilatation. Overall systolic function can be assessed from the difference between end-diastolic and peak systolic dimensions as seen from several 2-D views. Cardiac clinicians have been trained to think in terms of LV volumes and the LV ejection fraction in evaluating LV performance. Multiple methods have been used to simplify LV three-dimensional anatomy to convert echocardiographic measurements to the more-familiar LV volumes and ejection fraction (Feigenbaum, 1994).

Coronary Artery Disease

By convention, echocardiographic images of the LV are divided into 16 segments (Fig. 16–12). Individual segments of the myocardium may show reduced contractility in ischemia or nontransmural infarction (*hypokinesis*) no contractility in transmural infarction, severe ischemia or myocardial "stunning" (*akinesis*), or movement opposite the adjacent segments in LV aneurysms (*dyskinesis*). Myocardial thinning and reduced thickness occurs in chronic transmural infarction. Global left ventricular contractility can be reduced due to extensive coronary artery disease and may mimic cardiomyopathy from nonischemic causes. It is important to recognize that normal images of the LV on a resting echocardiogram in no way exclude even severe coronary artery disease. A difference in myocardial function before and after stress utilizing exercise or pharmaceuticals is required to exclude CAD.

Cardiomyopathy

Cardiomyopathy is a general term that indicates pathologic changes involving the heart muscle. These changes are almost always associated with systolic or diastolic dysfunction or both. These abnormalities are usually easily appreciated on standard echocardiography.

Dilated Cardiomyopathy

Dilated cardiomyopathy can occur in response to alcohol or other toxins such as anthracycline drugs used in cancer chemotherapy, or in a variety of degenerative, metabolic, nutritional, infectious, and genetic disorders involving the myocardial cells. Dilated cardiomyopathy can be seen in the later stages of some valvular heart diseases such as aortic and mitral insufficiency and aortic stenosis. Most patients with dilated cardiomyopathy that is not due to CHD or valvular disease have no specific etiology identified. The diagnosis of congestive cardiomyopathy is supported by an echocardiogram that shows increased LV intracavitary dimensions with a decrease in ventricular wall motion. Segmental wall motion abnormalities are occasionally seen when cardiomyopathy is of a non-CHD etiology. The mitral valve shows decreased opening amplitude due to reduced rate and volume of flow, reflecting the small difference in pressure between left atrium and left ventricle during diastole, which is in turn due to high left ventricular

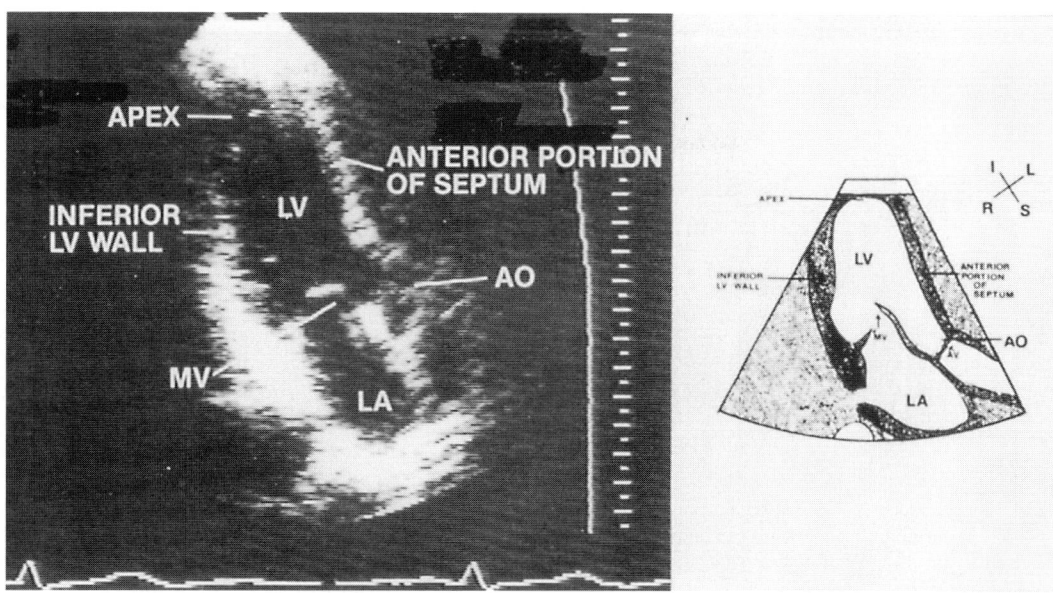

■ **Figure 16–9.** Apical long-axis view. Still frame (*left*) with schematic drawing (*right*) of the apical long-axis view of the left ventricle. The apex of the left ventricle is seen at the top of the screen with the left atrium (LA) at the bottom. The anterior portion of the septum is on the right, and the inferior left ventricular wall is on the left. The anterior mitral valve leaflet and posterior mitral valve leaflet are clearly demonstrated. The aortic root (AR) and aortic valve (AV) are seen on the right and inferiorly. MV, mitral valve. (From Levine, R.B., Brown, S.A., Janko, C. et al. [1984]. *Two-dimensional and Doppler echocardiographic technique* [p. 30]. Seattle, WA: University of Washington.)

diastolic pressure. The left atrium is often dilated. LV outflow tract velocity on Doppler imaging may be reduced, reflecting decreased cardiac output. Doppler assay of the atria may show mitral or tricuspid regurgitation related to dilatation of the valve annulus as the chamber enlarges. Small pericardial effusions are occasionally seen. The presence of poor LV function with good RV function usually indicates a CHD etiology.

Hypertrophic Cardiomyopathy

Hypertrophic cardiomyopathy occurs in conditions of increased LV afterload (aortic stenosis or systemic hypertension) but may also occur as an idiopathic or genetic disorder or in conjunction with rare systemic diseases such as progressive systemic sclerosis. The echocardiographic findings are increased wall

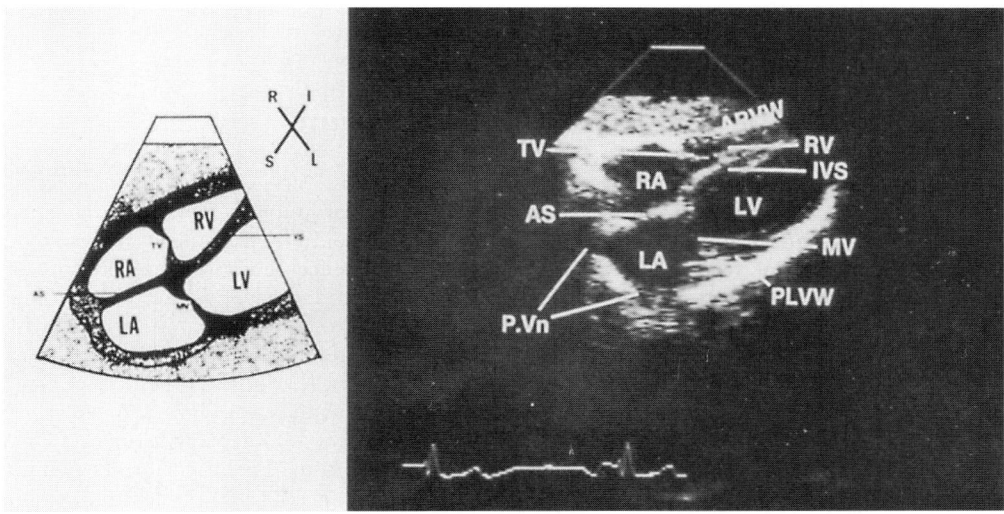

■ **Figure 16–10.** Subcostal four-chamber view. Still frame (*right*) with schematic drawing (*left*) of the subcostal four-chamber view. The right ventricle (RV) is seen at the top of the screen, with the left ventricle (LV) at the bottom toward the right. The ventricles are slightly foreshortened in this view. The interventricular septum (IVS), atrial septum (AS), mitral valve (MV), and tricuspid valve (TV) are readily apparent. The right atrium (RA) is seen at the left, with the left atrium (LA) below it. ARVW, anterior right ventricular wall; PLVW, posterior left ventricular wall; P.Vn, pulmonary veins. (From Levine, R.B., Brown, S.A., Janko, C. et al. [1984]. *Two-dimensional and Doppler echocardiographic technique* [p. 33]. Seattle, WA: University of Washington.)

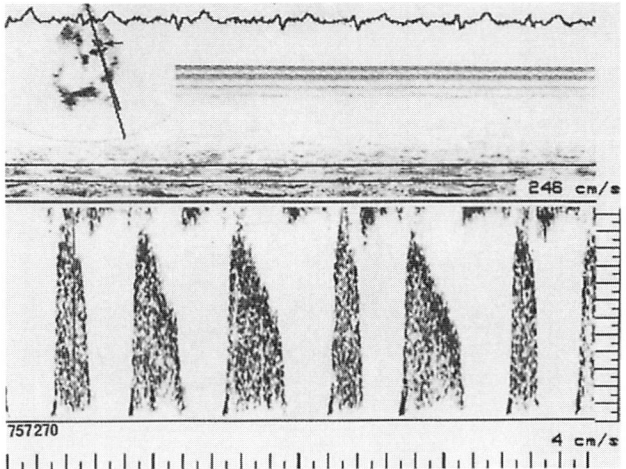

■ **Figure 16–11.** Doppler spectral display taken from the area of the mitral orifice, apical four-chamber view, in a patient with mitral stenosis. (From Feigenbaum, H. [1986]. *Echocardiography* [4th ed.]. Philadelphia: Lea & Febiger.)

thickness, usually with normal or reduced intracavitary dimensions. Diastolic flow velocity across the mitral valve may be low in early diastole and high with atrial systole (the opposite of that normally seen). LA enlargement is usually present. A subtype of hypertrophic cardiomyopathy is *idiopathic hypertrophic subaortic stenosis (IHSS)*. In this disorder, the ventricular septum is disproportionately thick and may cause obstruction of the LV outflow tract during systole. Echocardiographic findings include disproportionate septal thickening, narrowing of the outflow tract, abnormal motion of the anterior mitral leaflet during systole, and mid-systolic closure of the aortic valve as the obstruction begins. There is usually an acceleration in Doppler velocity between the LV cavity and outflow tract, which reflects the pressure gradient across the obstruction. The display of this acceleration can take several different forms depending on the patient hemodynamic factors and the severity of the obstruction.

Infiltrative Cardiomyopathy

Infiltrative cardiomyopathy is characterized by increased or irregular echocardiographic reflectance of the LV muscle giving it a bright or speckled appearance, normal or increased LV wall thickness, normal or reduced LV intracavitary dimension, often LA enlargement, and correlative findings of the infiltrative substance (e.g., amyloid, iron) by endomyocardial biopsy or examination of other tissues.

Interventricular Septum

The interventricular septum (IVS) should be assessed for both thickness (particularly as related to LV posterior wall thickness) and motion. Because the septum is normally functionally part of the left ventricle, it should move posteriorly in systole and anteriorly in diastole. A number of pathologic conditions can alter septal motion, including right ventricular (RV) volume or pressure overload and intraventricular conduction defects (left bundle-branch block). Interventricular septal motion is also

altered after any sort of cardiac surgery involving opening of the pericardium.

In the absence of aortic insufficiency or outflow tract narrowing or obstruction, the Doppler velocity of blood flow in the LV outflow tract can be a rough guide to cardiac output. Because the dimensions of the LV outflow tract change minimally throughout systole, the Doppler flow velocity in this area is primarily a reflection of the volume of blood ejected.

Septal Hypertrophy

Septal hypertrophy may occur pathologically, as described above. Focal proximal septal thickening may occur as a senile change without obstruction or pathologic implication in the elderly.

Ventricular Septal Defects

Ventricular septal defects can occur as congenital abnormalities or as a potentially catastrophic complication following septal MI. In the latter case, they are diagnosed by the presence of a high-velocity Doppler signal across the IVS from the LV to the RV. There may be accompanying dropout of echo signals in the region of the defect and dilatation of the RV may be seen.

Right Ventricle

As with the left ventricle, the right ventricle can be assessed for wall thickness, systolic function, and intracavitary dimensions. Because the anatomy of the right ventricle is much more complicated than the left ventricle, much of the evaluation of this structure is qualitative. Right ventricular infarction is suggested by the presence of hypokinesis and dilatation of the right ventricle in the setting of inferior MI. Right ventricular clots or masses may be imaged. Pacemaker leads are incidentally imaged and are often associated with small amounts of tricuspid regurgitation.

Left Atrium

The anteroposterior left atrial (LA) dimension is assessed from the parasternal long-axis view, but this chamber is also seen well on the apical four-chamber view. Increases in LA dimension usually reflect increases in LA pressure or volume, as may occur with mitral valve disease (either stenosis or regurgitation), increased LV pressure, or normally with advancing age. Rarely, echo-producing structures, such as clot or tumor, can be seen in the left atrium. The TEE is particularly effective for imaging the LA and the left atrial appendage. This is frequently done to look for a cardiac source for a systemic embolus. Clots may develop in the LA or its appendage during atrial fibrillation or in the presence of mitral stenosis.

Aortic Valve

The aortic valve can be visually assessed from parasternal long and short-axis views as well as from the apical two and four

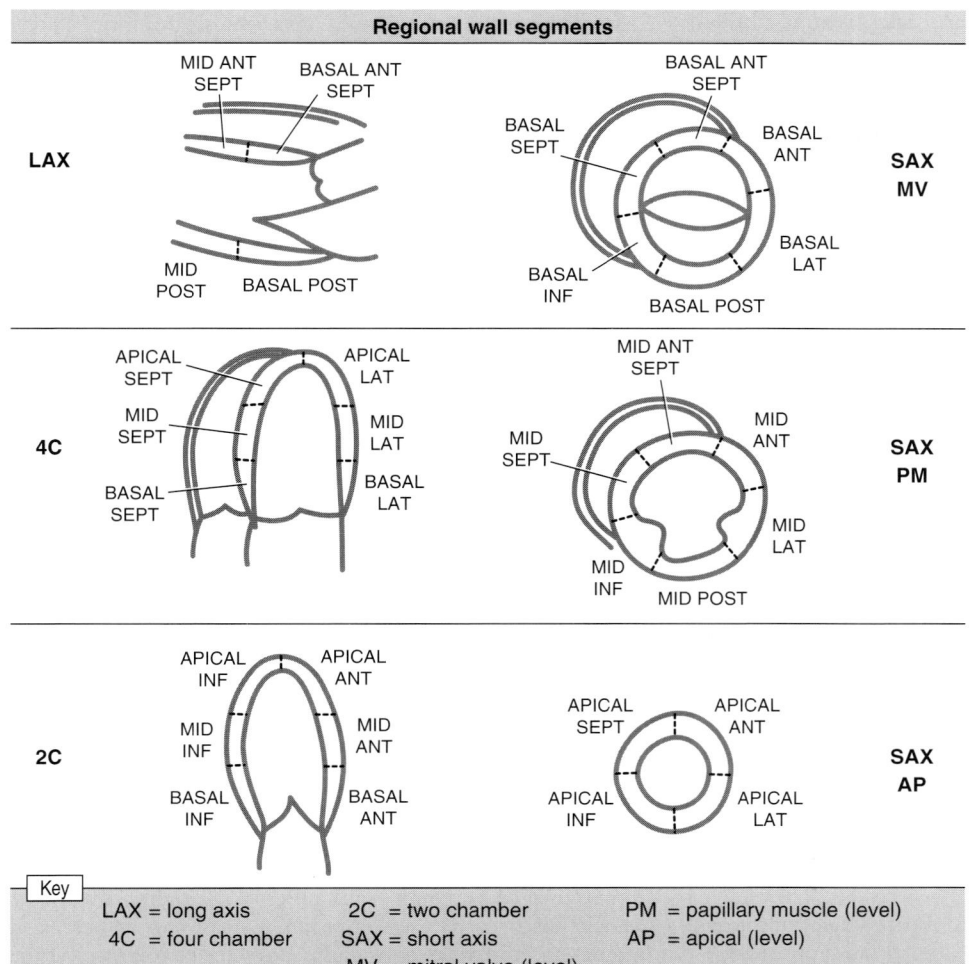

Regional wall segments

■ **Figure 16–12.** Schematic for the 16 conventional 2-D echocardiographic myocardial segments. (From Schiller, N.B., Shah, P.M., Crawford, M. et al. [1989]. Recommendations for quantitation of the left ventricle by two-dimensional echocardiography. *Journal of the American Society of Echocardiography,* 2, 358.)

Key

LAX = long axis	2C = two chamber	PM = papillary muscle (level)
4C = four chamber	SAX = short axis	AP = apical (level)
	MV = mitral valve (level)	

chamber views. It should be thin, pliable, and trileaflet. Calcification, valve thickening, and mild limitation in mobility are commonly seen with advancing age. The TEE typically provides higher resolution images of the aortic valve. More subtle abnormalities may be detected by TEE than TTE.

Aortic Stenosis

Aortic stenosis can be suspected, but not quantified, on M-mode and 2-D studies by the presence of a thickened, immobile aortic valve. The Doppler velocity in the LV outflow tract compared with that in the ascending aorta can be used in the above Doppler pressure formula ($\Delta P = 4V^2$) to estimate the aortic valve area. In most cases, this correlates closely with invasively determined valve area. Associated findings may include aortic insufficiency, LV hypertrophy, and a bicuspid rather than tricuspid valve.

Aortic Insufficiency

Aortic insufficiency can be determined from the presence of characteristic Doppler flow disturbance in the LV outflow tract during diastole. Associated findings include LV dilatation with

or without systolic dysfunction and dilatation of the aorta. Fluttering of the anterior mitral leaflet on 2-D and M-mode studies occurs in cases in which the regurgitant jet strikes the leaflet during diastole. When aortic regurgitation occurs acutely, as in aortic dissection or endocarditis, the LV may not be dilated, the regurgitant jet may be recorded in early diastole only, and the mitral valve may close prematurely owing to the rapid rise in LV end-diastolic pressure in the noncompliant left ventricle.

Mitral Valve

The mitral valve is usually the most vigorously moving structure on both the 2-D and M-mode echocardiogram and can serve as a marker for orienting the novice observer. The motion of the mitral valve is determined by the difference in pressure between the left atrium and the LV over the course of the cardiac cycle. Doppler LV inflow velocity as recorded at the mitral orifice parallels the motion of the mitral valve. Altered motion and Doppler flow are seen in many conditions not related to disease of valve itself. Decreased or increased cardiac output, LV diastolic noncompliance (a normal finding in the elderly), and cardiac rhythm disturbance such as atrial fibrillation can all alter mitral valve motion and the Doppler signal. Increased echogenicity in the valve, the mitral annulus or the chordae indicates thickening or calcification of these structures. This change occurs to some extent with aging.

Mitral Stenosis

Mitral stenosis almost always occurs secondary to rheumatic disease and is characterized by calcification of the leaflet tips, fusion of the valve commissures, variable mobility of the leaflet bellies, thickening and fusion of the chordae tendineae, and LA enlargement due to chronic LA pressure overload. The LV cavity is often small, and measurements reflective of cardiac output (LV outflow velocity) may be reduced. Doppler shows increased velocity through the mitral orifice. The pressure difference between the LA and LV persists at a higher than normal level and remains high longer in diastole than normal. These changes increase with increasing stenosis severity. The mitral valve orifice area, as would be measured at cardiac catheterization, can be estimated from the time required for the velocity of the Doppler signal to diminish by half. This measurement is termed the *mitral pressure half time*. Calculation of valve area using this measurement correlates well with invasive assessment and is independent of flow across the valve, which is affected by many variables including loading conditions, heart rate, rhythm and cardiac output. Patients with mitral stenosis often have associated mitral regurgitation. They may also have pulmonary hypertension (discussed later).

Mitral Regurgitation

Mitral regurgitation occurs in a variety of pathologic conditions that involve the mitral valve, its annulus, or its support apparatus. No 2-D or M-mode findings are pathognomonic for mitral regurgitation unless it is the result of chordal rupture and flail mitral leaflet. In this instance, the mitral leaflet or portions of its support apparatus may be seen flickering into the left atrium during ventricular systole. LA enlargement is common when mitral regurgitation is moderate or severe. The degree of LA enlargement is a function of the chronicity and severity of mitral regurgitation as well as the presence of associated conditions (LV diastolic dysfunction, mitral stenosis). Mitral regurgitation can be roughly quantified by the area of the left atrium over which the mitral regurgitation Doppler signal can be recorded as well as a number of other characteristics of the regurgitant Doppler signal. Because this represents a chronic volume overload for the left ventricle, LV dilatation with increased LV wall motion may be found with moderate or severe mitral regurgitation. Small amounts of mitral regurgitation are often seen in normal people.

Mitral Valve Prolapse

Mitral valve prolapse is a condition in which diagnosis depends primarily on physical examination findings but in which the echocardiographic findings provide strong supportive data. The 2-D images are characterized by posterior motion of one or both of the mitral leaflets into the left atrium during ventricular systole. The leaflets may be large, thickened, or redundant; mitral regurgitation of variable degree may be present. Abnormal valve motion with minimal or no structural change may be seen in otherwise normal young adults; the distinction between this relatively benign condition and true myxomatous degeneration of the valve should be made when possible. Mitral valve prolapse is associated with acute chordal rupture and mitral regurgitation in rare instances. Myxomatous mitral valves are susceptible to endocarditis.

Aortic Root

Measurements of the diameter of the aortic root are made from the parasternal long-axis view. Aortic root dilatation occurs to some extent with aging and in some pathologic conditions such as Marfan's syndrome. It can also occur in conjunction with aortic stenosis or insufficiency. The amplitude of the aortic root excursion is a reflection of the force and volume of LV systolic ejection. Aortic root dissection can be diagnosed from the presence of an additional linear structure moving parallel to the anterior and posterior aortic walls. The aortic root shows an increase in echogenicity with atherosclerosis. The abnormal anatomic relation of the aortic root to other cardiac structures helps define some forms of congenital heart disease.

Tricuspid and Pulmonic Valves

The tricuspid valve can be seen well from a modification of the parasternal long-axis view and also from the apical four chamber view. It should be thin and pliable. *Tricuspid regurgitation* can be imaged by Doppler sampling in the right atrium. The velocity of tricuspid regurgitation increases with increasing pulmonary artery pressure. Pulmonary artery pressure can be estimated by the formula $4V^2 + CVP$, where V = the Doppler velocity of the tricuspid regurgitation jet and CVP is the clinically estimated right atrial pressure in cmH_2O. The tricuspid valve may become involved with endocarditis.

The pulmonic valve can often be imaged from a modification of the parasternal short-axis view. Its motion resembles that of the aortic valve. The Doppler waveform is altered in pulmonary hypertension.

Pulmonic insufficiency of a minor degree is observed frequently in otherwise normal individuals when pulsed Doppler imaging of the RV outflow tract is carefully performed. Pathologically, it may occur in conjunction with congenital pulmonary valve abnormalities, pulmonary hypertension, and, rarely, endocarditis.

Pericardium

The posterior parietal pericardial echo is a thin line behind the epicardial LV posterior wall and is often the brightest interface seen on the echocardiogram. Multiple dense echoes arising from this structure can be seen with pericardial thickening; however, echocardiography is usually somewhat insensitive to this pathology unless it is severe. An echolucent space between the epicardium and pericardium anteriorly, inferiorly, or posteriorly can be seen with a pericardial effusion. A pericardial fat pad may be indistinguishable from a small pericardial effusion. Tiny pericardial effusions without tamponade are frequent in congestive heart failure, renal failure, and reduced serum proteins of any cause (e.g., severe extracellular volume excess, malnutrition).

Pericardial effusion (with or without tamponade) is a diagnosis best made by 2-D echocardiography showing the echolucent space in the area of the effusion. Abnormalities in the pattern of RV and right atrial wall motion indicating chamber collapse occur when tamponade is present, but clinical correlation is always needed. The echocardiogram can be used to direct pericardiocentesis. Hemopericardium, infectious pericarditis with effusion and pericardial tumors can all be seen with TTE.

Special Clinical Conditions

Prosthetic Cardiac Valves

All prosthetic heart valves can be imaged using TTE and TEE. The movement of mechanical parts or the leaflets of tissue valves can frequently but not always be imaged. Metal valve parts reflect back nearly 100% of the echo pulses, thus causing "shadows" or acoustic impedance preventing evaluation of structures or Doppler flow in structures behind the valve. For this reason, a prosthetic mitral valve is more accurately assessed with TEE where the transducer is nearer to the left atrium. Prosthetic dysfunction can be diagnosed from the combined echo and Doppler information.

Bacterial Endocarditis

Bacterial endocarditis can be identified from a TTE showing highly mobile echogenic structures moving with the valve, particularly when associated with valvular incompetence. The absence of obvious vegetations on TTE does not exclude the diagnosis of endocarditis. TEE has a higher sensitivity for this diagnosis and can also be used serially to follow the course of the disease (Ryan & Bolger, 2000).

Intracardiac Masses, Tumors and Foreign Bodies

Intracardiac tumors and masses, LA myxomata, intraventricular or intra-atrial thrombi, intracavitary catheters, electrodes or other foreign bodies, and intramyocardial or intrapericardial tumors can be imaged with 2-D and M-mode echocardiography. When the abnormality involves the atria, TEE almost always supplies much more diagnostic information than TTE. The presence of flow disturbance or hemodynamic effect from this group of abnormalities may be suggested by the presence of abnormal Doppler flow signals.

Intracardiac Source of Embolus

The heart is a prime suspect for origin of embolus in embolic stroke. Many such strokes arise in the left atrium in the presence of atrial fibrillation without other cardiac abnormalities. Unsuspected endocarditis or mural thrombi may occasionally be seen from a TTE and intravenously injected bubbles may show a patent foramen ovale, however, the TEE is much more helpful in evaluating the patient with stroke or systemic embolus. Interatrial septal abnormalities including interatrial septal aneurysm and patent foramen ovale have both been associated with stroke (Overell et al., 2000). Diagnostic yield, however, is much higher with transesophageal echocardiography, which may identify LA appendage clot, interatrial septal aneurysm with or without atrial septal defect, or unidentified vegetations of endocarditis.

Echocardiographic contrast using a 10-mL bolus of agitated saline improves the possibility of identifying intracardiac shunts compared with Doppler interrogation alone. A patent foramen ovale (PFO) or small atrial septal defect with right to-left shunt can be the cause of a "paradoxical" cerebral or systemic embolus. The presence of an atrial septal aneurysm with PFO in a patient with stroke or transient ischemic attack strongly suggests a cardioembolic etiology (Pearson et al., 1991).

NEWER TECHNIQUES

Contrast Echocardiography

Contrast echocardiography using intravenous bolus injection of albumin microbubbles or, more commonly, agitated saline has been in common and widespread usage for many years to evaluate the patency of the interatrial septum (see above, intracardiac source of embolus). This is a routine part of TEE and can also be employed with TTE. Myocardial perfusion can be assessed by 2D echocardiographic imaging of the left ventricular segments after intracoronary injection of echocardiographic contrast. This technique is obviously labor intensive, requiring not only standard coronary arteriography techniques but also requiring the presence in the cath lab of the sonographer and the echocardiographic equipment. Newer echocardiographic techniques called *second harmonic imaging* have made it possible to employ intravenous injection of contrast media in the echocardiographic laboratory or the hospital unit to image both the myocardium as well as the left ventricular intracavitary blood pool (Colonna et al., 2001). This technique greatly improves delineation of the endocardial surface and provides improved information in patients with suboptimal standard 2D images. It can be used in conjunction with stress testing to assess myocardial blood flow and segmental wall motion simultaneously. Development of this technique has required extensive revision of imaging techniques because the ultrasound beam quickly degrades the contrast bubbles.

Three-Dimensional Echocardiography

Three-dimensional echocardiography is a technique in development, which uses computer reconstruction of multiple 2-D echo images, which may be "gated" for both for respiration, and timing in the cardiac cycle to provide a reconstruction of the heart, which can be displayed in 2-D images, which can be rotated and manipulated. This technique has already yielded extensive new information about true in vivo appearance of cardiac structures in health and disease, and about the ways in which structures change in shape over the course of the cardiac cycle.

Much work has been done to validate the accuracy of these techniques in measuring left and right ventricular volumes and in correlating this information with other imaging techniques such as cardiac myocardial resonance imaging (MRI). The techniques remain quite cumbersome both for the operator and the patient and are not yet in widespread clinical use (Lange et al., 2001).

Digital Video Imaging and Storage

A technique that is in more widespread clinical use is digital image acquisition and storage. In this technique 2-D and Doppler information is obtained in standard fashion. Instead of storage on VHS videotape the images are transferred to computer files, which are data compressed and then available for viewing, transfer and storage using standard computer technology. Some of the advantages of this technique include the ability to store large numbers of studies without the space required for videotape, the ability to transfer studies electronically from one location to another, the ability to "cut and paste" images into other portions of the medical record and the ability to easily access prior studies in the same patient for easy side-by-side comparison. This method of acquisition and storage is likely to become the standard over the next several years (Soble et al., 1998).

■ CONCLUSION

Cardiac imaging is a rapidly expanding field of both clinical and research endeavor. Advances will continue to make the rapid, safe, and accurate identification of cardiac lesions easier. The clinician will ultimately have many testing modalities available, and intelligent use of the potential of these examinations, as well as the need for overall cost containment in the current health care milieu, will guide practice into the new century.

REFERENCES

Colonna, P. et al. (2001). Clinical applications of contrast echocardiography. *American Heart Journal,* 141, S36–44.

De Albuquerque, F.L., & Picano, E. (2001). Comparison of dipyridamole and exercise stress echocardiography for the detection of coronary artery disease (a meta-analysis). *American Journal of Cardiology,* 87, 1193–1196.

Ehler, D. et al. (2001). Guidelines for cardiac sonographer education: Recommendations of the American Society of Echocardiography Sonographer Training and Education Committee. *Journal of the American Society of Echocardiography,* 14, 77–84.

Feigenbaum, H. (1994). *Echocardiography* (5th ed.). Philadelphia, Lea & Febiger.

Lange, A. et al. (2001). Three-dimensional echocardiography: Historical development and current applications. *Journal of the American Society of Echocardiography,* 14, 403–412.

Mandavia, D.P., Hoffner, R.J., Mahaney, K., & Henderson, S.O. (2001). Bedside echocardiography by emergency physicians. *Annals of Emergency Medicine,* 38, 377–382.

Overell, J. R., Bone, I., & Lees, K. R. (2000). Interatrial septal abnormalities and stroke. *Neurology,* 55(8).

Pearson, A.C. et al. (1991). Superiority of transesophageal echocardiography in detecting cardiac source of embolism in patients with cerebral ischemia of uncertain etiology. *Journal of the American College of Cardiology,* 17(1), 66–72

Quinones, M.A., Douglas, P.S., & Foster, E. (2003). ACC/AHA clinical competence statement on echocardiography. A Report of the American College of Cardiology/American Hear Association/American College of Physicians—American Society of Internal Medicine Task Force on Clinical Competence. *Journal of the American Society of Echocardiography,* 16, 379–402.

Ryan, E.W., & Bolger, A.F. (2000). Transesophageal echocardiography (TEE) in the evaluation of infective endocarditis. *Clinical Cardiology,* 18(4), 773–87.

Soble, J. S. et al. (1998). Comparison of MPEG digital video with super VHS tape for diagnostic echocardiographic readings. *Journal of the American Society of Echocardiography,* 11, 819–825.

BIBLIOGRAPHY

Freeman, W. K. et al. (1994) *Transesophageal echocardiography.* Boston: Little, Brown and Company.

Otto, C. M. (2000). *Textbook of clinical echocardiography* (2nd ed.). St. Louis: W. B. Saunders Company.

Woods, S. L., Froelicher, E., & Motzer, S. (Eds.) (2000). *Cardiac nursing* (4th ed.). Philadelphia: Lippincott Williams & Wilkins.

17

Nuclear and Other Imaging Studies

LAURIE SOINE • MARGARET HANRAHAN

NUCLEAR STUDIES OF THE HEART

Radionuclides, substances that emit radioactivity, have been used as tracer in the body for more than 65 years. Over the past 30 years, since the development of the gamma ray camera by Anger and the introduction of radioactive potassium analogues, the use of radionuclides (radiotracers) to study the heart has been the subject of much research and increasing clinical application. The great interest in these techniques has been stimulated by scientific advances in the fields of myocardial biochemistry, nuclear engineering, computer technology, and radiopharmaceuticals. The introduction of new and improved radioisotopes and tomographic imaging techniques in the 1980s led to further clinical application of these studies.

Radioisotope Pharmaceuticals

Radionuclides are atoms in an unstable form. They have a finite probability of spontaneously converting to a more stable configuration. When they do so, small amounts of energy in the form of gamma rays are emitted. The rate at which atoms in a given sample undergo this conversion is denoted by the half-life, the time required for one half of the sample to undergo the conversion. Half-lives of radioactive substances may vary from a fraction of a second to a millennia; the half-life for any given radionuclide is always the same. The characteristics of an ideal radiotracer to assess myocardial blood flow are: have a half-life long enough to allow for convenient imaging, be easily combined with biologic substances, have 100% myocardial extraction across the entire spectrum of achievable or inducible coronary blood flow states, have instantaneous intracellular binding, have low extraction and clearance by organs adjacent to the heart, and be extracted by only viable cells. To date, no commercially available radiotracer of myocardial perfusion meets all of these criteria. The three most common radiotracers used in myocardial perfusion imaging are thallium 201 (^{201}Tl) and the technetium 99m-labeled tracers: ^{99m}Tc-sestamibi (Cardiolite) and ^{99m}Tc-tetrofosmin (Myoview).

The radioactive decay of these tracers is detected outside the body as scintillation (flash of light) by a gamma scintillation camera. The camera functions as a scanning device to detect the distribution of radioactivity in relatively stationary struc-tures (as in a lung scan), or when used with cardiac rhythm gating, to examine cardiac function and structure. Most examinations of the heart are performed as single-photon emission computed tomography (SPECT), which yields imaging information in a format somewhat similar to radiographic computed tomography.

Injection and detection of these radiotracers allow for the measurement of relative myocardial blood flow. ^{201}Tl is a potassium analogue. Because of the dynamic equilibrium for potassium between cells and the blood pool, potassium, and therefore ^{201}Tl, distributes in the myocardium in proportion to the blood flow. Myocytes with an intact sodium-potassium pump will takeup ^{201}Tl. However, the relatively low energy (60 KEV) emitted by ^{201}Tl makes imaging of this tracer at times suboptimal in patients with an increased body mass index. The technetium 99m-labeled radiotracers passively distribute across sarcolemmal and mitochondrial membranes and remain intracellularly bound. The relatively higher energy (140 KEV) emitted by this group of tracers allows for improved transmission through the chest tissue resulting in improved image quality.

Radionuclide Ventriculogram

A radionuclide ventriculogram (RNVG), also known as a MUGA (multiple gated acquisition) study, is a procedure in which a small amount of the patient's blood is withdrawn, labeled with a technetium 99m-labeled radionuclide, and then reinjected. Using the ECG signal for timing (gating), images are acquired at various points in the cardiac cycle. Radioactive scintillation counts from corresponding time segments are summed to augment image clarity. In this way, the manner in which the radioactivity (and hence the blood pool) changes over the cardiac cycle is demonstrated (Kostuk, et al., 1973). This summed cardiac cycle can be played back as a cine loop video display of a normally recurring cardiac cycle. LVEF, RVEF, and segmental wall motion can be calculated (Fig. 17-1). The video display resembles a contrast LV or RV angiogram. Variation in radioactive counts over time is analyzed to provide information about diastolic and systolic function. Rhythm disturbances such as atrial fibrillation or frequent premature contractions altering beat-to-beat filling and cycle length may decrease quantitative accuracy. This study is commonly used to evaluate cardiac function in

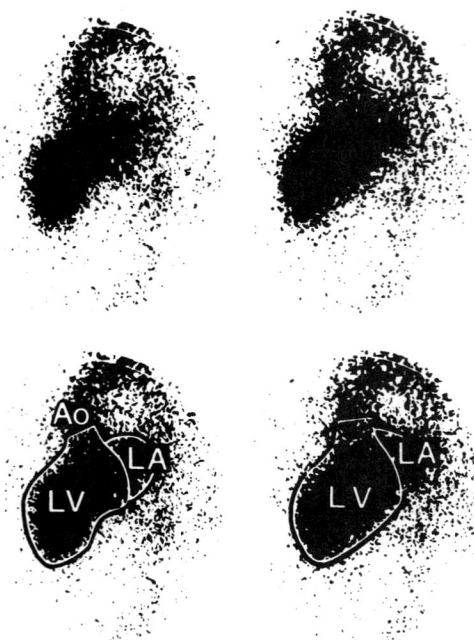

■ **Figure 17–1.** Systolic and diastolic frames from a radioisotope angiogram. Ao, aorta; LA, left atrium; LV, left ventricle. (Adapted from Kostuk, W.L., Ehsani, A.A., Karliner, J.S. et al. [1973]. Left ventricular performance after myocardial infarction assessed by radioisotope angiocardiography. *Circulation, 47,* 244.)

patients with heart failure or valvular heart disease or to monitor the potential cardiotoxic effects of commonly used chemotherapeutic agents.

There is no special patient preparation for this study. The patient may continue to take all medications. The entire study usually takes approximately 30 minutes.

Myocardial Perfusion Imaging

Stress myocardial perfusion imaging has become a very useful clinical study for the detection of coronary artery disease and risk stratification for patients with known coronary heart disease (Beller et al., 2000). Myocardial perfusion images provide the clinician and patient with important predictive and prognostic information, including LV chamber size, and global and regional LV function; location, size, and extent of impairment of coronary flow reserve (myocardial ischemia); and location, size, and extent of myocardial infarction (Hachamovitch et al., 2002).

Stress myocardial perfusion imaging involves comparing the pattern of myocardial blood flow in the resting state with the pattern of blood flow in the hyperemic or stress state. The goal of stress perfusion imaging is creating heterogeneity of myocardial blood flow and marking this effect with a radiotracer. In patients with normal coronary arteries, as the heart rate and blood pressure rise in response to exercise, normal coronary arteries dilate. Coronary flow reserve is maintained in arteries with less than 70% stenosis. In contrast, regions of the myocardium supplied by an artery with more than 70% stenosis, unable to appropriately dilate in response to increasing

myocardial work, resulting in a relative reduction in blood flow to this region of the myocardium (Gould et al., 1974).

The most common stress myocardial perfusion study is the "dual" (two) isotope imaging protocol. This protocol uses ^{201}Tl to evaluate the pattern of myocardial blood flow at rest and a technetium 99m-labeled product (Sestamibi or Myoview) for the stress images. Patients receive an intravenous injection of ^{201}Tl while sitting quietly at rest. A gated set of SPECT myocardial perfusion images are then immediately acquired. After the resting images of the myocardium, the patient is "stressed," or rather a hyperemic state of coronary blood flow is created. On the treadmill, this state is achieved by a patient exercising and achieving 85% of maximal predicted heart rate for given age. Studies of myocardial blood flow have demonstrated that at this workload, blood flow through a normal coronary artery increases two-fold, thereby creating heterogeneity of coronary blood flow, in which regions of the myocardium supplied by a normal coronary artery receives two-fold the amount of radiotracer compared to regions of the myocardium supplied by a diseased vessel. In patients unable to exercise adequately, an intravenous infusion of dipyridamole (0.57 mg/kg infused over 4 minutes) or adenosine (140mcg/kg per minute) reproduce this hyperemic state. These agents do not stress the myocardium but rather dilate normal coronary arteries having little effect on diseased vessels. At the standard infusion doses and rates, these agents dilate normal coronary arteries 4-fold to 5-fold (Iskandrian et al., 1994). After the stress study, a second set of gated SPECT images are acquired (Fig. 17-2).

The rest and post-stress gated SPECT images when processed and reconstructed reflect the pattern of myocardial blood flow in the two states. The images are reconstructed in three standardized views: short axis, vertical long axis, and horizontal long axis. Patterns of blood flow are compared between the two data sets. A segmental scoring system has become a widely applied quantitative tool to integrate the extent and severity of perfusion abnormalities (Cerqueira et al., 2002). Summed stress score is a quantitative tool used to evaluate the extent and severity of myocardium at risk (Germano et al., 2000). The score is determined by dividing the myocardium

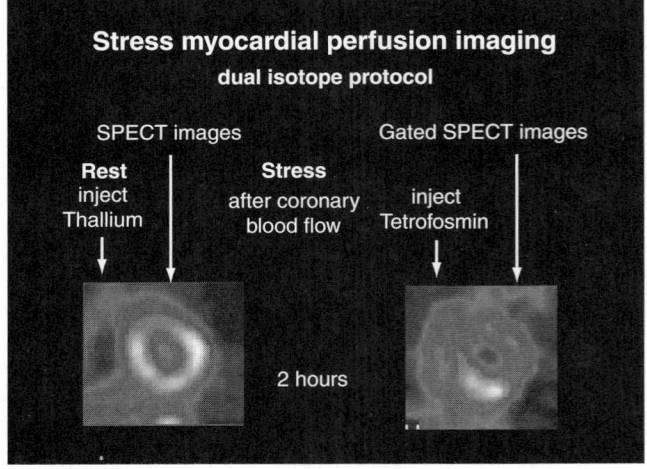

■ **Figure 17–2.** Dual isotope imaging protocol. SPECT, single-photon emission computed tomography.

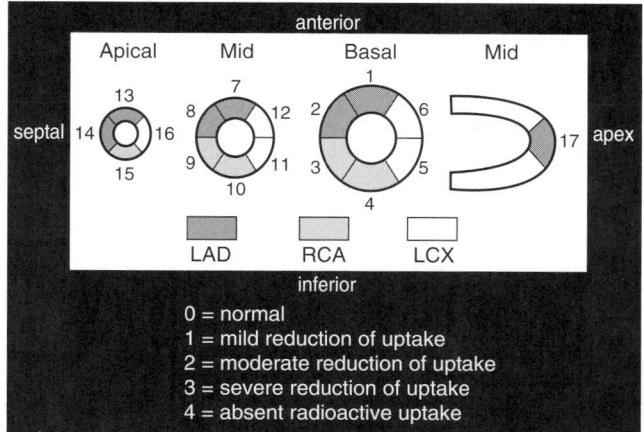

■ Figure 17–3. Coronary artery territories and perfusion SPECT 17-segment scoring (Adapted from Cerqueira, M.D., Weissman, N.J., Dilsizian, V. et al. [2002]. Standardized myocardial segmentation and nomenclature for tomographic imaging of the heart. *Circulation,* 105, 542.)

into 17 segments, scoring the percent reduction in radiotracer uptake, and adding the segments (Fig. 17-3).

A segment or region of the myocardium that has reduced radiotracer uptake on the stress images that appears more uniform (improved) on the resting images is consistent with myocardial ischemia. The severity of the impairment of coronary flow reserve can be qualitatively estimated by the degree of reduction of radiotracer uptake (i.e., mildly reduced, moderately reduced, or severely reduced uptake). A segment or region of the myocardium with a fixed reduction in radiotracer uptake on both stress and rest images is most consistent with myocardial injury or infarction (Fig. 17-4). An alternative explanation of an apparent fixed region of reduced radiotracer uptake that thickens and moves normally on gated cines may be attenua-

tion artifact. The most common attenuating structures include breast tissue (anterior wall) and diaphragm (inferior wall).

The summed stress score (extent and severity of ischemia and infarction) when combined with Duke Treadmill Score has been shown to an independent predictor of cardiac death in many high-risk patient populations (Hachamovitch et al., 1996) (Fig. 17-5). In addition to increasing the clinical identification and quantification of coronary artery disease, stress myocardial perfusion data have been shown to be an independent additive predictor of serious cardiac events in the ensuing year in many patient populations, including men and women of all ages as well as many high-risk groups, such as diabetic patients (Hachamovitch, Berman, Kiat, Cohen, Friedman and Shaw, 2002; Kang et al., 1999; Hachamovitch et al., 1996; Hachamovitch et al., 1997; Giri et al., 2002).

^{201}Tl is the most common radionuclide used for distinguishing viable or hibernating myocardium from scar. It is well established that chronic myocardial ischemia is associated with a severe reduction in contractile function. However, in contrast to infarct-related scar, dysfunctional but viable myocardium has the potential to regain function (Alderman et al., 1983). ^{201}Tl is injected in the resting state; gated SPECT images immediately acquired reflect myocardial perfusion. Delayed images acquired 4 to 24 hours later represent tissue viability. A region of the myocardium with reduced perfusion but preserved viability on delayed images is consistent with viable myocardium (Ragosta et al., 1993).

Myocardial viability studies with ^{201}Tl have been proved clinically helpful in patients with multivessel coronary artery disease and LV dysfunction. Potential reversibility of LV dysfunction is an important clinical consideration in these patients. Multiple studies have demonstrated that patients with viable myocardium benefit from revascularization versus augmented medical therapy. Alternatively, patients without evidence of viability do not show this same improvement after revascularization (Pagley et al., 1997; Imamaki et al., 2002).

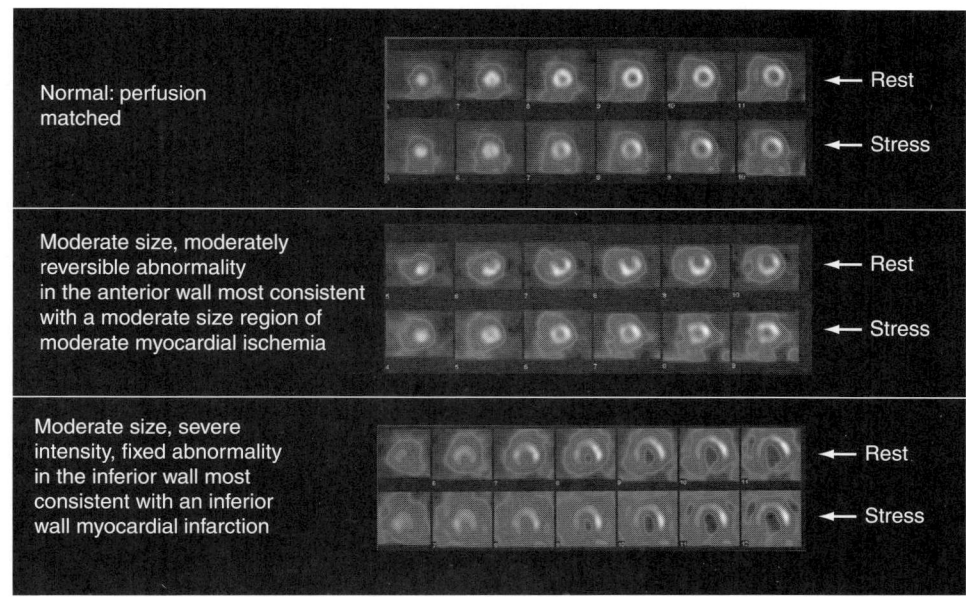

■ Figure 17–4. Stress myocardial perfusion images. LAD, left anterior descending artery; RCA, right coronary artery; LCX, left circumflex artery.

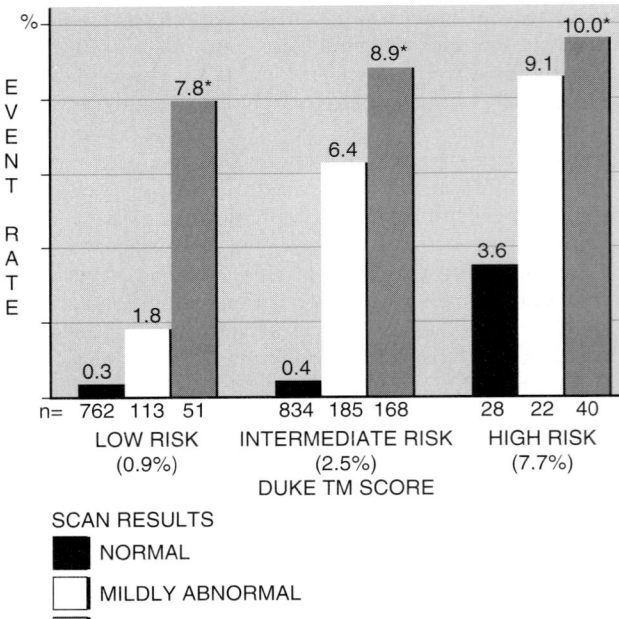

■ **Figure 17–5.** Myocardial perfusion scan results add incremental prognostic data when combined with Duke Treadmill (TM) score. Event rates for myocardial infarction or cardiac death are shown in parentheses under Duke Treadmill subgroups. *p < .05 across scan results. (Adapted from Hachamovitch, R., Berman, D.S., Kiat, H. et al. [1996]. *Circulation*, 93, 905.)

It is recommended that patients fast for 6 hours before injection of radionuclides. This preparation minimizes gastrointestinal blood flow, resulting in reduced gastric uptake of radionuclides. Consider holding cardiac medications, particularly nitrates, beta-blockers, and calcium channel blockers before stress studies, because these agents have been shown to reduce the sensitivity of the study for the detection of myocardial ischemia (Sharir et al., 1998).

Positron Emission Tomography

Positron emission tomography (PET), like other nuclear medicine studies, is based upon the radiotracer concept. Small quantities of a positron-emitting radiotracer are injected into a patient. Subsequent mapping of the tracer allows for quantitative and tomographic imaging of myocardial perfusion and metabolism without intrinsically altering these processes. Nitrogen-13-Ammonia, Oxygen-15 Labeled Water, and Rubidium-82 are the most common tracers of myocardial perfusion; Fluorine-18-2-Fluoro-2-Deoxyglucose (FDG) is used for myocyte metabolism. A positron-emitting radiotracer travels only a short distance in tissue prior to encountering an electron. This interaction causes annihilation of both particles, producing two high-energy photons that depart at an angle of 180 degrees from each other. PET imaging systems are designed to detect the two photons, which travel in opposite directions at essentially the speed of light (511-keV). By measuring the time that it takes for each photon to

encounter the circumferential ring of detectors, localization of the event can be mathematically derived.

Stress myocardial PET imaging using positron-emitting radiotracers allows for quantitative measurement of coronary blood flow. By comparing absolute blood flow at rest with a hyperemic state created by an intravenous infusion of either adenosine or dipyridamole, impairment of coronary flow reserve can be measured. The most common cause of impaired coronary flow reserve is atherosclerosis. PET imaging is also used to detect myocardial viability. FDG used to document myocyte metabolism and Nitrogen-13-Ammonia as a flow tracer is a highly sensitive study for differentiating viable myocardium from scar (Sharir et al., 1998). A flow-metabolism mismatch pattern has become synonymous with reversible contractile dysfunction and thus prediction of improvement in LV function after revascularization (Allman et al., 2002).

This technology requires a cyclotron for radiotracer generation. These tracers usually have very short half-lives, making imaging challenging; thus, widespread application of PET imaging is limited by the cost of the required generating and detection equipment.

Risks of Radionuclides

In contrast to radioactive substances used for therapeutic (tissue ablation) purposes, radiopharmaceuticals used for imaging have short half-lives (minutes to several hours), contributing to their decay in the body. They are used in very small amounts. Thus, there is no need to isolate patients who have had these studies, and no particular precautions are needed for disposal of body substances (including blood, urine, or stool). The risk to a fetus is small, but it is recommended that patients who are pregnant or breast-feeding should not undergo injection of radionuclides. Personnel should remember that radioactivity decreases dramatically with distance from the source and that prolonged close-range contact with patients soon after a study should be avoided. Personnel who work in nuclear medicine departments wear detecting badges like those worn by radiology personnel to monitor their exposure.

▓ OTHER IMAGING STUDIES OF THE HEART

Magnetic Resonance Imaging

Magnetic resonance imaging (MRI) is a diagnostic imaging modality that uses strong magnets and low-energy radio frequency signals to obtain information about the anatomy and function of the heart. Atomic particles in organic tissue absorb and release energy according to their specific chemical composition. Atomic particles, such as hydrogen, carbon-13, sodium, and phosphorus, contain electrically charged ionic particles that spin. Hydrogen is the most abundant atom in the body. When subjected to the strong magnetic field of the MRI scanner, the hydrogen ions align with the magnetic field and spin parallel with the field (a lower energy state) or antiparallel (a higher energy state). An applied radio frequency pulse causes resonance of the hydrogen ions. When the applied radiofrequency is turned off, there are two distinct relaxation parameters that are measured as the ions return to their original state. These relaxation parameters are known as T1 and T2. T1 relaxation is the phase when the ion transfers its spin energy to surrounding structures. T2 relaxation is the progressive loss of phase coherence of the magnetic spin. The imager's receiver coils that surround the patient detect this release of energy and a computerized image is created.

Spatial localization is a process that occurs when three gradient magnets, aligned on the x, y, and z axes of the scanner, are rapidly turned on and off to create local variations in a specific area of the body. Through this fluctuation in these gradient magnets, axial, sagittal, coronal, and oblique slices of any of the planes of the body can be examined. The timing of the excitation pulses and the successive magnetic field gradients determine the image contrast (Fayad et al., 2002).

Tissues of various types have different T1 and T2 relaxation times. The water content, physical state, and molecular motion affect the tissue's relaxation times and allow for differentiation of tissue structure and function.

Types of MRI Techniques

MRI techniques are evolving as technologic advances improve the quality and speed of image acquisition. Timing of radiofrequency and gradient magnetic applications allow for the creation of spin-echo imaging, gradient-echo imaging, MR angiography, high-speed MRI imaging, and MR spectroscopy. (van der Wall et al., 1999).

Spin-echo imaging, the first MRI techniques to be used clinically, is the most commonly used method for defining the structure of the heart and great vessels. With this technique, a static image is created along the transverse, coronal, and sagittal axial planes of the heart. Blood flow through the heart appears as natural contrast and appears black on imaging. Because spin-echo images highlight morphologic detail, these images are used to evaluate the size of vascular structures and cardiac chambers, ventricular wall thickness, left ventricular mass, pericardial thickness, cardiac and paracardiac masses, and congenital anomalies. It is also used to identify the fatty infiltration seen in arrhythmogenic right ventricular dysplasia.

Gradient-echo imaging provides dynamic information on cardiac function and blood flow. Moving blood creates a bright image as compared with spin-echo imaging. Turbulent blood will be seen less bright or even as a black image. Visualization of flow disturbances associated with valvular stenoses and insufficiencies can be seen as low-signal turbulent jet effects contrasting with the bright flow of normal blood. Gradient echo images are not based in real time and are images created with cardiac gating.

Coronary MR angiography (CMRA) is a phase contrast method that visualizes and quantifies blood flow based on the velocity-induced phase shifts of spins created in the presence of magnetic field gradients. High-resolution MR has the potential to image plaque composition including the assessment of fibrous cap thickness and vessel wall morphology.

MR spectroscopy is an evolving technique to quantify cardiac metabolism through measurement of changes in the high-energy phosphate ions in the myocardium. A decrease in phosphocreatine-to-adenosinetriphosphate (ATP) ratio is seen with myocardial ischemia.

MRI is a noninvasive technique that does not require use of radiation. Blurring of images can result from motion artifact caused by the beating of the heart or with breathing. Obtaining gated images in mid to late diastole minimizes the artifact in imaging. Breath holding or respiratory gating techniques can minimize respiratory motion artifact in acquiring images. Ultrafast MRI techniques have resulted in the reduction of acquisition times to 50 milliseconds or less per image. Motion artifacts from breathing are significantly reduced because of high-speed acquisition.

MR images can be captured in two-dimensional (2-D) imaging (slice acquisition) or three-dimensional (3-D) imaging (volume acquisition) techniques. The 2-D techniques may be limiting because it may be difficult to capture a picture of the coronary tree in one slice. Coronary arteries are better visualized in 3-D imaging, but 3-D imaging requires a longer scanning time and has an increased likelihood of motions artifact. Fat also creates artifact that can be eliminated by suppressing its signal by saturating it with a stronger radiofrequency pulse. This saturation affects the fat-bound hydrogen ions but does not affect the water bound hydrogen ions found in coronary blood.

Diagnostic Uses of MRI

Currently, the primary indications for MRI include diagnosing and monitoring complex congenital heart disease, diseases of the aorta, arrhythmogenic right ventricular dysplasia, and pericardial disease, along with paracardiac and intracardiac masses (White, 1996). MRI has been proven superior over computed tomography and transthoracic echo cardiography for the detection of aortic dissection in stable patients, allowing for the visualization of the intravascular and extravascular spaces and the walls of the aorta (Flamm et al., 1996). MRI can allow for better visualization of a cardiac mass that extends or arises from pericardial tissue. Spin-echo MRI can provide anatomic details of masses while gradient-echo MRI allows for the assessment of the hemodynamic effects of tumors throughout the cardiac cycle. The contrast resolution of MRI allows for the differentiation between an intact pericardial line and surrounding paracardiac tissues. Emerging uses for cardiac MRI include defining and assessing coronary artery lumen and vessel wall structure, determining myocardial perfusion, infarct size, metabolism, and spectroscopy, and as a source of imaging in interventional cardiology procedures.

Established uses of CMRA include the evaluation of patency of coronary artery bypass grafts and imaging of anomalous coronary arteries (Fayad et al., 2002). CMRA is an evolving technique because image quality is affected by motion artifacts from respiratory and cardiac cycles, along with the contractions of the coronary artery wall. While respiratory and cardiac gating and ultrafast image acquisition have improved this technique, it still lacks the sensitivity and specificity to detect coronary artery disease as traditional contrast coronary x-ray angiography does (Duerincks, 1996).

Patient Preparation

Most patients tolerate MRI procedures without need of sedation. Because patients need to remain motionless through most of the scanning, light sedation may be required. Ways to reduce patient anxiety include having a friend or family member positioned at the head of the machine to talk to the patient during scanning. Earphones can also be used to minimize the noise of the scanner.

MRI scanning can take between 30 minutes to 1 hour and is dependent on the complexity of the test. Scans determining ventricular function may take 30 minutes, whereas scans to assess congenital heart disease may take more than an hour. If a mild-to-moderate sedative is given before MRI, patients should avoid eating for 1 to 2 hours before testing. Patients should void before the testing. Patients with severe cyanosis or hemodynamic instability may need an inpatient procedure with anesthesia back-up if needed.

The most commonly implanted cardiac devices that exclude a patient from having MRI scan include temporary and permanent pacemakers, automatic implantable cardioverter defibrillators, or internal hemodynamic monitoring catheters. Prosthetic heart valves and annular rings are safe with the exception of the pre-6000 Starr-Edwards valves (Boxt, 1996). Sternal wires and bypass graft clips are safe but may result in signal artifact on the MRI scan. Intravascular coils, stents, and filters are unlikely to dislodge within several weeks of implantation but may create an MR signal artifact (Foster, 1998). Patients with other implanted metallic devices, such as electrical stimulators or intracerebral aneurysm clips, and patients who have free iron particulate matter in their eyes should avoid MRI scanning. Pregnancy is a relative contraindication to MR scanning.

The ECG tracing obtained for gating with MRI is useless for diagnosing ischemic changes during an examination but may be analyzed for extrasystolic beats and changes in cardiac rhythm. Electrocardiogram cables and external devices such as pulse oximetry devices must be MR-safe.

Electron Beam Computed Tomography and Computed Tomography Angiography

Electron beam computed tomography (EBCT), also known as ultrafast or cine computed tomography, uses an electron beam that sweeps across the patient and obtains x-ray images in 50 to 100 milliseconds. The very short image acquisition time of EBCT can virtually freeze cardiac motion and provides high-resolution three-dimensional images of the heart. Scanning of the heart can be achieved in one to two breath holds.

EBCT can be used to evaluate specific cardiac disease such as ischemic heart disease, pericardial disease, congenital abnormalities, diseases of the aorta, and masses of the pericardium, and myocardium. EBCT is the gold standard to detect and quantify the amount of calcium in coronary plaques.

The detection and quantification of atherosclerotic plaque burden can be detected by EBCT before the development of significant stenotic lesions. The use of EBCT to detect calcified coronary plaques may be considered in patients with atypical chest pain. It is also used to assess the rate of progression of calcified coronary plaque burden over time in asymptomatic patients with cardiovascular risk factors.

A high calcium score is a sensitive but not specific marker for obstructive coronary artery disease. A calcium score can be calculated for a given coronary segment, a specific coronary artery, or for the entire coronary system (Rumberger, 1999). In assessing plaque burden, the patient's age, gender, symptoms, risk factors, and number of calcified vessels are considered in interpreting this test. A calcium score of zero denotes a lack of identifiable atherosclerotic plaques and a very low risk for cardiovascular disease. Calcium scores have a greater significance if they are in the 75th percentile for the age and gender of the patient or if calcium is present in two or more vessels. Scores of 11 to 100 are consistent with a mild degree of atherosclerotic plaque burden. Calcium scores of 101 to 400 indicate a moderate atherosclerotic plaque burden, and aggressive risk factor modification is indicated. Scores of more than 400 indicate an extensive plaque burden and a high likelihood of at least one stenotic lesion of 90% or greater. It is strongly recommended that patients in this group undergo nuclear perfusion imaging or echocardiographic stress testing to rule out ischemia (Rumberger et al., 2003).

Race may affect the amount of calcification found in coronary arteries. A review of subjects between the ages of 40 to 45 undergoing EBCT to detect calcification revealed that blacks were significantly less likely than whites to have coronary artery calcification. Further outcome studies are needed to determine the use of coronary artery calcification for risk assessment in blacks (Lee et al., 2003) and other races.

A direct one-to-one correlation between coronary calcium as detected by EBCT and luminal disease is not possible (Rumberger et al., 1999). A high coronary calcium score is a sensitive but not specific marker for obstructive CAD. Currently, large randomized trials are underway to determine if coronary calcium scoring is an independent and superior predicator for future cardiac events.

EBCT with use of intravenous iodinated contrast agents is currently being investigated for direct visualization of coronary arteries. This technique, known as computed tomography coronary angiography (CTCA), involves scanning the heart during an injection of the iodinated contrast material through a peripheral intravenous catheter. The contrast agent renders the cardiac chambers, large vessels, and coronary arteries opaque on x-ray. The circulation time of the contrast agent is noted from the time of injection to peak enhancement. Limitations of this technique include coronary calcification, poor opacification because of vessel size, arrhythmias, and motion artifacts (Gerber et al., 2002).

REFERENCES

Alderman, E. L., Fisher, L. D., Litwin, P., Kaiser, G. C., Myers, W. O., Maynard, C., Levine, F. & Schloss, M. (1983). Results of coronary artery surgery in patients with poor left ventricular function (CASS). *Circulation,* 68, 785–795.

Allman, K. C., Shaw, L. J., Hachamovitch, R. & Udelson, J. E. (2002). Myocardial viability testing and impact of revascularization on prognosis in patients with coronary artery disease and left ventricular dysfunction: a meta-analysis. *Journal of American College Cardiology,* 39, 1151–1158.

Beller, G. A. & Zaret, B. L.(2000). Contributions of nuclear cardiology to diagnosis and prognosis of patients with coronary artery disease. *Circulation,* 101, 1465–1478.

Boxt, L.M. (1996). How to perform cardiac MR imaging. *MRI Clinics of North America-Cardiac Imaging,* 4(2), 191–216.

Cerqueira, M. D., Weissman, N. J., Dilsizian, V., Jacobs, A. K., Kaul, S., Laskey, W. K., Pennell, D. J., Rumberger, J. A., Ryan, T. & Verani, M. S. (2002). Standardized myocardial segmentation and nomenclature for tomographic imaging of the heart. A statement for healthcare professionals from the Cardiac Imaging Committee of the Council on Clinical Cardiology of the American Heart Association. *International Journal Cardiovascular Imaging,* 1, 539–42.

Danias, P G., Edelman, R. C., & Manning, W. J. (1999). MR Coronary angiography. *Critical Care Nursing Clinics of North America,* 11, 383–404.

Duerincks, A. J. (1996) Coronary MR angiography. *Critical Care Nursing Clinics of North America,* 11, 361–418.

Fayad, Z., Fuster, V., Nikolaou, K, & Becker, C. (2002). Computed tomography and magnetic resonance imaging for noninvasive coronary angiography and plaque imaging –Current and Potential Future Concepts. *Circulation,* 106, 2026–2034.

Flamm, S. D., VanDyke, C. W., & White, R. D. (1996). MR imaging of the thoracic aorta. *MRI Clinics of North America-Cardiac Imaging,* 4(2), 217–235.

Fuisz, A. R., Pohost, G. M., & Iqbal, U. (2003). Clinical utility of cardiovascular magnetic resonance imaging. . [On-line]. Available:http://www.uptodateonline.com.

Gerber, T. C., Kuzo, R. S., Karstaedt, N., Lane, G. E., Morin, R. L., Sheedy, P. F., Safford, R. E., Blackshear, J. L., & Pietan, J. H. (2002). Current results and new developments of coronary angiography with use of contrast-enhanced computed tomography of the heart. *Mayo Clinic Proceedings,* 77, 55–71.

Germano, G., Kavanagh, P. B., Waechter, P., Areeda, J., Van Kriekinge, S., Sharir, T., Lewin, H. C. & Berman, D. S. (2000). A new algorithm for the quantification of myocardial perfusion SPECT. I: technical principles and reproducibility. *Journal of Nuclear Medicine,* 41, 712–9.

Giri, S., Shaw, L. J., Murthy, D. R., Travin, M. I., Miller, D. D., Hachamovitch, R., Borges-Neto, S., Berman, D. S., Waters, D. D. & Heller, G. V. (2002). Impact of diabetes on the risk stratification using stress single-photon emission computed tomography myocardial perfusion imaging in patients with symptoms suggestive of coronary artery disease. *Circulation,* 105, 32–40.

Gould, K. L. & Lipscomb, K. (1974). Effects of coronary stenoses on coronary flow reserve and resistance. *American Journal of Cardiology,* 34, 48–55.

Hachamovitch, R., Berman, D. S., Kiat, H., Bairey, C. N., Cohen, I., Cabico, A., Friedman, J., Germano, G., Van Train, K. F. & Diamond, G. A (1996). Effective risk stratification using exercise myocardial perfusion SPECT in women: gender-related differences in prognostic nuclear testing. *Journal of the American College of Cardiology,* 28, 34–44.

Hachamovitch, R., Berman, D. S., Kiat, H., Cohen, I., Cabico, J. A., Friedman, J. & Diamond, G. A. (1996). Exercise myocardial perfusion SPECT in patients without known coronary artery disease: incremental prognostic value and use in risk stratification. *Circulation,* 93, 905–914.

Hachamovitch, R., Berman, D. S., Kiat, H., Cohen, I., Friedman, J. D. & Shaw, L. J. (2002). Value of stress myocardial perfusion single photon emission computed tomography in patients with normal resting electrocardiograms: an evaluation of incremental prognostic value and cost-effectiveness. *Circulation,* 105, 823–829.

Hachamovitch, R., Berman, D. S., Kiat, H., Cohen, I., Lewin, H., Amanullah, A., Kang, X., Friedman, J. & Diamond, G. A. (1997). Incremental prognostic value of adenosine stress myocardial perfusion single-photon emission computed tomography and impact on subsequent management in patients

with or suspected of having myocardial ischemia. *American Journal of Cardiology,* 80, 426–433.

Imamaki, M., Maeda, T., Tanaka, S., Sugawara, Y. & Shimakura, T. (2002). Prediction of improvement in regional left ventricular function after coronary artery bypass grafting: quantitative stress-redistribution 201Tl imaging in detection of myocardial viability. *J Cardiovascular Surgery (Torino),* 43, 603–607.

Iskandrian, A. S., Verani, M. S. & Heo, J (1994). Pharmacologic stress testing: mechanism of action, hemodynamic responses, and results in detection of coronary artery disease. *Journal of Nuclear Cardiology,* 1, 94–111.

Kang, X., Berman, D. S., Lewin, H., Miranda, R., Erel, J., Friedman, J. D. & Amanullah, A. M. (1999). Comparative ability of myocardial perfusion single-photon emission computed tomography to detect coronary artery disease in patients with and without diabetes mellitus. *American Heart Journal,* 137, 949–957.

Kostuk, W. J., Ehsani, A. A., Karliner, J. S., Ashburn, W. L., Peterson, K. L., Ross, J., Jr. & Sobel, B. E. (1973). Left ventricular performance after myocardial infarction assessed by radioisotope angiocardiography. *Circulation,* 47, 242–249.

Lee, T., O'Malley, P., Feuerstein, I., & Taylor, A. (2003). Prevalence and severity of coronary artery calcification in black and white subjects. *Journal of American College of Cardiology,* 41, 39–44.

Link, K. & Lesion, N. (1996). Congenital heart disease. In R. R. Edelman, J. R. Hesselink, & M. B. Zlatkin (Eds.), *MRI clinical magnetic resonance imaging* (2nd ed., pp.1683–1710) Philadelphia: W.B. Saunders.

Pagley, P. R., Beller, G. A., Watson, D. D., Gimple, L. W. & Ragosta, M.(1997). Improved outcome after coronary bypass surgery in patients with ischemic cardiomyopathy and residual myocardial viability. *Circulation,* 97, 793–800.

Ragosta, M., Beller, G. A., Watson, D. D., Kaul, S. & Gimple, L. W.(1993). Quantitative planar rest-redistribution 201Tl imaging in detection of myocardial viability and prediction of improvement in left ventricular function after coronary bypass surgery in patients with severely depressed left ventricular function. *Circulation,* 87, 1630–1641.

Rumberger, J. A.(2003). Electron beam (ultrafast) computed tomography for the evaluation of cardiac disease and function. [Online]. Available at: http://www.uptodateonline.com.

Rumberger, J. A., Brundage, B. H., Rader, D. J. & Kondos, G. (1999). Electron beam computed tomographic coronary calcium scanning: A review and guidelines for use in asymptomatic persons *Mayo Clinic Proceedings,* 74, 243–252.

Sharir, T., Rabinowitz, B., Livschitz, S., Moalem, I., Baron, J., Kaplinsky, E. & Chouraqui, P. (1998). Underestimation of extent and severity of coronary artery disease by dipyridamole stress thallium-201 single-photon emission computed topographic myocardial perfusion imaging in patients taking antianginal drugs. *Journal of the American College of Cardiology,* 31, 1540–1546.

Van der Wall, E. E. & Bax, J. (1996). Current clinic relevance of cardiovascular magnetic resonance and its relationship to nuclear cardiology. *Journal of Nuclear Cardiology,* 6(4), 462–469.

Van Geuns, R. M., Wielopolski, P. A., de Bruin, H. G., Rensing, B. J., van Ooijen, P. M., Hulshoff, M. Oudkerk, M. & de Feyter, P. J. (1999). Basic principals of magnetic resonance imaging. *Progress in Cardiovascular Disease,* 42(2), 149–156.

Van Geuns, R. M., Wielopolski, P. A., de Bruin, H. G., Rensing, B. J., van Ooijen, P. M., Hulshoff, M. Oudkerk, M. & de Feyter, P. J. (1999). Magnetic resonance imaging of the coronary arteries: Techniques and Results. *Progress in Cardiovascular Disease,* 42(2), 157–166.

White, C. S. (1996). MR evaluation of the pericardium and cardiac malignancies. *MRI Clinics of North America-Cardiac Imaging,* 4(2), 237–252.

Electrocardiography

CAROL JACOBSON

Electrocardiography is the graphic display of the changing potentials of the electrical field generated by the heart as recorded by electrodes placed on the body surface. Recording of the 12-lead electrocardiogram (ECG) is the most frequently used procedure for the diagnosis of heart disease. It is noninvasive, safe, simple to perform, reproducible, and relatively inexpensive. The 12-lead ECG can record changes indicative of primary myocardial disease such as coronary artery disease, cardiomyopathy, hypertension, or infiltrative diseases. It can also reflect changes associated with electrolyte abnormalities, metabolic disorders, drug effect, and other disease processes such as pulmonary embolism or pulmonary hypertension, renal failure, and central nervous system disease. The ECG is the gold standard for noninvasive diagnosis of cardiac arrhythmias and conduction abnormalities (see Chapter 19) and is a useful tool in evaluating function of implanted devices such as pacemakers and implantable cardioverter defibrillators (see Chapter 32) (Kadish et al., 2001).

This chapter discusses the electrocardiographic features of various cardiac conditions and other disease processes that may causes changes on the ECG. Specific information on the pathophysiology and treatment of cardiac disease and other medical conditions that may affect the ECG can be found in other chapters in this book or in medical textbooks.

ELECTRICAL CONDUCTION THROUGH THE HEART

The electrical impulse of the heart is the stimulus for cardiac contraction. The conduction system (Fig. 18-1) is responsible for the initiation of the electrical impulse and its sequential spread through the atria, atrioventricular (AV) junction, and ventricles.

The Cardiac Conduction System

The conduction system of the heart consists of the following structures.

Sinus Node

The sinus or sinoatrial (SA) node is a small group of cells in the high right atrium that functions as the normal pacemaker of the heart because it has the fastest rate of automaticity. The SA node normally depolarizes between 60 and 100 times per minute.

Atrioventricular Node

The AV node is a small group of cells in the low right atrium near the tricuspid valve. The AV node has three main functions:

1. Its major job is to slow conduction of the impulse from the atria to the ventricles to allow time for the atria to contract and empty their blood into the ventricles.
2. It has automaticity at a rate of 40 to 60 beats per minute and can function as a backup pacemaker if the SA node fails.
3. It screens out rapid atrial impulses to protect the ventricles from dangerously fast rates when the atrial rate is very rapid.

Bundle of His

The bundle of His is a short bundle of fibers at the bottom of the AV node leading to the bundle branches. Conduction velocity accelerates in the bundle of His, and the impulse is transmitted to both bundle branches.

Bundle Branches

The bundle branches are bundles of fibers that rapidly conduct the impulse into the right and left ventricles. The *right bundle* branch travels along the right side of the interventricular septum and carries the impulse into the right ventricle. The *left bundle branch* has two main divisions, the anterior fascicle and the posterior fascicle, which carry the impulse into the left ventricle.

Purkinje Fibers

The Purkinje fibers are hairlike fibers that spread out from the bundle branches along the endocardial surface of both ventricles and rapidly conduct the impulse to the ventricular muscle cells. Cells in the Purkinje system have automaticity at a rate of 20 to 40 beats per minute and can function as a backup pacemaker if all other pacemakers fail.

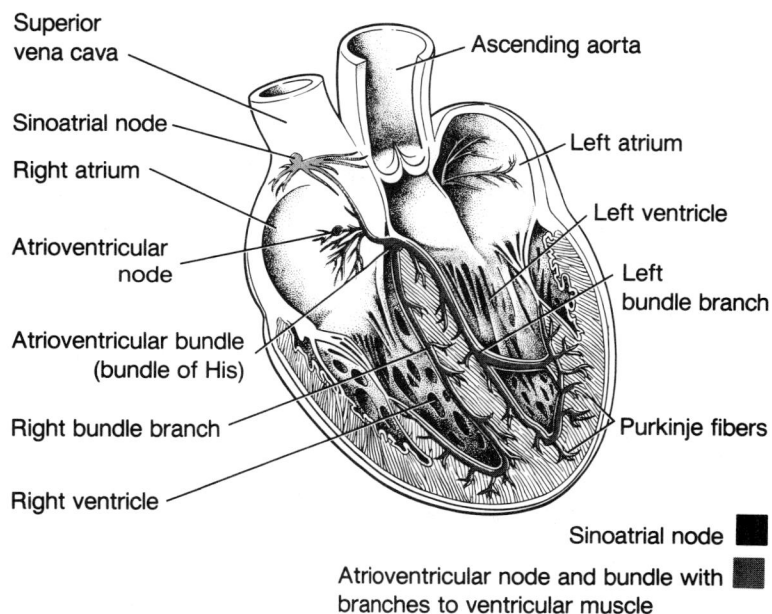

Superior vena cava

Sinoatrial node

Right atrium

Atrioventricular node

Atrioventricular bundle (bundle of His)

Right bundle branch

Right ventricle

Ascending aorta

Left atrium

Left ventricle

Left bundle branch

Purkinje fibers

Sinoatrial node

Atrioventricular node and bundle with branches to ventricular muscle

■ **Figure 18–1.** Cardiac conduction system. (From Jacobson, C. [1991]. Cardiac arrhythmias and conduction abnormalities. In M. L. Patrick, S. L. Woods, R. F. Craven, et al. [Eds.], *Medical-surgical nursing* [2nd ed., pp. 648–693]. Philadelphia: J. B. Lippincott.)

Origin and Spread of the Electrical Impulse Through the Heart

The impulse normally begins in the SA node, located in the high right atrium, because the SA node has the fastest rate of automaticity of all potential pacemaker cells in the heart. The impulse spreads from the SA node through both atria in an inferior and leftward direction, resulting in depolarization of the atrial muscle. When the impulse reaches the AV node, its conduction velocity is slowed before it continues into the ventricles. The slowing in the AV node is necessary to allow time for the atria to contract and empty their blood into the ventricles before the ventricles contract. When the impulse emerges from the AV node, it travels rapidly through the bundle of His and down the right and left bundle branches into the Purkinje network of both ventricles, and results in depolarization of the ventricular muscle. The spread of this wave of depolarization through the heart produces the classic surface ECG, which can be recorded by an electrocardiograph (ECG machine) or monitored continuously on a bedside cardiac monitor.

Waves, Complexes, and Intervals of the Cardiac Cycle

The ECG waves, complexes, and intervals are illustrated in Figure 18-2. Table 18-1 summarizes normal waveform configurations in each of the 12 ECG leads.

P Wave

The P wave represents atrial muscle depolarization. It is normally small, smoothly rounded, and no taller than 2.5 mm or wider than 0.11 second.

QRS Complex

The QRS complex represents ventricular muscle depolarization. The shape of the QRS complex depends on the lead being recorded and the ventricular activation sequence; not all leads record all waves of the QRS complex. A Q wave is an initial negative deflection from baseline and should be less than 0.03 second in duration and less than 25% of the R-wave amplitude. An R wave is the first positive deflection from baseline. An S wave is a negative deflection that follows an R wave. When a complex is all positive, it is just an R wave; when it is all negative, it is called a QS. Regardless of the shape of the complex, ventricular depolarization waves are called QRS complexes (Fig. 18-3). The width of the QRS complex represents intraventricular conduction time and is measured from the point at which it first leaves the baseline to the end of the last appearing wave. Normal QRS width is 0.04 to 0.10 second.

T Wave

The T wave represents ventricular muscle repolarization. It follows the QRS complex and is normally in the same direction as the QRS complex. The T wave is usually rounded and slightly asymmetric, rising more slowly than it descends. T waves are not normally taller than 5 mm in any limb lead or 10 mm in any precordial lead.

U Wave

The U wave is a small, rounded wave that sometimes follows the T wave and is most prominent in leads V_2–V_4. The U wave is normally in the same direction as the T wave but is only approximately 10% of its amplitude. The U wave is thought to be part of the ventricular repolarization process and may represent repolarization of the Purkinje network or certain cells in the

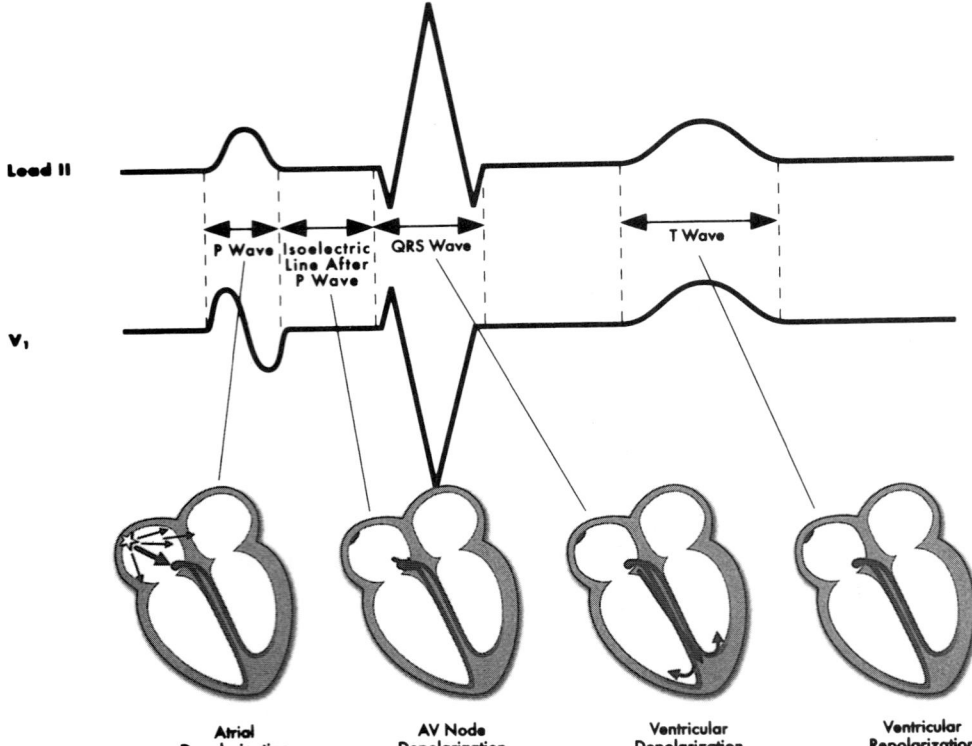

■ **Figure 18–2.** Waves, complexes, and intervals of the cardiac cycle in Leads II and V_1 (From Woods, S. L. [1997]. Interpretation and management of basic cardiac rhythms. In M. Chulay, C. Guzzetta, B. Dossey [Eds.], *AACN handbook of critical care nursing* [pp. 55–82]. Stamford, CT: Appleton & Lange.)

deep subepicardial layer of the ventricle (M cells), or summation of ventricular afterdepolarizations (Antzelevitch et al, 1995).

PR Interval

The PR interval is measured from the beginning of the P wave to the beginning of the QRS complex and represents the time required for the impulse to travel through the atria, AV junction, and Purkinje system. The normal PR interval is 0.12 to 0.20 second.

ST Segment

The ST segment represents the period of time when the ventricle is still depolarized. It begins at the end of the QRS complex (J point) and extends to the beginning of the T wave. The ST segment should be at the isoelectric line and gently curve up into the T wave.

QT Interval

The QT interval measures the duration of ventricular activation and recovery and varies with age, gender, and heart rate. The QT interval is measured from the beginning of the QRS complex to the end of the T wave, and, because it varies inversely with the heart rate, it must be corrected to a heart rate of 60 after measurement (QTc interval). Because the QT interval adjusts gradually to a change in heart rate, accurate measurement of the QTc can be done only after several regular and equal cardiac cycles. The normal QTc is usually less than half the preceding RR interval at normal heart rates, but a more accurate evaluation can be done using the nomogram for rate correction of the QT interval (Fig. 18-4) or by calculating the QTc using Bazett's formula: $QTc = QT / \sqrt{RR}$ interval, where QT and RR intervals are in seconds (Bazett, 1920). The upper limit of normal QTc is generally considered to be <0.43 second in adult males and <0.45 second in adult females (Moss, 1995).

BASIC ELECTROCARDIOGRAPHY

The ECG is the graphic record of the electrical activity of the heart. The spread of the electrical impulse through the heart produces weak electrical currents through the entire body, which can be detected and amplified by the ECG machine and recorded on calibrated graph paper. These amplified signals form the ECG tracing, consisting of the waveforms and intervals described previously, and are inscribed onto grid paper that moves beneath the recording stylus (pen) at standard speed of 25 mm per second. The grid on the paper consists of a series of small and large boxes, both horizontally and vertically; horizontal boxes measure time, and vertical boxes measure voltage (Fig. 18-5). Each small box horizontally is equal to 0.04 second, and each large box horizontally is equal to 0.20 second. On the vertical axis, each small box measures 1 mm and is equal to 0.1 mV; each large box measures 5 mm and is equal to 0.5 mV. In addition to the grid, most ECG paper places a vertical line in the top margin at 3-second intervals or places a mark at 1-second intervals.

Table 18-1 ■ NORMAL ELECTROCARDIOGRAM WAVEFORM CONFIGURATION IN EACH OF THE 12 LEADS

Lead	P Wave	Q Wave	R Wave	S Wave	T Wave	ST Segment
I	Upright	Small	Largest wave of complex	Small (less than R or none)	Upright	May vary from +1 to −0.5 mm
II	Upright	Small or none	Large (vertical heart)	Small (less than R or none)	Upright	May vary from +1 to −0.5 mm
III	Upright, diphasic, or inverted	Usually small or none (for large Q to be diagnostic, a Q must also be present in a VF)	None to large	None to large (horizontal heart)	Upright, diphasic, or inverted	May vary from +1 to −0.5 mm
aVR	Inverted	Small, none, or large	Small or none	Large (may be QS complex)	Inverted	May vary from +1 to −0.5 mm
aVL	Upright, diphasic, or inverted	Small, none, or large (to be diagnostic, Q must also be present in 1 or precordial leads)	Small, none, or large (horizontal heart)	None to large (vertical heart)	Upright, diphasic, or inverted	May vary from +1 to −0.5 mm
aVF	Upright	Small or none	Small, none, or large (vertical heart)	None to large (horizontal heart)	Upright, diphasic, or inverted	May vary from +1 to −0.5 mm
V_1	Upright, diphasic, or inverted	None or QS complex	Less than S wave or none	Large (may be QS)	Upright, diphasic, or inverted	May vary from 0 to +3 mm
V_2	Upright	None (rare QS)	Less than S wave, or none (larger than V_1)	Large (may be QS)	Upright	May vary from 0 to +3 mm
V_3	Upright	Small or none	Less, greater, or equal to S wave; (larger than V_2)	Large (greater, less, or equal to R wave)	Upright	May vary from 0 to +3 mm
V_4	Upright	Small or none	Greater than S (larger than V_3)	Smaller than R (smaller than V_3)	Upright	May vary from +1 to −0.5 mm
V_5	Upright	Small	Larger than R in V_4; less than 26 mm	Smaller than S in V_4	Upright	May vary from +1 to −0.5 mm
V_6	Upright	Small	Large; less than 26 mm	Smaller than S in V_5	Upright	May vary from +1 to −05 mm

U waves may follow T waves, particularly in leads V_2 to V_4 are upright, and are of lower amplitude than T waves.
Adapted from Goldschlager, & Goldman M. J. (1989). *Principles of clinical electrocardiography* (13th ed.). Norwalk, CT. Appleton & Lange.

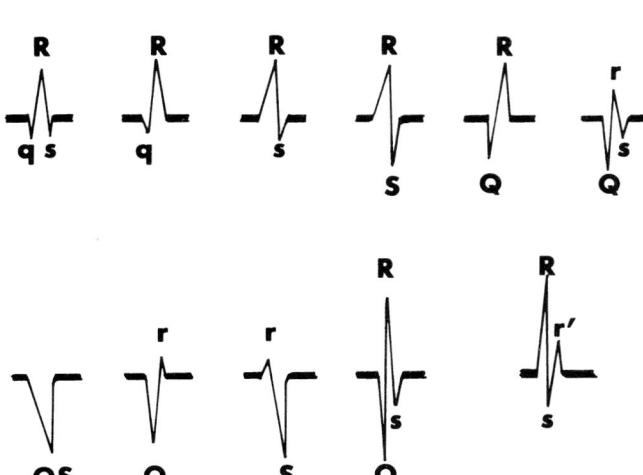

■ **Figure 18-3.** Examples of various QRS complexes. (From Jacobson, C. [2000]. Electrocardiography. In S. L. Woods, E. S. Froelicher, & S. Motzer [Eds.], *Cardiac nursing* [4th ed., pp. 263–296]. Philadelphia: Lippincott.)

The waveforms of the cardiac cycle can be recorded by a bedside cardiac monitor and displayed continuously on an oscilloscope or recorded on a rhythm strip, which consists of the same grid as described previously. The standard 12-lead ECG simultaneously records 12 different views of electrical activity as it travels through the heart and displays all 12 views on a full-page layout, which consists of the same grid. The 12 leads of the ECG are described in detail in following sections.

Determining Heart Rate on the Electrocardiogram

Heart rate can be determined from the ECG strip by several methods. An easy method that can be used for both regular and irregular rhythms is to count the number of RR intervals (not R waves) in a 6-second strip and multiply that number by 10, because there are ten 6-second intervals in 1 minute (Fig. 18-6A).

Another method that can be used only if the rhythm is regular is to count the number of large boxes between two R waves and divide that number into 300, because there are 300 large boxes in a 1-minute strip. The most accurate method to use for a regular rhythm is to count the number of small boxes between

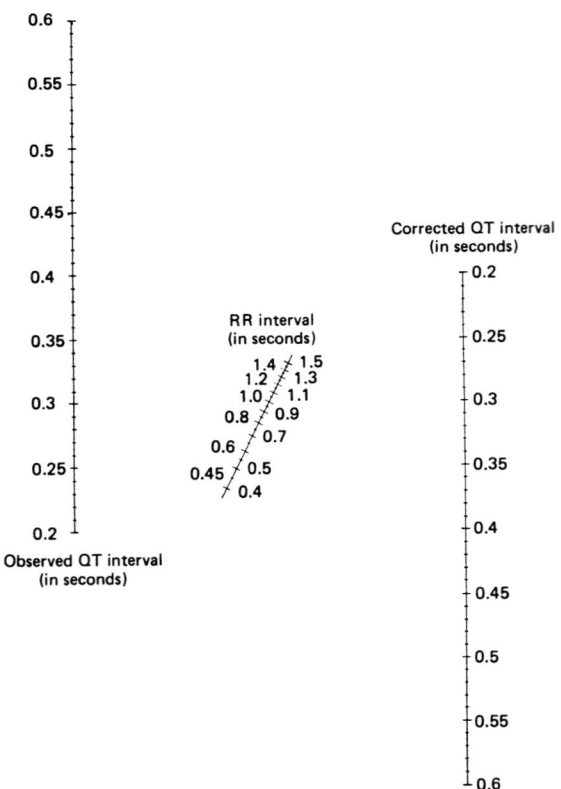

■ **Figure 18–4.** Nomogram for rate correction of QT interval. Measure the observed QT interval and the RR interval. Mark these values in the respective columns of the chart (left and middle). Place a ruler across these two points, The point at which the extension of this line crosses the third column is the corrected QT interval (QTc). (From Kissin, M., Schwarzschild, M. M., & Bakst, H. [1948]. A nomogram for rate correction of the QT interval in the electrocardiogram. *American Heart Journal,* 35, 991.)

two R waves and divide that number into 1,500, because there are 1,500 small boxes in a 1-minute strip. The easiest way to do either of these methods is to use the rate ruler in Figure 18-6*B*.

Determining the Cardiac Rhythm on the Electrocardiogram

The first step in interpreting a 12-lead ECG is to determine the cardiac rhythm. A rhythm strip should be analyzed in a systematic manner to aid in rhythm interpretation until the learner is able to identify arrhythmias by scanning the strip. See Chapter 19 for detailed information on the normal cardiac rhythm and both basic and advanced arrhythmias. The following steps provide a systematic approach to rhythm interpretation:

Regularity: First determine if the rhythm is regular or irregular because this information determines the method of heart rate calculation. If the rhythm is irregular, determine if the irregularity is random or if it occurs in a pattern (i.e., repetitive groups of beats separated by a pause).

Rate: Determine the heart rate as described previously. Determine both atrial and ventricular rates if they are not the same.

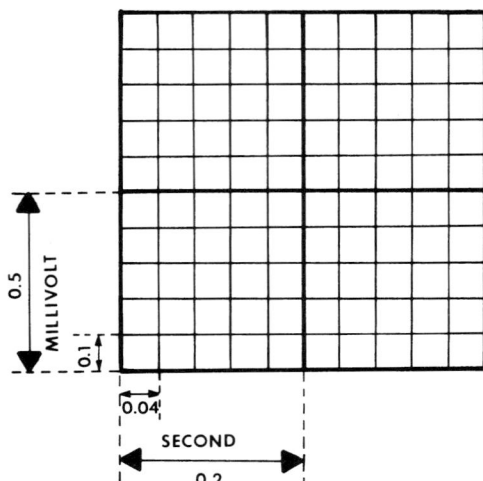

■ **Figure 18–5.** Time and voltage lines on ECG pager at standard paper speed of 25 mm/sec. Horizontal axis measures time: each small box = 0.04 second, one large box = 0.20 second. Vertical axis measures voltage: each small box = 1 mm or 0.1 mV, one large box = 5 mm or 0.5 mV. (From Jacobson, C. [2000]. Electrocardiography. In S. L. Woods, E. S. Froelicher, & S. Motzer [Eds.], *Cardiac nursing* [4th ed., pp. 263–296]. Philadelphia: Lippincott.)

P waves: Locate P waves and note their shape and relationship to QRS complexes. Determine if all P waves look alike and if they have a consistent relationship to QRS complexes (i.e., one P wave before every QRS, two or more P waves before each QRS) or if they occur randomly and are unrelated to QRS complexes.

PR interval: Measure the PR interval of several complexes in a row to determine if it is of normal duration and consistent for all complexes.

QRS width: Measure the QRS complex and determine if it is normal or wide.

Determine the rhythm based on an analysis of the information obtained in these steps. See Chapter 19 for details on arrhythmia analysis.

THE 12-LEAD ELECTROCARDIOGRAM

The 12-lead ECG records electrical activity as it spreads through the heart from 12 different leads that are recorded through electrodes placed on the arms, legs, and specific spots on the chest. Each lead represents a different view of the heart and consists of two electrodes with opposite polarity (bipolar) or one electrode and a reference point (unipolar). A *bipolar* lead has a positive pole and a negative pole, with each contributing equally to the recording. A *unipolar* lead has one positive pole and a reference pole in the center of the chest that is algebraically determined by the ECG machine. The reference pole represents the center of the electrical field of the heart and has a zero potential, so only the positive pole of a unipolar lead contributes to the tracing.

The standard 12-lead ECG consists of six limb leads that record electrical activity in the frontal plane—traveling up/down and

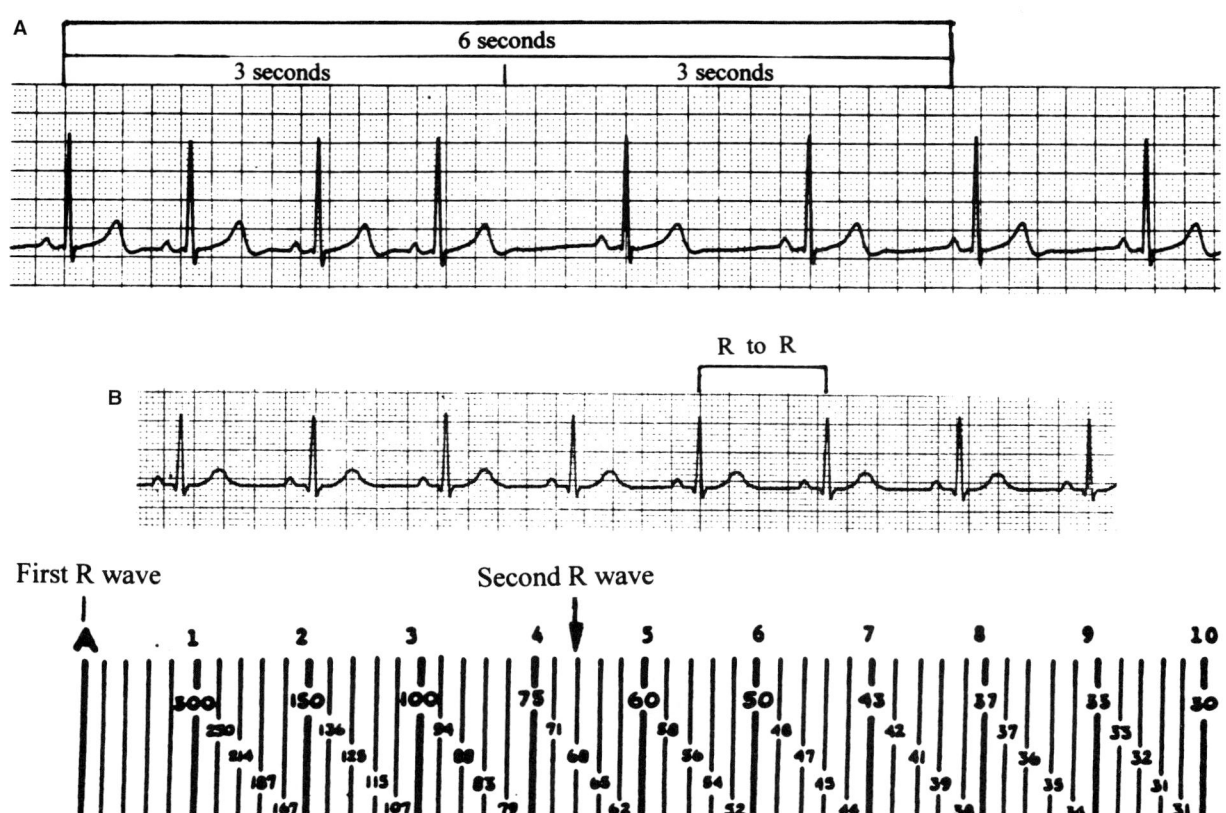

■ **Figure 18–6.** Heart rate determination for an irregular rhythm. Count the number or RR intervals in a 6 second strip and multiply by 10. In (A) there are almost 6 complete RR intervals in a 6 second strip; the heart rate is 60 beats/minute. (B) Heart rate determination for a regular rhythm using the rate ruler. Count the number of large and small boxes between R waves on the rhythm strip. In B there are four large boxes and two small boxes between the R waves marked on the strip. On the rate ruler, the first R wave is represented by the thick line marked "A". Each large box on the ECG paper is represented by a thick line on the rate ruler and is numbered at the top; each small box on the strip is represented by a thin line on the ruler. The number on the line on the ruler that corresponds to the second R wave on the strip represents the heart rate. In B, count four large boxes at the top of the ruler and then two small boxes; the heart rate is 68 beats/minute (represented by the *arrow*). (From Jacobson, C. [2000]. Electrocardiography. In S. L. Woods, E. S. Froelicher, & S. Motzer [Eds.], *Cardiac nursing* [4th ed., pp. 263–296]. Philadelphia: Lippincott.) (Rate ruler in *B* from Marriott, H. J. L. [1988]. *Practical electrocardiography* [8th ed., p 15]. Baltimore: Williams & Wilkins.)

right/left in the heart—and six precordial leads that record electrical activity in the horizontal plane—traveling anterior/posterior and right/left. Limb leads are recorded by electrodes placed on the arms and legs, whereas precordial leads are recorded by electrodes placed on the chest (Fig. 18-7). For convenience in continuous bedside monitoring, arm electrodes can be placed on the shoulders and leg electrodes on the lower part of the rib cage rather than on the limbs without significantly altering the signals recorded.

A camera analogy makes the 12-lead ECG easier to understand. Each lead of the ECG represents a picture of the electrical activity in the heart taken by the camera. In any lead, the positive electrode is the recording electrode or the camera lens. The negative electrode tells the camera which way to "shoot" its picture and determines the direction in which the positive electrode records. When the positive electrode sees electrical activity traveling toward it, it records an upright deflection on the ECG. When the positive electrode sees electrical activity traveling away from it, it records a negative deflection (Fig. 18-8). If the electrical activity travels perpendicular to a positive electrode, either a diphasic deflection or no activity is

recorded. The ECG records three bipolar frontal plane leads—lead I, lead II, and lead III—and three unipolar frontal plane leads—aVR, aVL, and aVF. In addition, there are six unipolar precordial leads: V_1, V_2, V_3, V_4, V_5, and V_6.

Bipolar Leads

Figure 18-9*A* illustrates the three bipolar frontal plane leads. In each lead, the camera represents the positive pole of the lead. In lead I, the positive electrode is on the left arm and the negative electrode is on the right arm. Any electrical activity in the heart that travels toward the positive electrode (camera lens) on the left arm is recorded as an upright deflection and any traveling away from it is recorded as a negative deflection. In lead II, the positive electrode is on the left leg and the negative electrode is on the right arm. Any electrical activity traveling toward the left leg electrode (camera lens) is recorded as an upright deflection and any traveling away from it toward the right arm electrode is recorded as a negative deflection. In lead III, the positive electrode is on the left leg and the negative electrode is on the left

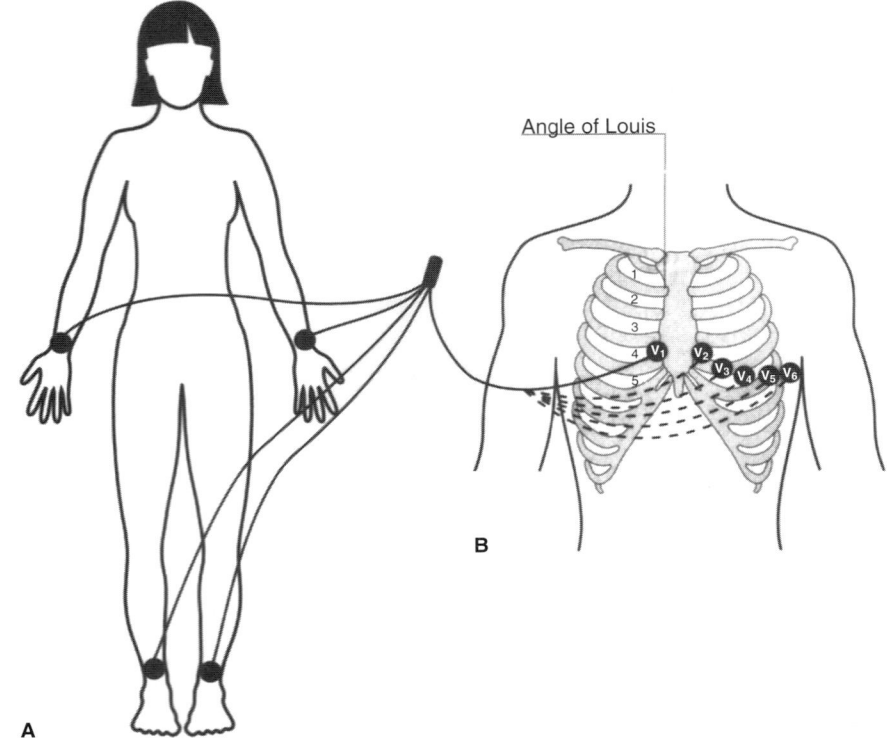

■ **Figure 18–7.** Electrode placement for limb leads and precordial leads. (*A*) Limb electrodes can be places anywhere on the arms and legs. (*B*) Chest electrode placement. V_1 = fourth intercostal space at right sternal border; V_2 = fourth intercostal space at left sternal border; V_3 = halfway betwen V_2 and V_4 in a straight line: V_4 = fifth intercostals space at midelavicular line; V_5 = same level as V_4 at anterior axillary line, V_6 = same level as V_4 at midaxillary line. (From Jacobson, C. [1997]. Advanced ECG concepts. In M. Chulay, C. Guzzetta, B. Dossey [Eds.], *AACN handbook of critical care nursing* [pp. 415–454]. Stamford, CT: Appleton & Lange.)

arm. Any electrical activity coming toward the left leg electrode (camera lens) is recorded as an upright deflection and any traveling away from it toward the left arm is recorded as a negative deflection. The right leg electrode serves as a ground and does not contribute to the signals recorded. The electrical sum of the voltages in the three bipolar frontal plane leads equals zero potential and forms a virtual ground in the center of the triangle used by the unipolar leads as their reference point.

Unipolar Leads

Figure 18-9*B* illustrates the three unipolar frontal plane leads, aVR, aVL, and aVF. The camera represents the location of the positive electrode: on the right shoulder for aVR, on the left shoulder for aVL, and at the foot (left leg) for aVF. The "negative end" of the unipolar lead is the reference point in the

center of the chest that is obtained as described previously. The same recording principles apply to unipolar leads: any electrical activity traveling toward the positive electrode is recorded as an upright deflection and any traveling away from it is recorded as a negative deflection. Figure 18-9*C* shows the six unipolar precordial leads recording from their locations on the chest and "shooting" toward the reference point in the center of the heart.

Right Chest and Posterior Leads

Additional leads can be recorded on the right chest or posterior thorax to gain additional information about right ventricular or posterior infarction or right ventricular hypertrophy (RVH). Figure 18-10 shows lead placement for obtaining right chest leads and posterior leads.

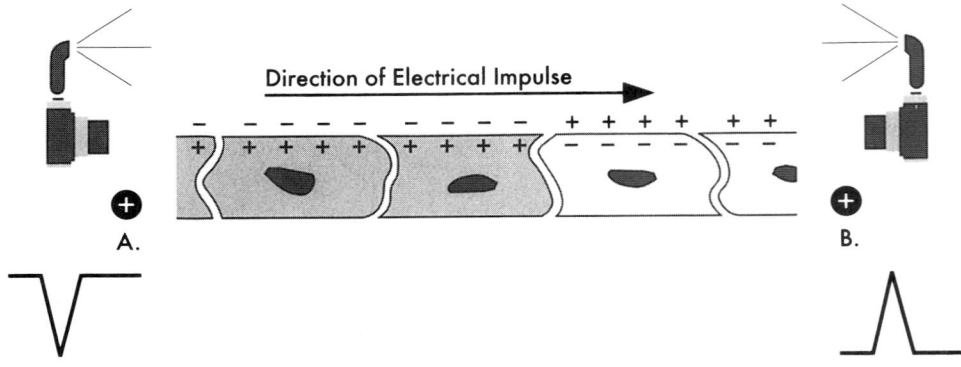

■ **Figure 18–8.** A strip of cardiac muscle depolarizing in the direction of the arrow. A positive electrode at *B* sees depolarization coming toward it and records an upright deflection. A positive electrode at *A* sees depolarization going away from it and records a negative deflection. (From Jacobson, C. [1997]. Advanced ECG concepts. In M. Chulay, C. Guzzetta, & B. Dossey [Eds.], *AACN handbook of critical care nursing* [pp. 415–454]. Stamford, CT: Appleton & Lange.)

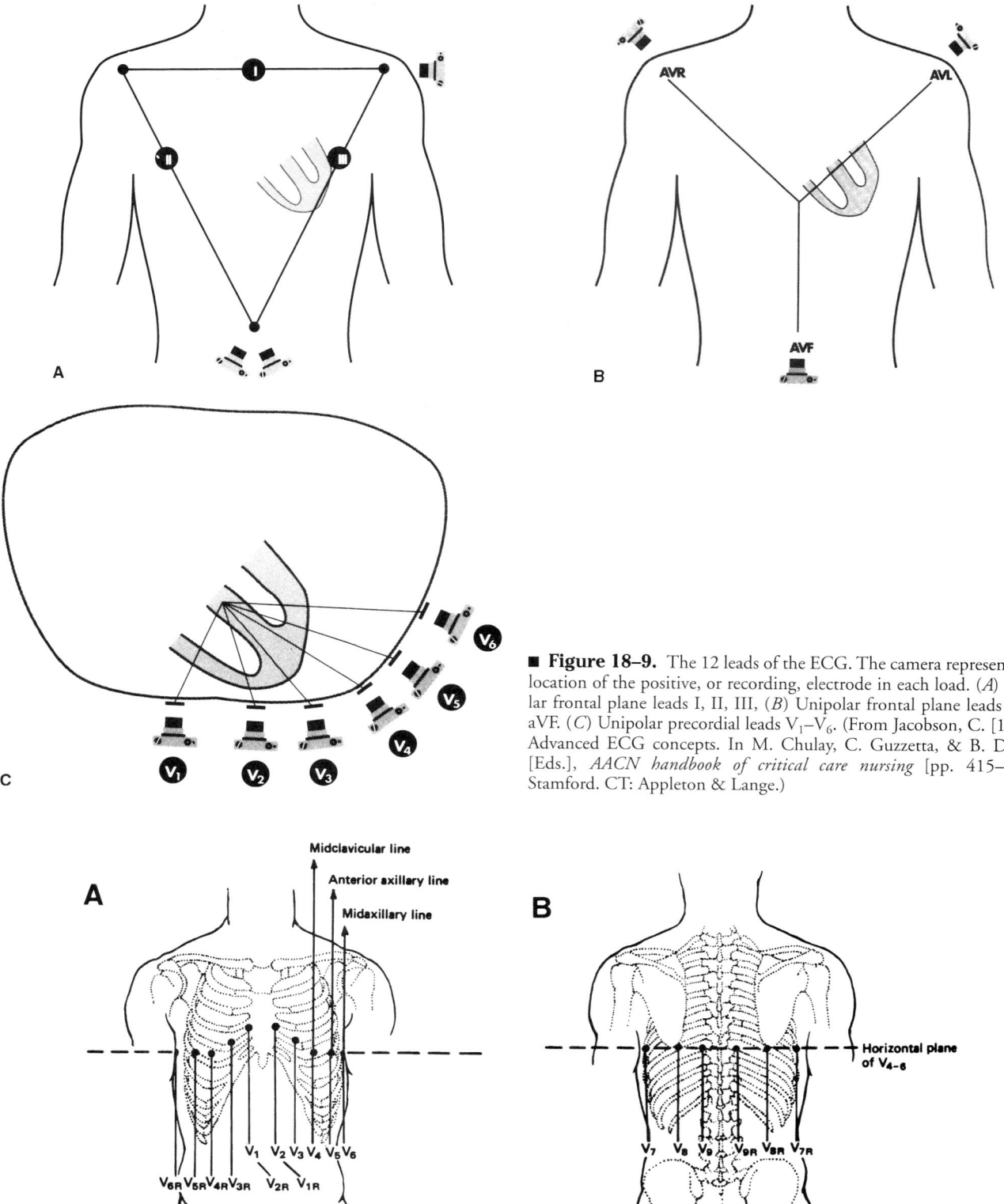

■ **Figure 18–9.** The 12 leads of the ECG. The camera represents the location of the positive, or recording, electrode in each load. (*A*) Bipolar frontal plane leads I, II, III, (*B*) Unipolar frontal plane leads aVR, aVF. (*C*) Unipolar precordial leads V_1–V_6. (From Jacobson, C. [1997]. Advanced ECG concepts. In M. Chulay, C. Guzzetta, & B. Dossey [Eds.], *AACN handbook of critical care nursing* [pp. 415–454]. Stamford. CT: Appleton & Lange.)

■ **Figure 18–10.** (*A*) Electrode placement for the six standard precordial leads and for right precordial leads. Right chest leads are a mirror image of left chest leads: V_{1R} is same as standard V_2, V_{2R} is the same as standard V_1, V_{3R} is halfway between V_{2R} and V_{4R}, V_{4R} is fifth intercostals space at right midclavicular line, V_{5R} is same level as V_{4R} in right anterior axillary line, V_{6R} is same level in right midaxillary line. (*B*) Electrode placement for left posterior leads: V_7, posterior axillary line; V_8, posterior scapular line; V_9, left border of spine. All three are in the same horizontal plane of V_4 to V_6. (Goldman, M. J. [1986]. *Principles of clinical electrocardiography* [12th ed.] Los Altos, CA: Lange Medical Publications.)

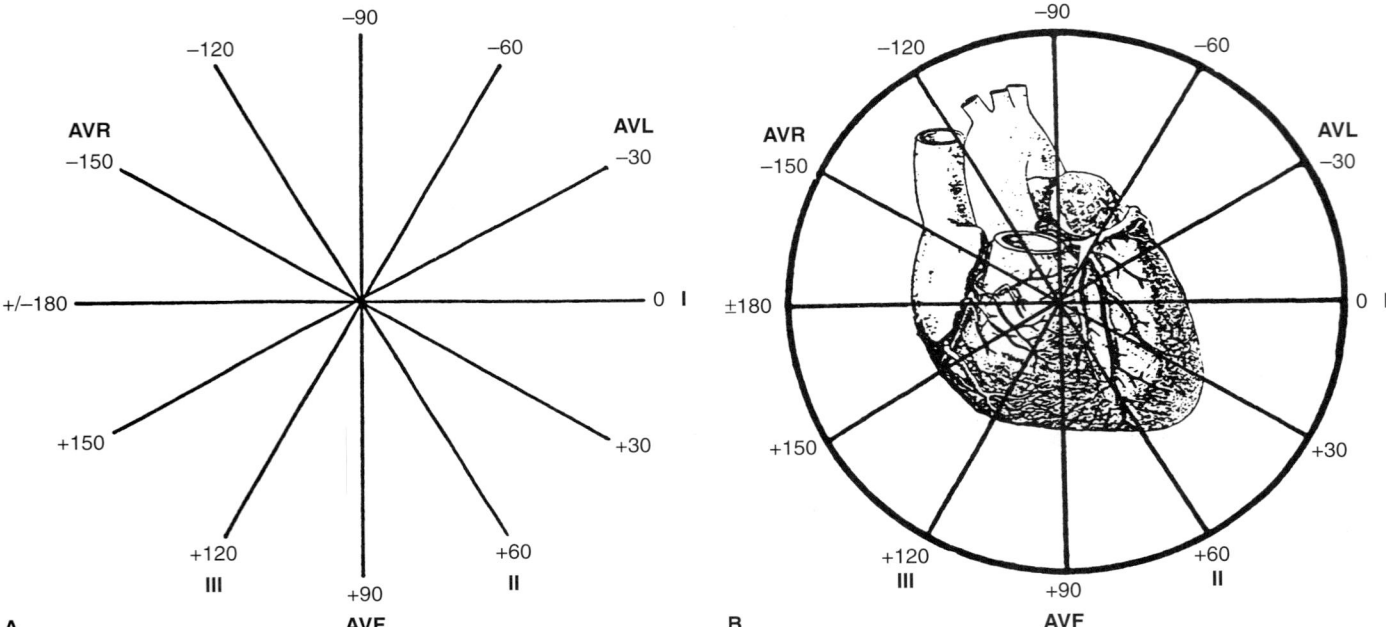

■ **Figure 18–11.** Hexaxial reference system (or axis wheel). Each lead is labeled at its positive end in both examples. (*A*) All six frontal plane leads bisect each other. The degrees of the axis wheel are shown. (*B*) The axis wheel superimposed on the heart to demonstrate each lead's of the heart. Leads I and a VL face the left lateral wall, leads II, III, and a VF face the inferior surface. (From Jacobson, C. [1997]. Advanced ECG concepts. In M. Chulay, C. Guzzetta, & B. Dossey [Eds.], *AACN handbook of critical care nursing* [pp. 415–454]. Stamford, CT: Appleton & Lange.)

The Hexaxial Reference System

Figure 18-11*A* shows the *hexaxial reference system* that is formed when the six frontal plane leads are moved together in such a way that they bisect each other in the center. Each lead is labeled at its positive end to make it easy to remember where the positive electrode is. In Figure 18-11*B*, the hexaxial reference system is superimposed over a drawing of the heart to illustrate how each frontal plane lead views the heart. The reference system forms a 360-degree circle surrounding the heart with 180 positive degrees and 180 negative degrees. By convention, the positive end of lead I is designated 0 degrees and the six leads divide the circle into 30-degree segments, as labeled in the figure.

The 12 Views of the Heart

The normal sequence of depolarization through the heart and the resulting P, QRS, and T waves for each frontal plane lead are illustrated in Figure 18-12*A*. The impulse normally originates in the SA node high in the right atrium and spreads leftward through the left atrium and downward toward the AV node low in the right atrium. Leads I and aVL, with their positive electrode (camera lens) on the left side of the body, record this leftward electrical activity as an upright P wave because the positive electrode sees atrial depolarization coming toward it. Leads II, III, and aVF, with their positive electrode at the bottom of the heart, record the downward spread of atrial activity as upright P waves for the same reason. Lead aVR, with its positive electrode on the right shoulder, sees the electrical activity moving away from it and records a negative P wave.

As the impulse spreads through the AV node, no electrical activity is recorded because the AV node is too small to be recorded by surface leads. As the impulse exits the AV node, it moves through the bundle of His and enters the right and left bundle branches. The left bundle branch sprouts some Purkinje fibers high on the left side of the septum that carry the impulse into the septum and cause it to depolarize first in a left-to-right direction. The electrical impulse then enters the Purkinje system of both ventricular free walls simultaneously and depolarizes them from endocardium to epicardium (indicated by the small arrows through the ventricles in Fig. 18-12*A*). Millions of electrical impulses travel through the ventricles in three dimensions simultaneously, but, if averaged together, they move downward, leftward, and posterior toward the large left ventricle, as indicated by the large arrow in the same figure. This large arrow represents the *mean axis,* which is the net direction of electrical depolarization through the ventricles when all the smaller arrows are averaged together.

The QRS complex is recorded as the ventricles depolarize. Leads I and aVL, with their positive electrodes on the left side of the body, see the septum depolarizing away from them in a left-to-right direction and record a small negative deflection (Q wave). They then see the large left ventricular free wall depolarizing toward them and record an upright deflection (R wave). Leads II, III, and aVF, with their positive electrodes at the bottom of the heart, may not see septal activity at all and not record any deflection. If these leads see septal activity coming slightly toward them, they record a positive deflection. They all then see the forces moving downward through the left ventricle toward them and record an upright deflection (R wave). Lead aVR, positive on the right shoulder, sees all activity moving away from it and records a negative deflection (QS complex).

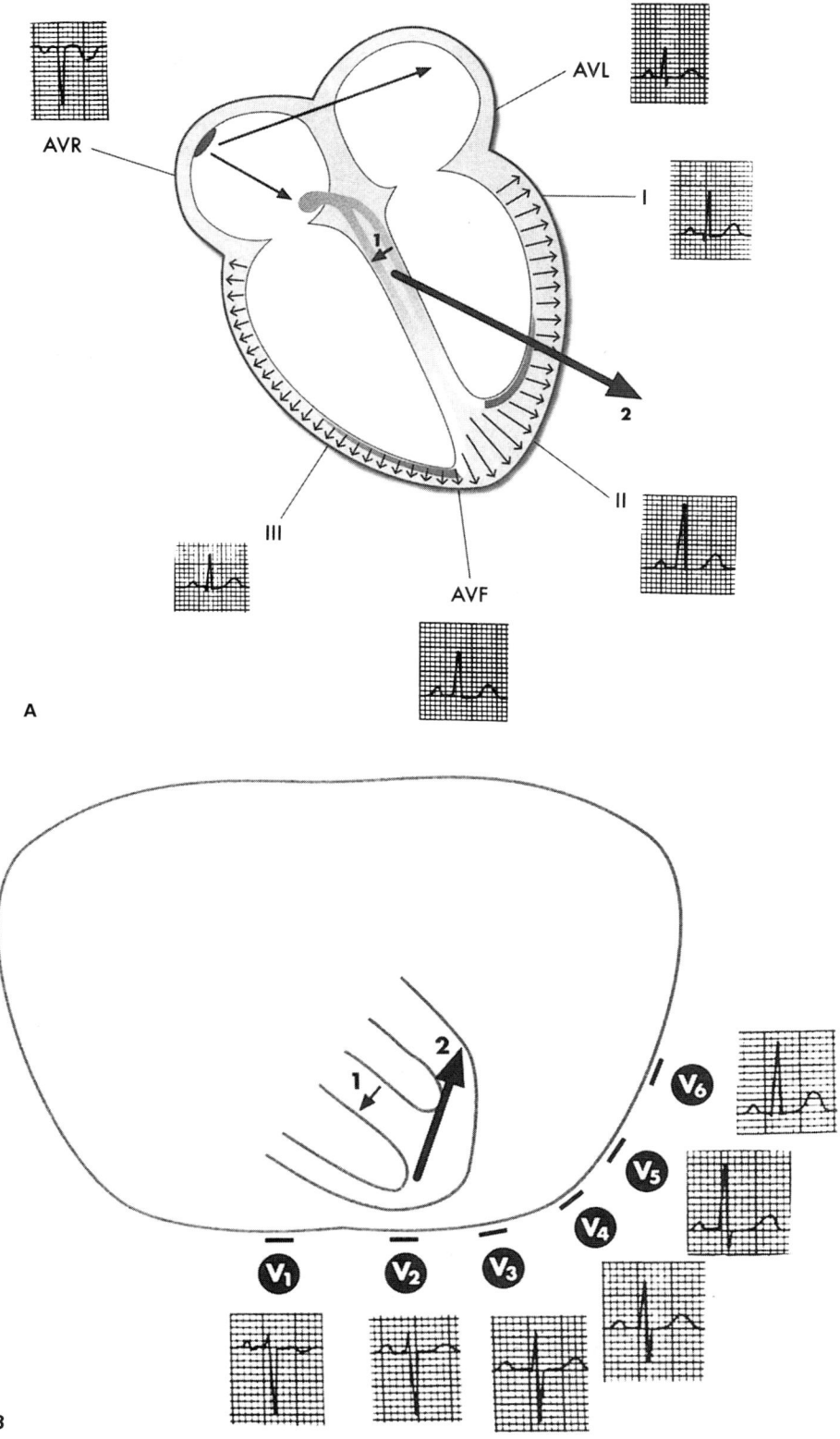

■ Figure 18–12. (*A*) Normal sequence of depolarization through the heart as recorded by each of the frontal plane leads. (*B*) Cross section of the thorax illustrating how the six precordial leads record normal electrical activity in the ventricles. In both examples, the small arrow (1) shows the initial direction of depolarization through the septum, followed by the mean direction of ventricular free wall depolarization, larger arrow (2). (From Jacobson, C. [1997]. Advanced ECG concepts. In M. Chulay, C. Guzzetta, & B. Dossey [Eds.] *AACN handbook of critical care nursing* [pp. 415–454]. Stamford, CT: Appleton & Lange.)

The six precordial leads record electrical activity traveling in the horizontal plane. Figure 18-12*B* illustrates the position of the precordial leads and how they record electrical activity as it spreads through the ventricles in the horizontal plane. Lead V_1 is located on the front of the chest and records a small R wave as the septum depolarizes toward it from left to right. It then records a deep S wave as depolarization spreads away from it through the thick left ventricle. As the positive electrode is moved across the precordium from the V_1 to the V_6 position, it records progressively more left ventricular forces and the R wave gets progressively larger. Lead V_6 is located on the left side of the chest and usually records a small Q wave as the septum depolarizes from left to right away from the positive electrode, and a large R wave as electrical activity spreads toward the positive electrode through the thick left ventricle. Normal R-wave progression means that the R wave gets progressively larger from V_1 to V_6, or that V_6 is predominantly an R wave compared with V_1, which is predominantly an S wave. Sometimes the largest precordial R wave is recorded in lead V_4 or V_5, which is a normal variant.

The Normal Adult 12-Lead Electrocardiogram

Table 18-1 lists normal waveform configurations for each of the 12 leads, and Figure 18-13 shows a normal 12-lead ECG. Normal sinus rhythm is present at a rate of 62 beats per minute, and the axis is approximately +10 degrees. P waves are normal (they are flat in aVL, but this is a normal variant), and T waves are normal (flat or slightly inverted in lead aVL and V_1 is a normal variant). The QRS complex is normal (0.08 second wide), there are no abnormal Q waves, and R-wave progression is normal across the precordium. The ST segment is at baseline in all leads. This ECG can be used for comparison as abnormalities are discussed throughout this chapter.

AXIS DETERMINATION

Conduction of a wave of depolarization through the myocardium results in propagation of thousands of electrical potentials in multiple directions. Over 80% of these potentials are balanced by similar instantaneous charges moving in opposite directions. Balanced alterations in electrical potentials result in an algebraic "canceling out" of these instantaneous vectors. What remains as the detected and amplified ECG tracing is the net vector, which reveals the magnitude, direction, and polarity of the mean electrical force as it travels through the myocardium. Frontal plane axis can be determined for P waves, QRS complexes, and T waves. This section deals only with QRS axis determination.

The normal QRS axis is defined as −30 to +110 degrees because most of the electrical forces in a normal heart are directed downward and leftward toward the large left ventricle. Left axis deviation is defined as −31 to −90 degrees and occurs when most of the forces move in a leftward and superior direction, as can happen in left ventricular hypertrophy (LVH), left anterior fascicular block (LAFB), inferior myocardial infarction (MI), left bundle-branch block (LBBB), several congenital defects, and some arrhythmias, especially ventricular tachycardia and Wolff-Parkinson-White syndrome. Right axis deviation is defined as +110 to +180 degrees and occurs when most of the forces move rightward, as can happen in RVH, left posterior fascicular block (LPFB), right bundle-branch block (RBBB), dextrocardia, ventricular tachycardia, and Wolff-Parkinson-White syndrome. When most of the forces are directed superior and rightward between −90 and −180 degrees, the term *indeterminate axis* is used. This axis can occur with ventricular tachycardia and occasionally with bifascicular block. Figure 18-14 shows the axis wheel divided into its normal, left deviation, right deviation, and indeterminate sections.

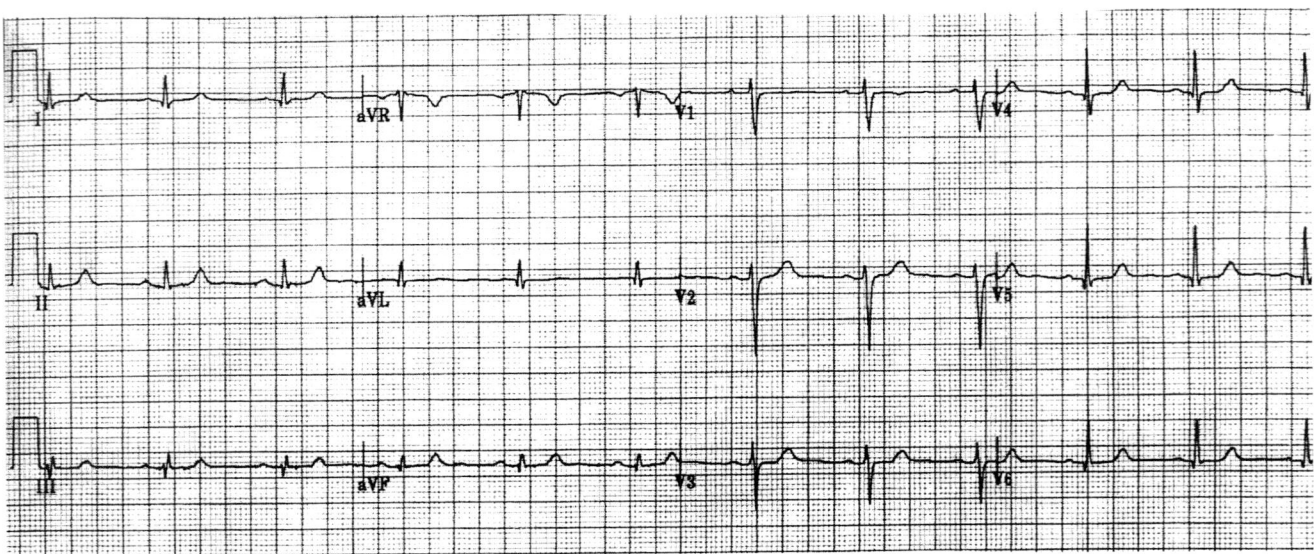

■ **Figure 18–13.** Normal 12-lead ECG.

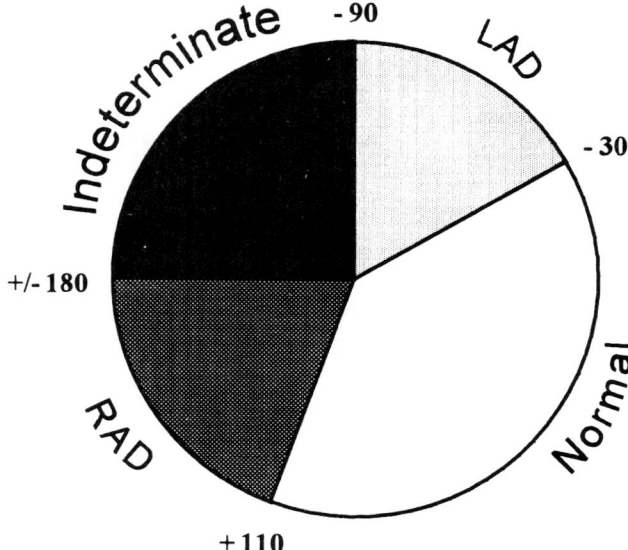

■ **Figure 18–14.** Normal axis = −30° to +110°, LAD = −30° to −90°, LAD = +110° to +180°, indetermnant axis = −90° to −180°. (From Jacobson, C. [1997]. Advanced ECG concepts. In M. Chulay, C. Guzzetta, & B. Dossey [Eds.], *AACN handbook of critical care nursing* [pp. 415–454]. Stamford, CT: Appleton & Lange.)

The mean frontal plane QRS axis can be determined in a number of ways. The most accurate method is to average the forces moving right and left with those moving up and down because this represents the frontal plane. Because lead I is the most direct right/left lead and lead aVF is the most direct up/down lead, it is easiest to use these two perpendicular leads to calculate the mean axis. Figure 18-15A shows the frontal plane leads of a 12-lead ECG. In Figure 18-15B, leads I and aVF are shown enlarged along with the axis wheel with small hash marks along the axes of lead I and lead aVF. These hash marks represent the small 1-mV boxes on the ECG paper. To determine the mean QRS axis, follow these steps:

1. Look at the QRS complex in lead I and count the number of positive and negative boxes. Mark the net vector along the appropriate end of lead I on the axis wheel. In Figure 18-15B, the QRS complex in lead I is five boxes positive and two boxes negative, resulting in a net three boxes positive, or +3. Count three hash marks toward the positive end of lead I and put a mark on the axis wheel at that spot.

2. Look at the QRS complex in aVF and follow the same procedure as before. In this example, the QRS complex in aVF is eight boxes positive and has two very small negative deflections that equal approximately one box when added together, resulting in a net +7. Count seven hash marks along the positive end of the aVF axis and place a mark at that spot.

3. Draw a perpendicular line down from the mark on the lead I axis and a perpendicular line across from the mark on the aVF axis.

4. Draw a line from the center of the axis wheel to the spot where these two perpendicular lines meet. This line is the mean QRS axis—approximately +65 degrees.

A quick but less accurate method of axis determination is to place the axis in its proper quadrant of the axis wheel by

looking at lead I and aVF, because these leads divide the wheel into four quadrants. As illustrated in Figure 18-16, if both of these leads are positive, the axis falls in the normal quadrant, 0 to +90 degrees. If lead I is positive and aVF is negative, the axis falls in the left quadrant, 0 to −90 degrees. If lead I is negative and aVF is positive, the axis falls in the right quadrant, +90 to +180 degrees. If both leads are negative, the axis falls in the indeterminate quadrant or "no-man's land," −90 to −180 degrees. Locating the correct quadrant is often adequate, but, because the portion of the left quadrant for 0 to −30 degrees is considered normal, it is necessary to be more precise in describing the axis when it falls in the left quadrant. To fine-tune the axis quickly, find the limb lead with the smallest or most equiphasic QRS complex. This lead is not seeing much electrical force if it is equiphasic or very small, and, therefore, its perpendicular lead must be seeing most of the forces. Locate the perpendicular lead (lead I and aVF are perpendicular, lead II and aVL are perpendicular, lead III and aVR are perpendicular), and see if the QRS is positive or negative in that lead. If it is positive, the axis is directed toward the positive end of the lead, and, if it is negative, the axis is directed toward the negative end of the lead. Using the ECG in Figure 18-15A, do the following:

1. Place the axis in its correct quadrant by looking at lead I and aVF. *Because both leads are positive, the axis is in the normal quadrant.*

2. Find the smallest or most equiphasic limb lead. *Lead aVL is the most equiphasic lead in this example.*

3. Find the lead that is perpendicular to the equiphasic lead and note if it is positive or negative. *Lead II is perpendicular to aVL and lead II is positive in this example. Therefore the axis is directed toward the positive end of lead II, which is +60 degrees.*

Using the ECG in Figure 18-17A, first place the axis in the appropriate quadrant by using lead I and aVF. Lead I is upright and aVF is negative, placing the axis in the left quadrant. However, because 30 degrees of the left quadrant is considered normal, we need to fine-tune the axis to determine where in the left quadrant it actually falls. Lead aVR is the most equiphasic lead in this ECG, which means that most of the electrical force is moving perpendicular to aVR. Lead III is perpendicular to aVR, and lead III is negative in this ECG, indicating that the axis is directed toward the negative pole of lead III. The axis is −60 degrees. The axis wheel shows how to count boxes in this example.

Using the ECG in Figure 18-17B, place the axis in the appropriate quadrant. Because lead I is negative and aVF is positive, the axis is in the right quadrant. The most equiphasic lead is aVR, and lead III is perpendicular to aVR. Because lead III is positive, the axis is directed toward the positive pole of lead III, or +150 degrees. The axis wheel shows how boxes are counted in this example.

INTRAVENTRICULAR CONDUCTION ABNORMALITIES

The intraventricular conduction system consists of the right bundle branch and the left main bundle branch, which fans out into septal fascicles, an anterior fascicle, and a posterior fascicle. There are numerous individual anatomic variations, but

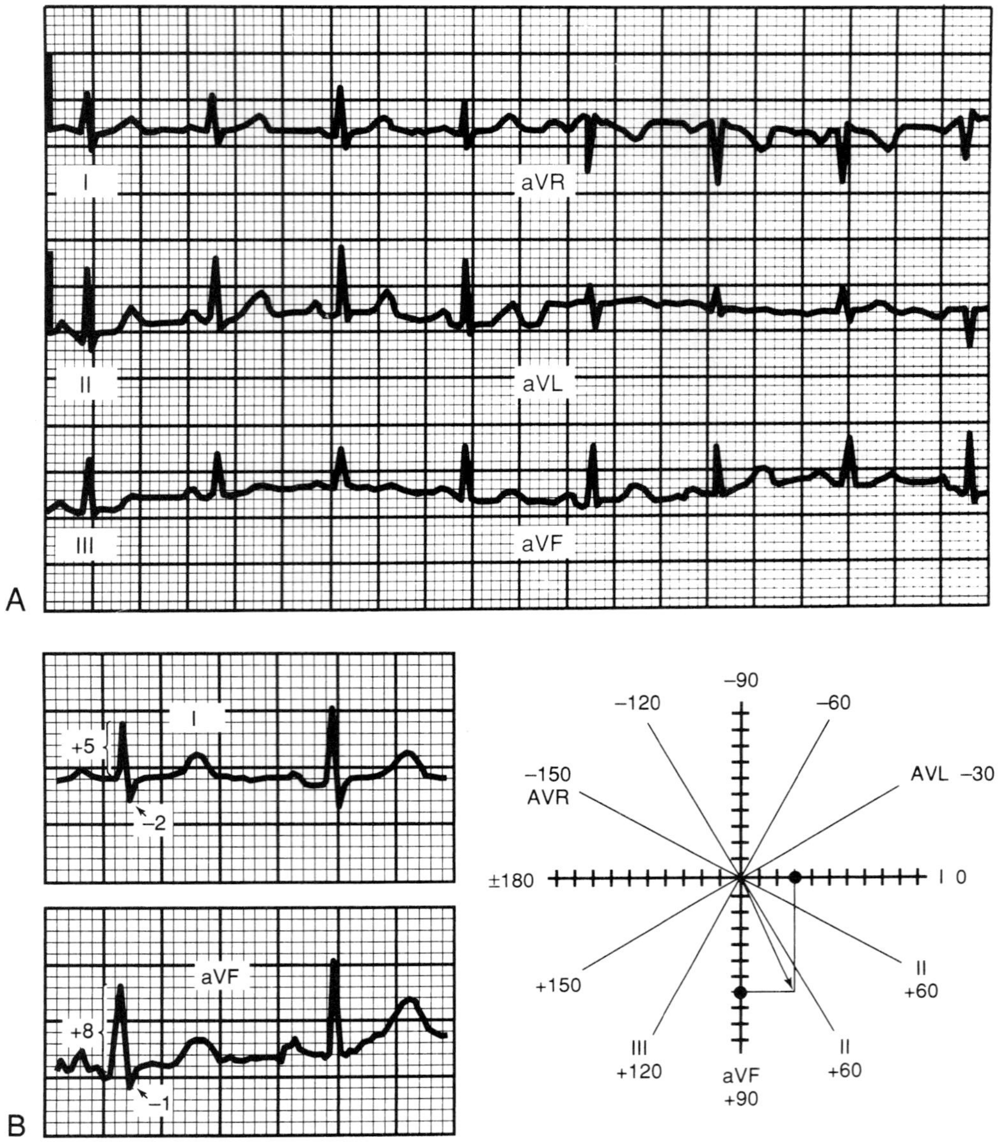

■ **Figure 18–15.** Calculating the mean QRS axis. (*A*) The six frontal plane leads of an ECG. (*B*) Lead I and lead a VF enlarged. See text for instructions on calculating the axis using leads I and a VF on the axis wheel. (From Jacobson, C. [1997]. *Advanced ECG concepts.* In M. Chulay, C. Guzzetta, & B. Dossey [Eds.], *AACN handbook of critical care nursing* [pp. 415–454]. Stamford, CT: Appleton & Lange.)

the intraventricular conduction system is generally regarded to consist of three major fascicles that diverge from the bundle of His: (1) the right bundle branch, (2) the anterior division of the left bundle branch (left anterior fascicle), and (3) the posterior division of the left bundle branch (left posterior fascicle; Fig. 18-18). Block may occur in any part of this conduction system. Monofascicular block is block in only one of the three major fascicles. Bifascicular block can mean block in both divisions of the left bundle branch, but it is more commonly used to describe the combination of RBBB and either LAFB or LPFB. Trifascicular block means block in all three major divisions.

Bundle-Branch Block

When one of the bundle branches is blocked, the ventricles depolarize asynchronously. Bundle-branch block is character-

ized by a delay of excitation to one ventricle and abnormal spread of electrical activity through the ventricle whose bundle is blocked. This delayed conduction results in widening of the QRS complex to 0.12 second or greater and a characteristic pattern best recognized in precordial leads V_1 and V_6 and limb leads I and aVL.

Normal ventricular depolarization as recorded by leads V_1 and V_6 is illustrated in Figure 18-19. The positive electrode for V_1 is located on the front of the chest at the fourth intercostal space to the right of the sternum, close to the right ventricle. The positive electrode for V_6 is located in the left mid-axillary line at the fifth intercostal space, close to the left ventricle. Lead V_1 records a small R wave as the septum depolarizes from left to right toward the positive electrode. It then records a negative deflection (S wave) as the main forces travel away from the positive electrode toward the left ventricle, resulting in the normal rS complex in V_1. Lead V_6 records a small Q wave as the septum depolarizes left to right away from the positive electrode.

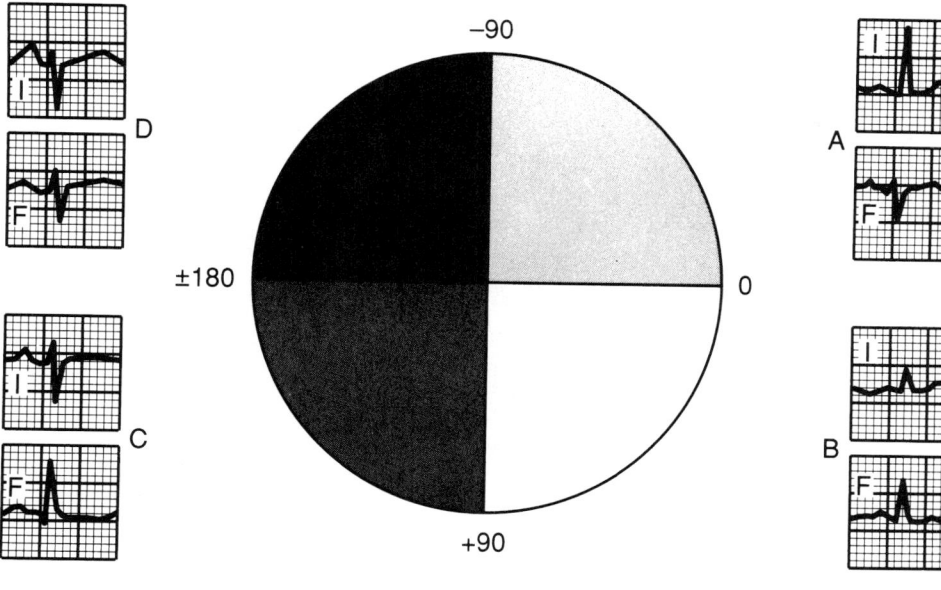

■ **Figure 18–16.** The four quadrants of the axis wheel. (*A*) Left quadrant, lead I is positive and lead a VF is negative. (*B*) Normal quadrant, both leads I and a VF are positive. (*C*) Right quadrant, lead I is negative and lead a VF is positive. (*D*) Indeterminate quadrant, both leads I and a VF are negative. (From Marriott, H. J. L. [1988]. *Practical electrocardiography* [8th ed.]. Philadelphia: Williams & Wilkins.)

It then records a tall R wave as the main forces travel toward the left ventricle, resulting in the normal qR complex in V_6. When both ventricles depolarize together, the QRS width is less than 0.12 second.

Right Bundle-Branch Block

Figure 18-20*A* illustrates the spread of electrical forces in the ventricles when the right bundle branch is blocked. Three separate forces occur:

1. Septal activation occurs first from left to right, resulting in the normal small R wave in V_1 and small Q wave in V_6.
2. The left ventricle is activated next through the normally functioning left bundle branch. Depolarization spreads normally through the Purkinje fibers in the left ventricle, causing an S wave in V_1 as the impulse travels away from its positive electrode and an R wave in V_6 as the impulse travels toward the positive electrode in V_6.
3. The right ventricle depolarizes late and abnormally as the impulse spreads by cell-to-cell conduction through the right ventricle. This abnormal activation causes a wide second R wave (called R') in V_1 as it travels toward the positive electrode in V_1, and a wide S wave in V_6 as it travels away from the positive electrode in V_6. Because muscle cell-to-cell conduction is much slower than conduction through the Purkinje system, the QRS complex widens to 0.12 second or greater.

Typical uncomplicated RBBB can be recognized by a wide rSR' pattern in V_1 and a wide qRs pattern in V_6 and in leads I and aVL, because the positive electrode in these two limb leads is located on the left side of the body. Figure 18-20*B* illustrates three variations of the RBBB pattern most commonly seen. If a patient with RBBB has a septal MI, the initial small R wave usually seen in lead V_1 in RBBB disappears because the septum no longer depolarizes normally from left to right, resulting in a qR pattern as seen in the second example in Figure 18-20*B*. Sometimes RBBB presents as a wide R wave in lead V_1 that

may or may not be notched, as shown in the third example of Figure 18-20*B*. The ECG in Figure 18-20*C* is an example of typical RBBB.

Left Bundle-Branch Block

Figure 18-21*A* illustrates the spread of electrical forces through the ventricles when the left bundle branch is blocked. In LBBB, the septum does not depolarize in its normal left-to-right direction because the block occurs above the Purkinje fibers that normally activate the left side of the septum. This causes the loss of the normal small R wave in V_1 and loss of the Q wave in V_6, lead I, and aVL. The loss of normal initial QRS forces in LBBB makes identification of MI more difficult. Two main forces occur in LBBB.

1. The right ventricle is activated first through the Purkinje fibers. Because the right ventricular free wall is so much thinner than the left ventricle, forces traveling through it are often not recorded in V_1. Sometimes a small, narrow R wave is recorded in V_1 during LBBB, and this is most likely the result of forces traveling through the right ventricular free wall.
2. The left ventricle depolarizes late and abnormally as the impulse spreads by cell-to-cell conduction through the thick left ventricle. This causes V_1 to record a wide negative QS complex as the impulse travels away from its positive electrode. The lateral leads V_6, I, and aVL record a wide R wave as the impulse travels through the large left ventricle toward their positive electrodes. The QRS widens to 0.12 second or greater due to the slow cell-to-cell conduction in the left ventricle.

Left bundle-branch block is recognized by a wide QS complex in V_1 and wide R waves with no Q waves in V_6, lead I, or aVL. Figure 18-21*B* shows two commonly seen LBBB patterns, the most common being the QS in lead V_1; the rS pattern is seen in approximately 30% of LBBB (Marriott, 1988). The ECG in Figure 18-21*C* illustrates LBBB.

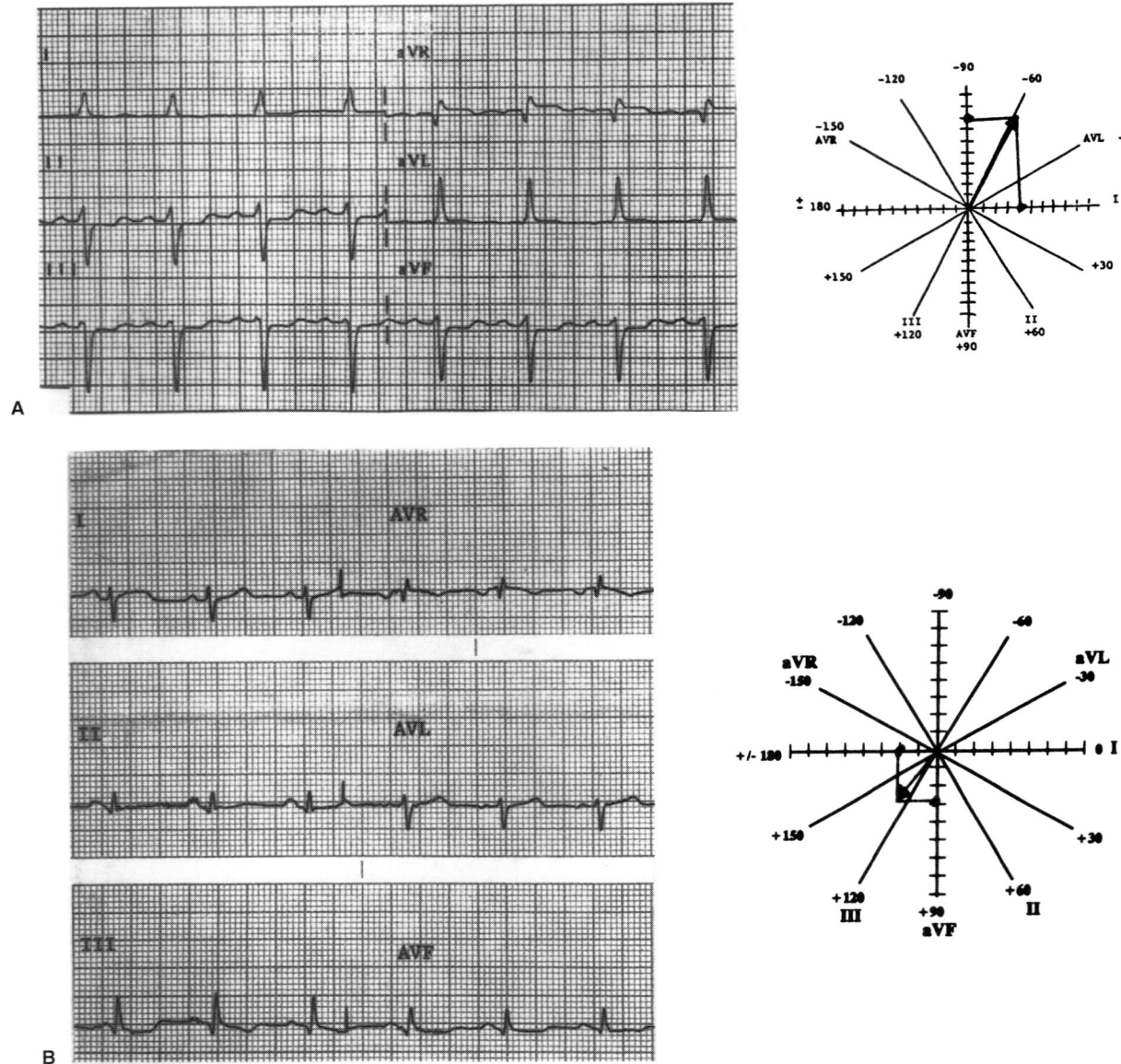

■ Figure 18–17. (*A*) Frontal plane leads demonstrating left axis deviation. Lead I is 5 boxes positive, a VP is 2 boxes positive and 10 boxes negative for a net of –8. The axis is −60°. This is an example of left anterior fascicular block. (*B*) Frontal plane leads demonstrating right axis deviation. Lead I is 2 boxes positive and 5 boxes negative for a net –3. Lead a VF is 2 boxes positive. The axis is +150°. This is an example of left posterior fascicular block. (From Jacobson, C. [1997]. Advanced ECG concepts. In M. Chulay, C. Guzzetta, & B. Dossey [Eds.], *AACN handbook of critical care nursing* [pp. 415–454]. Stamford, CT: Appleton & Lange.)

Fascicular Blocks

The term *fascicular block* or *hemiblock* is used to describe block in either division of the left bundle branch. In fascicular block, both ventricles depolarize simultaneously so the QRS remains narrow, but the direction of left ventricular depolarization is altered. The most useful ECG leads for recognizing fascicular block are leads I and aVF for the axis, and leads I and III for the typical pattern of fascicular block.

Figure 18-18*A* illustrates the normal intraventricular conduction system and the relationship between the anterior and posterior divisions of the left bundle. In Figure 18-18*B*, imagine the

apex of the left ventricle cut away and tipped toward you as you look up the barrel of the left ventricle. The main left bundle is seen coming from the septum into the left ventricle and dividing into the anterior and posterior fascicles, which course toward the anterior and posterior papillary muscles, respectively. When the left ventricular free wall is activated normally, the anterior fascicle carries the electrical impulse in a superior and leftward direction and the posterior fascicle carries it downward and rightward. Because free wall activation proceeds in both directions simultaneously, most of the forces cancel each other and result in the normal QRS shape seen in leads I and III and a normal QRS axis as the combined forces proceed downward and leftward through the left

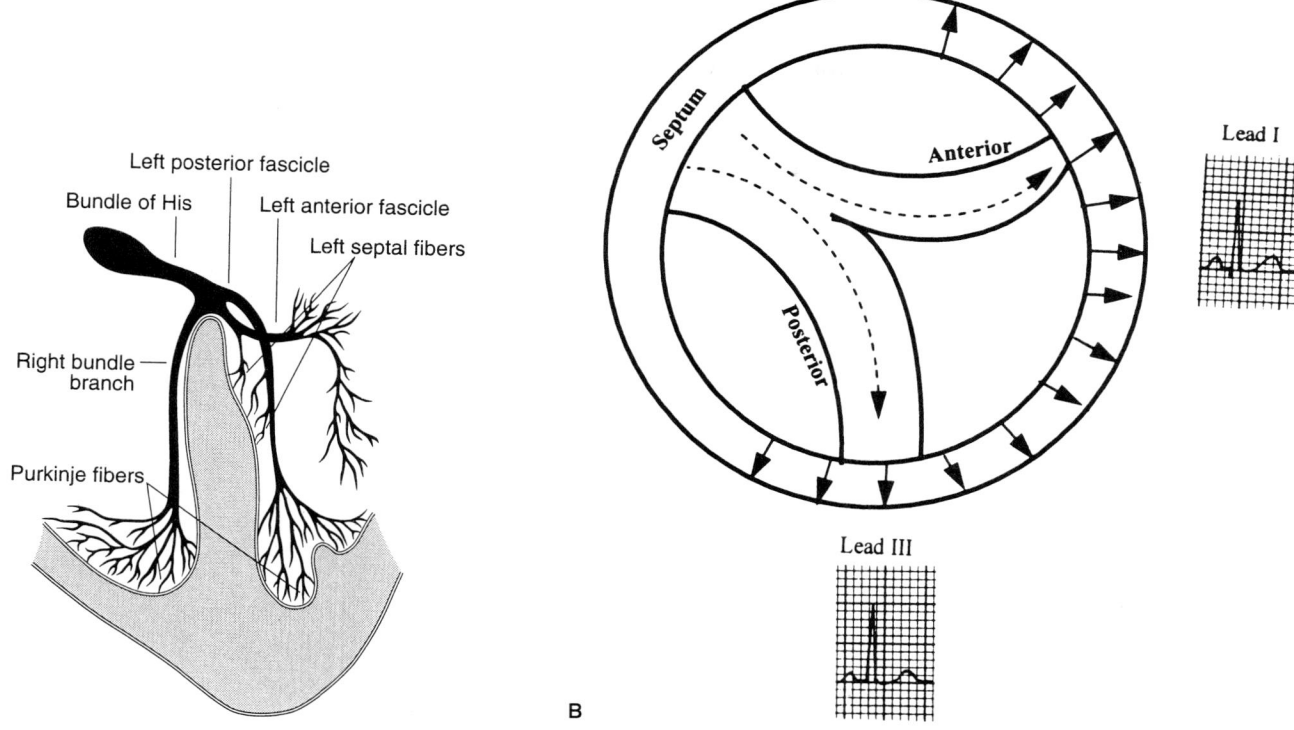

■ **Figure 18–18.** (*A*) Intraventricular conduction system. Right bundle branch carries impulse into right ventricle. Left main bundle branch divides into anterior and posterior fascicles which carry impulse into left ventricle. (*B*) Diagram of left ventricle as seen looking up from apex toward base. Anterior fascicle carries impulse upward and leftward, whereas posterior fascicle carries impulse downward and rightward in the left ventricle. QRS complexes in leads I and III are shown. (From Jacobson, C. [2000]. Electrocardiography. In S. L. Woods, E. S. Froelicher, & S. Motzer [Eds.], *Cardiac nursing* [4th ed., pp. 263–296]. Philadelphia: Lipincott.)

ventricle. When fascicular block occurs, left ventricular activation proceeds from one site instead of both simultaneously, removing the cancellation and altering the shape of the QRS in leads I and III. Because the left ventricle is depolarized in an abnormal direction, an axis deviation always results from fascicular block.

Left Anterior Fascicular Block

In LAFB (also called *anterior hemiblock*), the impulse conducts through the posterior fascicle and begins depolarizing the ventricle in an inferior and rightward direction. It then travels through the left ventricular free wall in a superior and leftward direction, resulting in a left axis deviation. The degree of left axis deviation required to diagnose LAFB is controversial, with some experts stating −45 to −90 degrees, and others at least −60 degrees. The initial forces are directed inferiorly and rightward, causing a small Q wave in lead I and a small R wave in lead III. The forces then travel superiorly and leftward, causing a normal R wave in lead I and an abnormally deep S wave in lead III. There may or may not be a Q wave in lead I, depending on whether initial septal activation is directed to the left or to the right. Figure 18-17*A* is an example of LAFB. The ECG characteristics of LAFB are (see also Fig. 18-22*A*):

1. Left axis deviation (-45 degrees or more)
2. Small Q in lead I, large S in lead III (QI, SIII), or an rS pattern in II, III, aVF

3. QRS duration not prolonged more than 0.11 second
4. Increased QRS voltage in limb leads due to loss of cancellation of forces in left ventricle

Left Posterior Fascicular Block

In LPFB (also called *posterior hemiblock*), the impulse conducts through the anterior fascicle and begins depolarizing the ventricle in a superior and leftward direction. It then travels through the left ventricular free wall in an inferior and rightward direction, resulting in a right axis deviation. The initial forces are directed superiorly and leftward, causing a small R wave in lead I and a small Q wave in lead III. The forces then travel inferiorly and rightward, causing a deep S wave in lead I and a tall R wave in lead III. Before diagnosing LPFB, the clinician must rule out RVH because RVH can cause the identical frontal plane picture. Figure 18-17*B* is an example of LPFB. The ECG characteristics of LPFB are (see also Fig. 18-22*B*):

1. Right axis deviation (.110 degrees)
2. Small R in lead I and aVL, small Q in II, III, aVF (SI, QIII), or an rS pattern in leads I and aVL
3. Normal QRS duration (not >0.11 second)
4. Increased QRS voltage due to loss of cancellation of QRS forces
5. No evidence of RVH

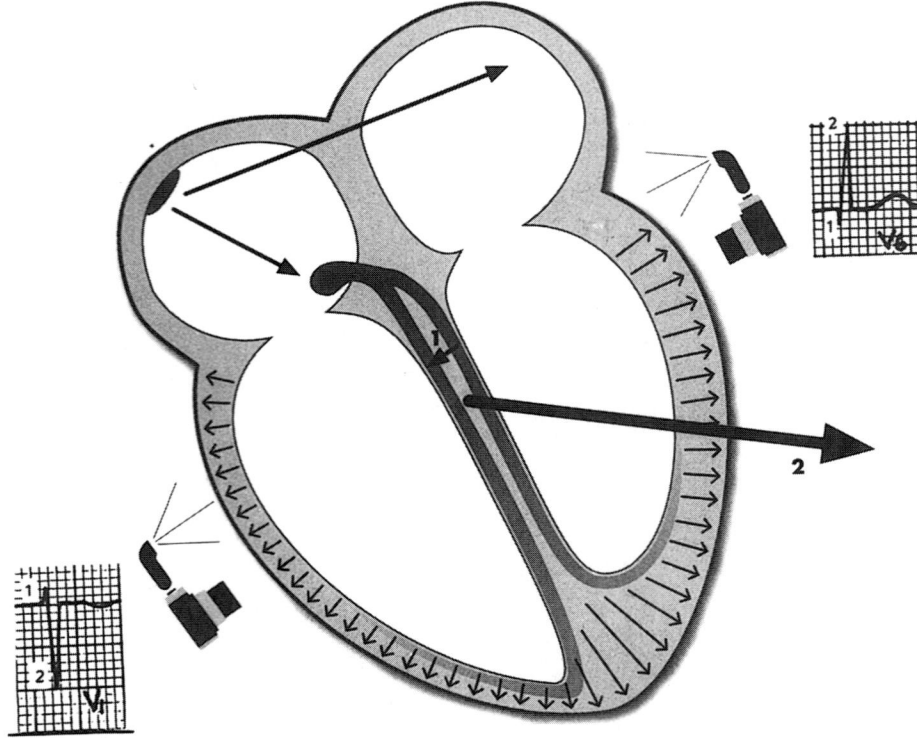

■ **Figure 18–19.** Normal ventricular activation as recorded by leads V_1 and V_6. (From Jacobson, C. [1997]. Advanced ECG concepts. In M. Chulay, C. Guzzetta, & B. Dossey [Eds.], *AACN handbook of critical care nursing* [pp. 415–454]. Stamford, CT: Appleton & Lange.)

Bifascicular Block

Bifascicular block means that two of the three major fascicles are blocked. Because block in both divisions of the left bundle branch presents as complete LBBB, the term *bifascicular block* is usually used to refer to block in the right bundle branch along with block in either the anterior or posterior divisions of the left bundle branch. The ECG displays the typical RBBB morphology (wide QRS and rsR' pattern, or one of its variants) along with an axis deviation consistent with the fascicular block. Figure 18-23 is an example of RBBB and LAFB. Figure 18-24 shows RBBB and LPFB.

ISCHEMIA, INJURY, AND INFARCTION

Myocardial ischemia is the result of an imbalance between myocardial O_2 supply and demand and is a reversible process if blood flow is restored before permanent cellular damage occurs. Ischemia can result from increased myocardial O_2 demands or from decreased myocardial O_2 supply. If ischemia is severe and blood flow is not restored relatively soon, cellular injury and eventually necrosis (cell death) result.

The term *acute coronary syndrome* (ACS) is used to refer to the pathophysiologic continuum that begins with plaque rupture in a coronary artery and ultimately results in permanent cell damage (infarction) if the process is not arrested (see Chapters 25 and 26). ACS encompasses three distinct phases of this continuum: (1) unstable angina (UA), (2) non-ST elevation MI

(NSTEMI), and (3) ST elevation MI (STEMI; Braunwald et al., 2002). Once an infarction has occurred, as indicated by elevated biochemical cardiac markers, it is classified electrocardiographically as either a Q-wave or a non-Q wave MI based on the presence or absence of Q waves on the ECG.

Myocardial infarction can occur because of blockage of a coronary artery with thrombus or from severe and prolonged ischemia due to coronary artery spasm or unrelieved obstruction of a coronary artery. When infarction does occur, there are varying degrees of damage to cells involved in the process, ranging from ischemia to injury to cell death. This has traditionally been described as three "zones" of tissue damage, each of which produces characteristic changes on the ECG (Fig. 18-25). Although this is an oversimplification of what actually happens, the concept is still useful in understanding the ECG changes that occur with myocardial infarction.

Myocardial ischemia can result in several changes on the ECG (Fig. 18-26). The most familiar pattern of ischemia is T-wave inversion, although T-wave inversion is often a nonspecific finding and can be due to a variety of causes other than ischemia. Other indicators of ischemia include ST-segment depression of 0.5 mm or more; an ST segment that remains on the baseline longer than 0.12 second; an ST segment that forms a sharp angle with the upright T wave; tall, wide-based T waves; and inverted U waves (Goldschlager & Goldman, 1989; Jaffe & Davidenko, 2001; Marriott, 1988; Mirvis & Goldberger, 2001; Surawicz & Knilans, 2001). Display 18-1 lists several causes of ST-segment and T-wave changes.

Myocardial injury is most often indicated by ST-segment elevation of 1 mm or more above the baseline. Other signs of acute injury include a straightening of the ST segment that

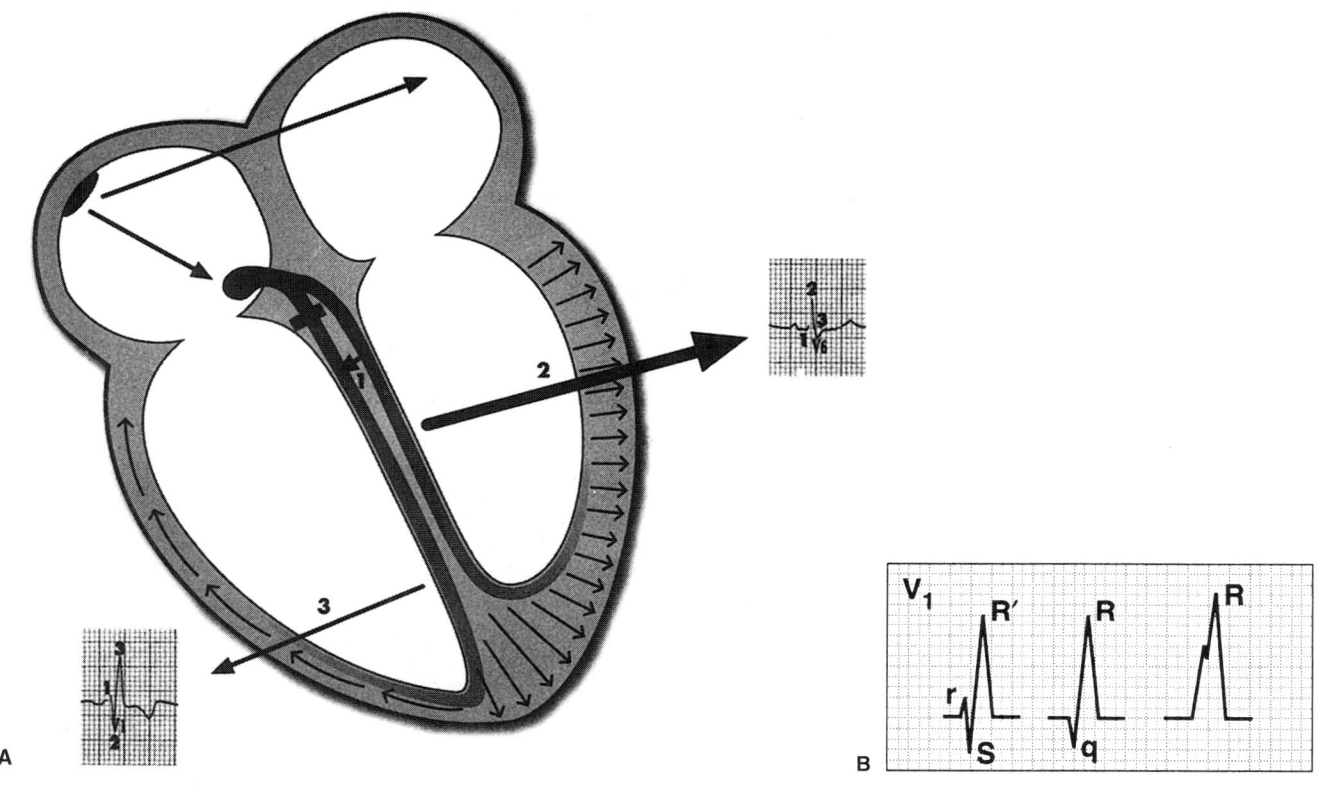

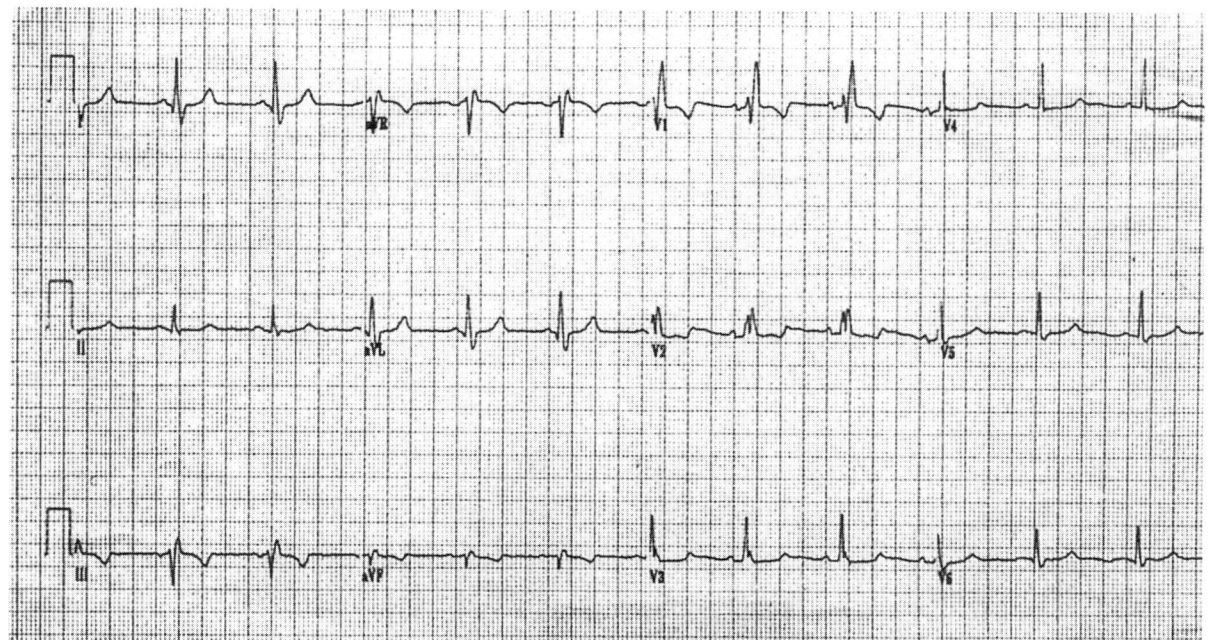

■ **Figure 18–20.** (*A*) Ventricular depolarization with right bundle branch block as recorded by leads V₁ and V₆. See text for details. (*B*) Three commonly seen variations of RBBB pattern. (*C*) 12-lead ECG illustrating RBBB. (Adapted from Jacobson, C. [1997]. Advanced ECG concepts. In M. Chulay, C. Guzzetta, & B. Dossey [Eds.], *AACN handbook of critical care nursing* [pp. 415–454]. Stamford, CT: Appleton & Lange.)

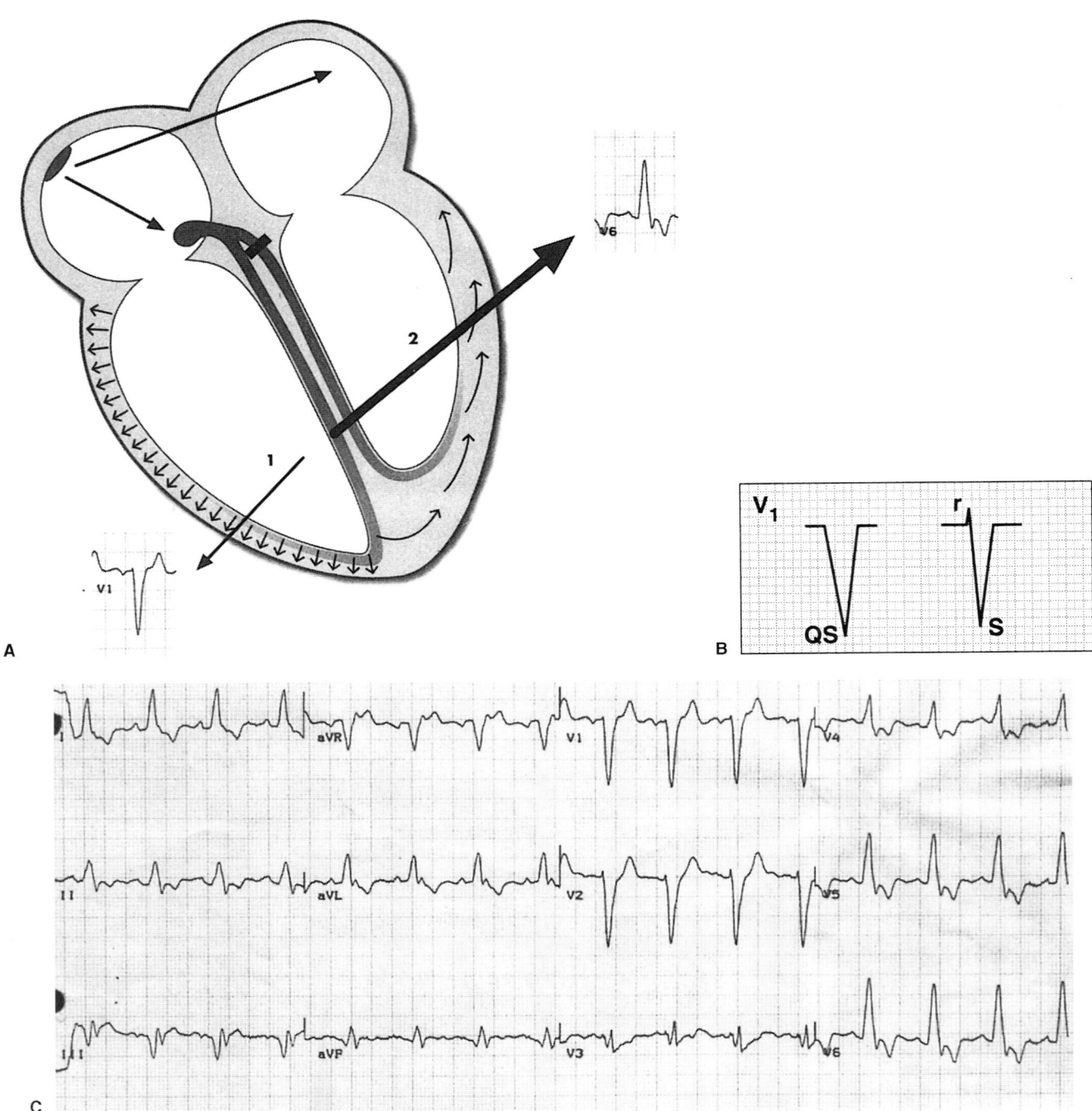

■ **Figure 18–21.** (*A*) Ventricular depolarization with left bundle branch block as recorded by leads V$_1$ and V$_6$, (*B*) Two commonly seen patterns of LBBB. (*C*) 12-lead ECG illustrating LBBB. (Adapted from Jacobson, C. [1997]. Advanced ECG concepts. In M. Chulay, C. Guzzetta, & B. Dossey [Eds.], *AACN handbook of critical care nursing* [pp. 415–454]. Stamford, CT: Appleton & Lange.)

slopes up to the peak of the T wave without spending any time on the baseline; tall, peaked T waves; and symmetric T-wave inversion (Goldschlager & Goldman, 1989; Jaffe & Davidenko, 2001; Marriott, 1988; Mirvis & Goldberger, 2001; Surawicz & Knilans, 2001; Fig. 18-27).

Necrosis or death of myocardial tissue is indicated on the ECG by development of new Q waves or deepening of preexisting Q waves. Abnormal Q waves are greater than 0.03 second

wide or 25% of the ensuing R-wave amplitude. (See Figs. 18-12 and 18-13 for examples of normal Q waves; Figs. 18-28, 18-29, and 18-30 show examples of abnormal Q waves.) Display 18-2 lists conditions other than infarction that can result in development of Q waves (Marriott, 1988; Mirvis & Goldberger, 2001). Traditionally, it was taught that the presence of Q waves indicates transmural MI extending through the entire thickness of the muscle, and that nontransmural (subendocardial)

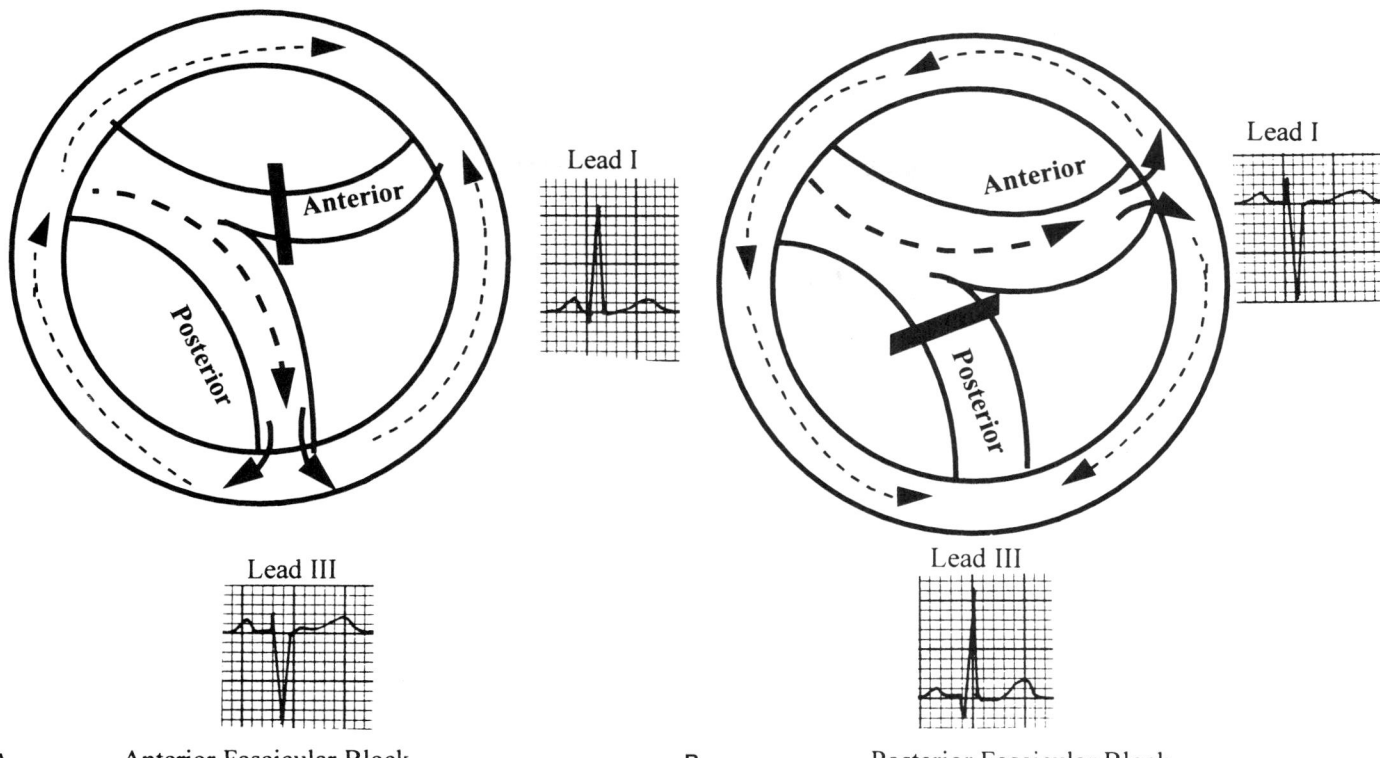

A   Anterior Fascicular Block   **B**   Posterior Fascicular Block

■ **Figure 18–22.** (*A*) Anterior fascicular block. Impulse depolarizes left ventricle in downward and rightward direction first through posterior fascicle, then travels upwards and to the left, resulting in left axis deviation, Q wave in lead I, S wave in lead III. (*B*) Posterior fascicular block. Impulse depolarizes left ventricle in upward and leftward direction first through anterior fascicle, then travels downward and rightward, resulting in right axis deviation, S wave in lead I, Q wave in lead III. (From Jacobson, C. [2000]. Electrocardiography. In S. L. Woods, E. S. Froelicher, & S. Motzer [Eds.], *Cardiac nursing* [4th ed., pp. 263–296]. Philadelphia: Lippincott.)

infarction involving less than the entire thickness of the muscle does not produce Q waves. It is now known that Q waves can develop transiently with severe ischemia and with nontransmural MI, and that transmural infarction can occur without the development of Q waves (Jaffe & Davidenko, 2001; Mirvis & Goldberger, 2001; Surawicz & Knilans, 2001). Therefore, the newer terms *Q wave* and *non-Q wave* MI are preferred over the older terms *transmural* and *non-*

transmural infarction. In any case, the presence of abnormal Q waves is still considered to be ECG evidence of myocardial necrosis.

The ECG reflects the progression of the infarction from the acute stage through the fully evolved stage. Very early MI often causes peaking and widening of the T waves followed within minutes by ST-segment elevation. ST-segment elevation can persist for hours to several days but resolves more

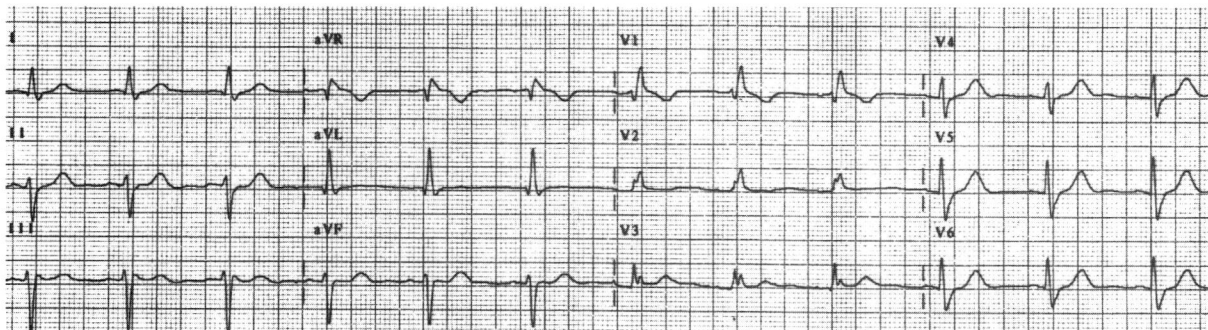

■ **Figure 18–23.** ECG of RBBB and LAFB. Rhythm is sinus, QRS width is 0.12 second, there is left axis deviation (−60°) due to LAFB, and V₁ shows the typical rsR' pattern of RBBB. (From Jacobson, C. [2000]. Electrocardiography. In S. L. Woods, E. S. Froelicher, & S. Motzer [Eds.], *Cardiac nursing* [4th ed., pp. 263–296] Philadelphia: Lippincott.)

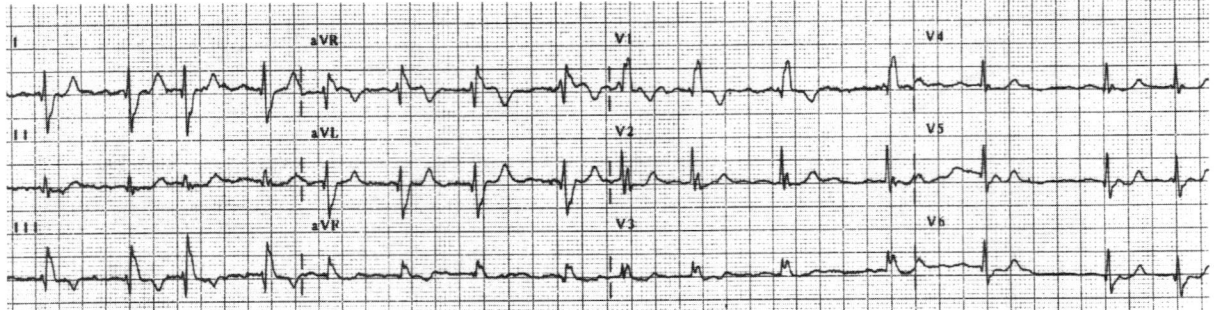

■ **Figure 18–24.** ECG of RBBB and LPFB. Rhythm is atrial fibrillation, QRS width is 0.12 second, there is right axis deviation (About +150°) due to LPFB, and V1 shows the typical rsR′ pattern of RBBB. (From Jacobson, C. [2000]. Electrocardiography. In S. L. Woods, E. S. Froelicher, & S. Motzer [Eds.], *Cardiac nursing* [4th ed., pp. 263–296]. Philadelphia: Lippincott.)

quickly with successful reperfusion. Once the ST segment has returned to baseline, ECG evidence of the acute stage is lost. Q waves appear within hours of pain onset and usually remain forever, although sometimes Q waves disappear over the years after infarction. T-wave inversion occurs within hours after infarction and can last for months. T waves often return to their previous upright position within a few months after acute MI. Thus, an *evolving infarct* is one in which serial ECGs show ST segments returning toward baseline, the development of Q

waves, and T-wave inversion. The term *old infarction* or *infarct of undetermined age* is used when the first ECG recorded shows Q waves, ST segment at baseline, and T waves either inverted or upright, indicating that an MI occurred at some point in the past.

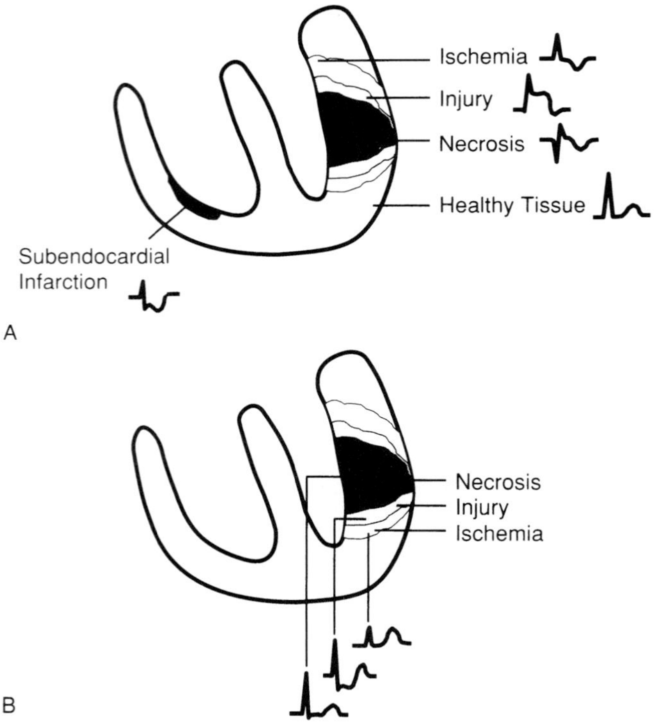

Locating the Infarction from the Electrocardiogram

ST-segment elevation, Q waves, and T-wave inversion are recorded in leads facing the damaged myocardium and are called the *indicative changes* of infarction. Other leads not facing the involved tissue are often affected by the loss of electrical forces in damaged tissue and record mirror-image changes called *reciprocal changes*. Figure 18-25 illustrates indicative and reciprocal changes associated with MI, and Table 18-2 lists leads in which indicative and reciprocal changes are found in each of the major types of MI. Figure 18-31 illustrates how to localize ischemia, injury, and infarction using the 12-lead ECG.

Anterior Myocardial Infarction

Anterior wall MI (see Fig. 18-28) is due to occlusion of the left anterior descending coronary artery and is recognized by indicative changes in leads facing the anterior wall (V_{1-4}). Reciprocal changes are often recorded in the lateral leads I and aVL and the inferior leads II, III, and aVF. Loss of normal R-wave progression or development of Q waves and ST elevation in V_{1-4} are seen in anterior infarction. If only the septum is infarcted, changes occur only in leads V_{1-2}, but, if the entire anterior wall is involved, changes are seen in V_{1-4}. Anterior wall infarction that extends laterally and involves leads I and aVL is often referred to as *extensive anterior* or *anterolateral* infarction (Fig. 18-32).

Inferior Myocardial Infarction

Inferior wall MI (see Fig. 18-29) is usually due to occlusion of the right coronary artery and is diagnosed by indicative changes in

■ **Figure 18–25.** Zones of ischemia, injury and infarction with associated ECG changes. (*A*) Indicative changes of ischemia, injury, and necrosis seen in leads facing the injured area. (*B*) Reciprocal changes often seen in leads not directly facing the involved area. (From Jacobson, C. [1997]. Advanced ECG concepts. In M. Chulay, C. Guzzetta, & B. Dossey [Eds.], *AACN handbook of critical care nursing* [pp. 415–454]. Stamford, CT: Appleton & Lange.)

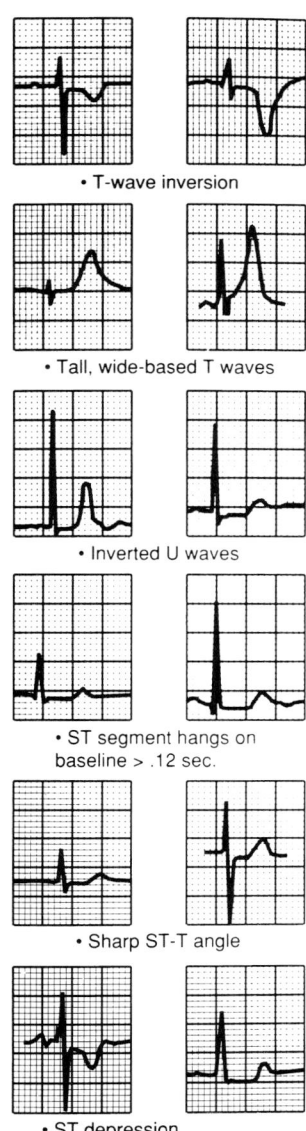

Figure 18–26. ECG patterns associated with myocardial ischemia. (From Jacobson, C. [1997]. Advanced ECG concepts. In M. Chulay, C. Guzzett, & B. Dossey [Eds.], *AACN handbook of critical care nursing* [pp. 415–454]. Stamford, CT: Appleton & Lange.)

leads II, III, and aVF. Reciprocal changes are often seen in leads I, aVL, or the V leads. In people with left dominant coronary circulation, the circumflex artery supplies the inferior surface of the heart and circumflex occlusion is the cause of inferior MI. Lead III can have a Q wave normally, but if the Q wave is large and accompanied by Q waves in leads II or aVF, it is considered indicative of inferior MI. Approximately 40% of inferior MIs involve the right ventricle (Fig. 18-33).

Lateral Myocardial Infarction

Lateral wall MI is due to circumflex artery occlusion and presents with indicative changes in leads I, aVL, and sometimes V₅₋₆, with reciprocal changes in inferior or anterior leads (see

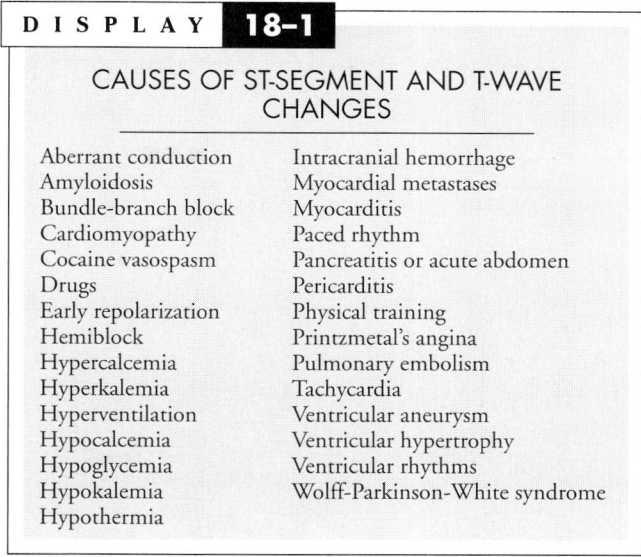

Fig. 18-30). Lateral wall MI does not often occur alone but commonly accompanies anterior MI, as it does in Figure 18-32.

Posterior Myocardial Infarction

Posterior wall MI (Fig. 18-34) is due to right coronary artery occlusion or to circumflex occlusion in left-dominant

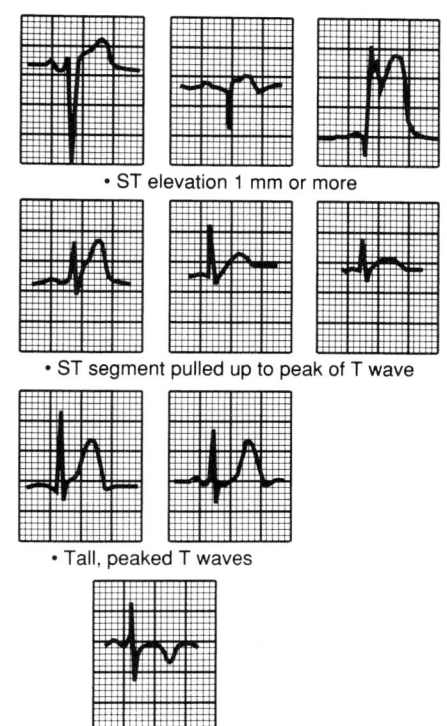

Figure 18–27. ECG patterns associated with acute myocardial injury. (From Jacobson, C. [1997]. Advanced ECG concepts. In M. Chulay, C. Guzzetta, & B. Dossey [Eds.], *AACN handbook of critical care nursing* [pp. 415–454] Stamford, CT: Appleton & Lange.)

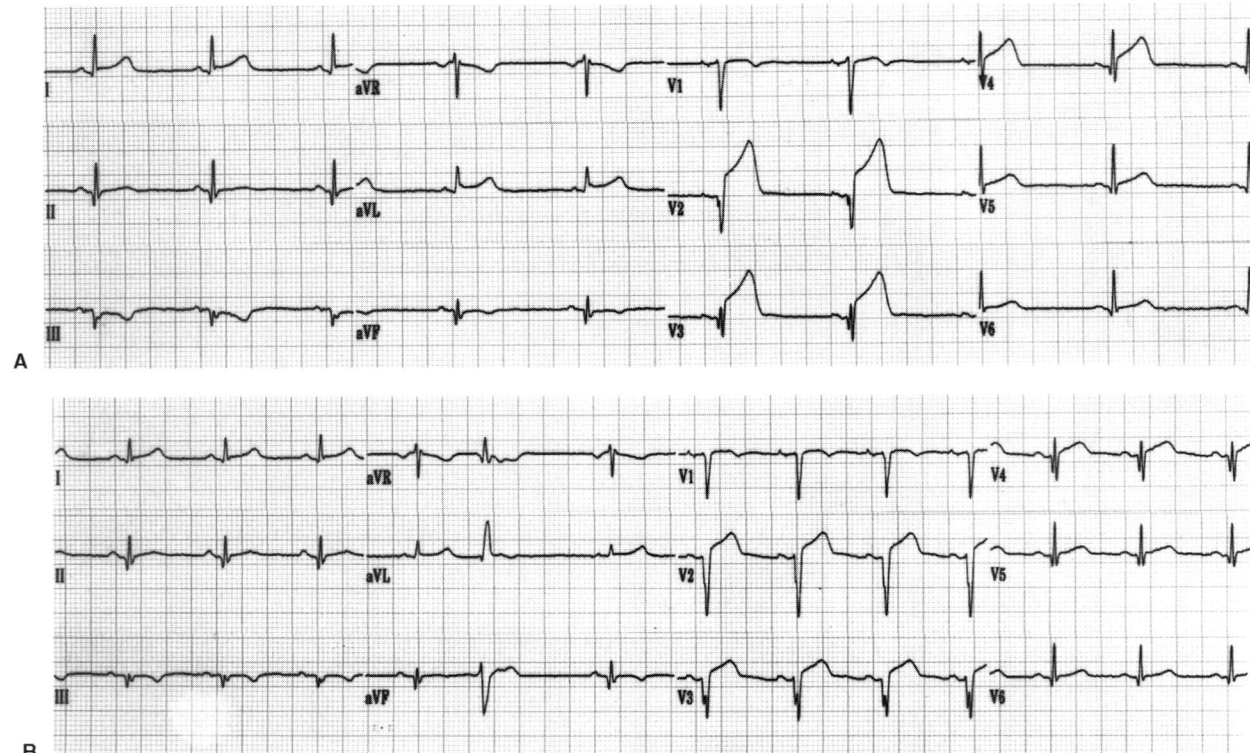

■ **Figure 18–28.** (*A*) Early acute anterior wall MI. Note abnormal R wave progression in V_{1-3} and ST elevation with tall wide-based T waves in V_{2-4}. Q waves are present in inferior leads indicating prior inferior wall MI. (*B*) Same patient 9 hours later. Q waves have developed in V_{1-4} and ST segments are still elevated.

circulation and usually occurs in conjunction with inferior MI. ECG changes of posterior MI are less obvious because in the standard 12-lead ECG there are no leads that face the posterior wall, and, therefore, no indicative changes are recorded. The diagnosis is made by observing reciprocal changes in the anterior leads, especially V_1 and V_2, but often all the way to V_4. Reciprocal changes seen in these leads include a taller R wave than normal (mirror image of the Q wave that would be recorded over the posterior wall), ST-segment depression (mirror image of the ST-segment elevation from the posterior wall), and upright, tall T waves (mirror image of the T-wave inversion from the posterior wall). The diagnosis can be confirmed by recording posterior leads (see Fig. 18-10) and observing ST elevation and Q waves.

Right Ventricular Myocardial Infarction

Right ventricular MI (RVMI; see Fig. 18-33) occurs in up to 45% of inferior MIs, and, therefore, it usually is associated with indicative changes in the inferior leads II, III, and aVF. In addition, it is not uncommon to see ST-segment elevation in V_1 as well, because V_1 is the chest lead that is closest to the right ventricle. ST-segment elevation in V_1 together with ST-segment elevation in the inferior leads is suspect for RVMI. Another clue is discordance between the ST segment in V_1 and the ST segment in V_2. Discordance means that the ST segments do not

point in the same direction—V_1 shows ST-segment elevation, whereas V_2 is either normal or shows ST-segment depression. This finding is highly likely to indicate RVMI, although rarely the ST segment will be elevated in V_1–V_4 in RVMI. When RVMI is suspected, right-sided chest leads should be obtained as soon as possible because the changes seen in right-sided leads may disappear within 24 hours (see Fig. 18-10). Leads V_{3R} through V_{6R} develop ST-segment elevation when acute RVMI is present. Lead V_{4R} is the most sensitive and specific lead for recognition of RVMI.

Non-Q Wave Myocardial Infarction

Non-Q wave myocardial infarction (NQMI) has traditionally been considered to involve necrosis of the subendocardial layer of the ventricle and not the entire thickness of the ventricular wall. Necrosis of sufficient myocardium can lead to loss of R-wave amplitude rather than to development of Q waves in leads facing the infarcted area (see Fig. 18-25). NQMI may present with either ST elevation or depression in leads facing the infarcted area, and T-wave inversion is common. NQMI is a common cause of giant negative T waves (Surawicz & Knilans, 2001). Most patients who present with ischemic chest pain and ST elevation ultimately develop a Q-wave MI, whereas most patients with no ST elevation are experiencing either unstable angina or NSTEMI. The distinction between these two conditions is

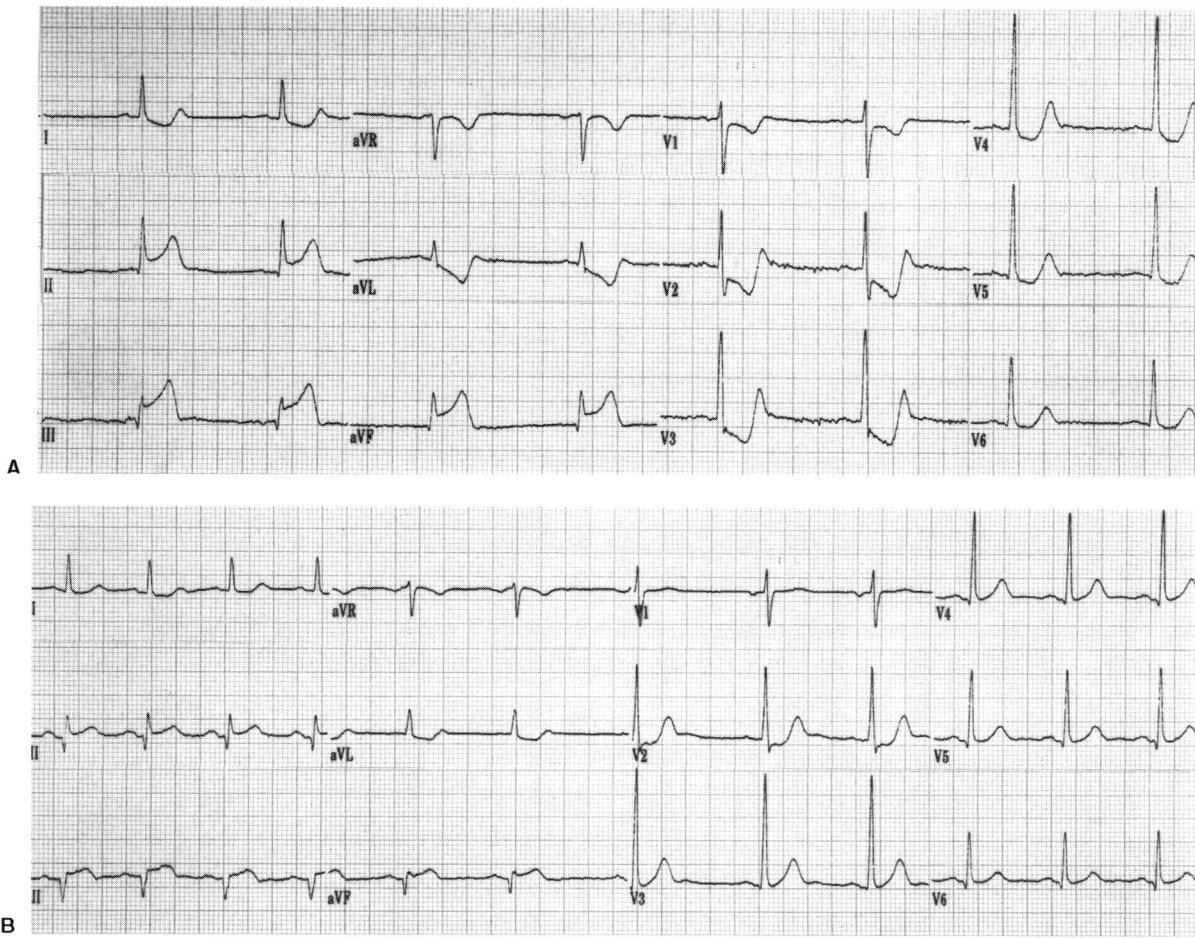

■ **Figure 18–29.** (*A*) Early acute inferior wall MI. Note ST elevation in leads II, III, a VF and reciprocal ST depression in V$_{1-6}$ I, and a VL. (*B*) Same patient next day. Q waves have developed and ST segments are coming down in inferior leads, and most of the reciprocal ST depression has resolved.

made based on the presence of cardiac markers in the blood. Most patients with NSTEMI do not develop Q waves on the ECG and are diagnosed as having a NQMI. (Braunwald et al., 2002). Figure 18-35 illustrates two examples of NQMI.

ATRIAL AND VENTRICULAR ENLARGEMENT

Each of the four heart chambers can enlarge because of increased pressure or volume overload. The thin-walled atria usually respond to both pressure and volume overload by dilating, whereas the thicker-walled ventricles tend to dilate with volume overload and hypertrophy (increase wall thickness) with pressure overload (Wagner, 2001).

Atrial Enlargement

Atrial enlargement is reflected on the ECG as changes in P wave size and morphology. Normal P waves are no wider than

0.11 second or taller than 2.5 mm. They are usually upright in leads I, II, and V$_{4-6}$ and diphasic with the initial portion upright and the terminal portion negative in V$_1$. Right atrial depolarization forms the first half of the P wave, and left atrial depolarization forms the second half (Fig. 18-36). Atrial enlargement usually accompanies ventricular enlargement, so the presence of ECG signs of atrial enlargement is suggestive of ventricular enlargement as well.

Left Atrial Enlargement

Left atrial enlargement is caused by conditions that increase pressure or volume in the left atrium, such as mitral stenosis, mitral regurgitation, systemic hypertension, and left heart failure. Left atrial enlargement can be manifested on the ECG in the following ways (Fig. 18-37):

1. The P wave is wider than 0.12 second and often notched in leads I, II, aVL, and V$_{4-6}$ (termed P mitrale). The interval between the notches is >0.04 second, and the P wave may encroach into the PR segment, making the PR segment appear shorter than normal.

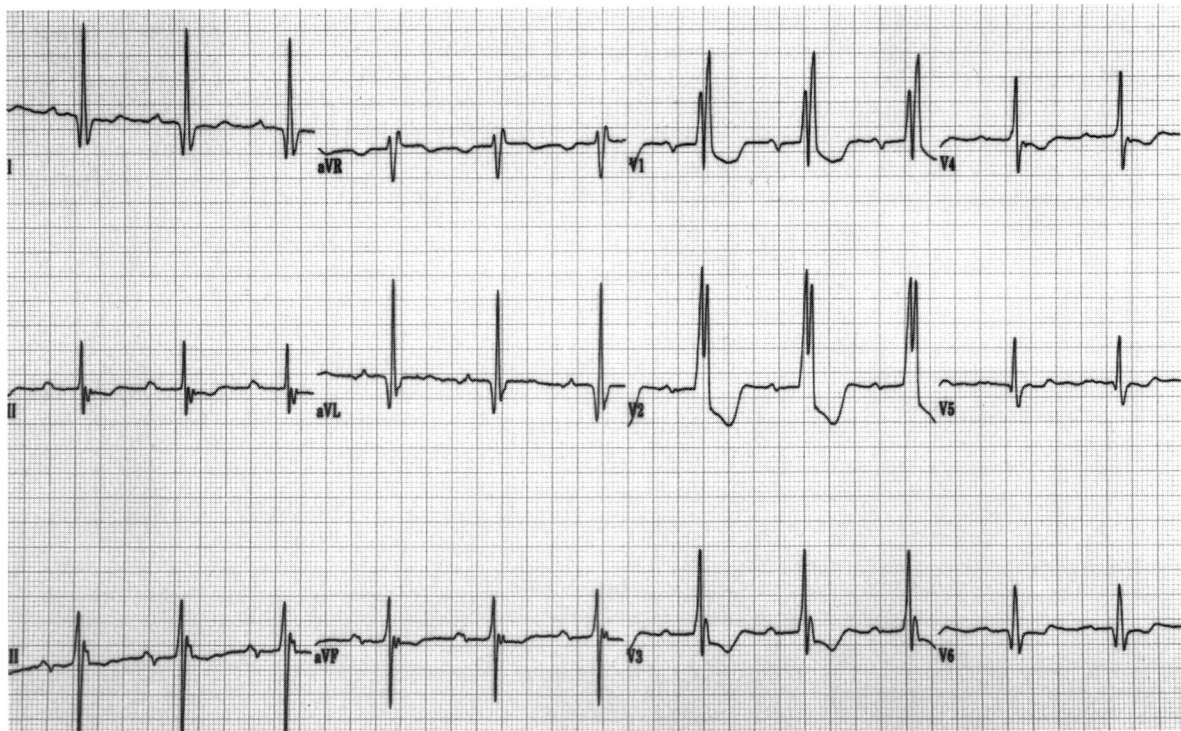

■ **Figure 18–30.** Lateral wall infarction. Note deep Q waves in leads I, aVL, and V6. ST segments are at baseline, indicating that this is an old MI. RBBB is also present.

2. Increased width and depth of the terminal negative component of the P wave in lead V_1 or V_2.
3. Leftward shift of P wave axis to between −30 and +45 degrees.

Right Atrial Enlargement

Right atrial enlargement is commonly caused by conditions that increase the work of the right atrium, such as pulmonary hypertension, pulmonary or tricuspid stenosis or regurgitation, and congenital heart disease. Right atrial en-

largement can be manifested on the ECG in the following ways (see Fig. 18-37):

1. The P waves are tall and peaked (>2.5 mm) in leads II, III, and aVF (termed *P pulmonale*).
2. P waves in leads V_{1-3} are sharp and pointed, increasing the area under the positive portion of the P wave.
3. Rightward shift of P wave axis to greater than +75 degrees.
4. If the right atrium gets large enough to extend leftward across the front of the heart, the P wave in V_1 may be inverted (Marriott, 1988).

Biatrial Enlargement

Biatrial enlargement occurs when both atria become enlarged. It is sometimes seen in mitral valve disease, atrial septal defect, multiple

---

DISPLAY 18-2

CAUSES OF NONINFARCTION Q WAVES

Anterior and posterior hemiblock
Cardiac amyloidosis
COPD
Hypertrophic cardiomyopathy
Incomplete left bundle-branch block
Myocarditis
Neuromuscular disorders
Pneumothorax
Pulmonary embolism
Sarcoidosis
Ventricular hypertrophy
Ventricular preexcitation (Wolff-Parkinson-White syndrome)

Table 18–2 ■ ELECTROCARDIOGRAPHIC CHANGES ASSOCIATED WITH MYOCARDIAL INFARCTION (MI)

Location of MI	Indicative Changes	Reciprocal Changes
Anterior	V_1 to V_4	I, aVL, II, III, aVF
Septal	V_1, V_2	I, aVL
Inferior	II, III, aVF	I, aVL, V_1 to V_4
Posterior	None	V_1 to V_4
Lateral	I, aVL, V_5, V_6	II, III, aVF, V_1, V_2
Right ventricle	V_3 R to V_6R	

From Chulay, M., Guzzetta, C., & Dossey, B. [Eds.] (1997). *AACN handbook of critical care nursing* (p. 430). Stanford, CT: Appleton & Lange.

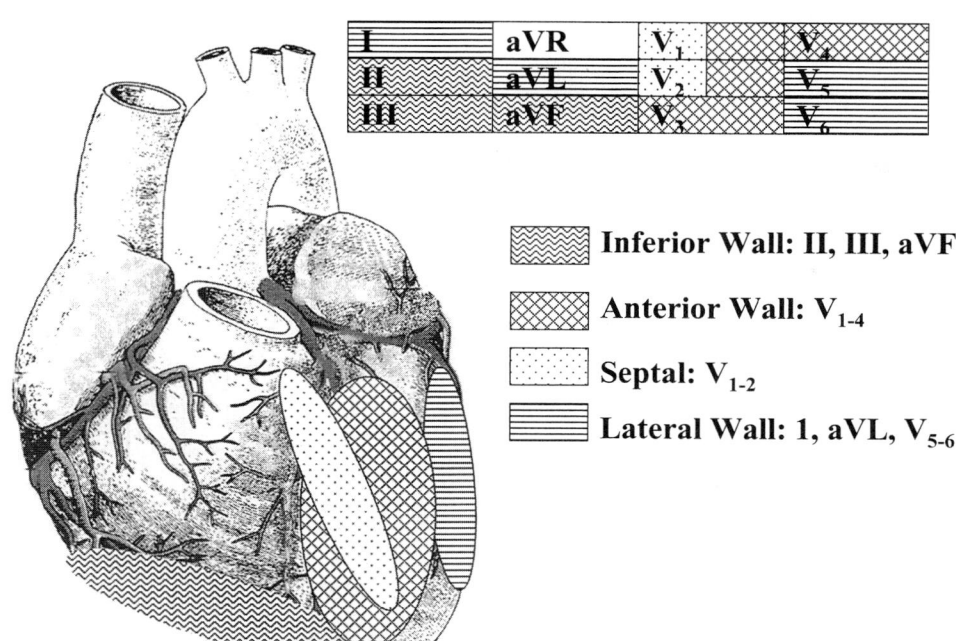

I	aVR	V₁	V₄
II	aVL	V₂	V₅
III	aVF	V₃	V₆

Inferior Wall: II, III, aVF

Anterior Wall: V₁₋₄

Septal: V₁₋₂

Lateral Wall: 1, aVL, V₅₋₆

■ **Figure 18–31.** Localizing myocardial ischemia, injury or infarction using the 12-lead ECG. The different areas of the heart are pattern-coded. Standard 12-lead ECG format is illustrated at upper right with leads pattern-coded to correspond to the area of the heart that each lead faces. (Adapted from Cummins, R. O. [2000]. *ACLS provider manual* [p. 129.]. Dallas, TX: American Heart Association.)

valvular defects, and biventricular failure. Biatrial enlargement is manifested on the ECG in the following ways (see Fig. 18-37):

1. The P wave is taller than 2.5 mm and wider than 0.11 second in lead II.
2. P waves may be notched.
3. Both the positive and negative components of the P wave in V₁ may be enlarged.

Ventricular Enlargement

The ventricles can enlarge because of increased pressure or volume in the chamber. Ventricular enlargement affects the size of the QRS complex and often causes ST segment and T wave changes as well (Fig. 18-38). Enlargement of the right and left ventricles is discussed separately.

Left Ventricular Enlargement

Left ventricular enlargement (LVE) caused by increased volume (diastolic overload or increased preload) or increased pressure (systolic overload or increased afterload) can be expressed on the ECG. The most characteristic effect of LVH is increased amplitude of the R wave in leads facing the left ventricle (leads I, aVL, V₅, and V₆) as more forces travel through the enlarged left ventricle. There is a concurrent decrease in R-wave amplitude and increase in S-wave amplitude in leads facing the right ventricle (leads V₁ and V₂). The intrinsicoid deflection (the time from the beginning of the QRS complex to the peak of the R wave) is slightly delayed in leads facing the left ventricle, and the QRS width approaches the upper limit of normal because of the increased time required for electrical forces to travel through the thick left ventricular muscle. Figure 18-39 is an example of LVH.

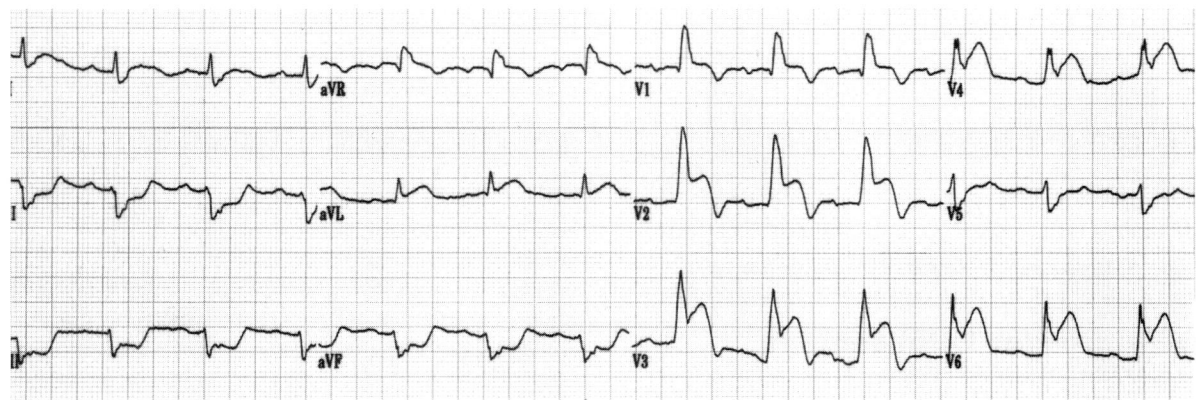

■ **Figure 18–32.** Acute anterolateral wall MI. ST elevation is present in I, aVL, and V₂–V₆. Reciprocal ST depression is present in III, aVF, and aVR.

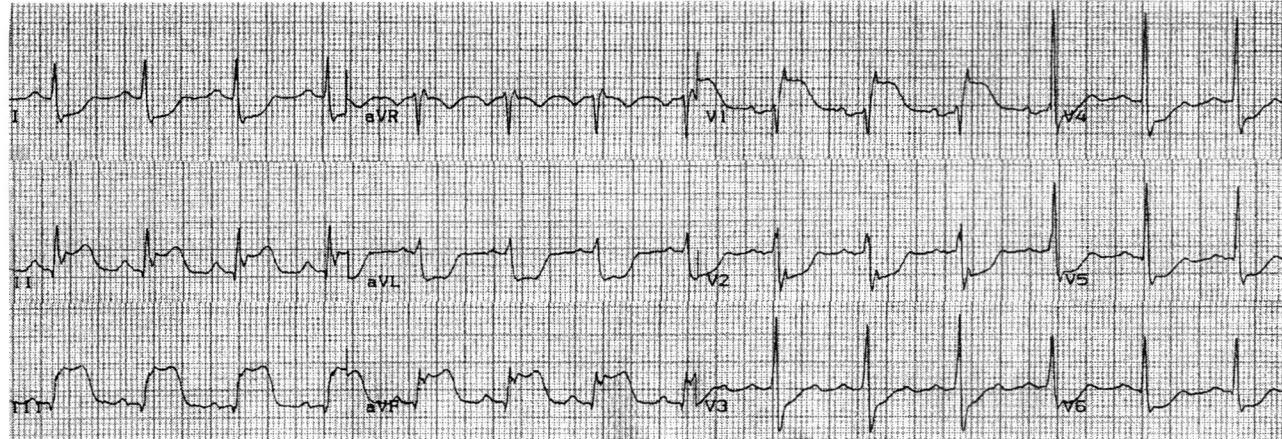

■ **Figure 18–33.** (*A*) Acute right ventricular MI. ST elevation is present in II, III, aVF, and V$_1$; reciprocal ST depression in all other leads. Note the discordant ST elevation in V$_1$ and depression in V$_2$. (*B*) Right-sided chest leads in a patient with acute RVMI. Note ST elevation in leads V$_{3R-6R}$. Note also that standard V$_1$ shows ST elevation while standard V$_2$ shows a normal ST segment (a form of "discordance").

The ST-T-wave changes that occur reflect repolarization abnormalities and may be due to hypertrophy or may be secondary consequences of dilation or ischemia. The term *strain* is often used to describe the ST-T-wave changes that commonly occur with LVH. ST-segment depression, often downsloping, with T-wave inversion commonly develops in left chest leads. Increased T-wave amplitude may be found in leads that show large R waves, and ST segments may be elevated in leads that show deep S waves. ST-segment depression and T-wave inversion accompany more severe hypertrophy and increased risk of cardiovascular events. (Mirvis & Goldberger, 2001) A variety of methods have been proposed to help diagnose LVH on the ECG, and Table 18-3 lists several of these methods.

Right Ventricular Enlargement

Right ventricular hypertrophy (RVH) may be caused by any condition that produces a sufficient load on the right ventricle,

such as pulmonary disease or congenital or acquired heart disease, particularly mitral valve disease. The electrical events of the right ventricle are normally masked by the events taking place nearly simultaneously in the dominant left ventricle. As the right ventricle enlarges, these right-sided (or anterior) forces are revealed and may become the dominant forces if the right ventricle becomes as large or larger than the left. The normal sequence of depolarization is altered, resulting in ECG changes in axis, QRS morphology and voltage, and ST-T waves (Fig. 18-40).

The most obvious ECG change with RVH is a reversal of normal R-wave progression in precordial leads. R waves become dominant and the S wave shrinks in right chest leads, whereas R waves shrink and S waves dominate in left-sided leads. The same "strain" pattern described previously with ST-segment depression and T-wave inversion occurs in right chest leads and in leads II, III, and aVF. Ten ECG features commonly seen with RVH are listed in Display 18-3. The presence of one of the criteria listed is highly indicative of RVH.

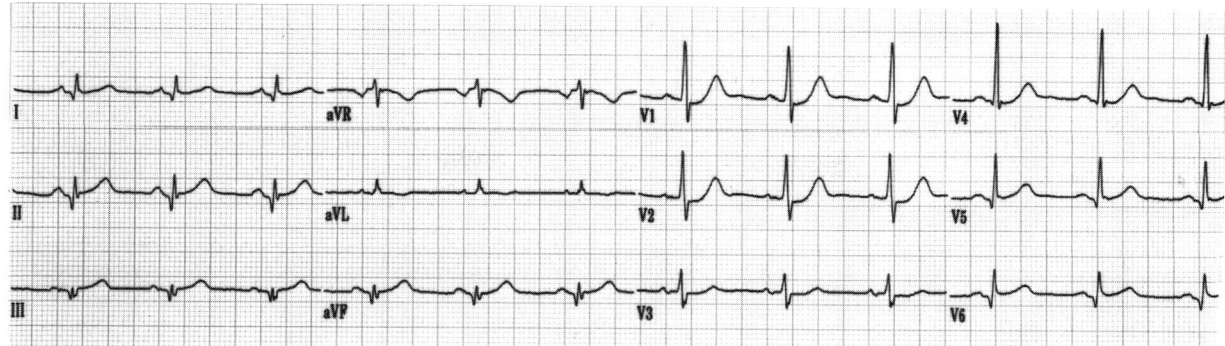

■ **Figure 18–34.** Posterior wall MI. Large R waves and ST depression are present in V_1 and V_2. Q waves and wide-based T waves in II, III, and aVF indicate probable inferior infarction as well.

ELECTROLYTE IMBALANCES

Hypokalemia (serum potassium <3 mEq/L) may produce ECG changes involving the ST segment, T waves, and U waves (Fig. 18-41). As potassium levels drop, the ST segment becomes progressively more depressed, T waves flatten, and prominent U waves develop. With advanced hypokalemia, the T and U waves often merge together and the U wave becomes larger than the T wave. These ST-T and U-wave changes correlate fairly well with serum potassium levels but are not specific for hypokalemia because they can also result from administration of certain drugs and from ventricular hypertrophy (Surawicz & Knilans, 2001). P waves usually widen, and the PR interval may prolong. Hypokalemia promotes atrial and ventricular ectopy and rhythms commonly seen in digitalis toxicity, such as atrial tachycardia with block and AV dissociation (see Chapter 19). Severe hypokalemia can cause ventricular tachycardia, torsades de pointes, and ventricular fibrillation.

Hyperkalemia (serum potassium >5.5 mEq/L) produces characteristic ECG changes involving the T wave and QRS complexes (Fig 18-42). When the serum K^+ level is about 5.5 mEq/L, T waves become tall and peaked with a narrow base (tented) and the QT interval shortens. As the potassium level rises, the QRS complex widens and ST-segment elevation may occur, simulating the injury current seen in acute MI. Typically, both the initial and terminal portions of the QRS are widened in hyperkalemia, unlike bundle-branch block

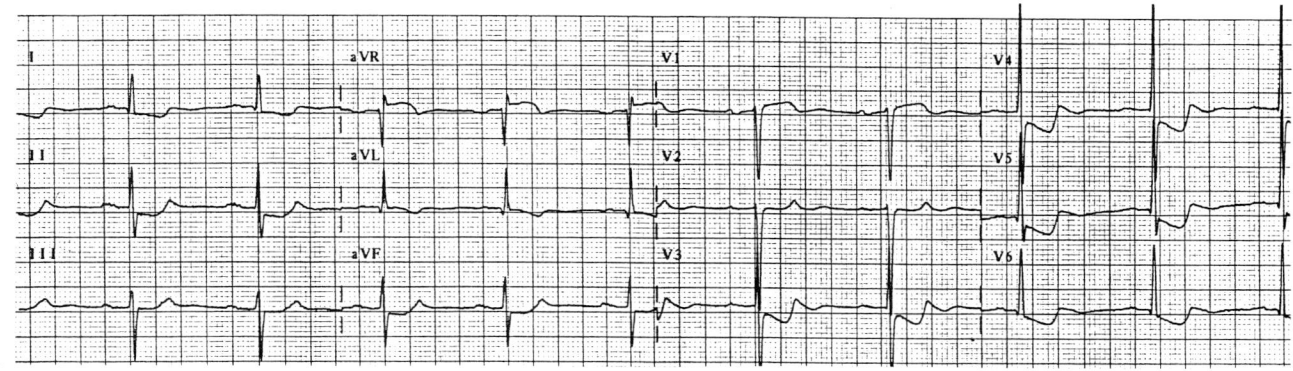

A

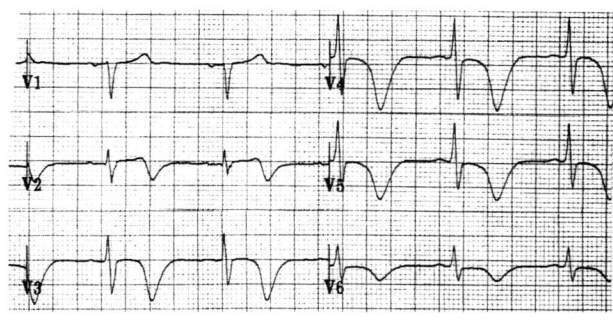

B

■ **Figure 18–35.** (*A*) Non-Q-wave MI. Note widespread ST depression in leads II, aVF, V_{3-6}. Cardiac enzymes were elevated, but no Q waves developed in any leads. (*B*) Precordial leads showing deep T wave inversion in a patient with elevated cardiac enzymes. No Q waves developed in these leads on serial tracings.

■ **Figure 18–36.** (*A*) Right and left atrial components of a normal P wave. (*B*) P mitrale pattern associated with enlargement of the left atrial component of the P wave. (*C*) P pulmonale pattern resulting from right atrial enlargement with increased amplitude of the right atrial component of the P wave. (Adapted from Surawicz B., & Knilans T. K. [2001]. *Chou's electrocardiography in clinical practice* [5th ed., p. 35]. Philadelphia: W. B. Saunders.)

A

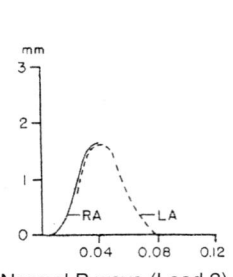

Normal P wave (Lead 2)

B

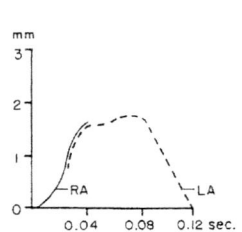

"P mitrale" due to left atrial enlargement

C

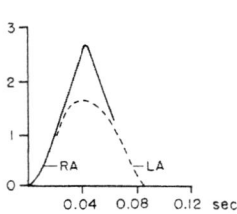

"P pulmonale" due to right atrial enlargement

where only the terminal QRS is affected (Surawicz & Knilans, 2001). First-degree AV block often occurs, and, as K$^+$ levels rise above 7 mEq/L, P waves flatten and eventually may disappear. With severe hyperkalemia, the QRS complex becomes broad and bizarre with a sine wave formation, and, when K$^+$ levels reach 12 mEq/L, ventricular fibrillation or asystole often occurs. These ECG changes are typical of hyperkalemia but do not correlate well with the actual serum potassium level. Some people do not show ECG changes until serum levels are quite high, whereas others show changes at lower potassium levels.

Hypocalcemia (serum calcium <6.1 mg/dL) prolongs the ST segment and the QT interval (Fig. 18-43). The prolonged QT interval is due to the abnormally long ST segment rather than to widening of the T wave as is seen with abnormal repolarization due to drugs. T waves are usually unchanged, but they may become flat or sharply inverted. With the possible exception of hypothermia, there is nothing other than hypocalcemia that prolongs the duration of the ST segment without changing T-wave duration (Surawicz & Knilans, 2001). Arrhythmias are uncommon in hypocalcemia.

Hypercalcemia (serum calcium >12mg/dL) shortens the QT interval, especially the distance from the beginning of the QRS to the peak of the T wave (Fig. 18-44). The ST segment practically disappears, and the proximal limb of the T wave takes off from the end of the QRS complex. P waves, T waves, and

QRS in hypertrophy

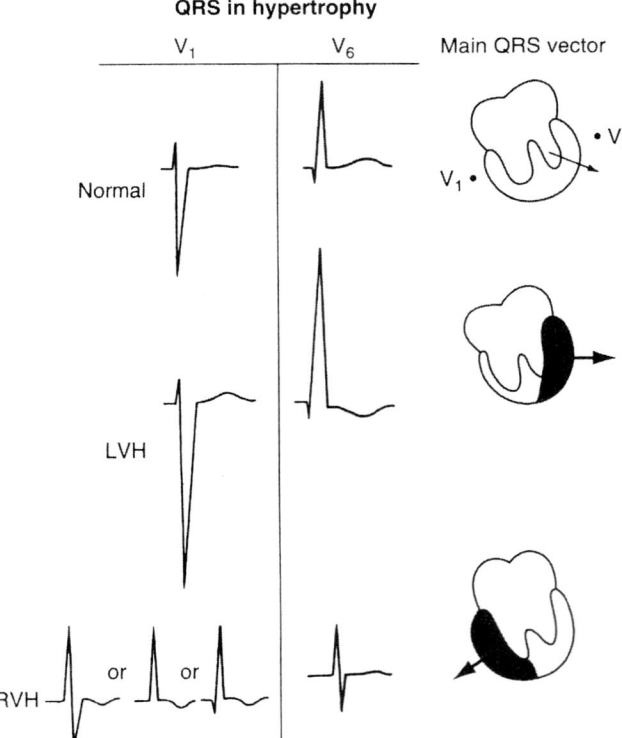

■ **Figure 18–38.** Normal ventricular size results in a dominant S wave in V$_1$, a dominant R wave in V$_6$, and a normal QRS axis. LVH increases the amplitude of forces directed to the left and posteriorly toward the enlarged left ventricle, resulting in large voltage S waves in V$_1$ and R waves in V$_6$, and shifting the axis leftward. RVH increases the amplitude of forces directed rightward and anteriorly through the enlarged right ventricle, causing large R waves in V$_1$ (usually R, RS or qR pattern) and deep S waves in V$_6$. (From Mirvis, D. M., & Goldberger, A. L. [2001]. Electrocardiography. In E. Braunwald, D. P. Zipes, & P. Libby [Eds.], *Heart disease: A textbook of cardiovascular medicine* [6th ed., p. 96]. Philadelphia: W. B. Saunders.)

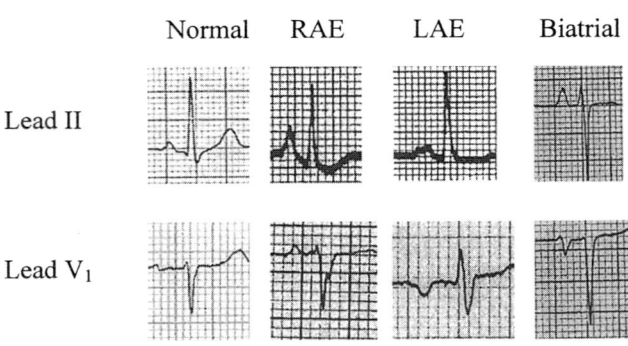

■ **Figure 18–37.** Normal P waves compared to those of left atrial enlargement, right atrial enlargement, and biatrial enlargement in Lead II and V$_1$. LAE causes widening and notching of P waves in many leads, and enlargement of the terminal negative portion of the P wave in V$_1$. RAE causes tall peaked P waves in many leads and enlargement of the initial upright portion of the P wave in V$_1$.

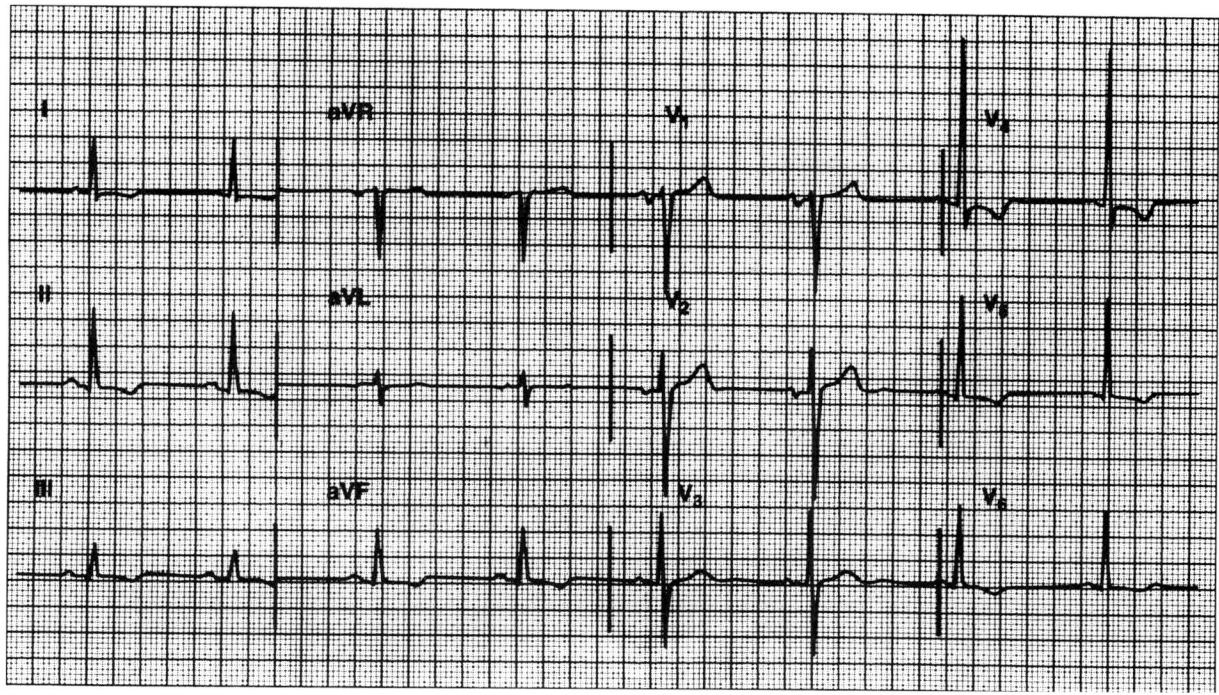

■ **Figure 18–39.** Left ventricular hypertrophy with deep S waves in V_{1-2} and large-voltage R waves in V_{4-6}. ST depression and T wave inversion (strain pattern) are seen in V_{4-6}. (From Mirvis, D. M., & Goldberger, A. L. [2001]. Electrocardiography. In E. Braunwald, D. P. Zipes, & P. Libby [Eds.] *Heart disease: A textbook of cardiovascular medicine* [6th ed., p. 96]. Philadelphia: W. B. Saunders.)

Table 18–3 ■ METHODS TO DIAGNOSE LEFT VENTRICULAR ENLARGEMENT (LVE) ON THE ELECTROCARDIO-GRAM (ECG)

Author/Method	ECG Criteria Favoring LVE	
Dubin, 1988	R wave in lead I + S wave in lead III > 26 mm	
	S wave in lead V_1 + R wave in lead V_5 or V_6 > 35 mm	
Sokolow and Lyon, 1949	R wave in VL ≥ 11 mm	
	S wave in lead V_1 + R wave in lead V_5 or V_6 > 35 mm	
	R wave in V_5 or V_6 > 26 mm	
Estes' Scorecard	*Criteria*	Points*
	1. R or S wave in limb lead 20 mm or more	
	⎫ S wave in lead V_1, V_2 or V_3 25 mm or more ⎫	
	⎭ R wave in lead V_4, V_5, or V_6 25 mm or more ⎭	3
	2. Any ST shift (without digitalis)	3
	Typical ST strain (with digitalis)	1
	3. Left axis deviation −30 degrees or more	2
	4. QRS interval 0.09 second or more	1
	5. Intrinsicoid deflection in V_5 and V_6 0.05 second or more	1
	6. P-wave terminal force in V_1 > 0.04 second	3
	Total possible	14
Scotts Criteria	Limb leads	
	R in 1 + S in 3 > 25 mm	
	R in aVL > 7.5 mm	
	R in aVF > 20 mm	
	S in aVR > 14 mm	
	Chest leads	
	S in V_1 or V_2 + R in V_5 or V_6 > 35 mm	
	R in V_5 or V_6 > 26 mm	
	R + S in any V lead > 45 mm	
Cornell Index	Women: R in aVL + S in V_3 > 20 mm	
	Men: R in aVL + S in V_3 > 28 mm	

* 5 = LVE; 4 = probable LVE.

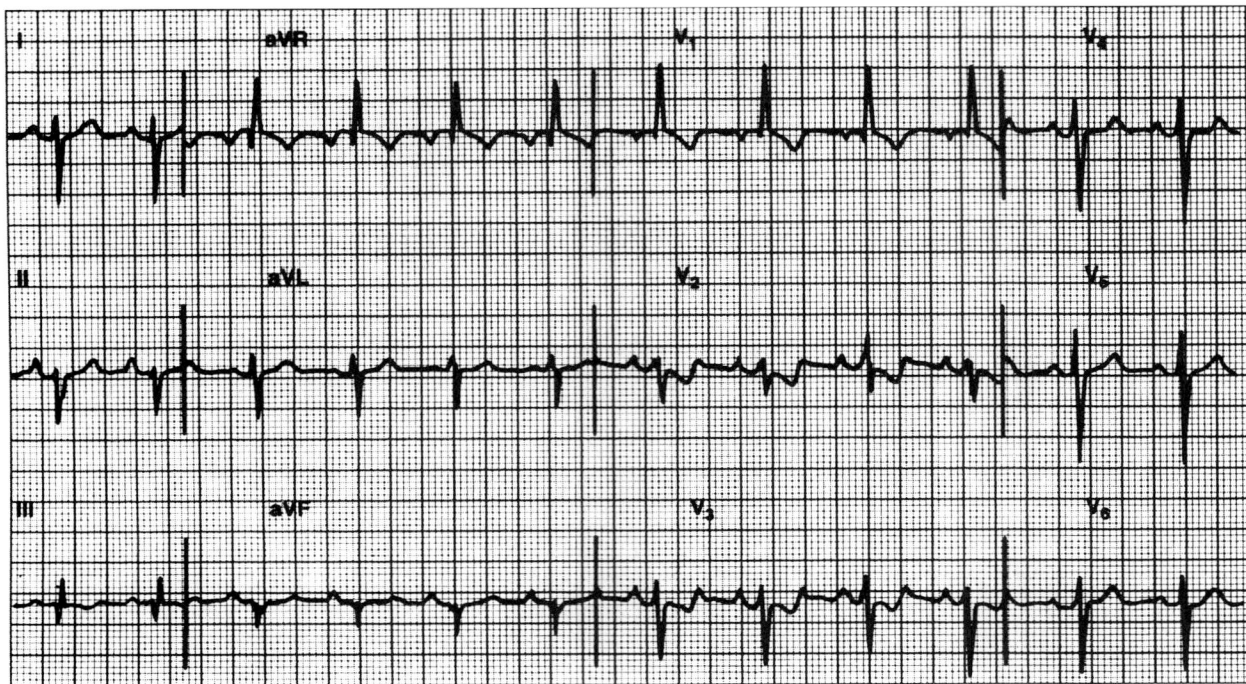

■ **Figure 18–40.** Right ventricular hypertrophy. Note marked right axis deviation and reversal of normal R wave progression across the precordium, with large R wave in V_1 and deep S wave in V_6. (From Mirvis, D. M., & Goldberger, A. L. [2001]. Electrocardiography. In E. Braunwald, D. P. Zipes, & P. Libby [Eds.], *Heart disease: A textbook of cardiovascular medicine* [6th ed., p. 98]. Philadelphia: W. B. Saunders.)

U waves are usually unchanged, and arrhythmias are uncommon in hypercalcemia.

Magnesium imbalances do not produce specific ECG changes. However, hypomagnesemia may contribute to arrhythmias caused by digitalis toxicity, ischemia, drugs, or potassium imbalances (Mirvis & Goldberger, 2001). Severe hypermagnesemia

has been associated with AV block and intraventricular conduction disturbances (Mirvis & Goldberger, 2001; Surawicz & Knilans, 2001).

▓ **WELLENS SYNDROME**

Wellens syndrome is a characteristic ECG pattern seen in patients with critical stenosis of the left anterior descending (LAD) coronary artery and is a warning of impending acute anterior wall MI. Recognition of Wellens syndrome indicates the need for immediate cardiac catheterization to intervene in the LAD with angioplasty or stenting before an acute MI occurs. These patients usually present with a diagnosis of unstable angina, and no or minimal cardiac enzyme elevation, and they exhibit the following ECG changes during pain-free periods (Conover, 1996; de Zwaan, Bar & Wellens, 1981):

1. ST segments: either normal or slightly elevated (no more than 1 mm), usually in leads V_2 and V_3, although this can be seen in V_{1-4}.
2. T waves: often start upright but the terminal portion dips below the baseline (*terminal T-wave inversion*) in V_{2-3} (may also appear in V_{1-4}). There is often progressive, symmetric, deep T-wave inversion in leads V_{1-4}.
3. R waves: there is no loss of R waves in V_{1-4} because there is no infarction yet.

Figure 18-45 illustrates an example of Wellens syndrome.

DISPLAY 18–3

DIAGNOSTIC CRITERIA FOR RIGHT VENTRICULAR ENLARGEMENT

R/S radio in V_5 or $V_6 \leq 1$
S wave in V_5 or $V_6 \geq 7$ mm
S_1, S_2, S_3 pattern
S_1, Q_3 pattern
Right axis deviation + 110 degrees ($\geq +90$ degrees)
R/S ratio in $V_1 > 1$ (with R wave > 5 mm)
R wave in $V_1 \geq 7$ mm
P pulmonale
QR in V_1
R wave in V_5 or $V_6 \leq 4$ mm (with S in $V_1 \leq 2$ mm)

Presence of one criterion indicates right ventricular enlargement with 95% specificity; two criteria indicate 99% specificity or higher.
Data from Mirvis, D.M. (1993). *Electrocardiography: A physiologic approach.* St. Louis, CV Mosby, 1993; and Murphy, MI. Thenabadu, P. N., Blue, L. R. et al. (1983). Descriptive characteristic of the electrocardiogram from autopsied men free of cardiopulmonary disease: A basis for evaluating criteria for ventricular hypertrophy. *American Journal of Cardiology,* 52, 1275–1280.

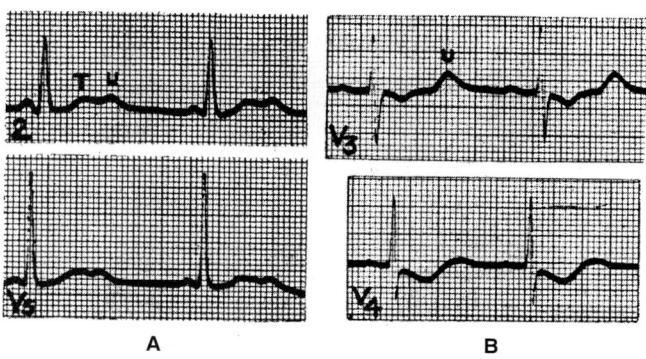

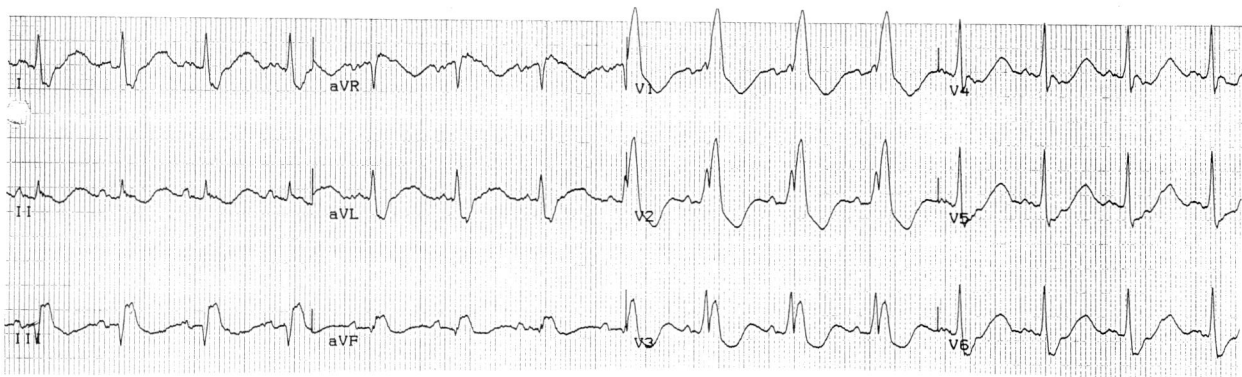

■ **Figure 18–41.** ECG effects of hypokalemia. (*A*) Early changes of hypokalemia with prminent U waves merging to form continuous undulating wave with T wave. (*B*) Advanced hypokalemia (1.8 mEq/L). Note ST-T depression with very prominent U waves in V₃ and the "roller coaster" pattern in V₄. (*C*) 12 lead ECG from patient with K 1.4mEq/L. Note "roller coaster" pattern, especially in lead II. RBBB is present, which widens the QRS. (*A* and *B* from Marriott, H. J. L. [1988]. *Practical electrocardiography* [8th ed., p. 523]. Baltimore: Williams & Wilkins.)

BRUGADA SYNDROME

In 1992, Brugada & Brugada described eight cases of aborted sudden cardiac death in patients with the following ECG findings (Brugada & Brugada, 1992):

1. Pattern of RBBB in V_1 to V_3: a late R wave (frequently small and called an "epsilon" wave), often without the corresponding deep S wave in left ventricular leads that is seen with true RBBB.
2. J point elevation in V_1 to V_3.
3. ST elevation in V_1 to V_3 that is unrelated to ischemia, electrolyte abnormalities, or structural heart disease.
4. Normal QT interval.

The ECG can be transiently normal, but patients with Brugada syndrome are prone to develop life-threatening ventricular arrhythmias leading to sudden death. It is now known that Brugada syndrome is an autosomal dominant inherited disease involving a genetic defect that causes abnormal cardiac sodium channel function (Antzelevitch & Burashnikov, 2001). Figure 18-46 illustrates an example of Brugada syndrome.

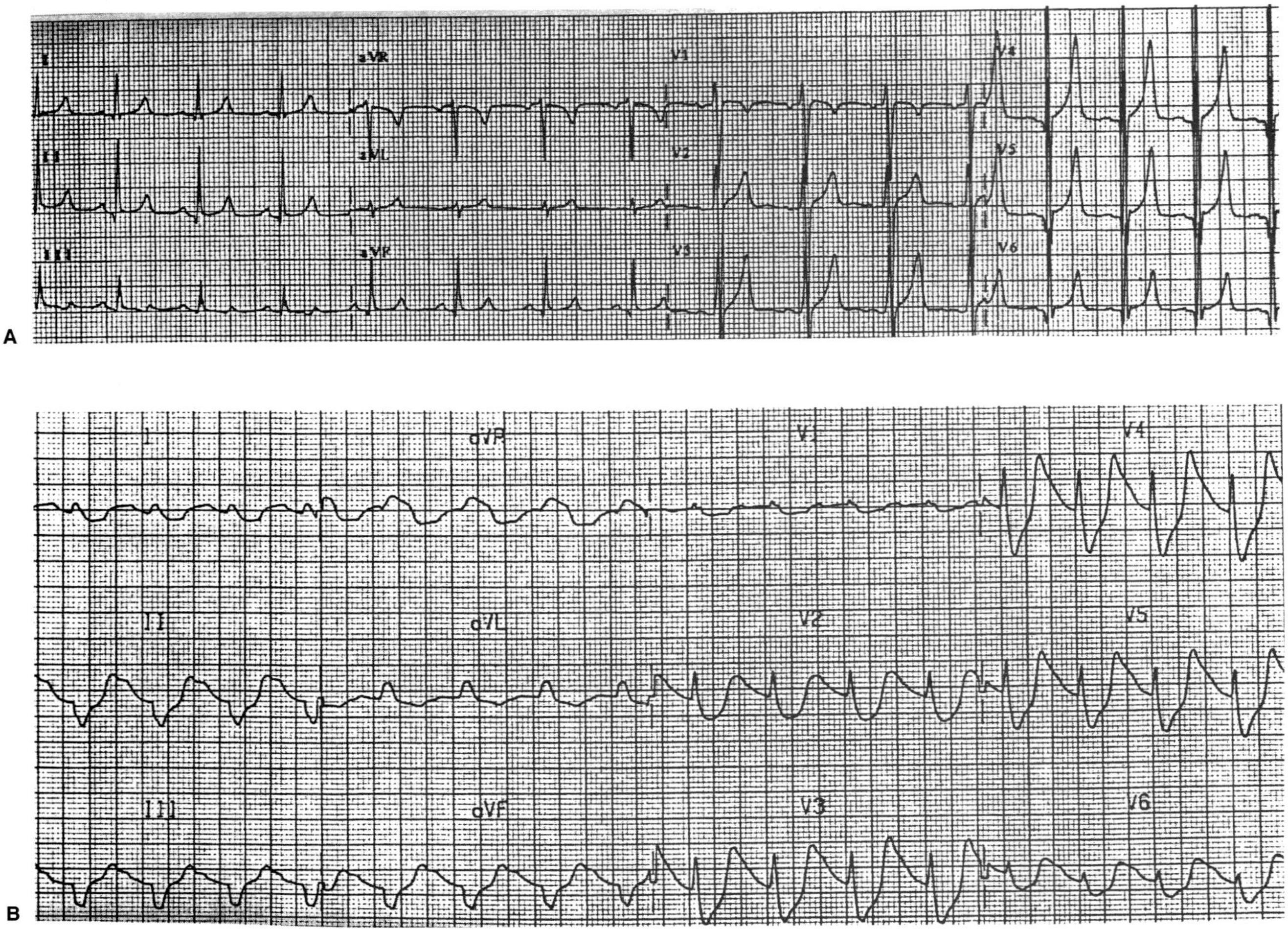

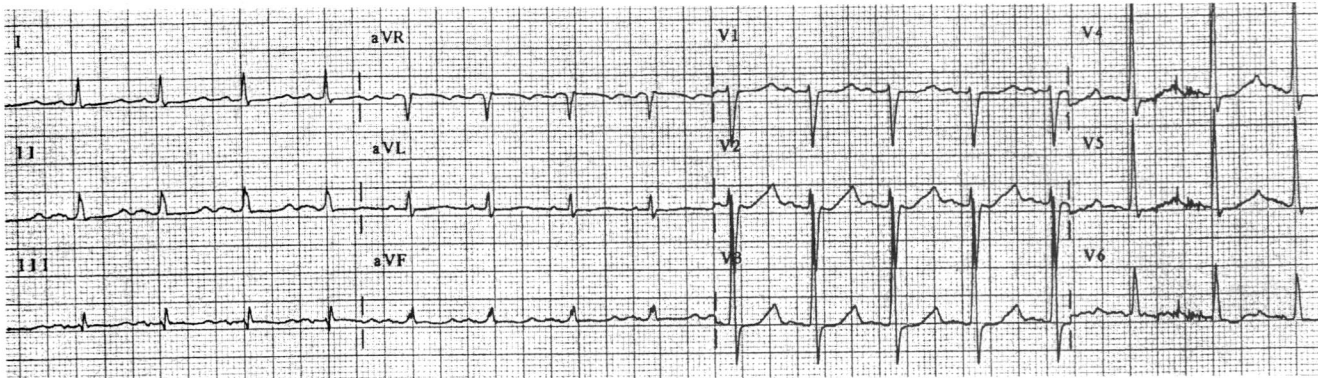

■ **Figure 18–42.** ECG effects of hyperkalemia. (*A*) Tall, peaked, narrow-based T waves typical of hyperkalemia. (*B*) Advanced hyperkalemia (K = 9.2 mEq/L). Note very wide QRS and almost sine-wave look in lead I and aVR.

■ **Figure 18–43.** ECG effects of hypocalcemia. Note the long ST segment that contributes to a prolonged QT interval.

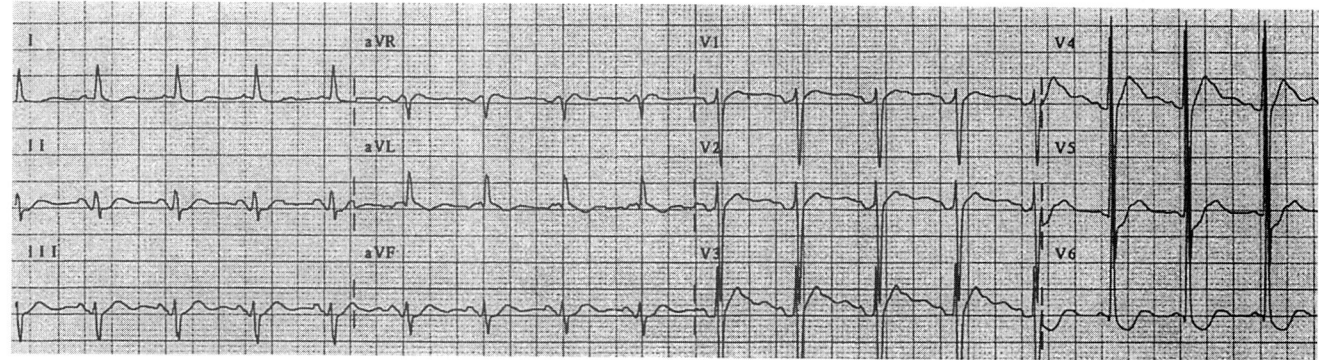

■ **Figure 18–44.** ECG effects of hypercalcemia. Note the short QT interval and how the T wave seems to take off from the end of the QRS in V$_{3-4}$.

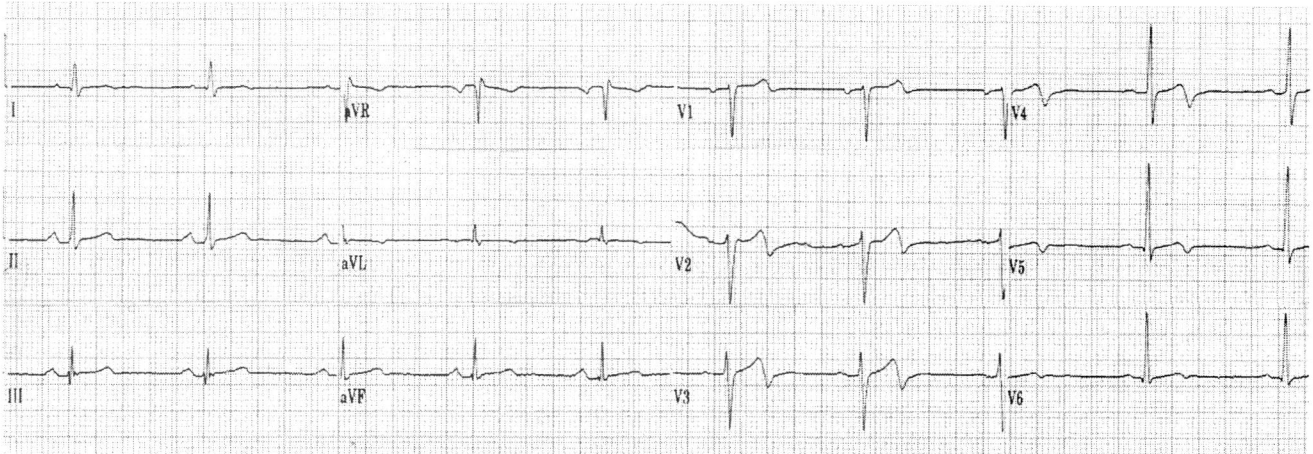

■ **Figure 18–45.** Wellens syndrome. Note terminal T wave inversion in leads V$_{1-5}$. The ST segment is not elevated, and there is normal R wave progression in the V leads. At cardiac catheterization the proximal LAD was found to be 90% occluded.

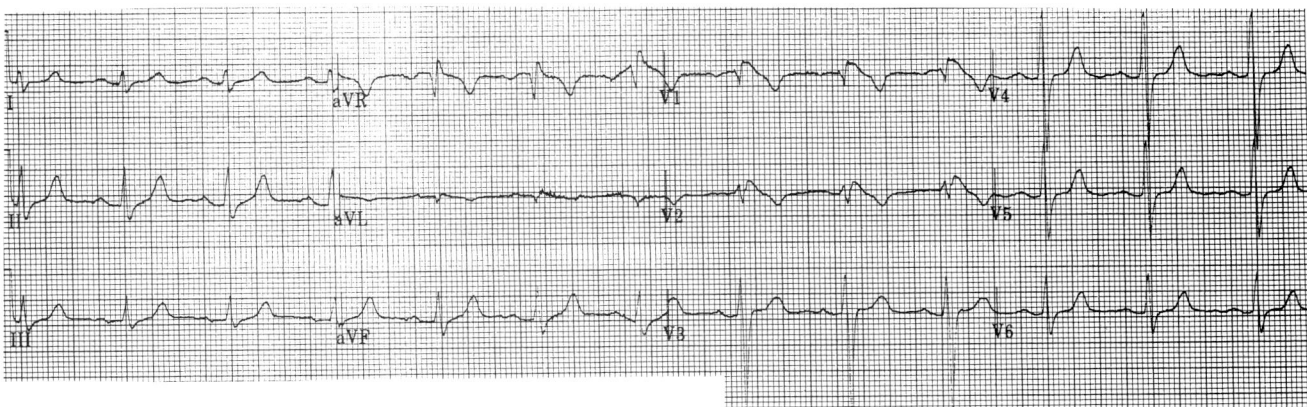

■ **Figure 18–46.** Brugada syndrome.

REFERENCES

Antzelevitch, C., et al. (1995). Clinical implications of electrical heterogeneity in the heart: The electrophysiology and pharmacology of epicardial, M, and endocardial cells. In P. J. Podrid & P. R. Kowey (Eds.), *Cardiac arrhythmia: Mechanisms, diagnosis, and management* (pp. 88–107). Baltimore: Williams & Wilkins.

Antzelevitch, C., & Burashnikov, A. (2001). Mechanisms of arrhythmogenesis. In P. J. Podrid & P. R Kowey (Eds.), *Cardiac arrhythmia: Mechanisms, diagnosis and management* (2nd ed., pp. 51–79). Philadelphia: Lippincott Williams & Wilkins.

Bazett, H. C. (1920). An analysis of the time relations of electrocardiograms. *Heart, 7,* 353–370.

Braunwald, E., Antman, E. M., Beasley, J. W., Califf, R. M., Cheitlin, M. D., Hochman, J. S., Jones, R. H., Kereiakes, D., Kupersmith, J., Levin, T. N., Pepine, C. J., Schaeffer, J. W., Smith, E. E., Steward, D. E., & Theroux, P. (2002). *ACC/AHA 2002 guideline update for the management of patients with unstable angina and non-ST-segment elevation myocardial infarction: A report of the American College of Cardiology/American Heart Association Task Force on Practice Guidelines (Committee on the Management of Patients With Unstable Angina).* Available: http://www.acc.org/clinical/guidelines/unstable/unstable.pdf.

Brugada, P., & Brugada, J. (1992). Right bundle branch block, persistent ST segment elevation and sudden cardiac death: A distinct clinical and electrocardiographic syndrome. *Journal of the American College of Cardiology, 20,* 1391–1396.

Castellanos, A., Interian, I., & Myerburg, R. J. (2001). The resting electrocardiogram. In V. Fuster, R. W. Alexander & R. A. O'Rourke (Eds.), *Hurst's the heart* (10th ed.). New York: McGraw-Hill.

Conover, M. B. (1996). *Understanding electrocardiography* (7th ed.). St. Louis: Mosby.

Cummins, R. O. (2001). *ACLS provider manual.* Dallas, TX: American Heart Association.

deZwaan, C., Bar, F., & Wellens, H. (1981). Characteristic electrocardiographic pattern indicating a critical stenosis high in left anterior descending coronary artery in patients admitted because of impending myocardial infarction. *American Heart Journal, 103,* 730–736.

Dubin, D. (1988). *Rapid interpretation of EKGs* (3rd ed.). Tampa, FL: Cover.

Goldman, M. J. (1986). *Principles of clinical electrocardiography* (12th ed.). Los Altos, CA: Lange Medical.

Goldschlager, N., & Goldman, M. J. (1989). *Principles of clinical electrocardiography* (13th ed.). Norwalk, CT: Appleton & Lange.

Jacobson, C. (2000). Electrocardiography. In S. L. Woods, E. S. Froelicher & S. Motzer (Eds.), *Cardiac nursing* (4th ed., pp. 263–296). Philadelphia: Lippincott.

_____. (1997). Advanced ECG concepts. In M. Chulay, C. Guzzetta & B. Dossey (Eds.), *AACN handbook of critical care nursing* (pp. 415–454). Stamford, CT: Appleton & Lange.

_____. (1991). Cardiac arrhythmias and conduction abnormalities. In M. L. Patrick, S. L. Woods, R. F. Craven, et al. (Eds.), *Medical-surgical nursing* (2nd ed., pp. 648–693). Philadelphia: J. B. Lippincott.

Jaffe, A. S., & Davidenko, J. (2001). Diagnosis of acute myocardial ischemia and infarction. In M. H. Crawford & J. P. Dimarco (Eds.), *Cardiology.* New York: Mosby.

Kadish, A. H., Buxton, A. E., Kennedy, H. L., Knight, B. P., Mason, J. W., Schuger, C. D., & Tracy, C. M. (2001). ACC/AHA clinical competence statement on electrocardiography and ambulatory electrocardiography: A report of the American College of Cardiology/American Heart Association/American College of Physicians-American Society of Internal Medicine Task Force on Clinical Competence (ACC/AHA Committee to Develop a Clinical Competence Statement on Electrocardiography and Ambulatory Electrocardiography). *Circulation, 104,* 3169–3178.

Marriott, H. J. L. (1988). *Practical electrocardiography* (8th ed.). Baltimore: Williams & Wilkins.

Mirvis, D. M.(1993). *Electrocardiography: A physiologic approach.* St. Louis: CV Mosby.

Mirvis, D. M., & Goldberger, A. L. (2001). Electrocardiography. In E. Braunwald, D. P. Zipes & P. Libby (Eds.), *Heart disease: A textbook of cardiovascular medicine* (6th ed., pp 82–128). Philadelphia: W. B. Saunders.

Moss, A. J. (1995). Long QT syndrome. In P. J. Podrid & P. R. Kowey (Eds.), Cardiac arrhythmia: Mechanisms, diagnosis, and management (pp. 1110–1120). Baltimore: Williams & Wilkins.

Murphy, M. I., Thenabadu, P. N., Blue, L. R., et al. (1983). Descriptive characteristics of the electrocardiogram from autopsied men free of cardiopulmonary disease: A basis for evaluating criteria for ventricular hypertrophy. *American Journal of Cardiology, 52,* 1275–1280.

Sokolow, M., & Lyon, T. P. (1949). The ventricular complex in left ventricular hypertrophy as obtained by unipolar precordial and limb leads. *American Heart Journal, 37,* 161–186.

Surawicz, B., & Knilans, T. K. (2001). *Chou's electrocardiography in clinical practice* (5th ed.). Philadelphia: W. B. Saunders.

Wagner, G. S. M. (2001). *Marriott's practical electrocardiography* (10th ed.). Philadelphia: Lippincott Williams & Wilkins.

Woods, S. L. (1997). Interpretation and management of basic cardiac rhythms. In M. Chulay, C. Guzzetta & B. Dossey (Eds.), *AACN handbook of critical care nursing* (pp. 55–82). Stamford, CT: Appleton & Lange.

SUGGESTED READING

Crawford, M. H., & Dimarco, J. P. (Eds.). (2001). *Cardiology.* New York: Mosby.

Fuster, V., Alexander, R. W., & O'Rourke, R. A. (Eds.). (2001). *Hurst's the heart* (10th ed.). New York: McGraw-Hill.

Marriott, H. J. L. (1997). *Emergency electrocardiography.* Naples, FL: Trinity Press.

Arrhythmias and Conduction Disturbances

CAROL JACOBSON

MECHANISMS OF ARRHYTHMIAS

Cardiac arrhythmias result from abnormal impulse initiation, abnormal impulse conduction, or both mechanisms together. Abnormal impulse initiation includes enhanced normal automaticity, abnormal automaticity, and triggered activity resulting from afterdepolarizations; abnormal impulse conduction includes conduction block and reentry (Antzelevitch & Burashinikov, 2001; Peters, Cabo & Wit, 2000; Rubart & Zipes, 2001; Waldo & Wit, 2001). Although all of these mechanisms have been shown to cause arrhythmias in the laboratory, it is not possible to prove which mechanism is responsible for a particular arrhythmia using currently available diagnostic tools in the clinical setting. However, it is possible to postulate the mechanism of many clinical arrhythmias based on their characteristics and behavior and to list rhythms most consistent with known electrophysiologic mechanisms (Bharucha & Podrid, 2001; Rubart & Zipes, 2001; Waldo & Wit, 2001). Some arrhythmias, such as atrioventricular nodal reentry tachycardia (AVNRT), atrial flutter, some ventricular tachycardias (VT), and reentry tachycardias involving accessory pathways, have been proven to be caused by reentry. This section describes the major mechanisms of arrhythmias and lists arrhythmias suggested or proven to be caused by each mechanism whenever possible. Knowledge of the cardiac action potential is essential in understanding concepts presented here (see Chapter 1).

Abnormal Impulse Initiation

Abnormal impulse initiation can be due to enhanced normal automaticity, abnormal automaticity, or afterdepolarizations. It is important to understand the property of normal automaticity before considering these other mechanisms.

Automaticity

Automaticity is the ability of certain cardiac cells to spontaneously depolarize and initiate an electrical impulse without external stimulation. The sinus node (or sinoatrial node) is the normal pacemaker of the heart because it has the fastest rate of automaticity. Other cells in the heart also have the property of automaticity, including cells in several areas of the atria, coronary sinus, pulmonary veins, atrioventricular (AV) junction, AV valves, and Purkinje system. The rates of these other pacemakers are slower than the rate of the sinus node; therefore, they are suppressed by the sinus node under normal conditions, a phenomenon known as *overdrive suppression*. The site of fastest impulse initiation is referred to as the *dominant pacemaker*, whereas sites of impulse formation that are suppressed by the dominant site are called *subsidiary* or *latent pacemakers*.

Enhanced Normal Automaticity

Impulse initiation can be shifted from the sinus node to other parts of the heart if the rate of the sinus node drops below that of a subsidiary pacemaker or if the automatic rate of a subsidiary pacemaker rises above that of the sinus node. Increased vagal tone, drugs, electrolyte abnormalities, or disease of the sinus node can decrease its rate of automaticity or can cause exit block of its impulse, thus allowing subsidiary pacemakers to assume control of the heart. Examples of clinical arrhythmias due to shifting of the pacemaker from the sinus node include atrial, junctional, or ventricular escape rhythms that occur due to sinus bradycardia or AV block. Such "escape" pacemaker activity cannot be considered abnormal because it is a manifestation of the normal automaticity of these cells.

Subsidiary pacemaker activity can be enhanced by factors that decrease the transmembrane resting potential (TRP), decrease the threshold potential, or increase the rate of diastolic phase 4 depolarization of the subsidiary pacemaker cells. Figure 19-1 illustrates how these mechanisms can change the rate of firing of pacemaker cells.

Enhanced normal automaticity can occur with sympathetic stimulation, drugs such as digitalis and sympathomimetic agents, or with disease states such as coronary heart disease or chronic pulmonary disease (Goldberger & Kadish, 2001). Clinical arrhythmias that may be due to enhanced normal automaticity include sinus tachycardia, wandering atrial pacemaker (WAP), some atrial tachycardias (AT), junctional tachycardia, some accelerated ventricular rhythms, and ventricular parasystole. The rate of arrhythmias due to enhanced normal automaticity is slower than those caused by abnormal automaticity, therefore

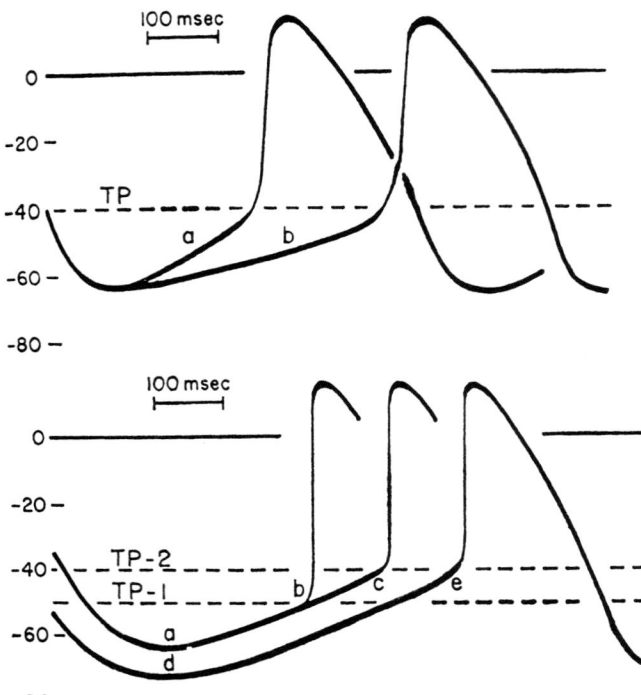

■ **Figure 19–1.** Diagram illustrating the principal mechanisms underlying changes in the frequency of discharge of a pacemaker fibre. The upper diagram shows a reduction in rate caused by a decrease in the slope of diastolic, or pacemaker, depolarization from a to b, and thus an increase in the time required for the membrane potential to decline to the threshold potential (TP) level. The lower diagram shows the reduction in the rate associated with a shift in the level of the threshold potential from TP-1 to TP-2, and a corrresponding increase in cycle length (*b* to *c*); also illustrated is a further reduction in rate due to an increase in the maximal diastolic potential level (Compare *a* with *c* and *d* with *e*). (From Hoffman, B. F., & Cranefield, P. F. [1960]. *Electrophysiology of the heart.* New York: McGraw-Hill. Used with permission of the McGraw-Hill Book Company.)

it is unlikely that tachycardias near 200 beats per minute or faster are due to enhanced normal automaticity (Antzelevitch & Burashinikov, 2001; Rubart & Zipes, 2001).

Abnormal Automaticity

Atrial and ventricular myocardial cells that do not normally have automaticity can develop abnormal automaticity when their TRP is reduced. Subsidiary pacemakers like those in the Purkinje system that are normally overdrive suppressed by the faster sinus node can also develop abnormal automaticity when their TRP is reduced. This abnormal automaticity is thought to be mediated by the slow inward current carried mainly by calcium (*slow channels*) because the normal fast sodium channels are inactivated at reduced membrane potentials (Antzelevitch & Burashinikov, 2001; Peters et al., 2000; Rubart & Zipes, 2001; Waldo & Wit, 2001). However, both sodium and calcium channels may play a role in the development of abnormal automaticity. Abnormal automaticity that develops at more negative diastolic potentials, between −70 and −50 mV, can be suppressed by sodium channel blockers, indicating that a sodium

current is involved; whereas automaticity that develops at less negative diastolic potentials, from −50 to −30 mV, can be suppressed by calcium channel blockers (Peters et al., 2000).

The resting potential of a cell can be reduced (e.g., from −90 to −70 mV) and the cell partially depolarized by anything that increases the extracellular potassium concentration, decreases the intracellular potassium concentration, increases the permeability of the membrane to sodium, or decreases the membrane permeability to potassium (Antzelevitch & Burashinikov, 2001; Gadsby, Karagueuzian & Wit, 1995; Peters et al., 2000; Rubart & Zipes, 2001; Waldo & Wit, 2001). Ischemia, hypoxia, acidosis, hyperkalemia, digitalis toxicity, chamber enlargement or dilation, stretch, and other metabolic abnormalities or drugs can reduce the resting potential and result in abnormal automaticity. Hypoxia and ischemia affect the TRP by decreasing the amount of oxygen available to supply adenosine triphosphate in amounts sufficient to operate the sodium-potassium pump efficiently. Anything that interferes with proper operation of this pump, such as digitalis, reduces normal resting ionic gradients across the cell membrane and results in reduction of the resting potential. When the TRP is reduced at rest, the cell is partially depolarized and the time required for spontaneous diastolic depolarization to reach threshold is reduced, thus increasing pacemaker activity (see Fig. 19-1). For the same reason, automaticity is increased when the threshold potential is reduced (e.g., from −40 to −50 mV) by ischemia or drug effects because less time is required for phase 4 depolarization to reach the lower threshold. The rate of phase 4 depolarization can be increased by several factors, including local norepinephrine release at ischemic sites, systemic catecholamine release, reduced vagal tone, and drugs.

Clinical arrhythmias that may be due to abnormal automaticity include some AT, accelerated ventricular rhythm, and some VT associated with acute myocardial infarction (MI; Antzelevitch & Burashinikov, 2001; Goldberger & Kadish, 2001; Peters et al., 2000; Rubart & Zipes, 2001; Waldo & Wit, 2001). The rate of a rhythm due to abnormal automaticity is related to the membrane potential from which it arose: the less negative the membrane potential (i.e., the greater the depolarization), the faster the rate. Rhythms due to abnormal automaticity tend to occur at faster rates than rhythms due to normal automaticity (Antzelevitch & Burashinikov, 2001; Peters et al., 2000).

Triggered Activity Due to Afterdepolarizations

Afterdepolarization is a transient depolarization of the cell membrane that occurs at some time during or right after repolarization of an action potential. Early afterdepolarizations (EAD) occur during the repolarization of an action potential. Delayed afterdepolarizations (DAD) occur after repolarization is complete but before the next action potential is due to occur. Figure 19-2 shows both EAD and DAD.

Early Afterdepolarizations. EAD occur during phase 2 or phase 3 of an action potential that was initiated from a high resting membrane potential (−75 to −90 mV). EAD that occur during phase 2 or early in phase 3 are thought to result from activation of the slow calcium channels because they arise at a time when the fast channels are largely inactivated

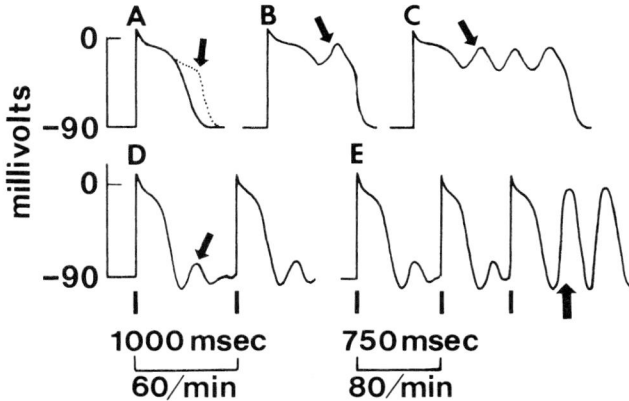

■ **Figure 19–2.** (*A*) An early afterpolarization (*arrow*). (*B*) A single triggered action potential caused by this afterdepolarization (*arrow*). (*C*) A train of triggered action potentials (*arrow*). (*D,E*) Action potentials caused by propagating impulses (indicated by *vertical lines*), followed by delayed afterdepolarization (arrow in *D*). (*E*) Triggered activity caused by the afterdepolarization (*arrow*). (From Wit, A., & Rosen, M. [1981]. Cellular electrophysiology of cardiac arrhythmias: J. Arrhythmis caused by abnormal impulse generation. *Modern Concepts in Cardiovascular Disease,* 50, 5. By permission of the American Heart Association, Inc.)

(Antzelevitch & Burashinikov, 2001; Gadsby et al., 1995; Peters et al., 2000). EAD that occur during the later part of phase 3 are probably due to current flowing through partially reactivated sodium channels (Peters et al., 2000; Waldo & Wit, 2001). If an EAD is large enough to reach threshold, a second upstroke occurs, causing an "early" beat. This second upstroke is called a *triggered beat* because it depends on and arises as a result of the preceding action potential. The triggered beat may be followed by its own afterdepolarization, which initiates yet another upstroke. This activity may be sustained for several beats and may terminate only when the membrane finally repolarizes to a high enough level to extinguish the rhythmic activity. This mechanism of abnormal impulse formation differs from abnormal automaticity in that automatic beats result from spontaneous initiation of each impulse, whereas beats due to afterdepolarizations depend on a preceding impulse.

EAD have been shown to occur most often in Purkinje fibers and mid-myocardial M cells in the ventricles (Antzelevitch & Burashinikov, 2001). EAD are caused by conditions that delay repolarization of the action potential and occur in the presence of hypoxia, acidosis, hypokalemia, hypomagnesemia, hypothermia, high pCO_2, and high concentrations of catecholamines, and in areas of stretch or mechanical injury (Antzelevitch & Burashinikov, 2001; Peters et al., 2000). Gene mutations that alter sodium and potassium ion channel activity and result in prolonged action potential duration have been identified and shown to cause EAD. The congenital long QT syndrome associated with torsades de pointes, a polymorphic VT associated with sudden cardiac death, has been shown to be due to genetic mutations that affect ion channel function and prolong repolarization, thus leading to EAD formation. Triggered activity due to EAD is enhanced by slow heart rates, and arrhythmias thought to be due to EAD often occur during bradycardia or after a pause in rhythm. The proarrhythmic effects of many drugs, especially class IA and III antiarrhythmics, are thought to be due to their ability to prolong repolarization in cardiac cells

and cause EAD. Clinical arrhythmias thought to be due to EAD include both acquired and congenital types of torsades de pointes, and many arrhythmias that occur with hypertrophy and heart failure (Antzelevitch & Burashinikov, 2001; Peters et al., 2000; Rubart & Zipes, 2001; Waldo & Wit, 2001).

Delayed Afterdepolarizations. DAD occur after the membrane has repolarized to its original level after an action potential. Subthreshold afterdepolarizations do not result in triggered activity, but, if the DAD is large enough to reach threshold, a triggered impulse arises. This triggered impulse may also be followed by its own afterdepolarization, leading to trains of triggered beats. Again, the mechanism differs from automaticity in that afterdepolarizations depend on and arise as a result of preceding action potentials. DAD occur in association with increased intracellular calcium levels, which commonly occur with digitalis toxicity. There is a direct relation between amplitude of DAD and heart rate: as the heart rate increases, so does afterdepolarization amplitude. Thus, triggered activity tends to occur after premature beats or at rapid heart rates. Factors that increase delayed afterdepolarization amplitude and contribute to triggered arrhythmias include high concentrations of catecholamines and digitalis, and hypokalemia (Antzelevitch & Burashinikov, 2001; Gadsby et al., 1995; Peters et al., 2000; Rubart & Zipes, 2001). Clinical arrhythmias that may be due to DAD include digitalis toxic rhythms like accelerated junctional rhythm and AT, idiopathic VT originating in the right ventricular outflow tract, accelerated idioventricular rhythm after MI, and tachycardias originating in the coronary sinus (Antzelevitch & Burashinikov, 2001; Rubart & Zipes, 2001; Waldo & Wit, 2001).

Abnormal Impulse Conduction

Abnormal impulse conduction can result in bradyarrhythmias or aberrancy when impulses are blocked, or premature beats and tachyarrhythmias when reentrant excitation occurs.

Conduction Block

The electrical impulse can be prevented from propagating through the heart for a variety of reasons. If the propagating impulse is not strong enough to excite the tissue ahead of it, conduction will fail (see section below on Decremental Conduction). If an impulse arrives at an area where the tissue is still refractory after a previous depolarization, it will not be able to conduct further (see section below on Phase 3 Block). If an impulse reaches tissue that is abnormally depolarized due to ischemia, disease, or drugs, it may not be able to conduct at all or will conduct with delay (see section below on Phase 4 Block). Scar tissue from previous MI, surgery, or catheter ablation also prevents conduction.

Decremental Conduction. Decremental conduction is the progressive decrease in conduction velocity of an impulse as it travels through a region of myocardium. Decremental conduction is a normal function of the AV node, delaying the impulse in the AV node long enough for atrial contraction to contribute to ventricular filling. Decremental conduction normally occurs in areas of the heart where resting potentials are low and action potentials depend on slow channels, such as the AV and sinus nodes. It can also occur in areas where resting potentials are low due to ischemia, disease, or drugs. Under

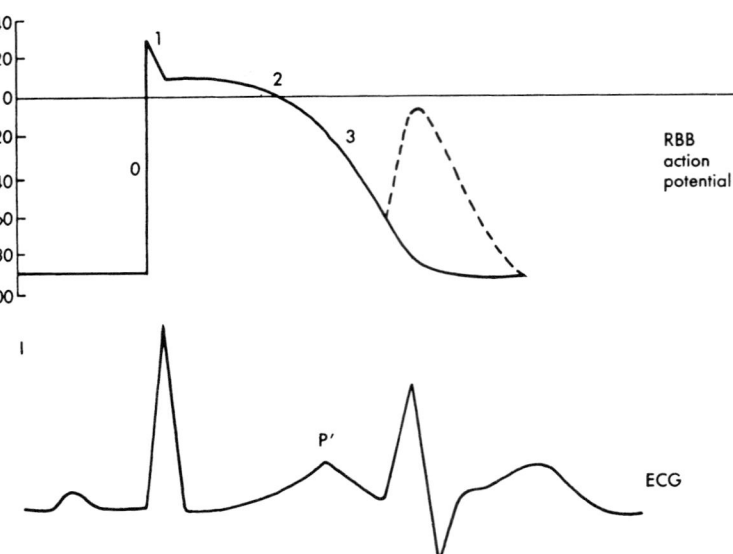

■ **Figure 19–3.** Phase 3 block. The electrocardiogram on the bottom shows a normal beat followed by a premature atrial beat that conducts with right bundle-branch block. The action potentials on top illustrate that the early beat entered the right bundle during phase 3, when the membrane potential was still reduced. The resulting action potential is a slow channel response, and conduction fails. (From Marriott, H. I. L., & Conover, M. [1998]. *Advanced concepts in arrhythmias* [3rd ed., p. 217]. St. Louis: CV Mosby.)

such circumstances, conduction velocity is slow because of the slower rate of rise of the action potential that occurs when cells are stimulated at reduced resting potentials. At times, decremental conduction can be so pronounced that the impulse fails to conduct, thus leading to block. This failure of conduction can occur in the sinus node, leading to sinus exit block; in the AV node, leading to AV block; or in the bundle-branch system, causing bundle-branch block (Waldo & Wit, 2001).

Phase 3 Block. When a cell is stimulated during phase 3 of the action potential, conduction is impaired because the membrane has not yet returned to its resting level. Whenever a cell is stimulated at a less negative membrane potential, the rate of rise of the action potential, and thus conduction velocity, is slow because most sodium channels are inactivated at reduced membrane potentials. Figure 19-3 illustrates phase 3 block occurring in the right bundle branch, resulting in aberrant conduction of the impulse with a right bundle-branch block (RBBB) pattern.

Phase 3 block, also called short-cycle aberrancy (Singer & Cohen, 1995), can occur in normal hearts if impulses are premature enough to reach fibers during their normal refractory period, resulting in aberrant conduction of premature beats. It is also responsible for rate-dependent bundle-branch blocks and for the aberration that commonly occurs when cycle lengths are very irregular, as in atrial fibrillation. Phase 3 block can occur pathologically if the refractory period is abnormally prolonged by drugs or disease.

Phase 4 Block. Phase 4 block, also called long-cycle aberrancy (Singer & Cohen, 1995), occurs late in diastole when fibers are stimulated at reduced membrane potentials secondary to spontaneous phase 4 depolarization (Waldo & Wit, 2001). In this case, the membrane has begun to depolarize spontaneously during its normal phase 4. By the time a stimulus arrives, the resting potential has been reduced enough to cause slow conduction. Again, whenever a cell is stimulated at a reduced membrane potential, only some of the sodium channels are available, and slow conduction results. Figure 19-4 shows a normal right bundle-branch action potential followed by spontaneous phase 4 depolarization. By the time the second impulse arrives in that bundle, membrane potential has been reduced enough to cause slow conduction and RBBB.

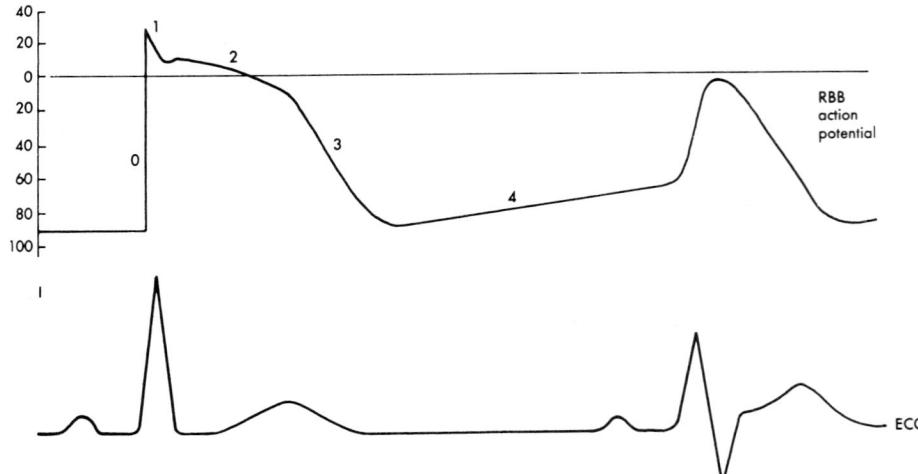

■ **Figure 19–4.** Phase 4 block. The electrocardiogram on the bottom shows a normal beat followed by a pause and a second beat that conducts with right bundle-branch (RBB) block. The action potential on top illustrates that the pause after the first normal action potential allowed sufficient time for spontaneous phase 4 depolarization to occur in the RBB. The impulse after the pause enters the RBB at a time when its membrane potential is reduced, resulting in conduction failure. (From Marriott, H. J. L., & Conover, M. [1989]. *Advanced concepts in arrhythmias* [3rd ed., p. 219]. St. Louis: CV Mosby.)

Table 19–2 ■ DRUGS USED FOR HEART RATE AND RHYTHM CONTROL.

Drug (Class)	Indication	Dose/Administration Therapeutic Level/Half Life	Side Effects	Comments
Adenosine (unclassified) (Adenocard)	First-line therapy to terminate AV nodal active SVT(AVNRT, AVRT). Can be diagnostic in AV nodal passive rhythms by causing AV block and revealing underlying atrial mechanism, and in wide complex tachycardias of uncertain origin. VT arising in the right ventricular outflow tract that is due to after depolarizations may respond to adenosine.	6 mg given very rapidly IV followed by rapid saline flush. May follow with 12 mg if needed and repeat 12 mg if no effect. Half life = 9 seconds	Acute onset of AV block usually lasting a few seconds. May result in brief period of asystole or bradycardia that is not responsive to atropine. Torsades can occur in patients who are susceptible to bradycardia-dependent arrhythmias. Flushing, hot flash, acute dyspnea lasting a few seconds, chest pressure. Can precipitate bronchoconstriction in asthmatic patients.	Very short half-life so side effects are transient. Warn patients about side effects before giving drug—especially dyspnea. It may be helpful to have patient take a deep breath while injecting drug to ↓ dyspneic sensation. Should not be used when arrhythmia is known to be atrial fib or flutter. Monitor ECG during administration and be prepared for cardioversion. May accelerate accessory pathway conduction and should not be used when antegrade conduction is occurring over accessory pathway. May rarely accelerate ventricular rate in atrial flutter. **Drug interactions:** Theophylline (and related drugs) and caffeine antagonize effects of adenosine and make it ineffective. Dipyridamole and carbamazepine potentiate effects of adenosine.
Amiodarone (III) (Cordarone)	Life-threatening ventricular arrhythmias: recurrent VF, recurrent hemodynamically unstable VT. Also used for: Conversion of atrial fib to sinus rhythm and maintenance of NSR. Treatment of atrial tachycardia, AVRT. Slows conduction through accessory pathways in atrial fib or AVRT.	**PO:** 800–1600 mg qd for 1–3 weeks, then 400–800 mg qd for 1–3 weeks. Maintenance: 100–400 mg/day. May be given as single daily dose or bid if GI intolerance occurs. **IV:** 1000 mg over first 24 hours given as follows: **First rapid infusion:** 150 mg over first 10 minutes (15 mg/min) [Add 3 mL (150 mg) to 100 mL D5W] Infuse 100 mL over 10 minutes. **Followed by slow infusion:** 360 mg over next 6 hours (1 mg/min) [Add 18 mL (900 mg) to 500 mL D5W] Infuse at 33.6 mL/h **Maintenance infusion:** 540 mg over next 18 hours (0.5 mg/min). [Decrease rate of slow loading infusion to 0.5 mg/min] Infuse at 16.8 mL/h May continue with 0.5 mg/min for 2–3 weeks if needed. Central line recommended for long-term infusions. If breakthrough VT occurs, may give supplemental doses of 150 mg over 10 min. [150 mg added to 100 mL D5W]	Bradycardia, heart block. Proarrhythmia (VF; incessant VT, torsades) Hypotension with IV form. Pulmonary fibrosis, corneal microdeposits, photosensitivity, blue skin, thyroid dysfunction (hypo and hyper), liver dysfunction. Tremor, malaise, fatigue, GI upsets, dizziness, poor coordination, peripheral neuropathy, involuntary movements. Liver enzyme elevations are common but occur in patients with MI, CHF, shock, multiple defibrillations, and so forth. It is unknown if elevations in liver enzymes are due to amiodarone or to associated conditions commonly present in these patients. Hepatocellular necrosis has occurred in patients who received IV amiodarone at rates higher than recommended.	Give with meals to ↓ GI intolerance. Baseline chest x-ray, renal, liver, thyroid function tests. Takes several weeks to achieve therapeutic blood levels and for effects to decrease after stopping drug. Is not dialyzable. Monitor K^+ and Mg^{++} levels. Monitor QTc interval. **Drug interactions:** Additive proarrhythmic effects with many drugs (1A antiarrhythmics, phenothiazines, tricyclic antidepressants, thiazide diuretics, sotalol) ↑ protime with coumadin. ↑ serum levels of digoxin, quinidine, procainamide, cyclosporine. May double flecainide level. Cimetidine ↑ serum amiodarone levels. Cholestyramine and phenytoin (Dilantin) ↓ serum amiodarone levels. Additive effects on ↓ HR and ↓ AV conduction with beta blockers and Ca^{++} blockers.

(continued)

Table 19–2 ■ DRUGS USED FOR HEART RATE AND RHYTHM CONTROL (Continued)

Drug (Class)	Indication	Dose/Administration Therapeutic Level/Half Life	Side Effects	Comments
		IV to PO transition: Duration of IV / <1 week PO dose 800–1600 mg qd / 1–3 weeks 600–800 mg qd / >3 weeks 400 mg qd / Therapeutic level = 1–2.5 mcg/mL / Very long half-life (26–107 days; average 53 days).		**Special precautions with IV form:** Physically incompatible with aminophylline, heparin, cefamandole, cefazolin, mezlocillin, sodium bicarbonate. Must be delivered using a *volumetric pump* (not drop counter) because drop size is altered by drug.
Atenolol (beta blocker) (Tenormin)	Ventricular rate control in atrial fib/flutter. Slow conduction through AV node in AVNRT and AVRT.	Initial dose: 12.5–25 mg PO qd Maintenance dose: 50–100 mg PO qd IV: 5 mg over 5 minutes, may repeat in 5 minutes Beta blocking plasma concentration = 0.2–5 mcg/mL Half life = 6–7 hours	Hypotension, bradycardia, AV block. Diarrhea, wheezing, CHF	Cardioselective beta blocker used primarily for hypertension and angina. **Drug interactions:** Additive effects on HR, AV conduction, BP, and ↑ potential for CHF when given with negative inotropic drugs, Ca++ blockers, digoxin.
Atropine (Anticholinergic, parasympatholytic)	Treatment of symptomatic bradycardia (sinus, junctional, AV block) and asystole	Symptomatic bradycardia: 0.5–1 mg IV. May repeat q 3–5 minutes to total of 0.04 mg/kg. Asystole: 1 mg IV, repeat q 3–5 minutes to total vagolytic dose of 0.04 mg/kg. May be given down ET tube during cardiac arrest if no IV available: use 2–2.5 mg. Half life = 2–5 hours	CV: tachycardia, chest pain, ventricular tachycardia/fibrillation (rare) CNS: drowsiness, confusion, dizziness, insomnia, nervousness GI: dry mouth, ↓ GI motility, constipation, nausea Other: urinary retention, hot flushed skin, rash	Doses <0.5 mg may cause paradoxical bradycardia. Causes pupils to dilate (significant when checking pupils during cardiac arrest situation). **Drug interactions:** Incompatible with aminophylline, metaraminol, norepinephrine, pentobarbitol, sodium bicarbonate.
Digoxin (unclassified)	Ventricular rate control in atrial fib/flutter. Also used as an inotropic agent in CHF.	PO loading dose: 0.5–1 mg divided into 3 or 4 doses at 6–8 hour intervals. PO maintenance dose: 0.125–0.5 mg qd. IV loading dose: 0.5–1 mg divided into 3 or 4 doses given at 4–8 hour intervals Therapeutic level = 0.8–2 ng/mL Half life = 36–48 hours	CV: bradycardia, AV block Digoxin toxicity: sinus exit block, AV block, atrial tachycardia with block, bidirectional tachycardia, fascicular tachycardia, accelerated junctional rhythm, regularization of ventricular fib response to atrial fib. Visual disturbances (halo vision), anorexia, nausea, vomiting, malaise, headache, weakness, disorientation, seizures.	Contraindicated in patients with WPW. Digoxin toxicity is more common in the presence of hypokalemia, renal failure, pulmonary or thyroid disease and in older people. **Drug interactions:** The following drugs ↓ digoxin levels: cholestyramine, antacids, kaopectate, neomycin, sulfasalazine, PAS. The following drugs ↑ digoxin levels: Erythromycin, tetracycline, quinidine, amiodarone, verapamil, spironolactone, nicardipine, indomethacin.
Diltiazem (Ca++ blocker) (Cardizem)	Ventricular rate control in atrial fib/flutter. Slow conduction through AV node in AVNRT and AVRT.	180–360 mg/day in divided doses. IV: 0.25 mg/kg bolus over 2 min. If needed, repeat with 0.35 mg/kg over 2 min. IV infusion: 10–15 mg/h Therapeutic level = 50–200 ng/mL Half life = 4–6 hours	Bradycardia, heart block, CHF, hypotension, flushing, angina, syncope, insomnia, ringing ears, edema, headache, nausea. Less depression of contractility than with verapamil but watch for CHF.	Contraindicated in patients with accessory pathways (WPW, short PR syndrome) **Drug interactions:** Additive effects on HR, AV conduction, BP, and ↑ potential for CHF when given with negative inotropic drugs, beta blockers, digoxin.
Disopyramide (IA) (Norpace)	Effective in treating PVC but not recommended due to proarrhyth-	Total daily dose = 400–800 mg in divided doses, usually 150 mg q6h.	Anticholinergic effects: dry mouth, urinary retention, constipation, precipi-	Monitor QT interval. **Drug Interactions:** May potentiate

(continued)

Drug	Action/Indication	Dose	Adverse Effects	Notes/Drug Interactions
	mic effects. Suppresses sustained VT Effective in preventing atrial fib and flutter. Slows conduction through accessory pathways.	divided doses, usually 150 mg q6h. SR form = 300 mg q12h. Therapeutic level = 3–6 mcg/mL Half life = 4–10 hours	nary retention, constipation, precipitation or exacerbation of glaucoma. CV: marked negative inotropic effects, CHF; prolongs QT interval, proarrhythmic (less than quinidine or procainamide), ↑ SVR	effect of coumadin. Additive negative inotropic effects with beta blockers or Ca^{++} blockers. Phenobarbitol, dilantin, rifampin ↓ disopyramide levels. Quinidine ↑ disopyramide level.
Dofetilide (III) (Tikosyn)	Conversion of atrial fibrillation or flutter to NSR and maintenance of NSR after conversion.	Dose based on creatinine clearance: if normal renal function, 500 mcg bid. If abnormal renal function, 250 mcg bid. Do not give if creatinine clearance <20 mL/min. Half life = 9.5 hours	Torsade de pointes (1.3%–4% incidence), usually occurs within 3 days after initiating therapy. Has no negative inotropic effects and does not lower BP.	Patient must be on telemetry during initiation of therapy or with increase in dosage (recommendation is for 3 days monitoring). Monitor QT interval every 2–3 hours: if QTc increases >15% or if QTc is >500 ms, reduce dose. If QTc after second dose is >500 ms, drug should be discontinued. **Drug Interactions:** Drugs that increase dofetilide levels include verapamil, ketoconazole, cimetidine, macrolide antibiotics, ritonavir, prochlorperazine, magesterol.
Epinephrine (Adrenalin)	Treatment of any cardiac arrest situation requiring CPR: VF, pulseless VT, asystole, PEA	1 mg IV bolus every 3–5 minutes during resuscitation efforts. May be given by way of ET tube if IV access not available: use 2–2.5 mg Alternative dosing can be used for cardiac arrest but has not been shown to improve outcomes. Intermediate dose: 2–5 mg IV every 3–5 minutes Escalating dose: 1 mg, 3 mg, 5 mg, 3 minutes apart. High dose: 0.1 mg/kg q 3–5 minutes May be infused at 2–10 mcg/min to maintain BP during symptomatic bradycardia	CV: tachycardia, hypertension, arrhythmias, angina CNS: restlessness, headache, tremor, stroke Other: nausea, ↓ urine output, transient tachypnea	Maintain normal K^+ and Mg^{++} levels. **Drug Interactions:** Has potential to cause arrhythmias when given with bretylium, digoxin, other sympathomimetic agents. Physically incompatible with aminophylline, ampicillin, cephapirin, sodium bicarbonate, and other alkaline solutions.
Esmolol (beta blocker) (Brevibloc)	Rapid control of ventricular rate in atrial fib/flutter.	Loading infusion: 500 mcg/kg/min for 1 min. Maintenance infusion: 50–100 mcg/kg/min. Use dosing chart that comes with drug. Beta blocking plasma concentration = 0.15–1 mcg/mL Half-life = 9 minutes	Hypotension, dizziness, diaphoresis, nausea.	Cardioselective beta blocker. Short half-life so effects reversed within 10–20 minutes after stopping drug. **Drug interactions:** May increase digoxin level.
Flecainide (IC) (Tambocor)	In absence of structural heart disease: Conversion of atrial fib to sinus and maintenance of NSR. Treatment of SVT: AVNRT, AVRT Slow conduction through accessory pathways in atrial fib or AVRT.	100–200 mg PO q12h Therapeutic level = 0.2–1 mcg/mL (Plasma levels do not correlate with efficacy, but incidence of CV toxicity greater when levels >1 mcg/mL)	CV: marked proarrhythmia, marked negative inotropic effects (CHF), bradycardia, heart block CNS: blurred vision, dizziness, flushing, ringing ears, drowsiness,	Additive effects on HR, AV conduction, BP, and ↑ potential for CHF when given with negative inotropic drugs, Ca^{++} blockers, digoxin. Incompatible with sodium bicarbonate, Lasix, Valium, thiopental. Higher mortality rate in post-MI patients when studied in CAST. Safest in patients with normal LV function. Should not be used in patients with recent MI.

Table 19-2 ■ DRUGS USED FOR HEART RATE AND RHYTHM CONTROL (Continued)

Drug (Class)	Indication	Dose/Administration Therapeutic Level/Half Life	Side Effects	Comments
	Life-threatening ventricular arrhythmias (sustained VT).		Other: bad taste, constipation, edema, abdominal pain	Prolongs QT interval, potential for proarrhythmia (torsades de pointes). Monitor for CHF. Full therapeutic effect may take up to 5 days. **Drug Interactions:** ↑ digoxin levels. Cimetidine, amiodarone, propranolol increase flecainide levels. Additive negative inotropic effects with beta blockers, Ca^{++} blockers, disopyramide.
Ibutilide (III) (Corvert)	Conversion of atrial fib or flutter to sinus. First drug approved by FDA specifically for this indication.	IV infusion of 1 mg over 10 minutes. May repeat same dose in 10 minutes if needed. In patients <60 kg: 0.01 mg/kg Half life = 6 hours	Hypotension, VT, bundle-branch block, AV block, nausea, headache.	Prolongs QT interval and may be proarrhythmic. Proarrhythmia usually occurs within 40 minutes. Monitor ECG continuously during administration and at least 4 hours after. Conversion to NSR usually occurs within 20–30 minutes of infusion. **Drug interactions:** Do not give other class I or class III agents within 4 hours.
Lidocaine (IB)	Treatment of ventricular arrhythmias: VT, VF. Effective for PVC suppression but PVC suppression not usually recommended.	For VT: 1 mg/kg IV bolus over 3 minutes followed by infusion at 2–4 mg/min. Repeat bolus of 0.5 mg/kg in 10 minutes to maintain therapeutic level. May repeat to total of 3 mg/kg. For VF or pulseless VT: 1.5 mg/kg IV bolus. May repeat with same amount and follow with infusion at 2–4 mg/min. May be given down ET tube during cardiac arrest if no IV available. Therapeutic level = 1.4–5 mcg/mL. Half-life of bolus = 10 minutes. Half-life once therapeutic level reached = 1.5–2 hours	Side effects relatively rare. CNS: lightheadedness, dizziness, tremor, agitation, tinnitus, blurred vision, convulsions, respiratory depression and arrest. CV: bradycardia, asystole, hypotension, shock.	↓ dose to half if liver disease or low liver blood flow (shock). **Drug Interactions:** Beta blockers and cimetidine increase lidocaine levels. Glucagon and isoproterenol may increase liver blood flow and ↓ lidocaine levels.
Magnesium	May be useful for treatment or prevention of both supraventricular and ventricular arrhythmias after MI or cardiac surgery. Treatment of choice for torsades de pointes and VF or pulseless VT refractory to other drugs.	1–2 g diluted in 10 mL D5W over 1–2 minutes. May be given IV push for VF or torsades. Infusion of 0.5–1 g/h for up to 24 hours.	CV: hypotension, bradycardia, heart block, cardiac arrest. CNS: weakness, drowsiness, peripheral neuromuscular blockade, absent deep tendon reflexes. Other: ↓ respiratory rate, respiratory paralysis.	**Drug Interactions:** CNS depression when used with general anesthetics, barbiturates, opiate analgesics. Additive effects with neuromuscular blocking agents. Incompatible with calcium, sodium bicarbonate, ciprofloxacin.
Metoprolol (beta blocker) (Lopressor)	Ventricular rate control in atrial fib/flutter. Slow conduction through AV node in	PO: 100–450 mg qd. IV: 5 mg q 2–5 minutes for three doses (used in acute MI)	Hypotension, bradycardia, AV block	Cardioselective beta blocker. **Drug interactions:** Additive effects on HR, AV conduction, BP, and ↑

Drug	Indications	Dosing / Pharmacokinetics	Side Effects	Comments / Drug Interactions
Mexiletine (IB) (Mexitil)	AVRT and AVRT. Acute and chronic treatment of symptomatic VT	Beta blocking plasma concentration = 50–100 ng/mL. Half-life = 3–4 hours. PO loading dose = 400 mg. Maintenance dose = 200–400 mg q8h. Therapeutic level = 0.5–2 mcg/mL. Half life = 10–17 hours	GI: nausea, vomiting, heartburn, anorexia, diarrhea. CNS: tremor, dizziness, ataxia, slurred speech, paresthesias, seizures, hallucinations, emotional instability, insomnia, memory impairment. CV: bradycardia, hypotension, CHF, proarrhythmia (rare compared to other agents). Other: thrombocytopenia, fever, rash, positive ANA.	potential for CHF when given with negative inotropic drugs, Ca^{++} blockers, digoxin. Often given in combination with other antiarrhythmics with increased effectiveness (quinidine, disopyramide, propafenone, amiodarone). **Drug interactions:** Phenobarbitol, dilantin, rifampin ↓ mexiletine levels. Cimetidine ↑ mexiletine levels. Mexiletine ↑ theophylline levels.
Procainamide (IA) (Pronestyl)	Conversion of atrial fib to sinus and maintenance of NSR. Suppresses PAC, atrial tachycardia, atrial flutter and fib. Slows conduction through accessory pathways. Effective in terminating and preventing VT. Effective in treating PVC but not recommended due to proarrhythmic effects.	PO dose 3–7.5 g qd in divided doses 3–4 times a day (never more than 6 h between doses) SR forms q6h. IV loading dose: 17 mg/kg at 20 mg/min. If rapid loading is needed, give 100-mg doses over 5 minutes to total of 1–1.5 g. IV drip 2–4 mg/min. Therapeutic level = 4–10 mcg/mL (may be as high as 5–32 mg/L to prevent sustained VT). Half-life = 3–4 hours. Active metabolite is NAPA: therapeutic level = 9–12 mg/L	GI: nausea, vomiting, anorexia. CV: bradycardia, heart block, proarrhythmia (less than with quinidine). Prolongs QT interval. Hypotension with IV use. CNS: headache, insomnia, dizziness, psychosis, hallucinations, depression. Lupuslike syndrome with long-term use (15%–25% of patients who take drug >1 year). Other: rash, fever, swollen joints, agranulocytosis, pancytopenia.	Monitor QT interval, QRS width, PR. Monitor NAPA level (active metabolite). Watch for hypotension with IV use. **Drug Interactions:** Amiodarone, cimetidine, ranitidine increase procainamide levels. Alcohol ↓ procainamide levels. Additive effects on conduction system disease when given with other class IA, class IC, tricyclic antidepressants, or Ca^{++} blockers.
Propafenone (IC) (Rhythmol) Also has beta blocker effects	Conversion of atrial fib to sinus and maintenance of NSR. Slow conduction through accessory pathways. Life-threatening ventricular arrhythmias (sustained VT).	150–300 mg tid. Therapeutic level = 0.2–3 mcg/mL. Half life = 2–10 hours in normal metabolizers, up to 32 hours in slow metabolizers.	GI: nausea, anorexia, constipation, metallic taste. CNS: dizziness, headache, blurred vision. CV: CHF, bradycardia, AV block, bundle-branch block, proarrhythmia	Was not included in CAST but is same class as drugs shown to cause higher mortality post MI. Watch for proarrhythmia. **Drug interactions:** ↑ digoxin levels. Potentiates coumadin. Has mild beta blocker and Ca^{++} blocker effects. ↑ cyclosporin levels. Quinidine and cimetidine increase propafenone levels.
Propranolol (beta blocker) (Inderal)	Ventricular rate control in atrial fib/flutter. Treatment of SVT (slow AV node conduction): AVNRT, AVRT. Effective in some types of VT: exercise induced, digitalis induced. Effective in reducing incidence of VF and sudden death post MI.	PO: 10–30 mg 3–4 times a day. IV: 1–3 mg at rate of 1 mg/min. Beta-blocking plasma concentration = 50–100 ng/mL. Half life = 3–5 hours	CV: bradycardia, heart block, hypotension, CHF. GI: nausea, vomiting, stomach discomfort, constipation, diarrhea. CNS: dreams, hallucinations, insomnia, depression. Other: bronchospasm, exacerbation of peripheral vascular disease, fatigue, hypoglycemia, impotence	Non-cardioselective beta blocker. **Drug interactions:** Additive effects on HR, AV conduction, BP, and ↑ potential for CHF when given with negative inotropic drugs, Ca^{++} blockers, digoxin.
Quinidine (IA)	Conversion of atrial fib to sinus and maintenance of NSR. May be used for other SVT: atrial tachycardia, AVNRT, accessory pathways.	Sulfate: 200–400 mg q6–8h. Gluconate: 324 mg SR tabs, 1–2 q8–12h. Therapeutic level = 2–5 µg/mL. Half-life = 7–9 hours	GI: nausea, diarrhea, abdominal pain. CV: hypotension, bradycardia, tachycardias, torsades de pointes, CHF. Prolongs QTc interval, proarrhythmia. CNS: cinchonism (tinnitus, hearing	Give with food. Monitor QT interval, QRS width, PR. Watch for proarrhythmia (torsades). IV use rare (hypotension).

(continued)

Table 19–2 ■ DRUGS USED FOR HEART RATE AND RHYTHM CONTROL (Continued)

Drug (Class)	Indication	Dose/Administration Therapeutic Level/Half Life	Side Effects	Comments
	Effective in treating PVC and VT but not recommended due to proarrhythmic effects.		loss, confusion, delirium, visual disturbances, psychosis) Other: fever, headache, rashes, leukopenia, thrombocytopenia	**Drug Interactions:** ↑ Digoxin levels. Increased bleeding when used with coumadin. Dilantin, phenobarb, rifampin, nifedipine, sodium bicarbonate, thiazide diuretics all ↓ quinidine levels. Cimetidine, amiodarone, verapamil all increase quinidine levels.
Sotalol (III) **(Betapace)** Has beta blocker effects	Conversion of atrial fib to sinus and maintenance of NSR. Treatment of SVT. Slow conduction through accessory pathways.	80 mg bid × 3 days, then 160 mg bid × 3 days. 240–320 mg bid if necessary Therapeutic level = 1–4 µg/mL (not clinically useful) Half life = 10–20 hours	CV: bradycardia, heart block, CHF, proarrhythmia. Other: bronchospasm, fatigue, weakness, GI symptoms, dizziness, dyspnea, hypotension.	Prolongs QT interval, potential for proarrhythmia. Watch for bradycardia, AV block and new or worsening CHF. No known drug interactions.
Tocainide (IB) **(Tonocard)**	Life-threatening VT, VF. Acute and chronic treatment of symptomatic VT	400–600 mg q8h PO Therapeutic level = 4–10 µg/mL Half life = 11–19 hours	GI: nausea, vomiting, heartburn, anorexia, diarrhea CNS: tremor, dizziness, ataxia, slurred speech, paresthesias, seizures, hallucinations, emotional instability, insomnia, memory impairment. CV: bradycardia, hypotension, CHF, proarrhythmia (rare compared to other agents) Other: agranulocytosis, fever, rash, positive ANA, pulmonary fibrosis	Give with food to ↓ GI effects. Can cause blood dyscrasias: monitor blood counts weekly for first 12 weeks of therapy and frequently thereafter. No known drug interactions.
Verapamil (Ca⁺⁺ blocker) **(Calan)**	Ventricular rate control in atrial fib/flutter. Slow conduction through AV node in AVNRT and AVRT.	PO: 80–120 mg tid or qid IV: 2.5–5 mg over 2 min. May repeat with 5–10 mg if needed Therapeutic level = 80–400 ng/mL Half life = 3–7 hours	Bradycardia, heart block, CHF, hypotension, fatigue, headache, edema, constipation.	Contraindicated in patients with accessory pathways (WPW, short PR syndrome) **Drug interactions:** Additive effects on HR, AV conduction, BP, and ↑ potential for CHF when given with negative inotropic drugs, Ca⁺⁺ blockers, digoxin.

AVNRT = atrioventricular nodal reentry tachycardia, CAST = Cardiac Arrhythmia Suppression Trial, AVRT = atrioventricular reentry tachycardia using an accessory pathway, ET = endotracheal, NSR = normal sinus rhythm, PEA = pulseless electrical activity, SVT = supraventricular tachycardia, SVR = systemic vascular resistance, SR = sustained release, WPW = Wolff-Parkinson-White syndrome.
↑ = increases, ↓ = decreases

Table 19–3 ■ COMMON THERAPIES FOR TACHYARRHYTHMIAS

Treatment	Atrial Fibrillation or Flutter Atrial Tachycardia	AVNRT	AVRT	VT
Adenosine 6 mg very rapidly IV. May repeat with 12 mg very rapidly IV if no effect within 2–3 minutes. May repeat 12-mg dose once more.	Slows AV conduction and unmasks atrial mechanism. (If atrial rate <250 = atrial tachycardia. If atrial rate >250 = atrial flutter. If atrial rhythm very rapid and chaotic with no formed P waves = atrial fibrillation.) Temporary slowing of ventricular rate only. Does not terminate atrial arrhythmia. Should not be used when mechanism is known to be atrial flutter, atrial fibrillation or ectopic atrial tachycardia or if atrial fibrillation with accessory pathway conduction is suspected.	**Drug of choice for treatment of PSVT when mechanism is unknown or if known AVNRT.** Terminates rhythm by blocking conduction through AV node. Does not prevent recurrence.	**Drug of choice for treatment of PSVT if mechanism unknown or if known CMT.** Terminates rhythm by blocking conduction through AV node. Does not prevent recurrence.	Usually no effect but also no harm. VT originating in the RVOT may terminate with adenosine.
Beta Blockers Esmolol (brevebloc) Atenolol (tenormin) Metoprolol (Lopressor)	Slow AV conduction and provide long-term control of ventricular rate. Usually do not convert atrial arrhythmias to sinus rhythm.	May terminate AVNRT by blocking conduction through slow pathway in AV node. Do not prevent recurrence unless they suppress initiating PAC.	May terminate CMT by blocking conduction through AV node. Do not prevent recurrence unless they suppress initiating PAC or PVC.	Not indicated for acute treatment of VT episode. May be used for prevention of some types of VT.
Calcium Channel Blockers Diltiazem (Cardizem) Verapamil (Calan)	Slow AV conduction and provide long-term control of ventricular rate. Usually do not convert atrial arrhythmias to sinus rhythm. **Do not use in atrial fibrillation with accessory pathway conduction.**	May terminate AVNRT by blocking conduction through slow or fast pathway in AV node. Do not prevent recurrence unless they suppress initiating PAC.	May terminate CMT by blocking conduction through AV node. Do not prevent recurrence unless suppress initiating PAC or PVC.	**Do not use for wide QRS tachycardia of uncertain type.** Generally not indicated for VT (except for "verapamil sensitive" types of VT)
Cardioversion (First choice for hemodynamically unstable tachycardias)	If rapid ventricular response results in hemodynamic instability. Terminates individual episode but does not prevent recurrence.	If rapid rate results in hemodynamic instability. Terminates individual episode but does not prevent recurrence.	If rapid rate results in hemodynamic instability. Terminates individual episode but does not prevent recurrence.	If rapid rate results in hemodynamic instability. Terminates individual episode but does not prevent recurrence.
Ibutilide (Corvert) 1 mg diluted in 50 mL over 10 minutes. May repeat same dose in 10 minutes if needed.	**Used to convert atrial fibrillation or flutter to NSR.** Usually converts within 20 minutes. Causes prolonged QT interval and may cause torsades.	Not indicated	Not indicated	Not indicated
Procainamide IV loading dose 17 mg/kg at 20 mg/min. PO sustained release up to 1000–1300 mg/day	**Commonly used for atrial fibrillation with accessory pathway conduction** because it prolongs refractory period of pathway and slows ventricular rate. May also convert atrial arrhythmias to sinus rhythm.	May terminate AVNRT by slowing conduction through fast pathway in AV node. May prevent recurrence by suppressing initiating PAC.	May terminate CMT by slowing conduction through accessory pathway. May prevent recurrence by suppressing initiating PAC or PVC.	May terminate VT or slow its rate. **Good choice for treating wide QRS tachycardias of unknown type or known VT.**

(continued)

Table 19–3 ■ COMMON THERAPIES FOR TACHYARRHYTHMIAS *(Continued)*

Treatment	Atrial Fibrillation or Flutter Atrial Tachycardia	AVNRT	AVRT	VT
Radiofrequency Catheter Ablation	Ablation of reentry circuit in right atrium frequently done to treat and prevent recurrence of atrial flutter. Ablation to create linear lesions in the atria (similar to surgical Maze procedure) and ablation around pulmonary veins successful in curing atrial fibrillation in many patients. Ablation of AV node in drug refractory atrial fibrillation and implantation of permanent pacemaker is often done when ventricular rate control not possible with drugs.	Ablation of slow pathway in AV node prevents recurrence of AVNRT and has become standard treatment for this arrhythmia.	Ablation of accessory pathway prevents recurrence of AVRT and has become standard treatment for this type of arrhythmia.	Ablation of VT focus may be helpful in VT originating in RVOT. Ablation of RBB sometimes successful in bundle-branch reentry VT.

Sinus Bradycardia

Sinus bradycardia is discharge of the sinus node at a rate slower than 60 beats per minute. It can be a normal variant, especially in athletes and during sleep. Sinus bradycardia may be a response to vagal stimulation, such as carotid sinus massage (CSM), ocular pressure, or vomiting. Disease processes that can cause sinus bradycardia include inferior wall MI, myxedema, obstructive jaundice, uremia, increased intracranial pressure, glaucoma, anorexia nervosa, and sick sinus syndrome (Olgin & Zipes, 2001; Reiffel, 2001; Robles de Medina & Wilde, 2000). Sinus bradycardia can be a response to several medications, including digitalis, beta blockers, calcium channel blockers, and antiarrhythmics.

The following are ECG characteristics of sinus bradycardia:

Rate: Less than 60 beats per minute
Rhythm: Regular
P waves: Precede every QRS, consistent shape
PR interval: Usually normal (0.12 to 0.20 second)
QRS complex: Usually normal (0.04 to 0.10 second)
Conduction: Normal through atria, AV node, bundle branches, and ventricles
Example: Sinus bradycardia, rate 40 beats per minute

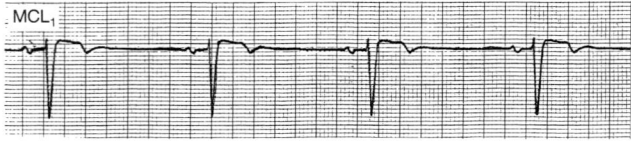

Sinus bradycardia does not require treatment unless the patient is symptomatic. If the arrhythmia is accompanied by hypotension, restlessness, diaphoresis, chest pain, or other signs of hemodynamic compromise or by ventricular ectopy, atropine, 0.5 to 1 mg intravenously (IV) is the treatment of choice. Attempts should be made to decrease vagal stimulation, and, if bradycardia is due to medications, they should be held until their need has been reevaluated. See Chapter 31 for the ACLS algorithm for treatment of symptomatic bradycardia.

Sinus Tachycardia

Sinus tachycardia is sinus rhythm at a rate faster than 100 beats per minute. It is a normal response to anything that stimulates the sympathetic nervous system, including sympathomimetic drugs, exercise, and emotion. Sinus tachycardia that persists at rest usually indicates some underlying problem, such as fever, blood loss, anxiety, heart failure, hypermetabolic states, or anemia (Olgin, 2000; Olgin & Zipes, 2001; Reiffel, 2001). Sinus tachycardia is a normal physiologic response to a decrease in cardiac output. Drugs that can cause sinus tachycardia include atropine, isoproterenol, epinephrine, dopamine, dobutamine, norepinephrine, nitroprusside, and caffeine.

The ECG characteristics of sinus tachycardia include the following:

Rate: Greater than 100 beats per minute
Rhythm: Regular
P waves: Precede every QRS; have consistent shape; may be buried in the preceding T wave
PR interval: Usually normal; may be difficult to measure if P waves are buried in T waves

Table 19-4 ■ COMMON THERAPIES FOR BRADYARRHYTHMIAS

Treatment	Sinus Bradycardia Junctional Bradycardia	Second-Degree AV Block Type I Wenckebach	Second-Degree AV Block Type II	Third-Degree AV Block	Asystole
Atropine 0.5–1 mg IV	↑ sinus rate, may ↑ rate of junctional pacemaker. May stimulate sinus rhythm when junctional pacemaker in control of ventricles. Usually very effective, especially for sinus bradycardia.	↑ sinus rate and ↑ AV nodal conduction. Usually very effective	Should be used with caution in type II block—may cause slowing of ventricular rate. Type II block is due to pathology below the AV node where atropine has no effect. Atropine ↑ sinus rate and AV conduction, thus ↑ number of impulses reaching diseased bundle branches.	Usually has no effect on complete AV block. If junctional rhythm is controlling ventricles, atropine may increase rate of junctional focus.	Given in addition to epinephrine to treat asystole. Give 1 mg IV every 3 minutes to total vagolytic dose of 0.04 mg/kg.
Epinephrine	May be infused at 2–10 mcg/min to maintain BP while waiting for pacing to be instituted.	May be infused at 2–10 mcg/min to maintain BP while waiting for pacing to be instituted.	May be infused at 2–10 mcg/min to maintain BP while waiting for pacing to be instituted.	May be infused at 2–10 mcg/min to maintain BP while waiting for pacing to be instituted.	IV bolus of 1 mg every 3–5 minutes during resuscitation efforts.
Transcutaneous pacing	Not usually needed but may be used for severe bradycardia until transvenous pacing wire can be placed.	Not usually needed. May be used temporarily until transvenous pacing can be instituted if symptomatic bradycardia is unresponsive to atropine.	May be used temporarily until transvenous pacing can be instituted if symptomatic bradycardia.	May be required in symptomatic patients until transvenous pacing wire can be placed.	May be helpful if instituted early in resuscitation efforts.
Temporary transvenous pacing	May be necessary on short-term basis if symptomatic bradycardia is unresponsive to atropine, especially in presence of inferior MI. Usually not needed for more than a few days, because sinus node function usually improves.	May be necessary on short-term basis if symptomatic bradycardia is unresponsive to atropine, especially in presence of inferior MI. Usually not needed for more that a few days, because block usually resolves.	May be necessary to stabilize patient with symptomatic bradycardia, especially in anterior MI. Often used as bridge to permanent pacemaker insertion if block does not resolve.	May be necessary to stabilize patient with symptomatic third-degree block regardless of cause. Often used as bridge to permanent pacemaker insertion if block does not resolve.	Not usually attempted during resuscitation due to difficulties placing wire during CPR unless transcutaneous pacing not available. If used, success rate better if instituted early in resuscitation attempt.

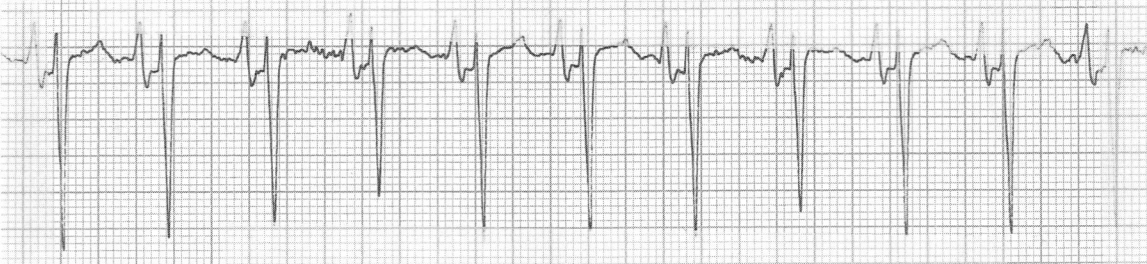

QRS complex: Usually normal
Conduction: Normal through atria, AV node, bundle branches, and ventricles
Example: Sinus tachycardia-rate, 107 beats per minute (see above)

Treatment of sinus tachycardia is directed at the cause. Because this arrhythmia is a physiologic response to a decrease in cardiac output, it should never be ignored, especially in the cardiac patient. Because the ventricles fill with blood and the coronary arteries perfuse during diastole, persistent tachycardia can cause decreased stroke volume, decreased cardiac output, and decreased coronary perfusion secondary to the decreased diastolic time that occurs with rapid heart rates. Carotid sinus pressure may slow the heart rate temporarily and thereby help in ruling out other arrhythmias. Beta blockers are used to treat tachycardia in patients with acute MI without signs of heart failure or contraindications to beta blocker therapy.

Sinus Arrhythmia

Sinus arrhythmia occurs when the sinus node discharges irregularly. It occurs as a normal phenomenon, especially in the young, and decreases with age. Sinus arrhythmia is commonly associated with the phases of respiration: during inspiration, the sinus node fires faster; during expiration, it slows. Other than this phasic increase and decrease in rate, sinus arrhythmia looks like normal sinus rhythm. The following characteristics are typical of sinus arrhythmia:

Rate: 60 to 100 beats per minute
Rhythm: Irregular; phasic increase and decrease in rate, which may be related to respiration
P waves: Precede every QRS; have consistent shape
PR interval: Usually normal
QRS complex: Usually normal
Conduction: Normal through atria, AV node, bundle branches, ventricles
Example: Sinus arrhythmia

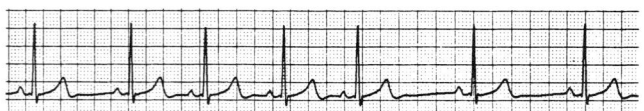

Sinus Arrest

Sinus arrest occurs when sinus node automaticity is depressed and impulses are not formed when expected. This results in the absence of a P wave at the time it is expected to occur, and unless there is escape of a junctional or ventricular pacemaker, the QRS complex is also missing. If only one sinus impulse fails to form, the term *sinus pause* is usually used, whereas if more than one sinus impulse in a row fails to form, sinus arrest has occurred. Because the sinus node has depressed automaticity and does not form impulses regularly as expected, the P-P interval in sinus arrest is not an exact multiple of the sinus cycle. Causes of sinus arrest include vagal stimulation, carotid sinus sensitivity, MI interrupting the blood supply to the sinus node, and drugs such as digitalis, beta blockers, and calcium channel blockers. Sinus arrest is characterized by the following ECG changes.

Rate: Atrial—usually within normal range but may be in bradycardic range if several sinus impulses fail to form. Ventricular—usually within normal range but may be in bradycardic range if several sinus impulses fail to form and there are no junctional or ventricular escape beats. Occasionally, the ventricular rate may be faster than the atrial rate because of junctional or ventricular escape beats that occur during the period of sinus arrest.
Rhythm: Irregular due to absence of sinus node discharge
P waves: Present when sinus node is firing and absent during periods of sinus arrest. When present, they precede every QRS complex and are consistent in shape. If junctional escape beats occur, P waves may be inverted either before or after the junctional QRS.
PR interval: Usually normal when P waves are present. If junctional escape beats occur, the PR interval is short when the P wave precedes the junctional QRS.
QRS complex: Usually normal when sinus node is functioning and absent during periods of sinus arrest unless escape beats occur. If ventricular escape beats occur, QRS complex is wide.
Conduction: Normal through atria, AV node, bundle branches, and ventricles when sinus node is firing. When the sinus node fails to form impulses, there is no conduction through the atria. If a junctional escape beat occurs, ventricular conduction is usually normal, whereas if a ventricular escape beat occurs, conduction through the ventricles is abnormally slow.

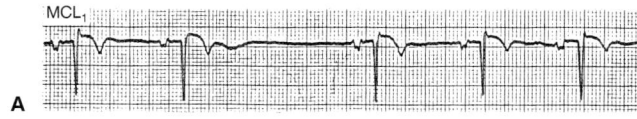

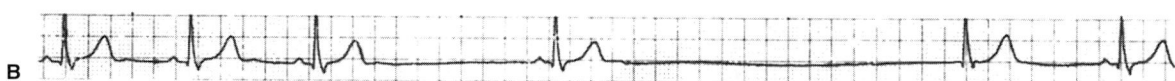

Examples: (A) Sinus pause. (B) Sinus pause and sinus arrest with a junctional escape beat (see above)

Treatment of sinus arrest is aimed at the cause and at increasing ventricular rate if the patient is symptomatic. Any offending drugs should be discontinued, and vagal stimulation should be minimized. If periods of sinus arrest are frequent and causing hemodynamic compromise, atropine, 0.5 to 1 mg IV, may increase the rate. Pacemaker therapy may be necessary if all other forms of management fail.

Treatment of sinus arrhythmia is usually not necessary, but the administration of atropine may increase the rate or abolish the irregularity.

Sinus Exit Block

Sinus exit block occurs when the impulse is formed in the sinus node normally but fails to exit the node to excite atrial tissue. Sinus exit block can be type I, type II, or complete. The section of this chapter on Complex Arrhythmias and Conduction Disturbances contains a discussion of sinus Wenckebach, which is type I sinus exit block. Type II sinus exit block looks exactly like sinus arrest except for the P-P intervals, which are multiples of the basic sinus cycle length. Complete sinus exit block exists when no impulses reach the atria from the sinus node and no P waves occur. In this case, either a junctional or ventricular pacemaker emerges to take over pacing duties, or asystole occurs.

Rate: Atrial—usually within normal range but may be in bradycardic range if several sinus impulses fail to exit the sinus node. Ventricular—usually in normal range but may be in bradycardic range if no junctional or ventricular escape beats occur during periods of sinus exit block.

Rhythm: Irregular due to pauses caused by sinus exit block

P waves: Present except when impulse fails to exit sinus node. When present, they precede every QRS and are consistent in shape. The P-P interval is an exact multiple of the sinus cycle because impulses are formed regularly but occasionally fail to exit the sinus node.

PR interval: Usually normal when P waves are present but may be prolonged if AV node conduction is slow.

QRS complexes: Usually normal when sinus impulse conducts and absent when exit block occurs. If ventricular escape beats occur, QRS is wide.

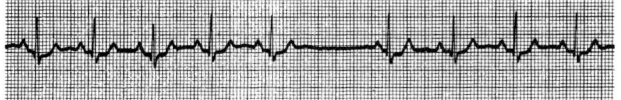

Conduction: Normal through atria, AV node, bundle branches, and ventricles when impulse exits sinus node normally.

Example: Sinus exit block. The length of the pause is exactly double the sinus rate (Huff, Doernbach, & White, 1993).

Treatment of sinus exit block depends on the resulting ventricular rate and its hemodynamic significance. Atropine may cause an increase in rate if bradycardia is symptomatic. Pacing may be necessary, especially with complete sinus exit block. Otherwise, the treatment is similar to that of sinus arrest.

Sick Sinus Syndrome

The term *sick sinus syndrome* is used to describe rhythms in which there is marked sinus bradycardia, sinus pauses, or periods of sinus arrest alternating with paroxysms of rapid atrial arrhythmias, especially atrial flutter or atrial fibrillation. The term *brady-tachy syndrome* is commonly used to describe the same arrhythmias. During periods of sinus bradycardia or arrest, junctional escape rhythms commonly occur, and AV block is also often associated with the sinus node dysfunction that causes sick sinus syndrome. Causes of sick sinus syndrome include inflammatory cardiac disease, cardiomyopathy, sclerodegenerative processes involving both the sinus and AV nodes, and drugs such as beta blockers, calcium channel blockers, digitalis, amiodarone, propafenone, and adenosine (Olgin & Zipes, 2001; Reiffel, 2001; Robles de Medina & Wilde, 2000). ECG characteristics of sick sinus syndrome include:

Rate: Varies from bradycardic to tachycardic rates depending on sinus node function, rate of escape pacemakers, and presence of atrial tachyarrhythmias

Rhythm: Irregular. Pauses of 3 seconds or more can occur during periods of sinus arrest. Regularity of rhythm depends on reliability of sinus node and escape pacemakers, and on type of tachyarrhythmia present (e.g., atrial fibrillation is very irregular).

P waves: Usually normal during periods of sinus rhythm. Absent during periods of sinus arrest or atrial fibrillation, inverted with junctional rhythms. Flutter waves are present during periods of atrial flutter.

PR interval: May be normal or prolonged depending on state of AV conduction

QRS complex: Usually normal unless there is associated bundle-branch block or ventricular escape rhythms

Conduction: Normal through the atria when the sinus node is in control, abnormal through atria during

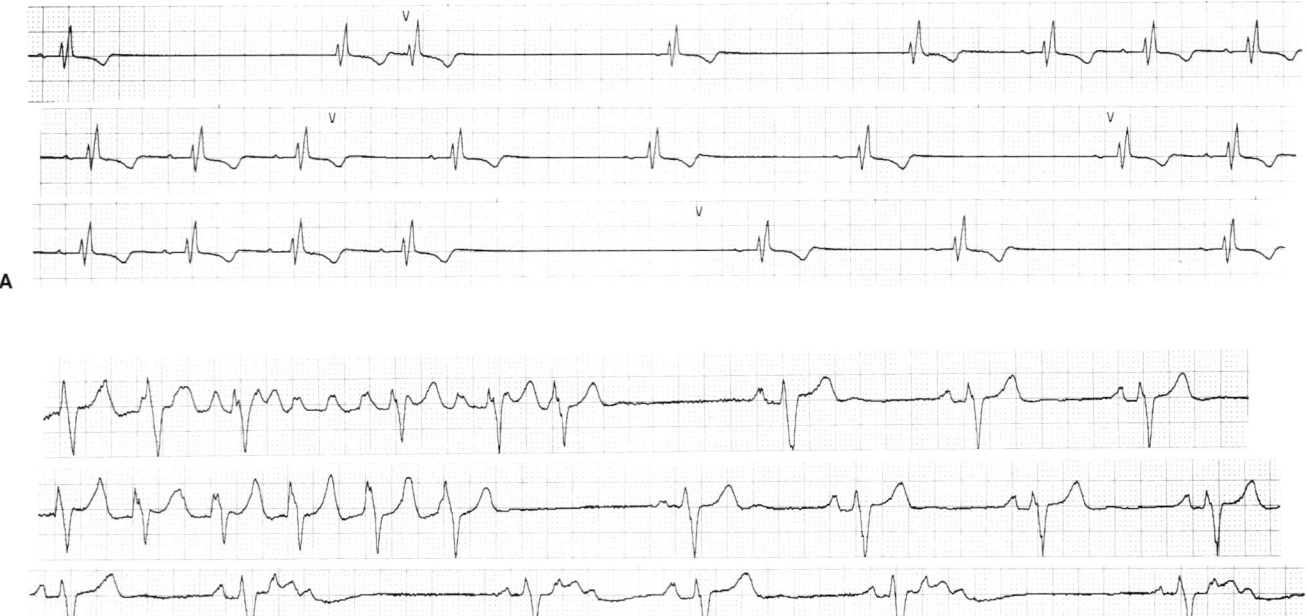

A

B

periods of atrial tachyarrhythmias. AV conduction may be normal or abnormal depending on degree of AV node disease. Conduction through ventricles normal unless bundle branch block is present or a ventricular escape rhythm occurs.

Examples: (A) Sick sinus syndrome presenting with extreme variation in sinus rate. (B) Brady-tachy syndrome. Rhythm changes back and forth from atrial fibrillation and flutter to sinus (see above).

Treatment of sick sinus syndrome may include atropine or pacing for bradyarrhythmias and antiarrhythmics for tachyarrhythmias. Permanent pacing is usually necessary because drugs used to treat the tachyarrhythmias aggravate bradycardia and often further depress sinus node function.

Rhythms Originating in the Atria

Ectopic impulses or reentry circuits can occur in the atrial myocardium, resulting in several atrial arrhythmias: premature atrial complex (PAC), WAP, AT, multifocal atrial tachycardia (MAT), atrial flutter, and atrial fibrillation. See Chapter 31 for the ACLS algorithm for treatment of tachycardias.

Premature Atrial Complexes

PAC occurs when an irritable focus in the atria fires before the next sinus impulse is due. PAC can be caused by caffeine, alcohol, nicotine, stretch on the atria (as in congestive heart failure [CHF] or pulmonary disease), interruption of atrial blood supply by myocardial ischemia or MI, anxiety, and hypermetabolic states. PAC often occur in normal hearts.

The ECG characteristics of PAC include the following:

Rate: Usually within normal range
Rhythm: Usually regular except when PAC occur, resulting in early beats. PAC often have a noncompensatory pause (interval between the complex before and that after the PAC is less than two normal R-R intervals) because premature depolarization of the atria by the PAC usually causes premature depolarization of the sinus node, thus causing the sinus node to "reset" itself.
P waves: Precede every QRS. The configuration of the premature P wave differs from that of the sinus P waves because the premature impulse originates in a different part of the atria and depolarizes them in a different way. Very early P waves may be buried in the preceding T wave.
PR interval: May be normal or long depending on the prematurity of the beat. Very early PAC may find the AV junction still partially refractory and unable to conduct at a normal rate, resulting in a prolonged PR interval.
QRS complex: May be normal, aberrant (wide), or absent, depending on the prematurity of the beat. If the ventricles have repolarized completely, they are able to conduct the early impulse normally, resulting in a normal QRS. If the PAC occurs during the relative refractory period of the bundle branches or ventricles, the impulse conducts aberrantly and the QRS is wide. If the PAC occurs very early during the complete refractory period of the AV node, bundle branches or ventricles, the impulse does not conduct to the ventricles and the QRS is absent.
Conduction: PAC travel through the atria differently from sinus impulses because they originate from a different spot. Conduction through the AV node, bundle branches, and ventricles is usually normal unless the PAC

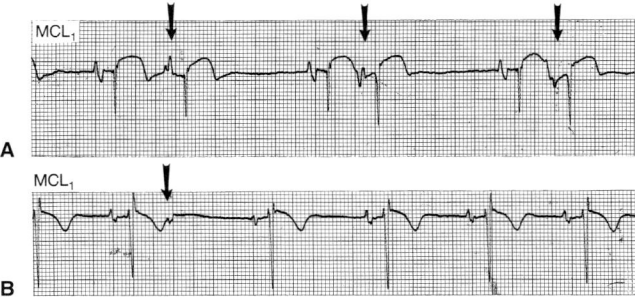

A

B

is very early (see previous discussion of PR interval and QRS complex).

Examples: (A) Sinus rhythm with PAC. (B) Sinus rhythm with a nonconducted PAC.

Treatment of PAC is rarely necessary because they do not cause hemodynamic compromise. Frequent PAC may precede more serious arrhythmias such as atrial fibrillation. Drugs such as beta blockers, calcium channel blockers, or procainamide can be used to suppress atrial activity if necessary.

Wandering Atrial Pacemaker

Wandering atrial pacemaker refers to rhythms that exhibit varying P-wave morphology as the site of impulse formation shifts from the sinus node to various sites in the atria to the AV junction and back (Olgin & Zipes, 2001). This occurs when two (usually sinus and junctional) or more supraventricular pacemakers compete with each other for control of the heart. Because the rates of these competing pacemakers are almost identical, it is common to have atrial fusion occur as the atria are activated by more than one wave of depolarization at a time, resulting in varying P-wave morphology. WAP can be due to increased vagal tone that slows the sinus pacemaker or to enhanced automaticity in atrial or junctional pacemaker cells, causing them to compete with the sinus node for control.

WAP is characterized as follows:

Rate: 60 to 100 beats per minute
Rhythm: May be slightly irregular
P waves: Exhibit varying shapes (upright, flat, inverted, notched) as impulses originate in different parts of the atria or junction and as atrial fusion occurs. At least three different P-wave configurations should be seen.
PR interval: May vary depending on proximity of the pacemaker to the AV node
QRS complex: Usually normal
Conduction: Conduction through the atria varies as it is depolarized from different spots. Conduction through the bundle branches and ventricles is usually normal.
Example: WAP

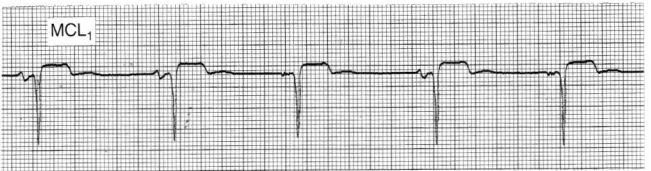

Treatment of WAP is not usually necessary. If heart rate is slow enough to be symptomatic, atropine can be given.

Multifocal Atrial Tachycardia

MAT (also known as chaotic atrial tachycardia) is rapid firing of several ectopic atrial foci at a rate faster than 100 beats per minute. MAT is most commonly associated with chronic pulmonary disease but can also occur in the presence of CHF, hypokalemia, hypomagnesemia, hypoxia, acute MI, and mitral stenosis (Goldberger & Kadish, 2001; Myerburg, Kloosterman & Castellanos, 2001; Olgin & Zipes, 2001).

The ECG characteristics of MAT include the following:

Rate: Usually 100 to 130 beats per minute
Rhythm: Usually irregular
P waves: Vary in shape because they originate in different spots in the atria. At least three different P waves are seen. They usually precede each QRS complex, but some may be blocked in the AV node.
PR interval: May vary depending on proximity of each ectopic atrial focus to the AV node and the prematurity of atrial impulses
QRS complex: Usually normal
Conduction: Usually normal through the AV node and ventricles. Aberrant ventricular conduction may occur if an impulse is conducted into the ventricles while they are partially refractory.
Example: MAT

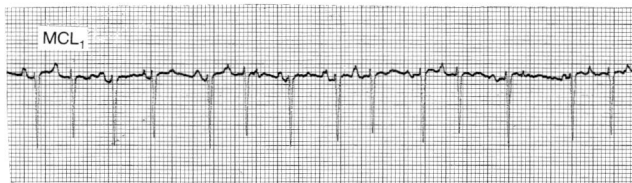

Treatment of MAT is directed toward eliminating the cause, including hypoxia and electrolyte imbalances. Antiarrhythmic therapy is often ineffective. Beta blockers, verapamil, flecainide, amiodarone, and magnesium have been reported to be successful (Goldberger & Kadish, 2001; Olgin & Zipes, 2001). Beta blockers seem to work best but must be used with caution because pulmonary disease is usually associated with MAT. Theophylline may need to be discontinued. If MAT is chronic and unresponsive to drug therapy, radiofrequency ablation of the AV node and insertion of a permanent pacemaker may be necessary to control the ventricular rate (Goldberger & Kadish, 2001).

Atrial Tachycardia and Paroxysmal Atrial Tachycardia

AT is a rapid atrial rhythm at a rate of 120 to 250 beats per minute. This rhythm may be due to rapid firing of an ectopic atrial focus (automaticity), an atrial reentry circuit that allows an impulse to travel rapidly and repeatedly around a pathway in the atria, or to afterdepolarizations resulting in a triggered AT (Goldberger & Kadish, 2001; Myerburg et al., 2001; Olgin & Zipes, 2001). The term *paroxysmal atrial tachycardia* is used to describe AT that begins and ends suddenly, and can occur in short bursts of several beats or be sustained for longer periods of time. Incessant AT is less common and lasts for more than half the day. AT has been associated with caffeine, tobacco, alcohol, mitral valve disease, rheumatic heart disease, chronic obstructive pulmonary disease, acute MI, theophylline administration, and digitalis toxicity.

If the atrial rate is very rapid, the AV node begins to block some of the impulses attempting to travel through it to protect the ventricles from excessively rapid rates. In normal, healthy hearts, the AV node can usually conduct each atrial impulse up to rates of approximately 180 beats per minute. In patients with cardiac disease or in those who take drugs that slow AV conduction or are digitalis toxic, the AV node cannot conduct each impulse, and AT with block occurs.

The ECG characteristics of AT include the following:

Rate: Atrial rate is 120 to 250 beats per minute. The ventricular rate depends on the amount of block at the AV node and may be the same as the atrial rate or slower.

Rhythm: Regular unless there is variable block at the AV node

P waves: Differ in configuration from sinus P waves because they are ectopic. Precede each QRS complex but may be hidden in preceding T wave. When block is present, more than one P wave appears before each QRS complex.

PR interval: May be shorter or longer than normal but often difficult to measure because of hidden P waves.

QRS complex: Usually normal but may be wide if aberrant conduction is present

Conduction: Usually normal through the AV node and into the ventricles. In AT with block, some atrial impulses do not conduct into the ventricles. Aberrant ventricular conduction may occur if atrial impulses are conducted into the ventricles while the bundle branches are still partially refractory.

Examples: AT. Both strips are from the same patient. (A) AT at a rate of 187 beats per minute. (B) AT with block, occurring after administration of propranolol.

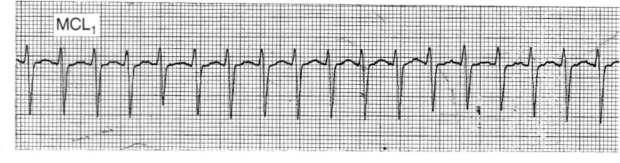

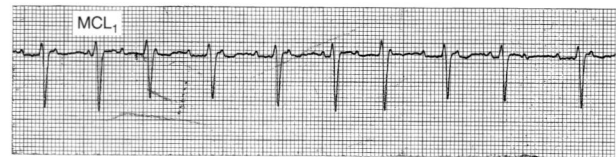

Treatment of AT is directed toward eliminating the cause and decreasing the ventricular rate. Sedation alone may terminate the rhythm or slow the rate. If the patient is severely symptomatic, cardioversion may be necessary to terminate the episode. Vagal stimulation, either through CSM or Valsalva maneuver, or adenosine may terminate some episodes of AT. Beta blockers, verapamil, and diltiazem increase block at the AV node and may slow ventricular response or terminate the tachycardia. Digitalis slows ventricular rate by increasing block at the AV node, but it can also be the cause of AT with block and should be discontinued if that is the case. Type IA, IC, and III antiarrhythmics may be effective in reducing the number of tachycardia episodes but can also be proarrhythmic. Radiofrequency catheter ablation of the ectopic focus or reentry circuit is successful in many cases (Lesh, 2000; Palma & Scheinman, 2001).

Atrial Flutter

In atrial flutter, the atria are depolarized at rates of 250 to 450 times per minute. Classic or typical atrial flutter (type I) is due to a fixed reentry circuit in the right atrium around which the impulse circulates in a counterclockwise direction, resulting in negative flutter waves in leads II and III and an atrial rate between 250 and 350 beats per minute (most commonly 300 beats per minute). Occasionally, the impulse reverses direction and circulates in a clockwise direction, resulting in positive flutter waves in leads II and III, and is called "atypical" flutter. Atrial flutter can also result from reentry around surgically created scars within the atria and is still considered to be type I flutter (Waldo, 2000). Less is known about type II flutter, which is more rapid (with atrial rates greater than 350 beats per minute), less stable than type I, and more likely to revert to atrial fibrillation (Kastor, 2000; Waldo, 2001).

At such rapid atrial rates, the AV node usually blocks at least half of the impulses to protect the ventricles from excessive rates. Because atrial flutter most often occurs at a rate of 300 beats per minute, and because the AV node usually blocks half of those impulses, a ventricular rate of 150 beats per minute is common. Therefore, whenever a ventricular rate of 150 beats per minute is seen, the diagnosis of atrial flutter with 2 : 1 conduction should be suspected until proved otherwise. Causes of atrial flutter include rheumatic heart disease, atherosclerotic heart disease, thyrotoxicosis, CHF, cardiac surgery, and myocardial ischemia or MI (Kastor, 2000; Olgin & Zipes, 2001; Waldo, 2001; Waldo 2000).

Atrial flutter is characterized as follows:

Rate: Atrial rate varies between 250 and 450 beats per minute, most commonly 300 beats per minute. Ventricular rate varies depending on the amount of block at the AV node, most commonly 150 beats per minute and rarely 300 beats per minute. Ventricular rates can be within the normal range when atrial flutter is treated with appropriate drugs. Rarely, 1 : 1 conduction results in a ventricular rate of 300 beats per minute.

Rhythm: Atrial rhythm is regular. Ventricular rhythm may be regular or irregular because of varying AV block.

P waves: F waves (flutter waves) are seen, characterized by a regular, sawtooth pattern thought to be composed of the atrial depolarization wave followed by the atrial repolarization, or atrial T wave. One F wave is usually hidden in the QRS complex, and when 2 : 1 conduction occurs, F waves may not be readily apparent. Flutter waves are best seen in the inferior leads (II, III, and avF) and may appear more like individual P waves in lead V_1.

PR interval: May be consistent or may vary in a Wenckebach-type pattern (see section on Multilevel Atrioventricular Block, under Complex Arrhythmias and Conduction Disturbances)

QRS complex: Usually normal; aberration can occur

Conduction: Usually normal through the AV node and ventricles. Multilevel AV block commonly occurs (see section on Complex Arrhythmias and Conduction Disturbances).

Examples: Atrial flutter. All strips are from the same patient. (A) Atrial flutter with 2 : 1 conduction. (B) Ventricular rate slows momentarily, and flutter waves are clearly visible at a rate of 300 beats per minute. (C) Atrial flutter with variable conduction.

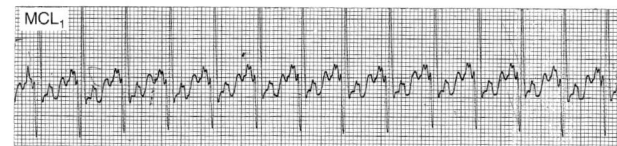

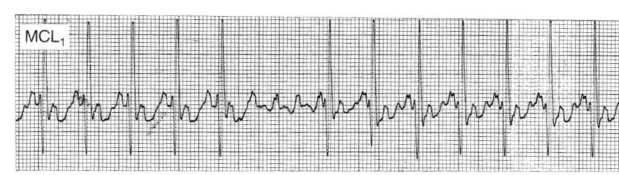

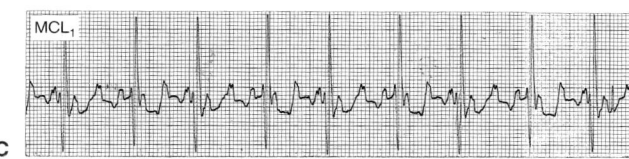

Because the ventricular rate in atrial flutter can be rapid, symptoms associated with decreased cardiac output can occur. Mural thrombi may form in the atria because there is no strong atrial contraction and blood stasis occurs, leading to a risk of systemic or pulmonary emboli. Persistent atrial flutter is uncommon; it usually converts to either sinus rhythm or atrial fibrillation spontaneously or as a result of drug therapy.

The immediate goal of treatment depends on the hemodynamic consequences of the arrhythmia. Ventricular rate control is the immediate goal of therapy if cardiac output is significantly compromised due to rapid ventricular rates. Electrical (direct current) cardioversion may be necessary as an immediate treatment, especially if 1 : 1 conduction occurs. IV calcium channel blockers (verapamil or diltiazem) or beta blockers can be used for ventricular rate control. Conversion to sinus rhythm can be accomplished by electrical cardioversion, drug therapy, or overdrive atrial pacing. Class IA (quinidine, disopyramide, and procainamide), type IC (flecainide, propafenone), or type III antiarrhythmics (sotalol, amiodarone) may convert flutter to sinus. These agents are also useful in maintaining sinus rhythm after conversion. Drugs that slow the atrial rate, like class IA or IC drugs, should not be used unless the ventricular rate has been controlled with an AV nodal blocking agent (i.e., calcium channel blocker, beta blocker, or digitalis). The danger

of giving class IA or IC agents alone is that, as atrial rate slows from 300 to 200 beats per minute, for example, it is possible for the AV node to conduct each impulse rather than block impulses, thus leading to even faster ventricular rates.

Newer type III antiarrhythmic agents, ibutilide (Corvert) and dofetilide (Tikosyn), can be given IV and are often successful in converting atrial flutter to sinus rhythm if flutter is recent in onset. Rapid atrial pacing can also be used to terminate atrial flutter, especially when it occurs after cardiac surgery. Radiofrequency catheter ablation of the flutter reentry circuit is the treatment of choice for chronic or recurrent atrial flutter and is an alternative to chronic drug therapy (Lesh, 2000; Palma & Scheinman, 2001).

Atrial Fibrillation

Atrial fibrillation is an extremely rapid and disorganized pattern of depolarization in the atria. The mechanism of this arrhythmia is most likely multiple random reentry circuits in the atria (Jahangir, Munger, Packer & Crijns, 2001; Janse, 2000; Myerburg, et al., 2001). Atrial fibrillation is the most common rhythm seen (next to sinus rhythm) and can be chronic or occur in paroxysms. Atrial fibrillation commonly occurs in the presence of atherosclerotic or rheumatic heart disease, thyrotoxicosis, CHF, cardiomyopathy, valve disease, pulmonary disease, MI, congenital heart disease, and after cardiac surgery.

Atrial fibrillation is characterized as follows:

Rate: Atrial rate is 400 to 600 beats per minute or faster. Ventricular rate varies depending on the amount of block at the AV node. In new-onset atrial fibrillation, the ventricular response is usually rapid, 110 to 160 beats per minute; in treated atrial fibrillation, the ventricular rate is controlled in the normal range of 60 to 100 beats per minute.

Rhythm: Irregular. One of the distinguishing features of atrial fibrillation is the marked irregularity of the ventricular response because of concealed conduction in the AV junction (see section on Complex Arrhythmias and Conduction Disturbances). If the ventricular response is ever regular in the presence of atrial fibrillation, AV dissociation should be suspected.

P waves: Not present. Atrial activity is chaotic, with no formed atrial impulses visible. Irregular F waves are often seen and vary in size from coarse to very fine.

PR interval: Not measurable because there are no P waves

QRS complex: Usually normal; aberration is common, especially at faster ventricular rates

Conduction: Intra-atrial conduction is disorganized and irregular. Most of the atrial impulses are blocked in the AV junction; those impulses that are conducted through the AV junction are usually conducted normally through the ventricles. If an atrial impulse reaches the bundle branch system during its refractory period, aberrant intraventricular conduction can occur.

Examples: (A) Atrial fibrillation. (B) Alternating coarse and fine atrial fibrillation (sometimes called *atrial fib-flutter*). (C) Fine atrial fibrillation. (D) Atrial fibrillation with a slow and regular ventricular response, most likely due to complete AV block.

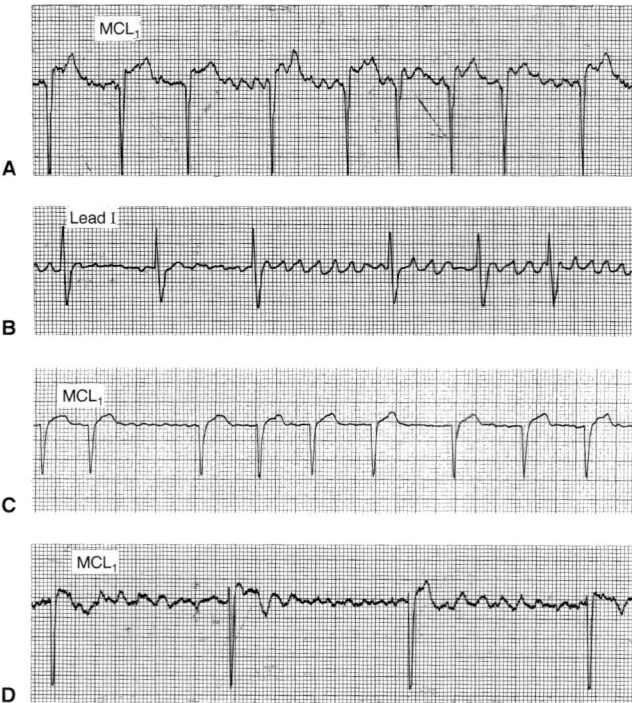

If the ventricular response to atrial fibrillation is rapid, cardiac output can be reduced secondary to decreased diastolic filling time in the ventricles. Because the atria quiver rather than contract, atrial kick is lost, which can also reduce cardiac output. Another possible complication is mural thrombus formation in the atria due to stasis of blood. This can lead to pulmonary or systemic embolization if clots dislodge spontaneously or with conversion to sinus rhythm.

Treatment of atrial fibrillation is directed toward eliminating the cause, controlling ventricular rate, restoring and maintaining sinus rhythm, and preventing thromboembolism. Electrical cardioversion may be necessary if the patient is hemodynamically unstable because of rapid ventricular rates. IV calcium channel blockers (diltiazem, verapamil) and beta blockers are commonly used in the acute situation for ventricular rate control. Beta blockers, calcium channel blockers, and digitalis can be used orally for long-term rate control. Atrial antiarrhythmic drugs used to convert atrial fibrillation to sinus rhythm and to maintain sinus rhythm include class IA agents (quinidine, procainamide, disopyramide), class IC agents (flecainide, propafenone), and class III agents (amiodarone, sotalol). Ibutilide and dofetilide are newer class III antiarrhythmic agents used for conversion of atrial fibrillation to sinus rhythm and work best in new-onset atrial fibrillation. Anticoagulation with warfarin is necessary if atrial fibrillation is chronic.

Nonpharmacologic therapies used for treatment of atrial fibrillation include implantable atrial defibrillators and radiofrequency catheter ablation. Atrial defibrillators detect the onset of atrial fibrillation and deliver a shock between two intracardiac leads to terminate atrial fibrillation (Jahangir et al., 2001). Ablation to create linear lesions within the atria (similar to the surgical Maze procedure) has been reported to be successful, as well as

focal ablations around the orifice of the pulmonary veins in the left atrium (Haissaguerre, Jais, Shah & Clementy, 2000; Jahangir et al., 2001). A new procedure called PLAATO (percutaneous left atrial appendage transcatheter occlusion) is being tried in an effort to prevent embolic stroke in patients with nonrheumatic atrial fibrillation. The PLAATO procedure is done in a cardiac catheterization laboratory by way of a right heart catheterization and transseptal puncture to place an occluder device into the left atrial appendage to seal it off and prevent embolization of clots that tend to form in the appendage (Reisman et al., 2003).

Supraventricular Tachycardia

The term *supraventricular tachycardia* (SVT) is used to describe a regular, narrow QRS tachycardia in which the exact mechanism cannot be identified from the ECG. Sinus node reentry, AT, atrial flutter, and junctional tachycardia can all cause SVT. AVNRT and AVRT using an accessory pathway are two of the most common mechanisms of SVT. (See section on Complex Arrhythmias and Conduction Disturbances for discussion of these two causes of SVT.) SVT is characterized by the following:

Rate: Greater than 100 beats per minute; can be as fast as 280 beats per minute
Rhythm: Regular
P waves: Usually not visible, making the exact mechanism of the tachycardia uncertain
PR interval: Not measurable if P waves cannot be seen
QRS complex: Usually narrow; may be wide if aberrant ventricular conduction occurs
Conduction: Conduction through the atria varies depending on the mechanism of tachycardia. Atria may depolarize in a retrograde direction when the mechanism is AVNRT or AVRT. Conduction through ventricles is normal unless bundle-branch block is present or there is anterograde conduction through an accessory pathway.
Example: SVT with a narrow QRS and no identifiable P waves

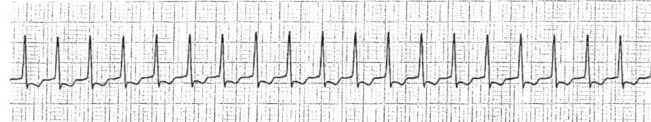

Treatment of SVT depends on the patient's tolerance of the arrhythmia. If the ventricular rate is fast enough to cause hemodynamic instability, cardioversion is the treatment of choice. Drugs such as adenosine, beta blockers, calcium channel blockers, and digitalis can slow ventricular rate or terminate many SVT. (See section on Complex Arrhythmias and Conduction Disturbances for more detailed information on treating SVT.)

Rhythms Originating in the Atrioventricular Junction

Cells surrounding the AV node in the AV junctional area have automaticity and are capable of initiating impulses and controlling the heart rhythm. Junctional arrhythmias include premature junctional complex (PJC), junctional rhythm, and junctional tachycardia.

Junctional beats and junctional rhythms can appear any of three ways on the ECG depending on the location of the junctional pacemaker and the speed of conduction of the impulse into the atria and ventricles:

1. When a junctional focus fires, the wave of depolarization spreads backward (retrograde) into the atria as well as forward (anterograde) into the ventricles. If the impulse arrives in the atria before it arrives in the ventricles, the ECG shows a P wave (inverted in inferior leads because the atria are depolarized from bottom to top) followed immediately by a QRS complex as the impulse reaches the ventricles. In this case, the PR interval is short, usually 0.10 second or less.

2. If the junctional impulse reaches both the atria and the ventricles at the same time, only a QRS is seen on the ECG because the ventricles are much larger than the atria, and only ventricular depolarization is seen, even though the atria are also depolarizing.

3. If the junctional impulse reaches the ventricles before it reaches the atria, the QRS precedes the P wave on the ECG. Again, the P wave usually is inverted because of retrograde atrial depolarization, and the RP interval (distance from the beginning of the QRS to the beginning of the following P wave) is short, 0.10 second or less.

Premature Junctional Complexes

Premature junctional complexes are due to an irritable focus in the AV junction. Irritability can be due to coronary heart disease (CHD) or MI disrupting blood flow to the AV junction, nicotine, caffeine, catecholamines, or drugs such as digitalis.

Premature junctional complexes have the following ECG characteristics:

Rate: 60 to 100 beats per minute or the rate of the basic rhythm
Rhythm: Irregular because of the early beats
P waves: May occur before, during, or after the QRS complex and are inverted in the inferior leads (II, III, aVF)
PR interval: Short, 0.10 second or less when P waves precede the QRS
QRS complex: Usually normal but may be aberrant if the PJC occurs very early and conducts into the ventricles during the refractory period of a bundle branch
Conduction: Retrograde through the atria, usually normal through the ventricles
Example: Sinus rhythm with two PJC

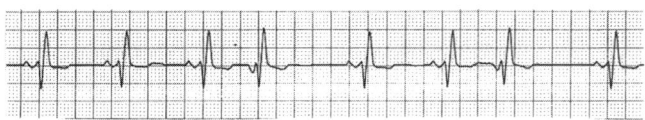

No treatment is necessary for PJC.

Junctional Rhythm and Junctional Tachycardia

Junctional rhythm can occur if the sinus node rate falls below the automatic rate of an AV junctional pacemaker, or in the presence of digitalis toxicity. Junctional rhythms commonly occur after inferior wall MI because the blood supply to the sinus node and the AV junction is disrupted. The rhythms are classified according to their rate; junctional rhythm usually occurs at a rate of 40 to 60 beats per minute, accelerated junctional rhythm occurs at a rate of 60 to 100 beats per minute, and junctional tachycardia occurs at a rate of 100 to 250 beats per minute.

Junctional rhythm has the following ECG characteristics:

Rate: Usually 40 to 60 beats per minute; accelerated junctional rhythm, 60 to 100 beats per minute; junctional tachycardia, 100 to 250 beats per minute
Rhythm: Regular
P waves: May precede or follow QRS
PR interval: Short, 0.10 second or less
QRS complex: Usually normal
Conduction: Retrograde through the atria, normal through the ventricles
Examples: (A) Junctional rhythm (rate, 43 beats per minute). (B) Accelerated junctional rhythm (rate, 84 beats per minute). Junctional rhythm rarely requires treatment unless the rate is too slow or too fast to maintain cardiac output. If the rate is slow, atropine can be given to increase the sinus rate and override the junctional focus or increase the rate of firing of the junctional pacemaker. If the rate is fast, drugs such as verapamil, beta blockers, or digitalis may be effective in slowing the rate or terminating the arrhythmia. Cardioversion may be necessary if the rate is so rapid that cardiac output is severely limited. Because digitalis toxicity is a common cause of junctional rhythms, the drug should be held until serum levels return to normal and the arrhythmia stops.

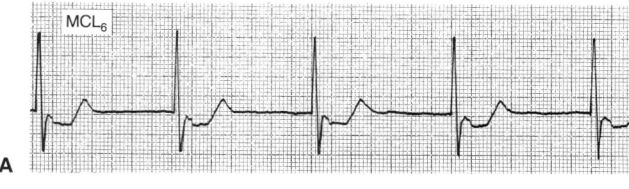

A

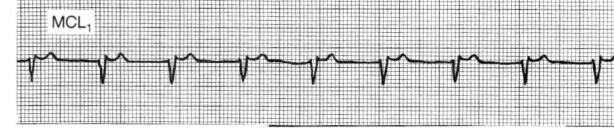

B

Rhythms Originating in the Ventricles

Ventricular arrhythmias originate in the ventricular muscle or Purkinje system and are considered to be more dangerous than other arrhythmias because of their potential to limit cardiac output severely. However, as with any arrhythmia, ventricular rate is a key determinant of how well a patient can tolerate a ventricular rhythm. Ventricular arrhythmias include premature ventricular complex (PVC), accelerated ventricular rhythm, VT, ventricular flutter, ventricular fibrillation, and ventricular asystole. See Chapter 31 for the ACLS algorithm for treatment of ventricular fibrillation and pulseless VT.

Premature Ventricular Complexes

Premature ventricular complexes (ventricular premature depolarizations [VPD]) are caused by premature depolarization of cells in the ventricular myocardium or Purkinje system due to enhanced normal automaticity or abnormal automaticity, reentry in the ventricles, or afterdepolarizations (Buxton & Duc, 2001; Olgin & Zipes, 2001). PVC can be caused by hypoxia, myocardial ischemia, hypokalemia, acidosis, exercise, increased levels of circulating catecholamines, digitalis toxicity, caffeine, alcohol, and other causes. PVC increase with aging and are more common in people with coronary heart disease, valve disease, hypertension, cardiomyopathy and other forms of heart disease. PVC are not dangerous in people with normal hearts but are associated with higher mortality rates in patients with structural heart disease or acute MI, especially if left ventricular function is reduced. PVC are considered potentially malignant when they occur more frequently than 10 per hour or are repetitive (i.e., occur in pairs, triplets, or more than three in a row) in patients with coronary disease, previous MI, cardiomyopathy, and with reduced ejection fraction (Bigger, 1983; Myerburg et al., 2001).

Premature ventricular complexes have the following ECG characteristics:

Rate: 60 to 100 beats per minute or the rate of the basic rhythm

Rhythm: Irregular because of the early beats

P waves: Not related to the PVC. Sinus rhythm is often not interrupted, so sinus P waves can frequently be seen occurring regularly throughout the rhythm. P waves may follow PVC because of retrograde conduction from the ventricle backward through the atria; these P waves are inverted in the inferior leads (II, III, aVF).

PR interval: Not present before most PVC. If a P wave happens, by coincidence, to precede a PVC, the PR interval is short.

QRS complex: Wide and bizarre, usually greater than 0.12 second in duration. May vary in morphology if PVC originate from more than one focus in the ventricles. T waves are usually in the opposite direction from the QRS complex.

Conduction: Impulses originating in the ventricles conduct through the ventricular myocardium from muscle cell to muscle cell rather than through Purkinje fibers, resulting in wide QRS complexes. Some PVC may conduct retrograde into the atria, resulting in inverted P waves that follow the PVC. When the sinus rhythm is undisturbed by PVC, the atria depolarize normally.

Examples: (A) Normal sinus rhythm with PVC. (B) Sinus rhythm with multifocal PVC. (C) Paired PVC. (D) R-on-T PVC, resulting in short runs of VT.

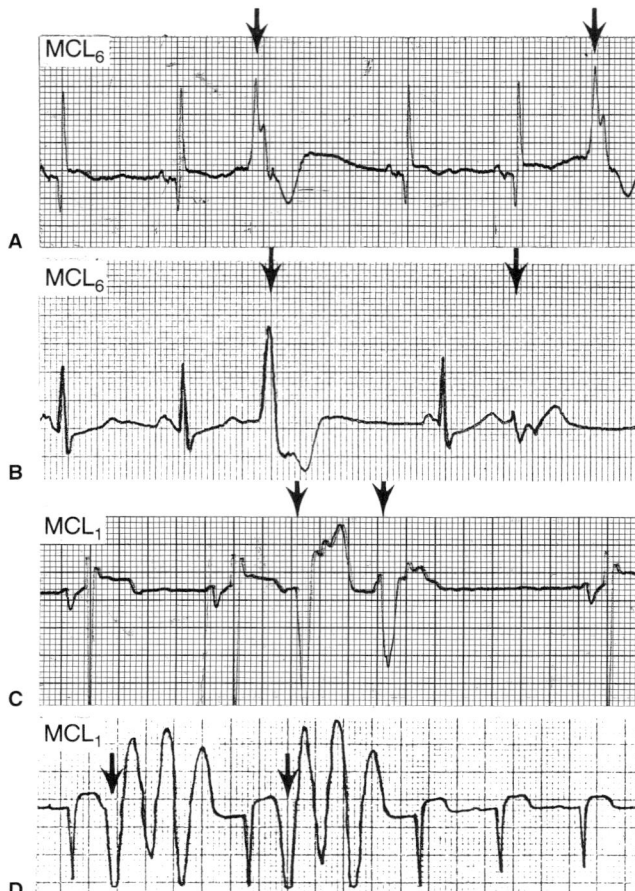

The significance of PVC depends on the clinical setting in which they occur. Many people have chronic PVC that do not need to be treated, and most of these people are asymptomatic. There is no evidence that suppression of PVC reduces mortality, especially in patients with no structural heart disease. If PVC cause bothersome palpitations, patients should be told to avoid caffeine, tobacco, other stimulants, and try stress reduction techniques. Low-dose beta blockers may reduce PVC frequency and the perception of palpitations and can be used for symptom relief. In the setting of an acute MI or myocardial ischemia, PVC may be precursors of more dangerous ventricular arrhythmias, especially when they occur near the apex of the T wave (R-on-T PVC; Buxton & Duc, 2001). Unless PVC result in hemodynamic instability or symptomatic VT, most physicians elect not to treat them, although some prefer to treat PVC that occur in the first 24 to 48 hours after acute MI or after cardiac surgery.

If PVC are to be treated, IV lidocaine is usually the recommended drug. Other antiarrhythmic agents such as procainamide or amiodarone can be used IV for acute control. Beta blockers are often effective in suppressing repetitive PVC and have become the drugs of choice for treating post-MI PVC that are symptomatic. Many other drugs effectively reduce the frequency of PVC, including quinidine, disopyramide, flecainide, mexiletine, tocainide, moricizine, propafenone, and sotalol; but are rarely used for this purpose due the potential for proarrhythmia and increased incidence of sudden death demonstrated by the CAST study (Cardiac Arrhythmia Suppression Trial Investigators, 1989).

Accelerated Idioventricular Rhythm

Accelerated idioventricular rhythm occurs when an ectopic focus in the ventricles fires at a rate of 50 to 100 beats per minute. Accelerated idioventricular rhythm commonly occurs in the presence of inferior MI and during reperfusion with thrombolytic therapy, when the rate of the sinus node slows below the rate of the latent ventricular pacemaker. (See section on Complex Arrhythmias and Conduction Disturbances for a discussion of AV dissociation.) The ECG characteristics of accelerated ventricular rhythm include the following:

Rate: 50 to 100 beats per minute

Rhythm: Usually regular

P waves: May be seen but are dissociated from the QRS. If retrograde conduction from the ventricle to the atria occurs, P waves follow the QRS complex.

PR interval: Not present

QRS complex: Wide and bizarre

Conduction: If sinus rhythm is the basic rhythm, atrial conduction is normal. Impulses originating in the ventricles conduct through the ventricular myocardium by cell-to-cell conduction, resulting in the wide QRS complex.

Example: Sinus rhythm with accelerated ventricular rhythm at a rate of 70 beats per minute. Note sinus P waves that continue uninterrupted during the period of accelerated ventricular rhythm (an example of AV dissociation). (N = arrhythmia computer's interpretation of normal beat, V = computer's interpretation of ventricular beat.)

The treatment of accelerated ventricular rhythm depends on its cause and how well it is tolerated by the patient. This arrhythmia alone is usually not harmful because the ventricular rate is within normal limits and usually adequate to maintain cardiac output. If the patient is symptomatic because of the loss of atrial kick, atropine can be used to increase the rate of the sinus node and overdrive the ventricular rhythm. Suppressive therapy is rarely used because abolishing the ventricular rhythm may leave an even less desirable heart rate. Usually, accelerated ventricular rhythm is transient and benign and does not require treatment.

Ventricular Tachycardia

Ventricular tachycardia is a rapid ventricular rhythm most likely due to reentry in the ventricles, although automaticity of an ectopic focus and afterdepolarizations may also be mechanisms of VT (Kastor, 2000; Martin & Wharton, 2001; Olgin & Zipes, 2001). VT can be classified according to (1) duration—*nonsustained* (lasts <30 seconds), *sustained* (lasts >30 seconds), *incessant* (VT present most of the time); (2) morphology (ECG appearance of QRS complexes)—*monomorphic* (QRS complexes have the same shape during tachycardia), *polymorphic* (QRS complexes vary randomly in shape), *bidirectional* (alternating upright and negative QRS complexes during tachycardia). The terms *salvos* and *bursts* are often used to describe short runs of VT (i.e., 5 to 10 or more beats in a row).

The most common cause of VT is coronary heart disease, including acute ischemia and MI, prior MI, and chronic coronary disease (Kastor, 2000; Martin & Wharton, 2001). The next most common cause is cardiomyopathy, both dilated and hypertrophic. Other causes include valvular heart disease, congenital heart disease, arrhythmogenic right ventricular dysplasia, cardiac tumors, cardiac surgery, and the proarrhythmic effects of many drugs (Kastor, 2000; Martin & Wharton, 2001; Olgin & Zipes, 2001). Idiopathic VT is VT that occurs in patients with no known structural heart disease. These patients tend to be younger than patients with VT who have structural heart disease, and the arrhythmia may be asymptomatic and present for years before they present for evaluation. These patients do not have "normal" hearts but are often found to have electrophysiologic abnormalities that may be associated with subtle structural abnormalities that are not detectible by current diagnostic tests (Kastor, 2000; Martin & Wharton, 2001). VT that occurs in the presence of left ventricular dysfunction and reduced ejection fraction is associated with a higher incidence of adverse cardiac events, including an increased risk of sudden cardiac death. (See section on Complex Arrhythmias and Conduction Disturbances later in this chapter for more information on monomorphic and polymorphic VT.) ECG characteristics of monomorphic VT include the following:

Rate: Ventricular rate is usually 100 to 220 beats per minute

Rhythm: Usually regular but may be slightly irregular

P waves: Often dissociated from QRS complexes. If sinus rhythm is the underlying basic rhythm, regular P waves may be seen but are not related to QRS complexes. P waves are often buried in QRS complexes or T waves. VT

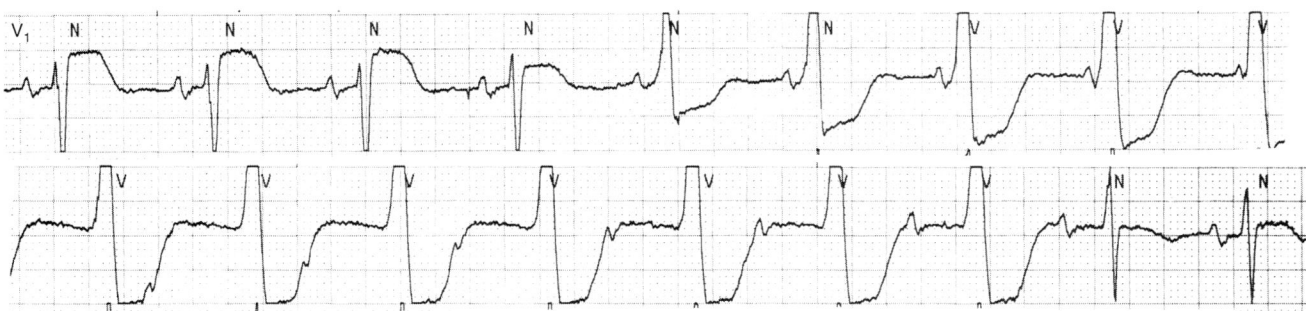

may conduct retrograde to the atria with P waves visible after each QRS.

PR interval: Not measurable because of dissociation of P waves from QRS complexes

QRS complex: Wide and bizarre, greater than 0.12 second in duration

Conduction: Impulse originates in one ventricle and spreads by muscle cell-to-cell conduction through both ventricles. There may be retrograde conduction through the atria, but often the sinus node continues to fire regularly and depolarizes the atria normally. Rarely, one of these sinus impulses may conduct normally through the AV node and into the ventricle before the next ectopic ventricular impulse fires, resulting in a normal QRS complex, called a *capture beat*. Occasionally, a *fusion beat* may occur as the ventricles are depolarized by a descending sinus impulse and the ventricular ectopic impulse simultaneously, resulting in a QRS complex that looks different from both the normal beats and the ventricular beats.

Examples: (A) Sinus rhythm with a PVC and a run of VT. (B) VT. AV dissociation is evidenced by independently occurring P waves. (C) VT with a fusion beat (fourth complex).

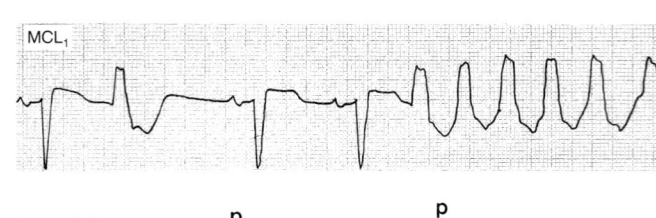

A

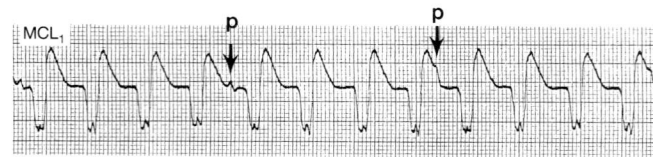

B

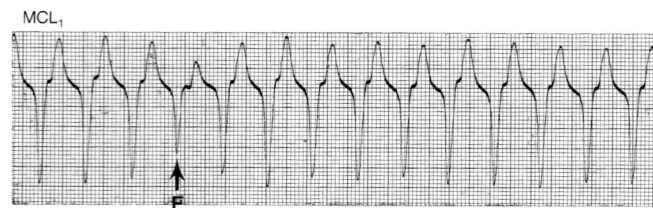

C

Immediate treatment of VT depends on how well the rhythm is tolerated by the patient. The two main determinants of patient tolerance of any tachycardia are ventricular rate and underlying left ventricular function. VT can be an emergency if cardiac output is severely decreased because of a very rapid rate or poor left ventricular function. The preferred immediate treatment for severely symptomatic VT is cardioversion, but defibrillation can be performed if there is not time to synchronize the shock. If the patient is not severely symptomatic, lidocaine is the drug often used for acute treatment of VT. IV procainamide, amiodarone, or magnesium sulfate can also be used for acute treatment. Maintenance therapy may be prescribed with the same drugs used for PVC, with increasing emphasis on class III agents with beta blocker effects, like

amiodarone and sotalol. See Chapter 31 for the ACLS algorithm for treatment of VT. Nonpharmacologic therapy for recurrent VT includes radiofrequency catheter ablation and the implantable cardioverter defibrillator (see Chapter 32).

Ventricular Flutter

Ventricular flutter is similar to VT, but the rate is faster. Hemodynamically, ventricular flutter is more dangerous because there is virtually no cardiac output. ECG characteristics of ventricular flutter are as follows:

Rate: Ventricular rate is usually 220 to 400 beats per minute

Rhythm: Usually regular

P waves: None seen

PR interval: None measurable

QRS complex: Very wide, regular, sine-wave type of pattern

Conduction: Originates in the ventricle and spreads through muscle cell-to-cell conduction, resulting in very wide, bizarre complexes

Example: Ventricular flutter

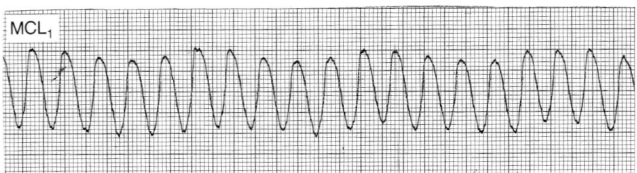

Ventricular flutter is fatal unless treated immediately by defibrillation. If a defibrillator is not immediately available, cardiopulmonary resuscitation (CPR) should be started. After the rhythm is converted, antiarrhythmic drug therapy should be initiated to prevent recurrence. Drug therapy is similar to that used for VT.

Ventricular Fibrillation

Ventricular fibrillation is rapid, ineffective quivering of the ventricles; is fatal without immediate treatment; and is the most frequent cause of sudden cardiac death (Kastor, 2000; Podrid & Kowey, 2001b). Electrical activity originates in the ventricles and spreads in a chaotic, irregular pattern throughout both ventricles. There is no cardiac output or palpable pulse with ventricular fibrillation. ECG characteristics of ventricular fibrillation include the following:

Rate: Rapid, uncoordinated, ineffective

Rhythm: Chaotic, irregular

P waves: None seen

PR interval: None

QRS complex: No formed QRS complexes seen; rapid, irregular undulations without any specific pattern. This erratic electrical activity can be coarse or fine.

Conduction: Random electrical activity in ventricles depolarizes them irregularly and without any organized pattern. There is no organized conduction and the ventricles do not contract.

Examples: Two examples of ventricular fibrillation (see p. 387).

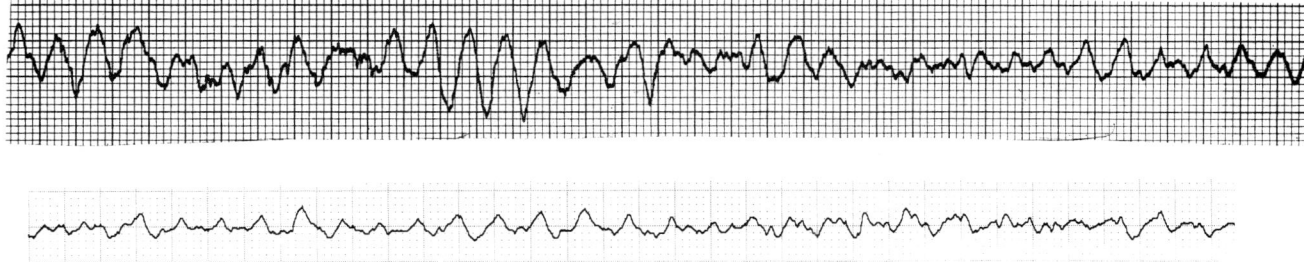

Ventricular fibrillation requires immediate defibrillation. Synchronized cardioversion is not possible because there are no formed QRS complexes on which to synchronize the shock. CPR must be performed if a defibrillator is not immediately available. The American Heart Association guidelines for ventricular fibrillation and pulseless VT call for CPR until a defibrillator is available, then defibrillation at 200 J (Cummins, 2000). If ventricular fibrillation continues, an immediate second shock at 300 J and a third shock at 360 J, if necessary, are recommended. If ventricular fibrillation does not convert after three shocks, CPR needs to be continued and drug therapy initiated. Antiarrhythmic agents such as lidocaine, procainamide, amiodarone, or magnesium are commonly used in an effort to convert ventricular fibrillation. Once the rhythm has converted, maintenance therapy with IV antiarrhythmic agents is continued. The implantable cardioverter defibrillator is becoming the standard of care for survivors of VF that occurs in the absence of acute ischemia (Kastor, 2000; Myerburg et al., 2001; Olgin & Zipes, 2001; Podrid & Kowey, 2001b). Beta blockers and amiodarone appear to be the most effective agents for long-term drug therapy options.

Ventricular Asystole

Ventricular asystole is the absence of any ventricular rhythm; there is no QRS complex, no pulse, and no cardiac output. This is always fatal unless treated immediately. Ventricular asystole has the following characteristics:

Rate: None
Rhythm: None
P waves: May be present if the sinus node is functioning
PR interval: None
QRS complex: None
Conduction: Atrial conduction may be normal if the sinus node is functioning. There is no conduction into the ventricles.
Example: Ventricular asystole. Two P waves are seen at the beginning of the strip.

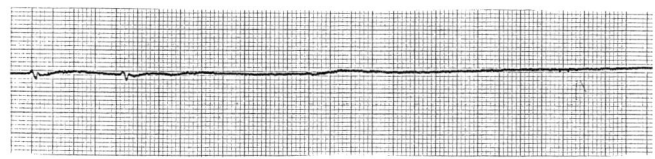

CPR must be initiated immediately if the patient is to survive. IV epinephrine and atropine may be given in an effort to stimulate a rhythm. If pacing is to be used, external pacing should be instituted early in the resuscitation attempt. Asystole has a very poor prognosis despite the best resuscitation efforts because it usually represents extensive myocardial ischemia or severe underlying metabolic problems. See Chapter 31 for the ACLS algorithm for treatment of asystole.

Conduction Abnormalities

The term *AV block* is used to describe arrhythmias in which there is delayed or failed conduction of supraventricular impulses into the ventricles. AV blocks have been classified according to location of the block and severity of the conduction abnormality. The following classification of AV blocks is discussed in this section:

First-degree AV block
Second-degree AV block
    Type I
    Type II
    2 : 1 conduction (can be type I or type II)
High-grade AV block (or advanced AV block)
    Type I
    Type II
Third-degree AV block

AV block can be caused by disease processes that either interrupt the blood supply to structures in the conduction system or otherwise interfere with the function of these structures, or by drugs that slow conduction through the AV node. It can also occur in normal hearts and be a result of normal physiologic variations (e.g., vagal tone) that affect conduction through the AV node, or in athletes or people who exercise regularly; and it can occur during sleep when sympathetic tone is reduced or vagal tone is enhanced. One of the main functions of the AV node is to block rapid atrial impulses to prevent dangerously fast ventricular rates in response to rapid atrial rhythms such as rapid AT, atrial flutter, or atrial fibrillation. In this case, the block is physiologic and must not be confused with pathologic block due to abnormal AV node function. For example, a sinus rate of 80 should be conducted through a normally functioning AV conduction system in a 1 : 1 fashion, so, if any of those sinus impulses are blocked, that is abnormal AV node function and the term *block* appropriately applies. However, a rapid AT at a rate of 180 might well result in block of some of those impulses in the AV node in an attempt to keep ventricular rate reasonable, in which case the conduction failure is physiologic and not due to abnormal AV node function. In such a case, the term *conduction* might be a better one to use than *block* (i.e., "AT with variable conduction" rather than "AT with block").

Myocardial ischemia and infarction can cause AV block by disrupting the blood supply to the AV node (common with inferior MI) or to the bundle of His or bundle branches (more common with anterior MI). Rheumatic heart disease, inflammatory diseases, infectious diseases (Lyme disease, endocarditis, myocarditis), collagen diseases, idiopathic fibrosis of the conduction system (Lev's disease or Lenègre's disease), valve disease (usually aortic or mitral), atrial septal defects, congenital heart disease, and infiltrative cardiomyopathies (amyloidosis, sarcoidosis) can all cause varying degrees of AV block (Arnsdorf & Verdino, 2001; Kastor, 2000; Myerburg et al., 2001; Olgin & Zipes, 2001). Drugs that slow conduction through the AV node and are often associated with development of intranodal block include digitalis, beta blockers, and calcium channel blockers. AV block can also be a temporary or permanent result of cardiac surgery (especially aortic valve surgery) and can occur with AV node ablation, either intentionally (i.e., ablation of the AV node in chronic atrial fibrillation) or as a complication of ablation for SVT.

First-degree Atrioventricular Block

First-degree AV block is defined as prolonged AV conduction time of supraventricular impulses into the ventricles. This delay usually occurs in the AV node, and all impulses conduct to the ventricles, but with delayed conduction times. First-degree AV block can be recognized by the following ECG characteristics:

Rate: Can occur at any sinus rate, usually 60 to 100 beats per minute
Rhythm: Regular
P waves: Normal, precede every QRS
PR interval: Greater than 0.20 second. PR intervals as long as 1 second or more have been reported (Olgin & Zipes, 2001; Rusterholz & Marriott, 1994).
QRS complex: Usually normal unless bundle-branch block exists
Conduction: Normal through the atria, delayed through the AV node, normal through the ventricles
Example: First-degree AV block (PR interval, 0.44 second)

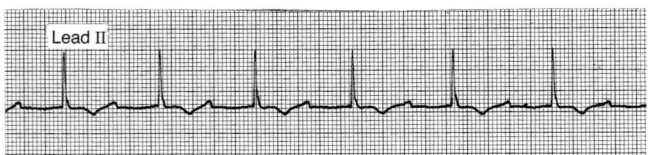

First-degree AV block does not require any specific treatment, but it should be observed for progression to more serious block.

Second-degree Atrioventricular Block

Second-degree AV block occurs when one atrial impulse at a time fails to be conducted to the ventricles. Second degree AV block can be divided into two distinct categories: type I block, occurring in the AV node, and type II block, occurring below the AV node in the bundle of His or bundle-branch system.

Type I (Wenckebach). Type I second-degree AV block, often referred to as *Wenckebach* or *Mobitz I,* is a progressive increase in conduction times of consecutive atrial impulses into the ventricles until one impulse fails to conduct, or is "dropped." This appears on the ECG as gradually lengthening PR intervals until one P wave fails to conduct and is not followed by a QRS complex, resulting in a pause, after which the cycle repeats itself. (See section on Complex Arrhythmias and Conduction Disturbances for a more detailed discussion of Wenckebach conduction.)

Type I second-degree AV block can be recognized by the following ECG characteristics:

Rate: Can occur at any sinus or atrial rate
Rhythm: Irregular unless 2 : 1 conduction is present. Overall appearance of the rhythm demonstrates group beating (i.e., groups of beats separated by pauses).
P waves: Normal. Some P waves are not conducted to the ventricles, but only one at a time fails to conduct.
PR interval: Gradually lengthens in consecutive beats. The PR interval preceding the pause is longer than that following the pause. When 2 : 1 conduction is present, PR intervals are constant.
QRS complex: Usually normal unless there is associated bundle-branch block
Conduction: Normal through the atria, progressively delayed through the AV node until an impulse fails to conduct. Ventricular conduction is normal. Wenckebach conduction ratios describe the number of P waves to QRS complexes: 6 : 5 conduction means six P waves resulted in five QRS complexes, or every sixth P wave is blocked. Conduction ratios can vary from low (e.g., 2 : 1, 3 : 2) to high (e.g., 12 : 11, 15 : 14).
Examples: (A) Second-degree AV block, type I (Wenckebach) with 3 : 2 conduction. (B) Second-degree AV block, type I. Note that the PR interval preceding the pause is longer than the PR interval after the pause.

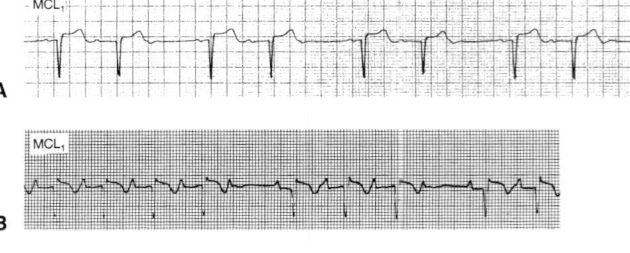

The treatment of type I second-degree AV block depends on the conduction ratio, the resulting ventricular rate, and, most important, the patient's tolerance for the rhythm. If ventricular rates are slow enough to decrease cardiac output, the treatment is atropine to increase the sinus rate and speed conduction through the AV node. At higher conduction ratios, where the ventricular rate is within a normal range, no treatment is necessary. If the block is due to digitalis or beta blockers, those drugs should be held. This type of block is usually temporary and benign and seldom requires pacing, although temporary pacing may be needed when the ventricular rate is slow.

Type II. Type II second-degree AV block, also called *Mobitz II,* is sudden failure of conduction of an atrial impulse to the ventricles without progressive increases in conduction time of consecutive P waves. Type II block occurs below the AV node and is usually associated with bundle-branch block; therefore, the dropped beats are usually a manifestation of bilateral bundle-branch block. This form of block appears on the ECG much the same as type I block, except that there is no progressive increase in PR intervals before the blocked beats. Type II block is less common but more serious than type I block. Type II second-degree AV block can be recognized by the following ECG characteristics:

Rate: Can occur at any basic rate

Rhythm: Irregular due to blocked beats unless 2 : 1 conduction is present

P waves: Usually regular and precede each QRS. Periodically, a P wave is not followed by a QRS complex.

PR interval: Constant before all conducted beats. The PR interval preceding the pause is the same as that after the pause.

QRS complex: Almost always wide because of associated bundle-branch block

Conduction: Normal through the atria and through the AV node but intermittently blocked in the bundle-branch system and fails to reach the ventricles. Conduction through the ventricles is abnormally slow because of associated bundle-branch block. Conduction ratios can vary from 2 : 1 to only occasional blocked beats.

Example: Second-degree AV block, type II. All PR intervals are constant. (From Conover, 1996.)

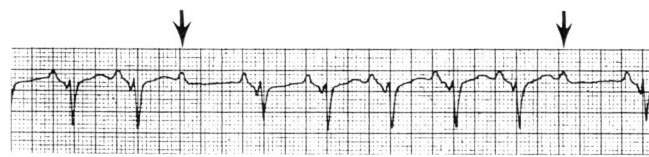

Type II block is more dangerous than type I because of a higher incidence of associated symptoms and progression to complete AV block. When it occurs in the presence of anterior wall MI, it is associated with a high mortality rate because of the extent of muscle damage necessary to produce this degree of block below the AV node.

Treatment usually includes pacemaker therapy because this type of block is often permanent and progresses to complete block. External pacing can be used for treatment of symptomatic type II block until transvenous pacing can be initiated. Atropine is not recommended because it may result in further slowing of ventricular rate by increasing the number of

impulses conducting through the AV node and bombarding the diseased bundles with more impulses than they can handle, resulting in further conduction failure.

2 : 1 Conduction. The 2 : 1 conduction ratio deserves special mention because it continues to be the source of much confusion and disagreement among electrocardiographers. The 2 : 1 block is failure of conduction of every other atrial impulse. Because only one P wave at a time is blocked, it is by definition a second-degree block. If the lesion causing conduction failure is in the AV node, it is type I block; if it is below the AV node, it is type II block. One source of confusion is the lack of progressive prolongation in PR intervals in type I block with 2 : 1 conduction, which has led educators for years to teach that all 2 : 1 block was "Mobitz II" block. Type I block with 2 : 1 conduction does not present with progressively prolonging PR intervals because there are no *consecutively conducted* beats in 2 : 1 block. The progressive prolongation of PR interval that characterizes Wenckebach behavior occurs on consecutively conducted P waves in type I block; so, when there is block of every other P wave, this typical behavior is not seen. However, the location of the lesion does not change; so, if the lesion is in the AV node, it is type I block regardless of the conduction ratio.

When a patient presents with a 2 : 1 conduction ratio, it is sometimes impossible to determine whether the block is type I or II without intracardiac recordings. However, an educated guess can be made depending on the length of the PR interval, the QRS width, and the clinical situation. The following ECG findings can be very helpful in determining the type of block in 2 : 1 conduction in the absence of intracardiac recordings:

PR interval: Often longer than normal (more than 0.20 second) in type I and normal in type II. Sometimes, the PR in type I is normal on conducted beats because the blocked P wave allows enough time for the AV node to recover so that it is able to conduct every other P wave with a normal PR interval. If there are any periods of typical Wenckebach conduction with progressive lengthening of the PR interval on consecutively conducted P waves (even if it only happens once), it is type I block.

QRS complex: Usually narrow in type I and almost always wide in type II. Exceptions can occur in type I when there is a coincidental bundle-branch block that widens the QRS, and in type II when the block is in the His bundle (still below the AV node, thus type II), resulting in a narrow QRS. Type II block is rare compared with type I, and intra-His type II block is even more rare, so the odds are greatly in favor of type I block when the QRS is narrow.

Examples: (A) Top strip shows 2 : 1 conduction that can be assumed to be type I because of the narrow QRS complex. Second strip proves that it is type I when consecutive P waves conduct with increasing PR intervals. (B) Top strip shows 2 : 1 conduction that can be assumed to be type II because of wide QRS. Second strip proves that it is type II when consecutively conducted PR intervals remain constant. (See below.)

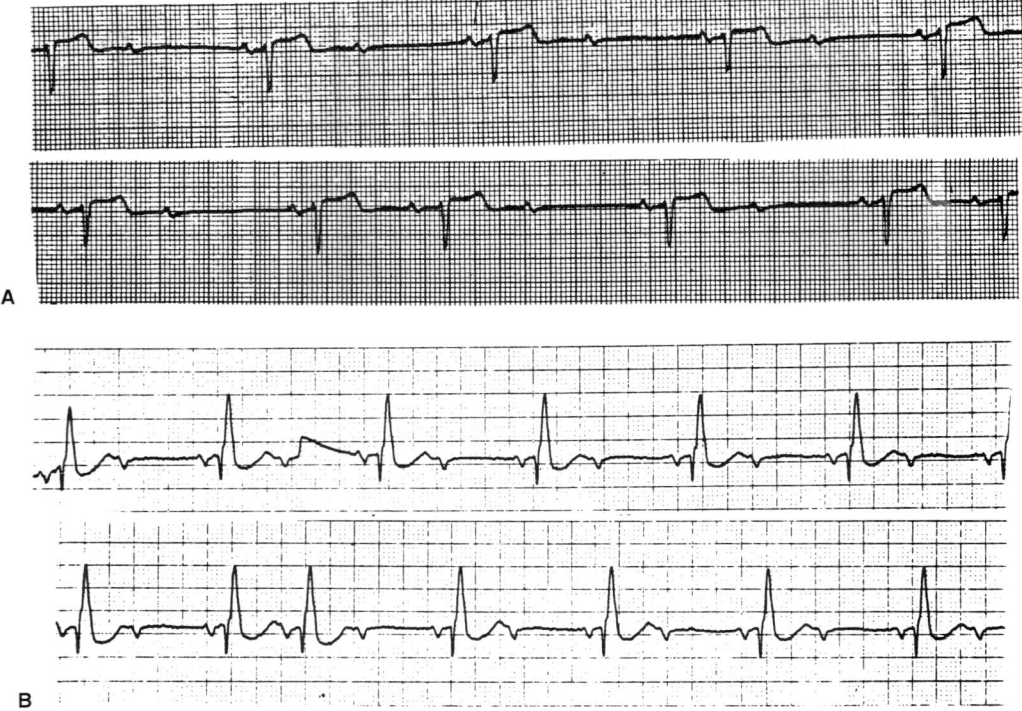

High-grade Atrioventricular Block

High-grade AV block (also called advanced AV block) is present when two or more consecutive atrial impulses are blocked, the atrial rate is reasonable (less than 135 beats per minute), and conduction fails because of the block itself and not because of interference from an escape pacemaker (Marriott, 1988). If the atrial rate is very fast, as in atrial flutter with rates of 300 beats per minute, physiologic AV block occurs as a normal function of the AV node and, therefore, cannot be called high-grade block; hence, the arbitrary atrial rate limit of 135 beats per minute. If a junctional or ventricular escape beat or rhythm occurs as a result of failed conduction of impulses into the ventricles and interferes with the ability of atrial impulses to conduct by causing refractoriness in the AV node or ventricles, high-grade block cannot be diagnosed; the mere presence of the escape beat or rhythm may be the cause of failed conduction, rather than a true block in the AV node or bundle-branch system.

High-grade AV block may be type I, occurring in the AV node, or type II, occurring below the AV node. High-grade block can be recognized by these ECG characteristics:

Rate: Atrial rate less than 135 beats per minute
Rhythm: Regular or irregular, depending on conduction pattern
P waves: Normal, present before every conducted QRS, but several P waves may not be followed by QRS complexes
PR interval: Constant before conducted beats; may be normal or prolonged
QRS complex: Usually normal in type I block and wide in type II block
Conduction: Normal through the atria. Two or more consecutive atrial impulses fail to conduct to the ventricles.

Ventricular conduction is normal in type I and abnormally slow in type II block.
Example: High-grade (advanced) AV block

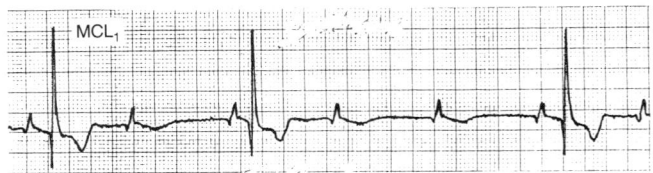

The significance of high-grade block depends on the conduction ratio and the resulting ventricular rate. Because ventricular rates tend to be slow, this arrhythmia is frequently symptomatic and requires treatment. Atropine can be given and is usually more effective in type I block. External cardiac pacing may be necessary until a temporary transvenous pacemaker can be inserted, and permanent pacing is usually necessary in type II high-grade block.

Third-degree Atrioventricular Block (Complete Block)

Third-degree AV block is complete failure of conduction of all atrial impulses to the ventricles. In third-degree AV block, there is complete AV dissociation; the atria are usually under the control of the sinus node, although complete block can occur with any atrial arrhythmia; and either a junctional or ventricular pacemaker controls the ventricles. The ventricular rate is usually less than 45 beats per minute; a faster rate could

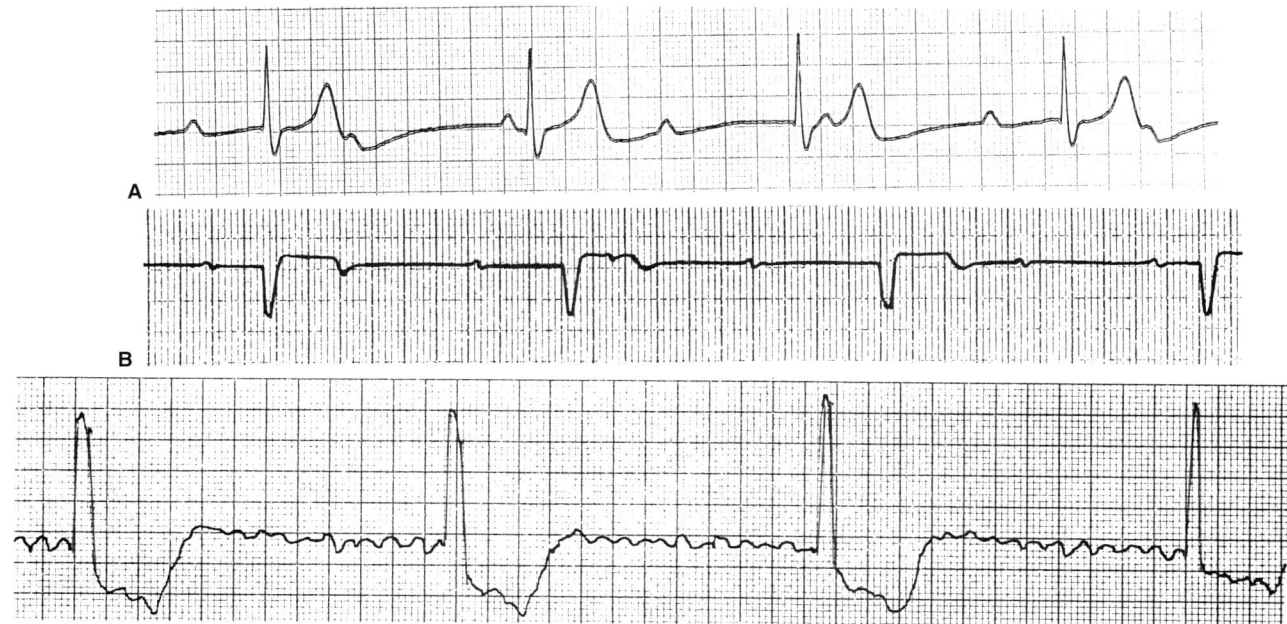

indicate an accelerated junctional or ventricular rhythm that interferes with conduction from the atria into the ventricles by causing physiologic refractoriness in the conduction system, thus causing a physiologic failure of conduction that must be differentiated from the abnormal conduction system function of complete AV block. Third-degree AV block can be recognized from the following ECG criteria:

Rate: Atrial rate is normal when sinus rhythm is present; ventricular rate is less than 45 beats per minute

Rhythm: Regular

P waves: Normal but dissociated from QRS complexes

PR interval: No consistent PR intervals because there is no relation between P waves and QRS complexes

QRS complex: Normal if ventricles controlled by a junctional pacemaker, wide if controlled by a ventricular pacemaker

Conduction: Normal through the atria. All impulses are blocked at the AV node or in the bundle branches, so there is no conduction to the ventricles. Conduction through the ventricles is normal if a junctional escape rhythm occurs and is abnormally slow if a ventricular escape rhythm occurs.

Examples: (A) Third-degree AV block with a junctional pacemaker at a rate of 36 beats per minute. (B) Third-degree AV block with a ventricular pacemaker at a rate of 32 beats per minute. (C) Atrial fibrillation with third-degree block and ventricular escape pacemaker at rate of 25 beats per minute. (See above)

Third-degree AV block can occur without significant symptoms if it is of gradual onset and the heart has time to compensate for the slow ventricular rate. If it occurs suddenly in the presence of acute MI, its significance depends on the resulting ventricular rate and the patient's tolerance. If symptoms of decreased cardiac output occur, external cardiac pacing can be used to maintain a ventricular rate until transvenous pacing can be initiated. Dopamine or epinephrine infusions can be used to maintain blood pressure and CPR should be performed until a pacemaker can be inserted if cardiac output is severely decreased.

COMPLEX ARRHYTHMIAS AND CONDUCTION DISTURBANCES

Abnormalities of cardiac rhythm can range from simple to advanced to complex. Disorders of the heart beat provide a constant challenge to those interested in the study of arrhythmias. This section discusses advanced concepts in arrhythmia interpretation and provides clues to aid in the recognition of selected advanced arrhythmias.

Preexcitation Syndromes

Preexcitation refers to early activation of the ventricular myocardium by supraventricular impulses entering the ventricles through accessory pathways. These pathways are capable of carrying the impulse directly into the ventricle, bypassing all or part of the normal AV conduction system. The most common accessory pathway is an AV bypass tract, the bundle of Kent, which originates in the atrium and inserts in the ventricle, bypassing the entire conduction system. Other accessory pathways include AV nodal bypass tracts, which carry the impulse from the atrium into the distal or compact AV node or from the atrium to the bundle of His (sometimes called *James fibers* or *atriohisian fibers*), and nodoventricular connections, which originate in or below the AV node and carry the impulse directly into the ventricular myocardium (*Mahaim fibers*; Kastor, 2000; Marinchak & Rials, 2001; Wellens et al., 1995). Other authors state that these latter fibers have been shown to originate in the right atrial free wall and insert into the right bundle branch and refer to them as atriofascicular fibers (Miles & Zipes, 2000). In any case, all of these bypass tracts have the potential to cause AVRT.

The most common type of preexcitation syndrome is Wolff-Parkinson-White (WPW) syndrome, in which the impulse is transmitted down the bundle of Kent directly from the atrium into the ventricles, bypassing the AV node.

Wolff-Parkinson-White

In WPW, during sinus rhythm, the ventricle is stimulated prematurely through the Kent bundle while the impulse is simultaneously conducted through the normal AV junctional conduction system. Impulses travel faster down the accessory pathway because they bypass the normal AV node delay. Part of the ventricle receives the impulse early through the accessory pathway and begins to depolarize before the rest of the ventricle is activated through the His-Purkinje system. Early stimulation of the ventricle results in a short PR interval and a widened QRS complex as the impulse begins to depolarize the ventricle through muscle cell-to-cell conduction. Premature ventricular stimulation forms a characteristic slurring of the initial portion of the QRS complex, called a *delta wave*. The remainder of the QRS complex is normal because the rest of the ventricle is then activated normally through the Purkinje system. This type of preexcitation results in fusion beats in the ventricles as they are depolarized simultaneously by the impulse coming through the accessory pathway and through the AV node.

The degree of preexcitation can vary depending on the relative rates of conduction through the bypass connection and the AV node, and it determines the length of the PR interval and the size of the delta wave (Fig. 19-6). Maximal preexcitation occurs when the ventricles are activated totally by the accessory pathway, resulting in an extremely short PR interval and uniformly wide QRS complex. Less than maximal preexcitation occurs when the impulse enters the ventricle through both pathways simultaneously, and the length of the PR interval and size of delta wave depend on how much of the ventricle is depolarized through the bypass connection. A concealed pathway is present when the ventricles are depolarized exclusively through the normal conduction system even though a bypass tract exists. In this case, the PR interval and QRS complex are normal because the accessory pathway is not being used for anterograde conduction.

Accessory pathways can be located in multiple places around the valve rings, the septum, and the free walls of both ventricles (Fig. 19-7). The ECG can be helpful in identifying location of accessory pathways: atrial origin can be deduced from polarity of the P waves during orthodromic tachycardia, and the ventricular insertion site can be inferred from the polarity of delta waves during sinus rhythm (Gallagher et al., 1978; Marinchak & Rials, 2001). Approximately 46% to 60% are in left lateral, 25% posterolateral, 2% anteroseptal, and 13% to 21% in right

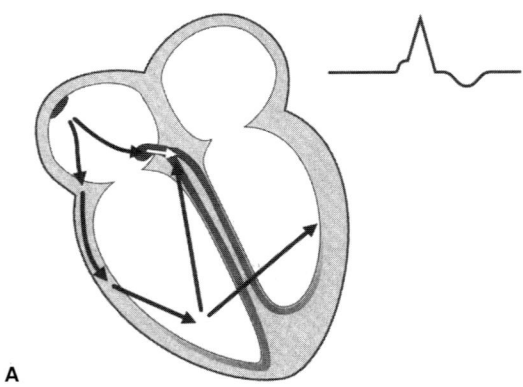

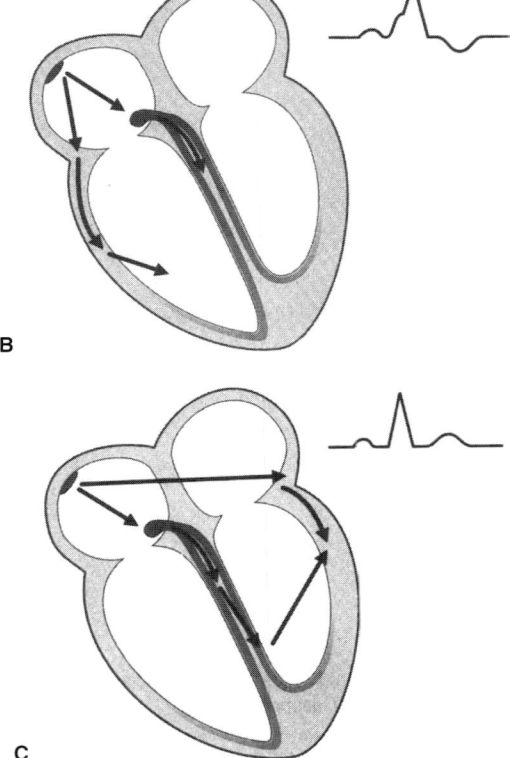

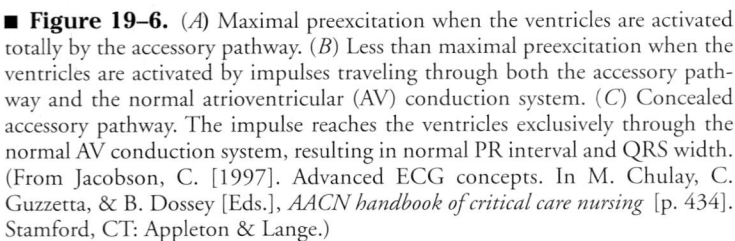

■ **Figure 19–6.** (*A*) Maximal preexcitation when the ventricles are activated totally by the accessory pathway. (*B*) Less than maximal preexcitation when the ventricles are activated by impulses traveling through both the accessory pathway and the normal atrioventricular (AV) conduction system. (*C*) Concealed accessory pathway. The impulse reaches the ventricles exclusively through the normal AV conduction system, resulting in normal PR interval and QRS width. (From Jacobson, C. [1997]. Advanced ECG concepts. In M. Chulay, C. Guzzetta, & B. Dossey [Eds.], *AACN handbook of critical care nursing* [p. 434]. Stamford, CT: Appleton & Lange.)

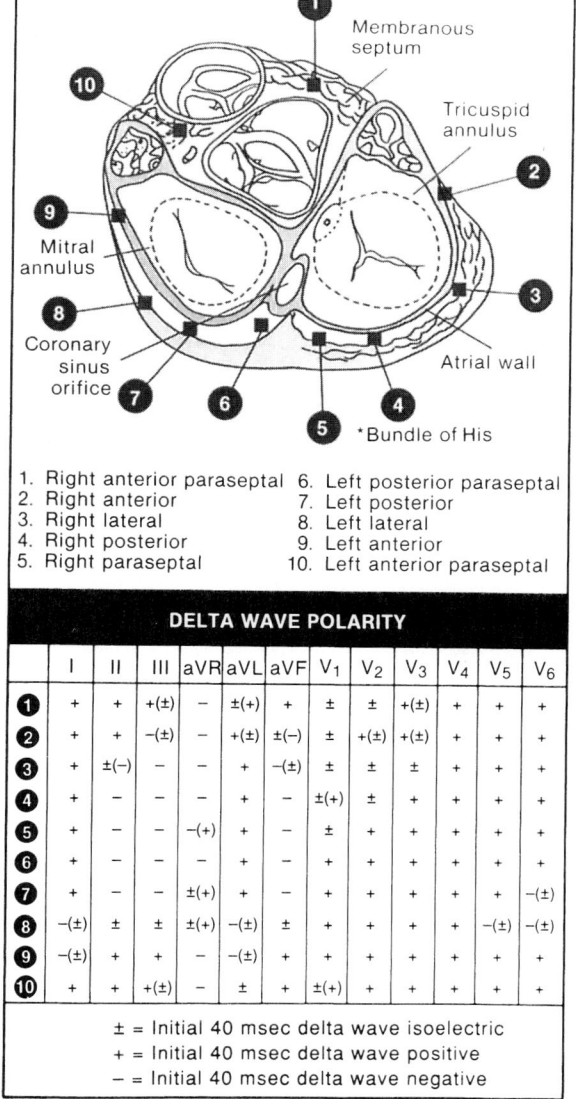

1. Right anterior paraseptal 6. Left posterior paraseptal
2. Right anterior   7. Left posterior
3. Right lateral   8. Left lateral
4. Right posterior   9. Left anterior
5. Right paraseptal   10. Left anterior paraseptal

DELTA WAVE POLARITY

	I	II	III	aVR	aVL	aVF	V₁	V₂	V₃	V₄	V₅	V₆
❶	+	+	+(±)	−	±(+)	+	±	±	+(±)	+	+	+
❷	+	+	−(±)	−	+(±)	±(−)	±	+(±)	+(±)	+	+	+
❸	+	±(−)	−	−	+	−(±)	±	±	±	+	+	+
❹	+	−	−	−	+	−	±(+)	±	+	+	+	+
❺	+	−	−	−(+)	+	−	±	+	+	+	+	+
❻	+	−	−	−	+	−	+	+	+	+	+	+
❼	+	−	−	±(+)	+	−	+	+	+	+	+	−(±)
❽	−(±)	±	±	±(+)	−(±)	±	+	+	+	+	−(±)	−(±)
❾	−(±)	+	+	−	−(±)	+	+	+	+	+	+	+
❿	+	+	+(±)	−	±	+	±(+)	+	+	+	+	+

± = Initial 40 msec delta wave isoelectric
+ = Initial 40 msec delta wave positive
− = Initial 40 msec delta wave negative

■ **Figure 19–7.** Sites of the potential position of accessory pathways. Delta-wave polarity in the 12-lead electrocardiogram is shown in the table at the bottom, (From Gallagher, J. J., Pritchell, E. L., Sealy, W. C., et al. [1982]. The preexcitation syndromes. *Progress in Cardiovascular Disease, 20,* 285, and adapted from Zipes D. P. [1992]. Specific arrhythmias: Diagnosis and treatment. In E. Braunwald [Ed.], *Heart disease* [4th ed., p. 697]. Philadelphia: WB Saunders.

lateral locations (Marinchak & Rials, 2001). Figure 19-8 illustrates two examples of preexcitation during sinus rhythm.

WPW is clinically significant because the presence of two pathways provides the opportunity for reentry of the impulse and may result in rapid reentrant tachycardias. When tachycardias accompany the WPW pattern described above, the term *WPW syndrome* is used. The most commonly occurring tachyarrhythmia in WPW is AVRT, which accounts for about 80% of tachycardias in patients with WPW syndrome (Olgin & Zipes, 2001). The incidence of atrial fibrillation occurring

in the presence of WPW is estimated to be around 40%, which is higher than its incidence in people without WPW and no structural heart disease (Marinchak & Rials, 2001). (See section on Supraventricular Tachycardia below for information on reentrant arrhythmias associated with accessory pathways.)

Atrial fibrillation and atrial flutter that occur in the presence of an accessory pathway are particularly dangerous because of the extremely rapid ventricular rate that can result from conduction of the atrial impulses directly into the ventricle through the bypass track. The ventricular rate can be as fast as 250 to 300 beats per minute and can deteriorate into ventricular fibrillation, resulting in sudden death. Atrial fibrillation with anterograde conduction over an accessory pathway presents on the ECG as a very rapid, irregular, wide QRS rhythm. The irregularity of the ventricular response helps to differentiate this rhythm from other wide QRS tachycardias.

The ECG characteristics of atrial fibrillation with anterograde conduction through an accessory pathway are as follows (Fig. 19-9):

Rate: Ventricular rates up to 300 beats per minute
Rhythm: Irregular. Often appears as groups of very short R-R intervals alternating with groups of longer R-R intervals. The longest R-R intervals are often more than twice the shortest R-R intervals.
P waves: None, because atria are fibrillating
PR interval: None
QRS complex: Wide, bizarre due to abnormal depolarization of ventricles through accessory pathway
Conduction: Disorganized and chaotic through atria. Atrial impulses conduct into ventricles through accessory pathway, resulting in muscle cell-to-cell conduction through ventricles.

Immediate treatment of atrial fibrillation with anterograde conduction through an accessory pathway depends on ventricular rate and the patient's tolerance of the arrhythmia. Cardioversion is the treatment of choice when severe hemodynamic impairment occurs. Drug treatment is directed at slowing conduction through the accessory pathway and restoring and maintaining sinus rhythm. Drugs that increase the refractory period and depress conduction in the bypass tract include quinidine, procainamide, flecainide, propafenone, amiodarone, and sotalol (Miles & Zipes, 2000; Opie, 2001). Many of these drugs are also effective in preventing recurrences of atrial fibrillation. Digoxin and calcium channel blockers, commonly used to treat atrial fibrillation that conducts through the AV node, are contraindicated whenever the tachycardia is due to anterograde conduction through an accessory pathway because they shorten the refractory period and accelerate conduction through the bypass tract (McGovern, Garan & Ruskin, 1986; Miles & Zipes, 2000; Opie, 2001).

WPW syndrome can resemble other conditions usually diagnosed by ECG. The presence of anteriorly directed delta waves can simulate RBBB, posterior or inferior MI, right ventricular hypertrophy, or posterior fascicular block. Posteriorly directed delta waves can simulate left bundle-branch block (LBBB), anterior MI, anterior fascicular block, and left ventricular hypertrophy (Gallagher et al., 1978; Marriott, 1988; Olgin & Zipes, 2001).

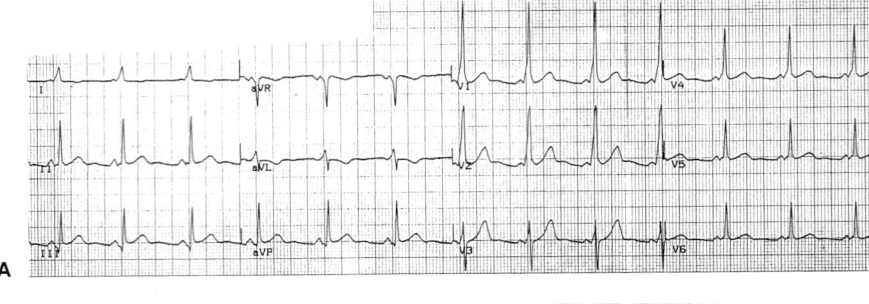

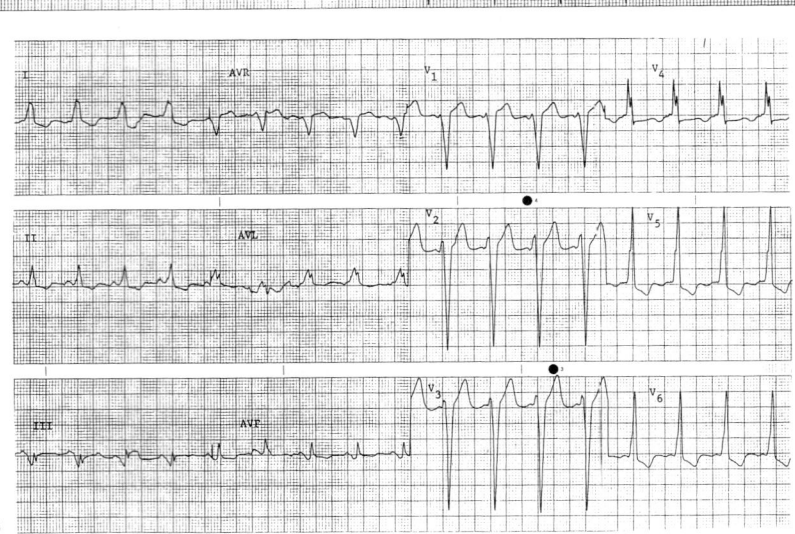

■ **Figure 19–8.** (*A*) Wolff-Parkinson-White (WPW) pattern of short PR interval and delta waves. Lead V_1 is positive, indicating a left lateral or posterior accessory pathway. (*B*) WPW pattern with short PR, delta waves, and a negative V_1, indicating an anterior or right-sided pathway.

Variants of Preexcitation Syndromes

In addition to the Kent bundle described above, which is responsible for WPW syndrome, other anatomical connections exist that can bypass the normal AV node delay or create connections between different parts of the conduction system and the ventricles and cause variations of the preexcitation pattern. Fibers originating in the atria and inserting into the His bundle (atriohisian fibers) have been demonstrated anatomically and can result in a short PR interval and normal QRS complex. This pattern used to be called Lown-Ganong-Levine (LGL) syndrome (Fig. 19-10), but evidence does not support a specific syndrome consisting of short PR, normal QRS, and tachycardias that can be proven to be related to these fibers (Olgin & Zipes, 2001). It is thought that the short PR interval

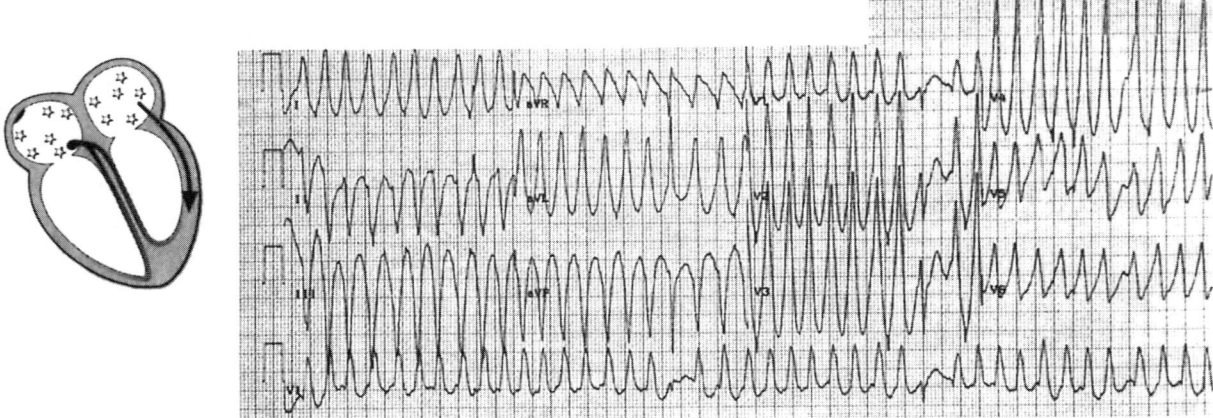

■ **Figure 19–9.** Atrial fibrillation conducting anterograde through an accessory pathway. Note the extremely short R-R intervals in the V leads. QRS is fast, wide, and irregular. (From Jacobson, C. [1997]. Advanced ECG concepts. In M. Chulay, C. Guzzetta, & B. Dossey [Eds.], *AACN handbook of critical care nursing* [p. 440]. Stamford, CT: Appleton & Lange.)

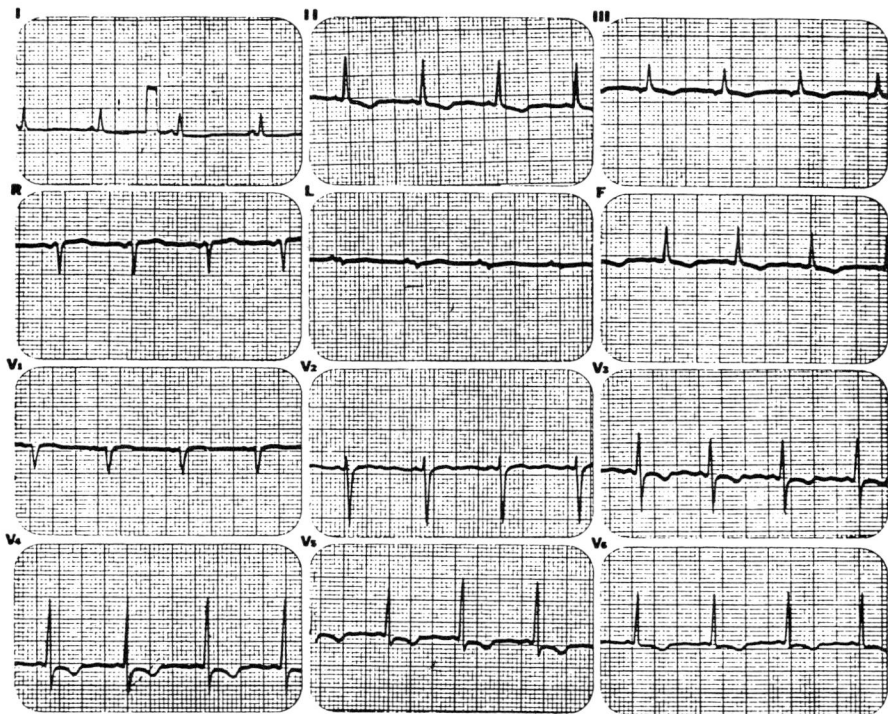

■ **Figure 19–10.** Lead ECG showing a short PR interval and normal QRS (formerly called Lown-Ganong-Levine syndrome). Upright P waves in inferior leads and negative P wave in a VR indicate a sinus origin, not junctional rhythm.

may be due to enhanced AV node conduction through an intranodal fast pathway and simply represents faster-than-normal AV node conduction that is not necessarily pathologic (Kastor, 2000). Some more recent textbooks do not even mention LGL in their discussions of preexcitation syndromes (Fuster, Alexander & O'Rourke, 2001; Podrid & Kowey, 2001a), whereas others continue to at least acknowledge the prior existence of the syndrome (Kastor, 2000; Braunwald et al., 2001).

Another variant of preexcitation involves conduction over a pathway that originates in either the atrium or the AV node and inserts into the right bundle branch (atriofascicular or nodofascicular fibers, also called Mahaim fibers), resulting in a wide QRS (usually LBBB morphology). In these variants, the PR interval may be normal or short. Reentrant tachycardias can occur with any of these variations in anatomy, and the QRS may be normal or wide during tachycardia, depending on the location of the accessory pathways responsible.

Treatment

Preexcitation syndromes do not require treatment unless they are associated with symptomatic tachyarrhythmias. Ideally, specific therapy should be based on a known mechanism of the arrhythmia and knowledge of a drug's effect on that mechanism in both conduction pathways. This knowledge is best gained through electrophysiologic study, which is done to (1) confirm the presence of preexcitation, (2) identify the mechanism of the associated tachyarrhythmia, (3) localize the site of the accessory pathway, (4) confirm participation of the accessory pathway in maintenance of the tachycardia, (5) determine the functional behavior of the accessory pathway, and (6) determine the effects of different drugs on conduction velocity

and refractoriness in both pathways. If the arrhythmia is due to reentry, therapy is directed toward changing the conduction time or the refractory period in the AV node or in the accessory pathway, or both, so that reentry is abolished. Prolonging the refractory period in the AV node or in the bypass tract or inducing block in either of these pathways can interrupt reentry and stop the tachycardia. If atrial fibrillation is the mechanism, treatment is aimed at preventing the occurrence of the arrhythmia and slowing conduction through the accessory pathway. Radiofrequency catheter ablation of the bypass tract offers a cure for tachycardias associated with accessory pathways. The reported success rate for controlling preexcitation tachycardias using radiofrequency ablation is >90% (Cappato, Schluter & Kuck, 2000; Palma & Scheinman, 2001). (See Chapter 20 for more information about electrophysiology studies and ablation in management of arrhythmias. The section below on supraventricular tachycardias covers drug therapy of specific tachycardias in more detail.)

Supraventricular Tachycardia

The term *supraventricular tachycardia* (SVT) is used for all tachycardias that originate above the bifurcation of the bundle of His (i.e., AT, atrial flutter, sinus node reentry) or incorporate tissues proximal to the bifurcation to the bundle of His in a reentrant circuit (i.e., AVNRT or AVRT using an accessory pathway; Myerburg et al., 2001). Usually, SVT is used to describe narrow QRS tachycardias because the narrow QRS denotes normal intraventricular conduction through the His-Purkinje system from a supraventricular focus. It is possible for an SVT to conduct with bundle-branch block, which would result

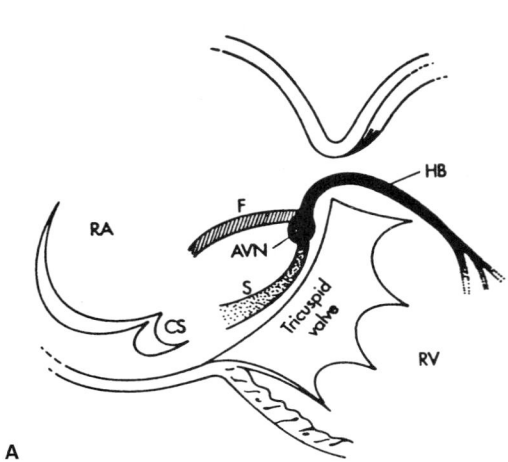

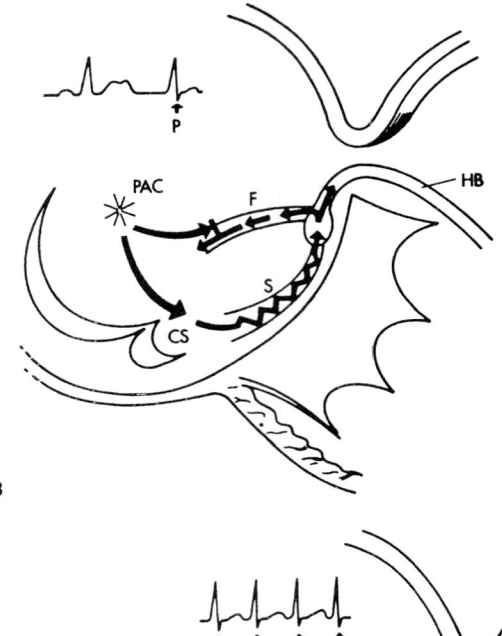

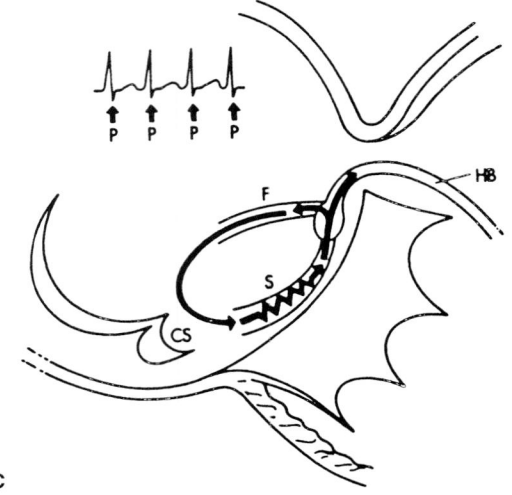

■ **Figure 19–11.** (*A*) Schematic showing cutaway view of right atrium (RA) and right ventricle (RV) to illustrate the two atrioventricular (AV) nodal pathways responsible for AV nodal reentry tachycardia (AVNRT). The fast pathway (F) has a long refraetory period, the slow pathway (S) has a short refractory period. AVN, body of AV node; CS, coronary sinus os. (*B*) A premature atrial complex is unable to conduct down the fast pathway because it is still refractory, so it conducts to the AV node through the slow pathway and into the ventricle with a long PR interval. In the node, the impulse is able to turn around and conduct back up the fast pathway, which has now recovered, and reenter the atrium. (*C*) AVNRT results when the impulse continues to circulate down the slow and up the fast pathways. Note the inverted P wave at the end of the QRS complex as the atria and ventricles depolarize simultaneously. (From Conover, M. B. [1996]. *Understanding electrocardiography* [7th ed.]. St. Louis: Mosby; and adapted from Keim, S., Werner, P., & Jazayeri, M., et al. [1992]. Localization of the fast and slow pathways in antrioventricular nodal reentrant tachycardia by intraoperative ice mapping. *Circulation, 86*[3], 919–925.)

in a wide QRS but would not change the fact that the rhythm is supraventricular. Thus, SVT can be used for wide QRS rhythms that are known to be coming from above the ventricles.

SVT can be classified into those that are AV nodal passive and those that are AV nodal active. AV nodal passive SVT are those in which the AV node does not play a part in the maintenance of the tachycardia but serves only to conduct passively the supraventricular rhythm into the ventricles. AV nodal passive SVT include AT, atrial flutter, and atrial fibrillation, all of which arise from within the atria and do not need the AV node's participation to sustain the atrial arrhythmia. AV nodal active tachycardias require participation of the AV node in the maintenance of the tachycardia. The two most common causes of a regular, narrow QRS tachycardia are AVNRT and AVRT using an accessory pathway, both of which require the AV node as part of the reentry circuit that sustains the tachycardia.

Atrial fibrillation is usually easily recognized owing to its irregularity, but AT, atrial flutter, junctional tachycardia, AVNRT, and AVRT can all present as a regular, narrow QRS tachycardia whose mechanism often cannot be determined

from the ECG. Because AVNRT and AVRT are responsible for most regular, narrow QRS tachycardias, these two are discussed in detail here.

Atrioventricular Nodal Reentry Tachycardia

AVNRT is the most common mechanism of SVT and is responsible for up to 60% of regular, narrow QRS tachycardias (Fogel & Prystowsky, 2001; Miles & Zipes, 2000; Myerburg et al., 2001; Olgin & Zipes, 2001). This rhythm involves dual AV nodal pathways: a fast-conducting pathway with a long refractory period and a slow-conducting pathway with a short refractory period. In AVNRT, a reentry circuit is set up in the AV node, using one pathway (usually the slow pathway) for the anterograde limb and the other pathway (usually the fast pathway) as the retrograde limb (Fig. 19-11).

Normally, the sinus impulse conducts down the fast pathway into the ventricles, resulting in a normal PR interval of 0.12 to 0.20 second. If a PAC occurs before the fast pathway with its long refractory period has recovered, the impulse conducts down the slow pathway because of its shorter refractory period, resulting in a PAC with a long PR interval. The long conduction time through the slow pathway allows the fast pathway time to recover, making it possible for the impulse to conduct backward into the fast pathway. The returning impulse can then reenter the slow pathway and initiate a circuit in the AV node, resulting in AVNRT. Figure 19-11 illustrates the most common mechanism of AVNRT. The resulting rhythm is usually a narrow QRS tachycardia because the ventricles are activated through the normal His-Purkinje system. P waves are either not visible at all or are seen peeking out at the end of the QRS complex because the atria are activated in a retrograde direction at the same time as the ventricles are being depolarized in an anterograde direction (Fig. 19-12). In the presence of preexisting bundle-branch block or rate-dependent bundle-branch block, the QRS in AVNRT is wide.

In approximately 10% of cases of AVNRT, the fast pathway is used as the anterograde limb and the slow pathway is used as the retrograde limb of the circuit (Otomo, Wang, Lazzara & Jackman, 2000). This results in a long R-P tachycardia in which the P wave appears in front of the QRS because atrial activation is delayed owing to slow conduction backward through the slow pathway. These P waves are inverted in inferior leads because the atria are depolarized in a retrograde direction.

AVNRT is an AV nodal active SVT because the AV node's participation is required to maintain the tachycardia. Therefore, anything that blocks the AV node, such as vagal stimulation or drugs like adenosine, beta blockers, or calcium channel blockers, can terminate the rhythm. AVNRT is usually well tolerated unless the rate is extremely rapid. Many people with this arrhythmia learn to stop it by coughing or breath holding, which stimulates the vagus nerve. Adenosine is the most effective agent for terminating AVNRT, but it does not prevent its recurrence. Radiofrequency ablation of the slow pathway has become the treatment of choice for all forms of AVNRT (Fogel & Prystowsky, 2001; Otomo et al., 2000; Strickberger & Morady, 2000).

Atrioventricular Reciprocating Tachycardia

Atrioventricular reciprocating tachycardia (AVRT) is SVT that occurs in people who have accessory pathways, also called *bypass tracts,* that allow impulses to conduct directly from atria to ventricles (see section on Preexcitation Syndromes, earlier). Approximately 30% of regular, narrow QRS tachycardias are due to AVRT using an accessory pathway (Kastor, 2000; Marinchak & Rials, 2001; Miles & Zipes, 2000; Myerburg et al., 2001).

In AVRT, the reentry circuit involves the atria, AV node, ventricle, and accessory pathway. The term *orthodromic* is used to describe the most common type of AVRT, in which the AV node is used as the anterograde limb and the accessory pathway is used as the retrograde limb of the circuit. This results in a narrow QRS tachycardia because the ventricles are depolarized through the His-Purkinje system. If bundle branch block is present, the QRS is wide. Because the atria and ventricles depolarize

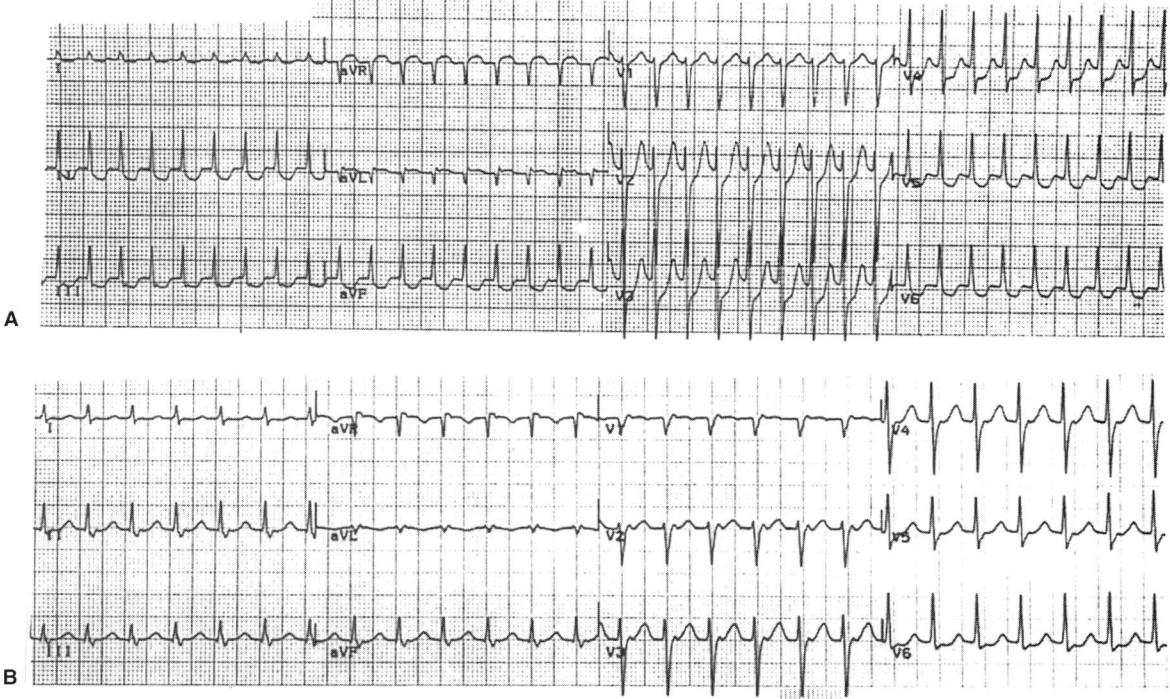

■ **Figure 19–12.** (*A*) Atrioventricular nodal reentry tachycardia (AVNRT); rate—214 beats/min. No P waves are visible. (*B*) AVNRT; rate—150 beats/min. P waves distort the end of the QRS complex in leads II, III, aVF, and V$_{1-3}$.

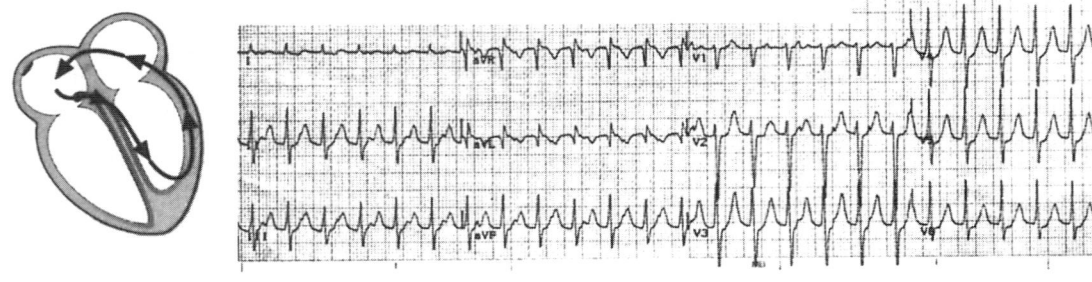

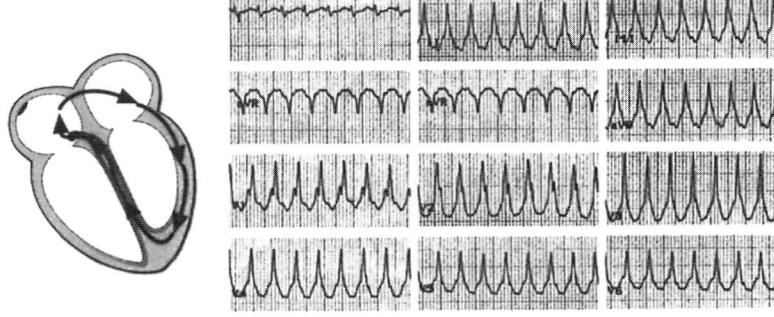

■ **Figure 19–13.** (*A*) Orthodromic AVRT using the atrioventricular (AV) node as anterograde limb and accessory pathway as retrograde limb of the reentry circuit. P waves are visible on the upstroke of the T wave in most leads. (*B*) Antidromic AVRT using the accessory pathway as the anterograde limb and the AV node as the retrograde limb of the reentry circuit. (From Jacobson, C. [1997]. Advanced ECG concepts. In M. Chulay, C. Guzzetta, & B. Dossey, [Eds.], *AACN handbook of critical care nursing* [p. 439]. Stamford, CT: Appleton & Lange.)

separately, the P waves in AVRT, if visible, are often seen in the ST segment or between the QRS complexes, usually closer to the preceding QRS than the following QRS (Fig 19-13*A*).

The term *antidromic* is used to describe a rare form of AVRT in which the accessory pathway is used as the anterograde limb of the circuit and the AV node is used as the retrograde limb. This results in a wide QRS tachycardia because the ventricles are depolarized abnormally through the accessory pathway, and it is often indistinguishable from VT (see Fig. 19-13*B*).

Like AVNRT, AVRT is an AV nodal active tachycardia because the AV node is necessary for maintenance of the tachycardia; therefore, vagal maneuvers or any drug that blocks the AV node can terminate the tachycardia. Alternatively, drugs that increase refractoriness or slow conduction in the accessory pathway can also be used to terminate tachycardia. Cardioversion is the treatment of choice for any tachycardia causing severe hemodynamic impairment.

If the patient is not seriously symptomatic and has a regular, narrow QRS tachycardia, indicating conduction down the AV node, vagal maneuvers such as CSM or Valsalva's maneuver, or the administration of adenosine, may terminate the arrhythmia by causing conduction delay in the AV node. Adenosine is very effective in this situation because of its immediate and short-term effect of slowing conduction in the AV node, and is effective about 95% of the time in terminating the arrhythmia (Miles & Zipes, 2000). Beta blockers and calcium channel blockers can also be used to slow AV node conduction. IV procainamide is an alternative choice for acute therapy because it prolongs the refractory period in all parts of the circuit (atrium, AV node, ventricle, and accessory pathway).

Tachycardias with wide QRS complexes, indicating conduction down the accessory pathway, are best treated acutely with IV procainamide, which increases the refractory period and depresses conduction in the bypass tract. Digitalis, verapamil, and diltiazem are contraindicated in this setting because they may

shorten the refractory period in the accessory pathway and facilitate conduction through it (McGovern et al., 1986; Miles & Zipes, 2000; Opie, 2001). Chronic therapy with class IC drugs (moricizine, flecainide, propafenone) or amiodarone can be used to slow conduction through the accessory pathway and the AV node, and may also suppress PAC and PVC that initiate the tachycardia (Miles & Zipes, 2000). Radiofrequency ablation of the accessory pathway has become the first-line treatment for tachycardias due to AVRT (Cappato et al., 2000; Marinchak & Rials, 2001; Myerburg et al., 2001).

Ventricular Tachycardia

VT can be one of the most serious arrhythmias encountered in cardiac patients and often requires immediate treatment to prevent hemodynamic collapse and possible deterioration into ventricular fibrillation. Three types of VT are commonly seen in patients with cardiac disease: (1) monomorphic VT, (2) polymorphic VT, and (3) torsades de pointes (Td).

Monomorphic Ventricular Tachycardia

Monomorphic VT, the most common type, refers to VT in which all of the QRS complexes are of the same morphology, indicating that they originate from the same spot in the ventricles (Fig. 19-14). Monomorphic VT occurs most often in patients with a history of MI, especially in those with an ejection fraction of less than 40%; most of these VT occur within 1 year of the infarct, but many patients present with their first episode many years after MI (Callans & Josephson, 2000; Martin & Wharton, 2001). This type of VT is treated acutely with the usual antiarrhythmic therapy used for ventricular arrhythmias: lidocaine, procainamide, and IV amiodarone. Amiodarone and

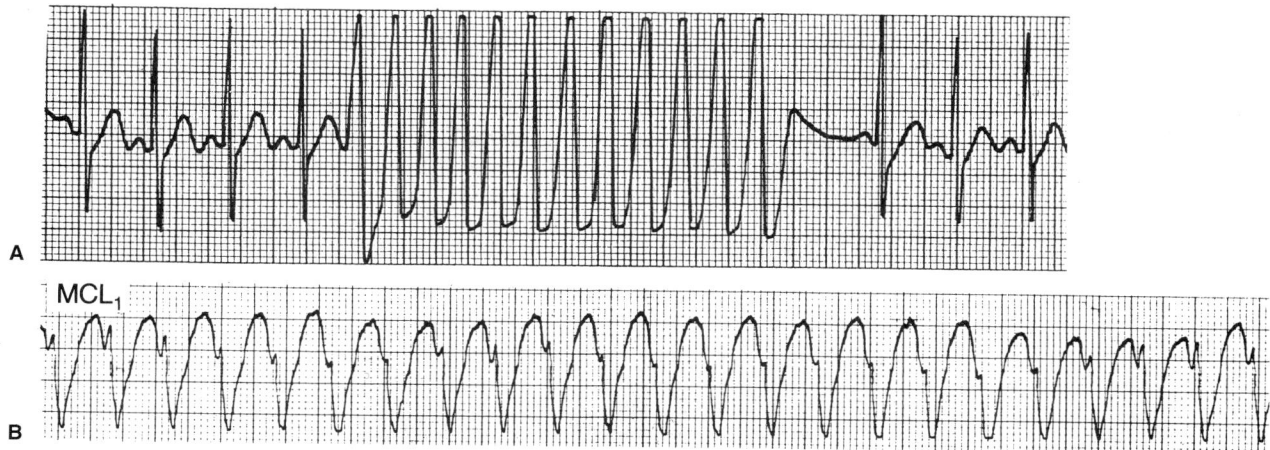

■ **Figure 19–14.** Monomorphic ventricular tachycardia. Tracings show two different examples, each with QRS complexes of one morphology.

sotalol are more effective than other types of antiarrhythmics for chronic therapy. An implantable cardioverter-defibrillator is often required in patients with recurrent VT that is resistant to drug therapy (see Chapter 32).

Another type of monomorphic VT arises in the right ventricular outflow tract (RVOT), occurs in patients with no structural heart disease, and is often induced by exercise (Martin & Wharton, 2001). RVOT tachycardia presents with LBBB morphology and inferior or rightward axis. RVOT tachycardia may respond to vagal maneuvers or adenosine. Beta blockers seem to work best for chronic therapy, and calcium channel blockers have been successful in some patients. Radiofrequency catheter ablation is often successful in destroying the focus in this type of VT.

Monomorphic VT arising in the left ventricle in young people with no structural heart disease presents with RBBB morphology and superior axis. This VT is often sensitive to verapamil or other calcium channel blockers but not to beta blockers. Radiofrequency catheter ablation has a success rate of about 90% in this type of tachycardia (Martin & Wharton, 2001).

Polymorphic Ventricular Tachycardia

Polymorphic VT refers to VT with unstable, continuously varying QRS morphology often occurring at rates of approximately 200 beats per minute (Hohnloser, 2001; Kastor, 2000; Myerburg et al., 2001; Fig. 19-15). Polymorphic VT is classified based on whether it is associated with normal or prolonged QT or QTU intervals. If a long QT interval is present, it is called TdP (see below). Polymorphic VT with a normal QT or QTU interval is thought to be due to reentry and occurs most often during acute ischemia or coronary vasospasm. The varying QRS morphologies can be explained by beat-to-beat variations in ventricular activation pattern due to changing sites and configuration of reentry circuits (El-Sherif & Turitto, 2000). Polymorphic VT with a normal QT interval tends to be initiated by the R-on-T closely coupled PVC without a preceding change in cycle length. Polymorphic VT may respond to the same antiarrhythmic drugs used to treat monomorphic VT, especially beta blockers and amiodarone, or to revascularization by surgery or angioplasty when associated with ongoing ischemia. (See Chapter 31 for ACLS recommendations for treatment of polymorphic VT.)

Torsades De Pointes

Torsades de pointes means "twisting of the points" and describes a special type of polymorphic VT in which the QRS complexes display continuously changing morphologies and seem to twist

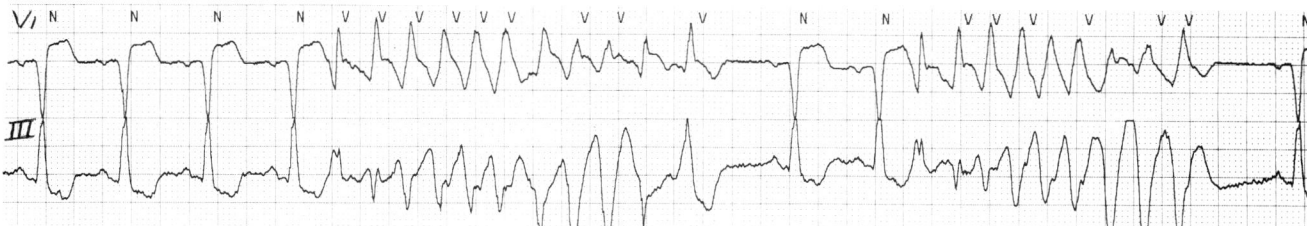

■ **Figure 19–15.** Polymorphic ventricular tachycardia recorded in two leads (V_1 and lead III). Note the normal QT interval. (N = arrhythmia computer's determination of a normal beat; V = computer determination of ventricular beat.)

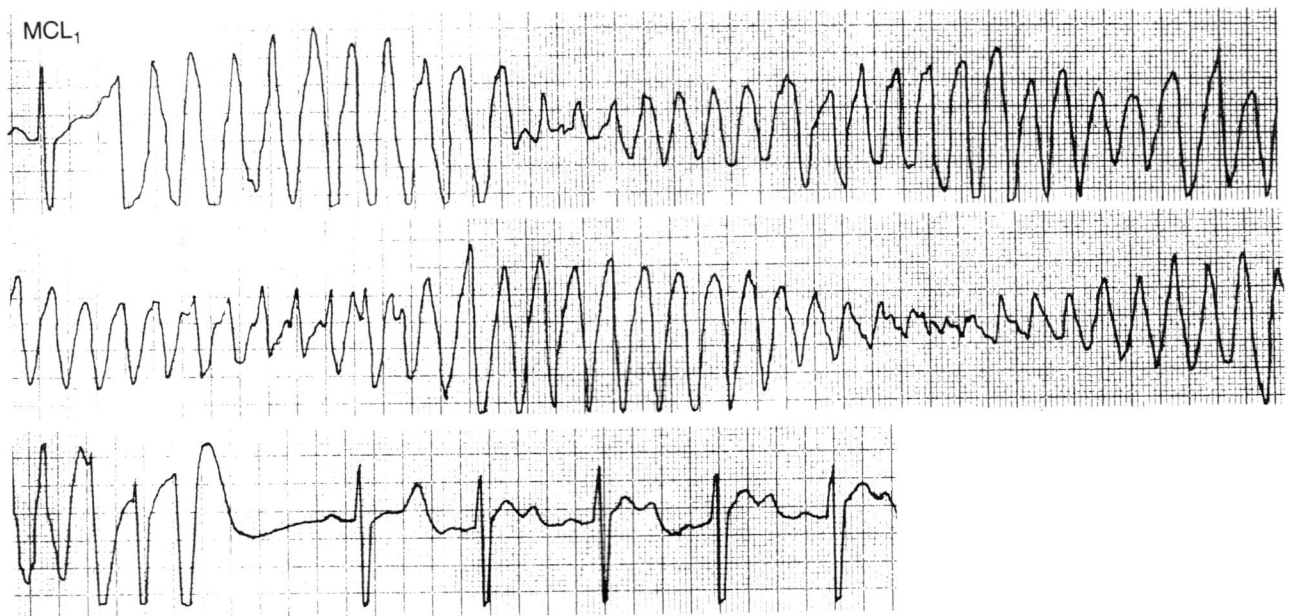

■ **Figure 19–16.** Torsades de pointes. Note characteristic features: (1)multiform RS complexes that twist and around the baseline, (2) initiation by a premature ventricular complex with a long coupling interval, and (3) associated long QT interval and wide TU waves during sinus rhythm.

around an imaginary line, often resembling ventricular fibrillation (Figs. 19-16 and 19-17). The underlying cause of this type of VT is delayed ventricular repolarization, which is manifested on the ECG as an abnormally prolonged QT or QTU interval; a large U wave after the T wave or merging with the T wave; wide, notched or biphasic T waves; and often associated with T wave alternans (Kastor, 2000; El-Sherif & Turitto, 2000; Hohnloser, 2001; Schwartz, Priori & Napolitano, 2000).

QT prolongation can be acquired or congenital. The acquired type is most often due to repolarization abnormalities induced by drugs, including class IA and class III antiarrhythmics, many antibiotics, antifungals, psychotropic drugs, some antihistamines, and others. Hypokalemia and hypomagnesemia are the electrolyte abnormalities most often associated with QT prolongation. Other factors that can lead to delayed repolarization include cerebral events such as cerebral vascular accidents and subarachnoid hemorrhage; and liquid protein weight-loss diets or starvation (El-Sherif & Turitto, 2000; Hohnloser, 2001; Kastor, 2000; Myerburg et al., 2001; Olgin & Zipes, 2001; Schwartz et al., 2000).

The congenital type of long QT syndrome (LQTS) is an inherited condition associated with TdP and sudden cardiac death. Evidence gathered in the past several years indicates that congenital LQTS is due to mutations of at least five genes identified so far, all of which modulate the function of sodium or potassium ion channels in the cardiac cell membrane (El-Sherif & Turitto, 2000; Hohnloser, 2001; Priori & Napolitano, 2001; Schwartz et al., 2000). (See Chapter 5 for more detailed information on genetics related to cardiac diseases.)

The electrophysiologic mechanism of TdP is thought to be EAD, which arise during the prolonged phase 2 of the cardiac action potential, leading to triggered beats and runs of TdP (El-Sherif et al., 1995; El-Sherif et al., 1988; Priori et al., 1995;

Schwartz et al., 2000). The notch commonly seen on the T wave of patients with TdP and long QT intervals may be a manifestation of these EAD arising during the repolarization phase of the action potential.

Characteristic ECG findings of TdP include (1) markedly prolonged QT intervals with wide TU waves; (2) initiation of the arrhythmia by an R-on-T PVC with a long coupling interval; and (3) wide, bizarre, multiform QRS complexes that change direction frequently, appearing to twist around the isoelectric line (see Figs. 19-16 and 19-17). TdP is usually associated with bradycardia and is "pause dependent," meaning that it tends to occur after pauses produced by PVC or sudden slowing of the heart rate. TdP is often initiated by a "long–short" cycle sequence in which episodes begin on the T wave of a beat that terminates a long cycle. Ventricular rate during TdP is commonly 200 to 250 beats per minute. TdP is usually self-terminating and occurs in repeated episodes, but it can deteriorate into ventricular fibrillation.

The differentiation of TdP from polymorphic VT and ventricular fibrillation is extremely important because TdP does not respond to conventional antiarrhythmic therapy and is usually made worse by the drugs used to treat ordinary VT. Treatment of TdP is aimed at shortening the refractory period and unifying repolarization by increasing the heart rate and correcting any contributing causes, such as electrolyte imbalances, or discontinuing causative drugs. Cardiac pacing at rates of 100 to 110 beats per minute can be instituted until the underlying cause is corrected. Magnesium can suppress the arrhythmia in both the acquired and congenital forms by reducing the amplitude of afterdepolarizations thought to cause TdP. Drugs such as quinidine, procainamide, disopyramide, sotalol, and amiodarone are contraindicated because they prolong the refractory period and contribute to the abnormal repolarization that causes TdP.

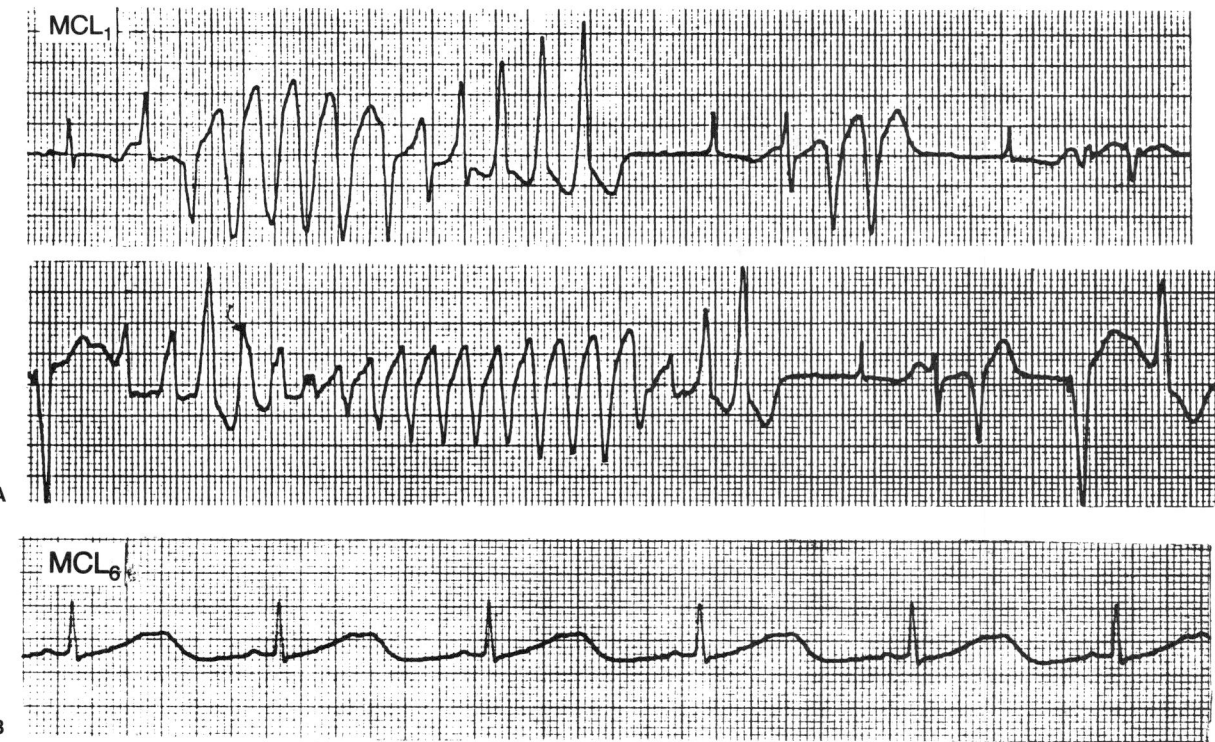

■ **Figure 19–17.** (*A*) Torsades de pointes. Note occurrence of frequent self-terminating runs of ventricular tachycardia initiated by premature ventricular complexes with long coupling intervals. QT is difficult to measure because of frequency of ventricular beats, but it appears long. (*B*) Sinus rhythm with very long QT interval and TU waves typical of abnormal repolarization. Torsades de pointes developed in the patient shortly after this strip was taken.

Differential Diagnosis of Wide QRS Beats and Tachycardias

One of the most frequently encountered problems in working with cardiac patients is differentiating ventricular tachycardia from aberrantly conducted supraventricular rhythms, both of which can cause a wide QRS complex. Establishing the correct diagnosis is important in choosing the correct therapy for the acute event as well as determining long-term therapy for the arrhythmia. Because aberrantly conducted supraventricular beats and tachycardias can look almost identical to ventricular ectopic beats or VT, it is sometimes impossible to tell them apart.

There are three major causes of wide QRS beats or tachycardias: (1) ventricular origin of the beat or rhythm, (2) aberrant conduction of a supraventricular beat or tachycardia through the bundle branch system (temporary or permanent bundle branch block), (3) preexcitation of the ventricle through an accessory pathway. VT is the most common cause of a wide complex tachycardia (WCT), accounting for approximately 80% of cases; aberrant conduction of a SVT occurs in 15% to 30% of cases of WCT; and accessory pathway conduction accounts for 1% to 5% of cases (Miller, Hsia, Rothman & Buxton, 2000). Other conditions that can also cause the QRS to widen include antiarrhythmic drugs; electrolyte abnormalities, especially hyperkalemia; and ventricular paced rhythms.

Although many criteria have been proposed to aid in differentiating wide QRS beats and rhythms, this section concentrates

only on selected criteria that seem to be the most helpful in the everyday clinical situation. Table 19-5 lists the ECG clues most helpful for differentiating wide QRS rhythms.

Mechanisms of Aberration

Aberrancy can occur whenever the His-Purkinje system is still partly or completely refractory when a supraventricular impulse attempts to traverse it. The refractory period of the conduction system is directly proportional to preceding cycle length. Long cycles (slow heart rates) are followed by long refractory periods, whereas short cycles (fast heart rates) are followed by short refractory periods. Supraventricular beats that occur early in the cycle, like PAC, may enter the conduction system during its refractory period and be conducted aberrantly. Similarly, beats that follow a sudden lengthening of the cycle may be conducted aberrantly because of the increased length of the refractory period that occurs when the cycle lengthens. There are three situations in which aberration is likely to occur (Singer & Cohen, 1995): (1) early supraventricular beats (e.g., PAC), (2) rapid heart rates where the supraventricular focus conducts into the intraventricular conduction system so rapidly that the bundles do not have time to repolarize completely, and (3) irregular rhythms where cycle lengths are constantly changing (e.g., atrial fibrillation). Because the right bundle branch has a longer refractory period than the left, aberrant beats tend to be conducted most often with an RBBB

Table 19–5 ■ ELECTROCARDIOGRAPHIC CLUES FOR DIFFERENTIATING WIDE QRS RHYTHMS

Electrocardiogram Feature	Aberrancy	Ventricular Ectopy
P waves	Precede QRS complexes (may be hidden in T waves)	Dissociated from QRS or occur at rate slower than QRS. If 1:1 ventriculoatrial conduction is present, retrograde P waves follow every QRS.
Right bundle-branch block QRS morphology	Triphasic rsR′ in V_1 Triphasic qRs in V_6	Monophasic R wave or diphasic qR complex in V_1 Left "rabbit ear" taller in V_1 Monophasic QS or diphasic rS in V_6
Left bundle-branch block QRS morphology	Narrow R wave (<0.04 s) in V_1 Straight downstroke of S wave in V_1 (often slurs or notches on upstroke) Usually no Q wave in V_6	Wide R wave (>0.03 s) in V_1 Slurring or notching on downstroke of S wave in V_1 Delay of >0.06 s to nadir of S wave in V_1 Any Q wave in V_6
Precordial QRS concordance	Positive concordance may occur with WPW	Negative concordance favors VT Positive concordance favors VT if WPW ruled out
Fusion or capture beats		Strong evidence in favor of VT
QRS axis	Often normal May be deviated to right or left	Indeterminate axis favors VT Often deviated to left or right
QRS width	Usually <0.14 s unless preexisting bundle-branch block	QRS >0.16 s favors VT

VT = ventricular tachycardia; WPW = Wolff-Parkinson-White syndrome.

pattern. Figures 19-18 and 19-19 illustrate these principles of refractory periods and cycle lengths.

Electrocardiographic Criteria

P Waves. When trying to make the distinction between aberrancy and ventricular ectopy, a helpful first step is to search for P waves and note their relation to QRS complexes. Atrial activity (represented by a P wave) preceding a wide beat or a run of tachycardia strongly favors a supraventricular origin of

that beat or tachycardia. Figure 19-20 illustrates an early ectopic P wave initiating three beats of a wide QRS rhythm that could easily be mistaken for PVC.

An exception to the preceding P wave rule is the case of end-diastolic PVC that occur after the sinus P wave has occurred.

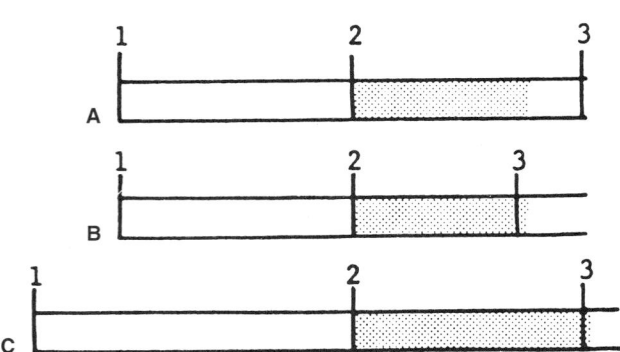

■ **Figure 19–18.** In the diagrams, 1, 2, and 3 are consecutive beats, and the shaded area represents the refractory period of some part of the conducting system after the second beat. (*A*) There are two regular cycles with normal conduction. The length of the refractory period is directly proportional to preceding cycle length. (*B*) Beat 3 occurs early and enters part of the conduction system during its refractory period, thus conducting aberrantly. (*C*) The first cycle is lengthened, resulting in a longer refractory period after beat 2. Beat 3 occurs no earlier than it did in *A*, but conducts aberrantly because the refractory period is prolonged. (From Marriott, H. J. L. [1988]. *Practical electrocardiography* [8th ed., p. 236]. Baltimore: Williams & Wilkins.)

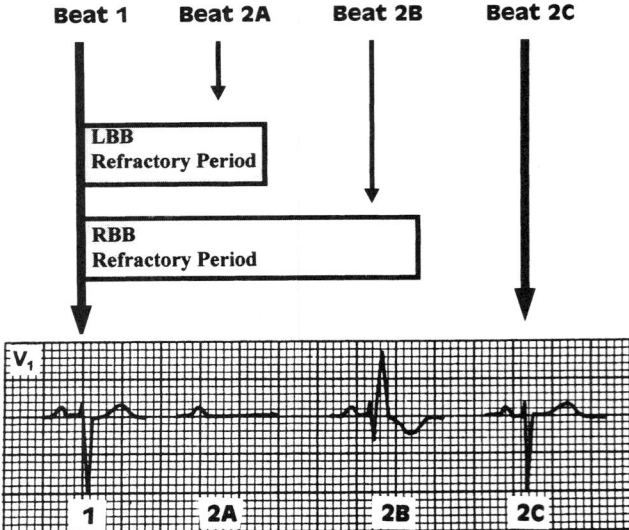

■ **Figure 19–19.** Diagram of refractory periods in the bundle branches and the effect of cycle length on conduction. The right bundle has a longer refractory period than the left. Beat 2A occurs so early that it cannot conduct through either bundle branch. Beat 2B encounters a refractory right bundle and conducts with right bundle-branch block. Beat 2C falls outside the refractory period of both bundles and is able to conduct normally. (From Jacobson, C. [1997]. Advanced ECG concepts. In M. Chulay, C. Guzzetta, & B. Dossey [Eds.], *AACN handbook of critical care nursing* [p. 440]. Stamford, CT: Appleton & Lange.)

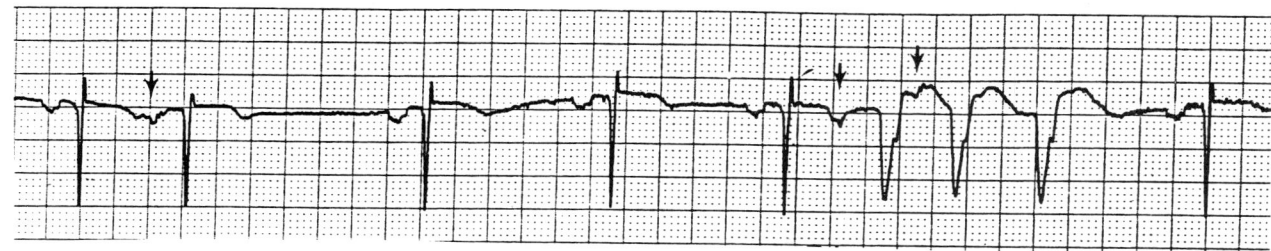

■ **Figure 19–20.** Sinus rhythm with premature atrial complexes (PACs) and three wide QRS beats that could be mistaken for ventricular tachycardia. The second beat in the strip is a PAC that conducts normally. Note the P waves preceding the wide QRS complexes, indicating aberrant conduction.

Figure 19-21 shows sinus rhythm with an end-diastolic PVC occurring immediately after the sinus P wave. In this case, the P wave preceding the wide QRS is merely a coincidence and does not represent aberrant conduction; the PR interval is much too short to have conducted that beat. In addition, the P wave preceding the wide QRS is not early; it is the regularly scheduled sinus beat coming on time. Thus, early P waves that precede early wide QRS complexes are usually related to those QRS, whereas "on time" P waves in front of end-diastolic PVC are not early and do not cause the wide QRS, although they may result in ventricular fusion beats.

P waves seen during a wide-complex tachycardia can be very helpful in making the differential diagnosis between SVT with aberration and VT. It is common for the sinus node to continue to fire regularly and independently of the ventricular focus when VT occurs. By noting the relationship between P waves and QRS complexes, it is sometimes possible to demonstrate AV dissociation, which means that the atria and ventricles are under the control of separate pacemakers (Fig. 19-22). Therefore, the presence of independent P waves in a wide QRS tachycardia indicates AV dissociation and is diagnostic of VT, whereas P waves seen before each QRS complex indicate a supraventricular origin of the rhythm. Figure 19-23 illustrates how P waves can be useful in differentiating two similar wide QRS tachycardias due to two different mechanisms.

QRS Morphology. The shape of the QRS complexes in a wide QRS tachycardia can be helpful in determining the mechanism of the arrhythmia. The following sections discuss the morphologic clues for wide-complex tachycardias with RBBB and LBBB morphologies.

Right Bundle-branch Block Pattern (Qrs Upright In V_1). Because the right bundle has a longer refractory period than the left, an impulse entering the conduction system early or at very rapid rates is more likely to encounter a still-refractory right bundle branch; therefore, most (80% to 85%) aberrantly conducted beats conduct with RBBB. However, approximately 60% of ventricular ectopic beats simulate an RBBB pattern (Marriott & Sandler, 1966; Sandler & Marriott, 1965). During normal ventricular depolarization, the septum depolarizes from left to right and creates a small initial r wave in V_1 (see Chapter 18). In the absence of septal infarction, the initial forces remain undisturbed during RBBB and beats that conduct with RBBB aberration have the same initial r wave in V_1 as during normal intraventricular conduction. Studies have shown that, of those beats presenting with an RBBB pattern in lead V_1, most aberrantly conducted supraventricular beats (70%) show a triphasic rsR′ pattern, whereas almost all ectopic ventricular beats (92%) show a monophasic (R) or biphasic (qR) pattern in V_1 (Fisch, 1991; Marriott & Sandler, 1966; Miller et al., 2000; Sandler & Marriott, 1965; Wellens, Frits & Lie, 1978). Therefore, a wide QRS complex with a triphasic pattern of RBBB in lead V_1 strongly favors aberrancy, whereas a monophasic or biphasic complex of RBBB type favors ventricular ectopy.

Other morphologic clues are presented in Figure 19-24. A monophasic or biphasic complex of RBBB type in lead V_1 with a taller left "rabbit ear" favors ectopy, whereas a taller right "rabbit ear" favors neither. Often V_6 is as helpful as V_1; a triphasic qRs complex in V_6 favors RBBB aberrancy, whereas a monophasic QS complex or a biphasic rS complex favors ventricular ectopy. Figure 19-25*A* shows VT with RBBB morphology.

Left Bundle-branch Block Pattern (qrs Negative In V_1). Leads V_1 or V_2 and V_6 also offer morphologic clues for tachycardias with LBBB morphology (Kindwall, Brown & Josephson, 1988; see Fig. 19-24). Three characteristics of the QRS complex in V_1 or V_2 favor a ventricular origin: a wide initial r wave of greater than 0.03 second, slurring or notching on the downstroke of the S wave, and a delay of 0.06 second or more from the beginning of the QRS to the nadir (deepest part) of the S wave. In addition, any q wave (qR or QS) in V_6 favors a ventricular origin. Figure 19-25*B* shows VT with LBBB morphology.

Brugada and colleagues (1991) suggest that additional morphologic clues in the precordial leads V_1 through V_6 can also be helpful. They suggest that a helpful first step in diagnosing a wide QRS rhythm is to scan the precordial leads to see if any lead shows an rS complex. If no precordial lead shows an rS pattern, VT is the likely diagnosis. If any precordial lead displays an rS pattern in which the measurement from onset of the r wave

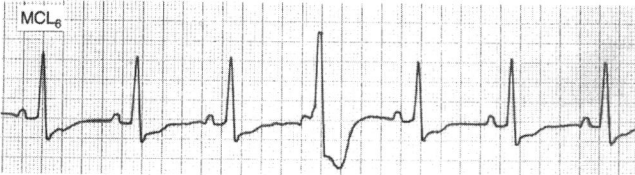

■ **Figure 19–21.** Sinus rhythm with one end-diastolic premature ventricular complex (PVC). The P wave preceding the PVC is the sinus P wave that coincidentally occurred just before the PVC.

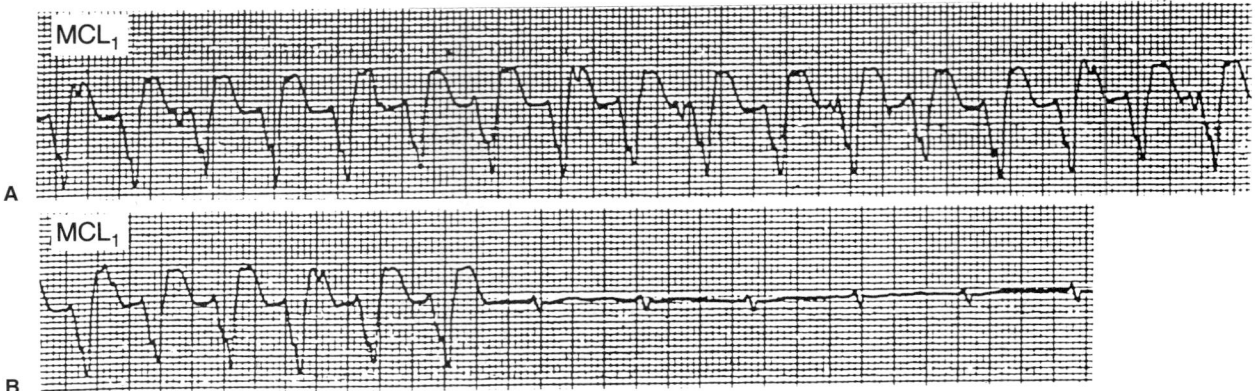

■ **Figure 19–22.** (*A*) Ventricular tachycardia (VT) at a rate of 136 beats/min. Independent P waves can be seen throughout the strip. (*B*) Sudden termination of VT, revealing the underlying sinus rhythm at a rate of 94 beats/min.

to nadir of the S wave exceeds 100 milliseconds (0.10 second), it favors the diagnosis of VT. They also emphasize that the presence of AV dissociation or any of the morphologic clues found in leads V_1, V_2, or V_6 discussed previously favor the diagnosis of VT (Fig. 19-26).

Lead V_6 or MCL_6 can be useful in differentiating supraventricular rhythms with aberrancy from ventricular ectopy (Drew & Scheinman, 1991; Drew, Scheinman & Dracup, 1991). In wide QRS rhythms of either RBBB or LBBB pattern, an interval of 50 milliseconds (0.05 second) or less from the onset of the QRS to the tallest peak of the R wave or nadir of the S wave favors a supraventricular origin, whereas an interval of 70 milliseconds (0.07 second) or more favors a ventricular origin (Fig. 19-27).

Fusion and Capture Beats. Ventricular fusion beats are produced when a supraventricular impulse and an ectopic ventricular impulse both contribute to ventricular depolarization. The resulting QRS complex does not look like a normally conducted beat or like the pure ventricular ectopic beat because it is formed by a combination of both depolarization waves (e.g., a "hybrid" morphology). The shape and width of fusion beats vary depending on the relative contributions of both the supraventricular and the ventricular impulses. The presence of fusion beats indicates AV dissociation; the atria and the ventricles

are under the control of separate pacemakers. Capture beats occur when, in the presence of AV dissociation, a supraventricular impulse manages to conduct into the ventricles and "capture" them, resulting in a normally conducted QRS complex. Thus, the presence of fusion or capture beats in a run of wide QRS tachycardia

RBBB PATTERN

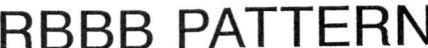

rsR' pattern in V1		ABERRATION
qRs in V6		ABERRATION
R or qR in V1 with taller LEFT rabbit ear		VT
QS or rS in V6		VT

LBBB PATTERN

In Leads V1 or V2:

Wide R, Slurred downstroke, >.06 sec to nadir of S   VT

Any Q (qR or QS) in V6   VT

■ **Figure 19–24.** Morphology clues for wide QRS beats and rhythms with right bundle-branch block (RBBB) pattern and left bundle-branch block (LBBB) pattern.

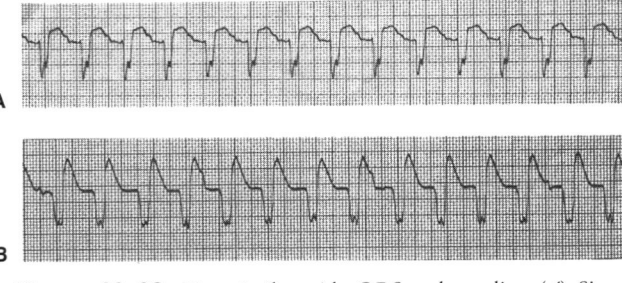

■ **Figure 19–23.** Two similar wide QRS tachycardias. (*A*) Sinus tachycardia; rate—115 beats/min. P waves can be seen preceding each QRS, indicating a supraventricular origin of the tachycardia. (*B*) P waves are independent of QRS complexes, indicating atrioventricular dissociation that favors ventricular tachycardia.

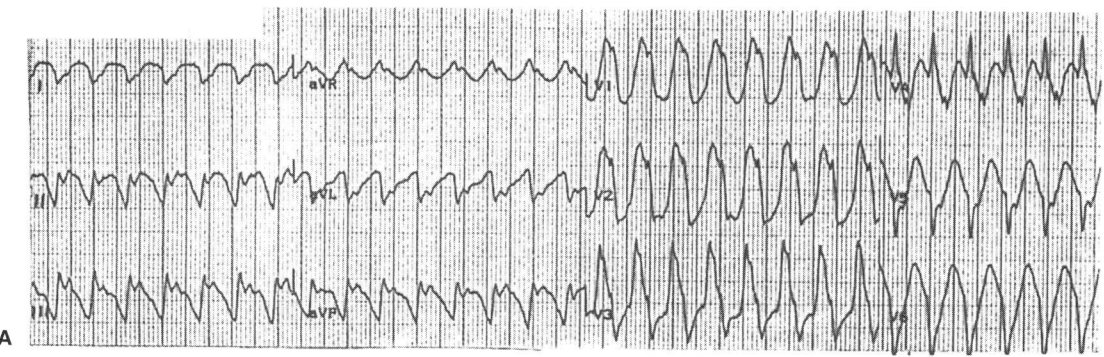

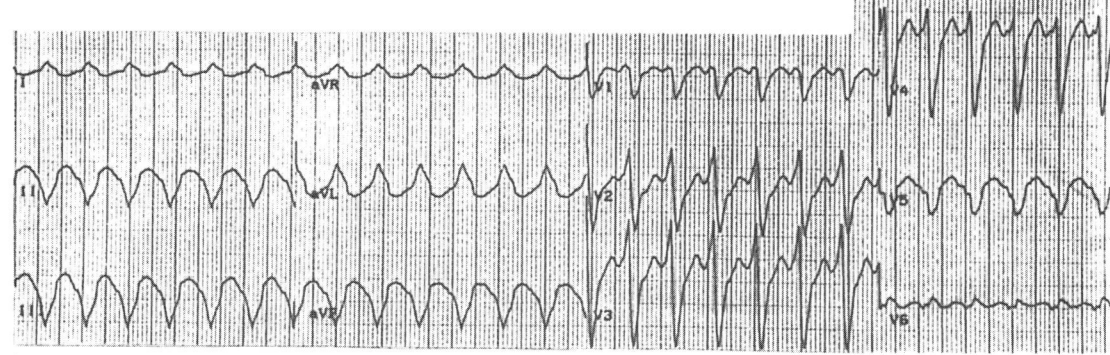

■ **Figure 19–25.** (*A*) Twelve-lead electrocardiogram (ECG) of ventricular tachycardia (VT) with right bundle-branch block morphology. Note monophasic R wave with taller left rabbit ear in V_1 and QS complex in V_6. The indeterminate QRS axis also favors VT. (*B*) Twelve-lead ECG of VT with left bundle-branch block morphology. Note wide R waves in V_1 and V_2, and qR pattern in V_6. (From Jacobson, C. [1997]. Advanced ECG concepts. In M. Chulay, C. Guzzetta, & B. Dossey [Eds.], *AACN handbook of critical care nursing* [p. 444]. Stamford, CT: Appleton & Lange.)

is diagnostic of VT, but, unfortunately, capture beats are rare and cannot be counted on to make the diagnosis (Fig. 19-28).

Cycle Length Variations. Ashman's phenomenon states that a beat that terminates a short cycle after a long cycle tends to be aberrantly conducted (Marriott, 1988). Because the refractory period of the conduction system varies with preced-

ing cycle length, a beat that terminates a long cycle has a long refractory period, causing the next beat to conduct aberrantly if it occurs early (i.e., terminates a short cycle). This aberrant conduction usually occurs with RBBB because the right bundle branch has a longer refractory period than the left. Thus, aberration tends to occur in early beats that cause a shortening of the

THE NETHERLANDS CLUES
Any of the following = VT

No RS in any precordial lead

R to S interval > 100ms in any precordial lead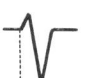

AV dissociation

Morphology criteria for VT present in V1-2 and V6

■ **Figure 19–26.** The Netherlands clues (so named because these clues originated in the Netherlands from research done by Brugada and colleagues). In a wide QRS tachycardia, if no precordial lead displays an RS complex, or if any precordial lead displays an RS complex that measures greater than 100 milliseconds from onset to nadir, ventricular tachycardia (VT) is the favored diagnosis. Atrioventricular dissociation and the morphology clues favoring VT in V_{1-2} and V_6 are also helpful.

THE SAN FRANCISCO CLUE
In either RBBB or LBBB morphologies

In V6 or MCL6:

Onset of QRS to tallest peak or to nadir < 50 ms   ABERRATION

Onset of QRS to tallest peak or to nadir > 70ms   VT

■ **Figure 19–27.** The San Francisco clue (so named because these clues originated from research done in San Francisco by Drew and Scheinman). In wide QRS tachycardias of either right or left bundle-branch block morphology, if measurement from beginning of QRS to tallest peak or to nadir of S wave is less than 50 milliseconds (ms) in V_6 or MCL_6, aberration is favored. It the measurement is more than 70 ms, VT is favored.

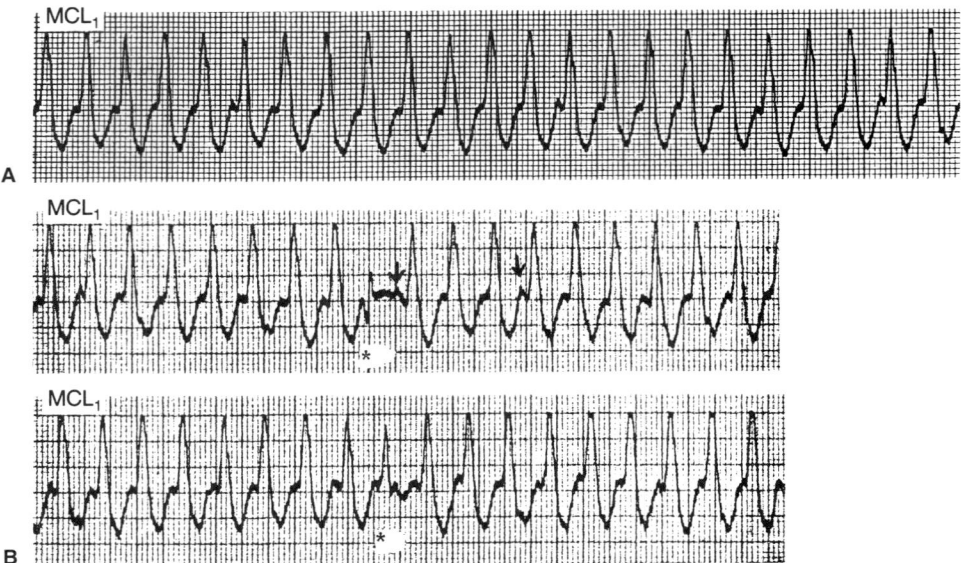

■ Figure 19–28. (*A*) Wide QRS tachycardia at a rate of approximately 200 beats/min. P waves are not easily recognizable, but the monophasic upright QRS morphology in V_1 favors ventricular tachycardia (VT). (*B*) Same patient with fusion beats among the wide QRS complexes (*asterisks*). *Arrows* point to P waves occurring independently of QRS complexes. Fusion beats and independent P waves are diagnostic of VT.

cycle, such as PAC, or only in the first beat of a run of SVT. Ashman's phenomenon does not prove aberration, it merely explains it if it occurs. Therefore, the presence of a beat that meets Ashman criteria (i.e., terminates a short cycle that follows a long cycle) does not prove that the wide beat is aberrant, because a PVC could just as easily have occurred in the same spot.

Depending only on cycle lengths to aid in the differentiation of aberration from ectopy is unreliable for another reason as well. By the "rule of bigeminy," a long cycle can also precipitate a PVC (Langendorf, Pick & Winternitz, 1955; Marriott & Conover, 1998). The mechanism responsible for this seems to be that the area of unidirectional block that allows the reentry of the impulse in the ventricular myocardium is able to conduct the impulse in a retrograde direction only after a certain rest period (i.e., a long cycle). Once a PVC has occurred, the pause that follows results in

another long cycle, which allows another PVC; thus, ventricular bigeminy tends to perpetuate itself. Because a long preceding cycle can occur in both aberration and ectopy, it alone cannot be used with certainty in differentiating the two mechanisms. However, the absence of a long preceding cycle favors ectopy and is evidence against aberration (Marriott, 1988).

Atrial fibrillation presents special difficulties in the differentiation of wide QRS complexes. The absence of P waves prevents the use of P-wave clues, and the variations in cycle length that are common in atrial fibrillation or atrial flutter provide a perfect set-up for both aberrant conduction and ventricular reentry. It is necessary to rely heavily on QRS morphology and it is helpful to compare cycle lengths. When comparing cycle sequences in atrial fibrillation or flutter, it is important to look at several sequences and not only at the sequence containing the beat with the wide QRS. Figure 19-29*A* shows atrial flutter

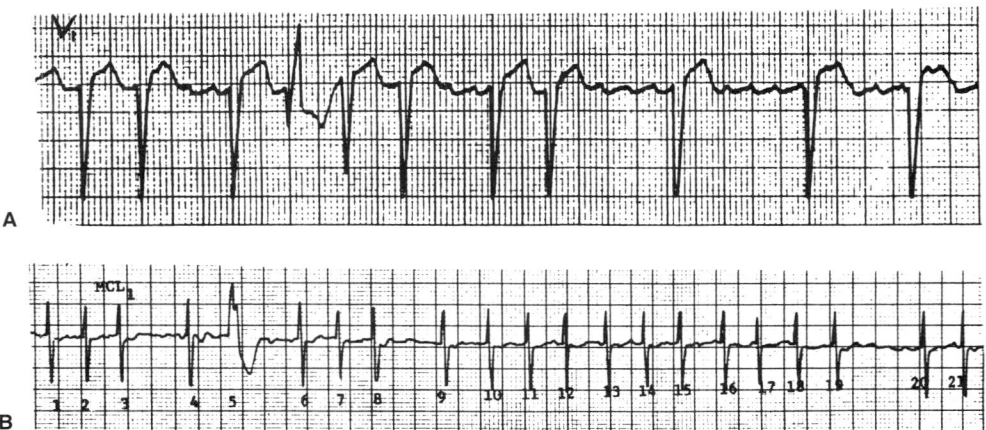

■ Figure 19–29. (*A*) Atrial flutter with one aberrantly conducted beat. Note the triphasic rSR′ complex of right bundle-branch block in V_1. (*B*) Atrial fibrillation with a premature ventricular complex (beat no. 5). The monophasic QRS with taller left "rabbit ear" favors a ventricular origin. Comparison of cycle lengths indicates that if any beat in this strip should be conducted aberrantly, it is beat no. 21, which terminates a short cycle after the longest cycle in the strip. If the heart can conduct beat 21 normally, there is no reason why it would conduct beat no. 5 aberrantly.

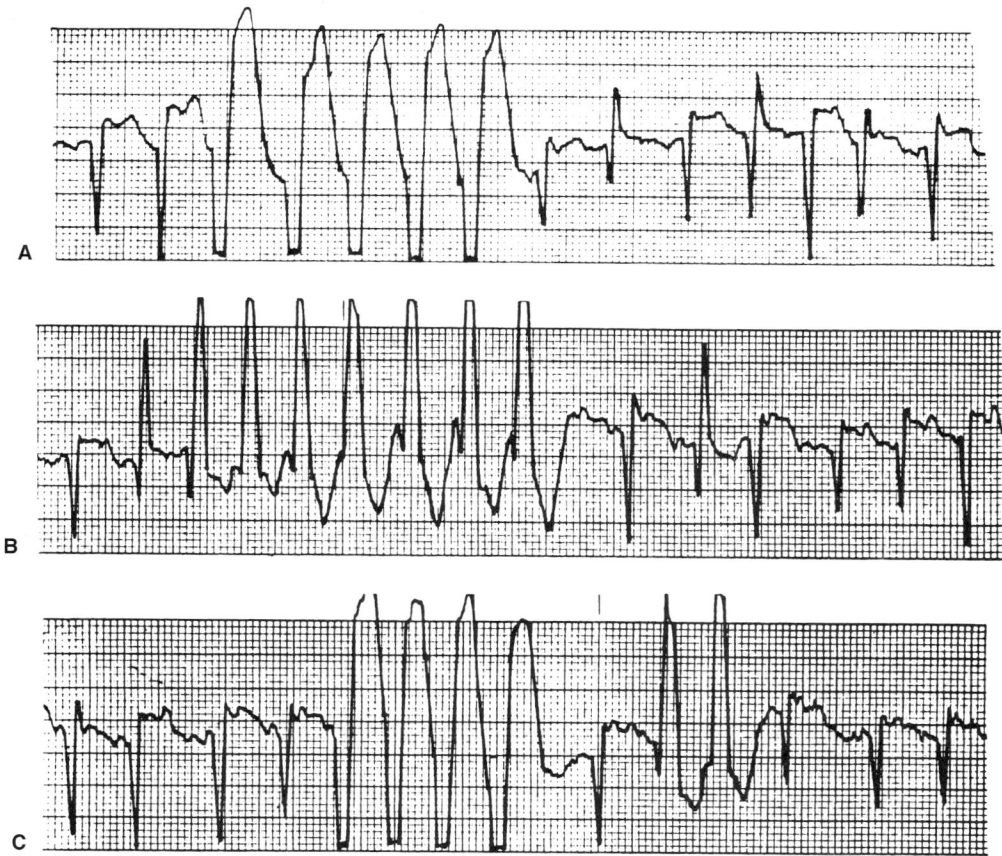

■ **Figure 19–30.** Atrial fibrillation with both left (*A*) and right (*B*) bundle-branch block aberration. (*C*) Left bundle-branch block aberration and right bundle-branch block aberration are separated by a single normal beat.

with an aberrantly conducted beat that terminates a short cycle after a long cycle (i.e., Ashman's phenomenon). In Figure 19-29*B*, beat 5 terminates a cycle that is shorter than the preceding cycle, but, in comparing other cycle sequences in the same strip, note that beat 21 terminates an even shorter cycle that follows the longest cycle in the strip and still conducts normally. The absence of aberration in beat 21 where it would be expected because of cycle lengths helps to identify beat 5 as a PVC.

It is common in the presence of atrial fibrillation to see both RBBB and LBBB aberration in the same patient. An interesting finding in many cases is that the two forms of aberration are often separated from one another by one normally conducted beat (Marriott, 1988; Marriott & Conover, 1998). The mechanism of this phenomenon is not understood, but it occurs often enough to make it a useful clue in differentiating aberration from bifocal ventricular ectopy (Fig. 19-30).

Whenever possible, it is useful to compare conduction during atrial fibrillation with conduction that occurs in the same patient during sinus rhythm. Figure 19-31*A* is from a patient in atrial fibrillation with many episodes of LBBB aberration resembling VT. Note that, whenever the ventricular response to atrial fibrillation slows even slightly, normal conduction resumes. Also note that the aberrantly conducted beats occur in an irregular pattern, just as the ventricular response to atrial

fibrillation typically occurs, and that the morphology favors LBBB rather than VT. The irregularity is a helpful observation because VT, although it does not have to be perfectly regular, is seldom as irregular as the ventricular response to atrial fibrillation. Figure 19-31*B* is from the same patient during one of his frequent episodes of sinus rhythm. Note that during the sinus rhythm, there are no aberrantly conducted beats. When sinus rhythm is restored, the ventricular rate slows and the cycle lengths become regular, both of which remove the opportunity for aberration to occur. If the wide beats that occur during atrial fibrillation were ventricular ectopic beats, they would be just as likely to occur during sinus rhythm. The disappearance of the wide QRS complexes every time sinus rhythm is restored helps make the diagnosis of aberration in Figure 19-31*A*.

Intra-atrial Electrograms and Esophageal Leads. Recording the electrogram from a lead in or on the right atrium or from a lead positioned behind the atria in the esophagus is a useful technique for demonstrating the relationship between atrial and ventricular electrical activity. When the lead is positioned in or very near the atria, atrial activity records as a large deflection and ventricular activity records as a smaller deflection, making it easier to see if P waves are associated with or dissociated from the QRS complexes. Figure 19-32 shows an intra-atrial recording from a patient with a wide QRS tachycardia in

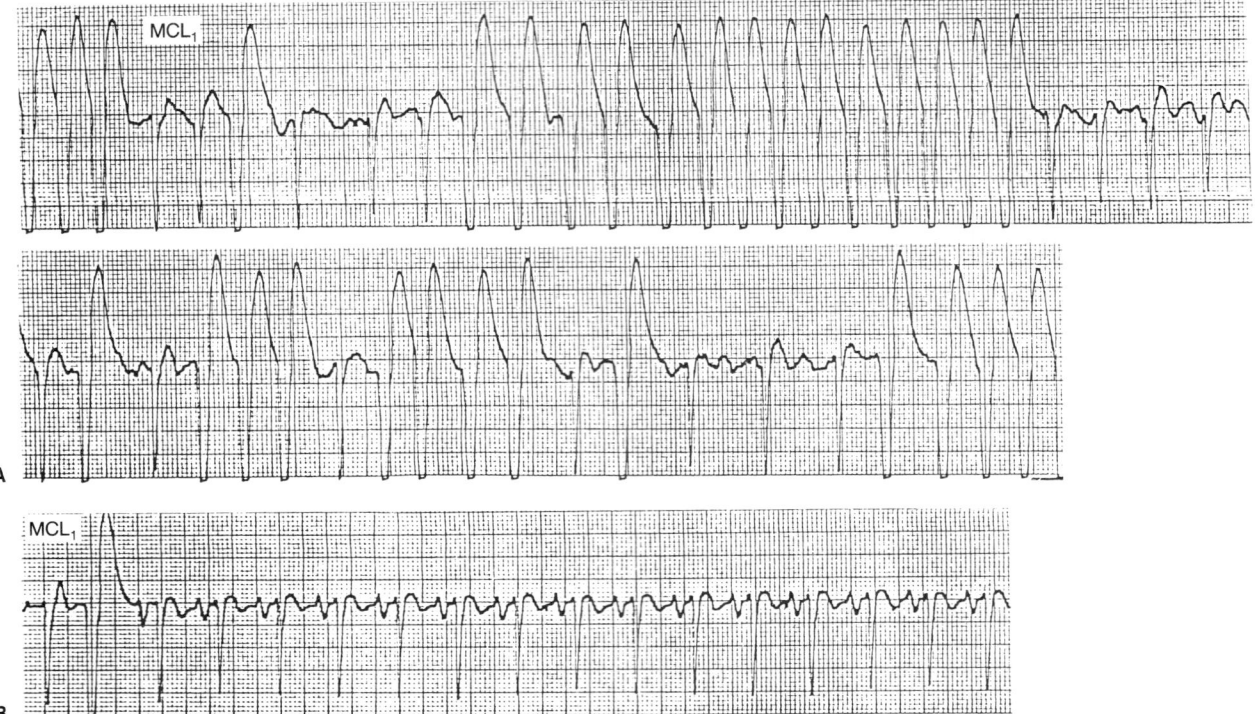

■ **Figure 19–31.** (*A*) Atrial fibrillation with frequent left bundle-branch block aberration resembling ventricular tachycardia. Normal conduction resumes whenever the ventricular rate slows even slightly. (*B*) Same patient during one of his frequent episodes of sinus tachycardia, restored after the second beat. During sinus tachycardia, no aberration occurs because the rate is slower and cycle lengths are regular, removing the opportunity for aberration.

whom the diagnosis was uncertain. AV dissociation is clearly present, as demonstrated by very large "P" waves and smaller QRS deflections. When recording an atrial electrogram, the recorder should be run at double the normal paper speed (i.e., at 50 mm per second instead of the usual 25 mm per second) to make it easier to differentiate atrial and ventricular activity.

Clinical Criteria

Several clinical criteria can be used to aid in the differentiation of aberration from ectopy.

Heart Sounds. Varying intensity of the S_1 heart sound occurs whenever the atrial activity is dissociated from ventricular

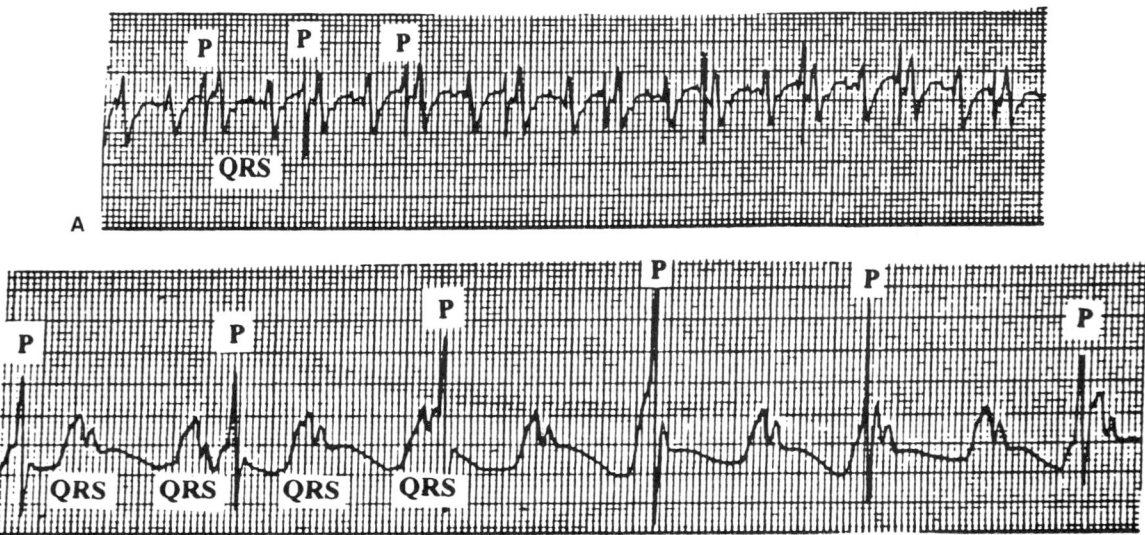

■ **Figure 19–32.** Intra-atrial recording of a wide QRS tachycardia at regular paper speed (*A*) and double paper speed (*B*). Atrioventricular dissociation is apparent and is diagnostic of ventricular tachycardia.

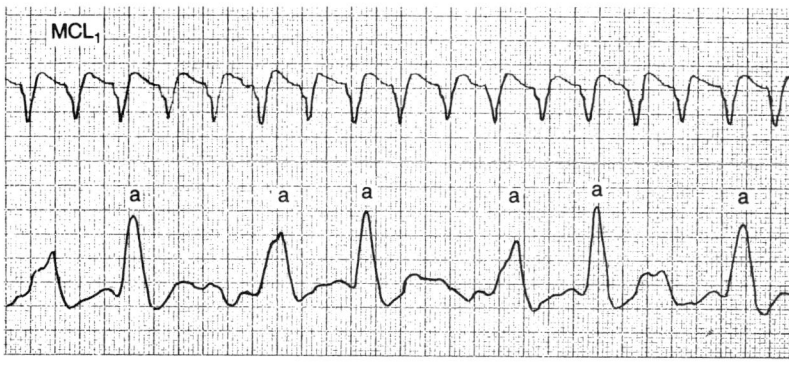

■ **Figure 19–33.** Electrocardiogram (ECG) and a central venous pressure (CVP) tracing of a patient in ventricular tachycardia. No P waves can be seen for certain in the ECG, but the CVP shows exaggerated a waves when the right atrium contracts against the closed tricuspid valve during atrioventricular dissociation.

activity, as frequently occurs in VT. The S_1 sound is produced by the closure of the AV valves, and its intensity depends on the proximity of the valve leaflets to one another at the time of ventricular systole. When atrial activity and ventricular activity are dissociated, the atria contract in variable relationship to the ventricles and the valve leaflets are at times wide open when ventricular systole occurs, causing a loud sound when they close. At other times, the leaflets have drifted closer together before ventricular systole and the resulting sound is softer. When there is a 1 : 1 relation between atrial and ventricular contraction, as occurs in a supraventricular rhythm, the intensity of S_1 is constant because the valve leaflets are in the same position every time they close. Thus, variable intensity of S_1 favors VT when AV dissociation is present.

Neck Veins. When AV dissociation is present, atrial and ventricular contraction is asynchronous and the atria and the ventricles occasionally contract simultaneously. When this occurs, the atria contract against closed AV valves, and blood from the right atrium has no place to go except back up into the neck veins. Observation of the patient's neck veins during AV dissociation reveals irregularly occurring "cannon a waves," which are large pulsations seen in the neck veins as blood is forced backward during atrial contraction. When atrial activity precedes ventricular activity, as it does in some SVT (e.g., sinus or AT), cannon a waves are not seen. When atrial activity occurs simultaneously with or after ventricular activity in a 1 : 1 relationship (as it may in junctional tachycardia or VT with retrograde conduction, AVNRT, or in AVRT due to an accessory pathway), cannon a waves are often seen with each beat. No a waves at all occur in the presence of atrial fibrillation because the atria do not contract. Therefore, the presence of *irregularly occurring* cannon a waves in the jugular pulse or in the central venous pressure or pulmonary wedge pressure tracing in the presence of a wide QRS tachycardia favors VT (Fig. 19-33).

Response to Vagal Maneuvers. Carotid sinus massage or other vagus-stimulating maneuvers, such as the Valsalva maneuver, are often used in the presence of a rapid heart rate either to terminate a supraventricular rhythm or diagnose the mechanism of the tachycardia. A sinus tachycardia usually responds to CSM by slowing its rate, whereas some SVT (especially AVNRT or AVRT) may convert to sinus rhythm. Atrial rhythms, such as AT, flutter, or fibrillation, usually respond with a slowing of the ventricular response but not by conversion to sinus rhythm. VT typically does not respond to CSM, and, occasionally, there is no response from a supraventricular

rhythm. Therefore, if the rate of the tachycardia slows in response to CSM or the rhythm converts to sinus rhythm, a supraventricular origin of the tachycardia is favored; if there is no response, neither aberration nor ectopy is favored.

Wenckebach Conduction

Wenckebach conduction is a progressive increase in conduction time of an impulse from its site of origin to its site of termination. AV Wenckebach is a common clinical occurrence and is easily recognized. It is known that Wenckebach conduction can occur in other areas of the heart (Peter, Harper, Vohra & Hunt, 1976), including the sinus node (Shamroth & Dove, 1966), various levels of the AV node (Halpern et al., 1973; Kosowsky, Latif & Radoff, 1976), the bundle branches (Rosenbaum et al., 1969; Sclarovsky, Strasberg & Agmon, 1978b), and reentry loops in the ventricles (Carleton, 1977), as well as from ectopic foci (Mirvis, Bandura & Brody, 1976). Recognition of Wenckebach conduction from these other sites is not as easy as recognizing AV Wenckebach, although Wenckebach conduction occurring anywhere in the heart follows the same rules as AV Wenckebach conduction. Therefore, a thorough understanding of typical AV Wenckebach conduction is necessary as a basis for recognizing Wenckebach conduction in other areas of the heart. This section describes the characteristics of typical AV Wenckebach conduction, the most commonly occurring atypical types of AV Wenckebach conduction, and Wenckebach conduction in other areas of the heart.

Atrioventricular Wenckebach

Wenckebach (type I) AV block is a progressive increase in conduction time of consecutive impulses from atria to ventricles until an impulse fails to be conducted, or is "blocked." It is characterized by progressive lengthening of the PR interval on consecutively conducted beats until the final P wave of the sequence is followed by a pause rather than by a QRS; then the cycle repeats itself (Fig. 19-34). The following are characteristics of typical AV Wenckebach conduction:

1. The PR interval progressively increases with each consecutively conducted beat.
2. The largest increment in PR interval usually occurs between the first and second beats in the cycle.

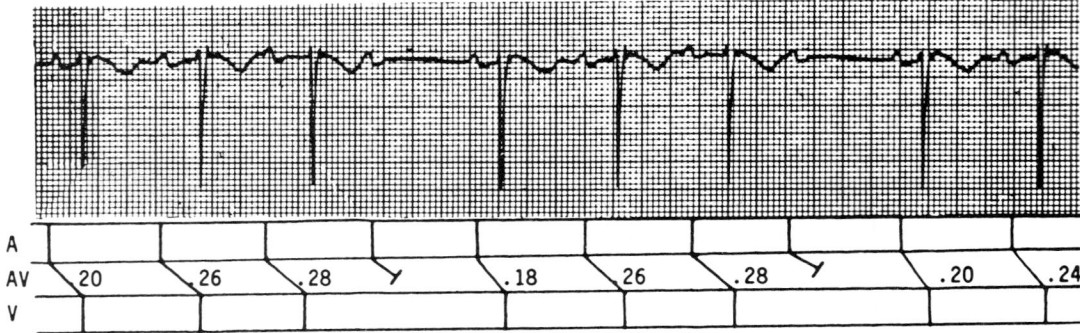

■ **Figure 19–34.** Typical atrioventricular (AV) Wenckebach conduction: The PR intervals gradually increase before the pause; R-R intervals shorten before the pause; the pause measures less than twice any R-R interval; the overall appearance is one of group beating. (In this and all other ladder diagrams, A, atria; AV, AV junction; V, ventricles. The slant of the line through the AV area represents conduction time through the AV junction. PR intervals are measured in seconds.) (From Jacobson, C. [1983]. Interpretation of complex arrhythmias. In S. L. Woods [Ed.], *Cardiovascular critical care nursing* [p.194]. New York: Churchill Livingstone. By permission.)

3. R-R intervals gradually shorten before the pause.
4. The pause is less than twice the length of any other cycle.
5. The overall appearance of the rhythm demonstrates group beating.

Typical AV Wenckebach conduction occurs most often at lower conduction ratios, such as 4 : 3 (four P waves to three QRS complexes), whereas atypical forms tend to be more common at higher conduction ratios, such as 8 : 7 conduction (Cabeen, Roberts & Child, 1978; El-Sherif et al., 1978; Watanabe, Dreifus & Mazgalev, 1995).

The gradual shortening of R-R intervals before the pause occurs because, although PR intervals gradually increase, they increase by decreasing amounts each time (Watanabe et al., 1995). Figure 19-35 illustrates this concept with a ladder diagram showing each beat of a Wenckebach cycle as a solid line compared with the previous beat as a dotted line. It can be readily seen that the AV conduction time progressively increases from 0.18 second to 0.30, 0.36, and 0.38 second, but the amount of increase decreases from 0.12 to 0.06 to 0.02 second, which causes the R-R intervals to shorten. Note also that the length of the pause is less than twice the length of any other cycle in the sequence. Figure 19-34 illustrates these common characteristics of typical AV Wenckebach conduction.

Atypical AV Wenckebach conduction occurs when the conduction delay is inconsistent and not all the usual features of typical Wenckebach conduction are present (Cabeen et al., 1978; Watanabe et al., 1995). The following are some commonly occurring atypical patterns:

1. The last PR interval of the cycle increases in length more than expected (Fig. 19-36A). A possible explanation for this unexpected lengthening of the last PR interval is that prolonged conduction time of the next-to-last beat in the cycle allows the AV node to recover some of its conductivity, thus enabling the impulse to reenter the AV node and propagate back toward the atria at the same time as it proceeds into the ventricles. This retrograde conduction through the AV node causes the node to be more refractory when the next sinus impulse arrives, thus prolonging conduction time of the last impulse in the cycle more than would normally be expected, resulting in the excessive length of the last PR interval (El-Sherif et al., 1978).

2. Conduction times can increase so gradually that the changes in PR intervals are not easily seen on the ECG (see Fig. 19-36B). For this reason, it is important to compare the PR interval preceding the pause with the PR interval after the pause. When Wenckebach conduction is present, the PR interval preceding the pause is longer than the PR interval after the pause.

3. Conduction times can remain the same for several beats within a cycle or can vary within a cycle. In these cases, PR

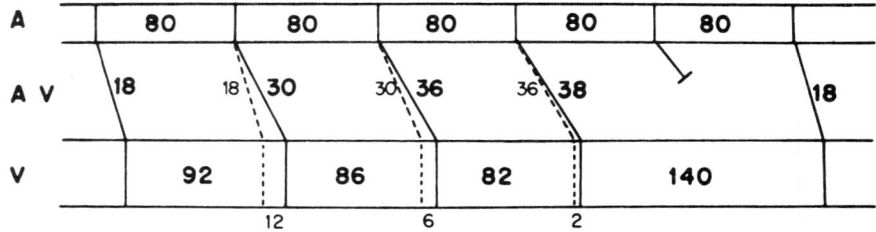

■ **Figure 19–35.** Diagram of typical Wenckebach cycle. Numbers are hundredths of a second. *Solid lines* represent the current cycle, compared with *dotted lines* representing the previous cycle. Note that atrioventricular conduction time gets longer with each cycle, but each increase is smaller than the preceding increase, causing R-R intervals to shorten. (From Watanabe, Y., & Driefus, L. [1995]. Atrioventricular block: Basic concepts. In W. J. Mandel [Ed.]. *Cardiac arrhythmias: Their mechanisms, diagnosis, and management* [p. 420]. Philadelphia: J. B. Lippincott.)

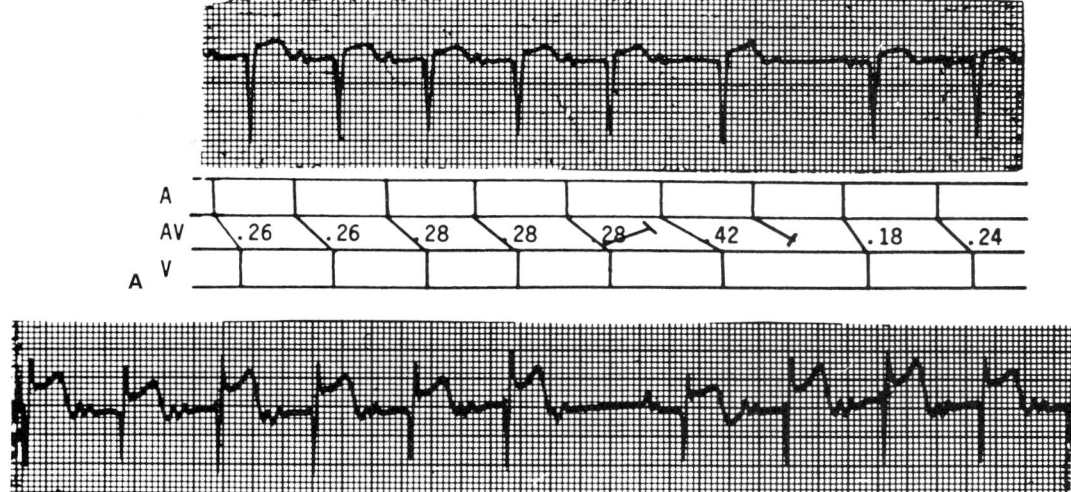

■ **Figure 19–36.** Atypical Wenckebach conduction. (*A*) Gradual lengthening of PR intervals until the sixth beat of the cycle, when the PR interval is suddenly longer than expected. The ladder diagram illustrates a possible explanation for the suddenly prolonged PR interval: reentry of the impulse back into the atrioventricular node causes it to be more refractory than expected to the next sinus impulse. PR intervals are shown in seconds. (*B*) Very gradual increases in PR intervals from 0.28 second in the first beat to 0.30 second in the last beat of the cycle. Note that the PR interval that follows the pause is 0.24 second. (From Jacobson, C [1983]. Interpretation of complex arrhythmias. In S. L. Woods [Ed.], *Cardiovascular critical care nursing* [p. 196]. New York: Churchill Livingstone. By permission.)

intervals may remain constant for several beats or may actually get smaller at one point in the cycle. Again, it is important to compare the PR interval preceding the pause with the PR interval after the pause to help establish the presence of Wenckebach conduction.

Wenckebach conduction can occur through the AV node in rhythms other than normal sinus rhythm. Figure 19-37*A* shows AT with a gradual Wenckebach conduction pattern. Figure 19-37*B* shows a rhythm that could be mistaken for atrial fibrillation with a rapid ventricular response. The overall appearance

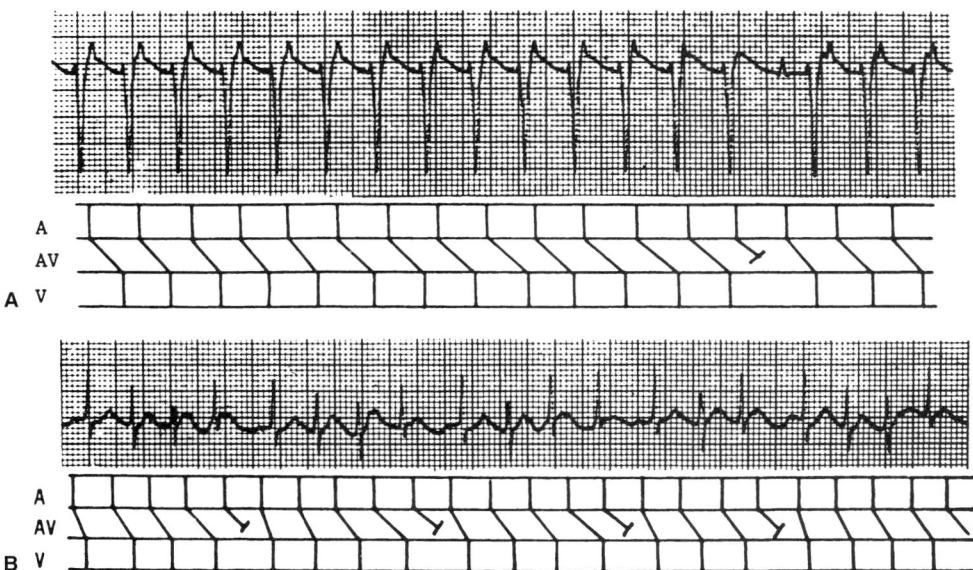

■ **Figure 19–37.** Atrial tachycardia with Wenckebach conduction. (*A*) P waves visible at a rate of 167 beats/min. The PR interval increase gradually from the first beat to the beat preceding the pause, and the PR interval that follows the pause is the shortest one in the strip. (*B*) P waves are visible at a rate of 214 beats/min, and PR intervals gradually increase before the pause. (From Jacobson, C. [1983]. Interpretation of complex arrhythmias. In S. L. Woods [Ed.], *Cardiovascular critical care nursing.* New York: Churchill Livingstone. By permission.)

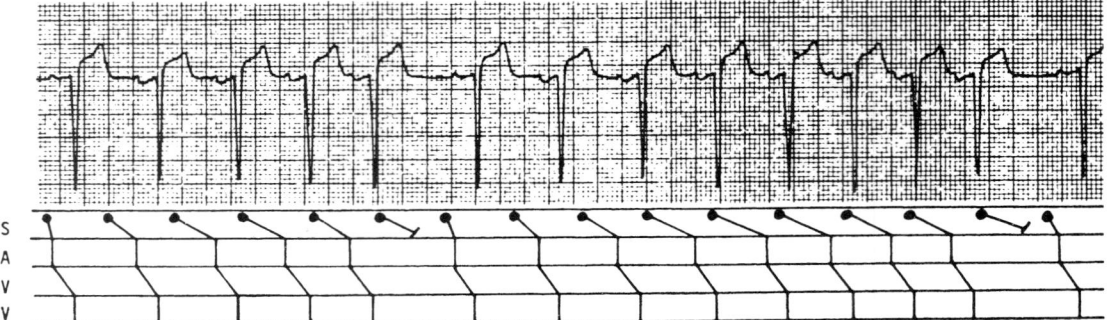

■ **Figure 19–38.** Sinus Wenckebach conduction. S indicates the sinus node, which is not visible on the electrocardiogram. The slant of the line through the S level indicates conduction time from sinus node to the atria. Note that sinoatrial conduction times progressively increase until a sinus impulse is completely blocked. PR intervals are constant, and P-P intervals gradually shorten before each pause. (From Jacobson, C. [1983]. Interpretation of complex arrhythmias. In S. L. Woods [Ed.], *Cardiovascular critical care nursing* [p.199]. New York: Churchill Livingstone. By permission.)

of the rhythm reveals group beating, and P waves occurring at a rate of 214 beats per minute can be seen in the pauses. Once P waves have been identified, it is easy to see that PR intervals progressively increase until a P wave fails to conduct to the ventricles, resulting in the pause.

Wenckebach Conduction in the Sinus Node

Sinus Wenckebach conduction is a form of sinus exit block in which sinus impulses are formed normally in the sinus node but take progressively longer to exit from the sinus node into the atria, until finally one impulse is completely blocked and fails to reach the atria. It is impossible to see this progressive prolongation of sinoatrial conduction time directly because the ECG does not show sinus node activity. What is seen on the ECG is the P wave as the atria depolarize in response to the sinus impulse. Therefore, sinus Wenckebach conduction appears on the ECG as progressive shortening of the P-P intervals until a P wave fails to appear. The length of the P-P interval that includes the pause is less than twice the length of any other P-P interval in the sequence. After the pause, the cycle repeats itself, thus giving the appearance of group beating (Fig. 19-38).

Sinus Wenckebach conduction is more easily understood if compared with typical AV Wenckebach conduction. In AV Wenckebach conduction, the progressive conduction delay takes place across the AV node and can be measured in the PR interval. In sinus Wenckebach conduction, the progressive conduction delay takes place across the sinoatrial junction and cannot be directly measured. AV Wenckebach conduction displays progressive shortening of R-R intervals until a P wave fails to conduct to the ventricles, resulting in a pause. This cycle then repeats itself, giving the appearance of group beating. Sinus Wenckebach conduction displays progressive shortening of the P-P intervals until an impulse fails to reach the atria, resulting in a pause and the absence of the next expected P wave. The cycle then repeats itself, giving the appearance of group beating. The P-P intervals shorten in sinus Wenckebach conduction for the same reason the R-R intervals shorten in AV Wenckebach conduction; although the impulse takes

progressively longer to exit from the sinus node, it takes longer by a smaller amount each time (see Fig. 19-35). The PR intervals remain constant in sinus Wenckebach conduction because the conduction delay is from sinus node to atria, not through the AV node.

Wenckebach Conduction in the Bundle Branches

Wenckebach conduction in the bundle-branch system is a progressive delay in conduction of the impulse down a bundle branch into its ventricle until an impulse is totally blocked in that bundle branch. The ECG demonstrates progressive widening of the QRS complex in successive beats until the last beat in the Wenckebach cycle shows complete bundle-branch block. Figure 19-39 shows Wenckebach conduction in the left and right bundle branches. The QRS complex gradually widens as the impulse is conducted progressively more slowly through the involved bundle branch. The first beat in the sequence is conducted normally because the impulse in the preceding beat is completely blocked in the affected bundle, allowing a prolonged recovery time in that bundle branch. This prolonged recovery time allows the next beat to travel without delay through the affected bundle branch, resulting in a normal QRS complex. Figure 19-40 shows Wenckebach conduction in the left anterior fascicle of the left bundle branch. The ECG shows progressive left axis deviation as the impulse is conducted progressively more slowly through the anterior fascicle.

Wenckebach Conduction In Reentrant Pathways

Ectopic beats can be caused by reentry of an original stimulus into previously depolarized areas of the heart through reentry pathways. Reentry can occur in various parts of the heart and is postulated to be a common cause of PVC when it occurs in the ventricles. One of the hallmarks of reentry in the ventricles is the presence of constant coupling intervals between the normal beat and the PVC (Carleton, 1977). The coupling interval represents conduction time through the ventricular reentry path-

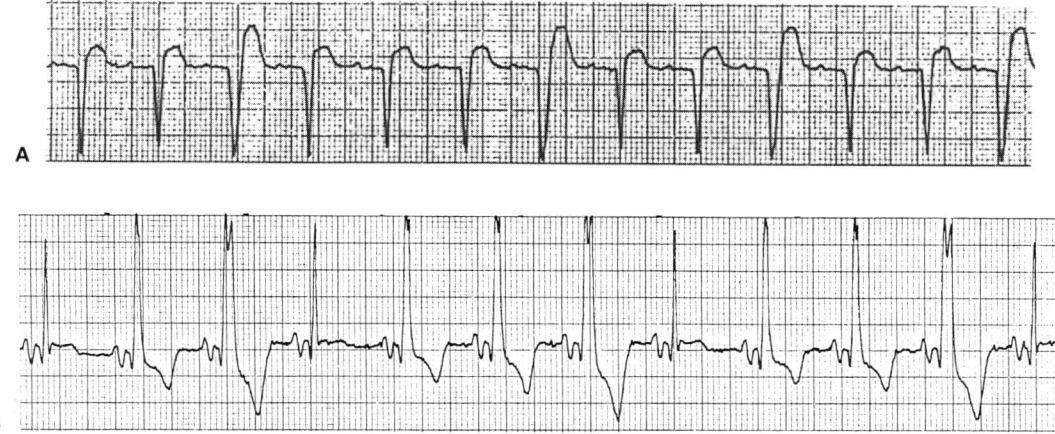

■ **Figure 19–39.** Wenckebach conduction in the bundle branches. (*A*) Sinus rhythm with Wenckebach conduction in the left bundle branch. QRS complexes gradually widen until complete left bundle-branch block occurs. (*B*) Sinus rhythm with Wenckebach conduction in the right bundle branch. QRS complexes gradually develop a wider terminal R wave until complete right bundlebranch block occurs.

way and is usually fixed or constant, indicating that reentering impulses take the same amount of time to travel the reentry loop each time they occur. Fixed coupling has been one of the main criteria used in differentiating randomly occurring PVC from ventricular parasystole.

Wenckebach conduction through the reentry pathway is postulated to be responsible for variable coupling intervals in the absence of parasystole (Carleton, 1977). Figure 19-41 shows sinus rhythm with ventricular bigeminy. The coupling intervals gradually increase until finally a PVC fails to appear. The ladder diagram illustrates progressively prolonged conduction times through the reentry loop until the fifth reentering impulse fails to travel through the loop, resulting in the absence of a PVC. Typically, conduction times through the reentry pathway increase by decreasing increments, just as PR intervals do in AV Wenckebach, and interectopic intervals decrease before the blocked impulse, just as R-R intervals do in AV Wenckebach conduction. Figure 19-41 illustrates an atypical case of Wenckebach conduction because the last conduction time through the reentry pathway is longer than would be expected; conduction times increase by decreasing

amounts during the first three trips around the loop, then increase by a longer amount for the final circuit.

Wenckebach Exit Block from an Ectopic Focus

Wenckebach exit block can occur from an ectopic atrial, junctional, or ventricular focus just as it can from the sinus node. Wenckebach conduction from an ectopic focus is a progressive increase in conduction time of an impulse from its site of origin into surrounding tissue. Figure 19-42*A* shows atrial fibrillation with a regular junctional rhythm controlling the ventricles, a sign of digitalis toxicity. In Figure 19-42*B*, note the group beating and gradually shortening R-R intervals typical of Wenckebach conduction. The ladder diagram illustrates that the ectopic junctional focus is firing regularly, but the impulse takes progressively longer to exit into the AV junctional tissue until, finally, an impulse fails to exit from its site of origin, resulting in a pause. The sequence repeats itself, giving the appearance of group beating. In Figure 19-42*C*, the conduction ratio changes to 3 : 2, resulting in groups of two beats.

Figure 19-43*A* is a 12-lead ECG tracing showing multiple runs of VT. Note that, in each lead, the R-R intervals gradually decrease during the runs of tachycardia, as happens in typical Wenckebach conduction. Figure 19-43*B* shows an enlarged lead II with a ladder diagram illustrating that the ectopic ventricular focus fires regularly, but conduction times from the ectopic focus into the ventricle gradually increase until an impulse finally fails to exit from its site of origin, resulting in the termination of the tachycardia.

Multilevel Atrioventricular Block

A block in impulse conduction can exist at more than one level in the AV conduction system, including multiple levels in the AV node (upper, middle, or lower parts of the AV node), His-Purkinje system, and AV bypass tracts (Castellanos et al., 1978; Castellanos et al., 1977; Halpern et al., 1973;

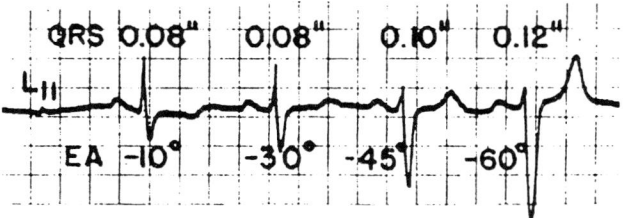

■ **Figure 19–40.** Wenckebach conduction in the left anterior fascicle of the left bundle branch. Lead II shows progressive left axis deviation from -10 to -60 degrees as conduction is progressively delayed through the left anterior fascicle. EA, electrical axis. The QRS gradually widens, possibly because of progressive right bundle-branch block. (From Sclarovsky, S., Strasberg, B., & Agmon, J. [1978]. Coexistent Wenckebach phenomenon in the distal branches of the specialized conduction system. *Chest, 73,* 534.)

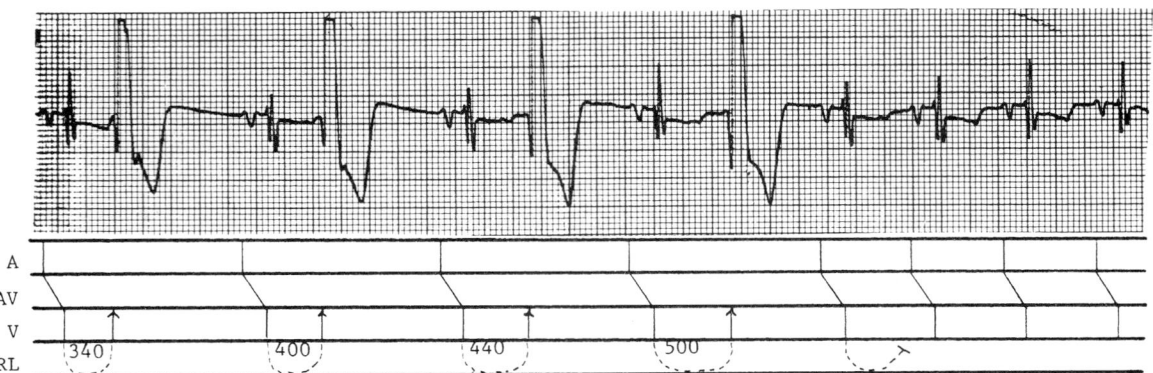

■ **Figure 19–41.** Wenckebach conduction through the reentry loop. Coupling intervals gradually increase from 340 to 500 millisceconds until the fifth reentering impulse is blocked in the loop. Interectopic intervals decrease slightly before the blocked impulse. Coupling intervals are shown in milliseconds. RL, reentry loop.

Kosowsky et al., 1976; Leon et al., 1975; Watanabe et al., 1995). *Alternating Wenckebach* is a term used to describe rhythms that demonstrate Wenckebach conduction of alternate atrial impulses (i.e., sinus or atrial rhythms with 2 : 1 conduction, in which the PR intervals of conducted beats progressively increase until two or more P waves are blocked). Alternating Wenckebach conduction can occur in the presence of sinus rhythm, AT, or atrial flutter and can be explained by postulating block at two or more levels in the AV conduction system. For the purposes of this discussion, the term *multilevel block* refers to two levels of block in the AV node.

In multilevel AV block, conduction in the upper level of the AV node can be either Wenckebach or 2 : 1 block, as can conduction in the lower level. Rhythms in which Wenckebach conduction is present in the upper level display a variety of patterns depending on the length of the Wenckebach cycle and the type of block in the lower level. These rhythms may contain one, two, or more consecutively blocked P waves. Rhythms in which there is 2 : 1 conduction in the upper level and Wenckebach conduction in the lower level demonstrate the group beating of typical Wenckebach conduction and progressive prolongation in the PR interval of conducted beats, terminating in three blocked P waves.

Figure 19-44*A* illustrates sinus tachycardia with 2 : 1 and 3 : 1 conduction and could be mistaken for complete AV block because PR intervals are so inconsistent, except that the ventricular response is not regular, as would be expected to occur in the presence of complete block. Note that the PR intervals before the conducted beats gradually increase until two P waves are completely blocked after the third QRS complex. The ladder diagram below illustrates two levels of block in the AV node: 7 : 6 Wenckebach conduction is present in the upper

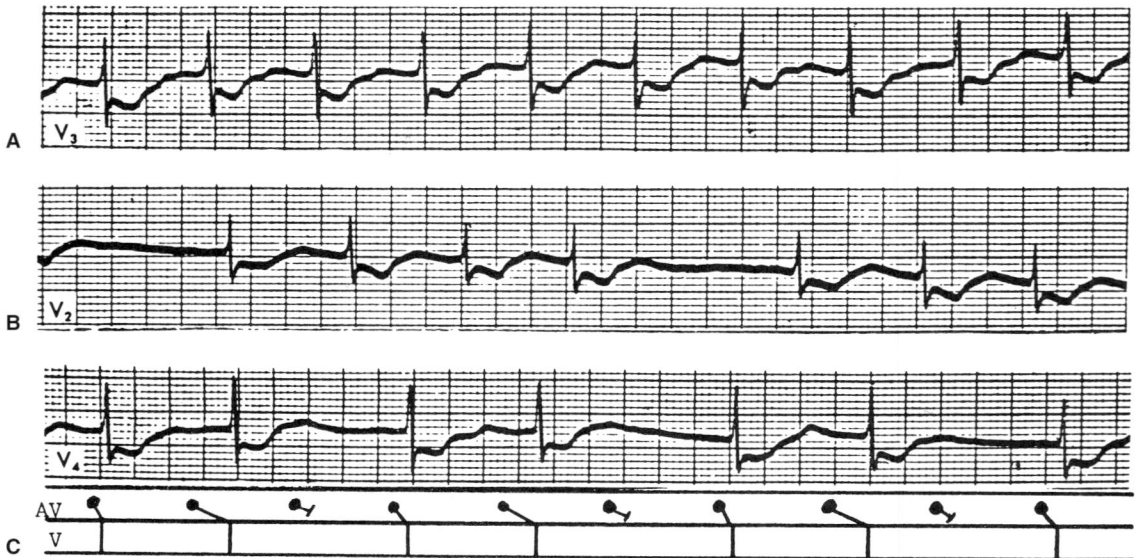

■ **Figure 19–42.** Wenckebach exit block from an atrioventricular junctional focus. (*A*) Atrial fibrillation with an accelerated junctional rhythm controlling the ventricles. (*B*) A 5 : 4 Wenckebach exit block from the junctional focus. Note group beating and gradual shortening of R-R intervals. (*C*) A 3 : 2 Wenckebach exit block from the junctional focus. (From Marriott, H. J. L., & Conover, M. [1989]. *Advanced concepts in arrhythmias* [2nd ed., p. 79]. St. Louis: CV Mosby.)

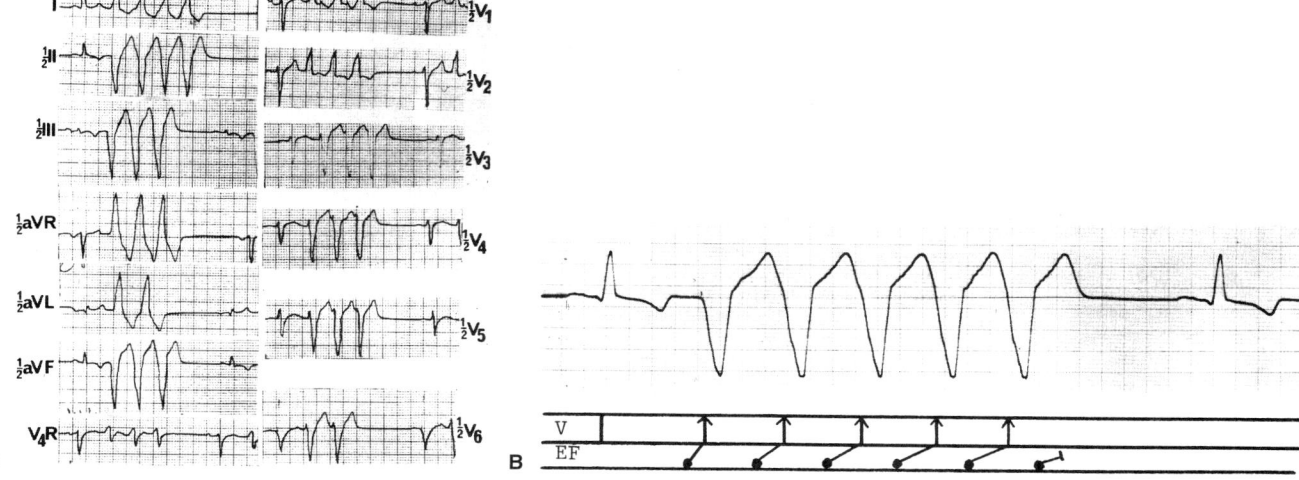

■ **Figure 19–43.** Ventricular tachycardia (VT) with Wenckebach exit block. (*A*) A 12-lead electrocardiogram (ECG) showing runs of VT. Note that R-R intervals decrease progressively in each lead. (*B*) Enlarged lead II from ECG in *A*. Ladder diagram illustrates a VT Wenckebach conduction from the ventricular focus. EF, ectopic focus. (From Peter, T., Harper, R. W., Vohra, J. K. et al. [1976]. The electrocardiographic recognition of Wenckebach phenomenon in sites other than the atrioventricular junction. *Heart & Lung*, 5, 747.)

level, 2 : 1 conduction is present in the lower level, and two consecutive P waves are blocked at the end of the Wenckebach cycle. This conduction pattern, ending with two blocked P waves, occurs when there is an odd number of P waves in the Wenckebach cycle in the upper level (Kosowsky et al., 1976; Leon et al., 1975).

The strip in Figure 19-44*B* shows sinus tachycardia with varying PR intervals and frequent nonconducted P waves. Note that the PR intervals of alternate beats are progressively

prolonged and that only one P wave at a time is blocked. The ladder diagram shows two levels of block in the AV node, with Wenckebach conduction in the upper level, an even number of atrial complexes in each Wenckebach cycle, and 2 : 1 conduction in the lower level. When there are even numbers of atrial beats in the Wenckebach cycle, the P wave blocked in the upper level follows a beat that has been conducted in the lower level; therefore, the beat blocked in the upper level would have been blocked in the lower level if it had been conducted that

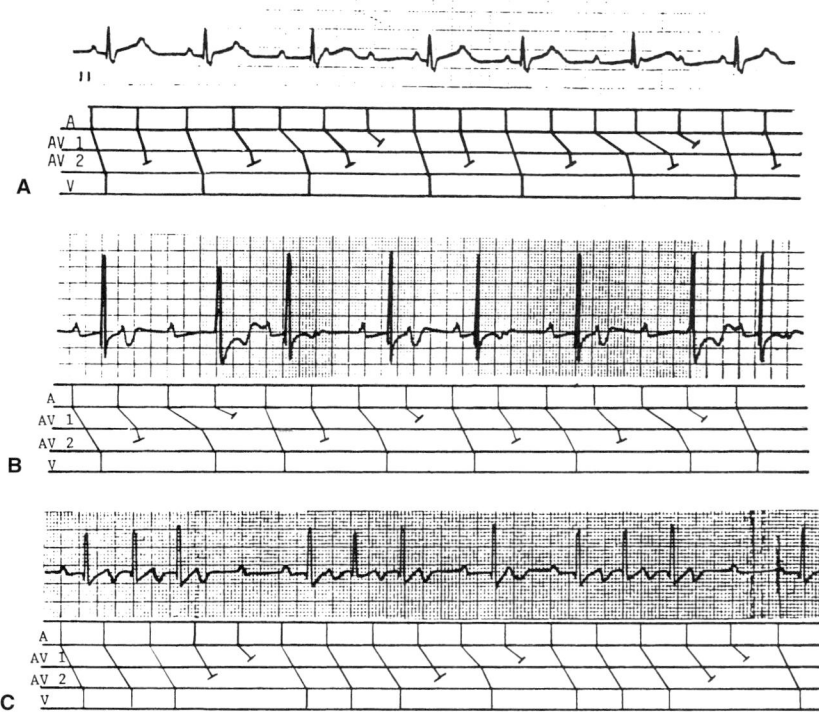

■ **Figure 19–44.** Multilevel atrioventricular (AV) block. The AV area in the ladder diagrams is divided into two levels to show conduction patterns in each level. (*A*) Sinus tachycardia with 7 : 6 Wenckebach conduction in the upper level of the AV junction and 2 : 1 conduction in the lower level. (*B*) Wenckebach conduction. 4 : 3 and 6 : 5, in the upper level and 2 : 1 conduction below. (*C*) Wenckebach conduction in both levels. (*A* adapted from Halpeern, M. S., Nau, G. J., Levi, R. J. et al. [1973]. Wenckebach periods of alternate beats: Clinical and experimental observations. *Circulation,* 48, 42; *B* and *C* adapted from Kosowsky, B., Latif, P., & Radoff, A. M. [1976]. Multilevel atrioventricular block. *Circulation,* 54, 918. By permission of the American Heart Association, Inc.)

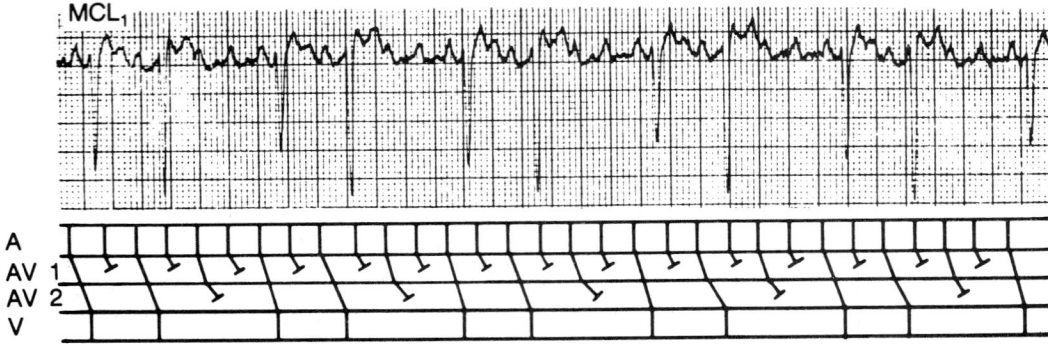

■ **Figure 19–45.** Atrial flutter and multilevel AV block with 2 : 1 conduction in the upper level and 3 : 2 Wenckebach conduction in the lower level. Note group beating and progressive increase in alternate FR intervals.

far (Kosowsky et al., 1976). Thus, P waves 5, 9, and 15 are conducted through the lower level of 2 : 1 block even though the previous P wave was not blocked on that level.

Figure 19-44*C* demonstrates sinus tachycardia with periods of 1 : 1 conduction, progressive prolongation of successive PR intervals, and a varying number of blocked P waves. This pattern could be mistaken for typical AV Wenckebach conduction except that there are times when more than one P wave in a row is blocked. In addition, the PR intervals that follow the pauses are not necessarily the shortest PR intervals and at times are longer than the PR intervals preceding the pauses. The ladder diagram illustrates two levels of AV block with Wenckebach conduction in both levels.

When 2 : 1 conduction is present in the upper level and Wenckebach conduction occurs in the lower level, the rhythm presents with the overall appearance of group beating and progressive prolongation of alternate PR intervals and ends with three blocked atrial impulses. Figure 19-45 shows atrial flutter with a ventricular response that occurs in groups of two. Note that the FR intervals (the distance from the beginning of a flutter wave to the beginning of the QRS complex) of alternate atrial beats gradually prolong and that the cycle ends with three blocked atrial impulses. The ladder diagram illustrates two levels of AV block with 2 : 1 conduction in the upper level and Wenckebach with 3 : 2 conduction in the lower level.

Figure 19-46 shows atrial flutter with a variable ventricular response. Note that the QRS complexes occur in groups, the FR interval of alternate beats is gradually prolonged, and the cycle ends with three blocked atrial impulses. These are all signs of multilevel block with 2 : 1 conduction in the upper level and Wenckebach conduction in the lower level. Note also that the flutter waves occur in groups of two with alternately longer and shorter F-F intervals, a sign of Wenckebach conduction. The ladder diagram illustrates Wenckebach exit block from the flutter focus in the atrium, leading to the grouping of flutter waves. There are two levels of block in the AV node, with 2 : 1 conduction in the upper level and Wenckebach with 5 : 4 conduction in the lower level, causing the grouping of QRS complexes.

The mechanism of multilevel AV block is not known but is thought to involve concealed conduction of impulses to various depths in the AV node or His-Purkinje system, affecting the conduction of subsequent impulses through those regions (Kosowsky et al., 1976). This type of block has been shown to be a common response to rapid atrial pacing, AT or flutter, and administration of digitalis for treatment of atrial flutter (Castellanos et al., 1977; Castellanos et al., 1978; Kosowsky et al., 1976). It has also been shown to be a sign of advanced digitalis toxicity (Castellanos et al., 1978) and to occur in patients with primary disease of the conduction system or with inferior MI (Castellanos et al., 1978;

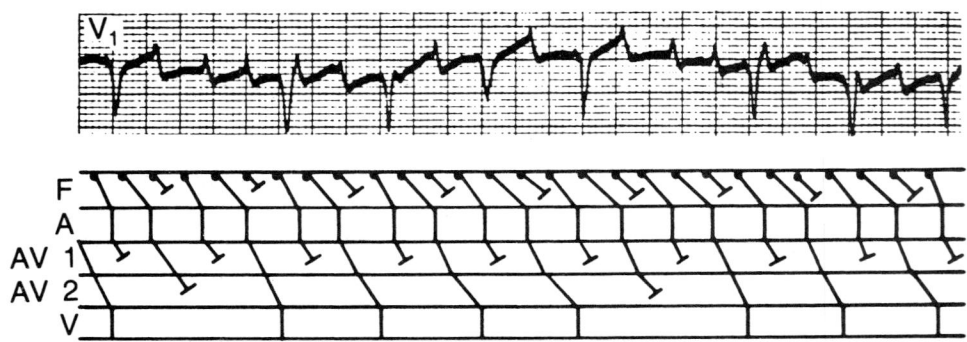

■ **Figure 19–46.** Atrial flutter with 3 : 2 Wenckebach exit block out of the flutter focus. In the atrioventricular junction, there are two levels of block: 2 : 1 conduction in the upper level and 5 : 4 Wenckebach conduction in the lower level. (Adapted from Marriott, H. J. L., & Conover, M. [1989]. *Advanced concepts in arrhythmias* [2nd ed., p. 344]. St. Louis: CV Mosby.)

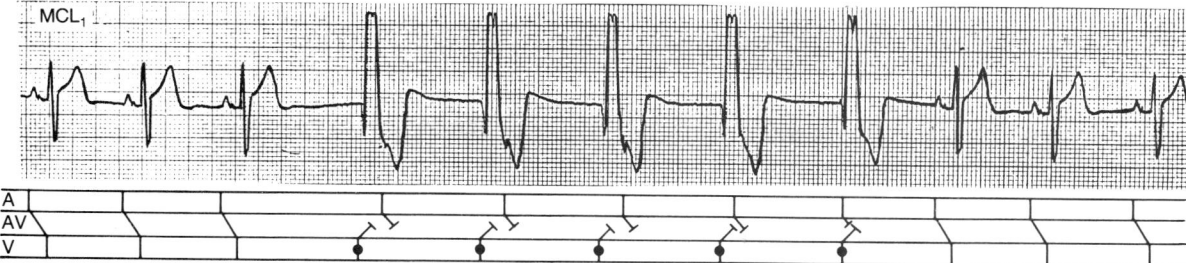

■ **Figure 19–47.** Atrioventricular (AV) dissociation due to slowing of the primary pacemaker. Sinus arrhythmia is present; the sinus rate slows after the third beat, allowing a ventricular escape pacemaker to take control of the ventricles at a rate of 60 beats/min. AV dissociation lasts until the rate of the sinus node becomes faster than the rate of the ventricular pacemaker.

Sclarovsky et al., 1978a). The clinical significance of multi-level AV block appears to depend on whether the sites of block are in the AV node, considered to be common and benign, or below the AV node in the His-Purkinje system, thought to be more dangerous; or whether the block is tachycardia dependent, thus benign, or associated with MI and possibly more dangerous.

Atrioventricular Dissociation

Atrioventricular dissociation means that the atria and ventricles are under the control of separate pacemakers and are beating independently of each other. Usually, the atria are controlled by the sinus node, but they can also be under the control of an atrial focus, as in AT, flutter, or fibrillation. The ventricles can be under the control of a junctional pacemaker or a ventricular pacemaker. AV dissociation is not a primary arrhythmia but is always secondary to some other disturbance that results in dissociation. Complete AV dissociation means that the atria and ventricles are always controlled by separate pacemakers and that the two different pacemakers never conduct into the other chamber to "capture" it. Incomplete dissociation occurs when one chamber is occasionally depolarized by the other chamber's pacemaker.

AV dissociation can be secondary to (1) slowing of the primary pacemaker (sinus node), (2) acceleration of a subsidiary pacemaker (AV junction or ventricle), (3) AV block, or (4) interference, or can result from a combination of these causes (Marriott, 1988; Myerburg et al., 2001; Olgin & Zipes, 2001).

If the rate of the sinus node slows below the rate of a subsidiary pacemaker in the AV junction or in the ventricles, the subsidiary pacemaker assumes control of the ventricles whereas the atria are still under the control of the sinus node. This dissociation, sometimes called *dissociation by default,* lasts until a sinus impulse occurs at a time when it can be conducted into the ventricles and regain control of them or until it speeds up enough to override the subsidiary pacemaker (Fig. 19-47).

AV dissociation can result from the acceleration of a subsidiary pacemaker, either junctional or ventricular, that fires faster than the sinus node and thus assumes control of the ventricles (*dissociation by usurpation*). Dissociation lasts until the rate of the subsidiary pacemaker slows below the rate of the sinus node or the sinus accelerates to a rate faster than that of the subsidiary pacemaker (Fig. 19-48). VT is an example of AV dissociation due to acceleration of a ventricular pacemaker; VT can be diagnosed by demonstrating independently occurring P waves, thus proving AV dissociation (see Fig. 19-22). Complete AV block is a form of AV dissociation because none of the atrial impulses conducts to the ventricles and the atria and ventricles are under the control of separate pacemakers (Fig. 19-49). Remember: every complete AV block is AV dissociation, but not every AV dissociation is complete AV block!

AV dissociation can result when an ectopic impulse, usually junctional or ventricular, makes the AV node refractory to the next sinus impulse, interfering with the conduction of the sinus impulse and allowing another pacemaker to control the ventricles (Fig. 19-50). Anything that causes a pause in the rhythm, like a premature beat, a blocked P wave, or sudden

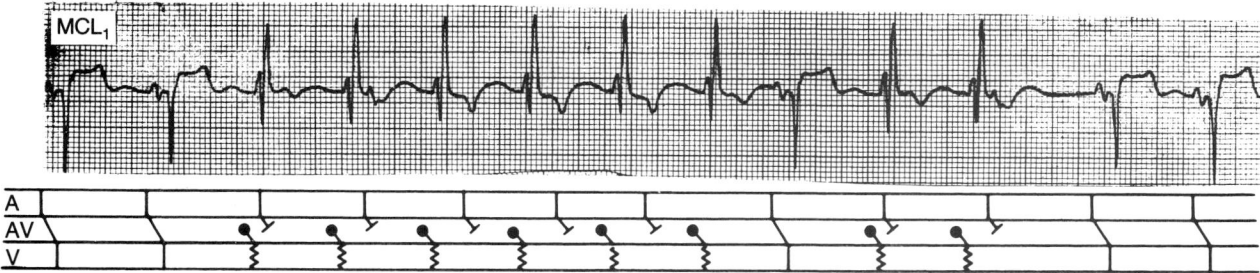

■ **Figure 19–48.** Atrioventricular dissociation due to acceleration of a subsidiary pacemaker. An accelerated junctional pacemaker assumes control of the ventricles and conducts aberrantly (right bundle-branch block) at a rate of 88 beats/min. Sinus arrhythmia is present at a rate in the 70s. Vertical wavy line indicates aberrant conduction.

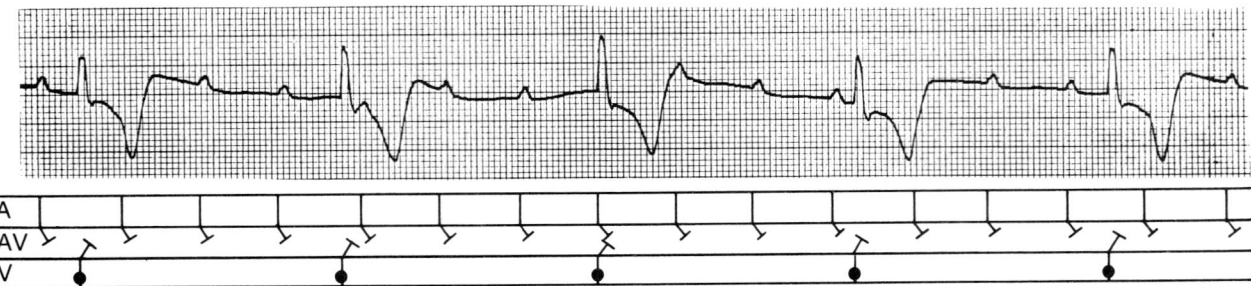

■ **Figure 19–49.** Atrioventricular (AV) dissociation due to complete AV block. Sinus tachycardia at a rate of 115 beats/min with third-degree AV block and a ventricular pacemaker controlling the ventricles at a rate of 34 beats/min. (From Jacobson, C. [1983]. Interpretation of complex arrhythmias. In S. L. Woods [Ed.], *Cardiovascular critical care nursing.* [p. 216]. New York: Churchill Livingstone. By permission.)

termination of a tachycardia can allow the escape of a subsidiary pacemaker and result in AV dissociation.

The term *isorhythmic dissociation* refers to AV dissociation with the atrial focus and the focus that controls the ventricles firing at almost identical rates. It is characterized by P waves that move into and out of the QRS complex, always staying close on either side or in the middle of the QRS (Fig. 19-51).

Parasystole

Parasystole is an ectopic focus that fires regularly and independently of the dominant cardiac rhythm and is protected from being depolarized by impulses from the dominant pacemaker.

Parasystole can occur in the atria, AV junction, or ventricles, but it occurs most often in the ventricles, where it is most easily recognized. The parasystolic focus is an automatic focus that spontaneously depolarizes but is surrounded by tissue with low excitability, causing decremental conduction of impulses coming from the dominant pacemaker and entrance block of outside stimuli. This same tissue may prevent conduction of the parasystolic impulse into surrounding tissue, causing exit block from the parasystolic focus (Castellanos, Saoudi, Moleiro & Myerburg, 2000; Conover, 1996; Fisch, 2000; Kinoshita, 1978; Marriott, 1988).

Parasystole is diagnosed from the ECG by the following criteria: (1) marked variation in coupling intervals of ectopic beats; (2) presence of interectopic intervals (the distance from one

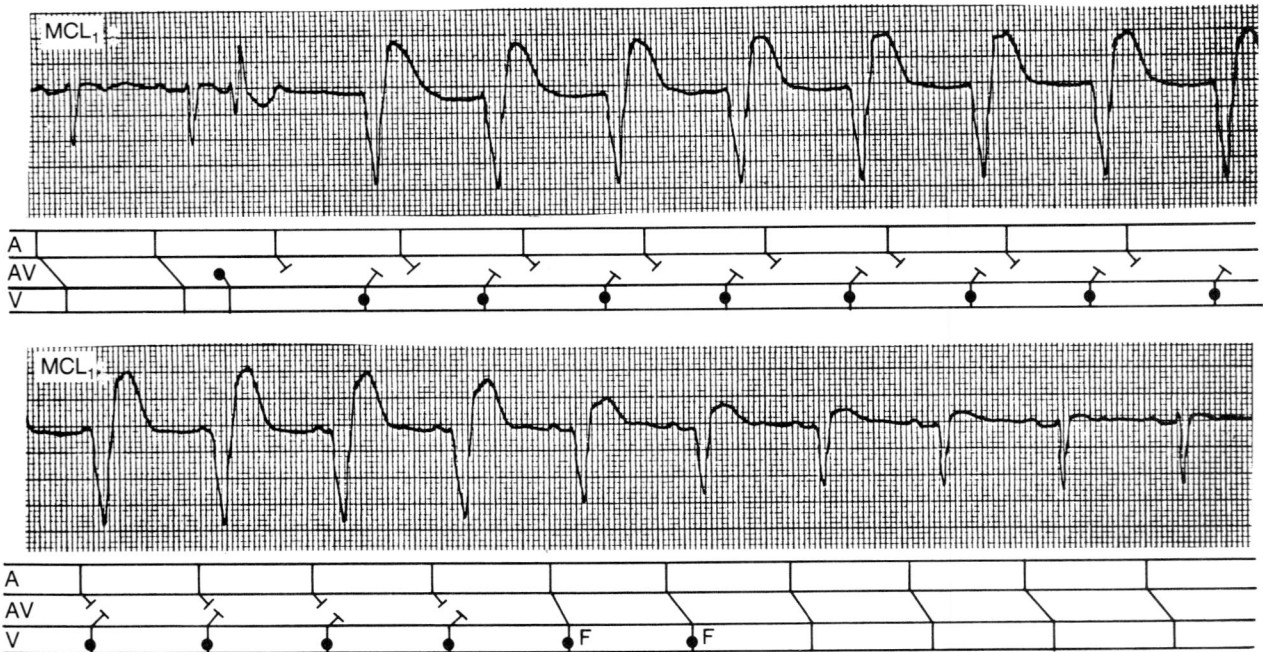

■ **Figure 19–50.** Atrioventricular (AV) dissociation due to interference. Strips are continuous. Sinus rhythm is present at a rate of 68 beats/min. The third beat in the top strip is a premature junctional beat that interferes with conduction of the next sinus impulse, which in turn is not conducted through the AV node. The resulting pause allows a ventricular rhythm to emerge at a rate of 65 beats/min. The bottom strip shows the slightly faster sinus P waves emerging in front of the QRS until ventricular capture occurs in the seventh beat. F, fusion beats. (From Jacobson, C. [1983]. Interpretation of complex arrhythmias. In S. L. Woods [Ed.], *Cardiovascular critical care nursing.* New York: Churchill Livingstone. By permission.)

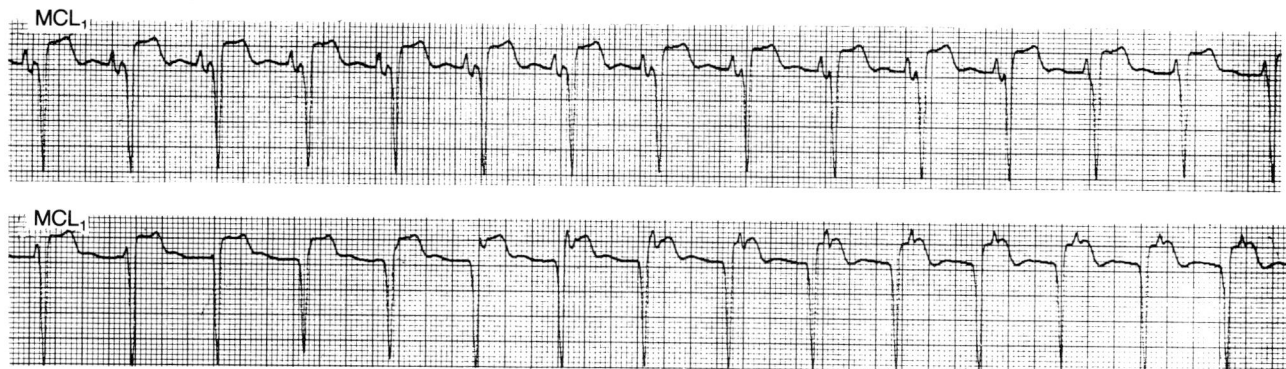

■ Figure 19–51. Isorhythmic dissociation. There is dissociation between a sinus rhythm and a junctional rhythm, both at a rate of approximately 88 beats/min. P waves disappear into the QRS complex toward the end of the top strip and emerge on the other side of the QRS in the bottom strip, always staying close to the QRS or in the middle of it.

ectopic beat to the next) that are multiples of a common denominator; and (3) the presence of fusion beats resulting from the simultaneous depolarization of a chamber, either atria or ventricles, by the dominant rhythm and the parasystolic focus. A simple ventricular parasystole appears on the ECG as PVC occurring at a regular rate, or a multiple of the rate, whenever the ventricular focus fires at a time when the ventricle is not refractory as a result of depolarization by the dominant pacemaker (Fig. 19-52). When the parasystolic focus fires during the refractory period of the ventricle, its impulse is unable to excite surrounding refractory tissue and it cannot be seen on the ECG. Coupling intervals vary because the parasystolic focus is an independently firing automatic focus that is not related to the sinus rhythm and, therefore, does not depend on the sinus rhythm for its existence. PVC due to reentry have fixed coupling intervals because they depend on the preceding impulse for their existence. Ventricular fusion beats occur whenever the parasystolic focus fires at the same time that the dominant focus enters the ventricles and begins to depolarize them. Atrial or

junctional parasystole behaves the same way, with coupling intervals measured from normal P wave to ectopic P wave and fusion beats occurring in the atria (Fig. 19-53).

A parasystolic focus usually fires at rates between 38 and 60 beats per minute but has been reported to occur at rates up to 300 beats per minute. The focus may fire regularly, exhibiting regular interectopic intervals or intervals that are exact multiples of its basic interval (a variation of 0.10 second is allowed before intervals are considered irregular); it may fire irregularly, resulting in irregular interectopic intervals. Several factors responsible for variance in parasystolic firing rate have been identified (Castellanos et al., 2000; Conover, 1996; Kinoshita, 1978; Lightfoot, 1978; Pick & Langendorf, 1976).

1. Intermittent firing of the parasystolic focus.
2. Change in the firing rate of the parasystolic focus secondary to ischemia, drug effects, electrolyte imbalances, autonomic influences, or any factor known to influence phase 4 depolarization of automatic cells.

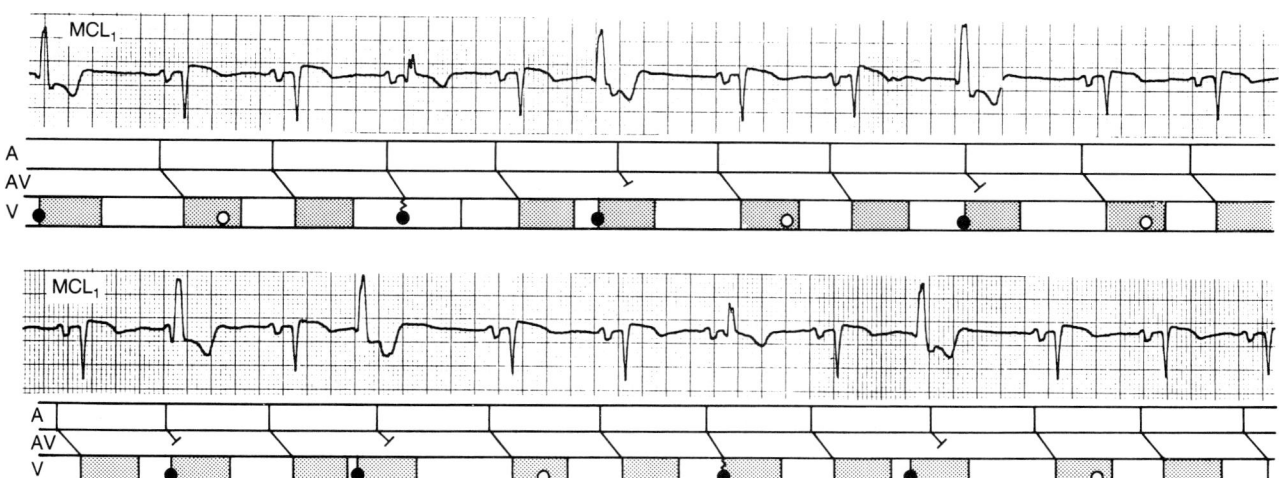

■ Figure 19–52. Ventricular parasystole. Sinus arrhythmia is present at a rate in the 60s with multiple premature ventricular complexes. Note the following characteristics of ventricular parasystole: (1) marked variation in coupling intervals. (2) presence of fusion beats, and (3) interectopic intervals that are a multiple of the basic parasystolic rate of 38 beats/min. The ladder diagram illustrates the parasystolic focus firing regularly at a rate of 38 beats/min. *Solid circles* indicate the parasystolic focus that is seen on the electrocardiogram (ECG); *open circles* indicate the focus firing but not seen on the ECG; the *shaded area* represents ventricular refractory period.

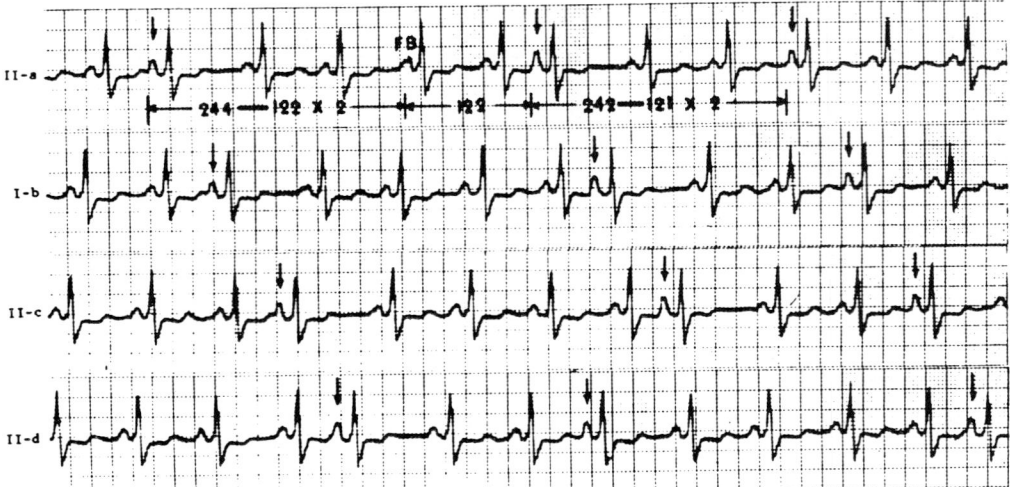

■ **Figure 19–53.** Sinus rhythm at a rate of 75 beats/min with atrial parasystole at a rate of 50 beats/min. Strips are continuous. *Arrows* indicate the atrial parasystolic P waves. Note an atrial fusion beat (FB). The numbers represent hundredths of a second. (From Chung, E. K. [1980]. *Electrocardiography: Practical applications with vectorial principles* [2nd ed., p. 552]. Hagerstown, MD: Harper & Row.)

3. Varying degrees of exit block from the parasystolic focus. Block can be type I (Wenckebach exit block), with impulses taking progressively longer to exit from the parasystolic focus into surrounding tissue, or type II, with sudden absence of an impulse where it would otherwise be expected. Exit block from a parasystolic focus is presumed to be present whenever the focus fires but fails to appear on the ECG when the refractory period of the ventricles is over.

4. Varying degrees of entrance block of the dominant impulse into the parasystolic focus. Although entrance block is the protective mechanism that allows the parasystolic focus to continue firing regularly without interference from the dominant pacemaker, a temporary loss of this protection can occur, and the dominant impulses can enter and reset the parasystolic focus.

Although simple parasystole can be recognized by the usual ECG criteria, more complicated forms of parasystole can occur when entrance or exit block is present, fixed coupling occurs, or more than one parasystolic focus fires at the same time.

Concealed Conduction

Concealed conduction is conduction of an impulse into a part of the conduction system but not completely through it, causing refractoriness that affects conduction or formation of subsequent impulses. Concealed conduction can occur in an anterograde direction from supraventricular impulses into the AV junction or His-Purkinje system, or in a retrograde direction from the ventricles backward into the AV junction. Because the original impulse never reaches its final destination, there is no evidence on the ECG that concealed conduction has occurred other than its influence on the conduction or formation of subsequent impulses.

Three types of concealed conduction are discussed next: (1) concealed conduction affecting subsequent impulse conduction, (2) concealed conduction affecting subsequent impulse formation, and (3) concealed impulse formation affecting subsequent impulse conduction (Fisch, 2000; Watanabe, 1978).

Concealed Conduction Affecting Subsequent Impulse Conduction

The most common example of concealed conduction occurs in atrial fibrillation, when the AV node is bombarded with hundreds of impulses each minute, most of which are blocked in the AV node. Many of these impulses are conducted to various depths in the AV node, leaving it refractory to following impulses and causing the characteristic irregular ventricular response in atrial fibrillation. Because the impulses that incompletely penetrate the AV node never reach the ventricles, there is no evidence on the ECG that they conducted at all, other than their effect on preventing conduction of following impulses.

Another common example of concealed conduction is illustrated in Figure 19-54. Figure 19-54A shows sinus tachycardia with ventricular bigeminy. The sinus beat that follows each PVC is not conducted, presumably because of concealed conduction of the PVC backward into the AV node, causing it to be refractory and preventing the conduction of the next sinus impulse. Figure 19-54B shows sinus rhythm with frequent PVC that conduct retrograde into the AV node, causing varying degrees of refractoriness that impede conduction of following sinus beats. Some PVC are followed by sinus beats with prolonged PR intervals and others by beats that are completely blocked; both situations are due to retrograde concealed conduction of the ventricular impulse into the AV node.

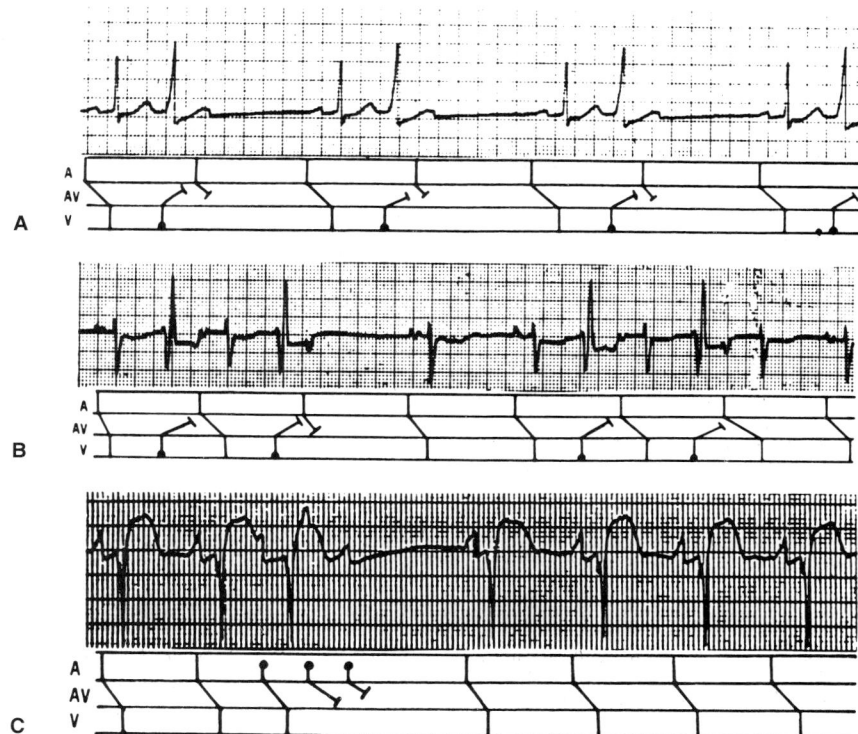

■ **Figure 19–54.** Concealed conduction affecting conduction of subsequent impulses. (*A*) Concealed conduction of premature ventricular complexes (PVCs) into the atrioventricular (AV) node, causing block of subsequent P waves. (*B*) Concealed conduction of PVCs into the AV node, causing varying degrees of conduction delay of subsequent sinus beats with a pseudo Wenckebach pattern. (*C*) Sinus rhythm with three premature atrial complexes (PACs). The first is conducted with delay; the second is not conducted completely through to the ventricles but is conducted for enough into the AV node to cause complete block of the third PAC. (From Jacobson, C. [1983]. Interpretation of complex arrhythmias. In S. L. Woods [Ed.], *Cardiovascular critical care nursing* [p. 207]. New York: Churchill Livingstone. By permission.)

Figure 19-54*C* shows sinus rhythm with three PAC. The first PAC conducts with delay; the second is not conducted completely into the ventricle but is conducted far enough into the AV node to prevent the conduction of the third PAC.

Concealed Conduction Affecting Subsequent Impulse Formation

In the presence of AV dissociation between a sinus pacemaker and an AV junctional pacemaker controlling the ventricles, the sinus impulse may occasionally conduct far enough into the AV junction to reset the junctional pacemaker and prevent the formation of the next expected junctional impulse. Figure 19-55 shows AV dissociation between a junctional rhythm at a rate of 64 beats per minute and a slightly slower sinus rhythm. The pause that occurs near the end of the strip is due to concealed conduction of the sinus impulse into the AV junctional focus, preventing the formation of the next expected junctional beat.

Concealed Impulse Formation Affecting Subsequent Impulse Conduction

If an impulse is formed in the AV junction but is blocked in both the anterograde and retrograde directions, there is no evidence on the ECG that the impulse ever existed unless it interferes with conduction of a following impulse. Such concealed junctional beats can imitate type I and II AV block, and their recognition may prevent misdiagnosis of a nonexistent conduction disturbance (Watanabe, 1978; Conover, 1996). Figure 19-56 illustrates sinus rhythm with junctional parasystole at a rate of approximately 50 beats per minute. The sinus impulse that follows beat 11 is blocked, simulating type II second-degree AV block, but this can be explained by concealed formation of the junctional parasystolic focus that fails to reach the ventricles but causes refractoriness in the AV node, preventing conduction of the next sinus impulse.

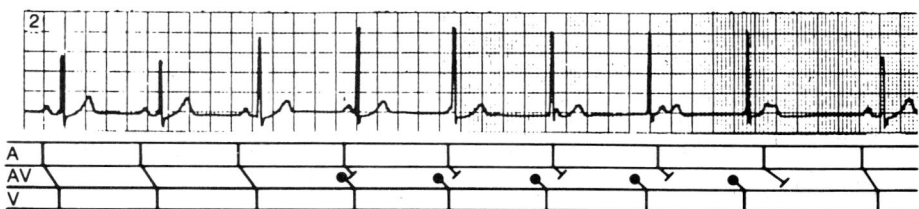

■ **Figure 19–55.** Concealed conduction affecting subsequent impulse formation. Atrioventricular (AV) dissociation between a junctional rhythm at a rate of 64 beats/min and a slightly slower sinus rhythm. The sinus P wave that follows the eighth QRS complex conducts far enough into the AV node to depolarize the junctional focus before it is due to fire again, causing the pause after the eighth beat. (Adapted from Marriott, H. J. L., & Conover, M. [1989]. *Advanced concepts in arrhythmias* [2nd ed., p. 321]. St. Louis: CV Mosby.)

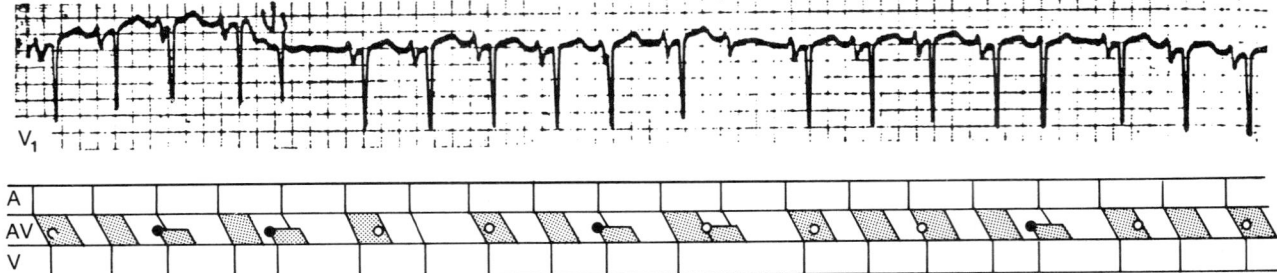

■ **Figure 19–56.** Concealed impulse formation affecting subsequent conduction. Sinus rhythm is present at a rate of 84 beats/min; an atrioventricular (AV) junctional parasystolic focus is firing at a rate of 48 beats/min. Concealed formation of the junctional focus after the 11th beat prevents conduction of the next sinus impulse, simulating type II second-degree AV block. *Solid circles* indicate the junctional parasystolic focus seen on the electrocardiogram (ECG); open circles indicate the focus firing but not seen on the ECG; the *shaded area* indicates the refractory period in the AV junction. (Adapted from Watanabe, Y. [1978]. Terminology and electrophysiologic concepts in cardiac arrhythmias: II. Concealed conduction. *Pacing and Clinical Electrophysiology*, 1, 354.)

REFERENCES

Antzelevitch, C., & Burashinikov, A. (2001). Mechanisms of arrhythmogenesis. In P. J. Podrid & P. R. Kowey (Eds.), *Cardiac arrhythmia: Mechanisms, diagnosis & management* (2nd ed., pp. 51–79). Philadelphia: Lippincott Williams & Wilkins.

Arnsdorf, M. F., & Verdino, R. (2001). Atrioventricular nodal conduction abnormalities. In P. J. Podrid & P. R. Kowey (Eds.), *Cardiac arrhythmia: Mechanisms, diagnosis & management* (2nd ed., pp. 671–691). Philadelphia: Lippincott Williams & Wilkins.

Bharucha, B., & Podrid, P. J. (2001). Use of the electrocardiogram in the diagnosis of arrhythmia. In P. J. Podrid & P. R. Kowey (Eds.), *Cardiac arrhythmia: Mechanisms, diagnosis & management* (2nd ed., pp. 127–164). Philadelphia: Lippincott Williams & Wilkins.

Bigger, T. J. (1983). Definition of benign versus malignant ventricular arrhythmias: Targets for treatment. *American Journal of Cardiology*, 52, 47C–54C.

Braunwald, E., Zipes, D. P., & Libby P. (2001). *Heart disease: A textbook of cardiovascular medicine* (6th ed.). Philadelphia: W. B. Saunders.

Brugada, P., Brugada, J., Mont, L., et al. (1991). A new approach to the differential diagnosis of a regular tachycardia with a wide QRS complex. *Circulation*, 83, 1649–1659.

Buxton, A. E., & Duc, J. (2001). Ventricular premature depolarizations and nonsustained ventricular tachycardia. In P. J. Podrid & P. R. Kowey (Eds.), *Cardiac arrhythmia: Mechanisms, diagnosis & management* (2nd ed., pp. 549–572). Philadelphia: Lippincott Williams & Wilkins.

Cabeen, W. R., Roberts, N. K., & Child, J. S. (1978). Recognition of Wenckebach phenomenon. *Western Journal of Medicine*, 129, 521–526.

Callans, D. J., & Josephson, M. E. (2000). Ventricular tachycardia in patients with coronary artery disease. In D. P. Zipes & J. Jalife (Eds.), *Cardiac electrophysiology: From cell to bedside* (3rd ed., pp. 530–536). Philadelphia: W. B. Saunders.

Cappato, R., Schluter, M., & Kuck, K. H. (2000). Catheter ablation of atrioventricular reentry. In D. P. Zipes & J. Jalife (Eds.), *Cardiac electrophysiology: From cell to bedside* (3rd ed., pp. 1035–1048), Philadelphia: W. B. Saunders.

Cardiac Arrhythmia Suppression Trial Investigators. (1989). Preliminary report: Effect of encainide and flecainide on mortality in a randomized trial of arrhythmia suppression after myocardial infarction. *New England Journal of Medicine*, 321, 406–411.

Carleton, R. A. (1977). Wenckebach (type I) behavior of ventricular reentry. *Chest*, 71, 740–745.

Castellanos, A., Saoudi, N., Moleiro, F., & Myerburg, R. J. (2000). Parasystole. In D. P. Zipes & J. Jalife (Eds.), *Cardiac electrophysiology: From cell to bedside* (3rd ed., pp. 690–695), Philadelphia: W. B. Saunders.

Castellanos, A., Sung, R. J., Aldrich, J. L., et al. (1978). Electrocardiographic manifestations and clinical significance of atrioventricular nodal alternating Wenckebach periods. *Chest*, 73, 69–74.

Castellanos, A., Sung, R. J., Aldrich, J. L., et al. (1977). Alternating Wenckebach periods occurring in the atria, His-Purkinje system, ventricles and Kent bundle. *American Journal of Cardiology*, 40, 853–859.

Chung, E. K. (1980). *Electrocardiography: Practical applications with vectorial principles* (2nd ed.). Hagerstown, MD: Harper & Row.

Conover, M. B. (1996). *Understanding electrocardiography* (7th ed.). St. Louis: Mosby.

Cummins, R. O. (Ed.). (2000). *Advanced cardiac life support*. Dallas, TX: American Heart Association.

Drew, B. J., & Scheinman, M. M. (1991). Value of electrocardiographic leads MCL_1, MCL_6 and other selected leads in the diagnosis of wide QRS complex tachycardia. *Journal of the American College of Cardiology*, 18, 1025.

Drew, B. J., Scheinman, M. M., & Dracup, K. (1991). MCL_1 and MCL_6 compared to V_1 and V_6 in distinguishing aberrant supraventricular from ventricular ectopic beats. *Pacing and Clinical Electrophysiology*, 14, 1375.

El-Sherif, N. (1995). Polymorphic ventricular tachycardia. In P. J. Podrid & P. R. Kowey (Eds.), *Cardiac arrhythmia: Mechanisms, diagnosis, and management* (pp. 936–950). Baltimore: Williams & Wilkins.

El-Sherif, N., Aranda, J., Befeler, B., et al. (1978). Atypical Wenckebach periodicity simulating Mobitz II AV block. *British Heart Journal*, 40, 1376–1383.

El-Sherif, N., & Turitto, G. (2000). Torsade de pointes. In D. P. Zipes & J. Jalife (Eds.), *Cardiac electrophysiology: From cell to bedside* (3rd ed., pp. 662–673), Philadelphia: W. B. Saunders.

El-Sherif, N., Zeiler, R. H., Craelius, W., et al. (1988). QTU prolongation and polymorphic tachyarrhythmias due to bradycardia dependent early afterdepolarizations: Afterdepolarizations and ventricular arrhythmias. *Circulation Research*, 63(2), 286–305.

Fisch, C. (2000). Electrocardiographic manifestations of exit block and supernormal and concealed conduction. In D. P. Zipes & J. Jalife (Eds.), *Cardiac electrophysiology: From cell to bedside* (3rd ed., pp. 685–689). Philadelphia: W. B. Saunders.

Fisch, C. (1991). Differential diagnosis of wide QRS tachycardia. In C. Fisch & B. Surawicz (Eds.), *Cardiac electrophysiology and arrhythmias* (pp. 199–209). New York: Elsevier.

Fogel, R. I., & Prystowsky, E. N. (2001). Atrioventricular nodal reentry. In P. J. Podrid & P. R. Kowey (Eds.), *Cardiac arrhythmia: Mechanisms, diagnosis & management* (2nd ed., pp. 433–456). Philadelphia: Lippincott Williams & Wilkins.

Fuster, V., Alexander, R. W., & O'Rourke, R. A. (Eds.). (2001). *Hurst's the heart* (10th ed.). New York: McGraw-Hill.

Gadsby, D. C., Karagueuzian, H. S., & Wit, A. L. (1995). Normal and abnormal electrical activity in cardiac cells. In W. J. Mandel (Ed.), *Cardiac arrhythmias: Their mechanisms, diagnosis, and management* (3rd ed., pp. 55–82). Philadelphia: J. B. Lippincott.

Gallagher, J. J., Pritchett, E. L., Sealy, W. C., et al. (1978). The preexcitation syndromes. *Progress in Cardiovascular Diseases*, 20, 279.

Goldberger, J. J., & Kadish, A. H. (2001). Sinoatrial/atrial tachyarrhythmias. In P. J. Podrid & P. R. Kowey (Eds.), *Cardiac arrhythmia: Mechanisms, diagnosis & management* (2nd ed., pp. 411–431), Philadelphia: Lippincott Williams & Wilkins.

Haissaguerre, M., Jais, P., Shah, D. C., & Clementy, J. (2000). Catheter ablation for atrial fibrillation: Clinical electrophysiology of linear lesions. In D. P. Zipes & J. Jalife (Eds.), *Cardiac electrophysiology: From cell to bedside* (3rd ed., pp. 994–1007), Philadelphia: W. B. Saunders

Halpern, M. S., Nau, G. J., Levi, R. J., et al. (1973). Wenckebach periods of alternate beats: Clinical and experimental observations. *Circulation*, 48, 41.

Hoffman, B. F., & Cranefield, P. F. (1960). *Electrophysiology of the heart.* New York: McGraw-Hill.

Hohnloser, S. H. (2001). Polymorphous ventricular tachycardia, including torsades de pointes. In P. J. Podrid & P. R. Kowey (Eds.), *Cardiac arrhythmia: Mechanisms, diagnosis & management* (2nd ed., pp. 604–619). Philadelphia: Lippincott Williams & Wilkins.

Huff, J., Doernback, D. C., & White, R. D. (1993). *ECG workout* (2nd ed., p. 53). Philadelphia: J. B. Lippincott.

Jacobson, C. (1997). Advanced ECG concepts. In M. Chulay, C. Guzzetta, & B. Dossey (Eds.), *AACN handbook of critical care nursing* (pp. 415–445). Stamford, CT: Appleton & Lange.

Jahangir, A., Munger, T. M., Packer, D. L., & Crijns, H. J. G. M. (2001). Atrial fibrillation. In P. J. Podrid & P. R. Kowey (Eds.), *Cardiac arrhythmia: Mechanisms, diagnosis & management* (2nd ed., pp. 457–499). Philadelphia: Lippincott Williams & Wilkins.

Janse, M. J. (2000). Mechanisms of atrial fibrillation. In D. P. Zipes & J. Jalife (Eds.), *Cardiac electrophysiology: From cell to bedside* (3rd ed., pp. 476–481). Philadelphia: W. B. Saunders.

Kastor, J. A. (2000). *Arrhythmias.* Philadelphia: W. B. Saunders.

Kindwall, K. E., Brown, J., & Josephson, M. E. (1988). Electrocardiographic criteria for ventricular tachycardia in wide complex left bundle branch block morphology tachycardia. *American Journal of Cardiology,* 61, 1279–1283.

Kinoshita, S. (1978). Mechanisms of ventricular parasystole. *Circulation,* 58, 715–722.

Kosowsky, B. D., Latif, P., & Radoff, A. M. (1976). Multilevel atrioventricular block. *Circulation,* 54, 914–921.

Langendorf, R., Pick, A., & Winternitz, M. (1955). Mechanisms of intermittent ventricular bigeminy: I. Appearance of ectopic beats dependent upon length of the ventricular cycle, the "rule of bigeminy." *Circulation,* 11, 422.

Leon, A., Chuquimia, R., Wu, D., et al. (1975). Alternating Wenckebach periodicity: A common electrophysiologic response. *American Journal of Cardiology,* 36, 757–764.

Lesh, M. D. (2000). Catheter ablation of atrial flutter and tachycardia. In D. P. Zipes & J. Jalife (Eds.), *Cardiac electrophysiology: From cell to bedside* (3rd ed., pp. 1009–1027). Philadelphia: W. B. Saunders.

Lightfoot, P. R. (1978). Parasystole simulating ventricular bigeminy with Wenckebach type coupling prolongation. *Journal of Electrocardiology,* 11, 385–390.

Marinchak, R. A., & Rials, S. J. (2001). Tachycardias in Wolff-Parkinson-White syndrome. In P. J. Podrid & P. R. Kowey (Eds.), *Cardiac arrhythmia: Mechanisms, diagnosis & management* (2nd ed., pp. 517–548). Philadelphia: Lippincott Williams & Wilkins.

Marriott, H. J. L. (1988). *Practical electrocardiography* (8th ed.). Baltimore: Williams & Wilkins.

Marriott, H. J. L., & Conover, M. (1998). *Advanced concepts in arrhythmias* (3rd ed). St. Louis: Mosby.

_____. (1989). *Advanced concepts in arrhythmias* (2nd ed.). St. Louis: Mosby.

Marriott, H. J. L., & Sandler, A. (1966). Criteria, old and new for differentiating between ectopic ventricular beats and aberrant ventricular conduction in the presence of atrial fibrillation. *Progress in Cardiovascular Diseases,* 9, 18–28.

Martin, D., & Wharton, J. M. (2001). Sustained monomorphic ventricular tachycardia. In P. J. Podrid & P. R. Kowey (Eds.), *Cardiac arrhythmia: Mechanisms, diagnosis & management* (2nd ed., pp. 573–601). Philadelphia: Lippincott Williams & Wilkins.

McGovern, G., Garan, H., & Ruskin, J. N. (1986). Precipitation of cardiac arrest by verapamil in patients with Wolff-Parkinson-White syndrome. *Annals of Internal Medicine,* 104, 791.

Miles, W. M., & Zipes, D. P. (2000). Atrioventricular reentry and variants: Mechanisms, clinical features, and management. In D. P. Zipes & J. Jalife (Eds.), *Cardiac electrophysiology: From cell to bedside* (3rd ed., pp. 488–504). Philadelphia: W. B. Saunders.

Miller, J. M., Hsia, H. H., Rothman, S. A., & Buxton, A. E. (2000). Ventricular tachycardia versus supraventricular tachycardia with aberration: Electrocardiographic distinctions. In D. P. Zipes & J. Jalife (Eds.), *Cardiac electrophysiology: From cell to bedside* (3rd ed., pp. 696–705). Philadelphia: W. B. Saunders.

Mirvis, D. M., Bandura, J. P., & Brody, D. A. (1976). Wenckebach-type exit block from an ectopic focus as a cause of variable coupling. *Journal of Electrocardiology,* 9, 365–370.

Myerburg, R. J., Kloosterman, E. M., & Castellanos, A. (2001). Recognition, clinical assessment, and management of arrhythmias and conduction disturbances. In V. Fuster, R.W. Alexander, & R. A. O'Rourke (Eds.), *Hurst's the heart* (10th Ed., pp. 797–874). New York: McGraw-Hill.

Olgin, J. E. (2000). Sinus tachycardia and sinus node reentry. In D. P. Zipes & J. Jalife (Eds.), *Cardiac electrophysiology: From cell to bedside* (3rd ed., pp. 459–468). Philadelphia: W. B. Saunders.

Olgin, J. E., & Zipes, D. P. (2001). Specific arrhythmias: Diagnosis and treatment. In E. Braunwald, D. P. Zipes, & P. Libby (Eds.), *Heart disease* (6th ed., pp. 659–699). Philadelphia: W. B. Saunders.

Opie, L. H., & Gersh, R. J. (2001). *Drugs for the heart* (5th ed.). Philadelphia: W. B. Saunders.

Otomo, K., Wang, Z., Lazzara, R., & Jackman, W. M. (2000). Atrioventricular nodal reentrant tachycardia: Electrophysiological characteristics of four forms and implications for the reentrant circuit. In D. P. Zipes & J. Jalife (Eds.), *Cardiac electrophysiology: From cell to bedside* (3rd ed., pp. 504–521). Philadelphia: W. B. Saunders.

Palma, E. C., & Scheinman, M. M. (2001). Treatment of cardiac arrhythmias with catheter-ablative techniques. In V. Fuster, R. W. Alexander & R. A. O'Rourke (Eds.), *Hurst's the heart* (10th ed., pp. 925–932). New York: McGraw-Hill.

Peter, T., Harper, R. W., Vohra, J. K., & Hunt, D. (1976). The electrocardiographic recognition of the Wenckebach phenomenon in sites other than the atrioventricular junction. *Heart and Lung,* 5, 747–754.

Peters, N. S., Cabo, C., & Wit, A. L. (2000). Arrhythmogenic mechanisms: Automaticity, triggered activity, and reentry. In D. P. Zipes & J. Jalife (Eds.), *Cardiac electrophysiology: From cell to bedside* (3rd ed., pp. 340–355). Philadelphia: W. B. Saunders.

Pick, A., & Langendorf, R. (1976). Parasystole and its variants. *Medical Clinics of North America,* 60, 125–147.

Podrid, P. J., & Kowey, P. R. (Eds.). (2001a). *Cardiac arrhythmia: Mechanisms, diagnosis & management* (2nd ed.). Philadelphia: Lippincott Williams & Wilkins.

_____. (2001b). Sudden cardiac death. In P. J. Podrid & P. R. Kowey (Eds.), *Cardiac arrhythmia: Mechanisms, diagnosis & management* (2nd ed., pp. 621–652). Philadelphia: Lippincott Williams & Wilkins.

Priori, S. G., Diehi, L., & Schwartz, P. J. (1995). Torsade de pointes. In P. J. Podrid & P. R. Kowey (Eds.), *Cardiac arrhythmia: Mechanisms, diagnosis, and management* (pp. 957–963). Baltimore: Williams & Wilkins.

Priori, S. G., & Napolitano, C. (2001). Genetics of arrhythmogenic disorders. In P. J. Podrid & P. R. Kowey (Eds.), *Cardiac arrhythmia: Mechanisms, diagnosis, and management* (pp. 81–107). Philadelphia: Lippincott Williams & Wilkins.

Reiffel, J. A. (2001). Sinus node function and dysfunction. In P. J. Podrid & P. R. Kowey (Eds.), *Cardiac arrhythmia: Mechanisms, diagnosis, and management* (pp. 653–670). Philadelphia: Lippincott Williams & Wilkins.

Reisman, M., Gray, W., Sievert, H., et al. (2003). An endovascular approach to stroke prevention in atrial fibrillation: Results of the multicenter PLAATO (percutaneous left atrial appendage transcatheter occlusion) feasibility trial. *Journal of the American College of Cardiology* (Suppl. A), 41(6), 103A.

Robles de Medina, E. O., & Wilde, A. M. (2000). Sinus bradycardia, sinus arrest, and sinoatrial exit block: Pathophysiological, electrocardiographic, and clinical considerations. In D. P. Zipes & J. Jalife (Eds.), *Cardiac electrophysiology: From cell to bedside* (3rd ed., pp. 447–451). Philadelphia: W. B. Saunders.

Rosen, M. R., & Danilo, P. (1979). Electrophysiological basis for cardiac arrhythmias. In O. S. Narula (Ed.), *Cardiac arrhythmias: Electrophysiology, diagnosis, management* (pp. 9–13). Baltimore: Williams & Wilkins.

Rosenbaum, M. B., Nau, G. J., Levi, R. J., et al. (1969). Wenckebach periods in the bundle branches. *Circulation,* 40, 79–86.

Rubart, M., & Zipes, D. P. (2001). Genesis of cardiac arrhythmias: Electrophysiological considerations. In E. Braunwald, D. P. Zipes, & P. Libby (Eds.), *Heart disease* (6th ed., pp. 659–699). Philadelphia: W. B. Saunders.

Rusterholz, A. P., & Marriott, H. J. L. (1994). How long can the P-R interval be? *American Journal of Noninvasive Cardiology,* 8, 11–13.

Samuels, F., Hessen, S. E., & Dreifus, L. S. (1995). Reentry and development of arrhythmias: Preclinical and clinical data. In P. J. Podrid & P. R. Kowey (Eds.), *Cardiac arrhythmia: Mechanisms, diagnosis, and management* (pp. 60–69). Baltimore: Williams & Wilkins.

Sandler, I. A., & Marriott, H. J. L. (1965). The differential morphology of anomalous ventricular complexes of RBBB-type in lead V_1: Ventricular ectopy versus aberration. *Circulation,* 31, 551–556.

Schamroth, L., & Dove, E.(1966). The Wenckebach phenomenon in sino-atrial block. *British Heart Journal,* 28, 350–358.

Schwartz, P. J., Priori, S. G., & Napolitano, C. (2000). The long QT syndrome. In D. P. Zipes & J. Jalife (Eds.), *Cardiac electrophysiology: From cell to bedside* (3rd ed., pp. 597–615). Philadelphia: W. B. Saunders.

Sclarovsky, S., Lervin, R., Strasberg, B., et al. (1978a). Dissociation of the atrioventricular node in acute inferior wall infarction: Transverse dissociation (alternate Wenckebach periods). *Chest, 73,* 634–637.

Sclarovsky, S., Strasberg, B., & Agmon, J. (1978b). Coexistent Wenckebach phenomenon in the distal branches of the specialized conduction system. *Chest, 73,* 534–536.

Singer, D. H., & Cohen, H. C. (1995). Aberrancy: Electrophysiologic mechanisms and electrocardiographic correlates. In W. J. Mandel (Ed.), *Cardiac arrhythmias: Their mechanisms, diagnosis, and management* (3rd ed., pp. 461–511). Philadelphia: J. B. Lippincott.

Strickberger, S. A., & Morady, F. (2000). Catheter ablation of atrioventricular nodal reentrant tachycardia. In D. P. Zipes & J. Jalife (Eds.), *Cardiac electrophysiology: From cell to bedside* (3rd ed., pp. 1028–1034). Philadelphia: W. B. Saunders.

Waldo, A. L. (2001). Atrial flutter. In P. J. Podrid & P. R. Kowey (Eds.), *Cardiac arrhythmia: Mechanisms, diagnosis & management* (2nd ed., pp. 501–516). Philadelphia: Lippincott Williams & Wilkins.

_____. (2000). Atrial flutter: Mechanisms, clinical features, and management. In D. P. Zipes & J. Jalife (Eds.), *Cardiac electrophysiology: From cell to bedside* (3rd ed., pp. 468–476). Philadelphia: W. B. Saunders.

Waldo, A. L., & Wit, A. L. (2001). Mechanisms of cardiac arrhythmias and conduction disturbances. In V. Fuster, R. W. Alexander, & R. A. O'Rourke (Eds.), *Hurst's the heart* (10th ed., pp. 751–796). New York: McGraw-Hill.

Watanabe, Y. (1978). Terminology and electrophysiologic concepts in cardiac arrhythmias: II. Concealed conduction. *Pacing and Clinical Electrophysiology, 1,* 345–356.

Watanabe, Y., Dreifus, L. S., & Mazgalev, T. (1995). Atrioventricular block: Basic concepts. In W. J. Mandel (Ed.), *Cardiac arrhythmias: Their mechanisms, diagnosis, and management* (3rd ed., pp. 417–434). Philadelphia: J. B. Lippincott.

Wellens, H. J., Frits, W. H., & Lie, K. I. (1978). The value of the electrocardiogram in the differential diagnosis of a tachycardia with a widened QRS complex. *American Journal of Medicine, 64,* 27–33.

Wellens, H. J. J., Smeets, J., Gorgels, A., et al. (1995). Wolff-Parkinson-White syndrome. In W. J. Mandel (Ed.), *Cardiac arrhythmias: Their mechanisms, diagnosis, and management* (3rd ed., pp. 389–413). Philadelphia: J. B. Lippincott.

Wit, A. L., & Rosen, M. R. (1981). Cellular electrophysiology of cardiac arrhythmias: Part I: Arrhythmias caused by abnormal impulse generation. *Modern Concepts in Cardiovascular Disease, 50,* 1–8.

Zipes, D. P. (1992). Specific arrhythmias: Diagnosis and treatment. In E. Braunwald (Ed.), *Heart disease: A textbook of cardiovascular medicine* (4th ed.). Philadelphia: W. B. Saunders.

Zipes, D. P., & Jalife, J. (Eds.). (2000). *Cardiac electrophysiology: From cell to bedside* (3rd ed.). Philadelphia: W. B. Saunders.

DRUG TABLES AND DRUG THERAPY REFERENCES

Anderson, J. L. (1995). Sotalol, bretylium, and other class 3 antiarrhythmic agents. In P. J. Podrid & P. R. Kowey (Eds.). *Cardiac arrhythmia: Mechanisms, diagnosis, and management* (pp. 450–466). Baltimore: Williams & Wilkins.

Campbell, R. W. F. (1995). Class 1B antiarrhythmic agents. In P. J. Podrid & P. R. Kowey (Eds.), *Cardiac arrhythmia: Mechanisms, diagnosis, and management* (pp. 391–404). Baltimore: Williams & Wilkins.

DiMarco, J. P. (1995). Adenosine. In P. J. Podrid & P. R. Kowey (Eds.), *Cardiac arrhythmia: Mechanisms, diagnosis, and management* (pp. 488–498). Baltimore: Williams & Wilkins.

Frishman, W. H., & Cavusoglu, E. (1995). Beta-adrenergic blockers and their role in the therapy of arrhythmias. In P. J. Podrid & P. R. Kowey (Eds.), *Cardiac arrhythmia: Mechanisms, diagnosis, and management* (pp. 421–434). Baltimore: Williams & Wilkins.

Giardina, E. V., & Lipka, L. J. (1995). Class 1A antiarrhythmic agents: Quinidine, procainamide, disopyramide. In P. J. Podrid & P. R. Kowey (Eds.), *Cardiac arrhythmia: Mechanisms, diagnosis, and management* (pp. 369–391). Baltimore: Williams & Wilkins.

Hondeghem, L. M. (1995). Receptor physiology and its relationship to antiarrhythmic drugs. In P. J. Podrid & P. R. Kowey (Eds.), *Cardiac arrhythmia: Mechanisms, diagnosis, and management* (pp. 347–354). Baltimore: Williams & Wilkins.

Johnson, J. H., Jadonath, R. L., & Marchlinski, F. E. (1995). Digoxin. In P. J. Podrid & P. R. Kowey (Eds.), *Cardiac arrhythmia: Mechanisms, diagnosis, and management* (pp. 478–488). Baltimore: Williams & Wilkins.

Keen, J. H., Baird, M. S., & Allen, J. H. (1996). *Critical care and emergency drug reference* (2nd ed.). St. Louis: Mosby.

Naccarelli, G. V., & Dougherty, A. H. (1995). Amiodarone: A review of its pharmacologic, antiarrhythmic, and adverse effects. In P. J. Podrid & P. R. Kowey (Eds.), *Cardiac arrhythmia: Mechanisms, diagnosis, and management* (pp. 434–449). Baltimore: Williams & Wilkins.

Naccarelli, G. V., Sager, P. T., & Singh, B. N. (2001). Antiarrhythmic agents. In P. J. Podrid & P. R. Kowey (Eds.), *Cardiac arrhythmia: Mechanisms, diagnosis & management* (2nd ed.). Philadelphia: Lippincott Williams & Wilkins.

Opie, L. H., & Gersh, B. J. (2001). *Drugs for the heart* (5th ed.). Philadelphia: W. B. Saunders.

Podrid, P. J. (1995). Aggravation of arrhythmia by antiarrhythmic drugs. In P. J. Podrid & P. R. Kowey (Eds.), *Cardiac arrhythmia: Mechanisms, diagnosis, and management* (pp. 507–522). Baltimore: Williams & Wilkins.

Pratt, C. M. (1995). Class 1C antiarrhythmic agents: Propafenone, flecainide, and ethmozine. In P. J. Podrid & P. R. Kowey (Eds.), *Cardiac arrhythmia: Mechanisms, diagnosis, and management* (pp. 404–421). Baltimore: Williams & Wilkins.

Siddoway, L. A. (1995). Pharmacologic principles of antiarrhythmic drugs. In P. J. Podrid & P. R. Kowey (Eds.), *Cardiac arrhythmia: Mechanisms, diagnosis, and management* (pp. 355–368). Baltimore: Williams & Wilkins.

Singh, B. N. (1995). Controlling cardiac arrhythmias with calcium channel blockers. In P. J. Podrid & P. R. Kowey (Eds.), *Cardiac arrhythmia: Mechanisms, diagnosis, and management* (pp. 466–478). Baltimore: Williams & Wilkins.

Woosley, R. L. (2001). Antiarrhythmic drugs. In V. Fuster, R. W. Alexander, & R. A. O'Rourke (Eds.), *Hurst's the heart* (10th ed., pp. 899–924). New York: McGraw-Hill.

20

Cardiac Electrophysiology Procedures

SUSAN BLANCHER

The use of cardiac electrophysiology (EP) procedures includes diagnostic testing and interventional treatment procedures. In general, diagnostic EP studies are performed to determine an arrhythmia diagnosis or EP mechanism of a known arrhythmia. Interventional or therapeutic EP studies include endocardial catheter ablation and surgical procedures for supraventricular and ventricular arrhythmias. The placement of implantable cardioverter defibrillators for management of ventricular tachycardia (VT) and ventricular fibrillation (VF) is also an interventional EP procedure and is discussed in Chapter 32. A knowledge of electrocardiography (see Chapter 18), normal cardiac activation (see Chapter 1), and cardiac activation during arrhythmias (see Chapter 19) is needed to understand EP studies.

DIAGNOSTIC ELECTROPHYSIOLOGY STUDIES

Before an EP study, a patient needs to be prepared for the procedure. This preparation and the techniques, complications, and indications of EP studies are presented here.

Patient Preparation

Preparation for EP procedures is similar to that for cardiac catheterization (see Chapter 22). Patients are fasting and usually sedated during EP studies. The degree of sedation depends on the type of study being performed and the preferences of the center performing the procedures. A peripheral intravenous line is required for medication administration. Systemic anticoagulation may be used during EP studies to decrease the incidence of thromboembolic complications (Horowitz, 1986). Appropriate emergency and resuscitation equipment is required for all EP procedures.

Techniques

During invasive EP testing, spontaneous and pacing-induced intracardiac and surface electrical signals are recorded. The normal timing and sequence of electrical activation can be observed and measured during a normal or baseline rhythm. Abnormal timing and electrical activation sequences are recorded and studied during tachyarrhythmias. Programmed electrical stimulation (PES) may also be used to induce and analyze paroxysmal arrhythmias that are the same as or similar to a patient's clinical arrhythmia (Josephson, 1993).

Flexible catheters with at least two and up to 10 electrodes are introduced percutaneously. The catheters are advanced using fluoroscopy into the heart. The right and left femoral, subclavian, internal jugular, and median cephalic veins are the most commonly used venous access sites. One to several catheters may be placed depending on the type of study to be performed (Fig. 20-1). The usual intracardiac recording sites include the high right atrium, right atrial appendage, right ventricular apex, right ventricular outflow tract, coronary sinus, and the His bundle region. In addition, a roving catheter can be used to map intracardiac electrograms arising from different regions of the heart during tachycardia. Occasionally, the left ventricle is used during a diagnostic study for PES if VT cannot be induced from the right ventricle.

After the catheters are in place and connected to the physiologic recording equipment, intervals are measured from both the 12-lead electrocardiogram (ECG) and the intracardiac electrograms in the baseline state (Fig. 20-2). The AH interval is a measurement of conduction time from the low right atrium through the atrioventricular (AV) node to the His bundle and is an approximation of AV node conduction time. The AH interval can vary a great deal depending on the patient's autonomic state and measures approximately 55 to 120 ms (Josephson, 1993). The HV interval represents conduction time from the onset of His bundle depolarization to the onset of ventricular activity. The normal HV interval measurement is 35 to 55 ms (Hammill et al., 1986). After baseline recordings, various pacing techniques may be performed to assess the patient's electrical conduction system. Refractory periods for the atrium, AV node, and ventricle are recorded. The presence of retrograde or ventricular-atrial (VA) conduction is noted as is the activation sequence. Attempts to induce and document the arrhythmia using the introduction of extrastimuli in either the atrium or the ventricle

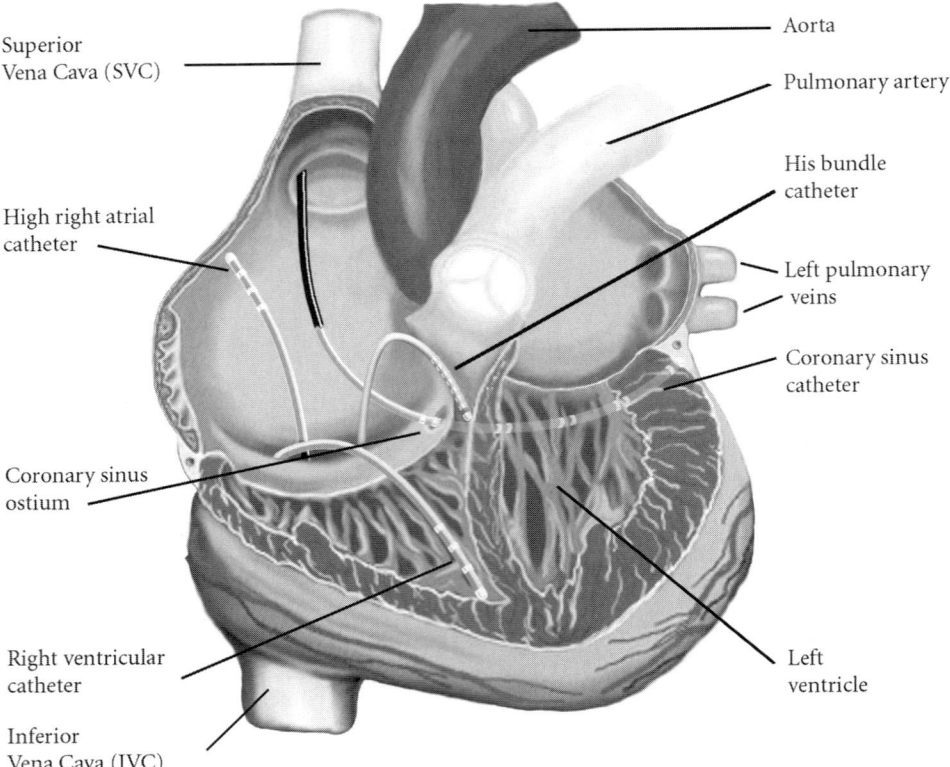

Superior
Vena Cava (SVC)

Aorta

Pulmonary artery

His bundle
catheter

High right atrial
catheter

Left pulmonary
veins

Coronary sinus
catheter

Coronary sinus
ostium

Right ventricular
catheter

Left
ventricle

Inferior
Vena Cava (IVC)

■ **Figure 20–1.** Diagram of intracardiac placement of catheters. 1, right atrial recording catheter; 2, right ventricular recording catheter; 3, His recording catheter; 4, coronary sinus catheter.

are then made. Intravenous isoproterenol or epinephrine may be used to help induce arrhythmias or reveal accessory pathway or slow AVN pathway conduction.

The patient must be adequately prepared before the study and should understand that arrhythmia induction is often one of the primary goals of the study. The electrophysiologist attempts to gather as much information as possible depending on the type of arrhythmia induced and how well it is hemodynamically tolerated. If the patient is hemodynamically unstable, such as during VF or rapid VT, then documentation of the arrhythmia with a 12-lead ECG is obtained before termination attempts. It is important to note the method of arrhythmia termination. Tachycardias may be self-terminating or require antitachycardia pacing to stop them. Occasionally, it is necessary to cardiovert or defibrillate the patient to stop the arrhythmia. It is usually necessary to wait until the patient loses consciousness before defibrillation to prevent painful shock in an awake state.

If the patient is hemodynamically stable during a ventricular arrhythmia, attempts to map its origin can be performed, particularly if ablation is planned (see Interventional Electrophysiology and Catheter Ablation). Atrial arrhythmias are usually well tolerated and allow for extensive mapping. Recordings are made at various locations in the heart and compared with a reference signal, either a surface ECG lead or stable intracardiac electrogram. The site of earliest activation is closest to the site where the arrhythmia originates. Occasionally, the clinical

arrhythmia cannot be induced or is not sustained long enough for adequate mapping.

Complications

Horowitz reviewed the experience of his EP laboratory and the laboratories of five others. During a 4-year period, 8,545 EP studies were performed on 4,015 patients. Five deaths (0.12%) occurred, all caused by intractable VF. The complications that occurred most frequently after EP studies were cardiac perforation (0.5%) and major venous thrombosis (0.5%). Cardiac perforation and pericardial effusion resolved without treatment in most patients; five patients required pericardial drainage or open repair. The femoral catheter site was the location of thrombosis for 95% of the 20 patients with venous thrombosis. Pulmonary emboli followed venous thrombosis in nine patients (0.2%) (Horowitz, 1986). A slightly higher incidence of venous thrombosis (1.1%) and pulmonary emboli (1.6%) was found in a study by DiMarco and others of 359 patients during 1,062 EP studies (DeMarco et al., 1982). They reported a 10% incidence of the use of countershock to terminate unstable VT; all patients returned to their original rhythm without complications. Systemic or catheter site infections were reported in 1.7% of patients in the study by DiMarco and colleagues but were not reported in Horowitz's study. Major hemorrhage and arterial injury are uncommon complications

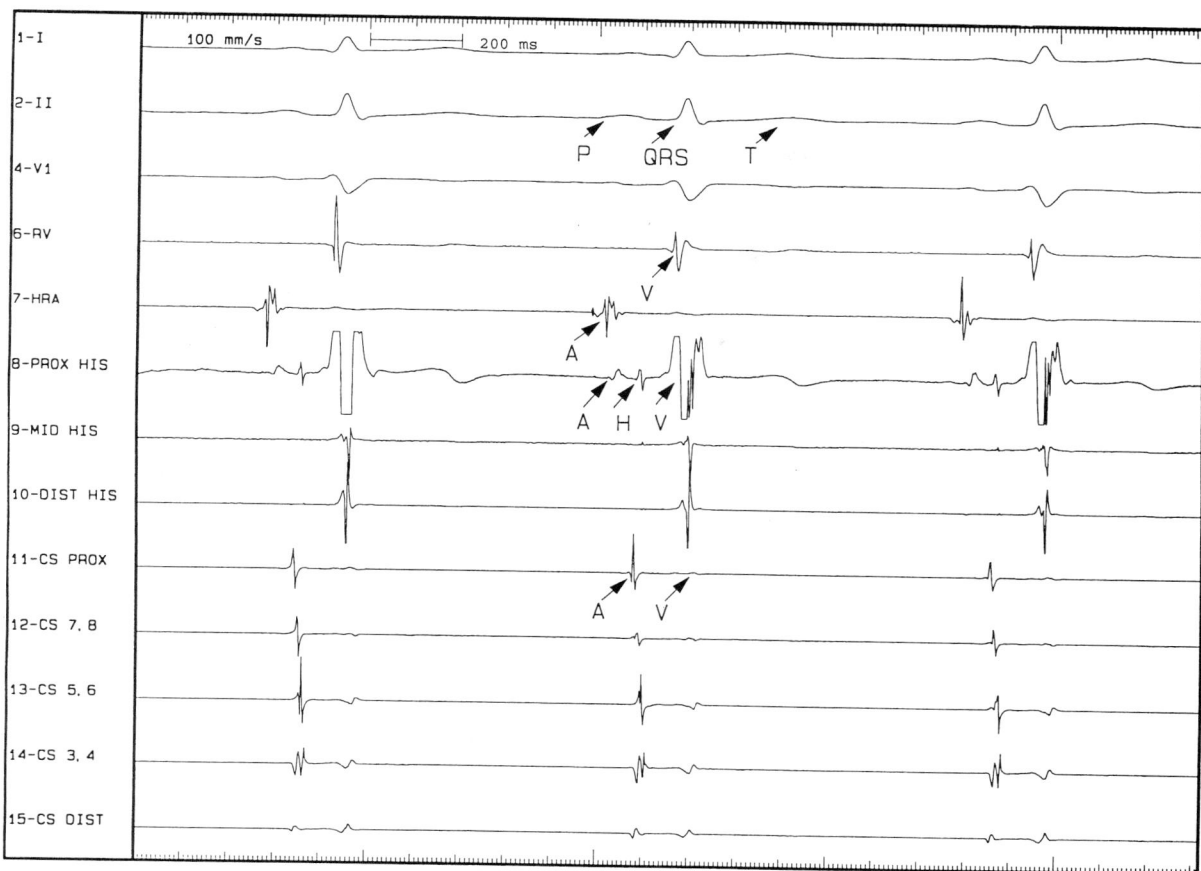

■ **Figure 20–2.** Basic intervals. Channel 1-I is lead I; channel 2-II is lead II; channel 4-V1 is lead V_1; channel 6-RV is a right ventricular tracing (V); channel 7-RA is a right atrial tracing (A); channel 8HIS PROX is a tracing from the proximal portion of the His bundle; channel 9-HIS MID is a tracing from the middle portion of the His bundle; channel 10-HIS DIST is a tracing from the distal portion of the His bundle. On channel 8-HIS PROX, the first waveform represents atrial depolarization (A) and occurs slightly later than the P wave on lead II. The next waveform is the His bundle deflection (H). The last waveform represents ventricular depolarization (V), corresponding to the QRS complex. Atrial and ventricular tracings are also recorded on channels 11-15-CS and reflect proximal to distal coronary sinus electrograms.

of EP studies and are substantially less than with standard cardiac catheterization. In general, the actual risk of death from EPS procedures approaches zero because reentrant ventricular tachycardia or fibrillation induced under controlled conditions can be quickly terminated (Fogoros, 1999).

Indications

A list of indications for EP testing is provided in Display 20-1. Specific clinical indications are discussed in the subsequent sections. Indications for testing supraventricular tachyarrhythmias are discussed in the section on Interventional Electrophysiology and Catheter Ablation.

Cardiac Arrest Survivors

People who survive a cardiac arrest not associated with an acute transmural myocardial infarction are at high-risk for recurrence. The 2-year recurrence rate has been reported at 47% (Schaffer, 1975). VF was the rhythm most commonly found at

the time of cardiac arrest (Cobb et al., 1977; Greene, 1990). VT and VF were induced during EP testing in a baseline, antiarrhythmic, drug-free state in 70% to 80% of patients resuscitated from cardiac arrest (Wilber et al., 1988; Skale et al., 1986). A full discussion of sudden cardiac death can be found in Chapter 31.

Serial, EP-guided, antiarrhythmic drug testing was once common practice in EP laboratories. The goal was to identify a drug that was effective in suppressing inducible VT or VF and subsequent recurrent cardiac arrest. VT or VF suppression with EP guided antiarrhythmic drug therapy has been reported in 26% to 80% of cardiac arrest survivors (Wilber et al., 1988; Skale et al., 1986). Antiarrhythmic medications may also provoke or exacerbate arrhythmias; this situation is referred to a proarrhythmic effect.

In recent years, several studies have shown implantable cardioverter defibrillator (ICD) therapy as superior to EP-guided antiarrhythmic drugs in reducing all-cause mortality (Moss et al., 1996, 2002; Buxton et al., 1999; Connolly et al., 2000; Kuck et al., 2000; AVID investigators, 1997). Therefore, ICD therapy is usually recommended as first-line

CLASS I INDICATIONS FOR ELECTROPHYSIOLOGY STUDY

Class I: Conditions for which there is general agreement that EPS provide information that is useful and important for patient treatment. Class II: Conditions for which EPS are frequently performed, but there is less certainty about the usefulness of the information that is obtained. Class III: Conditions for which there is general agreement that EPS do not provide useful information. EPS not warranted in patients with these conditions.

1. Sinus Node Function
   Symptomatic patients in whom sinus node dysfunction is suspected as the cause of symptoms but a causal relation between an arrhythmia and the symptoms has not been established after appropriate evaluation
2. Acquired AV Block
   Symptomatic patients in whom His-Purkinje block, suspected as a cause of symptoms, has not been established
3. Chronic Intraventricular Conduction Delay
   Symptomatic patients in whom the cause of symptoms is not known
4. Narrow QRS Complex Tachycardias
   Patients with frequent or poorly tolerated episodes of tachycardia that do not adequately respond to drug therapy and for whom information about site of origin, mechanism, and electrophysiological properties of the pathways of the tachycardia is essential for choosing appropriate therapy (drugs, catheter ablation, pacing, or surgery); patients who prefer ablative therapy to pharmacological treatment
5. Wide QRS Complex Tachycardias
   Patients with wide QRS complex tachycardia in whom correct diagnosis is unclear after analysis of available ECG tracings and for whom knowledge of the correct diagnosis is necessary for patient care
6. Prolonged QT Intervals
   None*
7. Wolff-Parkinson-White Syndrome
   Patients being evaluated for catheter ablation or surgical ablation of an accessory pathway; patients with ventricular preexcitation who have survived cardiac arrest or who have unexplained syncope; symptomatic patients in whom determination of the mechanism of arrhythmia or knowledge of the electrophysiological properties of the accessory pathway and normal conduction system would help in determining appropriate therapy.
8. Premature Ventricular Complexes, Couplets, and Nonsustained Ventricular Tachycardia
   None*
9. Unexplained Syncope
   Patients with suspected structural heart disease and syncope that remains unexplained after appropriate evaluation
10. Survivors of Cardiac Arrest
    Patients surviving cardiac arrest without evidence of an acute Q-wave MI; patients surviving cardiac arrest occurring more than 48 hours after the acute phase of MI in the absence of a recurrent ischemic event
11. Unexplained Palpitations
    Patients with palpitations who have a pulse rate documented by medical personnel as inappropriately rapid and in whom ECG recordings fail to document the cause of the palpitations; patients with palpitations preceding a syncopal episode
12. Guiding Drug Therapy
    Patients with sustained VT or cardiac arrest, especially those with prior MI; patients with AVNRT, AV reentrant tachycardia using an accessory pathway, or atrial fibrillation associated with an accessory pathway, for whom chronic drug therapy is planned
13. Candidates for or Who Have Implantable Electrical Devices
    Patients with tachyarrhythmias, before and during implantation, and final (predischarge) programming of an electrical device to confirm its ability to perform as anticipated; patients with an implanted electrical antitachyarrhythmia device in whom changes in status or therapy may have influenced the continued safety and efficacy of the device; patients who have a pacemaker to treat a brady arrhythmia, and receive a cardioverter-defibrillator, to test for device interactions

---

*Patients with prolonged QT intervals or patients with premature ventricular complexes, couplets, and nonsustained ventricular tachycardia have Class II and III indications only.
Zipes, D. P., et al. (1995). ACC/AHA guidelines for clinical intracardiac electrophysiological and catheter ablation procedures. *Circulation, 92,* 673–691.

therapy for patients with inducible VT or survivors of cardiac arrest.

Electrophysiology testing is often recommended for patients who receive nonpharmacologic drug therapy. Implantation of combination antitachycardia pacemakers and ICDs usually requires a baseline EP test and may require testing after implantation to allow for correct programming of the device. Knowledge of baseline conduction and the presence of concurrent atrial arrhythmias are also helpful for appropriate device selection (see Chapter 32). In the near future, patients with reduced left ventricular ejection fractions and coronary heart disease may be eligible to undergo prophylactic ICD implantation without previous EP evaluation (Moss et al., 2002).

Wide-Complex Tachycardias

Wide-complex tachycardias can be caused by VT, supraventricular tachycardia with aberration, or preexcitation syndromes

DISPLAY 20-2

CLASSIFICATION OF SYNCOPE

Cardiovascular

Reflex

Vasovagal
Vagovagal (situational)
  Micturition
  Deglutition
  Defecation
  Glossopharyngeal neuralgia
  Postprandial
  Tussive
  Supine hypotensive syndrome of near-term pregnancy
  Valsalva
  Oculovagal
  Sneeze
  Instrumentation
  Diving
  Jacuzzi
  Weight lifting
  Trumpet playing
Orthostatic
  Hyperadrenergic (e.g., volume depletion)
  Hypoadrenergic
    Primary autonomic insufficiency
    Secondary autonomic insufficiency (e.g., neurologic
      disorders or drugs)
Carotid sinus syncope
  Cardioinhibitory
  Vasodepressor
  Mixed
  Central

Cardiac

Mechanical (obstructive)
  Aortic stenosis
  Hypertrophic cardiomyopathy
  Pulmonary embolism
  Aortic dissection
  Myocardial infarction
  Mitral stenosis
  Left atrial myxoma

Cardiovascular *(continued)*

Cardiac

  Pulmonic stenosis
  Cardiac tamponade
  Prosthetic valve malfunction
  Global myocardial ischemia
  Tetralogy of Fallot
  Pulmonary hypertension
Electrical (dysrhythmic)
  Atrioventricular block
  Sick sinus syndrome
  Supraventricular or ventricular arrhythmias
  Long QT syndrome
  Pacemaker related

NonCardiovascular

Neurologic

Vertebrobasilar transient ischemic attack
  Atherosclerosis
  Mechanical
Subclavian steal syndrome
Takayasu disease
Normal pressure hydrocephalus
Unwitnessed seizure
Orthostatic syncope

Metabolic

Hypoxia
Hypoglycemia
Hyperventilation

Psychiatric

Panic disorders
Major depression
Hysteria

Unexplained

From Manolis, A. S., Linzer, M., Salem, D. et al. (1990). Syncope: Current diagnostic evaluation and management. *Annals of Internal Medicine, 112,* 850–863.

such as antidromic reciprocating tachycardia, in which an accessory bypass tract is the antegrade limb and the AV node is the retrograde limb of the tachycardia. Although guidelines and criteria have been established to help practitioners diagnose wide-complex tachycardias using the 12-lead ECG, necessary criteria may be difficult to identify, and the diagnosis may not be certain (Dongas et al., 1985; Wellens et al., 1984). In these cases, EP studies are necessary to confirm or establish a diagnosis so that proper safe treatment can be initiated (Zipes et al., 1995).

During invasive EP testing for wide-complex arrhythmias, the timing and sequence of atrial activation in relation to ventricular activation are recorded. Although it may be difficult to distinguish the various preexcitation syndromes from VT, the presence of AV dissociation favors a diagnosis of VT.

Syncope

Syncope is defined as a sudden, transient loss of consciousness accompanied by loss of postural tone (Hess et al., 1982). Syncope is a common medical problem with many potential causes (Display 20-2). The cause is unclear in approximately half the patients who present with syncope (Kapoor et al., 1983). Some cases may be benign and self-limiting. The 1-year mortality rate for presumed cardiac causes of syncope has been reported at 20% to 30% (Eagle et al., 1984; Kapoor et al., 1983, 1986). Even though patients are routinely referred to EP centers for syncope evaluation, invasive EP testing is not always indicated. A thorough history, physical examination, and noninvasive testing can frequently uncover the mechanism and direct treatment.

The history, including observers' statements, is extremely important to assist in directing the syncope evaluation. A description of onset and recovery can provide clues for the cause. For example, sudden onset without any warning signs or symptoms suggests a cardiac arrhythmia. Recovery from syncope caused by cardiac causes is usually rapid, without neurologic sequelae, whereas recovery from a seizure is usually associated with a period of drowsiness and confusion.

The physical examination should include orthostatic vital signs and carotid sinus pressure in patients who do not have cerebrovascular disease or carotid bruits (Nelson et al., 1987). A positive carotid sinus test is documented by recording a pause of 3 seconds or longer or a blood pressure decrease of greater than 50 mm Hg without symptoms. A 30 mm Hg blood pressure decrease with symptoms is also considered an abnormal t est result (Sugrue et al., 1984). Reproduction of symptoms may suggest the cause of syncope, especially if other causes are ruled out.

Once the practitioner determines that a cardiac cause is most likely, a series of noninvasive tests may be indicated. The 12-lead ECG should be evaluated for arrhythmias, long QT syndrome, left ventricular hypertrophy, preexcitation, conduction abnormalities, and ischemia or infarction. An echocardiogram helps to rule out or confirm the presence of structural heart disease and to evaluate left ventricular function. EP study results suggest that an arrhythmia is more likely to be the cause of syncope in patients who have structural heart disease and reduced left ventricular function. When ventricular arrhythmias are suspected, hospitalization with immediate EP testing is indicated because these patients are presumed to be at high-risk for sudden cardiac death until proven otherwise (Fogoros, 1999). Ambulatory monitoring for 24 to 48 hours may be helpful if the patient is having frequent symptoms and is not considered to be at high-risk for ventricular arrhythmias. If symptoms are not frequent enough, patient-activated transtelephonic event recorder (Linzer, 1988) or a subcutaneously implanted loop recorder system (Medtronic, Inc., Bedford, NH) may be helpful in documenting the presence or absence of arrhythmia during symptoms of pre-syncope or syncope (Krahn et al., 1995). The signal-averaged ECG has been reported as useful in screening patients at risk for VT-induced syncope (Gang et al., 1986; Winters et al., 1987). This technique involves recording, amplifying, and filtering the surface ECG. Low-amplitude, high-frequency signals called late potentials are detected at the terminal portion of the QRS (Berbari et al., 1988; Hall et al., 1989). Delayed myocardial activation in areas of scar tissue represented by late potentials is thought to be the cause of ventricular arrhythmias. Prediction of VT by signal-averaged ECG is more accurate in patients with coronary heart disease (Kuchar et al., 1986). A positive test in a patient with known heart disease is an indication for invasive EP testing (Nalos et al., 1987).

The head-upright tilt test is a noninvasive, provocative test used to try to reproduce and diagnose neurally mediated syncope (NMS). NMS is manifested by a combination of vasodilation and bradycardia, which occurs when the feedback mechanisms between the parasympathetic nervous system and sympathetic nervous system break down. Both systems are thought to activate alternately or simultaneously. Normal circulatory function is interrupted when both systems discharge rapidly. Vagal stimulation becomes exaggerated and causes bradycardia, vasodilation, or both in the presence of sympathetic nervous system stimulation (Clutter, 1991; Purcell, 1992). During the head-upright tilt test, the patient is placed on a tilt table with a footboard. There are various protocols for inducing NMS. Basically, an upright tilt at 60 to 80 degrees for 10 to 60 minutes is performed. Isoproterenol is administered in increasing doses until a positive result or until the end of the protocol is reached without documentation of syncope. A positive response reproduces the patient's symptoms along with documentation of bradycardia, hypotension, or both (Almquist et al., 1998; Fitzpatrick et al., 1991; Sheldon et al., 1992).

Invasive EP studies are indicated when a noninvasive evaluation for syncope is negative and the suspicion for a cardiac cause remains high (Bass et al., 1988; Denes et al., 1988; Teichman et al., 1985). Sinus node function is evaluated by measuring the sinus node recovery time. Overdrive pacing is performed in the high right atrium for 30 to 60 seconds (Yee et al., 1987). A prolonged sinus node recovery time may be an indication of sick sinus syndrome. The His-Purkinje system is evaluated by measuring the HV interval during sinus rhythm, and during incremental atrial pacing and atrial refractory period determinations. A prolonged HV interval is an indication of infrahisian disease (Zipes et al., 1995). AV node function is also evaluated by incremental atrial pacing and refractory period determinations. The Wenckebach point is recorded during incremental pacing, whereas the effective refractory periods of the atrium and AV node are recorded with the introduction of atrial extrastimuli. The atrium is refractory when the atrial extrastimuli fail to capture the atrium. The AV node is refractory when the atrial extrastimuli capture the atrium but fail to result in a His bundle depolarization (AV block). Permanent pacing may be indicated if abnormalities are found. Attempts are also made to induce ventricular and supraventricular tachycardia during EP testing for syncope.

In all cases, the findings of the EP study along with reproduction of the patient's symptoms and other findings in the work-up must be evaluated carefully to determine the appropriate course of therapy. Syncope remains unexplained in approximately half of all cases (Kapoor et al., 1984). The prognosis for this latter group of patients is good (DiMarco et al., 1981).

INTERVENTIONAL ELECTROPHYSIOLOGY AND CATHETER ABLATION

This interventional procedure includes a diagnostic EP study and catheter ablation. The mechanism of the arrhythmia is confirmed during the first part of the procedure, and the ablation takes place during the second part. Most centers combine the diagnostic and therapeutic segments of the study into one procedure (Calkins et al., 1992).

Radiofrequency Catheter Ablation

Catheter ablation techniques have been in use for more than 15 years. High-energy, direct-current shocks were delivered through catheters, using a standard defibrillator, to the endocardial ablation site (Gallagher et al., 1982; Scheinman et al., 1982). The technique was not widely used, however, because of the high complication rate, including cardiac tamponade and immediate and late sudden death (Evans et al., 1989; Hauer et al., 1988). As a result, efforts to find a safer energy source were pursued. In 1986, radiofrequency (RF) energy was applied through catheters to create endocardial lesions (Langberg et al., 1989; Huang et al., 1987). RF energy is a form of electrical energy that is produced by high-frequency alternating current. As the current passes through tissue, heat is created. RF current is used in the operating room to coagulate blood vessels and to ablate abnormal tissue during neurosurgery. RF current used during endocardial catheter ablation is alternating current with a 500,000- to 750,000-Hz frequency range. The current passes from the electrode tip to a large surface-area skin patch. The current is typically applied for 10 to 60 seconds at a time using 45 to 55 W. Catheter delivery of RF energy causes tissue heating in a small area around the electrode. The typical lesion is $3 \times 4 \times 5$ mm (Huang et al., 1987). Alternate forms of energy for lesion generation are currently under investigation. These include cryoablation, ultrasound, laser, and microwave energy sources.

Techniques

The first part of the procedure, the diagnostic phase, was described previously. After a diagnosis is made, an ablating catheter is positioned at the targeted area. The ablating catheter can be steered and has four to six electrodes 2 to 5 mm apart. The catheter tip is 4 to 8 mm long and serves as the electrode through which RF current is applied. The targeted area is located using fluoroscopy and by observing the electrogram patterns recorded by the distal mapping electrode pair. Recently developed three-dimensional mapping systems have vastly improved the precision and efficiency of mapping (Fisher & Swartz, 1992).

Complications

Two of the most common complications associated with catheter ablation are inadvertent complete heart block when ablating in close proximity to the conduction system and cardiac perforation with tamponade when ablating within the atria, coronary sinus or other cardiac veins, or right ventricle. Less than 1% to 2% of the occurrences of these complications have been reported. Rare complications include creating inadvertent arrhythmogenic foci, producing mitral or tricuspid regurgitation when ablating at or near valves, systemic embolization and stroke (particularly when ablating in the left heart), the creation of fixed lesions in coronary arteries when RF is applied in an adjacent area, and pulmonary vein stenosis when performing focal AF ablation (Fogoros, 1999; Robbins et al., 1998).

Indications

Combination EP study and catheter ablation procedures are indicated for patients with supraventricular tachycardias caused by accessory pathways (APs), AV nodal reentry tachycardia, intra-atrial tachycardias caused by either automatic or reentrant mechanism, atrial fibrillation, and atrial flutter. These procedures are also indicated for some patients with certain types of VT (Display 20-3).

Atrioventricular Nodal Reentrant Tachycardia

Dual AV nodal pathways are the substrate for AV nodal reentrant tachycardia (AVNRT). This arrhythmia is responsible for 60% to 70% of paroxysmal supraventricular tachycardias (PSVTs) (Calkins et al., 1992). The fast pathway has a longer effective refractory period and the slow pathway has a shorter refractory period. The typical form of AVNRT is initiated when a premature beat from the atrium is blocked in the fast pathway. The early beat conducts down the slow pathway and then reenters back into the atrium through the fast pathway. This impulse continues to conduct down the slow pathway and up the fast pathway, thus perpetuating the reentry circuit and the tachycardia. Uncommon or atypical forms of AVNRT can be found and consist of antegrade fast and retrograde slow pathway conductions, or antegrade and retrograde slow pathway conduction over multiple fibers. Ablation of all forms of AVNRT is generally the same and is accomplished by mapping the slow pathway region, which extends from the posterior/inferior interatrial septum near the coronary sinus ostium to the anterior/superior interatrial septum. After characteristic electrograms are recorded, RF energy is applied through the distal mapping and ablating electrode (Fig. 20-3). Repeat programmed stimulation is performed after the ablation in an attempt to induce the tachycardia. The procedure is considered successful when AVNRT cannot be induced and/or when there is no evidence of slow pathway conduction. Complete heart block is a potential serious complication because of the close proximity of the slow pathway to the compact AV node and has been reported 1.3% to 3% of the time. The success rate is reported between 96% and 100% (Scheinman, 1992; Jackman et al., 1992).

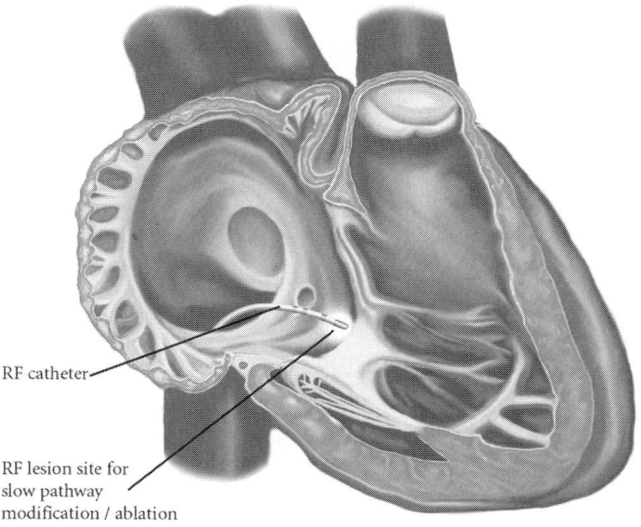

RF catheter

RF lesion site for slow pathway modification / ablation

■ **Figure 20–3.** Diagram of slow pathway catheter ablation for treatment of atrioventricular nodal reentrant tachycardia (AVNRT).

DISPLAY 20–3

INDICATIONS FOR CATHETER ABLATION PROCEDURES

Class I: Conditions for which there is general agreement that ablation procedure is beneficial for patient treatment.

Class II: Conditions for which ablation procedure is frequently performed, but there is less certainty about the benefit and experts are divided in their opinion as to whether patients with these conditions are likely to benefit from ablation.

Class III: Conditions for which there is general agreement that ablation procedure does not provide benefit for the patient and procedure is not warranted in patients with these conditions.

1. Modification of Atrioventricular Junction for Ventricular Rate Control of Atrial Tachyarrhythmias

   Class I: Patients with symptomatic atrial tachyarrhythmias who have inadequately controlled ventricular rates unless primary ablation of the atrial tachyarrhythmia is possible; Patients with symptomatic atrial tachyarrhythmias such as those above but when drugs are not tolerated or the patient does not wish to take them, even though the ventricular rate can be controlled; Patients with symptomatic nonparoxysmal junctional tachycardia that is drug resistant, drugs are not tolerated, or the patient does not wish to take them; Patients resuscitated from sudden cardiac death due to atrial flutter or atrial fibrillation with a rapid ventricular response in the absence of an accessory pathway.

   Class II: Patients with a dual-chamber pacemaker and pacemaker-mediated tachycardia that cannot be treated effectively by drugs or by reprogramming the pacemaker.

   Class III: Patients with atrial tachyarrhythmias responsive to drug therapy acceptable to the patient.

2. Atrioventricular Nodal Reentrant Tachycardia

   Class I: Patients with symptomatic sustained AVNRT that is drug resistant (DR) or the patient is drug intolerant (DI) or does not desire long-term drug (LTD) therapy.

   Class II: Patients with sustained AVNRT identified during electrophysiological study or catheter ablation of another arrhythmia: the finding of dual AV nodal pathway physiology and atrial echoes but without AVNRT during electrophysiological study in patients suspected of having AVNRT clinically

   Class III: Patients with AVNRT responsive to drug therapy that is well tolerated and preferred by the patient to ablation; the finding of dual AV nodal pathway physiology (with or without echo complexes) during electrophysiological study in patients in whom AVNRT is not suspected clinically.

3. Atrial Tachycardia, Flutter, and Fibrillation

   Class I: Patients with atrial tachycardia that is DR or the patient is DI or does not desire LTD therapy; patients with atrial flutter that is DR or the patient is DI or does not desire LTD therapy.

   Class II: Atrial flutter/atrial tachycardia associated with paroxysmal atrial fibrillation when the tachycardia is DR or the patient is DI or does not desire LTD; patients with atrial fibrillation and evidence of a localized site(s) of origin when the tachycardia is DR or the patient is DI or does not desire LTD therapy.

   Class III: Patients with atrial arrhythmia that is responsive to drug therapy, well tolerated, and preferred by the patient to ablation; patients with multiform atrial tachycardia.

4. Accessory Pathways

   Class I: Patients with symptomatic AV reentrant tachycardia that is DR or the patient is DI or does not desire LTD therapy; patients with atrial fibrillation (or other atrial tachyarrhythmia) and a rapid ventricular response via the accessory pathway when the tachycardia is DR or the patient is DI or does not desire LTD therapy.

   Class II: Patients with AV reentrant tachycardia or atrial fibrillation with rapid ventricular rates identified during electrophysiological study of another arrhythmia; asymptomatic patients with ventricular preexcitation whose livelihood or profession, important activities, insurability, or mental well being or the public safety would be affected by spontaneous tachyarrhythmias or the presence of the ECG abnormality; patients with atrial fibrillation and a controlled ventricular response via the accessory pathway; patients with a family history of sudden cardiac death.

   Class III: Patients who have accessory pathway-related arrhythmias that are responsive to drug therapy, well tolerated, and preferred by the patient to ablation.

5. Ventricular Tachycardia

   Class I: Patients with symptomatic sustained monomorphic VT when the tachycardia is DR or the patient is DI or does not desire LTD therapy; patients with bundle branch reentrant ventricular tachycardia; patients with sustained monomorphic VT and an ICD who are receiving multiple shocks not manageable by reprogramming or concomitant drug therapy.

   Class II: Nonsustained VT that is symptomatic when the tachycardia is drug resistant or the patient is drug intolerant or does not desire long-term drug therapy.

   Class III: Patients with VT that is responsive to drug, ICD, or surgical therapy and that therapy is well tolerated and preferred by the patient to ablation; unstable, rapid, multiple, or polymorphic VT that cannot be adequately localized by current mapping techniques; asymptomatic and clinically benign nonsustained VT.

Zipes, D. P., et al. (1995). ACC/AHA guidelines for clinical intracardiac electrophysiological and catheter ablation procedures. *Circulation, 92,* 673–691.

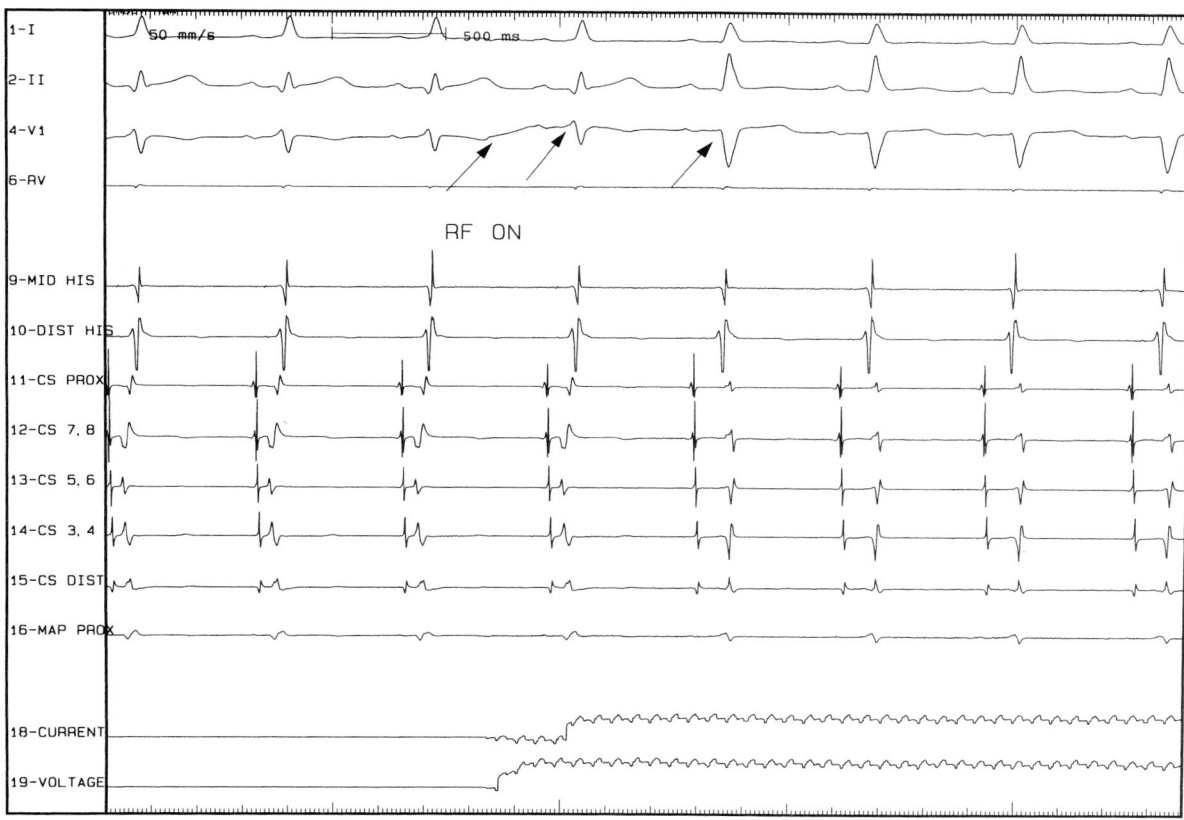

■ **Figure 20–4.** Loss of delta wave after onset of radiofrequency (RF) energy application. Channel 1, lead I; channel 2, lead II; channel 4, lead V_1; channel 6, right ventricular tracing; channels 9 and 10, His bundle electrograms; channels 11-15, coronary sinus (CS) electrograms. Notice that before RF energy is applied, the earliest ventricular depolarization occurs on the CS electrogram labeled CS 5, 6, corresponding to the left posterior septal position. This location is where the mapping and ablating catheter was positioned under the mitral valve annulus. After RF energy application, the delta wave disappears (leads I, II_1, V_1), and the ventricular activation sequence changes to normal on all coronary sinus electrograms.

Atrioventricular Reentrant Tachycardia

Both Wolff-Parkinson-White (WPW) syndrome and concealed AV bypass tracts are responsible for 30% to 40% of PSVTs (Calkins et al., 1991). The anatomy is basically the same. The AP is a small bundle of muscle fibers that crosses the AV groove on either the right or left side of the heart, creating an extra electrical connection that can conduct in one or both directions. When the AP conducts in an anterograde direction, a delta wave can be observed on the ECG and is characteristic of WPW syndrome. PSVT is initiated in the same manner as described for AVNRT. The AV node serves as the antegrade limb of the tachycardia and the AP serves as the retrograde limb of the tachycardia. This conduction pattern results in a narrow QRS complex and is known as orthodromic reciprocating tachycardia. If conduction travels antegrade over the AP and retrograde up the AV node, then a wide QRS complex is observed and is known as antidromic reciprocating tachycardia. If atrial fibrillation occurs in a patient with WPW syndrome, then a life-threatening situation may develop if conduction over the AP is rapid enough to induce VF. Less common forms of APs are the Mahaim fiber, which slowly conducts only antegrade and is found on the right side of the heart, and the permanent form

of junctional reciprocating tachycardia (PJRT), which slowly conducts only retrograde and is located very near or within the coronary sinus ostium (McClelland et al., 1994; Ticho et al., 1992).

Catheter ablation of AV bypass tracts on the left side of the heart involves one of two techniques. The mapping and ablating catheter can be advanced from the femoral artery retrograde across the aortic valve. The catheter is then positioned under or on the mitral valve annulus. When the catheter is positioned properly, the AP activation can be recorded (Calkins et al., 1992; Jackman et al., 1991). RF current is then applied. If the patient has WPW syndrome, the delta wave on the ECG disappears during RF energy application (Fig. 20-4). It is necessary to ablate so that both antegrade and retrograde conduction over the bypass tract are abolished. Testing is performed after ablating to assess for retrograde conduction and to try to induce tachycardia. Another approach to the mitral annulus is by means of transseptal catheterization. In this approach, the ablating and mapping catheter is advanced to the left atrium through the right heart using a special sheath assembly to cross the interatrial septum (Fig. 20-5). Both approaches have an 85% success rate (Lesh, 1993). Catheter ablation of right-sided and septal APs are somewhat more difficult because there is no structure analogous to the coronary

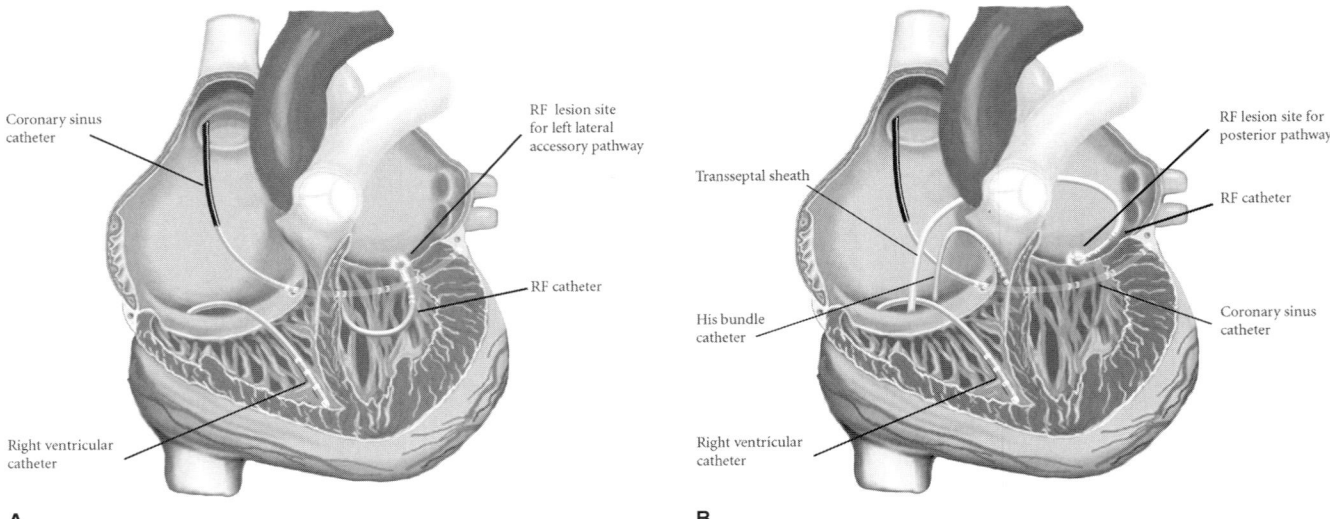

■ **Figure 20–5.** Diagram of catheter ablation of (*A*) left lateral accessory pathway using aortic approach associated radiograph in the left anterior oblique view and (*B*) left posterior lateral accessory pathway using transeptal approach. (A redrawn from Fellows, C. L., Brett, C., & Main, C. C. [1992]. Radio-frequency catheter ablation of Wolff-Parkinson-White syndrome. *Virginia Mason Clinic Bulletin,* 46, 45–51.)

sinus to aide in mapping the atrial- ventricular groove. Specialized multi-electrode, steerable catheters and long guiding sheaths have proven useful in providing catheter stability for mapping and ablating on the right side of the heart.

Atrial Fibrillation and Flutter

Complete AV node ablation is indicated for patients who have chronic or paroxysmal atrial fibrillation or flutter with a rapid ventricular response. This procedure should be performed only in patients for whom conventional antiarrhythmic drug therapy has failed or for whom the side effects from effective doses of medication are intolerable. This procedure is performed by advancing the ablating catheter from the right femoral vein to the area of the AV node (Fig. 20-6). Complete heart block or a junctional escape rhythm is the result. Permanent, rate-responsive pacing is indicated after AV node ablation, and the patient may discontinue all antiarrhythmic medications (Langberg et al.,

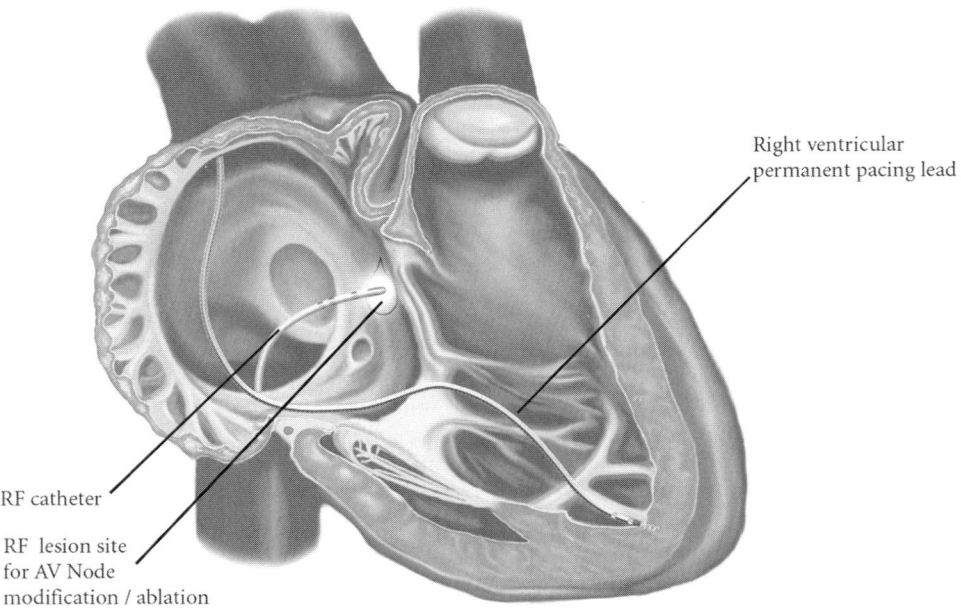

■ **Figure 20–6.** Diagram of catheter ablation of AV node and right ventricular pacemaker lead.

1989; Jackman et al., 1991). Continuous anticoagulation is recommended because the underlying arrhythmia is still present. Left ventricular dysfunction caused by chronic, rapid heart rates in atrial fibrillation has been reported to improve after AV node ablation (Rodriguez et al., 1993). In addition, more than 80% of patients report improved quality of life with increased exercise tolerance after this procedure (Fitzpatrick et al., 1996).

Recent ablation techniques for atrial fibrillation have focused on the ablation of triggers or ectopic beats that arise from the pulmonary veins within the left atrium. In the mid 1990s, Haissaguerre and colleges observed that isolated or multiple focal discharges emanated from sleeves of atrial myocardium, which encased the pulmonary veins. These discharges often led to the initiation of atrial fibrillation (Haissaguerre et al., 1996). Catheter ablation of these triggers involves puncture of the intra-atrial septum and placement of the ablation and mapping catheters within the left atrium. Pulmonary vein potentials can be mapped at the ostium of the pulmonary veins and RF current is applied at sites with early potentials (Fig. 20-7). The goal is to electrically isolate all four pulmonary veins, thereby eliminating the ability for these discharges to enter the left atrium and trigger atrial fibrillation. An alternative ablation technique involves the creation of linear lesions within the left atrium that encircle the atrial tissue around the pulmonary vein ostia. This approach is primarily anatomic, and mapping of electrogram is not necessary. A three-dimensional electro-anatomic mapping system is used as a guide (Pappone et al., 2000). Other lesion sets and ablation techniques for atrial fibrillation are currently under development. Potential complications include stroke, pulmonary vein stenosis, phrenic nerve injury, esophageal perforation, pericardial perforation and tamponade, as well as the usual complications associated with EP and catheter ablation

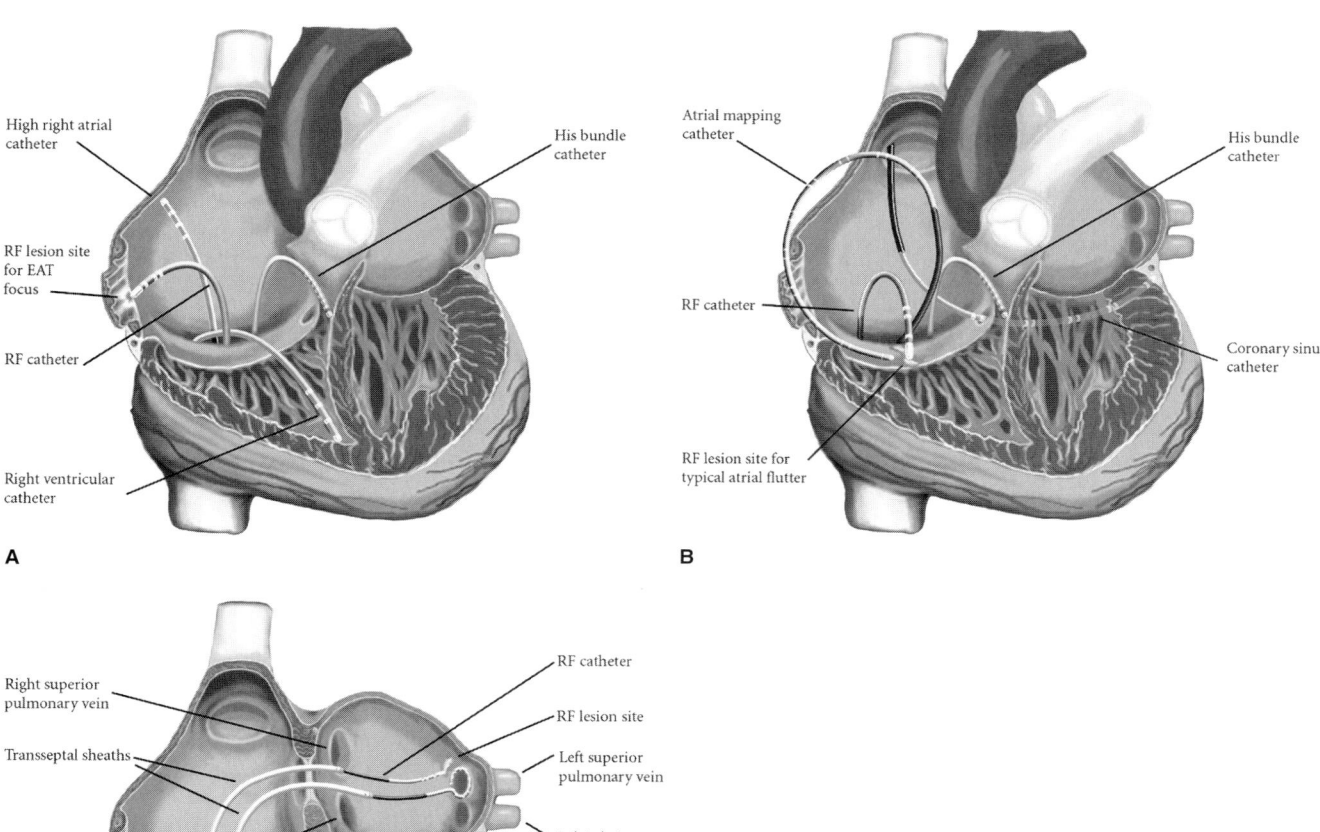

■ **Figure 20–7.** Diagram of catheter ablation of (*A*) ectopic atrial tachycardia with focus on lateral wall of right atrium, (*B*) right atrial isthmus dependent flutter, and (*C*) pulmonary vein ostium for atrial fibrillation.

procedures. The risk of major complications appears to be approximately 1% to 2%. Success rates vary with the experience of the centers performing this procedure and range from 70% to 80% (Haissaguerre et al., 2000; Chen et al., 1999; Pappone et al., 2000).

Primary ablation of typical or type 1 atrial flutter is being performed in many centers. This procedure involves ablation of a discrete anatomic region thought to be responsible for the arrhythmia. Ablation in the lower right atrium within a zone of critical slow conduction creates a line of block that prevents perpetuation of the arrhythmia (Figure 20- 7). Success rates in an experienced center were reported to be 88% (n = 51). Although the procedure was safe, with an extremely low complication rate, the recurrence of atrial flutter or the development of new-onset or recurrent atrial fibrillation was not uncommon. Repeat ablation was successful in most cases (Saxton et al., 1996).

Atrial Arrhythmias

Arrhythmias that originate in the atria and arise from either reentrant circuits or abnormal foci can often be treated with catheter ablation. Patients who have undergone atrial surgery for congenital heart disease may have fixed anatomic barriers within scar tissue, which facilitate a reentrant tachycardia. Arrhythmias that arise from abnormal atrial foci have increased automaticity as their mechanism and can be found in either the left or right atrium. The effective site for ablation in both cases is determined by methodically mapping the appropriate atrium during tachycardia (see Fig. 20-7). The earliest atrial endocardial electrogram marks the origin of the tachycardia (Lesh et al., 1994).

Ventricular Tachycardia

Ablation of paroxysmal VT can be a challenging therapy for patients whose tachycardia is suited to study and ablation. For a VT focus to be ablated, the tachycardia must be inducible, monomorphic, and tolerated for long enough periods to enable accurate mapping. The advent of electro-anatomic and non-contact three-dimensional mapping systems have greatly facilitated mapping and ablation of VT (Kautzner et al., 2003). For a successful ablation, the type of VT must be determined.

Bundle-branch reentrant tachycardia conducts antegrade over the right bundle and retrograde over the left bundle. This type of VT occurs in patients who have severe ischemic or idiopathic cardiomyopathy. The VT is rapid because it uses the His–Purkinje system. Ablation of the right bundle usually abolishes this VT (Cohen et al., 1991).

Benign monomorphic VT (idiopathic VT) typically occurs in young people with no structural heart disease. The VT can arise from the right ventricular outflow tract or from the inferior left ventricular septum. Various EP techniques are used to map the presumed site of origin before ablating. RF ablation is most often successful in this group of patients.

VT associated with coronary heart disease is usually caused by a reentrant mechanism in an area of patchy fibrosis or scar. One of the problems encountered with ablating in this situation is that these patients may have multiple tachycardia circuits (Lesh, 1993). Ablation can be attempted if a single monomorphic VT is identified. Three-dimensional mapping systems can be used to reconstruct the region of scar within the ventricle and to identify the critical zones of conduction delay responsible for reentrant VT. The earliest site of activation during VT can also be located using these mapping systems (Kautzner et al., 2003). Techniques to identify the best ablation site are still undergoing development.

NURSING CARE OF THE PATIENT UNDERGOING ELECTROPHYSIOLOGY PROCEDURES

Health care professionals caring for arrhythmia patients play a pivotal role for the patient undergoing an EP and/or catheter ablation procedure. The need for patient education throughout all phases of the arrhythmia experience has been well documented (Berry, 1993; Connelly, 1992; Moulton et al., 1993). Teaching before the study must include discussions about the nature of the test, a description of the procedure, procedure length, success rates, and complication rates. Nurses must also include postprocedure instructions and discharge instructions. After the procedure, the patient must keep the affected leg(s) straight for 3 to 4 hours to allow the venous puncture site to heal and for 4 to 6 hours if the femoral artery was punctured. The preliminary results of the procedure should be shared immediately with the patient and family. Frequent explanations may be required at first if the patient is recovering from heavy sedation. After a successful ablation, patients have no restrictions and antiarrhythmic medications are usually discontinued.

Most of the intraprocedure and postprocedure nursing care is centered on monitoring the patient for potential complications related to the procedure. In most instances, patients are anxious before and during EP procedures. Adequate sedation to allow for patient comfort should be provided. Oversedation must be prevented. Nurses must be alert for major complications directly related to placement of catheters inside the heart. Bleeding from catheter insertion sites, tamponade from perforation, and tachyarrhythmias and bradyarrhythmias can all occur during and after the EP procedure. Nurses who care for patients with arrhythmias in any setting should be prepared to handle any emergency that may arise. Other potential problems to monitor for include thrombophlebitis, thromboembolism, and infection.

The North American Society of Pacing and Electrophysiology (NASPE) has recently developed standards of professional practice for allied professionals (nurses, nurse practitioners, physician assistants, technicians) caring for patients with cardiac rhythm disorders. The standards for EP procedures are three-fold and include: (1) the application of scientific principals related to clinical electrophysiology to provide technical support and patient care services; (2) the demonstration of technical knowledge and clinical skills to operate laboratory equipment and troubleshoot equipment malfunction; and (3) the integration of cardiovascular and electrical knowledge to effectively monitor the patient throughout the procedure (Gure et al., 2003).

Acknowledgment: *The St. Jude Medical images were created by Claude Rickerd.*

REFERENCES

Almquist, A., Goldenberg, I. F., & Milstein, S., et al. (1989). Provocation of bradycardia and hypotension by isoproterenol and upright posture in patients with unexplained syncope. *New England Journal of Medicine, 320,* 346–351.

AVID Investigators. (1997). A comparison of antiarrhythmic drug therapy with implantable defibrillators in patients resuscitated from near-fatal ventricular arrhythmias. *New England Journal of Medicine, 337,* 1576–1583.

Bass, E. B., Elson, J. J., Fogoros, R. N., et al. (1988). Long-term prognosis of patients undergoing electrophysiology studies for syncope of unknown origin. *American Journal of Cardiology, 62,* 1186–1191.

Berbari, E. J., & Lazzara, R. (1988). An introduction to high resolution ECG recordings of cardiac late potentials. *Archives of Internal Medicine, 148,* 1859–1863.

Berry, V. A. (1993). Wolff-Parkinson-White syndrome and the use of radiofrequency catheter ablation. *Heart & Lung, 22,* 15–25.

Buxton, A. E., Lee, K. L., Fisher, J. D., et al. (1999). A randomized study of prevention of sudden death in patients with coronary artery disease: Multicenter Unsustained Tachycardia Trial Investigators. *New England Journal of Medicine, 341,* 1882–1890.

Calkins, H., Kim, Y. N., Schmaltz, S., et al. (1992). Electrogram criteria for identification of appropriate target sites for radiofrequency catheter ablation of accessory connections. *Circulation, 85,* 565–573.

Calkins, H., Sousa, J., El-Atassi, R., et al. (1991). Diagnosis and cure of the Wolff-Parkinson-White syndrome or paroxysmal supraventricular tachycardias during a single electrophysiologic test. *New England Journal of Medicine, 324,* 1612–1618.

Chen, S. A., Hsieh, M. H., Tai, C. T., et al. (1999). Initiation of atrial fibrillation by ectopic beats originating from the pulmonary veins: electrophysiological characteristics, pharmacological responses, and effects of radiofrequency ablation. *Circulation, 100,* 1879–1886.

Clutter, C. (1991). Neurally mediated syncope. *Journal of Cardiovascular Nursing, 5,* 65–73.

Cobb, L., & Hallstrom, A. P. (1977). Clinical predictors and characteristics of the sudden cardiac death syndrome. In *Proceedings USA/USSR First Joint Symposium on Sudden Death.* DHEW Publication no. (NIH) 78–1470. Washington, DC: National Institutes of Health.

Cohen, T. J., Chien, W. U., Lurie, K. G., et al. (1991). Radiofrequency catheter ablation for treatment of bundle branch reentrant VT: results and long-term follow-up. *Journal of the American College of Cardiology, 18,* 1767–1773.

Connelly, A. G. (1992). An examination of stressors in the patient undergoing cardiac electrophysiologic studies. *Heart Lung, 21,* 335–342.

Connolly, S. J., Gent, M., Roberts, R. S., et al. (2000). Canadian implantable defibrillator study (CIDS): A randomized trial of the implantable cardioverter defibrillator against amiodarone. *Circulation, 101,* 1297–1302.

Denes, P., Uretz, E., Ezri, M. D., et al. (1988). Clinical predictors of electrophysiologic testing in patients with syncope of unknown origin. *Archives of Internal Medicine, 148,* 1922–1928.

DiMarco, J. P., Garan, H., & Ruskin, J. N. (1982). Complications in patients undergoing electrophysiologic procedures. *Annals of Internal Medicine, 97,* 490–493.

Dongas, J., Lehman, M. H., Mahmud, R., et al. (1985). Value of preexisting bundle branch block in the ECG differentiation of supraventricular from ventricular origin of wide QRS tachycardia. *American Journal of Cardiology, 55,* 717–721.

Eagle, K. A., Black, H. R., Cook, E. F., et al. (1984). Evaluation of prognostic classifications for patients with syncope. *Annals of Internal Medicine, 100,* 755–757.

Evans, G. J., Scheinman, M. M., Zipes, D. P., et al. (1989). The percutaneous cardiac mapping and ablation registry: Final summary of results. *Journal of Pacing and Clinical Electrophysiology, 11,* 1621–1626.

Fisher, W. G., & Swartz, J. F. (1992). Three-dimensional electrogram mapping improves ablation of left sided accessory pathway. *Journal of Pacing and Clinical Electrophysiology, 15,* 2344–2356.

Fitzpatrick, A. P., Kourouyan, H. D., Siu, A., et al. (1996). Quality of life and outcomes after radiofrequency His-bundle ablation and permanent pacemaker implantation: Impact of treatment in paroxysmal and established atrial fibrillation. *American Heart Journal, 121,* 499–507.

Fitzpatrick, A. P., Theodorakis, G., Vardas, P., et al. (1991). Methodology of head-up tilt testing in patients with unexplained syncope. *Journal of the American College of Cardiology, 17,* 125–130.

Fogoros, R. N. (1999). Principles of the electrophysiology study. *Practical cardiac diagnosis series: Electrophysiologic testing* (3rd ed., pp. 37–60). Blackwell[AQ1] Science.

Gallagher, J. J., Svenson, R. H., Kasell, J. H., et al. (1982). Catheter technique for closed-chest ablation of the atrioventricular conduction system. *New England Journal of Medicine, 306,* 194–200.

Gang, E. S., Peter, T., Rosenthal, M. E., et al. (1986). Detection of late potentials on the surface electrocardiogram in unexplained syncope. *American Journal of Cardiology, 58,* 1014–1020.

Greene, H. L. (1990). Sudden arrhythmic cardiac death: Mechanisms, resuscitation, and classification. *American Journal of Cardiology, 65,* 4B–12B.

Gure, M. T., Bubien, R. S., Belco, K. M., et al. (2003). Policy statement: North American Society of Pacing and Electrophysiology: Standards of professional practice for the allied professional in pacing and electrophysiology. *Journal of Pacing and Clinical Electrophysiology, 26*(1), 127–131.

Haissaguerre, M., Jais, P., Shah, D. C., et al. (1998). A focal source of atrial fibrillation by ectopic beats originating in the pulmonary veins. *New England Journal of Medicine, 339,* 659–666.

Haissaguerre, M., Jais, P., Shah, D. C., et al. (2000). Electrophysiological end point for catheter ablation of atrial fibrillation initiated from multiple pulmonary venous foci. *Circulation, 101,* 1409–1417.

Hall, P. A., Atwood, J. E., Myers, J., et al. (1989). The signal averaged surface electrocardiogram and the identification of late potentials. *Progress in Cardiovascular Disease, 31,* 195–217.

Hammill, S. C., Sugrue, D. D., Gersh, B. J., et al.[AQ2] Clinical intracardiac electrophysiologic testing: Technique, diagnostic indications, and therapeutic uses. *Mayo Clinic Proceedings, 61,* 478–503.

Hauer, R., Straks, W., Borst, C., et al. (1988). Electrical catheter ablation in the left and right ventricular wall in dogs: Relation between delivered energy and histopathologic changes. *Journal of the American College of Cardiology, 8,* 637–643.

Hess, D. S., Morady, F., & Scheinman, M. M. (1982). Electrophysiologic testing in the evaluation of patients with syncope of undetermined origin. *American Journal of Cardiology, 50,* 1309–1315.

Horowitz, L. H. (1986). Safety of electrophysiologic studies. *Circulation, 73,* II-28–II-30.

Huang, S., Bharati, S., Graham, A., et al. (1987). Closed chest catheter desiccation of the atrioventricular junction using radiofrequency energy: A new method of catheter ablation. *Journal of the American College of Cardiology, 9,* 349–358.

Jackman, W. M., Beckman, K. J., McClelland, J. H., et al. (1992). Treatment of supraventricular tachycardia due to atrioventricular nodal reentry, by radiofrequency catheter ablation of slow-pathway conduction. *New England Journal of Medicine, 327,* 313–318.

Jackman, W. M., Wang, X., Friday, K. J., et al. (1991). Catheter ablation of atrioventricular junction using radiofrequency current in 17 patients. *Circulation, 83,* 1562–1576.

Jackman, W. M., Wang, X., Friday, K. J., et al. (1991). Catheter ablation of atrioventricular pathways (Wolff-Parkinson-White syndrome) by radiofrequency current. *New England Journal of Medicine, 324,* 1605–1611.

Josephson, M. E. (1993). Electrophysiologic investigation: General concepts. In M. E. Josephson (Ed.), *Clinical cardiac electrophysiology techniques and interpretations* (2nd ed., pp. 22–70). Philadelphia: Lea & Febiger.

Kapoor, W. N., Karpf, M., Wieand, S., et al. (1983). A prospective evaluation and follow-up of patients with syncope. *New England Journal of Medicine, 309,* 197–204.

Kapoor, W. N., Snustad, D., Peterson, J., et al. (1986). Syncope in the elderly. *American Journal of Medicine, 80,* 419–428.

Kautzner, J., Cihak, R., Peichl, P., et al. (2003). Catheter ablation of ventricular tachycardia following MI using 3-Dimensional electroanatomic mapping. *Journal of Pacing and Clinical Electrophysiology, 26*(1), 342–347.

Krahn, A. D., Klein, G. J., Norris, C., & Yee, R. (1995). The etiology of syncope in patients with negative tilt table and electrophysiology testing. *Circulation, 92,* 1819–1824.

Kuchar, D. L., Thorburn, C. W., & Sammel, N. L. (1986). Signal-averaged electrocardiogram for evaluation of recurrent syncope. *American Journal of Cardiology, 58,* 949–953.

Kuck, K., Cappato, R., Siebels, J., et al. (2000). Randomized comparison of antiarrhythmic drug therapy with implantable defibrillators in patients resuscitated from cardiac arrest: the Cardiac Arrest Study Hamburg (CASH). *Circulation, 102,* 748–754.

Langberg, J. J., Chin, M. C., Rosenqvist, M., et al. (1989). Catheter ablation of the atrioventricular junction with radiofrequency energy. *Circulation, 80,* 1527–1535.

Lesh, M. D. (1993). Interventional electrophysiology: State-of-the-art 1993. *American Heart Journal, 126,* 686–698.

Lesh, M. D., Van Hare, G. F., Epstein, L. M., et al. (1994). Radiofrequency catheter ablation of atrial arrhythmias results and mechanisms. *Circulation, 89,* 1074–1089.

Linzer, M., Prystowsky, E. N., Brunetti, L. L., et al. (1988). Recurrent syncope of unknown origin diagnosed by ambulatory continuous loop ECG recording. *American Heart Journal, 116,* 1632–1634.

McClelland, J. H., Wang, K., Beckman, K. J., et al. (1994). Radiofrequency catheter ablation of right atriofascicular (Mahiam) accessory pathways guided by accessory pathway activation potentials. *Circulation, 89,* 2655–2666.

Moss, A. J., Hall, W. J., Cannom, D. S., et al. for the Madit Investigators. (1996). Improved survival with an implantable defibrillator in patients with coronary artery disease at high risk of ventricular arrhythmia. *New England Journal of Medicine, 335,* 1933–1940.

Moss, A. J., Zareba, W., Hall, J., et al. (2002). Prophylactic implantation of a defibrillator in patients with myocardial infarction and reduced ejection fraction. *New England Journal of Medicine, 346,* 877–883.

Morady, F., Scheinman, M. M., Hess, D. S., et al. (1983). Electrophysiologic testing in the management of survivors of out-of-hospital cardiac arrest. *American Journal of Cardiology, 51,* 85–89.

Moulton, L., Grant, J., Miller, B., et al. (1993). Radiofrequency catheter ablation for supraventricular tachycardia. *Heart and Lung, 22,* 3–14.

Nalos, P. C., Gang, E. S., Mandel, W. J., et al. (1987). The signal averaged electrocardiogram as a screening test for inducibility of sustained ventricular tachycardia in high risk patients: A prospective study. *Journal of the American College of Cardiology, 9,* 539–548.

Nelson, S. D., Kou, W. H., De Buitleir, M., et al. (1987). Value of programmed ventricular stimulation in presumed carotid sinus syndrome. *American Journal of Cardiology, 60,* 1073–1077.

Pappone, C., Rosanio, S., Oreto, G., et al. (2000). Circumferential radiofrequency ablation of pulmonary vein ostia: a new anatomic approach for curing atrial fibrillation. *Circulation, 104,* 2539–2544.

Purcell, J. A. (1992). Provoking vasodepressor syncope with head-up tilt-table testing. *Progress in Cardiovascular Nursing, 7,* 15–18.

Robbins, I. M., Colvin, E. V., Doyle, T. P., et al. (1998). Pulmonary vein stenosis after catheter ablation of atrial fibrillation. *Circulation, 98,* 1769–1775.

Rodriguez, L. M., Smeets, J. L. R. M., Xie, B., et al. (1993). Improvement of left ventricular function by ablation of atrioventricular nodal conduction in selected patients with lone atrial fibrillation. *American Journal of Cardiology, 72,* 1137–1141.

Saxon, L. A., Kalman, J. M., Olgin, J. E., et al. (1996). Results of radiofrequency catheter ablation for atrial flutter. *American Journal of Cardiology, 77,* 1014–1016.

Schaffer, W. A., & Cobb, L. A. (1975). Recurrent ventricular fibrillation and modes of death in survivors of out-of-hospital ventricular fibrillation. *New England Journal of Medicine, 293,* 259–262.

Scheinman, M. M. (1994). Patterns of catheter ablation practice in the United States: results of 1992 NASPE survey. *Journal of Pacing and Clinical Electrophysiology, 17,* 873–875.

Scheinman, M. M., Morady, F., Hess, D., et al. (1982). Catheter induced ablation of the atrioventricular junction to control refractory supraventricular arrhythmias. *Journal of the American Medical Association, 248,* 851–855.

Sheldon, R., & Killam, S. (1992). Methodology of isoproterenol-tilt table testing in patients with syncope. *Journal of the American College of Cardiology, 19,* 773–779.

Skale, B. T., Miles, W. M., Heger, J. J., et al. (1986). Survivors of cardiac arrest: Prevention of recurrence by drug therapy as predicted by electrophysiologic testing or electrocardiographic monitoring. *American Journal of Cardiology, 57,* 113–119.

Sugrue, D. D., Wood, D. L., & McGoon, M. D. (1984). Carotid sinus hypersensitivity and syncope. *Mayo Clinic Proceedings, 59,* 637–640.

Teichman, S. L., Felder, S. D., Matos, J. A., et al. (1985). The value of electrophysiologic studies in syncope of undetermined origin: Report of 150 cases. *American Heart Journal, 110,* 469–479.

Ticho, B. S., Saul, J. P., Hulse, J. E., et al. (1992). Variable location of accessory pathways associated with PJRT and confirmation with radiofrequency ablation. *American Journal of Cardiology, 70,* 1559–1564.

Wellens, H. J. J., Brugada, P., & Heddle, W. F. (1984). The value of the 12 lead ECG in diagnosis type and mechanism of a tachycardia: A survey among 22 cardiologists. *Journal of the American College of Cardiology, 4,* 176–179.

Wilber, D. J., Garan, H., Finkelstein, D., et al. (1988). Use of electrophysiologic testing in the prediction of long-term outcome. *New England Journal of Medicine, 318,* 19–24.

Yee R., & Strauss H. C. (1987). Electrophysiologic mechanisms: Sinus node dysfunction. *Circulation, 75*(Suppl. III), 12–18.

Zipes, D. P., DiMarco, J. P., Gillette, D. C., et al. (1995). American College of Cardiology/American Heart Association guidelines for clinical intracardiac electrophysiological and catheter ablation procedures. *Circulation, 92,* 673–691.

21

Exercise Testing

JONATHAN MYERS

Exercise testing is a widely used, noninvasive procedure that provides diagnostic, prognostic, and functional information for a wide spectrum of patients with cardiovascular, pulmonary, and other disorders. Graded exercise tests are used to assess a patient's ability to tolerate increased physical activity, while electrocardiographic, hemodynamic, and symptomatic responses are monitored in a controlled environment. Graded, progressive exercise can produce abnormalities that are not present at rest, the most important of which are manifestations of myocardial ischemia, including ST segment changes on the electrocardiogram, symptoms, and electrical instability. The test is also commonly used to evaluate other system disorders, such as gas exchange abnormalities in patients with pulmonary disease or chronic heart failure, symptoms associated with peripheral vascular disease, and even neurologic disorders.

In cardiovascular medicine, the exercise test is commonly used for evaluating the efficacy of medical therapy, for the assessment of interventions, and as a first-choice diagnostic tool in patients with suspected coronary artery disease (CAD), a role in which it functions as a "gatekeeper" to more expensive and invasive procedures (Marcus et al., 1995). In the latter role, the test has become even more important in the current era of health care cost containment. Although originally developed as a diagnostic tool, recent studies have established the role of the exercise test in the selection of patients for cardiac transplantation, risk stratification after a myocardial infarction (MI), and the assessment of disability (American Thoracic Society/American College of Chest Physicians, 2003; Chang & Froelicher, 1994; Costanzo et al., 1995; Gibbons et al., 2002; Myers & Gullestad, 1998).

Because of the need to standardize the implementation and interpretation of the exercise test, professional organizations such as the American Heart Association (AHA), the American College of Cardiology (ACC) (Gibbons et al., 2002), the American College of Sports Medicine (ACSM) (American College of Sports Medicine: Guidelines, 2001), the American Thoracic Society (American Thoracic Society/ American College of Chest Physicians, 2003), and the American Association of Cardiovascular and Pulmonary Rehabilitation (American Association of Cardiovascular and Pulmonary Rehabilitation, 1999) have developed guidelines designed to optimize the test's safety, methodology, and objectives. The ACSM has developed certification programs for professional competency in exercise testing (American

College of Sports Medicine: Guidelines, 2001; American College of Sports Medicine: Resource, 2001). ACSM certification has been strongly recommended for nurses, technicians, or physiologists who oversee exercise testing in clinical settings (American College of Sports Medicine: Resource, 2001; Herbert & Herbert, 1993; Rogers et al., 2000). This chapter describes the applications, methodology, and principles of exercise testing for the cardiovascular nurse and the professional standards for exercise testing described in the aforementioned guidelines.

INDICATIONS AND OBJECTIVES

The exercise test has numerous indications. Surveys have shown that the most common reason patients are referred for exercise testing is for the evaluation of chest pain (Miranda et al., 1989; Myers et al., 2000) or, more generally, to assess signs and symptoms of coronary disease. Other common clinical objectives include the following:

- Physiologic response of post-MI and post-revascularization patients to exercise
- Functional capacity for the purpose of exercise prescription
- Exercise capacity for the purpose of work classification (disability evaluation) and risk stratification (prognosis)
- The efficacy of medical, surgical, or pharmacologic treatment
- The presence and severity of arrhythmias
- Preoperative physiologic status
- Intermittent claudication

SAFETY AND PERSONNEL

Provided that contraindications to exercise testing are considered and patients who undergo exercise testing are appropriate, the test has been shown to be extremely safe. Widely cited data from the Cooper Clinic in Dallas (Gibbons et al., 1989) suggest that an event serious enough to require hospitalization (e.g., sustained arrhythmia, heart attack, or death) occurs at a rate of 0.8 per 10,000 tests. This was recently confirmed in a survey of 71 medical centers within the Veterans Affairs Health Care System, in which an event rate of 1.2 per 10,000 tests was

439

reported (Myers et al., 2000). Earlier surveys conducted in the 1970s suggested a somewhat higher event rate, ranging from 1 to 4 per 10,000 (Franklin et al., 1997; Froelicher & Myers, 2000; Rochmis & Blackburn, 1971; Thompson, 1993). It has been suggested that the apparent improvement in the safety of the test reflected in the more recent surveys is because of a significantly better understanding of when to and when not to perform the test, when to terminate the test, and better preparation for any emergency that may arise (Franklin et al., 1997; Gibbons et al., 2002).

Clinical judgment is the most important consideration when deciding which patients should undergo exercise testing. Contraindications to testing usually describe conditions of cardiovascular instability, such as unstable angina, uncontrolled heart failure, and arrhythmias. A listing of the absolute and relative contraindications to testing is provided in Display 21-1.

DISPLAY 21-1

CONTRAINDICATIONS TO EXERCISE TESTING

Absolute

1. A recent change in the resting electrocardiogram suggesting infarction or other acute cardiac event
2. Recent complicated myocardial infarction
3. Unstable angina
4. Uncontrolled ventricular arrhythmia
5. Uncontrolled atrial arrhythmia that compromises cardiac function
6. Third-degree atrioventricular heart block without pacemaker
7. Acute congestive heart failure
8. Severe aortic stenosis
9. Suspected or known dissecting aneurysm
10. Active or suspected myocarditis or pericarditis
11. Thrombophlebitis or intracardiac thrombi
12. Recent systemic or pulmonary embolus
13. Acute infections
14. Significant emotional distress (psychosis)

Relative

1. Resting diastolic blood pressure >115 mmHg or resting systolic blood pressure >200 mmHg
2. Moderate valvular heart disease
3. Known electrolyte abnormalities (hypokalemia, hypomagnesemia)
4. Fixed-rate pacemaker
5. Frequent or complex ectopy
6. Ventricular aneurysm
7. Uncontrolled metabolic disease (e.g., diabetes, thyrotoxicosis, or myxedema)
8. Chronic infectious disease (e.g., mononucleosis or myxedema)
9. Neuromuscular, musculoskeletal, or rheumatoid disorders exacerbated by exercise
10. Advanced or complicated pregnancy

From American College of Sports Medicine (2001). *Guidelines for exercise testing and prescription* (6th ed.). Philadelphia: Lippincott Williams & Wilkins.

Historically, professional guidelines have suggested that physician supervision was necessary for all exercise testing in the clinical setting. Given the remarkable safety record of exercise testing, particularly in recent years (Franklin et al., 1997; Thompson, 1993), there is now some debate regarding the need for physician supervision for exercise testing (Franklin et al., 1997). This has important implications for nursing because the nurse is frequently the person who prepares the patient and serves as the technician conducting the test, and in many centers the nurse may supervise the test as a surrogate for the physician. Although the recent AHA/ACC guidelines (Gibbons et al., 2002) continue to recommend physician supervision when testing patients with heart disease in a clinical setting, the guidelines also state that ". . . exercise testing in selected patients can be safely performed by properly trained nurses, exercise physiologists, physical therapists, or medical technicians working directly under the supervision of a physician, who should be in the immediate vicinity and available for emergencies." The ACSM has outlined general guidelines for when physician supervision is recommended (American College of Sports Medicine: Guidelines, 2001). The nurse, physiologist, or technician conducting the test should have a comprehensive knowledge of the indications, contraindications, equipment, physiologic responses to exercise, and clinical condition of the patient to optimize the information yield and conduct the test safely.

A recent joint statement by the American College of Physicians, the ACC, and the AHA regarding clinical competence in exercise testing outlined the cognitive skills needed to perform exercise testing (Rogers et al., 2000). These include knowledge of indications and contraindications to testing, basic exercise physiology, principles of interpretation, and emergency procedures. The committee suggested that at least 50 procedures were required during training to achieve these skills. ACSM certification (American College of Sports Medicine: Guidelines, 2001; American College of Sports Medicine: Resource, 2001) is widely used to establish competency for technicians, nurses, or physiologists who oversee exercise testing and training.

PRETEST CONSIDERATIONS

Before an exercise test, all patients should undergo a complete medical history and a physical examination to identify contraindications to exercise testing (Froelicher & Myers, 2000; Gibbons et al., 2002). If the reason the patient was referred for the test in unclear, it should be postponed until this is clarified. The medical history should include any remote or recent medical problems, symptoms, medication use, and findings from previous examinations and tests. Major CAD risk factors and signs and symptoms suggesting cardiopulmonary disease should be identified. Physical activity patterns, vocational requirements, and family history of cardiopulmonary and metabolic disorders should also be assessed. Identification of absolute contraindications (see Display 21-1) should result in cancellation of the test and referral of the patient to the primary physician for further medical management. Patients with relative contraindications may be tested only after careful evaluation of the risk-to-benefit ratio.

Detailed verbal and written instructions, provided to the patient in advance, should include a request that the patient refrain from ingesting food, alcohol, and caffeine or using tobacco products within 3 hours of testing. Patients should be well rested and avoid vigorous activity the day of the test. Clothing should be comfortable and provide freedom of movement as well as allow access for electrode and blood pressure cuff placement. Properly fitting shoes with rubber soles should be worn to ensure good traction, particularly if a treadmill is the mode of testing. A thorough explanation of the potential risks and discomforts associated with exercise testing should be provided. Written informed consent has important ethical and legal implications and ensures the patient knows and understands the purposes and risks associated with the exercise test. There is sufficient case law to suggest that informed consent should always be obtained before beginning a test, although this issue has also been debated (Herbert & Herbert, 1993). A demonstration of how to get on and off the testing apparatus should be given, what is expected of the patient should be described (reporting of symptoms, level of exertion, testing endpoints), and any questions the patient has should be answered.

Whether patients should remain on all cardiovascular medicines for exercise testing has been the source of some debate. Many commonly used drugs can influence hemodynamic and electrocardiographic responses to exercise (Froelicher & Myers, 2000; Gibbons et al., 2002) (Table 21-1), but removing patients from their usual medicines can cause instability of symptoms, rhythm, blood pressure, and other problems. Recent versions of the aforementioned exercise testing guidelines (American Association of Cardiovascular and Pulmonary Rehabilitation, 1999; American College of Sports Medicine: Guidelines, 2001; Gibbons et al., 2002; Rogers et al., 2000) suggest that most patients can remain on their medical regimen for testing without greatly compromising the diagnostic performance of the test. Tapering beta-blockers or discontinuing antianginal medications for several days before testing should be reserved for particular patients in whom diagnostic sensitivity is paramount, and the tapering process should be carefully supervised by a physician.

Preparation for Electrocardiogram

Diagnostically, the electrocardiographic response is the cornerstone of the clinical exercise test. Thus, reliable test interpretation and patient safety mandate a high-quality exercise electrocardiogram. Critical to obtaining a high-quality electrocardiogram tracing are proper skin preparation and precise electrode placement. The goal of skin preparation is to decrease resistance at the skin-electrode interface and thus improve the signal-to-noise ratio. After removing hair from the general areas of placement, each site should be vigorously rubbed with an alcohol pad to remove skin oil. To reduce resistance further, the skin should be lightly abraded using an abrasive pad or other product designed for this purpose. Finally, each electrode should be carefully placed in the proper location to ensure good skin contact with both the conducting gel and adhesive surfaces of the electrode.

The Mason-Likar limb lead placement (Mason & Likar, 1966) (Fig. 21-1) is the standard configuration clinically because it provides a 12-lead electrocardiogram with less artifact and less restriction to movement than the standard limb placement. However, the Mason-Likar placement can result in differences in electrocardiographic amplitude and axis compared with the standard limb placement (Gamble et al., 1984; Kleiner et al., 1978; Rautaharju et al., 1982). Because these shifts may be misinterpreted as diagnostic changes, it is often recommended that a resting supine electrocardiogram be recorded using the standard limb lead placement. It is also important to note that position changes may alter the electrocardiogram. For this reason, diagnostic ST segment changes should always be made relative to the resting baseline position (i.e., upright rather than supine for treadmill and cycle ergometry).

Table 21–1 ▪ COMMON DRUGS AND THEIR IMPACT ON EXERCISE TESTING

Drug	Indications	Heart Rate	Blood Pressure	Electrocardiogram	Exercise Capacity
Beta blockers	Angina, hypertension, myocardial infarction, arrhythmias, tremors, migraine headache	Rest: ↓ Exercise: ↓	Rest: ↓ Exercise: ↓	↓ Signs of ischemia	↑ in those with angina, ↓ in those without angina
Calcium channel	Angina, coronary artery spasm, hypertension	Rest: ↓, Exercise: ↓	Rest: ↓ Exercise: ↓	↓ Signs of ischemia	↑ In those with angina, ↓ in those without angina
Digoxin	CHF, arrhythmias	No change	Rest: ↓ Exercise: ↓	Delayed signs of ischemia	↑ In those with angina (and CHF)
Nitrates	Angina	No change	Rest: ↓ Exercise: ↓	Delayed signs of ischemia	↑ In those with angina (and CHF)

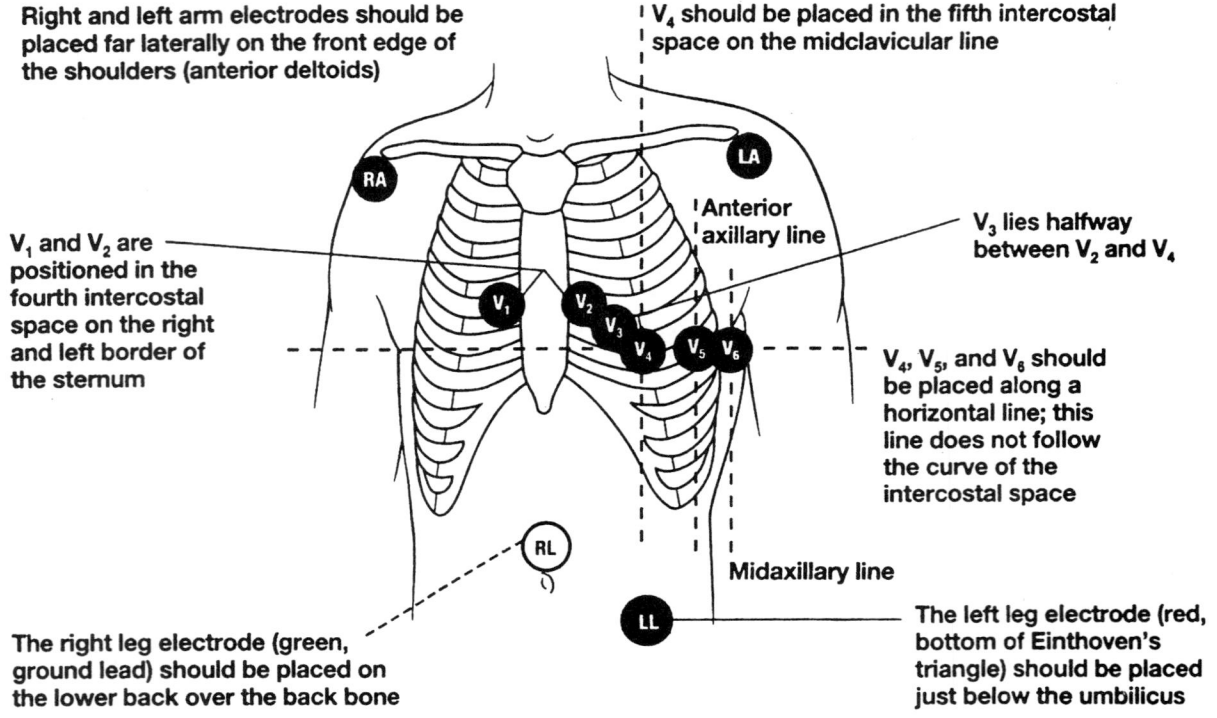

Right and left arm electrodes should be placed far laterally on the front edge of the shoulders (anterior deltoids)

V₄ should be placed in the fifth intercostal space on the midclavicular line

V₁ and V₂ are positioned in the fourth intercostal space on the right and left border of the sternum

Anterior axillary line

V₃ lies halfway between V₂ and V₄

V₄, V₅, and V₆ should be placed along a horizontal line; this line does not follow the curve of the intercostal space

Midaxillary line

The right leg electrode (green, ground lead) should be placed on the lower back over the back bone

The left leg electrode (red, bottom of Einthoven's triangle) should be placed just below the umbilicus

■ **Figure 21–1.** The Mason-Likar simulated 12-lead electrocardiogram electrode placement for exercise testing. (From Froelicher, V. F. & Myers, J. [2000]. *Exercise and the heart.* Philadelphia: W.B. Saunders, with permission.)

■ EXERCISE TEST SELECTION

The purpose of the test, the health and fitness of the patient, the exercise modality, and the exercise protocol are fundamental considerations when selecting the appropriate test for a given patient. In many exercise laboratories, these issues are determined by custom and the availability of equipment, but each can have a profound effect on the response to the exercise test. For example, a treadmill test may be inappropriate for a patient who has difficulty with balance or gait, such as someone who has had a stroke or is otherwise neurologically impaired, or someone who has severe peripheral vascular disease that prevents walking. A bicycle ergometer would be a more appropriate choice for such patients. Test specificity should also be considered. For example, it would be more appropriate to use a cycle ergometer to assess physiologic responses to a cycling program. Likewise, if a person is being assessed for readiness for return to work that requires arm strength, an arm ergometer test may give more appropriate information than a treadmill test.

Modalities

An ideal exercise mode increases total body and myocardial oxygen demand to its highest level safely and in moderate, continuous, and equal increments. This requires a dynamic exercise device that uses major muscle groups, permitting large increases in cardiac output, oxygen delivery, and gas exchange. Many modalities have been used for diagnostic testing, including cycle ergometers, treadmills, arm ergometers, steps, and, more recently, pharmacologic agents. Isometric, or static exercise, which involves muscle contraction without movement of the corresponding joint, causes a greater increase in systolic blood pressure and heart rate in relation to total body oxygen uptake and therefore a greater pressure load on the heart compared to dynamic exercise. Thus, it is not preferred for diagnostic exercise testing. However, isometric exercise has been used to provide occupation-specific information for patients whose job requires an extensive amount of isometric activity.

The bicycle ergometer and the treadmill are the most commonly used dynamic exercise devices. Bicycle ergometer testing is more commonly used in Europe, whereas the treadmill is more often used in the United States. The bicycle is usually less expensive, occupies less space, and is quieter. Upper body motion is decreased, making blood pressure and electrocardiographic recordings easier. The workload administered by simple, mechanically braked bicycle ergometers is not always accurate and depends on pedaling speed, causing variations in the work performed. These have largely been replaced by electronically braked bicycle ergometers, which maintain the workload at a specified level over a wide range of pedaling speeds, and are therefore more accurate. Bicycle ergometer work is commonly expressed in kilogram-meters per minute (kgm/min) or watts. The treadmill is usually more expensive than the cycle ergometer, is relatively immobile, and makes more noise. Studies comparing treadmill and bicycle ergometer exercise tests have reported maximal oxygen uptake to be approximately 10% to 20% higher and maximal heart rate 5% to 20% higher on the treadmill (Buchfuhrer et al., 1983; Hambrecht et al., 1992; Hermansen &

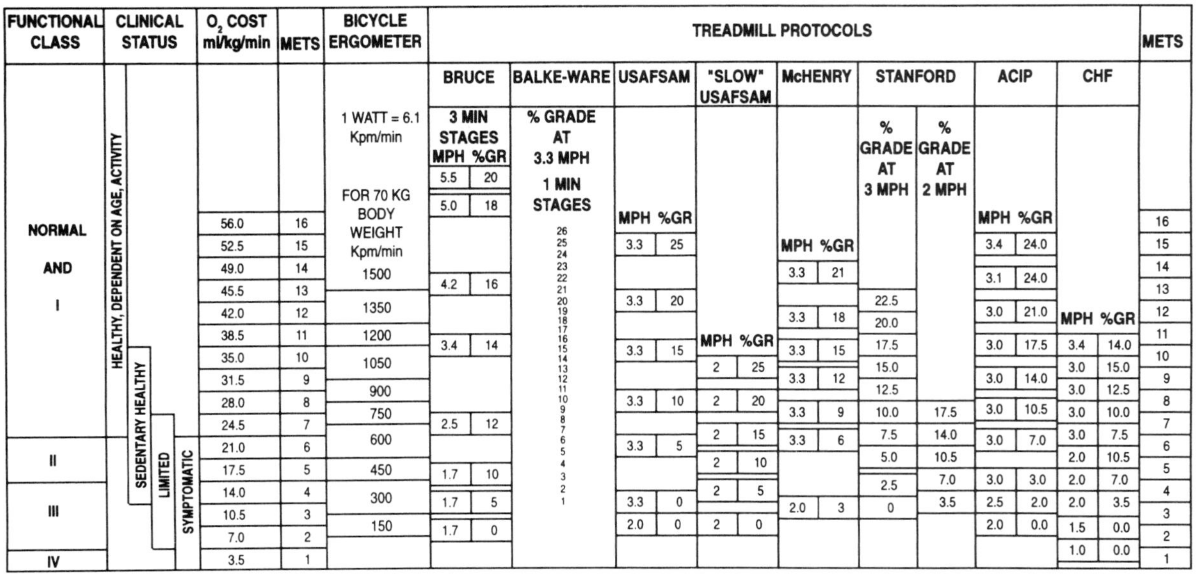

FUNCTIONAL CLASS	CLINICAL STATUS	O₂ COST ml/kg/min	METS	BICYCLE ERGOMETER (1 WATT = 6.1 Kpm/min; for 70 kg body wt, Kpm/min)	BRUCE 3 MIN STAGES (MPH / %GR)	BALKE-WARE % GRADE AT 3.3 MPH, 1 MIN STAGES	USAFSAM (MPH / %GR)	"SLOW" USAFSAM (MPH / %GR)	McHENRY (MPH / %GR)	STANFORD %GRADE AT 3 MPH	STANFORD %GRADE AT 2 MPH	ACIP (MPH / %GR)	CHF (MPH / %GR)	METS
					5.5 / 20									
					5.0 / 18									
NORMAL AND I	HEALTHY, DEPENDENT ON AGE, ACTIVITY	56.0	16			26						3.4 / 24.0		16
		52.5	15			25 / 24	3.3 / 25		3.3 / 21					15
		49.0	14	1500		23 / 22						3.1 / 24.0		14
		45.5	13		4.2 / 16	21				22.5		3.0 / 21.0		13
		42.0	12	1350		20 / 19	3.3 / 20		3.3 / 18	20.0				12
		38.5	11	1200	3.4 / 14	18 / 17			3.3 / 15	17.5		3.0 / 17.5	3.4 / 14.0	11
	SEDENTARY HEALTHY	35.0	10	1050		16 / 15	3.3 / 15	2 / 25	3.3 / 12	15.0			3.0 / 15.0	10
		31.5	9	900		14 / 13			3.3 / 9	12.5		3.0 / 14.0	3.0 / 12.5	9
		28.0	8	750		12 / 11	3.3 / 10	2 / 20		10.0	17.5	3.0 / 10.5	3.0 / 10.0	8
		24.5	7		2.5 / 12	10 / 9			3.3 / 6	7.5	14.0	3.0 / 7.0	3.0 / 7.5	7
II	LIMITED	21.0	6	600		8 / 7	3.3 / 5	2 / 15		5.0	10.5		2.0 / 10.5	6
		17.5	5	450	1.7 / 10	6 / 5		2 / 10				3.0 / 3.0	2.0 / 7.0	5
III	SYMPTOMATIC	14.0	4	300		4 / 3		2 / 5		2.5	7.0	2.5 / 2.0	2.0 / 3.5	4
		10.5	3		1.7 / 5	2	3.3 / 0	2 / 0	2.0 / 3	0	3.5	2.0 / 0.0	1.5 / 0.0	3
		7.0	2	150	1.7 / 0	1	2.0 / 0						1.0 / 0.0	2
IV		3.5	1											1

USAFSAM = United States Air Force School of Aerospace Medicine
ACIP = Asymptomatic Cardiac Ischemia Pilot
CHF = Congestive Heart Failure (Modified Naughton)
Kpm/min = Kilopond meters/minute
%GR = percent grade
MPH = miles per hour

■ **Figure 21–2.** Stages, workloads, and oxygen cost per stage of some commonly used protocols.

Saltin, 1969; Myers et al., 1991; Wicks et al., 1978). Significant ST segment changes are reported more frequently and angina is elicited more frequently during treadmill testing compared with the cycle ergometer (Myers et al., 1991; Wicks et al., 1978). In addition, exercise-induced myocardial ischemia by thallium scintigraphy was reported to be greater after treadmill testing than cycle ergometry (Hambrecht et al., 1992). Although most of these differences are minor, if assessing the functional limits of the patient and eliciting subjective or objective signs of ischemia are important goals of the test, the treadmill may be preferable.

Protocols

The purpose of the test and the person tested are important considerations in selecting the protocol. Exercise testing may be performed for diagnostic purposes, for functional assessment, or for risk stratification. An often ignored but nevertheless consistent recommendation in the recent exercise testing guidelines is that the protocol be individualized for the patient being tested (American College of Sports Medicine: Guidelines, 2001; Gibbons et al., 2002; Myers & Froelicher, 1994; Webster & Sharpe, 1989). For example, a maximal, symptom-limited test on a relatively demanding protocol would not be appropriate (or very informative) for a severely limited patient. Likewise, a very gradual protocol might not be useful for an apparently healthy, active person. Use of submaximal testing, gas exchange techniques, the presence of a physician, and the exercise mode and protocol should be determined by considering the person being tested and the goals of the test.

The most commonly used exercise protocols, their stages, and the MET level (metabolic equivalents; an estimated value representing a multiple of the resting metabolic rate) for each stage are outlined in Figure 21-2. The most suitable protocols for clinical testing should include a low-intensity warm-up phase followed by progressive, continuous exercise in which the demand is elevated to a patient's maximal level within a total duration of 8 to 12 minutes (American College of Sports Medicine: Guidelines, 2001; American Thoracic Society/American College of Chest Physicians, 2003; Buchfuhrer et al., 1983; Gibbons et al., 2002; Myers et al., 1991). In the absence of gas exchange techniques, it is important to report exercise capacity in METs rather than exercise time, so that exercise capacity can be compared uniformly between protocols. METs can be estimated from any protocol using standardized equations that have been put into tabular form (American College of Sports Medicine: Guidelines, 2001; Gibbons et al., 2002; Myers, 1996). In general, 1 MET represents an increment on the treadmill of approximately 1 mph or 2.5% grade. On a cycle ergometer, 1 MET represents an increment of approximately 20 W (120 kgm/min) for a 70-kg person. The assumptions necessary for predicting MET levels from treadmill or cycle ergometer work rates (including not holding the handrails, that oxygen uptake is constant [i.e., steady-state exercise is performed], that the subject is healthy, and that all people are similar in their walking efficiency) raise uncertainties as to the accuracy of estimating the work performed for an individual patient. For example, the steady-state requirement is rarely met for most patients on most exercise protocols; most clinical testing is performed among patients with varying degrees of cardiovascular or pulmonary disease; and people vary widely in their walking efficiency (Myers, 1996). It has therefore been recommended that a patient be ascribed a MET level only for stages in which all or most of a given stage duration has been completed.

Bruce Treadmill Protocol. Surveys have shown that the Bruce protocol is the most widely used in North America (Myers et al., 2000; Stuart & Ellestad, 1980). An advantage of using this test is that a great deal of functional and prognostic data have been generated over several decades using the Bruce protocol, and many published normative values have been derived from it. For example, some of the most robust databases on the use of the exercise test for assessing prognosis, such as those from the Coronary Artery Surgery Study (CASS) (Weiner et al., 1987) and the Duke Treadmill Score (Mark et al., 1987) were generated from patients who underwent exercise testing using the Bruce test. Numerous studies have shown that patients who are unable to complete the first stage of this protocol (approximately 5 METs) have an extremely poor prognosis (Morris et al., 1991; Myers & Gullestad, 1998; Weiner et al., 1987). However, the disadvantages of the Bruce protocol include its large and unequal increments in work, which have been shown to result in less accurate estimates of exercise capacity, particularly for patients with cardiac disease. Investigations have demonstrated that work rate increments that are too large or rapid result in a tendency to overestimate exercise capacity, less reliability for studying the effects of therapy, and possibly even lowered sensitivity for detecting coronary disease (Buchfuhrer et al., 1983; Myers et al., 1991; Myers & Froelicher, 1994; Panza et al., 1991; Redwood et al., 1971).

Balke Treadmill Protocol. The Balke protocol, and modifications of it, have been widely used for clinical exercise testing. It uses constant walking speeds (2.0 or 3.0 mph) and modest increments in grade (2.5% or 5.0%), and it has been used particularly often in studies assessing angina responses. Modifications of the original Balke treadmill protocol have become widespread. One modification, developed by the United States School of Aerospace Medicine (Balke-Ware) (Wolthius et al., 1977) consists of 5% grade increases every 2 minutes and a constant brisk walking speed of 3.3 mph (after an initial warm-up of 2.0 mph), which has been considered the most efficient speed for walking. The constant speed is advantageous in that it requires only an initial adaptation in stride.

Naughton Treadmill Protocol. The Naughton treadmill protocol (Naughton & Haiden, 1973) is a low-level test that has become common for multicenter trials in patients with chronic heart failure. The test begins with 2-minute stages at 1 and 2 mph and 0% grade, then continually increases grade in approximately 1-MET increments at a constant speed of 2 mph for the next 8 minutes. Speed then increases to 3 mph with a slight decrease in grade, followed by increases in grade equivalent to approximately 1 MET. The Naughton protocol provides reasonable and gradual work rate increases for patients with more advanced heart disease. Because this protocol has been used extensively in patients with chronic heart failure, it provides a substantial amount of functional and prognostic comparative data. The Naughton test, however, can result in tests of excessive duration among more fit subjects.

Cycle Ergometer Protocols

Although there are specific bicycle protocols named for early researchers in Europe, such as Astrand (Astrand & Rodahl, 1986), bicycle ergometer protocols tend to be more generalized than for the treadmill. For example, 15- to 25-W increments per 2-minute stage are commonly used for patients with cardiovascular disease, whereas for apparently healthy adults or athletic individuals, appropriate work rate increments might typically be between 40 and 50 W/stage. Most modern, electronically braked cycle ergometers have controllers that permit ramp testing, in which the work rate increments can be individualized in continuous fashion (see next section).

Ramp Testing

An approach to exercise testing that has gained interest in recent years is the ramp protocol, in which work increases constantly and continuously. In 1981, Whipp and colleagues (Whipp et al., 1981) first described cardiopulmonary responses to a ramp test on a cycle ergometer, and many of the gas exchange equipment manufacturers now include ramp software. Treadmills have also been adapted to conduct ramp tests (Myers et al., 1992; Myers et al., 1991). The ramp protocol uses a constant and continuous increase in metabolic demand that replaces the "staging" used in conventional exercise tests. The uniform increase in work allows for a steady increase in cardiopulmonary responses and permits a more accurate estimation of oxygen uptake (Myers et al., 1991). The recent call for "optimizing" exercise testing (Buchfuhrer et al., 1983; Gibbons et al., 2002; Myers & Froelicher, 1994; Webster & Sharpe, 1989) would appear to be facilitated by the ramp approach, because large work increments are avoided and increases in work are individualized, permitting test duration to be targeted. Because there are no stages per se, the errors associated with predicting exercise capacity alluded to previously are lessened (American College of Sports Medicine Guidelines, 2001; Gibbons et al., 2002; Myers et al., 1991).

Submaximal Testing

In general, maximal, symptom-limited tests are not considered appropriate until 1 month after MI or surgery. Thus, submaximal exercise testing has an important role clinically for pre-discharge, post-MI, or post-bypass surgery evaluations. Submaximal tests have been shown to be important in risk stratification (Chang & Froelicher, 1994; Sivarajan Froelicher, 1994; Olona et al., 1995) for making appropriate activity recommendations, for recognizing the need for modification of the medical regimen, or for further interventions in patients who have sustained a cardiac event. A submaximal, pre-discharge test appears to be as predictive for future events as a symptom-limited test among patients less than 1 month after MI. Submaximal testing is also appropriate for patients with a high probability of serious arrhythmias. The testing endpoints for submaximal testing have traditionally been arbitrary but should always be based on clinical judgment. A heart rate limit of 140 beats/min and a MET level of 7 are often used for patients younger than age 40 years, and limits of 130 beats/min and a MET level of 5 are often used for patients older than 40 years. For those using beta-blockers, a Borg perceived exertion level in the range of 7 to 8 (1 to 10 scale) or 15 to 16 (6 to 20 scale) are conservative endpoints. The initial onset of symptoms, including fatigue, shortness of breath, or angina, is also an indication to stop the test. A low-level protocol should be used, that is, one that uses no more than 1-MET increments per stage. The Naughton protocol (Naughton et al., 1964; Naughton & Haiden, 1973) is commonly used for submaximal testing. Ramp testing is also ideal for this purpose because the ramp rate (such as 5 METs achieved over a 10-minute duration) can be individualized depending on the patient tested (Myers et al., 1991).

INTERPRETATION OF EXERCISE TEST RESPONSES

The important exercise test responses that should be monitored and recorded are heart rate, blood pressure, electrocardiographic changes, exercise capacity, and subjective responses, including chest discomfort, undue fatigue, shortness of breath,

leg pain, and rating of perceived exertion. Each of these responses should be described in a comprehensive test report. Useful programs have been developed that automatically summarize the test responses and apply published regression equations that report pre-test and post-test risks of coronary disease, and some provide mortality estimates (Froelicher, 1996). An example of one such report is presented in Display 21-2.

Heart Rate

Heart rate increases linearly with oxygen uptake during exercise. Of the two major components of cardiac output, heart rate and stroke volume, heart rate is responsible for most of the increase in cardiac output during exercise, particularly at higher levels. Thus, maximal heart rate achieved is a major determinant of exercise capacity (Froelicher & Myers, 2000; Hammond & Froelicher, 1985). The inability to appropriately increase heart rate during exercise (chronotropic incompetence) has been associated with the presence of heart disease

---

DISPLAY 21-2

EXAMPLE OF AN AUTOMATED EXERCISE TEST SUMMARY REPORT WITH DIAGNOSTIC AND PROGNOSTIC PROBABILITIES GENERATED FROM A COMPUTER PROGRAM

Pretest Information

This patient is a 74-year-old active white male outpatient 70 inches tall, weighing 180 lbs, who underwent a treadmill test on April 12,2001. This exercise test was performed to evaluate symptoms/signs of possible heart disease or elevated risk factors.

Current Cardiac Medications

The patient is not taking any cardiac medications.

Medical History

The patient has the following symptoms: uncertain chest pain. The patient has no history of dysrhythmias.

Risk Factors

The patient is currently not smoking but has 15 pack-years of smoking. The patient is 8 lbs over the average appropriate body mass index. Other risk factors include low high-density lipoprotein level (31 mg/dL) and non-insulin-dependent diabetes mellitus.

History of Cardiac Events

No previous myocardial infarction. No bypass surgery performed. No percutaneous transluminal coronary angioplasty performed. No catheterization performed.

Resting ECG

The resting ECG is abnormal because of the following: left ventricular hypertrophy. The ejection fraction is approximately 45% based on the resting ECG.

Pulmonary Function

Forced vital capacity was 3.4 L (90.4% of expected), and the forced expiratory volume was 76.2% (normal is >75%).

Exercise Test Information

Exercise Capacity

The patient achieved 4.3 estimated METs and 4.1 measured METs at a perceived exertion level of 18 of 20 on the Borg scale. The test was terminated because of ST changes.

Hemodynamic Data	Heart Rate	Blood Pressure	Double Product (x1,000)
Resting:	65 bpm	146/70 mm Hg	9.5
At Max Exercise:	116 bpm	122/70 mm Hg	14.1

Chest Pain

Typical angina occurred during exercise.

(Continued)

DISPLAY 21-2 *(Continued)*

EXAMPLE OF AN AUTOMATED EXERCISE TEST SUMMARY REPORT WITH DIAGNOSTIC AND PROGNOSTIC PROBABILITIES GENERATED FROM A COMPUTER PROGRAM

Exercise ECG Response

The resting ECG shows no ST depression in V_5.

At maximal exercise, the ST segments showed 4 mm of downsloping depression in the lateral and inferior leads. In recovery, the ST segments showed 3 mm of downsloping depression in the lateral and inferior leads. No significant dysrhythmias occurred in response to exercise. No bundle-branch blocks or conduction defects were present at rest or developed during exercise.

Conclusions

ST segments exhibited abnormal depression during exercise and abnormal depression in recovery (abnormal ST response).

Exertional hypotension occurred (systolic blood pressure dropped below pretest standing SBP).

The exertional hypotension could be due to ischemia (ST depression).

The patient achieved 66% of normal exercise capacity for age, and 90% of normal maximal heart rate for age.

The patient has a high probability of having severe coronary artery disease.

Estimated prognosis from treadmill scores may be worse than expected for age, sex, and race.

Prognostic Addendum

Cardiovascular Mortality Prediction

The Framingham score (age, sex, cholesterol, diabetes, smoking, left ventricular hypertrophy, SBP) estimates a 5-year incidence of cardiovascular events (angina, myocardial infarction, or death) of 11% (as expected for age and gender). For comparison with the treadmill scores, the age-expected annual mortality rate from any cause is 5.1% (National Center for Health Statistics, 1990).

The Duke Score (METs, ST depression, and angina) estimates an annual cardiovascular mortality of 9.5% (not greater than two times the age-expected mortality). The Froelicher score (METs, congestive heart failure, SBP rise, and ST depression) estimates an annual cardiovascular mortality of 15.7% (three times the age-expected mortality).

Angiographic Coronary Artery Disease Prediction

The patient has no recorded history of coronary disease. Pretest probabilities for any significant coronary disease are 50% (CASS, 1981 [chest pain, age, gender]), 71% (Morise, 1992), and 51% (Do/Froelicher, 1995). Pretest probabilities for severe coronary disease are 22% (Duke, 1993), 52% (Morise, 1992), and 17% (Do/Froelicher, 1995).

The post-test probabilities for any clinically significant coronary artery disease are 99% (Detrano, 1992), 98% (Morise, 1992), and 94% (Do/Froelicher, 1995) due to age, diabetes mellitus, symptoms, and abnormal ST depression.

The probabilities of having severe coronary artery disease are 75% (Detrano, 1992) due to abnormal ST depression, 91% (Morise, 1992) due to age abnormal ST depression, and 74% (Do/Froelicher, 1995) due to abnormal ST depression.

Operative Mortality Prediction

If the patient would be selected for non-emergent bypass surgery and no renal dysfunction was present, the estimated operative morality rates are 9% (Parsonnet, 1989), 2% (NY State Dept. of Health, 1992), and 3% (VA, 1993). This is partially based on an estimated EF of 45%, so compare to measured EF.

Treadmill Report: Department of Cardiology

Disclaimer: This report was computer generated and the results are dependent on rules and correct data entry. It must be overread by a physician.

EF, ejection fraction; ECG, electrocardiographic; METs, metabolic equivalents; SBP, systolic blood pressure.
From Froelicher, V. F. (1996). *Exercise test reporting aid (EXTRA) software.* St. Louis: Mosby-Year Book.

and a worse prognosis (Hammond & Froelicher, 1985; Lauer et al., 1996). Although maximal heart rate has been difficult to explain physiologically (Graettinger et al., 1995), it is affected by age, gender, health, type of exercise, body position, blood volume, and environment. Of these factors, age is the most important. There is an inverse relationship between maximal heart rate and age, with correlation coefficients typically in the order of -0.40. However, the scatter around the regression line is quite large, with standard deviations ranging from 10 to 15 beats/min (Fig. 21-3). Thus, age-predicted "target" maximal heart rate is a limited measurement for clinical purposes and should not be used as an endpoint for exercise testing (American College of Sports Medicine Guidelines, 2001; Gibbons et al., 2002; Hammond & Froelicher, 1985).

Blood Pressure

Assessment of systolic and diastolic blood pressure at rest and during the exercise test is important for patient safety and can provide important diagnostic and prognostic information. Properly trained personnel can obtain accurate and reliable blood pressures using noninvasive auscultatory techniques, and guidelines have been developed for this purpose (Bailey & Bauer, 1993; Iyriboz & Hearon, 1992). Blood pressure should be measured at rest before the test in the supine and standing positions. Resting blood pressure, when measured before an exercise test, may be elevated compared to normal resting conditions because of pretest anxiety. Uncontrolled hypertension is a relative contraindication to exercise testing (American College

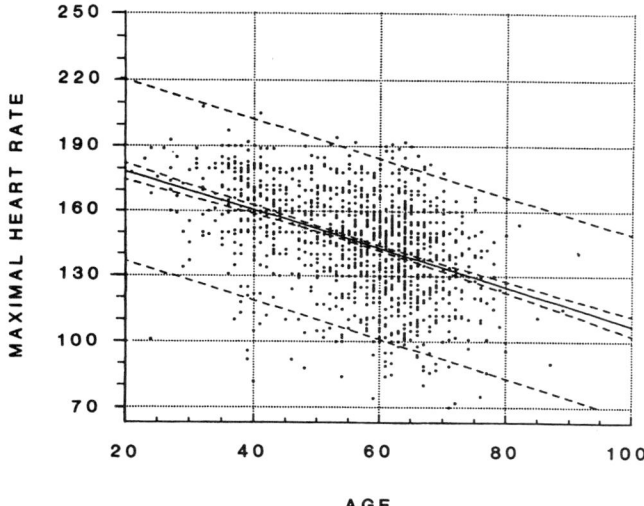

■ **Figure 21–3.** The relationship between maximal heart rate and age among patients referred for exercise testing. Inner lines represent the standard error; outer lines represent 95% confidence limits. (From Morris, C. K. et al. [1994]. *Journal of the American College of Cardiology,* 22, 175–182, with permission.)

modest decreases, in the order of 10 to 20 mm Hg, are associated with severe ischemia, left ventricular impairment, a high incidence of future cardiac events, or all three (San Marco et al., 1980; Weiner, 1982).

Exercise Capacity

Exercise capacity can be an extremely important test response to document because it has important implications concerning the efficacy of current therapies, the assessment of disability, and risk stratification. A patient's exercise capacity says a great deal about overall cardiovascular health. The most accurate method of measuring exercise capacity is with the use of ventilatory gas exchange techniques, but this requires specialized equipment and is not available in many clinical laboratories. Exercise capacity is therefore usually expressed as exercise duration, watts achieved (on a bicycle ergometer), maximal exercise stage, or METs. In the absence of gas exchange techniques, it is preferable to express exercise capacity in METs rather than exercise time. This is because a MET value can be ascribed to any speed and grade on a treadmill or workload achieved on a cycle ergometer; therefore, exercise capacity can be compared uniformly between protocols.

As mentioned previously in the discussion on protocols, there can be a great deal of uncertainly in predicting a person's energy cost from the treadmill or cycle ergometer workload. How accurately a MET level predicts a person's true oxygen uptake depends on several factors. For most patients with cardiovascular or pulmonary disease, there is a substantial over-prediction of the MET level (American College of Sports Medicine Guidelines, 2001; Foster et al., 1996; Myers, 1996; Myers et al., 1991). The error associated with this prediction is accentuated when rapidly incremented protocols are used, when patients are unaccustomed to walking on a treadmill or pedaling a cycle ergometer, and when patients are allowed to use handrail support (American College of Sports Medicine Guidelines, 2001; Foster et al., 1996; Myers, 1996).

Exercise capacity should be expressed as both an absolute value and as a relative percentage of normal for age and gender. The latter can be important because exercise capacity declines with increasing age and higher values are observed in men. Thus, when measuring or estimating oxygen uptake or MET levels, it is useful to have reference values for comparison. Normal reference values can facilitate communication with patients and between physicians regarding levels of exercise capacity in relation to a given patient's peers. Figures 21-4 and 21-5 are illustrations of nomograms for male patients referred for exercise testing. Expressing relative exercise capacity using a nomogram is advantageous because it offers a simple visual method of classifying a patient's response, without having to make cumbersome calculations from a particular regression equation. However, there are numerous available regression equations for "normal." All are population-specific, and numerous factors affect a person's exercise tolerance other than age and gender, including height, weight, body composition, activity status, and exercise test mode used, in addition to many clinical factors such as smoking history, heart disease, and medications (American College of Sports Medicine Resource, 2001; Myers, 1996).

of Sports Medicine Guidelines, 2001; Gibbons et al., 2002). However, if blood pressure is elevated because of anxiety, it is not uncommon or of concern to observe a slight decrease in blood pressure during the initial stage of an exercise test when the workloads are light.

The increase in systolic blood pressure during exercise reflects the inotropic reserve of the left ventricle. Systolic and diastolic blood pressure should be assessed during the last minute of each exercise stage and more frequently if hypotensive or hypertensive responses are observed. Normally, systolic blood pressure increases in parallel with an increase in work rate, and it is not uncommon in healthy people to exceed 200 mm Hg. In general, a value above 250 mm Hg is an indication to terminate the exercise test (American College of Sports Medicine Guidelines, 2001; Gibbons et al., 2002). Diastolic pressure normally stays the same or increases slightly during exercise. The fifth Korotkov sound, however, can frequently be heard all the way to zero in a young, healthy person. A diastolic blood pressure exceeding 115 mm Hg is an indication to terminate the exercise test (American College of Sports Medicine Guidelines, 2001; Gibbons et al., 2002). A decrease in systolic blood pressure with progressive exercise suggests that cardiac output is unable to increase in accordance with the work rate and is usually a reflection of severe ischemia. If systolic blood pressure appears to decrease, it should be re-measured immediately, and if the decrease is confirmed, the test should be terminated. The clinical consequences of abnormal blood pressure responses to exercise range from modest (Sivarajan Froelicher, 1994; Mazzotta et al., 1987) to severe, in which decreases in systolic blood pressure have been associated with ventricular fibrillation in the laboratory (Irving & Bruce, 1977). Dubach and colleagues (Dubach et al., 1988) have observed that systolic blood pressure must drop below the standing resting value to be prognostically valuable, whereas others have suggested that more

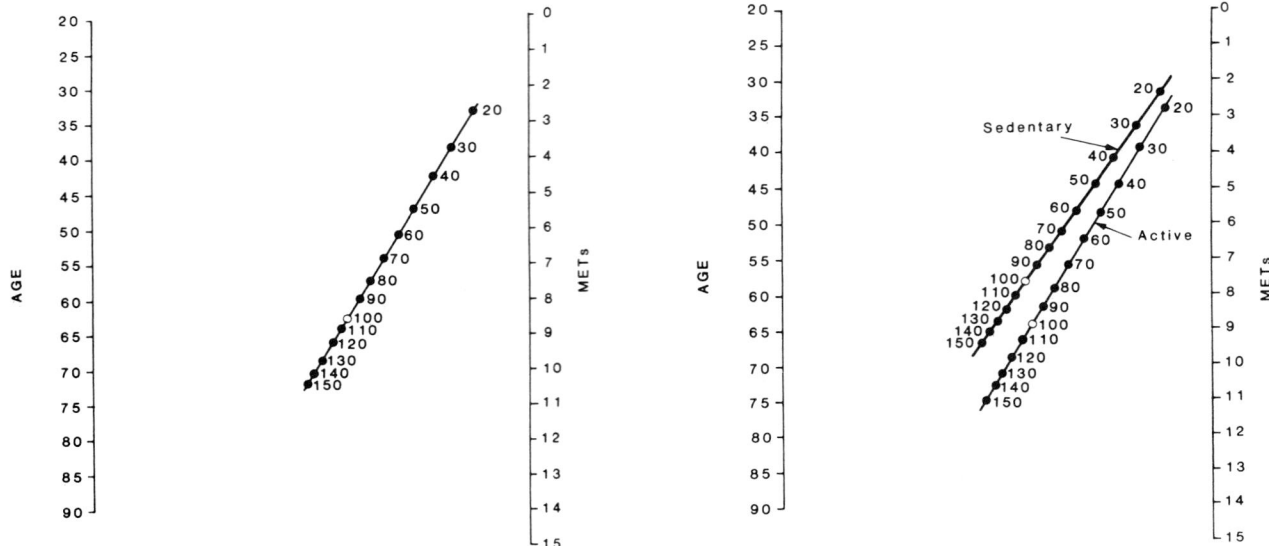

■ **Figure 21–4.** Nomogram of percentage normal exercise capacity for age in 1,388 male veterans referred for exercise testing (based on metabolic task equivalents [METs]). (From Morris, C. K. et al. [1994]. *Journal of the American College of Cardiology,* 22, 175–182, with permission.)

■ **Figure 21–5.** Nomogram of percentage normal exercise capacity for age among active and sedentary men referred for exercise testing (based on metabolic equivalents [METs]). (From Morris, C. K. et al. [1994]. *Journal of the American College of Cardiology,* 22, 175–182, with permission.)

Electrocardiographic Responses

In patients with CAD, exercise can cause an imbalance between myocardial oxygen supply and demand (ischemia), which can result in an alteration (decrease or elevation relative to the baseline) in the ST segment of the electrocardiogram. These changes are the foundation of the exercise test clinically. Normal and abnormal ST segment responses to exercise are illustrated in Figure 21-6. Ever since electrocardiographic changes were first associated with myocardial ischemia in the 1920s, the diagnostic electrocardiographic criteria and leads that exhibit abnormalities during exercise have been the source of significant debate. Numerous electrocardiographic criteria, including complex mathematical constructs, combined scores, and ST areas during exercise and recovery, have been proposed

to optimally diagnose the presence of CAD. Few of these studies, however, have followed accepted rules for evaluating a diagnostic test (Philbrick et al., 1989). Virtually every edition of exercise testing guidelines that has been published suggests the application of a traditional diagnostic criterion: 1 mm or greater ST segment depression that is horizontal or downsloping 60 to 80 milliseconds after the J-point (a "positive" response). ST segment depression greater than 1 mm that is down-sloping is generally indicative of more severe CAD. Most (probably 90%) ischemic ST changes occur in the lateral precordial leads (Gibbons et al., 2002). Although it has historically been thought that the diagnostic performance of the test was incomplete without all 12 leads, more recent studies suggest that ST segment changes isolated to the inferior leads are frequently false-positive responses (Miranda et al., 1992).

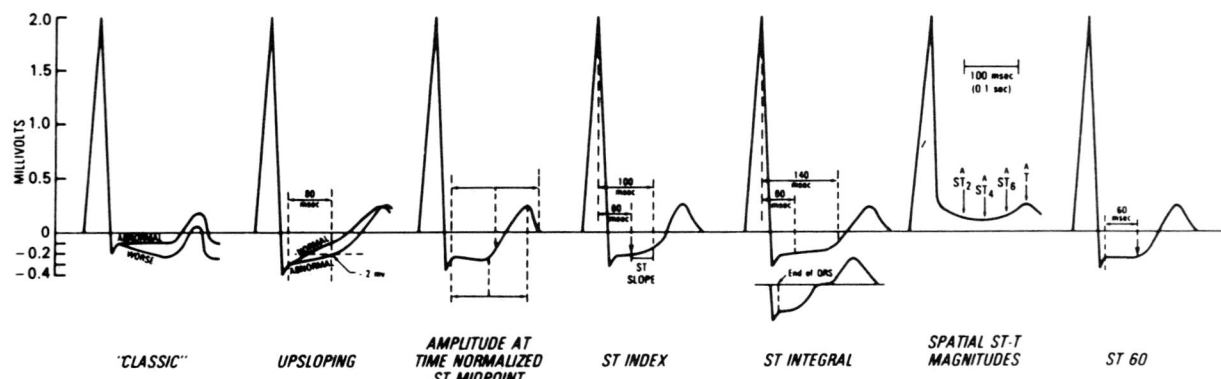

■ **Figure 21–6.** Normal and abnormal ST segment responses to exercise and the various criteria for ST segment depression. (From Froelicher, V. F., & Myers, J. [2000]. *Exercise and the heart.* Philadelphia: W.B. Saunders, with permission.)

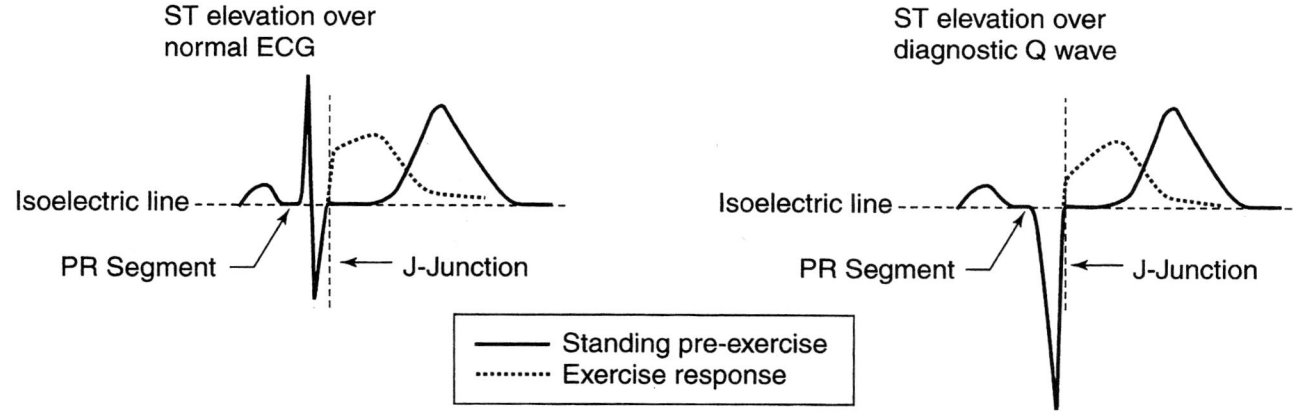

Figure 21–7. Example of exercise-induced ST segment elevation when the resting electrocardiogram is normal (*left*) and when the resting ECG has a diagnostic Q wave (*right*).

The significance of ST segment elevation depends on the presence or absence of Q waves. When ST elevation occurs in the presence of a normal resting electrocardiogram, it is usually indicative of severe transmural ischemia, it can be arrhythmogenic, and it localizes the ischemia. Conversely, exercise-induced ST segment elevation occurring in leads with Q waves is more common and is related to the presence of dyskinetic areas. This response is relatively common in patients after an MI and is of much less concern. Examples of these two responses are illustrated in Figure 21-7.

There are several important nuances concerning the proper measurement of exercise-induced ST segment changes. ST segment depression is measured as a change from the isoelectric line (PR segment) and is considered abnormal if the next 60 to 80 milliseconds after the J-point is flat

or down-sloping (Fig. 21-6). However, in patients who exhibit ST segment depression at rest, exercise-induced ST depression is measured from the baseline (resting) level (Fig. 21-8). In contrast, ST segment elevation is measured from the level at which the ST segment starts, and slope is not considered. The significance of up-sloping or horizontal ST segment depression with T-wave inversion has been debated. Infarction, ventricular aneurysm, bundle-branch block, hypokalemia, ventricular hypertrophy, abnormal oxygen-carrying capacity of blood caused by anemia, pulmonary disease, and drugs such as digoxin and quinidine may all influence the ST segment response; these and other conditions may cause exercise-induced ST segment depression that is not caused by CAD (see section on False-Positive and False-Negative Responses).

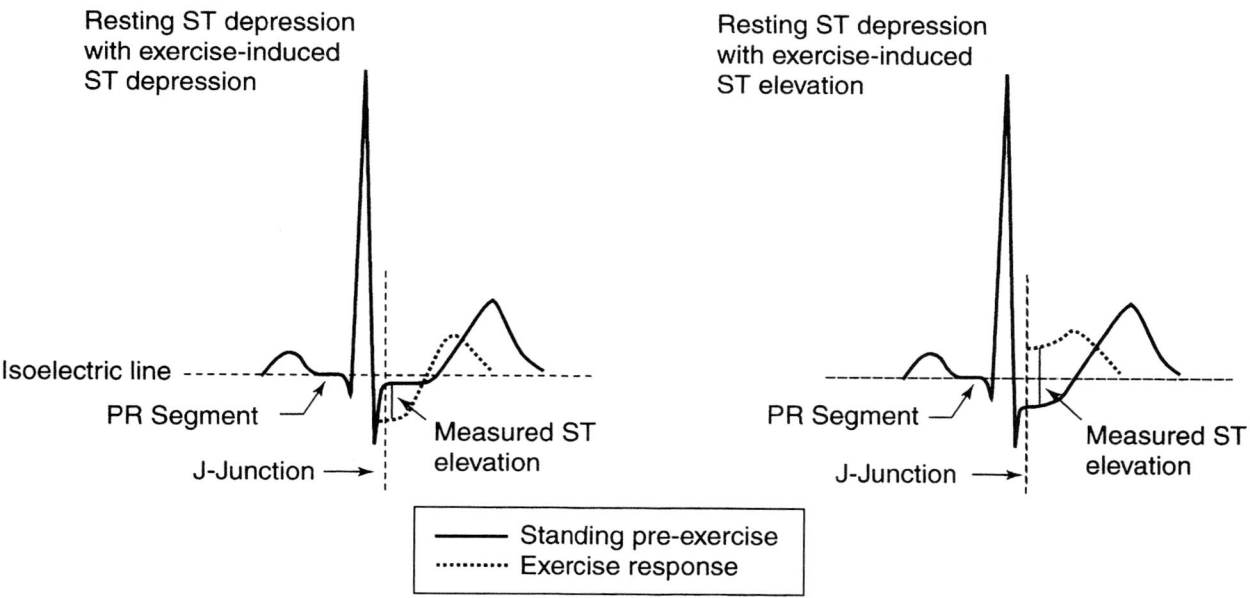

Figure 21–8. Example of how exercise-induced ST segment depression (*left*) and elevation (*right*) are measured when the electrocardiogram shows ST depression at rest.

Arrhythmias During Exercise Testing

Arrhythmias can occur during the exercise test or recovery period and can range in severity from life threatening to benign. There has been a great deal of debate about the importance of arrhythmias during exercise. The occurrence of "serious" arrhythmias during exercise, although rare, is an indication to terminate the exercise test. Arrhythmias may be overt, such as ventricular tachycardia, or subtle, such as unifocal premature ventricular complexes (PVCs) increasing in frequency, or a period of supraventricular tachycardia. Arrhythmias for which there should be no debate about stopping the test include second or third degree heart block and ventricular tachycardia of any duration. Other arrhythmias that have been generally classified as "significant" or "complex" include R-on-T PVCs, frequent unifocal or multifocal PVCs (constituting 30% or more of the beats per minute), and coupling of PVCs (two in succession) (American College of Sports Medicine: Guidelines, 2001; Gibbons et al., 2002). On rare occasion, any of these complex arrhythmias can be a precursor to a life-threatening sustained rhythm disturbance. When there is doubt as to the nature or origin of the arrhythmia, the test should be stopped. Electrophysiologic testing is commonly used to more fully evaluate complex arrhythmias and direct appropriate treatment.

The prognostic significance of exercise-induced PVCs, even when they occur frequently, has varied widely in the literature. This variation is most likely because of differences in how exercise-induced arrhythmias have been defined. Some studies have demonstrated that the occurrence of PVCs during an exercise test has minimal prognostic impact and should be interpreted in the context of "the company they keep" (Gibbons et al., 2002; Yang et al., 1991), such that the decision to terminate the test should be made based on the patient's history and whether the patient remains hemodynamically stable or the arrhythmias are accompanied by symptoms. Other studies have shown a clear association between PVCs that occur during exercise, recovery, or both, and increased mortality (Froelicher & Myers, 2000).

Subjective Responses

Assessment of symptoms and perception of effort during the exercise test are important to maximize safety, and these subjective measures yield valuable diagnostic information. Obtaining careful assessments of subjective measures during the exercise test requires thorough explanations to ensure the patient understands what is expected and how to communicate these responses to those conducting the test. Angina and dyspnea are the most common cardiopulmonary symptoms elicited during exercise and each is typically evaluated using a four-point scale (American College of Sports Medicine Guidelines, 2001; Myers, 1994) (Display 21-3). These scales should be carefully explained to the patient before the exercise test. Patients should be encouraged to report any and all symptoms during exercise.

It is important to distinguish between typical and atypical angina, because they have quite different diagnostic implications. Typical angina tends to be consistent in its presentation and location, is brought on by physical or emotional stress, and is relieved by rest or nitroglycerin. Atypical angina refers to pain

---

| DISPLAY | 21-3 |

ANGINA AND DYSPNEA SCALES

Angina Scale

1+	Onset of discomfort
2+	Moderate, bothersome
3+	Moderately severe
4+	Severe; most pain ever experienced

Dyspnea Scale

1+	Mild, noticeable to patient but not observer
2+	Mild, some difficulty, noticeable to observer
3+	Moderate difficulty, but can continue
4+	Severe difficulty, patient cannot continue

---

that has an unusual location, prolonged duration, or inconsistent precipitating factors that are unresponsive to nitroglycerin. Exercise-induced chest discomfort that has the characteristics of stable, typical angina provides better confirmation of the presence of significant CAD than any other test response. A patient exhibiting the combination of typical angina and an abnormal ST response has a 98% probability of having significant CAD. An important indication to stop the exercise test is moderately severe angina (level 3 on a scale of 1 to 4; see Display 21-3), which should correspond with pain that would normally cause the patient to stop daily activities or take a sublingual nitroglycerin pill (Myers & Froelicher, 1994; Myers, 1994).

Dyspnea may be the predominant symptom in some patients with CAD, but it is more often associated with reduced left ventricular function or chronic obstructive pulmonary disease. In both conditions, it may be the predominant factor causing poor exercise capacity. Dyspnea is also commonly quantified using a scale of 1 to 4 (see Display 21-3). Claudication is indicative of peripheral vascular disease. If peripheral vascular disease is known or suspected, pre-test determination of the presence and strength of peripheral pulses should be made so that post-test comparisons are possible. Leg fatigue not related to claudication is often experienced at maximum exercise; a careful distinction should be made between these two symptoms.

Dizziness and lightheadedness may reflect cerebral hypoxia and may coincide with a feeling of exhaustion at maximum exercise. Lightheadedness can also be a sign of left ventricular dysfunction or hypotension. Dizziness may be accompanied by signs of gray or ashen pallor, diaphoresis, ataxic gait, dyspnea, and strained appearance as blood is maximally shunted to the exercising muscles. Trained observers should be able to recognize these responses and make a determination as to when the test should be stopped.

■ TEST TERMINATION

The usual goal of the exercise test in patients with known or suspected disease is to achieve a maximal level of exertion. This permits the greatest information yield from the test. However,

DISPLAY 21-4

INDICATIONS FOR STOPPING AN EXERCISE TEST

Absolute

- Drop in systolic blood pressure of >10 mm Hg from baseline despite an increase in workload, when accompanied by other evidence of ischemia
- Moderate to severe angina
- Increasing nervous system symptoms (e.g., ataxia, dizziness, or syncope)
- Signs of poor perfusion (cyanosis or pallor)
- Technical difficulties in monitoring electrocardiogram or systolic blood pressure
- Subject's desire to stop
- Sustained ventricular Tachycardia
- ST elevation ($\geq$1.0 mm) in leads without diagnostic Q waves (other than V_1 or aVR)

Relative

- Drop in systolic blood pressure of $\geq$10 mm Hg from baseline blood pressure despite an increase in workload, in the absence of other evidence of ischemia
- ST or QRS changes such as excessive ST depression (>2 mm of horizontal or downsloping ST segment depression) or marked axis shift
- Arrhythmias other than sustained ventricular tachycardia, including multifocal PVCs, triplets of PVCs, supraventricular tachycardia, heart block, or bradyarrhythmias
- Fatigue, shortness of breath, wheezing, leg cramps, or claudication
- Development of bundle-branch block or intraventricular conduction delay that cannot be distinguished from ventricular Tachycardia
- Increasing chest pain
- Hypertensive response*

PVC, premature ventricular complex.
*In the absence of definitive evidence, the Committee suggests systolic blood pressure of >250 mm Hg or a diastolic blood pressure of 115 mm Hg.
From Gibbons, R. J., Balady, G. J., Bricker, J. T. et al. (2002). ACC/AHA 2002 guideline update for exercise testing. A report of the ACC/AHA Task Force on Practice Guidelines (Committee on Exercise Testing). *Journal of the American College of Cardiology* 40, 1531–40.

because of fatigue, dyspnea, or other symptoms. They should be informed that the test will be terminated if abnormal responses are observed by the operators. Although patients should be encouraged to exercise as long as possible, they should not be pushed beyond their capacity and any request to stop the test should be honored. Inability to fully monitor the patient's responses because of technical difficulties should result in immediate termination of the test. Most problems can be avoided by having an experienced physician, nurse, or exercise physiologist standing next to the patient, measuring blood pressure and assessing patient appearance during the test. The exercise technician should operate the recorder and treadmill, take appropriate tracings, enter data on a form, and alert the physician to any abnormalities that may appear on the monitor.

Although many efforts have been made to objectify maximal effort, such as age-predicted maximal heart rate, a plateau in oxygen uptake, exceeding the ventilatory threshold, or a respiratory exchange ratio greater than unity, all have considerable measurement error and intersubject variability (Hammond & Froelicher, 1985; Myers et al., 1989; Myers et al., 1990; Noakes, 1988; Stachenfeld et al., 1992). This variability occurs regardless of the population tested. The 95% confidence limits for maximal heart rate based on age, for example, range considerably (see Fig. 21-3); therefore, this endpoint is maximal for some and submaximal for others (Froelicher & Myers, 2000). The classic index of cardiopulmonary limits, a plateau in oxygen uptake, is not observed in many patients, is poorly reproducible, and has been confused by the many different criteria applied (Myers et al., 1989; Myers et al., 1990; Noakes, 1988; Stachenfeld et al., 1992). Although subjective, the Borg perceived exertion scale is helpful for assessing exercise effort (Borg, 1982) (Display 21-5). Good judgment on the part of the physician remains the most effective criterion for terminating exercise.

achieving a maximal effort should be superseded by any of the clinical indications to stop the test (Display 21-4), by clinical judgment, or by the patient's request to stop. The reason for stopping the test should be carefully recorded because the symptoms or signs manifested by exercise often relate to the mechanism of impairment.

Determining the endpoint of an exercise test can be problematic. It requires integration of objective physiologic data and termination criteria with subjective judgment based on clinical experience. Some patients may be unable or unwilling to exercise to an adequate level. In patients with suspected coronary disease, a symptom-limited, maximal test is usually more diagnostic. Thus, patients should be instructed to exercise to the point at which they can no longer continue

DISPLAY 21-5

BORG RATING OF PERCEIVED EXERTION SCALE

6	
7	Very, very light
8	
9	Very light
10	
11	Fairly light
12	
13	Somewhat hard
14	
15	Hard
16	
17	Very hard
18	
19	Very, very hard
20	

From Borg, G. A. V. (1985). *An Introduction to Borg's RPE scale.* Ithaca, NY: Movement Publications.

RECOVERY PERIOD

Some debate exists as to whether the post-exercise recovery period should be an active or passive process. This decision should be made based on the purpose of the exercise test. If the test is performed for diagnostic purposes, then it appears to be of value to place the patient in the supine position immediately after stopping exercise. The increase in venous return to the heart observed in the supine position results in increases in ventricular volume, wall stress, and, consequently, myocardial oxygen demand. Several studies have shown that ST segment abnormalities are enhanced in the supine position and that an active recovery may attenuate the magnitude of these changes (Gibbons et al., 2002; Lachterman et al., 1990). Once thought to be false-positive responses, ST segment changes 2 to 4 minutes into recovery are now known to be particularly important for the detection of ischemia. Patients with symptom-limiting angina or dyspnea may become more uncomfortable in the supine position and should recover in a seated upright or semi-recumbent position. If the test is performed for nondiagnostic purposes such as for a fitness evaluation in a healthy or athletic person, then an active recovery may be safer and more comfortable.

Typically, an active recovery period consists of walking on the treadmill at a speed of 1.5 to 2.0 mph or continuing to pedal the cycle ergometer slowly at a work rate ranging from 0 to 25 W. An active recovery decreases the risk of hypotension and may minimize the risk of dysrhythmias secondary to elevated catecholamines in the post-exercise period. Standing recovery should be avoided because of potential complications associated with venous pooling. Regardless of the method of recovery, patients should be monitored for at least 6 to 8 minutes into the post-exercise period. Blood pressure, the electrocardiogram, and symptoms should be monitored and recorded at 2-minute intervals for the duration of the recovery period. The recovery period should be extended as long as necessary to resolve symptoms or abnormal hemodynamic or electrocardiographic responses. After completion of the recovery portion of the test, patients should be given post-test instructions that include avoidance of long, hot showers or baths. In addition, patients should be told they may experience fatigue and muscle soreness and to avoid any heavy exertion that day. Any pain or discomfort during the day after the test should be reported to their physician immediately.

ASSESSING TEST ACCURACY

All diagnostic tests misclassify patients a certain percentage of the time. In the context of the exercise test, this is not a trivial issue, because people who are inaccurately identified as having disease may be subjected unnecessarily to additional, more invasive, and costly procedures. When the test is performed properly, it commonly serves the very important purpose of screening those who should or should not undergo these additional procedures. However, a patient with significant CAD who is incorrectly classified as normal may not receive appropriate medical therapy. How accurately the exercise test distinguishes people with disease from those without disease depends on the population tested, the definition of disease, and the criteria used for an abnormal test.

The most common terms used to describe test accuracy are sensitivity and specificity. Sensitivity is the percentage of times a test correctly identifies those with CAD. Specificity is the percentage of times a test correctly identifies those without cardiovascular disease. Sensitivity and specificity are inversely related and are affected by the choice of discriminant value for abnormal, the definition of disease, and, most importantly, by the prevalence of disease in the population tested. For example, if the population has a greater prevalence or severity of disease (such as coronary disease in multiple vessels), the test will have a higher sensitivity. Alternatively, the test will have a higher specificity (and low sensitivity) when performed in a group of younger, healthier subjects.

Meta-analysis of the exercise testing literature indicates that the exercise test has, on the average, a sensitivity of approximately 68% and a specificity of approximately 77% (Gianrossi, 1989). However, these values range widely in the various studies; sensitivity can be as low as 40% among patients with single-vessel disease, but greater than 90% among those with triple-vessel disease. Conversely, the specificity of the test is usually quite low (i.e., 50% to 60%) in patients who have more severe CAD but is quite high in populations that are relatively healthy. These values reported in the literature and the inverse relationship between sensitivity and specificity underscore the importance of considering the patient's pre-test characteristics (chest pain and CAD risk factors) before beginning the test. No test result can be interpreted accurately without considering the patient in the context of his or her pre-test characteristics.

Another important term that helps define the diagnostic value of a test is the predictive value. The predictive value of an abnormal test (positive predictive value) is the percentage of people with an abnormal test result who have disease. Conversely, the predictive value of a normal test (negative predictive value) is the percentage of people with a normal test result who do not have disease. The predictive value of a test cannot be determined directly from the sensitivity and specificity but is strongly associated with the prevalence of disease in the population tested. The calculations used to determine sensitivity, specificity, and predictive value are presented in Display 21-6.

DISPLAY   21-6

TERMS USED TO DEMONSTRATE THE DIAGNOSTIC VALUE OF A TEST

Sensitivity $\dfrac{TP}{TP + FN} \times 100$

Specificity $\dfrac{TP}{TN + FP} \times 100$

Positive predictive value $\dfrac{TP}{TP + FP} \times 100$

Negative predictive value $\dfrac{TN}{TN + FN} \times 100$

TP, true positives, or those with abnormal test results and with disease; FN, false-negatives, or those with normal test results with disease; FP, false-positives, or those with abnormal test results and no disease; TN, true negatives, or those with normal test results and no disease.

DISPLAY **21-7**

CAUSES OF FALSE-NEGATIVE AND FALSE-POSITIVE TEST RESULTS

False-Positive

1. Resting repolarization abnormalities (e.g., left bundle-branch block)
2. Cardiac hypertrophy
3. Accelerated conduction defects (e.g., Wolfe-Parkinson-White syndrome)
4. Digitalis
5. Nonischemic cardiomyopathy
6. Hypokalemia
7. Vasoregulatory abnormalities
8. Mitral valve prolapse
9. Pericardial disease
10. Coronary spasm in absence of coronary artery disease
11. Anemia
12. Female gender

False-Negative

1. Failure to reach ischemic threshold secondary to medications (e.g., beta blockers)
2. Monitoring an insufficient number of leads to detect electrocardiographic changes
3. Angiographically significant disease compensated by collateral circulation
4. Musculoskeletal limitations preceding cardiac abnormalities

False-Positive and False-Negative Responses

The factors associated with false-positive or false-negative responses should also be considered before the test. A false-positive response is defined as an abnormal exercise test response in a person *without* significant heart disease and causes the specificity to be decreased. A false-negative response occurs when the test is normal in a person *with* disease and causes the sensitivity of the test to be reduced. Factors associated with false-positive and false-negative responses are listed in Display 21-7. In people in whom the probability of a false-positive or false-negative test is high, an alternative procedure (exercise or pharmacologic echocardiogram or radionuclide test) may be appropriate.

ANCILLARY METHODS FOR THE DETECTION OF CORONARY ARTERY DISEASE

Several ancillary imaging techniques have been shown to provide a valuable complement to exercise electrocardiography for the evaluation of patients with known or suspected CAD. These techniques are particularly helpful among patients with equivocal exercise electrocardiograms or those likely to exhibit false-positive or false-negative responses. They are frequently used to clarify abnormal ST segment responses in asymptomatic people or those in whom the cause of chest discomfort remains uncertain. When exercise electrocardiography and an imaging technique are combined, the diagnostic and prognostic accuracy is enhanced (Borges-Neto et al., 1997). For example, patients exhibiting both a positive exercise electrocardiogram and a positive radionuclide scan have been shown to have a 2.6-fold increased risk for subsequent coronary events (Kotler & Diamond, 1990).

The major imaging procedures are myocardial perfusion and ventricular function studies using radionuclide techniques, exercise echocardiography, and pharmacologic stress testing. Because these techniques are often used in conjunction with or as a surrogate for standard exercise testing, they are briefly discussed here. Detailed reviews of these topics are available elsewhere (Froelicher & Myers, 2000; Ritchie et al., 1995).

Myocardial Perfusion Imaging

The most commonly used technique to evaluate myocardial perfusion is the application of the radionuclide thallium-201 (Berger et al., 1981; Ritchie et al., 1995). When thallium-201 is injected intravenously at maximal exercise, it is rapidly extracted from the blood by living cells in the myocardium. Uptake of thallium-201 is similar to that of potassium in living cells. Radiologic images are then taken, which reveal areas of absent, poor, or moderately poor uptake of thallium-201. When exercise images are compared with rest images, the differences in uptake of thallium-201 indicate areas of decreased blood flow. At the same time, if areas absent of thallium-201 uptake occur at rest, it can be assumed that this represents areas of myocardial scarring and not ischemia with exercise. This information, along with the exercise test, can be more definitive in the evaluation of the extent and localization of ischemia.

Perfusion imaging with technetium-99m sestamibi has become common. This imaging agent permits higher dosing with less radiation exposure than thallium, resulting in improved images that are sharper and have less artifact and attenuation. Sestamibi is the preferred imaging agent for obtaining tomographic images of the heart using single photon emission computed tomography (SPECT). SPECT images are obtained with a gamma camera, which rotates 180 degrees around the patient, stopping at preset angles to record the image. Cardiac images are then displayed in slices from three different axes to allow visualization of the heart in three dimensions. Thus, multiple myocardial segments can be viewed individually, without the overlap of segments that occurs with planar imaging (Berger et al., 1981). As with thallium-201 imaging, perfusion defects that are present during exercise but not seen at rest suggest ischemia. Perfusion defects that are present during exercise and persist at rest suggest previous MI or scar. In this manner, the extent and distribution of ischemic myocardium can be identified.

Perfusion imaging of the coronary anatomy has been shown to be somewhat more sensitive and specific than the exercise electrocardiogram for detecting CAD. An extensive review of the literature suggested the sensitivity and specificity of exercise thallium scintigraphy for detecting coronary disease were in the order of 84% and 87%, respectively (Kotler & Diamond, 1990). This modality also permits the localization of ischemia, which is not possible with ST segment depression on the electrocardiogram. This technique is especially helpful in patients with equivocal exercise electrocardiograms, those using digoxin, or those with left bundle-branch block, in whom the interpretation of electrocardiographic changes is more problematic (Froelicher & Myers, 2000; Gibbons et al., 2002).

Ventricular Function Studies

Ventricular function is commonly evaluated with the use of the radioisotope technetium-99m. This radioisotope is administered as an intravenous bolus, and its transit through the ventricles is measured by special cameras. Technetium-99m is also used to label red blood cells for equilibrium blood pool studies. Both of these methods have been used extensively in the evaluation of left and right ventricular function after acute MI and other cardiac events. This technique can be performed at rest as well as at maximal exercise. When performed at maximal exercise, it has the capability of determining decreased ventricular function compared to rest measures. This can help in the diagnosis of ischemic abnormalities as well as exercise-induced ventricular dysfunction. In addition to measures of ejection fraction, measures of specific regional wall motion can also be taken (Borges-Neto, 1997; Gibbons, 1991).

The limitations of thallium, sestamibi SPECT, and technetium imaging include their higher cost and exposure of the patient to ionizing radiation. Additional equipment and personnel are also required for image acquisition and interpretation, including a nuclear technician to administer the radioactive isotope and acquire the images, and a physician trained in nuclear medicine to reconstruct and interpret the images.

Exercise Echocardiographic Imaging

Echocardiographic imaging of the heart is being increasingly used during exercise and pharmacologic stress testing. This technique is frequently combined with an exercise electrocardiogram to increase the sensitivity and specificity of exercise testing. Typically, a resting two-dimensional image is taken, and repeat images are obtained at peak exercise or immediately afterward. If images are taken after exercise, they must be obtained within 1 to 2 minutes because abnormal wall motion begins to normalize after this point. Rest and stress images are compared side-by-side in a cine-loop display that is gated during systole from the QRS complex. Myocardial contractility normally increases with exercise, whereas ischemia causes hypokinesis, akinesis, and dyskinesis of the affected segments. Therefore, a test is considered positive if wall motion abnormalities develop in previously normal territories with exercise or worsen in an already abnormal segment (Armstrong & Marcovitz, 1993).

Some advantages of exercise echocardiography over nuclear imaging include the absence of exposure to ionizing radiation and a shorter amount of time required for testing. Like standard exercise testing and radionuclide techniques, the diagnostic accuracy of echocardiography depends primarily on the specific methodology used and the pretest probability of CAD in the subjects tested. The accuracy of echocardiographic testing also depends on observer experience. Reviews of studies published

since the advent of exercise echocardiography in the early 1980s suggest that the average sensitivity and specificity of this technique for detecting coronary disease are both approximately 85% (Armstrong et al., 1998). The limitations of exercise echocardiography include dependence on the operator for obtaining adequate, timely images, and some variation exists in image interpretation. In addition, as much as 20% of patients have inadequate echocardiographic windows secondary to body habitus or lung interference (Schmidt et al., 1995).

Pharmacologic Stress Techniques

It is advantageous to use pharmacologic stress techniques for patients who are unable to exercise on a treadmill or cycle ergometer to an adequate level. These include patients who have orthopedic limitations, peripheral vascular disease, and chronic obstructive pulmonary disease or other limiting pulmonary diseases; elderly patients with low functional capacity; diabetic patients with severe neuropathy; and patients with neuromuscular conditions. For these patients, pharmacologic methods can be extremely useful for evaluating coronary blood flow and myocardial function. Pharmacologic stress is a relatively new area with important applications for echocardiographic and nuclear techniques, but only limited data are available directly comparing pharmacologic stress testing with standard exercise testing.

Two types of pharmacologic stress agents have been used: those that increase coronary blood flow through coronary vasodilation and those that increase myocardial oxygen demand by increasing heart rate. The commonly used coronary vasodilators are adenosine and dipyridamole (Persantine), whereas dobutamine is used to increase myocardial oxygen demand. The vasodilators cause greatly increased endocardial and epicardial blood flow in normal coronary arteries but not in stenotic segments, whereas dobutamine can create an imbalance between myocardial oxygen supply and demand by increasing heart rate and contractility. These drugs are administered intravenously and, when associated with an imaging technique such as thallium-201 scintigraphy, sestamibi, or echocardiography, can provide important information about coronary artery stenosis. Comparisons between dipyridamole and standard exercise testing have demonstrated dipyridamole to have a diagnostic accuracy similar to or slightly better than that of standard exercise testing (Bolognese et al., 1989; Severi et al., 1994). The disadvantages of dipyridamole and adenosine stress testing include side effects (40% to 50% of patients have minor side effects) and lack of cardiovascular response (approximately 10% of patients) (Iskandrian, 1991; Ranhosky & Kempthorne-Rawson, 1990).

GAS EXCHANGE TECHNIQUES

Because of the inaccuracies associated with estimating oxygen uptake and METs from work rate (i.e., treadmill speed and grade), many laboratories directly measure expired gases. The measurement of gas exchange and ventilatory responses provides an added dimension to the exercise test by increasing the information obtained concerning a patient's cardiopulmonary function. The direct measurement of VO_2 has been shown to be more reliable and reproducible than estimated values from treadmill or cycle ergometer work rate (Myers, 1996). Peak VO_2 is the most accurate measurement of functional capacity and is a useful reflection of overall cardiopulmonary health. Measurement of expired gases is not considered necessary for all clinical exercise testing, but the additional information provides important physiologic data. Heart and lung diseases frequently manifest themselves through gas exchange abnormalities during exercise, and the information obtained is increasingly used in clinical trials to objectively assess the response to interventions. Moreover, a growing body of literature suggests that exercise capacity measured directly by gas exchange techniques provides superior prognostic information relative to exercise time or estimated METs (Mancini et al., 1991; Myers, 1996; Myers & Gullestad, 1998). Situations in which gas exchange measurements are appropriate include the following (American College of Sports Medicine Guidelines, 2001; Gibbons et al., 2002):

- When a precise response to a specific therapeutic intervention is needed for a particular patient
- When a research question is being addressed
- When the cause of exercise limitation or dyspnea is uncertain
- To evaluate exercise capacity in patients with heart failure to assist in the estimation of prognosis and assess the need for transplantation
- To assist in the development of an appropriate exercise prescription for cardiac rehabilitation

The use of these techniques, however, requires added attention to detail and a working knowledge of the equipment and basic physiology. This is particularly important given advances in automation for the collection and calculation of expired gases.

PROGNOSIS

The exercise test has been shown to be of value for estimating prognosis in patients with a wide range of severity of cardiovascular diseases (Froelicher & Myers, 2000; Gibbons et al., 2002; Mark et al., 1987; Morris et al., 1991; Myers & Gullestad, 1998; Myers et al., 2002; Roger et al., 1998; Weiner et al., 1987). One of the most important clinical applications of the exercise test is the identification of low-risk patients in whom catheterization (and revascularization) can be safely deferred. There are several reasons why accurately establishing prognosis is important. An estimate of prognosis provides answers to patients' questions regarding the probable outcome of their illness, which may be useful to the patient in planning return to work or making decisions regarding disability, recreational activities, and finances. A second reason to estimate prognosis is to identify patients for whom interventions might improve outcome. Combining clinical and exercise test information into scores has been shown to improve the estimation risk among men and women undergoing exercise testing (Ashley et al., 2002; Chang & Froelicher, 1994; Mark et al., 1987).

Although there are many exercise test variables known to be of value for estimating prognosis, including exercise capacity, maximal heart rate, a hypotensive response, ST depression, and symptoms, the most powerful predictor of risk appears to be exercise capacity. Recent studies from Duke University, the

Mayo Clinic, the Cleveland Clinic, and the Veterans Administration have confirmed the value of including exercise capacity in the risk paradigm among patients referred for exercise testing (Ashley et al., 2002; Mark et al., 1987; Myers et al., 2002; Roger et al., 1998). It has also been recently demonstrated that the rate in which heart rate recovers from exercise, long known to be associated with higher levels of fitness, is an important risk marker among patients undergoing exercise testing (Cole et al., 1999; Cole et al., 2000). For example, patients who fail to decrease heart rate more than 12 beats/min 1 minute after completing the exercise test have four-times the risk of mortality over the subsequent 6 years (Cole et al., 1999).

EXERCISE TESTING IN SPECIAL POPULATIONS

Women

The interpretation of exercise testing results in women is more challenging than that in men (Bryant & Limacher, 1994; Gibbons et al., 2002). Exercise-induced ST segment depression is less sensitive among women compared with men (Hlatky et al., 1984; Morise & Diamond, 1995). Test specificity is also thought to be lower among women, although there is a wide variation in the reported studies (Gibbons et al., 2002). Some of these differences may be explained by differences in the meaning of chest pain presentation between men and women, although typical angina is as meaningful in women older than age 60 years as it is in men. Nearly half the women with anginal symptoms in the CASS study (who were younger than age 65 years) had normal coronary arteries (Kennedy et al., 1977). Other possible explanations for the lower test accuracy in women include lower disease prevalence, higher incidence of mitral valve prolapse and syndrome X (chest pain without coronary disease), differences in microvascular function, and possibly hormonal differences (Cerqueira, 1995; Gibbons et al., 2002).

The accuracy for diagnosing CAD in women has been shown to be improved by the use of multivariate methods (Robert et al., 1991) and by the addition of nuclear or echocardiographic imaging techniques (Cerqueira, 1995; Marwick et al., 1995; Morise et al., 1995). Thus, when exercise testing is performed in women, factors that may affect test accuracy should be carefully considered; if the exercise test results are uncertain or when otherwise appropriate, a radionuclide imaging procedure should be considered. The optimal strategy for circumventing false-positive test results in women remains to be defined. Nevertheless, the current AHA/ACC guidelines suggest that there are insufficient data to justify routine radionuclide imaging procedures as the initial test for CAD in women (Gibbons et al., 2002).

The Elderly

The prevalence of CAD increases with increasing age, and the exercise test can be an extremely useful tool for diagnosing CAD in the elderly. However, exercise testing in the elderly can be problematic given their frequently compromised ability to exercise in the context of an increased prevalence of CAD. The occurrence of fatigue and lightheadedness caused by muscle weakness and deconditioning, vasoregulatory abnormalities, and difficulties with gait are important concerns in these patients. Thus, a test modality and protocol should be chosen that provides the highest degree of safety. For instance, cycle ergometry may be more appropriate for elderly patients who have a residual deficit from a cerebral vascular accident. In addition, the testing protocol should be modified considering the expected levels of exercise tolerance. More gradually incremented protocols, such as the Balke, ramp, or Naughton, are usually more suitable in the elderly population. The elderly are more likely to present with more complex medication regimens, more co-morbidities, and increased prevalence of aortic stenosis and other valvular diseases, in addition to more severe CAD. For these reasons, the elderly require particularly close evaluation before clearance for exercise testing, a modified testing protocol, and particular attention to appropriate endpoints (Bryant & Limacher, 1994; Gibbons et al., 2002).

Interpretation of the exercise test in the elderly can also differ significantly from that in younger people. Resting electrocardiographic abnormalities, including previous MI, left ventricular hypertrophy, and intraventricular conduction delays, may compromise the diagnostic accuracy of the exercise test. Nevertheless, the application of standard ST segment criteria among elderly subjects has been shown to have similar diagnostic characteristics as in younger subjects (Hlatky et al., 1984). No doubt because of the higher prevalence of CAD in the elderly, test sensitivity has even been shown to be comparatively higher among the elderly (84%), although specificity is somewhat lower when compared to younger populations (70%) (Kasser & Bruce, 1969). Thus, despite several problems posed by elderly subjects that require additional attention, exercise testing is not contraindicated in this group (Gibbons et al., 2002).

Patients after Cardiac Transplantation

Over the past two decades, transplantation has become a widely used and successful treatment option for patients with end-stage heart failure. The 1-year survival rate for patients who undergo this procedure is now approximately 90%, compared with only 50% to 60% in patients with severe heart failure who receive medical treatment (Costanzo et al., 1995). The hemodynamic response to exercise in patients who have undergone cardiac transplantation has been characterized since the early 1970s (Savin et al., 1980; Schroeder, 1979; Stinson, 1972). Because the heart is denervated, some intriguing hemodynamic responses are observed. Orthotopic transplantation removes the nervous system connections to the heart. Thus, the heart is not responsive to the normal actions of the parasympathetic and sympathetic systems. The absence of vagal tone explains the high resting heart rates in these patients (100 to 110 beats/min) and the relatively slow adaptation of the heart to a given amount of submaximal work (Stinson, 1972). This slows the delivery of oxygen to the working tissue, contributing to an earlier than normal metabolic acidosis and hyperventilation during exercise (Brubaker et al., 1993; Degre et al., 1987; Marzo et al., 1992; Savin et al., 1980; Schroeder, 1979). Although transplantation significantly improves the

hemodynamic and ventilatory response to exercise, the transplanted patient still exhibits many of the responses typical of the patient with chronic heart failure (Marzo et al., 1992). These include heightened ventilatory responses attributable to uneven matching of ventilation to perfusion and an increase in physiologic dead space. Maximal heart rate is lower in transplant recipients compared to normal subjects, which contributes to a reduction in cardiac output and peak VO_2; the arteriovenous oxygen difference widens as a compensatory mechanism.

The exercise test in patients who have undergone cardiac transplantation is less a diagnostic and more a functional tool. In the latter role, it is useful for assessing and modifying therapy in these patients, in addition to evaluating the appropriateness of daily activities and return to work. Although rare cases of chest pain associated with accelerated graft atherosclerosis have been reported in transplant recipients, decentralization of the myocardium usually eliminates anginal symptoms. Exercise electrocardiography is also inadequate in terms of assessing ischemia, as evidenced by its low sensitivity (21% or less) (Ehrman et al., 1993). Thus, radionuclide testing may be more useful for assessing ischemia in these patients.

■ SUMMARY

Although there have been advances in technologies related to the diagnosis of CAD, the numerous applications and widespread availability of the exercise test continue to make it one of the more important tools in cardiovascular medicine. The test is increasingly being supervised by non-physicians, (Franklin et al., 1997), and the cardiovascular nurse's role has expanded in many centers to include exercise test supervision. Thus, an understanding of proper methodology, conduct, indications, and the physiology related to exercise testing are increasingly recognized skills. A good understanding of these principles can also assist the nurse in applying the information gained from the exercise test to patients with various cardiovascular diseases. In addition to diagnostic and prognostic information, these applications include the assessment of therapy, exercise prescription, and helping to guide medical/surgical management decisions for the patient.

REFERENCES

American Association of Cardiovascular and Pulmonary Rehabilitation. (1999). *Guidelines for cardiac rehabilitation programs* (3rd ed.). Champaign, IL: Human Kinetics.

American College of Sports Medicine. (2001). *Guidelines for exercise testing and exercise prescription* (6th ed.). Baltimore: Lippincott Williams & Wilkins.

American College of Sports Medicine. (2001). *Resource manual for guidelines for exercise testing and prescription* (4th ed.). Baltimore: Lippincott Williams & Wilkins.

American Thoracic Society/American College of Chest Physicians. (2003) Statement on Cardiopulmonary Exercise Testing. *American Journal of Respiratory and Critical Care Medicine, 167*, 211–277.

Armstrong, W., & Marcovitz, P. A. (1993). In E. Braunwald (Ed.), *Stress echocardiography: Heart disease updates* (pp. 1–10). Philadelphia: WB Saunders.

Armstrong, W. F., Pellikka, P. A., Ryan, T. et al. (1998). Stress echocardiography: Recommendations for performance and interpretation of stress echocardiography. *Journal of the American Society of Echocardiography, 11*, 97–104.

Ashley, E., Myers, J., & Froelicher, V. (2002) Exercise testing scores as an example of better decisions through science. *Medicine and Science in Sports Exercise*, 34, 1391–1398.

Åstrand, P.-O., & Rodahl, K. (1986) *Textbook of work physiology* (3rd ed.). New York: McGraw-Hill.

Bailey, R. H., & Bauer, J. H. (1993). A review of common errors in the indirect measurement of blood pressure. *Archives of Internal Medicine*, 153, 2741–2748.

Berger, B. C., Watson, D. D., Taylor, G. J., et al. (1981). Quantitative thallium-201 exercise scintigraphy for detection of coronary artery disease. *Journal of Nuclear Medicine*, 22, 585–593.

Bolognese, L., Sarasso, G., Aralda, D., et al. (1989). High dose dipyridamole echocardiography early after uncomplicated acute myocardial infarction: Correlation with exercise testing and coronary angiography. *Journal of the American College of Cardiology*, 14, 357–363.

Borg, G. A. V. (1982). Psychophysical bases of perceived exertion. *Medicine and Science in Sports Exercise*, 14, 377–381.

Borges-Neto, S. (1997). Perfusion and function assessment by nuclear cardiology techniques. *Current Opinion in Cardiology*, 12, 581–586.

Borges-Neto, S., Shaw, L. J., Kesler, K. L., et al. (1997). Prediction of severe coronary artery disease by combined rest and exercise radionuclide angiocardiography and tomographic perfusion imaging with technetium 99m-labeled sestamibi: A comparison with clinical and electrocardiographic data. *Journal of Nuclear Cardiology*, 4, 189–194.

Brubaker, P. H., Berry, M. J., Brozena, S. C., et al. (1993). Relationship of lactate and ventilatory thresholds in cardiac transplant patients. *Medicine and Science in Sports Exercise*, 25, 191–196.

Bryant, B. A., & Limacher, M. C. (1994). Exercise testing in selected patient groups: Women, the elderly, and the asymptomatic. *Primary Care*, 21, 517–534.

Buchfuhrer, M. J., Hansen, J. E., Robinson, T. E., et al. (1983). Optimizing the exercise protocol for cardiopulmonary assessment. *Journal of Applied Physiology*, 55, 1558–1564.

Cerqueira, M. D. (1995). Diagnostic testing strategies for coronary artery disease: Special issues related to gender. *American Journal of Cardiology*, 75, 52D–60D.

Chang, J. A., & Froelicher, V. F. (1994). Clinical and exercise test markers of prognosis in patients with stable coronary artery disease. *Current Problems in Cardiology*, 19, 533–538.

Cole, C. R., Blackstone, E. H., Pashkow, F. J., et al. (1999). Heart rate recovery immediately after exercise as a predictor of mortality. *New England Journal of Medicine*, 341, 1351–1357.

Cole, C. R., Foody, J. M., Blackstone, E. H., et al. (2000). Heart rate recovery after submaximal exercise testing as a predictor of mortality in a cardiovascularly healthy cohort. *Annals of Internal Medicine*, 132, 552–555.

Costanzo, M. R., Augustine, s., Bourge, R., et al. (1995). Selection and treatment of candidates for heart transplantation: A statement for health professionals from the Committee on Heart Failure and Cardiac Transplantation of the Council on Clinical Cardiology, American Heart Association. *Circulation*, 92, 3593–3612.

Degre, S. G. L., Niset, G. L., DeSmet, J. M., et al. (1987). Cardiorespiratory response to early exercise testing after orthotopic cardiac transplantation. *Am J Cardiol*, 60, 926–928.

Dubach, P., Froelicher, V. F., Klein, J., et al. (1988). Exercise induced hypotension in a male population: Criteria, causes, and prognosis. *Circulation*, 78, 1380–1387.

Ehrman, J. K., Keteyian, S. J., Levine, A. B., et al. (1993). Exercise stress tests after cardiac transplantation. *American Journal of Cardiology*, 71, 1372–1373.

Foster, C., Crowe, A. J., Danies, E., et al. (1996). Predicting functional capacity during treadmill testing independent of exercise protocol. *Medicine and Science in Sports Exercise*, 28, 752–756.

Franklin, B. A., Gordon, S., Timmis, G. C., et al. (1997). Is direct physician supervision of exercise stress testing routinely necessary? *Chest*, 111, 262–264.

Froelicher, V. F. (1996). *Exercise test reporting aid (EXTRA) software*. St. Louis: Mosby-Year Book.

Froelicher, V. F., & Myers, J. (2000). *Exercise and the heart* (4th ed.). Philadelphia: W.B. Saunders.

Sivarajan Froelicher, E. (1994). Usefulness of exercise testing shortly after acute myocardial infarction for predicting 10-year mortality. *American Journal of Cardiology*, 74, 318–323.

Gamble, P., McManus, H., Jensen, D., et al. (1984). A comparison of the standard 12 lead electrocardiogram to exercise electrode placement. *Chest*, 85, 616–622.

Gianrossi, R., Detrano, R., Mulvihill, D., et al. (1989). Exercise-induced ST depression in the diagnosis of coronary artery disease: A meta analysis. *Circulation*, 80, 87–98.

Gibbons, L., Blair, S. N., Kohl, H. W., et al. (1989). The safety of maximal exercise testing. *Circulation*, 80, 846–852.

Gibbons, R. J., Balady, G. J., Bricker, J. T., et al. (2002). ACC/AHA 2002 Guideline Update for Exercise Testing. A report of the ACC/AHA Task Force on Practice Guidelines (Committee on Exercise Testing). *J Am Coll Cardiol*, 40, 1531–1540.

Gibbons, R. J. (1991). Nuclear cardiology. In E. R. Guiliani, V. Fyster, & B. J. Gersh, et al. (Eds.), *Cardiology: Fundamentals and Practice*, (2nd ed., pp. 161–180). St. Louis: CV Mosby.

Gibbons, R. J. (1991). Rest and exercise radionuclide angiography for diagnosis in chronic ischemic heart disease. *Circulation*, 84(Suppl 1), I–93–I–99.

Graettinger, W., Smith, D., Neutel, J. et al. (1995). Relationship of left ventricular structure to maximal heart rate during exercise. *Chest*, 107, 341–345.

Hambrecht, R., Schuler, G. C., Muth, T., et al. (1992). Greater diagnostic sensitivity of treadmill versus cycle exercise testing of asymptomatic men with coronary artery disease. *American Journal of Cardiology*, 70, 141–146.

Hammond, K., & Froelicher, V. F.AQ1 Normal and abnormal heart rate responses to exercise. *Prog Cardiovasc Dis*, 27, 271–296.

Herbert, D. L., & Herbert, W. G. (1993). *Legal aspects of preventive, rehabilitative, and recreational exercise programs* (3rd ed.). Canton: PRC.

Hermansen, L., & Saltin, B. (1969). Oxygen uptake during maximal treadmill and bicycle exercise. *Journal of Applied Physiology*, 26, 31–37.

Hlatky, M. A., Pryor, D. B., Harrell, F. E. Jr., et al. (1984). Factors affecting sensitivity and specificity of exercise electrocardiography: Multivariable analysis. *American Journal of Medicine*, 77, 64–71.

Irving, J. B., & Bruce, R. A. (1977). Exertional hypotension and postexertional ventricular fibrillation in stress testing. *American Journal of Cardiology*, 39, 849–851.

Iskandrian, A. S. (1991). Single-photon emission computed tomographic thallium imaging with adenosine, dipyridamole, and exercise. *American Heart Journal*, 122, 279–284.

Iyriboz, Y., & Hearon, C. M. (1992). Blood pressure measurement at rest and during exercise: Controversies, guidelines, and procedures. *Journal of Cardiopulmonary Rehabilitation*, 12, 277–287.

Kasser, I. S., & Bruce, R. A. (1969). Comparative effects of aging and coronary heart disease on submaximal and maximal exercise. *Circulation*, 39, 759–774.

Kennedy, H., Killip, T., Fischer, L., et al. (1977). The clinical spectrum of coronary artery disease and its surgical and medical management: 1974–1979, the Coronary Artery Surgery Study. *Circulation*, 56, 756–761.

Kleiner, J. P., Nelson, W. P., & Boland, M. J. (1978). The 12 lead electrocardiogram in exercise testing. *Archives of Internal Medicine*, 138, 1572–1573.

Kotler, T. S., & Diamond, G. A. (1990). Exercise thallium-201 scintigraphy in the diagnosis and prognosis of coronary artery disease. *Annals of Internal Medicine*, 113, 684–702.

Lachterman, B., Lehmann, K. G., Abrahamson, D., et al. (1990). "Recovery only" ST segment depression and the predictive accuracy of the exercise test. *Annals of Internal Medicine*, 112, 11–16.

Lauer, M. S., Okin, P. M., Larson, M. G., et al. (1996). Impaired heart rate response to graded exercise: Prognostic implications of chronotropic incompetence in the Framingham Heart Study. *Circulation*, 93, 1520–1526.

Levites, R., Baker, T., & Anderson, G. J. (1978). The significance of hypotension developing during treadmill exercise testing. *American Heart Journal*, 95, 747–753.

Mancini, D. M., Eisen, H., Kussmaul, W., et al. (1991). Value of peak oxygen consumption for optimal timing of cardiac transplantation in ambulatory patients with heart failure. *Circulation*, 83, 778–786.

Marcus, R., Lowe, R., Froelicher, V. F., et al. (1995). The exercise test as gatekeeper: Limiting access or appropriately directing resources? *Chest*, 107, 1442–1446.

Mark, D. B., Hlatky, M. A., Harell, F. E., et al. (1987). Exercise treadmill score for predicting prognosis in coronary artery disease. *Annals of Internal Medicine*, 106, 793–800.

Marwick, T. H., Anderson, T., Williams, M. J., et al. (1995). Exercise echocardiography is an accurate and cost-efficient technique for detection of coronary artery disease in women. *Journal of the American College of Cardiology*, 26, 335–341.

Marzo, K. P., Wilson, J. R., & Mancini, D. M. (1992). Effects of cardiac transplantation on ventilatory response to exercise. *American Journal of Cardiology*, 69, 547–553.

Mason, R. E., & Likar, I. (1966). A new system of multiple-lead exercise electrocardiography. *American Heart Journal*, 71, 196–205.

Mazzotta, G., Scopinaro, G., Falcidieno, M., et al. (1987). Significance of abnormal blood pressure response during exercise-induced myocardial dysfunction after recent acute myocardial infarction. *American Journal of Cardiology, 59*, 1256–1260.

Miranda, C. P., Lehmann, K. G., & Froelicher, V. F. (1989). Indications, criteria for interpretation, and utilization of exercise testing in patients with coronary disease: Results of a survey. *Journal of Cardiopulmonary Rehabilitation, 9*, 479–484.

Miranda, C. P., Liu, J., Kadar, A., et al. (1992). Usefulness of exercise induced ST segment depression in the inferior leads during exercise testing as a marker for coronary artery disease. *American Journal of Cardiology, 69*, 303–307.

Morise, A. P., & Diamond, G. A. (1995). Comparison of the sensitivity and specificity of exercise electrocardiography in biased and unbiased populations of men and women. *American Heart Journal, 130*, 741–747.

Morise, A. P., Diamond, G. A., Detrano, R., et al. (1995). Incremental value of exercise electrocardiography and thallium-201 testing in men and women for the presence and extent of coronary artery disease. *American Heart Journal, 130*, 267–276.

Morris, C. K., Ueshima, K., Kawaguchi, T., et al. (1991). The prognostic value of exercise capacity: A review of the literature. *American Heart Journal, 122*, 1423–1431.

Myers, J. (1996). *Essentials of cardiopulmonary exercise testing.* Champaign, IL: Human Kinetics.

Myers, J., Buchanan, N., Smith, D., et al. (1992). Individualized ramp treadmill: Observations on a new protocol. *Chest, 101*, 2305–2415.

Myers, J., Buchanan, N., Walsh, D., et al. (1991). Comparison of the ramp versus standard exercise protocols. *Journal of the American College of Cardiology, 17*, 1334–1342.

Myers, J., & Froelicher, V. F. (1994). Optimizing the exercise test for pharmacologic studies in patients with angina pectoris. In D. Ardissino, S. Savonitto, & L. H. Opie (Eds.), *Drug evaluation in angina pectoris* (pp. 41–52). Pavia, Italy: Kluwer Academic.

Myers, J., & Gullestad, L. (1998). The role of exercise testing and gas exchange measurement in the prognostic assessment of patients with heart failure. *Current Opinion in Cardiology, 13*, 145–155.

Myers, J., Prakash, M., Froelicher, V. F., et al. (2002). Exercise capacity and mortality in men referred for exercise testing. *New England Journal of Medicine, 346*, 793–801.

Myers, J., Walsh, D., Buchanan, N., et al. (1989). Can maximal cardiopulmonary capacity be recognized by a plateau in oxygen uptake? *Chest, 96*, 1312–1316.

Myers, J., Walsh, D., Sullivan, M., et al. (1990). Effect of sampling on variability and plateau in oxygen uptake. *Journal of Applied Physiology, 68*, 404–410.

Myers, J. N. (1994). Perception of chest pain during exercise testing in patients with coronary artery disease. *Medicine and Science in Sports Exercise, 26*, 1082–1086.

Myers, J., Voodi, L., Umann, T., & Froelicher, V. F. (2000). A survey of exercise testing: Methods, utilization, interpretation, and safety in the VAHCS. *Journal of Cardiopulmonary Rehabilitation, 20*, 251–258.

Naughton, J., Balke, B., & Nagle, F. (1964). Refinements in methods of evaluation and physical conditioning before and after myocardial infarction. *American Journal of Cardiology, 14*, 837–843.

Naughton, J. P., & Haiden, R. (1973). Methods of exercise testing. In J. P. Naughton, H.K. Hellerstien, & L.C. Mohler (Eds.), *Exercise testing and exercise training in coronary heart disease* (pp. 79–91). New York: Academic Press.

Noakes, T. (1988). Implications of exercise testing for prediction of athletic performance: A contemporary perspective. *Medicine and Science in Sports Exercise, 20*, 319–330.

Olona, M., Candell-Riera, J., Permanyer-Miralda, G., et al. (1995). Strategies for prognostic assessment of uncomplicated first myocardial infarction: 5-year follow-up study. *Journal of the American College of Cardiology, 25*, 815–822.

Panza, J., Quyyumi, A. A., Diodati, J. G., et al. (1991). Prediction of the frequency and duration of ambulatory myocardial ischemia in patients with stable coronary artery disease by determination of the ischemia threshold from exercise testing: Importance of the exercise protocol. *Journal of the American College of Cardiology, 17*, 657–663.

Philbrick, J. T., Horowitz, & Feinstein, A. R. (1989). Methodological problems of exercise testing for coronary artery disease: Groups, analysis and bias. *American Journal of Cardiology, 64*, 1117–1122.

Ranhosky, A., Kempthorne-Rawson, J., & the Intravenous Dipyridamole Thallium Imaging Study Group. (1990). The safety of intravenous dipyridamole thallium myocardial perfusion imaging. *Circulation, 81*, 1205–1209.

Rautaharju, P. M., Prineas, R. J., Crow, R. S., et al. (1980). The effect of modified limb positions on electrocardiographic wave amplitudes. *Journal of Electrocardiology, 13*, 109–114.

Redwood, D. R., Rosing, D. R., Goldstein, R. E., et al. (1971). Importance of the design of an exercise protocol in the evaluation of patients with angina pectoris. *Circulation, 43*, 618–628.

Ritchie, J. L., Bateman, T. M., Bonow, R. O., et al. (1995). Guidelines for clinical use of cardiac radionuclide imaging: Report of the American College of Cardiology/American Heart Association Task Force on Assessment of Diagnostic and Therapeutic Cardiovascular Procedures (Committee on Radionuclide Imaging, developed in conjunction with the American Society of Nuclear Cardiology). *Journal of the American College of Cardiology, 25*, 521–547.

Robert, A. R., Melin, J. A., & Detry, J. M. (1991). Logistic discriminant analysis improves diagnostic accuracy of exercise testing for coronary artery disease in women. *Circulation, 83*, 1202–1209.

Rochmis, P., & Blackburn, H. (1971). Exercise tests: A survey of procedures, safety, and litigation experience in approximately 170,000 tests. *JAMA, 217*, 1061–1066.

Roger, V. L., Jacobsen, S. J., Pellikka, P. A., Miller, T., Bailey, K. R., & Gersh, B. J. (1998). Prognostic value of treadmill exercise testing. A population-based study in Olmstead County, Minnesota. *Circulation, 98*, 2836–2841.

Rogers, G. P., Ayanian, J. Z., Balady, G. J., et al. (2000). American College of Cardiology/American Heart Association Clinical Competence Statement on Stress Testing. A report of the ACC/AHA and American Society of Internal medicine Task Force on Clinical Competence. *Circulation, 102*, 1726–1738.

San Marco, M., Pontius, S., & Selvester, R. (1980). Abnormal blood pressure response and marked ischemia by ST segment depression as predictors of severe coronary artery disease. *Circulation, 61*, 572–578.

Savin, W., Haskell, W. L., Schroeder, J. S., et al. (1980). Cardiorespiratory responses of cardiac transplant patients to graded, symptom limited exercise. *Circulation, 62*, 55–60.

Schmidt, D. H., Port, S. C., & Gal, R. A. (1995). Nuclear cardiology and echocardiography: Noninvasive tests for diagnosing patients with coronary artery disease. In M. Pollack & D. H. Schmidt (Eds.), *Heart disease and rehabilitation* (3rd ed., pp 81–94). Champaign, IL: Human Kinetics.

Schroeder, J. S. (1979). Hemodynamic performance of the human transplanted heart. *Transplant Proceedings, 11*, 304–308.

Severi, S., Picano, E., Michelassi, C., et al. (1994). Diagnostic and prognostic value of dipyridamole echocardiography in patients with suspected coronary artery disease: Comparison with exercise electrocardiography. *Circulation, 89*, 1160–1173.

Stachenfeld, N. S., Eskenazi, M., Gleim, G. W., et al. (1972). Predictive accuracy of criteria used to assess maximal oxygen consumption. *American Heart Journal, 123*, 922–926.

Stinson, E. B., Griepp, R. L., Schroeder, J. S., et al. (1972). Hemodynamic observations one and two years after cardiac transplantation in man. *Circulation, 14*, 1181–1193.

Stuart, R. J., Ellestad, M. H. (1980). National survey of exercise stress testing facilities. *Chest, 77*, 94–97.

Thompson, P. (1993). The safety of exercise testing and participation. In J. L. Durstine, A. C. King, P. L. Painter, J. L. Roitman, L. D. Zwirin, & W. L. Kenney (Eds.), *Resource manual for guidelines for exercise testing and prescription* (2nd ed., pp. 359–363). Philadelphia: Lea & Febiger.

Webster, M. W. I., & Sharpe, D. N. (1989). Exercise testing in angina pectoris: The importance of protocol design in clinical trials. *American Heart Journal, 117*, 505–508.

Weiner, D. A., McCabe, C. H., Cutler, S. S., et al. (1982). Decrease in systolic blood pressure during exercise testing: Reproducibility, response to coronary artery bypass surgery and prognostic significance. *American Journal of Cardiology, 49*, 1627–1632.

Weiner, D. A., Ryan, T. J., McCabe, C. H., et al. (1987). Value of exercise testing in determining the risk classification and the response to coronary artery bypass grafting in three-vessel coronary artery disease: A report from the Coronary Artery Surgery Study (CASS) registry. *American Journal of Cardiology, 60*, 262–266.

Whipp, B. J., Davis, J. A., Torres, F., et al. (1981). A test to determine parameters of aerobic function during exercise. *Journal of Applied Physiology, 50*, 217–221.

Wicks, J. R., Sutton, J. R., Oldridge, N. B., et al. (1978). Comparison of the electrocardiographic changes induced by maximum exercise testing with treadmill and cycle ergometer. *Circulation, 57*, 1066–1069.

Wolthius, R. A., Froelicher, V. F., Fischer, J., et al. (1997). New practical treadmill protocol for clinical use. *American Journal of Cardiology, 39*, 697–700.

Yang, J. C., Wesley, R. C., & Froelicher, V. F. (1991). Ventricular tachycardia during routine treadmill testing: Risk and prognosis. *Archives of Internal Medicine, 151*, 349–353.

Cardiac Catheterization

MICHAELENE HARGROVE DEELSTRA • CAROL JACOBSON

Cardiac catheterization is widely used for diagnostic evaluation and therapeutic intervention in the management of patients with cardiac disease. Nurses have an important role in pre-catheterization teaching, intracatheterization and postcatheterization care. The many nursing responsibilities related to cardiac catheterization are outlined in the American College of Cardiology/Society for Cardiac Angiography and Interventions (ACC/SCA&I) Clinical Expert Consensus Document on Cardiac Catheterization Laboratory Standards (Bashore et al., 2001).

Cardiac catheterization developed as a result of 50 years of clinical effort. Werner Forssman performed the first documented cardiac catheterization in 1929. Guided by fluoroscopy, Forssman passed a catheter into his own right heart through an antecubital vein. He then walked upstairs to the radiology department and confirmed the catheter position by radiograph. The techniques of right and left heart catheterization were developed during the 1940s and 1950s (Cournand & Ranges, 1941; Cournand & Riley, 1945; Richards, 1945). In 1953, the percutaneous techniques of arterial catheterization were introduced by Seldinger, and, in 1959, selective coronary arteriography was introduced by Sones and colleagues (1959). Important advances related to cardiac catheterization included the development of the Swan-Ganz catheter in 1970 for measuring right heart pressures and the thermodilution method for determination of cardiac output (CO); catheter-based coronary revascularization, including percutaneous transluminal coronary angioplasty (PTCA), atherectomy, laser therapy, and stent placement; electrophysiologic mapping and catheter ablation for the management of arrhythmias; valvuloplasty; and patent foramen, ovale (PFO) and atrial septal defect (ASD) closure (Grossman, 2000b; Pepine, Hill & Lambert, 1989).

Although noninvasive diagnostic techniques have an important role, cardiac catheterization remains the most definitive procedure for the diagnosis and evaluation of coronary disease. Angiography and intravascular ultrasound provide quantitative information of coronary anatomy, and newer techniques including fractional flow reserve and coronary flow reserve can provide direct measurement of coronary blood flow to evaluate significance of coronary lesions. This chapter describes cardiac catheterization procedures and their possible complications. It also describes the nursing care given before and after catheterization and the interpretation of data as they relate to coronary heart disease (CHD).

INDICATIONS

Cardiac catheterization is indicated in a wide variety of circumstances. The most frequent use of cardiac catheterization is to confirm or define the extent of suspected CHD. Anatomical and physiologic severity of disease is determined, and the presence or absence of related conditions is explored.

Cardiac catheterization is essential in evaluating patients with congenital or valvular heart disease for surgery (see Chapter 29), and the catheterization laboratory is also the site for interventional cardiology techniques (see Chapter 27). The American College of Cardiology (ACC) and the American Heart Association (AHA) have published guidelines for coronary angiography and indications for cardiac catheterization (Scanton et al., 1999). Indications for coronary angiography are classified for specific clinical presentations, including asymptomatic patients, atypical chest pain of uncertain origin, symptomatic patients, and acute myocardial infarction (MI). Class I indications are those for which there is general agreement that coronary angiography is indicated. Class II indications are conditions for which coronary angiography is frequently performed, but there is a divergence of opinion with respect to its justification in terms of value and appropriateness. Class I indications are summarized here. The reader is referred to the ACC/AHA guidelines for a more complete discussion. (Scanlon et al., ACC/AHA, 1999).

Recommendations for coronary angiography in patients with known or suspected CAD who are currently asymptomatic or have stable angina, such as patients without symptoms after MI or those with exercise-induced electrocardiogram (ECG) abnormalities without accompanying angina pectoris

In asymptomatic patients, class I indications include:

1. Canadian Cardiovascular Society (CCS) class III and IV on medical treatment.
2. High-risk criteria on noninvasive testing regardless of anginal severity (Table 22-1).
3. Patients who have been successfully resuscitated from sudden cardiac death or have sustained (>30 seconds) monomorphic ventricular tachycardia or nonsustained (<30 seconds) polymorphic ventricular tachycardia.

Recommendations for coronary angiography in patients with nonspecific chest pain:

Table 22–1 ■ NONINVASIVE TESTS RESULTS PREDICTING HIGH RISK FOR ADVERSE OUTCOME

1. Severe resting left ventricular dysfunction (LVEF <.35)
2. High-risk treadmill score
3. Severe exercise left ventricular dysfunction (exercise LVEF <.35)
4. Stress-induced large perfusion defect (particularly if anterior)
5. Stress-induced moderate-size multiple perfusion defects
6. Large, fixed perfusion defect with left ventricular dilatation
7. Stress-induced moderate-size perfusion defect with left-ventricular dilatation
8. Echocardiographic wall motion abnormality (involving >2 segments) developing at low-dose dobutamine or at low heart rate
9. Stress echocardiographic evidence of extensive ischemia

Adapted from Scanlon et al. (1999). ACC/AHA guidelines for coronary angiography: Executive summary and recommendations: A report of the American College of Cardiology Task Force on Practice Guidelines. *Circulation*, 99, 2345–2357.

In patients with nonspecific chest pain, class I indications include:

1. High-risk findings on noninvasive testing (see Table 22-1).
   Recommendations for coronary angiography in unstable coronary syndromes
   In patients with unstable angina, class I indications include:

1. High or intermediate risk for adverse outcome in patients with unstable angina (Table 22-2) refractory to initial adequate medical therapy, or recurrent symptoms after initial stabilization. Emergent catheterization is recommended.
2. High risk for adverse outcome in patients with unstable angina. Urgent catheterization is recommended (see Table 22-2).
3. High- or intermediate-risk unstable angina that stabilizes after initial treatment.
4. Initially low short-term risk unstable angina that is subsequently high risk on noninvasive testing (see Table 22-1).
5. Suspected Prinzmetal's variant angina.

Recommendations for coronary angiography in patients with postrevascularization ischemia

In patients who have had percutaneous revascularization, class I indications include:

1. Suspected abrupt closure or subacute stent thrombosis after percutaneous revascularization (see Chapter 27).
2. Recurrent angina or high-risk criteria on noninvasive evaluation within 9 months of percutaneous revascularization (see Table 22-1).

Recommendations for coronary angiography during the initial management of acute MI

In patients presenting with an acute MI, class I indications include:

1. An alternative to thrombolytic therapy in patients who can undergo angioplasty of the infarct artery within 12 hours of the onset of symptoms or beyond 12 hours if symptoms persist.
2. In patients who are within 36 hours of an acute ST elevation/Q wave or new left bundle branch block (LBBB) MI who develop cardiogenic shock, are <75 years of age, and in whom revascularization can be performed within 18 hours of the onset of shock.

Table 22–2 ■ SHORT-TERM RISK OF DEATH OR NONFATAL MI IN PATIENTS WITH UNSTABLE ANGINA

High Risk
≥ 1 of the following features must be present:
Prolonged ongoing (>20 min) pain at rest
Pulmonary edema, most likely related to ischemia
Angina at rest with dynamic ST changes ≥ 1 mm
Angina with new or worsening MR murmur
Angina with S_3 or new/worsening crackles
Angina with hypotension

Intermediate Risk
No high-risk feature but must have any of the following features:
Prolonged (>20 min) angina at rest, now resolved, with moderate or high likelihood of CAD
Angina at rest (>20 min or relieved with rest or sublingual nitroglycerin)
Nocturnal angina
Angina with dynamic T-wave changes
New-onset CCS class III or IV angina in the past 2 weeks with moderate or high likelihood of CAD
Pathologic Q waves or resting ST depression ≤ 1 mm in multiple lead groups (anterior, inferior, lateral)
Age > 65 years

Low Risk
No high- or intermediate-risk feature but may have any of the following features:
Increased frequency, severity, or duration of angina
Angina provoked at a lower threshold
New onset angina with onset 2 weeks to 2 months before presentation
Normal or unchanged ECG

Adapted from Scanlon et al. (1999). ACC/AHA guidelines for coronary angiography: Executive summary and recommendations: A report of the American College of Cardiology Task Force on Practice Guidelines. *Circulation*, 99, 2345–2357.

Recommendations for coronary angiography during the hospital management phase of patients with Q-wave and non-Q-wave MI

In patients hospitalized with MI, class I indications include:

1. Spontaneous myocardial ischemia or myocardial ischemia provoked by minimal exertion during recovery from infarction.
2. Before definitive therapy of a mechanical complication of infarction such as acute mitral regurgitation, ventricular septal defect, pseudoaneurysm, or left ventricular aneurysm.
3. Persistent hemodynamic instability.

Recommendations for coronary angiography during risk stratification phase

In patients with all types of MI for risk stratification, class I indications include:

1. Ischemia at low levels of exercise with ECG changes (=1 mm ST-segment depression with symptoms, functional capacity <5 metabolic equivalents (METS), inadequate blood pressure response to exercise and/or imaging abnormalities (Gibbons et al., 1997).

CONTRAINDICATIONS

Cardiac catheterization has relatively few contraindications. Any correctable illness or condition that, if corrected, would improve the safety of the procedure should be managed before catheterization. These conditions include uncontrolled ventricular irritability, uncorrected hypokalemia or digitalis toxicity, decompensated congestive heart failure (CHF), and severe renal insufficiency or anuria unless dialysis is planned after the procedure. Preexisting renal insufficiency, particularly in patients with diabetes, and patients with prior anaphylactic reaction to contrast medium require special treatment before the procedure. Other relative contraindications are recent stroke (within 1 month); active gastrointestinal bleeding; active infection; severe, uncontrolled hypertension; and the patient's refusal of the therapeutic procedures to be directed by the catheterization results (Grossman, 2000b; Pepine et al., 1989). The ACC/AHA Task Force agrees that coronary angiography is generally not indicated for the following conditions:

1. Patients asymptomatic after coronary artery bypass surgery or percutaneous transluminal coronary angioplasty (PTCA) and with no evidence of ischemia, unless they provide informed consent for institutionally approved research purposes
2. Symptomatic patients with mild, clinically stable angina pectoris who do not have impaired ventricular function or exercise studies suggesting high risk
3. Symptomatic patients with well-controlled angina pectoris or patients after MI who are not candidates for either coronary artery bypass surgery or angioplasty because of advanced age or a life expectancy limited by other illness
4. Completed MI with uncomplicated infarction without prior thrombolytic therapy
5. Patients with severe left ventricular dysfunction in the absence of angina pectoris or evidence of ischemia

Anticoagulation is a relative contraindication. Routinely, oral anticoagulants should be withheld for 48 hours before catheterization to achieve an international normalized ratio (INR) below 2.0. In patients who must remain on anticoagulants, the use of heparin is favored because its effects may be quickly reversed with protamine sulfate if bleeding or hemorrhage occurs (Grossman, 2000b).

PATIENT PREPARATION

Patients are usually admitted for cardiac catheterization the day of the procedure. The physician performing the catheterization explains the procedure and obtains informed consent before procedure admission.

Precatheterization orders usually include the following:

1. Standard 12-lead ECG.
2. Laboratory tests: Complete blood count including platelets and differential, electrolytes, BUN, and creatinine.
3. Nothing by mouth after midnight (or after a light breakfast if catheterization is to be in the afternoon).
4. Premedication with mild sedative may be given. During the procedure, a procedural sedation protocol should be followed.
5. Patients with renal insufficiency should be adequately hydrated before and after the procedure. A minimum of

radiographic nonionic contrast should be used. Clinical studies have indicated a positive impact after pretreatment with fenoldopam or acetylcysteine in prevention of nephrotoxicity (Asif, Preston & Roth, 2003).

6. Patients with a history of allergy to iodine-containing substances, such as seafood or contrast agents, should receive nonionic contrast and pretreatment with steroids, antihistamine, (diphenhydramine) and H2 blocker (cimetidine or ranitidine).
7. Patients who are fasting should take a reduced dose of insulin or hold dose as directed by physician. Oral diabetic agents are usually held the morning of the procedure. Metformin is held the day of the procedure and 48 hours after the catheterization.
8. Anticoagulation issues are directed by the physician. Acetylsalicylic acid (ASA) and antiplatelet medications are usually given before catheterization. Warfarin is generally discontinued 2 to 3 days before the procedure until the INR is <2.0. Warfarin can be reversed with vitamin K or fresh frozen plasma. If the patient is receiving heparin therapy, this can be continued during the catheterization and discontinued for sheath removal.
9. Patient to void before going to catheterization laboratory.
10. Use of prophylactic antibiotics is not recommended.
11. Patients who wear dentures, glasses, or hearing aids should be sent to the laboratory wearing them. The patient is better able to communicate when dentures and hearing aids are in place. Glasses allow the patient to view the angiogram on the monitor and help keep the patient oriented to the surroundings.

Nursing Assessment and Patient Teaching

Nursing assessment and teaching are important parts of patient preparation. The nursing assessment includes the patient's heart rate and rhythm, blood pressure, evaluation of the peripheral pulses of the arms and legs, and assessment of heart and lung sounds. The sites for best palpation of the patient's dorsalis pedis and posterior tibial pulses are marked on the skin. This information will be used for comparison in evaluating peripheral pulses after the catheterization procedure. A procedural sedation assessment is performed, including assessment of the patient's cardiovascular, respiratory, and renal systems. Care is taken to identify characteristics or conditions that may cause the patient to be at greater risk for complications associated with procedural sedation, such as a history of difficult intubation; history of difficulty with sedation; morbid obesity; sleep apnea; extremes of age; severe cardiac, respiratory, renal, hepatic, or central nervous system disease; and history of substance abuse (Kixmiller & Schick, 1997). The nursing assessment also includes an evaluation of the patient's emotional status and attitude toward catheterization.

- Is this the patient's first cardiac catheterization?
- What are the patient's apprehensions about the procedure?
- What has the patient heard about cardiac catheterization? (Patients have sometimes heard "horror stories" from friends or acquaintances about catheterization experiences and

may, therefore, need reassurance about the safety of the procedure.)

■ What decisions are being faced? (Patients may be facing good or bad news about the absence or presence and extent of disease. Thus, the period before catheterization most likely is a time of anxiety and fear for a variety of reasons. Discussion and reassurance may help to relieve some of these feelings.)

The catheterization laboratory confronts the patient with new sights, sounds, and experiences that may be intimidating and frightening. Teaching is aimed at preparing the patient for this experience and should begin in the physician's office. In some institutions, patients are given a video to view before the procedure. A printed booklet to which the patient can refer is also helpful. The following points should be covered in patient teaching:

1. The patient is given nothing by mouth for 6 to 8 hours before the catheterization and is asked to void before leaving the unit.
2. Medication is given before or during the procedure, if prescribed, but the patient is awake during the procedure.
3. The patient should be instructed in deep breathing or stopping the breath without bearing down and in coughing on request. With deep inspiration, the diaphragm descends, preventing it from obstructing the view of the coronary arteries in some radiographic projections. Bearing down (Valsalva maneuver) increases intra-abdominal pressure and may raise the diaphragm, obstructing the view. After the injection of contrast medium, coughing is requested to help clear the material from the coronary arteries. The rapid movement of the diaphragm also acts as a mechanical stimulant to the heart and helps prevent the bradycardia that may accompany the injection of contrast medium (Owens & Bashore, 1990; Schultz & Olivas, 1986).
4. The appearance of the laboratory should be explained to the patient, including the general function of the equipment.
5. The patient wears a gown to the laboratory.
6. The patient lies on a table that is hard and narrow.
7. The catheter insertion site is washed with an antibacterial scrub and hair is removed using clippers. Usually, both groins are prepped to provide easy access to the other side for patients with peripheral vascular disease and obstructive disease preventing catheter advancement or sudden instability during procedure requiring an intra-aortic balloon pump (Heupler et al., 1992). The right groin is generally used because the operator standing on that side of the table has easier access.
8. The expected length of the procedure should be explained to the patient.
9. The patient is given a local anesthetic at the catheter entry site.
10. The patient may have hot flashes or experience nausea during injection of the coronary arteries with contrast medium, most commonly occurring with the injection of the ventricle during ventriculogram.
11. The patient should report angina, shortness of breath (SOB), and other symptoms to the staff.
12. The patient should be told the expected length of bed rest after the catheterization.

Outpatient Cardiac Catheterization

Improvements in cardiac procedures and decline in risk associated with diagnostic cardiac catheterizations have increased the number of outpatient procedures. Advantages include decreased costs and avoidance of an unnecessary overnight hospital stay. Patients considered for outpatient cardiac catheterization are those with stable coronary symptoms. Patients in whom the outpatient procedure is contraindicated include those with unstable, accelerated, crescendo, or preinfarction angina pectoris; uncompensated CHF; severe aortic stenosis; suspected left main coronary disease; known bleeding disorders; and metabolically unstable patients.

Patients needing preadmission to the hospital for cardiac catheterization include those who require continuous anticoagulation or who have significant renal insufficiency or brittle diabetes mellitus. Noninvasive testing may identify patients with high-risk coronary or valvular disease before catheterization who should be studied in settings with cardiac surgery capacity. Additional considerations include the distance the patient lives from the hospital and the availability of someone to drive the patient home (Clark, Moscovich, Vetrovec & Wexler, 1992; Montes, 1997).

Freestanding cardiac catheterization laboratories that are not physically attached to a hospital facility are becoming common and are used primarily for diagnostic studies. It is the responsibility of each freestanding laboratory to have a formal relationship with a referral hospital for emergency services. Patients studied at freestanding laboratories require thorough screening. High-risk patients must be excluded to avoid complications that require emergency services (Bashore et al., 2001).

Preprocedure teaching is best done before hospital admission. The content is similar to that for patients undergoing an inpatient procedure. Patients who have significant CHD or left main coronary disease or complications during the procedure are usually admitted to the hospital for overnight observation (Table 22-3).

Table 22–3 ■ GENERAL EXCLUSION CRITERIA FOR EARLY (<2–6 HOUR) DISCHARGE AFTER INVASIVE CARDIAC PROCEDURE IN ADULTS

High risk due to identification of left main disease
NYHA class III or IV heart failure
Unstable ischemic symptoms at any time after the procedure
Recent MI with postinfarction ischemia
Pulmonary edema thought to be caused by ischemia
Severe aortic stenosis with LV dysfunction
Severe aortic insufficiency with a pulse pressure >80 mm Hg
Poorly controlled systemic hypertension
Inadequate or unreliable follow-up over the next 24 hours
Generalized debility or dementia
Renal insufficiency (creatinine >1.8 mg/dL)
Need for continuous anticoagulation therapy or treatment of a bleeding diathesis
Large hematoma or vascular complication

Adapted from Bashore, T. M., et al. 2001. Cardiac Catheterization Laboratory Standards: a report of the American College of Cardiology Task Force on Clinical Expert Consensus Documents (ACC/SCA&I Committee to Develop an Expert Consensus Document on Cardiac Catheterization Laboratory Standards). *Journal of the American College of Cardiology, 37,* 2170–2214.

After a diagnostic procedure, the patient spends 3 to 6 hours in a short-stay unit, ambulatory recovery, or similar setting. Postprocedure orders are the same for inpatient and outpatient cardiac catheterization. After the required period of bed rest, the patient is observed for 30 to 60 minutes while sitting, standing, and walking. During this time, discharge instructions are reviewed. The patient is then allowed to leave. Results of the catheterization are reviewed with the patient by the cardiologist before discharge. Patients who have had percutaneous intervention often stay overnight for observation and to receive antiplatelet drugs and are discharged the following morning.

PROCEDURE

Cardiac Catheterization Laboratory

The cardiac catheterization laboratory is a specially equipped radiologic laboratory for the study of children and adults with known or suspected heart disease. The primary technical focus is the generation, recording, and display of high-quality x-ray images during diagnostic and interventional procedures. The ongoing trend toward more complex interventional procedures results in greater exposure to radiation for the patient and laboratory staff. This radiation exposure is monitored for safety (Limacher et al., 1998).

The technique of imaging has moved away from cineangiographic to digital images in most laboratories. The laboratory usually has the following equipment:

1. A patient support table, adjustable height, flat top whose locks can be released to allow the table top to move horizontally head to toe and side to side for "panning."
2. Equipment for monitoring intracardiac pressures, cardiac output (CO) determination, and physiologic recordings.
3. A suspended C-arm that rotates around the patient and allows variable angulations of the x-ray beam.
4. The image chain consists of a generator and cine pulse system, an x-ray tube, an image intensifier, an optical distributor, a 35-mm cine camera, and a television camera and monitor. The image chain produces fluoroscopy, which is the continuous presentation of an x-ray image on a fluorescent screen. This allows the viewing of structures in motion. The image intensifier receives the fluoroscopic image and increases its brightness, permitting filming (cinefluoroscopy) or digital acquisition of motion pictures and viewing of the image with a television camera, television screen, and videotape recorder. Although 35-mm film was originally used for recording, since 1998 all new images are permanently recorded digitally (Grossman, 2000b).
5. Single or biplane imaging system can be used. Biplane imaging provides simultaneous viewing of cardiac structures from two angles, which is helpful for congenital heart disease, transseptal punctures, and electrophysiology ablations.
6. Advanced cardiac life support drugs and equipment with a cardioverter-defibrillator available for emergency treatment.
7. Monitoring electrocardiographic activity with continuous ECG monitor display.
8. A standby pacemaker, either a temporary transvenous electrode and pulse generator system or an external transthoracic pacemaker.
9. Intra-aortic balloon pump.

Catheterization Approach

Percutaneous Catheterization

Percutaneous catheterization is accomplished using the modified technique initially described by Seldinger (Seldinger, 1953; Fig. 22-1). The same technique is used for both arterial and venous entry. Using the modified Seldinger technique, the vessel is located and a local anesthetic is used to numb the puncture area. The percutaneous needle, with fluid-filled syringe attached, is inserted through the skin nearly parallel to the vessel and enters the front wall of the vessel. Entry of the needle into the vessel is verified by blood return into the syringe with aspiration. The syringe is removed, and a guide wire is passed through the needle into the vessel. The needle is then removed, and a nick is made in the skin with a #11 blade to create a hole large enough for a hemostatic introducer sheath to be advanced over the guide wire and placed within the vessel. Catheters are exchanged by inserting a guide wire into the catheter and inserting the catheter with the guide wire through the introducer sheath, into the vessel. Four to 6 cm of the guide wire is advanced past the distal end of the catheter so the wire leads as the catheter and wire are advanced to the aortic arch. The guide wire is removed from the catheter completely before catheter placement.

The femoral approach is the preferred site for catheterization. Location of the femoral stick is important to avoid vascular complications. The ideal puncture site should be in the common femoral artery (Fig. 22-2B). Puncture of the artery at or above the inguinal ligament makes catheter advancement difficult and predisposes to inadequate compression, hematoma formation, and retroperitoneal bleeding. Puncture of the artery more than 3 cm below the inguinal ligament increases the chance that the femoral artery will divide into its profunda and superficial branches. Puncture into these branches can cause development of a pseudoaneurysm or thrombotic occlusion of a small vessel (Spector & Lawson, 2001).

Alternative arterial puncture sites include the brachial and radial arteries (Fig. 22-2A). The brachial artery may be used in cases of known vascular disease of the abdominal aorta or iliac or femoral arteries. Before using the radial artery, an Allen test is performed to verify patency of the ulnar artery to ensure circulation to the hand. The small caliber of the radial artery mandates the use of small catheters. Injection of lidocaine, nitroglycerin, or calcium channel blocker through the sheath arm is usually necessary to control local spasm in the radial artery. Use of the radial or brachial approach allows for easier control of bleeding at the access site, eliminates the need for bed rest after the procedure, and facilitates earlier discharge of outpatients. Radial artery thrombosis is a potential complication of this approach.

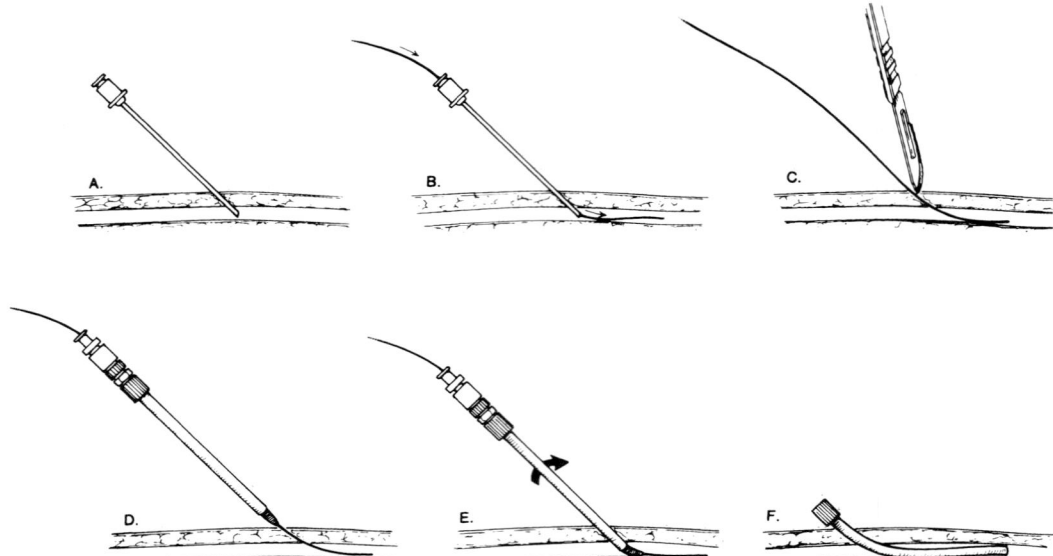

■ **Figure 22–1.** Modified Seldinger technique for percutaneous catheter sheath introduction. (*A*) Vessel is punctured by needle. (*B*) Flexible guidewire placed in vessel through needle. (*C*)Needle removed, guidewire left in place, and hole in skin around wire enlarged with scalpel. (*D*) Sheath and dilator placed over guidewire. (*E*) Sheath and dilator advanced over guidewire and into vessel. (*F*) Dilator and guidewire removed while sheath remains in vessel. (From Hill, J. A. et al. [1998]. Review of Techniques. In J. C. Pepine, J. A. Hill, C. R. Lambert (Eds.), *Diagnostic and therapeutic cardiac catheterization* [3rd ed., p. 107]. Baltimore: Williams & Wilkins.)

Direct Brachial Approach

The direct brachial approach requires a cutdown in the antecubital fossa to isolate the brachial artery and vein and is rarely used. A cardiologist trained in brachial cutdown and vascular repair of the artery and vein is required for this procedure. An incision is made over the medial vein for right heart catheterization or over both the vein and the brachial artery if right and left heart catheterization is planned. The vein and artery are approached by blunt dissection and are brought to the surface and tagged with surgical tape. Venotomy and arteriotomy are performed using scissors or a scalpel. The distal segment of the artery is flushed with heparinized saline to prevent clotting from distal arterial stasis. The catheterization is performed. After catheterization, the distal brachial artery is aspirated until a forceful backflow is achieved, and heparinized saline is injected. The arterial incision is then sutured (Grossman, 2000a). The patient may sit up in chair or bed after the procedure with arm held straight on an arm board. Distal pulses, sensation, and motor function are checked every 15 minutes for 2 hours.

Right Heart Catheterization

Right heart catheterization (Fig. 22-3) is used to obtain right heart pressures, to evaluate the pulmonic and tricuspid valves, to sample blood oxygen content of right heart chambers for detection of left-to-right shunt, to determine CO, and to evaluate mitral valve stenosis or mitral valve insufficiency by the transseptal approach.

The right heart can be approached through the femoral, internal jugular or subclavian veins. Once the inferior vena cava or superior vena cava is reached, the catheter is advanced through the right atrium, right ventricle, and pulmonary artery to a distal pulmonary vessel. Right ventricular irritability may be noted when the catheter tip passes through the right ventricle. The course of the catheter is followed with pressure monitoring through the catheter and with fluoroscopy. When indicated, blood samples are taken, and pressures are recorded as the catheter is advanced. If left heart catheterization is planned, the catheter may be left in the distal pulmonary vessel, so that simultaneous left ventricular and pulmonary artery wedge pressure waveforms can be recorded. As the catheter is removed, pull-back pressures can be recorded from the pulmonary artery to the right ventricle and from the right ventricle to the right atrium. These pressures are used to determine valve gradients and to evaluate pulmonic and tricuspid valve function. Blood samples can also be taken as the catheter is withdrawn for detection of left-to-right shunts. If pulmonic or tricuspid valve disease is suspected, contrast can be injected for digital imaging of the right atrium, right ventricle, or pulmonary artery (Grossman, 2000c).

Left Heart Catheterization

Left heart catheterization (see Fig. 22-2A) is used to perform coronary angiography for evaluation of coronary anatomy, to obtain pressure measurements to evaluate mitral and aortic valve function, and to perform left ventriculography to evaluate left ventricular function.

The two main approaches into the left heart are retrograde entry through the aortic valve by either the percutaneous femoral or brachial approach, and transseptal entry from the right atrium. The progress of the catheter in both approaches is

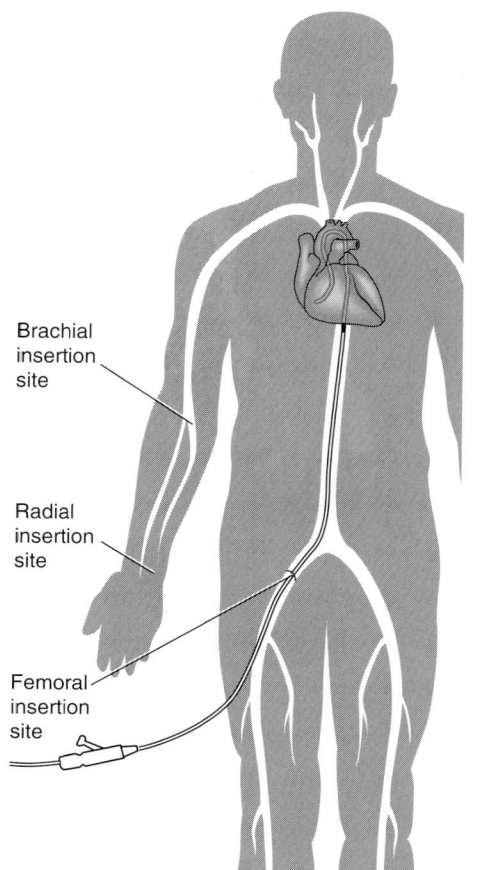

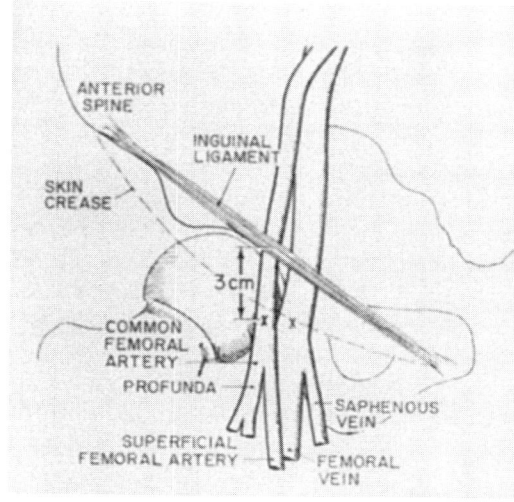

A   B

■ **Figure 22–2.** (*A*) Commonly used catheterization sites. The femoral approach is preferred, and the catheter is advanced in a retrograde direction up the aorta, around the aortic arch, and then into the ostia of the coronary arteries or across the aortic valve into the left ventricle. (*B*) Schematic diagram showing the right femoral artery and vein coursing underneath the inguinal ligament. The arterial skin nick (indicated by X) should be placed approximately 3 cm below the ligament and directly over the femoral arterial pulsation. The venous skin nick should be placed at the same level but approximately one fingerbreadth more medial. (*B* from Baim, D. S. [2000]. Percutaneous approach, including transseptal and apical puncture. In D. S. Baim & W. Grossman [Eds.], *Grossman's cardiac catheterization, angiography, and intervention* [6th ed., p. 71]. Philadelphia: Lippincott Williams & Wilkins.)

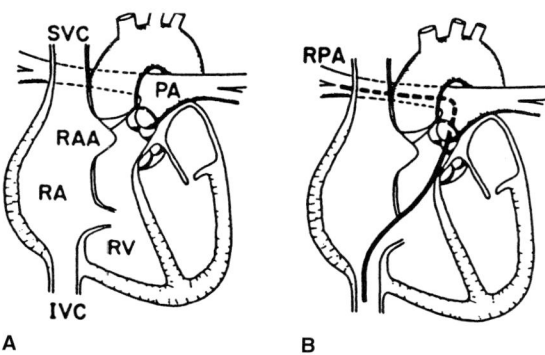

A   B

■ **Figure 22–3.** Right heart catheterization from the femoral approach. (*A*) Right heart chambers and pulmonary artery labeled. RA = right atrium, RAA = right atrial appendage, RV = right ventricle, PA = pulmonary artery. (*B*) Catheter shown entering the RA via the inferior vena cava, crossing the pulmonic valve and positioned in the right pulmonary artery (RPA). (Modified from Baim, D. S. [2000]. Percutaneous approach, including transseptal and apical puncture. In D. S. Baim, & W. Grossman [Eds.]. *Grossman's cardiac catheterization, angiography, and intervention* [6th ed., p. 78]. Philadelphia: Lippincott Williams & Wilkins.)

followed by fluoroscopy and pressure measurement. In the retrograde approach, the catheter is threaded along the aorta and across the aortic valve to the left ventricle. For mitral valve studies, simultaneous pulmonary artery wedge and left ventricular pressures or simultaneous left atrial and left ventricular pressures are recorded to evaluate pressure differences across the valve. To evaluate aortic valve function, pull-back pressure is recorded as the catheter is withdrawn from the left ventricle to the aorta. Digital imaging may be performed during contrast injection of the left atrium, left ventricle, or aortic root to evaluate valve function further.

Transseptal Left Heart Catheterization

The transseptal approach to left heart catheterization involves crossing from the right atrium to the left atrium through the fossa ovalis. This is infrequently done for diagnostic catheterizations but can be used in the rare situation when retrograde left heart catheterization is not possible due to severe aortic stenosis or a prosthetic valve that cannot be

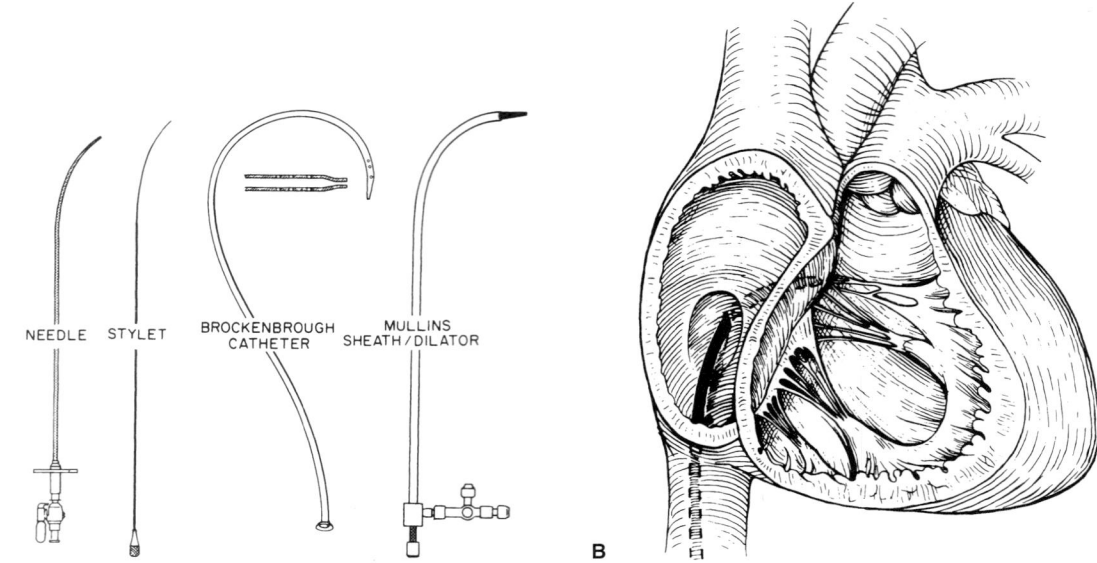

■ **Figure 22–4.** Transseptal catheterization. (*A*) Equipment for transseptal puncture. From left to right: the Brokenbrough needle, Bing stylet, Brokenbrough catheter, Mullins sheath/dilator system. (*B*) Front of right atrium and ventricle cut away to show the catheter entering the right atrium via the inferior vena cava and crossing the septum into the left atrium. (*A* from Baim D. S. [2000]. Percutaneous approach, including transseptal and apical puncture. In D. S. Baim, & W. Grossman [Eds.], *Grossman's cardiac catheterization, angiography, and intervention* [6th ed., p. 95]. Philadelphia: Lippincott Williams & Wilkins. *B* from Hill, J. A. et al. [1998]. Review of techniques. In J. C. Pepine, J. A. Hill, & C. R. Lambert [Eds.], *Diagnostic and therapeutic cardiac catheterization* [3rd ed., p. 116]. Baltimore: Williams & Wilkins.)

adequately evaluated by echocardiogram or transesophageal echocardiography (TEE). More common uses of the transseptal approach include mitral valvuloplasty, electrophysiology studies requiring access to the left atrium or left ventricle, and transcatheter closure of patent foramen ovale (PFO) or atrial septal defects (ASD).

Transseptal catheterization is done only through the right femoral vein and inferior vena cava, using percutaneous techniques and the needle and catheter described by Brockenbrough and Braunwald (1960; Fig. 22-4). The transseptal catheter is threaded into the right atrium over a guide wire, which is then removed. The transseptal needle, with a blunt stylet extending beyond its tip to prevent the needle from puncturing the catheter, is threaded up the catheter, the stylet is withdrawn, and the needle is connected to a pressure transducer. The catheter and needle are guided together to the fossa ovalis, where the needle is advanced to perforate the atrial septum. After perforation of the septum, left atrial pressure is recorded and a blood sample is drawn to confirm the catheter location. The catheter and needle are advanced well into the left atrium, the needle is withdrawn, and the desired studies are performed. The catheter may also be advanced to enter the left ventricle.

Transseptal puncture of the fossa ovalis is safe, but the danger in this approach is that the needle or catheter will inadvertently puncture an adjacent structure such as the posterior free wall of the right atrium, the coronary sinus, or the aortic root causing myocardial hemorrhage, tamponade, or death. The risk is higher in patients who are taking anticoagulants. If the patient is not taking anticoagulants and the perforation is limited to the needle puncture, it is usually benign. However, if the catheter is advanced into the

pericardium or aortic root, potentially fatal complications can occur. To minimize risk, the operator must have a detailed familiarity of the regional anatomy of the atrial septum, which can be distorted in aortic and mitral valve disease. When location of the necessary anatomic landmarks is impossible, as in patients who have severe chest deformities, abnormal heart position, or a huge right atrium, or in those who cannot lie flat, the transseptal approach is not recommended (Baim, 2000).

Ventriculography

Ventriculography is performed to evaluate valve structure or function, to define ventricular anatomy, and to evaluate ventricular function. Ventriculography is accomplished by opacifying the ventricular cavity with contrast medium and filming ventricular motion (Fig. 22-5). Digital image acquisition by biplane or single-plane left ventriculography provides information on the location and severity of segmental wall motion abnormalities. The ventriculogram may be performed before the coronary arteriogram because intracoronary contrast medium may have a depressant effect on ventricular function. In very sick patients, coronary angiography may be performed first because it is usually better tolerated than ventriculogram.

The catheter used for contrast injection during ventriculography delivers a large amount of contrast medium (30 to 36 mL) in a short period (10 to 12 mL per second). Many types of catheters are available for ventricular injections (Fig. 22-6). Catheters with side holes, with or without an end hole, are preferred to end-hole catheters because they have less tendency to

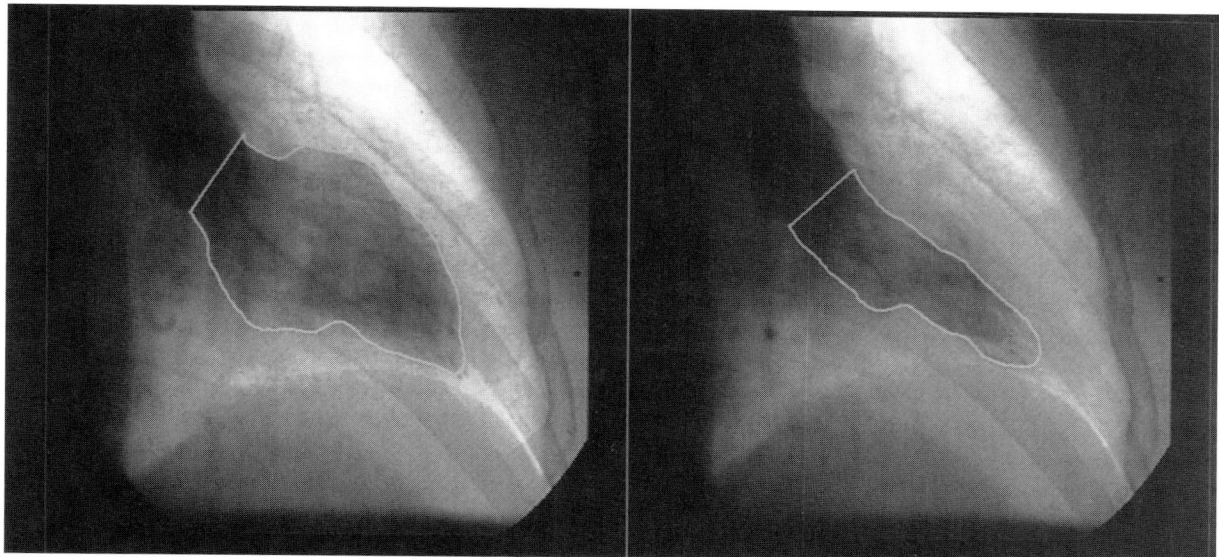

■ **Figure 22–5.** Left ventriculogram. Two frames in right anterior oblique projection showing the left ventricle in diastole (*left*) and in systole (*right*).(Courtesy of Swedish Medical Center, Seattle, WA.)

recoil. Catheter stability is also important to minimize the risk of ventricular arrhythmias during injection. Arrhythmias change the quality of contraction and, thus, make it impossible to use ventriculography for studies of ventricular function (Baim & Hillis, 2000).

Contrast injection is accomplished by power injection. Before the power injection is performed, it is important to

verify that the injection syringe is free of air to prevent air embolism. A low-pressure injection is done to ensure proper catheter placement, then the power injection is done. Patients often feel a hot flash for 30 seconds after injection, resulting from the vasodilatation caused by the contrast agent throughout the arterial system. Occasionally, the patient may experience nausea with the injection, or may vomit. The principal

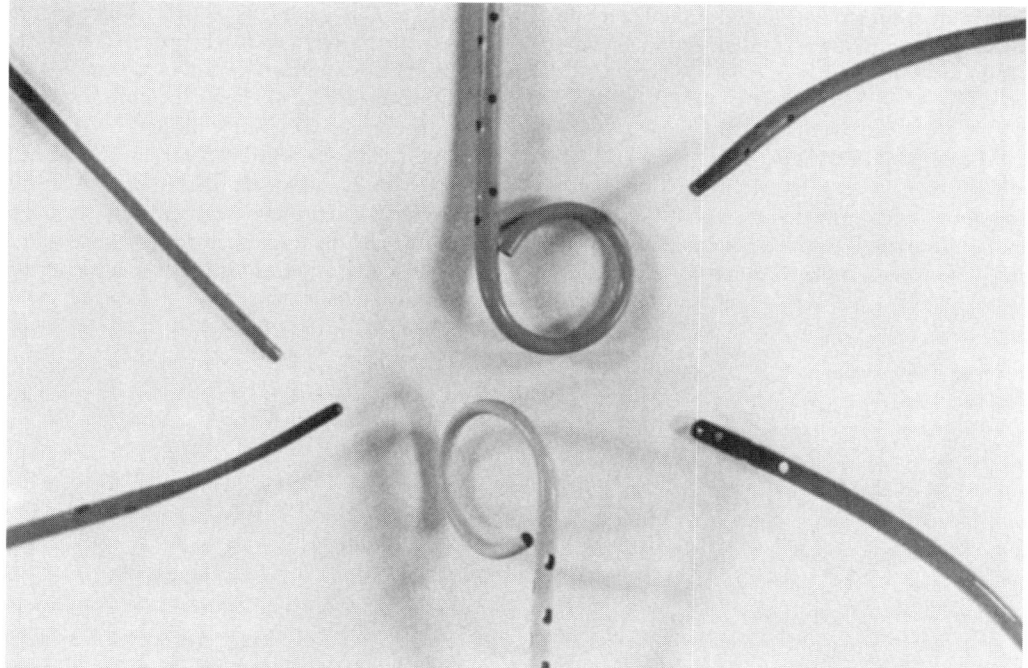

■ **Figure 22–6.** Examples of ventriculographic catheters in current use (clockwise from the top): pigtail 8F (Cook); Gensini 7F; NIH 8F; pigtail 8F (Cordis); Lehman ventriculographic 8F; Sones 7.5F tapering to a 5.5F tip. (From Baim, D. S., & Hill, L. D. [2000]. Cardiac ventriculography. In D. S. Baim, & W. Grossman [Eds.], *Grossman's cardiac catheterization, angiography, and intervention* [6th ed., p. 258]. Philadelphia: Lippincott Williams & Wilkins.)

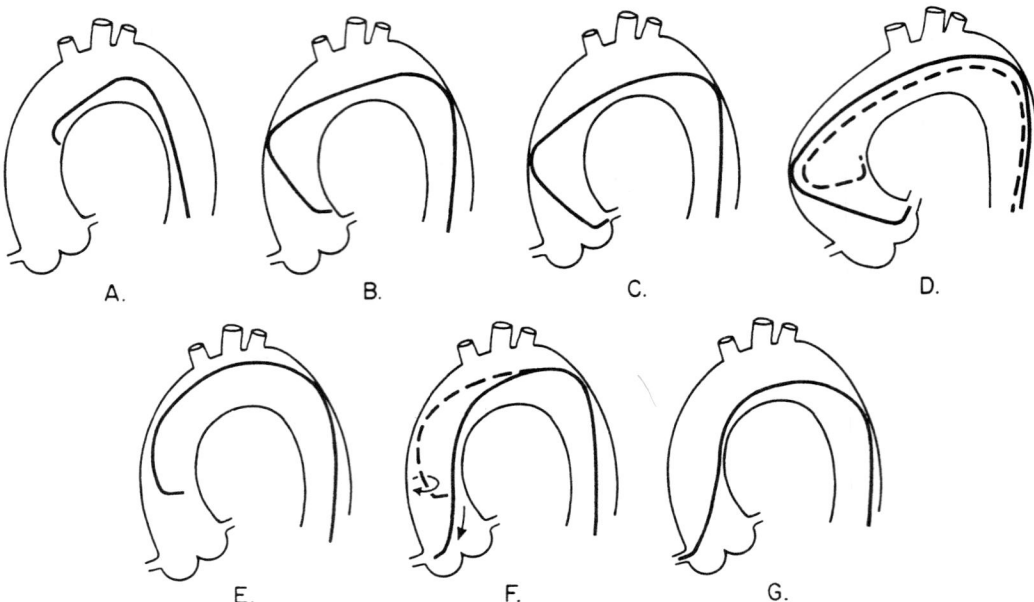

■ **Figure 22–7.** Judkins technique for catheterization of the left and right coronary arteries as viewed in the left anterior oblique projection. In a patient with a normal size aortic arch, advancement of a JL4 catheter leads to intubation of the left coronary ostium (*A, B,* and *C*). In a patient with an enlarged aortic root (*D*) the arm of the JL4 may be too short, causing the catheter tip to point upward or even flip back into its packaged shape (*dotted line*). A catheter with an appropriately longer arm (a JL5 or JL6) is required. To catheterize the right coronary ostium, the Judkins catheter is advanced around the aortic arch with its tip directed leftward, as viewed in the LAO projection, until it reaches a position 2–3 cm above the level of the left coronary ostium (*E*). Clockwise rotation causes the catheter tip to drop into the aortic root and point anteriorly (*F*). Slight further rotation causes the catheter tip to enter the right coronary ostium (*G*). (From Baim, D. S., & Grossman, W. [2000]. Coronary angiography. In D.S. Baim, & W. Grossman [Eds.], *Grossman's cardiac catheterization, angiography, and intervention* [6th ed., p. 218]. Philadelphia: Lippincott Williams & Wilkins.)

complications of injection are arrhythmias, intramyocardial or endocardial injection of contrast medium, transient left anterior fascicular block, and embolism from injection of air or thrombi (Baim & Hillis, 2000).

Coronary Arteriography

Coronary arteriography is performed most commonly by the percutaneous femoral approach. Preformed polyurethane catheters (most commonly Judkins or Amplatz catheters) are used for catheterization of the right and left coronary arteries (Judkins, 1968; Figs. 22-7 and 22-8). The catheters are guided over a guide wire through the distal aortic arch to the coronary ostium, the guide is withdrawn, and the catheter is filled with contrast medium. Figure 22-9 shows the coronary anatomy as viewed from the right anterior oblique (RAO) and left anterior oblique (LAO) projections. Images of both the right and left coronary arteries are recorded in the LAO and RAO views to ensure that all coronary segments are seen. The image intensifier can also be angulated toward the head (cranial) or the foot (caudal) to better visualize specific lesions (Figs. 22-10

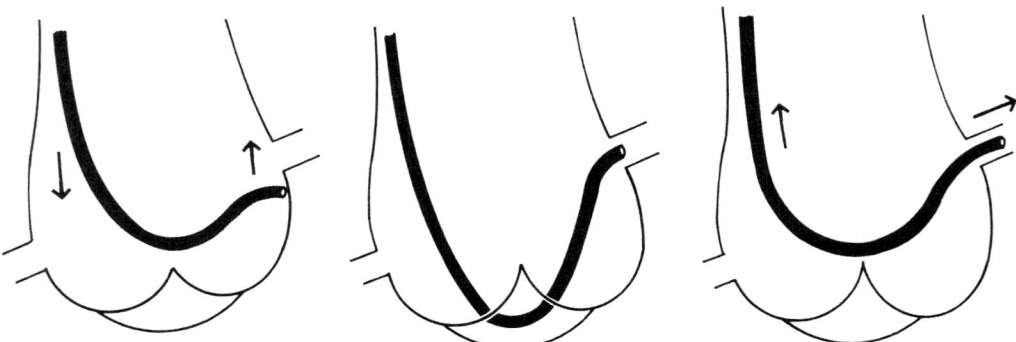

■ **Figure 22–8.** Catheterization of the left coronary artery with an Amplatz catheter. The catheter is advanced into the ascending aorta with its tip pointing downward. As the catheter is advanced into the left sinus of Valsalva, its tip initially lies below the left coronary ostium (*left*). Further advancement causes the tip to ride up the aortic wall and enter the ostium (*center*). Subsequently, slight withdrawal of the catheter causes the tip to seat more deeply in the ostium (*right*). (From Baim, D. S., & Grossman, W. [2000]. Coronary angiography. In D. S. Baim, & W. Grossman [Eds.], *Grossman's cardiac catheterization, angiography, and intervention* [6th ed., p. 219]. Philadelphia: Lippincott Williams & Wilkins.)

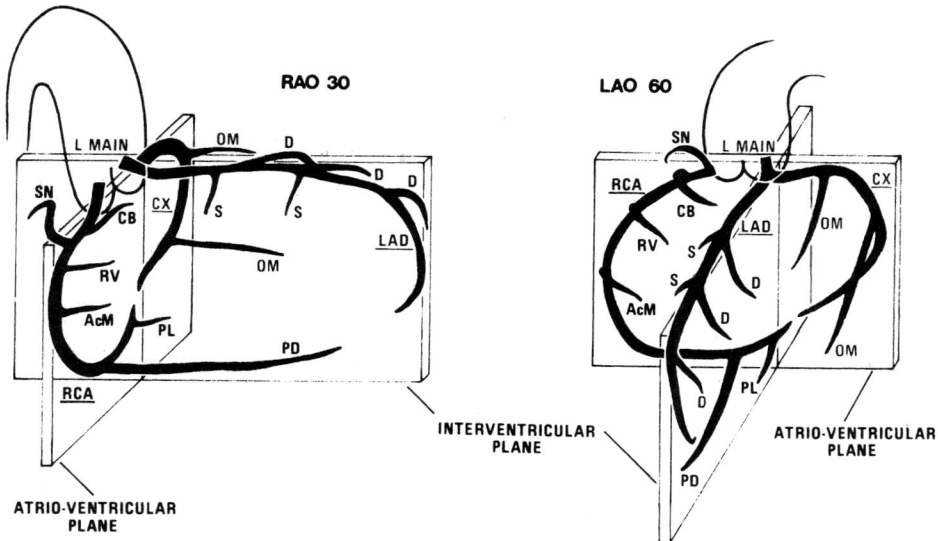

■ **Figure 22–9.** Representation of coronary anatomy in relation to the interventricular and atrioventricular valve planes. Coronary branches are as indicated: L Main = left main, LAD = left anterior descending, D = diagonal, S = septal, CX = circumflex, OM = obtuse marginal, RCA = right coronary artery, CB = conus branch, SN = sinus node, AcM = acute marginal, PD = posterior descending, PL = posterolateral left ventricular. (From Baim, D. S., & Grossman, W. (2000). Coronary angiography. In D. S. Baim, & W. Grossman [Eds.], *Grossman's cardiac catheterization, angiography, and intervention* [6th ed., p. 233]. Philadelphia: Lippincott Williams & Wilkins.)

and 22-11). A common sequence of angiographic views for the left coronary artery include:

■ RAO-caudal: to visualize the left main, proximal left anterior descending (LAD) and proximal circumflex coronary arteries
■ RAO-cranial: to visualize the middle and distal LAD without overlap of septal or diagonal branches
■ LAO-cranial: to visualize the middle and distal LAD in an orthogonal projection
■ LAO-caudal: to visualize the left main and proximal circumflex
■ Left lateral: to visualize the LAD

A common sequence of angiographic views for the right coronary includes:

■ LAO: to visualize the proximal right coronary artery
■ RAO-cranial: to visualize the posterior descending and posterolateral branches
■ Right lateral: to visualize the middle right coronary artery

The patient is asked to take a deep breath and hold it without bearing down, just before the injection, to clear the diaphragm from the field. After the injection, the patient is told to breathe and cough, which helps clear the contrast medium from the coronary arteries. Imaging of the coronary arteries may also be performed after the administration of nitroglycerin or other vasodilators to evaluate possible vasospasm effects on the coronary circulation, including the collateral vessels.

Cardiac Output Studies

The methods of CO determination include the Fick oxygen method, indicator dilution technique, and the thermodilution method. The thermodilution method uses a pulmonary artery catheter for CO determination (see Chapter 23). An older technique, the direct Fick method is still used to a limited extent in some institutions.

Direct Fick Method

The direct Fick method, which has historically been used in the catheterization laboratory for calculation of CO determination, is rarely used today in the original technique, but the theoretical principle has been maintained. The Fick method requires measurement of arterial oxygen saturation and mixed venous (pulmonary artery) oxygen saturation. Oxygen consumption ideally is a measured value obtained during catheterization. The methods of measuring oxygen consumption are extremely cumbersome and time consuming and, in general, not routinely employed in modern catheterization laboratories. Alternatively, oxygen consumption can be assumed based on the patient's body surface area (BSA). This is not as accurate a measurement, but it is acceptable. The Fick method of CO determination is helpful in cases where the patient is in atrial fibrillation, has significant tricuspid regurgitation, or a low CO state. It has largely been replaced by the thermodilution method for CO determination.

Thermodilution and Indicator Dilution Methods

Thermodilution and indicator dilution methods are based on the principle that, if a known amount of an indicator is added to an unknown quantity of flowing liquid, and the concentration of the indicator is then measured downstream, the time course of its concentration gives a quantitative index of the flow. Applied to the circulatory system, the amount of indicator, its dilution within the circulation, and the time during which the first circulation of the substance occurs can be used to compute CO (Grossman, 2000c).

The thermodilution technique using cold or room temperature dextrose or saline injectate solution is the most frequently used CO determination method in cardiac catheterization

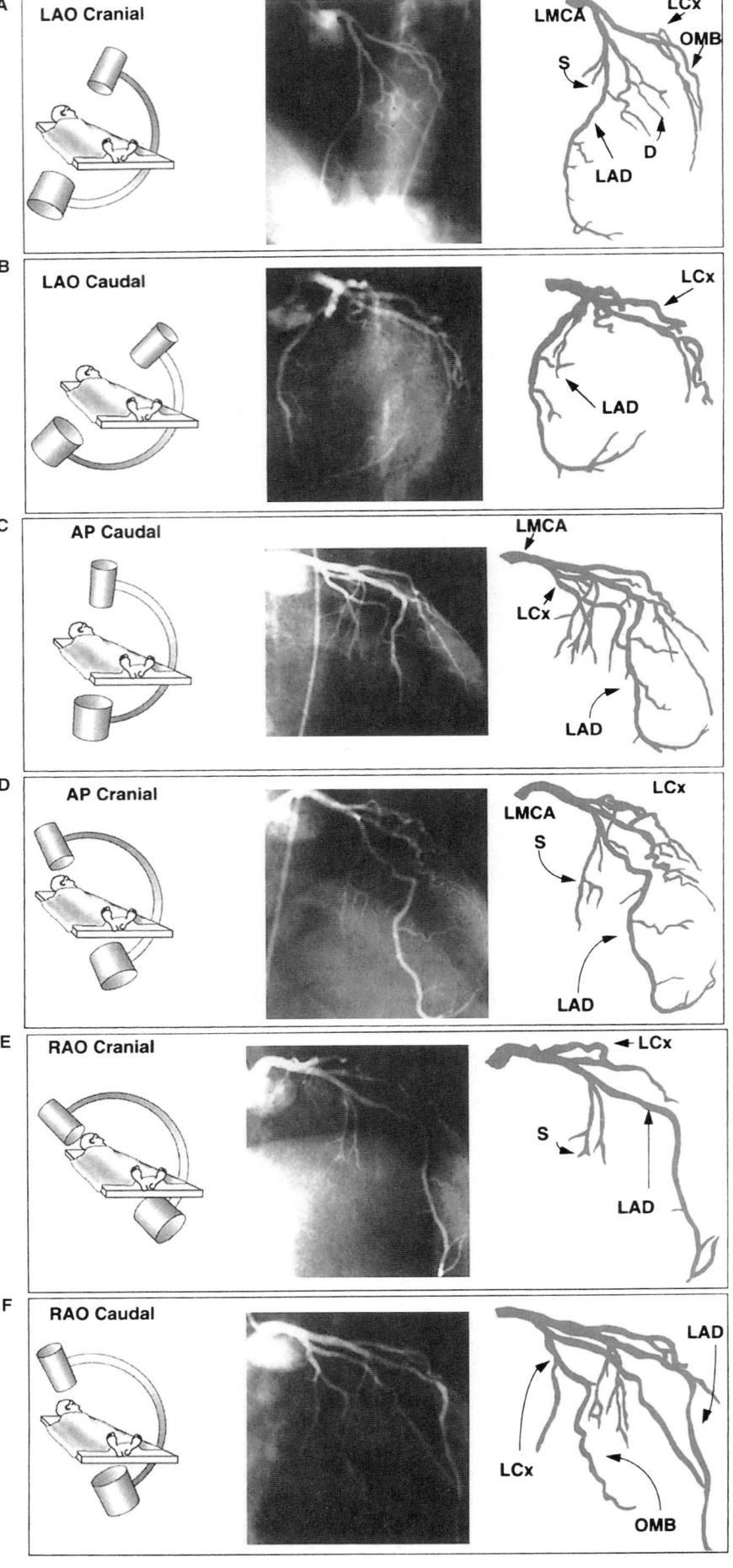

■ **Figure 22–10.** Angiographic views of the left coronary artery. The approximate position of the x-ray tube and image intensifier are shown for each of the commonly used angiographic views. (*A*). 60-degree LAO view with 20 degrees of cranial angulation (LAO cranial) shows the ostium and distal portion of the left main coronary artery (LMCA), the middle and distal portions of the left anterior descending artery (LAD), septal perforators (S), diagonal branches (D), and the proximal left circumflex (LCx) and superior obtuse marginal branch (OMB). (*B*). 60-degree LAO with 25 degrees of caudal angulation (LAO caudal) shows the proximal LMCA and the proximal segments of the LAD and LCx. (*C*) Anteroposterior projection with 20 degrees of caudal angulation (AP caudal) shows the distal LMCA and proximal segments of the LAD and LCx. (*D*). Anteroposterior projection with 20 degrees cranial angulation (AP cranial) also shows the midportion of the LAD and its septal (S) branches. (*E*). 30-degree RAO with 20 degrees of cranial angulation (RAO cranial) shows the course of the LAD and its septal (S) and diagonal branches. (*F*). 30-degree RAO with 25 degrees of caudal angulation (RAO caudal) shows the LCx and obtuse marginal branches (OMB). (From Popma, J. J., & Bittl, J. [2001]. Coronary angiography and intravascular ultrasonography. In E. Braunwald, D. P. Zipes, & P. Libby [Eds.], *Heart disease: A textbook of cardiovascular medicine* [6th ed., p. 395]. Philadelphia: W. B. Saunders.)

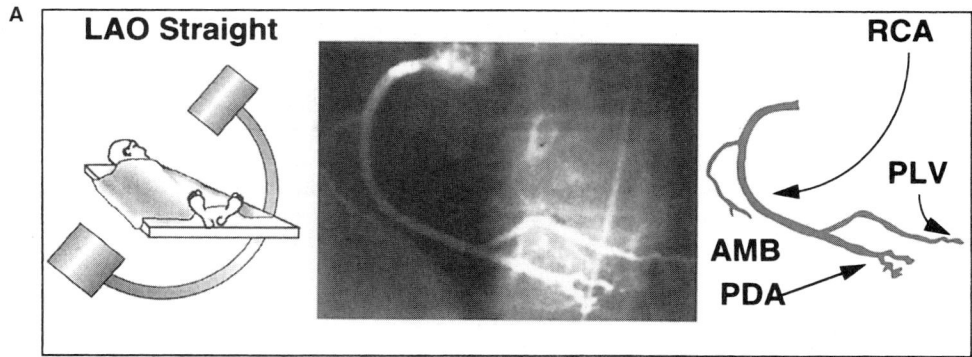

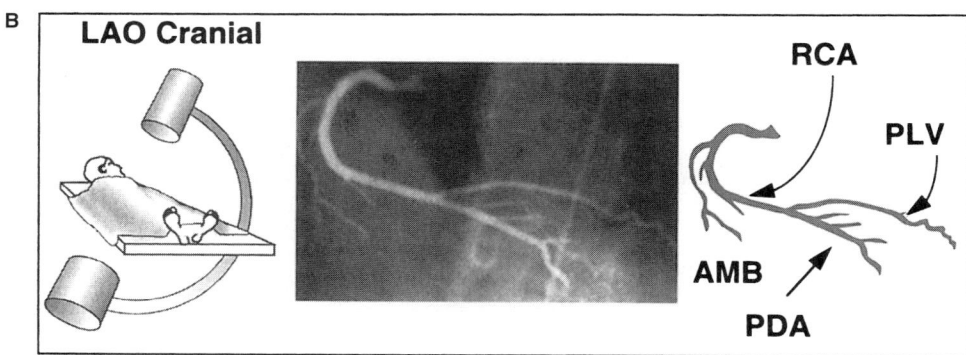

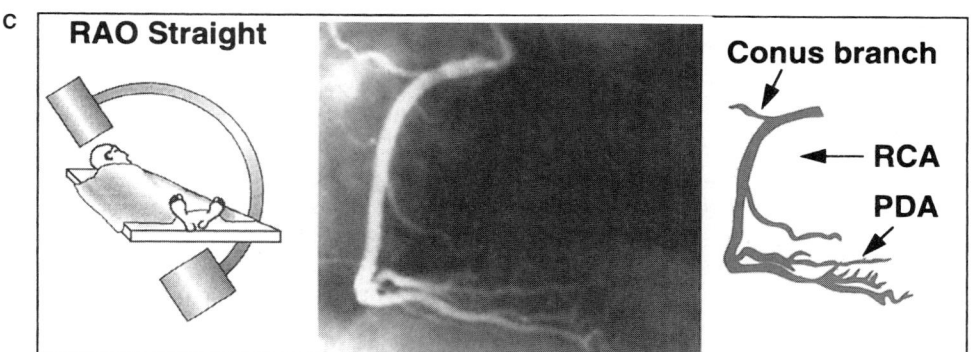

■ **Figure 22–11.** Angiographic views of the right coronary artery. The approximate position of the x-ray tube and image intensifier are shown for each of the commonly used angiographic views. (*A*). 60-degrees LAO view shows the proximal and midportions of the right coronary artery (RCA) as well as the acute marginal branches (AMB) and termination of the RCA in the posterior left ventricular branches (PLV). (*B*). 60-degree LAO view with 25 degrees of cranial angulation (LAO cranial) shows the midportion of the RCA and the origin and course of the posterior descending artery (PDA). (*C*) 30-degree RAO view shows the midportion of the RCA, the conus branch, and the course of the PDA. (From Popma, J. J., & Bittl, J. [2001]. Coronary angiography and intravascular ultrasonography. In E. Braunwald, D. P. Zipes, & P. Libby [Eds.], *Heart disease: A textbook of cardiovascular medicine* [6th ed., p. 396]. Philadelphia: W. B. Saunders.)

laboratories. The benefits of the thermodilution technique are that (1) it is performed over a short period and is, therefore, more likely to be recorded during a period of steady state; (2) it is most accurate in patients with normal or high CO; (3) the indicator used is inert and inexpensive; (4) it does not require an arterial puncture; and (5) the computer analysis curve is reasonably simple to interpret (Grossman, 2000c). Drawbacks of this method include its unreliability in the presence of atrial fibrillation, significant tricuspid regurgitation, and its tendency to overestimate CO in patients with low CO.

Radiographic Angiographic Contrast Agents

The two types of contrast agents are the high- and low-osmolar ionic agents and low-osmolar nonionic agents. Both types of agents contain iodine, which absorbs x-rays and, thus, provides their imaging properties. The hemodynamic and other side effects of contrast agents are related to their osmolality and their chemical and pharmacologic differences. Ionic agents have osmolalities as high as six times that of blood, whereas the low-osmolar ionic contrast and the nonionic agents have an osmolality approximately two to three times that of blood. Nonionic agents are associated with fewer side effects and less dramatic hemodynamic reactions than ionic agents, particularly in high-risk patients. Nonionic agents are more costly than ionic agents (Barrett et al., 1992).

Most catheterization laboratories use nonionic agents. Specific indications for use of nonionic agents include unstable ischemic syndromes including acute MI, CHF with hemodynamic instability, diabetes mellitus, ejection fraction less than 30%, acute or chronic renal insufficiency, severe bradycardia, history of contrast allergy, internal mammary artery injection, and PTCA (Baim, 2000; Brinker,1990).

The hemodynamic effects of contrast agents are well documented. These effects vary with the site and volume of the injection as well as with the osmolality, sodium content, and calcium concentration of the agent used. Immediate effects (10 to 120 seconds) are seen with both ventriculography and coronary angiography, whereas long-term effects are seen primarily with ventriculography or other injections that require large amounts of contrast medium (Hirshfeld, 1990).

After left ventricular injection, there is depression of left ventricular contractility and an increase in intravascular volume, and left ventricular end-diastolic pressure rises. As contrast reaches the systemic arterial system, there is arteriolar vasodilation; this response increases with the osmolality of the agent used. There is a corresponding decrease in arterial pressure. These effects peak within 2 to 3 minutes, and values return to normal within 5 minutes (Hirshfeld, 1990).

With coronary arteriography, immediate effects of contrast may include sinus bradycardia, systemic arterial hypotension, an increase in left ventricular end-diastolic pressure, arrhythmias, myocardial ischemia, and T-wave changes on the ECG. Usually, these changes revert quickly to normal when the catheter is withdrawn from the coronary ostia and the patient coughs, clearing the contrast medium from the coronary arteries.

The high osmolality of contrast medium raises serum osmolality. In response, plasma volume increases when water moves from the extravascular to the intravascular space. Both hematocrit and hemoglobin levels fall, whereas left atrial and left ventricular end-diastolic pressures increase in response to the increased intravascular volume. CO and stroke volume increase as a secondary response to the reduced systemic vascular resistance (afterload) and increased filling volume and pressures (preload).

Contrast agents act as an osmotic diuretic (Hirshfeld, 1990). The diuresis that occurs after catheterization may result in water and saline deficits, which precipitate hypotension. For this reason, patients should be given intravenous (IV) replacement or be encouraged to drink liquids on returning from the laboratory. Hydration is also important for patients with preexisting renal insufficiency.

THE NURSE IN THE CARDIAC CATHETERIZATION LABORATORY

Nurses working in cardiac catheterization laboratories fill many roles. The basic roles needed in a catheterization laboratory during a procedure are scrubber, recorder, and circulator.

In some laboratories, the nurses scrub and assist in the procedure; in others, they are responsible for monitoring pressure and cardiac rhythm, assisting with hemodynamic studies such as CO determination, and administering IV procedural sedation. The nurse may visit the patient before the procedure to teach and help in preparing the patient or after the procedure to evaluate puncture site stability. Ideally, the nurse has a background in intensive or coronary care and a thorough knowledge of cardiovascular drugs, arrhythmias, the principles of IV procedural sedation, sterile technique, cardiac anatomy and physiology, pacemakers, and the concepts of catheter management for coronary angiography and intervention. Changes in the patient's emotional status, alertness, vocal responses, and facial expressions are important indices of the patient's tolerance of the procedure. The nurse's alertness to these clues and early intervention with reassurance or appropriate medication may help to prevent more serious events, such as vasovagal reactions and coronary artery spasm. Training in advanced cardiac life support (ACLS) is often a requirement for catheterization laboratory nurses and those caring for patients after the procedure.

Complications and Nursing Care During Cardiac Catheterization

The nursing care of patients both during and after cardiac catheterization is directed toward the prevention and detection of complications. Extensive analysis of complications has been performed in the 1980s and 1990s with major complications reported less than 1%. A recent registry of consecutive diagnostic cardiac catheterizations performed between 1990 and 2000 indicated an overall complication rate of 0.8%, with a mortality rate of 0%. Lower complication rates were noted with experienced operators and the use of a smaller catheter size of 6 Fr. or less. Higher complication rates were noted in patients having right and left heart catheterizations, use of catheters greater than 6 Fr., and increased vascular complications in patients with higher body weight (Ammann et al., 2003). Although complications are rare, they do occur and may be life threatening. Early detection and intervention are essential in prevention.

Local problems at the catheter entry site are the most commonly seen complications after cardiac catheterization procedures. These problems include vessel thrombosis, distal embolization, dissection, or poorly controlled bleeding at the puncture site. Other vascular complications are less common. A complete list of complications is discussed in Chapter 27.

Ventricular arrhythmias often occur in response to catheter manipulation or contrast medium injection and tend not to recur after the predisposing stimulus is removed. Atrial and junctional arrhythmias and varying degrees of blocks also occur in response to these stimuli. Bradycardia is common in response to injection of the coronary arteries with contrast or during sheath insertion or removal.

Allergic reactions to the contrast medium may occur. Sneezing, itching of the eyes or skin, urticaria, bronchospasm, or other beginning signs of allergy are treated with antihistamines and corticosteroids. Full-blown anaphylactic reactions are treated with intramuscular (IM) or subcutaneous (SQ) epinephrine (1 : 10,000 concentration) and wide open normal saline IV to support blood pressure. Patients with known or suspected allergies to iodine-containing substances such as seafood or with a prior allergic reaction to radiographic contrast should be pretreated with prednisone 24 to 48 hours before procedure or IV steroids. An antihistamine and an H2 blocker are also given, and nonionic contrast should be used.

The catheterization laboratory nurse must be familiar with intra-aortic balloon pump (IABP) set-up and management, because the IABP is often used when patients become hemodynamically unstable during a catheterization procedure. The nurse must also be familiar with other equipment used in the laboratory, such as intravascular ultrasound (IVUS), pressure wire, thrombectomy and atherectomy equipment, and other specialized equipment. Additional skills include access site management, including sheath removal, manual pressure for hemostasis, and use of closure devices or Femostop for hemostasis; and a thorough knowledge of drugs commonly used during a procedure, such as heparin, bivalirudin (Angiomax), IIb/IIIa platelet inhibitors, antiarrhythmics, vasoactive drugs, and drugs used for procedural sedation.

Postprocedure Care

After the procedure, the patient may be transferred to an observation unit, telemetry unit, interventional cardiology unit, or intensive care unit depending on the type of procedure done and the patient's condition. In most facilities, diagnostic catheterization patients are cared for in an observational unit, such as an ambulatory care unit or same-day surgery unit, for up to 6 hours and then discharged if stable. Patients who have undergone interventional procedures often stay overnight and are cared for in a telemetry unit or interventional cardiology unit where nurses are specially trained and experienced in postprocedure care and have more in-depth knowledge of cardiovascular drugs, arrhythmia interpretation, ACLS skills, and management of access sites. If the patient is hemodynamically unstable or has a complication of the procedure such as MI, severe respiratory distress, coronary artery dissection, tamponade, unstable arrhythmias, or requires close observation or intensive nursing care, he or she is transferred to an intensive care unit.

After a diagnostic procedure, the femoral arterial or venous introducer sheaths are removed and manual or mechanical pressure is applied to the access site until hemostasis is achieved. Compression devices or vascular closure devices may be used to achieve hemostasis after a diagnostic or interventional procedure (see Chapter 27). For interventional procedures in which extensive anticoagulation was used or IV antiplatelet therapy (i.e., IIb/IIIa inhibitors) is to be continued for several hours, the sheath is often left in place until the activated clotting time (ACT) is below a critical level and then removed by either catheterization laboratory staff or nurses in the postprocedure unit. Nurses caring for patients after cardiac catheterization must be prepared to perform sheath removal according to institutional policies and guidelines, and must be able to recognize complications associated with this procedure

Table 22–4 ■ POSTCATHETERIZATION PROTOCOLS

General Guidelines
1. Assess vital signs, function every 15 min for 1 h, every 30 min for 1 h, and hourly for 4 h or until discharge.
2. Assess catheterization site for bleeding, hematoma formation, and swelling. Assess peripheral pulses and neurovascular status every 15 min for 1 h, every 30 min for 1 h, and hourly for 4 h or until discharge.
3. Resume precatheterization diet and medications.
4. Administer analgesic agents as needed.
5. Notify physician if any of the following occur:
   a. Decrease in peripheral pulses
   b. New hematoma or increase in size of existing hematoma
   c. Unusually severe catheter insertion site pain or affected extremity pain
   d. Onset of chest discomfort or shortness of breath

Femoral Approach
6. Place patient on bed rest for 4–6 depending on sheath size. The head of the bed may be raised to 30 degrees.
7. Instruct patient not to flex or hyperextend the hip joint of the affected leg for 4–6 h, and to use the bed controls to elevate the head of the bed or lower feet.
8. Compression device may be applied. Monitor peripheral pulses as per protocol.

Brachial or Radial Approach
9. Place patient on bed rest for 2–3 h. The patient may sit up in bed. Pressure dressing or Ace bandage may be applied to affected arm.
10. Monitor distal pulses every 15 min for 1 h, every 30 min for 1 h, and hourly for 4 h until discharge or stable.
11. Instruct patient not to keep the arm in a flexed position for an extended period of time, hyperextend or lie on the affected arm for 24 h.
12. Instruct patient in observation for bleeding or hematoma. If sutures were used, instruct patient regarding suture removal.

(Bogart , 1995; Juran et al., 1999; Lazzara, Pfersdorf & Sedlacek, 1997; Schickel et al., 1996).

After returning from the laboratory, the patient must be thoroughly assessed. Information about the approach used, the procedures performed, and any complications experienced during the catheterization should be obtained from the physician, nurse, or technician. Table 22-4 lists typical postcatheterization protocols, which may vary among institutions. The elements of the nursing assessment and intervention and potential findings are listed and explained in the following sections.

Psychological Assessment and Patient Teaching. Patients are often tired, hungry, and uncomfortable when they return from the laboratory. They are usually relieved that the procedure is over and may already know the preliminary findings of their study. This news may be good or bad, and it is important to find out what the patient has been told and what this means. The patient may have questions about surgery or about what to expect next. Some patients are anxious or depressed. Giving patients the opportunity to express their feelings about the procedure helps to calm and relax them. Reassure the patient by describing the sensations that can be expected, such as thirst and the frequent need to urinate although the patient has had nothing to eat or drink for several hours. Reemphasize the need for bed rest and the need to keep the catheterized limb immobile. Let the patient know that frequent checking of vital signs is routine and not a cause for alarm. Before hospital discharge, the patient should be instructed regarding symptoms for which to call the physician and site care (Table 22-5).

Table 22–5 ■ PATIENT DISCHARGE INSTRUCTIONS FOR INPATIENT AND OUTPATIENT CATHETERIZATION

1. Report the following symptoms to your physician if they occur:
   a. New bleeding or swelling at the catheterization site. (If marked bleeding occurs, press hand firmly over the area of bleeding and call 911.)
   b. Increased tenderness, redness, drainage, or pain at the catheterization site
   c. Fever
   d. Change in color (pallor), temperature (coolness), or sensation(numbness) in the leg or arm used for catheterization
2. Acetaminophen or other non-aspirin-containing analgesic may be taken every 4 h as needed for pain unless contraindicated.
3. If stitches are present, wear an adhesive bandage and remove as directed by physician. Otherwise, cover site with an adhesive bandage for 24 h.
   a. Patient may shower the day after the procedure.
   b. Tub bath should be avoided for 3 days after the procedure.
4. Patient to see physician for follow-up appointment _____ .
5. Continue prescribed medications as before unless otherwise indicated by your physician.
6. Avoid strenuous activity for 48 h. Do not lift anything heavier than 5 pounds for next 48 h.
7. Limit excessive stair climbing.
8. Patient must be driven home and be accompanied by a responsible adult until the following morning.
9. If pain or pressure occurs in chest, arms, shoulders, neck or jaw:
   a. Take nitroglycerin if it is prescribed for the patient.
   b. Notify cardiologist of chest pain if it is relieved with nitroglycerin.
   c. If chest pain is not relieved, call 911.
10. Follow diet as prescribed by cardiologist, usually a low-salt, low-fat diet.

Circulatory Integrity of Access Site. Careful assessment of the access site and limb is an important element of postcatheterization nursing care. The site should be checked for visible bleeding, swelling, or tenderness. The arterial pulse at the site and at points distal to it should be compared with pulses on the opposite limb and those recorded before the procedure. Capillary filling and the warmth of the limb should also be evaluated. Blanching, cramping, coolness, pain, numbness, or tingling may indicate reduced perfusion and must be carefully evaluated. A diminished or absent pulse is a sign of serious arterial occlusion, which often constitutes a surgical emergency. The first step, if any of these signs occur, is to check the compression device if used and release pressure. If symptoms do not resolve, the physician should be notified immediately and steps taken to preserve the limb.

Manual pressure or pressure with a compression device, such as C-clamp or Femostop, is used for hemostasis at the time of sheath removal and when bleeding continues or recurs after initial hemostasis. When pressure is applied at an arterial site, the pulse distal to the site may be safely occluded for 2 to 5 minutes, then pressure is released until the pulse returns. Distal pulses should remain palpable during the remainder of pressure application, which continues for 15 to 20 minutes. If oozing from the sheath insertion tract continues after initial hemostasis, infiltration of the tract with a solution of lidocaine and epinephrine (1 : 100,000 strength) followed by 2 to 5 minutes of light manual pressure is usually effective to control bleeding.

Blood Pressure Findings. Evaluation of the blood pressure after cardiac catheterization should include comparison of preprocedure and postprocedure pressures, checking for orthostatic hypotension once the bed rest period is over, and monitoring for

paradoxical pulse. Mild systolic hypotension frequently occurs after cardiac catheterization and is usually not of concern. Angiographic contrast medium acts as an osmotic diuretic, and patients frequently return with signs of volume depletion, including orthostatic hypotension. Therefore, patients are kept on bed rest until fluid balance is restored with oral liquids or by IV replacement. *Hypotension* may also be a response to the drugs given during the procedure. Vasodilators may be administered during coronary arteriography. If the blood pressure is less than 75% to 80% of baseline, other causes such as blood loss or arrhythmias must be considered and assessed, and the physician notified. *Paradoxical pulse* suggests pericardial tamponade, which may occur as a result of perforation of a coronary artery or the myocardium. In patients with known perforation, this sign should be specifically assessed with each blood pressure measurement, and, if it occurs, the physician should be notified. *Hypertension* can also occur and may contribute to access site bleeding if not controlled.

Heart Rate and Rhythm. Patients who have had an interventional procedure should be on a cardiac monitor for rhythm and ST-segment monitoring. A mild sinus tachycardia (100 to 120 beats per minute) is not unusual after catheterization and may be a sign of anxiety, an indication of saline and water loss due to diuresis, or a reaction to medication such as atropine. Fluids, time, and reassurance often bring the heart rate down to more normal levels. Heart rates above 120 beats per minute should be evaluated for other causes such as hemorrhage, more severe fluid imbalance, fever, or arrhythmias. Bradycardia may indicate vasovagal responses, arrhythmias, or infarction and should be assessed by 12-lead ECG and correlated with other clinical signs such as pain and blood pressure. Vasovagal reactions are fairly common and can occur immediately or hours after sheath removal. Cardiac monitoring for ST-segment displacement is useful to detect acute reocclusion of the artery or MI after an interventional procedure (Drew & Tisdale, 1993; Jacobson, 1996).

Temperature. Early increases in temperature may occur because of the fluid loss that occurs with catheterization. More persistent elevations may indicate infection or pyrogenic reactions.

Urinary Output. Because angiographic contrast medium acts as an osmotic diuretic, patients have an increase in urine output for a short time after catheterization. IV fluids are often continued for a variable time after the procedure, and oral fluids should be encouraged unless the patient is NPO for some reason.

Other Possible Problems. MI, stroke, and CHF are all potential complications after cardiac catheterization. The nurse caring for patients after cardiac catheterization should be aware of the signs and symptoms of these complications.

INTERPRETATION OF DATA

Table 22-6 lists normal ranges for some of the data gathered during cardiac catheterization. The assessment of coronary artery disease involves evaluation of the coronary vasculature and left ventricular function.

The first step in evaluating the coronary arteriogram is to determine whether the coronaries are unobstructed and free of lesions. Each major artery is traced along its entire length, and branches and collaterals are noted and evaluated for irregularities

Table 22–6 ▪ NORMAL ADULT VALUES FOR DATA COLLECTED DURING CARDIAC CATHETERIZATION

Pressures	(mm Hg)
Systemic arterial	
Peak-systolic	100–140
End-diastolic	60–90
Mean	70–105
Left ventricular	
Peak-systolic	100–140
End-diastolic	3–12
Left atrial	
Left atrial mean (or PAWP)	1–10
a wave	3–15
v wave	3–12
Pulmonary artery	
Peak-systolic	15–30
End-diastolic	3–12
Systolic Mean	9–16
Right ventricular	
Peak-systolic	15–30
End-diastolic	0–8
Right atrial	
Mean	0–8
a wave	2–10
v wave	2–10
Left Ventricular Volumes	
End-systolic volume (mL/m^2)	20–30
End-diastolic volume (mL/m^2)	70–79
Ejection fraction (%)	58–72
Resistance (dynes/s/cm^{-5})	
Total systemic resistance	900–1440
Pulmonary arteriolar (vascular) resistance	37–97
Flow	
Cardiac output (L/min)	4.0–8.0
Cardiac index (L/min/m^2)	2.5–4.0
Stroke index (mL/beat/m^2)	35–70
Stroke volume (mL/beat)	60–130
Oxygen consumption (mL/min/m^2)	125
Oxygen Saturation(%)	
Right atrium	60–75
Right ventricle	60–75
Pulmonary artery	60–75
Left atrium	95–99
Left ventricle	95–99
Aorta	95–99

PAWP = pulmonary artery wedge pressure.
From Fifer & Grossman, 2000; Grossman, 2000; Lumbert, Pepine & Nichols, 1989.

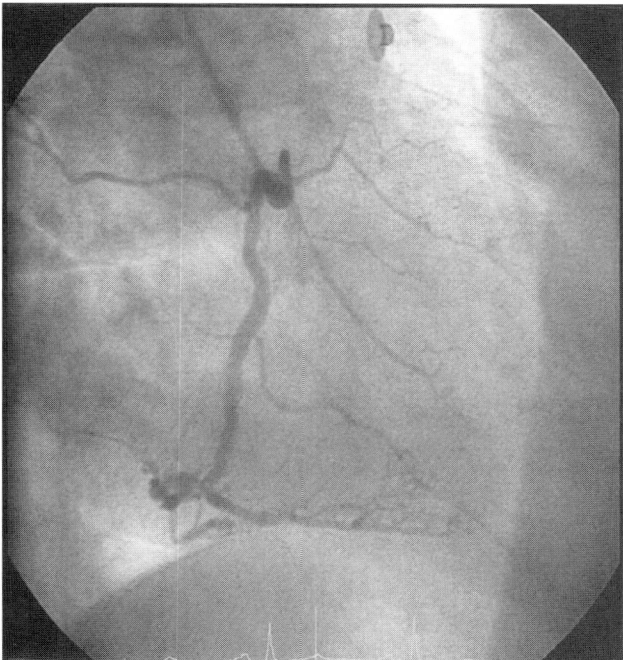

A

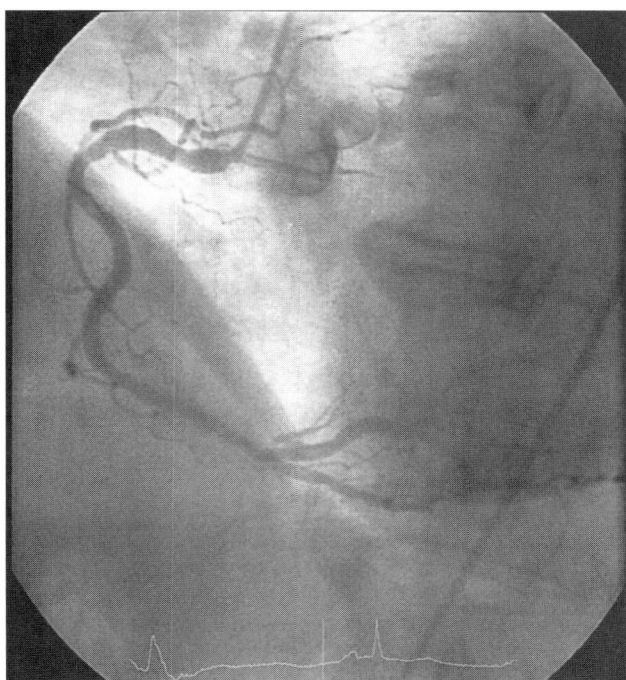

B

▪ **Figure 22–12.** Normal RCA shown in RAO projection (*A*) and LAO projection (*B*). (Courtesy of Swedish Medical Center, Seattle, WA.)

or narrowing. When occlusion is present, the degree of disease and the suitability of the artery for revascularization are of primary concern.

In addition to grading the occlusion, the condition of the distal artery must be evaluated. The distal artery may be identified by antegrade or collateral flow, and its caliber and suitability as a recipient for bypass grafting are evaluated. Arteries with diffuse atherosclerotic plaquing and small distal targets are less suitable for bypass grafting. The proximity of the occlusion determines the amount of myocardium in jeopardy. A subjective evaluation of the degree of arterial flow is made by observing the time required for perfused arteries to fill and clear. Contrast medium clears faster with higher flow rates. Intermittent luminal obstruction due to systolic constriction from encircling muscle bands or to coronary

artery spasm is also observed, and its degree, distribution, and pattern are evaluated. If bypass grafts have been injected, they are evaluated in the same manner for patency, flow indices, and the condition of the perfused artery. Figures 22-12 and 22-13 show normal angiograms of the right and left coronary arteries.

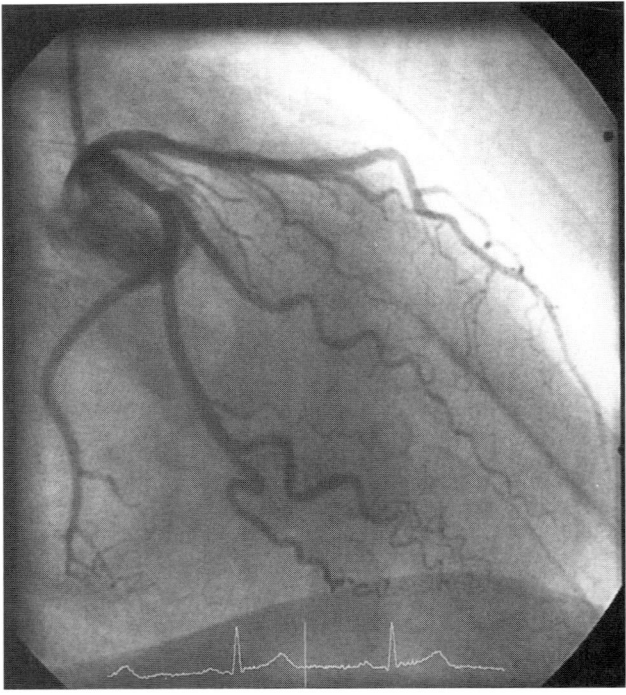

A

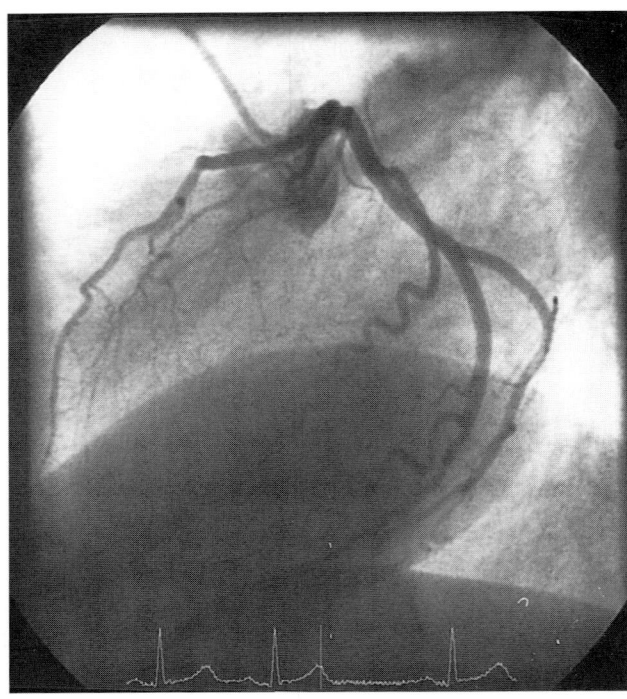

B

■ **Figure 22–13.** Normal left coronary arteries shown in RAO projection (*A*) and LAO projection (*B*). (Courtesy of Swedish Medical Center, Seattle, WA.)

Evaluation of myocardial function is an important part of the evaluation of coronary artery disease. Patterns of ventricular contraction are evaluated by ventriculography and estimated ejection fraction. The anteriolateral, apical, inferior, and posterobasal segments of the left ventricle can be examined in the RAO projection. In the LAO projection, the basal septal, apical septal, apical lateral, and basal lateral segments can be evaluated. Regional contraction may be classified as follows:

1. Normal
2. Mild hypokinesis—mild reduction in myocardial contraction
3. Severe hypokinesis—more severe reduction in myocardial contraction
4. Akinesis—total absence of wall motion in a discrete area
5. Dyskinesis—disturbance causing abnormal movement of left ventricular wall contraction
6. Aneurysm—paradoxical systolic expansion of a portion of the left ventricular wall

The reversibility of myocardial contraction abnormalities is an important consideration in the decision for surgery and long-term prognosis. Improved function is more common with hypokinesis than with akinesis or dyskinesis. The presence of collateral vessels and the lack of Q waves favor the reversibility of hypokinesis. (Fifer & Grossman, 2000)

REFERENCES

Ammann, P., Brunner-La Rocca, H. P., Angehrn, W., Roelli, H., Sagmeister, M., & Rickli, M. D. (2003). Procedural complications following diagnostic coronary angiography are related to the operator's experience and the catheter size. *Catheterization and Cardiovascular Intervention*, 59(1), 13–18.

Asif, A., Preston, R. A., & Roth, D. (2003). Radiocontrast-induced nephropathy. *American Journal of Therapeutics*, 10(2), 137–147.

Baim, D. S. (2000). Percutaneous approach, including transseptal and apical puncture. In D. S. Baim & W. Grossman (Eds.), *Grossman's cardiac catheterization, angiography, and intervention* (6th ed., pp. 669–101). Philadelphia: Lippincott Williams & Wilkins.

Baim, D. S., & Grossman, W. (2000a). Complications of cardiac catheterization. In D. S. Baim & W. Grossman (Eds.), *Grossman's cardiac catheterization, angiography, and intervention* (6th ed., pp. 35–69). Philadelphia: Lippincott Williams & Wilkins.

_____. (2000b). Coronary angiography. In D. S. Baim & W. Grossman (Eds.), *Grossman's cardiac catheterization, angiography, and intervention* (6th ed., pp. 211–257). Philadelphia: Lippincott Williams & Wilkins.

Baim, D. S., & Hillis, L. D. (2000). Cardiac ventriculography. In D. S. Baim & W. Grossman (Eds.), *Grossman's cardiac catheterization, angiography, and intervention* (6th ed., pp. 257–271). Philadelphia: Lippincott Williams & Wilkins.

Barrett, B. J., Parfrey, P. S., Vavasour, H. M., et al. (1992). A comparison of nonionic, low-osmolality radiocontrast agents with ionic, high-osmolality agents during cardiac catheterization. *New England Journal of Medicine*, 326, 431.

Bashore, T. M., Bates, E. R., Kern, H. J., et al. (2001). Cardiac catheterization laboratory standards: A report of the American College of Cardiology Task Force on Clinical Expert Consensus Documents (ACC/SCA&I Committee to Develop an Expert Consensus Document on Cardiac Catheterization Laboratory Standards). *Journal of the American College of Cardiology*, 37, 2170–2214.

Bogart, M. A. (1995). Time to hemostasis: A comparison of manual versus mechanical compression of the femoral artery. *American Journal of Critical Care*, 4, 149–156.

Braunwald, E., Mark, D. B., Jones, R. H., et al. (1994). *Unstable angina: Diagnosis and management* (86th ed., AHCPR publication 94-0602). Rockville, MD.

Brinker, J. A. (1990). Selection of a contrast agent in the cardiac catheterization laboratory. *American Journal of Cardiology*, 66, 26F–33F.

Brockenbrough, E. C., & Braunwald, E. (1960). A new technique for left ventricular angiography and transseptal left heart catheterization. *American Journal of Cardiology*, 6, 1062–1064.

Clark, D. A., Moscovich, M. D., Vetrovec, G. W., & Wexler, L. (1992). Guidelines for the performance of outpatients catheterization and angiographic procedures. *Catheterization and Cardiovascular Diagnosis*, 27, 5–7.

Cournand, A. F., & Ranges, C. S. (1941). Catheterization of the right auricle in man. *Proceedings of the Society for Experimental Biology and Medicine, 46,* 462.

Cournand, A. F., & Riley, R. L. (1945). Breed ES et al: Measurement of cardiac output in man using the technique of catheterization of the right auricle or ventricle. *Journal of Clinical Investigation, 24,* 106–116.

Davidson, C. J., & Bonow, R. O. (2001). Cardiac catheterization. In E. Braunwald, D. P. Zipes, & P. Libby (Eds.), *Heart disease: A textbook of cardiovascular medicine* (6th ed., pp. 359–386). Philadelphia: W. B. Saunders.

Drew, B., & Tisdale, L. A. (1993). ST segment monitoring for coronary artery reocclusion following thrombolytic therapy and coronary angioplasty: Identification of optimal bedside monitoring leads. *American Journal of Critical Care, 2,* 280–292.

Fifer, M. A., & Grossman, W. (2000). Measurement of ventricular volumes, ejection fraction, mass, wall stress, and regional wall motion. In D. S. Baim & W. Grossman (Eds.), *Grossman's cardiac catheterization, angiography, and intervention* (6th ed., pp. 353–367). Philadelphia: Lippincott Williams & Wilkins.

Franch, R. H., Douglas, J. S., King, S. B., et al. (2001). Cardiac catheterization, coronary arteriography, and coronary blood flow and pressure measurements. In V. Fuster, R. W. Alexander, & R. A. O'Rourke (Eds.), *Hurst's the heart* (10th ed., pp. 479–518). New York: McGraw-Hill.

Gibbons, R. J., Balady, G. J., Beasssley, J. W., et al. (1997). ACC/AHA guidelines for exercise testing: A report of the American College of Cardiology/American Heart Association Task Force on Practice Guidelines (Committee on Exercise Testing). *Journal of the American College of Cardiology, 30,* 260–311.

Grossman, W. (2000a). Brachial cutdown approach. In D. S. Baim & W. Grossman (Eds.), *Grossman's cardiac catheterization, angiography, and intervention* (6th ed., pp.101–125). Philadelphia: Lippincott Williams & Wilkins.

_____. (2000b). Cardiac catheterization: Historical perspective and present practice. In D. S. Baim & W. Grossman (Eds.), *Grossman's cardiac catheterization, angiography, and intervention* (6th ed., pp. 3–15). Philadelphia: Lippincott Williams & Wilkins.

_____. (2000c). Shunt detection and measurement. In D. S. Baim & W. Grossman (Eds.), *Grossman's cardiac catheterization, angiography, and intervention* (6th ed., pp.179–193). Philadelphia: Lippincott Williams & Wilkins.

Heupler, F. A., Heisler, M., Keys, T. F., et al. (1992). Infection prevention guidelines for cardiac catheterization laboratories. *Catheterization and Cardiovascular Diagnosis, 25,* 260–263.

Hill, J. A., Lambert, C. R., Vlietstra, R. E., & Pepine, C. J. (1998). Review of techniques. In J. C. Pepine, J. A. Hill, & C. R. Lambert (Eds.), *Diagnostic and therapeutic cardiac catheterization* (3rd ed., pp.106–128). Baltimore: Williams & Wilkins.

Hirshfeld, J. W. (1990). Cardiovascular effects of iodinated contrast agents. *American Journal of Cardiology, 66,* 9F–17F.

Jacobson, C. (1996). Bedside cardiac monitoring. In M. Chulay & S. Burns (Eds.), *Research-based practice protocols: Technology series.* Aliso Viejo, CA: American Association of Critical Care Nurses.

Judkins, M. P. (1968). Percutaneous transfemoral selective coronary arteriography. *Radiology Clinics of North America, 6,* 467–492.

Juran, N. B., Rouse, C. L., Smith, D. D., O'Brien, M. A., DeLucca, S. A., Sigmon, K., et al. (1999). Nursing interventions to decrease bleeding at the femoral access site after percutaneous coronary intervention. *American Journal of Critical Care, 8*(5), 303–313.

Kixmiller, J. M., & Schick, L. (1997). Procedural sedation in cardiovascular procedures. *Critical Care Nursing Clinics of North America, 9,* 301–312.

Lambert, C. R., Pepine, C. J., & Nichols, W. W. (1989). Pressure measurement. In C. J. Pepine, J. A. Hill & C. R. Lambert (Eds.), *Diagnostic and therapeutic cardiac catheterization* (pp. 283–297). Baltimore: Williams & Wilkins.

Lazzara, D., Pfersdorf, P., & Sedlacek, M. (1997). Femoral compression. *Nursing, 97,* 27(12), 54–57.

Limacher, M. C., Douglas, P. S., Germano, G., et al. (1998). ACC expert consensus document. Radiation safety in the practice of cardiology. *Journal of the American College of Cardiology, 31,* 892–913.

Montes, P. (1997). Managing outpatient catheterization. *American Journal of Nursing, 97,* 34–37.

Owens, P., & Bashore, T. M. (1990). The preparation and care of the patient and the laboratory. In T. M. Bashore (Ed.), *Invasive cardiology principles and techniques* (pp. 19–39). Toronto: B. C. Decker.

Pepine, C. J., Hill, J. A., & Lambert, C. R. (Eds.). (1998). *Diagnostic and therapeutic cardiac catheterization* (3rd ed.). Baltimore: Williams & Wilkins.

_____. (1989). History of the development and application of cardiac catheterization. In C. J. Pepine, J. A. Hill & C. R. Lambert (Eds.), *Diagnostic and therapeutic cardiac catheterization* (pp 3–10). Baltimore: Williams & Wilkins.

Peterson, K. L., & Nicod, P. (Eds.). (1997). *Cardiac catheterization: Methods, diagnosis, and therapy.* Philadelphia: W. B. Saunders.

Popma, J. J., & Bittl, J. (2001). Coronary angiography and intravascular ultrasonography. In E. Braunwald, D. P. Zipes, & P. Libby (Eds.), *Heart disease: A textbook of cardiovascular medicine* (6th ed., pp. 387–421). Philadelphia: W. B. Saunders.

Richards, D. W. (1945). Cardiac output by catheterization technique in various clinical conditions. *Federal Proceedings, 4,* 215–220.

Scanlon, P. J., Faxon, D. P., Audet, A.-M., et al. (1999). ACC/AHA guidelines for coronary angiography: Executive summary and recommendations: A report of the American College of Cardiology/American Heart Association Task Force on Practice Guidelines (Committee on Coronary Angiography) developed in collaboration with the Society for Cardiac Angiography and Interventions. *Circulation, 99,* 2345–2357.

Schickel, S., Cronin, S. N., Mize, A., et al. (1996). Removal of femoral sheaths by registered nurses: Issues and outcomes. *Critical Care Nursing, 16,* 32–36.

Schultz, D. D., & Olivas, G. S. (1986). The use of cough cardiopulmonary resuscitation in clinical practice. *Heart and Lung, 5,* 273–280.

Seldinger, S. I. (1953). Catheter replacement of the needle in percutaneous arteriography. *Acta Radiologica, 29,* 368–376.

Sones, F. M., Shirey, E. K., Prondfit, W. L., et al. (1959). Cine-coronary arteriography. *Circulation, 20,* 773.

Spector, K. S. & Lawson, W. E. (2001). Optimizing safe femoral access during cardiac catheterization. *Catheterization and Cardiovascular Interventions, 53*(2), 209–212.

23

Hemodynamic Monitoring

ELIZABETH J. BRIDGES

Cardiovascular support of critically ill patients requires noninvasive and invasive monitoring of physiological indicators of cardiovascular function, including factors that affect cardiac performance (preload, afterload, contractility, and heart rate) and the balance between O_2 supply and demand. This chapter reviews the most commonly used technologies for hemodynamic monitoring (arterial blood pressure monitoring, CVP/PA catheterization, and CO and $S\overline{v}O_2$ monitoring) and discusses the current recommendations for the effective use of hemodynamic monitoring in optimizing patient outcomes. New hemodynamic monitoring techniques (e.g., central venous oxygenation, functional hemodynamic monitoring) and new technologies such as transpulmonary indicator dilution (TPID) CO, pulse contour analysis, transesophageal Doppler, partial CO_2 rebreathing, sublingual capnography, and tissue oxygenation monitoring techniques are introduced.

TECHNICAL ASPECTS OF INVASIVE PRESSURE MONITORING

Referencing

Pressure in blood vessels has three components: dynamic blood pressure (i.e., the blood pressure generated by the heart), hydrostatic pressure (related to fluid density, gravitational acceleration, and height of the column of blood between the heart and the vessels), and static pressure (related to the volume of blood in the vascular system at zero flow) (Bridges et al., 1997). The blood pressure is the same at all points along a horizontal level. However, pressure at different vertical levels reflects not only the dynamic pressure but also the hydrostatic pressure.

Correct referencing of the pressure monitoring system is crucial to ensure the accuracy of pressure measurements. Referencing, which is performed to correct for the change in hydrostatic pressure in vessels above and below the heart, is accomplished by placing the air–fluid interface (stopcock) of the catheter system at the level of the heart to negate the weight effect of the catheter tubing. All invasive cardiovascular pressure monitoring systems (PA, CVP, and arterial) are referenced to the heart, not to the catheter tip or the site of insertion (Bridges et al., 1997; Courtois et al., 1995; McCann et al., 2001).

The reference points for the mid-RA are referred to as the phlebostatic axis and phlebostatic level (Fig. 23-1). As the patient moves from the flat to the upright position, the phlebostatic level rotates on the axis and remains horizontal (Fig. 23-2). The phlebostatic axis is also the reference for the left atrium (Kee et al., 1993). In patients with normal chest wall configuration, the mid-axillary line (MAL) is a valid reference level for the right and left atrium; however, use of the MAL in patients with varied chest configuration may result in a potential pressure difference of up to 6 mm Hg (Bartz et al., 1988). Therefore, use of the MAL as a reference is not recommended.

Previous research on the effect of position on hemodynamic pressure measurements has been limited by the use of incorrect reference points. In many of these studies, attainment of valid and reliable PA pressures was not possible because the use of a reference point above or below the left atrium resulted in the inclusion of hydrostatic pressure component; thus, the measured pressures were underestimated or overestimated (Bridges, 2000a). The effect of varying reference levels on pressures recorded was demonstrated in a study in which patients were placed in the 30-degree right and left lateral positions and then various reference points were used (Fig. 23-3) (Ross & Jones, 1995). These results demonstrate that for every 1 cm the reference point is above the left atrium, the measured pressure decreases by 0.73 mm Hg. Conversely, for every 1 cm the reference point is below the left atrium, the measured pressure increases by 0.73 mm Hg. The position-specific reference points are summarized in Table 23-1.

In the lateral position, reference points have only been validated for the 30-degree and 90-degree lateral positions with a 0-degree backrest elevation. Further study of the lateral position with varying degrees of backrest elevation is needed. Recommendations cannot be made for measurement of hemodynamic indices in the prone position because of contradictory results (Pelosi et al., 1998; Vollman & Bander, 1996). Evaluation of research using CT scans of the thorax in the prone position may provide insight into the anatomical shifts in the cardiovascular structures in the prone position. Research, which uses a validated reference and also controls for abdominal compression in the prone position, is needed.

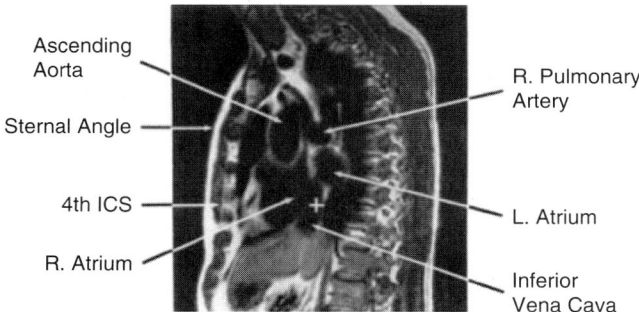

■ **Figure 23–1.** Magnetic resonance image of a 43-year-old man. White cross marks the phlebostatic axis. (Reproduced from McGee, S. R. [1998]. Physical examination of venous pressure. *American Heart Journal*, 136 [1], 10–18.)

Zeroing Versus Referencing

Zeroing is performed by opening the system to air to establish atmospheric pressure as zero and to compensate for offset caused by hydrostatic pressure or offset in the pressure transducer, amplifier, oscilloscope, recorder, or digital delays. The disposable transducer–catheter systems currently in use demonstrate minimal zero drift (Ahrens et al., 1995). Zero drift is related to the offset in the electrical and plumbing components of the system; thus, zeroing is primarily performed to correct for the offset caused by hydrostatic pressure. Calibration of disposable pressure transducers and fixed-calibration bedside pressure monitoring systems is no longer recommended (Gardner, 1996). The act of simulta-

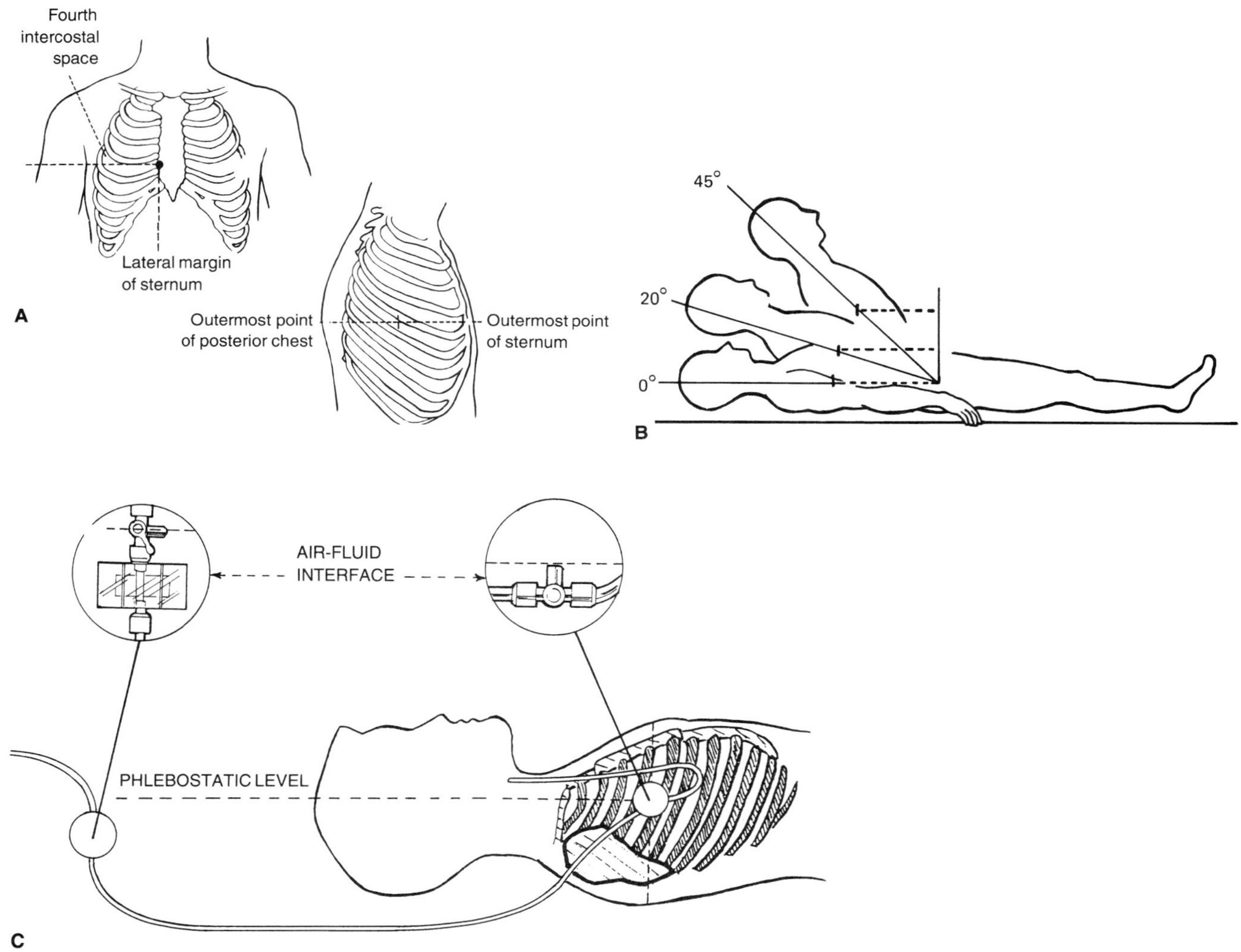

■ **Figure 23–2.** The phlebostatic axis and the phlebostatic level. (*A*) The *phlebostatic axis* is the intersection of two reference lines: first, an imaginary line from the fourth intercostal space (ICS) at the point where it joins the sternum, drawn out to the side of the body; second, a line drawn *midway* between the anterior and posterior surfaces of the chest (*B*) The phlebostatic level is a horizontal line through the phlebostatic axis. The air-fluid interface of the stopcock of the transducer or the zero mark on the manometer must be level with this axis for accurate measurements. Moving from the flat to erect positions, the patient moves the chest and therefore the reference level; the phlebostatic level stays horizontal through the same reference point. (Adapted from Shinn, J. A., Woods, S. L., Huseby, J. S. [1979]. Effect of intermittent positive pressure ventilation upon pulmonary capillary wedge pressures in acutely ill patients. *Heart & Lung*, 8, 324.) (*C*) Two methods for referencing the pressure system to the phlebostatic axis. The system can be referenced by placing the air-fluid interface of either the in-line stopcock or the stopcock on top of the transducer at the phlebostatic level. (From Bridges, E. J., & Woods, S. L. [1993]. Pulmonary artery pressure measurement: State of the art. *Heart & Lung*, 22, 101.)

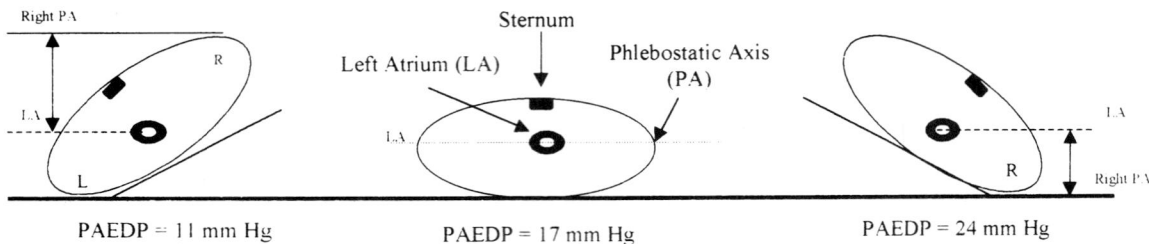

Left 30°-Lateral
Position

Supine Position

Right 30°Lateral
Position

PAEDP = 11 mm Hg   PAEDP = 17 mm Hg   PAEDP = 24 mm Hg

■ **Figure 23–3.** Based on work by Ross and Jones (1995) demonstrates the effect of varying references on measured pressures. The PAEDP in the supine/flat position using the phlebostatic axis as the reference was 17 mm Hg. When the phlebostatic axis was used with the patient in the 30° left-lateral position, the PAEDP was 11 mm Hg because the reference was above the left atrium (LA). With the patient in the right 30° lateral position, using the phlebostatic axis, the PAEDP was 24 mm Hg, reflecting the inclusion of hydrostatic pressure from a reference point below the left atrium. The reference point in the 30° lateral position is one-half the distance from the left sternal border to the surface of the bed. (Bridges et al., 2000; VanEtta et al., 1993.)

neously zeroing and referencing ensures that the pressures being measured are intracardiac (Display 23-1).

Infection Control

Catheter-related infection remains the leading cause of nosocomial infections, particularly in critical care. Migration of organisms along the catheter and contamination of the catheter hub are the primary causes of infection in short- and long-term catheters, respectively. Catheter-related infections are associated with increased length of hospital stay and resource use (Dimick et al., 2001). In 2002, the CDC published guidelines for the prevention of intravascular catheter-related infections (O'Grady et al., 2002). A summary of the recommendations is presented in Table 23-2. Staff education focused on catheter insertion techniques and maintenance as outlined in the CDC guidelines significantly decreases the incidence of primary blood stream infections (Coopersmith et al., 2002; Eggimann & Pittet, 2002).

Table 23–1 ■ POSITION-SPECIFIC REFERENCES

Position	Reference
Supine with backrest elevation up to 45°	Phlebostatic level (4th ICS at ¹/₂ AP diameter of chest)
Lateral	
30° (Bridges et al., 2000; VanEtta et al., 1993)	¹/₂ vertical distance from surface of bed to left sternal border
90° (Paolella et al., 1988)	
• Left lateral decubitus	• 4th ICS/left parasternal border
• Right lateral decubitus	• 4th ICS/midsternum

Dynamic Response Characteristics

The dynamic response characteristics of the catheter-transducer system reflect the system's ability to faithfully reproduce a pressure waveform. The dynamic response can be determined by evaluating the system's damping coefficient and natural (resonant) frequency (Fig. 23-4). The damping coefficient is a measure of how quickly the system dampens and eventually arrests the oscillations. A certain degree of damping is desirable for optimal fidelity and suppression of unwanted high-frequency vibration or noise. The natural frequency (Fn) refers to the frequency at which the system oscillates when shock excited (Gardner, 1981). As seen in Figure 23-4, the higher the Fn, the greater the range of acceptable damping. The Fn can be quickly assessed by measuring the horizontal distance between the points of two oscillations (each small box equals 1 mm) and dividing the paper speed (25 mm/sec) by this value. For example, if there are two small boxes between oscillations, then the Fn = 25/2 = 12.5 Hz, which is marginally acceptable. Optimizing the Fn has the greatest effect on the reproduction of a waveform. The most demanding waveforms (increased blood pressure and tachycardia >120 bpm) require an Fn greater than 20Hz to be faithfully reproduced. The Fn of the catheter–transducer system decreases over time (Promonet et al., 2000), indicating the need to routinely evaluate the dynamic response characteristics of the system.

An underdamped system results in falsely high systolic (15 to 30 mm Hg) and low diastolic pressures. An overdamped system loses its characteristic landmarks, and the waveform appears unnaturally smooth with a diminished or absent dicrotic notch (Gardner, 1981). An overdamped system causes falsely low systolic and high diastolic pressure readings. PA catheters have a decreased Fn compared to arterial pressure lines (Promonet et al., 2000); thus, taking steps to optimize the system is imperative (see Fig. 23-4). The simpler the system (shorter tubing, fewer stopcocks), the better its ability to

D I S P L A Y   23–1

PROTOCOL FOR OBTAINING PULMONARY ARTERY AND PULMONARY ARTERY WEDGE PRESSURES

1. Explain procedure to patient
2. Position patient in
   a. Supine position with backrest up to 60°
   b. Lateral position at 30° or 90°
3. Allow 5 minutes for pressure stabilization after position change
4. Reference and zero the pressure-transducer system
   a. Locate the reference point
      (1) Supine: line bisecting fourth ICS at the sternum and one-half anteroposterior diameter
      (2) 30-degree lateral (right and left): 1/2 distance from left sternal border to surface of bed
      (3) 90° lateral (right): fourth ICS at the midsternum
      (4) 90° lateral (left): fourth ICS left parasternal border
   b. Level the air-fluid interface with the reference level (use either the in-line stopcock or the stopcock on the top of the transducer)
   c. Remove the cap from the stopcock using aseptic technique
   d. Turn stopcock "off" to the patient and "open" to air
   e. Activate the "Zero" button on the monitor
   f. Close stopcock and replace cap

   g. Reference and zero the system anytime the patient's position changes
5. Check and troubleshoot the dynamic response characteristics of the system every shift, if the waveform characteristics change, or if the system has been disturbed (see Fig. 23-4)
6. Confirm Zone 3 catheter placement
   a. Review anteroposterior chest radiograph to ensure catheter is below left atrium (left atrium is ~ 3 cm below the carina (Fig. 23-16).
   b. During wedging the PA waveform should (1) flatten into a characteristic atrial waveform (distinct a and v waves may not be discernible), (2) immediately return to a PA configuration with balloon deflation, and (3) PAWP < mean PA in absence of large V wave.
   c. PAEDP-PAWP gradient > 4 mm Hg (may indicate Zone 1 or 2 placement).
7. Identify end-expiratory waveform
   a. Determine pressures using analog (graphic) tracing
   b. Record end-expiratory pressures

(1) Spontaneous: Immediately before inspiratory trough

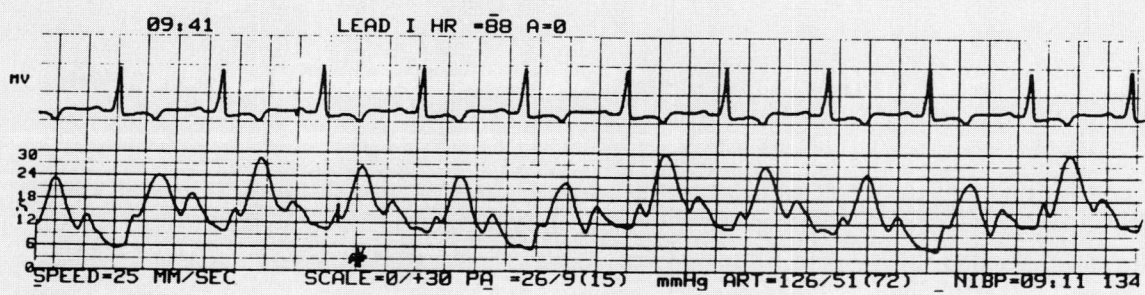

Interpretation: PA Systolic = 27 mm Hg; PAEDP = 13 mm Hg; PA mean = 19 mm Hg

(2) Mechanical ventilation: Immediately before inspiratory rise

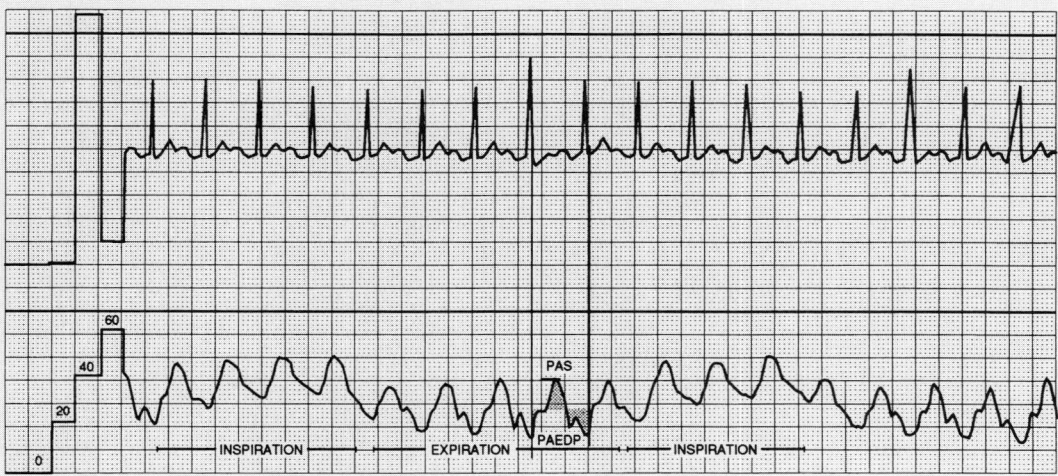

Interpretation: PA Systolic = 38 mm Hg; PAEDP = 16 mm Hg; PA mean = 27 mm Hg

(Continued)

DISPLAY   23–1(CONTINUED)

PROTOCOL FOR OBTAINING PULMONARY ARTERY AND PULMONARY ARTERY WEDGE PRESSURES

8. If digital data are the only available method, record the PAWP using the following:
   a. Controlled mechanical ventilation: diastolic mode (lowest pressure)
   b. Assisted ventilation: digital mean
   c. Spontaneous ventilation: systolic mode (highest pressure)
9. Evaluate pressures for normal fluctuation and trends
   a. PA systolic: 4–7 mm Hg
   b. PA mean: 4–5 mm Hg
   c. PAEDP: 4–7 mm Hg
   d. PAWP: 4 mm Hg
10. Improve accuracy of PAWP as an indicator of LAP with high levels of PEEP (> 10 cm H_2O)
    a. Position catheter tip dependent to the left atrium (Zone 3 – See #6) or position patient so catheter tip is below left atrium (e.g., if catheter tip is in right PA, positioning the patient in right lateral position places the tip below the left atrium). Use angle-specific reference.

b. Analyze the pulmonary capillary wedge blood. This confirms correct wedging but does not confirm that PAWP is an accurate indicator of LAP.
d. Estimate effect of increased transmural pressure on PAWP. Subtract $^1/_2$ applied PEEP (1 cm H_2O = 0.73 mm Hg) from measured PAWP (Marini et al., 1982). Example: 15 cm H_2O PEEP; measured PAWP = 18 mm Hg:

$$15 \text{ cm } H_2O \times 0.74 = 11.1 \text{ mm Hg}$$

$$18 \text{ mm Hg} - 5.6 \text{ mm Hg}$$

$$\textit{Estimated } \text{PAWP} = 12.4 \text{ mm Hg}$$

This is the largest pressure correction possible (less effect may occur).
e. Suspect non-zone 3 placement if with an increase in PEEP, the PAWP increases greater than $^1/_2$ the applied PEEP increment (i.e., PEEP increased by 5 cm H_2O (3.7 mm Hg), and PAWP increases greater than 1.8 mm Hg (3.7 mm Hg/2 = 1.8 mm Hg).

Table 23–2 ■ INFECTION CONTROL

	Comments
Skin antisepsis	• Skin antisepsis with a 2% chlorhexidene preparation is superior to 10% povidone–iodine or 70% alcohol in preventing catheter colonization
Insertion technique	• Central venous catheter: maximum sterile technique for insertion (cap, mask, sterile gloves, sterile gown, large sterile drapes) • Arterial line (not specifically addressed): technique similar to short term central venous catheter
Hand hygiene	• Perform hand-hygiene before and after manipulating catheters/catheter site • Use of gloves does not obviate the need for good hand washing
Location of insertion site	• Higher BSI rates associated with internal jugular or femoral insertion site compared to subclavian vein insertion site • Increased BSI with reinsertion over a guidewire at old insertion site • Avoid lower extremity insertion if possible
Antimicrobial catheters	• Catheters coated with chlorhexidene/silver sulfadiazine decrease the risk of catheter-related blood stream infections compared with standard catheters (Mermel, 2001) • Heparin bonding decreases risk of infection versus non-heparin bonded catheters (Marin et al., 2000) • Consider use of antimicrobial catheters if catheter is to remain in place > 5 days and current hospital BSI rate exceeds NNIS standards (3.3 infections per 1000 catheter days)
Catheter sleeve (PA catheter)	• Use sterile sleeve during PA catheter insertion
Frequency of catheter change	• Routine catheter replacement is not recommended (Timsit, 2000) • Change PA catheters no more frequently than every 7 days (Chen et al., 2003) • Arterial line (similar to short-term central venous catheters)—no specific recommendations for catheters that need to be in place > 5 days
Dressing	• Use sterile gauze or sterile, transparent semi-permeable membrane dressing • Change gauze dressing every 2 days and transparent dressing at least every seven days, when the dressing becomes, damp, loose or soiled or for site inspection
Flush solution	• Do not administer dextrose-containing solutions through the pressure monitoring system
Administration set	• Continuous-flush device • Replace pressure transducers and all tubing and flush solution every 96 hours
Obtaining cultures from central venous and arterial catheters	• Drawing cultures from only one lumen of a multilumen catheter has a 60% chance of detecting significant colonization. If only one lumen is sampled a negative culture does not necessarily rule out the CVC as a source of infection (Dobbins et al., 2003) • Cultures obtained through a central venous or arterial catheter are less specific than venipuncture specimens, with higher false-positives from central line cultures compared to arterial line/peripheral cultures (Martinez et al., 2002)

Decision Making Algorithm

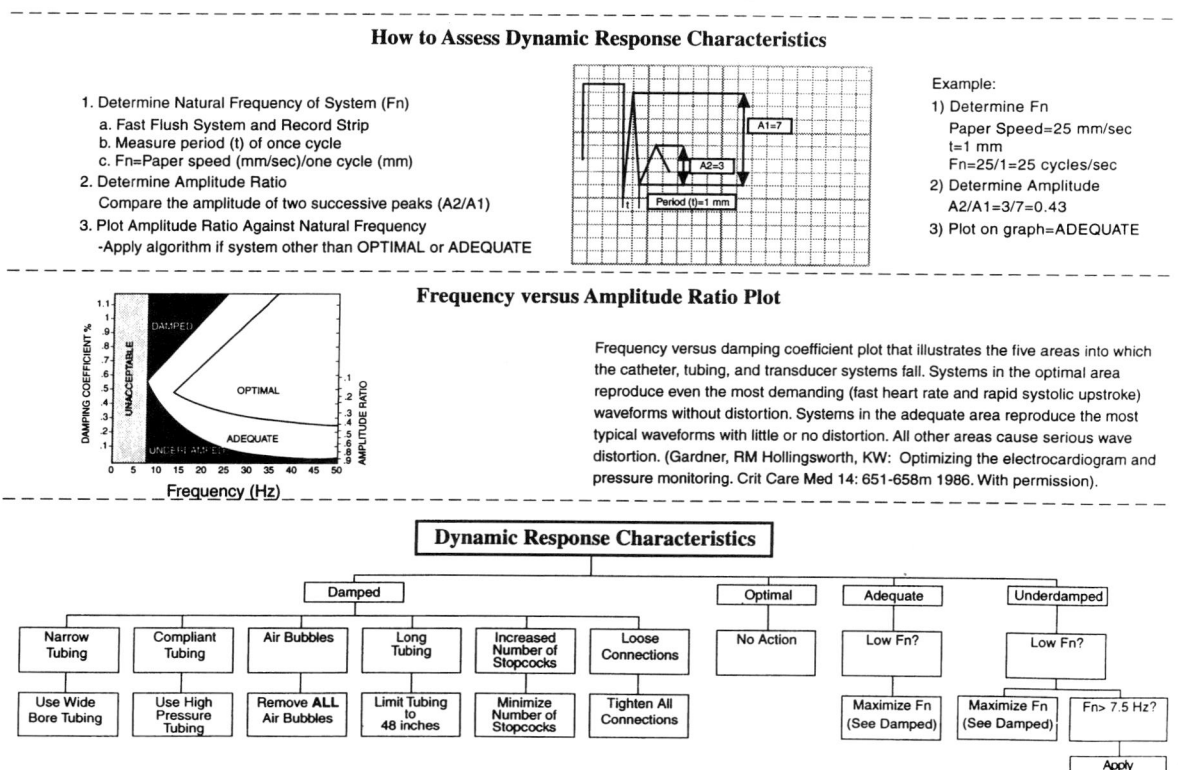

How to Assess Dynamic Response Characteristics

1. Determine Natural Frequency of System (Fn)
   a. Fast Flush System and Record Strip
   b. Measure period (t) of once cycle
   c. Fn=Paper speed (mm/sec)/one cycle (mm)
2. Determine Amplitude Ratio
   Compare the amplitude of two successive peaks (A2/A1)
3. Plot Amplitude Ratio Against Natural Frequency
   -Apply algorithm if system other than OPTIMAL or ADEQUATE

Example:
1) Determine Fn
   Paper Speed=25 mm/sec
   t=1 mm
   Fn=25/1=25 cycles/sec
2) Determine Amplitude
   A2/A1=3/7=0.43
3) Plot on graph=ADEQUATE

Frequency versus Amplitude Ratio Plot

Frequency versus damping coefficient plot that illustrates the five areas into which the catheter, tubing, and transducer systems fall. Systems in the optimal area reproduce even the most demanding (fast heart rate and rapid systolic upstroke) waveforms without distortion. Systems in the adequate area reproduce the most typical waveforms with little or no distortion. All other areas cause serious wave distortion. (Gardner, RM Hollingsworth, KW: Optimizing the electrocardiogram and pressure monitoring. Crit Care Med 14: 651-658m 1986. With permission).

■ **Figure 23–4.** Dynamic response characteristics. (From Bridges, E. J., & Middleton, R. [1997]. Direct arterial vs. oscillometric monitoring of blood pressure: Stop comparing and pick one [a decision making algorithm]. *Critical Care Nurse,* 17[3], 58–72. With permission.)

reproduce faithfully the pressure waveforms (Bridges & Middleton, 1997; Gardner, 1981; Gore et al., 1995). Use of in-line blood conservation devices decrease the Fn of the system, resulting in an underdamped system (Woda et al., 1999).

Blood Drawing from Arterial and Central Venous Catheters

Arterial blood gases, serum electrolytes, and coagulation studies can be drawn from an arterial line. To avoid contamination of the specimen with saline and/or heparin, two-times the deadspace volume (volume from the catheter tip to the aspiration site) or two-times the deadspace plus 2 mL (approximately equivalent to six-times the deadspace) should be withdrawn for ABGs and electrolytes (Rickard et al., 2003). For coagulation studies (e.g., PT/PTT) the discard volume should be four-times to six-times the deadspace volume (Heap et al., 1997; Laxson & Titler, 1994). Commercially available in-line blood conservation sets have a discard volume ranging from four-times to 13-times the deadspace volume (see manufacturer's information).

Serum sodium and glucose can be obtained from the infusion port of the PA catheter if the dwell volume plus 2 mL of additional blood is discarded (Carlson et al., 1990). Coagulation studies (ACT) drawn from heparin-bonded PA catheters

are significantly increased compared to specimens obtained from an arterial catheter (McNulty et al., 1998), although baseline specimens can be obtained from the introducer before placement of the PA catheter (Haering et al., 2000). No published research was found regarding measurement of potassium or other electrolytes from PA catheters; however, in a recent study of central venous lines, a discard volume of 3 mL (corresponding to six-times the catheter deadspace) was sufficient after initially flushing the line with 5 ml of saline (Odum & Drenck, 2002).

DIRECT ARTERIAL PRESSURE MONITORING

Indications

Intraarterial monitoring is indicated when precise and continuous monitoring is required. Examples of clinical conditions warranting direct arterial pressure monitoring include acute hypertensive crises, hypotension, any shock state, frequent drawing of arterial blood samples, monitoring of vasoactive pharmacologic support and, during aggressive respiratory support (e.g., high positive end-expiratory pressures [PEEP]).

Table 23–3 ■ MODIFIED ALLEN TEST

1. Compress both the radial and ulnar arteries
2. Have patient squeeze hand to remove blood from hand
3. Release ulnar artery only
4. Normal (negative) Allen test: return of normal or slightly red color to palm of hand in < 10 seconds (note: use of 6 seconds as cut-off point provides maximal sensitivity/specificity of test) (Jarvis et al., 2000)

* Avoid complete extension of the wrist with wide spreading of the fingers, because this will occlude the transpalmar arch

Catheter Placement

Sites for intraarterial catheterization include the radial, brachial, femoral, dorsalis pedis, and axillary arteries (Scheer et al., 2002). Important considerations in site selection include adequate collateral circulation, patient comfort, and avoidance of areas at increased risk for infection. The most common insertion site is the radial artery because of the presence of collateral circulation, which decreases the risk of vascular complications. The radial and ulnar artery/superficial palmar arteries provide a dual blood supply to the hand, which is important if radial artery perfusion becomes temporarily or permanently compromised because of catheter placement. Before radial artery cannulation is attempted, collateral circulation to the hand must be assessed. The most common test used clinically to evaluate collateral circulation is the modified Allen test (Table 23-3).

Harvesting of the radial artery for cardiac surgery has led to increased interest in the evaluation of collateral circulation to the hand. A cut-off of 6 seconds for the Allen test had a sensitivity of 55%, specificity of 92%, and diagnostic accuracy of 79% for adequate collateral circulation (Jarvis et al., 2000). Given this limited diagnostic accuracy newer technologies including digit pressure measurement and plethysmography and Doppler ultrasonography have been recommended for patients undergoing radial harvesting, particularly those with a positive Allen test.

The brachial artery is used less frequently because it does not have good collateral circulation, which in theory increases the risk for diffuse distal ischemia. Regardless of the insertion site, ongoing assessment of collateral circulation must be made while the catheter is in place. Another option is the dorsalis pedis artery (DPA). Complication rates associated with the DPA are comparable to radial artery insertion (Martin et al., 2001). However, the DPA pressures are significantly higher than radial pressures, even in the supine position (Parry et al., 1995).

Arterial Pressure Wave

The contour or the aortic pressure wave is illustrated in Figure 23-5. The initial sharp upstroke reflects the pressure increase during the rapid ejection phase of ventricular systole and a slower rise during later systole. The upstroke of the waveform is referred to as the anacrotic limb, which is followed by a brief, peaked, sustained pressure (anacrotic shoulder). At the end of systole, the pressure falls in the aorta and left ventricle and the downstroke of the pressure wave corresponds to the decrease in

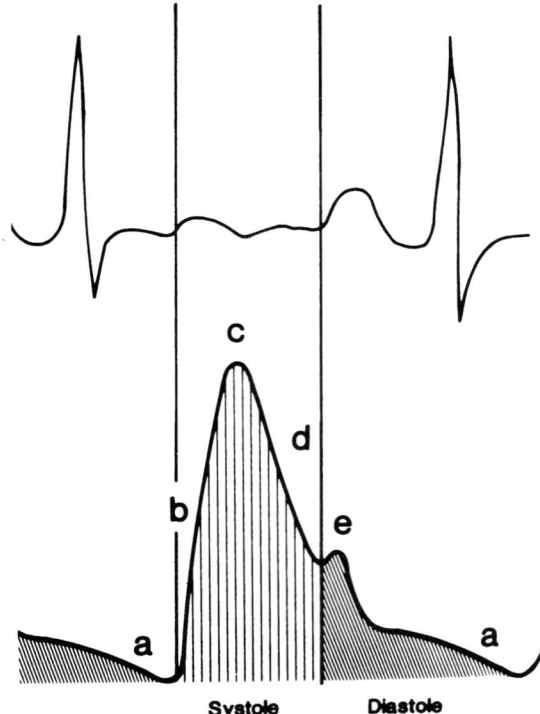

■ **Figure 23–5.** Components of arterial waveform during cardiac cycle. The pulse wave a to c waveform occurs as blood is ejected into the aorta from the ventricle during systole. Volume displacement occurs at point c. Segment d occurs during late systole as the ventricles empty and forward movement slows. Closure of the aortic valve is reflected as the dicrotic notch, point e. At point e, the pulmonic valve is also closed and the atrioventricular valves are opening. Upstroke of the arterial waveform begins approximately 0.2 seconds after the QRS complex. (From Campbell, B. [1997]. Arterial waveforms: Monitoring changes in figuration. *Heart & Lung, 26,* 204–214.)

aortic pressure during decreased ventricular ejection and the continued flow of blood into the periphery. The downstroke of the wave is interrupted by a sharp notch or incisura, denoting a transient reversal of blood flow just before aortic valve closure. Pressure in the aorta continues to decrease and is reflected on the arterial pressure waveform as a gradual downslope until the next ventricular systole. The interval after the incisura when the aortic pressure continues to decrease is referred to as the diastolic run-off period, and the slope of this period is affected by arterial stiffness and the rate at which the blood flows into the periphery (vascular resistance) (O'Rourke & Mancia, 1999).

The shape of the arterial waveform reflects the cushioning and conduit functions of the arterial system. Normally, approximately 50% to 60% of the SV is stored in the capacitive vessels and the remaining 40% to 50% is forwarded to the peripheral vessels (Belz, 1995). During diastole, the energy stored by the distention of the capacitive vessels is released as the aorta recoils, and the remaining blood moves into the periphery (Windkessel effect) (Fig. 23-6A). With increased arterial stiffness, a smaller amount of the SV can be stored in the capacitive vessels and a greater proportion of the SV is

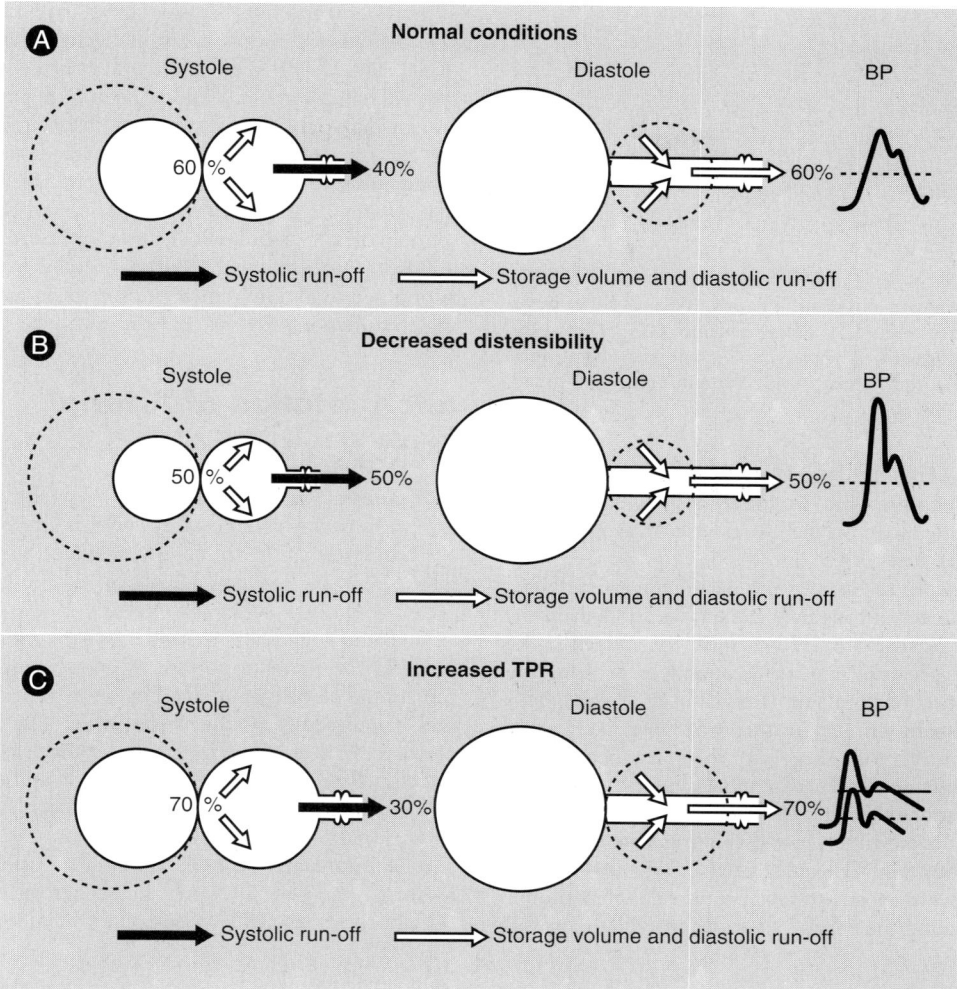

■ **Figure 23–6.** Diagrammatic representation of the cushioning effect of arteries on storage volume, systolic run-off, diastolic run-off, and arterial pulse wave. (*A*) Normal conditions. (*B*) Conditions of decreased arterial distensibility. (*C*) Conditions of increased total peripheral resistance. (From London, G. M., & Guérin, A. [1999]. Influence of arterial pulse and reflective waves on SBP and cardiac function. *Journal of Hypertension,* 17[Suppl. 2], S4–S5.)

transferred directly into the peripheral circulation. The increased arterial stiffness is manifested as an increased systolic pressure and a rapid decrease to the diastolic pressure (caused by greater run-off) (Fig. 23-6B). If the SVR is increased, the amount of blood stored in the capacitive vessels remains normal or increased; however, there is a decrease in the run-off of blood into the periphery. The increased SVR is manifested by an increased diastolic and mean blood pressure (Fig. 23-6C).

The arterial pressure waveform changes its contour when recorded at different sites along the arterial circuit (O'Rourke et al., 1993; Rowell et al., 1968) (Fig. 23-7). The pulse pressure and the systolic pressure increase, and the ascending limb of the waveform becomes steeper. In addition, the incisura is gradually replaced by a later diastolic wave (dicrotic notch). The change in amplitude and contour of the arterial waveform is primarily caused by peripheral pulse wave reflection (O'Rourke, 1993). Reflection occurs when flow is impeded (i.e., when low-resistance arteries terminate in high-resistance

vessels) and the pressure wave is reflected in a retrograde (backward) fashion. This retrograde pressure wave combines with the antegrade (forward) pressure pulse, and the arterial pressure is augmented.

The timing of the return of the reflected pressure wave from the periphery is important because if the reflected wave arrives during systole, it increases LV workload (O'Rourke & Kelly, 1993; Westerhof & O'Rouke, 1995). In young individuals, the reflected waves arrive at the heart after closure of the aortic valves, which beneficially augments the DBP and thus coronary perfusion. In young healthy individuals, the radial pressure exceeds central aortic pressure by 5 to 20 mm Hg. However, with aging or increased stiffness of the arteries (i.e., hypertension), the retrograde pulse wave arrives back at the heart during systole, which increases the SBP, and is the reason that the central aortic SBP is similar to peripheral systolic pressure (O'Rourke et al., 1993). Clinically, the increased systolic and pulse pressures are important as they are predictive of

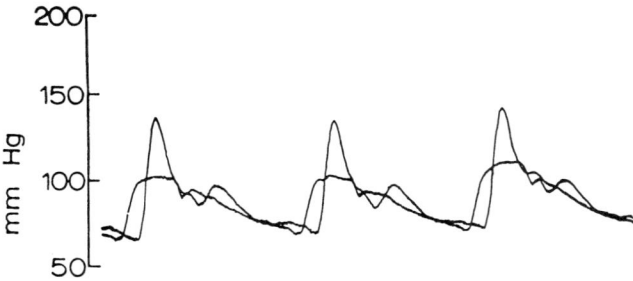

■ **Figure 23–7.** Simultaneous recordings of aortic and radial arterial pressure waves. (From Rowell, L. D., Brengelmann, G. L., Blackmon, R. J. et al. [1968]. Disparities between aortic and peripheral pulse pressures induced by upright exercise and vasomotor changes in man. *Circulation, 37,* 954–964.)

cardiovascular risk (Franklin et al., 1999). Additionally, in the presence of heart failure, the augmented systolic pressure, which causes increased load on the heart, has a greater deleterious effect on cardiac function.

The relation between the central and peripheral arterial pressure is also altered in conditions such as exercise, shock, and the administration of vasoactive medications. In exercise, the peripheral systolic pressure may be as much as 80 mm Hg greater than central aortic pressure (Rowell et al., 1968). This finding has important clinical implications for exercise in patients who have undergone surgery of the aorta, because the peripheral pressure is not necessarily reflective of the pressure stress being applied to the aorta. In shock, the peripheral systolic pressure may overestimate the ascending aortic pressure by as much as 20 mm Hg (O'Rourke et al., 1993).

Recognition of central aortic systolic pressure augmentation is important in evaluating the effects of various vasodilator agents.

Nitroglycerin and nitroprusside substantially decrease aortic pressure without a clinically measurable change in brachial pressure (Kelly et al., 1990). This effect, which is the result of the reduction in pulse–wave reflection (Fig. 23-8), may explain why a patient may "look better" after the initiation of vasodilator therapy even though there has been no marked decrease in peripheral blood pressure or preload. Conversely, vasoconstrictive agents (e.g., norepinephrine) increase peripheral pulse pressure and central aortic pressure, with femoral pressure higher than radial pressure (Dorman et al., 1998). Clinically, use of radial pressure as opposed to a more central pressure (e.g., femoral) may lead to underestimation of central pressure and excessive dosing.

Interpretation of Arterial Pressure Data

The mean arterial pressure (MAP), which represents the average pressure through a cardiac cycle, is affected by the CO and SVR as described by the following equation:

$$MAP = CO \times SVR$$

Recall of the factors that affect systolic, diastolic, and mean arterial pressures is important when assessing changes in blood pressure. The SBP is affected by LV SV, peak rate of ejection, and distensibility of the vessel walls. The DBP is primarily affected by arterial peripheral resistance. The pulse pressure, which is the difference between systolic and diastolic pressures, is determined by SV, peak rate of ventricular ejection, and the distensibility of the arterial walls.

The important point is that the peripheral SBP may be as much as 5 to 20 mm Hg higher than the aortic SBP (O'Rourke et al., 1993). Both peripheral wave reflection and

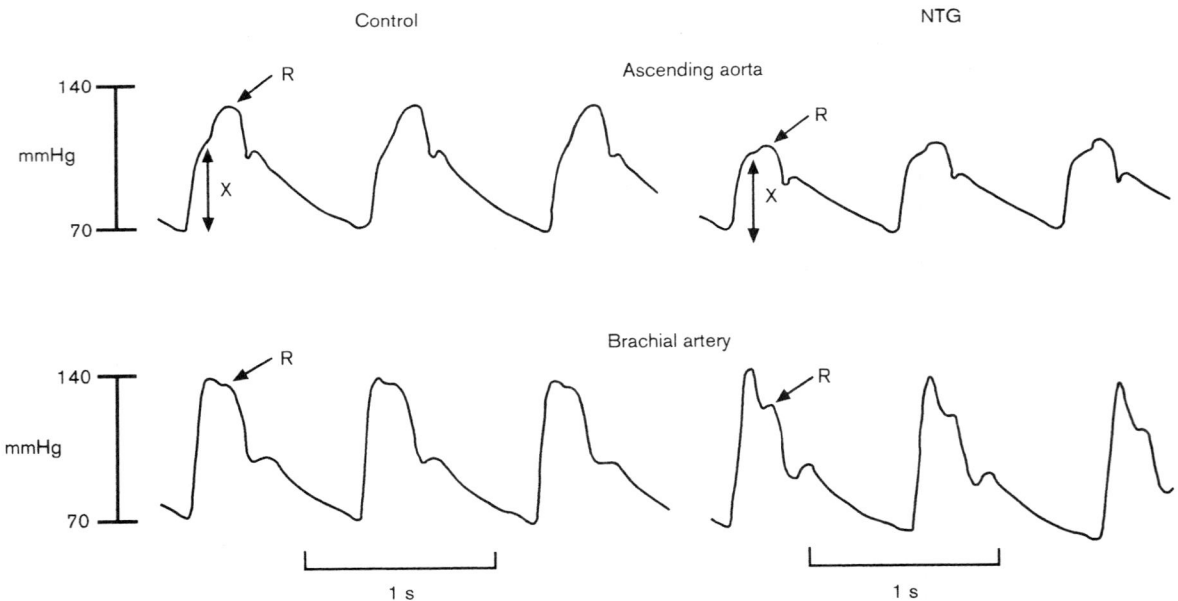

■ **Figure 23–8.** Pressure wave recorded directly in a central and peripheral artery. Nitroglycerine 0.3 mg (SL) on average caused a fall of 11 mm Hg in aortic systolic pressure more than the decrease in the brachial systolic pressure. Note the effect on the reflected (R) wave. (From Kelly, R. P., Gibbs, H. H., O'Rourke, M. F. et al. [1990]. Nitroglycerine has more favourable effects on left ventricular afterload than apparent from measurement of pressure in a peripheral artery. *European Heart Journal,* 11, 138–144.)

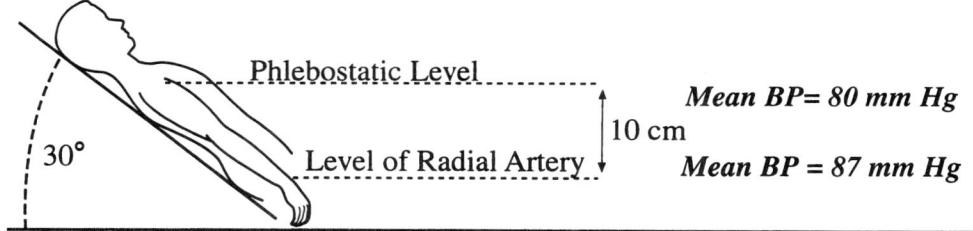

■ **Figure 23–9.** Effect of two reference points on the measured mean arterial pressure (MAP) in a patient in the 30-degree supine position. If the distance between the phlebostatic level and the radial insertion site is 10 cm, the MAP measured by the arterial line referenced to the radial insertion site will be 7.3 mm Hg higher than the pressure measured in the arterial line referenced to the phlebostatic level (1 cm = 0.73 mm Hg). (From Bridges, E. J., & Middleton, R. [1997]. Direct arterial vs oscillometric monitoring of blood pressure: Stop comparing and pick one [a decision making algorithm]. *Critical Care Nurse, 17*[3], 66.)

the end-pressure product, which is the result of the conversion of kinetic energy from flowing blood into pressure as the blood strikes the upstream-looking arterial catheter, cause augmentation of the SBP (Grossman, 1996). However, the MAP and the DBP are relatively unchanged in the periphery, and the MAP provides a more consistent value to evaluate and guide therapy.

Evaluation of the pulse pressure has taken on greater importance with its identification as a risk factor for cardiovascular disease. Recent research has demonstrated an increased relationship between pulse pressure and myocardial infarction, stroke, congestive heart failure, and total mortality (Haider et al., 2003; Psaty et al., 2001). The Framingham Study found that in patients with hypertension, the brachial pulse pressure is a stronger risk factor than SBP for myocardial infarction (Franklin et al., 1999).

Alterations in pulse pressure may be diagnostic. An increased pulse pressure is commonly seen with fever, anemia, exercise, and hyperthyroidism. Aortic regurgitation is associated with increased pulse pressure (Kern & Aguirre, 1992). In this case, the increased pulse pressure is caused by the rapid ejection of a large SV ("water-hammer pulse"), which increases the SBP, and a rapid and marked decrease in diastolic pressure ("collapsing pulse") secondary to flow back through the insufficient valve and peripheral vasodilation. An increase in pulse pressure also occurs with bradycardia because of an increase in SV. With aging (i.e., age older than 50 to 60) the arterial tree stiffens, and the pulse pressure increases because of an increase in pressure wave reflection from the periphery and the subsequent increase in SBP. The early wave reflection also decreases the normal peripheral to central gradient for pulse pressure. The implication of this decreased gradient is that brachial cuff pressures become a more accurate measure of central pulse pressure, and thus a more accurate indicator of cardiovascular risk. An acute decrease in pulse pressure is not a normal finding and may indicate an increase in vascular resistance, decreased SV (e.g., aortic stenosis); or decreased intravascular volume.

Direct Arterial Versus Cuff Pressure

There is no basis for the practice of comparing the intra-arterial blood pressure with the auscultatory or oscillometric blood pressure to assess if the systolic and diastolic pressures are similar. The direct method is based on pressure, whereas the oscillometric methods depends on flow-induced oscillations in the arterial wall (Ramsey, 1991). An erroneous assumption is that pressure equals flow. As described by a derivation of Ohm's law (pressure = flow × resistance), if resistance remains constant, there is a direct relationship between pressure and flow. However, clinically, resistance is seldom constant. Thus, blood pressure may appear adequate while flow is decreased, or conversely pressure may be low although perfusion remains adequate. Whereas the SBP varies depending on the measurement method used, the MAP is a relatively stable value across a wide variety of patients and methods and may provide a better means of monitoring the patient.

In addition to the physical factors that cause the differences in arterial pressure measured in various locations in the body, there are also technical factors that affect measurement accuracy (see Fig. 23-4). The accuracy of direct arterial pressure is affected by excessive tubing length (>4 feet), air bubbles in the tubing, and incorrect referencing. Oscillometric measurement is affected by the cuff size (bladder width 40% of the circumference of the limb at the point of measurement and sufficient to encircle 80% of the limb), loose cuff application (should only be able to slide one finger under the cuff), the presence of intrinsic (shivering, arm motion) and extrinsic movement (external compression of the cuff, passive arm motion), and variations in anatomy and physiology (respiratory variation, arrhythmias, patient talking, conically shaped arms) (Bridges & Middleton, 1997; Bur et al., 2003; Fonseca-Reyes et al., 2003). Additionally, the oscillometric system directly measures the mean pressure and extrapolates the systolic and diastolic pressure based on an algorithm, which may affect the accuracy of the systolic and diastolic pressure measurements.

Referencing to the right atrium is important for direct and oscillometric blood pressure monitoring. If the transducer or the arm is positioned above the right atrium, there will be a decrease in the measured pressure (Fig. 23-9). Conversely, if the transducer/arm is positioned below the atrium, there will be an increase in the measured pressure (Kirchoff et al., 1984; Netea et al., 2003). Algorithms have been developed to guide assessment of the physiological and technical factors that affect direct and oscillometric arterial pressure measurements, and to aid in answering the question, "Which do you believe, the arterial line or the cuff?" (Bridges & Middleton, 1997; Gore et al., 1995).

Table 23–4 ■ MOST FREQUENT COMPLICATIONS ASSOCIATED WITH ARTERIAL CATHETERIZATION

Complication	Risk Factors	Preventive Actions
Arterial occlusion/distal ischemia	• Catheter >20 gauge • Catheter in place >3 days • Female • Low CO/hypotension • Peripheral vascular disease • Vasopressor agents • Anticoagulation (↓ risk) • Femoral (↓ risk) • Systemic antithrombotics or anticoagulants (↓ risk) • Catheter length sheaths/arterial lines (↓ risk)	• Use heparinized flush solution (AACN, 1993; Randolph et al., 1998b) • Aspirate clot or discontinue line if thrombosis is suspected • Perform Allen test before insertion • Perform routine monitoring of distal perfusion (skin color, temperature and capillary refill) and after line manipulation • No beneficial effect from repeated flushes • No effect from method of blood sampling (waste versus nonwaste) (Kaye et al., 2001)
Bleeding	• Insertion site (femoral or axillary)	• Maintain system integrity • Monitor waveform for damping (may indicate loose connections)
Infection	• Insertion site preparation • Catheter in place >5–7 days • Insertion site	• See Table 23–1

Complications Related to Arterial Catheterization

The most common sites for arterial catheterization are the radial and femoral arteries. The most common complication associated with these sites is temporary occlusion of the artery (radial 19.7%; femoral 1.5%), although permanent occlusion of the artery is rare (0.09% and 0.18%, respectively). The axillary artery is a less common insertion site, with complication rates similar to radial and femoral insertions. Bleeding is a rare complication for all insertion sites (0.6%–1.6%), with increased incidence in femoral and axillary lines (Scheer et al., 2002). A summary of risk factors and actions to prevent complications is presented in Table 23-4.

CENTRAL VENOUS PRESSURE MONITORING

The central venous pressure (CVP) directly reflects right atrial pressure (RAP) and indirectly reflects the preload of the right ventricle or RV end-diastolic pressure. The CVP is determined by vascular tone, the volume of blood returning to the heart, the pumping ability of the heart, and patient position (supine, standing).

The CVP is measured in the superior vena cava and the RAP is measured from the proximal port of the PA catheter. Normally, the CVP ranges from 3 to 8 cm H_2O or 2 to 6 mm Hg (1 mm Hg = 1.36 cm H_2O). In the supine/flat position, a CVP of less than 2 mm Hg may indicate hypovolemia, vasodilation, or increased myocardial contractility. An increased CVP may indicate increased circulatory blood volume, vasoconstriction, or decreased myocardial contractility. An increased CVP is also observed in RV failure, tricuspid insufficiency, positive-pressure breathing, pericardial tamponade, pulmonary embolus, and obstructive pulmonary disease.

Indications

The placement of a central venous or RA catheter is indicated to secure venous access, to administer vasoactive drugs and parenteral nutrition, and to monitor right heart preload. Hemodynamic monitoring using a CVP is most often performed when cardiopulmonary function is relatively normal. Monitoring the CVP has regained importance with the recognition of the importance of right heart function on left heart function.

Catheter Placement

Insertion of a CVP catheter is achieved percutaneously or by venous cut-down through a central or peripheral vein. Selection of the appropriate site depends on the skill of the clinician inserting the catheter, physical structure and age of the patient, thoracic deformities, and clinical circumstances.

The CVP can also be monitored via a peripherally inserted central venous catheter (PICC). Measurements from the PICC overestimate measurements from a central catheter (1 ± 3 mm Hg). Passive hydrostatic pressure equilibration across the PICC line takes approximately 60 minutes, but this pressure gradient can be overcome immediately with a pressure line infusing fluid at 3 mL/hr (Black et al., 2000; Lopez et al., 2003). Measurements obtained via tunneled catheters are also comparable to direct RA pressure measurements (Blot et al., 2000)

Limitations

The CVP is not an accurate indicator of LV function or left heart preload (Forrester et al., 1971). In the presence of normal right heart function, severe deterioration of LV function may not be reflected by a change in RAP or CVP. An increased CVP is usually an indication of later stages of LV failure, although the CVP may remain normal even in the presence of high PA pressures and pulmonary edema.

Complications

Complications associated with CVP monitoring include localized infection, arrhythmias, vessel laceration, RV perforation, thrombophlebitis, hematoma formation at the insertion site, and pneumothorax or a malpositioned catheter (Timsit et al., 1998). There is an increased risk of arterial puncture, but fewer malpositioned catheters, with the jugular approach. Conversely, there may be a decreased risk of infection with a subclavian versus jugular or femoral insertion (Ruesch et al., 2002). Correct catheter placement is essential as intracardiac positioning of the catheter increases the risk for tamponade, whereas positioning of the catheter tip high in the superior vena cava is associated with increased thrombosis caused by vascular damage (Jones & Bodenham, 2002). Use of a portable ultrasound to place a central venous catheter decreases insertion failure rate and the incidence of insertion-related complications (Hind et al., 2003; Keenan, 2002). The use of heparin decreases thrombus formation and may also decrease the risk of infection (Randolph et al., 1998a).

Measurement Technique

The CVP system is referenced by placing the air–fluid interface of the stopcock at the level of the phlebostatic axis (+ in Fig. 23-1). With correct referencing, the hemodynamically stable patient can be positioned up to 45° for CVP measurements (Potger & Elliott, 1994).

An area of confusion when measuring the CVP is which port to transduce from a triple-lumen catheter. There are no research-based, standardized recommendations regarding port selection. The pressures measured from the various ports are small but different (<1.5 mm Hg) (Scott et al., 1998). Because of the potential for a clinically significant change in pressure depending on the port transduced, it seems prudent to transduce consistently one port, and if a change in the site of monitoring is necessary, to annotate the change on the flowsheet.

Interpretation of Data

Useful clinical information can be obtained by examining the CVP/RAP waveforms. There are five mechanical components of the RAP waveform. The mean RAP is determined by bisecting the a, c, and v waves so that there are equal areas above and below the bisection. A dual-channel strip chart recorder should be used to identify the corresponding venous pressure waves (a, c, and v waves) with the electrical events on the ECG (Display 23-2). The RAP tracing may be useful in the diagnosis of wide-complex tachyarrhythmias of unknown origin, tricuspid insufficiency, pericardial tamponade (Fig. 23-10), and constrictive pericarditis.

Assessment of the RAP is useful in guiding differential diagnosis. For example, if the PAWP is increased and greater than the RAP, the differential diagnosis should focus on the left heart. If both the PAWP and RAP are increased, the differential diagnosis should include diffuse coronary artery disease or cardiomyopathy, pericardial constriction or tamponade, or overdistention of the right heart. If the RAP is increased and

greater than the PAWP, consideration should be given to right heart failure or pulmonary vascular disease (Magder, 1998). In patients with severe heart failure, RAP ≥10 mm Hg had a positive predictive value of 85% for a PAWP ≥22 mm Hg and was useful in evaluating 80% of the patients studied (Drazner et al., 1999). Additionally, as described below, assessment of the dynamic changes of the RAP may be an indicator of fluid responsiveness.

PULMONARY ARTERY PRESSURE MONITORING

Indications

Since its introduction in 1970 (Swan et al., 1970), invasive hemodynamic monitoring with a PA catheter has become one of the most commonly used diagnostic tools in critical care (Ginosar & Sprung, 1996). In response to a study that suggested increased mortality associated with PA catheterization (Connors et al., 1996), there was a call for a reduction or restriction in the use of PA catheters. Since then, consensus statements have been issued by a number of professional organizations (Bernard et al., 2000; Pulmonary Artery Consensus; 1997). The consensus statements indicate that PA catheterization may decrease complications or improve outcomes in patients with hypotension and cardiogenic shock, mechanical complications, right heart failure, peripheral vascular disease, and trauma. Areas given high priority for further research related to PA catheter use include refractory congestive heart failure, acute respiratory distress syndrome, severe sepsis, and septic shock (Bernard et al., 2000). There is also a general consensus that standardized education is needed for critical care providers. This latter recommendation is based on studies that have demonstrated a lack of knowledge of technical and clinical aspects of PA catheterization by critical care physicians and nurses (Burns et al., 1996).

Since the consensus conferences, several randomized control trials have been initiated. A recent multicenter study found no improvement in patient outcomes from PA-catheter guided therapy in older (older than age 60 years) surgical patients (Sandham et al., 2003). The results of this study have been challenged because of possible methodological limitations (De Backer et al., 2003). Other studies and meta-analysis found conflicting results regarding complications and mortality associated with PA catheterization (Afessa et al., 2001; Barone et al., 2001; Polanczyk et al., 2001). Thus, the question regarding the usefulness of PA catheterization remains unanswered.

Description of the Pulmonary Artery Catheter

The PA catheter is a multilumen, polyvinylchloride catheter with a variable external diameter. Many models of PA catheters are available (Fig. 23-11). The standard thermodilution catheter is 7.5 French in diameter and 110 cm long and is marked in 10-cm increments. The balloon is inflated with a

DISPLAY 23-2

RELATION OF RIGHT ATRIAL AND PULMONARY ARTERY PRESSURES TO ECG FINDINGS

Pressures/waveforms	Mechanical Event	ECG Findings	Example

RA Pressure (2–6 mm Hg)

a wave	RA systole	80–100 msec after P wave (Downslope of the a wave)
x descent	RA relaxation	
c wave	Tricuspid valve closure	After the QRS (follows the a wave by a time interval = PR)
v wave	RA filling against closed tricuspid valve	Peak of the T wave
y descent	RA emptying with opening of tricuspid valve (onset of RV diastole)	(Downslope of the v wave)

Interpretation: RAP tracing from patient on mechanical ventilation. The RAP is a mean pressure (bisect an end-expiratory waveform so that the areas above and below are equal). RAP = 15 mm Hg

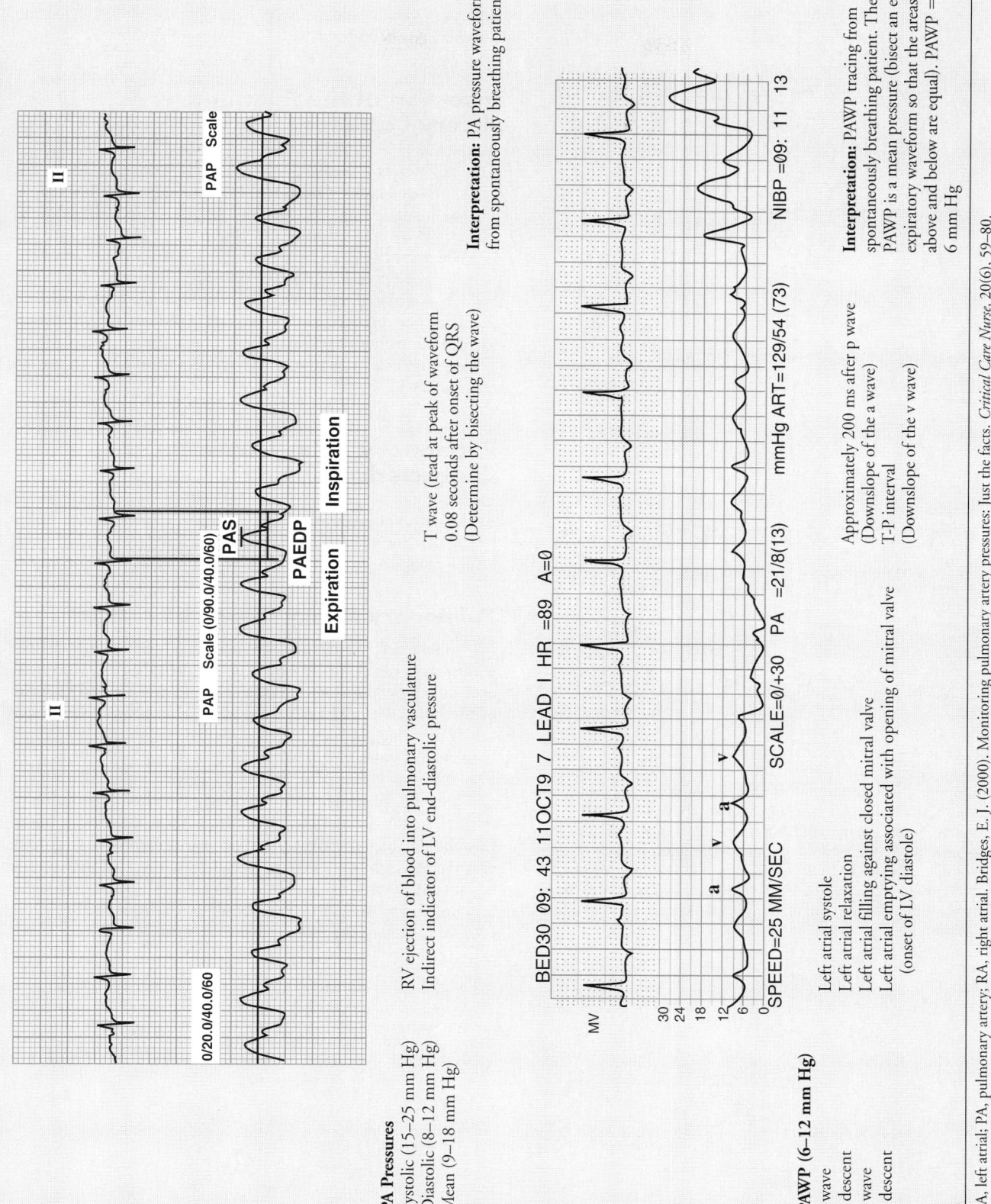

II

II

PAP   Scale (0/90.0/40.0/60)

PAP   Scale

0/20.0/40.0/60

PAS

PAEDP

Expiration   Inspiration

PA Pressures

Systolic (15–25 mm Hg)
Diastolic (8–12 mm Hg)
Mean (9–18 mm Hg)

RV ejection of blood into pulmonary vasculature
Indirect indicator of LV end-diastolic pressure

T wave (read at peak of waveform
0.08 seconds after onset of QRS
(Determine by bisecting the wave)

Interpretation: PA pressure waveform
from spontaneously breathing patient

BED30 09: 43 11OCT9 7 LEAD I HR =89   A=0

MV

30
24
18
12
6
0

a   v   a   v

SPEED=25 MM/SEC   SCALE=0/+30   PA =21/8(13)   mmHg ART=129/54 (73)   NIBP =09: 11 13

PAWP (6–12 mm Hg)

a wave   Left atrial systole
x descent   Left atrial relaxation
v wave   Left atrial filling against closed mitral valve
y descent   Left atrial emptying associated with opening of mitral valve
                (onset of LV diastole)

Approximately 200 ms after p wave
(Downslope of the a wave)
T-P interval
(Downslope of the v wave)

Interpretation: PAWP tracing from
spontaneously breathing patient. The
PAWP is a mean pressure (bisect an end-
expiratory waveform so that the areas
above and below are equal). PAWP =
6 mm Hg

LA, left atrial; PA, pulmonary artery; RA, right atrial. Bridges, E. J. (2000). Monitoring pulmonary artery pressures: Just the facts. *Critical Care Nurse*, 20(6), 59–80.

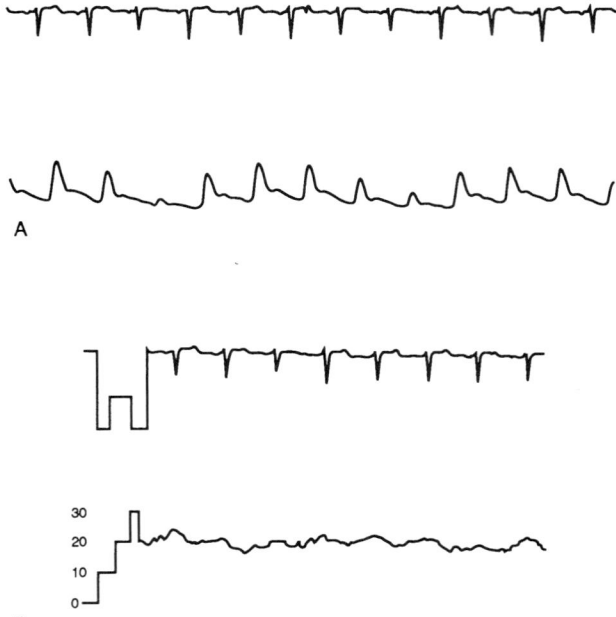

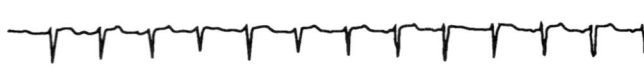

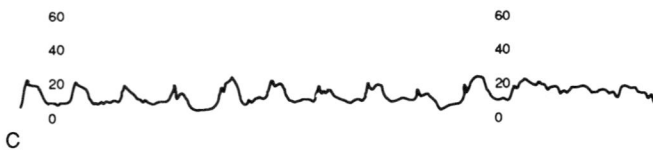

■ **Figure 23–10.** Pericardial tamponade in a spontaneously breathing patient. (*A*) Arterial waveform. Note the electrical alternans, alternating height or duration of the QRS complex, and pulsus paradoxus on the arterial waveform. (*B*) Right atrial pressure (RAP) = 20 mm Hg. (*C*) Pulmonary artery (PA) to PA wedge pressure. Pulmonary artery systolic (PAS) pressure = 26 mm Hg; pulmonary artery end-diastolic pressure (PAEDP) = 17 mm Hg; PA mean pressure = 19 mm Hg; PA wedge pressure = 20 mm Hg. Equalization of the diastolic pressures is the result of circumferential compression of all cardiac chambers.

maximum of 1.5 mL of air. Catheter patency is maintained with a heparinized solution, although research suggests that there is no difference in the patency rate between PA catheters maintained with saline versus a heparinized (1 U/mL) solution (Zevola et al., 1997).

Insertion of the Pulmonary Artery Catheter

The catheter is inserted percutaneously, with or without the use of fluoroscopy. Once the RA is reached, the balloon, located on the distal end of the catheter, is inflated and the catheter is "floated" through the RA and RV and out into the PA, where it occludes a branch of the PA. After the characteristic PA wedge pressure (PAWP) tracing has been obtained, the balloon is deflated, allowing the catheter to recoil slightly into the PA. The catheter is left in the balloon-down position to prevent pulmonary infarction. The nursing responsibilities during insertion of the PA catheter are summarized in Display 23-3.

Pulmonary Artery Waveform Characteristics

As the catheter passes through the heart, three pressure waveforms can be visualized using a PA catheter: RA, PA, and PAWP (Fig. 23-12B).

Pulmonary Artery Pressure

Pulmonary artery pressures provide an index of the pressure within the pulmonary vasculature and are affected by compliance of the LV, pulmonary vascular pressure, CO, and the state of the lung tissue. The PA pressure increases slightly with age (older than age 60 years, PA mean ≅ 16 ± 3 mm Hg; younger than age 60 years, PA mean ≅ 12 ± 2 mm Hg) (Davidson & Fee, 1990).

Three PA pressures are measured: systolic, diastolic, and mean. The PA systolic (PAS) pressure reflects the flow of blood into the PA from the RV. In the absence of elevated pulmonary vascular pressure or RV outflow obstruction, PAS pressure is equal to RV systolic pressure. During diastole, the mitral valve is open, and a continuous column of blood from the PA to the LA and LV exists; therefore, the pressure just before contraction

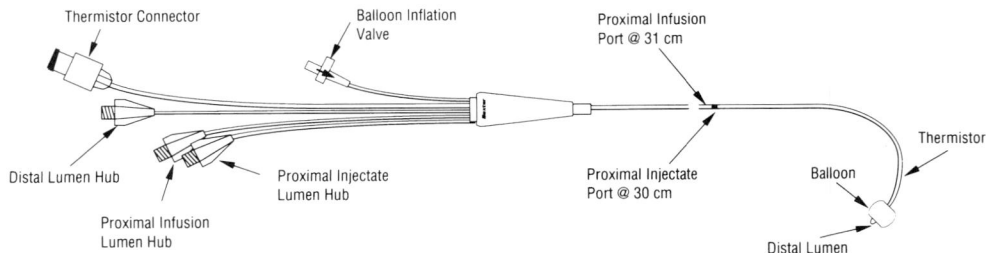

■ **Figure 23–11.** Venous infusion port PA catheter. (Courtesy of Baxter Healthcare Corporation, Edwards Critical Care Division, Santa Ana, CA.)

NURSING RESPONSIBILITIES DURING PULMONARY ARTERY CATHETER INSERTION

1. Prepare equipment
   a. Flush solution: 1–4 U heparin/mL of 5% dextrose in water or normal saline; remove all air from bag.
   b. Attach to pressure tubing with macrodrip chamber.
   c. Place flush solution in pressure bag and inflate to 50 mm Hg (low pressure minimizes microbubble formation during line preparation)
   d. Gently flush transducer/pressure tubing/stopcocks using aseptic technique. Avoid creation of microbubbles. Ensure all air bubbles are removed.
   e. Inflate pressure bag to 300 mm Hg (delivers solution at 3 mL/h)
   f. Attach pressure tubing to transducer system or cable, and reference system to patient's phlebostatic axis and zero system.
2. Assist during insertion
   a. Attach pressure tubing to proximal and distal ports and flush system.
   b. Determine integrity of balloon-provider inserting PA catheter by inflating the balloon; the balloon should be symmetric and not cover the tip.
   c. Transduce the distal lumen on monitor
   d. Inflate balloon at physician's direction (generally after catheter reaches right atrium).
   e. Monitor oscilloscope for characteristic waveform changes (see Fig. 23–12B) and ectopy.
   f. Record waveforms and pressures as catheter passes from right atrium to PAWP position.
   g. Deflate balloon once PAWP has been obtained, and note return of characteristic PA waveform.
   h. Secure catheter and note insertion distance.
   i. Apply sterile occlusive dressing (see infection control guidelines—Table 23–2).
   j. Obtain chest radiograph to confirm catheter placement.

(end-diastole) is approximately equal in the PA, left atrium, and left ventricle. As a result of the diastolic equalization, the PA end-diastolic pressure (PAEDP) is often used as an indirect indicator of PAWP and LV end diastolic pressure (LVEDP) (Bouchard et al., 1971). The difference between the RV end-diastolic pressure and PAEDP (an increase in the diastolic pressure as the catheter passes across the pulmonic valve) is an important characteristic in determining whether the catheter tip is correctly positioned in the PA or has flipped back into the right ventricle (Fig. 23-12B).

Pulmonary Artery Wedge Pressure

The PAWP is obtained by inflation of the balloon on the distal end of the PA catheter, which allows the catheter to float forward to occlude a segment of the PA. The occluded catheter creates a static column of blood through the pulmonary vasculature (Fig. 23-12A). This static column acts as an extension of the fluid within the catheter system and allows retrograde transmission of left heart pressures to the distal port of the catheter.

There is, in general, a good relationship between the mean PAWP and mean LAP. At end-diastole, pressure equalizes between the left atrium and ventricle; thus, the PAWP is used as an indirect measure of LV pressure. The assumption in using pressure as surrogate indicator of volume (preload) is that an increase in pressure indicates an increase in volume, and as described by Starling's Law of the Heart, an increase in CO. However, there are several factors that limit the use of pressure as an indicator of volume. First, the relationship between pressure and volume is curvilinear, not linear; thus, an absolute change in pressure (e.g., PAWP) is not associated with an absolute change in volume. Second, any alteration in myocardial compliance may affect the pressure–volume relation and limit the usefulness of the PAWP as an indicator of left heart preload. Absolute PAWP values should be used with caution in any situation that alters myocardial compliance, such as LV dysfunction or MI (particularly involving the posteroinferior surface of the heart) (Pinsky, 2003a). Third, the PAWP is affected by changes in pericardial pressure; thus the PAWP may not accurately reflect transmural pressure. Newer techniques, collectively referred to as functional hemodynamic monitoring, and more direct volumetric measures may address some of the limitations of the PAWP as an indicator of preload and fluid responsiveness.

In addition to being an indirect indicator of LVEDP, the PAWP is also an *estimate* of the capillary pressure (P_{cap}), which is the most important factor in the development of hydrostatic pulmonary edema (Cope et al., 1992). Assuming a close relationship between the PAWP and P_{cap}, in patients with MI, an increase in PAWP more than 18 mm Hg is associated with the onset of pulmonary congestion (Forrester et al., 1977). In contrast to patients with an acute MI, patients with chronic heart failure tolerate a substantially higher PAWP without the development of pulmonary edema (Chakko et al., 1991). This latter finding is thought to be caused by pulmonary vascular remodeling with increased wall thickness, increased arterial and venous resistance, and decreased capillary filtration (Huang, Kingsbury et al., 2001).

The close relationship between the PAWP and P_{cap} is based on the assumption that approximately 60% of the resistance across the pulmonary system occurs in the arterial (precapillary) vasculature and 40% is caused by venous resistance. When there is increased postcapillary resistance, the PAWP underestimates the actual P_{cap} and the patient may present with hydrostatic pulmonary edema despite a low PAWP (Cope et al., 1992). Caution must be taken in assuming that the PAWP is equivalent to the P_{cap} under conditions, such as sepsis or acute respiratory distress syndrome, in which there is an increase in pulmonary venous vascular resistance (Pinsky, 2003a, 2003c). Pulmonary edema may also occur with a normal PAWP if there is altered capillary or alveolar membrane permeability.

Pulmonary Artery Waveform Interpretation

Pulmonary artery waveform interpretation can be simplified by remembering that electrical activity, as indicated by the ECG, precedes mechanical activity (see Display 23-2) (Bridges, 2000b). Pulmonary artery pressure waveforms are useful in the diagnosis of various cardiac abnormalities.

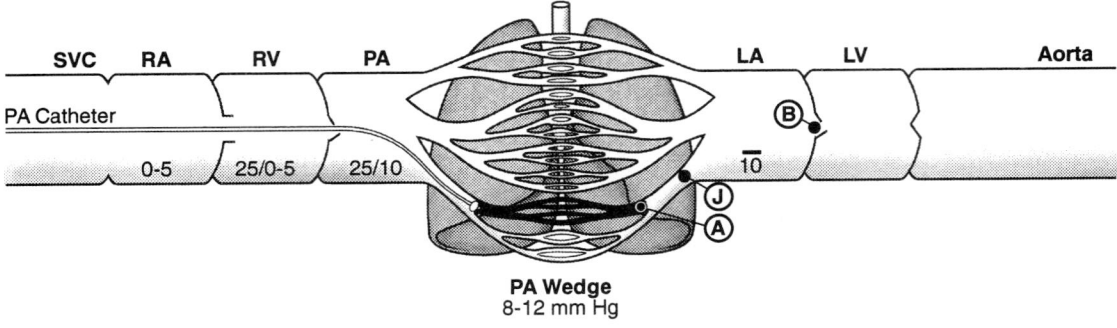

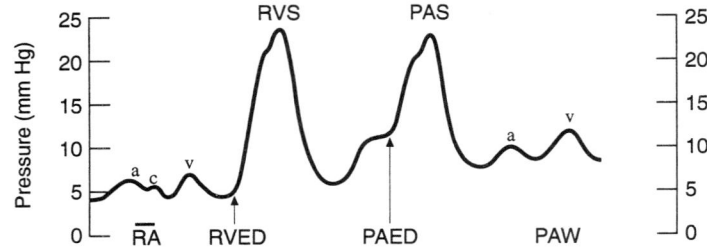

■ **Figure 23–12.** (*A*) Schema of the principle underlying the use of the PAWP as an indicator of LV preload. When the inflated balloon on the catheter obstructs arterial flow, the catheter records the pressure at the junction of the static column of fluid and flowing venous channels (J-point). The J-point occurs in the venous system, approximately 1.5 cm from the LA. The PAWP underestimates P$_{cap}$ when there is increased resistance in the postcapillary vessels proximal to the J-point (point A). The PAWP overestimates LV end-diastolic pressure (LVEDP) if there is obstruction distal to the J-point (point B; e.g., mitral stenosis, left atrial myxoma), whereas the PAWP underestimates the LVEDP in the presence of premature closure of the mitral valve as a result of aortic insufficiency. (*B*) Characteristic waveforms observed as the PA catheter is "floated" from the right atrium through the right ventricle and into the PA, where it wedges. Note that the mean RAP is similar to the RVEDP, the RV systolic and PAS pressures are similar, and there is a step-up in pressure as the catheter crosses the pulmonic valve and enters the PA. In a correctly positioned catheter, the PAWP is lower than the mean PA pressure and has a waveform that is relatively similar to the RAP (although slightly delayed relative to the ECG).

Pulmonary Artery Wedge Pressure

The PAWP waveform is similar to the LAP waveform but is slightly damped and phase delayed (50 to 70 milliseconds) because of pulmonary vascular transmission (Fig 23-13A). The PAWP is a mean pressure and is determined by bisecting the a and v waves, so there is an equal area above and below the bisection (see Display 23-2).

1. Elevated a wave: conditions that increase resistance to LV filling
   a. Mitral stenosis
   b. LV failure (Fig. 23-13B)
   c. Acutely ischemic left ventricle
2. Elevated v wave: conditions that cause increased LA filling during ventricular systole
   a. Acute mitral insufficiency (Fig. 23-13C)
   b. Ventricular septal defect
   c. Aortic regurgitation

The giant v wave in acute mitral regurgitation and ventricular septal defect is caused by augmented LA filling. The height of the v wave is determined by LA loading volume and compliance and LV afterload, and is not a consistent indicator of disease severity (Haskell & French, 1988). In the presence of a large v wave associated with mitral regurgitation (v wave 10 mm Hg greater than a wave), LVEDP is best correlated (*r* = 0.89) with the trough or nadir of the *x* descent (Haskell &

French, 1988) (Fig. 23-13C). The mean PAWP and peak of the a wave overestimate the LVEDP. The clinical importance of the giant v wave, regardless of cause, is the marked increase in P$_{cap}$, with the potential development of pulmonary edema. The ECG is useful in differentiating a bifid PA waveform from a PA wedge with a large v wave (Fig. 23-14).

3. Elevated a and v waves
   a. Cardiac tamponade (Fig. 23-10)
   b. Hypervolemia
   c. Constrictive pericarditis
   d. LV failure (Fig. 23-13B)
   e. Mitral stenosis

Although the mean PAWP is similar to LAP, in mitral stenosis, a pressure gradient develops between the LA and LV; therefore, the PA and PAWP are not accurate indices of LV pressure (Lange et al., 1989).

Pulmonary Artery Pressure

The PA systolic pressure is represented by a steep rise during RV ejection and usually occurs after the QRS complex or near the T wave of the ECG (Display 23-2). The PAEDP is measured 0.08 second after the onset of the QRS (Lipp-Ziff & Kawanishi, 1991), and the PA mean is determined by bisecting the end-expiratory waveform, so there is an equal area above and below the bisection. In the presence of LV dysfunction, the

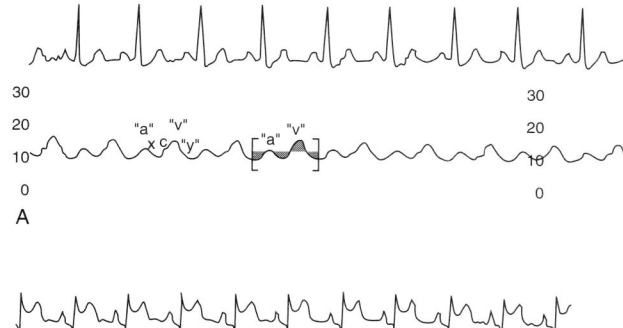

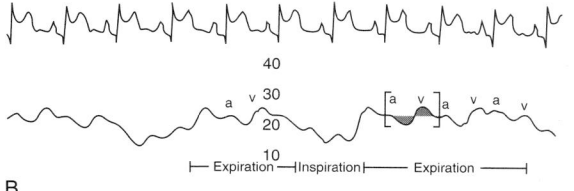

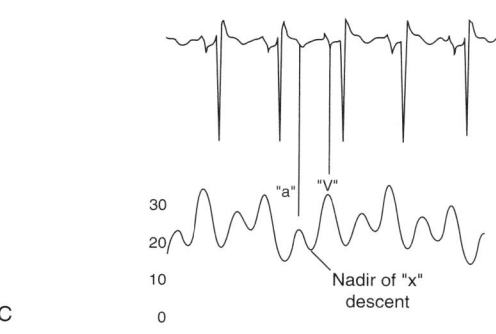

■ **Figure 23–13.** Pulmonary artery (PA) wedge pressure determination. (*A*) Normal PA wedge pressure tracing. The mean PA wedge pressure is read on an end-expiratory waveform and is determined by bisecting the a and v waves so there is an equal area above and below the bisection. PA wedge pressure = 12 mm Hg. (*B*) Elevated a and v waves. Patient with a history of an inferolateral myocardial infarction with congestive heart failure. The increased a and v waves are consistent with LV failure. PA wedge pressure = 24 mm Hg. (*C*) PA wedge pressure with elevated V wave in a spontaneously breathing patient who was complaining of chest pain. The PA wedge pressure is read at the nadir of the *x* descent. Note the relation of the v wave to the TP interval of the electrocardiogram. PA wedge pressure = 17 mm Hg.

presystolic a wave may provide a more consistent index of LVEDP than PAEDP or PAWP; however, the presence of this wave is variable (Rahimtoola et al., 1972).
Elevated PA pressures occur with:

1. Increased PVR (Fig. 23-15A)
   a. Pulmonary hypertension
   b. Chronic obstructive pulmonary disease
   c. Acute respiratory distress syndrome
   d. Hypoxia
   e. Pulmonary embolus
2. Increased pulmonary venous pressure
   a. LV failure
   b. Mitral stenosis
3. Increased pulmonary blood flow
   a. Hypervolemia
   b. Atrial and ventricular septal defects
4. Mitral insufficiency (Fig. 23-15B)

Technical Aspects of Pulmonary Artery Pressure Monitoring

Numerous research studies have evaluated the technical aspects of PA pressure measurement (Bridges, 2000b; Keickeisen, 1998; Quaal, 2001). Incorrect techniques may introduce error into pressure measurements and potentiate therapeutic mismanagement of critically ill patients.

Positioning

Traditionally, PA and PAWP measurements have been obtained with the patient supine and flat; however, this position may be poorly tolerated in patients with increased intracranial pressure or cardiopulmonary dysfunction. Research has shown that in a wide variety of critically ill patients, accurate PA pressures can be obtained in the supine position with legs extended and a backrest elevation up to 60° (Bridges, 2000a). Measurement of PA pressures in the sitting position (legs dependent) is not recommended. In the lateral position, PA and PAWP can be obtained in the 30° and 90° lateral positions, as long as an angle-specific reference is used (Table 23-1). Because some patients respond differently to position change, pressure measurements obtained in the flat, supine position should be compared with those measurements obtained with backrest elevation or lateral position before assuming no difference.

Pulmonary Effects

Correct function of the PA catheter requires a continuous column of fluid between the catheter tip and the left atrium. There are three physiologic zones in the lung that depend on the interaction of alveolar, arterial, and venous pressures (West et al., 1964). Alteration in any of these pressures may affect the fluid column between the catheter tip and the left atrium and alter the accuracy of PA pressure measurements. However, the delineation of the various lung zones is not clear-cut. Within any given level of the lung, all three zone conditions may coexist (Glenny et al., 1999). Because the presence of a zone-3 vascular bed is crucial for accurate PA pressure measurements, assessment of this factor should be performed routinely (Display 23-1 and Fig. 23-16).

PAEDP–PAWP Gradient

Assessment of the PAEDP–PAWP gradient provides information about pulmonary vascular resistance, incorrect catheter position in nonzone 3 location, a partial wedge, or venous obstruction. Normally, there is a 0- to 5-mm Hg pressure gradient between the PAEDP and the PAWP, which is consistent with the forward flow of blood from the PA to the LA. An increase in this gradient of more than 5 mm Hg may indicate increased PVR associated with such conditions as pulmonary hypertension, cor pulmonale, pulmonary embolus, hypoxia, Eisenmenger's syndrome, or inadequate time for diastolic equalization of pressures (tachycardia). In these clinical situations, the PAEDP is not an accurate indicator of LA pressure, and the PAWP should be used.

A PAWP that is greater than the PAEDP indicates some form of obstruction between the PA catheter and the LA, such as mitral stenosis, LA myxoma, mitral valve regurgitation,

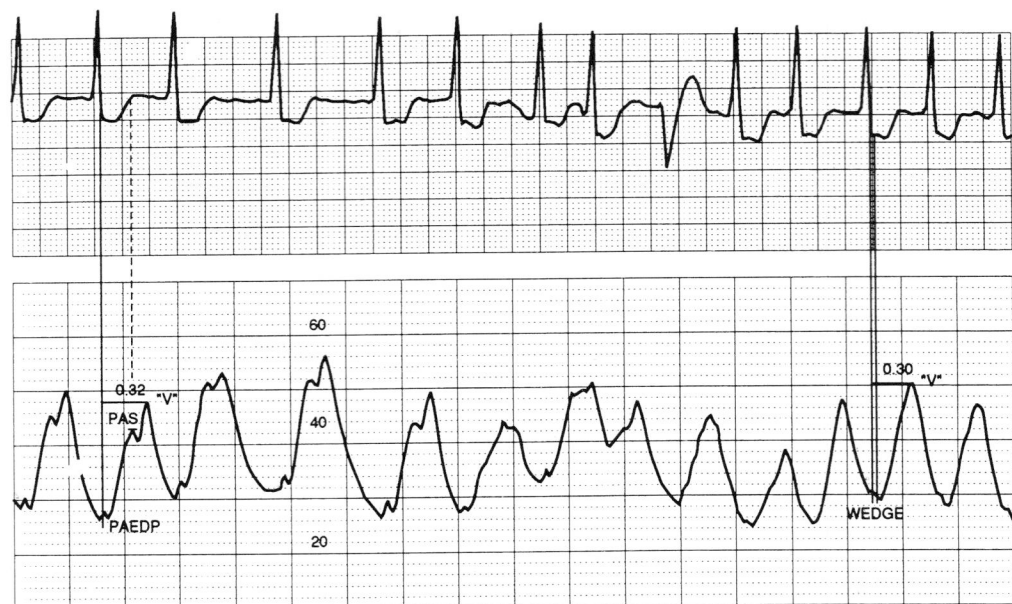

■ **Figure 23–14.** Pulmonary artery (PA) pressure or PA wedge pressure? In the presence of a large V wave, the PA wedge pressure tracing may mimic a PA tracing. Comparison of the PA and PAWP relative to the ECG reveals the following: (1) the v wave of the PA wedge pressure occurs during the TP interval, whereas the initial systolic upstroke of PA waveform is closely related to the end of the QRS complex; and (2) the PA v wave is a sharp upward deflection on the descending limb of the PA pressure curve, having the same temporal relation as the v wave in the PA wedge pressure tracing. PA wedge pressure = 30 mm Hg.

nonzone 3 catheter placement or a partial wedge. In these clinical situations, the PAWP is of limited use as an indicator of LA pressures.

Evaluation of the PAEDP–PAWP gradient is useful in differentiating cardiac and pulmonary pathology:

1. PAEDP = 30 mm Hg; PAWP = 22 mm Hg; PAEDP–PAWP = 8 mm Hg (increased LV preload and PVR, e.g., LV failure with pulmonary edema)
2. PAEDP = 35 mm Hg; PAWP = 13 mm Hg; PAEDP–PAWP = 19 mm Hg (increased PVR without an increase in LV volume, e.g., acute pulmonary embolus, addition of PEEP, hypoxia)
3. PAEDP = 23 mm Hg; PAWP = 20 mm Hg; PAEDP–PAWP = 3 mm Hg (LV overload without pulmonary involvement; in this situation, the PAEDP is an accurate indirect indicator of LV preload)

Spontaneous Versus Mechanical Ventilation

During spontaneous ventilation, the alveolar pressure decreases during inspiration and increases during expiration. Conversely, during positive-pressure ventilation, intrathoracic pressure increases during inspiration and decreases during expiration. The changes in intrathoracic pressure are transmitted to the cardiovascular structures in the thorax and are reflected by corresponding changes in PA pressures. At end-expiration, when no airflow occurs, pleural pressure equals atmospheric pressure regardless of the mode of ventilation and does not affect intracardiac pressures.

In patients with respiratory variation in the PA waveform tracing, the use of digital readings is unreliable because of the unselective nature of electrical averaging (Johnson & Schumann, 1995; Lundstedt, 1997). In addition, the "stop cursor" method (freezing the monitor screen) is less reliable than the graphic method (Lundstedt, 1997). The analysis of graphic recordings to identify the end-expiratory phase remains the recommended method for interpreting PA waveforms (Ahrens & Schallom, 2001). The addition of an airway pressure tracing may further improve the accuracy of the measurements (Rizvi et al., 2003). Display 23-1 reviews guidelines for recording PA pressure measurements.

Manipulation/Removal of PA Catheter

In a 1997 survey by the American Association of Critical Care Nurses, 54% of the respondents indicated they were removing or discontinuing PA catheters and 28% were advancing the catheters (AACN, 1997). Written protocols were available for withdrawal of catheters from a wedge position (61%), discontinuation of catheters (82%), and advancing catheters (22%). These procedures are not risk-free. Potential complications during repositioning include PA rupture, cardiac perforation or tamponade, thrombus formation, sepsis or catheter-related infection, and cardiac arrhythmias.

To safely manipulate or discontinue the catheter, critical care nurses must have knowledge of the correct technique for catheter insertion, be able to interpret waveforms (normal and

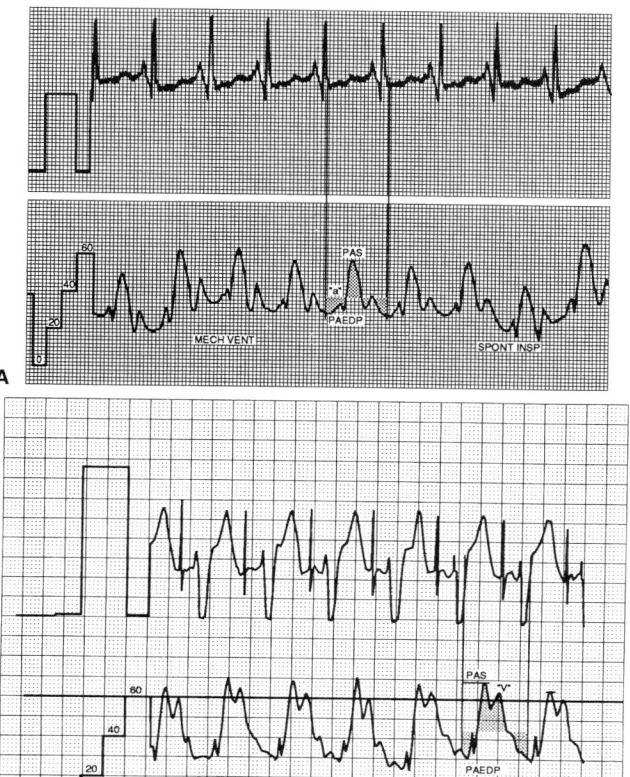

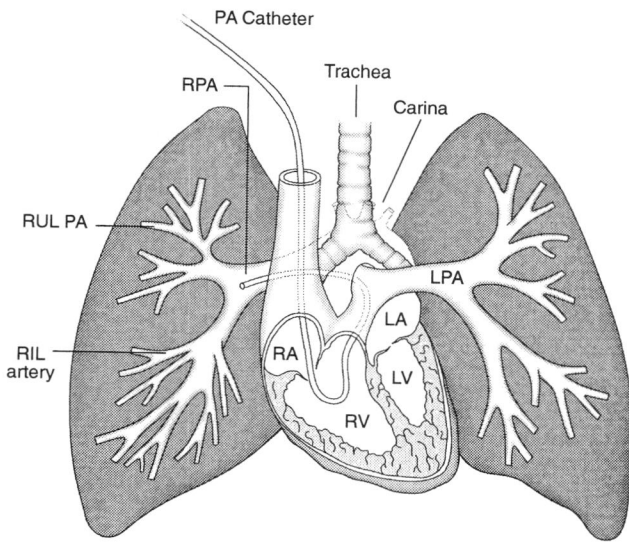

■ **Figure 23–16.** Schema of the cardiopulmonary structures demonstrating the relationship between the left atrium, pulmonary artery (PA), and pulmonary vasculature, with a correctly positioned PA catheter. RUL PA, right upper lobe PA; RIL, right interlobar PA; RPA, right PA; LPA, left PA; RA, right atrium; LA, left atrium; RV, right ventricle; LV, left ventricle.

■ **Figure 23–15.** Pulmonary artery (PA) pressure determination. (*A*) Elevated PA pressure related to LV failure and acute respiratory distress syndrome (ARDS). Patient is on intermittent mandatory ventilation. PAS = 58 mm Hg; PAEDP = 30 mm Hg; PA mean = 38 mm Hg. (*B*) Patient with vegetation on mitral valve resulting in acute mitral insufficiency. Note the v wave on the downstroke of the PA waveform (bifid waveform). PAS = 68 mm Hg; PAEDP = 32 mm Hg; PAM = 48 mm Hg.

abnormal) to confirm catheter position, have knowledge of the appropriate action required should an abnormal waveform occur, and be able to troubleshoot the catheter system (Antle, 2000) (Table 23-5).

Factors that contribute to PA rupture include balloon hyperinflation, peripheral location of the catheter tip, and hypothermia. Steps to avoid these risks are to slowly inflate the balloon to volume (1.25–1.5 mL of air, never fluids), at which time the pressure tracing should change from a PA to a PAWP waveform, and to limit inflation time to less than 15 seconds. If an overwedge is observed, stop immediately. To avoid distal migration of the catheter, the PA tracing should be continuously monitored and the chest radiograph should be assessed to determine if the tip of the catheter is correctly positioned within 5 cm of the mediastinum.

During PA catheter removal (Display 23-4), additional risks include air embolism, arrhythmias, and myocardial or valvular damage. Risk factors for air embolization include a decreased intravascular pressure (hypovolemia, tachycardia),

negative intrathoracic pressure (tachypnea, upright position, catheter removal during deep inspiration), an incompetent diaphragm on the introducer, and right to left intracardiac shunt. To minimize the risk of an air embolism, the patient should be placed in a supine/flat position and the catheter removed during breath holding at the end of a deep inspiration or positive pressure ventilation (to increase central venous pressure). After removal of the catheter the introducer should be sealed with a sterile obturator or a male cap. The incidence of cardiac arrhythmias during catheter removal ranges from 5% to 19%, with a small percentage of arrhythmias considered life threatening (Baldwin & Heland, 2000). Patients at increased risk for arrhythmias are those with electrolyte imbalances myocardial ischemia or infarction, CI < 2.5 L/min per square meter, or prolonged manipulation time (Bridges, 2000a). The use of a steady, continuous withdrawal of the catheter may decrease the incidence of arrhythmias. Myocardial or valvular damage can occur because of kinking or knotting of the catheter around cardiac structures or failure to deflate the balloon before withdrawal of the catheter. Caution should be taken if the patient has another cardiac catheter (i.e., transvenous pacemaker) or excessive catheter length (dilated heart).

Despite the potential complications associated with manipulating and removing the PA catheter, properly educated and qualified nurses can safely and successfully manipulate and remove PA catheters (Zevola & Maier, 1999). In a study of 125 patients with PA catheters, 39 (31%) of the catheters were incorrectly positioned (35 required advancement, 4 required withdrawal), of which 36 were repositioned by a critical care nurse (without complication) (Antle, 2000).

Table 23–5 ■ TROUBLESHOOTING THE PA CATHETER AND MEASUREMENT PROBLEMS

Clinical Problem	Implications	Possible Causes	Interventions
Overdamped pressure tracing	Falsely low systolic readings Falsely increased diastolic readings	Air bubbles in the pressure tubing or transducer More than three stopcocks between catheter and transducer Loose connections Collection of blood in tubing or in and around transducer Catheter kinked internally or at insertion site Catheter wedged against vessel wall Excessive tubing length (>4 feet) Clot or fibrin deposition on catheter tip	Flush all air from system (including microbubbles). Remove excess stopcocks. Tighten all connections. Flush tubing of all blood (if unable to clear, change transducer-tubing set-up). Maintain pressure in infusion bag at 300 mm Hg. Aspirate blood from catheter if clot suspected (*do not* flush). If PA catheter kinked-notify MD to reposition. If fibrin occluding catheter-catheter may need to be replaced.
Underdamped pressure tracing	Overestimation of systolic pressure Underestimation of diastolic pressure	Air bubbles in tubing, stopcocks, or transducer Excessive tubing length (>4 feet) Excess number of stopcocks	Use noncompliant/wide-bore tubing. Remove all air bubbles from system. Limit tubing to 4 feet maximum. Remove unnecessary stopcocks. If all attempts to resolve unsuccessful, consider the addition of an in-line damping device.
Catheter whip (fling) or artifact	Overestimation of systolic pressure Underestimation of diastolic pressure Difficult interpretation of waveform	Location of distal tip of PA catheter near pulmonic valve Hyperdynamic heart Looping of PA catheter in RV External disruption of PA catheter system	Assess dynamic response characteristics (troubleshoot system). Notify MD or qualified RN to reposition PA catheter. If fling fails to resolve, use mean pressure.
Absence of PA wedge tracing	Potential for air embolism or blood leaking from balloon port	Balloon rupture Improper positioning of PA catheter	If balloon is inflated without return of air into syringe on passive deflation, assess for signs of air embolism (if present, place in Trendelenburg in left lateral decubitus position-treat symptoms-notify MD). If stable-label balloon port "DO NOT WEDGE." Notify MD of need to replace catheter. If balloon is inflated to 1.5 mL, without change in waveform from PA to PA wedge pattern, notify MD or qualified RN of need to reposition catheter. Once catheter is repositioned, assess amount of air required for wedge (ideal volume 1.25–1.5 mL).
Migration of the PA catheter into the RV	Presence of RV arrhythmias Decreased diastolic pressure (equal to RAP)	Accidental or spontaneous withdrawal of catheter into the RV	Inflate the balloon fully to engulf the tip of the catheter and reduce ectopy. Notify MD or, if approved for RN, reposition catheter into PA. If compromised by arrhythmias, ensure balloon is deflated and withdraw catheter into RA (15–20 cm marking on PA catheter and RAP waveform observed from distal port).
Overwedging	Overwedging (eccentric balloon inflation or inflation in a small vessel) is a potential risk for PA perforation and rupture	Catheter migration Balloon position in small pulmonary vessel	Slowly inflate balloon while constantly observing the waveform. If overwedge pattern observed, immediately stop inflation and allow balloon to deflate passively. Notify MD or, if approved for RN, reposition catheter.
Spontaneous wedge	Potential for loss of blood supply to branch of pulmonary vessel and risk of PA infarction	Catheter migration (Patient movement, warming up of catheter after placement)	Turn patient to side opposite catheter placement. Have patient straighten arm or turn head to dislodge catheter. Have patient gently cough. Notify MD or RN, reposition catheter.

PA, pulmonary artery; RAP, right atrial pressure; RV, right ventricle.
Modified from Gardner, P. E. (1993). Pulmonary artery pressure monitoring. *AACN Clinical Issues in Critical Care Nursing*, 4, 98-119.

D I S P L A Y   23–4

REMOVAL OF PULMONARY ARTERY CATHETER

1. Verify the order to remove the catheter
2. Assemble necessary equipment
3. Document on the flow sheet the ECG rhythm and vital signs before initiating the procedure
4. Explain the procedure to the patient
5. Transfer IV infusions from PA catheter ports to side port of introducer or discontinue IV solutions if appropriate
6. Ensure that the patient remains in hemodynamically stable condition after transfer of infusions to side port
7. Turn off any remaining infusions to distal and proximal ports
8. Ensure that the balloon is deflated by lining up the red lines on the balloon port, drawing back on the syringe, and then discontinuing the syringe
9. Place the patients supine and turn the patient's head away from the insertion site
10. Open the sterile obturator/introducer cap, ensuring that sterility of the cap is maintained
11. Put on examination gloves
12. If the catheter dressing is nonocclusive or covers the introducer, after putting on a mask, remove the dressing
13. Instruct the patients to inspire deeply and hold their breath (or apply positive pressure breath on ventilator) during withdrawal of the catheter
14. Unlock the catheter shield from the introducer
15. While securing the introducer with nondominant hand, withdraw the catheter with dominant hand, using a constant steady continuous motion
16. Observe the ECG continuously during withdrawal of the catheter
17. If any resistance is met, do not continue to remove the catheter, and notify the physician immediately
18. Once the PA catheter has been removed, don sterile gloves and insert a sterile adaptor cap into the diaphragm site of the introducer
19. If necessary reapply a sterile dressing to the catheter site according to policy
20. Elevate HOB and return patient to position of comfort
21. Examine balloon and catheter to ensure that they are intact. If they are not intact, notify the physician immediately
22. Document on flow sheet the patient's response to procedure, including vital signs and ECG rhythm

Zevola, D. R., & Maier, B. (1999). Improving the care of cardiothoracic surgery patients through advanced nursing skills. *Critical Care Nurse*, 19(1), 34–44.

Right Ventricular Volumetric Measures

Although the focus of hemodynamic monitoring has been predominantly on left heart function, there has been a resurgence in awareness of the important role of RV function on overall cardiac function (Leeper, 2003; Safcsak & Nelson, 1999). Right ventricular function is altered in sepsis, acute respiratory distress syndrome, traumatic myocardial contusion, and with the application of positive end-expiratory pressure (PEEP) (Diebel et al., 1993; Theres et al., 1999).

Right ventricular end-diastolic volume (RVEDV) is measured using a modified PA catheter with a rapid-response thermistor located 4 cm from the catheter tip and a thermal filament approximately 14 to 25 cm from the catheter tip, which emits pulses of thermal energy that act as the indicator for thermodilution CO. Simultaneous recording of the CO curve and an ECG signal allows for the measurement of the RV ejection fraction (RVEF), CO, and SV and derived values: RV end-diastolic volume (RVEDV = SV/RVEF) and RV end-systolic volume (RVESV = RVEDV − SV) (Table 23-6).

The RVEDV is more closely related to the CI than the PAWP or CVP particularly in patients with acute respiratory failure, increased intrathoracic pressure, or intraabdominal hypertension (Cheatham, Safcsak et al., 1998; Diebel et al., 1997). In patients receiving various levels of PEEP (5 to 50 cm H_2O), the RVEDI was more significantly correlated with changes in the CI than the PAWP regardless of the degree of ventricular dysfunction (Cheatham, Nelson et al., 1998).

The RVEDVI may be an indicator of preload dependence. In patients with an RVEDVI < 90 mL/m² the CI increased in response to fluid volume in 64% of patients studied versus 0% for those with an RVEDVI > 140 mL/m² (Diebel et al., 1994). The criticism of the RVEDVI as a functional indicator is that there is no cut-off point for responders versus nonresponders between 90 and 140 mL/m² and patients with an RVEDVI > 140 mL/m² may respond to volume administration (Wagner & Leatherman, 1998). Although the RVEDVI tends to be lower in responders than nonresponders (Rezende et al., 2003), no specific value is indicative of preload dependence.

The RVEDVI may also be a useful endpoint for resuscitation. Trauma patients who were resuscitated to an RVEDVI greater than 120 mL/m² had a lower incidence of multisystem organ failure, better intestinal perfusion, and improved survival

Table 23–6 ■ RIGHT HEART FUNCTION VARIABLES

Variable	Normal
Stroke volume	60–100 mL/beat
Stroke volume index	33–46 mL/beat/m²
Right ventricular ejection fraction	40%–60% (0.4–0.6)
Right ventricular end-systolic index	30–60 mL/m²
Right ventricular end-diastolic volume index	60–100 mL/m²

compared to patients maintained with an RVEDVI between 90 and 100 mL/m² (Chang & Meredith, 1997; Miller, Meredith et al., 1998). Rather than aiming therapy to achieve a specific RVEDVI, consideration should be given to assessing the RVEDVI along with the RVEF with a goal of achieving an optimal SV.

With tricuspid regurgitation associated with pulmonary hypertension, the REF catheter consistently underestimates the RVEF and overestimates RV volumes (Hoeper et al., 2001). Continuous REF monitoring is not accurate when there are large changes in venous return (coughing, shivering, or changes in intrathoracic pressure), large deviations in body temperature (hypothermia or hyperthermia), tachycardia (HR > 150 bpm), or with significant cardiac arrhythmias.

FUNCTIONAL HEMODYNAMIC INDICES

The administration of fluids to augment preload and thus increase CO is a mainstay of the treatment of shock. However, the administration of fluids is not risk-free, because excessive volume administration may cause pulmonary edema. Therefore, a key clinical question is whether a patient will respond to volume loading with increased SV or whether volume administration will cause or worsen cardiopulmonary compromise?

Static preload indices (e.g., CVP or PAWP) are not good indicators of fluid responsiveness, that is, will the SV increase in response to volume resuscitation? Fluid responsiveness depends not only on the baseline preload but also on ventricular contractility and the slope of the ventricular function curve (Fig. 23-17). For example, if the preload is very low or if the heart is on the steep portion of the curve, an increase in volume should increase the SV (preload dependent). However, if the preload is in an intermediate range or the slope of the curve is depressed (indicative of failure), there may only be a small change in the SV (preload independent), and interpretation of a given preload value as predictive of fluid responsiveness will be difficult (Michard & Reuter, 2003). Patients will be "responders" to volume expansion only if both ventricles operate on the ascending portion of the curve. In contrast if one or both of the ventricles is operating on the flat portion of the curve, the patient will be a "nonresponder" (Michard & Teboul, 2000). Assessment of fluid responsiveness provides insight into ventricular function; however, the finding that a patient is fluid responsive does not necessarily mean that the patient requires fluids. The decision to administer fluids should be based on indications of altered cardiovascular function that would benefit from increased preload versus the risk for the development of pulmonary edema.

An alternative to static preload measures is "functional" or dynamic hemodynamic indices. These functional indices, which have been demonstrated to predict which patients will respond to volume loading, reflect spontaneous and mechanical ventilation-induced changes in intrathoracic pressure, with subsequent changes in measured RA and arterial blood pressure. To understand why dynamic measurements may be more accurate indicators of preload dependence, a review of the relationship between ventilatory-induced changes in intrathoracic pressure and right and left heart SV is provided.

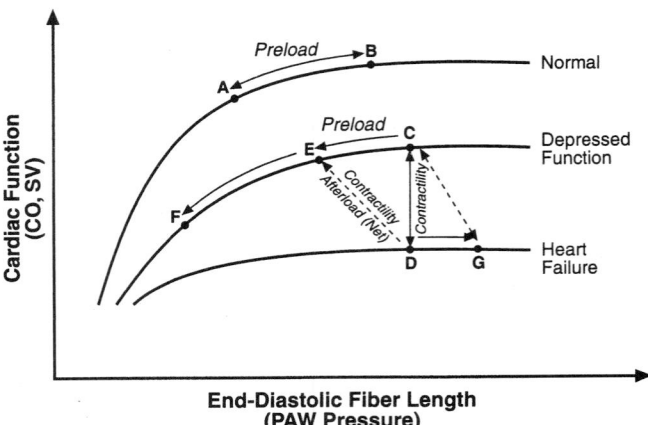

■ **Figure 23–17.** Family of ventricular function curves representing normal, depressed, and severely depressed function. A change in preload is represented by a move up or down a single curve (Frank-Starling principle). Point A to Point B and Point B to Point A reflect an increase and decrease, respectively, in preload. The response to volume loading is dependent on the position on the ventricular function curve. If the ventricles are on the steep portion of the curve the CO will increase in response to volume (responder). In contrast if the heart is on the flat portion of the curve the CO will not increase (nonresponder). A change in afterload results in a shift in the curve that appears similar to that caused by contractility, although the mechanism is different. Point D to E reflects the net effect of a decrease in afterload on a failing heart. This upward and lateral shift is the result of two actions. Point D to C reflects an increase in force of contraction and Point C to E a decrease in preload due to increased systolic ejection. A change in contractility is represented by an upward or downward shift of the curve, that is, for any given preload and afterload, the CO is increased or decreased. In a failing heart, an additional effect of decreased contractility is an increase in preload due to decreased systolic ejection; thus, the net effect of a decrease in contractility is to shift the curve down and to the left (Point C to G).

Spontaneous Ventilation

During spontaneous inspiration, pleural and intrathoracic pressure decreases with a resultant decrease in RAP. With a decrease in RAP, which is the backpressure to venous filling, venous return increases transiently. This increase in venous return results in an inspiratory increase in RV preload and output (assuming the right ventricle is on the steep portion of the ventricular function curve). However, if the right ventricle cannot dilate further (i.e., RV failure), the RAP will not decrease during inspiration, which indicates that the right atrium/ventricle are on the flat portion of the cardiac function curve, and the administration of additional volume will not increase RV output (Magder et al., 1992; Pinsky, 2002).

Mechanical Ventilation

During positive pressure mechanical ventilation, the inspiratory increase in intrathoracic pressure decreases venous return to the heart and increases RV afterload. These changes lead to a decrease in RV SV during inspiration. The decreased RV output causes a decrease in LV preload, which subsequently decreases

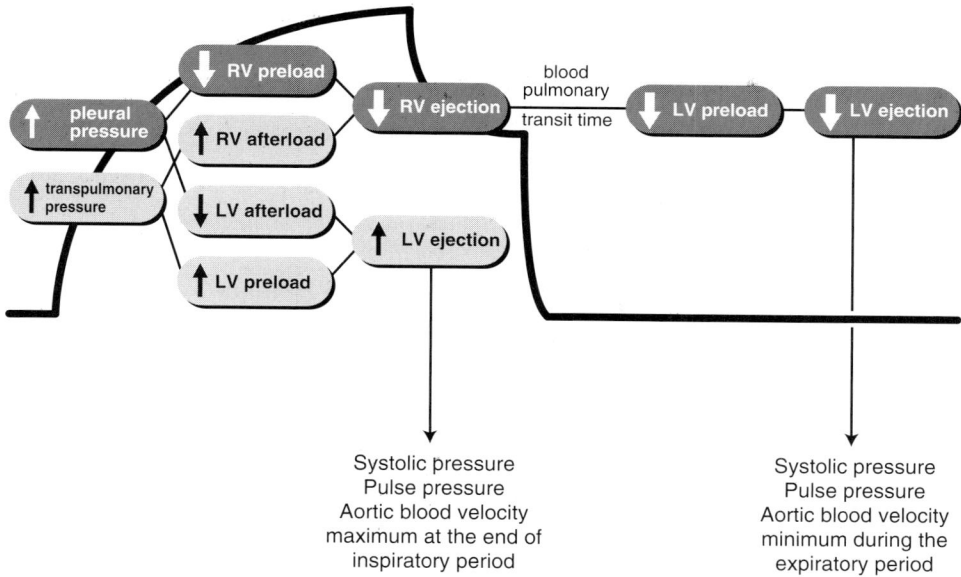

■ **Figure 23–18.** Hemodynamic effects of mechanical insufflation. The LV stroke volume is maximum at the end of inspiratory period and minimum two to three heart beats later (i.e., during expiratory period). The cyclic changes in LV stroke volume are mainly related to the expiratory decrease in LV preload due to the inspiratory decrease in RV filling and output. (From Michard, F., & Teboul, J. L. [2000]. Using heart-lung interactions to assess fluid responsiveness during mechanical ventilation. *Critical Care, 4,* 282–289.)

LV SV during expiration. Thus, the LV SV increases during inspiration because of compression of the pulmonary bed and decreases during expiration, primarily because of decreased RV output (Fig. 23-18) (Michard & Teboul, 2000, 2002). Observation of the ventilatory-induced changes in SV can be exploited based on the finding that RV preload and SV changes are greater when the ventricle is on the steep versus the flat portion of ventricular function curve (Magder, 1997). The increased RV output is transmitted to the left heart, and if both ventricles are preload-dependent, the increased LV preload will be observed as a cyclic change in LV SV. The assumption underlying the interpretation of the cyclic SV changes is that a greater cyclic change is indicative of preload dependence (i.e., a patient that will respond to volume loading with an increase in SV), whereas a smaller SV change indicates preload independence. Patients who are preload-independent will not increase their SV in response to volume loading and may be compromised by the excess fluid. The cyclic changes in LV SV are important, because the SV is a primary contributor to the SBP and pulse pressure. Variations in these hemodynamic indices may indicate preload dependence or independence. A number of functional hemodynamic indices have been evaluated (Table 23-7).

Respiratory Variation in Right Atrial Pressure

Although the absolute RAP is not predictive of which patients will respond to a volume challenge (Magder et al., 1992; Michard et al., 2000), the inspiratory change in RAP (ΔRAP) may be a useful predictor. In medical and cardiac surgery patients with an adequate spontaneous inspiratory effort (i.e.,

an inspiratory decrease in PAWP > 2 mm Hg), a spontaneous inspiratory decrease in RAP ≥ 1 mm Hg was a positive response (responder), whereas a decrease <1 mm Hg was a negative response (nonresponder) (Fig. 23-19) (Magder & Lagonidis, 1999). The value of the ΔRAP is the identification of patients who will not respond to fluids. Unlike other functional indices, the ΔRAP can be evaluated in spontaneously breathing patients.

Respiratory Variation in Systolic Blood Pressure

In mechanically ventilated patients, during expiration the SBP normally decreases 5 to 6 mm Hg from an end-expiratory baseline (ΔDown) and increases 2 to 4 mm Hg during inspiration (ΔUp). The difference between ΔDown and ΔUp is the systolic pressure variation (ΔPs), which is normally 8 to 10 mm

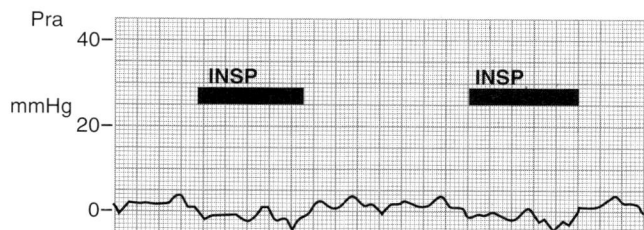

■ **Figure 23–19.** An example of a patient with a positive respiratory response in RAP. (From Magder, S., Georgiadis, G., & Cheong, T. [1992]. Respiratory variation in right atrial pressure predict the response to fluid challenge. *Journal of Critical Care, 7,* 76–85.)

Table 23–7 ■ FUNCTIONAL AND VOLUMETRIC INDICES

Indices/Definition	Predictive Value	Notes
RAP variation (ΔRAP)	ΔRAP > 1	• Spontaneous inspiratory decrease in RAP > 1 mm Hg predictive of volume response • ΔRAP > 1 does not predict a decrease in CO in response to an increase in PEEP • Measurement can be obtained on spontaneously breathing patients (on or off mechanical ventilation) • Patient must be able to generate adequate inspiratory effort (inspiratory ↓ PAWP > 2 mm Hg) to apply measurement
Systolic pressure variation (ΔPs) $\Delta Ps\% = 100 \times (Ps_{max} - Ps_{min})/$ $[(PS_{max} + Ps_{min})/2]$ ΔDown	• >12–15 mm Hg associated with hypovolemia • Increase in ΔPs > 4 mm Hg indicative of blood loss • >10% predictive in one study • >2–5 mm Hg* indicative of hypovolemia • No absolute predictive value identified	• Reported as an absolute amount (i.e., 5 mm Hg) or percentage (i.e., 15%) • Not solely affected by SV. Changes in chest wall and lung compliance, transmural pressure and tidal volume affect variation (increased Vt − increased variation). Comparison is possible if these pulmonary variables remain stable • Increased ΔPs associated with increased ΔCI for any given volume infused • More reliable indicator of preload dependence than CVP or PAWP • Patient must be on mechanical ventilation with a stable tidal volume • Not evaluated in patients with cardiac arrhythmias • *Absolute value depends on lung compliance and tidal volume • Patient must be on mechanical ventilation and heavily sedated and/or paralyzed • Requires creation of an end-expiratory apneic period • Not evaluated in patients with cardiac arrhythmias

Pulse pressure variation (ΔPp)
 	
$(Pp\% = [(PP_{max} - PP_{min})/(PP_{max} + PP_{min})/2] \times 100$
	>13%	• Affected only by change in SV (assuming arterial resistance and compliance do not acutely change during a single breath)
		• More reliable indicator of preload dependence than ΔPs (improved bias and precision), RAP, or PAWP
		• Patient must be on mechanical ventilation and heavily sedated and/or paralyzed
		• Affected by tidal volume (Vt)
		  ○ Vt must be remain unchanged for comparison of sequential values
		  ○ The cutoff point varies with changes in Vt
		• Not evaluated in patients with cardiac arrhythmias

Stroke volume variation (SVV) $SVV = SVV_{max} - SVV_{min}/SVV_{mean}$	>Neurosurgical patients 9.5% (Vt = 10 ml/kg) >13% (septic shock)	• More sensitive indicator of change in volume status than PAWP, CVP, ITBVI • Patient must be on mechanical ventilation and heavily sedated and/or paralyzed • SVV values change based on VT—cut points can only be applied to patients receiving similar VT
Aortic blood flow velocity $\Delta Vpeak (\%) = 100 \times (Vpeak_{max} - Vpeak_{min})/[Vpeak_{max} + Vpeak_{min})/2]$	>12% (septic shock)	• Patient must be on mechanical ventilation

Hg (Fig. 23-20) (Magder, 2001). The ΔPs is equivalent to or more sensitive to volume-induced changes in CI than the PAWP (Bennett-Guerrero et al., 2002; Tavernier et al., 1998). In patients with acute circulatory failure caused by sepsis, ΔPs% greater than 10% was predictive of fluid responsiveness (Michard et al., 2000; Tavernier et al., 1998).

The ΔPs may also be a useful indicator of hemorrhage or occult blood loss (Preisman et al., 2002). In experimental hemorrhage in cardiac surgery patients, ΔPs more than 4 mm Hg was indicative of a significant blood loss (Ornstein et al., 1998). Conversely, in patients undergoing therapeutic phlebotomy, ΔPs less than 5 mm Hg was considered to indicate an absence of hypovolemia (Rooke et al., 1995). Absolute ΔPs must be interpreted cautiously because it is affected by V_T (increased V_T causes increased ΔPs), lung and chest wall compliance, and transmural pressure (Denault et al., 1999).

ΔDown

A subset of the systolic pressure change is the delta Down (ΔDown), which is the difference between the SBP during a 5- to 15-second end-expiratory pause (apnea) and the minimum

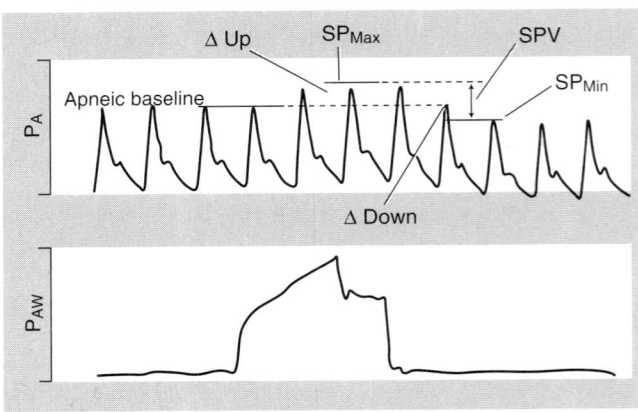

■ **Figure 23–20.** Systolic pressure variation associated with positive pressure variation. ΔDown: decrease in systolic pressure from an apneic baseline; ΔUp: increase in systolic pressure from an apneic baseline; P_{aw}: airway pressure; SP_{min}: minimum systolic pressure after a positive pressure breath; SP_{max}: maximum systolic pressure after a positive pressure breath; SPV (ΔPs): the difference between the SP_{max} and the SP_{min} or the sum of ΔUp plus ΔDown. (From Gunn, S., & Pinsky, M. [2001]. Implications of arterial pressure variation in patients in the intensive care unit. *Current Opinions in Critical Care, 7*, 212–217.)

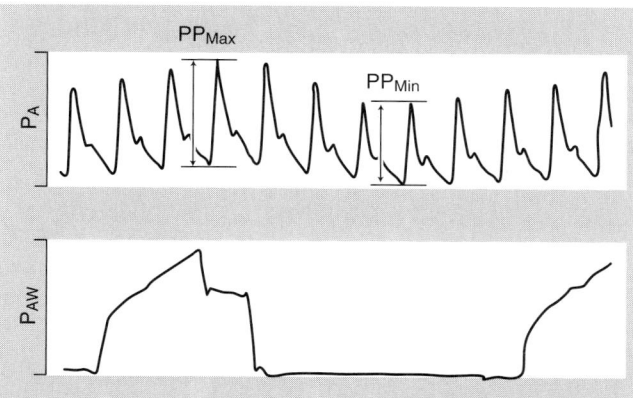

■ Figure 23–21. Pulse pressure variation related to positive pressure ventilation. PA: arterial pressure; PAW, airway pressure; PPmax: maximum pulse pressure after a positive pressure breath; PPmin: minimum pulse pressure after a positive pressure ventilation. (From Gunn, S., & Pinsky, M. [2001]. Implications of arterial pressure variation in patients in the intensive care unit. *Current Opinions in Critical Care, 7,* 212–217.)

SBP over a single respiratory cycle. Depending on the patient population, a ΔDown of 2 to 5 mm Hg is indicative of fluid responsiveness (Rooke et al., 1995; Tavernier et al., 1998). As with changes in the ΔPs, a change in the magnitude of the ΔDown is an early indicator of blood loss, with changes occurring markedly earlier than changes in HR or BP or traditional preload indices (CVP and PAWP) (Preisman et al., 2002). Clinically, use of the ΔDown is more difficult because of the requirement to create a 5- to 15-second apneic period and the absolute value is affected by changes in lung compliance.

Pulse Pressure Variation

Arterial pulse pressure is the difference between the arterial systolic and diastolic pressure (Fig. 23-21). Three factors affect the pulse pressure: LV SV, arterial resistance, and arterial compliance. Of note, the latter two factors do not change significantly during a single breath (Pinsky, 2002; Preisman et al., 2002); therefore, the beat-to-beat changes in pulse pressure reflect changes in LV SV. Unlike the SBP, which is affected by pleural pressure changes, the pulse pressure is affected by only the SV, because the pleural pressure equally affects the systolic and diastolic pressure.

Pulse pressure variation (ΔPp) is the variability in the pulse pressure during mechanical ventilation. In patients with septic shock on mechanical ventilation, a ΔPp of 13% of the baseline pulse pressure (e.g., if the baseline pulse pressure = 40 mm Hg, a 13% change $\cong$ 5 mm Hg) discriminated between responders and nonresponders to a 500-mL colloid bolus with 94% sensitivity and 96% specificity and was a more sensitive indicator than a change in ΔPs, PAWP, or RAP (Michard et al., 2000). An important finding in this study was that the greater the ΔPp before volume expansion, the greater the CI response to the fluid bolus. After volume expansion, the ΔPp decreased, indicating less preload dependence (a shift up the ventricular function curve).

Limitations of Functional Measures

There are limitations to the use of functional measurements. The ΔPs, ΔDown, and ΔPp can be determined only in patients who are on controlled ventilation and deeply sedated and/or paralyzed. Additionally, changes in tidal volume and pulmonary compliance will alter the magnitude of the response. Patients with cardiac arrhythmias have been excluded from all studies; thus, the use of these measures cannot be recommended for in this population. Finally, a majority of the studies were conducted in patients with relatively normal ventricular function; therefore, recommendations for patients with decreased LV function are limited.

Stroke Volume Variation

A volumetric measure has also been suggested as an indicator of fluid responsiveness. Stroke volume variation (SVV), which can be continuously measured using pulse contour analysis or esophageal Doppler, is defined as the change in SV over a 30-second period. The assumption underlying SVV is that the observed SV changes are respiratory-induced variations. Stroke volume variation values of 9.5% and 13.5% were predictive of fluid responsiveness in neurosurgical and septic shock patients, respectively (Berkenstadt et al., 2001; Cope et al., 2002).

As with other volumetric measurements, the SVV is more closely associated with changes in SV than are changes in PAWP and CVP (Cope et al., 2002; Reuter et al., 2002). Unlike other functional (ΔPs or ΔDown) or volumetric indices (intrathoracic blood volume), in patients with decreased LV function, changes in SVV were related to changes in SVI, although no predictive cut-off value has been identified.

Concern has been voiced regarding the method used to measure the SVV (direct measurement versus pulse contour analysis) (Pinsky, 2003b) as reflected in the contradictory results of the usefulness of SVV to predict fluid responsiveness (Reuter et al., 2002; Wiesenack et al., 2003). The contradictory results may reflect differences in the tidal volume, which affects the absolute SVV (Reuter et al., 2003), the hemodynamic status of the patients studied (stable versus hypovolemic), or the yet-to-be-described respiratory-induced changes in vascular impedance, which may affect pulse contour measurements. There is also significant operator variability in the SVV measurements obtained by esophageal Doppler; demonstrating the need for extensive training before using this method of monitoring. Finally, to achieve a stable tidal volume, SVV analysis can be performed only in patients who are on controlled mechanical ventilation and are heavily sedated/paralyzed.

CARDIAC OUTPUT MEASUREMENT

Measurement of CO by the thermodilution method (TDCO) is based on the injection of a known volume of cold or room temperature sterile D5W through the proximal port of the PA

DISPLAY   23–5

ASSESSMENT OF TDCO CURVES

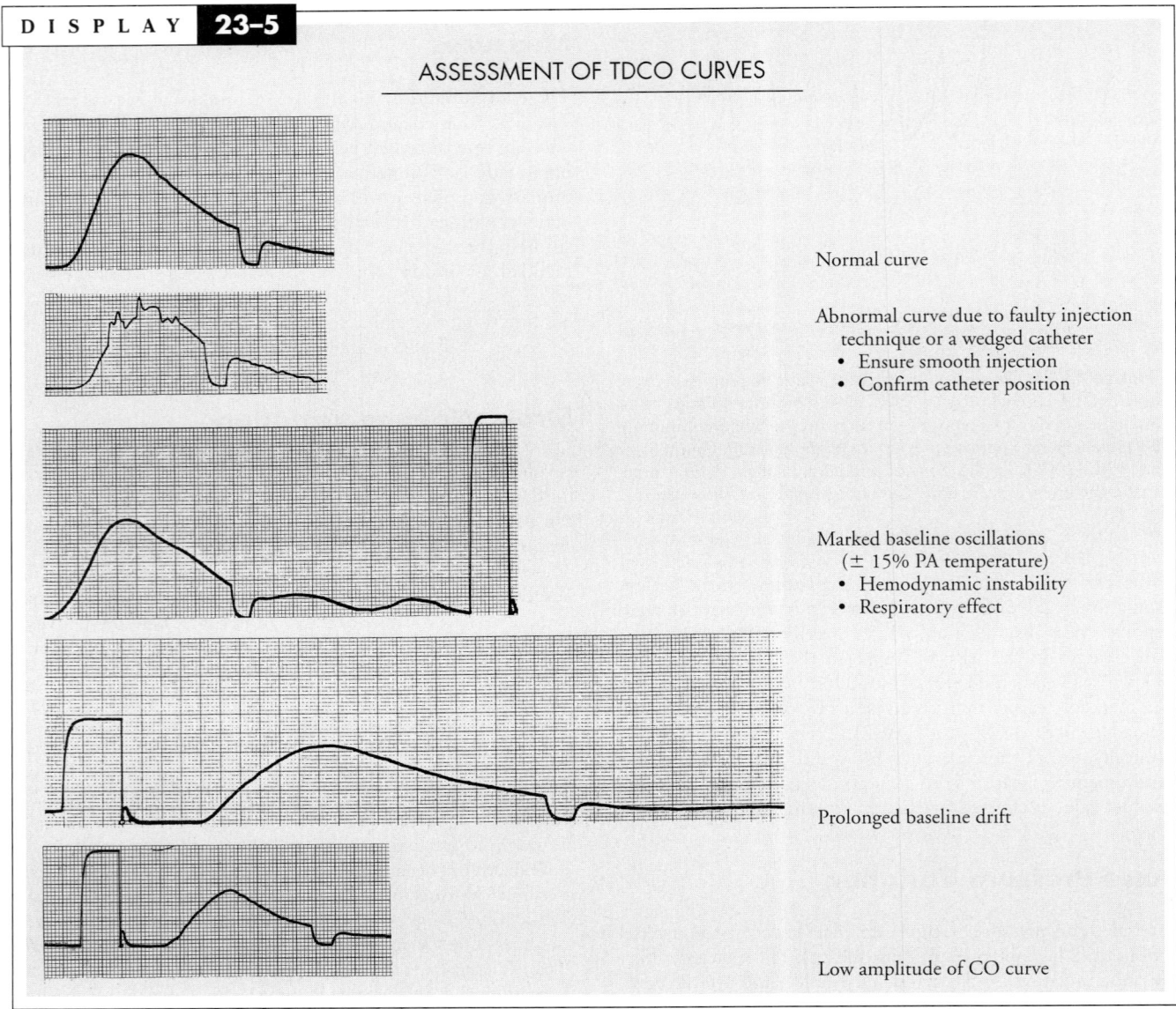

Normal curve

Abnormal curve due to faulty injection
   technique or a wedged catheter
   • Ensure smooth injection
   • Confirm catheter position

Marked baseline oscillations
   (± 15% PA temperature)
   • Hemodynamic instability
   • Respiratory effect

Prolonged baseline drift

Low amplitude of CO curve

catheter into the RA. The blood is temporarily cooled by the injectate, and the change in temperature is sensed by a thermistor on the distal end of the PA catheter. A computer connected to the PA catheter calculates the CO based on the area under the curve using the Stewart-Hamilton equation. The temperature of the blood is assumed to be stable; thus, theoretically any change in blood temperature is caused by the injectate. This assumption may be incorrect, particularly if a patient is on mechanical ventilation, which causes a ventilatory-induced variability in blood temperature. Most CO computers display the CO time–temperature curve, which allows for confirmation of a correct waveform (Display 23-5). A study using a modified catheter with a thermistor mounted in the right atrium found that 31% of the injections were in error (injection > 4.5 seconds, prolonged downslope and increased variability in baseline). Of note, these errors were not detected by the distal waveform and caused increased variability in CO measures (Stites et al., 1998).

Factors Influencing Thermodilution Cardiac Output Measurement

Factors that affect the accuracy of thermodilution CO measures include the catheter position, site of injection, use of the correct calibration constant, injection technique, and volume and temperature of the injectate. These factors are summarized in Display 23-6.

Pathophysiological Factors

Adequate mixing of the thermal indicator and blood must occur before sensing by the distal thermistor of the PA catheter. Pathophysiological conditions, such as tricuspid insufficiency and ventricular septal defect, inhibit adequate mixing of indicator and blood and may interfere with accurate TDCO

D I S P L A Y 23–6

PULMONARY ARTERY THERMODILUTION CARDIAC OUTPUT

Factor	Notes
Catheter position	• Distal port (catheter tip) must be in the pulmonary artery (confirm by observing PA waveform) • Proximal port should be positioned in RA (verify by observing RA waveform) • Ensure catheter not wedged
Injection port	• Inject into proximal port (RA), venous infusion port, or RV port • Injections through side-port less accurate than injections through infusion port • Ensure exit of proximal port is outside of introducer sheath
Calibration constant (CC) (see manufacturer's insert for catheter-specific CC)	• A factor that corrects for the gain of heat from the tubing and thermistor • Specific to (1) catheter type, (2) volume (5 vs 10 mL), (3) temperature (iced vs room temp), (4) solution type (D5W vs NS)
Injection technique • Injection rate of 4 seconds for 5-10 ml injectate • Use manual or automatic injector • Avoid handling syringe barrel • Inject at end-expiration or throughout respiratory cycle • Allow ~ 60 seconds between measures (monitor will indicate "READY")	• Injection rate demonstrated to produce accurate results • CO from manual method not significantly different from automatic injector • Heat transfer from hands will alter accuracy of measurements • Respiratory-induced changes in CO, with up to 30% variability between inspiration/expiration • Measurements obtained at end-expiration decrease variability in measures (may overestimate CO by 1–1.5 times) • Measurements obtained with random injection throughout respiration increases validity of measures *Obtain three measurements that are within 10% of median value (e.g., if median value = 5 L/min, include all measures 4.5–5.5 L/min)

Injectate temperature/volume • Temperature between injectate and blood should be ≥ 10°C • There is increased variability in CO measurements between cold and room temperature injectate particularly in patients with a low EF (<30%) (McCloy et al., 1999)	Iced injectate (0–5°C) • 5 mL ≅ 10 mL • Low and high CO • Hyperdynamic patients • 10 mL iced is considered the standard *It is not necessary to prime the catheter with cold solution before CO measurements	Room temperature (19–25°C) • 10 ml RT ≅ 10 mL IT • CO within normal limits (5 mL IT ≅ 10 mL RT) • Normothermia (5 mL if fluid restricted) • Hyperdynamic patients • Hypothermia

| Concomitant infusion | • Increased variability with concomitant infusion
 ○ Consider discontinuation of infusion if there is not risk to the patient
 ○ Avoid performance of TDCO during bolus infusion (Griffin et al., 1997)
• Remove all vasoactive medications from proximal port to avoid inadvertent bolus | |
| Patient position | • Reproducible measures with backrest up to 20 degrees
• 250–500 mL position related change CO in 20–degree sidelying position
 ○ Compare sidelying CO to supine CO | |

See *Cardiac nursing* (4th ed.) for review of literature (Bridges, 2000a).

---

measurements. Tricuspid regurgitation leads to overestimation of CO when the CO is low and underestimation of CO when the CO is increased (Heerdt et al., 2001).

Clinically Important Changes in Cardiac Output

In general, a change in CO of greater than 10% to 15% is considered to be physiologically important. The 10% value is based on studies that demonstrate that normal physiological variability is approximately 6.4% in patients with stable ($\pm$5% of the mean value) covariables (HR, respiratory rate, MAP, PA mean) and 9.9% in "covariable unstable" patients (Huang, Tsai et al., 2001; Sasse et al., 1994; Sasse et al., 1996). In assessing changes in CO, it is important to evaluate technical, physiological, and pathophysiological (Table 23-8) factors related to the CO. If the change in CO is determined to be clinically important, a sys-

tematic approach should be undertaken to determine the probable cause. The direct and derived indices used in a comprehensive hemodynamic assessment are outlined in Table 23-9.

VENTRICULAR FUNCTION CURVES

The preload indices discussed can be used to plot a family of ventricular function curves, which demonstrate the interaction between preload, afterload, and contractility and the effects of various disease processes (heart failure, hemorrhage) and therapeutic actions (vasodilator or inotropic drug therapy) on CO (see Fig. 23-17). The family of curves varies for each patient but is useful in predicting and evaluating the effects of various therapeutic interventions. The curves are constructed by plotting the PAWP (or some measure of end-diastolic volume) on the horizontal axis and the CO, CI, or SV on the vertical axis.

Table 23–8 ■ HEMODYNAMIC CHARACTERISTICS OF VARIOUS PATHOLOGICAL CONDITIONS

Pathophysiology	Hemodynamic Findings					Additional Findings
	RAP	PA	PAWP	SV	CO	
Pericardial tamponade	↑	↑	↑	↓	↓	Equalization (within 5 mm Hg) of RAP = PAEDP = PAWP; RAP waveform: prominent *x* descent with attenuated or absent *y* descent (d/t decreased ventricular filling); pulsus paradoxus (↓SBP > 10 mm Hg and ↓pulse pressure during inspiration; diastolic blood pressure unchanged); pulsus alternans (Fig. 23-10); absent S_3 heart sound; cardiac pressures may be normal if the patient is hypovolemic
Pericardial constriction	↑	↑	↑	↓	N/↓	RAP waveform: steep *x* and *y* descent resulting in an "M" or "W"-shaped waveform; RAP ≅ PAEDP ≅ PAWP (if no tricuspid or mitral regurgitation); decreased respiratory variation in RAP; Kussmaul's sign (inspiratory increase in RAP in severe pericardial constriction); pulsus paradoxus (approximately 33% of cases). CO maintained by tachycardia
Massive pulmonary embolism	↑	↑	↑/N/↓	↓	↓	Increased RA v wave with steep *y* descent due to tricuspid regurgitation, increased alveolar–arterial oxygen gradient (normal value does not rule out pulmonary embolism), tachypnea, dyspnea, increased pulmonic component of S_2, pleuritic chest pain
Mitral regurgitation			↑			If amplitude of V wave 10 mm Hg or more than a wave amplitude, read PAWP at nadir (base) of the *x* descent (Fig. 23-13*C*); PAWP > PAEDP (regurgitant v wave)
Left ventricular failure	N/↑	↑	↑	↓	↓	Pulmonary congestion or edema, S_3 or S_4, increased a wave height (due to decreased ventricular compliance); increased v wave height due to mitral regurgitation, pulsus alternans
Right ventricular infarction	↑	↑/↓	↑/↓	N/↓	N/↓	RAP > PAWP or RAP 1 to 5 mm Hg > PAWP, or RAP > 10 mm Hg, RA tracing with prominent *x* and *y* descent (M configuration), increased jugular venous pressure, systemic venous congestion, RV gallop, split S_2, positive hepatojugular reflux, increased RA a wave, positive Kussmaul's sign (increased RAP with inspiration), RV S_3 or S_4
Acute ventral septal defect	↑	↑	↑	↓	↓	Acute hypotension and pulmonary congestion, systolic thrill, holosystolic murmur, acute right heart failure with increased jugular venous pressure, late PAWP v wave, oxygen step up of >10% right atrium and PA
Hypovolemia	↓	↓	↓	↓	↓/N	Increased SVR (compensatory), decreased SvO_2
Septic shock (hyperdynamic)	↓	↓	↓/N/↑	N/↑	N/↑	Systemic hypotension, SBP < 90 mm Hg, metabolic acidosis with compensatory hyperventilation (respiratory alkalosis), decreased SVR, increased SvO_2
Septic shock (hypodynamic)	↑↓	↑↓	↑↓	↓	↓	Systemic hypotension, SBP < 90 mm Hg, systemic vasoconstriction (increased SVR), decreased SvO_2

N, normal; ↓, decreased; ↑, increased; CO, cardiac output; PA, pulmonary artery; PAEDP, pulmonary artery end diastolic pressure; PAP, pulmonary artery pressure; PAWP, pulmonary artery wedge pressure; RA, right atrial; RAP, right atrial pressure; SBP, systolic blood pressure; SV, stroke volume; SVR, systemic vascular resistance.

■ CONTINUOUS CARDIAC OUTPUT

Continuous CO (CCO) is performed using a PA catheter with a heating filament located in the RA or RV (14 to 25 cm from the catheter tip) that produces pseudorandom heat pulses in an on/off pattern. The heat pulses (0.02°C to 0.07°C) are detected by a thermistor on the distal end of the catheter (Yelderman, 1993). The heat pulses replace the cold bolus injection that is normally used for TDCO measurements. The CCO measurements are comparable with TDCO over a wide range of COs and temperatures, although increased variability exists between the two methods of measurements (Mets et al., 2002; Sun et al., 2002; Zollner et al., 2001).

The CCO measurements can be obtained with blood temperatures between 31°C and 41°C, although there is decreased accuracy above 38.5°C (Luchette et al., 2000). The CCO is accurate at low flow rates (0.5 to 3 L/min) (O'Malley et al., 2000), at increased HR, and during atrial fibrillation (Boyle et al., 1997), and it is less affected by external warming than TDCO (Spackman & Abenstein, 1993). However, at higher flow rates, there is an increased difference between CCO and TDCO and dye-dilution measurements (Jacquet et al., 1996). The displayed CO is updated every 30 seconds and represents

Table 23-9 ■ STANDARD HEMODYNAMIC INDICES

Indices/Equations	Normal Values	Interpretation
Preload		
Right atrial pressure (RAP or central venous pressure (CVP)	2–6 mm Hg	RV filling pressure
Pulmonary artery end-diastolic pressure (PAEDP)	8–12 mm Hg	Indirect indicator of LV filling pressure and capillary filling pressure (P_{cap})
Pulmonary artery wedge pressure (PAWP)	6–12 mm Hg	Indirect indicator of LV filling pressure and capillary filling pressure (P_{cap})
Afterload		
Systolic blood pressure (SBP)	120 mm Hg	Clinical indicator of pressure that must be overcome during ejection phase of cardiac cycle
Systemic vascular resistance (SVR) $$SVR = \frac{MAP - RAP}{CO} \times 80$$	800–1200 dynes/sec/cm^{-5}	Measure of systemic vascular tone (one factor that affects afterload; increased SVR manifested by increased MAP)
Systemic vascular resistance index (SVRI) $$SVRI = \frac{MAP - RAP}{CI} \times 80$$	1900–2400 dynes/sec/cm^{-5}/m^2	SVRI indexed to BSA
Force of Contraction		
Stroke volume (SV) $$SV = \frac{CO \times 1000}{HR}$$	60–180 mL/beat	Amount of blood ejected during each ventricular contraction
Stroke Volume Index $$SVI = \frac{CI \times 1000}{HR}$$	33–47 mL/beat/m^2	SVR indexed to BSA
Right ventricular stroke work index (RVSWI) RVSWI = SVI(MAP − CVP) × 0.0136	5–10 g-m/m^2/beat	Work performed by the right ventricle to eject blood into the pulmonary vasculature. Stroke work determines the energy expenditure (oxygen consumption) of the heart
Left ventricular stroke work index (LVSWI) LVSWI = SVI(MAP − PAWP) × 0.0136	45–65 g-m/m^2/beat	Work performed by the left ventricle to eject blood into the aorta. The factor 0.0136 is used to convert pressure and volume to units of work. With high filling pressures or hypotension, this equation may underestimate the amount of work performed.

BSA, body surface area, CI, cardiac index; CO, cardiac output; CVP, central venous pressure; MAP, mean arterial pressure; RAP, right atrial pressure

the average CO over the previous 3 to 6 minutes. A limitation of the CCO system is the delay between a change in CO and display of the change (Lazor et al., 1997). For example, the average time to report 75% of a 1-L change in CO was 10.5 minutes, and 90% of the change was reported in 11.8 minutes (Haller et al., 1995). Although newer technology has decreased the response time, when the two systems most commonly used in practice were exposed to a 4-L/min CO change, they detected 20% of the change in 5.3 to 6.5 minutes, 50% change in 7.6 to 8.8 minutes, and 80% change in 10.8 to 11.1 minutes. When flow was changed by 1 L every 2 minutes, neither system detected the change (Aranda et al., 1998). The observed changes in CO also lag behind changes in MAP, HR, and $S\overline{v}O_2$ (Poli de Figueiredo et al., 1999). The use of the STAT mode may be an option. Contrary to the concern that more frequent measurements may result in increased "noise", the bias (−0.04 to 0.18 L/min) and precision (0.61 to 0.84 L/min) of STAT mode versus TDCO were comparable to values comparing the TDCO with normal CCO (Singh et al., 2002).

The CCO system has several limitations. The infusion of a cold solution may cause overestimation of CCO measurements, although CCO measurements are minimally affected by fluctuations in PA temperatures (Haller et al., 1995). In addition, fluid boluses cause an underestimation of CO in low flow states (CO <4 L/min). Intracardiac shunt, tricuspid regurgitation, and incorrect catheter placement (thermal

filament in the vena cava or in contact with the heart) decrease the accuracy of CCO measures.

New continuous CO technology (truCCOMS; Aortech International, Bellshill, Scotland) that provides beat-to-beat CO measurement is being evaluated. The system uses a standard PA catheter with a temperature sensor at 10 cm and thermal coil located in the main PA (7.5 cm from the catheter tip). Unlike the described CCO systems, this system evaluates the amount of energy required to maintain the coil temperature at 1°C above the blood temperature. The amount of energy required to maintain a constant gradient between the coil and the blood temperature is directly related to the CO (i.e., increased blood flow causes increased heat dissipation, thus increased energy is required to maintain the temperature differential). During cardiac surgery and in critically ill ICU patients, the truCCOMS CO was comparable to CO measurements obtained with an aortic flow probe (Thierry et al., 2003).

LESS INVASIVE METHODS FOR CARDIAC OUTPUT MONITORING

Over the past decade, there has been increased emphasis on developing less invasive methods for CO monitoring. The validity and reliability of these measures compared with

Table 23–10 ■ VALIDATION OF LESS INVASIVE CO MEASUREMENTS

Instrument	Comments	Selected References
Transpulmonary indicator dilution (TPID)	Both TPID methods (PulseCO/PiCCO) are comparable, but consistently higher than PATD CO (bias 0.16–0.32 L/min; precision 0.37–1.3 L/min)	(Della Rocca et al., 2002; Linton et al., 1997; Zollner et al., 2000)
Pulse contour	Both methods are comparable to PATD CO and CCO measurements (bias: 0.003–0.4 L/min; precision: 0.1–1.2 L/min)	(Buhre et al., 1999; Felbinger et al., 2002; Godje et al., 2002; Rauch et al., 2002)
	Research is needed to validate these methods under conditions of decreased LV function.	
Doppler ultrasound	EDM CO is comparable to PATD, CCO, and Fick. The EDM tends to underestimate the CO compared to PATD CO (0.1–0.24 L/min).	(Turner, 2003; Valtier et al., 1998)
	Decreased agreement between EDM and PATD at higher COs.	(Moxon et al., 2003)
	Excellent agreement between EDM and CCO measures of CO and SVR.	(Baillard et al., 1999; Su et al., 2002)
Impedance cardiography	Meta-analysis: ICG and "gold standard" (single measure $r^2 = 0.53$; repeated measures $r^2 = 0.67$). Healthy individuals ($r^2 = 0.71$), critically ill patients ($r^2 = 0.67$), cardiac patients ($r^2 = 0.59$).	(Raaijmakers et al., 1999)
	Emergency department patients (ICG-PATD: bias -0.12 L/min/m^2; precision 0.75 L/min/m^2). Similar results in intraoperative critically ill patients.	(Shoemaker et al., 1998; Shoemaker, Thangathurai et al., 1999)
	The ICG tends to underestimate CO and has comparable or greater variability compared to other CO measures. New technology has decreased the bias and variability of ICG CO; however, the interpretation of absolute values must be performed with caution.	(Drazner et al., 2002; Sageman et al., 2002; Spiess et al., 2001; Van De Water et al., 2003)
Non-invasive partial CO$_2$ rebreathing system	Partial rebreathing CO measurements are comparable to other methods (PATD/CCO) during OPCAB, cardiac surgery, aortic reconstructive surgery, and manipulation of PEEP and CO.	(Kotake et al., 2003; Nilsson et al., 2001).
	Trauma victims NICO-CCO ($r^2 = 0.54$). Underestimated CCO by 27%.	(Maxwell et al., 2001)
	Overestimates actual CO when pulmonary blood flow is low and overestimates CO during hyperdynamic CO states and with increased alveolar deadspace.	(Gama de Abreu et al., 2003; Haryadi et al., 2000)

PATD-CO or Fick are summarized in Table 23-10. A majority of the research involving these new techniques has been to validate the method. Research is needed to demonstrate the usefulness of these methods in guiding therapy and in improving patient outcomes.

Transpulmonary Indicator Dilution (TPID) Techniques

Intermittent CO measurements using the transpulmonary indicator dilution technique (TPID) involve injection of an indicator into the venous circulation with a sensor in the systemic arterial circulation. There are currently two TPID techniques available for the measurement of CO. One uses cold temperature as the indicator (transpulmonary thermodilution [TPTD]) (PiCCO; Pulsion Medical Systems, Munich, Germany) and the other uses lithium as the indicator (LiDCO; LiDCO, London, UK).

Transpulmonary Thermodilution

The TPTD technique involves the administration of a single bolus injection of 10 to 15 mL of iced 5% glucose or saline over one ventilatory cycle via a central venous catheter with an in-line thermistor. A 4-Fr thermistor-tipped arterial catheter is placed in the femoral, brachial, or axillary artery (Segal et al., 2002). Use of the radial artery is not recommended because of vasoconstrictive changes in the waveform. The CO is calculated using a modified Stewart-Hamilton equation.

The TPTD curve is affected by respiratory variations. Use of a corrective algorithm may decrease variability compared with PATD measurements (Jansen et al., 2001). Partial or spontaneous ventilation increases the variability in the TPTD CO measures; thus, the effects of various ventilatory modes on the reliability and validity of TPTD-CO needs to be studied. The use of room temperature versus iced injectate also increases TPTD to CO variability. This latter effect along with the effect of varying injectate volumes (5 vs. 10 mL) requires additional study.

TPID-Lithium

The TPID-lithium (LiDCO) technique involves the injection of 150 mM (0.002–0.004 mM/kg) bolus injection of lithium into a peripheral or central venous site (Jonas et al., 1999), and a time curve is created by a lithium-sensitive electrode attached to an arterial pressure monitoring line. The CO is derived from the lithium dose, the area under the curve (AUC), and the packed cell volume (PCV = Hgb [g/dL]): CO = lithium dose (mmol) × 60/AUC × (1 − PCV). The dose of lithium is too small to create a pharmacological effect (Linton et al., 1993); however, LiDCO measurements cannot be performed in patients receiving lithium. In the presence of a ventricular shunt, the curve will be distorted and accurate CO measurements cannot be obtained.

Pulse Contour Analysis

The TPID techniques described were initially designed for the measurement of CO; however, with the development of continuous CO measurement via pulse contour analysis, these two TPID methods are now used primarily to calibrate the pulse

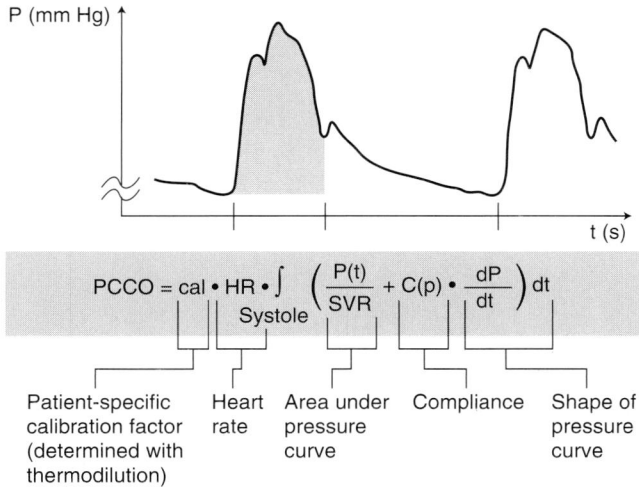

■ Figure 23–22. Calculation of pulse contour CO (PCCO). (Reproduced courtesy of Pulsion Medical Systems, Munich, Germany.)

contour system and to calculate intrathoracic blood volume (ITBV) and extravascular lung water (EVLW). Both methods have been studied primarily to validate the TPID methods. Research is needed to evaluate the usefulness of TPID in guiding therapy. One example of the clinical usefulness of TPID is in optimizing resynchronization pacemaker therapy (Roberts et al., 2002).

Thermodilution TPID

For thermodilution pulse contour analysis, the thermistor-tipped arterial catheter is attached to a high-fidelity transducer and a bedside computer for pulse contour analysis. The arterial waveform is digitized and the CO is derived using an algorithm (Fig. 23-22), which includes a measurement of the area under the systolic portion of the curve and a coefficient characterizing vascular compliance.

To calibrate the TPTD system (PiCCO), the arterial impedance is determined by simultaneously measuring arterial pressure wave and the TPTD CO. The TPTD CO is performed in triplicate using 10 mL of iced or 15 mL of room temperature injectate, with injections randomly spaced over the respiratory cycle. The injectate volume varies based on body weight and the temperature of the injectate. Once calibrated the system provides a beat-to-beat analysis of CO. The lithium-based system (PulseCO) uses a mathematical technique known as autocorrelation to transform the arterial waveform into a derived CO (Jonas & Tanser, 2002). A single TPID CO (LiDCO) is then used to calibrate the system and convert the derived CO into a patient-specific CO. The LiDCO system does not require a central venous catheter (Garcia-Rodriguez et al., 2002).

A concern regarding pulse contour analysis is that changes in vascular resistance may require recalibration of the system. While small changes in SVR (<20%) do not affect the pulse contour measurements, a greater than 50% increase in SVR increases the bias between PCCO and PATD CO measurements (Rodig et al., 1999). An algorithm that accounts for vascular compliance

and resistance was studied in postoperative cardiac surgery patients with CO changes greater than 20% (ΔCO 40%±27%) and a wide range of SVRs (450–2360 dynes/sec/cm^{-5}). The PiCCO CO measurement using this new algorithm, was closely correlated ($r = 0.88$) and similar to PATD CO measures (bias = -0.2 ± 1.2 L/min), although there was increased variability in the CO in contrast to hemodynamically stable patients (Godje et al., 2002). Recalibration of the two pulse contour systems is required every 4 to 8 hours or with marked changes in hemodynamic status (Hamilton et al., 2002; Pittman et al., 2002).

A concern about not using a PA catheter may be the lack of information about the risk for pulmonary edema. Pulse contour analysis allows for the measurement of both intrathoracic blood volume and extravascular lung water. Extravascular lung water (>7 ml/kg ideal body weight) was a better indicator of pulmonary edema than chest radiograph or PAWP (Bindels et al., 1999), and increased EVLW is associated with increased mortality (Mitchell et al., 1992). Fluid management guided by EVLW compared to PA pressure indices has been shown to reduce ventilator days, length of ICU stay, and mortality (Mitchell et al., 1992).

Limitations of Pulse Contour Analysis

A decrease in the accuracy of pulse contour measurements occurs with any condition that alters the transfer of the indicator across the heart and lungs (e.g., intracardiac shunts, aortic aneurysm/stenosis, pneumonectomy, and pulmonary embolism), arrhythmias, rapidly changing temperature, and during extracorporeal circulation or IABP. A relative contraindication to pulse contour analysis is the presence an extremely damped arterial waveform (Rodig et al., 1999). Of interest, a study of PulseCO catheters found that although 68% of the catheters had underdamped dynamic response characteristics, this did not affect the relationship between PulseCO and intermittent CO measurements (Pittman et al., 2002). Similar research is needed on PiCCO.

Doppler Ultrasound

Doppler ultrasound is performed using an internal probe (esophagus or endotracheal tube) or via a transcutaneous approach via the suprasternal notch. This section focuses on the esophageal Doppler monitor (EDM). Blood flow measurements using ultrasound are based on the Doppler principle. The system emits an ultrasound beam that is directed toward flowing blood. The ultrasound wave is reflected by the blood moving toward the signal, causing the signal to shift in frequency. The magnitude of the frequency shift is proportional to blood flow velocity. Blood flow is equal to the cross-sectional area of the column (i.e., the aorta) times the flow velocity (Gan, 2000; Singer, 1993). Stroke volume is derived by multiplying the cross-sectional area times the area under the flow curve. There are currently two methods used to measure the cross-sectional area: use of a nomogram based on age, weight, and height or direct measurement using an M-mode transducer embedded in the EDM probe (Boulnois & Pechoux, 2000). Inaccurate cross-sectional area measurement leads to underestimation of the CO. The calculation of systemic CO from aortic blood flow is based on the assumption that there is a constant division of blood flow between the aorta (70%) and brachiocephalic vessels (30%). This distribution may change under pathophysiological conditions and invalidate the CO measurement (Cariou et al., 1998).

The EDM probe, which is embedded in a 6- to 7-mm diameter tube, is positioned at the mid-thoracic level (approximately 30–40 cm from the teeth) and measures blood flow in the descending aorta (Fig. 23-23A). Correct positioning of the probe is determined by the observation of an optimal cardiac signal.

Clinical Applications of EDM

In addition to measuring the CO, the indices obtained from the Doppler flow wave also provide information regarding preload, contractility, and afterload (Table 23-11 and Fig. 23-23B, C). The intraoperative use of the EDM to guide optimization of volume status and SV has been shown to decrease postoperative morbidity and mortality (Sinclair et al., 1997). For example, in patients undergoing major surgery, optimizing preload using EDM-derived indices compared to standard monitoring was associated with decreased length of hospitalization (6 vs. 7 days), earlier tolerance of a solid diet (3 vs. 5 days), and decreased postoperative nausea and vomiting (Gan et al., 2002).

In patients undergoing emergent cardiac surgery, the best indicators of postoperative morbidity and mortality were the SV (<60 mL) and increased HR (>90 beats per minute) at the time of admission to the ICU, both of which can be effectively monitored with EDM (Poeze et al., 1999). Interim analysis of data from 39 critically ill patients treated in accordance with a nurse-driven algorithm demonstrated a 19% decrease in hospital length of stay for those patients who received aggressive volume resuscitation as guided by EDM during the first 4 hours after cardiac surgery (Saberi et al., 2000). Additionally in critically ill patients, the use of EDM, improved diagnostic accuracy by ICU physicians (the physicians correctly predicted the CI in only 44% of patients) and led to a change in therapy in 54% of the patients. This study demonstrated the safety of the EDM and the ability of critical care nurses to place and monitor the patient using this technology (Iregui et al., 2003). Use of EDM is contraindicated in patients with pathology of the aorta or intraaortic balloon pump.

Echocardiography

Doppler echocardiography provides information on CO, global and regional left and RV systolic and diastolic function, end-diastolic area (preload), and regional wall motion abnormalities.

■ **Figure 23–23.** (*A*) Correct positioning of the esophageal Doppler probe. (Reproduced courtesy of Deltex Medical.) (*B*) Doppler flow velocity waveform. (*C*) waveforms of EDM. The first graph shows the components of the normal Doppler waveform and the effect of increasing preload, which corresponds to an increased FT_c. The second graph displays poor contractility (decreased PV), which responds to inotropes by increasing PV. The last graph displays increased afterload (decreased FT_c and decreased PV) and the effects of afterload reduction (increased FT_c and increased PV) (Gan, T. [2000]. The esophageal Doppler as an alternative to the pulmonary artery catheter. *Current Opinion in Critical Care*, 6, 214–221.)

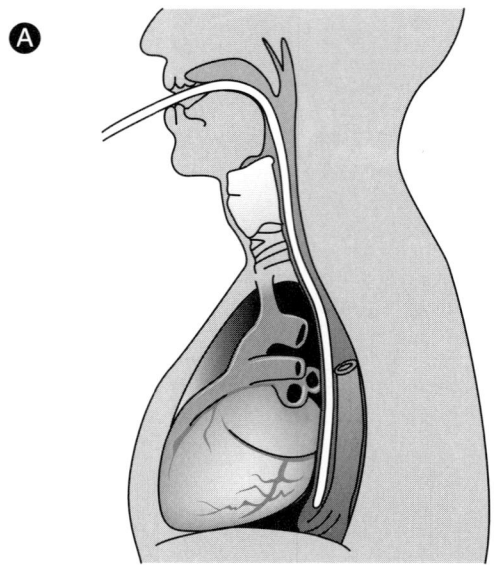

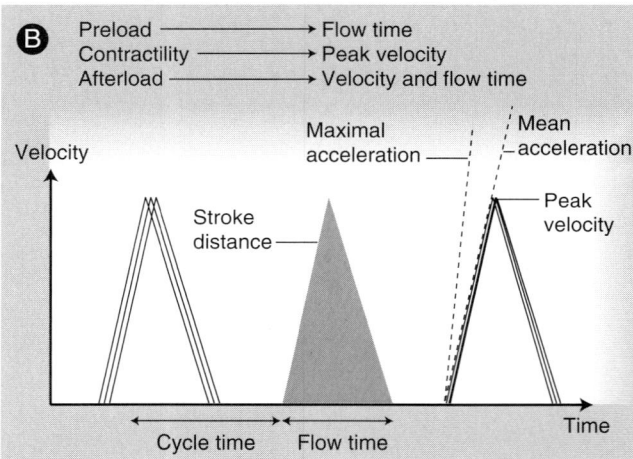

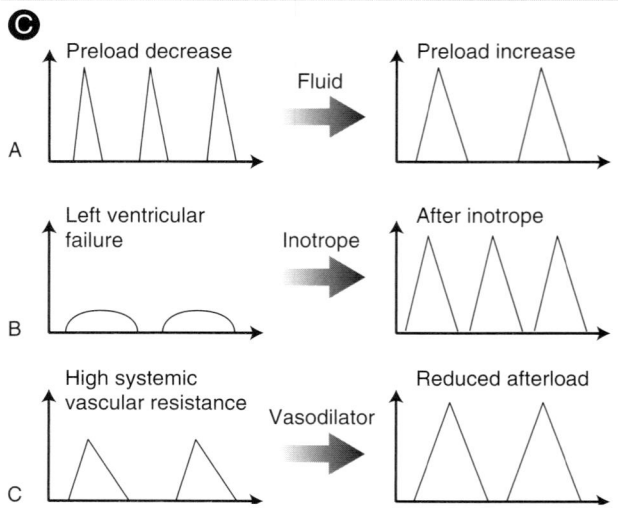

Table 23–11 ▪ DOPPLER INDICES

Indices	Normal Value			Interpretation
Flow time corrected (FTc)	330–360 msec			Correction in flow time for heart rate. The FT$_c$ provides an indicator of alterations in ventricular filling or preload. ↓ FTc (narrow base of waveform)—hypovolemia/decreased preload. ↑ FTc—increased preload. (DiCorte et al., 2000; Madan et al., 1999)
Peak velocity (PV) (Gardin et al., 1987)	Age	PV (cm/sec)	MA	Peak velocity of blood (apex of waveform) during the systolic ejection phase. Provides an index of contractility. ↑ PV—increased contractility
	20	90–120	15.6	
	30	85–115	14.9	
Mean acceleration (MA)	40	80–110	14.1	
	50	70–100	12.7	MA: Maximum slope of the velocity curve as a function of time (derivative of the velocity). Indicator of contractility.
	60	60–90	11.2	
	70	50–80	9.7	
	80	40–70	8.2	*↑ afterload: ↓ PV (decreased contractile force) and ↓ FTc
	90	30–60	6.7	(decreased ejection time)

Echocardiography is also useful in the diagnosis of traumatic aortic injury after blunt chest trauma, cardiac tamponade, and mechanical complications after an acute MI (e.g., mitral valve dysfunction, free wall rupture, septal defect) (Patel et al., 2003; Peterson et al., 2003).

Clinical Usefulness of TEE in The ICU

In the ICU, transesophageal echocardiography (TEE) rather than transthoracic echocardiography (TTE) may be necessary when there is interference with imaging caused by subcutaneous air, chest wall edema, the presence of mediastinal or pleural tubes, mechanical ventilation, or surgical dressings. Use of TEE in the ICU is recommended in the management of hemodynamic instability of unknown cause (Practice Guidelines, 1996).

Transesophageal echocardiography is typically used for a single monitoring event in sedated/anesthetized patients, although there is limited research demonstrating its usefulness for continuous monitoring during the postoperative period (4 hours). The use of TEE improves diagnostic accuracy in critically ill patients compared to PA catheter derived diagnosis, particularly in cases of unexplained hypotension, abnormal ventricular function, cardiac tamponade, and the determination of preload status (hypo- or hypervolemia) (Colreavy et al., 2002; Fontes et al., 1999). TEE–CO is only moderately correlated with PATD–CO and Fick–CO measurements (Jaeggi et al., 2003); thus CO–TEE can be used to follow trends, but caution must be taken when interpreting absolute values. TEE can be used to monitor respiratory-induced changes in peak aortic flow velocity as an indicator of preload responsiveness (Feissel et al., 2001) (see Table 23-7).

Complications and Limitations of TEE

Although TEE is a relatively safe procedure, complications can occur (major complications <0.02%) (Peterson et al., 2003). The patient should be monitored for hypotension, arrhythmias, and vomiting and aspiration during placement of the probe (Gendreau et al., 1999). Additional complications include pharyngeal, laryngeal, or esophageal trauma and dental damage. The use of TEE in the ICU is limited by the need for extensive training to perform this technique and the lack of research supporting its use for continuous monitoring. The TEE provides different information than standard hemodynamic monitoring and should be used to augment rather than replace standard monitoring.

Impedance Cardiography

Impedance cardiography (ICG) or thoracic electrical bioimpedance (TEB) measures the electrical resistance of the thorax to high-frequency low-amplitude current. The current is passed through the thorax and the voltage change with each systole is measured. This change in voltage is the result of a change in TEB, which corresponds with systole (Gendreau et al., 1999). The TEB is inversely proportional to the content of thoracic fluids (i.e., when thoracic fluids increase the TEB decreases). Three factors affect TEB: (1) change in tissue fluid volume; (2) respiratory-induced changes in pulmonary and venous volume; and (3) changes in aortic blood flow. The change in aortic blood flow can be measured by the change in TEB, assuming the other factors remain stable or are filtered (Chaney & Derdak, 2002).

The system consists of eight specialized electrodes, with two pairs placed laterally on the neck and two pairs at the lateral aspect of the lower thorax (at the level of the xiphosternal junction) (van der Meer et al., 1996). The electrical voltage (2 to 4 mA), which is safe and not felt by the patient, is passed longitudinally through the thorax between electrodes.

Factors that affect the accuracy of ICG measures include the positioning of the electrodes (i.e., the electrodes must be in exactly same position for each measurement) (van der Meer et al., 1996), any factor that interferes with electrode contact (e.g., perspiration), an irregular heart rhythm, or altered tissue water content (chest wall edema, pulmonary edema, or pleural effusions). Obesity (>15% of ideal body weight) (van der Meer et al., 1997) and breath holding also decrease the accuracy of the measure. ICG CO measurements cannot be obtained in patients with abnormal chest morphology (kyphoscoliosis), intraoperatively during electrocautery, low blood flow (<2 L/min), during mechanical ventilation (particularly with PEEP in conjunction with high CO), or an open thorax (Doering et al., 1995; Genoni et al., 1998).

Clinical Applications of ICG

Despite the concerns regarding the comparability of ICG CO with other CO measures, ICG has been used for intraoperative monitoring and in outpatient and emergency department settings for the diagnosis and management of patients. A unique variable provided by ICG is a measure of fluid status (Zo), which is a composite measure of interstitial, alveolar, and intracellular fluid (Lasater & Von Rueden, 2003). A normal Zo is 20 to 30 Ω for males and 25 to 30 Ω for females. In heart failure patients, there was an inverse relationship between Zo and chest radiograph findings of pulmonary edema, and a Zo less than 19 Ω is highly sensitive and specific for identifying radiographic findings of pulmonary edema. Interstitial edema was present at Zo = 18.5 ± 7.1 Ω and alveolar edema was present at 14.8 ± 5 Ω (Milzman et al., 1997). Use of ICG may aid in the differential diagnosis of shortness of breath. In patients with suspected heart failure and shortness of breath, the Zo was significantly different in patients with radiographic evidence of cardiomegaly (17.5 ± 5 Ω) and pulmonary edema (17.2 ± 4.2 Ω) than those with normal radiographs (23.4 ± 5.4 Ω) (Peacock et al., 2000). A second unique measure is the dZ/dt, which reflects the force of LV contraction and can be visualized on an impedance waveform. A less acute rise in the dZ/dt waveform may indicate decreased contractility and is useful in the differential diagnosis of systolic versus diastolic failure (Summers et al., 1999a, 1999b).

ICG monitoring has also been effectively used for the outpatient management of patients with heart failure. For detection of a CI ≤ 2.2 L/min/m² as determined by PATD, the ICG had a sensitivity of 62%, specificity of 79%, and a positive predictive values of 68%, highlighting the limitations in using absolute ICG values rather than following trends (Drazner et al., 2002). Several excellent nursing articles provide case studies of the usefulness of ICG to manage patients with heart failure and inotropic therapy (Gilbert & Lazio, 1999; Lasater, 1999; Lasater & Von Rueden, 2003). In patients with resistant hypertension, therapy guided by ICG monitoring resulted in a greater improvement in control rates compared to management by an experienced clinician (56% vs. 34%, $p < 0.05$) (Taler et al., 2002). The ICG can also be used to optimize pacemaker therapy (Johnson et al., 2001). However ICG monitoring is *absolutely contraindicated* in patients who have pacemakers that use "minute ventilation" to guide the firing rate. In this case, the ICG signal will interfere with the pacemaker signal and potentially cause a rapid increase in firing rate (Belott, 1999).

ICG monitoring has also been performed extensively in the emergency department to describe cardiopulmonary and tissue perfusion patterns in survivors and nonsurvivors of trauma or septic shock (Shoemaker et al., 1998; Shoemaker et al., 2001; Shoemaker et al., 2000). The early identification and treatment of patients with septic shock decreases morbidity and mortality (Rivers, Nguyen et al., 2001). ICG monitoring may aid in this early diagnosis and treatment.

Noninvasive Partial CO$_2$ Rebreathing System

Noninvasive partial CO$_2$ measurement uses a modified Fick equation to calculate CO. Simply stated, the system answers the question, "How much pulmonary capillary blood flow is necessary to effect an observed change in CO$_2$?" Measurements are obtained at baseline and after a short period of partial CO$_2$ rebreathing. The rebreathing phase is created by the automated addition of deadspace (120 mL) into the ventilator circuit, which causes rebreathing of exhaled gas. The system cycles every 3 minutes with 50-second rebreathing periods, thus updating the CO value every 4 minutes (Jaffe, 1999). The changes in CO$_2$ elimination and end-tidal CO$_2$, which are measured by a mainstream CO$_2$ analyzer, are used to derive the CO as described by the following equation

$$CO = \frac{\Delta \dot{V}CO_2}{\Delta CaCO_2}$$

where $\Delta \dot{V}CO_2$ is the change in CO$_2$ production and $\Delta CaCO_2$ is the change in CO$_2$ content.

A limitation of this technique is that it measures nonshunted pulmonary blood flow and requires a correction based on pulse oximetry data to estimate the shunt fraction and to calculate the CO. In the case of increased shunt (>15%), increased deadspace ($V_D/V_T > 0.6$), or abnormal arterial hemoglobin (Hgb <9 or >16 g/dL), the PaO$_2$ values from an ABG should be used to calculate the shunt fraction (Gama de Abreu et al., 2003). The accuracy of NICO CO measurements is also decreased under conditions of unstable ventilation (that is, with decreased V_T or minute ventilation) during spontaneous versus controlled ventilation and if the patient is hyperventilating (PCO$_2$ <30 mm Hg) (Gamma de Abreu et al., 2000; Tachibana et al., 2003). There is also an increased difference in CO measurements compared to PATD CO in patients with more severe lung disease. This technique must be used with caution in patients with head trauma because the rebreathing cycle causes an intermittent increase in PCO$_2$ of 2 to 5 mm Hg (Guzzi et al., 1998). Based on these findings, partial rebreathing CO$_2$ appears to be best used in patients with limited pulmonary compromise, receiving controlled ventilation, or in sedated patients on mechanical ventilation with limited variability in pulmonary indices (e.g., rate, V_T, minute ventilation) and a relatively normal hemodynamic profile.

■ OXYGEN SUPPLY AND DEMAND

In critically ill patients, the monitoring and evaluation of specific indicators of tissue hypoxia is warranted, because the standard indices of hemodynamic stability (i.e., BP, HR, and UOP) may be normal in the presence of continued tissue hypoxia. For example, 36 critically ill patients who despite being resuscitated to a HR of 50 to 120 bpm and a MAP of 70

Table 23–12 ■ OXYGEN TRANSPORT EQUATIONS

Variables	Equation/Example	Normal
Arterial oxygen content (CaO_2)	$(Hgb \times 1.36 \times SaO_2) + (0.003 \times PaO_2)$	20 mL/dL
	$(15 \times 1.36 \times 0.99) + (0.003 \times 100)$	
Venous oxygen content (CvO_2)	$(Hgb \times 1.36 \times S\bar{v}O_2) + (0.003 \times PvO_2)$	15 mL/dL
	$(15 \times 1.36 \times 0.75) + (0.003 \times 40)$	
Oxygen Delivery (DO_2)	$CO \times CaO_2 \times 10$	1000 mL/min
	$5 \times (15 \times 1.36 \times 0.99) \times 10$	
Oxygen Delivery Index (DO_2I)	$CI \times CaO_2 \times 10$	600 mL/min/m²
	$3.5 \times (15 \times 1.36 \times 0.99) \times 10$	
Oxygen Consumption (VO_2)	$CO \times 1.36 \times Hgb (SaO_2 - S\bar{v}O_2)$	250 mL/min
	$5 \times 1.36 \times 15 (1.0 - 0.75)$	
Oxygen Consumption Index (VO_2I)	$CI \times 1.36 \times Hgb (SaO2 - S\bar{v}O_2)$	125 mL/min/m²
	$3.5 \times 1.36 \times 15 (1.0 - 0.75)$	
Oxygen Extraction Ratio (O_2ER)	DO_2/VO_2	25%
Cardiac Index/Oxygen Extraction Ratio	CI/O_2ER	10–12
	3.0/0.25	

to 110 mm Hg continued to have signs of tissue hypoxia (lactate >2 mmol/L and a central venous oxygen saturation [$ScvO_2$] <65%). Although interventions were undertaken to improve tissue oxygenation for these patients (as indicated by a decrease in lactate and an increase in $ScvO_2$), there were no changes in the BP or HR (Rady et al., 1996). Similar results were observed in patients with cardiogenic shock (Ander et al., 1998) and trauma victims (Wo et al., 1993). Use of standard endpoints (e.g., MAP >60 mm Hg) may also be insufficient in ensuring adequate tissue perfusion. For example, in patients with septic shock whose MAP was increased with norepinephrine from 65 to 85 mm Hg, although the CI increased there was no improvement in indicators of tissue perfusion (lactate, gastric intramucosal PCO_2) (LeDoux et al., 2000). Therefore, standard hemodynamic indices may not be sensitive to changes in tissue oxygenation, and the use of global (O_2 delivery and consumption, serum lactate, and venous O_2 saturation) and regional indices (gastric tonometry, sublingual capnometry) may be needed. A discussion of the basic principles underlying the monitoring of each of these indices along with examples of the utility of the measurements follows.

Global Indicators of Oxygen Supply and Demand

Systemic Oxygen Consumption and Delivery

Oxygen delivery depends on the amount of O_2 in the blood and how much blood is delivered to the tissues (CO). The derivation of the O_2 delivery equations was outlined in Chapter 2. The other half of the delivery/consumption equation is O_2 consumption (VO_2). The normal (VO_2) is approximately 250 mL/min, with an indexed value of 115 to 165 mL/min/m² and an average of 125 mL/min/m². The (VO_2) cannot be directly measured at the bedside; therefore, derived values are often used (Table 23-12). The use of derived values must be undertaken with caution, because large individual variability (10%–25%) may exist (Grossman, 2000). A limitation of solely monitoring the (VO_2) is that it is affected by factors such

as core body temperature, nursing activities, and disease states (Table 23-13). A complete assessment requires knowledge of the DO_2 or an indicator of the balance between O_2 supply and demand (e.g., O_2ER, SvO_2, and ScvO2).

Response to Alterations in Oxygen Delivery

In response to an increase in O_2 demand or a decrease in Hgb or SaO_2, the normal compensatory response is to increase CO, such that VO_2 is not affected. As the result of this compensation, a change in DO_2 does not normally result in a decrease in VO_2. However, when the DO_2 decreases below a critical level (4 to 8 mL O_2/kg per min), the VO_2 also decreases (Ronco et al., 1993). This latter state is referred to as supply dependent O_2 consumption.

Of the three factors that affect delivery (CO, Hgb, SaO_2), changes in CO and Hgb have the greatest effect, with the changes in Hgb better tolerated than changes in CO (Reed, 1993). It is estimated that for every 1 g of Hgb lost, the CO must increase

Table 23–13 ■ PERCENTAGE INCREASE IN RESTING $S\bar{v}O_2$ ASSOCIATED WITH CONDITIONS AND ACTIVITIES

Conditions	%	Activities	%
Fever (each 1°C)	10	Dressing change	10
Fractures (each)	10	Electrocardiogram	10
Agitation	18	Physical examination	20
Chest trauma	25	Visitors	22
Work of breathing	40	Bath	23
Severe infection	60	Chest radiograph	25
Shivering	50–100	Endotracheal suctioning	27
Sepsis	50–100	Nasal intubation	25–40
Head injury, sedated	89	Turn to side	31
Head injury, not sedated	138	Chest physiotherapy	35
Burns	100	Weight on sling scale	36

White, K. M. (1993). Using continuous $S\bar{v}O_2$ to assess oxygen supply/demand balance in the critically ill patient. *AACN Clinical Issues in Critical Care Nursing, 4,* 134–147. With permission.

Table 23–14 ■ SYSTEMATIC APPROACH TO OXYGEN TRANSPORT GOALS (based on Yu, 1999)

	Recommendation

Optimize SaO_2	• Maintain $SaO_2 \geq 90\%$ with an $FiO_2 < 0.5$ to 0.6 with lowest airway pressure possible
	• Rule out pulmonary causes of hypoxia
	   • Hypoventilation
	   • Ventilation/perfusion mismatch
	   • Shunt
	• Rule out nonpulmonary causes of decreased SaO_2
	   • Increased shunt in presence of decreased Hgb or CO and/or increased VO_2
	*Accuracy of SaO_2 measures are affected by low CO, ambient temperature, vasoconstriction

Optimize Hgb	• Assess patients ability to increase CO to offset decreased O_2 carrying capacity along with indications of tissue hypoxia (e.g., lactate, base excess, $S\overline{v}O_2$, $ScvO_2$)
	• Transfusion triggers (Hebert, 1998)
	   • Significant cardiac disease (MI or unstable angina)
	     ◦ Transfuse at 10 g/dL
	     ◦ Maintain Hgb at 10–12 g/dL
	   • No cardiac disease
	     ◦ Transfuse at 8 g/dL
	     ◦ Maintain Hgb at 8–10 g/dL

Optimize CO	• Preload
	   • Evaluate preload indices (CVP, PAWP, functional indices)
	   • Goal: PAWP 12–15 mm Hg or no further improvement in functional indices
	• Afterload
	   • Ensure adequate preload before afterload manipulation
	   • Goal maintain MAP 65–90 mm Hg
	   • Vasoactive agent may vary depending on disease process (i.e., norepinephrine versus dopamine in septic shock)
	• Contractility
	   • Monitor effect of inotropic agents on myocardial O_2 consumption
	   • Optimize preload and afterload before initiation of inotropic therapy
	   • Agents: dobutamine (3–5 μg/kg/min and titrate up to 20 μg/kg/min)
	   • Titrate therapy based on MAP and $S\overline{v}O_2$/$ScvO_2$

9% to maintain a similar $\dot{D}O_2$. This is important in developing a plan of care to optimize O_2 delivery. A systematic approach (Table 23-14) that addresses all the factors that affect O_2 delivery should be taken to achieve O_2 transport goals (Yu, 1999).

Optimization of Oxygen Delivery

Previous research suggested that achieving optimal or supranormal O_2 supply and demand ($\dot{D}O_2 > 600$ mL/min per m², $\dot{V}O_2 > 170$ mL/min per m², CI > 4.5 L/min per m²) improved outcomes in patients at high risk (Boyd et al., 1993; Shoemaker et al., 1993). The rationale for these goals was that an O_2 debt develops when there is an imbalance between O_2 supply and consumption. This O_2 debt is a major determinant of mortality (Shoemaker et al., 1992). The goal of normal or "supranormal" O_2 delivery was to reverse the O_2 debt. However, clinical trials failed to demonstrate any benefit from this therapy, and attempts to achieve a supranormal state in patients who do not demonstrate a physiological reserve may be harmful (Velmahos et al., 2000; Yu et al., 1998).

In trauma victims in shock, patients who achieved optimal physiological levels either spontaneously or with therapeutic interventions (fluids, inotropes, blood) had improved survival compared to patients who did not achieve these levels (0% vs. 30% mortality) (McKinley et al., 2002; Velmahos et al., 2000). These results highlight the current interpretation of the literature that it is not the achievement of the optimal levels, but rather it is the ability to achieve optimal levels as an indicator of physiological reserve, which is predictive of survival.

A major criticism of the research related to optimization is that in many cases resuscitation was not initiated until after organ failure had occurred. Evidence suggests that although achieving normal O_2 delivery is important (Heyland et al., 1996), the timing of the initiation of goal-directed therapy may be the more critical factor in decreasing morbidity and mortality (Kern & Shoemaker, 2002; Rivers, Nguyen et al., 2001). A meta-analysis found no decrease in mortality if attempts to improve tissue perfusion were taken after the onset of organ failure (Alia et al., 1999; Gattinoni et al., 1995; Hayes et al., 1994; Yu et al., 1998; Yu et al., 1993). In contrast, beneficial effects were observed when attempts to improve oxygenation were taken before the onset of organ failure (Boyd et al., 1993; Lobo et al., 2000; Tuchschmidt et al., 1992; Wilson et al., 1999).

In a recent study, patients who presented to the emergency department with severe sepsis or septic shock received 6 hours of early goal-directed therapy, including volume resuscitation, blood transfusions, and vasopressor therapy, aimed at optimizing tissue oxygenation (CVP 8—12 mm Hg, MAP $\geq$ 65 mm Hg, UOP $\geq$ 0.5 mL/kg per hr, and $ScvO_2 > 70\%$). An interesting finding is this study was that on admission, despite relatively normal vital signs in both the control and experimental groups, both groups had indications of tissue hypoxia. Early goal-directed therapy was associated with a 16% absolute reduction in mortality compared to standard care. Although there was no difference between the routine care and experimental group in length of ICU stay, the experimental group was also less acutely ill during the first 3 days in the ICU and had a shorter length of hospitalization (Rivers, Nguyen et al., 2001).

Mixed Venous Oxygen Saturation

Although CO provides important information about the capacity of the cardiopulmonary system to deliver O_2 to the tissues, it does not necessarily depict the adequacy of O_2 supply at the tissue level. The $S\bar{v}O_2$, which is a global measure of the balance between total body O_2 delivery and consumption, is affected by factors that affect O_2 delivery and consumption. The assumption is that if the Hgb and SaO_2 are not changing; the change in $S\bar{v}O_2$ reflects a change in CO. However, a decreased $S\bar{v}O_2$ may also be caused by arterial hypoxemia, increased $\dot{V}O_2$, or a decreased Hgb; and in patients with severe heart failure (EF <30%), the $S\bar{v}O_2$ was not an adequate indicator of changes in CO (Gawlinski, 1998).

Technical Aspects of $S\bar{v}O_2$ Monitoring

Components of the $S\bar{v}O_2$ monitoring system include the fiberoptic PA catheter, the optical module, and the microprocessor. The fiberoptic catheter is a quadruple-lumen PA catheter with fiberoptic channels running the length of the catheter. The optical module contains diodes that emit light pulses at two or three wavelengths through one of the fiberoptic channels in the tip of the catheter. The second fiberoptic channel returns reflected light to a photodetector in the optical module. The amount of light reflected depends on the amount of saturated Hgb, because oxygenated and deoxygenated Hgb have different reflections. The light is relayed electronically to the microprocessor, which interprets the light signal and determines the ratio between oxygenated and deoxygenated blood. The $S\bar{v}O_2$ is based on this ratio.

Indications

Continuous $S\bar{v}O_2$ monitoring has been recommended for monitoring and as an outcome measure in patients with sepsis/septic shock, cardiac surgery, complicated MI (i.e., cardiogenic shock), or patients with respiratory failure requiring PEEP. However, changes in $S\bar{v}O_2$ are only moderately related to changes in CO in critically ill patients (cardiac, respiratory, surgical), postcardiac surgery patients, and patients with advanced heart failure (Gawlinski, 1998).

Clinical Application

The $S\bar{v}O_2$ normally ranges from 60% to 80% (average 75%), which is associated with a PvO_2 of 40 mm Hg. An $S\bar{v}O_2$ of less than 40% is usually accompanied by anaerobic metabolism, and an $S\bar{v}O_2$ between 40% and 60% indicates inadequate $\dot{D}O_2$ or excessive O_2 demand (Cernaianu & Nelson, 1993). In response to increased O_2 demand, the body either increases CO to deliver more O_2 or increases the extraction of O_2 from the blood. When the SaO_2 is maintained at a high level (near 100%), there is a strong relationship between the $S\bar{v}O_2$ and the O_2 extraction ratio (O_2ER), as defined by the equation: $S\bar{v}O_2 = 1 - O_2ER$. Increased O_2 extraction decreases Hgb saturation, which is reflected as a decrease in $S\bar{v}O_2$. As long as O_2 delivery is adequate to meet tissue O_2

demands, the $S\bar{v}O_2$ remains within 60% to 80%. Decreases in $S\bar{v}O_2$ occur with an increase in O_2 demand (e.g., fever, shivering, pain, seizures, sepsis) or decreased O_2 delivery (e.g., cardiac failure, hemorrhage, hypoxia, hypovolemia, arrhythmias). Conversely, increased $S\bar{v}O_2$ (>80%) is the result of decreased O_2 demand (e.g., hypothermia, sedation, neuromuscular blockade) or is an indicator of maldistribution or impaired cellular use of O_2 in sepsis. Technical causes of a high $S\bar{v}O_2$ include a wedged PA catheter or deposits of fibrin on the tip of the catheter, or during manual sampling when the rapid withdrawal of blood from the catheter results in a contaminated specimen.

Continuous $S\bar{v}O_2$ is useful in evaluating the effect of O_2-sensitive nursing and interdisciplinary interventions. Interventions such as a bed bath, positioning, or chest physiotherapy increase O_2 consumption (Table 23-13) (Atkins et al., 1994; Banasik & Emerson, 2001; Horiuchi et al., 1997). For example, in patients with low EF ($\leq$ 30%), the $S\bar{v}O_2$ decreased immediately after turning (Gawlinski & Dracup, 1998). The decrease was caused by increased $\dot{V}O_2$ in contrast to decreased delivery. In patients with anemia (Hgb <10 g/dL) and low $\dot{D}O_2I$ (<500 mL/min per m^2), the $S\bar{v}O_2$ decreased acutely with turning and remained lower for 10 minutes than in patients with Hgb more than 10 g/dL (Reed et al., 2003). These latter results are important given current recommendations to liberalize the trigger for blood transfusions to 8 g/dL for patients without cardiac disease and 10 g/dL for patients with cardiac disease (Hebert, 1998). Modification of the plan of care may be particularly important in patients with increased baseline ($\dot{V}O_2$) (sepsis, trauma, pain) who also have limited capacity to increase O_2 delivery (heart failure). An interdisciplinary plan of care aimed at balancing O_2 supply and demand may include actions to decrease ($\dot{V}O_2$) (antipyretics, pain medications, sedation) and limit or reorganize nursing activities (i.e., avoiding clustering of activities) in high-risk patients (Manthous et al., 1995). Interventions to improve $\dot{D}O_2$ have been previously described (see Table 23-14).

In cardiac surgery patients, continuous $S\bar{v}O_2$ was considered useful (i.e., triggered an intervention that would not have been initiated based on routine monitoring) in 57% of patients studied, with increased usefulness in the most critically ill (ASA Class 4, NYHA score $\geq$3) (Vedrinne et al., 1997). The $S\bar{v}O_2$ may also be predictive of cardiopulmonary compromise after cardiac surgery. An $S\bar{v}O_2$ of less than 55% on arrival to the ICU after cardiac surgery was predictive of a perioperative myocardial infarction, additional ventilatory support, and prolonged ICU stay (Keech & Reed, 2003). Continuous $S\bar{v}O_2$ monitoring is also useful in evaluating a patient's tolerance to ventilator weaning. Patients who failed to wean demonstrated a progressive decrease in $S\bar{v}O_2$ (Jubran et al., 1998).

The interpretation of CO should include a systematic assessment of the $S\bar{v}O_2$ and the (O_2ER) (Fig. 23-24). Vincent suggests that $S\bar{v}O_2$ is the most important factor in the determination of adequate hemodynamic status, particularly if it is low (Vincent & De Backer, 2002). In the presence of anemia, when the $S\bar{v}O_2$ is low, the creation of CI/O_2ER diagram may also be helpful (Yalavatti et al., 2000).

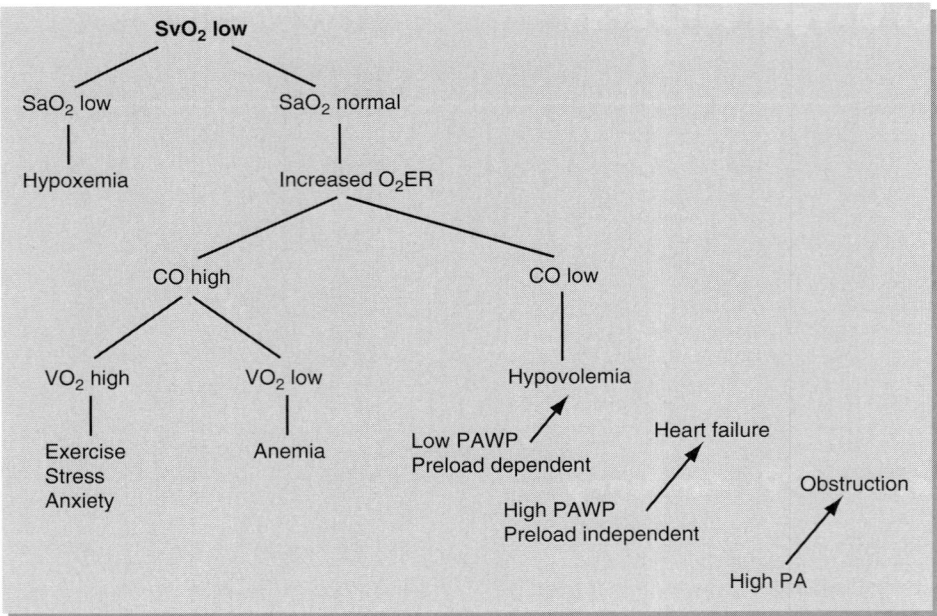

■ **Figure 23–24.** Interpretation of hemodynamic data starting with mixed venous O_2 saturation (SvO_2), O_2ER, O_2 extraction ratio; VO_2, O_2 uptake. (Vincent, J.L., De Backer, D. [2002]. Cardiac output measurement: Is least invasive always the best? *Critical Care Medicine*, 30 [10], 2381.

Central Venous Oxygen Saturation

An alternative to the $S\bar{v}O_2$ is the central venous O_2 saturation ($ScvO_2$), which is obtained from an oximetric catheter or PICC line positioned in the superior vena cava (Lopez et al., 2003; Rivers, Ander et al., 2001). In general, changes in the $ScvO_2$ match changes in $S\bar{v}O_2$. However, the $ScvO_2$ tends to overestimate the $S\bar{v}O_2$ by approximately 1% to 3% and wide individual variability can occur, thus the values are not interchangeable (Edwards & Mayall, 1998; Martin et al., 1992; Rivers, Ander et al., 2001; Turnaoglu et al., 2001).

Clinically, the $ScvO_2$ can be used to track changes, and low $ScvO_2$ (<60%), which indicates an even lower $S\bar{v}O_2$, can be used as an indicator of impaired O_2 delivery. The $ScvO_2$ may be a marker of unresolved tissue hypoxia, despite normalization of vital signs. For example, in critically ill patients who were resuscitated to normal vital signs, 50% continued to have increased lactate levels and decreased $ScvO_2$ levels (Rady et al., 1996). Similar results were observed in patients with acutely decompensated heart failure. In this latter group, the $ScvO_2$ increased with treatment to improve cardiac function (Ander et al., 1998). Most recently, $ScvO_2$ was used as a goal for resuscitation ($ScvO_2$ >70%) for patients with severe sepsis and septic shock. Patients in the early goal-directed therapy group had a significant reduction in mortality compared to patients who received standard care. The authors of this study advocate use of $ScvO_2$ because placement of a central venous catheter can be accomplished early in therapy, in contrast to the potential delay in placement of a pulmonary artery catheter for $S\bar{v}O_2$ monitoring (Rivers, Nguyen et al., 2001; Rivers, Ander et al., 2001).

Oxygen Extraction Ratio

Rather than simply evaluating the $\dot{D}O_2$ and ($\dot{V}O_2$), a more sensitive indicator of the adequacy of the balance between O_2 delivery and demand is the O_2 extraction ratio (O_2ER), which is described by the following equation:

$$O_2ER = (CaO_2 - C\bar{v}O_2/CaO_2$$
$$= (Hgb \times 1.36 \times SaO_2) - (Hgb \times 1.36 \times S\bar{v}O_2)/$$
$$(Hgb \times 1.36 \times SaO_2)$$
$$= (SaO_2 - S\bar{v}O_2)/SaO_2$$

The latter equation is particularly useful because the SaO_2 and $S\bar{v}O_2$ values can be measured at the bedside. A normal O_2ER is approximately 25% (i.e., 25% of the O_2 delivered is consumed). Under normal conditions, as the $\dot{D}O_2$ varies, the $\dot{V}O_2$ remains stable because of variations in O_2 extraction, that is, the $\dot{V}O_2$ is independent of the $\dot{D}O_2$. However, if the $\dot{D}O_2$ decreases to below a critical level, then the $\dot{V}O_2$ becomes dependent on the amount of O_2 delivered. An O_2ER greater than 30% requires further assessment because it indicates compensation for decreased O_2 delivery (Weissman et al., 1994).

Monitoring the O_2ER may be a more useful clinical endpoint than systemic O_2 delivery indices. For example, in elderly patients (older than age 75 years) whose normal $\dot{D}O_2I$ may only be 450 to 550 mL/min/m², maintaining an O_2ER less than 25% rather than aiming for an "optimal" $\dot{D}O_2$ may be a more appropriate clinical target (Yu, 1996; Yu et al., 1998). An increased O_2ER may also be prognostic. In critically ill surgical patients, an increased O_2ER was observed in patients with increased length of ICU stay (Polonen et al., 1997) and decreased survival (Shoemaker, Wo et al., 1999). Similar results were seen in patients with severe sepsis or septic shock (Shoemaker et al., 2000).

Lactate

Lactate is an end product of anaerobic metabolism, and an increased level (>2 mmol/L) is considered a surrogate indicator of tissue hypoxia. Although an increased lactate is indicative of tissue hypoxia because the liver has a large capacity to oxidize lactate, a normal serum lactate level does not mean that tissue hypoperfusion and anaerobic metabolism are not occurring. As long as hepatic function is relatively normal and the CO can increase in response to increased O_2 demands, there will be limited accumulation of lactate, even with a PaO_2 less than 30 mm Hg or with severe anemia (Mizock, 1998). In addition, localized hypoperfusion may be insufficient to increase systemic levels. Therefore, lactate is a late, and often insensitive, indicator of hypoperfusion. Conversely, increased lactate production occurs with factors other than hypoxia, including increased glycolysis (e.g., hypermetabolic state, catecholamine administration, diabetes mellitus, trauma, burns) and hepatic dysfunction. Tissue hypoxia should be ruled out before assuming that other factors are contributing to the increased levels.

Hyperlactatemia (lactate >2 mmol/L) persisting for more than 6 hours after admission is predictive of increased mortality in ICU and trauma patients (Suistomaa et al., 2000). Although increased levels of lactate (>4 mmol/L), particularly levels that do not decrease with treatment, are prognostic of organ failure and poor outcomes in these patients, the use of lactate levels as an indicator of tissue hypoxia is complicated in patients with septic shock (Venkatesh & Morgan, 2002). In septic shock, increased lactate levels occurred when there was adequate O_2 delivery, and, conversely, when the $\dot{D}O_2$ was increased, the lactate levels did not decrease (Vincent, 2002). One factor that may contribute to this effect is increased levels of endogenous epinephrine or the administration of exogenous epinephrine (James et al., 1999).

General recommendations for the use of lactate are to follow trends rather than a single measurement. A decrease in lactate of 5% to 10% per hour is usually indicative of adequate response to treatment, whereas no change or an increase in lactate level is an ominous sign (Takala et al., 1996). The use of gastric tonometry and, more recently, sublingual capnography demonstrate the delay between the onset of tissue hypoxia and increased levels of serum lactate and, conversely, the delay in a decrease in lactate with the resolution of hypoxia. Therefore, a high index of suspicion should be maintained despite a normal lactate level.

Regional Indicators

Monitoring of regional indices of oxygenation (gut mucosa, subcutaneous and muscle tissue) is based on the assumption that these areas serve as early markers of systemic hypoperfusion, because hypoperfusion results in the movement of blood away from these areas to more vital areas (i.e., heart, brain).

Gastric Tonometry

Gastric tonometry was originally designed to measure the intramucosal pH (pHi), which was shown to be a better predictor of organ dysfunction and mortality than O_2-derived variables. Because of limitations in this technique, the use of gastric mucosal pCO_2 ($PiCO_2$)–arterial CO_2 ($PaCO_2$) gap is now recommended. The $PiCO_2$ is obtained by aspirating gas samples from an air-filled balloon on the end of gastric tube. Currently, there is no standardized normal value for the $PiCO_2$–$PaCO_2$ gap, with recommended values ranging from 2 to 10 mm Hg (i.e., $PaCO_2 = 40$ mm Hg, $PiCO_2 = 50$ mm Hg) (Uhlig et al., 2002). While a $PiCO_2$–$PaCO_2$ gap greater than 25 to 35 mm Hg is indicative of the onset of anaerobic metabolism, a $PiCO_2$–$PaCO_2$ gap of 40 mm Hg is neither a sensitive nor a specific indicator of severe splanchnic hypoperfusion (Kellum et al., 2000). Of clinical usefulness, an increase in the $PiCO_2$–$PaCO_2$ gap greater than 20 mm Hg was associated with increased complications and mortality (Levy et al., 2003). In trauma patients, a value greater than 18 mm Hg was predictive of multiorgan dysfunction syndrome and death (Miller, Kincaid et al., 1998). The current recommendation is to maintain a gap less than 25 mm Hg to avoid anaerobic metabolism (Uhlig et al., 2002; Vallet et al., 2000), although there are no clinical trials demonstrating the usefulness of the measurement as an endpoint of resuscitation.

Although gastric tonometry provides potentially useful clinical information, its use at the bedside is limited. This semi-invasive system requires up to 90 minutes for equilibration, and for accurate measurements the patient must have feedings withheld for a minimum of 1 hour, or aspiration of the gastric contents, before measurements are obtained (Levy et al., 1998; Marik & Lorenzana, 1996). Recent research suggests that the $PiCO_2$ stabilizes after 24 to 48 hours of enteral nutrition, and stopping the nutrition may not be necessary after this point (Marshall & West, 2003). In light of these limitations, other areas along the gastrointestinal tract (esophagus and sublingual mucosa) have been considered for monitoring.

Sublingual Capnography

The intermittent measurement of sublingual CO_2 ($P_{SL}CO_2$) is being studied as a surrogate marker of gastrointestinal perfusion. The $P_{SL}CO_2$ is measured by using a sublingual measurement device (Capnoprobe; Nellcor, Pleasanton, CA), which consists of a disposable sensor covered with a membrane that is permeable to CO_2. The sensor contains a fluorescent dye, which emits a light in direct proportion to the amount of CO_2 present. Fiberoptic technology is used to detect the changes in the fluorescence, and these light signals are converted into numeric values. The probe is placed under the tongue in contact with the sublingual mucosa, with a measurement available in approximately 2 to 4 minutes.

In both hemorrhagic shock and septic shock models, the $P_{SL}CO_2$ measurements are comparable to those obtained by gastric tonometry, and the $P_{SL}CO_2$ closely follows changes in blood flow to the GI tract (Povoas et al., 2001). In hemorrhagic shock and septic shock, the $P_{SL}CO_2$ rapidly increased in contrast to lactate levels, which remained unchanged for

1 to 6 hours (Rackow et al., 2001); after replacement of blood in the hemorrhage model, the $P_{SL}CO_2$ rapidly returned to baseline in contrast to lactate, which did not begin to decrease for 1 hour.

A $P_{SL}CO_2$ greater than 70 mm Hg was 100% predictive of the circulatory shock, whereas a $P_{SL}CO_2$ less than 70 mm Hg predicted survival (Marik, 2001; Weil et al., 1999). Although the absolute $P_{SL}CO_2$ value may have prognostic implications, interpretation of this value is difficult because there is a direct relationship between the $PaCO_2$ and the $P_{SL}CO_2$.

The $P_{SL}CO_2$–$PaCO_2$ gradient is considered a more useful indicator of hypoperfusion than the $P_{SL}CO_2$ alone, because the tissue PCO_2 is not affected by alveolar ventilation ($PaCO_2$) unless the CO is decreased. When the O_2 supply to the tissues begins to decrease, the tissue PCO_2 will increase slightly relative to the $PaCO_2$. However, when perfusion decreases below a critical level, there will be a marked increase in tissue PCO_2, which reflects the generation of CO_2 from bicarbonate as it buffers the hydrogen ions produced by anaerobic metabolism (Bernardin et al., 1999). The increased tissue PCO_2 relative to the $PaCO_2$ results in an increased $P_{SL}CO_2$–$PaCO_2$ gradient.

A normal $P_{SL}CO_2$–$PaCO_2$ gradient is less than 10 mm Hg (e.g., $P_{SL}CO_2 = 50$ mm Hg; $PaCO_2 = 40$ mm Hg). In critically ill patients (a majority with severe sepsis), the $P_{SL}CO_2$–$PaCO_2$ gradient was significantly different between survivors (9.2 ± 5.0 mm Hg) and nonsurvivors (17.8 ± 11.5 mm Hg) (Marik, 2001). Current evidence suggests that the clinical usefulness of $P_{SL}CO_2$ monitoring is in the rapid detection of changes in gastric perfusion as an indicator of circulatory shock. However, the prognostic value of $P_{SL}CO_2$, along with its use as an endpoint of resuscitation, remains to be demonstrated, particularly in patients with septic shock.

Tissue Perfusion Monitoring

Clinically, hypovolemia is manifested by a decrease in subcutaneous and muscle tissue O_2 pressure ($P_{sq}O_2$ and $P_{m}O_2$) and increased P_mCO_2 (Drucker et al., 1996). The subcutaneous and muscle tissues regain normal perfusion after restoration of circulation in other areas, and monitoring of these areas may be useful in determining the adequacy of resuscitation. Tissue perfusion monitoring suggests a greater severity of hemorrhage and prolonged resuscitation of hemorrhagic shock than indicated by gastric mucosal or systemic indices. Noninvasive tissue perfusion monitoring may also replace invasive systemic O_2 monitoring (Table 23-15).

Near-Infrared Spectroscopy

Near-infrared spectroscopy (NIRS), which emits a light beam that is capable of penetrating skin, muscle, and bone, provides continuous, noninvasive, semiquantitative measurement of tissue O_2 saturation and the oxidation—reduction (redox) state of cytochrome a,a3. NIRS monitoring is based on the finding that hemoglobin, myoglobin, and cytochrome a,a3 alter their absorption of NIR light with changes in oxygenation.

Cytochrome a,a3, which is the terminal cytochrome of the respiratory chain, catalyzes the reduction of O_2 and generates ATP. This reaction is the major source of O_2 consumption in the body (Taylor & Simonson, 1996). The redox state of cytochrome a,a3 is determined primarily by the availability of O_2. Thus, a decrease in O_2 delivery, either because of hypoxic hypoxia or because of local ischemic hypoxia, causes a decrease in cellular oxidative phosphorylation and subsequently a decrease in the oxidative levels of cytochrome a,a3 (Guery et al., 1999). Monitoring cytochrome a,a3 provides insight into the O_2 available at the mitochondria.

Table 23–15 CLINICAL USEFULLNESS OF TISSUE OXYGENATION MONITORING

Variable/Condition	Findings
NIRS	
Hemorrhagic shock (Beilman et al., 1999; McKinley & Butler, 1999)	↓ visceral/muscle VO_2; ↑ P_mCO_2; ↓ pH_m Cytochrome a,a3 correlates with systemic DO_2
Cardiac surgery (Puyana et al., 2000; Soller et al., 2003)	pH_m and P_mO_2 sensitive indicators of perfusion
Transcutaneous Tissue Monitoring (Shoemaker, 1996; Shoemaker et al., 1998)	
Normal $P_{tc}O_2$	80% of PaO_2
Satisfactory perfusion	> 65 mm Hg
Marginal perfusion	40–65 mm Hg
Impaired Perfusion	25–40 mm Hg
Shock	< 25 mm Hg
Blunt/penetrating trauma victims (Tatevossian, Shoemaker et al., 2000; Tatevossian, Wo et al., 2000; Velmahos et al., 1999)	*Survivors:* Higher $P_{tc}O_2$ and $P_{tc}O_2$/FiO_2 on admission *Survivors with organ failure:* $P_{tc}O_2$/FiO_2 < 50 mm Hg, $P_{tc}O_2$ > 60 mm Hg *Nonsurvivors:* Higher $P_{tc}CO_2$, longer periods with $P_{tc}CO_2$ > 60 mm Hg *Predictors of poor outcome:* $P_{tc}O_2$/FiO_2 < 50 mm Hg for 60 minutes; $P_{tc}CO_2$ > 60 mm Hg for 30 minutes; $P_{tc}O_2$/$P_{tc}CO_2$ < 1 for 30 minutes

The use of NIRS as either an indicator of perfusion/resuscitation or as a guide to therapy remains experimental. NIRS may be a useful indicator of blood loss and the need for transfusion or to guide resuscitation in hemorrhagic shock and in evaluating perfusion during cardiac surgery. In postresuscitation hemorrhagic shock and postcardiac surgery, the pHm and PmO_2 failed to return to normal despite normalization of other oxygenation indices, possibly indicating incomplete resuscitation (Puyana et al., 2000; Soller et al., 2003).

Transcutaneous Tissue Monitoring

Transcutaneous tissue monitoring uses an electrode that heats the skin (44°C–45°C) and changes the structures of the stratum corneum from the gel to the sol state, which allows rapid diffusion of O_2 from the subcutaneous tissue to the probe. Calibration of the system requires approximately 20 minutes. The probe must be moved every 4 hours to avoid electrode-induced tissue damage. The transcutaneous O_2 ($P_{tc}O_2$) and transcutaneous CO_2 ($P_{tc}CO_2$) values may be early indicators of hypoxia and have prognostic implications (see Table 23-15). Use of $P_{tc}O_2$ and $P_{tc}CO_2$ values in goal-directed therapy remains to be studied.

REFERENCES

AACN. (1993). Evaluation of the effects of heparinized and nonheparinized flush solutions on the patency of arterial pressure monitoring lines: The AACN Thunder Project. *American Journal of Critical Care,* 2(1), 3–15.

AACN. (1997). *Clinical practice. The polling corner: Chest tubes/PA catheters.* Aliso Viejo, CA: American Association of Critical Care Nurses.

Afessa, B., Spencer, S., Khan, W., LaGatta, M., Bridges, L., & Freire, A. X. (2001). Association of pulmonary artery catheter use with in-hospital mortality. *Critical Care Medicine,* 29(6), 1145–1148.

Ahrens, T., Penick, J., & Tucker, M. (1995). Frequency requirements for zeroing transducers in hemodynamic monitoring. *American Journal Critical Care,* 4(6), 466–471.

Ahrens, T. S., & Schallom, L. (2001). Comparison of pulmonary artery and central venous pressure waveform measurements via digital and graphic measurement methods. *Heart and Lung,* 30(1), 26–38.

Alia, I., Esteban, A., Gordo, F., Lorente, J. A., Diaz, C., Rodriguez, J. A., et al. (1999). A randomized and controlled trial of the effect of treatment aimed at maximizing oxygen delivery in patients with severe sepsis or septic shock. *Chest,* 115(2), 453–461.

Ander, D. S., Jaggi, M., Rivers, E., Rady, M. Y., Levine, T. B., Levine, A. B., et al. (1998). Undetected cardiogenic shock in patients with congestive heart failure presenting to the emergency department. *American Journal Cardiology,* 82(7), 888–891.

Antle, D. (2000). Ensuring competency in nurse repositioning of pulmonary artery catheters. *Dimensions of Critical Care Nursing,* 19(2), 44–52.

Aranda, M., Mihm, F. G., Garrett, S., Mihm, M. N., & Pearl, R. G. (1998). Continuous cardiac output catheters: delay in in vitro response time after controlled flow changes. *Anesthesiology,* 89(6), 1592–1595.

Atkins, P., Hapshe, E., & Riegel, B. (1994). Effects of bedbath on mixed venous oxygen saturation and heart rate in coronary artery bypass graft patients. *American Journal of Critical Care,* 3, 107–115.

Baillard, C., Cohen, Y., Fosse, J. P., Karoubi, P., Hoang, P., & Cupa, M. (1999). Haemodynamic measurements (continuous cardiac output and systemic vascular resistance) in critically ill patients: transoesophageal Doppler versus continuous thermodilution. *Anaesthesia and Intensive Care,* 27(1), 33–37.

Baldwin, I. C., & Heland, M. (2000). Incidence of cardiac dysrhythmias in patients during pulmonary artery catheter removal after cardiac surgery. *Heart and Lung,* 29(3), 155–160.

Banasik, J. L., Emerson, R. J. (2001). Effect of lateral positions on tissue oxygenation in the critically ill. *Heart and Lung,* 30(4), 269–276.

Barone, J. E., Tucker, J.B., Rassias, D., & Corvo, P .R. (2001). Routine perioperative pulmonary artery catheterization has no effect on rate of complications in vascular surgery: a meta-analysis. *American Surgeon,* 67(7), 674–679.

Bartz, B., Maroun, C., & Underhill, S. (1988). Differences in midanteroposterior level and midaxillary level of patients with a range of chest configurations. *Heart and Lung,* 17(3), 309.

Beilman, G. J., Groehler, K. E., Lazaron, V., & Ortner, J. P. (1999). Near-infrared spectroscopy measurement of regional tissue oxyhemoglobin saturation during hemorrhagic shock. *Shock,* 12(3), 196–200.

Belott, P. (1999). Bioimpedance in the pacemaker clinic. *AACN Clinical Issues,* 10(3), 414–418.

Belz, G. G. (1995). Elastic properties and Windkessel function of the human aorta. *Cardiovascular Drugs and Therapy,* 9(1), 73–83.

Bennett-Guerrero, E., Kahn, R.A., Moskowitz, D. M., Falcucci, O., & Bodian, C. A. (2002). Comparison of arterial systolic pressure variation with other clinical parameters to predict the response to fluid challenges during cardiac surgery. *Mount Sinai Journal of Medicine,* 69(1–2), 96–100.

Berkenstadt, H., Margalit, N., Hadani, M., Friedman, Z., Segal, E., Villa, Y., et al. (2001). Stroke volume variation as a predictor of fluid responsiveness in patients undergoing brain surgery. *Anesthesia Analgesia,* 92(4), 984–989.

Bernard, G. R., Sopko, G., Cerra, F., Demling, R., Edmunds, H., Kaplan, S., et al. (2000). Pulmonary artery catheterization and clinical outcomes: National Heart, Lung, and Blood Institute and Food and Drug Administration Workshop Report. Consensus Statement. *JAMA,* 283(19), 2568–2572.

Bernardin, G., Lucas, P., Hyvernat, H., Deloffre, P., & Mattei, M. (1999). Influence of alveolar ventilation changes on calculated gastric intramucosal pH and gastric-arterial PCO2 difference. *Intensive Care Medicine,* 25(3), 269–273.

Bindels, A.J., van der Hoeven, J.G., & Meinders, A.E. (1999). Pulmonary artery wedge pressure and extravascular lung water in patients with acute cardiogenic pulmonary edema requiring mechanical ventilation. *American Journal of Cardiology,* 84(10), 1158–1163.

Black, I. H., Blosser, S. A., & Murray, W. B. (2000). Central venous pressure measurements: peripherally inserted catheters versus centrally inserted catheters. *Critical Care Medicine,* 28(12), 3833–3836.

Blot, F., Laplanche, A., Raynard, B., Germann, N., Antoun, S., & Nitenberg, G. (2000). Accuracy of totally implanted ports, tunnelled, single- and multiple-lumen central venous catheters for measurement of central venous pressure. *Intensive Care Medicine,* 26(12), 1837–1842.

Bouchard, R., Gault, J., & Ross, J. (1971). Evaluation of pulmonary arterial end-diastolic pressure as an estimate of left ventricular end-diastolic pressure in patients with normal and abnormal left ventricular performance. *Circulation,* 44, 1072–1079.

Boulnois, J. L., & Pechoux, T. (2000). Non-invasive cardiac output monitoring by aortic blood flow measurement with the Dynemo 3000. *Journal of Clinical Monitoring and Computing,* 16(2), 127–140.

Boyd, O., Grounds, R. M., & Bennett, E. D. (1993). A randomized clinical trial of the effect of deliberate perioperative increase of oxygen delivery on mortality in high-risk surgical patients. *JAMA,* 270(22), 2699–2707.

Boyle, M., Jacobs, S., Torda, T. A., & Shehabi, Y. (1997). Assessment of the agreement between cardiac output measured by bolus thermodilution and continuous methods, with particular reference to the effect of heart rhythm. *Australian Critical Care,* 10(1), 5–8, 10–11.

Bridges, E. (2000a). Hemodynamic monitoring. In S. Woods, E. Sivarajan Froelicher, & S. Underhill Motzer (Eds.), *Cardiac nursing* (4th ed., pp. 427–478). Philadelphia: Lippincott.

Bridges, E. (2000b). Monitoring pulmonary artery pressures: just the facts. *Critical Care Nurse,* 20(6), 59–78.

Bridges, E., Bond, E., Ahrens, T., Daly, E., & Woods, S. (1997). Ask the Experts: Direct arterial vs oscillometric monitoring of blood pressure: stop comparing and pick one. *Critical Care Nurse,* 17(6), 96–97, 101–102.

Bridges, E., & Middleton, R. (1997). Direct arterial vs oscillometric monitoring of blood pressure: stop comparing and pick one (A decision-making algorithm). *Critical Care Nurse,* 17(3), 58–72.

Bridges, E. J., Woods, S. L., Brengelmann, G.L., Mitchell, P., & Laurent-Bopp, D. (2000). Effect of the 30 degree lateral recumbent position on pulmonary artery and pulmonary artery wedge pressures in critically ill adult cardiac surgery patients. *American Journal Critical Care,* 9(4), 262–275.

Buhre, W., Weyland, A., Kazmaier, S., Hanekop, G. G., Baryalei, M. M., Sydow, M., et al. (1999). Comparison of cardiac output assessed by pulse-contour analysis and thermodilution in patients undergoing minimally invasive direct coronary artery bypass grafting. *Journal of Cardiothoracic and Vascular Anesthesia,* 13(4), 437–440.

Bur, A., Herkner, H., Vlcek, M., Woisetschlager, C., Derhaschnig, U., Delle Karth, G., et al. (2003). Factors influencing the accuracy of oscillometric blood pressure measurement in critically ill patients. *Critical Care Medicine,* 31(3), 793–799.

Burns, D., Burns, D., & Shively, M. (1996). Critical care nurses' knowledge of pulmonary artery catheters. *American Journal of Critical Care,* 5(1), 49–54.

Cariou, A., Monchi, M., Joly, L. M., Bellenfant, F., Claessens, Y. E., Thebert, D., et al. (1998). Noninvasive cardiac output monitoring by aortic blood flow determination: evaluation of the Sometec Dynemo-3000 system. *Critical Care Medicine,* 26(12), 2066–2072.

Carlson, K., Snyder, M., LeClair, H., Underhill, S., Ashwood, E., & Detter, J. (1990). Obtaining reliable sodium and glucose determinations from pulmonary artery catheters. *Heart and Lung,* 19(6), 613–619.

Cernaianu, A., Nelson, L. (1993). The significance of mixed venous oxygen saturation and technical aspects of continuous measurement. In J. D. Edwards, W. Shoemaker, & J.-L. Vincent (Eds.), *Oxygen transport: Principles and practice* (pp. 99–124). London: WB Saunders.

Chakko, S., Woska, D., Martinez, H., de Marchena, E., Futterman, L., Kessler, K. M., et al. (1991). Clinical, radiographic, and hemodynamic correlations in chronic congestive heart failure: conflicting results may lead to inappropriate care. *American Journal of Medicine,* 90(3), 353–359.

Chaney, J. C., & Derdak, S. (2002). Minimally invasive hemodynamic monitoring for the intensivist: current and emerging technology. *Critical Care Medicine,* 30(10), 2338–2345.

Chang, M. C., & Meredith, J. W. (1997). Cardiac preload, splanchnic perfusion, and their relationship during resuscitation in trauma patients. *Journal of Trauma,* 42(4), 577–582.

Cheatham, M., Nelson, L., Chang, M., & Safcsak, K. (1998). Right ventricular end-diastolic volume index as a predictor of preload status in patients on positive end-expiratory pressure. *Critical Care Medicine,* 26(11), 1801–1806.

Cheatham, M., Safcsak, K., Zoha, Z., Block, E., & Nelson, L. (1998). Right ventricular end-diastolic volume index as a predictor of preload status in abdominal compartment syndrome. *Critical Care Medicine,* 26(Suppl), A38.

Chen, Y. Y., Yen, D. H., Yang, Y. G., Liu, C. Y., Wang, F.D., & Chou, P. (2003). Comparison between replacement at 4 days and 7 days of the infection rate for pulmonary artery catheters in an intensive care unit. *Critical Care Medicine,* 31(5), 1353–1358.

Colreavy, F. B., Donovan, K., Lee, K. Y., & Weekes, J. (2002). Transesophageal echocardiography in critically ill patients. *Critical Care Medicine,* 30(5), 989–996.

Connors, A., Speroff, T., Dawson, N., Thomas, C., Harrell, F., Wagner, D., et al. (1996). The effectiveness of right heart catheterization in the initial care of critically ill patients. *JAMA,* 276, 889–897.

Coopersmith, C. M., Rebmann, T. L., Zack, J. E., Ward, M. R., Corcoran, R.M., Schallom, M.E., et al. (2002). Effect of an education program on decreasing catheter-related bloodstream infections in the surgical intensive care unit. *Critical Care Medicine,* 30(1), 59–64.

Cope, D. K., Grimbert, F., Downey, J. M., & Taylor, A. E. (1992). Pulmonary capillary pressure: a review. *Critical Care Medicine,* 20(7), 1043–1056.

Cope, T., Marx, G., McCrossan, L., Swaraj, S., Cowan, C., Mostafa, S., et al. (2002). Stroke volume variation for assessment of cardiac responsiveness to volume loading in severe sepsis. *Intensive Care Medicine,* 28(Suppl 1), S81.

Courtois, M., Fattal, P., Kovacs, S., Tierenbrunn, A., & Ludbrook, P. (1995). Anatomically and physiologically based reference level for measurement of intracardiac pressures. *Circulation,* 92(7), 1994–2000.

Davidson, W., & Fee, E. (1990). Influence of aging on pulmonary hemodynamics in a population free of coronary artery disease. *American Journal of Cardiology,* 65(22), 1454–1458.

De Backer, D., Creteur, J., & Vincent, J.L. (2003). Perioperative optimization and right heart catheterization: what technique in which patient. *Critical Care,* 7, 201–202.

Della Rocca, G., Costa, M. G., Pompei, L., Coccia, C., & Pietropaoli, P. (2002). Continuous and intermittent cardiac output measurement: pulmonary artery catheter versus aortic transpulmonary technique. *British Journal of Anaesthesia,* 88(3), 350–356.

Denault, A. Y., Gasior, T.A., Gorcsan, J., 3rd, Mandarino, W. A., Deneault, L. G., & Pinsky, M. R. (1999). Determinants of aortic pressure variation during positive-pressure ventilation in man. *Chest,* 116(1), 176–186.

DiCorte, C. J., Latham, P., Greilich, P. E., Cooley, M. V., Grayburn, P. A., & Jessen, M. E. (2000). Esophageal Doppler monitor determinations of cardiac output and preload during cardiac operations. *Annals of Thoracic Surgery,* 69(6), 1782–1786.

Diebel, L., Wilson, R. F., Heins, J., Larky, H., Warsow, K., & Wilson, S. (1994). End-diastolic volume versus pulmonary artery wedge pressure in evaluating cardiac preload in trauma patients. *Journal of Trauma,* 37(6), 950–955.

Diebel, L. N., Myers, T., & Dulchavsky, S. (1997). Effects of increasing airway pressure and PEEP on the assessment of cardiac preload. *Journal of Trauma,* 42(4), 585–590.

Diebel, L. N., Tagett, M. G., & Wilson, R. F. (1993). Right ventricular response after myocardial contusion and hemorrhagic shock. *Surgery,* 114(4), 788–792.

Dimick, J. B., Pelz, R.K., Consunji, R., Swoboda, S. M., Hendrix, C. W., & Lipsett, P. A. (2001). Increased resource use associated with catheter-related bloodstream infection in the surgical intensive care unit. *Archives of Surgery,* 136(2), 229–234.

Dobbins, B. M., Catton, J. A., Kite, P., McMahon, M. J., Wilcox, & M. H. (2003). Each lumen is a potential source of central venous catheter-related bloodstream infection. *Critical Care Medicine,* 31(6), 1688–1690.

Doering, L., Lum, E., Dracup, K., & Friedman, A. (1995). Predictors of between-method differences in cardiac output measurement using thoracic electrical bioimpedance and thermodilution. *Critical Care Medicine,* 23(10), 1667–1673.

Dorman, T., Breslow, M. J., Lipsett, P. A., Rosenberg, J. M., Balser, J. R., Almog, Y., et al. (1998). Radial artery pressure monitoring underestimates central arterial pressure during vasopressor therapy in critically ill surgical patients. *Critical Care Medicine,* 26(10), 1646–1649.

Drazner, M. H., Hamilton, M. A., Fonarow, G., Creaser, J., Flavell, C., & Stevenson, L.W. (1999). Relationship between right and left-sided filling pressures in 1000 patients with advanced heart failure. *Journal of Heart and Lung Transplantation,* 18(11), 1126–1132.

Drazner, M. H., Thompson, B., Rosenberg, P. B., Kaiser, P. A., Boehrer, J. D., Baldwin, B. J., et al. (2002). Comparison of impedance cardiography with invasive hemodynamic measurements in patients with heart failure secondary to ischemic or nonischemic cardiomyopathy. *American Journal of Cardiology,* 89(8), 993–995.

Drucker, W., Pearce, F., & Glass-Heidenreich, L. (1996). Subcutaneous tissue oxygen pressure: A reliable index of peripheral perfusion in humans after injury. *Journal of Trauma,* 40, S116–S122.

Edwards, J. D., & Mayall, R. M. (1998). Importance of the sampling site for measurement of mixed venous oxygen saturation in shock. *Critical Care Medicine,* 26(8), 1356–1360.

Eggimann, P., & Pittet, D. (2002). Overview of catheter-related infections with special emphasis on prevention based on educational programs. *Clinical Microbiology and Infection,* 8(5), 295–309.

Feissel, M., Michard, F., Mangin, I., Ruyer, O., Faller, J. P., & Teboul, J. L. (2001). Respiratory changes in aortic blood velocity as an indicator of fluid responsiveness in ventilated patients with septic shock. *Chest,* 119(3), 867–873.

Felbinger, T. W., Reuter, D. A., Eltzschig, H. K., Moerstedt, K., Goedje, O., & Goetz, A. E. (2002). Comparison of pulmonary arterial thermodilution and arterial pulse contour analysis: evaluation of a new algorithm. *Journal of Clinical Anesthesia,* 14(4), 296–301.

Fonseca-Reyes, S., De Alba-Garcia, J. G., Parra-Carrillo, J. Z., & Paczka-Zapata, J. A. (2003). Effect of standard cuff on blood pressure readings in patients with obese arms. How frequent are arms of a 'large circumference'? *Blood Pressure Monitoring,* 8(3), 101–106.

Fontes, M. L., Bellows, W., Ngo, L., & Mangano, D.T. (1999). Assessment of ventricular function in critically ill patients: limitations of pulmonary artery catheterization. *Journal of Cardiothoracic and Vascular Anesthesia,* 13(5), 521–527.

Forrester, J., Diamond, G., Mchugh, T., & Swan, H. (1971). Filling pressures in the right and left sides of the heart in acute myocardial infarction. A reappraisal of central-venous pressure monitoring. *New England Journal of Medicine,* 285(4), 190–192.

Forrester, J., Diamond, G., & Swan, H. (1977). Correlative classification of clinical and hemodynamic function after acute myocardial infarction. *American Journal of Cardiology,* 39(2), 137–145.

Franklin, S. S., Khan, S. A., Wong, N. D., Larson, M. G., & Levy, D. (1999). Is pulse pressure useful in predicting risk for coronary heart disease? The Framingham heart study. *Circulation,* 100(4), 354–360.

Gama de Abreu, M., Winkler, T., Pahlitzsch, T., Weismann, D., & Albrecht, D. M. (2003). Performance of the partial CO_2 rebreathing technique under different hemodynamic and ventilation/perfusion matching conditions. *Critical Care Medicine,* 31(2), 543–551.

Gamma de Abreu, M., Melo, M. F., & Giannella-Neto, A. (2000). Pulmonary capillary blood flow by partial CO2 rebreathing: importance of the regularity of the respiratory pattern. *Clinical Physiology, 20*(5), 388–398.

Gan, T. (2000). The esophageal Doppler as an alternative to the pulmonary artery catheter. *Current Opinion in Critical Care,* 6, 214–221.

Gan, T. J., Soppitt, A., Maroof, M., el-Moalem, H., Robertson, K. M., Moretti, E., et al. (2002). Goal-directed intraoperative fluid administration reduces length of hospital stay after major surgery. *Anesthesiology,* 97(4), 820–826.

Garcia-Rodriguez, C., Pittman, J., Cassell, C. H., Sum-Ping, J., El-Moalem, H., Young, C., et al. (2002). Lithium dilution cardiac output measurement: A clinical assessment of central venous and peripheral venous indicator injection. *Critical Care Medicine,* 30(10), 2199–2204.

Gardin, J. M., Davidson, D. M., Rohan, M. K., Butman, S., Knoll, M., Garcia, R., et al. (1987). Relationship between age, body size, gender, and blood pressure and Doppler flow measurements in the aorta and pulmonary artery. *American Heart Journal,* 113(1), 101–109.

Gardner, R. (1981). Direct blood pressure measurement. Dynamic response requirements. *Anesthesiology,* 54, 227–236.

Gardner, R. (1996). Accuracy and reliability of disposable pressure transducer coupled with modern pressure monitoring. *Critical Care Medicine,* 24(5), 879–882.

Gattinoni, L., Brazzi, L., Pelosi, P., Latini, R., Tognoni, G., Pesenti, A., et al. (1995). A trial of goal-oriented hemodynamic therapy in critically ill patients. SvO2 Collaborative Group. *New England Journal of Medicine,* 333(16), 1025–1032.

Gawlinski, A. (1998). Can measurement of mixed venous oxygen saturation replace measurement of cardiac output in patients with advanced heart failure? *American Journal of Critical Care,* 7(5), 374–380.

Gawlinski, A., & Dracup, K. (1998). Effect of positioning on SvO2 in the critically ill patient with a low ejection fraction. *Nursing Research,* 47(5), 293–299.

Gendreau, M. A., Triner, W.R., & Bartfield, J. (1999). Complications of transesophageal echocardiography in the ED. *American Journal of Emergency Medicine,* 17(3), 248–251.

Genoni, M., Pelosi, P., Romand, J. A., Pedoto, A., Moccetti, T., & Malacrida, R. (1998). Determination of cardiac output during mechanical ventilation by electrical bioimpedance or thermodilution in patients with acute lung injury: effects of positive end-expiratory pressure. *Critical Care Medicine,* 26(8), 1441–1445.

Gilbert, J., & Lazio, L. (1999). Managing congestive heart failure with thoracic electrical bioimpedance. *AACN Clinical Issues,* 10(3), 400–405.

Ginosar, Y., & Sprung, C. (1996). The Swan-Ganz catheter: Twenty-five years of monitoring. *Critical Care Clinics,* 12, 771–776.

Glenny, R. W., Bernard, S., Robertson, H. T., & Hlastala, M. P. (1999). Gravity is an important but secondary determinant of regional pulmonary blood flow in upright primates. *Journal of Applied Physiology,* 86(2), 623–632.

Godje, O., Hoke, K., Goetz, A. E., Felbinger, T.W., Reuter, D. A., Reichart, B., et al. (2002). Reliability of a new algorithm for continuous cardiac output determination by pulse-contour analysis during hemodynamic instability. *Critical Care Medicine,* 30(1), 52–58.

Gore, S., Middleton, R., & Bridges, E. (1995). Analysis of an algorithm to guide decision making regarding direct and oscillometric blood pressure measurement. *American Journal of Respiratory and Critical Care Medicine,* 151, A331.

Griffin, K., Benjamin, E., DelGiudice, R., Schechter, C., & Iberti, T. J. (1997). Thermodilution cardiac output measurement during simultaneous volume infusion through the venous infusion port of the pulmonary artery catheter. *Journal of Cardiothoracic and Vascular Anesthesia,* 11(4), 437–439.

Grossman, W. (1996). Pressure measurement. In D. S. Baim, & W. Grossman (Eds.), *Cardiac catheterization, angiography, and intervention* (5th ed., pp. 125–141). Baltimore: Williams & Wilkins.

Grossman, W. (2000). Blood flow measurement: Cardiac output and vascular resistance. In D. Baim, & W. Grossman (Eds.), *Grossman's cardiac catheterization, angiography and intervention* (6th ed., pp. 159–178). Philadelphia: Lippincott.

Guery, B. P., Mangalaboyi, J., Menager, P., Mordon, S., Vallet, B., & Chopin, C. (1999). Redox status of cytochrome a,a3: a noninvasive indicator of dysoxia in regional hypoxic or ischemic hypoxia. *Critical Care Medicine,* 27(3), 576–582.

Guzzi, L., Jaffe, M. B., & Orr, J. (1998). Clinical evaluation of a new noninvasive method of cardiac output measurement: Preliminary results in CABG patients. *Anesthesiology,* 89(3A), 543A.

Haering, J., Maslow, A., Parker, R., Lowenstein, E., & Comunale, M. (2000). The effect of heparin-coated pulmonary artery catheters on activated coagulation time in cardiac surgical patients. *Journal of Cardiothoracic and Vascular Anesthesia,* 14(3), 260–263.

Haider, A. W., Larson, M. G., Franklin, S.S., & Levy, D. (2003). Systolic blood pressure, diastolic blood pressure, and pulse pressure as predictors of risk for congestive heart failure in the Framingham Heart Study. *Annals of Internal Medicine,* 138(1), 10–16.

Haller, M., Zollner, C., Briegel, J., & Forst, H. (1995). Evaluation of a new continuous thermodilution cardiac output monitor in critically ill patients: a prospective criterion standard study. *Critical Care Medicine,* 23(5), 860–866.

Hamilton, T. T., Huber, L. M., & Jessen, M. E. (2002). PulseCO: a less-invasive method to monitor cardiac output from arterial pressure after cardiac surgery. *Annals of Thoracic Surgery,* 74(4), S1408–1412.

Haryadi, D. G., Orr, J. A., Kuck, K., McJames, S., & Westenskow, D. R. (2000). Partial CO2 rebreathing indirect Fick technique for non-invasive measurement of cardiac output. *Journal of Clinical Monitoring and Computing,* 16(5–6), 361–374.

Haskell, R., & French, W. (1988). Accuracy of left atrial and pulmonary artery wedge pressure in pure mitral regurgitation in predicting left ventricular end-diastolic filling pressure. *American Journal Cardiology,* 61, 136–141.

Hayes, M. A., Timmins, A. C., Yau, E.H., Palazzo, M., Hinds, C. J., & Watson, D. (1994). Elevation of systemic oxygen delivery in the treatment of critically ill patients. *New England Journal of Medicine,* 330(24), 1717–1722.

Heap, M. J., Ridley, S. A., Hodson, K., & Martos, F. J. (1997). Are coagulation studies on blood sampled from arterial lines valid? *Anaesthesia,* 52(7), 640–645.

Hebert, P.C. (1998). Transfusion requirements in critical care (TRICC): a multicentre, randomized, controlled clinical study. Transfusion Requirements in Critical Care Investigators and the Canadian Critical care Trials Group. *British Journal of Anaesthesia,* 81 Suppl 1, 25–33.

Heerdt, P. M., Blessios, G. A., Beach, M. L., & Hogue, C. W. (2001). Flow dependency of error in thermodilution measurement of cardiac output during acute tricuspid regurgitation. *Journal of Cardiothoracic and Vascular Anesthesia,* 15(2), 183–187.

Heyland, D. K., Cook, D. J., King, D., Kernerman, P., & Brun-Buisson, C. (1996). Maximizing oxygen delivery in critically ill patients: a methodologic appraisal of the evidence. *Critical Care Medicine,* 24(3), 517–524.

Hind, D., Calvert, N., McWilliams, R., Davidson, A., Paisley, S., Beverley, C., et al. (2003). Ultrasonic locating devices for central venous cannulation: meta-analysis. *British Medical Journal,* 327(7411), 361.

Hoeper, M., Tongers, J., Leppert, A., Baus, S., Maier, R., & Lotz, J. (2001). Evaluation of right ventricular performance with a right ventricular ejection fraction thermodilution catheter and MRI in patients with pulmonary hypertension. *Chest,* 120(2), 502–507.

Horiuchi, K., Jordan, D., Cohen, D., Kemper, M. C., & Weissman, C. (1997). Insights into the increased oxygen demand during chest physiotherapy. *Critical Care Medicine,* 25(8), 1347–1351.

Huang, C., Tsai, Y., Chen, N., Lin, M., Tsao, T., Lee, C., et al. (2001). Spontaneous variability of cardiac output in ventilated critically ill patients. *Critical Care Medicine,* 29(1), 220–221.

Huang, W., Kingsbury, M. P., Turner, M. A., Donnelly, J. L., Flores, N. A., & Sheridan, D. J. (2001). Capillary filtration is reduced in lungs adapted to chronic heart failure: morphological and haemodynamic correlates. *Cardiovascular Research,* 49(1), 207–217.

Iregui, M. G., Prentice, D., Sherman, G., Schallom, L., Sona, C., & Kollef, M. H. (2003). Physicians' estimates of cardiac index and intravascular volume based on clinical assessment versus transesophageal Doppler measurements obtained by critical care nurses. *American Journal of Critical Care,* 12(4), 336–342.

Jacquet, L., Hanique, G., Glorieux, D., Matte, P., & Goenen, M. (1996). Analysis of the accuracy of continuous thermodilution cardiac output measurement. Comparison with intermittent thermodilution and Fick cardiac output measurement. *Intensive Care Medicine,* 22(10), 1125–1131.

Jaeggi, P., Hofer, C. K., Klaghofer, R., Fodor, P., Genoni, M., & Zollinger, A. (2003). Measurement of cardiac output after cardiac surgery by a new transesophageal doppler device. *Journal of Cardiothoracic and Vascular Anesthesia,* 17(2), 217–220.

Jaffe, M.B. (1999). Partial CO2 rebreathing cardiac output—operating principles of the NICO system. *Journal of Clinical Monitoring and Computing,* 15(6), 387–401.

James, J.H., Luchette, F.A., McCarter, F.D., & Fischer, J.E. (1999). Lactate is an unreliable indicator of tissue hypoxia in injury or sepsis. *Lancet,* 354(9177), 505–508.

Jansen, J.R., Schreuder, J.J., Punt, K.D., van den Berg, P.C., & Alfieri, O. (2001). Mean cardiac output by thermodilution with a single controlled injection. *Critical Care Medicine,* 29(10), 1868–1873.

Jarvis, M.A., Jarvis, C. L., Jones, P. R., & Spyt, T.J. (2000). Reliability of Allen's test in selection of patients for radial artery harvest. *Annals of Thoracic Surgery, 70*(4), 1362–1365.

Johnson, M., & Schumann, L. (1995). Comparison of three methods of measurement of pulmonary artery catheter readings in critically ill patients. *American Journal of Critical Care, 4*(4), 300–307.

Johnson, W., Voegtlin, L., Bailin, S., & Hoyt, R. (2001). Impedance cardiography for acute AV pacing optimization. *Journal of Cardiac Failure, 7*(3, Suppl. 2), 52.

Jonas, M. M., Kelly, F. E., Linton, R. A., Band, D. M., O'Brien, T. K., & Linton, N. W. (1999). A comparison of lithium dilution cardiac output measurements made using central and antecubital venous injection of lithium chloride. *Journal of Clinical Monitoring and Computing, 15*(7–8), 525–528.

Jonas, M. M., & Tanser, S. J. (2002). Lithium dilution measurement of cardiac output and arterial pulse waveform analysis: an indicator dilution calibrated beat-by-beat system for continuous estimation of cardiac output. *Current Opinion in Critical Care, 8*(3), 257–261.

Jones, D., & Bodenham, A. (2002). Toward safer central venous access. In J. L. Vincent (Ed.), *Intensive care medicine* (pp. 417–426). Berlin: Springer.

Jubran, A., Mathru, M., Dries, D., & Tobin, M. J. (1998). Continuous recordings of mixed venous oxygen saturation during weaning from mechanical ventilation and the ramifications thereof. *American Journal of Respiratory and Critical Care Medicine, 158*(6), 1763–1769.

Kaye, J., Heald, G. R., Morton, J., & Weaver, T. (2001). Patency of radial arterial catheters. *American Journal of Critical Care, 10*(2), 104–111.

Kee, L., Simonson, J., Stotts, N., Skov, P., & Schiller, N. (1993). Echocardiographic determinations of valid zero reference levels in supine and lateral positions. *American Journal Critical Care, 2*(1), 72–80.

Keech, J., & Reed, R. L., 2nd. (2003). Reliability of mixed venous oxygen saturation as an indicator of the oxygen extraction ratio demonstrated by a large patient data set. *Journal of Trauma, 54*(2), 236–241.

Keenan, S.P. (2002). Use of ultrasound to place central lines. *Journal of Critical Care, 17*(2), 126–137.

Keickeisen, M. (1998). *Pulmonary artery pressure monitoring.* Aliso Viejo, CA: American Association of Critical Care Nurses.

Kellum, J. A., Rico, P., Garuba, A. K., & Pinsky, M.R. (2000). Accuracy of mucosal pH and mucosal-arterial carbon dioxide tension for detecting mesenteric hypoperfusion in acute canine endotoxemia. *Critical Care Medicine, 28*(2), 462–466.

Kelly, R., Gibbs, H., O'Rourke, M., Daley, J., Mank, D., Morgan, J., et al. (1990). Nitroglycerin has more favourable effects on left ventricular afterload than apparent from measurement of pressure in a peripheral artery. *European Heart Journal, 11*, 138–144.

Kern, J., & Aguirre, F. (1992). Aortic regurgitation. *Journal of Catheterization and Cardiovascular Diagnosis, 26*, 232–240.

Kern, J., & Shoemaker, W. (2002). Meta-analysis of hemodynamic optimization in high-risk patients. *Critical Care Medicine, 30*, 1686–1692.

Kirchoff, K., Rebenson-Piano, M., & Patel, M. (1984). Mean arterial pressure readings: Variations with positions and transducer level. *Nursing Research, 33*(6), 343–345.

Kotake, Y., Moriyama, K., Innami, Y., Shimizu, H., Ueda, T., Morisaki, H., et al. (2003). Performance of noninvasive partial CO2 rebreathing cardiac output and continuous thermodilution cardiac output in patients undergoing aortic reconstruction surgery. *Anesthesiology, 99*(2), 283–288.

Lange, R., Moore, D., & Cigarroa, R. (1989). Use of pulmonary capillary wedge pressure to assess severity of mitral stenosis: Is true left atrial pressure needed in this condition. *Journal American College of Cardiology, 13*(4), 825–829.

Lasater, M. (1999). Managing inotrope therapy noninvasively. *AACN Clinical Issues, 10*(3), 406–413.

Lasater, M., & Von Rueden, K. T. (2003). Outpatient cardiovascular management utilizing impedance cardiography. *AACN Clinical Issues, 14*(2), 240–250.

Laxson, C. J., & Titler, M.G. (1994). Drawing coagulation studies from arterial lines: an integrative literature review. *American Journal of Critical Care, 3*(1), 16–22.

Lazor, M. A., Pierce, E. T., Stanley, G. D., Cass, J. L., Halpern, E. F., & Bode, R. H., Jr. (1997). Evaluation of the accuracy and response time of STAT-mode continuous cardiac output. *Journal of Cardiothoracic and Vascular Anesthesia, 11*(4), 432–436.

LeDoux, D., Astiz, M. E., Carpati, C. M., & Rackow, E. C. (2000). Effects of perfusion pressure on tissue perfusion in septic shock. *Critical Care Medicine, 28*(8), 2729–2732.

Leeper, B. (2003). Monitoring right ventricular volumes: a paradigm shift. *AACN Clinical Issues, 14*(2), 208–219.

Levy, B., Gawalkiewicz, P., Vallet, B., Briancon, S., Nace, L., & Bollaert, P. E. (2003). Gastric capnometry with air-automated tonometry predicts outcome in critically ill patients. *Critical Care Medicine, 31*(2), 474–480.

Levy, B., Perrigault, P. F., Gawalkiewicz, P., Sebire, F., Escriva, M., Colson, P., et al. (1998). Gastric versus duodenal feeding and gastric tonometric measurements. *Critical Care Medicine, 26*(12), 1991–1994.

Linton, R., Band, D., O'Brien, T., Jonas, M., & Leach, R. (1997). Lithium dilution cardiac output measurement: a comparison with thermodilution. *Critical Care Medicine, 25*(11), 1796–1800.

Linton, R.A., Band, D.M., & Haire, K.M. (1993). A new method of measuring cardiac output in man using lithium dilution. *British Journal of Anaesthesia, 71*(2), 262–266.

Lipp-Ziff, E., & Kawanishi, D. (1991). A technique for improving the accuracy of the pulmonary artery diastolic pressure as an estimate of left ventricular end-diastolic pressure. *Heart and Lung, 20*(2), 107–115.

Lobo, S. M., Salgado, P. F., Castillo, V.G., Borim, A.A., Polachini, C. A., Palchetti, J.C., et al. (2000). Effects of maximizing oxygen delivery on morbidity and mortality in high-risk surgical patients. *Critical Care Medicine, 28*(10), 3396–3404.

Lopez, A., Thompson, D., Dauenhauer, C., Helmers, R., Johnson, D., Larson, J., et al. (2003). Accuracy of peripherally inserted central catheters (PICCs) for hemodynamic monitoring and central venous oximetry. Paper presented at the 2003 American Thoracic Society, Seattle, WA.

Luchette, F. A., Porembka, D., Davis, K., Jr., Branson, R. D., James, L., Hurst, J.M., et al. (2000). Effects of body temperature on accuracy of continuous cardiac output measurements. *Journal of Investigative Surgery, 13*(3), 147–152.

Lundstedt, J. (1997). Comparison of methods measuring pulmonary artery pressure. *American Journal Critical Care, 6*(4), 324–332.

Madan, A. K., UyBarreta, V. V., Aliabadi-Wahle, S., Jesperson, R., Hartz, R. S., Flint, L.M., et al. (1999). Esophageal Doppler ultrasound monitor versus pulmonary artery catheter in the hemodynamic management of critically ill surgical patients. *Journal of Trauma, 46*(4), 607–611.

Magder, S. (1997). The cardiovascular management of critically ill patients. In M. Pinsky (Ed.), *Applied cardiovascular physiology* (pp. 164–171). Berlin: Springer.

Magder, S. (1998). More respect for the CVP. *Intensive Care Medicine, 24*(7), 651–653.

Magder, S. (2001). Diagnostic information from the respiratory variations in central hemodynamic pressures. In S. Scharf, M. Pinsky, & S. Magder (Eds.), *Respiratory-circulatory interactions in health and disease* (pp. 861–882). New York: Marcel Dekker.

Magder, S., Georgiadis, G., & Cheong, T. (1992). Respiratory variation in right atrial pressure predict the response to fluid challenge. *Journal of Critical Care, 7*(2), 76–85.

Magder, S., & Lagonidis, D. (1999). Effectiveness of albumin versus normal saline as a test of volume responsiveness in post-cardiac surgery patients. *Journal of Critical Care, 14*(4), 164–171.

Manthous, C., Hall, J., Olson, D., Singh, M., Chatila, W., Pohlman, A., et al. (1995). Effect of cooling on oxygen consumption in febrile critically ill patients. *American Journal Respiratory Critical Care Medicine, 151*, 10–14.

Marik, P., & Lorenzana, A. (1996). Effect of tube feedings on the measurement of gastric intramucosal pH. *Critical Care Medicine, 24*(9), 1498–1500.

Marik, P. E. (2001). Sublingual capnography: a clinical validation study. *Chest, 120*(3), 923–927.

Marin, M. G., Lee, J. C., & Skurnick, J. H. (2000). Prevention of nosocomial bloodstream infections: effectiveness of antimicrobial-impregnated and heparin-bonded central venous catheters. *Critical Care Medicine, 28*(9), 3332–3338.

Marini, J., O'Quin, R., Culver, B., & Butler, J. (1982). Estimation of transmural cardiac pressure during ventilation with PEEP. *Journal of Applied Physiology, 53*(2), 384–391.

Marshall, A., & West, S. (2003). Gastric tonometry and enteral nutrition: a possible conflict in critical care nursing practice. *American Journal of Critical Care, 12*(4), 349–356.

Martin, C., Auffray, J.P., Badetti, C., Perrin, G., Papazian, L., & Gouin, F. (1992). Monitoring of central venous oxygen saturation versus mixed venous oxygen saturation in critically ill patients. *Intensive Care Medicine, 18*(2), 101–104.

Martin, C., Saux, P., Papazian, L., & Gouin, F. (2001). Long-term arterial cannulation in ICU patients using the radial artery or dorsalis pedis artery. *Chest, 119*(3), 901–906.

Martinez, J. A., DesJardin, J. A., Aronoff, M., Supran, S., Nasraway, S. A., & Snydman, D.R. (2002). Clinical utility of blood cultures drawn from central venous or arterial catheters in critically ill surgical patients. *Critical Care Medicine, 30*(1), 7–13.

Maxwell, R. A., Gibson, J. B., Slade, J. B., Fabian, T. C., & Proctor, K. G. (2001). Noninvasive cardiac output by partial CO2 rebreathing after severe chest trauma. *Journal of Trauma, 51*(5), 849–853.

McCann, U., Schiller, H., Carney, D., Kilpatrick, J., Gatto, L., Paskanik, A., et al. (2001). Invasive arterial BP monitoring in trauma and critical care. *Chest, 120*(4), 1322–1326.

McCloy, K., Leung, S., Belden, J., Castenada, J., Erickson, V., Koch, K., et al. (1999). Effects of injectate volume on thermodilution measurements of cardiac output in patients with low ventricular ejection fraction. *American Journal of Critical Care, 8*(2), 86–92.

McKinley, B. A., & Butler, B. D. (1999). Comparison of skeletal muscle PO2, PCO2, and pH with gastric tonometric P(CO2) and pH in hemorrhagic shock. *Critical Care Medicine, 27*(9), 1869–1877.

McKinley, B. A., Kozar, R. A., Cocanour, C. S., Valdivia, A., Sailors, R. M., Ware, D. N., et al. (2002). Normal versus supranormal oxygen delivery goals in shock resuscitation: The response is the same. *Journal of Trauma, 53*(5), 825–832.

McNulty, S., Maguire, D., & Thomas, R. (1998). Effect of heparin-bonded pulmonary artery catheters on activated coagulation time. *Journal of Cardiothoracic and Vascular Anesthesia, 12*, 533–535.

Mermel, L. A. (2001). New technologies to prevent intravascular catheter-related bloodstream infections. *Emerging Infectious Diseases, 7*(2), 197–199.

Mets, B., Frumento, R.J., Bennett-Guerrero, E., & Naka, Y. (2002). Validation of continuous thermodilution cardiac output in patients implanted with a left ventricular assist device. *Journal of Cardiothoracic and Vascular Anesthesia, 16*(6), 727–730.

Michard, F., Boussat, S., Chemla, D., Anguel, N., Mercat, A., Lecarpentier, Y., et al. (2000). Relation between respiratory changes in arterial pulse pressure and fluid responsiveness in septic patients with acute circulatory failure. *American Journal of Respiratory and Critical Care Medicine, 162*(1), 134–138.

Michard, F., & Reuter, D. A. (2003). Assessing cardiac preload or fluid responsiveness? It depends on the question we want to answer. *Intensive Care Medicine, 29*(8), 1396.

Michard, F., & Teboul, J. L. (2000). Using heart-lung interactions to assess fluid responsiveness during mechanical ventilation. *Critical Care, 4*(5), 282–289.

Michard, F., & Teboul, J. L. (2002). Predicting fluid responsiveness in ICU patients: a critical analysis of the evidence. *Chest, 121*(6), 2000–2008.

Miller, P., Meredith, J., & Chang, M. (1998). Randomized, prospective comparison of increased preload versus inotropes in the resuscitation of trauma patients: effects on cardiopulmonary function and visceral perfusion. *Journal of Trauma, 44*(1), 107–113.

Miller, P. R., Kincaid, E. H., Meredith, J. W., & Chang, M.C. (1998). Threshold values of intramucosal pH and mucosal-arterial CO2 gap during shock resuscitation. *Journal of Trauma, 45*(5), 868–872.

Milzman, D. P., Hogan, C., Han, C., Desai, S., & Wood, B. (1997). Continuous, noninvasive cardiac output monitoring quantified acute congestive heart failure in the ED. *Critical Care Medicine, 25*(1), 17/A47.

Mitchell, J. P., Schuller, D., Calandrino, F. S., & Schuster, D. P. (1992). Improved outcome based on fluid management in critically ill patients requiring pulmonary artery catheterization. *American Review of Respiratory Disease, 145*(5), 990–998.

Mizock, B. A. (1998). Lactate and point-of-care testing. *Critical Care Medicine, 26*(9), 1474–1476.

Moxon, D., Pinder, M., van Heerden, P. V., & Parsons, R. W. (2003). Clinical evaluation of the HemoSonic monitor in cardiac surgical patients in the ICU. *Anaesthesia and Intensive Care, 31*(4), 408–411.

Netea, R. T., Lenders, J. W., Smits, P., & Thien, T. (2003). Both body and arm position significantly influence blood pressure measurement. *Journal of Human Hypertension, 17*(7), 459–462.

Nilsson, L. B., Eldrup, N., & Berthelsen, P. G. (2001). Lack of agreement between thermodilution and carbon dioxide-rebreathing cardiac output. *Acta Anaesthesiologica Scandinavica, 45*(6), 680–685.

Odum, L., & Drenck, N. (2002). Blood sampling for biochemical analysis from central venous catheters: minimizing the volume of discarded blood. *Clinical Chemistry and Laboratory Medicine, 40*(2), 152–155.

O'Grady, N. P., Alexander, M., Dellinger, E. P., Gerberding, J. L., Heard, S.O., Maki, D.G., et al. (2002). Guidelines for the prevention of intravascular catheter-related infections. Centers for Disease Control and Prevention. *Morbidity and Mortality Weekly Report. Recommendations and Reports, 51*(RR-10), 1–29.

O'Malley, P., Smith, B., Hamlin, R., Nickel, J., Nakayama, T., MacVicar, M., et al. (2000). A comparison of bolus versus continuous cardiac output in an experimental model of heart failure. *Critical Care Medicine, 28*(6), 1985–1990.

Ornstein, E., Eidelman, L. A., Drenger, B., Elami, A., & Pizov, R. (1998). Systolic pressure variation predicts the response to acute blood loss. *Journal of Clinical Anesthesia, 10*(2), 137–140.

O'Rourke, M. (1993). Wave travel and reflection in the arterial system. In M. O'Rourke, M. Safar, & V. Dzau (Eds.), *Arterial vasodilation* (pp. 10–22). Philadelphia: Lea & Febiger.

O'Rourke, M., Avolio, A., Kellly, R., & Karamonoglu, M. (1993). Difference between central and upper limb pressure wave forms in man. In M. O'Rourke, M. Safar, & V. Dzau (Eds.), *Arterial vasodilation. Mechanisms and therapy*. Philadelphia: Lea & Febiger.

O'Rourke, M., & Kelly, R. (1993). Wave reflection in the systemic circulation and its implications in ventricular function. *Journal of Hypertension, 11*(4), 327–337.

O'Rourke, M. F., & Mancia, G. (1999). Arterial stiffness. *Journal of Hypertension, 17*(1), 1–4.

Paolella, L., Dortman, G., Cronan, J., & Hasan, F. (1988). Topgraphic location of the left atrium by computed tomography: Reducing pulmonary artery catheter calibration errors. *Critical Care Medicine, 16*(11), 1154–1156.

Parry, T., Hirsch, N., & Fauvel, N. (1995). Comparison of direct pressure measurement at the radial and dorsalis pedis arteries during surgery in the horizontal and reverse Trendelenburg positions. *Anaesthesia, 50*, 553–555.

Patel, N. H., Hahn, D., & Comess, K. A. (2003). Blunt chest trauma victims: role of intravascular ultrasound and transesophageal echocardiography in cases of abnormal thoracic aortogram. *Journal of Trauma, 55*(2), 330–337.

Peacock, W. I., Albert, N. M., Kies, P., White, R. D., & Emerman, C. L. (2000). Bioimpedance monitoring: better than chest x-ray for predicting abnormal pulmonary fluid? *Congestive Heart Failure, 6*(2), 86–89.

Pelosi, P., Yubiolo, D., Mascheroni, D., Vicardi, P., Crotti, S., Valenza, F., et al. (1998). Effects of the prone position on respiratory mechanics and gas exchange during acute lung injury. *American Journal of Respiratory and Critical Care Medicine, 157*(2), 387–393.

Peterson, G. E., Brickner, M. E., & Reimold, S. C. (2003). Transesophageal echocardiography: clinical indications and applications. *Circulation, 107*(19), 2398–2402.

Pinsky, M. (2002). Functional hemodynamic monitoring: Applied physiology at the bedside. In J. L. Vincent (Ed.), *Intensive care medicine. Annual update 2002* (pp. 537–552). Berlin: Springer-Verlag.

Pinsky, M. R. (2003a). Clinical significance of pulmonary artery occlusion pressure. *Intensive Care Medicine, 29*(2), 175–178.

Pinsky, M. R. (2003b). Probing the limits of arterial pulse contour analysis to predict preload responsiveness. *Anesthesia Analgesia, 96*(5), 1245–1247.

Pinsky, M. R. (2003c). Pulmonary artery occlusion pressure. *Intensive Care Medicine, 29*(1), 19–22.

Pittman, J., Sum-Ping, J., Sherwood, M., El-Moalem, H., & Mark, J. B. (2002). Continuous cardiac output monitoring by arterial pressure waveform analysis: A 24-hour comparison with the lithium dilution indicator method. Paper presented at the Society of Cardiovascular Anesthesia, New York.

Poeze, M., Ramsay, G., Greve, J. W., & Singer, M. (1999). Prediction of postoperative cardiac surgical morbidity and organ failure within 4 hours of intensive care unit admission using esophageal Doppler ultrasonography. *Critical Care Medicine, 27*(7), 1288–1294.

Polanczyk, C. A., Rohde, L.E., Goldman, L., Cook, E. F., Thomas, E. J., Marcantonio, E. R., et al. (2001). Right heart catheterization and cardiac complications in patients undergoing noncardiac surgery: an observational study. *JAMA, 286*(3), 309–314.

Poli de Figueiredo, L. F., Malbouisson, L. M., Varicoda, E. Y., Carmona, M. J., Auler, J. O., Jr., & Rocha e Silva, M. (1999). Thermal filament continuous thermodilution cardiac output delayed response limits its value during acute hemodynamic instability. *Journal of Trauma, 47*(2), 288–293.

Polonen, P., Hippelainen, M., Takala, R., Ruokonen, E., & Takala, J. (1997). Relationship between intra- and postoperative oxygen transport and prolonged intensive care after cardiac surgery: a prospective study. *Acta Anaesthesiologica Scandinavica, 41*(7), 810–817.

Potger, K. C., & Elliott, D. (1994). Reproducibility of central venous pressures in supine and lateral positions: a pilot evaluation of the phlebostatic axis in critically ill patients. *Heart and Lung, 23*(4), 285–299.

Povoas, H. P., Weil, M. H., Tang, W., Sun, S., Kamohara, T., & Bisera, J. (2001). Decreases in mesenteric blood flow associated with increases in sublingual PCO2 during hemorrhagic shock. *Shock, 15*(5), 398–402.

Practice guidelines for perioperative transesophageal echocardiography. A report by the American Society of Anesthesiologists and the Society of

Cardiovascular Anesthesiologists Task Force on Transesophageal Echocardiography. (1996). *Anesthesiology, 84*(4), 986–1006.

Preisman, S., DiSegni, E., Vered, Z., & Perel, A. (2002). Left ventricular preload and function during graded haemorrhage and retranfusion in pigs: analysis of arterial pressure waveform and correlation with echocardiography. *British Journal of Anaesthesia, 88*(5), 716–718.

Promonet, C., Anglade, D., Menaouar, A., Bayat, S., Durand, M., Eberhard, A., et al. (2000). Time-dependent pressure distortion in a catheter-transducer system: correction by fast flush. *Anesthesiology, 92*(1), 208–218.

Psaty, B. M., Furberg, C. D., Kuller, L. H., Cushman, M., Savage, P. J., Levine, D., et al. (2001). Association between blood pressure level and the risk of myocardial infarction, stroke, and total mortality: the cardiovascular health study. *Archives of Internal Medicine, 161*(9), 1183–1192.

Pulmonary Artery Catheter Consensus Conference: Consensus statement. (1997). *New Horizons, 5*(3), 175–194.

Puyana, J. C., Soller, B. R., Parikh, B., & Heard, S.O. (2000). Directly measured tissue pH is an earlier indicator of splanchnic acidosis than tonometric parameters during hemorrhagic shock in swine. *Critical Care Medicine, 28*(7), 2557–2562.

Quaal, S. J. (2001). Improving the accuracy of pulmonary artery catheter measurements. *Journal of Cardiovascular Nursing, 15*(2), 71–82.

Raaijmakers, E., Faes, T. J., Scholten, R. J., Goovaerts, H.G., & Heethaar, R. M. (1999). A meta-analysis of three decades of validating thoracic impedance cardiography. *Critical Care Medicine, 27*(6), 1203–1213.

Rackow, E. C., O'Neil, P., Astiz, M. E., & Carpati, C. M. (2001). Sublingual capnometry and indexes of tissue perfusion in patients with circulatory failure. *Chest, 120*(5), 1633–1638.

Rady, M. Y., Rivers, E. P., & Nowak, R. M. (1996). Resuscitation of the critically ill in the ED: responses of blood pressure, heart rate, shock index, central venous oxygen saturation, and lactate. *American Journal of Emergency Medicine, 14*(2), 218–225.

Rahimtoola, S., Loeb, H., & Ehsani, A. (1972). Relationship of pulmonary artery to left ventricular diastolic pressures in acute myocardial infarction. *Circulation, 46*, 283–290.

Ramsey, M. (1991). Blood pressure monitoring: automated oscillometric devices. *Journal of Clinical Monitoring, 7*, 56–67.

Randolph, A. G., Cook, D. J., Gonzales, C. A., & Andrew, M. (1998a). Benefit of heparin in central venous and pulmonary artery catheters: a meta-analysis of randomized controlled trials. *Chest, 113*(1), 165–171.

Randolph, A. G., Cook, D. J., Gonzales, C. A., & Andrew, M. (1998b). Benefit of heparin in peripheral venous and arterial catheters: systematic review and meta-analysis of randomised controlled trials. *British Medical Journal, 316*(7136), 969–975.

Rauch, H., Muller, M., Fleischer, F., Bauer, H., Martin, E., & Bottiger, B. W. (2002). Pulse contour analysis versus thermodilution in cardiac surgery patients. *Acta Anaesthesiologica Scandinavica, 46*(4), 424–429.

Reed, R. I. (1993). Oxygen consumption and delivery. *Current Opinion in Anesthesiology, 6*, 329–334.

Reed, S., Jesurum-Urbaitis, J., Kumpula, J., Motzer, S., Simpson, T., Burr, R., et al. (2003). The effect of lateral positioning on tissue oxygenation in cardiovascular surgical patients with anemia. *American Journal of Critical Care, 12*(3), 279–280.

Reuter, D. A., Bayerlein, J., Goepfert, M., Weis, F., Kilger, E., & Goetz, A. E. (2003). Functional preload monitoring by arterial pulse contour analysis: Influence of tidal volume on left ventricular stroke volume variations (abstract). *Critical Care Medicine, 30*(12 suppl.), A19.

Reuter, D. A., Felbinger, T. W., Schmidt, C., Kilger, E., Goedje, O., Lamm, P., et al. (2002). Stroke volume variations for assessment of cardiac responsiveness to volume loading in mechanically ventilated patients after cardiac surgery. *Intensive Care Medicine, 28*(4), 392–398.

Rezende, E., Assuncao, M., Manetta, J., Lopes, J., & Periera, R. (2003). Fluid challenge in spontaneous breathing patients: Is the right ventricular end-diastolic volume measurement important? *Critical Care Medicine, 31*(2 Suppl.), A63.

Rickard, C. M., Couchman, B. A., Schmidt, S. J., Dank, A., & Purdie, D. M. (2003). A discard volume of twice the deadspace ensures clinically accurate arterial blood gases and electrolytes and prevents unnecessary blood loss. *Critical Care Medicine, 31*(6), 1654–1658.

Rivers, E., Nguyen, B., Havstad, S., Ressler, J., Muzzin, A., Knoblich, B., et al. (2001). Early goal-directed therapy in the treatment of severe sepsis and septic shock. *New England Journal of Medicine, 345*(19), 1368–1377.

Rivers, E.P., Ander, D.S., & Powell, D. (2001). Central venous oxygen saturation monitoring in the critically ill patient. *Current Opinion in Critical Care, 7*(3), 204–211.

Rizvi, K., deBoisblanc, B., Dhillon, G., Arroliga, A., Fuchs, B., Guntupalli, K., et al. (2003). Effect of airway pressure display on inter-observer variability in assessment of vascular pressure in the ARDSnet Fluids & Catheters Treatment Trial (FACTT). Paper presented at the American Thoracic Society, Seattle, WA.

Roberts, P., Allen, S., Robinson, S.W., Tanser, S.J., Jonas, M., & Morgan, J. (2002). Use of lithium dilution assessment of cardiac output to optimise right/left ventricular activation in resynchronisation therapy. *Heart, 87*(Supplement II), A146.

Rodig, G., Prasser, C., Keyl, C., Liebold, A., & Hobbhahn, J. (1999). Continuous cardiac output measurement: pulse contour analysis vs thermodilution technique in cardiac surgical patients. *British Journal of Anaesthesia, 82*(4), 525–530.

Ronco, J. J., Fenwick, J. C., Tweeddale, M. G., Wiggs, B. R., Phang, P. T., Cooper, D. J., et al. (1993). Identification of the critical oxygen delivery for anaerobic metabolism in critically ill septic and nonseptic humans. *JAMA, 270*(14), 1724–1730.

Rooke, G. A., Schwid, H. A., & Shapira, Y. (1995). The effect of graded hemorrhage and intravascular volume replacement on systolic pressure variation in humans during mechanical and spontaneous ventilation. *Anesthesia Analgesia, 80*(5), 925–932.

Ross, C., & Jones, R. (1995). Comparisons of pulmonary artery pressure measurements in supine and 30 degree lateral positions. *Canadian Journal of Cardiovascular Nursing, 6*(3–4), 4–8.

Rowell, L., Brengelmann, G., Blackmon, J., Bruce, R., & Murray, J. (1968). Disparities between aortic and peripheral pulse pressures induced by upright exercise and vasomotor changes in man. *Circulation, 37*(954–964).

Ruesch, S., Walder, B., & Tramer, M.R. (2002). Complications of central venous catheters: internal jugular versus subclavian access—a systematic review. *Critical Care Medicine, 30*(2), 454–460.

Saberi, D., Caudwell, L., McGloin, H., et al. (2000). Proactive circulatory management in the 1st 4 hours post-cardiac surgery: Interim analysis of a nurse-led, oesophageal Doppler-guided protocol. *Intensive Care Medicine, 26*(3 (Suppl)), S220.

Safcsak, K., & Nelson, L. D. (1999). Right heart volumetric monitoring: measuring preload in the critically injured patient. *AACN Clinical Issues, 10*(1), 22–31.

Sageman, W. S., Riffenburgh, R. H., S& piess, B. D. (2002). Equivalence of bioimpedance and thermodilution in measuring cardiac index after cardiac surgery. *Journal of Cardiothoracic and Vascular Anesthesia, 16*(1), 8–14.

Sandham, J. D., Hull, R. D., Brant, R. F., Knox, L., Pineo, G. F., Doig, C. J., et al. (2003). A randomized, controlled trial of the use of pulmonary-artery catheters in high-risk surgical patients. *New England Journal of Medicine, 348*(1), 5–14.

Sasse, S., Chen, P., Berry, R., Sassoon, C., & Mahutte, C. (1994). Variability of cardiac output over time in medical intensive care unit patients. *Critical Care Medicine, 22*(2), 225–232.

Sasse, S. A., Chen, P. A., & Mahutte, C. K. (1996). Relationship of changes in cardiac output to changes in heart rate in medical ICU patients. *Intensive Care Medicine, 22*(5), 409–414.

Scheer, B., Perel, A., & Pfeiffer, U. J. (2002). Clinical review: Complications and risk factors of peripheral arterial catheters used for haemodynamic monitoring in anaesthesia and intensive care medicine. *Critical Care, 6*(3), 199–204.

Scott, S., Guiliano, K., Pysznik, E., Elliott, S., Welsh, K., & Delbuono, N. (1998). Influence of port site on central venous pressure measurements from triple-lumen catheters in critically ill adults. *American Journal of Critical Care, 7*(1), 60–63.

Segal, E., Katzenelson, R., Berkenstadt, H., & Perel, A. (2002). Transpulmonary thermodilution cardiac output measurement using the axillary artery in critically ill patients. *Journal of Clinical Anesthesia, 14*(3), 210–213.

Shoemaker, W. (1996). Temporal physiologic patterns of shock and circulatory dysfunction based on early descriptions by invasive and noninvasive monitoring. *New Horizons, 4*(2), 300–318.

Shoemaker, W., Appel, P., & Kram, H. (1992). Role of oxygen debt in the development of organ failure sepsis and death in high risk surgical patients. *Chest, 102*, 208–215.

Shoemaker, W.C., Appel, P.L., & Kram, H.B. (1993). Hemodynamic and oxygen transport responses in survivors and nonsurvivors of high-risk surgery. *Critical Care Medicine, 21*(7), 977–990.

Shoemaker, W. C., Belzberg, H., Wo, C. C., Milzman, D. P., Pasquale, M. D., Baga, L., et al. (1998). Multicenter study of noninvasive monitoring systems as alternatives to invasive monitoring of acutely ill emergency patients. *Chest, 114*(6), 1643–1652.

Shoemaker, W. C., Thangathurai, D., Wo, C. C., Kuchta, K., Canas, M., Sullivan, M.J., et al. (1999). Intraoperative evaluation of tissue perfusion in high-risk patients by invasive and noninvasive hemodynamic monitoring. *Critical Care Medicine,* 27(10), 2147–2152.

Shoemaker, W. C., Wo, C. C., Chan, L., Ramicone, E., Kamel, E. S., Velmahos, G.C., et al. (2001). Outcome prediction of emergency patients by noninvasive hemodynamic monitoring. *Chest,* 120(2), 528–537.

Shoemaker, W. C., Wo, C. C., Thangathurai, D., Velmahos, G., Belzberg, H., Asensio, J. A., et al. (1999). Hemodynamic patterns of survivors and nonsurvivors during high risk elective surgical operations. *World Journal of Surgery,* 23(12), 1264–1270.

Shoemaker, W. C., Wo, C. C., Yu, S., Farjam, F., & Thangathurai, D. (2000). Invasive and noninvasive haemodynamic monitoring of acutely ill sepsis and septic shock patients in the emergency department. *European Journal of Emergency Medicine,* 7(3), 169–175.

Sinclair, S., James, S., & Singer, M. (1997). Intraoperative intravascular volume optimisation and length of hospital stay after repair of proximal femoral fracture: randomised controlled trial. *British Medical Journal,* 315(7113), 909–912.

Singer, M. (1993). Esophageal Doppler monitoring of aortic blood flow: beat-by-beat cardiac output monitoring. *International Anesthesiology Clinics,* 31(3), 99–125.

Singh, A., Juneja, R., Mehta, Y., & Trehan, N. (2002). Comparison of continuous, stat, and intermittent cardiac output measurements in patients undergoing minimally invasive direct coronary artery bypass surgery. *Journal of Cardiothoracic and Vascular Anesthesia,* 16(2), 186–190.

Soller, B. R., Idwasi, P. O., Balaguer, J., Levin, S., Simsir, S. A., Vander Salm, T.J., et al. (2003). Noninvasive, near infrared spectroscopic-measured muscle pH and PO2 indicate tissue perfusion for cardiac surgical patients undergoing cardiopulmonary bypass. *Critical Care Medicine,* 31(9), 2324–2331.

Spackman, T., & Abenstein, J. (1993). Continous cardiac output may be more accurate than bolus thermodilution output during the use of an upper-body warming blanket. *Anesthesiology,* 79(3A), A473.

Spiess, B. D., Patel, M. A., Soltow, L. O., & Wright, I. H. (2001). Comparison of bioimpedance versus thermodilution cardiac output during cardiac surgery: evaluation of a second-generation bioimpedance device. *Journal of Cardiothoracic and Vascular Anesthesia,* 15(5), 567–573.

Stites, S., Barnes, J., Overman, J., & O'Boynick, P. (1998). Impact of injection technique on variability in thermodilution cardiac output. *Critical Care Medicine,* 26(1 (Suppl)), A67.

Su, N. Y., Huang, C. J., Tsai, P., Hsu, Y. W., Hung, Y. C., & Cheng, C. R. (2002). Cardiac output measurement during cardiac surgery: esophageal Doppler versus pulmonary artery catheter. *Acta Anaesthesiologica Sinica,* 40(3), 127–133.

Suistomaa, M., Ruokonen, E., Kari, A., & Takala, J. (2000). Time-pattern of lactate and lactate to pyruvate in the first 24 hours of intensive care emergency admissions. *Shock,* 14(1), 8–12.

Summers, R. L., Kolb, J. C., Woodward, L. H., & Galli, R. L. (1999a). Diagnostic uses for thoracic electrical bioimpedance in the emergency department: clinical case series. *European Journal of Emergency Medicine,* 6(3), 193–199.

Summers, R. L., Kolb, J. C., Woodward, L. H., & Galli, R. L. (1999b). Differentiating systolic from diastolic heart failure using impedance cardiography. *Academic Emergency Medicine,* 6(7), 693–699.

Sun, Q., Rogiers, P., Pauwels, D., & Vincent, J.L. (2002). Comparison of continuous thermodilution and bolus cardiac output measurements in septic shock. *Intensive Care Medicine,* 28(9), 1276–1280.

Swan, H., Ganz, W., Forrester, W., Marcus, H., Diamond, G., & Chonette, D. (1970). Catheterization of the heart in man with use of a flow-directed balloon-tipped catheter. *New England Journal of Medicine,* 283(9), 447–451.

Tachibana, K., Imanaka, H., Takeuchi, M., Takauchi, Y., Miyano, H., & Nishimura, M. (2003). Noninvasive cardiac output measurement using partial carbon dioxide rebreathing is less accurate at settings of reduced minute ventilation and when spontaneous breathing is present. *Anesthesiology,* 98(4), 830–837.

Takala, J., Uusaro, A., Parviainen, I., & Ruokonen, E. (1996). Lactate metabolism and regional lactate exchange after cardiac surgery. *New Horizons,* 4(4), 483–492.

Taler, S. J., Textor, S. C., & Augustine, J. E. (2002). Resistant hypertension: comparing hemodynamic management to specialist care. *Hypertension,* 39(5), 982–988.

Tatevossian, R. G., Shoemaker, W. C., Wo, C. C., Dang, A.B., Velmahos, G. C., & Demetriades, D. (2000). Noninvasive hemodynamic monitoring for early warning of adult respiratory distress syndrome in trauma patients. *Journal of Critical Care,* 15(4), 151–159.

Tatevossian, R. G., Wo, C. C., Velmahos, G. C., Demetriades, D., & Shoemaker, W. C. (2000). Transcutaneous oxygen and CO2 as early warning of tissue hypoxia and hemodynamic shock in critically ill emergency patients. *Critical Care Medicine,* 28(7), 2248–2253.

Tavernier, B., Makhotine, O., Lebuffe, G., Dupont, J., & Scherpereel, P. (1998). Systolic pressure variation as a guide to fluid therapy in patients with sepsis-induced hypotension. *Anesthesiology,* 89(6), 1313–1321.

Taylor, D. E., & Simonson, S. G. (1996). Use of near-infrared spectroscopy to monitor tissue oxygenation. *New Horizons,* 4(4), 420–425.

Theres, H., Binkau, J., Laule, M., Heinze, R., Hundertmark, J., Blobner, M., et al. (1999). Phase-related changes in right ventricular cardiac output under volume-controlled mechanical ventilation with positive end-expiratory pressure. *Critical Care Medicine,* 27(5), 953–958.

Thierry, S., Thebert, D., Brocas, E., Razzaghi, F., Van De Louw, A., Loisance, D., et al. (2003, Sep 10). *Evaluation of a new invasive continuous cardiac output monitoring system: The truCCOMS system,* from http://www.springer-link.com/app/home/issue.asp

Timsit, J. F. (2000). Scheduled replacement of central venous catheters is not necessary. *Infection Control and Hospital Epidemiology,* 21(6), 371–374.

Timsit, J. F., Farkas, J. C., Boyer, J. M., Martin, J. B., Misset, B., Renaud, B., et al. (1998). Central vein catheter-related thrombosis in intensive care patients: incidence, risks factors, and relationship with catheter-related sepsis. *Chest,* 114(1), 207–213.

Turnaoglu, S., Tugrul, M., Camci, E., Cakar, N., Akinci, O., & Ergin, P. (2001). Clinical applicability of the substitution of mixed venous oxygen saturation with central venous oxygen saturation. *Journal of Cardiothoracic and Vascular Anesthesia,* 15(5), 574–579.

Turner, M. A. (2003). Doppler-based hemodynamic monitoring: a minimally invasive alternative. *AACN Clinical Issues,* 14(2), 220–231.

Uhlig, T., Pestel, G., & Reinhart, K. (2002). Gastric mucosal tonometry in daily ICU practice. In J. L. Vincent (Ed.), *Intensive care medicine: Annual update 2002* (pp. 632–637). New York: Springer.

Vallet, B., Tavernier, B., & Lund, N. (2000). Assessment of tissue oxygenation in the critically-ill. *European Journal of Anaesthesiology,* 17(4), 221–229.

Valtier, B., Cholley, B. P., Belot, J. P., de la Coussaye, J. E., Mateo, J., & Payen, D.M. (1998). Noninvasive monitoring of cardiac output in critically ill patients using transesophageal Doppler. *American Journal of Respiratory and Critical Care Medicine,* 158(1), 77–83.

Van De Water, J. M., Miller, T. W., Vogel, R. L., Mount, B. E., & Dalton, M. L. (2003). Impedance cardiography: the next vital sign technology? *Chest,* 123(6), 2028–2033.

van der Meer, B. J., de Vries, J. P., Schreuder, W.O., Bulder, E. R., Eysman, L., & de Vries, P. M. (1997). Impedance cardiography in cardiac surgery patients: abnormal body weight gives unreliable cardiac output measurements. *Acta Anaesthesiologica Scandinavica,* 41(6), 708–712.

van der Meer, B. J., Woltjer, H. H., Sousman, A. M., Schreuder, W. O., Bulder, E. R., Huybregts, M. A., et al. (1996). Impedance cardiography. Importance of the equation and the electrode configuration. *Intensive Care Medicine,* 22(11), 1120–1124.

VanEtta, D., Gibbons, E., & Woods, S. (1993). Estimation of left atrial location in supine and 30° lateral position. *American Journal Critical Care,* 2(3), 264.

Vedrinne, C., Bastien, O., De Varax, R., Blanc, P., Durand, P. G., Du Gres, B., et al. (1997). Predictive factors for usefulness of fiberoptic pulmonary artery catheter for continuous oxygen saturation in mixed venous blood monitoring in cardiac surgery. *Anesthesia Analgesia,* 85(1), 2–10.

Velmahos, G. C., Demetriades, D., Shoemaker, W. C., Chan, L. S., Tatevossian, R., Wo, C.C., et al. (2000). Endpoints of resuscitation of critically injured patients: normal or supranormal? A prospective randomized trial. *Annals of Surgery,* 232(3), 409–418.

Velmahos, G. C., Wo, C. C., Demetriades, D., & Shoemaker, W. C. (1999). Early continuous noninvasive haemodynamic monitoring after severe blunt trauma. *Injury,* 30(3), 209–214.

Venkatesh, B., & Morgan, T. (2002). Tissue lactate concentrations in critical illness. In J. L. Vincent (Ed.), *Intensive care medicine* (pp. 587–599). New York: Springer.

Vincent, J. L. (2002). The available clinical tools—Oxygen-derived variables, lactate and pH. In J. L. Vincent (Ed.), *Tissue oxygenation in acute medicine* (pp. 193–203). New York: Springer.

Vincent, J.- L., & De Backer, D. (2002). Cardiac output measurement: Is least invasive always the best? *Critical Care Medicine,* 30(10), 2380–2382.

Vollman, K., & Bander, J. (1996). Improved oxygenation using a prone positioner in patients with acute respiratory distress syndrome. *Intensive Care Medicine,* 22(10), 1105–1111.

Wagner, J. G., & Leatherman, J. W. (1998). Right ventricular end-diastolic volume as a predictor of the hemodynamic response to a fluid challenge. *Chest,* 113(4), 1048–1054.

Weil, M. H., Nakagawa, Y., Tang, W., Sato, Y., Ercoli, F., Finegan, R., et al. (1999). Sublingual capnometry: a new noninvasive measurement for diagnosis and quantitation of severity of circulatory shock. *Critical Care Medicine,* 27(7), 1225–1229.

Weissman, C., Kemper, M., & Harding, J. (1994). Response of critically ill patients to increased oxygen demand: hemodynamic subsets. *Critical Care Medicine,* 22(11), 1809–1816.

West, J., Dollery, C., & Naimark, A. (1964). Distribution of blood flow in isolated lung; relation to vascular and alveolar pressures. *Journal Applied Physiology,* 19(4), 713–724.

Westerhof, N., & O'Rouke, M. (1995). Hemodynamic basis for the development of left ventricular failure in systolic hypertension and its logical therapy. *Journal of Hypertension,* 13(9), 943–952.

Wiesenack, C., Prasser, C., Rodig, G., & Keyl, C. (2003). Stroke volume variation as an indicator of fluid responsiveness using pulse contour analysis in mechanically ventilated patients. *Anesthesia Analgesia,* 96(5), 1254–1257.

Wilson, J., Woods, I., Fawcett, J., Whall, R., Dibb, W., Morris, C., et al. (1999). Reducing the risk of major elective surgery: randomised controlled trial of preoperative optimisation of oxygen delivery. *British Medical Journal,* 318(7191), 1099–1103.

Wo, C. C., Shoemaker, W. C., Appel, P. L., Bishop, M. H., Kram, H. B., & Hardin, E. (1993). Unreliability of blood pressure and heart rate to evaluate cardiac output in emergency resuscitation and critical illness. *Critical Care Medicine,* 21(2), 218–223.

Woda, R. P., Dzwonczyk, R., Buyama, C., Bernacki, B. L., & Kelly, W. B. (1999). In the dynamic performance of the Abbott Safeset blood-conserving arterial line system. *Journal of Clinical Monitoring and Computing,* 15(3-4), 215–221.

Yalavatti, G. S., DeBacker, D., & Vincent, J.L. (2000). Assessment of cardiac index in anemic patients. *Chest,* 118(3), 782–787.

Yelderman, M. (1993). Continuous cardiac output by thermodilution. *International Anesthesiology Clinics,* 31(3), 127–140.

Yu, M. (1996). Invasive and noninvasive oxygen consumption and hemodynamic monitoring in elderly surgical patients. *New Horizons,* 4(4), 443–452.

Yu, M. (1999). Oxygen transport optimization. *New Horizons,* 7(1), 46–53.

Yu, M., Burchell, S., Hasaniya, N. W., Takanishi, D. M., Myers, S. A., & Takiguchi, S.A. (1998). Relationship of mortality to increasing oxygen delivery in patients > or = 50 years of age: a prospective, randomized trial. *Critical Care Medicine,* 26(6), 1011–1019.

Yu, M., Levy, M. M., Smith, P., Takiguchi, S. A., Miyasaki, A., & Myers, S. A. (1993). Effect of maximizing oxygen delivery on morbidity and mortality rates in critically ill patients: a prospective, randomized, controlled study. *Critical Care Medicine,* 21(6), 830–838.

Zevola, D. R., Dioso, J., & Moggio, R. (1997). Comparison of heparinized and nonheparinized solutions for maintaining patency of arterial and pulmonary artery catheters. *American Journal of Critical Care,* 6(1), 52–55.

Zevola, D. R., & Maier, B. (1999). Improving the care of cardiothoracic surgery patients through advanced nursing skills. *Critical Care Nurse,* 19(1), 34–44.

Zollner, C., Goetz, A. E., Weis, M., Morstedt, K., Pichler, B., Lamm, P., et al. (2001). Continuous cardiac output measurements do not agree with conventional bolus thermodilution cardiac output determination. *Canadian Journal of Anaesthesia,* 48(11), 1143–1147.

Zollner, C., Haller, M., Weis, M., Morstedt, K., Lamm, P., Kilger, E., et al. (2000). Beat-to-beat measurement of cardiac output by intravascular pulse contour analysis: a prospective criterion standard study in patients after cardiac surgery. *Journal of Cardiothoracic and Vascular Anesthesia,* 14(2), 125–129.

Heart Rate Variability

DIANA MCMILLAN • ROBERT BURR

Heart rate variability (HRV) is the beat-to-beat variation of the cardiac cycle that results, in large part, from the interaction of sympathetic and parasympathetic inputs to the sinus node. The term "arrhythmia" often carries negative connotations, and many serious disturbances of heart rhythm and waveform morphology are malignant. However, some variation in the time between successive beats is normal, reflecting a healthy heart and healthy autonomic nervous system (ANS). A moderate amount of respiratory sinus arrhythmia (RSA), for example, is viewed as evidence of good cardiovascular health. In addition to short-term or beat-to-beat variation, a healthy individual also exhibits a marked circadian or 24-hour variation in heart rate.

Measures of HRV provide clinicians and researchers with a noninvasive, practical, reproducible, sensitive, and dynamic insight into the autonomic neural regulation of the heart. These measures are gaining popularity in cardiac care and are recognized as important diagnostic tools for risk identification in a wide range of cardiovascular conditions and health conditions that predispose cardiac complications.

This chapter provides a basic overview of the mechanisms of HRV, the approaches used in measuring HRV, and guidance for the interpretations of these measurements. Current research related to HRV patterns in common cardiovascular conditions and in health conditions predisposing cardiac complications is presented. General health history factors that can influence HRV patterns are discussed. The chapter concludes with a brief review of pharmacological and nonpharmacological interventions and their impact on HRV patterns.

MECHANISMS OF HEART RATE VARIABILITY

The beat-to-beat variation of the cardiac electrical signal expressed in normal sinus rhythm is termed HRV and is considered to be an index of ANS balance and imbalance. The time between successive beats is governed by the intrinsic firing rate of the sino-atrial (SA) node and the modulation of the SA node firing rate by input from the ANS. The input of the ANS is based on the relative contributions of the two ANS branches: the sympathetic nervous system (SNS) and the parasympathetic nervous system (PSNS). Thus, HRV does not reflect absolute sympathovagal input, but rather the relative dominance and interaction of these two ANS branches. PSNS activity normally dominates under conditions of rest and restoration. SNS activity predominance is associated with increased physiological arousal.

Complicating the interpretation of HRV indices aimed at identification of these respective ANS inputs are neural and non-neural factors that can modify the SA node firing rate. These factors include the central nervous system integration of cardiac neural input, positive feedback from sympathetic afferents, and negative feedback from baroreceptors and vagal afferents (Malliani et al., 1991). Despite our incomplete understanding of the physiological mechanisms associated with specific HRV measures, analysis of HRV provides significant clinical predictive usefulness within cardiac care.

HEART RATE VARIABILITY MEASUREMENT

Heart rate variability measures are statistical or mathematical summaries of within-subject variation in beat-to-beat heart period or instantaneous heart rate (Appel et al., 1989). This section summarizes the principles behind some of the more common HRV measures.

General Considerations

The current diversity of HRV measures and nomenclature is partially caused by the relative novelty and rapid proliferation of these methods. It also reflects simultaneous independent development in several distinct disciplines by clinical researchers with very different purposes and very different typical sources of heart rhythm information. Most HRV measures are so strongly correlated with each other that they are nearly redundant. However, no subset of HRV measures so consistently outperforms all the others in all circumstances that clear choices can be made. There have been several attempts at standardization of HRV measures and nomenclature (Task Force, 1996), but the recommendations have not been universally accepted, particularly in the interdisciplinary literature relevant to nursing.

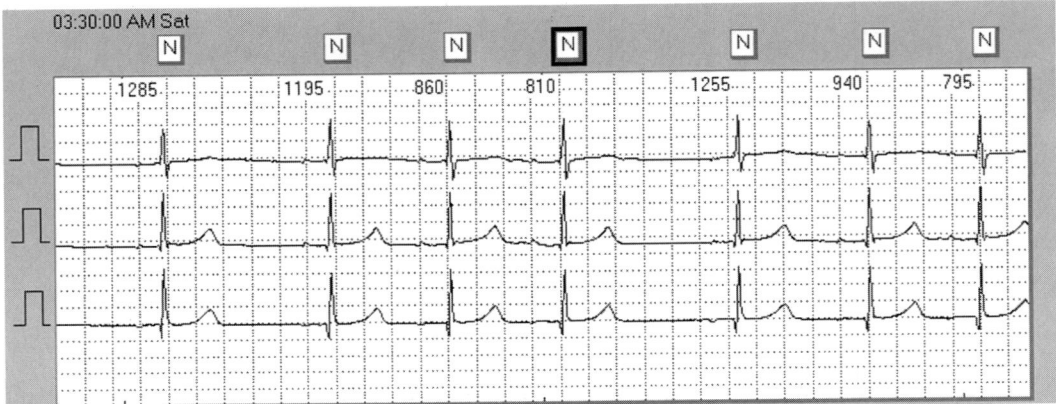

■ **Figure 24–1.** Example strip of ambulatory Holter ECG recorded during sleep. The beats are coded as Normal ("N"), and the RR intervals (in milliseconds) for each overlapping pair of beats are displayed above and slightly to the left of the R-wave that terminates the interval. Two respiratory cycles of probable respiratory arrhythmia (RSA) are visually apparent in the strip. Note that the measured sequential RR intervals vary considerably within a few seconds for this high HRV subject.

Practically, the instantaneous heart period must be defined from a series of discrete events corresponding to the beating of the heart. This discrete event series itself is usually derived from fiducial features of the raw electrocardiograph (ECG) waveform. The arrival time of a beat, in particular the time interval from the previous beat, provides us with somewhat irregularly spaced information about short-term fluctuations in heart rhythm, and by inference, the dynamic autonomic control of the heart (Coenen et al., 1977; Rompelman et al., 1977).

Despite the variety of purposes motivating HRV analysis, the primary goal is usually to compute some within-subject or within-condition indices of heart rhythm variation to make some qualified inferences, not about the heart organ itself, but about the sympathetic and parasympathetic neural traffic impinging on the sino-atrial node of the heart. Thus it would be ideal to base the definition of the inter-beat heart period on the interval between adjacent P-waves to reflect as closely as possible the statistics of the firing of the sino-atrial pacemaker node (Leffler et al., 1994; Takei, 1992). However, the P—P interval is much harder to empirically define than the RR interval, particular from noisy low-frequency Holter recordings of ambulatory subjects. Most heart rate variability studies, and essentially all of those performed using ambulatory ECG monitoring technology, use the RR interval as the fundamental metric. Although it is conventional to speak of heart period as specific to a particular beat, an RR interval is actually a measurement of the time interval between the R-waves of two successive normal beats, sometimes called an NN doublet (Fig. 24-1).

The quality of HRV indices is ultimately dependent on the consistency of the basic measurement of each RR interval. In modern digital applications, this is partially determined by the sampling rate of the raw ECG, and also by characteristics of the R-wave location finding algorithm. Typical sampling rates may vary from approximately 100 Hz (samples per second), still common in long time scale ambulatory monitoring, to 1,000 Hz or faster in laboratory studies. In general, a higher digital waveform sampling rate allows proportionally more precision in the estimation of the location of the R-waves at the cost of greater processing and memory requirements. However, the resulting apparent gain in precision may be illusory in ambulatory ECG recordings that contain noise and morphologies that vary slightly with posture and activity.

The RR intervals thus decoded from the raw ECG can be placed into an ordered temporal sequence to form a time series, in which the continuous length of each cardiac cycle is an interval measure of time, usually reported in units of milliseconds (ms). Each RR interval may be inverted to a beat-specific instantaneous equivalent heart rate, which can be considered the heart rate in beats per minute that would have been observed if all the heart beats in a 60-second period had exactly the length of that specific individual interval (Rompelman et al., 1977).

HRV Measures

Although there are a variety of approaches used to analyze HRV, the two major procedures are time domain analysis and frequency domain analysis. Definitions for HRV measures based on these approaches are presented in Tables 24-1 and 24-2, respectively.

Table 24–1 ■ DESCRIPTION OF TIME DOMAIN MEASURES OF HRV

Measure	Units	Description
Mean RR	ms	Mean of all NN intervals
SDNN	ms	Standard deviation of all NN intervals
CoV		Coefficient of variation, equal to $100 \times$ SDNN/(mean RR)
SDANN	ms	Standard deviation of the averages of NN intervals in all 5-minute segments of the recording
SDNN index	ms	Mean of the standard deviations of all NN intervals in all 5-minute segments of the recording
rmsSD	ms	Square root of the mean squared differences between successive NN intervals
pNN50	%	Number of successive NN intervals differing by more than 50 ms divided by the total number of successive NN intervals, expressed as a percentage

Table 24–2 ■ DESCRIPTION OF FREQUENCY DOMAIN MEASURES OF HRV

Measure	Units	Description
PSD plot	ms²/Hz	Plot of power spectral density (PSD) versus frequency; frequency range is generally less than 0.4 Hz
Total power	ms²	Area under PSD curve, equal to the variance of the segment; segment length can be short (5 min) or entire recording
LF	ms²	Power in the low-frequency band between 0.04 Hz and 0.15 Hz; it reflects both sympathetic and parasympathetic activity
HF	ms²	Power in the high-frequency band between 0.15 Hz and 0.4 Hz; it predominantly reflects parasympathetic activity
LF/HF		Ratio of LF power to HF power; a higher number indicates increased sympathetic activity or reduced parasympathetic activity
LFnu	%	Low-frequency power in normalized units, LF/(LF + HF), expressed as a percentage
HFnu	%	High-frequency power in normalized units, HF/(LF + HF), expressed as a percentage

Time Domain Analysis

Time domain analysis is based on the statistical interpretation of RR time interval values. Time domain measures of HRV (Table 24-1) are closely related to the total variance of the heart signal (Task Force, 1996). The most common index of overall HRV is the standard deviation of all RR intervals (SDNN), typically involving 80,000 to 150,000 heart period values in a 24-hour recording. Long-term variability, such as that reflecting normal circadian influence over a 24-hour period, is best reflected by two measures based on partitioning the full recording into sequential 5-minute segments. Each segment typically contains 300 to 500 RR intervals, and there would be 288 such segments in a 24-hour recording. The SDANN is defined as the standard deviation of the means of the RR intervals in each 5-minute segment, whereas the complementary SDNN Index is the mean of the standard deviations of the RR intervals in each 5-minute segment.

Short-term time domain measures of HRV are derived from the differences of successive normal RR intervals. They are highly correlated and are considered to provide good estimates of PSNS activity (Task Force, 1996). Short-term measures include the square root of the mean squared difference of successive normal RR intervals (rmsSD), and the percentage of successive normal RR intervals that change by more than 50 ms compared to the total number of RR intervals (pNN50).

Frequency Domain Analysis

Frequency domain analysis, or spectral analysis, is an elegant method for studying the rhythmic components in a RR interval sequence and presents intriguing possibilities for disentangling PSNS and SNS influences on the heart (Öri et al., 1992). A plot of the power spectral density (PSD) of HRV versus frequency describes how the variances of the frequency components of the heart signal are distributed (Task Force, 1996).

Both parametric and nonparametric methods common to time series analysis have been used to estimate the PSD. The most common methods are the Discrete Fourier Transform (DFT) (nonparametric), and autoregressive (AR) (parametric) time series models. The AR model-based spectrum is usually less computationally efficient than the DFT, but it can be applied to data sequences of arbitrary length, including very short segments. The AR approach tends to produce a spectrum that is statistically more stable than the DFT but requires assumptions about the time series model (Task Force, 1996).

The total area under the curve of the PSD versus frequency plot is equal to the total statistical variance, or the power of the signal. These power (variance) distributions are calculated for defined frequency bands and are interpreted as an estimate of the variance of the HRV signal within that band (Table 24-2). There are two major spectral components seen in HRV data: the high-frequency (HF) (0.15–0.40 Hz) component and the low-frequency (LF) (0.04–0.15 Hz) component (Fig. 24-2). The HF component is associated with respiration (Pagani et al., 1986) and is considered to reflect the relative input of the PSNS. The basis of the LF component is more controversial and may be the result of both SNS and PSNS activity input (Akselrod et al., 1981). The ratio of LF to HF (LF:LH) ratio has been regarded as reflecting the balance between the mixed PSNS and SNS activity input to the PSNS activity input (Task Force, 1996). The spectral HF and the LF:LH ratio are often reported together in nursing research studies seeking to explore the joint contribution of the SNS and the PSNS branches to HRV phenomena. Studies of very-low-frequency and ultra-low-frequency ranges have also been conducted but require long uninterrupted sampling periods and specialized methods of analysis. In addition, the clinical interpretation of findings in these frequency ranges remains controversial (Task Force, 1996).

In common with other variance-like measures, the within-subject HRV band power estimates are often re-expressed using the natural logarithm transform to reduce distributional skewness before use in statistical procedures. HRV quantitative band power summary indices (LF, HF, etc.) computed using the AR or DFT methods should be virtually identical (Cowan et al., 1992).

Several derived measures can easily be computed from these spectral band summaries (see Table 24-2). Normalized variants of the LF and HF indices are often defined by dividing the power in each band by the total power, with the result expressed as a percentage.

It should be pointed out that the HRV spectrum and spectrum-based band power (variance) summary statistics, like all HRV measures, are defined over blocks of RR intervals; thus, their meaning is not localized to a particular instant in time or to a particular beat. Typical block window lengths in clinical and research applications range from 2 minutes to 24 hours. Spectra derived from shorter blocks are more localized in time and are more likely to be internally stationary but may have less frequency resolution, especially with respect to slower rhythm patterns. HRV spectra based on very long individual blocks (for example, 24 hours) will have the ability to resolve very slow rhythmic patterns but will almost certainly span nonstationary data segments and heterogeneous latent autonomic states.

■ **Figure 24–2.** Two 5-minute HRV power/variance spectra based on data collected on a single male diabetic subject during sleep between 3 and 4 A.M. The top figure is based on data collected in 1992 when the subject was 42 years of age. The average heart rate of the analysis segment is 61 beats per minute, and the HRV spectrum demonstrates high total power/variance with a well-developed mid-frequency peak at 0.25 Hz, probably reflective of vagally mediated RSA. The lower figure is based on data collected from the same subject a decade later in 2002, when he was 52 years old. The average heart rate of the nocturnal analysis segment is 70 beats per minute. The total power of the HRV spectrum is an order of magnitude less, and while the low frequency peak has diminished, the high frequency peak is significantly attenuated. The quantitative band power and derived measure summaries appear in the table to the right of each figure, and document that the HF power is lower and the LF:HF ratio much increased in the lower figure. The changes over time may reflect the joint influence of aging and diabetes.

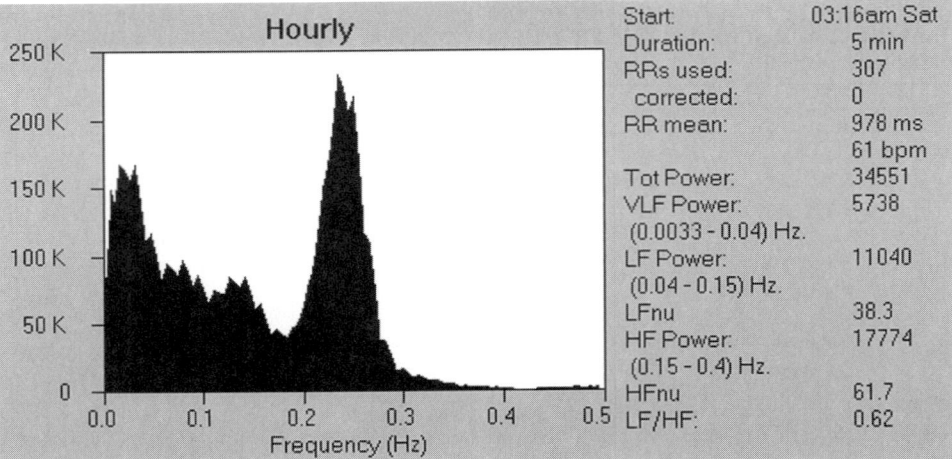

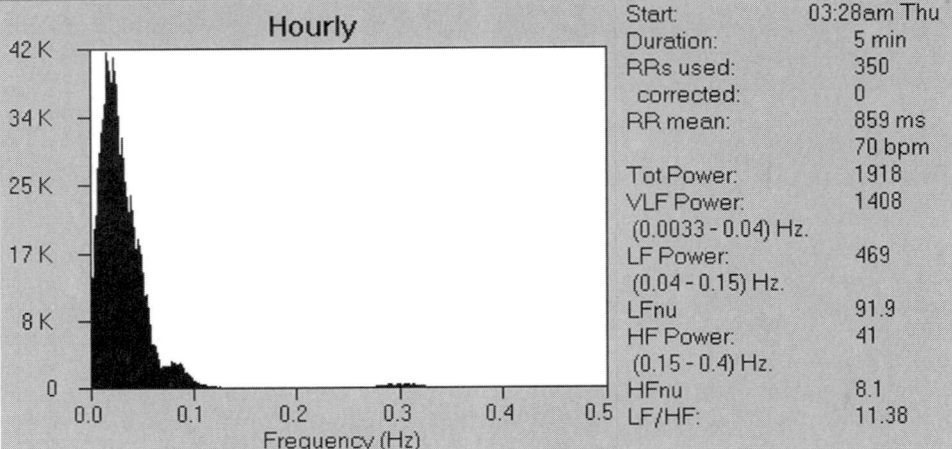

HRV PATTERNS IN COMMON CARDIOVASCULAR CONDITIONS

The following section provides a summary of HRV research findings in myocardial infarction; arrhythmias and sudden death; angina; hypertension; heart failure; and cardiac surgery, heart transplant, and other invasive procedures. The reader is referred to related chapters for more detailed descriptions of these conditions and interventions.

Myocardial Infarction

It is well established that HRV patterns are disturbed in patients who have experienced MI (Bigger et al., 1995; Liao et al., 1996; Sosnowski et al., 2002). In post-MI patients, those with restrictive left ventricular filling have been reported to have especially reduced HRV patterns compared to those without this disorder (Poulsen et al., 2001).

Decreased HRV after MI is viewed as a significant risk factor for cardiac death (Sosnowski et al., 2002) or subsequent nonfatal MI within 12 months (Kennon et al., 2003). HRV

measures of total variability, such as SDNN and SDANN, are viewed as the most useful predictors of mortality (Sosnowski et al., 2002; Task Force, 1996). Results from a landmark study, the Multicenter Post-Infarction Project (MPIP), indicate that patients with a SDNN of less than 50 ms (24-hour recording), measured within 11 days of the MI, have a risk of mortality at 1 year that is 5.3-times higher than do patients with a SDNN greater than 100 ms (Kleiger et al., 1987). Predicted risk is also increased for patients with below-normal SDNN and SDANN values in the chronic phase after MI. Reported normal lower limits for patients measured at least 3 months after MI range between 63 ms to 89 ms for SDNN and between 57 ms and 79 ms for SDANN (Ramaekers et al., 1998; Sosnowski et al., 2002). Reduced circadian variation in the cardiac signal, reduced total power, and a shift toward sympathetic predominance as reflected by an increased LF:HF ratio are also seen after MI (Task Force, 1996).

While HRV measures can provide independent risk prediction, the combination of HRV indices with other cardiovascular risk factors can enhance prediction of cardiac events. In a prospective study of 304 patients with acute coronary syndrome without ST elevation, a combination of risk factors including clinical data, troponin T concentrations, ST monitoring, and HRV provided a prediction of risk for ischaemic death or nonfatal MI of 40% in the first 30 days and of 46.9% in the first 12 months (Kennon et al., 2003).

Arrhythmias and Sudden Death

HRV studies indicate autonomic disturbance before arrhythmia, although the pattern of disturbance varies. Clinical research supports that reduced parasympathetic tone and increased sympathetic tone predisposes ventricular fibrillation and ventricular tachycardia (La Rovere, 2001). The onset of paroxysmal atrial fibrillation has been reported to follow autonomic changes characterized by an initial steady increase in SNS activity and a subsequent sharp predominance in PSNS activity (Bettoni & Zimmermann, 2002).

Reduced HRV is a consistent finding in a review of studies monitoring sudden death or sudden death and malignant arrhythmias (Stein & Kleiger, 1999). In a prospective study (N = 1071) of post-MI patients, reduced HRV independently contributed to the risk of sudden death and or sustained ventricular tachycardia (La Rovere et al., 2001). The combination of low HRV, nonsustained ventricular tachycardia, and baroreflex sensitivity led to a 22-fold increase in the risk for sudden death or sustained VT.

Sudden unexpected death syndrome is a leading cause of death in young men of Southeast Asian descent. Although nighttime ventricular fibrillation typically precedes the cardiac arrest, the pathophysiology of this disorder is not known. HRV analysis indicates reduced 24-hour HRV and reduced circadian variation in HRV, with very low nighttime HRV in survivors of this syndrome compared to controls (Krittayaphong et al., 2003).

Angina

Low HRV is associated with poor prognosis in stable angina (Forslund et al., 2002) and unstable angina (Kennon et al., 2003). Low HRV, including reduced total power and reduced HF, LF, and VLF components, provide strong and independent predictors of cardiac death but not nonfatal MI in stable angina pectoris (Forslund et al., 2002). Low HRV in patients presenting with unstable angina increases the risk of either cardiac death or nonfatal MI within 12 months (Kennon et al., 2003).

Hypertension

Individuals with hypertension (HTN) (Lucini et al., 2003) and those at high risk for HTN (Lucini et al., 2002; Singh et al., 1998) exhibit abnormal HRV patterns. HRV is reduced in individuals with essential HTN compared to healthy control subjects, as reflected in significantly reduced values for SDNN, SDANN, pNN50, and rmsSD (Kaftan & Kaftan, 2000). These findings are consistent with results from the Framingham Heart Study (N = 1919), a prospective epidemiological study of coronary risk factors (Singh et al., 1998). Singh et al. found significant reductions in time domain measures of HRV in men and women with HTN compared to normotensive subjects. Hypertensive patients also exhibit a lower than normal

vagal tone (low HF) (Kaftan & Kaftan, 2000; Singh et al., 1998).

Some HTN studies indicate a significant increase in mixed SNS and PSNS activity, reflected by increased resting LF power (Guzzetti et al., 1994; Kaftan & Kaftan, 2000). However, results from the Framingham Heart Study indicate reduced LF activity in patients with HTN and suggest that low vagal tone is a strong risk factor for the development of HTN in men (Singh et al., 1998). Methodological differences in covariate adjustment may have contributed to inconsistent study findings.

The normal circadian pattern of HRV is disturbed in patients with HTN. In normotensive individuals, the nighttime fall in blood pressure is paralleled by a corresponding reduction in the mixed PSNS and SNS activity marker LF. This nocturnal drop in LF power is not as large in subjects with HTN (Lucini et al., 2003).

Heart Failure

Patients with congestive heart failure (CHF) have reduced HRV (Kingwell et al., 1994). The most consistently reported finding is a reduction in SDNN (Bilchick et al., 2002; Krüger et al., 2002; La Rovere et al., 2003; Nolan et al., 1998). Some researchers report a significant early increase in sympathetic predominance (high LF:HF ratio) using a paced canine model of CHF (Eaton et al., 1995). This initial SNS surge appears to be lost as the condition worsens (Kingwell et al., 1994). Reduced vagal activity (low HF) and reduced total power have also been reported in patients with CHF (Kingwell, 1994).

Although the derangement of ANS function in heart failure is well recognized, the ability of HRV measures to aid in the risk assessment of patients with this disorder is mixed (Notarius & Floras, 2001). One of the factors complicating the interpretation of HRV patterns in heart failure is the impact of respiratory patterns. Cheyne-Stokes respiration and oscillatory breathing pattern (characterized by cyclic changes in ventilation without apnea) are common in CHF and are associated with significant reductions in mixed SNS and PSNS activity (low LF power) (Ponikowski et al., 1999). Interestingly, this severe LF power decrease contrasts with the increase in SNS activity found in patients with obstructive sleep apnea, hypoxia, and hypercapnia.

Despite these confounding factors, the use of HRV measures in heart failure is reported to be helpful in the evaluation of risk for malignant cardiac events. HRV is a significant predictor for sudden death (Bilchick et al., 2002; Krüger et al., 2002; La Rovere et al., 2003; Nolan et al., 1998). Based on a multivariate survival model, risk of sudden death in patients with CHF was strongly predicted by HRV (La Rovere et al., 2003). Researchers collected ECG data during 8 minutes of controlled breathing and found that reduced sympathetic predominance (LF power ≤ 13 ms^2) in patients with CHF was associated with a relative risk for sudden death of 3.7 compared to patients with sympathetic input above this level. Of patients with CHF, those presenting with values of SDNN less than 65.3 ms were reported to be at significantly greater risk for sudden death (Bilchick et al., 2002). In another study, mortality and hospitalization caused by deterioration of CHF were predicted by HRV. In this case, SDNN (<75 ms) provided significant and independent predictive value in addition to the standard risk indices of left ventricular ejection fraction and peak oxygen intake (Krüger et al., 2002).

Another cardiac condition exhibiting disturbed ANS functioning is aortic regurgitation. Low SDANN significantly predicted risk of death or progression to aortic valve repair in a study of 50 asymptomatic or minimally symptomatic patients with chronic severe aortic regurgitation (Freed et al., 1997).

Cardiac Surgery, Heart Transplantation, and Other Invasive Procedures

Cardiovascular surgery has been shown to impact HRV patterns. Results from the Cardiac Arrhythmia Suppression Trial (CAST) indicate that HRV is significantly reduced in post-MI patients after CABG surgery and that this reduction in HRV is not associated with increased mortality (Stein et al., 2000b). This finding contrasts with the increased risk of mortality seen in post-MI CAST patients who did not undergo CABG surgery but who did exhibit reduced HRV, specifically reduced SDANN. This is an important finding that may help to explain the lower than predicted mortality rates seen in some post-CABG surgery patients. Similar reductions in HRV were reported in a Danish study of CABG patients without a recent MI and with ejection fractions of $36 \pm 7\%$ (Wiggers et al., 2002). These researchers found significantly reduced HRV immediately post-CABG and at the 6-month follow-up. Furthermore, improvement in myocardial function seen after surgery was not associated with post-CABG measures of HRV.

Heart transplant patients exhibit significantly reduced HRV immediately after surgery (Kingwell et al., 1994). This reduction continues to be significantly reduced 2 years after surgery despite evidence of a return to near-normal cardiac-specific sympathetic nerve firing. This finding suggests insufficient or dysfunctional reinnervation of the cardiac muscle, and particularly the SA node with respect to ANS nerve fiber communication (Kingwell et al., 1994).

Biventricular pacing enhanced ANS functioning in a study of 13 patients with heart failure and ventricular conduction disturbances (Livanis et al., 2003). In this surgical procedure, chronic cardiac resynchronization is achieved through the permanent implanting of a pacemaker. Significant increases were found in several measures of HRV, although not in LF power. Larger samples and survival impact analysis are needed to confirm these early but positive findings.

Other cardiac procedures have been explored with respect to HRV. Transmyocardial laser revascularization (Brunner et al., 2002) and percutaneous transluminal angioplasty (Osterhues et al., 1998) are not associated with a significant change in HRV after procedure, but left ventricular reduction is associated with significant reduction in HRV (Brunner et al., 2002).

Noncardiac surgeries can also impact on postoperative HRV patterns. Reduced 24-hour HRV is found in the postoperative period after major abdominal surgery (Gogenur et al., 2002).

Significantly improved HRV has been noted in patients receiving kidney transplants and for those with kidney-pancreas transplants (Cashion et al., 1999). Measures of HRV may provide an indication of recovery in transplantation associated with disorders of autonomic neuropathy.

FACTORS INFLUENCING HEART RATE VARIABILITY

Several factors have been found to influence HRV and are important considerations for HRV interpretation. The following section provides a summary of the influences on HRV by age, gender, genetics, sleep and wake, body position, general health, and acute and chronic disorders. Readers should refer to Chapter 11 for a detailed review of sleep.

Age

HRV tends to decrease with increasing age (Cowan et al., 1994; Jensen-Urstad et al., 1997; Stein et al., 1997). This decline is caused by decreases in absolute PSNS and SNS activity and by reductions in their relative dominance (Liao et al., 1995; Öri et al., 1992). Stimulus challenge tests, such as active standing, are frequently included in assessments of ANS function. Test results should be interpreted within the context of the patient's age because responses to sympatho-excitatory (i.e., active standing) and sympatho-inhibitory (i.e., cold face challenge) stimuli decrease with age (Lucini et al., 1993).

Gender and Sex Hormones

Gender and the interaction of gender and age appear to influence HRV. Healthy women typically have higher heart rates and less HRV than healthy men (Bonnemeier et al., 2003; Fagard et al., 1999; Stein et al., 1997). Young men are reported to exhibit particularly high values in vagal-related indices (rmsSD, SDNN) (Bonnemeier et al., 2003). Other studies support that lower sympathetic predominance (low LF) and higher vagal activity (high HF) are seen in women in their mid-life years (Kuo et al., 1999; Liao et al., 1995). Gender disparities in HRV values diminish with increasing age (Bonnemeier et al., 2003), disappearing entirely by age 60 (Fagard et al., 1999; Kuo et al., 1999), and possibly as early as age 40 (Ramaekers et al., 1998).

The impact of endogenous sex hormones on ANS activity has been explored. HRV is not significantly different across menstrual phases, although heart rate is increased at ovulation. Positive correlations between peak estrogen levels at ovulation and LF power ($p = 0.05$), HF power ($p = 0.05$), and total power ($p = 0.05$) lend modest support for the claim that estrogen has cardioprotective effects (Leicht et al., 2003).

Genetics

Genetic factors influence many aspects of health, including HRV (Busjahn et al., 1998; Singh et al., 2001; Singh et al.,

2002). Genetic components are estimated to contribute 13% to 23% of the variance in HRV measures (Singh et al., 2001). Genetic testing provides suggestive but nonsignificant evidence linking LF power to chromosome 2 at 153 cM and linking VLF power to chromosome 15 at 62 cM (Singh et al., 2002). Increased HRV is also associated with the genotype factor described as polymorphisms in angiotensin-converting enzyme gene (Busjahn et al., 1998).

Sleep and Wake

Significant autonomic activity differences between wake and sleep and within different sleep states have been identified. HRV is normally characterized by greater variability during sleep than wake in adults (Malpas & Purdie, 1990) and children (Massin et al., 2000). This sleep-associated increase in variability persists even after controlling for behavioral rhythms (Aoyagi et al., 2000), daytime physical activity, posture (Van de Borne et al., 1994), and shift work (Ito et al., 2001).

Sleep is characterized by two major states: nonrapid eye movement (NREM) sleep and rapid eye movement (REM) sleep. NREM sleep is further divided into four stages, generally characterized by progressively slower frequency and higher amplitude brain wave activity. Low-voltage mixed-frequency brain wave activity, rapid saccadic eye movements, and CNS-invoked low skeletal muscle tone denote REM sleep. Individuals typically cycle between NREM and REM sleep approximately five times over the course of the night, with the proportion of REM sleep increasing across the night.

Not surprisingly, HRV patterns differ between NREM and REM sleep. NREM sleep is characterized by a low LF:HF ratio, interpreted to reflect PSNS predominance (Elsenbruch et al., 1999; Scholz et al., 1997; Vanoli et al., 1995). Researchers report a progressive increase in vagal activity across NREM sleep stages 1 to 4 (Toscani et al., 1996). The higher LF:HF ratio seen during REM sleep is similar to that of wakefulness and reflects a higher sympathetic tone (Elsenbruch et al., 1999; Scholz et al., 1997; Vanoli et al., 1995).

Sleep is scored in terms of discrete stages in 30-second epochs, but there is a range in the amount of delta (slow wave) activity present within these stages. Findings suggest that mixed SNS and PSNS activity (LF:HF ratio) is negatively dependent on the amount of delta activity, whereas PSNS activity (HF) is independent of delta activity (Yang et al., 2002).

A final consideration for HRV patterns in sleep is arousal activity. EEG defined arousals occur with a movement to a lower sleep stage or to wake. These arousals are associated with increased LF power in the cardiac signal (Bonnet & Arand, 1997). Although more subtle, NREM sleep is also characterized by two arousal rhythms. These NREM rhythms include a state of sustained arousal instability known as cyclic alternating pattern (CAP) and a stable arousal condition known as non-CAP. The percentage of LF power is greater in CAP, and HF power is greater in non-CAP within NREM stage 2 sleep and NREM slow-wave sleep (Ferri et al., 2000).

Body Position

Body position and the frequency of positional change are closely related to whether the person is awake or asleep. During sleep, an individual usually exhibits fewer and less dramatic changes in body position. Whether the patient is asleep or awake, body position should be considered in the interpretation of HRV. Comparative evaluations for treatment or intervention should be based on assessment that is consistent for positioning.

In terms of vertical positioning, HRV is significantly reduced from supine to sitting and further decreased from sitting to standing (Brguljan et al., 1993). In healthy subjects, change from supine to standing also reduces vagal input (low HF), increases the LF-to-HF ratio, and reduces LF power (Fagard et al., 1999). Postural changes evoke a greater HRV response in women than in men (Stolarz et al., 2003), although this difference was not found elsewhere (Fagard et al., 1999). ANS postural change responses are blunted with increased age (Fagard et al., 1999; Stolarz et al., 2003).

Recumbent positioning that enhances vagal tone in the cardiac care patient could promote recovery by reducing cardiac demand and, subsequently, the risk of malignant cardiac events. The right lateral position is associated with a higher vagal tone (higher HF) than either the left lateral or the supine positions. This position-based vagal enhancement is consistently found in individuals with coronary artery disease (Kuo & Chen, 1998), in patients during the acute phase of a MI (Kuo et al., 2000), and in patients with CHF (Fujita et al., 2000). Healthy individuals also show vagal predominance with the right lateral position (Kuo & Chen, 1998), although this observation is not reported consistently (Fujita et al., 2000).

Position-related differences in HRV may be an important factor in sudden infant death syndrome (SIDS). Compared to sleeping in the supine position, sleeping prone is recognized as a significant risk factor for SIDS and is associated with lower HRV in term infants at ages 1 and 3 months (Galland et al., 1998). Preterm infants are especially at risk for SIDS. HRV assessment of these high-risk patients measured during a daytime nap showed significantly reduced HRV and reduced PSNS activity in the prone versus supine position at 1 and 3 months corrected age (Ariagno et al., 2003). These results lend support for promoting sleep in the supine position.

General Health

Results from the Atherosclerosis Risk in Communities (ARIC) Study, a large population-based study of middle-aged men and women, support that low HRV is associated with increased mortality rates that are not attributable to cardiovascular risk factors or to other disease conditions (Dekker et al., 2000). This suggests that low HRV may be a sensitive indicator for poor general health in addition to an index of cardiovascular risk.

A major contributor to general health is lifestyle. Many aspects of lifestyle have been explored with respect to impact on HRV patterns. These include physical activity, obesity and diet, smoking, and alcohol and coffee consumption.

Physical Activity

Physically active individuals tend to have lower heart rates and increased HRV compared to those with a sedentary lifestyle (Ueno & Moritani, 2003). The difference in HRV between active and inactive individuals is particularly large in older individuals (Ueno & Moritani, 2003). Also, type of activity is important. Endurance (aerobic) training significantly increases HRV but resistance (weight) training does not (Grund et al., 2001).

Obesity and Diet

Obese individuals, as measured by body mass index (BMI), are characterized by increased resting sympathetic tone: faster heart rates, higher LF power, and lower HF power (Stolarz et al., 2003). Other researchers have not found significant associations between BMI and HRV in healthy adolescents (Faulkner et al., 2003) or between BMI and SNS activity markers in mild to moderately obese healthy adults (Kageyama et al., 1997). Rabbia et al. (2003) suggest that ANS function is dependent on duration of obesity. Specifically, compared to lean adolescents, measures of SNS activity were increased in subjects with recent (<4 years) obesity but not chronic obesity. HRV reduced significantly with duration of obesity. Orthostatic (lying to standing) stress testing indicates a blunted autonomic response in obese individuals (Stolarz et al., 2003).

The relationship of diet to HRV has received some attention. Levels of total cholesterol and low-density lipoprotein cholesterol are significant predictors of reduced HRV in "healthy" individuals with hypercholesterolemia (Danev et al., 1997). However, short-term dietary changes appear to have little immediate impact on HRV patterns. Individuals that are chronically underweight and undernourished show reduced total power, LF power, and HF power compared to underweight well-nourished or normal-weight well-nourished individuals (Vaz et al., 2003).

Smoking

Smoking has an immediate impact on HRV, characterized by an acute decrease in cardiac PSNS activity and a surge in systemic SNS activity, including increased heart rate (Hayano et al., 1990: Zhang & Kesteloot, 1999). The long-term and dose-related effects of smoking on HRV are less clear. Some researchers report that smoking, and especially chronic heavy smoking (>25 cigarettes per day), reduces HRV and vagal activity (Hayano et al., 1990). However, a significant association is not found consistently (Fagard et al., 1999; Kageyama et al., 1997; Stolarz et al., 2002).

Alcohol

HRV is one approach used to explore the cardioprotective and cardioputative effects of alcohol. Although population-based study results indicate that alcohol is not a significant lifestyle factor affecting HRV in healthy adults (Fagard et al., 1999; Kageyama et al., 1997), other research supports that the relationship is more complex. In one study involving a randomized crossover design, findings suggest that moderate regular alcohol consumption in healthy individuals enhances vagal activity (increased HF, reduced LF, increased HF:LF ratio) (Flanagan et al., 2002).

Alcohol restriction also impacts HRV patterns. Compared to their usual drinking patterns (70.1 ± 4.6 mL/day), 3 weeks of alcohol restriction (19.1 ±2.5 mL/day) in habitual drinkers led to reduced heart rate, increased HRV, and increased indices of PSNS activity (Minami et al., 2002). Findings support ANS activity recovery even after chronic high alcohol consumption.

Caffeine

Caffeine causes an acute increase in systemic vascular resistance through the blocking of central anti-adrenergic adenosine receptors. This acute increase in blood pressure is compensated for by a brief reduction in heart rate and a probable increase in vagal predominance. This prediction is in keeping with findings of a sympathetic rebound (higher LF:HF ratio) in coffee drinkers after at least 2 hours of abstinence from caffeine compared to individuals who regularly do not consume caffeine (Stolarz et al., 2003). More work is needed to fully determine the short-term and long-term impact of caffeine on HRV.

Acute and Chronic Conditions

Pain

Acute pain is clinically seen to increase heart rate and decrease HRV. Interventions that foster good pain management are expected to enhance HRV and reflect a decreased activation of the SNS. Exploration of HRV patterns related to chronic pain is limited and frequently confounded by cardiac pathology. HRV patterns across sleep cycles are not different between patients with chronic low back pain and healthy controls (Pivik et al., 1997). Standard measures of HRV are not significantly different for patients characterized by either successful or unsuccessful pain reduction after treatment for a herniated disc (Storella et al., 1999). These findings suggest that pain is not a modifying factor for HRV. More work is needed, however, before conclusions regarding the relationship between HRV patterns and chronic pain can be drawn.

Brain Injury

The ability to perform continuous and noninvasive assessments of ANS function with HRV has made this a valued additional approach for neurological injury assessment and prognosis.

Traumatic brain injury is associated with ANS dysfunction marked by reduced HRV and reduced LF and HF power (King et al., 1997). Biswas et al. (2000) studied children with brain injury. Factors that predicted poorer outcome, such as a low Glasgow Coma Scale score (3–4 versus 5–8), higher intracranial pressure (>30 mm Hg), and decreased cerebral perfusion pressure (<40 mm Hg) were associated with PSNS dominance as reflected by low LF:HF ratios. Profound vagal dominance is characteristic of patients with brain injury who progress to brain death (Biswas et al., 2000; Baillard et al., 2002).

Stroke patients exhibit cardiovascular regulatory impairment in both ANS branches. Total power, LF power, and HF power are all reduced (Arad et al., 2002; Meglic et al., 2001; Tokgözoglu et al., 1999), although an increase in the LF:HF ratio supports relative sympathetic dominance (Tokgözoglu et al., 1999). Injury in the region of the insula (especially the right) is strongly associated with ANS instability and sudden death (Tokgözoglu et al., 1999). Within the brainstem, only medullary stroke injury is associated with depressed ANS activity (reduced LF and HF power) (Meglic et al., 2001).

Depression

Depression is a significant risk factor for the development of cardiovascular disease and for the increased risk of cardiac mortality and morbidity in those with existing cardiovascular conditions (see reviews by Carney et al., 2002; Musselman, Evans & Nemeroff, 1998). One possible explanation is that depressive disorders may stimulate harmful influences on the ANS by increasing SNS activity and/or reducing vagal tone (Carney et al., 2002). Consistent with this hypothesis, lower HRV and reduced vagal tone (low HF) are found in depressed compared to nondepressed individuals with CHD (Stein et al., 2000a). The severity of depression in cardiac patients is negatively associated with HRV (Carney et al., 2000; Hallas et al., 2003; Stein et al., 2000a). Cardiac care patients successfully treated for severe depression exhibit enhanced HRV and reduced heart rate (Carney et al., 2000). Collectively, these findings underscore the need for prompt assessment and treatment of depression in cardiac care.

Diabetes

Autonomic neuropathy is a common and serious complication of diabetes. Measures of HRV can aid in the early diagnosis, and treatment of this ANS dysfunction and are recommended as components of standard diabetic care. Findings from the Framingham Heart Study indicate that individuals with diabetes mellitus have significantly lower HRV (SDNN), LF and HF power, and LF:HF ratios compared to those with normal fasting glucose ($p < 0.005$) (Singh et al., 2000). Results also show a strong negative association between these HRV measurements and the level of fasting blood glucose across all subjects. These findings support a blunting of ANS activity and a relative SNS dominance in patients with diabetes and in those with impaired blood glucose regulation.

Not surprisingly, diabetic patients exhibiting low HRV have an increased risk for CHD (Liao et al., 2002). Based on a 9-year follow-up, diabetic subjects with impaired autonomic function have nearly double the risk of mortality than the general population (Gerritsen et al., 2001). Thus, diabetes and poor glucose regulation signal serious risk for the development and or exacerbation of cardiovascular conditions.

Chronic Obstructive Pulmonary Disease

Individuals with COPD exhibit ANS disturbance as measured by HRV, although the nature of the dysfunction reported is not consistent (Stein et al., 1998; Tükek et al., 2003; Volterrani et al., 1994). Stein et al. (1998) studied young PiZ α_1-antitrypsin–deficient COPD patients and found significant decreases in almost all HRV parameters. Severity of ANS disturbance was directly related to clinical severity as measured by FEV_1. Vagal activity was significantly reduced during the daytime only. Other researchers report that compared to control subjects, COPD patients exhibit increased HF activity during the daytime (Volterrani et al., 1994) or abnormally reduced nocturnal vagal activity (Tükek et al., 2003). Stein et al. (1998) studied younger patients with more severe cases and, unlike the two other studies cited, did not wean them from any medications complicating interpretation.

Huntington and Parkinson Diseases

Analysis of HRV indicates disturbed ANS function in Huntington disease (Andrich et al., 2002). Compared to matched healthy controls, genetically and symptomatically positive patients at the mid-stage of Huntington disease progression exhibit significantly reduced vagal tone (low HF) and a shift toward sympathetic predominance (high LF). Degree of disturbance is significantly related to the severity of clinical symptoms.

Little research has been conducted to explore autonomic activity in patients with Parkinson disease. Further research is needed to determine the representativeness of reported trends of increased SNS tone and reduced HRV (Akincioğlu et al., 2003).

IMPACT OF INTERVENTIONS ON HRV

Although decreased HRV is strongly linked with poor prognosis, the increase of HRV does not directly appear to improve health outcomes (Stein & Kleiger, 1999). Still, there is support for improved health outcomes for pharmacologic and nonpharmacologic interventions that are also associated with increased HRV.

Several pharmacologic therapies are known to increase HRV and reduce mortality. These include beta-blockers after MI (primarily through the enhancement of vagal tone) (Lampert et al., 2003), ACE inhibitors and carvedilol in CHF, sotalol in the treatment of ventricular arrhythmias, and estrogen replacement therapy in postmenopausal women (Leicht et al., 2003; Stein & Kleiger, 1998, p. 256).

Nonpharmacologic interventions, such as physical training (Grund et al., 2001; Takeyama et al., 2000) and psychosocial therapy (Carney et al, 2000), increase HRV and improve cardiovascular status. One nursing study combined approaches in a randomized control trial of a psychosocial therapy targeting survivors of sudden cardiac arrest (N = 129) (Cowan et al., 2001). Therapy included three components: physiologic relaxation with biofeedback; cognitive behavioral therapy aimed at enhancing mental health; and health education targeting cardiovascular risk factors. Based on a 2-year follow-up period, this comprehensive psychosocial therapy significantly reduced cardiovascular death.

SUMMARY

In summary, HRV is disturbed in a number of cardiovascular disorders and health conditions that predispose cardiac complications. Clinicians and researchers who have knowledge of these HRV pattern anomalies and the factors that shape them will be able to include this approach in their work, strengthening their assessment and evaluation of the cardiovascular patient.

REFERENCES

Akincioğlu, Ç., Ünlü, M., & Tunç, T. (2003). Cardiac innervation and clinical correlates in idiopathic Parkinson's disease. *Nuclear Medicine Communications, 24,* 267–271.

Akselrod, S. Gordon, D., Ubel, F. A., Shannon, D. C., Berger, A. C., & Cohen, R. J. (1981). Power spectrum analysis of heart rate fluctuations: A quantitative probe of beat to beat cardiovascular control. *Science, 213,* 220–222.

Andrich, J., Schmitz, T., Saft, C., Postert, T., Kraus, P., Epplen, J. T., Przuntek, H., & Agelink, M. W. (2002). Autonomic nervous system function in Huntington's disease. *Journal of Neurology, Neurosurgery & Psychiatry, 72*(6), 726–731.

Aoyagi, N., Ohashi, K., Tomono, S., & Yamamoto, Y. (2000). Temporal contribution of body movement to very long-term heart rate variability in humans. *American Journal of Physiology. Heart Circulation Physiology, 278*(4), H1035–H1041.

Appel, M. L., Berger, R. D., Saul, J. P., Smith, J. M., & Cohen, R. J. (1989). Beat to beat variability in cardiovascular variables: noise or music? *Journal of the American College of Cardiology, 14*(5), 1139–1148.

Arad, M., Abboud, S., Radai, M. M., & Adunsky, A. (2002). Heart rate variability parameters correlate with functional independence measures in ischemic stroke patients. *Journal of Electrocardiology, 35,* 243–246.

Ariagno, R. L., Mirmiran, M., Adams, M. M., Saporito, A. G., Dubin, A. M., & Baldwin, R. B. (2003). Effect of position on sleep, heart rate variability, and QT interval in preterm infants at 1 and 3 months' corrected age. *Pediatrics, 111*(3), 622–625.

Baillard, C., Vivien, B., Mansier, P., Mangin, L., Jasson, S., Riou, B., Swynghedauw, B. (2002). Brain death assessment using instant spectral analysis of heart rate variability. *Critical Care Medicine, 30,* 306–310.

Bettoni, M. & Zimmermann, M. (2002). Autonomic tone variations before the onset of paroxysmal atrial fibrillation. *Circulation, 105,* 2753–2759.

Bigger, J. T. Jr., Fleiss, J. L., Steinman, R. C., Rolnitzky, L. M., Schneider, W. J., Stein, P. K. (1995). RR variability in healthy, middle-aged persons compared with patients with chronic coronary heart disease or recent acute myocardial infarction. *Circulation, 91,* 1936–1943.

Bilchick, K. C., Fetics, B., Djoukeng, R., Fisher, S. G., Fletcher, R. D., Singh, S. N., Nevo, E., & Berger, R. D. (2002). Prognostic value of heart rate variability in chronic congestive heart failure (Veterans Affairs' Survival Trial of Antiarrhythmic Therapy in Congestive Heart Failure). *American Journal of Cardiology, 90*(1), 24–28.

Biswas, A. K., Scott, W. A., Sommerauer, J. F., & Luckett, P. M. (2000). Heart rate variability after acute traumatic brain injury in children. *Critical Care Medicine, 28*(12), 3907–3912.

Bonnemeier, H., Richardt, G., & Potratz, J. (2003). Circadian profile of cardiac autonomic nervous modulation in healthy subjects. *Journal of Cardiovascular Electrophysiology, 14*(8), 791–799.

Bonnet, M. H. & Arand, D. L. (1997). Heart rate variability: sleep stages, time of night, and arousal influences. *Electroencephalography and Clinical Neurophysiology, 102*(5), 390–396.

Brguljan, J., Fagard, R., Macor, F., & Amery, A. (1993). The sympathetic response to different orthostatic challenges and its daytime variation, assessed by power spectral analysis of heart rate. *Journal of Hypertension Supplement, 11*(suppl 5), S150–S151.

Brunner, M., Hess, B., Lutter, G., Zipfel, M., Grom, A., Beyersdorf, F., Bode, C., & Zehender, M. (2002). Transmyocardial laser revascularization and left ventricular reduction surgery affect ventricular arrhythmias and heart rate variability. *American Heart Journal, 143,* 1012–1016.

Busjahn, A., Voss, A., Knoblauch, H., Knoblauch, M., Jeschke, E., Wessel, N., Bohlender, J., McCarron, J., Faulhaber, J., Schuster, J., Dietz, R., & Luft, F. C.

(1998). Angiotensin-converting enzyme and angiotensinogen gene polymorphisms and heart rate variability in twins. *American Journal of Cardiology, 81*(6), 755–760.

Carney, R. M., Freedland, K. E., Miller, G. E., & Jaffe, A. S. (2002). Depression as a risk factor for cardiac mortality and morbidity. A review of potential mechanisms. *Journal of Psychosomatic Research, 53,* 897–902.

Carney, R. M., Freedland, K. E., Stein, P. K., Skala, J. A., Hoffman, P., & Jaffe, A. S. (2000). Change in heart rate and heart rate variability during treatment for depression in patients with coronary heart disease. *Psychosomatic Medicine, 62,* 639–647.

Cashion, A. K., Hathaway, D. K., Milstead, E. J., Reed, L., & Gaber, A. O. (1999). Changes in patterns of 24-hr heart rate variability after kidney and kidney-pancreas transplant. *Transplantation, 68,* 1846–1850.

Coenen A. J., Rompelman, O., & Kitney, R. I. (1977). Measurement of heart-rate variability: Part 2- Hardware digital devices for the assessment of heart-rate variability. *Medical and Biological Engineering and Computing, 15*(4), 423–430.

Cowan, M. J., Pike, K. C., Budzynski, H. K. (2001). Psychosocial nursing therapy following sudden cardiac arrest: impact on two-year survival. *Nursing Research, 50*(2), 68–76.

Cowan, M. J., Burr, R. L., Narayanan, S. B, Buzaitis, A., Strasser, M., & Busch, S. (1992). Comparison of autoregression and fast Fourier transform techniques for power spectral analysis of heart period variability of persons with sudden cardiac arrest before and after therapy to increase heart period variability. *Journal of Electrocardiology, 25*(Suppl.), 234–239.

Cowan, M. J., Pike, K., Burr, R. L. (1994). Effects of gender and age on heart rate variability in healthy individuals and in persons after sudden cardiac arrest. *Journal of Electrocardiology, 27*(Suppl.), 1–9.

Danev, S., Nikolova, R., Kerekovska, M., & Svetoslavov, S. (1997). Relationship between heart rate variability and hypercholesterolaemia. *Central European Journal of Public Health, 5*(3), 143–146.

Dekker, J. M., Crow, R. S., Folsom, A. R., Hannan, P. J., Liao, D., Swenne, C. A., Schouten, E. G. (2000). Low heart rate variability in a 2-minute rhythm strip predicts risk of coronary heart disease and mortality from several causes. The ARIC study. *Circulation, 102,* 1239–1244.

Eaton, G. M., Cody, R. J., Nunziata, E., & Binkley, P. F. (1995). Early left ventricular dysfunction elicits activation of sympathetic drive and attenuation of parasympathetic tone in the paced canine model of congestive heart failure. *Circulation, 92,* 555–561.

Elsenbruch, S., Harnish, M. J., & Orr, W. C. (1999). Heart rate variability during waking and sleep in healthy males and females. *Sleep, 22*(8), 1067–1071.

Fagard, R. H., Pardaens, K., & Staessen, J. A. (1999). Influence of demographic, anthropometric and lifestyle characteristics on heart rate and its variability in the population. *Journal of Hypertension, 17*(11), 1589–1599.

Faulkner, M. S., Hathaway, D., & Tolley, B. (2003). Cardiovascular autonomic function in healthy adolescents. *Heart & Lung, 32,* 10–22.

Ferri, R., Parrino, L., Smerieri, A., Terzano, M. G., Elia, M., Musumeci, S. A., & Pettinato, S. (2000). Cyclic alternating pattern and spectral analysis of heart rate variability during sleep. *Journal of Sleep Research, 9,* 13–18.

Flanagan, D. E. H., Pratt, E., Murphy, J., Vaile, J. C., Petley, G. W., Godsland, I. F., & Kerr, D. (2002). Alcohol consumption alters insulin secretion and cardiac autonomic activity. *European Journal of Clinical Investigation, 32,* 187–192.

Forslund, L. Björkander, I., Ericson, M., Held, C., Kahan, T., Rehnqvist, N., & Hjemdahl, P. (2002). Prognostic implications of autonomic function assessed by analyses of catecholamines and heart rate variability in stable angina pectoris. *Heart, 87,* 415–422.

Freed, L. A., Stein, K., Borer, J. S., Hochreiter, C., Supino, P., Devereux, R. B., Roman, M. J., & Kligfield, P. (1997). Relation of ultra-low frequency heart rate variability to the clinical course of chronic aortic regurgitation. *American Journal of Cardiology, 79*(11), 1482–1487.

Fujita, M., Miyamoto, S., Sekiguchi, H., Eiho, S., & Sasayama, S. (2000). Effects of posture on sympathetic nervous modulation in patients with chronic heart failure. *Lancet, 356,* 1822–1823.

Galland, B. C., Reeves, G., Taylor, B. J., Bolton, D. P. (1998). Sleep position, autonomic function, and arousal. Archives of Disease in Childhood. *Fetal and Neonatal Edition, 78,* F189–F194.

Gerritsen, J., Dekker, J. M., TenVoorde, B. J., Kostense, P. J., Heine, R. J., Bouter, L. M., Heethaar, R. M., & Stehouwer, C. D. A. (2001). Impaired autonomic function is associated with increased mortality, especially in subjects with diabetes, hypertension, or a history of cardiovascular disease. *Diabetes Care, 24*(10), 1793–1798.

Gogenur, I., Rosenburg-Adamsen, S., Lie, C., Rasmussen, V., & Rosenberg, J. (2002). Lack of circadian variation in the activity of the autonomic nervous system after major abdominal operations. *European Journal of Surgery,* 168(4), 242–246.

Grund, A., Krause, H., Kraus, M., Siewers, M., Rieckert, H., & Müller, M. J. (2001). Association between different attributes of physical activity and fat mass in untrained, endurance- and resistance-trained men. *European Journal of Applied Physiology,* 84, 310–320.

Guzzetti, S., Dassi, S., Balsama, M., Ponti, G. B., Pagani, M., & Malliani, A. (1994). Altered dynamics of the circadian relationship between systematic arterial pressure and cardiac sympathetic drive early on in mild hypertension. *Clinical Science (London),* 86(2), 209–215.

Hallas, C. N., Thornton, E. W., Fabri, B. M., Fox, M. A., & Jackson, M. (2003). Predicting blood pressure reactivity and heart rate variability from mood state following coronary artery bypass surgery. *International Journal of Psychophysiology,* 47, 43–55.

Hayano, J., Yamada, M., Sakakibara, Y., Fujinami, T., Yokoyama, K., Watanabe, Y., & Takata, K. (1990). Short- and long-term effects of cigarette smoking on heart rate variability. *American Journal of Cardiology,* 65(1), 84–88.

Ito, H., Nozaki, M., Maruyama, T., Kaji, Y., & Tsuda, Y. (2001). Shift work modifies the circadian patterns of heart rate variability in nurses. *International Journal of Cardiology,* 79, 231–236.

Jensen-Urstad, K., Storck, N., Bouvier, F., Ericson, M., Lindblad, L. E., & Jensen-Urstad, M. (1997). Heart rate variability in healthy subjects is related to age and gender. *Acta Physiologica Scandinavica,* 160(3), 235–241.

Kaftan, A. H. & Kaftan, O. (2000). QT intervals and heart rate variability in hypertensive patients. *Japanese Heart Journal,* 41(2), 173–182.

Kageyama, T., Nishikido, N., Honda, Y., Kurokawa, Y., Imai, H., Koboayashi, T., Kaneko, T., & Kabuto, M. (1997). Effects of obesity, current smoking status, and alcohol consumption on heart rate variability in male white-collar workers. *International Archives of Occupational and Environmental Health,* 69, 447–454.

Kennon, S., Price, C. P., MacCallum, P. K., Cooper, J., Hooper, J., Clarke, H., & Timmis, A. D. (2003). Cumulative risk assessment in unstable angina: clinical, electrocardiographic, autonomic, and biochemical markers. *Heart,* 89, 36–41.

King, M. L., Lichtman, S. W., Seliger, G., Ehert, F. A., & Steinberg, J. S. (1997). Heart-rate variability in chronic traumatic brain injury. *Brain Injury,* 11(6), 445–453.

Kingwell, B. A., Thompson, J. M., Kaye, D. M., McPherson, G. A., Jennings, G. L., Esler, M. D. (1994). Congestive heart failure/hypertension/hypertrophy: heart rate spectral analysis, cardiac norepinephrine spillover, and muscle sympathetic nerve activity during human sympathetic nervous activation and failure. *Circulation,* 90(1), 234–240.

Kleiger, R. E., Miller, J. P., Bigger, J. T., Moss, A. J. (1987). Decreased heart rate variability and its association with incrased mortality after acute myocardial infarction. *American Journal of Cardiology,* 59, 256–262.

Krittayaphong, R., Veerakul, G., Bhuripanyo, K., Jirasirirojanakorn, K., & Nademanee, K. (2003). Heart rate variability in patients with sudden unexpected cardiac arrest in Thailand. *American Journal of Cardiology,* 91, 77–81.

Krüger, C., Lahm, T., Zugck, C., Kell, R., Schellberg, D., Schweizer, M. W. F., Kübler, W., & Haass, M. (2002). Heart rate variability enhances the prognostic value of established parameters in patients with congestive heart failure. *Zeitschrift für Kardiologie,* 91, 1003–1012.

Kuo, C. D. & Chen, G. Y. (1998). Comparison of three recumbent positions on vagal and sympathetic modulation using spectral heart rate variability in patients with coronary artery disease. *American Journal of Cardiology,* 81, 392–396.

Kuo, C. D., Chen, G. Y., & Lo, H. M. (2002). Effect of different recumbent positions on spectral indices of autonomic modulation of the heart during the acute phase of myocardial infarction. *Critical Care Medicine,* 28, 1283–1289.

Kuo, T. B., Lin, T., Yang, C. C., Li, C. L., Chen, C. F., & Chou, P. (1999). Effect of aging on gender differences in neural control of heart rate. *American Journal of Physiology,* 277(6 pt 2), H2233–H2239.

Lampert, R., Ickovics, J. R., Viscoli, C. J., Horwitz, R. I., & Lee, F. A. (2003). Effects of propranolol on recovery of heart rate variability following acute myocardial infarction and relation to outcome in the beta-blocker heart attack trial. *American Journal of Cardiology,* 91, 137–142.

La Rovere, M. T., Pinna, G. D., Maestri, R., Mortara, A., Capomolla, S., Febo, O., Ferrari, R., Franchini, M., Gnemmi, M., Opasich, C., Riccardi, P. G., Traversi, E., & Cobelli, F. (2003). Short-term heart rate variability strongly predicts sudden cardiac death in chronic heart failure patients. *Circulation,* 107, 565–570.

La Rovere, M. T., Pinna, G. D., Hohnloser, S. H., Marcus, F. I., Mortara, A., Nohara, R., Bigger, J. T. Jr., Camm, A. J., & Schwartz, P. J., on behalf of the Autonomic Tone and Reflexes After Myocardial Infarction (ATRAMI) Investigators. (2001). Baroreflex sensitivity and heart rate variability in the identification of patients at risk for life-threatening arrhythmias. *Circulation,* 103, 2072–2077.

Leffler, C. T., Saul, J. P., Cohen, R. J. (1994). Rate-related and autonomic effects on atrioventricular conduction assessed through beat-to-beat PR interval and cycle length variability. *Journal of Cardiovascular Electrophysiology,* 5(1), 2–15.

Leicht, A. S., Hirning, D. A., & Allen, G. D. (2003). Heart rate variability and endogenous sex hormones during the menstrual cycle in young women. *Experimental Physiology,* 88(3), 441–446.

Liao, D., Barnes, R. W., Chambless, L. E., Simpson, R. J. J., Sorlie, P., & Heiss, G. (1995). Age, race, and sex differences in autonomic cardiac function measured by spectral analysis of heart rate variability–The ARIC study. Atherosclerosis Risk in Communities. *American Journal of Cardiology,* 76(12), 906–912.

Liao, D., Carnethon, M., Evans, G. W., Cascio, W. E., & Heiss, G. (2002). Lower heart rate variability is associated with the development of coronary heart disease in individuals with diabetes: the atherosclerosis risk in communities (ARIC) study. *Diabetes,* 51(12), 3524–3531.

Liao, D., Evans, G. W., Chambless, L. E., Barnes, R. W., Sorlie, P., Simpson, R. J. Jr., & Heiss, G. (1996). Population-based study of heart rate variability and prevalent myocardial infarction. The Atherosclerosis Risk in Communities Study. *Journal of Electrocardiology,* 29(3), 189–198.

Livanis, E. G., Flevari, P., Theodorakis, G. N., Kolokathis, F., Leftheriotis, D., & Kremastinos, D. T. (2003). Effect of biventricular pacing on heart rate variability in patients with chronic heart failure. *European Journal of Heart Failure,* 5, 175–178.

Lucini, D., Bertoni, L., Pitto, G., Frassetto, G., Pagani, M., & Malliani, A. (1993). Reduced response with ageing to sympatho-excitatory and sympatho-inhibitory stimuli in humans. *Journal of Hypertension. Supplement,* 11(Suppl. 5), S170–S171.

Lucini, D., Melas, G. S., Malliani, A., & Pagani, M. (2002). Impairment in cardiac autonomic regulation preceding arterial hypertension in humans: insights from spectral analysis of beat-by-beat cardiovascular variability. *Circulation,* 106(21), 2673–2679.

Lucini, D., Porta, A., & Pagani, M. (2003). Assessing autonomic disturbances of hypertension in the general practitioner's office: a transtelephonic approach to spectral analysis of heart rate variability. *Journal of Hypertension,* 21, 755–760.

Malliani, A., Pagani, M., Lombardi, F., & Cerutti, S. (1991). Cardiovascular neural regulation explored in the frequency domain. *Circulation,* 84(2), 482–492.

Malpas, S. C. & Purdie, G. L. (1990). Circadian variation of heart rate variability. *Cardiovascular Research,* 24(3), 210–213.

Massin, M. M., Maeyns, K., Withofs, N., Ravet, F., & Gérard, P. (2000). Circadian rhythm of heart rate and heart rate variability. *Archives of Disease in Childhood,* 83, 179–182.

Meglic, B., Kobal, J., Osredkar, J., & Pogacnik, T. (2001). Autonomic nervous system function in patients with acute brainstem stroke. *Cerebrovascular Diseases,* 11(1), 2–8.

Minami, J., Yoshii, M., Todoroki, M. Nishikimi, T., Ishimitsu, T., Fukunaga, T., & Matsuoka, H. (2002). Effects of alcohol restriction on ambulatory blood pressure, heart rate, and heart rate variability in Japanese men. *American Journal of Hypertension,* 15, 125–129.

Musselman, D. L., Evans, D. L., & Nemeroff, C. B. (1998). The relationship of depression to cardiovascular disease. *Archives in General Psychiatry,* 55, 580–592.

Nolan, J., Batin, P., Andrews, R., Lindsay, S. J., Brooksby, P., Mullen, M., Baig, W., Flapan, A. D., Cowley, A., Prescott, R. J., Neilson, J. M. M., & Fox, K. A. A. (1998). Prospective study of heart rate variability and mortality in chronic heart failure: results of the United Kingdom Heart Failure Evaluation and Assessment of Risk Trial (UK-Heart). *Circulation,* 98(15), 1510–1516.

Notarius, C. F. & Floras, J. S. (2001). Limitations of use of spectral analysis of heart rate variability for the estimation of cardiac sympathetic activity in heart failure. *Europace,* 3, 29–38.

Öri, Z., Monir, G., Weiss, J., Sayhouni, X., & Singer, D. H. (1992). Heart rate variability. Frequency domain analysis. *Cardiology Clinics,* 10(3), 499–537.

Osterhues, H., Kochs, M., & Hombach, V. (1998). Time-dependent changes of heart rate variability after percutaneous transluminal angioplasty. *American Heart Journal,* 135, 755–761.

Pagani, M., Lombardi, F., Guzzetti, S., Rimoldi, O., Furlan, R., Pizzinelli, P., Sandrone, G., Malfatto, G., Dell'Orto, S., Piccaluga, E., et al. (1986). Power spectral analysis of heart rate and arterial pressure variabilities as a marker of sympatho-vagal interaction in man and conscious dog. *Circulation Research*, 58, 178–193.

Pivik, R. T., Haman, K., & Matsunga, L. (1997). Variations in heart rate across sleep cycles in chronic low back pain subjects: *Implications for nonrestorative sleep complaints*. San Francisco, CA: APSS.

Ponikowski, P., Anker, S. D., Chua, T. P., Francis, D., Banasiak, W., Poole-Wilson, P. A., Coats, A. J. S., & Piepoli, M. (1999). Oscillatory breathing patterns during wakefulness in patients with chronic heart failure: clinical implications and role of augmented peripheral chemosensitivity. *Circulation*, 100(24), 2418–2424.

Poulsen, S. H., Jensen, S. E., Moller, J. E., & Egstrup, K. (2001). Prognostic value of left ventricular diastolic function and association with heart rate variability after a first acute myocardial infarction. *Heart*, 86(4), 376–380.

Rabbia, F., Silke, B., Conterno, A., Grosso, T., De Vito, B., Rabbone, I., Chiandussi, L., & Veglio, F. (2003). Assessment of cardiac autonomic modulation during adolescent obesity. *Obesity Research*, 11(4), 541–548.

Ramaekers, D., Ector, H., Aubert, A. E., Rubens, A., & Van de Werf, F. (1998). Heart rate variability and heart rate in healthy volunteers. Is the female autonomic nervous system cardioprotective? *European Heart Journal*, 19, 1334–1341.

Rompelman, O., Coenen, A. J., & Kitney, R. I. (1977). Measurement of heart-rate variability: Part 1-Comparative study of heart-rate variability analysis methods. *Medical and Biological Engineering and Computing*, 15(3), 233–239.

Scholz, U. J., Bianchi, A. M., Cerutti, S., & Kubicki, S. (1997). Vegetative background of sleep: spectral analysis of the heart rate variability. *Physiology & Behavior*, 62(5), 1037–1043.

Singh, J. P., Larson, M. G., O'Donnell, C. J., & Levy, D. (2001). Genetic factors contribute to the variance in frequency domain measures of heart rate variability. *Autonomic Neuroscience*, 90(1-2), 122–126.

Singh, J. P., Larson, M. G., O'Donnell, C. J., Tsuji, H., Corey, D., & Levy, D. (2002). Genome scan linkage results for heart rate variability (The Framingham Heart Study). *American Journal of Cardiology*, 90, 1290–1293.

Singh, J. P., Larson, M. G., O'Donnell, C. J., Wilson, P. F., Tsuji, H., Lloyd-Jones, D. M., & Levy, D. (2000). Association of hyperglycemia with reduced heart rate variability (The Framingham Heart Study). *American Journal of Cardiology*, 86, 309–312.

Singh, J. P., Larson, M. G., Tsuji, H., Evans, J. C., O'Donnell, C. J., & Levy, D. (1998). Reduced heart rate variability and new-onset hypertension. Insights into pathogenesis of hypertension: The Framingham Heart Study. *Hypertension*, 32, 293–297.

Sosnowski, M., MacFarlane, P. W., Czyz, Z., Skrzypek-Wanha, J., Boczkowska-Gaik, E., & Tendera, M. (2002). Age-adjustment of HRV measures and its prognostic value for risk assessment in patients late after myocardial infarction. *International Journal of Cardiology*, 86, 249–258.

Stein, P. K., Carney, R. M., Freeland, K. E., Skala, J. A., Jaffe, A. S., Kleiger, R. E., & Rottman, J. N. (2000a). Severe depression is associated with markedly reduced heart rate variability in patients with stable coronary heart disease. *Journal of Psychosomatic Research*, 48, 493–500.

Stein, P. K., Domitrovich, P. P., Kleiger, R. E., Schechtman, K. B., & Rottman, J. N. (2000b). Clinical and demographic determinants of heart rate variability in patients post myocardial infarction: insights from the cardiac arrhythmia suppression trial (CAST). *Clinical Cardiology*, 23(3), 187–194.

Stein, P. K. & Kleiger, R. E. (1999). Insights from the study of heart rate variability. *Annual Reviews in Medicine*, 50, 249–261.

Stein, P. K., Kleiger, R. E., & Rottman, J. N. (1997). Differing effects of age on heart rate variability in men and women. *American Journal of Cardiology*, 80(3), 302–305.

Stein, P. K., Nelson, P., Rottman, J. N., Howard, D., Ward, S. M., Kleiger, R. E., & Senior, R. M. (1998). Heart rate variability reflects severity of COPD in PiZ α_1-Antitrypsin Deficiency. *Chest*, 113, 327–333.

Stolarz, K., Staessen, J. A., Kuznetsova, T., Tikhonoff, V., State, D., Babeanu, S. et al. (2003). Host and environmental determinants of heart rate and heart rate variability in four European populations. *Journal of Hypertension*, 21, 525–535.

Storella, R. J., Shi, Y., O'Connor, D. M., Pharo, G. H., Abrams, J. T., & Levitt, J. (1999). Relief of chronic pain may be accompanied by an increase in a measure of heart rate variability. *Anesthesia Analogs*, 89(2), 448–450.

Takei, Y. (1992). Relationship between power spectral densities of P-P and R-R intervals. *Annals of Physiological Anthropology*, 11(3), 325–32.

Takeyama, J., Itoh, H., Kato, M., Koike, A., Aoki, K., Fu, L. T., Watanabe, H., Nagayama, M. & Katagiri, T. (2000). Effects of physical training on the recovery of the autonomic nervous activity during exercise after coronary artery bypass grafting. *Japanese Circulation Journal*, 64, 809–813.

Task Force of the European Society of Cardiology and the North American Society of Pacing and Electrophysiology. (1996). Heart rate variability: standards of measurement, physiological interpretation and clinical use. *Circulation*, 93(5), 1043–1065.

Tokgözoglu, S. L., Batur, M. K., Topçuoglu, M. A., Sariabas, O., Kes, S., & Oto, A. (1999). Effects of stroke localization on cardiac autonomic balance and sudden death. *Stroke*, 30, 1307–1311.

Toscani, L., Gangemi, P. F., Parigi, A., Silipo, R., Ragghianti, P., Sirabella, E., Morelli, M., & Bagnoli, L. (1996). Human heart rate variability and sleep stages. *Italian Journal of Neurological Sciences*, 17, 437–439.

Tükek, T., Yildiz, P., Atilgan, D., Tuzcu, V., Eren, M., Erk, O., Demirel, S., Akkaya, V., Dilmener, M., & Korkut, F. (2003). Effect of diurnal variability of heart rate on development of arrhythmia in patients with chronic obstructive pulmonary disease. *International Journal of Cardiology*, 88, 199–206.

Ueno, L. M. & Moritani, T. (2003). Effects of long-term exercise training on cardiac autonomic nervous activities and baroreflex sensitivity. *European Journal of Applied Physiology*, 89, 109–114.

Van de Borne, P., Nguyen, H., Biston, P., Linkowski, P., Degaute, J. P. (1994). Effects of wake and sleep stages on the 24-h autonomic control of blood pressure and heart rate in recumbent men. *American Journal of Physiology*, 266(2 pt 2), H548–H554.

Vanoli, E., Adamson, P. B., Ba-Lin, Pinna, G. D., Lazzara, R., & Orr, W. C. (1995). Heart rate variability during specific sleep stages. A comparison of healthy subjects with patients after myocardial infarction. *Circulation*, 91, 1918–1922.

Vaughn, B. V., Quint, S. R., Messenheimer, J. A., & Robertson, K. R. (1995). Heart period variability in sleep. *Electroencephalography and Clinical Neurophysiology*, 94(3), 155–162.

Vaz, M., Bharathi, A. V., Sucharita, S., & Nazareth, D. (2003). Heart rate variability and baroreflex sensitivity are reduced in chronically undernourished, but otherwise healthy, human subjects. *Clinical Science (London)*, 104(3), 295–302.

Volterrani, M., Scalvini, S., Mazzuero, G., Lanfrachi, P., Colombo, R., Clark, A. L., & Levi, G. (1994). Decreased heart rate variability in patients with chronic obstructive pulmonary disease. *Chest*, 106, 1432–1437.

Wiggers, H., Bøtker, H. E., Egeblad, H., Christiansen, E. H., Nielsen, T. T., & Mølgaard, H. (2002). Coronary artery bypass surgery in heart failure patients with chronic reversible and irreversible myocardial dysfunction: effect on heart rate variability. *Cardiology*, 98, 181–185.

Yang, C. C. H., Lai, C., Lai, H. Y., Kuo, T. B. J. (2002). Relationship between electroencephalogram slow-wave magnitude and heart rate variability during sleep in humans. *Neuroscience Letters*, 329, 213–216.

Zhang, J. & Kesteloot, H. (1999). Anthropometric, lifestyle and metabolic determinants of resting heart rate. *European Heart Journal*, 20, 103–110.

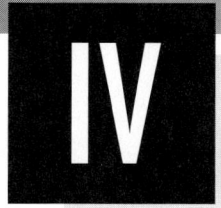

PART

IV

Pathophysiology and Management of Heart Disease

Pathophysiology of Acute Coronary Syndromes

POLLY GARDNER • GAYLENE ALTMAN

Acute coronary syndrome encompasses the clinical entities of myocardial ischemia and myocardial infarction. The diagnosis of acute coronary syndrome is based on history, risk factors, diagnostic laboratory tests, functional studies, and, to a lesser extent, the electrocardiogram. This chapter focuses primarily on the incidence, mechanisms, causes, and pathophysiology, including the cellular and metabolic changes of myocardial ischemia and infarction. Hemodynamic mechanisms affecting the balance of oxygen supply and demand are addressed. Clinical manifestations are briefly discussed and are fully detailed in Chapter 26.

INTRODUCTION

Many factors affect the pathophysiologic events that lead to ischemia, infarction, and injury of myocardial muscle. Injury to the myocardium can range from reversible to permanent damage of cellular components in localized tissue. Ischemia occurs from a transient imbalance of blood supply to an area of tissue, with the chief result being tissue hypoxia. Ischemia can be a sudden event or a gradual occurrence from a partial or totally occluded coronary vessel or vessels. The burden of the ischemic event depends on the sensitivity of the tissue to hypoxia, the degree and duration of ischemia, and the ability of the tissue to regenerate when conditions improve (Baxter et al., 1996; Virchow, 1858).

Myocardial ischemia is a condition that results from diminished oxygen supply coupled with inadequate removal of metabolites because of reduced perfusion to the heart muscle (Boersma et al., 2003; Bolli & Marban, 1999). Pure anoxia or hypoxia, without metabolic clearance, can occur in patients with congenital heart disease, severe anemia, asphyxiation, carbon monoxide poisoning, or cor pulmonale (Feigl, 1989). Myocardial ischemia can occur as a result of reduced oxygen and nutrient *supply* or increased metabolic *demand* to meet tissue demands (Opie, 1989) (Fig. 25-1). In the presence of coronary artery occlusion, an increase in oxygen demand requirements from exercise or emotional stress can cause a transitory imbalance known as *demand ischemia*. Angina pectoris is a condition

characterized by chest pain or discomfort, which results from myocardial ischemia. Patients with chronic stable angina experience this *demand ischemia* when they exert themselves yet obtain relief with rest. An abrupt or acute reduction in blood flow to myocardium is termed *supply ischemia*. This abrupt imbalance is caused by an increase in coronary vascular tone, such as coronary vasospasm, or by a marked reduction or cessation of blood flow caused by thrombi or platelet aggregation. *Supply ischemia* is seen in patients with unstable angina or myocardial infarction (Hackam & Anand, 2003). Unstable angina is not relieved with rest. Crescendo angina, a worsening chest pain that may lead to myocardial infarction or pre-infarct angina, can develop in some patients with unstable angina (Boersma et al., 2003; Braunwald, 2000; Cohen, 1978).

The coronary arteries supply blood flow to meet the specific demands of the myocardium under varying workloads such as stress, sleep, or exercise. If oxygen needs are not met, then normal coronary arteries dilate to increase delivery of oxygenated blood to the myocardium (Feigl, 1989). Various pathologic states can affect the endothelium of the epicardial arteries impairing and impacting the normal vasomotor response of vasodilatation when myocardial demand increases. Atherosclerotic plaques are the primary cause of endothelial injury and dysfunction interfering with normal vasomotor response causing a paradoxical response of vasoconstriction (Corti et al., 2003; Davies & Thomas, 1984; Falk et al., 1995; Houston et al., 1986; Kullo et al., 1998; Lee & Libby, 1997).

The heart is an aerobic organ that relies on oxidation of substrates for maximal efficiency. The myocardium has a small margin of oxygen debt to maintain normal function. Myocardial oxygen consumption ($M\dot{V}O_2$) is a measure of the heart's total metabolism and is used to determine myocardial oxygen consumption (Braunwald, 2000). Factors that determine myocardial oxygen consumption are heart rate, contractility, systolic wall tension, and metabolic and vasomotor regulation of coronary blood flow (Bolli & Marban, 1999; Braunwald, 2000).

Heart rate has a linear relationship with myocardial oxygen consumption. The faster the heart rate, the greater the myocardial oxygen consumption. Myocardial contractility is influenced by different stimuli. Positive inotropes such as epinephrine or

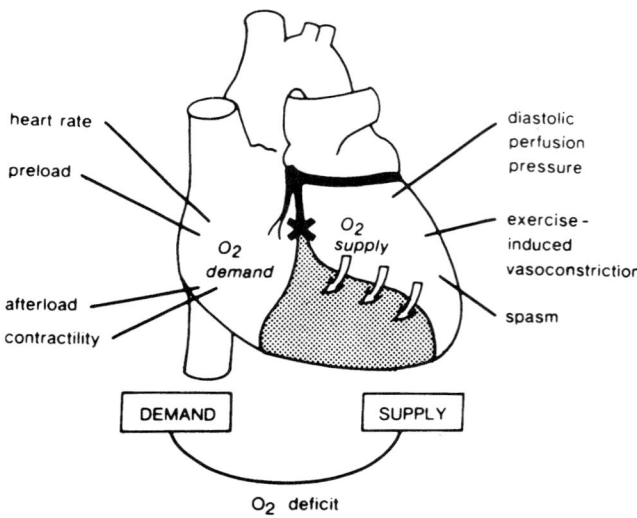

■ **Figure 25–1.** Myocardial oxygen balance. When the oxygen demand is increased, as in exercise, in the face of coronary artery disease, angina may be precipitated. When the supply is decreased abruptly, as in angina caused by coronary artery spasm or when a thrombus occludes the artery, angina at rest may be precipitated. (From Opie, L. H. [1991]. *The heart: physiology and metabolism* [p. 18]. New York: Raven Press.

dobutamine augment the contractile forces of the myocardium increasing myocardial oxygen consumption. Researchers believe the increase in MV̇O₂ may result from enhanced excitation-contraction coupling or more rapid uptake of calcium by the sarcoplasmic reticulum (Braunwald, 2000; Feigl, 1989).

Evans and Matsuoka, who concluded that a relationship exists between myocardial tension during systole and metabolism of contractile tissue, described myocardial systolic wall tension in 1915 (as cited in Braunwald, 2000). For every heart beat there is a generated ventricular tension or pressure, as measured in the area under the left ventricular curve. Refer to Chapter 1 for discussion of the Starling mechanism. Increases in myocardial tension or pressure increase myocardial oxygen consumption (Braunwald, 2000).

MECHANISMS THAT REGULATE CORONARY BLOOD FLOW

Mechanisms that determine coronary blood flow can be divided into mechanical factors and metabolic mediators. *Mechanical factors* affect blood flow by a driving force or resistance to pressure. Blood flow is directly related to the driving pressure and inversely related to the arteriolar resistance. Driving pressure, the mean arterial pressure less the central venous pressure, is influenced by volume, contractility, heart rate, and, hence, cardiac output. Any clinical state that reduces cardiac output to below the tissue's ability to compensate leads to ischemia. Examples are hypovolemia (reduction in the total vascular volume), decreased pumping efficiency of the heart, or increased vascular space secondary to systemic vasodilatation. Pumping action of the heart is decreased in the presence of ventricular arrhythmias,

heart failure, and direct trauma to the myocardium. In addition, the circular events of ischemia to the myocardium, decreased perfusion, and decreased contractility lead to decreased output. Vascular resistance is the result of obstruction of vessels, shunting of blood flow, or increased vascular resistance. Local trauma, vasoconstriction, calcific changes, or thrombus can enhance resistance. Obstruction can result from vasospastic stimuli, such as thermal changes, tissue edema, or injury leading to compression of vessels. Shunting of blood flow is the result of vasoactive substances that cause shunting, congenital malformations, or trauma to vessels. Arteriolar resistance is dependence on the effects of systemic mediators, which are locally released in response to the tissue energy, and oxygen needs.

Metabolic and vasoactive mediators influence the regulation of coronary blood flow. These metabolic mediators include adenosine, serotonin, acetylcholine, carbon dioxide, bradykinin, histamine, substance P, and prostaglandins (Feigl, 1989; Houston et al., 1986; Mombouli & Vanhoutte, 1999). Stimulation of the metabolic mediators induces arterial vasodilatation, thereby increasing coronary blood flow and subsequent increase in myocardial oxygen consumption (Feigl, 1989; Gibson et al., 2002; Mombouli & Vanhoutte, 1999). An imbalance of oxygen supply and demand of less than 1 second leads to changes in coronary vascular resistance or tone. When a coronary vessel is occluded and then released, coronary blood flow increases, causing a response called coronary reactive hyperemia (Gorlin, 1982). Metabolic mediators are released to relax vasomotor tone and improve blood flow to reestablish homeostasis. The vascular endothelium located between the vascular lumen and smooth muscle cells also release vasoactive substances that ultimately regulate vascular tone. These substances are known as prostacyclin, nitric oxide, endothelial-derived relaxing factor, and hyperpolarizing factor are potent vasodilators (Houston et al., 1986; Lee et al., 2000; Libby, 1995; Libby, 2000; Opie, 1989; Raines et al., 1989). In addition, endothelin-1 (ET-1), a potent vasoconstrictor, causes a reduction of Na⁺-/K⁺-ATPase activity. ATPases are impaired by anoxia and produce superoxides and free radicals. Thus, decreased oxygen leads to a production of superoxides and hydrogen peroxide, which are highly diffusible and induce cell damage. Early or chronic atherosclerosis and factors such as dyslipidemia, hypertension, diabetes mellitus, cigarette smoking, menopause, hyperhomocystinemia, and mutations in nitric oxide synthetase, may inhibit mediator effects and impair arterial endothelial function, causing increased permeability of blood lipids and monocytes (Libby, 1995; Libby, 2000; Mombouli & Vanhoutte, 1999; Opie, 1989; Ross, 1999). For further discussion of atherosclerosis, please refer to Chapter 7.

CAUSES OF MYOCARDIAL ISCHEMIA AND INFARCTION

The most predominant cause of myocardial ischemia is atherosclerotic plaque or atheroma disease (Fuster et al., 1992; Hackam & Anand, 2003; Lee & Libby, 1997; Libby, 2000; Ross, 1999). Atherosclerosis is a disease of the large and medium arteries, especially the aorta and arteries supplying the heart, brain, kidneys, and lower extremities (Libby, 2000).

The intima or innermost arterial layer is thickened by the development of fibrous tissue and the accumulation of lipid-forming atheromatous plaques (Lendon et al., 1991). These plaques or atheromas continue to develop and grow over the years, resulting in a narrowed arterial lumen. Blood flow through the coronary arteries is lessened, and some patients may begin to experience angina.

The degree of luminal narrowing by an atheroma has little relation to whether thrombosis will occur. Myocardial infarctions of most patients often result from atheromas of less than 50% luminal narrowing or occlusion (Davies & Thomas, 1984; Gibson et al., 2002; Jennings et al., 1990). Fissuring and disruption of atherosclerotic plaque can occur at any time during this chronic process (Falk et al., 1995; Kullo et al., 1998). The ability of the plaque to disrupt is a major factor in future ischemic events. Plaque composition, rather than the amount of narrowing, is a major determinant of the vulnerability of the plaque formation. Both mechanical and inflammatory changes affect the vulnerability of the plaque and propensity for thrombosis (Corti et al., 2003). Superimposed thrombosis on the ruptured, ulcerated plaque can impede blood flow and the delivery of nutrients to the myocardium.

Although plaque disruption and thrombosis can be separate processes, they appear to be interrelated. Thrombosis formation may be exacerbated by changes in the endothelium. Contractility, secretory, and mitogenic activities of the vessel wall all are factors that affect ischemia (Corti et al., 2003). A dysfunctional endothelium leads to the potential for thrombosis and the development of atherosclerotic lesions. Platelets migrate quickly to the site of plaque rupture and adhere. Platelet aggregation releases metabolic substances that cause vasoconstriction (Kullo et al., 1998). Thrombin formation is activated by factor XII, and the coagulation pathway results in the formation of fibrin. A fibrin mesh binds with the platelets and leads to formation of a clot (Boersma et al., 2003; Davies & Thomas, 1984; Fuster et al., 1992; Fuster et al., 1992; Ross, 1999).

The role of inflammation in weakening and disrupting the collagen matrix within the atherosclerotic plaque has been clearly established (Lee & Libby, 1997; Lee et al., 2000). Lipoproteins contribute to loss of smooth muscle cells through apoptosis (programmed cell death) (Dispersyn & Borgers, 2001; Isner et al., 1995). Metalloproteinases (MMP) activate macrophages that break-down collagen, thus weakening the atherosclerotic fibrous cap and making it prone to rupture (Dollery et al., 1995). Infectious agents have been associated in the development of coronary artery disease. *Chlamydia pneumoniae* and *Mycoplasma pneumoniae* have been implicated in the proliferation of inflammation and plaque instability (Higuchi & Ramires, 2002).

Biomarkers of vascular inflammation have been associated with the atherothrombogenic process. Several investigations have shown a positive relationship between high-sensitivity C-reactive protein, serum amyloid A, interleukin (IL)-6, fibrinogen, homocysteine, lipoprotein A, plasma protein A (pregnancy-associated), and the risk of acute coronary events (Higuchi & Ramires, 2002; Houston et al., 1986; Ishikawa et al., 2003; Klein et al., 1968; Nijmeijer et al., 2003; Pearson et al., 2003). For further discussion of these emerging inflammatory biomarkers for coronary heart disease, refer to Chapter 6.

Coronary artery spasm is a less common cause of ischemia (Gorlin, 1982). Ventricular hypertrophy from long-standing hypertension, valvular heart disease, or cardiomyopathy can cause ischemia because of increased left ventricular wall tension or pressure compressing the epicardial arteries (Bolli & Marban, 1999; Pfeffer, 1995). Embolic occlusion of the coronary arteries can impede blood flow to a tissue area. Cocaine and amphetamines cause ischemia because of increases in myocardial oxygen demand and may cause coronary artery spasm (Klein et al., 1968; Nademanee et al., 1989). Inflammation of the epicardial arteries from infectious diseases can impair blood flow to the myocardium.

Low blood pressure causing decreased blood return can lead to imbalances of oxygen supply and demand. Examples are hypotension or hypovolemia. Increased oxygen demand is caused by conditions such as hyperthyroidism, anemia, or hyperviscosity of the blood.

RISK FACTORS FOR CORONARY ARTERY DISEASE

Cardiac risk factors have been identified that precipitate and exacerbate the development of coronary artery disease (Dankner et al., 2003; Hackam & Anand, 2003; Pearson et al., 2003). Some modifiable risk factors can be altered to decrease one's risk of cardiovascular disease. These factors include hyperlipidemia, hypertriglyceridemia, hypertension, and cigarette smoking. Other modifiable risk factors include diabetes mellitus type 2, obesity, sedentary lifestyle, and ovarian hormone therapy. These factors remain controversial in the role of contributing to coronary artery disease. Non-modifiable risk factors are variables that cannot be altered and include age, being male and younger than age 70, genetic predisposition, and diabetes mellitus type 1. Nontraditional emerging risk factors include hyperhomocystinemia, hypoalphalipoproteinemia, high lipoprotein A, and high iron levels. Refer to Chapter 36 for a complete overview of coronary risk factors.

INCIDENCE OF MYOCARDIAL ISCHEMIA

The incidence of myocardial ischemia is difficult to ascertain because patients may have silent ischemia. Ischemic heart disease parallels that of coronary heart disease, with approximately 1 in 5 deaths per year (Braunwald, 2000; Braunwald et al., 2000). More than 16 million Americans had a history of myocardial infarction or experienced angina pectoris in 2000 (Boersma et al., 2003). Approximately every 1 minute, an American dies from a coronary event. In developed countries, the number of coronary events parallels the number of coronary events in the United States.

Racial and gender variations exist in the incidence, prevalence, presentations, and treatment responses (Dankner et al., 2003; Hackam & Anand, 2003). Blacks have higher morbidity and mortality rates from myocardial ischemia. They also have a higher incidence of hypertension, obesity, and metabolic syndrome. Their access to medical care often is delayed after a coronary event. Indian-Asians have twice the incidence of coronary heart disease than whites in the United States. Asians tend to have higher levels of lipoprotein A. People of Mediterranean descent have a much lower incidence of ischemic heart disease. The incidence of ischemic heart disease is equal in men and postmenopausal women. Older adults experience higher mortality and morbidity from ischemic heart disease and have more complications from multiple therapeutic interventions.

Cellular Mechanisms and Events Caused by Myocardial Ischemia

Myocardial ischemia develops if blood flow containing oxygen-rich nutrients is insufficient in meeting metabolic demands of the myocardial cells. Consequences of myocardial ischemia are depicted in Figure 25-2. Oxygen deprivation of the tissues caused by diminished blood flow can cause ischemia within 10 seconds (Libby, 1995). Myocardial oxygen reserves are used within 8 seconds. Myocardial function and contractility become profoundly depressed within 1 minute. The myocardium shifts from aerobic metabolism to anaerobic metabolism through the glycolic pathway. Glycolysis can supply only 65% to 70% of the total myocardial energy requirement. Anaerobic glycolysis will generate some ATP but is insufficient in maintaining homeostasis of myocardial cells. Phosphate production is markedly reduced. Intracellular hydrogen ions and lactic acid accumulate. Within a few minutes, ultrastructural changes can be seen, including cell swelling and depletion of glycolic stores. The combination of hypoxia, reduced energy reserves, and acidosis further hampers left ventricular function (Fuster et al., 1992). Myocardial cells remain viable for at least 20 minutes. After 20 minutes, irreversible injury begins to occur (Jennings et al., 1990). The actual events leading to cell death are unknown (Dispersyn & Borgers, 2001; Isner et al., 1995). It has been postulated that calcium overload may be a contributing factor because of the activation of various proteases and phospholipases (Libby, 1995; Libby, 2000). The integrity of the sarcoplasmic membrane is damaged by these enzymes, leading to eventual cell death. ATPases are impaired by anoxia, which results in the production of superoxides and hydrogen peroxide, both of which are highly diffusible and induce cell damage (Asano et al., 2003). In addition, oxidative stress causes a repertoire of cellular defenses to emerge. Ischemia can lead to endogenous antioxidant factors to modulate injury by enzymatic pathways of cellular signals, which may determine the outcome of injury (Marczin et al., 2003). For example, mitogen-activated protein kinase (MAPK) and nuclear factor (NF)-kappa B inhibit injury and signal intercellular adhesion molecule (ICAM-1) to mediate injury (Kaur et al., 2003; Squadrito et al., 2003).

Ischemic preconditioning, which refers to a state in which tissue is rendered resistant to deleterious prolonged ischemia and reperfusion before exposure of vascular occlusion, may be critical in determining the extent of injury that myocardial cells can sustain. Activation of adenosine receptors and protein kinase is essential to this preconditioning. A cascade of events including postischemic leukocyte rolling, which leads to adhesion and emigration, is dependent on expression

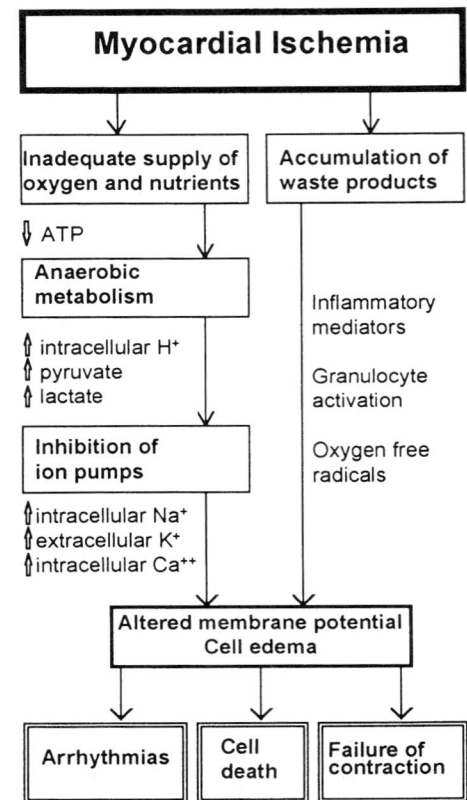

■ **Figure 25–2.** Consequences of ischemia.

of p-selectin on venular endothelium (Kubes et al., 1998). Another factor affecting endothelium may be the reduction in L-arginine availability, which has been identified with impairment of endothelium-dependent, nitric–oxide-mediated vasodilation by ischemia–reperfusion (Hein et al., 2003). Down-regulation of endothelial nitric oxide synthase may lead to the inability of arginase blockage or L-argine supplementation to completely restore vasodilatory function. In addition, activation of peroxisome proliferatory-activated receptor alpha, which regulates genes of myocardial fatty acid oxidation, may exhibit cardioprotection through metabolic mechanisms (Yue et al., 2003).

Restoration of oxygenated blood to the previously ischemic myocardium is called reperfusion (Braunwald & Kloner, 1985; Opie, 1989). Occlusion of coronary blood vessel followed by sudden release is called coronary reactive hyperemia (Kloner, 1993). Reperfusion of a tissue bed results in reversal of ischemia but also releases toxic free radicals and an overabundance of calcium. Although reperfusion is absolutely necessary to restoring cellular homeostasis, there are also detrimental effects that can result (Jennings et al., 1990). Myocardial stunning is a diminished contractile state in the non-infarcted myocardium from excess production of free radicals (Bolli & Marban, 1999; Fuster et al., 1992). Reperfusion arrhythmias are observed and are believed to be caused by fatally damaged myocardial cells by the previous ischemic event.

The hemodynamic effects of myocardial ischemia are reduced contractility and abnormal wall motion in the area of ischemia. Changes in wall compliance and stiffness are affected, thereby reducing cardiac output and stroke volume. Because of reduced emptying of the left ventricle, pressures within the heart become elevated. Pulmonary artery wedge pressure and left ventricular end diastolic pressure rise. Sympathetic compensatory mechanisms respond to the decreased myocardial function. Blood pressure and heart rate increase. A decreased blood pressure indicates a large area of myocardial ischemia or vasovagal response (Boersma et al., 2003).

The electrocardiographic findings with myocardial ischemia result from cellular changes. These changes may be reflected as ST-segment depression or T-wave inversion. Two conditions, Prinzmetal angina resulting from coronary artery spasm and pericarditis, are associated with ST-segment elevation. Refer to Chapter 18 for electrocardiographic examples of ischemic changes.

Clinical Manifestations of Myocardial Ischemia

Angina pectoris is the clinical description of chest pain or pressure that results from myocardial ischemia. Some patients describe a sensation of heaviness, tightness, or pressure to severe, clutching, grip-like pain. The pain or discomfort may be localized or radiate to the shoulder, neck, jaw, or right or left arms. Associated symptoms include lightheadedness, dyspnea, diaphoresis, and fatigue. Anginal pain is probably caused by extracellular accumulation of substances in the area of ischemia (Kullo et al., 1998). These substances include adenosine, potassium, lactic acid, and bradykinin. Abnormal stretching of the myocardium irritates afferent nerve fibers of the heart. Afferent nerve fibers that enter the spinal column from levels C3 to T4 account for the variety of locations and radiation patterns (Feigl, 1998).

There are three types of angina, including stable angina, unstable angina, and Prinzmetal angina (Braunwald et al., 2000). Stable angina is a condition in which there is chronic stable stenosis of one or more coronary arteries that are inefficient in supplying oxygenated during exertional or emotional stress. When the patient rests, the anginal pain resolves. Unstable angina is a condition characterized by pain that is not relieved with rest. This pain often indicates that there is an acute thrombosis of a coronary artery. Prinzmetal angina is a condition caused by vasospasm of one or more coronary arteries. It can occur at night during sleep and has a cyclical pattern to its occurrence. This condition may result from overstimulation of the sympathetic nervous system, increased flux of calcium in arterial smooth muscle cells, or impaired function of thromboxane or prostaglandins (Houston et al., 1986; Lee et al., 2000).

INCIDENCE OF MYOCARDIAL INFARCTION

Acute myocardial infarction is the leading cause of morbidity and mortality of women and men in the United States. There are 1.3 million reports of patients who experience non-fatal myocardial infarctions each year. For every 100,000 people,

there are at least 600 people who experience a coronary event (Braunwald & Kloner, 1985).

Approximately 500,000 to 700,000 deaths occur from coronary artery disease per year in the United States. More than half these deaths occur in the field or pre-hospital setting because of delay and access to medical treatment. Ten percent of patients die within the hospital setting. Another 10% of patients die within the first year after infarct (Dankner et al., 2003).

Myocardial infarction usually occurs in patients older than 45 years. Certain subpopulations of patients are at risk for myocardial ischemia and infarction, including insulin-dependent diabetic patients, cocaine and amphetamine users, and patients with hypercholesterolemia or a positive family history of early-onset (45 years old or younger) coronary artery disease.

The American College of Cardiology criteria for myocardial infarction are a typical rise and gradual fall of troponin or a rapid rise and fall of creatine kinase-MB, with at least one of the following: symptoms of ischemia, development of pathological Q-waves on the electrocardiogram (ECG), electrocardiographic changes of ST elevation or depression (Antman et al., 1996; Brogan et al., 1996; Pearson et al., 2003). In addition, patients qualify under the definition of myocardial infarction if they have any pathological findings of myocardial necrosis.

Cellular Mechanisms and Events Caused by Myocardial Infarction

Prolonged ischemia of more than 30 minutes will cause irreversible cellular damage of the myocardium and is termed myocardial infarction (Boersma et al., 2003; Jennings et al., 1990). Sudden occlusion of a coronary artery leads to an ischemic zone with potentially viable tissue that surrounds this zone. The size of this ischemic zone and the degree of blood flow within the area depends on the anatomy of the coronary circulation and the area of occlusion within the blood vessel. Collateral vessels, which form anastomoses or connections between major coronary branches, develop in some patients with long-standing atherosclerosis (Cohen, 1978). When a coronary branch is occluded, pressure changes occur in neighboring arteries that cause rapid recruitment of these collateral vessels to minimize this infarct zone. Ischemia is a major stimulus for angiogene, the growth of new capillaries (Lee et al., 2000). This revascularization occurs mainly by sprouting or intussusception. Many cytokines stimulate endothelial and smooth muscle cell proliferation with the migration or recruitment of activated monocytes (Falk et al., 1995). Once coronary blood flow is interrupted and the delivery of nutrients to the myocardium is blocked, the area of myocardium becomes depressed and hypokinetic. Gradually irreversible cardiac myocyte death occurs within the ischemic zone, leading to necrosis. The endocardial region is the first area of tissue that dies, followed by the mid-myocardium or subendocardium. If the ischemia persists, then eventually the infarct will be transmural, the full thickness of the myocardium. Loss of functional myocardium results in reduced left ventricular function affecting the patient's quality of life and morbidity and mortality (Pierard, 2003).

The development of infarction is a cascade of events including the migration and infiltration of leukocytes, release of metabolic mediators, cytokines, growth factors, and activation of coagulation and complement systems. Cellular edema and inflammatory response ensue (Libby, 2000). Myocardial necrosis activates the complement system, releases free radicals, triggers a cytokine cascade and chemokine upregulation, releasing IL-8, C5a, proteolytic enzymes, and adhesion molecules (Houston et al., 1986; Raines et al., 1989). Monocyte chemoattractant protein-1 may regulate mononuclear cell recruitment with accumulation of monocyte-derived macrophages, mast cells, growth factors, and fibroblasts (Libby, 2000). ET-1, IL-1 beta, and tumor necrosis factor (TNF) are a few of the inflammatory factors elevated with ischemia (Namiki et al., 2003). See Chapter 6 for further discussion of the inflammatory changes.

The cascade of inflammatory events along with angiogenesis and matrix MMPs may regulate extracellular matrix deposition and mediate ventricular remodeling (Jugdutt, 2003; Lee & Libby, 1997; Lee et al., 2000; Pfeffer, 1995). The inflammatory mediators lead to recruitment of blood-derived primitive stem cells, which differentiate into endothelial cells and lead to some myocardial regeneration (Ren et al., 2003). Certain MMPs are elevated in the blood of patients prone to rupture of atherosclerotic plaques (Ferroni et al., 2003).

In addition, the myocardial cells release catecholamines, placing the patient at risk for atrial and ventricular arrhythmias and heart failure. Catecholamines mediate the release of glycogen and glucose from the body's cell storage. Within 1 hour after a myocardial infarction, there is a rise in levels of free fatty acids and glycerol (Klein et al., 1968). Norepinephrine stimulates liver and skeletal muscle cells, elevating blood glucose levels and suppressing insulin production. The infarcted area is further complicated by coronary vasoconstriction and thrombi embolization. Cardiac myocyte cell death may activate the production of free radicals that plug the coronary capillaries causing the "no flow" phenomenon (Dispersyn & Borgers, 2001; Isner et al., 1995). The location of the infarction correlates with disease in a particular area of the coronary circulation. For example, disease in the proximal left anterior descending artery may cause wall motion abnormalities in the anterior or anterior-septal walls of the myocardium. Other common designated infarct areas include inferior, lateral, posterior, or septal sites.

Reperfusion of the infarcted area is necessary to alter the necrotic process. Re-establishment of coronary blood flow can be achieved by thrombolytics or catheter-based procedures (Gibson et al., 2002). Streptokinase, anistreplase, and tissue plasminogen activator are fibrinolytic agents that act as "clot busters" (Gershlick & More, 1998). Percutaneous coronary interventions are performed to place a wire across the blocked or stenosed coronary artery and inflate a balloon within the stenotic portion of the artery. This procedure is called percutaneous transluminal coronary angioplasty or PTCA. More often, a stent is placed in the coronary artery to ensure effective coronary artery blood flow to the myocardium. Some patients may have spontaneous reperfusion when a thrombus disperses naturally. See Chapter 27 for details outlining these interventional cardiology procedures. If patients are not amenable to these interventions, then they may undergo surgical revascularization with coronary artery bypass surgery (Chapter 29).

Evolution of Myocardial Infarction and Postinfarct Remodeling

The immediate and long-term consequences of acute myocardial infarction are determined by the size of the infarct zone and position of the infarct (Baxter et al., 1996; Galcera-Tomas et al., 2001). A large myocardial infarct, more than 40% damage of the myocardium, can cause markedly reduced left ventricular failure and circulatory failure. Cardiogenic shock will eventually occur if blood perfusion to the myocardium is not restored. The infarcted segment undergoes a series of changes during the process of healing and wound repair. Some of these changes can pose further risks to the patients. Initially, the infarct area is bruised and cyanotic from lack of nutrients and blood flow. Cardiac enzymes are released from the cells and can be detected in the blood stream (Libby, 2000). These biochemical markers of cellular injury include creatinine kinase (CK) and creatinine kinase-MB (CK-MB), which are the cardiac muscle enzymes sometimes present in skeletal muscle. They increase within 4 to 6 hours of cellular injury, peak in 18 to 24 hours, and last approximately 2 to 3 days (Brogan et al., 1996). The cardiac-specific troponins are regulatory proteins that control the calcium-mediated interaction of actin and myosin. Cardiac-specific troponin T (cTnT) and cardiac-specific troponin I (cTnI) elevate 4 to 6 hours after cellular injury, peak at 18 to 24 hours, and persist for at least 10 days (Antman et al., 1996). In addition, cardiotrophin-1 (CT-1), a member of the IL-6 family of cytokines, is elevated in ischemic heart disease and thought to have a role in post-MI wound healing. Occasionally, elevated troponins are seen in chronic dialysis patients and post-cardiac bypass patients (McDonough et al., 2001).

Biomarkers of myocardial injury can be measured and are discussed in Chapters 6 and 14. One of the most promising biomarkers is C-reactive protein, manufactured in the liver, which increases during inflammatory response to tissue injury (Ishikawa et al., 2003). Research is underway to determine if elevated levels of C-reactive protein are related to plaque instability and predictable of restenosis after percutaneous coronary intervention (Gibson et al., 2002; Hackam & Anand, 2003).

By the second or third day after myocardial infarction, leukocytes infiltrate the necrotic area and scavenger neutrophils release proteolytic enzymes to break down the necrotic tissue. The necrotic wall is very thin during this phase. Cardiac rupture can occur at any time after an infarction but most commonly within this first week. Rupture of the myocardial wall causes massive hemorrhage into the pericardial space, resulting in cardiac tamponade and pump failure. In the second week of the repair process, insulin secretion increases to mobilize glucose from the wound repairs. The initial phase of the collagen matrix is weak and vulnerable to re-injury (Libby, 2000). By the third week, scar formation has begun.

Postinfarct remodeling of the non-infarcted myocardium also begins (Pfeffer, 1995). The surviving myocytes hypertrophy because they cannot divide to make up for the loss of pump function of the dead myocytes. Fibrous connective tissue replaces necrotic tissue. There may be excessive deposition of collagen in the hypertrophied myocardium. Collagen is not a contractile protein and fibrosis may lead to a stiff or noncompliant ventricle and impaired contractility of the surviving myocardium. Current research has focused on early MMP activation and decreasing extracellular matrix (ECM) degradation (Dollery et al., 1995). After 6 weeks, the necrotic area is completely replaced by scar tissue, which is strong but ineffective in contributing to overall contractility of the myocardium. Myocardial infarction can result in abnormal wall motion abnormality, decreased myocardial function, reduced stroke volume, diminished ejection fraction, elevated ventricular filling pressures, and sinoatrial node dysfunction.

The degree of left ventricular functional impairment after a myocardial infarction depends on the size and location of the infarct, function of non-infarcted myocardium, collateral circulation, and compensatory mechanisms (Galcera-Tomas et al., 2001). These compensatory mechanisms operate to optimize cardiac output and peripheral perfusion. Impairment of left ventricular function with subsequent decreased cardiac output activates arterial vasoconstriction, which increases vascular resistance and mean arterial pressure. Venoconstriction increases venous return to the heart and ventricular filling. Higher diastolic filling pressures are necessary to maintain adequate stroke volume to a point. Increased ventricular pressure and volume stretches myocardial fibers to increase the force of contraction, according to the Starling law. Aldosterone is released to stimulate renal retention of sodium and water, thereby further increasing circulatory filling pressures. The depressed myocardium develops temporary left ventricular enlargement caused by cardiac dilatation from these compensatory mechanisms attempting to sustain cardiac output.

The hemodynamic effects of a myocardial infarction depend on the extensiveness and location of myocardial damage and restoration of coronary blood flow (Baxter et al., 1996; Boersma et al., 2003; Galcera-Tomas et al., 2001; Gershlick & More, 1998; Pfeffer, 1995; Pierard, 2003). Heart rate may be normal or borderline normal with mild myocardial depression. Tachycardia is observed in some patients with more extensive myocardial damage and is considered a poor clinical correlate. Blood pressure may be hypertensive in the initial phases of a myocardial ischemia. As myocardial depression worsens, hypotension ensues. Reflex sympathetic stimulation increases heart rate and contractility. Conversely, inferior wall myocardial infarctions may stimulate parasympathetic response of reduced heart rate and blood pressure, further compromising the depressed myocardium. As myocardial function worsens, contractility is reduced, wall compliance is altered, stroke volume is reduced, filling pressures including left ventricular end-systolic and end-diastolic volumes are elevated, resulting in pulmonary edema and circulatory failure. If the cycle is not reversed with restoration of coronary blood flow, then cardiogenic shock, cardiac rupture, and death ensue.

Clinical Manifestations of Myocardial Infarction

Acute myocardial infarction or acute coronary syndrome may present with a sudden onset of severe chest, jaw, back, or arm pain or pressure. The pain is described as heavy, crushing, and like a tight squeeze or elephant on the chest. Sometimes the pain will radiate to the shoulder, neck, and jaw and may be associated with symptoms of fatigue, lightheadedness, nausea, shortness of breath, or diaphoresis. At least 40% to 50% of individuals do not experience pain, especially in diabetic individuals or older adults (Fuster et al., 1992; Fuster et al., 1992). Some patients may have unrelenting gastric distress. Peripheral vasoconstriction may cause cool, clammy skin. Sometimes a low-grade fever may result from the inflammatory response within the myocardium.

The extent of complications after a myocardial infarction depends on the location and extent of necrosis and ischemia, the physiologic status of the patient before the event, and timing and availability of therapeutic interventions. Myocardial infarction can occur in the various regions of the heart muscle. An ECG is used in the diagnosis to localize the affected area. The zone of infarction and necrosis is surrounded the zone of hypoxia, which is surrounded by the zone of ischemia. Infarcted tissue is electrically silent and is not reflected on the ECG. Transmural infarctions reflect as a Q wave on the ECG in the region of infarction. Nontransmural or non-Q (zone of hypoxia) wave infarctions do not reflect a Q wave. Injured and ischemic tissues (zone of ischemia) are reflected as ST-segment depression or T-wave inversions, or as nonspecific ST-T wave changes. Refer to Chapter 18 for electrocardiographic examples of myocardial infarction.

IMPLICATIONS FOR NURSES

Acute coronary syndrome addresses both myocardial ischemia and myocardial infarction. Myocardial ischemia is a condition that results from reduced supply of oxygen and nutrients to the myocardium or increased demand of the myocardium for oxygen and nutrients. Myocardial infarction is a condition that results from an interruption in the normal coronary blood flow to the myocardium. Changes occur within seconds in the myocardium if ischemia persists, including shifting from aerobic metabolism to anaerobic metabolism through the glycolic pathway. Cell death occurs after 20 minutes if coronary blood flow is not restored. Nurses play a very important role in identifying patients through careful history taking and identifying early signs and symptoms of ischemia. Early intervention of establishing and restoring coronary blood flow will salvage myocardium and save the patient short-term and long-term postinfarction complications. Nurses can help patients identify risk factors that can be modified and promote positive outcomes and responses to lead healthy and productive lives.

REFERENCES

Antman, E.M., Tanasijevic, M. J., Thompson, B., Schactman, M., McCabe, C. H., Cannon, C. P., Fischer, G. A., Fung, A. Y., Thompson, C., Wybenga, D., & Braunwald, E. (1996). Cardiac-specific troponin I levels to predict the risk of mortality in patients with acute coronary syndromes. *New England Journal of Medicine,* 335(18), 1342–1349.

Asano, G., Takashi, E., Ishiwata, T., Onda, M., Yokoyama, M., Naito, Z., Ashraf, M., & Sugisaki, Y. (2003). Pathogenesis and protection of ischemia and reperfusion injury in myocardium. *Journal of the Nippon Medical School,* 70(5), 384–392.

Baxter, G. F., Sumeray, M. S., & Walker, J. M. (1996). Infarct size and magnesium: insights into LIMIT-2 and ISIS-4 from experimental studies. *Lancet,* 348(9039), 1424–1426.

Boersma, E., Mercado, N., Poldermans, D., Gardien, M., Vos, J., & Simoons, M. L. (2003). Acute myocardial infarction. *Lancet,* 361(9360), 847–858.

Bolli, R., & Marban, E. (1999). Molecular and cellular mechanisms of myocardial stunning. *Physiology Review,* 79(2), 609–634.

Braunwald, E. (2000). 50th anniversary historical article. Myocardial oxygen consumption: the quest for its determinants and some clinical fallout. *Journal of the American College of Cardiology,* 35(5 Suppl B), 45B–48B.

Braunwald, E., & Kloner, R. A. (1985). Myocardial reperfusion: a double-edged sword? *Journal of Clinical Investigation,* 76(5), 1713–1719.

Braunwald, E., Antman, E. M., Beasley, J. W., Califf, R. M., Cheitlin, M. D., Hochman, J. S., Jones, R. H., Kereiakes, D., Kupersmith, J., Levin, T. N., Pepine, C. J., Schaeffer, J. W., Smith, E. E., 3rd, Steward, D. E., Theroux, P., Alpert, J. S., Eagle, K. A., Faxon, D. P., Fuster, V., Gardner, T. J., Gregoratos, G., Russell, R. O., & Smith, S. C., Jr. (2000). ACC/AHA guidelines for the management of patients with unstable angina and non-ST-segment elevation myocardial infarction. A report of the American College of Cardiology/American Heart Association Task Force on Practice Guidelines (Committee on the Management of Patients With Unstable Angina). *Journal of the American College of Cardiology,* 36(3), 970–1062.

Brogan, G. X., Jr., Vuori, J., Friedman, S., McCuskey, C. F., Thode, H. C., Jr., Vaananen, H. K., Cooling, D. S., & Bock, J. L. (1996). Improved specificity of myoglobin plus carbonic anhydrase assay versus that of creatine kinase-MB for early diagnosis of acute myocardial infarction. *Annals of Emergency Medicine,* 27(1), 22–28.

Cohen, M. V. (1978). The functional value of coronary collaterals in myocardial ischemia and therapeutic approach to enhance collateral flow. *American Heart Journal,* 95(3), 396–404.

Corti, R., Fuster, V., & Badimon, J. J. (2003). Pathogenetic concepts of acute coronary syndromes. *Journal of the American College of Cardiology,* 41(4 Suppl S), 7S–14S.

Dankner, R., Goldbourt, U., Boyko, V., & Reicher-Reiss, H. (2003). Predictors of cardiac and noncardiac mortality among 14,697 patients with coronary heart disease. *American Journal of Cardiology,* 91(2), 121–127.

Davies, M. J., & Thomas, A. (1984). Thrombosis and acute coronary-artery lesions in sudden cardiac ischemic death. *New England Journal of Medicine,* 310(18), 1137–1140.

Dispersyn, G. D., & Borgers, M. (2001). Apoptosis in the heart: about programmed cell death and survival. *News in Physiological Science,* 16, 41–47.

Dollery, C. M., McEwan, J. R., & Henney, A. M. (1995). Matrix metalloproteinases and cardiovascular disease. *Circulation Research,* 77(5), 863–868.

Falk, E., Shah, P. K., & Fuster, V. (1995). Coronary plaque disruption. *Circulation,* 92(3), 657–671.

Feigl, E. O. (1989). Coronary autoregulation. *Journal of Hypertension (Suppl),* 7(4), S55–S58; discussion S59.

Feigl, E.O. (1998). Neural control of coronary blood flow. *Journal of Vascular Research,* 35(2), 85–92.

Ferroni, P., Basili, S., Martini, F., Cardarello, C. M., Ceci, F., Di Franco, M., Bertazzoni, G., Gazzaniga, P. P., & Alessandri, C. (2003). Serum metalloproteinase 9 levels in patients with coronary artery disease: a novel marker of inflammation. *Journal of Investigational Medicine,* 51(5), 295–300.

Fuster, V., Badimon, L., Badimon, J. J., & Chesebro, J. H. (1992). The pathogenesis of coronary artery disease and the acute coronary syndromes (2). *New England Journal of Medicine,* 326(5), 310–318.

Fuster, V., Badimon, L., Badimon, J. J., & Chesebro, J. H. (1992). The pathogenesis of coronary artery disease and the acute coronary syndromes (1). *New England Journal of Medicine,* 326(4), 242–250.

Galcera-Tomas, J., Castillo-Soria, F. J., Villegas-Garcia, M. M., Florenciano-Sanchez, R., Sanchez-Villanueva, J. G., de La Rosa, J. A., Martinez-Caballero, A., Valenti-Aldeguer, J. A., Jara-Perez, P., Parraga-Ramirez, M., Lopez-Martinez, I., Inigo-Garcia, L., & Pico-Aracil, F. (2001). Effects of early use of atenolol or captopril on infarct size and ventricular volume: A double-blind comparison in patients with anterior acute myocardial infarction. *Circulation,* 103(6), 813–819.

Gershlick, A. H., & More, R. S. (1998). Treatment of myocardial infarction. *BMJ,* 316(7127), 280–284.

Gibson, C. M., Dotani, M. I., Murphy, S. A., Marble, S. J., Dauterman, K. W., Michaels, A. D., & Dodge, J. T., Jr. (2002). Correlates of coronary blood flow before and after percutaneous coronary intervention and their relationship to angiographic and clinical outcomes in the RESTORE trial. Randomized Efficacy Study of Tirofiban for Outcomes and REstenosis. *American Heart Journal,* 144(1), 130–135.

Gorlin, R. (1982). Role of coronary vasospasm in the pathogenesis of myocardial ischemia and angina pectoris. *American Heart Journal,* 103(4 Pt 2), 598–603.

Hackam, D. G., & Anand, S. S. (2003). Emerging risk factors for atherosclerotic vascular disease: a critical review of the evidence. *JAMA,* 290(7), 932–940.

Hein, T. W., Zhang, C., Wang, W., Chang, C. I., Thengchaisri, N., & Kuo, L. (2003). Ischemia-reperfusion selectively impairs nitric oxide-mediated dilation in coronary arterioles: counteracting role of arginase. *FASEB Journal,* 17(15), 2328–2330.

Higuchi Mde, L., & Ramires, J. A. (2002). Infectious agents in coronary atheromas: a possible role in the pathogenesis of plaque rupture and acute myocardial infarction. *Revista do Instituto de Medicina Tropical de Sao Paolo,* 44(4), 217–224.

Houston, D. S., Shepherd, J. T., & Vanhoutte, P. M. (1986). Aggregating human platelets cause direct contraction and endothelium-dependent relaxation of isolated canine coronary arteries. Role of serotonin, thromboxane A2, and adenine nucleotides. *Journal of Clinical Investigation,* 78(2), 539–544.

Ishikawa, T., Hatakeyama, K., Imamura, T., Date, H., Shibata, Y., Hikichi, Y., Asada, Y., & Eto, T. (2003). Involvement of C-reactive protein obtained by directional coronary atherectomy in plaque instability and developing restenosis in patients with stable or unstable angina pectoris. *American Journal of Cardiology,* 91(3), 287–292.

Isner, J. M., Kearney, M., Bortman, S., & Passeri, J. (1995). Apoptosis in human atherosclerosis and restenosis. *Circulation,* 91(11), 2703–2711.

Jennings, R. B., Murry, C. E., Steenbergen, C., Jr., & Reimer, K. A. (1990). Development of cell injury in sustained acute ischemia. *Circulation,* 82(3 Suppl.), II2–II12.

Jugdutt, B. I. (2003). Ventricular remodeling after infarction and the extracellular collagen matrix: when is enough enough? *Circulation,* 108(11), 1395–1403.

Kaur, J., Woodman, R. C., & Kubes, P. (2003). P38 MAPK: critical molecule in thrombin-induced NF-kappa B-dependent leukocyte recruitment. *American Journal of Physiology Heart Circulation Physiology,* 284(4), H1095–H1103.

Klein, R. F., Troyer, W. G., Thompson, H. K., Bogdonoff, M. D., & Wallace, A. G. (1968). Catecholamine excretion in myocardial infarction. *Archives of Internal Medicine,* 122(6), 476–482.

Kloner, R. A. (1993). Does reperfusion injury exist in humans? *Journal of the American College of Cardiology,* 21(2), 537–545.

Kubes, P., Payne, D., & Ostrovsky, L. (1998). Preconditioning and adenosine in I/R-induced leukocyte-endothelial cell interactions. *American Journal of Physiology,* 274(4 Pt 2), H1230–H1238.

Kullo, I. J., Edwards, W. D., & Schwartz, R. S. (1998). Vulnerable plaque: pathobiology and clinical implications. *Annals of Internal Medicine,* 129(12), 1050–1060.

Lee, R. T., & Libby, P. (1997). The unstable atheroma. *Arteriosclerosis Thrombosis Vascular Biology,* 17(10), 1859–1867.

Lee, S. H., Wolf, P. L., Escudero, R., Deutsch, R., Jamieson, S. W., & Thistlethwaite, P. A. (2000). Early expression of angiogenesis factors in acute myocardial ischemia and infarction. *New England Journal of Medicine,* 342(9), 626–633.

Lendon, C. L., Davies, M. J., Born, G. V., & Richardson, P. D. (1991). Atherosclerotic plaque caps are locally weakened when macrophages density is increased. *Atherosclerosis,* 87(1), 87–90.

Libby, P. (1995). Molecular bases of the acute coronary syndromes. *Circulation,* 91(11), 2844–2850.

Libby, P. (2000). Changing concepts of atherogenesis. *Journal of Internal Medicine,* 247(3), 349–358.

Marczin, N., El-Habashi, N., Hoare, G. S., Bundy, R. E., & Yacoub, M. (2003). Antioxidants in myocardial ischemia-reperfusion injury: therapeutic potential and basic mechanisms. *Archives of Biochemistry and Biophysiology,* 420(2), 222–236.

McDonough, J. L., Labugger, R., Pickett, W., Tse, M. Y., MacKenzie, S., Pang, S. C., Atar, D., Ropchan, G., & Van Eyk, J. E. (2001). Cardiac troponin I is modified in the myocardium of bypass patients. *Circulation,* 103(1), 58–64.

Mombouli, J. V., & Vanhoutte, P. M. (1999). Endothelial dysfunction: from physiology to therapy. *Journal of Molecular and Cellular Cardiology,* 31(1), 61–74.

Nademanee, K., Gorelick, D. A., Josephson, M. A., Ryan, M. A., Wilkins, J. N., Robertson, H. A., Mody, F. V., & Intarachot, V. (1989). Myocardial ischemia during cocaine withdrawal. *Annals of Internal Medicine,* 111(11), 876–880.

Namiki, A., Kubota, T., Fukazawa, M., Ishikawa, M., Moroi, M., Aikawa, J., Ebine, K., & Yamaguchi, T. (2003). Endothelin-1 concentrations in pericardial fluid are more elevated in patients with ischemic heart disease than in patients with nonischemic heart disease. *Japanese Heart Journal,* 44(5), 633–644.

Nijmeijer, R., Lagrand, W. K., Lubbers, Y. T., Visser, C. A., Meijer, C. J., Niessen, H. W., & Hack, C. E. (2003). C-reactive protein activates complement in infarcted human myocardium. *American Journal of Patholgy,* 163(1), 269–275.

Opie, L. H. (1989). Reperfusion injury and its pharmacologic modification. *Circulation,* 80(4), 1049–1062.

Pearson, T. A., Mensah, G. A., Alexander, R. W., Anderson, J. L., Cannon, R. O., 3rd, Criqui, M., Fadl, Y. Y., Fortmann, S. P., Hong, Y., Myers, G. L., Rifai, N., Smith, S. C., Jr., Taubert, K., Tracy, R. P., & Vinicor, F. (2003). Markers of inflammation and cardiovascular disease: application to clinical and public health practice: A statement for healthcare professionals from the Centers for Disease Control and Prevention and the American Heart Association. *Circulation,* 107(3), 499–511.

Pfeffer, M. A. (1995). Left ventricular remodeling after acute myocardial infarction. *Annual Review of Medicine,* 46, 455–466.

Pierard, L. A. (2003). Assessing perfusion and function in acute myocardial infarction: how and when? *Heart,* 89(7), 701–703.

Raines, E. W., Dower, S. K., & Ross, R. (1989). Interleukin-1 mitogenic activity for fibroblasts and smooth muscle cells is due to PDGF-AA. *Science,* 243(4889), 393–396.

Ren, G., Dewald, O., & Frangogiannis, N. G. (2003). Inflammatory mechanisms in myocardial infarction. *Current Drug Targets Inflammation Allergy,* 2(3), 242–256.

Ross, R. (1999). Atherosclerosis–an inflammatory disease. *New England Journal of Medicine, 340*(2), 115–126.

Squadrito, F., Deodato, B., Squadrito, G., Seminara, P., Passaniti, M., Venuti, F. S., Giacca, M., Minutoli, L., Adamo, E. B., Bellomo, M., Marini, R., Galeano, M., Marini, H., & Altavilla, D. (2003). Gene transfer of IkappaBalpha limits infarct size in a mouse model of myocardial ischemia-reperfusion injury. *Laboratory Investiation,* 83(8), 1097–1104.

Virchow, R. (1858). *Cellular pathology.* London: John Churchill.

Yue, T. L., Bao, W., Jucker, B. M., Gu, J. L., Romanic, A. M., Brown, P. J., Cui, J., Thudium, D. T., Boyce, R., Burns-Kurtis, C. L., Mirabile, R. C., Aravindhan, K., & Ohlstein, E. H. (2003). Activation of peroxisome proliferator-activated receptor-alpha protects the heart from ischemia/reperfusion injury. *Circulation,* 108(19), 2393–2399.

Acute Coronary Syndromes

SHERRI DEL BENE AND ANNE VAUGHAN*

In the year 2000, the prevalence of coronary heart disease in the United States was 12,900,000, and there were 1,100,000 new and recurrent cases of myocardial infarction (MI) and 515,204 deaths (American Heart Association, 2003). The acute coronary syndromes (ACS) include a spectrum of atherosclerotic, vasospastic, and thrombotic conditions that cause myocardial ischemia. These conditions range from unstable angina (UA) and non-Q wave to Q wave MI. In UA, a thrombus may partially occlude the coronary artery resulting in episodes of coronary occlusion interspersed with reperfusion. ST-segment depression and T-wave inversion on the electrocardiogram (ECG) are common. Chest pain may be intermittent and occur at rest and may become progressively more frequent and persistent. Complete occlusion of the coronary artery, seen as ST elevation on the 12-lead ECG, leads to cell death and Q wave MI. Early reperfusion has emerged as the primary treatment modality for selected patients with acute MI.

ANGINA PECTORIS

Myocardial oxygen demand is increased by exercise, emotional stress, smoking tobacco, eating heavy meals, and exposure to cold weather or extreme humidity (Shub, Click & McGoon, 1996). As long as coronary vasodilation increases blood supply, this extra demand can be met. Coronary atherosclerosis causes progressive, fixed narrowing of the arterial lumen and stenosis, which prevents the affected arteries from dilating in response to an increase in myocardial oxygen demand, which may result in myocardial ischemia. Vasospasm may also cause myocardial ischemia. Ischemia is reversible, but, if myocardial blood flow is not increased or myocardial oxygen demands are not reduced, the ischemia can progress to cell death (i.e., MI; Fig. 26-1).

Stable (Classic) Angina

Angina pectoris, literally "a strangling of the chest" is a clinical syndrome characterized by transient episodes of substernal chest pain or discomfort caused by myocardial ischemia. It may be

accompanied by arm, jaw, back or neck pain, dyspnea, nausea, vomiting, and/or diaphoresis, and it usually occurs in predictable patterns. Chronic, stable angina is the most common manifestation of ischemic heart disease (IHD) and is the initial manifestation of IHD in approximately 50% of patients (Gibbons et al., 1999). Anginal pain is usually aggravated by physical exertion or emotional stress and is relieved by rest and/or nitrates. If relief is not obtained, it may indicate that myocardial ischemia is progressing to infarction.

Anginal equivalents are characterized by a sensation of dyspnea, excessive fatigue or weakness, or isolated arm or jaw pain, without experiencing chest discomfort as the major manifestation of cardiac ischemia. The elderly are likely to experience the anginal equivalents already described or may experience palpitations, excessive sweating, dizziness, or syncope as the major manifestations of angina (Olson & Aronow, 1996). Myocardial ischemia can also occur without angina or equivalents and is referred to as *silent ischemia,* which also tends to occur more frequently in the older population.

History

Angina is a subjective symptom that usually lasts 2 to 5 minutes if the precipitating factor is relieved. It can occasionally last 5 to 15 minutes, and up to 30 minutes. Angina is commonly described as a sensation of substernal heaviness, tightness, squeezing, pressing, or burning. A person may clench his or her fist over the sternum when describing the discomfort (Levine's sign). A circumscribed painful area smaller than the size of a fingertip usually does not indicate myocardial ischemia. Typically, angina occurs in people with coronary artery disease (CAD) involving one or more coronary arteries, although it can also occur in people with valvular heart disease, hypertrophic cardiomyopathy, or uncontrolled hypertension (Gibbons et al., 1999).

Stable angina occurs during physical exertion, usually at a defined exercise level, and is relieved by rest or nitroglycerin. Occasionally, a patient may experience a second-wind phenomenon, characterized by discomfort that develops during exertion but disappears while the activity is continued. In the early morning, angina may be precipitated by a level of activity that would not produce angina later in the day.

Angina may result from eating a heavy meal because of increased gastrointestinal (GI) oxygen demand. Smoking tobacco

---

*The section on Thrombolytics was updated from the fourth edition work of Michaelene Deelstra.

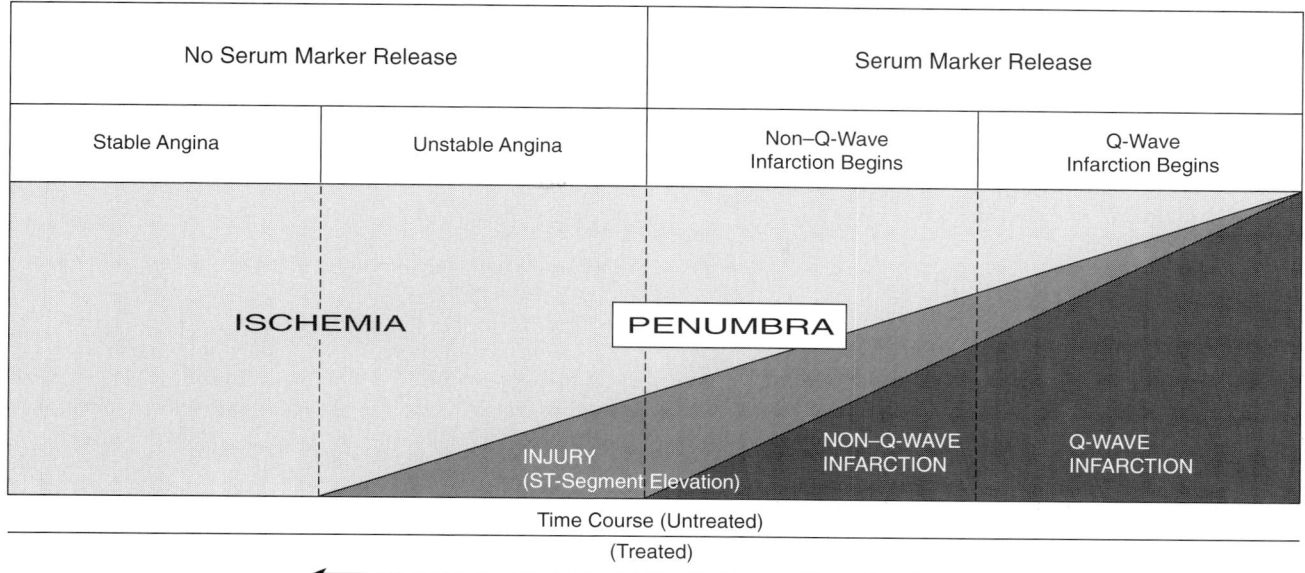

No Serum Marker Release		Serum Marker Release	
Stable Angina	Unstable Angina	Non–Q-Wave Infarction Begins	Q-Wave Infarction Begins

ISCHEMIA   PENUMBRA

INJURY (ST-Segment Elevation)

NON–Q-WAVE INFARCTION

Q-WAVE INFARCTION

Time Course (Untreated)

(Treated)

■ **Figure 26–1.** Schematic drawing showing the overlapping relationships of the acute coronary syndromes. The areas of ischemia and injury represent compromised but salvageable tissue in zones of reduced blood flow. In this zone, called the *penumbra*, the blood supply is inadequate to maintain normal myocardial functions. The penumbra is viable up to several hours from the primary onset of artial occlusion. The myocardium in the penumbra dies (infarcts) if not salvaged by reperfusion strategies such as thrombolytic agents or angioplasty. (From Cummins, R. O., Field, J. & Hazinski, M. [2001]. Acute coronary syndromes: Patients with acute ischemic chest pain. In *Advanced cardiac life support.* Dallas: American Heart Association.)

may result in angina by increasing myocardial work from the release of endogenous catecholamines, or by causing coronary artery spasm.

Emotional tension is a frequent precursor of angina. Catecholamine release increases heart rate and systemic BP, thereby increasing the work of the heart. Chest discomfort from emotional stress tends to persist longer than that produced by physical stress, probably because emotions are not as easily controlled or abated as activity (Shub et al., 1996).

Stable angina is often relieved by rest. Nitroglycerin also often relieves angina, and relief by nitroglycerin may help in diagnosing the cause of chest pain. However, these features alone are not sufficient for diagnosis because chest pain caused by esophageal spasm may also be relieved by nitroglycerin.

Risk Factors

There are multiple known risk factors for developing IHD. Age is the single most important with a fourteenfold increased risk in patients over 70 years of age (Selwyn & Braunwald, 2001). Other common risk factors include hyperlipidemia, hypertension, diabetes, obesity, and cigarette smoking. Hyperlipidemia adds to the development of atherosclerosis and ischemic syndromes. Hypertension that is not well controlled, and the left ventricular (LV) hypertrophy that can result from sustained hypertension, can aggravate ischemia. Diabetes mellitus accelerates coronary and peripheral atherosclerosis, as does cigarette smoking. Obesity increases the risk of coronary events by increasing the work of the heart, oxygen consumption, and predisposing a person to hypertension and impaired glucose toler-

ance. Heavy alcohol use is known to increase triglyceride levels and systolic BP, and also may ultimately impair LV function.

Although the pathophysiology is not clearly understood at this time, hyperhomocysteinemia appears to have toxic effects on the vascular endothelium. Homocysteine is both prothrombotic and atherogenic. An elevated homocysteine level is an independent risk factor for CAD (Bozkurt et al., 2002).

The risk for adverse outcomes in IHD is increased two to three times in patients whose troponin I level is elevated, regardless of when the level was obtained related to the cardiac event (Pepine, 2000).

Physical Assessment

A generalized physical assessment in the patient with stable angina is likely to be normal, although it may provide some signs of risk factors associated with coronary atherosclerosis. The presence of xanthomas, for example, especially in a young client, may indicate the presence of hypercholesterolemia. Systemic hypertension is known to accelerate the development of atherosclerosis. Carotid or femoral bruits may indicate diffuse atherosclerosis. The skin should be inspected for nicotine stains on the fingertips, as well as diabetic skin lesions. Auscultation may reveal a third or fourth heart sound, or the murmur of mitral regurgitation.

Physical examination may also aid in excluding some diagnoses from the list of differential diagnoses for IHD, which includes aortic stenosis, aortic regurgitation, pulmonary hypertension, and hypertrophic cardiomyopathy.

During an anginal event, the patient may exhibit pallor; cold, clammy skin; an increased heart rate; and pulsus alternans. Systemic BP may be elevated at the onset of the event. Myocardial ischemia can cause transient LV failure, producing a third or fourth heart sound. The murmur of mitral regurgitation secondary to papillary muscle ischemia might also appear during an event. The presence of any of these findings may assist the examiner in making the diagnosis of IHD.

Diagnostic Testing

Laboratory Testing

There are some basic laboratory tests that may aid in the diagnosis of IHD. Blood tests should include an evaluation of lipids, glucose, creatinine, and hematocrit. Urine should also be examined for ketones and glucose. Primarily, these tests will serve to assess kidney function, because renal disease can accelerate atherosclerosis. They also provide information about lipids and metabolic syndrome (Kastelein et al., 2000).

Electrocardiogram (ECG)

The ECG remains a standard diagnostic test for patients with angina, as recommended by the 2001 Advanced Cardiac Life Support guidelines (Cummins et al., 2001). Possible abnormal findings include pathologic Q waves, indicative of prior MI; ST-T abnormalities, indicative of ischemia; and conduction abnormalities, such as AV block or bundle-branch blocks (Shub et al., 1996). However, these findings are not specific for IHD. For example, ST-T abnormalities can also be seen in mitral valve prolapse, another common cause of chest pain. An ECG that shows ST-T abnormalities during an episode of chest pain can be extremely helpful in diagnosing angina due either to IHD or coronary spasm. ST-segment depression of at least 1 mm is evidence of ischemia and does occur during most anginal events, although ST elevation may be seen in Prinzmetal's angina (Selwyn & Braunwald, 2001). T-wave flattening or inversion is a more nonspecific diagnostic finding (Chapter 18). In approximately half the patients with chronic, stable angina, the resting ECG will be normal. Ambulatory ECG monitoring (Holter monitoring) can also be used to aid in diagnosing ischemia or IHD and may be particularly helpful in patients who have pain only at rest or are suspected of having silent ischemia (Schroeder, 1996).

Stress Testing

In the patient with a normal ECG, who is not taking digoxin, the exercise ECG, or stress test, is the next diagnostic tool used to determine whether the patient has IHD. The purpose of the stress test is to increase cardiac workload under direct observation and controlled conditions, using a treadmill or stationary bike, with the patient's ECG and blood pressure (BP) monitored before, during, and after the test. The variables assessed include ST-segment and T-wave changes, heart rate and BP response, and the presence or absence of arrhythmias and anginal symptoms (Shub et al., 1996; see Chapter 21). For patients unable to exercise due to obesity, chronic obstructive pulmonary disease (COPD), degenerative joint disease, or deconditioning, pharmacologic stress testing can be carried out with intravenous (IV) infusions of dipyridamole, adenosine, or dobutamine. Each of these medications increases the work of the heart, thereby increasing myocardial oxygen demand, while the patient remains stationary.

Cardiac Imaging

Cardiac imaging techniques are described in detail in Chapters 15, 16, and 17.

Chest radiographs are usually the initial imaging tests obtained in patients with suspected IHD. Radiography is of limited value in the diagnosis of IHD, but is of great value in excluding other potential causes of chest pain such as pneumonia, pneumothorax, or congestive heart failure (CHF; see Chapter 15).

Radionuclides such as thallium-201 or technetium-99m sestamibi can be used in association with exercise or pharmacologic stress testing to detect myocardial perfusion defects. The radionuclide is injected IV during maximal stress. Its distribution in the myocardium is proportional to myocardial blood flow. These examinations are highly sensitive and accurate, especially when evaluating ischemic areas in a heart with resting LV abnormalities. Thallium or sestamibi *single-photon emission computed tomography* (SPECT) provides a multiplanar evaluation of myocardial perfusion and may reveal areas of stress-induced ischemia. When this information is combined with the hemodynamic and ECG data, it offers a more complete evaluation of the patient (see Chapter 17).

Positron emission tomography (PET) may also be used to differentiate ischemic from infarcted myocardium. Cardiac PET uses radiolabeled glucose, which may provide more specific information about myocardial viability than thallium or sestamibi. PET has the significant disadvantages of very high cost and very limited availability.

Two-dimensional echocardiography can be used to detect transient or permanent segmental ventricular wall motion abnormalities or reduced ejection fractions associated with IHD. It may also detect areas of myocardial thinning from old MI, ventricular aneurysms, or valvular heart disease that may contribute to angina. Stress (induced by exercise or pharmacologically) echocardiography can detect the presence of akinesis or dyskinesis not visible or present at rest. Stress echocardiography has the advantages of higher sensitivity than stress ECG, and has higher specificity and is more readily available than radionuclide perfusion imaging (Selwyn & Braunwald, 2001; see Chapter 16).

Cardiovascular magnetic resonance imaging/angiography (Cardiac MRI/MRA) is a promising emerging noninvasive technology that may eventually replace conventional coronary angiography. Whereas cardiac MRI is gaining fairly widespread application in the assessment of wall motion and contractility in patients with nondiagnostic echocardiograms, cardiac MRA remains in the development phase, and is primarily a research application (Nagel et al., 2003).

Coronary Angiography

Coronary angiography is both the most accurate and the most invasive procedure to diagnose obstructive coronary atherosclerosis as well as other nonatherosclerotic possible causes of stable angina, such as coronary artery spasm. Coronary angiography is indicated to confirm or exclude the diagnosis of CAD when noninvasive tests have been equivocal, when disabling angina has been unresponsive to medical therapy, in UA, postinfarction angina, recurrent angina at rest, or with ischemia accompanied by an S₃ gallop or definite ECG changes, as well as in patients who are being considered for revascularization (Gibbons et al., 1999). In many centers, angiography offers the significant advantage of endovascular intervention (angioplasty, stenting), which may help to avoid surgery in selected cases.

Complications may occur with coronary angiography. Ventricular dysrhythmias are the most common and are usually easily treated, as is hematoma formation at the puncture site. Allergic reactions to the contrast are uncommon and are usually easily avoided by premedicating patients with known iodine allergy. Aortic rupture is an infrequent complication. These complications and the nursing care associated with coronary angiography are discussed in Chapter 22.

Prognosis

The most important determinants of outcome are the severity of LV dysfunction and the extent of myocardial ischemia. The presence of hypertension, resting ECG abnormalities, marked ST-segment changes during an anginal episode, cardiomegaly, and three-vessel or left main disease are indicators of adverse prognosis in the patient with angina. Patients with normal LV function and coronary arteries who have chest discomfort have an excellent prognosis. Elevations of cardiac troponins T or I are also prognostic indicators in patients with acute coronary syndrome. Troponin T, specifically, is a sensitive marker of underlying pathology and aids in identifying patients most likely to benefit from therapy (Pepine, 2000) (see Chap. 14).

Treatment

The goals of therapy in managing chronic, stable angina are to prolong survival, reduce disease progression, alleviate symptoms, and decrease the risk of MI. Treatment is based on increasing myocardial oxygen supply or decreasing myocardial oxygen demand. Lifestyle adjustment may be necessary in most patients with angina. This adjustment may include an individually prescribed exercise program, a decrease in dietary intake of cholesterol and saturated fats, smoking cessation, control of hypertension, weight reduction, and stress management. Other medical conditions that may exacerbate angina, such as anemia or COPD, may also warrant treatment. Medical conditions that may cause angina, such as aortic valve disease or hypertrophic cardiomyopathy, should also be treated. Hypertension and diabetes mellitus must be well managed, because both contribute to coronary atherosclerosis.

Medical management is the initial treatment for most patients with chronic, stable angina. Treatment may include the nonpharmacologic interventions mentioned previously, and the use of one or more medications, including nitrates, beta blockers, or calcium antagonists (presented later in this chapter). If medical therapy is unsuccessful, myocardial revascularization may be necessary.

Table 26–1 ■ CANADIAN CARDIOVASCULAR SOCIETY CLASSIFICATION FOR ANGINA PECTORIS

Class I	- Ordinary physical activity (such as walking or climbing stairs) does not cause angina. Angina may occur with strenuous, rapid, or prolonged exertion (work or recreation).
Class II	- There is slight limitation of ordinary activity. Angina may occur with walking or climbing stairs rapidly; walking uphill; walking or stair-climbing after meals, or in the cold, or in the wind, or under emotional stress; walking more than two blocks on the level and climbing one flight of stairs at a normal pace under normal conditions.
Class III	- There is marked limitation of ordinary physical activity. Angina may occur after walking one or two blocks on the level, or climbing one flight of stairs in normal conditions at a normal pace.
Class IV	- There is inability to carry on any physical activity without discomfort; angina may be present at rest.

From Canadian Cardiovascular Society classification for angina pectoris. Courtesy of the Canadian Cardiovascular Society. Shub, C., Click, P. L., & McGoon, M. D. (1996). *Myocardial ischemia clinical syndromes. Mayo Clinic practice of cardiology* (3rd ed.). St. Louis: Mosby.

Myocardial Revascularization

Revascularization procedures include percutaneous transluminal coronary angioplasty and/or stenting (PTCA), and coronary artery bypass grafting (CABG). Stable or UA with a positive exercise test is an indication for PTCA. The primary goal of PTCA (Chapter 27) is to increase blood flow to ischemic areas by dilating coronary artery stenoses. The long-term efficacy of balloon angioplasty in patients with chronic IHD is well documented (Juergens, Whitbourn, Yeung & Oesterle, 1997). However, the long-term efficacy in patients with multivessel disease remains controversial and continues to be studied.

Intracoronary stenting during PTCA can be used to dilate lesions resistant to balloon angioplasty. It involves insertion of a wire mesh stent that holds open the stenotic segment.

CABG is the most widely accepted treatment for patients with severe anginal symptoms unrelieved by medical therapy, although its role remains controversial in stable angina (see Chap. 29). It is primarily indicated for patients with left main CAD, three-vessel disease with LV dysfunction, worsening angina, or disabling symptoms (Gibbons et al., 1999) The more severe the heart disease, the greater the survival advantage of CABG over PTCA (Petticrew, Turner-Boutle & Sheldon, 1997). Potential complications of CABG include bleeding, failure of the bypass graft, and graft stenosis. Potential complications of PTCA and intracoronary stenting include acute vessel occlusion, groin hematomas, and progressive restenosis of the stented or angioplastied segment.

(See Table 26-1 for Canadian Cardiovascular Society Classification for Angina Pectoris.)

Unstable Angina and Non–ST-segment Elevation Myocardial Infarction

UA and non–ST-segment elevation MI are acute coronary syndromes, usually resulting from luminal narrowing due to rupture of an atherosclerotic plaque, which partially thromboses

Table 26–2 ■ CLASSIFICATION OF UNSTABLE ANGINA

Severity	A—Develops in the Presence of Extracardiac Condition That Intensifies Myocardial Ischemia (Secondary UA)	B—Develops in the Absence of Extracardiac Condition (Primary UA)	C—Develops Within 2 Weeks of AMI
I—New onset of severe angina or accelerated angina (no rest pain)	IA	IB	IC
II—Angina at rest within past month, but not within past 48 hours (angina at rest, subacute)	IIA	IIB	IIC
III—Angina at rest within past 48 hours (angina at rest, acute)	IIIA	IIIB-T$_{neg}$ IIIB-T$_{pos}$	IIIC

UA = unstable angina; AMI = acute myocardial infarction; T$_{neg}$ = troponin negative; T$_{pos}$ = troponin positive.
From Hamm, C. W. & Braunwald, E. (2000). A classification of unstable angina revisited. *Circulation*, 102, 120.

a coronary artery. UA is defined as (1) new onset angina that is severe or frequent (three or more times per day), (2) angina that is becoming more severe (in frequency, duration, or precipitated by less activity than usual), or (3) patients with angina at rest (Hamm & Braunwald, 2000; Table 26-2).

The 2000 American College of Cardiology (ACC)/American Heart Association (AHA) Guidelines (Braunwald et al., 2000) state that UA and non–ST-segment elevation myocardial infarction (NSTEMI) have similar pathogenesis and clinical presentations, but differ in severity. Initially, the severity of injury is determined by the amount of detectable quantities of myocar-

dial injury markers (i.e., cardiac troponins T [cTnT] and I [cTnI], and creatinine phosphokinase, muscle bands isoenzyme [CKMB]). If no serum biochemical marker is present, the patient with ACS is diagnosed with UA, whereas the patient who has myocardial injury markers present is diagnosed with NSTEMI (see Chapter 14). Patients with chest pain can be stratified into low- or high-risk categories for myocardial ischemia on the basis of history and laboratory findings (Table 26-3).

A 12-lead ECG is obtained immediately, along with a medical history and physical examination to allow the clinician to establish risk and select the level of care (intensive care versus

Table 26–3 ■ SHORT-TERM RISK OF DEATH OR NONFATAL MI IN PATIENTS WITH UNSTABLE ANGINA

Feature	High Risk (At least one of the following features must be present)	Intermediate Risk (No high-risk feature, but must have one of the following features)	Low Risk (No high- or intermediate-risk feature, but may have any of the following features)
History	Accelerating tempo of ischemic symptoms in preceding 48 h	Prior MI, peripheral or cerebrovascular disease or CABG; aspirin use	New onset CCS class III or IV angina in the past 2 weeks with moderate or high likelihood of CAD
Character of pain	Prolonged (>20 min) ongoing rest pain	Prolonged (>20 min) rest angina, now resolved, with moderate or high likelihood of CAD Rest angina, <20 min or relieved by rest of SL NTG	
Clinical findings	Pulmonary edema, most likely related to ischemia New/worsening MR murmur S$_3$ or new/worsening rales Hypotension, bradycardia, tachycardia Age >75 years	Age >70 years	
ECG findings	Angina at rest with transient ST-segment changes >0.05 mV Bundle-branch block, new or presumed new Sustained ventricular tachycardia	T-wave inversion >0.2mV Pathologic Q waves	Normal or unchanged ECG during an episode of chest discomfort
Cardiac markers	Markedly elevated (e.g., TnT or TnI >0.1 ng/mL)	Slightly elevated (e.g., TnT >0.01 but <0.1 ng/mL)	Normal

An estimation of the short-term risks of death and nonfatal cardiac ischemic events in UA is a complex multivariable problem that cannot be fully specified in a table such as this. Therefore, the table is meant to offer general guidance and illustration rather than rigid algorithms.
TnT = troponin T; TnI = troponin I; MI = myocardial infarction; CABG = coronary artery bypass graft; SL = sublingual; NTG = nitroglycerin; CCS = Canadian Cardiovascular Society; CAD = coronary artery disease; ECG = electrocardiogram.
From Braunwald, E., Antman, E. M., Beasley, J. W., et al. (2000). ACC/AHA guidelines for the management of patients with unstable angina and non ST segment elevation myocardial infarction: Executive summary and recommendations. *Circulation*, 102, 1195.

stepdown versus observation area) and therapy. The patient should also be placed on bed rest with continuous ECG monitoring because sudden ventricular fibrillation is the major preventable cause of death in the early period (Braunwald et al., 2000). Correction of reversible precipitating factors (e.g., hypertension, anemia, heart failure) is imperative.

Treatment

Once the physician has assigned the patient a diagnosis, if there are no further symptoms for 12 to 24 hours and the patient falls into the low-risk category, he or she may be scheduled for a stress ECG. If symptoms persist, or if there is a change in the ECG, or if cardiac markers are present, then the patient will remain on bed rest, with continuous ECG monitoring, and will be given supplemental oxygen and nitroglycerin (sublingually until IV is available). Morphine sulphate may be administered if the discomfort is still unrelieved or if there is acute pulmonary congestion. An IV beta blocker may be added if chest pain continues. If ischemia persists and beta blockers are contraindicated, a nondihydropyridine calcium antagonist can be given IV (unless contraindicated, as in LV failure). If hypertension persists despite nitroglycerin and beta blocker therapy in patients with LV dysfunction or CHF, an angiotensin-converting enzyme (ACE) inhibitor is the treatment of choice. ACE inhibitors are also recommended for diabetics (Braunwald et al., 2000).

The 2001 Advanced Cardiac Life Support Guidelines (Cummins et al., 2001) recommend that antiplatelet therapy also be initiated, beginning with aspirin, unless the patient experiences or has a history of GI intolerance or hypersensitivity, in which case, a thienopyridine (clopidogrel, ticlopidine) would be administered. There is more recent evidence to suggest, however, that clopidogrel significantly reduces risk of MI in both high- and low-risk patient groups, and suggests its use as opposed to aspirin (Cannon, 2002). Parenteral anticoagulation therapy with unfractionated heparin (UFH) or subcutaneous low-molecular-weight-heparin (LMWH) will also be administered at this point. Although the current guidelines call for the use of either UFH or LMWH, the latter has recently become more widely used because research has shown it to be at least equal to, and in some cases superior to UFH (Ibbotson & Goa, 2002).

Cardiac catheterization may also be considered after symptoms are controlled because there is a high prevalence of left main and three-vessel CAD in patients with UA. If either is demonstrated by cardiac catheterization, PTCA, stenting, or CABG is indicated.

Investigational Procedures

Procedures under investigation include laser angioplasty, transmyocardial revascularization (TMR) and percutaneous transmyocardial revascularization (PTMR). Laser angioplasty is under investigation as adjunctive therapy to PTCA and CABG. It involves the use of a laser to vaporize coronary obstruction during CABG or PTCA and can be used to treat in-stent restenosis. TMR is being researched as a treatment for medically refractory angina that is not amenable to the current established treatment methods. In TMR, a high-powered carbon dioxide laser is used to create transmural channels that directly perfuse the ischemic

myocardium, leading to the creation of new blood vessels (Ballard, Wood & Lansing, 1997). PTMR is also under investigation, one of the differences being that, in PTMR, channels are created on the inner surface of the ventricle. Both the latter procedures are treatment options for patients with chronic class III or IV angina for whom repeat CABG or PTCA is not feasible due to their unsuitable coronary anatomy (Dudek, 1999).

Variant Angina (Prinzmetal's Angina)

Variant angina, a less common form of angina, is characterized by episodes of chest pain that occur at rest. This discomfort tends to be prolonged, severe, and not readily relieved by nitroglycerin. Variant angina is caused by spasm of the coronary arteries and can be accompanied by transient elevation of the ST segment. The *transient* multilead ST-segment elevation recorded during an episode of variant angina should not be confused with the ST-segment elevation recorded in the acute phase of MI.

Recommendations for Variant Angina

Patients with variant (Prinzmetal's) angina usually require hospitalization and intense medical therapy, initially. Both nitrates and calcium antagonists are effective in controlling symptoms, although calcium antagonists are sometimes more successful. If symptoms are not controlled adequately with these medications, beta-adrenergic blocking agents may be beneficial. The response to beta blockers is variable because blockade of the beta-2 receptors may allow unopposed alpha-receptor-mediated coronary vasoconstriction (Shub et al., 1996). Surgery and PTCA usually are not indicated in patients with isolated coronary artery spasm unless it occurs in conjunction with marked coronary atherosclerosis (Selwyn & Braunwald, 2001).

Nursing Management

Nursing care in the acute situation should be aimed toward minimizing or eliminating myocardial ischemia and preventing progression to infarction. This includes administering supplemental oxygen, administering the prescribed medications in the appropriate routes (nitrates, beta blockers, GP IIb/IIIa inhibitors), and caring for the patient before and after procedures. The nurse also must aid in reducing the patient's anxiety related to the anginal episode.

In the chronic situation, nurses must assist the patient and family to identify lifestyle changes to reduce or eliminate angina. Sudden bursts of activity should be avoided, particularly after prolonged rest periods, because they may precipitate an anginal episode, although a mild to moderate exercise regimen may be prescribed. Patients should be educated in ways to control emotional reactions to stressful situations by way of biofeedback or relaxation therapy. Paradoxically, sexual activity may be encouraged, perhaps with prophylactic use of sublingual nitroglycerin (Riegel, Thomason & Carlson, 1997).

Patients should be instructed in the importance of adhering to the prescribed medication regimen to minimize pain and myocardial damage. The proper use of sublingual nitroglycerin should be stressed. The patient should be taught to recognize symptoms of worsening ischemia, and instructed to seek prompt medical assistance if indicated.

MYOCARDIAL INFARCTION

Acute MI occurs as a result of thrombotic occlusion of the coronary artery and causes irreversible cell injury and necrosis. Chest pain is associated with MI in a majority of cases. The pain of an acute MI is severe and typically lasts longer than 30 minutes. The diagnosis of acute MI is based on patient history, the presence of characteristic ECG changes on the 12-lead ECG, and serial markers of myocardial necrosis (Gibler, 1998). Mortality from an MI is the greatest within the first 24 to 48 hours after onset of symptoms. Early diagnosis and treatment of MI with reperfusion therapies, such as thrombolytics and primary angioplasty, are critical to preserve myocardial function and prevent complications.

Classification

Classification of MI is based on the location of the infarction and the layers of the heart involved. Because the three major branches of the coronary arteries almost always supply the regions of the left ventricle that have the greatest oxygen need, most MI involve the left ventricle. Coronary occlusions that also jeopardize perfusion of other cardiac structures, such as the right ventricle and AV node, may cause more extensive damage and conduction abnormalities such as heart block, ventricular tachycardia (VT), or atrial fibrillation. LV infarctions are typically classified as anterior, inferior, and posterior or lateral based on the site of tissue damage. MI may involve the subendocardial layer of the heart (non Q-wave MI) or may involve all layers of the heart (Q wave MI). Heart failure may result when large areas of the myocardium are damaged.

Anterior Myocardial Infarction

Anterior MI result from the occlusion of the left anterior descending coronary artery (LAD). The LAD supplies blood to the anterior wall of the left ventricle and the anterior two thirds of the intraventricular septum. Complications of an anterior MI include severe LV dysfunction resulting in CHF and cardiogenic shock. Occlusion of the LAD may also produce variable degrees of AV or fascicular heart block resulting from infarction of the intraventricular septum. Sinus tachycardia is a common finding and may be related to a neurohormonal sympathetic response to reduced cardiac output or BP.

Inferior and Posterior Myocardial Infarction

Inferior and posterior MI occurs from the occlusion of the right coronary artery (RCA) that supplies these regions of the heart in 80% to 90% of patients. In the remaining 10% to 20% of patients, inferior and posterior MI result from the occlusion of the left circumflex artery. The extent of LV damage ranges from apical diaphragmatic to posterobasal involvement. Sinus node block and atrial arrhythmias may develop. Varying degrees of heart block, especially second-degree AV block type I, are common as is hypotension. These symptoms are usually transient and related to heightened parasympathetic nervous system activity. Other symptoms of parasympathetic activity, such as hiccoughing, nausea, vomiting, and an urge to defecate, are seen frequently in the patient with an inferior or posterior MI.

Lateral Myocardial Infarction

Lateral MI results from the occlusion of coronary branches supplying the lateral wall of the left ventricle. These branches include the left circumflex branch of the left coronary artery, the diagonal branches of the LAD, and the terminal branches of the RCA. Because the left circumflex artery supplies the AV junction, the His bundle, and anterior and posterior papillary muscles in 10% of the population, its occlusion may be associated with conduction abnormalities or with mitral valve insufficiency due to papillary muscle dysfunction.

Right Ventricular Myocardial Infarction

Although right ventricular (RV) MI occurs chiefly in correlation with an inferior MI, it has important clinical features and consequences that are distinct from an LV infarction. One third to one half of inferior MIs are complicated by RV infarction (Bueno et al., 1997). Concomitant RV infarction is associated with greater risk of complications and higher mortality than the presence of inferior MI alone (Kinch & Ryan, 1994) . When RV infarction is present in patients with inferior MI, their in-hospital mortality may reach 31% compared with 6% of patients with inferior MI alone (p<0.001; Kinch & Ryan, 1994). Elderly patients with RV MI are at higher risk of major complications, including cardiogenic shock, mechanical complications, and complete AV block compared to elderly patients without RV MI (Bueno et al., 1997). In most cases, RV MI results from an occlusion of the RCA proximal to the acute marginal branches (Isner & Roberts, 1978). However, in patients with left dominant coronary circulation, isolated RV infarct results from the occlusion of the nondominant right coronary artery (Kinch & Ryan, 1994).

Q-Wave and Non–Q-Wave Myocardial Infarction

Damage to the heart occurs in a continuum that progresses from the subendocardium to the epicardium. The subendocardium is particularly vulnerable to changes in LV dynamics. As the damage approaches the full thickness of the myocardium, Q waves appear on the 12-lead ECG. Q wave MI results from a thrombus that occludes the coronary artery for a prolonged period. A non–Q-wave MI occurs when a thrombus, rich in platelets, partially occludes the coronary vessel. A thrombus that intermittently occludes the coronary artery may cause subendocardial necrosis and a non–Q-wave MI. Non–Q-wave MI may be associated with nondiagnostic ECG changes such as ST-segment depression and T-wave abnormalities. Forty percent of patients who develop an MI present with ST-segment depression, T-wave abnormalities, or other nonspecific ECG changes (Ryan et al., 1996a). Q-wave MI are associated with higher in-hospital mortality and may result in signs and symptoms of heart failure, mural thrombi, and pericarditis. However, people with non–Q-wave MI frequently experience recurrent ischemia, MI, and death in the weeks and months after discharge (Berger et al., 1992). Indeed, the cumulative mortality after non–Q-wave MI is comparable to that of Q-wave MI after 2 years (Rogers, 1995).

Diagnosis

The diagnosis of acute MI is based on the patient's clinical presentation, history, serial ECG, and cardiac specific enzyme changes indicative of myocardial necrosis. The diagnosis of acute MI is confirmed by cardiac enzyme changes and reinforced by the clinical presentation of persistent chest pain and ST-segment elevation in patients with Q-wave MI and ST-segment depression and T-wave inversion in patients with non–Q-wave MI.

History

The presence of chest pain is a hallmark symptom in the diagnosis of acute MI. Ninety-nine percent of patients in The Myocardial Infarction Triage and Intervention (MITI) Registry presented with chest pain initially, although, by the time of hospital admission, 78% of women were experiencing chest pain compared with 84% of men (Kudenchuk et al., 1996). The pain may resemble classic angina pectoris but occurs at rest or with less than usual activity or at rest (Antman & Braunwald, 2001a, b). Typically, the pain is severe and prolonged and may be described as crushing, constricting, or oppressive. The pain may radiate down the ulnar aspect of the left arm. The pain may also radiate into the neck, jaw, and interscapular region. Pain may occur in the epigastric region and may simulate GI disorders. Chest discomfort may be associated with indigestion, nausea and vomiting, diaphoresis, palpitations, or dyspnea. Some patients, however, may not experience chest pain. In a sample of patients enrolled in the National Registry of Myocardial Infarction 2, 30% of subjects diagnosed as having acute MI did not experience chest pain. In this study, patients without chest pain tended to be over 75 years of age and to be female. Patients without chest pain also had an increased incidence of diabetes, hypertension, prior heart failure, and stroke (Canto et al., 2000). Patients who do not present with chest pain may present with "angina equivalent" symptoms such as dyspnea, palpitations, or arrhythmias. Women with acute MI may present with jaw and back pain, nausea and vomiting, and dyspnea (DeVon & Zerwic, 2002). Older patients more often experience symptoms of stroke, confusion, and syncope with acute MI (Gibler, 1998).

Physical Assessment

The patient experiencing acute MI may appear pale, anxious, and in distress. Cold perspiration may be present on the skin. Depending on the degree of LV dysfunction and sympathetic stimulation, the patient may be cool and clammy to the touch. The patient may exhibit a productive cough with pink, frothy, or blood-tinged sputum. An S_3 gallop may be present as well as crackles in the lower lung fields, indicating LV failure. An S_4 heart sound may also be present and indicates decreased LV compliance. In the setting of worsening LV failure and cardiogenic shock, hypotension, oliguria, pallor, and confusion may become evident. Many patients experience a fever in the first 24 to 49 hours after acute MI as a response to tissue necrosis. The fever typically resolves within 4 to 6 days after acute MI.

The patient's heart rate may range from bradycardia to tachycardia depending on the level of pain, location of the infarct, and degree of autonomic stimulation. Many patients initially demonstrate tachycardia related to pain and anxiety. The patient with an anterior MI may experience tachycardia due to excess sympathetic stimulation. In contrast, the patient experiencing an inferior MI may present with bradycardia as a result of excess parasympathetic stimulation. The rhythms typically associated with excess parasympathetic stimulation include sinus bradycardia, first-degree heart block, and second-degree heart block type I.

In RV infarction, the abnormalities noted on physical examination depend on the degree of RV dysfunction. RV failure produces signs of systemic venous congestion and poor systemic perfusion (Table 26-4). Jugular venous distention is a sign of elevated RV filling pressure. An inspiratory rise in jugular venous pressure (Kussmaul's sign) and pulsus paradoxus may be present. In RV infarction, Kussmaul's sign reflects the inability of the right ventricle to manage the augmented venous return that normally accompanies inspiration. Hepatomegaly and peripheral edema may develop from persistently elevated systemic venous pressure. The lung fields are usually clear, a finding in sharp contrast to the pulmonary congestion usually noted with LV dysfunction.

Diagnostic Testing

Electrocardiographic Changes with Myocardial Infarction

The ECG is central to the diagnosis of acute MI and should be obtained within 10 minutes of presentation. Diagnostic criteria on the ECG for transmural ischemia and injury include ST-segment elevation of greater than 0.1 mV in two or more contiguous leads (Fig. 26-2). ST-segment elevation indicates myocardial injury that occurs when ischemia is prolonged. Patients with ST-segment elevation or new left bundle-branch block (LBBB) should be evaluated for immediate reperfusion therapy. Unequivocal ECG changes include the development of abnormal, persistent Q waves; presence of a QS complex in two or more leads; or an evolving injury current pattern lasting longer than 1 day. The presence of Q waves indicates infarcted tissue that extends at least halfway through the myocardial wall.

Table 26–4 ■ MAJOR DIFFERENCES IN THE LOW CARDIAC OUTPUT SYNDROMES OF PREDOMINANT RIGHT VENTRICULAR VERSUS LEFT VENTRICULAR INFARCTION

	Right Ventricle	Left Ventricle
Physical examination	Clear lungs	Crackles, pulmonary edema
	Systemic venous congestion	No systemic venous congestion
	Jugular venous distention	Normal jugular veins
	S_3 or S_4 may be present	S_3 or S_4
	Tricuspid regurgitation	Mitral regurgitation
Hemodynamic profile	Cl <2.2 L/min/m^2	Cl <2.2 L/min/m^2
		PAWP >18 mm Hg
		Decreased preload
Treatment	Increase preload	Decrease preload
	Volume load	Limit volume administration
	Avoid diuretics and nitrates	Give diuretic therapy
	Give inotropes (dobutamine)	Give nitrates
	Maintain AV synchrony	Give arterial vasodilators (sodium nitroprusside,
	Reduce RV afterload in setting of LV failure with	hydralazine)
	IABP, vasodilators (sodium) nitroprusside, hydralazine)	Give inotropes
	Reperfuse	Use IABP
		Reperfuse

CI = cardiac index; PAWP = pulmonary artery wedge pressure.

Q waves may appear within hours of MI. The presence of Q waves, however, does not indicate when an MI has occurred.

Equivocal ECG changes are not diagnostic but suggestive of MI. These changes include ST-segment depression, T-wave inversion in the leads facing the damaged zone, and conduction disturbances. The diagnosis of acute MI becomes difficult or impossible in the presence of preexisting ECG abnormalities such as LBBB, a previous MI in the same area, ventricular hypertrophy and Wolff-Parkinson-White syndrome. Other disorders, such as cardiomyopathies, pulmonary embolism, pericarditis, and subarachnoid hemorrhage, may mimic the ST-segment and T-wave abnormalities of acute MI.

The standard 12-lead ECG does not provide specific diagnostic clues to acute RV infarction. Frequently, the ECG demonstrates the evolution of a concomitant acute inferior or posterior LV infarction. A right precordial ECG should be performed in patients with suspected inferior and/or posterior MI and with signs and symptoms of an RV MI. ST-segment elevation of more than 1 mm in lead V4R with an upright T wave in the same lead is the most sensitive electrocardiographic sign of RV infarction

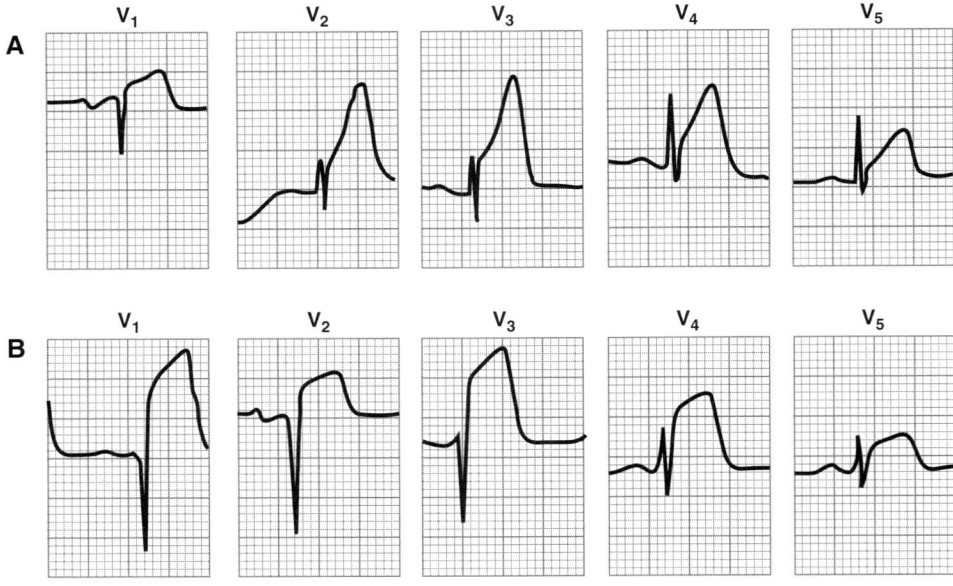

■ **Figure 26–2.** Chest leads from a patient with acute anterior wall infarction. (*A*) In the earliest phase of the infarction, tall, positive (hyperacute) T waves are seen in leads V_2 to V_5. (*B*) Several hours later, marked ST segment elevation is seen in the same leads and abnormal Q waves are seen in leads V_1 and V_2. (From Goldberger, A. L. [1999]. *Clinical electrocardiography: A simplified approach* [6th ed.]. St. Louis: Mosby, Inc.)

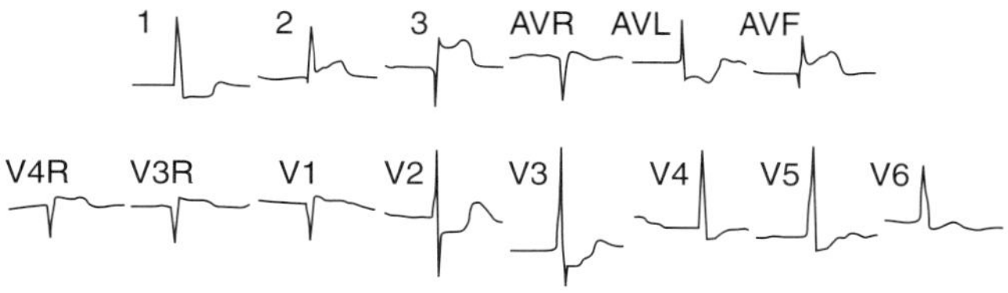

■ Figure 26–3. Electrocardiogram demonstrating an evolving inferior myocardial infarction with ST segment elevation and QS pattern in leads V₃R and V₄R suggestive of right ventricular involvement. (From Morgera, T., Alberti, E., Silvestri, F. et al. [1984]. Right precordial ST and QRS changes in the diagnosis of right ventricular infarction. *American Heart Journal*, 108, 13.)

(Zehender & Kaspar, 1993; Zimetbaum & Josephson, 2003). However, ST-segment elevation in lead V4R rarely lasts more than 12 hours after infarction (Zimetbaum & Josephson, 2003). On the standard ECG, ST-segment elevation in lead V1 in the presence of ST-segment elevation in leads II, III, and aVF may indicate the presence of RV MI. An ECG pattern seen in inferior MI with posterior LV and RV involvement is illustrated in Figure 26-3 (Morgera, Alberti & Silvestri, 1984).

Serum Markers Associated with Myocardial Infarction

The World Heath Organization (WHO) has identified three criteria for the diagnosis of acute MI. These criteria include patient history of severe and prolonged chest pain, unequivocal ECG changes that include the development of abnormal and persistent Q waves, and changes in serial enzymes that indicate myocardial injury and infarction. An increase in the level of biomarkers in the blood is indicative of myocardial injury but should be considered in light of other criteria in making a final diagnosis of acute MI (Jaffe et al., 2000).

The measurement of CK and CK-MB has been the gold standard for serum markers of MI. CK and CK-MB enzymes are released with tissue necrosis and rise 4 to 6 hours after MI (see Chapter 14).[AQ20] Recently, biochemical markers have emerged that are not enzymes. These markers include troponin I (cTnT), troponin T (cTnT), and myoglobin. The troponins are emerging as the preferred biochemical indicator of MI due to improved tissue specificity and sensitivity as well as a prolonged time window that the marker will be elevated (Jaffe et al., 2000). In one study, an elevated troponin T level and ST-segment elevation predicted a threefold increase in mortality during the first 30 days after MI (Ohman & Armstrong, 1996). The troponins appear within 4 to 12 hours after onset of symptoms and remain abnormal for 4 to 10 days (Wu et al., 1999). Troponin I has demonstrated 93% specificity for cardiac tissue injury and sensitivity of 96%. However, these percentages have not been realized until 18 hours after onset of chest pain (Zimmerman et al., 1999).

Biochemical markers that aid in early diagnosis of acute MI include myoglobin and CK-MB subforms. Myoglobin, a heme protein, found in all striated tissue and released from myocytes after injury, rises within 1 to 2 hours after onset of symptoms. Myoglobin, however, is not specific to cardiac tissue and may be elevated for reasons other than acute MI. CK-MB subforms increase within 6 hours of onset of symptoms and, in one study, detected 80% of patients who had an MI (Zimmerman et al., 1999).

Hemodynamic Monitoring

Hemodynamic monitoring of pulmonary artery pressures is not indicated in patients with uncomplicated MI. However, for patients with complicated MI, knowledge of pulmonary artery and pulmonary artery wedge pressures (PAWP) is important for prescribing treatment. Indications for placement of a pulmonary artery catheter include (1) severe or progressive CHF or pulmonary edema; (2) cardiogenic shock or progressive hypotension; and (3) suspected mechanical complications of acute MI such as ventricular septal defect (VSD), papillary muscle rupture, or pericardial tamponade (Ryan et al., 1996a). The central venous pressure (CVP), PAWP, and cardiac output guide treatment decisions by helping distinguish the patient with inadequate intravascular volume with low filling pressures who may require fluid administration from the patient with LV dysfunction with high filling pressures who may require diuresis, inotropes, and/or afterload reduction (see Chapter 23).

Echocardiography

Echocardiography (echo) is useful in the diagnosis and evaluation of acute MI. Regional wall motion abnormalities are associated with MI in 90% to 100% of patients with a transmural MI (Kontos et al., 1998). Echocardiography allows for identification of regions of abnormal wall motion and is also useful in ruling out other causes for hemodynamic compromise such as a pericardial effusion and mitral insufficiency. In some cases, two-dimensional (2-D) echo has been found to be significantly more sensitive in detecting MI than the initial ECG (Kontos et al.,1998). Echo may facilitate the diagnosis of MI in cases where the ECG is nondiagnostic. The echocardiogram may further provide information about the location and extent of the MI and thereby impact treatment. Absence of regional wall motion abnormalities on echo may also provide data needed to rule out the diagnosis of MI (Sobel, Dittrich & Keen, 1998; see Chapter 16).

Cardiac Imaging

Radionuclide studies may be performed to identify areas of myocardium at risk as well as tissue necrosis. Technetium-99 sestamibi is a radioisotope that is taken up by myocardial tissue in proportion to blood flow in the region and may be used to identify areas of tissue viability (Marcassa et al., 1995). As with echo, the technetium-99 sestamibi study may be useful as an aid to rule out the diagnosis of acute MI when the ECG is normal or nondiagnostic. The patient may be injected with the isotope during an episode of chest pain, and imaging can be delayed for several hours because the scan reflects myocardial perfusion at the time of injection (Arrighi & Dilsizian, 1998). Sestamibi scans, performed before and after reperfusion therapies, may also be used to evaluate the effectiveness of reperfusion strategies on regional blood flow to the myocardium (see Chapter 17).

Complications of Acute Myocardial Infarction

Patients with acute MI are prone to a variety of complications. Some of these (e.g., sudden death) may occur before the patient reaches the hospital. Additional complications may occur simply as a result of the hospitalization itself (nosocomial infection) or may be more likely in elderly patients, particularly those requiring intensive care (delirium, pressure ulcers; Malone, Rosen & Goodwin, 1998). This section discusses only those complications occurring during the initial hospitalization.

Infarct Expansion/Left Ventricular Remodeling

Through mechanisms that are not completely understood, the infarcted segment of myocardium may increase its surface area, thereby increasing LV volume (Hochman & Gerch, 1998). LV volume may also increase in an attempt to preserve stroke volume (SV) despite a falling ejection fraction. Increased LV volume increases the oxygen requirement of the remaining viable tissue and requires gradual lengthening of the remaining muscle, placing it at a mechanical disadvantage. The use of inotropic agents and afterload reduction may help optimize myocardial performance, but this can become a progressive cycle, leading to a dilated, poorly contractile LV. ACE inhibitors are particularly beneficial to those patients whose ejection fraction has fallen below 40% (Antman & Braunwald, 2001a, b).

Left Ventricular Aneurysms

In addition to global ventricular dilation, more localized dilation or aneurysm formation can occur. The two types of aneurysms are termed *true* and *false*.

True Aneurysms

True LV aneurysms are broad-necked, localized dilations of the left ventricle. The LV wall segment, although likely a noncontractile fibrous scar, remains intact. They tend to involve the apex, may calcify over time, and may accumulate thrombus, although clinically recognized embolization is uncommon. They are not prone to rupture, but cause morbidity and mortality because of recurrent ventricular arrhythmias, thought to be incited at the junction of the aneurysm with adjacent, normal myocardium.

False Aneurysms

False aneurysms (pseudoaneurysms) result from myocardial ruptures that are contained by the pericardium. The wall of these narrow-necked aneurysms is composed of pericardium and adhesions, and they are usually lined by thrombus (Hochman & Gerch, 1998). These aneurysms have a tendency to rupture, with a uniformly fatal outcome. Surgical repair is always recommended.

Left Ventricular Failure

LV failure ranges from mild decreases in LV ejection fraction to cardiogenic shock, which may occur in 5% to 20% of patients with acute MI. The degree of hemodynamic compromise parallels the degree of LV dysfunction, as do the clinical manifestations.

Left Ventricular Dysfunction

Ischemic myocardial segments have diminished (or absent) contractility, and, depending on the size of the segment and the degree of decreased contractility, LV ejection fraction is compromised. Diminished contractility places an increased burden on the remaining functioning myocardium, some of which may also be supplied by stenotic coronary vessels. The left ventricle may dilate in an effort to preserve SV despite a decrease in ejection fraction, which, in turn, increases oxygen demand and LV end-diastolic pressure. Increases in LV end-diastolic pressure lead to varying degrees of pulmonary interstitial edema.

Myocardial ischemia not only impairs LV contraction and, therefore, peripheral perfusion (systolic dysfunction), but the ischemic segment may initially become stiff and noncompliant (diastolic dysfunction), which also increases the LV end-diastolic pressure (Hochman & Gerch, 1998).

Hemodynamic Alterations

Some investigators have grouped patients with acute MI into clinical subsets based on the predominance of peripheral hypoperfusion or pulmonary venous hypertension (Antman & Braunwald, 2001a, b), those with no significant manifestation of either (subset 1), those with primarily pulmonary manifestations (subset 2), those with primarily peripheral hypoperfusion (subset 3), and those with manifestation of both (subset 4). These subsets may be separately recognized by physical examination and monitored by specific hemodynamic parameters, and each requires different treatment.

Subset 1: Up to 50% of patients with acute MI may have no clinical evidence of LV dysfunction. They require no additional hemodynamic monitoring.

Subset 2: Patients with primarily pulmonary manifestations can be further divided according to the severity of pulmonary symptoms. Those with mild venous congestion can be managed with supplemental oxygen, diuretics, morphine, and careful use of vasodilators, without invasive monitoring. Those with more severe manifestations may require ventilatory support, and invasive hemodynamic monitoring (which usually reveals a pulmonary artery wedge pressure (PAWP) of 25 mm Hg) to guide vasodilator and other pharmacotherapy.

Subset 3: Signs and symptoms of peripheral hypoperfusion (hypotension, peripheral vasoconstriction, impaired mental status, and decreased urine output) without pulmonary symptoms usually occur in the setting of RV infarction or hypovolemic shock. These patients require invasive monitoring to guide the use of rehydration and inotropics or vasodilators.

Subset 4: Patients with signs of hypoperfusion and pulmonary venous congestion require use of invasive monitoring to guide the use of inotropics, diuretics, and possibly vasodilators.

Hypovolemia, usually related to reduced fluid intake early in the illness, or diuretic use, is a relatively easily corrected complication of acute MI. Because hypovolemia can lead to hypotension and vascular collapse, volume should be cautiously restored to facilitate adequate LV filling pressures.

Cardiogenic shock is a clinical syndrome characterized by hypoperfusion and hypotension in conjunction with pulmonary edema. Clinical evaluation of these patients reveals signs and symptoms of decreased peripheral perfusion, including marked hypotension (systolic pressure <80 mm Hg), impaired mental status, decreased urine output, and peripheral vasoconstriction. Cardiac index is markedly diminished [<1.8 L/(min/m^2)], PAWP is elevated (>18 mm Hg), and systemic vascular resistance (SVR) may be elevated or remain within the normal range. Cardiogenic shock results from severe LV dysfunction, usually caused by large infarcts with transmural necrosis (35% to 40% of LV mass), and is highly correlated with three-vessel disease. Cardiogenic shock may occur at the onset or within a few hours of acute MI, or later as a consequence of mechanical complications. Mortality rates in patients with early cardiogenic shock may be >70% without aggressive revascularization (Antman & Braunwald, 2001a, b). Therapy includes cautious use of sympathomimetics, vasodilators, and intraaortic balloon counterpulsation. Aggressive revascularization, with either percutaneous coronary intervention (PCI) or surgery, may decrease the mortality rate to 25% to 50%.

Right Ventricular Myocardial Infarction

RV MI may occur to some degree in patients with inferior wall MI, but hemodynamically significant RV infarction occurs in less than 10% of patients with inferior wall MI. RV failure results in underfilling of the left atrium and ventricle, reducing pump efficiency and SV. Resultant peripheral hypoperfusion may be exacerbated by concomitant bradyarrhythmia. It is recognized clinically as a triad of hepatomegaly, jugular venous pressure that rises with inspiration (Kussmaul's sign), and clear lungs, in a patient with inferior wall MI (Antman & Braunwald, 2001a, b). Hypotension may or may not be present. ST-segment elevation may be seen in lead V4R in the first 24 hours of the RV infarction, and RV dysfunction can be confirmed by echocardiography. Because these patients require fluid resuscitation, invasive hemodynamic monitoring may be required. PAWP is usually low, and fluid resuscitation is continued until PAWP reaches 18 to 20 mm Hg. Diuretics and afterload-reducing agents must be avoided. Aggressive reperfusion is first-line strategy in management of patients with acute MI.

Mechanical Complications

Ventricular Free Wall Rupture

Free wall rupture complicates anterior and inferior MI with equal frequency, occurring typically within the first week after infarction, although up to 30% may develop in the first 24 hours. It may account for up to 10% of acute MI-associated mortality. The risk for myocardial rupture increases with the age of the patient (Antman & Braunwald, 2001a, b). Clinically, it manifests as pulseless electrical activity (PEA) and sudden death, with attempts at resuscitation being futile. Rarely, patients present with a syndrome of subacute rupture, with pericardial pain,

ECG evidence of pericarditis, and echocardiographic evidence of localized pericardial effusion or even pseudoaneurysm. Such a scenario is, unfortunately, uncommon, and accurately identifying patients at high risk for rupture is extremely difficult, although large Q-wave infarcts are associated with higher risk of myocardial rupture (Antman & Braunwald, 2001a, b).

Ventricular Septal Rupture

Septal rupture may occur with anterior MI, producing apical septal rupture, or with inferior wall MI, with rupture occurring at the base of the septum. It is seen with transmural infarction and occurs in 1% to 3% of acute MI (Hochman & Gerch, 1998). It tends to occur between 3 and 7 days after infarction. Patients present with sudden, severe LV failure; a loud, holosystolic murmur; and systemic hypoperfusion due to left-to-right shunting. Diagnosis may be made with color-flow Doppler echocardiography (Antman & Braunwald, 2001a, b). Prompt diagnosis and early intervention (intra-aortic balloon counterpulsation and nitroprusside infusion until prepared for surgical intervention) are required because the mortality rate is >20% in 24 hours and >40% in 1 week.

Mitral Regurgitation

Mitral regurgitation may occur early in the course of acute MI secondary to ischemia of the valve itself, or due to ischemia and dysfunction (or necrosis and rupture) of one of the papillary muscles that support the chordae tendineae of the mitral valve. It occurs most frequently with inferior wall or subendocardial (non–Q-wave) MI (Hochman & Grech, 1998) and tends to occur within the first week after MI. With mitral valve dysfunction, the resultant pulmonary congestion may be intermittent or persistent, and the diagnosis can be confirmed by echocardiography. A small percentage of these patients require relatively prompt revascularization.

Papillary muscle rupture can be a catastrophic event, leading to a rapid decline in LV function, which may necessitate surgical repair. Intra-aortic balloon counterpulsation and an infusion of nitroglycerin or sodium nitroprusside may be used for interim management, if it is necessary, for example, to allow pulmonary congestion to clear before surgery (Antman & Braunwald, 2001a, b).

Arrhythmias. Dysrhythmias may occur early in the course of the event because of electrophysiologic alterations in ischemic myocardium, pharmacotherapy, electrolyte disturbances, or endogenous epinephrine release. Arrhythmias that occur later may be secondary to other complications (e.g., CHF or ventricular aneurysm). The majority of arrhythmia-related deaths occur in the hours immediately after MI, so it is critical to begin continuous ECG monitoring as quickly as possible in the course of treatment of MI.

Tachyarrhythmias

Ventricular Tachyarrhythmias. Many patients with acute MI experience premature ventricular contractions, which in themselves do not require therapy but may herald the onset of more dangerous arrhythmias. Approximately 7% of patients with acute MI experience ventricular fibrillation, and a similar number experience recurrent VT. Hypokalemia and hypomagnesemia are also important risk factors for ventricular fibrillation in patients with MI. The use of lidocaine is no longer standard in the treatment of premature ventricular beats and is indicated only in the presence of sustained ventricular arrhythmias (Antman & Braunwald, 2001a, b) because lidocaine may actually increase the mortality rate. This is due to the widespread use of beta-adrenergic blockers and the great success of cardioversion and defibrillation (Antman & Braunwald, 2001a, b).

Accelerated Idioventricular Rhythm (AIVR). AIVR occurs in up to 25% of patients with acute MI, and often transiently during reperfusion after thrombolytic therapy (Antman & Braunwald, 2001a, b). AIVR is generally not a herald of lethal arrhythmias and most times can go untreated. If symptomatic, atropine may be administered to increase the sinus rate.

Supraventricular Arrhythmias. Sinus tachycardia, atrial fibrillation, and atrial flutter are included in this subgroup. These arrhythmias may exacerbate myocardial ischemia by increasing the heart rate. If the primary cause for sinus tachycardia is suspected to be something other than cardiac (fever, anemia), the primary cause should be treated first. Atrial fibrillation and atrial flutter, which may be a result of LV failure, are generally treated successfully with digoxin. If heart failure is not present, beta blockers or certain calcium channel agents are the treatment of choice. In the case of sustained supraventricular tachyarrhythmia (>120 beats per minute for >2 hours), synchronized cardioversion may be used.

Bradyarrhythmias

Bradyarrhythmias are, in general, more common with inferior wall MI, with sinus bradycardia, sinus arrest, second- and third-degree AV block occurring more commonly in RV infarction. Complete heart block occurs in up to 20% of patients with acute RV infarcts. These bradyarrhythmias are usually treated with atropine, although they may also require transvenous pacing. A sinus bradycardia would only be treated if the patient is symptomatic, in which case atropine would be the drug of choice.

Anterior wall MI is much more likely to cause infranodal conduction disturbances. These patients experience wide complex idioventricular rhythms, which carry a much worse prognosis because they are associated with large infarcts. They are typically treated temporarily with transvenous pacing, although the prognosis for anterior wall MI remains quite poor.

Pericarditis

Pericarditis most commonly occurs several weeks after MI (Dressler's syndrome). However, in some patients, it may occur acutely, within 3 days of the event, and sometimes as early as the first day. In these cases, it is often localized to the pericardium adjacent to the infarcted segment and results from transmural infarction extending to the epicardial surface, inciting a localized inflammatory response. The diagnosis is made clinically by history, physical examination, and ECG. The pain is typically sharp, severe, and substernal, radiating to the neck, shoulders, and back. The pain is exacerbated with inspiration and with reclining. A pericardial friction rub may be present on auscultation. The classic ECG changes (ST-segment elevation in multiple chest leads) are not usually present with localized

pericarditis. Typically, pericarditis can be managed with aspirin. The incidence of acute pericarditis has decreased by almost 50% with the use of thrombolytic therapy (Hochman & Grech, 1998).

Medical Management

Goals for treatment of acute MI include (1) restoring coronary blood flow and minimizing infarct size, (2) maintaining adequate oxygenation, (3) administering appropriate fluid therapy, (4) improving ventricular performance to maximize oxygen supply and demand ratio, (5) administering the appropriate adjunctive drug therapy, (6) detecting and managing complications early, and (7) assessing risk after infarction. A calm, quiet atmosphere should be maintained, and explanations should be given to the patient with the goal of reducing anxiety. Early reperfusion of the occluded artery with thrombolytics therapy or with PCI can substantially reduce infarct size. These two approaches have emerged as the standard of care for patients who experience acute MI with ST-segment elevation. Figure 26-4 illustrates the American Heart Association's recommended algorithm for management of ischemic chest pain (Cummins, Field & Hazinski, 2001).

Thrombolytic Therapy

In 1980, DeWood and colleagues (DeWood et al., 1980) reported a high prevalence of coronary artery thrombosis in acute MI, establishing the pathophysiologic basis for thrombolytic therapy of patients with acute MI. The success of thrombolytic therapy is based on the pathophysiology of acute MI; a large occlusive thrombus is commonly found adherent to an underlying ruptured mild or moderate atherosclerotic plaque (Brown et al., 1986). Subsequently, research has attempted to determine the most efficacious means of early clot lysis, including studies of exogenously administered thrombolytic agents.

Thrombolytic Agents

Thrombolytic agents can be divided into two major categories: *fibrin selective,* characterized by activation of fibrin-bound plasminogen and a high velocity of clot lysis, and *nonselective,* characterized by systemic plasminogenolysis and fibrinogenolysis, somewhat slower clot lysis, and a more prolonged systemic lytic state (Topol, 1990). Fibrin-selective agents include tissue-type plasminogen activator (t-PA), recombinant tissue plasminogen activator, recombinant plasminogen activator (reteplase; r-PA), and single-chain urokinase plasminogen activator (scu-PA or prourokinase). Nonselective agents include streptokinase (SK), anisoylated plasminogen streptokinase activator complex (APSAC), and urokinase (UK). The most commonly used thrombolytics for IV administration in the setting of acute MI are discussed in the following sections.

Streptokinase is a nonenzymatic protein product of hemolytic streptococci. Exogenously administered SK combines with circulating plasminogen, forming complexes that catalyze plasmin formation. The resultant excessive circulating plasmin then creates a systemic lytic state, with dissolution of all recent

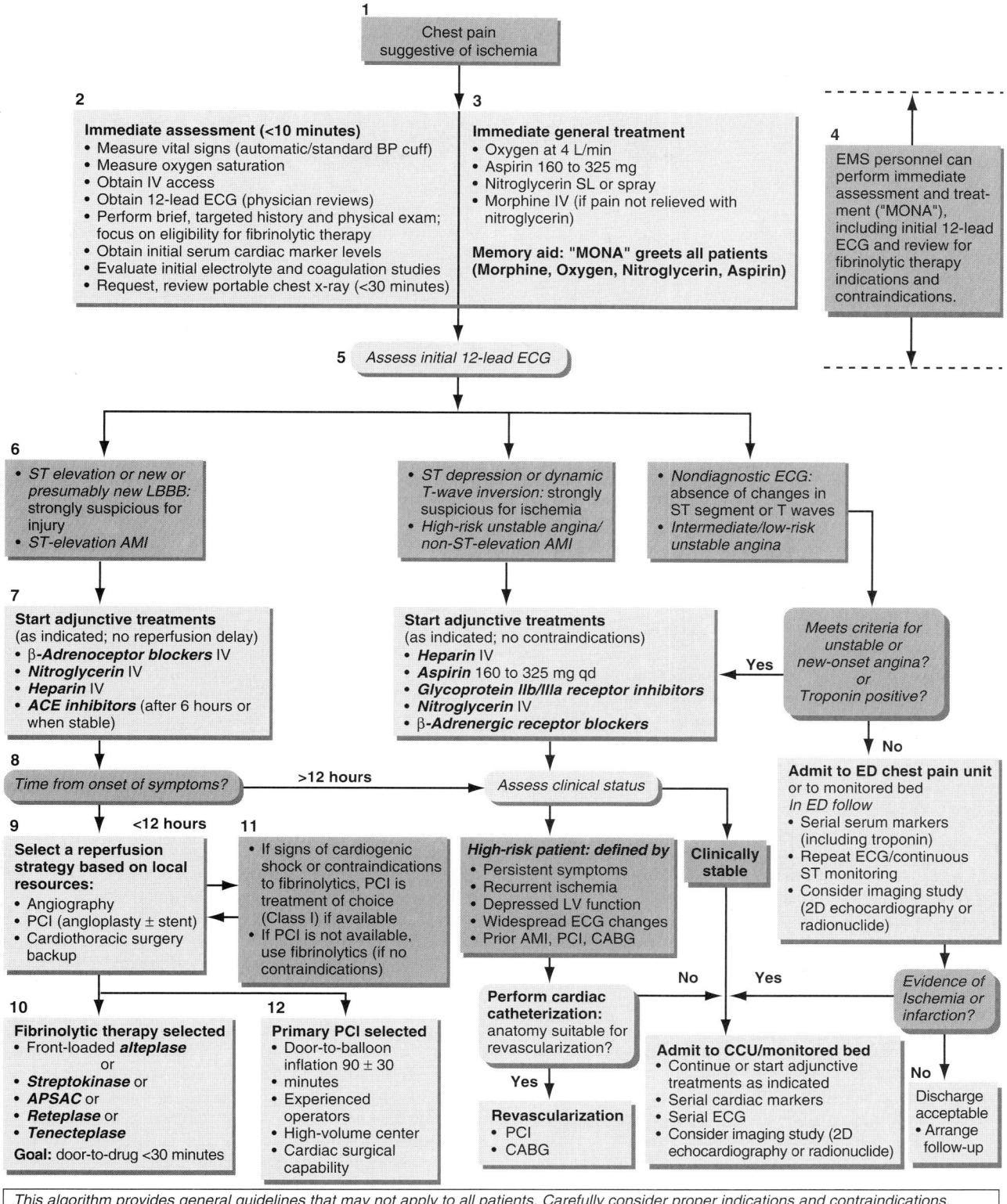

Figure 26–4. Ischemic chest pain algorithm. (From Cummins, R. O., Field, J. & Hazinski, M. [2001]. Acute coronary syndromes: Patients with acute ischemic chest pain. In *Advanced cardiac life support.* Dallas: American Heart Association.)

thrombi, depletion of circulating fibrinogen, plasminogen, factors V and VIII, and accumulation of fibrin(ogen) degradation products.

Streptokinase is given in a dose of 1.5 million units infused over 30 to 60 minutes. Reported 90-minute angiographic patency of the infarct-related artery after this dose of SK ranges from 42% to 58%. Because of its foreign protein origins, SK may trigger an antigenic response. Some type of allergic reaction was reported to occur in 3.6% of patients receiving SK in a large, multicenter study (Litvak, Marglis & Cummins, 1992). Pruritus, fever, nausea, flushing, urticaria, headache, and malaise are common symptoms, with bronchospasm and angioedema rarely reported.

People with anti-SK antibodies may not attain full therapeutic benefit from the SK, and, therefore, patients with known recent streptococcal infection or those who received SK within the last 5 days to 6 months should not be treated with an SK-based drug. Variable degrees of hypotension may also occur with administration of SK, presumably owing to plasmin-mediated activation of kinins and the complement system (Topol, 1990), although hypotension may also be related to hemodynamic changes associated with acute myocardial ischemia. The Third International Study of Infarct Survival (ISIS-3) investigators reported hypotension in 11.8% of patients receiving SK, with 6.7% requiring pharmacologic intervention for hypotension (ISIS-3:Third International Study of Infarct Survival Collaborative Group, 1992).

Anisoylated plasminogen streptokinase activator complex (APSAC) is a chemically altered form of SK, created by the addition of an acyl group to an SK and lys-plasminogen activator complex. In the circulation, the activator complex converts circulating and fibrin-bound plasminogen into plasmin. APSAC has a relatively long half-life and results in pronounced fibrinogenolysis.

APSAC is administered as a bolus of 30 U over 2 to 5 minutes. The reported 90-minute angiographic patency from APSAC ranges from 72% to 90% (Brochier, Quillet, & Kulbertus, 1987; Lopez-Sendon, Seabra-Bomes, & Santos, 1988). Because APSAC is a form of SK, it possesses the same antigenic properties of SK. Allergic symptoms occurred in 5.1% of patients receiving APSAC in the ISIS-3 study (ISIS-3, 1992). Hypotension may occur in about 12% of patients and is more pronounced if the drug is administered rapidly (Litvak et al., 1992). Because of side effects, APSAC is infrequently used in current clinical practice.

Endogenous *tissue-type plasminogen activator (t-PA)* is a serine protease produced by vascular endothelial cells. t-PA exhibits marked affinity for fibrin, primarily activating fibrin-bound plasminogen. Exogenously administered t-PA for clinical use is produced by recombinant DNA techniques. Alteplase (rt-PA) standard dose accelerated regimen includes a 15-mg bolus, 50 mg or 0.75 mg/kg body weight over 30 minutes, and 35 mg or 0.50 mg/kg body weight over 60 minutes for a total maximum dose 100 mg (De Jaegere, Serruys & Bertrand, 1992). Weight adjustment for patients who weigh less than 65 kg is recommended (Hirschfeld, Schwartz & Jugo, 1991). The half-life is 5 minutes. The reported 90-minute angiographic patency from 100 mg of rt-PA ranges from 61% to 89% (Simoons, Phillips & Myoung-Mook, 1988; Verstraete, Brower & Collen, 1985).

Newer drugs such as reteplase and tenecteplase that are derived from tPA are administered as one or two bolus doses. Reteplase (r-PA) is a modified recombinant form of rtPA with a longer half-life (15 minutes) that can be given as two 10-megaunit (MU) bolus doses 30 minutes apart. In a randomized trial that compared double-bolus reteplase with front-loaded accelerated alteplase in patients with acute MI, double-bolus reteplase achieved higher patency rates than alteplase at 60 and 90 minutes. However, follow-up angiography indicated similar overall patency rates in the alteplase and reteplase groups and did not show differences in mortality and patient outcome (Bode et al., 1996).

The unique activity and short half-lives of rt-PA and r-PA result in an increased likelihood of arterial reocclusion. Systemic anticoagulation with continuous IV heparin to maintain the activated partial thromboplastin time (aPTT) within a therapeutic range is recommended to sustain arterial patency after rt-PA and r-PA (Hsia, Hamilton & Kleiman, 1990). Allergic symptoms and hypotensive events have also been reported with t-PA (ISIS-3, 1992).

Tenecteplase (Cannon et al., 1998) is derived from a modification of native tPA. This modification results in decreased clearance of the drug from the plasma, enhanced fibrin specificity, and increased resistance to inhibition by plasminogen activator inhibitor-1 (PAI 1; Llevadot, Giugliano & Antman, 2001). The goal in the development of TNK-tPA was to design a drug that was very fibrin specific and would allow selective clot lysis with minimal systemic effects, including intracranial bleeding.

The TIMI 10B trial compared TNK-tPA with front loaded tPA (alteplase) in acute MI. In this study, 886 patients were randomized to receive either a 50-mg bolus or a 30-mg bolus of TNK-tPA or front-loaded tPA. The 50-mg dose was replaced with a 40-mg dose due to increased bleeding with the higher dose. The 40-mg dose of TNK-tPA and tPA resulted in similar rates of TIMI grade 3 flow at 90 minutes. Lower rates of serious bleeding and intracranial hemorrhage were seen with both drugs when the accompanying heparin dose was decreased and the initiation of heparin was delayed by 6 hours. The study suggests that weight-based dosing of TNK-tPA and appropriate heparin dosing are key safety factors in the use of both drugs (Cannon et al., 1998).

The therapeutic index for the thrombolytic drugs is narrow: a dose that is too low may result in MI whereas a dose that is too high may lead to major bleeding, including an intracerebral bleed. Medication errors related to thrombolytic therapy have been associated with increased mortality. In the Global Utilization of SK and rt-PA in Occluded Coronary Arteries (GUSTO) I trial, 13.5% of patients treated with SK and 11.5% of patients treated with tPA experienced a medication error related to thrombolytic therapy (Cannon, 2000). The 30-day mortality was significantly higher in patients for whom the administration of SK or tPA was associated with a medication error (Cannon, 2000). Bolus dosing of thrombolytics may be associated with fewer medication errors than the bolus and drip dosing. Investigators in the inTIME-II study compared administration errors between tPA (bolus and 90-minute infusion) and a single bolus dose of lanoteplase (nPA) and found that the correct dose of tPA was administered 80% of the time whereas the correct dose of lanoteplase was given in 94% of cases (p<0.0001; Coulter et al., 1999).

Table 26–5 ■ CONTRAINDICATIONS AND CAUTIONS FOR THROMBOLYTIC USE IN MYOCARDIAL INFARCTION

Contraindications
- Previous hemorrhagic stroke at any time: other strokes or cerebrovascular events within 1 year
- Know intracranial neoplasms
- Active internal bleeding (does not include menses)
- Suspected aortic dissection

Cautions/Relative Contraindications
- Severe, uncontrolled hypertension on presentation (blood pressure >180/110 mm Hg). Could be low risk in low-risk patients with MI
- History of prior cerebrovascular accident or known intracerebral pathology not covered in contraindications
- Current use of anticoagulants in therapeutic doses (INR ≥2 – 3); known bleeding diathesis
- Recent trauma (within 2–4 weeks), including head trauma or traumatic or prolonged (>10 min) CPR or major surgery (<3 weeks)
- Noncompressible vascular punctures
- Recent (within 2–4 weeks) internal bleeding
- For streptokinase/anistreplase: prior exposure (especially within 5 days–2 years) or prior allergic reaction
- Pregnancy
- Active peptic ulcer
- History of chronic severe hypertension

Adapted from Ryan, T., Anderson, J., Antman, E. et al. (1996b). ACC/AHA Task Force Report on Practice Guidelines: Management of acute myocardial infarction. *Journal of the American college of cardiology,* 28, 1328–1428.

Patient Selection

The accepted indication for IV thrombolysis is chest pain suggestive of myocardial ischemia associated with acute ST-segment elevation on 12-lead electrocardiogram (ECG) or a presumed new LBBB. The duration of symptoms or "window of opportunity" has been an issue of controversy. In the 1986 GISSI study, patients who received SK 6 hours or more after the onset of symptoms had no improvement in mortality compared with patients who received placebo (GUSTO Investigators, 1993). In contrast, patients who received SK within 6 hours of symptom onset demonstrated reduced mortality compared to placebo, with the greatest mortality difference noted in patients treated within 1 hour of symptom onset. These findings were consistent with a general belief that there is a limited time before the myocardium supplied by the occluded artery suffers irreversible ischemic damage and that thrombolytic reperfusion is of no benefit after that time. Consequently, many thrombolytic trials and institutional protocols excluded patients who presented 4 to 6 hours or more after symptom onset. The ISIS-2 studies, however, which admitted patients up to 24 hours after symptom onset, demonstrated treatment benefit in patients presenting 6 to 24 hours after symptoms began (ISIS-2: Second International Study of Infarct Survival Collaborative Group, 1988).

The original investigations of thrombolytic agents in acute MI excluded patients deemed at risk for bleeding, including patients with previous cerebrovascular accident, patients with severe hypertension, patients who received cardiopulmonary resuscitation, and patients older than 75 years of age. Strict application of these contraindications excludes approximately 30% of patients from consideration for thrombolytic therapy despite proven mortality reduction (Topol, 1990). Therefore, many of the contraindications have been challenged, particularly the upper age limit and hypertension. In general, the risk of uncontrollable bleeding is weighed against the potential benefit of thrombolytic therapy to the patient with acute MI. The established absolute and relative contraindications to the drugs are outlined in Table 26-5 (Ryan et al., 1996b).

The prevailing goal when treating a patient with acute MI is to attempt rapid reperfusion by the best means available. To this end, most institutions have developed protocols, checklists, or standing orders to facilitate patient selection and reduce delays in thrombolytic treatment (Daily, 1991). At minimum, institutions must (1) establish patient selection criteria; (2) delineate the medical staff responsible for the decision to administer a thrombolytic agent; (3) determine which agent or agents will be available in the institution; (4) determine where thrombolytic drugs will be stored; (5) delineate responsibility for mixing, delivering, and administering the drug; and (6) establish the parameters of monitoring and intervention during and after thrombolytic administration.

Before thrombolysis, a brief, focused history and physical examination are necessary to establish the presence of any absolute or relative contraindications to thrombolytic therapy and to determine the characteristics and duration of symptoms. A 12-lead ECG should be performed. In some cases, the emergency medical technician (EMT) or paramedic personnel may obtain and transmit the initial ECG to the emergency department and screen for thrombolytic therapy in the field. ECG criteria indicative of acute myocardial injury include >0.1 mV of ST-segment elevation in two or more contiguous leads, new or presumed new LBBB, or ST-segment depression with a prominent R wave in precordial leads V_2 and V_3 if thought to be indicative of posterior infarction (Anderson & Willerson, 1993). Sublingual nitroglycerin may be administered to rule out myocardial ischemia primarily due to spasm. Baseline laboratory tests are obtained, including complete blood count, chemistry profile, aPTT, cardiac enzymes, and type and crossmatch (patient specific). The treatment is explained to the patient, and thrombolytics are administered as prescribed. Chewable aspirin (acetylsalicylic acid [ASA]), 160 or 325 mg, is given with the thrombolytic drug and continued orally on a daily basis. Continuous IV heparin is initiated during or after infusion of the thrombolytic agent, adjusted to maintain a therapeutic aPTT and continued for 48 hours. Additional therapies such as IV nitroglycerin, antiarrhythmic agents, atropine, morphine sulfate, and beta blockers may be given. Continuous ECG monitoring in a lead appropriate for identification of ongoing cardiac ischemia and arrhythmia detection aids in monitoring response to thrombolysis as well as identification of reocclusion.

Patient Outcomes

Mortality studies have evaluated the efficacy of thrombolysis for acute MI. Topol performed a meta-analysis of trials comparing SK, t-PA, or APSAC to placebo and noted that the reported mortality risk reductions in the various studies overlap at 27% (Topol, 1990). In ISIS-3, patients were randomized to receive SK, double-chain t-PA, or APSAC with and without subcutaneous heparin to determine if one thrombolytic agent offered a clear benefit in mortality reduction (ISIS-3, 1992). The mortality rates in the groups were 10.6%, 10.3%, and 10.5%, respectively. These differences were not statistically significant. The ISIS-3 trial has been criticized for not using continuous, monitored IV heparin therapy after thrombolysis, which may have introduced bias in favor of the nonselective agents SK and APSAC. The GUSTO trial randomized 41,021 patients to one of four treatment arms: accelerated-dose rt-PA plus IV heparin, SK plus IV heparin, SK plus subcutaneous heparin, or a combination of rt-PA, SK, and IV heparin (GUSTO Investigators, 1993). The 30-day mortality rate of the accelerated rt-PA group was 6.3%, compared with 7.2% for the SK plus subcutaneous heparin group ($P = 0.009$), 7.4% for the SK plus IV heparin group ($P = 0.003$), and 7% for the rt-PA plus SK plus IV heparin group ($P = 0.04$). This was a significant reduction in mortality with the accelerated-dose rt-PA, suggesting rapid and complete reperfusion improves overall outcome and survival.

Bleeding is the most serious complication from thrombolytic therapy and relates to the dissolution of protective vascular thrombi as well as the delayed blood coagulation from circulating fibrin(ogen) degradation products and heparin. Most commonly, bleeding occurs at vascular access sites. In one study of 20,768 patients receiving SK or t-PA with or without subcutaneous heparin, major bleeds (bleeding requiring transfusion of 2 U or more) occurred in approximately 0.8% of patients. Hemorrhagic stroke occurred in approximately 0.4% (International Study Group, 1990). Hemorrhagic stroke was more common in patients receiving t-PA than in patients receiving either SK or APSAC in the ISIS-3 trial (0.66% vs. 0.24% vs. 0.55% in ISIS-3; ISIS-3, 1992). In the GUSTO trial, clinically important bleeding (bleeding requiring transfusion, intracerebral bleeding, or bleeding causing hemodynamic compromise) occurred in 5.4% to 6.8% of patients. Hemorrhagic stroke was significantly more common in the accelerated t-PA plus heparin group compared with both SK groups (0.72% accelerated t-PA plus heparin, 0.49% SK plus subcutaneous heparin, 0.54% SK plus IV heparin; $P = 0.03$). The combined t-PA, SK, and IV heparin group had the highest overall rate of hemorrhagic stroke at 0.94% (GUSTO Investigators, 1993).

Reocclusion: Because most patients presenting with acute MI have a coronary stenosis with underlying thrombosis and ongoing stimulus to form clot, reocclusion is a risk and

occurs in approximately 12% to 29% of patients, depending on the timing of follow-up angiography (Ohman & Armstrong, 1996). Reinfarction due to reocclusion was reported to occur in 2.9% to 3.6% of patients in the ISIS-3 trial (ISIS-3, 1992).

Unfortunately, no reliable noninvasive means of early determination of thrombolytic success has been established. The clinical events of relief of chest pain and resolution of ST-segment elevations and arrhythmia were noted to occur with reperfusion, but lack adequate predictive value (Califf, O'Neill, & Stack, 1988). Early peaking of the plasma level of the myocardial band of creatine kinase (CK-MB) is associated with reperfusion (Puleo & Perryman, 1991).

Agent Selection: Selection of a thrombolytic agent is based on its adverse effects as well as its efficacy. The tPA type of thrombolytic has a more rapid rate of reperfusion but a higher frequency of hemorrhagic stroke compared with SK. The higher cost of tPA over SK must also be considered. Patients who present early with large areas of affected myocardium and with low risk in intracranial bleed may benefit most from the tPA type of thrombolytic. Simplicity of bolus dosing may also factor into choice of thrombolytics because it may result in fewer medication errors and lead to faster administration of the drug.

Percutaneous Coronary Intervention

PCI of the occluded coronary artery has emerged as the therapy of choice for selected patients with acute MI as described in greater detail in Chapter 27. PCI should be considered in patients with a diagnosis of acute MI only if it can be performed in a timely manner by professionals highly skilled in the procedure in centers that perform angioplasty in a high percentage of patients. PCI has been associated with lower early mortality and better long-term outcome compared with thrombolysis (Stone et al., 1997). However, these results have been obtained only when the delay is minimal. The 2000 AHA Emergency Cardiac Care (ECC) guidelines acknowledge that PCI is an equivalent therapy to thrombolysis if: (1) PCI can be performed within 90 minutes of presentation; (2) PCI operators are highly experienced; (3) the PCI center performs a high number of procedures per year; and (4) the PCI center achieves a documented TIMI grade II or III flow in 90% of cases without emergency CABG, stroke, or death (Cummins et al., 2001; Ryan et al., 1999).

Prehospital Care

Prehospital treatment includes reducing mortality from MI, reducing infarct size, and preserving LV function. Availability of 911 access is of central importance in prompt response and treatment of patients with ACS. An Emergency Medical Services (EMS) system strives to minimize the delay between onset of symptoms in a person and initiation of reperfusion strategies such as thrombolysis or PCI. Early initial intervention can be achieved by a prehospital community system of cardiac life support. The AHA guidelines strongly support availability of an EMS system staffed by persons trained to treat cardiac arrest with defibrillation and to triage patients with ischemic chest pain (Ryan et al., 1999). Basic to an effective community-wide emergency cardiac care (ECC) system is an informed public, an efficient communication center, trained medical and paramedical teams, and appropriate vehicles with appropriate equipment.

Although an effective ECC system is an important factor in reducing the delay between the patient's onset of symptoms and treatment, the patient and family play an important role. Of all patients with MI, one fourth to one half delay longer than 6 hours from onset of symptoms (Dracup & Moser, 1997). Dracup found that the mean time from onset of symptoms until arrival in the emergency department averaged 110 minutes. Patients who are most likely to delay seeking treatment include the elderly, persons with lower incomes, persons with diabetes, those who experienced symptoms at home, those who did not appraise symptoms as serious or heart related and those who had intermittent symptoms. Analysis of the data on delay from the GUSTO I and GUSTO III trials also found that women and African Americans were also more likely to delay seeking treatment for symptoms of ischemia (Gibler et al., 2002). Furthermore, in-hospital and overall mortality tended to be significantly higher in patients who delayed seeking treatment (Gibler et al., 2002). Interventions, such as teaching the patient and family about symptoms of MI and initial steps to take with onset of symptoms, should target groups who delay (Dracup & Moser, 1997).

The Rapid Heart Attack Alert Program focused on the effects of a community-wide education program designed to reduce patient delay from symptom onset to hospital presentation (Luepker et al., 2000). Although education resulted in increased EMS use, time from symptom onset to hospital presentation did not change.

Emergency Department Care

Treatment in the Emergency Department (ED) focuses on a rapid, targeted history and physical assessment, initial treatment, and risk stratification of the patient with an acute MI. Figure 26- 4 outlines the algorithm for ischemic chest pain recommended by the AHA subcommittee on Advanced Cardiac Life Support (Cummins et al., 2001). Continuous cardiac monitoring should be started upon arrival. The targeted history and physical examination and a 12-lead ECG should be performed and interpreted within 10 minutes of arrival in the ED on all patients with suspected MI (Ryan et al., 1999). Serum cardiac markers should be drawn as a part of the initial assessment. The AHA Committee on Emergency Cardiovascular Care recommends stratifying patients into one of three categories based on the 12-lead ECG: (1) ST-segment elevation; (2) ST-segment depression or T-wave inversion, or (3) nondiagnostic ECG findings. If the ECG shows ST-elevation of 1 mm or more in two contiguous leads or LBBB, screening for contraindications to thrombolytic therapy should be initiated. If the patient is eligible for thrombolytic therapy, it should be started within 30 minutes of arrival in the hospital (Gershlick & More, 1998).

Patients without contraindications should receive four agents upon arrival: morphine for pain relief, nitroglycerin, oxygen, and aspirin. Beta-blocker therapy should also be initiated in the

patient without contraindications within 12 hours of infarction (Ryan et al., 1999). Clinicians should also consider initiating IV nitroglycerin and IV heparin (Cummins et al., 2001). At least one IV line should be started. Two IV lines should be started if the patient is a candidate for thrombolytic therapy. In patients with nondiagnostic ECG changes, without ST-segment elevation, consideration should be given to IV GPIIb/IIIa inhibitors to stabilize the patient and reduce acute events.

The recent development of the "chest pain" emergency department represents an attempt to balance the risk of unnecessary and costly admissions of patients to the cardiac intensive care unit (CICU) who eventually "rule out" for an MI with the risk of sending the patient experiencing an MI home. Of the patients admitted to the hospital for suspected MI, 70% eventually rule out for an MI (Bahr, 1998). On the other hand, 2.9% to 10% of patients who present with chest pain with acute MI are sent home (Gibler, 1998). The chest pain unit focuses on rapid diagnosis of the patient experiencing chest discomfort with nondiagnostic ECG changes and low risk of having acute MI. Rapid diagnosis is accomplished by assessment of serial markers of myocardial necrosis such as CK-MB. With more rapid testing of CK-MB available, the diagnosis of an acute MI can be determined within 4 to 5 hours after onset of symptoms (Gibler, 1998). Other tests used in the early diagnosis of an acute MI include 2-D echocardiography and radionuclide scanning.

Cardiac Care Unit (CCU) Treatment

Since its inception in the early 1960s, the focus of the CCU has evolved from monitoring and rapid treatment of arrhythmias to aggressive intervention and alteration of the underlying disease process (Fleischmann & Lee, 1998). The CCU environment provides capacity for arrhythmia monitoring as well as invasive cardiac monitoring with arterial lines and pulmonary artery catheters. Intervention with the intra-aortic balloon pump (IABP) and, in some cases, a left ventricular assist device (LVAD) is possible in the CCU because of highly skilled nursing staff and the availability of equipment. Nursing staffing ratios and competencies support the ability to provide intensive monitoring and rapid intervention for patients with acute MI. Since the advent of the CCU, mortality of cardiac patients has decreased dramatically; initially due to the early detection and treatment of arrhythmias, and later to advanced hemodynamic monitoring, and the use of cardiac medications such as thrombolytics and vasoactive drips (Armstrong et al., 1998; Braunwald & Antman, 1997).

Standard admission orders for patients with suspected MI should facilitate early, rapid decision making, monitoring the patient's response to acute interventions and observing for and treating complications. Data considerations in the admission orders should focus on continuous ECG monitoring, invasive cardiac monitoring depending on patient acuity, frequency of vital sign measurement, intake and output, and daily weights. Appropriate diagnostic and laboratory tests may include a 12-lead ECG, chest radiograph, serum markers of MI, electrolytes, glucose, creatinine, BUN, a baseline lipid panel, coagulation studies, arterial blood gases, and urinalysis. Standard therapies should include IV fluids, nutrition, management of pain and anxiety, anticoagulation if indicated, treatment of nausea or vomiting, stool softeners, and ensuring adequate sleep cycles. The patient should remain NPO until pain free and then progress to a Healthy Heart diet. Emergency drugs, such as epinephrine, a defibrillator, and pacemakers should be available at all times. ACE inhibitors are usually started early to prevent LV remodeling and decrease sudden death and recurrent MI (Ryan et al., 1996a). The patient should also continue on beta blockers and daily aspirin. Although physical activity should be limited for at least 12 hours, a plan should be made to increase activity gradually based on the patient's condition and functional status. The interdisciplinary team should ask the patient about his or her preferences for resuscitation and life support in the event of a cardiac arrest and should ask whether the patient has an advance directive.

Continuous cardiac monitoring, which includes ST-segment monitoring if available, should be initiated immediately and continued for at least 24 to 48 hours or until the patient is event free for 12 to 24 hours (Drew & Krucoff, 1999). The risk of reinfarction and death in the patient with acute MI is highest in the first 24 hours after infarction (Ryan et al., 1996a). Five lead wires are typically used to monitor the patient. An electrode is placed on the right arm, the left arm, the right leg, the left leg, and the chest. Accurate lead placement is illustrated in Figure 26- 5 (Drew, 1993). When five leads are used, only one precordial lead can be selected. This lead may be either V1 or V6. V1 is the preferred choice of precordial leads because it allows for detection of right bundle-branch block (RBBB) and the distinction between ventricular tachycardia (VT) and supraventricular tachycardia (SVT) (Drew, 1993). Many cardiac monitors have the capability to display two leads simultaneously. In this case, a precordial lead and a limb lead, such as lead II, may be monitored.

ST-segment abnormalities may be seen in select leads depending on the area of ischemia and injury. The lead chosen for monitoring in the patient with an MI should reflect area of ischemia and location of the coronary artery occlusion (Drew, 1991). The 12-lead ECG, taken during the initial period after an MI, provides the best information about which leads to monitor. For example, the most sensitive leads in detecting ischemia caused by an occlusion of the right coronary artery are leads II, III, and aVF (Tisdale & Drew, 1993).

Many monitors provide capability for ST-segment monitoring at the bedside. ST-segment deviation is the number of millimeters the ST segment is displaced from the isoelectric line. ST-segment displacement of a minimum of 1 mm from the patient's baseline or isoelectric line for at least 1 minute is indicative of ischemia (Tisdale & Drew, 1993). ST-segment monitoring may assist in detecting silent ischemia, recurrent ischemia after an MI as well as the effectiveness of reperfusion therapy. ST-segment monitoring may also provide the means to assess the effect of nursing care and self-care activities on the incidence of ischemia (Bell, 1992). Moreover, absence of ischemic events during activities may support transfer from ICU or early discharge from the hospital (Drew & Krucoff, 1999).

IV access is required for drug administration and blood draws if the patient has received thrombolytic therapy. As one or more stable IV lines are established, blood for laboratory tests can be obtained through the IV catheter to prevent additional venipuncture sites that may bleed after thrombolytic therapy. One IV catheter may be capped to provide access for direct blood sampling and a saline flush can be injected every 8 hours and after medication administration to maintain patency. If thrombolytic or vasoactive agents are infusing, an additional IV catheter is needed for administration of pain medications and emergency cardiac drugs. For the patient admitted to the CCU with an IV line in place, the line's patency, the conditions under which it was inserted, and the appropriateness of the site should be assessed. The insertion site should be inspected daily for signs of infection.

Oxygen therapy is beneficial for MI patients who are hypoxemic. Hypoxia is common in patients with acute MI and is usually the result of ventilation-perfusion abnormalities (Fillmore, Shapiro & Killip, 1970). Some evidence suggests that oxygen therapy may reduce ischemia and limit infarct size (Maroko, Radvany, Braunwald, & Hale, 1975). If the patient's oxygen saturation is less than 90% or if overt pulmonary edema is present, supplemental oxygen therapy should be given (Ryan et al., 1996a, b).

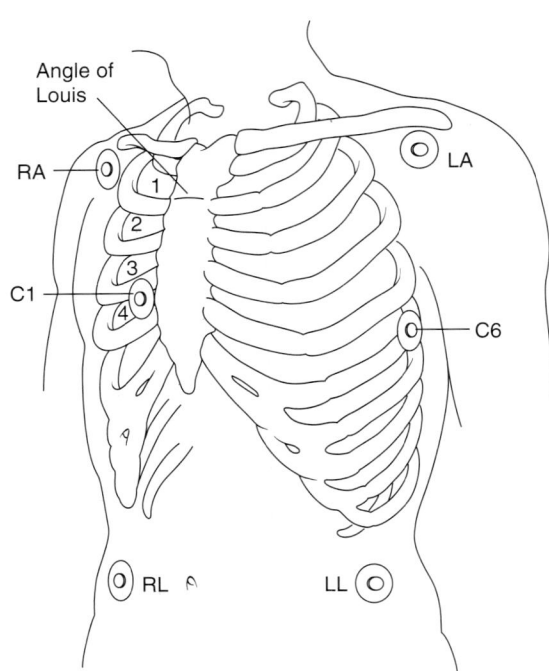

■ **Figure 26–5.** Proper electrode placement for obtaining V_1, as well as the six limb leads. Electrodes designated for the limbs are placed close to where each limb joins the torso, and the chest electrode is placed in the fourth intercostal space at the right sternal border (C_1). Because patients vary with respect to body shape, it is difficult to palpate the first intercostal space with any accuracy. Thus, the fourth intercostal space is located by first palpating the little bony prominence, called the angle of Louis, where the body of the sternum joins the manubrium. This rise in the sternum identifies the second rib, and the space below it is the second intercostal space. To obtain V_6, the chest electrode is moved to the mid-axillary line at the level of the fifth intercostal space (C_6). (From Drew, B. J. [1993]. Bedside electrocardiogram monitoring. *AACN Clinical Issues,* 4[1], 26.)

Although the CCU may have limited access for visitors, family presence is frequently important to the patient's recovery and provides continuity for care at home. Liberalized visiting policies can be helpful for many patients. Family visits have not been found to have a greater negative impact on heart rate, BP, or the occurrence of ventricular ectopy than other social situations (Simpson, 1990).

Length of stay in the CCU is based on the patient's condition. Patients without history of previous MI and without complications such as CHF, postinfarction angina, hypotension, and heart block, may transfer out of the ICU in 24 to 36 hours (Antman & Braunwald, 2001a, b). After the stay in the CCU, the patient may be transferred to a telemetry unit where they may gradually increase their physical activity with close monitoring of heart rate, BP, and symptoms. Low-risk patients without ECG changes and ongoing chest pain may be admitted directly to an intermediate or general telemetry unit.

The development and implementation of clinical pathways and practice guidelines represent an attempt to provide high-quality care and to reduce the costs associated with unnecessary tests and treatments. Clinical pathways and care maps reflect optimal management strategies as defined by a consensus of "experts" in a particular health care organization and outline goals for the patient as well as ideal sequencing and timing of interventions to meet goals with maximal efficiency (Pearson, Goulart-Fischer & Lee, 1995). The purpose of critical pathways is to (1) reduce practice variation; (2) minimize delay in treatment; (3) decrease resource use; and (4) improve or maintain the quality of care (Ireson, 1997). The critical pathway also serves as a tool for planning interdisciplinary care. An example of a critical pathway for complicated acute MI can be seen in Table 26-6 (Becker, 2001).

Clinical practice guidelines provide evidence-based recommendations for care of patients with specific conditions. These clinical practice guidelines provide a framework for the standardization of care for patients with acute MI, based on clinical evidence of effective diagnosis and treatment as well as expert opinion. Guidelines are "evidence based" and define optimal care in terms of quality and cost. The American Heart Association and the American College of Cardiology initially developed practice guidelines for the management of patients with acute MI in 1990, and the guidelines have been updated every 5 years. The guidelines are intended as a guide for management rather than a strict prescription and are to be altered based on clinical judgment, individual patient needs, and new findings (Ryan et al., 1996b).

Pain Management

Pain management is a priority for the patient with acute MI. Pain management strategies focus on increasing oxygen supply to the heart and reducing oxygen demand. Interventions include nitrates, narcotic analgesics, oxygen therapy, and beta blockers in conjunction with reperfusion therapies such as thrombolysis and PCI. Sublingual nitroglycerin may be tried first if the patient's systolic BP is greater than or equal to 90 and the heart rate is between 50 and 100 beats per minute (Ryan et al., 1996a). Nitrates cause dilation of the coronary arteries, enhance collateral flow to the ischemic myocardium, and dilate the venous bed, which decreases ventricular preload

and reduces coronary spasm. Long-acting nitrates should be avoided in the management of early MI; therefore, an IV nitroglycerin drip may be initiated. Nitroglycerin, however, should not be used as a substitute for narcotic analgesics (Ryan et al., 1996b). Morphine sulfate relieves pain and anxiety and reduces the patient's restlessness. Morphine also reduces the activity of the sympathetic nervous system with a resultant decrease in myocardial oxygen consumption by a decrease in heart rate and BP. It also dilates the venous and arterial bed, reduces ventricular preload, and may relieve symptoms of pulmonary edema (Abrams, 1995). Morphine sulfate may be given in doses of 2 to 4 mg IV every 5 minutes until the pain is relieved or problematic side effects such as respiratory depression or hypotension occur. Some patients require as much as 25 to 30 mg IV to relieve pain and anxiety. Morphine-related hypotension is mainly seen in the setting of orthostatic volume depletion and may be prevented by maintaining the patient in a supine position as tolerated (Antman & Braunwald, 2001a). In patients with morphine sensitivity, the patient may receive IV meperidine.

Physical Activity

The plan for physical activity after acute MI should be individualized based on the patient's condition. Specific activities should be stopped for increasing shortness of breath, patient's perception of fatigue, or increase in heart rate of greater than 20 to 30 beats per minute (Antman & Braunwald, 2001a). In general, patients with uncomplicated MI should not be confined to bed for more than 12 hours if they are hemodynamically stable. After 12 hours, the patient who is hemodynamically stable may transfer from bed to chair and remain in the chair for 1 to 2 hours per day. The patient without complications may bathe and perform personal care activities within the first 24 hours and may shower after the third day (Antman & Braunwald, 2001a).

The patient should use a bedside commode rather than a bedpan (Winslow, Lane, & Gaffney, 1984). The position one assumes when using a commode is more natural and allows for appropriate and optimal use of the muscles of defecation (abdominal and rectal), which may reduce the resultant straining usually associated with the Valsalva maneuver. Therefore, the use of the commode is recommended for patients without specific contraindications to postural change. Stool softeners should also be given to avoiding straining while defecating.

Coronary Precautions

"Coronary precautions," introduced in the 1960s, have been widely practiced despite a lack of literature to support their use (Riegel, Thomason, Carlson & Gocka, 1996). Examples of coronary precautions include the limitation of hot and iced fluids, avoidance of rectal temperatures, limitation of caffeine beverage, and avoidance of the Valsalva maneuver. The only "coronary precaution" supported by literature is avoidance of the Valsalva maneuver. In the Valsalva maneuver, air is trapped in the lungs by a closed glottis and intrathoracic pressure increased by expiratory mechanisms, causing sudden and intense changes in systolic BP and heart rate. Increased intrathoracic pressure results in a decreased venous return to

Table 26–6 ▪ ACUTE CARDIAC CARE-INTERDISCIPLINARY MANAGEMENT PATHWAY

Diagnosis	ST Segment Elevation/Bundle Block MI					
	Day 0 Emergency Department	**Day 0 CCU**	**Day 1 CCU**	**Day 2* Step Down Unit**	**Day 3* Step Down Unit**	**Pre-Discharge***
Assesment	• Vitals • Continuous ECG monitoring • Secure venous access	• Vitals q2-4° • Continuous ECG monitoring	• Vitals q4° • Continuous ECG monitoring	• Vitals q8°	• Vitals q8°	• Vitals AM
Benchmark	• Reperfusion Rx* • Salvage myocardium • Treat arrhythmias • Maintain hemodynamic stability	• Pain relief* • Hemodynamically stable • Oxygenating	• Afebrile* • Hemodynamically stable • Oxygenating	• No recurrent chest pain++ • No sign of CHF • No arrhythmias	• Ambulating without difficulty	• Discuss EMS options • Discuss recommendation for seeking medical care
Medication	• ±fibrinolytic • β-blocker • Aspirin • Unfractionated Heparin	• Hepanin • Aspirin • β-blocker • ACE-Inhibitor • Statin	• Heparin (SC) • Aspirin • β-blocker • ACE-Inhibitor • Statin	• Aspirin • β-blocker • ACE-Inhibitor • Statin	• Aspirin • β-blocker • ACE-Inhibitor • Statin	• Medication education • Prescriptions (Including sublingual nitroglycerin)
Laboratory Tests	• CBC • Chemistry profile • CK, CK-MB ±Troponin • Lipid profile • INR/aPTT	• CBC • Selected chemistries • CK, CK-MB q8° × 3 • aPTT	• CBC • Selected chemistries	• Selected chemistries	• Selected chemistries	• Fasting lipid profile • CRP 4 weeks post-discharge
Diagnostic/ Interventional Procedures	• 12-lead ECG • ±echocardiogram • ±coronary anglography • ±IABP (for shock)	• 12-lead ECG • ±echocardiogram • ±coronary anglography • ±IABP (for shock)	• 12-lead ECG	• 12-lead ECG	• Modified ETT • ± coronary anglography • ±echocardiogram	• Standard ETT 2 weeks post-discharge
Nutrition Activity Case Management	• NPO • Bed rest • Notify primary care physician • Notify case manager	• NPO • Bed rest • Notify social services	• AHA Step II • Bed to chair • Cardiac rehabilitation consult	• AHA Step II • Ambulate • Lipid management • Family education • Smoking cessation	• AHA Step II • Routine activity • Nutrition consult	• AHA Step II • Routine activity • Discuss medication/ Insurance coverage • Notify primary care physician • Schedule return visit

From Becker, R. L. (2001). Complicated myocardial infarction. In C. P. Cannon, & P. T. O' Gana (Eds.). *Critical pathways in cardiology* (p. 115). Philadelphia: Lippincott Williams & Wilkins.
* = Noncomplicated MI.
CBC = Complete blood count; CK = creatine kinase; IABP = intra-aortic balloon pump; NPO = nothing by mouth; aPTT = activated partial thromboplastin time; CHF = congestive heart failure; ACE = angiotensin converting enzyme; ETT = exercise tolerance test; CRP = C-reactive protein.

the heart (decreased preload), decreased stroke volume, decreased cardiac output, and increased heart rate and peripheral vasoconstriction. When the forced air is released, the intrathoracic pressure is decreased, and preload is increased, resulting in increased workload for the heart.

Diet

The patient may eat unassisted with his or her back and arms supported. Eating, and other low-level activities such as toileting and positioning are safe for most patients after acute MI because they require low energy expenditure (Reigel, Thomason & Carlson, 1996). The patient should follow the AHA Step II

diet, which is low in saturated fat (Ryan et al., 1996a; Ryan et al., 1999). The patient's diet should consist of foods high in fiber, potassium, and magnesium (except in the presence of renal failure) and low in sodium, and should include plenty of fresh fruits and vegetables.

The literature does not support limiting beverages containing caffeine. BP changes related to caffeine consumption are not significant until at least 400 mg of caffeine is consumed. Moderate consumption of caffeine does not increase the likelihood of ventricular arrhythmias or coronary events (Lynn & Kissinger, 1992). People who routinely drink caffeinated beverages develop a tolerance, and withdrawal from caffeine can cause headaches and an increase in heart rate (Ryan et al., 1996b).

Treatment of Hemodynamic Disturbances

Treatment of hemodynamic disturbances is critical in the management of the patient with MI. After acute MI, patients may be classified into one of four hemodynamic subsets: (1) normal perfusion (cardiac output) and no pulmonary congestion (normal PAWP); (2) normal perfusion and pulmonary artery congestion (high PAWP); (3) low perfusion (low cardiac output) without pulmonary congestion; and (4) low perfusion (low cardiac output) and pulmonary congestion (high PAWP; Forrester, Diamond, & Chatterjee, 1976a; 1976b). Therapy is tailored to the patient's hemodynamic profile, and the patient may move between hemodynamic subsets as a result of therapy. In all cases, therapies are designed to maintain ventricular performance, support hemodynamics, and protect the ischemic myocardium by decreasing the workload on the heart and optimizing oxygen delivery.

Right heart catheterization at the bedside with a pulmonary artery catheter may provide valuable diagnostic information in select patients with hemodynamic disturbances. Indications for insertion of a pulmonary artery catheter in the patient after acute MI include (1) hypotension not corrected by volume administration; (2) hypotension in the presence of CHF; (3) hemodynamic compromise requiring vasoactive drugs or balloon counterpulsation; (4) mechanical lesions such as cardiac tamponade, severe mitral valve regurgitation, RV infarction, or ruptured ventricular septum (Antman & Braunwald, 1997; Mueller et al., 1998). Use of a pulmonary artery catheter may also be helpful in distinguishing between cardiac and noncardiac etiologies of pulmonary edema.

Limitation of Infarct Size

Strategies to limit infarct size and decrease morbidity and mortality after acute MI include early reperfusion and reducing myocardial oxygen demands (Antman & Braunwald, 2001).[AQ58] Early reperfusion with thrombolytics, primary PTCA, or CABG results in restored blood flow to the myocardium and improved hemodynamics. Restored blood flow prevents the extension of the existing infarction and reinfarction. Therapies that reduce myocardial oxygen demands include beta blockers, pain relief and sedation, and providing the patient with a restful quiet environment. Hypertension and tachycardias increase myocardial oxygen demand and place the patient at risk. Associated clinical conditions that increase myocardial oxygen demand, such as fever and infection, should be treated.

Other therapies may improve the supply of oxygen to the myocardium. Supplemental oxygen has been shown to decrease acute ischemia injury and development of myocardial necrosis in an experimental model (Maroko et al., 1975). Supplemental oxygen is recommended for all patients with acute MI for the first 2 to 3 hours and in patients with arterial oxygen saturation levels less than 90% and overt pulmonary congestion (Ryan et al., 1996b). Anemia may reduce oxygen delivery to the heart and should be treated promptly. The administration of IV nitroglycerin during acute MI has also been found to limit infarct size and improve LV function (Hennekens, Albert, Godfried, Gaziano & Burning, 1996).

Treatment of Right Ventricular Infarction

The presence of RV infarction associated with inferior MI has been associated with an in-hospital mortality seven to eight times that of patients with inferior MI alone (Zehender & Kaspar, 1993). RV infarction is also an independent predictor of mortality in elderly patients with the first inferior MI (Bueno et al., 1997). Early diagnosis is key to effective treatment. A right precordial ECG should be obtained on all patients presenting with signs and symptoms of an inferior MI because RV involvement has been associated with inferior MI in up to 50% of cases (Kinch & Ryan, 1994).

The treatment of RV MI differs in some aspects from that of LV MI and may include (1) early reperfusion with thrombolytics or PCI; (2) volume administration to maintain RV preload; (3) the administration of inotropic medications such as dobutamine; (4) the reduction of RV afterload; and (5) the insertion of a pacemaker in cases of AV block. The administration of fluids increases cardiac output by increasing RV preload. Drugs that are typically used in the setting of LV infarction, such as nitroglycerin and diuretics, may decrease cardiac output and cause hypotension and should be avoided (Ryan et al., 1999). If the cardiac output has not improved after 1 to 2 L of fluid, inotropic drugs such as dobutamine or dopamine should be administered (Ryan et al., 1996). Dobutamine may markedly improve RV and LV systolic performance through improved contractility of hypokinetic wall segments (Dell' Italia, Starling, & Blumhardt 1985).

The reduction of RV afterload, in the setting of LV dysfunction, by reducing LV afterload may also improve cardiac output. Judicious use of vasodilators such as sodium nitroprusside has been recommended to increase the pressure gradient from the right to left side of the heart, thereby promoting passive flow through the pulmonary vascular system and increasing LV filling (Cohn, Guiha, Broder, & Limas, 1974; Kinch & Ryan, 1994). Sodium nitroprusside dilates both the pulmonary and the systemic vascular bed and decreases LV and RV afterload (Yager, 1996). In the setting of LV dysfunction, the use of an IABP may improve cardiac output by decreasing LV afterload and improving LV performance, thereby decreasing RV afterload and improving forward flow (Ryan et al., 1996).

Patients with RV infarction are predisposed to sinus bradycardia and high-grade AV block (Wellens, 1993). AV pacing is considered optimal. An external pacemaker may be used in emergency situations. Preservation of synchronous atrial contraction ("atrial kick") is considered especially important in RV infarction for three reasons: (1) to maintain adequate RV preload by maximizing presystolic stretch of damaged RV myocardial fibers, (2) to propel blood forward into the pulmonary circuit in the absence of effective RV contraction, and (3) to avoid further pericardial restriction by preventing simultaneous atrial and ventricular diastole. Up to one third of patients with RV infarction my experience atrial fibrillation due to atrial infarction or right atrial chamber enlargement (Kinch & Ryan, 1994). These patients should be cardioverted as soon as possible to preserve atrial function and optimize cardiac output.

Discharge Planning

Discharge planning and teaching should begin early in the patient's hospital stay. Before discharge, patients should receive detailed instructions regarding follow-up medical care, including activity and exercise, diet, medications, risk factor modification, and when to seek help. The patient should receive extensive education about discharge medications. Discharge medications for patients without contraindications should include a beta blocker, aspirin, and an ACE inhibitor. A lipid-lowering medication (a statin, a bile acid sequestrant, or nicotinic acid) may be prescribed in patients with a low density lipoprotein (LDL) greater than 130mg/dL with the goal of reducing the LDL to below 100mg/dl (Grundy et al., 1997). Patients should be counseled to follow an AHA step II diet, which is low in saturated fat and cholesterol. The diet should also consist of foods high in potassium (fruits and vegetables), magnesium (green, leafy vegetables, whole grains, beans, seafood), and fiber (fresh fruit and vegetables, whole grain breads and cereals). The nurse should advise patients to avoid lifting and any activity that elicits symptoms. During the acute phase, the nurse may also begin teaching about risk factor modification including smoking cessation (see Chapters 36 through 44).

The ACC/AHA guidelines for treatment of acute MI recommend a stress ECG before discharge for individual risk and functional assessment. The patient may undergo submaximal exercise testing at 4 to 6 days after AMI or symptom limited at 10 to 14 days (Gibbons et al., 2002). Many patients are referred to a cardiac rehabilitation program. Cardiac rehabilitation is the process of actively assisting the cardiac patient to achieve and maintain optimal health. Components of a cardiac rehabilitation program include a specific and individualized plan for and close monitoring of physical activity. Many cardiac rehabilitation programs include education and support for patient and family education and risk factor modification (see Chapters 36 through 44).

Pharmacologic Management

Aspirin

Actions/Indications. Platelet activity is increased in the setting of acute MI. Platelets are initially involved in thrombus at the site of the ruptured atherosclerotic plaque (Anderson & Willerson, 1993). Aspirin inhibits cyclooxygenase-dependent aggregation and inhibits platelet activity (ISIS-4 Collaborative Group, 1995). Moreover, aspirin appears to damage platelets permanently, and restoration of normal hemostatic function occurs only after the damaged platelets have been replaced by normal ones (2 to 7 days).

The International Study of Infarct Survival (ISIS-4 Collaborative Group, 1995) trial found that the administration of 162 mg of enteric-coated aspirin alone resulted in a 23% reduction in the odds of death compared with placebo in the setting of acute MI. The risk of reinfarction, cardiac arrest, and stroke were also significantly reduced in the group receiving aspirin alone. This study demonstrated reduced mortality rates when aspirin was used in conjunction with streptokinase. Aspirin is commonly given at 81 to 325 mg per day. Patients with suspected MI or UA should receive aspirin immediately upon presentation and should continue to take it indefinitely. Chewing the aspirin tablet in the acute phase of MI can accelerate absorption into the blood and hasten the antiplatelet effect (Feldman & Cryer, 1999). In

patients who are allergic to aspirin or who fail to achieve platelet inhibition with aspirin, clopidogrel (Plavix), a thienopyridine platelet inhibitor, can be prescribed (see Chapter 27).

Contraindications/Adverse Reactions. Aspirin is contraindicated for patients with known sensitivity to the drug, history of GI bleeding and intrinsic coagulation defects.

Nursing Implications. Aspirin may be taken with meals to avoid gastric irritation. The nurse should teach the patient to monitor possible sites for bleeding. The clinician may follow the patient's hemoglobin and/or hematocrit levels on a periodic basis.

Heparin

Action/Indications. Heparin is an antithrombotic agent that prevents coagulation by interfering with the formation of thrombin from prothrombin, and preventing thrombin from supporting or allowing the conversion of fibrinogen to fibrin. Although it has no effect on existing clots, heparin does interfere with platelet function and is the anticoagulant of choice to treat MI as well as IHD, pulmonary emboli, and deep vein thrombosis (Casey, Bedker & Roussel-McElmeel, 1998). The accumulation of thrombin at sites of endothelial injury promotes platelet aggregation, vasoconstriction, and the conversion of fibrinogen to fibrin. When administered in conjunction with aspirin, heparin has been shown to reduce the frequency of MI when given to patients in the acute phase of UA (Antman & Braunwald, 2001a; Willerson, 1998). The goal of heparin therapy is to prevent the extension of thrombus. With UFH administered IV, the therapeutic activated partial thromboplastin time (aPTT) threshold (1.5 to 2.0 times the control value) should be reached within 24 hours of initiating therapy.

Heparin is used in non–ST-segment elevation MI, and acute MI. Standard unfractionated heparin (UFH) has pharmacokinetic limitations that LMWH does not. For example, UFH has a variable anticoagulant response, requiring frequent monitoring of the aPTT, hemoglobin, hematocrit, and platelets, and is more commonly associated with heparin-induced thrombocytopenia (Ibbotson & Goa, 2002). There is no need to monitor coagulation values while using LMWH because it has a more stable, reliable anticoagulant effect (Antman & Braunwald, 2001a, b; Braunwald et al., 2000). Another advantage to LMWH is that it is administered subcutaneously, twice daily, as compared with the continuous IV infusion required for UFH. LMWH is, however, associated with a higher incidence of minor bleeding than UFH (Ibbotson & Goa, 2002).

Contraindications/Adverse Reactions. Heparin may be contraindicated in patients with heparin allergy, acute cerebrovascular accident, or a history of life-threatening GI bleeding, or who are thrombocytopenic or coagulopathic on another basis. Heparin can induce thrombocytopenia, and patients should be monitored for this. LMWH can also produce minor bleeding.

Nursing Implications. A baseline aPTT should be obtained before therapy with UFH is begun, 6 hours after therapy is initiated, any time a dose change occurs, and every 6 hours until the therapeutic level is obtained on two consecutive aPTTs. The aPTT may then be drawn every 24 hours for 3 days. Therapy should be discontinued after 3 to 5 days or if bleeding occurs. Patients receiving heparin, particularly UFH, therapy should be frequently assessed for hemorrhage and thrombocytopenia. A baseline platelet count and hemoglobin and hematocrit should be obtained and monitored daily with the use of UFH. Hemodynamic monitoring may aid in the early detection of occult hemorrhage. Heparin should not be abruptly discontinued because MI can develop quickly, especially in the absence of aspirin.

There is no routine monitoring associated with the use of LMWH.

Nitrates

In the setting of acute MI, nitrates are effective in treating ischemic chest pain and hypertension and reducing pulmonary congestion. Nitrates decrease preload by peripheral vasodilatation and decrease afterload at higher doses by arterial vasodilatation. In the coronary circulation, nitrates dilate the coronary arteries and collateral vessels. Nitroglycerin may also inhibit platelet activation and aggregation (Abrams, 1995). Despite the effectiveness of nitrates in the treatment of ischemic chest pain, at least two large studies have failed to find a reduction in mortality associated with the use of nitrates after acute MI. In ISIS-4, patients who presented within 24 hours of onset of symptoms were randomized to oral controlled-release isosorbide mononitrate or placebo. A nonsignificant 3% reduction in mortality was found at 35 days (ISIS-4 Collaborative Group, 1995). In GISSI 3, patients were randomized to IV nitroglycerin for 24 hours followed by transdermal nitroglycerin or usual care. Mortality in the nitrate group was reduced by 6%, which was not significant. However, patients experienced lower rates of postinfarction angina (p = 0.033) and reduced rates of cardiogenic shock (p = 0.009) (Gruppo Italiano per lo Studio della Sopravvivenza nell' Infarto Miocardico, 1994). Nitroglycerin is recommended for the first 24 to 48 hours in patients with acute MI and CHF, persistent ischemia, or hypertension and beyond 48 hours in patients with recurrent angina or persistent pulmonary congestion (Ryan et al., 1996a). Nitroglycerin should be used with caution in patients with RV MI because it may cause a reduction in preload with associated reduction in cardiac output.

Nitrates come in a variety of preparations including IV, topical, spray, sublingual, and oral forms. IV nitroglycerin may cause severe headache and hypotension. Tolerance, which requires increased dosage of medication, may develop as soon as 12 hours after the start of the infusion. Providing a period of time without nitrates may reduce the effects of tolerance. For example, a nitroglycerin patch should be worn for only 12 to 14 hours followed by a patch-free interval of 10 to 12 hours (Abrams, 1995).

Beta-blocking Agents

Action/Indications. The cardiovascular system's response to catecholamines is mediated by specific cell membrane receptors. The action of a specific beta blocker is determined by the type and site of receptor with which it interacts. Stimulation of β_1 receptors, which are located primarily in the myocardium, increases cardiac contractility, sinus discharge rate, and AV node conduction velocity, and decreases AV node refractoriness. Stimulation of β_2 receptors, the predominant β-adrenergic receptor in vascular and bronchial tissue, mediates arteriolar dilation and bronchial smooth muscle relaxation. Beta blockers are used in the management of angina and after MI because of their ability to inhibit the chronotropic and inotropic responses to catecholamines. Their use has been shown to improve postinfarction survival rates, and decrease infarct size when administered immediately after MI (Andresen, Ehlers, Wiedman & Bruggemann, 1999; Antman & Braunwald, 2001; Gibbons et al., 1999).

Blocking sympathetic stimulation of beta-adrenergic receptors decreases myocardial contractility, slows the heart rate, and decreases systolic BP, decreasing myocardial oxygen demand (Casey et al., 1998). A slower heart rate also provides a longer diastole, thereby increasing coronary artery blood flow and myocardial oxygen supply. Beta blockers are classified by cardioselectivity, duration of action, membrane-stabilizing activities, and lipophilic properties. β_1-selective beta blockers, such as atenolol, esmolol, and metoprolol, are considered "cardioselective" and are recommended for use in patients who have a history of obstructive pulmonary disease or mild CHF because they are less likely to cause bronchospasm. Certain beta blockers (i.e., propranolol and metoprolol) have the secondary properties of inhibiting platelet aggregation and desensitizing activated platelets. Beta blockers are classified as class II antiarrhythmics according to the Vaughn Williams' classification (see Chapter 19) and are initial therapy in stable angina (Gibbons et al., 1999). Propranolol, nadolol, timolol, atenolol, esmolol, and labetalol are a few examples of beta-adrenergic receptor blocking agents.

Contraindications/Adverse Reactions. The use of beta blockers is contraindicated in patients with moderate to severe CHF, pulmonary edema, LV dysfunction, obstructive pulmonary disease, cardiogenic shock, severe peripheral vascular disease, and in patients with a history of depression (Andresen et al., 1999; Antman & Braunwald, 2001a, b). In patients with impaired LV function, CHF may occur or intensify, although it may be controlled with the use of digitalis or diuretics. The use of beta blockers is contraindicated in variant angina because coronary artery spasm is likely to worsen. Caution should be used when administering beta blockers to patients with first-degree AV block, a bifascicular block, or sick sinus syndrome. Chronic administration of beta blockers has been associated with unfavorable effects on plasma lipid and lipoprotein levels, including a decrease in high-density lipoprotein cholesterol. Some adverse reactions associated with beta-blocker therapy include bradycardia, heart block, bronchospasm, fatigue, dyspepsia, diarrhea or constipation, mental disturbances such as mood changes, and nightmares. Beta blockers can also intensify the hypoglycemia produced by insulin and oral hypoglycemic agents (Gibbons et al., 1999).

Nursing Implications. When beta blockade is initiated, a patient should have continuous ECG monitoring. The target heart rate is 50 to 60 beats per minute, although the medication should not be initiated if the heart rate is less than 60 beats per minute. Beta blockers should be avoided if the PR interval is more than 0.24 second, or if second- or third-degree AV block is present. Because a major effect of beta blockade is a decrease in systolic BP, patients must be monitored for hypotension, and therapy should not be initiated if systolic BP is less than 90 mm Hg. Beta blockers should not be administered to patients with known or suspected coronary artery vasospasm because they allow unopposed alpha-adrenergic stimulation and may intensify the frequency and severity of coronary artery spasm. Nurses must be aware that sudden withdrawal of beta blockers may result in exaggerated cardiac beta-adrenergic responsiveness, producing an exacerbation of angina and precipitating arrhythmias or acute MI. The mechanism for the rebound effect after abrupt withdrawal is unknown, although it is likely related to increased myocardial sensitivity to catecholamines on the removal of beta blockade. Elderly patients may have occult sinus or AV node disease unmasked by the use of beta blockers and, therefore, must be monitored carefully on initiation of therapy and followed closely for signs of conduction delay (Olson & Aronow, 1996). Patients of Chinese descent tend to have an increased sensitivity to beta blockers and, therefore, may have good results achieved with lower-than-expected doses. Beta blockers are generally avoided in people with insulin-dependent diabetes mellitus because symptoms of hypoglycemia may be masked or hypoglycemia may be intensified by their use. Their use in non–insulin-dependent diabetes mellitus is considered more appropriate because hypoglycemia is less of a threat.

Angiotensin-Converting Enzyme (ACE) Inhibitors

Action/Indications. Angiotensin-converting enzyme inhibitors are a class of drug that blocks the conversion of angiotensin I, which is a weak vasoconstrictor, to angiotensin II, a potent vasoconstrictor. Their use in acute MI has been shown to reduce postinfarction mortality rates if therapy is begun within 24 hours of hospital admission (Casey et al., 1998), and their effects are even better when administered in conjunction with aspirin and beta blockers (Antman & Braunwald, 2001a, b). Their vasodilating effects help to reduce afterload, thereby reducing the work of the heart. They have also been shown to prevent or retard development of LV dysfunction. They show maximum benefit in high-risk patients, and short-term benefits when administered to all hemodynamically stable acute MI patients. The use of ACE inhibitors has been shown to decrease ventricular remodeling that occurs with MI, and decrease the risk of CHF, and possibly even recurrent infarction (Antman & Braunwald, 2001a, b). Pepine (2000) suggests the use of ACE inhibitors in patients with CAD for long-term prophylaxis, and states that diabetics and those with LV dysfunction can also benefit from their use. Long-term use (6 to 12 months) of ACE inhibitors may improve the endothelium in abnormal segments of coronary arteries. There is little evidence to support their use in UA or NSTEMI (Antman & Braunwald, 2001a, b). Examples of ACE inhibitors include captopril, enalapril, quinapril, and lisinopril.

Contraindications/Adverse Reactions. ACE inhibitors should be used very cautiously in patients who are hemodynamically unstable, particularly in the presence of hypovolemia, because the vasodilation caused with ACE inhibitor therapy can produce a marked hypotension. If diuretic dosages are decreased during the first 48 to 72 hours of initiating ACE inhibitor therapy, hypotension can often be avoided. Cautious use of ACE inhibitors is recommended for patients with renal insufficiency. Therapy is contraindicated in patients with renal artery stenosis because very rapid and significant elevations of creatinine levels may occur. In general, therapy can be initiated safely if serum creatinine is less than 2.5 mg/dL.

Nursing Implications. Before initiation of therapy, a baseline serum creatinine level should be drawn and baseline BP obtained. It is of utmost importance that patients receiving ACE inhibitor therapy be monitored closely for hypotension, especially on initiation of therapy. Serum creatinine levels should also be monitored closely, and a significant elevation in serum creatinine should receive prompt attention.

Calcium Antagonists

Action/Indications. Calcium antagonists, or calcium channel blockers, are sometimes considered for patients with stable angina, UA or NSTEMI, and contraindications to beta blockers. They are potent vasodilators that block the calcium inflow in smooth muscle cells, dilating coronary arteries and thereby increasing myocardial oxygen supply. Some calcium antagonists decrease heart rate and AV node conduction rate, increasing diastolic filling time and thereby increasing myocardial oxygen supply. They effectively decrease myocardial oxygen demand by decreasing SVR and myocardial contractility. Calcium antagonists are also thought to interfere with thrombus formation by reducing platelet aggregation.

Calcium antagonists are usually considered a better choice than beta blockers for patients with asthma or COPD. Diltiazem and verapamil should be avoided in patients with bradycardia or heart block because of their negative chronotropic effects, but remain good choices for patients with tachycardia (Braunwald et al., 2000). The relaxation of coronary arteries may be especially beneficial in patients with Prinzmetal's angina, and short-acting nifedipine is used acutely in conjunction with nitroglycerin in this population. They are also beneficial in the long-term management of Prinzmetal's angina (Antman & Braunwald, 2001a, b). Nifedipine, amlodipine, nicardipine, verapamil, and diltiazem are a few examples of calcium channel blocking agents.

Calcium antagonists are not recommended in acute MI because, in multiple clinical trials, they have not shown a decrease in morbidity and mortality in this population (Antman & Braunwald, 2001a, b). Calcium antagonists are only used in stable angina when beta blockers are contraindicated, or when unacceptable side effects of beta blockers have occurred (Gibbons et al., 1999). In UA and NSTEMI, they are used to control persistent ischemia in patients who are already receiving beta blockers and nitrates, or in patients who are unable to tolerate one or both of those medications (Braunwald et al., 2000).

Contraindications/Adverse Reactions. Calcium channel agents should be avoided in patients with evidence of significant LV dysfunction (LV ejection fraction <40%), and pulmonary edema. There is an increase in adverse reactions in patients receiving short-acting dihydropyridines (nifedipine) if adequate beta blockade is not present (Braunwald et al., 2000). Adverse reactions include dizziness, headache, flushing, peripheral edema, bradycardia, or LV dysfunction.

Nursing Implications. As with beta blockers, when therapy with calcium antagonists is initiated, patients should receive continuous ECG monitoring and be closely monitored for hypotension and conduction disturbances. Unlike beta blockers, calcium channel agents can be used safely in patients with COPD, and their vasodilating effects may be critical in patients with Prinzmetal's angina.

Glycoprotein IIb/IIIa Receptor Antagonists

Action/Indications. Glycoprotein (GP) IIb/IIIa receptor antagonists are a class of drug that prevents platelet aggregation by preventing fibrinogen binding. They facilitate thrombolysis and reduce the rate of reocclusion of reperfused vessels. GPIIb/IIIa inhibitors are particularly useful in patients with acute MI undergoing PCI, and they reduce mortality and recurrent acute MI in patients with NSTEMI (Antman & Braunwald, 2001a, b). The addition of a GPIIb/IIIa receptor antagonist (tirofiban) to standard antithrombotic therapy with aspirin and heparin in UA/NSTEMI patients was associated with a marked reduction in the rate of ischemic events in the acute phase, and there was continued benefit during the 6-month follow-up period. The benefit was greatest in those patients undergoing revascularization procedures (Theroux et al., 2000).

The currently available antagonists differ greatly in their pharmacokinetics, and there is, as yet, no study comparing one to the others, although there are large studies demonstrating the effectiveness of each of them, individually. Each trial, PURSUIT, PRISM-PLUS, and CAPTURE, studying eptifibatide, tirofiban, and abciximab, respectively, has demonstrated a statistically significant reduction in mortality rate as well as the rate of MI during the phase of medical management, although the reduction in event rates was greatest at the time of PCI (Braunwald et al., 2000). Aspirin has been administered with the GPIIb/IIIa inhibitor in all trials, and LMWH is currently being studied for use with these agents.

Contraindications/Adverse Reactions. The risk of bleeding is increased, particularly at the vascular access site. The risk of thrombocytopenia is rare, but present.

Nursing Implications. Monitoring of hemoglobin, hematocrit, and platelet counts should be carried out daily during therapy. The vascular access site (typically the groin) should be carefully monitored for bleeding because this is one of the major adverse effects of therapy with this class of medication.

Warfarin Sodium

Actions/Indications. Warfarin sodium (Coumadin) is an oral anticoagulant that competes with vitamin K, which is essential for the liver to manufacture clotting factors II, VII, IX, and X. Warfarin is bound to albumin in the blood, with very little of the drug remaining "free." It is this free warfarin, however, that provides the drug's therapeutic effect. When initiating warfarin therapy, it is important to know that a lag time of 48 to 72 hours occurs between initiation of therapy and the achievement of therapeutic levels. This lag time signifies the gradual disappearance of the clotting factors. Warfarin is prescribed for patients who have sustained a large anterior MI with demonstrated LV thrombus or who are in persistent atrial fibrillation and require long-term anticoagulation (Lee, 2001).

Contraindications/Adverse Reactions. Patients with a history alcohol abuse, those with malignant hypertension or active tuberculosis, and patients in a job with high risk for trauma should not receive warfarin because of an increased risk of bleeding.

Nursing Implications. The effectiveness of warfarin therapy should be measured by an international normalized ratio (INR). The INR standardizes different laboratory methods for determining PT values throughout the world. A baseline INR should be drawn before therapy is initiated, and levels should be checked daily. Once a patient's response to therapy has been established, the INR can be checked less frequently depending on individual response to therapy (see Chapter 14). In patients with anterior MI and demonstration of thrombus, the INR should be 2 to 3 and warfarin is typically continued for at least 6 months.

The patient should be counseled to follow standard safety precautions: these include (1) using electric shavers rather than razors; (2) wearing gloves while gardening; (3) using a soft bristle toothbrush, and (4) avoiding contact sports. The nurse should teach the patient to check urine and stool color daily, and report epistaxis, bleeding gums, and bruising immediately. The patient should also be counseled about any medications or foods that may interact with warfarin. Warfarin should be protected from light and stored in a cool, dry place because it loses its potency when exposed to high heat.

Nursing Management Plan

Nursing management of the patient with CHD or MI may involve caring for the patient in varying stages of the disease process: during the acute chest discomfort before or during CCU admission, as the diagnosis or angina pectoris or MI is confirmed, at hospital discharge, during convalescence, or on an ongoing basis with the goal of preventing episodes of angina or another MI. The focus of this section is on the nursing management of angina pectoris or during the acute phase of MI. This section includes examples of nursing diagnoses for problems associated with angina and MI.

Chest Discomfort

Diagnosis

Chest discomfort, related to an imbalance between myocardial oxygen supply and demand, manifested by patient complaints of chest discomfort, with or without radiation to arms, neck, back, or jaw, by nonverbal expressions of discomfort (facial grimacing, Levine sign), and by increases in heart rate, BP, and respiratory rate and by cool, clammy skin.

Goals

Goals for this diagnosis include:

1. To detect chest discomfort and associated electrocardiographic and hemodynamic changes early.
2. To reduce or eliminate chest discomfort.
3. To prevent the occurrence of chest discomfort.

Interventions

Interventions are directed toward assessment and improvement of the imbalance between myocardial supply and demand. The balance between myocardial supply and demand can be improved by interventions that decrease myocardial oxygen consumption or increase coronary blood flow. Examples of nursing interventions for the hospitalized patient with angina or acute MI follow.

For Goal 1

Teach the patient to report chest discomfort immediately (based on a scale of 1 to 10, with 10 being as bad as it could be); at onset of discomfort and,

1. Assess and document the patient's description of chest discomfort, including location, radiation, duration, and the factors that affect it.
2. Assess BP, heart rate, and rhythm, and respiratory rate and rhythm.
3. Assess the skin for temperature and moistness.
4. Obtain a 12-lead ECG during chest discomfort.
5. Consider ST-segment monitoring to detect silent ischemia or to evaluate relationship between patient care activities and ischemia.
6. Report the findings of the above assessment to the physician.

For Goal 2

1. Immediately reduce patient's physical activity to the level of activity before occurrence of chest discomfort.
2. Administer oxygen, morphine sulfate, nitroglycerin, or other medications as ordered, and continuously evaluate the patient's response to therapy.
3. Provide a restful environment; and promote the patient's physical comfort by elevating head of bed to 20 to 30 degrees or higher and by individualizing basic nursing care.

For Goal 3

1. Provide care in a calm, competent manner.
2. Provide a restful, quiet environment.
3. Provide small portions of easily digested food.
4. Assist the patient with activities of daily living.
5. Teach patient to exhale with physical movement, and, as necessary, offer stool softeners and laxatives to prevent straining with bowel movements.
6. Teach patient to recognize precipitating factors and alter behavior accordingly.
7. Teach patient to practice relaxation techniques.

Outcome Criteria

Outcome criteria are written for each goal statement.

For Goal 1

Chest discomfort, changes in the 12-lead ECG, and hemodynamic responses are detected at onset.

For Goal 2

Within 5 minutes of intervention: patient states that chest discomfort is relieved or reduced; patient appears comfortable; heart and respiratory rates and BP are returning or have

---

DISPLAY 26-1

SELECTED THERAPIES TO REDUCE ISCHEMIA

Decrease Myocardial O$_2$ Consumption

Narcotic analgesics
Beta-blocking agents
Maintain blood pressure within normal limits
Maintain normal sinus rhythm with medications, pacing, or cardioversion
Selected diet (initially clear liquids followed by small, frequent, easily digested meals)
Stress reduction techniques
Anxiolytics as indicated
Maintain quiet environment
Stool softeners and laxatives
Rest with backrest elevation 20–30 degrees
Gradually increase physical activity

Increase Myocardial O$_2$ Supply

Oxygen
Nitroglycerin
Aspirin
Anticoagulants such as hepain
Reperfusion
    Thombolytics
    Percultaneous coronary intervention(PCI)
    Coronary artery bypass graft (CABG)

Adapted from Woods, S. L., & Underhill, S. L. (1986). Coronary heart disease: Myocardial ischemia and infarction. In M. Patrick, S. L. Woods, R. F. Craven, et al. (Eds.), *Medical surgical nursing: Pathophysiological concepts* (p.522). Philadelphia: J. B. Lippincott.

---

returned to baseline level before the onset of chest discomfort; ST segments and T waves revert to pattern seen before onset of chest discomfort; and skin is warm and dry.

For Goal 3

Patient denies chest discomfort; patient appears comfortable; heart and respiratory rates and BP are within patient's normal range; and skin is warm and dry (Display 26-1).

Decreased Myocardial Tissue Perfusion

Diagnosis

Decreased myocardial tissue perfusion related to an imbalance between myocardial oxygen supply and demand and manifested by chest discomfort, arrhythmias, conduction disturbances, and/or heart failure. Refer to previous diagnosis of chest discomfort for goals, interventions, and outcome criteria for chest discomfort.

Goals

Goals for this diagnosis include:

1. To detect early manifestations (specify) and etiologies of decreased myocardial tissue perfusion.

2. To reduce or eliminate manifestations (specify) of decreased myocardial tissue perfusion.
3. To prevent, when possible, manifestations (specify) of decreased myocardial tissue perfusion and extension of MI or progression to infarction in patients with angina.

Interventions

Interventions are designed to detect the manifestations of the imbalance between myocardial oxygen supply and demand and to improve this imbalance. Interventions to meet each goal include:

For Goal 1

1. The patient's heart rate and rhythm should be monitored frequently during the acute phase of MI. Assess and document cardiac rhythm every 1 to 4 hours depending on patient condition, before and after each dose of antiarrhythmic or vasoactive drug (or any drug with cardiovascular effects), and when patient status indicates. Assess BP and obtain 12-lead ECG with changes in cardiac rhythm or if patient complains of palpitations.
2. If the patient experiences arrhythmias, perform a cardiovascular examination; obtain venous blood for electrolytes, hemoglobin, and, if appropriate, drug levels; obtain arterial blood for blood gas analysis; and obtain a chest radiograph as ordered by the physician.
3. Initially, every 4 to 8 hours, and during chest discomfort, assess, document, and report to the physician the following: new S_3 or S_4 gallops or a new murmur of mitral regurgitation; new or increasing crackles; and reduced activity tolerance.

For Goal 2

1. Immediately reduce patient's physical activity to the level of activity before occurrence of manifestations of decreased myocardial tissue perfusion.
2. Administer oxygen and antiarrhythmic and other medications (positive inotropic, afterload-reducing, and preload-reducing agents) as ordered and continuously evaluate the patient's response to therapy.
3. Provide a restful environment; and promote the patient's physical comfort by elevating head of bed to 20 to 30 degrees or higher and providing individualized basic nursing care.

For Goal 3

1. Provide small portions of easily digested, low-sodium, low saturated fat foods.
2. Provide a restful environment; as needed, assist the patient in a supportive, calm, competent manner with activities of daily living.
3. Teach patient to exhale with physical movement; as necessary.
4. Offer stool softeners and laxatives to prevent straining with bowel movements, and teach patient relaxation techniques.

Outcome Criteria

Outcome criteria are written for each goal statement.

For Goal 1

Arrhythmias and conduction disturbances and signs and symptoms of heart failure are detected at onset.

For Goal 2

Immediately after intervention, the patient's cardiac rate and rhythm return to patient's normal range. Patient states that palpitations are relieved or reduced; patient appears comfortable; BP is returning or has returned to baseline level. S_3 or S_4 gallops or the murmur of mitral regurgitation disappear or do not increase in intensity; crackles are eliminated or reduced; activity tolerance is maintained or improved.

For Goal 3

Patient denies chest discomfort. Patient appears comfortable. Heart and respiratory rates and BP are within patient's normal range. Skin is warm and dry. No S_3 or S_4 gallops; no murmur of mitral regurgitation; no crackles. Activity tolerance is maintained.

Decreased Systemic Perfusion

Diagnosis

Decreased systemic tissue perfusion related to a decrease in cardiac output from arrhythmias and conduction disturbances and from heart failure, manifested by abnormal pulse rate and rhythm; abnormal respiratory rate and rhythm; deterioration of other hemodynamic parameters; decreased mentation; decreased urine output; individually defined undue or excess fatigue; and moist, cool, cyanotic skin.

Goals

Goals for this diagnosis include:

1. Detect early manifestations and etiologies of decreased systemic tissue perfusion.
2. Reduce or eliminate manifestations of decreased systemic tissue perfusion.
3. Prevent manifestations of decreased systemic tissue perfusion.

Interventions

Interventions are designed to detect the manifestations of the imbalance between systemic oxygen supply and demand and to improve this imbalance by restoring the balance between myocardial oxygen supply and demand. Interventions to meet each goal include:

For Goal 1

1. On admission, every 4 hours, and during chest discomfort, assess, document, and report to the physician the following: abnormal heart rate and rhythm; hypotension; narrowing pulse pressure; abnormal respiratory rate and rhythm; decreased mentation; decreased urine output; increasing fatigue; and moist, cool, cyanotic skin.

For Goal 2

1. Immediately reduce patient's physical activity to the level of activity before occurrence of manifestations of decreased systemic tissue perfusion.
2. Administer oxygen and antiarrhythmic and other medications (positive inotropic, afterload-reducing, and preload-reducing agents) as ordered, and continuously evaluate the patient's response to therapy.
3. Provide a restful environment; and promote the patient's physical comfort by elevating head of bed to 20 to 30 degrees or higher, or by providing a cardiac chair (depending on BP response), and by giving individualized basic nursing care.

For Goal 3

1. Provide small portions of easily digested, low-sodium, low saturated fat foods. Provide a restful environment; as needed, assist the patient in a supportive, calm, competent manner with activities of daily living.
2. Teach patient to exhale with physical movement.
3. Offer stool softeners and laxatives to prevent straining with bowel movements. Teach patient to recognize precipitating factors of decreased systemic tissue perfusion and to alter behavior accordingly.

Outcome Criteria

Outcome criteria are written for each goal statement.

For Goal 1

Signs and symptoms of decreased systemic tissue perfusion are detected early.

For Goal 2

BP and pulse pressure are returning or have returned to baseline level. Respiratory rate and rhythm are returning or have returned to patient's baseline. Patient remains fully alert and oriented, without personality change. Urine output remains greater than 250 cc per 8 hours. Patient's complaints of fatigue are reduced. Patient is able to carry out activities of daily living within prescribed activity limits. Extremities remain warm, dry, and of normal color.

For Goal 3

Normal sinus rhythm without arrhythmia or conduction disturbance is maintained. BP and pulse pressure are maintained at patient's baseline level. Respiratory rate and rhythm are maintained at patient's baseline. Patient remains fully alert and oriented, without mental status change. Urine output remains greater than 250 cc per 8 hours. Patient does not complain of worsening fatigue. Patient is able to carry out activities of daily living within prescribed activity limits. Extremities remain warm, dry, and of normal color.

Fear or Anxiety

Diagnosis

Fear or anxiety related to diagnosis, treatment, and prognosis of angina or acute MI, manifested by abnormal rate and rhythm of pulse and respiration, elevated BP, subjective complaints of fear and anxiety from patient and family, restlessness, and sleeplessness.

Goals

Goals for this diagnosis include:

1. To detect early manifestations of fear and anxiety.
2. To reduce or eliminate fear and anxiety.
3. To prevent, when possible, fear and anxiety.

Interventions

Interventions are directed at reducing fear and anxiety in the patient and family. Patients with angina or acute MI are understandably frightened and concerned. They frequently associate the occurrence of chest pain or heart attack with impending death. Most people have had relatives or friends who died suddenly from heart problems. The acute onset of symptoms, the decision to seek medical help, transportation to the hospital, the admission procedure, and the rapid, frequently invasive therapeutics are extremely stressful. During this time, the patient is required to make rapid, important decisions regarding care. In addition, many patients need to make major lifestyle changes to manage manifestations of CHD. Fear and anxiety perpetuate the ischemic process by increasing sympathetic nervous system responses, resulting in elevated serum catecholamines, which increase myocardial oxygen consumption. The increased myocardial oxygen consumption can precipitate an attack of angina and jeopardizes ischemic myocardium in patients with acute MI, increasing pain and further increasing anxiety. The nursing role includes interventions aimed at reducing anxiety in the patient and family. Interventions to meet each goal include:

For Goal 1

1. Assess and document the patient's and family's level of fear and anxiety and effectiveness of coping mechanisms.

For Goals 2 and 3

1. Promptly treat chest discomfort or any other manifestations of angina or acute MI.
2. Provide a restful environment.
3. Provide individualized basic nursing care in a supportive, calm, and competent manner.
4. Provide a atmosphere conducive to communication and facilitate communication (listen, reflect, guide).
5. Discuss diagnostic procedures with patient, and describe sensations that patient may experience during procedures.
6. Teach stress reduction techniques.
7. Assess the need for spiritual counseling and refer as appropriate.

Outcome Criteria

Outcome criteria are written for each goal statement.

For Goal 1

Abnormal rate and rhythm of pulse and respiration, elevated BP, and subjective complaints of fear and anxiety, restlessness, and sleeplessness are detected early.

For Goal 2

Rate and rhythm of pulse and respiration and BP are normal or are approaching normal. Subjective complaints of fear, anxiety, restlessness, and sleeplessness are reduced or absent.

For Goal 3

Rate and rhythm of pulse and respiration and BP remain normal. Subjective complaints of fear, anxiety, restlessness, and sleeplessness are absent.

Knowledge Deficit

Diagnosis

Knowledge deficit about acute MI and CHD, medical or surgical management plan, risk factor modification, or return to usual activities of daily living; related to fear and anxiety, lack of recall, nonuse of information, misinterpretation, cognitive limitations, disinterest, lack of familiarity with available resources, or denial of angina or acute MI; manifested by the patient being unable to describe the disease process, unable to explain the rationale behind the diagnosis, treatment, and prognosis of acute MI and CHD, unaware of activity limitations and prescribed medications, unaware of cardiac risk factors in general, or unaware of specific risk factors and how to modify them.

Goals

Goals for this diagnosis include:

1. Early detection, reduction or elimination, and prevention of the specific knowledge deficit and maintenance of heart-healthy behaviors in the patient and family.
2. Specific goals should be based on each identified knowledge deficit.

Interventions

1. Development of a teaching plan enables the nurse to provide standardized content to each patient.
2. Teach patient to decrease activity and take nitroglycerin as prescribed during periods of angina.
3. Teach patient to seek medical attention immediately if relief of chest discomfort has not occurred within 30 minutes; and call the physician if there is a change in the pattern of angina.
4. Diagnostic procedures and interventions may be a source of anxiety and fear. Provide concrete information about procedures and describe sensory experiences that they may have. For example, "the dye (during cardiac catheterization) will make you feel hot and flushed for about 15 seconds" or "the room (cardiac catheterization laboratory) will be dimly lit and cool."
5. Teach the patient and family the content necessary for them to modify their lifestyles. Provide information about modi-

fication of risk factors such as elevated cholesterol levels, smoking, hypertension, and physical activity. Advise the patient to adhere to the prescribed therapeutic plan (diet, medication, and activity level).
6. Encourage active participation in cardiac rehabilitation programs.
7. To prevent myocardial ischemia from progressing to infarction or reinfarction, teach the patient to be aware of physiologic (such as activity during cold weather, after a heavy meal, or with sexual intercourse) and psychological (such as anger or grief) precipitating factors.
8. Teach the patient to reduce precipitating factors by taking prophylactic nitroglycerin, reducing specific physical activity and psychological stress that often result in chest discomfort, and countering emotional stress by regular physical exercise.

Outcome Criteria

The patient and family are able to describe the disease process and explain the rationale behind the diagnosis, treatment, and prognosis of acute MI and CHD. The patient and family describe activity limitations and prescribed medications. The patient and family list general and specific cardiac risk factors and describe strategies they will use to modify risk factors.

Nursing Management Plan for Patients With Right Ventricular Infarction: Analysis of Medical and Nursing Assessment Data and Formulation of Nursing Diagnoses

An important initial nursing consideration is to suspect RV infarction in any person admitted to an intensive care unit with an acute inferior or posterior LV infarction. A right precordial ECG should be obtained for any patient with evidence of an inferior MI. Initial clues to the development of RV dysfunction may be subtle. In addition, the low cardiac output syndrome may be thought secondary to primary LV dysfunction. The major differences between the low cardiac output state of predominant RV and LV infarction are listed in Table 26-4. Critical care nurses can facilitate the diagnosis and appropriate management of patients with RV infarction through awareness of the usual clinical features and electrocardiographic changes associated with RV infarction and the systematic and continual assessment of these features as well as the evaluation of the patient's response to therapy.

Patients with RV infarction experience similar alterations in functional health status as those with LV infarction. Nursing Care Plan 26-1 encompasses altered health patterns of patients with MI. In the setting of RV infarction, however, decreased cardiac output is a potential nursing problem that requires a different approach in terms of detection, assessment, and treatment.

Nursing Care Plan 26–1 ■ The Patient with Right Ventricular Infarction

Nursing Diagnosis
➤ Decreased cardiac output, related to dilated and noncompliant right ventricle, manifested by decreased blood pressure, decreased pulmonary artery wedge pressure (PAWP), decreased urine output, cool moist skin, cyanosis, mental confusion

Nursing Goal 1
➤ To detect early the signs of right ventricular (RV) dysfunction secondary to RV infarction

Outcome Criteria
➤ During hospitalization, the following signs are detected, documented, and immediately reported to the physician:

1. Physical assessment features: jugular venous distention, RV S_3 or S_4 gallop, systolic murmur of tricuspid regurgitation, hepatomegaly, peripheral edema, hypotension, urine output less than 0.5 mL/kg/h or 4 mL/k/8 h, cool, moist skin, cyanosis, mentation change

2. Right precordial electrocardiographic (ECG) features:
   ST elevation of $\geq$0.5 − 1 mm in lead V_4R
   ST elevation of $\geq$1 mm in lead $V_4R − V_6R$ or V_6R only
   QS pattern in lead V_4R or $V_3R − V_4R$
   ST elevation in lead V_4R that is greater than the ST elevation in $V_1 − V_3$
   ST depression in lead V_2 that is 50% or less than the magnitude of ST elevation in aVF

3. Hemodynamic profile characteristics:
   RA pressure >10 mm Hg and RA: PAWP ration $\geq$0.8
   RA waveform: prominent y descent that is at least as great as the x descent
   RV waveform: diastolic dip-plateau pattern ("square-root sign")
   Cardiac index <2.2 L/min/m^2

NURSING INTERVENTIONS	RATIONALE

1. On admission, every 4 hours, and with chest pain, assess, document, and report to the physician the following:
  a. Jugular venous distention
  b. RV S_3 or S_4 gallop
  c. Systolic murmur of tricuspid regurgitation
  d. Hepatomegaly
  e. Peripheral edema
  f. Clear lungs
  g. Hypotension
  h. Urine output less than 0.5 mL/kg/h or 4 mL/k/8 h
  i. Cool, moist, cyanotic extremities
  j. Mentation change
	1. Required to detect changes.

2. On admission, every 8 hours the first 25 hours, and every 24 hours for at least 3 days obtain standard 12-lead ECG and right precordial ECG.	2. ST segment elevation suggestive of RV infraction may disappear in less than 10 hours from onset of chest pain, necessitating frequent serial recordings to allow documentation.
3. Continually monitor the V_4R lead in addition to conventional leads, and record a rhythm strip every 4 hours and during chest discomfort.	3. ST segment and QRS morphologic changes thought to be indicative or RV infarction frequently involve lead V_4R. Continual monitoring of this lead may provide early ECG clues to the occurrence of RV infarction and subsequently expedite appropriate treatment.

4. Assess serial (as stated in number 2) right precordial ECG for the following changes:
  a. ST elevation of $\geq$0.5 − 1 mm is lead V_4R
  b. ST elevation of $\geq$1 mm is lead $V_4R − V_6R$ or V_6R only
  c. QS pattern in lead V_4R or $V_3 − V_4R$
  d. ST elevation in V_4R greater than the ST elevation in $V_1 − V_3$
  e. ST depression in V_2 that is 50% or less than the magnitude of ST elevation in aVF
	4. Clinical studies suggest that these ECG features may suggest an evolving RV infarction.

5. Record and document pressures and obtain pressure tracings as the pulmonary artery catheter is inserted into the RA, RV, pulmonary artery, and wedge position.	5. These measurements and tracings serve as a baseline for comparison of later data. Also, the hemodynamic diagnosis of RV infarction may be missed with exclusion of this step, precluding prompt treatment.

Nursing Care Plan 26–1 ■ The Patient with Right Ventricular Infarction (continued)

NURSING INTERVENTIONS	RATIONALE
6. Measure RA pressure, PAWP, and cardiac index, and derive pulmonary and systemic vascular resistance every hour.	**6.** Early frequent recordings of hemodynamic parameters may aid in the recognition of low cardiac output secondary to RV infarction.
7. Observe, document, and report the following hemodynamic patterns: **a.** RA pressure >10 mm Hg and RA:PAWP ration of ≥0.8 **b.** RA waveform: prominent *y* descent that is at least as great as the *x* descent **c.** RV waveform: diastolic dip-plateau pattern ("square-root sign") **d.** Cardiac index <2.2 L/min/m^2	**7.** Investigative reports suggest that these hemodynamic criteria may be indicative of RV infarction.

Nursing Goal 2	➤	To eliminate the signs of RV dysfunction secondary to RV infarction.
Outcome Criteria	➤	During hospitalization, the following signs are observed and documented: Systolic blood pressure >90 mm Hg PAWP of 15 − 20 mm Hg Urine output = at least 0.5 mL/kg/h or 4 mL/kg/8h Cardiac index >2.2 L/min/m^2 Skin pink, warm, dry Mentation unchanged

NURSING INTERVENTIONS	RATIONALE
1. Infuse intravenous fluid bolus per physician protocol to attain a PAWP of 15–20 mm Hg.	**1.** Initial rapid volume expansion increases RV end-diastolic volume, which may optimize contractility of a diastolic noncompliant RV.
2. Administer positive inotropic agents such as dobutamine or dopamine per physician protocol. Monitor heart rate and rhythm for development of tachycardia or tachyarrhythmias.	**2.** Dobutamine (2–20 μg/kg/min) and dopamine (2–10 υg/kg/min) directly stimulate β-adrenergic myocardial receptors, resulting in increased contractility and cardiac output. Although dobutamine is less arrhythmogenic than dopamine, both agents may precipitate tachycardia and tachyarrhythmias, resulting in decreased diastolic filling and reduced cardiac output.
3. Administer peripheral vasodilators such as nitroprusside or hydralazine per physician protocol. Monitor pulmonary and systemic vascular resistance at least every hour.	**3.** These agents decrease RV and LV afterload, thereby enhancing RV and LV stroke volume. Hydralazine may be preferable because it selectively vasodilates arterioles and should not decrease preload. Pulmonary and systemic vascular resistance parameters are necessary to optimize preload and afterload.
4. When pacing therapy is indicated, institute atrial or atrioventricular sequential method per physician protocol.	**4.** Preservation of atrioventricular synchronous contraction maximizes contractility and cardiac output.
5. Avoid administration of drugs and performance of maneuvers that decrease preload: **a.** Diuretics **b.** Venodilators (nitroglycerin, morphine) **c.** Sitting up in bed **d.** Valsalva meneuver	**5.** Filling of the left ventricle is dependent on distention of the right ventricle. These actions decrease preload, thereby reducing stretch of the RV myocardial fibers and further compromising the ability of the noncompliant chamber to propel blood forward. Reduced cardiac output results.

REFERENCES

Abrams, J. (1995). The role of nitrates in coronary heart disease. *Archives of Internal Medicine, 155*(4), 357.

American Heart Association. (2003). *Heart attack and angina statistics, 2003.* Dallas: AHA.

Anderson, H. V., & Willerson, J. T. (1993). Current concepts: Thrombolysis in acute myocardial infarction. *New England Journal of Medicine, 329*(10), 703–709.

Andresen, D., Ehlers, H., Wiedman, M., & Bruggemann, T. (1999). Beta blockers: Evidence versus wishful thinking. *American Journal of Cardiology, 83*(5B), 64D–66D.

Antman, E., & Braunwald, E. (2001a). Acute myocardial infarction. In E. Braunwald (Ed.), *Braunwald: Heart disease: A textbook of cardiovascular medicine* (6th ed., vol. 2, pp. 1114–1231). St. Louis: W. B. Saunders.

_____. (2001b). Acute myocardial infarction. In E. Braunwald, A. S. Fauci, S. L. Hauser, D. L. Longo & J. L. Jameson (Eds.), *Harrison's principles of internal medicine* (15th ed., pp. 1386–1399). New York: McGraw-Hill.

_____. (1997). Myocardial infarction. In E. Braunwald (Ed.), *Heart disease: A textbook of cardiovascular medicine* (5th ed., vol. 2, pp. 1184–1274). Philadelphia: W. B. Saunders.

Armstrong, P. W., Fu, Y., Chang, W.-C., Topol, E. J., Granger, C. B., Betriu, A., et al. (1998). Acute coronary syndromes in the GUSTO IIb trial: Prognostic insights and impact of recurrent ischemia. *Circulation, 98,* 1860–1868.

Arrighi, J. A., & Dilsizian, V. (1998). Identification of viable, nonfunctioning myocardium. In D. L. Brown (Ed.), *Cardiac intensive care* (pp. 307–327). Philadelphia: W. B. Saunders.

Bahr, R. (1998). The concept and development of chest pain emergency departments as a strategy in the war against heart attack. *Critical Care Nursing Clinics of North America, 4*(2), 41–51.

Ballard, J. C., Wood, L. L., & Lansing, A. M. (1997). Transmyocardial revascularization: criteria for selecting patients, treatment, and nursing care. *Critical Care Nurse, 17*(1), 42–49, 59.

Becker, R. C. (2001). Complicated myocardial infarction. In C. P. Cannon & P. O'Gara (Eds.), *Critical pathways in cardiology.* Philadelphia: Lippincott Williams & Wilkins.

Bell, N. N. (1992). Clinical significance of ST-segment monitoring. *Critical Care Nursing Clinics of North America, 4*(2), 313–323.

Berger, C., Murabito, J., Evans, J., Anderson, K., & Levy, D. (1992). Prognosis after first myocardial infarction: Comparison of Q-wave myocardial infarction in the Framingham Heart Study. *Journal of the American Medical Association, 268,* 1545–1551.

Bode, C., Smalling, R. W., Berg, G., Burnett, C., Lorch, G., Kalbfleisch, J. M., et al. (1996). Randomized comparison of coronary thrombolysis achieved with double-bolus reteplase (recombinant plasminogen activator) and front-loaded, accelerated alteplase (recombinant tissue plasminogen activator) in patients with acute myocardial infarction. *Circulation, 94*(5), 891–898.

Bozkurt, E., Erol, M. K., Keles, S., Acikel, M., Yilmaz, M., & Gurlertop, Y. (2002). Relation of plasma homocysteine levels to intracoronary thrombus in unstable angina pectoris and in non-Q-wave acute myocardial infarction. *American Journal of Cardiology, 90*(4), 413–415.

Braunwald, E., & Antman, E. M. (1997). Evidence-based coronary care. *Annals of Internal Medicine, 126*(7), 551–553.

Braunwald, E., Antman, E. M., Beasley, J. W., Califf, R. M., Cheitlin, M. D., Hochman, J. S., et al. (2000). ACC/AHA guidelines for the management of patients with unstable angina and non-ST-segment elevation myocardial infarction: Executive summary and recommendations. A report of the American College of Cardiology/American Heart Association Task Force on Practice Guidelines (Committee on the Management of Patients With Unstable Angina). *Circulation, 102*(10), 1193–1209.

Brochier, M., Quillet, L., & Kulbertus, H. (1987). Intravenous APSAC versus intravenous streptokinase in evolving myocardial infarction. *Drugs, 33*(Suppl 3), 140.

Brown, B., Gallery, C., Badger, R., Kennedy, J., Mathey, D., Bolson, E., et al. (1986). Incomplete lysis of thrombus in the moderate underlying atherosclerotic lesion during intracoronary infusion of streptokinase for acute myocardial infarction: Quantitative angiographic observations. *Circulation, 73*(4), 653–661.

Bueno, H., Lopez-Palop, R., Bermejo, J., Lopez-Sendon, J. L. M., & Delcan, J. (1997). In-hospital outcome of elderly patients with acute inferior myocardial infarction and right ventricular involvement. *Circulation, 96*(2), 436–441.

Califf, R., O'Neill, W., Stack, R., et al. (1988). Failure of simple clinical measurements to predict perfusion status after intravenous thrombolysis. *Annals of Internal Medicine, 108,* 658.

Cannon, C. P. (2002). Effectiveness of clopidogrel versus aspirin in preventing acute myocardial infarction in patients with symptomatic atherothrombosis (CAPRIE trial). *American Journal of Cardiology, 90*(7), 760–762.

_____. (2000). Thrombolysis medication errors: Benefits of bolus thrombolytic agents. *American Journal of Cardiology, 85*(1), 17–22.

Cannon, C. P., Gibson, C. M., McCabe, C. H., Adgey, A. A. J., Schweiger, M. J., Sequeira, R. F., et al. (1998). TNK–tissue plasminogen activator compared with front-loaded alteplase in acute myocardial infarction: Results of the TIMI 10B trial. *Circulation, 98*(25), 2805–2814.

Canto, J. G., Shlipak, M. G., Rogers, W. J., Malmgren, J. A., Frederick, P. D., Lambrew, C. T., et al. (2000). Prevalence, clinical characteristics, and mortality among patients with myocardial infarction presenting without chest pain. *Journal of the American Medical Association, 283*(24), 3223–3229.

Casey, M., Bedker, D. L., & Roussel-McElmeel, P. L. (1998). Myocardial infarction: Review of clinical trials and treatment strategies. *Critical Care Nurse, 18*(2), 39–52.

Cohn, J. N., Guiha, N. H., Broder, M. I., & Limas, C. J. (1974). Right ventricular infarction. Clinical and hemodynamic features. *American Journal of Cardiology, 33*(2), 209–214.

Coulter, S. A., McCabe, C. H., Giugliano, R. P., Culter, S. S., Charlesworth, A., Chew, P. H., et al. (1999). Dosing errors and outcomes in patients receiving single bolus compared to bolus + infusion thrombolytic regimens: An inTIME-II study. *Circulation, 100*(Suppl. I), I–791.

Cummins, R., Field, J., & Hazinski, M. (2001). *Acute coronary syndromes: Patients with acute ischemic chest pain: ACLS provider manual.* Dallas: American Heart Association.

Daily, E. (1991). Clinical management of patients receiving thrombolytic therapy. *Heart and Lung, 20,* 520–565.

De Jaegere, P., Serruys, P., & Bertrand, M. (1992). Wiktor stent implantation in patients with restenosis following angioplasty of a native coronary artery. *American Journal of Cardiology, 69*(598).

Dell' Italia, L., Starling, M., & Blumhardt, R. (1985). Comparative effects of volume loading, dobutamine and nitroprusside in patients with predominant right ventricular infarction. *Circulation, 72,* 1327.

DeVon, H., & Zerwic, J. (2002). Symptoms of acute coronary syndromes: Are there gender differences? A review of the literature. *Heart and Lung, 31*(4), 235–245.

DeWood, M., Spores, J., Notske, R., Mouser, L., Burroughs, R., Golden, M., et al. (1980). Prevalence of total coronary occlusion during the early hours of transmural myocardial infarction. *New England Journal of Medicine, 303*(16), 897–902.

Dracup, K., & Moser, D. K. (1997). Beyond sociodemographics: Factors influencing the decision to seek treatment for symptoms of acute myocardial infarction. *Heart and Lung, 26,* 253–262.

Drew, B. J. (1993). Bedside electrocardiogram monitoring. *AACN Clinical Issues, 4*(1), 25–33.

_____. (1991). Bedside electrocardiographic monitoring: State of the art for the 1990s. *Heart and Lung, 20,* 610–623.

Drew, B. J., & Krucoff, M. (1999). Multilead ST-segment monitoring in patients with acute coronary syndromes: A consensus statement for healthcare professionals. *American Journal of Critical Care, 8*(6), 372–388.

Dudek, A. A. (1999). Percutaneous transluminal myocardial revascularization. A new treatment for angina. *Critical Care Nursing Clinics of North America, 11*(3), 327–332.

Feldman, M., & Cryer, B. (1999). Aspirin absorption rates and platelet inhibition times with 325 mg buffered aspirin tablets (chewed or swallowed intact) and with buffered aspirin solution. *American Journal of Cardiology, 84*(4), 404–409.

Fillmore, S., Shapiro, M., & Killip, T. (1970). Arterial oxygen tension in acute myocardial infarction: Serial analysis of clinical state and blood gas changes. *American Heart Journal, 79,* 620.

Fleischmann, K. E., & Lee, T. H. (1998). The evolution of the coronary care unit: Past, present and future. In D. L. Brown (Ed.), *Intensive cardiac care* (pp. 3–5). Philadelphia: W. B. Saunders.

Forrester, J., Diamond, G., & Chatterjee, K. (1976a). Medical therapy of acute myocardial infarction by application of hemodynamic subsets. *New England Journal of Medicine, 295,* 1356.

_____. (1976b). Medical therapy of acute myocardial infarction by application of hemodynamic subsets. *New England Journal of Medicine, 295,* 1404.

Gershlick, H. G., & More, R. S. (1998). Recent advances: Treatment of myocardial infarction. *British Medical Journal, 316,* 280–284.

Gibbons, R. J., Balady, G. J., Bricker, J. T., Chaitman, B. R., Fletcher, G. F., Froelicher, V., et al. (2002). *ACC/AHA 2002 guideline update for exercise testing: A report of the American College of Cardiology/American Heart Association Task Force on Practice Guidelines—Committee on Exercise Testing.* Available: www.acc.org/clinical/guidelines/exercise/dirIndex.

Gibbons, R. J., Chatterjee, K., Daley, J., Douglas, J. S., Fihn, S. D., Gardin, J. M., et al. (1999). ACC/AHA/ACP-ASIM guidelines for the management of patients with chronic stable angina: Executive summary and recommendations. A report of the American College of Cardiology/American Heart Association Task Force on Practice Guidelines (Committee on Management of Patients with Chronic Stable Angina). *Circulation,* 99(21), 2829–2848.

Gibler, W. B. (1998). Diagnosis of acute coronary syndromes in the emergency department: Evolution of chest pain centers. In E. J. Topol (Ed.), *Acute coronary syndromes.* New York: Marcel Dekker.

Gibler, W. B., Armstrong, P. W., Ohman, E. M., Weaver, W. D., Stebbins, A. L., Gore, J. M., et al. (2002). Persistence of delays in presentation and treatment for patients with acute myocardial infarction: The GUSTO-I and GUSTO-III experience. *Annals of Emergency Medicine,* 39(2), 123–130.

Grundy, S. M., Balady, G. J., Criqui, M. H., Fletcher, G., Greenland, P., Hiratzka, L. F., et al. (1997). When to start cholesterol-lowering therapy in patients with coronary heart disease: A statement for healthcare professionals from the American Heart Association Task Force on Risk Reduction. *Circulation,* 95(6), 1683–1685.

Gruppo Italiano per lo Studio della Sopravvivenza nell' Infarto Miocardico. (1994). GISSI-3: Effects of lisinopril and transdermal glyceryl trinitrate singly and together on 6-week mortality and ventricular function after acute myocardial infarction. *Lancet,* 343(8906), 1115–1122.

GUSTO Investigators. (1993). An international trial comparing four thrombolytic strategies for acute myocardial infarction. *New England Journal of Medicine,* 329, 673.

Hamm, C. W., & Braunwald, E. (2000). A classification of unstable angina revisited. *Circulation,* 102(1), 118–122.

Hennekens, C. H., Albert, C. M., Godfried, S. L., Gaziano, J. M., & Burning, J. E. (1996). Adjunctive drug therapy of acute myocardial infarction: Evidence from clinical trials. *New England Journal of Medicine,* 335(22), 1660–1667.

Hirschfeld, J., Schwartz, S., & Jugo, R. (1991). Restenosis after coronary angioplasty: A multivariate statistical model to relate lesion and procedure variables to restenosis. *Journal of the American College of Cardiology,* 18(647).

Hochman, J. S., & Gerch, B. J. (1998). Acute myocardial infarction. In E. J. Topol (Ed.), *Textbook of cardiovascular medicine* (pp. 437–480). Philadelphia: Lippincott-Raven.

Hsia, J., Hamilton, W., & Kleiman, N. (1990). A comparison between heparin and low-dose aspirin as adjunctive therapy with tissue plasminogen activator for acute myocardial infarction. *New England Journal of Medicine,* 323, 1433.

Ibbotson, T., & Goa, K. L. (2002). Enoxaparin: An update of its clinical use in the management of acute coronary syndromes. *Drugs,* 62(9), 1407–1430.

International Study Group. (1990). In-hospital mortality and clinical course of 20,891 patients with suspected acute myocardial infarction randomized between alteplase and streptokinase with or without heparin. *Lancet,* 336, 71.

Ireson, C. L. (1997). Critical pathways: Effectiveness in achieving patient outcomes. *Journal of Nursing Administration,* 27, 6.

ISIS-2: Second International Study of Infarct Survival Collaborative Group. (1988). Randomized trial of intravenous streptokinase, oral aspirin, both or neither among 17,187 cases of suspected acute myocardial infarction. *Lancet* (2), 349.

ISIS-3: Third International Study of Infarct Survival Collaborative Group. (1992). A randomized comparison of streptokinase vs. tissue plasminogen activator vs. anistreplase and of aspirin plus heparin vs aspirin alone among 41,299 cases of suspected acute myocardial infarction. *Lancet,* 339, 753.

ISIS-4 Collaborative Group. (1995). ISIS-4: A randomized factorial trial assessing early oral captopril, oral mononitrate, and intravenous magnesium sulfate in 58,050 with suspected acute myocardial infarction. *Lancet,* 345(8951), 669–682.

Isner, J., & Roberts, W. (1978). Right ventricular infarction complicating left ventricular infarction secondary to coronary heart disease. *American Journal of Cardiology,* 42, 885.

Jaffe, A. S., Ravkilde, J., Roberts, R., Naslund, U., Apple, F. S., Galvani, M., et al. (2000). It's time for a change to a troponin standard. *Circulation,* 102, 1216–1220.

Juergens, C. P., Whitbourn, R. J., Yeung, A. C., & Oesterle, S. N. (1997). Primary angioplasty for acute myocardial infarction. *Vascular Medicine,* 2(4), 327–334.

Kastelein, J. J., Jukema, J. W., Zwinderman, A. H., Clee, S., van Boven, A. J., Jansen, H., et al. (2000). Lipoprotein lipase activity is associated with severity of angina pectoris. REGRESS Study Group. *Circulation,* 102(14), 1629–1633.

Kinch, J. W. M., & Ryan, T. J. (1994). Right ventricular infarction. *New England Journal of Medicine,* 330(17), 1211–1217.

Kontos, M. C., Arrowood, J., Paulsen, W. H., & Nixon, J. (1998). Early echocardiography can predict cardiac events in emergency department patients with chest pain. *Annals of Emergency Medicine,* 31(5), 550–557.

Kudenchuk, P. J., Maynard, C., Martin, J. S., Wirkus, M., & Weaver, W. D. (1996). Comparison of presentation, treatment, and outcome of acute myocardial infarction in men versus women (The Myocardial Infarction Triage and Intervention Registry). *American Journal of Cardiology,* 78, 9–14.

Lee, T. J. (2001). Guidelines, diagnosis and management of acute myocardial infarction. In E. Braunwald (Ed.), *Braunwald: Heart disease: Textbook of cardiovascular medicine* (pp. 1219–1231). St. Louis: W. B. Saunders.

Litvak, F., Marglis, J., & Cummins, R. (1992). Excimer laser coronary (ECLA) registry: Report of the first 2080 patients. *Journal of the American College of Cardiology,* 19, 276A.

Llevadot, J., Giugliano, R. P., & Antman, E. M. (2001). Bolus fibrinolytic therapy in acute myocardial infarction. *Journal of the American Medical Association,* 286(4), 442–449.

Lopez-Sendon, J., Seabra-Bomes, R., & Santos, M. (1988). Intravenous anisoylated plasminogen streptokinase complex (APSAC) versus intravenous streptokinase in acute myocardial infarction (AMI): A randomized trial. *European Heart Journal,* 9(Suppl. A), 10.

Luepker, R., Raczynski, J., Osganian, S., Goldberg, R., Finnegan, J., Hedges, J., et al. (2000). Effect of a community intervention on patient delay and emergency medical service use in acute coronary heart disease: The Rapid Early Action for Coronary Treatment (REACT) trial. *Journal of the American Medical Association,* 284(1), 60–67.

Lynn, L., & Kissinger, J. (1992). Coronary precautions: Should caffeine be restricted in patients after myocardial infarction? *Heart and Lung,* 21, 365–370.

Malone, M. L., Rosen, L. B., & Goodwin, J. S. (1998). Complications of acute myocardial infarction in patients > or =90 years of age. *American Journal of Cardiology,* 81(5), 638–641.

Marcassa, C., Galli, M., Temporelli, P., Campini, R., Orrego, P., Zoccarato, O., et al. (1995). Technetium-99m sestamibi tomographic evaluation of residual ischemia after anterior myocardial infarction. *Journal of the American College of Cardiology,* 25, 590–596.

Maroko, P., Radvany, P., Braunwald, E., & Hale, S. (1975). Reduction of infarct size by oxygen inhalation following acute coronary occlusion. *Circulation,* 52, 360–368.

Morgera, T., Alberti, E., & Silvestri, F. (1984). Right precordial ST and QRS changes in the diagnosis of right ventricular infarction. *American Heart Journal,* 108(1), 13–18.

Mueller, H., Chatterjee, K., Davis, K., Franklin, C., Greenberg, M., Labovitz, A., et al. (1998). Present use of bedside right heart catheterization in patients with cardiac disease. *Journal of the American College of Cardiology,* 32(3), 840–864.

Nagel, E., Klein, C., Paetsch, I., Hettwer, S., Schnackenburg, B., Wegscheider, K., et al. (2003). Magnetic resonance perfusion measurements for the noninvasive detection of coronary artery disease. *Circulation,* 108(4), 432–437.

Ohman, E. M., & Armstrong, P. W. (1996). Cardiac troponin t-levels for risk stratification in acute myocardial ischemia. *New England Journal of Medicine,* 335, 1333–1341.

Olson, H. G., & Aronow, W. S. (1996). Medical management of stable angina and unstable angina in the elderly with coronary artery disease. *Clinics in Geriatric Medicine,* 12(1), 121–140.

Pearson, T. A., Goulart-Fischer, D., & Lee, T. (1995). Critical pathways as a strategy for improving care: Problems and potential. *Annals of Internal Medicine,* 123, 941–948.

Pepine, C. J. (2000). An ischemia-guided approach for risk stratification in patients with acute coronary syndromes. *American Journal of Cardiology,* 86(12B), 27M–35M.

Petticrew, M., Turner-Boutle, M., & Sheldon, T. (1997). The management of stable angina. *Health Service Journal,* 107(5577), 36–37.

Puleo, P., & Perryman, M. (1991). Noninvasive detection of reperfusion in acute myocardial infarction based on plasma activity of creatine kinase subforms. *Journal of the American College of Cardiology,* 17, 1047.

Riegel, B., Thomason, T., & Carlson, B. (1997). Nursing care of patients with acute myocardial infarction: Results of a national survey. *Critical Care Nurse,* 17(5), 23–33.

Riegel, B., Thomason, T., Carlson, B., & Gocka, I. (1996). Are nurses still practicing coronary precautions? A national survey of nursing care of acute myocardial infarction patients. *American Journal of Critical Care,* 5(2), 91–98.

Rogers, W. J. (1995). Contemporary management of acute myocardial infarction. *American Journal of Medicine,* 99(2), 195–206.

Ryan, T. J., Anderson, J. L., Antman, E. M., Braniff, B. A., Brooks, N. H., Califf, R. M., et al. (1996a). ACC/AHA guidelines for the management of patients with acute myocardial infarction: Executive summary: A report of the American College of Cardiology/American Heart Association Task Force on Practice Guidelines (Committee on Management of Acute Myocardial Infarction). *Circulation,* 94(9), 2341–2350.

———. (1996b). ACC/AHA task force report on practice guidelines: Management of acute myocardial infarction. *Journal of the American College of Cardiology,* 28, 1328–1428.

Ryan, T. J., Antman, E. M., Brooks, N. H., Califf, R. M., Hillis, L. D., Hiratzka, L. F., et al. (1999). 1999 update: ACC/AHA guidelines for the management of patients with acute myocardial infarction: Executive summary and recommendations. *Circulation,* 100, 1016–1030.

Schroeder, J. S. (1996). Unstable angina and non-Q-wave myocardial infarction. In J. S. Alpert (Ed.), *Cardiology for the primary care physician.* St. Louis: Mosby.

Selwyn, A. P., & Braunwald, E. (2001). Ischemic heart disease. In E. Braunwald, A. S. Fauci, S. L. Hauser, D. L. Longo & J. L. Jameson (Eds.), *Harrison's principles of internal medicine* (15th ed., pp. 1399–1410). New York: McGraw-Hill.

Shub, C., Click, R. L., & McGoon, M. D. (1996). Myocardial ischemia clinical syndromes, angina pectoris, and coronary heart disease. In E. R. Giuliani, B. J. Gersh, M. D. McGoon, & V. Hartzell (Eds.), *Mayo Clinic practice of cardiology* (3rd ed., pp. 1160–1190). St. Louis: Mosby.

Simoons, M. L., Arnold, A. E., Betriu, A., et al. (1998). Thrombolysis with tissue plasminogen activator in acute myocardial infarction: No additional benefit from immediate percutaneous angioplasty. *Lancet,* 1(8579), 197–203.

Simpson, T. (1990). Cardiovascular responses to family visits in coronary care unit patients. *Heart and Lung,* 19, 344–351.

Sobel, J., Dittrich, H., & Keen, W. (1998). Echocardiography in the cardiac intensive care unit. In D. L. Brown (Ed.), *Cardiac intensive care.* Philadelphia: W. B. Saunders.

Stone, G. W., Grines, C. L., & O'Neill, W. W. (1997). Primary coronary angioplasty versus thrombolysis. *New England Journal of Medicine,* 337(16), 1168–1169.

Theroux, P., Alexander, J., Jr., Pharand, C., Barr, E., Snapinn, S., Ghannam, A. F., et al. (2000). Glycoprotein IIb/IIIa receptor blockade improves outcomes in diabetic patients presenting with unstable angina/non-ST-elevation myocardial infarction: results from the Platelet Receptor Inhibition in Ischemic Syndrome Management in Patients Limited by Unstable Signs and Symptoms (PRISM-PLUS) study. *Circulation,* 102(20), 2466–2472.

Tisdale, L., & Drew, B. J. (1993). ST segment monitoring for myocardial ischemia. *AACN Clinical Issues,* 4(1), 34–43.

Topol, E. J. (1990). Thrombolytic intervention. In E. J. Topol (Ed.), *Textbook of interventional cardiology.* Philadelphia: W. B. Saunders.

Verstraete, M., Brower, R., & Collen, D. (1985). Double-blind randomized trial of intravenous tissue-type plasminogen activator versus placebo in acute myocardial infarction. *Lancet* (2), 965.

Wellens, H. (1993). Right ventricular infarction. *New England Journal of Medicine,* 328(14), 1036–1038.

Willerson, J. T. (1998). Recognition and treatment of stable angina. In D. L. Brown (Ed.), *Cardiac intensive care.* Philadelphia: W. B. Saunders.

Winslow, E., Lane, L., & Gaffney, A. (1984). Oxygen uptake and cardiovascular response in patients and normal adults during in-bed toileting. *Journal of Cardiac Rehabilitation,* 4, 346–354.

Wu, A. H. V., Apple, F. S., Gibler, W. B., Jesse, R. L., Warshaw, M. M., & Valdes, R. Jr. (1999). National Academy of Clinical Biochemistry standards of laboratory practice: Recommendations for the use of cardiac markers in coronary artery disease. *Clinical Chemistry,* 45(7), 1104–1121.

Yager, M. (1996). Right ventricular infarction in the emergency department: A review of pathophysiology, assessment, diagnosis, treatment, and nursing care. *Journal of Emergency Nursing,* 22(4), 288–292.

Zehender, M., Kasper, W., Kauder, E., et al. (1993). Right ventricular infarction as an independent predictor of prognosis after acute inferior myocardial infarction. *New England Journal of Medicine,* 328(14).

Zimetbaum, P. J., & Josephson, M. E. (2003). Use of the electrocardiogram in acute myocardial infarction. *New England Journal of Medicine,* 348(10), 933–940.

Zimmerman, J., Fromm, R., Meyer, D., Boudreaux, A. C., Wun, C.-C., Smalling, R., et al. (1999). Diagnostic marker cooperative study for the diagnosis of myocardial infarction. *Circulation,* 99, 1671–1677.

27

Interventional Cardiology Techniques

MICHAELENE HARGROVE DEELSTRA

Interventional cardiology has expanded to include multiple techniques and procedures for percutaneous treatment of coronary heart disease (CHD) and treatment of other cardiac structural abnormalities, which previously required surgery. Since the early 1970s the goal of acute care for patients with myocardial ischemia caused by (CHD) has shifted from reducing risks associated with acute myocardial infarction (MI) to improving myocardial blood flow by reperfusion or revascularization of the myocardium. Restoration of perfusion to myocardial ischemic areas may be achieved through angioplasty, atherectomy, intracoronary stents, and pharmacological therapies, or a combination of these interventions. The major emphasis is the discussion of the treatment of CHD. The goal of this interventional cardiology chapter is to provide an understanding of the evolution of device technology and present the current trends and devices used in the catheterization laboratory today.

PERCUTANEOUS CORONARY INTERVENTIONS

The term percutaneous coronary intervention (PCI) refers to the group of procedures performed through a percutaneous approach used to treat coronary lesions. Although, initially limited to percutaneous transluminal coronary angioplasty (PTCA), new coronary devices have expanded the clinical and anatomical indications for PCI. The major procedures include angioplasty, atherectomy, and intracoronary stenting. The American College of Cardiology/American Heart Association task force provides board guidelines and recommendations for appropriate application of this PCI technology. More than 50,000 PCI procedures are performed yearly in the USA and more than 1,000,000 procedures are performed annually worldwide. (ACC/AHA, 2001)

Patient Selection

The patients treated with PCI include those with stable CAD, unstable angina, and patients presenting with an acute coronary syndrome. When the patient is considered for revascularization with PCI, the potential risks and benefits should be discussed in detail with the patient and family and be weighed against alternative therapies such as medical therapy or CABG surgery. Patients should understand the possible complications associated with the procedure, the possibility of restenosis (see late complications) after the procedure, and the potential for incomplete revascularization in patients with diffuse CHD. The clinical and angiographic variables associated with increased mortality include advanced age, female gender, diabetes mellitus, previous MI, multi-vessel disease, left main or equivalent (severe stenosis of the left anterior descending artery and circumflex arteries proximal to any major branch), a large area of myocardium at risk, preexisting impairment of LV function or renal function, and collateral vessels supplying significant areas of myocardium that originate distal to the segment to be treated.(ACC/AHA, 2001)

Special Subgroups With Coronary Heart Disease

Women presenting with CHD frequently have increased severity of disease at time of presentation. Women are generally older when they present with their first coronary event, with more diffuse disease, and a higher incidence of co-morbidities, including hypertension, diabetes mellitus, hypercholesteremia, peripheral vascular disease, and unstable angina. Women have an excellent long-term prognosis after a successful procedure, even though coronary vessel lumen size tends to be smaller and women have more ostial lesions that are difficult to treat with intervention. However, procedural and in-hospital morbidity and mortality for PTCA is three times higher for women. Women undergoing revascularization have a higher incidence of left ventricular hypertrophy and hypertensive heart disease compared to men contributing to congestive heart failure from diastolic dysfunction after the procedure. Although newer revascularization procedures such as stents and glycoprotein (GP) IIb/IIIa receptor inhibitors have shown similar benefit in women as men, these interventions have not eliminated the difference in mortality between women and men. The sex difference in mortality has persisted with device treatment in the setting of acute coronary syndrome and elective procedures. (Jacobs, 2003, Mosca et al., 1997)

Patients with diabetes mellitus account for 25% of revascularization procedures. Current guidelines have favored CABG surgery for diabetic patients with two- or three-vessel disease, because of the results of the Bypass Angioplasty Revascularization Investigation (BARI) study. This study showed significant and sustained survival benefit for CABG at 5 years in treated diabetic patients as compared to angioplasty (BARI Investigators, 1996; BARI Investigators, 2000). More recent studies using new device technology including stents and GP IIb/IIIa receptor-inhibitor agents (see anticoagulation options for PCI) have shown reduced restenosis and long-term mortality in diabetic patients with multi-vessel disease similar to CABG. Patients with refractory angina and who are at high risk for CABG because of a previous CABG, recent MI, poor left ventricular ejection fraction, or age older than 70 were found in the AWESOME trial to have similar survival rates with PCI versus CABG. (Sedlis et al., 2002)

Older patients who undergo PTCA are more likely to be women and to have multi-vessel CAD with increased hospital death and postprocedural MI. The newer transcatheter procedures, including stenting, have shown similar success rates for patients older than age 70 years compared with younger patients in the Newer Approaches to Coronary Interventions (NACI) registry. However, incidence of increase in non-ST elevation MI and vascular complications in the older patient group have been reported (Williams, 2002). Older adults are also at increased risk for neurological events secondary to diffuse atherosclerotic disease.

Management of Patient During PCI

Preprocedural Management

PCI may be scheduled electively and the patient admitted through same-day surgery or emergently in the case of an acute MI when the patient presents through the emergency room. Before the procedure, the patient must give informed consent. Consent for CABG is usually given provisionally at the same time. Patient education including the expectations of the procedure and the postprocedure care should be discussed. All patients receive aspirin before the PCI. If allergic to ASA, then an oral theinopyridine (adenosine diphosphate receptor antagonists) such as ticlopidine or clopidogrel should be administered. Other routine medications are adjusted individually. Generally, oral hypoglycemic agents are withheld before PCI and some (i.e., metformin) continue to be held for several days after the procedure. Insulin dosages are decreased while the patient is NPO. An insulin drop or sliding-scale insulin may be ordered. Diuretics may be withheld or administered depending on the patient's volume status. The patient's cardiologist will provide orders for individual adjustments. Baseline laboratory tests are evaluated to recognize potential problems associated with anemia, bleeding, or renal insufficiency.

Intraprocedural Management

The patient is prepared in the same way as the patient having a diagnostic cardiac catheterization (see Chapter 22). Conscious sedation is given at the discretion of the cardiologist and the patient monitored by the catheterization laboratory staff as per protocol. A sheath is placed in the femoral artery, which is the most common site for arterial access. Alternatively, the brachial or radial artery can also be used for arterial access.

A bolus of heparin is administered to maintain an activated clotting time (ACT) of 275 to 300 seconds. Lower levels of ACT below 250 seconds have been associated with thrombotic complications during PCI with multiple catheters, wires, or devices being placed in the aorta and coronary arteries (Baim, 2000). Use of low-molecular-weight heparin or direct thrombin inhibitors can be used as an alternative to heparin (see anticoagulation options for PCI). Baseline angiographic views are obtained of the coronary artery to be treated using the standard diagnostic catheter or the guiding catheter. Coronary injections may be repeated after administration of intracoronary nitroglycerin to exclude spasm as a significant component of the target stenosis and to minimize the occurrence of coronary spasm during the PCI. The appropriate guiding catheter is positioned in the coronary ostium and a guidewire is directed across the stenotic lesion. After the wire tip is confirmed to be in the distal portion of the coronary artery to be treated, the angioplasty balloon or other device is selected. The patient is monitored for hemodynamic stability and ECG changes during the procedure.

During the procedure, additional heparin or a direct thrombin inhibitor may be administered by the cardiologist. A GP IIb/IIIa receptor inhibitor may be selected for patients with an acute coronary syndrome or angiographic thrombus. After the procedure is complete, the patient is prepared for transfer to the postintervention ward. Vital signs are monitored and the patient placed on a portable monitor for transfer. The arterial access site is assessed for bleeding or hematoma before transfer. Report is called to the receiving staff, including type of procedure performed, specific artery treated, vital signs, status of the arterial sheath, and other pertinent information about the procedure. The sheath is usually removed by the nursing staff or catheterization technician on the nursing unit in approximately 4 hours, when the ACT is less than 180 seconds. Patient may have the sheath removed in the catheterization laboratory if the ACT is less than 180 seconds or a vascular closure device has been used (see vascular sheaths under post procedure management).

Postprocedural Management

The interventional patient is monitored for manifestations of myocardial ischemia such as chest pain, ECG changes, arrhythmias, or hemodynamic instability. A 12-lead ECG is obtained after the procedure to establish a baseline for comparison. Laboratory tests are obtained, such as CBC, electrolytes, BUN, creatinine, and cardiac enzymes, in patients with unstable angina or MI. Elective-surgery patients should have minimal blood tests including hematocrit, platelets, BUN, and creatinine after PCI. Patients may be relatively volume-depleted after PCI because of NPO status and radiographic contrast-induced diuresis. Hydration is maintained by intravenous fluids until oral intake is sufficient to meet patient requirements.

Anticoagulants, anti-thrombin agents, or GP IIb/IIIa receptor-inhibitor infusions are continued as per institutional protocol or physician orders.

Vascular sheath removal, mobilization, and ambulation protocols vary according to the device protocol and different management strategies as mandated by hospital policy. In general, the sheaths are removed 4 to 6 hours after the procedure, when the activated clotting time falls to less than 150 to 180 seconds. When using low-molecular-weight heparin, monitoring ACT and PTT are not helpful to access the patient's anticoagulation status (French & Faxon, 2002). A specific protocol has been developed for dosing in the catheterization laboratory. The sheath can usually be removed 4 hours after PCI (Collet, 2001; Kereiakes, 2002). Vascular sheaths are removed by manual pressure or compression device, with strict attention to the arterial site and distal circulation. Common practices after sheath removal include use of compression devices (c-clamp or Fem-Stop [RAD1]), pressure dressings, and sand bags to groin sites. Pressure is applied for at least 20 minutes or more, as warranted to provide homeostasis. Recognition and treatment of complications are essential to prevent peripheral vascular injuries. The vascular site is monitored for bleeding, hematoma formation, distal limb circulation, and sensation every 15 minutes initially, advancing to every hour until stable.

A nursing substudy from the randomized placebo-controlled trial of the effect of eptifibatide on complications of percutaneous coronary intervention (IMPACT II) trial called Standards of Angioplasty Nursing Techniques to Diminish Bleeding Around the Groin (SANDBAG) investigated nursing interventions to minimize vascular bleeding with PTCA. The patients were randomized to receive a GP IIb/IIIa receptor inhibitor (eptifibatide) or placebo. The IMPACT II trial did not show increased bleeding risk in patients with the GP IIb/IIIa receptor inhibitors allowing sheath removal while the agent is infusing (IMPACT II Investigators, 1997). Nursing care to prevent groin complications recommended by the Sandbag investigators include: (1) a nurse-to-patient ratio of 1:1.5 or less maintained during sheath removal; (2) sheaths should be removed within 4 to 6 hours; (3) patients should be medicated for comfort; head of bed can be raised to 30 degrees; (4) patients should be allowed to ambulate 8 hours after sheath removal; and (5) sandbags are not effective to minimize bleeding and cause discomfort (Juan et al., 1999).

Vascular closure devices for rapid hemostasis after femoral access became available in the early 1990s. Multiple invasive and noninvasive devices are available. The most common vascular closure devices for femoral artery puncture sites include the VasoSeal, Angio-Seal, Duett, and the Perclose.

Reasons for use of closure devices as supported by clinical trials include early sheath removal, increased patient comfort, decreased compression time by hospital staff, and early ambulation. The VasoSeal (Datascope Corp.) and Angio-Seal (St. Jude Medical) work primarily by collagen-induced thrombus generation. The Duett (Vascular Solutions, Inc.) uses a combination of collagen and thrombin. The Perclose (Abbott Laboratories) is a suturing device using nonabsorbable suture. The use of arterial closure devices requires specific training by the cardiologist and the catheterization staff. Major and minor complications up to 5% have been reported with these devices, including leg ischemia requiring vascular surgery, infection, and bleeding (Silber, 2000).

PERCUTANEOUS CORONARY PROCEDURES

Percutaneous Transluminal Coronary Angioplasty

Dotter and Judkins first proposed the concept of transluminal angioplasty in 1964. Andreas Gruentzig initially applied the technique of percutaneous transluminal coronary angioplasty (PTCA) to human coronary arteries in 1977. Since the first PTCA, advances in catheter and balloon technique and technology have improved immediate success rates to 90% to 98%, with low complication rates of 1% to 2% (Baim, 2000). Balloon angioplasty can be applied to patients with single coronary lesions or to patients with multi-vessel disease. Newer devices are now used in more than 80% of coronary interventions, so that plain old balloon angioplasty (POBA) is not frequently used as a stand-alone procedure. The role of angioplasty has changed to be an adjunctive technique.

The desired therapeutic effect of balloon angioplasty is the enlargement of the internal luminal diameter of the diseased artery. Balloon pressure to an area of atherosclerotic stenosis results in plaque rupture, disruption of the endothelium, and stretching of the vessel segment, enlarging the vessel lumen size.

Guiding catheters have large internal lumens, come with and without sideholes, have nontraumatic soft tips, are available in many shapes and French sizes, and are designed to provide support for the delivery of guidewires, balloons, and other devices. There is a wide range of intracoronary guidewires with different coating and characteristics such as flexibility, diameter, radio-opacity, and torquability for different coronary lesions. PTCA may be performed using monorail, rapid-exchange balloon catheters, or over-the-wire systems. Although the over-the-wire systems predominate in North America, in some parts of the world, rapid-exchange catheters are more popular because of their ease and speed of use.

In the catheterization laboratory, after the guide catheter is placed and the wire crosses the lesion, a balloon catheter is selected that most closely approximates the diameter of the nondiseased reference segment adjacent to the site to be treated. The prepared and flushed balloon is loaded onto the free end of the guidewire. The balloon is passed into the guide catheter, down the proximal vessel, and across the lesion. Once the balloon catheter is positioned across the lesion, the balloon is inflated using a handheld inflation device equipped with a pressure dial. Multiple balloon inflations of variable pressure and duration are used depending on the type of lesion and the physician preference. The response of the lesion to dilatation is assessed by repeat angiography through the guiding catheter with the guide wire in place. When the result is almost complete, normalization of the vessel lumen or less than a 30% residual stenosis after inflation the procedure is considered to be successful. The guidewire and guiding catheter are removed after an adequate result is obtained (Fig. 27-1).

Cutting balloon angioplasty uses a special designed balloon with three to four microscopic blades or atherotomes mounted on the surface of a balloon that protrude slightly above the

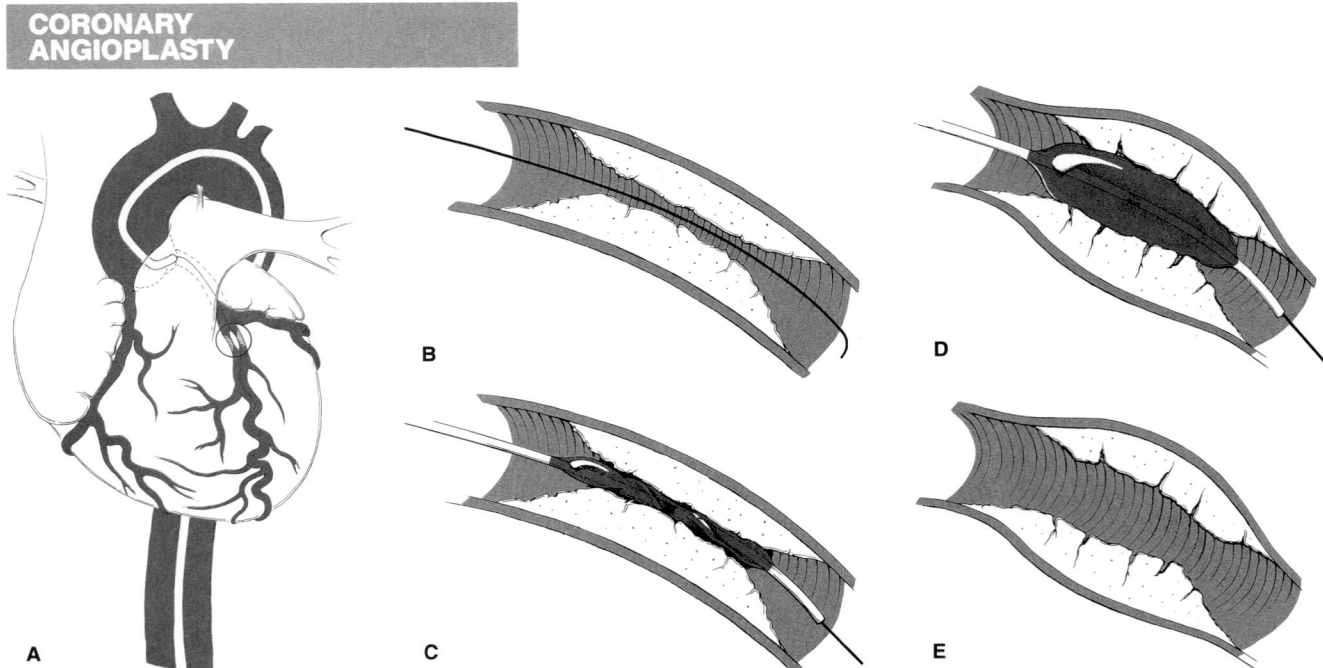

CORONARY ANGIOPLASTY

■ **Figure 27–1.** Mechanism of intracoronary balloon angioplasty. (***A***) A balloon catheter is introduced into the coronary artery through a guide catheter in the aorta. (***B***) A guide wire is advanced across the area of narrowing. (***C***) The balloon catheter is advanced over the wire across the lesion. (***D***) The balloon is inflated. (***E***) Coronary artery after PTCA. (Courtesy of Boston Scientific Corporation, Maple Grove, MN.)

balloon surface when inflated (Fig. 27-2). The mechanism of action referred to as atherotomy uses the balloon device to make three to four controlled incisions, which score the plaque in an atherosclerotic coronary artery. The noncompliant balloon then dilates the incised areas, resulting in more plaque[i]

compression and less vessel wall expansion. The cutting balloon is designed for lesions resistant to dilatation by traditional angioplasty balloons such as elastic and fibrotic lesions. The cutting balloon may be used alone or in combination with stents (Rizik et al., 1999).

Coronary Atherectomy

The atherectomy catheters reduce the severity of coronary stenosis by removing the atheromatous plaque rather than compressing or fracturing the plaque or stretching the arterial wall. In theory, this approach was developed to permit a more controlled vascular injury and to minimize the degree of arterial mural stretch. Removal of plaque creates a smoother surface by debulking the vessel and removes atherosclerotic plaque that is frequently resistant to balloon dilatation.

The atherectomy devices have been used successfully to remove atherosclerotic plaque but were associated with increased complication rates. The incidence of restenosis was found to be no better than with PTCA from neointimal hyperplasia. These devices have fallen out of favor but still provide a treatment option for difficult anatomical lesions such as calcific, long diffuse, and chronic occlusions. Stents are usually used in conjunction with the atherectomy devices.

Directional Coronary Atherectomy

The directional coronary atherectomy (DCA) catheter, or Simpson AtheroCath (Guidant Corporation, Santa Clara, CA), approved for treatment of coronary arteries and saphenous

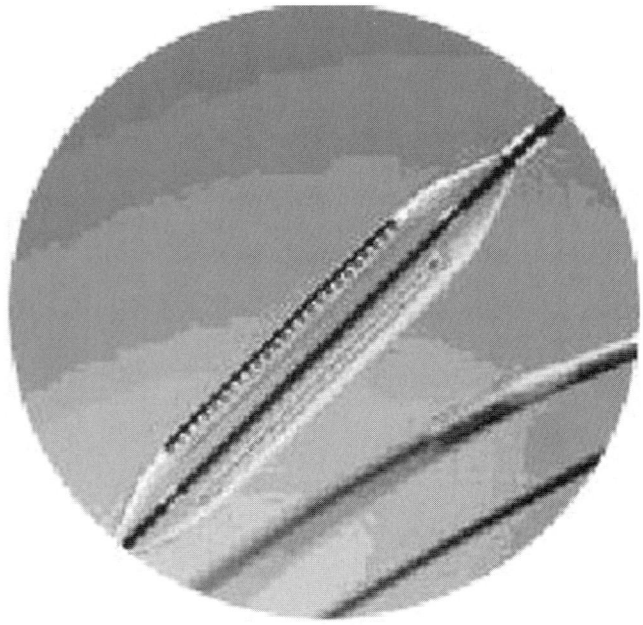

■ **Figure 27–2.** The cutting balloon. (Courtesy of Boston Scientific Corporation, Maple Grove, MN.)

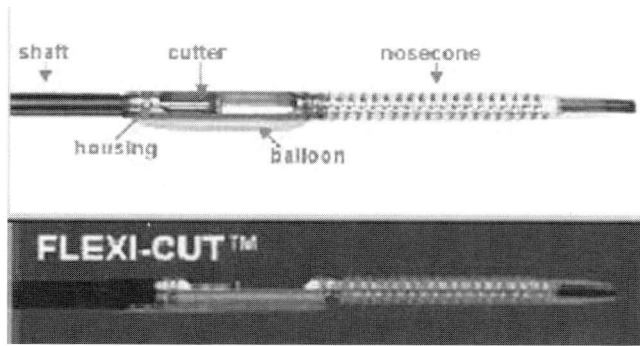

■ **Figure 27–3.** Directional coronary atherectomy catheter: FLEXI-CUT directional debulking system. (Courtesy of Guidant Corporation, Santa Clara, CA.)

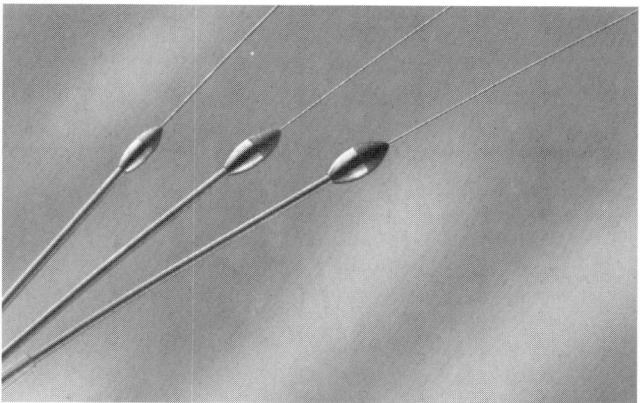

■ **Figure 27–4.** Rotational atherectomy catheters in different sizes. (Courtesy of Boston Scientific Corporation, Maple Grove, MN.)

vein grafts (SVG) in 1990, consists of a catheter-mounted, cylindrical, metallic housing unit (i.e., collection chamber, window, and cup-shaped cutter) and a small balloon attached to the housing. A handheld motor drive unit is attached to the proximal end of the catheter, and the cutter in the housing is rotated at 2,000 rpm through the driving cable. When this catheter is placed at the stenotic lesion, a balloon is inflated at low pressure against one wall of the vessel to stabilize the housing chamber and the window against the opposite vessel wall of atherosclerotic plaque. Plaque that protrudes into the housing unit through the window is then excised with the rotating cutter, which is advanced manually. The device is then rotated and plaque is excised from around the vessel lumen. (Topol et al., 1993; Holmes et al., 1994) (Fig. 27-3).

Rotational Atherectomy

The rotational atherectomy device (Rotablator/Boston Scientific, Maple Grove, MN) was approved for clinical use in 1993. The Rotablator is a flexible catheter-deliverable system that can be used transluminally. The Rotablator system uses a high-speed, rotating, elliptical burr coated with diamond chips 20 to 30 μm in diameter that form an abrasive surface. When the burr is spun at a high speed (140,000–180,000 rpm, depending on burr size), it preferentially removes atheroma because of its selective differential cutting of inelastic plaque rather than elastic normal tissue. The process involves a stepwise incremental increase in burr size to provide a "sanding effect" (Fig. 27-4). Gradual advancement and withdrawal of the burr in 2- to 5-second intervals for up to 20 to 30 seconds in the lesion allows for heat dissipation, improved distal perfusion, and washout of particulate debris. The postablation vessel diameter is equal to the largest burr size used. Adjunctive PTCA and stenting is frequently used to maximize final coronary artery luminal diameter. The debris emitted from the Rotablator ablation process is released into the coronary bloodstream as pulverized microparticles. Rotational atherectomy has been shown to be particularly effective in the treatment of calcified coronary lesions by ablating the fibrocalcific plaque, which is difficult to dilate with an angioplasty balloon. (Buchbinder et al., 1992; Hong, 1996).

Angiojet Thrombectomy

The angiojet is a rheolytic thrombectomy (Possis Medical Inc., Minneapolis, MN) catheter designed for the percutaneous disruption and removal of unorganized thrombus from native coronary arteries and bypass grafts using high velocity saline. It consists of a double-lumen catheter that is 140-cm long. The smaller lumen of the catheter is used to supply the catheter tip with saline jets. The saline jets that emerge at the tip of the catheter are generated by an external drive unit. These jets aid in the formation of a recirculation pattern that fragments the thrombotic material. An additional three saline jets are directed retrograde into the larger exhaust lumen of the catheter. These jets create a "Venturi effect" that aids in evacuation of the macerated thrombotic material (Silva, 2001).

Coronary Laser Angioplasty

The concept of applying laser energy to remove, in a percutaneous manner, atherosclerotic coronary obstructions first emerged in the late 1980s. Laser energy from the xenon chloride laser ablates inorganic material by photochemical mechanisms that involve breaking of molecular bonds without generation of heat. The mechanisms for tissue ablation are believed to consist of a combination of photochemical, localized thermal, and mechanical effects. A decline in laser angioplasty occurred because of significant dissections and perforations of the coronary artery with early techniques. The current generation of xenon chloride excimer lasers is occasionally being used for coronary angioplasty. Newer applications of the laser include pacemaker and implantable defibrillator lead extractions and myocardial laser revascularization (Ebersole, 1999; Saririan, 2003). Laser angioplasty has been used for treatment of in-stent restenosis with good procedural success but disappointing long-term results (Dahm et al., 2002).

Coronary Stents

The major portion of PCI, more than 80% worldwide, involves placement of intracoronary stents as a primary or an adjunctive

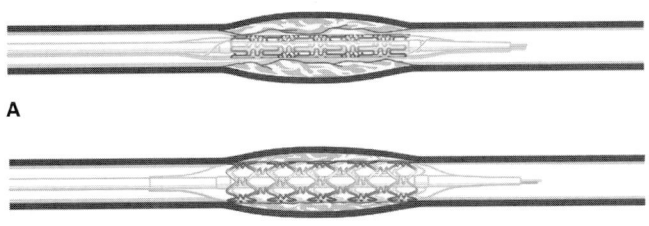

A

B

■ **Figure 27–5.** Stent deployment. (*A*) Stent in the closed position across lesion on the balloon delivery system. (*B*) Stent in open position in coronary artery after balloon inflation. (Courtesy of Cordis Corporation, a Johnson & Johnson Company, Miami Lakes, FL.)

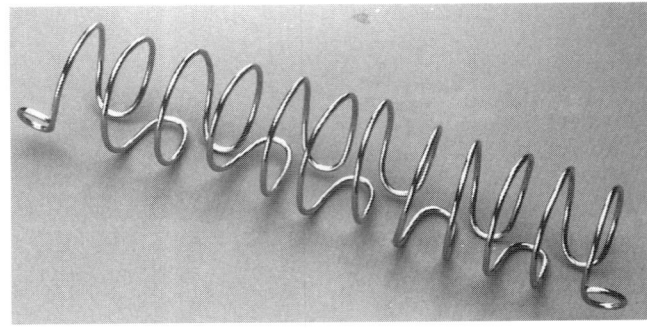

■ **Figure 27–6.** The Gianturco-Roubin Flex-Stent. (Courtesy of Cook, Inc., Bloomington, IN.)

procedure. With the approval of drug-eluting stents, the number of primary stent procedures is expected to increase. After the introduction of PTCA, the procedure was plagued by acute closure resulting from coronary dissection occurring in 5% to 10% of patients, depending on lesion characteristics in the acute phase and restenosis as a late complication. Dotter first demonstrated the concept of stenting an injured vessel in 1969. In 1986, percutaneous implantation of metallic stents in coronary vessels was first reported in humans by Sigwart and coworker with the Wallstent, a self-expanding stent (Sigwart et al., 1987). The development of intracoronary stents was initiated to provide structural support to an artery opposing elastic recoil, to prevent vasoconstriction, and to prevent or treat dissections of the arterial wall. The stent procedure is similar in preparation to PTCA with a guide catheter in the ostium of the coronary artery and a guide wire across the lesion. The lesion can be predilated with an angioplasty balloon or the stent placed without predilatation. The most commonly used balloon-expandable stents are delivered over a guide wire into the coronary artery in a collapsed state mounted on a balloon delivery system. Once the balloon is positioned correctly across the lesion, the balloon is inflated, expanding the stent. The balloon delivery system is removed. Frequently, a high-pressure balloon is then used to completely expand the stent (Fig. 27-5).

The other type of stents, used less often, is the self-expanding stents. The self-expanding stents are placed on the delivery system in a collapsed state with a retaining outer membrane.

Retraction of the membrane after the delivery system is across the lesion allows the stent to expand. A high-pressure balloon can be used after deployment to completely expand the stent.

The first stent approved by the FDA for clinical use was the Gianturco-Roubin Flex-Stent in June 1993 for acute and threatened closure of coronary arteries. This was successful in reducing the incidence of emergent CABG surgery associated with PTCA (Rubin et al., 1992). The Gianturco-Roubin coronary stent (Cook, Inc., Bloomington, IN) was balloon-expandable and consisted of surgical stainless steel that was wrapped cylindrically, with bends that make an inverted "U" configuration every 360 degrees (Fig. 27-6).

The second stent was the Palmaz-Schatz coronary stent approved for use in 1994. The original stent design, developed by Palmaz, consists of a single, rigid, slotted, stainless steel tube. The Palmaz-Schatz stent modified by Schatz for coronary arteries (Cordis, a Johnson & Johnson Company) consists of two 7-mm tubes connected by a central bridging 1-mm strut (Fig. 27-7). The stent fits over an angioplasty balloon for deployment. When the balloon is inflated, the struts of the stent take on a diamond configuration, with a high open space-to-metal ratio. The articulation point of the stent imparts longitudinal flexibility, which enhanced passage (Schatz et al., 1991).

These two stent designs are no longer used for coronary intervention but have provided the initial model from which to build and develop new stent designs with better success rates and long-term results.

■ **Figure 27–7.** The Palmaz-Schatz® balloon-expandable Stent. (Courtesy of Cordis Corporation, a Johnson & Johnson Company, Miami Lakes, FL.)

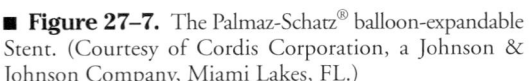
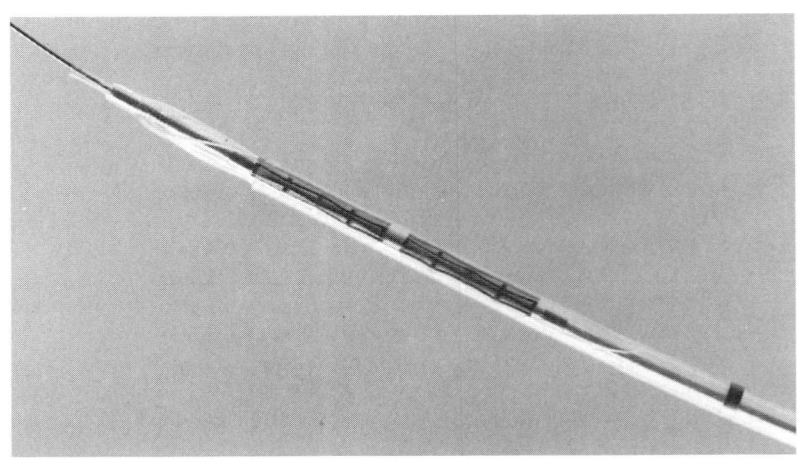

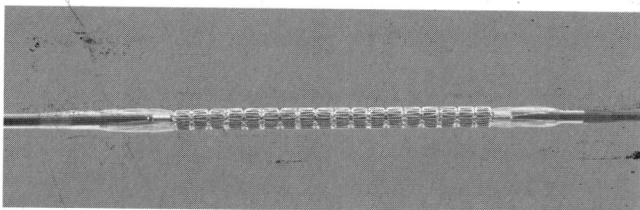

A

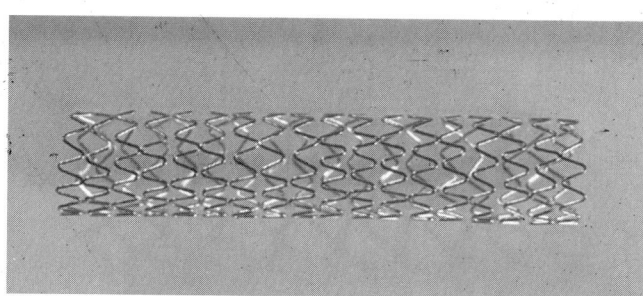

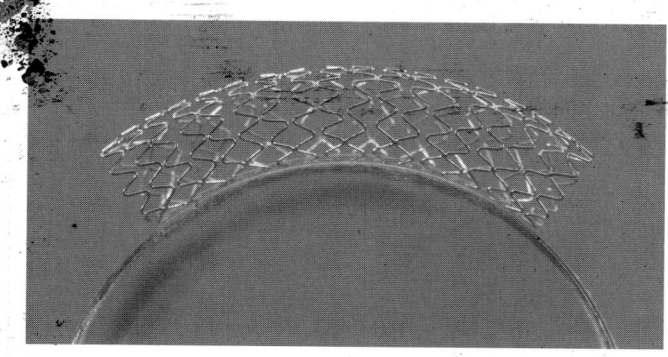

C

■ **Figure 27–8.** The S7 Stent (*A*) crimped on the balloon delivery system, (*B*) completely deployed, and (*C*) demonstrating the flexibility of the stent. (Courtesy of Medtronic AVE, Inc. Santa Rosa, CA.)

Two landmark clinical stent trials that empowered the stent revolution were randomized trials comparing the Palmaz-Schatz Stent with PTCA. The Stent Restenosis Trial (STRESS) found that patients with an intracoronary stent in a *de novo* lesion had a higher procedural success rate and a less frequent need for revascularization. The angiographic restenosis rate was 31.6% for stents and 42.1% for PTCA, with similar rates of clinical events after 6 months (Fischman et al., 1994). In the Belgium Netherlands Stent Trial (Benestent), over a 7-month follow-up, clinical and angiographic outcomes were better in patients who received a stent rather than PTCA, with restenosis rates of 22% for stents and 32% for PTCA (Serruys et al., 1994). However, this benefit was achieved at the cost of a significantly higher risk of vascular bleeding complications and a longer hospital stay. An aggressive regimen of adjunctive pharmacologic agents was used during these trials and during the initial experience of stenting, including ASA, dipyridamole, warfarin, heparin, and dextran. The initial stent trials were hindered by a high rate of subacute stent thrombosis, embolization of stents, difficulty in stent placement, and groin complications. Improvement in stent deployment, elimination of aggressive anticoagulation regimens, and

the introduction of antiplatelet therapy facilitated widespread acceptance of coronary stenting with less complications.

Stent technology has improved, leading to better stent designs and the availability of multiple products. The optimal stent should be easily and safely deliverable to various locations in coronary arteries. It should be flexible, low-profile, radiopaque, smooth-contoured, of sufficient radial strength, and tissue-and blood-compatible. Stents may be classified according to the following characteristics: mechanism of expansion—self-expanding or balloon-expandable; composition—stainless steel, cobalt alloy, tantalum, or nitinol; and design—mesh structure, coil, slotted tube, ring, multiple cell design, or custom design (Colombo et al., 2002). All stents are designed to be implanted into coronary arteries and some are specific for vein grafts. Most stents are premounted on a balloon delivery system (Fig. 27-8).

Drug-Eluting Stents

A new generation of drug-eluting stents designed to limit restenosis is now available for PCI. The concept of drug-eluting stents is to coat a stent with a drug or material that can be delivered locally to the coronary lesion with antiproliferative properties, preventing neointimal hyperplasia and restenosis. The stent design, type of drug, presence or absence of a polymer to absorb the drug, type of polymer, and release pattern of the drug is important to provide safety and prevent cell death and necrosis of the coronary vessel leading to vascular complications. The clinical success of this technology depends on the complex interaction between the stent, coating matrix, drug, and vessel wall. The first drug-eluting stent approved for use in PCI in the USA in April 2003 was the sirolimus-eluting stent. The BX VELOCITY stent is used as the stent platform and the drug sirolimus and polymer coating is placed on the stent (Cordis, a Johnson & Johnson Company) (Fig. 27-9). The dual mechanism of action includes inhibition of cell proliferation by targeting smooth muscle cells while simultaneously reducing cytokine production and inflammation in the vessel wall. Sirolimus allows normal development of endothelial lining on the stent struts, which is important for preventing direct contact between bare metal and circulating blood, a circumstance that can lead to clot formation and stent thrombosis. Two-year angiographic and intravascular ultrasound follow-up after implantation of the sirolimus stent has shown safety and efficacy with reduction in the restenosis phenomenon (Sousa et al., 2003). A second drug-eluting stent released for use in 2004 is a paclitaxel-eluting Taxus stent (Boston Scientific

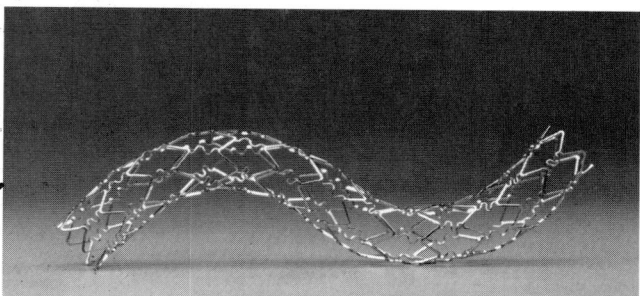

■ **Figure 27–9.** The BX VELOCITY® Coronary Stent used for delivery of sirolimus: The Cypher Sirolimus-Eluting Stent. (Courtesy of Cordis Corporation, a Johnson & Johnson Company, Miami Lakes, FL.)

Corporation). The Taxus stent has shown similar results as the Cypher stent. Clinical trials are ongoing with other drugs and polymers placed on stents. The economics associated with the cost of drug-eluding stents as compared to conventional stents has become a major issue in selecting a specific type of stent for PCI. With the current cost of drug-eluting stents up to $3,000, it is expected to have a dramatic impact on hospital budgets and medical costs of treatment. In Europe, where the drug-eluting stents became available in 2002, they have not had widespread application because of cost issues. The initial clinical trails with drug-eluting stents are limited and have concentrated on patients with short lesions and relatively large lumen arteries. The results of these trials do not reflect the broad range of patients treated on a daily basis with diffuse coronary artery disease, multi-vessel disease or small vessels. These patient subsets will be further evaluated in clinical trails and the information obtained will be needed before this new technology can be broadly applied. Concern about possible late thrombogenicity and impact on health care ecomonics are issues to be further investigated (Degertekin et al., 2003; Grube et al., 2002).

Radiation PCI: Brachytherapy

A PCI used to treat in-stent restenosis is brachytherapy in the coronary artery. This technique of brachytherapy involved local radiation treatment to the coronary vessel wall. The treatment of restenosis with vascular radiation has been very successful and appears to work through inhibition of smooth muscle cell proliferation. Two types of radiation devices are available for treatment using a gamma ray or beta particle emitting source. Patients presenting with in-stent restenosis undergo diagnostic angiography and placement of equipment as for PTCA. After dilatation of the target lesion, a catheter containing a closed-end source delivery lumen is advanced over a guide-wire and positioned across the target lesion. A wire containing radioactive sources at its distal tip is then loaded into the source lumen of the catheter and advanced distally until the radioactive sources span the lesion. This process, called afterloading, can be accomplished manually by the radiation oncologists advancing the source wire by hand or automatically by a motor-driven unit. Several multicenter trials have shown the effective anti-proliferative effect of brachytherapy on in-stent restenosis (Teirstein & Kuntz, 2001).

Early safety and efficacy have been demonstrated, but there were several concerns about long-term effects with initial trials. The first issue was late thrombosis that occurred after discontinuing thienopyridines (clopidogrel or ticlopidine). The current recommendation is for longer use of clopidogrel or ticlopidine for 9 to 12 months or indefinitely for some patients. Without immediate neointimal hyperplasia covering the stent, there is no longer a protection from platelets and thrombus accumulating on bare stent struts. The placement of additional stents with brachytherapy has been discouraged unless absolutely necessary to avoid late thrombosis. Anti-platelet medications have been successful in preventing late thrombosis when continued for longer period of time.

The second issue causing concern with brachytherapy was re-narrowing found at the treatment edges of the coronary lesion caused by radiation drop-off. This decrease in radiation at the edge of the lesion caused the delivering of a subtherapuetic

dose of radiation, leading to edge restenosis. Recommendations to avoid edge failure include accurate placement of radiation therapy and providing a wide margin of radiation source to either side of the injured vessel (Terstein & Kuntz, 2001).

COMPLICATIONS ASSOCIATED WITH PCI

Recurrent Chest Pain

Anatomic improvement after a PCI correlates with elimination of angina symptoms. Recurrent chest pain or persistent chest pain should be monitored and reported to a cardiologist. Some patients may have residual chest pain after the procedure secondary to vessel dilatation and stretch or distal embolization of embolic debris in the microcirculation. This discomfort should be transient and dissipate in severity over several hours of PCI. If ongoing angina persists, it may indicate untreated disease or a poor result at the site treated and requires further evaluation by the cardiologist.

Abrupt Closure

Coronary artery plaque disruption or dissection is caused by a controlled injury resulting from balloon dilatation with PTCA or atherectomy device. However, large progressive dissections may interfere with blood flow, cause compression of the true lumen by the dissection flap, have superimposed thrombus formation, platelet adhesion, or vessel spasm, and may lead to a total occlusion of the treated artery, which is a phenomenon known as abrupt closure. Vessel wall damage activates the GP IIb/IIIa receptor on the platelet surface, causing platelet aggregation and thrombosis. Abrupt or acute closure causes acute myocardial ischemia with chest pain and ECG changes. If the coronary artery is not successfully reopened percutaneously, the event may progress to MI, emergent CABG surgery, or death. With the use of stents and GP IIb/IIIa receptor inhibitors, there has been a decrease in the incidence of abrupt closure requiring emergent bypass surgery in less than 0.5% (Carrozza & Baim, 2000; Kong et al., 1998).

Acute Stent Thrombosis

Acute stent thrombosis can occur, resulting in acute closure of the coronary vessel. The metallic surface of the conventional stents contributes to the thrombogenic potential. Risk associated with this event includes stenting in acute coronary syndromes, inadequate deployment of stent, or propagation of thrombus from inadequate anticoagulation or anti-platelet therapies. Using the current antiplatelet regimen after the procedure has reduced the incidence of acute stent thrombosis. Intravascular ultrasound has provided invasive evaluation tool to assess stent expansion and full apposition of struts to the vessel wall preventing inflow or outflow obstruction in coronary artery leading to thrombus formation. Acute stent thrombosis has been reduced to approximately 1% with the current treatment regimens (Carrozza & Baim, 2000).

Vascular Spasm

Vascular spasm at the site or distal to the treated site is a potential cause of acute chest pain or ischemia during or after PCI. This is most common with atherectomy devices, particularly the high-speed rotation of the rotablator device. It may occur at the treated site, in the proximal vessel secondary to guide catheter-related injury, or in the distal vessels. Vascular spasm is usually transient, causing chest pain and hypotension, and most commonly occurs in the catheterization laboratory. Treatment includes nitroglycerin or a low-pressure balloon. If spasm is significant, the patient may be maintained on nitroglycerin and intravenous fluids overnight.

Non-ST Elevation MI

Elevation of cardiac enzymes after PCI is common, occurring in 10% to 30% of uncomplicated PCI. This is usually a result of distal microembolization or loss of small side branches. Distal embolization of friable plaque or thrombus can be released into the microcirculation during PCI. If a large amount of material is released into the coronary circulation as in rotational atherectomy with particulate debris, in an acute thrombus with acute coronary syndrome, or during treatment of an SVG, then a "no-flow" phenomenon can occur with transient occlusion of the coronary vessel and elevation of CPK-MB. Patients with CPK-MB elevations have shown increased incidence of adverse events at 3 to 5 years. Treatment with GP IIb/IIIa receptor inhibitor and distal protection devices are recommended to prevent microembolization in high-risk patients (Baim, 2000).

ST Elevation MI

MI, as documented by ECG including new Q waves or new LBBB pattern or cardiac enzyme elevation more than three-times the upper level of normal, occurs in approximately 1% of patients. It is usually caused by an acute coronary syndrome, abrupt closure, or loss of major side branch originating within or in close proximity to the lesion being treated.

Coronary Vessel Perforation

Perforation of a coronary artery is infrequent and rarely occurs with a guide wire alone. If a device is passed over a wire that is extraluminal, perforation of the vessel may occur. Frank rupture of the coronary artery from too large a balloon or atherectomy device can cause vessel perforation that leads to rapid hemodynamic collapse and cardiac tamponade. Management of coronary perforation includes reversal of anticoagulation with protamine if needed. Balloon inflation at the perforation site may occlude the perforation and prevent further extravasation of blood. A specific designed membrane-covered stent (JoStent Graft; JOMED Inc., San Diego, CA) can be used to tack-up the perforation and prevent further extravasation into the pericardium. Patients with limited pericardial blood can be managed conservatively, as identified by echocardiogram. If there is a significant leak into the pericardial space resulting in potential cardiac tamponade, then pericardiocentesis may be required. Perforation into the pericardium with cardiac tamponade may also result from the right ventricle during temporary pacemaker wire placement used for bradycardia during PCI. Patient anticoagulation state during PCI increases the risk of wire perforation. If unable to manage the bleeding in the catheterization laboratory, then emergent cardiac surgery may be necessary (Ellis et al., 1994; Hinoharo et al., 1998; Baim, 2000).

Arrhythmias and Conduction Disturbances

A variety of conduction abnormalities can occur during PCI. Ischemia during treatment can cause electrocardiographic changes, including transient heart block, atrial arrhythmias, or ventricular arrhythmias such as ventricular tachycardia. Severe bradycardia or ventricular fibrillation occurs in approximately 1% of PCI, usually as a result of prolonged ischemia during balloon inflation or luminal occlusion with devices (Baim, 2000). Vasovagal reaction can occur at time of sheath insertion or at time of sheath removal. Common symptoms associated with a vasovagal reaction include hypotension, nausea, vomiting, yawning, and diaphoresis. This syndrome is triggered by pain and anxiety, particularly in the setting of hypovolemia (Landau, 1993). Treatment includes cessation of painful stimuli, rapid volume administration, elevation of legs or Trendelenburg position, and atropine intravenously. If hypotension persists, additional pressor support with vasoactive drugs may be needed.

Failure of Device or Retained Equipment

Failure of a wire or device may occur when the equipment is stressed beyond their design parameters, causing knotting, entrapment, or fragmentation. The cardiologist should be familiar with retrieval devices and techniques to recover the fragments. If device or fragments cannot be retrieved in the catheterization laboratory, surgery may be necessary.

Contrast-Related Complications

Allergic reactions are triggered by iodinated contrast agents. Risk of allergic reactions is increased in patients allergic to seafood that contains organic iodine. Premedication with prednisone for 24 to 48 hours before the procedure or an intravenous steroid the day of the procedure, an H1 antihistamine (diphenhydramine), and H2 blocker (cimetidine or ranitidine) before the procedure has been effective in preventing anaphylaxis (Goss, 1995).

Contrast-induced nephropathy can cause temporary or permanent renal dysfunction. Older patients and patients with diabetes or preexisting real insufficiency are at highest risk. Limiting volume of contrast and hydration before PCI remains the best preventive strategy.

Volume overload can be caused by hypertonic contrast agents, myocardial depression secondary to ischemia, poor baseline ventricular function, supine position, and volume preloading. Prevention involves continued monitoring of fluid status before and after the procedure and possible need for diuretics.

Cerebrovascular Complications

Spontaneous intracerebral hemorrhage may occur with aggressive anticoagulation medications.

Transient ischemic attacks or cerebral vascular accidents secondary to plaque disruption may occur from manipulation of catheters and devices during intervention in patients with diffuse atherosclerotic disease (Lasky et al., 1993).

LATE COMPLICATIONS OF PCI

Subacute Occlusion

Subacute closure of stents is a potentially life-threatening complication that can occur with all stents, regardless of design or composition. This mechanism can lead to death or MI and occurs in approximately 1% of patients 1 to 2 days after stent implantation. Improved stent deployment, intravascular/ultrasound (IVUS), and antiplatelet medications have decreased the incidence (Carrozza & Baim, 2000).

Restenosis

A late-occurring complication is the process of restenosis that is a coronary luminal re-narrowing after a coronary intervention. This process occurs during a time interval of 3 to 6 months; it is unusual for this to occur after 12 months in PTCA, atherectomy, and conventional stents. Restenosis rates are variable from reports of clinical trials but have been reported from 20% to 45% with PTCA, 35% to 50% with atherectomy, and 22% to 35% with conventional stents (Ellis et al., 1992; Buchbinder et al., 1992; Sketch et al., 1992; Topol et al., 1993; Holmes et al., 1994). Restenosis after PTCA and atherectomy involves a series of mechanisms that involve a loss of vessel lumen size because of the elastic recoil; a wound healing process including thrombotic, inflammatory, and cell growth proliferation that form a neointimal hyperplasia; and a remodeling of the treated vessel causing shrinkage. When a conventional stent was used, the elastic recoil and shrinkage was prevented but neointimal hyperplasia was noted to still be present and responsible for restenosis. The smaller the vessel size, the higher incidence of restenosis. Patients with diffuse CHD and diabetes have also shown a higher incidence of restenosis.

A decrease in the incidence of restenosis has recently been seen in clinical trails with drug-eluting stents. The RAVEL (Randomized Comparison of a Sirolimus-eluting stent with a standard stent for coronary revascularization) trial investigators reported a significant reduction in angiographic restenosis rate at 6 months and target lesion revascularization at 1 year after implantation of the sirolimus-eluting stent (Morice et al., 2002). Sousa et al. in 2003 reported sustained lumen patency

at 2 years in patients receiving sirolimus-eluting stents, with restenosis rates at approximately 10%. The antiproliferative activity with drug-eluding stents has shown promise in eliminating the neointimal hyperplasia at the treatment site in PCI.

Groin Complications

The incidence of vascular complications has been as high as 21% in the early days of PCI. Decreased incidence of complications has been seen with the decrease in sheath size and the current standard drug regimen for stenting including ASA, clopidogrel, and GP IIb/IIIa receptor inhibitors.

Hematoma formation is frequent and self-limiting, and it usually requires no intervention.

Retroperitoneal bleeding caused by large hematomas dissecting into the retroperitoneum is life-threatening and need prompt attention by the nursing and medical staff. Inadvertent puncture of the artery proximal to the inguinal ligament while placing the arterial sheath, which involves the external iliac artery, is frequently the cause. There is less supporting tissue in this area, and it is more difficult to compress the puncture site. Retroperitoneal bleeding is characterized by lumbar or groin pain and a significant drop in hematocrit, hypotension, and possibly bradycardia or tachycardia. Diagnosis is confirmed by a computed tomography scan. Treatment involves transfusion and fluid resuscitation to maintain adequate blood pressure, reversal of anticoagulation, and occasionally surgical repair of the artery.

Arterial thrombosis at the puncture site may lead to occlusion of the artery or distal thrombosis into the extremity. Preexisting peripheral vascular disease increases the risk of a thromboembolic event. Surveillance of distal circulation and sensory checks should be continued after sheath removal. Signs of loss of pulse, color changes, decreased sensation, decreased temperature, or decreased motor function are potential indicators of thrombosis.

Pseudoaneurysm is an extraluminal cavity in communication with an adjacent artery, usually the femoral artery. Inadvertent puncture of the superficial femoral or profunda femoris artery increases the incidence of arterial complications. Contributing factors include inadequate compression of the puncture site, heparin use, intramural arterial calcifications, and hypertension. On physical examination, the patient may have a pulsatile mass, systolic bruit, normal distal arterial pulses, and pain in the groin. Doppler ultrasound and color flow imaging are used to confirm the diagnosis and delineate the location and size of the pseudoaneurysm. Although most small pseudoaneurysms spontaneously close in 4 to 8 weeks without sequelae, they may enlarge or hemorrhage, especially in patients with prolonged anticoagulation. Treatment includes ultrasound-guided compression, thrombin injection with ultrasound guidance, or surgical closure (Bogart et al., 1995).

Arteriovenous fistula is a communication between an artery and vein. The mechanism of injury involves a puncture through the femoral artery and vein, which results in a false communication. On physical examination, the patient may have a pulsatile mass in the groin and a continuous systolic–diastolic bruit; over time, temperature of the extremity may be decreased because of high flow through the fistula and ischemia of the extremity. A thrill may be present at the site,

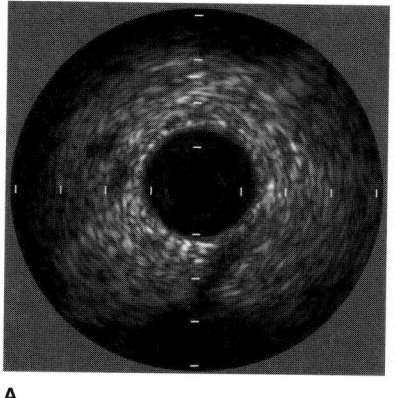 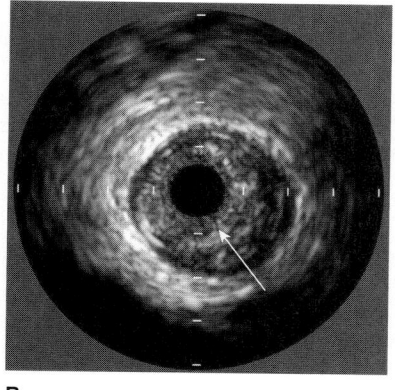 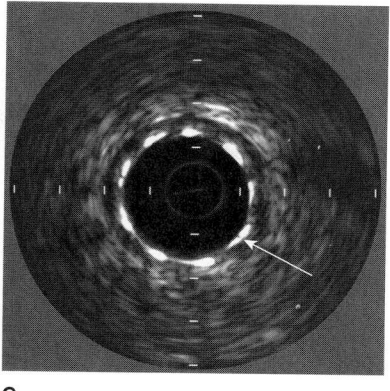

A   **B**   **C**

■ **Figure 27–10.** Intravascular ultrasound. (*A*) Normal coronary artery; (*B*) concentric atherosclerotic plaque inside coronary artery; *arrow* points to plaque; (*C*) coronary artery after stent placment; *arrow* points to stent struts. (Courtesy of JOMED, Inc., Rancho Cordova, CA.)

and congestive heart failure may result if the fistula is persistent. Doppler ultrasound and color flow imaging confirm diagnosis. Surgical treatment may be necessary for closure and repair of the peripheral vasculature.

Septic endarteritis is rare and has been implicated in chronic intimal damage and stasis caused by flow turbulence in the region of a pseudoaneurysm or AV fistula, multiple procedures through same access, obesity, or sheaths left in place for more than 24 hours. In high-risk patients, antibiotics are administered after the procedure and may be continued on an outpatient basis if warranted (Frazee et al., 1991).

ADJUNCTIVE MODALITIES

Coronary angiography alone sometimes does not provide enough information to distinguish ischemia-producing coronary lesion from nonischemic-producing intermediate coronary lesions. Nuclear perfusion imaging and stress echocardiography are noninvasive tests used to delineate ischemic areas that should be treated in patients with CHD. In the catheterization laboratory, invasive diagnostic procedures can be used to guide appropriate treatment. The following invasive modalities are used for diagnostic purposes.

Intravascular Ultrasound

Intravascular ultrasound (IVUS) imaging provides a detailed cross-sectional image of the vessel wall. This method of direct visualization of the arterial wall and lesion at the site of a planned intervention has improved clinical and angiographic outcomes. A miniaturized ultrasound transducer is placed on the distal end of a flexible catheter and advanced down the coronary artery. IVUS can be used during cardiac catheterization to evaluate plaque and tissue characteristics and during interventional procedures to verify adequate results and stent deployment. Colombo and associates (1995) recognized with the use of IVUS that stent deployment techniques were inadequate and that the stents frequently were not completely expanded in the vessel, contributing to subacute closure. As a result of these findings, the use of high-pressure balloon dilatation after stent deployment to ensure full stent expansion was instituted,

which had a significant effect on stenting practices and decreased thrombotic complications (Fig. 27-10).

Coronary Flow Reserve

Doppler wire-derived measurements can be obtained to assess coronary flow across a lesion to determine significance of blockage. The ability to increase coronary blood flow by reducing vasomotor tone to meet myocardial demand is called coronary flow reserve (CFR). Normal individuals can increase coronary blood flow by four- to six-fold to meet increased myocardial demand. In the presence of a physiologically significant lesion, the resistance vessel compensates by vasodilating. In a severe lesion, the resistance vessels are fully vasodilated. Use of this physiologic assessment can help guide interventional therapy (Hasdai et al., 2000).

Fractional Flow Reserve

Coronary pressure wire-derived fractional flow reserve is used to assess significance of coronary lesions. The pressure wire placed across the coronary lesion provides a pressure gradient measurement. The fractional flow reserve (FFR) is a ratio between the driving pressure distal to the lesion and the driving pressure in the aorta. The clinical use for FFR is for assessment of intermediate lesions and optimization of procedure outcomes (Okura et al., 2000). Information concerning ischemia-producing lesions obtained with the pressure wire in the catheterization laboratory is similar to results obtained by noninvasive testing.

Distal Protection Devices

Distal protection devices are designed to provide protection of the distal microcirculation during PCI. Several devices are available for use during PCI in patients at high risk for distal embolization. One device type is a balloon occlusive system that temporarily occludes the distal vessel during the intervention followed by the aspiration of liberated atheromatous and thrombotic material before it reaches that arteriolar and capillary bed. The other device type is a nonocclusive, filter-based system that preserves coronary blood flow through tiny pores, as low as 100 microns. Atheromatous and thrombotic material is trapped in the filter-based systems and then removed with the retrieval of the device through a retrieval catheter. These techniques can reduce the incidence of cardiac enzyme elevation after PCI.

ANTICOAGULATION OPTIONS FOR PCI

Anticoagulation during PCI is critical to prevent abrupt and subacute closure. Initial trials suggested the need for aggressive anticoagulation regimens. The Intracoronary Stenting and Antithrombotic Regimen trial compared the outcomes of two different antithrombotic regimens after placement of coronary stents. The combined antiplatelet therapy with ticlopidine plus aspirin (ASA) was superior to therapy with heparin, warfarin, and ASA alone in reducing cardiac events and hemorrhagic and vascular complications after stenting. This change in therapy decreased length of stay and cost of hospitalization (Schomig et al., 1996). Current management includes the pretreatment of patients with ASA and continuation indefinitely, the use of high-dose unfractionated heparin (UFH) during the procedure, and a thienopyridine (clopidogrel or ticlopidine). Clopidogrel is the preferred thienopyridine because of more rapid onset of action and better safety profile compared to ticlopidine. GP IIb/IIIa receptor inhibitors may be administered with PCI. Antiplatelet therapy with clopidogrel is continued for 4 weeks after conventional stenting, 6 to 12 months after brachytherapy, 3 to 6 months after drug-eluding stents, and possibly longer for high-risk patients. Recommendations for length of antiplatelet therapy in constantly changing and current protocol should be reviewed for patient teaching. Risk of thrombocytopenia with clopidogrel requires surveillance of platelet counts before and after PCI. When using ticlopidine, there is a risk of neutropenia requiring a complete blood count with differential checked before and after PCI and then again in 7 to 10 days (Leon et al., 1998).

Low-molecular-weight heparin (LMWH) (enoxaparin and dalteparin) has been recommended in the ACC/AHA guidelines for treatment in unstable angina as an alternative to UFH. UFH is associated with a prothrombotic rebound phenomenon, giving LMWH an advantage over heparin during intervention. However, the longer half-life and the difficulty with monitoring make LMWH less attractive with PCI and sheath management. Because enoxaparin binds factor Xa, monitoring ACT or PTT is not helpful (French & Faxon, 2002).

Another alternative to UFH is a direct thrombin inhibitor, bivalirudin, which has been approved for coronary intervention. One benefit of this agent is that it prolongs the ACT, allowing monitoring of the dose during PCI, similar to UFH. Bivalirudin inhibits bound and free thrombin, making it more effective in preventing thrombus formation. Clinical trials (REPLACE I and REPLACE II) indicated decreased ischemic events and decreased major bleeding with the use of bivalirudin (Lincoff et al., 2003) Antman, 2003).

Glycoprotein IIb/IIIa Receptor Inhibitors

The GP IIb/IIIa receptor inhibitors are a class of drugs used in interventional cardiology procedures and acute coronary syndromes. Platelet aggregation at the site of plaque rupture is a dominant feature in the pathophysiology of unstable angina, MI, and associated treatment with PTCA and interventional procedures. The final common pathway to platelet aggregation and coronary thrombus involves the activation of the platelet GP IIb/IIIa receptor. After platelet activation, GP IIb/IIIa becomes a receptor for fibrinogen and von Willebrand factor, increasing thrombus formation. There are three GP IIb/IIIa receptor inhibitors available for intravenous use to block platelet aggregation: abciximab, tirofiban, and eptifibatide. Clinical trials have indicated that use of GP IIb/IIIa receptor antagonists diminishes ischemic complications of PCI (Adgey, 1998).

Abciximab, the first agent approved for use by the FDA, is a human murine chimeric monoclonal antibody (7E3). Intravenous administration of a bolus dose of abciximab in the catheterization laboratory followed by a 12-hour infusion produces sustained GP IIb/IIIa receptor blockade and inhibition of platelets for the duration of the infusion with lower levels of GP IIb/IIIa receptor blockade present for more than 10 days after cessation of the infusion. Complications associated with administration include bleeding, thrombocytopenia, intracerebral hemorrhage, and allergic reactions. Platelet infusion may be needed in excess bleeding or for urgent surgery (The EPIC Investigators, 1994; The EPILOG Investigators, 1997).

Tirofiban is a tyrosine-derived, nonpeptide mimetic antagonist of the GP IIb/IIIa receptor, which competitively binds to the receptor in a rapidly reversible fashion. Tirofiban has a short plasma half-life of 1.6 hours (PRISM-PLUS Investigators, 1998).

Eptifibatide is a cyclic heptapeptide inhibitor of the GP IIb/IIIa receptor that is rapidly reversible, with a plasma half-life of 2.5 hours. The nonpeptide and peptide synthetic compounds (tibofiban and eptifibatide) have the advantage of a short half-life, rapid onset of action, and return of normal platelet function in 2 to 4 hours. This provides reversal of platelet function in the event of emergency surgery or significant bleeding (IMPACT II Investigators, 1997). The disadvantage is a shorter inhibition of platelet aggregation. Abciximab has the longest length of platelet inhibition.

NONCORONARY DEVICES

Patent Foramen Ovale/Atrial Septal Defect Devices

Transcatheter patent foramen ovale (PFO) and atrial septal defect (ASD) closure devices available for treatment in the catheterization laboratory have high success rates, low incidence of hospital complications, and low recurrent systemic thromboembolic events (Sanchez et al., 2002; Sacco et al., 2002).

King et al. documented initial techniques of percutaneous ASD closure in the 1970s. Bridges et al. (1992) first proposed that closure of PFOs would reduce the incidence of recurrent stroke events in patients after paradoxical embolism. Since that time, clinical studies have shown safety with current techniques for closure. However, the study results have been mixed in terms of the effectiveness and necessity of closure. A pooled analysis suggests that the presence of an ASD or a PFO alone increased risk for recurrent embolic event or stroke. Other studies have

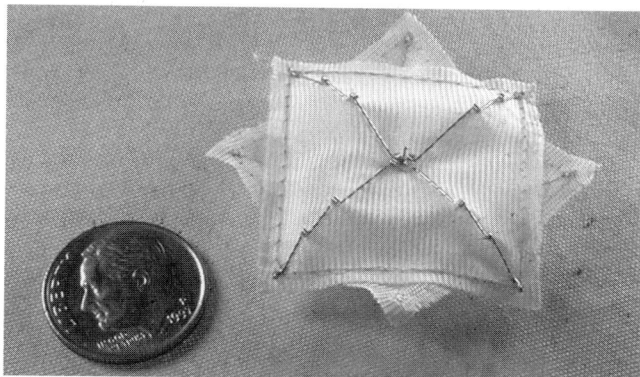

Figure 27–11. The CardioSeal PFO device. A dime is placed next to the device to represent size. (Courtesy of NMT Medical, Inc., Boston, MA.)

isolated PFO alone but a strong influence by a PFO association with an ASD in the presence of an atrial septal aneurysm.

The diagnosis of PFO or ASD is established by standard echocardiogram using a bubble study (an injection of agitated saline used in conjunction with echocardiogram) or transesophageal echocardiogram (TEE). Three devices available for closure include the Amplatzer Atrial Septal Occluder (AGA Medical), CardioSeal (NMT), and Starflex (NMT) (Fig. 27-11).

The implantation can be performed with a single femoral venous puncture under fluoroscopy. The PFO device can be passed by sliding along the septum primum, coming from the inferior vena cava, with a wire or a curved catheter. A transvenous sheath is placed in the left atrium. The left-sided disk is unfolded and pulled back against the septum, pulling the septum primum against the septum secundum and closing the slit valve. The right-sided disk is then deployed and the device released. Appropriate placement can be evaluated by TEE, intracardiac echocardiography, or injection of dye into the right atrium through the introducer. Medical treatment after implantation includes ASA, clopidogrel for 3 months, and antibiotics during the intervention and 6 months after the procedure for endocarditis prophylaxis (McGaw et al., 2003). Questions still remain about appropriate patient selection for PFO closure devices. Further studies are ongoing.

FUTURE RESEARCH

Interventional cardiology has expanded to provide the cardiologist with an array of options for treating CHD. Treatment of cardiac abnormalities noninvasively is possible, whereas previously surgery was required for correction. Devices play a complementary or synergistic role in allowing revascularization in the catheterization laboratory and treatment of CHD to be safer and successful with minimal complications. Restenosis is the most important problem that continues to complicate treatment with interventional devices. The release of drug-eluting stents shows great promise in the prevention of restenosis. We will continue to see more stent products on the market with drug-eluding properties. The cost for new technology and research will continue to be a challenge.

NURSING MANAGEMENT

Nursing management focuses on identification and preparation of eligible patients before treatment and on prevention, detection, and treatment of potential complications after interventional cardiology measures.

Analysis of Medical and Nursing Assessment Data and Formulation of Nursing Diagnoses

Based on the discussion of PCI and related areas of assessment, management, and complications, the following nursing diagnoses are derived and include the following:

Anxiety related to unfamiliar environment, unfamiliar treatment modality, and uncertainty of outcome manifested by restlessness or chest pain.

Risk of altered myocardial tissue perfusion related to myocardial ischemia; and reocclusion of a coronary artery secondary to abrupt closure, vascular spasm, loss of side branch, or distal microembolization after PCI.

Risk of decreased cardiac output related to arrhythmias, myocardial ischemia, or congestive heart failure.

Risk of altered cerebral tissue perfusion related to intracerebral hemorrhage or cerebral vascular accident.

Extracellular fluid volume deficit related to contrast-induced diuresis or restricted oral intake before elective procedures.

Risk of extracellular fluid volume deficit: hemorrhage related to delayed coagulation secondary to medications resulting in vascular access bleeding, retroperitoneal bleeding, or gastrointestinal bleeding.

Anxiety

Diagnosis. At the time of admission, anxiety may occur related to unfamiliar environment, unfamiliar treatment modality, and uncertainty of outcome. Chest pain related to myocardial ischemia if the patient is in the acute phase of MI or unstable angina may contribute to increased anxiety, causing increased pulse rate, respiratory rate, and blood pressure. Patient may exhibit inability to focus attention or signs of anxiety such as facial grimaces, hand clutched to chest, anger, and moaning.

Goals. The goals of nursing intervention are to provide the patient and family with sufficient information to allow decision-making and to reduce anxiety.

Interventions. Concise, precise explanations of all procedures and a calm, organized delivery of care aid in alleviation of anxiety. History and physical assessment of the patient under consideration for PCI. Baseline ECG and laboratory data are obtained. Conventional measures to relieve ischemic chest pain are implemented (see Chapter 26). Many indices of anxiety are also cues to pain, and skilled assessment is necessary to distinguish pain from anxiety. Anxiety also increases myocardial oxygen demand and may contribute to ischemic pain. For patients admitted for elective intervention, an assessment of the level of understanding is necessary to guide patient teaching. The focus of teaching is to enhance patient and family knowledge of the procedure and postprocedure care. Risks, potential complications, and alternative therapies are part of informed consent and should be addressed by the cardiologist.

Patients should be provided with alternative means of coping with stress and anxiety. Music therapy, meditation, and relaxation techniques should be presented.

Outcome Criteria. Outcome criteria to measure alleviation of anxiety include reduction in magnitude and numbers of verbal and nonverbal indices of anxiousness. The patient and family report that questions are satisfactorily answered, and informed decision-making occurs.

Risk of Altered Myocardial Tissue Perfusion Causing Chest Pain Related to Myocardial Ischemia

Diagnosis. If risk of recurrent chest pain related to ongoing ischemia and decreased myocardial tissue perfusion secondary to abrupt closure, vascular spasm, loss of side branch, distal microembolization, or slow flow secondary to thrombus burden in acute coronary syndrome are involved, then the patient may return to the floor with reports of chest pain that have continued or have reoccurred. Patient may still have residual chest pain related to MI, or procedural event.

Goals. Nursing goals are prevention, detection, and treatment of chest pain and inadequate myocardial tissue perfusion.

Interventions. Obtain baseline vital signs, ECG, and place patient on telemetry monitor with lead that reflects the lesion treated. Compare ECG to previous ECG performed before procedure. Nitroglycerin may be administered as needed. If patient had MI, vascular spasm, or a concern for distal microembolization, then a nitroglycerin drip should be continued until pain-free or directed by the cardiologist. If significant changes in vital signs, ECG, or escalation of chest pain pattern occur, the cardiologist should be notified. Prevention of myocardial ischemia requires maintenance of anticoagulant infusions as prescribed and monitoring of ordered coagulation tests. Reocclusion of the stenotic coronary artery or intracoronary stent is signaled by sudden onset of chest pain and return of ST segment elevation on the ECG. Lead selection for continuous ECG monitoring should be based on knowledge of the involved vessels to allow early detection of ST segment changes that may occur in the absence of chest pain. Treatment is the same as described for the patient with myocardial ischemia in Chapter 26.

Outcome Criteria. Outcome criteria for prevention of altered myocardial tissue perfusion are that coagulation tests remain within therapeutic range and that the patient remains free of chest pain and ECG manifestations of acute injury. Early detection necessitates that chest pain and ECG, and hemodynamic changes are noted and reported within 15 minutes of onset.

Risk of Decreased Cardiac Output Related to Arrhythmias

Diagnosis. Cardiac ischemia, reperfusion, injection of contrast, and fluctuating fluid and electrolyte status place patients receiving interventional cardiac therapies at risk for cardiac arrhythmias. The severity of the drop in cardiac output determines the patient's response to arrhythmias. Some arrhythmias are well tolerated and require only identification, assessment of hemodynamic response, and documentation.

Goals. Goals of nursing intervention are early detection, identification, and treatment of arrhythmias, and assessment and treatment of hemodynamic response to arrhythmias.

Interventions. Continuous cardiac monitoring is necessary to detect arrhythmias after interventional cardiac therapy. Appropriate assessment includes identification and documentation of the arrhythmia and the associated hemodynamic response. The most common reperfusion arrhythmia is a well-tolerated accelerated idioventricular rhythm requiring no additional intervention. Also common are ventricular tachycardia responsive to lidocaine or amiodarone infusion and cardioversion; ventricular fibrillation requiring countershock therapy; and bradyarrhythmia and atrioventricular blocks responsive to atropine. Specific therapies are determined by the type of arrhythmia and severity of alteration in cardiac output.

Outcome Criteria. Outcome criteria for the patient with decreased cardiac output caused by arrhythmias include the detection at onset of arrhythmias and accompanying hemodynamic response and immediate institution of appropriate interventions to stop the arrhythmia or stabilize hemodynamic parameters.

Risk of Altered Cerebral Tissue Perfusion Related to Intracerebral Hemorrhage or Cerebral Vascular Accident

Diagnosis. Although rare, cerebral bleeding is a potentially devastating complication of anticoagulation therapy. Elderly patients or patients with severe atherosclerosis are at risk for plaque disruption in the aorta releasing embolic material from manipulation of catheters. Severity of injury ranges from transient neurological dysfunction to permanent impairment or death.

Goals. Nursing interventions are directed at prevention, early detection, and treatment of cerebral hemorrhage.

Interventions. Interventions include careful monitoring of medication infusion with anticoagulants or GP IIb/IIIa receptor inhibitors. Monitor platelet counts. Careful patient selection and frequent assessment of central nervous system function are necessary for prevention and detection of cerebral bleeding. If signs and symptoms of neurological impairment are manifested, the anticoagulant therapies are discontinued.

Outcome Criterion. The outcome criteria for measurement of prevention of cerebral hemorrhage are the absence of subjective and objective indices of altered central nervous system function. Changes in neurological assessment are noted and reported within 30 minutes of onset, and treatment is initiated to control bleeding so that central nervous system function does not deteriorate.

Extracellular Fluid Volume Deficit Related to Contrast-induced Diuresis or Restricted Oral Intake

Diagnosis. Risk for fluid or volume deficit related to contrast-induced diuresis or restricted oral intake before elective procedures.

Goals. Nursing goals are prevention, early detection, and treatment of fluid volume deficit.

Interventions. Ongoing patient assessment is necessary to prevent and detect fluid volume deficit. Infuse hydrating intravenous fluids as ordered and provide plenty of fluid to drink unless contraindicated. Monitor patient response to oral and intravenous fluid by evaluating patient reports of thirst, intake and output, body weight, blood pressure, heart rate and rhythm, and pulmonary artery pressures if applicable. If parameters indicate inadequate intravascular volume, notify the physician and obtain a prescription for appropriate volume replacement. Check postural blood pressures before ambulating after the procedure.

Outcome Criteria. The outcome criteria for prevention of fluid volume deficit are the absence of subjective and objective indicators of volume deficit. Early detection of volume deficit is achieved when signs of volume deficit are recognized and reported within 60 minutes. Effectiveness of dependent nursing functions to treat volume deficit is determined by continued monitoring and reporting of indices of volume status.

Risk of Extracellular Fluid Volume Deficit: Hemorrhage Related to Delayed Coagulation

Diagnosis. Risk of bleeding or hemorrhage related to delayed clot formation secondary to anticoagulant and anti-platelet agents, or groin complications. Aggressive anticoagulation, anti-platelet agents, or direct thrombin inhibitors, and vessel trauma from the intravascular sheaths for mechanical interventions place the patient at risk for arterial access bleeding.

Goals. Goals of nursing interventions are early detection, identification, and treatment of ECF volume loss.

Interventions

Puncture Sites. Bleeding at puncture sites occurs from vascular trauma caused by diagnostic angiography or mechanical interventions. This type of peri-access bleeding is a risk for all patients receiving some type of interventional cardiac therapy, because aggressive postprocedure anticoagulation and antiplatelet therapies result in delayed clot formation. Peri-access bleeding ranges from oozing at the site of puncture to hematoma formation or retroperitoneal bleeding if the femoral approach is used.

Prevention of peri-access bleeding may involve leaving arterial and venous sheaths in place until heparin or a direct thrombin inhibitor can be interrupted or discontinued. Systematic monitoring and assessment of access sites and serial laboratory evaluation of patient platelet count and hemoglobin and hematocrit levels aid in detection of overt or occult peri-access bleeding. Care is also guided by institutional protocols and standing orders specific to each type of intervention.

Gastrointestinal Bleeding. Prevention of gastrointestinal bleeding is achieved by careful patient selection and minimization of procedural or pharmacologic trauma to the gastrointestinal tract. All nasogastric drainage and feces are tested to detect occult bleeding. Treatment depends on the severity of bleeding but may require discontinuance of anticoagulant therapy or antiplatelet therapy and transfusion of blood products. Treatment with proton pump inhibitors for a patient with history of gastrointestinal bleeding is recommended with long-term oral antiplatelet drugs.

Outcome Criteria. The outcome criteria for prevention of hemorrhage are absence of all subjective and objective signs of puncture site. Early detection of hemorrhage is achieved by recognition of subjective or objective indices of severe bleeding within 15 minutes of onset. Criteria for evaluation of treatment specify effectiveness of dependent and independent nursing functions in controlling hemorrhage and maintaining hemodynamic stability.

Summary of Nursing Diagnoses

The proceeding is a partial list of nursing diagnoses and management principles. Institutional protocols concerning interventional cardiac techniques vary; therefore, nurses must familiarize themselves with the protocols of their institution. Management of therapeutic regimens such as education on specific medications, activity, and diet must be provided for discharge planning.

REFERENCES

ACC/AHA guidelines for percutaneous coronary intervention (Revision of the 1993 PTCA Guidelines) Executive Summary. (2001). *Journal of the American College of Cardiology,* 37(8), 2215–2238.

Adgey, A. A. (1998). An overview of the results of clinical trials with glycoprotein IIb/IIIa inhibitors. *American Heart Journal,* 135, S43.

Agrawal, S. K., Pinheiro, L., Roubin, G. S., et al. (1992). Non-surgical closure of femoral pseudoaneurysms complicating cardiac catheterization and percutaneous transluminal coronary angioplasty. *Journal of the American College of Cardiology,* 20, 610.

Antman, E. M. (2003). Should bivalirudin replace heparin during percutaneous coronary interventions? *JAMA,* 289(7), 903–905.

Baim, D. S. (2000). Coronary angioplasty. In D. S. Baim, & W. Grossman (Eds.), *Grossman's cardiac catheterization, angiography, and intervention* (6th ed., pp. 547–599). Philadelphia: Lippincott Williams & Wilkins.

Baim, D. S., & Grossman, W. (2000). Complications of cardiac catheterization. In D. S. Baim, & W. Grossman (Eds.), *Grossman's cardiac catheterization, angiography, and intervention* (6th ed., pp. 35–65). Philadelphia: Lippincott Williams & Wilkins.

BARI Investigators. (1996). Comparison of coronary bypass surgery with angioplasty in patients with mutivessel disease. *New England Journal of Medicine,* 335, 217–225.

BARI Investigators. (2000). Seven-year outcome in the Bypass Angioplasty revascularization Investigation(BARI) by treatment and diabetic status. *Journal of the American College of Cardiology,* 35, 1122–1129.

Bogart, D. B., Bogart, M. A., Miller, J. T., Farrar, M. W., Barr, W. K., & Montgomery, M. A. (1995). Femoral artery catheterization complications: a study of 503 consecutive patients. *Catheter Cardiovascular Diagnosis,* 34, 8–13.

Bridges, N. D., Hellenbrand, W., Latson, L., et al. (1990). Transcatheter closure of patent foramen ovale after presumed paradoxical embolism. *Circulation,* 81, 1902–1908.

Buchbinder, M., Leon, M., Warth, D. C., et al. (1992). Multicenter registry of percutaneous coronary rotational ablation using the Rotablator. *Journal of the American College of Cardiology,* 19, 333A.

Carrozza, J. P., & Baim, D. S. (2000). Coronary stenting. In D. S. Baim, & W. Grossman (Eds.), *Grossman's cardiac catheterization, angiography, and intervention* (6th ed., pp. 637–666). Philadelphia: Lippincott Williams & Wilkins.

Carrozza, J. P., Kuntz, R. E., Levine, M. J., et al. (1992). Angiographic and clinical outcome of intracoronary stenting: Immediate and long-term results from a large single-center experience. *Journal of the American College of Cardiology,* 20, 328.

Collet, J. P., Montalescot, G., Lison, L., Choussat, R., Ankri, A., Drobinski, G., Sotirov, I., & Thomas, D. (2001). Percutaneous cororonary intervention after subcutaneous enoxaparin pretreatment in patients with unstable angina pectoris. *Circulation,* 103(5), 658–663.

Colombo, A., Hall, P., Nakamura, S., et al. (1995). Intracoronary stenting without anticoagulation accomplished with intravascular ultrasound guidance. *Circulation,* 91, 1676.

Colombo, A., Stankovic, G., & Moses, J. W. (2002). Selection of coronary stents. *Journal of the American College of Cardiology,* 40(6), 1021–1033.

Cowley, M. J., & DiSciascio, G. (1993). Directional coronary atherectomy for saphenous vein disease. *Catheter Cardiovascular Diagnosis,* Suppl. 1, 10.

Dahm, J. B., Kuon, E., Vogelgesang, D., Hummel, A., Mox, B., Staudt, A, & Felix, S. (2002). Relation of degree of laser debulking of in-stent restenosis as a predictor of restenosis rate. *American Journal of Cardiology*, 90, 68–70.

Degertekin, M., Regar, E., Tanabe, K., et al. (2003) Sirolimus-eluting stent for treatment of complex in-stent restenosis: the first clinical experience. *Journal of the American College of Cardiology*, 14, 41(2), 184–189.

Ebersole, D. G. (1999) Clinical applications for excimer laser. *Cardiovascular R & R*, June, 330–335.

Ellis, S. G., Savage, M., Fischman, D. et al. (1992). Restenosis after placement of Palmaz-Schatz stents in native coronary arteries. *Circulation*, 86, 1836.

The EPIC Investigators. (1994). Use of a monoclonal antibody directed against the platelet glycoprotein IIb/IIIa receptor in high-risk coronary angioplasty. *New England Journal of Medicine*, 330, 956.

The EPILOG Investigators. (1997). Platelet glycoprotein IIb/IIIa receptor blockade and low-dose heparin during percutaneous coronary revascularization. *New England Journal of Medicine*, 336, 1689.

The EPISTENT Investigators. (1998). Randomised placebocontrolled and balloon-angioplasty-controlled trial to assess safety of coronary stenting with use of platelet glycoprotein IIb/IIIa blockade. *Lancet*, 352, 87.

Fischman, D. L., Leon, M. B., Baim, D. S. et al. (1994). A randomized comparison of coronary-stent placement and balloon angioplasty in the treatment of coronary artery disease. *New England Journal of Medicine*, 331, 496.

Frazee, B. W., & Flajhert, J. P. (1991). Septic endarteritis of the femoral artery following angioplasty. *Review of Infectious Diseases*, 13, 620.

French, M. H., & Faxon, D. P. (2002). Current anticoagulation options in percutaneous intervention: Designing patient-specific strategies. *Reviews in Cardiovascular Medicine*, 3(4), 176–182.

Goss, J. E., Chambers, C. E., Heupler, F. A., et al. (1995). Systematic anaphylactoid reactions to iodinated contrast media during cardiac catheterization procedures—guidelines for prevention, diagnosis, and treatment. *Catheter Cardiovascular Diagnosis*, 34,99.

Grube, E., Gerckens, U., & Buellesfeld, L. (2002). Drug-eluting tents: clinical experiences and perspectives. *Minerva Cardioangiology*, 50(5), 469–473.

Harrington, R. (1997). Design and methodology of the PURSUIT trial: Evaluating eptifibatide for acute ischemic coronary syndromes. *American Journal of Cardiology*, 80(Suppl. 4A), 34B.

Hasdai, D., Holmes, D. R., & Lerman, A. (2000). Evaluating stenosis severity: Quantitative angiography, coronary flow reserve, and intravascular ultrasound. In S.G. Ellis & D. R. Holmes, Jr. (Eds.), *Strategic approaches in coronary intervention* (2nd ed., pp. 175–184). Philadelphia: Lippincott Williams & Wilkins.

Hinohara, T., Robertson, G. C., Selmon, M. R., et al. (1993). Directional coronary atherectomy complications and management. *Catheter Cardiovascular Diagnosis*, Suppl. 1, 61.

Holmes, D., Toprol, E., Califf, R., et al. (1994). A multicenter randomized trial of coronary angioplasty versus directional atherectomy for patients with saphenous vein bypass graft lesions. CAVEAT-II Investigators. *Circulation*, (7), 1966–1974.

Hong, M. K., Mintz, G. S., Popma, J. J., et al. (1996). Safety and efficacy of elective stent implantation following rotational atherectomy in large calcified coronary arteries. *Catheter Cardiovascular Diagnosis*, Suppl. 3, 50.

Jacobs, A. K. (2003). Coronary revascularization in women in 2003. *Circulation*, 107(3), 375–377.

Juran, N. B., Rouse, C. L., Smith, D. D., O'Brien, M. A., DeLuca, S. A., Sigmon, K., & the SANDBAG Nursing Coordinators. (1999). Nursing Interventions to decrease bleeding at the femoral access site after percutaneous coronary intervention. *American Journal of Critical Care*, 8(5), 303–3131.

Kereiakes, D. J., Montalescot, G., Antman, E. M., Cohen, M., Darius, H., Ferguson, J. J., et al. (2002). Low molecular weight heparin therapy for non-ST-elevation acute coronary syndromes and during percutaneous coronary interventions: An expert consensus. *American Heart Journal*, 144(4), 615–624.

King, T. D., Thompson, S. L., Steiner, C., & Mills, N. L. (1976). Secundum atrial septal defect: Nonoperative closure during cardiac catheterization. *JAMA*, 235, 2506–2509.

Kong, D. F., Califf, R. A., Miller, D. P., et al. (1998). Outcomes of therapeutic agents that block the platelet gycoprotein IIb/IIIa integrin in iscchemic heart disease. *Circulation*, 98, 2829.

Leon, M. B., Baim, D. S., Popma, J. J., et al. (1998). A clinical trial comparing three antithrombotic-drug regimens after coronary artery stenting. *New England Journal of Medicine*, 339, 1665–1671.

Lasky, W., Boyle, J., Johnson, L. W., & the Registry Committee of the Society for Cardiac Angiography and Intervention. (1993). Multivariable model for prediction of risk of significant complications during diagnostic cardiac catheterization. *Catheter Cardiovascular Diagnosis*, 30, 185.

Landau, C., Lange, R. A., Glamann, D. B., Willard, J. E., & Hillis, L. D. (1993). Vasovagal reactions in the cardiac catheterization laboratory. *American Journal of Cardiology*, 73, 95.

Lincoff, A. M., Bittl, J. A., Harrington, R. A., Feit, F., Kleiman, N. S., Jackman, J. D., et al. (2003). Bivalirudin and Provisional Glycoprotein IIb/IIa Blockade Compared with Heparin and Planned Glycoprotein IIb/IIIa Blockade during Percutaneous Coronary Intervention. *JAMA*, 289(7), 853.

Mosca, L., Manson, J. E., Sutherland, S. E., Langer, R. D., Manolio, T., & Barrett-Connor, E. (1997). Cardiovascular Disease in Women. *Circulation*, 96, 2468–2482.

Okura, H., Benneau, H. N., Yock, P. G., & Fitzgerald, P. J. (2000). Intravascular ultrasound: Practical use in the cardiac catheterization laboratory. In S.G. Ellis & D. R. Holmes, Jr. (Eds.), *Strategic approaches in coronary intervention* (2nd ed., pp. 175–184). Philadelphia: Lippincott Williams & Wilkins.

The PRISM-PLUS Investigators. (1998). Inhibition of the platelet glycoprotein IIb/IIIa receptor with tirofiban in unstable angina and non-Q wave myocardial infarction. *New England Journal of Medicine*, 338, 1488.

Rizik, D., Leon, M., Strumpf, R., Weiner, B., Cohen, E., et al. (1999). Benefits of cutting balloon after stenting *American Journal of Cardiology*, 84(6A), 16.

Roubin, G. S., Cannon, A. D., Agrawal, S. K., et al. (1992). Intracoronary stenting for acute and threatened closure complicating percutaneous transluminal coronary angioplasty. *Circulation*, 85, 916.

Sacco, R. L., Di Tullio, M. R., Sciacca, R. R., Mohr, J. P. (2002). Effect of medical treatment in stroke patients with foramen ovale: Patent foramen ovale in cryptogenic stroke study. *Circulation*, 105, 2625–2631.

Sanchez, P. L., Doherty, E., Colon-Hernandez, P. J., Delgado, G., Inglessis, I., Scott, N., et al. (2002). Percutaneous transcatheter closure of patent foramen ovale in patients with paradoxical embolism. *Circulation*, 106, 1121–1126.

Saririan, M., & Eisenberg, M. J. (2003). Myocardial laser revascularization for the treatment of end stage coronary artery disease. *Journal of the American College of Cardiology*, 41(2), 173–183.

Schatz, R. A., Baim, D. S., Leon, M., et al. (1991). Clinical experience with the Palmaz-Schatz coronary stent: Initial results of a multicenter study. *Circulation*, 83, 148.

Schomig, A., Neumnn, F. J., Kastrati, A., et al. (1996) A randomized comparison of antiplatelet and anticoagulant therapy after the placement of coronary-artery stents. *New England Journal of Medicine*, 34, 1084.

Sedlis, S. P., Morrison, D. A., Lorin, J. D., Esposito, R., Sethi, G., Sacks, J., Henderson, W., et al. (2002). Percutaneous coronary intervention versus coronary bypass graft surgery for diabetic patients with unstable angina and risk factors for adverse outcomes with bypass. *Journal of the American College of Cardiology*, 40(9), 1555–1566.

Serruys, P. W., De Jaegere, P., Kiemeneij, F., et al. (1994). A comparison of balloon-expandable-stent implantation with balloon angioplasty in patients with coronary artery disease. *New England Journal of Medicine*, 331, 489.

Sigwart, U., Puel, J., Mirkovitch, V., et al. (1987). Intravascular stents to prevent occlusion and restenosis after transluminal angioplasty. *New England Journal of Medicine*, 316, 13.

Silva, J. A., Ramee, S. R., Cohen, D. J., Carrozza, J. P., Popma, J. J., Lansky, A. A., Dandreo, K., et al. (2001). Reolytic thrombectomy during percutaneous revascularization for acute myocardial infarction: experience with the angiojet catheter. *American Heart Journal*, 141(3), 353–359.

Sketch, M. H., O'Neill, W. W., Galichia, J. P., et al. (1992). Restenosis following coronary transluminal extraction-endarterectomy: The final analysis of a multicenter registry. *Journal of the American College of Cardiology*, 19, 277A.

Sousa, J. E., Costa, M. A., Sousa, A. G., Abizaid, A. C., Seixas, A. C., Abizaid, A. S., Feres, F., et al. (2003). Two year angiographic and intravascular ultrasound follow-up after implantation of Sirolimus-eluting stents in human coronary arteries. *Circulation*, 107, 381–383.

Stevens, M. A., McCullough, P. A., Tobin, K. J., et al. (1999). A prospective randomized trial of prevention measures in patients at high risk for contrast nephropathy. *Journal of the American College of Cardiology*, 33, 403.

Teirstein, P. S., Kuntz, R. E. (2001). New frontiers in interventional cardiology: Intravascular radiation to prevent restenosis. *Circulation*, 104, 2620.

Terstein, P. S., Warth, D. C., Haq, N., et al. (1991). High speed rotational coronary atherectomy for patients with diffuse coronary artery disease. *Journal of the American College of Cardiology*, 18, 1694.

Topol, E. J., Leya, F., Pinkerton, C. A., et al. (1993). A comparison of directional atherectomy with comparison of coronary angioplasty in patients with coronary artery disease. *New England Journal of Medicine*, 329, 221.

Williams, M. A., Fleg, J. L., Ades, P. A., Chaitman, B. R., Miller, N. H., Mohiuddin, S. M., Ockene, I. S., et al. (2002). Secondary prevention of coronary heart disease in the elderly (with emphasis on patients >75 years of age). AHA scientific Statement. *Circulation*, 105(14), 1735.

Heart Failure

DEBRA LAURENT

Heart failure (HF) is the pathophysiologic state in which an abnormality of cardiac function is responsible for the failure of the heart to pump blood at a rate adequate to meet the requirements of the tissue or can do so only from an elevated filling pressure. Although this syndrome has been extensively researched and intensively treated, it remains a significant health problem in the United States and worldwide. There is an increasing incidence of HF in the aging population, with a prevalence of approximately 10% by age 70 years. For HF occurring in the absence of myocardial infarction, the lifetime risk is 1 in 9 for men and 1 in 6 for women; the increase in HF is largely attributable to hypertension (Lloyd-Jones et al., 2002). As many as 20 million people in the United States who have asymptomatic impairment of cardiac function are likely to have symptoms of HF within 5 years (American Heart Association.2002). In the past decade, experimental and clinical studies have demonstrated increased neurohormonal activity is a major pathophysiologic component of heart failure. The quality of life, exercise capacity, and perhaps the life expectancy of patients with HF may be altered by the introduction of appropriate medical and nursing therapy at the appropriate time in the course of the patient's heart disease. This chapter reviews major physiologic and pathophysiologic concepts of chronic HF as a basis for understanding its underlying causes as well as its clinical and physical findings. Emphasis also is placed on the various diagnostic tests, the vast array of pharmacologic agents, and other medical and nursing interventions in the adult patient with left ventricular systolic and/or diastolic dysfunction. With this knowledge, the nurse is able to implement a plan of care, which may involve restriction of activity and diet, medications, and coping strategies for patients and families to adapt effectively to a chronic illness.

ETIOLOGIES AND DEFINITIONS

Heart failure is a complex clinical syndrome manifested by shortness of breath, fatigue, and characterized by abnormalities of left ventricular function and neurohormonal regulation. HF is not a diagnosis, and its cause should be sought carefully. Any disorder that places the heart under an increased volume or pressure load or that produces primary damage or an increased metabolic demand on the myocardium may result in HF

(Table 28-1) (Michaelson, 1983; Givertz et al., 2001). It is helpful for the clinician to identify the underlying and the precipitating causes of HF. Coronary artery disease is the underlying cause of HF in two thirds of patients with systolic dysfunction. Hypertension is implicated in systolic and diastolic dysfunction. Arrhythmias are common in patients with underlying structural heart disease, and they commonly precipitate HF. These arrhythmias may take the form of tachyarrhythmias (most commonly atrial fibrillation), marked bradycardia, degrees of heart block, and abnormal intraventricular conduction such as left bundle branch block or ventricular arrhythmias. Other precipitating factors include systemic infections, anemias, and pulmonary emboli that all place increased metabolic and hemodynamic demand on the heart. Administration of cardiac depressants or salt-retaining drugs may precipitate HF; examples may include corticosteroids, nondihydropyridine calcium channel antagonists, and nonsteroidal anti-inflammatory agents. Alcohol is a potent myocardial depressant and may be responsible for the development of cardiomyopathy. Inappropriate reduction in therapy is perhaps the most common cause of decompensation in a previously compensated patient, with reduction in pharmacological therapy or dietary excess of sodium (Francis, 1998; Givertz, 2001). Clinical manifestations of HF have been described by different theories (Colucci and Braunwald, 2001). From a historical standpoint, these theories include backward and forward failure, left-sided and right-sided failure, acute and chronic HF, low-output and high-output syndrome, and systolic and diastolic dysfunction. Even though the neurohormonal pathogenesis of HF dominates our understanding of this clinical syndrome, it is also useful to review HF in the context of hemodynamic abnormalities.

Backward and Forward Failure

In 1832, James Hope first described *backward failure* as the failure that results as the ventricle fails to pump its volume, causing blood accumulation and subsequent increase in ventricular, atrial, and venous pressures. A primary cause of backward failure is mechanical cardiac obstruction.

The term *forward failure,* proposed by MacKenzie in 1913, is applied to a situation in which the primary pathologic process is decreased cardiac output, which ultimately leads to a

Table 28–1 ■ CONDITIONS UNDERLYING OR PRECIPITATING HEART FAILURE

Abnormal Volume Load	Abnormal Pressure Load	Myocardial Dysfunction	Filling Disorders	Increased Metabolic Demand
Aortic incompetence	Aortic stenosis	Cardiomyopathy	Mitral stenosis	Anemias
Mitral incompetence	Hypertrophic	Myocarditis	Tricuspid stenosis	Thyrotoxicosis
Tricuspid incompetence	cardiomyopathy	Coronary heart disease	Cardiac tamponade	Fever
Overtransfusion	Coarctation of the aorta	Ischemia	Restrictive pericarditis	Beriberi
Left-to-right shunts	Hypertension	Infarction	Restrictive	Paget's disease
Secondary hypervolemia	Primary	Arrhythmias	cardiomyopathy	Arteriovenous fistulas
	Secondary	Toxic disorders		Pulmonary emboli
		Alcohol		Systemic emboli
		Cocaine		
		Administration of cardiac depressants or salt-retaining drugs		

Adapted From Michaelson C.R. (Ed.). (1983). Congestive heart failure (p. 45). St Louis: CV Mosby.

decrease in vital organ perfusion and water and sodium retention (Colucci & Braunwald, 2001; Francis, 2001). Backward and forward failures are seen in most patients with chronic HF.

Left-Sided and Right-Sided Failure

Based on the backward failure theory, fluid can accumulate behind the specific cardiac chamber. The right and left sides of the heart are independent circuits and can fail independently. It is, however, unusual for left-sided failure not to progress to biventricular failure.

Left-sided HF exists when LV stroke volume is reduced and blood accumulates in the left ventricle, left atrium, and pulmonary circulation, which causes elevated pulmonary venous pressure and reduced cardiac output. LV failure is by far the more frequent of the two instances in which only one side of the heart is affected. Arterial high blood pressure, myocardial ischemia or MI, aortic valve incompetence or stenosis, or mitral valve incompetence or stenosis can cause it. People with chronic volume overload, high-output states, cardiomyopathies, or arrhythmias demonstrate signs of LV failure before those of right HF (Michaelson, 1983; Francis et al., 2001).

Inability of the right heart to empty its blood volume results in blood backing-up into the systemic circulation. LV failure is the most common cause of right ventricular (RV) failure. Sustained pulmonary hypertension also causes RV failure. Pulmonary hypertension occurs in patients with congenital anomalies (tetralogy of Fallot or ventricular septal defect), severe pulmonary infections, massive pulmonary embolization, or mitral or aortic stenosis (Francis et al., 2001).

Acute and Chronic Failure

The clinical manifestations of acute and chronic failure depend on how rapidly the syndrome of HF develops. *Acute HF* may be the initial manifestation of heart disease or may indicate exacerbation of a chronic cardiac condition. The marked decrease in left ventricular (LV) function may be caused by acute myocardial infarction (MI) or acute valvular dysfunction.

The events occur so rapidly that the sympathetic nervous system compensation is ineffective, resulting in the rapid development of pulmonary edema and circulatory collapse (cardiogenic shock) (see Chapter 30). *Chronic HF* develops over time and is usually the end result of an increasing inability of physiologic mechanisms to compensate. It can be caused by coronary artery disease, valvular disease, high blood pressure, cardiomyopathies, or chronic obstructive pulmonary disease (Colucci & Braunwald, 2001; Givertz et al., 2001).

Low and High Cardiac Output Syndromes

In response to high blood pressure and hypovolemia, low cardiac output syndrome appears. The word *syndrome* implies that the failure represents a reaction rather than a primary pathologic process. Low cardiac output syndrome is evidenced by impaired peripheral circulation and peripheral vasoconstriction (i.e., valvular, rheumatic, hypertensive, coronary artery disease).

Any condition that causes the heart to work harder to supply blood may be categorized as high cardiac output syndrome. High cardiac output states require an increased oxygen supply to the peripheral tissues, which can occur only with an increased cardiac output. Reduced systemic vascular resistance (SVR) is characteristic of this condition and augments peripheral circulation and venous return, which in turn increases stroke volume and cardiac output. High cardiac output states may be caused by increased metabolic requirements, as seen in hyperthyroidism, fever, and pregnancy, or may be triggered by hyperkinetic conditions such as arteriovenous fistulas, anemia, and beriberi (Givertz et al., 2001).

Systolic and Diastolic Dysfunction

A more useful classification than forward and backward failure is the difference between systolic and diastolic dysfunction. *Systolic dysfunction* is determined by an impaired pump function with reduced left ventricular ejection fraction ($<.40$) and an enlarged end-diastolic chamber volume. The ventricle is dilated, thin-walled, and often eccentrically hypertrophied. Systolic dysfunction can be regional, as in myocardial infarction, or global, as in dilated cardiomyopathy (Parmley, 1992; Federman & Hess, 1994). The principal clinical manifestations of left ventricular systolic dysfunction result from an inadequate cardiac output and fluid retention (forward failure). *Diastolic dysfunction* or heart failure with preserved ejection fraction implies normal systolic function in the presence of clinical HF and is characterized by an increased resistance to filling, with increased filling pressures with one or both ventricles becoming stiff or noncompliant. The ventricle is thickened and concentrically hypertrophied, with a normal or small cavity (Carelock, 2001; Francis et al., 2001). LV failure is caused by diastolic dysfunction in up to 40% of cases, mainly because of long-standing systemic hypertension. Other myocardial disorders include coronary artery disease, hypertrophic, infiltrative and restrictive cardiomyopathies, and primary valve disorders (e.g. aortic stenosis) (Katz, 2000). Pure diastolic dysfunction has also been observed immediately after cardiac surgery (McKinney et al., 1994). Changes that occur in the cardiovascular system as a result of aging have a greater impact on diastolic function than on systolic function. Consistency of the association of female gender with preserved LV function

across numerous subgroups of patients implies that gender itself is an important determinant of LV adaptation, regardless of the underlying pathophysiologic process (Kitzman, 2003; Masoudi, 2003). The major consequence of diastolic failure relate to elevation of ventricular filling pressures, causing pulmonary/and or systemic congestion (backward failure).

During the past 20 years, the role of diastolic dysfunction has been increasingly recognized. The different pathophysiologic processes behind systolic and diastolic dysfunction affect prognosis and treatment and are addressed in the following sections (Givertz et al., 2001).

PATHOPHYSIOLOGY AND PATHOGENESIS

When the heart is presented with an increased workload, by either pressure or volume overload, or by myocardial abnormality, a number of physiologic alterations are evoked in an attempt to maintain normal cardiac pumping function (Fig. 28-1) (Francis et al., 2001).

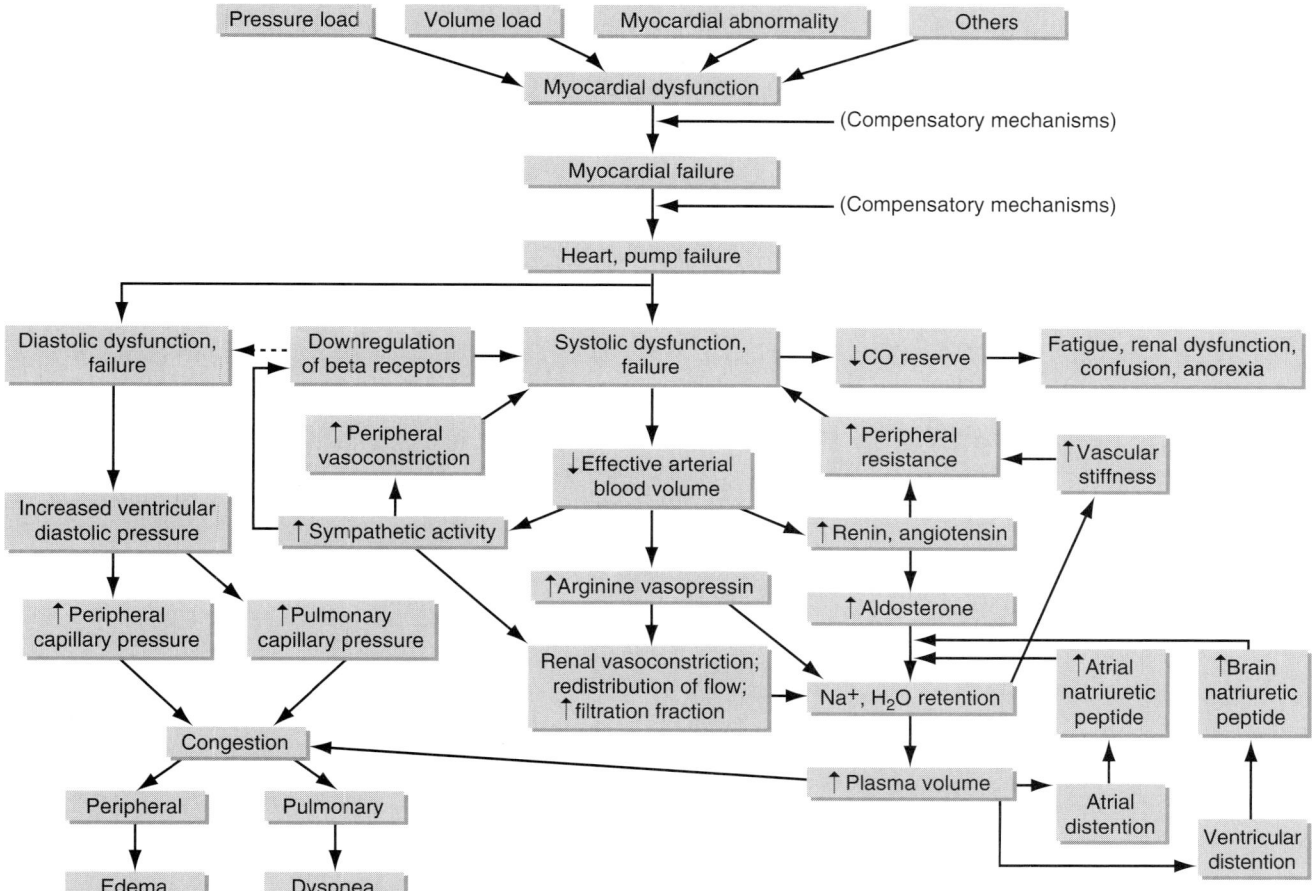

■ **Figure 28–1.** Sequence of events in heart failure. An increased load or myocardial abnormality leads to myocardial failure and eventually heart failure. This results in increased sympathetic activity, increased activity of the renin-angiotensin-aldosterone system, pulmonary and peripheral congestion and edema, and decreased cardiac output reserve. Both the atrial natriuretic and b-type natriuretic peptide are also released in response to increased plasma volume. (From Francis, G. S., Gassler, J. P., & Sonneblick, E. H. [2001]. Pathophysiology and diagnosis of heart failure. In J. W. Hurst [Ed.], *The heart* [10th ed.]. New York: McGraw-Hill.)

Regardless of the original cardiac abnormality, HF presents a complex picture including altered myocardial function, ventricular remodeling, altered hemodynamics, neurohormonal and cytokine activation, and vascular and endothelial dysfunction. Multiple alterations in organ and cellular physiology contribute to HF under various circumstances. Adaptive and maladaptive processes affect the myocardium, kidneys, peripheral vasculature, smooth and skeletal muscle, and multiple reflex control mechanisms (Drexler & Hasenfuss, 2001; Katz, 2000).

Hemodynamic Abnormalities

Myocardial contractility (inotropy) and relaxation (lusitropy) are impaired in most patients with HF. In addition, systemic hemodynamics, which include both preload and afterload, and ventricular architecture (shape, cavity size, and wall thickness) determine ejection and filling by a failing heart (Fig. 28-2) (Katz, 2000).

Impaired Ejection

As diastolic filling increases, ventricular dilatation occurs in response to maladaptive growth response and remodeling of the damaged or chronically overloaded heart. Renal compensatory mechanisms cause sympathetic stimulation, thus increasing the end-diastolic volume or preload. The Frank-Starling response is immediately activated as a consequence of increased diastolic volume. According to the Frank-Starling law of the heart, length-dependent changes in contractile performance during diastole increases the force of contraction during systole. The increased preload augmenting contractility is the major mechanism by which the ventricles maintain an equal output as their stroke volumes vary (Katz, 2000; Francis et al., 2001). It may be useful to consider normal and impaired myocardial function within the framework of the Frank-Starling mechanism, as illustrated by analysis of LV function curves (Fig. 28-3). Cardiac output or cardiac index is used as a measure of ventricular work; LV end-diastolic pressure or pulmonary artery wedge pressure (PAWP) is used as a reflection of

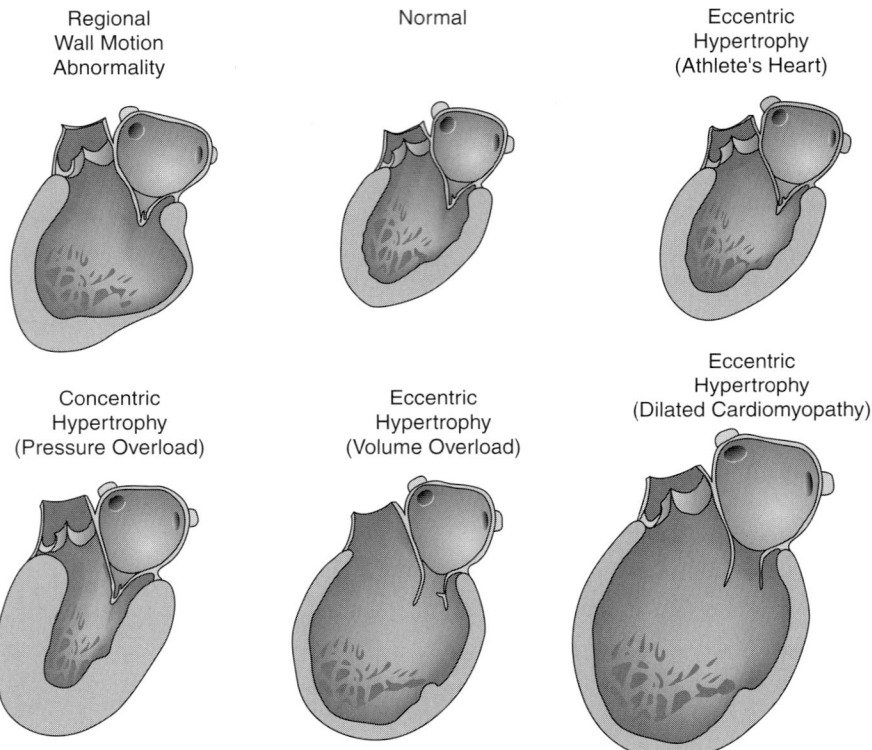

Regional
Wall Motion
Abnormality

Normal

Eccentric
Hypertrophy
(Athlete's Heart)

Concentric
Hypertrophy
(Pressure Overload)

Eccentric
Hypertrophy
(Volume Overload)

Eccentric
Hypertrophy
(Dilated Cardiomyopathy)

■ **Figure 28–2.** Five examples of the many architectural patterns of cardiac hypertrophy. A normal left ventricle is represented at the center top row. The eccentric hypertrophy seen in the "athletes heart" (*top right*) is a physiologic hypertrophy that differs from the pathologic eccentric hypertrophy of systolic dysfunction seen in dilated cardiomyopathy (*bottom right*) and following a chronic volume overload such as occurs in aortic insufficiency (*bottom center*). A regional wall abnormality (*top left*), commonly seen as a result of myocardial infarction, causes the noninfarcted regions of the ventricle to undergo eccentric hypertrophy as well. These pathologic forms of eccentric hypertrophy lead to the progressive dilatation called "remodeling." Deterioration is usually more rapid in dilated cardiomyopathy and regional wall abnormality than in chronic volume overload. All are different than the concentric hypertrophy (*bottom left*) caused by chronic pressure overload (diastolic dysfunction), as occurs in chronic hypertension and aortic stenosis. Progressive dilatation (remodeling) of a concentrically hypertrophied heart is uncommon, but diastolic dysfunction, like systolic dysfunction, leads to deterioration of the overloaded myocardium. (From Katz, A.M. [2000]. *Heart failure: Pathophysiology, molecular biology and clinical management.* Philadelphia: Lippincott Williams & Wilkins.)

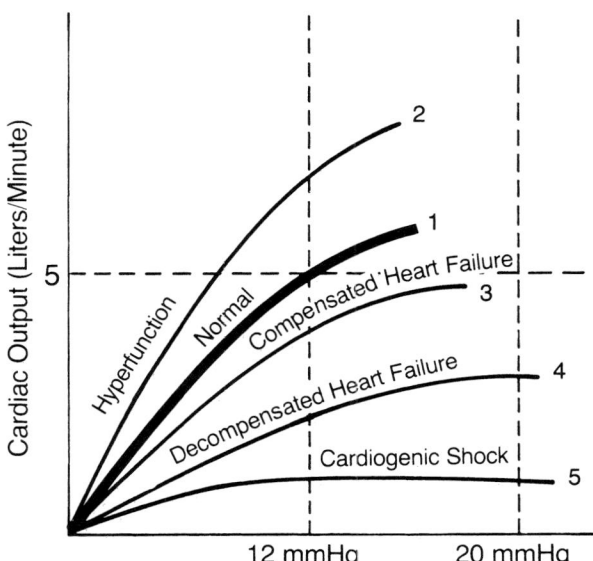

■ **Figure 28–3.** Left ventricular function curves. Curve 1: Normal function curve, with a normal cardiac output at optimal filling pressures. Curve 2: Cardiac hyperfunction, with an increased cardiac output at optimal filling pressures. Curve 3: Compensated heart failure, with normal cardiac outputs at higher filling pressures. Curve 4: Decompensated heart failure, with a decrease in cardiac output and elevated filling pressures. Curve 5: Cardiogenic shock, with extremely depressed cardiac output and marked increase in filling pressures. (Adapted from Michaelson, C.R. [1983]. *Congestive heart failure* [p 61]. St. Louis: CV Mosby.)

preload. The normal relation between ventricular end-diastolic volume and ventricular work is shown in Figure 28-3 by curve 1. Optimal contractility occurs at a diastolic volume of 12 to 18 mm Hg. If the heart is physiologically stressed, as occurs in acute MI, the initial drop in cardiac output stimulates the sympathetic nervous system. An increase in sympathetic tone elevates heart rate and contractility, illustrated in Figure 28-3 by curve 2. As the cardiac workload increases and myocardial dysfunction persists, HF progresses, which is reflected by further elevation of end-diastolic volume (preload) and ventricular dilatation. This increased preload, in turn, may further contribute to depressed ventricular contractility and the development of congestive symptoms (Fig. 28-3, curve 3) (Weil et al., 1998).

The normal left ventricle is able to adjust to large changes in aortic impedance (afterload) with small changes in output, in part by calling on the Frank-Starling response and, perhaps, by augmenting the contractile force as an intrinsic property of the normal myocardium. In contrast, the damaged left ventricle loses this compensatory ability and becomes sensitive to even small changes in impedance (Francis, 1998). Because increased activity of the sympathetic nervous system or the renin-angiotensin-aldosterone system results in vasoconstriction of the small arteries and arterioles, increased impedance of LV filling is imposed, decreasing the stroke volume and cardiac output. Because HF is characterized by heightened activity of

these neurohormonal vasoconstrictor systems, a positive-feedback loop can be generated in which impaired pump performance increases impedance to LV ejection, further impairing the pump performance.

Impaired Filling

Ventricular relaxation is a dynamic process that begins at the end of systole and occurs during isovolumetric relaxation. This is controlled by the uptake of calcium by the sarcoplasmic reticulum and the efflux of calcium from the myocyte (Colucci & Braunwald, 2001; Drexler & Hasenfuss, 2001). These active processes are regulated by the sarcoplasmic reticulum calcium ATP-ase pump (SERCA). The LV also has passive compliance or elastic property that characterizes wall stiffness. Diastolic function can be impaired by four types of lusitropic abnormalities: slowed relaxation with decreased rate of pressure fall (–dP/dt) during isovolumetric relaxation, delayed filling during early diastole, incomplete relaxation with reduced filling throughout diastole, and decreased compliance or increased stiffness in late diastole (Fig. 28-4). These cause abnormal pressure–volume relationships and produce a higher pressure for any given volume. The pressure is transmitted backwards to the atria, pulmonary, and systemic circulation and is noted with elevated pulmonary pressures and decreased cardiac output leading to dyspnea and fatigue during exercise (Katz, 2000).

Concentric and eccentric hypertrophy impair ventricular filling. Decreased cavity size as seen in concentric hypertrophy decreases compliance and thus impedes venous return. Eccentric hypertrophy, which increases end-diastolic volume and pressure, is also accompanied by a decrease in compliance (Fig. 28-5) (Drexler & Hasenfuss, 2001). Mechanisms responsible for diastolic dysfunction include hypertrophy, as described, which affects an increase in passive chamber stiffness (decreased compliance) and decreased active relaxation. Decreased levels of activity of SERCA to remove calcium from the cytosol and an increase in phospholamban (SERCA inhibitory protein) lead to a net effect of impaired relaxation. This net effect is also seen in myocardial ischemia, abnormal ventricular loading (as seen in hypertrophies or dilated cardiomyopathy), asynchrony, abnormal flux of calcium ions, and hypothyroidism. Of interest, SERCA decreases with age, coincident with impaired diastolic dysfunction (Colucci & Braunwald, 2001; Drexler & Hasenfuss, 2001; Francis et al., 2001).

Wall stiffness or decreased compliance is increased with age and is caused, in part, by diffuse fibrosis. Decreased compliance is also noted in patients with focal scar or aneurysm after myocardial infarction. Infiltrative cardiomyopathies (e.g., amyloidosis) can also increase wall stiffness. Pericardial constriction or tamponade causes mechanical increased resistance to filling of part or all of the heart (Angeja & Grossman, 2003). Interactions with left ventricular hypertrophy (LVH), ischemia, and diastolic dysfunction create a vicious cycle in which LVH predisposes to ischemia, the ischemia causes impairment of relaxation in the heart with LVH, and this worsens the severity of subendocardial ischemia. Several mechanisms appear to lower subendocardial perfusion pressure. Coronary vascular remodeling occurs with increased medial thickness and perivascular fibrosis. The increased LV mass and inadequate vascular growth result in a loss of coronary vasodilator reserve so that there is a limited ability to

A. Slowed relaxation: Decreased -dP/dt

B. Slowed relaxation: Delayed filling

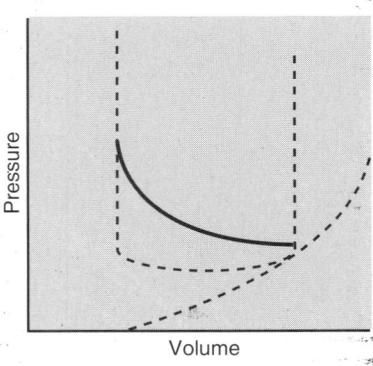

■ **Figure 28–4.** Pressure volume loop is depicted with dotted lines representing normal subjects; solid lines represent subjects with diastolic dysfunction. Ventricular filling can be impaired by four types of lusitropic abnormalities: (*A*) slowed relaxation with decreased rate of pressure fall (-dP/dt) during isovolumetric relaxation; (*B*) slowed relaxation with delayed filling during early diastole; (*C*) incomplete relaxation with impaired filling throughout diastole; (*D*) decreased compliance (increased stiffness). (From Katz, A.M. [2000]. *Heart failure: Pathophysiology, molecular biology and clinical management.* Philadelphia: Lippincott Williams & Wilkins.)

C. Incomplete relaxation

D. Decreased compliance

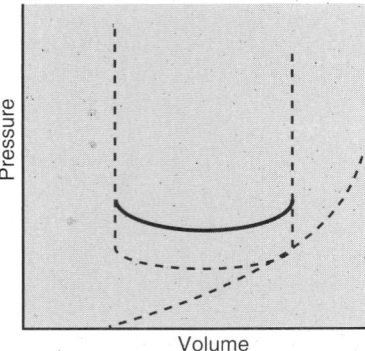

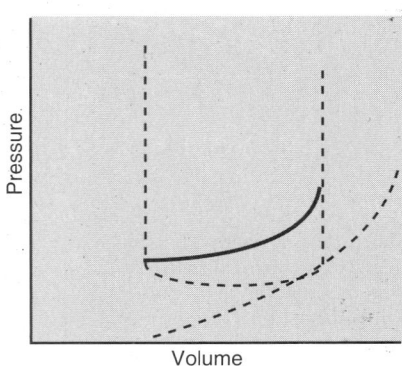

increase myocardial perfusion in response to an increased oxygen demand. In addition, increased diastolic pressure exerts a compressive force against the subendocardium and restricts subendocardial perfusion (Colucci & Braunwald, 2001).

Neurohormonal Response

The major elements of the neurohormonal response may be described as three categories: the hemodynamic defense reaction, the inflammatory reaction, and the growth or hypertrophic response. These homeostatic mechanisms represent a beneficial short-term response to impaired cardiac function but are associated with detrimental maladaptive long-term consequences (Table 28-2) (Katz, 2000).

Hemodynamic Defense Reaction

The neurohormonal response to a decrease in cardiac output accelerates heart rate, vasoconstricts arteries and veins, increases the ejection fraction and the capacity of the heart to fill, and, by promoting salt and water retention by the kidneys, increases blood volume. Salt and water retention, vasoconstriction, and cardiac stimulation are mediated by signaling molecules that play a regulatory and counter-regulatory role in HF (Table 28-3). The various mediators evoke similar and often overlapping responses. When a regulatory signal turns on

a process, counter-regulatory signals are released to turn off the process (Katz, 2000; Francis et al., 2001).

Fluid Retention. Renal compensation is triggered initially by a decrease in kidney perfusion, which decreases glomerular filtration and activates the renin-angiotensin-aldosterone system (RAAS), resulting in an increased SVR and increased sodium and water absorption. (Fig. 28-6) (Abraham & Schrier, 2000). Mediators of the selective vasoconstrictor response include norepinephrine (NE), arginine vasopressin or the antidiuretic hormone (ADH), angiotensin II, and endothelin. Aldosterone, a steroid hormone, increases tubular sodium along with angiotensin II and NE. Arginine vasopressin or ADH acts on the collecting ducts to promote water reabsorption. In early HF, catecholamines, ADH, and endothelin play the major role in stimulating aldosterone secretion. In patients with advanced HF, the most important stimulus for aldosterone release is angiotensin II, whose levels are increased with diuretic therapy (Cody, 2000; Katz, 2000). Natriuretic peptides are counter-regulatory mediators produced in the body. This family of peptides includes atrial natriuretic peptide (ANP), brain natriuretic peptide or b-type natriuretic peptide (BNP), and clearance natriuretic peptide (CNP). The heart itself produces two peptides, ANP and BNP. ANP is stored mainly in the right atria, and an increase in atrial distending pressure, however produced, leads to the release of ANP. BNP, identified initially in the brain, is synthesized in the ventricle and is released in response to increased ventricular pressure. CNP is produced in blood

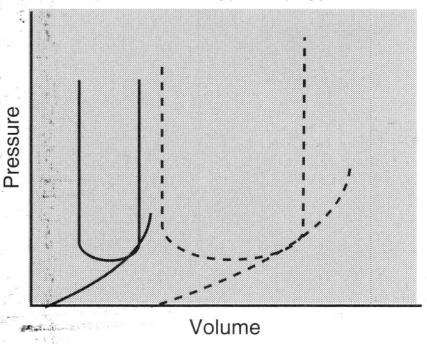

A. Decreased cavity size
(Concentric hypertrophy)

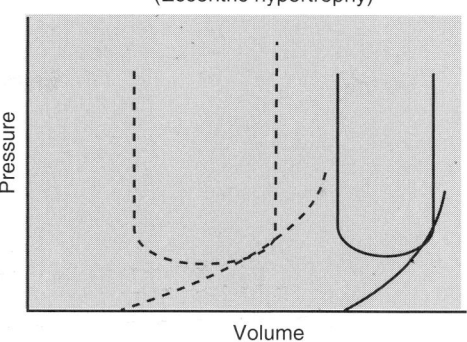

B. Increased cavity size, remodeling
(Eccentric hypertrophy)

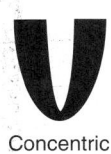 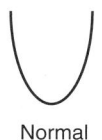

Concentric   Normal
hypertrophy

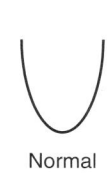 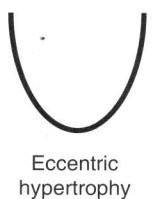

Normal   Eccentric
hypertrophy

■ **Figure 28–5.** Effects of different patterns of hypertrophy on diastolic function. Normal curves are shown in dotted line. (*A*) Concentric hypertrophy reduces both ventricular volume and compliance. (*B*) Eccentric hypertrophy, which increases ventricular volume, is also generally accompanied by a decreases in compliance. (From Katz, A.M. [2000]. *Heart failure: Pathophysiology, molecular biology and clinical management.* Philadelphia: Lippincott Williams & Wilkins.

vessels and in the brain. CNP appears to act primarily as a clearance receptor that regulates levels of the peptides and reduces vascular resistance but has no natriuretic property. Both ANP and BNP promote vasodilatation and sodium excretion (Anand et al., 2003). They may also attenuate sympathetic tone, RAAS activity (see Fig. 28-6), vasopressin (ADH), and the growth or hypertrophy of the ventricle (Cody, 2000; Colucci & Braunwald, 2001; Drexler & Hasenfuss, 2001; Francis et al., 2001). All three peptides are elevated in HF (Aronson et al., 2003).

Vasoconstriction. The most important stimulus for vasoconstriction in HF is sympathetic activation that releases catecholamines. Plasma levels of NE become elevated. Sympathetic effects on the peripheral vascular system by binding to alpha 1-adrenergic receptors increases vascular tone to raise SVR (afterload) and mean systemic filling pressure, thereby augmenting venous return or preload (Fig. 28-7) (Colucci, 2000). Other mediators include angiotensin II, vasopressin (ADH), and endothelin.

As described, the RAAS plays an important role in HF, and angiotensin II has a vast range of biologic activities (see Fig. 28-6). In addition to stimulating aldosterone, angiotensin II is a potent vasoconstrictor (Cody, 2000). There are four recognized angiotensin II (AT) receptor sites, but the AT1 receptors, which predominate in adult hearts, exert their regulatory effects, including vasoconstriction, increase in myocardial contractility, cell growth (hypertrophy), and apoptosis (programmed cell death) in myocytes. The AT2 receptor, a "fetal phenotype," promotes counter-regulatory effects, including vasodilatation and decrease in growth and proliferation of cells. The AT1 receptor is down-regulated in patients with HF (Zisman, 1995).

Table 28–2 ■ NEUROHORMONAL RESPONSE: SHORT- AND LONG-TERM RESPONSES

Mechanism	Short-Term Adaptive Response	Long-Term Maladaptive Response
Hemodynamic defense		
Fluid retention	↑Preload, ↑cardiac output	Pulmonary and systemic edema
Vasoconstriction	↑Afterload, maintain blood pressure	↓ Cardiac output, ↑energy expenditure, cardiac necrosis
Sympathetic stimulation of heart	↑Heart rate, ↑contractility, ↑relaxation, ↑cardiac output	↑Cardiac energy expenditure, arrhythmias, sudden death, cardiac necrosis
Inflammatory reaction		
Cytokine activation	Vasodilatation	Cardiac cachexia (skeletal catabolism)
Free radicals	Antiapoptosis (?)	↓Inotropy, LV remodeling, cardiac apoptosis, necrosis
Hypertrophy or growth response	Adaptive hypertrophy	Maladaptive hypertrophy
Early gene response	↓ Load, ↓ energy demand	Remodeling
Transcription factors	↑ Sarcomere number	↑ Energy demand
	↑Cardiac output	Cardiac apoptosis, necrosis

Adapted from Katz, A. M. (Ed.). (2000). *Heart failure:Pathophysiology, molecular biology, and clinical management* (p. 110). Philadelphia: Lippincott Williams & Wilkins.

Table 28–3 ■ SIGNALING MOLECULES IN THE HEMODYNAMIC DEFENSE REACTION

I. Signaling Molecules: Regulatory Role

Mediators

Catecholamines (norepinephrine, epinephrine)
  Heart—increased rate, contractility, relaxation (increased chronotrophy, inotropy, lusitrophy)
  Peripheral—arterial vasoconstriction (increased afterload), venous vasoconstriction (increased preload)
  Stimulates cell growth, fibrosis, progressive remodeling
Renin-angiotensin-aldosterone system (angiotensin II)
  Arterial vasoconstriction (increased afterload)
  Venous vasoconstriction (increased preload)
  Sodium and water retention (increased preload and afterload)
  Increased myocardial contractility (increased inotropy)
  Stimulates cell growth, fibrosis, progressive remodeling
Arginine vasopressin or ADH
  Sodium and water retention (increased preload and afterload)
  Stimulates cell growth, fibrosis, progressive remodeling
Endothelin
  Promotes aldosterone, ADH release thereby increasing sodium and water retention (increased preload and afterload)
  Peripheral–arterial vasoconstriction (increased afterload)
  Stimulates cell growth, fibrosis, progressive remodeling

II. Signaling Molecules: Counter-Regulatory Role

Mediators

Atrial and b-type natriuretic peptides (ANP, BNP)
  Vasodilatation, natriuresis, renin inhibition (decreased preload and afterload)
  Inhibit cell growth and proliferation
Nitric Oxide (NO)
  Mediator of endothelium dependent vasodilatation (decrease afterload)
  Sodium and water retention (increased preload and afterload)
  Inhibit cell growth and proliferation
Bradykinin
  Vasodilatation (decrease afterload)
  Inhibit cell growth and proliferation
Adrenomedullin
  Vasodilatation (decrease afterload)
  Increases levels of ANP, BNP
Catecholamine (Dopamine)
  Vasodilatation (decrease afterload)
Prostaglandins (Prostacyclin, Prostaglandin E2)
  Vasodilatation (decrease afterload; paracrine and autocrine effect)

Adapted from Katz, A. M. (Ed.). (2000). *Heart failure:Pathophysiology, molecular biology, and clinical management,* (p. 113.). Philadelphia: Lippincott Williams & Wilkins.

Arginine vasopressin (ADH) is a pituitary hormone that plays a central role in regulation of plasma osmolality and free water clearance. It is released into the circulation in response to hyperosmolarity and angiotensin II. It causes vasoconstriction via vasopressin 1 receptors (Fig. 28-8) (Colucci & Braunwald, 2001). Endothelin is also a potent vasoconstrictor, which is stimulated by vasopressin (ADH), catecholamines, angiotensin II, and growth factors. Two endothelin receptor sites, endothelin ET-A and ET-B, have been identified. The ET-A elicits, in addition to peripheral vasoconstriction, an increase in inotropy, fluid retention, and growth or hypertrophy. The ET-B receptor is less well understood, although it can mediate vasoconstriction and also a vasodilator effect through increased levels of NO and prostaglandins. Plasma endothelin correlates directly with pulmonary artery pressures and pulmonary artery resistance and may play a role in pulmonary hypertension seen in patients with HF (Cody, 2000; Johnson et al., 2000).

Counter-regulatory mediators that cause vasodilatation include the natriuretic peptides (see previous section), NO, bradykinin, dopamine, and some of the prostaglandins, all of which act directly to relax arteriolar smooth muscle. Nitric oxide (NO), a free-radical gas initially known as endothelial-derived relaxing factor (EDRF), is synthesized by the vascular endothelium. Inability of the endothelium to respond to vasodilator stimulus of NO may contribute to the exercise intolerance in patients with HF. Bradykinin and related peptides are vasodilators. Bradykinin is a substrate for angiotensin-converting enzyme that is also responsible for the production of angiotensin II. In addition, bradykinin also inhibits maladaptive growth (Cody, 2000; Katz, 2000; Colucci & Braunwald, 2001). Adrenomedullin is a peptide with vasodilating and natriuretic properties. It also has positive inotropic effects. The clinical importance of these effects on HF is not fully established (Szokosi et al., 1998). Dopamine, which is a precursor to NE, is a catecholamine that has central and peripheral effects. At low concentrations, dopamine relaxes smooth muscle; this vasodilatation lowers peripheral resistance and dilates renal blood vessels. Prostaglandin synthesis is stimulated by NE, angiotensin II, and vasopressin (ADH). The vasodilators are prostacyclin (PGI_2) and prostaglandin E_2. Because they are short-lived, they act locally to exert their effects, either released from one cell to work on another (paracrine effect) or binding to the same cell that released the prostaglandin (autocrine effect). In patients with HF, these counter-regulatory effects are often overwhelmed by the vasoconstrictor response (Cody, 2000; Katz, 2000; Colucci & Braunwald, 2001).

Stimulation of the Heart. Stimulation of the inotropic, lusitropic, and chronotropic (heart rate) properties of the heart is the third component of the hemodynamic defense reaction. In HF, stimulation of the sympathetic nervous system represents the most immediately responsive mechanism of compensation. Stimulation of the β-adrenergic receptors in the heart causes an elevation in heart rate and contractility to raise stroke volume and cardiac output. Sympathetic overactivity in HF may exert adverse effects on the structure and function of the myocardium by the process of remodeling. Myocardial remodeling involves hypertrophy and apoptosis of myocytes, regression to a cellular phenotype, and changes in the nature of the extracelluar matrix (see Fig. 28-7) (Katz, 2000; Colucci & Braunwald, 2001).

Weakening of the myocardial response to NE is an important counter-regulatory change in patients with HF. Chronic sympathetic stimulation inhibits β-receptor synthesis and reduces the ability of the β-receptor to respond to the stimulus of NE. Beta-receptor down-regulating reduces the amount of receptors available to bind to NE. Mechanisms responsible for β1-receptor down-regulation help protect the failing heart from the adverse effects of sustained sympathetic stimulation.

Inflammatory Response

Local and systemic inflammation plays an important role in HF, particularly in regard to disease progression (Mann, 2002). Cytokines are signaling peptides whose actions include cell growth and cell death through direct toxic effects on the heart and peripheral circulation. The proinflammatory or

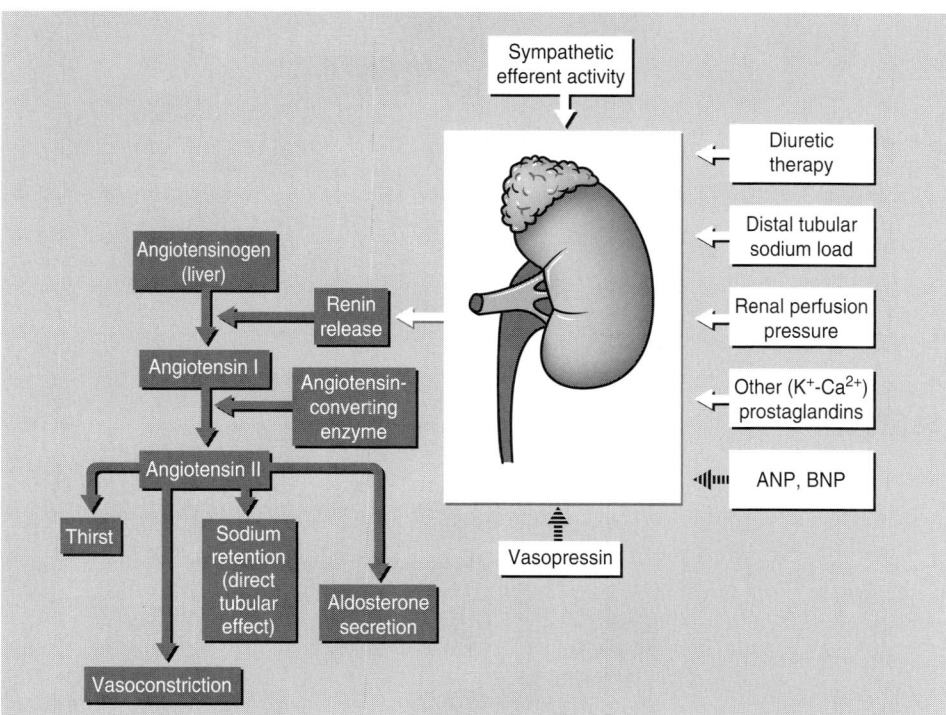

■ **Figure 28–6.** The renin-angiotensin-aldosterone system is activated in patients with heart failure. Multiple stimuli may contribute to renal release of renin into the systemic circulation, including increased sympathetic efferent activity, decreased tubular sodium delivery, reduced renal perfusion, and diuretic therapy. Natriuretic peptides (ANP, BNP), and vasopressin (ADH)(*dashed arrows*) may inhibit release of renin. Angiotensin I is converted to angiotensin II, which is a potent vasoconstrictor; it promotes sodium reabsorption by increasing aldosterone secretion, and by a direct effect on the tubules, stimulates water intake by acting on the thirst center. (Adapted from Paganelli, W.C., Craeger, M.A., & Dzau, V.J. [1986]. Cardiac regulation of renal function. In T.O. Cheung [Ed.], *International textbook of cardiology*. New York: Bergamman Press.)

"stress-activated" cytokines include tumor necrosis factor-alpha (TNF-α) and some interleukins. The cardiac myocytes themselves are capable of synthesizing these proinflammatory cytokines in response to various forms of cardiac injury (Mann, 2000). The local inflammatory response can appear within minutes of an abnormal stress. Local inflammation of the cytokines and other mediators includes deleterious effects of LV remodeling, which include myocyte hypertrophy, alteration in fetal gene expression, contractile defects, and progressive myocyte loss through apoptosis. In addition, there may be promotion of LV remodeling through alterations of the extracellular matrix. A number of studies have shown that the local proinflammatory molecules are activated as early as NYHA class II, which is before some of the classic neurohormonal responses, that tend to be activated in the latter stages (NYHA III and IV) (Mann, 2002). There are important signaling interactions between the RAAS and the sympathetic nervous system, along with the proinflammatory cytokines (Katz, 2000).

Activation of the systemic inflammatory response is found in advanced HF. Cardiac cachexia and skeletal muscle myopathy, which is responsible for the fatigue and muscle weakness seen in HF, is a part of the systemic inflammatory response, and the elevation of the proinflammatory cytokines correlates with the severity of the syndrome. The knowledge of the role of inflammation remains incomplete. As with the hemodynamic defense reaction, the inflammatory response may be initially beneficial, but when sustained becomes deleterious.

Hypertrophic Response

As discussed, the hypertrophic response is initially an important adaptive mechanism of the heart to an increased load, either pressure or volume. When the primary stimulus is pressure overload, there is increased systolic wall stress that leads to parallel replication of myofibrils, thickening of myocytes, and concentric hypertrophy. With a ventricular volume overload, increased diastolic wall stress leads to replication of sarcomeres in series, elongation of myocytes, and ventricular dilatation or eccentric hypertrophy. Maladaptive growth and changing myocyte phenotype leads to myocyte thickening (seen in diastolic dysfunction and concentric hypertrophy) and myocyte elongation (seen in systolic dysfunction and eccentric hypertrophy) (Drexler & Hasenfuss, 2001; Francis & Pathak, 2001). These large genetically abnormal cells cannot contract as efficiently as normal ones (Fig. 28-9).

Myocardial remodeling and transition from compensated hypertrophy to failure of the myocardium involves complex events at the molecular and cellular level (Hein et al., 2003). Increased pressure or volume reactivates growth factors present in the embryonic heart but dormant in the adult heart. This fetal gene expression stimulates the hypertrophy of the myocytes and the synthesis and degradation of the extracellular matrix. There is some evidence that extracellular matrix degradation may elicit side-to-side slippage of myocytes, perhaps caused by dissolution of collagen struts that normally hold cells together, whereas reparative and reactive fibrosis may represent a secondary event resulting in a stiffer ventricle. Myocyte slippage may also be caused by myocyte loss (Johnson et al., 2000).

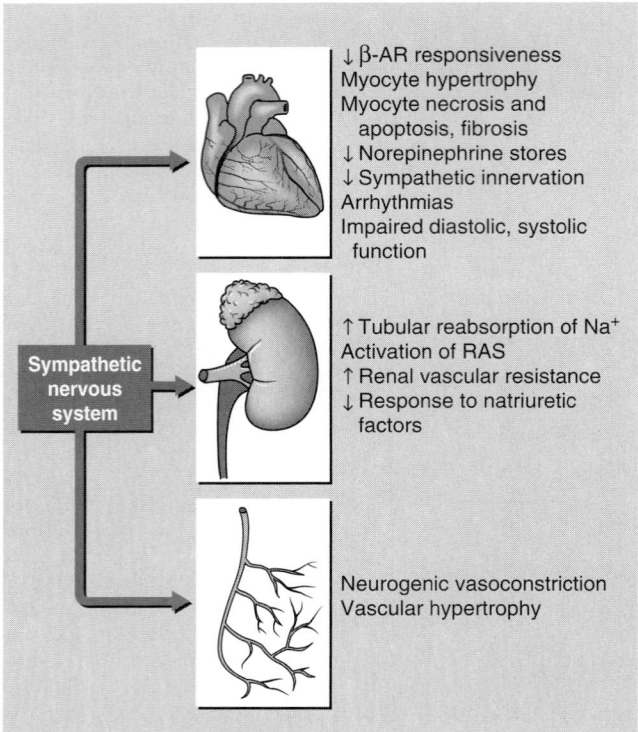

■ **Figure 28–7.** Increased sympathetic activity may contribute to the pathophysiology of HF by multiple mechanisms. (B-AR, postsynaptic beta adrenergic receptor; RAS, renin-angiotensin system.) (Adapted from Floras, J. S. [1993]. Clinical aspects of sympathetic activation and parasympathetic withdrawal in heart failure. *Journal of American College of Cardiology,* 22[72A].)

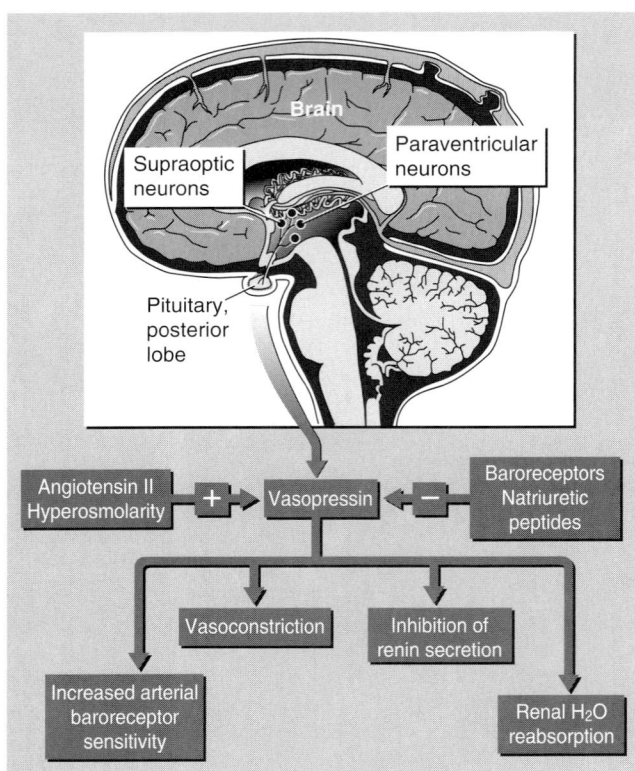

■ **Figure 28–8.** Arginine vasopressin (ADH) is a peptide released from the posterior pituitary gland. Angiotensin II and osmoreceptors stimulate vasopressin release; the natriuretic peptides (ANP, BNP) inhibit vasopressin secretion. Vasopressin causes vasoconstriction, renal reabsorption of water, and renal secretion of renin. (Cusco, J. A. & Creager, M. A. [1999]. Neurohumoral, renal, and vascular adjustments in heart failure. In W.S. Colucci & E. Braunwald, *Atlas of heart failure. Cardiac function and dysfunction* [2nd ed.]. Philadelphia: Blackwell Science.)

Myocyte loss may occur by one of two mechanisms: apoptosis or necrosis. Apoptosis is a programmed cell death that is energy-dependent, producing cell dropout. Apoptosis is a highly regulated process that causes the cell to shrink, yielding cell fragments that are surrounded by plasma membrane. This process does not invoke an inflammatory or fibrotic response. Apoptosis is stimulated by hypoxia, angiotensin II, TNF-α myocyte calcium overload, and mitochondrial or cell injury (Mani & Kitis, 2003). Two forms of apoptosis appear to affect the course of postinfarction remodeling: ischemic-driven apoptosis at the site of the infarction and load-dependent or receptor-dependent apoptosis at sites remote from the ischemic areas (Abbate et al., 2003). Necrosis or accidental cell death occurs when the myocyte is deprived of oxygen or energy. Energy starvation of the myocyte results from an increase in energy demand and a reduced capacity for energy production. The inflammatory response that is induced by overload elevates circulating levels of cytokines that in turn release reactive oxygen species and free radicals. Calcium overload increases energy expenditure and slows energy production. All these processes lead to the loss of cellular membrane integrity, causing the cell to swell and eventually burst. This releases proteolytic enzymes that cause cellular disruption. The release of cell contents initiates an inflammatory reaction that leads to scarring and fibrosis. Myocyte necrosis may be localized, as in a myocardial infarction, or diffuse, as from myocarditis or idiopathic cardiomyopathy (Katz, 2000; Colucci & Braunwald, 2001). The vicious cycle of the overloaded heart is depicted in Figure 28-10.

Alteration in expression and function of the contractile proteins is found in pathological hypertrophy that is signaled by mechanical wall stress, angiotensin II, NE, endothelin, TNF-α and some interlukins, and intracellular calcium signaling. There are changes in the sarcomeric proteins that lead to decrease in contraction velocity and lead to a decreased stroke volume and increased ventricular volume (Katz, 2000; Kearney et al., 2002).

■ CLINICAL MANIFESTATIONS

Most patients with HF have reduced LV systolic function and/or degrees of diastolic dysfunction. The predominant symptom of LV failure is breathlessness or dyspnea. Orthopnea and paroxysmal nocturnal dyspnea occur in the more advanced stages of HF. *Systolic dysfunction* is characterized by occurrence of HF as a result of a decreased cardiac output and secondary salt and water

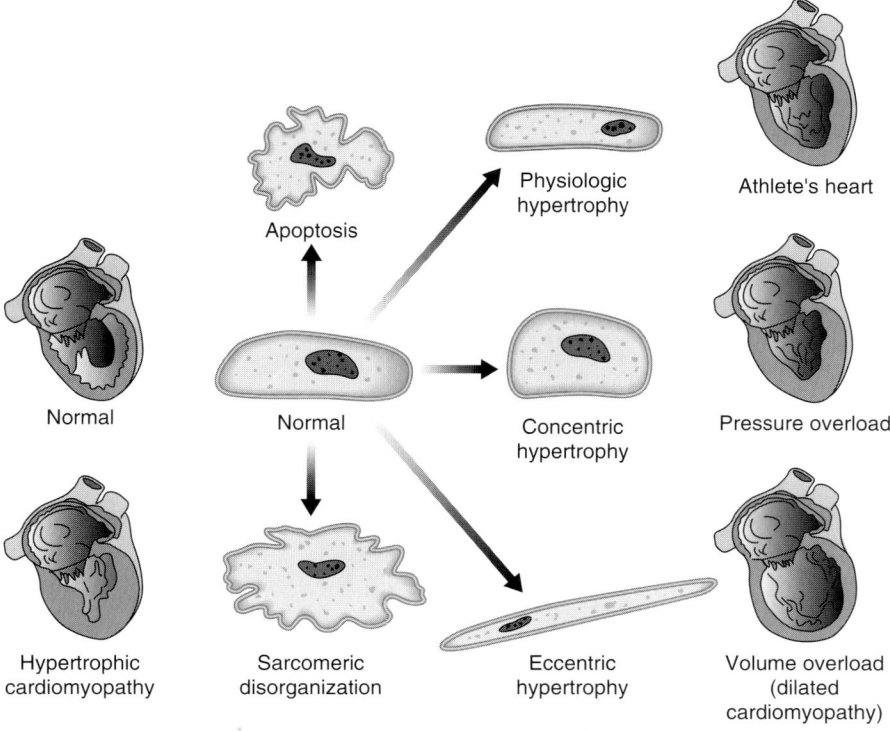

■ **Figure 28–9.** Phenotype change of the heart at the cellular and organ level. Normal muscle can grow in a physiologic way, as seen in the athlete's heart. Concentric hypertrophy can result from pressure overload; eccentric hypertrophy due to volume overload, or dilated cardiomyopathy. (From Drexler, H. & Hasenfuss, G. [2001]. Physiology of the normal and failing heart. In M. Crawford & J.P. DiMarco [Eds.], *Cardiology.* London: Mosby.)

retention. *Diastolic dysfunction* is associated with elevated ventricular filling pressures caused by an abnormality of diastolic function, which may be caused by slow or incomplete ventricular relaxation causing pulmonary and/or systemic congestion.

The signs and symptoms that characterize HF can be considered in the context of the four components of the syndrome:

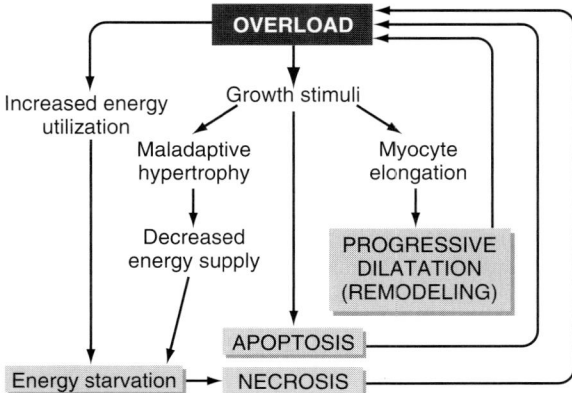

■ **Figure 28–10.** Vicious circle of the overloaded heart. Overload both increases energy utilization and stimulates growth. The former contributes directly to a state of energy starvation, which is made worse by several consequences of maladaptive hypertrophy. The later includes myocyte elongation, which causes remodeling, a progressive dilatation that increases wall tension so as to increase the overload. Growth stimuli also promotes apoptosis, which by decreasing the number of viable myocytes, increases the load on those that survive. (From Katz, A.M. [2000]. *Heart failure: Pathophysiology, molecular biology and clinical management.* Philadelphia: Lippincott Williams & Wilkins.)

failure of the left ventricle as a pump, failure of the right ventricle as a pump, pulmonary venous congestion, and systemic venous congestion (Givertz, 2001; Patel & Konstam, 2001). Symptoms are often described as those caused by left- or right-sided HF, and although the symptoms of both types overlap, they are addressed separately in the following discussion (Fig. 28-11).

Related to Left-Sided Heart Failure

Left-sided HF, associated with elevated pulmonary venous pressure and decreased cardiac output, appears clinically as breathlessness, weakness, fatigue, dizziness, confusion, pulmonary congestion, hypotension, and death.

Weakness or fatigue is precipitated by decreased perfusion to the muscles. Abnormalities of skeletal muscle histology and biochemistry also play a role, along with deficient endothelial function. Patients describe a feeling of heaviness in their arms and legs, and there is a reduction in exercise capacity. Cardiac cachexia is a severe complication of HF and is considered a terminal manifestation. The cytokines are known to be important in tissue catabolism.

Decreased cerebral perfusion caused by low cardiac output leads to changes in mental status, such as restlessness, insomnia, nightmares, or memory loss. Anxiety, agitation, paranoia, and fear of impending doom may develop as the syndrome progresses.

During the course of HF, pulmonary congestion progresses through three stages: stage 1, early pulmonary congestion; stage 2, interstitial edema; and stage 3, alveolar edema (Givertz, 2001; LeJemtel et al., 2001). During the early phase, little measurable increase in interstitial lung fluid is noted. There are few clinical manifestations during this phase.

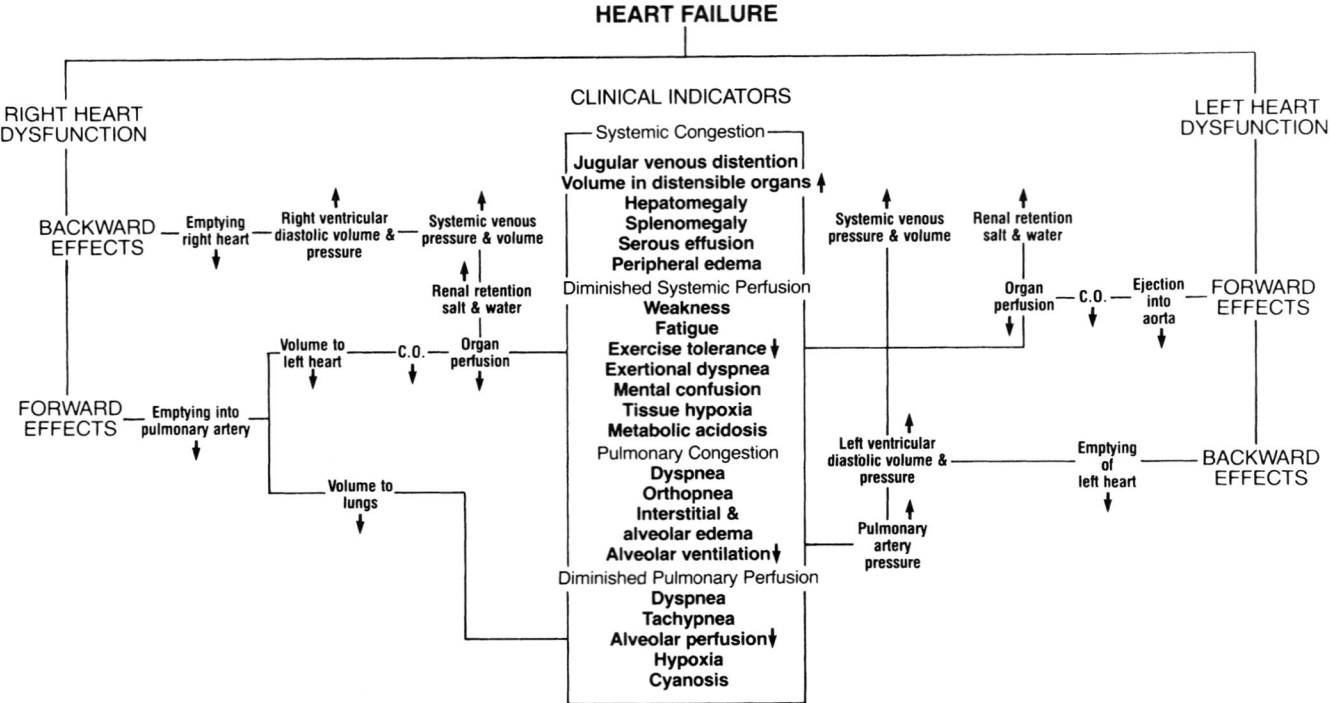

■ **Figure 28–11.** Heart failure flow chart, with complex interaction of forward and backward effects of right and left ventricular failure. The clinical indicators arise from systemic and pulmonary congestion and from diminished systemic and pulmonary perfusion. (From Michaelson, C.R. [1983]. *Congestive heart failure* [p. 52]. St Louis: CV Mosby.)

Interstitial edema occurs when the PAWP exceeds 18 mm Hg, leading to a net filtration of fluid into the interstitial space. Clinical manifestations of interstitial edema are varied. Engorged pulmonary vessels, elevated PA pressure, and reduced lung compliance cause increased exertional dyspnea. If the left ventricle is severely impaired, orthopnea or a nonproductive cough may be present. Paroxysmal nocturnal dyspnea may also occur because of postural redistribution of blood flow that increases venous return and pulmonary vascular pressure when the patient is in a recumbent position. Congestion of the bronchial mucosa that increases airway resistance and the work of breathing may also contribute to paroxysmal nocturnal dyspnea. Pulmonary crackles are first noted over the lung bases, and as the PAWP ranges between 18 and 25 mm Hg, they progress toward the apices.

Stage 3 occurs when the PAWP rises to 25 to 28 mm Hg, causing rapid movement of fluid out of the intravascular and interstitial spaces into the alveoli. As the edema progresses, the alveoli no longer remain open because of the large fluid accumulation. At this point, the alveolar–capillary membrane is disrupted, fluid invades the large airways, and the patient expectorates frothy, pink-tinged sputum. Acute pulmonary edema is a catastrophic indicator of HF.

Related to Right-Sided Heart Failure

Right-sided HF, associated with increased systemic venous pressure, gives rise to the clinical signs of jugular venous distention, hepatomegaly, dependent peripheral edema, and

ascites (Givertz et al., 2001; LeJemtel et al., 2001; Patel & Konstam, 2001). Dependent ascending peripheral edema is a manifestation in which edema begins in the lower legs and ascends to the thighs, genitalia, and abdominal wall. Patients may notice their shoes fitting tightly or marks left on the feet from their shoes or socks. Weight gain is what most patients recognize, and consistent morning daily weights help to detect any sudden weight gain. An adult may retain 10 to 15 pounds (4 to 7 L) of fluid before pitting edema occurs.

Congestive hepatomegaly characterized by a large, tender, pulsating liver and ascites also occur. Liver engorgement is caused by venous engorgement, whereas ascites results from transudation of fluid from the capillaries into the abdominal cavity. Gastrointestinal symptoms such as nausea and anorexia may be a direct consequence of the increased intra-abdominal pressure.

Another finding related to fluid retention is diuresis at rest. When at rest, the body's metabolic requirements are decreased, and cardiac function improves. This decreases systemic venous pressure, allowing edema fluid to be mobilized and excreted. Table 28-4 lists the various subjective and objective indicators for LV and RV failure.

■ CLASSIFICATION

The writing committee of the American College of Cardiology and the American Heart Association (ACC/AHA) Task Force decided to emphasize the evolution and progression of HF in their revision of the guidelines (Hunt et al., 2001).

Table 28–4 ▪ CLINICAL INDICATORS AND PHYSICAL FINDINGS OF LEFT AND RIGHT VENTRICULAR FAILURE

Left Ventricular Failure	Right Ventricular Failure
Subjective Findings	
Breathlessness	Weight gain
Cough	Transient ankle swelling
Fatigue and weakness	Abdominal distention
Memory loss and confusion	Gastric distress
Diaphoresis	Anorexia, nausea
Palpitations	
Anorexia	
Insomnia	
Objective Findings	
Tachycardia	Neck vein pulsations and distention
Decreased S_1	Increased jungular venous pressure
S_3 and S_4 gallops	(increased central venous pressure),
Crackles (rales)	direct and indirect measurement
Pleural effusion	Edema
Diaphoresis	Hepatomegaly
Pulsus alternans	Positive hepatojugular reflux
Increased pulmonary artery wedge pressure	Ascites
Decreased cardiac index	
Increased systemic vascular resistance	

This classification recognizes that HF, like coronary artery disease, has established risk factors, that the progression of HF has asymptomatic and symptomatic phases, and that treatments prescribed at each stage can reduce morbidity and mortality. The new guidelines complement the standard New York Heart Association Functional Classification (NYHA-FC) (Table 28-5).

Four stages of HF were identified. Stage A identifies the patient who is at high risk but has no structural heart disease; stage B refers to a patient with structural heart disease but no symptoms of HF; stage C denotes the patient with structural heart disease and current or previous symptoms of HF; and stage D describes the patient with end-stage disease that requires special interventions.

MEDICAL MANAGEMENT

Patients with LV dysfunction present with exercise intolerance, shortness of breath, and/or fluid retention. Incidental findings of left ventricular hypertrophy or dysfunction may be found in asymptomatic patients, also.

All patients presenting with HF should undergo a detailed evaluation to: (1) determine the type of cardiac dysfunction; (2) uncover correctable causative factors; (3) determine prognosis; and (4) guide treatment. Recognition of signs and symptoms resulting from an inadequate cardiac output and from systemic and pulmonary congestion is accomplished through a careful history, physical examination, routine laboratory analyses, and diagnostic studies (Francis, 1998; Hunt et al., 2001).

A careful history is important to ascertain possible causes of HF and those patients at increased risk, and should include past medical history and review of systems. This includes a history of coronary artery disease, hypertension, valvular heart disease, congenital heart defects, or diabetes. Other endocrine abnormalities include a history of thyroid disease. A family history of cardiomyopathy or coronary artery disease should be explored. Ascertain if the patient is using possible toxic agents such as alcohol

Table 28–5 ▪ HEART FAILURE CLASSIFICATION

New York Heart Association Classification	American College of Cardiology/American Heart Association Guidelines	Examples
	Stage A. Patients at high risk of developing HF but without structural heart disease or symptoms of HF.	Systemic hypertension; coronary artery disease; diabetes mellitus; cardiotoxic drug therapy or alcohol abuse; family history of cardiomyopathy
Class I. Patients with cardiac disease without limitations of physical activity.	*Stage B.* Patients who have structural heart disease but have no symptoms of HF.	Left ventricular hypertrophy; enlarged, dilated ventricle; asymptomatic valvular disease; previous myocardial infarction
Class II. Patients with cardiac disease who have slight limitations of physical activity. Ordinary physical activities cause symptoms.	*Stage C.* Patients who have structural heart disease with current or prior symptoms.	Dyspnea or fatigue due to left ventricular dysfunction; asymptomatic patients who are undergoing treatment for prior symptoms of HF
Class III. Patients with cardiac disease who have marked limitation to physical activity. Less than ordinary physical activities cause symptoms.		
Class IV. Patients with cardiac disease who cannot carry out any physical activity without symptoms. Symptoms may be present at rest.	*Stage D.* People with refractory heart failure that requires specialized intervention.	Patients who have marked symptoms at rest despite maximal medical therapy; who cannot be discharged from the hospital; who are recurrently hospitalized, awaiting heart transplantation, in hospice setting, receiving intravenous therapy for symptom relief, or being supported by mechanical assist device

Adapted from Hunt, S.A. et al. (2001). ACC/AHA guidelines for the evaluation and management of chronic heart failure in the adult: executive summary: A report of the American College of Cardiology and American Heart Association Task Force on Practice Guidelines. *Circulation, 104,* 2296–3007.

or cocaine or has been exposed to radiation of chemotherapy. Patients with a history of central sleep apnea may also have impaired autonomic control and increased cardiac arrhythmias (Lanfranchi et al., 2002). Precipitating factors for HF should be looked for, such as anemia, infection, or pulmonary embolism (Ezekowitz et al., 2002). Obtaining a description of a patient's exercise capacity and ability to perform activities of daily living may be useful in assessing their degree of limitation. Patients who describe symptoms of presyncope or syncope should be evaluated for arrhythmias, because atrial fibrillation and ventricular arrhythmias are found in this patient population. Sudden death is responsible for up to 40% to 50% of fatal events in HF (Myerburg, 2001). In patients with decompensation of existing HF, dietary or medication noncompliance or exacerbating mediations like nonsteroidal antiinflammatory agents should be addressed.

Physical Assessment

A major goal in assessing the patient with HF is to determine the type and severity of the underlying disease causing HF and the extent of the HF syndrome. Physical examination of the patient with HF focuses on the cardiovascular and pulmonary systems and relevant aspects of gastrointestinal and skin assessment (Francis, 1998).

Cardiovascular Assessment. Determination of the rate, rhythm, and character of the pulse is important in patients with HF. The pulse rate is usually elevated in response to a low cardiac output. Pulsus alternans (alternating pulse) is characterized by an altering strong and weak pulse with a normal rate and interval. Pulsus alternans is associated with altered functioning of the left ventricle causing variance in LV preload. An irregularly irregular pulse is usually indicative of atrial fibrillation. Increased heart size is common in patients with HF. This cardiac enlargement is detected by precordial palpation, with the apical impulse displaced laterally to the left and downward. In patients with HF, there is a third heart sound (S_3) that is associated with a reduced ejection fraction and impaired diastolic function as determined by the peak filling rate. A fourth heart sound (S_4) may occur, although it is not in itself a sign of failure but rather a reflection of decreased ventricular compliance associated with ischemic heart disease, high blood pressure, or hypertrophy. When the heart rate is rapid, these two diastolic sounds may merge into a single loud sound or summation gallop. Patients with HF frequently have a murmur of mitral regurgitation, which radiates to the axilla (Francis, 1998). Jugular venous pulses are a means of estimating venous pressure. The a and v waves rise as the mean right atrial pressure rises. The hepatojugular reflux is also assessed. When the abdomen of a patient with RV failure is compressed, there is an increase in the forward flow of blood to the right atrium, causing the right atrial pressure to rise (Chatterjee, 2000).

Pulmonary Assessment. Persistently elevated PA pressures result in the transudation of fluid from the capillaries into the interstitial spaces and, eventually, into the alveolar spaces. The accumulated fluid results in pulmonary crackles. Initially, the crackles are heard at the most dependent portions of the lungs; but later, as pulmonary congestion increases, crackles become diffuse and are heard over the entire chest. Respiratory rate and

pattern reflect the severity of the pulmonary compromise, with rapid breathing (tachypnea) or periodic respiratory (Cheyne-Stokes) being noted (Lanfranchi et al., 2002).

Integumentary Assessment. Patients with HF often present with dependent symmetric edema. It is most often detected in the feet, ankles, or sacral area. Color and temperature of the skin are also assessed, with major findings being pallor, decreased temperature, cyanosis, and diaphoresis. Cardiac cachexia, with a decrease in tissue mass, may be evident in patients with long-standing HF. Cachexia is defined as a documented, unintentional, nonedematous weight loss of 5 kilograms or more with a body mass index of less than 24 kg/m^2.

Gastrointestinal Assessment. Characteristically, HF results in hepatomegaly. The liver span is increased and the liver is usually palpable well below the right costal margin. An enlarged spleen may also be palpated in advanced HF.

Diagnostic and Laboratory Tests

Transthoracic Doppler two-dimensional echocardiography coupled with Doppler flow studies is the single most valuable tool and is of particular benefit for specifically assessing ventricular mass, chamber size, valvular changes, pericardial effusion, and systolic and diastolic dysfunction (Givertz et al., 2001; Hunt et al., 2001). Systolic dysfunction is defined as an ejection fraction of less than .35 to .40. Diastolic dysfunction appears with concentric LV hypertrophy, left atrial enlargement, an ejection fraction of .45 to .55, a reduced rate of LV filling, and a prolonged time to peak filling (Angeja & Grossman, 2003). More recent studies have shown increased left ventricular mass/volume were increased in diastolic dysfunction but not in those with systolic dysfunction (Kitzman et al., 2002). Radionuclide studies are a more precise and reliable measurement of ejection fraction (technetium pyrophosphate imaging, technetium sestamibi, or thallium scintigraphy) and have also become important in providing clues to the presence and cause of HF (Hunt et al., 2001). These noninvasive stress tests are also a valuable tool in assessing myocardial viability, detecting ischemia in patients without angina but with a high probability of coronary artery disease (CAD) who would be candidates for revascularization (Hunt et al., 2001; Francis et al., 2001; LeJemtel et al., 2001).

If systolic function is normal, additional steps must be taken to diagnose diastolic dysfunction. Exclusion of other significant causes of dyspnea is important, and appropriate studies may include pulmonary function testing, noninvasive testing, and cardiac catheterization/coronary arteriography. Noninvasive stress testing is used to detect ischemia in patients without angina but with high probability of coronary artery disease who would be candidates for revascularization. Cardiac catheterization/coronary arteriography is used in patients with angina or large areas of ischemic or hibernating myocardium. This is also the best quantitative evaluation of diastolic dysfunction and shows an increase in PAWP or LV end-diastolic pressure during exercise or volume loading (Francis et al., 2001; Hunt et al., 2001).

A number of routine laboratory tests useful in the evaluation of HF, including a chest radiograph, should also be included to assess the size of the heart and the pulmonic vascular markings. The ECG is not helpful in assessing the presence or degree of HF, but it demonstrates patterns of ventricular hypertrophy, arrhythmias, and any degree of myocardial ischemia, injury, or infarction (LeJemtel et al., 2001).

Laboratory tests include blood chemistries, complete blood count, and urinalysis. Measurement of hemoglobin and hematocrit is useful to exclude anemia in patients with HF (Kosiborod et al., 2003). Anemia was found to be a common factor in patients with HF and an independent prognostic factor for mortality (Ezekowitz, 2002). Electrolyte imbalances in HF reflect complications of failure as well as the use of diuretics and other drug therapy. Disturbances in sodium, potassium, and magnesium are particularly significant. In patients with severe HF, an increase in total-body water dilutes body fluid and is reflected by a decrease in the serum sodium. Diuretics may also contribute to this low-serum sodium if fluid intake is not restricted. Hypokalemia, or low-serum potassium level, and low-serum magnesium may complicate HF as the result of the use of diuretics such as thiazides and furosemides, because these diuretics may lead to excessive excretion of potassium and magnesium.

Hyperkalemia, or elevated potassium level, may occur secondary to depressed effective renal blood flow and low glomerular filtration rate (Givertz et al., 2001).

Any impairment of kidney function may be reflected by elevated blood urea nitrogen (BUN), creatinine, and uric acid (McClellan et al., 2002). Elevated levels of bilirubin, serum glutamic oxaloacetic transaminase, and lactate dehydrogenase result from hepatic congestion. Urinalysis may reveal proteinuria, red blood cells, and high specific gravity. Thyroid-stimulating hormone in patients with atrial fibrillation and unexplained HF may also be helpful. Diabetes and lipid abnormalities are risk factors, and these should also be measured (Bell, 2003).

In patients with decompensation of HF, arterial blood gases usually show a decrease in PaO$_2$ (hypoxemia) and a low PaCO$_2$. In the clinical situation of HF, the alveoli become filled with fluid, causing a decrease in PaO$_2$, whereas the compensatory attempt to increase the PO$_2$ by hyperventilating causes a decrease in the PCO$_2$, resulting in a mild respiratory alkalosis. Later changes caused by decreased peripheral perfusion result in a build-up of lactic acid, causing metabolic acidosis (LeJemtel et al., 2001).

Measurement of BNP has become a recent laboratory value that is measured as a means to identify those patients with elevated left ventricular filling pressures (Maisel et al., 2001; Anand et al., 2003). It is increased in systolic and diastolic dysfunction, and although it cannot distinguish between the two dysfunctions, it is being widely investigated as a biochemical marker for morbidity and mortality (Maisel et al., 2001; Bozkurt & Mann, 2003; Nielson et al., 2003). It is very helpful in differentiating dyspnea caused by HF from other causes. Normal level of BNP is less than 100 pg/mL (Fig. 28-12).

Although not a general test for HF, an additional laboratory value is measurement of plasma homocysteine level, which is associated with increased risk for vascular disease. A recent study showed that increased plasma homocysteine

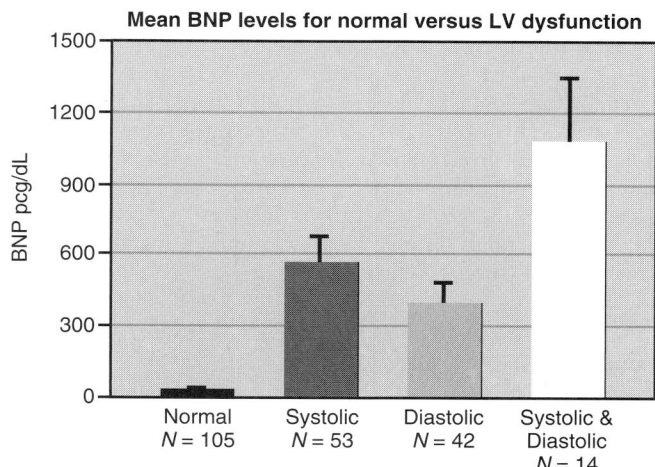

■ **Figure 28–12.** BNP values for the different subclasses of LV dysfunction. Normal BNP levels are less than 100 picograms/milliliter. (From Maisel, A.S., Koon, J., Krishnaswamy, P., Kazenegra, R et al. [2001]. Utility of B-natriuretic peptide as a rapid, point-of-care test for screening patients undergoing echocardiography to determine left ventricular dysfunction. *American Heart Journal,* 141, 369.)

level independently predicts risk of the development of HF in adults without previous myocardial infarction (Vasan et al., 2003).

Treatment

There are various principles that guide management of HF. The first is the treatment of the underlying disease or diseases, such as aggressive medical management of hypertension, coronary revascularization procedures for CAD for reversible myocardial ischemia, or surgical correction of structural abnormalities (Guidelines for coronary bypass graft surgery, 1991; Lejemtel et al., 2001). The second approach is the removal of the precipitating cause, such at infection, arrhythmia, and pulmonary emboli. The third is the treatment and control of HF. Therapy for HF is directed at reducing the workload of the heart and manipulating the various factors that determine cardiac performance, such as contractility, heart rate, preload, and afterload. The greatest advance has been in agents that inhibit harmful neurohormonal systems that are activated in support of the failing heart, specifically the renin-angiotensin system and sympathetic nervous system (Linseman & Bristow, 2003). Treatment of HF is based on the manner in which the patient clinically presents, which may encompass the extremes from asymptomatic left ventricular failure to acute cardiogenic shock (Ammon, 2001; LeJemtel et al., 2001).

Acute Heart Failure

Acute HF can be grouped clinically into acute cardiogenic pulmonary edema, cardiogenic shock, and acute decompensation of chronic left HF (Givertz et al., 2001). The goal of therapy is support of pump function, which may include positive inotropic agents, vasodilator therapy, and/or, if extremely severe, mechanical devices. A detailed section on specific management for these conditions is found in Chapter 30. In the case of ischemia caused by CAD, treatment of the underlying process is the management goal. The combination of ischemia and LV dysfunction carries a poor prognosis, and it is this patient group that may benefit from revascularization by percutaneous coronary intervention techniques (Chapter 27) or urgent cardiac surgery (Chapter 29).

Chronic and Stabilized Acute Heart Failure In Adults

Systolic Dysfunction. Coronary heart disease, hypertension, and dilated cardiomyopathy are the most commonly identified causes of LV systolic dysfunction. The writing committee of the ACC/AHA (Hunt et al., 2001) based the therapy guidelines on the four stages of evolution of HF (Table 28-6). *Stage A* includes patients who are at high risk for HF but do not have left ventricular dysfunction. Treatment is aimed at risk factor modification, including management of hypertension, diabetes and lipids, cessation of smoking, and counseling to avoid alcohol and illicit drugs. Patients are encouraged to exercise on a regular basis. Obesity increases the risk of diabetes and hypertension, and steps should be taken to promote strategies to maintain optimal weight. An angiotensin-converting enzyme (ACE) inhibitor is indicated in those with a history of atherosclerotic vascular

disease, hypertension, or diabetes (Heart Failure Society of American [HFSA], 1999).

Stage B includes patients who are asymptomatic but who have left ventricular systolic dysfunction and are at significant risk for HF. All of Stage A therapies are needed, with the addition of an ACE inhibitor and beta-blockers unless contraindicated (Gottlieb et al., 2002; Krum et al., 2003). Valve replacement or repair should be undertaken in patients with hemodynamcially significant valvular stenosis or regurgitation.

Stage C includes patients with left ventricular dysfunction with current or previous symptoms and who need to be treated with all measures used for Stages A and B. They should be routinely managed with four types of drugs: a diuretic, an ACE inhibitor, a beta-blocking agent, and digitalis. For those patients with an intolerance to ACE inhibitors, an angiotensin receptor blocker (ARB) can be used. For those patients with renal insufficiency or angioedema, a hydralazine/nitrate combination can be substituted (Dominiak, 2002). The use of an aldosterone antagonist, spironolactone, for NYHA Class III and IV symptoms should be considered (Rousseau et al., 2002). Avoid the use of antiarrhythmics, nonsteroidal antiinflammatories, and most calcium channel blockers. Calcium channel blockers are not of proven benefit for patients with systolic dysfunction and may be harmful. Such risks may not extend to the use of longer-acting calcium channel blockers (e.g., amlodipine), which are undergoing further evaluation. Nonpharmacologic therapies include a 2- to 3-g sodium diet, encouragement of physical activity with possible referral for cardiac rehabilitation

Table 28–6 ■ HEART FAILURE GUIDELINES AND RECOMMENDATIONS

New York Heart Association Classification	American College of Cardiology/American Heart Association Guidelines	Recommendations
	Stage A. Patients at high risk of developing HF but without structural heart disease or symptoms of HF.	Treat hypertension, lipid disorders, diabetes Encourage smoking cessation Encourage exercise and optimal weight Discourage usage of alcohol, illicit drugs ACE inhibitor
Class I. Patients with cardiac disease without limitations of physical activity.	*Stage B.* Patients who have structural heart disease but have no symptoms of HF.	All stage A therapies ACE inhibitor unless contraindicated Beta-blocker unless contraindicated

Class II. Patients with cardiac disease who have slight limitations of physical activity. Ordinary physical activities cause symptoms.	*Stage C.* Patients who have structural heart disease with current or prior symptoms.	All stage A and B therapies
		Drugs for routine use
		    Diuretic
		    ACE inhibitor
		    Beta-blockers
		    Digitalis

Class III. Patients with cardiac disease who have marked limitation to physical activity. Less than ordinary physical activities cause symptoms.		2-3 gm sodium restricted diet Consider aldosterone antagonist Avoid use of antiarrhythmic agents, most calcium channel blockers, and nonsteroidal anti-inflammatory agents
Class IV. Patients with cardiac disease who cannot carry out any physical activity without symptoms. Symptoms may be present at rest.	*Stage D.* People with refractory heart failure that requires specialized intervention	All stage A, B, and C therapies Mechanical assist devices Palliative continuous inotropic therapy Heart transplantation Hospice care

Adapted from Hunt, S.A. et al. (2001). ACC/AHA guidelines for the evaluation and management of chronic heart failure in the adult: executive summary: a report of the American College of Cardiology and American Heart Association Task Force on Practice Guidelines. *Circulation*, 104, 2296–3007.

and exercise training, and administration of influenza and pneumococcal vaccines.

Stage D includes patients with refractory end-stage HF, which responds to all measures used for stages A, B, and C. An overview of the specific pharmacologic therapy for systolic dysfunction is described in Table 28-7. It is critical in the group of patients to have meticulous control of fluid retention. Patients who are at the end stage of their disease are at particular risk for hypotension and may be able to tolerate only a smaller dose of ACE inhibitors or beta-blockers, or they may not be able to tolerate them at all (Packer et al., 2002). Despite optimal treatment, some patients do not improve. For these patients, specialized treatment strategies include mechanical circulatory support, continuous inotropic therapy, referral for cardiac transplantation, or hospice care.

Circulatory support may include left ventricular assistance devices (LVAD) or extracorporeal devices (Gorcsan et al., 2000). For patients who cannot be sustained on medical therapy, LVAD has been a successful bridge to transplantation. Portable devices have been approved by the FDA (refer to Chapter 30). Low-dose dopamine, dobutamine, or milrinone on an outpatient basis may benefit patients with refractory HF. However, the intermittent or chronic use of these positive inotropic agents remains an area of controversy. All of these agents have been associated with an increase in mortality as a result of markedly higher occurrences of sudden death (Ellis et al., 1998). Cardiac transplantation plays a role in end-stage patients without contraindications to this operation (Young, 1998). The goal of therapy with those patients not eligible for the procedure is symptom relief. End-of-life considerations deserve attention for this patient population as well, with the focus of hospice care extending to the relief of symptoms.

Diastolic Dysfunction. Several myocardial disorders are associated with diastolic dysfunction, including restrictive, infiltrative, and hypertrophic cardiomyopathy. The affects of aging that result in changes that occur in the cardiovascular system have a greater impact on diastolic function than on systolic performance. HF associated with preserved systolic function is predominantly a disease of elderly women, most with hypertension and left ventricular hypertrophy (Kitzman et al., 2003; Masoudi et al., 2003). In contrast to systolic dysfunction, there are few studies on therapy for diastolic dysfunction (Angeja & Grossman, 2003). The difference in pharmacologic therapy is that the goal of drug therapy in diastolic dysfunction is to reduce symptoms by lowering the elevated filling pressures without significantly reducing cardiac output (Table 28-8). The treatment of HF caused by diastolic dysfunction has similarities and dissimilarities to the treatment of HF caused by systolic dysfunction (Wigle, 1995; Cash, 1996; Hunt el al.,

Table 28-7 ■ SYSTOLIC DYSFUNCTION PHARMACOLOGIC THERAPIES

ACE inhibitor: Titrate to target dose as tolerated

Do not use if creatinine > 3.0 mg/dL or potassium > 5.5 mEq/L

Begin therapy if systolic blood pressure (SBP) > 90 mm Hg without vasodilator therapy or > 80 mm Hg and asymptomatic with other vasodilator therapy

Begin therapy if serum sodium > 134 mg/dL

Alternative to ACE inhibitor: angiotensin II receptor blocker or hydralazine/nitrate combination

Do not hold vasodilator unless SBP < 80 mm Hg or signs/symptoms of orthostasis, mental changes or ↓ urine output

IV/oral loop diuretics for volume overload

Maintenance dosing versus aggressive dosing with symptoms

Add thiazide diuretic for synergistic response as needed

Add aldosterone antagonist, spironolactone 25 mg qd (or less) for class III and IV

Beta-blocker: Titrate to target dose as tolerated

Use in NYHA II, III patients.* May use in NYHA class I patients with history of myocardial infarction or hypertension.†

May use in NYHA class IV patients* who are euvolemic without significant signs/symptoms of volume overload

Do not initiate therapy if history of bronchospasm, heart block or sick sinus syndrome without permanent pacemaker; hepatic failure; overt congestion; symptomatic hypotension

Digoxin: Dose is based on weight, age, gender, creatinine clearance, and concomitant medication

Given at a low dose of 0.125 mg qd. Maintain serum digoxin level of 0.8–2.0 ng/dL

* Coreg is the only beta-blocker indicated in mild, moderate, and severe HF and essential hypertension.
† Coreg is not indicated in NYHA class I.

Table 28-8 ■ DIASTOLIC DYSFUNCTION GENERAL TREATMENT

Goal	Treatment
Reduce venous pressure	Decrease central blood volume Salt restriction Diuretics Dialysis Tourniquets Venodilation ACE inhibitors ARBs Nitrates Morphine
Maintain atrial contraction, synchrony	Electrical or pharmacologic cardioversion Sequential A-V pacing Radiofrequency ablation of AV node Biventricular pacing
Prevent tachycardia and promote bradycardia	Digitalis in atrial fibrillation Beta-adrenergic blockers Calcium channel blockers (verapamil, diltiazem) Radiofrequency ablation
Treat and prevent ischemia	Nitrates, beta-adrenergic blockers, calcium channel blockers Coronary revascularization (percutaneous coronary intervention or bypass surgery)
Control hypertension and promote regression of hypertrophy	ACE inhibitors, other antihypertensive agents Surgical intervention (e.g., aortic valve repair)
Attenuate neurohormonal activation	ACE inhibitors, beta-adrenergic blockers
Prevent fibrosis and promote regression of fibrosis	ACE inhibitor or ARB Spironolactone Anti-anginal agents
Improve ventricular relaxation	Beta-adrenergic blocker Calcium channel blockers (in hypertrophic cardiomyopathy) Systolic unloading agents

Adapted from Gaasch, W.H., & Shick, E.C. (2000). Heart failure with normal left ventricular ejection fraction: a manifestation of diastolic dysfunction. In M.H. Crawford & J.P. DiMarco (Eds.), *Cardiology* (Section 5, pp 6.1–6.8). London: Mosby.

2001). The first step is the treatment of the underlying cause. Ischemia is relieved through standard medical management and revascularization for CAD (Hunt et al., 2001). Medical management extends to the use of nitrates, beta-blockers, and calcium channel blockers. Volume reduction with diuretics is used to control pulmonary congestion and peripheral edema, and these should be titrated carefully. Fluid and sodium restriction or dialysis for patients with renal failure is also needed (Golper et al., 2000). Control of systemic hypertension is important, with ACE inhibitors assisting in normalizing blood pressure and reducing LV mass in patients with hypertension-induced LV hypertrophy. Other antihypertensive agents may also be needed (Hunt et al., 2001; Angeja & Grossman, 2003).

Tachycardia is poorly tolerated, and atrial tachyarrhythmias and even sinus tachycardia have a negative impact on diastolic function. Allowing maximum time for diastolic filling and lowering diastolic filling pressure can be accomplished by rate-slowing agents. Benefit of bradycardia also increases coronary perfusion time, a decrease in myocardial oxygen requirements, and an increase in myocardial efficiency. Beta-blockers and calcium channel blockers (verapamil or diltiazem) have been used to prevent excessive tachycardia and also have been shown to improve some exercise parameters (Gaasch & Schick, 2001; Banerjee et al., 2003). Calcium channel blockers have important lusitropic effects that enhance ventricular relaxation, with verapamil usually the drug of choice, particularly in hypertrophic cardiomyopathy (Federman & Hess, 1994; Gaasch & Schick, 2001). β-adrenergic blockers also improve LV relaxation by decreasing myocardial oxygen consumption and ischemia (Cohn, 1998).

Atrial fibrillation is poorly tolerated, and electrical or chemical cardioversion should be performed to restore normal sinus rhythm. Beta-blockers and/or amiodarone may be required to control and prevent atrial fibrillation. Radiofrequency ablation and atrioventricular pacing may also be used. Agents with positive inotropic actions are not indicated if systolic function is normal, and these agents appear to provide little benefit and have the potential to worsen pathophysiologic processes, such as myocardial ischemia (Gaasch & Schick, 2001).

Adjunctive Therapy

Pharmacologic Therapy. Routine anticoagulation with warfarin is not recommended but is appropriate for patients with atrial fibrillation, a previous history of systemic pulmonary embolism, or mobile ventricular thrombi (HFSA, 1999; Bristow, 2001; Hunt et al., 2001). Use of warfarin for patients with LV ejection fraction of .35 or less may be considered, but careful assessment of the risks and benefits should be undertaken (HFSA, 1999).

Antiplatelet drugs include aspirin, clopidogrel, and ticlodipine. Strong evidence supports the clinical benefit of antiplatelet drug therapy in ischemic heart disease and atherosclerosis (Sharis et al., 1998) (see Chapter 7). Recently reported retrospective data show a potential interaction between ACE inhibitors and aspirin. In the presence of aspirin, the bradykinin-induced increase in protaglandins should attenuate or block the positive vasodilator properties of the prostaglandins, reducing the ben-

efit of the ACE inhibition (Al-Khadra et al., 1998; Nawarskas & Spinler, 1998). Definitive resolution of this issue of aspirin and ACE inhibitors and the appropriate alternative awaits the results of further clinical research (HFSA, 1999).

HF patients with depression have an increased mortality risk. Tricyclic antidepressants have been associated with myocardial depression and probably are contraindicated in HF. The selective serotonin reuptake inhibitors have a favorable risk profile in cardiac patients and can be considered as adjunctive therapy for depression (Lejemtel et al., 2001).

Device Therapy. Device therapy extends to biventricular pacing and implantable cardiac defibrillators. Cardiac resynchronization therapy (CRT) by simultaneous pacing of the left ventricle and right ventricle through biventricular pacing may be an advantageous therapy that, in patients with severe HF and intraventricular conduction delay, improves ventricular coordination and hemodynamics (Linde et al., 2002; Pinski, 2003; Ukkonen et al. 2003). By synchronizing left ventricular contraction, there is improvement of left ventricular dP/dT, ejection fraction, and cardiac output, as well as reduction of wall stress and left ventricular filling pressures (Bradley et al., 2003; Varma et al., 2003).

Implantable cardiac defibrillators (ICD) are the treatment of choice in patients with LV dysfunction who have documented ventricular tachycardia or ventricular fibrillation (Myerberg, 2001). Because HF patients are at high risk for sudden cardiac death, these patients should be evaluated for the presence of ICD indications, which include an ejection fraction less than .35, previous myocardial infarction, and nonsustained ventricular tachycardia (Klein et al., 1999). Combined device therapy includes ICD with pacemaker capabilities (see Chapter 32). However, for patients with standard indications for ICD therapy, no indication for cardiac pacing, and an ejection fraction of .40 or less, dual chamber backup pacing did not offer any clinical advantage over ventricular backup pacing and was potentially detrimental (DAVID Trial Investigators, 2002).

Surgical Therapy. When symptoms prove refractory to medical therapy, surgical therapy or invasive therapy may be considered. Mechanical removal of fluid may be required in chronic failure. If fluid collects in serous cavities, thoracentesis, paracentesis, or dialysis may be necessary. Mitral regurgitation occurs to some extent in the remodeled, dilated ventricle, and mitral valve reconstruction has been undertaken (Bolling et al., 1998). Ventricular reduction surgery, originally known as the Batista procedure, was a surgical approach to reverse remodeling by removing a large (20% to 40%) amount of LV and reshaping it. Unfortunately, there was an increase in mortality, cardiac transplantation, and need for a left ventricular assist device (Starling et al. 1997).

Specific Strategies

Inhibitors of the Renin-Angiotensin-Aldosterone System

Angiotensin-Converting Enzyme Inhibitors. The use of ACE inhibitors has been conclusively shown to improve long-term prognosis in HF. (CONSENSUS Trial Study Group, 1987; SOLVD Investigators, 1991; HFSA, 1999; Hunt et al., 2001). ACE inhibitors block the formation of angiotensin II, which

Table 28–9 PHARMACOLOGIC AGENTS

Angiotensin-Converting Enzyme Inhibitors and Vasodilators	Start (mg)	Target (mg)	Maximum (mg)
Captopril (Capoten)	6.25–12.5 tid	50 tid	100 tid
Enalapril (Vasotec)	2.5–5 bid	10 bid	20 bid
Lisinopril (Prinivil, Zestril)	2.5–5 qd	20 qd	40 bid
Ramipril (Altace)	1.25–2.5 bid	5 bid	10 bid
Quinipril (Accupril)	5 bid	20 bid	20 bid
Fosinorpil (Monopril)	2.5–5 bid	20 bid	20 bid
Hydralazine (Apresoline)	25 qid	50–75 bid to tid	100 qid
Isosorbide dinitrate (Isordil)	10–20 tid	20–80 tid	80 tid
Isosorbide mononitrate (Imdur)	30 qd	60–120 qd	240 qd
Diuretics			
Furosemide (Lasix)*	20–40 qd	As required	480 qd
Hydrochlorothiazide (Hydrodiuril)†	25 qd	As required	200 qd
Metolazone (Zaroxylyn)†	2.5 qd	As required	5 qd
Spironolactone (Aldactone)‡	25 qd	As required	50 bid
Beta Blockers			
Carvedilol (Coreg)	3.125 bid	6.35–25 bid	25 bid
Metoprolol succinate (Toprol XL)	12.5–25 qd	150–200 qd	200 qd
Bisoprolol (Zebeta)¶	1.25 qd	10 qd	20 qd
Angiotensin II Receptor Blockers			
Ibersartan (Avapro)	150 qd	300 qd	300 qd
Candesartan (Atacand)	16 qd	32 qd	32 qd
Losartan (Cozaar)	12.5–25	50 qd	50–100 qd
Valsartan (Diovan)	80 qd	160 qd	320 qd

* Watch potassium carefully; may cause hyponatremia
† Give 30 minutes before loop diuretic
‡ May increase serum potassium; do not give if serum potassium > 4.7 mEq/L
¶ Not indicated for use in heart failure
Adapted from The Cleveland Clinic Foundation Heart Failure Management Standards of Care, 2001.

reverses vasoconstriction (reducing afterload), and inhibit endocrine, paracrine, and cellular growth effect of angiotensin II. ACE inhibitors also diminish release of aldosterone (inhibiting sodium retention) and produce venodilation (reducing preload) (Hunt et al., 2001; Opie et al., 2001). In addition to blocking angiotensin II formation, this drug class increases levels of bradykinin that promote vasodilatation and also inhibits maladaptive growth that includes ventricular remodeling, hypertrophy, fibrosis, and endothelial and vascular function. The unique characteristics of this class of neurohormonal inhibitors support the use of ACE inhibitors as first-line drugs in all patients with HF or asymptomatic left ventricular systolic dysfunction. Clinical benefit also extends to patients with evidence of atherosclerotic disease (The Heart Outcomes Prevention Evaluation Study Investigators, 2000). The doses used should be titrated to target levels (Young, 1991; LeJemtel, 2001; Bohachick et al., 2002). Nonsteroidal antiinflammatory agents (NSAIDs) should be avoided in patients in HF, and particularly in those patients using ACE inhibitor therapy (LeJemtel et al., 2001).

Angiotensin II Receptor Blockers. Angiotensin II (AT) receptor blockers differ in their mechanism of action compared to ACE inhibitors. Rather than inhibiting the production of angiotensin by blockade of the angiotensin-converting enzyme, ARBs block the cell surface receptor for AT_1 (Opie et al., 2001). Hemodynamic effects are similar to those of ACE inhibitors with respect to reducing preload and afterload and increasing cardiac output (Pitt et al., 1997). The potential concern of this class of drug is that the blockade of AT_1 elevates serum angiotensin II, which, because the AT_2 receptors are not blocked, can increase counter regulatory actions of AT_2 activation (Katz, 2000; Opie et al., 2001).

There is ongoing interest and investigational studies in combination therapy with ACE inhibitors and ARBs (Baruch et al., 1999; Cohn, 2000; Greenberg, 2002; Hennig, 2002), but at the preset time this cannot be recommended as routine therapy. ACE inhibitors rather than ARBs continue to be the agent of choice for blockade of the RAAS in HF, and the use of ARBs should be reserved for patients truly intolerant to ACE inhibitor because of cough or angioedema (HFSA, 1999; Hunt et al., 2001).

Aldosterone Antagonists. It has been shown that ACE inhibitors do completely block the effect of the RAAS, and after several months of treatment there can be an increase in aldosterone levels (Opie et al., 2001). Aldosterone promotes sodium retention (edema), promotes the release of cytokines and growth factors, and causes myocardial and vascular fibrosis (autocrine or paracrine effects), baroreceptor dysfunction, and progressive remodeling. The addition of low-dose spironolactone to standard therapy in Stage C and or D (NYHA Class III and IV) promotes a therapeutic effect and reduces morbidity and mortality (Rosseau et al., 2002; Kasama et al., 2003). The benefit of this class of drug is not primarily a diuretic effect, and studies demonstrated that spironolactone lessens myocardial fibrosis, significantly reduces the plasma levels of BNP, improves LV remodeling, and improves cardiac sympathetic nerve activity (which may reduce ventricular arrhythmias in sudden cardiac death) (Opie et al., 2001; Rosseau et al., 2002; Kasama et al., 2003).

Beta-adrenergic Blockers

Cardiac myocytes have three adrenergic receptors (beta$_1$, beta$_2$, and alpha$_1$) that are coupled with positive inotropic and chronotropic response, cardiac myocyte growth, toxicity, and apoptosis. Although β_1 and β_2 receptors are present in the normal human myocardium, β_2 receptors predominate in the failing myocardium as β_1 receptors are down-regulated. Neurohormonal activity in HF can be blunted by β-adrenergic blockers (Cohn, 1998; Katz, 2000; Opie & Yusef, 2001; Bristow, 2003). Second- and third-generation β-adrenergic blockers have been used in HF. Metoprolol (MERIT-HF Study Group, 1999) and bisoprolol are second-generation selective β_1-adrenergic blockers (Kukin, 2002). Carvedilol is a nonselective β-adrenergic (blocking β_1 and β_2 receptors), as well as an alpha-blocking agent. At low doses, carvedilol exhibits β_1 selectivity; at higher target doses, it blocks all three adrenergic receptors, allowing for renal and systemic vasodilatation. Data to determine whether the benefits of beta-blockade are a class effect or if one beta-blocker is more efficacious than the other were recently completed (Poole-Wilson et al., 2003), which suggest that carvedilol extends survival compared with metoprolol. Beta-blockers should be routinely administered to clinically stable patients who are on standard therapy (usually ACE inhibitor and diuretic). ACC/AHA Stages B, C, and D (HFSA 1999; Hunt et al., 2001; Packer et al., 2002; Gattis et al., 2003) therapy should be initiated at low doses and up-titrated slowly, generally no sooner than at 2-week intervals (Table 28-10) (Cleland et al., 2002; Krum et al., 2003). The safety of beta-blockers in asymptomatic LV dysfunction has not been tested.

Diuretics

The kidney is the target organ of many of the neurohormonal and hemodynamic changes that occur in HF (Abraham & Schrier; Bristow et al., 2001). Diuretics and dietary salt restriction exert their primary benefit by decreasing extracellular water and intravascular blood volume (Opie et al., 2001). The elimination of dependent edema helps reduce tissue pressure, opposing venous pooling and therefore improving the capacitance of the venous system. Similarly, the decrease in intravascular volume also reduces ventricular preload directly and thereby helps to diminish the filling pressures in the pulmonary and systemic circulations. Thiazide diuretics may be helpful in patients with mild fluid overload and normal renal function, but most patients require loop diuretics (HFSA, 1999). Administration of the aldosterone antagonist spironolactone should be considered (see previous section). With advanced HF and compromised renal function, multiple diuretics with different sites of renal action are usually needed (HFSA, 1999; Lejemtel et al., 2001, Opie et al., 2001).

Digitalis Glycosides

The cardiac glycosides have important effects in HF, including augmenting contractility (positive inotropy), slowing of the sinus pacemaker and atrioventricular conduction (negative

Table 28–10 ■ MANAGING SIDE EFFECTS DURING TITRATION OF BETA BLOCKERS

VASODILATOR EFFECTS (dizziness or light headedness)
Give drug with food
Give drug 2 hours before vasodilator agents or stagger doses of vasodilator medications or other medications affecting blood pressure
Reduce diuretic or vasodilator therapy temporarily
Reduce beta-blocker dose if symptoms persist after diuretic and vasodilator decreased two times

SIGNIFICANT BRADYCARDIA (< 60–65 bpm with symptoms)
Reduce beta-blocker dose
Clarify digoxin dosage
    temporarily stop digoxin or reduce digoxin dose
    monitor digoxin levels
Clarify concomitant drug use
    Amiodarone
    Calcium channel blockers (verapamil or diltiazem)

WORSENING HEART FAILURE (dyspnea, weight gain, edema)
Increase diuretic dose (if qd increase to bid; if bid, double the dose)
Intensify salt restriction
Reduce beta-blocker dose (if symptoms persist after diuretic increased two times)

REINSTATING BETA BLOCKER AFTER DISCONTINUATION
If off < 72 hours and no cardiogenic shock, same dose as taking before discontinuation
If off > 72 hours and no cardiogenic shock, restart at ½ dose taken before discontinuation
If off > 7 days or episode of cardiogenic shock, restart at lowest dose and re-titrate

chronotropy and dromotrophy), and neurohormonal modulating effects including a sympathoinhibitory effect (Opie & Gersh, 2001; Yusef, 1997). Little controversy exists as to the benefit of digoxin in patients with symptomatic systolic dysfunction and concomitant atrial fibrillation, but the debate still continues over its current role in patients in normal sinus rhythm (HFSA, 1999; LeJemtel et al., 2001). Digoxin should be considered as a fourth-line medication in patients who have LV systolic dysfunction while receiving standard therapy (HFSA, 1999; Hunt et al., 2001). In the majority of patients with HF and normal sinus rhythm, the starting dosage should be 0.125 mg or 0.25 mg once daily (no loading dose) based on ideal body weight, age, and renal function. In patients with HF and rapid ventricular response, higher doses are not recommended (HFSA, 1999). If amiodarone is added, the dose of digoxin should be reduced. A recent study recommends prudent practice and supports a lower-serum digoxin concentration target in the range of 0.5 to 0.8 nanograms/deciliter, because higher concentrations were associated with increased mortality (Rathore et al., 2003).

Vasodilator Therapy

The venous and arterial beds are often inappropriately constricted. Venoconstriction tends to displace blood in the thorax, causing pulmonary congestion, whereas arteriolar constriction increases the impedance to LV emptying. Arteriolar dilatation results in a reduction of afterload and may augment cardiac output, whereas venodilatation tends to produce a reduction in preload, lowers ventricular filling pressure, and reduces symptoms of pulmonary congestion. Vasodilators may be separated into three categories: venous dilators (preload reducers), arterial dilators (afterload reducers), and mixed venous and arterial dilators (preload and afterload reducers) (Massie, 2001).

Venous Dilators. Nitroglycerin and the closely related isosorbide dinitrate are primarily reducers of preload because they dilate the systemic veins and reduce venous return, ultimately to reduce LV filling pressure. Nitrates are indicated for the treatment of angina in patients with HF (Hunt et al., 2001). A combination of hydralazine with isosorbide dinitrate combines the effect of improved preload and afterload (see next section on hydralazine) and may be administered to patients on standard therapy who cannot be administered an ACE inhibitor because of hypotension or renal insufficiency or true intolerance (Cohn et al., 1987; Cohn et al., 1991; HFSA, 1999; Hunt et al., 2001).

Arterial Dilator. As a direct arteriolar vasodilator with direct inotropic effects, hydralazine can improve LV function by reducing afterload and myocardial oxygen consumption, augmenting stroke volume, and improving cardiac output. It is used in combination as described in the previous section.

Calcium Channel Blockers

The net benefits of calcium channel blocker use lay in their ability to decrease afterload and their anti-ischemic effects. Calcium channel blockers are a diverse group of agents with complex actions. They do not seem to have a place in systolic dysfunction and may be harmful, although risks may not accompany the use of the longer-acting agents (e.g., amlodipine) in patients with concomitant hypertension or angina (Young, 1998; Lejemtel, 2001). Calcium channel blockers may be of benefit in diastolic dysfunction because of improvement of diastolic relaxation, control of blood pressure, and prevention of myocardial ischemia, and they may reverse LV hypertrophy (Wigle, 1995; Gasssch & Schick, 2000).

Antiarrhythmics

Heart failure is the most arrhythmogenic disorder in cardiovascular disease. Management of arrhythmias in this group of patients is difficult and remains far from satisfactory. Nearly all patients with HF experience frequent and complex ventricular tachyarrhythmias, and the imminent risk of sudden death appears to be present for all patients with HF. Experimental and clinical evidence indicates that circulatory neurohormonal and electrolyte deficits (potassium and magnesium) interact to provoke malignant ventricular ectopic rhythms. In general, antiarrhythmic therapy in HF patients is reserved for symptomatic arrhythmias or for control of ventricular responses to atrial fibrillation (Echt et al., 1991; HFSA, 1999; Hunt et al., 2001). Antiarrhythmic agent drug selection may best be guided with invasive electrophysiological testing. Class 1 antiarrhythmics demonstrated an increase in mortality in patients with ventricular arrhythmias in HF (Echt et al., 1991). Beta-blockers can prevent up to 40% to 50% of sudden cardiac death, which adds to their benefit in managing HF patients (Massie, 2001; Myerberg, 2001). Amiodarone has undergone the most extensive evaluation for efficacy and safety in left ventricular dysfunction, but has had equivocal effect on sudden cardiac

death. Survival of patients with life-threatening arrhythmias is improved with ICD placement as compared with antiarrhythmic therapy (DAVID Trial Investigators, 2002). Amiodarone is the preferred drug in patients with HF with supraventricular tachycardia not controlled by beta-blocker or digoxin, or for those patients who are not candidates for ICD placement (HFSA, 1999; Hunt et al., 2001).

Future Therapy

Several agents that block neurohormonal and inflammatory pathways are currently being studied for possible beneficial effects in patients with HF. These therapies may extend to AT_1 receptor blockers, endothelin (ET_1) receptor blockade, cyclooxygenase inhibition, inhibitors of apoptosis, and cytokine blockade (Luscher et al., 2002). In addition, gene therapy to prevent the loss of myocytes or even restore myocytes to the heart is in the future (Katz, 2000; Endoh, 2001; Massie, 2001).

NURSING MANAGEMENT

Whether the setting is a clinic, hospital, nursing home, or patient's home, the nurse cares for patients in some phase of HF. The nurse may be the first person to assess the presence of HF. The best means of controlling HF is through early detection and treatment of predisposing factors. The importance of early diagnosis is highlighted by evidence that treatment of asymptomatic patients can slow progression and improve clinical outcomes. Screening for high blood pressure, arteriosclerosis and atherosclerosis, diabetes, valvular disorders, and congenital anomalies may ensure aggressive treatment of the patient and prevention of complications.

A major goal of assessing the patient in HF is to determine the type and severity of the underlying disease and the extent of the syndrome. Identification of the early onset of HF may allow therapeutic means to be instituted on an ambulatory basis and prevent frequent hospital readmissions. Coordination of care by a nurse-directed multidisciplinary team including nursing, cardiologist, emergency room physician, case manager, dietician, pharmacist, and cardiac rehabilitation specialist can provide HF initiatives to guide evidence-based practice, enable self-care at home, and coordinate clinical care across the continuum (Miranda et al., 2002). A growing trend has been to have advanced practice nurses coordinate these programs (Dahl & Penque, 2002).

Patient related decompensation of chronic HF can be attributed to knowledge deficit of their disease, diet and medications; non-adherence to medication and diet; inability to recognize signs and symptoms of HF; inadequate social support; and inability to access health care providers. Several clinical studies have demonstrated a decline in hospital readmissions by as much as 50% with aggressive telephone follow-up care. Telemanagement of HF has been undertaken by advanced practice nurses (Paul, 1997; Mueller, et al., 2002), which helped promote consistency of care across health care sites. Adaptation of computer-based technology to closely monitor HF patients with an advanced practice nurse in collaboration with a cardiologist has been shown to be cost-effective and leads to improved outcomes of care (Benatar et al., 1999).

Similar to cancer centers, heart failure centers and clinics are being established to care for HF patients to oversee therapeutic options, including complex polypharmacy, device therapy and investigational agents (Fonarow et al., 2001). Nursing plays a key role in these centers and clinics, coordinating care that impacts the physical, psychological, and social challenges that these patients face. In addition to morbidity and mortality, quality of life is an equally important outcome in patients with HF (Moser & Dracup, 2001). Risk factor modification, management of nutrition, biobehavioral therapy, drug management, and exercise training are just some of the interventions for patients with HF (Bennett et al., 2001; Moser & Stevenson, 2001). Until recently, HF patients have been instructed to avoid exercise, and exercise intolerance and deconditioning were evident in this group of patients. In small controlled studies, neurohormonal activation, symptoms, resting cardiac function, and quality of life appear to improve with exercise (Bristow, 2001; Wilson et al., 2001).

Home management of HF may relate to stabilizing the patients' condition after hospital discharge, providing care before cardiac transplantation, or hospice care for those patients with end-stage HF (Bither, 2001).

When the patient is admitted to the hospital, the problems associated with HF may have become more advanced and may require supervised administration of medications as well as other measures to reduce edema and improve myocardial performance.

The overall plan of care for patients with HF is to reduce cardiac workload, improve cardiac output, prevent complications, and educate the patient regarding follow-up care. Display 28-1 presents topics for patient, family, and caregiver education (Konstam et al., 1994; Ammon, 2001).

Analysis of Medical and Nursing Assessment Data and Formulation of Nursing Diagnoses

Based on the assessment data, including medical and nursing histories, physical examination, hemodynamic monitoring, and diagnostic tests, the most common nursing diagnoses for the patient with HF are: (1) decreased cardiac output; (2) altered respiratory function, including ineffective breathing patterns, ineffective airway clearance, and impaired gas exchange; (3) extracellular fluid volume excess; and (4) knowledge deficit.

Decreased Cardiac Output

Diagnosis. This diagnosis can be stated as: decreased cardiac output, related to an inability of the heart to pump effectively associated with myocardial damage or hypertrophy, manifested by decrease in blood pressure; increase in heart rate; fatigue; cool, clammy skin; decreased urine output; and decreased level of consciousness.

Goals. Possible goals for this diagnosis include:

1. To detect specific early manifestations of decreased cardiac output

---

DISPLAY 28-1

SUGGESTED TOPICS FOR PATIENT, FAMILY, AND CAREGIVER EDUCATION AND COUNSELING

GENERAL COUNSELING

Explanation of heart failure and the reason for symptoms
Cause or probable cause of heart failure
Expected symptoms
Symptoms of worsening heart failure
What to do if symptoms worsen
Self-monitoring with daily weights
Explanation of treatment/care plan
Clarification of patient's responsibilities
Importance of cessation of tobacco use
Role of family members or other caregivers in the treatment/ care plan
Availability and value of qualified local support group
Importance of obtaining vaccinations against influenza and pneumococcal disease

PROGNOSIS

Life expectancy
Advance directives
Advice for family members in the event of sudden death

ACTIVITY RECOMMENDATIONS

Recreation, leisure, and work activity
Exercise
Sex, sexual difficulties, and coping strategies

DIETARY RECOMMENDATIONS

Sodium restriction
Avoidance of excessive fluid intake
Fluid restriction (if required)
Alcohol restriction

MEDICATIONS

Effects of medications on quality of life and survival
Dosing
Likely side effects and what to do if they occur
Coping mechanisms for complicated medical regimens
Availability of lower-cost medications or financial assistance

IMPORTANCE OF COMPLIANCE WITH THE TREATMENT/CARE PLAN

---

2. To reduce or eliminate specific manifestations of decreased cardiac output
3. To prevent symptoms of decreased cardiac output

Interventions. Interventions are designed to detect the manifestations of the imbalance between myocardial oxygen supply and demand and to improve cardiac output. Interventions to meet this goal include the following.

For Goal 1. Assess the blood pressure, apical-radial heart rate, cardiac rhythm, lung sounds, heart sounds, level of consciousness, urine output, and condition of the skin as indicated by the patient's condition. Monitor ECG readings, continuously assessing heart rate and rhythm, and document ECG rhythm strips every 4 hours and with conduction disturbances or arrhythmias. Obtain a chest radiograph. Assess, document, and report to the physician the following: drop of 20 mm Hg in systolic pressure, a systolic pressure below 80 mm Hg, or a mean arterial pressure less than 60 mm Hg; presence of new S_3 or S_4 gallops; new or increasing crackles; urine output less than 30 mL/h and significant change in mental status. For patients with hemodynamic monitoring with a PA catheter, assess the preload and afterload parameters by obtaining right atrial or PA diastolic or wedge pressures, and the derived parameters of SVR. Obtain cardiac output readings in relation to other physical findings and in relation to titration of vasoactive medications; decreased cardiac output (<4 L/min) or cardiac index (<2.2 L/min/m²); increased PAWP (>18 mm Hg);

For Goal 2. Perform actions to reduce cardiac workload. Place the patient in a semi to high Fowler's position; administer oxygen and other medications, including positive inotropic agents (to improve contractility), venodilators (to reduce preload), arterial dilators (to decrease afterload), balanced vasodilators (to decrease preload and afterload), and ACE inhibitors (to decrease SVR and venous tone) as ordered and evaluate the patient's response to therapy; and provide a restful environment.

For Goal 3. Instruct the patient to avoid activities that create a Valsalva response; provide frequent, small meals low in sodium; discourage smoking and intake of caffeine containing foods and beverages; and gradually increase activities of daily living.

Outcome Criteria. Outcome criteria are written for each goal statement.

For Goal 1. Signs and symptoms of HF are detected at onset.

For Goal 2. Immediately after intervention, the client has improved cardiac output as evidenced by blood pressure within normal range for patient; apical pulse audible, regular, and between 60 and 100 beats/min; resolution of S_3 or S_4 gallops, which disappear or do not increase in intensity; crackles absent or reduced; urine output at least 30 mL/h; decrease in peripheral edema; mental status improving; and hemodynamic parameters returning to a normal range.

For Goal 3. Patient appears comfortable; heart rate, respiratory rates, blood pressure, and hemodynamic parameters are within patient's normal range; no S_3 or S_4 gallops; skin is warm and dry and without edema; no crackles; and activity tolerance is maintained.

Altered Respiratory Function

Diagnosis. This diagnosis includes the following diagnostic labels: ineffective breathing pattern, ineffective airway clearance, and impaired gas exchange. This diagnosis can be stated three ways:

1. Ineffective breathing pattern related to loss of alveolar elasticity owing to vascular engorgement, restricted lung expansion from pleural effusion, and respiratory depressant effect of hypoxia or hypercapnia, as manifested by tachypnea, orthopnea, or hyperventilation
2. Ineffective airway clearance related to fluid accumulation associated with pulmonary edema, as manifested by ineffective cough, dyspnea, cyanosis, pallor, and abnormal breath sounds
3. Impaired gas exchange related to ineffective breathing patterns and airway clearance and decreased systemic tissue perfusion associated with decreased cardiac output, as man-

ifested by decreased oxygen content, increased PCO_2, cyanosis, lethargy, and fatigue

Goals. Goals for this diagnosis include:

1. To detect specific early manifestations and etiologies of altered respiratory function
2. To reduce or eliminate specific manifestations of altered respiratory function
3. To prevent when possible specific manifestations of altered respiratory function

Interventions. Interventions are designed to detect the manifestations of alterations in respiratory function and maintain adequate ventilatory exchange. Interventions to meet each goal include the following.

For Goal 1. Assess, document, and report to the physician the following: diminished or absent breath sounds; adventitious breath sounds (crackles, wheezes, rhonchi); dyspnea or orthopnea; decreased pulse oximetry; confusion or somnolence; and persistent cough or productive frothy or blood-tinged sputum; abnormal arterial blood gases.

For Goal 2. Immediately implement measures to improve respiratory status. Place the patient in a semi to high Fowler's position; administer oxygen; instruct patient to deep breathe every hour; and perform actions to improve cardiac status. (Refer to first diagnosis in this section.) Monitor for therapeutic and nontherapeutic effects of the following if administered: medications to improve cardiac output (refer to first diagnosis in this section); diuretics (decrease pulmonary fluid accumulation); morphine sulfate (decreases pulmonary vascular congestion); and possible administration of bronchodilators (decreases bronchoconstriction).

For Goal 3. To facilitate removal of pulmonary secretions: instruct and assist patient to cough every 1 to 2 hours; humidify inspired air as ordered; assist with administration of mucolytic agents by nebulizer; assist with or perform postural drainage; and perform tracheal suctioning if needed. Instruct the patient to avoid intake of gas-forming foods and large meals to prevent gastric distention and a further increase in pressure on the diaphragm.

Outcome Criteria. Specific outcome criteria are written for each goal statement.

For Goal 1. Specific signs and symptoms of alteration in respiratory function are detected within 4 hours of onset of respiratory distress.

For Goal 2. After interventions, the patient experiences adequate respiratory function as evidenced by normal rate, rhythm, and depth of respirations; decreased dyspnea; usual or improved breath sounds; and improving blood gases.

For Goal 3. Patient denies dyspnea, orthopnea, shortness of breath; patient appears comfortable; respiratory rate, rhythm, and depth are within normal range; no adventitious breath sounds are heard; skin color is normal, and skin is warm and dry; and blood gases are within normal range.

Extracellular Fluid (ECF) Volume Excess

Diagnosis. This diagnosis can be stated as: extracellular fluid volume excess related to high levels of aldosterone and antidiuretic hormone associated with decreased renal blood flow, manifested by edema, weight gain, increased venous filling pressures, and intake greater than output.

Goals. Goals for this diagnosis include:

1. To detect early specific manifestations and etiologies of ECF volume excess
2. To reduce or eliminate specific manifestations of ECF volume excess
3. To prevent when possible specific manifestations of ECF volume excess

Interventions. Interventions are designed to detect the manifestations of fluid volume overload and to stabilize the fluid volume. Interventions to meet each goal include the following.

For Goal 1. Assess, document, and report to the physician the following: history of significant weight gain (>0.5 kg/d); development of an S_3; intake greater than output; low serum osmolality; distended neck veins; dyspnea, orthopnea; rales and diminished or absent breath sounds; and peripheral edema. Assess for peripheral edema including legs, feet and abdomen; skin for evidence of breakdown; review and record daily weight, fluid intake and output.

For Goal 2. Implement measures to reduce ECF volume excess, including: maintain fluid restriction as ordered; and restrict sodium intake as ordered (usually 2 to 3 g/d). Monitor for therapeutic and nontherapeutic effects of diuretics (to increase excretion of water) and positive inotropic agents and arterial dilators (to improve renal blood flow).

For Goal 3. Teach dietary restrictions of sodium and fluid intake, provide a diet high in protein; instruct patient to record weight daily; and assist the patient with activities of daily living.

Outcome Criteria. Outcome criteria are written for each goal statement.

For Goal 1. Signs and symptoms of fluid overload are detected at onset.

For Goal 2. After intervention, the patient shows resolution of fluid imbalance as evidenced by decline in weight toward patient's normal; resolution of S_3; less labored respirations; improved breath sounds; further balancing of intake and output; resolution of peripheral edema and neck vein distention; and serum osmolality returning to normal range.

For Goal 3. Patient maintains normal weight; no S_3; no crackles; balanced intake and output; no peripheral edema; and normal serum osmolality.

Knowledge Deficit

Diagnosis. The diagnosis can be stated as: knowledge deficit: related to understanding of HF, management plan (medications and diet), risk factor modification, prognosis and return to activity of daily living.

Goals. Goals for this diagnosis include:

1. To detect specific knowledge deficits.
2. To reduce or eliminate specific knowledge deficits.
3. To promote quality of life for patients with HF.

Interventions. Development of a teaching plan to provide information for patients, family and caregivers. Suggested topics are listed in Display 28-1.

Outcome Criteria. This may include the patient and family being able to describe signs and symptoms and disease process of HF; explain the diagnosis, treatment, and prognosis of HF; relate their understanding of medications, activity and dietary recommendations; awareness of risk factor modification; and when to alert medical and nursing personnel with changes in their health status. This may also be reflected in a decrease in decompensation of HF, a decrease in readmission rate, or decreased length of hospital stay.

REFERENCES

Al-Khadra, A. S., Salem, D. N., Rand, W. M., et al. (1998). Antiplatelet agents and survival: a cohort analysis from the Studies of Left Ventricular Dysfunction (SOLVD) trial. *Journal of the American College of Cardiology,* 31, 419–425.

American Heart Association. (2002). Heart and stroke statistics update. 2001.http://www.americanheart.org/statistics/othercvd.html.)

Abbate, B., Biondi-Zoccai, G., Bussani, R., et al. (2003). Increased myocardial apoptosis in patients with unfavorable left ventricular remodeling and early symptomatic post-infarction heart failure. *Journal of the American College of Cardiology,* 41(4), 753–60.

Abraham, W. T., & Schrier, R. W. (2000). Renal salt and water handling in congestive heart failure. In J. D. Hosenpud & B. H. Greenberg (Eds.), *Congestive heart failure* (pp. 253–266). Philadelphia: Lippincott Williams & Wilkins.

Ammon, S. (2001). Managing patients with heart failure. *American Journal of Nursing.* 101, 34–40.

Anand, I. S., Fisher, L. D., Chian, Y. T., et al. (2003). Changes in brain natriuretic peptide and norepinephrine over time and mortality and morbidity in the valsartan heart failure trial (Val-HeFT). *Circulation,* 107, 11278–1283.

Angeja, B. G., & Grossman, W. (2003). Evaluation and management of diastolic heart failure. *Circulation,* 107, 659–663.

Aronson, D., & Burger, A. J. (2003). Neurohormonal prediction of mortality following admission for decompensated heart failure. *American Journal of Cardiology,* 91, 245–248.

Banerjee, P., Banerjee, T., Khand, A., et al. (2002). Diastolic heart failure: neglected or misdiagnosed? *Journal of the American College of Cardiology,* 39, 138–141.

Baruch, L., Anand, I., Cohen, I. S., et al. (1999). Vasodilator-Heart Failure Trial (V-HeFT) Study Group. Augmented and long-term hemodynamic and hormonal effects of an angiotensin receptor blocker added to angiotensin converting enzyme inhibitor therapy in patients with heart failure. *Circulation,* 99, 1658–1664.

Benatar, D., Bondmass, M., Ghitelman, J., & Avitall, B. (2003). Outcomes of chronic heart failure. *Archives of Internal Medicine.* 164, 347–352.

Bennett, S. J., Hackward, L., Blackburn, S. A. (2001). Nutritional management of the patient with heart failure. In D. K. Moser & B. Riegel (Eds), *Improving outcomes in heart failure: An interdisciplinary approach* (pp. 99–123). Gaithersburg, MD: Aspen Publication.

Bell, D. (2003). Heart failure: The frequent, forgotten and often fatal complication of diabetes. *Diabetes Care,* 26(5), 2433–2441.

Bither, C. J., & Aplles, S. (2001). Home management of the failing heart. *American Journal of Nursing,* 101(12), 41–45.

Bohachick, R., Burke, E., Sereika, S. et al. (2002). Adherence to angiotensin-converting enzyme inhibitor therapy for heart failure. *Progress in Cardiovascular Nursing,* 17(4), 1601–1606.

Bolling, S. F., Pagani, F. D., Deeb, G. M., & Bach, D. S. (1998). Intermediate-term outcome of mitral reconstruction in cardiomyopathy. *Journal of Thoracic Cardiovascular Surgery,* 115, 381–386.

Bozkurt, B., & Mann, D. (2003). Use of biomarkers in the management of heart failure. Are we there yet? *Circulation,* 107, 12231–1233.

Bradley, D. J., Bradley, E. A., Baughman, K. L., et al. (2003) Cardiac resynchronization and death from progressive heart failure: a meta-analysis of randomized controlled trials. *Journal of the American Medical Association,* 289, 730–740.

Bristow, M. (2003). Antiadrenergic therapy of chronic heart failure: surprises and new opportunities. *Circulation,* 107, 1100–1102.

Bristow, M. R. (2001). Management of heart failure. In E. Braunwald, D. P. Zipes, & P. Libby (Eds.), *Heart disease: A textbook of cardiovascular medicine* (6th ed., pp. 635–658).

Bristow, M. R., Port, J. D., Kelly, R. A. (2001). Treatment of heart failure: pharmacological methods. In E. Braunwald, D. P. Zipes, & P. Libby (Eds.), *Heart disease: A textbook of cardiovascular medicine* (6th ed. pp. 562–599).

Carelock, J., & Clark, A. P. (2001). Heart failure: Pathophysiologic mechanisms. *American Journal of Nursing, 101*(12), 26–33.

Cash, L. A. (1996). Heart failure from diastolic dysfunction. *Dimensions of Critical Care Nursing, 15*(4), 170–177.

Chatterjee, K. (2000). Physical examination in heart failure. In J. D. Hosenpud & B. H. Greenberg (Eds.), *Congestive heart failure* (pp. 615–627). Philadelphia: Lippincott Williams & Wilkins.

Cleland, J. G. F., Cohen-Solai, A., Aguilar, J. C., et al. (2002). Management of heart failure in primary care (the IMPROVEMENT of heart failure programme): an international survey. *Lancet, 360*, 1631–1638.

Cody, R. J. (2000). Hormonal alterations in heart failure. In J. D. Hosenpud & B. H. Greenberg (Eds.), *Congestive heart failure* (pp. 199–232). Philadelphia: Lippincott Williams & Wilkins.

Cohn, J. N. (2002). Lessons learned from the valsartan-heart failure trial (val-HeFT): angiotensin receptor blockers in heart failure. *American Journal of Cardiology, 90*(9), 1–3.

Cohn, J. N. (1998). Beta-blockers in heart failure. *European Heart Journal,* 19(Supplement F), F52–F55.

Cohn, J. N. (2000). Lessons learned from the Valsartan-Heart Failure (Val-HeFT): angiotensin receptor blockers in heart failure. *American Journal of Cardiology, 90*(9), 1–3.

Colucci, W. S. (2000). The sympathetic nervous system in heart failure. In J. D. Hosenpud & B. H. Greenberg (Eds.), *Congestive heart failure* (pp. 189–197). Philadelphia: Lipppincott Williams & Wilkins.

Cohn, J. N., Archibald, D. G., Francis, G. S. et al. (1987). Veterans Administration Cooperative Study on vasodilator therapy of heart failure: Influence of prerandomization variables on the reduction of mortality by treatment with hydralazine and isosorbide dinitrate. *Circulation, 75*(5) (Part II), 49–54.

Cohn, J. N., Johnson, G., Ziesche, S. et al. (1991). A comparison of enalapril with hydralazine-isosorbide dinitrate in the treatment of chronic congestive heart failure. *New England Journal of Medicine, 325*, 303–310.

Colluci, W. S., & Braunwald, E. (2001). Pathophysiology of heart failure. In Braunwald, E., Zipes, D. P., & Libby, P. (Eds.), *Heart disease: A textbook of cardiovascular Medicine* (pp. 503–533).

CONSENSUS Trial Study Group. (1987). Effects of enalapril on mortality of chronic congestive heart failure: Results of a Cooperative North Scandinavian Enalapril Survival Study. *New England Journal of Medicine, 316*, 1429.

Dahl, J., & Penque, S. (2002). APN spells success for a heart failure program. *Nursing Management* 33(2), 46–48.

DAVID Trial Investigators. (2002). Dual-chamber pacing or ventricular backup pacing in patients with an implantable defibrillator. The dual chamber and VVI implantable defibrillator (DAVID) trial. *Journal of the American Medical Association, 2888*(240), 3115–3123.

Dominiak, P. (2002). Pharmacotherapeutic strategy in heart failure. *Clinical Nephrology, 58*(Suppl. 10), S2–S6.

Drexler, H. & Hasenfuss, G. (2201). Physiology of the normal and failing heart. In M. Crawford & J. P. DiMarco (Eds.), *Cardiology* (pp. 5.1–5.15). London: Mosby.

Echt, D. S., Liebson, P. R., Mitchell, L. B. et al. (1991). Mortality and morbidity in patients receiving encainide, flecainide, or placebo. The Cardiac Arrhythmia Suppression Trial (CAST). *New England Journal of Medicine, 342*, 452–458.

Ellis, A., Bental, T., Kimochi, O., et al. (1998). Intermittent dobutamine treatment in patients with chronic refractory congestive heart failure: A randomized, double blind, placebo study. *Clinical Pharmacologic Therapy, (63)*, 682–685.

Endoh, M. (2001). Mechanisms of action of novel cardiotonic drugs. *Journal of Cardiovascuar Pharmacology, 40*(3), 323–338.

Ezekowitz, J. A., McAlister, F. A., & Armstrong, P. W. (2002). Anemia is common in heart failure and is associated with poor outcomes. *Circulation, 107*, 223–225.

Federman, M., & Hess, O. M. (1994). Differentiation between systolic and diastolic dysfunction. *European Heart Journal, 15*(Suppl D). D2–D6.

Francis, G. S. (1998). Pathophysiology of the heart failure clinical syndrome. In E. J. Topol (Ed.), *Textbook of cardiovascular medicine* (pp. 2179–2203). Philadelphia: Lippincott-Raven.

Francis, G. S., Gassler, J. P., & Sonneblick, E. H. (2001). Pathophysiology and diagnosis of heart failure. In J. W. Hurst (Ed.), *The heart* (10th ed., pp. 665–685). New York: McGraw-Hill.

Francis, G. S., Pathak, A. (2001). Congestive heart failure due to systolic dysfunction. In M. H. Crawford, & J. P. DiMarco (Eds.), *Cardiology* (Section 5, pp. 4.1–4.10). London: Mosby.

Gaasch, W. H., & Schick, E. C. (2000). Heart failure with normal left ventricular ejection fraction: a manifestation of diastolic dysfunction. In M. H. Crawford, & J. P. DiMarco (Eds.), *Cardiology* (Section 5, pp. 6.1–6.8). London: Mosby.

Gattis, W. A., O'Connor, C. M., Leimberger, J. D., et al. (2003). Clinical outcomes in patients on beta-blocker therapy admitted with worsening heart failure. *American Journal of Cardiology, 91*, 169–1174.

Givertz, M. M., Colucci, W. S., & Braunwald, E. (2001). Clinical aspects of heart failure: High-output failure: Pulmonary edema. In E. Braunwald, D. P. Zipes, & P. Libby (Eds.), *Heart disease: A textbook of cardiovascular medicine* (6th ed., pp. 534–561).

Golper, T. A., Glasco, G. B., & Canaud, B. J. (2000). Dialysis and hemofiltration for congestive heart failure. In J. D. Hosenpud & B. H. Greenberg (Eds.), *Congestive heart failure* (2nd ed., pp. 213–231). Philadelphia: Lippincot William & Wilkins.

Gottlieb, S. S., Fisher, M. L., Kjekshus, J., et al. (2002). Tolerability of beta-blocker initiation and titration in the Metoprolol CR.XL Randomized Intervention Trial in Congestive Heart Failure (MERIT-HF). *Circulation,* 105, 1182–1188.

Gorcsan, J. III, Crawford, L., Soran, O. et al. (2000) Improvement in left ventricular performance by enhanced external counterpulsation in patients with heart failure. *Journal of the American College of Cardiology, (35)*, 230 A.

Greenberg, B. H. (2002). Angiotensin receptor blockers in heart failure: A work in progress. *Journal of Cardiac Failure, 4*(5), 257–382.

Guidelines and indications for coronary artery bypass graft surgery: A report of the American College of Cardiology/American Heart Association Task Force on Assessment of Diagnostic and Therapeutic Cardiovascular Procedures. (1991). *Journal of the American College of Cardiology, 17*, 543–589.

Heart Failure Society of American. (1999). HFSA guidelines for management of patients with heart failure caused by left ventricular systolic dysfunction-pharmacologic approach. *Journal of Cardiac Failure, 4*(5), 357–382.

Hein, S., Arnon, E., Kostin, S., et al. (2003). Progression from compensated hypertrophy to failure in the pressure-overloaded human heart: Structural deterioration and compensatory mechanisms. *Circulation, 107*, 984–991.

Hennig, L. (2002). Clinical studies on the therapy of heart failure using ACE-inhibitors and AT_1 receptor blockers-does combination therapy make sense? *Clinical Nephrology, 58* (suppl 1), S1–S11.

The Heart Outcome Prevention Evaluation Study Investigators (HOPE). (2000). Effects of angiotensin-converting enzyme inhibitor, ramipril, on cardiovascular events in high-risk patients. *New England Journal of Medicine,* 342, 145–153.

Hunt, S. A., Baker, D. W., Chin, M. H., Cinquiergrani, M. P., Fledman, A. M., Francis, G. S., Ganiats, T. G., Goldstein, S., Gregoratos, G., Jessup, M. L., Noble, R. J., Packer, M., Silver, M. A., & Stevenson, L. W. (2001). ACC/AHA guidelines for the evaluation and management of chronic heart failure in the adult: executive summary: a report of the American College of Cardiology and American Heart Association Task Force on Practice Guidelines (Committee to Revise the 1995 Guidelines for the Evaluation and Management of Heart Failure). *Circulation, 104*, 2296–3007.

Johnson, W., Hirsch, A. T., & Creager, M. A. (2000). The peripheral circulation in heart failure. In J. D. Hosenpud & B. H. Greenberg (Eds.), *Congestive heart failure* (pp. 233–252). Philadelphia: Lippincott Williams & Wilkins.

Kasama, S., Toyoma, T., Kumakura, H et al. (2003). Effect of spironolactone on cardiac nerve activity and left ventricular remodeling in patients with dilated cardiomyopathy. *Journal of the American College of Cardiology, 41*, 574–581.

Katz, A. M. (2000). *Heart failure: Pathophysiology, molecular biology and clinical management.* Philadelphia: Lippincott Williams & Wilkins.

Kearney, M. T., Fox, K. A. A., Lee, A. J., et al. (2002). Predicting death due to progressive heart failure in patients with mild-to-moderate chronic heart failure. *Journal of the American College of Cardiology, 40*(10), 1801–1808.

Kitzman, D. W., Little, W. C., Brubaker, P. H., et al. (2003). Pathophysiological characterization of isolated diastolic dysfunction in comparison to systolic heart failure. *Journal of the American College of Cardiology, 40*(10), 1801–1808.

Klein, H., Auricchio, A., Reek, S., et al. (1999). New primary prevention trials of sudden cardiac death in patients with left ventricular dysfunction: SCD-HeFT and MADIT-II. *American Journal of Cardiology, 341*, 1882–1890.

Kosiborod, M., Smith, G. L., Radford, M. J., et al. (2003). The prognostic importance of anemia in patients with heart failure. *American Journal of Medicine, 114*(2), 1–10.

Kukin, M. L. (2002). Beta blockers in chronic heart failure; considerations for selecting an agent. *Mayo Clinic Proceedings, 77,* 1196–1206.

Krum, H., Roeker, E. B., Mohacsi, P., et al. (2003). Effects of initiating carvedilol in patients with congestive heart failure: results from the COPERNICUS study. *Journal of the American College of Cardiology, 289,* 712–718.

Lanfrnachi, P. A., Somer, V. K., Braghiroli, A., Cora, U., et al. (2002). Central sleep apnea in left ventricular dysfunction: Prevalence and implications for arrhythmic risk. *Circulation, 107,* 727–732.

LeJemtel, T. H., Sonneblick, E. H., & Frishman, W. H. (2001). Diagnosis and management of heart failure. In J. W. Hurst (Ed.), *The heart* (10th ed., pp. 655–685). New York: McGraw-Hill.

Linde, C., Leclercq, C., Rex, S., et al. (2002). Long-term benefits of biventricular pacing in congestive heart failure: Results from the Multisite Stimulation in Cardiomyopathy (MUSTIC) Study. *Journal of the American College of Cardiology,* 40(1),111–118.

Linseman, J. V., & Bristow, M. R. (2003). Drug therapy and heart failure prevention. *Circulation, 107,* 1234–1236.

Lloyd-Jones, D. M., Larson, M. G., Leip, E. P., et al. (2002). Lifetime risk for developing congestive heart failure: The Framingham heart study. *Circulation, 106,* 3068–3072.

Luscher, T. F., Enseleit, F., Pacher, R., et al. (2002). Hemodynamics and Neurohormonal effects of selective endothelin A (ET$_A$) receptor blockade in chronic heart failure. The heart failure ET$_A$ receptor blockade trial (HEAT). *Circulation, 106,* 2666–2672.

Maisel, A. S., Koon, J., Krishnaswamy, P., Kazenegra, R., et al. (2001). Utility of B-natriuretic peptide as a rapid, point-of-care test for screening patients undergoing echocardiography to determine left ventricular dysfunction. *American Heart Journal, 141,* 367–374.

Mani, K., & Kitis, R. N. (2003). Myocyte apoptosis: programming ventricular remodeling. *Journal of the American College of Cardiology,* 41(5), 761–764.

Mann, D. L. (2000). Cytokines as mediators of disease progression in the failing heart. In J. D. Hosenpud & B. H. Greenberg (Eds.), *Congestive heart failure* (2nd ed., pp. 213–231). Philadelphia: Lippincott William & Wilkins.

Mann, D. L. (2002). Inflammatory mediators and the failing heart: Past, present, and the foreseeable future. *Circulation Research, 91,* 988–998.

Masoudi, F. A., Havranek, E. P., Smith, G., et al. (2003). Gender, age and heart failure with preserved left ventricular systolic function. *Journal of the American College of Cardiology,* 41(3), 217–223

Massie, B. M. (2001). Management of the patient with chronic heart failure In M. H. Crawford & J. P. DiMarco (Eds.), *Cardiology* (Section 5, pp. 5.1–5.16). London: Mosby.

McClellan, W. M., Flanders, W. D., Langston, R. D., et al. (2002). Anemia and renal insufficiency are independent risk factors for death among patients with congestive heart failure admitted to community hospitals: a population-based study. *Journal of the American Society of Nephrology,* 40(7), 1248–1258.

McKenney et al. (1994). Diastolic function after bypass surgery. *JACC, 24,* 1189–1194.

MERIT-HF Study Group. (1999). Effect of metoprolol CR/XL in chronic heart failure: Metoprolol CR/XL Randomized Intervention Trial in Congestive Heart Failure (MERIT-HF). *Lancet, 353,* 20001–2006.

Metra, M., Nodari, S., D'Aloia, et al. (2002). Beta-blocker therapy influences the hemodynamic response to inotropic agents in patients with heart failure: A randomized comparison of dobutamine and enoximone before and after chronic treatment with Metoprolol or carvedilol. *Journal of the American College of Cardiology,* 40(7), L1248–L1258.

Michaelson, C. R. (1983). Pathophysiology of heart failure: A conceptual framework for understanding clinical indicators and therapeutic modalities. In C. R. Michaelson (Ed.), *Congestive heart failure* (pp. 44–83). St Louis: CV Mosby.

Miranda, M. B., Gorski, L. A., LeFevre, J. G., et al. (2002). An evidence-based approach to improving care of patients with heart failure across the continuum. *Journal of Nursing Care Quality,* 17(1), 1–14.

Moser, D. K., & Dracup, K. (2001). Impact of nonpharmacologic therapy on quality of life in heart failure. In D. K. Moser & B. Riegel (Eds.), *Improving outcomes in heart failure: An interdisciplinary approach* (pp. 77–96). Gaithersburg, MD: Aspen Publication.

Moser, D. K., & Stevenson, L. W. (2001). Biobehavioral therapy in the management of patients with heart failure In D. K. Moser & B. Riegel (Eds.), *Improving outcomes in heart failure: An interdisciplinary approach* (pp. 152–177). Gaithersburg, MD: Aspen Publication.

Mueller, T. M., Vuckovic, K. M., Knox, D. A., & Williams, R. E. (2002). Telemanagement of heart failure: A diuretic treatment algorithm for advanced practice nurses. *Heart and Lung,* 31(5), 340–347.

Myerburg, R. J. (2001). Sudden cardiac death: exploring the limits of our knowledge. *Journal of Electrophysiological,* 12, 369–391.

Nawarskas, J. J., & Spinler, S. A. (1998). Does aspirin interfere with the therapeutic efficacy of angiotensin-converting enzyme inhibitors in hypertension or congestive heart failure? *Pharmacotherapy,* 18, 1041–1052.

Nielson, O. W., McDonagh, T. A., Robb, S. D., & Dargie, H. J. (2003). Retrospective analysis of the cost-effectiveness of using plasma brain natriuretic peptide in screening fro left ventricular systolic dysfunction in the general population. *Journal of the American College of Cardiology,* 41(1), 113–120.

Opie, L. H., & Gersh, B. J. (2001). Digitalis, acute inotropes, and inotropic dilators. In L. H. Opie (Ed.), *Drugs for the heart* (5th ed., pp. 154–186). Philadelphia: WB Saunders.

Opie, L. H., & Yusef, S. (2001). Beta-blocking agents. In L. H. Opie (Ed.), *Drugs for the heart* (5th ed., pp. 107–153). Philadelphia: WB Saunders.

Opie, L. H., Yusef, S., Kaplan, N. M., & Poole-Wilson, P. A. (2001). Diuretics. In L. H. Opie (Ed.,: *Drugs for the heart* (5th ed., pp. 84–107). Philadelphia: WB Saunders.

Opie, L. H., Yusef, S., Poole-Wilson, P. A., & Pfeffer, M. (2001). Angiotensin converting enzyme (ACE) inhibitors, angiotensin-II receptor blockers (ARBs), and aldosterone antagonism. In L. H. Opie (Ed.), *Drugs for the heart* (5th ed., pp. 107–153). Philadelphia: WB Saunders.

Packer, M., Fowler, M. B., Roecker, E. B., Coats, A. J. S., et al. (2002). Effect of carvedilol on the morbidity of patients with severe chronic heart failure. Results of the carvedilol prospective randomized cumulative survival (COPERNICUS) study. *Circulation, 106,* 2194–2199.

Parmley, W. W. (1992). Pathophysiology of congestive heart failure. *Clinical Cardiology,*15(Suppl. I), I–5–I–12.

Patel, A. R., & Konstam, M. A. (2001). Assessment of the patient with heart failure. In M. Crawford & Z. J. P. DiMarco (Eds). *Cardiology* (Section 5, 2.1–2.9). London: Mosby.

Paul, S. (1997). Implementing an outpatient congestive heart failure clinic: the nurse practitioner role. *Heart and Lung,* 26, 486.

Pinski, S. (2003). Continuing progress in the treatment of severe congestive heart failure. *Journal of the American Medical Association,* 289(6), 747–756.

Poole-Wilson, P. A., Swedberg, K., Cleland, J. G. et al. (2003). Comparison of carvedilol and metoprolol on clinical outcomes in patients with chronic heart failure in the Carvedilol Or Metoprolol European Study (COMET): a randomized controlled trial. *Lancet,* 362(9377), 7–13.

Pitt, B., Segal, R., Martinez, F., et al. (1997). On behalf of the ELITE study investigators. Randomized trial of losartan versus captopril in patients over 65 with heart failure (Evaluation of Losartan in the Elderly Study ELITE).*Lancet,* 349, 747–752.

Rathore, S. S., Curtis, J. P., Wang, U., Bristow, M. R., & Krumholtz, H. M. (2003). Association of serum digoxin concentration and outcomes in patients with heart failure. *Journal of the American Medical Association,* 289 (7), 871–878.

Roussaeu, M. F., Gurne, O., & Duprez, D. (2002). Beneficial Neurohormonal profile of spironolactone in severe congestive heart failure: results from the RALES Neurohormonal substudy. *Journal of the American College of Cardiology,* 40(9), 1596–1601.

Sharis, P. J., Cannon, C. P., & Loscalzo, J. (1998). The antiplatelet effect of ticlodipine and clopidogrel. *Annals of Internal Medicine,* 129, 394–405.

SOLVD Investigators. (1991). Effect of enalapril on survival in patients with reduced left ventricular ejection fraction and congestive heart failure. *New England Journal of Medicine,* 325(5), 293–302.

Starling, R. C., Young, J. B., Scalia, G. M., et al. (1997). Preliminary observations with ventricular remodeling surgery for refractory congestive heart failure. *Journal of the American College of Cardiology.*

Szokosi, J., Kinnune, P., Weckstrom, M., et al. (1998). Evidence for camp-independent mechanisms mediating the effects of adrenomedullin, a new inotropic peptide. *Circulation,* 107, 28–31.

Ukkonene, H., Beanlans, R. S. B., Burwash, I. G., et al. (2003). Effect of cardiac resynchronization on myocardial efficiency and regional oxidative metabolism. *Circulation,* 107, 28–31.

Varma, C., Sharma, S., Firoozi, S., et al. (2003). Plasma homocysteine and risk for congestive heart failure in adults without prior myocardial efficiency and regional oxidative metabolism. *Circulation,* 107, 28–31.

Vasan, R. S., Beiser, A., D'Agostino, R. B., et al. (2003). Plasma homocysteine and risk for congestive heart failure in adults without prior myocardial infarction. *Journal of the American Medical Association.* 289(10), 1251–1257.

Weil, J., Eschenhagen, T., Hirt, S., Magnussen, O., Mittmann, C., Remmers, U., & Scholz, H. (1998). Preserved Frank-Starling mechanism in end stage heart failure. *Cardiovascular Research,* 37, 541–548.

Wigle, E. D. (1995). Diastolic dysfunction: Pathophysiology and treatment options. In N. S. Dhalla, R. E. Beamish, N. Takeda, et al. (Eds.), *The failing heart* (pp. 79–94). Philadelphia: Lippincott-Raven.

Wilson, J. R., Chomsky, D. B., Dahle, K. (2001). Exercise in heart failure. In D. K. Moser & B. Riegel (Ed.), *Improving outcomes in heart failure: An interdisciplinary approach* (pp. 124–135). Gaithersburg, MD: Aspen Publication.

Young, J. B. (1998). Chronic heart failure management. In E. J. Topol (Ed.), *Textbook of cardiovascular medicine* (pp. 2273–2307). Philadelphia: Lippincott-Raven.

Yusef, S. (1997). Digoxin in heart failure: Results of the recent digoxin investigation group trial I the context of other treatments for heart failure. *European Heart Journal, 18*, 1685–1688.

Zisman, L. S., Asano, K., Dutcher, D. L., et al. (1995). Differential regulation of cardiac angiotensin-converting enzyme binding sites and AT_1 receptor density in the failing human heart. *Circulation, 98*, 1735–1741.

29

Cardiac Surgery

DENISE LEDOUX* • HELEN LUIKART†

Surgical intervention continues to be a mainstay of treatment for acquired heart disease even though catheter-based interventional cardiology techniques have continued to expand and medical management has improved. This chapter focuses on surgical interventions for acquired heart disease, including coronary artery bypass grafting (CABG), minimally invasive cardiac surgery, transmyocardial revascularization, cardiomyoplasty, aortic surgery, and cardiac transplantation. Surgical intervention for valvular heart disease is briefly discussed in this chapter and is more extensively covered in Chapter 33.

EVOLVING TRENDS IN CARDIAC SURGERY

Cardiac surgical operative techniques continue to evolve. Myocardial protection approaches involve antegrade and retrograde delivery of cardioplegia solution as well as refined reperfusion strategies (Loop, 1998). Arterial bypass conduits such as the internal mammary artery (IMA) are the preferred graft because of excellent long-term patency. Additional arterial conduits have expanded to include radial artery grafts and the gastroepiploic artery (GEA). Spawned by laparoscopic approaches in other surgical subspecialties, minimally invasive cardiac surgery (with and without cardiopulmonary bypass [CPB]) has rapidly developed. Computer-assisted, robotic CABG, and mitral valve surgical procedures have been preformed world wide on highly selected patients (Diodato et al., 2003). Shorter intubation times and "rapid recovery" programs have led to shorter intensive care unit stays with overall reduced length of stay and decreased cost associated with cardiac surgery.

As cardiac surgery techniques evolve, the population changes as well. Interventional cardiology approaches such as coronary angioplasty, atherectomy, and stenting have delayed or replaced surgical revascularization in patients with coronary lesions amenable to catheter-based interventions. Many investigators have found an increase in the age of surgical candidates,

more women, less severe angina but greater incidence of recent myocardial infarction (MI), more left ventricular dysfunction, a higher rate of surgical candidates with three-vessel disease, and other comorbidity such as diabetes, arrhythmias, and heart failure (Loop & Muehrcke, 1998). The mean age of CABG surgical candidates has increased from 50 years in 1967 to 66 years today, and nearly 30% of patients are older than age 70 years (Loop, 1998).

PREOPERATIVE ASSESSMENT AND PREPARATION

Before referral for cardiac surgery, patients complete their cardiac work-up, which includes cardiac catheterization to define coronary artery anatomy and target vessels for revascularization; stress testing to verify areas of ischemia; nuclear scans to identify areas of myocardial viability and ventricular function; and echocardiography to delineate valvular lesions, ventricular function, and focal wall motion abnormalities. Usually, most of the preoperative medical evaluation is completed before the patient enters the hospital. Prior to cardiac surgery, the patient should have a complete physical examination with special attention given to the cardiovascular examination. A new history and physical examination, chest radiograph, electrocardiogram (ECG), complete blood count, serum electrolytes, coagulation screen, and typing and crossmatching of blood are performed. These data provide information about other disease conditions and cardiac problems. Patients are admitted to the hospital early on the morning of their surgery. Patients with symptomatic carotid bruits should undergo carotid duplex to assess for carotid stenosis. Patients with chronic lung disease should undergo pulmonary function testing and arterial blood gas testing because they may have difficulty weaning from the ventilator. Patients undergoing valve surgery should complete a dental evaluation and work before valve repair or replacement to reduce the chance of dental disease being a source of bacteremia and possible prosthetic valve endocarditis. Patients are maintained on antianginal, antihypertensives, and heart failure medications until surgery. Antiplatelet medications are usually discontinued before surgery: aspirin,

---

*Author of the section on cardiac surgery.
†Author of the section on cardiac transplantation.

clopidogrel, and nonsteroidal anti-inflammatory agents should be stopped 7 to 10 days before surgery to prevent perioperative bleeding. Patients on warfarin usually have their dose withheld 3 to 5 days preoperatively. Patients on warfarin for previous mechanical valve replacements may be admitted 1 to 2 days before surgery for intravenous heparin. Heparin is withheld 1 to 2 hours before surgery, whereas enoxaparin is usually stopped 12 hours beforehand. In a study by Jones and associates (Jones et al., 2002), patients on preoperative enoxaparin demonstrated a higher rate of bleeding requiring re-exploration for bleeding (7.9% versus 3.7% in the unfractionated heparin group, $P = 0.03$).

The preoperative nursing assessment should be thorough and well documented because it provides baseline data for postoperative comparison. The history should include a social assessment of family roles and support systems, and a description of the patient's usual functional level and typical activities. Elderly patients or those with limited social and emotional support may need additional assistance from social service for effective discharge and rehabilitation planning. The patient with acute coronary heart disease (CHD) may be hospitalized for only hours or days before surgery. A myocardial infarction may have occurred, or the patient may be experiencing unstable angina. In either case, if CABG surgery is being considered, then a cardiac catheterization must be performed to determine if surgery is indicated and to define coronary anatomy.

SURGICAL TECHNIQUES

Minimally Invasive Techniques

In standard cardiac surgery, the heart is arrested and circulation is maintained by placing the patient on CPB. Although this procedure has been used successfully for more than three decades, it has drawbacks such as physiologic derangements associated with CPB and long hospital stays. Minimally invasive cardiac surgery has evolved out of laparoscopic techniques originally used in general and gynecologic surgery. The term *minimally invasive* covers a variety of techniques rather than referring only to one surgical procedure. Minimally invasive techniques include CABG surgery performed by standard sternotomy but without the use of CPB (off-pump or OPCAB), CABG surgery performed off-pump through a small left anterior thoracotomy (minimally invasive direct coronary artery bypass [MIDCAB]), valve surgery performed on-pump but through "mini-sternotomy," and computer-enhanced robotic system techniques that allow CABG and valve surgery to be performed on-pump through a small incision with videoscopic assistance and femoral bypass (Falk et al., 2003). Techniques are rapidly evolving that are geared toward multivessel revascularization through port access on a beating heart. Rather than just one approach for all patients, cardiac surgeons have a variety of surgical techniques available depending on the patient's anatomy, medical history, and comorbid conditions. Further discussion of these surgical methodologies is found in the coronary bypass and valve surgery sections of this chapter.

Cardiopulmonary Bypass

Cardiopulmonary bypass (CPB) comprises an extracorporeal circuit that circulates systemic throughout the body during periods of time the heart and lungs are not functioning during cardiac surgical procedures. CPB has been the standard method used during cardiac surgery for diverting blood from the heart and lungs to provide a stationary, bloodless surgical field and to promote preservation of optimal organ function. Blood is removed from the right atrium or vena cava by one or two cannulae, routed through the CPB machine, and returned to the patient by a cannula in the ascending aorta or the femoral artery.

The CPB system has several components, including venous and arterial cannulae; a membrane or bubble oxygenator that oxygenates the blood, removal of carbon dioxide, and delivery of anesthetic gases; a heat exchanger that allows the blood to be either heated or cooled by conduction; a pump, which keeps the blood moving at a constant speed; filters, which remove particulate or gas emboli and plasma protein or platelet aggregates; a left ventricular vent to prevent distention of the left ventricle during aortic cross-clamp; cardiotomy suction to aspirate blood from the operative field; and sensors, which detect air bubbles, low levels of oxygen saturation, and low levels of blood in collection chambers (Seifert, 2002; Bojar, 1999). Heparin is used for anticoagulation during CPB to prevent clotting in the CPB circuit. Before initiation of CPB, a heparin dose of 3 mg/kg is administered through a central line. Activated clotting time is monitored a minimum of every 30 minutes during CPB. Once CPB is completed, heparin is reversed using protamine sulfate (Seifert, 2002). Care is taken to administer protamine slowly and watch for a possible protamine reaction, which may vary from mild hypotension to full-blown anaphylaxis. Patients at greater risk for protamine reaction include those with insulin-dependent diabetes and those with an allergy to fish. While the patient is connected to the CPB machine, the surgeon, anesthetist, and CPB perfusionists control many physiologic variables. Hemodilution with crystalloid solutions is used to reduce hematocrit and the blood's viscosity. CPB flow rates are controlled to maintain a cardiac index of $=2.2$ L/min per meters squared and a mean arterial pressure around 60 mm Hg. Blood may be cooled to reduce metabolic demands or warmed to normothermia towards the end of the procedure.

Blood passing through the CPB machine and extracorporeal circuit triggers a series of cascades mediated by proteolytic enzymes (Morris & St. Claire, 1999) as a result of the blood's contact with non-endothelial surfaces in the CPB circuit. CPB initiates an inflammatory state that involves platelet-endothelial interactions and vasoactive responses that may result in low-flow states within the coronary circulation (Morris & St. Claire, 1999). Cardiopulmonary bypass produces a systemic inflammatory response that releases biologically active substances that impair coagulation and the immune response. Pro-inflammatory cytokines contribute to neutrophil adhesion (Ng et al., 2002). Oxygen free radicals are released in response reperfusion injury, which contribute to transient ventricular dysfunction postoperatively (Morris & St. Claire, 1999). In response to the vascular permeability changes that occur with CPB and to the decrease in plasma oncotic pressure that occurs with hemodilution, large amounts of fluid move from intravascular to interstitial spaces. Movement of fluid into interstitial spaces causes postoperative edema. This generalized edema that occurs after CPB resolves after the first few days postoperative or fluid mobilization may be facilitated with the use of diuretics. The longer the CPB time, the more severe the physiologic derangements during the postoperative recovery.

Systemic warming is started approximately 30 minutes before the anticipated time of discontinuing CPB. If the left atrium, left ventricle, or aorta has been entered, air must be evacuated before aortic cross-clamp removal to prevent air embolism. The heart is warmed and resumes spontaneous rhythm or is paced with epicardial wires. Ventricular fibrillation may occur and is converted with internal defibrillation. Under the direction of the surgeon and anesthesiologist, CPB weaning begins by ventilation of the lungs. CPB is gradually weaned by decreasing the amount of blood diverted through the CPB circuit. When the heart is functioning normally with adequate blood pressure and adequate cardiac index, CPB is discontinued, heparin is reversed, and cannulae are removed. If the heart cannot support an adequate cardiac index and mean arterial pressure after weaning from CPB, the patient may have to be placed back on CPB to rest the heart, and other measures for heart failure may need to be instituted, such as inotropic treatment or intra-aortic balloon pump. In patients who continue to have severe hemodynamic compromise, ventricular assist devices may be used.

Myocardial Protection

Myocardial protection can be defined as the specific intraoperative strategies designed to protect the myocardium from tissue damage resulting from the ischemic state that occurs with extracorporeal circulation (Finkelmeier, 1995). In cardiac surgical procedure requiring CPB, cross clamping of the aorta without the use of myocardial protection would result in anaerobic metabolism and depletion of myocardial energy stores. Cross-clamping the aorta without protection for more than 15 to 20 minutes would result in profound myocardial dysfunction (Bojar, 1999). Advances in myocardial protection in cardiac surgery have been instrumental in achieving successful outcomes (Earp & Mallia, 1997). Cardioplegia is infused to arrest the heart and provide a bloodless, motionless operative field as well as protect the heart during cardiac surgery. Cardioplegic solution is infused into the aorta or coronary sinus or into the coronary arteries themselves to cause cardiac arrest. Debate continues over the best type of cardioplegia, what is the best temperature (hypothermic vs. normothermic), whether cardioplegia should be infused antegrade or retrograde, and timing of infusion (intermittent or continuous). Most cardiac surgery programs use a combination of the myocardial protection techniques discussed here.

Cardioplegia solutions are made of crystalloid, oxygenated crystalloid, or crystalloid-blood mixtures. Standard crystalloid solutions can deplete adenosine triphosphate stores because they carry insufficient oxygen and substrates to replenish myocardial stores (Seifert, 1998). Blood cardioplegia (one part cardioplegia to four parts blood) provides oxygen carrying capability and maintains oncotic pressure, resulting in less myocardial edema. Blood proteins furnish buffering and contain oxygen free radical scavengers that can decrease oxygen-mediated injury with reperfusion (Seifert, 1998). Although cardioplegic solutions vary widely, typical components include potassium, magnesium, or procaine to provide immediate diastolic arrest; oxygen, glucose, glutamate, or aspartate as energy substrate; bicarbonate or phosphate to buffer acidosis; and calcium, steroids, or procaine to stabilize membranes. The solution should be hyperosmolar to edema. Cardioplegia is infused continuously or intermittently. Generally, cardioplegia delivered by antegrade method is infused intermittently, and cardioplegia delivered retrograde is infused continuously (Earp & Mallia, 1997).

Cardioplegia can be normothermic or hypothermic. Hypothermic techniques were originally used as a means to reduce metabolic demands during arrest. A cooled nonbeating heart uses less oxygen than a warm beating or fibrillating heart. Cold cardioplegic solutions are commonly cooled to 15°C to 20°C to reduce oxygen demand. Deep hypothermia can increase edema because of activation of the sodium-potassium pump, alter function of platelets and leukocytes, produce arrhythmias, prolong bleeding times, alter membrane stability, and impair calcium influx, thus affecting systolic function (Seifert, 1998). Normothermic cardioplegia has been used at both the induction of cardioplegic arrest and at the termination of arrest. Warm, oxygenated, hyperkalemic blood cardioplegia maintains arrest while supplying oxygenated blood to myocardial cells. "Hot shots" are warm cardioplegic infusions administered at the end of the surgical procedure, before removal of the aortic cross-clamp. Warm cardioplegia has been associated with an increased incidence of total neurologic and perioperative cerebral vascular accidents (Martin et al., 1994). Because hypothermia reduces cerebral oxygen demand, cerebral protection is improved and transient injury from emboli and ischemia is better tolerated and less likely to result in permanent damage (Earp & Mallia, 1997).

Cardioplegia solution can be delivered antegrade into the ascending aorta proximal to the aortic cross-clamp (Seifert, 1998), after which it flows through the coronary circulation and returns to the heart through the coronary sinus. Although antegrade cardioplegia has been the standard in cardiac surgery for many years, its delivery may be inadequate. Antegrade cardioplegia infusion through coronary arteries that are severely stenosed or occluded is uneven. Hearts with left ventricular hypertrophy may receive incomplete delivery to the subendocardium. In patients with aortic insufficiency, the left ventricle may become distended because of the retrograde flow of cardioplegia across the valve. Although cardioplegia can be delivered through saphenous vein grafts, it cannot be delivered through IMA grafts. Insufficient delivery of cardioplegia results in poor myocardial protection, which results in postoperative myocardial damage and dysfunction. Because of inadequate delivery using antegrade techniques, retrograde delivery systems were developed. Retrograde cardioplegia is infused under low pressure through catheters inserted directly into the coronary sinus. Cardioplegia flows retrograde through the coronary veins to capillaries to the coronary arterial bed, and exits at the coronary ostia, where effluent is removed by vent and suction. Retrograde and combined retrograde-antegrade techniques allow for optimal delivery and myocardial protection.

Deep Hypothermic Circulatory Arrest

Circulatory arrest (interruption of circulation through the ascending aorta for an extended period of time) may be necessary in procedures involving the ascending aorta and aortic arch. Profound hypothermia is used to protect the brain and other vital organs. The patient's body temperature is lowered to 18° C and CPB is stopped. Operative procedures are performed expediently because of the interruption of circulation to vital organs. In general, deep hyperthermic arrest can be used up to 60 minutes (Heitmiller et al., 1994; Bojar, 1999). After repair, the patient is placed back on CPB and is gradually rewarmed.

CARDIAC SURGERY PROCEDURES FOR CORONARY ARTERY REVASCULARIZATION

Coronary Artery Bypass Surgery

Indications for Surgical Revascularization

Coronary artery bypass graft surgery is done primarily to alleviate anginal symptoms as well as improve survival. CABG surgery is among the most common surgical procedures preformed worldwide and accounts for more resources expended than in any other single procedure in cardiovascular medicine (Eagle et al., 1999). The American College of Cardiology and the American Heart Association Task Force on Practice Guidelines was formed to recommend appropriate use of diagnostic tests and therapies. Based on both literature review and expert opinion, the ACC/AHA revised the guidelines for CABG in 1999. Class I guideline indications for CABG are described as conditions for which there is evidence and/or general agreement that a given procedure or treatment is useful and effective. Class I recommendations for CABG surgery include: significant left main coronary artery stenosis or equivalent; three-vessel coronary disease; two-vessel coronary disease and an ejection fraction less than 50%; one- or two-vessel disease with a large amount of viable myocardium at risk; and one- or two-vessel disease with severe angina despite maximal medical therapy (Eagle et al., 1999).

Relative Contraindications

Conditions that greatly increase the mortality risk during surgery and anatomic limitations are relative contraindications to CABG surgery. Lack of adequate conduit, coronary arteries distal to the stenosis smaller than 1 to 1.5 mm, and severe aortic atherosclerosis are all anatomic abnormalities that may limit the success of the revascularization for technical reasons. Severe left ventricular failure and coexisting pulmonary, renal, carotid, and peripheral vascular disease may significantly increase the risk of surgery by predisposing to complications during the perioperative period.

Bypass Conduits

Coronary artery revascularization is accomplished most commonly with the IMA in combination with saphenous vein grafts. Because of the excellent patency associated with IMA grafts, other arterial conduits are now accepted for bypass surgery. Use of the right GEA as a pedicle graft to the right coronary or as a free graft to the left coronary system requires a more extensive surgery because the abdomen must be entered. Radial artery grafts were initially used in the early 1970s but were abandoned because of their tendency to spasm and their poor short-term patency. With the advent of calcium channel blockers, radial artery grafts have enjoyed renewed interest. Greater saphenous vein from the legs is the most commonly used venous conduit. Because of patient anatomy, history of vein stripping, or previous revascularizations, alternative conduits may be necessary. Veins harvested from the arms, such as the cephalic or basilic, make poor bypass conduits because of their caliber and high incidence of aneurysm formation. Lesser saphenous vein located on the posterior aspect of the lower leg may be used, but may be small caliber and difficult to harvest. Synthetic bypass grafts have also been used but are not in common use because of poor patency rates (Coleman et al., 1993). Cryopreserved vein grafts harvested from cadavers also appears to have high early and midterm occlusion rates (Cho et al., 1994). Although the choice of conduit has no effect on early patency of bypass grafts, IMA grafts have demonstrated longer patency rates (up to 96% at 10 years) than saphenous vein grafts (81% at 10 years) (Loop et al., 1986). Because of long-term patency, the left IMA is most commonly used to bypass the left anterior descending (LAD) artery. The right IMA may also be used to bypass the LAD artery as well as the posterior descending or right coronary artery (Shinn, 1992). When multiple grafts are required, single or bilateral IMA grafts in combination with other arterial conduit and saphenous vein grafts can be used to accomplish complete revascularization (Fig. 29-1). Many authors recommended complete arterial revascularization in young patients in hopes of avoiding additional revascularizations later in life.

Saphenous Vein Bypass Grafts. While the sternal incision is made and the patient is readied for CPB, the saphenous vein is prepared. Traditionally, saphenous vein is harvested using standard incisions. With the advent of minimally invasive surgery, saphenous vein can be harvested using endoscopic techniques and small incisions at the same time that the IMA graft is taken down from the retrosternal bed (Fig. 29-2). A long segment of vein is carefully exposed, the branches are ligated and divided, and the vein is removed. The vein is flushed with a cold heparinized solution and checked for leaks. One side of the untwisted vein is marked with a surgical pencil, and the vein is filled with and stored in a cold solution. CPB is instituted, a clamp is placed across the distal aorta, and cold cardioplegia is injected into the aortic root. Portions of saphenous vein are sutured to coronary arteries beyond the arterial stenoses. Distal anastomoses to the LAD artery are usually made first, followed by distal anastomoses to the coronary arteries located on the back of the heart. After all distal anastomoses are completed, the aortic cross-clamp is removed and patient warming is begun. Small openings in the ascending aorta are made with a punch, and the proximal end of the saphenous vein is anastomosed to

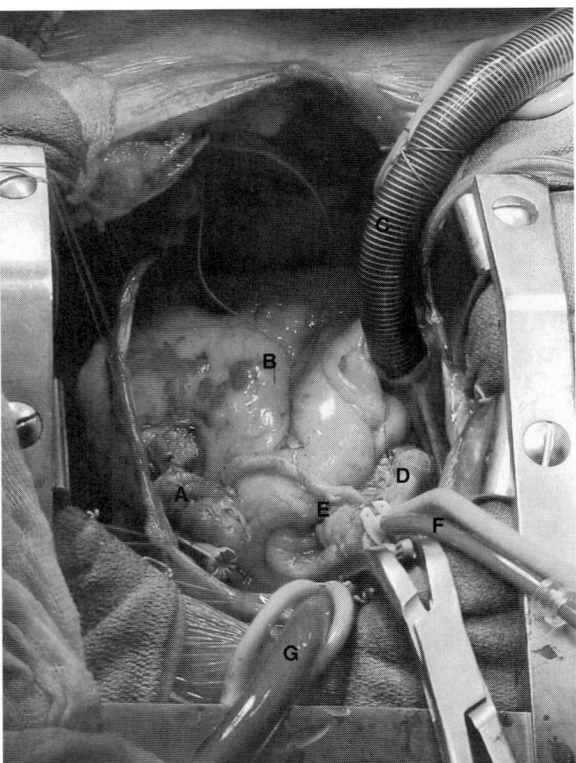

■ **Figure 29–1.** View of completed internal mammary and saphenous vein grafts. View from the head of the operating table shows (*A*) internal mammary graft to left anterior descending coronary artery; (*B*) temporary epicardial pacing wires inserted into the right ventricle; (*C*) venous cannula into right atrium; (*D*) ascending aorta; (*E*) saphenous vein graft; (*F*) cardioplegia delivery catheter; (*G*) aortic cannula. (Photo by D. LeDoux, 2003.)

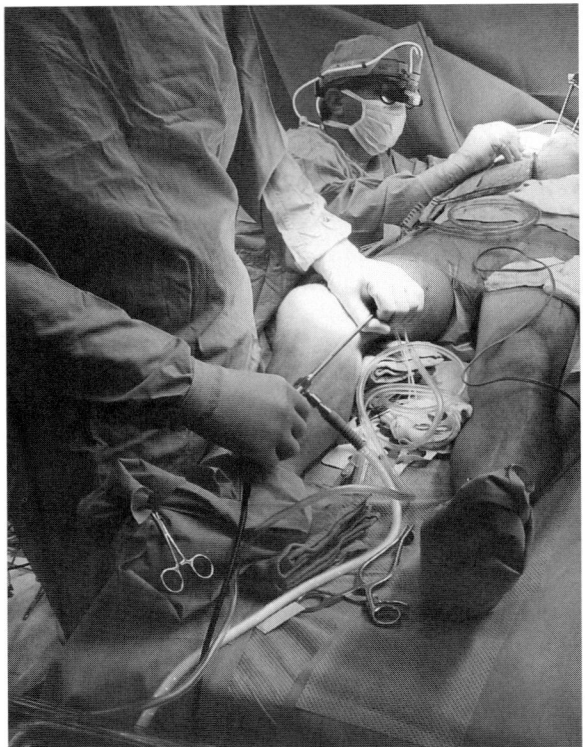

■ **Figure 29–2.** *Saphenous* vein is dissected out by video-assisted endoscopic approach while the internal mammary is dissected down from the retrosternal bed. (Photo by D. LeDoux, 2003.)

the aorta. After the proximal anastomoses are completed, CPB is discontinued and the chest is closed.

Internal Mammary Artery Bypass Grafts. Harvesting the IMA is technically more difficult than harvesting the saphenous vein graft. After the sternum is cut open, the IMA is dissected away from the chest wall. A special retractor is used to expose the IMA in the retrosternal bed (Seifert, 2002). A 2-cm-wide pedicle strip is removed from the chest wall muscle, fat, and pleura that surround the IMA. The pedicle strip, with the IMA lying in the center, is exposed from the IMA origin at the subclavian artery down to the level of the fourth to sixth intercostal space. The branches of the IMA are exposed, divided, and ligated. An incision is made into the coronary artery to be bypassed (usually the left anterior descending) and the distal end of the IMA is sutured into place. The IMA can be used as a free graft rather than a pedicle graft if it is not long enough to reach the target. Bilateral IMA grafting may also be used but has been associated with an increased incidence of sternal wound infection (Pym et al., 1997).

Radial Artery Bypass Grafts. The radial artery graft is used for bypass conduit only after collateral circulation of the ulnar artery has been assessed by vascular ultrasound or Allen's test. Although both radial arteries can be used, the radial artery from the patient's nondominant hand is the usual choice and can be harvested before the chest is opened. Because the radial artery is

very thick walled and prone to spasm, after harvesting, papaverine may be used to flush and dilate the artery before grafting. During and after surgery, nitrates and calcium channel blockers are used to prevent spasm, although duration of administration of these agents has not been standardized (Acorda, 2000). The radial graft is a desirable conduit because of its length and ability to reach most distal targets. Postoperative nursing care includes evaluation of ulnar pulse and distal circulation.

Gastroepiploic Graft. The right GEA is a branch of the gastroduodenal artery that supplies blood to the greater curvature of the stomach. The GEA can be used as an *in situ* graft on the posterior surfaces of the heart or as a free graft to other vessels. Harvesting of the GEA graft requires laparotomy in addition to the sternotomy or thoracotomy incisions required for CABG. Longer operative times and abdominal surgery increase the complexity of the surgery. Because of its excellent flow and resistance to atherosclerosis, it is hoped that the GEA will have long-term patency similar to that of IMA grafts (Rosborough, 1993). The inferior epigastric artery may also be used as bypass conduit. Because of its length (only 10 to 12 cm), it can be used only as a free graft (Pym et al., 1997).

Operative Results

Coronary bypass surgery is done to improve quality of life by relieving anginal symptoms, or to prolong life (Yusuf et al., 1994). Although angina pectoris is relieved in more than 90% of patients who undergo CABG surgery, Canadian Cardiovascular Society class III angina reoccurs in 5% to 10% of patients at 3 years and gradually increases because of graft stenosis or progression of native disease (Chatterjee, 1998). Though operative mortality rates in the 1980s were approximately 1%, operative mortality rates for CABG surgery approached 3% in the early 1990s, with rates of 1% to 1.5% for uncomplicated patients with stable angina (Chatterjee, 1998). The overall rate is thought to have increased because of the changing population referred for cardiac surgery. With the advent of interventional cardiology and improved medical management, patients now referred for CABG surgery are older, sicker, and have more complex disease.

Minimally Invasive Coronary Artery Bypass Surgery

Minimally invasive direct coronary artery bypass is CABG surgery performed through a left anterior small thoracotomy (LAST), a short parasternal incision, or small incisions using port access and video-assisted technology. Because the small incisions limit the surgical approach, MIDCAB is usually confined to proximal disease of the LAD or right coronary artery with IMA as conduits to these sites. Radial artery, GEA, and saphenous vein grafts have also been used if the IMA graft could not be used or if more distal targets required grafting. Surgery is performed on the beating heart. To allow suturing of the graft anastomosis to the beating heart, pharmacologic measures such as adenosine and beta-blockers are used to slow or temporarily stop the heart, in conjunction with mechanical stabilizers that immobilize the portion of the coronary artery where the graft anastomosis is sutured (Fig. 29-3). Blood flow through the target vessel is temporarily interrupted with padded snares or luminal occluders (Vitello-Cicciu et al., 1998). Transesophageal echocardiography is used to assess for wall motion abnormalities that would signal ischemia. CPB is on standby during each MIDCAB procedure if emergent conversion to standard sternotomy and CPB is required. The advantages of MIDCAB surgery are coronary revascularization without the physiologic derangements of CPB and avoidance of the traditional sternotomy incision. As a result, patients have less pain, need fewer blood transfusions, and have reduced overall length of hospital stay. With shortened length of stay, MIDCAB procedures have become a competitive alternative to PTCA or stenting of proximal coronary artery lesions.

Coronary artery bypass surgery performed by median sternotomy but without the use of CPB is known as off-pump CABG (OPCAB). Like MIDCAB, grafts are performed on the beating heart. Avoidance of CPB and aortic cross-clamping may be desirable in patients with poor ventricular function or severe atherosclerosis of the aorta who may not tolerate aortic cross-clamping. Median sternotomy allows for better exposure than in MIDCAB techniques. In a study by Tasdemir and colleagues (Tasdemir et al., 1998) that reviewed 2,052 CABG cases performed off-pump, 74.2% did not require transfusion, the overall mortality rate was 1.9%, and the perioperative MI rate was 2.9%. While it has been suggested that OPCAB offers neurologic protection, a randomized controlled trial comparing neurologic outcome of OPCAB to CABG with CPB demonstrated improved neurologic outcomes at 3 months but this difference became negligible at 12 months (Van Dijk et al., 2002).

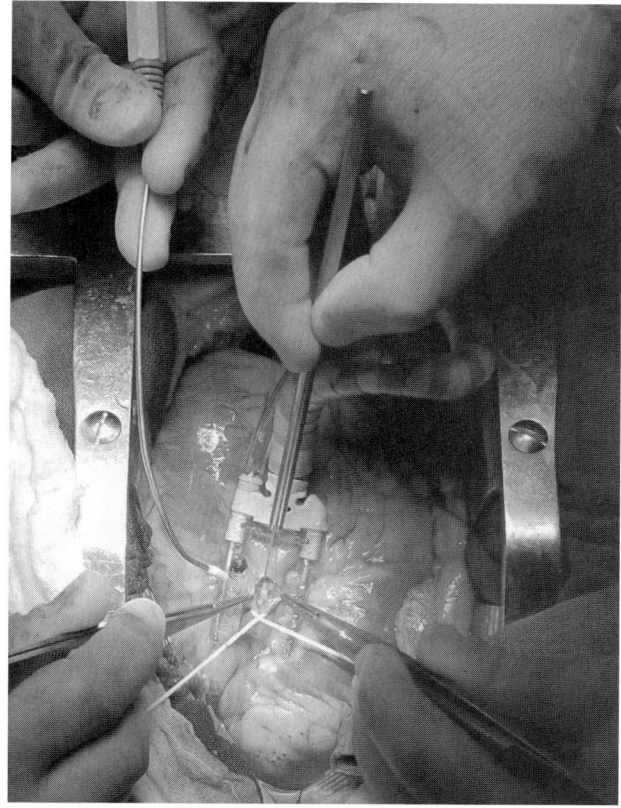

■ **Figure 29–3.** A two-pronged stabilizer immobilizes the surrounding myocardium and coronary artery in off-pump bypass surgery done on a beating heart. A snare is used proximal to the incision on the left anterior descending (LAD) coronary artery. Forceps hold open the incision on the LAD open, and the internal mammary pedicle will be sewn into place. (Photo by D. LeDoux, 2003.)

Despite comparable mortality results, a study by Gundry and colleagues (Gundry et al., 1998) suggested that off-pump CABG was twice as likely to require repeat catheterization (30% vs. 16%) and had a much higher rate of repeat intervention (20% vs. 7%).

Operative Results for MIDCAB and OPCAB

Midterm results in patients undergoing MIDCAB through LAST and using the left IMA and OPCAB have been encouraging. In a multicenter, randomized controlled trial comparing OPCAB and CABG with CPB (Van Dijk et al., 2001), the OPCAB group had less use of blood products ($p < 0.01$) and 41% less release of creatine kinase ($P < 0.01$), but otherwise there were no significant differences in complications, quality of life, length of stay, or recurrent angina. In a series by Calafiore and associates (Calafiore et al., 1998) (n = 460), 71.2% of patients were extubated by the second postoperative hour, the mean intensive care unit stay was 4.2 ± 4.5 hours, and the mean postoperative hospital length of stay was 66 ± 29 hours. In the study, 5.7% of patients required conversion from the LAST approach to standard sternotomy, the 30-day mortality rate was 1.1%, and the late mortality rate was 1.4%. At 29 months after surgery, the survival rate was 97.1% ± 0.7% (95% confidence interval, 90.5% to 100%), and the event-free survival rate was 89.4% ± 1.2% (95% confidence interval: 78.2% to 100%) (Calafiore et al., 1998). Ascione et al. reported OPCAB costs per patient as nearly $1,000 less ($P < 0.001$) (Ascione et al., 1999). A prospective randomized trial was conducted by Drenth et al. comparing coronary artery percutaneous transluminal coronary angioplasty with stenting (PCI) to OPCAB in patients for high-grade proximal LAD lesions (Drenth et al., 2002). In a mean follow-up time of 3 years, angina pectoris class was lower in the OPCAB group ($P = 0.02$) as well as the need for antianginal medication ($P = 0.01$) when compared to the PCI group. OPCAB is technically more difficult and demanding for surgeons (Mangino-Blanchard, 2002). Because operative techniques that involve minimally invasive incisions, port access, and operation on a beating heart have a learning curve, results associated with this newer operative technology are expected to continue to improve over time.

Transmyocardial Laser Revascularization

Transmyocardial laser revascularization (TMLR) is a technique under investigation in patients with refractory angina. In TMLR, carbon dioxide, holmium-YAG (yttrium-aluminum garnet), or excimer lasers (Frazier et al., 1998) are used to produce multiple channels from the endocardial surface of the ventricular wall in an effort directly to improve blood flow to areas of myocardium that cannot be revascularized using traditional techniques. It has also been postulated that myocardial blood flow is enhanced by angiogenesis that occurs with TMLR, although this is still unproven. Left anterolateral thoracotomy is most often used to provide exposure, although TMLR can also be done by standard median sternotomy if it is performed at the same time as standard CABG to other vessels. Clinical trials using the holmium-YAG are being carried out by cardiologists using transluminal catheter-based technology through a percutaneous approach (Leeper, 2000), creating laser channels from within the ventricular cavity. TMLR is done on a beating heart. The laser is synchronized with the patient's ECG to provide the laser pulse with the R wave so that firing occurs during end-diastole, thus minimizing the risk of ventricular arrhythmias (Lynn-McHale et al., 1998). Transesophageal echocardiography is used to detect steam or bubbles that verify channel creation. Epicardial surface seals off with gentle pressure, leaving an endocardial channel in which blood flows.

Patients selected for TMLR have severe CHD with Canadian Cardiovascular Society functional class III or IV (Lynn-McHale et al., 1998); viable myocardium with reversible ischemia as evidenced by radionuclide myocardial scan; left ventricular ejection fraction of 20% or more; diffuse coronary disease; or target vessels too small for catheter-based intervention or CABG. Research strategies are aimed at defining which laser works best and which patients benefit the most in terms of anginal relief, and developing transvenous approaches of TMLR. Nursing care and recovery after TMLR are similar to those in patients who have had MIDCAB.

Operative Results and Future Trends

Clinical studies involving TMLR have demonstrated a decrease in angina by more than two Canadian Cardiovascular Society classes, improved clinical status, mild to moderate improvement in regional cardiac perfusion, and exercise tolerance for more than 2 years (Frazier et al., 1998). Meta-analysis of TMR studies comparing those treated with laser to those with medical therapy demonstrated no significant statistical difference (Horvath, 2003). Although TMLR clinical trials have established it as a low-risk therapy for patients with end-stage ischemic CHD, it has been more effective in improving quality of life for these patients than in improving survival (Frazier et al., 1998). Recently in clinical trials, investigators have been combining the use of TMR with endothelial growth factor (Leeper, 2000). The ability to deliver TMLR by a less invasive means will broaden its applications and increase its availability to patients with depressed cardiac function who would not be eligible for the current thoracotomy approach.

CARDIAC SURGERY PROCEDURES FOR ACQUIRED STRUCTURAL HEART DISEASE

Acquired Valvular Heart Disease

Valvular Repair

Surgical repair of a stenotic or incompetent mitral valve is performed frequently. The reparative surgeries, mitral commissurotomy (in which the fused valve cusps are split open) and annuloplasty (in which the large orifice of an incompetent valve is made smaller) are discussed in Chapter 33. Care of the patient after surgical repair of valves is similar to that of the patient after CABG surgery.

Valvular Replacement

If a dysfunctional mitral or aortic valve is not suitable for repair, valve replacement is undertaken. Valvular heart surgery can be accomplished through a standard median sternotomy incision, through a small parasternal incision, or through port access using small incisions and endoscopic techniques. Because valve surgery requires an arrested, open heart, CPB must be used and can be done by the standard method or by femoro-femoral cannulation. Surgical techniques for mitral valve replacement (MVR) and aortic valve replacement (AVR), types of prosthetic heart valves, and indications for valvular replacement are discussed in Chapter 33.

Mitral Valve Repair or Replacement. The routine medical care after MVR surgery is similar to that after CABG surgery. Early after MVR surgery, a patient is more likely to have important cardiovascular or pulmonary dysfunction than a patient who has undergone CABG surgery. Late after surgery, problems related to the prosthetic device may occur. Prognosis and outcome after MVR are related to severity of the left ventricular and right ventricular dysfunction before surgery.

Aortic Valve Replacement. The routine medical care after AVR surgery is similar to that after CABG surgery. Early after AVR surgery, a patient is more likely to have arrhythmia, decreased cardiac output, or neurologic dysfunction than a patient who has undergone CABG surgery. Late after surgery, arrhythmia, heart failure, or problems related to the prosthetic device may occur. Prognosis and outcome after AVR are related to severity of left ventricular dysfunction before surgery.

Surgical Techniques for the Failing Heart

As an alternative to cardiac transplant, number surgical techniques are evolving. In the Dor procedure, the left ventricular cavity is opened and monofilament sutures placed circumferentially above the boarder of the diseased muscle, restoring the normal contour of the ventricle (Calafiore et al., 2003). The reduction ventriculoplasty was pioneered by Batitista as a surgical option for patients with cardiomyopathy who cannot undergo cardiac transplantation. To decrease wall tension and ventricular size in the dilated left ventricular, an oval-shaped portion of myocardium is removed from apex to base Although Batitista reported encouraging results in his own series, this procedure after being introduced in the United States has had mixed results (Calafiore et al., 2003). While the Cleveland Clinic series reported midterm results with a 30-day mortality rate of 3.2% (Franco-Cereceda et al., 2001), other series have reported high mortality rates (Calafiore et al., 2003).

Dynamic cardiomyoplasty is an alternative to heart transplantation for patients with end-stage heart failure. Skeletal muscle from the latissimus dorsi is wrapped around the weakened heart muscle and paced in synchrony with the heart to strengthen ventricular contraction (Vargo & Dimengo, 1993). Surgery is accomplished through a left thoracotomy incision, and CPB is not required. The latissimus dorsi muscle is placed into the thoracic cavity through a space where the second rib has been resected. Intramuscular pacing electrodes are inserted in the proximal portion of the muscle. The patient is then repositioned, and a sternal incision is made to complete the muscle wrap around the heart. A cardiomyostimulator (a pacemaker especially designed for cardiomyoplasty) is implanted beneath the rectus muscle and activated 2 weeks after surgery, allowing the muscle to rest and develop collateral circulation before pacing is started. Stimulation is gradually introduced by a stimulated pulse synchronized to every other cardiac cycle. Over the next 7 to 8 weeks, amplitude and number of pulses are increased to every cycle with clinical improvements appearing to plateau at 6 to 12 months (Futterman & Lemberg, 1996). The operative mortality rate with cardiomyoplasty has been reported at approximately 10%, with more than 80% of patients experiencing functional improvement greater than that of the control group, which was treated medically (Chiu, 1997). Long-term survival after cardiomyoplasty has been reported as high as 50% at 8 years (Chachques et al., 2003). Although cardiomyoplasty is not a replacement for cardiac transplantation, it may have a limited role in patients who would not be candidates for transplantation.

Acquired Ventricular Septal Defect Repair

Rupture of the intraventricular septum after MI is a rare complication that occurs in only 0.5% to 2% of patients with acute MI (Matlof, 1990). The infarct that accompanies ventricular septal defect (VSD) is usually extensive and transmural. Thinning and dilatation of the infarcted portion of septum, which evolves to rupture 1 to 7 days after MI, causes biventricular failure as the left ventricle shunts blood into the right ventricle, causing right-sided heart failure and pulmonary edema. Clinical signs of acquired VSD include rapid-onset biventricular failure or cardiogenic shock, pansystolic murmur, and a sequential increase in venous oxygen saturation from the right atrium to the pulmonary artery. Bedside cardiac output measures done with the pulmonary artery catheter by thermodilution are falsely elevated because of the left-to-right ventricular shunt. The anatomy and size of the septal rupture is diagnosed by echocardiography and cardiac catheterization.

Stabilization of the patient with septal rupture is aimed at afterload reduction. Using pharmacologic vasodilators and intra-aortic balloon pumping, forward flow is improved and the left-to-right shunt fraction is reduced. The VSD is repaired by patching the defect with a Dacron-covered patch, which is then lined, if possible, with pericardium to make it leak proof. In patients with significant coronary artery stenosis, CABG surgery may also be added to the operative procedure. Even with surgical repair, the hospital mortality rate after VSD repair remains 10% to 40% (King & Verrier, 2003). The important risk factors associated with early death are poor preoperative hemodynamic state and acute right ventricular dysfunction.

Repair of Ascending Aortic Aneurysm or Dissection

Aortic aneurysm is used to describe localized dilatation of the aorta. Causes of ascending aortic aneurysm include hypertension, Marfan's syndrome, and cystic medial necrosis. The likelihood of aortic aneurysm rupture is related to size. The more the aorta is stretched, the greater the tension and wall stress forces. If the ascending aorta is aneurysmal, the cusps of the aorta may be distorted, resulting in aortic insufficiency and acute or chronic heart failure.

Aortic dissection occurs secondary to disruption of the intimal layer of the aorta and is a true medical emergency. Blood enters the intimal tear and dissects a false lumen in the abnormal medial layer, with blood flowing retrograde and antegrade, separating layers of the intimal and adventitial layers. The dissection is propagated by hypertension and elevated force of contraction. In the Stanford classification, type A describes dissection of the ascending aorta and transverse arch, whereas type B is used to describe dissections of the descending thoracic aorta. Aortic dissection has a grave prognosis and requires prompt surgical intervention.

Ascending aortic dissection and aneurysm are treated with surgical resection of the involved portion of aorta and replacement with prosthetic tubular graft. In ascending aortic aneurysm or type A dissection, if the aortic valve is regurgitant, it is replaced. In the case of aneurysm alone, it may be possible to spare the aortic valve by re-suspending it within the prosthetic graft of the ascending aorta (David procedure). If surgery involves the aortic arch, deep hypothermic circulatory arrest is used (see section on Surgical Techniques).

Routine Postoperative Care

Immediate postoperative care is similar for patients undergoing any cardiac surgical procedure, including CABG, MIDCAB, valve repair or replacement, and cardiac transplantation. After cardiac surgery, the patient is admitted to an intensive care unit for close monitoring for 6 to 24 hours after surgery. On arrival in the intensive care unit, the critical care nurse performs a number of rapid assessments to ensure patient stability. Routine care includes continuous ECG monitoring, measurement of blood pressure by arterial line, pulse oximetry, pulmonary artery pressures, and body temperature measurement. Intermittent parameters may include cardiac output measurement as well as calculation of derived hemodynamic parameters, such as afterload, cardiac index, and contractility indices. Specialty pulmonary artery catheters, such as the continuous cardiac output pulmonary artery catheter, may be used to evaluate minute-to-minute changes in cardiac output. Oximetry pulmonary artery catheters may be used continuously to monitor mixed venous oxygen concentration, and values can be used to calculate oxygen consumption and delivery parameters during periods of critical illness.

Sinus bradycardia or other hemodynamically significant bradycardic dysrhythmias such as accelerated junctional rhythm can occur postoperatively and may be treated with an atrial or atrioventricular pacemaker set at a rate of 70 or 100 beats/min. Heart block may occur after valve repair or replacement because of edema and trauma at the suture lines close to the conduction system. Postoperative hypertension may be related preoperative hypertension or to elevated vascular resistance, endogenous catecholamines, and renin levels (Morris & St. Claire, 1999). Hypertension may be treated with either intravenous nitrates or sodium nitroprusside. Hypotension occurs often during the first 12 hours after surgery as the patient warms and as systemic vascular resistance decreases to normal levels. Hypovolemia (right or left atrial or pulmonary artery wedge pressure of less than 8 to 10 mm Hg) may be present because of the fluid volume alterations that occur with CPB or if diuretic was administration at the end of CPB. Hypovolemia may be treated with crystalloid or colloid volume expanders such as 5% albumin or hetastarch, or with crystalloid. If the patient's hemoglobin is less than 8 g/dL, packed red blood cells or whole blood may be administered. In a prospective randomized trial of 428 consecutive patients undergoing CABG surgery, the threshold for red blood cell transfusion was decreased to 8 g/dL. While there was no significant morbidity or mortality between the two groups (Bracey et al., 1999), self-assessment of fatigue and anemia were also reported as similar. Blood may be recovered through the chest tubes for autotransfusion during the first 4 to 12 hours after surgery. If patients are normovolemic, they are usually placed on a salt and free-water restriction. Potassium replacement is often necessary.

Patients are usually maintained on a respirator for the first 1 or 2 hours after surgery, until the effects of anesthesia have reversed. Patients are on prophylactic antibiotics, usually a second-generation cephalosporin, to prevent wound infection. Antibiotic prophylaxis beyond 48 hours is not associated with decreased infections (Kreter & Woods, 1992).

Because of improved anesthesia and surgical techniques and a shift from acute care resulting from changes in reimbursement, cardiac surgery has evolved to include same day admission and shortened length of stay. Stable, uncomplicated patients are earmarked to "fast track" by extubating early and minimizing their intensive care unit and hospital stay. Patient care is directed by an established care map or "roadmap." In the operating room, patients receive lower doses of opioids with the aim of extubation within 1 or 2 hours after arrival in the intensive care unit. The patient is kept sedated with short-acting agents such as propofol or midazolam intravenous infusions. When the patient is hemodynamically stable, awake and responsive without neurologic complications, pain is controlled, and mediastinal bleeding is minimal, the patient is extubated (Staples & Ramsay, 1997). As a result, cardiac surgery patients may stay in the intensive care unit as little as 8 to 12 hours, thus freeing up critical care beds and reducing costs to the patient. Patients who are "fast tracked" in rapid recovery programs are discharged 3 to 5 days after surgery. While earlier discharge originally raised cause for concern, in a study by Lahey and colleagues (Lahey et al., 1998), patients discharged 7 or more days postoperatively represented the greatest risk for readmission. Nurse practitioners or physician assistants in collaboration may manage cardiac surgery patients with the physician. Atrial arrhythmias and pulmonary complications are the most common variances that keep patients in hospital longer than planned by the care map. Elderly patients may be difficult to discharge within 5 days after surgery because of comorbid conditions and social issues related to discharge (Verrier et al., 1995).

Early Complications After Cardiac Surgery

Cardiovascular

Cardiovascular dysfunction or low cardiac output syndrome can occur after cardiac surgery. Low cardiac output syndrome may be related to reduced preload, increased afterload, arrhythmias, cardiac tamponade, or myocardial depression with or without myocardial necrosis. Excessive bleeding can occur secondary to coagulopathy, uncontrolled hypertension, or inadequate hemostasis. Perioperative MI and pericarditis can occur as a result of cardiac surgery.

Postoperative Bleeding. Pleural and mediastinal tubes are attached to water-seal and 20-cm suction to drain mediastinal shed blood. Although blood may clot in these chest tubes, they should not be stripped because stripping may cause excessive suction, which may increase bleeding or cause damage to grafts (Duncan & Erickson, 1982). Excessive postoperative bleeding (mediastinal drainage of more than >500 mL for the first hour after surgery or drainage, totaling >200 mL/h thereafter) usually is mechanical in nature and caused by bleeding from suture lines, but it may be caused by the presence of pericardial adhesions from an earlier surgery or to a coagulopathy. Postoperative bleeding is usually venous rather than arterial. Coagulopathies may occur in patients with prolonged CPB times or excessive intraoperative bleeding. Coagulation panels should be obtained immediately in patients with excessive bleeding. Ideally, platelet counts should be kept higher than 100,000, and prothrombin time and partial prothrombin time should be less than 1.2-times the control value (Czer, 1990). The thromboelastogram is used as a measure of whole blood clotting and is abnormal if there are qualitative or quantitative coagulation disorders of any kind. Bleeding in the face of a normal thromboelastogram suggests surgical bleeding rather than coagulopathy (Staples & Ramsay, 1997). Coagulopathies caused by depletion of factors should be treated with administration of depleted factors, such as fresh-frozen plasma, platelets, and cryoprecipitate. Autotransfusion may be used to replete red blood cells, but filtered blood lacks adequate clotting factors.

Pharmacologic means of controlling postoperative hemorrhage include a variety of nonhematogenous therapies. Aprotinin, a serine protease inhibitor, inhibits plasmin. Aprotinin also preserves platelet function during bypass and, like the antifibrinolytics, has been shown to reduce postoperative bleeding (Staples & Ramsay, 1997) and decrease the need for blood transfusion. Aprotinin is used in high-risk operations in which bleeding is anticipated (such as re-operations or when prolonged CPB is expected), and may be used in the Jehovah's Witness patient to reduce blood loss. Prophylactic administration of Aprotinin has been shown to reduce blood loss and transfusions requirements (Nuttall et al., 2000). Aminocaproic acid is an antifibrinolytic medication that inhibits conversion of plasminogen to plasmin. Aminocaproic acid is loaded intravenously in a 5-g dose over 5 minutes and is then followed by a 1-g/h infusion for up to 6 hours (Czer, 1990). Desmopressin (DDAVP) may be infused intravenously in patients with severe platelet dysfunction after prolonged CPB or uremia. DDAVP shortens bleeding time and improves platelet function by increasing circulating levels of von Willebrand factor. DDAVP also increases factor VIII C levels, which shorten the partial prothrombin time. Protamine also may be administered intravenously in patients who had inadequate reversal of heparin or in those with heparin rebound. Protamine must be administered as a slow intravenous infusion to prevent hypotension. Patients with insulin-dependent diabetes or allergy to fish are more likely to have allergic reactions to protamine. If postoperative bleeding continues and coagulation tests are normal, bleeding may be mechanical or may result from suture line or venous bleeding. By increasing the patient's positive end-expiratory pressure on the ventilator, diffuse mediastinal bleeding may be reduced (Banasik & Tyler, 1986). Adequate control of hypertension with sodium nitroprusside may also help control bleeding. If coagulopathies were corrected and bleeding continues, mediastinal re-exploration is advised to decrease the risk of cardiac tamponade.

Cardiac Tamponade. Cardiac tamponade is a life-threatening emergency that may occur immediately postoperative. Compression of the right heart with blood and/or clot decreases left ventricular preload and consequently, cardiac output that results in causes hemodynamic deterioration (Braile & Petrucci, 2000). Cardiac tamponade is suspected as a cause of low cardiac output if right and left heart pressures increase and equalize. Physical exam findings, hemodynamic parameters, and diagnostic tests for tamponade include: decreased cardiac index; mediastinal drainage that may increase as well as decrease or stop; radiography shows widening of the cardiac silhouette; neck vein distention; a pulsus paradoxus is noted by arterial line or by auscultation; or narrow pulse pressure is present. Although tachycardia is a sign of classic tamponade, the cardiac surgical patient may be unable to generate a compensatory tachycardia because of heart block or previously administered beta-blockers or calcium channel blockers. Symptoms and physical findings may be nonspecific and inadequate for diagnosis and intervention (Tsang et al., 1999). Echocardiography provides rapid confirmation of pericardial fluid and tamponade physiology, facilitating intervention with echo-guided pericardiocentesis or open pericardial drainage in the operating room.

Myocardial Depression. Myocardial depression (impaired myocardial contractility) may be reversible or irreversible after cardiac surgery. If a patient is not acidotic or hypoxemic and has evidence of decreased cardiac contractility, myocardial cell dysfunction or necrosis is suspected. Treatment of low cardiac output secondary to myocardial dysfunction first involves treatment of hypoxemia, acidosis, heart rate and rhythm abnormalities, decreased preload, and increased afterload. If a patient continues to have a low cardiac output after these maneuvers, inotropes or intraaortic balloon pump therapy is instituted. A variety of inotropes and vasoactive medications may be employed postoperatively (Table 29-1). Dobutamine, dopamine, epinephrine, norepinephrine, and milrinone intravenous infusions are frequently used for inotropic support of myocardial depression after cardiac surgery. If the patient's cardiac index is normal to high and hypotension is related to vasodilation, pressers such as vasopressin and phenylephrine may be used A variety of vasodilating agents such as sodium nitroprusside, nitroglycerin, and angiotensin-converting enzyme inhibitors may be used to reduce afterload in low cardiac output syndrome as well as hypertension. Intra-aortic balloon pump therapy is frequently used in patients with severe cardiac dysfunction that is not adequately supported with medications alone.

Perioperative Myocardial Infarction. Despite improved methods of myocardial protection, perioperative MI continues to be a serious complication. At the consensus meeting of the National Institutes of Health, it was determined that the rate of perioperative MI may be expected to be as high as 5% for patients with stable angina and 10% for those with unstable angina (Bateman & Gray, 1990). Diagnosis of perioperative MI is made from a variety of diagnostic tests including ECG, echocardiography, and cardiac enzymes. Mechanisms of MI include graft spasm, embolization of air or debris into coronary artery or graft, and inadequate myocardial protection (Bateman & Gray, 1990). Creatine kinase (CK) is routinely elevated immediately after cardiac surgery and usually drops after 12 to 16 hours. CK peaks associated with perioperative MI occur 16 to 24 hours after surgery. CK-MB levels that indicate possible MI is established by individual institutions based on average CK elevations on uncomplicated, consecutively operated cohorts with no ECG abnormalities (Bateman & Gray, 1990). More recently, troponin I has been used for the diagnosis of perioperative MI. Postoperative troponin I levels in patients

Table 29–1 ■ INOTROPES AND VASODILATOR INTRAVENOUS INFUSIONS COMMONLY USED AFTER CARDIAC SURGERY

Medication	Dose Range	Mechanism of action	Indications	Heart Rate	Blood Pressure	Cardiac Output
Dobutamine	2–15 mcg/kg/min	Primarily beta-1 adrenergic receptor stimulation	Low cardiac output after cardiac surgery	+	+/0/-	++
Dopamine	1–2 mcg/kg/min for renal effect 5–20 mcg/kg/min for inotropy and increased vascular resistance	Stimulation of dopaminergic and a drenergic receptors	Treatment of shock and hypotension after cardiac surgery in patient who has been volume resuscitated	+	++	++
Epinephrine	0.01–0.1 mcg/kg/min to high dose 0.3–0.3 mcg/kg/min	Stimulation of alpha and beta-1, beta-2 adrenergic receptors	Treatment of low cardiac output and shock after cardiac surgery	++	++	++
Isoproterenol	0.01–0.1 mcg/kg/min	Stimulation of beta-1 and beta-2 adrenergic receptors	Used after heart transplantation and in patients with severe bradycardia to stimulate heart rate	+++	+	++
Milrinone	0.25–0.75 mcg/kg/min	Phosphodiesterase inhibition resulting in increase inotropy and vasodilation	Low cardiac output after cardiac surgery; may require use of adrenergic agent to maintain blood pressure	0/+	−	+
Nitroglycerin	5–200 mcg/min	Dilates coronary arteries and reduces myocardial oxygen demand, reduce ventricular pressures	Used to prevent spasm in arterial grafts after cardiac surgery as well as may be used to reduce preload and afterload	−/+	−	−
Nitroprusside	0.3–5 mcg/kg/min (high doses may result in thiocyanate toxicity)	Cause peripheral vasodilation by acting directly on smooth muscle in the venous and arterial circulation	Used to decreased blood pressure and afterload	−	—	0/+
Norepinephrine	0.01–0.1 mcg/min	Stimulation of alpha and beta adrenergic receptors (alpha effects are predominate)	Used for shock and low systemic vascular resistance after cardiac surgery	+/-	++	+
Phenylephrine	0.1–0.3 mcg/kg/min	Potent alpha adrenergic stimulator	Used to increase systemic vascular resistance and blood pressure cardiac output is maintained but blood pressure is low	O/−	++	−
Vasopressin	0.01–0.1 units/min	Potent vasoconstrictor	Used to treat shock and increase systemic vascular resistance and blood pressure cardiac output is maintained but blood pressure is low	−	++	−

+ = increase; 0 = no change; − = decrease.

without perioperative MI peak at 8 to 10 hours, whereas in patients with perioperative MI, troponin I levels peak in 20 hours and at higher concentrations (Dehoux et al., 2001). A study by Lasocki and associates found that elevated troponin I levels more than 13 ng/mL was an independent predictor of in-hospital mortality (Lasocki et al., 2002). New wall motion abnormalities noted on echocardiography are another way to verify perioperative MI. Postoperative pericarditis may mimic myocardial ischemia with chest pain and widespread ST segment elevation. ECG changes associated with pericarditis are J-point changes, concave rather than convex, and do not result in pathologic Q waves.

Arrhythmias. Arrhythmias are common after cardiac surgery and are a prevalent cause of increased length of stay after cardiac surgery. Brady arrhythmias are common after CABG and valve surgeries and may require temporary pacing via epicardial pacing wires placed at the time of surgery. Hemodynamically significant bradycardia or heart block may require placement of permanent transvenous pacers before discharge (Chung, 2000). Atrial arrhythmias are the most common after cardiac surgery, occurring in approximately 20% to 40% of

patients (Kern, 1998). Contributing factors of atrial fibrillation (AF) may include electrolyte or metabolic disturbances, increased circulating catecholamines, volume overload, hypoxia, and myocardial ischemia or MI. The association of tachyarrhythmias and the severity of cardiac dysfunction suggest a causal relationship between catecholamines therapy and development of tachyarrhythmias (Knotzer et al., 2001). Although atrial tachyarrhythmias may occur any time during the first few days to weeks after cardiac surgery, they frequently peak around the second or third day postoperative. Risk factors for postoperative atrial fibrillation include advanced age, history of congestive heart failure or atrial fibrillation, chronic obstructive lung disease, male sex, history of rheumatic heart disease, prolonged aortic cross-clamp time, and bicaval cannulation (Cleveland & Grover, 2003). The onset of tachyarrhythmias is often preceded by frequent premature atrial contractions. Medications commonly used to control the ventricular response in atrial fibrillation and flutter include diltiazem (either intravenous drip or orally), digoxin, and beta-blockers (orally or by intravenous drip, such as esmolol). Medications used to promote conversion of atrial fibrillation include procainamide,

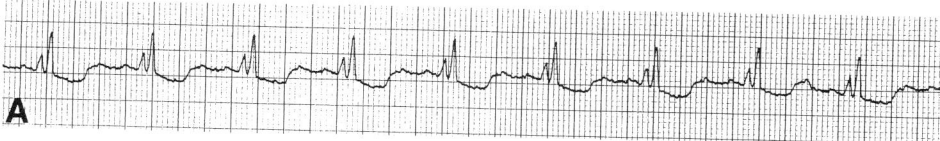

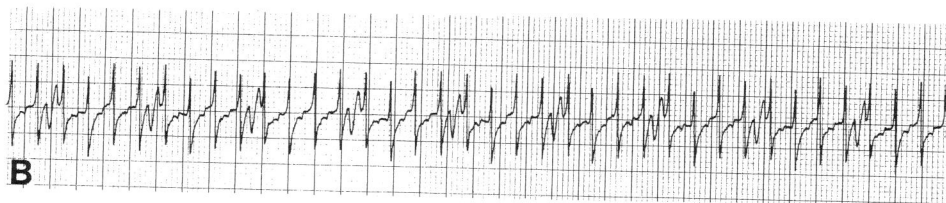

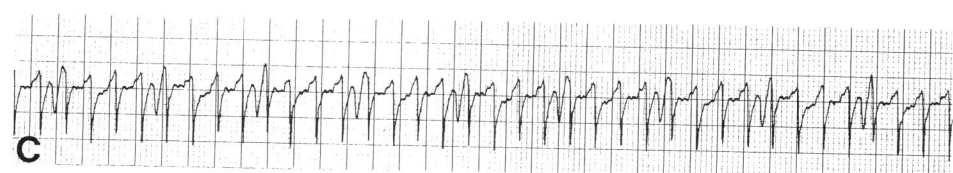

■ **Figure 29–4.** Atrial electrocardiography (ECG) is done by attaching limb leads and V_1 in standard fashion and then attaching V_2 and V_3 directly to the atrial pacing wires with alligator clips. Simultaneous surface lead and unipolar atrial lead ECG recordings are obtained. (*A*) Lead V_1 is the surface or reference lead. There is no atrial enhancement. (*B, C*) Leads V_2 and V_3 are unipolar atrial leads that accentuate the atrial activity and demonstrate an atrial rate of approximately 300 beats/min that was not apparent on the surface lead or standard 12-lead ECG.

amiodarone, and sotalol. While multiple medications have been studied, beta-blockers have been the only medication consistently shown across clinical studies that reduce the frequency of postoperative AF (Hill et al., 2002). Beta-blockers should be considered early during the postoperative course, especially if the patient was on beta-blockers preoperatively. Although beta-blockers, atrial pacing, anti-arrhythmic medications, or a combination of these therapies may reduce the incidence or duration of AF, optimal strategies are still being defined (Maisel et al., 2001).

Postoperative arrhythmia diagnosis and treatment is facilitated by the presence of atrial epicardial pacemaker wires. Atrial activity is more pronounced when recorded in atrial ECGs than when recorded in a normal surface ECG (Fig. 29-4). When atrial activity is accentuated, differentiation between supraventricular and ventricular arrhythmias, and atrial fibrillation and flutter is made easier. If the ventricular response to atrial fibrillation exceeds 110 beats/min, then the patient's rate should be controlled.

If pharmacologic modalities fail to convert the patient to a sinus rhythm, electrical therapies may be used. Atrial flutter may be converted using rapid atrial pacing. To perform rapid atrial pacing, both atrial epicardial wires are connected to the rapid atrial pacemaker. The pacemaker output is set between 10 and 20, and the pacemaker rate is set approximately 20% faster than the existing atrial rate (atrial rate can be determined on the atrial ECG). Rapid atrial pacing continues for 30 seconds or until the atrial ECG complex changes from a negative to a positive deflection in lead II. Rapid atrial pacing is then abruptly discontinued, which allows the atria to resume a normal sinus rhythm (Fig. 29-5). Patients with chronic atrial fibrillation may be refractory to either pharmacologic or electrical conversion. If the atrial fibrillation is new in onset (<1 year), the patient may be successfully cardioverted by synchronized cardioversion. If the patient has been in atrial fibrillation or flutter longer than 48 hours or the atrial fibrillation remains paroxysmal, it is desirable to anticoagulate for 3 to 4 weeks to prevent thromboembolism, and then have the patient return for elective cardioversion if they remain in atrial fibrillation or flutter.

While premature ventricular contractions (PVCs) and non-sustained runs of ventricular tachycardia (NSVT) may occur commonly after cardiac surgery, sustained ventricular tachycardia (VT), and ventricular fibrillation (VF) are rare but associated with a poor prognosis (Rho et al., 2000). Risk factors for

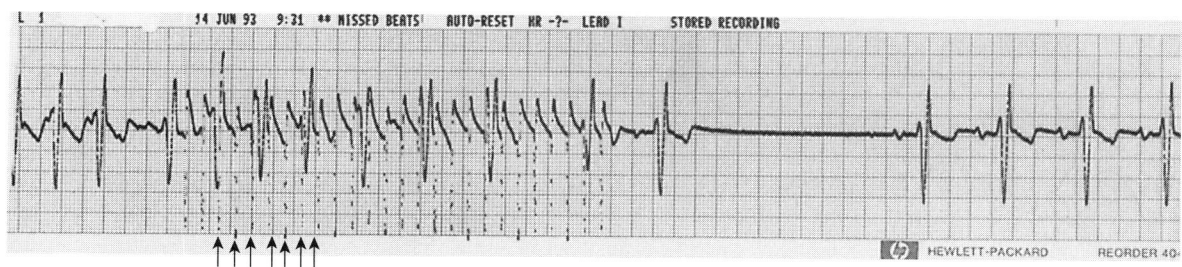

■ **Figure 29–5.** Recording of a burst of rapid atrial pacing used to overdrive and convert this atrial flutter to sinus rhythm. *Arrows* denote atrial pacing spikes.

VT include previous myocardial infarction, ejection fraction less than 40%, and severe heart failure (Steinberg et al., 1999). PVC's and NSVT should be treated with correction of electrolytes, reduction or elimination of arrhythmogenic drugs such as catecholamines, and ruled out for ischemia. Sustained VT should be cardioverted and antiarrhythmic agents such as amiodarone or lidocaine should be instituted (Rho et al., 2000). In CABG after recent myocardial infarction, reperfusion via new bypass grafts may restore electrical activity to an infarct zone creating reentrant circuits and the possible development of VT (Steinberg et al., 1999). Electrophysiology studies and implantable defibrillators may be used in selected cases.

Pulmonary

Respiratory dysfunction is the most significant cause of morbidity after cardiac surgery (Morris & St. Claire, 1999). Routinely, patients are intubated and ventilated for 2 to 4 hours after cardiac surgery. Pulmonary function is monitored with continuous pulse oximetry as well as intermittent arterial blood gases and chest radiographs. Mild pulmonary dysfunction is common after cardiac surgery. Pathophysiologic changes that occur after CPB include increased capillary permeability, increased pulmonary vascular resistance, and intrapulmonary aggregation of leukocytes and platelets. A noncardiac pulmonary edema may occur immediately after CPB or during the first several days after surgery. Comparative studies between OPCAB and CABG with CPB suggest that CPB alone may not be the major cause of the development of postoperative pulmonary dysfunction (Ng et al., 2002). In a prospective, controlled trial by Roosens et al., both patients with and without CPB had dramatic impairment of respiratory system mechanic postoperatively (Roosens et al., 2002). Severe pulmonary dysfunction is uncommon and may be related to preexisting lung disease. Although severe lung injury after cardiac surgery is rare, it continues to be a major impact on morbidity and mortality as well as related cost of hospitalization (Ng et al., 2002). In a case controlled study by Milot and collegues in 3,278 patients, adult respiratory distress syndrome (ARDS) after cardiac surgery was rare (0.4%) but carried a 15% mortality rate (Milot et al., 2001). Independent predictors of ARDS in cardiac surgery patients include number of blood products transfused, shock, and previous cardiac surgery (Milot et al., 2001). Chest radiographs should be performed as part of the fever work-up to rule out atelectasis and pneumonia. Bronchial breath sounds may reflect atelectasis, which occurs in up to 70% of patients (Morris et al., 1998). Atelectasis may occur secondary to hypoventilation related to sternal incision discomfort. Pain from chest tubes and sternotomy incision interferes with normal respiration and pulmonary toilet, making adequate pain control a high priority. Diminished breath sounds and lung fields at the bases that are dull to percussion indicate significant pleural effusions. Pneumothorax may occur any time during the postoperative period or at the time of pleural chest tube removal. Phrenic nerve damage may result in diaphragmatic paralysis or dysfunction but is uncommon with today's surgical techniques.

Pulmonary embolism (PE) is uncommon after cardiac surgery. While the incidence of fatal PE after cardiac surgery is only 0.5%, clinical recognition is extremely low (<2%) given its often-silent presentation (Shammas, 1999). Factors associated with a higher incidence of pulmonary emboli include atrial fibrillation, heart failure, obesity, hypercoagulable states, and immobilization. Diagnostic work-up for pulmonary emboli includes arterial blood gas, ventilation perfusion scan, CT scan, or pulmonary angiogram. Treatment with continuous intravenous heparin is begun once the diagnosis of pulmonary emboli is established, and warfarin is started for long-term anticoagulation. In patients in whom anticoagulation is contraindicated, an inferior vena caval filter may be placed. Surgical pulmonary embolectomy may be used in patients with large pulmonary emboli and associated clinical presentation of right-side heart failure.

Renal

Renal impairment after cardiac surgical procedures results in increased morbidity, mortality, and prolonged length of stay (Mangano et al., 1998). While the pathogenesis of renal failure after cardiac surgery is multifactorial, CPB represents a specific risk factor (Loef et al., 2002). CPB results in reduced glomerular filtration rate, reduced renal blood flow, and redistribution of blood flow from the cortex to the outer medulla (Young & Dai, 2000). Radiocontrast used during coronary angiography before cardiac surgery can further reduce renal function. Nonoliguric renal failure after cardiac surgery occurs most commonly after cardiac surgery. If renal dysfunction progresses to oliguric renal failure, serum potassium levels may rise rapidly and maintenance of normovolemia may be difficult without hemofiltration or dialysis. While the incidence of renal failure requiring dialysis after cardiac surgery ranges from 2% to 3%, mortality associated with new oliguric renal failure after cardiac surgery has been reported as high as 65% (Alfieri & Kotler, 1990). The best way to prevent renal failure postoperatively is by early recognition and measures to insure adequate volume, pressure, and cardiac output (Morris & St. Claire, 1999). Nephrotoxic medications such as aminoglycoside antibiotics, radiographic contrast, and nonsteroidal anti-inflammatory drugs must be avoided in postoperative renal failure, and many other medications, such as antibiotics and digoxin, must be adjusted for decreased renal clearance.

Gastrointestinal

Although infrequent after cardiac surgery, serious gastrointestinal (GI) complications may impose a high risk of morbidity and mortality as well as prolonged hospitalization and increased costs (Yilmaz et al., 1996). The overall incidence of GI complications after cardiac surgery is usually quoted as 1% to 2%, with most of these complications being related to ischemia after CPB (Sakorafas & Tsiotos, 1999). Abdominal distention can occur during the first days after surgery secondary to decreased motility related to anesthesia, narcotics, and diabetic gastroparesis. If ileus and abdominal distention do not resolve with fasting and suppository or enema treatments, the etiology of the distention should be explored further. GI bleeding is the most common serious complication after cardiac surgery (Halm, 1996; Mercado et al., 1994). Gastroduodenal bleeding can result from erosive gastritis or esophagitis, or frank ulceration, especially in patients with a previous history of peptic ulcer disease. Patients after cardiac surgery usually are placed on prophylactic gastrointestinal agents such as antacids, sucralfate, histamine blockers such as famotidine or ranitidine, or proton pump inhibitors such as pantoprazole. Cholecystitis presents with right upper quadrant pain and can be evaluated with abdominal ultrasound. After cardiac surgery or critical illness, cholecystitis commonly occurs in its acalculous (no stones) form. Mild elevations of hepatic transaminases also occur commonly after CPB. Severe hepatic dysfunction or "shock liver syndrome" with massive increases in liver enzymes most often occurs as a result of global hypoperfusion and end-organ damage. Acute hemorrhagic pancreatitis is uncommon after CABG surgery, but it has high rates of mortality and morbidity. If the patient continues to remain acidotic and the diagnostic work-up fails to identify another cause, abdominal exploration is done in the hope of finding a correctable source such as necrotic bowel. Diarrhea may occur with enteral feedings and medications such as quinidine or procainamide, or may be the result of *Clostridium difficile* infection. Patients with diarrhea should have stool samples sent to test for *C. difficile* toxin and are treated with oral administration of metronidazole or vancomycin.

Neuropsychological

Neuropsychological dysfunction after cardiac surgery can be either central or peripheral. Cognitive decline after CPB has been estimated from 3% to 50%, depending on definitions and time of assessment and stroke in approximately 3% of patients undergoing CABG surgery (Van Dijk et al., 2002). Central neurologic complications are among the most devastating after cardiac surgery because they may have long-lasting effects on the patient and family and may require lengthy hospitalization and rehabilitation (Mravinac, 1991). In the elderly, neurologic complications increase disproportionately to cardiac risk with advancing age (Tuman et al., 1992). Signs of focal or generalized neurologic damage usually are apparent soon after surgery, usually within the first 24 to 48 hours after surgery (Morris & St. Claire, 1999). Embolization is the most common etiology of stroke during cardiac surgery but hypoperfusion may also play a role (Lopes, 2000).

Two types of peripheral neurologic deficits, brachial plexus injury and ulnar nerve injury, are described after cardiac surgery. The brachial plexus is susceptible to stretch injury and sternal retraction is a key factor responsible for injury (Sharma et al., 2000). This neurologic dysfunction involves the C8 and T1 vertebral levels and results from mechanical trauma caused by sternal retraction, but may also be caused by penetration by a posterior fractured segment of the first rib during cannulation of the internal jugular vein (Morris et al., 1998). In addition to a history of upper extremity pain and paresthesia, examination for brachial plexus injury includes evaluation of motor function of muscle groups innervated by the brachial plexus and sensation to pin prick (Sharma et al., 2000). Ulnar nerve injury, a result of nerve compression, is frequently described by patients after cardiac surgery as paraesthesias in the affected arm below the elbow in the ulnar distribution involving the third, fourth, and fifth digits.

Postcardiotomy delirium occurs 2 to 5 days after cardiac surgery and is manifested as mild confusion, somnolence, agitation, or hallucinations. Memory and alertness are frequently preserved but psychosis may occur (Lopes, 2000). While postcardiotomy delirium is usually self-limiting, it may put the patient at increased risk for self-injury and prolonged hospitalization. Haloperidol is often used for sedation.

Late Postoperative Complications

After the fourth postoperative day, most cardiac surgery patients have short, uncomplicated hospital stays and are discharged to home. However, postpericardiotomy syndrome, cardiac tamponade, or incisional wound infection may occur during the last postoperative period.

Postpericardiotomy syndrome occurs when traumatized tissue in the pericardial cavity triggers an autoimmune response. Postpericardiotomy syndrome usually occurs weeks to months after surgery and results from inflammation of the pleura and pericardium causes aching pericardial pain and severe pleuritic pain. Pleural and pericardial effusions may accompany the inflammation. Treatment is with ibuprofen, indomethacin, or a brief course of prednisone. Large or symptomatic pleural effusions should be drained by thoracentesis (Fig. 29-6).

Late Cardiac tamponade may occur several days to weeks after surgery and is seen more frequently in patients on warfarin or other anticoagulants. The incidence ranges from 0.5% to 2.0% of cardiac surgeries and late tamponade may be related or unrelated to postpericardiotomy syndrome (Braile & Petrrucci, 2000). While the clinical findings of tachycardia, decreased cardiac output, and enlarged cardiac silhouette may be present, late tamponade may present with patient symptoms of increasing shortness of breath, decreased exercise tolerance, and near syncope. Late tamponade is most often treated with pericardiocentesis.

Wound infection after CABG surgery occurs despite perioperative antibiotics and aseptic technique. Sternal wound infections and mediastinitis occur in 0.4% to 5% of patients after sternotomy, associated with risk factors such as prolonged intubation, bilateral IMA grafting, pneumonia, diabetes, emergency surgery, postoperative bleeding, and surgical re-exploration (Morris et al., 1998). Deep infections involving the mediastinum and sternum cause high morbidity, with increased cost of care and prolonged hospital stays (Ridderstolpe et al., 2001). Sternal wound infections typically present 4 to 14 days after surgery with fever, leukocytosis, and inflammatory wound with purulent drainage. Sternal wounds are often associated with a sternal click and sternal instability. Staphylococci, both *Staphylococcus aureus* and coagulase-negative staphylococcus, are the most common causative organism (Gardlund et al., 2002). Superficial chest wounds are treated with antibiotics and local drainage. Deep sternal wounds and mediastinitis are treated with surgical débridement and closure or plastic surgical closure with muscle flap. Infections at the venectomy donor sites may also occur and are usually treatable with oral antibiotics, but severe infections may require open drainage and intravenous antibiotics.

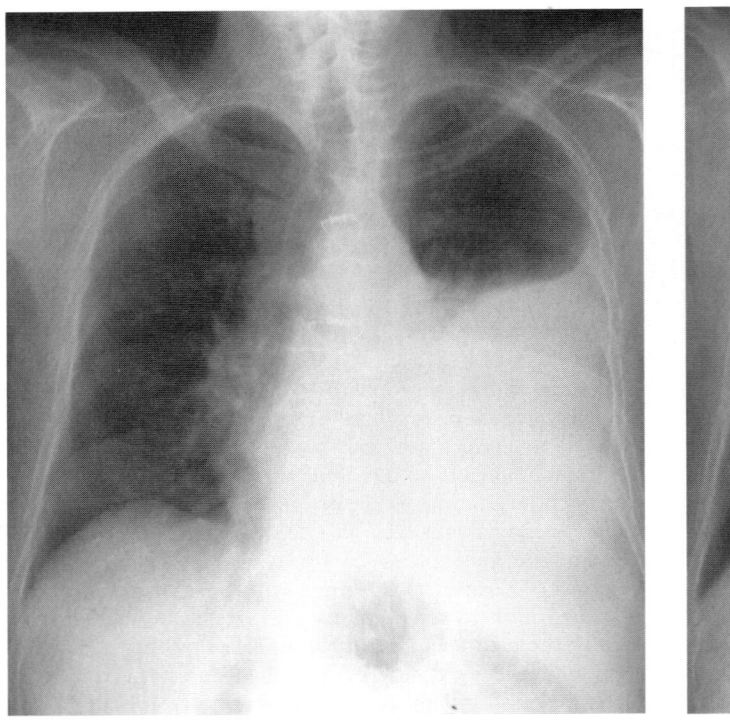
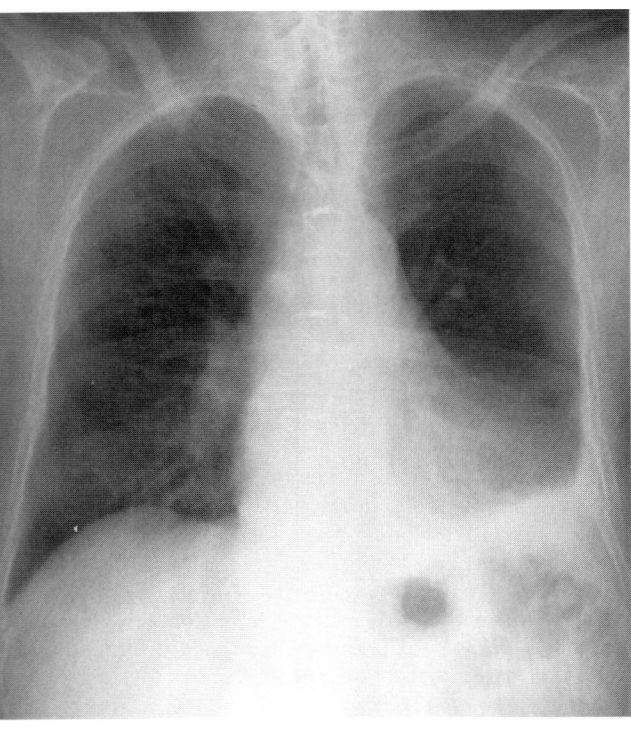

A   B

■ **Figure 29–6.** Left pleural effusion after coronary bypass surgery. (*A*) Chest radiograph shows large pleural effusion obscuring the left heart border. (*B*) Chest radiograph film shows decrease in effusion after 1,500 mL of serosanguineous fluid was aspirated by thoracentesis.

CARDIAC TRANSPLANTATION

Cardiac transplantation is an accepted therapy for end-stage heart disease. Impressive improvements in survival, refinement of immunosuppressive therapy, and improvements in monitoring techniques have prompted many new centers to initiate cardiac transplantation programs. Worldwide, 61,533 heart transplantations have been performed, with 3,122 performed in 2001 (Hertz et al., 2002). The 1-year actuarial survival rate for patients after heart transplantation is 85%, the 5-year survival rate is 68%, and the 10-year survival rate is 48% (Hertz et al., 2002). These figures represent patients who underwent transplantation from 1987 through 2001. This section outlines expectations, therapeutic treatment regimes, and a plan of nursing care.

Progress in Cardiac Transplantation

One-year survival rates after cardiac transplantation have improved from 22% in 1968 to more than 83% in 2001 (Hertz et al., 2002). In 1974, major changes in survival were attributed to the introduction of the endomyocardial biopsy technique for monitoring rejection, to the treatment of rejection, and to the introduction of polyclonal antibodies. Survival results took another upward leap after the introduction of

cyclosporine therapy in 1980. We are now benefiting from better prevention, diagnosis, and management of rejection and the complications of immunosuppressive therapy.

The calcinurin inhibitor, cyclosporine, is one of the most effective immunosuppressant drugs available and is capable of specific immunosuppressant activity to control rejection without totally suppressing the body's ability to fight infection (Baren et al., 2002; Taylor, 2000). It contributed to an approximate 20% increase in 1-year patient survival in the early 1980s. This is caused in large part by its superior ability selectively to inhibit T-cell proliferation and reduce the incidence of rejection.

Improved survival has led to alterations in patient selection criteria with respect to age. Other selection criteria have changed little since the earlier years of cardiac transplantation. Before the introduction of cyclosporine therapy, an upper age limit of 50 years and a lower age limit of adult sized adolescence were followed. Earlier data indicated that patients older than age 50 years did not tolerate immunosuppression and had poorer survival (Kirklin et al., 1994). Because cyclosporine does not totally suppress the entire immune system, older patients are considered for transplantation. The general trend is to define the upper age limit as 60 to 65 years. The current age range is from newborn to 75.3 years, with a mean age of 45 years (Hertz et al., 2002). Before 1980, children younger than 10 years of age were not considered to be transplantation candidates. This criterion was reevaluated. Before 1980, each year, fewer than five children (18 years of age or younger) underwent heart transplantation. In 2001, 78 transplantations were performed in children from newborn to 1 year of age, and 170 transplantations were performed in children between 1 and 18 years of age (*2002 Annual Report*). Actuarial 1-year survival for pediatric patients is slightly less than 90%, the primary causes of death for patients surviving greater than 1 year are coronary vasculopathy, acute rejection, and malignancy (including lymphoma) (Boucek et al., 2003).

Distant organ procurement enables transplantation centers to increase the number of transplantations performed. A surgical team can be dispatched from the transplantation center and can travel up to 500 miles to retrieve the needed heart. An ischemic time of up to 4 hours is considered acceptable. This allows for an approximate travel time of 2.5 hours, with the remaining time required to implant the heart into the patient. Greater public awareness and media attention focused on the need for donors have also contributed to an increase in the available donor pool and transplantation activity. Legislation in some states requires that a family of a potentially eligible donor be asked if that person wished organ donation. However, the limiting factor in solid organ transplantation continues to be organ donation. The success of heart transplantation has created an ever-increasing gap between the number of transplantation candidates and usable heart donors. In 2001, there were 4,096 patients waiting for a heart donor and 2,343 transplantations in the United States (*2002 Annual Report*). Transplant centers and organ procurement organizations work together to promote organ donation by public and health care professional education (Brown, 1995).

With a greater number of centers involved in transplantation and listing potential recipients in organ registries, the average wait for a donor heart has increased dramatically. As a result, the patients often become sicker while waiting. Because of the increasingly sophisticated management of the patient with heart failure, the use of beta blockers to produce hemodynamic and symptomatic improvement, and the pressure for transplant physicians to manage patients on an outpatient basis, patients are put on an acuity scale (status) of need which includes strict definitions of illness. Medical review boards are used to monitor transplant centers listing criteria.

Evaluation of Recipients

Patients who are acceptable candidates for cardiac transplantation must have end-stage cardiac disease not amenable to further medical or surgical therapy (Deng, 2002; Packer et al., 1996). The prognosis for these patients must be limited to 6 to 12 months to live without transplantation. The most frequent medical diagnoses of these patients are cardiomyopathy of various origins (idiopathic, viral, or valvular) and ischemic heart disease (Hertz et al., 2002). Candidate criteria have been established for use in the evaluation process to identify patients most likely to benefit from the operation. Table 29-2 outlines contraindications to cardiac transplantation.

Pediatric patients who may benefit from cardiac transplantation include those with cardiomyopathy and those with structural heart disease without severe pulmonary vascular disease (Boucek et al., 2003). These patients might have been treated surgically initially, but progressive, severe ventricular dysfunction or progressive pulmonary vascular disease limits further therapeutic

Table 29–2 ▪ CONTRAINDICATIONS TO CARDIAC TRANSPLANTATION

Condition	Rationale
Age older than 65 years	Older patients do not tolerate immunosuppression well, and poor survival is likely.
Severe pulmonary vascular hypertension	Normal transplanted right ventricle fails when faced with acute, severe increase in workload.
Irreversible renal and hepatic failure	Organs are damaged further by immunosuppressive therapy; poor survival is likely.
Malignancy, severe peripheral or cerebrovascular disease	These conditions limit long-term survival.
Active peptic ulcer disease and insulin-dependent diabetes	Conditions are exacerbated by steroid therapy. Diabetic patients are prone to poor wound healing and may be more prone to infection.
Active infection	Infection is exacerbated by immunosuppression; poor risk for survival.
Potential sites of infection (recent pulmonary infarction, embolus, open wounds)	High risk of infection.
History of substance abuse that resulted in previous noncompliance with a medical regime or interfered with work performance or family relationships. Careful individual evaluation indicated.	A history of poor compliance and disruption of work and family relationships may indicate the patient is at high risk for future noncompliance. This may not be a contraindication if patient has successfully recovered from previous substance abuse problem.

options. A child with severe pulmonary vascular disease is not a cardiac transplant candidate because of the likelihood of irreversible right ventricular failure after transplantation. Pediatric transplantation has been at a plateau since the early nineties. Neonatal transplantation is performed on a smaller scale. In 2001, 64 children younger than age 1 year underwent transplantation; 1% of this donor population cause of death was form sudden infant death syndrome (*2002 Annual Report*). Once a child reaches late adolescence, it becomes feasible to use adult donor hearts, and organ procurement is no more difficult than it is with adults. However, there has been a trend over the past 10 years to transplant pediatric donor hearts into children because the allocation policy gives preference for the pediatric recipient to receive the pediatric donor organ (*2002 Annual Report*).

As previously indicated, the potential transplant recipient must not have fixed irreversible pulmonary hypertension. This is defined as a pulmonary vascular resistance greater than 6 to 8 Wood units. The presence of severe pulmonary hypertension would result in certain right ventricular failure in a newly transplanted heart. The transplanted heart is developed normally and not accustomed to pumping against such elevated pressures. Irreversible hepatic and renal failure also may preclude transplantation. Some dysfunction may exist, but this should be because of the patient's low cardiac output and is expected to reverse with replacement with a healthy heart. Cyclosporine, tacrolimus, and azathioprine have untoward side effects on renal and hepatic function, respectively. Irreversible failure in either organ limits the possibility of survival.

Other systemic conditions that contraindicate transplantation include malignancy, severe peripheral or cerebrovascular disease, and active peptic ulcer disease. Insulin-dependent diabetes does not appear to effect outcome and does not contraindicate transplantation unless associated with severe end-organ disease (Frazier, 1996). Patients with mild diabetes may be candidates. Most centers also view cured (no evidence of disease for more than 5 years), nonmetastatic malignancies as a relative contraindication (Deng, 2002). All these conditions may limit long-term survival, and the required steroid therapy would exacerbate active peptic ulcer disease and insulin-dependent diabetes. Any active infection would progress rapidly after immunosuppression; patients with active infection are excluded for that reason. Any patient with a condition that places him or her at high risk for infection is also excluded. Because the lungs are the most frequent site of infections, patients who had a recent pulmonary infarction or embolus are excluded until these conditions resolve.

Donor Characteristics

It is widely recognized that pronouncement of death can be based on neurologic criteria (Veith et al., 1978). People who have sustained complete and irreversible destruction of the brain and have met the criteria for brain death may become heart donors. The most common causes of brain death among heart donors are blunt head trauma, gunshot wounds, intracerebral hemorrhage, and cerebral anoxia. Donors are typically men younger than 30 years of age. Donor age ranges from newborn to 70 years of age, with the average being 26.7 years. Seventy percent of donors are men (Hertz et al., 2002). Male heart donors may be considered up to the age of 40 to 45 years, however older donors are considered based on need, negative cardiac history, negative echocardiogram and/or negative preprocurement coronary angiography (Zaroff et al., 2001).

Nurses play an important role in managing the care of heart donors. Once brain death has occurred, hemodynamic instability potentially can develop in donors because of several factors. Hypotension in a donor may be caused by multiple contributing clinical conditions. Preexisting fluid deficits may be present in donors who were treated with diuretics to decrease cerebral edema and may precipitate hypotension. In addition, with the death of the brainstem and loss of the vasomotor center, vascular tone is lost, resulting in vascular dilatation and subsequent hypotension. It is crucial to restore intravascular volume to avoid serious hypotension. With loss of pituitary function, antidiuretic hormone secretion ceases. This change contributes to the development of diabetes insipidus and subsequent decreased intravascular volume. After correcting intravascular volume deficits with fluid administration, vasomotor tone may be supported with a vasopressor agent. Dopamine hydrochloride is used most often because of its property of renovascular dilatation and its beneficial effects on renal perfusion. Diabetes insipidus is treated with aqueous vasopressin, which increases reabsorption of water by the renal tubules.

Surgical Procedure

Once accepted into a transplantation program, the recipient must wait for the donor heart. This requires a residence close to the hospital. Recipients often carry telepagers or beepers and are "on call" for a donor heart. When a donor is available, the recipient is admitted rapidly to the hospital and prepared for surgery. Because little time is available for preoperative teaching and preparation for the recovery process, the major portion of that is performed during the initial candidacy evaluation and during the process of informed consent.

Donor and recipient are matched by ABO blood group, weight, and body size. Lymphocyte crossmatch is necessary for those recipients whose lymphocytes react to crossmatch testing (performed when recipients are accepted as transplantation candidates) against standard pools of lymphocytes from multiple serum donors.

The original surgical technique for orthotopic heart transplantation described by Shumway and colleagues in 1960 has remained the standard procedure (Shumway & Lower, 1966). After a median sternotomy and the initiation of CPB, the recipient's heart is removed, leaving the posterior walls of the atria intact (Fig. 29-7). The inflows of the two venae cavae and the pulmonary veins are left in place and unaltered. Both the aorta and pulmonary artery are transected. Then the atrial walls of the donor heart are anastomosed to the recipient atria, with care taken to avoid injury to the donor heart's sinus node. After atrial anastomosis, the donor pulmonary artery and aorta are anastomosed to the recipient vessels. On completion of the procedure, temporary epicardial atrial and frequently ventricular pacing wires are placed. Before closing the chest, mediastinal drainage tubes are secured as with any cardiac surgical procedure.

An alternative technique is referred to as total orthotopic heart transplantation or the bicaval and pulmonary venous anastomosis. The basic features of the bicaval method are complete excision of the recipient atria and donor heart implantation with bicaval end-to-end anastomosis. Proponents of this technique cite the potential for more synchronous atrial contraction, reduction of pacemaker implantation, and atrioventricular valve regurgitation (Trento et al.,1996).

Medical Management

In the immediate postoperative period, postoperative care is similar to that of any cardiac surgical patient. Transplant recipients are intubated and mechanically ventilated for 12 to 24 hours and require hemodynamic stabilization. Differences in care revolve around the patient's likely debilitated preoperative status, potential manifestations of ischemia in the donor heart, potential cardiac rejection, and immunosuppression.

Impact of Preoperative Status

Cardiac transplant recipients were in chronic low cardiac output states before transplantation surgery. They likely had poor nutritional status and were relatively immobile. Many were hospitalized with an acute exacerbation of heart failure and, in some cases, cardiogenic shock. Maintenance of adequate nutrition during the preoperative phase is difficult because of the anorexia, nausea, and impaired digestion and absorption associated with serious cardiac failure.

After transplantation, interventions to improve nutritional status are important because the patient is immunosuppressed. Postoperative basal metabolic requirements are increased at the same

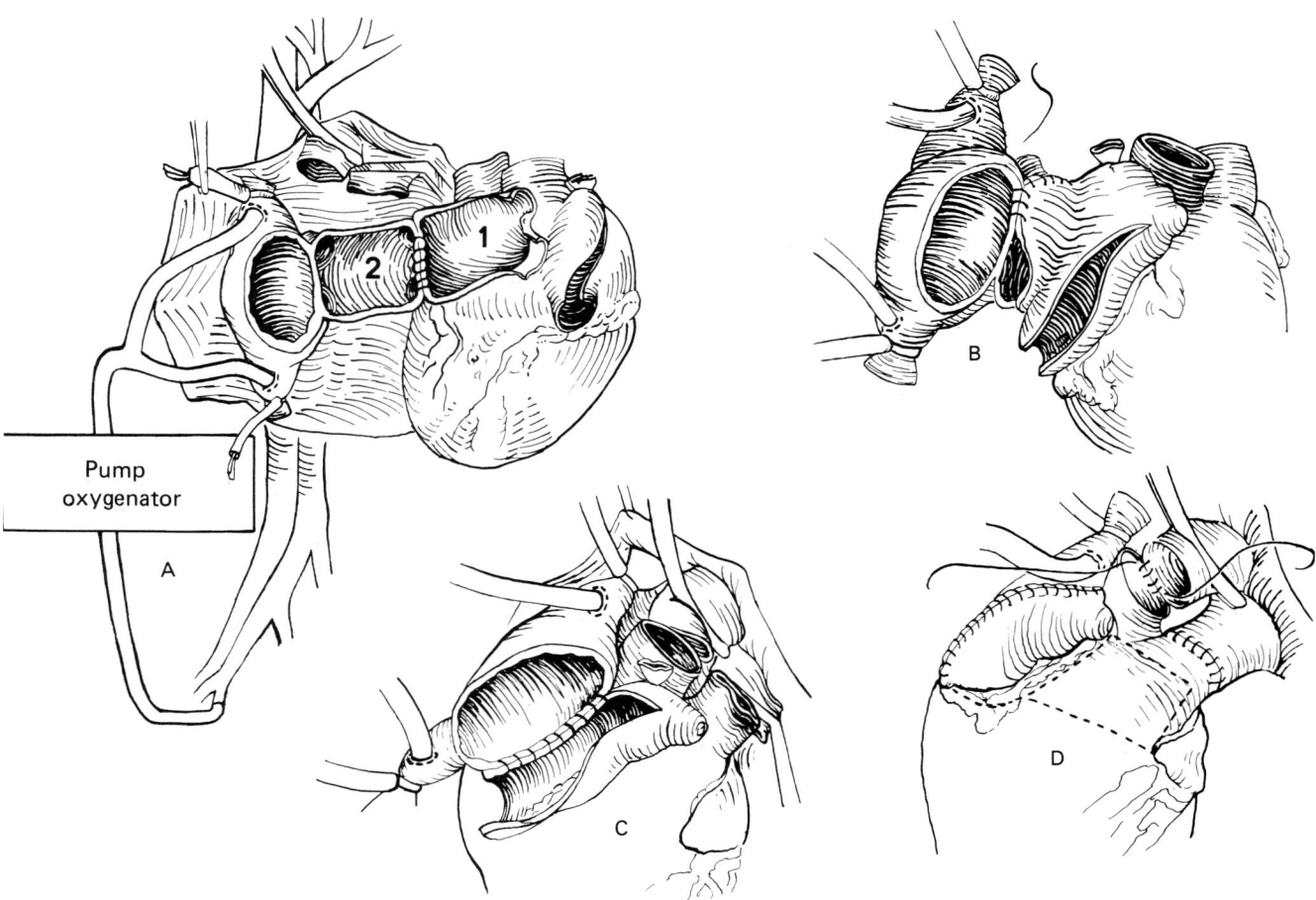

■ Figure 29–7. (*A*) Cardiac transplantation begins by suturing the donor left atrium (1) to the posterior wall of the recipient left atrium (2). (*B*) The intra-atrial septa are anastomosed, followed by (*C*) anastomosis of the right atrial wall. (*D*) The final step is the anastomosis of the donor and recipient great vessels. (Adapted from Cooley, D. A., & Norman, J. L. [1975]. *Techniques in cardiac surgery* [p. 220]. Houston: Texas Medical Press.)

time corticosteroid therapy is accelerating protein catabolism. Maintaining adequate nutrition is important to minimize postoperative complications and to facilitate recovery and rehabilitation (Frazier et al., 1995). Diet becomes an important factor in minimizing some of the side effects of corticosteroid therapy (Shinn, 1985). Diet can be supplemented with hyperalimentation and intravenous lipid preparations in sicker patients.

Preoperative cardiac failure potentially contributes to postoperative renal and hepatic dysfunction as a result of the chronic low cardiac output state. Elevated serum creatinine levels are evidence of renal dysfunction. Because cyclosporine and tacrolimus may induce nephrotoxicity, careful attention must be given to monitoring renal status. An elevated preoperative serum creatinine may be an indication to reduce cyclosporine/tacrolimus dosage or even delay by a few days postoperative administration of the drug. Weekly urine creatinine clearance tests may be ordered to follow postoperative renal function closely.

Preoperative hepatomegaly from chronic heart failure may precipitate postoperative bleeding due to clotting deficiencies associated with compromised hepatic function. Vitamin K deficiency also may contribute to the problem. It is fairly routine to administer fresh-frozen plasma and vitamin K

before transplantation to minimize the expected coagulopathy. The risk of bleeding is increased slightly in patients who have had previous cardiac surgery. Previous surgery usually requires more dissection through adhesions that formed during the previous healing process. Coagulation status and blood loss are monitored carefully during the postoperative period. Treatment of coagulopathy is usually addressed with the administration of fresh-frozen plasma and platelets. Autotransfusion is the preferred approach to blood replacement. If additional replacement is required, consideration is given to the recipient's cytomegalovirus (CMV) status. If the titer is negative, the patient should receive only blood that also has a negative CMV titer to avoid the possibility of introducing an opportunistic infection.

Cardiac Function

Although the donor heart is protected from ischemia with cold saline immersion and cardioplegia, it may still incur some ischemia that is evident during the immediate postoperative period. The transplanted heart benefits from pharmacologic ß-receptor stimulation in the early postoperative period. Isoproterenol is used routinely for up to 4 days to augment contractility,

Table 29–3 ■ HEMODYNAMIC SUPPORT IN THE IMMEDIATE POSTOPERATIVE PERIOD

Heart rate and rhythm	Isoproterenol titrated to maintain heart rate >100 beats/min; range 0.5 to 1 μg/min
	Atrial pacing to maintain sinus rhythm
Contractility	Isoproterenol as above maintained for 4 postoperative days
Renal perfusion	Dopamine hydrochloride 3 μg/kg/min
	May be increased for inotropic effect
Blood pressure control	Sodium nitroprusside titrated to maintain mean arterial pressure between 65 and 85 mm Hg; maximum dose 5 μg/kg/min
Volume therapy	Normal saline, plasma expanders, or blood products to maintain central venous pressure 8–12 mm Hg
Pulmonary vasodilation	Prostaglandin E_1 used for elevated pulmonary vascular resistance or long donor ischemic times associated with right ventricular dysfunction

atrioventricular conduction, and heart rate. The denervated heart cannot respond to the autonomic nervous system and depends on circulating catecholamines. Unfortunately, isoproterenol is no longer widely available. Atrial pacing is now commonly used to support heart rate and dopamine to support contractility. Underlying bradycardia and junctional rhythms are not uncommon during this time. Because node dysfunction can occur as a result of injury during procurement, surgery, or distortion of the atria with transplantation, or it may be acquired as the result of cardiac rejection (Bexton et al., 1984). Temporary atrial pacing may also be used for arrhythmia issues during the immediate postoperative period. Once the heart has recovered from the trauma of surgery, a normal intrinsic heart rate of approximately 100 beats/min becomes evident. Sinus node dysfunction is common, and 6% to 10% of patients may require permanent pacemaker implantation (DiBiase et al., 1991).

Blood pressure control with sodium nitroprusside therapy is usually required for the first 24 to 48 hours after surgery. In patients with high preoperative pulmonary artery pressures, inhaled nitric oxide therapy may be used to dilate the pulmonary vascular bed and reduce afterload in the graft right ventricle. Pulmonary artery pressures decrease over the next few days, while the right ventricle adjusts to its new workload. Dopamine hydrochloride is administered at doses of 3 mcg/kg per minute or less to enhance renal vascular blood flow. This drug is usually discontinued after the first 24 to 48 hours. Table 29-3 outlines hemodynamic support in the immediate postoperative period.

Monitoring Rejection

Rejection of the heart is triggered by the presence of antigens on the surface of the cells of the transplanted heart. There are three forms of rejection: hyperacute, acute, and chronic.

Hyperacute rejection occurs when the recipient has preformed cytotoxic antibodies to the donor antigens (Rose, 1986). Hyperacute rejection may result from ABO blood group incompatibility. Matching the donor and recipient ABO blood group prevents this origin of rejection. The potential recipient is screened for the presence of preformed cytotoxic antibodies by mixing the recipient's serum with a known pool of different antigens. Results of the antibody screening are reported as percentage of reactive antibody (%PRA). If the recipient has cytotoxic antibodies present, more specific testing for compatibility with a specific donor heart can be done by mixing recipient serum with that donor's lymphocytes. This testing identifies if the potential recipient has cytotoxic antibodies that will react to that specific donor heart. Hyperacute rejection results in immediate, irreversible heart failure and can be treated only by re-transplantation.

Acute rejection is the most frequently occurring form of rejection and is a major cause of death within the first year after transplantation (Hertz et al., 2002). Preoperative immunosuppressive therapy is begun in anticipation of acute cardiac rejection. Routine monitoring for acute rejection is centered around endomyocardial biopsy. With cyclosporine/tacrolimus therapy, there are few clinically evident signs and symptoms of acute rejection. The objective is to detect acute rejection in its early stages at a time when the process can be reversed, thus preventing serious, permanent damage to the new heart. Therefore, biopsy remains the gold standard for monitoring and early detection of acute rejection. Because acute rejection is expected to occur during the first 3 months after surgery, biopsy is performed within the first 14 days after transplantation, and then up to once per week during this crucial time interval. Any time that rejection is suspected, biopsies are performed frequently to monitor the progress of antirejection treatment. By 1 month, the biopsy schedule is tapered to every other week, then once per month after the third month. Patients are then monitored indefinitely by biopsy every 4 months to annually, depending on the transplant center.

The biopsy procedure is routinely performed in the catheterization laboratory but may be performed in the operating room or echocardiography laboratory. It can be performed in 15 to 30 minutes and requires only local anesthesia. Figure 29-8 illustrates the technique of endocardial specimen retrieval

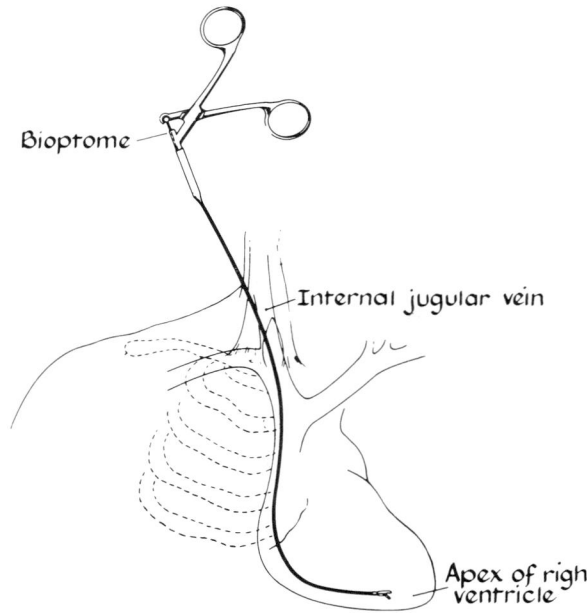

■ **Figure 29–8.** To perform a biopsy, a bioptome is introduced by way of the internal jugular vein and advanced to the right ventricular apex, where several pieces of tissue are retrieved for analysis.

Table 29-4 ■ INTERNATIONAL SOCIETY OF HEART AND LUNG TRANSPLANTATION STANDARD GRADING OF CARDIAC REJECTION

Grade	Nomenclature
0	No rejection
1	A, Focal, mild
	B, Diffuse, mild
2	One aggressive infiltrate, focal moderate
3	A, Multifocal aggressive, moderate
	B, Diffuse inflammatory process
4	Diffuse, aggressive, with necrosis, severe acute rejection

from the right ventricle. Mild rejection may resolve spontaneously and is often not treated. It is characterized by endocardial and interstitial infiltrate, International Society of Heart and Lung Transplantation (ISHLT) grade 1A, 1B, and 2. Moderate rejection is characterized by the presence of myocyte necrosis and perivascular, endocardial, and interstitial infiltration of immunoblasts (ISHLT grade 3A, 3B). Severe rejection results in myocyte and vascular necrosis with hemorrhage and a mixed infiltrate of immunoblasts and neutrophils (ISHLT grade 4) (Rose, 1986). Resolving rejection is evidenced by active fibrosis, which represents reparative changes. Table 29-4 outlines the heart biopsy grading system adopted by the ISHLT in 1990 (Billingham et al., 1990). Treatment of rejection depends on the grade of rejection, length of time from transplantation, clinical findings, symptoms, and the presence or absence of hemodynamic compromise.

Accelerated graft coronary heart disease or graft atherosclerosis, often referred to as chronic rejection, may be present in up to 50% of patients 5 years after transplantation (Gao et al., 1995). This type of rejection is thought to be caused by a complex combination of immunologic and non-immunologic injury to the coronary arteries and results in diffuse obliterative vascular lesions (Deng, 2002). Severe myocardial fibrosis occurs as a result and can cause serious myocardial dysfunction. Occlusive lesions also may precipitate MI. Exercise stress testing, annual cardiac catheterization, and intravascular coronary ultrasound are used to monitor for the development or progression of this condition. These are necessary because of the denervated state of the heart. The patient does not experience the early warning signs of angina if arterial occlusions are causing ischemia. Chronic rejection is treated with retransplantation. The diffuse nature of the condition usually precludes the use of CABG or angioplasty as treatment options (Aranda & Hill, 2000).

Monitoring for Infection

Infection is an ever-present threat to the immunosuppressed cardiac transplant recipient and is almost inevitable at some point during the postoperative course. It is a major cause of morbidity and mortality (Deng, 2002; Hertz et al., 2002). Patients on multiple immunosuppressants at high doses are at greater risk. Bacterial infections are the most common form of infection. Fungal, viral, and protozoan infections are the most difficult to treat. Prophylactic regimes have been shown to be

effective in transplant recipients to prevent or attenuate opportunistic infections. Trimethoprim-sulfamethoxazole is used against *Pneumocystis carinii*, and intravenous ganciclovir is used after surgery for 4 to 6 weeks against CMV activation or reactivation; in addition, hyperimmune globulin may be used in CMV-seronegative recipients of a seropositve donor (Valantine, 1995; Deng, 2002).

Hand washing and universal precautions are used as the mainstays of protection in the hospitalized patient. Infection is monitored for closely. Because the lungs are the primary site of infection, daily chest radiographs are performed immediately after surgery, as well as chest auscultation every 4 hours. Good pulmonary assessment is extremely important. Incentive spirometry, early mobility, and coughing and deep breathing are used to minimize atelectasis and possible infection. A temperature rise over 37°C, changes on the chest radiograph, or development of a cough are indications for obtaining sputum cultures. A temperature increase more than 38°C is an indication for blood cultures. Otherwise, routine laboratory screening for infection is performed on a weekly basis, except white blood cell counts, which are performed daily.

Monitoring for Immunosuppressive Drug Side Effects

Specific adverse effects and clinical manifestations of common immunosuppressive drugs are outlined in Table 29-5. Several side effects have implications for patient teaching and coaching and warrant further discussion. Nurses play a key role in providing patients with knowledge of drug side effects and methods of self-monitoring. It is important that patients are able to detect problems that can be injurious to their health and know when to seek medical attention. A knowledgeable patient also can take steps to minimize some of these problems. Some of the drug side effects may be particularly emotionally troublesome for patients. Nurses can do much to prepare them for this and assist them with strategies for coping with these side effects.

Calcineurin Inhibitors

Cyclosporine. Cyclosporine (Sandimmune, Neoral, Gengraf, Eon) is a natural metabolite found in a fungus. It is a lymphokine synthesis inhibitor that profoundly inhibits cell-mediated immunity. It also impairs interleukin secretion by macrophages. Cyclosporine selectively interferes in the immune system, specifically targeting T cells; this specificity allows the body to retain some ability to protect itself from infection (Baran et al., 2002; Taylor, 2000). The drug must be used cautiously and monitored closely. Cyclosporine is nephrotoxic, leading to a decrease in glomerular filtration rate, renal plasma, and blood flow (Meyers et al., 1984; Moran et al., 1985). Cyclosporine-induced arterial hypertension has been reported to be as high as 100% and is a difficult problem to control in the long-term survivor (Thompson et al., 1983). It is important to maintain a consistent administration time for cyclosporine. Equally important is timely acquisition of blood specimens for cyclosporine levels after the last dose of the drug. Cyclosporine has numerous drug interactions with common medications. Cyclosporine is metabolized by the cytochrome P-450 system,

Table 29–5 ■ MAJOR ADVERSE SIDE EFFECTS OF IMMUNOSUPPRESSIVE AGENTS AND CLINICAL MANIFESTATIONS

Drug	Adverse Effects	Clinical Manifestations
Cyclosporine	Nephrotoxicity	Elevated BUN and creatinine.
		Decreased urine output
		Weight gain, edema
	Hypertension	Elevated blood pressure
	Hepatotoxicity	Elevated bilirubin
		Elevated alkaline phosphatase, AST, and ALT levels
		Jaundice
	Hypertrichosis	Excessive hair growth all over body
	Tremors, seizures	Fine motor tremors, especially hands
		Associated paresthesias
		Seizure activity
	Increased risk of malignancy when associated with high doses of multiple agents	Dependent on type and location of malignancy
	Gingival hyperplasia	Growth of gums over teeth
		Bleeding of gums
Tacrolimus	Nephrotoxicity associated with high doses	Elevated BUN and creatinine
		Decreased urine output
	Hyperkalemia	Elevated potassium levels
	Insomnia	Sleep disturbances
	Malaise	Headaches, nausea, and vomiting associated with IV administration
Corticosteroids	Aseptic necrosis of bone, osteoporosis	Pain in weight-bearing joints
		Pathologic fractures
	Hyperglycemia, steroid-induced diabetes mellitus	Elevated serum glucose
		Polydipsia, polyuria
	Salt and water retention	Weight gain or fluctuations associated with edema
	Hypertension	Elevated blood pressure
	Skin alterations	
	Acne	Rash or pimples on face and trunk
	Sun sensitivity	Susceptibility to sunburn
		Skin malignancies
	Hirsutism	Excessive hair growth on face, trunk, and extremities
	Growth retardation in children	Failure to reach normal height for age
	Gastritis/gastrointestinal ulcerations	Abdominal pain, dysphagia
		Hematemesis, guaiac-positive stools
	Cataracts	Visual acuity problems
Azathioprine	Bone marrow depression	Leukopenia, thrombocytopenia, anemia
	Hepatotoxicity	Elevated bilirubin
		Elevated alkaline phosphatase, AST, and ALT levels
		Jaundice
	Increased risk of malignancy when associated with high doses of multiple agents	Dependent on type and location of malignancy
	Sun sensitivity of skin	Susceptibility to sunburn
		Skin malignancies
Orthocione OKT3	Pyrexia, malaise	Fever, chills, influenza-like symptoms
		Headache, diarrhea
	Respiratory distress associated with intial doses and fluid overload	Chest tightness, dyspnea, wheezing
	Increased risk of malignancy when associated with high doses of multiple agents	Dependent on type and location of malignancy
Antithymocyte preparations	Anaphylactic reactions	Hypotension, dyspnea, wheezing, fever, chills
	Serum sickness associated with antibody formation to foreign protein	Fever, joint pain
		Elevation of BUN and creatinine
	Bone marrow depression associated with prolonged use in conjunction with azathioprine	Leukopenia
		Thrombocytopenia
		Anemia
	Local inflammatory reactions associated with intramuscular administration	Pain, redness, extreme muscle soreness, swelling
	Increased risk of malignancy when associated with high doses of multiple agents	Dependent on type and location of malignancy
Mycophenolate mofiteil	Bone marrow suppression	Neutropenia
	Gastrointestinal disturbance	Nausea, vomiting, diarrhea, constipation
	Malaise	Headache, nausea
Rapammune	Bone marrow suppression	Anemia, thrombocytopenia
	Hypercholesteremia	Elevated serum cholesterol, elevated triglycerides
	Hyperlipidemia	Elevated serum lipid levels
	Hypertension	Elevated blood pressure

ALT, alanine aminotransferase; AST, aspartate aminotransferase; BUN, blood urea nitrogen. (Urden, L. D., Stacy, K. M., & Lough, M. E. [Eds.]. [2002]. *Critical care nursing: Diagnosis and management* [4th ed., pp. 998–1001]. St. Louis: Mosby; Micromedex Healthcare Series: Micromedex, Inc. Breenwood Village, CO (edition expires 9/03). Available: http://hcs.mdx.com (accessed April 2003); Luikart, H. [2001]. Pediatric transplantation: Management issues. *Journal of Pediatric Nursing, 16*, 320–331.)

so drugs that affect the P-450 system alter the metabolism of cyclosporine (Wagoner, 1997). It is extremely important for nurses to know most of these interactions to avoid adverse side effects, in addition to understanding the pharmacology of cyclosporine. Patients are taught to take this drug after meals to decrease the possibility of gastrointestinal intolerance and to promote absorption.

Hypertension is a serious side effect that often is difficult to control. Patients need to monitor their hypertension and should be taught how to take an accurate blood pressure. They are also sent home with an understanding of what symptoms, such as headaches, may indicate their hypertension has become uncontrolled.

Cyclosporine therapy does result in changed bodily appearance, particularly diffuse increased hair growth. Changed bodily appearance was reported in 34% of 44 patients on cyclosporine and corticosteroid protocols (Lough et al., 1987). Excessive hair growth was reported in 45% of the patients. Nurses can coach patients to prepare for this side effect and provide ideas for managing this problem. Cyclosporine can also cause neurotoxicity, and patients may exhibit tremors and report headache.

Tacrolimus. Tacrolimus (Prograf), formally referred to as FK506, is a potent immunosuppressive macrolide antibiotic. Tacrolimus acts by inhibition of the earliest steps of T-cell activation in a manner similar to that of cyclosporine. It was initially used in liver and kidney transplantation with successful results, and it is now used as a frequent alternative to cyclosporine. It is used as an effective agent for rescue therapy in refractory cardiac rejection and as a primary immunosuppressant in some centers (Przepiorka, 1992).

Tacrolimus has demonstrated that it is well tolerated in general. It is nephrotoxic, as is cyclosporine, and has a slightly higher diabetogenic effect (DrugPoints, 2003). Tacrolimus does not cause hirsutism, gingival hyperplasia, or facial dysmorphism as cyclosporine can. Its primary side effects are headache, nausea, and tremors. It is important to monitor patient blood levels, kidney function, and blood glucose. Tacrolimus is also similar to cyclosporine in that it is metabolized through the P-450 system; therefore, similar drug interactions are present (Wagoner, 1997).

Corticosteroids. The anti-inflammatory actions of corticosteroids provide important protection of the transplanted heart against damage from rejection. Steroids impair the sensitivity of T cells to the foreign antigen, decrease proliferation of sensitized T cells, and decrease macrophage mobility. Long-term corticosteroid therapy may be associated with several side effects that require monitoring. Glucose intolerance may develop during hospitalization and persist long enough to require insulin therapy. Insulin coverage is initiated for serum glucose levels in excess of 200 to 250 mg/dL. This necessitates patient instruction on diet management and self-administration of insulin. Weight gain is problematic for many patients. Diet instruction and initiation of exercise programs may help minimize this problem. Regular exercise is also thought to be important in minimizing the calcium loss from bone associated with long-term corticosteroid therapy. Stress ulceration is a concern in patients on higher doses of corticosteroid therapy for long periods. Nurses need to be aware of the possibility and be alert to signs or symptoms that may indicate a problem. It is also necessary to teach the importance of good skin care. Fragile skin that heals poorly may become a problem with the long-term patient. Patients should be taught to monitor the condition of their skin and be alert for lesions that do not heal well or that become infected.

Fragile skin and bruising were reported to occur often or always in up to 60% of patients on corticosteroid and azathioprine protocols. Changed facial and bodily appearance was reported by 43%. Poor vision, a problem associated with corticosteroid therapy, was "quite a bit" or "extremely" upsetting to 30% of patients (Lough et al.,1987; Lough et al., 1985).

Azathioprine. Azathioprine (Imuran) is used as a maintenance drug to prevent activation and proliferation of T cells in response to the foreign antigen or the transplanted heart. It is an antimetabolite that interferes with purine synthesis. Purine synthesis is necessary for antibody production and for synthesis of nucleic acids in rapidly proliferating cells, such as the cells of the immune system (Crandell, 1990). Prevention of this cell proliferation can also impair other rapidly proliferating cells in the body and cause conditions such as leukopenia, thrombocytopenia, and anemia. It is important to monitor the patient's white blood cell count closely and titrate the dose of the drug accordingly.

Mycophenolate Mofetil. Mycophenolate mofetil (Cell-Cept) is an immunosuppressive agent that inhibits the *de novo* pathway of purine synthesis in activated lymphocytes. Mycophenolate mofetil works at a late stage in T-cell activation, in contrast to cyclosporine and tacrolimus, which inhibit the earliest events. Mycophenolate mofetil has been shown to have activity against B cells; therefore, it may have a role in preventing graft atherosclerosis (Wagoner, 1997).

Multicenter trials have shown that mycophenolate mofetil is an effective immunosuppressant, safe and well tolerated in kidney and heart transplant recipients. It is less myelosuppressive than azathioprine, thereby avoiding the neutropenia and anemia, and less hepatotoxic as well. Its major side effects are gastrointestinal disturbances. Nausea, vomiting, and diarrhea are the most frequently reported symptoms. These symptoms are usually self-limiting and dose-dependent (Kirklin et al., 1994).

Antilymphocyte Antibodies

Orthoclone OKT3. Orthoclone OKT3 is a monoclonal antibody that is targeted to remove T cells from circulation through the formation of antigen-antibody complexes (Crandell, 1990). It can be used initially after transplantation to eliminate the T-cell response in the first 14 postoperative days, or can be used to treat a later rejection episode. Patients can acquire sensitivity to the drug and form antibodies against the foreign protein. For that reason, usually only one 7-day course of the drug is given. Adverse effects are caused by the massive lysis of T cells, resulting in general malaise, fever, and chills.

Antithymocyte Preparations. Like orthoclone OKT3, antithymocyte preparations are antibodies produced by animals in response to foreign human T cells. They are polyclonal preparations pooled from multiple animals, however, with much variation in potency, and are not specific for the T cell most important in the rejection process. These preparations are used only to treat severe rejection after standard antirejection therapy has failed. The course of therapy is typically 5 days. As with orthoclone OKT3, adverse effects are associated with the massive lysis of T cells, causing fever and chills (Crandell, 1990). Although rare, patients can have anaphylactic reactions to the foreign animal protein.

Sirolimus and Everolimus

Sirolimus. Sirolimus (Rapamune) and its derivative Everolimus (Certican, Rad) is an antibiotic similar to tacrolimus except that it has a different mechanism of action. Sirolimus prevents cell cycle activation and t-cell proliferation. Sirolimus and its derivatives may be synergistic with the calcineuron inhibitors. These drugs are dosed orally once or twice daily. Blood trough levels are measured for dose monitoring. Research studies suggest that Rapamycin treatment may prevent or even reverse allograft vascular disease (Taylor, 2000). The common side effects of sirolimus are increased levels of triglycerides, decrease in hemoglobin and platelet count, tremors, and arthralgias (Baran et al., 2002).

Daclizumab and Basiliximab. Daclizumab and Basiliximab are newer monoclonal antibodies. They are hybrid, humanized interleukin-2 receptor antibodies. The advantage of these agents is the minimal administration side effects that other monoclonal have exhibited, and the apparent usefulness in preventing early rejection (Taylor, 2000; Baren et al., 2002).

Complications

Hypertension

Hypertension is a long-term, ever-present complication that requires considerable attention. Hypertension is caused in large part by the calcineurin inhibitors that are known to cause chronic nephropathy; in addition, cyclosporine is implicated in the activation of the sympathetic nervous system, resulting in hypertension (Eisen, 2003). Patients are managed on one, two, or three agents because of the tenacity of the hypertension.

Transplant Vasculopathy

Cardiac allograft vasculopathy (CAV) is an accelerated and diffuse form of coronary heart disease unique to the transplanted heart. It is the major cause of death in the long-term heart transplant patient (Deng, 2002). CAV is a peculiar kind of vasculopathy characterized by diffuse and concentric vascular inflammation and smooth muscle proliferation. It results in coronary lumen loss, ischemia, silent MI, and graft loss, which can present as a sudden death (Aranda & Hill, 2000).

Treatment of CAV is limited because of the diffuse nature of the disease, and it is not typically amenable to usual palliative interventions such as angioplasty, atherectomy, or coronary artery bypass. Re-transplantation is the only definitive treatment, and it is fraught with high morbidity and mortality rates, and brings fourth the debate regarding the use of limited donor supply.

Sexual Dysfunction

Sexual dysfunction is a prevalent problem in cardiac transplantation recipients. Impotence is not uncommon, and much of it

can be attributed to the requirement for antihypertensive therapy. Patients would benefit from knowing that these occurrences are not uncommon. They need to feel comfortable voicing concerns and reporting future problems so that appropriate counseling or other assistance can be provided.

Conditioning and Exercise Training

Physical rehabilitation is a necessary part of the posttransplantation patient recovery program. Physical therapy is needed to ameliorate the deconditioning of the pre-transplantation, heart failure state and to decrease the sequelae of the immunosuppressants and surgical procedure (Sadowsky, 1996). Low-level exercise is begun with extremity and shoulder flexion, extension, and abduction exercises. The intensity and duration are progressed to the patient's tolerance (Sadowsky, 1986). These low-level exercises serve as warm-up for more intensive exercises once the patient can complete the low-level program without undue fatigue or balance loss.

Bicycle ergometry is usually introduced within 3 days. Intensity and duration are gradually progressed according to patient response. By discharge, most patients are able to cycle for 20 minutes without resistance and for 5 minutes with resistance. With cardiac denervation, heart rate response to exercise is abnormal.

The ability to perform any exercise beyond mild in intensity depends on circulating catecholamines to increase heart rate, contractility, and cardiac output. The normal, immediate increase in heart rate induced by exercise is absent in the denervated heart, and several minutes are required before heart rate can increase. Warm-up exercise is necessary before vigorous activity, and its duration should be approximately 5 minutes. Deceleration of heart rate after exercise is prolonged. The patient's heart rate may not return to resting levels for up to 20 minutes after cessation of the activity. Prolonged cool-down periods are also necessary. Figure 29-9 illustrates a typical response to exercise.

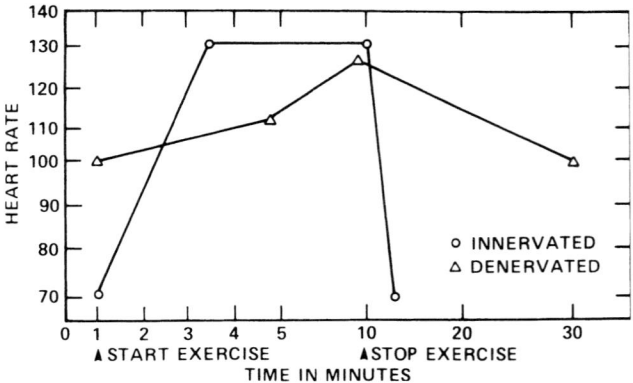

■ **Figure 29–9.** Sample differences in response to exercise between an innervated and denervated heart. (From McKelvey, S.A. [1985]. Effects of denervation in the cardiac transplant recipient. In M. K. Douglas, & J. A. Shinn [Eds.], *Advances in cardiovascular nursing* [p. 201]. Rockville, MD: Aspen Systems.)

Table 29–6 CARDIAC TRANSPLANT RECIPIENTS'
DYSPNEA INDEX FOR EXERCISE TRAINING

Level 0	No shortness of breath
	Can count to 15 without taking a breath
Level 1	Mild shortness of breath
	Counts to 15 and requires one breath in the sequence: continue at this intensity
Level 2	Moderate shortness of breath Counts to 15 and requires two breaths in the same sequence; this is the desired level of intensity
Level 3	Definite shortness of breath
	Must take three breaths in the sequence of counting to 15; reduce the intensity of exercise
Level 4	Severe shortness of breath
	Unable to count or speak; cease activity

Adapted with permission from Sadowsky, H. S. Rohrkemper, K. F. & Quon, S. (1986). *Rehabilitation of cardiac and cardiopulmonary recipients,* appendix 1. Stanford, CA: Stanford University Hospital.

Patients need to understand how their response to exercise is different after transplantation. Self-monitoring techniques are taught before discharge, and continued regular exercise is encouraged. Patients are taught to use dyspnea as a guide for activity intensity rather than heart rate. The dyspnea index is presented in Table 29-6. Patients are coached not to exceed a dyspnea index greater than level 2. The rating of perceived exertion is a widely used self-monitoring tool for transplant recipient. The Borg scale is a rating of perceived exertion that is scaled from 6 (very, very easy) to 12 to 14 (somewhat hard), to 15 to 20 (very, very difficult). Patients are instructed to continue their exertion until they perceive their exercise has become somewhat hard (Sadowsky, 1996). Patients are also counseled to decrease their duration of exercise if they experience excessive fatigue during or after exercise.

Corticosteroid therapy, cyclosporine, and tacrolimus are detrimental to bone density and structure. Potential corticosteroid-induced osteoporosis puts the patient in greater jeopardy of bone fractures. Several types of medications are available to treat transplantation osteoporosis such as bisphosphonates, calcitonin, estrogen, and vitamin D. Bisphosphonates, such as alendronate, inhibit bone resorption and can prevent bone loss. Calcitonin is another antiresorptive drug. Estrogen therapy effectively prevents bone loss related to estrogen deficiency (Rodino & Shane, 1998).

Regular exercise programs help patients to control weight and to minimize calcium loss from bone. Approximately 86% of transplant recipients are considered to have class I New York Heart Association functional status. More than 90% of the recipients report having no activity limitations up to 5 years post transplant (Hertz et al., 2002). They are capable of performing most recreational activities and are advised against contact sports or other sports with high risk of injury, such as alpine skiing, unless the recipient was previously accomplished in the sport. Physician approval is recommended if patients wish to pursue vigorous running or jogging. The additional benefit of improved collateral circulation is important if chronic rejection develops at a later time.

Preparation for Discharge

Patient preparation for discharge begins in the intensive care unit and continues until discharge. It is important that patients fully understand their condition and the implications of cardiac denervation. They need to adapt to a new medical regime and must understand its importance in maintaining their state of health. Patients are discharged with multiple medications and must understand their purpose, actions, and side effects. By discharge, it is important that they assume total responsibility for self-care. Bedside flow sheets can be used by the nursing staff to indicate the progress of the patient's learning. Patients are taught how to detect signs of infection and to monitor their temperature. Cardiac risk factors should be evaluated with the patient so that strategies can be outlined to decrease risk. In addition to the primary nurse, dietitians, social workers, physical therapists, and the nurse transplantation coordinators can all contribute to patient instruction. It is important for a nurse to have good teaching skills, sensitivity to the patient's psychological needs, and an ability to communicate. These skills can greatly enhance the patient's success in learning.

Nursing Management Plan

Nursing care of the transplant recipient is, for the most part, interdependent with medical management. The exception to this is the provision of patient teaching. Nonetheless, several nursing diagnoses can be identified for the patient after cardiac transplantation. This management plan focuses on diagnoses, goals, and interventions unique to the transplant recipient. Because this patient has undergone cardiac surgery, many diagnoses used for the cardiac surgical patient can be used with the transplant recipient. Nursing Care Plan 29-1 is an outline of a nursing management plan for an uncomplicated cardiac transplantation recipient. Sample nursing diagnoses are presented. Not all possibilities have been discussed. Other diagnoses that the nurse may assess for include:

Potential fluid volume excess related to sodium and water retention from corticosteroid therapy

Potential altered nutrition: more than body requirement related to appetite increase from corticosteroid therapy

Potential fear or anxiety related to the possibility of rejection and death from complications

Altered family processes related to disruption of family life from prolonged hospitalization and need to reside in the local area for 2 to 3 months after discharge

Potential for noncompliance related to the complexity of the prescribed medical regime

Nursing Care Plan 29–1 ■ The Patient With Uncomplicated Cardiac Transplantation

Nursing Diagnosis 1 ➤ Decreased cardiac output in the immediate postoperative period related to cardiac denervation and ischemia during transplantation, manifested by bradycardia and hypotension.

Nursing Goal 1 ➤ To detect early manifestations of decreased cardiac output.

Outcome Criteria ➤
1. Patient will maintain a mean arterial blood pressure (MAP) between 70 and 90 mm Hg.
2. Patient will maintain a sinus rhythm with a heart rate (HR) of 100 to 110 beats/min.
3. Changes in above conditions will be detected within 20 minutes of occurrence.
4. Patient's skin will be warm, dry, and normal in color.
5. Nail beds will return to normal color after blanching from pressure over the capillary bed.
6. All peripheral pulses will be palpable. Urine output will be >30 mL/h.
7. Changes in 4, 5, and 6 above will be detected within an hour of occurrence.

NURSING INTERVENTIONS	RATIONALE
1. Assess and document MAP, HR, and rhythm continuously. 2. Report any HR < 100, loss of sinus rhythm, or MAP < 70 mm Hg to physician. 3. Evaluate volume status; a central venous pressure (CVP) < 8 mm Hg may indicate need for fluid. If MAP < 60 mm Hg with an adequate CVP, hypotension may be a result of decreased contractility. Notify physician if these findings occur. 4. Assess and document skin temperature, color, moisture, capillary filling, quality of peripheral pulses, and urine output hourly as needed. Report abnormal findings to physician.	1. Required to detect changes. 2. An HR < 100 may be considered bradycardic for the immediate postoperative transplantation period and may indicate the need for more isoproterenol support. Myocardial edema and manipulation of the heart during surgery increase the risk of bradycardia. Junctional rhythms occur at lesser degrees of bradycardia in the transplant recipient and loss of sinus rhythm may indicate the need for atrial pacing. Loss of blood pressure may be a result of bradycardia or loss of sinus rhythm. 3. Hypotension also may be an indication of hypovolemia or a depressed inotropic state related to ischemia incurred during surgery and organ donation. Further evaluation is required. 4. Low cardiac output will be manifested by decreased peripheral perfusion and decreased renal vascular blood flow, resulting in decreased glomerular filtration and subsequent urine output.

Nursing Goal 2 ➤ To reduce or eliminate manifestations of decreased cardiac output specifically bradycardia or hypotension

Outcome Criteria ➤
1. Within 15 minutes of intervention, HR returns to > 100 beats/min.
2. Within 15 minutes of intervention, MAP returns to > 70 mm Hg.
3. Within 30 minutes of intervention, good peripheral pulses are present, skin is warm, dry, and of normal color.

NURSING INTERVENTIONS	RATIONALE
1. Connect pacing wires to a temporary pacemaker. Obtain an order for pacing support and appropriate settings. HR is usually maintained at 100 beats/min minimum. 2. Notify physician if a junctional rhythm develops and results in bradycardia or hypotension. 3. Verify that CVP is between 8 and 12 mm Hg and administer ordered replacement fluid if CVP is below ordered minimum (usually < 8 mm Hg). 4. Notify physician if hypotension does not respond to volume therapy or is present with an adequate CVP.	1. Temporary pacing may be indicated to maintain an HR in the prescribed parameters. 2. Sinus node function may be impaired due to myocardial edema in the area of the sinus node. Atrial pacing may be indicated. 3. Hypotension may be the result of hypovolemia: a denervated heart depends on a large stroke volume to stretch myocardial fibers (Starling mechanism) and produce a strong contraction. 4. Hypotension may be the result of decreased contractility, and further inotropic support is needed.

(continued)

Nursing Care Plan 29–1 ■ (Continued)

Nursing Diagnosis 2 ➤ Potential for infection related to immunosuppression manifested by a temperature > 37.5°C, a *rising* white blood cell count, or a change in pulmonary secretions.

Nursing Goal 1 ➤ To prevent conditions and situations that predispose the patient to increased risk of infection.

Outcome Criteria ➤
1. Patient will maintain a temperature , 37°C.
2. Patient will maintain a white blood cell count between 5,000 and 10,000.
3. Patient will have normal breath sounds without cough and a clear chest radiograph.

NURSING INTERVENTIONS	RATIONALE
1. Maintain protective protocols and monitor protective technique of all visitors and staff entering the patient's room.	1. Poor technique may put the patient at risk for infection by organisms carried in the room from the outside environment.
2. Restrict plants, flowers, and unpeeled fruit from the room.	2. Plants, flowers, and unpeeled fruit, such as oranges, may harbor fungus and put the patient at risk for fungal infection.
3. Teach each patient technique for wearing mask when leaving the room. Explain rationale. (May not be required in all institutions.).	3. It is important for the patient to begin to assume responsibility for health maintenance. The hospital environment is contaminated with multiple organisms and potentially resistant strains that may jeopardize the patient not knowledgeable in precautionary techniques.
4. Monitor visitors and personnel for signs of infection and decline entry into room.	4. Some visitors and personnel may be unaware of the potential threat of a seemingly benign infection. Viral infections such as herpes simplex or colds, or infected cuts and other skin lesions, are of particular concern.
5. Change all wound, CVP insertion site, and pacemaker wire exit site dressings daily. Use absolute sterile technique.	5. Conscientious attention to potential ports of entry reduces the potential for wound, systemic, or pacemaker wire–borne infection.
6. Change all intravenous solutions, tubings, stopcocks, and any heparin-locked lines daily. (Individual program guidelines may vary from 24 to 48 hours.)	6. Intravenous lines that are frequently accessed for specimens and medications increase risk of introducing organisms into the bloodstream.
7. Monitor patient technique of self-administration of antibiotic and antifungal mouthwashes. Ensure that mouthwashes are swished throughout the mouth, are allowed to linger, and are taken after meals. Teach patient not to perform toothbrushing or eat immediately after the administration of mouthwashes.	7. The patient is at risk for opportunistic oral infection, and care must be taken to ensure that medications are used appropriately. Mouthwashes should be allowed to linger and not be followed by eating, drinking, or other rinsing, which reduce mouthwash effectiveness.
8. Restrict patient to room during rejection or if daily white blood cell count returns below target suppression level (less than 5,000). Notify physician if white blood cell count falls below 5,000.	8. Patient is at greatest risk for infection during augmented immunosuppression and any time the white blood cell count falls below target suppression level. A fall in this count indicates a need for adjustment of azathioprine dosage.
9. Provide aggressive pulmonary care, including inspirometers, deep breathing, coughing, and early mobility to prevent atelectasis.	9. Atelectasis is a risk after surgery, and its development increases the risk of pulmonary infection.

Nursing Goal 2 ➤ To detect early manifestations of infection to ensure prompt medical attention and interventio

Outcome Criteria ➤
1. Patient will have negative cultures 7 days after course of antimicrobial therapy.
2. Patient will have a white blood cell count between 5,000 and 10,000 after antimicrobial therapy.
3. Patient's temperature will return to less than 37°C after antimicrobial therapy.

NURSING INTERVENTIONS	RATIONALE
1. Obtain weekly urine, sputum, and viral cultures as ordered. Ensure that daily white blood cell counts and chest radiographs are obtained.	1. Absolute vigilance in monitoring for infection a fying organisms is crucial to successful, early tre infection.
2. Auscultate breath sounds every 4 hours. Document and immediately report changes in secretions or aeration.	2–4. Nurses are often the first to identify changes i status. The lungs are a likely site of infection, medical evaluation is important. Cultures are
3. Monitor for and report any productive or nonproductive cough.	identify appropriate antimicrobial therapy.

Nursing Care Plan 29–1 ■ (Continued)

NURSING INTERVENTIONS	RATIONALE
4. Obtain sputum cultures if quantity, composition, color, or odor changes dramatically. 5. Observe all wound, intravenous, and pacemaker wire sites daily for signs of suspect drainage, redness, swelling, or heat, and report any of these findings to the physician. 6. Obtain cultures of any suspicious drainage. 7. Obtain temperature every 4 hours. Immediately document and report any temperature greater than 37°C. 8. Obtain aerobic and anaerobic blood cultures if temperature is greater than 37°C.	5–6. Wound and insertion site infections can be well established by the time overt signs are present in the immunosuppressed patient. Prompt treatment and insertion site changes are indicated. 7–8. Corticosteroid therapy reduces normal basal and maximal body temperature. A temperature rise greater than 37°C may indicate the presence of systemic infection. It is important to obtain cultures when the temperature elevation occurs to identify possible organisms and appropriate antimicrobial therapy.

Nursing Diagnosis 3 ➤ Activity intolerance related to preoperative deconditioned state manifested by easy fatigue, decreased muscle strength, and inability to ambulate outside of room without assistance.

Nursing Goal 1 ➤ To increase activity intolerance and muscle strength to level compatible with requirements for activities of daily living and recreational exercise

Outcome Criteria ➤
1. Patient will be able to ambulate independently in room by fourth postoperative day and out of room by sixth postoperative day.
2. Patient will be able to cycle on stationary bicycle for 20 minutes at dyspnea level 2 by discharge.
3. Patient will self-monitor exercise tolerance by discharge.

NURSING INTERVENTIONS	RATIONALE

1. Obtain physical therapy consult and evaluation 2 days after transplantation.
   Begin supine in-bed exercises on first postoperative day after extubation (one session per day).
   Progress patient activity to include shoulder circles, trunk _____on, and knee flexion and extension when stable in a ____ position (one session per day).
   ____ patient is able to stand with sufficient balance, include ____ trunk lateral flexion, backward and forward bends, ____rcles in the exercise program (one session per day).
   ____ to complete previous activities without undue ____ance loss, initiate light weight resistance exer-____onary cycling (two sessions per day).
   ____cument blood pressure, dyspnea, and heart ____ercise. Monitor and document symptom ____ercise. Stop exercise:
   ____sure increases greater than 40 mm Hg ____han 15 mm Hg from baseline.
   ____ than 30 beats/min over baseline.
   ____r than level 2.
   ____ssive fatigue, or ST segment in-____than 1 mm. Report any findings ____ exercise progression with
   ____oderate or severe rejection ____uidelines.
   ____d how to obtain a pulse.
   ____.
	1. Reconditioning exercises can begin as soon as the patient is alert, extubated, and hemodynamically stable. Further inactivity may contribute to existing deconditioned state.
	2. Patients are mobile enough to perform ankle pumps and flexion and abduction of hips and shoulders.
	3–6. Slow progression of conditioning can coincide with increasing patient strength and endurance. Progression can be guided by patient tolerance and is only decreased during rejection episodes. Once rejection resolves, activity progression resumes.
	
	7. It is important to limit the amount of stress on the rejecting heart. Exercise capacity is decreased during this time.
	8. Patient must acquire self-monitoring skills for continuation of safe exercise after discharge.
	
	(continued)

d identi-
atment of
pulmonary
and prompt
necessary to
(continued)

Nursing Care Plan 29–1 ■ *(Continued)*

Nursing Diagnosis 4 ➤ Potential disturbance in self-concept related to changes in facial appearance secondary to immuno-suppressive drug therapy, manifested by subjective complaints.

Nursing Goal 1 ➤ To assist patient with identifying strategies to enhance appearance and self-esteem

Outcome Criteria ➤ 1. Patient will identify methods to minimize hirsutism and increased body hair.
2. Patient will identify methods to deemphasize cushingoid facial features.
3. Patient will remain socially involved.
4. Patient will take initiative to seek resources for enhancing appearance if desired.

NURSING INTERVENTIONS	RATIONALE
1. Introduce patient to a transplantation support group or to other patients who have had a cardiac transplantation.	1. Transplant recipients achieve a better understanding of positive adaptive measures used by other patients who have experienced transplantation.
2. Allow male patients time to shave more frequently if bothered by increased facial hair growth. Allow female patients extra time for grooming.	2–3. Cyclosporine stimulates hair follicles, causing a diffuse increase in hair growth (hypertrichosis). Corticosteroid steroid therapy contributes to the development of hirsutism. Male patients may not view this as problematic, but female patients may find this side effect to be troublesome.
3. Offer female patients possible solutions to increased body hair growth and hirsutism if perceived as disturbing. Shaving, bleaching, and cream hair removers may be suggested. Caution patient not to apply to inflamed, broken, or chapped skin.	
4. In response to expressed concerns, arrange for patients to meet with other patients or hairstyle and makeup experts to provide possible suggestions for enhancing facial features. Seek patient's agreement before initiating.	4. Hairstyle and makeup application changes can deemphasize cushingoid facial features and enhance self-confidence and self-esteem. Men may choose to grow a beard to mask cushingoid features.
5. Allow patients to initiate any changes; merely offer ideas and resources that have been helpful to others. Avoid introducing personal values and feelings about patient's change in appearance.	5. Patients are likely to have different values about their appearance, and changes may not be problematic to all. A nurse's eagerness to intervene may hinder a patient's adaptation to this alteration in appearance.

Nursing Diagnosis 5 ➤ Potential knowledge deficit about medications related to lack of familiarity, manifested by inability to self-administer medications correctly.

Nursing Goal 1 ➤ To provide patient with knowledge and skills that will allow patient to self-administer medications correctly by discharge.

Outcome Criteria ➤ 1. Patient will identify each medication by name, proper dose, dosae schedule, and potential side effects by discharge.
2. Patients will self-administer medications at correct time on a consistent basis by discharge.

NURSING INTERVENTIONS	RATIONALE
1. Set realistic goals for self-administration. Consider patient's previous experience with self-medication, present state of recovery, ability to concentrate and read printed material. Include patient in planning realistic time frames.	1. It is unrealistic to expect patients to learn multiple medications in a short time. They also may not be feeling well and may not be able to concentrate on instruction while still experiencing discomforts from surgery. Rushing learning may only increase anxiety about their capabilities.
2. Tape sample medications to a poster accompanied by the medication's name. Once the patient learns this, add side effects of the medication. Progressive information can be added as patient accomplishes learning of previous material.	2–3. A poster allows the patient visual and written information about medications. Its format allows for independent review at the patient's directed pace. Learning is more successful when a variety of materials are used.
3. Provide patient with a variety of materials to assist with learning, such as flashcards, posters, and written material.	

(continued)

Nursing Care Plan 29–1 ■ *(Continued)*

NURSING INTERVENTIONS	RATIONALE
4. Allow patient to assume gradually total responsibility for self-administration of medication. Acknowledge accomplishments. 5. Monitor patient's progress in ability to self-administer medications and document.	

NOTE: There are many other areas of potential knowledge deficit. These include:
   Prevention of infection
   Signs and symptoms of infection
   Monitoring activity progression at home
   Diet
   Treatment of rejection
   Seeking medical attention for illness or unusual symptoms
   Follow-up care
   Management of health care insurance and other financial issues
   Return to work

REFERENCES FOR CARDIAC SURGERY

Acorda, R., Kraus, T., & Casey, P. E. (2000). Advances in surgical treatment of coronary artery disease. *Nursing Clinics of North America*, 35, 913–932.

Alfieri, A., & Kotler, M. N. (1990). Noncardiac complications of open-heart surgery. *American Heart Journal*, 119, 149–157.

Antman, E. M. (1992). Medical management of the patient undergoing cardiac surgery. In E. Braunwald (Ed.), *Heart disease* (4th ed., pp. 1670–1693). Philadelphia: WB Saunders.

Ascione, R., Lloyd, C. T., & Underwood, M. J. (1999). Economic outcome of off-pump coronary artery bypass surgery: A prospective randomized controlled trial. *Annals of Thoracic Surgery*, 68, 2237–2242.

Banasik, J. L., & Tyler, M. L. (1986). The effect of prophylactic positive end expiratory pressure on mediastinal bleeding after coronary revascularization surgery. *Heart and Lung*, 15, 43–48.

Bateman, T. M., & Gray, R. J. (1990). Perioperative myocardial infarction. In R. J. Gray & J. M. Matlof (Eds.), *Medical management of the cardiac surgical patient* (pp. 12–26). Baltimore: Williams & Wilkins.

Bojar, R. M. (1999). Intraoperative considerations in cardiac surgery. In R. M. Bojar & K. G. Warner, *Manual of perioperative care in cardiac surgery* (3rd ed., pp. 93–106). Malden: Blackwell Science.

Bracey, A. W., Radovancevic, R., Riggs, S. A., et al. (1999). Lowering the threshold for transfusion in coronary bypass procedures: effect on patient outcome. *Transfusion*, 10, 1070–1077.

Braile, D., & Petrucci, O. (2000). Cardiac tamponade. In P. P. Soltoski, H. L. Karamanoukian, & T. A. Salerno, *Cardiac surgery secrets* (pp. 228–229). Philadelphia: Hanley & Belfus.

Calafiore, A. M., Di Mauro, M., & Contini, M. (2003). Left ventricular volume reduction for dilated cardiomyopathy. In K. L. Franco & E. D. Verrier (Eds.), *Advanced therapy in cardiac surgery* (pp. 415–430). Hamilton, Ontario: BC Decker.

Calafiore, A. M., Giammarco, G. D., Teodori, G., et al. (1998). Midterm results after minimally invasive coronary surgery (LAST operation). *Journal of Thoracic Cardiovascular Surgery*, 115, 763–771.

Chachques, J. C., Cattadori, B, & Carpentier, A. (2003.) Dynamic to cellular cardiomyoplasty. In K. L. Franco & E. D. Verrier (Eds.), *Advanced therapy in cardiac surgery* (pp. 431–438). Hamilton, Ontario: BC Decker.

Chatterjee, K. (1998). Recognition and management of patients with stable angina pectoris. In L. Goldman & E. Braunwald (Eds), *Primary cardiology* (pp. 234–256). Philadelphia: WB Saunders.

Chiu, R. C. (1997). Cardiomyoplasty. In L. H. Edmunds (Ed.), *Cardiac surgery in the adult* (pp. 1491–1504). New York: McGraw-Hill.

Cho, P. W., Finney, R. C. S., & Gardner, T. J. (1994). Ischemic heart disease and its complications. In W. A. Baumgartner, S. G. Owen, D. E. Cameron, et al. (Eds.), *The Johns Hopkins manual of cardiac surgical care* (pp. 335–364). St. Louis: Mosby.

Chung, M. K. (2000). Cardiac surgery: postoperative arrhythmias. *Critical Care Medicine*, 28[Suppl.], N136–N144.

Cleveland Jr., J. C., & Grover, F. L. (2003). Prophylaxis against atrial fibrillation following open heart surgery. In K. L. Franco & E. D. Verrier (Eds.), *Advanced therapy in cardiac surgery* (pp. 22–26). Hamilton, Ontario: BC Decker.

Coleman, B., Coughlan Lavieri, M., & Gross, S. (1993). Patients undergoing cardiac surgery. In J. M. Clochesy, C. Breu, S. Cardin, et al. (Eds.), *Critical care nursing* (pp. 385–436). Philadelphia: WB Saunders.

Czer, L. S. C. (1990). Mediastinal bleeding, blood conversation techniques, and transfusion practices. In R. J. Gray & J. M. Matlof (Eds.), *Medical management of the cardiac surgical patient* (pp. 55–68). Baltimore: Williams & Wilkins.

Dehoux, M., Provenchere, S., Benessiano, J., et al. (2001). Utility of cardiac troponin measurement after cardiac surgery. *Clinica Chimica Acta*, 311, 41–44.

Diodato Jr., M. D., Maniar, H. S., Prasad, S. M., et al. (2003). Robotics in cardiac surgery. In K. L. Franco & E. D. Verrier (Eds.), *Advanced therapy in cardiac surgery* (pp. 102–114). Hamilton, Ontario: BC Decker.

Drenth, D. J., Veeger, N. J., & Winter, J. B. (2002). A prospective randomized trail comparing stenting with off-pump coronary surgery for high-grade stenosis of the left anterior descending coronary artery: Three-year follow-up. *Journal of the American College of Cardiology*, 40, 1955–1960.

Duncan, C., & Erickson, R. (1982). Pressures associated with chest tube stripping. *Heart and Lung*, 11(2), 166–171.

Eagle, K. A., Guyton, R. A., Davidoff, R., et al. (1999). ACC/AHA guidelines for coronary artery bypass graft surgery: Executive summary and recommendations. *Circulation*, 100, 1464–1480.

Earp, J. K., & Mallia, G. (1997). Myocardial protection for cardiac surgery: The nursing perspective. *AACN Clinical Issues*, 8, 20–32.

Elefteriades, J. A., & Zaret, B. L. (1998). Coronary bypass: The bad ventricle. In L. R. Kaiser , I. L. Kron, & T. L. Spray (Eds.), *Mastery of cardiothoracic surgery* (pp. 409–419). Philadelphia: Lippincott-Raven.

Falk, V., Jacobs, S., Walther, T., et al. (2003). Total endoscopic bypass grafting. In K. L. Franco & E. D. Verrier (Eds.), *Advanced therapy in cardiac surgery* (pp.119–123). Hamilton, Ontario: BC Decker.

Finkelmeier, B. A. (1995a). Myocardial preservation. In B. A. Finkelmeier (Ed.), *Cardiothoracic surgical nursing* (pp. 121–125). Philadelphia: JB Lippincott.

Finkelmeier, B. A. (1995b). Cardiopulmonary bypass. In B. A. Finkelmeier (Ed.), *Cardiothoracic surgical nursing* (pp. 113–120). Philadelphia: JB Lippincott.

Franco-Cereceda, A., McCarthy, P. M., & Blackstone, E. H. (2001). Partial left ventriculectomy for dilated cardiomyopathy: is this an alternative to transplantation? *Journal of Thoracic Cardiovascular Surgery*, 121, 879–893.

Frazier, O. H., Kadipasaoglu, K. A., & Cooley, D. A. (1998). Transmyocardial laser revascularization: Does it have a role in treatment of ischemic heart disease? *Texas Heart Institute Journal*, 25, 24–29.

Futterman, L. G., & Lemberg, L. (1996). Cardiomyoplasty. A potential alternative to cardiac transplantation. *American Journal of Critical Care*, 5, 80–86.

Gardlund, B, Bitkover, C. Y., & Vaage, J. (2002). Postoperative mediastinitis in cardiac surgery— microbiology and pathogenesis. *European Journal of Cardio-thorac Surgery*, 21, 825–830.

Gray, R. J., & Mandel, W. J. (1990). Management of common postoperative arrhythmias. In R. J. Gray & J. M. Matlof (Eds.), *Medical management of the cardiac surgical patient* (pp. 12–26). Baltimore: Williams & Wilkins.

Gundry, S. R., Romano, M. A., Shattuck, O. H., et al. (1998). Seven-year follow-up of coronary artery bypasses performed with and without cardiopulmonary bypass. *Journal of Thoracic Cardiovascular Surgery*, 115, 1273–1278.

Halm, M. A. (1996). Acute gastrointestinal complications after cardiac surgery. *American Journal of Critical Care*, 5, 109–118.

Heitmiller, E. S., Thompson, S., Michael, K., et al. (1994). Multidisciplinary care in conducting the operation. In W. A. Baumgartner, S. G. Owen, D. E. Cameron, et al. (Eds.), *The Johns Hopkins manual of cardiac surgical care* (pp. 335–364). St. Louis: Mosby.

Hill, L. L., DeWat, C., & Hogue Jr, C. W. (2002). Management of atrial fibrillation after cardiac surgery, part II: prevention and treatment. *Journal of Cardiothoracic and Cardiovascular Anesthesia*, 16, 626–637.

Horvath, J. A. (2003). Transmyocardial laser revascularization. In K. L. Franco & E. D. Verrier (Eds.), *Advanced therapy in cardiac surgery* (pp. 131–137). Hamilton, Ontario: BC Decker.

Jones, H. U., Muhlestein, J. B., Jones, K. W., Bair, T. L., et al. (2002). Preoperative use of enoxaparin compared with unfractionated heparin increases the incidence of re-exploration for post-operative bleeding after open-heart surgery in patients who present with an acute coronary syndrome. *Circulation*, 106(Suppl. I), I-19–I-22.

Kern, L. S. (1998). Management of postoperative atrial fibrillation. *Journal of Cardiovascular Nursing*, 12(3), 57–77.

King, R. C., & Verrier, E. V. (2003). Postinfarction ventricular septal defect repair. In K. L. Franco & E.D. Verrier (Eds.), *Advanced therapy in cardiac surgery* (pp. 83–88). Hamilton, Ontario: BC Decker.

Knotzer, A. M. H., Pajk, W., Luckner, G., et al. (2001). Risk factors associated with new onset tachyarrhythmias after cardiac surgery—a retrospective analysis. *Acta Anaesthesiology Scandinavia*, 25, 543–549.

Kreter, B., & Woods, M. (1992). Antibiotic prophylaxis for cardiothoracic operations. *Journal of Thoracic Cardiovascular Surgery*, 104(3), 590–599.

Lahey, S. J., Campos, C. T., & Jennings, B. (1998). Hospital readmission after cardiac surgery: Does "fast track" cardiac surgery result in cost saving or cost shifting? *Circulation*, 98, II-35–II-40.

Lasocki, S., Provenchere, S., Benessiano, J., et al. (2002) Cardiac troponin I is an independent predictor of in-hospital death after cardiac surgery. *Anesthesiology*, 97, 405–411.

Leeper, B. (2000). Transmyocardial laser revascularization. *Nursing Clinics of North America*, 4, 933–943.

Loef, B. G., Epema, A. H., Navi, G., et al. (2002). Off-pump coronary revascularization attenuates transient renal damage compared to on-pump revascularization. *Chest*, 121, 1190–1194.

Loop, F. D. (1998). Coronary artery bypass surgery. In E. J. Topol (Ed.), *Textbook of cardiovascular medicine* (pp. 2011–2030). Philadelphia, PA: Lippincott-Raven.

Loop, F. D., Lytle, B. W., Cosgrove, D. M., et al. (1986). Influence of the internal-mammary-artery graft on 10-year survival and other cardiac events. *New England Journal of Medicine*, 314(1), 1–6.

Loop, F. D, & Muehrcke, D. D. (1998). Surgical treatment of atherosclerotic coronary heart disease. In R.W. Alexander, R.C. Schlant, & V. Fuster (Eds.), *Hurst's the heart, arteries, and veins* (9th ed., pp. 1473–1487). New York: McGraw-Hill.

Lopes, D. K. (2000). Neurologic complications of cardiac surgery. In P. P. Soltoski, H. L. Karamanoukian, & T. A. Salerno, *Cardiac surgery secrets* (pp. 253–257). Philadelphia: Hanley & Belfus.

Lynn-McHale, D. J., Hambach, C., Carter, T., et al. (1998). Transmyocardial laser revascularization. *Journal of Cardiovascular Nursing*, 12(3), 17–28.

Maisel, W. H., Rawn, J. D., & Stevenson, W. G. (2001). Atrial fibrillation after cardiac surgery. *Annals of Internal Medicine*, 135, 1061–1073.

Mangano, C. M. Diamondstone, L. S., Ramsay, J. G., et al. (1998). Renal dysfunction after myocardial revascularization: risk factors, adverse outcomes, and hospital resource utilization. *Annals of Internal Medicine*, 128, 194–203.

Mangino-Blanchard, L. (2002). Off-pump coronary revascularization: Is it all that it's cracked up to be? *Dimensions of Critical Care Nursing*, 21(5), 190–194.

Martin, T., Craver, J., Gott, J., et al. (1994). Prospective randomized trial of retrograde warm blood cardioplegia: Myocardial benefit and neurological threat. *Annals of Thoracic Surgery*, 57, 298–304.

Matlof, J. M. (1990). Current indications for coronary pass and/or valvular surgery. In R. J. Gray & J. M. Matlof (Eds.), *Medical management of the cardiac surgical patient* (pp. 12–26). Baltimore: Williams & Wilkins.

Mercado, P. D., Farid, H., O'Connell, T. X., et al. (1994). Gastrointestinal complications associated with cardiopulmonary bypass procedures. *American Surgeon*, 60, 789–792.

Milot, J., Perron, J., Lacasse, Y., et al. (2001). Incidence and predictors of ARDS after cardiac surgery. *Chest*, 119, 884–888.

Morris, D. C., Clements, S. D., & Hug Jr., C. C. (1998). Management of the patient after cardiac surgery. In R. W. Alexander, R. C. Sclant, & V. Fuster (Eds.), *Hurst's the heart, arteries, and veins* (9th ed, pp. 1489–1500). New York: McGraw-Hill.

Morris, D. C., & St. Claire Jr., D. (1999). Management of patients after cardiac surgery. *Current Problems in Cardiology*, April, 166–228.

Mravinac, C. M. (1991). Neurologic dysfunctions following cardiac surgery. *Critical Care Nursing Clinics of North America*, 3, 691–697.

Ng, C. S. H., Wan, S., Yim, A. P. C., et al. (2002). Pulmonary dysfunction after cardiac surgery. *Chest*, 121(4), 1269–1277.

Nuttall, G. A. Oliver Jr., W. C., & Ereth, M. H. (2000). Comparison of blood-conservation strategies in cardiac surgery patients at high risk for bleeding. *Anesthesiology*, 92(3), 674–682.

Pym, J., Luffman, B., & Parry, M. (1997). Total arterial revascularization of the heart: Intentional or inevitable. *AACN Clinical Issues*, 8, 9–19.

Rho, R. W., Bridges, C. R., & Kocovic, D. (2000). Management of postoperative arrhythmias. *Seminars in Thoracic and Cardiovascular Surgery*, 12, 349–361.

Ridderstolpe, L., Gill, H., Grandfeldt, H., et al. (2001). Superficial and deep sternal wound complications: incidence, risk factors, and mortality. *European Journal of Cardio-thoracic Surgery*, 20, 1168–1175.

Roosens, C., Heerman, J., DeSomer, F., et al. (2002). Effects of off-pump coronary surgery on the mechanics of the respiratory system, lung, and chest wall: Comparison with extracorporeal circulation. *Critical Care Medicine*, 30, 2430–2437.

Rosborough, D. (1993). Surgical myocardial revascularization in the 1990's. *AACN Clinical Issues*, 4, 219–226.

Sakorafas, G. H., & Tsiotos, G. G. (1999). Intra-abdominal complications after cardiac surgery. *European Journal of Surgery*, 165, 820–827.

Seifert, P. C. (1998). Advances in myocardial protection. *Journal of Cardiovascular Nursing*, 12(3), 29–38.

Seifert, P. C. (2002a). Basic cardiac surgical procedures. In P. C. Seifert, *Cardiac surgery: Perioperative patient care* (pp. 213–257). St Louis: Mosby.

Seifert, P. C. (2002b). Surgery for coronary artery disease. In P. C. Seifert, *Cardiac surgery: Perioperative patient care* (pp. 258–306). St Louis: Mosby.

Shammus, N. W. (1999). Pulmonary embolus after coronary artery bypass surgery; a review of the literature. *Clinical Cardiology*, 23, 637–644.

Sharma, A. D., Parmley, C. L., & Sreeram, G. (2000). Peripheral nerve injuries during cardiac surgery: risk factors, diagnosis, prognosis, and prevention. *Anesthesia and Analgesia*, 91, 1358–1369.

Shinn, J. (1992). Management of a patient undergoing myocardial revascularization: Coronary artery bypass graft surgery. *Nursing Clinics of North America*, 27, 243–256.

Staples, J. R., & Ramsay, J. G. (1997). Advances in anesthesia for cardiac surgery: An overview for the 1990's. *AACN Clinical Issues*, 8, 41–49.

Steinberg, J. S., Gaur, A., & Sciacca, R. (1999). New-onset sustained ventricular tachycardia after cardiac surgery. *Circulation*, 99, 903–908.

Tasdemir, Q., Vurnal, K. M., Karagoz, H., et al. (1998). Coronary artery bypass grafting on the beating heart without use of extracorporeal circulation: Review of 2052 cases. *Journal of Thoracic Cardiovascular Surgery*, 116, 68–73.

Tsang, T. S. M., Barnes, M. E., & Hayes, S. N. (1999). Clinical and echocardiographic characteristics of significant pericardial effusions following cardiothoracic surgery and outcomes of echo-guided pericardiocentesis for management. *Chest*, 116, 322–331.

Tuman, K. J., McCarthy, R. J., Najafi, H., et al. (1992). Differential effects of advanced age on neurologic and cardiac risks of coronary artery operations. *Journal of Thoracic Cardiovascular Surgery*, 104(6), 1510–1517.

Van Dijk, D., Jansen, E. W., Hijman, R., et al. (2002). Cognitive outcomes after off-pump and on-pump coronary artery bypass surgery. *JAMA*, 287, 1405–1412.

Van Dijk, D., Nierch, A. P., & Jansen, E. W. L. (2001). Early outcomes after off-pump coronary bypass surgery. *Circulation*, 104, 1761–1766.

Vargo, R., & Dimengo, J. (1993). Surgical alternatives for patients with heart failure. *AACN Clinical Issues*, 4, 244–259.

Verrier, E. D., Wright, I. H., Cochran, R. P., et al. (1995). Changes in cardiovascular surgical approaches to achieve early extubation. *Journal of Cardiothoracic Vascular Anesthesiology*, 9(Suppl. 1), 10–15.

Vitello-Cicciu, J., Fitzgerald, C., & Whalen, D. (1998). On the horizon: Minimally invasive cardiac surgery. *Journal of Cardiovascular Nursing, 12*(3), 1–16.

Yilmaz, A. T., Arslan, M., & Demirkilic, U. (1996). Gastrointestinal complications after cardiac surgery. *European Journal of Cardio-thoracic Surgery,* 10, 763–767.

Young, Z., & Dai, B. (2000). Complications of cardiopulmonary bypass. In P. P. Soltoski, H. L. Karamanoukian, & T. A. Salerno, *Cardiac surgery secrets* (pp. 253–257). Philadelphia: Hanley & Belfus.

Yusuf, S., Zucker, D., Peduzzi, P., et al. (1994). Effect of coronary bypass graft surgery on survival: Overview of 10-year results from randomized trials by the Coronary Artery Bypass Graft Surgery Trialists Collaboration. *Lancet,* 344, 563–570.

REFERENCES FOR CARDIAC TRANSPLANTATION

2002 annual report of the U.S. Organ Procurement and Transplantation Network and the Scientific Registry of Transplant Recipients: Transplant data 1992–2001. Department of Health and Human Services, Health Resources and Services Administration. Office of Special Programs, Division of Transplantation, Rockville, MD; United Network for Organ Sharing, Richmond, VA; University Renal Research and Education Association, Ann Arbor, MI.

Aranda, J. M., & Hill, J. (2000). Cardiac transplant Vvsculopathy. *Chest,* 118, 1792–1800.

Baran, D. A., Galin, I. D., & Gass, A. L.(2002). Current practices: Immunosuppression induction, maintenance, and rejection regimens in contemporary post-heart transplant patient treatment. *Current Opinion in Cardiology,* 17,165–170.

Bexton, R. S., Nathan, A. W., Hellestrand, K. J., et al. (1984). Sinoatrial function after cardiac transplantation. *Journal of the American College of Cardiology,* 13, 712–723.

Billingham, M. E., Cary, N. R. B., Hammond, M. E., et al. (1990). A working formulation for the standardization of nomenclature in the diagnosis of heart and lung rejection: Heart rejection study group. *Journal of Heart Transplantation,* 9, 587–591.

Boucek, M. M., Edwards, L. B., Keck, B. M., et al. (2003). The Registry of the International Society for Heart and Lung Transplantation: Sixth Official Pediatric Report-2003. *Journal of Heart and Lung Transplantation,* 22, 636–652.

Brown, M. (1995). Thoracic transplantation: Procurement and organization. In N. E. Shumway & S. J. Shumway (Eds.), *Thoracic transplantation* (pp. 79–83). Cambridge: Blackwell Science.

Crandell, B. (1990). Immunosuppression. In K. M. Sigardson-Poor., & L. M. Haggerty (Eds.), *Nursing care of the transplant recipient* (pp 53–85). Philadelphia: WB Saunders.

Deng, M. C. (2002). Cardiac transplantation. *Heart,* 87, 177–184.

DiBiase, A., Tse, T. M., Schnittger, I., et al. (1991). Frequency and mechanism of bradycardia in cardiac transplant recipients and need for pacemakers. *American Journal of Cardiology,* 67, 1385–1389.

DrugPoints System: Thomson MICROMEDEX(R) Healthcare series vol. 116 expires 6/2003.

Eisen, H. J. (2003). Hypertension in heart transplant recipients: more than just cyclosporine. *Journal of the American College of Cardiology,* 41(3), 433–434.

Frazier, O. H.(1996). Patient selection for heart transplantation. In O. H. Frazier, M. P. Macris, & B. Radovancevic (Eds.), *Support and replacement of the failing heart* (pp. 59–68). Philadelphia: JB Lippincott.

Frazier, D. H., VanBuren, C. T., & Poindexter, S. M. (1985). Nutritional management of the heart transplant recipient. *Heart Transplantation,* 4, 450–452.

Gao, S., Hunt, S. A., & Schroeder, J. S. (1995). Accelerated graft coronary artery disease. In N. E. Shumway, & S. J. Shumway (Eds.), *Thoracic transplantation* (pp. 273–289). Cambridge: Blackwell Science, 1995.

Hertz, M. I, Taylor, D. O., Trulock, E. P., et al. (2002). The Registry of the International Society for Heart and Lung Transplantation: Nineteenth Official Report—2002. *Journal of Heart and Lung Transplantation,* 21, 950–970.

Kirklin, J. K., Bourge, R. C., & Naftel, D. C. (1994). Treatment of recurrent heart rejection with mycophenolate mofetil (RS-61443): Initial clinical experience. *Journal of Heart and Lung Transplantation,* 13, 444–450.

Lough, M. E., Lindsey, A. M., Shinn, J. A. (1987). Impact of symptom frequency and symptom distress on self-reported quality of life in heart transplant recipients. *Heart and Lung,* 16, 193–200.

Lough, M. E., Lindsey, A. M., & Shinn, J. A. (1985). Life satisfaction following heart transplantation. *Heart Transplantation,* 4, 446–449.

Luikart, H. (2001). Pediatric transplantation: Management issues. *Journal of Pediatric Nursing,* 16, 320–331.

Micromedex Healthcare Series: Micromedex, Inc. Breenwood Village, CO (edition expires 9/13). Available: http://hcs.mdx.com (accessed April 2003).

Moran, M., Tomlanovich, S., & Myers, B. D. (1985). Cyclosporin-induced nephropathy in human recipients of cardiac allografts. *Transplant Proceedings,* 17(Suppl. 1), 185–190.

Myers, B. D., Ross, J., Newton, L., et al. (1984). Cyclosporin associated chronic nephrotoxicity. *New England Journal of Medicine,* 311, 699–705.

Packer, M., Bristow, M. R., Cohn, J. N., et al. (1996). The effect of carvedilol on morbidity and mortality in patients with chronic heart failure. *New England Journal of Medicine,* 334, 1349–1355.

Przepiorka, D. (1992). Tacrolimus: Preclinical and clinical experience. In D. Przepioka & H. Sollinger (Eds.), *Recent developments in transplantation medicine: New immunosuppressive drugs* (pp. 29–50). Glenview, IL: Physicians and Scientist Publishing.

Rodino, M. A., & Shane, E. (1998). Osteoporosis after organ transplantation. *American Journal of Medicine,* 104 (5), 459–469.

Rose, A. G. (1986). Endomyocardial biopsy diagnosis of cardiac rejection. *Heart Failure,* 2 (2), 64–72.

Sadowsky, H. S. (1996). Cardiac transplantation: A review. *Physical Therapy,* 76, 498–515.

Sadowsky, H. S. & Fries, K. (1986) *Introduction to the treatment of cardiac and cardiopulmonary transplant patients.* Stanford, CA: Stanford University Hospital, Department of Physical and Occupational Therapy.

Shinn, J. A. (1985). New issues in cardiac transplantation. In M. K. Douglas & J. A. Shinn (Eds.), *Advances in cardiovascular nursing* (pp. 185–195). Rockville: Aspen Systems.

Shumway, N. E., Lower, R. R., & Stofer, C. (1966). Transplantation of the heart. *Advances in Surgery,* 2, 265–284.

Starnes, V. A., Bernstein, D., Oyer, P. E., et al. (1989). Heart transplantation in children. *Journal of Heart Transplantation,* 8, 20–26.

Stevenson, L. W., Laks, H., Terasaki, P. I., et al. (1988). Cardiac transplant selection, immunosuppression and survival. *Western Journal of Medicine,* 149, 572–582.

Taylor, D. O.(2000). Immunosuppressive therapies after heart transplantation: best, better, and beyond. Current Opinion Cardiology, 15, 108–114.

Thelan, L. A., Urden, L. D., Lough, M. E,. et al. (Eds.) (1998). *Critical care nursing: Diagnosis and management* (3rd ed., pp. 1179–1184). St. Louis: Mosby.

Thompson, M. E., Shapiro, M. E., Johnsen, A. M., et al. (1983). New onset of hypertension following cardiac transplantation. *Transplant Proceedings,* 25(Suppl. 1), 2573–2577.

Trento, A., Takkenberg, J. M., Czer, L. S. C., et al. (1996). Clinical experience with one hundred consecutive patients undergoing orthotopic heart transplantation with bicaval and pulmonary venous anastomosis. *Journal of Thoracic Cardiovascular Surgery,* 112, 1496–1503.

Valantine, H. A. (1995). Prevention and treatment of cytomegalovirus disease in thoracic organ transplant patients: Evidence for a beneficial effect of hyperimmune globulin. *Transplant Proceedings,* 27, 49–57.

Veith, F. J., Fein, J. M., Tendler, M. D., et al. (1978). Brain death: I. A status report of medical and ethical considerations. *JAMA,* 238, 1651–1655.

Wagoner, L. W. (1997). Management of the cardiac transplant recipient: Roles of the transplant cardiologist and primary care physician. *American Journal of Medical Science,* 324, 173–184.

Zaroff, J. G., Rosengard, B. R., Armstrong, W. F., et al. (2002). Consensus Conference Report. Maximizing use of organs recovered from the cadaver donor: Cardiac recommendations. *Circulation,* 106, 836–841.

Acute Heart Failure and Shock

DEBRA LAURENT • JULIE A. SHINN

DATABASE FOR NURSING MANAGEMENT

Shock is a complex clinical syndrome characterized by impaired cellular metabolism caused by decreased tissue perfusion. The inadequacy of tissue perfusion results in cellular hypoxia, the accumulation of cellular metabolic wastes, cellular destruction, and, ultimately, organ and system failure. The syndrome begins as an adaptive response to some insult or injury and progresses to multiple organ system failure (Shuster & Lefrak, 1992; Mouchawar & Rosenthal, 1995). The pathophysiologic mechanisms of shock include decreased circulating blood volume, decreased cardiac contractility, and increased venous capacitance. One of these mechanisms predominates in each type of shock; however, the mechanisms are interactive, with more than one occurring in each of the shock syndromes.

Classification

This chapter discusses three basic types of shock: cardiogenic, hypovolemic, and distributive. Cardiogenic shock (pump failure) is characterized by a decreased strength of contraction of myocardial fibers, leading to a decreased cardiac output. The decrease in myocardial contractile strength may be caused by myocardial ischemia, myocardial infarction (MI), trauma, myocarditis, or cardiomyopathy. Extracardiac form of shock is obstructive shock as seen in patients with pericardial tamponade or pulmonary embolism. Hypovolemic shock (preload failure) exists when there is a decrease in the circulating blood volume. Losses of blood volume may be external (e.g., hemorrhage) or internal (e.g., sequestration of fluid in the abdomen secondary to intestinal obstruction). Distributive shock (afterload failure) is characterized by vasodilatation in response to neurological or hormonal stimuli. Profound vasodilatation results in an inequality between the circulating blood volume and the capacity of the vascular bed. Septic shock is the most often encountered form of distributive shock and is the representative form discussed in this chapter. Two other forms of distributive shock are anaphylactic and neurogenic (Rice, 1991a; Shuster & Lefrak, 1992; Mouchawar & Rosenthal, 1995).

Pathophysiology

Although the clinical syndrome of shock has various causes and basic pathophysiologic defects, all three types are characterized by tissue hypoperfusion, which, if untreated or inadequately treated, results in generalized cellular and systemic dysfunction. In response to tissue hypoperfusion, compensatory mechanisms are activated and are directed at the restoration and maintenance of adequate blood volume and pressure and at the adequate perfusion of the heart and brain. If the basic physiologic defect is not corrected, compensatory mechanisms become counterproductive, resulting in the vicious cycle of irreversible shock (Rice, 1991a; Saltzberg et al., 2001)

Clinical shock is a dynamic continuum. The prominence of its features and compensatory mechanisms varies with time and with treatment. Although other features (e.g., low blood pressure or decreased cardiac output) are present, the basic problem is acute, generalized tissue hypoperfusion. The pathophysiology and clinical presentations of shock are listed in Table 30-1.

Cardiogenic Shock

Acute heart failure (HF) is a true medical emergency that warrants an expedient diagnosis, and if appropriate treatment is not instituted within a short time course, then irreversible decompensation may ensue, leading to a progressive syndrome of shock (Haas & Young, 1998). As the endpoint on the clinical continuum of left ventricular (LV) failure, cardiogenic shock includes shock caused by ineffective cardiac contractility and myocardial failure. The complexity of acute heart failure has diverse potential etiologies making a precise definition difficult, but in clinical practice it is recognized within hours to days in patients without previous history of cardiac decompensation.

Atherosclerotic heart disease and the complications of ischemia and infarction is the most common cause of acute HF (Chatterjee et al., 1996). Acute coronary occlusion first impairs diastolic function, with later diminished systolic function, stoke volume, and blood pressure. This begins a downward spiral leading to progressive myocardial dysfunction and possibly death (Fig. 30-1) (Hollenberg, 2001). Shock occurs in approximately 8% of patients with acute MI of the left ventricle. It is most associated with anterior wall MI. Angiographic findings

Table 30–1 ■ PATHOPHYSIOLOGY AND CLINICAL PRESENTATION OF SHOCK

Type of Shock			Forward Cardiac Output	CVP	PAWP	SVR	Clinical Findings
Cardiogenic shock	Pump failure	Left ventricle MI	↓↓↓	↑↑	↑↑↑	↑↑	S3, S4
		Right ventricle MI	↓↓	↑↑↑	↑or↔	↑or↔	Right sided S3, S4
		Non-ischemic cardiomyopathy	↓↓↓	↑↑	↑↑↑	↑↑	S3, S4
		Infiltrative disease (late)	↓↓↓	↑↑	↑↑↑	↑or↔	S4
	Mechanical failure	Trauma	↓↓	↑or↔	↑↑	↑or↔	Variable
		Acute AI, native or prosthetic valve	↓↓	↔	↑↑ or ↑↑↑	↑↑	Early diastolic murmur
		Acute MR, native or prosthetic valve	↓↓	↑or ↔	↑↑↑↑	↑↑	Holosystolic murmur apex anterior axillary
		Aortic stenosis	↔	↑or↔	↑↑	↑↑	Systolic ejection murmur, LSB
		Mitral stenosis	↔	↑or↔	↑↑↑	↑↑	Diastolic rumbling murmur apex
		VSD (acute post-MI)	↓ or ↓↓	↑or ↑↑	↑ or ↑↑	↑↑	Holosystolic murmur
		Free wall rupture	↓ or ↓↓	↑or ↑↑	↑ or ↑↑	↑↑	Silent
Extracardiac	Obstructive shock	Pericardial tamponade	↓↓ (LV)	↑↑↑	↑↑	↑↑	Silent or rub
		Pulmonary embolism	↓↓ (RV)	↑↑↑	↔	↑or ↑↑	Right sided S3, S4
Hypovolemic shock		Blood or volume loss	↓	↓↓↓	↓↓↓	↑or ↔	Silent
Distributive shock		Septic shock	↑or ↑↑ ↓↓(10-15%)	Initial ↓↓	↓↓	↓↓↓↓	Hyperdynamic precordium
		Anaphylactic shock	↔ or ↑	↓↓	↓↓	↓↓↓↓	None

CVP, central venous pressure; PAWP, pulmonary artery wedge pressure; SVR, systemic vascular resistance; MI, myocardial infarction; LSB, left sternal border; RV, right ventricle.
Adapted from Saltzberg, M. T., Soble, J. S., & Parrillo, J. E. (2001). Acute heart failure and shock. In M. H. Crawford & J. P. DiMarco (Eds.), *Cardiology* (Section 5, 3.2). London: Mosby.

of the SHOCK trial showed left main occlusion in 20% of patients, three-vessel disease in 64%, two-vessel disease in 23%, and single-vessel disease in 13% of patients (Hochman et al., 1999). Some patients may present in cardiogenic shock on admission, but shock often evolves over several hours. The median delay from onset of MI to development of cardiogenic shock in the randomized SHOCK trial was 5.6 hours (Hochman et al., 1999).

Shock with a delayed onset may result from infarct expansion, reocclusion of a previously patent infarct artery, or decompensation of myocardial function in the noninfarct zone caused by metabolic abnormalities (Hollenberg, 2001; Saltzberg et al., 2001). Ischemia-related systolic dysfunction also could contribute to the development of cardiogenic shock. One pattern is the "hibernating" myocardium, seen with low tissue perfusion states matched by a decline in compensatory function. The second pattern is the "stunned" myocardium, which is a more prolonged (hours to days) myocardial dysfunction after a relatively brief interruption of myocardial perfusion. These patterns have been reported after percutaneous coronary interventions, cardioplegic arrest, and unstable angina (Bonow, 1995; Bolli, 1998; Saltzberg et al., 2001).

Right ventricular infarction occurs after occlusion of the proximal right coronary artery and is identified in the setting of concomitant infero-posterior left ventricular dysfunction. There is up to a 32% incidence of shock with clinically evident right ventricular systolic dysfunction and secondary to right and left ventricular interaction (Saltzberg et al., 2001).

Complications of MI include mitral regurgitation, ventricular septal defect (VSD), and free-wall rupture. Significant mitral regurgitation patterns are seen clinically: papillary muscle (usually the posterior papillary muscle) or chordal rupture caused by MI, and mitral regurgitation associated with left ventricular dilatation (Gorman et al., 1997). Acute VSD abruptly increases pulmonary blood flow and leads to symptoms of biventricular failure within hours to days if not corrected. Left ventricular free wall rupture occurs in less than 1% of acute MIs but carries a high mortality rate (Hochman et al., 1995).

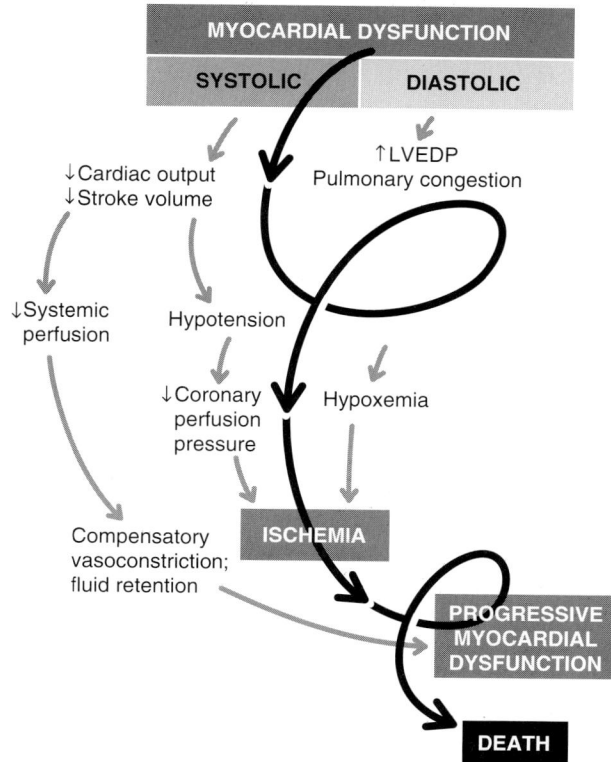

■ **Figure 30–1.** The downward spiral in cardiogenic shock. LVEDP = left ventricular end-diastolic pressure. (From Hollenberg, S. M. [2001]. Cardiogenic shock. *Critical Care Clinics,* 17[2],395.)

Non—MI-related acute valvular problems involve the mitral and aortic valve. Acute mitral regurgitation can be caused by spontaneous chordal rupture, infective endocarditis, inflammatory disorders (e.g. rheumatic fever), or trauma. Acute aortic insufficiency may caused by infective endocarditis with leaflet destruction (most common), acute aortic

dissection, or traumatic injury. Shock may be caused by aortic stenosis with increasing metabolic demands or with concomitant LV failure. Mitral stenosis rarely causes shock without rapid atrial fibrillation (Saltzberg et al., 2001). Prosthetic valve dysfunction, especially left-sided, most often causes shock because of valvular insufficiency. Acute prosthetic valvular insufficiency occurs because of dehiscence of the sewing ring, infective endocarditis, or catastrophic mechanical failure.

Infiltrative disease, such as amyloidosis, sarcoidosis, and hemochromatosis are examples of infiltrative diseases in their later stages that may be associated with shock. Shock caused by trauma is usually seen secondary to myocardial or aortic rupture, or caused by acute volume loss secondary to hemorrhage.

Acute decompensation of chronic HF represents a different pathophysiologic state, because these patients have a marked reduction in LV systolic function at baseline as compared to those patients with acute HF without prior LV dysfunction (Haas & Young, 1998). Patients with chronic HF are likely to be using combination therapy, usually and angiotensin-converting enzyme inhibitor (ACE), diuretic, beta-blocker, and/or digoxin. There is already activation of the neurohormonal compensatory mechanisms, including increased sympathetic stimulation of the heart, activation of the renin-angiotensin-aldosterone system (RAAS), increased vasoconstriction, fluid retention by the kidneys, increased ventricular preload, and LV hypertrophy and remodeling (Francis et al., 2001) (see Chapter 28). When a precipitating event occurs, there is further derangement of these compensatory mechanisms. Factors leading to acute decompensation in chronic HF may include the following: acute myocardial ischemia; poorly treated or untreated hypertension; new-onset atrial fibrillation; concurrent infections (e.g. pneumonia, influenza); medication noncompliance; dietary excess of sodium; administration of cardiac depressant drugs; use of nonsteroidal antiinflammatory drugs; and endocrine abnormalities (poorly controlled diabetes, hyperthyroidism) (Francis, 2000). Table 30-2 compares clinical and pathophysiologic features of acute and chronic HF (Saltzberg et al., 2001).

Table 30–2 ■ COMPARISON OF ACUTE VERSUS CHRONIC HEART FAILURE

Feature	Acute Heart Failure	Decompensated Chronic Heart Failure	Stable Chronic Heart Failure
Symptom severity	Marked	Marked	Mild to moderate
Pulmonary edema	Frequent	Frequent	Rare
Peripheral edema	Rare	Frequent	Occasional
Weight gain	None to mild	Frequent	Frequent
Total body volume	No change of mild increase	Markedly increased	Increased
Cardiomegaly	Uncommon	Usual	Common
LV systolic function	Hypo-, normo- or hypercontractile	Reduced	Markedly reduced
L V wall stress	Elevated	Markedly elevated	Elevated
Activation of sympathetic nervous system	Marked	Marked	Mild to marked
Activation of RAAS	Markedly elevated	Marked	Mild to moderate
Acute ischemia	Common	Occasional	Rare
Hypertensive crisis	Common	Occasional	Rare
Repairable, remedial causes*	Common	Occasional	Occasional

L V, left ventricle; RAAS, renin-angiotensin-aldosterone system.
*E.g., acute coronary syndrome, acute mitral regurgitation, ventricular septal defect.
Adapted from Leier, C. V. (1995). Unstable heart failure. In E. Braunwald (W. S. Colucci, Vol. ed.) *Atlas of the heart* (Vol. 4.). St Louis: CV Mosby.

Extracardiac Obstructive Shock

Pericardial Tamponade. The accumulation of fluid within the pericardial sac increases pressure, causing extracardiac obstruction to filling that results in a decrease in ventricular preload and cardiac output. What determines whether pericardial effusion will cause shock is how rapidly the fluid accumulates. Patients at risk for shock caused by tamponade are those with malignancy (especially lung and breast cancer, lymphoma, leukemia, melanoma), infection, aortic dissection, or severe pericarditis (Brown et al., 1992).

Pulmonary Embolism. When embolic material, such as thrombus, fat, tumor, or air, obstructs 30% or more or the pulmonary vasculature, the right ventricle cannot provide adequate pressure to compensate for the increased resistance to blood flow. Right ventricular failure ensues, with increased right ventricular end-diastolic and right atrial pressures, and finally a decrease in cardiac output and shock (Saltzberg et al., 2001).

Hypovolemic Shock

Hypovolemic shock exists when the volume of blood is inadequate to fill the intravascular space. A significant reduction in the venous return to the right heart results in a decreased cardiac output, a reduced mean arterial blood pressure (MAP), and renal hypoperfusion. A 10% reduction in blood volume initiates compensatory mechanisms, and a rapid reduction of 20% of blood volume produces the clinical signs and symptoms of hypovolemic shock (Rice, 1991a).

Distributive Shock

Massive peripheral vasodilatation causes shock because the blood volume, although within normal limits, is insufficient to fill the enlarged vascular capacity. This leads to decreased venous return and a diminished cardiac output (Mouchawar & Rosenthal, 1995). Several types of distributive shock exist, including septic, anaphylactic, and neurogenic shock.

Septic Shock. In septic shock, cellular derangements precede and contribute to cardiovascular abnormalities (Shuster & Lefrak, 1992). Any type of microorganism can produce septic shock, including gram-negative bacteria, gram-positive bacteria, viruses, fungi, and rickettsiae; however, gram-negative bacteria are the most common cause, producing more than two thirds of the reported cases (Rice, 1991a). The gram-negative bacteria include *Escherichia coli, Klebsiella, Enterobacter,* and *Serratia* species, *Pseudomonas aeruginosa,* and *Bacteroides* and *Proteus* species. A complex hormonal and chemical release of substances is produced through the body's immune system in response to the adverse effects of endotoxins. The invading microorganisms elaborate vasoactive toxins (histamine, kinins, prostaglandins, oxygen free radicals), which results in selective but profound vasodilatation. Tumor necrosis factor (TNF-α) has also been elevated in this patient population. In addition, the pathogens create a focus of inflammation, which creates a high-flow, low-resistance state (Shuster & Lefrak, 1992).

There is a persistent decreased ability to extract oxygen from inspired air and from the blood, which results in tissue hypoxia. These abnormalities in oxygen diffusion result from destruction of pulmonary alveolar type I and II cells, a reduction in

2,3-diphosphoglycerate, and a shift of the oxyhemoglobin dissociation curve to the left. In late stages (see section on Irreversible Stage), septic shock is remarkably similar to cardiogenic and hypovolemic shock, with hypotension, vasoconstriction, decreased cardiac output, hypoxia, and acidosis (Rice, 1991a; Shuster & Lefrak, 1992).

Anaphylactic Shock. Anaphylactic shock is the result of a severe allergic, antigen-antibody reaction producing large amounts of histamine, prostaglandins, kinins, and other mediators, resulting in widespread microvascular leak and peripheral vasodilatation. Tumor necrosis factor has been shown to be another important mediator. Examples of substances that can act as antigens include drugs, contrast media, transfused blood and blood products, and insect venoms (Rice, 1991a; Saltzberg et al., 2001). Slow-reacting substances of anaphylaxis are also released, causing bronchoconstriction.

Neurogenic Shock. In neurogenic shock, there is a reduction of vasomotor tone, which occurs at the level of the vasomotor centers in the brainstem and causes decreased vasoconstriction, resulting in generalized systemic vasodilatation. This form of shock can develop with spinal anesthesia, spinal cord injury, or altered function of the vasomotor center in response to low blood sugar or drugs, including sedatives, barbiturates, and narcotics (Schuster and Lefrak, 1992).

Compensatory Mechanisms

The following equations illustrate the physiologic relation of the hemodynamic variables. Here, CO = cardiac output, SV = stroke volume, HR = heart rate, MAP = mean arterial pressure, and SVR = systemic vascular resistance:

$$CO = SV \times HR$$
$$MAP = CO \times SVR$$

In the pathophysiologic state of shock, the decrease in MAP is brought about by an alteration in one of the variables. In hypovolemic and cardiogenic shock, the reduction in MAP results from a decrease in stroke volume, whereas in distributive shock the reduction in MAP results from a decrease in systemic vascular resistance:

1. Hypovolemic:

$$CO = {\downarrow}SV \times HR; {\downarrow}MAP = {\downarrow}CO \times SVR$$

2. Cardiogenic:

$${\downarrow}CO = {\downarrow}SV \times HR; {\downarrow}MAP = {\downarrow}CO \times SVR$$

3. Vasogenic:

$$CO = SV \times HR; {\downarrow}MAP = CO \times {\downarrow}SVR$$

Compensatory mechanisms consist of reflex reactions to an initial fall in blood pressure. They are activated immediately and increase in intensity in an attempt to restore adequate tissue perfusion (Rice, 1991b). The compensatory mechanisms are directed at the restoration and maintenance of adequate blood volume, cardiac output, and vascular tone. The initial compensatory mechanisms vary with the primary pathophysiologic derangement, but the intermediate and final stages are similar. The initial compensatory mechanisms in hypovolemic

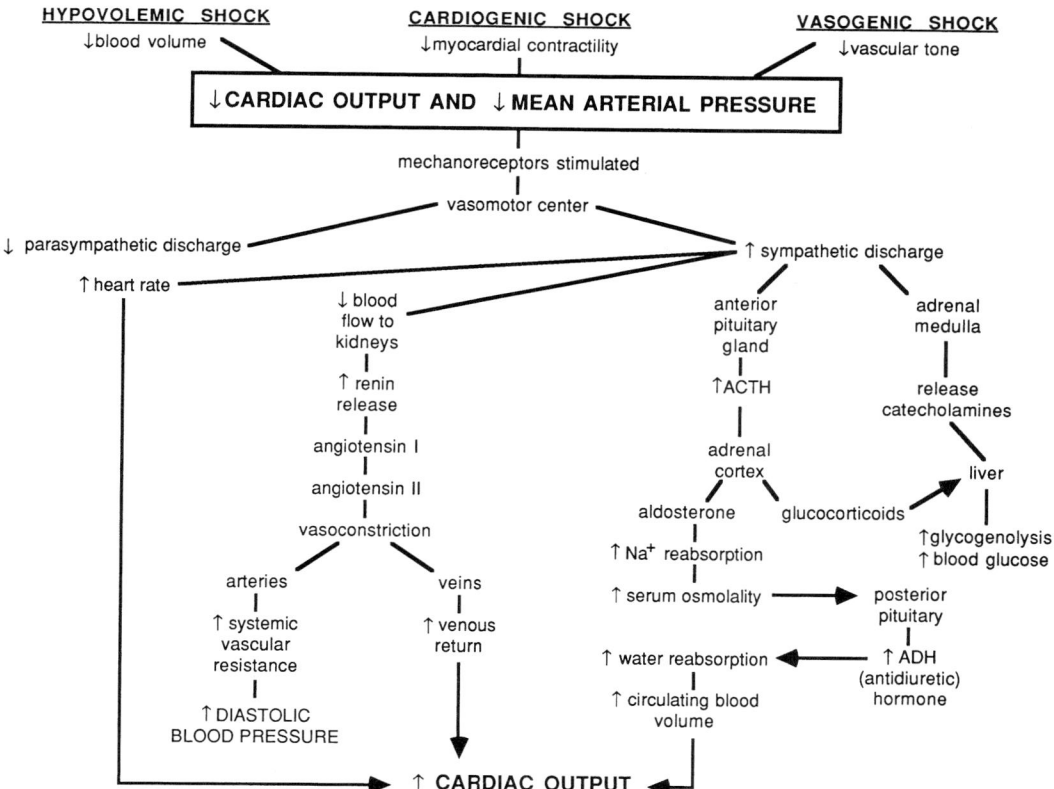

■ **Figure 30–2.** In the initial stage of shock, all three types of shock lead to a decrease in mean arterial pressure. Compensatory mechanisms attempt to reduce the effects of this decreased mean arterial pressure and, if successful, lead to an increase in cardiac output and mean arterial pressure.

and cardiogenic shock are increased heart rate and increased systemic vascular resistance. In vasogenic shock, the initial compensatory mechanism is increased heart rate and cardiac output (Shuster & Lefrak, 1992; Mouchawar & Rosenthal, 1995).

Initial Stage

In cardiogenic shock, the decreased coronary blood flow results in profound local compensatory events. There is an increase in myocardial oxygen extraction and dilatation of the coronary arteries. The myocardial cells shift to anaerobic metabolism and use glycolysis in the production of adenosine triphosphate (ATP) (Francis et al., 2001; Hollenberg et al., 1997; Hollenberg, 2001). These events occur immediately in response to myocardial ischemia. If inadequate, myocardial contractility decreases, leading to a decrease in cardiac output and systemic hypoperfusion. The initial stage of hypovolemic shock is characterized by selective venoconstriction of the renal, cutaneous, muscular, and splanchnic beds, with preservation of circulation to the heart and brain (Rice, 1991b).

The initial stage of septic shock is characterized by a hyperdynamic cardiovascular and metabolic state. This hyperdynamism results from the interrelation between the inflammatory responses and those caused by the endotoxins. Various vasoactive substances (e.g., vasodilators, histamine, and kinins) are released early in septic shock (Mouchawar & Rosenthal, 1995; Rice, 1991b). It is in the late stages of sepsis that a hypodynamic state characterized by reduced cardiac output,

vasoconstriction, and additional blood shunting occurs and initiates compensatory mechanisms similar to those in cardiogenic and hypovolemic shock (Fig. 30-2).

A reduction in arterial blood pressure secondary to decreased blood volume, decreased cardiac output, or increased venous capacitance initiates the body's compensatory mechanisms to maintain adequate tissue perfusion. These mechanisms serve to increase cardiac output and arterial blood pressure through increasing heart rate, enhancing myocardial contractility, providing selective vasoconstriction, conserving sodium and water, and shifting fluid from the interstitial to the intravascular space.

Specialized nerve endings (mechanoreceptors) in the carotid sinus, aortic arch, heart, and lungs sense the decrease in blood pressure and transmit their impulses to the vasomotor center. The vasomotor center stimulates the sympathetic nervous system, inhibits the parasympathetic, and initiates the secretion of catecholamines from the adrenal gland. Sympathetic nervous system stimulation unopposed by parasympathetic effects results in increased heart rate, increased myocardial contractility, and selective vasoconstriction. Reflexes of the sympathetic nervous system are active within 30 seconds of an acute decrease in circulating blood volume and are able to compensate for a 20% loss in blood volume by increasing cardiac output by 20% to 25% (Rice, 1991b; Mouchawar & Rosenthal, 1995). In response to ischemia and sympathetic stimulation, hormones are released from the adrenal medulla, adrenal cortex, anterior and posterior pituitary gland, and kidney, which further compensate for decreased circulating blood volume.

The adrenal medulla releases epinephrine and norepinephrine, which enhance vasoconstriction, myocardial contractility, and heart rate (Francis et al., 2001). Epinephrine and norepinephrine also stimulate glycogenolysis, thus increasing serum glucose. The adrenal cortex releases glucocorticoids, which also increase serum glucose. Decreased renal blood flow results in the release of renin, which initiates a series of reactions in the liver and elsewhere, resulting in the production of angiotensin. Angiotensin promotes the release of aldosterone by the adrenal cortex and, in situations of hypovolemia, promotes profound vasoconstriction. Aldosterone enhances renal sodium reabsorption accompanied by increased water reabsorption. Antidiuretic hormone is released from the posterior pituitary and further enhances renal water reabsorption. Thirst is stimulated and also causes increased fluid intake (Francis, 1998; Francis et al., 2001). As a result of decreased capillary pressure, Starling capillary balance is shifted, and fluid is transferred from the interstitial space to the capillary.

Intermediate Stage

If shock is not recognized and reversed in the initial compensatory stage, it progresses (Fig. 30-3). Compensatory mechanisms are no longer able to maintain homeostasis and may become counterproductive. For example, continued profound vasoconstriction in the presence of decreased MAP promotes inadequate tissue perfusion and cellular hypoxia (Rice, 1991b).

Decreased delivery of oxygen and nutrients causes cells to shift to anaerobic metabolic pathways (Hollenberg et al., 1997). Increasing amounts of lactic acid are produced and accumulate in the cells because of decreased perfusion. Because anaerobic metabolism is less efficient in meeting the energy requirements of the cells, ATP is depleted. Reduction in the available ATP results in failure of the membrane transport mechanisms, intracellular edema, and rupture of the cell membrane. Progressive tissue ischemia results in increased anaerobic metabolism and the further production of metabolic acidosis (Hollenberg et al., 1997).

Impairment of cellular function disrupts all body organs and organ systems. Splanchnic ischemia results in the release of endotoxin from the intestine. The reticuloendothelial (tissue macrophage) system (RES) is suppressed by splenic and hepatic ischemia. The continued renal response to ischemia leads to further vasoconstriction, stimulating the release of aldosterone from the adrenal gland and promoting the reabsorption of sodium in the kidney. This response is no longer useful because the increased volume cannot be pumped by the failing heart and results in ventilatory failure. The increased volume begins to pool in tissues secondary to profound venoconstriction and increased capillary permeability (Rice, 1991b).

If the myocardial ischemia is severe and prolonged enough, myocardial cellular injury becomes irreversible (Hollenberg et al., 1997). Cytokines are signaling peptides whose actions include cell growth and cell death through direct toxic effects on the heart and peripheral circulation. The proinflammatory

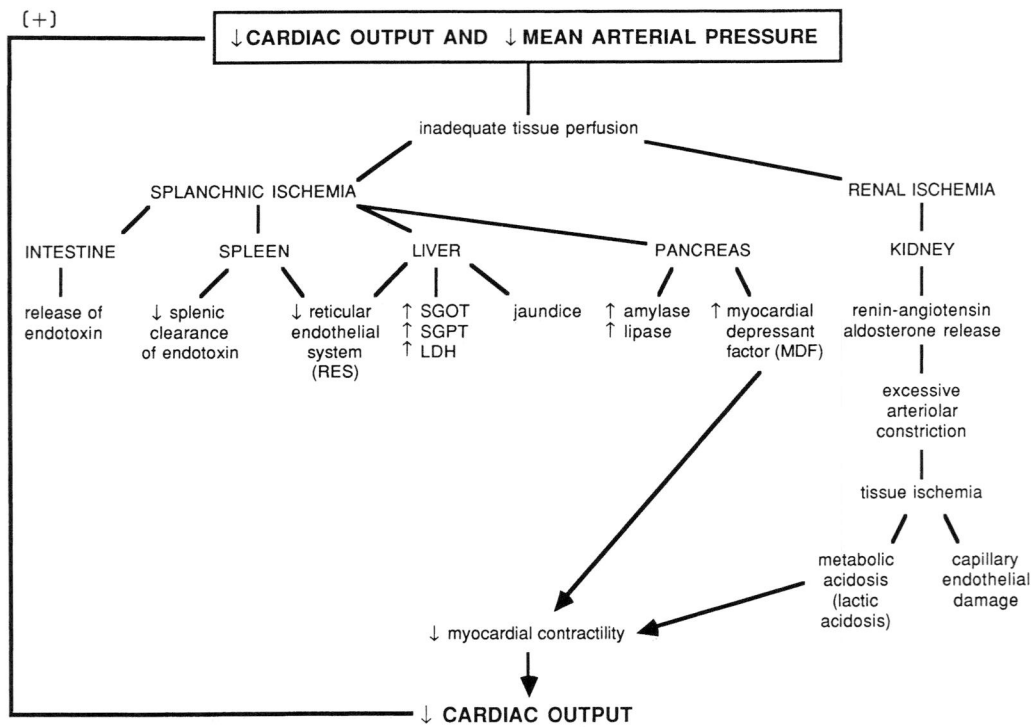

■ **Figure 30–3.** In the intermediate stage of shock, compensatory mechanisms fail, resulting in decreased tissue perfusion and organ function. Decreased myocardial contractility leading to a decrease in cardiac output sets up a positive feedback mechanism (+) to decrease further cardiac output and mean arterial pressure. SGOT, serum glutamic oxaloacetic transaminase; SGPT, serum glutamic pyruvic transaminase; LDH, lactate dehydrogenase.

or "stress-activated" cytokines include the tumor necrosis factor alpha (TNF-α) and the interleukin family. The cardiac myocytes themselves are capable of synthesizing these proinflammatory cytokines in response to various forms of cardiac injury (Mann, 2000). The local inflammatory response can appear within minutes of an abnormal stress. Local inflammation of the cytokines and other mediators includes deleterious effects of LV remodeling, which include myocyte hypertrophy, alteration in fetal gene expression, contractile defects, and progressive myocyte loss through apoptosis (Mann, 2000; Mann, 2002). Apoptosis (programmed cell death) contributes to myocyte loss, and evidence for apoptosis has been found consistently in the border zone of infarcts after ischemia and reperfusion, and also in areas remote from the ischemic area (Bartling et al., 1998; Katz, 2000). In addition to the direct detrimental effects of myocardial ischemia, there is some evidence that a peptide secreted by the pancreas, the myocardial depressant factor (MDF), may further depress myocardial function (Schuster & Lefrak, 1992). MDF has been identified in the serum of patients in the early stages of septic shock. Its presence in other forms of shock remains controversial.

Irreversible Stage

In this stage, the compensatory mechanisms are nonfunctioning or no longer effective, and hypotension has reached the critical level of adversely affecting the heart and brain (Fig. 30-4). Myocardial hypoperfusion, resulting from hypotension and tachycardia, produces acidosis, which leads to further depression of myocardial function. Decreased cerebral blood flow leads to depressed neuronal function and activity and loss of the central neuronal compensatory mechanisms (Rice, 1991b; Hollenberg et al., 1997).

The progressive general hypoxia and reduction in cardiac output further deprive body cells of oxygen and nutrients needed for cell growth and result in microcirculatory insufficiency. The microcirculation responds by vasodilatation to secure the necessary nutrients and oxygen for the deprived cells. Microcirculatory vasodilatation in association with systemic vasoconstriction results in the sequestration of blood in the capillary beds, further limiting the volume of blood returning to the systemic circulation. This loss of circulating blood volume and impaired capillary flow result in reduced venous return, further reducing cardiac output and arterial pressure. This situation creates a positive feedback mechanism in which the low-flow state produces a further reduction in flow (Rice, 1991b; Schuster & Lefrak, 1992; Hollenberg et al., 1997).

Clinical Manifestations

Patients in the initial stages of shock exhibit a variety of behavioral and physiologic symptoms, depending on the cause of shock. Changes noted on physical examination during the initial stages are primarily caused by sympathetic stimulation. Regardless of the classification of shock, the principal physiologic defect remains the same: reduced cellular perfusion. Continued tissue hypoxia and acidosis affect specific vital organs in specific ways (Astiz & Rackow, 1993).

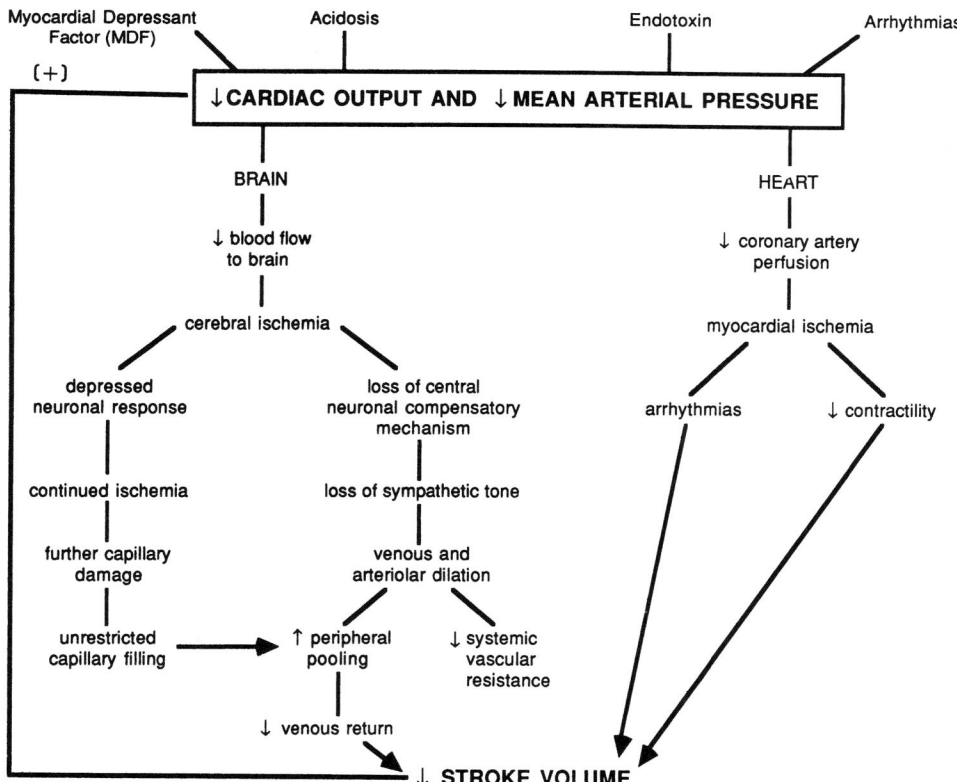

■ **Figure 30–4.** In the irreversible stage of shock, a prolonged decrease in cardiac output and mean arterial pressure leads to cellular necrosis and multiple organ failure.

Brain. Decreased cerebral blood flow and coagulopathy can lead to a cerebral infarction or cerebral thrombus formation. Alterations in cellular metabolism throughout the body, metabolic acidosis, and the accumulation of toxins further depress cerebral function. Lethargy, stupor, and coma develop as shock progresses. Finally, in the irreversible stage of shock, the vasomotor center in the brain is disrupted, causing failure of the circulatory mechanisms (Rice, 1991b; Hollenberg et al., 1997).

Myocardium. Because it cannot greatly increase oxygen extraction as other organs and tissues can, the myocardium is more vulnerable to the effects of decreased blood flow. A decrease in aortic pressure decreases coronary perfusion pressure. Myocardial cells convert to anaerobic metabolism because of the underperfused hypoxic myocardium, and lactate production increases. The normal functioning of the sodium-potassium pump is disrupted. Apoptosis promotes further myocyte loss (see previous section). Because of ischemia and necrosis of the pancreas, MDF is released and has a direct negative inotropic effect on the myocardium, contributing to further ischemia. MDF is thought to interfere with calcium in coupling electrical excitation with contraction of the heart (Parrillo et al., 1985).

Kidney. Adequate renal perfusion produces a minimum of 400 mL urine/24 hours, or 20 mL/h. Impaired renal perfusion in shock results in hourly urine outputs of less than 20 mL/h (Rice, 1991b; Hollenberg et al., 1997). The excretion of high volumes of low solute urine may also represent renal hypoperfusion. Prolonged hypoperfusion may lead to acute tubular necrosis and acute renal failure.

Gastrointestinal Tract. Compensatory vasoconstriction in shock may result in mucosal ischemia, an ileus, and full-thickness gangrene of the bowel. If the bowel wall becomes disrupted, the normal bacterial flora of the intestines enters the abdomen and can then enter the circulation. Gastrointestinal bleeding may also occur.

Liver. Factors that cause damage to the liver include decreased blood flow, splanchnic vasoconstriction, pooling of blood in the microcirculation, right HF, and bacterial invasion. The subsequent changes include a loss of RES function, increasing the risk of infection; a decreased lactic acid conversion, contributing to metabolic acidosis; altered protein, fat, and carbohydrate metabolism; and altered bilirubin function (Hollenberg et al., 1997). Jaundice, increased serum bilirubin levels, and increased serum enzymes are early indicators of liver damage associated with shock. Serum globulin is increased, and serum albumin is decreased (Rice, 1991b; Hollenberg et al., 1997).

Lungs. The lung is fairly resistant to short-term ischemia. Thus, it is unlikely that low blood flow is the sole cause of pulmonary insufficiency associated with shock. Other contributory factors have been implicated, including thromboemboli or fat emboli in the pulmonary tree, the toxic effect of fibrin degradation products resulting from intravascular coagulation, serum complement depletion with sequestration of granulocytes in the lung, and sepsis. These factors lead to increased pulmonary capillary permeability. As the ensuing alveolar edema impairs surfactant production, massive atelectasis develops. Clinically, this is called shock lung, systemic inflammatory response syndrome (SIRS), adult respiratory distress syndrome (ARDS), or primary pulmonary edema, and it is characterized by severe hypoxemia, dyspnea, a marked reduction in lung compliance, and the presence of extensive lung infiltrates (Baue et al., 1998).

In cardiogenic shock, failure of the left ventricle leads to acute cardiogenic pulmonary edema. Because of the increase in LV end-diastolic pressure, there is an increase in left atrial pressure and dilation. Pressure is increased within the pulmonary capillary bed, forcing plasma or whole blood into the pulmonary interstitial compartment and, finally, into the pulmonary alveoli.

Coagulation. Disseminated intravascular coagulation is a disorder characterized by simultaneous thrombosis and hemorrhage, which occurs in the stage of irreversible shock. Procoagulants initiate uncontrolled microcirculatory clotting. The rapid thrombin formation causes three major problems: fibrin deposits in the microcirculation, consumption of clotting factors, and provocation of the fibrinolytic system. The prothrombin time and the partial thromboplastin time are prolonged, the platelet count and fibrinogen levels are decreased, and the fibrin degradation products are increased. Diffuse bleeding, which may ultimately lead to massive bleeding, may occur from the mucosal surfaces in the trachea, gastrointestinal tract, or urinary tract.

Immune System. Patients sustaining shock or trauma are at heightened risk of serious infection. The RES function is depressed in shock. The ability of the RES to clear damaged red cells, fibrin degradation products, and bacteria is impaired and contributes to the increased susceptibility to infection (Hollenberg et al., 1997).

Physical Assessment

Ongoing assessment of the patient at risk for or in shock, with early detection of subtle changes in the patient's condition, is essential. Subjective and objective data must be correlated with adjunctive clinical measurements such as the measurement of cardiac output and oxygen consumption. The clinical assessment of the patient provides the basis for medical and nursing intervention.

Integumentary

Skin appearance and temperature provide a clinical measure of peripheral circulation. Progressive peripheral vasoconstriction results in a change from the initial normal skin appearance to cool, moist, pale skin with mottling. In cardiogenic shock, cool, moist skin with barely perceptible peripheral pulses is commonly observed. Patients with vasogenic shock initially appear flushed, followed by pallor and mottling as shock progresses. Capillary refill and peripheral pulses are other indicators of the relative adequacy of cardiac output. Normal capillary refill is almost instantaneous; in cardiogenic and hypovolemic shock, capillary refill is often prolonged. Dry mucous membranes and thirst may be seen in association with elevated serum sodium (Rice, 1991d; Schuster & Lefrak, 1992).

Circulatory

Blood pressure is one of the defining characteristics of shock. A MAP of 65 to 75 mm Hg is required to maintain myocardial and renal perfusion. Shock is defined clinically as the pathophysiologic state that results from a MAP of less than 65 mm Hg over time. Narrowing of the pulse pressure indicates arteriolar vasoconstriction and a decreasing cardiac output (Francis et al., 2001; Hollenberg, 2001).

Pulse rate usually increases in response to sympathetic stimulation to compensate for decreased stroke volume and to maintain cardiac output. In vasogenic shock, the pulse may be full and bounding; in hypovolemic and cardiogenic shock, the pulse is weak and thready.

Jugular veins are flat in hypovolemic and vasogenic shock. Distended neck veins may be seen with cardiogenic shock associated with right ventricular failure (Givertz et al., 2001). The presence of a right ventricular heave, jugular venous V waves, and right-sided S3 or S4 may suggest pulmonary emboli. Distant heart sounds and an exaggerated pulsus paradoxus (>10 mm Hg) suggest cardiac tamponade. A laterally displaced and sustained left ventricular apical impulse with left-sided S3 and/or S4 suggests LV dysfunction (Saltzberg et al., 2001).

Neuroregulatory

Level of consciousness is an indicator of the adequacy of cerebral blood flow. With cerebral ischemia, the patient initially exhibits hypervigilance, restlessness, agitation, and mild confusion. Persistent cerebral hypoxia results in progressive unresponsiveness to verbal stimuli with eventual coma.

Renal

Urine output is an indicator of the adequacy of renal perfusion and may decrease early in hypovolemic and cardiogenic shock. Distributive shock may initially cause polyuria. Oliguria is defined by a urine output of less than 20 mL/h. Urine osmolarity and specific gravity increase, and urine sodium decreases with decreased urine output. Nonoliguric renal insufficiency is characterized by the output of large volumes of urine with low specific gravity. An elevated serum creatinine is an early, nonspecific indicator of impaired renal perfusion.

Pulmonary

Respiratory rate and depth are initially increased in all forms of shock, and patients may experience dyspnea or air hunger. This increased ventilation represents the body's attempt to eliminate lactic acid resulting from decreased tissue perfusion. Increased respiratory depth also enhances blood return to the right heart. Arterial blood gases initially reveal respiratory alkalosis. As shock progresses, this is followed by a combined metabolic and respiratory acidosis.

Medical Management Plan

Diagnosis

The diagnosis of shock is made by the history, physical examination, and collection of data from adjunctive diagnostic tests. The first priority is to differentiate low from high cardiac output. Physical examination of cool extremities, a narrow pulse pressure, and poor peripheral perfusion is characteristic of low output failure. Normal or high output shock is characterized by warm extremities, widened pulse pressure, and fever (if septic). The primary measurements that document the relative adequacy of blood flow include continuous monitoring of arterial blood pressure and monitoring of the electrocardiogram (ECG) and rhythm analysis. The ECG can be diagnostic in the setting of MI. Most patients in shock are tachycardic and may show evidence of supraventricular or ventricular arrhythmias. Low QRS voltage and/or electrical alternans can be seen in cardiac tamponade (Saltzbert et al., 2001).

Echocardiography is an excellent tool to obtain noninvasive information regarding the overall and regional systolic and diastolic function, intravascular volume, and cardiac hemodynamics (Stein et al., 1997). Echocardiography can rapidly assess for mechanical causes such as severe mitral regurgitation and papillary muscle rupture, acute ventricular septal defect, free wall rupture, and tamponade. Predictors of short-term and long-term mortality from cardiogenic shock relate to the LV ejection fraction and mitral regurgitation on presentation, supporting early use of echocardiography in the course of cardiogenic shock (Picard et al., 2002).

Chest radiography may suggest a specific diagnosis. Continuous measurement of urine output and urine studies is the best indicator of adequate organ perfusion, because the kidney is sensitive to decreased blood flow. A complete blood count and serial cardiac enzymes should be obtained. Serial measurements of arterial blood gases reflect the overall metabolic state of the patient, the adequacy of ventilation, and the adequacy of the circulation in providing for oxygen and metabolic needs. Measurement of mixed venous oxygen content (Sv^-O_2) by direct blood sampling or by continuous invasive monitoring reflects peripheral oxygen extraction and use. Serial arterial lactate levels can also be measured because the presence of lactic acidosis helps identify critical hypoperfusion as marked by anaerobic metabolism (Mizock & Falk, 1992; Rady, 1992; Astiz & Rackow, 1993).

Measurement of brain natriuretic peptide (BNP) has become a recent laboratory value that is measured as a means to identify those patients with elevated left ventricular dysfunction (Maisel et al., 2001; Anand et al., 2003). An elevated BNP correlates with increased LV end-diastolic pressure and volume, New York Heart Association classifications, and PAWP. Normal BNP level is less than 100 picograms/mL, and levels greater than 100 picograms/mL are a primary indication of HF. Elevation of other substances in the blood that reflect the function of specific organs, such as blood urea nitrogen, creatinine, bilirubin, aspartate aminotransferase, and lactate dehydrogenase, may be useful in the diagnosis of shock.

In seriously ill patients, direct determination of intra-arterial pressure with an arterial line is necessary because systemic arterial pressure determines the perfusion pressure of various organ systems and is predominantly the product of the cardiac output and systemic vascular resistance (SVR). In HF, a drop in cardiac output is compensated for by an increased SVR in an attempt to maintain the arterial blood pressure in normal range. SVR is also elevated in hypovolemic shock. Low SVR is initially found in septic shock because of the profound vasodilatation.

Right-sided heart catheterization with a pulmonary artery (PA) quadruple lumen thermodilution catheter can aid in the diagnosis and assessment of the severity of HF. This invasive hemodynamic monitoring can be useful in excluding volume depletion, right ventricular infarction, and mechanical problems (e.g., acute mitral regurgitation). It is also useful for monitoring the response to treatment (including volume, diuretics, inotropic support, vasoactive agents, natriuretic peptide) and manipulation of the variables of cardiac output, preload, and afterload (Ryan et al., 1997). The hemodynamic variables measured by this catheter are cardiac output by thermodilution, right atrial pressure, and PA systolic, diastolic, and wedge pressures (Woods, 1976). The cardiac output is decreased in HF, whereas the right atrial pressure or central venous pressure is either normal in LV failure or elevated in right HF. The PAWP indirectly measures the LV end-diastolic pressure, which is a measure of end-diastolic volume or preload and is elevated in HF.

Derived parameters that may be obtained by the use of the PA catheter include cardiac index (CI) and SVR. Body surface area (BSA), measured in square meters, is correlated with the volume of cardiac output (CO) to establish the CI:

$$CI = \frac{CO}{BSA}$$

Systemic vascular resistance (SVR), measured in dynes/second per centimeter^{-5}, reflects the pressure difference of the systemic arteries to the veins.

$$SVR = \frac{MAP - RAP}{CO} \times 80$$

where MAP is mean arterial pressure and RAP is right atrial pressure.

Besides offering diagnostic information, hemodynamic variables show a strong prognostic value for short-term survival. Forrester and colleagues (Forrester et al., 1976) classified patients with acute MI into four subsets with different mortality rates (Fig. 30-5). They showed that clinical signs of hypoperfusion occur with a cardiac index of less than 2.2 L/min per meter^2 and clinical signs of pulmonary congestion occur with a PAWP greater than 18 mm Hg. Subset I shows a patient with normal cardiac index and normal PAWP with no evidence of pulmonary congestion or peripheral hypoperfusion (warm and dry). Subset III shows a patient with a low cardiac index and PAWP reflecting peripheral hypoperfusion without pulmonary congestion (cool and dry) as seen in patients with hypovolemia. Subset II describes the patient with pulmonary edema with an elevated PAWP but without peripheral hypoperfusion (warm and wet), which may be seen in acute heart failure or decompensated chronic HF. Subset IV describes the patient with pulmonary edema with hypoperfusion (cold and wet), as seen in cardiogenic shock (Forrester & Walter, 1978).

Assessment of tissue metabolism, which is determined by mixed venous oxygen saturation, conventionally required sending a PA blood sample to the laboratory for interpretation. Some PA catheters are designed with a fiberoptic photometric lumen, allowing for continuous monitoring of mixed venous oxygen saturation.

Although PA catheters have been widely used for almost 30 years, there has been controversy because of retrospective studies that reported increased mortality in critically ill patients (Connors et al., 1996; Taylor, 1997). Current consensus is that

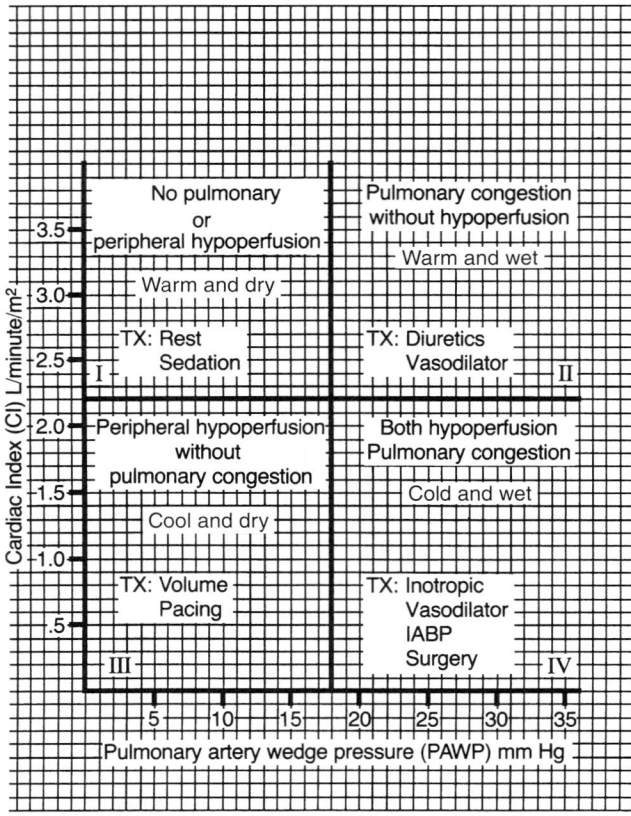

■ **Figure 30–5.** Forrester subsets: clinical states and therapy. IABP, intra-aortic balloon pumping.

PA catheters are useful in settings of myocardial infarction and cardiogenic shock and in those patients who do not respond to standard resuscitative measures for noncardiogenic shock (Mimoz et al., 1994; Ryan et al., 1996).

Acute Heart Failure, Acute Decompensated Chronic Heart Failure, and Cardiogenic Shock. The diagnosis of cardiac failure is seen on a continuum and is diagnosed by the presence of systemic and pulmonary hemodynamic alterations and neurohormonal mechanisms that reflect ventricular failure and result in an inadequate cardiac output and the retention of sodium and water. Noninvasive assessments of a rapid, thready pulse, elevated jugular venous pressure, arrhythmias, presence of and S3 and /or S4, oliguria, and decreased mentation are important clinical indices of an inadequate cardiac output and alterations in preload and afterload (Hass and Young, 1998; Francis, 2000). Primary indicators of acute heart failure or decompensated chronic heart failure may show an elevated PAWP greater than 18 mm Hg, but an initial normal cardiac index (Forrester subset II; see Fig. 30-5). The patient shows signs of pulmonary congestion without peripheral hypoperfusion (warm and wet). Primary indicators of cardiogenic shock include a systolic blood pressure less than 85 mm Hg or a MAP less than 65 mm Hg; cardiac index less than 2.2 L/min per meter^2; and an elevated PAWP greater than 18 mm Hg (Forrester subset IV; see Fig. 30-5). The patient shows signs of pulmonary congestion with peripheral hypoperfusion (cold and wet) (Forrester & Walter, 1978). Radiographically, the heart may be enlarged, and there may be evidence of pulmonary congestion.

The arterial blood gases frequently show a decreased PaO$_2$, which provides an important indicator of intrapulmonary shunting.

Hypovolemic Shock. Hypovolemic shock is a diagnosis based on the history and clinical assessment. Patients admitted after injury or surgery and those experiencing dehydration, gastrointestinal hemorrhage or obstruction, burns, liver disease, or peritonitis are all at risk for development of hypovolemic shock. In the initial stages of hypovolemia, interstitial fluids tend to move into the capillaries. The hematocrit value reflects the relation between red cells and intravascular fluid and decreases 6 to 8 hours after hemorrhage. Hematocrit initially is stable in hemorrhage, because red cells and plasma are lost. It is elevated in situations in which intravascular fluid is sequestered in the abdomen or selectively lost from the body, as in burns. If the fluid volume is monitored invasively, a worsening fluid volume deficit is indicated by a sustained decrease in CVP or PAWP (Gould et al., 1993; Rice, 1991c).

Distributive Shock. Septic shock has no universal pattern of signs and symptoms. Its many variations make it difficult to diagnose. The diagnosis is confirmed by microbiologic data, usually from two sets of blood cultures and cultures of sputum and urine (Eskridge, 1982).

Prognosis

The stages of shock depict a series of pathophysiologic changes that occur if medical and nursing interventions are delayed or inappropriate. The stages do not progress at the same speed in all patients. The length of time tissues are hypoxic is a major factor in determining the occurrence of complications. The early and intermediate stages of shock are reversible with aggressive management. The irreversible stage, caused by cellular necrosis and multiple organ failure, is not. The chance of recovery in the irreversible stage without permanent injury is low. In cardiogenic shock, patients with a cardiac index less than 1.81 L/min per meter^2 have a 70% mortality rate (Forrester et al., 1976). Patients with Sv$^-$O$_2$ less than 55% also have a high mortality rate (Mizock & Falk, 1992). Patients in septic shock are at greater risk for development of disseminated intravascular coagulation and ARDS than are patients with cardiogenic or hypovolemic shock. The survival rate with ARDS varies from 50% to 70% and depends on early recognition and management (Baue et al., 1998).

Treatment

The main goal of treatment of the metabolic defects produced by shock is the restoration of adequate tissue perfusion. Treatment should be aimed at: (1) restoring the blood volume; (2) strengthening the heart; and (3) restoring the normal luminal size of blood vessels. Depending on the cause of shock, treatment must revolve around the manipulation of one or more of these three mechanisms (Imm & Carlson, 1993; Mouchawar et al., 1993; Rice, 1999c; Hollenberg, 2001). Initial general management for patients is placement of large-bore venous catheters, continuous ECG, and blood pressure and pulse oximetry monitoring. If respiratory failure is imminent with patients with severe hypoxemia, hypercarbia or metabolic acidosis, then endotracheal intubation may be required with mechanical ventilation. A pulmonary artery catheter may be placed. Volume expansion may be needed to restore adequate circulation to maintain a PAWP of 14 to 16 mm Hg. Vasopressor support should be used only after preload is adequate to restore the blood pressure. The choice of a particular vasopressor/inotropic agent depends on the clinical circumstance (Table 30-3).

Table 30–3 ■ VASOPRESSORS AND INOTROPES USED IN SHOCK

Feature	Dopamine		Dobutamine	Norepinephrine	Epinephrine	Phenylephrine	Milrinone
Dosage mcg/kg/min	1–4	4–20	2.5–20	0.05–1	0.05–2	0.5–5	0.375–0.750
Receptor							
α	+	+++	+	++++	++++	++++	0
β$_1$	+	++	+++	+	++++	0	0
β$_2$	0	0	++	0	++	0	0
Dopaminergic	+++	++	0	0	0	0	0
Chronotropic (HR)	+	++	++	+	+++	0	+
Inotropic (stroke volume/ cardiac output)	+	++/+++	+++	+	+++	0	+++
SVR (afterload)	↓	↑↑	↓↓	↑↑↑↑	↓↓↑↑	↑↑↑↑	↓↓↓
Filling pressure (preload)	↓	↔↑↑	↓↓	↔↑↑	↔	↔	↓↓
Comments	Improves renal flow in low dose; first-line drug to restore BP		First-line agent to improve CO, but arrhythmogenic	Pure vasoconstrictor compared to dopamine	Increases MVO$_2$; avoid in cardiogenic shock	Purest vasoconstrictor	Inotrope of choice in pulmonary hypertension or failed dobutamine

Acute Heart Failure, Acute Decompensated Chronic Heart Failure, and Cardiogenic Shock

Acute manifestations of HF can be either in the setting of a new onset or in patients with established chronic HF, and further decompensation can lead to cardiogenic shock. It is critical to establish the diagnosis and determine the hemodynamic status: pulmonary congestion without peripheral hypoperfusion versus shock/hypoperfusion (Fig. 30-6). The three major goals of treatment are: (1) to increase the oxygen supply to the myocardium; (2) to maximize the cardiac output; and (3) to decrease the workload of the left ventricle.

1. *Increase the oxygen supply to the myocardium.* Increased inspired oxygen concentrations, including the institution of mechanical ventilation with positive end-expiratory pressure, may be required to maintain arterial blood gases within normal limits. Narcotic analgesics are used to control the patient's pain and aid in reducing myocardial oxygen demands.

   Aggressive reperfusion of the coronary arteries can be undertaken by invasive and noninvasive approaches, including percutaneous transluminal coronary angioplasty, atherectomy or stent placement, use of adjunctive antiplatelet therapy, thrombolytic therapy, and coronary artery bypass grafting (CABG), which were all associated with lower in-hospital mortality rates than treatment with standard medical therapy (Hochman et al., 1999; Urban et al., 1999; IAGS Proceedings, 2002). Studies suggest that immediate revascularization with percutaneous intervention (PCI), which may include angioplasty, stent placement, and atherectomy, along with adjunctive antiplatelet therapy, improves outcomes in patients with cardiogenic shock (Hochman et al., 1995; Hochman et al., 1999; Dauerman et al., 2002). Improvement is seen in wall motion in the infarct territory, with increased perfusion of the infract zone augmenting contraction of remote myocardium, possibly because of recruitment of collateral blood flow (Hochman et al., 1999). Reperfusion therapy with thrombolytic agents has decreased the occurrence of cardiogenic shock in patients with persistent ST segment elevation myocardial infarction, but thrombolytic therapy for patients in whom shock has already developed is disappointing and may be attributed to low perfusion pressure (Prewitt et al., 1992; GUSTO –IIb Angioplasty Substudy, 1997). For hospitals without revascularization capability, early thrombolytic therapy along with intra-aortic balloon pumping followed by immediate transfer for PCI or CABG may be appropriate (Sanborn et al., 2000). Several trials have reported favorable outcomes for patients undergoing emergent coronary artery bypass grafting (Hochman et al., 1999).

2. *Maximize the cardiac output.* Because the cardiac output is already compromised, arrhythmias, which occur as a result of ischemia, acid–base alterations, or MI, can cause a further decline in cardiac output. Electrolyte abnormalities should be corrected, because hypokalemia and hypomagnesemia predispose to ventricular arrhythmias. Antiarrhythmic agents, pacing, or cardioversion may be used to maintain a stable heart rhythm (Hass & Young 1998; Francis, 2000). Volume loading is undertaken with caution and in the presence of adequate hemodynamic monitoring. Optimal preload (LV end-diastolic pressure or PAWP) ranges between 14 and 18 mm Hg. However, fluid loading must be abandoned when the increase in filling pressure occurs without increase in cardiac output.

   Patients with chronic HF are usually using chronic pharmacologic therapy, which usually includes a diuretic, angiotensin-converting enzyme inhibitor (ACE inhibitor), beta-blocker, and digitalis, whereas acute HF patients are not. Treatment of acute episodes in these two scenarios are similar, with the exception of the higher incidence of reparable lesions in acute HF (e.g., acute occlusion of major coronary artery, ruptured chordae tendineae) (Hass & Young 1998; Francis, 2000). The Forrester subsets (see Fig. 30-5) can be used as guidelines for these patients in pulmonary edema (warm and wet) (Forrester & Walter, 1978). In subset II, the goal of therapy is to reduce the PAWP below a level that causes pulmonary congestion but above a level that causes a deleterious reduction in cardiac output by the Starling mechanism (Coombs, 1993). There are several options, because diuretics, peripheral vasodilators, and inotropic agents all reduce PAWP (Tables 30-3 and 30-4). The management strategy for the patient in acute cardiogenic pulmonary edema is outlined in Display 30-1.

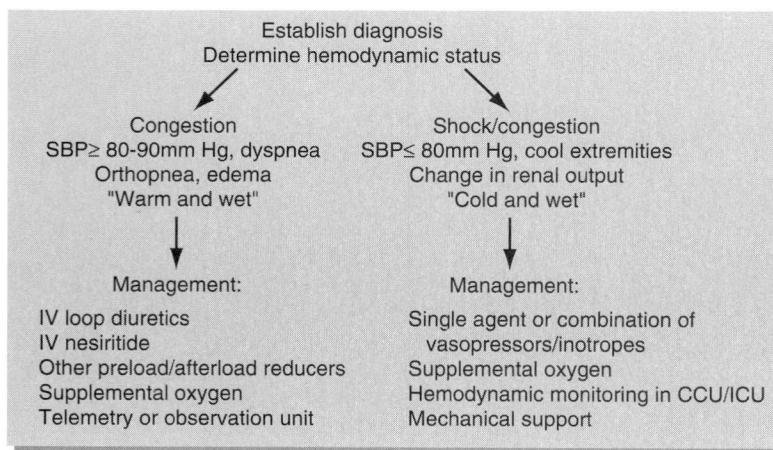

■ **Figure 30–6.** Algorithm for establishing the diagnosis of acute heart failure/ acute decompensation of chronic heart failure with pulmonary congestion versus cardiogenic shock with hypoperfusion and pulmonary congestion. General management principles for each diagnosis are listed. SBP, systolic blood pressure; IV, intravenous, IABP, intra-aortic balloon pump. (From Hass, G. J., & Young, J. B. [1998]. Acute heart failure management. In E. J. Topol [Ed.], *Textbook of cardiovascular medicine* [p. 2262]. Philadelphia: Lippincott-Raven.)

Table 30–4 ■ PRELOAD AND AFTERLOAD-REDUCING AGENTS FOR ACUTE/DECOMPENSATED HEART FAILURE

Drug	Dosing	Advantages	Disadvantages
Nitroglycerine	Sublingual:0.4 mg (or 1–2 sprays) at 5-minute intervals Intravenous: 0.4 μg/kg/min initially; increase as needed	+ Effect on coronary vasculature and in myocardial ischemia infarction	Hypotension Drug tolerance Inadequate afterload reduction in catastrophic disorders (e.g., acute valve insufficiency)
Nitroprusside	Intravenous: 0.1 μg/kg/min initially; increase as needed	Powerful afterload reducer	Hypotension Infusion needs to be watched closely; less favorable effects on coronary vasculature and myocardial ischemia; thiocyanate or cyanide toxicity during high-dose or prolonged infusion; particularly in renal failure
Nesiritide	Intravenous: bolus of 2 μg/kg, followed by 0.01 μg/kg/min infusion; may rebolus 1 μg/kg 1, and increase infusion up to maximum, which is 0.03 μg/kg/min	Favorable renal profile; use in decompensated heart failure	Hypotension; not to be used in patients in cardiogenic shock, systolic BP <90 mm Hg

D I S P L A Y   30-1

INITIAL MANAGEMENT OF ACUTE OR DECOMPENSASTED HEART FAILURE WITH PULMONARY EDEMA

Low Severity

Oxygen
Sublingual nitroglycerin 0.4 mg every 5 min or nitropaste
Intravenous nitroglycerin Start at 0.2 to 0.4 μg/kg/min
Intravenous furosemide (loop diuretic) 20 to 40 mg
    intravenously

Moderate Severity

Oxygen
Loop diuretic as above
Nesiritide bolus of 2μg/kg, followed by 0.01 μg/kg/min infusion
Nitroglycerin sublingual, paste
Consider intravenous morphine (2 to 6 mg) if no pulmonary
    contraindication

Critical Severity

Oxygen
Loop diuretic
Nesiritide
Nitroglycerin
Nitroprusside if further afterload reduction required
Mechanical ventilation as guided by arterial blood gas analysis
Electrocardiogram—exclude myocardial infarction
Echocardiography—evaluate ventricular function, valvular status
Proceed with urgent coronary angiography if reperfusion
    therapy indicated

Adapted from Hass, G. J., & Young, J. B. (1998). Acute heart failure management. In E. J. Topol (Ed.), *Textbook of cardiovascular medicine* (p. 2247–2271). Philadelphia: Lippincott-Raven.

An intravenous diuretic such as furosemide is administered when symptoms of pulmonary edema occur. A most recent new pharmacologic agent is nesiritide (B-type natriuretic peptide [BNP]; Natrecor), which represents a new drug class for acute decompensated HF. Nesiritide affords a unique combination of hemodynamic effects as a venous and arterial vasodilator, reducing preload and afterload while increasing cardiac output (indirectly) without increasing heart rate. It also has neurohormonal (inhibition of the RAAS and norepinephrine) and renal (diuresis and natreiuresis) effects (Colucci et al., 2000; Publication Committee for the VMAC Investigators, 2002). Nesiritide is best used early in conjunction with intravenous diuretics. ACE inhibitors and/or beta-blocker therapy may be continued for those patients with decompensated chronic HF. Many patients are also receiving digoxin, and digoxin levels should be measured because they may be abnormally increased during acute decompensation. Adjustments of the daily digoxin dose may be necessary (Francis, 2000). Once the patient is compensated and free from congestion, the nesiritide can be discontinued, and oral medications for HF should be optimally maximized. Nesiritide should not be used in cardiogenic or distributive shock, severe valvular stenosis, restrictive or obstructive cardiomyopathy, or constrictive pericarditis and pericardial tamponade.

Because patients in cardiogenic shock are in the high-risk Forrester subset IV (see Fig. 30-5), simultaneous improvement of both cardiac index and PAWP is the goal of therapy (Hollenberg, 2001; Francis, 1998; Hass & Young, 2000). These patients are hypoperfused and have pulmonary congestion (cold and wet). For patients with adequate intravascular volume, inotropic agents should be initiated. Inotropic agents are used to increase systemic and coronary artery perfusion pressure. Dobutamine can improve myocardial contractility and increase cardiac output and is usually the agent of choice in patients with systolic pressures greater than 80 mm Hg. Dobutamine can precipitate tachyarrhythmias and exacerbate hypotension. Dopamine is preferable in patients with systolic pressures less than 80 mm Hg. Tachycardia and increased peripheral resistance is dose-dependent, and can exacerbate myocardial ischemia (Francis, 2000; Opie & Gersh, 2001). In some situations, a combination of dopamine and dobutamine can be more effective than one agent alone (Francis, 2000; Hollenberg, 2001). When hypotension remains refractory, norepinephrine may be necessary. Other agents used for positive inotropic effect include phosphodiesterase inhibitors, such as amrinone or milrinone (Opie & Gersh, 2001).

Afterload reduction by peripheral vasodilators appears particularly well suited to reducing PAWP and SVR and improving CI. Inotropic agents are also used to increase systemic and coronary artery perfusion pressure. IABP counterpulsation may also be indicated (Francis, 2000; Saltzberg et al., 2001).

3. *Decrease the LV workload.* The efficacy of vasodilators has been shown in the treatment of cardiogenic shock. The major

physiologic effect of vasodilators is a reduction in LV end-diastolic pressure and systemic vascular resistance, with a subsequent increase in stroke volume and improved LV function (Chatterjee et al., 1993; Francis, 2000). Intravenous nitroprusside remains the drug of choice in cardiogenic shock, because it acts rapidly and has a balanced effect, dilating both veins and arterioles, thereby reducing both preload and afterload. Nitroglycerin can also be used, but it predominantly is a venous vasodilator, and large doses are sometimes required to reduce SVR (afterload). Intravenous nitroglycerin may be preferred in patients with acute MI because of its favorable effect on coronary blood flow (Francis, 2000).

Mechanical support of circulation may be used in the reduction of LV workload in cardiogenic shock. The intra-aortic balloon pump (IABP) is used to reduce afterload and improve cardiac output at the time of systolic contraction and to increase myocardial perfusion during diastole (Hochman et al., 1995; Hollenberg, 2001). Other mechanical assist devices may be used. Display 30-2 reviews the hemodynamically

---

DISPLAY   30–2

HEMODYNAMICALLY DIRECTED PROTOCOL FOR ACUTE HEART FAILURE/CARDIOGENIC SHOCK THERAPY

I. General hemodynamic goals
RAP $\leq$ 7 mm Hg
PAWP $\geq$ 15 mm Hg
SVR 1,000 to 1,200 dyne/sec/cm^5
CI > 2.5 L/min/m^2
"Optimum" systolic or mean BP is the lowest pressure that adequately supports renal function and central nervous system activity without significant orthostatic symptoms (systolic BP usually > 80 to 90 mm Hg)

II. Patient-specific hemodynamic goals
"Optimum filling pressure" (PAWP): lowest PAWP that can be maintained without preload-related decline in systolic BP or CI. A higher PAWP (18 to 20 mm Hg) is usually required in acute myocardial injury
"Optimum afterload" (SVR): lowest SVR that leads to reasonable cardiac index while maintaining adequate systolic BP (usually > 80 mm Hg) and renal perfusion (urine output > 0.5 mL/kg/h)

III. Specific intravenous pharmacologic therapy
Nitroprusside: begin when combined preload and afterload reduction is most important hemodynamic goal
Start at 0.1 to 0.2 µg/kg/min
Titrate upward by 0.2 µg/kg/min at 3- to 5-min intervals
Target hemodynamics (Section I)
Hemodynamic effects resolve rapidly when infusion stopped
Nitroglycerin: begin when preload reduction is primarily desired
Start at 0.2 to 0.3 µg/kg/min
Titrate at 3- to 5-min intervals
Be aware of tolerance
Target hemodynamics (Section I)
Effects resolve rapidly when infusion stopped
Dobutamine: begin when both inotropic and vasodilating effects desired but inotropic effects most important
Start at 2.5 µg/kg/min
Attempt to keep dose <15 µg/kg/min; avoid significant tachycardia
Consider adding low-dose dopamine or milrinone to assist with augmenting renal perfusion or achieving hemodynamic endpoints
Hemodynamic effects resolve over minutes to hours when infusion stopped, but benefits occasionally persist longer
Milrinone: begin when both vasodilating and inotropic effects desired
Dose range is 0.375 to 0.75 µg/kg/min (usual is 0.5 µg/kg/min)
Target hemodynamics (Section I)
Excessive hypotension with loading dose; would avoid loading in acute heart failure
Prolonged hemodynamic effects after drug is stopped

BP, blood pressure; CI, cardiac index; PAWP, pulmonary artery wedge pressure; RAP, right atrial pressure; SVR, systemic vascular resistance
From Hass G. J., & Young J. B. (1998). Acute heart failure management. In E. J. Topol (Ed.), *Textbook of cardiovascular medicine* (p. 2247–2271). Philadelphia: Lippincott-Raven.

directed pharmacologic protocol for acute heart failure and cardiogenic shock therapy. An in-depth discussion of circulatory assist devices follows this treatment section.

Specific Strategies

Right Ventricular Infarction. Interventions include correction of hypovolemia with fluid administration and maintaining right ventricular preload to a mean right atrial pressure of 15 mm Hg. Inotropic therapy with dobutamine can be used to support cardiac output (Kinch & Ryan, 1994; Mehta et al., 2001). Atrioventricular (AV) synchrony is also important, and AV sequential pacing can improve blood pressure and cardiac output. Reperfusion of the occluded coronary artery is also crucial (Hollenberg, 2001).

Acute Mitral Regurgitation. Management includes afterload reduction, usually with nitroprusside, and IABP as temporizing measures. Inotropic or vasopressor support may also be needed to support blood pressure and cardiac output. Surgical valve repair or replacement is the definitive treatment (Khan & Gray, 1991).

Ventricular Septal Wall Rupture. IABP and supportive pharmacologic agents are necessary. Operative repair is the only option. The timing of the repair remains controversial, although most feel repair should be undertaken within 48 hours of the rupture (Killen et al., 1997).

Cardiac Free Wall Rupture. This condition usually occurs during the first week after myocardial infarction, and the classic patient is an elderly woman with hypertension. This is a catastrophic event. Possible salvage is possible with rapid recognition, pericardiocentesis to relieve acute tamponade, and thoracotomy with repair (Reardon et al., 1997; Slater et al., 2000).

Valvular Heart Disease. Emergency surgery is indicated for aortic dissection that results in acute aortic regurgitation. In cases of severe mitral stenosis, decreasing the heart rate to improve diastolic filling time improves cardiac output. Mitral valvuloplasty or surgical intervention is indicated (Saltzberg et al., 2001).

Extracardiac Obstructive Shock. Pulmonary embolism is best treated with thrombolytic therapy (Meneveau et al., 1998). Cardiac tamponade initially needs volume support, but definitive therapy is pericardiocentesis and possible pericardial window (Slater et al., 2000; Saltzberg et al., 2001).

Hypovolemic Shock. Hypovolemic shock requires restoration of fluids and the circulating plasma volume. The amount of fluids and the speed at which they are infused is dictated by the severity of the loss and clinical status of each patient. Parental fluids used in shock include blood and blood products, colloids (e.g., dextran, hetastarch, albumin, plasma protein fraction [Plasmanate], modified fluid gelatins), and crystalloids (e.g., normal saline or lactated Ringer's solution) (Haljamae, 1993; Kuhn, 1993; Wu, Huang, Tan et al., 2001). After severe hypotension from massive hemorrhage, volume replacement should be administered rapidly enough to maintain the systolic pressure greater than 100 mm Hg and the MAP greater than 80 mm Hg. To maximally augment stroke volume, the CVP should be raised to 15 cm H_2O or the PAWP to 16 to 20 mm Hg.

The type of fluid to be administered is determined by the type lost, although opinions vary as to the amount and type

(Griffel & Kaufman, 1992; Gould et al., 1993). Crystalloid solutions, such as lactated Ringer's, are the most appropriate replacement solutions in hypovolemia because of vomiting, intestinal obstruction, or other sequestration of fluids (Drobin & Hahn, 1999). Crystalloid solutions can be administered initially while blood is being crossmatched for the patient who has hemorrhaged, and resuscitation with Ringer's alone may be adequate if blood loss is 20% or less (Kuhn, 1993). When acute hemorrhage reaches 20% to 50% blood loss, colloid solutions (e.g., 5% albumin, dextran) may be indicated. Major losses of whole blood (>50%) should be replaced with whole blood and fresh or frozen plasma to maintain a hematocrit of at least 24% and a hemoglobin of 8 g/dL (Nacht, 1992; Gould et al., 1993). Packed cells should be used if the CVP is high or if myocardial failure limits the amount and speed of fluid resuscitation. If the blood loss exceeds 80%, for every 5 units of blood, 1 to 2 units of fresh-frozen plasma and 1 to 2 units of platelets should be given to prevent hemodilution of clotting factors and bleeding (Imm & Carlson, 1993; Gould et al., 1993).

Much work has focused on the efficacy of hypertonic saline solutions (3%, 5%, and 7.5%) for fluid resuscitation in various forms of circulatory shock (Younes et al., 1992; Imm & Carlson, 1993). The amount of volume replacement with hypertonic solutions was reduced, but careful monitoring was essential to avoid complications. An infusion of hypertonic saline should always be accompanied by endogenous infusion of free water into the extracellular fluid space. They should not be considered for widespread clinical use (Younes et al., 1992; Gould et al., 1993).

Septic Shock. Treatment of septic shock has two primary therapeutic goals: (1) to eradicate the causative organism; and (2) to support vital life functions compromised by circulatory failure (Mouchawar & Rosenthal, 1993; Rice, 1991c). Interventions directed at identifying, localizing, and controlling the microorganisms include surgery, removal of the source of the contaminating organisms, and antimicrobial drugs.

Fluid replacement is the most common therapy used to support vital functions in septic shock. As with hypovolemic shock, there is disagreement about which fluid to use. Advantages of one fluid type over another have not been conclusively demonstrated (Imm & Carlson, 1993; Kuhn, 1993). Two types of fluids are used: crystalloids (e.g., lactated Ringer's, normal saline) and colloids (e.g., albumin, hetastarch, or dextran) (Haupt et al., 1992). Weil and Shubin advocate a "7/3 rule" for fluid replacement. They give fluid challenges of 5 to 20 mL/min for 10 minutes. If the PAWP reading is elevated more than 7 mm Hg above the beginning level, the infusion is stopped. If the PAWP or pulmonary artery diastolic pressure increases only 3 mm Hg above the starting point or if it decreases, another fluid challenge is given (Weil & Shubin, 1969).

Vasopressor agents are sometimes indicated to maximize cardiac output (see Table 30-4). The most commonly recommended inotropic agent in septic shock is norepinephrine. Alternatively, phenylephrine may be considered when the duration of vasodilatation is expected to be short and no cardiac dysfunction is present (Levy et al., 1999; LeDoux et al., 2000; Kellum & Pinsky, 2002). If patients are refractory to these agents, epinephrine should be used.

Clinical research studies report conflicting results from the use of steroids in septic shock. Steroids at high doses appear to block inhibition of gluconeogenesis by endotoxin and thus prevent intracellular hypoglycemia. Other actions of steroids include reduction of lactic acid concentration and stabilization of the endothelial wall of the pulmonary microcirculation. Stress doses of steroids are indicated mainly when there is suspicion of adrenal insufficiency (Bollaert et al., 1998; Briegal et al., 1999). Future therapies will focus on the immune system, with interferon and the prostaglandins as agents involved in the immune response (Mouchawar and Rosenthal, 1992; Shuster & Lefrak, 1992; Kellum & Pinsky, 2002).

One of the greatest challenges in septic shock is maintaining adequate tissue oxygenation. A recent study addressed the optimization of oxygen delivery (DO_2) to "supranormal" levels, with the DO_2 indexed goal of 600 mL/min/m^2 (Yu et al., 1993). This study suggested that the standard of care of treating these critically ill patients to a normal indexed DO_2 of 450 to 550 mL/min/m^2 should be reconsidered.

NURSING MANAGEMENT PLAN FOR THE PATIENT IN SHOCK

When caring for the acutely ill patient in shock, the goals of nursing and medicine merge to preserve life through the maintenance of oxygenation and circulation. In addition, the nurse considers the human responses to shock and the extent to which normal daily activities must be supplemented by nursing care. A through functional assessment of the individual patient is needed. Cues are collected within functional categories, and patterns are recognized, which provide the basis for nursing diagnosis and intervention. Altered tissue perfusion, self-care deficit, and altered family processes are among the nursing diagnoses encountered in association with shock.

Decreased Cardiac Output

Decreased cardiac output is a clinical problem requiring the specialized intervention of nursing and medicine for resolution. Both disciplines possess the knowledge necessary to recognize the signs and symptoms and to diagnose the problem. The accepted therapy (e.g., fluid replacement, inotropes, vasopressors, IABP) legally falls within the definition of medical practice. The physician must define the parameters of therapy. The nurse uses knowledge and judgment in administering the prescribed therapy (Coombs, 1993). In addition, the nurse considers the impact that a reduction in cardiac output has on other functional categories, such as perceptual awareness or activity tolerance. After confirming the specific response of the patient, the nurse intervenes directly to foster a salutary response.

Decreased Tissue Perfusion

Decreased tissue perfusion requires further specification to provide direction for nursing care. Because a nursing diagnosis must describe a problem for which nurses are educated and licensed to treat, use of the customary "related to" clause is inappropriate. Instead, the nurse must specify the impact of decreased tissue perfusion on the health of the patient, for example, altered tissue perfusion: decreased, cerebral, resulting in restlessness and agitation. The independent nursing interventions are then directed toward patient protection, the maintenance of the current level of function, and early recognition and prevention of further deterioration.

Self-Care Deficit

A self-care deficit exists when an individual experiences impaired motor function or cognitive function, resulting in a decreased ability to feed, bathe, dress, or toilet his or herself. Critical illness implies the inability to meet one's care needs. Self-care requires energy and endurance, which may surpass the strengths of the critically ill patient. Detailed assessment is required to determine the scope and extent of the deficit and to provide appropriate supportive or supplemental intervention. Nursing activities designed to meet these needs include turning, positioning, bathing, massaging, and communicating. Knowing when to help and when to refrain from helping are equally important. There is an interrelatedness among the self-care deficits—feeding, bathing, toileting—and interventions instituted in one category may affect other categories.

Altered Family Processes Related to an Ill Family Member

This nursing diagnosis refers to the state in which a normally supportive family experiences a stressor that challenges its previously effective functioning ability. It is frequently seen in caring for people who are critically ill, with the stressors being the critical illness and the intensive care environment. Defining characteristics include a family system that cannot or does not: (1) meet the physical, emotional, or spiritual needs of its members; (2) accept or express a full range of feelings; (3) seek or accept help appropriately; (4) communicate openly with its members; or (5) adapt constructively to crisis. Nursing interventions must be individualized but may include actions such as conducting family orientation to the hospital, providing a private place for family to wait, providing information regarding changes in the patient's condition or treatment, acknowledging family strengths, and facilitating the expression of feelings.

Circulatory Assist Devices

Circulatory assist devices have been clinically used, in various forms, since the mid 1960s. IABP counterpulsation is now commonly used in a variety of hospital centers for medical and surgical patients. Temporary circulatory support devices, once restricted to a few large centers, are now used with increasing frequency in most larger hospitals as an adjunct to cardiovascular surgery programs. Such devices are used to support circulation temporarily when the injured myocardium cannot generate adequate cardiac output. In centers with heart transplantation programs, these devices are accepted therapy for temporarily supporting patients with end-stage HF until a donor heart becomes available (Stevenson & Kormos, 2001). One such device has been used successfully to support a patient

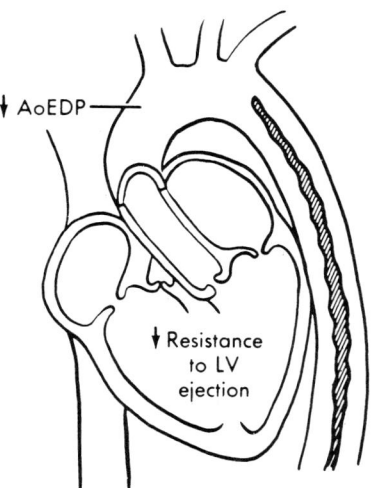

■ **Figure 30–10.** Impedence or resistance to left ventricular (LV) ejection is decreased by abrupt balloon deflation before systole. Properly timed deflation decreases aortic end-diastolic pressure (A₀EDP), which decreases the workload of the left ventricle. (From Quaal, S. J. [1984]. *Comprehensive intra-aortic balloon pumping* [p. 83]. St. Louis: C.V. Mosby.)

contributes to decreasing LV workload. Improved forward flow results in increased cardiac output with a resultant increase in blood pressure. Tachycardia that resulted from decreased stroke volume in the shock state is not necessary for compensation as forward flow (stroke volume) improves. As a result, rapid heart rate should diminish, decreasing oxygen demand. Better systemic perfusion helps to reverse the acidosis often seen in shock states and improves secondary organ dysfunction related to the previous hypoperfused state. Displays 30-4 and 30-5 summarize the physiologic effects of IABP therapy.

Contraindications. Inflation of the balloon during diastole dictates that the aortic valve be competent. If aortic regurgitation is present, then inflation serves to generate more aortic regurgitation because of the increased pressure and retrograde

---

DISPLAY 30-4

PHYSIOLOGIC EFFECTS AND EXPECTED CLINICAL OUTCOMES OF BALLOON INFLATION

PHYSIOLOGIC EFFECTS

Increased early diastolic pressure
Diastolic augmentation
Increased aortic root pressure
Enhanced coronary artery perfusion pressure
Improved oxygen delivery
Decreased ischemia

CLINICAL OUTCOME

Early diastolic pressure ≥ systolic pressure
Decreased angina
Decreased signs of ischemia on the electrocardiogram
Decreased ventricular ectopy of ischemic origin

DISPLAY 30-5

PHYSIOLOGIC EFFECTS AND EXPECTED CLINICAL OUTCOMES OF BALLOON DEFLATION

PHYSIOLOGIC EFFECTS

End-diastolic drop in aortic pressure
Decreased afterload requirement
Lower systolic pressure requirement
Improved contractility
Increased forward flow during systole
Improved secondary organ perfusion
Increased efficiency of left ventricular work (decreased oxygen demand)

CLINICAL OUTCOMES

Improved forward flow
Decreased preload
Decreased pulmonary artery wedge pressure
Decreased crackles in the lung fields
Increased cardiac output
Increased mean blood pressure
Improved urine output
Improved peripheral pulses and warm skin temperature
Clearer sensorium
Decreased heart rate

---

flow against the aortic valve. This effect actually increases the workload of the ventricle. Thus, IABP therapy is of no benefit to this patient and actually may contribute to further deterioration of the patient's condition.

The presence of an aortic aneurysm also contraindicates IABP therapy. First, the tip of the catheter may advance into the aneurysm during insertion, resulting in perforation of the weakened wall or dislodgement of thrombus. A second concern is the effect of inflation and deflation adjacent to the thrombotic debris that accumulates in the aneurysm. There is a great potential for thrombus material to break free, resulting in emboli and possibly precipitating a catastrophic event.

Severe peripheral vascular occlusive disease is considered a contraindication to IABP therapy. More accurately, a femoral or iliac artery insertion site is the actual contraindication. Catheter insertion may be difficult or impossible in this situation. There is a potential for dislodgement of plaque from the vessel wall, which can embolize and totally disrupt distal flow. Dissection of the vessel is also possible in this situation. Another possibility is disruption of flow caused by the presence of the catheter in an already compromised vessel. Such a situation jeopardizes the distal extremity by depriving it of blood flow. This potential problem can be avoided by selecting an alternate method of insertion. In the cardiac surgery patient, the catheter may be inserted directly into the thoracic aorta. The obvious disadvantage of this approach is the requirement for reopening the sternotomy incision to remove the catheter. Another, less conventional approach is antegrade aortic insertion of the balloon catheter by way of the right subclavian artery (McBride et al., 1989). This approach requires a subperiosteal clavicular resection to access the artery, but is less invasive than a sternotomy incision. Newer catheters of smaller diameter minimize the risk of occluding distal blood flow. A final contraindication is balloon catheter insertion in any patient who has a terminal condition in which no medical or surgical therapy exists that might alter the outcome. It would serve no purpose to introduce more aggressive therapy to support such a patient. The only time this may be considered is when the patient meets the criteria for heart transplantation.

Proper Timing to Achieve Expected Clinical Outcomes.
Proper timing of IABP therapy is crucial to achieving the beneficial hemodynamics previously outlined. Proper timing requires coordination of inflation and deflation of the balloon with the patient's cardiac cycle. The R wave from the ECG, pacemaker spikes on the ECG, or the arterial systolic pressure is used to identify individual cardiac cycles. All these act as signals to the IABP console to discriminate systole from diastole. The R wave signals the onset of electrical depolarization, which precedes mechanical systole. A ventricular pacemaker spike essentially represents the same event. Arterial systolic pressure signals the onset of mechanical systole. Any of these can be used as a reference point to determine when deflation of the balloon should optimally occur. An arterial waveform is necessary to determine the onset of mechanical diastole and systole and to verify timing. Diastole has begun when the dicrotic notch appears on the arterial waveform. Balloon inflation is timed to occur at this point in the cardiac cycle. The deflation point can be optimally adjusted by observing the end-diastolic drop in pressure created by balloon deflation. The goal is to create the greatest pressure drop possible. Ideally, the difference between end-diastolic pressure without the balloon effect and end-diastolic pressure created by balloon deflation is at least 10 mm Hg. Evidence that afterload reduction has occurred is seen in the following systolic pressure. With afterload reduction, the next systolic pressure after balloon deflation is lower than the systolic pressure with no balloon effect. This is evidence that LV workload has been decreased. To evaluate balloon timing properly, the assist ratio is set at 1:2, meaning the balloon is assisting every other cardiac cycle. In this way, the observer can compare the effect of balloon inflation and deflation with unassisted beats. Most patients tolerate this well for a brief period. Five criteria can be used to determine the effectiveness of IABP timing, as illustrated on the arterial pressure tracing (Fig. 30-11).

The first step is to ensure that inflation occurs at the dicrotic notch, the beginning of diastole. Inflation should actually be timed to obliterate the notch. The interval between the onset of systolic upstroke and the point of balloon inflation should not be shorter than the interval between the systolic upstroke and dicrotic notch on the unassisted beat. Inflation that occurs too early is detrimental to the patient because the abrupt increase in diastolic pressure may force the aortic valve closed prematurely. Complete ejection may be impaired. Late inflation, past the dicrotic notch, does not harm the patient, but the duration of assistance is unnecessarily shortened so that maximal benefit from augmented pressure is not achieved.

Next, the upstroke of balloon inflation should be sharp and parallel with the preceding systolic upstroke. This creates a V-shaped appearance, with the nadir of the V being the point of inflation. The sharp upslope ensures that maximal early augmentation is occurring. A slope that is not straight may indicate that the balloon is inflating late, perhaps off of some

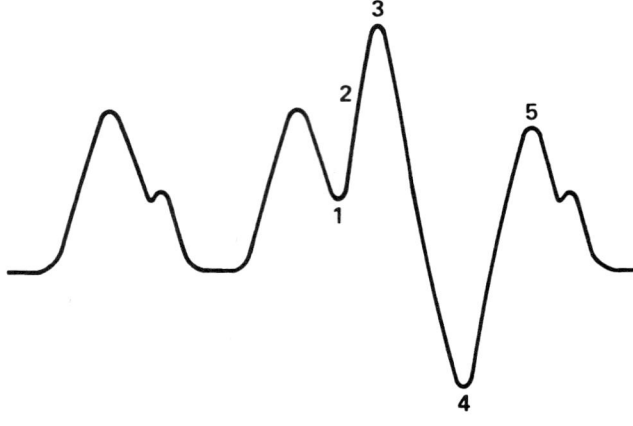

IABP ON

■ **Figure 30–11.** Criteria for effective intra-aortic balloon pump (IABP) timing: (1) inflation occurs at the dicrotic notch; (2) the slope of rise of balloon inflation is straight and runs parallel with the preceding systolic upstroke; (3) augmented diastolic pressure is at least equal to the preceding systolic pressure; (4) end-diastolic pressure at balloon deflation is lower than the preceding unassisted end-diastolic pressure; (5) the next systolic pressure is assisted systole and is lower than the preceding systole, which was not affected by balloon deflation. (From Shinn, J. A. [1990]. Intra-aortic balloon pump counterpulsation. In C. M. Hudak, B. M. Gallo, & T. S. Lohr [Eds.], *Critical care nursing: A holistic approach* [5th ed., p. 213]. Philadelphia: J. B. Lippincott.)

other artifact during early diastole. In this case, the loss of the V configuration also is evident.

The third criterion is that the augmented diastolic pressure peak be at least equal to the preceding systolic pressure peak. A decrease in this pressure peak may indicate gas loss from the balloon. This loss can occur by natural diffusion. A balloon normally requires refilling every 1 to 2 hours because of natural diffusion of gas through the membrane. Most consoles automatically purge and refill the balloon and catheter at least every 2 hours. An abrupt loss of the pressure peak may indicate the development of a leak in the balloon or the catheter. Occasionally, augmentation greater than the systolic pressure is not achievable because of the size of the balloon relative to the size of the aorta. To fit properly, the balloon should occlude 85% to 90% of the aorta when inflated. If a smaller balloon was used because of insertion difficulties, or if the aorta is dilated, diastolic augmentation pressure may be less than the patient's systole. In this instance, balloon inflation does not generate as much volume displacement or rise in aortic pressure during diastole.

The fourth point to evaluate is balloon deflation at the end of diastole. Proper deflation results in a drop in pressure at the end of diastole. This drop in pressure creates an end-diastolic pressure much lower than diastolic pressure without the balloon effect. Timing is adjusted so that the lowest pressure possible is achieved. It is important to make sure that the systolic upstroke that follows is straight and that a sharp, V-shaped configuration is present. The V shape indicates that systole began immediately after deflation. Any plateau indicates that deflation occurred too early. In this case, early deflation does not relieve the ventricle of impedance, and afterload reduction does not occur. Late deflation results in higher impedance because the balloon remains inflated at the onset of systolic ejection. An end-diastolic pressure that is the same or greater than the end-diastolic pressure without balloon assistance is evidence of late deflation. The following systolic pressure is the same as the unassisted systole because no afterload reduction has occurred. It can also be lower than the unassisted systole because of the inability of the failing ventricle to work against the higher impedance to ejection.

Finally, the observer should note what effect balloon deflation has on the next systolic pressure, for reasons just described. The goal is to ensure that the lower systolic pressure that follows balloon deflation is caused by afterload reduction and not by improper timing, which resulted in late deflation. Proper balloon fit has an impact on the ability to achieve afterload reduction. If the balloon size is small, then volume displacement may have less of an effect on lowering end-diastolic pressure. Figure 30-12 illustrates the four possible errors that can occur with timing.

Complications. Intra-aortic balloon pump therapy carries a relatively low risk of morbidity given the clinical condition of the patient. Most complications are vascular. The incidence has been reported to be approximately 15% (Arafa et al., 1999; Cohen et al., 2000). Vascular injuries that may occur during insertion include plaque dislodgement, dissection, laceration, and compromised circulation to the distal extremity. If a cutdown was used during insertion, then peripheral nerve injury is another complication that may be incurred during the insertion procedure. Compromised circulation can occur any time during IABP therapy as a result of the presence of the indwelling catheter, compartment syndrome, or embolus from thrombus formation along the catheter or on the balloon (Cohen et al., 2000). The incidence of limb ischemia ranges from 5% to 35% (Arafa et al., 1999; Cohen et al., 2000). These complications occur with greater frequency in patients with peripheral vascular occlusive disease, in women with small vessels, in smaller patients (BSA < 1.8 m2), and in patients

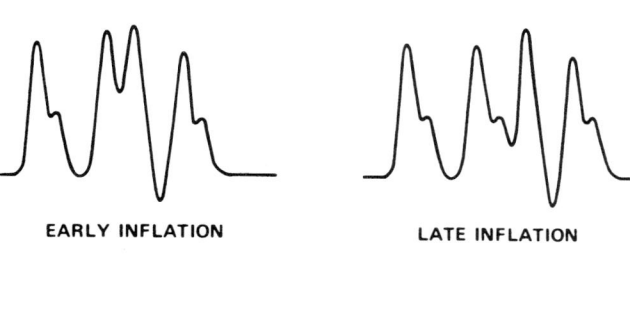

EARLY INFLATION   LATE INFLATION

EARLY DEFLATION   LATE DEFLATION

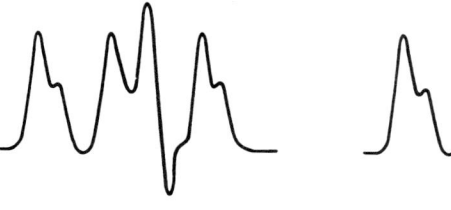

■ **Figure 30–12.** Possible errors in balloon timing. (From Shinn, J. A. [1986]. Intra-aortic balloon pump counterpulsation. In C. M. Hudak, B. M. Gallo, & T. S. Lohr [Eds.], *Critical care nursing: A holistic approach* [4th ed., p. 198]. Philadelphia: J. B. Lippincott.)

with a history of stroke, transient ischemic attacks, and diabetes (Cohen et al., 2000). Nursing functions involved in monitoring or preventing compromised circulation include careful assessment of peripheral perfusion; preventing the patient from flexing the hip of the affected extremity, which may compromise blood flow; and maintaining coagulation times within prescribed parameters by careful titration of anticoagulants. The nurse should be aware that multiple or prolonged attempts at insertion increase the risk of vascular injury and thrombus formation. Infection at the insertion site is reported to occur in less than 5% of patients. Insertion site infections may dictate the removal of the IABP catheter. Careful efforts must be made to maintain the sterility of insertion site dressings. Other problems that may be encountered include thrombocytopenia; compromised circulation to the left subclavian, renal, or mesenteric arteries because of balloon malposition; and bleeding from the insertion site or other line insertion sites. Mechanical problems related to the balloon include improper timing or a leak or perforation in the balloon, necessitating its removal. A leak in the balloon becomes evident as augmentation becomes less effective. Eventually, blood backs up in the catheter and can be detected. When a leak has occurred, the balloon must be removed immediately to avoid the possibility of gas embolus or balloon entrapment. Entrapment occurs when blood enters the balloon and becomes a large, hardened mass. The size makes it difficult to remove without a surgical intervention.

Nursing Management Plan. Good cardiovascular assessment of the patient provides indicators that IABP therapy is effectively assisting LV function. Assessment includes vital signs, cardiac output, heart rhythm, heart regularity, heart ischemia, urine output, color, peripheral perfusion, and mentation. All these parameters should reflect an improvement in the patient's condition. The patient using IABP therapy is relatively immobile because of the need to avoid hip flexion and to multiple invasive monitoring and infusion lines. Often, the patient requires endotracheal intubation and ventilator support. Care must be taken to prevent or minimize extensive atelectasis. These patients also are at greater risk for respiratory tract infection. Careful suctioning technique and prevention of aspiration reduce this risk.

Prolonged hypotension from the shock state may jeopardize renal function. Monitoring urine output and quality closely may contribute to early recognition and treatment of renal dysfunction, thus avoiding acute renal failure. Psychosocial support of the patient and family is important. The patient requires interventions that minimize stress, disorientation, and sleep deprivation. Families benefit from honest communication and help with the interpretation of the patient's condition. Nursing Care Plan 30-1 outlines a plan of care for the patient on IABP therapy. Because this patient is experiencing acute LV failure or cardiogenic shock, many nursing diagnoses used for those conditions apply. The plan of care that is outlined focuses on issues unique to IABP therapy.

Left Ventricular Assist Devices. In patients who have catastrophic myocardial injury or deteriorating end-stage HF, IABP therapy may provide inadequate support. IABP therapy depends on ventricular function to maintain systemic blood pressure. The IABP is not capable of contributing to cardiac output directly. With profound ventricular failure, mean blood pressure is less than 60 mm Hg, systolic blood pressure is less

Nursing Care Plan 30–1 ■ The Patient with an Intra-aortic Balloon Pump

Nursing Diagnosis 1 ➤ Potential decreased tissue perfusion in the lower extrenities related to possible catheter obstruction, emboli, or thrombosis, manifested by signs and symptoms of decreased perfusion in legs.

Nursing Goal 1 ➤ To minimize risk of decreased tissue perfusion in lower extremities

Outcome Criteria ➤ 1. Appropriate level of anticoagulation will be maintained as prescribed.
2. Dorsalis pedis and posterior tibial pulses will be palpable and of equivalent strength of baseline assessment.
3. Patient's skin will be warm, dry, and of normal color.
4. Patient will be knowledgeable about proper hip position.

NURSING INTERVENTIONS	RATIONALE
1. Record quality of peripheral pulses before insertion of the intra-aortic balloon pump (IABP) catheter.	1. Required to establish a baseline so changes will be detectable.
2. Evaluate quality of peripheral pulses, skin color, capillary refill, and temperature at least hourly.	2. Required to detect changes.
3. Maintain anticoagulation level at prescribed range by accurate monitoring or heparin or dextran infusion.	3. Thrombus could form along catheter or on balloon if anticoagulation falls below therapeutic range. Any thrombus may potentially break loose with balloon movement, causing emboli
4. Assist patient with ankle flexion and extension every 1 to 2 hours.	4. Exercise of calf muscles will minimize venous stasis and potential for deep venous thrombosis.
5. Maintain cannulated extremity in a straight position, avoiding hip flexion. Use a brace or soft restraint as needed.	5–7. Hip flexion will decrease flow in the cannulated artery, potentially compromising distal circulation.
6. Keep head of bed at a 15-degree backrest position or lower. If it is desirable to elevate the head of the bed for pulmonary care issues, put the patient in reverse Trendelenburg to achieve the desired elevation without hip flexion.	
7. If patient is alert, instruct patient in importance of avoiding hip flexion.	
8. Maintain continuous alternating inflation and deflation of the balloon.	8. Continuous motion minimizes the possibility of thrombus formation on the balloon. Thrombus can occur rapidly on a motionless balloon, with subsequent risk of vascular occlusion or embolization.

Nursing Goal 2 ➤ To detect early manifestations of decreased tissue perfusion in lower extremities

Outcome Criteria ➤ 1. Patient will maintain palpable dorsalis pedis and posterior tibial pulses equivalent to baseline.
2. Patient's skin will be warm, dry, and of normal color.
3. These changes will be detected within 1 hour of occurence.

NURSING INTERVENTIONS	RATIONALE
1. Monitor quality of peripheral pulses, capillary refill, skin temperature, and color hourly.	1. Required to detect changes.
2. Notify physician if pulses diminish or become absent in the cannulated extremely.	2. Circulatory compromise may progress slowly as thrombus grows larger or rapidly as a result of an embolus.
3. If patient complains of leg pain, promptly evaluate peripheral perfusion. Notify physician of any changes.	3. Leg pain may be occurring as a result of ischemia. Ischemia is an indication for removal of the IABP catheter.
4. Monitor for swollen limb that is tense on palpation, patient complaints of continuous pressure, and pain induced with passive stretching of the affected muscle.	4. These signs and symptoms may indicate the presence of compartment syndrome.

(continued)

Nursing Care Plan 30–1 ■ The Patient with an Intra-aortic Balloon Pump *(Continued)*

Nursing Diagnosis 2 ➤ Decreased cardiac output related to suboptimal IABP therapy, manifested by lowered mean arterial blood pressure with requirement for high-dose inotropic support.

Nursing Goal 1 ➤ To prevent decreases in cardiac output as a result of suboptimal IABP therapy

Outcome Criteria ➤ 1. Mean arterial blood pressure will be 60 to 70 mm Hg or better.
2. IABP timing will be correct with:
   Inflation occuring at the dicrotic notch
   Optimal diastolic augmentation
   Deflation at end-diastole wit a drop in pressure of at least 8 to 10 mm Hg below unassisted end-diastole.
3. Balloon will be refilled before large gas losses secondary to diffusion.
4. Patient will have decreasing requirements for inotropic support over the course of IABP assistance.

NURSING INTERVENTIONS	RATIONALE
1. Verify correct timing of IABP hourly. Make correction as needed.	1. Timing may be altered if the heart rate changes or systolic function improves.
2. Document settings for inflation, deflation, and systolic, end-diastolic, and mean arterial pressures with IABP assistance.	2. Documentation will illustrate trends, improvement, and necessary interventions to achieve optimal assistance.
3. Document level of diastolic augmentation, Evaluate for a decrease in augmentation.	3–4. A decrease in diastolic augmentation indicates a need to refill the balloon. A major loss of diastolic augmentation in a short time may indicate a tear or leak in the balloon (Check catheter for evidence of blood backing up from aorta.)
4. Maintain proper volume of balloon to ensure optimal diastolic augmentation.	
5. Ensure that the balloon is refilling every 1–2 hours, depending on the type of machine.	5. An optimally filled balloon is necessary for optimal diastolic augmentation.

Nursing Goal 2 ➤ To reduce or eliminate situations that will interfere with maintenance of proper IABP timing assist ratio (i.e., assistance of every beat).

Outcome Criteria ➤ 1. Patient will have a regular heart rhythm.
2. There will be no interference of trigger signal to IABP console.
3. Timing will be corrected with changes in heart rate.
4. Balloon will be free of kinking.

NURSING INTERVENTIONS	RATIONALE
1. Reevaluate timing anytime there is greater than a 10- to 20-beat change in heart rate on onset of new arrhythmias. Use the automatic timing feature on the IABP console if available	1. A 10- to 20-beat or greater change in heart rate alters the systole-to-diastole ratio in each cardiac cycle. Previous inflation and deflation settings may be inappropriate for a change in this ratio (i.e., the time spent in diastole is longer at slower heart rates and shorter at rapid heart rates) unless the IABP console has an automatic timing feature.
2. Maintain adequate electrocardiogram (ECG) trigger signals to IABP console. Change any ECG electrodes that become loose, placing new ones on clean, dry skin.	2. Loss of trigger signals impairs IABP ability to assist the heart with each cardiac cycle.
3. Notify physician of any dysrhythmias. Secure cardiac pacing parameters if dysrhythmia is irregular and is impairing IABP tracking. Administer antiarrhythmic agents as ordered.	3. Irregular arrhythmias may impair IABP ability to assist each cardiac cycle. Pacing can stabilize this situation so that systole-to diastole ratio is the same for each cardiac cycle. The pacemaker spike may be used as the trigger for IABP timing.
4. Maintain patient in proper body position (head of bed 15 degrees and no hip flexion). Use leg brace and soft restraint as necessary. Log roll patient when turning.	4–5. Sitting the patient upright or elevating head of bed may cause hip flexion and subsequent catheter kinking. Kinking impairs the flow of gas in and out of balloon. An upright position also may cause the catheter to advance up the aorta with potential migration into an aortic arch vessel.
5. Instruct X-ray technicians and other personnel not to sit patient upright.	

(continued)

Nursing Care Plan 30–1 ■ The Patient with an Intra-aortic Balloon Pump *(Continued)*

Nursing Diagnosis 3 ➤ Sensory/perceptual alterations: sensory overload related to intensive care unit environment and the need for frequent monitoring, manifested by disorientation, anxiety, restlessness, and sleeplessness.

Nursing Goal 3 ➤ To reduce or eliminate excessive sensory stimuli that might impair sleep-wake cycles

Outcome Criteria ➤ 1. There will be no excessive or unnecessary noise in patient's environment.
2. Patient will have progressive blocks of undisturbed time for sleep.

NURSING INTERVENTIONS	RATIONALE
1. Maintain monitor "bleep" volume at lowest audible level. 2. Minimize amount of extraneous noise from other equipment in patient's room. 3. Minimize unnecessary noise caused by staff conversations in patient's room. 4. Turn down lights in patient's room during the night. 5. Organize nursing care so patient has uninterrupted time for sleep during the night, amount to be determined by patient's condition.	1–3. Unnecessary noise disturbs patient's sleep and creates higher levels of stress during wakefulness. 4. Darkening the room during the night helps patient distinguish day from night and provides a better environment for sleep at night. 5. Organized care can provide patients with up to 2-hour periods when it is unnecessary directly to touch the patient. As the patient's condition improves, longer blocks of time are feasible.

Nursing Goal 2 ➤ To assist patient with maintaining orientation and some degree of control of self

Outcome Criteria ➤ 1. Patient will be oriented to date, time, and place.
2. Patient will be able appropriately to interpret his or her environment.

NURSING INTERVENTIONS	RATIONALE
1. Talk with patient while administering care. Explain noises, activity, and procedures to be done. 2. Involve patient in decision making about care if possible (e.g., which direction to turn next). When patient is able, teach patient to do ankle flexion exercises and deep breathing exercises, which can be done independently by patient. 3. Frequently inform patient of the time and date and orient to surroundings. 4. Place familiar objects such as pictures within patient view; involve family in the process.	1. Explanations assist the patient to interpret the environment appropriately and minimize stress and anxiety associated with a fear of the unknown. 2. Involvement in decisions helps the patient maintain some degree of control. 3. Frequently reorienting the patient helps prevent disorientation. 4. Familiar objects may help maintain orientation.

Nursing Diagnosis 4 ➤ Ineffective family coping related to inadequate support, knowledge deficit, fear of patient dying, and fear of the intensive care unit environment, manifested by requests for help or inappropriate behavior.

Nursing Goal ➤ To assist family with development of ability to cope.

Outcome Criteria ➤ 1. The family members will acknowledge their fears and concerns.
2. The family will verbalize a decrease in their level of fear and will appear calmer.
3. The family will demonstrate an ability to cope effectively.

(continued)

Nursing Care Plan 30-1 ■ The Patient with an Intra-aortic Balloon Pump *(Continued)*

NURSING INTERVENTIONS	RATIONALE
1. Encourage family members to express feelings, and convey understanding of their concerns and emotional stress.	1. Expression of concerns promotes effective coping.
2. Provide the family with honest information about the patient's condition to reduce fears. Keep the family informed of changes.	2–3. Fear is reduced by clarifying misunderstandings. Information decreases fear of the unknown.
3. Set aside time during visiting hours to spend with the family, and encourage family members to ask questions. Offer explanations about the intensive care unit environment.	
4. Encourage realistic hope based on the patient's progress. Point out progress to the family.	4. Hope helps the family with coping.
5. Allow family to participate in care as appropriate.	5. Participation decreases feelings of helplessness in aiding the recovery of the patient.
6. Determine how the family has coped with previous stressful situations.	6. It is important to identify previous effective coping mechanisms and to promote the use of these mechanisms.

than 90 mm Hg, and the cardiac index typically is less than 2.0 L/min/m^2 (Leh, 1991; Maroney & Reedy, 1994). IABP therapy increases cardiac output only marginally (500 to 800 mL/min), and the expectation of long-term support in this scenario is unrealistic (Copeland et al., 1985). Therefore, more aggressive therapy with an LVAD, which can provide a physiologic cardiac output, is warranted.

Patient Indications. The most frequent indications for use of an LVAD are to support a patient awaiting a donor for heart transplantation or for patients who cannot be weaned from cardiopulmonary bypass after conventional treatment, including IABP therapy. Approximately 1% to 4% of cardiac surgery patients cannot be weaned from cardiopulmonary bypass after major myocardial injury (Magovern et al., 1985; Miller et al., 1990). Between 25% and 50% of those patients may survive with LVAD support (Jett, 1994; Rose et al., 1983). Some centers use LVADs to support the patient in cardiogenic shock after MI. The LVAD is used to decrease LV work and to maintain systemic blood pressure while the left ventricle recovers from injury. If allowed to rest for 48 to 96 hours, there is potential for myocardial function to return. Indications of initial ventricular recovery should appear within 30 hours (Magovern et al., 1985). The decision to insert an LVAD must be made quickly but carefully. The longer the patient remains on cardiopulmonary bypass, the more likely the patient is to have profound coagulopathy, which may become difficult or impossible to amend.

Situations that may contraindicate LVAD placement include preexisting disease states, severe debilitation making recovery unlikely, massive myocardial injury in which recovery is not possible, multisystem organ failure, and prolonged cardiac arrest associated with neurologic damage (Macgovern et al., 1985). Unless cardiac transplantation is an option, a major factor in the decision-making process is to select patients in whom recovery is possible, thus avoiding a situation in which the patient becomes totally LVAD-dependent without potential for weaning.

Mechanism of Support. Left ventricular assist devices are designed temporarily to replace the pumping function of the left ventricle by being placed in the circuit of normal blood flow.

Blood is diverted from the left atrium or left ventricle and shunted to the LVAD by the pressure gradient between those chambers and the LVAD. Blood is returned to the aorta with continuous flow from the LVAD or in a pulsatile fashion with pump ejection occurring during the patient's diastole or asynchronous to the patient's cardiac cycle. Available pumps are divided into two categories: continuous-flow pumps and pulsatile pumps. They may also be thought of as temporary, short-term pumps or as pumps capable of providing long-term support.

Continuous-flow pumps are continuously filled by left atrial blood flow, and blood is returned to the aorta at a continuous rate. There is no ability to mimic systole or diastole, but constant flow rates and mean blood pressure are maintained. Left atrial blood flow is captured by a cannula placed in the left atrial chamber. As a result, LV preload is markedly diminished, and LV workload is reduced. Continuous-flow pumps are capable of flow rates of up to 6 L/min (Maroney & Reedy, 1994; Miller et al., 1990). Pulsatile pumps are generally filled at anytime throughout the cardiac cycle. They may also fill over more than one cardiac cycle. LV pressures as low as 10 mm Hg may be all that is required to fill the LVAD. These pulsatile pumps are totally dependent on the patient's adequate preload for their filling. Anything that decreases the patient's preload will decrease the output from the pumps. If the LV is cannulated to bring flow to the pump, then the LV is basically now acting as an "atrium" for the pump. The trigger for ejection from this type of pump is the actually fully filled state of the pump. This type of mode is called fill-to-empty or automatic. Filling of the LVAD can occur during the patient's native systole if the pump is synchronized to the patient's cardiac cycle. In that case, the LVAD is empty before LV contraction, impedance to LV ejection is reduced dramatically, and minimal work is required to fill the LVAD. The aortic valve remains closed, and no blood is ejected from the ventricle into the aorta during systole. Once the LVAD is filled, ejection from the LVAD pump into the aorta occurs, which coincides with the patient's native diastole. The LVAD is in counterpulsation with the patient's heart. It is in its filling phase during LV contraction and is ejecting during LV relaxation. Pumps can also be set to run at fixed specific rates that may or may not be the same as the patient's heart rate. In general, the operation mode of choice is fill-to-empty or automatic. This mode insures that the blood sac is fully filled with each beat, minimizing the chances for thrombus to develop in the pump. The pulsatile LVADs are capable of assuming total responsibility for maintaining physiologic cardiac output.

Types of Continuous-flow Devices. One type of device provides continuous flow by means of a roller pump. This pump is filled from a left atrial cannula, and flow is returned to the ascending aorta after passing through a roller pump. Cannulas must exit the chest to connect to the pump and the chest is left open. Maximal heparinization is required to prevent thrombus formation within the cannulas. Roller pumps also traumatize blood cells, causing hemolysis. This device is only indicated for short-term situations after cardiac surgery. After long periods, hemolysis and coagulopathies become problematic. An example of this support would be the maintenance of partial cardiopulmonary bypass after a cardiac surgical procedure. Roller pumps represent the first attempts to provide circulatory assist outside of the operating room.

The centrifugal–kinetic energy pump is an example of a frequently used continuous-flow LVAD (Fig. 30-13). The Bio-Medicus pump (Medtronic, Minneapolis) is an example of this type of device. With this system, blood is taken from the left atrium and returned to the aorta. The major advantage of such a device is the ability to function at low pressure while delivering high volume or flow. As blood enters the pump, it is whirled by centrifugal force, creating a vortex or tornado effect, which is the energy needed to propel the blood forward (Maroney & Reedy, 1994; Marchetta & Stennis, 1988). The centrifugal force is created by a revolving magnet on the pump console. The pump also contains a magnet that will spin according to the revolutions per minute that are set on the pump consol. Trauma to blood cells is markedly decreased, compared to cardiopulmonary bypass or roller pumps. Heparinization is not required for up to 48 hours, as long as flow rates are kept at greater than 1 L/min. This pump also minimizes the buildup of excessive outflow pressure that can result in tubing disconnections. These devices can support patients for longer periods of time than roller pump designs, primarily because of the decreased trauma to blood cells. However, they, too, require that the chest be left open in many cases. Another advantage of this pump is that it can be used for almost any size patient. This pump is only indicated for postcardiotomy support.

New devices undergoing clinical trials also work in series with the native heart. These devices are called axial flow pumps and are capable of generating up to 10 L/min of continual, nonpulsatile blood flow, which more effectively rests the left ventricle (Frazier et al., 2002). The Jarvik Heart 2000 (Jarvik Heart Inc., New York) is an example of this type of pump. The pump is mounted on a conduit that is inserted directly into the LV. Axial flow is achieved by rotating blades contained within the pump housing, which rotate at speeds of up to 12,000 rpm (Frazier et al., 2002). This action draws blood from the left ventricle and propels it through a conduit that is anastomosed either to the ascending aorta or to the descending aorta, where blood can be returned to the systemic circulation. The anastomoses will determine whether the incision for the operation will be a sternotomy or a left thoracotomy. Power to run the motor comes via a percutaneous lead that exits the body in the right upper quadrant of the abdomen. Placement of the pump is an elective procedure for patients with end-stage heart failure. It has been developed currently as a bridge to transplantation, but the eventual design goal is for it to be an alternative to transplantation. A major benefit of the pump is its small size. It is small enough for women and small men who presently are excluded as candidates for implantable pumps because their body size is too small to accommodate the larger size of the implantable pumps. Another advantage of this pump design is that it does not have to be synchronized with the heart. The flow through the pump is governed by the revolutions per minute that the propellers in the pump spin, which is controlled by the pump operator. If the patient wants to increase activity level, the patient can actually adjust the pump to provide more flow for activity and decrease the flow for lighter activity. The Jarvik Heart 2000 is currently in clinical trials and not available for general use because it is not FDA-approved.

Types of Pulsatile Pumps. Pulsatile LVAD pumps are either pneumatic (air driven) or electric. Either can be used as temporary support, but the electrically driven pump has the potential to be totally implantable and is more convenient for patients. Pneumatic pumps require compressors, which means that patients are always tethered to a consol. A major advantage of these pumps is their pulsatile flow, which allows for longer-term support. Pulsatile flow provides better kidney perfusion, decreases peripheral vascular resistance, and increases systemic perfusion.

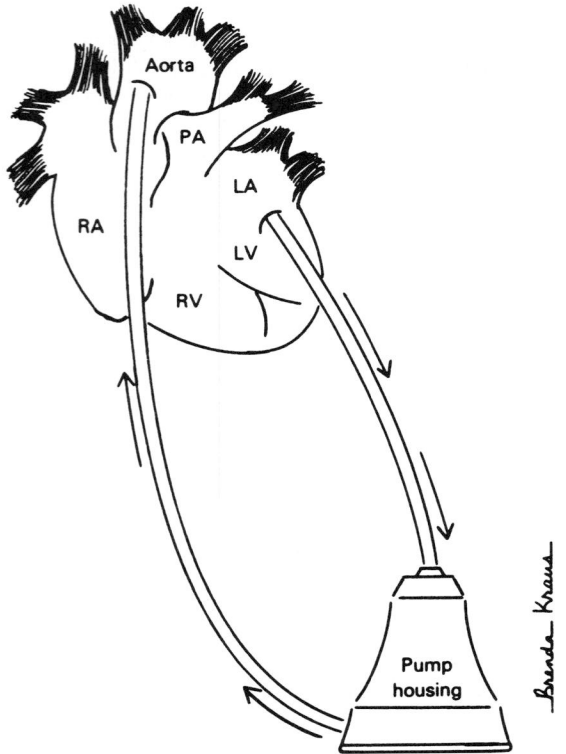

■ **Figure 30–13.** Continuous-flow centrifugal-kinetic energy pump. PA, pulmonary artery; LA, left atrium; LV, left ventricle; RA, right atrium; RV, right ventricle. (From Marchetta, S., & Stennis, E. [1988]. Ventricular assist devices: Applications for critical care. *Journal of Cardiovascular Nursing,* 2[2], 45.)

The Thoratec pump (Thoratec Laboratories Inc., Pleasanton, CA) is an example of a pneumatic system. Pulsatile flow is created by air compression of a polyurethane sac that contains 65 mL of blood. Positive air pressure compresses the sac, causing ejection from the LVAD to the aorta. Negative pressure is applied after ejection, causing the blood sac to fill. Backward flow is prevented by placement of inflow and outflow disk valves in the pump. The blood sac is filled by means of a cannula placed in either the left atrium or the left ventricle. It can be controlled by three modes: (1) a fixed rate that is asynchronous with the patient's heart and delivers variable stroke volumes; (2) triggering of the pump by the R wave of the ECG (not practical for long-term support or in ambulatory patients); or (3) triggering of pump ejection by reaching full-fill (also called *fill-to-empty mode*) (Maroney & Reedy, 1994; Ley, 1991). A major advantage is pulsatile flow, which allows for longer-term support. A major disadvantage is the risk of infection associated with a pump that is placed externally. Conduits from the atrium or ventricle and the return conduits to the aorta are tunneled through the chest and connected to the external pump (Fig. 30-14). For longer-term support, the preference is to cannulate the ventricle as larger flows can be obtained. Epithelial cells ingrow into the Dacron-covered conduits and protect the patient from infection. Tissue growth acts as a seal from the surface of the body. Another pulsatile pump is the Novacor pump (World Heart Corp, Oakland, CA). This electrically driven pump is designed to be totally implanted in a preperitoneal pocket just anterior to the posterior rectus sheath. Chronic support is possible because electrical energy can be stored in battery cells that are small enough to implant, although the electric power unit currently used is an exchangeable 5-hour battery. Filling of the pump occurs from a cannula that is placed in the LV apex. The cannula is tunneled through to the preperitoneal pocket, where the pump is implanted. Blood is returned to the ascending aorta through another cannula. The device also uses inflow and outflow tissue valves. Ejection is triggered by a fixed rate, changes in the velocity of filling, or in a fill-to-empty mode. When the blood sac is filled, or when the trigger is recognized, two electrically powered pusher plates compress the blood sac, which is located between the two plates. Ejection occurs when the sac is compressed (Shinn & Oyer, 1993). The major advantage of this system is the ability to implant the device, eliminating much of the risk of infection. Another major advantage is patient mobility and the capacity for rehabilitation from their previous state of heart failure making discharge from the hospital possible. Figure 30-15 illustrates the appearance of the device. In the device's current configuration, patients must wear a controller on a belt and carry two sources of power with them. The controller and

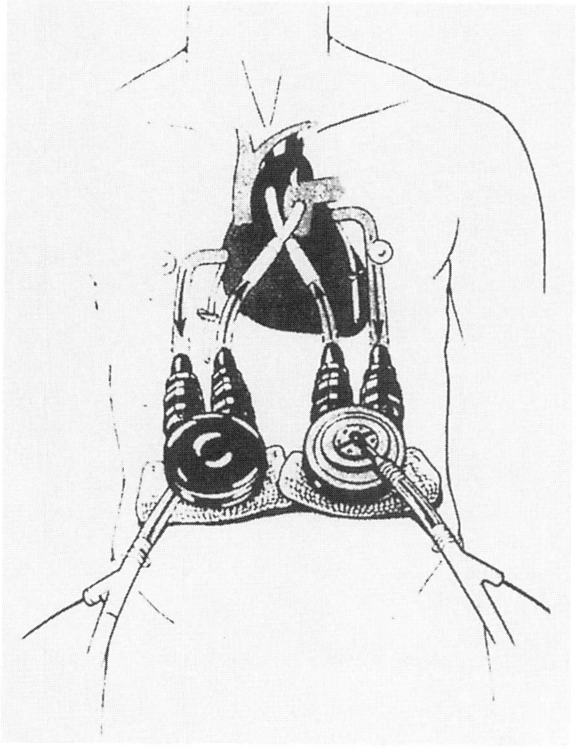

■ **Figure 30–14.** Cannula placement of two Thoratec pumps during support of both right and left ventricles. Arrows indicate direction of blood flow. (From Ruzevich, S. A., Swartz, M. I., & Pennington, D. G. [1988]. Nursing care of the patient with a pneumatic ventricular assist device. *Heart & Lung, 17,* 399–405.)

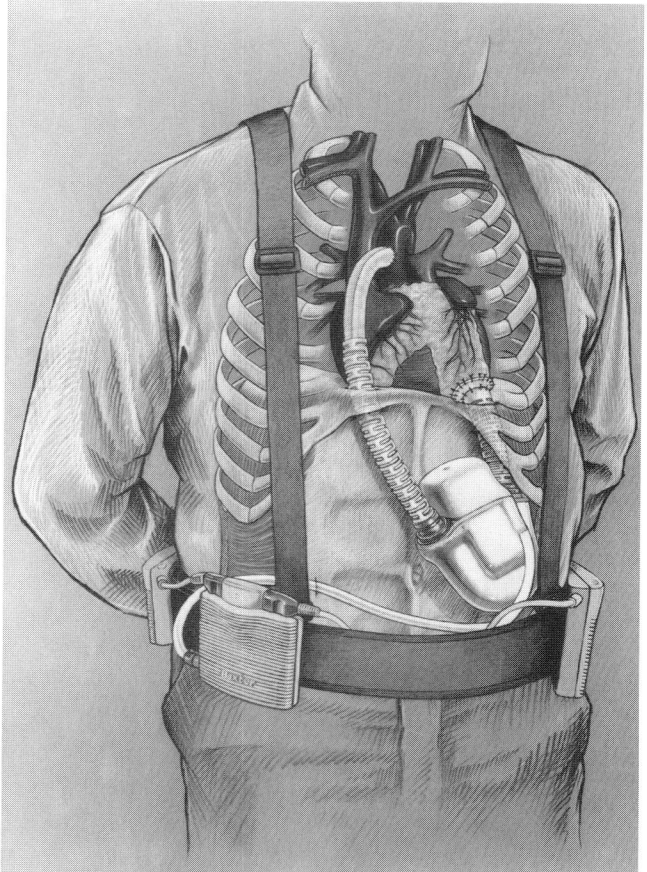

■ **Figure 30–15.** Illustration of the Novacor left ventricular assist device shows the design of the implanted system. Power is transmitted through a percutaneous lead to the implanted pump. The patient either wears portable batteries or can be connected to an AC power source when at rest. (Courtesy of World Heart Inc. Oakland, CA.)

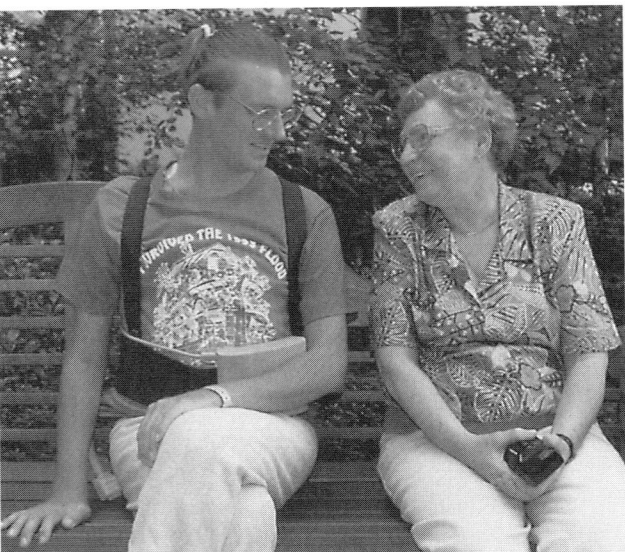

■ **Figure 30–16.** A patient with the wearable Novacor left ventricular assist system. The patient carries a 5-hour battery pack on a specially designed belt, allowing him to be totally untethered to a heavy operating console, as with many other types of devices. This patient is shown at approximately 3 weeks after implantation and is waiting for a donor heart.

battery packs can also be carried in a shoulder bag or in specially designed vests that have pockets for the controller and two battery packs. One battery serves as a reserve supply when the patient switches from AC power to battery operation, and vice versa. The other primary battery pack can supply power for up to 5 hours, allowing the patient freedom from a tethered set-up. Figure 30-16 shows the first patient in the United States to receive the wearable system. Another pump that can also be totally implanted is the HeartMate vented electric system (Thoratec, Pleasanton, CA). The Heartmate pump is electrically driven, with a controller and battery pack system similar to those of the Novacor pump. Ejection occurs as a result of compression of the blood sac by a single, motor-driven pusher plate (Hunt et al., 1998). Both the Novacor and Heartmate systems can support patients for extended periods with a relatively low risk of thromboembolism or mechanical problems. All are used to support patients awaiting heart transplantation. The portability of the systems allows patients to be ambulatory and to care for themselves. As a result, these patients are now routinely discharged from the hospital while they wait for suitable donor hearts (McGovern, 1998; Moroney & Powers, 1997; Myers et al., 1996).

REFERENCES FOR ACUTE HEART FAILURE AND CARDIOGENIC SHOCK

Anand, I. S., Fisher, L. D., Chian, Y. T., et al. (2003). Changes in brain natriuretic peptide and norepinephrine over time and mortality and morbidity in the valsartan heart failure trial (Val-HeFT). *Circulation, 107*, 11278–1283.

Astiz, M. E, & Rackow, E. C. (1993). Assessing perfusion failure during circulatory shock. *Critical Care Clinics, 9*, 299–309.

Bartling, B., Holtz, J., & Darmer, D. (1998). Contribution of myocyte apoptosis to myocardial infarction. *Basic Research in Cardiology, 93*, 71–84.

Baue, A. E., Durham, R., & Faist, E. (1998). Systemic inflammatory response syndrome (SIRS), multiple organ dysfunction (MODS), multiple organ failure (MOF): are we winning the battle? *Shock, 10*(2), 79–89.

Bollaert, P. E., Charpentier, C., Levy, B., et al. (1998). Reversal of late septic shock with supraphysiologic doses of hydrocortisone. *Critical Care Medicine, 26*, 645–650.

Bolli, R. (1998). Basic and clinical aspects of myocardial stunning. *Progress in Cardiovascular Disease, 40*, 477–516.

Bonow, R. O. (1995). The hibernating myocardium: Implications for management of congestive heart failure. *American Journal of Cardiology, 75*, 17A–25A.

Briegel, J., Forst, H., Haller, M., et al. (1999). Stress doses of hydrocortisone revere hyperdynamic septic shock: a prospective, randomized, double-blind, single center study. *Critical Care Medicine, 27*, 723–732.

Brown, J., MacKinnon, D., King, D., et al. (1992) Elevated arterial blood pressure in cardiac tamponade. *New England Journal of Medicine, 327*, 463–466.

Chatterjee, K., Hutchinson, S. J., & Chou, T. M. (1996) Acute ischemic heart failure: Pathophysiology and management. In P. Poole-Wilson, W. Colucci, K. Chatterjee, et al. (Eds.), *Heart failure: Scientific principles and clinical practice* (pp. 523–549). New York: Churchill Livingstone.

Chatterjee, K., Parmly, W. W., Swan, W., et al. (1973). Hemodynamic and metabolic responses of vasodilator therapy in acute myocardial infarction. *Circulation, 48*(6), 1183–1193.

Colucci, W. S., et al. (2000). Intravenous nesiritide: a natriuretic peptide, in the treatment of decompensated heart failure. *New England Journal of Medicine, 343*(4), 246–253.

Connors, A. F. Jr, Speroff, T., Dawson, N. V., et al. (1996) The effectiveness of right heart catheterization in the initial care of critically ill patients. SUPPORT investigators. *JAMA, 276*, 889–897.

Coombs, M. (1993) Hemodynamic profiles and the critical care nurse. *Intensive Critical Care Nurse* 9(1), 11–26.

Dauerman, H. L., Goldberg, R. J., White, K., et al. (2002). Revascularization, stenting, and outcomes of patients with acute myocardial infarction complicated by cardiogenic shock. *American Journal of Cardiology*, (90), 838–842.

Drobin, D., & Hahn, R. G. (1999). Volume kinetics of Ringer's lactated solution in hypovolemic volunteers. *Anesthesiology, 90*, 10, 81–91.

Eskridge, R. A. (1982). Septic shock. *Critical Care Quarterly, 4*, 55–68.

Forrester, J. S., & Walter, D. (1978). Hospital treatment of congestive heart failure: management of hemodynamic profile. *American Journal of Medicine, 65*, 173–179.

Forrester, J. S., Diamond, G., Chatterjee, K., et al. (1976). Medical therapy of acute myocardial infarction by application of hemodynamic subsets. *New England Journal of Medicine, 295*, 1362-1386; 1404–1413.

Francis, G. S. (2000). Management of acute and decompensated heart failure. In J. D. Homespun & B. H. Greenberg (Eds.), *Congestive heart failure* (2nd ed., pp. 553–569). Philadelphia: Lippincott-Raven.

Francis, G. S. (1998). Pathophysiology of heart failure clinical syndrome. In E. J. Topol (Ed.), *Textbook of cardiovascular medicine* (pp. 2179–2203). Philadelphia: Lippincott-Raven.

Francis, G. S., Galler, J. P., & Sonnelbick, E. H. (2001). Pathophysiology and diagnosis of heart failure. In J. W. Hurst (Ed.), *The heart* (10th ed., pp. 655–685). New York: McGraw-Hill.

Givertz, M. M., Colucci, W. S., & Braunwald, E. (2001). Clinical aspects of failure: high output failure; pulmonary edema. In E. Braunwald, D. P. Zipes, & P. Libby (Eds.), *Heart disease: A textbook of cardiovascular medicine* (6th ed., pp. 534-561). Philadelphia: W. B. Saunders.

Gorman, J. H., 3rd, Gomar, R. C., Jackson, B. M., et al. (1997). Distortion of the mitral valve in acute ischemic mitral regurgitation. *Annals of Thoracic Surgery, 64*, 1026–1031.

Gould, S. A., Sehgal, L. R., Sehgal, H. L., & Moss, G. S. (1993). Hypovolemic shock. *Critical Care Clinics, 9*(2), 239–259.

Griffel, M. I., & Kaufman, B. S. (1992). Pharmacology of colloids and crystalloids. *Critical Care Clinics, 8*, 235–248.

GUSTO-IIb Angioplasty Substudy Investigators. (1997). An international randomized trial of 1138 patients comparing primary coronary angioplasty versus tissue plasminogen activator for acute myocardial infarction. *New England Journal of Medicine, 336*, 1621–1628.

Haas, G. J., & Young, J. B. (1998). Acute heart failure management. In E. J. Topol (Ed.), *Textbook of cardiovascular medicine* (pp.2247–2271). Philadelphia: Lippincott-Raven.

Haas, G. J., & Young, J. B. (1998). Acute heart failure management. In E. J. Topol (Ed.), *Textbook of cardiovascular medicine* (pp. 2247–2271). Philadelphia: Lippincott-Raven.

Haljamae, H. (1993). Volume substitution in shock. *Acta Anaesthesiol Scandinavia (Suppl.)*, 98, 25–28.

Haupt, M. I., Kaufman, B. S., & Carlson, R. (1992). Fluid resuscitation in patients with increased vascular permeability. *Critical Care Clinics* 8, 341–352.

Hochman, J. S., Boland, J., Sleeper, L. A., et al. (1995). Current spectrum of cardiogenic shock and effect of early revascularization on mortality. Results of an International Registry. *Circulation*, 91, 873–881.

Hochman, J. S., Sleeper, L. A., Webb, J. G., et al. (1999). Early revascularization in acute myocardial infarction complicated by cardiogenic shock. *New England Journal of Medicine*, 341, 625–634.

Hollenberg, S. M. (2001). Cardiogenic shock. *Critical Care Clinics*, 17(2), 391–411.

Hollenberg, S. M., & Parrillo, J. E. (1997). Shock. In A. S. Fauci, E. Braunwald, K. J. Isselbacher, et al. (Eds.), *Harrison's principles of internal medicine* (pp. 214–222). New York: McGraw-Hill.

IAGS Proceedings (2002). Supporting patients in shock. The high mortality among patients in cardiogenic shock "LV or RV infarcts": What have we learned and have we made a difference? *Journal of Invasive Cardiology*, 14(8), 483–491.

Imm, A., & Carlson, R. W. (1993). Fluid resuscitation in circulatory shock. *Critical Care Clinics* 9(2), 313–333.

Katz, A. M. (2000). *Heart failure: Pathophysiology, molecular biology and clinical management*. Philadelphia: Lippincott Williams & Wilkins.

Kellum, J. A., & Pinsky, M. R. (2002). Use of vasopressor agents in critically ill patients. *Current Opinion in Critical Care*, 8, 236–241.

Khan, S. S., & Gray, R. J. (1991). Valvular emergencies. *Cardiology Clinics*, 9(4), 689–710.

Kinch, J. W., & Ryan, T. J. (1994). Right ventricular infarction. *New England Journal of Medicine*, 330, 1211–1217.

Killen, D. A., Piehler, J. M., Borkon, A. M., et al. (1997). Early repair of postinfarction ventricular septal rupture. *Annals of Thoracic Surgery*, 63, 138–142.

Kuhn, M. M. (1993). Colloids versus crystalloids. *Critical Care Nurse*, 11(5), 37–52.

LeDoux, D., Astiz, M. E., Carpati, C. M., et al. (2000). Effects of perfusion pressure on tissue perfusion in septic shock. *Critical Care Medicine*, 28, 2729–2732.

Levy, B., Bollaert, P. E., Charpentier, C., et al. (1997). Comparison of norepinephrine and dobutamine to epinephrine for hemodynamics, lactate metabolism, and gastric tonometric variables in septic shock: a prospective, randomized study. *Intensive Care Medicine*, 23, 282–287.

Maisel, A. S., Koon, J., Krishnaswamy, P., Kazenegra, R., et al. (2001). Utility of B-natriuretic peptide as a rapid, point-of-care test for screening patients undergoing echocardiography to determine left ventricular dysfunction. *American Heart Journal*, 141, 367–374.

Mann, D. L. (2000). Cytokines as mediators of disease progression in the failing heart. In J. D. Hosenpud, & B. H. Greenberg (Eds.), *Congestive heart failure* (2nd ed., pp.213–231). Philadelphia: Lippincott William & Wilkins.

Mann, D. L. (2002). Inflammatory mediators and the failing heart: Past, present, and the foreseeable future. *Circulation Research*, 91, 988–998.

Mehta, S. R., Eikelboom, J. W., Natarajan, M. K., et al. (2001). Impact of right ventricular involvement on mortality and morbidity in patients with inferior wall myocardial infarction. *Journal of the American College of Cardiology*, 37(1), 37–43.

Meneveau, N., Schiele, F., & Metz, D. (1998). Comparative efficacy of a two-hour regimen of streptokinase versus atelplase in acute massive pulmonary embolism: immediate clinical and hemodynamic outcome and one-year follow-up. *Journal of the American College of Cardiology*, 31, 1057–1063.

Mizock, B. A., & Falk, J. L. (1992). Lactic acidosis in critical illness. *Critical Care Medicine* 20, 80–91.

Mouchawar, A., & Rosenthal, M. (1993). A pathophysiologic approach to the patient in shock. *Anesthesioly Clinics* 31, 1–17.

Nacht, A. (1992). The use of blood products in shock. *Critical Care Clinics* 8, 255–291.

Opie, L. H., & Gersh, B. J. (2001). Digitalis, acute inotropes, and inotropic dilators. In L. H. Opie (Ed.), *Drugs for the heart* (5th ed., pp. 154–186). Philadelphia: WB Saunders.

Parrillo, J. E., Burch, C., Shelhamer, J. H., et al. (1985). A circulating myocardial depressant substance in humans with septic shock. *Journal of Clinical Investigation*, 76(4), 1539–1553.

Picard, M. H., Davidoff, R., Sleeper, L. A., et al. (2002). Echocardiographic predictors of survival and response to early revascularization in cardiogenic shock. *Circulation*, 107, 279–284.

Prewitt, R. M., Gu, S., Schick, U., & Ducas, J. (1994). Intraaortic balloon counterpulsation enhances coronary thrombolysis induced by intravenous administration of a thrombolytic agent. *Journal of the American College of Cardiology*, 23, 794–798.

Publications Committee for the VMAC (Vasodilatation in the Management of Acute Congestive Heart Failure) Trial. (2002). Intravenous nesiritide versus nitroglycerin for treatment of decompensated heart failure. *JAMA*, 287, 1531–1540.

Rady, M. Y. (1992). The role of central venous oximetry, lactic acid concentration and shock index in the evaluation of clinical shock: A review. *Resuscitation* 24, 55–60.

Reardon, M. I., Carr, C. L., Diamond, A., et al. (1997). Ischemic left ventricular free wall rupture: prediction, diagnosis, and treatment. *Annals of Thoracic Surgery*, 64, 1509–1513.

Rice, V. (1991a). Shock, a clinical syndrome: An update. Part one: An overview of shock. *Critical Care Nurse*, 11(4), 20–27.

Rice, V. (1991b). Shock, a clinical syndrome: An update. Part two: The stages of shock. *Critical Care Nurse*, 11(5), 75–85.

Rice, V. (1991c). Shock, a clinical syndrome: An update. Part three: Therapeutic management. *Critical Care Nurse*, 11(6), 34–39.

Rice, V. (1991d). Shock, a clinical syndrome: An update. Part four: Nursing care of the shock patient. *Critical Care Nurse*, 11(7), 28–39.

Ryan, T. J., Anderson, J. L., Antman, E. M., et al. (1996). ACC/AHA guidelines for the management of patients with acute myocardial infarction. A report of the American College of Cardiology/American Heart Association Task Force on Practice Guidelines (Committee on Management of Acute Myocardial Infarction). *Journal of the American College of Cardiology*, 28, 1328–1428.

Saltzberg, M. T., Soble, J. S., & Parrillo, J. E. (2001). Acute heart failure and shock. In M. H. Crawford & J. P. DiMarco (Eds.), *Cardiology* (Section 5, pp. 3.1–3.12). London: Mosby.

Sanborn, T. A., et al. (2000). Impact of thrombolysis, intra-aortic balloon pump counterpulsation, and their combination in cardiogenic shock complicating acute myocardial infarction: a report from the SHOCK trial registry. *Journal of the American College of Cardiology*, 36, 1123–1129.

Schuster, D. P., & Lefrak, S. S. (1992). Shock. In J. M. Civetta, R. W. Taylor, & R. R. Kirby (Eds.), *Critical care* (2nd ed., pp. 407–422). Philadelphia: JB Lippincott.

Slater, J., Brown, R. J., Antonelli, T. A., et al. (2000). Cardiogenic shock due to cardiac free-wall rupture or tamponade after acute myocardial infarction; A report from the SHOCK trial registry. *Journal of the American College of Cardiology*, 36(3), Supplement A, 1117–1122.

Stein, J. H., Neuman, A., Preston, L. M., et al. (1997). Echocardiography for hemodynamics assessment of patients with advanced heart failure and potential heart transplant recipients. *Journal of the American College of Cardiology*, 30, 1765–1772.

Taylor, R. W. (1997). Controversies in pulmonary artery catheterization. *New Horizons*, 5, 173–296.

Weil, M. H., & Shubin, H. (1969). The "VIP" approach to the bedside management of shock. *JAMA*, 207(2), 337–340.

Woods, S. L. (1976). Monitoring pulmonary artery pressure. *American Journal of Nursing*, 76, 1766–1771.

Wu, J. J., Huang, M., Tang, G., et al. (2001). Hemodynamic response of modified gelatin compared with lactated Ringer's solution fro volume expansion in emergency resuscitation of hypovolemic shock patients: preliminary report of a prospective, randomized trial. *World Journal of Surgery*, 25,598–602.

Younes, R. N., Aun, F., Accioly, C. Q., et al. (1992). Hypertonic solution in the treatment of hypovolemic shock: A prospective, randomized study in patients admitted to the emergency room. *Surgery* 111, 380–385.

Yu, M., Levy, M. M., Smith, P., et al. (1993). Effect of maximizing oxygen delivery on morbidity and mortality rates in critically ill patients: A prospective randomized, controlled study. *Critical Care Medicine*, 21, 834–838.

REFERENCES FOR IABP AND LVAD

Arafa, O. E., Pedersen, T. H., Svennevig, J. L., Foss, E., & Geiran, O. (1999). Vascular complications of the intra-aortic pump in patients undergoing open heart operations: 15 year experience. *Annual Thoracic Surgery*, 67, 645–651.

Bates, E. R., Stomel, R. J., Hochman, J. S., & Ohman, E. M. (1998). The use of intra-aortic balloon counter pulsation as an adjustment to reperfusion therapy in cardiogenic shock. *International Journal of Cardiology,* 65(Supplement I), 537–542.

Casarotto, D., Bottio, T. Gambino, A., Testolin, L., & Gerosa, G. (2003). The last to die is hope: Prolonged mechanical circulatory support with a Novacor left ventricular assist device as a bridge to transplantation. *Journal of Thoracic Cardiovascular Surgery,* 125 (2), 417–418.

Cohen, M., Dawson, M. S., Kopistansky, C., & McBride, R. (2000). Sex and other predictors of intra-aortic balloon counter pulsation-related complications: Prospective study of 1119 consecutive patients. *American Heart Journal,* 139, 282–287.

Deng, M. C., Young, J. B., Stevenson, L. W., Oz, M. C., Rose, E. A., Hunt, S. A., Kirklin, J. K., Kobashigawa, J., Miller, L., Saltzberg, M., Konstam, M., Portner, P. M., & Kormos, R. (2003). Destination mechanical circulatory support: Proposal for clinical standards. *Journal of Heart-Lung Transplant,* 22(4), 365–369.

Frazier, O. H., Myers, T. J., Gregoric, I. D., Kahn, T., Delgado, R., Croitoru, M., Miller, R., Jarvik, R., & Westaby, S. (2002). Initial clinical experience with the Jarvik 2000 implantable axial-flow left ventricular assist system. *Circulation,* 105, 2855–2860.

Hunt, S. A., Frazier, O. H., & Myers, T. J. (1998). Mechanical circulatory support and cardiac transplantation. *Circulation,* 97, 2079–2090.

Jett, G. K. (1994). Post-cardiotomy support with ventricular assist devices: Selection of recipients. *Seminars in Thoracic and Cardiovascular Surgery,* 6(3), 136–139.

Kantrowitz, A. (1990). Origins of intra-aortic balloon pumping. *Annual Thoracic Surgery,* 50, 672–674.

Liy, S. J. (1991). The thoracic ventricular assist devices: Nursing, technical and educational considerations. *American Journal of Critical Care.* 5, 355–362.

Magovern, G. J., Park, S. B., & Maher, T. D. (1985). Use of the centrifugal pump without anticoagulants for post-operative left ventricular assist. *World Journal of Surgery,* 9(1), 25–36.

Marchetta, S., & Stennis, E. (1988) Ventricular assist devices: Applications for critical care. *Cardiovascular Nursing,* 2(2), 39–51.

Maroney, D. A., & Reedy, J. E. (1994). Understanding ventricular assist devices: A self study guide. *Journal of Cardiovascular Nurse,* 8(2), 1–12.

Maroney, D. A., & Powers, K. (1997). Outpatient use of left ventricular assist devices: Nursing, technical and educational considerations. *American Journal of Critical Care,* 6(5), 355–362.

McBride, L. R., Miller, L. W., & Nauheim, K. S. (1989). Auxiliary artery insertion of an intra-aortic balloon pump. *Annual of Thoracic Surgery,* 48, 874–875.

McGovern, K. J. (1998) Developing an outpatient ventricular assist device program to meet the needs of a "too successful" heart transplant program. *Journal of Cardiovascular Management,* 9(5), 19–22.

Miller, C. A., Pae, W. E., & Pierce, W. S. (1990) Combined registry for the clinical use of mechanical ventricular assist devices: Post-cardiotomy cardiogenic shock. *Transactions of the American Society for Artificial Internal Organs,* 36, 43–46.

Rose, D. M., Culliford, A., Cunningham, J. et al. (1983). Late functional and hemodynamic status of surviving patients following insertion of a left heart assist device. *Journal of Thoracic Cardiovascular Surgery,* 86, 639–645.

Shinn, J. A., & Oyer, P. E. (1993). Novacor ventricular assist system. In S. Quaal (Ed.), *Cardiac mechanical assist beyond balloon pumping* (pp.99–115). St. Louis: C. V. Mosby.

Stevenson, L. W., & Kosmos, R. L. (2001). Mechanical cardiac support 2000: Current applications and future trial design. *Journal of Thoracic Cardiovascular Surgery,* 121(3), 418–424.

Van Citters, R. L., Bauer, C. B., Christopherson, L. K., et al. (1985). Artificial heart and assist devices: Directions, needs, costs, special and ethical issues. *Artificial Organs,* 9, 375–415.

31

Sudden Cardiac Death and Cardiac Arrest

DONNA GERITY

Sudden cardiac death (SCD) is a major clinical and public health problem in the United States, accounting for approximately 400,000 deaths annually. Even with significant advances in management of coronary artery disease, and the treatment of heart failure, the overall incidence has remained unchanged as our population ages (Zheng et al., 2001). Coronary artery disease is present in nearly 80% of those individuals who experience sudden cardiac death. Autopsy studies show that 50% of these sudden death patients have acute changes in coronary status, such as plaque, rupture, or thrombus (Callans, 2002). Survival rates for out-of-hospital sudden cardiac arrest victims are low, with only 2% to 25% surviving to discharge in the United States. Those survivors of sudden cardiac arrest have a high risk for future events. Therefore, the aim at decreasing sudden cardiac death is to better identify and treat potential victims of SCD. Future events will be minimized if the incidence of CAD is reduced and primary and secondary prevention is provided (Prystowsky, 2001).

DEFINITION OF SUDDEN DEATH

Sudden cardiac death is defined as an unexpected death caused by cardiac causes that occurs within 1 hour of symptom onset. The person may or may not have known of preexisting heart disease. Cardiac arrest, usually caused by cardiac arrhythmias, is the term used to describe the sudden collapse, loss of consciousness, and loss of effective circulation that precedes biologic death (Myerburg & Castellanos, 1997). A subclassification of sudden death uses the term *instantaneous death,* a death with immediate collapse without preceding symptoms. Other causes of death may also be instantaneous, such as stroke, massive pulmonary embolism, or rupture of an aortic aneurysm. It is also important to note that not all arrhythmic deaths are sudden. A patient may be successfully resuscitated from a cardiac arrest but may die days later from complications (Dimarco, 2003).

PATHOPHYSIOLOGY AND CAUSE OF SUDDEN CARDIAC ARREST

The epidemiology of sudden cardiac death tends to follow that of coronary heart disease patients. The incidence of SCD increases with the aging population in both men and women, whites and nonwhites, just as ischemic heart disease increases. Sudden cardiac death occurs 75% more often in men. Hypertension, left ventricular hypertrophy, intraventricular conduction disease, hypercholesterolemia, vital capacity, smoking, relative weight, and heart rate were all noted as risk factors per the 26-year follow-up of the Framingham Study (Zipes & Wellens, 1998).

There are several different arrhythmia mechanisms responsible for sudden cardiac death. Holter monitor recordings from patients who experienced out-of-hospital cardiac arrest show that ventricular fibrillation (VF) and rapid ventricular tachycardia are the most commonly documented arrhythmias (Dimarco, 2003). However, the mechanism that produces the potentially fatal arrhythmia among patients with coronary artery disease is difficult to define. The episode could be caused from pure ischemic injury because of occlusion of a major artery in a patient with a normal ventricle in whom VF develops in the first minutes of an acute infarction. The other type of mechanism is one in which a patient with a previous MI has postinfarction scarring that provides the anatomic substrate for VT that leads to hemodynamic collapse and SCD. Patients could also have complex substrates consisting of dense scar tissue with aneurysms or other areas where disorganized arrhythmias predominate. This complex interaction and multiplicity of influences that occur in a cardiac arrest episode differ for all patients (Dimarco, 2003; Callans, 2002).

Structural Abnormalities

Coronary Heart Disease

Coronary heart disease (CHD) is the major structural abnormality found in most sudden cardiac arrest victims (Myerburg

& Castellanos, 1997; Zipes & Wellens, 1998). In an early study of cardiac arrest survivors, 78% of patients with CHD reported histories of previous MI, angina, congestive heart failure, or hypertension before the arrest. For the remaining 22% of survivors, the sudden cardiac arrest was their first manifestation of CHD (Cobb & Werner, 1982). In another study, 81% of 220 sudden cardiac arrest victims had CHD as a major causative factor (Liberthson et al., 1974). Previous healed MI has been reported in as many as 75% of hearts examined at autopsy after SCD (Myerburg & Castellanos, 1997; Reichenbach et al., 1977).

Up to 75% of SCD victims have been reported as having advanced, chronic, atherosclerotic coronary artery lesions. Severe CHD is defined as one or more coronary vessels with 75% or more stenosis. In a sample of 87 people who died suddenly, 59% had a previous complete occlusion in one or more coronary vessels; 8% had single-vessel stenosis of more than 90%; 18% had double-vessel stenosis of more than 90%; and 13% had triple-vessel stenosis of more than 90%. Only 8% did not have significant CHD (Reichenbach et al., 1977). No correlation has been demonstrated between the anatomic pattern or distribution of the coronary artery lesion and the risk for SCD (Warnes & Roberts, 1984). There is some evidence that acute thrombotic coronary lesions may be related to the occurrence of sudden cardiac arrest (Zipes & Wellens, 1998; Davies & Thomas, 1984). Acute coronary lesions are defined as plaque fissuring, platelet aggregation, acute thrombi, or any combination of these. Changes in coronary artery blood flow from other causes such as spasm can also provoke ischemia and create myocardial electrical disturbances and the development of VF (Davies & Thomas, 1984). Sudden cardiac arrest also may be part of a spectrum of unstable angina and acute MI. Therefore, if the plaque were restabilized and antegrade blood flow through the coronary artery was maintained or rapidly restored, evidence for a transmural MI would not necessarily be present (Davies, 1992).

Cardiomyopathy

The second largest group of patients who experience SCD includes those with cardiomyopathy (Zipes & Wellens, 1998). Severely depressed left ventricular function is an independent predictor of SCD in patients with ischemic and nonischemic cardiomyopathy. An ejection fraction of less than .30 is the most powerful predictor of sudden cardiac death. Better treatment options for heart failure patients provide better long-term survival of such patients. However, there is an increasing proportion of heart failure patients who die suddenly (Myerburg & Castellanos, 1997). The Multicenter Automatic Defibrillator Implantation Trial (Madit II) has shown that the implantable cardiac defibrillator (ICD) will reduce total mortality in ischemic cardiomyopathy patients with ejection fractions less that .30. The Sudden Cardiac Death in Heart Failure Trial (SCD-HeFT) will help answer this question with the nonischemic cardiomyopathy patient. Nonischemic dilated cardiomyopathy is present in approximately 10% of all sudden cardiac arrest patients (Dimarco, 2003).

Left ventricular hypertrophy has been established as an independent risk factor for SCD (Zipes & Wellens, 1998). Increased ventricular ectopy has also been associated with electrocardiographic patterns of LV hypertrophy as well as increased myocardial mass documented by echocardiography (Lenachen et al., 1987). The underlying causes for myocardial hypertrophy include hypertensive or valvular heart disease, obstructive and nonobstructive hypertrophic cardiomyopathy, and right ventricular hypertrophy secondary to pulmonary hypertension or congenital heart disease. All of these conditions are associated with increased risk of SCD, but it has been suggested that people with severely hypertrophic ventricles are especially susceptible to SCD (Zipes & Wellens, 1998; Myerburg & Castellanos, 1997; Anderson, 1984).

Hypertrophic cardiomyopathy is often seen in young adults with no previous cardiac history. Sudden death often occurs with vigorous exercise is this group of patients. Various risk factors for sudden death with hypertrophic cardiomyopathy include: family history of sudden death, documented nonsustained ventricular tachycardia, and recurrent and unexplained syncope. Polymorphic ventricular tachycardia and ventricular fibrillation are thought to be the initial rhythm for patients with hypertrophic cardiomyopathy who experience sudden cardiac death (Dimarco, 2003). Currently, the genetics of hypertrophic cardiomyopathy are being studied. It is hoped that specific genetic patterns will be able to predict either a high or a low risk of sudden cardiac death (Dimarco, 2003; Myerburg & Spooner, 2001).

Valvular Heart Disease

The risk of sudden death in patients with valve disease is low, but present. After prosthetic or heterograft aortic valve replacements, patients are at risk for SCD caused by arrhythmias, prosthetic valve dysfunction, or existing coronary heart disease. The risk of SCD after surgery peaks at 3 weeks and plateaus after 8 months (Zipes & Wellens, 1998; Myerburg & Castellanos, 1997). Sudden death can also occur with exertion in young adults with congenital aortic stenosis. The mechanism is uncertain but thought to be from sudden changes in ventricular filling or aortic obstruction with secondary arrhythmias (Dimarco, 2003). Mitral valve prolapse is associated with a high incidence of symptomatic atrial and ventricular arrhythmias; however, whether it causes SCD is unresolved (Zipes & Wellens, 1998).

Sudden Cardiac Death Without Structural Heart Disease

Nearly 5% of those patients who experience SCD have no demonstrable structural heart disease (Callans, 2002). There are many potential causes (Display 31-1) of SCD in this small percentage of patients, but there are three important electrophysiological abnormalities to be considered. Long QT syndrome, either congenital or acquired by use of drugs, often antiarrhythmic and psychotropic drugs (Display 31-2), can result in torsades de pointes type of polymorphic VT. Congenital long QT is hereditary and two forms have been reported, the Romano Ward syndrome and the Jervell and Lange-Nielsen syndrome (Zipes & Wellens, 1998; Callans, 2002). Brugada's syndrome is also an inherited disease that is caused by a mutation of a particular cardiac sodium channel gene. The Brugada

CAUSES OF SUDDEN DEATH

Cardiac Causes

Acute myocarditis
Aortic or ventricular aneurysm with dissection or rupture
Aortic stenosis
Cardiomyopathies
    Ischemic cardiomyopathy
    Nonischemic dilated cardiomyopathy
    Hypertrophic cardiomyopathy
    Alcoholic cardiomyopathy
Chagas disease
Congenital heart disease
Coronary artery abnormalities
    Myocardial infarction
    Coronary artery spasm
    Coronary artery embolism
    Prosthetic aortic or mitral valves
Endocarditis
Electrophysiologic abnormalities
    Brugada syndrome
    Complete AV block
    Wolff Parkinson White
    Long QT syndrome—congenital and acquired
Prolapsed mitral valve syndrome
Right ventricular dysplasia
Sarcoidosis

Noncardiac Causes

Cerebral or subarachnoid hemorrhage
Choking
Dissecting aneurysm of the aorta
Electrolyte abnormalities
Metabolic disturbances
Pulmonary hypertension (primary, particularly during
    pregnancy)
Pulmonary embolism
Sudden infant death syndrome (should at least in part be
    included in cardiac causes)

syndrome is confirmed with ST segment elevation in the precordial leads, RBBB conduction pattern, and history of sudden cardiac death (Callans, 2002). Wolff-Parkinson-White (WPW) syndrome is associated with an accessory pathway that allows for conduction between the atria and ventricles. Normally, WPW is associated with nonlethal arrhythmias. However, if atrial fibrillation develops and conduction is rapid over the accessory pathway, the ventricular rate can become so fast that the rhythm degenerates into ventricular fibrillation (Zipes & Wellens, 1998).

MANAGEMENT OF SUDDEN CARDIAC ARREST

Ventricular fibrillation is the initial rhythm most often identified by rescuers in cardiac arrest. The outcome of cardiac arrest is determined by how promptly treatment is initiated (advanced cardiac life support [ACLS]). To improve outcome from sudden cardiac arrests, the following must occur as rapidly as possible: (1) early recognition of warning signs; (2) early activation of the emergency medical system; (3) early basic cardiopulmonary resuscitation (CPR); (4) early defibrillation; and (5) early ACLS. These events have been described as "links in a chain of survival," because they are all connected and indispensable to the overall success of emergency cardiac care (American Heart Association, 2003; Cummins et al., 1991).

Although this section summarizes ACLS recommendations for the adult patient, it is not a complete reference. For each cardiac nurse, participation in an ACLS provider course by the American Heart Association is strongly recommended. In addition, the most current version of *Emergency Cardiac Care, Basic Life Support for Healthcare Providers,* and *The Textbook of Advanced Cardiac Life Support* should be used as definitive references.

Adult Advanced Cardiac Life Support

ACLS teaches the appropriate skills and knowledge, as determined by leaders in emergency cardiovascular care (ECC), to treat cardiopulmonary arrest. Advanced cardiac life support includes early recognition of prearrest, basic life support, the use of airway and circulation adjuncts, cardiac monitoring, and defibrillation and other arrhythmia control techniques. ACLS also includes establishment of intravenous access, drug therapy, and postresuscitation care (American Heart Association, 2003) (Fig. 31-1). This section focuses on defibrillation and ACLS management of cardiac arrest caused by VF and VT. Postresuscitation management of sudden cardiac arrest survivors is also included. For discussions of basic and complex arrhythmia and conduction disturbances, electrophysiology studies, acute coronary syndrome, hemodynamic monitoring, pacemakers, and implantable defibrillators, respectively, refer to Chapters 19, 20, 25, 26, 23, and 32.

Electrical Therapy of Malignant Arrhythmia

Defibrillation and cardioversion are a delivery of electrical energy that totally depolarizes and stuns the myocardium, which allows the sinus node to resume its function as the pacemaker for the heart. Defibrillation is, by definition, the therapy for VF. Cardioversion, which is a synchronized shock, is the electrical therapy for all other tachyarrhythmias. Transcutaneous and transvenous pacing are additional types of electrical therapy used in ACLS for patients with hemodynamically compromised bradycardias (see Chapter 32).

Early Defibrillation

Ventricular tachycardia (VT) and VF cause 80% to 90% of nontraumatic adult cardiac arrests (Greene, 1990). Defibrillation is the definitive therapy for cardiac arrest caused by VF. Rapid, early defibrillation is a key step and the most important intervention likely to save lives (Cummins, 1989; Cummins & Thies, 1990). A major obstacle to rapid, early defibrillation is

DISPLAY 31-2

DRUGS THAT POTENTIALLY PROLONG THE QT INTERVAL

Antiarrhythmic Agents

Class I

Disopyramide/Norpace
Flecainide/Tambocor
Moricizine/Ethmozine
Procainamide/Pronestyl
Propafenonel/Rhythmol
Quinidine/Quinidex
Tocainide/Tonocard

Class III

Amiodarone/Cordarone
Ibutilide/Corvert
Sotalol/Betapace
Dofetilide/Tikosyn

Class IV

Bepridil/Vascor

Antihistamines

Terfenadine/Seldane (Off U.S. Market)
Astemizole/Histamil (Off U.S. Market)

Antimicrobials

Ampicillin/Polycillin
Clarithromycin/Biaxin
Erythromycin/E-Mycin
Pentamidine/Pentam
Trimethoprim-sulfamethoxazole/Bactrim

Antidepressants

Amitriptyline/Elavil
Amoxapine/Asendin
Clomipramine/Anafranil
Desipramine/Norpramin
Imipramine/Tofranil
Maprotiline/Ludiomil
Nortriptyline/Pamelor
Protriptyline/Vivactil

Antipsychotics

Chlorpromazine/Thorazine
Perphenazine/Trilafon
Risperidone/Risperdal
Thioridazine/Mellaril
Thiothixene/Navane
Trifluoperazine/Stelazine

Antiemetics

Droperidol/Inapsine
Prochlorperazine/Compazine

Gastrointestinal Agents

Cisapride/Propulsid
Ipecac Syrup

Lipid-Lowering Agents

Probucol/Lorelco

---

that most cardiac arrests occur outside of the hospital, indicating a need for public health initiatives to improve early recognition of heart attack symptoms and signs (Zheng et al., 2001). The widespread use of automated external defibrillators (AEDs) assists in making early defibrillation a reality by expanding the number of rescuers available to treat SCD. The American Heart Association has now integrated the use of AEDs into the *Textbook of Basic Life Support for Healthcare Providers,* acknowledging the importance of early defibrillation and the increased availability of AEDs (American Heart Association, 2000).

Defibrillators. Defibrillators are the power source used to deliver the electrical therapy. Defibrillators typically include a capacitor charger, a capacitor to store energy, a charge switch, and discharge switch to complete the circuit from the capacitor to the electrodes. The capacitor charger converts power from a low-voltage source, such as direct current, to a voltage level sufficient for a shock. Portable defibrillators derive their power from a battery, which must be kept charged. Electrical output of defibrillators is quantified in terms of joules (J), or watt-seconds, of energy (American Heart Association, 2003).

Defibrillators deliver energy to the electrode in either a biphasic or a monophasic waveform. Biphasic waveforms deliver current in a positive direction for a specific duration, and then reverse the current to a negative direction for the remaining discharge. A monophasic waveform delivers the current in one polarity or direction. Studies show that biphasic waveforms achieve shock success rates at lower energies, 150 joules compared to 200 joules, and produce less ST segment change than shocks delivered with monophasic waveforms (Bardy et al., 1997; Schneider et al., 2000). Lower energy requirements reduce the size and weight of the defibrillator, which in turn increases public access to AEDs because they are easier to handle, less expensive, and more convenient to keep available (Weisfeldt et al., 1995).

Rapid defibrillation can be performed with manual, automatic, or semiautomatic external defibrillators. Manual defibrillators must be operated by well-trained personnel, often ACLS responders, who are able to interpret cardiac rhythms on a rhythm strip or monitor. Automatic advisory or semiautomatic external defibrillators have been developed for use by first responders. AEDs are accurate and easy to use and, unlike standard defibrillators, have detection systems that analyze the rhythm and advise the operator to shock when VF/VT characteristics are determined. Thus, successful defibrillation can be achieved without requiring the operator to have rhythm recognition skills. AEDs are attached to the patient with the use of adhesive sternal and apex pads that are connected to a cable, allowing for "hands-free defibrillation" (American Heart Association, 2003). AEDs were shown to help emergency personnel deliver the first shock on an average of 1 minute sooner than personnel using conventional defibrillators (Stults et al., 1986).

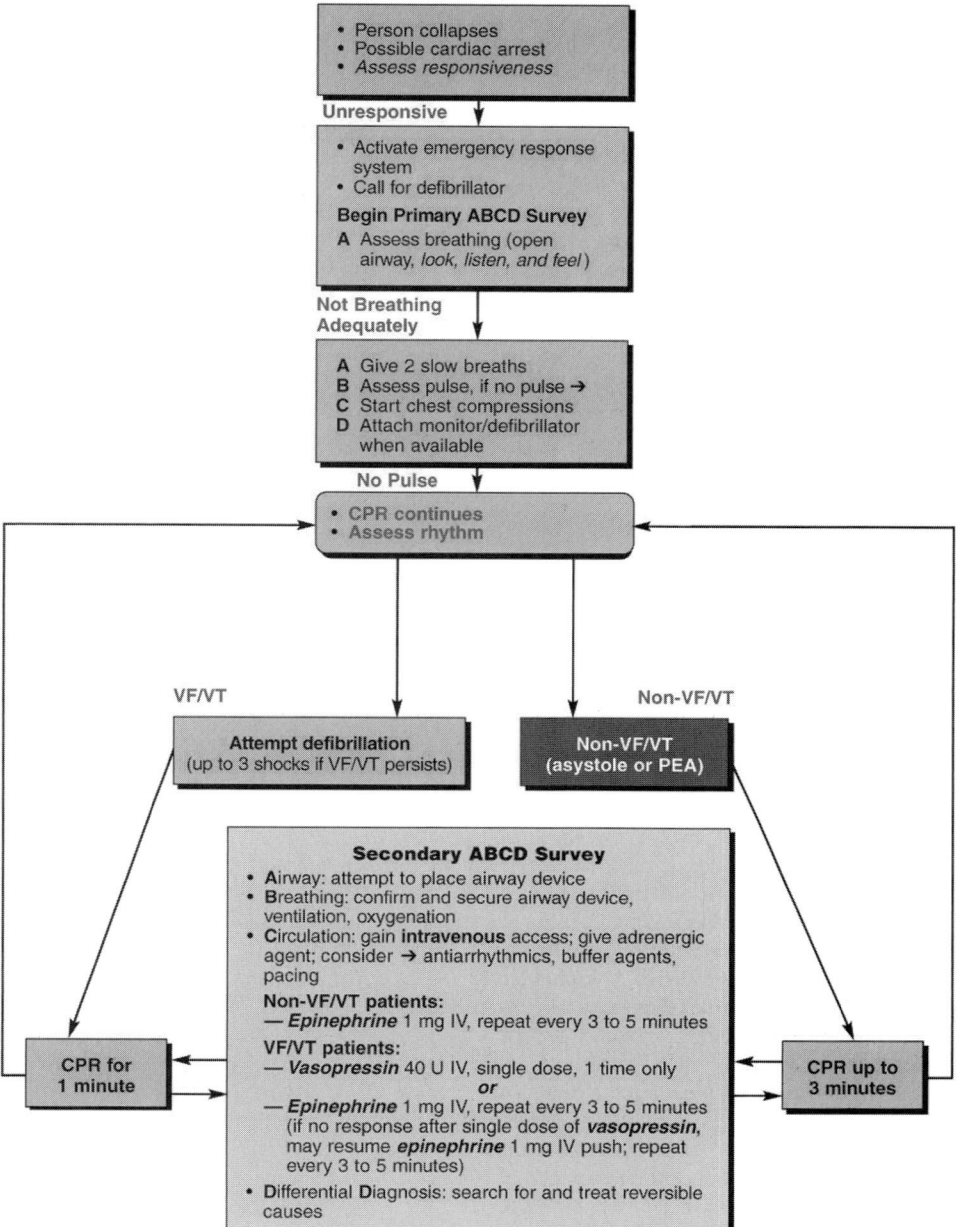

■ **Figure 31–1.** Comprehensive ECC algorithm recommending the steps ACLS providers should follow during resuscitation attempts. (From American Heart Association. [2003]. *ACLS—The reference textbook: Principles and practice* [p. 10]. Dallas: AHA.)

Many experts believe that the AED is the most important development in the management of SCD in the past quarter century (American Heart Association, 2003).

Transthoracic Impedance. The ability to defibrillate requires the passage of sufficient electric current through the heart. Current flow is determined by transthoracic impedance, or resistance to current flow, and the selected energy (joules). If transthoracic impedance is high, a low-energy shock may fail to produce enough current to defibrillate. The factors that determine transthoracic impedance include energy setting, electrode size and composition, electrode–skin interface, number of and time interval between previous electrical discharges, electrode

pressure, ventilation phase, and electrode placement (Thomas et al., 1977; Kerber et al., 1981).

Resistance between the electrode and the chest wall must be minimized. Bare electrodes produce high resistance to electrical flow (Ewy & Taran, 1977). Defibrillation electrode gel or paste, made specifically for defibrillation will help to decrease impedance. Self-adhesive monitor or defibrillator pads are also available and very effective. The adhesive defibrillator pads are thought to be more convenient and safer, as they reduce the possibility of arcing (American Heart Association, 2003).

Repeat defibrillator shocks decrease transthoracic impedance (Sima, 1989). Transthoracic impedance is lowered by approximately 8% after the second shock. In hand-held paddles, the amount of paddle pressure applied to the chest influences the transthoracic impedance by ensuring good electrode–skin contact (Kerber et al., 1981). Current recommendations are to apply 25 pounds of pressure per paddle (American Heart Association, 2003). Minimum transthoracic impedance occurs in the end-expiratory phase of the respiratory cycle. Proper paddle positioning will maximize current flow and decrease transthoracic impedance. The optimal paddle size for adults in hand-held and self-adhesive electrodes is 8.5 to 12 cm in diameter (Kerber et al., 1981).

Energy Requirements. Selection of the appropriate energy is one of the factors that determines success of defibrillation. A shock with insufficient energy and current fails to defibrillate. Myocardial damage may occur if energy and current are too high (American Heart Association, 2003).

Once VF or pulseless VT has been identified (Fig. 31-2), immediate defibrillation must be performed. Three shocks at 200 J, 200 to 300 J, and up to 360 J, or equivalent biphasic shocks, are delivered one after the other. The defibrillator paddles should be left on the chest between shocks. The rescuers should *not* perform CPR between shocks. While the defibrillator is recharging, the rhythm should be rechecked. It is not necessary to perform pulse checks between shocks if a properly connected monitor shows persistent VF and VT. Rescuers who perform defibrillation must announce that they are about to deliver a shock. They must then check that all personnel are clear of the patient and stretcher before defibrillating. If the first or second shocks are successful, but the patient subsequently goes back to VF, the energy should be kept at the last successful level rather than increased to 360 J. Because the most important determinant of survival in VF is *rapid* defibrillation, the shocks should be given as soon as the defibrillator arrives (Cummins & Thies, 1990).

Electrode Position. Electrode placement is critical in ensuring that a critical mass of myocardium is depolarized. Any of three electrode positions may be used. *Standard* or *anterolateral* electrode placement involves one electrode being placed to the right of the upper sternum just below the right clavicle. The other electrode is placed just to the left of the left nipple, with the center of the electrode in the mid-axillary line (Fig. 31-3). *Anterior–posterior* electrode placement involves one paddle positioned anteriorly over the precordium, just to the left of the lower sternal border. The other electrode is positioned posteriorly behind the heart (American Heart Association, 2003). A third alternative for paddle placement is to place the posterior paddle in the right infrascapular location and the anterior paddle over the left apex (Kerber et al., 1981). In patients with permanent pacemakers, electrode placement should be as far as possible from the pacemaker pulse generator, and when possible the anterior–posterior position is preferred (Hayes et al., 2000). Refer to Chapter 32 for information on paddle placement for patients with implantable cardioverter defibrillators (ICDs).

Defibrillation Procedure. Identify the rhythm as VF. If the rhythm appears to be asystole, check the rhythm in another lead to confirm that the rhythm is not fine VF.

- Apply conductive material to electrodes, unless using conductive pads. Position electrodes on the chest.
- Turn on the defibrillator.
- Set energy level to 200 J.

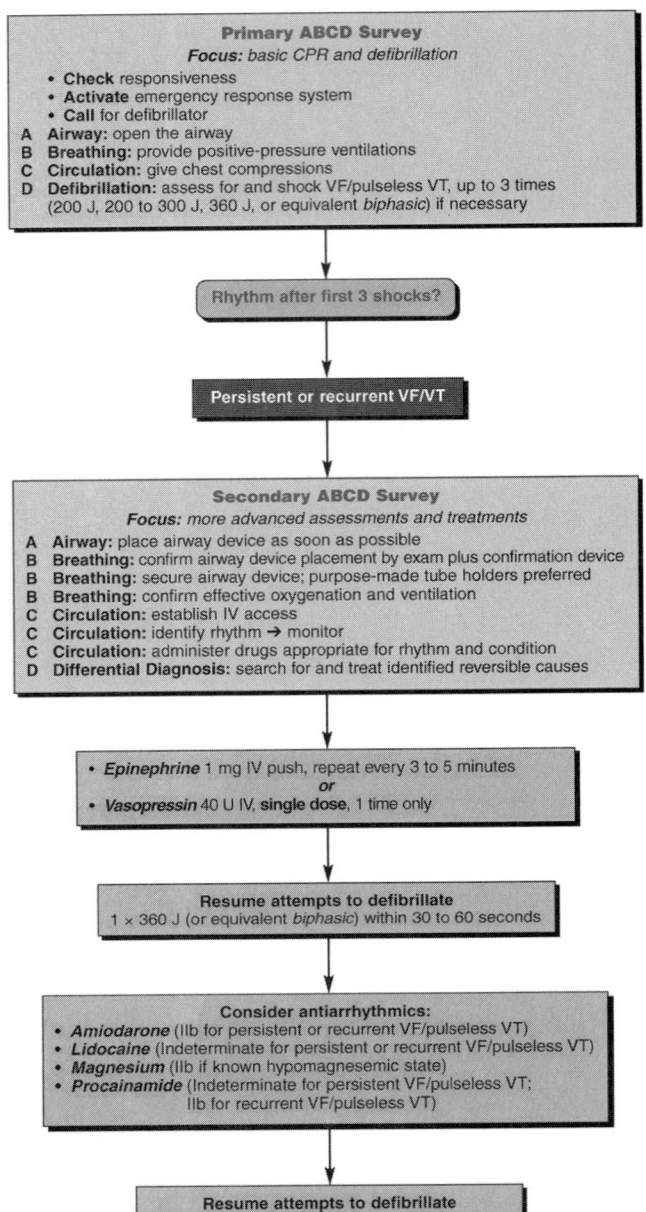

■ **Figure 31–2.** Algorithm for ventricular fibrillation and pulseless ventricular tachycardia (*VF* and *VT*). IIb refers to the classification of interventions that are acceptable and possibly effective. (From American Heart Association. [2003]. *ACLS—The reference textbook : Principles and practice* [p. 60]. Dallas: AHA.)

- Charge capacitors. Charging may take several seconds. Many defibrillators emit a sound or light signal, or both, to indicate that the unit has charged.
- Ensure proper electrode placement on chest.
- Apply pressure of 25 pounds per paddle. Do not lean forward because of the danger of the paddles slipping.
- Scan the area to ensure that no personnel are in contact directly or indirectly with the patient. Make sure there is no flowing oxygen source in electrical field.
- State firmly, "all clear" or other warning chant

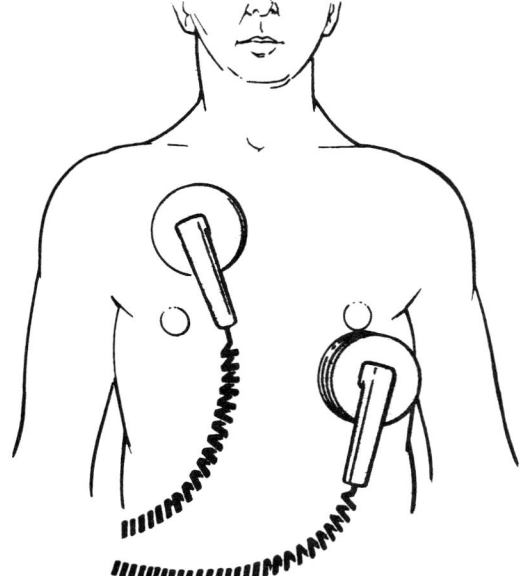

- Check rhythm—if patient remains in VF, deliver shock by depressing both buttons simultaneously on the paddles.
- Reassess rhythm. Do not remove the paddles from the chest. If VF persists, shock a second time at 200 to 300 J. Scan for personnel in contact with the patient, State, *"all clear,"* and re-shock immediately.
- Repeat assessment procedure. If necessary, increase the energy to 360 J. Scan for personnel in contact with the patient, state, *"all clear,"* and re-shock immediately.
- Repeat assessment procedure. If VF continues or if the patient has no pulse, start (or resume) CPR (see Fig. 31-2).

■ Figure 31–3. Standard positioning of defibrillator paddles. (From Underhill, S. L., & Woods, S. L. [1986]. Nursing strategies for common cardiac problems. In M. L. Patrick, S. L. Woods, R. F. Craven, et al. [Eds.], *Medical–surgical nursing: Pathophysiological concepts* [p. 498]. Philadelphia: J. B. Lippincott.)

Management of Cardiac Arrest—ACLS Algorithms

A general framework for the use of ACLS algorithms in outlined in Display 31-3. The initial approach to the management of SCD is outlined in the ECC Universal algorithm (see Fig 31-1). ACLS providers must always start with this algorithm by activating the emergency medical system and beginning basic life support. The basics of airway, breathing, and circulation remain important during the entire resuscitation continuum. Once the patient is attached to a monitor, determine the rhythm and potential cause for the arrest. If VF or pulseless VT is present, go to the VF and pulseless VT algorithm (see Fig. 31-2). If electrical activity is present without a pulse, go to the pulseless electrical activity (PEA) algorithm (Fig. 31-4). If the monitor displays asystole, go to the asystole algorithm (Fig. 31-5).

D I S P L A Y 31–3

THE ALGORITHM APPROACH TO EMERGENCY CARDIAC CARE

The American Heart Association guidelines use algorithms as an educational tool. They are an illustrative method to summarize information. Providers of emergency care should view algorithms as a summary and a memory aid. They provide ways to treat a broad range of patients. Algorithms by nature oversimplify. The effective teacher and care provider uses them wisely, not blindly. Some patients may require care not specified in the algorithms. When clinically appropriate, flexibility is accepted and encouraged. Many interventions and actions are listed as "considerations" to help providers think. These lists should not be considered endorsements or requirements or "standard of care" in a legal sense. Algorithms do not replace clinical understanding. Although the algorithms provide a good "cookbook," the patient always requires a "thinking cook."

The following clinical recommendations apply to all treatment algorithms:

- First, treat the patient, not the monitor.
- Algorithms for cardiac arrest presume that the condition under discussion continually persists, that the patient remains in cardiac arrest, and that CPR is always performed.
- Apply different interventions whenever appropriate indications exist.
- The flow diagrams present mostly class I (acceptable, definitely effective) interventions. The footnotes present class IIa (acceptable, probably effective), class IIb (acceptable, possibly effective), and class III (not indicated, may be harmful) interventions.
- Adequate airway, ventilation, oxygenation, chest compressions, and defibrillation are more important than administration of medications and take precedence over initiating an intravenous line or injecting pharmacologic agents.
- Several medications (epinephrine, lidocaine, and atropine) can be administered by the endotracheal tube, but the dosage should be 2 to 2.5 times the intravenous dose.
- With a few exceptions, intravenous medications should always be administered rapidly, by a bolus method.
- After each intravenous medication, give a 20- to 30-mL bolus of intravenous fluid and immediately elevate the extremity. This will enhance delivery of drugs to the central circulation, which may take 1–2 minutes.
- Last, treat the patient, not the monitor.

From American Heart Association: *Supplement to Circulation.* Guidelines 2000 for Cardiopulmonary Resuscitation and Emergency Cardiovascular Care. International Consensus on Science, pp. 1–141. Copyright 2000, AHA.

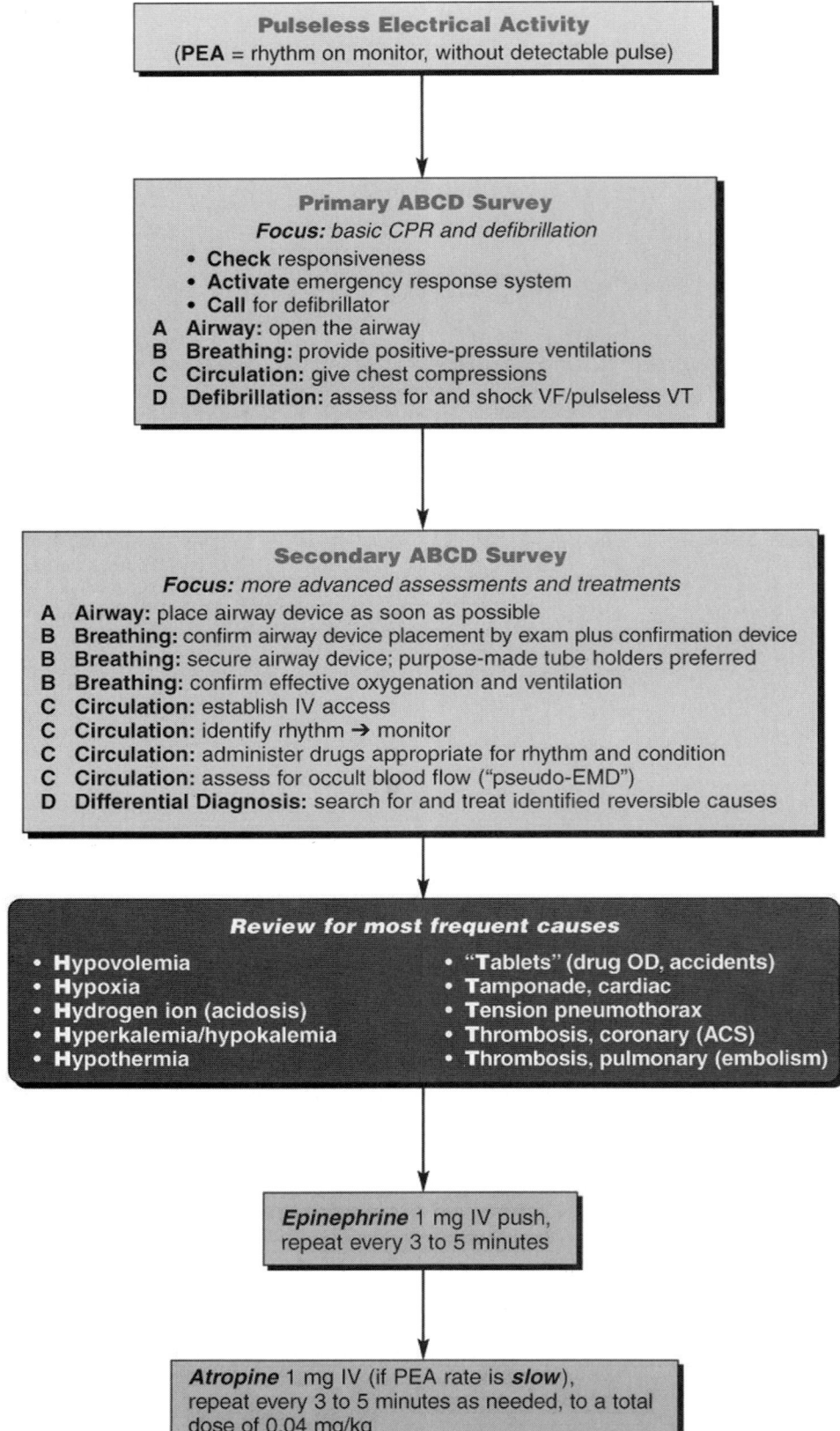

■ **Figure 31–4.** Algorithm for pulseless electrical activity (PEA). (From American Heart Association. [2003]. *ACLS—The reference textbook: Principles and practice* [p. 80]. Dallas: AHA.)

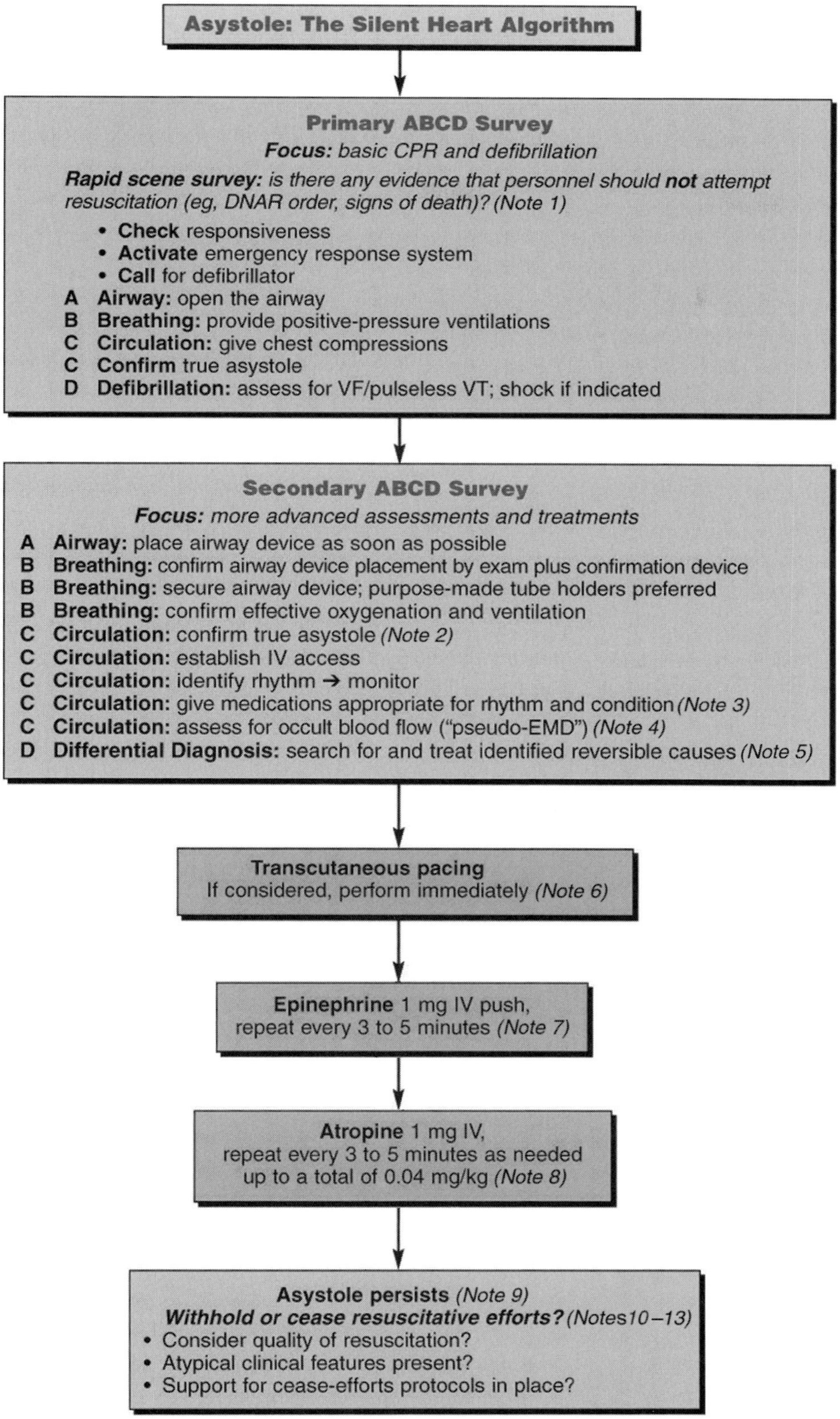

Figure 31–5. Asystole treatment algorithm. (From American Heart Association. [2003]. *ACLS—The reference textbook : Principles and practice* [p. 74]. Dallas: AHA.)

Note 1—Reasons to not start CPR: valid DNAR order, the patient has signs of irreversible death, no physiologic benefit can be expected.

Note 2—Confirm true asystole: check monitor (batteries and gain), check ECG leads and lead select.

Note 3—In the absence of a known, specific cause of asystole, resuscitation guidelines recommend two drugs: epinephrine and atropine.

Note 4—The use of cardiac ultrasound to identify cardiac contraction is becoming a standard in most emergency departments.

Note 5—PEA and asystole share the same possible reversible causes. Identification of reversible cause for asystole is uncommon.

Note 6—To have any success at treating asystole, you must perform transcutaneous pacing (TCP) early.

Note 7—The recommended dose of epinephrine is 1 mg IV push every 3 to 5 minutes. If this approach fails, higher doses of epinephrine (up to but no higher than 0.1 mg/kg) are acceptable but not recommended. There is no current evidence to support use of vasopressin for asystole.

Note 8—The recommendation for atropine in asystole is based on the assumption that the arrest is due to vagal stimulation. Avoid atropine when the lack of cardiac activity has a clear reason, such as hypothermia.

Note 9—If TCP, epinephrine and atropine fail to convert asystole, it is time to ask if it is time to cease efforts.

Notes 10—13—What has the quality of the resuscitation attempt been? Was there effective BLS and ACLS? Are there any atypical features present that would justify prolonging the resuscitation: such as young age, profound hypothermia, family expressing opposition to stopping efforts? Are there *cease-efforts protocols* in place? How will you support family presence?

Cardiac arrest should be managed by an ACLS team composed of a team leader and one or more team members. Priorities for resuscitation are (American Heart Association, 2003):

- Rapid, early defibrillation for VF or pulseless VT
- Effective CPR with endotracheal intubation and 100% oxygen delivery
- Vasopressin single dose or epinephrine given every 3 to 5 minutes to maintain coronary and cerebral perfusion
- Differential diagnosis: search for and treat any reversible causes.

Ventricular Fibrillation and Pulseless Ventricular Tachycardia

Rapid defibrillation is the determinant of survival in VF and pulseless VT. If the arrest was witnessed and a defibrillator is not immediately available, a precordial thump may be effective in terminating VT and, rarely, VF (Caldwell et al., 1985). A precordial thump must never be allowed to delay defibrillation when a defibrillator is available. Because a precordial thump may convert VT to VF, asystole, or electromechanical dissociation, it should not be used in a patient who has VT with a pulse unless a defibrillator and external pacemaker are present (Miller et al., 1984).

If three shocks fail to convert the patient, the VF and pulseless VT algorithm directs rescuers to give either a one-time dose of vasopressin or epinephrine. Vasopressors remain an extremely important drug for patients in cardiac arrest. The beneficial effects of both vasopressin (nonadrenergic vasopressor) and epinephrine (adrenergic vasopressor) during cardiac arrest come from vasoconstriction, which increases aortic diastolic pressure, coronary perfusion pressure, and coronary blood flow (American Heart Association, 2003). Defibrillation at 360 J should be performed within 30 to 60 seconds after administration of all drugs in ACLS. If VF and VT are still present after CPR, intubation, ventilation, four shocks, and vasopressor administration, then rescuers are dealing with refractory VF. An antiarrhythmic drug should be considered at this time and would include amiodarone, lidocaine, magnesium, or procainamide (Display 31-4). Antiarrhythmic drugs are delivered in bolus form during cardiac arrest; however, after a return of spontaneous circulation, they are often converted to infusions.

Asystole

The prognosis for patients in asystole is extremely poor. Asystole usually is the result of end-stage heart disease or prolonged cardiac arrest. CPR, intubation, epinephrine, and atropine are the treatment options in cardiac arrest with asystole (see Fig. 31-5). Shocking asystole has been discouraged. Electric shocks can cause parasympathetic discharge and may, in fact, prevent a return of spontaneous cardiac electrical activity (Vassalle, 1985). There have been no studies that have documented an improvement in survival by shocking asystole.

Transcutaneous pacing must be performed early. It is rarely effective in the out-of-hospital setting (Cummins et al., 1989). Transcutaneous pacing is most likely to benefit those patients in whom a bradysystolic arrest or asystole develops from vagal discharge after defibrillation (Bocka, 1989).

Pulseless Electrical Activity

Pulseless electrical activity includes electromechanical dissociation, pseudo-electromechanical dissociation, idioventricular

---

D I S P L A Y   31-4

ARREST AND ALIVE—SCIENTIFIC EVIDENCE FOR USE OF AMIODARONE

ARREST Trial – **A**miodarone in Out-of-Hospital **R**esuscitation of **RE**fractory **S**ustained Ventricular **T**achyarrhythmias

Methods: Patients were enrolled if they had three or more unsuccessful shocks for VF or pulseless VT in an out-of-hospital cardiac arrest. In a randomized, double-blind, placebo controlled study patients were either randomly assigned to receive 300mg of IV amiodarone (246 patients) or placebo (258 patients).

Results: Patients in the amiodarone group were more likely to survive to be admitted to the hospital. 44% of patients in the amiodarone group survived to hospital admission compared to 34% in the placebo group. There was no statistical difference in survival to hospital discharge between the two groups.

Conclusion: Patients in refractory VT/VF treated with amiodarone in out-of-hospital cardiac arrests have a higher rate of survival to hospital admission. Further investigation is warranted to see if the benefits extend to hospital discharge. (Kudenchuk et al., [1999]. *New England Journal of Medicine*, 341, 871–878.)

ALIVE –**A**miodarone versus **Li**docaine in Prehospital **V**entricular Fibrillation **E**valuation.

Methods: Patients were enrolled if they had an out-of-hospital VF arrest resistant to total of four shocks and one dose of epinephrine; or if they had a recurrence of VF after initial success. Patients were randomized in a double-blind manner to receive either IV amiodarone plus lidocaine placebo (179 patients) or IV lidocaine plus amiodarone placebo (165 patients). The primary endpoint was survival to hospital admission.

Results: Those patients receiving amiodarone had a higher rate of survival to hospital admission than those receiving lidocaine (22.8 % in amiodarone group vs. 12.0% in lidocaine group). However only 5 % of amiodarone group survived to hospital discharge, and 3 % of lidocaine group survived to hospital discharge.

Conclusion: Amiodarone shows clinical effectiveness in the early stages of resuscitation. There appears to be no indication for the administration of lidocaine in the out-of-hospital setting for shock-resistant ventricular fibrillation. (Dorian et al., [2002]. *New England Journal of Medicine*, 346, 884–890.)

rhythms, ventricular escape rhythms, postdefibrillation idioventricular rhythms, and bradysystolic rhythms (American Heart Association, 2003) (see Fig. 31-4). Prognosis of patients with electromechanical dissociation is very poor unless the underlying cause can be identified and treated appropriately. Therefore, the highest priority is to find the correctable cause while maintaining the patient's airway, breathing, and circulation. Common correctable causes of electromechanical dissociation include hypovolemia, cardiac tamponade, tension pneumothorax, hypoxemia, and acidosis. Massive damage from MI, prolonged ischemia during resuscitation, and pulmonary embolism are less correctable causes. Patients in profound shock of any cause initially may present with PEA. Hypovolemia is assessed by history and lack of neck vein distention; it is treated by volume replacement. Tension pneumothorax is assessed by history and neck vein distention; it is treated by needle aspiration, chest tube insertion, or both. Cardiac tamponade is assessed by history and neck vein distention; it is treated by pericardiocentesis or thoracotomy. Hypoxemia is assessed by history and arterial blood gases; it is treated by improving oxygenation and ventilation. Acidosis is assessed by history and arterial blood gases; it is treated by improving CPR technique and hyperventilating the patient. If bradycardia is present, then atropine may be administered in an attempt to increase heart rate (American Heart Association, 2003).

Management of Impending Cardiac Arrest

Ventricular and Supraventricular Tachycardia

The linked tachycardia treatment algorithm (Figs. 31-6, 31-7, and 31-8) directs rescuers to focus on the patient and determine the hemodynamic stability of the patient. The tachycardia algorithm is "linked" with different interventions for narrow-complex tachycardia and wide-complex tachycardia. Electrical cardioversion is the therapy of choice for unstable ventricular and supraventricular tachyarrhythmias with a heart rate greater than 150 beats/min. When the patient is in stable wide-complex or narrow-complex tachycardia, a specific diagnosis should be made. A 12-lead ECG should be obtained along with clinical information, and vagal maneuvers should be considered before administration of medications.

With R-wave synchronous cardioversion, the defibrillator is programmed to deliver therapy on the R wave, thus avoiding the vulnerable period of cardiac repolarization, which is the downslope of the T wave. If the electrical shock were delivered on the downslope of the T wave, then the patient's rhythm probably would deteriorate into VF.

When pulseless, the patient is treated as if in VF; thus, R-wave asynchronous cardioversion is not used (refer to Fig. 31-2 and the procedure for defibrillation). If the patient is severely unstable (e.g., in acute pulmonary edema, having chest pain, or is unconscious or hypotensive), then unsynchronized cardioversion is recommended. There can be considerable time delays with synchronized cardioversion, but in patients with extremely rapid VT, asynchronous cardioversion actually may be safer, because at rapid rates the synchronizer may not be able to distinguish the T wave from the QRS complex. In this instance, an asynchronous shock may have less likelihood of falling on the T wave than a synchronous shock (American Heart Association, 2003).

Energy Requirements. Energy requirements are variable depending on the rhythm and the number of cardioversion attempts. Rhythms that tend to be organized (i.e., VT, atrial flutter) usually require less energy than unorganized rhythms (i.e., VF, atrial fibrillation).

The energy requirements for cardioverting VT depend on the rate and morphology of the arrhythmia. The operator should start at 100 J for an organized, monomorphic VT with or without a pulse. Polymorphic VT requires initial shock energy of 200 J. The electrical cardioversion algorithm recommends a 100-, 200-, 300-, and 360-J sequence for synchronized cardioversion (Display 31-5).

Procedure for Urgent Synchronized Cardioversion. Because the patient is conscious, anesthesia or analgesia is necessary. Except for the following points, the procedure for urgent synchronized cardioversion is the same as for defibrillation:

- Turn on the synchronizer.
- Select the appropriate energy level.

DISPLAY **31-5**

ARRHYTHMIAS AND RECOMMENDED ENERGY LEVELS FOR CARDIOVERSION

Acceptable Starting Energy Levels for Arrhythmia	50 Joules	100 Joules	200 Joules	≥300 Joules
Give stepwise ↑ if 1st shock fails	Atrial flutter	Monomorphic VT	Polymorphic VT	For additional shocks
	PSVT	SVT		
		Atrial fibrillation		

Starting energy levels for cardioversion vary with different arrhythmias. Atrial flutter and paroxysmal supraventricular tachycardia (PSVT) can convert to sinus rhythm with energy levels as low as 50 joules (J). If unsuccessful, increase energy level to 100 J for 2nd shock, 200 J for 3rd shock, and 300 J or higher for additional shocks. Start energy level at 100 J for monomorphic VT, SVT, and atrial fibrillation, increasing energy level as needed. Polymorphic VT often requires 200 J for beginning shock, increasing as needed if unsuccessful. (American Heart Association, 2003.)

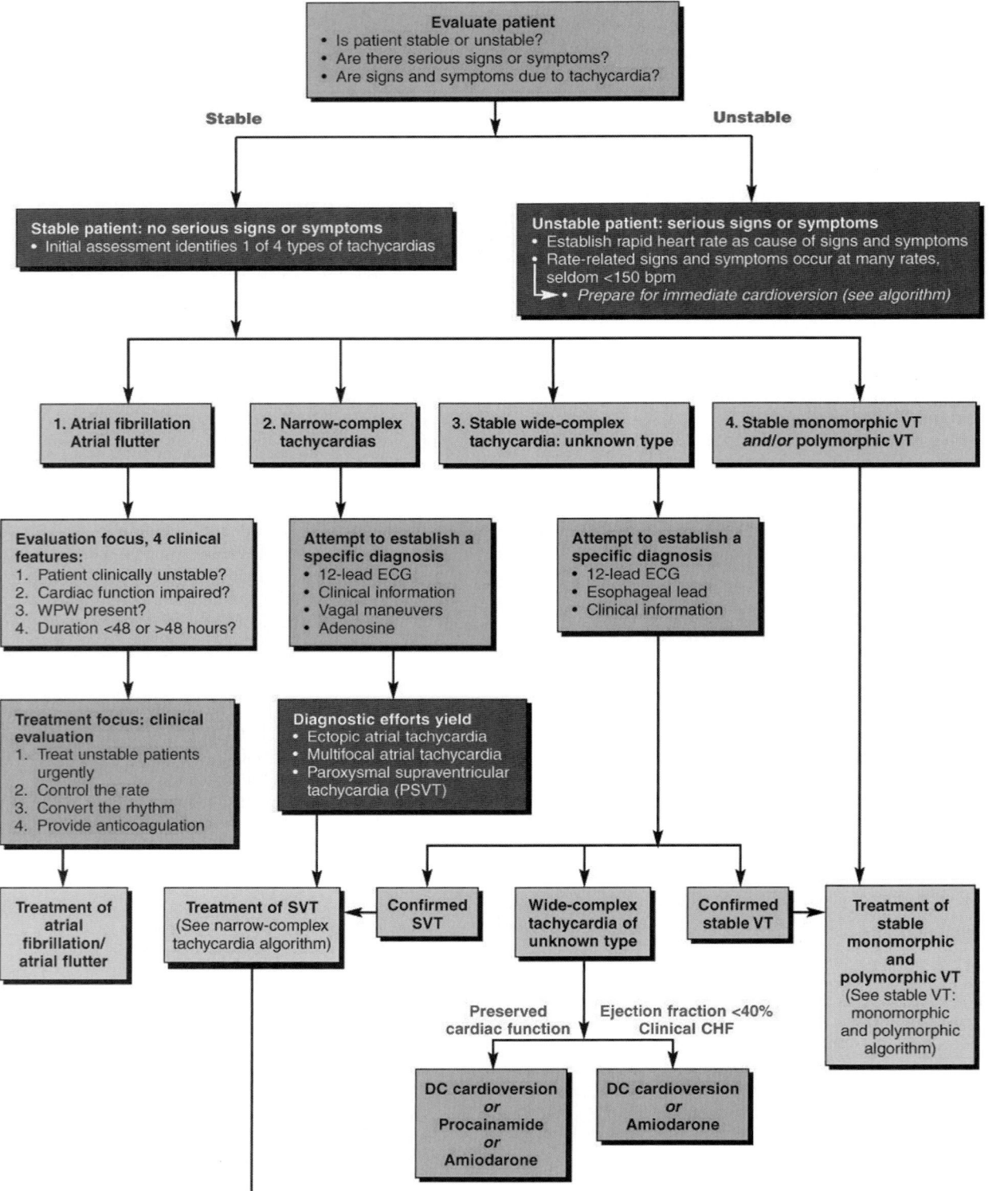

■ **Figure 31–6.** The "linked" tachycardia algorithms. The tachycardia algorithm is designed to first focus on the patient and determine if he or she is stable or unstable. If unstable, treat immediately. If stable, make a rhythm diagnosis. The diagnosis will fall into a particular rhythm category: (1) atrial fibrillation/atrial flutter; (2) narrow-complex tachycardia; (3) stable wide-complex tachycardia: unknown type; and (4) stable monomorphic VT and/or polymorphic VT. (From American Heart Association. [2003]. *ACLS – The reference textbook : Principles and practice* [p. 314]. Dallas: AHA.)

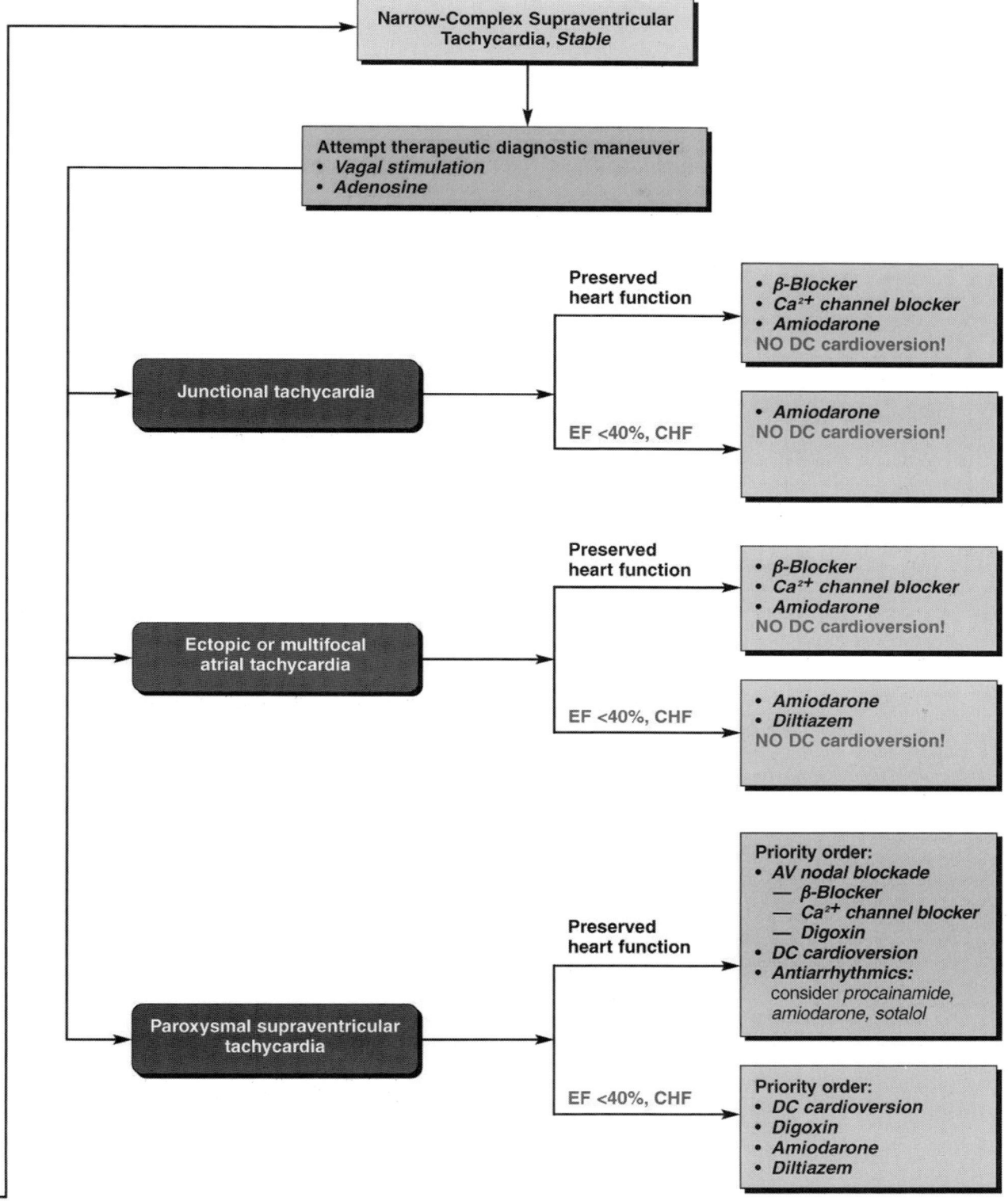

■ **Figure 31–7.** The "linked" tachycardia algorithm—narrow complex SVT—stable. In the narrow complex rhythm category, the emphasis should be to obtain diagnosis if at all possible. Follow algorithm for specific treatment of junctional tachycardia, atrial tachycardia, and PSVT. ACLS guidelines also focus on normal ventricular function and decreased left ventricular function when prioritizing treatment. (From American Heart Association. [2003]. *ACLS — The reference textbook : principles and practice* [p. 315]. Dallas: AHA.)

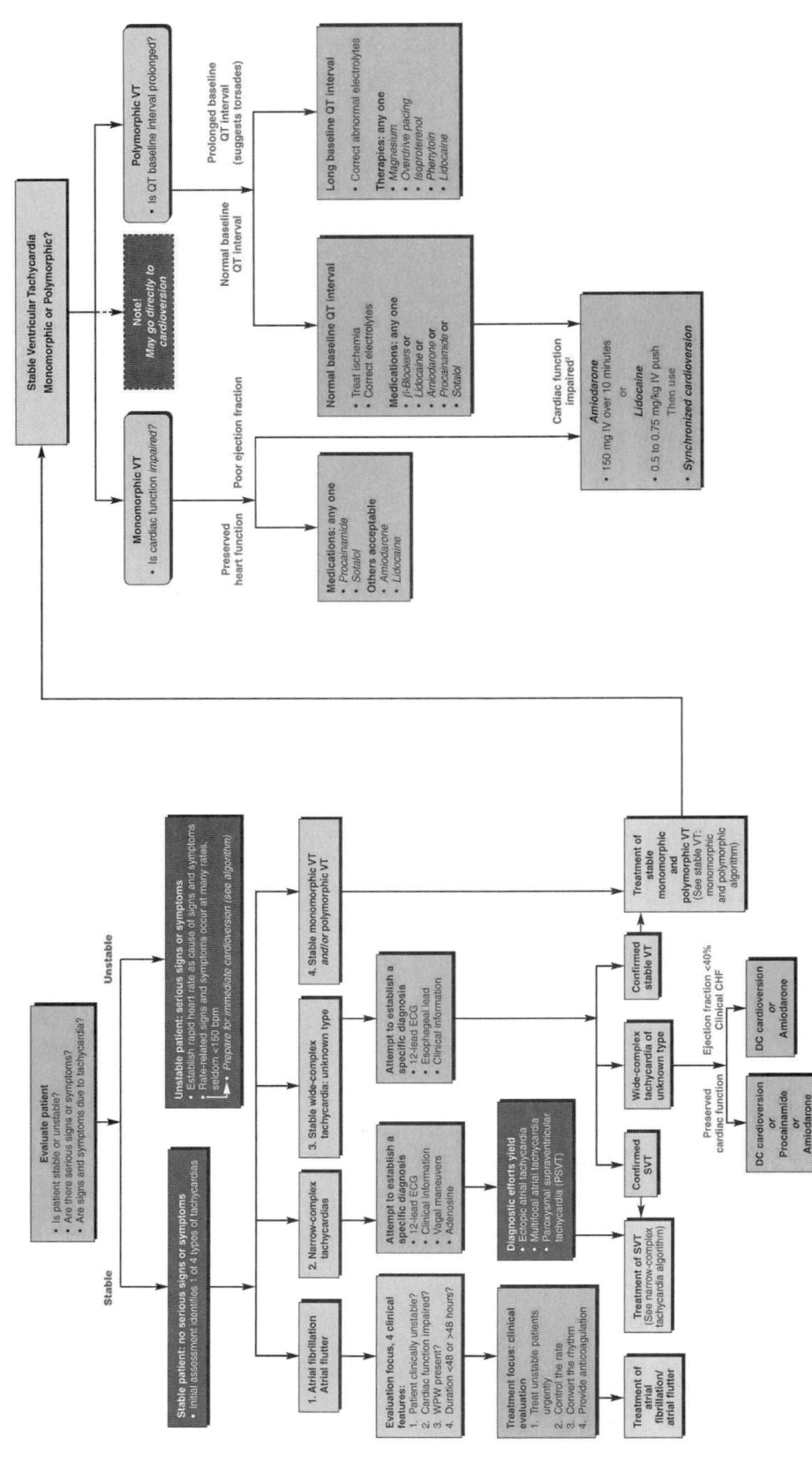

■ **Figure 31-8.** The "linked" tachycardia algorithm—monomorphic or polymorphic VT. If unstable, go directly to cardioversion. Treat stable VT per monomorphic or polymorphic guidelines. (From American Heart Association. [2003]. *ACLS— The reference textbook : Principles and practice* [p. 361]. Dallas: AHA.)

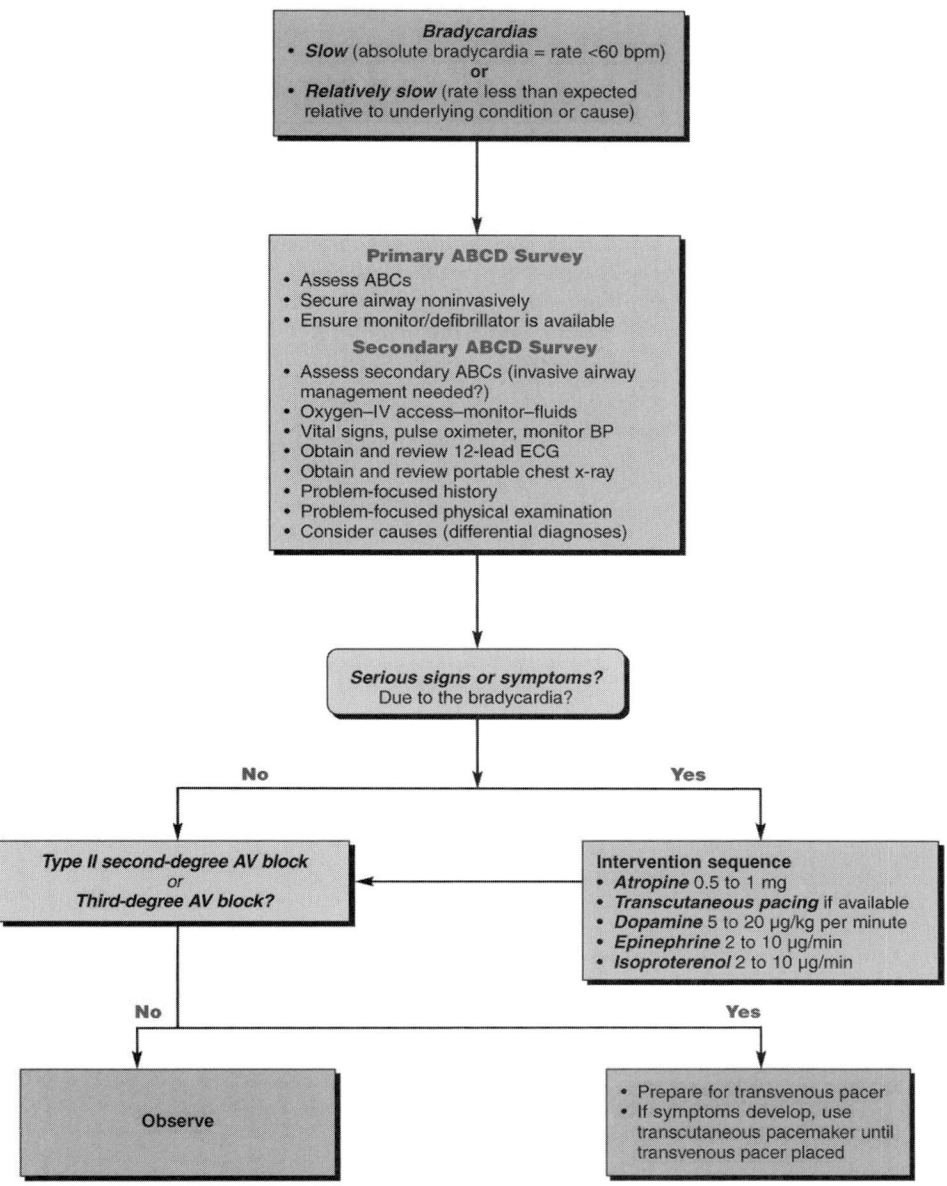

Figure 31–9. Bradycardia algorithm: atrioventricular blocks and emergency pacing. (From American Heart Association. [2003]. *ACLS — The reference textbook : Principles and practice* [p. 291]. Dallas: AHA.)

- Look for the synchronizer indicator on the screen, usually a spike or dot highlighted on the R wave. If you are unable to get a highlighted indicator, consider switching leads. Some older defibrillator or cardioverter units require an upright R wave for synchronization.
- Reassess rhythm.
- Expect a slight delay (milliseconds) from the time the buttons are pushed to the delivered shock
- If the defibrillator does not fire, reassess rhythm. If the patient has reverted to VF, there is no R wave with which to synchronize. Therefore, the unit will not fire. Immediately turn the synchronizer off, adjust the energy level, and proceed to defibrillate the patient.
- If VF develops in the patient after the synchronous shock, immediately turn the synchronizer off, adjust the energy level, and proceed to defibrillate the patient.

Symptomatic Bradycardia

The bradycardia algorithm (Fig. 31-9) outlines the approach to management of symptomatic bradyarrhythmias. Symptoms resulting from bradycardia (heart rate <60 beats/min) include chest pain, dyspnea, lightheadedness, hypotension, or ventricular ectopy. An external pacemaker is always appropriate for use in symptomatic bradycardias and should be used immediately for patients who do not respond to atropine. Atropine must be used with caution in patients with acute MI who have third-degree heart block and ventricular escape beats or Mobitz type II heart block. Dopamine and epinephrine should be added as the patient's condition worsens. Isoproterenol increases myocardial oxygen consumption and peripheral vasodilatation. It should be used only with extreme caution. Cardiac arrest from bradycardias, asystole, and pulseless electrical activity

(PEA) appear to occur more often in patients with severely diseased hearts, most likely representing more global cardiac dysfunction (Stevenson, 1993).

■ SURVIVORS OF CARDIAC ARREST

Prognosis

Prognosis of survivors is affected by how promptly definitive therapy is initiated, the rhythm or conduction disturbance initially recognized after cardiac arrest, and whether the patient also has sustained an acute MI. For patients whose initially recognized rhythm is asystole or PEA, prognosis is dismal. Survival rates for patients found in asystole or PEA are only 1% to 6%, compared with 25% for those patients found in VT/VF (Deshpande et al., 1998). Despite early CPR and advanced life support, which have substantially improved initial resuscitation success rates up to 50%, only approximately half of these patients are discharged home. Most of these patients die of cardiogenic shock, congestive heart failure, respiratory complications, or sepsis (Deshpande et al., 1998).

Survivors of SCD are at high risk for future events. An epidemiologic study reported recurrence rates of 30% to 50% during a 2-year follow-up (Myerburg et al., 1992). However, in recent years, SCD survivors have received benefits from AEDs, revascularization procedures, ICDs, antiarrhythmic drugs, radiofrequency ablation of VT, or any combined therapies. Research has focused on providing primary prevention with prophylactic ICD therapy for patients with history of previous MI and LV dysfunction, improving the survival rate by 31% (Moss, 2002) (Display 31-6).

Medical Management of Survivors of Cardiac Arrest

Immediate Postresuscitation Goals

- Provide cardiac and respiratory support for optimal tissue perfusion, especially to the brain.
- Transfer the patient to the nearest appropriately equipped emergency department and then to a critical care unit.
- Identify the causes of the arrest.
- Institute medical therapy to prevent arrhythmia recurrence, such as antiarrhythmic drug therapy and correction of underlying abnormalities that may have precipitated the cardiac arrest.
- Treat complications of resuscitation.

Cerebral Resuscitation

The primary goal of cardiopulmonary–cerebral resuscitation is to retain healthy brain function. Unfortunately, neurologic recovery is incomplete after a successful cardiac resuscitation. Cessation of circulation for 10 to 20 seconds results in loss of consciousness caused by lack of oxygen. Within 2 to 4 minutes, glucose and glycogen stores are used up, and after 4 to 5 minutes ATP is exhausted. Hypoxemia and hypercarbia cause loss of cerebral blood flow autoregulation, the brain then becomes dependent on cerebral perfusion pressure (Holzer, 2002, & Holzer, 2003). Cerebral perfusion pressure is equal to mean arterial pressure minus intracranial pressure (CPP = MAP − ICP). After return of spontaneous circulation (ROSC), a brief period of hyperemia occurs along with global hypoperfusion resulting in a "no-reflow phenomenon" (Holzer & Sterz, 2003; American

---

DISPLAY   31-6

PRIMARY VERSUS SECONDARY PREVENTION OF SCD

Primary prevention of SCD is aimed at preventing the first potentially fatal arrhythmic event. Primary prevention is an elusive goal. It has been difficult to show that therapy directed at any single risk factor is effective. Beta-blockers, ACE inhibitor therapy, and lipid management aimed at stabilizing plaque formation have been shown to decrease sudden and nonsudden deaths in patients with heart failure or after myocardial infarction.

Several ICD trials have shown that ICD therapy provides primary protection in a will-defined high-risk subgroup of patients. The MADIT II Trial, for patients with prior myocardial infarction and ejection fraction ≤.30, showed a 30% reduction in overall mortality compared to "conventional antiarrhythmic therapy (Moss et al., 2002).

There is a role for home AEDs in preventing SCD. The Home AED trial (HAT) is currently underway and is testing the effectiveness of widespread use of Home AEDs in the post-MI patient.

Current research that is looking at predicting SCD susceptibility includes testing for markers of inflammation, most notably C-reactive protein (CRP) and homocysteine levels, which may be useful indicators for long-term risk of SCD (Albert et al., 2002).

There is also accumulating research evidence to suggest that there may be molecular, genetic, and biochemical indicators of

SCD. Genetic mutations have been identified in individuals with rare inherited arrhythmias (long QT syndrome and Brugada's syndrome) (Myerburg & Spooner, 2001).

Secondary prevention of SCD is aimed at preventing a recurrence of a potentially fatal arrhythmia or cardiac arrest among patients who have survived a sudden cardiac arrest or arrhythmic event. Patients who have experienced one sudden cardiac arrest are at high risk for recurrent cardiac arrest.

The ICD is superior to any other treatment and is the only evidence-based therapeutic strategy for secondary prevention.

Three randomized trials—the Antiarrhythmic versus Implantable Defibrillators (AVID), Cardiac Arrest Study Hamburg (CASH), and the Canadian Implantable Defibrillator Study (CIDS)—all found the ICD to be superior to antiarrhythmic drugs. AVID was terminated early because the overall survival rate, for 3 years, in the ICD group was 32% higher than the drug group (AVID Investigators, 1997). The CASH study showed a 23% lower mortality rate in the ICD group compared to the patients randomized to amiodarone/metoprolol (Kuck et al., 2000). The CIDS trial showed similar results, with a 19% reduction in mortality in the ICD group compared to patients taking amiodarone (Connolly et al., 2000).

DISPLAY **31-7**

RELEVANT RESEARCH:
PROTECTING THE BRAIN—HYPOTHERMIA AFTER CPR

Cooling the body to protect the brain has been used for many years during cardiac surgery in association with cardiopulmonary bypass. Recently two studies were completed on two different continents (Europe and Australia) using therapeutic hypothermia to prevent neurologic injury in comatose survivors of cardiac arrest. The Hypothermia after Cardiac Arrest Study Group enrolled VF survivors to a blinded assessment of outcome study. The patients were randomly assigned to a hypothermia group (temperature maintained at 32–34° Celsius per bladder temperature for a 24-hour period) or to receive standard treatment with normothermia. The primary end point was favorable neurologic outcome within 6 months of cardiac arrest. Study results showed mortality in the hypothermia group was 41% and mortality in the normothermia group was 55%. The conclusions of this European study were that therapeutic mild hypothermia increased the rate of favorable neurologic outcome and reduced mortality.

Researchers in Australia randomized cardiac arrest survivors to either a hypothermia or normothermia group. In the hypothermia group body temperature was reduced to 33° Celsius within 2 hours of return of spontaneous circulation and maintained at 33° C for 12 hours. Similar results were noted to the above study. Preliminary observations suggest that lowering the body temperature to 33° C for 12 hours in comatose survivors of cardiac arrest improves neurologic outcomes.

From Holzer et al. (2002) and Bernard et al. (2002).

Heart Association, 2000). Improvement in cerebral recovery after cardiac arrest results when cardiac arrest and CPR times are short, and ROSC is restored quickly.

Treatment for the unresponsive patient should include optimizing cerebral perfusion pressure by maintaining a normal or slightly elevated mean arterial pressure and reducing intracranial pressure. Hyperthermia and seizures increase the oxygen requirements of the brain; therefore, all attempts at maintaining normothermia should be made. Recent research has shown induced hypothermia improves outcomes in comatose survivors of cardiac arrest; however, optimal duration and temperature range remain under further investigation (Holzer & Sterz, 2003) (Display 31-7).

Seizure activity should be controlled with use of phenobarbital, dilantin, or diazepam. The patient's head should be maintained in a midline position and elevated to 30 degrees to increase cerebral venous drainage. Vigilant attention should be made at maintaining oxygenation and perfusion to the brain to maximize the chance for full neurological recovery (American Heart Association, 2000).

Ongoing Medical Care

The medical management for survivors of cardiac arrest depends on the patient's central nervous system function and known preexisting factors. Management includes diagnostic evaluation and therapy directed toward ischemia, LV dysfunction, structural abnormalities, arrhythmias, and other concurrent medical conditions. The evaluation process for the SCD survivor is summarized in Figure 31-10. In the evaluation of

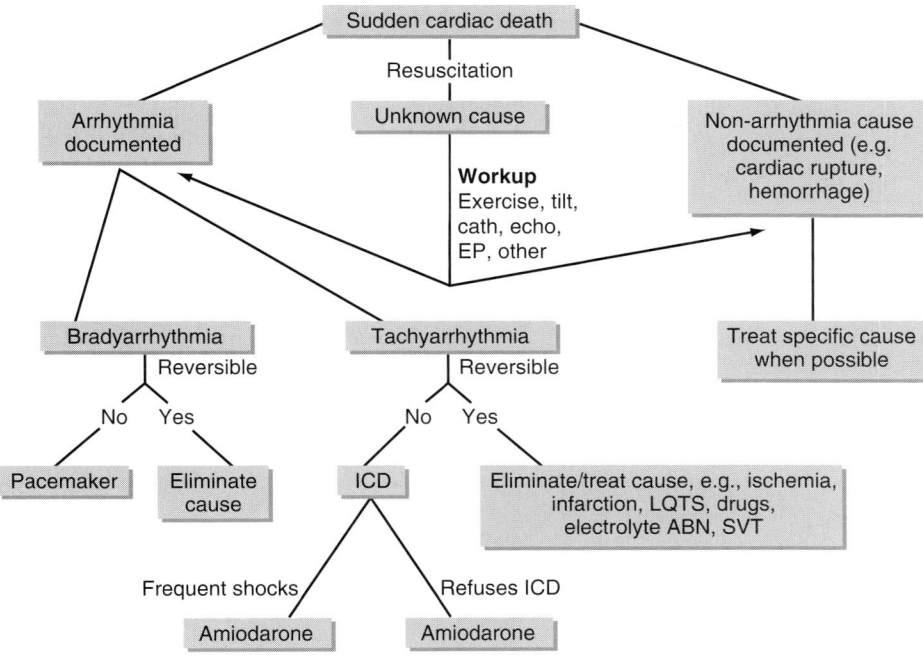

■ **Figure 31–10.** Treatment algorithm for patient resuscitated from SCD. Cath indicates catherization; echo, echocardiography; EP, electrophysiologic study; LQTS, long QT syndrome; ABN, abnormality; SVT, supraventricular tachycardia; ICD, internal cardioverter defibrillator. (From Zipes, D. P. & Wellens, H. J. J. [1998]. Sudden cardiac death. *Circulation,* 98, 2334–2351.)

the SCD patient, the electrophysiology study, the degree and type of underlying structural heart disease, and the status of the LV function are used to determine further management and therapies (Zipes & Wellens, 1998).

Diagnostic Evaluation. If the central nervous system function is limited, extensive evaluation usually is deferred. If the patient sustained cardiac arrest as a result of acute MI, evaluation and treatment are no different from those in any other patient with acute MI. The cardiac arrest produces a period of global ischemia and stunning to the myocardium; potentially, there is a need for either inotropic or intraaortic counterpulsation to maintain perfusion. Often, ventricular dysfunction improves after the initial injury, and the initial low ejection fraction may not represent a true reading (Dimarco, 2003). If the arrest is attributable to proarrhythmic drug effects or electrolyte disturbances, extensive evaluation usually is not indicated. Aggressive evaluation is warranted for most patients whose cardiac arrest was precipitated by coronary atherosclerosis not associated with acute transmural MI, or with other heart disease that can be managed medically or surgically. Diagnostic tests include cardiac catheterization, radionuclide stress testing, echocardiography, electrophysiologic studies, and possibly magnetic resonance imaging if arrhythmogenic right ventricular dysplasia is suspected (Dimarco, 2003; Zipes & Wellens, 1998).

Reduction of Ischemia. Depending on the anatomy and physiology of the disease process, either medical or surgical therapy is indicated. Medical therapy includes β-adrenergic blocking agents, calcium channel blocking agents, and angiotensin-converting enzyme (ACE) inhibitors, alone or in combination. One important study, the Beta-blocker Heart Attack Trial (BHAT), a randomized, double-blind, placebo-controlled study, tested whether the use of beta-blockers in patients with a history of at least one MI could reduce subsequent mortality (Woods et al., 1998). The study was stopped 9 months early because of significant improvement in total mortality in the beta-blocker treatment group. SCD was significantly less frequent in the beta-blocker group (3.3% vs. 4.6%). Patients with a history of congestive heart failure who were treated with beta-blockers experienced a more dramatic reduction in SCD (10.4% vs. 4.4%). ACE inhibitor use also may reduce SCD, as evidenced by the Trandolapril Cardiac Evaluation Trial (TRACE) (Kober et al., 1995).

Myocardial revascularization has been shown to reduce the incidence of SCD in patients with heart disease, both in primary and secondary prevention of SCD. The greatest benefits are seen in those patients with multivessel disease and decreased left ventricular function (Dimarco, 203). Surgery is indicated for those patients with conventional criteria (i.e., uncontrolled angina or left main or multiple-vessel CHD) or with specific criteria for antiarrhythmic surgery (i.e., discrete ventricular aneurysms or inducible, potentially lethal, arrhythmias not controlled by medication) (Dimarco, 2003).

Because of the complexity of sudden cardiac death mechanisms, treatment is geared at delaying further progression of coronary heart disease in those patients with known cardiac disease. Long-term treatments include preventing thrombus formation and plaque rupture, preventing arrhythmias, stabilizing autonomic balance, improving pump function, and correcting ischemia (Zipes & Wellens, 1998).

Antiarrhythmic Therapy. The use of antiarrhythmic drugs are valuable in the immediate period after resuscitation. Intravenous amiodarone and beta-blockers are the most effective antiarrhythmics in the early phase. However, unlike beta-blockers and ACE inhibitors, certain antiarrhythmics, particularly class I drugs, have been associated with increased mortality rates despite suppressing ventricular ectopy (Dimarco, 2003). Increased mortality was seen in the CAST study with the use of encainide and flecainide in the patient after acute MI. CAST II showed increased mortality rates in this same group with the use of moricizine (Echt et al., 1991). In contrast, several trials have shown a beneficial effect on mortality with the use of amiodarone, a class III drug, in patients after MI. Properties of amiodarone that may help reduce mortality after MI are coronary vasodilation and heart rate reduction, which serve to reduce ischemia (Zipes & Wellens, 1998).

Implantable Cardioverter–Defibrillators. ICD therapy has emerged as the therapy of choice for secondary prevention of sudden cardiac death in patients with preexisting heart disease. Three large multicenter trials compared ICD therapy versus antiarrhythmic drug therapy in survivors of sudden cardiac arrest and demonstrated ICD therapy was superior to best antiarrhythmic drug therapy (see Display 31-6). Recent years have produced dramatic technological improvements in ICDs. Devices are smaller, implantation has been greatly simplified, and therapy options are greater, which help to reduce the number of unnecessary shocks. Treatment of life-threatening ventricular arrhythmias will most likely remain the domain of the ICD in the future. Antiarrhythmic drugs and catheter ablation will continue to complement the ICD, decreasing the frequency of ICD discharges and, hopefully, improving quality of life (see Chapter 32 for additional ICD information).

Nursing Management of Sudden Cardiac Death Survivors

Survivors of cardiac arrest and their families have physiologic, psychological, and educational needs that differ from those of the patient with acute myocardial ischemia and infarction. However, if the underlying cause includes ischemia, management of the patient with ischemia and infarction should be included in nursing care.

Physiologic Nursing Management

After cardiac arrest, patients are admitted to the cardiac care unit. A complete evaluation for heart disease will be obtained on all patients. Treatment goals are dependent on the underlying heart disease. Occasionally, patients present with an "arrhythmia storm" and are in danger of recurrent VF. The patient will need aggressive correction for acute ischemia, and possibly hemodynamic support (Callans, 2002). The patient will require continuous ECG monitoring until an ICD is placed. An intravenous line is left in place for immediate venous access. Time of hospital discharge is related to the cause of the cardiac arrest, the type of diagnostic studies required, and the eventual therapies selected by the patient and family. If the patient will be receiving an ICD, the implications of having an ICD must be discussed thoroughly. As much education and support as possible should be provided about the ICD (see Chapter 32).

Emotional Support

Emotional support given to patients and their families affects their quality of life. Fear of recurrent cardiac arrest is experienced by patients and their families. Fear is exacerbated further at the time of transfer out of the cardiac care unit to a telemetry unit, and further still at the time of discharge from the hospital. Patients who experience cardiac arrest with no known (and, therefore, treatable) cause may require more emotional support than do patients who can receive treatment to correct or modify the causative factor (Druss & Kornfeld, 1967). Anxiety, fear, memory difficulties, loss of sexual interest, trouble concentrating, and perceived lifestyle changes have also been reported in the cardiac arrest survivor (Finkelmeier et al., 1984). Several researchers have reported that cardiac arrest survivors about to receive an ICD, or newly implanted with an ICD, are often depressed or show depressive symptoms (Thomas et al., 2001). Denial, isolation, projection, and hallucinatory or delusional behavior have been identified as coping mechanisms used by survivors (Druss & Kornfeld, 1967).

Should VF recur in the hospital, it is important to realize that some patients retain auditory function during cardiac arrest. Therefore, refrain from negative, ominous, or derogatory remarks during the arrest. If the family members are present at the time of arrest, direct someone to take them to a private waiting room, stay with them, and, if requested, help them to contact a member of the clergy. After a successful resuscitation, allow family members to see the patient as soon as possible (Tuggle, 1982). Nurses play a major therapeutic role in the management of the sudden cardiac arrest survivor and their family.

Patient and Family Education

Next to competent resuscitative and emotional care, education of the patient and family may do the most to relieve fear of, and prevent death from, recurrent cardiac arrest. Assess readiness to learn. Teach at an appropriate level, taking into account any learning disabilities from central nervous system dysfunction that may have resulted from the arrest. Content that should be presented and understood before discharge includes normal cardiac anatomy and physiology; pathophysiology related to CHD in general and to the arrest in particular; ICD teaching for those patients who receive an ICD, including implications, follow-up care, and what to do if they receive an ICD shock; CHD risk factor modification; medications; activity prescription; importance and dates of return appointments; how to activate the emergency medical system; and CPR. Specific recommendations about teaching CPR to families have been made: teach only one-rescuer CPR; teach CPR in short segments, with reinforcement of each segment before progression to the next; and emphasize the need to teach neighbors and coworkers (Dracup & Breu, 1987).

All of this information is overwhelming and almost impossible to remember without teaching aids such as booklets, charts, videotapes, and pictures. Family members may also feel particularly overwhelmed by the thought of recurring episodes. Support groups provide invaluable services to patients and their families. They allow the patient and family members to ask questions and discuss issues related to devices and heart disease, as well as provide the chance for them to meet and talk to others with similar circumstances. Another avenue for patients to explore is Internet web sites. It is best to provide the patient with a list of suggested web sites that have been prescreened to ensure accuracy and appropriateness of content. Patients need to be warned of potential misinformation from obtaining information through Internet web sites.

SUMMARY

Sudden cardiac death remains the primary cause of cardiac death in the United States, despite advances in therapy and technology. At present, the mechanisms for SCD are not clearly understood. Primary prevention of SCD will remain a challenge until there is a better understanding of the pathophysiology of ventricular fibrillation, along with risk factor stratification. Until we understand the pathophysiology and identify high-risk individuals, public education and training should continue to focus on initiating the "chain of survival" and increasing the number of willing and able CPR providers.

REFERENCES

ACLS: Principles and Practice (2003). *ACLS -Reference Textbook.* Dallas, TX: American Heart Association.

Albert, C. M., Jing, M., Nader, R., et al. (2002). Prospective sudy of C-reactive protein, Homocysteine, and plasma lipid levels as predictors of sudden cardiac death. *Circulation, 105,* 2595–2599.

Anderson, K. P. (1984). Sudden death, hypertension, and hypertrophy. *Journal of Cardiovascular Pharmacology, 6,* S498–S503.

The Antiarrhythmics vs. Implantable Defibrillators (AVID) Investigators (1997). A comparison of antiarrhythmic drug therapy with implantable defibrillators in patients resuscitated from near fatal ventricular arrhythmias. *New England Journal of Medicine, 337,* 1576–1583.

Bocka, J. J. (1989). External transcutaneous pacemakers. *Annuals of Emergency Medicine, 18,* 1280–1286.

Bardy, G. H., Marchlinski, F. Sharma, A., et al. (1996). For the Transthoracic Investigators. Multicenter comparison of truncated biphasic shocks and standard damped sine wave monophasic shocks for transthoracic ventricular fibrillation. *Circulation, 94,* 2507–2514.

Bernard, S. A., Gray, T. W., Buist, M. D., et al. (2002). Treatment of comatose survivors of out-of-hospital cardiac arrest with induced hypothermia. *New England Journal of Medicine, 346(8),* 557–563.

Caldwell, G., Miller, G, Quinn, E., et al. (1985). Simple mechanical methods for cardioversion: Defense of the precordial thump and cough version. *British Medical Journal, 291,* 627–630.

Callans, D. J. (2002). Management of the patient who has been resuscitated from sudden cardiac death. *Circulation, 105,* 2704–2707.

Cobb, L. A., & Werner J. A. (1982). Predictors and prevention of sudden cardiac death. In J. W. Hurst (Ed.), *The heart* (pp. 538–546). New York: McGraw-Hill.

Connolly, S. J., Gent, M., Roberts, R. S., et al. (2000). Canadian Implantable Defibrillator Study (CIDS): a randomized trial of the implantable cardioverter defibrillator against amiodarone. *Circulation, 101,* 1297–1302.

Cummins, R. O., Graves, J., Horan, S., et al. (1989). Prehospital transcutaneous pacing of significant bradycardias by paramedics: clinical and system effectiveness. *Prehospital Disaster Medicine, 4,* 70.

Cummins, R. O., Ornato J. P., Thies, W. H., & Pepe, P. H. (1991). Improving survival from sudden cardiac arrest: the "chain of survival" concept. A statement for health professionals from the Advanced Cardiac Life Support

Subcommittee and the Emergency cardiac Care Committee, American Heart Association. *Circulation, 83,* 1832–1847.

Cummins, R. O., & Thies, W. H. (1990). Encouraging early defibrillation: The American Heart Association and automated external defibrillators. *Annals of Emergency Medicine, 19,* 1245–1248.

Davies, M. J. (1992). Anatomical features in victims of sudden coronary death. *Circulation,* 85(Suppl. I), I–19–I–24.

Davies, M. J. & Thomas, A. (1984). Thrombosis and acute coronary lesions in sudden cardiac ischemic death. *New England Journal of Medicine, 310,* 1137–1140.

Deshpande, S., Vora, A., Axtell, K., et al. (1998). Sudden cardiac death. In D. Brown (Ed.), *Cardiac intensive care* (pp. 391–404). Philadelphia: W. B. Saunders.

Dimarco, J. P. (2003). Sudden cardiac death. In M. H. Crawford (Ed.), *Current diagnosis and treatment in cardiology* (2nd ed., Chapter 24). New York: Lange Medical Books/McGraw-Hill.

Dorian, P., Cass, D., Schwartz, B., et al. (2002) Amiodarone as compared with lidocaine for shock-resistant ventricular fibrillation. *New England Journal of Medicine, 346,* 884–890.

Dracup, K. & Breu, C. (1987). Teaching and retention of cardiopulmonary resuscitation skills for families of high-risk patients with cardiac disease. *Focus on Critical Care, 14*(1), 67–72.

Druss, R. G. & Kornfeld, D. S. (1967). The survivors of cardiac arrest. *JAMA, 201,* 297.

Echt, D. S., Liebson, P. R., Mitchell, L. B., et al. (19XX). [AQ1] Mortality and morbidity in patients receiving encainide, flecainide, or placebo: The Cardiac Arrhythmia Suppression Trial. *New England Journal of Medicine, 324,* 781–788.

Ewy, G. A., & Taren, D. T. (1977). Comparison of paddle electrode pastes used for defibrillation. *Heart and Lung, 6,* 847.

Finkelmeier B. A., Kenwood, N. J., & Summers, C. (1984). Psychologic ramifications of survival from sudden cardiac death. *Critical Care Quarterly, 7,* 71–79.

Greene, H. L. (1990). Sudden arrhythmic cardiac death: Mechanisms, resuscitation, and classification. *American Journal of Cardiology, 65:* 4B–12B.

Hayes, D. L., Lloyd, M. A., & Friedman, P. A. (2000). *Cardiac pacing and defibrillation: A clinical approach.* Elmsford, NY: Blackwell Publishing.

Holzer, M. & Sterz, F. (2003). Hypothermia after CPR. *Currents in Emergency Cardiovascular Care, 14* (2), 10–12.

Holzer, M. & The Hypothermia After Cardiac Arrest Study Group (2002). Mild therapeutic hypothermia to improve the neurologic outcome after cardiac arrest. *New England Journal of Medicine, 346,* (8), 549–556.

Kerber, R. E., Grayzel, J. Hoyt, R., et al. (1981). Transthoracic resistance in human defibrillation: Influence of body weight, chest size, serial shocks, paddle size, and paddle contact pressure. *Circulation, 63,* 676–682.

Kerber, R. E., Jensen, S. R., Grayzel, J., et al. (1981). Elective cardioversion: Influence of paddle-electrode location and size on success rates and energy requirements. *New England Journal of Medicine, 305,* 658–662.

Kober, L. Torp-Pederson, C., Carlsen J. E., et al. (1995). A clinical trial for the Ace inhibitor Trandolapril in patients with left ventricular dysfunction after myocardial infarction. *New England Journal of Medicine, 333,* 1670–1676.

Kuck, K., Cappato, R., Siebels, J., et al. (2000). Randomized comparison of antiarrhythmic drug therapy with implantable defibrillators in patients resuscitated from cardiac arrest: the Cardiac Arrest Study Hamburg (CASH). *Circulation, 102,* 748–754.

Kudenchuk, P. J., Cobb, L.A., Copass, M. K., et al. (1999). Amiodarone for resuscitation after out-of-hospital cardiac arrest due to ventricular fibrillation. *New England Journal of Medicine, 341,* 871–878.

Lenachen, J. M., Henderson, E., Morris, K.I., et al. (1987) Ventricular arrhythmias in patients with hypertensive left ventricular hypertrophy. *New England Journal of Medicine, 317,* 787.

Liberthson, R. R., Nagel E. L., Hirschman, J. C., et al. (1974). Pathophysiologic observations in prehospital ventricular fibrillation and sudden cardiac death. *Circulation, 49,* 790–798.

Miller J., Tresch D., et al. (1984). The precordial thump. *Annals of Emergency Medicine, 13,* 791–794.

Moss, A. J., Zareba, W., Hall, W. J., et al. (2002). Prophylactic implantation of a defibrillator in patients with myocardial infarction and reduced ejection fraction. *New England Journal of Medicine, 346*(12), 877–883.

Myerburg, R. J., Kessler, K. M., & Castellanos, A. (1992). Sudden cardiac death: Structure, function and time-dependence of risk. *Circulation,* 85(Suppl. I), I–2–I–10.

Myerburg, R. J, & Castellanos A. (1997). Cardiac arrest and sudden cardiac death. In E. Braunwald (Ed.), *Heart disease: A textbook of cardiovascular medicine* (5th ed., pp. 742–779). Philadelphia: WB Saunders.

Myerburg, R. J. & Spooner, P. M. (2001). Opportunities for sudden death prevention: Direction for new clinical and basic research. *Cardiovascular Research, 50,* 177–185.

Prystowsky, E. N. (2001). Primary and secondary prevention of sudden cardiac death: The role of the implantable cardioverter defibrillator. *Reviews in Cardiovascular Medicine, 2*(4), 197–205.

Reichenbach, D., Moss, N., & Meyer, E. (1977). Pathology of the heart in sudden cardiac death. *American Journal of Cardiology, 39,* 865–872.

Schneider, T., Martens, P. R., Paschen, H., et al. (2000). Multicenter, randomized, controlled trial of 150-J biphasic shocks compared with 200 to 360-J monophasic shocks in the resuscitation of out-of-hospital cardiac arrest victims. Optimized Response to Cardiac Arrest (ORCA) Investigators. *Circulation, 102,* 1780–1787.

Sima, S. J., Kieso, R. A., Fox-Eastham, K. J., et al. (1989). Mechanisms responsible for decline in transthoracic impedance after DC shocks. *American Journal of Physiology, 257,* H1180–H1183.

Stevenson, W. G., Stevenson L.W., Middlekauff H.R., & Saxon, L.A. (1993) Sudden death prevention in patients with advanced ventricular dysfunction. *Circulation ,88,* 2953–2550.

Stults, K. R., Brown, D.D., Kerber, R. E., et al. (1986). Efficacy of an automated external defibrillator in the management of out-of-hospital cardiac arrest: Validation of the diagnostic algorithm and initial experience in a rural environment. *Circulation, 73,* 701–709.

Thomas, E. D., Ewy, G. A., Dahl, C. F., et al. (1977). Effectiveness of direct current defibrillation; role of paddle electrode size. *American Heart Journal, 93,* 463–467.

Thomas, S. A., Friedmann, E., Kelley, F. J., et al. (2001). Living with an implantable cardioverter-defibrillator: A review of the current literature related to psychosocial factors. *AACN Clinical Issues, 12,* 156–163.

Vasselle, M. (1985). On the mechanisms underlying cardiac standstill: Factors determining success or failure of escape pacemakers in the heart. *Journal of the American College of Cardiology, 5,* 35B–42B.

Warnes, C. A., & Roberts, W. C. (1984). Sudden coronary death: Relation of amount and distribution of coronary narrowing at necropsy to previous symptoms of myocardial ischemia, left ventricular scarring and heart weight. *American Journal of Cardiology, 54,* 65.

Weisfeldt, M. L., Kerver, R.E., McGoldrick, R. P., et al. (1995). American Heart Association Report on Public Access Defibrillation Conference, December 8-10, 1994. *Circulation, 92,* 2740–2747.

Woods, K. L., Ketley, D., Lowy, A., et al. (1998). Beta blockers and antithrombotic treatment for secondary prevention after acute myocardial infarction: towards an understanding of factors influencing clinical practice. *European Heart Journal, 19,* 774–779.

Zheng, Z.J., Croft, J.B, Giles, W.H., & Mensah, G.A. (2001). Sudden cardiac death in the United States, 1989-1998. *Circulation, 104,* 2158–2163.

Zipes, D. P., & Wellens, H. J. (1998). Clinical cardiology: New frontiers–sudden cardiac death. *Circulation, 98,* 2334–2351.

32

Pacemakers and Implantable Defibrillators*

CAROL JACOBSON • DONNA GERITY

PACEMAKERS

Arrhythmia device therapy has become common and very complex, requiring clinicians to have more knowledge and greater responsibilities than ever before. Early pacemakers were single-chamber devices designed to pace only in the ventricle, and the only programmable parameters were pacing rate and output. With the introduction of dual-chamber pacemakers with the capability of pacing the atria and the ventricles, the number of programmable parameters increased dramatically. Rate-responsive pacemakers came next and are capable of increasing the pacing rate in response to the body's need for increased cardiac output. Antitachycardia devices were developed to terminate supraventricular and ventricular tachyarrhythmias using pacing techniques, cardioversion, or defibrillation. Most recently, the development of biventricular pacing capability allows for pacing to improve hemodynamics and left ventricular function in patients with heart failure and cardiomyopathy. There have been tremendous advances in technology of devices for both bradycardia and antitachycardia therapy in recent years, with even more complex devices coming in the future. Given the number of companies in the arrhythmia device market and the increasing complexity of the devices themselves, it has become very difficult for clinicians to stay abreast of device features and function. The goal of this chapter is to present generic concepts of pacemaker and implantable defibrillator functions to provide a basic knowledge background on which cardiac nurses can build to enhance their understanding of antiarrhythmia devices.

Indications for Pacing

Pacemakers were originally designed to treat disorders of impulse initiation or impulse conduction resulting in symptomatic bradycardia. *Symptomatic bradycardia* is a term used to define a bradycardia that is directly responsible for symptoms such as syncope, near syncope, transient dizziness or light-headedness,

and confusion resulting from cerebral hypoperfusion caused by slow heart rate (Gibbons et al., 2002). Other symptoms such as fatigue, exercise intolerance, congestive heart failure (CHF), dyspnea, and hypotension can also result from bradycardia. Symptomatic bradycardia can be caused by sinus node dysfunction or by conduction failure in or below the AV node. Sinus node dysfunction is the most common indication for permanent pacing, followed by AV node dysfunction (Hayes & Zipes, 2001; Mitrani et al., 2001; Shanker & Saksena, 2001).

In addition to treating symptomatic bradycardia, pacemaker therapy can have beneficial effects on hemodynamics and clinical status by providing rate response for patients whose sinus node is not capable of increasing its rate appropriately in response to the body's need for increased cardiac output (chronotropic incompetence). Dual-chamber pacemaker therapy can preserve stroke volume in patients with left ventricular dysfunction, hypertrophic cardiomyopathy, or dilated cardiomyopathy by ensuring AV synchrony and providing optimal AV intervals to enhance ventricular filling (Atlee & Bernstein, 2001; Bourke & Healey, 2002; Fananapazir et al., 1998; Gilligan et al., 1998; Hayes & Friedman, 2000; Shanker & Saksena, 2001). Cardiac resynchronization therapy (CRT) with biventricular pacing improves septal wall motion, mitral valve function, and the dynamics of left ventricular contraction in patients with severe heart failure or dilated cardiomyopathy (Abraham, 2002; Atlee & Bernstein, 2001; Cazeau et al., 1998; Daubert et al., 2000; Daubert et al., 1998; Luck et al., 2002). The use of pacemaker therapy to prevent atrial fibrillation is an area of intense interest and investigation and has proven successful in many patients (Bourke & Healey, 2002; Daubert et al., 2000; Hayes & Zipes, 2001; Mitrani et al., 2001; Saksena et al., 1998; Spurrell & Sulke, 2000). Other indications for cardiac pacing include hypersensitive carotid sinus syndrome, neurocardiogenic syncope (vasovagal syncope), and long QT syndrome (Bourke & Healey, 2002; Grubb, 1998; Hayes & Zipes, 2001; Mitrani et al., 2001; Shanker & Saksena, 2001). There is even evidence that atrial pacing may be helpful in preventing sleep apnea (Bourke & Healey, 2002; Garrigue et al., 2002).

The American College of Cardiology and American Heart Association task force on pacemaker implantation has published guidelines for implantation of permanent pacemakers

---

*Carol Jacobson wrote the section on pacemakers. Donna Gerity wrote the section on implantable defibrillators.

CLASS I INDICATIONS FOR PERMANENT PACING IN ADULTS

Acquired Atrioventricular Block

1. Third-degree and advanced second-degree AV block at any anatomic level, associated with any one of the following conditions:
   a. Bradycardia with symptoms (including hear failure) presumed to be due to AV block.
   b. Arrhythmias and other medical conditions that require drugs that result in symptomatic bradycardia.
   c. Documented periods of asystole greater than or equal to 3.0 seconds or any escape rate less than 40 bpm in awake, symptom-free patients.
   d. After catheter ablation of the AV junction.
   e. Postoperative AV block that is not expected to resolve after cardiac surgery.
   f. Neuromuscular diseases with AV block, such as myotonic muscular dystrophy, Kearns-Sayre syndrome, Erb's dystrophy (limb-girdle), and peroneal muscular atrophy, with or without symptoms, because there may be unpredictable progression of AV conduction disease.
2. Second-degree AV block regardless of type or site of block, with associated symptomatic bradycardia.

Pacing for Chronic Bifascicular and Trifascicular Block

1. Intermittent third-degree AV block
2. Type II second-degree AV block
3. Alternating bundle branch block.

Pacing for Atrioventricular Block Associated with Acute Myocardial Infarction

1. Persistent second-degree AV block in the His-Purkinje system with bilateral bundle branch block or third-degree AV block within or below the His-Purkinje system after AMI.
2. Transient advanced (second or third-degree) infranodal AV block and associated bundle branch block. If the site of block is uncertain, an electrophysiologic study may be necessary.
3. Presistent and symptomatic second or third-degree AV block.

Pacing in Sinus Node Dysfunction

1. Sinus node dysfunction with documented symptomatic bradycardia, including frequent sinus pauses that produce symptoms. In some patients, bradycardia is iatrogenic and will occur as a consequence of essential long-term drug therapy of a type and dose for which there are no acceptable alternatives.
2. Symptomatic chronotropic incompetence.

Pacemakers That Automatically Detect and Pace to Terminate Tachycardias

1. None (all past recommendations for antitachycardia pacing have been moved to Class IIa in the 2002 guidelines).

Pacing to Prevent Tachycardia

1. Sustained pause-dependent VT, with or without prolonged QT, in which the efficacy of pacing is thoroughly documented.

Pacing in Hypersensitive Carotid Sinus Syndrome and Neurocardiogenic Syncope

1. Recurrent syncope caused by carotid sinus stimulation; minimal carotid sinus pressure induces ventricular asystole of more than 3 seconds' duration in the absence of any medication that depresses the sinus node or AV conduction.

Pacing for Hypertrophic Cardiomyopathy

1. Class I indications for sinus node dysfunction or AV block as described previously.

Pacing for Dilated Cardiomyopathy

1. Class I indications for sinus node dysfunction or AV block as described previously.

(Gibbons R. J., et al. [2002]. ACC/AHA/NASPE 2002 Guideline Update for Implantation of Cardiac Pacemakers and Antiarrhythmia Devices. A report of the American College of Cardiology/American Heart Association task force on practice guidelines [ACC/AHA/NASPE committe on pacemaker implantation].)

and antiarrhythmia devices (Gibbons et al., 2002). Display 32-1 lists the class I indications for permanent pacing according to the guidelines. Refer to the guidelines for class II indications.

Temporary pacing is indicated to treat symptomatic bradycardia after AMI or when associated with hyperkalemia or drug toxicity; bradycardia-dependent ventricular tachycardia (VT); before permanent pacemaker implantation in symptomatic patients; and in reversible conditions that will not likely result in the need for permanent pacing, such as bacterial endocarditis, Lyme disease, or cardiac trauma (Shanker & Saksena, 2001). Temporary pacing in acute MI is still controversial. Inferior MI results in intranodal block that is usually benign and temporary and requires pacing only if it results in symptomatic bradycardia or bradycardia dependent VT. When AV block occurs in anterior MI, it is usually infranodal, involves a large amount of myocardium, and is often symptomatic. Second- or third-degree AV block associated with anterior MI and bundle-branch block usually requires temporary pacing, but the mortality rate is high because of left ventricular dysfunction secondary to the large infarction rather than to the conduction

disturbance. Prophylactic temporary pacing is often performed in the presence of new right bundle-branch block with either anterior or posterior hemiblock, in left bundle-branch block with first-degree AV block, and in alternating right and left bundle-branch block (Shanker & Saksena, 2001).

Temporary pacing is often used after cardiac surgery to treat or prevent or treat symptomatic bradycardia and is sometimes used prophylactically in high-risk patients during cardiac catheterization, or with electrical or chemical cardioversion. Overdrive atrial pacing is sometimes used in an attempt to terminate atrial flutter or fibrillation after cardiac surgery when atrial epicardial leads are in place.

Types of Pacemakers

Refer to Displays 32-2 and 32-3 for definitions of single- and dual-chamber pacemaker terminology. The terms defined there are used throughout the pacemaker section of this chapter and are not defined in the text unless necessary.

SINGLE CHAMBER PACING TERMINOLOGY

Asynchronous (fixed rate) pacing—the pacemaker releases a pacing stimulus at the programmed rate regardless of the heart's intrinsic activity. No sensing occurs so the pacemaker fires in competition with the heart's natural rhythm. Examples of asynchronous modes are AOO, VOO, DOO.

Automatic interval—the time period between two consecutive paced events without an intervening sensed event. Also known as the **basic interval** or **pacing interval.**

Base rate—the rate at which the pacemaker paces when no intrinsic cardiac activity is present. Also called the **minimum rate** or **lower rate.**

Bipolar—having two poles. (1) A pacing lead with two electrical poles. The negative pole is the distal tip of the lead and the positive pole is a metal ring located a few millimeters proximal to the distal tip. The stimulating pulse is delivered through the distal tip electrode. (2) A pacing system with both electrical poles in or on the heart.

Capture—ability of the pacing stimulus to depolarize the chamber being paced. Capture is recognized on the ECG whenever the pacing spike is followed immediately by the appropriate waveform: an atrial spike followed by a P wave or a ventricular spike followed by a wide QRS.

Demand pacing—the pacemaker only paces when the heart's intrinsic rate is below the pacemakers programmed rate (only when necessary or on demand). This mode means that the pacemaker senses intrinsic cardiac activity and inhibits its output when intrinsic activity is present.

Electrode—the exposed metal tip of a pacing lead that contacts myocardium and directly transmits the pacing stimulus to cardiac tissue.

Electromagnetic, interference—electrical signals from the environment (i.e. radiofrequency waves) which can be sensed by the pacemaker and interfere with pacer function. Abbreviated **EMI.**

Escape interval—the period of time between a sensed cardiac event and the next pacemaker output. The escape interval is usually equal to the basic pacing rate but it can be programmed longer in some pacemakers (hysteresis).

Fusion beat—a cardiac depolarization (either atrial or ventricular) that results from two foci both contributing to depolarization of the chamber. In pacing, a fusion beat results when an intrinsic depolarization and a pacing stimulus occur simultaneously and both contribute to depolarization (usually seen in the ventricle).

Hysteresis—a programmable feature in some pacemakers that allows the escape interval to be programmed longer than the basic pacing interval (the pacing interval following a sensed beat is longer than the basic pacing interval). This allows more time for the heart's intrinsic activity to occur.

Inhibited response—a type of response to sensing that inhibits pacemaker output when an intrinsic beat is sensed. This results in demand pacing, or pacing only when the heart's intrinsic activity is slower than the basic pacing rate.

Lead—the insulated wire and it's electrode that transmits the pacing stimulus from the pulse generator to the heart and relays sensed intrinsic activity back to the pulse generator. A single chamber pacemaker uses on lead and a dual chamber pacemaker usually uses two leads, one in the atrium and one in the ventricle.

Magnet mode—a term used for the pacemaker's response when a magnet is placed over the pulse generator. A magnet inactivates the sensing circuitry and causes a pacemaker to function asychronously at a predetermined rate and in a preset manner. The magnet mode differs among manufacturers in pacing rate and number of impulses delivered with the magnet in place. A change is magnet-induced pacing rate is often an indicator of battery depletion and warrants pulse generator replacement.

Myopotential—an electrical signal generated by muscle movement. Myopotentials are sometimes sensed by the pacemaker and cause inhibition of pacemaker output.

Output—the electrical stimulus delivered by the pulse generator, usually defined in terms of pulse amplitude (V = volts) and pulse width (milliseconds = ms).

Oversensing—detection of inappropriate electrical signals by the pacemaker's sensing circuit, resulting in inappropriate inhibition of pacer output. Sources of oversensing can include electromagnetic interference, myopotentials, T waves, or crosstalk between atrial and ventricular channels in dual chamber pacemakers.

Pacemaker syndrome—adverse clinical signs and symptoms due to inadequate timing of atrial and ventricular contraction. The syndrome can be due to loss of AV synchrony in VVI pacing, inappropriate AV interval in dual chamber pacing, or inappropriate rate modulation. Symptoms include fatigue, confusion, unpleasant pulsations in neck or chest, limited exercise capacity, CHF, hypotension, syncope or near syncope.

Pacing interval—the time between two consecutive paced events without an intervening sensed event. Measured in milliseconds (ms). AA interval = atrial pacing interval, VV interval = ventricular pacing interval.

Pacer spike—term used to describe the small vertical "blip" recorded on the ECG with every pacemaker output pulse. The presence of a pacer spike indicates that a stimulus was released by the pacemaker.

Pseudofusion beat—an electrocardiographic phenomenon resulting from delivery of a pacemaker spike into an intrinsic event. In the ventricle, it appears as a pacer spike in an intrinsic QRS complex, but since the ventricle is already depolarized the spike is ineffective but may distort the QRS complex on the ECG.

Pulse generator—the device that contains the power source (battery) and the electronic circuits that control pacemaker function. The term "pacemaker" is commonly used for the pulse generator.

Rate modulation—the ability of a pacemaker to increase the pacing rate in response to physical activity or metabolic demand. The pacemaker uses some type of physiologic sensor to determine the need for increased pacing rate. The most commonly used sensors at the present time are motion sensors and minute ventilation sensors. Also called **rate adaptation** or **rate response.**

Refractory period—(1) In the heart, the period of time that the myocardium is incapable of responding to a stimulus. (2) In the pacemaker, an interval or timing cycle following a sensed or paced event during which the pacemaker will not respond to incoming signals. A single chamber pacemaker has one refractory period, a dual chamber pacemaker has an atrial refractory and a ventricular refractory period.

Sensing—the ability of the pacemaker to recognize and respond to intrinsic cardiac depolarization.

Sensing threshold—the smallest intrinsic atrial or ventricular signal (measured in mV) that can be consistently sensed by the pacemaker.

(continued)

D I S P L A Y **32–2 (Continued)**

SINGLE CHAMBER PACING TERMINOLOGY

Stimulation threshold—the minimum amount of voltage necessary to capture the heart consistently. Also called **capture threshold** or **pacing threshold.**

Undersensing—failure of a pacemaker to sense intrinsic cardiac depolarizations. This can result in competition between the pacemaker and the intrinsic rhythm.

Unipolar—having one pole. (1) A unipolar lead has only one pole, located at the distal tip. (2) A pacing system with one pole in or on the heart and the second pole located remote from the heart to complete the circuit. Permanent unipolar systems utilize the back of the pulse generator as the second pole. Temporary epicardial pacing systems utilize a ground wire in subcutaneous tissue as the second pole.

D I S P L A Y **32–3**

DUAL CHAMBER PACEMAKER TERMINOLOGY

Adaptive AV delay (or rate adaptive AV delay)—see AV Interval.

Alert period—the portion of the pulse generator's timing cycle during which it can sense and respond to intrinsic cardiac activity. The alert period follows the refractory period.

Atrial escape interval—period of time from a sensed or paced ventricular event to the next paced atrial event. Also called the **V-A interval.**

Atrial refractory period—period of time during which the atrial channel is unable to respond to sensed signals. In dual chamber pacemakers, the total atrial refractory period is divided into two parts: the AV Interval and the post ventricular atrial refractory period (PVARP).

Atrial tracking—a state of pacing in which sensed atrial activity triggers a ventricular pacing output at the end of the programmed AV delay. Also known simply as **tracking.**

AV interval (or AV delay)—the "electronic PR interval", or the length of time between a sensed or paced atrial event and the delivery of the ventricular pacing output. The AV intercal is programmable and is measured in milliseconds (e.g. an AV interval of 120 ms = a PR interval of .12 second). Many pacemakers have an **adaptive AV delay,** meaning that the AV delay can be programmed to shorten when the intrinsic atrial rate increases, thus mimicking the heart's own physiological increase in AV conduction as heart rate increases. Many devices also have a **differential AV delay,** meaning that the AV interval can be programmed to be longer on an atrial paced beat than on an atrial sensed beat (e.g., 200 ms when the atrium is paced and 150 ms when P waves are sensed).

Blanking period—a very short ventricular refractory period that occurs simultaneously with every atrial pacing output to prevent the ventricle from sensing the atrial stimulus. It is intended to prevent inhibition of ventricular output due to crosstalk (see definition below). Many pacemakers allow the blanking period to be programmed longer to prevent crosstalk.

Crosstalk—the sensing of a signal in one chamber by the sensing circuit in the other chamber, usually used in reference to the sensing of the atrial output pulse by the ventricular channel. Crosstalk due to sensing of atrial signals by the ventricular channel causes inhibition of ventricular pacing output because the ventricular channel thinks that the atrial output is a ventricular event.

Differential AV delay—see AV Interval.

Endless loop tachycardia—see Pacemaker Mediated Tachycardia.

Maximum tracking rate (MTR)—the programmable upper rate limit of a dual chamber pacemaker that determines the fastest rate at which 1:1 tracking of atrial sensed events will occur. The

MTR prevents the ventricular channel from pacing faster than the upper rate limit when the intrinsic atrial rate exceeds the programmed MTR. When the intrinsic atrial rate is faster than the upper rate limit, the pacemaker reverts to its "upper rate response" (see below) to prevent the ventricular rate from exceeding the MTR. Also called the **ventricular tracking limit** or **upper rate limit.**

Mode switching—ability of a dual chamber pacemaker to switch from an atrial tracking mode (e.g., DDD) to a non-tracking mode (e.g., DDI or VVI) when rapid atrial impulses are sensed by the atrial channel. This prevents the pacemaker from pacing the ventricle rapidly and erractically when atrial fibrillation or flutter occur.

Non-competitive atrial pace (NCAP)—a feature in some dual chamber pacemaker that delays the delivery of the next atrial output when an atrial signal is sensed in the atrial channel's refractory period (e.g., a PAC that occurs in PVARP delays the delivery of the next atrial pacing output). This prevents the delivery of an atrial output during the atrial refractory period in an attempt to prevent induction of atrial fibrillation.

Pacemaker mediated tachycardia—a tachycardia induced by competition between the pacemaker and the intrinsic rhythm and sustained by the continued participation of the pacemaker. Most commonly used to describe the endless loop tachycardia that results when there is retrograde conduction from the ventricle to the atria, sensing of the retrograde P wave by the atrial channel, and pacing in the ventricle in response to the sensed P wave. This results in a reentry tachycardia in which the pacemaker serves as the antegrade limb of the circuit and the intrinsic conduction system serves as the retrograde limb. Also known as **endless loop tachycardia** or **pacemaker reentry tachycardia.**

Psuedopseudofusion beat—an electrocardiographic phenomenon in which an atrial pacing spike is superimposed on a native QRS complex. The atrial pacing spike cannot contribute to ventricular depolarization, but the presence of the spike can distort the native QRS complex on the ECG.

PVARP (post-ventricular atrial refractory period)—part of the total atrial refractory period that begins with a sensed or paced ventricular event. PVARP is a programmable parameter and is intended to prevent the atrial channel from sensing far-field ventricular signals, such as T waves or local myocardial potentials. PVARP can also be programmed to prevent the atrial channel from sensing retrograde P waves, thus preventing PMT.

Rate drop response—pacing at a rate faster than the programmed pacing rate when the patient's intrinsic heart rate

(continued)

DUAL CHAMBER PACEMAKER TERMINOLOGY

drops suddenly, as in vasovagal syncope or hypersensitive carotid sinus syndrome. Pacing is initiated at a rate up to 110 beats per minute if bradycardia suddenly occurs.

Rate response—ability of the pacemaker to increase its pacing rate in response to physical activity or increased metabolic demand. Rate responsive pacemakers have some type of sensor that detects physical activity or a physiological parameter that indicates the need for increased heart rate. Currently, the sensors most commonly used are vibration or motion sensors and minute ventilation sensors. Other sensors being evaluated include blood temperature, blood oxygen content, QT interval, and stroke volume. Also known as **rate modulation** or **rate adaptation.**

Rate smoothing—a programmable function that prevents excessive cycle-to-cycle changes in pacing rate. Atrial tracking and rate response can occur but no sudden acceleration or deceleration in pacing rate can occur.

Safety pacing—the delivery of a ventricular output at a short AV interval whenever a signal is sensed early in the AV delay. The

purpose of safety pacing is to prevent crosstalk inhibition of ventricular output. Also called **non-physiological AV delay** or **ventricular safety standby.**

Sleep rate—the pacemaker is programmed to gradually decrease the base pacing rate to a lower limit (e.g., a sleep rate of 50 beats per minute) at bedtime and gradually increase the base pacing rate when the patient awakens.

Total atrial refractory period (TARP)—timing cycle that determines the total length of time that the atrial channel is unresponsive to signals (in effect, "has its eyes closed"). TARP is composed of two seperately programmable timing cycles during which the atrial channel is refractory: the AV interval and PVARP.

Ventricular refractory period—the amount of time following a ventricular sensed or paced event during which the ventricular channel cannot respond to signals (in effect, "has its eyes closed"). The purpose is to prevent the ventricular channel from seeing large repolarization signals (T waves) or other local myocardial signals.

Permanent Pacemakers

Permanent pacemakers are usually implanted under local anesthesia in the operating room, electrophysiology laboratory, or cardiac catheterization laboratory. The pulse generator is placed in a subcutaneous pocket in the pectoral area and the pacing lead is inserted either through the cephalic vein or through the subclavian vein into the right ventricular apex (Fig. 32-1). If a dual-chamber pacemaker is implanted, then a second lead is placed in the right atrial appendage. Permanent pulse generators are powered by lithium batteries with a lifespan of approximately 10 years, depending on many factors, including how the pacemaker is programmed and the percentage of time that it paces.

Temporary Pacemakers

Temporary pacing can be accomplished with transvenous, epicardial, or transcutaneous methods. Temporary pacing can be performed in emergency and elective situations, and it is usually

performed in a monitored unit such as critical care or telemetry unit. Transcutaneous pacing can also be performed by paramedics or other trained personnel in emergency response vehicles or in the field.

Transvenous Pacing. Transvenous pacing is usually performed by percutaneous puncture of the internal jugular, subclavian, antecubital, or femoral vein and threading a pacing lead into the apex of the right ventricle for ventricular pacing, the right atrium for atrial pacing, or both chambers for dual-chamber pacing (Fig. 32-2). The transvenous pacing

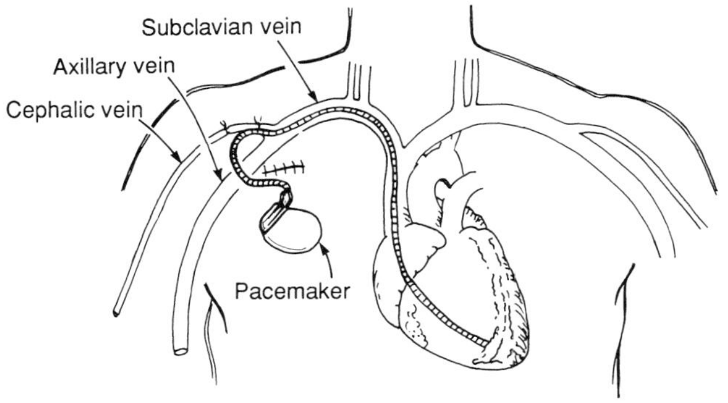

■ **Figure 32–1.** Transvenous installation of a permanent pacemaker. For dual-chamber pacing, a separate pacing lead would be in the atrium.

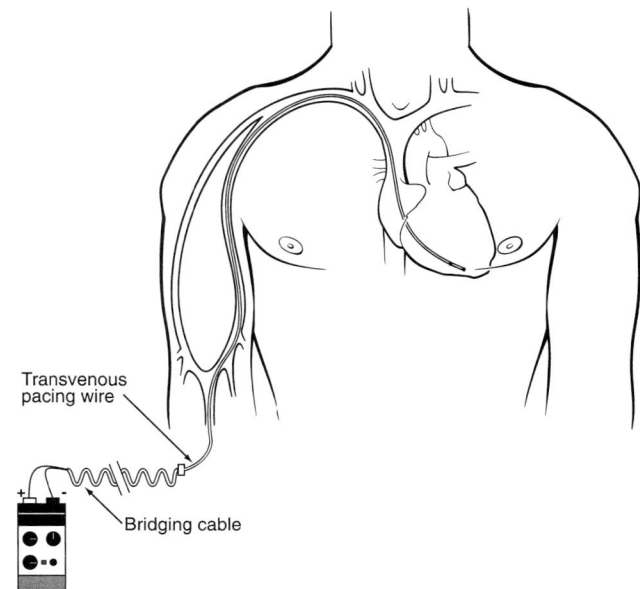

■ **Figure 32–2.** Temporary transvenous pacing lead in right ventricle inserted through antecubital vein.

lead is attached to an external pulse generator that is kept either on the patient or at the bedside. The procedure can be performed under fluoroscopy in a cardiac catheterization laboratory or without fluoroscopy at the bedside. Transvenous pacing is usually necessary only for a few days until the rhythm returns to normal or a permanent pacemaker is inserted. Instructions for initiating transvenous pacing are covered later in this chapter.

Epicardial Pacing. Epicardial pacing is performed through electrodes placed on the atria or ventricles during cardiac surgery. The pacing electrode end of the lead is looped through or loosely sutured to the epicardial surface of the atria or ventricles and the other end is pulled through the chest wall, sutured to the skin, and attached to an external pulse generator. A ground wire is often placed subcutaneously in the chest wall and pulled through with the other leads. The number and placement of leads varies with the surgeon; there may be one or two atrial leads, one or two ventricular leads, and one, two, or no ground leads (Fig. 32-3). Instructions for initiating epicardial pacing are covered later in this chapter.

Transcutaneous Pacing. Transcutaneous pacing is a noninvasive method of pacing used as a temporary measure in emergency situations for treatment of asystole, severe bradycardia, or overdrive pacing for tachyarrhythmias until a transvenous pacing lead can be inserted. Large-surface adhesive electrodes are attached to the anterior and posterior chest wall and connected to an external pacing unit (Fig. 32-4). The pacing current passes through skin and chest wall structures to reach the heart; therefore, large energies are required to achieve capture and sedation is usually needed to minimize the discomfort felt during pacing.

Single-Chamber Pacing

Single-chamber pacing means that only the atria or the ventricles, but not both, are paced. This requires only one pacing lead inserted into the desired chamber. Single-chamber ventricular pacing is the most frequently used temporary transvenous type of pacing and is also often used for permanent pacing. Single-chamber atrial or ventricular pacing can be performed using epicardial pacing leads.

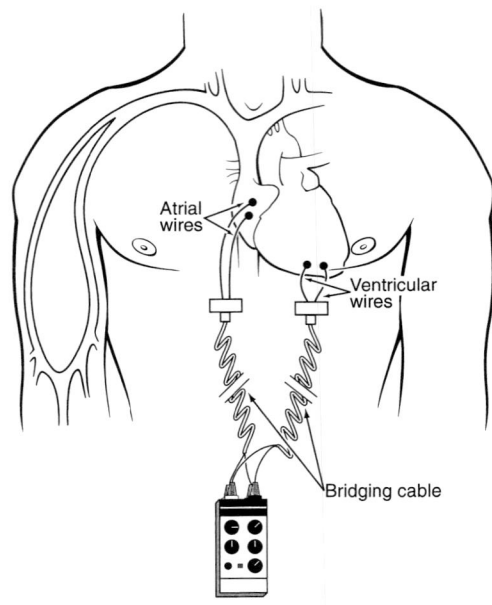

■ **Figure 32–3.** Epicardical pacing using atrial and ventricular pacing leads attached to a dual-chamber pacemaker.

Dual-Chamber Pacing

Dual-chamber pacing means that both the atria and the ventricles can be paced. Dual-chamber pacing is a frequently used method of permanent pacing and can also be performed via epicardial pacing leads. Temporary transvenous dual chamber pacing can be performed, but it is difficult to place temporary atrial leads and it is not as reliable as ventricular pacing.

Biventricular Pacing

Biventricular pacing means that both ventricles are simultaneously paced via a lead in the right ventricular apex for RV pacing and a lead threaded through the coronary sinus into a

■ **Figure 32–4.** Transcutaneous pacing. Electrodes are placed on anterior and posterior chest wall and attached to the external pacing unit.

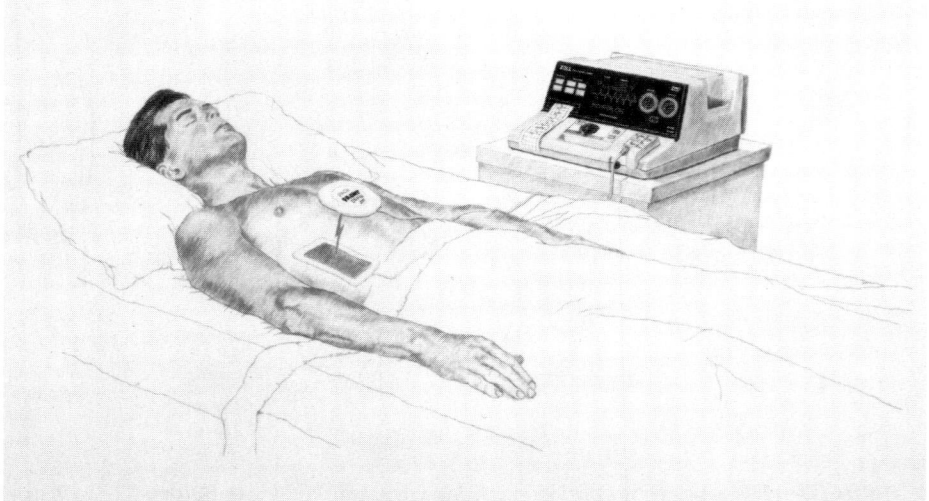

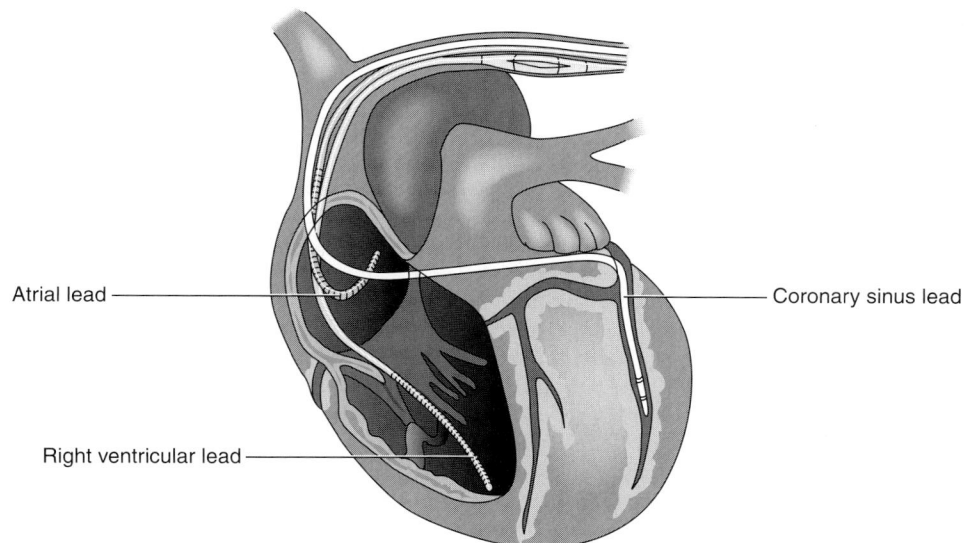

■ **Figure 32–5.** Biventricular pacing. There is a lead in the atrium and a lead in the right ventricle for dual chamber pacing. The left ventricle is paced via a lead threaded through the coronary sinus and down a lateral cardiac vein in the left ventricle.

lateral cardiac vein (or less commonly via an epicardial left ventricular lead) for LV pacing. Figure 32-5 illustrates dual-chamber biventricular pacing leads, and this topic is discussed in more detail later in this chapter.

Classification of Pacemakers

The current nomenclature used to describe the expected function of a pacemaker was established by members of the North American Society of Pacing and Electrophysiology (NASPE) and the British Pacing and Electrophysiology Group (BPEG) and is designated the NBG code for pacing nomenclature (Bernstein et al., 1987). The code describes the expected function of the device according to the site of the pacing electrodes and the mode of pacing. The first letter describes the chamber that is paced: A = atrium, V = ventricle, D = dual (both atrium and ventricle), O = none. The second letter describes the chamber where intrinsic electrical activity is sensed: A = atrium, V = ventricle, D = dual (both atrium and ventricle), O = none. The third letter describes the pacemaker's response to sensing of intrinsic electrical activity: I = inhibited, T =

triggered, D = dual (inhibits or triggers), O = none. The fourth and fifth letters describe additional functions but are not usually used, except for the letter R in the fourth position, which indicates that the pacemaker is a rate-adaptive device. Table 32-1 illustrates the pacemaker code in detail.

The most commonly used pacing modes are VVI and DDD. The VVI mode means that the electrode is in the ventricle and paces the ventricle (first V), senses ventricular activity (second V), and inhibits its output when it senses intrinsic ventricular depolarization (I in third position). VVI is the most commonly used mode of pacing with temporary transvenous leads because it is the quickest and easiest method of pacing in an emergency, and it is difficult to get a temporary atrial lead to stay in place. VVI is also often used with epicardial leads after cardiac surgery, especially if third-degree AV block is present, and is the mode that has to be used for permanent pacing in patients with chronic atrial fibrillation. The DDD mode means that both atrial and ventricular electrodes are present and both chambers are paced (first D), both chambers are sensed (second D), and the device either inhibits or triggers an output in response to sensed intrinsic activity (D in third position means dual-response to sensing). DDD is the most

Table 32–1 ■ 5-LETTER PACEMAKER CODE

First Letter: Chamber Paced	Second Letter: Chamber Sensed	Third Letter: Response to Sensing	Fourth Letter: Programmability, Rate Modulation	Fifth Letter: Antitachycardia Pacing Functions
O = None	O = None	O = None	O = None	O = None
A = Atrium	A = Atrium	I = Inhibited	P = Simple programmable	P = Pacing
V = Ventricle	V = Ventricle	T = Triggered	M = Multi-programmable	(Antitachcardia)
D = Dual (A & V)	D = Dual (A & V)	D = Dual (I & T)	C = Communicating	S = Shock
			R = Rate modulation	D = Dual (P & S)

frequently used permanent pacing mode, unless the patient has chronic atrial fibrillation or flutter.

Other pacing modes that are sometimes used are AOO, AAI, DVI, DDI, and VDD.

Basics of Pacemaker Operation

Electrical current flows in a closed-loop circuit between two pieces of metal (poles). For current to flow, there must be conductive material (i.e., a lead, muscle, or conductive solution) between the two poles. In the heart, the pacing lead, cardiac muscle, and body tissues serve as conducting material for the flow of electrical current in the pacing system. The pacing circuit consists of the pacemaker (the power source), the conducting lead (pacing lead), and the myocardium. The electrical stimulus travels from the pulse generator through the pacing lead to the myocardium, through the myocardium, and back to the pulse generator, thus completing the circuit.

Components of a Pacing System

The three basic components of a cardiac pacing system are the pulse generator, the pacing lead, and the myocardium. The *pulse generator* contains the power source (battery) and all of the electronic circuitry that controls pacemaker function. Most pacemakers are powered by a lithium battery. The pulse generator of a permanent pacemaker is small and thin and is implanted in the pectoral area or sometimes in the abdominal area (see Fig. 32-1). Once a permanent pulse generator is implanted, the only way to alter its pacing parameters is with a programmer that communicates with the pacemaker through a wand placed over the pulse generator. A temporary pulse generator is a box that is kept at the bedside of the patient and is usually powered by a regular 9-volt battery. It has controls on the front that allow the operator to set certain pacing parameters easily (Fig. 32-6).

The *pacing lead* is an insulated wire used to transmit the electrical current from the pulse generator to the myocardium. A unipolar lead contains a single wire and a bipolar lead contains two wires that are insulated from each other. In a unipolar lead, the electrode is an exposed metal tip at the end of the lead that contacts the myocardium and serves as the negative pole of the pacing circuit. In a bipolar lead, the end of the lead is a metal tip that contacts myocardium and serves as the negative pole, and the positive pole is an exposed metal ring located a few millimeters proximal to the distal tip. Permanent pacing leads can be unipolar or bipolar, but bipolar is more commonly used. Permanent leads have some type of fixation device on the end of the lead that helps keep the tip in contact with myocardium. Passive-fixation leads usually have tines on the end that get caught in the trabeculae of the right ventricle and keep the lead in position. Active-fixation leads have a screw on the end that is screwed into the ventricular muscle to hold the lead in place (Fig. 32-7). Occasionally, epicardial leads with a screw-type fixation are used in permanent pacing, especially in children and with implantable defibrillators. Temporary transvenous pacing leads are insulated wires (usually bipolar) with no-fixation device, making them more prone to dislodgment. Temporary epicardial pacing leads are unipolar or bipolar wires with one end looped through the myocardium and the leads then pulled through the chest wall for easy access.

A *bridging cable* is usually used to connect a temporary pacemaker pulse generator to the pacemaker lead, similar to an extension cord. This enhances patient comfort by allowing the pulse generator to be kept at the bedside rather than being strapped to the patient.

Bipolar Pacemaker Operation

In any pacing system, there are two metal poles that make up the pacing circuit. The term *bipolar* means that both of these poles are in or on the heart. In a bipolar system, the pulse generator initiates the electrical impulse and delivers it out the negative terminal of the pacemaker to the pacing lead. The impulse travels down the lead to the distal electrode (negative pole or cathode) that is in contact with myocardium. As the impulse reaches the tip, it travels through the myocardium and returns to the positive pole (or anode) of the system, completing the circuit. In a bipolar system, the positive pole is the proximal ring located a few millimeters proximal to the distal tip. As illustrated in Figure 32-8, the circuit over which the electrical impulse travels in a bipolar system is small because the two poles are located close together. This results in a small pacing spike on the electrocardiogram (ECG) as the pacing stimulus travels between the two poles. If the stimulus is strong enough to depolarize the myocardium, then the pacing spike is immediately followed by a P wave if the lead is in the atrium, or a wide QRS complex if the lead is in the ventricle.

Unipolar Pacemaker Operation

A unipolar system has only one of the two poles in or on the heart. In a permanent unipolar pacing system, the back of the pulse generator serves as the second pole. In a temporary epicardial pacing system, a ground lead placed in the subcutaneous tissue in the mediastinum serves as the second pole. Unipolar pacemakers work the same way as bipolar systems, but the circuit over which the impulse travels is much larger because of the distance between the two poles (Fig. 32-9). This results in a large pacing spike on the ECG as the impulse travels between the two poles.

Asynchronous (Fixed-Rate) Pacing Mode

A pacemaker programmed to an asynchronous mode paces at the programmed rate regardless of intrinsic cardiac activity. This can result in competition between the pacemaker and the heart's own electrical activity. Asynchronous pacing in the ventricle is unsafe because of the potential for pacing stimuli to fall in the vulnerable period of repolarization and cause ventricular fibrillation (VF). Asynchronous pacing in the atria is less dangerous but can cause atrial fibrillation.

Demand Mode

The term *demand* means that the pacemaker paces only when the heart fails to depolarize on its own, that is, the pacemaker

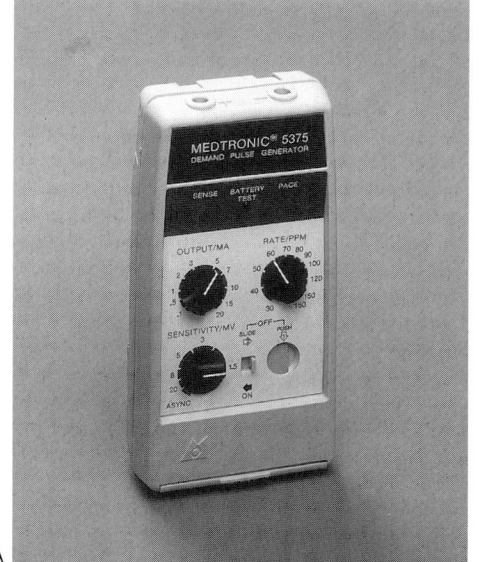

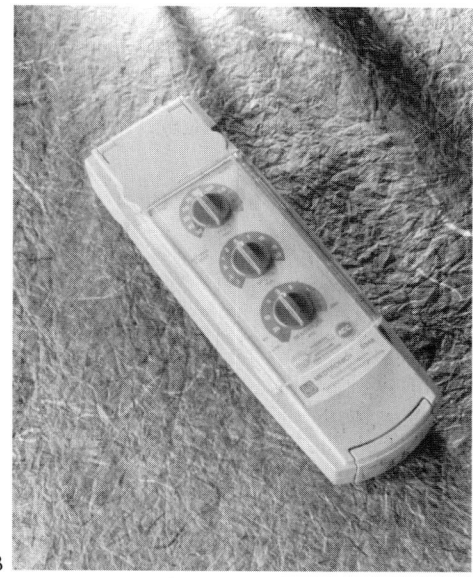

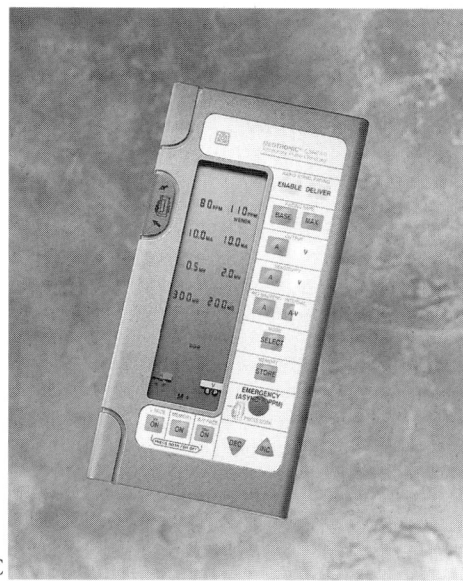

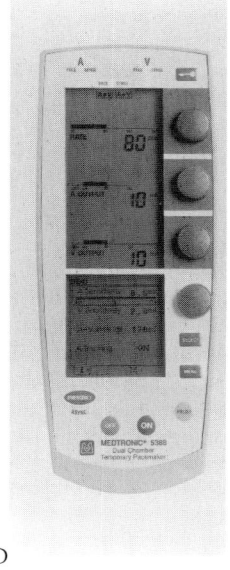

A   B

C   D

■ **Figure 32–6.** Examples of temporary pulse generators. (A, B) Single-chamber pulse generators. (C, D) Dual-chamber pulse generators.

fires only "on demand." In the demand mode, the pacemaker's sensing circuit is capable of sensing intrinsic cardiac activity and inhibiting pacer output when intrinsic activity is present. Sensing takes place between the two poles of the pacemaker. A bipolar system senses over a small area because the poles are close together, and this can result in "undersensing" of intrinsic signals. A unipolar system senses over a large area because the poles are far apart, and this can result in "oversensing." A unipolar system is more likely to sense myopotentials caused by muscle movement and inappropriately inhibit pacemaker output, potentially resulting in periods of asystole if the patient has no underlying cardiac rhythm. The demand mode should always be used for ventricular pacing to avoid the possibility of VF.

Capture

Capture means that a pacing stimulus results in depolarization of the chamber being paced. Capture is determined by the strength of the stimulus, which is measured in milliamperes (mA), the amount of time the stimulus is applied to the heart (pulse width), and by contact of the pacing electrode with the myocardium. Capture cannot occur unless the distal tip of the pacing lead is in contact with healthy myocardium that is capable of responding to the stimulus. Pacing in infarcted tissue usually prevents capture. Similarly, if the catheter is floating in the cavity of the ventricle and not in direct contact with myocardium, capture will not occur.

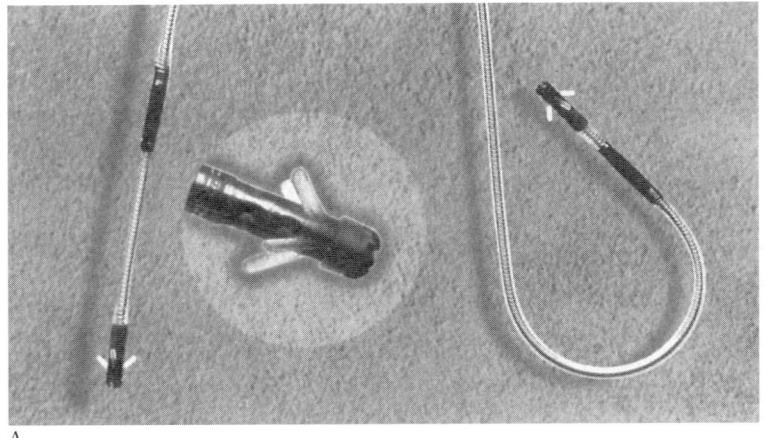
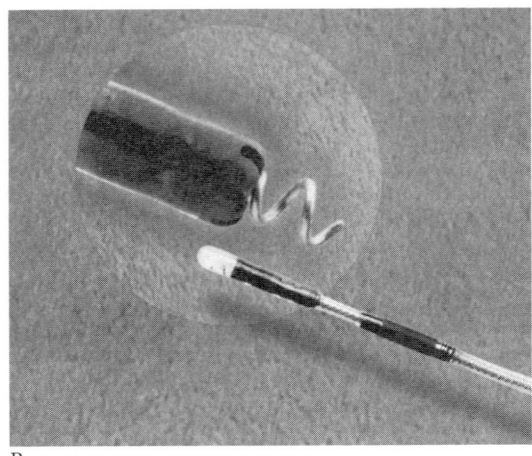

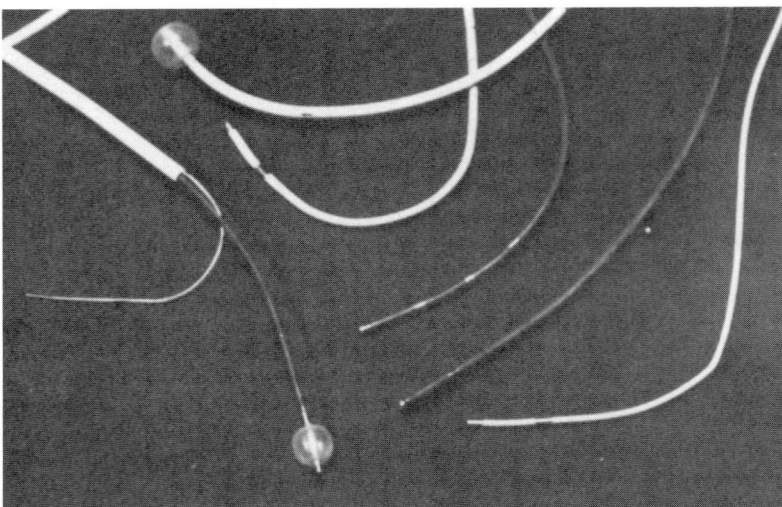

■ **Figure 32–7.** Pacing leads. (*A*) Passive fixation leads with silicone or polyurethane tines that help hold the lead in place. (*B*) Active fixation lead with screw tip to secure lead to myocardium. (*C*) Temporary transvenous pacing leads. Atrial leads are J-shaped. Some leads have a balloon tip for flotation. (*A* and *B* are from Sultzer Intermedics, Angleton, TX, *Concepts of cardiac pacing*, p. 7, 1998. *C* is from Furman, S., Hayes, D. L., & Holmes D. R. [1989]. *A practice of cardiac pacing* [2nd ed., p. 216]. Armonk, NY: Futura Publishing Co.)

In permanent pacing systems, stimulus strength is programmed at implant and can be changed as necessary by using a pacemaker programmer. In temporary pacing, the output dial on the face of the pulse generator controls stimulus strength and can be set and changed easily by the operator. Temporary pulse generators usually are capable of delivering a stimulus of from 0.1 to 20 mA.

Sensing

The sensing circuit controls how sensitive the pacemaker is to intrinsic cardiac depolarizations. Intrinsic activity is measured in millivolts (mV), and the higher the number, the larger the intrinsic signal. For example, a 10-mV QRS complex is larger than a 2-mV QRS. When pacemaker sensitivity needs to be increased to make the pacemaker "see" smaller signals, the sensitivity number must be decreased. For example, a sensitivity of 2 mV is more sensitive than one of 5 mV.

A fence analogy may help explain sensitivity. Think of sensitivity as a fence standing between the pacemaker and what it

wants to see—the ventricle, for example. If there is a 10-foot-high fence (or a 10-mV sensitivity) between the two, then the pacemaker may not see what the ventricle is doing. To make the pacemaker able to see, the fence needs to be lowered. Lowering the fence to 2 feet would probably enable the pacemaker to see the ventricle. Changing the sensitivity from 10 to 2 mV is like lowering the fence—the pacemaker becomes more sensitive and is able to "see" intrinsic activity more easily. Thus, to increase the sensitivity of a pacemaker, the millivolt number (fence) must be decreased.

Initiating Temporary Pacing

Transvenous Ventricular Pacing

A transvenous pacing lead is inserted through a peripheral vein, either antecubital or femoral, or through the internal jugular or subclavian vein, and threaded into the apex of the right ventricle. The lead is sutured in place at its insertion site and a dressing is applied. Temporary transvenous pacing leads are bipolar

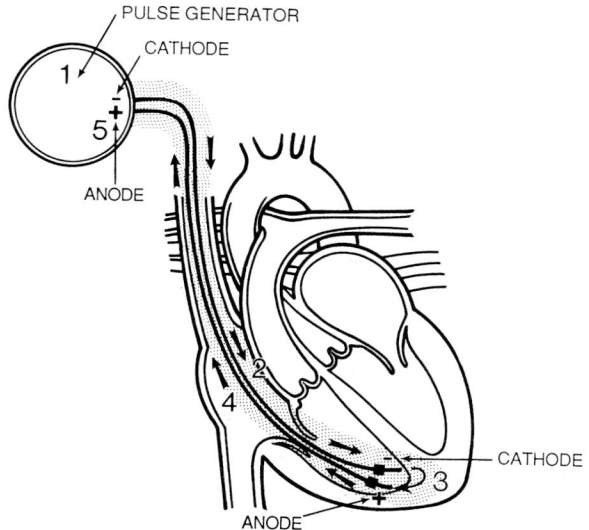

■ **Figure 32–8.** Bipolar pacing system. (1) The pulse generator delivers an electrical stimulus at a predetermined rate. (2) The stimulus travels down the negative electrode lead. (For learning purposes, the positive and negative leads are exposed; normally, they are insulated from each other and encased in a single catheter.) (3) The electrical stimulus is delivered to the myocardium. (The catheter is positioned at the apex of the right ventricle.) (4) Current spreads through cardiac muscle and then to the positive electrode lead. (5) Current returns to the pulse generator, completing the circuit. (From Purcell, J. A., & Burrows S. G. [1985]. A pacemaker primer. *American Journal of Nursing,* 85, 553–568.)

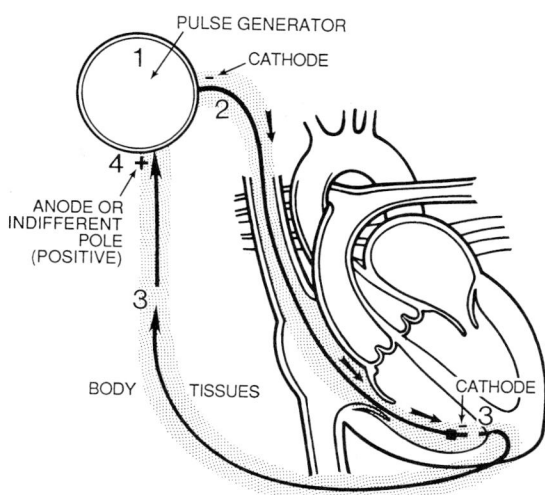

■ **Figure 32–9.** Unipolar pacing system. (1) The pulse generator delivers an electrical impulse. (2) The stimulus travels from the negative terminal to the electrode at the tip of the catheter. (3) Current exits through the electrode tip, stimulates the myocardium, and completes the circuit by traveling through body tissues to the positive terminal. (4) A metal plate on the pulse generator serves as the positive terminal (From Purcell J.A., & Burrows S. G. [1985]. A pacemaker primer. *American Journal of Nursing,* 85, 553–568.)

and have two tails, one marked "positive" or "proximal" and the other marked "negative" or "distal," that are connected to the pulse generator. To initiate ventricular pacing using a transvenous lead (Fig. 32-10):

1. Connect the negative terminal of the pulse generator to the distal end of the pacing lead
2. Connect the positive terminal of the pulse generator to the proximal end of the pacing lead
3. Set the rate at 70 to 80 beats/min or as ordered by physician
4. Set the output at 5 mA and adjust according to stimulation threshold
5. Set the sensitivity at 2 mV and adjust according to sensitivity threshold.

See the section on Nursing Considerations for the procedure for performing stimulation and sensitivity threshold tests.

Epicardial Pacing

The number and location of epicardial leads placed in surgery determine connections for epicardial pacing. There may be one or two atrial or ventricular leads with a ground or no ground lead. If only one lead is on a chamber, then unipolar pacing is performed. If there are two leads on a chamber, then bipolar pacing can be performed.

To initiate unipolar atrial or ventricular pacing (Fig. 32-11*A*):

1. Connect the negative terminal of the pulse generator to the lead on the chamber to be paced (atrial lead for atrial pacing, ventricular lead for ventricular pacing)

2. Connect the positive terminal of the pulse generator to the ground lead
3. Set the rate at 70 to 80 beats/min or as ordered by physician
4. Set the output at 10 mA for atrial pacing and 5 mA for ventricular pacing, then determine stimulation threshold and set two- to three-times higher
5. Set the sensitivity at the lowest possible number for atrial pacing and at 2 mV for ventricular pacing.

To initiate bipolar atrial or ventricular pacing (see Fig. 32-11*B*):

1. Connect the negative terminal of the pulse generator to one of the leads on the chamber to be paced (atrial lead for atrial pacing, ventricular lead for ventricular pacing)
2. Connect the positive terminal of the pulse generator to the other lead on the chamber to be paced
3. Set the rate at 70 to 80 beats/min or as ordered
4. Set the output at 10 mA for atrial pacing and 5 mA for ventricular pacing, then determine stimulation threshold and set two- to three-times higher
5. Set the sensitivity at the lowest possible number for atrial pacing and at 2 mV for ventricular pacing.

Dual-Chamber Temporary Pacing

Dual-chamber pacing can be performed through epicardial pacing leads or with transvenous atrial and ventricular leads. Transvenous dual-chamber pacing is not often performed because of difficulties in placing temporary atrial leads and the unreliable stability of atrial leads. Epicardial dual-chamber pacing is often performed after cardiac surgery, but should be performed only when there are two ventricular leads in place. Two ventricular leads allow for bipolar ventricular pacing and sensing, thus reducing the possibility that the ventricular lead

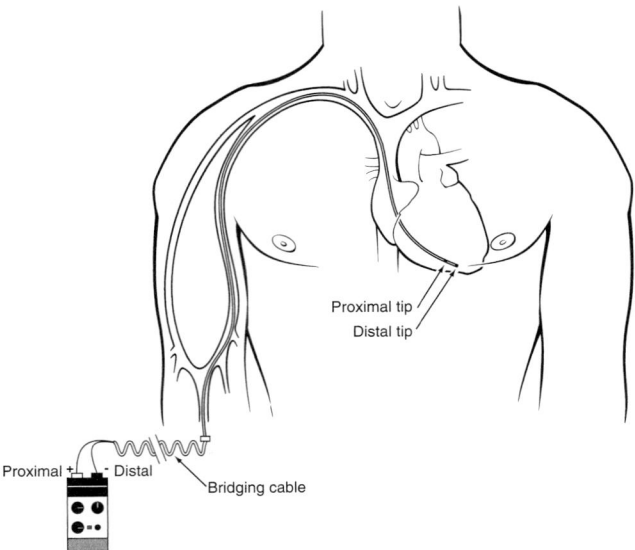

■ Figure 32–10. Initiating temporary transvenous pacing. The distal tail of the pacing lead is connected to the negative terminal of the pacemaker, and the proximal tail of the pacing lead is connected to the positive terminal of the pacemaker.

will sense atrial output and inappropriately inhibit ventricular pacing (crosstalk).

Dual-chamber pacing modes available depend on the type of pulse generator used for pacing. Older dual-chamber temporary pulse generators (like that shown in Fig. 32-6A) allow only DVI pacing. The newer dual-chamber units allow for DDD, DVI, DDI, and VDD pacing in addition to the single-chamber options AAI, AOO, and VVI.

To initiate dual-chamber pacing with epicardial leads:

1. Connect atrial leads:
   a. If two atrial leads are present, then connect one to the positive atrial terminal and the other to the negative atrial terminal on the pulse generator
   b. If only one atrial lead is present, then connect it to the negative atrial terminal on the pulse generator.
2. Connect ventricular leads:
   a. Connect one ventricular lead to the negative ventricular terminal and the other ventricular lead to the positive ventricular terminal on the pulse generator.
3. Select dual-chamber pacing mode desired (if option is provided): DDD, DDI, DVI, VDD. The DDD mode is almost always used.
4. Set AV delay at 150 milliseconds or as ordered.
5. Set atrial output at 10 mA and ventricular output at 5 mA, then determine stimulation thresholds for both chambers and set output two- to three-times higher than threshold.
6. Set atrial or ventricular sensitivity as necessary, depending on pacing mode selected (Atrial sensing occurs only in DDD, DDI, and VDD dual-chamber modes.)
   a. Set atrial sensitivity as 0.5 mV
   b. Set ventricular sensitivity at 2 mV.

Nursing Considerations

Nursing care of patients with pacemakers requires an understanding of how pacemakers work and what to expect the pacemaker to do depending on how it is programmed. Clinicians working in pacemaker follow-up clinics or physician offices have the advantage of being able to use the pacemaker programmer and view intracardiac electrograms and marker

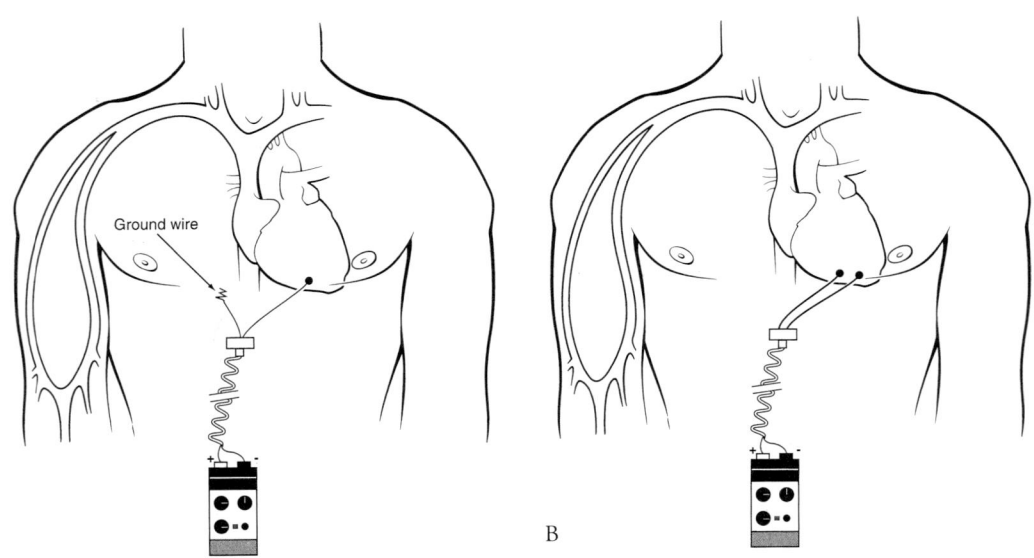

A   B

■ Figure 32–11. Initiating epicardial pacing. (*A*) Unipolar epicardial pacing. The ventricular lead (or atrial lead for atrial pacing) is connected to the negative terminal of the pacemaker and the ground lead is connected to the positive terminal. (*B*) Bipolar epicardial pacing. One ventricular lead is connected to the positive terminal and one to the negative terminal of the pacemaker. (For atrial pacing, either atrial lead is connected to the positive terminal and the other atrial lead to the negative terminal of the pacemaker.)

channels to help evaluate pacemaker function. Bedside nurses in most acute care facilities do not have access to programmers and must be able to evaluate appropriate pacemaker function by looking at the ECG or rhythm strips. The next section of this chapter covers ECG analysis of pacemaker rhythm strips to assist bedside practitioners in evaluating pacemaker function. It is beyond the scope of this chapter to discuss pacemaker follow-up in a clinic or office setting.

An important function for nurses or monitor technicians is to document significant bradycardias that may require pacemaker therapy and to relate these bradycardia events with clinical symptoms whenever possible. The guidelines for pacemaker insertion state, "definite correlation of symptoms with a bradyarrhythmia is required to fulfill the criteria that define symptomatic bradycardia" (Gibbons et al., 2002). Many insurance companies will not cover the cost of pacemaker insertion without good clinical documentation of the need. Nurses and monitor technicians are in a prime position to be able to document the bradycardia event, by mounting rhythm strips in the patient's chart or getting a 12-lead ECG, and symptoms that occur in conjunction with the bradycardia. Documentation of hypotension, syncope or near syncope, dizziness or light headedness, confusion, fatigue, exercise intolerance, and development of symptoms of CHF associated with bradycardia is an important nursing function.

Permanent Pacemakers

Implantation of a permanent pacemaker is often performed on an outpatient basis, but many patients are kept overnight for observation. The procedure is performed under local anesthesia in the cardiac catheterization laboratory, electrophysiology laboratory, or the operating room, and it takes from 1 to 5 hours to complete depending on the number and location of pacing leads being inserted. In addition to routine postoperative care given to any surgical patient, permanent pacemaker insertion usually requires that the patient immobilize the operative arm in a sling for the first 24 hours to prevent lead dislodgment. The nurse must be aware of the potential complications of pacemaker insertion, including the potential for cardiac perforation leading to tamponade, and monitor for those complications. Patient teaching includes information about pacemaker function, how to count the pulse, and importance of follow-up visits to the physician. Because patients are discharged so soon after the procedure, they should be told to take their temperature and monitor the insertion site for signs of infection.

Using a Magnet With a Permanent Pacemaker

Occasionally, the nurse is asked to place a pacemaker magnet over the permanent pulse generator. Use of a magnet usually requires a physician's order or is covered by a written protocol detailing conditions under which a magnet can be used without a direct order.

A magnet inactivates the sensing circuit of a permanent pacemaker and causes it to revert to the asynchronous mode of pacing. This may be performed to verify a pacemaker's ability to pace when it is being inhibited by a patient's own natural rhythm. With a magnet in place, the pacemaker paces at a fixed rate in competition with the patient's rhythm, thus verifying the pacemaker's ability to deliver pacing stimuli. When a paced impulse happens to fall at a time when the ventricle is able to respond, capture should occur, verifying the pacemaker's ability to capture. A magnet may also be used to evaluate battery status if a pacemaker is nearing its end of service. Often the primary indicator of battery depletion is a change in the magnet-induced pacing rate. Some models of pacemakers pace at a faster rate for the first several beats after magnet application and then pace at a slower rate. Some pacemakers remain in the asynchronous pacing mode for the entire duration that the magnet is in place, whereas others only pace asynchronously for a certain number of beats and then revert to normal operation. It is possible to program the magnet operation off in some pacemakers, although this is rarely performed. Because of the wide variety of potential responses to magnet application, it is advisable to know what pacemaker is present and what the programmed parameters are whenever possible when using a magnet.

Another indication for magnet use is to terminate a pacemaker-mediated tachycardia (PMT) in a dual-chamber pacemaker (see section on Dual-Chamber Pacing). When using the magnet, the nurse should have the patient on a cardiac monitor and must be aware of the potential danger of a pacing spike falling in the vulnerable period and causing ventricular arrhythmias. A defibrillator should be immediately available whenever a magnet is used on a permanent pacemaker.

Pacemakers in the Operating Room

The biggest concern regarding pacemakers in the operating room (OR) is the potential effect of electromagnetic interference (EMI) on pacemaker operation. Cautery used during surgery is a type of EMI that can cause abnormal behavior of the pacemaker. Although modern pacemakers are heavily shielded and protected from many sources of EMI, it is still possible for extraneous signals to enter the pacemaker when detected by the pacing leads. Bipolar pacing systems are less likely to be affected than unipolar systems because the sensing circuit in a bipolar system is much smaller than that in a unipolar system. Possible responses to EMI include: (1) inhibition of pacemaker output; (2) triggering of pacemaker output at rapid rates; (3) asynchronous pacing; (4) mode resetting; (5) damage to the circuitry in the pacemaker; or (6) delivery of inappropriate shocks if the device is an ICD (Atlee & Bernstein, 2001; Kusumoto & Goldschlager, 1998). The most common responses to EMI in the OR are inhibition of pacing or reversion to a "noise mode," usually VOO or DOO pacing (asynchronous pacing). Inhibition of pacing occurs when the pacemaker senses the cautery and interprets those signals as intrinsic ventricular activity. This can result in asystole if the patient is pacemaker-dependent with no reliable underlying rhythm and is the most worrisome concern when dealing with pacemakers in the OR. Many pacemakers revert to asynchronous pacing when they sense electrical "noise" from cautery or other sources of EMI. This allows pacing to occur in an asynchronous mode, creating the potential problem of pacemaker output occurring during the vulnerable period of ventricular repolarization and resulting in VF.

Several things can be performed to reduce the potential adverse effects of EMI during surgery. If cautery is to be used, then place the grounding pad as far away from the pulse generator as possible (e.g. on a leg rather than on the chest or back), and place it on the opposite side of the body from the pacemaker. Use cautery in short bursts rather than long, continuous applications. Observe the monitor for pacemaker response to cautery, and if cautery appears to cause inhibition of pacing place a magnet over the pacemaker while cautery is being applied. A defibrillator and other emergency equipment should be immediately available during surgery. It is advisable to interrogate a pacemaker both before and after surgical procedures involving cautery or other sources of EMI (i.e. high intensity radiation, radiofrequency ablation, lithotripsy) to verify programmed parameters before surgery and make sure they have not changed after surgery. If the pacemaker is programmed to a rate modulated mode (VVIR, DDDR), then it is wise to disable rate modulation by programming to VVI or DDD before surgery, because mechanical ventilators, bone hammers, surgical saws, and other equipment in the surgical environment may trigger the physiological sensors and result in rapid pacing.

Non-medical Sources of EMI

Pacemakers can be adversely affected by EMI in the environment, and patients should be taught about potential pacemaker interactions with common sources of EMI. Security systems or antitheft devices in department stores can potentially interact with pacemakers and cause intermittent inhibition of pacing output, although this is not a common problem. Patients should be cautioned not to linger close to a security system but to pass through it and then move away. Cell phones (especially digital phones) are a potential source of EMI that can inhibit pacemaker output, cause asynchronous pacing, or cause inappropriate ventricular tracking in a dual-chamber device (Mitriani et al., 2001; Kusomoto & Goldschlager, 1998). Patients should avoid carrying their cell phone in a pocket near the pulse generator and should use the ear opposite the pacemaker when talking on a cell phone. Patients who are totally pacemaker-dependent should consider not using digital cell phones at all until improvements are made in both pacemaker shielding and cell phone technology to eliminate possible interference from EMI.

Household appliances are safe for use by patients with pacemakers, as are other commonly used electrical or motor-driven appliances like lawn mowers, leaf blowers, and small tools (drills, saws, etc.).

Cardioversion and Defibrillation

Patients with pacemakers can be safely cardioverted or defibrillated if precautions are taken to protect the pacemaker from high-energy electrical forces. Paddles or defibrillation pads should not be placed directly over the pulse generator. Placing the paddles or pads in the anterior-posterior position is preferred over the standard transthoracic placement (refer to Fig. 32-4, which illustrates anterior-posterior pad placement for external pacing). Whenever possible the pacemaker should be interrogated after cardioversion or defibrillation to make sure it is still programmed and functioning as intended.

Temporary Pacemakers

In the care of patients with temporary pacemakers, the following additional considerations become important.

Insertion Site Care. A temporary pacing catheter is usually inserted through a venous sheath that is sutured to the skin and treated as any central venous catheter. Maintaining a clean, dry insertion site is important to prevent infection, and hospital policies governing the care of central venous catheters and dressings should be followed. If the pacing catheter is placed via a femoral vein, then the patient needs to be on bedrest with the affected leg straight and head of bed elevated no more than 20 degrees while the femoral sheath is in place.

Care of Epicardial Leads. Epicardial leads exit through the chest and unless they are being used for pacing, they are usually coiled and placed in a gauze dressing until needed. The exit site should be kept clean and dry according to established hospital policies on exit site care. Epicardial leads are easily dislodged, so care must be taken when handling them so as not to pull them out. Use of a bridging cable is recommended to prevent the need to strap the temporary pacemaker directly to the patient's body. The leads and bridging cable must be securely taped to the chest to prevent dislodgement of epicardial leads. Because the exposed metal end of the leads is a direct route for electrical current from the environment to conduct directly to the heart, care must be taken to insulate the leads to prevent cardiac arrhythmias, especially VF (see the section on Electrical Safety, next, for more information).

Electrical Safety. A temporary pacing lead provides a direct pathway for stray electrical current to reach the heart without the protective resistance of the skin. Even a very small electrical current can initiate atrial fibrillation or VF if it is conducted directly to the heart by pacing leads.

Some considerations for electrical safety when caring for patients with temporary pacing leads include:

1. Wear gloves when handling pacing leads
2. Make sure that all connections between the pulse generator and bridging cable and between bridging cable and pacing leads are tight and inserted completely into their receptacles so no metal is exposed
3. If using a bridging cable with an alligator clip connector, then wrap a glove around the connections in such a way that they are separated and insulated from each other and from the environment
4. Cover exposed metal ends of pacing leads that are not in use with some type of insulating material
   a. Wrap a glove around the ends of transvenous leads and tape loosely
   b. Place the ends of epicardial leads in a glove (or cut a finger from a glove and place them inside) or place the metal end of each individual lead in a needle cover, small syringe, or some other insulating material.
5. Keep dressings over pacing lead insertion sites dry; wet dressings conduct electricity more easily
6. Make sure all electrical equipment in the room is grounded and in good working order
7. Be aware of your own body's static electricity, especially if your unit is carpeted
   a. Never let the pacing system be the first thing you touch when entering a patient's room

b. Be especially careful when using slider boards to transfer patients into and out of bed, because they generate static electricity.

Stimulation Threshold Test. The stimulation threshold is the minimum pacemaker output necessary to capture the heart consistently. The contact of the pacing lead with the myocardium causes local tissue edema and inflammation that impedes the delivery of current to the myocardium. Peak thresholds occur approximately 3 to 4 weeks after permanent lead placement, and chronic stable thresholds are usually reached at approximately 3 months. Stimulation threshold testing with a temporary pacing system should be performed every shift to ensure an adequate safety margin for capture. The procedure for performing a stimulation threshold test is as follows:

1. Verify that the patient is in a paced rhythm; pacing rate may need to be temporarily increased to override an intrinsic rhythm
2. Watch the cardiac monitor continuously while gradually decreasing output
3. Note when loss of capture occurs (pacing spike not followed by appropriate waveform: P wave for atrial pacing, QRS for ventricular pacing)
4. Gradually turn output up until 1:1 capture resumes—this is the stimulation threshold
5. Set the output two- to three-times higher than threshold to ensure adequate safety margin; for example, if consistent capture is regained at 2 mA, then set the output at 4 to 6 mA.

Sensitivity Threshold Testing. The sensitivity threshold is the minimum voltage of intrinsic cardiac activity that can be sensed by the pacemaker. The pacemaker becomes more sensitive (can sense smaller signals) as the number on the sensitivity control gets smaller (see section on Sensing, previously, for further explanation).

Sensitivity testing can be performed only if the patient has a hemodynamically stable underlying rhythm. If the patient is completely pacemaker-dependent or has a very slow underlying rate, then do not perform sensitivity threshold testing. The procedure for performing a sensitivity threshold test is as follows:

1. Verify that the patient has an intrinsic rhythm (is not being paced); this may require temporarily decreasing the pacing rate to allow the underlying rhythm to emerge
2. Slowly decrease the pacemaker's sensitivity (by *increasing* the number on the sensitivity control) while watching the sense indicator light on the pulse generator or watching the cardiac monitor
   a. The sense indicator light flashes with each sensed P wave (for atrial sensing) or QRS (for ventricular sensing)
   b. Pacing remains inhibited and there are no pacing spikes seen on the monitor as long as sensing continues.
3. Note when the sense indicator fails to flash with each P wave or QRS and when pacing spikes begin to appear in competition with the intrinsic rhythm; this is the sensitivity threshold
4. Set the sensitivity at one-half the identified threshold to ensure an adequate safety margin; for example, if the threshold is 5 mV, then set the sensitivity at 2.5 mV.

Evaluating Pacemaker Function

This section is directed primarily at temporary pacemakers because nurses can interact more directly with them than with permanent pacemakers. The same concepts apply to permanent pacemakers, but corrective measures require the use of a pacemaker programmer or an actual surgical procedure to reposition pacing leads or replace the pulse generator.

Evaluation of pacemaker function requires knowledge of the mode of pacing expected (e.g., VVI, AAI, DDD); the minimum rate of the pacemaker, or pacing interval; and any other programmed parameters in the pacemaker. The basic functions of a pacemaker include stimulus release, capture, and sensing, and they should be evaluated for both temporary and permanent pacemakers. *Stimulus release* refers to pacemaker output, or the ability of the pacemaker to generate and release a pacing impulse. *Capture* is the ability of the pacing stimulus to cause depolarization of the chamber being paced. *Sensing* is the ability of the pacemaker to recognize and respond to intrinsic electrical activity in the heart. Pacemaker operation is evaluated by assessing these three functions. Single-chamber pacemaker evaluation is much less complicated than dual-chamber evaluation. Because ventricular pacing is the most common type of single-chamber pacing, evaluation of VVI pacemakers is discussed here. The concepts presented for ventricular pacemaker evaluation can also be applied to atrial pacemaker evaluation.

A VVI pacemaker is expected to pace the ventricle at the set rate unless spontaneous ventricular activity occurs to inhibit pacing. The minimum rate of the pacemaker, or pacing interval, is measured from one pacing stimulus to the next consecutive pacing stimulus with no intervening sensed beats between the two. In a normally functioning VVI pacemaker, pacing spikes occur at the preset pacing interval and each spike results in a ventricular depolarization (capture). If spontaneous ventricular activity occurs (either a normally conducted QRS or a PVC), that activity is sensed, the next pacing stimulus is inhibited, and the pacing interval timing cycle is reset. If no intrinsic ventricular activity occurs, a pacing stimulus is released at the end of the timing cycle. Figure 32-12 shows normal VVI pacemaker function.

The pacemaker has a *refractory period*, which is a period of time after either pacing or sensing in the ventricle during which the pacemaker is unable to respond to intrinsic activity. During the refractory period, the pacemaker in effect has its "eyes closed" and is not able to sense spontaneous activity. If an intrinsic QRS should occur during the pacemaker's refractory period, it is not sensed because the pacemaker is "blind" at that time.

Stimulus Release

Stimulus release is verified on the ECG by the presence of a pacing spike. A pacing spike indicates that the pacemaker battery has enough power to initiate a stimulus and that the stimulus was delivered into the body. When evaluating a temporary pacing system, the presence of a pacing spike indicates that the connections between the pulse generator and the bridging cable and between the bridging cable and the pacing leads are intact. If any part of the system becomes disconnected, the stimulus

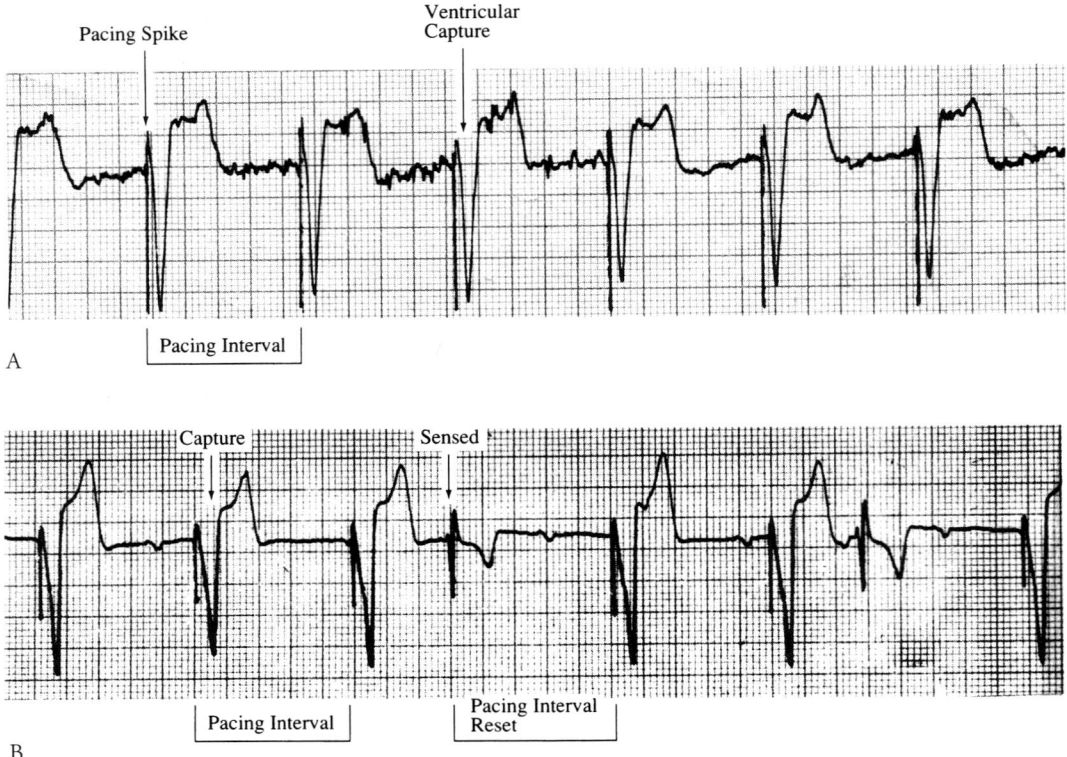

■ **Figure 32–12.** Normal VVI pacemaker function. (*A*) Capture is good, but sensing cannot be evaluated because no intrinsic QRS complexes are present. (*B*) Capture and sensing both normal. The two intrinsic QRS complexes are sensed, inhibit ventricular pacing output, and reset the pacing interval. (From Chulay, M., Guzzetta, C., & Dossey, B. [1997]. *AACN handbook of critical care nursing* [p. 448]. Stamford, CT: Appleton Lange.)

cannot reach the body and a pacing spike is not seen. The presence of a pacing spike alone does not indicate where the stimulus was delivered, only that it entered the body somewhere.

Absence of pacing stimuli when they should be present can indicate a faulty pulse generator or battery, or a break or disconnection in the lead system. Pacing stimuli can also be absent when pacing is inhibited by the sensing of extraneous electrical signals, such as electromagnetic interference (EMI) or myopotentials. Figure 32-13 illustrates total loss of stimulus release in a patient whose permanent pacemaker battery was dead.

Capture

Capture is indicated by a wide QRS complex immediately after the pacemaker spike and represents the ability of the pacing stimulus to depolarize the ventricle. Loss of capture is recognized by

the presence of pacing spikes that are not followed by paced ventricular complexes (Fig. 32-14). Causes of loss of capture include:

1. Inadequate stimulus strength, which can be corrected by increasing the electrical output of the pacemaker (turning up the milliamperage)
2. Pacing lead out of position and not in contact with myocardium, which can sometimes be corrected by repositioning the patient; repositioning the pacing lead is usually not a nursing function and must be performed by a physician or someone trained in intracardiac catheter manipulation
3. Pacing lead positioned in infarcted tissue, which can be corrected by repositioning the lead to a place where myocardium is healthy and capable of responding to the stimulus
4. Electrolyte imbalances or drugs that alter the ability of the heart to respond to the pacing stimulus

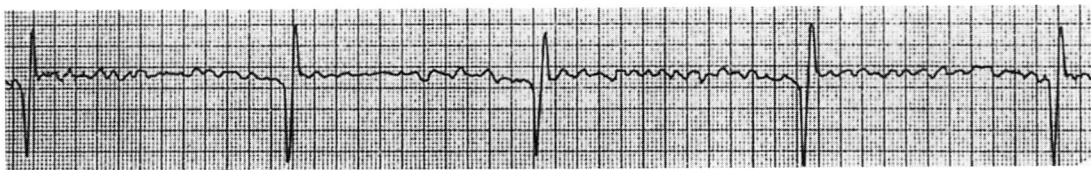

■ **Figure 32–13.** Absence of stimulus release in a patient with a permanent pacemaker. Underlying rhythm is atrial fibrillation with complete atrioventricular block and a very slow ventricular rate. The battery in the pacemaker generator was at end of service. (From Chulay, M., Guzzetta, C., & Dossey, B. [1997]. *AACN handbook of critical care nursing* [p. 448]. Stamford, CT: Appleton Lange.)

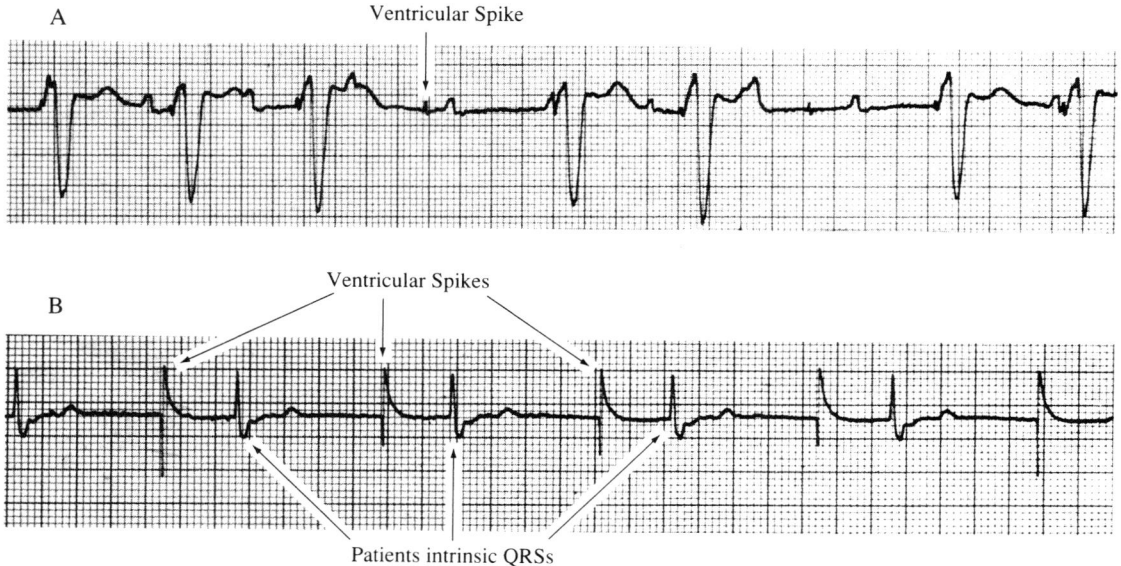

A   Ventricular Spike

Ventricular Spikes

B

Patients intrinsic QRSs

■ **Figure 32–14.** (*A*) VVI pacemaker with intermittent loss of capture. (*B*) VVI pacemaker with total loss of capture. (From Chulay, M., Guzzetta, C., & Dossey, B. [1997]. *AACN handbook of critical care nursing* [p. 449]. Stamford, CT: Appleton Lange.)

5. Delivery of a pacing stimulus during the ventricle's refractory period when the heart is physiologically unable to respond to the stimulus; this problem occurs with loss of sensing (undersensing) and can be prevented by correcting the sensing problem (Fig. 32-15*A*).

Loss of capture in a totally pacemaker-dependent patient is an emergency because without an effective underlying rhythm, the patient may be asystolic or severely symptomatic because of slow, ineffective rate. If the underlying rhythm is ineffective or absent, cardiopulmonary resuscitation must be performed until the capture problem is corrected or until emergency transcutaneous pacing can be instituted. If loss of capture is intermittent, it may not result in symptoms but should be corrected as soon as possible.

Sensing

Sensing of intrinsic ventricular electrical activity inhibits the next pacing stimulus and resets the pacing interval. Sensing cannot occur unless the pacemaker is given the opportunity to sense. It must be in the demand mode and there must be intrinsic ventricular activity for the pacemaker to have an opportunity to sense. In Figure 32-12*A*, sensing cannot be evaluated because there is no intrinsic ventricular activity; therefore, the pacemaker is not given an opportunity to sense. In Figure 32-12*B*, the occurrence of two spontaneous QRS complexes provides the opportunity to sense. In this example, sensing occurred normally, as indicated by the absence of the next expected pacing stimulus and resetting of the pacing interval from the intrinsic QRS complex.

Undersensing. *Undersensing* means that the pacemaker fails to sense intrinsic activity that is present (Fig. 32-15A and Fig. 32-16A). This can be caused by:

1. Asynchronous (fixed-rate) pacing mode in which the sensing circuit is off; this problem can be corrected by turning the sensitivity control to the demand mode

2. Pacing catheter out of position or lying in infarcted tissue, which can be corrected by repositioning the lead; lead repositioning must be performed by a physician; however, turning the patient to the side sometimes temporarily works when the pacing lead loses contact with the ventricle

3. Intrinsic QRS voltage may be too low to be sensed by the pacemaker; increasing the pacemaker's sensitivity (by decreasing the number on the sensitivity control) allows it to see smaller intrinsic signals and may solve the problem

4. Break in connections, battery failure, or faulty pulse generator; check and tighten all connections along the pacing system, and replace the battery if it is low; a chest radiograph may detect lead fracture; change the pulse generator if problems cannot be corrected any other way

5. Intrinsic ventricular activity falling in the pacemaker's refractory period; if a spontaneous QRS complex occurs during the time the pacemaker has its "eyes closed," then the pacemaker cannot see it; this may occur when the pacemaker fails to capture, which can allow an intrinsic QRS to occur during the pacemaker's refractory period; this problem is caused by loss of capture and does not reflect a sensing malfunction (see Fig. 32-15*B*).

Oversensing. *Oversensing* means that the pacemaker is so sensitive that it inappropriately senses internal or external signals as QRS complexes and inhibits its output. Common sources of external signals that can interfere with pacemaker function include electromagnetic or radiofrequency signals or electronic equipment in use near the pacemaker. Internal sources of interference can include large P waves, large T-wave voltage, local myopotentials in the heart, or skeletal muscle potentials. Figure 32-16B illustrates oversensing in a temporary pacemaker. Because a VVI pacemaker is programmed to inhibit its output when it senses, oversensing can be a dangerous situation in a pacemaker-dependent patient, resulting in a dangerously slow rate or ventricular asystole. Oversensing is

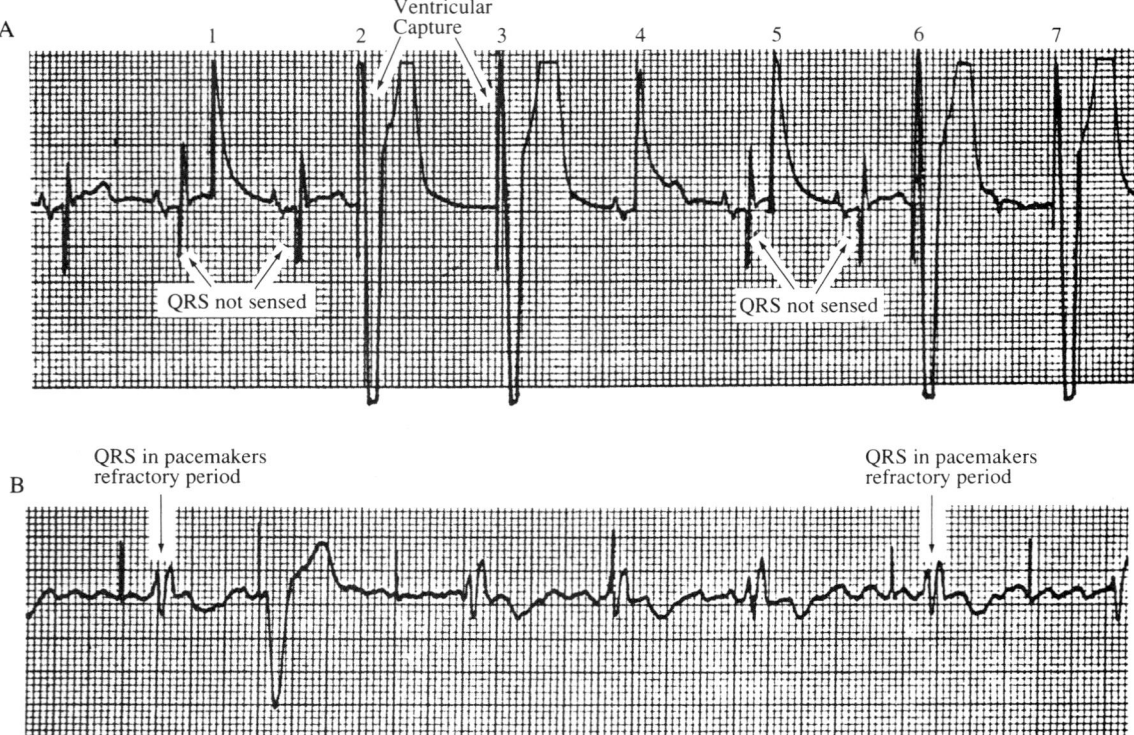

■ **Figure 32–15.** (*A*) Intermittent loss of sensing in a VVI pacemaker. Delivery of the pacing stimulus during the heart's refractory period makes it appear that capture is lost as well. Because the heart is physiologically unable to respond to the pacing stimulus when it falls in the refractory period, this is not a problem. Pacing spikes 1, 2, 5, and 6 should not have occurred; their presence is due to loss of sensing. Pacing spike 4 occurred coincident with the normal QRS complex, resulting in a "pseudofusion" beat, and does not represent loss of sensing. (*B*) Loss of capture in a VVI pacemaker. Only one pacing spike captures the ventricle. Two QRS complexes occur during the pacemaker's refractory period and thus are not sensed. This does not represent loss of sensing because the pacemaker has its "eye closed" during the time intrinsic ventricular activity occurred. (From Chulay, M., Guzzetta, C., & Dossey, B. [1997]. *AACN handbook of critical care nursing* [p. 451]. Stamford, CT: Appleton Lange.)

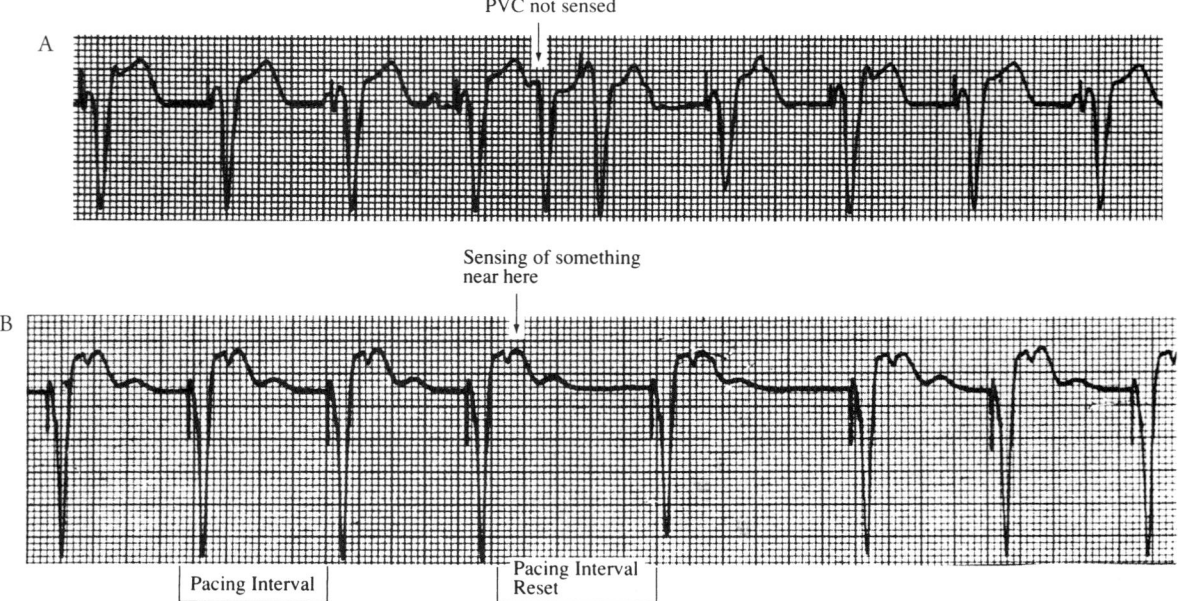

■ **Figure 32–16.** (*A*) Undersensing in a VVI pacemaker. The premature ventricular contraction (PVC) is not sensed and pacing occurs at the programmed pacing interval, resulting is a spike on the T wave of the PVC. (*B*) Oversensing in a VVI pacemaker. The pacing rate slows for two intervals, presumably because the device sensed something near the T wave that reset the pacing interval from the point where sensing occurred. (From Chulay, M., Guzzetta, C., & Dossey B. [1997]. *AACN handbook of critical care nursing* [p. 450]. Stamford, CT: Appleton Lange.)

Table 32–2 ■ DUAL-CHAMBER PACING MODES

Mode	Chamber(s) Paced	Chamber(s) Sensed	Response to Sensing
DVI	Atrium & ventricle	Ventricle	Ventricular sensing inhibits atrial & ventricular pacing
VDD	Ventricle	Atrium & ventricle	Atrial sensing—triggers ventricular pacing Ventricular sensing—inhibits ventricular pacing
DDI	Atrium & ventricle	Atrium & ventricle	Atrial sensing inhibits atrial pacing Ventricular sensing inhibits ventricular pacing
DDD	Atrium & ventricle	Atrium & ventricle	Atrial sensing—inhibits atrial pacing, triggers ventricular pacing Ventricular sensing—inhibits atrial & ventricular pacing

usually caused by the sensitivity being set too high, which can be corrected by reducing the pacemaker's sensitivity by increasing the number on the sensitivity control. For example, if sensitivity is set at 0.5 mV, changing it to 2 mV decreases the sensitivity of the pacemaker. For ventricular pacing, a sensitivity of 2 mV is usually safe and can always be changed if needed to correct sensing problems.

Dual-Chamber Pacemaker Operation

Dual-chamber pacemakers have become very complicated, with multiple programmable parameters and varying functions, depending on the manufacturer. Because it is impossible to present a detailed explanation of all aspects of dual chamber pacing in a single chapter, this section concentrates on basic dual-chamber pacing concepts that apply to all manufacturers' products. More detailed information is best obtained by attending a formal pacing program sponsored by a pacemaker manufacturer or from a pacemaker technical manual. Dual-chamber pacemakers can function in a variety of modes, depending on how they are programmed (Table 32-2). Because the DDD mode is most commonly used, basic DDD function is described here. Display 32-3 defines terms commonly used in dual-chamber pacing.

Dual-Chamber Timing Cycles

According to the pacemaker code, DDD means that both chambers (atria and ventricles) are paced, both chambers are sensed, and the mode of response to sensed events is either inhibited or triggered, depending on which chamber is sensed. When atrial activity is sensed, atrial pacing is inhibited and ventricular pacing is triggered at the end of the programmed AV delay. When ventricular activity is sensed, all pacemaker output is inhibited. The following timing cycles determine how a dual-chamber pacemaker functions, and Figure 32-17 illustrates many of these timing cycles:

1. Pacing interval (or lower rate limit)—the base rate of the pacemaker, measured between two consecutive atrial pacing stimuli with no intervening sensed events; the pacing interval is a programmable parameter and determines the minimum rate at which the pacemaker paces in the absence of intrinsic cardiac activity

2. AV delay (or AV interval)—the amount of time between atrial and ventricular pacing, or the "electronic PR interval;" this is measured from the atrial pacing spike to the ventricular pacing spike and is a programmable parameter; the AV delay timer is initiated by a paced or sensed atrial event, and if no intrinsic conduction occurs to the ventricle within that time, a ventricular pacing spike occurs at the end of the programmed AV delay

3. Atrial escape interval (or ventriculoatrial [VA] interval)—the interval from a sensed or paced ventricular event to the next atrial pacing output; the VA interval represents the amount of time the pacemaker waits after it paces in the ventricle or senses ventricular activity before pacing the atrium; the atrial escape interval is not a programmed parameter, but rather is derived by subtracting the AV delay from the pacing interval; its length can be estimated by measuring from a ventricular spike to the next atrial pacing spike

4. Total atrial refractory period—the period of time after a sensed P wave or a paced atrial event during which the atrial channel does not respond to sensed events; the total atrial refractory period consists of the AV delay and the postventricular atrial refractory period (PVARP)

5. PVARP—the period of time after an intrinsic QRS or a paced ventricular beat during which the atrial channel is refractory and does not respond to sensed atrial activity; PVARP is a programmable parameter but is not evident on a rhythm strip

6. Blanking period—the very short ventricular refractory period that occurs with every atrial pacemaker output; the ventricular channel "blinks its eyes" so it will not sense the atrial output and inappropriately inhibit ventricular pacing; the blanking period is a programmable parameter but is not evident on a rhythm strip

7. Ventricular refractory period—the period of time after a ventricular pacing output or a sensed QRS during which the ventricular channel ignores intrinsic ventricular activity; ventricular refractory period is a programmable parameter but is not evident on a rhythm strip

8. Maximum tracking interval (or upper rate limit)—the maximum rate at which the ventricular channel tracks atrial activity; the upper rate limit prevents rapid ventricular pacing in response to very rapid atrial activity, such as atrial tachycardia or atrial flutter; the maximum tracking interval is a programmable parameter and usually is set according to how active a patient is expected to be and how fast a ventricular rate is likely to be tolerated.

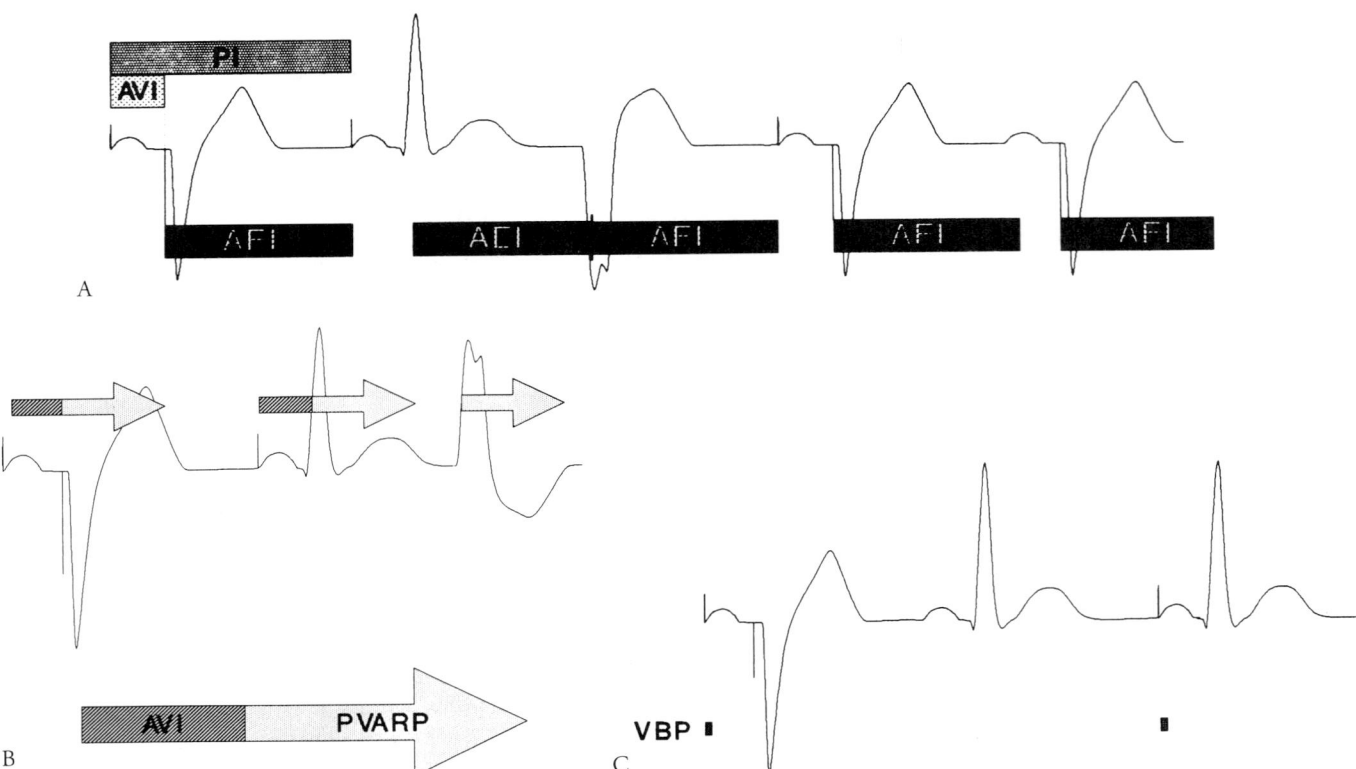

■ **Figure 32–17.** Dual-chamber pacemaker timing cycles. (*A*) The pacing interval (PI) represents the minimum pacing rate and is measured from one atrial pacing spike to the next consecutive atrial pacing spike. The atrioventricular interval (AVI) is measured from the atrial pacing spike to the ventricular pacing spike. The atrial escape interval (AEI) is the interval from a sensed or paced ventricular event to the next atrial pacing output and determines when the next atrial output is due. (*B*) The arrows represent the total atrial refractory period, which is composed of the AVI, begins with an atrial output or sensed P wave, and the post ventricular atrial refractory period (PVARP) begins with a paced or sensed ventricular event. (*C*) The ventricular blanking period (VBP) is a brief ventricular refractory period that occurs with every atrial pacer output to prevent sensing of atrial output by the ventricular channel (crosstalk). The ventricular refractory period (VRP) begins with a paced or sensed ventricular event. (From *Pacemaker technology for nurses and allied health professionals*, p. 71, 54, 66, with permission from St. Jude Medical Cardiac Rhythm Management Division, Sylmar, CA.)

The Four States of Dual-Chamber Pacing

When programmed to the DDD mode, dual-chamber pacemakers are capable of functioning in four main ways, depending on intrinsic cardiac activity and conduction capability. Each of the four states of pacing is described in the following sections.

Atrioventricular Sequential Pacing State (Atrial and Ventricular Pacing). Atrial and ventricular pacing (AV sequential pacing state) occurs at the minimum rate (Fig. 32-18A). Atrial pacing occurs at the lower rate limit, followed by ventricular pacing at the end of the programmed AV delay. This type of pacing would occur if the underlying cardiac rhythm were sinus bradycardia with AV block or asystole.

Atrial Pacing State (Atrial Pacing With Ventricular Sensing). Atrial pacing occurs at the minimum rate, but normal conduction to the ventricle occurs before the AV delay times out, resulting in intrinsic QRS complexes after the paced atrial beats (see Fig. 32-18B). This type of pacing would occur if the underlying rhythm were sinus bradycardia with normal conduction through the AV node.

Atrial Tracking State (Atrial Sensing With Ventricular Pacing). Intrinsic P waves are followed by paced ventricular beats (see Fig. 32-18C). Intrinsic atrial activity is sensed by the pacemaker and starts the AV delay. No intrinsic ventricular activity occurs before the AV delay times out, so a ventricular output is released at the end of the programmed AV delay. This type of pacing would occur if the underlying rhythm were sinus rhythm with complete AV block.

Inhibited State (Atrial and Ventricular Sensing). No pacing occurs in either chamber because intrinsic atrial and ventricular activity is present at a rate faster than the minimum pacing rate (see Fig. 32-18D). This occurs when the underlying rhythm is normal sinus rhythm.

The pacemaker is capable of switching from one state of pacing to another on a beat-to-beat basis depending on intrinsic activity. Figure 32-19 illustrates a DDD pacemaker operating in all four pacing states within a short period of time.

Evaluating Dual-Chamber Pacemaker Function

Because a dual-chamber pacemaker has both atrial and ventricular pacing and sensing functions, evaluation includes assessing atrial capture, atrial sensing, ventricular capture, and ventricular sensing. To evaluate pacemaker function, it is necessary to

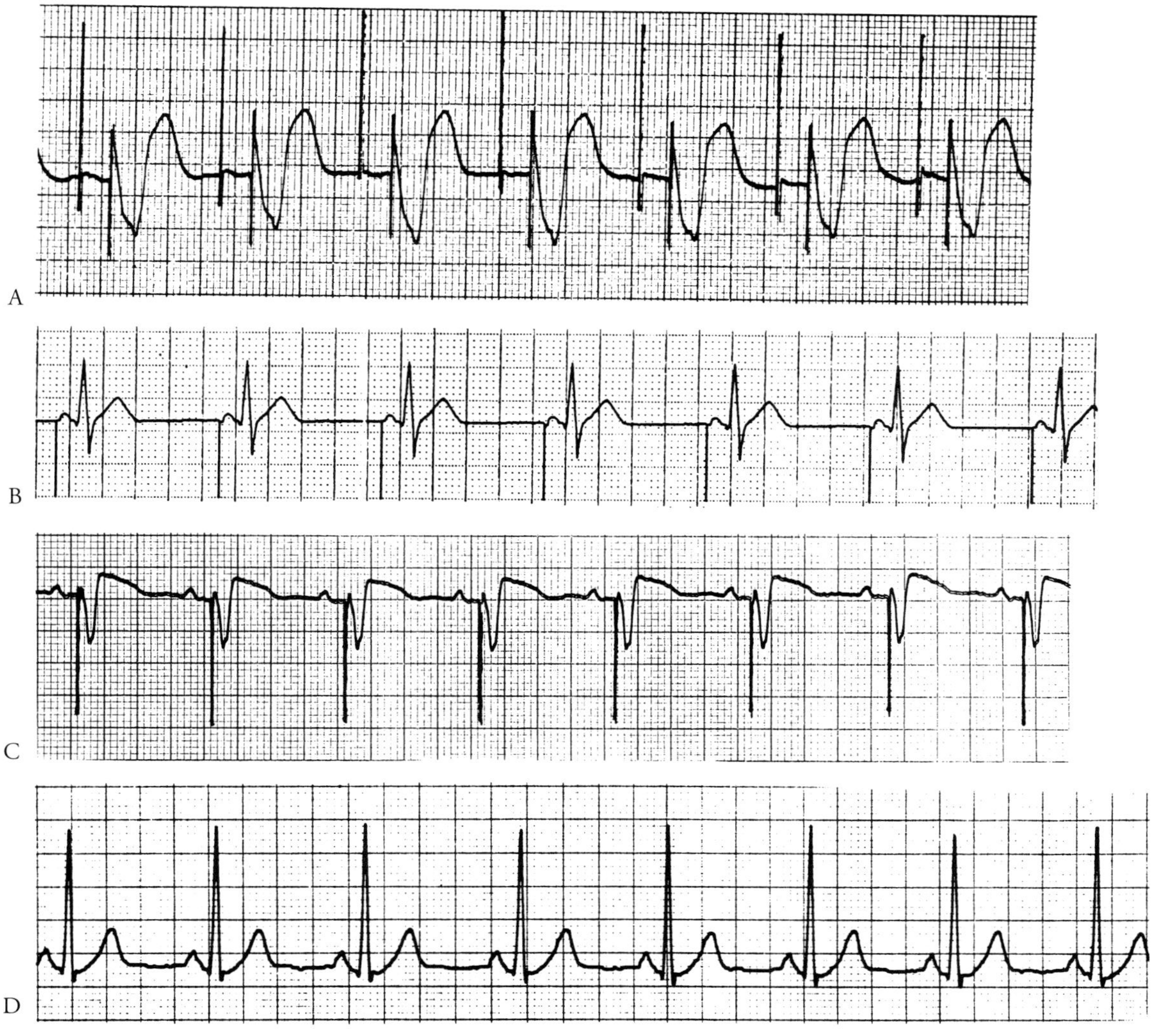

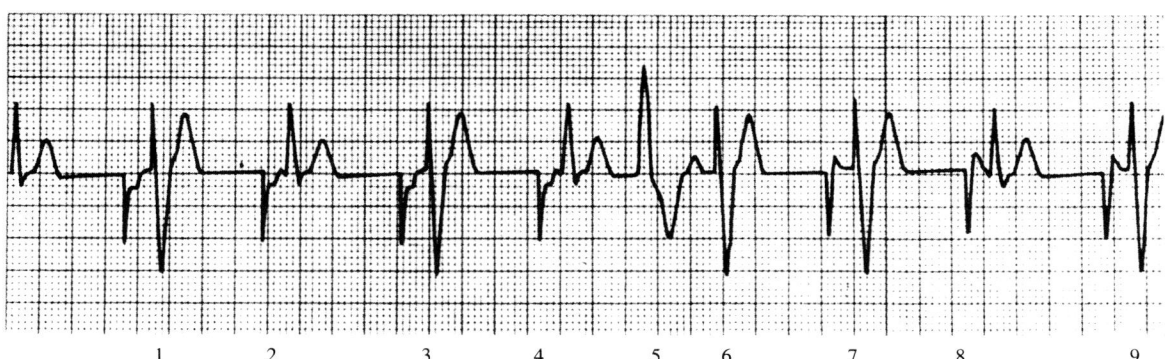

■ **Figure 32–18.** The four states of dual-chamber pacing. (*A*) Atrioventricular (AV) sequential pacing state with atrial and ventricular pacing at the minimum pacing rate. (*B*) Atrial pacing state with atrial pacing at the minimum rate and normal conduction to the ventricles, which inhibits ventricular output and terminates the AV delay. (*C*) Atrial tracking state. The pacemaker senses the patient's intrinsic P waves and paces the ventricle at the end of the AV delay. (*D*) Inhibited state with all pacing inhibited by normal sinus rhythm.

■ **Figure 32–19.** DDD pacemaker operating in all four states of pacing (stimulated strip). Beat 1 = atrioventricular (AV) sequential pacing; beat 2 = atrial pace, ventricular sense; beat 3 = AV sequential pacing; beat 4 = atrial pace, ventricular sense; beat 5 = premature ventricular contraction; beat 6 = atrial sense, ventricular pace; beat 7 = AV sequential pacing; beat 8 = atrial pace, ventricular sense; beat 9 = AV sequential pacing. Atrial capture is proven by beats 2, 4, and 8 (atrial spike followed by normal QRS within the programmed AV delay). Atrial sensing is proven by beat 6 (normal P followed by paced V at end of AV delay). Ventricular capture is verified by beats 1, 3, 6, 7, and 9 (wide paced QRS following ventricular pacing spike). Ventricular sensing is proven by beats 2, 4, and 8 (atrial spike followed by normal QRS, which inhibited ventricular pacing spike).

know the programmed mode (e.g., DDD, DVI), the minimum rate, the upper rate limit, the programmed AV delay, and refractory periods for both channels. In reality, the only time all of this information is available is immediately after an implantation, when the final programmed parameters are in the current patient chart, or in the physician's office records. Therefore, in the real world of bedside nursing, we have to rely on a basic understanding of the issues involved in pacemaker evaluation, often without having all of the necessary information at hand. Some of the needed information can be determined by measuring intervals on a rhythm strip. For example, the AV delay can be measured from atrial spike to ventricular spike if there are any AV sequentially paced beats present. The minimum rate can be determined by measuring the interval between two consecutive atrial pacing spikes, if present. The following sections briefly discuss the issues of assessing atrial and ventricular capture and sensing in a dual-chamber pacing system.

Atrial Capture

Atrial capture can be verified by seeing a P wave in response to every atrial pacing spike, although this is not always easy to see. The atrial response to pacing is often so small that it cannot be seen in many monitoring leads, so we cannot rely on the presence of a P wave after atrial pacing spikes as evidence of atrial capture. In the absence of a clear P wave, atrial capture can be assumed only when an atrial pacing spike is followed by a normally conducted QRS complex within the programmed AV delay. If the atrial spike captures the atrium and there is intact AV conduction, the presence of the normal QRS indicates that the atrium must have been captured for conduction to have occurred in the ventricles before the ventricular pacing stimulus was delivered. Because a DDD pacemaker paces the ventricle at a preset AV delay after atrial pacing, the presence of a ventricular paced beat after an atrial paced beat does not verify atrial capture, because the ventricle paces at the end of the AV delay regardless of whether atrial capture occurs. Therefore, atrial capture can be assumed only when there is an obvious P wave after every atrial pacing spike or when an atrial pacing spike is followed by a normal QRS within the programmed AV delay (see Figs. 32-18B and 32-19).

Atrial Sensing

Atrial sensing is verified by the presence of an intrinsic P wave that is followed by a paced ventricular beat at the end of the programmed AV delay. If a P wave is sensed, it starts the AV delay and ventricular pacing is triggered at the end of the AV delay, unless AV conduction is intact and results in a normal QRS. The presence of a normal P wave followed by a normal QRS proves only that AV conduction is intact, not that the P wave was sensed by the pacemaker. Therefore, atrial sensing is verified by an intrinsic P wave followed by a paced QRS (see Figs. 32-18C and 32-19).

Ventricular Capture

Ventricular capture is recognized by a wide QRS immediately after a ventricular pacing spike. Ventricular capture is much easier to recognize than atrial capture and is the same as with single-chamber ventricular pacing (see Figs. 32-18A and C and 32-19).

Ventricular Sensing

Ventricular sensing can be assessed only if there is intrinsic ventricular activity present for the pacemaker to sense. Ventricular sensing is verified by an atrial pacing spike followed by a normal QRS that inhibits the ventricular pacing spike, which is the same event that proves atrial capture (see Figs. 32-18B and 32-19). If a QRS is sensed before the next atrial pacing spike is due, both the atrial and ventricular pacing stimuli are inhibited and the VA interval (atrial escape interval) is reset.

Other Functions of Dual-Chamber Pacemakers

Upper-Rate Behavior

To avoid rapid ventricular pacing in response to atrial arrhythmias, dual-chamber pacemakers have an *upper rate limit* or *maximal tracking rate* that limits the rate at which ventricular pacing occurs in response to sensed atrial activity. This upper rate limit applies only to paced tachycardias, not to intrinsic tachycardias. That is, tachycardias that are caused by ventricular pacing in response to rapid atrial rhythms should not exceed the upper rate limit of the pacemaker. However, spontaneous VT or supraventricular tachycardia that conducts to the ventricle through the normal AV node or across an accessory pathway may result in ventricular rates that exceed the upper rate limit of the pacemaker. When an atrial rate being tracked by the ventricular channel of the pacemaker exceeds the upper rate limit, the pacemaker is programmed to limit the ventricular rate. Upper rate responses can be used alone or in combination and include Wenckebach response, block response, fallback, or rate smoothing.

Wenckebach response is the most commonly used upper rate response. As the atrial rate increases above the upper rate limit, P waves fall progressively closer to the preceding ventricular paced beat and the AV interval gets progressively longer. Eventually, a P wave falls in PVARP, where it cannot be sensed. The unsensed P wave does not start an AV delay; therefore, there is no ventricular paced beat after that P wave, and the resulting pause causes the ventricular paced rate to remain at or below the upper rate limit. The ECG shows a gradual lengthening of the AV interval and pauses whenever a P wave falls in PVARP (Fig. 32-20). This pattern presents as group beating just like AV Wenckebach, but the R-R intervals are constant instead of getting shorter. The atrial rate, the upper rate limit, and the PVARP determine the degree of block (e.g., 3:2, 5:4).

In *block response,* 1:1 tracking occurs at a constant AV delay until the atrial rate reaches a critical rate at which a P wave falls in PVARP and sudden block develops. As the atrial rate increases, P waves fall closer to the preceding ventricular paced beat, and eventually a P wave lands in PVARP where it cannot be sensed. The unsensed P wave does not start an AV delay; therefore, there is no ventricular paced beat after that P wave and the resulting pause keeps the ventricular paced rate below

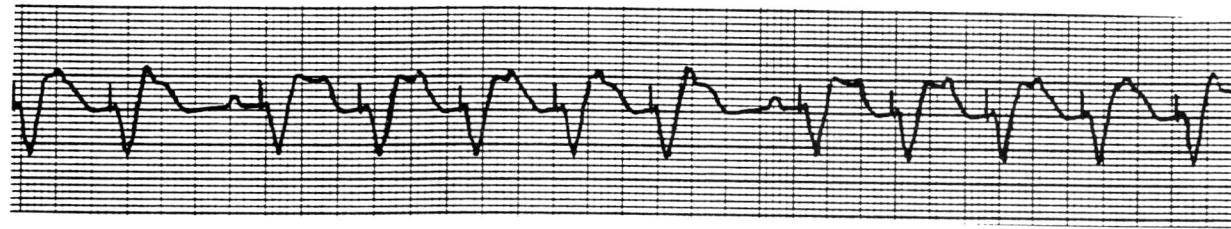

■ **Figure 32–20.** Wenckebach upper-rate response. Sinus tachycardia at a rate of 115 beats/min is present and the upper rate limit programmed in the pacemaker is 110 beats/min. The pacemaker tracks the intrinsic P waves and ventricular pacing occurs at the upper rate limit of 110, with occasional pauses. Note that the atrioventricular delay prolongs on consecutive beats until a P wave falls in the postventricular atrial refractory period, causing a pause in the ventricular paced rhythm. (From *Pacemaker technology for nurses and allied health professionals* p. 119, with permission from St. Jude Medical Cardiac Rhythm Management Division, Sylmar, CA.)

the upper rate limit. The ECG shows constant AV intervals with sudden block, often in a 2:1 ratio (Fig. 32-21). This type of response causes an abrupt rate change rather than a more gradual rate change, as occurs with other upper rate responses.

Fallback response is believed to be a more physiologic, but also more complex, type of response. When atrial tachycardia is first recognized by the atrial channel, ventricular pacing synchronizes with atrial activity for a programmable amount of time, after which the atrial and ventricular channels dissociate. From then on, the ventricular pulse interval (distance between two paced beats) lengthens. The pacing rate eventually slows down to the programmed fallback rate, which is a process taking as long as several minutes. While the ventricular rate slows gradually, the atrial rate is still monitored. When the atrial rate falls below the upper rate limit, the pacemaker returns to its original mode of pacing. This type of rate response provides a more comfortable hemodynamic transition from a rapid to a lower rate of ventricular pacing. AV synchrony, however, is not maintained by the fallback response (Fig. 32-22).

Rate smoothing is not truly an upper-rate response but rather a programmed parameter used to prevent the ventricular pacing rate from changing by more than a predetermined percentage from one cardiac cycle to the next. This response prevents the pacemaker from tracking rapid atrial rates at the onset or if the rapid atrial rate stops abruptly. With this type of response, when the atrial rate exceeds the upper rate limit, a Wenckebach response is observed. When the tachycardia stops abruptly, pacing resumes at a rate faster than the lower rate limit to prevent an abrupt decrease in ventricular rate (Fig. 32-23).

Pacemaker-Mediated Tachycardia

Pacemaker-mediated tachycardia (PMT, also called *endless loop tachycardia* or *pacemaker reentry tachycardia* [PRT]) is rapid ventricular pacing, usually at the upper rate limit, that can occur in patients with dual-chamber pacemakers when retrograde conduction is present in the normal conduction system or in an accessory pathway. Retrograde conduction means that impulses can conduct backward from ventricle to atrium. Pacemaker units that detect intrinsic atrial activity and stimulate the ventricle after an appropriate AV delay (VDD and DDD modes) can participate in the maintenance of a PMT. The tachycardia circuit consists of the patient's normal AV conduction system (or an accessory pathway) that is capable of retrograde conduction, and the pacemaker's atrial sensing and ventricular output circuits (Fig. 32-24*A*). Retrograde conduction results in a sensed atrial depolarization, which in turn triggers the ventricular output channel. If this sequence is repeated, a tachycardia is maintained indefinitely until the retrograde pathway fatigues or until the tachycardia is terminated by inactivating the atrial sensing circuit (see Fig. 32-24*B*). Placing a magnet over the pulse generator inactivates the atrial sensing circuit and terminates PMT.

Conditions necessary for initiation of PMT include loss of AV synchrony, intact retrograde conduction, and VA conduction times longer than PVARP. Any condition that results in the atrium being repolarized and ready to respond to retrograde conduction can initiate PMT. Common initiators include loss of atrial capture, PVCs with retrograde conduc-

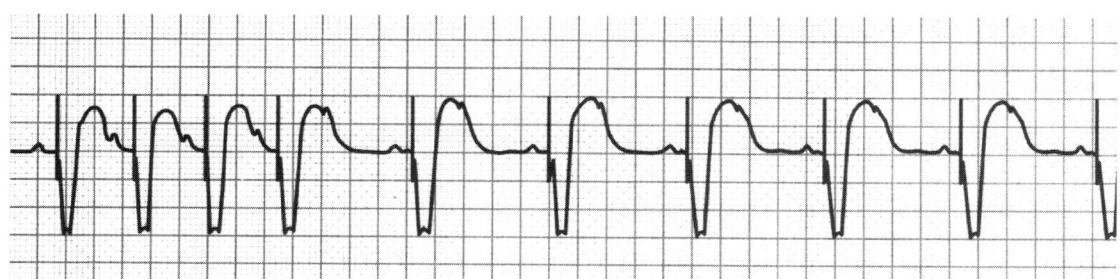

■ **Figure 32–21.** Atrioventricular block upper-rate response (simulated strip). Sinus tachycardia is present at a rate of approximately 120 beats/min and the upper rate limit is 120 beats/min. Atrial tracking occurs at the beginning of the strip. As the sinus rate increases slightly, 2 : 1 block develops as every other P wave falls in the postventricular atrial refractory period. (From Sultzer Intermedics, Angleton, TX, *Concepts of permanent cardiac pacing*, p. 144, 1998).

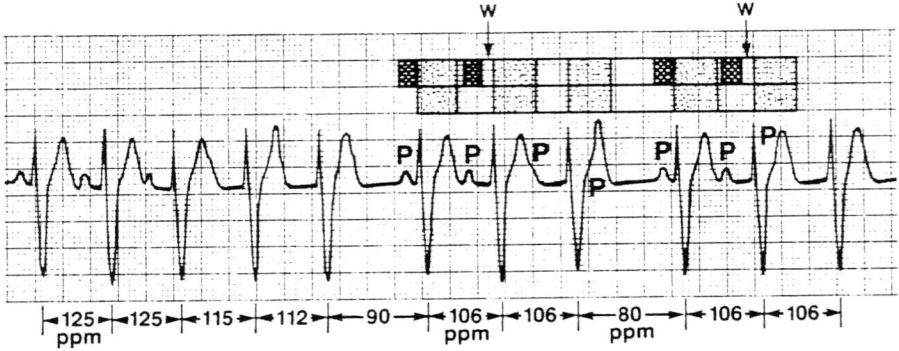

■ **Figure 32–22.** Fall-back response from an atrial tachycardia of 125 pulses/min to the nominal programmed fall-back rate of 100 pulses/min seen in the strip as falling between 80 to 106 pulses/min. P, P waves; heavy stippling, atrioventricular delay; light stippling, post ventricular refractory periods; no stippling, alert periods; W, ventricular channel wall, cannot pace in the ventricle faster than the nominal fallback rate (From Isicoff C. [1985]. Understanding upper rate responses of DDD pacers. *Heart & Lung*, 14, 327–334.)

tion, premature atrial contractions, myopotential or EMI tracking, magnet application and removal, and reprogramming from asynchronous to synchronous mode (Barold, 1997). Most newer dual-chamber pacemakers incorporate PMT prevention algorithms, such as extending PVARP after a PVC or temporarily inactivating the atrial sensing circuit after a PVC, in an attempt to prevent the initiation of PMT. Many devices also have PMT termination algorithms that attempt to break the tachycardia if it occurs.

Crosstalk

Crosstalk refers to the sensing of activity in one channel of the pacemaker by the other channel's sensing circuit. The most common and potentially dangerous type of crosstalk is sensing of the atrial output pulse by the ventricular channel, resulting in inhibition of ventricular output. If the ventricular channel senses the atrial pacing stimulus, it thinks it sees a ventricular event and thus inhibits its next output. This could result in total ventricular asystole in a patient who has no underlying ventricular rhythm (Fig. 32-25A, middle section of top strip). Other manifestations of crosstalk include atrial pacing at a rate faster than the programmed rate and a longer distance from the

atrial pacing spike to the conducted QRS than is programmed for the AV delay (see Fig. 32-25). Atrial pacing at a rate faster than the programmed rate occurs because the ventricular channel sees every atrial output spike and interprets it as a QRS, thus inhibiting ventricular output and resetting the VA interval from the atrial spike instead of from a subsequent ventricular beat. When this occurs, the VA interval times out sooner than it would have if it had been reset by a ventricular event, causing the next atrial output to occur sooner than the programmed pacing rate (see Fig. 32-25A, top strip). An increase in the AR interval (longer distance from the atrial output spike to a conducted QRS than is programmed for the AV delay) occurs when ventricular output is inhibited by crosstalk (so there is no paced ventricular beat at the end of the programmed AV interval), and normal conduction occurs to the ventricle but takes longer than the programmed AV delay (see Fig. 32-25A, first two beats in top strip).

Blanking Period. The ventricular blanking period is one method of trying to eliminate crosstalk. The blanking period is a very short refractory period that occurs on the ventricular channel during delivery of the atrial output pulse (see Figs. 32-17C and 32-25A). The blanking period "blinds" the ventricular channel for a short time so it cannot see the atrial pacing output. This

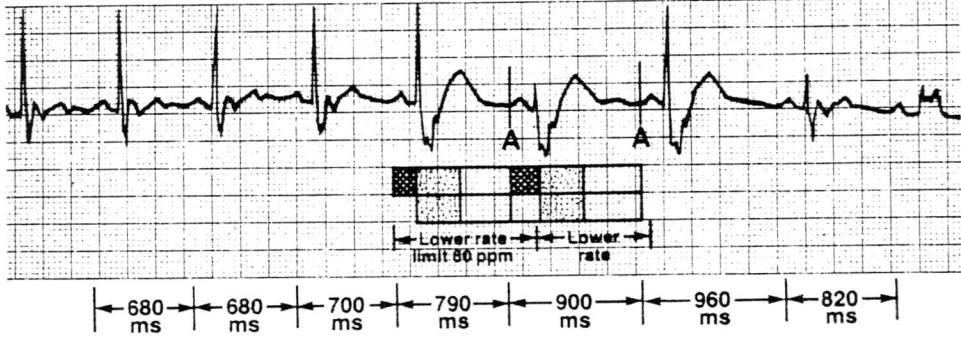

■ **Figure 32–23.** Electrocardiogram strip and timing cycle of rate smoothing as the intrinsic rate decreases. Atrial pacing is seen before the programmed lower rate limit of 60 pulses/min because the pacer does not allow P-P or R-R intervals to change by more than 12.5% (program smoothing constant) from one beat to the next. ms, milliseconds; A, atrial output pulse; heavy stippling, atrioventricular delay; light stippling, post ventricular refractory periods; no stippling, alert periods. (From Isicoff, C. [1985]. Understanding upper rate responses of DDD pacers. *Heart & Lung*, 14, 327–334.)

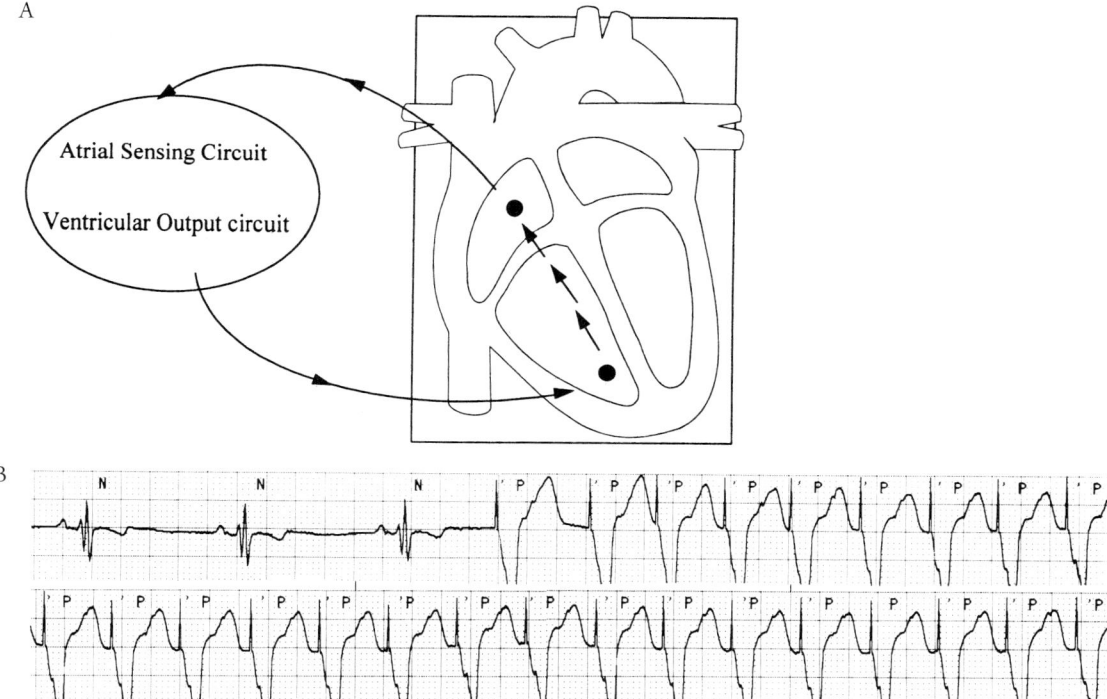

■ **Figure 32–24.** (*A*) Diagram illustrating the mechanism of pacemaker-mediated tachycardia (PMT). Retrograde ventriculoatrial conduction is representd by the dashed line. The retrograde P wave is sensed by the atrial channel of the pacemaker and a ventricular output is delivered at the end of the programmed atrioventricular delay. The reentry circuit consists of the intrinsic conduction system as the retrograde limb and the pacemaker as the antegrade limb. (*B*) Rhythm strip of PMT. Sinus rhythm is present, and then a ventricular paced beat occurs, probably in response to and extraneous signal (e.g., myopotential or electromagnetic interference from something in the environment). Retrograde conduction occurs to the atria (seen as a P wave after the first ventricular paced beat), which then initiates PMT. On the rhythm strip, N is the rhythm strip recorder's annotation of a "normal" beat, and P is the annotation of a "paced" beat (however, the Ps happen to coincide with the retrograde P waves seen on the rhythm strip.)

should prevent crosstalk, but if the blanking period is too short, it may still be possible for the ventricular channel to sense the end of the atrial output pulse. In most pacemakers, the blanking period is programmable and can be made longer if necessary to prevent crosstalk.

Safety Pacing (Nonphysiologic AV Delay). Safety pacing is a mechanism used to prevent the inhibition of ventricular output when crosstalk occurs. Safety pacing results in the delivery of a ventricular pacing spike at a short AV delay (e.g., 100 milliseconds) whenever the ventricular channel senses any signal immediately after the blanking period. Safety pacing prevents inhibition of ventricular pacing and the short AV delay prevents delivery of the ventricular pacing spike on a T wave (Fig. 32-26). Safety pacing presents on the ECG as a shorter than programmed AV interval, and is another way to verify that ventricular sensing is intact, because safety pacing only occurs when the ventricular channel senses something right after the end of the blanking period.

Rate-Adaptive Pacing

Rate-adaptive pacing is used when the heart is unable to increase its rate appropriately when the body's need for cardiac output increases (chronotropic incompetence). The pacing system contains a physiologic sensor that tells the pacemaker

to pace faster in response to the sensed parameter. The most frequently used sensors at this time are motion sensors and minute ventilation sensors. Motion sensors are activated by body movement, such as occurs with exercise, and signal the pacemaker to pace faster. Minute ventilation sensors measure transthoracic impedance and increase the pacing rate when the respiratory rate is increased in response to exercise, emotional states, fever, etc. Other technologies being investigated include sensors for metabolic parameters like blood temperature and venous oxygen saturation, and sensors of cardiac indices like QT interval, ventricular depolarization gradient, pre-ejection interval, stroke volume, and rate of myocardial wall tension development (Grubb, 1998; Hayes & Zipes, 2001; Mitrani et al., 2001; Shanker & Saksena, 2001). It is likely that future pacemakers will combine two or more sensors to get the most physiologic response to the body's needs for increased cardiac output. Figures 32-27 and 32-28 illustrate ECG examples of rate adaptive pacing, which can appear as pacemaker malfunction if the observer is unaware of the rate response feature.

Atrial Overdrive Pacing

Atrial pacing at rapid rates of 200 to 500 impulses/min is used in an attempt to terminate atrial tachyarrhythmias such as atrial

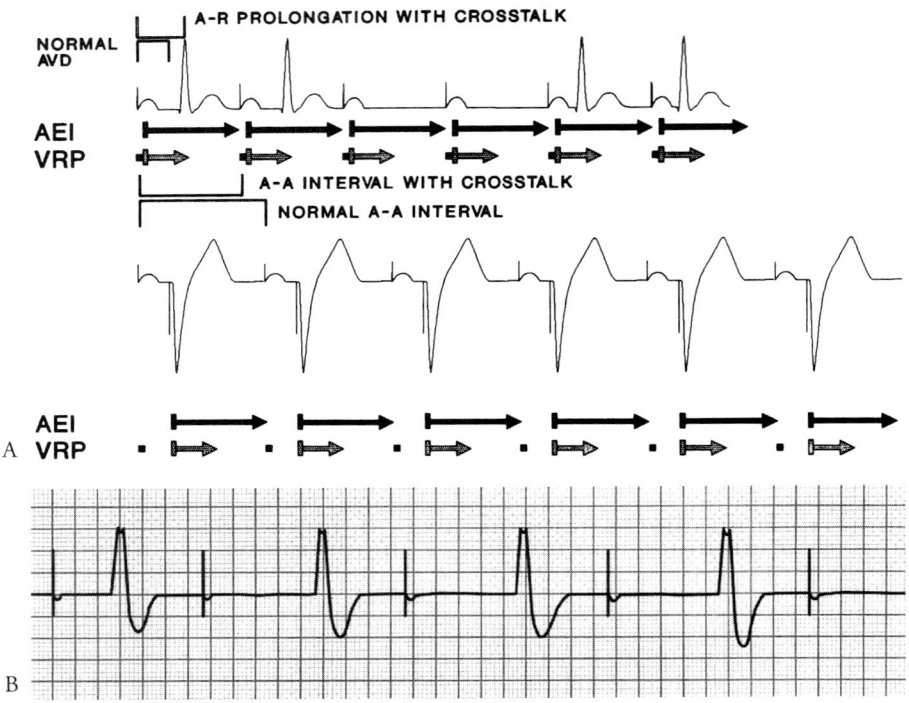

■ **Figure 32–25.** Crosstalk. (*A*) Lower diagram illustrates the normal programmed AA interval (minimum pacing rate), atrioventricular (AV) delay (measure from A spike to V spike), atrial escape interval (AEI), ventricular refractory period (VRP), and ventricular blanking period (small square in front of the VRP arrows). The upper diagram shows possible manifestations of crosstalk due to ventricular sensing of atrial output: (1) shortening of the A-A interval, seen as atrial pacing at a rate faster than programmed, (2) prolongation of the A-R interval (time from atrial pace to intrinsic R wave) seen in the first two beats, and (3) inhibition of ventricular output, seen in the middle of the strip. (*B*) Crosstalk inhibition of ventricular pacing. Atrial pacing spikes are present followed by paced P waves. No ventricular output is delivered at the end of the AV delay because the ventricular channel senses the atrial output, interprets it as a ventricular event, and inhibits ventricular output. The wide QRS complexes represent an underlying ventricular escape rhythm. (*A* from *Pacemaker technology for nurses and allied health professionals,* p. 75, with permission from St. Jude Medical Cardiac Rhythm Management Division, Sylmar, CA. *B* from Sultzer Intermedics, Angleton, TX, *Concepts of cardiac pacing,* p. 131, 1998.)

tachycardia, atrial flutter, and atrial fibrillation (Fig. 32-29). This type of pacing is most frequently performed using a temporary pulse generator and pacing through epicardial leads in cardiac surgery patients. It can also be performed with a transvenous atrial lead, but this is less effective. Newer dual-chamber temporary pulse generators have overdrive pacing capability. It is extremely important to accurately identify the atrial pacing

wires and make sure that rapid pacing is not performed through ventricular leads, because that would most likely result in VF.

Antitachycardia Pacing

Antitachycardia pacing involves the delivery of one to several paced impulses to the atria or the ventricles in an attempt to

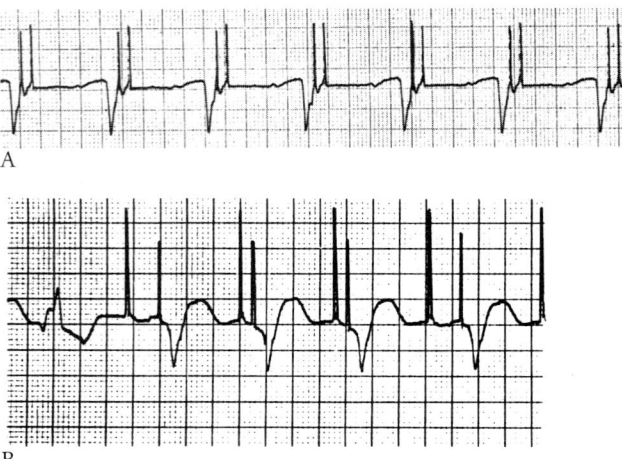

■ **Figure 32–26.** (*A*) Safety pacing due to crosstalk. The programmed atrioventricular (AV) interval is 150 milliseconds (ms). The pacemaker is in the AV sequential pacing state with an AV delay of approximately 100 ms due to crosstalk. (*B*) Safety pacing due to sensing early in the AV delay. The first two beats are AV sequential paced beats with an AV delay of approximately 150 ms. The ventricular channel blanking period occurs with the delivery of each atrial pacing spike and prevents the ventricular channel from sensing atrial output. The third beat is a premature ventricular contraction (PVC) that occurs immediately after the atrial pacing spike. When the ventricular channel "opened its eyes" after the blanking period, it saw the PVC very early in the AV delay, and rather than inhibit its output, it paced at the safety pacing AV delay of approximately 100 ms. Safety pacing prevents inappropriate inhibition of ventricular pacing but delivers the ventricular output early enough to avoid the T wave of the PVC. (B, from Furman, S., Hayes, D. L., & Holmes, D. R., [1989]. *A practice of cardiac pacing.* Armonk, NY: Futura Publishing Co.)

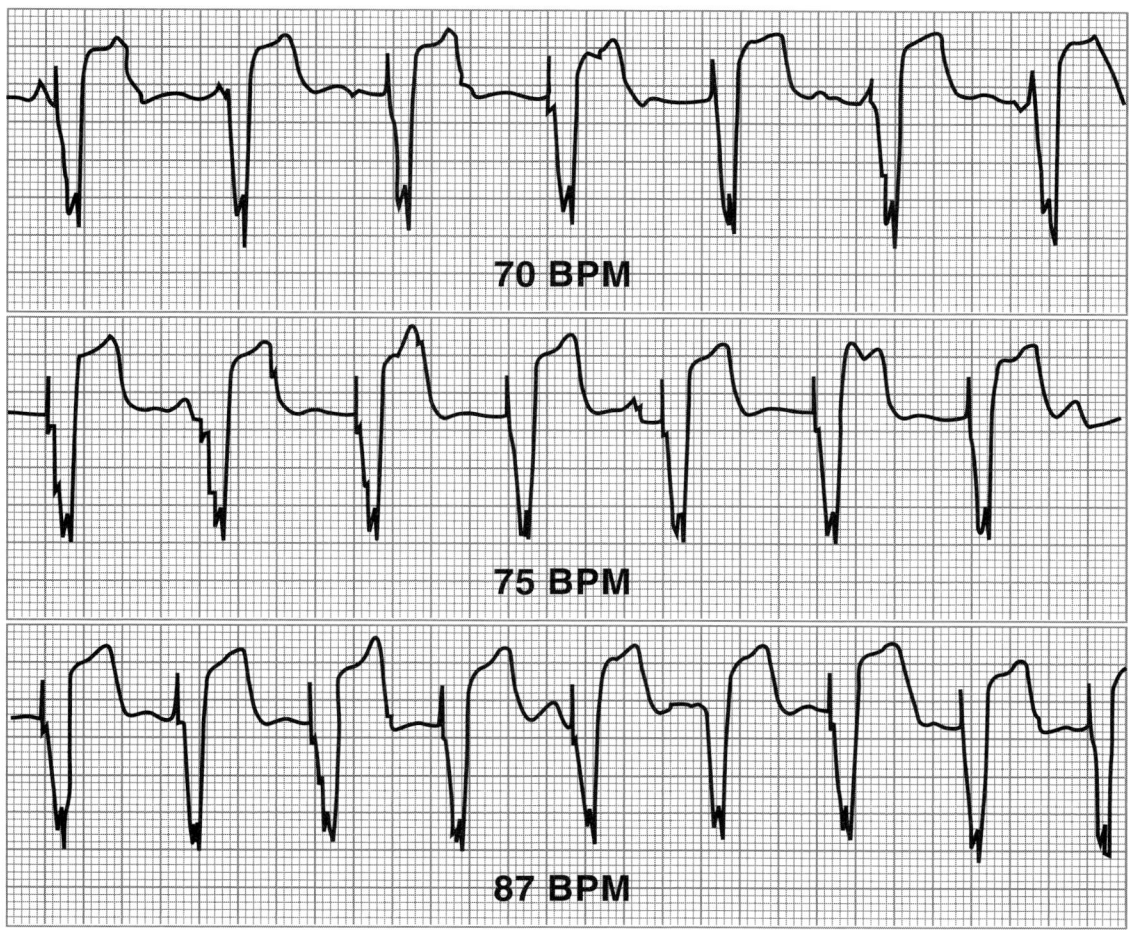

■ **Figure 32–27.** ECG example of VVIR pacing in an elderly patient with complete heart block. Note the increase in VVI pacing rate from 70 bpm to 87 bpm with activity. (Modified from Furman, S., Hayes, D. L., & Holmes D. R. [1989]. *A practice of cardiac pacing* [2nd ed., p. 414]. Armonk, NY: Futura Publishing Co.)

terminate tachycardias. This type of pacing is most often performed in the ventricle to terminate VT, and most antitachycardia pacing is incorporated into implantable defibrillator devices, which are covered later in this chapter. Figure 32-30 is an example of antitachycardia pacing during VT in a patient with an ICD.

Cardiac Resynchronization Therapy (CRT) with Biventricular Pacing

Many patients with advanced systolic heart failure have delays in AV conduction (long PR intervals that result in reduced ventricular filling), interventricular conduction (usually LBBB that causes the right ventricle to contract before the left and results in abnormal septal depolarization), and intraventricular conduction (abnormal spread of the electrical impulse through the LV that causes abnormal contraction of that chamber), which combine to reduce LV function in several ways. The term *ventricular dysynchrony* is used to describe the delayed electrical activation and mechanical contraction abnormalities that result in reduced LV performance in patients with advanced heart failure, specifically (Abraham,

2002; Cazeau et al., 1998; Daubert et al., 2000; Daubert et al., 1998; Luck et al., 2002):

1. Paradoxical septal wall motion in which the septum contracts early compared to the LV and is finished repolarizing by the time LV contraction begins; this results in the septum moving away from the LV instead of participating in LV ejection
2. Prolonged mitral regurgitation caused by delayed activation of the LV; the abnormal spread of electrical activation to the lateral wall of the LV that occurs with a wide QRS and LBBB causes delayed activation of the papillary muscle that is supposed to hold the mitral valve closed during LV systole
3. Septal dyskinesis in which the septum moves away from the LV and into the RV during LV contraction; late activation of the LV allows the septum to finish repolarizing at a time when LV pressure is rising because of delayed LV contraction; the resulting abnormal septal wall motion decreases the septum's contribution to stroke volume and impairs mitral valve function (see Chapter 28 for more detailed information on heart failure).

The use of AV sequential biventricular pacing, in which both ventricles are paced simultaneously, can correct the electrical

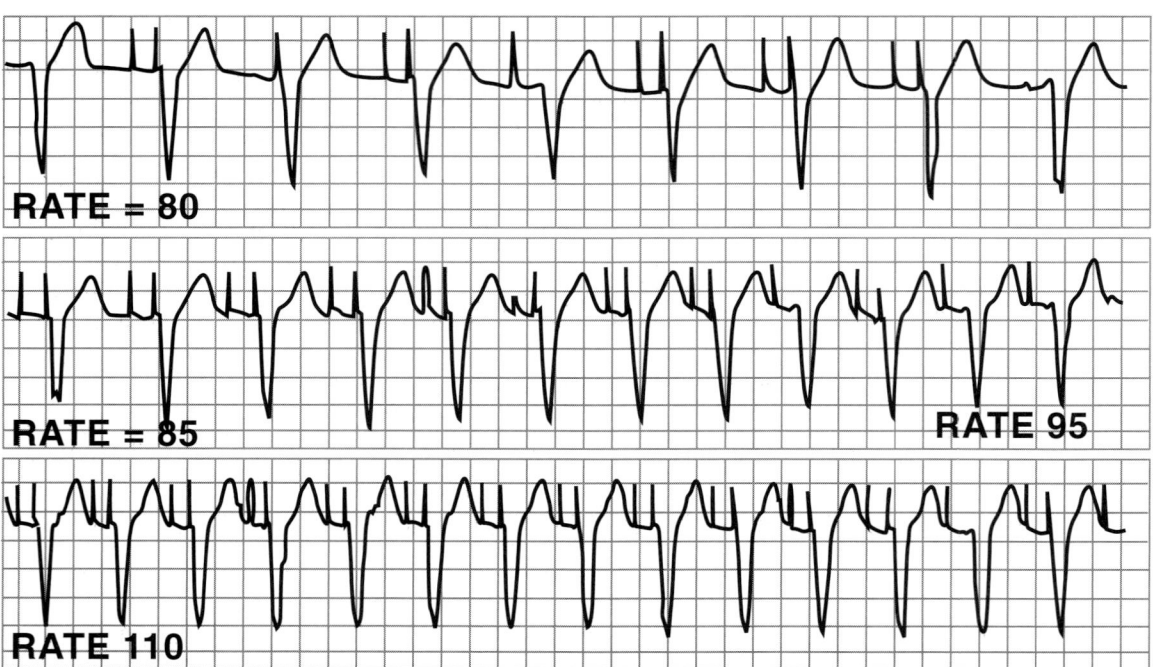

RATE = 80

RATE = 85   **RATE 95**

RATE 110

■ **Figure 32–28.** ECG example of DDDR pacing, with a gradual increase in pacing rate from 60 bpm at rest to 110 bpm with activity. This also illustrates the feature of adaptive AV delay in which the AV interval gradually shortens as the pacing rate increases, mimicking normal AV node physiology. (Modified from Furman, S., Hayes, D. L., & Holmes D. R. [1989]. *A practice of cardiac pacing* [2nd ed., p. 420]. Armonk, NY: Futura Publishing Co.)

abnormalities that cause mechanical dysfunction and "resynchronize" ventricular contraction to improve LV function, exercise capacity, and quality of life (Abraham et al., 2002; Luck, 2002). Simultaneous electrical activation of the ventricles with biventricular pacing allows ejection to occur in both ventricles before repolarization of the septum and reduces the adverse effects of paradoxical septal wall motion on stroke volume. Control of the AV interval with dual chamber pacing improves mitral valve motion and facilitates ventricular filling by optimizing atrial kick. Results of the MIRACLE trial (Abraham et al., 2002) demonstrated significant clinical improvement in patients with moderate to severe heart failure and an intraventricular conduction delay.

CRT with biventricular pacing is indicated for the reduction of symptoms of moderate to severe heart failure (NYHA class III or IV) in patients who remain symptomatic despite stable, optimal medical therapy and have a LV ejection fraction of 35% or less and a QRS duration of 130 ms or more (Indications for the InSync System, Medtronic, 2001). AV sequential biventricular pacing (also called *atriobiventricular pacing*) is

accomplished by inserting a standard atrial pacing lead in the right atrium, a ventricular lead in the RV apex, and a special lead threaded into the coronary sinus and down a lateral cardiac vein in the LV (see Fig. 32-5).

Evaluating Ventricular Capture in a Biventricular Pacemaker

Evaluating ventricular capture in a biventricular pacemaker is complicated and requires that the clinician be attuned to changes in the shape and width of the QRS complex. Because both ventricles are paced simultaneously, the paced QRS in biventricular pacing is usually narrower than ordinary paced QRS complexes, although in some patients there is not much noticeable difference. As capture is lost in one or the other ventricle, the QRS changes shape and becomes much wider because one ventricle depolarizes before the other. When capture is lost in both ventricles, the QRS resumes its pre-paced shape and width, usually a pattern of LBBB. Lead V_1 should be the best lead for evaluating ventricular capture in a

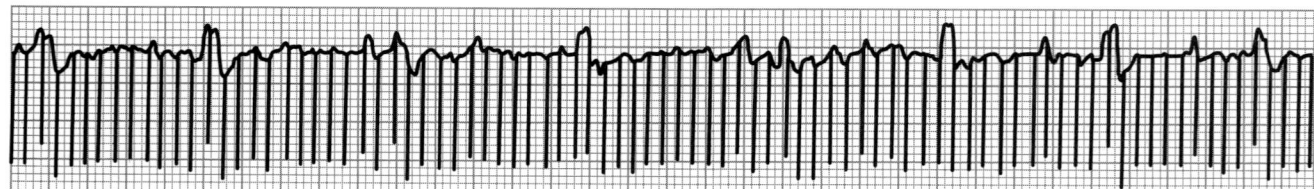

■ **Figure 32–29.** Atrial overdrive pacing in attempt to terminate atrial flutter using atrial epicardial wires in a post cardiac surgery patient.

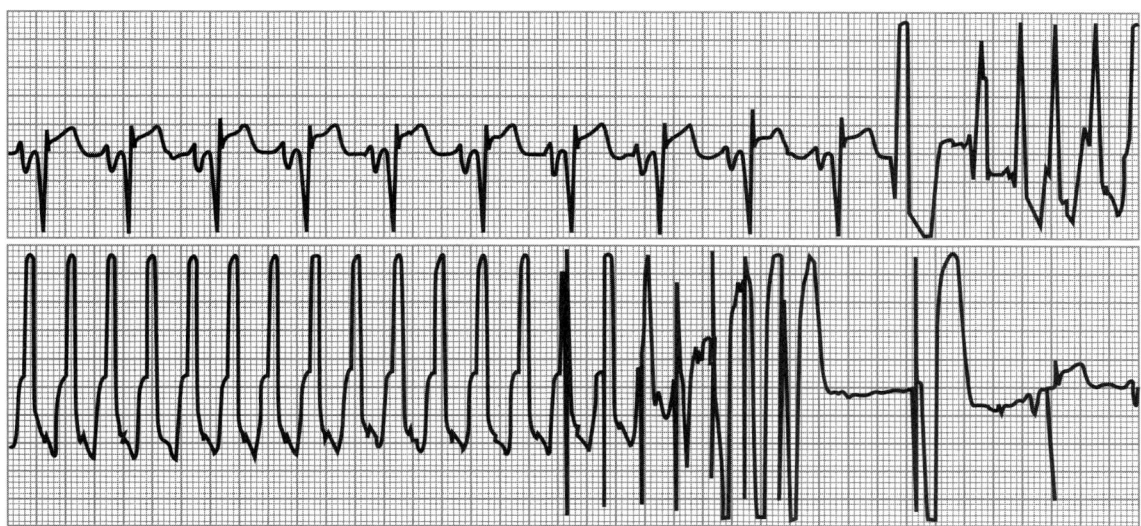

■ **Figure 32–30.** Antitachycardia pacing into VT in a patient with an ICD. The onset of VT is seen in the top strip and continues into the bottom strip. In the bottom strip, a train of seven pacing spikes is delivered, which successfully terminate the VT. One backup bradycardia paced beat occurs following termination of the VT before sinus rhythm resumes.

biventricular pacemaker because of its ability to differentiate RV from LV activation (see discussion of bundle-branch block patterns in Chapter 18), and the following concepts should apply:

1. Biventricular capture in lead V_1 usually presents with a negative QRS that is narrower than a paced QRS resulting from right ventricular pacing alone
2. When capture is lost in the RV but is present in the LV, the QRS widens and becomes upright in V_1 (assumes a RBBB morphology)
3. When capture is lost in the LV but present in the RV, the QRS widens and becomes negative in V_1 (assumes a LBBB morphology), and looks like an ordinary RV paced beat

4. When capture is lost in both ventricles, the QRS resumes its pre-paced shape and width, usually LBBB with a QRS more than 120 ms.

Research is needed in this area to verify the accuracy of lead V_1 in biventricular pacemaker evaluation and to determine if other leads are helpful. Figure 32-31 is an example of loss of capture in a biventricular pacemaker.

Potential Complications of Pacing

Pacemaker complications can be caused by implant-related problems or by malfunction of any part of the pacemaker system

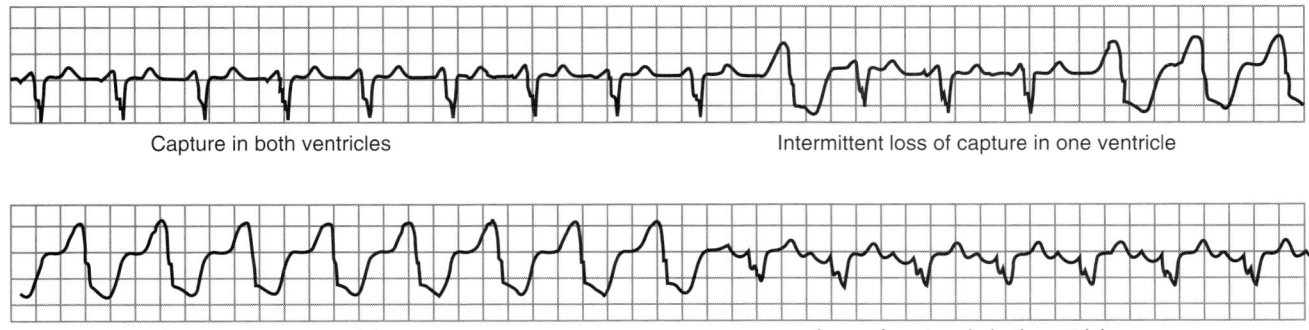

Capture in both ventricles   Intermittent loss of capture in one ventricle

Loss of capture in one ventricle   Loss of capture in both ventricles

■ **Figure 32–31.** Continuous strips showing loss of capture in one and then both ventricles in a biventricular pacemaker. The lead is not known, but assuming it is lead V1, the first half of the top strip illustrates biventricular capture, although pacing artifacts are very small and not easily seen. The second half of the top strip shows intermittent loss of capture, presumably in the RV, since the QRS complexes have a very wide RBBB morphology. The first half of the bottom strip continues to show loss of RV capture. The last half of the bottom strip shows loss of capture in both ventricles, with a very wide LBBB morphology. This morphology could be compared to the pre-paced QRS in this lead to verify that it is the same. (Modified from Medtronic [2001]. Cardiac resynchronization therapy for heart failure management. Powerpoint/Slide Presentation available from Medtronic, Minneapolis, MN or at *www.medtronic.com.*)

(e.g. lead problems or generator problems). The pacing lead must be in firm contact with the pulse generator for the system to work correctly. In a permanent pacing system, good contact between the lead connector pin and the pulse generator at the connector block of the pulse generator is dependent on a setscrew being tightened adequately during implantation; a loose setscrew can create problems with pacemaker output or sensing. In addition, normal pacemaker function can appear to be abnormal because of idiosyncrasies of specific devices or unusual programming, resulting in what appears to be abnormal pacing rates or changes in the AV interval.

Early complications of temporary or permanent pacemaker insertion are usually related to lead insertion and include pneumothorax or hemothorax, lead perforation (subclavian vein or myocardium), air embolus, and ventricular arrhythmias. Complications occurring later can include infection at the insertion site, endocarditis, hematoma formation, venous thrombosis, skin erosion over a permanent pulse generator, lead dislodgment or fracture, Twiddler syndrome, symptoms from pacemaker syndrome, and pacemaker failure (Hayes & Zipes, 2001; Hayes & Spittell, 1998; Kusumoto & Goldschlager, 1998; Mitrani et al., 2001; Shanker & Saksena, 2001).

Pneumothorax can occur when the subclavian vein is used for lead insertion because the apex of the lung is located very near the subclavian vein, and lung injury is a possibility when accessing the vein. Pneumothorax may become manifest immediately or as long as 48 hours after implantation (Furman, 1989). Clinical signs of pneumothorax can include respiratory distress, absence of lung sounds on the affected side, chest pain, hypotension, elevated neck veins, and hypoxia.

Lead perforation may be asymptomatic or it can lead to cardiac tamponade if there is rapid accumulation of blood in the pericardium secondary to perforation of the right ventricular wall. If the pacing lead perforates the septum and enters the left ventricle, the ECG may show a right bundle-branch block pattern rather than the usual left bundle-branch block pattern that results from pacing the right ventricular apex. Intercostal muscle or diaphragmatic stimulation by a perforated lead can cause hiccups or muscle twitching in the chest wall. The presence of a friction rub after implantation can indicate pericarditis or pericardial effusion caused by lead perforation.

Ventricular arrhythmias, either PVCs or runs of VT, can result from irritation of the ventricle by the pacing lead. PVCs that are caused by pacing lead irritation have the same morphology as paced beats because they originate from the same spot (see Fig. 32-16A). Lead-induced arrhythmias most often occur within 24 to 48 hours of lead placement and usually resolve spontaneously (Furman, 1989).

Pacemaker system infection can involve just the pacemaker pocket or the entire generator and lead system and can occur early or late after implant. The use of prophylactic antibiotics and irrigation of the pacemaker pocket with antibiotics at the time of implant can reduce the incidence of infection. Infections involving the lead system can lead to endocarditis and usually require removal of the entire pacing system until the infection is resolved. Because patients are discharged so soon after implantation, they need to be taught to look for and report signs of infection: redness, swelling, or weeping of fluid from the pacemaker pocket; erosion of the pacemaker; and fever that is not related to the flu or other identifiable illness.

Twiddler syndrome is manipulation of a permanent pulse generator within its pocket by the patient. This can lead to rotation of the pacemaker and twisting of the leads, which can result in lead fracture or dislodgment. Patients should be cautioned to keep their hands away from the pacemaker pocket and to avoid manipulating the pulse generator.

Pacemaker syndrome refers to a constellation of symptoms resulting from inadequate timing of atrial and ventricular contraction. Symptoms include fatigue, jugular venous distention and pulsations in the neck, weakness, dizziness or near-syncope, hypotension, CHF, and pounding in the chest. Symptoms may occur during periods of VVI pacing because of loss of AV synchrony or when retrograde conduction to the atria occurs, causing the atria to contract against closed AV valves. Contraction of the atria at a time when the AV valves are closed because ventricular systole can activate stretch receptors in the atrial wall and pulmonary veins, resulting in a reflex vasodilation that causes hypotension and dizziness. The loss of AV synchrony causes loss of atrial contribution to ventricular filling and may be another cause of symptoms.

IMPLANTABLE CARDIOVERTER DEFIBRILLATORS

Sudden cardiac death (SCD) continues to claim approximately 400,000 lives each year, with most deaths related to VF or VT (Myerburg & Castellanos, 1997; Zheng, 2001). The implantable cardioverter defibrillator (ICD) terminates VT/VF automatically, preventing sudden death. ICD implants have increased exponentially since first implanted in 1980. A further increase in ICD therapy is expected, with expansion of indications for the ICD. Clinical trials have shown that the ICD is better than antiarrhythmic therapy in preventing sudden death from ventricular arrhythmias (Moss et al., 2002; AVID Investigators, 1997).

Development

The implantable defibrillator was the brainstorm of Dr. Michel Mirowski. In the late 1960s, Mirowski conceived the idea of an automatic implantable defibrillator after a close friend died from repeated episodes of ventricular arrhythmias. The first experimental model was tested successfully in 1969 in a dog. After many years, and much refining, the ICD was first implanted in humans in 1980 (Mirowski, 1985). The device was experimental until 1985, when it gained full U.S. Food and Drug Administration approval. The first generation devices were large (weighing 250 g and occupying a volume of 145 mL), requiring implantation in a subcutaneous abdominal pocket.

The earliest ICD systems required a thoracotomy, because patch electrodes were sutured to the pericardium over the apex of the heart, and either epicardial screw-in leads or an endocardial lead was placed for rate sensing and pacing (Fig. 32-32).

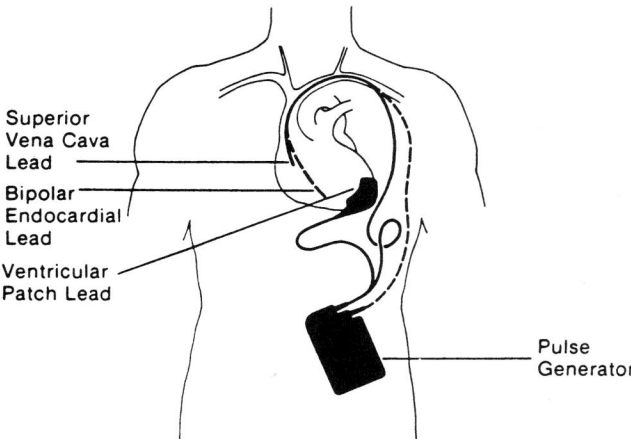

■ **Figure 32–32.** ICD. Diagram of automatic implantable cardioverter defibrillator with placement in abdominal region. (*Physician's manual for the automatic implantable cardioverter defibrillator*, p. 1. St. Paul, Cardiac Pacemaker, Inc., 1986.)

The leads were then tunneled to the pulse generator in the abdominal pocket (Gold, 2000; O'Callaghan & Ruskins, 1997). The need for thoracotomy increased morbidity and mortality associated with ICD implantation and limited use in high-risk patients.

The first ICD was a non-programmable, committed, shock-only device intended to treat VF but was quickly modified to a second-generation device that had cardioversion capabilities (O'Callaghan & Ruskins, 1997; Wolfe et al., 1998). The current generations of defibrillators have evolved into a smaller, sophisticated device, much like a pacemaker (Fig. 32-33). ICDs can deliver either high-energy or low energy shocks, demand and rate-responsive pacing, anti-tachycardic pacing, and noninvasive electrical stimulation for electrophysiology studies (EPS), have extensive programmability allowing for tiered therapy, and have the ability to record and store electrograms of tachycardic episodes. Lead technology and the use of biphasic waveforms have made transvenous, nonthoracotomy systems the standard, eliminating the need for open-heart surgery (Gold, 2000).

Indications for Use

Initial indications for an ICD during clinical trials in 1980 were quite stringent. To meet criteria for receiving an ICD, the patient had to have survived at least two episodes of cardiac arrest not associated with an acute MI. Documentation of VF had to occur on at least one occasion, and the patient had to have been treated with antiarrhythmics on one episode (O'Callaghan & Ruskin, 1997). Since 1980, guidelines have been updated several times by expert panels of the American College of Cardiology (ACC), American Heart Association Task Force (AHA), and the North American Society of Pacing and Electrophysiology (NASPE). The current guidelines were published in 2002 and are no longer based on the assumption that first-line therapy for VF or symptomatic sustained VT should be guided by drug therapy. Current recommendations are evidence-based whenever possible and are given rankings based on current ACC/AHA format (class I-III indications). Class I indication means that evidence supports an ICD to be beneficial, useful, and effective. Class II means there is conflicting evidence about usefulness/efficacy for an ICD. Class II is broken-down further: class IIa indicates weight of evidence in favor of ICD and class IIb indicates evidence is less established for ICD implantation. Class III indication means there is evidence to suggest the ICD would *not be* useful and in some cases may be harmful. The indications are then given level A, B, and C rankings (Gregoratos et al., 2002). Level A indicates that data were derived from multiple, randomized, clinical trials involving a large number of subjects. Level B indicates data were derived from a limited number of trials involving comparatively small numbers of patients or from well designed, nonrandomized studies or observational data registries. Level C indicates that the consensus opinion of experts was the primary source of the recommendation (Gregoratos et al., 2002) (Display 32-4).

The rapid evolution of ICD technology, with the results of studies documenting efficacy of the ICD over drugs in both secondary and primary prevention of SCD, has led to the expansion of indications for the ICD (Saksena, & Madan, 2002). Patients who receive an ICD usually fall into one of four

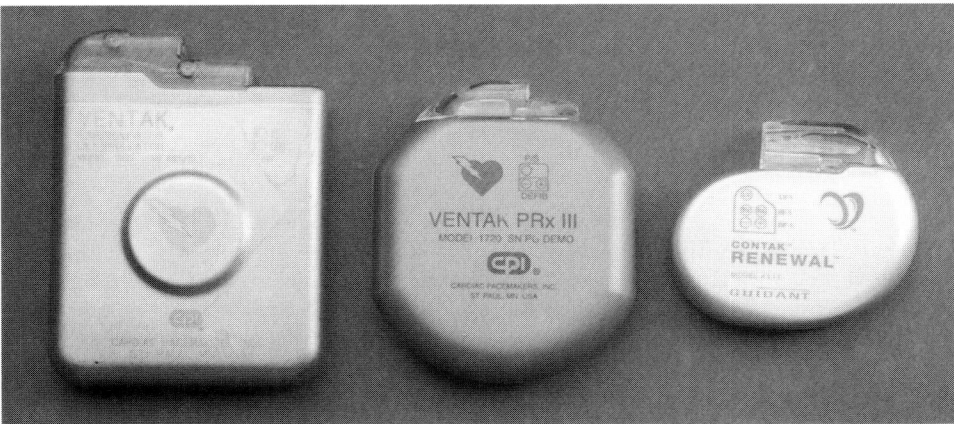

■ **Figure 32–33.** ICD. Assortment of Guidant ICDs, showing the evolution in size. The largest one was the first-generation series; the smallest is the current Biventricular ICD.

DISPLAY 32–4

2002 INDICATIONS FOR IMPLANTABLE CARDIOVERTER-DEFIBRILLATOR THERAPY (ACC/AHA/NASPE) PRACTICE GUIDELINES

Class I Indications

Indications per level of evidence-A, B, or C

A: Data were derived from multiple *randomized* clinical trials involving a large number of subjects.
B: Data were derived from a limited number of trials involving comparatively small numbers of patients from well designed data analysis of *nonrandomized* studies or *observational* data registries.
C: Consensus of expert opinion was the primary source or recommendation.
1. Cardiac arrest due to VF or VT-not due to a transient or reversible cause. *(Level A)*
2. Spontaneous sustained VT in association with structural heart disease. *(Level B)*
3. Syncope of undetermined origin with sustained VT or VF induced with EP study when drug therapy is ineffective, not tolerated, or not preferred. *(Level B)*
4. Nonsustained VT with coronary disease, prior MI, LV dysfunction, and inducible VF or sustained VT at EP study that is not suppressible by class I antiarrhythmic drug. *(Level A)*

Class IIA Indications (New for 2002)

1. Patients with LV ejection fraction $\leq$ 30%, at least one month post myocardial infraction and three months post coronary artery revascularization surgery. *(Level B)*

Class IIB Indications

1. Cardiac arrest presumed to be due to VF when EP testing is precluded by other medical conditions. *(Level C)*
2. Severe symptoms (syncope) attributable to VT/VF while waiting heart transplantation. *(Level C)*
3. Familial or inherited conditions with a high risk for life-threatening arrhythmias such as long QT syndrome or hypertrophic cardiomyopathy. *(Level B)*
4. Nonsustained VT with CAD, prior MI, and LV dysfunction, with EP-induced VT or VF. *(Level B)*
5. Recurrent syncope of undetermined etiology in the presence of ventricular dysfunction and inducible EP study, when other causes of syncope have been excluded. *(Level C)*
6. Syncope of unexplained etiology or family history of unexplained SCD in association with RBBB and ST-segment elevations (Brugada syndrome). *(Level C)*
7. Syncope in patients with advanced structural heart disease in which a full workup has failed to define a cause. *(Level C)*

Class III Indications*

1. Syncope of undetermined cause in patient without EP-induced arrhythmais, and no structural heart disease. *(Level C)*
2. Incessant VT or VF. *(Level C)*
3. VF or VT resulting from arrhythmias that are amenable to ablation (e.g., Wolff-Parkinson-White syndrome, right ventricular outflow tachycardia, fascicular VT). *(Level C)*
4. Ventricular arrhythmias due to transient or reversible causes. *(Level B)*
5. Significant psychiatric illnesses that may be aggravated by ICD implantation, or systematic follow-up. *(Level C)*
6. Terminal illness with life expectancy <6 months. *(Level C)*
7. Patients with CAD and LV dysfunction with prolonged QRS duration in the absence of spontaneous or inducible VT who are undergoing coronary artery bypass surgery. *(Level B)*
8. New York Heart Association class IV drug-refractory congestive heart failure in patients who are not candidates for heart transplantation. *(Level C)*

CAD, coronary artery disease; EP, electrophysiology; ICD, implantable cardioverter-defibrillator; LV, left ventricle; MI, myocardial infraction; RBBB, right bundle branch block VF, ventricular fibrillation; VT, ventricular tachycardia.

*Class III indications are patients in whom ICD therapy is not appropriate.

(Adapted from Guidelines for Implantation of Cardiac Pacemakers and Antiarrhythmia Devices-ACC/AHA Practice Guidelines, 2002.)

---

categories: cardiac arrest survivors; those with spontaneous sustained VT; those with syncope of unknown origin with inducible VT/VF per electrophysiologic testing; and patients at high risk for future life-threatening arrhythmic events.

Sudden Cardiac Death Survivors

Ventricular arrhythmias are the cause of most sudden cardiac arrests (Engelstein, 2003). Survivors of cardiac arrest, in the absence of acute MI, are at risk for a future event. Cobb and associates report a 36% 1-year mortality rate in untreated patients who were successfully resuscitated, hospitalized, and discharged home. Follow-up data on ICD patients have shown that 42% to 60% of them have received ICD discharges for VT or VF in a follow-up period of 2 to 3 years (Cappato,1999). Three landmark trials have shown the benefit of ICD therapy for the prevention of SCD in those patients who have experienced a cardiac arrest or have had documented hemodynamically significant VT (see Display in Chapter 31, Primary vs. Secondary Prevention of SCD). The Antiarrhythmics Versus Implantable Defibrillator (AVID) trial (AVID Investigators, 1997), the Cardiac Arrest Study Hamburg (CASH) (Kuck et al., 2000), and the Canadian Implantable Defibrillator Study (CIDS) (Connolly et al., 2000) all established the benefit of ICD therapy as the first line treatment option for patients with life-threatening arrhythmias. Before these studies, the ICD was used as a therapy option only for patients who continued to have life-threatening arrhythmias in combination with antiarrhythmic drug therapy.

Sustained Ventricular Tachycardia

The ICD is also first line therapy in the patient who has spontaneous sustained monomorphic VT with structural heart disease. The ICD is most efficacious in patients with impaired left ventricular function. In patients without structural heart disease, the ICD is also a therapy option when alternative options have failed (Gregoratos et al., 2002). Patients with VT and who have an ICD may have other treatments options combined with ICD therapy, which include: (1) antiarrhythmic drug therapy to decrease ICD discharges; (2) surgical aneurysmectomy when a ventricular aneurysm is the substrate for VT; (3) radiofrequency catheter ablation (RFA) of the VT foci; and (4) combination of anti-arrhythmic drugs and RFA (Engelstein, 2003; O'Callaghan & Ruskin, 1997).

Therapy options with current ICDs are very beneficial in the VT patient. The anti-tachycardic pacing mode (ATP) delivers an effective therapy in terminating monomorphic VT. ATP is particularly effective with slower VT and, when delivered, is usually imperceptible to the patient. Low-energy cardioversion or high-energy cardioversion-defibrillation is also programmed into the ICD. With ATP, the patient has fewer shocks, the therapy is not painful, and the patient's acceptance of the device is enhanced (Wathen et al., 2001).

Syncope of Unknown Origin

Syncope in the setting of structural heart disease and inducible VT per electrophysiologic testing carries a high risk of SCD. Bass and colleagues reported a sudden death rate of 48% at 3 years in patients with syncope of unknown origin and inducible sustained VT, compared with only 9% in patients with a negative EP study (Bass et al., 1988). Syncope with induced VT/VF is considered a class I indication for an ICD. Syncope in patients with structural disease in which all invasive and noninvasive examinations have failed to define a cause are likely to have an arrhythmic event. New recommendations for ICD therapy were applied to this group of patients with the 2002 implant guidelines. Syncope of unexplained cause or family history of sudden death in association with Brugada syndrome (RBBB and ST segment elevation) is a new recommendation for ICD implantation with the 2002 implant guidelines (Gregoratos et al., 2002).

High-Risk Patients

The most notable change in the revised guidelines for ICDs is that prophylactic ICD implantation is now justified in patients who are considered at high risk but have never had a spontaneous episode of sustained VT or VF. The goal is to prevent sudden death in the patient with LV ejection fraction of less than or equal to 30% and with history of myocardial infarction (1 month after acute MI and 3 months after coronary artery revascularization surgery). The first randomized study to report primary prevention of SCD with direct comparison between the ICD and antiarrhythmic drugs was the Multicenter Automatic Defibrillator Implantation Trial (MADIT). MADIT was designed as a prophylactic trial to determine if patients with coronary heart disease, left ventricular dysfunction, and inducible VT, per electrophysiological testing, would have a better survival rate than those patients who were treated with conventional medical therapy. MADIT established that the incidence of cardiac arrest and total mortality were markedly reduced in the group of patients who received an ICD. The study was actually stopped early on advice of the Data and Safety Monitoring Board because the patients randomized to the ICD arm were found to have a 54% reduction in all-cause mortality compared with the patients receiving conventional therapy (Moss et al., 1996).

Given the results of MADIT, Moss and colleagues reasoned that patients with previous history of myocardial infarction and advanced LV dysfunction had substrate for life-threatening cardiac arrhythmias and would benefit from a prophylactic ICD without electrophysiological testing to confirm inducible VT. MADIT II, a randomized, controlled, clinical trial was designed to evaluate the benefit of the ICD in patients with a previous MI and a left ventricular ejection fraction of 0.30 or less. The study began in 1997 and was stopped in November of 2001. Analysis revealed a 31% decrease in mortality among the ICD group (Moss et al., 2002).

Results of these studies have expanded ICD indications for the patient with previous myocardial infarction and advanced LV dysfunction, who definitely benefit from ICD therapy before sustaining a sudden cardiac arrest. Other groups of patients may also benefit from prophylactic ICD therapy. Those patients with idiopathic dilated cardiomyopathy, hypertrophic cardiomyopathy, long QT syndrome, Brugada syndrome, and arrhythmogenic right ventricular dysplasia have been shown to have better survival rates when treated with an ICD (Gregoratos, 2002).

Functional Characteristics

The ICD system consists of a pulse generator and defibrillation lead electrodes for arrhythmia detection and therapy delivery. ICD systems are implanted transvenously, like pacemakers, and no longer require cardiac surgery. However, devices that use defibrillation patches on the ventricle are still in use, and if these leads are still functional at the time of generator change for depleted battery, the original leads are retained and used (Groh et al., 1998). The ICD systems consist of a unipolar system that uses the pectorally implanted pulse generator as part of the electrical circuit, simplifying implantation (Fig. 32-34). In addition to internal defibrillation, today's ICD can provide all of the following: synchronized cardioversion, ATP, VVI, DDDR, and cardiac re-synchronization (CRT) pacing, telemetry, episode history logs, electrograms, and handheld activators for termination

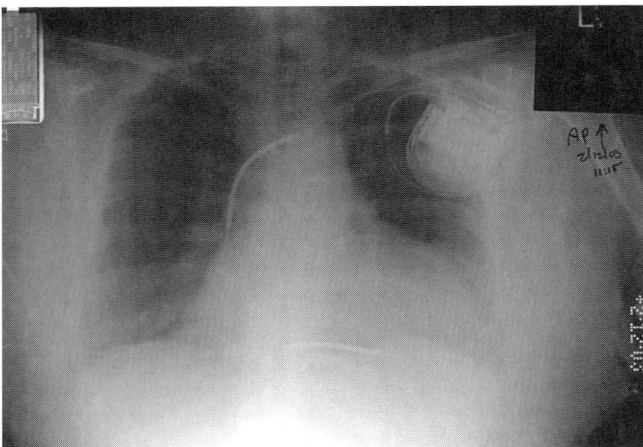

■ **Figure 32–34.** ICD. Radiograph of transvenous lead placed in the right ventricle and a pectoral implant of ICD.

of atrial fibrillation. An example of device diagnostics is shown in Figure 32-35. Defibrillators for CRT (CRT-D) (Fig. 32-36) and for atrial arrhythmias are the newest type of defibrillators (read about them in Displays 32-5 and 32-6).

The pulse generator is essentially a self-powered computer in a hermetically sealed titanium can. The operational circuitry consists of a battery, sense amplifier, control circuits (microprocessors, logic, and memory), high-voltage charging circuits, defibrillation energy-storing capacitor, and a high-voltage output switch circuit. A header made of epoxy is the interface between the generator and the leads (Kuck et al., 1996) (Display 32-7).

The lead system connects the generator to the heart. Lead technology has markedly improved; however, the lead system is the most vulnerable aspect of the ICD system and the most frequent cause of system failure. ICD leads are now smaller, come with steroid elution to help achieve lower pacing thresholds, and provide better sensing, which is a critical function of the ICD (Hayes et al., 2000). If a single-chamber ICD is placed, only one lead is required and it is placed into the right ventricle in the same manner as a pacemaker lead. The ventricular lead has sensing and pacing capabilities similar to pacing leads but also has a large electrical surface area for delivering high-energy shocks. If a dual-chamber ICD is placed, a second lead is placed in the atrium, and if CRT therapy is required, a third lead is placed into the coronary sinus (Hayes et al., 2000). The defibrillation pathway that is used with all ICD implants today is a unipolar defibrillation system, and the titanium case of the pulse generator becomes part of the lead system. The generator is often referred to as an "active can" or "hot can." Using the generator to complete the defibrillation circuit has helped lower defibrillation thresholds known as DFTs (Gold, 2000).

Early ICDs delivered shocks with a monophasic waveform, which was a single pulse at a given polarity and duration. Today's ICDs deliver shocks with a biphasic waveform. A biphasic shock has a negative and positive pulse, which lowered DFTs significantly. Lower thresholds result in higher rates of successful defibrillation, a higher margin of safety, and prolonged battery life (Bardy et al., 1993).

Sensing and Detection Enhancements

Recognizing ventricular arrhythmias is essential for the ICD; it is the *sensing* that measures the intracardiac electrogram signal from the lead electrodes. The sensing electrodes transmit each ventricular depolarization (R-wave) signal to the sense amplifier of the ICD. The main challenge for the sensing system is

Therapy History:			03-MAR-2003 to 30-JUN-2003
No New Episodes Since Counters Last Reset			

Episode Counters - Tachy		
03-MAR-2003 to 30-JUN-2003		
	Since Last Reset	Device Totals
Treated		
VF Therapy	0	2
VT Therapy	0	0
VT-1 Therapy	0	0
Commanded Therapy	0	0
Nontreated		
No Therapy Programmed	0	0
Nonsustained Episodes	0	0
Total Episodes	0	2

Device Parameter Summary		
VF 180 bpm		26J/ 31J/ 31J
1.0 sec		# of Additional Max Shocks 3

Brady Parameters		
	Normal Brady	Post-shock Brady
Mode	VVIR	VVIR
Lower Rate Limit	60 ppm	50 ppm
Max Sensor Rate	120 ppm	120 ppm
VRP	240–250 ms	240–250 ms
Ventricular	2.6 V & 0.5 ms	7.5 V & 1.0 ms
Enable Magnet Use		On
Change Tachy Mode with Magnet		Off
Beep During Capacitor Charge		Off
Beep on Sensed and Paced Ventricular Events		Off
Beep when ERI is Reached		On
Electrogram Storage Source		
Ventricular		On
Shock		On
Onset EGM Storage		On
EGM Storage		9:30 m:s

AICD Device Data	
Last Interrogation	30-JUN-2003 11:48
Last Re-programming	21-OCT-2002 10:50
Last Delivered Shock	13-AUG-2002 11:11
Energy	17 J
Charge Time	5.4 sec
Shock Impedance	33 Ω
Auto Capacitor Re-form	90 days
Last Capacitor Re-form	11-MAY-2003 09:04
Charge Time	13.8 sec
Cumulative Charge Time	01:43 m:s
Time Since Implant	11 months
Battery Status	BOL
Monitoring	3.22 V
Charging	2.34 V

Lead System Data			
	Implant Date 13-AUG-2002	Previous Follow-up	This Follow-up
Ventricular			
Intrinsic Ampl	8 mV	12.5 mV 03-MAR-03	12.3 mV
Impedance	750 Ω	655 Ω 03-MAR-03	647 Ω
Threshold	0.4V 0.5 ms	0.4V 0.5ms 03-MAR-03	0.4V 0.5 ms
Shock			
Impedance	N/R Ω	39 Ω 03-MAR-03	39 Ω

■ **Figure 32–35.** ICD. Printout of Guidant's Quick Notes Report from a Prizm VR, Model 1855. The episode log shows no arrhythmias in a 4-month period. AICD device and lead data show normal variation from previous follow-up. ICD has been in 11 months; battery status remains at beginning of life (BOL).

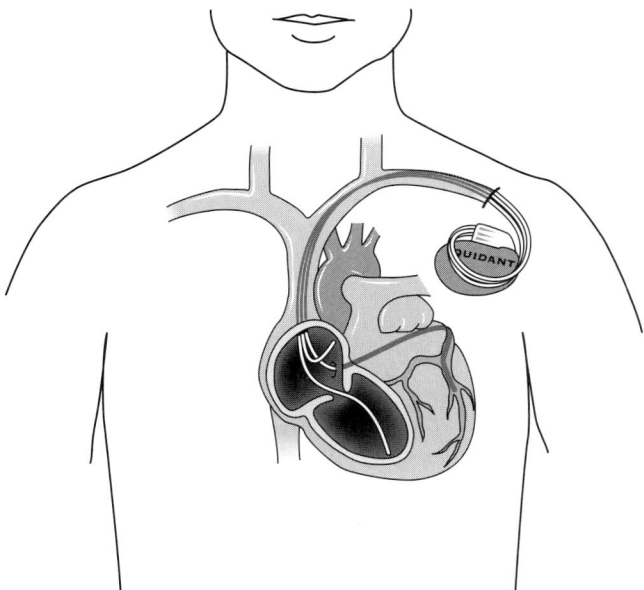

■ **Figure 32–36.** ICD. Diagram showing lead placement for cardiac resynchronization device. Three leads are placed into the heart. Right atrial lead, right ventricular lead, and left ventricular lead are placed into the coronary sinus and positioned into a lateral vein.

two-fold. It must detect the very low amplitudes of VF while avoiding oversensing of T waves during repolarization and P waves during atrial depolarization. Other incoming signals that can be sensed include low-frequency noise, skeletal myopotentials, and EMI. ICD systems have either an automatic gain

control or an auto-adjusting threshold feature that helps with proper sensing (Groh, 1998).

The ICD primarily *detects* arrhythmias by looking at the cycle length, which is the time between R waves produced by ventricular depolarization. The cycle length represents the heart rate. The ICD can also be programmed to look at signal morphology, which helps in arrhythmia detection (Wolfe et al., 1998). For VF, ICD devices use rate criteria as the sole detection method. The use of rate criteria results in maximal sensitivity. The ICD charges the capacitor once the programmed amount of intervals is met (e.g., 8 to 12 intervals of a rate of 180 beats/min). The ICD then delivers the shock after reconfirming the rate. If rate criteria are not met, the shock is aborted. The reconfirmation prevents unnecessary shocks for nonsustained events.

A VT zone can also be programmed into the ICD. Once again, rate is the primary detection method, but other detection enhancements can be programmed to increase specificity of VT detection, thus decreasing inappropriate shocks for supraventricular tachycardia and atrial fibrillation (Hayes et al., 2000). These optional detection features include a sudden-onset criterion, an R-R interval stability criterion, an electrogram width criterion, and sustained rate duration. Dual-chambered pacemaker defibrillators also looks at atrial rate data (Fig. 32-37) and have a V-rate greater than A-rate override feature to help deliver appropriate therapy (Mortensen & Pedersen, 1997).

Onset criterion is a feature used to distinguish sinus tachycardia from VT. When the patient is exercising and the ventricular rate increases gradually and subsequently goes into the VT zone, the ICD does not classify the tachycardia as VT. The ICD compares each cycle length interval and determines if the rate has increased faster than would be expected for a sinus increase (O'Callaghan & Ruskin, 1997).

D I S P L A Y | 32–5

WHAT'S NEW WITH ICDS ... CARDIAC RESYNCHRONIZATION THERAPY—DEFIBRILLATORS (CRT-D)

CRT is a term used to describe biventricular pacing. Biventricular pacing is used to improve mechanical efficiency of the heart. When both the left and right side of the heart are paced simultaneously contraction of the ventricles become coordinated overcoming the inefficiency associated with large conduction delays, particularly left bundle branch block (LBBB). When LBBB is present there is a delay in the electrical conduction. This effects the mechanical action of the left ventricle and impairs systolic and diastolic function, CRT devices are placed in Class III and Class IV heart failure patients. Since left ventricular (LV) function and heart failure are predictors of sudden cardiac death the combination of CRT with implantable defibrillators provide additional benefit.

The most common lead placement for CRT-D devices is a right atrial lead, a coronary sinus pacing lead inserted into a distal coronary sinus tributary, which supplies the LV free wall, and a standard right ventricular ICD lead (Fig. 32-36) CRT involves sensing or pacing the right atrium followed by simultaneous pacing of the right and left ventricle. CRT-D devices combine all the pacing therapies of standard biventricular pacemakers with all the standard defibrillator therapies into one device.

The first controlled randomized study that clearly demonstrated improvement with heart failure patients was the Multicenter InSync Randomized Clinical Evaluation Trial (MIRACLE). When patients received biventricular pacing there were significant improvements in all three primary endpoints: the six minute walk, New York Heart Association class (NYHA), and quality of life. Beneficial remodeling of the heart was also seen. LV size decreased and there was an increase in LV ejection fraction.

The COMPANION Trial, Comparison of Medical Therapy, Pacing, and Defibrillation in Chronic Heart Failure released preliminary data showing:

1) A 19 percent reduction in combined all cause mortality for heart failure patients who received CRT-P (pacemakers) plus optimal medical therapy.

2) A 43 percent reduction in combined all cause mortality for heart failure patients with CRT-D plus optimal medical therapy. Full report of the Companion Trial was not available at the time of this writing, but will be available in 2004.

(Abraham, W. T. et al., [2002]. Cardiac resynchronization in chronic heart failure. *Guidant New Bulletin,* Preliminary results of COMPANION Trial, 2003.)

DISPLAY 32-6

WHAT'S NEW WITH ICDS ... ATRIAL DEFIBRILLATORS

Atrial defibrillators are relatively new, unlike the typical ventricular defibrillators that are programmed to withhold therapy for atrial fibrillation, atrial defibrillators detect and deliver specific atrial therapies. Atrial defibrillators are used to improve quality of life and reduce symptoms associated with atrial arrhythmias. Atrial defibrillators all have back up ventricular therapies, which are programmed separately.

At the time of this writing the two FDA approved atrial defibrillators being used are the *Medtronic Gem III AT ICD System* and the *Guidant Vitality AVT.* In addition to the standard ventricular therapies discussed in this chapter (ATP, cardioversion, and defibrillation) these devices have atrial prevention and termination therapies.

Medtronic's ICD offers *atrial rate stabilization* to prevent onset of atrial arrhythmias by preventing long pauses after premature atrial contractions by pacing faster than the intrinsic heart rate, gradually slowing back down to the intrinsic or lower pacing rate. Therapies designed to terminate atrial arrhythmia include: (1) atrial ATP using burst, ramp or 50 Hz (high-frequency) trains. The ATP therapies are effective for organized atrial arrhythmias like atrial flutter. (2) Atrial defibrillation shocks which can actually be programmed to occur at a specific time of day for patient comfort and acceptance, as atrial fibrillation is not life theatening like

ventricular fibrillation. (3) A handheld patient activator for delivery of a shock on command by either the patient or physician. The handheld device also allows the patient to query the defibrillator to confirm they are in atrial fibrillation.

Guidant's ICD offers *dynamic overdrive pacing* designed to pace the atrium at a slightly higher rate than the intrinsic rate after sensing an atrial event. Overdrive pacing at a higher rate following a PAC is also available. Therapies include: (1) atrial ATP using burst, ramp or scan pacing methods; (2) automatic cardioversion that can be programmed for a certain amount of time after initial onset of the atrial arrhythmia; (3) patient-controlled cardioversion, which gives the patient the option to interrogate the ICD and deliver a shock.

Atrial defibrillators for primary management of atrial fibrillation are for a small percentage of atrial fibrillation patients in whom traditional medial therapy has failed. However use of atrial defibrillators in the patient population receiving ICDs is higher as atrial fibrillation and flutter is a common arrhythmia in conjunction with advanced age and heart disease. Atrial defibrillators provide management of both atrial and ventricular arrhythmias.

(Medtronic—Gem III Dual ICD Therapies Flipbook [2001]; Guidant—Vitality AVT, Atrial Features Reference Guide [2003].)

The rate stability criterion is used to help differentiate atrial fibrillation from VT. Atrial fibrillation has large cycle length variability, whereas VT cycle length varies minimally. When a fast ventricular response from atrial fibrillation meets the VT criteria and rate stability is programmed on, the ICD does not classify the fast rate as VT because it varies

more than a monomorphic VT would (O'Callaghan & Ruskin, 1997).

The electrogram width criterion (EGM width) measures the intracardiac electrogram and inhibits the ICD from detecting sinus tachycardia as VT. The ICD compares the width of the R wave with a programmed value. This algorithm uses digital

DISPLAY 32-7

FYI: THE MAKINGS OF AN ICD

Leads: Leads are insulated wires made from either silicone rubber or polyurethane, they connect the ICD to the patient's heart. There are five major components to a lead: (1) the electrode(s); (2) the conductor(s); (3) insulation; (4) connector pins; and (5) the fixation mechanism. The ICD system can have up to three leads placed, dependent on the system.

Casing: The casing, or outer shell of the ICD is made from titanium. Titanium is biocompatible, and highly resistant to penetration by body fluids. Titanium is stronger than steel, but up to 45% lighter.

Header: The top portion of the ICD is called the header; it is made of a see–through epoxy. The header has ports, which the connector pins of the lead(s) are inserted. The lead is secured into the header with the setscrew.

Setscrews: The leads are connected seeurely to the ICD with a small screw to ensure electrical contact between the lead and the ICD. At implant, a small sterile screwdriver is packaged with the ICD.

Circuitry: The ICD contains complex micro-electronics (very small computer chips) that allows the ICD to process incoming signals, store information, and produce a response dependent on the signals that are processed. The microprocessors can

respond to programming instructions that allow for changes after implantation. The circuits contain both read only memory (ROM) and random access memory (RAM). Just as in new computers, the amount of RAM in new ICDs is increasing rapidly, allowing for increased diagnostic information to be stored.

Battery: The internal power source for the ICD is the battery. Most ICD batteries are made from lithium silver vanadium oxide. The battery longevity is close to 5 years for most ICDs. Battery depletion is monitored regularly at follow-up visits. Once the battery reaches the elective replacement indicator (ERI), the entire ICD is replaced, not just the battery.

Capacitors: The ICD is able to generate enough energy to deliver a shock because the capacitors store an electrical charge. The capacitor is made of multiple conductors separated by insulators. Capacitors with high-voltage capabilities can charge up to 830 volts in order to deliver a high-energy shock. It can take up to 15 seconds for the device to fully charge to the highest energy level, usually around 35 joules.

(Ellenbogen, K. A. & Wood, H. A. [2002]. *St. Jude Medical What's inside an ICD?*)

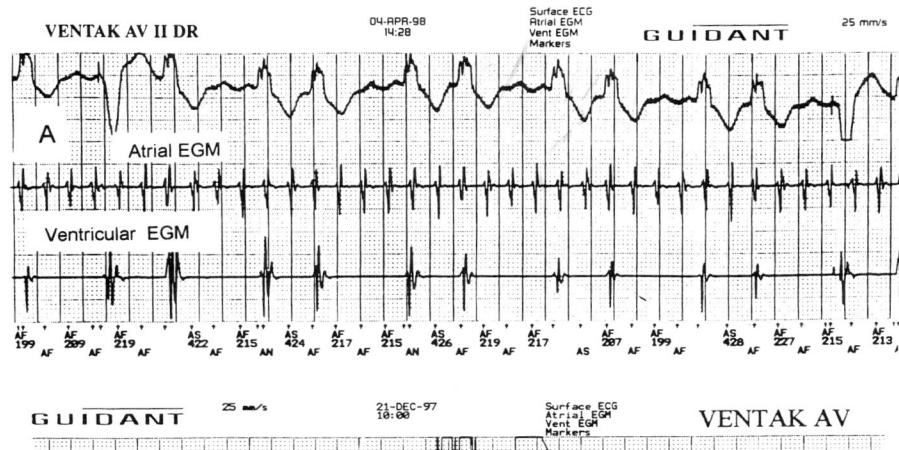

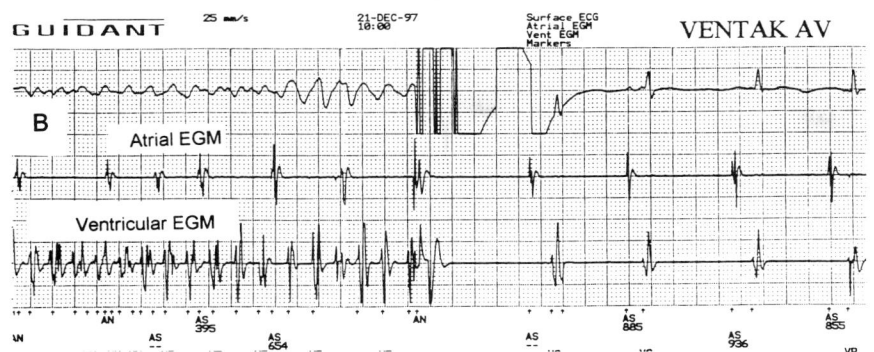

■ **Figure 32–37.** ICD. Panel *A* shows tracing of atrial fibrillation (AF); the atrial electrogram (EGM) shows the rapid atrial response of AF and the much slower ventricular response. Panel *B* shows a tracing of induced ventricular fibrillation VF with the ventricular rate being much faster than the atrial rate. (Marker annotation for Guidant AV II DR ICD; AF = atrial fibrillation, AS = atrial sense, AN = atrial noise, VF = ventricular fibrillation, VN = ventricular noise, VP = ventricular pace.)

signal processing to measure each beat and defines the rhythm as wide or narrow on the basis of its intracardiac morphology. If the R wave is narrow, the ICD classifies the tachycardia as sinus. If the R wave is wide, the ICD treats the tachycardia as VT. Electrogram width should be used cautiously or avoided in patients with a bundle-branch block or surface QRS width that exceeds 100 milliseconds (Hayes et al., 2000). Patients who have had inappropriate shocks for SVT should have detection enhancements programmed on (Hayes et al., 2002).

The Wavelet Dynamic Discrimination Criterion, known as "Wavelet," is a new SVT discrimination algorithm in Medtronic Marquis VR ICD. Wavelet is an electrogram template algorithm that automatically compares the morphology of tachycardia to the morphology of normal sinus beats. If the morphology is similar to the normal beat, the tachycardia would be classified as SVT. However, if the morphology of the tachycardia differs from the normal beat, then the tachycardia is classified as VT/VF. The Wavelet will replace EGM width on all new Medtronic single-chamber ICDs (Medtronic, 2002).

Dual-chamber ICDs have additional detection enhancements. Guidant devices have two additional programmable detection enhancements: (1) V rate greater than A rate and (2) atrial fibrillation rate threshold. Both of these detections work with stability and onset and are only applied in the VT zone. The V rate greater than A rate is based on the premise of AV dissociation and can only be VT. When V rate greater than A rate is programmed "on" and a VT occurs, other therapy inhibitors are bypassed and the ICD delivers therapy immediately. The AF rate threshold increases specificity by confirming AF from the atrial electrograms and withholding therapy for irregular ventricular rhythms.

Medtronic devices have PR logic pattern and rate analysis for SVT detection. The algorithm uses rate cut-off and stability and then applies PR logic to further categorize the arrhythmia. PR logic has three programmable parameters: (1) atrial fibrillation/atrial flutter; (2) sinus tachycardia; and (3) other 1:1 SVTs; each parameter must be programmed "on" or "off." Once tachycardia is detected, the PR logic algorithm uses six elements in identification of VT versus SVT. The algorithm relies on rate (atrial and ventricular), pattern, regularity, AV dissociation, far-field R wave, and AF evidence (Hayes et al., 2000).

Modes of Operation

Implantable cardioverter defibrillators can be programmed to detect one to three zones, one zone for VF and two different zones for VT. Therapies are programmed according to the detection zone. ICDs offer different types of tachyarrhythmia therapy depending on the manufacturer, including burst pacing, adaptive burst pacing or ramp pacing, incremental/decremental bursts, low-energy cardioversion, and defibrillation. Different zones allow the ICD to be programmed in a tiered or staged-therapy approach, allowing for maximum safety in the VF zone and less aggressive and less painful therapies in the VT zones. In addition to VT/VF therapy, the ICD has pacing abilities. Depending on the ICD system implanted, VVI pacing or DDDR pacing with mode switching is available (Hayes et al., 2000).

All ICDs have a magnet mode, a feature that is activated when a magnet is placed over the pulse generator. Magnet modes allow for therapy to be suppressed in emergency situations when the patient is receiving inappropriate shocks. Some

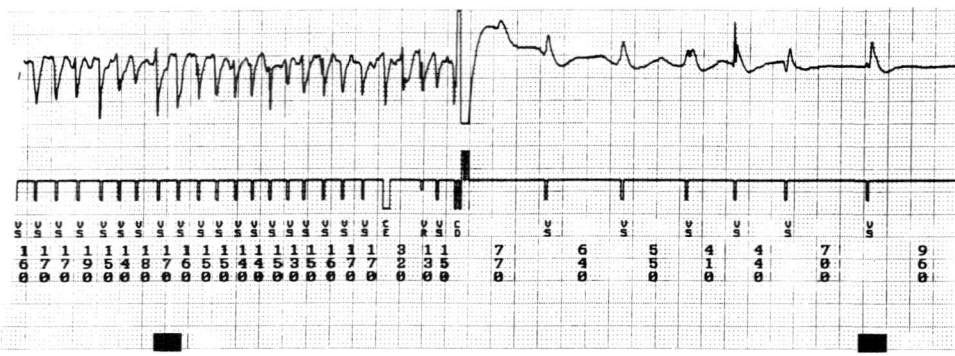

```
SUMMARY
-------
  Type:                           VF
  Average Cycle(ms):              160
  Last Therapy:                   VF  Rx 1, Successful
  Duration:                       11 sec

DETECTION SETTINGS
------------------
  Detection Intervals(ms): VF=310        VT=400
  NID Initial:             VF=18         VT=16
  NID Redetect:            VF=12         VT=12

  Stability:               ON
  Onset:                   OFF
```

■ **Figure 32–38.** ICD. Electrogram tracing showing an episode of VF that is detected and successfully converted with a 33 J shock. Total duration 11 seconds. Device summary shows that device is set as a two-zone device with the VT zone at 400 ms (150 bpm) and the VF zone set at 310 ms (194 bpm). The arrhythmia was rapid—140–170 ms (400bpm–VF); therefore, it was detected and treated in the VF zone.

generators emit audible tones when a magnet is placed over the unit. Some of the newer devices offer the option of programming the device temporarily to inhibit therapy, or turn off therapies with magnet application. ICDs also provide noninvasive EPS capabilities that help confirm the inducibility of the patient's clinical arrhythmia and evaluate the effectiveness of various therapies.

All newer devices have memory and electrogram storage capability. The ICD continuously stores parameter setting, device status, and significant information about the patient's arrhythmia. When the ICD programmer retrieves the data, it summarizes the data for display and printout. For each episode, up to maximum storage capacity, the ICD stores the ventricular electrogram for the single-chamber devices and stores atrial and ventricular electrograms for the dual-chamber devices. The ability to review stored electrograms from an episode has been especially helpful in differentiating between appropriate and inappropriate shocks. Once a cause has been determined, optimal programming can be performed to help eliminate inappropriate shocks (Groh et al., 1998; Hayes et al., 2000).

Ventricular Fibrillation Therapy

Implantable cardioverter defibrillators use defibrillation as the sole therapy option for arrhythmias in the VF zone (Fig. 32-38). Programming of the shock energy is based on DFT testing. The DFT is the minimum effective energy required to defibrillate the heart. To ensure that the ICD is effective, ICD shocks must be programmed above the DFT. Historically, a safety margin of 10 joules (J) has been used; therefore, the first therapy is usually set between 20 and 34 J in the VF zone (Hayes, et al., 2000). The ICD reconfirms that the patient is still in VF before delivering the first shock. If the patient has returned to sinus rhythm during the charging time, the first VF therapy is aborted. The ICD attempts to deliver a synchronized shock to the R wave if at all possible.

Ventricular Tachycardia Therapy

In contrast to treating arrhythmias in the VF zone, there are many more options when the ICD is programmed in the VT zone. Each VT episode can be treated with multiple therapies and is often treated in a step-wise fashion. The first therapy is often ATP, followed by low-energy cardioversion and, finally, by defibrillation if necessary to terminate the episode (O'Callaghan & Ruskin, 1998). Most sustained monomorphic VTs are caused by reentry and can be terminated by a timed pacing sequence. Pacing at a faster rate than the VT increases the probability of VT termination. ATP offers the patient the ability to terminate a tachycardia without a shock. ATP has shown to be effective in terminating VT 90% of the time when the heart rate is less than 188 bpm, and 89% effective when the VT rate is between 188 and 250 bpm (Wathen et al., 2001). The downside of ATP is the risk of acceleration to a faster rhythm. That is the reason shocks are necessary in the VT zone, as shown in Figure 32-39. Wathen et al. reported a 4% chance of VT acceleration with the use of ATP for fast VT, with

Parameter Summary

Type	Detection		Rx1	Rx2	Rx3	Rx4	Rx5	Rx6
VF	On	200-500 bpm	15 J	30 J	30 J	30 J	30 J	30 J
FVT	via VT	176-200 bpm	Ramp(3)	5 J	20 J	30 J	30 J	30 J
VT	On	109-200 bpm	Ramp(3)	10 J	30 J	30 J	30 J	30 J

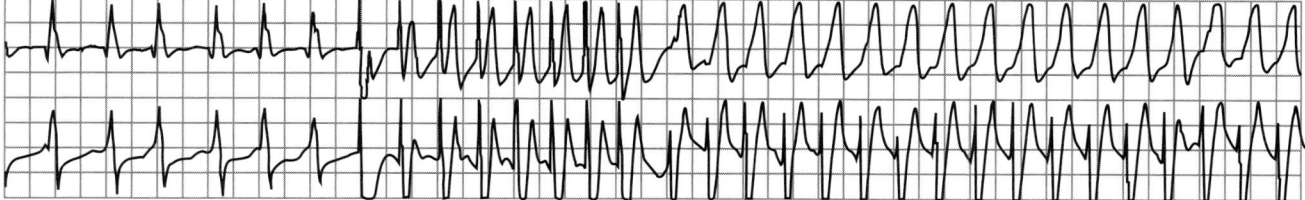

VT Detected in Slow VT Zone Ramp pacing for 8 beats accelerates VT to VF zone (HR > 200)

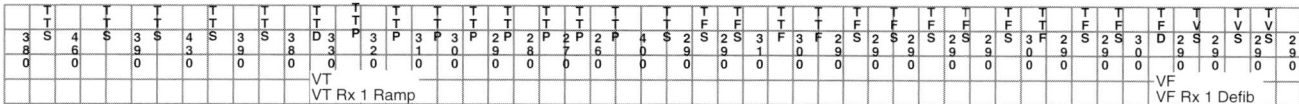

Ventricular EGM
Farfield recording (HVA to HVB)

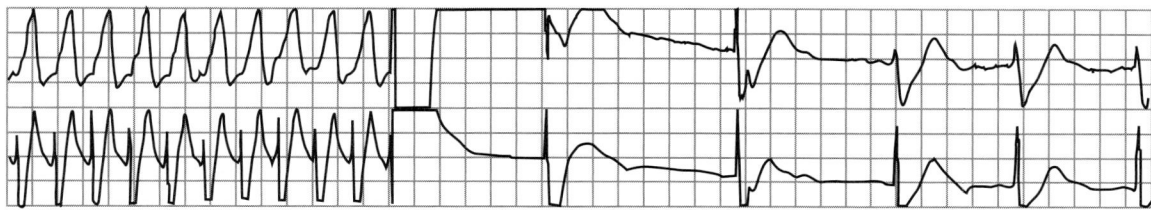

Ventricular EGM
Nearfield recording (Vtip to Vring)

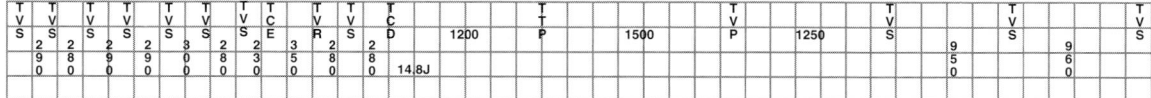

■ **Figure 32–39.** ICD. Electrogram printout from a Medtronic Gem III VR model 7231, showing an onset of slow VT. The ICD appropriately detected the VT and attempted to Ramp pace to SR; however, the pacing accelerated the rhythm to a rapid VT, requiring a 15-Joule cardioversion. Cardioversion therapies are included with ATP features for this reason.

syncope occurring in 2% of the patients. Reviewing stored electrograms confirm that the onset of arrhythmias is primarily VT; when 1100 episodes were reviewed, 97% started as VT. VF as the onset arrhythmia occurred only 3% of the time (Wathen et al., 2001).

Anti-tachycardic pacing mode therapies can be set in the electrophysiology laboratory after VT has been induced and a specific ATP therapy has been proven successful in terminating the tachycardia. Another approach is programming the ICD empirically, modifying it if needed, after the patient has a spontaneous VT event (O'Callaghan & Ruskin, 1998; Wathen et al., 2001). A variety of pacing modes can be used to terminate the tachycardia. Each manufacturer has a slightly different approach to programming ATP. A common form of ATP is burst pacing, in which a group of paced beats is delivered at equal or fixed-cycle intervals that exceed the rate of the tachycardia. The number of beats in each burst and the number of burst sequences are programmed and vary from device to device. Adaptive bursts, also called *ramp pacing,* is another frequently used ATP method. A ramp sequence consists of a set of pulses delivered at decreasing intervals to treat a detected episode of VT. Incremental/decremental bursts are another form of burst pacing in which the bursts alternate between incremental and decremental cycle lengths (O'Callaghan & Ruskin, 1998).

Low-energy cardioversion is available on all devices and can be set as low as 0.1 J. The very-low-energy therapies are often determined by electrophysiology testing. Shocks that are under 2 J are much more comfortable for the patient and usually are perceived as small shocks (Davidson, et al., 1994). Low-energy shocks often are delivered after ATP therapy has failed but may also be programmed as the initial therapy to terminate the tachycardia. Another advantage of cardioversion is that it can be delivered more rapidly than repeated ATP sequences. If low-energy cardioversion is unsuccessful, a high-energy shock is delivered (O'Callaghan & Ruskin, 1998; Hayes et al., 2000).

Bradycardia Pacing

Bradycardia pacing (VVI) is a standard feature available on all ICDs. Dual-chamber pacing has become available as well, reducing the need for separate pacemaker implantation in pacemaker-dependent patients. Dual-chamber ICD systems are placed in approximately 40% of patients receiving ICDs (Gold, 2000). Pacing rate, hysteresis, sensitivity, pulse width, pulse amplitude, and blanking after pace are all programmable. In the dual-chamber device, atrial tachycardia rate and mode-switch capabilities can also be programmed. Pacing thresholds during VT and after defibrillation are usually higher than needed for bradycardia pacing, and they can be independently programmed in some of the devices.

Device Implantation

ICD implants are preferably implanted in the left pectoral region. The ICD in the unipolar system is known as the *active can* or *hot can*. There is more surface area covered with a shock when the system is placed on the left side and the current travels from the right ventricle to the active can on the left side. The lead is inserted in either the subclavian vein or the cephalic vein and advanced to the right ventricular apex, using techniques similar to those for permanent pacemaker implantation. Defibrillation testing is completed once the lead is in place and secured. Delivering a small shock, approximately 1 joule, to the vulnerable part of the T wave induces VF. Induction of VF is necessary to test whether the ICD can detect the fine fibrillatory waves of VF and if the programmed energy level of the ICD can convert the VF to sinus rhythm. If the first shock fails, a second shock at maximum output is delivered. If the second shock fails, a 360-J external shock is delivered. The ICD is implanted only if sensing during sinus rhythm and VF is acceptable, if pacing thresholds and impedances are within normal limits, and if an adequate safety margin is demonstrated by DFT testing (Singer, 1997). With the current unipolar pectoral ICDs and biphasic waveform, it is very rare for implant criteria not to be met (Singer, 1997; Hayes et al., 2000). The ICD may be implanted in the electrophysiology laboratory, catheterization laboratory, or operating room. Anesthesia can be local or general, and the device can be placed subcutaneously or submuscularly (O'Callaghan & Ruskin, 1997). Most patients with an ICD placed transvenously in the pectoral position are discharged on the day after surgery. A postimplantation noninvasive study is often performed before discharge to verify proper functioning of the device and to "fine-tune" the device programming (Wolbrette & Naccarelli, 2001).

Complications

Postoperative complications have been reduced with the advent of the transvenous pectoral technique for ICD implantation. Complications after implantation resemble those observed with permanent pacemaker implantation (Hayes et al., 2000). Potential complications of ICD implantation are listed in Display 32-8. One of the most serious complications is infection of the ICD system. Removal of the entire ICD system is mandatory, and a long course of antibiotics is necessary. Surgical

---

DISPLAY 32–8

POTENTIAL COMPLICATIONS OF IMPLANTABLE CARDIOVERTER-DEFIBRILLATOR

Adverse Events Associated With Surgery

Subclavian stick complications
  Pneumothorax
  Hemothorax
  Air embolism
  Subclavian artery puncture
Bleeding
Right ventricular perforation
Thromboemboli
Venous occlusion
Pericardial effusion/tamponade
Pocket hematoma
Hypotension—hemodynamic compromise
Cerebrovascular accident
Proarrhythmia

Adverse Events After System In Place

System related
  Lead dislodgement
  Loose setscrew
  Lead fracture
  Lead insulation defect
  Exit block
  Premature battery depletion
Chronic nerve damage
Diaphragmatic stimulation
Erosion of pulse generator
Fluid accumulation/seroma
Infection of the pocket/system
Keloid formation
Venous thromboembolism
Endocarditis

---

revision of the ICD system may be necessary after lead dislodgment in the early recovery period (24 to 72 hours) or lead fracture, which is seen in long-term follow-up. Lead-related problems have been reported to occur in 5.8% to 7.8% of patients with transvenous ICD implants (Lawton, et al., 1996).

Electromagnetic interference can result in inappropriate discharge or inhibition of the ICD. These problems can be temporary or permanent (O'Callaghan & Ruskin, 1997). The delivery of inappropriate therapy can actually produce tachyarrhythmias. Sources of interference include, but are not limited to, electrocautery, diathermy, hydraulic shock-wave lithotripsy, current-carrying conductors, arc welders, electrical smelting furnaces, and radiofrequency transmitters such as radar, high-voltage systems, theft prevention equipment, and high-powered electromagnetic fields. Magnetic resonance imaging is contraindicated because it may cause permanent damage to the ICD. Inadvertent contact between the generator and magnets should be avoided because changes in the magnetic field may inactivate the pulse generator or cause erratic functioning (Hayes, et al., 2000). Tachyarrhythmia detection must be programmed *OFF* before subjecting the patient to procedures that induce strong EMI. If detections are turned OFF, the patient should be monitored.

CRITICAL CONCEPTS: ICDS AND MAGNETS

Magnets affect all ICDs. Magnets open the reed switch within the ICD, suspending detections or inhibiting therapy without a programmer. In an emergency place the magnet directly over the ICD if it needs deaetivated. *All* ICDs that are manufactured can be disabled while the magnet is applied.[*] Call to have the ICD checked with the programmer once the Magnet is removed. This will assure all settings have been returned to normal programmed parameters.

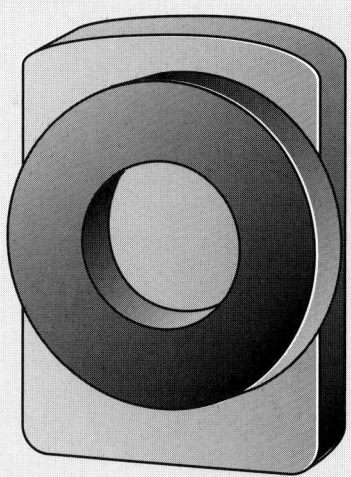

- Cautery and other sources of strong EMI can be interpreted as an arrhythmia leading to shocks.
- Placing a magnet over the ICD for surgical procedures is an excellent way to ensure patient safety. In the event of a dangerous arrhythmia during surgery removing the magnet will usually return the ICD to normal function, treating the arrhythmia. It may not be possible to place the magnet over the ICD for all surgeries (shoulder, neck, and chest) as the magnet would be in the sterile field, in that setting the ICD needs to be programmed off.
- Inappropriate shocks can occur with lead damage. The ICD detects the noise from the damaged lead as an arrhythmia and can deliver multiple inappropriate shocks.
- In the event of an inappropriate shock confirmed by ECG monitoring, a magnet should be placed over the ICD to prevent further shocks until the device can be turned off.
- A Magnet can be used to prevent further inappropriate shocks from rapid atrial fibrillation or SVT. Once it is determined that the patient is receiving shocks for atrial fib place a magnet over the ICD until the fast rates are controlled, or the ICD is programmed to detect the atrial arrhythmia and withhold therapy.

[*]Magnet response is a programmable feature in *Guidant & St. Jude Devices.* Only on rare occasion would the ICD be programmed to ignore magnets, or permanently disable therapies. Biotronik, Ela. & Medtronic ICD's *always* suspend therapy when a magnet is applied; once the magnet is removed normal function returns. *Magnet information obtained by personal communication of all ICD company technical service departments, listed above.* (Medtronic Magnet Image courtesy of Medtronic, Inc.)

Once the procedure is completed, the ICD should be reprogrammed to the active mode. Placing a magnet over the ICD will inactivate it temporarily in most cases (Display 32-9). This is actually a safer option for turning off the ICD. If a patient has a VT or VF episode, removing the magnet will allow the ICD to treat the arrhythmia. If the ICD were programmed off, it takes a programmer and extra time to reactivate the ICD, delaying treatment time of the arrhythmia. Close communication with the patient's implanting physician should be made before deactivating the ICD. This will help determine the best approach for deactivating the device (magnet vs. programmer).

Antiarrhythmic medications can result in complications by changing the appearance or rate of the arrhythmia or by altering the DFT. The arrhythmia rate also may be slowed below the cut-off rate so that the ICD fails to identify VT. Drugs could change the DFT, resulting in ineffective shocks. Amiodarone, for example, increases the threshold. Repeat EPS testing is often performed after the addition of class I or class III antiarrhythmic drugs (Hayes et al., 2000).

Standard Precautions

External Defibrillation

Implantable cardioverter defibrillators are designed to withstand external defibrillation. However, possible circuit damage or loss of output may occur if the external paddle is placed to close to the device. If at all possible, the anterior-posterior approach should be used for external paddle placement (Fig. 32-40). Direct defibrillation could cause permanent damage to the ICD or the implanted leads. Effectiveness of transthoracic defibrillation may also be affected by the implanted ICD system. Therefore, standard defibrillator protocols may need to be altered depending on the type of lead system used. If the patient has an older system with patches, paddle electrode placement should be perpendicular to an imaginary line drawn between the patches. The silicone rubber insulation on the back of the defibrillating patches effectively blocks current from passing through them (O'Callaghan, & Ruskin, 1997). After any external defibrillation, the ICD should be interrogated and checked to ensure proper function.

Pacemaker Interaction

With the advent of dual-chamber ICDs, the problems with device interactions between separate systems has been eliminated. If a patient has an older-model ICD in place and requires a temporary or permanent pacemaker in conjunction with the ICD, special care is required. For those patients who may still have an older system in place, unipolar pacemakers are contraindicated because the larger pacing pulse associated with unipolar lead systems may be mistaken by the ICD for the

Anterior-Apex   Anterior-Posterior

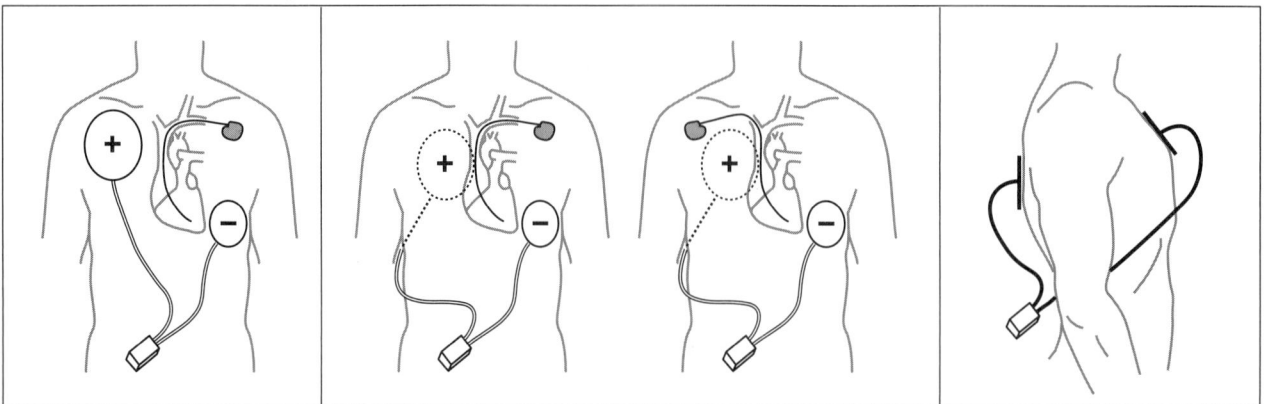

■ **Figure 32–40.** ICD. For external cardioversion or defibrillation, the paddles should be positioned in the anterior-posterior position if at all possible. Ideally the external paddles should be kept 4–6 inches away from the pulse generator. When the patient has a device in the left pectoral region, the anterior-apex position is acceptable.

patient's intrinsic rhythm (Gold, 2000). Three unique complications have been observed in patients with *both* a permanent pacemaker and an ICD: (1) failure of the ICD to detect and treat VT/VF, as the ICD is counting pacer spikes only; (2) double counting of pacing spikes and QRS complexes, because the ICD thinks it is seeing VT and delivers a discharge; and (3) misinterpretation of ST segment elevation as a sinusoid pattern, resulting in discharge. To avoid potential complications with older-generation ICDs, single-chamber pacemakers with bipolar leads and lower voltages have been used (Hayes et al., 2000).

Preoperative and Postoperative Nursing Care

Consideration of the emotional response of the patient and family to the ICD is an important part of nursing care. Before surgery, an assessment of the patient's (and family's) knowledge level, support systems, and usual coping mechanisms should be made. Patients may have a high anxiety level because of categorization as a high-risk patient, EPS, impending surgery, and the ICD unit. Anxiety may be reduced through provision of competent care, education, and permission to express feelings.

Patient education is very important. The patient should understand why the ICD is recommended and how it functions. ICD system models and patient education videotapes are available from the ICD manufacturers and are useful tools in providing visual and general information (Shaffer, 2002). The surgical procedure, where the ICD is placed, and the need to restrict overhead arm movements after surgery should be reviewed with the patient. The patient and family members should also understand that the ICD does not prevent arrhythmias from occurring, but is there to correct the arrhythmia.

After the ICD is implanted, anxiety is common. As many as 87.5% of patients were reported to experience increased symptoms of anxiety by Sears and colleagues. Other psychosocial concerns reported are feelings of powerlessness and a component of

depression or sadness (Sears, 1999; Dougherty, 1995). The majority of patients generally accept the ICD. Quality of life may temporarily decline in the first 6 months, but by 12 months returns to pre-implant levels (May et al, 1995). In heart failure patients with the addition of CRT, in conjunction with their ICD, quality of life may significantly improve (Abraham et al., 2002).

Postoperative care of the patient with an ICD is similar to the care of the patient after permanent pacemaker implantation. The patient should be informed that mild or moderate pain will be felt at the incision site. The patient's pain level and the incision site should be assessed and pain medications administered as needed. The patient should be instructed to minimize arm movements for the first 24 hours after implantation. Discharge instructions are an important aspect of postoperative nursing care. With transvenous ICD implants, hospital stays are much shorter, which limits the time available to teach patients. Written discharge instructions should be supplied to the patient and should include instructions about pain management, site assessment and care, what to do in the event of receiving a shock, when to notify the physician, the importance of carrying proper identification that allows medical personnel quickly to check the ICD with the correct programmer, avoiding magnetic fields, and cardiopulmonary resuscitation, as well as information regarding support groups (Wolbrette & Naccarelli, 2001) (Display 32-10).

Instructions regarding ICD discharges should be thoroughly reviewed and understood, because at least one spontaneous discharge occurs in approximately 50% of patients during the first year after receiving an ICD (Bocker et al., 1993). With ICD discharges, the patient will often have a sensation of their arrhythmia and wait for the ICD to deliver therapy. Patient perceptions of the discharge vary from none to very painful. The ICD shock is often described as a feeling of being punched in the chest or kicked by a horse (Thomas et al., 2001). Patients with VF or a rapid VT may experience a syncopal event by the time the generator discharges (Wathen et al., 2001). Routine emergency protocols should be administered as

PATIENT DISCHARGE INSTRUCTION SHEET FOR IMPLANTABLE CARDIOVERTER DEFIBRILLATOR (ICD)

Topic	Instruction/Information
Site care	• Keep site dry for 4 days. • Change dressing daily. • Report drainage, redness, swelling, and symptoms of infection to your doctor.
Activity restriction	• Avoid lifting arm on ICD side overhead, and no lifting with that arm until approved by your doctor. • Avoid pushing, pulling, or twisting. • Discuss resuming sexual activity with your doctor. Most patient resume sexual activity when their incisions heal.
Driving	• No driving until your doctor gives his approval.
ICD discharges	• If you get a shock, call your doctor immediately.
Your ICD will shock for fast rate>	• If you get a shock, and do not feel well, call 911. • If you get two or more shocks, call 911.
The pacemaker in your ICD will pace for slow rate <	
ICD identification	• Always carry your ICD identification card with you. Use the temporary card for now; your ICD Company will mail you a permanent one. • It is advisable to wear a Medic Alert ID bracelet or necklace.
Medical information	• Keep a current list of the medication you take.
Magnetic fields	• Avoid large magnets and strong electromagnetic fields. • Review your patient booklet about EMI. • You cannot have a magnetic resonance imaging scan (MRI). • Always tell medical personnel that you have an ICD. Your ICD will need to be turned off for some medical procedures.
CPR	• In the event of future emergencies, family members should learn CPR.
Emergency numbers	• Doctor _____ • Family member _____

CPR, cardiopulmonary resuscitation; EMI, electromagnetic interference.

needed. People who touch the patient as the unit discharges will feel the shock, but it will not be dangerous (AHA, 2003).

Psychosocial Issues

Automobile Driving

Patients with an ICD who are SCD survivors may be restricted from driving for at least 6 months. The main concern is the risk of an arrhythmic event or the delivery of a shock while driving. The length of the driving restriction depends on where the patient resides and state/country regulations. Patients with ICDs are prohibited from driving commercially. Driving restrictions can cause feelings of isolation, anger, and loss of autonomy, because driving is an important part of maintaining independence (Cambre & Sullivan, 1993). It is important for the patient to realize that the symptoms are associated with ventricular arrhythmias, not the ICD, which makes driving potentially dangerous. After 6 months, if the patient has not had an ICD discharge, he or she may resume noncommercial driving. Patients who have had their ICD placed for prophylactic reasons and have not had a documented spontaneous episode of ventricular tachyarrhythmia should not be prohibited from driving (O'Callaghan & Ruskin, 1997; Hayes et al., 2000).

All patients should be restricted from driving for the first 1 to 2 weeks after an initial implant or revision, until the site is healed. Patients may report discomfort with using a seatbelt, because the shoulder strap comes across the ICD implant site for a driver with a left pectoral implant and for a passenger with a right pectoral implant. Seatbelt shoulder protectors are recommended and can be found in stores selling auto parts. Simple padding can also be placed over the ICD. Patients should be encouraged to continue using seatbelts.

Quality of Life

Implantable cardioverter defibrillator therapy may be the primary treatment for life-threatening ventricular arrhythmias, but its impact on quality of life should be considered. Factors that affect quality of life include frequent or inappropriate shocks, device malfunction, or product recall (Thomas et al., 2001; Sneed et al., 1994). Sometimes, patients may think that they have received a shock, but when the ICD is interrogated, there is no record that a discharge has occurred. This phenomenon is known as a *phantom shock*. Phantom shocks are fairly common, often occurring as the patient is drifting off to sleep and more commonly in patients with previous ICD discharges (Hayes et al., 2000). It is important to spend time reassuring the patient and family and reviewing the interrogated follow-up

Initial Report

ICD Model: Gem 7227   Serial Number: PIP106863H   Date of Visit: Jun 02, 2003

Quick Look

ICD and Lead Information

ICD	Medtronic		Gem 7227		PIP106863H		

ICD Status

Battery Voltage (ERI=2.55 V, EOL=2.40 V)				2.57 V		Jun 02, 2003	
Last Full Energy Charge				14.32 sec		May 31, 2003	
Last Capacitor Formation (Interval=1 month)						May 31, 2003	

Lead Performance   Ventricular

Pacing Impedance				349 ohms		Jun 02, 2003	
Defibrilltation (HVB) Impedance				12 ohms		Jun 02, 2003	

Parameter Summary

Type	Detection		Rx1	Rx2	Rx3	Rx4	Rx5	Rx6
VF	On	188-500 bpm	30 J	35 J	35 J	35 J	35 J	35 J
FVT	via VF	188-231 bpm	Burst(3)	35 J	35 J	35 J	35 J	35 J
VT	Off		Burst(4)	30 J	35 J	35 J	35 J	35 J

SVT Criteria On: EGM Width, VT Stability

Modes   Rates

Mode	VVIR	Lower	60 ppm		
		Upper Sensor	120 ppm		

Lead Parameters   Ventricular

Amplitude			3 V		
Pulse Width			0.3 ms		
Sensitivity			0.3 mV		

Clinical Status: Since May 09, 2003

Episodes		% Pacing			
VF	0	Sensed		1 %	
FVT	0	Paced		98 %	
VT	0				
SVT/NST	0				

Observations (2)

- Patient Alert triggered – Battery was 2.55 Volts.
- VT detection is Off but some VT therapies are On.

■ **Figure 32–41.** ICD. Quick Look Report from a Medtronic Gem 7227. Report shows battery at 2.57, on day of interrogation. The patient came in for follow-up because *Patient Alert Alarm* was triggered when battery dipped to 2.55. The alarm was programmed off, and the patient was scheduled for elective replacement of the ICD. Other information gleaned from Quick Look report: no episodes of VT, VF, or nonsustained events since last interrogated; 98% paced since last interrogated. Note VT detection is off—purposely programmed off; device prints out useful observations.

printouts with them. An ICD discharge can be frightening for both the patient and spouse, particularly if the shock occurs with sexual activity. The patient may need to have the tachycardia detection rate increased if sexual activity increases the heart rate enough to meet the detection criteria. Education and support regarding shocks should be provided to the patient. Professional counseling should be recommended for the patient and spouse with emotional concerns. Many implanting centers have ICD support groups that can be very helpful to the ICD recipient and family. The support group provides a forum for the patients to discuss their concerns and fears with one another and provides the nurse with an excellent opportunity for patient education (Shaffer, 2002).

If the patient has had multiple ICD discharges during an occurrence of an "ICD storm," in which they experience three or more shocks in a 24-hour period, they will most likely experience symptoms of anxiety. These patients should be reassured, but if symptoms persist, then referral to psychiatric specialists or the use of antidepressant or antianxiety drugs should be considered (Shaffer, 2002).

Follow-up Care

Regular ICD follow-up is necessary to assess the patient's clinical status, ICD battery status, and device function. Review of stored electrograms provides diagnostic information for treated episodes of tachyarrhythmias. In general, there are two components of the follow-up: (1) assessment of the patients status, reviewing the cardiovascular-medical condition of the patient as well as screening for medication changes and (2) the defibrillator and lead are assessed for normal device function (Hayes et al., 2000).

The ICD pulse generator is highly reliable but must be observed for battery status and charge times. When pulse generator defects do occur, they can be manifested by early battery depletion. Battery status is monitored at each follow-up visit (Fig. 32-41). If the device is close to its elective replacement indicator (ERI), more frequent visits may be required. Episode data are reviewed and compared with the patient's clinical symptoms. Stored electrograms provide trending information on the frequency and severity, if any, of spontaneous ventricular arrhythmias (see Display 32-11 for information regarding Internet follow-up).

The lead system is evaluated by testing lead impedance, completing pacing thresholds, and determining appropriate R-wave sensing. Evaluating the marker channel and real-time electrograms will identify appropriate R-wave sensing. Potential for lead problems can be identified if inappropriate sensing is noted. Chest radiographs should be used periodically for evaluation of system integrity (Hayes et al., 2000).

Episode data are reviewed and compared with the patient's clinical symptoms. Stored electrograms provide trending information on the frequency and severity, if any, of spontaneous ventricular arrhythmias.

Troubleshooting

Differentiating appropriate from inappropriate device function when a patient receives an ICD discharge or experiences symptoms such as syncope or palpitations can be challenging. Evaluation of a single ICD shock is usually performed in the outpatient clinic. Multiple successive shocks constitute a medical emergency and require a hospital admission for evaluation (Groh et al., 1998). The initial approach is to *identify* the problem, placing the problem in one of five categories: (1) appropriate therapy; (2) suspected inappropriate therapy; (3) failure to deliver therapy; (4) ineffective therapy; and (5) device deactivation. The second step is to *analyze* the problem by completing a full interrogation of the device to determine if the therapy was appropriate or inappropriate. The third step is

to use a *systematic approach* to determine the cause for device deactivation or failure (Singer, 1997).

Approximately 20% of patients with ICDs that use heart rate only as the detection criterion receive an inappropriate shock, most commonly from atrial fibrillation or sinus tachycardia (O'Callaghan & Ruskin, 1998; Singer, 1997). The newer devices that provide detection enhancement criteria can reduce this problem considerably. When stored electrograms are available, the appropriateness of ICD therapy can be checked immediately. The ICD also tracks nonsustained episodes, allowing the health care provider to know the frequency and severity of arrhythmias.

If the patient is receiving multiple ICD discharges and not having clinical symptoms, then dislodged lead, fractured lead, or double counting of QRS and T waves should be suspected. The patient should be instructed to call emergency medical services for transport to the hospital if having multiple shocks. When electrograms are available, interrogation of ICD can confirm fractured lead artifact (Fig. 32-42). In an emergency situation, placing a large ICD/pacemaker magnet over the

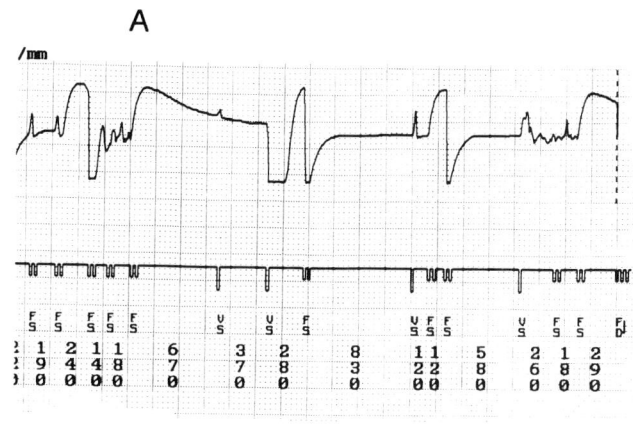

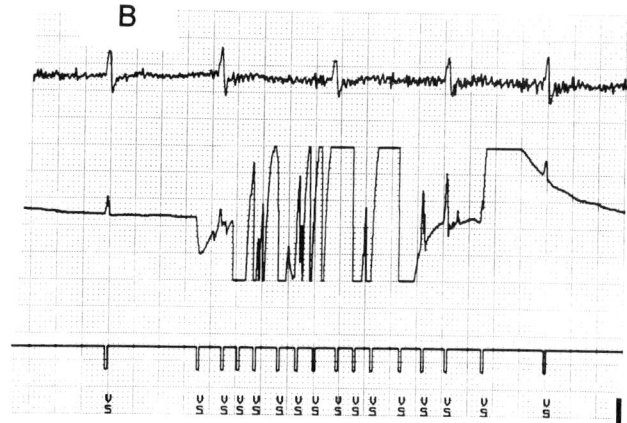

■ **Figure 32–42.** ICD. Electrogram tracings showing artifact from fractured lead. Panel *A* shows intracardiac signal from stored electrograms, artifact signals and irregular cycle length confirm fracture. Panel *B* shows real-time recording while having patient move arm with detections suspended to reproduce artifact. This was from an older epicardial patch lead system and abdominal implant. The patient was admitted to hospital for placement of new ICD system. Marker annotation for Medtronic Jewel 7202: VS=ventricular sense, FS=fibrillation sense, FD=fibrillation detection–charge initiated.

ICD can deactivate the ICD, as mentioned. Magnets do not inhibit the bradycardia therapy that is programmed into the ICD. A chest radiograph may be able to provide information on lead fracture or insulation breaks and can diagnose a dislodged lead (Hayes et al., 2000; Groh et al., 1998).

Failure to deliver therapy is caused by failure to detect the arrhythmia. This could be caused by a sensitivity problem, a change in VT rate, deactivation of the device, or system failure. Inadvertent deactivation of the ICD is rare but potentially devastating (Hayes et al., 2000; Singer, 1997). The device could be inadvertently deactivated during a programming session. Therefore, a final interrogation with a printout should always be performed. Some ICDs (Guidant-CPI; St. Paul, MN) can be programmed to turn *off* after a magnet has been placed over the ICD for approximately 30 seconds. Rarely, exposure to a strong magnetic field results in deactivation. Battery depletion and circuit failure could be other causes of the ICD failing to deliver therapy.

Frequent and thorough follow-up care can help detect potential problems early, preventing devastating results. ICDs have become sophisticated and complex, providing information on patient activity, heart rate, frequency of arrhythmia, as well as ICD status. ICDs have continued to improve, enhancing patient safety and comfort.

CONCLUSION

Tremendous technological advances have been made in the ICD since first implanted in 1980. The ICD is no longer a simple shock box. With the introduction of dual-chamber ICDs, many new programmable features are available. The ICD provides high-energy shocking capabilities for VF, ATP features for VT, atrial therapies for atrial arrhythmias, and CRT for heart failure patients. Detection enhancements have improved dramatically. Inappropriate shocks have gone from common to rare. ICDs provide diagnostic data to assist the clinician in providing cardiac care to their patients. Diagnostic data such as activity levels, minimum and maximum heart rates, and heart rate variability monitor patient trends.

ICDs are not just for cardiac arrest survivors. They are being used as primary prevention in the postmyocardial infarction patient with decreased LV function. ICDs will become common in cardiac patients as the first-line defense in preventing sudden death. Health care providers must become comfortable with the ICD and its capabilities and limitations.

REFERENCES FOR PACEMAKERS

Abraham, W. T., Fisher, W. G., Smith, A. L., et al. for the MIRACLE Study Group (2002). Cardiac resynchronization in chronic heart failure. *New England Journal of Medicine, 346,* 1845–1853.

Abraham, W. T. (2002). Cardiac resynchronization therapy for heart failure: biventricular pacing and beyond. *Current Opinion in Cardiology,* 17(4), 346–352.

Atlee, J. L., & Bernstein, A. D. (2001). Cardiac rhythm management devices (Part I): indications, device selection, and function. *Anesthesiology,* 95(5), 1265–1280.

Atlee, J. L., & Bernstein, A. D. (2001). Cardiac rhythm management devices (Part II): Perioperative management. *Anesthesiology,* 95(6), 1492–1506.

Barold, S. S. (1997). Complications of pacemaker implantation and troubleshooting. In I. Singer (Ed.), *Interventional electrophysiology.* Baltimore: Williams & Wilkins, 935–1054.

Bernstein, A. D., Camm, A. J., Fletcher, R. D., et al. (1987). The NASPE/BPEG generic pacemaker code for antibradyarrhythmia and adaptive-rate pacing and antitachyarrhythmia devices. *Pacing and Clinical Electrophysiology,* 10, 794.

Bourke, M. E., & Healey, J. S. (2002). Pacemakers, recent directions and developments. *Current Opinion in Anaesthesiology,* 15(6), 681–686.

Cazeau, S., Ritter, P., Lazarus, A., Gras, D., Mabo, P., Daubert, J. C., & Jugica, J. (1998). Multisite pacing for heart failure. In S. S. Barold & J. Mugica (Eds.), *Recent advances in cardiac pacing* (pp. 81–88). Armonk, NY: Futura Publishing Company.

Daubert, J. C., D'allonnes, G. R., Pavin, D., & Mabo, P. (2000). Prevention of atrial fibrillation by pacing. In I. E. Ovsyshcher (Ed.), *Cardiac arrhythmias and device therapy: Results and perspectives for the new century* (pp. 155–166). Armonk, NY: Futura Publishing Co.

Daubert, J. C., Leclercq, C., Alonso, C., & Cazeau, S. S. (2000). Long-term experience with biventricular pacing in refractory heart failure. In I. E. Ovsyshcher (Ed.), *Cardiac arrhythmias and device therapy: Results and perspectives for the new century* (pp. 385–392). Armonk, NY: Futura Publishing Co.

Daubert, J. C., Leclercq, C., Pavin, D., & Mabo, P. (1998). Pacing therapy in congestive heart failure: present status and new perspectives. In S. S. Barold, & J. Mugica (Eds.), *Recent advances in cardiac pacing* (pp. 50–80). Armonk, NY: Futura Publishing Company.

Fananapazir, L., Atiga, W., Tripodi, D., Steele, S., & McAreavey, D. (1998). Obstructive hypertrophic cardiomyopathy: therapeutic options. In S. S. Barold, & J. Mugica (Eds.), *Recent advances in cardiac pacing* (pp. 35–50). Armonk, NY: Futura Publishing Company.

Furman, S., Hayes, D. L., & Holmes, D. R. (1989). *A practice of cardiac pacing* (2nd ed.). Armonk, NY: Futura Publishing Co.

Garrigue, S., Bordier, P., Jais, P., et al. (2002). Benefit of atrial pacing in sleep apnea syndromes. *New England Journal of Medicine,* 412.

Gibbons, R. J., Antman, E. M., & Task Force on Practice Guidelines (ACC/AHA/NASPE Committee on Pacemaker Implantation) (2002). ACC/AHA/NASPE 2002 Guideline Update for Implantation of Cardiac Pacemakers and Antiarrhythmia Devices. [On-line]. Available at www.acc.org, www.americanheart.org, or www.naspe.org.

Gilligan, D. M., Morillo, C. A., Wood, M. A., & Ellenbogen, K. A. (1998). Hemodynamics of pacing: new aspects and unresolved issues. In S. S. Barold, & J. Mugica (Eds.), *Recent advances in cardiac pacing* (pp. 3–34). Armonk, NY: Futura Publishing Company.

Grubb, B. P. (1998). Permanent cardiac pacing: new and emerging indications other than cardiomyopathies. In S. S. Barold, & J. Mugica (Eds.), *Recent advances in cardiac pacing* (pp. 89–100). Armonk, NY: Futura Publishing Company.

Grubb, B. P. (1998). Update on new concepts in sensor technology for rate-adaptive pacing: base principles. In S. S. Barold, & J. Mugica (Eds.), *Recent advances in cardiac pacing* (pp. 283–294). Armonk, NY: Futura Publishing Company.

Hayes, D. L., & Friedman, P. A. (2000). Implantable device therapy for patients with hypertrophic cardiomyopathy. In I. E. Ovsyshcher (Ed.), *Cardiac arrhythmias and device therapy: Results and perspectives for the new century* (pp. 393–400). Armonk, NY: Futura Publishing Co.

Hayes, D. L., & Spittell, P. C. (1998). Thrombotic venous complications of permanent pacing. In S. S. Barold, & J. Mugica (Eds.), *Recent advances in cardiac pacing* (pp. 214–236). Armonk, NY: Futura Publishing Company.

Hayes, D. L., & Zipes, D. P. (2001). Cardiac pacemakers and cardioverter-defibrillators. In E. Braunwald, D. P. Zipes, & P. Libby (Eds.), *Heart disease* (6th ed., Vol. 1). Philadelphia: W.B. Saunders.

Isicoff, C. (1985). Understanding upper rate responses of DDD pacers. *Heart and Lung,* 14, 327–334.

Kusumoto, F. M., & Goldschlager, N. (1998). Unusual complications of cardiac pacing. In S. S. Barold, & J. Mugica (Eds.), *Recent advances in cardiac pacing* (pp. 237–282). Armonk, NY: Futura Publishing Company.

Luck, J., Wolbrette, D. L., Boehmer, J. P., Ulsh, P. J., Silber, D., & Nacarelli, G. V. (2002). Biventricular pacing in congestive heart failure: a boost toward finer living. *Current Opinion in Cardiology,* 17(1), 96–101.

Mitrani, R. D., Myerburg, R. J., & Castellanos, A. (2001) Cardiac pacemakers. In V. Fuster, R. W. Alexander, & R. A. O'Rourke (Eds.), *Hurst's the heart* (10th ed.). New York: McGraw-Hill.

Purcell, J. A., & Burrows, S. G. (1985). A pacemaker primer. *American Journal of Nursing, 85,* 553–568.

Saksena, S., Prakash, A., Madan, N., Giorgberidze, I., Munsif, A. N., Mathew, P., & Krol, R. B. (1998). Prevention of atrial fibrillation by pacing. In S. S. Barold, & J. Mugica (Eds.), *Recent advances in cardiac pacing* (pp. 101–114). Armonk, NY: Futura Publishing Company.

Shanker, A., & Saksena, S. (2001). Cardiac pacemakers. In P. J. Podrid, & P. R. Kowey (Eds.), *Cardiac arrhythmia: Mechanisms, diagnosis, and management* (2nd ed., pp. 323–356), Philadelphia: Lippincott Williams & Wilkins.

Spurrell, P., & Sulke, N. (2000). Pacing and defibrillation for the prevention and termination of atrial fibrillation. In I. E. Ovsyshcher (Ed.), *Cardiac arrhythmias and device therapy: Results and perspectives for the new century* (pp. 181–190). Armonk, NY: Futura Publishing Co.

St. Jude Medical & Cardiac Rhythm Management Division (originally Siemens Pacesetter). *Pacemaker technology for nurses and allied health professionals.* Sylmar, CA.

Sulzer Intermedics Educational Services (1998). *Concepts of permanent cardiac pacing.* Angleton, TX.

REFERENCES FOR IMPLANTABLE DEFIBRILLATORS

ACLS: Principles and Practice (2003). *ACLS reference textbook.* Dallas, TX:American Heart Association.

Abraham, W. T., Westby, F. G., Smith, A. L., et al. (2002). Cardiac resynchronization in chronic heart failure. *New England Journal of Medicine, 346,* 1845–1853.

The Antiarrhythmics vs. Implantable Defibrillators (AVID) Investigators (1997). A comparison of antiarrhythmic drug therapy with implantable defibrillators in patients resuscitated from near fatal ventricular arrhythmias. *New England Journal of Medicine, 337,* 1576–1583.

Bardy G. H., Johnson G., Poole J. E., et al. (1993). A simplified, single-lead unipolar transvenous cardioversion-defibrillation system. *Circulation* 88: 543–547.

Bass, E. B., Elson, J. J., Fogoros, R. N., et al. (1988). Long-term prognosis of patients undergoing electrophysiologic studies for syncope of unknown origin. *The American Journal of Cardiology, 62,* 1186–1191.

Bocker, D., Block. M., Isbruch, F., et al. (1993). Do patients with an implantable defibrillator live longer? *Journal of the American College of Cardiology, 21,* 1638–1644.

Cambre, S., & Silverman, M. E. (1993). Is it safe to drive with an automatic implantable cardioverter defibrillator or a history of recurrent symptomatic ventricular arrhythmias? *Heart Disease and Stroke, 2,* 179–181.

Cappato, R. (1999). Secondary prevention of sudden death: The Dutch Study, the Antiarrhythmic Versus Implantable Defibrillator Study. *American Journal of Cardiology, 83*(Suppl.), 68D–73D.

Cobb L. A., Baum R. S., Alvarez, H., et al. (1975). Resuscitation from out-of-hospital ventricular fibrillation: 4-year follow-up. *Circulation, 52*(Suppl. III), 23.

Connolly, S. J., Gent, M., Roberts, R. S. et al. (2000). Canadian Implantable Defibrillator Study (CIDS): a randomized trial of the implantable cardioverter defibrillator against amiodarone. *Circulation, 101,* 1297–1302.

Davidson T., Van Riper, S. Harper, P., et al. (1994). Implantable cardioverter defibrillators: A guide for clinicians. *Heart and Lung, 23,* 205–215.

Dougherty, C. M. (1995). Psychological reactions and family adjustment in shock versus no shock groups after implantation of internal cardioverter defibrillator. *Heart and Lung, 24,* 281–291.

Ellenbogen, K. A., & Wood, M. A. (2002). *Cardiac pacing and ICDs* (3rd ed.). Malden, Massachusetts: Blackwell Science Inc.

Engelstein, E. D. (2003). Prevention and management of chronic heart failure with electrical therapy. *American Journal of Cardiology, 91*(9A), 62–73.

Gold, M. R. (2000). ICD therapy in the new millennium. *Cardiology Clinics, 18,* No. 2, 375–389.

Gregoratos, G., Abrams, J., Epstein, A. E., et al. (2002). ACC/AHA/NASPE 2002 Guidelines for Implantation of Cardiac Pacemakers and Antiarrhythmia Devices: Summary Article: A report of the American College of Cardiology/American Heart Association Task Force on Practice Guidelines (ACC/AHA/NASPE Committee to update the 1998 Pacemaker Guidelines). *Circulation, 106,* 2145–2161.

Groh, W. J., Foreman, L. D., & Zipes, D. P. (1998). Advances in the treatment of arrhythmias: Implantable cardioverter-defibrillators. *American Family Physician, 57,* 297–307.

Harper, P. & VanRiper, S. (1993). Implantable cardioverter defibrillator: A patient education model for the illiterate patient. *Critical Care Nurse* 13(2), 55–59.

Hayes, D, L., Lloyd, M. A., & Friedman, P. A. (2000). *Cardiac pacing and defibrillation: A clinical approach.* Elmsford, NY: Blackwell Publishing Inc.

Kuck, K. H., Cappato, R., Siebels, J., et al. (2000). Randomized comparison of antiarrhythmic drug therapy with implantable defibrillators in patients resuscitated from cardiac arrest: the Cardiac Arrest Study Hamburg (CASH). *Circulation, 102,* 748–754.

Kuck, K. H., Cappato, R., & Siebels J. (1996). ICD therapy. In J. A. Camm (Ed.), *Clinical approaches to tachyarrhythmias* (pp. 1–69). New York: Futura Publishing Co.

Lawton, J. S., Wood, M. A., Gilligan, D. M., et al. (1996). Implantable transvenous cardioverter defibrillator leads: The dark side (Guest Editorial). *Pacing and Clinical Electrophysiology (PACE), 19,* 1273–1278.

Medtronic Inc. Wavelet Dynamic Discrimination Criterion in the Marquis VR ICD Model 7230. *Tachyarrhythmia Technical Concept Paper,* V, No. II, 1–4.

May, C. D., Smith, P. R., Murdock, C. J. & Davis, M. J. (1995). The impact of the implantable cardioverter defibrillator on the quality of life. *PACE—Pacing and Clinical Electrophysiology, 18,* 1411–1418.

Mirowski, M. (1985). The automatic implantable cardioverter-defibrillator: An overview. *American Journal of Cardiology, 6,* 461–466.

Mortensen, P. T., & Pedersen, K. A. (1997) An overview of the Ventak AV AICD European Clinical Review. *Guidant AICD Technology and Therapy Advances,* fall issue, 2–5.

Moss, A., Hall, J., Cannom, D. et al., for the Multicenter Automatic Defibrillator Implantation Trial. (1996) Improved survival with an implanted defibrillator in patients with coronary disease at high risk for ventricular arrhythmia. *New England Journal of Medicine, 335,*1933–1940.

Moss, A. J., Zareba, W., Hall, W. J., et al. (2002). Prophylactic implantation of a defibrillator in patients with myocardial infarction and reduced ejection fraction. *New England Journal of Medicine, 346,* No. 12, 877–883.

Myerburg, R. J., & Castellanos A. (1997). Cardiac arrest and sudden cardiac death. In E. Braunwald (Ed.), *Heart disease: A textbook of cardiovascular medicine* (5th ed., pp. 742–779). Philadelphia: WB Saunders.

O'Callaghan, P. & Ruskin, J. (1997). Current status of implantable cardioverter-defibrillators. *Current Problems in Cardiology, 22,* 645–707.

Sears, S. F., Conti, J. B., Curtis, A. et al. (1999). Affective distress and implantable cardioverter defibrillators: cases for psychological and behavioral interventions. *PACE—Pacing and Clinical Electrophysiology, 22,* 1831–1834.

Saksena, S., & Madan, N. (2002). Management of the patient with an implantable cardioverter-defibrillator in the third millennium. *Circulation, 106,* 2642–2646.

Shaffer, R. (2002). ICD therapy: The patient's perspective: The device saves lives by creates new psychosocial concerns for its recipients. *American Journal of Nursing, 102*(2), 4649.

Sneed, N. V., Finch, N. J., & Leman, R. B. (1994). The impact of device recall on patients and family members of patients with automatic implantable cardioverter defibrillators. *Heart and Lung, 23,* 317–322.

Singer, I. (1997). Defibrillation threshold testing and intraoperative ICD evaluation. In I. Singer (Ed.), *Interventional electrophysiology* (pp. 741–762). Baltimore: Williams & Wilkins.

St. Jude Medical. Patient educational information, Cardiac Rhythm Management Division: *What's inside and ICD?* Catalog no. J0086.

Thomas, S. A., Friedmann, E., Kelley, F. J., et al. (2001). Living with an implantable cardioverter-defibrillator: A review of the current literature related to psychosocial factors. *AACN Clinical Issues, 12,* 156–163.

Wathen, M. S., Sweeney, M. O., Degroot, P. J., et al. (2001). Shock reduction using antitachycardia pacing for spontaneous rapid ventricular tachycardia in patients with coronary artery disease. *Circulation, 104,* 796–801.

Wolbrette, D. L., & Naccarelli, G. V. (2001). Management of implantable cardioverter defibrillator patients: role of predischarge electrophysiologic testing and proper patient instruction before hospital discharge. *Current Opinion in Cardiology, 16*(1), 72–75.

Wolfe, D. A., Kosinski, D., & Grubb, B. P. (1998). Update on implantable cardioverter-defibrillators: New, safer devices have led to changes in indications. *Postgraduate Medicine, 103,* 115–130.

Zheng, Z. J., Croft, J. B, Giles, W. H., & Mensah, G. A. (2001). Sudden cardiac death in the United States, 1989-1998. *Circulation, 104,* 2158–2163.

Acquired Valvular Heart Disease

DENISE LEDOUX

DATABASE FOR NURSING MANAGEMENT

Definition, Classification, and Epidemiology

Valvular heart disease continues to be a common source of cardiac dysfunction and mortality. Competent cardiac valves maintain a unidirectional flow of blood through the heart as well as to the pulmonary and systemic circulations. Diseased cardiac valves that restrict the forward flow of blood because they are unable to open fully are referred to as *stenotic*. Stenotic valves elevate afterload and cause hypertrophy of the atria or ventricles pumping against the increased pressure. Cardiac valves that close incompetently and permit the backward flow of blood are referred to as *regurgitant, incompetent,* or *insufficient*. Regurgitant valves cause an elevated volume load and dilation of the cardiac chambers receiving the blood reflux. Valvular dysfunction may be primarily stenotic or regurgitant, or it is a "mixed" lesion, a valve that neither opens nor closes adequately. Valvular heart disease is usually described by the duration of the dysfunction (acute vs. chronic), the valves involved, and the nature of the valvular dysfunction (stenosis, insufficiency, or a combination of stenosis and insufficiency). The degree of cardiac dysfunction is defined by the New York Heart Association's (NYHA) Functional and Therapeutic Classification. Acquired valvular heart disease most commonly affects, and is most symptomatic with, the aortic and mitral valves. This chapter focuses on the mitral and aortic valves, with a brief discussion of tricuspid valve disease. Because the cause of pulmonic disease is primarily congenital, it is not presented (see Chapter 35).

Causes of Acquired Valvular Heart Disease

Rheumatic Heart Disease

Rheumatic fever is the most commonly acquired cause of valvular heart disease in childhood (Khan, 1996). Tissues involved in rheumatic fever include the lining and valves of the heart, skin, and connective tissue (Fig. 33-1). Rheumatic fever results as a complication of group A streptococcal upper respiratory tract infections, occurring in approximately 3% of those with streptococcal pharyngitis 2 to 3 weeks after acute rheumatic fever. Rheumatic fever is an acute systemic, inflammatory disease that occurs as a response to streptococcal infections (Bhola & Gill, 2001). Group A streptococcal throat infection is responsible for initial and recurrent attacks of rheumatic fever. Lymphatic channels from the tonsils are thought to transmit group A streptococci to the heart.

Although acute rheumatic fever is still common in other countries, it has declined in frequency in the United States since mid century, even though there is a persistently high frequency of streptococcal pharyngitis (Burge & DeHoratius, 1993). Reasons for the decline in rheumatic fever include the use of antibiotics to treat and prevent streptococcal infections, as well as improved social conditions such as decreased crowding, better housing and sanitation, and access to health care. Rheumatic fever persists in underdeveloped countries in which socioeconomic conditions enable the spread of streptococcal bacteria and limit access to adequate health care.

Acute rheumatic fever involves diffuse exudative and proliferative inflammatory reactions in the heart, joints, and skin. Major diagnostic criteria include carditis, polyarthritis, chorea, subcutaneous nodules, and erythema marginatum (pink, circinate skin rash). Manifestations with minor diagnostic importance include arthralgias, fever, acute-phase reactants in the blood (C-reactive protein), elevated erythrocyte sedimentation rate, and a prolonged PR interval on the electrocardiogram (Kaplan, 1998).

Carditis is the most important clinical manifestation of acute rheumatic fever, causing inflammation of the endocardium, myocardium, and pericardium. Myocarditis is characterized by interstitial inflammation that may affect cardiac conduction. Pericardial inflammation may result in a fibrinous exudate and small to moderate amounts of serous fluid in the pericardial sac (Abraham et al., 1991). Endocarditis causes extensive inflammatory changes, resulting in scarring of the heart valves and acute heart failure. Warty lesions of eosinophilic material build-up at the bases and edges of the valves. As the lesions progress, granulation tissue and subsequent vascularization develop, and fibrosis occurs. The annulus, cusps, and chordae tendineae are scarred and, as a

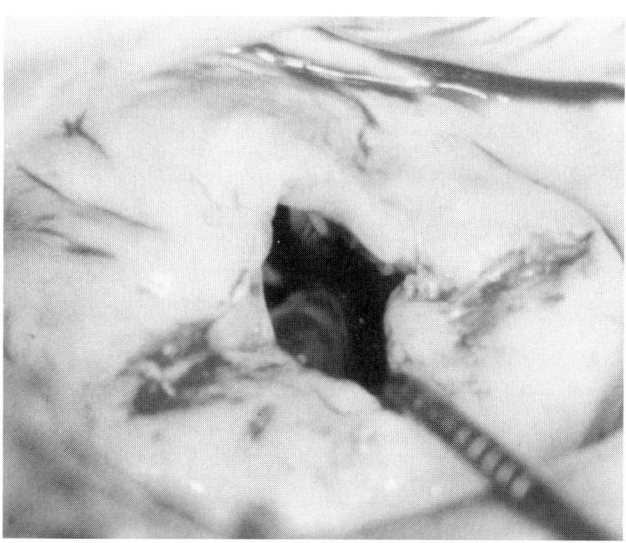

■ **Figure 33–1.** Rheumatic mitral valve with leaflet thickening and commissural fusion. (From Alpert, J. S., Sabick, J., & Cosgrove, D. M. [1998]. Mitral valve disease. In E. J. Topol , R. M. Califf, J. M. Isner et al. [Eds.], *Textbook of cardiovascular medicine* [p. 511]. Philadelphia: Lippincott-Raven.)

result, they thicken and shorten. Acute heart failure develops because of interstitial myocarditis. Fibrinoid degeneration develops, followed by the appearance of Aschoff nodules, the characteristic pathologic lesion of acute rheumatic fever. As Aschoff nodules heal, fibrous scars remain. In severe cases, death from acute heart failure may result. Carditis frequently does not cause any symptoms and is detected only when the patient seeks help because of arthritis or chorea.

Auscultatory signs of aortic and mitral insufficiency are frequently apparent. In more than 90% of patients with carditis, the mitral valve is affected. When the mitral valve is affected, there may be a high-pitched, blowing, pansystolic murmur. A Carey-Coombs murmur, a low-pitched, mid-diastolic murmur of short duration, may be noted at the apex. The Carey-Coombs murmur may be attributed to swelling and stiffening of mitral valve leaflets, increased flow across the valve, and alteration in left ventricular compliance. The regurgitation of the aortic valve results in diastolic murmurs, whereas involvement of the tricuspid valve is rarely appreciated during the acute phase (Abraham et al., 1991).

Rheumatic fever can be prevented by aggressive treatment of the initial episode of streptococcal pharyngitis: penicillin G, 500 mg as the first dose and then 250 mg four times daily for a duration of 10 days. If a patient is penicillin allergic, then clarithromycin 500 mg twice daily for 7 to 14 days or clindamycin 150 mg every 8 hours can be substituted (Khan, 1996).

Infective Endocarditis

Infective endocarditis is an endovascular infection that supports continuous bacteremia from the source of the infection, usually a vegetation on a heart valve (Towns & Reller, 2003). Although incidence of infective endocarditis is low, between 1.5 and 6 cases per 100 cases per year, morbidity and mortality are high (Sexton & Spelman, 2003). Rheumatic heart disease, as well as other cardiac lesions such as calcific aortic stenosis, hypertrophic cardiomyopathy, and congenital heart disease, and the presence of prosthetic heart valves predispose to endocarditis. Intravenous drug abusers are at risk for infective endocarditis caused by recurrent bacteremias related to injection from contaminated needles and localized infections at injection sites. Patients with long-term intravenous lines or dialysis catheters are also at increased risk. Acute endocarditis can also occur in normal heart valves from infection somewhere else in the body. In patients with community-acquired, native valve endocarditis, *Staphylococcus aureus* is the predominant cause of acute disease (Karchmer, 1998). Pathogens that are most commonly responsible for subacute endocarditis include streptococci, enterococci, coagulase-negative staphylococci, and the HACEK group of organisms (*Hemophilus* species, *Actinobacillus actinomycetemcomitans, Cardiobacterium hominis, Eikenella* species, and *Kingella kingae*). The *S. aureus* infecting intravenous drug users is frequently methicillin-resistant (Karchmer, 1998). Clinical presentations of endocarditis range from fever and malaise to symptoms related to systemic emboli (Table 33-1).

The pathologic process of endocarditis requires that several conditions exist to permit infection to grow in the heart and to promote an environment that supports growth on the endocardial surface. For endocarditis to occur, there must be: (1) endocardial surface injury; (2) thrombus formation at the site of injury; (3) bacteria in the circulation; and (4) bacterial adherence to the injured endocardial surface (Chan et al., 1993). The complications of infective endocarditis include congestive heart failure, paravalvular abscess formation, and embolic events to the brain or other organs, sepsis, pericarditis, renal failure, and metastatic abscesses (Sexton & Spelman, 2003). The reduction in mortality for infective endocarditis over the past 30 years from 25% to 30% down to 10% to 20% may be largely related to aggressive surgical intervention in cases complicated by congestive heart failure, invasive abscesses, and prosthetic valve infections (Olaison & Pettersson, 2003).

Blood cultures are an essential diagnostic tool in infective endocarditis. Three separate sets of blood cultures drawn from different venipuncture sites, obtained over 24 hours, usually identify the organism. Patients with infective endocarditis that

Table 33–1 ■ CLINICAL MANIFESTATIONS OF INFECTIVE ENDOCARDITIS

Symptoms	Physical Examination Findings
Fever	Fever
Chills and sweats	Changing or new heart murmur
Malaise	Evidence of systemic emboli
Weight loss	Splenomegaly
Anorexia	Janeway lesions (small
Stroke symptoms	hemorrhages on palms or soles
Myalgias	of feet)
Arthralgias	Splinter hemorrhages (hemorrhagic
Confusion	streaks at fingernail tips)
Congestive heart failure	Osler's nodules (small, tender
	nodules on finger or toe pads)

CLINICAL APPROACH TO ENDOCARDITIS

Establish diagnosis
  Blood cultures
  Physical examination findings
  Echocardiography
  Establish source that seeded endocarditis
Start appropriate antibiotics based on blood cultures
Monitor telemetry for conduction defects
Treat valvular regurgitation with afterload reduction agents
Repeat blood cultures 3 days after antibiotics started to ensure
  response
Insert long-term intravenous access for antibiotics
Monitor drug levels when appropriate
Monitor for systemic emboli

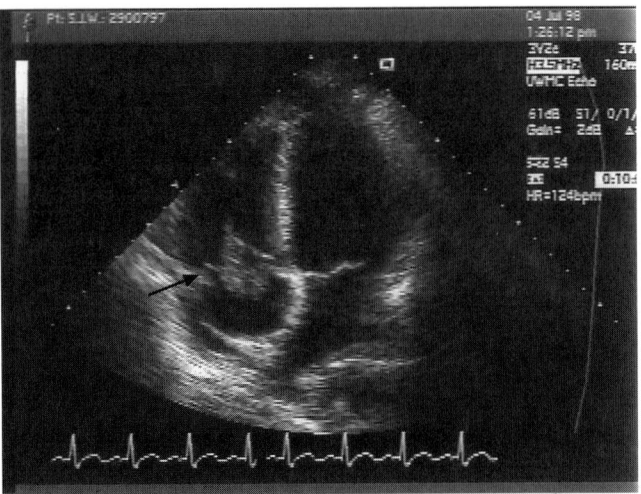

■ **Figure 33–2.** Two-dimensional echocardiogram view of vegetation on tricuspid valve in 27-year-old woman with endocarditis (*arrow*).

remain culture-negative may have fastidious organisms or may have received intravenous antibiotics before blood samples were drawn. In acute endocarditis, antibiotic therapy should be started after blood cultures have been obtained using strict aseptic technique and optimal skin prep (Towns & Reller, 2003). The clinical approach in acute endocarditis includes appropriate antibiotics and monitoring for complications (Display 33-1). The usual course is 6 full weeks of intravenous antibiotics. Patients who do not respond well to standard antibiotic therapy may be referred for surgical valve replacement (Display 33-2).

Echocardiography is frequently used to verify the presence of vegetations on the valves (Fig. 33-2). Transthoracic echocardiography (TTE) is less sensitive than transesophageal (TEE) echocardiography in identifying vegetations (45% to 75% vs. 90% to 94%) (Karchmer, 1998). Transesophageal echocardiography is also useful to identify paravalvular leaks and annular abscesses seen in prosthetic valve endocarditis. Although TEE is more sensitive, some clinicians recommend that TTE be obtained first and to perform TEE only if the TTE images are inadequate or suspicion of infective endocarditis remains high and the initial TTE was negative (Sachdev et al., 2003).

Prevention of endocarditis in high-risk populations, such as those with rheumatic heart disease or structural valve disease, is essential. Patients at risk (Display 33-3) who are undergoing procedures that may cause a transient bacteremia, such as dental or genitourinary procedures, should be treated prophylactically using recommended guidelines (for complete guidelines, refer to *Prevention of Bacterial Endocarditis: Recommendations by the American Heart Association*) (Dajani et al., 1997). The treatment for infective endocarditis is prolonged high-dose antibiotic therapy and valve replacement for those who have evidence of severe valve dysfunction (Chan, 1993).

Miscellaneous Causes of Valvular Disease

In addition to rheumatic fever and endocarditis, there are other causes of acquired valvular heart disease. Degenerative changes of the tissue, such as myxomatous degeneration, calcification, and those associated with Marfan syndrome, can cause valvular dysfunction. Trauma or infection may affect the supportive or subvalvular apparatus. Dilation of the ventricles caused by chronically elevated preloading may dilate an atrioventricular valve opening to the point that the leaflets no longer

INDICATIONS FOR CARDIAC SURGERY IN INFECTIVE ENDOCARDITIS

Heart failure with hemodynamic instability
Persistent bacteremia and fever despite optimal antibiotic
  therapy
Paravalvular abscess or fistula
Recurrence of endocarditis after full course of antibiotics
Systemic emboli
Heart failure due to prosthetic valvular dysfunction
Valve dehiscence (in prosthetic valvular endocarditis)
New conduction system defects
Fungal endocarditis

RISK FACTORS FOR INFECTIVE ENDOCARDITIS

Recent dental procedure or periodontal disease
History of congential heart disease
History of valvular heart disease
Long-term in-dwelling intravenous line
Genitourinary infections or instrumentation
Prosthetic valve (mechanical or biologic)
History of intravenous drug abuse
Hemodialysis

approximate and the valve becomes incompetent. Coronary heart disease (CHD) and myocardial infarction (MI) can affect the papillary muscles of the right and left ventricles, causing either dysfunction caused by ischemia or frank flail of atrioventricular valve leaflets caused by papillary muscle rupture. Systemic diseases such as lupus erythematosus and scleroderma may also cause valvular dysfunction.

Diagnostic Testing for Valvular Heart Disease

The diagnosis of valvular heart disease is based on patient history, physical assessment, and diagnostic testing. Some tests, such as the ECG and the chest radiograph, may be relatively insensitive in diagnosing valvular heart disease, even though they are part of standard screening tests in patients with heart dysfunction. Diagnostic tests that are more specific and quantitative for valvular dysfunction include echocardiography (M-mode, two-dimensional, Doppler ultrasonography, or transesophageal), right and left heart catheterization, nuclear imaging, and exercise testing (Buccino et al., 1993). Diagnostic findings for specific valvular lesions are noted in the sections discussing each abnormality.

Mitral Stenosis

Cause

The predominant cause of mitral stenosis is rheumatic fever. The mitral valve is the valve most often damaged by rheumatic carditis (Dalen & Fenster, 2000). Rheumatic fever causes thickening and decreased mobility of the mitral valve leaflets associated with fusion of the commissures. Uncommon, nonrheumatic causes of mitral stenosis include malignant carcinoid syndrome, severe mitral annular or leaflet calcification, congenital absence of one of the papillary muscles resulting in a parachute deformity of the mitral valve, neoplasm, endocardial vegetations, and degenerative calcification of an implanted tissue prosthetic heart valve (Fann et al., 1997).

Pathology

The rheumatic process causes the mitral valve to become fibrinous, resulting in leaflet thickening, commissural or chordal fusion, and calcification. As a result, the mitral valve apparatus becomes funnel-shaped with a narrowed orifice. Fusion of the mitral valve commissures results in narrowing of the principal orifice, whereas interchordal fusion obliterates the secondary orifices.

Pathophysiology

The normal mitral valve area is 4 to 6 cm^2. Once the cross-sectional area of the mitral valve is reduced to 2 cm^2 or less, a pressure gradient between the left atrium and left ventricle occurs. The reduced orifice impedes left atrial emptying. Increased left atrial pressure and dilation occurs along with left atrial hypertrophy in an attempt to maintain normal diastolic

flow into the left ventricle. Increased left atrial pressure is transmitted to the pulmonary circuit, resulting in pulmonary hypertension and pulmonary congestion. As the left atrium distends and pressure rises, atrial conduction fibers are stretched, stimulating onset of atrial fibrillation (Chan et al., 1993). Patients have left-sided congestive heart failure (CHF) without left ventricular dysfunction. Mitral stenosis has a sparing effect on the left ventricle. Symptoms of mitral stenosis are usually related to obstruction of the mitral valve rather than ventricular dysfunction. As pulmonary pressure increases, right-sided heart failure may occur.

Clinical Manifestations

Women have mitral stenosis four-times more frequently than men do (Braunwald, 1998). Women who had previously been asymptomatic with mitral stenosis may become symptomatic and even experience severe hemodynamic decompensation during pregnancy (Teerlink & Foster, 1998). Most patients remain asymptomatic for several years and may not have symptoms until the fourth or fifth decades of life (Carabello, 1998).

Mild dyspnea on exertion occurs as the most common symptom of mild mitral stenosis (valve area of 1.6 to 2.0 cm^2). As mitral stenosis becomes more severe (valve area of 1 to 1.5 cm^2), dyspnea, fatigue, paroxysmal nocturnal dyspnea, and atrial fibrillation may occur. When mitral stenosis becomes severe (valve area of 1 cm^2 or less), symptoms include fatigue and dyspnea with mild exertion or rest. Patients often have a cough or hoarseness and may have hemoptysis (Khan, 1996). With advanced mitral stenosis, pulmonary hypertension and symptoms of right-sided heart failure occur (i.e., edema, hepatomegaly, ascites, elevated jugular venous pressure). Increased left atrial pressure, atrial fibrillation, and stagnation of left atrial blood flow can result in formation of mural thrombi, with resultant embolic events, including cerebral vascular accidents.

Physical Assessment

In severe mitral stenosis, on auscultation, there are four typical findings, including: (1) an accentuated S$_1$; (2) an opening diastolic snap; (3) a mid-diastolic rumble noted best at the apex (in sinus rhythm, followed by presystolic accentuation); and (4) an increased pulmonic S$_2$ intensity associated with pulmonary hypertension (Table 33-2). It usually takes 2 or more years after the rheumatic episode for development of the typical murmur of mitral stenosis (Khan, 1996).

Patients with mitral stenosis may exhibit malar blush (pink discoloration of the cheeks). Patients with severe mitral stenosis may have weak pulses secondary to reduced cardiac output. The apical pulse is tapping in quality and is nondisplaced. A lower left parasternal lift or heave caused by right ventricular hypertrophy may be present. Cardiac rhythm is often irregular, indicating atrial fibrillation.

Diagnostic Tests

Echocardiography is used in the evaluation of mitral stenosis to: (1) quantify the valve area and gradient; (2) quantify the degree of mitral insufficiency; (3) define the degree of left atrial

Table 33–2 ■ DIASTOLIC MURMURS IN ACQUIRED VALVULAR HEART DISEASE

Origin of Murmur	Auscultatory Location and Radiation	Configuration	Quality and Frequency	Maneuvers That Alter Intensity
Aortic insufficiency	Third and fourth left intercostal spaces	Decrescendo S_1 S_2 S_1	Blowing High pitched	Increases with isometric exercise and squatting Decreases with amyl nitrate and Valsalva maneuver
Mitral stenosis	Apex	Decrescendo Opening snap OS S_1 S_2 S_1	Rumbling Low pitched	Increases with expiration, squatting, amyl nitrate, and isometric exercise Decreases with Valsalva maneuver
Pulmonic insufficiency	Second left intercostal space	Crescendo-decrescendo S_1 S_2 S_1	Blowing High pitched	Increases with inspiration and amyl nitrate Decreases with Valsalva maneuver
Tricuspid stenosis	Parasternal at left fourth and fifth intercostal spaces	Decrescendo S_1 S_2 S_1	Rumbling Low pitched	Increases with inspiration, squatting, and amyl nitrate Decreases with Valsalva maneuver

enlargement; (4) assess mitral annular calcification; (5) assess pulmonary artery pressures and degree of pulmonary hypertension; and (6) evaluate right- and left-sided ventricular function. Transesophageal echocardiography provides better detail of the mitral valve and provides better visualization of atrial thrombus (Brady, 2003).

Cardiac catheterization is used less in diagnosis of mitral stenosis as echocardiography techniques improve. Cardiac catheterization does allow for accurate assessment of valve area and can also identify associated mitral regurgitation. For patients with known or suspected CHD, coronary angiography can delineate coronary anatomy. Right heart catheterization can evaluate right heart and pulmonary artery pressures.

Electrocardiography is nonspecific and does not indicate the severity of mitral stenosis. If the patient remains in sinus rhythm and left atrial enlargement has occurred, characteristic P mitrale (broad, bifid P waves in leads II and V_1) may be identified. Right axis deviation and right ventricular hypertrophy may be noted in severe mitral stenosis. Atrial fibrillation is common in patients with long-standing mitral stenosis and is usually coarse in appearance.

Chest radiography correlates with the degree of mitral stenosis. As mitral stenosis becomes more severe, the chest radiograph demonstrates straightening of the left heart border caused by left atrial enlargement, elevation of the left mainstem bronchus caused by distention of the left atrium, and distribution of blood flow from the lower to upper lobes. Although heart size remains normal, central pulmonary arteries become prominent. Kerley B lines and interstitial edema are often present.

Medical Management

Medical therapy for mitral stenosis is aimed at preventing the complications of systemic embolization and bacterial endocarditis, as well as atrial fibrillation if it occurs (Dalen & Fenster, 2000). Patients who have asymptomatic mitral stenosis require only antibiotic prophylaxis. Patients with mild pulmonary congestion can be managed with diuretics alone. Beta-blockers can be used to reduce heart rate and improve diastolic filling time. When patients have atrial fibrillation, digoxin, beta-blockers, or calcium channel blockers can be used for ventricular response rate control. Patients with atrial fibrillation require anticoagulation to prevent thrombus formation in the atrium. Once the patient has symptoms of NYHA functional class III or IV despite adequate medical management, mechanical correction of mitral stenosis by balloon valvuloplasty or surgery should be performed.

Interventional and Surgical Management

Percutaneous Mitral Catheter Balloon Valvuloplasty. Percutaneous mitral catheter balloon valvuloplasty is an alternative, less invasive procedure than surgical treatment for mitral stenosis. Balloon valvuloplasty is performed in the cardiac catheterization laboratory by a cardiologist experienced with invasive techniques. A small balloon valvuloplasty catheter is introduced percutaneously at the femoral vein and passed into the right atrium. The catheter is then directed transseptally and positioned across the mitral valve.

Inflation of either one large balloon (23 to 25 mm) or two smaller balloons (12 to 18 mm) stretches the valve leaflets (Fig. 33-3). Separation of the commissures and fracture of nodule calcium are the apparent mechanisms that improve valve movement and function (Braunwald, 1992). The best results from this technique to date have been in patients with rheumatic mitral stenosis with commissural fusion. An echocardiographic scoring system rates leaflet thickening, leaflet mobility,

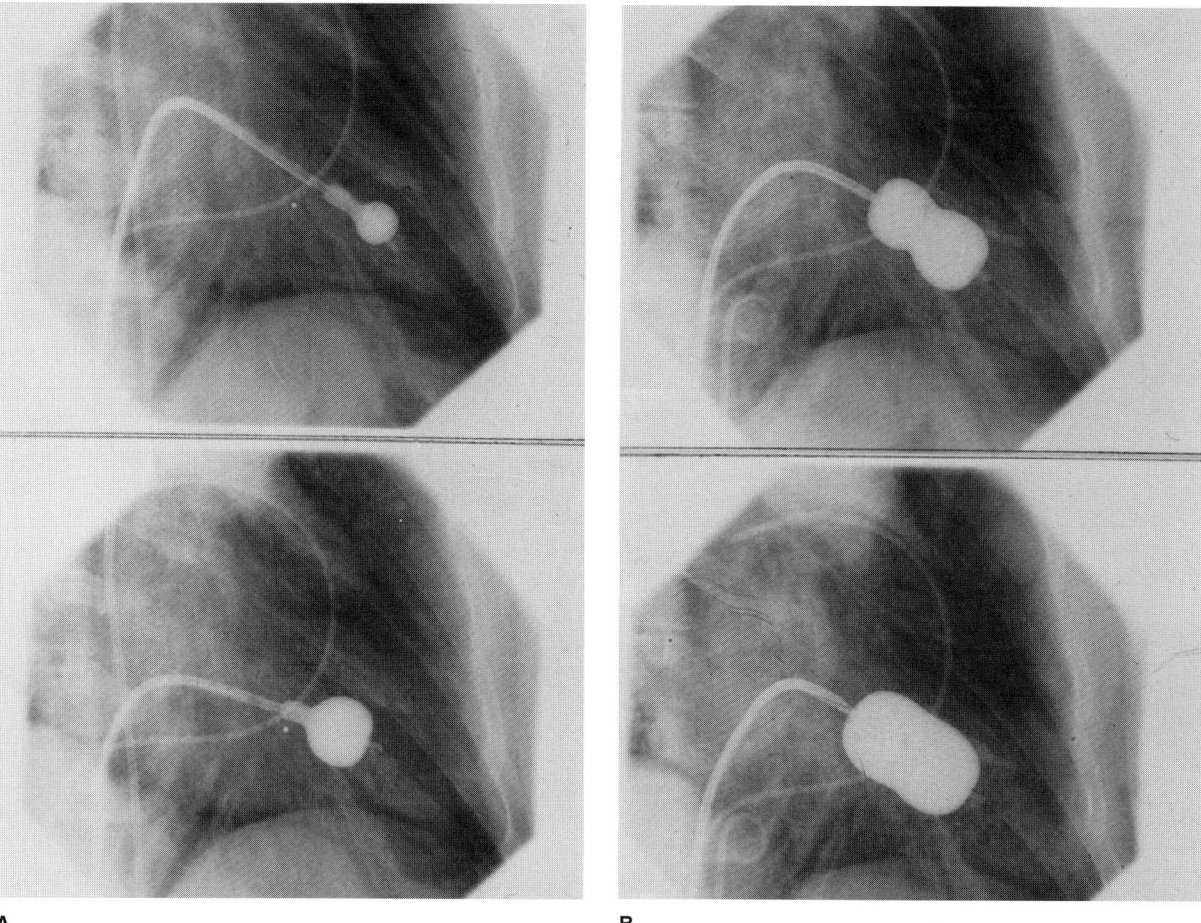

A   B

■ **Figure 33–3.** Mitral valvuloplasty: Inoue's technique. (*A*) Inflation of distal portion of balloon, which is then pulled back and anchored at the mitral valve. (*B*) Inflation of proximal and middle portions of balloon. At full inflation, the narrowed "waist" of the balloon has disappeared. (From Vahanian, A. S. [1998]. Valvuloplasty. In E. J. Topol , R. M. Califf, J. M. Isner et al. [Eds.], *Textbook of cardiovascular medicine* [p. 2157]. Philadelphia: Lippincott-Raven.)

calcification, and subvalvular deformity, with a maximum score of 4 in each division. Patients with a total echo score of ≤8 respond most favorably (Palacios et al., 2002). Balloon valvuloplasty has been associated with complications including systemic embolization (1% to 3%), severe mitral regurgitation (3% to 5%), and death (0% to 1%) (Mayes et al., 1999). An atrial septal defect may also occur in as many as 10% of patients undergoing balloon valvuloplasty as a result of the transseptal approach, but this closes or decreases in most patients (Mazur et al., 1999). Results have been promising, with the average gradient reduction being approximately 18 to 6 mm Hg and, on the average, an increase in calculated valve area of 50% to 100%. Mitral balloon valvuloplasty is reserved for patients who continue to be symptomatic despite adequate medical therapy.

Balloon valvuloplasty has become increasingly useful in women who experienced hemodynamic decompensation during pregnancy (Teerlink & Foster, 1998).

Surgical Treatment. Surgical replacement of the mitral valve is required when there is severe mitral regurgitation coexisting with mitral stenosis or if the mitral stenosis is not amenable to percutaneous balloon valvuloplasty. Although some valves with mitral stenosis may be repaired by open commissurotomy and

reconstruction, heavily calcified rheumatic mitral valves often are beyond the point of repair. The usual prosthetic valve of choice in mitral stenosis is a mechanical prosthesis, because patients already require life-long anticoagulation because of atrial fibrillation. For young women who wish to become pregnant, a bioprosthesis may be recommended.

Tricuspid Valve Disease

Tricuspid regurgitation is primarily "functional" rather than structural and occurs secondary to dilation of the right ventricle and the annulus of the tricuspid valve. Functional tricuspid regurgitation frequently accompanies mitral stenosis and pulmonary hypertension because of the increased pressure and volume load on the right ventricle. Symptoms include signs of right-sided heart failure, large V waves in their right atrial or central venous pressure trace, and pulsatile neck veins. Other causes of tricuspid regurgitation include trauma, infective endocarditis, right atrial tumor, and tricuspid valve prolapse. The murmur of tricuspid regurgitation is a holosystolic murmur heard along the left sternal border and may extend over

Table 33–3 ■ SYSTOLIC MURMURS RELATED TO ACQUIRED VALVULAR HEART DISEASE

Origin of Murmur	Auscultatory Location and Radiation	Configuration	Quality and Frequency	Maneuvers That Alter Intensity
Aortic stenosis	Right second intercostal space Radiates to carotid arteries and apex	Crescendo-decrescendo "Diamond shaped" ◆ S₁ S₂	Harsh High pitched	Increases with squatting, amyl nitrate Decreases with standing, Valsalva maneuver, and isometric exercise
Mitral regurgitation	Apex Radiates to axilla and back	Holosystolic S₁ S₂	Harsh or blowing High pitched	Increases with expiration, squatting, and isometric exercise Decreases with Valsalva maneuver, standing, and amyl nitrate
Mitral valve prolapse	Apex Radiates to axilla and back	Mid- to late systolic, with systolic click S₁ click S₂	Harsh High pitched	Increases with Valsalva maneuver, amyl nitrate, and inspiration Decreases with squatting, standing, and isometric exercise
Tricuspid regurgitation	Fourth and fifth left intercostal spaces Radiates to right parasternal border	Holosystolic S₁ S₂	Harsh High pitched	Increases with amyl nitrate and inspiration Decreases with Valsalva maneuver and standing
Pulmonic stenosis	Second left intercostal space Radiates to back	Crescendo-decrescendo "Diamond shaped" ◆ S₁ S₂	Harsh High pitched	Increases with amyl nitrate, squatting, and inspiration Decreases with Valsalva maneuver and standing

the precordium, sounding like the murmurs of mitral regurgitation and ventricular septal defect (Table 33-3). Patients with mild tricuspid regurgitation normally do not require treatment. Medical treatment is aimed at reducing pulmonary artery pressures and right heart afterload. If tricuspid regurgitation is severe and symptomatic, surgical intervention with annuloplasty repair may be performed. Tricuspid valve replacement is performed only if repair is not feasible or fails (Otto, 1999).

Acquired tricuspid stenosis is uncommon, recognized in approximately 5% of patients with rheumatic heart disease, and usually does not occur without involvement of the mitral valve (Ewy, 2000). Tricuspid stenosis has a pathologic process similar to that of mitral stenosis. The murmur of tricuspid stenosis is comparable to the murmur of mitral stenosis, including an opening snap followed by a diastolic rumble. The murmur of tricuspid stenosis is a diastolic decrescendo murmur along the left sternal border (see Table 33-2). Common symptoms of tricuspid stenosis include fatigue, minimal orthopnea, paroxysmal nocturnal dyspnea, hepatomegaly, and anasarca. Although there is limited experience with balloon valvuloplasty, when tricuspid stenosis is severe, surgical repair with direct commissurotomy

and annuloplasty is usually performed at the same time as mitral valve intervention (Otto, 1999).

Prosthetic Valves

Prosthetic cardiac valves have been used since the mid 1960s to treat acquired valvular heart disease. Because no "perfect" prosthetic valve exists, the patient with valvular heart disease is managed medically as long as it is safely feasible. Timing of valve replacement depends on the patient's functional status, ventricular dysfunction, and the natural course of the lesion.

Before a decision is made to use a particular valve, factors in valve design, specifically durability, thrombogenic potential, and hemodynamic properties, are weighed against annulus size and certain clinical conditions such as the desirability of long-term anticoagulation. Table 33-4 summarizes the characteristics considered in selection of prosthetic valves. Because of their proven durability, mechanical valves are most often chosen for patients younger than age 65 to 70 years, unless contraindicated (e.g., previous bleeding

Table 33–4 ■ SELECTION OF TYPE OF PROSTHETIC VALVE BASED ON PATIENT CHARACTERISTICS

Biologic Valve	Mechanical Valve
History of bleeding	Age <65 years
Inability to take warfarin	Already on anticoagulation
Desire to become pregnant	History of embolic cerebral
History of thrombosis with	vascular accident
mechanical valve	History of atrial fibrillation
Age >65 years	

problems, desire to become pregnant, or poor compliance with medication and follow-up). Prosthetic heart valves differ in design, echocardiography image, and radiologic appearance (Fig. 33-4).

Mechanical Valves

Although the age of patients undergoing valve replacement in the United States continues to increase, mechanical valves dominate the market with a 60% to 40% market share advantage over biological valves (Wernly & Crawford, 1998). Mechanical (nonbiologic) valves have excellent durability but are usually thrombogenic. Bileaflet and tilting-disk valves are the

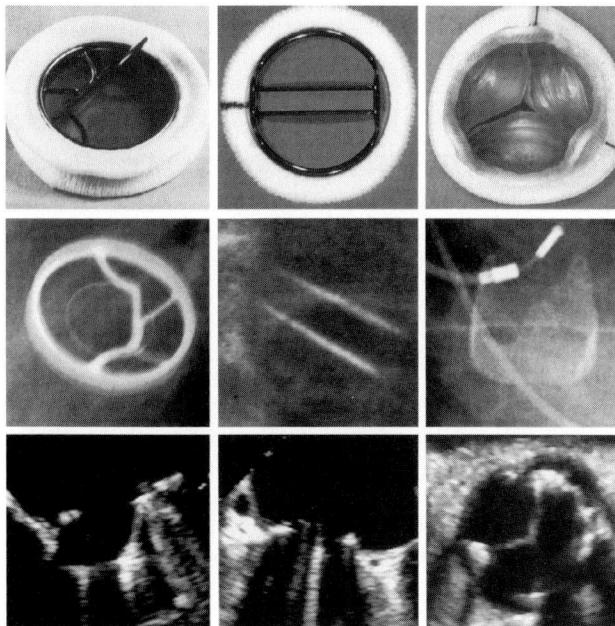

■ **Figure 33–4.** Photographic (*top row*), radiographic (*middle row*), and echocardiographic (*bottom row*) appearance of prosthetic valves. From left to right: Bjork-Shiley single tilting disk, St. Jude's Medical bileaflet mechanical valve, and Carpentier-Edwards xenograft (radiographs courtesy of Dr. Carolyn van Dyke). (Adapted from Garcia, M. L. [1998]. Prosthetic valve disease. In E. J. Topol, R. M. Califf, J. M. Isner et al. [Eds.], *Textbook of cardiovascular medicine* [p. 580]. Philadelphia: Lippincott-Raven.)

mechanical valves in common use today. Caged-ball valves are used less frequently in the United States but may be used in other areas of the world. In patients with aneurysm or dissection of the ascending aorta, composite grafts of conduit and mechanical valves may be used.

Bileaflet valves, such as St. Jude, ATS (advancing the standard), and the CarboMedic are low-profile valves that have centrally mounted leaflets attached to the seating ring with butterfly hinges. These hinges allow the leaflets to open to 85 degrees, making these valves the least obstructive of the mechanical valves. Made of pyrolytic carbon, these valves produce nearly central flow with little turbulence (Edmunds et al., 1991). The two leaflets swing open in systole, resulting in three separate flow areas (Grunkemeier et al., 1994). With adequate anticoagulation, thromboembolic risk is low with bileaflet valves.

The *tilting-disk valve* is a low-profile valve consisting of a disk that sits in a seating ring; the flat or convexoconcave disk tilts in response to pressure changes. The Medtronic Hall valve is a tilting-disk valve commonly used today. Tilting-disk valves open to an angle of 60 to 75 degrees in relation to the seating ring. When open, tilting-disk valves produce a minor and major orifice for blood to pass through. Tilting disks have more central flow, but usually more turbulence, than caged-ball valves.

Tilting disks close with an audible click. The technology for production of tilting-disk valves has evolved so that a single piece of metal is used to avoid welded struts. In the past, welded struts fractured and caused fatal results, as did the older Bjork-Shiley convexoconcave valve, which is no longer, manufactured or implanted (Edmunds et al., 1991).

Caged-ball valves have been used since the 1960s and have an excellent durability record. Changes in pressure cause the ball to move forward and back within its caged structure. Flow is directed laterally through the valve rather than centrally. Because of its high profile, the caged-ball valve prosthesis can become obstructive, especially when used in patients with small aortic roots or small left ventricles. The Starr-Edwards and the Sutter (formerly SmeloffCutter) are two of the most common caged-ball valves used. Caged-ball prostheses have been largely abandoned in favor of lower-profile bileaflet valves.

Tissue Valves

Tissue (biologic) valves are characterized by having low rates of thrombotic episodes associated with their use. Porcine or bovine tissue is strengthened and made nonviable by treatment with glutaraldehyde. Homografts are tissue valves from cadavers. They are preserved cryogenically, but are difficult to procure, and their longevity has not been well proven. The main advantages of tissue valves are the associated low rates of thromboembolism and the subsequent decrease in patient morbidity when anticoagulant therapy is not required. Nonthrombogenicity is particularly important for those patients in whom long-term anticoagulation should be avoided, such as children, young adult women, patients older than age 70 years, or people with a history of bleeding.

The Hancock porcine valve, the Medtronic Mosaic porcine bioprosthesis (treated with alpha oleic acid to retard calcification), and the Carpentier-Edwards porcine valve are xenografts using porcine aortic valves preserved with glutaraldehyde under pressure, mounted on a stent (Jamieson, 2003). The Carpentier-Edwards pericardial bioprosthesis is made of leaflets fashioned from bovine pericardium fixed without pressure in glutaraldehyde.

Stentless bioprosthetic porcine xenograft valves such as the St. Jude Medical-Toronto, the Medtronic Freestyle Stentless, and the Edwards Prima Plus porcine bioprosthesis have been developed to improve the durability and enhance the hemodynamic performance of porcine aortic valves. Stentless aortic biological valves were developed secondary to the recognition that conventional bioprosthesis have limitations of long-term durability and residual obstruction that may impede left ventricular mass regression (Goldman & Mallidi, 2003). Because of the structural similarity to aortic allografts, stentless bioprostheses adapt to the aortic root and reproduce the anatomy of the native aortic valve (Luciani et al., 1998). Use of the stentless aortic bioprosthesis has resulted in enhanced survival and hemodynamic superiority (David, 1998). It is expected that reducing mechanical stress on valve leaflets, and the associated degeneration of the bioprosthesis, may be slowed. Thus, stentless xenografts may prove more durable than commonly used stented valves (Luciani et al., 1998).

Homografts or *allografts* from human cadavers are virtually free of any associated thrombosis. They are especially useful in patients with small aortic roots or in patients with active endocarditis. Earlier homografts were preserved with glutaraldehyde and demonstrated early failure. Homografts are now stored "fresh" after harvesting in an antibiotic solution and are then cryopreserved, increasing their longevity to at least 10 years. Valve failure is uncommon and usually the result of progressive valve incompetence (Doty et al., 1998). Even though the homografts are human tissue, there does not appear to be any problem with antigenicity (Whittlesay & Geha, 1991). Aortic allografts have demonstrated excellent freedom from thromboembolism, endocarditis, and progressive valve incompetence (Doty et al., 1998). Because of lack of availability, use of homografts has been limited.

In the *Ross procedure* (also known as pulmonary autograft), the aortic valve is replaced with a pulmonary autograft, and the native pulmonary valve is replaced with a pulmonic allograft. Although this procedure introduced by Donald Ross in 1967 (Elkins, 2003) was originally developed for pediatric application, it has been expanded to adult surgery as well. In patients undergoing the Ross procedure, the native pulmonary valve is excised and then implanted in the aortic position (autograft); a pulmonary homograft (allograft) is implanted into the pulmonic position (Fig. 33-5). The pulmonary autograft has been shown to be resistant to degeneration and calcification (Ross, 1987). Potential clinical and hemodynamic advantages of the pulmonary autograft over the aortic homograft include potential for growth when used in the pediatric population, increased cellular viability, enhanced durability, and possibly internal innervation of the cusps (Santini, 1997). The 30-day mortality for the Ross procedure as reported by the International Ross Registry is 3.3% (140 of 4,197 patients) (International Ross Registry, 2003). The actuarial freedom from pulmonary autograft valve replacement is 90% ± 3% at 13 years (Elkins, 2003). Although the Ross procedure is gaining

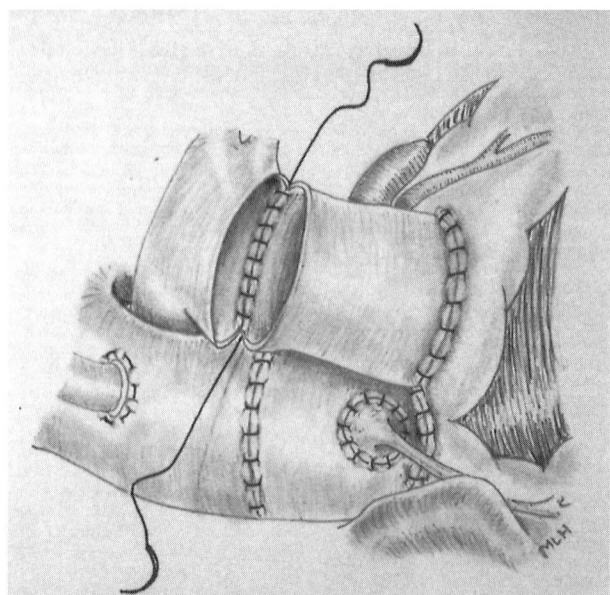

■ **Figure 33–5.** Illustration of Ross procedure. Suture line of pulmonary homograft is shown. (From Elkins, R. C. [1998]. Valve repair and valve replacement in children, including the Ross procedure. In L. R. Kaiser, I. L. Kron, & T. L. Spray [Eds.], *Mastery of cardiothoracic surgery* [p. 947]. Philadelphia: Lippincott-Raven.)

acceptance, especially in young adults who wish to avoid anticoagulation, there is concern that it offers no better result than the aortic homograft, which is a simpler procedure, with less morbidity. Pulmonary autografts require significantly longer operating time but do not seem to affect early and midterm outcomes compared with aortic homografts (Santini, 1997).

Minimally Invasive Valve Surgery

Minimally invasive valve surgery is now used for both aortic valve replacement and mitral valve repair and replacement. Minimally invasive surgical approaches are possible because a wide assortment of technological advances, such as endoscopic and surgical equipment, have been developed. Although patients undergoing minimally invasive valve surgery still require cardiopulmonary bypass, classic median sternotomy may be avoided, thus reducing pain, improving cosmetic results, and expediting recovery. These patients have a lower requirement for erythrocytes, express greater satisfaction, and have lower hospital charges (approximately 20% less than in patients with standard mitral valve and aortic valve approaches) (Cohn et al., 1997). As minimally invasive valve surgery continues to evolve, it will likely become a mainstay in the treatment of valvular heart surgery.

Aortic valve replacement can be performed through an upper "T" mini-sternotomy without intraoperative difficulties. Postoperative pain is reduced and recovery is expedited, with patients discharged to home as early as postoperative day 3 (Izzat et al., 1998). Two minimally invasive techniques for mitral valve surgery have been used: a right parasternal approach (Fig. 33-6) developed at the Cleveland Clinic and a mini-thoracotomy (Chitwood et al., 1997). Compared with

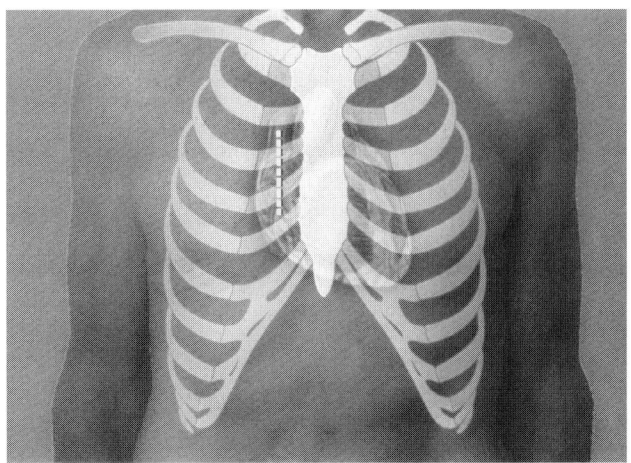

■ **Figure 33–6.** Example of one approach to minimally invasive mitral valve surgery. An 8- to 10-cm incision is made from the lower border of the second costal cartilage to the upper border of the fifth costal cartilage. (From Alpert, J. S., Sabick, J., & Cosgrove, D. M. [1998]. Mitral valve disease. In E. J. Topol, R. M. Califf, J. M., Isner et al. [Eds.], *Textbook of cardiovascular medicine* [p. 526]. Philadelphia: Lippincott-Raven.)

patients with median sternotomy, patients undergoing mitral valve replacement through the right parasternal approach had a shortened length of stay and reduced direct hospital costs (Cosgrove et al., 1998). The mini-thoracotomy approach with video assistance can be used safely in patients undergoing mitral valve repair or replacement; compared with standard techniques, the mini-thoracotomy resulted in less morbidity, earlier discharge, and lower cost (Chitwood et al., 1997). The majority of clinical series demonstrates that minimally invasive port-access approach to mitral valve surgery has low morbidity and mortality, with echocardiographic outcomes equivalent to conventional mitral valve surgery (Sharony et al., 2003). More recently, minimally invasive mitral valve surgery has evolved to include computed-assisted robotic techniques in current clinical trials. The daVinci Surgical System allows the surgeon to operate from a console through an end-affector using micro wrist instruments, which are mounted on robotic arms, inserted through the chest wall (Chitwood, 2003).

Complications of Prosthetic Valves

Thromboembolism remains the most common complication of patients with prosthetic valves. Anticoagulant therapy with warfarin is begun in all patients 48 hours after surgery and is continued for 6 to 12 weeks. All patients with mechanical valves require life-long anticoagulation because of the risk of thrombosis and embolization. The highest thromboembolic risk for mechanical and biologic valves occurs in the first few days to months after implantation, before the valve is fully endothelialized. Even with anticoagulation, the risk of thromboembolism is 1% to 2% per year for patients with mechanical valves (McAnulty & Rahimtoola, 1998). The American Heart Association and the American College of Cardiology recommend INR of 2.0 to 3.0 for mechanical aortic valves and INR of 2.5 to 3.5 for mechanical mitral valves (Goldsmith et al., 2002).

Of mechanical valves, the caged-ball valves have the highest rate of thromboembolism, and the St. Jude valves have the lowest (Garcia, 1998). Tissue valves other than homografts also usually require anticoagulation for 6 to 12 weeks after surgery, after which patients have their therapy converted to aspirin. The overall risk of thromboembolism with biologic valves is 0.6% to 0.7% per year (McAnulty & Rahimtoola, 1998). Homografts or the Ross procedure require no anticoagulation.

Prosthetic valvular thrombosis is a serious complication and can result in severe hemodynamic compromise. In patients with prosthetic valves who are not anticoagulated into a therapeutic range, thrombosis of the prosthetic valve can occur. Valve thrombosis can occur with either mechanical or bioprosthetic heart valves but occurs most often in prosthetic valves in the mitral position (Garcia, 1998). Thrombus or pannus formation on the valve may occlude the orifice or entrap the pivoting mechanisms, causing acute stenosis or regurgitation. Symptoms of valve thrombosis include embolic events and CHF. Valve thrombosis can be diagnosed with transesophageal echocardiography (McAnulty & Rahimtoola, 1998). Emergent valve replacement usually is indicated for large thrombi, but if the patient is not a surgical candidate, thrombolytic agents may be used (Garcia, 1998).

The rate of *bacterial endocarditis* is approximately 3% the first year after valve replacement and 0.5% each year thereafter (McAnulty & Rahimtoola, 1998). Although symptoms of prosthetic valve endocarditis are similar to those of native valve endocarditis, the infection may be difficult to control with antibiotics alone because of prosthetic material involved.

Early prosthetic valve endocarditis (within the first 60 days) carries a high mortality rate of 20% to 70% (Garcia, 1998). Early prosthetic valve endocarditis occurs in less than 1% of valve replacement patients and frequently requires the patient to undergo additional operations (Crawford & Durack, 2003). The most common organism in early prosthetic valve endocarditis is *Staphylococcus epidermidis*. Eighty percent of these staphylococci are methicillin-resistant, suggesting that these infections may be nosocomial in nature (Garcia, 1998). Fever, heart failure, new murmur, and embolic events are common manifestations.

Late prosthetic valve endocarditis (more than 60 days after surgery) occurs most commonly in patients with bioprosthetic valves in the aortic position. Urinary infection, dental procedures, and urologic procedures are the most common sources identified (Garcia, 1998). The incidence is less than 1% per year and is generally caused by the same bacterial species that cause subacute bacterial endocarditis (Crawford & Durack, 2003). For patients who do not respond to antibiotic therapy or who have local invasion of the annulus, embolic events, fungal infection, heart failure, or prosthetic valve dysfunction, repeat valvular replacement is indicated (McAnulty & Rahimtoola, 1998).

Prosthesis malfunction is uncommon for the first 10 years after mechanical valve implantation. The best-known problems with mechanical failures were those affecting the Bjork-Shiley convexoconcave tilting-disk valves first manufactured in 1978, with the peak incidence of valve failure in the 1981 to 1982 models. Subsequent modifications improved the valve area but also increased stress forces. As a result, by 1994, 564 strut fractures were reported in these Bjork-Shiley valves; two thirds of those strut fractures were fatal (Garcia, 1998). Although these valves have been withdrawn from the market, approximately 40,000 had been implanted worldwide. Because acute valve strut fracture can be fatal, patients with these valves should be evaluated for partial strut fracture using high-resolution cineradiography. Prophylactic replacement of these valves is not advocated (Wernly & Crawford, 1998).

Valve degeneration is the primary complication of patients with tissue prostheses. Degeneration of biologic prostheses can occur as lipid or calcium deposits cause valve cusps to stiffen and stenose. The incidence of structural failure requiring replacement is approximately 30% at 10 years after valve replacement (Garcia, 1998). Failure of tissue valves often occurs slowly over months to years and presents as progressive heart failure. Prosthetic valve degeneration and failure are most easily diagnosed with echocardiography.

Paravalvular leaks between the prosthetic ring and the annulus occur because of tearing of the suture line, spontaneously or after infection. Presence of a new murmur and signs of heart failure alert the clinician to paravalvular leaks. The patient's clinical course should be followed up; when the leak becomes significant, surgical repair or replacement is indicated. Hemolysis may also accompany paravalvular leaks.

Hemolytic anemia is a consequence of shortened red cell survival time in all patients with prosthetic valves. Movement of the valve ball or disk causes varying degrees of destruction of the red blood cells. Hemolysis may also occur with paravalvular leak. Commonly, hemolysis is mild and the patient can compensate by increasing red blood cell production. Rarely, hemolytic anemia occurs. Chronic intravascular hemolysis results in loss of iron in the urine; iron deficiency anemia may result after several years.

Mitral Insufficiency

Cause

Mitral insufficiency (also termed *regurgitation*) may be either chronic or acute (Table 33-5). Acute mitral regurgitation is caused by chordal rupture, MI, trauma, myxomatous valvular degeneration, mitral valve prolapse, or endocarditis (Carabello, 2000). Chronic mitral regurgitation may be the result of a number of abnormalities including, but not limited to, rheumatic heart disease, injury after radiation, cardiomyopathies, infiltrative disease, ischemic damage to the subvalvular apparatus, infective endocarditis, myxomatous degeneration, hypertrophic cardiomyopathy, diet-drug–induced lesions, or marked left ventricular dilation (Enriquez-Sarano et al, 2000).

Pathology

Primary mitral regurgitation occurs when the mitral valve annulus, leaflets, chordae, or papillary muscles are affected by ischemia, collagen disease, infection, calcification, trauma, or degenerative changes, causing incompetent coaptation of the mitral leaflets. Secondary mitral regurgitation occurs with ventricular dilation when ventricular geometry is changed, causing malalignment of the papillary muscles. Although it is sometimes difficult to distinguish between primary and secondary

Table 33–5 ■ ETIOLOGIES OF ACQUIRED MITRAL REGURGIATION

Chronic Mitral Regurgitation	Acute Mitral Regurgitation
Rheumatic heart disease	Myocardial infarction causing:
Ischemia to subvalvular apparatus	Papillary muscle rupture or dysfunction
Infective endocarditis	Rupture of chordae
Myxomatous degeneration	Infective endocarditis
Hypertrophic cardiomyopathy	Trauma
Left ventricular dilation	Myxomatous degeneration with chordal rupture
Systemic lupus erythematosus	
Marfan's syndrome	
Calcification of annulus	
Ankylosing spondylitis	
Scleroderma	
Ehlers-Danlos syndrome	
Prosthetic paravalvular leak	
Deterioration of prosthetic mitral valve	

regurgitation, primary regurgitation is often more severe than insufficiency secondary to annular dilation (Braunwald, 1992).

Pathophysiology

Mitral regurgitation occurs as the result of inadequate closure of the mitral valve, allowing regurgitant flow back into the left atrium during each left ventricular systole. Its severity depends on the volume of regurgitant flow. Regurgitant flow into the left atrium reduces forward flow, stroke volume, and cardiac output (Khan, 1996). Regurgitant flow also increases left atrial pressure, causing left atrial dilation and pulmonary congestion. During diastole, the regurgitant volume returns to the left ventricle and increases its volume load.

In chronic mitral regurgitation, persistent volume overload results in progressive ventricular dilation and mild hypertrophy. Although ventricular dilation and hypertrophy are initially compensatory, over time, chronic volume overload may result in decreased systolic function of the left ventricle and lead to heart failure (Khan, 1996). In acute mitral regurgitation, neither the left atrium nor the ventricle has had sufficient time to adjust to the increased volume load. Left atrial pressure rises quickly, resulting in pulmonary congestion and edema.

Clinical Manifestations

Patients with acute versus chronic mitral regurgitation vary in clinical presentation and physical examination findings. In acute mitral regurgitation, symptoms progress rapidly. Symptoms are typically those of left ventricular failure. The patient is usually tachycardic to compensate for the reduced forward stroke volume. Patients are dyspneic secondary to pulmonary congestion and edema; they are often orthopneic and have paroxysmal nocturnal dyspnea and poor exercise tolerance. Patients may also have signs of biventricular failure because right-sided failure may occur secondary to pulmonary hypertension. Patients in acute mitral regurgitation often present to the emergency room with reports of sudden inability to breathe. New-onset atrial fibrillation can occur. Patients with ischemic mitral insufficiency or papillary muscle rupture may also report chest pain.

During the compensatory phase of chronic mitral regurgitation, patients may be relatively asymptomatic for years. Initial signs of mitral regurgitation include exertional dyspnea, orthopnea, paroxysmal nocturnal dyspnea, cough, palpitations, new atrial fibrillation, and lower extremity edema. Symptoms may occur so gradually that patients may present subacutely to the clinic with symptoms as vague as fatigue and inability to sleep.

Physical Assessment

On examination, the most easily noted characteristic of either chronic or acute mitral regurgitation is the holosystolic murmur, which is heard best at the apex and radiates to the axilla (see Table 33-3). The murmur of mitral regurgitation may vary somewhat depending on the underlying cause. Patients may have an S_3 gallop in moderate to severe regurgitation caused by high diastolic flow into the ventricle. An S_4 gallop is uncommon in chronic mitral regurgitation. However, in acute mitral regurgitation, an S_4 gallop is common because the left atrium and ventricle are noncompliant. The patient with rheumatic heart disease may also have a diastolic murmur related to coexisting mitral stenosis.

Because of left ventricular dilation, patients with chronic mitral regurgitation have an easily palpated, left laterally displaced point of maximal impulse. Patients with a markedly enlarged left atrium may have a left parasternal lift because of anterior displacement of the apex. Patients with acute or decompensated chronic mitral regurgitation may be anxious and diaphoretic because of left ventricular failure. Blood pressure may be normal to low and pulse pressure may be narrowed secondary to decreased stroke volume. Jugular venous pressure can be normal or elevated in the patient with right-sided heart failure. Breath sounds can range from basilar crackles to dullness secondary to pleural effusion. In addition, hepatosplenomegaly, hepatojugular reflux, peripheral edema, and ascites may be present in the patient with right-sided heart failure.

Diagnostic Tests

Transthoracic echocardiography can identify the structural cause of the mitral regurgitation as well as gauge left atrial size, left ventricular dimensions and performance, pulmonary artery pressures, and right heart function. Color flow Doppler allows for assessment of severity of regurgitation. *Transesophageal echocardiography* is better than transthoracic echocardiography for defining mitral valve anatomy and discriminating prosthetic valves and paravalvular leaks.

Cardiac catheterization is used to identify coexisting coronary artery disease and to grade the severity of mitral regurgitation. Left ventriculography can assess left ventricular function and distinguish any wall motion abnormalities. Right heart catheterization quantifies pulmonary artery pressures and allows for evaluation of the large V waves in the pulmonary artery wedge tracing.

Electrocardiography in chronic mitral regurgitation may demonstrate left ventricular hypertrophy and left atrial enlargement or P mitrale (characterized by M-shaped P waves). Atrial fibrillation may occur with acute and chronic mitral regurgitation. Patients with ischemic papillary muscle dysfunction may demonstrate ischemic changes, and patients with papillary muscle rupture can show acute inferior, posterior, or anterior MI.

Chest radiography in chronic mitral regurgitation shows left ventricular hypertrophy and left atrial enlargement. Calcification of the mitral valve annulus and apparatus may also be seen. In acute or decompensated chronic mitral regurgitation, pulmonary vascular redistribution and pulmonary edema can be observed. If the heart is of normal size, the degree of mitral regurgitation is so mild or so acute that eccentric left ventricular hypertrophy has not had time to develop.

Medical Management

Medical therapy for mitral regurgitation is geared toward afterload reduction to promote forward flow and minimize regurgitation back into the left atrium and pulmonary vasculature. In patients with acute or decompensated chronic mitral regurgitation, intravenous vasodilators such as nitroprusside can reduce filling pressures and ventricular cavity size and promote forward flow with afterload reduction. Intravenous diuretics are used to reduce volume overload. In acutely ill patients refractory to medications, intra-aortic balloon counterpulsation can be used further to reduce afterload while maintaining coronary perfusion with diastolic augmentation.

In patients with chronic mitral regurgitation or those in acute heart failure who are being weaned from intravenous inotropes and vasodilators, other afterload-reducing agents, such as angiotensin-converting enzyme (ACE) inhibitors, nitrates, or hydralazine, may be used. Diuretics can treat chronic and acute volume overload. Some practitioners continue to advocate the use of digoxin, especially for patients in atrial fibrillation. In the patient with chronic but compensated mitral valve regurgitation, mitral surgery can be safely deferred or avoided. The patient should be carefully monitored, however, and referred for mitral valve repair or replacement before significant left ventricular dysfunction or pulmonary hypertension occurs.

Surgical Management

Surgical Intervention. Two surgical approaches are used to treat mitral regurgitation. Mitral valve repair uses reconstructive techniques as well as a rigid prosthetic ring to repair the mitral valve apparatus, thus sparing the valve and avoiding the consequences of valve replacement (Fig. 33-7). Mitral valve replacement involves implantation of a prosthetic valve with attempted preservation of at least part of the mitral valve apparatus (Reardon & David, 1998), which contributes to left ventricular function (Fig. 33-8).

In patients with chronic mitral regurgitation, mitral replacement should occur before the patient has had irreversible left ventricular dysfunction. Mitral valve replacement or repair can preserve left ventricular function and ejection fraction. Patients with NYHA class II symptoms should be considered for surgery. Factors contributing to increased operative risk

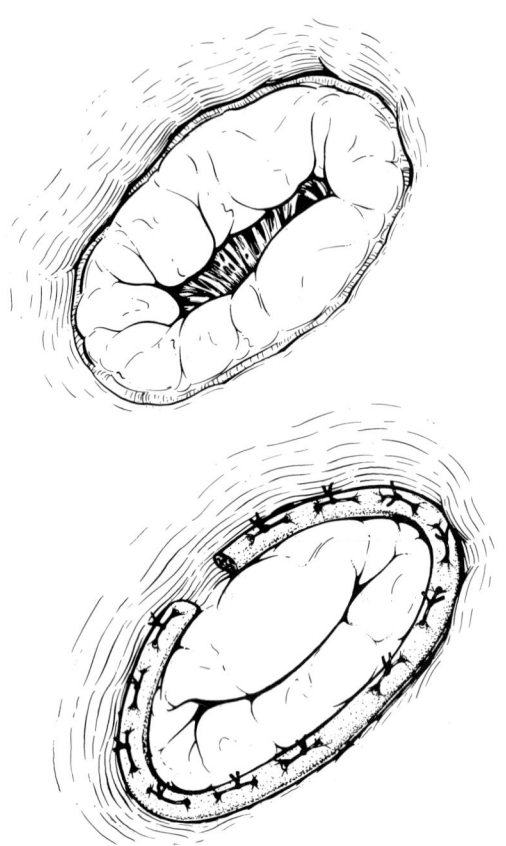

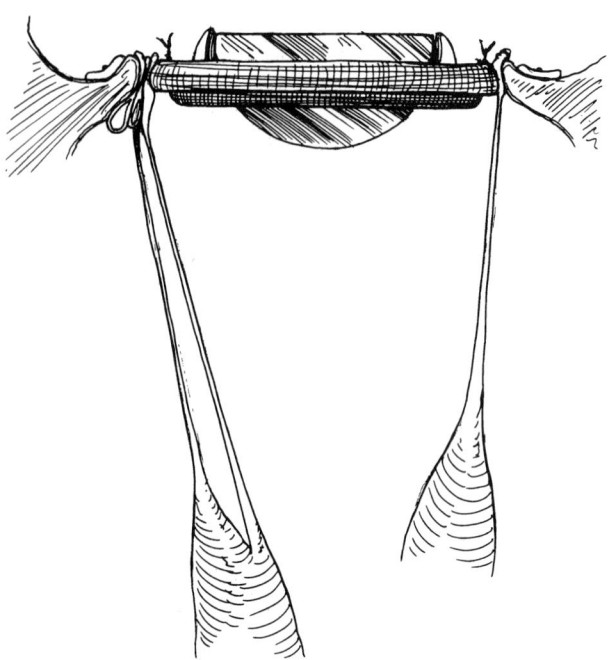

■ **Figure 33–8.** Valve replacement with chordal preservation. (From Chitwood, W. R. [1998]. Mitral valve repair: Ischemic. In L. R. Kaiser, I. L. Kron, & T. L. Spray [Eds.], *Mastery of cardiothoracic surgery* [p. 321]. Philadelphia: Lippincott-Raven.)

■ **Figure 33–7.** (*Top*) Regurgitant mitral valve (note large primary orifice). (*Bottom*) Completed mitral valve annuloplasty with ring sutured in place.

include reduced left ventricular ejection fraction, increased left ventricular end-systolic volume, older age, concomitant coronary artery disease, previous cardiac surgery, and pulmonary hypertension (Fann et al., 1997).

Mitral Valve Repair. In selected patients, mitral valve repair may be undertaken for patients with mitral insufficiency as an alternative to replacement. Surgical techniques involve reconstructing the leaflets and annulus in such a way as to narrow the orifice. These procedures consist of direct suture of the valve cusps, repair of the elongated or ruptured chordae tendineae (chordoplasty), or repair of the valve annulus (annuloplasty). With an annuloplasty, the incompetent valve is remodeled using a ring prosthesis that is attached to the leaflets and the annulus. Mitral valve repair has demonstrated excellent short-term and long-term results with low perioperative mortality rate (not >2% in most reported series). Carpentier and associates report 94% and 92% freedom from re-operations at 10 and 20 years, respectively (Hampton & Verrier, 2003).

Mitral Valve Replacement. In patients with acute mitral regurgitation secondary to MI, coronary angiography should be performed to define coronary anatomy for concomitant coronary bypass surgery at the time of mitral valve repair or replacement. In patients with acute mitral regurgitation secondary to MI, the mortality rate can be as high as 50% secondary to acute left ventricular failure (Fann et al., 1997).

Mitral Valve Prolapse

Cause

Mitral valve prolapse refers to a number of conditions in which one or both of the mitral valve leaflets becomes superior to the plane of the annulus during systole (Braunwald, 1998). The posterior leaflet is most often affected. Mitral valve prolapse (MVP) is also known as Barlow syndrome or click-murmur syndrome. It is the most common cause of significant isolated mitral regurgitation (Karon, 1997) and has been reported to be one of the most common heart disorders, with an overall prevalence of 2.4% (Playford & Weyman, 2001). Although MVP occurs most commonly in women, with a peak incidence in the fourth decade of life, severe mitral regurgitation associated with mitral valve prolapse is more common in men (Fann et al., 1997). The most common cause of MVP is myxomatous degeneration. Marfan syndrome, Ehlers-Danlos syndrome, rheumatic heart disease, and ischemic papillary muscle dysfunction also cause mitral valve prolapse. In addition, MVP has a hereditary component transmitted as an autosomal dominant trait (Braunwald, 1992).

Pathology

Patients with MVP have redundant myxomatous tissue with excess deposits of proteoglycans in the middle or spongiosa layer of the valve.

Histologically, collagen fragmentation and disorganization as well as elastic fiber are present. Acid mucopolysaccharide material accumulates in the valve leaflets. The mitral valve leaflets, annulus, and chordae tendineae may also demonstrate disrupted collagen structure and extensive myxomatous change. Myxomatous changes may also occur in the tricuspid, aortic, and pulmonic valves (Alpert et al., 1998).

Pathophysiology

Enlargement of the valve leaflets related to myxomatous degeneration causes systolic prolapse of one or both leaflets into the left atrium. Patients with MVP may have mitral regurgitation ranging in severity from none to severe. Persistent billowing of the valve causes stress to the underlying chordae and papillary muscles. Progressive mitral valvular degeneration can result in increasingly severe mitral regurgitation. If chordal rupture occurs, severe mitral regurgitation develops.

Supraventricular tachycardias (i.e., premature atrial contractions and paroxysmal supraventricular tachycardias) and ventricular arrhythmias may occur in patients with MVP. Although some patients with MVP have had sudden cardiac death, it is unclear what role MVP has in the cause. Some investigators believe that patients with MVP, history of syncope, complex ventricular arrhythmias, significant mitral regurgitation, and prolonged QT interval are at increased risk for sudden death (Kligfield & Devereux, 1995). Patients with MVP may also have autonomic nervous system dysfunction; specifically, mid-brain control of adrenergic and vagal responses may be abnormal. Heightened sympathetic nervous system tone may lead to a decease in left ventricular preload, resulting in MVP (Alpert et al., 1998).

Clinical Manifestations

Most patients with MVP are asymptomatic. Patients may have sharp, localized chest pain that is usually brief in duration. Although the cause of this chest pain is unclear if the patient does not have CHD, some authorities have suggested that the chest pain is cardiac in origin and is related to abnormal traction and tension on the papillary muscles (O'Rourke, 1998). Patients may have equivocal symptoms of anxiety, fatigue, palpitations, and orthostatic hypotension. As mitral regurgitation progresses, patients may note increasing dyspnea, fatigue, decreased exercise tolerance, orthopnea, and paroxysmal nocturnal dyspnea. Ruptured chordae with leaflet flail and acute mitral regurgitation result in symptoms of severe left ventricular failure.

Physical Assessment

The classic auscultatory finding of mitral valve prolapse is midsystolic click with mid to late systolic murmur (see Table 33-3). The click of MVP occurs when the elongated mitral valve apparatus reaches the end of its tether in mid systole (Carabello, 1998). The murmur occurs secondary to regurgitant flow when the mitral valve leaflets fail to approximate. Patients with mitral valve prolapse may have the murmur or click, or both. Findings may also vary over time. When the degree of mitral regurgitation is mild to moderate or less, heart rate and blood pressure may be normal. Additional physical findings may

include thin body habitus, pectus excavatum, straight-back syndrome, and scoliosis.

Diagnostic Tests

Echocardiography plays a key role in the diagnosis of MVP. Abnormal systolic motion of one or both of the mitral valve leaflets superior to the annular plane can be seen (Fig. 33-9). Doppler echocardiography gives additional evidence of valve regurgitation. *Transesophageal echocardiography* provides a more detailed look at the mitral valve and chordal structures (Brady, 2003).

Cardiac catheterization can be used to rule out CHD as the origin of chest pain. Left ventriculography can demonstrate

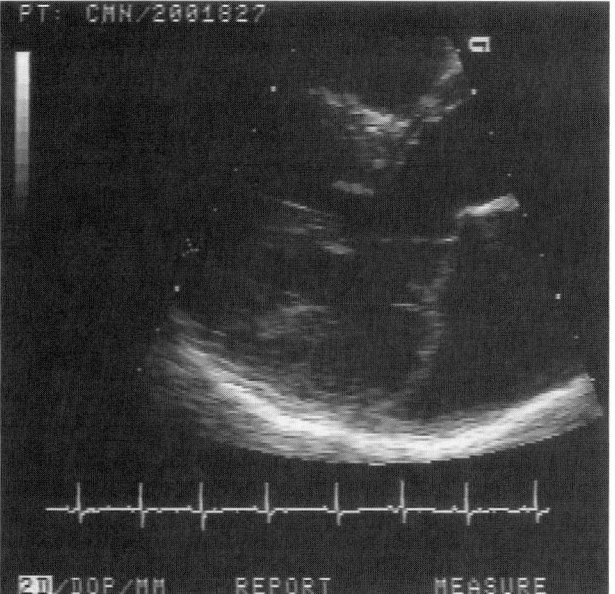

A

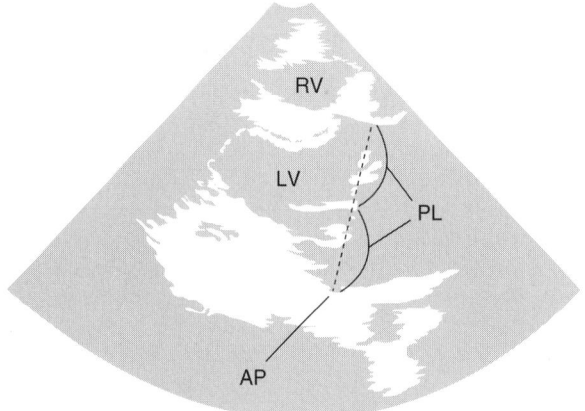

B

■ **Figure 33–9.** (*A*) Long-axis echocardiographic view of mitral valve with bileaflet prolapse above the annular plane into the left atrium. (*B*) Illustration corresponding to echocardiogram. RV, right ventricle; LV, left ventricle; AP, annular plane; PL, prolapsing leaflet.

abnormal motion of the mitral valve and help determine the degree of regurgitation.

Electrocardiography is nondiagnostic. The ECG may be normal or have nonspecific ST-T-wave changes in the inferior leads (II, III, and aVF) and occasionally in the anterolateral leads (V_4 through V_6). The ST-T-wave changes may become more notable with exercise. Premature atrial and ventricular complexes may also be identified. *Exercise testing* may be used to help rule out the cause of the chest pain.

Chest radiography is often normal and is usually nondiagnostic for MVP. Patients with acute mitral regurgitation secondary to chordal rupture have pulmonary congestion but not cardiomegaly. Patients with chronic severe mitral regurgitation have an enlarged cardiac silhouette secondary to left atrial and left ventricular enlargement in addition to pulmonary congestion (Fig. 33-10).

Medical and Surgical Management

Medical Treatment. Asymptomatic patients with MVP require no therapy other than antibiotic prophylaxis. Opinions remain divided on whether patients with isolated click without murmur require antibiotic prophylaxis. Patients with the murmur of mitral regurgitation or echocardiographic evidence of mitral regurgitation are recommended to have antibiotic prophylaxis. Beta-blockers or calcium channel blockers may be used to help alleviate palpitations or chest pain syndrome.

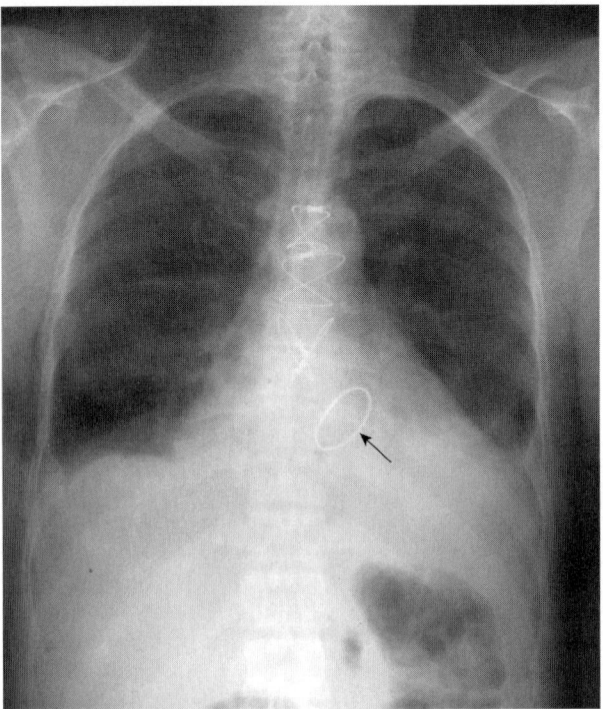

■ **Figure 33–10.** Chest radiograph of 51-year-old man with history of mitral valve prolapse and repair (note annuloplasty ring marked with *arrow*). Patient's valve repair has failed and his mitral regurgitation is now severe. Patient is now in severe heart failure with notable bilateral pleural effusions and cardiomegaly.

Surgical Treatment. Patients with MVP and severe mitral regurgitation or flail leaflets should be evaluated for surgery. They can often undergo repair rather than replacement. For discussion of surgical options, refer to the section on surgical intervention for mitral regurgitation.

Prognosis. MVP is usually a benign condition. Most patients remain asymptomatic for their entire lives. However, in a small subset of patients, sudden cardiac death may occur secondary to arrhythmias. Patients with palpitations, syncope, or dizziness should be further evaluated and considered for treatment of arrhythmias (Shah, 1991).

Aortic Stenosis

Cause

Aortic stenosis is characterized by obstruction of the left ventricular outflow tract. Most commonly, left ventricular outflow obstruction is valvular, but it may be either supravalvular or subvalvular. The age at which aortic stenosis becomes symptomatic is determined by the underlying cause. Aortic stenosis occurring from ages 1 to 30 years usually represents congenital aortic stenosis. Aortic stenosis presenting at the ages of 40 to 60 years is primarily rheumatic in origin or secondary to calcific aortic stenosis in a congenitally bicusp aortic valve. Past the age of 60 to 70 years, calcific degenerative stenosis is the most prevalent cause. Of the causes of aortic stenosis, senile/degenerative calcific aortic stenosis is most common.

Pathology

In senile/degenerative calcific aortic stenosis, cumulative wear and tear leads to calcification on an otherwise normal aortic valve. Calcific deposits prevent the cusps from opening normally in systole, resulting in stenosis. Risk factors for development of calcific aortic stenosis include male gender, elevated lipoprotein(a), height, hypertension, smoking, elevated low-density lipoprotein cholesterol, raised serum calcium, raised serum creatinine, and diabetes (Rajamannan et al., 2003). In patients with congenitally bicuspid aortic valves, abnormal flow through the valve leads to calcium deposition and restriction of cusp opening. In rheumatic aortic stenosis, inflammation and fibrosis of the valve result in fusion of the commissures as well as calcified masses in the aortic cusp (Chan, 1993).

Pathophysiology

Aortic stenosis typically progresses over a period of years. As the valve cusps become less mobile, the valve orifice decreases in size, resulting in an increasingly higher left ventricular systolic pressure necessary to eject blood across the stenosed valve. This increased left ventricular afterload results first in compensatory concentric left ventricular hypertrophy. Although initially adaptive in aortic stenosis, left ventricular hypertrophy leads to decreased ventricular compliance and diastolic dysfunction. As aortic stenosis becomes severe, left ventricular systolic function may also decline, resulting in

CHF. Late in the course, any coexisting mitral regurgitation increases because of an increased pressure gradient, which drives blood from the left ventricle into the left atrium (Braunwald, 1992).

Angina may result even in the absence of CHD because of an imbalance in myocardial oxygen supply and demand. Myocardial oxygen demand is increased secondary to increased left ventricular wall stress and muscle mass. Myocardial oxygen delivery is reduced as a result of decreased coronary perfusion pressure.

Syncope or near syncope can result secondary to reduced cerebral perfusion pressure, inappropriate left ventricular baroreceptor response, or arrhythmia. Orthostatic blood pressure changes may occur during exertion when arterial pressure drops because of systemic vasodilation in the setting of a fixed cardiac output. Increased left ventricular pressure may result in inappropriate baroreceptor response. Rapid atrial arrhythmias or ventricular arrhythmias may also cause "graying out" spells or frank syncopal episodes (Braunwald, 1992).

Clinical Manifestations

Patients with mild to moderate aortic stenosis are usually asymptomatic. As severe aortic stenosis develops, the most common initial symptom is dyspnea on exertion, followed by angina and near syncope or syncope. CHF also may occur as a result of ventricular dysfunction or increasing mitral regurgitation. Less commonly, sudden death, probably caused by ventricular fibrillation, may be the presenting clinical feature.

Physical Assessment

Aortic stenosis is most readily detected by auscultation of its classic mid-systolic (systolic ejection) murmur (see Table 33-3). As aortic stenosis progresses, the murmur peaks progressively later in systole and decreases in intensity as cardiac output falls. The murmur may decrease or disappear over the sternum and reappear at the apex, causing the incorrect impression of mitral regurgitation (Gallavardin phenomenon) (Carabello, 1998). An S_4 gallop is usually present. The point of maximal intensity is sustained but may not be displaced. Blood pressure is normal to hypertensive until late in the disease progress. Jugular venous pressure is normal in most patients except those with severe aortic stenosis associated with heart failure. Reduction in stroke volume and cardiac output may cause diminished carotid upstrokes and late systolic peak (tardus) in severe or critical aortic stenosis.

Diagnostic Tests

Echocardiography is the principal modality used to diagnose and quantify aortic stenosis. Two-dimensional echocardiography defines valve leaflet thickening and cusp movement restriction as well as gauging left ventricular hypertrophy and evaluating ventricular function (Carabello, 1998). Aortic valve pressure gradient can be measured, aortic valve area calculated, and pulmonary artery pressures estimated. Echocardiography is the most important diagnostic imaging technique used to diagnose and follow aortic stenosis (Brady, 2003).

Cardiac catheterization is performed in patients with aortic stenosis primarily to rule out concomitant CHD. Left ventriculography can quantify the left ventricular ejection fraction. The transvalvular gradient can be established by direct pressure measurement. Right heart catheterization can better quantify pulmonary artery pressures and cardiac output.

Electrocardiography often shows a pattern of left ventricular hypertrophy, although its absence does not exclude the presence of critical aortic stenosis. In addition to QRS amplitude changes typically associated with left ventricular hypertrophy, the patient with aortic stenosis may demonstrate ST-T-wave changes typical of left ventricular strain (Braunwald, 1992).

Exercise testing in patients with mild to moderate aortic stenosis with equivocal symptoms may be cautiously accomplished in the hands of a cardiologist and can provide relevant information regarding exercise tolerance. In patients with known severe aortic stenosis and classic symptoms such as syncope, dyspnea, and chest pain, exercise testing carries increased risk of ventricular tachyarrhythmias and ventricular fibrillation and should not be preformed.

Gated blood pool radionuclide scans provide information regarding ventricular function similar to echocardiography and left ventriculography. Gated pool scans may be useful in patients in whom left ventriculography cannot be performed (i.e., patients with elevated creatinine), or in those in whom the left ventricle cannot be clearly imaged with echocardiography.

Chest radiography may be negative even in advanced disease. Heart size may be normal or only minimally enlarged. The left ventricular border and apex may be rounded, demonstrating a boot-shaped silhouette. Identifiable calcification of the aortic valve and aorta may be present. As disease progresses, left atrial enlargement, pulmonary hypertension, and CHF may become evident. Poststenotic dilation of the proximal ascending aorta may be noted along the right heart border in the posteroanterior chest radiograph (Fig. 33-11).

Medical Management

Aside from antibiotic prophylaxis to prevent endocarditis, there is no effective medical management of aortic stenosis (Carabello, 1998). Because the course of aortic stenosis varies in its progression, patients should be carefully followed-up by their health care providers with serial physical examinations and periodic echocardiography. Patients with mild aortic stenosis undergo echocardiography every 2 years. Patients with asymptomatic severe aortic stenosis are followed-up with serial echocardiograms every 6 to 12 months. Patients are instructed regarding symptoms of aortic stenosis, including dyspnea, decreased exercise tolerance, shortness of breath, chest pain, near syncope, and syncope (Braunwald, 1992). Beta-blockers, diuretics, nitrates, and ACE inhibitors must be used with caution, because they may precipitate syncope or even cardiovascular collapse in the patient with severe aortic stenosis (Carabello, 1998).

Interventional and Surgical Management

Percutaneous Aortic Catheter Balloon Valvuloplasty. Percutaneous aortic catheter balloon valvuloplasty is accomplished by passing a guide wire across the stenotic aortic valve into

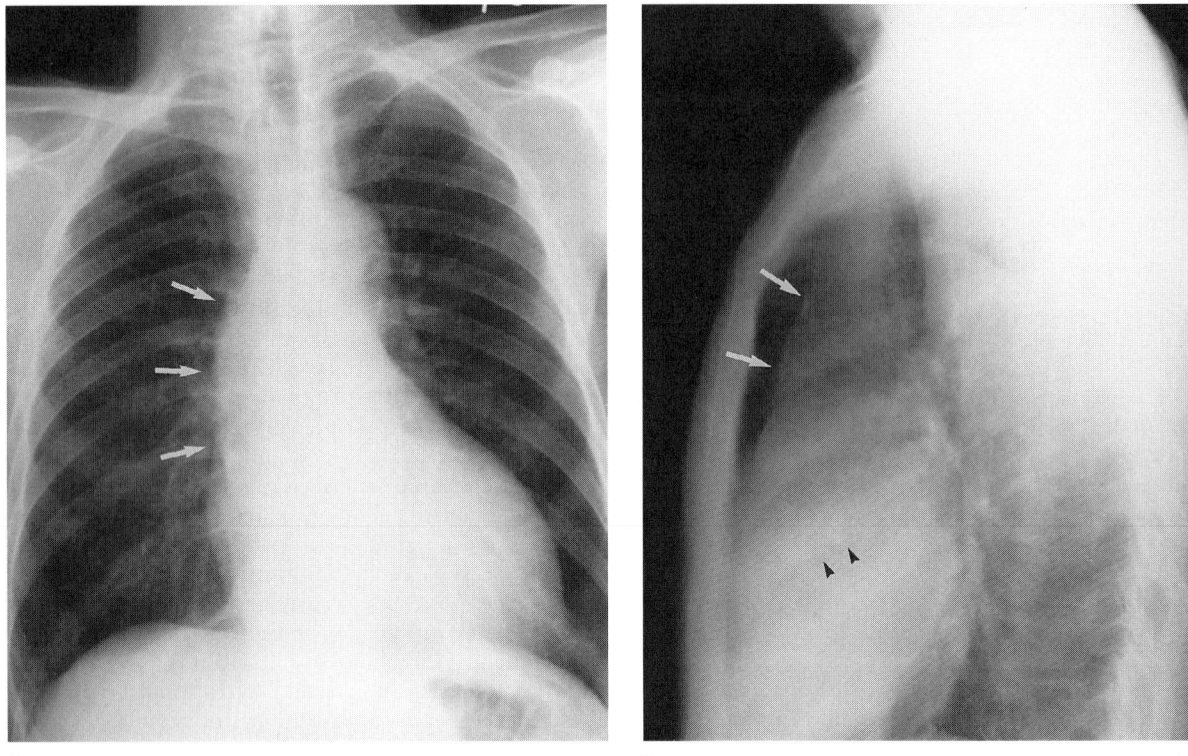

A **B**

■ **Figure 33–11.** (*A*) Posteroanterior chest radiograph showing rounded border of left ventricle (*arrows*). (*B*) Lateral chest radiograph showing calcified aortic valve (*arrowheads*) and filling of the retrosternal airspace with dilated ascending aorta (*arrows*). (From Boxt, L. M. [1998]. Plain film examination of the chest. In E. J. Topol, R. M. Califf, J. M. Isner et al. [Eds.], *Textbook of cardiovascular medicine* [p. 511]. Philadelphia: Lippincott-Raven.)

the apex of the left ventricle. A balloon-tipped catheter is advanced retrograde across the stenotic valve. The balloon is inflated, fracturing calcified nodules and separating the fused commissures. The aortic valve ring is also stretched to increase the size of the aortic valve orifice. Although results vary, aortic balloon valvuloplasty has been shown, on average, to increase aortic valve area from 0.5 to 0.8 cm^2 and to decrease the gradient from 60 to 30 mm Hg. In addition, left ventricular ejection fraction tends to rise in those patients with depressed left ventricular function (Braunwald, 1992).

Restenosis is a major problem in balloon aortic valvuloplasty in adults, occurring in approximately half of the patients within 6 months. Approximately one third of patients have recurrence of symptoms within 6 months. Because of the high restenosis rate, aortic balloon valvuloplasty in adults is reserved for those candidates unsuitable for surgery (i.e., the elderly with heart failure or pregnant women). Aortic balloon valvuloplasty may be used as a bridge or palliative procedure in these populations, and surgical replacement may be considered for a later time (Braunwald, 1992).

Aortic Valve Replacement. Aortic valve replacement is the only effective treatment for advanced aortic stenosis (Chan, 1993). The natural history of aortic stenosis is used as a guide to determine the timing of aortic valve replacement surgery. Patients with asymptomatic aortic stenosis have nearly the same survival rate as the age-matched general population. Once the patient experiences symptoms of angina, syncope,

or heart failure, there is an abrupt decline in survival rate. In patients presenting with CHF, only 50% survive 2 years. For patients who present with syncope, the 3-year survival rate is only 50% without aortic valve replacement. The average life expectancy of patients with apnea is only 5 years without aortic valve replacement (Ross, 1968). Aortic valve replacement is recommended in all patients with severe, symptomatic aortic stenosis. Although the average perioperative mortality rate in most centers ranges from 2% to 8% (Braunwald, 1992), perioperative mortality rates range from less than 5% in young, healthy patients to as high as 30% in the frail elderly (Nishimura, 1997). Factors that increase the mortality risk at the time of aortic valve replacement include class III or IV heart failure, emergency surgery, aortic insufficiency, and cardiomegaly (Shine & Howland-Gradman, 1996). Even in patients with severe left ventricular dysfunction, improvement of symptoms and left ventricular ejection fraction occurs in most (Connolly et al, 1997). Selection of aortic valve prostheses was discussed earlier in this chapter.

Aortic Insufficiency

Cause

Aortic regurgitation may be caused by either intrinsic abnormalities of the aortic valve leaflets or disease of the aortic root. In rheumatic fever and endocarditis, the aortic leaflets are directly affected. In congenitally bicuspid valves, the larger cusp may become redundant, resulting in diastolic prolapse and progressive aortic regurgitation. The aortic valve may also become incompetent because of aortic root dilation. As the aortic root dilates, the aortic annulus becomes so large that the valve cusps no longer approximate, resulting in regurgitation.

Aortic root dilation is seen in patients with Marfan syndrome, rheumatic arthritis, ankylosing spondylitis, annuloaortic ectasia (associated with hypertension and aging), aortic dissection, syphilitic aortitis, and collagen vascular disease.

Pathology

Rheumatic fever leads to fibrinous infiltrates on the valve cusps, causing them to contract and become malaligned and incompetent. Patients with rheumatic disease may have a "mixed lesion" that includes both aortic regurgitation and aortic stenosis. In acute or subacute infective endocarditis of the aortic valve, tissue destruction of the leaflets causes cusp perforation or prolapse. Vegetations adherent to the aortic valve may also interfere with valve closure, causing incompetence. In patients with aortic root dilation or ascending aortic dissection, the aortic annulus becomes greatly enlarged, the aortic leaflets separate, and aortic incompetence follows.

Pathophysiology

Volume overload occurs secondary to regurgitant volume reentering the left ventricle from the aorta through the incompetent aortic valve. Retrograde flow occurs during diastole when left ventricular pressure is low and aortic pressure is high. The left ventricle is forced to pump the normal volume received from the left atrium as well as the regurgitant volume from the aorta.

Similar to mitral regurgitation, the hemodynamic presentation and the heart's ability to compensate differ depending on whether the aortic insufficiency is acute or chronic. In chronic aortic regurgitation, the left ventricle is subjected to pressure and volume overload. As a result, the left ventricle develops mild concentric hypertrophy to accommodate the pressure load and eccentric hypertrophy to compensate for the increased volume load. Patients with chronic aortic regurgitation may remain asymptomatic for years, until progressive left ventricular dilation and dysfunction result in CHF. In patients with acute aortic regurgitation, the left ventricle has not had time to compensate with either concentric or eccentric hypertrophy and cannot accommodate the large volume caused by acute aortic regurgitation. As a result, left ventricular and left atrial pressures rise sharply, causing acute CHF and pulmonary edema. Patients with acute aortic regurgitation usually require surgical intervention.

Clinical Manifestations

Patients with chronic aortic regurgitation are often asymptomatic for many years. Common symptoms of aortic regurgitation include fatigue and exertional dyspnea. Patients may report palpitations, dizziness, and the sensation of a forceful heartbeat, especially when lying on their left side. Angina may also be noted, but it occurs less frequently in aortic regurgitation than in aortic stenosis. As heart failure ensures, patients experience orthopnea, paroxysmal nocturnal dyspnea, and cough related to

Table 33–6 ■ SPECIFIC PHYSICAL EXAMINATION FINDINGS IN AORTIC REGURGITATION

Sign	Physical Description
Quincke's sign	Pulsatile flushing/blanching of nail bed with application of gentle pressure
de Musset's sign	Bobbing of head with each pulse
Corrigan's pulse (waterhammer)	Sharp systolic upstroke and diastolic collapse of pulse
Müller's sign	Bobbing of uvula with each pulse
Traube's sign	"Pistol shot" sound auscultated over the femoral arteries
Duroziez's sign	Biphasic femoral bruit auscultated with mild pressure
Hill's sign	Blood pressure higher in arms than legs

left-sided heart failure. With acute aortic regurgitation, symptoms of left-sided heart failure develop rapidly.

Physical Assessment

The typical murmur of aortic regurgitation is a high-pitched, early diastolic decrescendo murmur with a blowing quality (see Table 33-2). Patients may also have a physiologic murmur of mitral stenosis caused by the regurgitant aortic jet, which partially prevents mitral valve closure (Austin Flint murmur). As the severity of aortic regurgitation increases, the murmur becomes louder and longer. In chronic aortic regurgitation, the point of maximal impulse is displaced laterally. Systolic hypertension and decreased diastolic pressure create a widened pulse pressure. Patients with chronic aortic regurgitation may have a host of other physical findings that may not be present in acute aortic regurgitation (Table 33-6).

Diagnostic Tests

Echocardiography is helpful in identifying the cause of aortic regurgitation. Echocardiography can indicate left ventricular volume overload by the increased internal diameter of the ventricular chamber during systole and diastole. Doppler echocardiography is the best noninvasive means to detect aortic regurgitation. Transesophageal echocardiography is especially useful in imaging the ascending and descending aorta in patients with suspected aortic dissection.

Cardiac catheterization should be performed to visualize and quantify the extent of regurgitation before surgery. However, physical findings and noninvasive tests are sufficient to establish the diagnosis of aortic insufficiency. In patients with known or suspected CHD, coronary angiography should be performed. In patients with aortic root dilation, aortic root angiography may be performed concurrently with coronary angiography.

Radionuclide imaging can be used to estimate ejection fraction and determine myocardial perfusion defects in patients with concomitant CHD.

Exercise testing may be used to establish exercise tolerance and to evaluate asymptomatic patients.

Electrocardiography may be normal in patients with acute aortic regurgitation or in patients with mild to moderate chronic regurgitation. Patients with moderate to severe chronic regurgitation may have left-axis deviation and a pattern of left ventricular strain (Q waves in I, aVL, and V_3 to V_6, with small R wave in V_1). Intraventricular conduction defects may occur with left ventricular dysfunction or annular abscess.

Chest radiography may show only CHF in the patient with acute aortic regurgitation because compensatory left ventricular dilation has not yet occurred. In chronic aortic regurgitation, the chest radiograph demonstrates marked cardiomegaly with inferior and leftward displacement of the apex (Braunwald, 1992). Dilation of the ascending aorta and a widened mediastinum may be noted in patients with aortic dissection. In patients with a dilated aortic root or dissection, computed tomography or magnetic resonance imaging may be necessary to better-delineate the ascending aorta, transverse arch, and proximal descending aorta.

Medical Management

Patients who have asymptomatic aortic regurgitation should receive appropriate antibiotic prophylaxis as well as afterload reduction with vasodilators. In patients with asymptomatic, chronic, or severe aortic regurgitation and normal left ventricular function, nifedipine reduced left ventricular size and mass and further improved left ventricular function (Scognamiglio et al., 1994), thus reducing and delaying the need for aortic valve replacement. Nifedipine is superior to hydralazine, which does not decrease left ventricular mass or reduce left ventricular dimension (Khan, 1996). Diltiazem and verapamil are contraindicated in aortic regurgitation because they have a more potent negative inotropic effect and may produce bradycardia, which may worsen heart failure. It is probably reasonable to substitute other dihydropyridine calcium channel blockers if nifedipine is poorly tolerated (Carbello, 1998). ACE inhibitors may be used to reduce afterload, although they are not as well studied in this population of patients.

Patients with moderate to severe aortic regurgitation should not participate in vigorous exercise or competitive sports. Patients with chronic severe aortic regurgitation should be followed-up with physical examination and echocardiography every 6 to 12 months (Rahimtoola, 1998). Sodium nitroprusside reduces preload and afterload and can be used to stabilize patients with acute aortic regurgitation before surgery. Intra-aortic balloon counterpulsation cannot be used because inflation of the balloon during diastole would increase the regurgitant volume into the left ventricle, which acutely worsens left ventricular dilation and heart failure.

Surgical Management

Acute aortic regurgitation requires urgent aortic valve replacement. Without adequate time for compensatory mechanisms to develop, aortic regurgitation triggers rapid onset of CHF, tachycardia, and diminished cardiac output. It is desirable to treat patients with acute aortic regurgitation secondary to infective endocarditis with a minimum of 48 hours of appropriate intravenous antibiotics before implanting a prosthetic valve. In patients with active endocarditis who are hemodynamically unstable, use of cadaveric human aortic homografts may mini-

mize the risk of prosthetic valve endocarditis. Patients who have aortic regurgitation caused by ascending aortic dissection or dilation require replacement of the ascending aorta as well.

In chronic aortic regurgitation, the aortic valve must be replaced before irreversible left ventricular dysfunction. In asymptomatic patients, it is usually recommended that the aortic valve be replaced when left ventricular function begins to deteriorate. Surgery is recommended when the echocardiographic left ventricular ejection fraction is .55 or less, the end-diastolic diameter approaches 75 mm, or the end-systolic diameter reaches 50 mm. When symptoms of heart failure develop, aortic valve surgery should be performed regardless of echocardiography findings, because new-onset heart failure indicates that the heart has met the limits of compensation (Carbello, 1998).

REFERENCES

Alpert, J. S., Sabick, J., & Cosgrove, D. M. (1998). Mitral valve disease. In E. J. Topol, R. M. Califf, J. M. Isner et al. (Eds.), *Textbook of cardiovascular medicine* (pp. 503–532). Philadelphia: Lippincott-Raven.

Abraham, M. T., & Cherin, G. (1991). Rheumatic fever. In K. Chatterjee, M. D. Cheitlin, J. Karliner et al. (Eds.), *Cardiology: An illustrated text/reference* (pp. 10.98–10.106). Philadelphia: JB Lippincott.

Bhola, R., & Gill, E. (2001). Rheumatic heart disease and mitral stenosis. In O. V. Adair, *Cardiology secrets* (2nd ed., pp. 226–235).

Brady, T. J., Grist, T. M., Westra, S. J., et al. (2003). Valvular. In T. J. Brady, T. M. Grist, S. J. Westra, et al, *Pocket radiologist: Cardiac top 100 diagnoses* (pp. 53–75). Salt Lake, UT: Amirsys.

Braunwald, E. (1992). Valvular heart disease. In E. Braunwald (Ed.), *Heart disease: A textbook of cardiovascular medicine* (4th ed., pp. 1007–1077). Philadelphia: WB Saunders.

Braunwald, E. (1998). Valvular heart disease. In A. S. Fauci, E. Braunwald, & K. J. Isselbacher (Eds.), *Harrison's principles of internal medicine* (14th ed., pp. 1311–1324). New York: McGraw-Hill.

Buccino, D., Tu, A. S., & Come, P. C. (1993). Diagnostic imaging and catheterization techniques. In L. S. Lilly (Ed.), *Pathophysiology of heart disease* (pp. 130–146). Philadelphia: Lea & Febiger.

Burge, D. J., & DeHoratius, R. J. (1993). Acute rheumatic fever. In A. N. Brest (Ed.), *Valvular heart disease: Comprehensive evaluation and treatment* (2nd ed., pp. 3–7). Philadelphia: F. A. Davis.

Carabello, B. A. (1998). Recognition and management of patients with valvular heart disease. In L. Goldman, & E. Braunwald (Eds.), *Primary cardiology* (pp. 370–389). Philadelphia: WB Saunders.

Carabello, B. A. (2000). Acute mitral regurgitation. In J. S. Alpert, J. E. Dalen, & S. H. Rahimtoola (Eds.), *Valvular heart disease* (3rd ed., pp. 143–155). Philadelphia: Lippincott Williams & Wilkins.

Chan. E., Duh, E., Stidham, B. et al. (1993). Valvular heart disease. In L. S. Lilly (Ed.), *Pathophysiology of heart disease* (pp. 130–146). Philadelphia: Lea & Febiger.

Chitwood, W.R., Wixon, C. L., & Elbeery, J. R. (1997). Video-assisted minimally invasive mitral valve surgery. *Journal of Thoracic & Cardiovascular Surgery,* 114, 773–781.

Chitwood, W. R. (2003). Robot-assisted mitral valve surgery. In K. L. Franco, & E. D. Verrier (Eds.), *Advanced therapy in cardiac surgery* (pp. 220–229). Hamilton, Ontario: BC Decker.

Cohn, L. H., Adams, D. H., Couper, G. S., et al. (1997). Minimally invasive cardiac valve surgery improves patient satisfaction while reducing costs of cardiac valve replacement and repair. *Annals of Surgery,* 226, 421–426.

Connolly, H. M., Oh, J. K., Orszulak, T. A., et al. (1997). Aortic valve replacement for aortic stenosis with severe left ventricular dysfunction: Prognostic Indicators. *Circulation,* 95, 2395–2399.

Cosgrove, D. M., Sabik, J. F., & Navia, J. L. (1998). Minimally invasive valve operations. *Annals of Thoracic Surgery,* 65, 1538–1539.

Crawford, M. H. & Durack, D. T. (2003). Clinical presentation of infective endocarditis. *Cardiology Clinics,* 21, 159–166.

Dajani, A. S., Taubert, K. A., Wilson, W., et al (1997). Prevention of bacterial endocarditis: Recommendations by the American Heart Association. *Circulation,* 96, 358–366.

Dalen, J. E., & Fenster, P. E. (2000). Mitral stenosis. In J. S. Alpert, J. E. Dalen, & S. H. Rahimtoola (Eds.), *Valvular heart disease* (3rd ed., pp. 75–112). Philadelphia: Lippincott Williams & Wilkins.

David, T. E., Puschmann, R., Ivanov, J., et al. (1998). Aortic valve replacement with the stentless and stented porcine valves: A case-match study. *Journal of Thoracic & Cardiovascular Surgery*, 116, 236–240.

Doty, J. R., Salazar, J. D., Liddicoat, J. R., et al. (1998). Aortic valve replacement with cryopreserved aortic allograft: Ten year experience. *Journal of Thoracic Cardiovascular Surgery*, 115, 371–379.

Edmunds, L. H., Addonizio, V. P., & Tepe, N. A. (1991). Valvular heart disease: Prosthetic valve replacement. In K. Chatterjee, M. D. Cheitlin, & J. Karliner et al. (Eds.), *Cardiology: An illustrated text/rReference* (pp. 940–941). Philadelphia: JB Lippincott.

Elkins, R. C. (2003). Pulmonary autograft. In K. L. Franco & E. D. Verrier (Eds.), *Advanced therapy in cardiac surgery* (pp. 156–167). Hamilton, Ontario: BC Decker.

Enriquez-Sarano, M., Schaff, H. V., Tajik, A. J. & Frye, R. L. (2000). Chronic mitral regurgitation. In J. S. Alpert, J. E. Dalen, & S. H. Rahimtoola (Eds.), *Valvular heart disease* (3rd ed., pp. 113–141). Philadelphia: Lippincott Williams & Wilkins.

Ewy, G. A. (2000). Tricuspid valve disease. In J. S. Alpert, J. E. Dalen, & S. H. Rahimtoola (Eds.), *Valvular heart disease* (3rd ed., pp. 377–392). Philadelphia: Lippincott Williams & Wilkins.

Fann, J. I., Ingels, N. B., & Miller, D. C. (1997). Pathophysiology of mitral valve disease and operative indications. In L. H. Edmunds (Ed.), *Cardiac surgery in the adult* (pp. 959–990). New York: McGraw-Hill.

Garcia, M. J. (1998). Prosthetic valve disease. In E. J. Topol, R. M. Califf, J. M. Isner et al. (Eds.), *Textbook of cardiovascular medicine* (pp. 579–605). Philadelphia: Lippincott-Raven.

Goldman, B. S., & Mallidi, H. (2003). Update on Stentless valves. In K. L. Franco & E. D. Verrier (Eds.), *Advanced therapy in cardiac surgery* (pp. 196–206). Hamilton, Ontario: BC Decker.

Goldsmith, I., Turpie, A. C. G., & Lip, G. Y. (2002). ABC of Antithrombotic therapy: valvular heart disease and prosthetic heart valves. *BMJ*, 325, 1228–1231.

Grunkemeier, G. L., Starr, A., & Rahimtoola, S. H. (1994). Replacement heart valves. In R. A. O'Rourke (Ed.), *Hurst's the heart: Update I* (pp. 98–123). New York: McGraw-Hill.

Hamptom, C. R., & Verrier, E. D. (2003). Mitral valve repair. In K. L. Franco & E. D. Verrier (Eds.), *Advanced therapy in cardiac surgery* (pp. 207–219). Hamilton, Ontario: BC Decker.

International Ross Registry. (2003). Follow-up data. [Online]. Available: http://www.rossregistry.com (Accessed 8/28/03).

Izzat, M. B., Yim, A. P., El-Zufari, et al. (1998). Upper T mini-sternotomy for aortic valve operations. *Chest*, 114, 291–294.

Jamieson, W. R. E. (2003). Update on new tissue valves. In K. L. Franco & E. D. Verrier (Eds.), *Advanced therapy in cardiac surgery* (pp. 177–195). Hamilton, Ontario: BC Decker.

Kaplan, E. L. (1998). Acute rheumatic fever. In R. W. Alexander, R. C. Sclant, & V. Fuster (Eds.), *Hurst's the heart* (9th ed., pp. 1759–1787). New York: McGraw-Hill.

Karchmer, A. W. (1998). Approach to the patient with infective endocarditis. In L. Goldman & E. Braunwald (Eds), *Primary cardiology* (pp. 201–218). Philadelphia: WB Saunders.

Karon, B. L. (1997). Valvular regurgitation. In J. G. Murphy (Ed.), *Mayo Clinic cardiology review* (pp. 533–554). Armonk, NY: Futura.

Khan, M. G. (1996). Valvular heart disease and rheumatic fever. In M. G. Khan (Ed), *Heart Disease Diagnosis and Therapy: A Practical Approach* (pp. 415–460). Baltimore: Williams & Wilkins.

Kligfield, P., & Devereux, R. B. (1995). Arrhythmia in mitral valve prolapse. In P. R. Podrid & P. R. Kowey (Eds.), *Cardiac arrhythmia: Mechanisms, diagnosis, and management* (pp. 1253–1260). Baltimore: Williams & Wilkins.

Luciani, G. B., Bertolini, P., Vecchi, B. et al. (1998). Midterm results after aortic valve replacement with freehand stentless xenografts: A comparison of three prostheses. *Journal of Thoracic and Cardiovascular Surgery*, 115, 1287–1296.

Mayes, C. E., Cigarroa, J. E., Lange, R. A., et al. (1999). Percutaneous mitral balloon valvuloplasty. *Clinics in Cardiology*, 22, 501–503.

Mazur, W., Parilak, L. D., Kaluza, G., et al. (1999). Balloon valvuloplasty for mitral stenosis. *Current Opinion in Cardiology*, 14, 95–103.

McAnulty, J. H., & Rahimtoola, S. H. (1998). Antithrombotic therapy and valvular heart disease. In R. W. Alexander, R. C. Sclant, & V. Fuster (Eds.), *Hurst's the heart* (9th ed., pp. 1759–1787). New York: McGraw-Hill.

Nishimura, R. A. (1997). Valvular stenosis. In J. G. Murphy (Ed.), *Mayo Clinic cardiology review* (pp. 521–532). Armonk, NY: Futura.

Olaison, L., & Pettersson, G. (2003) Current best practices and guidelines: Indications for surgical intervention in infective endocarditis. *Cardiology Clinics*, 21, 235–251.

O'Rourke, R. A. (1998). Mitral valve prolapse syndrome. In R. W. Alexander, R. C. Sclant, & V. Fuster (Eds.), *Hurst's the heart* (9th ed., pp. 1821–1831). New York: McGraw-Hill.

Otto, C. M. (1998). Aortic stenosis: Clinical evaluation and optimal timing of surgery. *Cardiology Clinics*, 16(3), 353–373.

Otto, C. M. (1999). Right-sided valve disease. In C. M. Otto, *Valvular heart disease* (pp. 362–379). Philadelphia: W.B. Saunders.

Palacios, I. F., Sanchez, P. L. Harrell, L. C., et al. (2002). Which patients benefit from percutaneous mitral balloon valvuloplasty? *Circulation*, 105, 1465–1471.

Playford, D., & Weyman, A. E. (2001). Mitral valve prolapse: time for a fresh look. *Reviews in Cardiovascular Medicine*, 2(2), 73–81.

Rahimtoola, S. H. (1998). Aortic valve disease. In R. W. Alexander, R. C. Sclant, & V. Fuster (Eds.), *Hurst's the heart* (9th ed., pp. 1759–1787). New York: McGraw-Hill.

Rajamannan, N. M., Gersh, B., & Bonow, R. O. (2003). Calcific aortic stenosis: from bench to bedside- emerging clinical and cellular concepts. *Heart*, 89, 801–805.

Reardon, M. J., & David, T. E. (1998). Mitral valve replacement with preservation of the subvalvular apparatus. *Current Opinion in Cardiology*, 14, 104–110.

Ross, J. Jr., & Braunwald, E. (1968). Aortic stenosis. *Circulation* (Suppl. V), 38, 61–67.

Ross, D. N., Jackson, M., & Davies, J. (1987). Pulmonary autograft aortic valve replacement. *Circulation*, 75, 895–901.

Sachdev, M., Peterson, G. E., & Jollis, J. G. (2003). Imaging techniques for diagnosis of infective endocarditis. *Cardiology Clinics*, 21, 185–195.

Santini, F., Dyke, C., Edwards, S., et al. (1997). Pulmonary autograft versus homograft replacement of the aortic valve: A prospective randomized trial. *Journal of Thoracic and Cardiovascular Surgery*, 113, 894–899.

Scognamiglio, R., Rahimtoola, S. H., Fasoli, G., et al. (1994). Nifedipine in asymptomatic patients with severe aortic regurgitation and normal left ventricular function. *New England Journal of Medicine*, 331, 689–694.

Sexton, D. J., & Spelman, D. (2003). Current best practices and guidelines: Assessment and management of complications in infective endocarditis. *Cardiology Clinics*, 21, 273–282.

Shah, P. M. (1991). Mitral valve prolapse. In K. Chatterjee, M. D. Cheitlin, J. Karliner et al. (Eds.), *Cardiology: An illustrated text/reference* (pp. 9.30–9.39). Philadelphia: JB Lippincott.

Sharony, R., Grossi, E. A. Ribakove, G. H., et al. (2003). Minimally invasive cardiac valve surgery. In K. L. Franco & E. D. Verrier (Eds.), *Advanced therapy in cardiac surgery* (pp.147–155). Hamilton, Ontario: BC Decker.

Shine, L., & Howland-Gradman, J. (1996). Aortic stenosis in the elderly: Valvuloplasty vs surgery. *American Journal of Nursing* (Suppl.), 7–11.

Teerlink, J. R., & Foster, E. (1998). Valvular heart disease in pregnancy. *Cardiology Clinics*, 16 (3), 573–594.

Towns, M. L., & Reller, L. B. (2003). Diagnostic methods: current best practices and guidelines for isolation of bacteria and fungi in infective endocarditis. *Cardiology Clinics*, 21, 197–205.

Wernly, J. A., & Crawford, M. H. (1998). Choosing a prosthetic heart valve. *Cardiology Clinics*, 16 (3), 491–504.

Whittlesay, D., & Geha, A. S. (1991). Selection and complications of cardiac valvular prosthesis. In A. E. Baue, A. S. Geha, G. L. Hammond et al. (Eds.), *Glenn's thoracic and cardiovascular surgery* (5th ed., pp. 1719–1728). Norwalk, CT: Appleton & Lange.

Pericardial, Myocardial, and Endocardial Disease

MARGARET M. MCNEILL

Diseases of the pericardium, myocardium, and endocardium have a major impact on cardiac function, and therefore on quality of life. For this reason, and because of wide-ranging economic ramifications, it is imperative that nurses have a comprehensive understanding of these conditions and provide care that optimizes outcomes for patients and families.

PERICARDIAL DISEASE

The pericardium is composed of two layers, the *serosa* and the *fibrosa,* which contain nerves, blood vessels, and lymphatics (Spodick, 1997j). The fibrous outer layer, also called the parietal pericardium, is discretely attached to the sternum, great vessels, and diaphragm (Shabetai, 1998; Spodick, 1997j). A serosal layer of cuboidal cells one-cell layer thick lines the pericardium. The monocellular serosa directly covers the heart surfaces and is also known as the *visceral pericardium* or the *epicardium.* The phrenic nerves supply most of the parietal pericardium. The pericardial space between the layers normally contains 15 to 35 mL of serous pericardial fluid, an ultrafiltrate of the blood plasma (Spodick, 1997j).

The pericardium serves several functions, yet cardiac activity is normal if it is missing because of congenital absence or surgical removal. The pericardium is a relatively inelastic covering and it exerts a powerful restraining effect on the size of the heart in situations of acute volume overload (Shabetai, 1998; Spodick, 1997k). The pericardium maintains the heart in a comparatively stable position and functionally optimum shape in the mediastinum. It acts as a barrier to inflammation from adjacent structures and contains defensive immunologic constituents. The pericardial fluid reduces friction on the pericardium.

Almost every known pathologic process, medical and surgical, can contribute to pericardial disease, either primarily involving the pericardium or with an indirect pericardial impact (Spodick, 1997a). For unknown reasons, there is a predominance of men with pericardial disease. The many types and descriptions of pericardial diseases are given in Table 34-1, and the major primary congenital abnormalities are listed in Display 34-1 (Spodick, 1997e).

Pericarditis

The clinically most significant pericardial condition is pericarditis, an inflammation of the pericardium.

Etiology

The major causes of pericarditis are given in Display 34-2 (Shabetai, 1998; Spodick, 1997a; Spodick, 2001; Johnson et al., 1999). Direct or indirect trauma to the chest, as well as injuries caused by pacing wires and migrating or misplaced central catheters, can lead to pericarditis (Karmy-Jones, 2002). Viral pathogens and diseases include but are not limited to coxsackievirus, infectious mononucleosis, influenza, chickenpox, and acquired immunodeficiency syndrome (AIDS). In AIDS, opportunistic infections, such as tuberculosis, or neoplasms are the most likely etiologies of pericardial disease. Some of the bacteria causing pericarditis include *Staphylococcus, Pneumococcus,* and *Streptococcus* species, and *Mycobacterium tuberculosis. Aspergillosis* and histoplasmosis are among the fungal infections that can cause pericarditis.

Abnormalities of the myocardium, pleura, lungs, diaphragm, esophagus, and mediastinal lymph nodes all may directly involve the pericardium because of its proximity or by transmission through lymphatic or blood circulation. Transmural myocardial infarction (MI) frequently involves the pericardium, but this is not detected in more than half of the cases (Spodick, 1997a). Metastatic cancers, including bronchogenic carcinoma, breast cancer, lymphoma, leukemia, and melanoma, can all cause pericarditis, as can some of the treatments for these conditions. Pericarditis has been linked to end-stage renal disease related to both uremia and dialysis. Uremic pericarditis is usually found in patients with newly diagnosed chronic renal failure who have never undergone dialysis. Dialysis-associated pericarditis could be related to infection, heparin, and elevations of blood urea nitrogen (BUN), creatinine, and uric acid (Berg, 1990).

Most chronic inflammatory disorders of the vasculitis connective tissue disease group, which share the common feature of inflammation tending to damage blood vessel walls, can cause pericarditis, pericardial effusion, pericardial adhesions, and constriction. The vasculitis seen in this group of diseases probably is primarily due to deposition of immune complexes resulting in

Table 34–1 ■ ACQUIRED PERICARDIAL DISEASE

Condition	Description
Pericarditis	Inflammation of the pericardium
Myopericarditis	Inflammation of both the myocardium and the pericardium
Pericardial fat necrosis	Rare condition sometimes causing chest pain
Pericardial effusion	Excess pericardial fluid produced by the pericardium
Polyserositis	Multiple serous membrane inflammation
Hemopericardium	Frank bleeding into the pericardium
Chylopericardium	Results from extravasation of chyle (milklike contents of the lacteals and lymphatic vessels, carried by the lymphatic vessels to the thoracic duct and to the left subclavian vein) due to a neoplasm or abnormal communication between pericardium and the thoracic duct
Cholesterol pericarditis	High concentration of cholesterol in the pericardial fluid
Lymphopericardium	Rare lesion related to lymphangiectasis, a dilation of the lymphatic vessels
Pneumopericardium	Air or gas in the pericardium caused by trauma or communication between the esophagus, stomach, or lungs and the pericardium
Pneumohydropericardium	Air and fluid accumulation in the pericardium

inflammatory cell infiltration in blood vessels and the pericardium (Spodick, 1997h). Systemic lupus erythematosus (SLE), rheumatoid arthritis, and progressive systemic sclerosis are just a few of the syndromes related to pericarditis. SLE causes many anatomic and pathophysiological pericardial abnormalities, including acute, clinically dry pericarditis and exudative (serous, serosanguineous, or hemorrhagic) pericardial effusions.

SLE should be suspected in all women with acute pericarditis until disproved, because this may be its first manifestation (Spodick, 1997h). Drug-induced SLE, caused by medications such as procainamide, isoniazid, hydralazine, methyldopa, or penicillin, also produces pericarditis.

Acute Clinically Noneffusive Pericarditis. Noneffusive or "dry" pericarditis refers to pericardial inflammation without a significant symptom-causing effusion. This is the most commonly recognized pericarditis. Frequently, the patient's history indicates that a viral infection preceded the pericarditis, or sometimes the pericarditis itself is the first presenting symptom of a systemic disease, as in SLE or malignancy. Viral infection is often presumed rather than definitively diagnosed, so many cases are classified as idiopathic (Shabetai, 1998). Acute

---

DISPLAY 34–1

MAJOR PRIMARY CONGENITAL ABNORMALITIES OF THE PERICARDIUM

Pericardial (celomic) cysts
Pericardial absence
   Complete
   Partial
Teratomas
Lymphangiomas
Diverticulum

DISPLAY 34–2

MAJOR CAUSES OF PERICARDITIS

Idiopathic
Trauma

- Direct
- Indirect

Infections

- Viral
- Bacterial
- Parasitic
- Fungal

Radiation
Immunologic conditions
Connective tissue diseases

- Systemic lupus erythematosus
- Vasculitis

Metabolic disorders

- Uremia

Myocardial infarction
Dissecting aneurysm
Drugs/anticoagulants

---

inflammatory pericarditis usually lasts one to three weeks and does not lead to further problems. Approximately 20 % of pericarditis patients have a recurrence within months, or rarely, within years (American Heart Association [AHA], 2002).

Assessment Findings. The onset of symptoms can be acute, as is commonly seen in viral pericarditis, or insidious, as in uremic pericarditis. Acute viral pericarditis is nearly always preceded by a recent respiratory, gastrointestinal, or "flu-like" illness. This prodromal illness may be characterized by fever and myalgia. The characteristic symptom of pericarditis is chest pain, although sometimes pain is absent. Initially, the pain of acute pericarditis tends to be sharp, precordial, and pleuritic, exacerbated by inspiration and lying down. The patient often sits up and leans forward to achieve relief. The pain can radiate in a manner similar to angina, confusing the diagnosis. Trapezius ridge pain is almost pathognomonic for pericardial irritation, and in some patients this is the only area of pain (Spodick, 1997b). The pain is transmitted through the phrenic nerves, and usually occurs on the left side. Shoulder pain should be distinguished from trapezius ridge pain by having the patient physically point to the specific site of pain. Frequently the chest pain caused by pericarditis induces shallow tachypnea as patients attempt to splint their chest movement (Spodick, 1997b). Fever, usually below 39°C, is also very common in acute pericarditis. The hallmark sign of acute pericarditis is the pericardial friction rub, a superficial, scratchy, or creaky, mostly high-pitched sound, most commonly heard between the middle to lower left sternal edge and the cardiac apex (Shabetai, 1998). The sounds can be very distant and faint, or loud and even palpable, especially in uremic pericarditis (Spodick, 1997c). Pericardial rubs are thought to be due to friction between pericardial surfaces. The sound can be heard throughout the cardiac cycle, can come and go, and can change in quality and intensity. Auscultation for a pericardial friction rub is accomplished with the diaphragm of the stethoscope at the left middle to lower sternal border during both inspiration and expiration, while the patient changes positions. Sometimes the rub can be heard best while the patient is in the sitting position. Rubs in acute pericarditis may disappear or persist regardless of the presence of a large effusion or tamponade. The classic pericardial friction rub is triphasic, with components during atrial systole, ventricular systole, and ventricular diastole (Klein, 1998; Spodick, 1997c).

The pericardium itself does not produce electrical activity. The ECG changes seen in pericarditis are a result of superficial inflammation of the myocardium underneath the pericardium. The ECG of a patient with pericarditis may be normal, atypically abnormal with nonspecific changes, or have a four-stage sequence that is diagnostic (Fig. 34-1). In stage I, there are ST segment deviations, primarily due to inflammation on the ventricular surfaces. PR segment deviations also usually are present. Stage I is virtually pathognomonic of acute pericarditis when it involves all or almost all leads with early ST junction elevations that produce an appearance of T waves "jacked-up" on the QRS interval, but that is otherwise normal (Spodick, 1997g). The ST segment is always depressed in aVR. In early stage II, the ST segments return to baseline, and PR segments may now be depressed. In late stage II, the T waves flatten and then invert. In stage III, the ECG is characteristic of diffuse myocardial injury. In stage IV, the ECG evolves back to the pre-pericarditis state (Shabetai, 1998; Spodick, 1997g). PR-segment deviation may be the initial electrocardiographic change in acute pericarditis, according to recent research (Baljepally & Spodick, 1998).

The changes seen in the ECG of a patient with pericarditis can occur over hours, particularly from stage I to II, or can take place over days or weeks, most often as stage III evolves to stage IV. The ST elevation seen in pericarditis is usually distinguished from that of acute MI by the absence of Q waves, upward ST segments, and the absence of associated T-wave inversion (Shabetai, 1998). In research examining the cause of ST segment abnormalities in emergency department chest pain patients, pericarditis was found in 1% of the study population (Brady et al., 2001).

Evaluation of laboratory results almost always reveals an elevated erythrocyte sedimentation rate. Leukocytosis is present early but, depending on etiology, may give way to lymphocytosis. Serum cardiac enzymes are frequently normal unless the myocardium is involved, and then they give some indication as to the degree of involvement. In recent studies, 49% to 71% of patients with pericarditis had elevations of Troponin I, and this was found more frequently than positive CK MB enzyme levels (Brandt et al., 2001; Bonnefoy et al., 2000). It is often difficult to differentiate pericarditis from MI. (Colletti, 1999). In some parts of the world, such as South Africa, tuberculosis is a major health problem, and can be complicated by tuberculosis pericarditis. The need for early diagnosis has led to emphasis on biochemical tests such as the pericardial adenosine deaminase (ADA) test, and the use of interferon as an indicator of pericardial disease due to tuberculosis (Burgess et al., 2002).

Medical Management. In pericarditis, the goal of treatment is to eliminate the underlying cause and relieve symptoms. Analgesics and bed rest are used to treat pain. Nonsteroidal anti-inflammatory drugs (NSAIDs) are the mainstay of treatment (Shabetai, 1998; Spodick, 1997b). Gastrointestinal mucosa protectants guard against the side effects, but close monitoring is essential. Colchicine, which is an anti-inflammatory agent, may

be added to an NSAID or given as monotherapy for both the initial attack and to prevent recurrences (Spodick, 1997b; Adler et al., 1998). Corticosteroids are used only if other treatments fail, and then only in minimally effective dosages. The use of these agents is controversial. The patient with pericarditis is also closely observed for development of the complications of pericardial effusion or cardiac tamponade.

Constrictive Pericarditis. In constrictive pericarditis, the pericardium loses its flexibility and elasticity and becomes scarred and rigid. As a result, the heart is compressed and its function is disturbed. Advances in diagnostic testing as well as in our understanding of hemodynamics have improved early diagnosis. Traditionally, constriction has been chronic, with sometimes surprising pericardial thickness. Recently, relatively thinner constricting pericardia are increasingly evident, perhaps because of earlier diagnoses and a shift in recognizable etiologies (Spodick, 1997f). In the U.S. tuberculosis was a major cause of this disease in the past, but the incidence has declined and previous mediastinal radiation and cardiac surgery have emerged as increasingly important causes. Tuberculosis is still the most common cause in developing countries (Ling et al., 1999; Mehta et al., 1999) The etiology of constrictive pericarditis is often undetermined, but it can result from almost all the conditions that also cause acute pericarditis.

Pathophysiology. The essential pathological process is healing, resulting in a scar, thick or thin, that restricts cardiac filling, particularly that of the ventricles. A constricting pericardial scar accentuates the ventricular pressure-volume relationship and increases ventricular coupling while restricting filling of the ventricles progressively earlier in diastole, until 70% to 80% of the reduced filling occurs in the first 25% to 30% of diastole (Spodick, 1997f). The filling pressures of the two sides of the heart equilibrate. Elevated pulmonary arterial pressures reflect elevated ventricular diastolic pressures. Because of constriction, CO decreases, and compensatory tachycardia ensues. The syndrome of increased ventricular diastolic pressure, low CO, and increased systemic vascular resistance mimics cardiac failure (Shabetai, 1998). The thickened pericardium effectively isolates the heart from normal respiratory swings in pressure (Klein & Scalia, 1998).

Assessment Findings. A history of antecedent pericarditis or drugs or procedures that induce pericarditis may indicate constrictive pericarditis. Many abnormal findings can be seen on the echocardiogram that indicate constrictive pericarditis, such as premature opening of the pulmonic valve and rapid posterior motion of the left ventricular posterior wall in early diastole, with little or no posterior motion during the rest of diastole. However, these findings are not specific for constrictive pericarditis and can be caused by other conditions, such as restrictive cardiomyopathy (Goyle & Walling, 2002; Nishimura, 2001).

Two-dimensional and Doppler transesophageal echocardiography (TEE) with respiratory monitoring have emerged as useful tools in categorizing patients with impaired diastolic function, primarily those with restrictive physiologic features or constrictive pericarditis (Klein et al., 1999). Recently, tissue Doppler echocardiography and color M-mode Doppler have been advanced as new methods of evaluating diastolic function in these diseases (Rajagopalan et al., 2001). Magnetic resonance imaging (MRI) enables accurate measurements of pericardial thickness, a hallmark of the disease (Myers & Spodick, 1999).

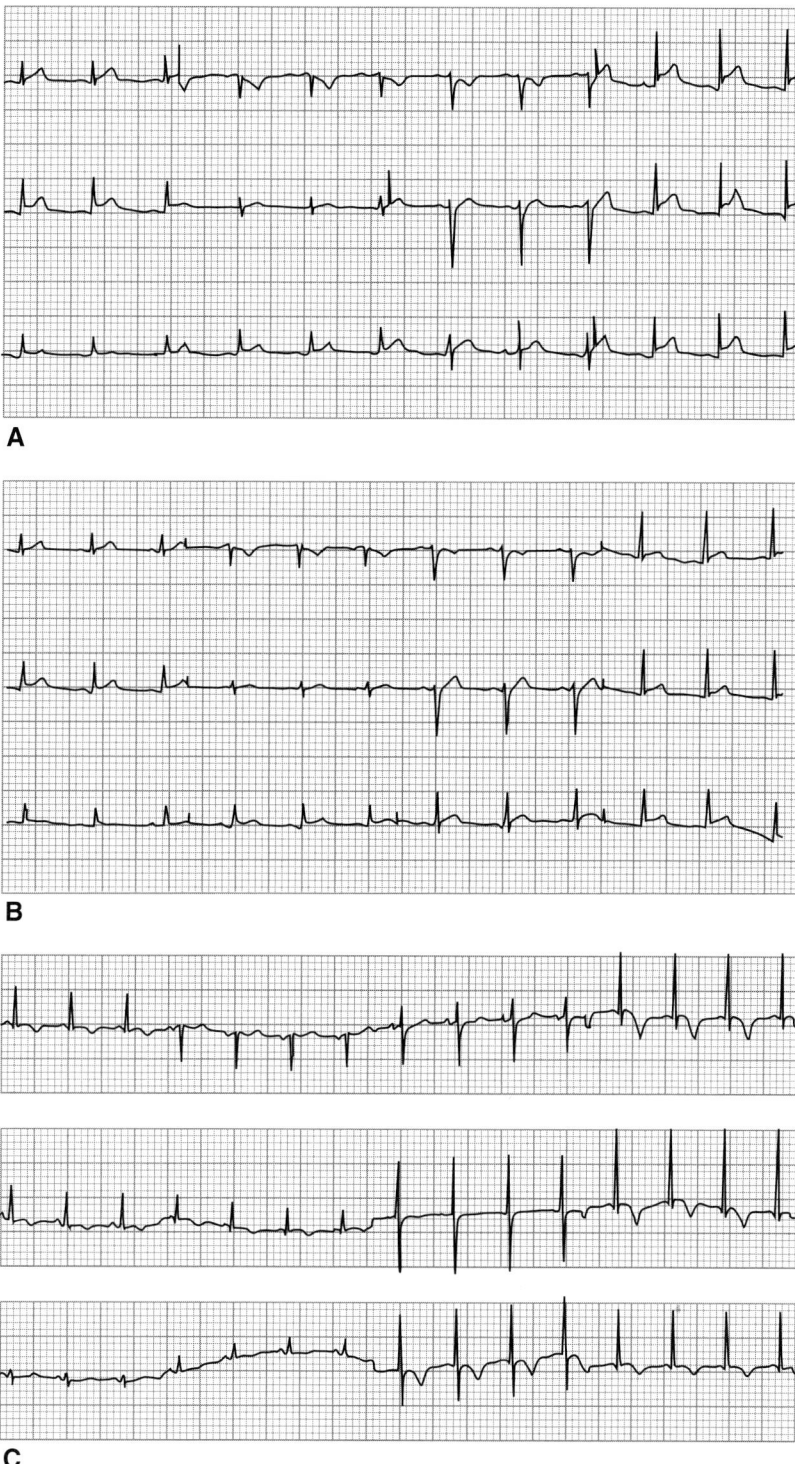

■ **Figure 34–1.** Electrocardiographic manifestations of pericarditis. (*A*) Typical, quasidiagnostic Stage I ECG: J (ST) elevated in all leads except AVL, depressed AVR and V1. PR segment deviated except in aVL where P is small. (*B*) Early stage II. J (ST) returning to baseline. (*C*) Stage III. T waves inverted in most leads and typically upright in aVR and V1. (From Spodick, D. H. [1997g]. Electrocardiographic abnormalities in pericardial disease. In D. H. Spodick [Ed.], *The pericardium: A comprehensive textbook* [pp. 40–64]. New York: Marcel Dekker.)

Pericardial thickness can also be detected on computed tomography (CT) (Song et al., 2002). The advances in imaging techniques have reduced the necessity of biopsy as a means to distinguish constrictive pericarditis and restrictive cardiomyopathy (Myers & Spodick, 1999). One study determined pericardial calcification is a common finding on chest radiography in patients with constrictive pericarditis (Ling et al., 2000).

On cardiac catheterization, the major finding is near equalization of all diastolic chamber pressures and venous pressures. Both left and right ventricular traces have a dip and plateau, the "square root" configuration, more pronounced in the right ventricle, because of the sharp, short, early diastolic decrease toward zero pressure (dip), increasing rapidly to a restrictive plateau as the relaxing ventricles rapidly reach the tight, limiting pericardium (Spodick, 1997f). There is equalization of the right atrial and pulmonary wedge pressures (Sexton, 1998). The central venous pressure is elevated and shows no respiratory deviation except in the depth of they descent. During classic constriction, Kussmaul's sign, inspiratory jugular venous distention, replaces the normal inspiratory venous "collapse" that reflects a normal inspiratory decrease of 3 to 7 mm Hg in right atrial pressure (Spodick, 1997f). This is a hallmark of constrictive pericarditis. Severe compression causes signs and symptoms of heart failure: dyspnea, ascites, leg edema, neck vein distention, organomegaly, and decreased coronary, cerebral, and renal perfusion (Rogers, 1990; Spodick, 1997f). The patient can display tachycardia, atrial fibrillation, and signs of decreased CO such as cool extremities, peripheral cyanosis, and jaundice due to liver involvement. Blood pressure may be normal, hypotensive, and sometimes hypertensive. An early diastolic thrust corresponds to a rapid ventricular filling pressure and coincides with a loud abnormal S-3 produced in both ventricles, sometimes with a "knocking" quality. S-1 and S-2 can be muted because of hemodynamic compromise.

Laboratory tests often reveal normocytic normochromic anemia, abnormal liver function tests, and hypoalbuminemia. The ECG is nonspecifically abnormal. The T waves are usually flat or low and sometimes inverted. The QRS interval and T waves may show decreased voltage. Interatrial block is common, indicated by widened, notched P waves.

Medical Management. Medical management does not relieve pericardial constriction. Surgical pericardectomy, which is the definitive treatment, is more easily accomplished if done relatively early in the course of the disease, when the patient has less systemic disease and before calcification and myocardial abnormalities develop (Klein and Scalia, 1998). Surgical pericardectomy is recommended for patients in NYHA class II or III functional status (Mahta, 1999). Preventing the development of constrictive pericarditis is the optimal method to combat this condition, through adequate treatment of pericarditis, and draining of fluid and pus if indicated.

Pericarditis Associated with Myocardial Infarction

Early Acute Postmyocardial Infarction Pericarditis. In the immediate period after MI, an early pericardial syndrome may develop and then resolve over a period of approximately one week. Patients with infarct pericarditis usually have a larger infarct size (Spodick, 2001). The ECG shows a typical pattern of pericarditis and should be helpful in differentiating between pericardial and ischemic pain. This early "infarct pericarditis," also known as epistenocardiac pericarditis, is confined to the infarct zone. It occurs in approximately 50% of transmural myocardial infarctions, although it is detected less often, and produces a precordial friction rub (Spodick, 2001). As in all pericarditis, rubs are virtually 100% specific, but sensitivity depends on frequency of auscultation, because they tend to come and go over hours (Spodick, 2003). The course is usually benign, and treatment consists of aspirin or other NSAIDs. Early thrombolytic therapy has decreased the incidence due to an unknown mechanism (Pierce, 1992).

Dressler's Syndrome. Dressler's syndrome of chest pain, pleurisy, pericarditis with friction rub, severe malaise, and moderate fever and leukocytosis occurs 3 weeks to several months post-MI. The underlying pathologic process is unknown, but many believe an autoimmune reaction occurs secondary to the infarct. Patients with Dressler's syndrome can have recurrent ischemia, significant pericardial effusion, bacterial superinfection, and hemorrhagic complications (Klein and Scalia, 1998).

Pericardial Effusion

Pericardial effusion is the excess accumulation of fluid, blood, pus, or a combination of all three, in the pericardium. If the rate of exudation is slow enough to allow the pericardium to stretch, even large amounts of fluid might not compromise cardiac function.

Etiology

Pericardial effusions are caused by pericardial irritation and inflammation. Congestive heart failure contributes to many small-and moderate-sized effusions. There is a high incidence of pericardial effusion in patients infected with the human immunodeficiency virus (HIV), and moderate or severe effusions have been found to be more frequent in patients at more advanced stages of HIV infection (Silva-Cardoso et al., 1999). Pericardial effusion is also a complication of chronic renal failure, especially untreated, advanced uremia (Wood et al., 2001). Hypothyroidism can also cause pericardial effusions (Gupta et al., 1999).

Assessment Findings

"Noncompressing" effusions do not produce changes in CO or pulsus paradoxus. If the effusions are caused by a systemic disease, then the symptoms are related to that disease. A pericardial rub may or may not be appreciated. The ECG shows reduced voltage, and these changes are nonspecific and unreliable for diagnosis. Electrical alternans is a marker of massive pericardial effusion (Klein & Scalia, 1998). Chest radiographs are at best suggestive and nonspecific, and the effusion may be only apparent as an enlarged cardiac silhouette. If the effusion is visible on radiography, then there is at least 250 mL of fluid accumulated (Spodick, 1997i).

On echocardiography, normal and excess fluid can be seen. The size of the effusion can be estimated, giving a powerful predictor of prognosis in hospitalized patients. Echocardiography is the mainstay of diagnosis and the tool of choice (Klein & Scalia, 1998; Spodick, 1997i). Computed tomography and MRI can also aid in diagnosis.

Medical Management

Patients presenting for the first time with pericardial effusion are usually hospitalized to determine the cause of the effusion and to observe for the development of cardiac tamponade (Hoit, 2002). In the absence of tamponade or pyopericardium, there are few absolute indications for drainage. Successful treatment of the cause should lead to resolution of the effusion. Persistent illness without etiologic diagnosis indicates need for surgical tissue and fluid sampling. Techniques include subxiphoid incision and video-assisted thoracoscopic pericardial resection and drainage, which allows for removal of thrombi, adhesions, and fibrinous material. Fluid can be drained by pericardiocentesis. However, when used for diagnostic purposes, pericardiocentesis often yields poor results (Spodick, 1997i). Patients must be monitored after drainage for decompensation secondary to cardiac dilation, which can take place once the effusion that was compressing the heart, is removed.

Cardiac Tamponade

Cardiac tamponade is defined as significant compression of the heart by accumulating pericardial content. Cardiac tamponade can be of varying degrees and can be caused by varying amounts of fluid. The speed of accumulation usually affects the severity of symptoms. Any scarring or thickening of the pericardium serves to amplify the effects of excess fluid on the heart.

Etiology

Any disease affecting the pericardium can cause effusion that can be complicated by cardiac tamponade. The common causes are idiopathic or viral pericarditis, neoplastic invasion of the pericardium, and nephrogenic pericardial disease. Acute tamponade is frequently caused by trauma, which may be iatrogenic, or by aortic rupture or rupture of the heart after MI (Shabetai, 1998).

Assessment Findings

Symptoms are related to the degree of cardiac impairment. It may be difficult to diagnose cardiac tamponade if the patient initially presents in cardiogenic shock or cardiopulmonary failure. Symptoms include tachypnea and dyspnea on exertion, progressing to air hunger at rest. Cough and dysphagia may be early symptoms but often are not recognized as indicating tamponade. Oliguria and acute renal failure can develop as the tamponade worsens in severity (Saklayen et al., 2002). Syncope and convulsions can develop. If the patient has pericarditis, a pericardial friction rub may be detectable. Heart sounds may be muffled because of excess fluid and impaired cardiac function. The venous pressure is elevated in all except the mildest cases of tamponade, or if hypovolemia is present. Jugular venous pressure is elevated. Central venous pressure can be as high as 30 mm Hg (Shabetai, 1998). Hypotension is produced by significant tamponade, leading to symptoms of poor perfusion.

Pulsus paradoxus develops when tamponade becomes moderately severe. Pulsus paradoxus is present when systemic arterial pressure drops 10 mm Hg or more during inspiration. It is easily observed on arterial line tracings and can be detected by using a sphygmomanometer. To measure the blood pressure change using a blood pressure cuff, inflate the cuff to 15 mm Hg above the highest systolic reading. The cuff is slowly deflated until the first Korotkoff sounds are heard. The sounds are heard only with some heart beats; these are the ones occurring during expiration at that pressure. The other sounds are heard at a lower pressure during inspiration. Slowly deflate the cuff until all of the Korotkoff sounds can be heard. The difference between these two readings gives the size of the pulsus (Spodick, 1997d). The pressure

also decreases during inspiration, reflecting decreased stroke volume (Shabetai, 1998).

The mechanism of pulsus paradoxus is related to competition between the two sides of the compressed heart for the severely restricted space. During inspiration, the expansion of the right heart volume impairs left heart stroke volume (Shabetai, 1998). Experimental observations indicate that this is only part of the explanation for pulsus paradoxus in cardiac tamponade (Shabetai, 1965). Pulsus paradoxus is multifactorial and still incompletely understood (Spodick, 1997l).

In moderate to severe tamponade, right atrial, right ventricular diastolic, and pulmonary artery wedge and diastolic pressures are all equal. Exceptions are commonly seen and are due to underlying cardiac disease. The ECG usually does not show diagnostic features. Electrical alternans of the P wave, QRS complex, and T wave are highly suggestive of cardiac tamponade, but are uncommon (Shabetai, 1998).

Medical Management

Cardiac tamponade is usually an indication for pericardiocentesis, drainage of the fluid accumulated in the pericardium. If tamponade recurs, open drainage may be indicated and is safer, particularly if tissue samples are needed (Shabetai, 1998).

If cardiac tamponade is caused by bleeding, the bleeding may actually be slowed by tamponade pressure. In this case, open surgical drainage and treatment of the bleeding source is superior to pericardiocentesis (Spodick, 1997l). Continuous hemodynamic monitoring of the effects of the procedure is critical.

Nursing Management in Pericardial Disease

The nurse is in a prime position to recognize the symptoms of pericardial disease and the complications that may develop. A careful and skilled assessment is critical and often crucial to the medical diagnosis. The nurse who is knowledgeable of pericardial disease is able to identify the patients most at risk, such as those with renal failure or MI. The subtle characteristics of pericardial pain, including the location, quality, and the effect of position changes, are aspects of the patient's condition that nurses are best suited to assess. As the member of the health care team who is consistently evaluating the patient, the nurse is most likely to find a pericardial friction rub because the sound is likely to come and go, and change in quality.

Evaluation of laboratory results, ECGs, and vital signs are key nursing interventions that have an enormous impact on the outcome of care. If the patient with pericardial disease is uremic, then he or she is prepared for increased dialysis. Emotional support and education can serve to decrease patient anxiety. Consistent care and a caring demeanor can encourage both the patient and family members to verbalize their fears. Listening to concerns and questions and providing information bolsters coping by patients and their family. Teaching about diagnostic tests can allay fears. The nurse intervenes with many measures that promote patient comfort, including narcotics and NSAIDs, positioning, diversion, and bed rest or limitation of activities.

It is critical that the patient maintain an adequate CO. The nurse evaluates the patient's hemodynamic state and implements any interventions that increase cardiac function, including vasoactive medications, decreasing anxiety and stress, and detection of pulsus paradoxus and jugular venous distension. Nurses monitor for cardiac arrhythmias and evaluate their effects on the patient. It is imperative that cardiac tamponade be diagnosed early, before a crisis ensues. If a patient is at risk, the nurse has the equipment readily available for an emergency pericardiocentesis. Monitoring the patient's condition during and after the procedure detects any other complications.

If a patient is to have surgery, preoperative teaching and preparation are a key nursing responsibility. Letting the patient and family know what to expect can help them deal with this frightening event. If a patient has a pericardectomy or a pericardial window, close monitoring of hemodynamics after surgery is important. Volume expanders and vasopressors may both be needed to maintain CO. Accurate hemodynamic readings are the nurse's responsibility and guide many treatment decisions. The nurse must provide respiratory care to prevent atelectasis and pneumonia and monitor the surgical incision for infection. The nurse also monitors the effects of any therapy, such as NSAIDs, and is vigilant for side effects such as gastrointestinal upset or bleeding. The physician is notified if the desired effects of medical interventions are not being achieved or if side effects or complications arise.

CARDIOMYOPATHIES

Cardiomyopathy is an irreversible primary disease of the heart muscle. Cardiomyopathy affects the myocardial layer of the heart, but it can also affect the endocardial, subendocardial, and pericardial layers. Cardiomyopathies used to be defined as heart muscle disease of unknown cause, but in recent years much has been learned about some of the etiologies of these diseases (Perloff, 1998). The condition is characterized by ventricle dilation, myocyte and wall thickening (hypertrophy), interstitial fibrosis, decreased contractility, and conduction disturbances (Fonarow, 2001). The end result is usually severe dysfunction of the heart muscle, resulting in terminal heart failure (Francis et al., 1998).

The most widely used functional classification of cardiomyopathy recognizes three disturbances of function: dilatation, hypertrophy, and restriction. Dilatation is dominated by left ventricular cavity enlargement and systolic failure. Hypertrophy includes both obstructive and non-obstructive forms. Restriction is characterized by inadequate compliance causing restriction of diastolic filling (Mason, 2001).

Dilated Cardiomyopathy

Dilated cardiomyopathy (DCM) is a primary disease of the ventricular myocardium characterized by decreased systolic function, ventricular dilation, and myocyte hypertrophy (Fonarow, 2001). Stroke volume is initially maintained despite a reduced ejection fraction because the decrease in systolic function is accompanied by an increase in end-systolic and end-diastolic volumes. Therefore, there is compensation early in the disease. Eventually, the ejection fraction deteriorates, myocardial contractility is further

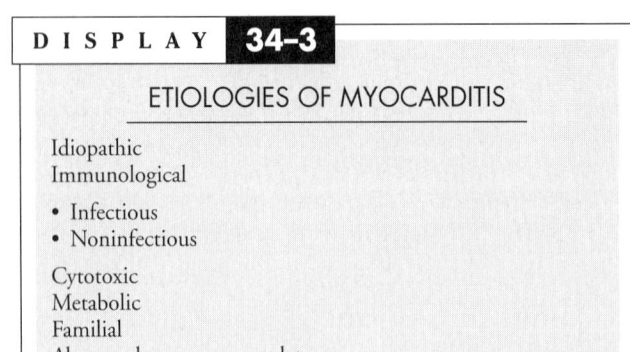

DISPLAY 34–3

ETIOLOGIES OF MYOCARDITIS

Idiopathic
Immunological

• Infectious
• Noninfectious

Cytotoxic
Metabolic
Familial
Abnormal coronary vasculature

depressed, and severe dysfunction of the heart muscle leads to heart failure (Francis et al., 1998, Fonarow, 2001).

Etiologies

Myocarditis, inflammation of the myocardium, is thought to be the major cause of DCM. Discussed in greater depth later in this chapter, the causes of myocarditis are many, and thus so are the causes of DCM. The etiologies are listed in Display 34-3 (Wynne and Braunwald, 2001). Half of the patients with DCM are diagnosed with idiopathic DCM, isolated heart failure of unknown etiology (Olson et al., 1998). This condition affects 5 to 8 of 100,000 people (Kasper et al., 1994; Manolio et al., 1992). Genetic factors make idiopathic DCM hereditary in approximately 20% of cases (Michels et al. 1992). Studies support the hypothesis that alcohol is one of many triggers for the development of DCM in a susceptible person or may aggravate a viral myocarditis that leads to DCM (Constant, 1999). Cocaine abuse can also lead to DCM, as well as CHF and endocarditis (Paul & York, 1992). Many chemotherapeutic agents, such as doxorubicin, daunorubicin, and idarubicin have been linked to DCM (Shanholtz, 2001).

The pathogenesis of DCM is controversial and is believed to include genetic factors, viral infection, autoimmune mediated inflammation, cytoskeletal contractile protein abnormalities, metabolic derangements and growth factor/cytokine signaling pathways (Fonarow, 2001; Mestroni et al., 1998; Bachinski & Roberts, 1998; Luppi et al., 1998). Further research in these areas may lead to new treatments. DCM is the principle indication for cardiac transplantation throughout childhood apart from infancy, when congenital heart disease is a more prevalent indication (Burch, 2002).

Assessment Findings

Clinical manifestations of DCM reflect right and left ventricular dysfunction, a combination of inadequate CO and perfusion, and excessive congestion of the pulmonary and systemic venous circulations. Orthopnea, nocturnal cough, and dyspnea may present if DCM progresses slowly. Abdominal distention, right upper quadrant pain, and nausea secondary to systemic congestion can be the dominant symptoms if DCM progresses rapidly. Physical signs often depend on how long the patient has had DCM, and this usually relates to the severity of the condition. Specific findings include a point of maximal intensity away from the normal position (i.e., at the fifth intercostal space mid-clavicular line). Auscultation of heart sounds may reveal an S-3, indicating failure, or a murmur, signifying mitral regurgitation or tricuspid regurgitation. Mitral regurgitation is common even if a murmur is not heard. Peripheral edema and jugular venous distention may be apparent.

Because stroke volume and CO are decreased, blood pressure may be low and pulse pressure may be narrow. Extremities are cool and clammy, and peripheral pulses are decreased. There may be evidence of systemic emboli secondary to endocardial thrombi that are most likely to lodge in the apex of the left ventricle. The ECG of a patient with DCM may show nonspecific ST segment and T-wave abnormalities or may indicate bundle-branch blocks and supraventricular and ventricular arrhythmias. Echocardiography reveals dilated chambers with normal or decreased wall thickness. Left ventricular ejection fraction is less that 45%, and symptomatic patients frequently have an ejection fraction of less than 30% (Fonarow, 2001). Radiography shows cardiomegaly with ventricular enlargement. Cardiac troponin I emerges as a superior marker to detect recent myocardial inflammation or injury in patients presenting with new onset heart failure (Chan et al., 2000). Other laboratory values reflect the impact of DCM on other organs. Liver functions test results are elevated, as are the BUN and creatinine.

Medical Management

Fifty percent of all deaths in patients with DCM occur suddenly. A 5-year mortality rate of 50% has been reported for DCM of various etiologies with ejection fractions below 50% (Stevenson & Perloff, 1988). In a recent report on 616 patients with idiopathic cardiomyopathy, the 5-year survival rate was 75% (Felker, 2000). Ventricular arrhythmias are possibly the major cause of death, but clots and hemorrhages secondary to treatment or bradyarrhythmias may also contribute to deaths in DCM. If the etiology of the DCM can be determined, treatment focuses on eliminating the cause, as specific treatment may reverse the cardiac dysfunction (Fonarow, 2001). Otherwise, general principles of medical care include maximizing ventricular function and exercise performance, reducing associated risks, and, late in the disease, consideration for cardiac transplantation (Stevenson & Perloff, 1988). The suppression of premature ventricular contractions may be associated with improvement of left ventricular function in patients with presumed idiopathic DCM (Duffee et al., 1998). Medications such as digoxin and dobutamine are administered to increase contractility. Vasodilators are administered to decrease afterload and therefore left ventricular work, and increase CO. Heparin and warfarin are used for long-term anticoagulant therapy to prevent clot formation in the dilated left ventricle or if atrial fibrillation is present. Fluid and sodium restriction, along with administration of diuretics, maintain fluid balance. Daily weights assist in monitoring fluid status.

The most important recent therapeutic advance for cardiomyopathy treatment has been the recognition that agents that inhibit neurohormonal activation relieve symptoms, improve functional status, reduce hospitalizations, and prolong survival (Fonarow, 2001). ACE-inhibitors have produced hemodynamic, symptomatic, and functional benefits. The addition of spironolactone has been shown to reduce risk of sudden death from heart failure (Pitt et al., 1999). Beta-blockers

have also been beneficial in patients with cardiomyopathy and are included in the recommended treatment.

A preliminary study on the intermittent home administration of the inotrope/vasodilator milrinone in patients with end-stage heart failure secondary to DCM showed multiple benefits (Cesario et al., 1998). Intermittent infusions limited the toxicity and tachyphylaxis seen previously in outpatient use. Another study found that continuous inotropic therapy was best suited to those patients with idiopathic DCM who were not able to be weaned while hospitalized, and helped to manage these patients at decreased hospital stays, until transplantation was available (Sindone et al., 1997).

Cardiac transplantation prolongs the lives of patients with DCM, but not every patient is a candidate for the procedure. Cardiac transplantation is performed approximately 2,300 times per year in the United States, but each year 3,700 people are on the waiting list (United Network for Organ Sharing [UNOS], 1997). Many patients die before a heart becomes available. Implantation of a ventricular assist device (VAD) is becoming more common for patients with end-stage disease awaiting transplantation. Patients with chronic advanced end-stage heart failure have been noted to improve cardiac function parameters to a point where removal of the VAD was possible (Young, 2001). This has led to study of how the heart can heal during the use of VAD therapy as a "bridge-to-recovery" (Kumpati et al., 2001). Dynamic cardiomyoplasty is another alternative to transplantation. The procedure involves the use of an autologous latissimus dorsi muscle graft that is wrapped around the ventricles by pericardial attachment. The muscle graft is then stimulated by specialized synchronous train impulses from a cardiomyostimulator; the resultant muscle graft contractions provide support for ventricular function (Vollman, 1995; Acker, 1999; Chacques et al., 2003). This procedure remains controversial. Partial left ventriculectomy (Batista procedure), also known as heart reduction surgery, removes a triangular wedge of the lateral wall of the left ventricle in an effort to decrease the size of the large dilated ventricle seen in DCM. The application of the revolutionary procedure remains under study (Starling and Young, 1998). Isolated mitral valve repair treats a key component of heart failure and has also been studied (Dreyfus & Mihealaino, 2001). Dual chamber pacing has been helpful to some patients with ventricular conduction delay and other electrical abnormalities, but evidence of long-term benefits is lacking (Wynne & Braunwald, 2001). Implantable cardioverter-defibrillators (ICD) have not proven to be beneficial in prevention of sudden death in idiopathic DCM (Bansch et al., 2002). High dose intravenous immunoglobulin has both antiviral and immune modulating effects. However, a prospective randomized study performed to evaluate the potential role in treatment of DCM failed to demonstrate benefit (McNamara et al., 2001).

Due to the genetic component of DCM, relatives of these patients should be systematically screened, and family members at risk can be identified (Mestroni, 1998).

Nursing Management in Dilated Cardiomyopathy

The nurse can help in identifying the cause of DCM through a careful and detailed nursing history. The nurse is also in the best position to monitor the patient for worsening of symptoms and for response to medical treatments. Evaluation of heart sounds, lung sounds, vital signs, and peripheral perfusion, as well as interpretation of laboratory results, are key nursing responsibilities. Signs of congestion and decreased CO must be detected and reported early to provide the most effective treatment. The nurse titrates medications to increase left heart function, monitoring the effects and side effects. If a ventricular assist device is used, the nurse monitors the effects of this therapy as well. Reduction of afterload and filling pressures is accomplished with diuretics and vasodilators given and monitored by the nurse. The nurse optimizes the patient's oxygenation through position changes, pulmonary toilet, monitoring and interpretation of arterial blood gases, and oxygen administration or ventilator management. Recognition of symptoms of excess use of cocaine or alcohol or withdrawal from these substances is necessary (Paul & York, 1992).

The patient and his or her family must be educated about DCM and its treatments and possible complications. Each test that is done should be explained to the patient. The plan of care needs to be discussed and agreed on. If anticoagulants are used, side effects and their symptoms, as well as dietary interactions, need to be explained. Other dietary considerations must be addressed, such as fluid and salt restriction, and the nurse as a leader of the multidisciplinary team can ensure that the patient's multiple needs are met Emotional needs are particularly significant in DCM because of its wide-ranging impact on the lives of both the patient and family. Physical limitation was a significant predictor of less effective psychosocial adjustment for patients studied with DCM (Bohachick & Anton, 1990; Frost et al., 1994). A study on couples dealing with severe cardiomyopathy found they experienced considerable psychosocial distress attributable to illness. DCM affects the entire family, and adequate information about the illness and treatment, along with emotional support, can facilitate adaptation and coping (Bohachick & Anton, 1990). Individual counseling, support groups, or both can be effective. When the patient is to have surgery, preoperative education can allay many fears if the patient and family have an opportunity to ask questions and are prepared for the postoperative course. Teaching needs to be individualized, with determination of the best method for the patient and family. The nurse is responsible for postoperative hemodynamic monitoring, pain control, and respiratory care. Infection control is also critical.

Hypertrophic Cardiomyopathy

Hypertrophic cardiomyopathy (HCM) is a disorder of cardiac muscle characterized by myocardial hypertrophy, most commonly affecting the intraventricular septum, and disorganization of the cardiac myocytes and myofibrils (McKenna & Elliot, 1998). HCM is the most common cause of sudden cardiac death in young competitive athletes (Drezner, 2000).

Etiology

The etiology of HCM is thought to be mutations in genes encoding several cardiac sarcomeric proteins (McKenna, 1998). As many as 60% to 80% of cases are inherited

through autosomal dominant transmission, but it is usually undetected until adulthood. Its prevalence is 1 per 500 in the general U.S. population and is higher in blacks (Maron, 1997).

Pathophysiology

Up to 80% of people with HCM have abnormalities of diastolic function that include slow and prolonged isovolumic relaxation, reduced rate of rapid filling, increased left ventricular stillness, and altered atrial contribution to stroke volume. Myocardial fibrosis, left ventricular hypertrophy, myocyte disarray and myocardial ischemia are likely contributory factors (McKenna & Elliot, 1998). Myocardial ischemia is common and related to impaired vasodilator reserve, increased oxygen demand, and increased filling pressures causing subendocardial ischemia (Wynne & Braunwald, 2001).

Approximately 25% of patients with HCM also have left ventricular outflow tract obstruction (LVOTO) caused by a markedly hypertrophic, asymmetric septal wall that is out of proportion to the remainder of the chamber. This changes the shape of the left ventricular cavity, causing the papillary muscles to become misaligned. During contraction, the papillary muscle abnormally pulls the anterior mitral leaflet toward the ventricular septum; this is known as systolic anterior motion of the mitral valve. Together, the displaced papillary muscle, mitral valve leaflet, and septal hypertrophy cause a left ventricular outflow gradient (Schactman et al., 1997). This pressure gradient increases myocardial oxygen demand and left ventricular systolic pressures. This condition is also known as idiopathic hypertrophic subaortic stenosis (IHSS).

Assessment Findings

Many patients with HCM are asymptomatic or have only mild symptoms. Often diagnosis is made during screening because a relative has been diagnosed. Sometimes the first sign is sudden death. The risk is often higher in children. The abnormality in diastolic relaxation produces increased left ventricular end diastolic pressure with resulting pulmonary congestion and dyspnea, the most common symptom in HCM (Wynne & Braunwald, 2001). Angina pectoris, fatigue, presyncope, and syncope are also common. In children and adolescents, presyncope and syncope identify patients at increased risk of sudden death. Heart sounds are abnormal, often with a split S-2. HCM with LVOTO produces a harsh systolic murmur heard between the apex and the left sternal border. Most patients have ECG abnormalities, but the changes are not specific to the disease. Most common are ST segment and T wave abnormalities. Q waves are seen in 20% to 50% of patients (Wynne & Braunwald, 2001). Patients have ventricular and supraventricular arrhythmias, including SVT and atrial fibrillation.

Left ventricular hypertrophy is the cardinal echocardiographic feature of HCM. It is usually of the septum and anterolateral free wall, but can be seen in the apex and free wall, also.

Medical Management

The main goals of management of patients with HCM are to alleviate symptoms, prevent complications, and decrease risk of sudden death (McKenna & Elliot, 1998; Wynne & Braunwald, 2001). There are few controlled studies on the pharmacological managements of patients with HCM, but beta-blockers are the main treatment. Patients without left ventricular outflow gradients taking beta-blockers have decreased oxygen consumption and chest pain (Spirito et al., 1997; Popjes & Sutton, 2003). However, in a review and analysis of the use of beta blockers in HCM, McKenna concluded that propranolol exerted no significant effect on the incidence of sudden death (McKenna, 1998). Calcium channel blockers as well as disopyramide both work to decrease left ventricular outflow gradient. Amiodarone is effective to suppress both atrial and ventricular tachyarrhythmias in HCM. An ICD should be inserted in patients at highest risk for sudden death. Strenuous activity is associated with sudden death and should be avoided. Patients with atrial fibrillation should be pharmacologically or electrically converted if possible because the atria provide an extremely important contribution to ventricular filling in this disorder (Spirito et al., 1997). Anticoagulants are necessary for the patients with chronic atrial fibrillation. Patients with HCM with left ventricular outflow track gradient are at increased risk of endocarditis and need antibiotic prophylaxis for certain procedures.

Dual-chamber pacing has been beneficial for some patients with an outflow track gradient. The exact mechanism for the improved clinical status in HCM is unknown, but remodeling of the myocardium is one possibility (Schactman et al., 1997). It is important that AV synchrony be maintained because although the left atrial contribution to CO is only 20% to 30% in the normal heart, it becomes a major factor to the total CO in a patient with LVOTO. Two recent studies have confirmed beneficial effects on the left ventricular outflow gradient, but could not demonstrate quantifiable improvement in exercise capacity (Kappenberger et al., 1997; Maron et al., 1999) This intervention is still under study, but may be best for patients refractory to drug therapy (Gadler et al., 1999).

Surgical procedures such as septal myectomy/myotomy, mitral valve replacement, and Morrow septal myectomy, have improved symptoms and exercise capacity (Wynne & Braunwald, 2001). A new procedure, ethanol-induced therapeutic myocardial infarction via the septal perforator arteries, is used to treat HCM with LVOTO by lessening the obstruction in the outflow track. The septal perforator arteries perfuse the anterior two-thirds of the intraventricular septum, most of the right bundle branch, and the anterosuperior fascicle of the left bundle branch. Many patients have experienced symptomatic relief, but long-term effects are to be determined (Lewis et al., 2001; Sherrid et al., 2003). A recent study compared left ventricular diastolic function in obstructive HCM in patients undergoing percutaneous septal alcohol ablation versus surgical myotomy/myectomy. The diastolic function indexes after each procedure were similar (Sitges et al., 2003).

Nursing Management in Hypertrophic Cardiomyopathy

HCM is a condition that limits activity and is potentially life threatening. It is associated with substantial restrictions in health-related quality of life (Cox et al., 1997). It is often diagnosed after another family member has died a sudden death. Genetic testing may identify those likely to develop the disease (Mogensen et al., 2003). While a patient is grieving for a family member, he may also be coping with his or her own new diagnosis. To make the diagnosis, the patient undergoes many tests, such as echocardiography and cardiac catheterization. Emotional support and education are key components of nursing care of patients with HCM. The other goals of nursing care for patients with HCM are to assess and observe for complications and to promote comfort. After surgery or pacemaker insertion, careful monitoring of hemodynamic status and prompt detection of decreased blood pressure and CO, CHF, arrhythmias, and bleeding are important. Conduction defects are common after surgery. After ethanol-ablation patients are also at risk for conduction problems such as RBBB, first-degree AV block, and third-degree heart block. A temporary pacemaker is in place for 24 hours, and persistent third-degree block necessitates permanent pacemaker placement. Cardiac enzymes are monitored frequently. Pain medicine consists of hydrocodone acetaminophen. It is crucial that the patient with HCM wear a medical alert bracelet in case of emergency and that family members be trained in basic life support techniques (Vollman, 1995). Young family members should be screened prior to participation in sports (Maron, 2001).

Restrictive Cardiomyopathy Pathophysiology and Etiology

Restrictive cardiomyopathy (RCM) is an uncommon heart muscle disorder characterized by impaired filling of the ventricles with reduced volume in the presence of normal or near normal wall thickness and systolic function. There is failure of the myocardium to relax in diastole (Davies, 2000). The disease is manifested by progressive left and right-sided heart failure (Morgensen et al., 2003). Diminished ventricular distensibility, caused by thickened rigid ventricular walls, is manifested functionally by a disproportionate increase in diastolic pressure for a given increased diastolic volume. The result is an abnormally steep slope of the diastolic pressure-volume curve known as the *square root* hemodynamic pattern (Child & Perloff, 1988; Klein & Scalia, 1998). RCM can be mistaken for constrictive pericarditis (Hancock, 2001). Although several inherited and acquired disorders may cause RCM, many cases remain idiopathic (Keren & Popp, 1992; Kushwaha et al., 1999). It is seen in amyloidosis, sarcoidosis, endomyocardial fibrosis, and other infiltrative diseases (Child and Perloff, 1988; Kabbani and Lewinter, 2000).

Assessment Findings

Clinical signs and symptoms are those of high systemic and pulmonary venous pressure. The most common symptoms in one study were dyspnea and edema (Ammash et al., 2000). Ascites may be evident. There is a normal left ventricular systolic impulse and a prominent S-3. Auscultation frequently reveals AV valve regurgitation. Biatrial enlargement due to rigid ventricular walls is seen, and atrial fibrillation is common (Child & Perloff, 1988; Klein & Scalia, 1998). PA systolic pressure often is greater than 50 mm Hg in patients with RCM (Kabbani & Lewinter, 2000).

Medical Management

There is no known treatment for RCM, so therapy is supportive. It includes diuretics, corticosteroids, or anticoagulants, depending on the etiology and manifestations. Fluid restriction, oxygen, and positive inotropes may also be used to treat the symptoms. Some patients may benefit from heart transplantation.

Myocarditis

Myocarditis is an inflammation of the myocardium. It is usually diagnosed when it leads to significant cardiac dysfunction. Myocarditis can cause considerable morbidity and mortality and is implicated in the development of DCM (Davis et al., 2002; D'Ambrosio et al., 2001; Kawai, 1999).

Etiology

Myocarditis can be caused by a variety of agents. Display 34-4 gives a list of the etiologies (Borczuk & van Hoeven, 1997; Brown & Bertolet, 1998; Friedrich et al., 1998; Galiuto et al., 1997; Mason, 1999). Viral myocarditis is considered the most common type and is estimated to affect at least 1 in 10,000 of the U.S. population each year, frequently striking children, young adults, and pregnant women (Suddaby, 1996).

DISPLAY 34-4

ETIOLOGIES OF MYOCARDITIS

Infections
Viral

- Coxsackievirus
- Poliomyelitis
- Mumps
- Rubella
- Epstein-Barr
- Human immunodeficiency virus

Bacterial

- Tuberculosis
- Tetanus
- Staphylococcal
- Pneumococcal

Fungal
Parasitic

- Toxoplasmosis
- Cytomegalovirus

Pharmacologic agents

- Inotropes

Cocaine
Radiation therapy
Chemical poisons
Peripartum condition
Autoimmune

- Eosinophilia
- Asthma

Pathophysiology

Myocarditis is usually characterized by necrosis and cell injury associated with inflammation of the heart muscle and lymphocytic inflammation in the absence of an ischemic episode (Carthy et al., 1997). As the myocardium becomes infected and necrosis occurs, an immune response is initiated and cytokines are produced. The viral infection persists, and an autoimmune response is initiated, causing the body to attack its own cells. These mechanisms and the viral attack of vascular endothelium, causing microvascular spasm and reperfusion injury, are thought to produce the myocardial damage that occurs in myocarditis. The histological hallmark of myocarditis is an inflammatory myocardial infiltrate with an associated evidence of myocyte damage (Pisani et al., 1997).

Assessment Findings

Myocarditis classically presents with nonspecific symptoms such as fatigue, dyspnea, and palpitations, along with viral illness symptoms, including fever. If the disease has progressed, symptoms of heart failure present, such as tachycardia, pulmonary edema, diaphoresis, neck vein distention, and cardiomegaly. Symptoms of poor perfusion or cardiogenic shock can also be manifested, such as hypotension, cool, clammy extremities, decreased urine output, and decreased level of consciousness. Cardiac function is evaluated through echocardiography, ECG, nuclear scans, and cardiac catheterization with endomyocardial biopsy. The latter test remains the gold standard for diagnosis of myocarditis, although results remain controversial and it is invasive and costly (Friedrich et al., 1998; James et al., 1997; Zales & Wright, 1997). Studies indicate that MRI may serve as a powerful, noninvasive diagnostic tool in myocarditis (Friedrich et al., 1998; Robiti et al., 2000). In myocarditis, the ECG can show low-voltage QRS complexes, ST segment elevation, or heart block. Nonsustained atrial or ventricular arrhythmias are common. An S-4 and systolic ejection murmurs may be heard on auscultation.

Medical Management

Management of myocarditis is focused on support. Heart failure, arrhythmias, and conduction abnormalities are treated. Inotropic support of cardiac function with amrinone, dopamine, or dobutamine may be used. Nitroprusside and nitroglycerin may be used to reduce afterload. Bed rest is used to promote healing and minimize myocardial oxygen consumption. Intubation, ventilation, and sedation may be necessary to decrease cardiac workload (Ledford, 1997; Stevenson & Perloff, 1988). Extracorporeal membrane oxygenation has been used in 50 cases of pediatric and neonatal myocarditis, with a 54% survival rate (Sandberg et al., 1995). It has also been used successfully in several adult cases (Acker, 2001). Mechanical assist devices such as intra-aortic balloon pulsation and left or bi-ventricular assist devices have been used to improve CO in myocarditis (Ueno et al., 2000). Some patients can even be treated on an outpatient basis (Schmid et al., 1999). Another important aspect of management is prevention of complications. If the ejection fraction is low and there is blood stasis in the chambers, anticoagulant therapy is necessary to prevent thrombus formation. The use of immunosuppression in the treatment of myocarditis is controversial. Some immunosuppressive therapy trials of myocarditis demonstrated no beneficial effects, but recent studies suggest that immunosuppression may be effective in certain adult subsets (Mason et al., 1995; Garg et al., 1998; James et al., 1997; Wojnicz et al., 2001; Parillo, 2001; Tedeschi et al., 1998).

Nursing Management in Myocarditis

Psychological support is an important aspect of care because the patient and family are faced with a sudden and devastating illness. They may need assistance coping with this stressful crisis. Providing education and accurate information on the condition, medications, test, and treatments is an important intervention (Lewandowski, 1999). Nutrition is another important aspect of care that the nurse must evaluate, along with the dietitian. As a leader of the health care team, the nurse can alert social workers, chaplains, mental health professionals, and others to the needs of the patient and coordinate the multidisciplinary care. The nurse is responsible for oxygenation and ventilation management, fluid balance and electrolyte monitoring, and prevention of infection. Accurate hemodynamic monitoring is essential. All of these nursing priorities are crucial in patients that have ventricular assist devices as well (Chillcott et al., 1998). Skin care of the patient on bed rest with decreased CO can be a difficult challenge (Baker, 1994). Because lethal arrhythmias can occur, emergency equipment should be readily available.

■ ENDOCARDIAL DISEASE

Infectious Endocarditis

Infectious endocarditis (IE) is a disease in which infective organisms invade the endothelial lining of the heart, usually involving one or more valves. This is the major endocardial disease. The endocardium covers the valves and surrounds the chordae tendineae. The infection that forms, usually on the valve of the heart, is called *vegetation*.

Epidemiology

The incidence of IE is not known accurately. The International Collaboration of Endocarditis has been conceived recently to develop a large global database of patients whose clinical, echocardiographic, and microbiological findings have been characterized by using standard methodology (Cabell & Abrutyn, 2002). One of the goals of this group is to facilitate randomized clinical trials to increase the evidence on diagnosis and medical treatment.

A study in the eastern United States showed the estimated rate was 11.6 cases per 100,000 per year (Berlin et al., 1995). This rate was influenced by a high number of intravenous drug users and may be somewhat lower in other areas (Durack, 1998). Current estimates suggest an incidence of 1.7-6.2 per 100,000 person years in the U.S. (Mylonakis & Calderwood, 2001). Since World War II, advances in the use of antibiotics, the evolution of cardiac

surgery, and the advent of improved diagnostic techniques have changed the trends of IE. Historically, three quarters of the patients have a structural cardiac abnormality. Rheumatic heart disease was the major risk factor, but this has been replaced by mitral valve prolapse with regurgitation, aortic valve disease, and congenital heart disease (Sexton & Bashore, 1998). The congenital heart defects of greatest risk are those in an area of high turbulence, such as septal defects, valvular abnormalities under high pressure, prosthetic valves and conduits, cyanotic defects, and palliative shunts. HCM with LVOTO also is a risk for IE (Spirito et al., 1999). Long-term dialysis and the presence of cardiovascular catheters are the only risk factors that were more prevalent in patients with no known predisposing cardiac disease (Castillo et al., 2002). The incidence of IE in children, though low, may be increasing possibly due to increasing use of invasive techniques in neonatal and pediatric medical management and increased survival rate of children with congenital heart disease (Cabell et al., 2002). Streptococcal cases have decreased, whereas staphylococcal cases have increased. Many more organisms have been found to cause IE, including rare and unusual microbes, and HIV infection has also been implicated, particularly in those with advanced immunosuppression (Durack, 1998; Wilson et al., 2002). Current social trends, such as tattooing and body piercing can be dangerous for those having heart defects or who have undergone surgery for congenital heart disease (Ochsenfahrt et al., 2001; Satchithananda, et al., 2001). Early in the 20th century, IE had a near 100% mortality rate. Despite many improvements in diagnostics and therapy, IE remains a disease with high morbidity and mortality (Sexton & Bashore, 1998). Display 34-5 lists predisposing factors for IE (Durack, 1998).

Types

In the past, IE has been divided into three categories, acute, subacute, and chronic, according to the presentation and condition

---

D I S P L A Y ■ **34-5**

PREDISPOSING FACTORS FOR INFECTIOUS ENDOCARDITIS

Male sex
Rheumatic heart disease
Degenerative valvular disease
Aortic or mitral valve disease

• Mitral valve prolapse

Prosthetic cardiac valve
Congenital heart disease

• Ventricular septal defect
• Coarctation of the aorta
• Patent ductus arteriosus

Hypertrophic cardiomyopathy with left ventricular outflow tract obstruction
Intravenous drug use
Diabetes mellitus
Pregnancy
Marfan's syndrome
Central venous and pulmonary artery catheters

of the patient. The lines separating these categories are blurred, and the same organisms can produce sudden, severe disease as well as slowly progressing disease in different cases (Durack, 1998). IE can be better classified by site of involvement, such as native valve versus prosthetic valve; by type of pathogen; and definitiveness of the diagnosis, such as possible, probable, or definite (Miner, 1994).

Native valve endocarditis (NVE), the most common type, is an infection seen in patients without prosthetic valves but who usually have valvular or heart disease that predisposes them to IE. NVE, a severe complication of IV drug use, is responsible for 5%-20% of hospital admissions, and 5%-10% of total deaths in this population (Miro et al., 2002). IE in injection drug users is presumed to be caused by trauma to heart valves from contaminated injections, paraphernalia, and skin bacteria at the injection site (Sexton & Bashore, 1998). IE in these patients often involves the tricuspid valve (Eyken, 2001).

The clinical index for suspicion is much higher for *prosthetic valve endocarditis* (PVE), which occurs more frequently than NVE. PVE is also much more likely to require surgery as part of the treatment.

Nosocomial endocarditis occurs late during hospitalizations, and is probably underdiagnosed. The primary pathogen is *Staphylococcus aureus*, secondary to vascular access or hemodialysis (Gouello et al., 2000; Eyken, 2001). Colonized intravascular catheters are the most common identified source of nosocomial endocarditis (Mermel et al., 2001).

Pathogenesis and Pathology

Based on results of experimental and clinical studies, it is known that IE results from a complex interaction between damaged vascular endothelium, local hemodynamic abnormalities, circulating bacteria, and local and systemic host defenses (Bansal, 1995). The pathophysiology of IE involves damage to the valvular endothelium, the formation of a platelet-fibrin thrombus and adherence of bacteria to the platelet thrombin plaque, followed by the proliferation of the infecting organism (Brown & Levine, 2002). The lesions formed are called *nonbacterial thrombotic endocarditis* (NBTE) lesions. Bacteremia often occurs after manipulation of the oropharyngeal, gastrointestinal, and genitourinary tracts. The bacteremia in postoperative and intensive care patients usually occurs secondary to intravenous lines, invasive monitoring devices, wound infections, pneumonia, and urinary tract infections (Miner, 1994). Bacteremia can occur after urethral catheterization, labor and delivery, and abortion. The ability of microbes to adhere to fibrin correlates with their ability to cause IE (Durack, 1998). Dextran-producing strains avidly bind to the fibrin-platelet aggregate on the cardiac valves. Damaged endothelial cells produce fibronectin. Fibronectin receptors have been demonstrated on the surface of several organisms that cause IE (Bansal, 1995). Once the bacteria adhere to the NBTE lesion and multiply, they stimulate inflammatory responses. Cytokines and tumor necrosis factor may be involved in the systemic manifestations of IE (Brown & Griffin, 1998).

Almost any type of bacteria can cause IE. Streptococci and staphylococci cause 80% to 85% of cases. *S. viridans* is being superceded by *S. aureus* as the main causative agent in more recent studies (Sexton et al., 2002). Fungal endocarditis is a rare illness but has a reported mortality of 56% (Pierrotti & Baddour, 2002).

Assessment Findings

In 1994, Durack and colleagues proposed a new set of diagnostic criteria for the diagnosis of IE that subsequently became known as the Duke criteria (Durack, et al., 1994). According to the Duke criteria, persistent bacteremia with organisms typical for endocarditis and an oscillating mass on a valve (vegetation) make a clinically definitive diagnosis of IE. In the course of clinical practice, the diagnosis is suspected more often than it is confirmed. The Duke criteria include several minor criteria that also suggest IE, such as predisposition, fever, vascular phenomena such as septic pulmonary infarcts, and immunologic phenomena such as Osler's nodes. In 2000, other researchers proposed modifications to the Duke criteria that include the use of TEE (Li et al. 2000). Transthoracic echocardiography with Doppler flow studies should be performed in everyone suspected of having endocarditis. If the clinical suspicion is high and the transthoracic echocardiogram is negative or inconclusive, a transesophageal echocardiogram should be obtained (Sexton & Bashore, 1998; Li et al., 2000).

Blood cultures should be drawn from three different sites with 1 hour between each draw or, if time is limited, a total of 1 hour between the first and the last draw. Blood cultures isolate the organism, and positive cultures over time demonstrate true persistence. Meticulous site preparation is essential to avoid contamination (Towns & Reller, 2002). Blood cultures can be negative in 5% to 10% of patients who satisfy diagnostic criteria for IE (Mylonakis & Calderwood, 2001). Other laboratory findings seen in IE can include normocytic anemia, elevated white blood cell count, elevated erythrocyte sedimentation rate in almost all cases, proteinuria, hematuria, elevated BUN and creatinine possibly secondary to embolization, and positive rheumatoid factor in approximately 50% of cases (Conlon et al., 1998).

The virulence of the organism usually determines the acuteness of the presentation. The illness may be characterized by subtle chronic fatigue with low-grade fevers, weight loss, and malaise, or abrupt fulminating and acute pulmonary edema brought on by massive acute aortic regurgitation (Scrima, 1987). The symptoms seen are a reflection of the effects of infective vegetations in the heart and throughout the body. Symptoms include fever, chills, rigors, weight loss, fatigue, loss of appetite, weakness, myalgias, arthralgias, and back pains. Splenomegaly and metastatic infections may become evident. The symptoms can be distinguished by the effect the IE has on the heart and the effect emboli from the vegetations have on the lungs or other organs. Intracardiac symptoms most often come from regurgitant aortic or mitral valves, on the most frequently affected left side of the heart. Tachycardia, gallop rhythm, dyspnea, crackles, and hypotension caused by decreased CO can result from left-side IE. Intracardiac complications of IE include valvular destruction with regurgitation and heart failure, ring abscesses with first- or second-degree heart block, and valve perforations. The complications from systemic emboli that can accompany left-sided IE include hemiplegia and paralysis, mental status changes, visual defects and blindness,

Table 34–2 ■ IMMUNOLOGIC MANIFESTATIONS OF INFECTIOUS ENDOCARDITIS

Finding	Description	Occurrence
Petechiae	Red, flat, 1– to 2–mm, nontender lesions	50% of patients
Splinter hemorrhages	Linear, black, longitudinal streaks on distal tip of nail bed	20% of patients with subacute IE
Osler's nodes	Red, swollen lesions with white centers 1 to 10 mm in size, most commonly found on the pads of the fingers or toes, palms, soles of feet or thighs	10%–20% of patients with subacute IE
Janeway lesions	Nontender, purple or red lesion 1 to 5 mm in size, found on arms, legs, palms, and soles of feet	Not known
Conjunctival petechiae	Caused by microemboli	Not known
Roth's spots	Small, 3– to 10-mm white spots in the retina close to the optic disc, often encircled by hemorrhages	Not known

IE, infectious endocarditis.

MI, intra-abdominal disaster, and renal failure. These symptoms are caused by infarcts of the spinal cord, brain, retina, heart, bowel, spleen, or kidney. When an arterial wall is damaged by septic emboli, mycotic aneurysms can form and are subject to sudden bleeding. Patients can have toxic metabolic encephalopathy, meningitis, brain abscesses, seizures, and headache from sepsis and septic emboli. Myocarditis and pericarditis can also result from IE.

Right-side IE is not as common as left-sided IE and is usually seen in intravenous drug users. When the tricuspid valve is affected, the symptoms that are produced include peripheral edema, neck vein distention, hepatomegaly, ascites, and atrial arrhythmias. Pulmonary emboli that accompany right-sided IE result in chest pain, cough, hemoptysis, tachycardia, pneumothorax, pleural effusions, and pneumonia. Early distribution to other sites was associated with adverse outcomes (Netzer et al., 1995). The circulating immune complexes in IE produce the symptoms of glomerulonephritis, petechiae, Osler's nodes, and arthritis (Bansal, 1995; Conlon et al., 1998; Durack, 1998). Age appears to predict adverse events in those surviving early stages of IE (Caball & Peterson, 2001). Table 34-2 lists the common immunologic manifestations of IE (Durack, 1998; Miner, 1994; Page & Hubble, 1996).

Medical Management

The cornerstone of treatment of IE is early recognition and elimination of the infecting organism. Timely surgical intervention and anticipation and treatment of complications are also key concepts in the care of these patients. Antibiotics are usually bactericidal. Published experience can guide specific therapeutic regimens (Simmons et al., 1998; Wilson et al., 1995). The American Heart Association plans to update the 1995 recommendations in the near future. Antibiotics often are given for 4 to 6 weeks, and longer courses are sometimes necessary. Outpatient intravenous antibiotic therapy has been successful in stable patients with endocarditis in limited trials (Brown, 1992). Others have experienced problems with safety and efficacy and have called for controlled clinical trials to determine if home versus hospital-based antimicrobial therapy have similar outcomes (Colford et al., 1993). IE still has a high mortality rate despite new and potent antibiotics, modern diagnostic tests, and advanced surgical techniques (Le et al., 2003).

Surgery is indicated in IE if the patient has heart failure that is not responding to medical management; recurrent infection;

infection of prosthetic valves, especially if the valve is malfunctioning; large aortic valve vegetations; or recurrent systemic embolization. Early surgical intervention improved long-term survival versus medical therapy alone (Bishara et al., 2002). Echocardiography provides direct visualization of cardiac anatomy, enhancing sensitivity for diagnosis and identifying complications that warrant valve surgery (Sachdev et al., 2002). Most patients with PVE require valve replacement. (Gillinov et al., 2002). Urgent surgery is indicated for severe CHF secondary to significant aortic regurgitation.

Valve replacement has become the routine in the management of patients with IE and should be undertaken as soon as signs and symptoms of failure appear (Sexton & Bashore, 1998). Surgical correction of tricuspid valves through valvuloplasty, which allows for débridement of vegetation, is usually successful, especially if a single leaflet is involved (Relf, 1993).

Prevention

Prevention of IE remains the standard of care. Meticulous dental hygiene may be just as important as antibiotic prophylaxis in the prevention of IE (Sexton & Bashore, 1998). The American Heart Association and European experts have published guidelines for antimicrobial prophylaxis for IE (Dajani et al., 1997; Rey et al., 1998). This is in spite of the fact that there has never been a controlled study in humans proving the benefit of antibiotic prophylaxis in the prevention of IE (Hartman, 1999). It is generally agreed that patients with prosthetic valves and a prior episode of IE are at increased risk for IE. Because patients who are at risk for development of IE have been identified, the usual practice is to prescribe prophylactic antibiotics if these patients are to undergo procedures that are likely to produce bacteremia. However, there is varied scientific evidence that antibiotic prophylaxis is effective (Sexton & Bashore, 1998). It is also critical that hospital personnel adhere to infection control guidelines when inserting and maintaining vascular access catheters and other invasive devices (Mermel et al., 2001; Schmid, 2000).

Nursing Management in Infectious Endocarditis

Nurses need to be knowledgeable about IE and its symptoms and complications, the difficulty in making the diagnosis, and its far-reaching effects. A detailed history reveals risk factors, symptoms, prodromal illness, recent antibiotic therapy, and preexisting renal disease. This information aids in the medical diagnosis. Determination of body piercing or tattooing is necessary. A careful physical examination may reveal the signs of IE, such as a murmur secondary to new-onset regurgitation.

Once the patient is diagnosed, the plan of care should be discussed with the patient and family. The nurse can be the leader on the health care team to make sure the multiple needs of the patient with IE are addressed and met by all disciplines (Marrie, 1997). A lengthy hospitalization is likely, and patients need assistance with coping with this and the illness.

This illness is life threatening, so information and emotional support are crucial in facilitating coping mechanisms (Traush, 1988). If it is indicated, a referral for drug addiction treatment should be completed. Drug addiction and alcohol abuse frequently engender strong negative feelings among nurses and physicians. The nurse must make care decisions in an ethical, professional manner, even when caring for patients who use intravenous drugs, do not follow recommendations, or do not take the prescribed medications (Maupin, 1995). Other issues in this population are an increased tolerance to analgesia, potential drug withdrawal, and behavior and adherence problems, and poly-substance abuse (Jenkins, 2000; Broyles & Korniewicz, 2002). The nurse manages oxygen therapy, ventilator care, and vasoactive medications and monitors fluid balance and ECGs. The nurse often obtains the blood for laboratory tests and blood cultures, and then interprets the results. The nurse is responsible for proper administration of antibiotics and monitoring for therapeutic levels and side effects. The nurse also manages the intravenous lines for the long course of antibiotics. If a pulmonary artery catheter is in place, accurate measurements and interpretations guide medical care. Meticulous handwashing, infection control and early removal of invasive lines help to prevent nosocomial IE.

Careful assessment facilitates early detection of complications. Knowing the indications for surgery may prove life saving (Snelson et al., 1993). Perivalvular abscesses may manifest as various forms of heart block when adjacent tissues containing conduction fibers become inflamed or directly damaged (Sexton & Spelman, 2002). Preoperative teaching is necessary to prepare the patient undergoing surgery. During surgery, it is desirable to keep the family informed of the progress. After surgery, pulmonary hygiene and close hemodynamic monitoring are crucial, as is monitoring for potential drug withdrawal if the patient is an intravenous drug user (Contoreggi, 1998). The signs include restlessness, insomnia, diaphoresis, chills, diarrhea, tachycardia, hypertension, pupillary dilation, and tachypnea (Relf, 1993). Once the patient is ready for discharge, education is critical because the patient must be knowledgeable about recurrence of symptoms, such as fever and weight loss, antibiotic prophylaxis for certain high-risk procedures, and the need for keeping all health care providers informed that he or she is at increased risk for IE. The nurse should stress the importance of postdischarge follow-up and inform the patient about the need to obtain medical alert identification. The importance of proper oral hygiene should also be stressed (DeJong, 1998).

REFERENCES

Acker, M. A. (2001). Mechanical circulatory support for patients with acute-fulminant myocarditis. *Annals of Thoracic Surgery,* 71(3 Suppl.), S73–6

Adler, Y., Finkestein, Y., Guindo, J., Rodrigues le la Serna, A., Shoenfeld, Y., Bayes-Genis, A., et al. (1998). Colchicine treatment for recurrent pericarditis: a decade of experience. *Circulation, 97,* 2183–2185.

American Heart Association (2003). Pericardium and pericarditis [On-line]. Available: http://americanheart.org.

Ammash, N. M., Seward, J. B., Baily, K. R., Edwards, W. D., & Tajik, J. (2000). Clinical profile and outcome of idiopathic restrictive cardiomyopathy. *Circulation, 101,* 2490–2496.

Bachinski, L. L., & Roberts, R. (1998). New theories: Causes of dilated cardiomyopathy. *Cardiology Clinics,* 16(4), 603–610.

Baker, A. (1994). Acquired heart disease in infants and children. *Critical Care Clinics of North America,* 6(1), 175–186.

Baljepally, R., & Spodick, D. H. (1998). PR-segment deviation as the initial electrocardiographic response in acute pericarditis. *American Journal of Cardiology,* 81(12), 1505–1506.

Bansch, D., Antz, M., Boczor, S., Volkmer, M., Tebbenjohanns, J., Seidl, K., Block, M., Gietzen, F., Berger, J., Kuck, K. H. (2002). Primary prevention of sudden cardiac death in idiopathic dilated cardiomyopathy. *Circulation, 105,* 1453–1458.

Berg, J. (1990). Assessing pericarditis in the end-stage renal disease patient. *Dimensions of Critical Care Nursing, 9,* 266–271.

Bishara, J., Beibovici, L., Gartma-Israel, D., Sagie, A., Kazakov, A., Miroshnik, E., et al. (2001). Long-term outcome of infective endocarditis: The impact of early surgical intervention. *Clinical Infectious Disease,* 33(10), 1636–1643.

Bohachick, P., & Anton, B. B. (1990). Psychosocial adjustment of patients and spouses to severe cardiomyopathy. *Research in Nursing and Health, 13,* 385–392.

Borczuk, A. C., van Hoeven, K. H., & Factors, M. (1997). Review and hypothesis: The eosinophil and peripartum heart disease (myocarditis and coronary artery dissection)–coincidence or pathogenetic significance? *Cardiovascular Research, 33,* 527–532.

Brady, W. J., Perron, A. D., Martin, M. L., Beagle, C., & Aufderheide, T. (2001). Cause of ST segment abnormality in ED chest pain patients. *American Journal of Emergency Medicine,* 19(1), 25–28.

Brandt, R., Filzmaier, K., & Hanrath, P. (2001). Circulating cardiac troponin I in acute pericarditis. *American Journal of Cardiology, 87,* 1326–1328.

Brown, C. S., & Bertolet, B. D. (1998). Peripartum cardiomyopathy: A comprehensive review. *American Journal of Obstetrics and Gynecology, 2,* 409–414.

Brown, M., & Griffin, G. E. (1998). Immune responses in endocarditis. *Heart, 79,* 1–2.

Brown, P. D., & Levine, D. P. (2002). Infective endocarditis in the injection drug user. *Infectious Disease Clinics of North America, 16,* 645–665.

Brown, R. B. (1991). Selection and training of patients for outpatient intravenous antibiotics. *Reviews in Infectious Disease,* 13(Suppl. 12), S147–151.

Broyles, L., & Korniewicz, D. (2002). The opiate-dependent patient with endocarditis: addressing pain and substance abuse withdrawal. *AACN Clinical Issues,* 13(3), 431–451.

Burch, M. (2002). Heart failure in the young. *Heart, 88,* 198–202.

Burgess l. J., Reuter, H., Carstens, M. E., Taljaard, F., & Doubell, A. F. (2002). The use of adenosine deaminase and interferon-γ as diagnostic tools for tuberculosis pericarditis. *Chest, 122,* 900–905.

Caball, C., & Abrutyn, E. (2002). Progress toward a global understanding of infectious endocarditis: Early lessons from the international collaboration on endocarditis investigation. *Infectious Disease Clinics of North America, 16,* 255–272.

Caball, C., Jollis, J., Peterson, G., Corey, G., Anderson, D., Sexton, D., et al. (2002). Changing patient characteristics and the effect on mortality in endocarditis. *Archives in Internal Medicine, 162,* 90–94.

Caball, C., & Peterson, G. (2001). Factors affecting long-term mortality in endocarditis: the bugs, the drugs, the knife...or the patients? *American Heart Journal, 141,* 6–8.

Carthy, C. M., Yang, D., Anderson, D. R., Wilson, J. E., & McManus, B. M. (1997). Myocarditis as systemic disease: New perspectives on pathogenesis. *Clinical Experiments in Pharmacology and Physiology, 24,* 997–1000.

Castillo, J., Anguita, M., Torres, F., Mesa, D., Franco, M., Gonzalez, E., et al. (2002). Comparison of features of active infective endocarditis involving native cardiac valves in nonintravenous drug users with and without predisposing cardiac disease. *American Journal of Cardiology,* 90(Dec 1), 1266–1269.

Cesario, D., Clark, J., & Maisel, A, (1998). Beneficial effects of intermittent home administration of the inotrope/vasodilator milrinone in patients with end-stage congestive heart failure: A preliminary study. *American Heart Journal,* 135, 121–129.

Chachques, J. C., Argyriadis, P. G., Fontaine, G., Hebert, J. L., Frank, R. A., D'Attellis, N., et al. (2003). Right ventricular cardiomyoplasty: 10-year follow-up. *Annals of Thoracic Surgery,* 75(5), 1464–1468.

Chan, A. W., McManus, B., & Ignaszewski, A. P. (2000). The enigma of recent onset dilated cardiomyopathy: What cause, what consequence, what control? *Canadian Journal of Cardiology,* 16(5), 641–652.

Child, J. S., & Perloff, J. K. (1998). The restrictive cardiomyopathies. Cardiology Clinics, 6, 289–316.

Chillcott, S. R., Atkins, P. J., & Adamson, R. M. (1998). Left ventricular assist is a viable alternative for cardiac transplantation. *Critical Care Nursing Quarterly,* 20(4), 64–79.

Colford, J. M., Corelli, R. L., & Ganz, J. W. (1993). Home antibiotic therapy for streptococcal endocarditis: A call for a controlled trial. *American Journal of Medicine,* 94, 111–112.

Colleti, C. (1999). Pericarditis: Is this a life-threatening myocardial infarction or something else? *American Journal of Nursing,* 99(10), 35.

Conlon, P. J., Jeffries, F., Krigman, H. R., Covey, G. R., Sexton, D. J., & Abramson, M. A. (1998). Predictors of prognosis and risk of acute renal failure in bacterial endocarditis. *Clinical Nephrology,* 49, 96–101.

Constant, J. (1999). The alcoholic cardiomyopathies-genuine and pseudo. *Cardiology,* 91, 92–95.

Contoreggi, C., Rexroad, V., & Lange, W. R. (1998). Current management of infectious complications in the injecting drug user. *Journal of Substance Abuse Treatment,* 15, 95–106.

Cox, S., O'Donoghue, A. C., McKenna, W. J., Steptoe, A.J. (1997). Health related quality of life and psychological wellbeing in patients with hypertrophic cardiomyopathy. *Heart,* 78, 182–187.

Dajani, A. S., Taubart, K. A., Wilson, W., Bolger A. F., Bayer A., Ferrieri, P., et al. (1997). Prevention of bacterial endocarditis. Recommendations by the American Heart Association. *Circulation,* 96, 358–366.

D'Ambrosio, A., Patti, G., Manzoli, A., Sinagra, G., DiLenarda, A., Silverstri, F., et al. (2001). The fate of acute myocarditis between spontaneous improvement and evolution to dilated cardiomyopathy: A review. *Heart,* 85, 499–504.

Davies, M. (2000). The cardiomyopathies: An overview. *Heart,* 83, 469–474.

Davis, J., Kirklin, J., Pearce, F., Rayburn, B., Winokur, T., & Holman, W. (2002). Mechanical circulatory support for myocarditis: How much recovery should occur before device removal? *Journal of Heart Lung Transplant,* 21, 1246–1249.

DeJong, M. J. (1998). Infectious endocarditis. *American Journal of Nursing,* 98(5), 34.

DeRose, J. J., Banas, J. S., & Winters, S. L. (1994). Current perspectives on sudden cardiac death in hypertrophic cardiomyopathy. *Progress in Cardiovascular Disease,* 36, 475–484.

Drezner, J. A. (2000). Sudden cardiac death in young athletes. *Post Graduate Medicine,* 108(5), 37–50.

Dreyfus, G., & Mihealaino, S. (2001). The Batista procedure. *Heart,* 85, 1–2.

Duffee, D. F., Shen, W. K., & Smith, H.C. (1998). Suppression of frequent premature ventricular contractions and improvement of left ventricular function in patients with presumed idiopathic dilated cardiomyopathy. *Mayo Clinic Proceedings,* 73, 430–433.

Dugan, K. J. (1998). Caring for patients with pericarditis. *Nursing,* 3, 50–351.

Durack, D. T., Bright, D. K., & Lukes, A. S. (1994). Duke endocarditis service new criteria for diagnosis of infective endocarditis: Utilization of specific echocardiographic findings. *American Journal of Medicine,* 96, 200–209.

Felker, G. M., Thompson, R. E., Hare, J. M., Hruban, R. H., Clemetson, D. E., Howard, D. L., et al. (2000). Underlying causes and long-term survival in patients with initially unexplained cardiomyopathy. *New England Journal of Medicine,* 342, 1077–1084.

Fonorow, G. C. (2001). Pathogenesis and treatment of cardiomyopathy. *Advances in Internal Medicine,* 47, 1–45.

Francis, S. E., Holden, H., Holt, C. M., & Duff, G. M. (1998). Interleukin-1 in myocardium and coronary arteries of patients with dilated cardiomyopathy. *Journal of Mollecular Cellular Cardiology,* 30, 215–223.

Friedrich, M. G., Strohm, O., Shulz-Menger, J., Marciniak, H., Luft, F. C., Dietz, R. (1998). Contrast media-enhanced magnetic resonance imaging visualizes myocardial changes in the course of viral myocarditis. *Circulation,* 97, 1802–1809.

Frost, M. H., Kelly, A. W., Mangan, D. B., & Zarling, K. K. (1994). An analysis of factors influencing psychosocial adjustment to cardiomyopathy. *Cardiovascular Nursing,* 30, 1–7.

Gadler, F., Linde, C., Duabert, C., Meisel, E., Aliot, E., Chojnowska, L., et al. (1999). Significant improvement in quality of life following AV synchronous pacing in patients with hypertrophic obstructive cardiomyopathy. *European Heart Journal,* 20, 1044–1055.

Gagliardi, J. P., Nettles, R. E., McCarty, D. E., Sanders, L. L., Corey, G. R., & Sexton, D. J. (1998). Native valve infectious endocarditis in elderly and younger adult patients: Comparison of clinical features and outcomes with the use of the Duke criteria and the Duke endocarditis database. *Clinics in Infectious Disease,* 26, 1165–1168.

Galiuto, L., Enriquez-Sarano, M., Reeder, G. S., Tazelaar, H. D., Li, J. T., Miller, F. A., et al. (1997). Eosinophilic myocarditis manifesting as myocardial infarction: Early diagnosis and successful treatment. *Mayo Clinic Proceedings,* 72, 603–610.

Garg, A., Shian, J., & Guyatt, G. (1998). The effectiveness of immunosuppressive therapy in lymphocytic myocarditis: An overview. *Annals of Internal Medicine,* 128, 317–322.

Gillinov, G., Faber, C., Sabil, J., Pettersson, G., Griffin, B., Gordon, S., et al. (2002). Endocarditis after mitral valve repair. *Annals of Thoracic Surgery,* 73, 1813–1816.

Goldrick, B. A. (2003). Endocarditis associated with body piercing. *American Journal of Nursing,* 103(1), 26–28.

Gouello, J., Asfar, P., Brenet, O., Kouatchet, A., Berthelot, G., & Alquier, P. (2000). Nosocomial endocarditis in the ICU: An analysis of 22 cases. *Critical Care Medicine,* 28(2), 377–382.

Goyle, K. K., & Walling, A. D. (2002). Diagnosing pericarditis. *American Family Physician,* 66(9), 1695–1702.

Gupta, R., Munyak, J., Haydock, T., & Gernsheimer, J. (1999). Hypothyroidism presenting as acute cardiac tamponade with viral pericarditis. *American Journal of Medicine,* 17(2), 176–178.

Hancock, E. (2001). Differential diagnosis of restrictive cardiomyopathy and constrictive pericarditis. *Heart,* 86, 343–349.

Hartman, B. (2002). Selective aspects of infective endocarditis: considerations on diagnosis, risk factors, treatment and prophylaxis. *Advances in Cardiology,* 39, 195–202.

Hoit, B. D. (2002). Management of effusive and constrictive pericardial heart disease. *Circulation,* 105, 2939–2942.

James, K. B., Ratliff, N., Starling, R., & Young, J. B. (1997). Inflammatory cardiomyopathy. *Rheumatic Disease Clinics of North America,* 23, 333–343.

Jenkins D.H. (2000). Substance abuse and withdrawal in the intensive care unit. *Surgical Clinics of North America,* 80, 1033–1053.

Johnson, S. D., Johnson, D. W., & O'Rourke, D. (1999). Carcinoid constrictive pericarditis. *Heart,* 82, 641–643.

Kabbani, S. S., & Lewinter, M. M. (2000). Diastolic heart failure: Constrictive, restrictive and pericardial. *Cardiology Clinics,* 18(3), 301–509.

Kappenberger, L., Linde, C., Daubert, C., McKenna, W., Meisel, E., Sadone, N., et al. (1997). Pacing in hypertrophic cardiomyopathy: A randomized crossover study. *European Heart Journal,* 18, 1249–1256.

Karmy-Jones, R., Yen, T., & Cornejo, C. (2002). Pericarditis after trauma resulting in delayed cardiac tamponade. *Annals of Thoracic Surgery,* 74, 239–249.

Kasper, E. K., Agema, W. R., Hutchins, G. M., Deckers, J. W., Hare, J. M., & Baughman, K. L. (1994). The causes of dilated cardiomyopathy: A clinicopathologic review of 673 consecutive patients. *Journal of the American College of Cardiology,* 23, 586–590.

Kawai, C. (1999). From myocarditis to cardiomyopathy: Mechanisms of inflammation and cell death. *Circulation,* 99, 1091–1100.

Keren, A., & Popp, R. L. (1992) Assignment of patients into the classification of cardiomyopathies. *Circulation,* 86, 1622–1633.

Klein, A. L., Canale, M. P., Rajagopalan, N., White, R. D., Murray, R. D., Wahi, S., et al. (1999). Role of transesophageal echocardiography in assessing diastolic dysfunction in a large clinical practive: A 9-year experience. *American Heart,* 138, 880–889.

Klein, A. L., & Scalia, G. M. (1998). Diseases of the pericardium, restrictive cardiomyopathy and diastolic dysfunction. In E. J. Topol (Ed.), *Comprehensive cardiovascular medicine* (pp. 639–705). Philadelphia: Lippincott-Raven.

Kumpati, G. S., McCarthy, P. M., & Hoercher, K. J. (2001). Left ventricular assist device bridge to recovery: A review of the current status. *Annals of Thoracic Surgery,* 71, S103–108.

Kushwaha, S.S., Fallon, J. T., & Fuster, V. (1999). Restrictive cardiomyopathy. *New England Journal of Medicine,* 336, 267–276.

Le, T., & Bayer, A. (2003). Combination antibiotic therapy for infective endocarditis. *Clinical Infectious Disease,* 36, 615–621.

Ledford, D. K. (1997). Immunologic aspects of vasculitis and cardiovascular disease. *Journal of the American Medical Association,* 278, 1962–1965.

Lewis, P., Boyd, C., Hubert, N., & Steele, M. (2001). Ethanol-induced therapeutic myocardial infarction to treat hypertrophic obstructive cardiomyopathy. *Critical Care Nurse,* 21(2), 20–34.

Li, J. S., Sexton, D. J., Mick N., Nettles R., Fowler, V. O., Ryan T., et al. (2000). Proposed modification to the Duke criteria for the diagnosis of infectious endocarditis. *Clinical Infectious Disease,* 30(4), 633–638.

Li, W., & Somerville, J. (1998). Infectious endocarditis in the grown-up congenital heart (GUCH) population. *European Heart Journal,* 19, 166–173.

Ling, L. H., Oh, J. K., Schaff, H. V., Danielson, G. K., Mahoney, D. W., Seward, J. B., et al. (1999). Constrictive pericarditis in the modern era: Evolving clinical spectrum and impact on outcome after pericardiectomy. *Circulation,* 100, 1380–1386.

Ling, L., Oh, J., Breen, J., Schaff, H., Danielson, G., Mahoney, D., et al. (2000). Calcific constrictive pericarditis: Is it still with us? *Annals of Internal Medicine,* 132(6), 444–450.

Luppi, P., Rudert, W.A., Zanone, M. M., Stassi, G., Trucco, G., Finegold, D., et al. (1998), Idiopathic cardiomyopathy: A superantigen-driven autoimmune disease. *Circulation,* 98, 777–785.

Manolio, T. A., Baughman, K. L., Rodeheffer, R., Pearson, T. A., Bristow, J. D., Michels, V. V., et al. (1992). Idiopathic dilated cardiomyopathy, prevalence and etiology: Summary of a National Heart, Lung, and Blood Institute workshop. *American Journal of Cardiology,* 69, 1458–1466.

Maron, B. J. (2001). Hypertrophic cardiomyopathy. In V. Foster, R. Alexander, R. O'Rourke (Eds.), *Hurst's the heart* (10th ed., pp. 1967–1987). New York: McGraw-Hill.

Maron, B. J. (1997). Hypertrophic cardiomyopathy. *Lancet,* 350 (907D), 127–133.

Maron, B. J., Nishimura, R.A., McKenna, B. J., Rakowski, H., Josephson, M. E., & Kieval, R. S. (1999). Assessment of permanent dual-chamber pacing as a treatment for drug-refractory symptomatic patients with obstructive hypertrophic cardiomyopathy. A randomized, double-blind crossover study (M-PATHY). *Circulation,* 99, 2927–2933.

Marrie, T. J. (1987). Infectious endocarditis: A serious and changing disease. *Critical Care Nurse,* 7(2), 31–46.

Mason, J. W. (1999). Myocarditis. *Advances in Internal Medicine, 44,* 293–310.

Mason, J. W. (2001). Classification of cardiomyopathies. In V. Foster, R. Alexander, & R. O'Rourke (Eds.), *Hurst's the heart* (10th ed., pp. 1941–1946). New York: McGraw-Hill.

Mason, J. W., O'Connell, J. B., Herskowitz, A., Rose, N.R., McManus, B. M., Billingham, et al. (1995). A clinical trial of immunosuppressive therapy for myocarditis. *New England Journal of Medicine, 333,* 269–275.

Maupin, C.R. (1995). The potential for noncaring when dealing with difficult patients: Strategies for moral decision making. *Journal of Cardiovascular Nursing, 9*(3), 11–22.

McKenna, W. J., Codd, M. B., McCann, H. A., & Sugrue, D. D. (1998). Alcohol consumption and idiopathic dilated cardiomyopathy: A case control study. *American Heart Journal, 135,* 833–837.

McKenna, W. J. (1998). The natural history of hypertrophic cardiomyopathy. *Cardiovascular Clinics, 19,* 135–145.

McKenna, W. J., & Elliot, P. M. (1998). Hypertrophic cardiomyopthy. In E. J. Topol (Ed.), *Comprehensive cardiovascular medicine* (pp. 745–768) Philadelphia: Lippincott-Raven.

McNamara, D. M., Holubkov, R., Starling, R. C., Dec, G. W., Loh, E., Torre-Amione, G., et al. (2001). Controlled trial of intravenous immune globulin in recent-onset dilated cardiomyopathy. *Circulation, 103,* 2254–2259.

Mehta, A., Mehta, M., & Jain A. (1999). Constrictive pericarditis. *Clinics of Cardiology, 22,* 334–344.

Mermel, L., Farr, B., Sherertz, R., Radd, I., O'Grady, N., Harris, J., et al. (2002). Guidelines for the management if intravascular catheter-related infections. *Journal of Intravascular Nursing, 24*(3), 180–205.

Mestroni, L., Rocco, C., Vatta, M., Miocic, S., & Giacca, M. (1998). Advances in molecular genetics of dilated cardiomyopathy. *Cardiology Clinics, 16,* 611–621.

Michels, V. V., Moll, P. P., Miller, F. A., Tajik, A. J., Chi, J. S., Driscoll, D. S., Burnett, J. C., Rodeneffer, R. J., Chesecro, J, H., & Tazelaar, H. D. (1992). The frequency of familial dilated cardiomyopathy in a series of patients with idiopathic dilated cardiomyopathy. *New England Journal of Medicine, 326,* 77–82.

Miner, P.D. (1994). Infective endocarditis: Implications for care of the adult with congenital heart disease. *Nursing Clinics of North America, 29,* 269–283.

Miro, J., del Rio, A., & Mestres, C. (2002). Infective endocarditis in intravenous drug abusers and HIV-infected patients. *Infectious Disease Clinics of North America, 16,* 273–295.

Mogensen J., Bahl, A., & McKenna, W. J. (2003) Hypertrophic cardiomyopathy-the clinical challenge of managing a hereditary heart condition. *European Heart Journal,* 24, 496–498.

Mogensen, J., Kubo, T., Duque, M., Uribe, W., Shaw, A., Murphy, R., et al. (2003). Idiopathic restrictive cardiomyopathy is part of the clinical expression of cardiac troponin I mutations. *Journal of Clinical Investigations,* 111(2), 209–216.

Myers, R. B., & Spodick, D. H. (1999). Constrictive pericarditis: Clinical and pathophysiologic characteristics. *American Heart Journal,* 138, 219–232.

Mylonakis E., & Calderwood, S. (2001). Endocarditis in adults. *New England Journal of Medicine,* 345, 1318.

Netzer, R., Zollinger, E., Seiler, C., & Cerny, A. (2000). Infective endocarditis: Clinical spectrum, presentation and outcome, an analysis of 212 cases 1980–1995. *Heart,* 84, 25–30.

Nishimura, R. A. (2001). Constrictive pericarditis in the modern era: A diagnostic dilemma. *Heart,* 86, 619–623.

Ochsenfahrt, C., Friedl, R., Hannekum, A., & Schumacker, B. (2001). Endocarditis after nipple piercing in a patient with a bicuspid aortic valve. *Annals of Thoracic Surgery,* 71, 1365–1366.

Olson, T. M., Michels, V. V., & Thibideau, S. N. (1998). Actin mutations in dilated cardiomyopathy: A heritable form of heart failure. *Science,* 280, 750–752.

Organ Procurement and Transplantation Network/SR 1996 Annual report. (April 15, 1997). United Network for Organ Sharing (UNOS) Scientific Registry. Richmond, VA. UNOS.

Page, J. G., & Hubble, M. W. (1996). Recognizing infectious endocarditis: Case study of a 28-year-old. *Journal of Emergency Nursing,* 22, 24–28.

Parillo, J. E. (2001). Inflammatory cardiomyopathy (myocarditis): Which patients should be treated with anti-inflammatory therapy? *Circulation,* 104, 4–6.

Paul, S., & York, D. (1992). Cocaine abuse: An expanding health care problem for the 1990s. *American Journal of Critical Care,* 1, 109–113.

Perloff, J. K. (1998). Cardiomyopathies: Introduction. *Cardiology Clinics,* 6, 185–195.

Pierce, C. D. (1992). Acute post-MI pericarditis. *Journal of Cardiovascular Nursing, 6*(4), 46–56.

Pierroti, L., & Baddour, L. (2002). Fungal endocarditis 1995–2000. *Chest,* 122, 302–310.

Pisani, B., Taylor, D. O., & Mason, J. W. (1997). Inflammatory myocardial diseases and cardiomyopathies, *American Journal of Medicine,* 102, 459.

Pitt, B., Zannad, F., Remme, W. J., Cody, R., Castaigne, A., Perez, A., Palensky, J., et al. (1999). The effect of spironolactone on morbidity and mortality in patients with severe heart failure. Randomized Aldactone evaluation study investigators. *New England Journal of Medicine,* 341, 709–717.

Rajagopalan, N., Garcia, M., Rodriguez, L., Murray, R. D., Apperson-Hansen, C., Stugaard, M., et al. (2001). Comparison of new Doppler echocardiographic methods to differentiate constrictive pericardial heart disease and restrictive cardiomyopathy. *American Journal of Cardiology,* 87, 86–94.

Relf, M. V. (1993). Surgical intervention for tricuspid valve endocarditis: Vegetectomy, valve excision, or valve replacement? *Journal of Cardiovascular Nursing,* 7(2), 71–79.

Rey, J. R., Axon, A., Budzynska, A., Kruse, A., & Nowak, A. (1998). Guidelines of the European Society of Gastrointestinal Endoscopy (ESGE): Antibiotic prophylaxis for gastrointestinal endoscopy. *Endoscopy,* 30, 318–324.

Robiti, G., Hartnell, G., & Cohen, M. (2001). MRI changes in myocarditis-evaluation with spin echo, cine MR angiography and contrast enhanced spin echo imaging. *Clinical Radiology,* 55, 752–758.

Rodgers, M. L. (1990). Pericarditis: A different kind of heart disease. *Nursing,* 2, 52–58.

Sachdev, M., Peterson, G., & Jollis, J. (2002). Imaging techniques for diagnosis of infectious endocarditis. *Infectious Disease Clinics of North America,* 16, 319–337.

Saklayen, M., Anne, V.V., & Lapuz, M. (2002). Pericardial effusion leading to acute renal failure. Two case reports and a discussion of pathophysiology. *American Journal of Kidney Diseases,* 40(4), 837–841.

Sandberg, M., Singh, A., & Graves, P. (1995). Extracorporeal membrane oxygenation as therapy in refractory reversible myocarditis. *Critical Care Nurse,* 15, 53–58.

Satchithananda, D., Walsj, J., & Schofield, P. (2001). Bacterial endocarditis following repeated tattooing. *Heart,* 85, 11–12.

Schactman, M., Cote, P. M., & Ramza B. (1997). The importance of atrial contribution: A case study of dual-chamber pacing in hypertrophic obstructive cardiomyopathy. *Heart Lung,* 26, 345–349.

Schmid, C., Hammel, D., Deng, M., Weyland, M., Baba, H., Tjan, T., et al. (1999). Ambulatory care of patients with left ventricular assist devices *Circulation,* 100(Suppl. II), 224–228.

Scrima, D.A. (1987). Infective endocarditis: Nursing considerations. *Critical Care Nurse,* 7(2), 47–56.

Sexton, D.J, & Bashore, T. M. (1998). Infectious endocarditis. In E. J. Topol (Ed.), *Comprehensive cardiovascular medicine* (pp. 607–637) Philadelphia: Lippincott-Raven.

Sexton, D. J., & Spelman, D. (2002). Current best practice and guidelines: assessment and management of complications of infectious endocarditis. *Infectious Disease Clinics of North America,* 16, 507–521.

Shabetai, R. (1998). Pericardial disease. In D. L. Brown (Ed.), *Cardiac intensive care* (pp. 469–475) Philadelphia: WB Saunders.

Shabetai, R., Fowler, N. O., Fenton, J.C., & Masangkay, M. (1965). Pulsus paradoxus. *Journal of Clinical Investigation,* 44, 1882–1898.

Shanholtz, C. (2001). Acute life-threatening toxicity of cancer treatment. *Critical Care Clinics,* 17(3), 483–502.

Sherrid, M., Chandhry, F., & Swistel, D. (2003). Hypertrophic cardiomyopathy: Echocardiography, pathophysiology, and the continuing evolution of surgery for obstruction. *Annals of Thoracic Surgery,* 75, 620–632.

Silva-Cardoso, J., Moura, B., Martins, L., Mota-Miranda, A., Rocha-Concalves, & Lecour, H. (1999). Pericardial involvement in human immunodeficiency virus infection. *Chest,* 115, 418–422.

Simmons, N. A., Ball, A. P., Eykyn, S. J., Littler, W.A., McGowan, D. A., Conlon, C., et al. (1998). Amoxycillin prophylaxis for endocarditis prevention. *British Dental Journal,* 184(5), 208–213.

Sindone, A. P., Keogh, A, M., MacDonald, P.S., McCosker, C. J., & Kaanaf, C. J. (1997). Continuous home ambulatory intravenous inotropic drug therapy in severe heart failure: Safety and cost efficiency. *American Heart Journal,* 134(5 pt 1), 889–900

Sitges, M., Shiota, T., Lever, H., Qin, J., Bauer, F., Drinko, J., et al. (2003). Comparison of left diastolic function in obstructive hypertrophic cardiomyopathy in patients undergoing percutaneous septal alcohol ablation versus surgical myotomy/myectomy. *American Journal of Cardiology,* 91, 817–821.

Snelson, C., Cline, B. A., & Luby, C. (1993). Infective endocarditis: A challenging diagnosis. *Dimensions of Critical Care Nursing,* 12(4), 4–16.

Song, H., Choi, Y. W., Jang, S., Jeon, S., Park, C. K., Lee, S., et al. (2002). Pericardium: Anatomy and spectrum of disease on computed tomography. *Current Problems in Radiology,* 31, 198–209.

Spodick, D. H. (1997a). Acquired pericardial disease: Pathogenesis and overview. In D. H. Spodick (Ed.), *The Pericardium: A Comprehensive Textbook* (pp. 76–93). New York, Marcel Dekker.

Spodick, D. H. (1997b). Acute, clinically noneffusive ("dry") pericarditis. In D. H. Spodick (Ed.), *The Pericardium: A Comprehensive Textbook* (pp. 94–113). New York, Marcel Dekker.

Spodick, D. H. (1997c). Auscultatory phenomena in pericardial disease. In D. H. Spodick DH (Ed.), *The Pericardium: A comprehensive textbook* (pp. 27–39). New York, Marcel Dekker.

Spodick, D. H. (1997d). Cardiac tamponade: Clinical characteristics, diagnosis, and management. In D. H. Spodick (Ed.), *The Pericardium: A comprehensive textbook* (pp. 153–179). New York, Marcel Dekker.

Spodick, D. H. (1997e). Congenital abnormalities of the pericardium. In D. H. Spodick DH (Ed.), *The Pericardium: A Comprehensive Textbook* (pp. 65–75). New York, Marcel Dekker.

Spodick, D. H. (1997f). Constrictive pericarditis. In D. H. Spodick (Ed.), *The pericardium: A comprehensive textbook* (pp. 214–259). New York: Marcel Dekker.

Spodick, D. H. (1997g). Electrocardiographic abnormalities in pericardial disease. In D. H. Spodick (Ed.), *The pericardium: A comprehensive textbook* (pp. 40–64). New York: Marcel Dekker.

Spodick, D. H. (1997h). Pericardial disease in the vasculitis-connective tissue disease group. In D. H. Spodick (Ed.), *The pericardium: A comprehensive textbook* (pp. 314–333). New York: Marcel Dekker.

Spodick, D. H. (1997i). Pericardial effusion and hydropericardium without tamponade. In D. H. Spodick (Ed.), *The pericardium: A comprehensive textbook* (pp. 126–152). New York: Marcel Dekker.

Spodick, D. H. (1997j). Pericardial macro- and microanatomy: A synopsis. In D. H. Spodick (Ed.), *The pericardium: A comprehensive textbook* (pp. 7–14). New York: Marcel Dekker.

Spodick, D. H. (1997k). Physiology of the normal pericardium: Functions of the normal pericardium. In D. H. Spodick (Ed.), *The pericardium: A comprehensive textbook* (pp. 15–26). New York: Marcel Dekker.

Spodick, D. H. (1997l). Pulsus paradoxus. In D. H. Spodick (Ed.), *The pericardium: A comprehensive textbook* (pp.191–199). New York: Marcel Dekker.

Spodick, D. H. (2001). Pericardial diseases. In E. Braunwald, D. Zipes, & P. Libby (Eds.), *Heart disease: A textbook of cardiovascular medicine* (6th ed., pp 1751–1806). Philadelphia: W. B. Saunders.

Spodick, D. H. (2003). Acute pericarditis: Current concepts and practice. *Journal of the American Medical Association, 289*(9), 1150–1153.

Starling, R. C., & Young, R. B. (1998). Surgical therapy for dilated cardiomyopathy. *Cardiology Clinics,* 16(4), 727–737.

Stevenson, L.W., & Perloff, J.K. (1988). The dilated cardiomyopathies: Clinical aspects. *Cardiology Clinics,* 6, 187–218.

Suddaby, E.C. (1996). Viral myocarditis in children. *Critical Care Nurse,* 16, 73–82.

Tedeschi, A., Airaghi, L., Giannini, S., Ciceri, L., & Massari, F. (2002). High-dose intravenous immunoglobulin in the treatment of acute myocarditis. A case report and review of the literature. *Journal of Internal Medicine,* 251, 169–173.

Towns, M., & Reller, L. (2002). Diagnostic methods current best practices and guidelines for isolation of bacteria and fungi in infective endocarditis. *Infectious Disease Clinics of North America,* 16, 363–376.

Trausch, P.A. (1988). Infective endocarditis: Nursing care and prevention. *Progress in Cardiovascular Nursing,* 3(2), 45–53.

Ueno, T., Bergin, P., Richardson, M., Esmore, D. (2000). Bridge to recovery with a left ventricular assist device for fulminant acute myocarditis. *Annals of Thoracic Surgery,* 69, 284–286.

Vollman, M.W. (1995). Dynamic cardiomyoplasty: Perspectives on nursing care and collaborative management. *Progress in Cardiovascular Nursing,* 10(2), 15–22.

Wilson, L., Thomas, D., Astemborski, J., Freedman, T., & Vlahav, D. (2002). Prospective Study of infective endocarditis among injection drug users. *Journal of Infectious Disease,* 185, 1761–1766.

Wilson, W. R., Karchmer, A. W., Dajani, A. S., Taubert, K., Bayer A., Kaye, D., et al. (1995) Adults with infective endocarditis due to streptococci, enterococci, staphylococci, and HACEK microorganisms. *Journal of the American Medical Association,* 274, 1706–1743.

Wojnicz, R., Nowalany-Kozielska, E., Wojciechowska, C., et al. (2001) Randomized, placebo-controlled study for immunosuppressive treatment of inflammatory dilated cardiomyopathy. Two-year follow-up results. *Circulation,* 104, 39–45.

Wood, J. E., & Mahnensmith, R. L. (2001). Pericarditis associated with renal failure: Evolution, and management. *Seminars in Dialysis,* 14, 61–66.

Wynne, J., & Braunwald, E. (2001). The cardiomyopathies. In E. Braunwald, D. Zipes, & P. Libby (Eds.), *Heart disease: A textbook of cardiovascular medicine* (6th ed., pp 1751–1806.). Philadelphia: W.B. Saunders.

Young, J. (2001). Healing the heart with ventricular assist device therapy: Mechanisms of cardiac recovery. *Annals of Thoracic Surgery,* 71, S210–219.

Zales, V.R., Wright, & K.L. (1997). Endocarditis, pericarditis, myocarditis. *Pediatric Annals,* 26, 116–121.

Congenital Heart Disease

MARY M. CANOBBIO

Over the past four decades, advances in diagnosis and therapy, including palliative or corrective surgery, have resulted in increased survival of adults with congenital heart disease. Surgical interventions not only have increased life expectancy of patients with defects that allow natural long-term survival but also have permitted survival of a large number of patients with disorders previously fatal in childhood. Appropriate long-term management of this population requires an understanding of the anomalies and the residual effects of the surgical repair.

INCIDENCE AND PREVALENCE

Precise incidence rates for congenital heart disease are difficult to estimate. It is generally accepted that approximately 1% of all live births are complicated by some cardiovascular malformation. (Mitchell et al., 1971) However, this figure is known to underestimate the true incidence of congenital heart disease because of the number of defects that go undiagnosed at birth.

Even less clear is the current prevalence of corrected and uncorrected congenital heart disease. Data gathered on the long-term survival of persons with congenital heart disease indicate that the greatest influences on the increasing prevalence of congenital heart disease are the successful palliative and surgical procedures routinely performed in infancy and early childhood (Perloff, 1991; Morris, Menasche, 1991). It has been estimated that currently there are approximately 750,000 adult survivors of CHD between the ages of 21 and 40 years with congenital heart disease (Warnes, 2001). Added to this fact is the knowledge that at least 85% of infants born with cardiovascular anomalies can expect to reach adulthood (Gillium, 1994; Warnes, 2001). Data reported by the Second Natural History Study (NHS-2) of Congenital Heart Disease have provided additional follow-up information on selected defects that extend from childhood to adulthood (Hayes, Gersony, Driscoll et al., 1993). Following a cohort of 2262 patients enrolled in the first NHS, the NHS-2 found that of the original cohort, 74.3% were known to be alive at 25 years. These data are important in that they are predictive of the increasing number of adults with congenital heart disease. In the future, we will be providing nursing care not only for the primary defect but also for the postoperative residua, sequelae, and complications, many of which become apparent in adulthood.

CONGENITAL HEART DEFECTS

Detailed review of all defects is beyond the scope of this chapter. Selected defects, however, in which natural survival to adulthood is possible and for which there are documented long-term residua, will be highlighted. Table 35-1 summarizes common and uncommon forms of congenital heart disease in which survival to adulthood can be expected or is considered exceptional. A variety of methods have been suggested in the classification of congenital heart disease (Emmanouilides et al., 1995; Perloff, 2003). A commonly used method is based on the presence or absence of cyanosis; however, to better understand the hemodynamic effects of various defects, it is preferable to classify congenital heart disease in terms of the direction and magnitude of pulmonary blood flow. Figure 35-1 demonstrates this method of classification and is the basis of this discussion.

NORMAL PULMONARY BLOOD FLOW-IMPAIRMENT OR OBSTRUCTION TO VENTRICULAR OUTFLOW

Pulmonic Valve Stenosis

Description. Right ventricular outflow obstructive lesions constitute a large percentage of congenital malformations of the heart. Pulmonic valve stenosis (PVS) can occur at the valvular, subvalvular (infundibular or subinfundibular), or supravalvular level (stenosis of the pulmonary artery and its branches). It may occur as an isolated defect or in combination with other congenital cardiac defects, including ventricular septal defects (VSD), atrial septal defects (ASD), or as part of the tetralogy of Fallot. Survival to adulthood with mild to moderate PVS that has not been repaired is common, involving men and women equally, and has been reported in siblings (Kaplan, 1979). Long-term follow-up of these patients shows a survival rate similar to that of the general population; morbidity

Table 35–1 ■ NATURAL SURVIVAL OF COMMON AND UNCOMMON FORMS OF CONGENITAL

Common congenital cardiac defects in which adult survival is expected:
Functionally normal bicuspid aortic valve
Congenital valvular aortic stenosis
Coarctation of the aorta
Valvular pulmonic stenosis
Atrial septal defect
Patent ductus arteriosus
Ventricular septal defect with pulmonic stenosis (Fallot tetralogy)

Uncommon congenital cardiac defects in which adult survival is expected:
Situs Inversus
Dextroversion of the heart
Congenital complete heart block
Congenitally corrected transposition of the great arteries
Idiopathic dilatation of the pulmonary trunk
Subvalvular pulmonic stenosis
Supravalvular pulmonic stenosis
Ebstein anomaly of the tricuspid valve
Congenital pulmonary arteriovenous fistula
Common atrium
Congenital aneurysms of the sinus of Valsalva
Vena caval to left atrial connection
Congenital pulmonary valve regurgitation
Primary pulmonary hypertension

Common congenital cardiac defects in which adult survival is exceptional:
Ventricular septal defect
Ventricular septal defect with aortic regurgitation
Endocardial cushion defect
Tricuspid atresia
Complete transposition of great arteries

Uncommon congenital cardiac defects in which postpediatric survival is exceptional:
Anomalous origin of the left coronary artery from pulmonary trunk
Cortriatriatum
Right ventricular origin of both great arteries (double outlet right ventricle)
Truncus arteriosus
Total anomalous pulmonary venous connection
Single ventricle
Discrete subvalvular aortic stenosis

Adapted from Canobblo, M. M., & Perloff, J. K. (1981). Critical care of the adult with congenital heart disease. *Critical Care Quarterly,* 4(3), 39.

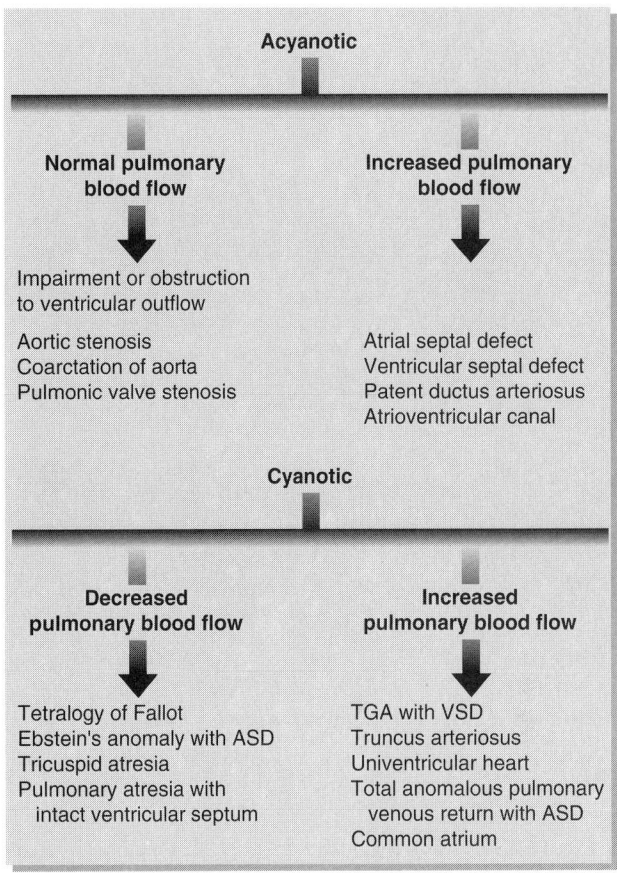

■ **Figure 35–1.** Classification of congenital heart disease based upon the direction of pulmonary blood flow. ASD, atrial septal defect; TGA, transposition of great arteries; VSD, ventricular septal defect.

is rare and risk of endocarditis is nonexistent (Fig. 35-2A) (Hayes, Gersony, Driscoll et al., 1993).

Pathophysiology. The clinical course of pure isolated PVS is dependent on the degree of right ventricular (RV) obstruction. Most patients with mild PVS (peak RV systolic outflow pressure gradients of 25 mm Hg) to moderate PVS (RV systolic pressures of 75 mm Hg) are asymptomatic. Varying degrees of RV hypertension may exist, but pulmonary blood flow remains normal. With moderate stenosis, easy fatigability may be the only symptom. The functional consequences of PVS are related to the degree of stenosis and the adaptive response of the RV. The RV hypertrophies in proportion to the degree of stenosis. Over time, changes in the RV, such as myocardial fibrosis, infundibular stenosis, and subvalvular muscular hypertrophy, can lead to alterations in RV function, which contributes further to the obstruction to RV outflow. Furthermore, with advancing age, a congenitally deformed pulmonic

valve can become thickened, fibrotic, and even calcified, thus reducing valve mobility and increasing the degree of obstruction. In more severe cases, right atrial hypertrophy must be present and be of sufficient degree to open a previously patent foramen ovale leading to right-to-left shunting. Severe PVS eventually leads to tricuspid regurgitation and frank RV failure.

Clinical Manifestations. Physical findings include a loud mid-systolic murmur heard along the left sternal border (LSB), at the second intercostal space, accompanied by a thrill during the ejection phase. A pulmonic ejection sound produced by the doming of the stenotic valve is present in mild to moderate cases but may be absent in severe PVS. Splitting of the pulmonic component of the second heart sound is present but diminished in intensity in mild stenosis. As the gradient increases, the pulmonic component becomes further delayed and softer or even inaudible.

Management. Patients with mild PS (RV-PA gradient 25 mm Hg) should be followed medically but have no restrictions. Patients with moderate gradients (50 to 79 mm Hg) or severe gradient (80 mm Hg) are managed with balloon angioplasty. Balloon valvuloplasty is successful in reducing the pulmonary gradient by at least 50% in the majority of patients (Hermann, Hill, Krol et al., 1991). Surgical valvotomy is indicated when the pulmonary valve is dysplastic rendering balloon valvuloplasty less effective. Valve replacement in the presence of significant

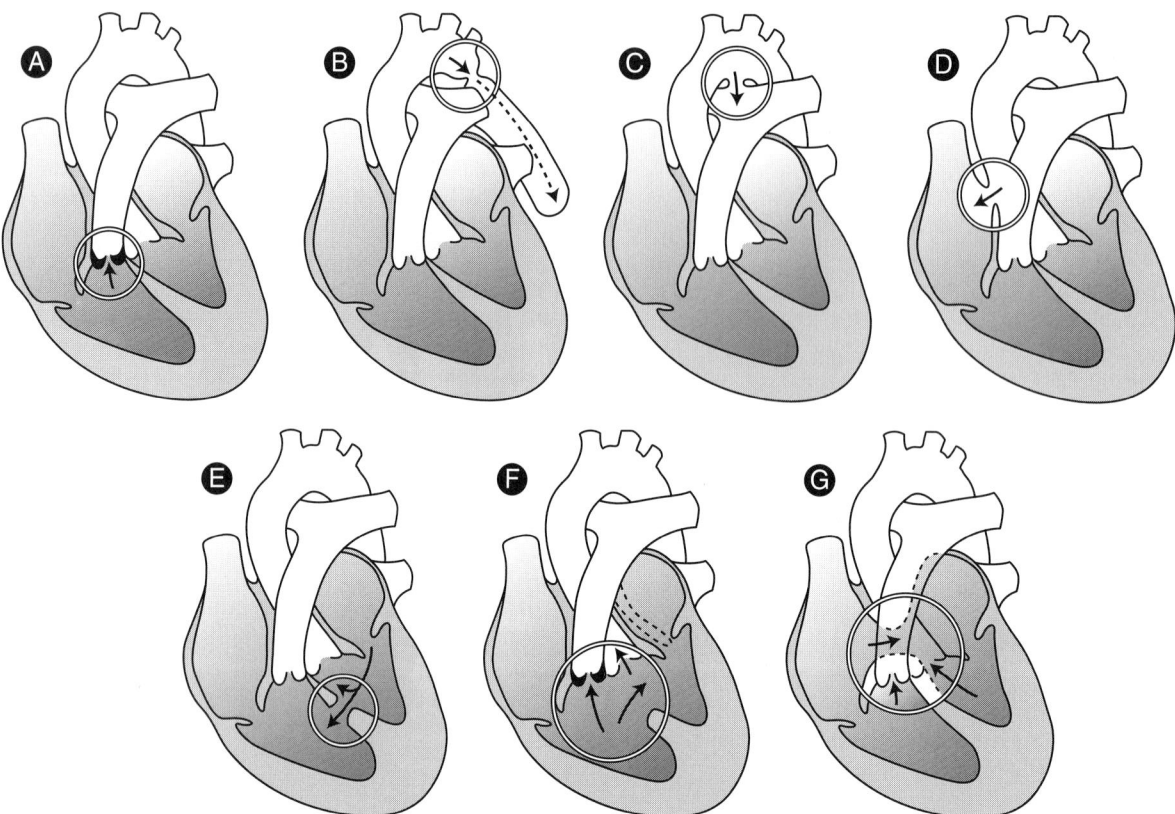

■ **Figure 35–2.** Congenital heart defects. (*A*) Pulmonic valve stenosis with increased pulmonary blood flow and right ventricular hypertrophy. (*B*) Postductal coarctation of the aorta. (*C*) Patent ductus arteriosus. The high pressure blood of the aorta is shunted back to the pulmonary artery. (*D*) Atrial septal defect. Blood is shunted from left to right. (*E*) Ventricular septal defect. Blood is usually shunted from left to right. (*F*) Tetralogy of Fallot. This involves a ventricular septal defect, dextroposition of the aorta, right ventricular hypertrophy. Blood is shunted from right to left. (*G*) Transposition of the great arteries. The pulmonary artery is attached to the left side of the heart and the aorta to the right side. (Adapted from Porth, C. M. [1999]. *Pathophysiology: Concepts of altered health states* [4th ed., p. 406]. Philadelphia: J.B. Lippincott.)

obstruction with calcification of the pulmonic valve is seen in older adults.

Aortic Stenosis

Description. Obstruction to left ventricular (LV) outflow can occur as a result of congenital valvular, supravalvular, or subvalvular aortic stenosis (AS). The most common form is valvular AS. Usually the result of a bicuspid aortic valve, it has been suggested that by age 60 years, 53% of bicuspid aortic valves will have become stenotic (Beppu, Suzuki, et al., 1993). Congenital AS, which accounts for 3% to 6% of all cases of congenital heart disease, occurs more frequently in males than females and may occur in association with coarctation of the aorta and patent ductus arteriosus (PDA) (Emmanouilies et al., 1995). The 25-year survival rate of patients with AS is 85%. The mortality rate is highest among patients with significant aortic valve obstruction, aortic regurgitation, or both. Long-term morbidity includes arrhythmias and endocarditis, the latter occurring more frequently in patients with severe AS (Keane, Driscoll, Gersony, et al., 1993).

Pathophysiology. Aortic stenosis is characterized by thickening and rigidity of the valve tissue with a varying degree of commissure fusion in childhood and adolescence and calcification in adults. The adaptation response of chronic AS is concentric hypertrophy, which can sustain large pressure gradients across the aortic valve without a decrease in cardiac output, LV dilatation, or development of symptoms. Peak systolic pressure gradients with a normal cardiac output (CO) reflect the severity of the obstruction. Mild obstruction produces a pressure gradient of less than 25 mm Hg (an aortic orifice of 0.8 cm^2/m^2 of body surface area); a moderate obstruction produces a gradient of 25 to 50 mm Hg (0.5 cm^2/m^2 to 0.8 cm^2/m^2); stenosis that produces gradients more than 75 mm Hg (a body surface area <0.5 cm^2/m^2) reflects severe obstruction to left ventricular outflow. Resting CO and stroke volume (SV) are generally within normal limits. With exercise, however, the CO increases, as does the gradient across the area of obstruction, causing the obstruction to become more severe.

In severe AS, the hemodynamic abnormalities produced by the obstruction to LV outflow increase myocardial oxygen demand, and the abnormally elevated pressure compressing the coronary perfusion pressure exceeds the coronary perfusion pressure, thereby interfering with coronary blood flow. As a result, significant stenosis may result in reduced subendocardial perfusion, particularly during exercise, leading to ischemia. Subendocardial ischemia plays a key role in the angina, syncope, ventricular arrhythmias, and sudden death reported in patients with AS (Perloff, 2003). Exertional syncope, which can occur in patients with gradients exceeding 50 mm Hg, is related to the inability of the LV to increase its output and to maintain cerebral flow during exercise. The onset of clinical symptoms in adults may not occur until the fourth or fifth decade and is usually the result of aortic valve calcification.

Clinical Manifestations. The symptoms of valvular AS may be inconspicuous. When they occur, those most noted are fatigue, exertional dyspnea, angina, and syncope. With significant stenosis, an LV lift may be palpable. A precordial systolic thrill is palpated over the base of the heart and is transmitted to the suprasternal notch and over both carotid arteries. The typical murmur of valvular AS is a harsh, loud systolic murmur that begins after the first heart sound, rising to a peak (crescendo), and declining (decrescendo) before the second heart sound. The murmur radiates to the suprasternal notch and carotid arteries. A systolic ejection sound, which may be heard at the cardiac apex, implies a mobile valve and is found in mild to moderate stenosis. As calcification impairs valve mobility, the ejection sound decreases or vanishes completely.

Management. Asymptomatic patients with mild AS and gradients less than 25 mm Hg may be treated medically; however, because AS is a progressive disease, these patients should be evaluated at regular intervals. Prophylaxis against endocarditis is required. With higher gradients more than 50 mm Hg, balloon vavuloplasty may be successfully performed, resulting in a 60% to 70% reduction in systolic gradient across the aortic valve. Balloon valvuloplasty is not recommended if aortic insufficiency is present, in patients with subvalvar stenosis, or in adults with heavily calcified valves (Gersony 2002). Patients with decrete subvalvar AS and mild gradients (<30 mm Hg) must be followed-up yearly to detect signs of progression. Symptomatic or asymptomatic patients with gradients more than 50 mm Hg are usually treated with surgical resection of subaortic fibrous ring, leaving the aortic valve intact. For patients with a narrowed LV outflow tract and small aortic valve annulus, the Ross-Konno surgical procedure may be performed to relieve left ventricular obstruction to outflow.

Coarctation of the Aorta

Description. Coarctation of the aorta is a deformity of the aortic isthmus, characterized by narrowing either proximal or distal to the left subclavian artery where the ductus arteriosus joins the descending aorta; it represents 5% to 10% of all congenital cardiac anomalies (Fig. 35-2B) (Perloff, 2003). Occasionally, the coarctation is located at or just proximal to the origin of the left subclavian artery and the zone of coarctation occurs above the origin of the right subclavian. Blood flow through the right subclavian artery results in decreased blood pressure in the right arm. Coarctation of the aorta occurs with greater frequency in males than in females and is strongly associated with bicuspid aortic valve, VSD, PDA, and initial valve abnormalities (Gersony, 1990). A noncardiac anomaly

associated with coarctation of the aorta is an aneurysm of the circle of Willis.

Pathophysiology. The physiologic consequences of coarctation stem primarily from systemic hypertension. The increased resistance produced by aortic narrowing results in increased pressure in the aorta proximal to the coarcted area and a decreased pressure distal to the narrowing. Because renal artery blood flow is decreased, plasma renin release is stimulated, contributing further to the regulation of systemic arterial pressure. Complications in late adolescence and adulthood may include rupture of the aorta, seen more commonly in the second and third decade; infective endocarditis of a susceptible bicuspid aortic valve or endarteritis at the site of the coarctation; cardiac failure, which increases in incidence after the fourth decade; and cerebral hemorrhage caused by rupture of an aneurysm of the circle of Willis. In pregnant women, the risk of heart failure or intracranial hemorrhage is low (Perloff & Koos, 1985). Whereas toxemia occurs with less frequency in pregnant women with coarctation than in pregnant women with other forms of hypertension, pregnancy does increase the risk of aortic rupture, particularly at the end of the third trimester (Table 35-2).

Clinical Manifestations. Coarctation of the aorta is characterized by systemic hypertension with abnormal differences in the upper and lower extremities, pulses, and systolic blood pressure. As the patient grows older, systolic pressures rise more than do diastolic pressures, resulting in a widened pulse pressure. Arterial pressures may also vary between right and left arms depending on the zone of coarctation relative to the subclavian artery. In the presence of an anomalous right subclavian artery, the BP in the right arm is lower than in the left. When the coarctation involves the origin of the left subclavian artery, the BP in the left arm is lower than the right. Differences between arm and leg BP are accentuated further by exercise, with the brachial BP rising, whereas the femoral pressure remains unchanged or may decrease. Often the patient exhibits forceful carotid and suprasternal pulsations resembling aortic regurgitation. Collateral arterial pulsations may be seen beneath the skin, particularly around the scapulae. Hypertensive retinopathy is rare. The femoral pulses may be delayed,

Table 35–2 ■ PREGNANCY RISKS IN CONGENITAL HEART DISEASE

Low	Intermediate	High
Postoperative with no residual: ASD, VSD, TOF. PDA	*Unrepaired:*	Cyanotic CHD
Isolated pulmonic stenosis	Aortic valve disease	Increased PVR
Small unrepaired VSD	Coarctation of aorta	Heart failure (NYHA III, IV)
	Ebstein anomaly	
	Congenital CTGA	
Functionally normal bicuspid AV	*Repaired with residuals:* Coarctation of aorta TOF, Ebstein	
	Postoperative*	
	Fontan, Mustard	

PDA, patent ductus arteriosus; ASD, atrial septal defect; VSD, ventricular septal defect; TOF, tetralogy of Fallot; AV, aortic valve; PVR, pulmonary vascular resistance; CTGA, corrected transposition of great arteries.
*Pregnancy data are limited but in early reports indicate that in clinically stable patients, pregnancy is well tolerated (Clarkson, 1998; Canobbio, 1996).

diminished, or absent. A suprasternal thrill is common, but precordial thrills are uncommon. Palpation of the precordium reveals an LV impulse that may vary from normal to the sustained heaving impulse of ventricular hypertrophy. Auscultatory signs consist of widespread, delayed systolic murmurs, caused by flow through collateral vessels, and the murmur at the site of coarctation. A mild late systolic murmur is heard best along the left sternal border toward the apex and in the suprasternal notch. An early diastolic murmur, suggestive of aortic regurgitation and an aortic ejection sound, may be heard, particularly with a bicuspid aortic valve.

Management. In the majority of cases, resection of the coarctation with end-to-end anastomosis of the proximal and distal aorta is currently the recommended choice of surgical treatment (Gersony,1990). Patients with mild coarctation pressure gradients (<30 mm Hg) may be treated medically but should be followed-up carefully to monitor for an increase in the gradient. Balloon angioplasty and stenting are being more commonly used for treatment of native and recurrent coarctation (Ebeid, Prieto & Latson, 1997). As the technology improves, reports of aneurysm formation and recurrent coarctation are decreasing and hold promise. Stenting for recoarcation is recommended for use in older patients to relieve obstruction.

Postoperative residual systemic hypertension, in the absence of a residual coarctation, appears to be related to the age of the patient at the time of surgery. For example, 50% of patients who undergo surgery during childhood are normotensive 20 years later (Perloff, 2003). By contrast, more than 50% of adults surgically repaired after age 40 years will have persistent postoperative hypertension (Salazar, Steinberger, & Carpenter, 1996). Long-term follow-up requires routine antibiotic prophylaxis for prevention of infective endocarditis and monitoring of blood pressure, because hypertension may persist in the absence of obstruction or may be a sign of a residual or recurrent coarctation.

LEFT-TO-RIGHT SHUNTS WITH INCREASED PULMONARY BLOOD FLOW

Patent Ductus Arteriosus (PDA)

Description. The ductus arteriosus is a vascular connection, which during fetal life directs blood flow from the pulmonary artery (PA) to the aorta, bypassing the lungs. Functional closure of the ductus occurs within hours or days after birth, in some cases taking 6 months to several years to close. If the ductus remains patent, the direction of blood flow is reversed to left-to-right because of high systemic pressure in the aorta. The hemodynamic changes and clinical manifestations depend on the magnitude of the pulmonary blood flow. The amount of left-to-right shunt is related to the size of the ductal lumen and the resistance in the pulmonary vascular bed. When the ductus is small, the pulmonary artery pressure remains normal; when larger, aortic pressure is transmitted into the pulmonary trunk. A patent ductus, which can escape recognition until adulthood, accounts for approximately 10% of all cases of congenital heart disease and predominates in females. The in-

cidence is reported to be six-times greater in persons born at higher elevations; if they continue to reside at higher elevations, there is a greater tendency for them to have pulmonary hypertension and reversed shunting (Coggin, Parke & Keith, 1970; Perloff, 2003).

Pathophysiology. A PDA functions as an arteriovenous fistula, increasing the work of the left ventricle (Fig. 35-2C). The major complications are ventricular failure, presence of increased pulmonary vascular disease, and infective endarteritis. Adults with small left-to-right shunts from a persistent ductus cause no symptoms and life expectancy is normal; however, they are at risk for infective endarteritis. Patients with large shunts and relatively low pulmonary vascular resistance (PVR) are at risk for left ventricular failure, pulmonary vascular disease, and reversed shunting. In such cases, operation is advised. Once pulmonary resistance exceeds systemic pressure, patients are rendered inoperable.

Clinical Manifestations. The clinical appearance characterizing a moderate or large PDA with normal PA pressure includes bounding peripheral pulses and a widened pulse pressure, with diastolic pressures as low as 30 to 50 mm Hg. The left ventricular impulse is hyperdynamic and, if present, a systolic thrill may be palpated over the suprasternal notch area. A continuous loud "machinery" murmur accentuated in late systole is heard best in the first or second left intercostal space. In the setting of increased PVR, the diastolic component of the murmur disappears, leaving only the systolic component.

Patients with a moderate shunt may have no symptoms during infancy but may begin to have fatigue, dyspnea, or palpitations during childhood or adulthood. Occasionally, the ductus arteriosus may become aneurismal, calcified, and rupture (Fisher, Moodie & Sterba, 1986).

Management. In the absence of pulmonary vascular disease, it is recommended that all PDAs be closed either by surgical ligation or by interventional catheterization using percutaneous closure devices (Khan, Youseff & Mullins, 1992). Once closed, long-term follow-up and endocarditis prophylaxis is not required. If a residual shunt remains, bacterial endocarditis prophylaxis is recommended.

Atrial Septal Defects

Description. Atrial septal defects (ASD), abnormal communications between the left and right atria, comprise 10% of all congenital heart anomalies (Fig. 35-2D). There is a female predominance (Perloff, 2003). They are differentiated by their occurrence within the septum. *Ostium secundum* ASD, the most common type, occurs in the central region of the fossa ovalis; *ostium primum,* which occurs low in the atrial septum, has an associated cleft anterior mitral valve with varying degree of mitral insufficiency; *sinus venosus* occurs in the upper part of the atrial septum near the entry of the superior vena cava and may be associated with the partial anomalous right pulmonary venous connection. Because of the trivial or absent physical signs, ASD may go undetected until the fourth or fifth decade.

Pathophysiology. The hemodynamic consequences of ASD are dependent on: (1) the size and direction of the shunt; (2) the compliance of the left and right ventricles; and (3) the responsive behavior of the pulmonary vascular bed. In infancy, the persistence of increased PVR and the relatively equally compliant left and right ventricles limit the amount of left-to-right shunting. With increasing age, PVR decreases, and the neonatal right ventricle becomes thinner, offering less resistance to filling than the left. Consequently, the conditions are appropriate for left-to-right flow across the defect. Although left atrial pressure is only slightly higher than right atrial pressure, a left-to-right shunt is present, and the pulmonary blood flow may exceed systemic blood flow by three to four times (Gersony, 2002).

Major problems of adults with unrepaired ASD include the development of atrial arrhythmias, which increase in frequency with age; a persistent increase in PVR leading eventually to reversed shunting and cyanosis, or the Eisenmenger reaction; and heart failure. The latter is usually the result of associated diseases affecting LV function, such as systemic hypertension or ischemic heart disease. Left ventricular failure reduces the distensibilty of the LV, increasing the volume of left atrial blood being shunted across the defect, thus adding to the burden of an already volume-overloaded right ventricle.

Clinical Manifestations. Characteristic of the increased pulmonary flow across the pulmonic valves is a soft mid-systolic pulmonic ejection murmur. If the shunt is large, a mild diastolic rumbling murmur is heard at the lower left sternal border (LSB), caused by increased blood flow across the tricuspid valve. A second sound, which is widely split and does not vary with respiration, is consistent with a low PVR. Prominent RV pulsations along the LSB and PA are palpable. The presence of a systolic thrill reflects a large shunt or coexisting pulmonic stenosis. In ostium primum, there is the addition of the murmur of mitral regurgitation, a left ventricular impulse, and systolic thrill. In sinus venosus, the clinical findings are similar to the ostium secundum. Most patients with ASD remain asymptomatic but may report easy fatigability and exertional dyspnea.

Management. Closure of ASD is recommended, particularly in those with large defects (Qp/Qs ratio >1.5:1). Most surgical repairs are performed in infancy by simple suture closure; in larger defects, a pericardial or prosthetic patch may be required to close the defect. For *ostium primum* defects, repair of the mitral valve cleft is also undertaken. If mitral insufficiency persists, the patient must be followed-up closely to determine need for further valve repair or even replacement.

Percutaneous ASD closure devices performed during cardiac catheterization are becoming increasing used in patients with *secundum ASD*. Although still in early stages, the preliminary reports are favorable (Buter, DeRosa et al., 2003). The major concerns for these devices include incomplete closure of the shunt, acute embolization of the devices, and the potential for thromboembolic complications.

Ventricular Septal Defects (VSD)

Description. An interventricular defect results in shunting of blood between right and left ventricles. Ventricular septal defects (VSD) are generally described as membranous or muscular. There are four types, each classified according to its location. Type I defects are the supracristal defects, found above the crista supraventricularis and just below the pulmonic valve.

Type II defects involve the outflow portion of the right ventricle and are located in the membranous portion of the septum (Fig. 35-2E). Perimembraneous defects are the commonest type of defect, accounting for 80% of all VSDs. Type III defects, which only account for a small percentage of defects, are located directly below the AV valves, occurring as part of an endocardial cushion defect. These are referred to as atrioventricular (AV) canal defects. The fourth type of VSD occurs in the muscular portion of the septum and accounts for approximately 15% of all VSD (Gersony, 2002). Ventricular septal defects, the most commonly occurring congenital heart defect, appear in 1 in 400 live births (Perloff, 2003). Isolated VSDs occur with equal frequency in males and females. Whereas the majority close spontaneously in childhood, small to moderate isolated VSDs account for 7% of congenital heart defects found in adults. The 25-year follow-up for patients, as reported in the NHS-2, indicated that the majority of patients managed medically or surgically who did not have Eisenmenger syndrome fared well. The NHS-2 reported, however, a higher-than-normal prevalence of serious arrhythmias and sudden death, even among patients with the smaller defects (Kidd, Driscoll & Gersony, 1993).

Pathophysiology. Defects may be single or multiple, with the degree of shunting dependent on the size of the defect rather than the anatomic location. Defects vary in size from 1 to 2 mm in diameter to large openings with little or no septal wall, which behave physiologically like a single ventricle. Small isolated defects (less than 7 mm in diameter) and moderate-size defects (7 mm to 1.25 cm), which are referred to as "restrictive," have minimal hemodynamic changes and produce little or no symptomatology. However, if moderate in size, it may be significant enough to produce some cardiac enlargement. If the defect is large (1.5 cm to 3 cm), systemic pressure in the RV is equal or slightly lower than the left ventricle, creating a left-to-right shunt and increased pulmonary blood flow. This increase in blood flow is returned to the left heart, creating volume overload of both right and left ventricles. In addition, increased pulmonary blood flow may produce pulmonary hypertension. Because of the open communication between the two ventricles, systolic blood pressure in the PA rises, equaling that in the aorta. If the PA pressure continues to increase and PVR approaches or exceeds systemic pressure, shunt reversal (right to left) occurs, rendering the patient cyanotic and no longer a candidate for surgical correction. This syndrome is referred to as Eisenmenger reaction.

Clinical Manifestations. Clinical features depend on the volume of pulmonary blood flow, which in turn depends on the size of the defect and the PVR. A harsh holosystolic murmur and palpable thrill along the lower LSB may be the only findings of a small or moderate defect. A normal splitting second sound indicates the PA pressure is below systemic pressure. In large shunts, the murmur is lower in intensity, a mid-diastolic "flow murmur" and third heart sound are heard at the apex, and an RV impulse is palpable.

Mangement. Patients with small VSD and normal pulmonary vascular resistance remain asymptomatic and do not require surgical intervention; however, they are at risk for endocarditis and require antibiotic prophylaxis. In the absence of high or fixed pulmonary vascular obstructive disease, surgical correction is indicated in patients with moderate to large left-to-right shunt.

Patients who have undergone successful repair require only periodic follow-up to assess for the development of any clinical sequelae, such as arrhythmias, or progression of any preoperative ventricular dysfunction (Gersony, 2002). Older patients operated on during early days of surgical development often present with complications of ventricular arrhythmias, conduction defects, and ventricular dysfunction (Kidd, Driscoll & Gersony, 1993).

CYANOTIC RIGHT-TO-LEFT SHUNTS WTH DECREASED PULMONARY BLOOD FLOW

Tetralogy of Fallot

Description. Tetralogy of Fallot (TOF) accounts for 10% of all congenital heart disease and has an equal sex distribution (Perloff, 2003). Whereas a wide anatomic and clinical spectrum exists, the classic cyanotic tetrad includes a nonrestrictive VSD, severe PS causing obstruction to pulmonary blood flow, RV hypertrophy, and various degrees of overriding or dextroposition of the aorta (Fig. 35-2F). Today, surgical repair is undertaken in early childhood; however, natural survival of an unoperated adult is possible. Morbidity and mortality in adults with unrepaired TOF result from cardiac failure; sudden death, presumably to arrhythmias; cerebral vascular accidents (CVA) or brain abscess; and infective endocarditis.

Pathophysiology. The physiologic consequences of TOF depend on the degree of PVS, which regulates pulmonary blood flow; the size of the VSD; and the systemic vascular resistance. The PVS is usually infundibular but may occur at the valvular level or in the pulmonary trunk and its branches. When the stenosis is mild, the shunt remains left-to-right with no cyanosis and is referred to as "acyanotic" TOF. As pulmonic obstruction increases, the shunt reverses to right-to-left. Right ventricular hypertrophy develops because of resistance to the outflow. When total obstruction to pulmonary flow exists, and when the pulmonary trunk and its branches are present, blood flow to the lung is mainly through enlarged bronchial arteries and, at times, also through a PDA. This severe form of TOF is referred to as pulmonary atresia.

Clinical Manifestations. Typically, the patient with TOF has mild to moderate cyanosis and clubbing. The hyperpneic episodes ("hypoxic spells") associated with TOF are virtually absent in the adult. The physical appearance is characterized by a small underdeveloped body size. If the patient has only mild cyanosis, development is normal. A loud systolic murmur over the third LSB with a thrill is characteristic; with severe tetralogy and marked decrease in pulmonary blood flow; the murmur may be short and of low intensity, caused by the absence of turbulent blood flow between the two high-pressure ventricles. When total obstruction (pulmonary atresia) is present, the murmur of the PVS vanishes and is replaced by a soft midsystolic murmur. Continuous murmurs, an auscultatory sign of pulmonary atresia, indicate collateral circulation by way of bronchial arteries or presence of a PDA.

Management. The majority of patients born with TOF have survived as a result of having undergone a series of surgical procedures. During infancy, a palliative systemic to pulmonary arterial shunt procedure would have been undertaken to permit pulmonary arterial blood flow and enhance oxygen saturation. Later in childhood, patients underwent complete surgical correction that included closure of the VSD and relief of the RV outflow obstruction. Today, although palliative shunt procedures are still performed in selected cases, the majority of patients born with TOF undergo reparative surgery in infancy.

Long-term survival after corrective repair is reportedly more than 90% (Murphy, Gersh & Mair et al., 1993; Rosenthal, Behrendt & Sloan et al., 1984). However, a number of residual complications must be monitored on a regular basis, including ventricular arrhythmias, which have been reported to occur particularly in patients who were older at the time of their surgical repair (Vaksmann, Fournier, Davignon et al., 1990), pulmonary regurgitation, ventricular dysfunction, and atrial arrhythmias (Zahka, Horneffer, Rowe et al., 1988; Roos-Hesselink, Perloroth, McGhie et al., 1995). A small number of patients with TOF remain cyanotic. These are usually patients who have pulmonary vascular obstructive disease and are no longer surgical candidates and are managed symptomatically. Patients, either repaired or unrepaired, are at risk for endocarditis and should received antibiotic prophylaxis.

Ebstein Anomaly

Description. Ebstein anomaly involves the tricuspid valve and is characterized by a downward displacement of portions of the tricuspid valve into the right ventricles (Celermajer, Bull & Till, 1994; Perloff, 2003). The portion of the normal RV that underlies the tricuspid valve becomes mechanically a part of the right atrium (atrialized RV). As a result, the right atrium (RA) is exceptionally large, the RV is small, and the tricuspid valve is incompetent.

Ebstein anomaly occurs in less than 1% of all congenital heart defects involving males and females equally. The anomaly is compatible with a relatively long and active life. Patients with Ebstein anomaly may live beyond age 50 years, although this group makes up less than 5% of the congenital heart disease found in adults (Cehermajer, Bull & Till, 1994). The most common cause of death attributed to the malformation is heart failure, hypoxia, and arrhythmia. Sudden unexpected death tends to occur in adults rather than in children and has been attributed to paroxysmal atrial arrhythmias, to which this population is prone.

Pathophysiology. Hemodynamically abnormal function of the right heart is related to three problems: a malformed tricuspid valve, the atrialized portion of the RV, and the reduced capacity of the pumping portion of the RV. Ineffective emptying of the RA may result in an increase in RA volume and a right-to-left shunt through a patent foramen ovale or ASD. Tricuspid regurgitation caused by the malformed leaflets adds to the hemodynamic burden. Important complications associated with Ebstein anomaly include supraventricular tachycardia resulting from Wolff-Parkinson White (WPW) bypass tracts.

Clinical Manifestations. Clinical features of Ebstein anomaly may include effort intolerance caused by dyspnea or fatigability. Progressive cyanosis and hypoxemia may occur as a result of a right-to left atrial shunt. Because of the thin toneless atrialized RV, the jugular pulse may be unimpressive despite tricuspid regurgitation. Auscultatory findings consist of a widely split first heart sound with a loud delayed second component. An S3 is common because of abnormal filling characteristics of the functional RV. In addition, an S4 may be present, causing a quadruple rhythm. Murmurs vary from early systolic to holosystolic and are of medium frequency.

Management. Medical management of patients with Ebstein anomaly is directed toward the prevention of complications and to the treatment of symptoms as they present themselves. Those patients with supraventricular tachycardia, or persistent atrial fibrillation or flutter, may be treated with radiofrequency catheter ablation, although complete ablation of accessory pathways has a lower rate of success in patients with Ebstein anomaly (Cappato, Schluter, Weiss et al., 1996). Surgical repair of the tricuspid valve and closure of the ASD is recommended in symptomatic patients. Valve repair using annuloplasty ring is preferred to replacement, which is reserved for non-reparable valves. When required, a bioprosthetic valve is preferred to mechanical prosthesis (Brickner, 2000).

Tricuspid Atresia

Description. Tricuspid atresia, which is reported to occur in 1% to 2% of all congenital heart defects, occurs equally in males and females. However, there is a male preponderance in patients with transposition of the great arteries (Rao, 1992). Tricuspid atresia involves the absence of a tricuspid valve, resulting in a total right-to-left shunt at the atrial level by way of an obligatory ASD or foramen ovale. In addition, there is a varying degree of hypoplasia of the RV and an enlargement of the mitral valve and LV. Although all types of tricuspid atresia have in common the absence of the tricuspid valve, various forms exist. One commonly used classification focuses on the relation of the great arteries, the degree of reduced pulmonary blood flow, and the size of the VSD (Table 35-3) (Edward & Burcheill, 1949). Patients with type I-b, with normally related great arteries, PVS, and VSD, characterize the most common form of tricuspid atresia.

Pathophysiology. In type I-b, the most common form of tricuspid atresia, the VSD is small, the RV is hypoplastic, and the great arteries are normally related. Because of the atretic

Table 35–3 ■ ANATOMIC CLASSIFICATION OF TRICUSPID ATRESIA BASED ON RELATIONSHIP WITH THE GREAT ARTERIES

Type I
  Normally related great arteries
  Subgroup a: pulmonary atresia; no VSD
  Subgroup b: pulmonary or subpulmonic stenosis; small VSD
  Subgroup c: no pulmonary hypoplasia; large VSD

Type II
  Complete transposition (D-transposition)
  Subgroup a: pulmonary atresia
  Subgroup b: pulmonary or subpulmonary stenosis
  Subgroup c: large pulmonary artery; no pulmonic stenosis

Type III
  Congenitally corrected (L-transposition)
  Subgroup a: pulmonic or subpulmonic stenosis
  Subgroup b: subaortic stenosis

tricuspid valve, systemic venous return crosses from the RA to the LA via an intra-atria communication. There, oxygenated and deoxygenated blood are mixed, then redirected to the LV, where blood is then ejected into the aorta, with some blood reaching the pulmonary circulation by way of the VSD. Survival is determined by the adequacy of pulmonary blood flow and the pressure in the pulmonary vascular bed (Perloff, 2003). In most cases, pulmonary blood flow is restricted because of subvalvular or valvular pulmonary stenosis. As a result, these patients are hypoxic and cyanosed.

Patients with normally related great arteries, a large VSD, and little or no pulmonary restriction (type I-c) may have congestive heart failure caused by the excessive pulmonary blood flow, which results in volume overload of the LV. In patients with transposed great arteries (type II), without pulmonary obstruction, the result is excessive pulmonary blood flow with pulmonary artery hypertension. The overload caused by the increased pulmonary blood flow often leads to congestive heart failure.

Clinical Manifestations. Clinically, the patient with type I-b is characterized by cyanosis, clubbing of the extremities, normal or reduced pulmonary blood flow, a dominant LV impulse, and a noticeably absent RV impulse. The dominant LV impulse occurs as a result of its handling both systemic and pulmonary circulation, despite a decreased pulmonary blood flow. The physical features are dependent on the anatomic findings. Because of the absence of the tricuspid valve, the first heart sound is single. The presence or absence of a systolic murmur depends on the size of the VSD. If significant, a holosystolic murmur may be heard at the mid-to-lower left sternal border and can generate a precordial thrill. If the size of the VSD decreases, the murmur may change from holosystolic to early systolic (Perloff, 2003).

Management. Survival beyond infancy without surgical intervention is rare. However, the palliative shunts such as Blalock-Taussig (subclavian artery to pulmonary artery) performed in infancy and the increasing success of the surgical procedures such as the Fontan, lateral tunnel, and bi-directional Glenn have contributed to an increasing number of patients reaching adulthood. Introduced in 1971, the Fontan procedure has undergone a number of modifications; however, each provides an aorticopulmonary (A-P) or atrioventricular (A-V) connection. Ten- and 15-year survival rates after modified Fontan repair are good (Driscoll, Offord, Feldt et al., 1992). However, the long-term concerns associated with these surgical procedures include the physiologic effects of persistent elevated RA pressure and elevated systemic venous pressure, and problems with stenosis or obstruction of the conduit used in the different connections.

CYANOTIC CONGENITAL HEART DEFECTS WITH INCREASED PULMONARY BLOOD FLOW

Truncus Arteriosus

Description. In this lesion, which occurs in less than 1% of all congenital heart diseases, the primitive trunk fails to divide into two great arteries. Thus, a single great vessel emerges from the base of the heart through a single semilunar valve, straddling both ventricles over a large VSD. The truncus, which is the aorta, receives blood from both ventricles and gives rise to both pulmonary and systemic circulations, as well as coronary arteries. The second semilunar valve is absent, but a short pulmonary trunk without a valve may emerge from the side of the truncus and give rise to the right and left pulmonary arteries (type I), or both pulmonary arteries may arise directly from the posterior or lateral walls of the truncus (type II). Pulmonary blood flow then arises entirely by way of collaterals from bronchial arteries or a PDA.

Survival to adulthood is exceptional; however, if the pulmonary arteries are small or absent, or if increased PVR is present, congestive heart failure caused by increased pulmonary blood flow is delayed. Patients with regulated pulmonary circulation have been reported to survive into the third and fourth decade (Gersony, 2002).

Pathophysiology. The hemodynamic consequences of truncus arteriosus depend on the magnitude of pulmonary blood flow, which reflects the presence and the size of the pulmonary arteries and the resistance to flow through the lungs (Perloff, 2003). In the types with large unobstructed pulmonary arteries arising from the arterial trunk, pulmonary blood flow is greatly increased, clinically resembling patients with large VSD with left-to-right shunts.

Clinical Manifestations. Cyanosis, which may be mild or absent, occurs with increased pulmonary blood flow. RV pressure is equal to systemic pressure, because both ventricles eject directly into the single trunk. The patient with mild cyanosis and a large pulmonary blood flow has a loud systolic murmur along the lower LSB. The second heart sound is single and loud. Diastolic flow murmurs may be present if truncus dilatation with resultant regurgitation is present. Variations may be caused by the resistance to flow into the pulmonary circuit (i.e., a higher resistance leads to shortening and softening of the murmur).

Management. Palliative procedures such as a bilateral pulmonary artery banding to restrict pulmonary blood flow have been performed with limited success in the past. Today, however, the majority of infants will undergo primary surgical repair, which includes closure of the VSD, committing the truncus valve to the left ventricle, and thus serving as an aortic valve. In the right ventricle, a homograft or conduit is constructed connecting the right ventricle to the pulmonary artery. Long-term survival after complete repair is determined by the degree of truncal valve insufficiency, residual VSD, and any right or left ventricular dysfunction (Bull, Macartaney, Horvath et al., 1987). In some cases, replacement of the RV-PA homograft may be required because the conduits are subject to calcification or valve degeneration.

Transposition of the Great Arteries

Transposition of the great arteries implies a reversal of the aorta and PA . It may be complete transposition, also referred to as *D-transposition* (Fig. 35-2G), or congenitally corrected, referred to as *L-transposition*.

Complete Transposition of the Great Arteries

In complete transposition, the aorta arises from the RV and is located anterior to the PA, with the PA arising from the LV.

Blood returning to the heart from the systemic circulation is ejected from the RV into the aorta, sending unoxygenated blood back into the systemic circulation. Survival is exceptional and necessitates some means of blood exchange between the pulmonary and systemic circulations. Infant survival beyond the first months of birth occurs only as a result of the presence of a large VSD, PDA, ASD, or patent foramen ovale, which permit varying degrees of arteriovenous mixing. Natural survival is extremely rare, and survival into adulthood is dependent on the early use of palliative shunting procedures (atrioseptectomy, atrioseptostomy), PA banding to regulate pulmonary flow, and, later, the atrial switch procedures known as the Mustard or Senning operation. Both of these procedures divert caval blood to the mitral valve and pulmonary venous blood to the tricuspid valve (Kidd & O'Neal, 1982). In the Mustard procedure, venous blood is diverted to the mitral valve by means of an intra-atrial baffle. In the Senning procedure a tunnel is created within the RA that carries caval blood to the mitral valve. Pulmonary venous blood then drains around this tunnel into the tricuspid valve and into the systemic circulation. Whereas the 20-year survival rates associated with the atrial switch procedures have been encouraging, progressive loss of sinus node function and the long-term complications of arrhythmias, baffle obstruction, and progressive failure of the systemic RV have caused renewed interest in the arterial switch procedure (Wilson & Clarkson et al., 1998; Puley & Sui et al., 1999). Performed in an infant's first few weeks of life, the arterial switch procedure involves surgically detaching the coronary arteries from the aorta, then separating the aorta and pulmonary arteries above the semilunar valves. The aorta is then reimplanted to the stump of the pulmonary trunk, and the pulmonary artery is reimplanted to the stump of the aortic root. The coronary arteries are then anastomosed to the new aorta. Although long-term survival data are limited, results appear to be very good. The majority of patients are asymptomatic, ventricular function is good and rhythm disturbances are uncommon. The major concern in the long-term is the status of coronary arteries. Earlier studies reported kinking and obstruction; however, in recent years the incidence of coronary insufficiency has been low (Gersony, 2002).

Congenitally Corrected Transposition of the Great Arteries

Similar to complete transposition in that the great vessels are reversed, corrected transposition is so-called because the ventricles are also inverted, with the anatomic RV being on the left side of the heart and the anatomic LV on the right side. The atrioventricular valves remain with the anatomic ventricular chamber with which they are associated (i.e., the mitral valve remains with the anatomic LV) (Connelly, Lie, et al., 1996). Physiologically, the flow of blood proceeds along normal pathways: RA to LV to PA to lungs to pulmonary veins to LA to RV to aorta to systemic circulation. Other defects commonly associated with this condition include VSD, PS, and single ventricle. Most cases are detected in childhood, but many do go unnoticed until clinical signs become apparent. Patients with corrected transposition without associated anomalies may reach adulthood and lead normal lives. The most common clinical sequelae associated with corrected transposition are arrhythmias, atrioventricular block, and the development of nonrheumatic mitral regurgitation.

Eisenmenger Reaction

Eisenmenger reaction occurs as a result of increased PVR and reversed or bidirectional shunts at the aorticopulmonary, ventricular, or atrial levels. It is associated with decreased oxygen saturation in the systemic circulation, cyanosis, and erthrocytosis. The term Eisenmenger reaction applies to a number of shunting defects that are hemodynamically similar because of the presence of pulmonary hypertension and an associated right-to-left shunt. It is usually a consequence of delayed operation and may go undetected until adolescence or adulthood, when operation is no longer possible. Most patients survive and live reasonably active and productive lives throughout the fourth, fifth, and sixth decades. Sudden death, presumably from arrhythmias, is the usual cause of death. Other causes of death include heart failure, pulmonary infarction from arterial thrombosis, and complications of cerebral abscesses and CVA (Canobbio, 1984; Cantor, Harrison & Moussadji, 1999).

▓ MEDICAL MANAGEMENT PLAN

The medical management of the adult with congenital heart disease is dictated by the signs and symptoms related to the natural sequelae, residual effects, and medical complications of the individual defects. In general, these include heart failure (see Chapter 28), arrhythmias (see Chapter 19), sudden death (Chapter 31), and infective endocarditis (Chapter 34). Additionally, there are issues of particular concern to the adult with congenital heart disease, including hematologic consequences of cyanotic heart disease, Eisenmenger reaction, and the special considerations related to contraception, pregnancy for women, and psychosocial issues, including activity allowances and limitation, employability, and insurability (Canobbio, 2002).

Erythrocytosis

The chronic hypoxemia associated with long-standing cyanotic congenital heart disease results in erythrocytosis, an adaptive increase in red blood cell ($>45\%$) production that is caused by increased erythropoietin production. Because of the viscous effects of excessive red cell volume, a minor increase in hematocrit above 65% to 75% may produce marked increase in whole blood viscosity that can lead to a number of symptoms including headache, lightheadedness, myalgias, and visual disturbances. Therapeutic phlebotomy is rarely required in stable "compensated" patients, but may be indicated in symptomatic patients with unstable hematocrits of 65% to 70%. When indicated, phlebotomy must be accompanied by crystalline or plasma exchange (Rosove & Perloff, 1986; Miner & Canobbio, 1994).

Nursing Management Plan

In caring for the patient with congenital heart disease, nurses must have a clear understanding of the underlying defect and the clinical sequelae that each patient presents and also must be sensitive to the potential impact that these defects may have on the individual's desired lifestyle. Assessment must include not only the presenting signs and symptoms of the primary defect and surgical interventions that may have taken place but also the questions related to issues such as activity levels, occupation, marital status, and childbearing. For females detail information regarding gynecologic history and contraception must be included (Canobbio, 1994). From the database, the nurse identifies the patient's actual or potential problems and the nursing diagnosis.

Whereas each cardiac defect has its own potential list of nursing problems, most are related to the complications cited earlier (the reader is again referred to those sections for appropriate nursing management). Three nursing diagnoses, specific to congenital heart disease in the adult, are listed in Nursing Care Plan 35-1. Most people with postoperative congenital heart disease assume lifestyles similar to the general population, but they require long-term surveillance.

Nursing Care Plan 35–1 ■ The Adult Patient With Congenital Heart Disease

Nursing Diagnosis 1	➤	Knowledge deficit related to specific deficit and clinical status
Nursing Goal	➤	To identify patient's knowledge base and increase level of understanding regarding clinical status
Outcome Criteria	➤	Patient verbalizes: Knowledge of individual anomaly, the prescribed treatment regimen, and need for regular return visits. Knowledge regarding endocarditis prophylaxis Knowledge regarding childbearing, pregnancy, and contraception

NURSING INTERVENTIONS	SCIENTIFIC RATIONALE

1. Develop a comprehensive teaching plan that includes:
  a. Description of primary defect
  b. Description of any palliative corrective surgical interventions and any residual effects.
  c. Importance of follow-up visits
	1. Serious gaps in health knowledge of young persons have been reported (Ferenencz et al., 1980). This lack of knowledge has potential serious consequences for long-term follow-up and care, particularly in those cases in which the long-term residua and sequelae are unknown.

Nursing Care Plan 35–1 ■ The Adult Patient With Congenital Heart Disease *(Continued)*

NURSING INTERVENTIONS	SCIENTIFIC RATIONALE
d. Functional status: Review allowances and limitations as indicated by defect **e.** Importance of understanding the need for endocarditis prophylaxis as indicated by defect. **f.** Information regarding childbearing: Risk of genetic transmission **2.** For women: **a.** Risks of pregnancy and delivery vary according to type of defect, surgical interventions, and NYHA classification **b.** Need for prepregnancy counseling for women who fall into moderate to high risk classification	**2.** a,b. To determine the potential risk to women with congenital heart disease during pregnancy, two factors must be considered. First, the primary defect of surgical interventions that have occurred, and second, the overall cardiovascular status of the patient. Pregnancy risks can be divided into low, intermediate, and high risk (Table 35-2). Women with mild unoperated acyanotic lesions present a maternal risk similar to the general population. Susceptibility to infective endocarditis is the only concern. Women considered at intermediate risk are those with both repaired and unrepaired anomalies with residual effects. Women who are cyanotic with increase PVR or functional class III, IV are considered high risk for both maternal and fetal mortality, and pregnancy is not advised.
c. Appropriate type of contraceptive use	**c.** Oral contraception, particularly the estrogenic type, is hazardous for women who are cyanotic and those with increased PVR, obstruction to LV outflow, heart failure, or arrhythmias. Intrauterine devices are contraindicated in patients at risk for developing infective endocarditis. The diaphragm with gel foam is currently the safest and most effective method of contraception. Other contraceptive methods that may be used but offer less security are spermicidal sponges and gel. Male contraception is an alternative. Sterilization, such as tubal ligation of the patient or vasectomy of the spouse, is suggested for women identified as high risk.

Nursing Diagnosis 2 ➤ Anxiety and fear related to actual or perceived: severity of condition, chronic disability, shortened lifespan

Nursing Goal: ➤ To identify and reduce patient's level of anxiety

Outcome Criteria: ➤ Patient is able to verbalize source of anxiety
Patient demonstrates a reduction in level of anxiety and fear

NURSING INTERVENTIONS	SCIENTIFIC RATIONALE
1. Assess level of anxiety and determine primary cause. Assess patient's information level to identify any misconceptions related to condition. Elicit questions and concerns. **2.** Provide or clarify information relative to condition, prognosis.	**1.** These date provide information about the patient's perception of the clinical condition, of their long-term survival, and of physical limitations imposed by diagnosis. **2.** Anxiety is often the result of an inadequate knowledge based or misinterpretation of what congenital heart disease means. If diagnosed in infancy or childhood, these patients are often products of parents who understandably protected them and may have imposed significant restrictions on physical and social activity.
3. Assess usual coping mechanisms for dealing with stress.	**3.** Patient's usually method of dealing with stress may be insufficient to control anxiety and fear.
4. Assist patient to deal realistically with anxiety, providing alternative methods for dealing with different types of stress. **5.** Provide positive reinforcement about their prognosis; assist them in attaining realistic goals and life-styles.	**4.** Patient's level of anxiety may require alternative methods of stress reduction suck as relaxation, imagery. **5.** Setting achievable goals promotes a sense of wellness and optimism.

Nursing Care Plan 35–1 ■ The Adult Patient With Congenital Heart Disease *(Continued)*

Nursing Diagnosis 3	➤	Ineffective family (spouse) coping: compromise actual or potential
Nursing Goal:	➤	To assess and identify stressors that may interfere with family coping mechanisms.
Outcome Criteria:	➤	Patient and family (spouse) are able to identify and verbalize stress or events that may be contributing to family stress.

NURSING INTERVENTIONS	SCIENTIFIC RATIONALE
1. Assess the family's perceptions of condition, identify any misconceptions, associated guilt, fears, or tendency for inappropriate overprotectiveness 2. Determine the degrees of emotional and financial stress placed on family by patient's condition. Refer to appropriate support services. 3. Include family/spouse in teaching plan. Acknowledge and encourage verbalization of feelings individually and together as a family. 4. Provide opportunity for family group sessions.	1. Poor emotional adjustment often seen in adults has been related more to parental anxiety than to degree of severity of disease. 2. Issues of occupation and insurability are often faced by these patients and present a source of constant strain on family. 3. It is important that each family member (including children and siblings) have an opportunity to express concerns without fear of recrimination. 4. Settings in which all members are present encourage open discussion about common fears and help to clarify any misconceptions.

REFERENCES

Allen, H. D., Gersony, W. M., & Taubert, D. A. (1992). Insurability of the adolescent and young adult with heart disease. *Circulation, 86,* 703.

Benson, L. V., Bonet, J., McLaughlin, P., et al. (1982). Assessment of right ventricular function during supine bicycle exercise after Mustard operation. *Circulation, 65,* 1052.

Beppu, S., Suzuki, S., Matsuda, H. et al. (1993). Rapidity of progression of aortic stenosis in patients with congenital bicuspid aortic valves. *American Journal of Cardiology, 71,* 322.

Bull, C., MacArtney, F. J., Horvath, P., et al. (1987). Evaluation of long-term results of homograft and heterograft values in extrocardiac conduits. *Journal of Thoracic Cardiovascular Surgery, 94,* 12.

Buckner, E. M., Hillis, L. D., & Lange, R. A. (2000). Congenital heart in adults. Second of Two Parts. *New England Journal of Medicine, 342,* 334–341.

Butera, G., De Rosa, G., Chessa, M., Rosti, L., Negura, D. G., Luciane, P., Giamberti, A., Bossone, E., & Carminati, M. (2003). Transcatheter closure of atrial septal defect in young children: results and follow-up. *Journal of the American College of Cardiology,* 116, 241–5.

Canobbio, M. M. (1986). Counseling the adult with congenital heart disease. In W. Roberts (Ed.), *Congenital heart disease in adults* (2nd ed.). Philadelphia: FA Davis.

Canobbio, M. M. (1984). The Eisenmenger syndrome. *Nursing Clinics of North America, 19,* 537–554.

Canobbio, M. M. (1994). Reproductive issues for women with congenital heart disease. *Nursing Clinics of North America, 29,* 285–297.

Canobbio, M. M., Mair, D. D., vander Velde, M., & Koos, B. J. (1996). Pregnancy outcomes after the Fontan repair. *Journal of the American College of Cardiology, 28,* 764–767.

Canobbio, M. M. (2001). Health care issues facing adolescents with congenital heart disease. *Journal of Pediatric Nursing, 16,* 363–370.

Cantor, W. J., Harrison, D. A., Moussadj, J. S., et al. (1999). Determinants of survival and length of survival in adults with Eisenmenger Syndrome. *American Journal of Cardiology, 84,* 677.

Cappato, R., Schluter, M., Weiss, C., et al. (1996). Radiofrequency current catheter ablation of accessory atrio ventricular pathways in Ebstein's Anomaly. *Ciculation* 94, 376.

Celermajer, D. S., Bull, C., Till, J. A., et al. (1994). Ebstein's anomaly: presentation and outcome from fetus adult. *Journal of the American College of Cardiology, 23,* 170–176.

Coggin, C. J., Parker, K. R., & Keith, J. D. (1970). Natural history of isolated patent ductus arteriosus and the effect of surgical correlation: twenty years experience at hospital for sick children. *Toronto Canadian Medical Association Journal, 102,* 718.

Clarkson, P. M., Wilson, N. J., Neutz, J. M., North, R. A., Calder, A. L., & Barratt-Boyes, B.G. (1994). Outcome of pregnancy after the Mustard operation for transposition of the great arteries with intact ventricular septum. *Journal of the American College of Cardiology, 24,* 190–193.

Connelly, M. D., Lie, P. P., Williams, W. G., et al. (1996). Congenitally corrected transposition in the adult. Functional status and complications. *Journal of the American College of Cardiology, 27,* 1238.

Driscoll, D. J., Offord, D. P., Feldt, R. H., et al. (1992). Five-to-fifteen year followup after Fontan operation. *Circulation, 86:* 469.

Emmanouilides, G. C., Riemenschneider, T.A., Allen, H. D., & Gutgesill, H. P. (1995). In Moss & Adams [AQ1] (Eds.), *Heart disease in infants, children and adolescents* (5th ed). Baltimore: Williams and Wilkins.

Edwards, J. E., & Burchell, H. B. (1949). Congenital tricuspid atresia: A classification. *Medical Clinics of North America, 33,* 1177.

Ferenencz, C., Wegmann, F. L., & Dunning, R. E. (1980). Medical knowledge of young persons with heart disease. *Journal of School Health, 50,* 133.

Fisher, R. G., Moodie, D. S., Sterba, R., & Gill, C. C. (1990). Patient ductus arteriosus in adults – long-term follow-up: nonsurgical versus surgical treatment. *Journal of the American College of Cardiology, 8,* 280–4.

Gersony, W. M. (1990). *Coarctation of aorta. Heart disease in infants, children, and adolescents.* Baltimore: William and Wilkins.

Gersony, W. M., & Rosenbaum, M. S. (2002). *Congenital heart disease in the adult.* NY: McGraw-Hill.

Gillum, R. F. (1994). Epidemiology of congenital heart disease in the US. *American Heart Journal, 127,* 919–27.

Graham, T., Burger, J., Bender, H.B., et al. (1985). Improved right ventricular function after intra-atrial repair of transposition of great arteries. *Circulation,* 72(suppl), II–45.

Hagler, D. J., Julsrud, P.R., et.al. (1991). Early and late results of the modified Fontan procedure for double-inlet left ventricle: the Mayo experience. *Journal of the American College of Cardiology, 18,* 727.

Hayes, C. H., Gersony, W. M., Driscoll, D. J., et al. (1993). Second natural history study of congenital heart defects: Results of treatment of patients with pulmonary valvar stenosis. *Circulation, 87*(suppl): I–27.

Hermann, H. C., Hill, J. A., Krol, J., et al. (1991). Effectiveness of percutaneous balloon valvuloplasty in adults with pulmonic valve stemosis. *American Journal of Cardiology, 68:*1111.

Kaplan, S., & Adolph, R. J. (1979). Pulmonic valve stenosis in adults. In W. C. Roberts (Ed.), *Congenital heart disease in the adult*. Philadelphia: FA Davis.

Keane, J. F., Driscoll, D. J., Gersony, W. M., et al. (1993). Second natural history study of congenital heart defects: Aortic stenosis. *Circulation,* 87(suppl), I–16.

Khan, A., Yousef, S. A., Mullins, C. E., & Sawyer, W. (1992). Experience with 205 procedures of transcatheter closure of ductus arteriosis in 182 patients with special reference to residual shunts and long-term follow-up. *Journal of Thoracic and Cardiovascular Surgery,* 104, 1721.

Kidd, L., Driscoll, D. J., Gersony, W. M., et al. (1993). Second natural history study of congenital heart defects: Results of treatment of patients with ventricular septal defects. *Circulation,* 87(suppl), I–38.

Kidd, L., O'Neil, H. (1982). Transposition of the great arteries in the adult. In W. C. Roberts (Ed.), *Congenital heart disease in adults.* Philadelphia: FA Davis.

Miner, P. D., & Canobbio, M. M. (1994). Care of the adult cyanotic congenital heart disease. *Nursing Clinics of North America,* 29, 249–267.

Mitchell, S. C., Korones, S.B., & Bererrdes, H. W. (1971). Congenital heart disease in 56, 109 births: Incidence and natural history. *Circulation,* 43, 323.

Morgan, B. C. (1978). Incidence, etiology, and classification of congenital heart disease. *Pediatric Clinics of North America,* 25, 700–721.

Morris, C. D., & Menashe, V. D. (1991). 25-year mortality after surgical repair of congenital heart defect in childhood: A population-based cohort study. *JAMA,* 266, 3447.

Murphy, J. G., Gersh, B. J., Mair, D. D., et.al. (1993). Long-term outcomes in patients undergoing surgical repair of tetralogy of Fallot. *New England Journal of Medicine,* 329, 593–9.

Ottenkamp, J., Rohmer, J., Mquaegebeur, J. M., et al. (1982). Nine years experience of physiological correction of tricuspid atresia: Long term results and current surgical approach. *Thorax,* 37, 718.

Perloff, J. K. (2003). *The clinical recognition of congenital heart disease* (5th ed.). Philadelphia: WB Saunders.

Perloff, J. K., & Koos, B. (1998). Pregnancy and congenital heart disease. In J. K. Perloff & J. S. Child (Eds.), *Congenital heart disease* (2nd ed., pp. 144–164). Philadelphia: WB Saunders.

Perloff, J. K. (1991). Congenital heart disease after childhood: An expanding patient population. *Journal of American Clinics in Cardiology,* 18, 311.

Puley, G., Sui, S., Connally, M., et al. (1991). Anhythmia and survival in patients >18 years of age after the Mustard procedure for complete transposition of great arteries. *American Journal of Cardiology,* 83, 1080.

Rao, P .S. (1992). Demographic features of tricuspid atresia. In P. S. Rao (Ed.), *Tricuspid atresia* (2nd ed.). New York: Futura Publishing Co.

Rosenthal, A., Behrendt, D., Sloan, H., et al. (1984). Long-term prognosis (15 to 26 years) after repair of tetralogy of Fallot. I. Survival and sympathetic status. *Annals of Thoracic Surgery,* 38, 151.

Report from the Joint Study on the Natural history of Congenital Heart Defects. (1993). *Circulation,* 87(suppl), I–I.

Roberts, N. K., & Cretin, S. (1995). The changing face of congenital heart disease. *Medical Care,* 28, 930.

Roos-Hesselink, J., Perlroth, M. G., McGhie, J., & Spitaels, S. (1995). Atrial arrhythmias in adults after repair of tetralogy of fallot: correlations with clinical, exercise, and echocardiographic findings. *Circulation,* 91, 2241–9.

Rosove, M. H., Perloff, Hocking, W. G., Canobbio, et al. (1986). Chronic hypoxaemia and decompensated erythrocytosis in cyanotic congenital heart disease. *Lancet,* 2, 313–315.

Sade, R. M., & Fyfe, D. A. (1990). Tricuspid atresia: Current concepts in diagnosis and treatment. *Pediatric Clinics of North America,* 37, 151.

Salazar, O., Steinberger, J., Carpenter, B., et al. (1996). Predictors of hypertension in long-term survivors of repaired coarctation of aorta. *Journal of the American College of Cardiology,* 27(Suppl A), 35A.

Trusler, G. A., Williams, W. G., Izukawa, T., et al. (1980). Current results with the Mustard operation in isolated transposition of the great arteries. *Journal of Thoracic and Cardiovascular Surgery,* 80, 381.

Vaksmann, G., Fournier, A., Davignon, A., Ducharmc, G., Houye, L., & Fouron, J. C. (1999). Frequency and prognosis of arrhythmias after operative "correction" of tetralogy of Fallot. *American Journal of Cardiology,* 66, 346–350

Warnes, C. A., Liberthson, R., Davidson, G. K., Dora, Harris, L., et al. (2001). Task Force 1: The changing profile of CHD in adult life. *Journal of the American College of Cardiology,* 37, 1161–98

Whittemore, R. (1982). Pregnancy and its outcome in women with and without surgical treatment of congenital heart disease. In J. K. Perloff & M. E. Engle (Eds.), *Congenital heart disease: Benefits, residua and sequelae.* New York: Yorke Medical Books.

Wilson, N. J., Clarkson, P. M., Barnett-Bayes, B. G., et al. (1998). Long-term outcome after the Mustard repair for simple transposition of great arteries: 28 years of old follow-up. *Journal of American Cardiology,* 32, 758.

Zahka, K. G., Horneffer, P. J., Rowe, S. A., et al. (1988). Long-term valvular function after total repair of tetrology of Fallot: relation to ventricular arrhythmias. *Circulation,* 78 Suppl III, III-14-III–19.

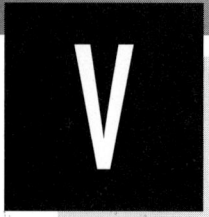

P A R T

V

Health Promotion and Disease Prevention

36

Coronary Heart Disease Risk Factors

KATHERINE M. NEWTON • ERIKA SIVARAJAN FROELICHER

Coronary heart disease (CHD) is usually associated with one or more characteristics known as risk factors. A risk factor is "an aspect of personal behavior or lifestyle, an environmental exposure, or an inborn or inherited characteristic, which on the basis of epidemiologic evidence is known to be associated with" the occurrence of disease (Last, 1988).

Several aspects of the association between a potential risk factor and the disease are evaluated before an association is considered causal. These include the strength or magnitude of the association, the consistency or repeatability of the association, temporality (the cause precedes the disease), dose response (greater dose leads to greater likelihood of disease), the biologic and epidemiologic plausibility of the association, coherence of the potential cause with what is known about the disease, a decrease in the incidence of disease when the potential cause is eliminated, and experimental evidence (Kelsey, 1986; Rothman, 1986). Although few potential risk factors meet all of these criteria, the goal of epidemiologic investigations is to establish these characteristics. The results of epidemiologic studies of disease cause are frequently presented either as disease rates or as a relative risk. Relative risk is the rate of disease in a group exposed to a potential risk factor, divided by the rate of disease in an otherwise similar group that is unexposed to the risk factor (Rothman, 1986). For example, if the rate of fatal myocardial infarction (MI) in a group of smokers was 120 per 100,000 per year, and the rate in comparable nonsmokers was 60 per 100,000 per year, then the relative risk associated with smoking would be:

$$
\begin{aligned}
\text{Relative risk} &= \text{rate in exposed} \div \text{rate in unexposed} \\
&= (120/[100,000/\text{yr}]) \div (60/[100,000/\text{yr}]) \\
&= 2.0
\end{aligned}
$$

The risk of MI is thus doubled in the smokers, or there is a 200% increase in risk compared with nonsmokers. A relative risk of 1.30 represents a 30% increase in risk; a relative risk of 3.0 represents a 300% increase, or a tripling of risk. United States death rates in 1998 from all cardiovascular diseases combined, acute MI, cancer, and other causes, for black and white women and men are presented in Figure 36-1 (Centers for Disease, 1998). Cardiovascular disease continues to be the leading cause of death for black and white men and women throughout their life spans. Death rates from MI

increase with age in men and women. CHD incidence in women lags approximately 10 years behind that in men, and there is approximately a 20-year lag for serious clinical events such as CHD mortality (Fig. 36-2) (American Heart Association, 2003). The rate of acute MI is higher in black women than white women throughout their life span, whereas MI rates in white and black men are similar until age 65 years, when the rate in white men exceeds that in black men. In the Third National Health and Nutrition Examination Survey (NHANES III), the prevalence of a personal history of MI was higher for men than women among whites and Mexican Americans, but this difference was less pronounced among blacks (Table 36-1).

Coronary heart disease mortality rates have declined steadily since the late 1960s. From 1968 to 1984, CHD mortality declined at an average rate of 2% to 3% per year in all age groups, in both sexes, and in blacks and whites (Sempos, 1988). From 1979 to 1985, the average annual percentage change in CHD mortality, for people aged 35 to 74 years, was −2.59% for white women, −3.37% for white men, −2.0% for black women, and −2.84% for black men (Sempos, 1988). From 1987 to 1994, the average annual percentage change in CHD mortality, for people aged 35 to 74 years, was −4.5% for white women, −4.7% for white men, −4.1% for black women, and −2.5% for black men (Rosamond, 1998). Overall, cardiovascular disease death rates declined 17.0% from 1990 to 2000 (American Heart Association, 2003). From 1990 to 1998 age-adjusted death rates for diseases of the heart declined 15% for non-Hispanic whites, 11% for non-Hispanic blacks, 17% for Hispanics, 14% for Asian/Pacific Islanders, and 8% for American Indians/Alaska Natives (American Heart Association, 2003). There is ongoing speculation as to the cause of this decline in cardiovascular disease mortality, although multiple causes are likely. Small, population-wide behavior changes leading to lower serum cholesterol, lower smoking rates, and lower blood pressure may account for as much as 50% of the decrease in coronary mortality (Sempos, 1988). Decreases in case fatality rates also have been documented. This indicates that changes in patient management, including more rapid access to emergency care and interventions that reduce infarct size and prevent death caused by arrhythmias, may account for some of the decline in CHD mortality (Pell & Fayerweather, 1985).

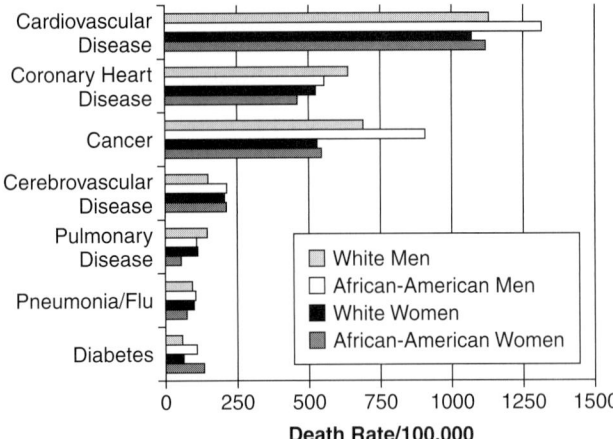

■ Figure 36–1. U.S. death rates per 100,000 population for major causes of death, by gender, and race/ethnicity. (From Centers for Disease Control and Prevention: CDC Wonder. Available: *http://wonder.cdc.gov/WONDER/mort.oo.ex./.*October, 1998.)

Table 36–1 ■ PERSONAL HISTORY OF MYOCARDIAL INFARCTION AMONG U.S. WOMEN AND MEN BY AGE AND RACE/ETHNICITY

Age Group	White Women (%)	White Men (%)	Black Women (%)	Black Men (%)	Mexican American Women (%)	Mexican American Men (%)
20–29	0.0	0.2	0.1	0.9	0.1	0.4
30–39	0.0	0.7	0.1	0.2	0.7	0.8
40–49	0.5	2.7	1.7	2.2	0.5	2.6
50–59	1.9	6.4	5.2	7.3	3.3	6.4
60–69	5.9	13.3	8.3	10.5	4.0	8.8
≥70	11.9	18.8	11.1	11.1	6.6	12.1

From the National Center for Health Statistics: *National Health and Nutrition Examination Survey, III. 1988–1994.* Rockville, MD.

Cardiovascular disease risk factors have additive effects. The MI risk in a person with three major risk factors is higher than that of a person with two or one (Kannell, 1984). Furthermore, for any given combination of risk factors, at a given age, the risk is lower in women than in men. In this chapter, the major known risk factors for cardiovascular disease are briefly reviewed. Data from NHANES III are used to demonstrate the prevalence of CHD risk factors in U.S. women and men.

■ DEMOGRAPHIC CHARACTERISTICS

Coronary heart disease mortality rates increase exponentially with age for men and women (see Fig. 36-2). Until the seventh decade of life, black men have the highest rates of CHD mortality, followed by white men, black women, and white women. The rates in men converge at approximately the sev-

enth decade, and those in women converge in the eighth decade. Further data about CHD rates by race/ethnicity come from analysis of death rates in California from 1985 to 1990 (Wild, 1995). The CHD death rates per 100,000 population were as follows: white women, 143; white men, 302; Hispanic women, 97; Hispanic men, 175; black women, 214; black men, 316; Chinese women, 73; Chinese men, 155; Japanese women, 67; Japanese men, 146; Asian-Indian women, 110; and Asian-Indian men, 258 (Wild, 1995).

Perceived financial status is associated with MI and coronary death in women (Eaker, 1992). Higher systolic blood pressure, higher low-density lipoprotein (LDL) cholesterol, higher fasting glucose levels and 2-hour insulin values, higher body mass index (BMI), and lower high-density lipoprotein (HDL) cholesterol are all associated with lower socioeconomic status (Matthews & Kelsey, 1989).

Educational attainment, which often determines socioeconomic status, is inversely related to CHD risk in black and white women and white men but is positively associated with CHD in black men (Eaker, 1992; Eaker, 1989; Keil, 1987; Kitagawa, 1973; Nyboe, 1989). Women of lower educational attainment are more often smokers, sedentary, angry, pessimistic, depressed, dissatisfied with their work, and have less social support and self-esteem (Matthews & Kelsey, 1989). Educational incongruity with the spouse is associated with increased risk of sudden cardiac death and MI in women (Szklo, 1976; Talbott, 1977). Among men, the 10-year incidence of CHD increases with the wife's education level for those whose wives are employed outside the home, but not for those whose wives are homemakers (Kannell, 1987).

■ FAMILY HISTORY OF CARDIOVASCULAR DISEASE

A family history of CHD puts women and men at increased risk for CHD, probably from a combination of genetic and environmental factors (Burke, 1991; Jousilahti, 1996; Nyboe, 1989; Roncaglioni, 1992). A history of MI in one first-degree relative doubles, and in two or more first-degree relatives it

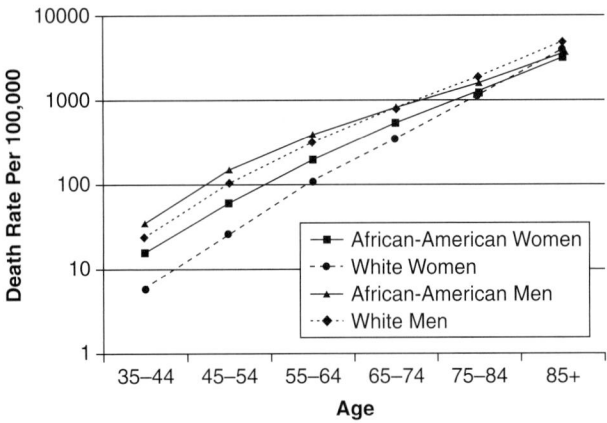

■ Figure 36–2. U.S. coronary heart disease death rate per 100,000 population by age, gender, and race/ethnicity. (From Centers for Disease Control and Prevention: CDC Wonder. Available: *http://wonder.cdc.gov/WONDER/mort.oo.ex./.*October, 1998.)

triples MI risk (Roncaglioni, 1992; Friedlander, 2001). MI risk is strongest when MI in relatives occurs before age 55 years but is still present when MI occurs after age 55 years (Roncaglioni, 1992). The risk associated with a positive family history is independent of other known CHD risk factors. In the Nurses Health Study, women with a family history of parental MI at age 60 years or younger had 2.8-times the risk of nonfatal MI, five-times the risk of fatal CHD, and 3.4-times the risk for angina pectoris compared with women without a history of parental MI (Stampfer, 1987). For women with a history of parental MI after age 60 years, there was no increase in risk for nonfatal CHD, compared with women with no family history of CHD (Stampfer, 1987). In contrast, a study of older women found no increase in CHD risk with a family history of heart attack. (Barrett-Connor, 1987).

Twin studies shed further light on the influence of family history on CHD risk. In a study of male and female Swedish monozygotic and dizygotic twins, among male twins the relative risk of CHD for monozygotic twins was 8.1, and the relative risk for dizygotic twins was 3.8 when one twin died of CHD before age 55 years (Marenberg, 1994). Among female twins, the relative risk of CHD for monozygotic twins was 15,

and the relative risk for dizygotic twins was 2.6 when one twin died of CHD before age 55 years. In monozygotic and dizygotic twins, as the age at which one twin died increased, the risk for CHD among the remaining twin decreased.

CIGARETTE SMOKING

In 2000, 46.5 million adults were current smokers, i.e., 23.3% of the adult U.S population (25.7% of men and 21.0% of women). Smoking prevalence varies markedly by race/ethnicity and age (Fig. 36-3). In 2000, smoking rates by race/ethnicity were as follows: Native Americans/Alaskan Natives, 36.0%; black, 23.2%; non-Hispanic whites, 24.1%; Hispanics, 18.6%; and Asians 14.4% (Epidemiology Branch, 2002). From 1965 to 1985, the prevalence of smoking in men and women decreased at a rate of 0.5% per year. From 1987 through 1990, smoking prevalence decreased at an even faster rate of 1.1% per year, although smoking prevalence was the same in 1991 as in 1990 for white men (Epidemiology Branch, 1994). From 1993 to 2000, smoking rates continued to

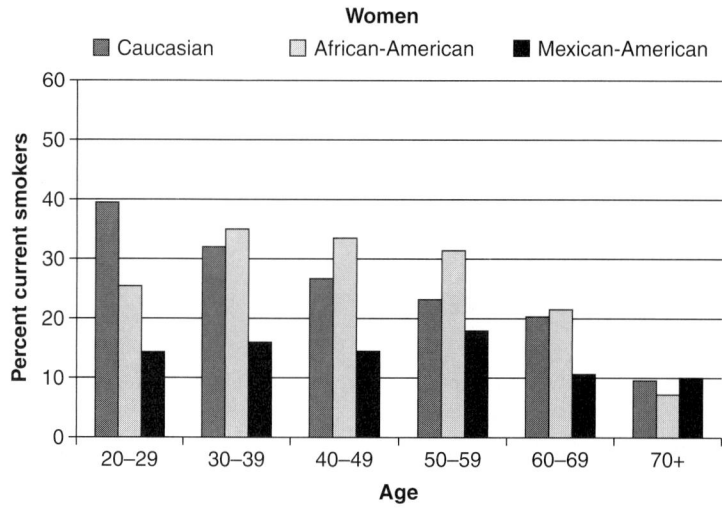

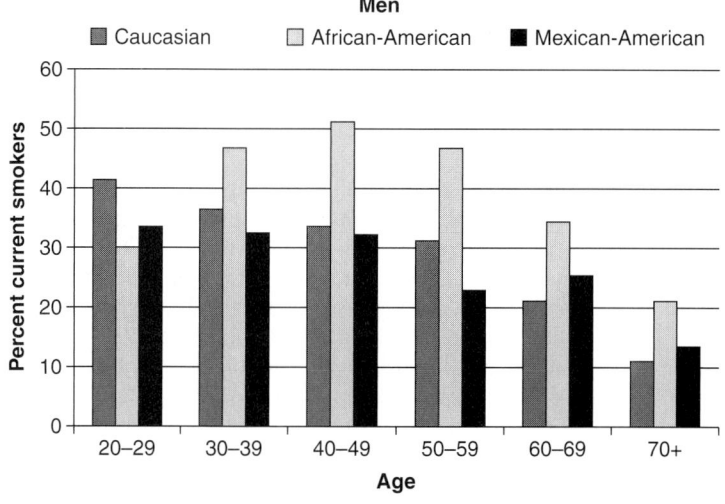

■ **Figure 36–3.** Prevalence of current smoking among U.S. women and men by age and race/ethnicity. (National Center for Health Statistics. *National Health and Nutrition Examination Survey, III, 1988–1994.*)

decline in all age groups except persons aged 18 to 24 years (Epidemiology Branch, 2002). For blacks and women, the smoking prevalence was actually higher in 1991 than in 1990 (Epidemiology Branch, 1993).

Smoking and Coronary Heart Disease

Cigarette smoking is perhaps the most preventable known cause of CHD today, leading to more deaths from CHD than from either lung cancer or chronic obstructive pulmonary disease (Glantz, 1991). CHD risk increases with number of cigarettes smoked, longer duration of smoking, and younger age at initiation of smoking (Jensen, 1991; Slone, 1978).

The CHD risk of male cigarette smokers is two (aged 60 years and older) to three (aged 30 to 59 years) times that of nonsmokers, (Dawber, 1980) whereas women who are current smokers have up to four-times the risk of first MI of those who have never smoked (Croft, 1989; LaVecchia, 1987; Rosenberg, Palmer, Shapiro, 1990). In the Nurses Health Study, cigarette smoking was associated with a five-fold increase in the risk for fatal CHD and nonfatal MI, and tripled the risk of angina (Willett, 1995). This elevation in risk of MI and CHD death is sustained from youth into advanced age for men and women (LaCroix, 1992; Slone, 1978). Smoking low-tar (<17.6 mg), low-nicotine (<1.2 mg), or filter cigarettes does not lower the risk of MI compared with high-tar, high-nicotine, or nonfiltered cigarettes (Kannell, 1984; Kaufman, 1983).

Smoking cessation confers benefit regardless of sex, age, or presence of CHD. Men and women of all ages with documented CHD who quit smoking have half the risk of mortality compared with those who continue to smoke (Hermanson, 1988; LaVecchia, Franceshi, 1987; Salonen, 1980). For women who quit smoking, MI risk is indistinguishable from that of nonsmokers within 3 to 5 years of smoking cessation (LaCroix, 1991; Rosenberg, 1990; Stampfer, 1987). There are many successful approaches to smoking cessation, and these interventions are less costly than many other preventive interventions (Cromwell, 1997). Smoking cessation should be encouraged regardless of age, sex, or the presence of established disease.

Environmental Tobacco Smoke

It is estimated that 53,000 deaths annually are attributable to environmental tobacco smoke (ETS), making it the third leading preventable cause of death in the Unites States (Glantz, 1991). Ten times as many of these deaths are caused by CHD as lung cancer. Exposure of nonsmokers to ETS from a spouse who smokes increases the risk of CHD death by 30% in men and women. This risk increases with the amount smoked by the spouse. (Glantz, 1991). ETS causes arterial endothelial damage, may initiate or accelerate the development of atherosclerosis, and increases platelet aggregation, which may result in coronary thrombosis (Glantz, 1991). Thus, the effects of ETS are similar to those of smoking cigarettes.

HYPERTENSION

Hypertension is defined as a systolic blood pressure of 140 mm Hg or more or diastolic blood pressure of 90 mm Hg or more. Hypertension carries particular importance as a cardiovascular risk factor for several reasons: it is highly prevalent, it is relatively simple to identify, it is a major risk for devastating cardiovascular outcomes, and control of hypertension is known to decrease its risk (Kannell, 1987). Prevalence of hypertension increases with age among whites, blacks, and Mexican Americans (Center for Disease Control 1998) (Fig. 36-4). The prevalence of hypertension is highest among blacks at all ages. Results of NHANES surveys conducted 1999 to 2000 indicate that hypertension prevalence has increased from 1988 to 2000 among women (5.6% increase) but not among men (Hajjar, 2003). Hypertension is associated with three- to four-fold increases in the risk of CHD, stroke, and MI (Dawber, 1980; Jensen, 1991; La Vecchia & Fransechi, 1987), and it increases the risk of peripheral vascular disease, renal failure, and congestive heart failure in men and women across the life span (Anastos, 1991; Dawber, 1980). The normalization of blood pressure dramatically decreases the risk of stroke, renal failure, cardiac failure, and coronary events (Hypertension Detection and Follow-up, 1988; Medical Research Council, 1992; Ramsay, 1991). Even in the elderly, control of hypertension confers major benefits against stroke, coronary events, and all cardiovascular events (Medical Research Council, 1985; SHEP, 1991). Hypertension and the nurse's role in its management are discussed in detail in Chapter 39.

SERUM LIPIDS AND LIPOPROTEINS

Elevated serum total cholesterol and LDL cholesterol are associated with an increased risk of CHD in men and women of all ages (Bush, 1988; Manolio, 1992; Wilson, 1990). The prevalence of hypercholesterolemia is higher in U.S. women than men, and higher in whites and blacks than in Mexican Americans (National Center, 1997) (Table 36-2). In the Framingham Heart Study, women and men with serum cholesterol concentrations greater than 295 mg/dL had more than three-times the risk of MI and definite coronary events than those with cholesterol concentrations less than 204 mg/dL (Bush, 1988). CHD rates are lower for women than men at any given level of serum cholesterol (Bush, 1988).

Serum HDL cholesterol has a protective effect against CHD. A 1-mg/dL increment in HDL is associated with a 2% (men) to 3% (women) decrement in total CHD risk, and a 3.7% (men) to 4.7% (women) decrement in CHD mortality (Gaziano, 1994). At any given level of LDL, higher levels of HDL confer protection against CHD (Kannel, 1987).

Attention has been focused on subfractions of HDL and LDL, the apolipoproteins (apo AI, apo AII, apo B), and lipoprotein(a) (Lp[a]). In a study of the predictors of premature CHD at coronary arteriography, Kwiterovich and associates (Kwiterovich, 1992) found that apo B was more strongly associated with an increase in CHD risk in women than in men,

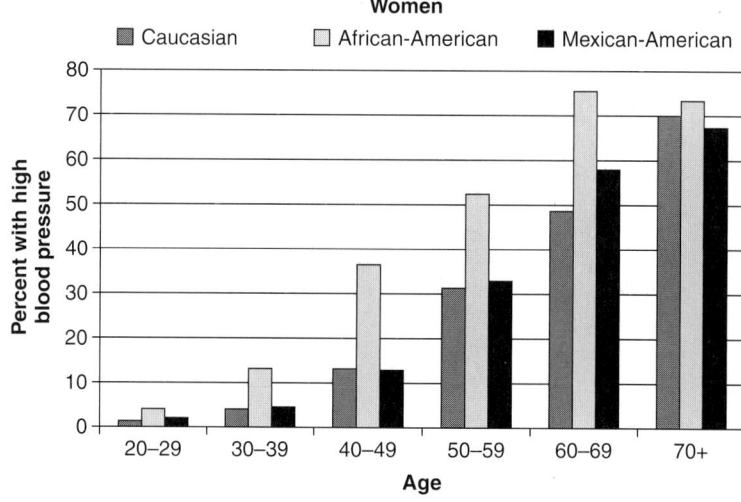

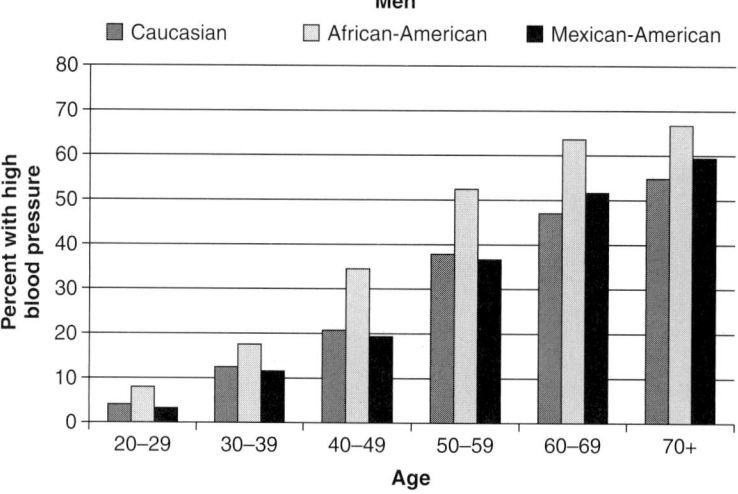

■ **Figure 36–4.** Prevalence of high blood pressure among U.S. women and men by age and race/ethnicity. (National Center for Health Statistics. *National Health and Nutrition Examinations Survey, III, 1988–1994.*)

whereas Apo AI was more strongly associated with a decrease in CHD risk in men than in women. Increasing levels of Lp(a) are also associated with an increase in CHD risk (Austin, 1988; Bostom, 1996; Bostom, 1994; Stein, 1997). In the Framingham

Table 36–2 ■ PREVALENCE OF HYPERCHOLESTEROLEMIA* AMONG U.S. WOMEN AND MEN BY AGE AND RACE/ETHNICITY

Age Group	White Women (%)	White Men (%)	Black Women (%)	Black Men (%)	Mexican American Women (%)	Mexican American Men (%)
20–29	6.9	4.6	7.3	7.3	7.2	7.7
30–39	7.8	17.8	7.3	9.7	8.8	18.0
40–49	20.3	25.0	16.4	19.2	16.8	20.6
50–59	39.1	26.6	35.1	26.9	27.3	26.9
60–69	44.2	29.4	47.8	28.3	39.7	33.8
≥70	43.4	23.6	39.6	23.6	28.9	18.1

* Based on self-reported use of cholesterol-lowering medication or a total serum cholesterol value of ≥240 mg/dL.
From the National Center for Health Statistics, U.S. Department of Health and Human Services (DHHS). *Third National Health and Nutrition Examination Survey, 1988–1994, NHANES III Data File (CD-ROM Series II, NO 1). Public Use Data File.* Hyattsville, MD: Centers for Disease Control and Prevention, 1997.

Heart Study, the relative risk for CHD associated with elevated Lp(a) was 1.6 in women (Bostom, 1996) and 1.9 in men (Bostom, 1994). LDL subclass patterns also influence CHD risk. Compared with light, buoyant LDL, small, dense LDL is associated with a three-fold increase in risk of MI (Austin, 1988).

Serum cholesterol levels influence prognosis after MI. The risk for reinfarction is 3.7- (men) to 9.2-times (women) as great when serum cholesterol levels are 275 mg/dL or greater, compared with levels of less than 200 mg/dL (Wong, 1991). There is evidence that normalization of serum lipids and lipoproteins reduces the CHD mortality rate (Brown, 1990). Hyperlipidemia and its management are discussed in more detail in Chapter 40.

PHYSICAL ACTIVITY

The roles of physical activity and physical fitness in preventing cardiovascular disease and controlling cardiovascular disease risk factors are well established. The 1996 Surgeon General's Report on Physical Activity and Health recommends that children and adults perform at least 30 minutes of moderate-intensity physical activity most days of the week (U.S. Department, 1996). Applying this definition to NHANES III data (Figs. 36-5 and

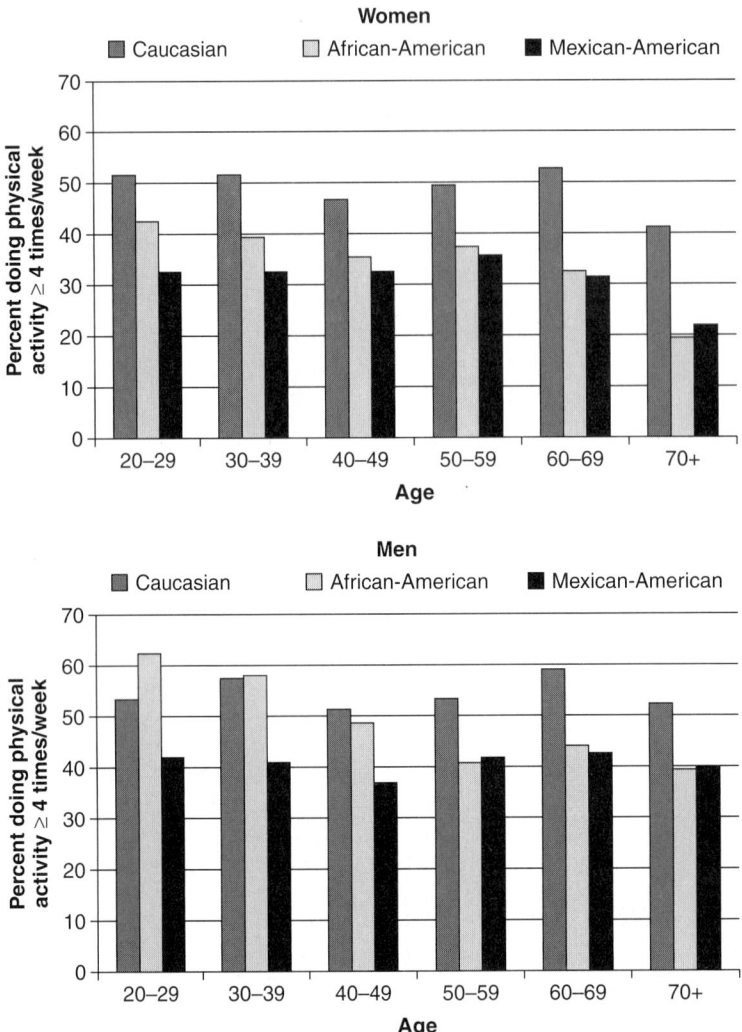

■ Figure 36–5. Prevalence of physical activity at least four times per week among U.S. women and men by age and race/ethnicity. Physical activity = walking, jogging or running, bicycling, swimming, aerobics, dancing, calisthenics, garden/yard work, and/or lifting weights. (National Center for Health Statistics. *National Health and Nutrition Examination Survey, III, 1988–1994.*)

36-6) shows that only approximately half of all white women and less than 40% of black and Mexican American women are physically active four or more times per week, and less than 25% of women walk at least four times per week. The proportions are only slightly higher for American men. Thus, a large proportion of the American public could be targeted for public health interventions to increase physical activity. Studies of the effects on cardiovascular disease of both on-the-job and leisure-time activity indicate that in general, people who are more physically active or physically fit tend to have CHD less often than sedentary or less fit people. CHD tends to be less severe and occurs at a later age among those who are physically active compared with those who are sedentary (Haskell, 1992). When data from cohort studies of occupational physical activity and CHD risk were pooled, the risk for CHD death for those with low-level occupational activity was almost twice that of those with high-level activity, and MI risk was 40% higher in the sedentary group (Berlin, 1990).

Analysis of studies of nonoccupational activity showed a 60% increase in risk of CHD death for low compared with high activity and a tripling of the risk of MI (Berlin, 1990). There was a 30% to 40% increase in risk of CHD death and MI for moderate occupational and nonoccupational activity compared with high activity (Berlin, 1990).

In the five studies that included women, the risk for angina pectoris, MI, and sudden death was two- to three-times higher among women in the lowest compared with the highest activity level (Douglas, 1992). An important addition to understanding the benefits of fitness has been made by studies that measure physical fitness using standardized exercise tests and then compare fitness with later cardiovascular outcomes (Blair, 1989; Ekelund, 1988; Slattery, 1988; Sobolski, 1987). In these studies, a higher level of fitness was associated with a significantly lower rate of cardiovascular disease mortality in men and women (Blair, 1989; Sobolski, 1987), all-cause mortality in men and women (Blair, 1989), and ischemic heart disease (fatal and nonfatal MI plus sudden death) in men (Solbolski, 1987). There are insufficient data to determine whether physical conditioning reduces reinfarction or mortality in people with

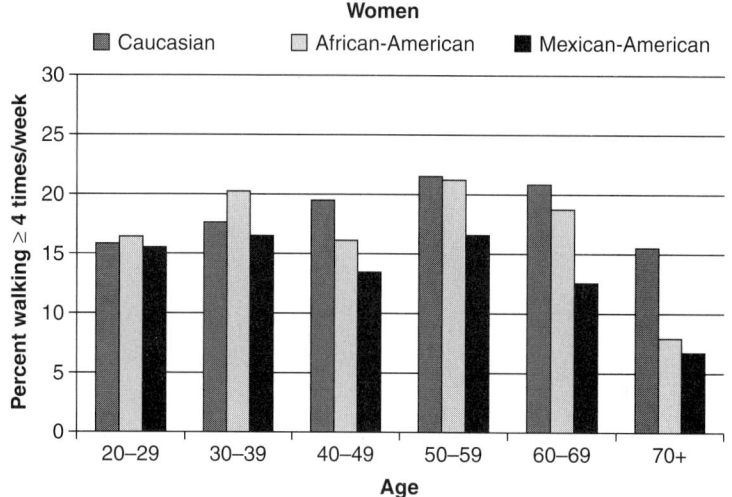

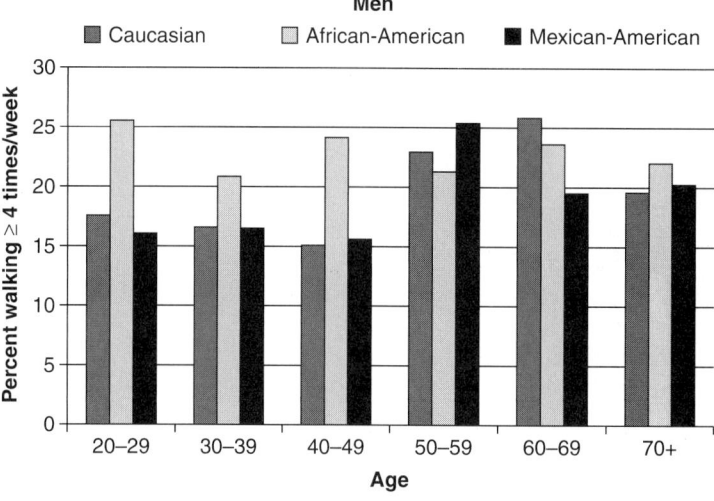

■ **Figure 36–6.** Prevalence of walking at least 1 mile without stopping at least four times per week among U.S. women and men by age and race/ethnicity. (National Center for Health Statistics. *National Health and Nutrition Examination Survey, III, 1988–1994.*)

established CHD (Haskell, 1992). Although pooled analyses from randomized trials of comprehensive cardiac rehabilitation suggest a 19% to 25% reduction in mortality rates associated with rehabilitation, it is difficult to dissociate the benefits of the exercise component of these programs from other lifestyle changes (Oldridge, 1988; Thompson, 1988). However, the potential benefits of a program of regular exercise after MI include an increase in exercise capacity, decrease in angina, improved control of other cardiovascular disease risk factors, decreased anxiety and depression, and increased self-esteem and sense of well-being (Thompson, 1988). Exercise training is also recognized as an important adjunctive therapy, with similar benefits for those with a history of congestive heart failure (Pina, 2003). Activity and exercise are discussed further in Chapter 41.

DIABETES MELLITUS

The American Diabetes Association diagnostic criteria for diabetes mellitus are random blood glucose of at least 200 mg/dL or fasting blood glucose of at least 126 mg/dL (Expert Committee, 1997). Approximately 17 million people in the United States

have diabetes, more than 5% of adults have type 2 diabetes, and the prevalence of diabetes is rapidly increasing (Howard 2002). Diabetes is more prevalent in minority populations. In the NHANES III study, using the criteria of self-reported diabetes or a fasting plasma glucose of at least 126 mg/dL, the prevalence of diabetes in black and Hispanic women was two- to three-times that of white women in the United States (Fig. 36-7). By 60 to 69 years of age, approximately 11% of white women, 13% of white men, 27% of black and Hispanic women, 18% of black men, and 24% of Hispanic men have diabetes.

Diabetes is associated with increased rates of virtually all forms of cardiovascular disease (Howard, 2002). In men, diabetes is associated with a doubling in CHD incidence, and in women with diabetes, CHD incidence is five- to seven-times that of women without diabetes (Dawber, 1980; Stampfer, 1987). Diabetes doubles the rate of MI in men and increases the rate of MI in women four- to six-fold (Dawber, 1980; Lavecchia, 1987; Stampfer, 1987). CHD and MI rates in diabetic women approach those of men of similar age, essentially eliminating the advantage found in nondiabetic women compared with men. This is true for white (Orchard, 1996), Mexican American (Mitchell, 1992), and Japanese (Kuczmarski, 1994) women. Ischemic heart disease mortality is doubled in men with diabetes and tripled in women with diabetes (Barrett-Connor, 1983).

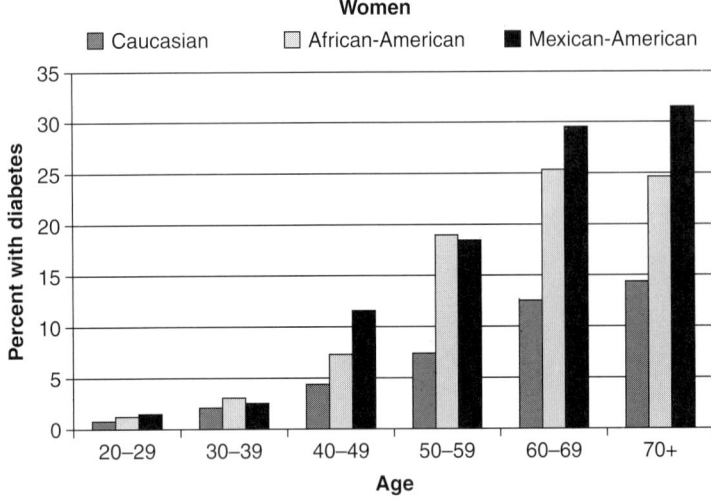

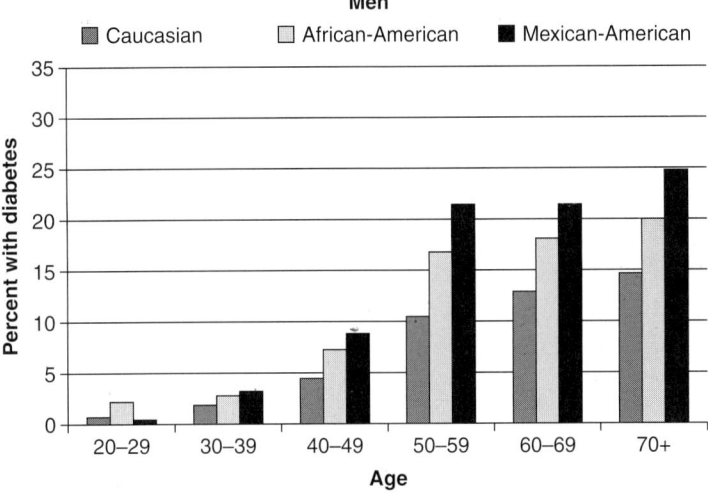

■ **Figure 36–7.** Prevalence of diabetes among U.S. women and men by age and race/ethnicity. (National Center for Health Statistics. *National Health and Nutrition Examination Survey, III, 1988–1994.*)

Rates of other atherosclerotic manifestations such as atherothrombotic stroke and peripheral vascular disease are also higher in diabetic people (Dawber, 1980). The incidence of peripheral vascular disease is five times higher in men and eight times higher in women with diabetes compared with nondiabetic people. Diabetes is associated with a three- to five-fold increase in the incidence of atherothrombotic stroke in men and women (Dawber, 1980; Manson, 1991).

After MI or the diagnosis of CHD, diabetic patients have a significantly poorer prognosis than nondiabetic patients, and this effect is particularly pronounced for women (Khaw, 1986; Wong, 1989). Diabetic patients with MI are two to four times as likely to die in hospital, more often have congestive heart failure and postinfarction angina pectoris, and more often extend their infarct than nondiabetic patients (Stone, 1989).

Among survivors of an initial MI, the incidence of recurrent MI is increased by 30% in diabetic men and almost tripled in diabetic women, whereas fatal CHD is doubled in men and women (Abbott, 1988). During follow-up after MI, total mortality among diabetic patients is 1.5-times to three-times that of nondiabetic patients (Stone, 1989). Whether the degree of control of diabetes after MI affects survival after MI is unknown. Insulin resistance, the primary pathologic process in

type II diabetes, is also associated with CHD. Among nondiabetic adults in the Atherosclerosis Risk in Communities Study (ARIC), women in the highest quintile of fasting insulin had a threefold increase in CHD risk compared with women in the lowest quintile of fasting insulin; however, fasting insulin was not associated with CHD risk in men (Folsom, 1997). In contrast, a study of Finnish men and women found that CHD prevalence increased with increasing fasting plasma insulin levels in diabetic and nondiabetic men and women (Rönnemaa, 1991). A prospective study in England found a 60% increase in risk of fatal and nonfatal MI among men in the tenth decile of serum insulin compared with the first to ninth deciles (Perry, 1996). The differences in these findings in men appear to be related to the degree of insulin elevation; only severe elevations are related to increased risk. The mechanisms responsible for the acceleration of myocardial dysfunction and atherosclerosis associated with diabetes are the subject of great scrutiny (Kaplan, 1989; Simonson, 1991). Diabetes, hyperinsulinemia, and insulin resistance are associated with higher relative weight (specifically with a central body fat distribution); higher systolic and diastolic blood pressure; lower levels of HDL; and higher total cholesterol, HDL, and triglyceride levels (Kaplan, 1989; Kannel, 1984; Manson, 1990; Simonson, 1991). These disturbances, sometimes called the "metabolic syndrome," appear to be linked through a complex set of genetic and environmental factors, and hypotheses about these associations are still being explored.

Although diabetes management has traditionally focused primarily on glycemic control, there is increasing recognition that interventions aimed at cardiovascular disease prevention, including behavioral interventions and pharmacotherapy aimed at treating overweight/obesity, hypertension, lipid disorders, and prothrombotic states, are critical in preventing cardiovascular complications among those with diabetes (Diabetes Control and Complications, 1993; Gaede, 2003; Grundy, 2002).

Recent trials have demonstrated that the onset of diabetes can be postponed or prevented through intensive lifestyle modification. In the Diabetes Prevention Program Study, an intensive lifestyle modification program aimed at modest weight loss (goal 7% loss in body weight) and physical activity (goal 150 minutes of brisk walking per week) in men and women at risk for diabetes decreased diabetes incidence by 58%. The average weight loss in the intervention group was 5.6 kg, versus 0.1 kg in the placebo group (Diabetes Prevention Program, 2002). Similar results were reported from a Finish study that used intensive lifestyle interventions to promote weight loss and increased physical activity in overweight persons with impaired glucose tolerance (Tuomilehto, 2001). These results provide some of the most dramatic and powerful endorsements to date for primary prevention of diabetes through intensive behavioral intervention (see Chapter 43 for further discussion of diabetes).

BODY WEIGHT

The proportion of U.S. adults characterized as overweight and obese is reaching epidemic proportions. Widely, NIH Clinical Guidelines suggest that overweight and obesity be defined as a body mass index of 25.0 to 29.9 kg/m^2 and 30 or greater kg/m^2, respectively (National Institutes of Health, 1998). For example, an individual who is 5 feet 8 inches tall would be overweight at 160 pounds and obese at 200 pounds. Using these definitions, the NHANES surveys show that compared to data collected in 1976 to 1980, in 1999 the age-adjusted prevalence of overweight and obesity increased from 47% to 61% (U.S. Department, 2001). Data from the 2001 Behavioral Risk Factor Survey show that overweight and obesity increase with age, peaking at mid-life, and that the prevalence of obesity is highest in African-American and multiracial individuals, and lowest in Caucasians and those classified as "other" (Fig. 36-8). Of grave concern is the increased prevalence of overweight among children and adolescents in the United States. Using a definition of overweight based on gender- and age-specific BMI >95th percentile, compared to data collected in 1963 to 1970, in 1999 the prevalence of overweight among children aged 6 to 11 years increased from 4% to 13%, and the prevalence among adolescents aged 12 to 19 years increased from 5% to 14% (U.S. Department, 2001). The potential long-term effects on diabetes and cardiovascular disease risks are staggering.

A positive association between obesity and CHD is expected. Hypertension, diabetes, and hypercholesterolemia are all more

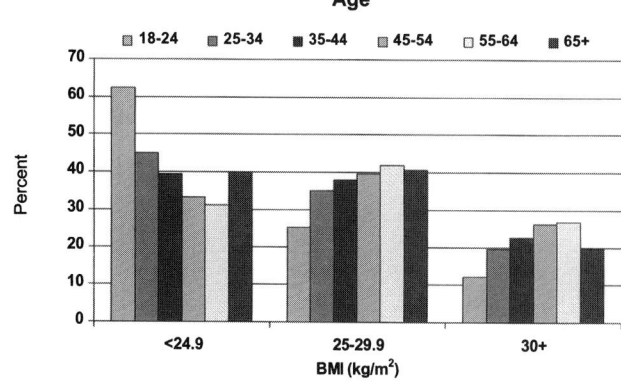

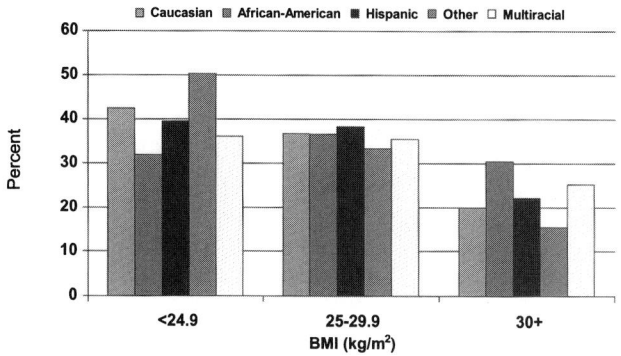

■ **Figure 36–8.** Prevalence of overweight and obesity among U.S. men and women (combined) by age and race/ethnicity. (National Center for Health Statistics.2001 Behavioral Risk Factor Survey. *http://apps.nccd.cdc.gov/brfss/display.asp? cat = RF&yr = 2001&qkey = 4409&state = US.*)

common in overweight people (Van Itallie, 1985), and weight reduction is an important therapy in the management of all CHD risk factors. Nevertheless, findings about the association between body weight and CHD risk are inconsistent. For example, despite the fact that body weight increased for black and white men and women from 1962 through 1980, cardiovascular mortality, stroke, and MI all decreased during this same time. (Barrett-Connor, 1985) In the Framingham Heart Study, men younger than age 50 years who were greater than 30% above ideal weight (determined by Metropolitan Life Insurance tables) had twice the incidence of CHD and acute MI compared with those less than 10% above ideal weight (Hubert, 1983). The findings were similar but of lower magnitude in those older than age 50 years (Hubert, 1983). In a Dutch study of BMI measured at age 18 years in men, the 32-year CHD mortality rate was more than doubled in those in the highest BMI category (Hoffmans, 1989).

Others have found no relationship between BMI and CHD mortality among white men, but a 70% increase in CHD mortality in black men in the 90th percentile of BMI compared with the 50th percentile. Still, other investigators have found no association between BMI and CHD death rates in black or white men (Keil, 1993).

In women, relative weight predicts angina pectoris, CHD other than angina, CHD death, stroke, and congestive heart failure (Hubert, 1983). In the Nurses Health Study, women in the highest quartile of BMI (>29 kg/m^2) had a relative risk of nonfatal MI and fatal CHD of 1.8 and double the risk of angina pectoris compared with women in the lowest BMI quartile (Manson, 1990). These relationships hold even among women of normal or near-normal weight; those with a BMI of 25 to 28.9 kg/m^2 and 23 to 24.9 kg/m^2 had a relative risk for CHD of 2.06 and 1.45, respectively, compared with women with a BMI less than 21 kg/m^2 (Willett, 1995). In the Framingham Heart Study, obese women (Metropolitan Relative Weight $>130\%$) aged 50 years or younger had a 2.4-fold increase in CHD risk over 26 years of follow-up compared with lean women (Metropolitan Relative Weight $<110\%$) (Hubert, 1983). The relationship between overweight and CHD is weaker among black women. In black women, BMI is unrelated to MI (Johnson, 1986; Keil, 1993; Stevens, 1992), CHD death (Keil, 1993; Stevens, 1992), or all-cause mortality (Johnson, 1986; Stevens, 1992).

Overweight also has a role in secondary prevention. Among women who have survived a first MI, a 1-unit increase in BMI is associated with a 3% increase in risk of reinfarction (Newton, 1996).

Overweight continues to play a role in the elderly. Among men and women aged 65 years and older, the total mortality rate is as much as doubled in those above the 70th percentile of BMI compared with those in the 10th to 29th percentile, and the CHD mortality rate is increased by 50% in men and doubled in women (Harris, 1988). Weight gain after the young adult years increases the risk of CHD in men and women (Hubert, 1983; Manson, 1990). In the Nurses Health Study, women who gained 20 to 35 kg after age 18 years had double the risk of nonfatal MI and fatal CHD compared with those who gained less than 3 kg (Manson, 1990).

The role of the distribution of body weight has attracted increasing attention. The primary hypothesis is that a central body weight distribution, often measured as waist-to-hip ratio, increases CHD risk to a greater degree than a more peripheral body weight distribution. In white men, abdominal girth was not associated with total or CHD mortality, although black men in the 90th percentile for abdominal girth had almost double the rate of CHD mortality compared with those in the 50th percentile (Stevens, 1992). These results were reversed in women. There was no association between abdominal circumference and all-cause or CHD mortality in black women, but white women in the 85th percentile of abdominal circumference had a 50% increase in all-cause and CHD mortality compared with those in the 15th percentile (see Chapter 42 for further discussion of obesity).

REPRODUCTIVE HORMONES

Reproductive History

Blood pressure and blood lipids change in relation to reproductive events. It is thus reasonable to investigate the potential impact of these events on the risk of CHD in women. Few studies have examined these factors, and their findings are contradictory. Nulliparous women appear to be at lower risk of CHD than parous women, and a woman's risk of CHD may increase with younger age at first birth (Beard, 1984; LaVecchia & DeCarli, 1987; Palmer, 1992). Increasing parity may also increase CHD risk, perhaps because of the large changes in hormones associated with pregnancy (Palmer, 1992). Others, however, have found no differences in risk with parity and number of births (Colditz, 1987).

Earlier age at menopause increases CHD risk regardless of the mechanism of menopause. Among women who undergo bilateral oophorectomy, those younger than age 35 years have almost eight-times the risk for nonfatal MI compared with natural menopause (Stampfer, 1990). Premenopausal women of any age who undergo bilateral oophorectomy without estrogen replacement therapy have twice the risk of nonfatal MI and fatal CHD compared with premenopausal women of the same age (Stampfer, 1991). At menopause, serum HDL levels decrease and LDL levels increase compared with premenopausal values (Lindquist, 1985; Matthews, 1989).

Oral Contraceptives

The increased risk for fatal and nonfatal MI in users of oral contraceptives (OC) was first established in the 1960s and early 1970s. In these early studies, OC use was associated with an increased risk of nonfatal and fatal MI in young women. In women aged 30 to 39 years, the risk of fatal and nonfatal MI among OC users was three-times that of nonusers. For women aged 40 to 44 years, risk of fatal MI was 5.7-times (Mann & Vesssey, 1975) and risk of nonfatal MI 4.7-times (Mann & Inman, 1975) that of nonusers. Concurrent cigarette smoking acts synergistically with the risk from OCs, with the greatest risk occurring in women who smoke and are older than age 35 years (Croft, 1989; Jick, 1978).

The risk in past users was similar to that in women who had never used OCs (Mann & Vessey, 1975; Mann & Innman, 1975; Slone, 1981; Stampfer, 1988). When duration of past use was examined, use of 5 to 9 years increased the risk of nonfatal MI by 50%, and 10 or more years of use more than doubled the risk. (Slone, 1981). Smoking did not amplify this effect of past use. There are at least two mechanisms for the risk of cardiovascular events associated with OCs. First, OCs increase the risk of arterial and venous thromboembolism. The risk of arterial and venous thrombosis increases with the dosage of estrogen, whereas higher dosages of progestogens increase only the risk of arterial thrombosis (Kelleher, 1990; Meade, 1988). The second possible mechanism for the association between OCs and CHD risk is the promotion of atherogenesis through unfavorable effects on blood pressure, serum lipids, and glucose tolerance (Rosenberg, Palmer, & Lesko, 1990).

Dosages of estrogen and progestin in current OCs are considerably lower than those of the 1970s, and there appears to be little or no risk of MI or CHD death among users of newer OC formulations (Mant, 1998; Sidney, 1998; Stampfer, 1988; Stampfer, 1990). The exception is the finding in some (Croft, 1989; Mant, 1998) but not all (Sidney, 1998) studies of continued high risk among women who are heavy cigarette smokers and OC users. A prospective cohort study in England and Scotland found a five-fold increase in risk of MI among current smokers who used OCs (Mant, 1998). It has been estimated that 9.7% of cases of nonfatal MI among women aged 35 to 44 years in the United States are caused by the combination of smoking and OC use (Goldbaum, 1987). However, a U.S. case-control study of low-dose OCs and MI risk in women aged 18 to 44 years found no increase in risk among smokers (Sidney, 1998). Overall, OCs appear to offer a safe contraceptive alternative in terms of cardiovascular disease risk.

Postmenopausal Hormone Replacement Therapy

The public health implications of HRT have shifted dramatically with the publication of the findings from two landmark randomized, clinical trials: the Heart and Estrogen/Progestin Replacement Study (HERS) and the Women's Health Initiative (WHI). Despite the consistent findings of observational studies that HRT is associated with a 30% to 50% reduction in CHD events in women with (Newton, 1997) and without (Grodstein, 1995; Stampfer, 1991) preexisting CHD, the results of the first randomized trial of the effects of HRT on CHD risk found no benefit (Hulley, 1998). The HERS randomized 2,763 women to placebo or 0.625 mg of conjugated equine estrogens plus 2.5 mg of medroxyprogesterone acetate daily. After 4.1 years of follow-up, the relative risk for MI or CHD death was 0.99, or no difference between the placebo and control groups. In their first year in the trial, women assigned to HRT had a 50% increase in MI and CHD death compared with women assigned to placebo. By years 4 and 5, these relationships were reversed and women assigned to HRT had a 33% reduction in CHD risk compared with women using placebo. The HERS study challenged our understanding of the effects of HRT in women with cardiovascular disease. There was a 50% increase in the relative risk of cardiovascular disease events in the first year of HRT use among women with established coronary disease. Overall, there was no difference in the likelihood of cardiovascular events between placebo and control. Because of the lack of overall benefit and the increased risk in the first year, the HERS investigators concluded that women with coronary disease should not initiate HRT.

In the WHI, the estrogen plus progestin arm (planned duration 8.5 years) was stopped after an average of 5.2 years of follow-up because the overall risks outweighed the benefits of therapy (Writing Group, 2002). Compared to women using placebo, women using estrogen plus progestin had a 29% increase in risk of CHD, a 26% increase in risk of breast cancer, a 41% increased in risk of stroke, a doubling of risk of pulmonary embolus, a 37% decrease in risk of colorectal cancer, and a 44% decrease in risk of hip fracture. Although many of these findings were in the expected direction, the increase in risk of CHD and stroke were unexpected. The study investigators concluded that HRT should not be used for the primary prevention of coronary disease. More recently, the WHI Memory Study reported that estrogen plus progestin was associated with a doubling in dementia risk and with an increased risk of having a significant decline ($\geq$2 SD) in cognitive function (Shumaker, 2003; Rapp, 2003).

Further evidence against a cardiovascular benefit of HRT comes from the ERA trial (Herrington, 2000). In this randomized, controlled trial, neither unopposed estrogen nor estrogen plus progestin altered the progression of angiographically verified coronary disease compared to placebo after a mean of 3.2 ± 0.6 years. A similar trial showed no effect of HRT on progression of carotid atherosclerosis (Angerer, 2001).

Thus, although trial data support a protective effect of HRT against fracture, and possibly colorectal cancer, concerns about breast cancer risk have been confirmed, and hopes that HRT would protect against cardiovascular disease and dementia have been reversed. The American College of Gynecology now recommends that HRT use should be limited to short-term therapy for vasomotor symptoms (ACOG, 2002).

FOLATE AND HOMOCYSTEINE

Homocysteine is an amino acid that is an intermediate byproduct of methionine metabolism. Homocysteine levels are higher in postmenopausal than premenopausal women, lower in women than in men, positively correlated with age, and negatively correlated with serum/plasma levels of folic acid, vitamin B6, and vitamin B12 (Bates, 1997; Dalery, 1995; Malinow, 1999; Selhub, 1993). Homocysteine levels of 5 to 15 μmol/L are considered normal, and elevations of 16 to 30, 31 to 100, and greater that 100 μmol/L are considered moderate, intermediate, or severe, respectively. Methylenetetrahydrofolate (MTHFR) is an enzyme that contributes to the remethylation of homocysteine to methionine. This reaction requires folate as the substrate, and levels of dietary and blood folate are strong determinants of homocysteine levels (Schwartz, 1997). Normally present in only small amounts ($<$10 μmol/L), homocysteine is highly toxic to the vascular endothelium. Homocysteine is associated with endothelial dysfunction, arterial intimal-medial thickening, wall stiffening, and a procoagulant activity (Mangoni, 2002). People with homocysteinuria, a rare autosomal recessive condition in which homocysteine levels are severely elevated, are at extremely high risk for premature atherosclerosis.

Even mild elevations in homocysteine appear to be associated with increased CHD risk, and there is no specific threshold for the association between homocysteine and CHD risk. Numerous observation cohort and case-control studies have been conducted to evaluate the association between homocysteine and various manifestations of cardiovascular disease, including coronary heart disease, stroke, and peripheral vascular disease. The majority of studies show a positive association between homocysteine levels and these conditions (Malinow, 1999; Mangoni, 2002). For example, in a case-control study of MI among women younger than age 45 years, those in the highest quartile ($>$15.6 $m$mol/L) of homocysteine had 2.3-times the risk of MI compared with those in the lowest quartile ($<$10 $m$mol/L). This relationship was reversed for serum folate; women in the highest quartile of folate had half the risk of those in the lowest quartile (Selhub, 1995). Among French Canadians with CHD, 44% of women and 18.1% of men had homocysteine levels greater than the 90th percentile of control levels (Dalery, 1995). Mean homocysteine levels of those with and without CHD were 12.0 ± 6.3 *m*mol/L versus 7.6 ± 4.1 *m*mol/L for women, and 11.7 ± 5.8 *m*mol/L versus 9.7 ± 4.9 *m*mol/L in men. Homocysteine levels are higher in women and men with angiographically confirmed obstruction of one or more major coronary arteries than in those with normal coronaries (Kang, 1986; Robinson, 1995). In the Framingham Heart Study, high plasma homocysteine concentrations and low concentrations of folate were associated with increased risk of extracranial carotid artery stenosis (Selhub, 1995). In ARIC, the relative risk for carotid artery intimal-medial wall thickening among participants in the highest versus the lowest quintiles of plasma homocysteine was 3.2 (Malinow, 1993).

In a 2-year prospective study, HRT was associated with an 11% decrease in homocysteine. The decrease was 17% in women with high homocysteine levels, whereas levels in women with low homocysteine did not change (Van Der Mooren, 1994). Increasing homocysteine after menopause may partially explain the increase in CHD risk associated with aging. Postmenopausal women have an excessive increase in homocysteine after a methionine load compared with premenopausal women, and folic acid supplementation decreases this increase in homocysteine after methionine loading (Brattstrom, 1985).

Despite evidence from observational studies that homocysteine is associated with an increased risk for cardiovascular disease, there is currently no evidence that lowering homocysteine levels will decrease coronary morbidity and mortality. Therefore, population-wide screening of homocysteine is considered inappropriate at this time (Malinow, 1999; Mangioni, 2002). Several randomized, controlled trials are currently underway that will examine the relationship between vitamin supplementation, homocysteine, and coronary and stroke risk.

ANTIOXIDANTS

Epidemiologic findings that antioxidants decrease CHD risk are supported by evidence that oxidized LDL is present in atherosclerotic lesions (Diaz, 1997; Steinbrecher, 1997). The accumulation of lipids in the arterial intima is the hallmark of early atherosclerotic lesions, and oxidation of LDL enhances its accumulation in the arterial wall lesions. Interest in the effects of antioxidants and CHD risk has centered on vitamins E and C and β-carotene (Diaz, 1997; Tribble, 1999). Although observational studies suggested that consumption of foods high in β-carotene might reduce CHD risk (Gaziano, 1994; Tavani, 1997), the results of randomized trials in men (Alpha Tocopheral, 1994; Hennekens, 1996) and men and women (Omenn, 1996) show no benefit of β-carotene supplementation on CHD risk. Similarly, evidence that vitamin C reduces CHD risk is weak or lacking (Gaziano, 1994; Kushi, 1996; Rimm, 1997).

There is evidence of cardiovascular benefit associated with vitamin E (Rimm, 1993; Rimm, 1997; Stampfer, 1993). In the Nurses Health Study, the rate of major CHD was 35% lower among women in the highest quintile of vitamin E consumption compared with women in the lowest quintile (Stampfer, 1993). The authors found that most of the variability in vitamin E consumption was caused by supplements. In the Iowa

Women's Health Study, among women who did not use supplements, women in the highest quintile of vitamin E intake had a 60% reduction in CHD death compared with women in the lowest quintile, but there was no association between vitamin A or vitamin C intake and CHD risk (Kushi, 1996). There is evidence from observational studies and randomized trials of a beneficial effect of increased vitamin E intake in men. Among U.S. male health professionals, there was a 36% reduction in CHD risk among those who consumed more than 60 IU vitamin E per day compared with those who consumed less than 7.5 IU per day (Rimm, 1993). There was a similar reduction in risk among men who took at least 100 IU per day in supplements compared with those who did not. These beneficial effects of vitamin E appear to reduce CHD risk even in the elderly. Users of vitamin E supplements in the Established Populations for Epidemiologic Studies of the Elderly had a 67% reduction in risk for CHD mortality compared with nonusers (Losonczy, 1996). Finally, a randomized trial of 50 mg of vitamin E in male smokers found only a 4% reduction in major coronary events (Vitamo, 1998), whereas in a trial of patients with angiographically proven CHD, supplementation with 400 to 800 IU of vitamin E resulted in a 75% reduction in nonfatal MI compared with placebo (Stephens, 1996). These trials imply that only supplementation at high doses may yield CHD protection. Further randomized trials of the effect of vitamin E on the primary and secondary prevention of CHD in women and men are underway. Recommendations about the use of vitamin E for CHD prevention should await the results of these trials.

CONCLUSIONS

Outstanding progress has been made in our understanding of CHD risk factors and their management. The evidence against cigarette smoking, elevated serum cholesterol, and high blood pressure is strong, and sustained campaigns are underway to prevent and appropriately manage them. The importance of adequate physical activity and weight control is acknowledged, and the American Heart Association now features sedentary lifestyle in its list of risk factors for CHD. Research continues on other emerging risk factors. The focus of future research will be on clarifying the role of these factors, particularly for women and ethnic minorities.

REFERENCES

Abbott, R. D., Donahue, R. P., Kannell, W. B., et al. (1988). The impact of diabetes on survival following myocardial infarction in men vs. women: The Framingham Study. *JAMA, 260*, 3456–3460.

ACOG. (2002). http: and www.acog.org/from_home/publications/press_releases/nr08-30-02.cfm..

Alpha Tocopherol, Beta Carotene Cancer Prevention Study Group (1994). The effect of vitamin E and beta carotene on the incidence of lung cancer and other cancers in male smokers. *New England Journal of Medicine, 330*, 1029–1035.

American Heart Association. (2002). *Heart disease and stroke statistics–2003 Update*. Dallas, Tx: American Heart Association.

Anastos, K., Charney, P., Charon, R. A. et al. (1991). Hypertension in women: What is really known? The Women's Caucus, Working Group on Women's

Health of the Society of General Internal Medicine. *Annals of Internal Medicine,* 115, 287–293.

Angerer, P., Strok, S., Kothny, W., et al. (2001). Effect of oral postmenopausal hormone replacement on progression of atherosclerosis: a randomized, controlled trial. *Arteriosclerosis Thrombosis Vascular Biology,* 21, 262–268.

Austin, M. A., Breslow, J. L., Hennekens, C. H., et al. (1988). Low-density lipoprotein subclass patterns and risk of myocardial infarction. *JAMA,* 260, 1917–1921.

Barrett-Connor, E., Khaw, K. T., & Wingard, D. L. (1987). A ten-year prospective study of coronary heart disease mortality among Rancho Bernardo women. In E. D. Eaker, B. Packard, & N. K. Wenger, et al. (Eds.), *Coronary heart disease in women* (pp. 117–121). New York: Haymarket Doyma.

Barrett-Connor, E., & Wingard, D. L. (1985). Sex differential in ischemic heart disease mortality in diabetics: A prospective population-based study. *American Journal of Epidemiology,* 118, 489–496.

Barrett-Connor, E. L. (1985). Obesity, atherosclerosis, and coronary artery disease. *Annals of Internal Medicine,* 103, 1010–1019.

Bates, C. J., Mansoor, M. A., van der Pols, J., et al. (1997). Plasma total homocysteine in a representative sample of 972 British men and women aged 65 and over. *European Journal of Clinical Nutrition,* 51, 691–697.

Beard, D. M., Fuster, V., & Annergers, J. F. (1984). Reproductive history in women with coronary heart disease: A case-control study. *American Journal of Epidemiology,* 120, 108–114.

Berlin, J. A., & Colditz, G. A. (1990). A meta-analysis of physical activity in the prevention of coronary heart disease. *American Journal of Epidemiology,* 132, 612–628.

Blair, S. N., Kohl, H. W., Paffenbarger, R. S., et al. (1989). Physical fitness and all-cause mortality: A prospective study of healthy men and women. *JAMA,* 262, 2395–2401.

Bostom, A. G., Cupples, L. A., Jenner, J. L., et al. (1996). Elevated plasma lipoprotein(a) and coronary heart disease in men aged 55 years and younger: A prospective study. *JAMA,* 276, 544–548.

Bostom, A. G., Gagnon, D. R., Cupples, L. A., et al. (1994). A prospective investigation of elevated lipoprotein(a) detected by electrophoresis and cardiovascular disease in women: The Framingham Heart Study. *Circulation,* 90, 1688–1695.

Brattstrom, L. E., Hultberg, B. L., & Hardebo, J. E. (1985). Folic acid responsive postmenopausal homocysteinemia. *Metabolism,* 34, 1073–1077.

Brown, G., Albers, J. J., Fisher, L. D., et al. (1990). Regression of coronary artery disease as a result of intensive lipid-lowering therapy in men with high levels of apolipoprotein B. *New England Journal of Medicine,* 323, 1289–1298.

Burke, G. L., Savage, P. J., Sprafka, J. M., et al. (1991). Relation of risk factor levels in young adulthood to parental history of disease. The CARDIA study. *Circulation,* 84, 1176–1187.

Bush, T. L., Fried, L. P., & Barrett-Connor, E. (1988). Cholesterol, lipoproteins and coronary heart disease in women. *Clinical Chemistry,* 34: 660–670.

Centers for Disease Control and Prevention. (1998). CDC Wonder. Mortality. Available: http://wonder.CDC.gov/WONDER.

Chandrashekhar, Y., & Amand, I. S. (1991). Exercise as a coronary protective factor. *American Heart Journal,* 122, 1723–1739.

Colditz, G. A., Willett, W. C., Stampfer, M. J., et al. (1987). A prospective study of age at menarche, parity, age at first birth, and coronary heart disease in women. *American Journal of Epidemiology,* 126, 861–870.

Croft, P., & Hannaford, P. C. (1989). Risk factors for acute myocardial infarction in women: Evidence from the Royal College of General Practitioners' oral contraception study. *BMJ,* 298, 165–168.

Cromwell, J., Bartosch, W. J., Fiore, M. C., et al. (1997). Cost-effectiveness of the clinical practice recommendations in the AHCPR guideline for smoking cessation. *JAMA,* 278, 1759–1766.

Dahlen, G. H., Guyton, J. R., Attar, M., et al. (1986). Association of levels of lipoprotein Lp(a), plasma lipids, and other lipoproteins with coronary artery disease documented by angiography. *Circulation,* 74, 758–765.

Dalery, K., Lussier-Cacan, S., Selhub, J., et al. (1995). Homocysteine and coronary artery disease in French Canadian subjects: Relation with vitamins B$_{12}$, B$_6$, pyridoxal phosphate, and folate. *American Journal of Cardiology,* 75, 1107–1111.

Dawber, T. R. (1980). *The Framingham Study: The epidemiology of atherosclerotic disease.* Cambridge, MA: Harvard University Press.

Diabetes Control and Complications Trial Research Group. (1993). The effect of intensive treatment of diabetes on the development and progression of long-term complications in insulin-dependent diabetes mellitus: The Diabetes Control and Complications Trial Research Group. *New England Journal of Medicine,* 329, 977–986.

Diabetes Prevention Program Research Group. (2002). Reduction in the incidence of type 2 diabetes with lifestyle intervention or metformin. *New England Journal of Medicine,* 346, 393–403.

Diaz, M. N., Frei, B., Vita J. A., et al. (1997). Mechanisms of disease, antioxidants and atherosclerotic heart disease. *New England Journal of Medicine,* 337, 408–416.

Douglas, P. S., Clarkson, T. B., Flowers, N. C., et al. (1992). Exercise and atherosclerotic heart disease in women. *Medical Science Sports Exercise,* 23(Suppl.), S266–S276.

Eaker, E. D., Pinsky, J., & Castelli, W. P. (1992). Myocardial infarction and coronary death among women: Psychosocial predictors from a 20-year follow-up of women in the Framingham Study. *American Journal of Epidemiology,* 135, 854–864.

Eaker, E. D. (1989). Psychosocial factors in the epidemiology of coronary heart disease in women. *Psychiatric Clinics of North America,* 12, 167–173.

Ekelund, L. G., Haskell, W. L., Johnson, J. L., et al. (1988). Physical fitness as a predictor of cardiovascular mortality in asymptomatic North American men: The Lipid Research Clinics mortality follow-up study. *New England Journal of Medicine,* 319, 1379–1384.

Epidemiology Branch, Office on Smoking and Health, National Center for Chronic Disease Prevention and Health Promotion, Division of Health Interview Statistics, National Center for Health Statistics. (1993). Cigarette smoking among adults: United States, 1991. *MMWR Morbidity and Mortality Weekly Report,* 42, 230–233.

Epidemiology Branch, Office on Smoking and Health, National Center for Chronic Disease Prevention and Health Promotion, Centers for Disease Control. (1994). Surveillance for selected tobacco-use behaviors: United States, 1900-1994. *MMWR Morbidity and Mortality Weekly Report,* 43, SS–3.

Epidemiology Branch, Office on Smoking and Health, National Center for Chronic Disease Prevention and Health Promotion, Centers for Disease Control. (2002). Cigarette smoking among adults: United States, 2000. *MMWR Morbidity and Mortality Weekly Report,* 642–1306.

Expert Committee on the Diagnosis and Classification of Diabetes Mellitus. (1997). Report of the Expert Committee on the Diagnosis and Classification of Diabetes Mellitus. *Diabetes Care,* 20, 1183–1197.

Folsom, A. R., Szklo, M., Stevens, J., et al. (1997). A prospective study of coronary heart disease in relation to fasting insulin, glucose, and diabetes. *Diabetes Care,* 20, 935–942.

Friedlander, Y., Arbogast, P., Schwwartz, S. M., et al. (2001). Family history as a risk factor for early onset myocardial infarction in young women. *Atherosclerosis,* 156, 2101–2207.

Gaede, P., Vedel, P., Larsen, N., et al. (2003). Multifactorial intervention and cardiovascular disease in patients with type 2 diabetes. *New England Journal of Medicine,* 348:383–393.

Gaziano, J. M. (1994). Antioxidant vitamins and coronary artery disease risk. *American Journal of Medicine,* 97, 3A-18S-3A-28S.

Glantz, S. A., & Parmleyn, W. W. (1991). Passive smoking and heart disease: Epidemiology, physiology and biochemistry. *Circulation,* 83, 1–12.

Goldbaum, G. M., Kendrick, J. S., Hogelin, G. C., et al. (1987). The relative impact of smoking and oral contraceptive use on women in the United States. *JAMA,* 258, 1339–1342.

Grodstein, F., & Stampfer, M. (1995). The epidemiology of coronary heart disease and estrogen replacement in postmenopausal women. *Progress in Cardiovascular Disease,* 38, 199–210.

Grundy, S. M., Garber, A., Goldberg, R., et al. (2002). Diabetes and Cardiovascular Disease Writing Group IV: Lifestyle and medical management of risk factors. *Circulation,* 105, e153–e158.

Hajjir, I., & Kotchen, T. A. (2003). Trends in prevalence, awareness, treatment, and control of hypertension in the United States, 1998-2000. *JAMA,* 290, 199–206.

Harris, T., Cook, E. F., Garrison, R. et al. (1988). Body mass index and mortality among nonsmoking older persons: The Framingham Heart Study. *JAMA,* 259, 1520–1524.

Haskell, W. L., Leon, A. S., Caspersen, C. J., et al. (1992). Cardiovascular benefits and assessment of physical activity and physical fitness in adults. *Medical Science Sports Exercise,* 24(Suppl.), S201–S220.

Hennekens, C. H., Buring, J. E., Manson, J. E., et al. (1996). Lack of effect of long-term supplementation with beta carotene on the incidence of malignant neoplasms and cardiovascular disease. *New England Journal of Medicine,* 334, 1145–1149.

Hermanson, B., Omenn, G. S., Kronmal, R. A., et al. (1988). Beneficial six-year outcome of smoking cessation in older men and women with coronary artery disease: Results from the CASS registry. *New England Journal of Medicine,* 319, 1365–1369.

Herrington, D. M., Reboussin, D. M., Brosnihan, K. B., et al. (2000). Effects of estrogen replacement on the progression of coronary-artery atherosclerosis. *New England Journal of Medicine, 343,* 522–9.

Hoffmans, M. D. A. F., Kromhout, D., & De Lezenne Coulander, C. (1989). Body mass index at the age of 18 and its effects on 32-yearmortality from coronary heart disease and cancer. *Journal of Clinical Epidemiology, 42,* 513–520.

Howard, B. V., Rodriques, B. L., Bennett, P. H., et al. (2002). Prevention Conference VI: Diabetes and Cardiovascular Disease Writing Group I: Epidemiology. *Circulation, 105,* e132–e137.

Hubert, H. B., Feinleib, M., McNamara, P. M., et al. (1983). Obesity as an independent risk factor for cardiovascular disease: A 26-year follow-up of participants in the Framingham Heart Study. *Circulation, 67,* 968–977.

Hulley, S., Grady, D., Bush, T., et al. (1998). Randomized trial of estrogen plus progestin for secondary prevention of coronary heart disease in postmenopausal women. Heart and Estrogen/progestin Replacement Study (HERS) Research Group. *JAMA, 280,* 605–13.

Hypertension Detection and Follow-up Program Cooperative Group. (1988). Persistence of reduction in blood pressure and mortality of participants in the hypertension detection and follow-up program. *JAMA, 259,* 2113–2122.

Jensen, G., Nyboe, J., Appleyard, M., et al. (1991). Risk factors for acute myocardial infarction in Copenhagen: II. Smoking, alcohol intake, physical activity, obesity, oral contraception, diabetes, lipids, and blood pressure. *European Heart Journal, 12,* 298–308.

Jick, H., Dinan, B., & Rothman, K. J. (1978). Oral contraceptives and nonfatal myocardial infarction. *JAMA, 239,* 1403–1406.

Johnson, J. L., Heineman, E. F., Heiss, G., et al. (1986). Cardiovascular disease risk factors and mortality among black women and white women aged 40–64 years in Evans County, Georgia. *American Journal of Epidemiology, 123,* 209–220.

Jousilahti, P., Puska, P., Vartiainen, E., et al. (1996). Parental history of premature coronary heart disease: An independent risk factor of myocardial infarction. *Journal of Clinical Epidemiology, 49,* 497–503.

Kang, S., Wong, P. W. K., Cook, H. Y., et al. (1986). Protein-bound homocysteine, a possible risk factor for coronary artery disease. *Journal of Clinical Investigation, 77,* 1482–1486.

Kannel, W. B., et al. (1984). Report of Inter-Society Commission for Heart Disease Resources: Optimal resources for primary prevention of atherosclerotic diseases. *Circulation, 70,* 181A.

Kannel, W. B. (1987). New perspectives of cardiovascular risk factors. *American Heart Journal, 114,* 213–219.

Kannel, W. B. (1987). Status of risk factors and their consideration in antihypertensive therapy. *American Journal of Cardiology, 59,* 80A–90A.

Kaplan, N. M. (1989). The deadly quartet: Upper-body obesity, glucose intolerance, hypertriglyceridemia, and hypertension. *Archives of Internal Medicine, 149,* 1514–1520.

Kaufman, D. W., Helmrich, S. P., Rosenberg, L. et al. (1983). Nicotine and carbon monoxide content of cigarette smoke and the risk of myocardial infarction in young men. *New England Journal of Medicine, 308:* 409–413.

Keil, J. E., Gazes, P. C., Loadholt, C. B., et al. (1987). Coronary heart disease mortality and its predictors among women in Charleston, South Carolina. In E. D. Eaker, B. Packard, & N. K. Wenger, et al. (Eds.), *Coronary heart disease in women* (pp. 90–98). New York: Haymarket Doyma.

Keil, J. E., Sutherland, S. E., Knapp, R. G., et al. (1993). Mortality rates and risk factors for coronary disease in black as compared with white men and women. *New England Journal of Medicine, 329,* 73–78.

Kelleher, C. C. (1990). Clinical aspects of the relationship between oral contraceptives and abnormalities of the hemostatic system: Relation to the development of cardiovascular disease. *American Journal of Obstetrics and Gynecology, 163,* 392–395.

Kelsey, J. L., Thompson, W. D., & Evans, A. S. (1986). *Methods in observational epidemiology.* New York: Oxford University Press.

Khaw, K. T., & Barrett-Connor, E. (1986). Prognostic factors for mortality in a population-based study of men and women with a history of heart disease. *Journal of Cardiopulmonary Rehabilitation, 6,* 474–480.

Kitagawa, W. M., & Hauser, P. M. (1973). *Differential mortality in the United States: A study of socioeconomic epidemiology.* Cambridge, MA: Harvard University Press.

Kraus, J. F., Borhani, N. O., & Franci, C. E. (1980). Socioeconomic status, ethnicity, and risk of coronary heart disease. *American Journal of Epidemiology, 111,* 407–414.

Kuczmarski, R. J., Flegal, K. M., Campbell, S. M. et al. (1994). Increasing prevalence of overweight among US adults: The National Health and Nutrition Examination Surveys, 1960 to 1991. *JAMA, 272,* 205–211.

Kushi, L. H., Folsom, A. R., Prineas, R. J., et al. (1996). Dietary antioxidant vitamins and death from coronary heart disease in postmenopausal women. *New England Journal of Medicine, 334,* 1156–1162.

Kwiterovich, P. O., Coresh, J., Smith, H. H., et al. (1992). Comparison of the plasma levels of apolipoproteins B and A-1, and other risk factors in men and women with premature coronary artery disease. *American Journal of Cardiology, 69,* 1015–1021.

LaCroix, A. Z., Lang, J., Scherr, P., et al. (1991). Smoking and mortality among older men and women in three communities. *New England Journal of Medicine, 324,* 1619–1625.

LaCroix, A. Z., & Omenn, G. S. (1992). Older adults and smoking. *Clinics in Geriatric Medicine, 8,* 69–87.

Last, J. M. (1988). *A dictionary of epidemiology* (2nd ed.). New York: Oxford University Press.

LaVecchia, C., DeCarli, A., Franceshi, S., et al. (1987). Menstrual and reproductive factors and the risk of myocardial infarction in women under fifty-five years of age. *American Journal of Obstetrics and Gynecology, 157,* 1108–1112.

LaVecchia, C., Franceshi, S., Decarli, A., et al. (1987). Risk factors for myocardial infarction in young women. *American Journal of Epidemiology, 125,* 832–843.

Lindquist, O., Bengtsson, C., & Lapidus, L. (1985). Relationships between the menopause and risk factors for ischaemic heart disease. *Acta Obstetrica Gynecologica Scandia Suppl, 130,* 43–47.

Losonczy, K. G., Harris, T. B., & Havlik, R. J. (1996). Vitamin E and vitamin C supplement use and risk of all-cause and coronary heart disease mortality in older persons: The Established Populations for Epidemiologic Studies of the Elderly. *American Journal of Clinical Nutrition, 64,* 190–196.

Malinow, M. R., Bostom, A. G., & Krauss, R. M. (1999). Homocyst(e)ine, diet, and cardiovascular diseases: a statement for healthcare professionals from the Nutrition Committee, American Heart Association. *Circulation, 99,* 178–82.

Malinow, M. R., Nieto, F. J., Szklo, M., et al. (1993). Carotid artery intimalmedial wall thickening and plasma homocysteine in asymptomatic adults. *Circulation, 87,* 1107–1113.

Mangoni, A. A., & Jackson, S. H. (2002). Homocysteine and cardiovascular disease: current evidence and future prospects. *American Journal of Medicine, 112,* 556–65.

Mann, J. I., & Inman, W. H. W. (1975). Oral contraceptives and death from myocardial infarction. *BMJ, 2,* 245–248.

Mann, J. I., Vessey, M. P., Thorogood, M., et al. (1975). Myocardial infarction in young women with special reference to oral contraceptive practice. *BMJ, 2,* 241–245.

Manolio, T. A., Pearson, T. A., Wenger, N. K., et al. (1992). Cholesterol and heart disease in older persons and women: Review of an NHLBI workshop. *Annals of Epidemiology, 2,* 161–176

Manson, J. E., Colditz, G. A., Stampfer, M. J., et al. (1991). A prospective study of maturity-onset diabetes mellitus and risk of coronary heart disease and stroke in women. *Archives of Internal Medicine, 151,* 1141–1147.

Manson, J. E., Colditz, G. A., Stampfer, M. J., et al. (1990). A prospective study of obesity and risk of coronary heart disease in women. *New England Journal of Medicine, 322,* 882–889.

Mant, J., Painter, R., & Vessey, M. (1998). Risk of myocardial infarction, angina and stroke in users of oral contraceptives: An updated analysis of a cohort study. *British Journal of Obstetrics and Gynaecology, 105,* 890–896.

Marenberg, M. E., Risch, N., Berkman, L. F., et al. (1994). Genetic susceptibility to death from coronary heart disease in a study of twins. *New England Journal of Medicine, 330,* 1041–1046.

Matthews, K. A., Kelsey, S. F., Meilhan, E, N., et al. (1989). Educational attainment and behavioral and biologic risk factors for coronary heart disease in middle-aged women. *American Journal of Epidemiology, 129,* 1132–1144.

Matthews, K. A., Meilhan, E., Kuller, L. H., et al. (1989). Menopause a risk factor for coronary heart disease. *New England Journal of Medicine, 321,* 641–646.

Meade, T. W. (1988). Risks and mechanisms of cardiovascular events in users of oral contraceptives. *American Journal of Obstetrics and Gynecology, 158,* 1646–1652.

Medical Research Council Working Party. (1992). Medical research council trial of treatment of hypertension in older adults: Principal results. *BMJ, 304,* 405–412.

Medical Research Council Working Party. (1985). MRC trial of treatment of mild hypertension: Principal results. *BMJ, 291,* 97–104.

Mitchell, B. D., Haffner, S. M., Huzuda, H. P., Patterson, J. K., et al. (1992). Diabetes and coronary heart disease risk in Mexican-Americans. *Annals of Epidemiology, 2,* 101–106.

National Center for Health Statistics, U.S. of Health and Human Services (DHHS). (1997). *Third National Health and Nutrition Examination Survey, 1988-1994, NHANES III Data File (CD-ROM Series II, No 1). Public Use Data File.* Hyattsville, MD: Centers for Disease Control and Prevention.

National Institutes of Health (NIH). (1998). *National Heart, Lung, and Blood Institute (NHLBI). Clinical guidelines on the identification, evaluation, and treatment of overweight and obesity in adults.* Bethesda, MD: HHS, Public Health Service (PHS).

Newton, K. M., LaCroix, A. Z., McKnight, B., et al. (1997). Estrogen replacement therapy and prognosis after first myocardial infarction. *American Journal of Epidemiology, 145,* 269–277.

Newton, K. M., & LaCroix, A. Z. (1996). Association of body mass index with reinfarction and survival after first myocardial infarction. *Journal of Women's Health, 5,* 433–444.

Nyboe, J., Jensen, G., Appleyard, M., et al. (1989). Risk factors for acute myocardial infarction in Copenhagen: I. Hereditary, educational and socioeconomic factors. Copenhagen City Heart Study. *European Heart Journal, 10,* 910–916.

Oldridge, N. B., Guyatt, G. H., Fischer, M. E., et al. (1988). Cardiac rehabilitation after myocardial infarction, combined experience of randomized clinical trials. *JAMA, 260,* 945–950.

Omenn, G. S., Goodman, G. E., Thornquist, M. D., et al. (1996). Effects of a combination of beta carotene and vitamin A on lung cancer and cardiovascular disease. *New England Journal of Medicine, 334,* 1150–1155.

Orchard, T. J. (1996). The impact of gender and general risk factors on the occurrence of atherosclerotic vascular disease in non-insulin-dependent diabetes mellitus. *Annals of Medicine, 28,* 323–333.

Palmer, J. R., Rosenberg, L., & Shapiro, S. (1992). Reproductive factors and risk of myocardial infarction. *American Journal of Epidemiology, 136,* 408–416.

Pell, S., & Fayerweather, W. E. (1985). Trends in the incidence of myocardial infarction and associated mortality and morbidity in a large employed population, 1957-1983. *New England Journal of Medicine, 312,* 1005–1011.

Perry, I. J., Wannamethee, S. G., Whincup, P. H., et al. (1996). Serum insulin and incident coronary heart disease in middle-aged British men. *American Journal of Epidemiology, 144,* 224–234.

Pina, I. L., Apstein, C. S., Balady, G. J., et al. (2003). Exercise and heart failure, a statement from the American Heart Association Committee on Exercise, Rehabilitation, and Prevention. *Circulation, 107,* 1210–1225.

Ramsay, L. E., & Yeo, W. W. (1991). Hypertension and coronary artery disease: An unsolved problem. *Journal of Cardiovascular Pharmacology, 18*(Suppl.), S31–S34.

Rapp, S. R., Espland, M. A., Shumaker, S. A., et al. (2003). Effect of estrogen plus progestin on global cognitive function in postmenopausal women, The Women's Health Initiative Memory Study: A Randomized controlled trial. *JAMA, 289,* 2663–2672.

Rimm, E. B., Stampfer, M., Ascherio, A., et al. (1993). Vitamin E consumption and the risk of coronary heart disease in men. *New England Journal of Medicine, 328,* 1450–1456.

Rimm, E. B., & Stampfer, M. J. (1997). The role of antioxidants in preventive cardiology. *Current Opinion in Cardiology, 12,* 188–194.

Robinson, K., Mayer, E. L., Miller, D. P., et al. (1995). Hyperhomocysteinemia and low pyridoxal phosphate, common and independent reversible risk factors for coronary artery disease. *Circulation, 92,* 2825–2830.

Roncaglioni, M. C., Santoro, L., D'Avanzo, B., et al. (1992). Role of family history in patient with myocardial infarction: An Italian case-control study. GISSI-EFRIM investigators. *Circulation, 85,* 2065–2072.

Rönnemaa, T., Kaakso, M., Pyörälä, K., et al. (1991). High fasting plasma insulin is an indicator of coronary heart disease in non—insulin-dependent diabetic patients and nondiabetic subjects. *Arteriosclerosis and Thrombosis, 11,* 80–90.

Rosamond, W. D., Chambless, L. E., Folsom, A. R., et al. (1998). Trends in the incidence of myocardial infarction and in mortality due to coronary heart disease, 1987 to 1994. *New England Journal of Medicine, 339,* 861–867.

Rosenberg, L., Palmer, J. R., Lesko, S. M., et al. (1990). Oral contraceptive use and the risk of myocardial infarction. *American Journal of Epidemiology, 131,* 1009–1016.

Rosenberg, L., Palmer, J. R., & Shapiro, S. (1990). Decline in the risk of myocardial infarction among women who stop smoking. *New England Journal of Medicine, 322,* 213–217.

Rothman, K. J. (1986). *Modern epidemiology.* Boston: Little, Brown.

Salonen, J. T. (1980). Stopping smoking and long-term mortality after acute myocardial infarction. *British Heart Journal, 43,* 463–469.

Schwartz, S. M., Siscovick, D. S., Malinow, M. R., et al. (1997). Myocardial infarction in young women in relation to plasma total homocysteine, folate, and a common variant in the methylenetetrahydrofolate reductase gene. *Circulation, 96,* 412–417.

Selhub, J., Jacques, P. F., Bostom, A. G., et al. (1995). Association between plasma homocysteine concentrations and extracranial carotid-artery stenosis. *New England Journal of Medicine, 332,* 286–291.

Selhub, J., Jacques, P. F., Wilson, P. W. F., et al. (1993). Vitamin status and intake as primary determinants of homocysteinemia in an elderly population. *JAMA, 270,* 2693–2698.

Sempos, C., Cooper, R., Kovar, M. G., et al. (1988). Divergence of the recent trends in coronary mortality for the four major racesex groups in the United States. *American Journal of Public Health, 78,* 1422–1427.

SHEP Cooperative Research Group. (1991). Prevention of stroke by antihypertensive drug treatment in older persons with isolated systolic hypertension: Final results of the systolic hypertension in the elderly program (SHEP). *JAMA, 265,* 3255–3264.

Shumaker, S. A., Legault, C. L., Rapp, S. R., et al. (2003). Estrogen plus progestin and the incidence of dementia and mild cognitive impairment in postmenopausal women, The Women's Health Initiative memory study: A randomized controlled trial. *JAMA, 289,* 2651–2662.

Sidney, S., Siscovick, D. S., Petitti, D. B., et al. (1998). Myocardial infarction and use of low-dose oral contraceptives: A pooled analysis of 2 US studies. *Circulation, 98,* 1058–1063.

Simonson, D. C., & Dzau, V. J. (1991). Workshop IX: Lipids, insulin, diabetes. *American Journal of Medicine, 90*(Suppl. 2A), 85S–86S.

Slattery, M. L., & Jacobs, D. R. (1988). Physical fitness and cardiovascular disease mortality: The US Railroad Study. *American Journal of Epidemiology, 127,* 571–580.

Slone, D., Kaufman, D. W., Shapiro, S., et al. (1981). Risk of myocardial infarction in relation to current and discontinued oral contraceptive use. *New England Journal of Medicine, 305,* 420–424.

Slone, D., Shapiro, S., Rosenberg, L., et al. (1978). Relation of cigarette smoking to myocardial infarction in young women. *New England Journal of Medicine, 298,* 1273–1276.

Sobolski, J., Kornitzer, M., Backer, G. D., et al. (1987). Protection against ischemic heart disease in the Belgian physical fitness study: Physical fitness rather than physical activity? *American Journal of Epidemiology, 125,* 601–610.

Stampfer, M. J., Colditz, G. A., Willett, W. C., et al. (1987). Coronary heart disease risk factors in women: The Nurses' Health Study experience. In E. D. Eaker, B. Packard, N. K. Wenger, et al. (Eds.), *Coronary heart disease in women* (pp. 112–116). New York: Haymarket Doyma.

Stampfer, M. J., Colditz, G. A., & Willett, W. C. (1990). Menopause and heart disease: A review. *Annals of the New York Academy of Scivience, 592,* 193–203.

Stampfer, M. J., & Colditz, G. A. (1991). Estrogen replacement therapy and coronary heart disease: A quantitative assessment of the epidemiologic evidence. *Preventive Medicine, 20,* 47–63.

Stampfer, M. J., Hennekens, C. H., Manson, J. E., et al. (1993). Vitamin E consumption and the risk of coronary heart disease in women. *New England Journal of Medicine, 328,* 1450–1456.

Stampfer, M. J., Willett, W. C., Colditz, G. C., et al. (1988). A prospective study of past use of oral contraceptive agents and risk of cardiovascular diseases. *New England Journal of Medicine, 319,* 1313–1317.

Stampfer, M. J., Willett, W. C., Colditz, G. C., et al. (1990). Past use of oral contraceptives and cardiovascular disease: A meta-analysis in the context of the Nurses' Health Study. *American Journal of Obstetrics and Gynecology, 163,* 285–291.

Stampfer, M. U., Hennekens, C. H., Manson, J. E., et al. (1993). Vitamin E consumption and the risk of coronary disease in women. *New England Journal of Medicine, 328,* 1444–1449.

Stein, J. H., & Rosenson, R. S. (1997). Lipoprotein Lp(a) excess and coronary heart disease. *Archives of Internal Medicine, 157,* 1170–1176.

Steinbrecher, U. P. (1997). Dietary antioxidants and cardioprotection: Fact or fallacy? *Canadian Journal of Physiology and Pharmacology, 75,* 228–233.

Stephens, N. G., Parsons, A., Schofiled, P. M., et al. (1996). Randomized controlled trial of vitamin E in patient with coronary disease: Cambridge Heart Antioxidant Study. *Lancet, 347,* 781–786.

Stevens, J., Keil, J. E., Rust, P. F., et al. (1992). Body mass index and body girths as predictors of mortality in black and white women. *Archives of Internal Medicine, 152,* 1257–1262.

Stone, P. H., Muller, J. E., Hartwell, T., et al. (1989). The effect of diabetes mellitus on prognosis and serial left ventricular function after acute myocardial infarction: Contribution of both coronary disease and diastolic left ventricular dysfunction to the adverse prognosis. *Journal of the American College of Cardiology, 12,* 49–57.

Szklo, M., Tonascia, J., & Gordis, L. (1976). Psychosocial factors and the risk of myocardial infarction in white women. *American Journal of Epidemiology,* 103, 312–320.

Talbott, E., Kuller, L. H., Detre, K., et al. (1977). Biologic and psychosocial risk factors for sudden death from coronary disease in white women. *American Journal of Cardiology,* 39, 858–864.

Tavani, A., Negri, E., Avanzo, B. D., et al. (1997). Beta-carotene intake and risk of nonfatal acute myocardial infarction in women. *European Journal of Epidemiology,* 13, 631–637.

Thompson, P. D. (1988). The benefits and risks of exercise training in patients with chronic coronary artery disease. *JAMA,* 259, 1537–1540.

Tribble, D. L. (1999). Antioxidant consumption and risk of coronary heart disease: Emphasis on vitamin C, vitamin E, and β-carotene. A statement from healthcare professionals from the American Heart Association. *Circulation,* 99, 591–595.

Tuomilehto, J., Lindstrom, J., Eriksson, J. G., et al. (2001). Finnish Diabetes Prevention Study Group. Prevention of type 2 diabetes mellitus by changes in lifestyle among subjects with impaired glucose tolerance. *New England Journal of Medicine,* 344(18), 1343–50.

U.S. Department of Health and Human Services. (2001). *The Surgeon General's call to action to prevent and decrease overweight and obesity.* Rockville, MD: U.S. Department of Health and Human Services, Public Health Service, Office of the Surgeon General. Available from: US GPO, Washington.

U.S. Department of Health and Human Services. (1996). *Physical activity and health: A report of the Surgeon General.* Atlanta, GA: U.S. Department of Health and Human Services, Centers for Disease Control and Prevention, National Center for Chronic Disease Prevention and Health Promotion.

Van Der Mooren, M. J., Wouters, M. G., Blom, H. J., et al. (1994). Hormone replacement therapy may reduce high serum homocysteine in postmenopausal women. *European Journal of Clinical Investigation,* 24, 733–736.

Van Itallie, T. B. (1985). Health implication of overweight and obesity in the United States. *Annals of Internal Medicine,* 103, 983–988.

Vitamo, J., Rapola, M. J., Ripatti, S., et al. (1998). Effect of vitamin E and beta carotene on the incidence of primary nonfatal myocardial infarction and fatal coronary heart disease. *Archives of Internal Medicine,* 158, 668–675.

Wild, S. H., Laws, A., Fortmann, S. P., et al. (1995). Mortality for coronary heart disease and stroke for six ethnic groups in California, 1985 to 1990. *Annals of Epidemiology,* 5, 432–439.

Willett, W. C., Green, A., & Stampfer, M. J. (1987). Relative and absolute excess risks of coronary heart disease among women who smoke cigarettes. *New England Journal of Medicine,* 317, 1303–1309.

Willett, W. C., Manson, J. E., Stampfer, M. J., et al. (1995). Weight, weight changes, and coronary heart disease in women, risk within the "normal" weight range. *JAMA,* 273, 461–465.

Wilson, P. W. F. (1990). High-density lipoprotein, low-density lipoprotein and coronary artery disease. *American Journal of Cardiology,* 66, 7A–10A.

Wong, N. D., Cupples, L. A., Ostfeld, A. M., et al. (1989). Risk factors for long-term coronary prognosis after initial myocardial infarction: The Framingham Study. *American Journal of Epidemiology,* 130, 469–480.

Wong, N. D., Wilson, P. W. F., & Kannel, W. B. (1991). Serum cholesterol as a prognostic factor after myocardial infarction: The Framingham Study. *Annals of Internal Medicine,* 115, 687–693.

Writing Group for the Women's Health Initiative Investigators. (2002). Risks and benefits of estrogen plus progestin in healthy postmenopausal women: principal results from the Women's Health Initiative randomized controlled trial. *JAMA,* 288, 321–33.

Psychosocial Risk Factors: Assessment and Management Interventions

SIMONE K. MADAN • ERIKA SIVARAJAN FROELICHER

Over the past several decades, much wisdom and knowledge have been gained about coronary heart disease (CHD). Despite enormous research efforts, traditional risk factors and genetics fail to fully explain either the development or the course of the disease. Consistent with biopsychosocial models of health, studies have now demonstrated that psychological and social factors are also related to the development of and recovery from heart disease. In health schemas that consider the mind and body, emotions and feelings have usually been linked to aspects of the body. Our language is full of expressions that describe this attachment, "feelings of joy that make your heart flutter" or anxiety that causes "butterflies in your stomach." Since early times, emotions have also been specifically attached to the heart. William Harvey (1578–1657), who first described the circulatory system, wrote "every affliction of the mind that is attended with either pain or pleasure, hope or fear, is the cause of an agitation whose influence extends to the heart" (Jenkins, 1978). In this chapter we summarize the evidence relating psychological and social factors to CHD and describe ways that nurses can assess and manage selected psychosocial risk factors to promote cardiovascular and psychosocial health.

PSYCHOSOCIAL RISK FACTORS AND CHD

Several psychosocial factors have been identified as risk factors or prognostic factors for CHD. These include depression, anxiety, social isolation, low perceived social support, socioeconomic status, type A personality, hostility, job stress, and acute life events (Lynch et al., 1995; Hemingway & Marmot, 1999; Bunker et al., 2003; ENRICHD Investigators, 2003). Among these, the association of depression and social support with CHD has been most well established as independent risk factors for CHD as shown in Table 37-1 (Hemingway et al, 2003).

Depression and CHD

Depression is a clinical diagnosis, defined by a complex classification system that includes major and minor depression

and takes into consideration the number, frequency and duration of symptoms and signs (American Psychiatric Association, 1994). In this chapter we use depression (major and minor) as all inclusive. There is substantial empirical evidence from well-designed population studies (Barefoot & Schroll, 1996; Pratt et al., 1996) and review papers (Hemingway & Marmot, 1999; Bunker et al., 2003) that depression is a risk factor for CHD. Furthermore, depression is also a prognostic factor for patients with CHD (Carney et al., 1987, 1988; Fielding, 1991; Frasure-Smith et al., 1996; Hemingway & Marmot, 1999; Bunker et al., 2003), as is supported by high prevalence rates of depression in CHD populations. Depression is found in about 6% of the general population, whereas 16%–25% of the CHD population are reported to have depression (Carney et al., 1987, 1988; Fielding, 1991; Frasure-Smith et al., 1996). Women are especially at a higher risk because they are twice more likely to be depressed than men in the general population (Nolen-Hokesema, 1990). In addition to women, depression is also significantly higher among individuals with low income and less education (Kessler et al., 2003). Regardless of the severity of the CHD, patients with depression are three- to four-times more likely to die in the first year after an MI compared to those with no depression (Frasure-Smith et al., 1993, 1995b). Patients who were depressed had a subsequent 17% event rate compared to 3% in non-depressed patients 6 months after an MI (Frasure-Smith et al., 1993).

Depression can lead to social withdrawal and lower participation in activities such as exercise (Beck et al., 1979; Cole et al., 1997). The combination of depression and CHD can therefore present a significant challenge for patients recovering from a cardiac event. Depressed patients have more difficulty adopting and maintaining healthy lifestyle behaviors (Allison et al., 1995). Depressed patients with CHD consistently report higher smoking rates compared with non-depressed patients with CHD (Carney et al., 1987; Littman, 1993). For example, in elderly patients after an MI, depression scores predicted the performance of self-care behaviors related to risk reduction (Conn et al., 1991). In patients attending cardiac rehabilitation, anxiety, depression, and coping abilities predicted 1-year leisure-time activity and higher smoking cessation

Table 37–1 ■ PSYCHOSOCIAL RISK FACTORS AND CHD: SUMMARY OF PROSPECTIVE STUDIES

	Number of Reports of Etiological Studies (n = 70)				Number of Reports of Prognostic Studies (n = 92)			
	−	0	+	++	−	0	+	++
Depression	0	8	5	9	0	16	7	11
Social support	0	3	4	2	0	7	4	10
Anxiety	0	4	1	3	1	9	4	4
Type A behavior/hostility	1	11	5	1	3	10	1	1
Work characteristics	0	3	5	5	0	2	2	0

− Finding counter to hypothesis; 0 Lack of clear association;
+ Moderate association (RR ≥ 1.50 and < 2.00); ++ Strong association (RR ≥ 2.00)
Borrowed with permission from Hemingway, H., Kuper, H., Marmot, M. (2003). Psychosocial factors in the primary and secondary prevention of coronary heart disease: a systematic review. In S. Yusuf, J. A. Cairns, E. Fallen, B. J. Gersch & A. J. Camm (Eds.), *Evidence based cardiology*. London: British Medical Journal Publishing.

(Guiry et al., 1987). In relation to functional impairments, only 38% of the patients with depression versus 63% of non-depressed returned to work within 3 months after a cardiac event (Wells et al., 1989). Depression is also associated with delay in seeking medical treatment due to minimization of cardiac symptoms (Finnegan & Suler, 1985; Blumenthal & Williams, 1982) and lower medication compliance (Carney et al., 1988, 1995). In addition to the individual health consequences of depression in CHD patients, there are tremendous economic costs affecting society. The economic cost of increased hospitalizations for recurrent cardiac events and longer hospital stays is also associated with higher emotional distress. The average cost for a depressed cardiac patient is more than four times the cost for a non-depressed patient (Allison et al., 1995).

Social Support and CHD

Social support is defined based on quality of the structure and function of social relationships. Structural support reflects the number and frequency of social interactions, social ties, and networks (Antonucci & Johnson, 1994; Smith et al., 1994). Functional support focuses on the type of function provided by the support such as tangible aid, emotional comfort and care as well as the value or importance the individual places on the support (Antonucci & Johnson, 1994; Smith et al., 1994). However, structural and functional support alone fails to account for individual perceptions and beliefs about the support, nor does it take into consideration the necessary social skills needed to elicit support from others; whether or how much support is needed or is acceptable and who should provide it, as well as whether one deserves to receive support or the concern for cost of seeking support (Vinokur et al., 1987). Individual differences need to be considered because what one person may consider as valuable support may in another person engender feelings of obligation or guilt. Gender or ethnic differences may influence attitudes and beliefs about support (Pitula et al., 1999). The definition of social support in research substantiating the social support association with CHD is highly varied, consisting of definitions being based on marital status, or being single, to measurement of social support that considers a high level of complexity.

Social support from others decreased the incidence of cardiac events in men without CHD (Ortho-Gomer et al., 1993).

One important form of social support can be derived from a marital relationship. Marital relationships perceived as satisfactory are associated with decreased mortality (Bretcht et al., 1994). However, marital problems are associated with poor health outcomes since social connections can also lead to stress if perceived needs or expectations are not met. Higher likelihood of mortality in cardiac patients has been associated with low perceived support or lack of support in case of a single marital status (Ebrahims et al., 1995; Gorkin et al., 1993; Williams et al., 1992).

In addition, it appears that lack of social support is also a risk factor if cardiac disease is already well established. Case and colleagues (1992) examined social networks by comparing recurrent cardiac events in post-MI patients. Patients who lived alone had a 50% increased risk for subsequent events. In patients with MI, CHF, or both, those with no sources of emotional support had a twofold risk of a subsequent event (Berkman et al., 1992; Krumholz et al., 1998). In examining gender differences, high marital distress in women was associated with three-times higher risk of recurrent coronary events (Ortho-Gomer et al., 2000)

Low social support seems to influence lack of necessary behavioral change after an MI. "Unmarried" patients with higher rates of smoking are less likely to stop smoking compared to married patients, and marital separation at the time of the MI decreases the likelihood of giving up smoking (Rankin-Esquer et al., 1997). Men who are cardiac patients receive more support for their participation from their spouses than women cardiac patients (Nyamathi et al., 1992). During or after a hospitalization, distress can surface even in a satisfactory relationship if coping resources get challenged or spouses become overprotective, which may be perceived as stressful for the patient (Coyne & Delongis, 1986). On the other hand, an MI can exacerbate existing distress in a high conflict relationship when there is lack of emotional or functional support in response to a time of high need for nurturing (Wishnie et al., 1971). In fact, a divorced or separated marital status has been suggested as an independent risk factor for a MI (Pratt et al., 1996). Perhaps social support influences physiological factors and behavioral factors that promote "heart healthy behaviors" which are reinforced by support and encouragement. These provide a sense of intimacy, belonging while promoting competence and self efficacy (Berkman, 1995). Although we lack a clear understanding of how social support protects the patient with CHD, it appears such protection exists.

Anxiety and CHD

High levels of anxiety are related to increased incidence of heart disease. Men who report two or more symptoms of anxiety are three times more likely to have a fatal CHD event than men without symptoms of anxiety (Kawachi et al., 1994). Similar associations have been reported for phobic anxiety symptoms and for high levels of chronic worry among patients with CHD (Kawachi et al., 1994a; Kubansky et al., 1997). The presence of symptoms of anxiety during a hospitalization increases the risk of recurrence of cardiac events independent of depression (Frasure-Smith et al., 1995b). In patients with acute MI, high levels of anxiety were associated with increased in-hospital complications, including acute ischemia, arrhythmias, functional impairments, re-infarction and sudden cardiac death (Ahern et al., 1990; Hayward, 1995; Kawachi et al., 1994a; Moser & Dracup, 1996). Anxious cardiac patients without adequate support and education are more likely to smoke, to have higher cholesterol, hypertension and diabetes mellitus (Kawachi et al., 1994a) and can be fearful of physical activity (Grace et al., 2002).

Hostility/Anger

After years of research examining the relationship between type A behavior and CHD, hostility and anger emerged as risk factors for CHD (King, 1997). Hostility has been redefined to include behavioral, affective, and cognitive components. *Expressive hostility* refers to the expression of overt behaviors, such as anger expression, aggressive or rude behaviors, or assaultive behaviors (Smith, 1992). *Potential for hostility* refers to the tendency to experience the emotion of anger and resentment in daily life (Smith, 1992). Hostile cognitions include appraisals/perceptions of others as distrustful and attributions of others as causing frustration and mistreatment. Studies of hostility in adults support the association between hostility and CHD morbidity and mortality. Men with high hostility, followed for 9 years, had a twofold risk for MI, even after controlling for behavioral risk factors such as smoking, alcohol intake, and body mass index (Everson et al., 1997; Julkunen et al., 1994; Kawachi et al., 1996; Mittleman et al., 1995). The link between anger and hostility with cardiac reactivity suggests an important physiologic pathway for triggering cardiovascular events. Expression of acute anger has been reported to lead to a coronary event within 2 hours (Follick et al., 1990); increased platelet aggregation and thrombogenesis (Malkoff et al., 1993), plaque rupture and occlusion have been hypothesized as the most likely mechanisms (Muller et al., 1994). High levels of hostility were also predictive of restenosis after angioplasty (Goodman et al., 1996). Whether hostility is also a prognostic factor for CHD is not known (Hemingway & Marmot, 1999; King 1997).

Acute Stress or Stressful Life Events

There is good evidence that acute stress or life events can trigger cardiac events. Observational studies have examined exposure to sudden stresses such as natural disasters on the incidence of cardiac events. The incidence of fatal and nonfatal myocardial infarction (MI) in Los Angeles County significantly increased on the day of the Northridge earthquake compared with rates before and after the earthquake (Kloner et al., 1997). In contrast, mortality rates for other types of heart disease, such as cardiomyopathy or cerebrovascular disease, were not increased. Similar increases were observed after major Japanese earthquakes and the 1991 Gulf War missile attacks in Israel. These studies are unable to exclude the effects of increased physical stress brought on by exertion. Interestingly, data from both the Israel missile attacks and from Japanese earthquakes suggest that the incidence of MI and CHD mortality was greater in women than in men. Post-traumatic stress scores were also higher in Japanese women than in men, suggesting that mental stress could be a trigger of these coronary events (Kark et al., 1995; Suzuki et al., 1997). There is some suggestive evidence that in the hour after high levels of negative emotions, the risk for ischemic episodes doubles (Gullette et al., 1997). Some have suggested that lower socioeconomic groups appear to have increased incidence of CHD because of the effects of exposure to stressful life events. It has been argued that lower social class reflects less dominance and control over one's environment that can be stressful; other factors, such as lack of access to medical care or engaging in unhealthy lifestyle behaviors, may be an alternative explanation.

Acute stress can also lead to arrhythmias and sudden cardiac death in patients with CHD (Goldstein & Niaura, 1992). The effects of mental stress (with a stimulus being arithmetic problems) have been evaluated during angiography: it found that stenosed coronary artery segments responded to mental stress by constricting, whereas normal segments typically responded by dilating (Yeung et al., 1991). Studies using challenging, timed video games have demonstrated similar results. Comparisons of mental and physical activity stress tests found that mental stress produces higher diastolic blood pressure and lower heart rate responses than physical activity (Rozanski et al., 1988). These studies suggest that ischemia occurring in response to mental stress might be accounted for by inappropriate vasoconstrictor responses. However, since the effects of exposure to severe stress cannot be ethically evaluated in experimental human studies, conclusive statements about its effects cannot be made.

Job Stress

Several observational studies have attempted to link chronic work stress with the precipitation of coronary events. Higher numbers of MI occur in the early morning hours and are associated with morning increases in catecholamines. Weekly patterns suggest approximately a 20% increase in MI incidence on Mondays, with the lowest rates occurring on Saturdays and Sundays (Spielberg et al., 1996). Some relate this increased incidence with return to a stressful workplace environment; others have suggested that lifestyle habits associated with work versus weekend leisure time account for this difference. Occupational stress has been posited as the explanation for the increase in CHD mortality observed among blue-collar workers. As more women enter the workforce, some have suggested that women will experience increased cardiovascular events.

When CHD risk factors were examined in middle-aged women in Rancho Bernardo, California, employed women had significantly lower lipids and glucose levels than unemployed women. In the same study, employed women tended to smoke fewer cigarettes and exercised more than unemployed women (Kritz-Silverstein et al., 1992). This suggests that factors other than employment status explain observed associations. Low levels of support from coworkers and supervisors have also been associated with elevated blood pressure after accounting for factors such as cigarette smoking (Matthews et al., 1987). Such findings led to the suggestion that workers who have job strain (high job demands and a low amount of control) would be more likely to acquire CHD (Schwartz et al., 1988). Studies using this assessment of "job strain" have, however, shown both positive and negative associations with CHD mortality (Hlatky et al., 1995; Karasek et al., 1981). Therefore, researchers suggest that other job factors, including support from coworkers, job security, and juggling family and job demands, likely influence whether employment is experienced as a stressor. Similarly, what one person experiences as stress, another may view as a stimulating and exciting experience. Overall, clearly substantiated evidence supporting the causal relationship between job stress and CHD is still absent (Bunker et al., 2003; Smith et al., 2002).

MECHANISMS FOR PSYCHOSOCIAL RISK FACTORS AND CHD

Two theories that offer the most likely explanation for the link between psychosocial risk factors and CHD are the neuroendocrine response theory and the behavioral mechanisms theory, or a combination of the two theories. Based on the neuroendocrine response theory, a state of physiologic arousal is engendered in response to real or imagined threats or stressors (Lazarus & Folkman, 1984). The physiologic responses to stressors have been described as the "fight-or-flight" responses (Selye, 1956). Neuroendocrine response systems are activated, triggering the release of cortisol and catecholamines (epinephrine [adrenaline] and norepinephrine) that initiate a variety of physiologic responses (Fig. 37-1).

Circulating levels of plasma lipids are also increased; platelet and macrophage cells are activated to release chemotactic and cytotoxic substances. Cardiovascular responses include increased heart rate, blood pressure, muscle and myocardial oxygen demands, and accelerated blood flow. Increased blood flow triggers a cascade of endothelial vascular responses, including release of nitric oxide to promote vasodilation, stimulation of platelets to release chemoattractants and promote thrombosis, and activation of macrophages. Activated macrophages enhance phagocytic activity and have been implicated in the development of atherosclerotic foam cells and the destabilization and rupture of the fibrous cap surrounding atherosclerotic plaque (for details see reviews by Adams, 1994, and McCarty & Gold, 1996).

The above theory leads to speculation about connection between physiological responses and behavioral responses to negative states. Negative affective states perpetuate behaviors such as social withdrawal, lack of pleasurable activities, chronic angry outbursts, and disconnection from support, which can have an adverse impact on cardiac physiology. Lower heart rate variability and decreased parasympathetic nervous system activity in depressed patients has been associated with ventricular fibrillation (Frasure-Smith et al., 1995). Those with hostile traits usually have higher blood pressure, heart rate, and neuroendocrine responses, such as cortisol release, in frustrating or harassing

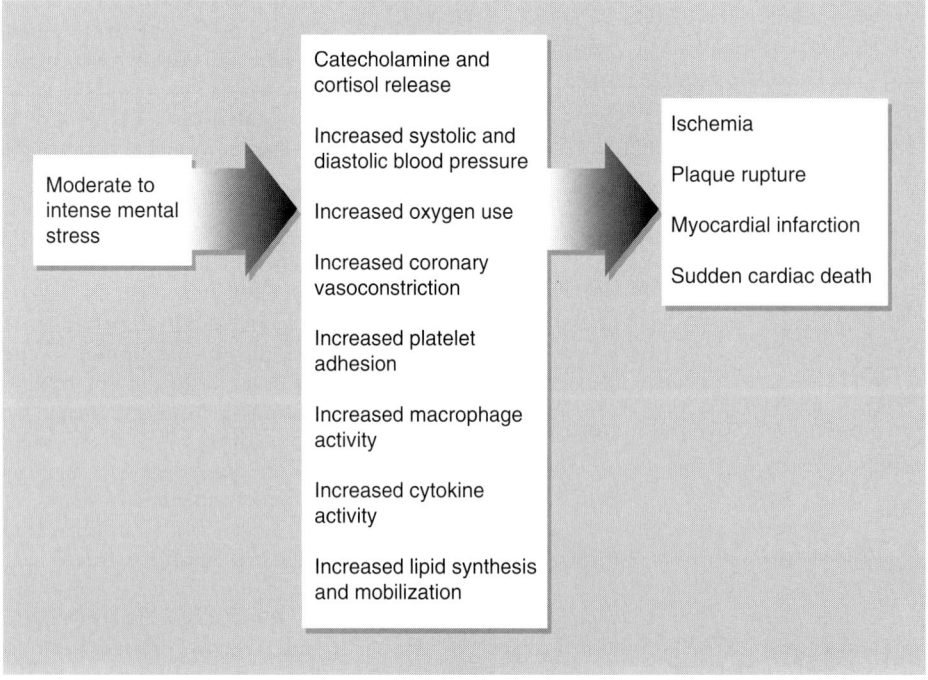

■ **Figure 37–1.** Physiologic mechanisms linking stress and coronary heart disease.

situations (Smith, 1992). When the negative emotions of depression, anger, and anxiety were simultaneously evaluated in the same group of patients with MI, both depression and anxiety were significant independent predictors of subsequent cardiac events (Frasure-Smith et al., 1996). In this study, the authors divided events into thrombogenic events (infarction or unstable angina) or arrhythmic events, and found that anxiety and a past history of depression were associated with thrombogenic events, whereas current depression and anger were associated with arrhythmic events. The study authors speculate that mechanisms such as enhanced platelet adhesion leading to plaque instability and thrombosis might account for these results. These biologic pathways have yet to be tested.

Alternatively, patients who experience psychosocial risk factors may be less compliant with risk reduction strategies, and it may be the non-compliant behaviors that are the mechanism associated with the development of CHD, and its prognosis. Longstanding negative behaviors such as inadequate self care, smoking, lack of exercise, high-calorie diet, and inadequate sleep are likely to contribute to development of CHD and unless modified following an MI continue to increase susceptibility towards future events. Both of these theories may explain the link between psychosocial risk factors and CHD.

ASSESSMENT OF PSYCHOSOCIAL RISK FACTORS

Nurses in any practice setting are encouraged to evaluate patients not only for the traditional risk factors but also for psychosocial risk factors. Next, a brief description of subjective and objective assessment of depression, low perceived social support, anxiety, and hostility and anger are given. It is important to note that several of these psychosocial risk factors may be present at the same time.

Depression

Depression is diagnosed by taking a constellation of symptoms in consideration and requires the skills of a licensed mental health practitioner. However, nurses are in a pivotal role through their extensive contact with cardiac patients to recognize or screen for depression. Several brief and reliable screening tools exist that can be used by nurses to identify patients at high risk for depression. Even in a busy clinic or hospital setting, two questions can be asked: "During the past month, have you often been bothered by feeling down, depressed, and hopeless?" and "During the past month, have you often been bothered by having little interest or pleasure in doing things?" These can identify depression (Whooley & Simon, 2000). For both questions the response options are yes/no. If "no" is given to both questions, then the patient is unlikely to have major depression; if "yes" is answered to either question, then perform a follow-up clinical interview. Other screening tools are the Beck Depression Inventory, the Center for Epidemiological Studies Depression Scale (CES-D), and the Geriatric Depression Scale (GDS). The Beck Depression Inventory is a self-report 21-item scale that has been used with cardiac and other medical patients

(Beck et al., 1961). It is a valid and reliable tool (Beck et al., 1988) that yields response scores ranging from 0 to 63, with a score of 10 to 16 being considered mildly depressed, 17 to 29 moderately depressed, and more than 30 as severely depressed. The CES-D is another 20-item self-report questionnaire based on the frequency of the symptom occurrence in the past week (Radloff, 1977). The Geriatric Depression Scale (GDS) is a 30-item screening instrument with yes/no responses and specifically developed for the elderly. It can be used in the presence of physical illness and is considered to be a reliable and valid instrument (Yesavage et al., 1983). The choice of screening instrument depends on clinician's skill and comfort, patient population, experience with the clinical interpretation of the instrument, and the available time and resources.

Social Support

The ENRICHD Social Support Instrument (ESSI) is a seven-item, five-point Likert scale developed using several other social support scales that are predictive of mortality. The first four questions use the stem, "Is there someone available to you: (1) whom you can count on to listen to you when you need to talk; (2) to give you advice about a problem; (3) who shows you love and affection; (4) to help you with daily chores?" The next two questions ask, "Can you count on anyone to provide you with emotional support (talking over problems or helping you make a difficult decision)?" and "Do you have as much contact as you would like with someone you feel close to, in someone you can trust in and confide?" (ENRICHD Investigators, 2001b). The Likert scale response options range from 1 to 5, in which 1 = none of the time, 2 = little of the time, 3 = some of the time, 4 = most of the time, and 5 = all of the time. The last question is a yes/no question: "Are you currently married or living with a partner?" Scoring needs to be added and the criteria for low perceived social support is based on five items (i.e., items 1, 2, 3, 5, and 6) of seven items. The criteria is met if the score is less than or equal to 2 on at least two of the five items listed and a total score of less than 18. The timing of the assessment of social support is crucial. Most individuals experience an artificial inflation of support at the time of the hospitalization as friends and family may mobilize to respond to the crisis. However a more realistic assessment of support is likely to occur after discharge from the hospital (Pitula & Daugherty, 1995). Because people with few social ties and little structural support have a significantly poorer prognosis than those with complex social networks, the size and quality of the patient's network should also be evaluated. If the patient lives alone, he or she should be asked if they have someone who usually provides support for them (e.g., driving them to a doctor's appointment). Questions such as, "how may times per week do you visit with friends or relatives," or "how many times per week do you attend a community or social event, such as church" can provide key information for evaluating social support.

Additional Assessments

If time allows one can also administer PRIME-MD, then a diagnostic two-part instrument that combines 27 self-report screening questions and short clinical interview modules (Spitzer et al., 1994). The interview modules are based on the psychiatric diagnostic criteria of the *Diagnostic and Statistical Manual of Mental Disorders, III-R* and can identify depressive disorders, panic disorder, generalized anxiety disorder, eating disorder and alcohol abuse. PRIME-MD is a practical and useful tool designed for medical practices (Table 37-2).

The brief self-report screen for depression has two yes/no items similar to the above-mentioned instrument. "During the past month, have you been bothered a lot by little interest or pleasure in doing things and feeling down, depressed or hopeless?" If either item is answered as a "yes," then a short interview module for depression can be conducted. The three screening items for anxiety are "During the past month, have you been often bothered by "nerves" or feeling anxious or on edge; worrying about a lot of different things" and "During the past month, have you had an anxiety attack (suddenly feeling

fear or panic)." A "yes" response to one of these leads to the anxiety interview module. Other screens for anxiety include the State Trait Anxiety Inventory, a 40-item standardized questionnaire that has been used in several nursing studies (Van Der Ploeg et al., 1980). Excessive anxiety or phobias can also be evaluated in CHD patients by using the Crown-Crisp Experiential Index (Kawachi et al., 1994). Hostility is frequently measured by a Cook-Medley Hostility Inventory, a 50-item questionnaire of the Minnesota Multiphasic Personality Inventory (MMPI). An adaptation of this questionnaire and scoring method is provided in a book by R. Williams for lay audiences (Williams & Williams, 1993). Patients could use this resource for self-assessment and education.

Patients may manifest one of more of the above psychosocial manifestations, one of the most important contributions that a nurse working with cardiac patients can make is to refer patients meeting the above diagnostic/assessment criteria to a licensed mental health professional for a complete professional evaluation and "work up" and initiation of a suitable treatment plan.

Table 37–2 ■ PRIME-MD (PRIMARY CARE EVALUATION OF MENTAL DISORDERS), DIAGNOSTIC ASSESSMENT FOR DEPRESSION AND ANXIETY—PATIENT QUESTIONNAIRE

Instructions: This questionnaire will help your health provider better understand problems that you may have.

During the PAST MONTH, have you often been bothered by....

1.	stomach pain	Y	N
2.	back pain	Y	N
3.	pain in your arms, legs, or joints (knees, hips etc.)	Y	N
4.	menstrual pain or problems	Y	N
5.	pain or problems during sexual intercourse	Y	N
6.	headaches	Y	N
7.	chest pain	Y	N
8.	dizziness	Y	N
9.	fainting spells	Y	N
10.	feeling your heart pound or race	Y	N
11.	shortness of breath	Y	N
12.	constipation, loose bowels or diarrhea	Y	N
13.	nausea, gas, or indigestion	Y	N
14.	feeling tired or having low energy	Y	N
15.	trouble sleeping	Y	N
16.	the thought that you have a serious undiagnosed disease	Y	N
17.	your eating being out of control	Y	N
18.	little interest or pleasure in doing things	Y	N
19.	feeling down depressed or hopeless	Y	N
20.	"nerves" or feeling anxious or on edge	Y	N
21.	worrying about a lot of different things	Y	N
22.	have you had an anxiety attack (suddenly feeling fear or panic)	Y	N
23.	have you thought you should cut down your drinking of alcohol	Y	N
24.	has anyone complained about your drinking	Y	N
25.	have you felt guilty or upset about your drinking	Y	N
26.	was there ever a single day in which you had five or more drinks of beer, wine, or liquor	Y	N

Overall would you say your health is:
　　Excellent
　　Very Good
　　Good
　　Fair
　　Poor

Borrowed with permission from: Spitzer, R., Williams, J.B., Linzer, M. et al. (1994). Utility of a new procedure for diagnosing mental disorders in primary care: The PRIME-MD 1000 study. *JAMA, 272,* 1749–1756.

MANAGEMENT INTERVENTIONS FOR PSYCHOSOCIAL RISK FACTORS

A majority of research on psychosocial interventions has examined its effects on decreasing cardiac morbidity and mortality. The mixed results or small effect sizes from such inquiries in the last decade have been attributed to many factors: insufficient sample sizes; individual versus group based interventions; heterogeneous targets of intervention: behavioral, physiological or emotional distress reduction; length of treatment; lack of biological or cardiac endpoints as outcome variables (Linden, 2000; Smith & Ruiz, 2002). Enhanced Recovery in Coronary Heart Disease (ENRICHD), a multi-center randomized controlled clinical trial, is the first large study to test if an intervention aimed to reduce depression and improve social support can reduce mortality and CHD morbidity. This was a study of 2481 MI patients that included a broad distribution of age, gender, ethnicity, and race. ENRICHD was unable to demonstrate that treatment had a mortality benefit (ENRICHD, 2003). However, ENRICHD did demonstrate a statistically significant reduction in depression and improvement in social support adding up to a better quality of life in patients who received psychosocial intervention. Another study, Sertraline Antidepressant Heart Attack Randomized Trial (SADHART), conducted concurrently to test if pharmacological management of depression alone can reduce CHD mortality, also failed to improve survival (Glassman et al., 2002). Despite these results, the role of depression and social support in the development and maintenance of cardiac disease is well established; hence, the interest in developing and implementing psychosocial interventions to modify behavioral risk factors, decrease emotional distress (particularly depression), and improve quality of life continues to be a focus of treatment delivery as an adjunct to cardiac medical and surgical procedures (Smith & Ruiz, 2002; ENRICHD, 2003).

During recovery from coronary events, nurses have many opportunities to educate, motivate, facilitate, and provide psychosocial interventions to their patients. It is highly desirable that nurses initiate such interventions while the patients are still in the hospital as the first few months are critical for survival after a coronary event. Also an acute medical crisis is often the time when patients are more willing and motivated to consider lifestyle changes. For example, in one study smoking cessation rates were 70% among patients after an MI versus 9% for smokers in the general population (Feinstein et al., 1999). Similarly they may be more receptive to treatment of their psychosocial risk factors. The experience of ENRICHD study was that patients' interest in treatment waned after some time and that they often wanted to put the experience of a cardiac event behind them (ENRICHD Investigators, 2001a). Therefore, the first few months after an event lend a window of opportunity for early and intense intervention while the patient might still be motivated to make lifestyle changes. Most patients are receptive to education and informational support during the acute phase of a cardiac event. These interventions can provide a sense of control, decrease anxiety and improve self-efficacy. The psychosocial management interventions described below target physiological arousal, negative behaviors and negative attitudinal cycles. Nurses can present these in an educational way.

Self-Monitoring of Negative Reactions/Responses

An important part of any intervention includes the recognition by the nurse of the degree of the patient's self-awareness of their behaviors and emotions. Acute coronary events are overwhelming and can initially invoke denial (ENRICHD, 2001a) making it difficult for patients to sort out their reactions to such an event. For many patients, even prior to such an acute event, there is lack of awareness or discomfort with emotional reactions if these are considered to be harmful or unimportant by them (Billings et al., 1996). Denial, a useful coping response in the short term, can lead to avoidance or minimization of symptoms and a lack of investment in making lifestyle changes in the long term (Hackett & Cassem, 1975; Mayou et al., 1978). It can lead to unchallenged negative assumptions and negative emotional states that foster increased helplessness and hopelessness, and thus impede problem solving and may lead to social disconnectedness. Cognitive behavioral treatment is useful in understanding one's reactions and modifying assumptions that lead to negative emotions and behaviors. It is a short-term structured treatment that collaboratively focuses on current problems to develop mood management skills, new strategies to handle difficult situations, self-therapy skills and can be applied to problems related to anxiety, anger, stress, social isolation and maladaptive behaviors in addition to depression (Beck, 1995). This can be administered as an individual or a group treatment. Cognitive behavioral therapy (Beck et al., 1979) has been well established as an effective treatment for depression (Elkin et al., 1989; Agency for Health Care Policy and Research, 1993). Evidence-based guidelines for treatment of depression recommend the use of cognitive behavioral therapy (CBT) for mild to moderate depression.

There are several studies of cardiac patients including ENRICHD (Allan & Scheidt, 1998; Billings et al., 1996; Burell, 1996; Bracke & Thoresen, 1996; Carney et al., 1987;

ENRICHD, 2003) that have used this treatment to increase the awareness of automatic assumptions about self, others and the world as well as implement strategies and skill building to improve mood by evaluating assumptions, engage in positive behaviors, practice behavior drills, improve interactions with others and to increase self-efficacy and self-esteem. CBT emphasizes that a major stressful event such as a CABG or everyday stressors associated with recovery can lead to negative reactions at multiple levels—attitudinal cognitions (thoughts), emotional, physiological and behavioral. For example, a successful entrepreneur who built his career at the expense of fostering relationships and who experiences significant physical weakness associated with recovery from his CABG, may react to it by having thoughts such as "I am useless or worthless, I will never be able to work like before, I will have to quit." This leads to depressed mood, fatigue and behaviors such as sleeping excessively, not initiating support and when at home not taking his medication that might worsen his physical symptoms. This may be followed by more negative thoughts (Fig. 37-2). If he becomes aware of his assumptions, it may help him to re-evaluate his cognitions and improve his mood by taking action such as seeking reliable information. However, the lack of awareness may lead to prolonged negative mood states and poor health outcome.

Another patient may experience chest tightness and aches associated with his surgery. He responds through negative thoughts such as "what if the doctor missed something" or "this could be another heart attack." This can lead to anxiety and worry. Worry may manifest in behaviors such as the patient seeking frequent reassurance. Once the patient is home, the manifestation of the anxiety can be in behaviors such as frequent phone calls to the physician, avoiding being alone, avoiding engaging in activities, or hyper-monitoring of physical sensations which further perpetuate anxiety states. A

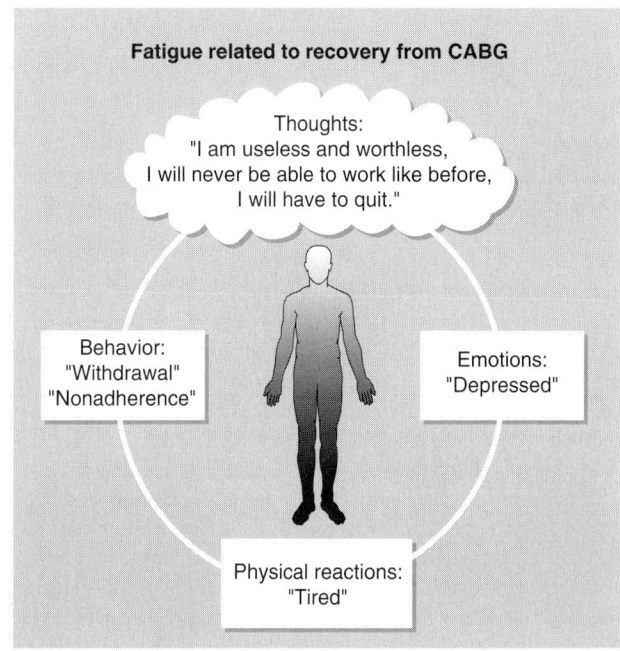

■ **Figure 37–2.** An example of cognitive and behavioral responses to stressful situations.

patient who is a sole provider for his large family may feel discouraged by his fatigue. He prematurely returns to work because of fear of losing his job as a waiter. He also takes back the responsibility of driving his children to three different schools before going to work because his wife does not drive. Engaging in these commitments without receiving social support while still in the recovery phase increases his fatigue, his fear, and possibly leads to slower recovery.

A woman patient anxious of losing affection from others because of her decreased ability to take care of others may dismiss indicators of fatigue or physical discomfort and push herself, overdo her activities, or postpone going to cardiac rehabilitation. Similarly, another woman patient trying to impress others and seek approval may make unrealistic demands on herself for her recovery and may also dismiss her need for rest when exhausted, reject offers for help, and may have setbacks and complications. These examples highlight the negative beliefs or thoughts that perpetuate negative "heart health" behaviors that are harmful during recovery from an acute coronary event.

For patients who are receptive, nurses can help them increase their awareness of automatic and often false appraisals of stressful events. Patients can be encouraged to journal these self-observations. If nurses have assessed the patient for psychosocial risk factors and are listening to patients' verbal and nonverbal communications, they can assist patients in increasing their awareness of automatic reactions through some gentle, non-confrontational questioning. This would be of great therapeutic value. They can also educate their patients about the impact of such automatic reactions on their recovery while normalizing these automatic reactions. It is also important to teach patients that such self-observation would be more effective if it is performed in a curious and respectful manner rather than with a self-critical or perfectionistic attitude. This has been promoted in several large research trials (Burell, 1996; Bracke & Thoresen, 1996).

Decreasing Physiological Arousal

Educating a CHD patient about the benefits of relaxation training and its direct impact on decreasing sympathetic nervous system arousal and increasing heart rate variability which is associated with increased parasympathetic activity is likely to be quite compelling. Relaxation training is a standard part of many large scale research trials, including (Recurrent Coronary Prevention Project (RCPP), Project New Life and ENRICHD (Burell, 1996; Bracke & Thoresen, 1996; Billings et al., 1996; ENRICHD, 2000) and can be used in clinical settings. This training can serve as a tool for increased self-awareness of responses to daily stressors and a method to decrease physiological arousal. Studies have demonstrated the beneficial effects of repeated practice of relaxation in decreasing cortical arousal, decreasing breathing rate, decreasing sympathetic nervous system activity, increasing heart rate variability, improving sleep and emotional states (Freidman et al., 1996). In addition, decreasing physiological arousal has the additional benefit of providing a neutral perspective for reevaluating stress-related perceptions (Benson, 1975*)*. A patient can be provided with a rationale that is followed by practice of a relaxation exercise. Relaxation techniques are

easily learned by most patients, can offer a sense of control, and can be an effective tool for managing pain while still in the acute setting (Stuart-Shor, 1996). There are several relaxation methods that vary in terms of a focal point of breath, muscle groups, image or phrase/word. Relaxation involves focused attention on one of these focal points. A common recommendation is to practice daily for approximately 20 minutes and have several repetitions of shorter versions throughout the day (Display 37-1). Many cardiac rehabilitation programs also include relaxation techniques as an integral part of the program that may be particularly useful for patients with high arousal states because of anxiety, anger, and depression.

Another method of managing physiological arousal is through exercise. However, the first step again is to educate the patients about the rationale for exercise. Physiological explanations can be compelling including role of exercise regimens in decreasing hypertension, decreasing weight, increasing heart rate variability, decreasing heart rate and thereby decreasing the oxygen demand that benefits the patient by raising the threshold for angina symptoms. This lesser need for oxygen and improvement in angina related to exercise training could motivate patients to make changes (Blumenthal et al., 2000; Stahle et al., 1999; Stein, 1996). Exercise also seems to improve a sense of self-efficacy and decreases negative mood states (Stein, 1996).

DISPLAY 37-1

A CLASSIC EXAMPLE OF A RELAXATION EXERCISE

Transcendental Meditation

1. Sit quietly in a comfortable position.
2. Close your eyes.
3. Deeply relax all your muscles, beginning at your feet and progressing up to your face. Keep them relaxed.
4. Breathe through your nose. Become aware of your breathing. As you breathe out, say the word, "ONE," silently to yourself. For example, breathe IN.... OUT, "ONE"; IN.... OUT, "ONE"; etc. Breathe easily and naturally.
5. Continue for 10–20 minutes. You may open your eyes to check the time, but do not use an alarm. When you finish, sit quietly for several minutes, at first with your eyes closed and later with your eyes opened. Do not stand up for a few minutes.
6. Do not worry about whether you are successful in achieving a deep level of relaxation. Maintain a passive attitude and permit relaxation to occur at its own pace. When distracting thoughts occur, try to ignore them by not dwelling upon them and return to repeating "ONE." With practice, the response should come with little effort. Practice the technique once or twice daily, but not within two hours after any meal, since the digestive processes seem to interfere with the elicitation of the Relaxation Response.

From Benson, H. (1975). *Relaxation response* (pp. 114–115). New York: William Morrow.

Interventions for Depression and Anxiety

In everyday life, chronic stress increases vulnerability toward developing negative emotional states of depression, anxiety, and anger. These are often accompanied by negative lifestyle behaviors that further contribute to the wear and tear of the cardiovascular system. Lack of exercise, lack of pleasant activities, and inadequate diet and sleep increase vulnerability to more stress, creating a vicious cycle (Buselli & Stuart, 1999). Treating depression and anxiety can improve compliance with medication and heart-healthy behaviors such as exercise and diet (Lane et al., 1999).

First and foremost, it is important to recognize that depression and anxiety are associated with negative lifestyle behaviors such as smoking, excessive drinking and eating, decreased exercise, hostile behaviors, and social withdrawal. Patients with moderate to severe depression are likely to have multiple negative behaviors and several unsuccessful attempts with changing their negative health behaviors. These patients require consultation from psychiatry services and are likely to need professional help. Some patients with less severe depression are likely to respond well to encouragement to engage in positive activities that increase connection with others or increase sense of accomplishment through activities or a combination of the two. For example, encourage initiating contact with family and friends, having a meal with a friend, exercising with a friend, going to a lecture, working on a home project etc. Such activity scheduling is a hallmark of cognitive behavioral treatment of depression (Beck et al., 1979). The rationale of such an intervention is that these activities are pleasant because they foster connections with others or give a sense of accomplishment, improving emotional states. However, the choice of satisfactory activity is individually based. In one exercise study, those who adhered to exercise had greater reductions in anxiety and depression than nonadherers (Fontana et al., 1986; Byrne & Byrne, 1993). The relationship between adherence to exercise and improvement in psychological variables was also seen in a community study of older adults (King et al., 1993). Participation in exercise was related to lower depression and anxiety (Stein, 1996). Thus exercise training as an intervention has the dual benefit of improved cardiovascular health and self-esteem (Benson, 1975) and important intervention for patients who are anxious or depressed. Patients and their families need to be educated about the benefits of exercise and referral to cardiac rehabilitation should be facilitated. For patients who are fearful of exercise, initial supervised trials of exercise would help build confidence and get them engaged in exercise.

Depression and anxiety are also self-perpetuated by the negative perceptions, beliefs and thoughts in response to stressful situations. The successful entrepreneur gets depressed when he perceives that his physical weakness after CABG reflects a "permanent situation" and that he will "never be able to work like before." He takes these thoughts or perceptions to be "facts." The nurses' role during patient education can focus on helping the patient replace several inaccurate and negative perceptions about his recovery and its implications on his future functioning. Patients can be encouraged to check out these automatic perceptions via questions and clarifications to test their hypotheses, challenge their concerns rather than taking these thoughts at face value. This intervention is called cognitive restructuring or, simply put, "realistic thinking." It uses the evaluation and testing of the actual evidence that supports or invalidates the depressive cognitions/assumptions (Beck et al., 1979). The patient who is anxious about another heart attack can be taught that his excessive scanning of physical symptoms and worry are likely to increase anxiety and physiological arousal, which is not beneficial during his recovery. He can be taught relaxation strategies along with methods of worry control to decrease his anxiety. Worry control methods include postponing of worry, postponing of checking of physical symptoms, and scheduling worry periods. These methods are outlined in a book by Bourne for lay audiences for management of anxiety and fears (Bourne, 1995).

Social Support Interventions

Nurses can provide functional support in terms of education and knowledge. Anticipatory guidance regarding the disease and recovery process can alleviate both patient and family stress. Benefits of support and the role it serves as a buffer against stress can be discussed. However, it is important to assess the patient's needs and desire for knowledge. This is illustrated by research observations of patients with a repressive coping style. Those who were provided high levels of information had a higher frequency of heart alarms and more medical complications (Ell & Dunkel-Schetter, 1994). Patients who actively deny they have had a heart attack are not ready to receive high levels of information. Open-ended questions that allow the patient to direct the flow of information should be used. The nurse is also in a position to provide emotional support through empathic listening and encouraging social interactions. Cardiac hospitalizations invoke apprehension and fear in most patients. Allowing the patient and spouses an opportunity to express these concerns can be beneficial for both the patient and their family. Such expressions can provide opportunities for educating the patient and his family. Encouraging meals with other patients, facilitating access to social visits, having family members cook can facilitate connections with others and enhance a sense of perceived support (Dossey, 1997). For patients with few social ties or existing ties that are perceived to be unsupportive, referral to cardiac rehabilitation programs or to Mended Hearts may provide increased community contacts. Patients referred to cardiac rehabilitation benefit from observing other patients' recoveries, and from the continuing contact with health care staff. Many patients in rehabilitation programs develop lasting friendships with their counterparts. Such ties serve as a buffer from the stresses of daily life. Patients with existing support networks are likely to benefit from the inclusion of family members or significant others during the course of the recovery in the hospital. Just like the patient, spouses and significant others are likely to distort and make false assumptions about the patient's recovery during a course of a medical emergency. Spouses can be significantly distressed by the hospitalization for several reasons such as lack of control, fear of the unknown, fear of change in roles, self-blame for the event and fear of loss (Bedsworth & Molen, 1982; Bramwell, 1986, Gillis, 1984). Also, providing information before procedures and rehabilitation can decrease fear of uncertainty. Educating the spouse about the MI, the course of treatment and recovery can decrease over-protectiveness and over-involvement when the patient goes home (Doerr & Jones, 1979). Behavioral strategies that allow the patient and family to rehearse or model experiences are useful. For example, treadmill exercise testing before discharge from the hospital if observed by the spouse has been shown to enhance the patient's self-esteem and to reduce spousal anxiety (Taylor et al., 1985). Rather than being overprotective in the recovery period, the spouse can provide positive support.

Intervention Strategies for Hostility and Anger

Hostility can often be a more longstanding trait and less responsive to change. In some cases, referral to mental health specialist may be required. Patients with these traits may be less compliant with risk factor modification and medical regimes. For example, when patients use smoking to relieve symptoms experienced during episodes of anger or frustration, quit rates are lower (Littman, 1993). Evaluating adherence and applying problem-solving strategies is important in all coronary patients, but may be particularly important in people with high hostility and anger ratings.

After establishing rapport with the patient, nurses can be instrumental in providing education about the physiological effects of hostility and anger to patients with these traits. It is often good to begin educating by first using gentle questioning ("Do you think that you often get more angry than others in similar situations or that you stay resentful for longer periods?" or "How do you think your anger and resentments effect your heart or your blood pressure?"), gaining insight into the patient's understanding. This also helps to assess how to approach the delivery of information so as not to provoke anxiety, and to assess patient readiness to receive information. It is also important to elicit feedback from the patients to assess how the information is being processed.

The patient can be informed about the effects of heightened cardiovascular and neuroendocrine responses that increase cortisol levels and plasma lipid levels. The impact of angry assumptions/thoughts and angry behaviors on decreasing parasympathetic response can be discussed. The benefits of exercise and relaxation training to decrease physiological arousal, decrease emotional arousal and increase parasympathetic response can be especially emphasized for patients with hostility and anger (Bracke & Thoresen, 1996). Patients can be encouraged to journal their thoughts and feelings to increase awareness of their hypercritical view of others as incompetent or untrustworthy. Such generalizations can be gently questioned to have them evaluate their assumptions from a neutral perspective. Also they can be questioned about the usefulness or function of their anger and hostility (Sotile, 1999). They can also learn to evaluate and distinguish between when anger is justified and when it is unjustified (Williams & Williams, 1993).

Most research interventions used group therapy programs with educational and behavioral strategies to assist patients in identifying and modifying their behaviors. One such strategy put forward by Powell is the Hook intervention (Powell, 1996) taught to patients with high level of autonomic reactivity to daily life hassles such as waiting in lines and being delayed in traffic. These patients frequently react to the unfairness of the external environment and unsuccessfully attempt to gain control over their environment through overt or covert impatient and hostile behaviors leading to further frustration and physiological arousal. Through practice, they can learn that the average thirty some daily hassles are "hooks/baits" thrown at them and they have a choice in terms of biting or letting go to manage their arousal levels. For example, a patient might identify routine time-urgent behaviors such as speeding up at a yellow light or passing cars or multitasking. These patients can be instructed to modify their behavior by purposefully driving in the slow lane, standing in a longer line, and performing one task at a time.

These patients also tend to have unsatisfactory relationships and may have difficulty maintaining relationships (Eriksen, 1994). Interventions have targeted ways to nurture social connectedness in these patients who either lack the skills to connect or are fearful of the cost of these social connections in terms of risk of rejection and time away from goal oriented activities (Bracke & Thoresen, 1996). These patients learn to recognize their own internal reactions in an interpersonal context followed by practice of expression of feelings, reflective and empathetic listening. They also practice assertiveness skills such as saying no and delegating to others while learning differences among assertive and aggressive responses (Sotile, 1996). These programs, although costly and time consuming, have shown reduction in hostility ratings (Nunes et al., 1987).

PHARMACOLOGICAL INTERVENTIONS

In addition to psychosocial interventions, patients should also be evaluated for psychopharmacological interventions after a thorough assessment particularly for depression. The efficacy of antidepressants in treatment of clinical depression is well established. The depression treatment guidelines (Agency for Health Care and Policy Research, 1993) recommend that moderate to severe depression and recurrent depression should be treated with the combination of antidepressants and psychotherapy. Antidepressant treatment in addition to depression, may also decrease anxiety, hostility, and is sometimes used to help with smoking cessation (Lesperance & Frasure–Smith, 2000; Strik et al., 2000; Sauer et al., 2001; Shapiro et al., 1999; Covey et al., 2002; ENRICHD, 2003). A consultation with a psychiatrist is recommended given the availability of wide range of antidepressants, implications related to potential side effects and drug interactions for CHD patients. The general empirically based consensus based on a review by Roose (2001) is that selective serotonin reuptake inhibitors (SSRI) have fewer side-effect contraindications for cardiac patients, unlike tricyclic antidepressants, which increase orthostatic hypotension, increase heart rate (Roose et al., 1998; Kannel et al., 1987) and slow conduction (lethal for those with conduction problems). However, while prescribing SSRI it is essential to be aware that these can inhibit cytochrome P450 enzymes which help in metabolizing drugs (such as antiarrhythmics) commonly given to CHD patients and change plasma levels of these drugs (Taylor & Cameron, 1999). It is important that nurses monitor whether patients are on these medications and consult pharmacology texts to identify specific side effects and contradictions. Generally, sertraline is considered a safe and effective antidepressant for treating recurrent depression in CHD (Glassman et al., 2002).

SUMMARY

A multifactorial program that includes both psychosocial and traditional risk reduction strategies may provide the greatest overall benefit for both men and women with CHD. Although behavioral strategies such as education, counseling, emotional support, and risk reduction may improve emotional states, all psychosocial interventions should be implemented only after fully assessing the needs and beliefs of the individual patient. In the final analysis, important components of psychosocial interventions relate first to the recognition of the psychological and social needs of each patient. Education, counseling, modifying of automatic assumptions, specific behavioral strategies, relaxation strategies and emotional support can influence a patient's response to psychosocial factors. Consistent with a nursing perspective, it is important to treat the person as a whole. Management of the coronary patient calls for attention to all cardiovascular risk factors, including psychosocial factors.

Acknowledgment: The authors would like to acknowledge the scholarly contribution of Joan M. Fair. She was one of the authors of this chapter for the previous edition.

REFERENCES

Adams, D.O. (1994). Molecular biology of macrophage activation: A pathway whereby psychosocial factors can potentially affect health. *Psychosomatic Medicine, 56,* 316–327.
Agency for Health Care Policy and Research. (1993). *Depression in primary care: Detection, diagnosis and treatment.* Rockville, MD: U.S. Department of Health and Human Services.
Ahern, D.K., Gorkin, L., Anderson, J.L., et al. (1990). Biobehavioral variables and mortality for cardiac arrest in the Cardiac Arrthymia Pilot Study (CAPS). *American Journal of Cardiology, 60,* 59–62.
Allan, R., & Scheidt, S. (1998). Group psychotherapy for patients with coronary heart disease. *International Journal of Psychotherapy, 48,* 187–214.
Allison, T.G., Williams, D.E., Miller, T.D., et al. (1995). Medical and economic costs of psychological distress in patients with coronary artery disease. *Mayo Clinic Proceedings, 70*(8), 734–742.
American Psychiatric Association. (1994). *Diagnostic and statistical manual of mental disorders* (4th ed.). Washington, DC: American Psychiatric Association.
Antonucci, T.C., & Johnson, E.H. (1994). Conceptualization and methods in social support theory and research as related to cardiovascular disease. In S.A.Shumacker & S.M. Czajkowski (Eds.), *Social support and cardiovascular disease* (pp. 21–39). New York: Plenum.
Barefoot, J.C., & Schroll, M. (1996). Symptoms of depression, acute myocardial infarction, and total mortality in a community sample. Circulation, 93, 1976–1980.
Beck, A.T., Ward, C.H., Mendelson, M., et al. (1961). An inventory for measuring depression. *Archives of General Psychiatry, 4,* 53–63.
Beck, A.T., Rush, A.J., Shaw, B.F., et al. (1979). *Cognitive therapy of depression.* New York: Guilford.

Beck, A.T., Steer, R.A., & Garbin, M.G. (1988). Psychometric properties of the Beck Depression Inventory: Twenty years of evaluation. *Clinical Psychiatry Review, 8,* 77–100.
Beck, J.S. (1995). *Cognitive therapy: Basics and beyond.* New York: Guilford.
Bedsworth, J.A., & Molen, M.T. (1982). Psychological stress in spouses of patients with myocardial infarction. *Heart Lung,* 11, 450–456.
Benson, H. (1975). *The relaxation response.* New York: William Morrow.
Benson, H., & Stuart, E.M. (1993). *The wellness book.* New York: Simon & Schuster.
Berkman, L.F., Leo-Summers, L., & Horwitz, R.I. (1992). Emotional support and survival after myocardial infarction. *Annals of Internal Medicine, 117,* 1003–1009.
Berkman, L.F. (1995). The role of social relations in health promotion. *Psychosomatic Medicine, 57,* 245–254.
Billings, J.H., Scherwitz, L.W., Sullivan, R., et al. (1996). The Lifestyle Heart Trial: Comprehensive treatment and group support study. In R. Allan & S. Scheidt (Eds.), *Heart and mind: The practice of cardiac psychology* (pp. 233–253). Washington, DC: American Psychological Association.
Blumenthal, J.A., Sherwood, A., & Gullette, E.C.D. (2000). Exercise and weight loss reduce blood pressure in men and women with mild hypertension. Effects on cardiovascular, metabolic, and hemodynamic functioning. *Archives of Internal Medicine, 160,* 1947–1958.
Blumenthal, J.A., & Williams, R.S. (1982). Physiological and psychological variables predict compliance to prescribed exercise therapy in patients recovering from myocardial infarction. *Psychosomatic Medicine, 44,* 519–527.
Bourne, E.J. (1995). The anxiety and phobia workbook. Oakland: New Harbinger.
Bracke, P.E., & Thoresen, C.E. (1996). Reducing Type A behavior patterns: A structured-group approach. In R. Allan & S. Scheidt (Eds.), *Heart and mind: The practice of cardiac psychology* (pp. 255–290). Washington, DC: American Psychological Association.
Bramwell, L. (1986). Wives' experiences in the support role after husbands' first myocardial infarction. *Heart Lung,* 15, 578–584.
Brecht, M.L., Dracup, K., Moser, D., et al. (1994). The relationship of marital quality and psychosocial adjustment to heart disease. *Journal of Cardiology Nursing,* 9, 74–85.
Bunker, S.J., Colquhoun, D.M., Esler, M.D., et al. (2003). Stress and coronary heart disease: psychosocial risk factors. *Medical Journal of Australia, 178,* 272–276.
Burell, G. (1996). Group psychotherapy in Project New Life: Treatment of coronary-prone behaviors for patients who have had coronary artery bypass graft surgery. In R. Allan & S. Scheidt (Eds.), *Heart and mind: The practice of cardiac psychology* (pp. 291–310). Washington, DC: American Psychological Association.
Buselli, E.F., & Stuart, E.M. (1999). Influence of psychosocial factors and biopsychosocial interventions on outcomes after myocardial infarction. *Journal of Cardiovascular Nursing,* 13, 60–72.
Byrne, A., & Byrne, D.G. (1993). The effect of exercise on depression, anxiety, and other mood states. *Journal of Psychosomatic Research, 37,* 565–574.
Carney, R.M., Freeland, K., Eisen, R., et al. (1995). Depression as a risk factor for cardiac events in established coronary heart disease: A review of possible mechanisms. *Annals of Behavioral Medicine, 17,* 142–149.
Carney, R.M., Rich, M.W., Freeland, K.E., et al. (1988). Major depressive disorder predicts cardiac events in patients with coronary artery disease. *Psychosomatic Medicine, 50,* 627–633.
Carney, R.M., Rich, M.W., Tevelde, A., et al. (1987). Major depressive disorder in coronary artery disease. *American Journal of Cardiology, 60,* 1273–1275.
Case, R.B., Moss, A.J., Care, N., et al. (1992). Living alone after myocardial infarction: Impact on prognosis. *JAMA, 267,* 515–519.
Cole, S.A., Christensen, J.F., Rajum, M.A., et al. (1997). Depression. In M.D. Feldman & J.F. Christensen (Eds.), *Behavioral medicine in primary care: A practical guide* (pp. 177–192). Norwalk, CT: Appleton & Lange.
Conn, V.S., Taylor, S.G., & Wiman, O. (1991). Anxiety, depression, quality of life, and self-care among survivors of myocardial infarction. *Issues in Mental Health Nursing,* 12, 321–331.
Covey, L.S., Glassman, A.H., Stetner, F., et al. (2002). A randomized trial of sertraline as a cessation aid for smokers a history of major depression. *American Journal of Psychiatry, 159,* 1731–1737.
Coyne, J.C., & DeLongis, A. (1986). Going beyond social support—the role of social relationships in adaptation. *Journal of Consulting Clinical Psychology,* 54, 545–560.
Doerr, B.C., & Jones, J.W. (1979). Effect of family preparation on the state of anxiety level in CCU patient. *Nursing Research, 28,* 315–316.

Dossey, B.M. (1997). *Core curriculum for holistic nursing.* Gaithersburg, MD: Aspen Publishers.

Ebrahims, S., Wannamethee, G., McCallum, A., et al. (1995). Marital status, change in marital status and mortality in middle-aged British men. *American Journal of Epidemiology,* 142, 834–842.

Elkin, I., Shea, M.T., Watkins, J.T., et al. (1989). National Institute of Mental Health Treatment of Depression Collaborative Research Program: general effectiveness of treatments. *Archives of General Psychiatry,* 46, 971–982.

Ell, K., & Dunkel-Schetter, C. (1994). Social support and adjustment to myocardial infarction, angioplasty and coronary artery bypass surgery. In S.A. Shumacker & S.M. Czajkowski (Eds.), *Social support and cardiovascular disease* (pp. 301–322). New York: Plenum.

ENRICHD Investigators. (2000). Enhancing recovery in coronary heart disease patients: ENRICHD study design and methods. *American Heart Journal,* 139, 1–9.

ENRICHD Investigators. (2001a). Enhancing recovery in coronary heart disease (ENRICHD) study intervention: Rationale and design. *Psychosomatic Medicine,* 63, 747–755.

ENRICHD Investigators. (2001b). Enhancing recovery in coronary heart disease (ENRICHD): Baseline characteristics. *American Journal of Cardiology,* 88, 316–322.

ENRICHD Investigators. (2003). Enhancing recovery in coronary heart disease patients (ENRICHD) randomized trial: Effects of treating depression and low perceived social support on clinical events after myocardial infarction. *JAMA,* 289(23), 3106–3116.

Eriksen, W. (1994). The role of social support in the pathogenesis of coronary heart disease—a literature review. *Family Practice,* 11, 201–209.

Everson, S.A., Kauhanen, J., Kaplan, G.A., et al. (1997). Hostility and increased risk of mortality and acute myocardial infarction: The mediating role of behavioral risk factors. *American Journal of Epidemiology,* 146, 142–152.

Feinstein, R.E., Carey, L., Rabinowitz, P.M., et al. (1999). Cardiovascular and psychosocial risk factors reduction: Office-based interventions. In R.E. Feinstein & A.A. Brewer (Eds.), *Primary care psychiatry and behavioral medicine* (pp. 299–329). New York: Springer.

Fielding, R. (1991). Depression and acute myocardial infarction: A review and reinterpretation. *Social Science Medicine,* 32, 1017–1027.

Finnegan, D.L., & Suler, J.R. (1985). Psychological factors associated with maintenance of improved health behavior in post coronary patients. *Journal of Psychology,* 119, 87–94.

Follick, M.J., Ahern, D.K., Gorkin, L., et al. (1990). Relation of psychosocial and stress reactivity variables to ventricular arrthymias in the cardiac arrthymia pilot study (CAPS). *American Journal of Cardiology,* 66, 63–67.

Fontana, A.F., Kerns, R., Rosenberg, R., et al. (1986). Exercise training for cardiac patients: Adherence, fitness and benefits. *Journal of Cardiopulmonary Rehabilitation,* 6, 4–15.

Frasure-Smith, N., Lesperance, F., & Talajic, M. (1993). Depression following myocardial infarction: impact on 6 month survival. *JAMA,* 270, 1819–1825.

Frasure-Smith, N., Lesperance, F., & Talajic, M. (1995a). Depression and 18 month prognosis after a myocardial infarction. *Circulation,* 91, 999–1005.

Frasure-Smith, N., Lesperance, F., & Talajic, M. (1995b). The impact of negative emotions on prognosis following myocardial infarction: Is it more than depression? *Health Psychology,* 14, 388–398.

Frasure-Smith, N., Lesperance, F., & Talajic, M. (1996). Major depression before and after myocardial infarction: Its nature and consequences. *Psychosomatic Medicine,* 58, 99–110.

Freidman, R., Myers, P., Krass, S., et al. (1996). The relaxation response: Use with cardiac patients. In R. Allan & S. Scheidt (Eds.), *Heart and mind: The practice of cardiac psychology* (pp. 363–384). Washington, DC: American Psychological Association.

Gillis, C.L. (1984). Reducing family stress during and after coronary artery bypass surgery. *Nursing Clinics of North America,* 19, 103–111.

Glassman, A.H., O'Connor, C.M., Califf, R.M., et al. (2002). Sertraline treatment of major depression in patients with acute MI or unstable angina. *JAMA,* 288, 701–709.

Goldstein, M.G. & Niaura, R. (1992). Psychological factors affecting physical condition: Cardiovascular disease literature review. *Psychosomatics,* 33, 134–154.

Goodman, M., Quigley, J., Moran, G., et al. (1996). Hostility predicts restenosis after percutaneous transluminal coronary angioplasty. *Mayo Clinic Proceedings,* 71, 729–734.

Gorkin, L., Schron, E.B., & Brooks, M.M. (1993). Psychosocial predictors of mortality in the Cardiac Arrthymia Supression Trial –1 (CAST-1). *American Journal of Cardiology,* 71, 263–267.

Grace, S.L., Abbey, S.E., Shnek, Z.M., et al. (2002). Cardiac rehabilitation I: Review of psychosocial factors. *General Hospital Psychiatry,* 24, 121–126.

Guiry, E., Conroy, R.M., Hickey, N., et al. (1987). Psychological response to an acute coronary event and its effect on subsequent rehabilitation and lifestyle change. *Clinical Cardiology,* 10, 256–260.

Gullette, E., Blumenthal, J., Babyak, M., et al. (1997). Effects of mental stress on myocardial ischemia during daily life. *JAMA,* 277, 1521–1526.

Hackett, T.P., & Cassem, N.H. (1975). Psychological management of the myocardial patients. *Journal of Human Stress,* 1(30), 25–38.

Hayward, C. (1995). Psychiatric illness and cardiovascular disease risk. *Epidemiology Review,* 17, 129–138.

Helmer, D.C., Ragland, D.R., & Syme, S.L. (1991). Hostility and coronary artery disease. *American Journal of Epidemiology,* 133, 112–122.

Hemingway, H., Kuper, H., & Marmot, M. (2003). Psychosocial factors in the primary and secondary prevention of coronary heart disease: a systematic review. In S. Yusuf, J.A. Cairns, E. Fallen, B.J. Gersch, & A.J. Camm (Eds.), *Evidence based cardiology.* London: British Medical Journal Publishing.

Hemingway, H. & Marmot, M. (1999). Psychosocial factors in the etiology and prognosis of coronary heart disease. Systematic review of prospective cohort studies. *British Medical Journal,* 381, 1460–1467.

Hlatky, M.A., Lam, L.C., Lee, K., et al. (1995). Job strain and the prevalence and outcome of coronary artery disease. *Circulation,* 92, 327–333.

Jenkins, C.D. (1978). Behavioral risk factors in coronary artery disease. *Annual Review of Medicine,* 29, 543–563.

Julkunen, J., Salonen, R., Kaplan, G.A., et al. (1994). Hostility and the progression of carotid atherosclerosis. *Psychosomatic Medicine,* 56, 519–525.

Kannel, W.B., Kannel, C., Pattenbarger Jr., R.S., et al. (1987). Heart rate and cardiovascular mortality rate—the Framingham Study. *American Heart Journal,* 113, 1489–1494.

Karasek, R., Baker, D., Marxer, F., et al. (1981). Job decision latitude, job demands and cardiovascular disease: A prospective study of Swedish men. *American Journal of Public Health,* 71, 694–705.

Kark, J.D., Goldman, S., & Epstein, L. (1995). Iraqi missile attacks on Israel. *JAMA,* 273, 1208–1210.

Kawachi, I., Colditz, G.A., Ascherio, A., et al. (1994a). Prospective study of phobic anxiety and risk of coronary heart disease in men. *Circulation,* 89, 1992–1997.

Kawachi, I., Sparrow, D., Spiro, A., et al. (1996). A prospective study of anger and coronary heart disease. *Circulation,* 94, 2090–2095.

Kawachi, I., Sparrow, D., Vokona, S.P.S., et al. (1994b). Symptoms of anxiety and risk of coronary heart disease: The Normative Aging Study. *Circulation,* 90, 2225–2229.

Kessler, R.C., Berglund, P., Demler, O., et al. (2003). The epidemiology of major depressive disorder. *JAMA,* 289, 3095–3105.

King, A., Taylor, C.B., & Haskell, W. (1993). The effects of differing intensities and formats of twelve months of exercise training on psychological outcomes. *Health Psychology,* 12, 292–302.

King, K.B. (1997). Psychologic and social aspects of cardiovascular disease. *Annals of Behavioral Medicine,* 19(3), 264–270.

Kloner, R.A., Leor, J., Poole, W.K., et al. (1997). Population-based analysis of the effect of the Northridge earthquake on cardiac death in Los Angeles County. *Journal of the American College of Cardiology,* 30, 1174–1180.

Kritz-Silverstein, D., Wingard, D., & Barrett-Connor, E. (1992). Employment status and heart disease risk factors in middle-aged women: The Rancho Bernardo Study. *American Journal of Public Health,* 82, 215–219.

Krumholz, H.M., Butler, J., Miller, J., et al. (1998). Prognostic importance of emotional support for elderly patients hospitalized with heart failure. *Circulation,* 97, 958–964.

Kubzansky, L.D., Kawachi, I., Spiro III, A., et al. (1997). Is worrying bad for your heart? *Circulation,* 95, 818–824.

Lane, D., Carroll, D., Lip, G.Y., et al. (1999). Psychology in coronary care. *Quarterly Journal of Medicine,* 92, 425–431.

Lazarus, R.S., & Folkman, S. (1984). *Stress, appraisal, and coping.* New York: Springer-Verlag.

Lesprance, F., & Frasure-Smith, N. (2000). Depression in patients with cardiac disease. The role of psychosomatic medicine. *Journal of Psychosomatic Research,* 48, 379–392.

Linden, W. (2000). Psychological treatments in cardiac rehabilitation: Review of rationales and outcomes. *Journal of Psychosomatic Research,* 48, 443–454.

Littman, A.B. (1993). Review of psychosomatic aspects of cardiovascular disease. *Psychothererapy and Psychosomatics,* 60, 148–167.

Lynch, J., Kaplan, G., Salonen, R., et al. (1995). Socioeconomic status and carotid atherosclerosis. *Circulation,* 92, 1786–1792.

Malkoff, S.B., Muldoon, M.F., Zeigler, Z.R., et al. (1993). Blood platelet responsivity to acute mental stress. *Psychosomatic Medicine, 55,* 477–482.

Matthews, K., Cottington, E., Talbot, E., et al. (1987). Stressful work conditions and diastolic blood pressure among blue collar factory workers. *American Journal of Epidemiology, 126,* 280–291.

Mayou, R.A., Foster, A., & Williamson, B. (1978). Psychosocial adjustment in patients after one year after myocardial infarction. *Journal of Psychosomatic Research, 22*(5), 447–453.

McCarty, R., & Gold, P.E. (1996). Catecholamines, stress, and disease: A psychobiological perspective. *Psychosomatic Medicine, 58,* 590–597.

Mittleman, M.A., Maclure, M., Sherwood, J.B., et al. (1995). Triggering of acute myocardial infarction onset by episodes of anger. *Circulation, 92,* 1720–1725.

Moser, D.K., & Dracup, K. (1996). Is anxiety after myocardial infarction associated with subsequent ischemic and arrhythmic events? *Psychosomatic Medicine, 58,* 395–401.

Muller, J.E., Abela, G.S., Nesto, R.W., et al. (1994). Triggers, acute risk factors and vulnerable plaques: The lexicon of a new frontier. *Journal of the American College of Cardiology, 23,* 809–813.

Nolen-Hokesema, S. (1990). *Sex differences in depression.* Stanford: Stanford University Press.

Nunes, E.V., Frank, K.A., & Kornfeld, D.S. (1987). Psychologic treatment for the type A behavior pattern and for coronary heart disease: A meta-analysis of the literature. *Psychosomatic Medicine, 48,* 159–173.

Nyamathi, A.M., Jacoby, [AQ1] Constancia, P., et al. (1992). Coping and adjustment of spouses of critically ill patients in cardiac disease. *Heart Lung, 21,* 160–166.

Ortho-Gomer, K., Rosengran, A., & Wilhelmsen, L. (1993). Lack of social support and incidence of coronary heart disease in middle-aged Swedish men. *Psychosomatic Medicine, 55,* 37–43.

Ortho-Gomer, K., Wamala, S.P., Horsten, M., et al. (2000). Marital stress worsens prognosis in women with coronary heart disease. The Stockholm Female Coronary Risk Study. *JAMA, 284,* 3008–3014.

Pitula, C.R., Burg, M.M., & Froelicher, E.S. (1999). Psychosocial risk factors: Assessment and intervention for social isolation. In *Cardiac rehabilitation: A guide to practice in the 21st century* (pp. 279–286). New York: Marcel Dekker.

Pitula, C.R., & Daugherty, S.R. (1995). Sources of social support and conflict in hospitalized depressed women. *Research in Nursing Health, 18,* 325–332.

Powell, L.H. (1996). The hook: A metaphor for gaining control of emotional reactivity. In R. Allan & S. Scheidt (Eds.), *Heart and mind: The practice of cardiac psychology* (pp. 313–327). Washington, DC: American Psychological Association.

Pratt, L.A., Ford, D.E., Crum, R.M., et al. (1996). Depression, psychotropic medication, and risk of myocardial infarction. Prospective data from Baltimore ECA follow-up. *Circulation, 94,* 3123–3129.

Radloff, L.S. (1977). The CES-D scale: A self-report depression scale for research in the general population. *Applied Psychological Measurement, 1,* 385–401.

Rankin-Esquer, L.A., Miller, N.H., Myers, D., et al. (1997). Marital status and outcome in patients with coronary heart disease. *Journal of Clinical Psychology in Medical Settings, 4,* 417–435.

Roose, S.P., Laghrissi-Thode, F., Kennedy, J.S., et al. (1998). Comparison of paroxetine and nortriptyline in depression patients with ischemic heart disease. *JAMA, 279,* 287–291.

Roose, S.P. (2001). Depression, anxiety and the cardiovascular system: The psychiatrist's perspective. *Journal of Clinical Psychiatry, 62*(8), 19–22.

Rozanski, A., Bairy, C.N., Krantz, D.S., et al. (1988). Mental stress and the induction of myocardial ischemia in patients with coronary artery disease. *New England Journal of Medicine, 318,* 1005–1012.

Schwartz, J., Pieper, C., & Krarasek, R.A. (1988). A procedure for linking psychosocial job characteristics data to health surveys. *American Journal of Public Health, 78,* 904–909.

Sauer, W.H., Berlin, J.A., & Kimmel, S.E. (2001). Selective serotonin reuptake inhibitors and myocardial infarction. *Circulation, 104,* 1894–1898.

Selye, H. (1956). *The stress of life.* New York: McGraw-Hill.

Shapiro, P.A., Lesperance, F., Frasure-Smith, N., et al. (1999). An open label preliminary trial of sertraline for treatment of major depression after acute myocardial infarction (the SADHART trial). *American Heart Journal, 137,* 1100–1106.

Smith, C.E., Fernengel, K., Holcroft, C., et al. (1994). Meta-analysis of the associations between social support and health outcomes. *Annals of Behavioral Medicine, 16,* 352–362.

Smith, T.W. (1992). Hostility and health: Current status of a psychosomatic hypothesis. *Health Psychology, 11,* 139–150.

Smith, T.W., & Ruiz, J.M. (2002). Psychosocial influences on the development and course of coronary heart disease: Current status and implications for research and practice. *Journal of Consulting Clinical Psychology, 70,* 548–568.

Sotile, W.M. (1996). *Psychosocial interventions for cardiopulmonary patients. A guide for health professionals.* Champaign, IL: Human Kinetics.

Sotile, W.M. (1999). Psychosocial risk factors: overview, assessment and intervention for anger and hostility. In *Cardiac rehabilitation: A guide to practice in the 21st century* (pp. 257–261). New York: Marcel Dekker.

Spielberg, C., Falkenhaln, D., Willich, S., et al. (1996). Circadian, day of week, and seasonal variability in myocardial infarction: Comparison between working and retired patients. *American Heart Journal, 132,* 579–585.

Spitzer, R., Williams, J.B., Linzer, M., et al. (1994). Utility of a new procedure for diagnosing mental disorders in primary care: The PRIME-MD 1000 study. *JAMA, 272,* 1749–1756.

Stahle, A., Nordlander, R., & Bergfeldt, L. (1999). Aerobic group training improves exercise capacity and heart rate variability in elderly patients with a recent coronary event. A randomized controlled study. *European Heart Journal, 20,* 1638–1646.

Stein, R.A. (1996). Exercise and patient with coronary heart disease. In R. Allan & S. Scheidt (Eds.), *Heart and mind: The practice of cardiac psychology* (pp. 385–396). Washington, DC: American Psychological Association.

Strik, J.J.M.H., Hong, A., Lousberg, R., et al. (2000). Efficacy and safety of fluoxetine in the treatment of patients with major depression after first myocardial infarction. Findings from a double blind, placebo controlled trial. *Psychosomatic Medicine, 62,* 783–789.

Stuart-Shor, E.M. (1999). Stress management. In *Cardiac rehabilitation: A guide to practice in the 21st century* (pp. 287–294). New York: Marcel Dekker.

Suzuki, S., Sakamotot, S., Koide, M., et al. (1997). Hanshi-Awaji earthquake as a trigger for acute myocardial infarction. *American Heart Journal, 134,* 974–977.

Taylor, C.B., Bandura, A., Ewart, C., et al. (1985). Exercise testing to enhance wives' confidence in their husbands' cardiac capacity soon after clinically uncomplicated myocardial infarction. *American Journal of Cardiology, 55,* 635–638.

Taylor, C.B., & Cameron, R.P. (1999). Psychosocial risk factors: Assessment and intervention for depression. In *Cardiac rehabilitation: A guide to practice in the 21st century* (pp. 263–277). New York: Marcel Dekker.

Van Der Ploeg, H., Defares, P., & Spielberger, C. (1980). *Manual for the State Trait Anxiety Inventory.* Lisee, The Netherlands: Swets & Zeitlinger.

Vinokur, A., Schul, Y., & Caplan, R.D. (1987). Determinants of perceived social support: Interpersonal transactions, personal outlook and transient affective states. *Journal of Personal and Social Psychology, 53,* 1137–1145.

Wells, K.B., Stewart, A., Hays, R.D., et al. (1989). The functioning and well being of depressed patients. *JAMA, 262,* 914–919.

Whooley, M.A., & Simon, G. (2000). Managing depression in medical outpatients. *New England Journal of Medicine, 343*(26), 1942–1950.

Williams, R.B., Barefoot, J.C., Califf, R.M., et al. (1992). Prognostic importance of social and economic resources among medically treated patients with angiographically documented coronary artery disease. *JAMA, 267,* 520–524.

Williams, R.B., & Williams, V.P. (1993). *Anger kills: Seventeen strategies for controlling the hostility that can harm your health.* New York: Times Books.

Wishnie, H.A., Hackett, T.P., & Cassem, N.H. (1971). Psychological hazards of convalescence following myocardial infarction. *JAMA, 215,* 1292–1296.

Yesavage, J.A., Brink, T.L., Rose, T.L., et al. (1983). Development and validation of a geriatric depression screening scale: A preliminary report. *Journal of Psychiatric Research, 17,* 37–49.

Yeung, A.C., Vekshtein, V.I., Krantz, D.S., et al. (1991). The effect of atherosclerosis on the vasomotor responses of coronary arteries to mental stress. *New England Journal of Medicine, 325,* 1551–1556.

Smoking Cessation: A Systematic Approach to Managing Patients With Coronary Heart Disease

KIRSTEN MARTIN • ERIKA S. SIVARAJAN FROELICHER

In the year 2000, 46.5 million adults in the United States were current smokers. This represents approximately 23.3% of the adult population (Centers for Disease Control and Prevention [CDCP], 2002a). Smoking is a known cause of cardiovascular disease, stroke, cancer, and obstructive pulmonary disease (Agency for Health Care Policy and Research, 1996). Between 1995 and 1999, smoking caused approximately 442,000 premature deaths in the United States annually, making cigarette smoking the principle cause of premature death in the United States. Male smokers lost an average of 13.2 years of life, whereas females lost an average of 14.5 years of life; 33.5% of the smoking-related deaths were the result of cardiovascular-related disease (CDCP, 2002b). Although this loss of life is tragic in and of itself, it must be noted that smoking has other costs. Cigarette smoking is responsible for approximately $157 billion annually in health-related economic losses, including $75.5 billion for medical expenses and $81.9 billion for losses in worker productivity. One fourth of the approximately 33 million hospital admissions annually involve smokers (Britton et al., 1991). Although these statistics are staggering, they do not fully reflect the risks for vulnerable populations like the uninsured, migrant, immigrant, and poor who are less likely to be represented because of limitations in surveillance and outreach efforts (Hutchinson & Froelicher, 2003). With all of this in mind, health and policy experts have continued to make cigarette smoking a major focus of risk factor modification. For example, the United States Department of Health and Human Services (USDHHS) has set a goal of reducing the prevalence of cigarette smoking to less than 12% in its *Healthy People 2010: National Health Promotion and Disease Prevention Objectives* (2000a) and has recently published a clinical practice guideline titled *Treating Tobacco Use and Dependence* (2000b). These guidelines are intended to provide a framework for intervention to all smokers no matter their intention to quit at the present time. The relevance of these new guidelines is particularly strong, because recent research indicates that when asked, 70% of smokers said they wanted to quit and 41% had tried to quit during the preceding year (CDCP, 2002a).

Although nurses know that smoking has a negative impact on health, especially cardiovascular health, most fail to provide a smoking cessation intervention. Smoking cessation has just recently become a focus of nursing research. For example, a review of data-based articles and research briefs published in the journal *Nursing Research* between 1952 and 2000, in which tobacco use was an issue, found that 53% of the articles were published after 1990 and that 71% of the studies, in which tobacco use was a potential study outcome, were published between 1995 and 2000 (Sarna & Lillington, 2003). One of the major responsibilities of the nurse is health promotion; therefore, it is important that nurses be aware that they can play a major role in smoking cessation. For example, there is a significant body of research that has documented the effectiveness of nurse-managed smoking cessation interventions, particularly in the hospitalized cardiovascular population (Taylor et al., 1990; Rice et al., 1994; Wewers et al., 1994; Taylor et al., 1996; Johnson et al., 1999; Froelicher & Christopherson, 2000; Martin et al., 2000; Froelicher & Kozuki, 2001; Froelicher, Christopherson et al., 2002; Froelicher, Houston Miller et al., 2002; Mahrer-Imhof et al., 2002; Smith et al., 2002).

Successful smoking cessation interventions usually have behavior modification as a core component. Behavioral modification skills include identifying areas of concern for patients, teaching patients strategies to cope with difficult situations, and role-playing strategies with patients to allow them to practice their new coping strategies. These behavioral modification skills usually are not part of most nursing school curricula (Sarna & Lillington, 2003). Even when they are taught, there is rarely an opportunity for practice, feedback, and development of confidence in performing these skills. This chapter focuses on the important steps in smoking cessation interventions that should be provided to patients with cardiovascular disease, with an emphasis on behavioral and pharmacologic approaches. After completing this chapter, the nurse, no matter what setting he or she practices in–intensive care unit, cardiac care unit, medical–surgical, labor and delivery, outpatient care–will posses the necessary knowledge to provide a smoking cessation intervention to every patient who smokes, every time the patient is encountered.

Permanent smoking cessation should be the goal for every intervention and every person who smokes. Achievement of this goal is difficult, however, because the nicotine in tobacco products is an addictive substance (USDHHS, 1988). Smokers are physically and emotionally compelled to continue smoking even in the face of serious adverse health consequences. In addition, multiple quit attempts and failure to quit smoking despite high levels of motivation are common. The presence of withdrawal symptoms is another indicator of the addictive properties of nicotine. The criteria for diagnosis of nicotine withdrawal are met when any four of the following symptoms commence within 24 hours of the abrupt cessation of nicotine use: dysphoric or depressed mood; insomnia; irritability, frustration, or anger; anxiety; difficulty concentrating; restlessness; decreased heart rate; or increased appetite or weight gain (American Psychiatric Association, 1994). Rapid identification of these withdrawal symptoms and prompt intervention are important skills for all nurses, particularly hospital-based nurses, because these withdrawal symptoms may be so intense for a given patient that he or she is unable to make rational health care decisions and may leave the hospital against medical advice to relieve them with a cigarette.

HARMFUL EFFECTS OF SMOKING

Cigarette smoking, hypercholesterolemia, hypertension, and physical inactivity are considered the four major risk factors for cardiovascular disease. What makes cigarette smoking unique among these is that it interacts synergistically with hypercholesterolemia and hypertension to increase greatly the risk for coronary heart disease (CHD). For example, in people who smoke and have hypercholesterolemia or hypertension, the risk for CHD is doubled. For people who have all three risk factors, the risk for CHD is quadrupled (USDHHS, 1989).

In general, cigarette smoking accelerates atherosclerosis throughout the body, but this effect is most important in the coronary arteries, the aorta, and the carotid and cerebral arteries. Several mechanisms have been described to explain how cigarette smoking leads to atherosclerosis. These include: (1) adverse effects on lipid profiles; (2) endothelial damage or dysfunction; (3) hemodynamic stress; (4) oxidant injury; (5) neutrophil activation; (6) enhanced thrombosis; and (7) increased blood viscosity (Benowitz & Gourlay, 1997).

Although the acceleration of atherosclerosis is a major contributor to cardiovascular morbidity (e.g., aggravation of stable angina pectoris, vasospastic angina, intermittent claudication), a major focus in the population of smokers with cardiovascular disease is how smoking mediates acute cardiovascular events (e.g., myocardial infarction [MI], sudden death, stroke) that

lead to hospitalization. The smoking related mechanisms thought to contribute to these events are: (1) induction of a hypercoagulable state; (2) increased myocardial workload; (3) reduced oxygen-carrying capacity of the blood; (4) coronary vasoconstriction; and (5) catecholamine release (Benowitz & Gourlay, 1997).

Nicotine and carbon monoxide, although only two of the more than 4,000 chemicals in cigarette smoke, are generally considered to be the major contributors to atherosclerotic disease (Stillman, 1995). Nicotine disrupts lipid metabolism, resulting in an increased level of low-density lipoprotein and a decreased level of high-density lipoprotein. Nicotine is also responsible for the increased platelet aggregation and hypercoagulability found in smokers. In addition, it leads to increased production of catecholamines, which in turn increase blood pressure, heart rate and contractility, and systemic vascular resistance, all of which result in increased myocardial oxygen demand (Benowitz & Gourlay, 1997; USDHHS, 1983). Unfortunately, meeting this demand is difficult because cigarette smoking constricts large and small epicardial arteries and coronary resistance vessels, leading to a decrease in coronary blood flow (Quillen et al., 1993). In fact, in a study of patients with established CHD, Barry and colleagues (1989) found that continued cigarette smoking was related to a 12-fold increase in the amount of total ischemia daily. Episodes of ischemic ST segment depression occurred three-times as often, and the duration was 12-times longer in smokers compared with nonsmokers (median duration of 24 min/24 hr vs. 2 min/24 hr). This increased ischemia may be related to the increased probability of recurrent coronary events in people who smoke. The increase in heart rate may also lead to endothelial injury, myocardial ischemia and MI, arrhythmias, and sudden death (Benowitz & Gourlay, 1997).

Carbon monoxide interferes with oxygen transport, leading to a reduced supply of oxygen to the tissues, and, more important, to the myocardium at a time when the demand is high because of a higher heart rate (Stillman, 1995). Carbon monoxide interferes with the oxygen-carrying capacity of red blood cells by binding to hemoglobin, thereby reducing the amount of hemoglobin available for binding with oxygen and by impeding oxygen release from hemoglobin (Benowitz & Gourlay, 1997). Carbon monoxide also increases the permeability of endothelial membranes, resulting in increased uptake of cholesterol that leads to atherogenesis (USDHHS, 1983).

When the number of cigarettes smoked daily, the total number of years of smoking, the degree of inhalation, and the age of smoking initiation are considered, the risk for development of CHD is found to increase with increasing exposure to cigarette smoke. Overall, cigarette smokers have a two- to four-fold greater incidence of CHD than do nonsmokers, and cigarette smokers have a 70% greater death rate caused by CHD than nonsmokers. Cigarette smokers also experience a two- to four-fold greater risk of sudden death than nonsmokers (USDHHS, 1983). The damage caused by cigarette smoking is not restricted to the heart alone. Cigarette smokers have a higher incidence of arteriosclerotic peripheral vascular disease and more severe atherosclerosis of the aorta than nonsmokers

(Stillman, 1995), as well as an increased rate of stroke and cerebrovascular disease (USDHHS, 1983).

BENEFITS OF SMOKING CESSATION

The health benefits of smoking cessation on the cardiovascular system are well documented. The increased tendency to thrombus formation, coronary artery spasm, arrhythmias, and reduced oxygen supply are likely to reverse in a short time (Samet, 1991). For example, evidence suggests that quitting smoking after an initial MI decreases a person's risk of death from CHD by at least 50% in the first year after quitting (Sparrow et al., 1978).

This decline in risk appears to be independent of the severity of the MI (Wilhelmsson et al., 1975). In addition, reports from the Coronary Artery Surgery Study (CASS) indicate that smoking cessation significantly improves survival for people of all ages, including those older than age 70 years (Hermanson et al., 1988). In fact, after 1 year of abstinence from smoking, the excess risk of CHD related to smoking is cut in half and then gradually continues to decline over time. After 15 years of abstinence, the former smoker has achieved a risk level similar to that of a person who has never smoked. Smoking cessation also lowers the overall risk for stroke to that of a nonsmoker within 5 to 15 years of abstinence (Stillman, 1995).

Because the overall death rate and rate of reinfarction is higher in patients with established CHD, intensive smoking cessation intervention should be directed to this population. Nurses who provide care for patients with cardiovascular disease in all practice settings must not miss the opportunity to encourage smokers to quit at every encounter. In addition to the smoking cessation efforts of public education, commercial programs, and worksite health promotion, efforts to assist patients who have manifestations of CHD in the primary care setting are worthwhile.

THEORETICAL FRAMEWORK FOR SMOKING CESSATION

Two theories are commonly cited in smoking cessation research. The Transtheoretical Model (DiClemente et al., 1991; Prochaska et al., 1994; Velicer et al., 1995) classifies smokers into four categories or stages based on their desire to quit smoking and their smoking status. The stages include precontemplation, contemplation, action, and maintenance. While this theory has received mounting popularity, it suffers from numerous deficiencies in its theoretical assumptions (Bandura, 1997); hence, the model we advocate and prefer to use is the self-efficacy model based on social cognitive learning theory by Bandura (1997).

Self-efficacy, in the case of smoking cessation, is defined as the smoker's level of confidence that he or she could refrain from smoking in various challenging or "risky" situations such as social situations (with friends in a cafe, when someone offers them a cigarette), emotional situations (when feeling tense or depressed), and habitual–addictive situations (when

desiring a cigarette or when they are experiencing withdrawal symptoms) (Dijkstra et al., 1996). The belief is that as risky situations are identified, strategies can be developed by the patient in conjunction with his/her health care provider that will help the patient to either avoid or cope with a given situation. Low self-efficacy is a strong predictor of relapse to smoking (Dornelas et al., 2000; Froelicher, Houston Miller, Li et al., 2002); therefore, it behooves the health care provider to assess self-efficacy and provide coping skills and strategies to help the smoker successfully navigate those situations where they are most at risk.

Research has identified a strong correlation between the stage a patient is in and his or her self-efficacy expectations. Smokers in the contemplation stage have significantly higher self-efficacy than those in the precontemplation stage, and those in the action and maintenance stages have significantly higher levels of confidence across the various situations compared with those in the contemplation or precontemplation stages (DiClemente et al., 1991; Dijkstra et al., 1996; King et al., 1996).

Self-efficacy in various situations, however, is easily assessed in the clinical setting. It has recently been hypothesized, however, that self-efficacy is intertwined with the patient's smoking behaviors and fluctuates over the course of the quit attempt. In other words, when the patient is initially attempting to quit, self-efficacy may be low to moderate; as the patient successfully abstains from smoking, self-efficacy increases; self-efficacy may then decrease with a relapse and increase with renewed cessation. This cycle would continue to fluctuate until permanent smoking cessation has been achieved which would lead, theoretically, to continuously high self-efficacy. Unfortunately, self-efficacy has rarely been measured more than once or twice in a clinical trial, so this hypothesis requires further testing (Froelicher & Kozuki, 2001). In the mean time, however, self-efficacy can be used clinically to help guide the intervention and is especially helpful in relapse prevention. The identification of risky situations, strategies to deal with risky situations, and relapse prevention are discussed in greater detail in the section titled Relapse Prevention.

SMOKING CESSATION INTERVENTIONS IN THE CORONARY HEART DISEASE POPULATION

The number of randomized clinical trials of smoking cessation interventions conducted in patients with established CHD continues to rise as the medical community recognizes that clinical studies on promotion of smoking cessation show positive smoking cessation rates and decreases in morbidity and mortality. In the past, most of the studies were observational or cross-sectional and used primarily physician advice, education, or group counseling to help patients quit smoking. These studies were usually limited by small sample size, lack of uniformity regarding the definition of abstinence, and reliance on self-report data for confirmation of smoking status (Burling et al., 1984). Recently, more and more trials have had larger study populations, used more clearly defined definitions for abstinence, and saliva or serum cotinine levels or expired carbon monoxide levels have been used to biochemically verify nonsmoking status. Another problem with many of the early studies in patients with CHD was a lack of significant numbers of women subjects and/or women only studies. Only recently have randomized clinical trials been conducted in women with CHD. Despite these early limitations and as a result of several more recent trials, it is apparent that physicians and other health care professionals can have a positive impact on smoking behavior (Pozen et al., 1977; Burt et al., 1974; Taylor et al., 1990; Miller et al., 1997; Froelicher, Houston Miller et al., 2002; Rice et al., 1994; Johnson et al., 1999; Dornelas et al., 2000). When the physician provides simple advice to the patient, the expected cessation rate in the general population is approximately 6% per year (Kottke et al., 1988), whereas group programs that use behavioral methods may achieve yearly cessation rates as high as 26% to 40% (Schwartz, 1987). In the CHD population in particular, the strong stimulus provided by a CHD event results in rates of smoking cessation that are higher than in most studies conducted in the general population (Burt et al., 1974; Mulcahy, 1983; Baile et al., 1982). In particular, studies on those patients having coronary artery bypass graft surgery show smoking cessation rates of approximately 50% (Crouse & Hagaman, 1991; Rigotti et al., 1994), whereas those undergoing coronary arteriography have smoking cessation rates of up to 62% (Ockene et al., 1992). Finally, studies of patients with an MI or angina pectoris reported smoking cessation rates of between 20% and 70% (Burt et al., 1974; Taylor et al., 1990; Baile et al., 1982; Havik & Maeland, 1988; Scott & Lamparski, 1985).

A significant body of research has also focused on nurse-managed smoking cessation interventions that begin in the hospital and then continue with telephone follow-up after discharge from the hospital. The effectiveness of this type of intervention has been demonstrated in patients after MI (Burt et al., 1974) and cancer surgery (Stanislaw & Wewers, 1993) and in patients admitted to the hospital (Miller et al., 1997).

In general, research indicates that those patients with high motivation or strong intention to quit (Rigotti et al., 1994; Ockene et al., 1992), more severe disease (Ockene et al., 1992), who were given strong advice to quit by their physician (Burt et al., 1974; Miller et al., 1997), who have cardiovascular disease (Miller et al., 1997), are male (Rice et al., 1994), have made fewer attempts to quit in the past, and who had no difficulty refraining from smoking while in the hospital (Rigotti et al., 1994) achieved the highest smoking cessation rates. Patients with CHD who continue to smoke are in general younger (Glasgow et al., 1991), female, unmarried/not living with a partner (Glasgow et al., 1991; Rice et al., 1994), belong to a lower socioeconomic (Ockene, 1985; Rice et al., 1994) and educational level, have a less negative attitude about smoking, smoke a greater number of cigarettes, and are more likely to be anxious or depressed (Ockene, 1985). Whereas effective interventions have been conducted to address some of these characteristics, interventions aimed at people of lower educational and socioeconomic status are still lacking (Hutchinson & Froelicher, 2003).

GENERAL TRENDS IN SMOKING CESSATION INTERVENTIONS

The public health approach to smoking cessation that has predominated in the smoking literature in the 1990s has primarily targeted populations or high-risk groups in their natural environments, such as worksites. Public health interventions are usually brief, low-cost, and are often provided by laypeople or through automated means (e.g., mail, contests).

Clinical approaches, however, are targeted to people who are self-referred or recruited, are most commonly applied in a medical or group setting, use trained professionals, and provide intensive multisession interventions. Because patients with CHD are at risk for recurrent cardiac events, such as another MI, a clinical approach is more cost-effective for this population–it is cheaper to help patients quit smoking than to hospitalize them for a repeat MI (Krumholz et al., 1993).

Many intensive group smoking cessation programs are offered, but most smokers prefer to quit on their own or with individualized support (Fiore et al., 1990). For example, in a study of cardiovascular patients admitted to the hospital who were smoking at the time of admission, 86% expressed an interest in quitting. However, of the 86% who were interested in quitting, 79% stated they were interested in quitting on their own, with 50% expressing interest in the use of self-help materials. Fewer than 10% of patients endorsed a formal treatment program (Emmons & Goldstein, 1992). The literature also supports the fact that 90% of all smokers eventually quit on their own, normally after three to four unsuccessful attempts (Pechacek, 1984). It therefore behooves nurses to consider methods that may be individualized to patient needs, combining a clinical approach with multicomponent strategies without requiring patients to attend a formal treatment program.

TREATING TOBACCO USE AND DEPENDENCE: CLINICAL PRACTICE GUIDELINE

As the body of knowledge about the health consequences of smoking and the health benefits of smoking cessation grow, smoking cessation interventions play an even greater role in decreasing smoking-related cardiovascular morbidity and mortality. After a thorough, evidence-based review of the available literature in 2000, the U.S. federal government concluded that tobacco dependence is a chronic condition of dependence frequently requiring repeated interventions, that these interventions (behavioral and pharmacologic) are cost-effective, and that every patient who uses tobacco should be offered at least brief treatment. To address these issues, the USDHHS convened an expert panel and charged it with identifying effective, experimentally validated smoking cessation treatments and practices through a systematic review and analysis of available scientific research. The resulting evidence-based document, *Treating Tobacco Use and Dependence: Clinical Practice Guideline* (USDHHS, 2000b), will be referred to as the *Guideline* throughout the remainder of this chapter. The *Guideline* provides recommendations for primary care clinicians, smoking cessation specialists, and health care administrators, insurers, and purchasers. These recommendations are pertinent to the cardiovascular nurse as well, especially because one of the primary roles of the cardiovascular nurse is risk factor modification.

So every smoker receives at least a brief smoking cessation intervention, the *Guideline* (USDHHS, 2000b) has established five major intervention steps also known as the "5As." These are: (1) ask about tobacco use; (2) advise the patient to quit; (3) assess willingness to make a quit attempt; (4) assist in the quit attempt; and (5) arrange follow-up. Examples of how to implement a brief smoking cessation intervention consistent with the *Guideline* (USDHHS, 2000b) follow.

Step 1: Ask—Systematically Identify All Tobacco Users at Every Visit

To identify every smoker every time he or she is seen by a clinician, a system-wide structure must be put in place. It can be as simple as adding assessment of smoking status to the routine vital signs (heart rate, blood pressure, respiratory rate, temperature) at every visit. To ensure that the smoking status question is asked every time, preprinted progress notes can be used, vital sign stamps can be made, special stickers indicating smoking status can be placed on the outside of charts, and for those with computer charting, a query of smoking status can be inserted into the data collection tool. To obtain this information on patients who are hospitalized, smoking status must be asked as part of the routine admission questionnaire or, as in the outpatient setting, assessed with initial vital signs. It is especially important to identify hospitalized smokers because hospitalization causes them to become ex-smokers because of no-smoking policies. If not identified, these patients may go through severe nicotine withdrawal unnecessarily, which may lead to noncompliance with treatments and, in the extreme case, a patient leaving against medical advice. Even though surveys indicate that physicians believe they have a responsibility to help smokers, only half of all physicians provide such advice (Frank et al., 1991). In addition, half of the nurses surveyed by Kviz and colleagues (1995) believe that the responsibility for advising patients age 50 years or older is equally divided between nurses and physicians. These statistics show how easily a smoker can slip through the cracks. Often, if a responsibility is shared, it never gets done because one person assumes the other person did it. Therefore, the roles of the nurse and the physician need to be clearly identified in each setting. However, in one study, 3% of nurses reported that they did not know how to counsel patients, 27% claimed it was not rewarding, 8% thought it was too time-consuming, and only 14% reported ever receiving formal training in smoking cessation counseling (Goldstein et al., 1987). In addition, Faulkner and Ward (1983) found that nurses' knowledge of the effects of smoking was limited because they were on average able to name only two physiologic effects and three disease processes related to smoking, even when given cues to correct answers. Lack of knowledge is not the only problem; attitudes and opinions must also be altered. For example, nurses in general believe that patients

---

D I S P L A Y 38-1

HOW TO ASK ABOUT SMOKING STATUS

Initial Assessment

"We're interested in knowing about your lifestyle and habits as they relate to your health. Have you ever smoked in your life? Are you still smoking?" *or* "Over the course of a lifetime, many people pick up the smoking habit. Have you ever smoked? Do you still smoke?"

Follow-Up

If the patient was not ready to quit at the last visit: "I'm sure it must be difficult, but have you seriously considered making an attempt to quit smoking since your last visit?"

If the patient was in the precontemplation stage at the last visit: "At your last visit, you were seriously thinking about quitting smoking. Were you able to cut down on the number of cigarettes you smoke, or were you successful at quitting since your last visit?"

If the patient was in the action stage at the last visit: "Have you had any problems in refraining from smoking since your last visit?"

---

who smoke are not concerned about the health consequences of smoking and do not have a strong desire to stop smoking. Furthermore, nurses believe that if they do advise a patient to stop smoking, the likelihood of the patient actually stopping is not very high (Kviz et al., 1995). It is thus critically important that physicians and nurses, as well as all other health care professionals, assess their level of comfort in offering advice and, if necessary, receive training on how to counsel people. Simply bringing up the subject may seem overwhelming to health care professionals. Simple ways to introduce the subject are shown in Display 38-1.

Step 2: Advise—Strongly Urge All Smokers to Quit

Smokers tend to deny anything but the most direct advice and clear-cut message about quitting. Therefore, the first step in the process of providing help to a smoker is to give him or her a clear, strong, and personalized message about quitting, such as "Your smoking is harming your health. As your nurse, I need to tell you that smoking is your major risk factor for cardiovascular disease. Continuing to smoke will lead to further cardiovascular disease and possibly death. Together, we must figure out how to help you become a non-smoker." Clear and strong, however, is not enough. The message must be personalized. Make your message relevant to the smoker's current concerns about his or her health, disease status, family or social situation, age, sex, and past smoking behaviors. For example, if a patient is hospitalized for a coronary angioplasty, it is necessary for him or her to know that continued smoking is associated with an increased restenosis rate. Follow this with information about the health risks associated with continuing to smoke (see section on Harmful Effects of Smoking) and the health and social benefits of smoking cessation (see section on Benefits of

DISPLAY **38-2**

HOW A SMOKER MAY INTERPRET AN INADEQUATE MESSAGE

If you say:	The smoker may think:
You probably should stop smoking.	I guess I don't have to stop smoking.
You are older, but stopping smoking may help anyway.	I don't have much time to live, so why stop smoking now?
The surgery has restored your circulation to normal.	Good. Now I don't have to quit smoking.

Smoking Cessation). Display 38-2 illustrates how a smoker may interpret an inadequate message.

Step 3: Assess—Identify Smokers Willing to Make a Quit Attempt

After providing advice, it is important to determine if the patient is willing to quit smoking at this time. Willingness to quit can be measured through a simple yes/no question, such as "Are you willing to quit smoking now?" Another measure of a patient's willingness to quit smoking can be assessed using an intention question, "Do you intend to stay off cigarettes or other tobacco products in the next month?" A response scale is shown in Display 38-3. Patients who score a three or less usually are not interested or ready to quit (Taylor et al., 1990). If the patient is willing to quit, provide a brief or more intensive intervention according to patient's preference.

If patients are unwilling to quit, it is important to determine why. In some cases, patients may not have been given enough information about associated risks. Whatever the barrier, providing help or solutions to anticipated problems may encourage the patient to think further about quitting, moving him or her from the precontemplation stage to the contemplation or action stage. If the patient is then willing to quit, move to step 4. If the patient clearly states that he or she is not willing to quit at this time, do not give up; instead, provide a motivational intervention. The *Guideline* (USDHHS, 2000b) recommends using the "5Rs": (1) relevance, (2) risks, (3) rewards, (4) roadblocks, and (5) repetition. To ensure that the 5Rs are as individualized and personally motivational as possible, it is important to have the patient self-identify in conjunction with the provider their own relevance, risks, rewards, and roadblocks. To make an intervention relevant and meaningful to a patient, discuss smoking cessation in light of the patient's disease status, family or social situation, age, sex, and other characteristics unique to the patient. Three types of risks should be addressed with the patient. Acute risks include shortness of breath and exacerbation of asthma. Long-term risks include heart attack, stroke, cancer, and chronic obstructive pulmonary disease. Environmental risks include risks that put the patient's children and other family members at risk for lung cancer, sudden infant death syndrome, and asthma (AHCPR, 1996). The rewards of smoking cessation should also be discussed with the patient. These include improved health, energy level, sense of smell and taste, and self-esteem, economic savings, reduced wrinkling/aging of skin, modeling nonsmoking for children, as well as freedom from worry about the effect the patient's smoking has on his or her children and other family members. Roadblocks or barriers to quitting that need to be identified with the patient include withdrawal symptoms, fear of failure, weight gain, lack of social support, living with a smoker, depression, and loss of tobacco. Finally, repetition is included because the relevance, risks, and rewards need to be reviewed with the patient every time he or she is seen because on any given visit, the patient may finally be receptive to a smoking cessation intervention.

Step 4: Assist—Aid the Patient in Quitting

Setting a Quit Date and Planning for an Intervention

The first step in assisting the patient ready to quit smoking involves establishing a quit plan. Components of a quit plan include: (1) setting a quit date; (2) telling family, friends, and coworkers about quitting and the desire for support; (3) anticipating challenges to remaining smoke-free; and (4) removing tobacco products from home and work settings. In regard to setting a quit date, if a patient is motivated, setting a quit date within 2 weeks of meeting with the health care provider is most appropriate. Some patients, however, prefer to quit suddenly, or "cold turkey." If the smoker is identified in the hospital, setting a quit date is not necessary because the patient has become an ex-smoker because of the hospital smoking ban. Some programs have patients monitor the situations that cause them to smoke before they quit or reduce the number of cigarettes in the weeks before quitting. These techniques, however, although helpful to some, may simply prolong the process of quitting. Signing a contract at this point is a behavioral technique that has proved effective in helping patients to quit smoking. This process helps to formalize the smoker's commitment

DISPLAY **38-3**

RESPONSE SCALE

1	2	3	4	5	6	7
Definitely No	Probably No	Possibly No	Maybe	Possibly Yes	Probably Yes	Definitely Yes

to quitting and can serve as a method by which the nurse extends support to the patient in this process. Contracts must be simple and explicitly written so that both parties agree with the stated terms, and they should specify the consequences of not adhering to the expected behavior (see Harmful Effects of Smoking) and the rewards of successful adherence (see Benefits of Smoking Cessation) (Taylor Houston-Miller, Haskell, DeBusk, 1988-1).

The *Guidelines* (USDHHS, 2000b) recommend that five major components be a part of a brief intervention. These include: (1) provision of practical counseling such as problem solving, skills training, relapse prevention, and stress management; (2) provision of social support directly by the provider (intra-treatment social support); (3) helping the patient obtain social support outside of the clinical setting (extra-treatment social support); (4) recommending the use of approved pharmacotherapy, except in special circumstances; and (5) provision of supplementary materials. Practical counseling components include helping patients identify and anticipate "danger situations," such as events, activities, and internal states that increase the risk for smoking relapse, for example, negative affect, being with or living with another smoker, drinking alcohol, and stress. Coping strategies to review with patients include anticipatory planning, avoidance, and stress reduction. When providing practical counseling, it is also imperative to advise patients that smoking, even one puff of a cigarette, increases the likelihood of a complete relapse to smoking. Other information that is useful to patients attempting to quit smoking includes the addictive nature of smoking (Sohn et al., 2003), potential withdrawal symptoms, and that they can expect withdrawal symptoms to reach maximal intensity within 24 to 48 hours and then gradually subside over a 1- to 2-week period. The provision of intra-treatment support is the simple act of providing the patient with encouragement, showing the patient that you care about them and their health, and giving the patient the opportunity to talk about their quit attempt (concerns, fears, successes). The provision of extra-treatment social support includes encouraging family members and significant others to support the patient in the quit attempt and, if appropriate, providing a simultaneous smoking cessation intervention to household members who smoke. It is especially important to address this with women living with another smoker, because living with a smoker is a strong predictor of relapse in women (Froelicher, Houston Miller, Christopherson, et al., 2002). It may also include role playing with the patient how he or she will ask for the support that is needed, identifying and referring patient to community resources such as hotlines, web sites, or group meetings, and helping patients find "cessation buddies" with whom they can work. Provision of effective pharmacotherapies is strongly recommended and is discussed in greater detail later. Finally, as the patient leaves the health care setting, it is strongly advised that they take with them supplemental information in the form of pamphlets that are culturally, racially, educationally, and age appropriate for the patient. Patients then need follow-up in the form of face-to-face or telephone contacts (USDHHS, 2000b).

When planning a smoking cessation intervention, the nurse should take into account the patient's desire for formal help. Literature on compliance suggests that when the patient participates in developing a personalized plan of action, greater follow-through is achieved. Because most people choose individual methods for cessation, providing self-help materials is a low-cost method of intervention. When combined with strong advice by the nurse, these materials often double success rates. For the cardiac patient, the American Heart Association's *An Active Partnership for the Health of Your Heart* offers effective multimedia materials, including a videotape, audiotape, and workbook (American Heart Association, 2002). Other self-help materials, like those from the American Cancer Society and the American Lung Association, along with information for the nurse, are listed at the end of this chapter.

Although most patients choose to quit on their own with minimal help, some patients prefer, and may benefit from, a group program that provides 8 to 10 weeks of behavior modification. Knowing available community resources and making them available to patients by providing them with a list of programs to choose from, including the intervention methods, costs, and a contact person, ensures that patients are adequately informed. The patient may also be encouraged to address the issue with his or her employer, because many larger employers offer smoking cessation programs as an employee benefit.

Occasionally, patients may decide that acupuncture or hypnosis is a viable alternative. The success rates of these types of smoking cessation interventions, however, have been shown to be no better than placebo (USDHHS, 2000b). Some patients, however, anecdotally report these methods to be helpful. If a patient chooses a group cessation program or an alternative intervention, referral should be made and follow-up scheduled to determine the success of the chosen intervention. It is important to note that although the majority of smokers will express the desire to quit on their own, this strategy has proven to be of limited success; therefore, it behooves the health care provider to encourage a combination of self-help and more intensive strategies including pharmacological therapy (Ockene et al., 2000).

Relapse Prevention

A major component of successful smoking cessation interventions for patients who have recently quit is relapse prevention training (Marlatt, 1982), which involves: (1) identifying the patient's high-risk situations; (2) providing skills training to help the patient cope with these situations; and (3) rehearsing the coping mechanisms. Relapse prevention is a key because the majority of relapses occur early after initiation of cessation, primarily within the first 3 months after treatment, but risk for relapse continues long after the initial quit date, leading many to conclude that there is no safe point beyond which relapse does not occur (Ockene et al., 2000). Although a variety of predictors for relapse have been identified, stress, high nicotine dependence, low self-efficacy, limited social support, etc., are the strongest clues to probable relapse within 60 days after cessation (Ockene et al., 2000).

The *Guideline* (USDHHS, 2000b) divides relapse prevention into two categories, minimal practice interventions and prescriptive interventions. A minimal practice intervention should be provided to the patient who has recently quit every time their health care provider sees them. The provider must congratulate the patient on his or her successes, assist in problem-solving and any difficulties that have occurred or are anticipated, and strongly encourage the patient to remain a non-smoker. A prescriptive relapse prevention intervention is a more in-depth evaluation of potential high-risk situations,

How confident are you that you can resist the urge to smoke in the 14 situations below?

Not at All Confident			Slightly Confident			Fairly Confident			Very Confident	
0%	10%	20%	30%	40%	50%	60%	70%	80%	90%	100%

1. When you feel bored or depressed   _____
2. When you see others smoking   _____
3. When you want to relax or rest   _____
4. When you just want to sit back and enjoy a cigarette   _____
5. When you are watching TV   _____
6. When you are driving or riding in a car   _____
7. When you have finished a meal or snack   _____
8. When you feel frustrated, worried, upset, tense, nervous, angry, anxious, or annoyed   _____
9. When you want to snack, but don't want to gain weight   _____
10. When you need more energy or can't concentrate   _____
11. When someone offers you a cigarette   _____
12. When you are drinking coffee or tea   _____
13. When you are in a situation where alcohol is involved   _____
14. When you feel smoking is part of your self-image   _____

■ **Figure 38–1.** The Confidence Questionnaire (Modified Form). (Reprinted with permission from Condiotte, M. M., & Lichtenstein, E. [1981]. Self-efficacy and relapse in smoking cessation programs. *Journal of Consulting and Clinical Psychology,* 49, 648–658).

support systems, depression, withdrawal symptoms, and motivation to remain a non-smoker and can be delivered in person or over the telephone.

Two useful ways to help patients identify their personal high-risk situations are self-monitoring and self-efficacy scales. Through self-monitoring, patients keep a record of each cigarette smoked, noting the time of day, situation during which they smoke, and a rating of mood. A thorough examination of this record can be used to identify patterns of smoking behavior. Self-efficacy scales, however, measure a patient's confidence to resist the urge to smoke in a variety of situations. Studies have shown that self-efficacy ratings in smoking are predictive of subsequent outcome and, when smoking is resumed, specific situations or contexts are frequently predictive of a relapse episode (Gwaltney et al., 2002: Condiotti & Lichtenstein, 1981). In fact, the specific context (negative affect, positive affect, restricted smoking, idle time, social/food situations, low arousal, craving) with the lowest self-efficacy rating proves to be the best predictor of relapse or a sort of "Achilles heel" (Gwaltney et al., 2001). A 14-item self-efficacy scale, which is a shorter version of the scale by Condiotte and Lichtenstein (1981), is illustrated in Figure 38-1.

Less than 70% confidence for a given efficacy item denotes a high-risk situation for which patients may require help (Taylor et al., 1990; Froelicher & Christopherson, 2000). Patients are taught to work on those situations in which they show the least confidence to resist smoking. After identification of high-risk situations, skills training helps people mobilize their resources by developing cognitive and behavioral strategies to cope with the situation. Tsoh and colleagues (1997) recommend teaching patients to cope with urges to smoke by using the ACE (avoid, cope, escape) strategies. For example, if a patient does not feel ready to handle a risky situation, encourage the patient to avoid it until the patient's confidence in his or her ability to handle that particular risky situation improves. If a patient routinely watches football at a smoke-filled sports bar, tell him or her to invite some nonsmoking friends over to his or her home to watch the game. If a patient is going to a restaurant, he or she can ask to sit in the nonsmoking section, thereby avoiding the option to smoke. If a patient cannot avoid a risky situation, then coping with it is the next step. Possible coping strategies include distraction, incompatible behaviors, and positive self-talk. Distraction from the urge to smoke can be achieved by going for a walk, telephoning a friend, reading, or any other activity that gets the patient's mind off smoking until the urge subsides. Behaviors that are incompatible with smoking include chewing gum, snacking on low-calorie, low-fat foods, or engaging in tasks that occupy the hands, like knitting, sewing, woodworking, or crossword puzzles. Positive self-talk involves the patient telling himself or herself that he or she can continue to be a non-smoker. For example, a patient may say, "I can do this. I am capable of remaining a non-smoker. I have the power to improve my health by remaining a non-smoker." Other things a patient can do include reminding himself or herself about the health risks of cigarette smoking, the health benefits of quitting, and the monetary savings.

If the patient cannot avoid or cope with a risky situation, escape is the next option. "Escape" means getting out of a risky situation without a puff. For example, if the patient is at a party with friends, the patient can socialize with non-smokers in attendance instead of stepping outside with smokers. When dining out with others, escape can mean stepping outside while the others smoke after-dinner cigarettes. It is important to stress to the patient that a combination of strategies (ACE) is essential. By having many strategies, the patient decreases the risk of being caught in a situation he or she is not prepared to handle. The last step in relapse prevention training is practicing the coping response through rehearsal. Even though an urge may occur, if the patient is prepared to handle the situation, it decreases the likelihood that he or she will pick up a cigarette. One nursing responsibility includes practicing the different strategies to strengthen coping responses by role-playing with the patient a solution to handle the high-risk situation.

In addition to the strategies developed for specific situations, relapse prevention training focuses on general lifestyle modifications that help to enhance the patient's self-control (Marlatt, 1982). Exercise and relaxation techniques are two such strategies that have been used successfully to help patients develop a greater sense of self-control. In a study of patients after MI, smokers participating in an exercise training program combined with smoking cessation had greater cessation rates and smoked significantly fewer cigarettes than those who did not participate in such a program (Taylor, Houston-Miller, Haskell, & DeBusk, 1988). Exercise may also help reduce weight gain after quitting smoking and may minimize some withdrawal symptoms. For these reasons, patients should be encouraged to increase their activity levels through walking or other forms of exercise. Finally, patients who enjoy occasional social drinking should be encouraged to avoid using alcohol while attempting to become a non-smoker, because alcohol consumption is an independent predictor of relapse to smoking (Shiffman, 1986). Alcohol consumption and its relationship to smoking cessation are further discussed later.

Pharmacologic Therapy

The *Guideline* (USDHHS, 2000b) recommends that *all* patients expressing the desire to quit smoking receive both counseling and pharmacotherapy, except in special situations like pregnant or breast-feeding women, adolescents, those smoking fewer than 10 cigarettes per day, and those with medical contraindications such as recent MI or worsening angina. Through meta-analysis, five first-line pharmacotherapies were determined to be safe and efficacious, leading to cessation rates approximately double those of placebo. These are nicotine patch, nicotine gum, nicotine inhaler, nicotine nasal spray, and bupropion SR. Each of these first-line agents has received US Food and Drug Administration approval for use in smoking cessation. Each of these pharmacotherapies

has demonstrated efficacy, but none stands out above the others as being more efficacious, so there is no recommendation of one agent over the others. The nicotine patch, gum, and lozenge are available over the counter. The other forms of NRT are available by prescription only. The first-line agents are discussed below.

Nicotine Replacement Therapy (NRT)

NRT is a pharmacologic therapy that provides either continuous or bolus dosing of nicotine through the skin (transdermal patch) or mucous membranes (gum, inhaler, nasal spray, lozenge). NRT has been used as a smoking cessation aid since the early 1990s and has consistently demonstrated an abstinence rate of approximately twice that of placebo (USDHHS, 2000b: Shiffman et al., 2002, Silagy et al., 2002, Glover et al., 2002). Previously, NRT was regularly offered only to those patients who were considered highly addicted to cigarettes and was contraindicated in patients with cardiovascular disease.

Currently, the only *Guideline* (USDHHS, 2000b) recommendation related to patients considered highly addicted is the preference for the use of 4-mg gum as opposed to 2-mg gum. Combination NRT is appropriate for those patients unable to quit using a single first-line pharmacotherapeutic; however, although there is early indication of efficacy in those patients considered highly addicted, there is, as yet, not enough evidence to formally recommend it as particularly efficacious in those patients (USDHHS, 2000b). Patients who have had severe withdrawal symptoms in the past on making an attempt to quit are likely to be highly addicted to nicotine. The Fagerstrom Test for Nicotine Dependence (Heatherton et al., 1991) (Fig. 38-2) is an eight-item tool commonly used to measure addiction to nicotine. Patients can administer this self-test to identify their degree of dependence. In a study of cardiovascular patients, Taylor and coworkers (1990) noted that patients who smoke more than 25 cigarettes per day, who

Question	Answers	Points
1. How soon after you wake up do you smoke your first cigarette?	Within 5 minutes	3
	6–30 minutes	2
	31–60 minutes	1
	After 60 minutes	0
2. Do you find it difficult to refrain from smoking in places where it is forbidden (e.g., in church, at the library, in the cinema, etc.)?	Yes	1
	No	0
3. Which cigarette would you hate most to give up?	The first on in the morning	1
	All others	0
4. How many cigarettes/day do you smoke?	10 or less	0
	11–20	1
	21–30	2
	31 or more	3
5. Do you smoke more frequently during the first hours after waking than during the rest of the day?	Yes	1
	No	0
6. Do you smoke if you are so ill that you are in bed most of the day?	Yes	1
	No	0

Total score ranges from 0 to 10.
Total score of greater than 7 indicates nicotine dependence.

■ **Figure 38–2.** The Fagerstrom tolerance test. (Reprinted with permission from Heatherton, T., Kozlowski, L. Frecker, R., & Fagerstrom K. O. [1991]. The Fagerstrom Test for Nicotine Dependence: A revision of the Fagerstrom Tolerance Questionnaire. *British Journal of Addiction*, 86, 1119–1127.)

smoke as soon as they get up in the morning, and who smoke when they are so ill they are in bed are highly addicted to nicotine. Patients who meet the criteria for nicotine dependence and/or have experienced particularly troublesome withdrawal symptoms may be more successful in quitting if they are provided NRT in the form of 4-mg nicotine gum or are given a combination of the nicotine patch and gum or nasal spray. In fact, the meta-analysis performed for the *Guideline* (USDHHS, 2000b) found the abstinence rate increased from 17.4 with a single form of NRT to 28.6 with the use of two forms of NRT.

Previously, the Agency for Health Care Policy and Research's expert panel (1996), concluded that an acute cardiovascular events was a relative contraindication for NRT, and NRT was particularly contraindicated in patients who had experienced an MI within 4 weeks, had serious arrhythmias, or had worsening angina pectoris. Now, however, NRT is *not* considered an independent risk factor for acute myocardial events and has been found to be safe for the population of smokers with CVD. It should be used with caution in those patients experiencing acute cardiovascular events such as recent MI (within the previous 2 weeks), serious arrhythmias, and serious or worsening angina pectoris (USDHHS, 2000b). Establishment of a favorable risk-to-benefit ratio for NRT was based in part on the work of Benowitz (1988), who found that blood levels obtained during the use of 2-mg nicotine gum average 12 mg/mL, compared with peak levels without the gum of 35 to 54 mg/mL during smoking (Benowitz, 1988). Moreover, in assessing the effects of transdermal nicotine in cardiac patients, multiple studies have found no association between the patch and acute cardiac events (USDHHS, 2000b; Rennard et al., 1991). A review found that NRT constricts coronary arteries and alters hemodynamic profiles, leading to increased myocardial workload and oxygen demand. Cigarette smoking, however, precipitates acute cardiac events by three mechanisms, which are: (1) it produces a hypercoagulable state and promotes thrombosis; (2) it delivers carbon monoxide, which limits oxygen delivery to the heart; and (3) it alters hemodynamic profiles. The reviewers also concluded that the alterations in hemodynamic profiles caused by NRT were less hazardous than those produced by cigarette smoking (Benowitz & Gourlay, 1997). Therefore, it appears that the effects of NRT on the cardiovascular system are no greater and are probably less than the effects of cigarette smoking (Stillman, 1995).

Currently, NRT takes many forms, patch, gum, nasal spray, inhaler, and the newest form to be introduced is the lozenge. All forms of NRT appear to result in similar cessation rates if used as prescribed or intended (USDHHS, 2000b; Shiffman et al., 2002; Lam et al., 1987; Abelin et al., 1989; Tonneson et al., 1988). The nicotine patch and gum are the most widely used forms. The choice of which agent to use can be made by determining patient preference; previous experience (good or bad) with a given form of NRT; whether the patient wears dentures, which precludes the use of nicotine gum; and whether the smoking habit is associated with oral gratification, which may favor the gum, lozenge, or inhaler. An alternative form of NRT that has not been widely used is the nicotine nasal spray. Widespread use may be prohibited by the common adverse effects of nicotine nasal spray, including headache, burning sensations in the nose or throat, watery eyes, nasal and throat irritation, sneezing, runny nose, cough, and sleep disturbances. These

adverse effects usually begin on the first day of use but diminish over time (Hurt et al., 1998). Nicotine nasal spray, however, may be especially helpful for the highly addicted smoker because of its rapid onset of action (Schneider et al., 1996). A recent randomized controlled trial found that in terms of preference, the patch was the most preferred form of NRT followed by the spray, inhaler, and gum. The effectiveness of the product randomly assigned to the test subjects without regard to their stated preference did not significantly influence quit rates. It was noted, however, that women were more successful quitters using the inhaler compared to the gum, and among those heavily addicted smokers the relapse rates to smoking were lower for those using the inhaler than any other form of NRT (West et al., 2001). The use of the nicotine patch and gum, the most commonly used forms of NRT, because of over-the-counter availability, are described in more detail in Display 38-4.

Although multiple studies have demonstrated the value of NRT in smoking cessation, the use of NRT remains relatively limited. As was stated, NRT should NOT be reserved for severely addicted smokers only or withheld until the patient has attempted to quit on his or her own in an effort to assess the level of withdrawal and determine the need for pharmacologic assistance. Studies, however, continue to document the underuse of NRT and several theories regarding potential barriers to prescription and use have been proposed. For example, the Women's Initiative for Nonsmoking (WINS) study revealed that of 142 women with CVD in the intervention group, 127 met the study criteria for NRT use, but the reported use of NRT by patients ranged from 9% (2-day follow-up) to 22% (90-day follow-up), even in light of the fact that NRT was available to the women free of charge. The researchers hypothesized that the intervention nurses may have been leery of recommending NRT because the AHCPR had previously cautioned against use of NRT in CVD patients, or because of lack of patient education regarding the myths of NRT such as trading one addiction for another (Mahrer-Imhof et al., 2002). Emmons et al. (2000) also demonstrated a low level of use of NRT in hospitalized patients of only 7.1% of patients in a sample of 580 men and women smokers who were hospitalized. Another potential explanation for lack of use of NRT is reluctance on the part of health care providers to recognize cigarette smoking as an addiction. Cigarette smoking has clearly been found to be an addiction because it fulfills the requirements for addiction of: (1) highly controlled or compulsive use; (2) psychoactive effects; and (3) drug-reinforced behavior (USDHHS, 1988).

Bupropion

Another alternative to NRT is sustained-release bupropion (Zyban SR; GlaxoSmithKline, Research Triangle Park, NC), an oral medication that comes in tablet form. This pharmacologic aid for smoking cessation has been used for many years to treat depression. The exact mechanism that promotes smoking cessation is unknown. Bupropion is, however a weak inhibitor of neuronal uptake of dopamine, serotonin, and norepinephrine (GlaxoSmithKline, 2003). It is believed to affect the mesolimbic dopaminergic system and, therefore, mediates reward for nicotine use (Hays & Ebbert, 2003). Like NRT, Bupropion produces cessation rates approximately double those of placebo

DISPLAY 38-4

NICOTINE REPLACEMENT THERAPY (NRT)

Nicotine Gum

Nicotine chewing gum has been available in the United States since 1984, and has been available over the counter since 1997. It comes in 2- and 4-mg doses. It is a resin-based gum that releases nicotine into the bloodstream through the buccal mucosa inside the mouth. The success of nicotine gum is highly dependent on its proper use. It has been shown to be highly ineffective when dispensed without proper chewing instruction. Moreover, when nicotine gum is prescribed without any counseling or strong advice, it has been shown to produce very low cessation rates (Cummings et al., 1988; Sachs, 1989).

Patients should start using the gum immediately as soon as they stop smoking. Although nicotine gum was originally prescribed to be taken on an as-needed basis, studies suggest that a regular schedule of taking the gum, normally one piece every 60 minutes during waking hours, ensures constant blood nicotine levels (Killen et al., 1990). Side effects are also minimal and transient if the gum is administered properly. Most often, these side effects are limited to local mouth irritation, some gastrointestinal distress such as nausea and heartburn, palpitations, and jaw ache from excessive chewing.

An acidic environment in the mouth blocks nicotine absorption. Because the use of beverages such as colas, coffee, tea, and juices changes the oral pH to an acidic environment, these agents should not be used within 15 minutes of using the gum or during the first 15 minutes of chewing the gum (Henningfield et al., 1990). Because nicotine gum is now available over the counter, it is imperative that teaching be done by the nurse or, alternatively, the patient should be encouraged to discuss proper use with a pharmacist. Nicotine chewing gum is normally used for a period of 3 to 6 months. A tapering schedule of at least 1 month is recommended. Weaning can be accomplished by decreasing the dosage, cutting gum pieces in half, and substituting sugarless gum for some of the doses. Nurses should also be aware that 8% to 25% of nicotine gum users who successfully quit smoking use the gum beyond the 6 months recommended for maximal use. Habitual use of the gum to deal with negative emotional states is often the cause of this prolonged use (Hajek et al., 1988). As noted previously, the prolonged use of the gum is preferred to smoking and has not been shown to be harmful (USDHHS, 2000b).

Nicotine Patch

The transdermal nicotine patch has been available in the United States by prescription since 1991 and over the counter since 1997. The nicotine patch produces a therapeutic effect by releasing a controlled amount of nicotine through the skin that is absorbed through the capillary bed. Studies have been con-

ducted in patients with coronary heart disease to ascertain the safety and efficacy of the patch, and current findings suggest that it is both safe and efficacious. The only subsets of the CHD population in which the patch should be used with caution are those in immediate postmyocardial infarction period, those with serious arrhythmias, and those with serious or worsening angina (USDHHS, 2000b). In general, the patch has been found to roughly double abstinence rates (USDHHS, 2000b) and success rates of NRT in the general population varies widely, from as high as 71% at 6 weeks (Hurt et al., 1990) after cessation to as low as 18% at 3 weeks after cessation (Rose et al., 1990).

Higher success rates have been achieved in patients who receive supportive counseling or therapy (Rennard et al., 1991; Hurt et al., 1990; Transdermal Nicotine Study Group, 1991; Krumpe et al., 1989; Mulligan et al., 1990; Draughton et al., 1991), but these rates have frequently been found to decrease to approximately half of the initial rates 6 to 12 months after beginning treatment.

Nicotine patches ameliorate some aspects of tobacco withdrawal but not all cravings or urges. Some studies have shown that self-reported cravings have been reduced (Abelin et al., 1989; Tonnesen et al., 1991), and negative affect and lethargic feelings are decreased (Rose et al., 1990). However, the nicotine patch has little effect on habit-based urges (Rose et al., 1990).

The nicotine patch is designed to be worn for a period of 16 to 24 hours depending on the brand, with a recommended dose of 21 mg/24 h, or 15 mg/16 h. Lower doses (10–14 mg) are recommended for some cardiovascular patients, see above. Patches are designed to be changed daily and are normally recommended to be used for 8 weeks, with weaning beginning at 4 weeks. During the weaning period, the dose is reduced in a stepwise manner (i.e., 21, 14, and 7 mg) to 7 mg/24 h, or 5 mg/16 h, and finally discontinued (AHCPR, 1996). The nicotine patch is often considered the preferred choice for patients because of ease of use. It requires little effort to apply the patch and coverage can be ensured for up to 24 hours.

The most frequent side effect of the nicotine patch is local skin redness, which occurs in approximately 35% to 54% of patients using the patch (Ciba-Geigy Corporation, 1992; Marion Merrell Dow, Inc., 1991; Lederele Laboratories, 1992; Parke-Davis, 1992). Severe skin reactions, which include rashes or eczema, have led to discontinuation of therapy in less than 7% of patients (Rose et al., 1990; Draughton et al., 1991). Other side effects reported, which occur much less frequently, include gastrointestinal problems of dyspepsia, abdominal pain, and diarrhea; muscle and limb weakness; paresthesia; nervousness; and vivid or disturbing dreams (Transdermal Nicotine Study Group, 1991).

(USDHHS, 2000b; Holm & Spencer, 2000; Tonstad, 2002; Tonstad et al., 2003). The recommended dosage of bupropion is 150 mg daily for 3 days, increased to 150 mg 2 times per day thereafter (USDHHS, 2002b).

Unlike NRT, bupropion treatment should be initiated while the patient is still smoking, because it takes approximately 1 week of treatment to achieve steady-state blood levels of bupropion. A target quit date should be established in the second week of treatment to promote the highest likelihood of cessation. Treatment with bupropion SR should last a minimum of 7 to 12 weeks. Longer treatment has been shown effective and should be guided by an evaluation of the risks and benefits for the individual patient. If smoking cessation has not been achieved by the seventh week, it is not likely to occur and therapy with bupropion SR should be discontinued (Glaxo-SmithKline, 2003).

Bupropion seems to have its highest level of success with women and the previously depressed. In a randomized, controlled clinical trial of 893 smokers using a combination of bupropion or placebo and 21-mg nicotine patch or placebo patch, bupropion was found to approximately triple 1-year smoking cessation in women and subjects with previous depression (Smith et al., 2003).

Bupropion is safe and effective for patients with CVD. Tonstad found in a randomized double-blind study of CVD patients that there were no clinically significant changes in heart rate or blood pressure during treatment with bupropion, and that it resulted in cessation rates of greater than twice that of placebo (2003). Likewise, in a literature review of the tolerability and safety of bupropion SR, Aubin (2002) found that mean values for heart rate, blood pressure, and routine laboratory values remained unchanged in those given bupropion relative to placebo.

Bupropion is contraindicated, however, in patients at high risk for seizure because of previous head trauma, central nervous system tumor, anorexia nervosa, bulimia, previous seizure, or concomitant use with another medication that lowers the seizure threshold (antipsychotics, antidepressants, theophylline, systemic steroids) (GlaxoSmithKline, 2003). Bupropion also interferes with the degradation of drugs such as tricyclic antidepressants, beta-blockers, and antiarrhythmics such as flecainide (Haustein, 2003). The most common side effects are insomnia and dry mouth; both symptoms are generally transient and usually resolve without intervention (GlaxoSmithKline, 2003; Holm & Spencer, 2000; Aubin, 2002; The Medical Letter, 1997). Thus, bupropion is generally well tolerated with discontinuation rates of 6% to 12% because of adverse events (Aubin, 2002).

Bupropion has been shown to decrease cravings associated with smoking cessation, which is an important piece of information to be aware of when considering pharmacologic interventions, because craving has been cited as a strong predictor of relapse to smoking cessation. For example, in a double-blind, placebo-controlled trial of bupropion SR, craving was cited as the impetus of relapse by 49.2% versus 22.4% of relapsers receiving placebo and bupropion SR, respectively (Durcan et al., 2002). Bupropion has also been deemed effective at prolonging the median time to relapse, 156 days versus 65 days, when compared to placebo and it has been found to delay weight gain when used long-term (Hays et al., 2001).

Step 5: Arrange–Schedule Follow-Up Contact

A meta-analysis conducted by Kottke and colleagues (1988) concluded that reinforcement by numerous contacts and health care professionals leads to greater smoking cessation rates. Ideally, follow-up contact should occur soon after the established quit date, preferably within the first week and then again within the first month. Follow-up can be performed in person or by telephone. Important components of follow-up include congratulations on success, support, reinforcement, and problem solving. If the patient slipped or relapsed, follow-up provides the opportunity to review the circumstances that led to the slip or relapse, create a new plan to deal with a similar situation in the future, and establish a new quit date. Follow-up

also allows the clinician to review and trouble-shoot any problems associated with the use of pharmacologic therapies.

Although a brief intervention is the minimum that all health care providers should offer their patients, the *Guideline* (USDHHS, 2000b) clearly points out that implementation of a more intensive intervention is the goal because there is a strong dose–response relation between counseling intensity and success in smoking cessation. The meta-analyses conducted for the current *Guideline* strongly indicate that there is a dose-response relationship between session length and abstinence rates, total amount of contact time and abstinence rates, and the number of sessions and treatment efficacy. In terms of session length, it was found that abstinence rates increase from 10.9 with NO contact to 22.1 with longer counseling sessions (lasting >10 minutes). In terms of contact time, it was found that abstinence rates increase from 11.0 with NO contact time to 28.4 with 91 to 300 minutes. In terms of number of sessions, abstinence rates double from 12.4 with no or one session to 24.7 with more than eight sessions. The *Guideline* thus recommends four or more sessions lasting longer than 10 minutes for a total contact time of more than 30 minutes.

■ SPECIAL AREAS ON WHICH TO FOCUS

Stress

Patients may often relapse to smoking during stressful times, especially those involving emotional circumstances, such as arguments or a crisis situation with a spouse, family members, or coworkers (Shiffman, 1986). The frequency and severity of distressing demands during everyday life have also been shown to be predictors of later relapse to smoking in both men and women (Romano et al., 1991; Gritz et al., 1996). Although some patients may need in-depth counseling to help them with such problems, simple relaxation training may produce a sense of increased control, which may in turn affect the patient's confidence to withstand the urge to smoke. Many patients can benefit from the use of inexpensive relaxation audiotapes that use simple instructions on how to use muscle tension and deep breathing exercises to achieve relaxation.

Depression

Current smokers have been found to have higher mean depression scores than never smokers in both men and women (Haukkala et al., 2000). Smokers, in general, have had a significantly greater number of past episodes of major depression than average, and smokers with a history of major depression who quit are seven-times more likely to have a recurrence of major depression than individuals who continue to smoke (Glassman et al., 2001). Depressive episodes occurring before smoking cessation have an inverse relationship with 6-month abstinence (Cinciripini et al., 2003). In other words, patients who have had a previous history of depression but are not depressed at the time smoking cessation is initiated have less success at quitting than do smokers who have never

	YES	NO
1. Have you ever felt you ought to CUT DOWN on your drinking?	☐	☐
2. Have people ANNOYED you by criticizing your drinking?	☐	☐
3. Have you ever felt GUILTY about your drinking?	☐	☐
4. Have you ever had a drink first thing in the morning (EYE OPENER) to steady your nerves or get rid of a hangover?	☐	☐

■ **Figure 38–3.** The CAGE questionnaire. (Reprinted with permission from Ewing, J. A. [1984]. Detecting alcoholism: The CAGE questionnaire. *JAMA,* 252, 1905–1907.)

experienced depression. Higher depression scores are also related to lower self-efficacy for quitting, especially among men (Haukkala et al., 2000), and decreases in self-efficacy, if they are going to occur, will most likely happen in the first 2 weeks after cessation (Cinciripini et al., 2003). Women experiencing depression were found to have more difficulty initiating a smoking cessation attempt, maintaining abstinence, and were likely to relapse to smoking significantly earlier than were non-depressed women (Pomerleau, Brouwer, & Pomerleau, 2001). Therefore, clinicians working with depressed smokers making a quit attempt may need to focus on enhancing self-efficacy and providing additional support in the first few weeks after cessation to prevent negative affect from significantly decreasing self-efficacy and increasing the likelihood of relapse. One thing that does bode well for smoking cessation is the finding that higher depression scores are related to a greater motivation to quit in women, a factor that clinicians must use in their favor (Haukkala et al., 2000). Although there are multiple depression screening tools available in the literature, Whooley and Simon (2000) have developed a very brief two-question case finding instrument that is quickly and easily used in the clinical setting to help guide plans for a smoking cessation intervention. The two questions are: (1) during the past month, have you often been bothered by feeling down, depressed, or hopeless?; and (2) during the past month, have you often been bothered by having little interest or pleasure in doing things? If the patient answers "no" to both questions, the patient is unlikely to have major depression. If the patient answers "yes" to either question, a follow-up clinical interview by a mental health professional is recommended; alternatively, a referral to either the primary care provider or a psychiatrist is indicated. Bupropion SR should be considered the first-line pharmacotherapeutic agent used in patients with current or past depression because it has been proven effective for both smoking cessation and depression therapy (USDHHS, 2000b).

Alcohol Use

Social situations that involve alcohol use are another predictor of relapse to smoking (Shiffman, 1986). For this reason, nurses need to determine whether the smoker attempting to quit consumes excessive alcohol regularly. This information can be ascertained while taking a smoking history by using the simple four-item CAGE questionnaire (Ewing, 1984) (Fig. 38-3), which is a screening tool for alcohol abuse. If a diagnosis of alcoholism is made, patients should be encouraged to seek treatment for alcoholism and smoking cessation simultaneously. Patients who are heavy social drinkers should also be encouraged

to avoid alcohol or decrease their consumption substantially until they feel successful in their smoking cessation efforts.

Loss

For many patients, giving up smoking is like "losing a best friend." Nurses must help patients to recognize and understand the magnitude of this loss. Helping patients acknowledge how they feel about their loss and working with them to select new activities that provide immediate gratification is important. For example, patients should be encouraged to focus on old, or select new, hobbies. They can also develop reward systems for their daily success in remaining nonsmokers. Nurses should also encourage patients to build new activities into their daily schedules that also increase confidence as their focus shifts to new behaviors.

Weight Gain

The average weight gain after smoking cessation is approximately 6 to 10 pounds, much of which is caused by metabolic changes that occur with cessation (Wack & Rodin, 1982). It appears weight gain is more often associated with those who smoke more cigarettes or have a history of weight problems (Hall et al., 1986). In addition, those who quit smoking often crave sweet foods (Grunberg, 1982).

Encouraging patients to be more active through daily exercise and helping them to identify low-calorie snacks and sweets can help patients avoid excessive weight gain. Patients must also be aware that the risks of continued smoking far outweigh the risks of gaining a few pounds. Weight gain cannot be treated lightly because 67% of women in one study stated that they were very concerned or somewhat concerned about weight gain after cessation (Pomerleau, Zucker, & Stewart, 2001). In another study, up to 75% of women and 35% of men reported an unwillingness to gain 5 or more pounds as a result of stopping smoking. In particular, more than half of women younger than age 25 years and 39% of women older than 40 years stated that they were unwilling to gain any weight (Tsoh et al., 1997). It is important to note that weight gain is not just a concern of women. Weight gain in the first 3 months after cessation was predictive of relapse to smoking for men. In fact, the risk of relapse increased by 17% for every kilogram of weight gained (Borrelli, 2001). Providers must therefore openly discuss the possibility of weight gain but stress to the patient that the amount of weight gained is usually limited and that a program of exercise and a healthy diet can control weight gain (USDHHS, 2000b). In addition, current

Please read the following questions and circle the response that most closely describes your current situation.

1. Is there someone available to you whom you can count on to listen to you when you need to talk?

None of the time	A little of the time	Some of the time	Most of the time	All of the time
1	2	3	4	5

2. Is there someone available to give you good advice about a problem?

None of the time	A little of the time	Some of the time	Most of the time	All of the time
1	2	3	4	5

3. Is there someone available to you who shows you love and affection?

None of the time	A little of the time	Some of the time	Most of the time	All of the time
1	2	3	4	5

4. Is there someone available to help you with daily chores?

None of the time	A little of the time	Some of the time	Most of the time	All of the time
1	2	3	4	5

5. Can you count on anyone to provide you with emotional support (talking over problems or helping you make a difficult decision)?

None of the time	A little of the time	Some of the time	Most of the time	All of the time
1	2	3	4	5

6. Do you have as much contact as you would like with someone you feel close to, someone in whom you can trust and confide?

None of the time	A little of the time	Some of the time	Most of the time	All of the time
1	2	3	4	5

7. Are you currently married or living with a partner?

Yes	No

■ **Figure 38–4.** ENRICHD Social Support Instrument (ESSI). (Reprinted with permission from Mitchell, P. H., Powell, L., Blumenthal, J., Norten, J., et al. [2003]. A short social support measure in patients reserving from myocardial infarction: The ENRICHD social support inventory. *Journal of Cardiac Rehabilitation*, in press.)

studies indicate that NRT, particularly the gum, and bupropion SR have been shown to at least delay post-cessation weight gain, (USDHHS, 2000b). In the case of bupropion SR, weight gain was actually significantly less compared to placebo, 3.8 kg versus 5.6 kg, respectively (Hays et al., 2001).

Social Support

Support from a spouse or family members is directly related to quitting smoking and short-term maintenance of the non-smoking behavior (Cohen et al., 1988). Women in particular give social support higher ratings of importance in smoking cessation than do men (Gritz et al., 1996). If family members or close friends smoke, it is important to initiate a plan to help the patient resist the temptation to smoke when around others who are smoking. It is imperative to prepare the patient for this situation if the family member or friend who smokes lives with the patient. Previous preparation is particularly important for women living with a smoker because the odds of relapsing are 2.5-times higher in this population (Froelicher, Houston-Miller, Christopherson, et al., 2002). The ideal situation, of course, is when the family member or friend attempts to quit at the same time the patient does; therefore, interventions that target other smokers in the household at the same time seem prudent. If this is not feasible, the nurse should counsel the family member or friend to: (1) not smoke in the presence of the patient if possible; (2) remove all cigarettes and other tobacco products from the household; and (3) refrain from offering cigarettes to the patient who is trying to quit. Family members and friends should also be encouraged to provide daily positive reinforcement for patients successful at quitting. It may also be appropriate for the nurse to teach the patient some basic assertiveness skills, so that the patient is prepared to ask assertively that the family member or friend not smoke in his or her presence, not offer him or her cigarettes, and so forth. The ENRICHD Social Support Instrument (ESSI) is a brief seven-item questionnaire that is useful in assessing social support in cardiac patients (ENRICHD Investigator Writing Group, 2001; Mitchell et al., 2003; ENRICHD Investigator Writing Group, 2003) and can help guide where emphasis should be placed when designing an individualized intervention when social support is low (Fig. 38-4).

Vulnerable Populations

Vulnerable populations include, but are not limited to, the economically disadvantaged, underinsured or uninsured, migrant workers, immigrants, incarcerated, homeless, lesbian, gay, bisexual, or transgender populations, ethnic minorities, and infants and young children. These populations are vulnerable because of inadequate, inappropriate, or unavailable resources and/or inadequate knowledge of the numbers and needs of these populations as a result of inadequate census and research data (Hutchinson & Froelicher, 2003). In general, smoking cessation interventions have, for the most part, been successful in a variety of different types of populations from blue collar workers (Gritz et al., 1998) to those enrolled in managed care medical programs (Smith et al., 2002); therefore, it is in the best interest of the smoker no matter his or her age, ethnicity, lifestyle, or occupation to receive a smoking cessation intervention that is as individually tailored as possible. With time and further research, the hope is that current intervention strategies are found to be effective in these populations or that new strategies will be developed and found efficacious.

Women

The most recent Surgeon General's Report, Women and Smoking, reiterates the need for smoking cessation efforts targeted directly at women because approximately three million women in the United States have died since 1980 from a smoking-related disease (CDCP, 2001). Of even further concern is that the World Health Organization's Report, Women and the Tobacco Epidemic: Challenges for the 21st Century, confirms that the problem is not restricted to the United States (World Health Organization, 2001). Some researchers have found that women are less likely to quit smoking than men are (Okene et al., 1992), whereas others have found similar cessation rates (Whitlock et al., 1997; Gritz et al., 1998). It is generally believed, however, that women respond differently to smoking cessation interventions. Some possible explanations are differences in physiology and behavioral and psychological factors. For example, the menstrual cycle may play a role in smoking cessation. The symptoms of menstrual distress include depression, irritability, anxiety, tension, decreased ability to concentrate, and weight changes, all of which are also symptoms of nicotine withdrawal. Withdrawal has been shown to be greater when the quit date is set during the luteal phase (ovulation to day before menses) of the menstrual cycle as opposed to the follicular phase (day 1 of menses to day 15). Therefore, it may be valuable to assess the menstrual cycle pattern before setting a quit date to reduce compounding withdrawal with normal menstrual distress (O'Hara et al., 1989). Behavioral and psychological factors that play a large role in smoking cessation for women are fear of weight gain, low social support, reliance on cigarettes for control of negative affect or stress management, and self-efficacy in quitting (Gritz et al., 1996). These areas must be addressed when implementing a smoking cessation intervention with a woman. For example, the Women's Initiative for Nonsmoking (WINS) study found that low self-efficacy and living with a smoker were predictive of smoking at 6 and 12 months of follow-up. In addition, women who perceived themselves to be in "fair" or "poor" health were more likely to be smokers at 12 months (Froelicher, Houston-Miller, Christopherson, et al., 2002). Gritz and colleagues also found that a higher education level and a "white collar" job classification were also predictive of smoking cessation in a workplace-based study (1998). As always, it is best to tailor the intervention to the individual patient when possible. It is important to note, however, that women preferred to use a greater number and variety of quitting strategies, including individual strategies, like reading cessation materials, smoking substitutes, relaxation techniques, seeking support, hypnosis, and acupuncture, than men (Whitlock et al., 1997). Specific benefits of smoking cessation we have found helpful to discuss with women include improved complexion, fewer wrinkles, no odor of cigarettes on their breath or in their hair or clothes, and better health for children and family members. Given the limited information on characteristics predictive of smoking cessation success in women and the limited number of women-only smoking cessation studies, the information on how specifically to support the female smoker in quitting is limited.

▪ SUMMARY

A systematic approach to smoking cessation leads to better outcomes. The measure of success should be based on the frequency with which the nurse asks about a patient's smoking status. Multicomponent strategies that include strong physician and nurse advice, self-help materials, behavioral counseling, pharmacologic therapy, and follow-up can be used to help the general population and those with CHD.

Acknowledgement: *We thank Nancy Houston Miller for contribution to the fourth edition of this chapter.*

REFERENCES

Abelin, T., Buehler, A., Miller, P., Vesanen, K., & Imhof, P. R. (1989). Controlled trial of transdermal nicotine patch in tobacco withdrawal. *Lancet*, 1, 7–10.

Agency for Health Care Policy and Research: U.S. Department of Health and Human Services. (1996). *Clinical Practice Guideline: Smoking cessation.* Publication no. 96-0692. Washington, DC: Government Printing Office.

American Heart Association. (2002). *An active partnership for the health of your heart.* Dallas, TX: American Heart Association.

American Psychiatric Association. (1994). *Diagnostic and statistical manual of mental disorders* (4th ed.). Washington, DC: American Psychiatric Association.

Aubin, H. J. (2002). Tolerability and safety of sustained-release bupropion in the management of smoking cessation. *Drugs, 62*(Suppl. 2), 45–52.

Baile, W. F., Bigelow, G. E., Gottlieb, S. H., & Sacktor, J. D. (1982). Rapid resumption of cigarette smoking following myocardial infarction: Inverse relation to myocardial infarction severity. *Addictive Behavior, 7*, 373–380.

Bandura, A. (1997). The anatomy of stages of change [editorial]. *American Journal of Health Promotion, 12*(1), 8–10.

Barry, .J, Mead, K., Nabel, E., Rocco, M. B., Campbell, S., Fenton, T., Mudge, G. H., & Selwyn, A. P. (1989). Effect of smoking on the activity of ischemic heart disease. *Journal of the American Medical Association, 261*, 398–402.

Benowitz, N. L. (1988). Pharmacological aspects of cigarette smoking and nicotine addiction. *New England Journal of Medicine, 319*, 1318–1329.

Benowitz, N., & Gourlay, S. (1997). Cardiovascular toxicity of nicotine: Implications for nicotine replacement therapy. *Journal of the American College of Cardiology, 29*, 1422–1431.

Borrelli, B., Spring, B., Niaura, R., Hitsman, B., & Papandonatos, G. (2001). Influences of gender and weight gain on short-term relapse to smoking in a cessation trial. *Journal of Consulting and Clinical Psychology, 69*(3), 511–515

Britton, R., McMahon, M., & Bryant, D. (1991). Smoking in hospitalized patients. *Addictive Behavior, 16*, 79–81.

Burling, T. A., Singleton, E. G., Bigelow, G. E., Baile, W. F., & Gottlieb, S. H. (1984). Smoking following myocardial infarction: A critical review of the literature. *Health Psychology, 3*, 83–96.

Burt, A., Thornley, R., Illingworth, D., White, P., Shaw, T. R. D., & Turner, R. (1974). Stopping smoking after myocardial infarction. *Lancet, 1*, 304–306.

Centers for Disease Control and Prevention. (2001). Surgeon General's Report: women and smoking 2001–at a glance. [On-line]. Available: http://www.cdc.gov/tobacco/sgr/sgr_forwomen/ataglance.htm.

Centers for Disease Control and Prevention. (2002a). Cigarette smoking among adults–United States, 2000. *Morbidity and Mortality Weekly Report, 51*(29), 642–645.

Centers for Disease Control and Prevention. (2002b). Annual smoking-attributable mortality, years of life lost, and economic costs–United States, 1995-1999. *Morbidity and Mortality Weekly Report*, 51(14), 300–303.

Ciba-Geigy Corporation (1992). *Habitrol (nicotine transdermal therapeutic system) prescribing information*. Edison, NJ: CibaGeigy.

Cinciripini, P. M., Wetter, D. W., Fouladi, R. T., Blalock, J. A., Carter, B. L., Cinciripini, L. G., & Baile, W. F. (2003). The effects of depressed mood on smoking cessation: mediation by postcessation self-efficacy. *Journal of Consulting and Clinical Psychology*, 71(2), 292–301.

Cohen, S., Lichtenstein, E., Mermelstein, R., et al. (1988). Social support interventions for smoking cessation. In B. H. Gottlieb (Ed.), *Marshaling social support: Formats, processes, and effects* (pp. 211–240). Newbury Park, CA: Sage.

Condiotte, M. M. & Lichtenstein, E. (1981). Self-efficacy and relapse in smoking cessation programs. *Journal of Consulting and Clinical Psychology*, 49, 648–658.

Crouse, J. & Hagaman, A. (1991). Smoking cessation in relation to cardiac procedures. *American Journal of Preventive Medicine*, 7, 131–135.

Cummings, S. R., Hansen, B., Richard, R. J., Stein, M. J., & Coates, T. J. (1988). Internists and nicotine gum. *Journal of the American Medical Association*, 260, 1565–1569.

DiClemente, C., Prochaska, J., Fairhurst, S. K., Velicer, W. F., Velasquez, M. M., & Rossi, J. S. (1991). The process of smoking cessation: An analysis of precontemplation, contemplation, and preparation stages of change. *Journal of Consulting and Clinical Psychology*, 59, 295–304.

Dijkstra, A., DeVries, H., & Baker, M. (1996). Pros and cons of quitting, self-efficacy, and the stages of change in smoking cessation. *Journal of Consulting and Clinical Psychology*, 64, 758–763.

Dornelas, E. A., Sampson, R. A., Gray, J. F., Waters, D., & Thompson, P. D. (2000). A randomized controlled trial of smoking cessation counseling after myocardial infarction. *Preventive Medicine*, 30, 261–268.

Draughton, D. M., Heatley, S. A., Prendergast, J. J., Causey, D., Knowles, M., Rolf, C. N., Cheney, R. A., Hatlelid, K., Thompson, A. B., & Rennard, S. I. (1991). Effect of transdermal nicotine delivery as an adjunct to low intervention smoking cessation therapy. *Archives of Internal Medicine*, 151, 749–752.

Durcan, M. J., Deener, G., White, J., Johnston, J. A., Gonzales, D., Niaura, R., Rigotti, N., & Sachs, D. P. (2002). *Clinical Therapeutics*, 24(4A), 540–551.

Emmons, K. M. & Goldstein, M. G. (1992). Smokers who are hospitalized: A window of opportunity for cessation interventions. *Preventive Medicine*, 21, 262–269.

Emmons, K. M., Goldstein, M. G., Roberts, M., Cargill, B., Sherman, C. B., Millman, R., Brown, R., & Abrams, D. B. (2000). The use of nicotine replacement therapy during hospitalization. *Annals of Behavioral Medicine*, 22(4), 325–329.

ENRICHD Investigator Writing Group. (2001). Enhancing recovery in coronary heart disease (ENRICHD): baseline characteristics. *American Journal of Cardiology*, 88, 316–322.

ENRICHD Investigator Writing Group. (2003). Effects of treating depression and low perceived social support on clinical events after myocardial infarction: the enhancing recovery in coronary heart disease patients (ENRICHD) randomized trial. *Journal of the American Medical Association*, 289(23), 3171–3173.

Ewing, J. A. (1984). Detecting alcoholism: The CAGE questionnaire. *Journal of the American Medical Association*, 252, 1905–1907.

Faulkner, A. & Ward, L. (1983). Nurses as health educators in relation to smoking. *Nursing Times*, 79(8), 47–48.

Fiore, M. C., Novotny, T. F., Pierce, J. P., Giovino, G. A., Hatziandreu, E. J., Newcomb, P. A., Surawicz, T. S., & Davis, R. M. (1990). Methods used to quit smoking in the United States: Do cessation programs help? *Journal of the American Medical Association*, 263, 2760–2765.

Frank, E., Winkleby, M. A., Altman, D. G., Rockhill, B., & Fortmann, S. P. (1991). Predictors of physician's smoking cessation advice. *Journal of the American Medical Association*, 266, 3139–3144.

Froelicher, E. & Christopherson, D. J. (2000). Women's initiative for nonsmoking (WINS) I: design and methods. *Heart & Lung*, 29(6), 429–437.

Froelicher, E. S., & Kozuki, Y. (2002). Theoretical applications of smoking cessation interventions to individuals with medical conditions: women's initiative for nonsmoking (WINS) – part III. *International Journal of Nursing Studies*. 39, 1–15.

Froelicher, E. S., Christopherson, D. J., Houston-Miller, N., & Martin, K. (2002). Women's initiative for nonsmoking (WINS) IV: Description of 277 women smokers hospitalized with cardiovascular disease. *Heart & Lung*, 31(1), 3–14.

Froelicher, E. S., Houston-Miller, N., Christopherson, D. J., Martin, K., Parker, K., Amonette, M., Benowitz, N., Taylor, C. B., & Bacchetti, P. (2002). Efficacy of smoking cessation intervention in women hospitalized

with cardiovascular disease: Women's Initiative for Nonsmoking (WINS). *Circulation*, 106(19), II–735.

Froelicher, E. S., Houston-Miller, N., Li, W., Mahrer-Imhof, R., Sohn, M. & Bacchetti, P. (2002). Predictors of smoking cessation in women with cardiovascular disease: the Women's Initiative for Nonsmoking (WINS). *Circulation*, 106(19), II–666.

Glasgow, R. E., Stevens, V. J., Vogt, T. M., Mullooly, J. P., & Lichtenstein, E. (1991). Changes in smoking associated with hospitalization: Quit rates, predictive variables, and intervention implications. *American Journal of Health Promotion*, 6(1), 24–29.

Glassman, A. H., Covey, L. S., Stetner, F., & Rivelli, S. (2001). Smoking cessation and the course of major depression: a follow-up study. *Lancet*, 357(9272), 1929–1932.

GlaxoSmithKline. (2003). *Zyban prescribing information*. [Online]. Available: http://us.gsk.com/products/assets/us_zyban.pdf.

Glover, E. D., Glover, P. N., Franzon, M., Sullivan, C. R., Cerullo, C. C., Howell, R. M., Keyes, G. G., Nilsson, F., & Hobbs, G. R. (2002). A comparison of a nicotine sublingual tablet and placebo for smoking cessation. *Nicotine & Tobacco Research*, 4(4), 441–450.

Goldstein, A. O., Hellier, A., Fitzgerald, S., Stegall, T. S., & Fischer, P. M. (1987). Hospital nurse counseling of patients who smoke. *American Journal of Public Health*, 77, 1333–1334.

Gritz, E. R., Nielsen, I. R., & Brooks, L. A. (1996). Smoking cessation and gender: The influence of physiological, psychological, and behavioral factors. *Journal of the American Medical Women's Association*, 51, 35–42.

Gritz, E. R., Thompson, B., Emmons, K., Ockene, J. K., McLerran, D. F., & Nielsen, I. R. (1998). Gender differences among smokers and quitters in the Working Well Trial. *Preventive Medicine*, 27, 553–561.

Grunberg, N. E. (1982). The effects of nicotine and cigarette smoking on food consumption and taste preferences. *Addictive Behavior*, 7, 317–331.

Gwaltney, C. J., Shiffman, S., Norman, G. J., Paty, J. A., Kassel, J. D., Gnys, M., Hickcox, M., Waters, A., & Balabanis, M. (2001). Does smoking abstinence self-efficacy vary across situations? Identifying context-specificity within the Relapse Situation Efficacy Questionnaire. *Journal of Consulting and Clinical Psychology*, 69(3), 516–527.

Gwaltney, C. J., Shiffman, S., Paty, J. A., Liu, K. S., Kassel, J. D., Gnys, M., & Hickcox, M. (2002). Using self-efficacy judgments to predict characteristics of lapses to smoking. *Journal of Consulting and Clinical Psychology*, 70(5), 1140–1149.

Hajek, P., Jackson, P., & Belcher, M. (1988). Long term use of nicotine chewing gum. *Journal of the American Medical Association*, 260, 1593–1596.

Hall, S. M., Ginsburg, D., & Jones, R. T. (1986). Smoking cessation and weight gain. *Journal of Consulting and Clinical Psychology*, 54, 342–346.

Haukkala, A., Uutela, A., Vartiainen, E., McAlister, A, & Knekt, P. (2000). Depression and smoking cessation: the role of motivation and self-efficacy. *Addictive Behaviors*, 25(2), 311–316.

Haustein, K. O. (2003). Bupropion: pharmacological and clinical profile in smoking cessation. *International Journal of Clinical Pharmacology*, 41(2), 56–66.

Havik, O. E. & Maeland, J. G. (1988). Changes in smoking behavior after a myocardial infarction. *Health Psychology*, 7, 403.

Hays, J. T., Hurt, R. D., Rigotti, N. A., Niaura, R., Gonzales, D., Durcan, M. J., Sachs, D. P., Wolter, T. D., Buist, A. S., Johnston, J. A., & White, J. D. (2001). Sustained-release bupropion for pharmacologic relapse prevention after smoking cessation: a randomized, controlled trial. *Annals of Internal Medicine*, 135(6), 423–433.

Hays, J. T. & Ebbert, J. O. (2003). Bupropion for the treatment of tobacco dependence: guidelines for balancing risks and benefits. *CNS Drugs*, 17(2), 71–83.

Henningfield, J. E., Radizius, A., Cooper, T. M., & Clayton, R. R. (1990). Drinking coffee and carbonated beverages blocks absorption of nicotine from nicotine polacrilex gum. *Journal of the American Medical Association*, 264, 1560–1564.

Heatherton, T., Kozlowski, L., Frecker, R., & Fagerstrom, K. O. (1991). The Fagerstrom Test for Nicotine Dependence: a revision of the Fagerstrom tolerance questionnaire. *British Journal of Addiction*, 86, 1119–27.

Hermanson, B., Omenn, G., Krommel, R., & Gersh, B. J. (1988). Beneficial six-year outcome of smoking cessation in older men and women with coronary artery disease: Results from the CASS registry. *New England Journal of Medicine*, 319, 1365–1368.

Holm, K. J. & Spencer, C. M. (2000). Bupropion: a review of its use in the management of smoking cessation. *Drugs*, 59(4), 1007–1024.

Hurt, R. D., Lauger, G. G., Offord, K. P., Kottke, T. E., & Dale, L. C. (1990). Nicotine replacement therapy with the use of a transdermal nicotine patch:

A randomized double-blind placebo-controlled trial. *Mayo Clinic Proceedings*, 65, 1529–1537.

Hurt, R. D., Lowell, C. D., Croghan, G. A., Croghan, I. T., Gomez-Dahl, L. C., & Offord, K. P. (1998). Nicotine nasal spray for smoking cessation: Patterns of use, side effects, relief of withdrawal symptoms, and cotinine levels. *Mayo Clinic Proceedings*, 73, 118–125.

Hutchinson, K. M. & Froelicher, E. (2003). Populations at risk for tobacco-related diseases. *Oncology Seminars*.^AQ1 In press.

Johnson, J. L., Budz, B., Mackay, M., & Miller, C. (1999). Evaluation of a nurse-delivered smoking cessation intervention for hospitalized patients with cardiac disease. *Heart & Lung*, (28)1, 55–64.

Killen, J. D., Fortmann, S. P., Newman, B., & Varady, A. (1990). Evaluation of a treatment approach combining nicotine gum and self-guided treatment for smoking relapse prevention. *Journal of Consulting and Clinical Psychology*, 58, 85–92.

King, T. K., Marcus, B. H., Pinto, B. M., Emmons, K. M., & Abrams, D. B. (1996). Cognitive-behavioral mediators of changing multiple behaviors: smoking and a sedentary lifestyle. *Preventive Medicine*, 25, 684–691.

Kottke, T. E., Battista, R. N., DeFriese, G. H., & Brekke, M. L. (1988). Attributes of successful smoking cessation interventions in medical practice: A meta-analysis of 39 controlled trials. *Journal of the American Medical Association*, 259, 2883–2998.

Krumholz, H. M., Cohen, B. J., Tsevat, J., Pasternak, R. C., & Weinstein, M. C. (1993). Cost-effectiveness of a smoking cessation program after myocardial infarction. *Journal of the American College of Cardiology*, 22, 1697–1702.

Krumpe, P., Malani, N., Adler, J., et al. (1989). Effects of transdermal nicotine administration as an adjunct for smoking cessation in heavily addicted smokers (Abstract). *American Review of Respiratory Diseases*, 139, 337.

Kviz, F. J., Clark, M. A, Prohaska, T. R., Slezak, J. A., Crittenden, K. S., Freels, S., & Campbell, R. T. (1995). Attitudes and practices for smoking cessation counseling by provider type and patient age. *Preventive Medicine*, 24, 201–212.

Lam, W., Sze, P. C., Sacks, H. S., & Chalmers, T. C. (1987). Meta-analysis of randomized controlled trials of nicotine chewing gum. *Lancet*, 2, 27–30.

Lederele Laboratories. (1992). *PROSTEP (nicotine transdermal system) prescribing information*. Wayne, NJ: Lederele Laboratories.

Mahrer-Imhof, R., Sivarajan Froelicher, E., Li, W., Parker, K. M., & Benowitz, N. (2002). Women's Initiative for Nonsmoking (WINS V): Under use of nicotine replacement therapy. *Heart & Lung*, 31(5), 368–373.

Marion Merrell Dow, Inc. (1991). *Nicoderm (nicotine transdermal system) prescribing information*. Kansas City, MO: Marion Merrell Dow, Inc.

Marlatt, A. G. (1982). Relapse prevention: A self control program for the treatment of addictive behaviors. In R. B. Stuart (Ed.), *Adherence, compliance and generalization in behavioral medicine* (pp. 329–378). New York: Brunnel/Mazel.

Martin, K., Froelicher, E. S., & Miller, N. H. (2000). Women's Initiative for Nonsmoking (WINS) II: the intervention. *Heart & Lung*. 29(6), 438–445.

Miller, N. H., Smith, P. M., DeBusk, R. F., Sobel, D. S., & Taylor, C. B. (1997). Smoking cessation in hospitalized patients: Results of a randomized trial. *Archives of Internal Medicine*, 157, 409–415.

Mitchell, P. H., Powell, L., Blumenthal, J., Norten, J., Ironson, G., Pitula, C. R., Froelicher, E. S., Czajkowski, S., Youngblood, M., Huber, M., & Berkman, L. F. (2003). A short social support measure in patients recovering from myocardial infarction: the ENRICHD social support inventory. *Journal of Cardiac Rehabilitation*,^AQ2 in press.

Mulcahy, R. (1983). Influence of cigarette smoking on morbidity and mortality after myocardial infarction. *British Heart Journal*, 49, 410–415.

Mulligan, S. C., Masterson, J. G., Devane, J. G., & Kelly, J. G. (1990). Clinical and pharmacokinetics of transdermal nicotine patch. *Clinical Pharmacology Therapeutics*, 47, 331–337.

O'Hara, P., Portser, S. A., & Anderson, B. P. (1989). The influence of menstrual cycle changes on the tobacco withdrawal syndrome in women. *Addictive Behavior*, 14, 595–600.

Ockene, J. K., Emmons, K. M., Mermelstein, R. J., Perkins, K. A., Bonollo, D. S., Voorhees, C. C., & Hollis, J. F. (2000). Relapse and maintenance issues for smoking cessation. *Health Psychology*, 19(1-Suppl.), 17–31.

Ockene, J. K., Hosmer, D., Rippe, J., Williams, J., Goldberg, R. J., DeCosimo, D., Maher, P. M., & Dalen, J. E. (1985). Factors affecting cigarette smoking status in patients with ischemic heart disease. *Journal of Chronic Disease*, 38, 985–994.

Ockene, J., Kristeller, J., Goldberg, R., Ockene, I., Merriam, P., & Barrett, S. (1992). Smoking cessation and severity of disease: The coronary artery smoking intervention study. *Health Psychology*, 11, 119–126.

Parke-Davis. (1992). *Nicotrol (nicotine transdermal system) prescribing information*. Morris Plains, NJ: Parke-Davis.

Pechacek, T. F. (1984). Modification of smoking behavior. In *Smoking and health: A report of the Surgeon General*. Washington, DC: Government Printing Office.

Pomerleau, C. S., Brouwer, R. J., & Pomerleau, O. F. (2001). Emergence of depression during early abstinence in depressed and non-depressed women smokers. *Journal of Addictive Diseases*, 20(1), 73–80.

Pomerleau, C. S., Zucker, A. N., & Stewart, A. J. (2001). Characterizing concerns about post-cessation weight gain: results from a national survey of women smokers. *Nicotine & Tobacco Research*, 3(1), 51–60.

Pozen, M. W., Stockmuller, J. A., Harris, W., Smith, S., Fried, D., & Voigt, G. C. (1977). A nurse rehabilitator's impact on patients with myocardial infarction. *Medical Care*, 15, 830–836.

Prochaska, J. O., Velicer, W. F., Rossi, J. S., Goldstein, M. G., Marcus, B. H., Rakowski, W., Fiore, C., Harlow, L. L., Redding, C. A., Rosenbloom, D., & Rossi, S. R. (1994). Stages of change and decisional balance for 12 problem behaviors. *Health Psychology*, 13, 39–46.

Quillen, J. E., Rossen, J. D., Oskarsson, H. J., Minor, R. L., Lopez, A. G., & Winniford, M. D. (1993). Acute effect of cigarette smoking on the coronary circulation: Constriction of epicardial and resistance vessels. *Journal of the American College of Cardiology*, 22, 642–647.

Rennard, S., Draughton, D., Fortman, S. P., et al. (1991). Transdermal nicotine enhances smoking cessation in coronary artery disease patients (Abstract). *Chest*, 100, 5S.

Rice, V. H., Fox, D. H., Lepczyk, M., Sieggreen, M., Mullin, M., Jarosz, P. & Templin, T. (1994). A comparison of nursing interventions for smoking cessation in adults with cardiovascular health problems. *Heart & Lung*, 23(6), 473–486.

Rigotti, N. A., McKool, K. M., & Shiffman, S. (1994). Predictors of smoking cessation after coronary bypass surgery: Results of a randomized trial with 5-year follow-up. *Annals of Internal Medicine*, 120, 287–293.

Romano, P. S., Bloom, J., & Syme, S. L. (1991). Smoking, social support, and hassles in an urban African American community. *American Journal of Public Health*, 81, 1415–1422.

Rose, J. E., Levin, E. D., Behm, F. M., Adivi, C., & Schur, C. (1990). Transdermal nicotine facilitates smoking cessation. *Clinical Pharmacology Therapeutics*, 47, 323–330.

Sachs, D. L. (1989). Nicotine polacrilex: Practical use requirements. *Current Pulmonology*, 10, 141–158.

Samet, J. (1991). Health benefits of smoking cessation. *Clinics in Chest Medicine*, 12, 669–679.

Sarna, L. & Lillington, L. (2002) Tobacco: an emerging topic in nursing research. *Nursing Research*, 51(4), 245–253.

Schneider, N. G., Lunell, E., Olmstead, R. E., & Fagerstrom, K. O. (1996). Clinical pharmacokinetics of nasal nicotine delivery. *Clinical Pharmacokinetics*, 31, 65–80.

Schwartz, J. L. (1987). *Review and evaluation of smoking cessation methods: The United States and Canada, 1978-1985*. DHHS publication No. (NIH) 87-2940. Washington, DC: Department of Health and Human Services, Public Health Service.

Scott, R. R. & Lamparski, D. (1985). Variables related to long-term smoking status following cardiac events. *Addictive Behavior*, 10, 257–264.

Shiffman, S. (1986). A cluster-analytic classification of relapse episodes. *Addictive Behavior*, 11, 295–307.

Shiffman, S., Dresler, C. M., Hajek, P., Gilburt, S. J., Targett, D. A. & Strahs, K. R. (2002). Efficacy of a nicotine lozenge for smoking cessation. *Archives of Internal Medicine*, 162(11), 1267–1276.

Silagy, C., Lancaster, T., Stead, L., Mant, D., & Fowler, G. (2002). Nicotine replacement therapy for smoking cessation. *Cochrane Database System Review*, 4, CD000146.

Smith, P. M., Reilly, K. R., Houston Miller, N., DeBusk, R. F., & Taylor, C. B. (2002). Application of a nurse-managed inpatient smoking cessation program. *Nicotine & Tobacco Research*, 4(2): 211–222.

Smith, S. S., Jorenby, D. E., Leischow, S. J., Nides, M. A., Rennard, S. I., Johnston, J. A., Jamerson, B., Fiore, M. C., & Baker, T. B. (2003). Targeting smokers at increased risk for relapse: treating women and those with a history of depression. *Nicotine & Tobacco Research*, 5(1), 99–109.

Sohn, M., Hartley, C., Froelicher, E. S., & Benowitz, N. L. (2003). Tobacco use and dependence. *Oncology Seminars*,^AQ3 in press.

Sparrow, D., Dawber, T., Colton, T. (1978). The influence of cigarette smoking on prognosis after a first myocardial infarction. *Journal of Chronic Disease*, 31, 425–432.

Stanislaw, A. E. & Wewers, M. E. (1993). A smoking cessation intervention with hospitalized surgical cancer patients: A pilot study. *Cancer Nursing*, 17, 81–86.

Stillman, F. A. (1995). Smoking cessation for the hospitalized cardiac patient: Rationale for and report of a model program. *Journal of Cardiovascular Nursing*, 9, 25–36.

Taylor, C..B., Houston-Miller, N., & Flora, J. (1988). Principles of health behavior change. In *Resource manual for guidelines for exercise testing and prescription* (pp. 323–328). Philadelphia: Lea & Febiger.

Taylor, C. B., Houston-Miller, N., Haskell, W. L., & DeBusk, R. F. (1988). Smoking cessation after acute myocardial infarction: The effects of exercise training. *Addictive Behavior*, 13, 331–335.

Taylor, C. B., Miller, N. H., Killen, J. D., & DeBusk, R. F. (1990). Smoking cessation after myocardial infarction: Effects of a nurse-managed intervention. *Annals of Internal Medicine*, 113, 118–123.

Taylor, C. B., Miller, N. H., Herman, S., Smith, P. M., Sobel, D., Fisher, L., & DeBusk, R. F. (1996). A nurse-managed smoking cessation program for hospitalized smokers. *American Journal of Public Health*, 86(11), 1557–1560.

The Medical Letter (1997). Bupropion (Zyban) for smoking cessation. *Medical Letter*, 39, 77–80.

Tönnesen, P., Nörregaard, J., Simonsen, K., & Sawe, U. (1991). A double blind trial of a 16 hour transdermal nicotine patch in smoking cessation. *New England Journal of Medicine*, 325, 311–315.

Tönneson, P., Fryd, V., Hansen, M., Helsted, J., Gunnersen, A. B., Forchammer, H., & Stockner, M. (1988). Effect of nicotine chewing gum in combination with group counseling and the cessation of smoking. *New England Journal of Medicine*, 318, 15–18.

Tonstad, S. (2002). Use of sustained-release bupropion in specific patient populations for smoking cessation. *Drugs*, 62(Suppl. 2), 37–43.

Tonstad, S., Farsang, C., Klaene, G., Lewis, K., Manolis, A., Perruchoud, A. P., Silagy, C., van Spiegel, P. I., Astbury, C., Hider, A., & Sweet, R. (2003). Bupropion SR for smoking cessation in smokers with cardiovascular disease: a multicenter, randomized study. *European Heart Journal*, 24(10), 946–955.

Transdermal Nicotine Study Group. (1991). Transdermal nicotine for smoking cessation: Six-month results from two multicenter controlled clinical trials. *Journal of the American Medical Association*, 266, 3133–3138.

Tsoh, J. Y., McClure, J. B., Skaar, K. L., Wetter, D. W., Cinciripini, P. M., Prokhorov, A. P., Friedman, K., & Gritz, E. (1997). Smoking cessation 2: Components of effective intervention. *Behavioral Medicine*, 23, 15–27.

U. S. Department of Health and Human Services. (1988). *The health consequences of smoking: Nicotine addiction. A report of the Surgeon General*. DHHS Publication no. (CDC) 888406. Washington, DC: Government Printing Office.

U. S. Department of Health and Human Services. (1983). *The health consequences of smoking: Cardiovascular disease. A Report of the Surgeon General*. Washington, DC: Government Printing Office.

U. S. Department of Health and Human Services. (1989). *Reducing the health consequences of smoking: 25 years of progress. A report of the Surgeon General*. DHHS Publication no. (CDC) 89–8411. Washington, DC: Government Printing Office.

U. S. Department of Health and Human Services. (2000a). *Healthy people 2010: Understanding and improving health, Volume 2*. [Online]. Available: http://www.healthypeople.gov/document/html/volume2/27 tobacco.htm.

U. S. Department of Health and Human Services. (2000b). *Treating tobacco use and dependence: Clinical practice guideline*. Washington, DC: Government Printing Office.

Velicer, W. F., Fava, J. L., Prochaska, J. O., Abrams, D.B., Emmons, K. M., & Pierce, J. P. (1995). Distribution of smokers by stage in three representative samples. *Preventive Medicine*, 24, 401–411.

Wack, J. T., & Rodin, J. (1982). Smoking and its effects on body weight and systems of caloric regulation. *American Journal of Clinical Nutrition*, 35, 366–380.

West, R., Hajek, P., Nilsson, F., Foulds, J., May, S., & Meadows, W. (2001). Individual differences in preferences for and responses to four nicotine replacement products. *Psychopharmacology*, 153(2), 225–230.

Wewers, M. E., Bowen, J. M., Stanislaw, A. E., Desimone, V. B. (1994). A nurse-delivered smoking cessation intervention among hospitalized postoperative patients-influence of smoking-related diagnosis: a pilot study. *Heart & Lung*, 23, 151–156.

Whitlock, E. P., Vogt, T. M., Hollis, J. F., & Lichtenstein, E. (1997). Does gender affect response to a brief clinic-based smoking intervention? *American Journal of Preventive Medicine*, 13(3), 159–166.

Wilhelmsson, L., Vedin, J. A., Elmfeldt, D., Tibblin, G. & Wilhelmsen, L., (1975). Smoking and myocardial infarction. *Lancet*, 1, 415–420.

Whooley, M. A. & Simon, G. E. (2000). Managing depression in medical outpatients. *New England Journal of Medicine*, 343(26), 1942–1950.

World Health Organization. (2001). *Women and the tobacco epidemic. Challenges for the 21st century*. Samet, J. M. & Yoon, S. (Eds.). Geneva: World Health Organization.

PATIENT AND NURSING REFERENCES

Patient Materials

How Can I Quit and *An Active Partnership for the Health of Your Heart*
American Heart Association
1-800-AHA-USA1 (242-8721)
www.AmericanHeart.org)

Complete Guide to Quitting
American Cancer Society
1599 Clifton Road NE
Atlanta, GA 30329
1(800) ACS-2345
www.Cancer.org

Freedom from Smoking
American Lung Association
1740 Broadway
New York, NY 10019
www.lungusa.org
(or call your local chapter of the American Lung Association)

Help for Smokers: Ideas to Help You Quit and *You Can Quit Smoking*
Agency for Healthcare Research and Quality
Office of Health Care Information
540 Gaither Road
Rockville, MD 20850.
http://www.ahcpr.gov/consumer/index.html#smoking

Materials and Websites for Nurses

Nurses: Help Your Patients Stop Smoking
National Heart, Lung, and Blood Institute
P.O. Box 30105
Bethesda, MD 20824-0105
NIH publication no. 92-2962
(301) 592-8573
www.nhlbi.nih.gov

Treating Tobacco Use and Dependence: Clinical Practice Guideline and *Treating Tobacco Use and Dependence: Quick Reference Guide for Clinicians*
Agency for Healthcare Research and Quality
Publications Clearinghouse
PO Box 8547
Silver Spring, MD 20907-8547
(800) 358-9295

The University of Wisconsin Center for Tobacco Research and Intervention
www.ctri.wisc.edu

Nursing Center for Tobacco Intervention
College of Nursing at Ohio State
www.con.ohio-state.edu/tobacco

39

Hypertension

SUSANNA CUNNINGHAM

High blood pressure (BP) is the most common risk factor for cardiovascular disease in developed and developing countries. Since the late 1960s there has been a dramatic decrease in the mortality rate from hypertensive heart disease in Europe and the United States, primarily because of the development of effective antihypertensive drugs. At least 58 million Americans have hypertension, and an additional large number have BPs at the upper level of the normal range, which puts them at greater risk for hypertension than people with lower BPs (Hajjar & Kotchen, 2003).

High BP is also known as hypertension. The National High Blood Pressure Program, since its inception in 1972, has intentionally used the phrase "high blood pressure" instead of the word hypertension. This choice was made because of the misconceptions that occur when the word hypertension is used. People think that because they are neither "tense" nor "hyper" that they will be unlikely to have hypertension. Among health care professionals, it is useful to use the word hypertension; however, it is important to remember that because this word can be confusing, high blood pressure is a better term to use when communicating with the public. High BP can be considered as a sign, a risk factor, and a disease. Because BP is a continuous variable, one of the challenging aspects is deciding the boundaries between normal and abnormal for the two components of BP: systolic and diastolic BP.

DATABASE FOR MANAGEMENT

Definitions

One problem with setting specific definitions of normal and high BP is that systolic and diastolic BPs are both continuous variables. Also, elevations of either systoli or diastolic pressure increase a person's risk for a clinical event. Because some of the early clinical trials looking at the efficacy of drug treatment of hypertension used diastolic BP as their main outcome variable, the misconception has arisen that elevations in diastolic BP are more serious than elevations in systolic pressure (Veterans Administration Cooperative Study Group on Antihypertensive Agents, 1967, 1970). The truth is that elevations in either diastolic or systolic pressure are associated with increased risk. The greater the elevation, the greater the risk. Conversely, it is

generally true that the lower the pressures, the lower the risk of morbidity and mortality, except in the relatively uncommon situations of sympathetic nervous system dysfunction or hypovolemia. The risks associated with elevations in systolic BP have been documented in the Whitehall Study as well as among the approximately 360,000 men screened for the Multiple Risk Factor Intervention Study (Lichtenstein, Shipley et al., 1985; J. Stamler, Stamler et al., 1993).

Adults

As new research has become available, many countries have established guidelines on the detection, evaluation, and treatment of high BP (Swales, 1993). The two most well known guidelines defining normal and elevated BP levels were developed by The Joint National Committee of the National High Blood Pressure Education Program and the Guidelines subcommittee of the World Health Organization and the International Society of Hypertension (WHO/ISH). Since 1977, The Joint National Committees have produced seven reports; the most recent, known as JNC 7, was produced in 2003 (Chobanian, Bakris et al., 2003). The most recent set of WHO/ISH guidelines were issued in 1999 (Guidelines Subcommittee, 1999). These committees agree that a systolic BP of greater than 140 mm Hg and a diastolic BP greater than 90 mm Hg should be defined as hypertensive. Both reports agree that BP should be considered together with other risk factors for atherosclerotic cardiovascular disease when making decisions about when to initiate treatment.

To reflect the curvilinear nature of the relationship between systolic and diastolic BP and risk, JNC 7 has defined two levels of BP with the "normal" range and two stages of hypertension as shown in Table 39-1 (Chobanian, Bakris et al., 2003). The two levels of normal pressure are normal and prehypertension. The term prehypertension was chosen to communicate the increasing risk that is associated with increasing pressures even though the pressures have not risen to a level that would be considered hypertensive (Vasan, Larson et al., 2001). Above the level of 140/90 mm Hg there are two stages of hypertension with defined ranges for systolic and diastolic pressures. The Joint National Committee chose to use the word stages to convey the seriousness of BP elevations by using terminology mirroring that used in other chronic diseases such as cancer. Isolated systolic hypertension is defined as the occurrence of a

Table 39–1 ■ CLASSIFICATION AND MANAGEMENT OF BLOOD PRESSURE FOR ADULTS*

BP Classification	SBP* MMHG	DBP* MMHG	Lifestyle Modification	Initial Drug Therapy Without Compelling Indication	Initial Drug Therapy With Compelling Indications (See Table 8)
Normal	<120	and <80	Encourage		
Prehypertension	120–139	or 80–89	Yes	No antihypertensive drug indicated.	Drug(s) for compelling indications.‡
Stage 1 Hypertension	140–159	or 90–99	Yes	Thiazide-type diuretics for most. May consider ACEI, ARB, BB, CCB, or combination.	Drug(s) for the compelling indications.‡ Other antihypertensive drugs (diuretics, ACEI, ARB, BB, CCB) as needed.
Stage 2 Hypertension	≥160	or ≥100	Yes	Two-drug combination for most† (usually thiazide-type diuretic and ACEI or ARB or BB or CCB).	

DBP, diastolic blood pressure; SBP, systolic blood pressure.
Drug abbreviations: ACEI, angiotensin converting enzyme inhibitor; ARB, angiotensin receptor blocker; BB, beta-blocker; CCB, calcium channel blocker.
*Treatment determined by highest BP category.
†Initial combined therapy should be used cautiously in those at risk for orthostatic hypotension.
‡Treat patients with chronic kidney disease or diabetes to BP goal of <130/80 mmHg.
(Chobanian, A. V., Bakris, G. L., Black, H. R., et al. [2003]. The Seventh Report of the Joint National Committee on Prevention, Detection, Evaluation, and Treatment of High Blood Pressure: the JNC 7 report. [Erratum in *JAMA*, 2003, 290[2]: 197] *JAMA*, 289[19], 2560–2572.)

systolic BP greater than 140 mm Hg with a diastolic pressure less than 90 mm Hg. The incidence of isolated systolic hypertension increases with age and thus is predominantly a problem of the elderly (National High Blood Pressure Education Program Working Group, 1994).

Previous classifications of high BP such as labile, benign, or malignant (accelerated) were confusing and often misleading (Labarthe, 1978). The term "benign" has a false association with lower morbidity; and "malignant" hypertension, often reversible with proper treatment, is not always fatal. The development of the JNC and WHO/ISH classification schemes as well as advances in the detection and treatment of high BP have made most of these terms obsolete. Types of high BP are classified as: (1) systolic and diastolic hypertension (either primary or secondary) and (2) isolated systolic hypertension caused by increased cardiac output or increasing rigidity of the aorta.

Children

Criteria used for categorizing BP in adults are not applicable to children. The level of BP that is considered normal increases gradually from infancy to adulthood. Systolic and diastolic BP levels correlate with height and weight, as well as age (Voors, Webber et al., 1978). BP for children is considered normal if it is less than the 90th percentile for age, sex, and height (National High Blood Pressure Education Program Working Group on Hypertension Control in Children and Adolescents, 1996). High normal BP refers to pressure measured on at least three occasions that falls between the 90th and 95th percentiles for age, height, and sex. See Tables 39-2 and 39-3 for the current BP levels for the 90th and 95 percentiles for boys and girls. Hypertension is defined as systolic or diastolic BP, or both, above the 95th percentile for age, height, and sex. Both the

JNC 7 Report and the 1996 Update on the 1987 Task Force Report on Blood Pressure in Children and adolescents recommend that the 5th Korotkoff sound can be used to define diastolic pressure in children and adolescents (Chobanian, Bakris et al., 2003; National High Blood Pressure Education Program Working Group on Hypertension Control in Children and Adolescents, 1996). However, data from the longitudinal Bogalusa Heart Study indicated that in children (up to age 13), the 4th Korotkoff sound may be a more reliable predictor of the risk for hypertension in adulthood than the 5th Korotkoff sound (Elkasabany, Urbina et al., 1998).

Epidemiology

Incidence and Prevalence of High BP

Based on the results of the United States National Health and Nutrition Examination Survey (NHANES), conducted between 1999 and 2000, it is estimated that approximately 29%, or just over 58 million, of Americans have hypertension (Hajjar & Kotchen, 2003). When the rates were categorized into three ethnic groups, non-Hispanic white, non-Hispanic black, and Mexican American, the prevalence of high blood pressure was highest in the non-Hispanic black category (29 percent) and lowest in the Mexican American category (17 percent). For the survey, an individual was considered to be hypertensive if the measured BP was 140/90 mm Hg or higher, or if the person reported using antihypertensive medications. Overall, 69% of the people who were found to have an elevated BP were aware of their condition, and 58% were using medications to control their pressure. Of those using medications, only 53% had their BPs under control, which was defined as having a BP less than 140/90 mm Hg. Only 25% of individuals with both diabetes mellitus and high blood pressure had achieved the recommended

Table 39–2 ■ BLOOD PRESSURE LEVELS FOR THE 90TH AND 95TH PERCENTILES OF BLOOD PRESSURE FOR BOYS AGED 1 TO 17 YEARS BY PERCENTILES OF HEIGHT

Age (y)	Blood Pressure Percentile[*]	Systolic Blood Pressure by Percentile of Height[†] (mm Hg)							Diastolic Blood Pressure by Percentile of Height[†] (mm Hg)						
		5%	10%	25%	50%	75%	90%	95%	5%	10%	25%	50%	75%	90%	95%
1	90th	94	95	97	98	100	102	102	50	51	52	53	54	54	55
	95th	98	99	101	102	104	106	106	55	55	56	57	58	59	59
2	90th	98	99	100	102	104	105	106	55	55	56	57	58	59	59
	95th	101	102	104	106	108	109	110	59	59	60	61	62	63	63
3	90th	100	101	103	105	107	108	109	59	59	60	61	62	63	63
	95th	104	105	107	109	111	112	113	63	63	64	65	66	67	67
4	90th	102	103	105	107	109	110	111	62	62	63	64	65	66	66
	95th	106	107	109	111	113	114	115	66	67	67	68	69	70	71
5	90th	104	105	106	108	110	112	112	65	65	66	67	68	69	69
	95th	108	109	110	112	114	115	116	69	70	70	71	72	73	74
6	90th	105	106	108	110	111	113	114	67	68	69	70	70	71	72
	95th	109	110	112	114	115	117	117	72	72	73	74	75	76	76
7	90th	106	107	109	111	113	114	115	69	70	71	72	72	73	74
	95th	110	111	113	115	116	118	119	74	74	75	76	77	78	78
8	90th	107	108	110	112	114	115	116	71	71	72	73	74	75	75
	95th	111	112	114	116	118	119	120	75	76	76	77	78	79	80
9	90th	109	110	112	113	115	117	117	72	73	73	74	75	76	77
	95th	113	114	116	117	119	121	121	76	77	78	79	80	80	81
10	90th	110	112	113	115	117	118	119	73	74	74	75	76	77	78
	95th	114	115	117	119	121	122	123	77	78	79	80	80	81	82
11	90th	112	113	115	117	119	120	121	74	74	75	76	77	78	78
	95th	116	117	119	121	123	124	125	78	79	79	80	81	82	83
12	90th	115	116	117	119	121	123	123	75	75	76	77	78	78	79
	95th	119	120	121	123	125	126	127	79	79	80	81	82	83	83
13	90th	117	118	120	122	124	125	126	75	76	76	77	78	79	80
	95th	121	122	124	126	128	129	130	79	80	81	82	83	83	84
14	90th	120	121	123	125	126	128	128	76	76	77	78	79	80	80
	95th	124	125	127	128	130	132	132	80	81	81	82	83	84	85
15	90th	123	124	125	127	129	131	131	77	77	78	79	80	81	81
	95th	127	128	129	131	133	134	135	81	82	83	83	84	85	86
16	90th	125	126	128	130	132	133	134	79	79	80	81	82	82	83
	95th	129	130	132	134	136	137	138	83	83	84	85	86	87	87
17	90th	128	129	131	133	134	136	136	81	81	82	83	84	85	85
	95th	132	133	135	136	138	140	140	85	85	86	87	88	89	89

[*] Blood pressure percentile was determined by a single measurement.
[†] Height percentile was determined by standard growth curves.
(National High Blood Pressure Education Program Working Group on Hypertension Control in Children and Adolescents [1996]. Update on the 1987 task force report on high blood pressure in children and adolescents: a working group report from the National High Blood Pressure Education Program. *Pediatrics*, 98, 649–658.)

BP of 130/95 or less (Hajjar & Kotchen, 2003) (Note: since the time of Hajjar and Kotchen's analysis of the NHANES data, the JNC 7 has recommended an even lower BP goal of 130/80 or less for persons with diabetes mellitus) (Chobanian, Bakris et al., 2003).

Age, Weight, and Gender

The evidence suggests that hypertension begins in childhood, perhaps even in utero, although a meta-analysis of 55 studies of birth weight and blood pressure later in life did not support this so-called fetal origins hypothesis (Falkner, 2002; Huxley, Neil et al., 2002; Law, de Swiet et al., 1993). Because hypertension in children is defined as a pressure greater than the 95th percentile for a child of any given age and height, the initial incidence of hypertension in children is automatically 5%. However, the recommendations suggest that before a child has high BP diagnosed, the measurement should be repeated for a total of three consecutive examinations, because the true incidence is usually found to be lower (National High Blood Pressure Education Program Working Group on Hypertension Control in Children and Adolescents, 1996). In a study of junior high school students, it was found that even by the second examination, the prevalence of persistent elevations in pressure had decreased to approximately 1% (Adrogue & Sinaiko, 2001). Both height and weight directly influence children's BPs.

Normally, BP increases in children at a rate of between 1 and 4 mm Hg per year for both SBP and DBP and then it levels off after age 18 to 20. Children whose BP consistently falls above the 95th percentile for height, gender, and age are at risk for sustained hypertension and should be evaluated and possibly treated (National High Blood Pressure Education Program Working Group on Hypertension Control in Children and Adolescents, 1996).

In adults, BP tends to increase with age (Dannenberg, Garrison et al., 1988; Hajjar & Kotchen, 2003; Kannel, Brand

Table 39-3 ■ IMPORTANT ASPECTS OF THE PATIENT'S HISTORY

Duration of the hypertension	Presence of other risk factors
Last known normal blood pressure	Smoking
Course of the blood pressure	Diabetes
Prior treatment of the hypertension	Dyslipidemia
Drugs: types, doses, side effects	Physical inactivity
Intake of agents that may interfere	Concomitant diseases
Nonsteroidal antiinflammatory drugs	Dietary history
Oral contraceptives	Weight change
Sympathomimetics	Fresh vs. processed foods
Adrenal steroids	Sodium
Excessive sodium intake	Saturated fats
Alcohol (>2 drinks/day)	Sexual function
Herbal remedies	Features of sleep apnea
Family history	Early morning headaches
Hypertension	Daytime somnolence
Premature cardiovascular disease or	Loud snoring
death	Erratic sleep
Familial diseases: pheochromocytoma,	Ability to modify lifestyle and
renal disease, diabetes, gout	maintain therapy
Symptoms of secondary causes	Understanding the nature of
Muscle weakness	hypertension and the need
Spells of tachycardia, sweating, tremor	for regimen
Thinning of the skin	Ability to perform physical
Flank pain	activity
Symptoms of target organ damage	Source of food preparation
Headaches	Financial constraints
Transient weakness or blindness	Ability to read instructions
Loss of visual acuity	Need for care providers
Chest pain	
Dyspnea	
Edema	
Claudication	

(Kaplan, N. M. [2002]. *Kaplan's clinical hypertension* [8th ed.]. Philadelphia. Lippincott Williams & Wilkins.)

et al., 1967). Overall, women have a higher prevalence of hypertension than do men. The age-adjusted percent for women is 30%; and for men, it is 27% (Hajjar & Kotchen, 2003). JNC 7 emphasizes the high risk for hypertension with aging and the importance of elevations of systolic pressure in persons older than age 50 (Chobanian, Bakris et al., 2003). Participants of the Framingham Cohort Study aged 55 to 65 years and without hypertension at baseline were found to have a 90% risk for hypertension or using antihypertensive medications in their remaining lifetime, indicating a major challenge for the national health care system (Vasan, Beiser et al., 2002).

Data from the Framingham and other epidemiologic studies have shown that as body weight increases, so do systolic and diastolic BP in adults and children (Brown, Higgins et al., 2000; Freedman, Dietz et al., 1999; Kannel, Brand et al., 1967; National High Blood Pressure Education Program Working Group on Hypertension Control in Children and Adolescents, 1996). In the Bogalusa Study, children and adolescents who were overweight (body mass index [BMI] >85 percentile) were 2.4-times more likely to have hypertension than those with a BMI less than the 85th percentile (Freedman, Dietz et al., 1999). An analysis of the NHANES III data revealed that the incidence of hypertension in men and women with a BMI of less than 25 was 15%, whereas in men and women with a BMI 30 or more the incidence was 42%

and 38%, respectively (Brown, Higgins et al., 2000). This relationship between weight and BP is thought to be one of the reasons that BP increases with age.

Family History and Genetic Factors

Family history of hypertension has been used as an indicator of the influence of genetics on the epidemiology of hypertension. With the progress on the human genome project, it is possible that we may be able to predict risk with more precision; however, expense and issues of privacy must also be considered. Depending on how a positive family history of hypertension is defined, a person with a positive history has a relative risk for hypertension of between 2.4 and 5.0 (Hunt & Williams, 1999). The risks are greater when more family members have high BP and if these family members had hypertension diagnosed before age 55. The risk associated with a positive family history is slightly greater for women than for men. The influence of family history is seen in children as well as adults (Burke, Beilin et al., 2001; Fuentes, Notkola et al., 2000).

Ethnic and Geographic Differences

Data from the 1999 to 2000 National Health and Nutrition Examination Survey show that non-Hispanic black men and women had higher age-adjusted prevalence rates of high BP than non-Hispanic white and Mexican American men and women (Hajjar & Kotchen, 2003). The same analysis also found that non-Hispanic black men and women had the highest systolic and diastolic BPs in almost all age groups. In an analysis of control rates of those known to have high blood pressure, persons who self-identified as Mexican American men and women had the lowest control rate of 18% compared with 28% for non-Hispanic blacks and 33% for non-Hispanics (Hajjar & Kotchen, 2003).

Geographic differences in the prevalence of high BP have been described for different parts of the world as well as within the United States. Around the world, the prevalence of hypertension is reported to be lowest in rural Africa and southern China and highest in Finland, Russia, and parts of the United States (Cooper, 1999). An analysis of national blood pressure surveys performed in six European countries, England, Finland, Germany, Italy, Spain, and Sweden, plus two North American countries, Canada and the United States, found that the average blood pressure in the European countries was 136/83 mm Hg and in North America it was 127/77 mm Hg (Wolf-Maier, Cooper et al., 2003). The researchers also found that the age- and sex-adjusted prevalence of hypertension was 44% in the European countries compared to 28% in North America. In all the countries studied, there was a high correlation (correlation coefficient 0.78) between the prevalence of high blood pressure and the incidence of stroke (Wolf-Maier, Cooper et al., 2003). It is not clear whether these data reflect an actual difference in the incidence of hypertension or perhaps a difference in the standards for the treatment of elevated blood pressures. The researchers note that the blood pressure differences between Europe and North American countries may also be caused by differences in blood pressure measurement, genetics, lifestyle choices, or other confounding variables.

Within the United States, a selection of states in the southeast has been designated as "the stroke belt," because of the high incidence of hypertension and strokes (Hall, 1999; Lackland, Bachman et al., 1998). It is not clear whether these geographic variations are caused by genetic, social, or environmental factors. Within the United States, the area known as the "stroke belt" is also an area with dietary, physical activity, low birth weight, obesity patterns, and social conditions that may account for most or all of the excess in hypertension prevalence (Hall, 1999).

Income and Education

An inverse relationship between socioeconomic status, including educational level and income, and the prevalence of high BP has been documented in some studies (Daugherty, 1983; Holme, Helgeland et al., 1976; Hypertension Detection and Follow-up Program Cooperative Group, 1987; Levenstein, Smith et al., 2001; Stamler, Shipley et al., 1992). The Atherosclerosis Risk in Communities Study of 10,091 black and white Americans has even found a relationship between the stretch capacity (elasticity) of the carotid arteries and socioeconomic status, with persons in the lowest socioeconomic stratum having the greatest impairment of carotid elasticity (Din-Dzietham, Liao et al., 2000). The impact of socioeconomic status on BP and other cardiovascular risk factors is thought to be related to social, financial, and political barriers to health care and to adoption of low-risk lifestyles (Bolen, Rhodes et al., 2000; Jones, 1999).

Hemodynamics of High Blood Pressure

Blood pressure is the product of the amount of blood pumped by the heart each minute (cardiac output) and the degree of dilation or constriction of the arterioles (systemic vascular resistance). Arterial BP is controlled over short time periods by the arterial baroreceptors that sense changes in the pressure within the major arteries and then through neurohumoral feedback mechanisms, which vary heart rate, myocardial contractility, and vascular smooth muscle contraction to maintain the BP within normal limits. Over longer time periods (hours to days), neurohumoral and direct renal regulation of vascular volume also play an important role in maintaining a normal BP. Baroreceptors in the low-pressure components of the cardiovascular system such as the veins, atria, and pulmonary circulation have a role in the neurohumoral regulation of vascular volume.

For an individual to have hypertension, there must be an increase in cardiac output and/or systemic vascular resistance (Julius, 1988; Lund-Johansen, 1977). It may be that either one is elevated or that both are elevated. Because BP can be measured relatively easily and because it is not easy to measure cardiac output or systemic vascular resistance, we identify dysfunction of these variables as disorders of BP regulation. As discussion in several chapters of this text reveal, each of these variables, cardiac output and systemic vascular resistance, are themselves influenced by many factors. Given all the factors that can influence it, BP needs to be considered as an extremely complex variable.

Two investigators, Stevo Julius and Per Lund-Johansen, are known for their studies of the hemodynamics of hypertension. In a longitudinal prospective study of a relatively small group of hypertensive men, Lund-Johansen found variability in hemodynamics (Lund-Johansen, 1991). In the younger men, the hypertension was caused either by an increased cardiac output or by an increase in systemic vascular resistance. Over 20 years of follow-up, he found that all subjects who were hypertensive at baseline, regardless of their initial hemodynamic pattern, had an increase in systemic vascular resistance plus a decrease in cardiac index and stroke index. Even subjects whose BP had been controlled with medications showed a significant increase in resistance. Similarly, Julius found that most people with borderline hypertension had an elevated cardiac output (Julius, 1988). Over time, the hypertension remained but transitioned from a high cardiac output state to a state of elevated total peripheral resistance. The data, therefore, indicate that initially an elevated pressure may be secondary to either elevated cardiac output or systemic vascular resistance, or to elevations in both. In long established hypertension, the usual hemodynamic finding is an elevated systemic vascular resistance.

Cause

Despite decades of research and countless publications, the underlying cause of most cases of high BP is not yet known. To distinguish between hypertension with a known cause and that with unknown cause, the terminology of primary and secondary hypertension or high BP is used. The terms primary or idiopathic high BP are used to indicate those cases of hypertension for which no cause can be identified. Approximately 90% to 95% of cases of hypertension fit within this category (Danielson & Dammstrom, 1981; Sinclair, Isles et al., 1987). The term secondary hypertension describes the 5% to 10% of cases of high BP for which a cause can be identified.

Primary High BP

Medical professionals originally thought that if no cause for a person's hypertension could be determined, then a higher BP must be necessary or "essential" for getting blood through arteries and arterioles that had become narrowed by disease or aging. In the first half of the twentieth century, clinicians believed that any attempt to lower the elevated pressure would result in inadequate tissue perfusion. It was subsequently demonstrated that this original hypothesis was in error; lowering BP reduces morbidity and mortality rates, even in the elderly (Amery, Birkenyhäger et al., 1985; Hypertension Detection and Follow-up Program Cooperative Group, 1979; Sagie, Larson et al., 1993; Veterans Administration Cooperative Study Group on Antihypertensive Agents, 1967, 1970).

The cause or causes of primary hypertension remain in question. Blood pressure is a complex variable involving mechanisms that influence cardiac output, systemic vascular resistance, and blood volume. Hypertension is caused by one or several abnormalities in the function of these mechanisms or the failure of other factors to compensate for these malfunctioning mechanisms. The current revolution in genetics and molecular biology have begun to shed light on some causes of high BP and to raise the hope that the more complex polygenic and environmental interactions that contribute to high BP will soon be understood (Lifton, 1996; Weder, 1998). Currently, the genetic basis for a few rare types of hypertension have been identified, but it is hoped that these discoveries will lead eventually to understanding the cause or causes of most or all types of high blood pressure (Wilson, Disse-Nicodeme et al., 2001).

Genetic predisposition; environmental factors such as stress, obesity, and excess sodium (Na^+) intake; and sympathetic nervous system dysfunction may all contribute to high BP. Several explanations regarding the cause of primary hypertension are currently being investigated. These explanations are not mutually exclusive and probably overlap. It is likely that the eventual understanding of the cause of hypertension will involve the integration of more than one of these hypotheses. Some of the hypotheses include:

1. Dysfunction of the autonomic nervous system–The influence of autonomic nervous system imbalance may be direct because of inheritance of genes that predispose the individual to having increased sympathetic nervous system activity or indirect through the effects of environment and lifestyle on sympathetic nervous system activity (Esler, 2000).
2. Variations in renal sodium reabsorption–An increase in blood volume secondary to an impaired ability to excrete extracellular fluid (saline) resulting in an increased blood volume is one of hemodynamic alterations that can result in high blood pressure. Identification of several genes involved in rare, inherited forms of hypertension support the hypothesis that primary hypertension may be related to mutations in several genes related that increase an individual's susceptibility to disorders of renal reabsorption of sodium, chloride, and water (Lifton, 1996). Gain- and loss-of-function mutations in the epithelial sodium channel (EnaC) found in the distal collecting duct of the kidney are associated, respectively, with inherited forms of hypertension and hypotension (Cruz, Simon et al., 2001; Schafer, 2002; Wong, Stebbing et al., 1999). A small postmortem study of 10 white subjects aged 35 to 59 years with primary hypertension who died accidentally found that compared to controls, the individuals with high blood pressure had approximately 50% fewer nephrons in their kidneys (Keller, Zimmer et al., 2003).
3. Dysfunction of the renin-angiotensin aldosterone (RAA) system–Increased RAA activity has long been known to result in extracellular fluid volume expansion and systemic vascular resistance. Over the past decade, research has revealed that aldosterone also acts as a paracrine (a cytokine that influences cells located near it) in tissues such as the vasculature, brain, and heart to cause collagen formation and vascular inflammation (Rocha & Funder, 2002; Tharaux, Chatziantoniou et al., 2000). This research has led to the development of a new selective aldosterone antagonist, eplerenone, which was first demonstrated to be effective in the treatment of heart failure and, more recently, in high blood pressure (Pitt, Zannad et al., 1999; Weber, 2002). Angiotensin II has also been recognized as acting like a growth factor and a cytokine resulting in growth, differentiation, and apoptosis in vascular tissues (Touyz & Berry, 2002). At the gene level, studies have identified variations in

the gene coding for components of the RAA and their roles in the development of high BP (Jeunemaitre, Soubrier et al., 1992; Zhu, Chang et al., 2003).

4. Impaired vascular responsiveness–Recent research has revealed impairments in vascular dilation and increased vascular contraction related to the function of the endothelium in persons with hypertension. It is not clear whether these changes in vascular reactivity and endothelial function precede or follow the onset of high BP (Bolen, Rhodes et al., 2000; Ferri, Bellini et al., 1998; Frostegard, Wu et al., 1998; Yukihito Higashi, Oshima et al., 1997; Krum, Viskoper et al., 1998).
5. Insulin resistance as a contributory factor in hypertension–Hypertension and diabetes frequently occur together. It has been hypothesized that insulin resistance may be a common factor that links hypertension, type II diabetes, and other metabolic abnormalities (Ferrannini & Natali, 1991; Fuenmayor, Moreira et al., 1998; Muller-Wieland, Kotzka et al., 1998; Reaven, Lithell et al., 1996). This clustering of cardiovascular risk factors is currently known as the metabolic syndrome and is sometimes also referred to as syndrome X, insulin resistance syndrome, and "the deadly quartet" (Chobanian, Bakris et al., 2003; Executive Summary of The Third Report of The National Cholesterol Education Program (NCEP) Expert Panel on Detection, Evaluation, And Treatment of High Blood Cholesterol In Adults (Adult Treatment Panel III), 2001; N. M. Kaplan, 1989). The metabolic syndrome is defined as including abdominal obesity, increased blood pressure, dyslipidemia, and insulin resistance with or without impaired glucose tolerance plus prothrombotic and proinflammatory states (Executive Summary of The Third Report of The National Cholesterol Education Program (NCEP) Expert Panel on Detection, Evaluation, And Treatment of High Blood Cholesterol In Adults (Adult Treatment Panel III), 2001).

Secondary High BP

Although secondary hypertension affects less than 10% of all hypertensive adults, the majority of the hypertension that occurs in children younger than age 10 years is secondary to a specific physiologic condition. The epidemic of obesity in children, however, is resulting in more primary hypertension in youth (Sinaiko, 1996; Sorof & Daniels, 2002). In children younger than 10, the most common causes of persistent hypertension are renal disease and vascular problems such as coarctation of the aorta. In adults, chronic renal disease, renovascular disease, primary aldosteronism, and use of oral contraceptives are the most common causes of secondary high BP (Danielson & Dammstrom, 1981; Sinclair, Isles et al., 1987). In one study of 3,783 persons referred to a specialty hypertension clinic in Scotland, these causes of secondary hypertension accounted for 7.8% of all cases of high BP, with all other secondary causes accounting for only 0.1% (Sinclair, Isles et al., 1987). Display 39-1 summarizes many of the secondary causes of hypertension in children and adults. The newest additions to this list are the relatively rare, but fascinating, genetic mutations that cause hypertension (Lifton, 1996; Wilson, Disse-Nicodeme et al., 2001). Sleep apnea is also increasingly being recognized as a cause of secondary hypertension (Chobanian, Bakris et al., 2003).

D I S P L A Y   39–1

SECONDARY CAUSES OF HIGH BLOOD PRESSURE IN ORDER OF FREQUENCY

Kidney Disorders

Renal artery stenosis
Unilateral
  Tumor
  Hypoplasia
  Renal tuberculosis
  Pyelonephritis
  Hydronephrosis
  Single cysts
Bilateral
  Acute or chronic renal failure
  Polycystic disease
  Pyelonephritis
  Glomerulonephritis
  Nephropathy from gout, diabetes, and phenacetin
    abuse
  Lupus erythematosus
  Progressive systemic sclerosis
  Periarteritis nodosa
  Amyloidosis
  Radiation nephritis
Renin-secreting tumors
  Wilms' tumor
    Nephroblastoma
    Paraganglioma
  Hemangiopericytoma
  Renin-producing pulmonary carcinoma

Endocrine Disorders

Adrenal cortex
  Primary aldosteronism
  Secondary aldosteronism
  Cushing's syndrome
  Excess deoxycortisol
  Congenital adrenal hyperplasia
  Adenoma
Adrenal medulla
  Pheochromocytoma
Hypothyroidism
Hyperparathyroidism
Acromegaly

Cardiovascular Disorders

Coarctation of the aorta
Patent ductus arteriosus
Polycythemia hypertonica

Neurologic Disorders

Autonomic hyperreflexia
Excessive rapid-eye-movement sleep
Increased intracranial pressure
Ganglioneuromas, neuroblastomas, and tumors
  of the posterior fossa
Sleep apnea syndrome

Surgical Procedures Involving The Cardiovascular System
Pregnancy

Preeclampsia
Eclampsia

Exogenous Compounds

Sympathomimetic agents
  Amphetamine
  Caffeine
  Adrenalin
  Dopamine
  Nicotine
  Methyldopa
  Tyramine
Tricyclic antidepressants
Phenacetin-containing analgesics
Licorice
Chewing tobacco
Steroid therapy
Monoamine oxidase inhibitors
  Isocarboxazid [Marplan]
  Isoniazid
  Nialamide (Niamid)
  Pargyline (Eutonyl)
  Phenelzine (Nardil)
  Procarbazine
  Tranylcypromine (Parnate)
Tryptophan- and tyramine-containing foods
  Chicken liver
  Pickled herring
  Yeast extract
  Broad beans
  Matured cheeses (especially cheddar)
  Beer
  Wines (especially Chianti)
Oral contraceptives
Trace metals, minerals, and electrolytes
  Cadmium
  Zinc
  Lead
  Selenium
  Mercury
  Calcium
  Magnesium
  Potassium
  Sodium
Cocaine
Cyclosporine
Erythropoietin

Genetic Disorders—Single-Gene Mutations

Glucocorticoid-remediable aldosteronism
Syndrome of apparent mineralocorticoid excess
Liddle's syndrome

Chronic Renal Disease. The relationship between the kidneys and hypertension is circular. Chronic renal disease causes hypertension and hypertension contributes to the development of chronic renal disease. Chronic renal disease causes between 2.5% and 5.6% of all hypertension and is the most common type of secondary high BP (Danielson & Dammstrom, 1981; Sinclair, Isles et al., 1987). In chronic renal disease, there are three major factors that contribute to the development of high BP: loss of nephrons leading to retention of sodium, chloride, and water; decreased release of vasodilator substances such as nitric oxide; and activation of the renin-angiotensin aldosterone system. Research has shown that treatment of hypertension with a low-protein diet and antihypertensive medications reduces the progression of chronic renal disease to end-stage renal disease (Lazarus, Bourgoignie et al., 1997; Peterson, Adler et al., 1995; Toto, Mitchell et al., 1995).

Renovascular Disorders. Renovascular hypertension occurs when there is disease of one or both of the renal arteries leading to decreased perfusion of the kidneys. The most common causes of renal artery stenosis are atherosclerosis, which can proceed to occlusion, and fibromuscular hyperplasia, which rarely causes occlusion (Pickering, 1989). Initially, hypertension is caused by activation of the renin-angiotensin aldosterone system, resulting in retention of sodium, chloride, and water. Renovascular hypertension is treated by angioplasty, stent placement, revascularization, or drug therapy with either angiotensin-converting enzyme (ACE) inhibitors or calcium-channel blockers. The longer that the underlying stenosis is not treated, the greater the secondary damage to the vasculature caused by the hypertension. In one study of 110 patients with renovascular hypertension, it was found that surgery on those with high BP less than 5 years resulted in a 78% success rate, whereas those with hypertension for more than 5 years had only a 25% success rate (Hughes, Dove et al., 1981). A meta-analysis of only three clinical trials comparing angioplasty with medical therapy found that angioplasty resulted in an average 7 mm Hg greater decrease in blood pressure than medical therapy (Nordmann, Woo et al., 2003).

Primary Aldosteronism. Primary aldosteronism, a disease characterized by excess secretion of aldosterone, can be caused by an adrenocortical adenoma, adrenal hyperplasia, adrenal carcinoma, or the cause may be unknown; in which case, it is diagnosed as idiopathic hyperaldosteronism (Young, 2003). With high circulating levels of aldosterone, there is retention of sodium, chloride, and water resulting in an expanded extracellular fluid volume. Use of a simple blood test, the plasma aldosterone concentration (PAC)-to-plasma renin activity (PRA) ratio has led to increased diagnosis of the occurrence of this condition. Recent sources estimate that primary aldosteronism may actually be the cause of between 5% and 13% of all cases of hypertension (Young, 2003). Although hypokalemia has historically been considered to be a key sign of aldosteronism, a recent series at the Mayo Clinic only found a low serum potassium in 37% of the cases of primary aldosteronism (Young, 2003). Clinicians should consider the possibility of primary aldosteronism in any patient with resistant hypertension, particularly if the person is younger than 50 years old or if they have hypertension with hypokalemia. Primary aldosteronism caused by adrenocortical adenoma is treated by surgical removal of the tumor if possible. If there is no tumor, then treatment with the aldosterone antagonists eplerenone or spironolactone is usually effective.

Use of Oral Contraceptives. Before the development of the new low-dose oral contraceptives, hypertension related to the use of oral contraceptives accounted for approximately 1% of the cases of secondary hypertension (Danielson & Dammstrom, 1981; Sinclair, Isles et al., 1987). A recent analysis of the data from the Nurses' Health Study found the rate of hypertension in users of low-dose contraceptive pills to be 41.5 cases per 10,000 years of follow-up (Chasan-Taber, Willett et al., 1996). The data indicated that cessation of the use of the pills resulted in a return to normal BP. Even though the low-dose pills do not cause hypertension, analysis of the circadian rhythm of BP of 20 women using oral contraceptives and 20 young women who were not showed that the women using oral contraceptives had significantly higher BPs (Heintz, Schmauder et al., 1996).

Coarctation of the Aorta. Coarctation, or narrowing of the lumen, of the aorta is a rare cause of hypertension in the adults, although it is relatively common in children (Sinaiko, 1996). The narrowing most commonly occurs distal to the origin of the left subclavian artery (de Leeuw & Birkenhäger, 1994). Individuals with coarctation of the aorta have hypertension above the lesion and reduced pressure below the lesion. If untreated, coarctation can cause left ventricular hypertrophy. The longer it is untreated, the worse the prognosis. Treatment is usually with surgical repair of the lesion or angioplasty (de Leeuw & Birkenhäger, 1994). A comparison of the blood pressure and left ventricular mass of patients who had surgical repair of a coarctation to controls found that the patients had significantly higher 24-hour ambulatory systolic pressures and LV mass than the controls (de Divitiis, Pilla et al., 2003). These results indicate the importance of continued follow-up in persons with a history of coarctation of the aorta.

Sleep Apnea. The JNC 7 is the first of the JNC reports to add sleep apnea to its list of possible causes for secondary hypertension (Chobanian, Bakris et al., 2003). The supporting reasons for adding it, however, were not included in the express edition of the report. Although the association between sleep-disordered breathing and systemic hypertension has been reported since the 1970s, a recent review concluded that although it was true that there was an increased incidence of sleep apnea in persons with hypertension, it was not clear that there was a causal relationship between the two conditions (Dart, Gregoire et al., 2003). Sleep-disordered breathing includes frequent episodes of hypopnea (reduced chest movement plus 4% or more decrease in oxyhemoglobin saturation) and/or apnea (cessation of airflow for 10 seconds or more) (Dart, Gregoire et al., 2003; Peppard, Young et al., 2000). Continuous positive airway pressure (CPAP) has been reported to reduce blood pressure in persons with sleep-disordered breathing, but many of the studies are of short duration and may be confounded by associated weight loss (Dart, Gregoire et al., 2003; Hla, Skatrud et al., 2002; Pepperell, Ramdassingh-Dow et al., 2002). One 7-year follow-up of 182 men from a sleep clinic found a significantly increased incidence of CVD in the men with obstructive sleep apnea, and a reduced incidence of CVD in the men whose sleep apnea had been successfully treated (Peker, Hedner et al., 2002). Assessment for sleep patterns and also snoring is indicated for persons with resistant hypertension. The client's sleeping partner may be an excellent source of information about a client's sleep habits.

Clinical Manifestations of High BP

Signs and Symptoms

Unfortunately, there are few signs and no symptoms of hypertension until it becomes very severe and target organ damage has occurred. The major sign, obviously, is the presence of elevated arterial BP based on the criteria for the definition and measurement of high BP (see Table 39-1). Other signs and symptoms are described in the next section on complications of hypertension.

The morbidity and mortality associated with elevations in BP are predominately a consequence of damage to a selected set of organs known as "target organs." These target organs are the blood vessels, heart, brain, kidneys, and eyes. When the influence of hypertension in manifested in any one of these organs, it is called target organ disease (TOD). When a clinician assesses a client with an elevated BP, the assessment will exclude examining for evidence of damage in one of these target organs. Evidence of TOD is considered a serious prognostic sign in a person with hypertension. JNC 7 included assessment of TOD along with risk factors for atherosclerotic disease as key components of the evaluation of persons with documented elevated blood pressures (Chobanian, Bakris et al., 2003). The major cardiovascular risk factors and TODs are shown in Display 39-2.

DISPLAY 39-2

CARDIOVASCULAR RISK FACTORS

Major Risk Factors

Hypertension*
Cigarette smoking
Obesity* (body mass index ≥ 30 kg/m²)
Physical inactivity
Dyslipidemia*
Diabetes mellitus*
Microalbuminuria or estimated GFR <60 mL/min
Age (older than 55 for men, 65 for women)
Family history of premature cardiovascular disease (men under age 55 or women under age 65)

Target Organ Damage

Heart

- Left ventricular hypertrophy
- Angina or prior myocardial infarction
- Prior coronary revascularization
- Heart failure

Brain

- Stroke or transient ischemic attack

Chronic kidney disease
Peripheral arterial disease
Retinopathy

GFR, glomerular filtration rate.
*Components of the metabolic syndrome.
(Chobanian, A. V., Bakris, G. L., Black, H. R., et al. [2003]. The Seventh Report of the Joint National Committee on Prevention, Detection, Evaluation, and Treatment of High Blood Pressure: the JNC 7 report. *JAMA*, 289(19), 2560–2572. [Erratum in *JAMA*, 2003, 290[2],197].)

Vascular Changes Associated with High BP

The blood vessels, specifically the arteries, are unique in that they are both a separate target organ as well as a part of the other major target organs. Hypertension can influence the endothelium, vascular smooth muscle, extracellular matrix, and connective tissue of the arteries. In addition, hypertension contributes to the rate at which atherosclerosis accumulates within the large elastic arteries and the intermediate-size muscular arteries and arterioles.

In a normal artery, the intima is composed of the endothelium, a smooth-surfaced inner lining, and the potential space between the endothelial cells and the internal elastic lamina. The media or middle layer consists of the internal elastic lamina, smooth muscle cells, elastin, collagen, and extracellular matrix. The smooth muscle cells control the beat-to-beat adjustment of vascular diameter by contracting and relaxing to dilate and constrict the vessel. The adventitia or outer layer, made up of connective tissue, fibroblasts, and a few smooth muscle cells, anchors the vessel to surrounding structures and supports the blood and lymph vessels that serve the artery. In the early stages of hypertension, hypertrophy of the large arteries and the arterioles is observed. This medial thickening results in a narrower vessel lumen and therefore higher vascular resistance (Lindop, 1994). Under conditions of sustained hypertension, the layers of the normal artery change. Advances in our understanding of signaling by the RAA system indicate that these vascular changes may be caused by angiotensin II acting on the AT_{1a} receptor (Touyz & Berry, 2002). The next sections discuss changes in endothelial function and then changes in artery structure, including atherosclerosis, arteriosclerosis, and fibrinoid arteriolar necrosis.

Changes in the Vascular Endothelium. Some experts consider the vascular endothelium to be the largest organ in the body (Sowers & Izzo Jr., 1999). The designation of the endothelium as a separate organ reflects the recent recognition that the endothelium is a highly dynamic interface between the blood and the rest of the body, not simply the smooth lining of the blood vessels. The endothelium regulates vasomotion; coagulation and fibrinolysis; the traffic of inflammatory and immune cells between the blood, lymph, and tissues; the movement of nutrients and waste products between the blood and tissues; and secretion of a wide variety of cytokines and growth factors (DiCorleto & Gimbrone Jr., 1996).

Impaired endothelial vasodilation has been identified in persons with hypertension and even in the normotensive children of hypertensive parents (Panza, 1997; Taddei, Virdis et al., 1996). Preliminary work with 33 subjects found evidence that the degree of endothelial impairment was negatively correlated with mean BP (Higashi, Oshima et al., 1997). This result indicates that the higher the BP, the greater the impairment in vascular dilation. Later work by the same research group found evidence of endothelial dysfunction in secondary hypertension when forearm blood flow was compared between 15 individuals with renovascular hypertension and 15 age- and sex-matched controls without disease (Higashi, Sasaki et al., 2002). Investigation has not yet revealed what aspect of the nitric oxide vasodilation system is dysfunctional in hypertension.

Other factors that cause endothelial dysfunction include aging, hypercholesterolemia, diabetes, smoking, physical inactivity, and homcysteinemia (Bataineh & Raij, 1998; Panza, 1997; Sowers & Izzo Jr., 1999). In a substudy of the Anglo-Scandinavian Cardiac Outcomes Trial (ASCOT), 76 subject with hypertension and other risk factors including dyslipidemia and diabetes mellitus were compared with matched controls before and after 6 months of intensive antihypertensive and lipid-lowering (if indicated) treatment. Before treatment, the hypertensive subjects had increased levels of markers of endothelial dysfunction and also prothrombotic factors. After treatment, all the indicators improved significantly, although they remained abnormal compared to the controls (Felmeden, Spencer et al., 2003). Researchers hope that understanding the molecular basis for endothelial dysfunction in hypertension will be the pathway to developing new therapies to reduce the impact of hypertension. It is not yet known whether endothelial dysfunction is truly a precursor of hypertension or a sequel. It is also not known whether improving endothelial function will improve hypertension and reduce morbidity and mortality, but researchers are hypothesizing that it will.

Atherosclerosis. Hypertension is one of the major modifiable risk factors for atherosclerosis. Atherosclerosis affects primarily the aorta and large and medium arteries. It develops in areas where pressure is high, such as the bronchial arteries, particularly at branch points, and not in areas where pressure is low, as in the pulmonary arteries. It is the most common vascular pathology associated with cerebral infarction, renovascular hypertension, and systolic hypertension in the elderly. The pathogenesis of atherosclerosis is discussed in Chapter 7.

Arteriosclerosis. Arteriosclerosis is described as the changes in the artery wall that occur as a result of aging (London, Guerin et al., 1998; O'Rourke, 1999). The literature on the subject reflects confusion in the use of this term because sometimes it is clearly used to mean atherosclerosis (Oh & Seo, 2001; Schmahl & Kahle, 1996), whereas in other situations the authors make a clear differentiation between arteriosclerosis and atherosclerosis (Zou, Hu et al., 1998). O'Rourke states that arteriosclerosis differs from atherosclerosis because it results in lesions that are concentric and dilated whereas atherosclerosis results in eccentric and constricting lesions (O'Rourke, 1999). Arteries with arteriosclerosis are stiff because of loss of elastin and an increase in collagen. In addition, hyaline, which is a glycoprotein plus a small amount of lipid, is found beneath the internal elastic lamina as a part of the arteriosclerosis. In the kidney, arteriosclerosis occurs most commonly in the afferent arterioles (Lindop, 1994).

Fibrinoid Arteriolar Necrosis. Fibrinoid necrosis occurs in the small arterioles in persons with accelerated (malignant) hypertension. The primary lesion in fibrinoid necrosis is accumulation of deposits of fibrin, fibrinogen, and other plasma proteins within the vessel wall. In addition, there is evidence of death of cells with the vessel wall. This lesion is most frequently seen in the kidney and may also be called malignant nephrosclerosis (Lindop, 1994). References to fibrinoid arteriolar necrosis are most often found in pathology reports and journals.

Heart

The cardiac sequelae of hypertension include left ventricular hypertrophy, heart failure, coronary artery disease, and myocardial infarction. Data from the Framingham study indicate that persons with hypertension have at least a two-times greater risk of coronary disease and heart failure than person who are normotensive (Kannel, 1996).

Chapters 25 and 28 discuss coronary heart disease and heart failure. Although left ventricular hypertrophy is most commonly seen in adults, it has also been found in children with hypertension (Daniels, Loggie et al., 1998; Schieken, Clarke et al., 1981).

There is a positive correlation between cardiovascular morbidity and mortality and left ventricular hypertrophy. The greater the left ventricular mass, the greater the risk of dying of heart disease (Kannel & Cobb, 1992). This risk is intensified if the person also has hypertension, glucose intolerance, dyslipidemia, and/or smokes cigarettes.

Although the mechanisms contributing to left ventricular hypertrophy are not well understood, recent studies have implicated angiotensin, aldosterone, and the atrial natriuretic peptides as potential causative factors(Muscholl, Schunkert et al., 1998; Ramirez-Gil, Delcayre et al., 1998). Other growth factors and cytokines are probably also involved in the development of hypertrophy (Susic, Nunez et al., 1995). Rossi and colleagues found increases in collagen, extracellular matrix, and myocyte diameter in hypertrophied human hearts studied at autopsy (Rossi, 1998). The putative role of the renin-angiotensin aldosterone system in the development of left ventricular hypertrophy is supported by the finding that treatment of hypertension with ACE inhibitors is associated with regression of the hypertrophy (Gottdiener, Reda et al., 1997; Schmieder, Martus et al., 1996). Other interventions that have also been associated with regression of left ventricular hypertrophy include weight loss, physical activity, and treatment with angiotensin II receptor blocking agents, calcium-channel antagonists, beta blockers, and diuretics (Gottdiener, Reda et al., 1997; Kokkinos, Narayan et al., 1995; S. W. MacMahon, Wilcken et al., 1986; Ofili, Cohen et al., 1998; Schmieder, Martus et al., 1996; Thurmann, Kenedi et al., 1998). It is assumed, but not yet demonstrated, that regression of left ventricular hypertrophy will be associated with reduced morbidity and mortality.

Kidney

There is a vicious, circular relationship between hypertension and renal disease. Persons with kidney disease and hypertension have a worse prognosis than those who are normotensive. In a follow-up study of the 339,544 middle-aged men at high risk screened for the Multiple Risk Factor Intervention Trial, a strong positive relationship was found between baseline BP and end-stage renal disease (Klag, Whelton et al., 1996). Compared to men with BPs less than 120/80 mm Hg, those with pressures from high-normal to severe hypertension had significantly elevated adjusted relative risks of end-stage renal disease ranging from 1.9 in the high-normals to 22.1 for those with pressures more than 210/120 mm Hg. Several studies have demonstrated that BP control, often using ACE inhibitors, can slow the progression of renal insufficiency (Bakris, Mangrum et al., 1997; Giatras, Lau et al., 1997; Lewis, Hunsicker et al., 1993; Maschio, Alberti et al., 1996).

In a healthy kidney, contraction of the afferent arterioles prevents variations in pressure from being transmitted to the glomerulus and thus influencing filtration. In persons with chronic renal failure or prolonged hypertension, it is thought

Table 39–4 ■ CLASSIFICATION OF HYPERTENSIVE RETINOPATHY

	Vasculopathy		Neuroretinal Changes		
Grade	Arterial Narrowing AV Ratio*	Focal Spasm†	Hemorrhage	Exudates	Papilledema
Normal	>3 : 4 (>75%)	None	0	0	0
Grade I	3 : 4–1 : 2 (75%–50%)	None	0	0	0
Grade II	<1 : 2–1 : 3 (49%–33%)	<1 : 1–2 : 3 (>66%)	0	0	0
Grade III	<1 : 3–1 : 4 (32%–25%)	<2 : 3–1 : 3 (66%–33%)	+	+	0
Grade IV	<1 : 4 (<25%) Thread-like	<1 : 3 (<33%) Fibrous cords	+	+	+

*Retinal artery diameter to vein diameter ratio.
†Arterial focal spasm diameter to proximal artery ratio.
(Patel, V., & Kohner, E. M. [1994]. The eye in hypertension. In J. D. Swales (Ed.), *Textbook of hypertension* [pp. 1015–1025]. Oxford: Blackwell.)

that there may be failure of the afferent arterioles to protect the glomerulus from elevated systemic arterial pressure. Proteinuria is a clinical manifestation of elevated glomerular filtration pressure. Microalbuminuria, defined as a daily urinary protein excretion of more than 20 mg, is found in approximately 15 % of persons with essential hypertension (Anderson, 1999).

Pathologists describe the renal lesions associated with hypertension as arteriosclerotic with patches of hyaline sclerosis. In addition, atherosclerosis of the renal arteries can have a contributing role as is seen in renovascular hypertension (Anderson, 1999; Kashgarian, 1990).

Eye

The retina is the only part of the body where arteries and arterioles can be seen easily without invasive methods. Evidence of vessel damage in the retina indicates blood vessel damage elsewhere.

Hypertensive changes in the retina include changes in the diameter of the arteries, focal spasms, hemorrhages, formation of exudates, local infarctions, and edema of the optic fundus. Various combinations of these changes have been used over the years to classify the condition of the retina as either normal or as one of several grades of hypertensive retinopathy. One recently recommended classification is shown in Table 39-4 (Patel & Kohner, 1994). In this classification, the major criteria that are used to grade retinopathy are the ratio of the retinal artery diameter to the diameter of the renal vein; the presence or absence of focal spasm of the retinal arteries; and then the presence of absence of hemorrhages, exudates, and papilledema. Grades I and II differ only in the degree of arterial narrowing. If either retinal hemorrhages or exudates are present, it is grade III retinopathy. The presence of edema of the optic fundus indicates grade IV.

Some criteria that are included in other classifications are the arterial light reflex and what is known as "A-V nicking." The arterial light reflex is an indicator of the amount of thickening of the walls of the retinal arteries. With moderate thickening, the arteries have a "copper wire" appearance, and with severe narrowing the arteries are thought to resemble "silver wire." A-V nicking occurs at locations where arteries and veins cross. When A-V nicking is present, it is an indentation in the outer contour of a vein secondary to compression caused by thickening of the walls of the crossing retinal artery.

Diagrams of the optic fundus and the changes associated with hypertension are included in Chapter 13. Research on pigs and rhesus monkeys has revealed that cotton–wool spots result from retinal ischemia and infarction (Hayreh, Servais et al., 1989; McLeod, Marshall et al., 1977; Murata & Yoshimoto, 1983). Infarction blocks axonal transport and the accumulation of material in the axon is seen as the white patches known as cotton–wool spots. The swelling of the optic nerve head that occurs with hypertension needs to be differentiated from the papilledema that occurs with increased intracranial pressure (Patel & Kohner, 1994). Some authorities refer the optic nerve edema in accelerated hypertension as papilledema whereas others are careful to use terminology like disc edema (Kaplan, 1998; Patel & Kohner, 1994). A controversy exists about the ability of clinicians to identify papilledema and whether it is a useful prognostic indicator (Ahmed, Walker et al., 1986; Frank, 1999; McGregor, Isles et al., 1986). In a 10-year follow-up of 96 persons with hypertension, McGregor and colleagues found that those with grades III and IV retinopathy had a survival rate of 46% and 48%, respectively (McGregor, Isles et al., 1986). Unfortunately, the sample size is small, which makes the clinical implications of these results uncertain.

Brain

Two changes occur in the cerebral arteries in response to chronic elevations in BP: remodeling and hypertrophy. Remodeling is a reduction in the outer diameter of an arteriole, whereas hypertrophy results in an increase in the thickness of the vessel wall. Both changes promote vasoconstriction and inhibit vasodilation, and they also support cerebral autoregulation. Autoregulation is a property of vascular beds that allows them to maintain a constant blood flow in response to a relatively wide range of perfusion pressure. With autoregulation, blood flow in an organ is held almost constant except at very low or high perfusion pressures. In hypertension, it has been demonstrated that cerebral autoregulation is maintained but the pressure–flow relationship is shifted to the right of what is seen with normotension (Baumbach & Heistad, 1999).

Stroke. Hypertension is a clearly identifiable risk factor for stroke and its precursor, transient ischemic attacks (TIAs) (Khaw, 1996). Stroke is the number one cause of marked disability and number three cause of death in the United States (Decline in deaths from heart disease and stroke–United States, 1900-1999, 1999). Research has documented the positive relationship between stroke and high BP as well as the reduction in stroke with BP control (Collins, Peto et al., 1990; Garraway & Whisnant, 1987; Gueyffier, Boutitie et al., 1997; Lewington, Clarke et al., 2002; MacMahon, Peto et al., 1990). When lipid-lowering with atorvastatin was compared to placebo in an arm of a clinical trial with 10,305 subjects, stroke incidence was significantly reduced even though blood pressure control was identical in both groups (Sever, Dahlof et al., 2003). This result differs from the cholesterol-lowering arm of the Antihypertensive and Lipid-Lowering Treatment to Prevent Heart Attack Trial (ALLHAT). Further study is required to clarify the role of lipid-lowering in stroke prevention (Major outcomes in moderately hypercholesterolemic, hypertensive patients randomized to pravastatin vs usual care: The Antihypertensive and Lipid-Lowering Treatment to Prevent Heart Attack Trial (ALLHAT-LLT), 2002).

Ischemic injury to the brain is caused by decreased cerebral perfusion as a consequence of thrombosis, embolism, or a decreased blood supply to an area. It is now recognized that small strokes can occur without complete occlusion of the cerebral arteries (Pullicino, 1999). Emboli from the left ventricle or from the peripheral veins via a patent foramen ovale cause approximately 20% of strokes. Another source of emboli may be atherosclerotic plaques in the carotid arteries. Hypertension increases the risk of stroke and transient ischemic attacks because it contributes to the formation and growth of atherosclerotic plaque. Hypertension also causes hypertrophy in arteriolar walls, luminal narrowing, and, therefore, decreased cerebral perfusion and ischemia. The accumulation of hyaline in cerebral arteries, secondary to hypertension, contributes to occlusion of the cerebral arteries. Hypertension also contributes to the rupture of cerebral arteries leading to hemorrhage and to the formation of aneurysms (Pullicino, 1999).

Hypertensive Encephalopathy. Cerebral encephalopathy is a consequence of accelerated or malignant hypertension. Encephalopathy occurs when the BP levels exceed the upper limit of autoregulation so that the cerebral arteries become dilated and the blood-brain barrier in the cerebral venules is disrupted (Baumbach & Heistad, 1999). This disruption of the blood-brain barrier is thought to contribute to the formation of cerebral edema; local changes in ion and cytokine concentrations; and/or alteration in neural function. Although rare, hypertensive encephalopathy occurs in children as well as in adults (Wright & Mathews, 1996).

MANAGEMENT OF HIGH BP

Assessment and Diagnosis

Diagnosis

Hypertension is relatively easy to diagnose. The fact that people with hypertension usually have no symptoms presents the greatest problem in establishing the diagnosis. Partly because of the lack of symptoms, in 1999 to 2000, approximately 30% of the hypertensive population in the United States were unaware of their condition (Chobanian, Bakris et al., 2003). The awareness, treatment, and control rates for hypertension in the United States between 1976 and 2000 are shown in Table 39-5. The hypertension control rate in 1999 to 2000 of 34% indicates a need for increased efforts on the part of health care professionals to manage the treatment of hypertension successfully.

Blood Pressure Measurement. The diagnosis of hypertension cannot be made from a single measurement because BP can vary markedly over weeks, days, and even minutes. In both hypertensive and normotensive people, there is diurnal variation in BP with the highest pressures occurring between 8:00 and 11:00 AM and lowest during sleep between 2:00 and 6:00 AM (Millar-Craig, Bishop et al., 1978). There can be a marked variation in BP during REM sleep and a substantial elevation when a person first awakens (de Leeuw, van Leeuwen et al., 1985; Lightman, James et al., 1981). Furthermore, a person's BP can be elevated during an office visit because of apprehension, pain, or preexisting illness. In view of the normal lability and biologic variations in BP, JNC 7 states that a diagnosis can only be established on the basis of an average of two or more BPs measured on two or more subsequent occasions. The reliability and accuracy of BP readings depend on good technique and standardization of the procedure. The American Heart Association pamphlet Recommendations for Human BP Determination by Sphygmomanometers (Perloff, Grim et al., 1993) can

Table 39–5 ■ TRENDS IN AWARENESS, TREATMENT, AND CONTROL OF HIGH BLOOD PRESSURE IN ADULTS AGES 18–74

	National Health And Nutrition Examination Survey, Percent			
	II (1976–80)	III (Phase 1 1988–91)	III (Phase 2 1991–94)	1999–2000
Awareness	51	73	68	70
Treatment	31	55	54	59
Control[†]	10	29	27	34

*High blood pressure is systolic blood pressure (SBP) ≥140 mm Hg or diastolic blood pressure (DBP) ≥90 mmHg or taking antihypertensive medication.
[†]SBP <140 mmHg and DBP <90 mm Hg.
Sources: Unpublished data for 1999–2000 computed by M. Wolz, National Heart, Lung, and Blood Institute; JNC 6.
(Chobanian, A. V., Bakris, G. L., Black, H. R., et al. [2003]. The Seventh Report of the Joint National Committee on Prevention, Detection, Evaluation, and Treatment of High Blood Pressure: the JNC 7 report. *JAMA*, 289[19], 2560–2572. [Erratum in *JAMA*, 2003, 290(2), 197].)

DISPLAY **39-3**

IMPORTANT ASPECTS OF THE HISTORY AND PHYSICAL EXAMINATION

History

Duration of the hypertension

Last known normal blood pressure
Course of the blood pressure

Prior treatment of the hypertension

Drugs: types, doses, side effects

Intake of agents that may cause hypertension

Oral contraceptives
Sympathomimetics
Adrenal steroids
Excessive sodium intake

Family history

Hypertension
Premature cardiovascular disease or death
Familial diseases: pheochromocytoma, renal disease,
   diabetes, gout

Symptoms of secondary causes

Muscle weakness
Spells of tachycardia, sweating, tremor
Thinning of the skin
Flank pain

Symptoms of target organ damage

Headaches
Transient weakness or blindness
Loss of visual acuity
Chest pain
Dyspnea
Claudication

Presence of other risk factors

Smoking
Diabetes

Dyslipidemia
Physical inactivity

Dietary history

Sodium
Alcohol
Saturated fats

Psychosocial factors

Family structure
Work status
Educational level

Sexual function

Features of sleep apnea

Early morning headaches
Daytime somnolence
Loud snoring
Erratic sleep

Physical Examination

Accurate measurement of blood pressure
General appearance: distribution of body fat, skin lesions,
   muscle strength, alertness
Funduscopy
Neck: palpation and auscultation of carotids, thyroid
Heart: size, rhythm, sounds
Lungs: rhonchi, rales
Abdomen: renal masses, bruits over aorta or renal arteries,
   femoral pulses
Extremities: peripheral pulses, edema
Neurologic assessment

(Kaplan, N. M. [2002]. *Clinical hypertension* [8th ed.]. Baltimore:
Williams & Wilkins.)

---

be found on the American Heart Associations web site: http://www.americanheart.org/presenter.jhtml?identifier= 3000894.

Clinical Evaluation. The objectives of the medical assessment for hypertension are to determine if there is/are: (1) target organ involvement; (2) other cardiovascular risk factors; (3) cardiovascular disease and any response to its treatment; (4) an identifiable cause for the elevated pressure; and (5) comorbid conditions. The assessment should include a careful history and physical examination. Display 39-3 lists many of the important variables to assess during the history and physical (Kaplan, 2002). It is also important to ask the client about any non-traditional remedies they may be using including herbs, vitamins, and other supplements (The reader is referred to Chapter 45). Table 39-6 lists the basic and optional laboratory tests recommended by JNC 7 for assessment of target organ damage.

Although secondary hypertension is rare (approximately 10% of all hypertension), practitioners should, nevertheless, attempt to rule out secondary causes. Additional evaluation is recommended in patients whose age, severity of hypertension,

history, physical examination, or laboratory findings are suggestive of secondary hypertension. Poor response to antihypertensive drug therapy, accelerated or malignant hypertension, or an accelerated phase of previously well-controlled

Table 39–6 ■ RECOMMENDED AND OPTIONAL LABORATORY TESTS AND DIAGNOSTIC PROCEDURES

Recommended

Urinalysis
Hematocrit
Blood chemistries
   Potassium, calcium, creatinine or estimated glomerular filtration rate,
   fasting glucose, fasting lipid profile
12-lead electrocardiogram

Optional

Urinary albumin excretion or
Albumin/creatinine ratio

(Chobanian, A. V., Bakris, G. L., Black, H. R., et al. [2003]. The Seventh Report of the Joint National Committee on Prevention, Detection, Evaluation, and Treatment of High Blood Pressure: the JNC 7 report. *JAMA,* 289(19), 2560–2572. [Erratum in *JAMA,* 2003, 290[2], 197].)

hypertension also indicates a need for further investigation (Chobanian, Bakris et al., 2003).

Prognosis

The Veterans Administration study documented a morbidity rate of 55% in people with an untreated diastolic pressure of 90 to 114 mm Hg (Veterans Administration Cooperative Study Group on Antihypertensive Agents, 1970). With untreated diastolic pressures more than 115 mm Hg, the morbidity rate was 80% (Veterans Administration Cooperative Study Group on Antihypertensive Agents, 1967). In the patients with diastolic pressure more than 115 mg Hg, there were four deaths in the placebo group compared with none in the treatment group. This and other studies have documented that treatment can prevent morbidity and mortality in persons with elevated BPs (Hypertension Detection and Follow-up Program Cooperative Group, 1982; Medical Research Council Working Party, 1985).

The strong, graded, independent, and continuous relationships between SBP, DBP, and cardiovascular risk were clearly illustrated by the analysis of 6 years of follow-up data from the screenings for the Multiple Risk Factor Intervention Trial (MRFIT) (Stamler, Stamler et al., 1993). Data from the 361,662 men screened for the study from 1973 to 1975 showed that relative risk of cardiovascular disease began increasing above a SBP of 120 mm Hg and a diastolic pressure of 90 mm Hg. Mortality rates were two- to three-times higher for men with systolic pressures greater than 120 mm Hg. Two meta-analyses by MacMahon, Peto, and Collins and associates explored the data documenting the nature and strength of the relationships between BP control, stroke incidence, and coronary heart disease (Collins, Peto et al., 1990; MacMahon, Peto et al., 1990). A meta-analysis of 61 observational studies of more than one million subjects found that even lowering blood pressure within the range that is usually considered normotensive down to a minimum pressure of 115/75 mm Hg would result in reductions in death from stroke and ischemic heart disease (Lewington, Clarke et al., 2002).

Treatment Options

Answers to a series of questions outline the progress in the treatment of high BP. In the 1950s, the initial question was whether any treatment for hypertension would reduce morbidity and mortality. Once clinical trials revealed that treatment was beneficial in reducing both morbid and mortal events, then the following questions became relevant. Did the benefits extend to persons different than those included in the initial clinical trials? What was the risk-to-benefit profile of different medications? How low should BP be lowered? Did the benefits extend to the elderly? Can high BP be prevented? What lifestyle or non-pharmacologic interventions are most effective? What is the best way to support people to follow the prescribed therapy, both changing their lifestyles to reduce risk and also using medications routinely? The current state of knowledge relating to these questions is discussed in the next sections, beginning with prevention of hypertension and then

moving to lifestyle and pharmacologic management, and then finally to management of hypertension in special populations.

The goal of therapy for patients with hypertension is the prevention of morbidity and mortality related to the elevated pressure, specifically the prevention of target organ damage and progression of atherosclerotic cardiovascular and renal disease (Chobanian, Bakris et al., 2003). Factors to consider in making treatment choices are any co-morbid conditions, cost of treatment, client preference, and potential impacts on the client's quality of life.

An important tool in the management of high BP is the concept of setting a "goal BP" for each client. This pressure is usually less than 140/90 mm Hg, although for patients with diabetes mellitus or renal disease a lower goal is recommended (see section on special populations for specific information on persons with renal disease and diabetes mellitus). The clinician may choose lower or higher goals depending on the individual client. The concept of goal BP has been demonstrated to be an effective tool in client management (Hypertension Detection and Follow-up Program Cooperative Group, 1979; Lazarus, Bourgoignie et al., 1997).

Prevention of High BP

The concept of hypertension prevention is relatively new. The sixth report of the Joint National Committee for the first time in 1997 included the word prevention in the title (The Joint National Committee on Prevention Detection Evaluation and Treatment of High Blood Pressure and the National High Blood Pressure Education Program Coordinating Committee, 1997). In 2002 the National High Blood Pressure Program released its second statement on the Primary Prevention of Hypertension (Whelton, He et al., 2002). This report points out the importance of beginning the lifestyle habits that prevent the development of high blood pressure during childhood.

Of the many interventions that have been studied in major clinical trials of hypertension prevention, only six have been demonstrated to be effective (Appel, Moore et al., 1997; Cushman, Cutler et al., 1998; Hypertension Prevention Trial Research Group, 1990; Stamler, Stamler et al., 1989; Trials of Hypertension Prevention Collaborative Research Group, 1992, 1997). The six interventions that have been shown to delay or prevent the onset of high BP are: weight loss, sodium restriction, a reduction in alcohol intake, increased exercise, potassium supplementation, and modified diets (see information on the DASH diet in the section on the non-pharmacologic management section) (He, Whelton et al., 2000; Stevens, Obarzanek et al., 2001; Whelton, He et al., 2002). The interventions that were not shown to be effective were: supplementation of calcium, magnesium, fiber, and fish oil administered in pill form; stress management; reduced alcohol intake; and alterations in macronutrients such as protein, carbohydrates, and fats (Batey, Kaufmann et al., 2000; Cushman, Cutler et al., 1998; National High Blood Pressure Education Program, 1993). In the Trial of Hypertension Prevention, one important finding was that the subjects had difficulty maintaining their changes in weight and sodium intake over prolonged periods of time (Trials of Hypertension Prevention Collaborative Research Group, 1997). Reductions in BP were greatest at 6 months and decreased over 3 to 7 years of follow-up (He, Whelton et al.,

2000; Stevens, Obarzanek et al., 2001). Even though the weight loss was not maintained, the odds of hypertension developing was 0.23 (95% confidence interval: 0.07–0.76) in the weight loss group compared to the control group at 7 years (Stevens, Obarzanek et al., 2001). There was no apparent benefit of the dietary sodium reduction at 7 years.

Two short-term dietary studies have provided evidence that a diet high in fruits and vegetables may be helpful in preventing high BP (Appel, Moore et al., 1997; John, Ziebland et al., 2002). After 8 weeks on a fruit and vegetable diet combined with low-fat dairy products and a reduction in saturated and total fat (DASH diet) the 326 normotensive subjects had significant greater reductions in their systolic and diastolic pressures (3.5 and 2.1 mm Hg, respectively; $p < 0.003$) than the control group (Lawrence J. Appel, Moore et al., 1997). A 6-month randomized controlled trial of increased fruit and vegetable intake in 690 healthy subject between the ages of 25 and 64 years resulted in lower systolic and diastolic pressures, $-4/-1.5$ mm Hg, in the group randomized to eat more fruits and vegetables (John, Ziebland et al., 2002). Even though these decreases are modest for an individual, they do have the potential of reducing the incidence of cardiovascular morbidity and mortality in a population.

Non-pharmacologic Management of High Blood Pressure

The non-pharmacologic or lifestyle measures that have been demonstrated to reduce blood pressure are three nutritional measures plus exercise or increased physical activity. The nutritional measures are sodium restriction and a diet high in fruits and vegetables. A combined approach that aims to balance energy intake with energy expenditure through a suitable dietary plan and physical activity/exercise is effective and an important component of weight loss and weight management. The JNC 7 recommendations for these lifestyle modifications are listed in Table 39-7 (Chobanian, Bakris et al., 2003). In addition, persons with high BP are encouraged to modify their other risk factors for cardiovascular disease such as dyslipi-demia and smoking because of their additive impact on the rate of development and progression of atherosclerosis.

Weight Control. The results of many studies indicate a direct relationship between hypertension and obesity (Garrison, Kannel et al., 1987; Huang, Willett et al., 1998; Kannel, Brand et al., 1967). There is also a correlation between the presence of excess abdominal adiposity (defined as an increased waist-to-hip ratio of more than 0.85 in women and 0.95 in men) and the development of hypertension, diabetes, dyslipidemia, and increased CHD mortality (Blair, Habicht et al., 1984; Despres, Moorjani et al., 1990; Folsom, Prineas et al., 1990; Haarbo, Hassager et al., 1989; Ostlund, Staten et al., 1990). Studies in Framingham, Massachusetts and Evans County, Georgia reveal that overweight people have from two- to three-times the risk for hypertension compared to persons who are not overweight (Kannel, Brand et al., 1967; Stamler, Stamler et al., 1978). The exact mechanism by which obesity contributes to hypertension is unclear. However, the influence of weight may be related to alterations in cardiovascular, endocrine, and metabolic factors caused by obesity. These alterations include increased cardiac output, increased blood volume, and sodium retention. There is also evidence that hyperinsulinemia, insulin resistance, decreased carbohydrate tolerance, and decreased insulin sensitivity occur in conjunction with obesity (Manolio, Savage et al., 1991; Muller-Wieland, Kotzka et al., 1998). This constellation of risk factors is known as the metabolic syndrome (Executive Summary of The Third Report of The National Cholesterol Education Program (NCEP) Expert Panel on Detection, Evaluation, And Treatment of High Blood Cholesterol In Adults (Adult Treatment Panel III), 2001). Recent research also indicates alterations in endothelial function in persons who are overweight (Muller-Wieland, Kotzka et al., 1998).

Weight loss has consistently been demonstrated to reduce BP more effectively than any other lifestyle measure (He, Whelton et al., 2000; Hypertension Prevention Trial Research Group, 1990; Langford, Blaufox et al., 1985; Stevens, Obarzanek et al., 2001; Trials of Hypertension Prevention Collaborative Research Group, 1992, 1997; Wassertheil-Smoller,

---

Table 39-7 ▪ LIFESTYLE MODIFICATIONS TO MANAGE HYPERTENSION[*][†]

Modification	Recommendation	Approximate SBP Reduction (Range)
Weight reduction	Maintain normal body weight (body mass index 18.5–24.9 kg/m^2).	5–20 mm Hg/10 kg weight loss
Adopt DASH eating plan	Consume a diet rich in fruits, vegetables, and lowfat dairy products with a reduced content of saturated and total fat.	8–14 mm Hg
Dietary sodium reduction	Reduce dietary sodium intake to no more than 100 mmol per day (2.4 g sodium or 6 g sodium chloride).	2–8 mm Hg
Physical activity	Engage in regular aerobic physical activity such as brisk walking (at least 30 min per day, most days of the week).	4–9 mm Hg
Moderation of alcohol consumption	Limit consumption to no more than 2 drinks (1 oz or 30 mL ethanol; e.g., 24 oz beer, 10 oz wine, or 3 oz 80-proof whiskey) per day in most men and to no more than 1 drink per day in women and lighter weight persons.	2–4 mm Hg

DASH, Dietary Approaches to Stop Hypertension.
[*]For overall cardiovascular risk reduction, stop smoking.
[†]The effects of implementing these modifications are dose and time-dependent, and could be greater for some individuals.
(Chobanian, A. V., Bakris, G. L., Black, H. R., et al. [2003]. The Seventh Report of the Joint National Committee on Prevention, Detection, Evaluation, and Treatment of High Blood Pressure: the JNC 7 report. *JAMA*, 289[19], 2560–2572. [Erratum in *JAMA*, 2003, 290[2], 197].)

Oberman et al., 1992; Whelton, Appel et al., 1998). The study by Langford and associates of subjects whose BP had been controlled with medications for 5 years found that an average weight loss of 10 pounds prevented 60% of the overweight subjects from having to return to taking medications (Langford, Blaufox et al., 1985). In addition, weight loss has been found to complement pharmacologic management of mild-high BP (Neaton, Grimm et al., 1993; Oberman, Wassertheil-Smoller et al., 1990). Counseling a hypertensive, overweight patient about weight reduction is important, both as a preventive measure as well as an independent or complementary treatment for high BP. The challenge for both clinicians and clients is supporting maintenance of weight loss, because longitudinal studies have shown that subjects who lose weight initially tend to gain back the weight over time (Whelton, Appel et al., 1998). In a study of male health professionals, Coakley and associates found that vigorous physical activity was associated with weight loss whereas eating between meals and watching television were associated with weight gain (Coakley, Rimm et al., 1998) (see Chapter 42 on obesity).

Sodium Restriction. The role of sodium in the development of hypertension and its efficacy as an intervention to treat or prevent high BP are controversial topics. It is clear that some, but not all, hypertensive persons respond to a reduction in sodium intake with a decrease in BP. Data from Ferri and colleagues indicate that there may be a relationship between damage to the vascular endothelium and salt sensitivity (Ferri, Bellini et al., 1998). What has been even more controversial is whether a public health approach that lowered the sodium intake of all members of a population would result in lower morbidity and mortality related to high BP (Cutler, Follmann et al., 1997; Luft, 1998; Midgley, Matthew et al., 1996).

Clinical trials of non-pharmacologic approaches to the treatment of hypertension have consistently shown that reduction of sodium intake is effective in reducing BP (Appel, Espeland et al., 2001; Cutler, Follmann et al., 1997; Hypertension Prevention Trial Research Group, 1990; Langford, Blaufox et al., 1985; Midgley, Matthew et al., 1996; Sacks, Svetkey et al., 2001; Trials of Hypertension Prevention Collaborative Research Group, 1992, 1997). In two separate meta-analyses of randomized trials of reduced sodium intake in persons with high BP, it was found that for a 100-mmol/d decrease in sodium intake, there was a −3.7 to −5.8 mm Hg decrease in systolic BP and a −0.9 to −2.5 mm Hg decrease in diastolic pressure (Cutler, Follmann et al., 1997; Midgley, Matthew et al., 1996). The impact of reducing sodium intake was greater in persons who were older and who had higher levels of BP. A randomized controlled trial of sodium reduction in 681 persons between ages 60 and 80 years found that reducing sodium intake resulted in lower blood pressures and a reduced need for antihypertensive medications (Appel, Espeland et al., 2001). Lowering salt intake is cheaper than antihypertensive medications and probably has markedly fewer side effects, especially in older persons.

JNC 7 recommends a goal sodium intake of no more than 100 mmol/d, which is equivalent to approximately 6 grams of sodium chloride or 2.4 grams of sodium per day (Chobanian, Bakris et al., 2003). In many of the clinical trials of sodium reduction, the goals levels of sodium intake were between 70 and 100 mmol/d, although the average intake for most subjects ranged between 104 and 124 mmol/d. The apparent difficulty in achieving this goal sodium intake underscores the challenge of reducing sodium intake. It is estimated that the average adult man uses approximately 3.9 grams of sodium daily whereas women take in approximately 2.8 grams (Engstrom, Tobelmann et al., 1997). It may help clients to know that it takes 8 to 12 weeks to adjust one's sense of taste to a lower intake of sodium (Mattes, 1997).

Sodium restriction has also been shown to be a beneficial adjunct to the pharmacologic treatment of high BP (Dustan, Schneckloth et al., 1958; Weinberger, Cohen et al., 1988). Weinberger and colleagues found that subjects who decreased their intake of sodium to between 50 and 100 mmol/d were able to decrease significantly their doses of diuretics and potassium-sparing agents (Weinberger, Cohen et al., 1988). Salt intake has also been found to influence the plasma concentration of medications such as verapamil (Darbar, Fromm et al., 1998). Plasma levels of verapamil were found to be lower when subjects ingested 400 mEq/d compared to 10 mEq/d of sodium. Sodium restriction (1–3 g/d) has been shown to restore the typical circadian rhythm of BP in persons with essential hypertension and primary aldosteronism (Uzu, Ishikawa et al., 1997; Uzu, Nishimura et al., 1998).

The variability of an individual's BP response to level of sodium intake has been called salt sensitivity (Fuenmayor, Moreira et al., 1998; Gonzalez-Albarran, Ruilope et al., 1998). Although it is known that some individuals have a decrease in BP when sodium intake is reduced whereas other persons have no change in pressure, there is not yet any test that allows the clinician to identify who is susceptible. Analysis of participants in the Trial of Hypertension Prevention study found differences in angiotensinogen genotype between those who were salt-sensitive and those who were not (Hunt, Cook et al., 1998). Subsequent research has found associations between two other genetic polymorphisms in the RAA system and salt sensitivity (Poch, Gonzalez et al., 2001). Until there is a test for sodium sensitivity, clinicians can do an "N of 1" study by trying a period of salt restriction with a client and measuring BP before and after to determine the individual's response. A useful measure of a client's sodium intake is a 24-hour urine sample analyzed for sodium content.

Diet High in Fruits and Vegetables. The Dietary Approaches to Stop Hypertension (DASH) study examined the effects of an 8-week dietary intervention on BP in normotensive and hypertensive subjects (Appel, Moore et al., 1997). In the 133 hypertensive subjects, the investigators found that adherence to a diet high in fruits, vegetables, and low-fat dairy products and low in saturated and total fat resulted in a marked decline in both systolic and diastolic BP. Compared to normotensive control subjects, those with a systolic pressure between 140 and 160 mm Hg and/or a diastolic pressure between 90 and 95 mm Hg had decreases in BP of −11.4/−5.5 mm Hg. There was no significant change in weight during the study in any of the study groups. The DASH diet included 8 to 10 servings per day of fruits and vegetables and 2.7 servings of low-fat dairy products. The subjects were either fed at the research center or were given their meals in coolers to eat at home or work. Subsequent clinical trials based on the DASH diets have shown that: (1) adding salt reduction results in a significantly greater decrease in systolic and diastolic

Table 39–8 ▦ THE DIETARY APPROACHES TO STOP HYPERTENSION (DASH) DIET*

Food Group	Daily Servings	Serving Sizes	Examples and Notes	Significance of Each Food Group to the DASH Diet Pattern
Grains and grain products	7–8	1 slice bread 1/2 cup dry cereal 1/2 cup cooked rice, pasta, or cereal	Whole-wheat bread, English muffin, pita bread, bagel, cereals, grits, oatmeal	Major sources of energy and fiber
Vegetables	4–5	1 cup raw leafy vegetable 1/2 cup cooked vegetable 6 oz vegetable juice	Tomatoes, potatoes, carrots, peas, squash, broccoli, turnip greens, collards, kale, spinach, artichokes, beans, sweet potatoes	Rich sources of potassium, magnesium, and fiber
Fruits	4–5	6 oz fruit juice 1 medium fruit 1/4 cup dried fruit 1/2 cup fresh, frozen, or canned fruit	Apricots, bananas, dates, grapes, oranges, orange juice, grapefruit, grapefruit juice, mangoes, melons, peaches, pineapples, prunes, raisins, strawberries, tangerines	Important sources of potassium, magnesium, and fiber
Low-fat or nonfat dairy foods	2–3	8 oz milk 1 cup yogurt 1.5 oz cheese	Skim or 1% milk, skim or low-fat buttermilk, nonfat or low-fat yogurt, part-skim mozzarella cheese, nonfat cheese	Major sources of calcium and protein
Meats, poultry, and fish	2 or less	3 oz cooked meats, poultry, or fish	Select only lean; trim away visible fats; broil, roast, or boil, instead of frying; remove skin from polutry	Rich sources of protein and magnesium
Nuts, seeds, and legumes	4–5 per week	1.5 oz or 1/3 cup nuts 1/2 oz or 2 Tbsp seeds 1/2 cup cooked legumes	Almonds, filberts, mixed nuts, peanuts, walnuts, sunflower seeds, kidney beans, lentils	Rich sources of energy, magnesium, potassium, protein, and fiber

*The DASH eating plan shown is based on 2,000 calories per day. Depending on an individual's caloric needs, the number of daily servings in a food group may vary from those listed. (The Joint National Committee on Prevention, Detection, Evaluation, and Treatment of High Blood Pressure and the National High Blood Pressure Education Program Coordinating Committee. [1997]. The sixth report of the Joint National Committee on Prevention, Detection, Evaluation, and Treatment of High Blood Pressure. *Archives of Internal Medicine, 157*, 2413–2446.)

pressures; and (2) the DASH diet can successfully be combined with other lifestyle modifications specifically limiting alcohol intake to 1 ounce or less per day and increasing physical activity to a minimum of 180 minutes (3 hours) each week (Appel, Champagne et al., 2003; Sacks, Svetkey et al., 2001). The diet can work, but the challenge will be finding a way to support adoption of the diet in a manner that fits with the individual's daily life. A description of the DASH diet is shown in Table 39-8 and a sample menu is shown in Table 39-9. Additional information on the DASH diet is available at http://www.nhlbi.nih.gov/health/public/heart/hbp/dash/. Further research is also needed to look at the impact of the DASH diet over extended time periods.

Physical Activity. A sedentary lifestyle is one of the risk factors for hypertension (Arakawa, 1993; Blair, Goodyear et al., 1984; Horan & Lenfant, 1990; Ledoux, Lambert et al., 1997; Westheim & Os, 1992). The results of three meta-analyses on the effect of physical activity on hypertension concluded that aerobic training does reduce BP (Fagard, 1993; Kelley & Kelley, 2000; Whelton, Chin et al., 2002). The data indicate that physical fitness training had a graded influence on BP from a small influence on normotensive individuals to a larger impact on those with hypertension. Additional studies have supported the conclusions of these meta-analyses (Kokkinos, Narayan et al., 1995; Melby, Goldflies et al., 1991). Other analyses of research data indicate that persons who are physically active experience reduced cardiovascular and all-cause mortality rates (S. N. Blair, Kohl et al., 1989; Ekelund, Haskell et al., 1988; Erikssen, Liestol et al., 1998; Ford & DeStefano, 1991; Fried, Kronmal et al.,

1998; Hakim, Petrovitch et al., 1998; Kujala, Kaprio et al., 1998; Kushi, Fee et al., 1997; Paffenbarger, Hyde et al., 1986; Salonen, Slater et al., 1988; Sandvik, Erikssen et al., 1993; Sherman, D'Agostino et al., 1994a, 1994b).

Physical activity is known to have a variety of metabolic and other effects that may partially explain its beneficial effects on BP. One confounding factor in some of these studies is that sometimes the physical activity intervention is combined with weight loss. Another problem is that the studies include only a small number of subjects because of the cost and complexity of performing invasive measurements. In a study of nine hypertensive and obese men with an average age of 62, it was found that a 6-month period of physical training improved glucose and lipid metabolism. The men lost 9% of their body weight and improved the exercise capacity (VO_2max) by 16% (Dengel, Hagberg et al., 1998). Two studies of 18 persons with high BP and left ventricular hypertrophy found that after 24 to 32 weeks of exercising at least three times per week, the participants had significant decreases in indices of left ventricular hypertrophy (Kokkinos, Narayan et al., 1995). The 1996 Surgeon General's Report on Physical Activity and Health documents the extent of the known benefits of physical activity for chronic disease prevention (US Department of Health and Human Services, 1996) (see Chapter 41 for physical activity and exercise).

JNC 7 recommends that persons with high BP should exercise moderately for a minimum of 30 minutes almost every day of the week (Chobanian, Bakris et al., 2003). Although the report does not mention the need for a physical examination before beginning a program of moderate aerobic activity, no

Table 39–9 ■ DIETARY APPROACHES TO STOP HYPERTENSION (DASH) DIET SAMPLE MENU (BASED ON 2,000 KCAL/D)

Food	Amount	Servings Provided
Breakfast		
Orange juice	6 oz	1 fruit
1% Low-fat milk	8 oz (1 cup)	1 dairy
Corn flakes (with 1 tsp sugar)	1 C	2 grains
Banana	1 medium	1 fruit
Whole-wheat bread (with 1 Tbsp jelly)	1 slice	1 grain
Soft margarine	1 tsp	1 fat
Lunch		
Chicken salad	3/4 cup	1 poultry
Pita bread	1/2, large	1 grain
Raw vegetable medley:		
Carrot and celery sticks	3–4 sticks each	
Radishes	2	1 vegetable
Loose-leaf lettuce	2 leaves	
Part-skim mozzarella cheese	1.5 slice (1.5 oz)	1 dairy
1% Low-fat milk	8 oz (1 cup)	1 dairy
Fruit cocktail in light syrup	1/2 cup	1 fruit
Dinner		
Herbed baked cod	3 oz	1 fish
Scallion rice	1 cup	2 grains
Steamed broccoli	1/2 cup	1 vegetable
Stewed tomatoes	1/2 cup	1 vegetable
Spinach salad:		
Raw spinach	1/2 cup	
Cherry tomatoes	2	1 vegetable
Cucumber	2 slices	
Light Italian salad dressing	1 Tbsp	1/2 fat
Whole-wheat dinner roll	1 small	1 grain
Soft margarine	1 tsp	1 fat
Melon balls	1/2 cup	1 fruit
Snacks		
Dried apricots	1 oz (1/4 cup)	1 fruit
Mini-pretzels	1 oz (3/4 cup)	1 grain
Mixed nuts	1.5 oz (1/3 cup)	1 nuts
Diet ginger ale	12 oz	0

Total number of servings in 2,000 kcal/d menu:

Food Group	Servings
Grains	=8
Vegetables	=4
Fruits	=5
Dairy foods	=3
Meats, poultry, and fish	=2
Nuts, seeds, and legumes	=1
Fats and oils	=2.5

Tips on Eating the DASH Way

- Start small. Make gradual changes in your eating habits.
- Center your meal around carbohydrates, such as pasta, rice, beans, or vegetables.
- Treat meat as one part of the whole meal, instead of the focus.
- Use fruits or low-fat, low-calorie foods such as sugar-free gelatin for desserts and snacks.

REMEMBER! If you use the DASH diet to help prevent or control high blood pressure, make it part of a lifestyle that includes choosing foods lower in salt and sodium, keeping a healthy weight, being physically active, and, if you drink alcohol, doing so in moderation

To learn more about high blood pressure, call 1-800-575-WELL or visit the NHLBI web site at http://www.nhlbi.nih.gov/nhlbi/nhlbi.htm. DASH is also on-line at http://www.nhlbi.gov/health/public/heart/hbp/dash/index.htm.
(The Joint National Committee on Prevention, Detection, Evaluation, and Treatment of High Blood Pressure and the National High Blood Pressure Education Program Coordinating Committee. [1997]. The sixth report of the Joint National Committee on Prevention, Detection, Evaluation, and Treatment of High Blood Pressure. *Archives of Internal Medicine,* 157, 2413–2446.)

patient with high BP or any other major cardiovascular risk factor should leave the care of their health provider without instructions on the signs and symptoms of heart attack and stroke and a discussion of what to do if symptoms occur (call 911 or its local equivalent).

Reduction of Alcohol Intake. The data from epidemiologic studies clearly indicate that an alcohol intake of more than three to four standard drinks per day is associated with high BP (Beilin & Puddey, 1992; Cushman, 1999; Klatsky, Friedman et al., 1977; Thun, Peto et al., 1997). A standard drink has been defined as approximately 14 grams of alcohol, which is the amount contain in 12 ounces of beer, 5 ounces of wine, or 1.5 ounces of distilled liquor such as vodka, gin, or scotch (Cushman, 1999). There is some dispute about whether persons who have a modest intake of alcohol, one to two drinks per day, may have a lower BP than non-drinkers. A recent case-control study of adults older than age 40 found a lower incidence of ischemic stroke in persons with an alcohol intake of one to two drinks per day compared to abstainers (Sacco,

Elkind et al., 1999). Some research has found a higher rate of hypertension and mortality in non-drinkers than in those who report one to two drinks per day. However, non-drinkers differ significantly from people who drink in relation to factors such as educational level and body weight (Potter, 1997).

Intervention studies have found that reducing alcohol intake results in lower systolic and diastolic pressures (Cushman, 1999; Cushman, Cutler et al., 1998; Puddey, Parker et al., 1992). Unfortunately, most of these studies have been of short duration (2 to 18 weeks), whereas the two studies of the longest duration (52 and 104 weeks) were only able to demonstrate marginally significant reductions in BP (Cushman, Cutler et al., 1998; Wallace, Cutler et al., 1988). The authors of the most recent of these studies, the Prevention and Treatment of Hypertension Study (PATHS), felt the most reasonable explanation for this small impact of reduced drinking was that there was only a reported intake difference of 1.3 drinks per day between their treatment and control groups (Cushman, Cutler et al., 1998). They also discussed the difficulty of motivating subjects to reduce alcohol intake. A meta-analysis of 15 randomized controlled trials of the impact of limiting alcohol intake on blood pressure found that this intervention resulted in small but significant decreases in systolic and diastolic pressures, $-3.3/-2.0$ mm Hg (Xin, He et al., 2001). JNC 7 recommends that men with hypertension should consume no more two drinks per day and women no more than one drink per day (Chobanian, Bakris et al., 2003).

Other Potential Interventions. A number of other interventions that were thought to have the potential to reduce BP have been studied but have not been found in large clinical trials to be effective (Allender, Cutler et al., 1996; Kotchen & McCarron, 1998; National High Blood Pressure Education Program, 1993; The Joint National Committee on Prevention Detection Evaluation and Treatment of High Blood Pressure and the National High Blood Pressure Education Program Coordinating Committee, 1997; Trials of Hypertension Prevention Collaborative Research Group, 1992). Some of the interventions that have been suggested include: stress reduction; reduced caffeine intake; increased garlic or onion intake; and increased intake of potassium, magnesium, or calcium (see Chapter 45 for complementary and alternative medicine). Even though clinical trials have not shown calcium to be very beneficial for BP reduction, it is important for the prevention of osteoporosis. There is insufficient scientific evidence at this time to recommend these therapies. However, further research on these factors may shown any one or more of them to have a role in the management of high BP at some time in the future, especially when more is learned about the causes of hypertension.

Control of Other Risk Factors. Any individual who has an elevated systolic or diastolic BP has an increased risk for atherosclerotic cardiovascular disease. In addition, longitudinal epidemiologic studies have shown that the major risk factors have an additive effect on the probability that an individual will have a morbid or mortal event (Kannel, McGee et al., 1976; Lerner & Kannel, 1986; Luria, Erel et al., 1991; Otten, Teutsch et al., 1990). Therefore, even though quitting smoking and improving dyslipidemia will not improve a client's BP, these interventions will reduce the risk of morbidity and mortality from atherosclerotic cardiovascular disease (Doll & Peto, 1976; Grover, Paquet et al., 1998; Hallstrom, Cobb et al., 1986; Hermanson, Omenn et al., 1988; Kawachi, Colditz et al., 1993; LaCroix, Lang et al., 1991; Shepherd, Cobbe et al., 1995) (see Chapter 38 for smoking cessation and Chapter 40 for lipid management).

Pharmacologic Management

Since the 1960s, randomized, placebo-controlled, clinical trials have provided evidence that pharmacologic treatment of high BP reduces mortality and morbidity. The Veterans Administration Cooperative Group Studies on Antihypertensive Agents were the first studies in the United States demonstrating that drug treatment was extremely beneficial in people with moderate and severe hypertension (Veterans Administration Cooperative Study Group on Antihypertensive Agents, 1967, 1970). Subsequent clinical trials have explored the benefits of treatment in more representative populations as well as at lower BP levels. The Hypertension Detection and Follow-up Program (HDFP), with a study population of 10,940, was one

of the first to demonstrate the benefits of hypertension treatment extended to persons with diastolic BPs between 90 and 105 mm Hg (Hypertension Detection and Follow-up Program Cooperative Group, 1979, 1982). Studies with varying approaches and in different countries have strengthened the conclusion that hypertension treatment reduces morbidity and mortality in men and women across the age span (Dahlof, Lindholm et al., 1991; Kostis, Davis et al., 1997; Management Committee of the Australian Therapeutic Trial in Mild Hypertension, 1982; Medical Research Council Working Party, 1985; 1992; Psaty, Smith et al., 1997).

Two issues remain controversial in the treatment of high BP. The first is how much should BP be lowered in the treatment of hypertension, and the second concerns the relative risks and benefits of the different classes of antihypertensive medications. Some specialists in the field of BP management have been concerned that excessive lowering of BP may increase the risk of cardiovascular mortality (Cruickshank, Thorp et al., 1987; Fletcher & Bulpitt, 1992; Lennart Hansson, 1990). The Hypertension Optimal Treatment (HOT) Study was designed to examine the optimal target diastolic pressure for persons with hypertension (Lennart Hansson, Zanchetti et al., 1998). The HOT randomized trial enrolled 18,790 men and women between ages 50 and 80 from 20 countries. One third of the subjects were randomized to one of three target diastolic pressures, 80, 85, or 90 mm Hg. Initial drug treatment was with felodipine, a calcium-channel antagonist, and other agents were added as needed according to a preset protocol. In the last 6 months of the study, the mean achieved BPs for the three target groups were, respectively, 81, 83, and 85 mm Hg. When the relationships between achieved BPs and the study outcomes were examined, the lowest risk for major cardiovascular events was at a pressure of 138.5/82.6 mm Hg, for stroke it was 142.2/<80 mm Hg, and for cardiovascular mortality it was 138.8/86.5 mm Hg. In hypertensive patients, lowering the BP below 140/85 mm Hg showed neither added risk nor benefit. Because the BPs achieved by the three groups in this study were similar, additional research will be needed to determine if lowering the BP further than 80 mm Hg would be beneficial or harmful (Kaplan, 1998). In diabetes and renal disease, there are data that support a lower target BP, as discussed later in the section on Special Populations.

The relative benefits and risks associated with the major classes of medications used to treat hypertension have been, and continue to be, controversial. Some experts and JNC 7 advocate the use of diuretics and beta-blockers because they are the drugs that have been used in the major randomized controlled trials that demonstrated reduced cardiovascular and all-cause mortality (Chobanian, Bakris et al., 2003; Furberg, Psaty et al., 1995; Psaty, Smith et al., 1997). This position was considered confirmed in 2002 when the results of the Antihypertensive and Lipid-Lowering Treatment to Prevent Heart Attack Trial (ALLHAT) were published. ALLHAT followed-up 33,357 subjects, aged 55 and older, from 18 countries, who were randomized to chlorthalidone, amlodipine, or lisinopril for an average of 4.9 years (Major outcomes in high-risk hypertensive patients randomized to angiotensin-converting enzyme inhibitor or calcium-channel blocker vs diuretic: The Antihypertensive and Lipid-Lowering Treatment to Prevent Heart Attack Trial (ALLHAT), 2002). There was no difference between the three treatment groups for the primary trial outcome, which was a combination of fatal coronary heart disease or non-fatal myocardial infarction. There was a significantly higher incidence of heart failure, one of the study's pre-designated secondary outcomes, in the amlodipine group as compared to the chlorthalidone groups, incidences of 10.2% and 7.7%, respectively. The authors' conclusion, and that of the experts who wrote the JNC 7, was that unless specifically contraindicated, thiazide-type diuretics are the preferred first-step drugs for the treatment of high blood pressure because they are equally effective and less expensive than other drug classes. Just 2 months after ALLHAT, the results of the Second Australian National Blood Pressure Study (ANBP2) were published with apparently contradictory results (Wing, Reid et al., 2003). ANBP2 compared the efficacy of the diuretic, hydrochlorothiazide, to an ACE inhibitor, enalapril, in 6,083 subjects (50% women) aged 65 to 84 years over a median follow-up period of 4.1 years. With identical reductions in blood pressure ($-26/-12$ mm Hg), the group treated with the ACE inhibitor had fewer cardiovascular events or deaths than the group treated with diuretic with a hazard ratio of 0.89 (95% confidence interval: 0.79 to 1.00). Separate analysis of the data from men and women showed that the difference was significant in men but not in women. It is difficult to compare these two studies directly because although both were well-designed clinical trials, there were differences in the details of the trial designs, study populations, medications, and designated endpoints. In the end, clinicians must consider co-existing conditions of their clients, health care resources, and the fact that most persons with hypertension will need at least two classes of medication to control BP (Frohlich, 2003).

Questions have been raised about the risks associated with the use of calcium-channel antagonists (Michael H. Alderman, Cohen et al., 1997; Buring, Glynn et al., 1995; Furberg, Psaty et al., 1995; McMurray & Murdoch, 1997; Psaty, Heckbert et al., 1995). The Syst-Eur Trial, which compared nitrendipine to placebo in the treatment of isolated systolic hypertension, found no evidence of a harmful effect of calcium-channel blockers (Staessen, Fagard et al., 1997). A large, randomized, clinical trial (CONVINCE) of 16,602 subjects with hypertension plus at least one other CVD risk factor comparing controlled-onset verapamil with hydrochlorothiazide and atenolol found no difference in blood pressure control or outcomes, except a significant increase in hemorrhagic stroke in the verapamil group (Black, Elliott et al., 2003). The researchers concluded that the trial did not demonstrate that the verapamil treatment was equivalent to the diuretic or beta-blocker treatment. JNC 7 does not recommend calcium-channel antagonist as initial therapy but does indicate that it may be appropriate to use as an additional drug in person with a high risk of CHD or with diabetes mellitus (Chobanian, Bakris et al., 2003).

JNC 7 Algorithm for Hypertension Treatment. The currently recommended algorithm for hypertension management is shown in Figure 39-1 (Chobanian, Bakris et al., 2003). Based on the results of many previous trials and the ALLHAT results, JNC 7 recommends that unless there are compelling reasons against them (summarized in Table 39-10), thiazide-type diuretic should be the initial therapy in most persons with high blood pressure (Chobanian, Bakris et al., 2003; Major outcomes in high-risk hypertensive patients randomized to

angiotensin-converting enzyme inhibitor or calcium-channel blocker vs diuretic: The Antihypertensive and Lipid-Lowering Treatment to Prevent Heart Attack Trial [ALLHAT], 2002). With the advent of new classes of antihypertensive medications and the recognition that co-existing conditions will influence the appropriateness of an individual's medication, the suggestions of the best drug for initial therapy have broadened. Table 39-10 includes the co-morbid conditions that need to be considered when selecting medications for the person with hypertension. Other factors that need to be considered in choosing therapy include cost, convenience, duration of action, frequency of adverse effects, client preference, quality of life, and other medications the client is using, both those available over-the-counter and those prescribed by a health care provider.

Seven classes of drugs are available for the treatment of hypertension: (1) diuretics; (2) adrenergic inhibitors, of which there are beta-adrenergic blocking agents, central-acting inhibitors, central alpha-agonists, alpha-adrenergic blockers, and combined alpha-adrenergic and beta-adrenergic blockers; (3) vasodilators; (4) calcium-channel blocking agents; (5) ACE inhibitors; (6) angiotensin II receptor blockers; and (7) aldosterone receptor blockers. Table 39-11 lists the generic and trade names, usual dose ranges, and selected side effects of most of the common antihypertensive agents. Some of the most commonly used combination medications are listed in Table 39-12. These combinations can be very useful in simplifying therapy once the clinician has titrated the dose of each medication for effectiveness in the individual client. Once an initial drug has been chosen, it is recommended that the client begin with a low dose, and then either the dose is increased or a new drug is added if the goal BP is not achieved after a period of 1 to 2 months (Chobanian, Bakris et al., 2003).

BP Management in Special Populations

The management of hypertension is modified depending on the characteristics of the individual plus additional knowledge about the care in specific groups. The following section outlines some additional information that guides the management of high BP in the elderly, in pregnancy, and in persons with other conditions, including diabetes, renal disease, hyperlipidemia, and hypertensive crises.

The Elderly. The elderly experience systolic diastolic hypertension and isolated systolic hypertension and are the population group in the United States who are most likely to be aware of their elevated BPs (Hyman & Pavlik, 2001). Isolated systolic hypertension is defined as a systolic BP greater than 160 mm Hg with a diastolic pressure less than 90 mm Hg (The Joint National Committee on Prevention Detection Evaluation and Treatment of High Blood Pressure and the National High Blood Pressure Education Program Coordinating Committee, 1997). Borderline isolated systolic hypertension is a systolic BP of 140 to 159 mm Hg with a diastolic below 90 mm Hg (Sagie, Larson et al., 1993). In Europe, the upper limit of diastolic pressure in isolated systolic hypertension is 95 mm Hg (Amery, Birkenhäger et al., 1985; Staessen, Fagard et al., 1997).

The incidence of isolated systolic hypertension increases with age, with the incidence in persons older than 70 years being 7%, and in persons older than 80 years the incidence was

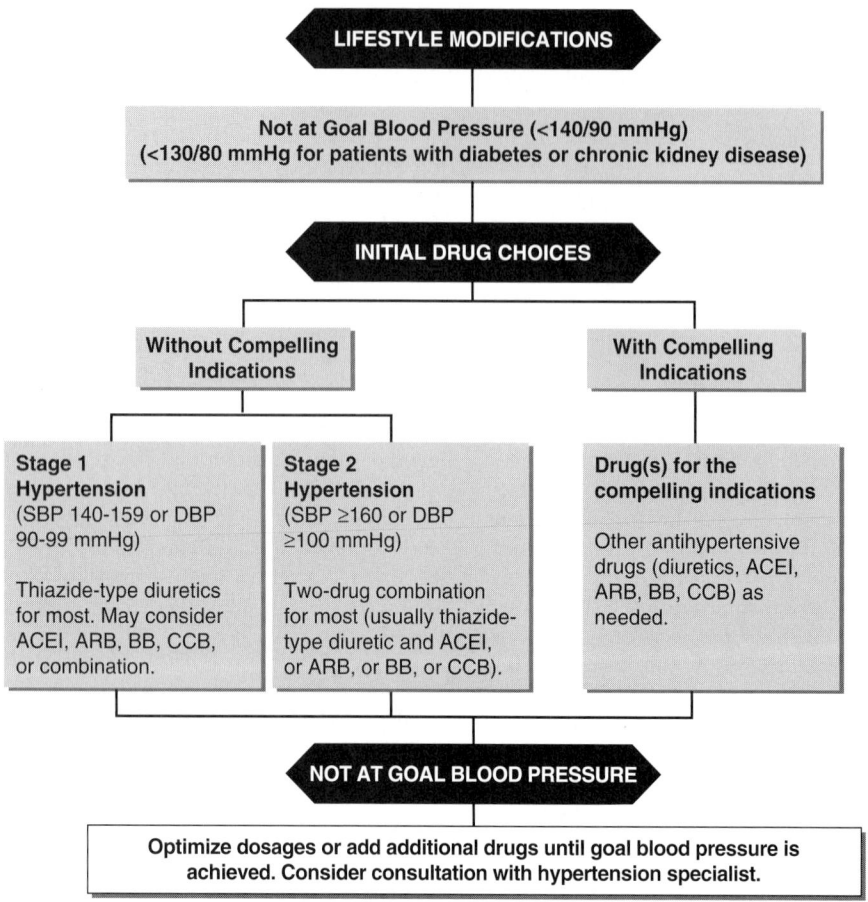

DBP, diastolic blood pressure; SBP, systolic blood pressure.
Drug abbreviations: ACEI, angiotensin converting enzyme inhibitor; ARB, angiotensin receptor blocker;
BB, beta-blocker; CCB, calcium channel blocker.

■ **Figure 39–1.** Treatment algorithm for patients with high blood pressure. (Chobanian, A. V., Bakris G. L., Black, H. R., et al. [2003]. The Seventh Report of the Joint National Committee on Prevention, Detection, Evaluation, and Treatment of High Blood Pressure: the JNC 7 report. *JAMA,* 289[19], 2560–2572. [Erratum in *JAMA,* 290(2), 197].)

more than 25% (Staessen, Amery et al., 1990). Analysis of data from the Framingham Study and a 20-year follow-up of NHANES I participants revealed even borderline systolic hypertension was associated with significant morbidity and mortality (Qureshi, Suri et al., 2002; Sagie, Larson et al., 1993). In the Framingham study, persons with borderline isolated systolic pressure had increased risks for all cardiovascular disease, coronary heart disease, stroke, transient ischemic attack, heart failure, and mortality from cardiovascular disease. The hazard ratios for each of these were significantly greater than 1.0 (range 1.42 to 1.60) after the data had been adjusted for sex, decade of age, cholesterol level, body mass index, cigarette smoking, and glucose intolerance. In a community study of BP in 3,657 elderly persons in East Boston, a linear relationship between systolic BP and mortality was identified. An individual's risk of cardiovascular and total mortality increased with their systolic BP (Glynn, Field et al., 1995).

Several large randomized trials have demonstrated the benefits of BP control in the elderly (Amery, Birkenyhäger et al., 1985; Dahlof, Lindholm et al., 1991; MRC Working Party, 1992;

SHEP Cooperative Research Group, 1991; Staessen, Fagard et al., 1997). Two meta-analyses of clinical trials on persons older than age 60 found that treatment reduced the incidence of coronary heart disease by between 18% and 19%, of stroke by 30% to 34%, and total mortality by 13% (MacMahon & Rodgers, 1993; Staessen, Gasowski et al., 2000). The largest study, the Systolic Hypertension in the Elderly Program (SHEP), had a population of 4,736 men and women older than age 60 years with a mean baseline BP of 170/70 mm Hg (SHEP Cooperative Research Group, 1991). The goal of this clinical trial was to determine drug efficacy, side effects, and eventual long-term outcomes related to morbidity and mortality from cardiovascular disease. When the 17-mm Hg reduction in mean systolic BP in the treatment group was compared with the control group, there was a significant decrease in stroke. No serious short-term side effects occurred as a result of treatment. The Swedish Trial in Old Patients with Hypertension (STOP Hypertension) studied a group of 1,627 with systolic and diastolic hypertension (mean entry BP 195/102 mm Hg) (Hansson, Lindholm et al., 1999). In the group treated with diuretics or beta-blockers, there was a

Table 39–10 ■ CLINICAL TRIAL AND GUIDELINE BASIS FOR COMPELLING INDICATIONS FOR INDIVIDUAL DRUG CLASSES

| | Recommended Drugs[†] | | | | | | |
Compelling Indication[*]	DIURETIC	BB	ACEI	ARB	CCB	ALDO ANT	Clinical Trial Basis[‡§]
Heart failure	●	●	●	●		●	ACC/AHA Heart Failure Guideline, MERIT-HF, COPERNICUS, CIBIS, SOLVD, AIRE, TRACE, ValHEFT, RALES
Postmyocardial infarction		●	●			●	ACC/AHA Post-MI Guideline, BHAT, SAVE, Capricorn, EPH ESUS
High coronary disease risk	●	●	●		●		ALLHAT, HOPE, ANBP₂ LIFE, CONVINCE
Diabetes	●	●	●	●	●		NKF-ADA Guideline, UKPDS, ALLHAT
Chronic kidney disease			●	●			NKF Guideline, Captopril Trial, RENAAL, IDNT, REIN, AASK
Recurrent stroke prevention	●		●				PROGRESS

[*]Compelling indications for antihypertensive drugs are based on benefits from outcome studies or existing clinical guidelines; the compelling indication is managed in parallel with the BP.

[†]Drug abbreviations: ACEI, angiotensin converting enzyme inhibitor; ARB, angiotensin receptor blocker; Aldo ANT, aldosterone antagonist; BB, beta-blocker; CCB, calcium channel blocker.

[‡]Conditions for which clinical trials demonstrate benefit of specific classes of antihypertensive drugs.

[§] See list of references for these trials at the end of the chapter.

(Chobanian, A. V., Bakris, G. L., Black, H. R., et al. [2003]. The Seventh Report of the Joint National committee on Prevention, Detection, Evaluation, and Treatment of High Blood Pressure: the JNC 7 report. *JAMA*, 289(19), 2560–2572.) [Erratum in: *JAMA*, 2003, 290[2], 197].

mean decrease in BP of 27/9 mm Hg, with statistically significant decreases in fatal and nonfatal strokes and congestive heart failure. This study showed the benefit of treating elderly patients with systolic and diastolic hypertension. In response to an ongoing concern in the health care community, a later report from the STOP Hypertension-2 study found no relationship between type of antihypertensive agent used and the incidence of cancer in the study participants (Lindholm, Anderson et al., 2001).

Treatment of the elderly is similar to that of younger clients. More emphasis can be put on the lifestyle management, including weight loss, sodium restriction, and exercise, because of the multiple benefits to the older person (Black, 1999). Physical activity, for example, offers not only reduction of BP but also weight management, reduced disability, and decreased mortality (Lakka, Venalainen et al., 1994; Vita, Terry et al., 1998). The same medications are used in the elderly, but smaller initial doses are recommended, and there may be more co-morbid conditions that will make one medication a better choice than another (Chobanian, Bakris et al., 2003). Cost will also be a factor because many elderly persons have a limited income. Because the elderly have an increased sensitivity to orthostatic hypotension, caution is required with drugs that may cause dizziness on standing, such as diuretics in large doses, peripheral adrenergic blockers, and alpha-blockers (Joint National Committee on Prevention Detection Evaluation and Treatment of High Blood Pressure and the National High Blood Pressure Education Program Coordinating Committee, 1997).

Hypertension in Pregnancy. High BP occurs in pregnancy either because of pre-existing chronic high BP or because of the development of pregnancy-induced hypertension including gestational hypertension, preeclampsia, and eclampsia. Elevated BP (>140/90 mm Hg) that a woman has before she becomes pregnant, that develops before the 20th week of pregnancy, or that persists more than 6 weeks after delivery is considered chronic hypertension (Report of the National High Blood Pressure Education Program Working Group on High Blood Pressure in Pregnancy, 2000). Gestational hypertension is defined as an elevated BP that usually occurs in the third trimester and is not accompanied by other signs and symptoms (Sibai, 1996). In preeclampsia and eclampsia, the elevated BP is considered as one of several signs and symptoms of an underlying disorder of organ perfusion. Edema and proteinuria usually occur with pregnancy-induced high BP. Although there has been controversy about whether the fourth or fifth Korotkoff sound should be used to indicate diastolic pressure in pregnant women, recent research indicates that the fifth sound is closer to actual intra-arterial pressure and should therefore be used (Brown, Buddle et al., 1998; Report of the National High Blood Pressure Education Program Working Group on High Blood Pressure in Pregnancy, 2000).

JNC 7 and the recent Working Group Report on High Blood Pressure in Pregnancy recommend the use of beta-blockers, methyldopa, or vasodilators for pregnant women (Chobanian, Bakris et al., 2003; Report of the National High Blood Pressure Education Program Working Group on High Blood Pressure in Pregnancy, 2000). ACE inhibitors are contraindicated because of their documented adverse effects on fetal growth and development. Because of the adverse effects of ACE inhibitors, angiotensin-receptor blockers have not been studied in pregnant women and their use is also contraindicated (Report of the National High Blood Pressure Education Program

Table 39–11 ■ ORAL ANTIHYPERTENSIVE DRUGS*

Drug	Trade Name	Usual Dose Range, Total mg/d* (frequency per day)	Selected Side Effects and Comments*
Diuretics (partial list)			Short term: increases cholesterol and glucose levels; biochemical abnormalities: decreases potassium, sodium, and magnesium levels, increases uric acid and calcium levels; rare: blood dyscrasias, photosensitivity, pancreatitis, hyponatremia
Chlorthalidone (G)†	Hygroton	12.5–50 (1)	
Hydrochlorothiazide (G)	HydroDIURIL, Microzide	12.5–50 (1)	
Indapamide	Lozol	1.25–2.5 (1)	(Less or no hypercholesterolemia)
Metolazone	Mykrox	0.5–1.0 (1)	
	Zaroxolyn	2.5–10 (1)	
Loop Diuretics			
Bumetanide (G)	Bumex	0.5–2 (2)	(Short duration of action, no hypercalcemia)
Furosemide (G)	Lasix	40–80 (2)	(Short duration of action, no hypercalcemia)
Torsemide	Demadex	2.5–10 (1)	
Potassium-Sparing Agents			Hyperkalemia
Amiloride hydrochloride (G)	Midamor	5–10 (1–2)	
Triamterene (G)	Dyrenium	50–100 (1–2)	
Adrenergic Inhibitors			
Central Alpha Agonists			Sedation, dry mouth, bradycardia, withdrawal hypertension
Clonidine hydrochloride (G)	Catapres	0.1–0.8 (2)	(More withdrawal)
Guanfacine hydrochloride (G)	Generic	0.5–2 (1)	(Less withdrawal)
Methyldopa (G)	Aldomet	250–1000 (2)	(Hepatic and "autoimmune" disorders)
Reserpine (G)	Generic	0.05–0.25 (1)	(Nasal congestion, sedation, depression, activation of peptic ulcer)
Alpha Blockers			Postural (orthostatic) hypotension
Doxazosin mesylate	Cardura	1–16 (1)	
Prazosin hydrochloride (G)	Minipress	2–20 (1–2)	
Terazosin hydrochloride	Hytrin	1–20 (1)	
Beta Blockers			Bronchospasm, bradycardia, heart failure, may mask insulin-induced hypoglycemia; less serious: impaired peripheral circulation, insomnia, fatigue, decreased exercise tolerance, hypertriglyceridemia (except agents with intrinsic sympathomimetic activity)
Acebutolol§‡	Sectral	200–800 (2)	
Atenolol (G)§	Tenormin	25–100 (1)	
Betaxolol§ hyperchloride	Kerlone	5–20 (1)	
Bisoprolol fumarate§	Zebeta	2.5–10 (1)	
Metoprolol tartrate (G)§	Lopressor	50–100 (1–2)	
Metoprolol succinate§	Toprol XL	50–100 (1)	
Nadolol (G)	Corgard	40–120 (1)	
Penbutolol sulfate‡	Levatol	10–40 (2)	
Pindolol (G)‡	Visken	10–40 (2)	
Propranolol hydrochloride (G)	Inderal	40–160 (2)	
	Inderal LA	40–180 (1)	
Timolol maleate (G)	Blocadren	20–40 (2)	
Combined Alpha and Beta Blockers			Postural hypotension, bronchospasm
Carvedilol	Coreg	12.5–50 (2)	
Labetalol hydrochloride (G)	Normodyne, Trandate	200–800 (2)	
Direct Vasodilators			Headaches, fluid retention, tachycardia
Hydralazine hydrochloride (G)	Apresoline	25–100 (2)	(Lupus syndrome)
Minoxidil (G)	Loniten	2.5–80 (1–2)	(Hirsutism)

Table 39–11 ■ ORAL ANTIHYPERTENSIVE DRUGS* *(Continued)*

Drug	Trade Name	Usual Dose Range, Total mg/d* (frequency per day)	Selected Side Effects and Comments*
Calcium antagonists			
Nondihydropyridines			Conduction defects, worsening of systolic dysfunction, gingival hyperplasia
Diltiazem hydrochloride	Cardizem LA	120–540 (1)	(Nausea, headache)
	Cardizem CD, Dilacor XR, Tiazac	180–240 (1)	
Mibefradil dihydrochloride (T-channel calcium antagonist)	Posicor	50–100 (1)	(No worsening of systolic dysfunction; contraindicated with terfenadine [Seldane], astemizole [Hismanal], and cisapride [Propulsid])
Verapamil hydrochloride	Isoptin SR, Calan SR Coer (Verelan PM, Covera HS)	120–360 (1–2) 120–360 (1)	(Constipation)
Dihydropyridines			Edema of the ankle, flushing, headache, gingival hypertrophy
Amlodipine besylate	Norvasc	2.5–10 (1)	
Felodipine	Plendil	2.5–20 (1)	
Isradipine	DynaCirc CR	2.5–10, 5–20 (1)	
Nicardipine	Cardene SR	60–120 (2)	
Nifedipine	Procardia XL, Adalat CC	30–60 (1)	
Nisoldipine	Sular	10–40 (1)	
Angiotensin-Converting Enzyme Inhibitors			Common: cough; rare: angioedema, hyperkalemia, rash, loss of taste, leukopenia
Benazepril hydrochloride	Lotensin	10–40 (1-2)	
Captopril (G)	Capoten	25–100 25-(2)	
Enalapril maleate	Vasotec	2.5–40 (1–2)	
Fosinopril sodium	Monopril	10–40 (1)	
Lisinopril	Prinivil, Zestril	10–40 (1)	
Moexipril	Univasc	7.5–30 7.5-(1)	
Quinapril hydrochloride	Accupril	10–40 (1)	
Ramipril	Altace	2.5–20 (1)	
Trandolapril	Mavik	1–4 (1)	
Angiotensin II Receptor Blockers			Angioedema (very rare), hyperkalemia
Candesartan	Atacand	8–32 (1)	
Epresartan	Tevetan	400–800 (1–2)	
Irbesartan	Avapro	150–300 (1)	
Losartan potassium	Cozaar	25–100 (1–2)	
Oimesartan	Benicar	20–40 (1)	
Telmisartan	Micardis	20–80 (1)	
Valsartan	Diovan	80–320 (1)	
Aldosterove Receptor Blockers			
Eplerenone	Inspra	50–100 (1–2)	Hyperkalemia
Spironolactone	Aldactone	25–50 (1–2)	Hyperkalemia, gynecomastia

*These dosages may vary from those listed in the *Physicians' Desk Reference* (51st edition), which may be consulted for additional information. The listing of side effects is not all-inclusive and side effects are for the class of drugs except where noted for individual drugs (in parentheses); clinicians are urged to refer to the package insert for a more detailed listing.
† (G) indicates generic available.
‡ Has intrinsic sympathomimetic activity.
§ Cardioselective.
¹¹ Also acts centrally.

Working Group on High Blood Pressure in Pregnancy, 2000). Methyldopa is considered the drug of choice because of the long experience with using it and the relative lack of adverse impacts on mother and infant (Report of the National High Blood Pressure Education Program Working Group on High Blood Pressure in Pregnancy, 2000). Treatment of hypertension in pregnancy is challenging because there are no clinical trials of antihypertensive agents in pregnant women.

Diabetes Mellitus and Hypertension. Risk factor clustering is found in individuals with diabetes mellitus (Berenson, Srinivasan et al., 1997; Cobbe, 1998; Dengel, Hagberg et al., 1998; Meigs, D'Agostino et al., 1997; Tsao, Niebauer et al., 1998). In one study, 57 % of persons with noninsulin-dependent diabetes were found to have hypertension (Bog-Hansen, Lindblad et al., 1998). Several clinical trials including the United Kingdom Prospective Diabetes Study Group Study 39 (UKPDS39), the Losartan Intervention for Endpoint reduction in hypertension

Table 39–12 ■ COMBINATION DRUGS FOR HYPERTENSION

Combination Type*	Fixed-dose Combination, Mg[†]	Trade Name
ACEIs and CCBs	Amlodipine/benazepril hydrochloride (2.5/10, 5/10, 5/20, 10/20)	Lotrel
	Enalapril maleate/felodipine (5/5)	Lexxel
	Trandolapril/verapamil (2/180, 1/240, 2/240, 4/240)	Tarka
ACEIs and diuretics	Benazepril/hydrochlorothiazide (5/6.25, 10/12.5, 20/12.5, 20/25)	Lotensin HCT
	Captopril/hydrochlorothiazide (25/15, 25/25, 50/15, 50/25)	Capozide
	Enalapril maleate/hydrochlorothiazide (5/12.5, 10/25)	Vaseretic
	Lisinopril/hydrochlorothiazide (10/12.5, 20/12.5, 20/25)	Prinzide
	Moexipril HCI/hydrochlorothiazide (7.5/12.5, 15/25)	Uniretic
	Quinapril HCI/hydrochlorothiazide (10/12.5, 20/12.5, 20/25)	Accuretic
ARBs and diuretics	Candesartan cilexetil/hydrochlorothiazide (16/12.5, 32/12.5)	Atacand HCT
	Eprosartan mesylate/hydrochlorothiazide (600/12.5, 600/25)	Teveten/HCT
	Irbesartan/hydrochlorothiazide (150/12.5, 300/12.5)	Avalide
	Losartan potassium/hydrochlorothiazide (50/12.5, 100/25)	Hyzaar
	Telmisartan/hydrochlorothiazide (40/12.5, 80/12.5)	Micardis/HCT
	Valsartan/hydrochlorothiazide (80/12.5, 160/12.5)	Diovan/HCT
BBs and diuretics	Atenolol/chlorthalidone (50/25, 100/25)	Tenoretic
	Bisoprolol fumarate/hydrochlorothiazide (2.5/6.25, 5/6.25, 10/6.25)	Ziac
	Propranolol LA/hydrochlorothiazide (40/25, 80/25)	Inderide
	Metoprolol tartrate/hydrochlorothiazide (50/25, 100/25)	Lopressor HCT
	Nadolol/bendrofluthiazide (40/5, 80/5)	Corzide
	Timolol mateate/hydrochlorothiazide (10/25)	Timolide
Centrally acting drug and diuretic	Methyldopa/hydrochlorothiazide (250/15, 250/25, 500/30, 500/50)	Aldoril
	Reserpine/chlorothiazide (0.125/250, 0.25/500)	Diupres
	Reserpine/hydrochlorothiazide (0.125/25, 0.125/50)	Hydropres
Diuretic and diuretic	Amiloride HCI/hydrochlorothiazide (5/50)	Moduretic
	Spironolactone/hydrochlorothiazide (25/25, 50/50)	Aldactone
	Triamterene/hydrochlorothiazide (37.5/25, 50/25, 75/50)	Dyazide, Maxzide

*Drug abbreviations: ACEI, angiotensin converting enzyme inhibitor; ARB, angiotensin receptor blocker; BB, beta-blocker; CCB, calcium channel blocker.
[†]Some drug combinations are available in multiple fixed doses. Each drug dose is reported in milligrams.
(Chobanian, A. V., Bakris, G. L., Black, H. R., et al. [2003]. The Seventh Report of the Joint National Committee on Prevention, Detection, Evaluation, and Treatment of High Blood Pressure: the JNC 7 report. *JAMA, 289*(19), 2560–2572. [Erratum in *JAMA,* 2003, 290 [2], 197].)

Study (LIFE), the Heart Outcomes Prevention Evaluation (HOPE) Study, ALLHAT, and the Appropriate Blood Pressure Control in Diabetes (ABCD) Study have documented the benefits of treating high blood pressure in persons who also have diabetes mellitus (Efficacy of atenolol and captopril in reducing risk of macrovascular and microvascular complications in type 2 diabetes: UKPDS 39. UK Prospective Diabetes Study Group, 1998; Lindholm, Ibsen et al., 2002; Major outcomes in high-risk hypertensive patients randomized to angiotensin-converting enzyme inhibitor or calcium-channel blocker vs diuretic: The Antihypertensive and Lipid-Lowering Treatment to Prevent Heart Attack Trial [ALLHAT], 2002; Mehler, Coll et al., 2003; Yusuf, Sleight et al., 2000). Because of this documented reduction in mortality and progression to end-stage renal disease from treating high blood pressure, both the American Diabetes Association and JNC 7 have set the goal BP for persons with both diabetes and hypertension at less than 130/80 mm Hg (Arauz-Pacheco, Parrott et al., 2003; Chobanian, Bakris et al., 2003). Lifestyle interventions are also recommended and include weight control and exercise, which are keys to BP control in persons with diabetes (Ikeda, Gomi et al., 1996; Lazarus, Bourgoignie et al., 1997; Perseghin, Price et al., 1996). JNC7 recommended the use of five drug classes, including diuretics, beta-blockers, ACE inhibitors, angiotensin-receptor blockers, and calcium-channel blockers for the treatment of hypertension plus diabetes (Chobanian, Bakris et al., 2003).

Renal Disease and Hypertension. Control of hypertension has been shown to be extremely effective in preventing the progression of renal failure in persons with renal disease (Klag, Whelton et al., 1996; Klag, Whelton et al., 1997; Lazarus, Bourgoignie et al., 1997). JNC 7 has set the goal BP for persons with renal disease at a minimum of 130/80 mm Hg (Chobanian, Bakris et al., 2003). The lifestyle interventions that have been shown to be effective in controlling BP in persons with renal disease are restriction of sodium intake to less than 100 mmol per day and restriction of dietary protein. One small study of 15 subjects with hypertensive diabetic nephropathy demonstrated that calcium-channel antagonist therapy with long-acting diltiazem was only effective in reducing albuminuria when sodium intake was also restricted to 50 mmol/d (Bakris & Smith, 1996). When the BP was lowered equivalently but the subjects were eating a high-sodium (250 mmol/d) diet, there was no decrease in albuminuria. JNC 7 recommended use of ACE inhibitors and ARBs in treating persons with hypertension and renal disease based on clinical trials demonstrating their effectiveness (Brenner, Cooper et al., 2001; Giatras, Lau et al., 1997; Lewis, Hunsicker et al., 1993; Lewis, Hunsicker et al., 2001; Maschio, Alberti et al., 1996; Randomised placebo-controlled trial of effect of ramipril on decline in glomerular filtration rate and risk of terminal renal failure in proteinuric, non-diabetic nephropathy. The GISEN Group [Gruppo Italiano di Studi Epidemiologici in Nefrologia], 1997).

Hyperlipidemia and Hypertension. Dyslipidemia is another of the cardiovascular risk factors that is known to cluster with hypertension and, along with obesity and insulin resistance, is considered the metabolic syndrome (Cobbe, 1998; Executive Summary of The Third Report of the National Cholesterol Education Program [NCEP] Expert Panel on Detection, Evaluation, and Treatment of High Blood Cholesterol in Adults [Adult Treatment Panel III], 2001). The dyslipidemia includes a low HDL cholesterol level and high levels of LDL cholesterol and triglycerides. In an analysis of the NHANES III database, body mass index, low HDL levels, and elevated blood pressures were found to be strongly associated with each other (Brown, Higgins et al., 2000). JNC 7 recommended the use of drugs from four classes: diuretics, beta-blockers, ACE inhibitors, and calcium-channel blockers for persons with a high risk for CHD (Chobanian, Bakris et al., 2003). Weight loss and physical activity are lifestyle interventions that have been shown to lower BP and to improve dyslipidemia (Executive Summary of The Third Report of The National Cholesterol Education Program [NCEP] Expert Panel on Detection, Evaluation, and Treatment of High Blood Cholesterol in Adults [Adult Treatment Panel III], 2001; Grimm, Flack et al., 1996; Stamler, Briefel et al., 1997).

Hypertensive Crisis. Acute hypertensive crises are rare situations in which patients require immediate intervention to reduce BP. These crises may occur either in persons whose hypertension was previously not diagnosed or in persons with known but poorly controlled high BP. Hypertensive crises have been classified into two types: hypertensive emergencies and urgencies. A hypertensive emergency occurs when end-organ damage is acute or imminent and immediate reduction in BP, usually via intravenous medication in an intensive care unit (ICU), is required. A hypertensive urgency occurs when the BP is critically high, with signs such as edema of the optic disk, but there is less evidence of target organ damage, so that BP reduction can occur over a longer period using oral antihypertensive medications (Chobanian, Bakris et al., 2003). There is a continuum from emergencies to urgencies and excellent assessment and judgment are required. Acute elevations of BP may occur after certain medications such as clonidine are discontinued or the client either forgets to take or runs out of medication (Neusy & Lowenstein, 1989).

The parenteral drugs that may be used in hypertensive emergencies are listed in Table 39-13. One drug that is not recommended because of the high rate of adverse events that accompany its use is sublingual nifedipine (Grossman, Messerli et al., 1996; Varon & Marik, 2000). Nitroprusside is also recognized as a medication with great potential toxicity that should used with great hesitancy (Varon & Marik, 2000). JNC 7 recommends that persons with a hypertensive urgency be treated immediately with oral combination therapy, but the report does not address the risks or benefits of any specific antihypertensive agent. In the management of hypertensive emergencies, the goal is to reduce the pressure so that target organ damage from the high pressure is prevented or minimized while preventing the cerebral or myocardial ischemia that could result from too rapid a reduction in pressure (Vidt, 1999). After the blood pressure has been brought under control, the client who has experienced a hypertension emergency or urgency will require extended expert outpatient blood pressure control management.

Achieving Blood Pressure Control

Despite the impressive array of lifestyle and pharmacologic treatments for high BP and the existence of the National High Blood Pressure Education Program since 1972, the awareness, treatment, and control rates are low. Table 39-5 shows the levels of these factors that have been measured in the National Health and Nutrition Examination Surveys at four times over the past 24 years in the United States (Chobanian, Bakris et al., 2003). In 1999 to 2000, only 60% of persons with hypertension were treated and only 34% had their BPs controlled to less than 140/90 mm Hg. A survey of 56,026 patients in The Netherlands found that BP was not controlled in 30% of the women and in 47% of the men with hypertension (Klungel, de Boer et al., 1998). This lack of success in managing high BP has many contributing factors (Ebrahim, 1998; Roter, Hall et al., 1998). These will be explored by looking at the groups who influence the management of hypertension, focusing on what each group can do to improve BP control. Some of the actions that care providers, patients, and health care organizations can use to improve BP control are listed in Table 39-14. Although the terms, adherence, and compliance are often used in discussions of BP control, they are not used here because their use usually carries the implication that the patient is mainly responsible for poor BP control.

Role of Health Care Professionals

Health care providers in partnership with clients hold the keys to BP control. The provider's responsibilities range from knowing and using the latest guidelines for BP control to motivating the client to follow the treatment plan. At a minimum, the challenges to a provider include correctly diagnosing the client's condition; communicating the importance of BP as a disease and as a risk factor for atherosclerosis; developing an effective treatment plan that fits the client's lifestyle and economic situation; and evaluating the results of the therapy. To achieve these goals, the care provider needs skills in assessment, diagnosis, communication, and behavioral counseling.

The care provider has the responsibility of assuring that the client is educated about the medical condition and the treatment plan. Display 39-4 summarizes strategies that health care providers can use to improve BP control. Some medical and nursing schools include courses in risk factor management and health promotion in their school curricula and offer students clinical opportunities to practice the skills required to support clients in effective disease prevention and risk factor management (Ockene & Ockene, 1992). There is a growing need for more research on effective methods to promote behavior change because the traditional professional approaches of screening, patient education, and counseling have had little impact on secondary risk factors such as obesity (Langeluddecke, 1986). The technique of motivational interviewing has been used by nutritionists working with the DASH diet program to help their clients adopt new dietary practices (Windhauser, Ernst et al., 1999). A meta-analysis of methods that clinicians could use to support their clients in using antihypertensive medications concluded that there were no particularly effective interventions available that were practical and simple enough to use (McDonald, Garg et al., 2002).

Table 39–13 ■ PARENTERAL DRUGS FOR TREATMENT OF HYPERTENSIVE EMERGENCIES*

Drug	Dose	Onset of Action	Duration of Action	Adverse Effects‡	Special Indications
Vasodilators					
Sodium nitroprusside	0.25–10 µg/kg/min as IV infusion‡ (maximal dose for 10 min only)	Immediate	1–2 min	Nausea, vomiting, muscle twitching, sweating, thiocyanate and cyanide intoxication	Most hypertensive emergencies; caution with high intracranial pressure or azotemia
Nicardipine hydrochloride	5–15 mg/h IV	5–10 min	1–4 h	Tachycardia, headache, flushing, local phlebitis	Most hypertensive emergencies except acute heart failure; caution with coronary ischemia
Fenoldopam mesylate	0.1–0.3 µg/kg/min IV infusion	<5 min	30 min	Tachycardia, headache, nausea, flushing	Most hypertensive emergencies; caution with glaucoma
Nitroglycerin	5–100 µg/min as IV infusion§	2–5 min	3–5 min	Headache, vomiting, methemoglobinemia, tolerance with prolonged use	Coronary ischemia
Enalaprilat	1.25–5 mg every 6 h IV	15–30 min	6 h	Precipitous fall in pressure in highrenin states; response variable	Acute left ventricular failure; avoid in acute myocardial infarction
Hydralazine hydrochloride	10–20 mg IV / 10–50 mg IM	10–20 min / 20–30 min	3–8 h	Tachycardia, flushing, headache, vomiting, aggravation of angina	Eclampsia
Diazoxide	50–100 mg IV bolus repeated, or 15–30 mg/min infusion	2–4 min	6–12 h	Nausea, flushing, tachycardia, chest pain	Now obsolete; when no intensive monitoring available
Adrenergic Inhibitors					
Labetalol hydrochloride	20–80 mg IV bolus every 10 min 0.5–2.0 mg/min IV infusion	5–10 min	3–6 h	Vomiting, scalp tingling, burning in throat, dizziness, nausea, heart block, orthostatic hypotension	Most hypertensive emergencies except acute heart failure
Esmolol hydrochloride	250–500 µg/kg/min for 1 min, then 50–100 µg/kg/min for 4 min; may repeat sequence	1–2 min	10–20 min	Hypotension, nausea	Aortic dissection, perioperative
Phentolamine mesylate	5–15 mg IV	1–2 min	3–10 min	Tachycardia, flushing, headache	Catecholamine excess

IV, intravenous; IM, intramuscular.
*These doses may vary from those in the *Physicians' Desk Reference* (51st edition).
‡Hypotension may occur with all agents.
§Require special delivery system.

The adequacy of the care of 800 hypertensive veterans with average age of 65.5 years was recently evaluated over a 2-year period (Berlowitz, Ash et al., 1998). The researchers found that less than 25% of the patients had BPs less than 140/90 mm Hg and 40% had BPs more than 160/90 mm Hg despite 2 years of treatment for high BP with an average of five medical clinic visits yearly. The patients who received the most intensive or aggressive treatment were most like to have their BPs controlled. The researchers interpreted their findings as indicating that physicians need to be more aggressive in their management of high BP. The clinical trials of BP control have demonstrated the potential impact of BP reduction on morbidity and mortality, but if health care providers do not prescribe adequate therapy to lower BP and follow-up with their clients, then this potential will be difficult to realize.

Although practice guidelines such as the JNC reports are prepared by groups of national experts, the evidence is that clinicians are often unaware of, or do not follow, them (Alderman, Furberg et al., 2002; Hyman & Pavlik, 2000; Tu, Mamdani et al., 2002). In response to a questionnaire mailed to a random sample of primary care physicians in the United States, of the 379 respondents (34% response rate), 41% were not aware of the contents of the JNC V report; of the 59% who had heard of the guidelines, approximately half had not read them (Hyman & Pavlik, 2000). Also many of the physicians, between 33% and 43%, had higher thresholds of diastolic and systolic pressure for beginning drug treatment than were recommended by the JNC report. A similar survey of primary care physicians working in a large Detroit health care organization found that the doctors were willing to tolerate a higher

Table 39–14 ■ ACTIONS TO INCREASE COMPLIANCE WITH PREVENTION AND TREATMENT RECOMMENDATIONS

Actions	Specific Strategies
Actions by Patients	
Patients must engage in essential prevention and treatment behaviors.	
Decide to control risk factors.	Understand rationale, importance of commitment.
Negotiate goals with provider.	Develop communication skills.
Develop skills for adopting and maintaining recommended behaviors.	Use reminder systems.
Monitor progress toward goals.	Use self-monitoring skills.
Resolve problems that block achievement of goals.	Develop problem-solving skills, use social support networks.
Patients must communicate with providers about prevention and treatment services.	Define own needs on basis of experience.
	Validate rationale for continuing to follow recommendations.
Actions by Providers	
Providers must foster effective communication with patients.	
Provide clear, direct messages about importance of a behavior or therapy.	Provide oral and written instruction, including rationale for treatments.
	Develop skills in communication/counseling.
Include patients in decisions about prevention and treatment goals and related strategies.	Use tailoring and contracting strategies.
	Negotiate goals and a plan.
	Anticipate barriers to compliance and discuss solutions.
Incorporate behavioral strategies into counseling.	Use active listening.
	Develop multicomponent strategies (ie., cognitive and behavioral).
Providers must document and respond to patient's progress toward goals.	
Create an evidence-based practice.	Determine methods of evaluating outcomes.
Assess patient's compliance at each visit.	Use self-report or electronic data.
Develop a reminder system to ensure identification and follow-up of patient status.	Use telephone follow-up.
Actions by Health Care Organizations	
Develop an environment that supports prevention and treatment interventions.	Develop training in behavioral science, office set-up for all personnel.
	Use preappointment reminders.
	Use telephone follow-up.
	Schedule evening/weekend office hours.
	Provide group/individual counseling for patients and families.
Provide tracking and reporting systems.	Develop computer-based systems (electronic medical records).
Provide education and training for providers.	Require continuing education courses in communication, behavioral counseling.
Provide adequate reimbursement for allocation of time for all health care professionals.	Develop incentives tied to desired patient and provider outcomes.
Adopt systems to incorporate innovations rapidly and efficiently into medical practice.	Incorporate nursing case management.
	Implement pharmacy patient profile and recall review systems.
	Use of electronic transmission storage of patient's self-monitored data.
	Obtain patient data on lifestyle behavior before visit.
	Provide continuous quality improvement training.

(Adapted from Miller, N. H., Hill, M. N., Kottke, T, & Ockene. I. S. [1997]. The multilevel compliance challenge: Recommendations for a call to action. *Circulation*, 95, 1085–1090. Reprinted with permission.)

systolic pressure (≤150 mm Hg) than was recommended by the JNC VI report (Oliveria, Lapuerta et al., 2002). In Ontario, Canada, an analysis of prescribing trends for patients who were starting treatment for high blood pressure revealed that the guidelines released by the provincial Ministry of Health had no noticeable impact on the prescribing practices of Ontario physicians (Tu, Mamdani et al., 2002). Alderman and colleagues recently published some strategies to improve hypertension guidelines but, interesting, they did not address the most basic problem of all, which is how to improve clini-cian awareness and use of the JNC reports (Alderman, Furberg et al., 2002).

Role of Clients

The challenge for clients in achieving BP control is to modify their lives in ways that support their treatment plan. Making the decision to control BP is the critical client factor that pre-cedes lifestyle modification and BP control (Working Group to Define Critical Patient Behaviors in High Blood Pressure

DISPLAY 39-4

PREVENTING, MONITORING, AND ADDRESSING PROBLEMS OF ADHERENCE

Educate About Conditions and Treatment

Assess patient's understanding and acceptance of the diagnosis and expectations of being in care.

Discuss patient's concerns and clarify misunderstandings.

Inform patient of blood pressure level.

Agree with patient on a goal blood pressure.

Inform patient about recommended treatment and provide specific written information.

Elicit concerns and questions and provide opportunities for patient to state specific behaviors to carry out treatment recommendations.

Emphasize need to continue treatment, that patient cannot tell if blood pressure is elevated, and that control does not mean cure.

Individualize the Regimen

Include patient in decision making.

Simplify the regimen.

Incorporate treatment into patient's daily lifestyle.

Set, with the patient, realistic short-term objectives for specific components of the treatment plan.

Encourage discussion of side effects and concerns.

Encourage self-monitoring.

Minimize cost of therapy.

Indicate you will ask about adherence at next visit.

When weight loss is established as a treatment goal, discourage quick weight loss regimens, fasting, or unscientific methods, because these are associated with weight cycling which may increase cardiovascular morbidity and mortality.

Provide Reinforcement

Provide feedback regarding blood pressure level.

Ask about behaviors to achieve blood pressure control.

Give positive feedback for behavioral and blood pressure improvement.

Hold exit interviews to clarify regimen.

Make appointment for next visit before patient leaves the office.

Use appointment reminders and contact patients to confirm appointments.

Schedule more frequent visits to counsel nonadherent patients.

Contact and follow up patients who missed appointments.

Consider clinician–patient contracts.

Promote Social Support

Educate family members to be part of the blood pressure control process and provide daily reinforcement.

Suggest small group activities to enhance mutual support and motivation.

Collaborate with Other Professionals

Draw on complementary skills and knowledge of nurses, pharmacists, dietitians, optometrists, dentists, and physician assistants.

Refer patients for more intensive counseling.

(National High Blood Pressure Education Program [1994]. *The Fifth Report of the Joint National Committee on Detection, Evaluation, and Treatment of High Blood Pressure.* NIH publication no. 93–1088. Bethesda, MD: US Department of Health and Human Services National Institutes of Health.)

Control, 1979). Depression has recently been reported as one possible factor that may underlie difficulty in complying with using antihypertensive medications (Wang, Bohn et al., 2002). Because this study was both cross-sectional and relatively small, the results will need to be replicated; however, clinicians can be thoughtful of the client's mood state when assessing for reasons for not following through with a treatment plan. Interviews with 525 hypertensive patients from three different care provider systems found that patients who were older, using multiple medications, unaware of their goal blood pressures, and who experienced more side effects were more likely to have uncontrolled blood pressures (Knight, Bohn et al., 2001). Chapters 44 and 46 include a review of strategies that have been demonstrated to be effective in helping patients control their risk factors for cardiovascular disease.

Role of Health Care Organizations

Some of the actions that health care organizations can take to improve BP control are included in Display 39-4. HealthSystem Minnesota has implemented a hypertension services program using a team approach, with nurse coordinators delivering primary care in partnership with patients and physicians (Christianson, Pietz et al., 1997). Health care organizations have the opportunity to: provide education for both providers and patients; set

standards to care; implement computerized data systems; document the impact of care on patient outcomes; and determine which types of care are cost-effective while maintaining quality of life (Bernard, Townsend et al., 1998).

Role of the Community and Public Health

Community-based interventions in the United States and Europe have demonstrated that community action can reduce the risks of cardiovascular disease (Farquhar, Fortmann et al., 1990; Puska, Tuomilehto et al., 1989). Recent data collected using a nationwide yearly telephone survey of adult risk factors and preventive practices indicate that there are geographic/regional variations in the prevalence of risk factors. It is believed that this regional variability is related to the local sociocultural environment, which may or may not promote risk factor reduction (Hahn, Heath et al., 1998). Such variability of risk, and the evidence that community programs can impact risk, challenge communities to initiate projects that promote healthy lifestyles. Kalamazoo, Michigan and the state of Kansas have developed programs to reduce chronic disease risk by promoting healthy diets and exercise (Diehl, 1998; Paine-Andrews, Harris et al., 1997). The National High Blood Pressure Program suggests that community programs should have the goals of promoting: the intake of foods lower in calorie and sodium content and higher in potassium; increased physical activity; and moderation in alcohol intake (National High Blood Pressure Education Program, 1993). Other community activities can include raising awareness of risk factors, supporting entry into the health care system, and supporting individuals after their treatment plans (Egan & Lackland, 1998). The National High Blood Pressure Education Program also has resources to support the development of community programs in schools, churches, sporting events, and workplaces, as well as in rural, suburban, urban, and inner city settings (Chobanian, Bakris et al., 2003).

In the early years of community programs, the emphasis was on screening to identify individuals with hypertension (Joint National Committee on Detection Evaluation and Treatment of High Blood Pressure, 1984). In subsequent years, the emphasis of community programs was shifted toward integrated cardiovascular risk factor management and screening was only recommended for populations considered to be at high risk for having large numbers of individuals with undetected high blood pressure (Fifth Report of the Joint National Committee on Detection, Evaluation, and Treatment of High Blood Pressure [JNC V], 1993; National Heart, 1988). Currently, blood pressure screenings may be performed as part of local events such as health fairs. It is important that if a blood pressure screening is included in such an event that there is a mechanism for follow-up of each person found to have an elevated BP.

Role of Policy

The impressive impact of legislation to reduce smoking in public places, such as airplanes, highlights the powerful role of policy in the reduction of cardiovascular risk. In the area of hypertension, national policy makers can encourage the food manufacturing and marketing industries to reduce the sodium, calorie, and saturated fat content of processed foods as well as make information about diet and risk available at points of food purchase (National High Blood Pressure Education Program, 1993). Another important policy arena is assurance of the provision of health care and payment for medications for persons without health insurance (Dustan, Francis et al., 1993). An analysis of data from NHANES III to identify factors that predicted blood pressure control revealed that having health insurance, consistency of care including seeing the same provider and going to the same facility, and having had a blood pressure check in the previous 6 months were significant predictors (He, Muntner et al., 2002). Finally, continuation of the policy of funding basic and applied research related to cardiovascular disease is important to unraveling the causes of primary hypertension.

Team Approach to Blood Pressure Management

The optimal management of high BP requires the collaboration of health care professionals (Coordinating Committee of the National High Blood Pressure Education Program, 1984; Miller, Hill et al., 1997). Team members include the client, health educator, nurse, nutritionist, pharmacist, and physician.

The Mayo Clinic has documented their successful use of a hypertension clinic that uses the team approach. In this setting, the patient's care is managed by the nurse clinician (Schultz &

Sheps, 1994). Successful teams require expertise in communication, coordination, and an appreciation of the skills of each team member (Coordinating Committee of the National High Blood Pressure Education Program, 1984).

The Role of Nursing in Blood Pressure Management

Nurses and nursing have a role in all aspects of hypertension management, from measuring BPs to research to setting national policy. The role of the individual nurse depends on his or her preparation and work experience. The successful use of nurses to manage patients with hypertension has been reported in the literature since the 1970s (Curzio, Rubin et al., 1990; Logan, Milne et al., 1979; Pheley, Terry et al., 1995; Schultz & Sheps, 1994; Smith, Merritt et al., 1997). The current era of cost containment and the preparation of advanced practice nurses (Clinical Nurse Specialists and Nurse Practitioners) create a receptive climate for further development of the nurses' role in hypertension management.

Nursing Diagnoses

The nursing diagnoses for the person with hypertension are derived from data collected to formulate a complete and accurate nursing assessment. These diagnoses may include the following:

1. Knowledge deficit about the disease process of high BP, its consequences, and treatment related to lack of effective teaching as manifested by verbal acknowledgement of a deficiency in knowledge, expressions of an inaccurate perception of health status, or incorrect performance of the desired or prescribed health behavior.
2. Potential noncompliance with the plan of therapy related to knowledge deficit, failure to follow a prescribed regimen, inadequate support system, or lack of involvement in the treatment plan.
3. Potential ineffective coping related to the lack of motivation to respond, depression in response to the stress of a chronic disease, or unsatisfactory support system.
4. Potential fluid volume deficit related to abnormal fluid loss caused by use of diuretics.
5. Potential alteration in tissue perfusion: cardiovascular, related to hypertension, and cerebrovascular blood flow.

Nursing Care Plan 39-1 summarizes care for two of the most important nursing diagnoses.

Goals

General goals for people who have hypertension are the following:

1. Achievement and maintenance of goal BP
2. Understanding, participating in, and implementing the prescribed treatment plan
3. Movement toward adaptation to having a chronic condition that increases their risk of atherosclerotic cardiovascular disease and stroke
4. Confidence in ability to cope with hypertension within the demands of daily life

Nursing Care Plan 39–1 ■ The Patient With Hypertension

Nursing Diagnosis 1   ➤   Knowledge deficit about the disease process, its consequences and treatment related to lack of effective teaching as manifested by verbal acknowledgment of knowledge deficit, inaccurate perception of health care status, and failure to perform the desired or prescribed health behaviors

Nursing Goal   ➤   To detect early and reduce signs and symptoms of knowledge deficit

Outcome Criteria   ➤   The patient will be able to
1. Describe the disease process and the causes and factors contributing to the course of the disease
2. Describe the procedure for hypertension control
3. Actively participate in health behaviors prescribed or desired
4. Experience less anxiety related to fear of loss of control, misconceptions, or misinformation
5. Blood pressure will be maintained within normal limits

NURSING INTERVENTIONS	RATIONALE
1. Assess, document, and report factors contributing to knowledge deficit. a. Level of knowledge b. Emotional readiness for learning c. Support system(s) d. Health beliefs e. Provider practices	1. Learning needs differ depending on the dispositions and conditions that influence patient's health behavior. Assessment before developing a teaching plan ensures greater efficiency, appropriateness, and success of teaching and learning process.
2. Provide patient with additional information regarding pathology, general well-being (dietary habits, weight control, alcohol, exercise, caffeine, smoking, stress management), and risks of uncontrolled high blood pressure.	2. Enables patient to make choices about lifestyle changes and adherence to medical regimen.
3. Develop an individualized teaching plan based on the individual's knowledge, habits, and experience.	3. Same rationale as no. 1 above.
4. Initiate behavior modification methods. a. Have patient keep written diary of activities, diet, and medication over a week's time. b. Ask patient to recall activities, dietary intake, and medication over a 2-day period. c. Teach patient to take and record own blood pressure, and to record factors of concern including medication side effects. d. Explore patient's beliefs in relation to his or her identified behaviors.	4. Patient education and opportunities to make voluntary adaptions of behavior will improve or maintain health. This implies active involvement of the patient in his or her own care and assumes that the patient takes responsibility for learning (Working Group to Define Critical Patient Behaviors in High Blood Pressure Control, 1979).
5. Discuss drug actions, interactions, and side effects. a. Discuss potential for sexual dysfunction. b. For women of reproductive age discuss risks and benefits of all birth control methods. c. Provide information about possibility of interactions with over-the-counter drugs such as cough or cold medications or herbals. d. Discuss general side effects of drugs: lightheadedness, lethargy, and orthostatic hypotension. e. If hypotensive effects occur teach patient to notify care provider and if feasible try to increase large muscle activity or lie down briefly.	5. Knowledge, attitudes, and skills of the four critical patient behaviors are essential to taking medication and ultimately to achievement of long-term blood pressure control (Working Group to Define Critical Patient Behaviors in High Blood Pressure Control, 1979). a. Antihypertensive medications affect the autonomic nervous system, which plays a part in libidinal reactions. Change in drug or dosage may relieve signs and symptoms. b. Oral contraceptives may increase renin production by the kidney and increase BP. c. May contain sympathomimetic agents, which may increase BP or counteract antihypertensive effects. d. Upright position produces decrease in venous return because of decreased BP, decreased systemic vascular resistance, and decreased cardiac output.

Nursing Care Plan 39–1 ■ The Patient With Hypertension *(continued)*

Nursing Diagnosis 2 ➤ Potential ineffective management of therapeutic regimen: noncompliance to long-term disease management, related to the chronic nature of the disease, knowledge deficit, inability to follow treatment regimens, lack of social support, or a lack of active involvement in self-care as manifested by verbalization of nonparticipation, missed appointments, partially used or unused medications, persistence of symptoms, or progression of the disease process

Nursing Goal ➤ To promote development of a treatment plan acceptable to the patient and understanding of disease control

Outcome Criteria ➤ The patient will
1. Assume responsibility for self-care as able
2. Develop personal and health care goals that contribute to following the treatment plan and control of high blood pressure

NURSING INTERVENTIONS

1. Assess patient's perception of his illness and its treatment.

2. Assess patient's self-care performance.
   a. Determine baseline actions regarding medications, diet, weight, exercise, stress management, smoking, and alcohol.
   b. Monitor and record improvement in following the treatment plan.
3. Develop a system for patient tracking.
   a. Patient contact system-mail, telephone, and personal contacts
   b. Record-keeping system-patient outcomes, teaching-plan, patient education, prescription refills, progress in adherence
   c. Alert system to signal need for patient contact using indicators such as missed appointments or laboratory results,
4. Encourage the patient to express any questions, concerns, fears or frustrations he or she has related to health needs.

5. Explain the regimen to the patient.
   a. Discuss benefits, problems, or inconvenience.
   b. Assist patient to incorporate regimen into everyday life (written medication schedule, diet, lifestyle modification, appointment keeping, multimedia information).

6. Provide continual feedback and reinforcement of treatment plan.
7. Simplify the therapeutic regimen.
   a. Encourage care provider to prescribe once-a-day medications.
   b. Provide written instructions with appropriate literacy level and/or language on medication dosage, schedule side effects, and goals of therapy.
   c. Schedule medication taking in association with daily activities.
   d. Stress not stopping or changing medication without calling clinician.

RATIONALE

1. Inaccurate perceptions held by the patient about his or her disease and its treatment must be identified and corrected. Misunderstandings of the nature and seriousness of the illness and susceptibility to complications can greatly affect compliance.
2. Assessment of patient participation is best accomplished by asking patients in a nonjudgmental way if they have problems in following the prescribed regimen.

3. A tracking system improves adherence and consequently BP control. Increased contact between the patient and the health care provider is essential to participation, communication, and learning.

4. Fears and frustrations about prescribed treatment (whether valid or not) can interfere with following the treatment plan and must be discussed openly for effective problem solving to take place.
5. Patient participation and satisfaction is enhanced when patient-clinician interaction is good and when patient is actively involved in decisions about self-care. Explicit instructions and focusing on one task or skill at a time help to ensure mastery of critical behaviors for BP control(Working Group to Define Critical Patient Behaviors in High Blood Pressure Control, 1979).
6. Same rationale as diagnosis no. 1, rationale no. 1.

7. Same rationale as no. 5 above.

(continued)

Nursing Care Plan 39–1 ■ The Patient With Hypertension *(continued)*

NURSING INTERVENTIONS	RATIONALE
8. People are more likely to take an active role in their care if they believe that they have control over treatment outcomes. Helps the patient to be more aware of BP and treatment trends and places emphasis on therapeutic goals. The focus is on the outcome as well as the problems encountered (Working Group to Define Critical Patient Behaviors in High Blood Pressure Control, 1979).	8. Encourage active participation by the patient and his or her family. a. Identify desirable self-care behaviors (make decision to control BP, follow treatment plan, monitor progress toward goal BP, resolve barriers blocking BP control). b. Take home BP measurements. c. Keep a graphic record of BP and medication schedule, dosage, and side effects. d. Assist in planning menus, shopping for and preparation of meals.
9. Contracting increases patient participation in care and encourages behavior modification.	9. Devise a verbal or written contract with the patient specifying each particular behavior to be changed.

Client Education

The nurse shares the responsibility for client teaching with other members of the care team. In individual situations, it may be either the nurse or the health educator who assumes responsibility for assuring that the client learns about his or her high blood pressure. Some of the barriers to successful client education are low literacy, lack of understanding of the importance of treating a condition without apparent symptoms, language differences, and great variability in health beliefs, perceptions, and priorities (Fouad, Kiefe et al., 1997; Williams, Baker et al., 1998). Researchers at The Johns Hopkins University have developed and validated a 14-item scale, the Hill–Bone Compliance to High Blood Pressure Therapy Scale, that clinicians can use to assess how patients are able to follow treatment recommendations (Kim, Hill et al., 2000). The National High Blood Pressure Education Program and the American Heart Association are good sources for patient education materials in English and also have some materials in Spanish. Both agencies maintain web sites with directions for downloading or acquiring their materials.

Evaluation

Evaluation of goal achievement is based on whether goal BP has been attained, whether the client's adherence to therapeutic regimens is improved, and whether the teaching goals for the patient with high BP are met. In essence, goal achievement consists of adaptation to, and the ability to cope with, a chronic, life-long condition.

Another aspect of evaluation is the nurse's evaluation of his or her performance as a care provider to persons with high BP. Is the nurse measuring blood pressure according to the recognized standards? Is the nurse explaining to every client the meaning of the systolic and diastolic blood pressure numbers? Does the nurse see every encounter with the client as an opportunity to learn and teach? The encounter can be an opportunity to learn how the client is managing, whether they are experiencing side effects, and whether the educational materials are in the relevant language and at the correct literacy level. If the nurse is directing the hypertension clinic, then what is the control rate for high blood pressure in the clinic? Are all clients leaving with a clear understanding of what they should do when they get home or why they are using certain types of medications? Because all clients with high blood pressure have at least one risk factor for atherosclerotic cardiovascular disease, do all clients know the signs and symptoms for heart attacks and stroke? What actions should be taken if they have these signs or symptoms?

REFERENCES

Adrogue, H. E., & Sinaiko, A. R. (2001). Prevalence of hypertension in junior high school-aged children: effect of new recommendations in the 1996 Updated Task Force Report. *American Journal of Hypertension, 14*(5 Pt 1), 412–414.

Ahmed, M. E., Walker, J. M., Beevers, D. G., & Beevers, M. (1986). Lack of difference between malignant and accelerated hypertension. *BMJ (Clinical Research Edition), 292*(6515), 235–237.

Alderman, M. H., Cohen, H., Roqué, R., & Madhavan, S. (1997). Effect of long-acting and short-acting calcium antagonists on cardiovascular outcomes in hypertensive patients. *Lancet, 349*, 594–598.

Alderman, M. H., Furberg, C. D., Kostis, J. B., Laragh, J. H., Psaty, B. M., Ruilope, L. M., et al. (2002). Hypertension guidelines: criteria that might make them more clinically useful. *American Journal of Hypertension, 15*(10 Pt 1), 917–923.

Allender, S. P., Cutler, J. A., Follmann, D., Cappuccio, F. P., Pryer, J., & Elliott, P. (1996). Dietary calcium and blood pressure: a meta-analysis of randomized clinical trials. *Annals of Internal Medicine, 124*, 825–831.

Amery, A., Birkenhäger, W., Brixko, P., Bulpitt, C., Clement, D., Deruyttere, M., et al. (1985). Mortality and morbidity results from the European working party on high blood pressure in the elderly trial. *Lancet, 1*, 1349–1354.

Anderson, S. (1999). Pathogenesis of hypertensive renal damage. In J. L. Izzo Jr. & H. R. Black (Eds.), *Hypertension primer* (Second ed., pp. 190–193). Baltimore: Lippincott, Williams & Wilkens.

Appel, L. J., Champagne, C. M., Harsha, D. W., Cooper, L. S., Obarzanek, E., Elmer, P. J., et al. (2003). Effects of comprehensive lifestyle modification on blood pressure control: main results of the PREMIER clinical trial. *JAMA, 289*(16), 2083–2093.

Appel, L. J., Espeland, M. A., Easter, L., Wilson, A. C., Folmar, S., & Lacy, C. R. (2001). Effects of reduced sodium intake on hypertension control in older individuals: results from the Trial of Nonpharmacologic Interventions in the Elderly (TONE). Archives of Internal Medicine, 161(5), 685–693.

Appel, L. J., Moore, T. J., Obarzanek, E., Vollmen, W. M., Svetkey, L. P., & Sacks, F. M., et al. (1997). A clinical trial of the effects of dietary patterns on blood pressure. *New England Journal of Medicine, 336*, 1117–1124.

Arakawa, K. (1993). Hypertension and exercise. *Clinical Experience in Hypertension,* 15(6), 1171–1179.

Arauz-Pacheco, C., Parrott, M. A., & Raskin, P. (2003). Treatment of hypertension in adults with diabetes. *Diabetes Care,* 26 Suppl. 1, S80–82.

Bakris, G. L., Mangrum, A., Copley, J. B., Vicknair, N., & Sadler, R. (1997). Effect of calcium-channel or beta-blockade on the progression of diabetic nephropathy in African Americans. *Hypertension,* 29(3), 744–750.

Bakris, G. L., & Smith, A. (1996). Effects of sodium intake on albumin excretion in patients with diabetic nephropathy treated with long-acting calcium antagonists. *Annals of Internal Medicine,* 125(3), 201–204.

Bataineh, A., & Raij, L. (1998). Angiotensin II, nitric oxide, and end-organ damage in hypertension. *Kidney Inernationalt Supplement,* 68, S14–19.

Batey, D. M., Kaufmann, P. G., Raczynski, J. M., Hollis, J. F., Murphy, J. K., & Rosner, B., et al. (2000). Stress management intervention for primary prevention of hypertension: detailed results from Phase I of Trials of Hypertension Prevention (TOHP-I). *Annals of Epidemiology,* 10(1), 45–58.

Baumbach, G. L., & Heistad, D. D. (1999). Cerebrovascular disease: A. Cerebrovascular disease in experimental models of hypertension. In J. D. Swales (Ed.), *Textbook of hypertension* (pp. 682–690). Oxford: Blackwell Scientific Publishing.

Beilin, L. J., & Puddey, I. B. (1992). Alcohol and hypertension. *Clinical Experience in Hypertension [A],* 14(1–2), 119–138.

Berenson, G. S., Srinivasan, S. R., & Bao, W. (1997). Precursors of cardiovascular risk in young adults from a biracial (black-white) population: the Bogalusa Heart Study. *Annals of the New York Academy of Science,* 817, 189–198.

Berlowitz, D. R., Ash, A. S., Hickey, E. C., Friedman, R. H., Glickman, M., Kader, B., et al. (1998). Inadequate management of blood pressure in a hypertensive population. *New England Journal of Medicine,* 339, 1957–1963.

Bernard, D. B., Townsend, R. R., & Sylvestri, M. F. (1998). Health and disease management: what is it and where is it going? What is the role of health and disease management in hypertension? *American Journal of Hypertension,* 11(8 Pt 2), 103S–108S.

Black, H. R. (1999). Management of hypertension in older persons. In J. L. Izzo Jr & H. R. Black (Eds.), *Hypertension primer* (Second ed., pp. 430–432). Baltimore: Lippincott, Williams & Wilkens.

Black, H. R., Elliott, W. J., Grandits, G., Grambsch, P., Lucente, T., White, W. B., et al. (2003). Principal results of the Controlled Onset Verapamil Investigation of Cardiovascular End Points (CONVINCE) trial. *JAMA,* 289(16), 2073–2082.

Blair, D., Habicht, J.-P., Sims, E. A., Sylwester, D., & Abraham, S. (1984). Evidence for an increased risk for hypertension with centrally located body fat and the effect of race and sex on this risk. *American Journal of Epidemiology,* 119, 526–540.

Blair, S. N., Goodyear, N. N., Gibbons, L. W., & Cooper, K. H. (1984). Physical fitness and incidence of hypertension in healthy normotensive men and women. *JAMA,* 252, 487–490.

Blair, S. N., Kohl, H. W., Paffenbarger, R. S., Clark, D. G., Cooper, K. H., & Gibbons, L. W. (1989). Physical fitness and all-cause mortality: a prospective study of healthy men and women. *JAMA,* 262, 2395–2401.

Bog-Hansen, E., Lindblad, U., Bengtsson, K., Ranstam, J., Melander, A., & Rastam, L. (1998). Risk factor clustering in patients with hypertension and non-insulin-dependent diabetes mellitus. The Skaraborg Hypertension Project. *Journal of Internal Medicine,* 243(3), 223–232.

Bolen, J. C., Rhodes, L., Powell-Griner, E. E., Bland, S. D., & Holtzman, D. (2000). State-specific prevalence of selected health behaviors, by race and ethnicity–Behavioral Risk Factor Surveillance System, 1997. *MMWR CDC Surveillance Summary,* 49(2), 1–60.

Braunwald, E., Antman, E. M., Beasley, J. W., Califf, R. M., Cheitlin, M. D., Hochman, J. S., et al. (2002). ACC/AHA 2002 guideline for the management of patients with unstable angina and non-ST-segment elevation myocardial infarction–summary article: a report of the American College of Cardiology/American Heart Association task force on practice guidelines (Committee on the Management of Patients With Unstable Angina). *Journal of the American College of Cardiology,* 40(7), 1366–1374.

Brenner, B. M., Cooper, M. E., de Zeeuw, D., Keane, W. F., Mitch, W. E., Parving, H. H., et al. (2001). Effects of losartan on renal and cardiovascular outcomes in patients with type 2 diabetes and nephropathy. *New England Journal of Medicine,* 345(12), 861–869.

Brown, C. D., Higgins, M., Donato, K. A., Rohde, F. C., Garrison, R., Obarzanek, E., et al. (2000). Body mass index and the prevalence of hypertension and dyslipidemia. *Obesity Research,* 8(9), 605–619.

Brown, M. A., Buddle, M. L., Farrell, T., Davis, G., & Jones, M. (1998). Randomised trial of management of hypertensive pregnancies by Korotkoff phase IV or phase V. *Lancet,* 352, 777–781.

Buring, J. E., Glynn, R. J., & Hennekens, C. H. (1995). Calcium-channel blockers and myocardial infarction: a hypothesis formulated but not yet tested. *JAMA,* 274, 654–655.

Burke, V., Beilin, L. J., & Dunbar, D. (2001). Tracking of blood pressure in Australian children. *Journal of Hypertension,* 19(7), 1185–1192.

Chasan-Taber, L., Willett, W. C., Manson, J. E., Spiegelman, D., Hunter, D. J., Curhan, G., et al. (1996). Prospective study of oral contraceptives and hypertension among women in the United States. *Circulation,* 94(3), 483–489.

Chobanian, A. V., Bakris, G. L., Black, H. R., Cushman, W. C., Green, L. A., Izzo, J. L., Jr., et al. (2003). The Seventh Report of the Joint National Committee on Prevention, Detection, Evaluation, and Treatment of High Blood Pressure: the JNC 7 report *JAMA,* 289(19), 2560–2572. (Erratum in *JAMA,* 2003, 290[2]:197.)

Christianson, J. B., Pietz, L., Taylor, R., Woolley, A., & Knutson, D. J. (1997). Implementing programs for chronic illness management: the case of hypertension services. *Jt Comm Journal of Quality Improvement,* 23(11), 593–601.

Coakley, E. H., Rimm, E. B., Colditz, G., Kawachi, I., & Willett, W. (1998). Predictors of weight change in men: results from the Health Professionals Follow-up Study. *International Journal of Obesity and Related Metabolic Disorders,* 22(2), 89–96.

Cobbe, S. M. (1998). Lipids in hypertensive patients. *American Journal of Hypertension,* 11(7), 887–889.

Cohn, J. N., & Tognoni, G. (2001). A randomized trial of the angiotensin-receptor blocker valsartan in chronic heart failure. *New England Journal of Medicine,* 345(23), 1667–1675.

Collins, R., Peto, R., MacMahon, S., Hebert, P., Fiebach, N. H., Eberlein, K. A., et al. (1990). Blood pressure, stroke, and coronary heart disease. Part 2, short-term reductions in blood pressure: overview of randomised drug trials in their epidemiological context. *Lancet,* 335, 827–838.

Cooper, R. S. (1999). Geographic patterns of hypertension: a global perspective. In J. L. Izzo Jr & H. R. Black (Eds.), *Hypertension primer* (Second ed., pp. 224–225). Baltimore: Lippincott Williams & Wilkins.

Coordinating Committee of the National High Blood Pressure Education Program. (1984). Collaboration in high blood pressure control: among professionals and with the patient. *Annals of Internal Medicine,* 101(3), 393–395.

Cruickshank, J. M., Thorp, J. M., & Zacharias, F. J. (1987). Benefits and potential harm of lowering high blood pressure. *Lancet,* 1, 581–584.

Cruz, D. N., Simon, D. B., Nelson-Williams, C., Farhi, A., Finberg, K., Burleson, L., et al. (2001). Mutations in the Na-Cl cotransporter reduce blood pressure in humans. *Hypertension,* 37(6), 1458–1464.

Curzio, J. L., Rubin, P. C., Kennedy, S. S., & Reid, J. L. (1990). A comparison of the management of hypertensive patients by nurse practitioners compared with conventional hospital care. *Journal of Human Hypertension,* 4(6), 665–670.

Cushman, W. C. (1999). Alcohol use and blood pressure. In J. L. Izzo Jr & H. R. Black (Eds.), *Hypertension primer* (2nd ed., pp. 263–265). Baltimore: Lippincott Williams & Wilkins.

Cushman, W. C., Cutler, J. A., Hanna, E., Bingham, S. F., Follmann, F., Harford, T., et al. (1998). Prevention and treatment of hypertension study (PATHS): effects of an alcohol treatment program on blood pressure. *Archives of Internal Medicine,* 158, 1197–1207.

Cutler, J. A., Follmann, D., & Allender, P. S. (1997). Randomized trials of sodium reduction: an overview. *American Journal of Clinical Nutrition,* 65(2 Suppl), 643S–651S.

Dahlof, B., Devereux, R. B., Kjeldsen, S. E., Julius, S., Beevers, G., Faire, U., et al. (2002). Cardiovascular morbidity and mortality in the Losartan Intervention For Endpoint reduction in hypertension study (LIFE): a randomised trial against atenolol. *Lancet,* 359(9311), 995–1003.

Dahlof, B., Lindholm, L. H., Hansson, L., Schersten, B., Ekbom, T., & Wester, P. O. (1991). Morbidity and mortality in the Swedish Trial in Old Patients with Hypertension (STOP-Hypertension). *Lancet,* 338(8778), 1281–1285.

Daniels, S. R., Loggie, J. M., Khoury, P., & Kimball, T. R. (1998). Left ventricular geometry and severe left ventricular hypertrophy in children and adolescents with essential hypertension. *Circulation,* 97(19), 1907–1911.

Danielson, M., & Dammstrom, B. (1981). The prevalence of secondary and curable hypertension. *Acta Medica Scandinavia,* 209(6), 451–455.

Dannenberg, A. L., Garrison, R. J., & Kannel, W. B. (1988). Incidence of hypertension in the Framingham Study. *American Journal of Public Health,* 78, 676–679.

Darbar, D., Fromm, M. F., Dell'Orto, S., Kim, R. B., Kroemer, H. K., Eichelbaum, M., et al. (1998). Modulation by dietary salt of verapamil disposition in humans. *Circulation, 98*(24), 2702–2708.

Dargie, H. J. (2001). Effect of carvedilol on outcome after myocardial infarction in patients with left-ventricular dysfunction: the CAPRICORN randomised trial. *Lancet, 357*(9266), 1385–1390.

Dart, R. A., Gregoire, J. R., Gutterman, D. D., & Woolf, S. H. (2003). The association of hypertension and secondary cardiovascular disease with sleep-disordered breathing. *Chest, 123*(1), 244–260.

Daugherty, S. A. (1983). Hypertension Detection and Follow-up: description of the enumerated and screened population. *Hypertension, 5*(Suppl. IV), IV 1–IV 43.

de Divitiis, M., Pilla, C., Kattenhorn, M., Donald, A., Zadinello, M., Wallace, S., et al. (2003). Ambulatory blood pressure, left ventricular mass, and conduit artery function late after successful repair of coarctation of the aorta. *Journal of the American College of Cardiology, 41*(12), 2259–2265.

de Leeuw, P. W., & Birkenhäger, W. H. (1994). Coarctation of the aorta. In J. D. Swales (Ed.), *Textbook of hypertension* (pp. 969–979). Oxford: Blackwell Scientific Publications.

de Leeuw, P. W., van Leeuwen, S. J., & Birkenhager, W. H. (1985). Effect of sleep on blood pressure and its correlates. *Clinical Experience in Hypertension [A], 7*(2–3), 179–186.

Decline in deaths from heart disease and stroke–United States, 1900–1999. (1999). *MMWR Morbidity and Mortality Weekly Report, 48*(30), 649–656.

Dengel, D. R., Hagberg, J. M., Pratley, R. E., Rogus, E. M., & Goldberg, A. P. (1998). Improvements in blood pressure, glucose metabolism, and lipoprotein lipids after aerobic exercise plus weight loss in obese, hypertensive middle-aged men. *Metabolism, 47*(9), 1075–1082.

Despres, J. P., Moorjani, S., Lupien, P. J., Tremblay, A., Nadeau, A., & Bouchard, C. (1990). Regional distribution of body fat, plasma lipoproteins, and cardiovascular disease. *Arteriosclerosis, 10*(4), 497–511.

DiCorleto, P. E., & Gimbrone Jr, M. A. (1996). Vascular endothelium. In V. Fuster, R. Ross & E. J. Topol (Eds.), *Atherosclerosis and coronary artery disease* (Vol. 1, pp. 387–399). Philadelphia: Lippincott-Raven.

Diehl, H. A. (1998). Coronary risk reduction through intensive community-based lifestyle intervention: the Coronary Health Improvement Project (CHIP) experience. *American Journal of Cardiology, 82*(10B), 83T–87T.

Din-Dzietham, R., Liao, D., Diez-Roux, A., Nieto, F. J., Paton, C., Howard, G., et al. (2000). Association of educational achievement with pulsatile arterial diameter change of the common carotid artery: the Atherosclerosis Risk in Communities (ARIC) Study, 1987–1992. *American Journal of Epidemiology, 152*(7), 617–627.

Doll, R., & Peto, R. (1976). Mortality in relation to smoking: 20 years' observations on male British doctors. *BMJ, 2,* 1525–1536.

Dustan, H. P., Francis, C. W., Allen, H. D., Cunningham, S. L., Dulany, W., Hay, J., et al. (1993). Principles of access to health care. Access to Health Care Task Force, American Heart Association. *Circulation, 87*(2), 657–658.

Dustan, H. P., Schneckloth, R. E., Corcoran, A. C., & Page, I. H. (1958). The effectiveness of long-term treatment of malignant hypertension. *Circulation,* 18, 644–651.

Ebrahim, S. (1998). Detection, adherence and control of hypertension for the prevention of stroke: a systematic review. *Health Technology Assessment,* 2(11), 1–78.

Effect of enalapril on survival in patients with reduced left ventricular ejection fractions and congestive heart failure. The SOLVD Investigators. (1991). *New England Journal of Medicine, 325*(5), 293–302.

Effect of ramipril on mortality and morbidity of survivors of acute myocardial infarction with clinical evidence of heart failure. The Acute Infarction Ramipril Efficacy (AIRE) Study Investigators. (1993). *Lancet, 342*(8875), 821–828.

Efficacy of atenolol and captopril in reducing risk of macrovascular and microvascular complications in type 2 diabetes: UKPDS 39. UK Prospective Diabetes Study Group. (1998). *BMJ, 317*(7160), 713–720.

Egan, B. M., & Lackland, D. T. (1998). Strategies for cardiovascular disease prevention: importance of public and community health programs. *Ethnic Disease,* 8(2), 228–239.

Ekelund, L., Haskell, W. L., Johnson, J. L., Whaley, F. S., Criqui, M. H., & Sheps, D. S. (1988). Physical fitness as a predictor of cardiovascular mortality in asymptomatic North American men. *New England Journal of Medicine,* 319, 1379–1384.

Elkasabany, A. M., Urbina, E. M., Daniels, S. R., & Berenson, G. S. (1998). Prediction of adult hypertension by K4 and K5 diastolic blood pressure in children: the Bogalusa Heart Study. *Journal of Pediatrics, 132*(4), 687–692.

Engstrom, A., Tobelmann, R. C., & Albertson, A. M. (1997). Sodium intake trends and food choices. *American Journal of Clinical Nutrition,* 65(2 Suppl), 704S–707S.

Erikssen, G., Liestol, K., Bjornholt, J., Thaulow, E., Sandvik, L., & Erikssen, J. (1998). Changes in physical fitness and changes in mortality. Lancet, 352, 759–762.

Esler, M. (2000). The sympathetic system and hypertension. *American Journal of Hypertension, 13*(6 Pt 2), 99S–105S.

Executive Summary of The Third Report of The National Cholesterol Education Program (NCEP) Expert Panel on Detection, Evaluation, And Treatment of High Blood Cholesterol In Adults (Adult Treatment Panel III). (2001). *JAMA, 285*(19), 2486–2497.

Fagard, R. H. (1993). Physical fitness and blood pressure. *Journal of Hypertension,* 11(Suppl 5), S47–S52.

Falkner, B. (2002). Birth weight as a predictor of future hypertension. *American Journal of Hypertension, 15*(2 Pt 2), 43S–45S.

Farquhar, J. W., Fortmann, S. P., Flora, J. A., Taylor, C. B., Haskell, W. L., Williams, P. T., et al. (1990). Effects of communitywide education on cardiovascular disease risk factors. The Stanford Five-City Project. *JAMA, 265,* 359–365.

Felmeden, D. C., Spencer, C. G., Chung, N. A., Belgore, F. M., Blann, A. D., Beevers, D. G., et al. (2003). Relation of thrombogenesis in systemic hypertension to angiogenesis and endothelial damage/dysfunction (a substudy of the Anglo-Scandinavian Cardiac Outcomes Trial [ASCOT]). *American Journal of Cardiology, 92*(4), 400–405.

Ferrannini, E., & Natali, A. (1991). Essential hypertension, metabolic disorders, and insulin resistance. *American Heart Journal,* 121, 1274–1282.

Ferri, C., Bellini, C., Desideri, G., Giuliani, E., De Siati, L., Cicogna, S., et al. (1998). Clustering of endothelial markers of vascular damage in human salt-sensitive hypertension: influence of dietary sodium load and depletion. *Hypertension, 32*(5), 862–868.

The fifth report of the Joint National Committee on Detection, Evaluation, and Treatment of High Blood Pressure (JNC V). (1993). Archives of Internal Medicine, 153(2), 154–183.

Fletcher, A. E., & Bulpitt, C. J. (1992). How far should blood pressure be lowered? *New England Journal of Medicine,* 326, 251–254.

Folsom, A. R., Prineas, R. J., Kaye, S. A., & Munger, R. G. (1990). Incidence of hypertension and stroke in relation to body fat distribution and other risk factors in older women. *Stroke,* 21, 701–706.

Ford, E. S., & DeStefano, F. (1991). Risk factors for mortality from all causes and from coronary heart disease among persons with diabetes. *American Journal of Epidemiology,* 133, 1220–1230.

Fouad, M. N., Kiefe, C. I., Bartolucci, A. A., Burst, N. M., Ulene, V., & Harvey, M. R. (1997). A hypertension control program tailored to unskilled and minority workers. *Ethnic Disease, 7*(3), 191–199.

Frank, R. N. (1999). The eye in hypertension. In J. L. Izzo Jr & H. R. Black (Eds.), *Hypertension primer* (2nd ed., pp. 194–196). Baltimore: Lippincott, Williams & Wilkens.

Freedman, D. S., Dietz, W. H., Srinivasan, S. R., & Berenson, G. S. (1999). The relation of overweight to cardiovascular risk factors among children and adolescents: the Bogalusa Heart Study. *Pediatrics, 103*(6 Pt 1), 1175–1182.

Fried, L. P., Kronmal, R. A., Newman, A. B., Bild, D. E., Mittelmark, M. B., Polak, J. F., et al. (1998). Risk factors for 5-year mortality in older adults: The Cardiovascular Health Study. *JAMA,* 279, 585–592.

Frohlich, E. D. (2003). Treating hypertension - what are we to believe? *New England Journal of Medicine, 348*(7), 639–641.

Frostegard, J., Wu, R., Gillis-Haegerstrand, C., Lemne, C., & de Faire, U. (1998). Antibodies to endothelial cells in borderline hypertension. *Circulation,* 98, 1092–1098.

Fuenmayor, N., Moreira, E., & Cubeddu, L. X. (1998). Salt sensitivity is associated with insulin resistance in essential hypertension. *American Journal of Hypertension,* 11(4 Pt 1), 397–402.

Fuentes, R. M., Notkola, I. L., Shemeikka, S., Tuomilehto, J., & Nissinen, A. (2000). Familial aggregation of blood pressure: a population-based family study in eastern Finland. *Journal of Human Hypertension, 14*(7), 441–445.

Furberg, C. D., Psaty, B. M., & Meyer, J. V. (1995). Nifedipine: dose-related increase in mortality in patients with coronary heart disease. *Circulation,* 92, 1326–1331.

Garraway, W. M., & Whisnant, J. P. (1987). The changing pattern of hypertension and the declining incidence of stroke. *JAMA,* 258, 214–217.

Garrison, R. J., Kannel, W. B., Stokes III, J., & Castelli, W. P. (1987). Incidence and precursors of hypertension in young adults: The Framingham Offspring Study. *Preventive Medicine,* 16, 235–251.

Giatras, I., Lau, J., & Levey, A. S. (1997). Effect of angiotensin-converting enzyme inhibitors on the progression of nondiabetic renal disease: a meta-analysis of randomized trials. Angiotensin-Converting-Enzyme Inhibition and Progressive Renal Disease Study Group. *Annals of Internal Medicine,* 127(5), 337–345.

Glynn, R. J., Field, T. S., Rosner, B., Hebert, P. R., Taylor, J. O., & Hennekens, C. H. (1995). Evidence for a positive linear relation between blood pressure and mortality in elderly people. *Lancet,* 345(8953), 825–829.

Gonzalez-Albarran, O., Ruilope, L. M., Villa, E., & Garcia Robles, R. (1998). Salt sensitivity: concept and pathogenesis. *Diabetes Research and Clinical Practice,* 39 Suppl, S15–26.

Gottdiener, J. S., Reda, D. J., Massie, B. M., Materson, B. J., Williams, D. W., & Anderson, R. J. (1997). Effect of single-drug therapy on reduction of left ventricular mass in mild to moderate hypertension: comparison of six anti-hypertensive agents. The Department of Veterans Affairs Cooperative Study Group on Antihypertensive Agents. *Circulation,* 95(8), 2007–2014.

Grimm, R. H., Jr., Flack, J. M., Grandits, G. A., Elmer, P. J., Neaton, J. D., Cutler, J. A., et al. (1996). Long-term effects on plasma lipids of diet and drugs to treat hypertension. Treatment of Mild Hypertension Study (TOMHS) Research Group. *JAMA,* 275(20), 1549–1556.

Grossman, E., Messerli, F. H., Grodzicki, T., & Kowey, P. (1996). Should a moratorium be placed on sublingual nifedipine capsules given for hypertensive emergencies and pseudoemergencies? *JAMA,* 276(16), 1328–1331.

Grover, S. A., Paquet, S., Levinton, C., Coupal, L., & Zowall, H. (1998). Estimating the benefits of modifying risk factors of cardiovascular disease: a comparison of primary vs secondary prevention *Archives of Internal Medicine,* 158(6), 655–662. (Published erratum appears in *Archives of Internal Medicine,* 1998, 158[11],1228.)

Gueyffier, F., Boutitie, F., Boissel, J. P., Pocock, S., Coope, J., Cutler, J., et al. (1997). Effect of antihypertensive drug treatment on cardiovascular outcomes in women and men. A meta-analysis of individual patient data from randomized, controlled trials. The INDANA Investigators. *Annals of Internal Medicine,* 126(10), 761–767.

Guidelines Subcommittee. (1999). 1999 Wordl Health Organization-International Society of Hypertension guidelines for the management of hypertension. *Journal of Hypertension,* 11, 905–918.

Haarbo, J., Hassager, C., Riis, B. J., & Christiansen, C. (1989). Relation of body fat distribution to serum lipids and lipoproteins in elderly women. *Atherosclerosis,* 80, 57–62.

Hager, W. D., Davis, B. R., Riba, A., Moye, L. A., Wun, C. C., Rouleau, J. L., et al. (1998). Absence of a deleterious effect of calcium-channel blockers in patients with left ventricular dysfunction after myocardial infarction: The SAVE Study Experience. SAVE Investigators. Survival and Ventricular Enlargement. *American Heart Journal,* 135(3), 406–413.

Hahn, R. A., Heath, G. W., & Chang, M. H. (1998). Cardiovascular disease risk factors and preventive practices among adults–United States, 1994: a behavioral risk factor atlas. Behavioral Risk Factor Surveillance System State Coordinators. *Morbidity and Mortality Weekly Report CDC Surveillance Summary,* 47(5), 35–69.

Hajjar, I., & Kotchen, T. A. (2003). Trends in prevalence, awareness, treatment, and control of hypertension in the United States, 1988–2000. *JAMA,* 290(2), 199–206.

Hakim, A. A., Petrovitch, H., Burchfiel, C. M., Ross, G. W., Rodriguez, B. L., White, L. R., et al. (1998). Effects of walking on mortality among non-smoking retired men. *New England Journal of Medicine,* 338, 94–99.

Hall, W. D. (1999). Geographic patterns of hypertension in the United States. In J. L. Izzo Jr & H. R. Black (Eds.), *Hypertension primer* (2nd ed., pp. 226–228). Baltimore: Lippincott Williams & Wilkins.

Hallstrom, A. P., Cobb, L. A., & Ray, R. (1986). Smoking as a risk factor for recurrence of sudden cardiac arrest. *New England Journal of Medicine,* 314, 271–275.

Hansson, L. (1990). How far should blood pressure be lowered? What is the role of the J-Curve? *American Journal of Hypertension,* 3, 726–729.

Hansson, L., Lindholm, L. H., Ekbom, T., Dahlof, B., Lanke, J., Schersten, B., et al. (1999). Randomised trial of old and new antihypertensive drugs in elderly patients: cardiovascular mortality and morbidity the Swedish Trial in Old Patients with Hypertension-2 study. *Lancet,* 354(9192), 1751–1756.

Hansson, L., Zanchetti, A., Carruthers, S. G., Dahlöf, B., Elmfeldt, D., Julius, S., et al. (1998). Effects of intensive blood-pressure lowering and low-dose aspirin in patients with hypertension: principal results of the Hypertension Optimal Treatment (HOT) randomised trial. *Lancet,* 351, 1755–1762.

Hayreh, S. S., Servais, G. E., & Virdi, P. S. (1989). Cotton-wool spots (inner retinal ischemic spots) in malignant arterial hypertension. *Ophthalmologica,* 198(4), 197–215.

He, J., Muntner, P., Chen, J., Roccella, E. J., Streiffer, R. H., & Whelton, P. K. (2002). Factors associated with hypertension control in the general population of the United States. *Archives of Internal Medicine,* 162(9), 1051–1058.

He, J., Whelton, P. K., Appel, L. J., Charleston, J., & Klag, M. J. (2000). Long-term effects of weight loss and dietary sodium reduction on incidence of hypertension. *Hypertension,* 35(2), 544–549.

Heintz, B., Schmauder, C., Witte, K., Breuer, I., Baltzer, K., Sieberth, H. G., et al. (1996). Blood pressure rhythm and endocrine functions in normotensive women on oral contraceptives. *Journal of Hypertension,* 14(3), 333–339.

Hermanson, B., Omenn, G. S., Kronmal, R. A., Gersh, B. J., & Study, P. C. (1988). Beneficial six-year outcome of smoking cessation in older men and women with coronary artery disease. *New England Journal of Medicine,* 319, 1365.

Higashi, Y., Oshima, T., Ozono, R., Matsuura, H., & Kajiyama, G. (1997). Aging and severity of hypertension attenuate endothelium-dependent renal vascular relaxation in humans. *Hypertension,* 30, 252–258.

Higashi, Y., Sasaki, S., Nakagawa, K., Matsuura, H., Oshima, T., & Chayama, K. (2002). Endothelial function and oxidative stress in renovascular hypertension. *New England Journal of Medicine,* 346(25), 1954–1962.

Hla, K. M., Skatrud, J. B., Finn, L., Palta, M., & Young, T. (2002). The effect of correction of sleep-disordered breathing on BP in untreated hypertension. *Chest,* 122(4), 1125–1132.

Holme, I., Helgeland, A., Hjermann, I., Lund-Larsen, P. G., & Leren, P. (1976). Coronary risk factors and socioeconomic status: the Oslo study. *Lancet,* 2, 1396–1398.

Horan, M. J., & Lenfant, C. (1990). Epidemiology of blood pressure and predictors of hypertension. *Hypertension,* 15(2 Suppl), I20–24.

Huang, Z., Willett, W. C., Manson, J. E., Rosner, B., Stampfer, M. J., Speizer, F. E., et al. (1998). Body weight, weight change, and risk for hypertension in women. *Annals of Internal Medicine,* 128, 81–88.

Hughes, J. S., Dove, H. G., Gifford, R. W., Jr., & Feinstein, A. R. (1981). Duration of blood pressure elevation in accurately predicting surgical cure of renovascular hypertension. *American Heart Journal,* 101(4), 408–413.

Hunt, S. A., Baker, D. W., Chin, M. H., Cinquegrani, M. P., Feldman, A. M., Francis, G. S., et al. (2001). ACC/AHA guidelines for the evaluation and management of chronic heart failure in the adult: executive summary. A report of the American College of Cardiology/American Heart Association Task Force on Practice Guidelines (Committee to revise the 1995 Guidelines for the Evaluation and Management of Heart Failure). *Journal of the American College of Cardiology,* 38(7), 2101–2113.

Hunt, S. C., Cook, N. R., Oberman, A., Cutler, J. A., Hennekens, C. H., Allender, P. S., et al. (1998). Angiotensinogen genotype, sodium reduction, weight loss, and prevention of hypertension: trials of hypertension prevention, phase II. *Hypertension,* 32(3), 393–401.

Hunt, S. C., & Williams, R. R. (1999). Genetics and family history of hypertension. In J. L. Izzo Jr & H. R. Black (Eds.), *Hypertension primer* (2nd ed., pp. 218–221). Baltimore: Lippincott Williams & Wilkins.

Huxley, R., Neil, A., & Collins, R. (2002). Unravelling the fetal origins hypothesis: is there really an inverse association between birthweight and subsequent blood pressure? *Lancet,* 360(9334), 659–665.

Hyman, D. J., & Pavlik, V. N. (2000). Self-reported hypertension treatment practices among primary care physicians: blood pressure thresholds, drug choices, and the role of guidelines and evidence-based medicine. *Archives of Internal Medicine,* 160(15), 2281–2286.

Hyman, D. J., & Pavlik, V. N. (2001). Characteristics of patients with uncontrolled hypertension in the United States. *New England Journal of Medicine,* 345(7), 479–486.

Hypertension Detection and Follow-up Program Cooperative Group. (1979). Five-year findings of the hypertension detection and follow-up program. I. Reduction in mortality of persons with high blood pressure, including mild hypertension. *JAMA,* 242, 2562–2571.

Hypertension Detection and Follow-up Program Cooperative Group. (1982). The effect of treatment on mortality in "mild" hypertension. Results of the Hypertension Detection and Follow-up Program. *New England Journal of Medicine,* 307, 976–980.

Hypertension Detection and Follow-up Program Cooperative Group. (1987). Educational level and 5-year all-cause mortality in the hypertension detection and follow-up program. *Hypertension,* 9, 641–646.

Hypertension Prevention Trial Research Group. (1990). The Hypertension Prevention Trial: three-year effects of dietary changes on blood pressure. *Archives of Internal Medicine,* 150, 153–162.

Ikeda, T., Gomi, T., Hirawa, N., Sakurai, J., & Yoshikawa, N. (1996). Improvement of insulin sensitivity contributes to blood pressure reduction after weight loss in hypertensive subjects with obesity. *Hypertension, 27*(5), 1180–1186.

Jeunemaitre, X., Soubrier, F., Kotelevtsev, Y. V., Lifton, R. P., Williams, C. S., Charru, A., et al. (1992). Molecular basis of human hypertension: role of angiotensinogen. *Cell, 71*(1), 169–180.

John, J. H., Ziebland, S., Yudkin, P., Roe, L. S., & Neil, H. A. (2002). Effects of fruit and vegetable consumption on plasma antioxidant concentrations and blood pressure: a randomised controlled trial. *Lancet, 359*(9322), 1969–1974.

Joint National Committee on Detection Evaluation and Treatment of High Blood Pressure. (1984). The 1984 Report of the Joint National Committee on Detection, Evaluation, and Treatment of High Blood Pressure. *Archives of Internal Medicine, 144*, 1045–1057.

Jones, D. W. (1999). Socioeconomic status and blood pressure. In J. L. Izzo Jr & H. R. Black (Eds.), *Hypertension primer* (2nd ed., pp. 242–243). Baltimore: Lippincott Williams & Wilkins.

Julius, S. (1988). Transition from high cardiac output to elevated vascular resistance in hypertension. *American Heart Journal, 116*, 600–606.

K/DOQI clinical practice guidelines for chronic kidney disease: evaluation, classification, and stratification. Kidney Disease Outcome Quality Initiative. (2002). *American Journal of Kidney Diseases, 39*(2 Suppl 2), S1–246.

Kannel, W. B. (1996). Blood pressure as a cardiovascular risk factor: prevention and treatment. *JAMA, 275*(20), 1571–1576.

Kannel, W. B., Brand, N., Skinner, J. J., Jr., Dawber, T. R., & P. M. McNamara. (1967). The relation of adiposity to blood pressure and development of hypertension: the Framingham study. *Annals of Internal Medicine, 67*, 48–59.

Kannel, W. B., & Cobb, J. (1992). Left ventricular hypertrophy and mortality–results from the Framingham Study. *Cardiology, 81*(4–5), 291–298.

Kannel, W. B., McGee, D., & Gordon, T. (1976). A general cardiovascular risk profile: the Framingham Study. *American Journal of Cardiology, 38*, 46–51.

Kaplan, N. (1998). J-curve not burned off by HOT study. *Lancet, 351*, 1748–1749.

Kaplan, N. M. (1989). The deadly quartet: upper-body obesity, glucose intolerance, hypertriglyceridemia, and hypertension. *Archives of Internal Medicine, 149*, 1514–1520.

Kaplan, N. M. (2002). *Kaplan's Clinical hypertension* (8th ed.). Philadelphia: Lippincott Williams & Wilkins.

Kashgarian, M. (1990). Hypertensive disease and kidney structure. In J. H. Laragh (Ed.), *Hypertension: pathophysiology, diagnosis and management* (pp. 389–398). New York: Raven Press.

Kawachi, I., Colditz, G. A., Stampfer, M. J., Willett, W. C., Manson, J. E., Rosner, B., et al. (1993). Smoking cessation in relation to total mortality rates in women: a prospective study. *Annals of Internal Medicine, 119*, 992–1000.

Keller, G., Zimmer, G., Mall, G., Ritz, E., & Amann, K. (2003). Nephron number in patients with primary hypertension. *New England Journal of Medicine, 348*(2), 101–108.

Kelley, G. A., & Kelley, K. S. (2000). Progressive resistance exercise and resting blood pressure : A meta-analysis of randomized controlled trials. *Hypertension, 35*(3), 838–843.

Khaw, K. T. (1996). Epidemiology of stroke. *Journal of Neurological and Neurosurgical Psychiatry, 61*(4), 333–338.

Kim, M. T., Hill, M. N., Bone, L. R., & Levine, D. M. (2000). Development and testing of the Hill-Bone Compliance to High Blood Pressure Therapy Scale. *Progress in Cardiovascular Nursing, 15*(3), 90–96.

Klag, M. J., Whelton, P. K., Randall, B. L., Neaton, J. D., Brancati, F. L., Ford, C. E., et al. (1996). Blood pressure and end-stage renal disease in men. *New England Journal of Medicine, 334*, 13–18.

Klag, M. J., Whelton, P. K., Randall, B. L., Neaton, J. D., Brancati, F. L., & Stamler, J. (1997). End-stage renal disease in African-American and white men. 16-year MRFIT findings. *JAMA, 277*(16), 1293–1298.

Klatsky, A. L., Friedman, G. D., Siegelaub, A. B., & Gerard, M. J. (1977). Alcohol consumption and blood pressure Kaiser-Permanente Multiphasic Health Examination data. *New England Journal of Medicine, 296*(21), 1194–1200.

Klungel, O. H., de Boer, A., Paes, A. H., Seidell, J. C., Nagelkerke, N. J., & Bakker, A. (1998). Undertreatment of hypertension in a population-based study in The Netherlands. *Journal of Hypertension, 16*(9), 1371–1378.

Knight, E. L., Bohn, R. L., Wang, P. S., Glynn, R. J., Mogun, H., & Avorn, J. (2001). Predictors of uncontrolled hypertension in ambulatory patients. *Hypertension, 38*(4), 809–814.

Kober, L., Torp-Pedersen, C., Carlsen, J. E., Bagger, H., Eliasen, P., Lyngborg, K., et al. (1995). A clinical trial of the angiotensin-converting-enzyme inhibitor trandolapril in patients with left ventricular dysfunction after myocardial infarction. Trandolapril Cardiac Evaluation (TRACE) Study Group. *New England Journal of Medicine, 333*(25), 1670–1676.

Kokkinos, P. F., Narayan, P., Colleran, J. A., Pittaras, A., Notargiacomo, A., Reda, D., et al. (1995). Effects of regular exercise on blood pressure and left ventricular hypertrophy in African-American men with severe hypertension. *New England Journal of Medicine, 333*, 1462–1467.

Kostis, J. B., Davis, B. R., Cutler, J., Grimm, R. H., Jr., Berge, K. G., Cohen, J. D., et al. (1997). Prevention of heart failure by antihypertensive drug treatment in older persons with isolated systolic hypertension. SHEP Cooperative Research Group. *JAMA, 278*(3), 212–216.

Kotchen, T. A., & McCarron, D. A. (1998). Dietary electrolytes and blood pressure: a statement for healthcare professionals from the American Heart Association Nutrition Committee. *Circulation, 98*, 613–617.

Krum, H., Viskoper, R. J., Lacourciere, Y., Budde, M., Charlon, V., & Investigators, f. t. B. H. (1998). The effect of an endothelin-receptor antagonist, Bosentan, on blood pressure in patients with essential hypertension. *New England Journal of Medicine, 338*, 784–790.

Kujala, U. M., Kaprio, J., Sarna, S., & Koskenvuo, M. (1998). Relationship of leisure-time physical activity and mortality: The Finnish Twin Cohort. *JAMA, 279*, 440–444.

Kushi, L. H., Fee, R. M., Folsom, A. R., Mink, P. J., Anderson, K. E., & Sellers, T. A. (1997). Physical activity and mortality in postmenopausal women. *JAMA, 277*, 1287–1292.

Labarthe, D. R. (1978). Problems in definition of mild hypertension. *Annals of the New York Academy of Science, 304*, 3–14.

Lackland, D. T., Bachman, D. L., Carter, T. D., Barker, D. L., Timms, S., & Kahli, H. (1998). The geographic variation in stroke incidence in two areas of the southeastern stroke belt: The Anderson and Pee Dee Stroke Study. *Stroke, 29*, 2061–2068.

LaCroix, A. Z., Lang, J., Scherr, P., Wallace, R. B., Coroni-Huntley, J., Berkman, L., et al. (1991). Smoking and mortality among older men and women in three communities. *New England Journal of Medicine, 324*, 1619–1625.

Lakka, T. A., Venalainen, J. M., Rauramaa, R., Salonen, R., Tuomilehto, J., & Salonen, J. T. (1994). Relation of leisure-time physical activity and cardiorespiratory fitness to the risk of acute myocardial infarction in men. *New England Journal of Medicine, 330*, 1549–1554.

Langeluddecke, P. M. (1986). The role of behavioral change procedures in multifactorial coronary heart disease prevention programs. *Progress in Behavior Modification, 20*, 199–225.

Langford, H. G., Blaufox, M. D., Oberman, A., Hawkins, C. M., Curb, J. D., Cutter, G. R., et al. (1985). Dietary therapy slows the return of hypertension after stopping prolonged medication. *JAMA, 253*, 657–664.

Law, C. M., M. de Swiet, Osmond, C., Fayers, P. M., Barker, D. J. P., Cruddas, A. M., et al. (1993). Initiation of hypertension in utero and its amplification throughout life. *BMJ, 306*, 24–27.

Lazarus, J. M., Bourgoignie, J. J., Buckalew, V. M., Greene, T., Levey, A. S., Milas, N. C., et al. (1997). Achievement and safety of a low blood pressure goal in chronic renal disease. The Modification of Diet in Renal Disease Study Group. *Hypertension, 29*(2), 641–650.

Ledoux, M., Lambert, J., Reeder, B. A., & Despres, J. P. (1997). Correlation between cardiovascular disease risk factors and simple anthropometric measures. Canadian Heart Health Surveys Research Group. *Canadian Medical Association Journal, 157* Suppl 1, S46–53.

Lerner, D. J., & Kannel, W. B. (1986). Patterns of coronary heart disease morbidity and mortality in the sexes: A 26-year follow-up of the Framingham population. *American Heart Journal, 111*, 383–390.

Levenstein, S., Smith, M. W., & Kaplan, G. A. (2001). Psychosocial predictors of hypertension in men and women. *Archives of Internal Medicine, 161*(10), 1341–1346.

Lewington, S., Clarke, R., Qizilbash, N., Peto, R., & Collins, R. (2002). Age-specific relevance of usual blood pressure to vascular mortality: a meta-analysis of individual data for one million adults in 61 prospective studies. *Lancet, 360*(9349), 1903–1913.

Lewis, E. J., Hunsicker, L. G., Bain, R. P., & Rohde, R. D. (1993). The effect of angiotensin-converting-enzyme inhibition on diabetic nephropathy. The Collaborative Study Group. *New England Journal of Medicine, 329*(20), 1456–1462.

Lewis, E. J., Hunsicker, L. G., Clarke, W. R., Berl, T., Pohl, M. A., Lewis, J. B., et al. (2001). Renoprotective effect of the angiotensin-receptor antagonist irbesartan in patients with nephropathy due to type 2 diabetes. *New England Journal of Medicine, 345*(12), 851–860.

Lichtenstein, M. J., Shipley, M. J., & Rose, G. (1985). Systolic and diastolic blood pressures as predictors of coronary heart disease mortality in the Whitehall Study. *British Heart Journal, 291*, 243–245.

Lifton, R. P. (1996). Molecular genetics of human blood pressure variation. *Science, 272*, 676–680.

Lightman, S. L., James, V. H., Linsell, C., Mullen, P. E., Peart, W. S., & Sever, P. S. (1981). Studies of diurnal changes in plasma renin activity, and plasma noradrenaline, aldosterone and cortisol concentrations in man. *Clinical Endocrinology (Oxford), 14*(3), 213–223.

Lindholm, L. H., Anderson, H., Ekbom, T., Hansson, L., Lanke, J., Dahlof, B., et al. (2001). Relation between drug treatment and cancer in hypertensives in the Swedish Trial in Old Patients with Hypertension 2: a 5-year, prospective, randomised, controlled trial. *Lancet, 358*(9281), 539–544.

Lindholm, L. H., Ibsen, H., Dahlof, B., Devereux, R. B., Beevers, G., de Faire, U., et al. (2002). Cardiovascular morbidity and mortality in patients with diabetes in the Losartan Intervention For Endpoint reduction in hypertension study (LIFE): a randomised trial against atenolol. *Lancet, 359*(9311), 1004–1010.

Lindop, G. B. M. (1994). The effects of hypertension on the structure of human resistance vessels. In J. D. Swales (Ed.), *Textbook of hypertension* (pp. 663–669). Oxford: Blackwell Scientific Publications.

Logan, A. G., Milne, B. J., Achber, C., Campbell, W. P., & Haynes, R. B. (1979). Work-site treatment of hypertension by specially trained nurses. A controlled trial. *Lancet, 2*(8153), 1175–1178.

London, G. M., Guerin, A. P., Pannier, B., Marchais, S. J., & Safar, M. E. (1998). Large artery structure and function in hypertension and end-stage renal disease. *Journal of Hypertension, 16*(12 Pt 2), 1931–1938.

Luft, F. C. (1998). Salt and hypertension at the close of the millenium. *Wien Klin Wochenschr, 110*(13-14), 459–466.

Lund-Johansen, P. (1977). Central haemodynamics in essential hypertenison. *Acta Medica Scandinavia, 603*(Suppl.1), 35–42.

Lund-Johansen, P. (1991). Twenty-year follow-up of hemodynamics in essential hypertension during rest and exercise. *Hypertension, 18*(Suppl. III), III-54–61.

Luria, M. H., Erel, J., Sapoznikov, D., & Gotsman, M. S. (1991). Cardiovascular risk factor clustering and ratio of total cholesterol to high-density lipoprotein cholesterol in angiographically documented coronary artery disease. *American Journal of Cardiology, 67*, 31–36.

MacMahon, S., Peto, R., Cutler, J., Collins, R., Sorlie, P., Neaton, J., et al. (1990). Blood pressure, stroke, and coronary heart disease. Part 1, prolonged differences in blood pressure: prospective observational studies corrected for dilution bias. *Lancet, 335*, 765–774.

MacMahon, S., & Rodgers, A. (1993). The effects of blood pressure reduction in older patients: an overview of five randomized controlled trials in elderly hypertensives. *Clinical Experience in Hypertension, 15*(6), 967–978.

MacMahon, S. W., Wilcken, D. E. L., & MacDonald, G. J. (1986). The effect of weight reduction on left ventricular mass. A randomized controlled trial in young, overweight hypertensive patients. *New England Journal of Medicine, 314*, 334–339.

Major outcomes in high-risk hypertensive patients randomized to angiotensin-converting enzyme inhibitor or calcium-channel blocker vs diuretic: The Antihypertensive and Lipid-Lowering Treatment to Prevent Heart Attack Trial (ALLHAT). (2002). *JAMA, 288*(23), 2981–2997.

Major outcomes in moderately hypercholesterolemic, hypertensive patients randomized to pravastatin vs usual care: The Antihypertensive and Lipid-Lowering Treatment to Prevent Heart Attack Trial (ALLHAT-LLT). (2002). *JAMA, 288*(23), 2998–3007.

Management Committee of the Australian Therapeutic Trial in Mild Hypertension. (1982). Untreated mild hypertension. *Lancet, 1*(8265), 185–190.

Manolio, T. A., Savage, P. J., Burke, G. L., Hilner, J. E., Liu, K., Orchard, T. J., et al. (1991). Correlates of fasting insulin levels in young adults: the CARDIA study. *Journal of Clinical Epidemiology, 44*(6), 571–578.

Maschio, G., Alberti, D., Janin, G., Locatelli, F., Mann, J. F., Motolese, M., et al. (1996). Effect of the angiotensin-converting-enzyme inhibitor benazepril on the progression of chronic renal insufficiency. The Angiotensin-Converting-Enzyme Inhibition in Progressive Renal Insufficiency Study Group. *New England Journal of Medicine, 334*(15), 939–945.

Mattes, R. D. (1997). The taste for salt in humans. *American Journal of Clinical Nutrition, 65*(2 Suppl), 692S–697S.

McDonald, H. P., Garg, A. X., & Haynes, R. B. (2002). Interventions to enhance patient adherence to medication prescriptions: scientific review. *JAMA, 288*(22), 2868–2879.

McGregor, E., Isles, C. G., Jay, J. L., Lever, A. F., & Murray, G. D. (1986). Retinal changes in malignant hypertension. *BMJ (Clinical Research Edition), 292*(6515), 233–234.

McLeod, D., Marshall, J., Kohner, E. M., & Bird, A. C. (1977). The role of axoplasmic transport in the pathogenesis of retinal cotton- wool spots. *British Journal of Ophthalmology, 61*(3), 177–191.

McMurray, J., & Murdoch, D. (1997). Calcium-antagonist controversy: the long and short of it? *Lancet, 349*, 585–586.

Medical Research Council Working Party. (1985). MRC trial of treatment of mild hypertension: principal results. *BMJ, 291*, 97–104.

Mehler, P. S., Coll, J. R., Estacio, R., Esler, A., Schrier, R. W., & Hiatt, W. R. (2003). Intensive blood pressure control reduces the risk of cardiovascular events in patients with peripheral arterial disease and type 2 diabetes. *Circulation, 107*(5), 753–756.

Meigs, J. B., D'Agostino, R. B., Sr., Wilson, P. W., Cupples, L. A., Nathan, D. M., & Singer, D. E. (1997). Risk variable clustering in the insulin resistance syndrome. The Framingham Offspring Study. *Diabetes, 46*(10), 1594–1600.

Melby, C. L., Goldflies, D. G., & Hyner, G. C. (1991). Blood pressure and anthropometric differences in regularly exercising and nonexercising black adults. *Clinical Experience in Hypertension [A], 13*(6-7), 1233–1248.

Midgley, J. P., Matthew, A. G., Greenwood, C. M., & Logan, A. G. (1996). Effect of reduced dietary sodium on blood pressure: a meta-analysis of randomized controlled trials. *JAMA, 275*, 1590–1597.

Millar-Craig, M. W., Bishop, C. N., & Raftery, E. B. (1978). Circadian variation of blood-pressure. *Lancet, 1*(8068), 795–797.

Miller, N. H., Hill, M., Kottke, T., & Ockene, I. S. (1997). The multilevel compliance challenge: recommendations for a call to action. A statement for healthcare professionals. *Circulation, 95*(4), 1085–1090.

MRC Working Party. (1992). Medical Research Council trial of treatment of hypertension in older adults: principal results. *BMJ, 304*(6824), 405–412.

Muller-Wieland, D., Kotzka, J., Knebel, B., & Krone, W. (1998). Metabolic syndrome and hypertension: pathophysiology and molecular basis of insulin resistance. *Basic Research in Cardiology, 93*(Suppl 2), 131–134.

Murata, M., & Yoshimoto, H. (1983). Morphological study of the pathogenesis of retinal cotton wool spot. *Japanese Journal of Ophthalmology, 27*(2), 362–379.

Muscholl, M. W., Schunkert, H., Muders, F., Elsner, D., Kuch, B., Hense, H. W., et al. (1998). Neurohormonal activity and left ventricular geometry in patients with essential arterial hypertension. *American Heart Journal, 135*(1), 58–66.

National Heart, L., and Blood Institute. (1988). 1988 Report of the Joint National Committee on detection, evaluation, and treatment of high blood pressure. *Archives of Internal Medicine, 148*, 1023–1038.

National High Blood Pressure Education Program. (1993). *National High Blood Pressure Education Program Working Group Report on Primary Prevention of Hypertension* (No. NIH publication no. 93–2669). Bethesda, MD: U.S. Department of Health and Human Services, National Institutes of Health.

National High Blood Pressure Education Program Working Group. (1994). National High Blood Pressure Education Program Working Group report on hypertension in the elderly. *Hypertension, 23*, 275–285.

National High Blood Pressure Education Program Working Group on Hypertension Control in Children and Adolescents. (1996). Update on the 1987 task force report on high blood pressure in children and adolescents: a working group report from the National High Blood Pressure Education Program. *Pediatrics, 98*, 649–658.

Neaton, J. D., Grimm, R. H., Prineas, R. J., Stamler, J., Grandits, G. A., Elmer, P. J., et al. (1993). Treatment of Mild Hypertension Study: final results. *JAMA, 270*, 713–724.

Neusy, A. J., & Lowenstein, J. (1989). Blood pressure and blood pressure variability following withdrawal of propranolol and clonidine. *Journal of Clinical Pharmacology, 29*(1), 18–24.

Nordmann, A. J., Woo, K., Parkes, R., & Logan, A. G. (2003). Balloon angioplasty or medical therapy for hypertensive patients with atherosclerotic renal artery stenosis? A meta-analysis of randomized controlled trials. *American Journal of Medicine, 114*(1), 44–50.

O'Rourke, M. F. (1999). Arterial stiffness and hypertension. In J. L. Izzo Jr & H. R. Black (Eds.), *Hypertension primer* (2nd ed., pp. 160–162). Baltimore: Lippincott, Williams & Wilkins.

Oberman, A., Wassertheil-Smoller, S., Langford, H. G., Blaufox, M. D., Davis, B. R., Blaszkowski, T., et al. (1990). Pharmacologic and nutritional treatment of mild hypertension: changes in cardiovascular risk status. *Annals of Internal Medicine, 112*, 89–95.

Ockene, J. K., & Ockene, I. S. (1992). Training program. In I. S. Ockene & J. K. Ockene (Eds.), *Prevention of coronary heart disease* (pp. 567–579). Boston: Little, Brown and Company.

Ofili, E. O., Cohen, J. D., St. Vrain, J. A., Pearson, A., Martin, T. J., Uy, N. D., et al. (1998). Effect of treatment of isolated systolic hypertension on left ventricular mass. *JAMA, 279*(10), 778–780.

Oh, H. S., & Seo, W. S. (2001). Development of a structural equation model for causal relationships among arteriosclerosis risk factors. *Public Health Nursing, 18*(6), 409–417.

Oliveria, S. A., Lapuerta, P., McCarthy, B. D., L'Italien, G. J., Berlowitz, D. R., & Asch, S. M. (2002). Physician-related barriers to the effective management of uncontrolled hypertension. *Archives of Internal Medicine, 162*(4), 413–420.

Ostlund, R. E., Staten, M., Kohrt, W. M., Schultz, J., & Malley, M. (1990). The ratio of waist-to-hip circumference, plasma insulin level, and glucose intolerance as independent predictors of the HDL_2 cholesterol level in older adults. *New England Journal of Medicine, 322*, 229–234.

Otten, M. W., Teutsch, S. M., Williamson, D. F., & Marks, J. S. (1990). The effect of known risk factors on the excess mortality of black adults in the United States. *JAMA, 263*, 845–850.

Packer, M., Coats, A. J., Fowler, M. B., Katus, H. A., Krum, H., Mohacsi, P., et al. (2001). Effect of carvedilol on survival in severe chronic heart failure. *New England Journal of Medicine, 344*(22), 1651–1658.

Paffenbarger, R. S., Jr., Hyde, R. T., Wing, A. L., & Hsieh, C.-C. (1986). Physical activity, all-cause mortality, and longevity of college alumni. *New England Journal of Medicine, 314*, 605–613.

Paine-Andrews, A., Harris, K. J., Fawcett, S. B., Richter, K. P., Lewis, R. K., Francisco, V. T., et al. (1997). Evaluating a statewide partnership for reducing risks for chronic diseases. *Journal of Community Health, 22*(5), 343–359.

Panza, J. A. (1997). Endothelial dysfunction in essential hypertension. *Clinical Cardiology, 20*(11 Suppl 2), II-26–33.

Patel, V., & Kohner, E. M. (1994). The eye in hypertension. In J. D. Swales (Ed.), *Textbook of hypertension* (pp. 1015–1025). Oxford: Blackwell Scientific Publications.

Peker, Y., Hedner, J., Norum, J., Kraiczi, H., & Carlson, J. (2002). Increased incidence of cardiovascular disease in middle-aged men with obstructive sleep apnea: a 7-year follow-up. *American Journal of Respiratory Critical Care Medicine, 166*(2), 159–165.

Peppard, P. E., Young, T., Palta, M., & Skatrud, J. (2000). Prospective study of the association between sleep-disordered breathing and hypertension. *New England Journal of Medicine, 342*(19), 1378–1384.

Pepperell, J. C., Ramdassingh-Dow, S., Crosthwaite, N., Mullins, R., Jenkinson, C., Stradling, J. R., et al. (2002). Ambulatory blood pressure after therapeutic and subtherapeutic nasal continuous positive airway pressure for obstructive sleep apnoea: a randomised parallel trial. *Lancet, 359*(9302), 204–210.

Perloff, D., Grim, C., Flack, J., Frohlich, E. D., Hill, M., Mcdonald, M., et al. (1993). Human blood pressure determination by sphygmomanometry. *Circulation, 88*, 2460–2470.

Perseghin, G., Price, T. B., Petersen, K. F., Roden, M., Cline, G. W., Gerow, K., et al. (1996). Increased glucose transport-phosphorylation and muscle glycogen synthesis after exercise training in insulin-resistant subjects. *New England Journal of Medicine, 335*, 1357–1362.

Peterson, J. C., Adler, S., Burkart, J. M., Greene, T., Hebert, L. A., Hunsicker, L. G., et al. (1995). Blood pressure control, proteinuria, and the progression of renal disease. The Modification of Diet in Renal Disease Study. *Annals of Internal Medicine, 123*(10), 754–762.

Pheley, A. M., Terry, P., Pietz, L., Fowles, J., McCoy, C. E., & Smith, H. (1995). Evaluation of a nurse-based hypertension management program: screening, management, and outcomes. *Journal of Cardiovascular Nursing, 9*(2), 54–61.

Pickering, T. G. (1989). Renovascular hypertension: etiology and pathophysiology. *Seminars in Nuclear Medicine, 19*(2), 79–88.

Pitt, B., Remme, W., Zannad, F., Neaton, J., Martinez, F., Roniker, B., et al. (2003). Eplerenone, a selective aldosterone blocker, in patients with left ventricular dysfunction after myocardial infarction. *New England Journal of Medicine, 348*(14), 1309–1321.

Pitt, B., Zannad, F., Remme, W. J., Cody, R., Castaigne, A., Perez, A., et al. (1999). The effect of spironolactone on morbidity and mortality in patients with severe heart failure. Randomized Aldactone Evaluation Study Investigators. *New England Journal of Medicine, 341*(10), 709–717.

Poch, E., Gonzalez, D., Giner, V., Bragulat, E., Coca, A., & de La Sierra, A. (2001). Molecular basis of salt sensitivity in human hypertension. Evaluation of renin-angiotensin-aldosterone system gene polymorphisms. *Hypertension, 38*(5), 1204–1209.

Potter, J. D. (1997). Hazards and benefits of alcohol. *New England Journal of Medicine, 337*(24), 1763–1764.

Psaty, B. M., Heckbert, S. R., Koepsell, T. D., Siscovick, D. S., Raghunathan, T. E., Weiss, N. S., et al. (1995). The risk of myocardial infarction associated with antihypertensive drug therapies. *JAMA, 274*, 620–625.

Psaty, B. M., Smith, N. L., Siscovick, D. S., Koepsell, T. D., Weiss, N. S., Heckbert, S. R., et al. (1997). Health outcomes associated with antihypertensive therapies used as first-line agents. A systematic review and meta-analysis. *JAMA, 277*(9), 739–745.

Puddey, I. B., Parker, M., Beilin, L. J., Vandongen, R., & Masarei, J. R. (1992). Effects of alcohol and caloric restrictions on blood pressure and serum lipids in overweight men. *Hypertension, 20*(4), 533–541.

Pullicino, P. (1999). Pathogenesis of stroke. In J. L. Izzo Jr & H. R. Black (Eds.), *Hypertension primer* (2nd ed., pp. 183–185). Baltimore: Lippincott, Williams & Wilkins.

Puska, P., Tuomilehto, J., Nissinen, A., Salonen, J. T., Vartiainen, E., Pietinen, P., et al. (1989). The North Karelia project: 15 years of community-based prevention of coronary heart disease. *Annals of Medicine, 21*(3), 169–173.

Qureshi, A. I., Suri, M. F., Mohammad, Y., Guterman, L. R., & Hopkins, L. N. (2002). Isolated and borderline isolated systolic hypertension relative to long-term risk and type of stroke: a 20-year follow-up of the national health and nutrition survey. *Stroke, 33*(12), 2781–2788.

Ramirez-Gil, J. F., Delcayre, C., Robert, V., Wassef, M., Trouve, P., Mougenot, N., et al. (1998). In vivo left ventricular function and collagen expression in aldosterone/salt-induced hypertension. *Journal of Cardiovascular Pharmacology, 32*(6), 927–934.

Randomised placebo-controlled trial of effect of ramipril on decline in glomerular filtration rate and risk of terminal renal failure in proteinuric, non-diabetic nephropathy. The GISEN Group (Gruppo Italiano di Studi Epidemiologici in Nefrologia). (1997). *Lancet, 349*(9069), 1857–1863.

Randomised trial of a perindopril-based blood-pressure-lowering regimen among 6,105 individuals with previous stroke or transient ischaemic attack. (2001). *Lancet, 358*(9287), 1033–1041.

A randomised trial of beta-blockade in heart failure. The Cardiac Insufficiency Bisoprolol Study (CIBIS). CIBIS Investigators and Committees. (1994). *Circulation, 90*(4), 1765–1773.

A randomized trial of propranolol in patients with acute myocardial infarction. I. Mortality results. (1982). *JAMA, 247*(12), 1707–1714.

Reaven, G. M., Lithell, H., & Landsberg, L. (1996). Hypertension and associated metabolic abnormalities - the role of insulin resistance and the sympathoadrenal system. *New England Journal of Medicine, 334*, 374–381.

Report of the National High Blood Pressure Education Program Working Group on High Blood Pressure in Pregnancy. (2000). *American Journal of Obstetrics and Gynecology, 183*(1), S1–S22.

Rocha, R., & Funder, J. W. (2002). The pathophysiology of aldosterone in the cardiovascular system. *Annals of the New York Academy of Science, 970*, 89–100.

Rossi, M. A. (1998). Pathologic fibrosis and connective tissue matrix in left ventricular hypertrophy due to chronic arterial hypertension in humans. *Journal of Hypertension, 16*(7), 1031–1041.

Roter, D. L., Hall, J. A., Merisca, R., Nordstrom, B., Cretin, D., & Svarstad, B. (1998). Effectiveness of interventions to improve patient compliance: a meta-analysis. *Medical Care, 36*(8), 1138–1161.

Sacco, R. L., Elkind, M., Boden-Albala, B., Lin, I. F., Kargman, D. E., Hauser, W. A., et al. (1999). The protective effect of moderate alcohol consumption on ischemic stroke. *JAMA, 281*(1), 53–60.

Sacks, F. M., Svetkey, L. P., Vollmer, W. M., Appel, L. J., Bray, G. A., Harsha, D., et al. (2001). Effects on blood pressure of reduced dietary sodium and the Dietary Approaches to Stop Hypertension (DASH) diet. DASH-Sodium Collaborative Research Group. *New England Journal of Medicine, 344*(1), 3–10.

Sagie, A., Larson, M. G., & Levy, D. (1993). The natural history of borderline isolated systolic hypertension. *New England Journal of Medicine, 329*, 1912–1917.

Salonen, J. T., Slater, J. S., Tuomilehto, H., & Rauramaa, R. (1988). Leisure time and occupational physical activity: risk of death from ischemic heart disease. *American Journal of Epidemiology, 127*, 87–94.

Sandvik, L., Erikssen, J., Thaulow, E., Erikssen, G., Mundal, R., & Rodahl, K. (1993). Physical fitness as a predictor of mortality among healthy, middle-aged Norwegian men. *New England Journal of Medicine, 328*, 533–537.

Schafer, J. A. (2002). Abnormal regulation of ENaC: syndromes of salt retention and salt wasting by the collecting duct. *American Journal of Physiology and Renal Physiology, 283*(2), F221–235.

Schieken, R. M., Clarke, W. R., & Lauer, R. M. (1981). Left ventricular hypertrophy in children with blood pressures in the upper quintile of the distribution. The Muscatine Study. *Hypertension, 3*, 669–675.

Schmahl, F. W., & Kahle, P. F. (1996). Screening for risk factors of arteriosclerosis in occupational medicine with special consideration of serum lipids: implications for health policy. *International Journal of Occupational Medicine and Environmental Health,* 9(2), 93–101.

Schmieder, R. E., Martus, P., & Klingbeil, A. (1996). Reversal of left ventricular hypertrophy in essential hypertension. A meta-analysis of randomized double-blind studies. *JAMA,* 275(19), 1507–1513.

Schultz, J. F., & Sheps, S. G. (1994). Management of patients with hypertension: a hypertension clinic model. *Mayo Clinic Proceedings,* 69(10), 997–999.

Sever, P. S., Dahlof, B., Poulter, N. R., Wedel, H., Beevers, G., Caulfield, M., et al. (2003). Prevention of coronary and stroke events with atorvastatin in hypertensive patients who have average or lower-than-average cholesterol concentrations, in the Anglo-Scandinavian Cardiac Outcomes Trial–Lipid Lowering Arm (ASCOT-LLA): a multicentre randomised controlled trial. *Lancet,* 361(9364), 1149–1158.

SHEP Cooperative Research Group. (1991). Prevention of stroke by antihypertensive drug treatment in older persons with Isolated Systolic Hypertension: Final results of the Systolic Hypertension in the Elderly Program (SHEP). *JAMA,* 265, 3255–3264.

Shepherd, J., Cobbe, S. M., Ford, I., Isles, C. G., Lorimer, A. R., Macfarlane, P. W., et al. (1995). Prevention of coronary heart disease with pravastatin in men with hypercholesterolemia. *New England Journal of Medicine,* 333, 1301–1307.

Sherman, S. E., D'Agostino, R. B., Cobb, J. L., & Kannel, W. B. (1994a). Does exercise reduce mortality rates in the elderly? Experience from the Framingham Heart Study. *American Heart Journal,* 128, 965–972.

Sherman, S. E., D'Agostino, R. B., Cobb, J. L., & Kannel, W. B. (1994b). Physical activity and mortality in women in the Framingham Heart Study. *American Heart Journal,* 128, 879–884.

Sibai, B. M. (1996). Treatment of hypertension in pregnant women. *New England Journal of Medicine,* 335(4), 257–265.

Sinaiko, A. R. (1996). Current concepts: hypertension in children. *New England Journal of Medicine,* 335, 1968–1973.

Sinclair, A. M., Isles, C. G., Brown, I., Cameron, H., Murray, G. D., & Robertson, J. W. (1987). Secondary hypertension in a blood pressure clinic. *Archives of Internal Medicine,* 147(7), 1289–1293.

Smith, E. D., Merritt, S. L., & Patel, M. K. (1997). Church-based education: an outreach program for African Americans with hypertension. *Ethnic Health,* 2(3), 243–253.

Sorof, J., & Daniels, S. (2002). Obesity hypertension in children: a problem of epidemic proportions. *Hypertension,* 40(4), 441–447.

Sowers, J. R., & Izzo Jr, J. L. (1999). Endothelial dysfunction. In J. L. Izzo Jr & H. R. Black (Eds.), *Hypertension primer* (2nd ed., pp. 167–169). Baltimore: Lippincott Williams & Wilkins.

Staessen, J., Amery, A., & Fagard, R. (1990). Isolated systolic hypertension in the elderly. *Journal of Hypertension,* 8, 393–405.

Staessen, J. A., Fagard, R., Thijs, L., Celis, H., Arabidze, G. G., Birkenhäger, W. H., et al. (1997). Randomised double-blind comparison of placebo and active treatment for older patients with isolated systolic hypertension. *Lancet,* 350, 757–764.

Staessen, J. A., Gasowski, J., Wang, J. G., Thijs, L., Den Hond, E., Boissel, J. P., et al. (2000). Risks of untreated and treated isolated systolic hypertension in the elderly: meta-analysis of outcome trials. *Lancet,* 355(9207), 865–872.

Stamler, J., Briefel, R. R., Milas, C., Grandits, G. A., & Caggiula, A. W. (1997). Relation of changes in dietary lipids and weight, trial years 1-6, to changes in blood lipids in the special intervention and usual care groups in the Multiple Risk Factor Intervention Trial. *American Journal of Clinical Nutrition,* 65(1 Suppl), 272S–288S.

Stamler, J., Stamler, R., & Neaton, J. D. (1993). Blood pressure, systolic and diastolic, and cardiovascular risks. *Archives of Internal Medicine,* 153, 982–988.

Stamler, R., Shipley, M., Elliott, P., Dyer, A., Sans, S., & Stamler, J. (1992). Higher blood pressure in adults with less education: some explanations from INTERSALT. *Hypertension,* 19, 237–241.

Stamler, R., Stamler, J., Gosch, F. C., Civinelli, J., Fishman, J., McKeever, P., et al. (1989). Primary prevention of hypertension by nutritional-hygienic means. Final report of a randomized, controlled trial [published erratum appears in JAMA 1989 Dec 8;262(22):3132]. *JAMA,* 262(13), 1801–1807.

Stamler, R., Stamler, J., Riedlinger, W. F., Algera, G., & Roberts, R. H. (1978). Weight and blood pressure. Findings in hypertension screening of 1 million Americans. *JAMA,* 240(15), 1607–1610.

Stevens, V. J., Obarzanek, E., Cook, N. R., Lee, I. M., Appel, L. J., Smith West, D., et al. (2001). Long-term weight loss and changes in blood pressure: results of the Trials of Hypertension Prevention, phase II. *Annals of Internal Medicine,* 134(1), 1–11.

Susic, D., Nunez, E., & Frohlich, E. D. (1995). Reversal of hypertrophy: an active biologic process. *Current Opinion in Cardiology,* 10(5), 466–472.

Swales, J. D. (1993). Guidelines on guidelines. *Journal of Hypertension,* 11, 899–903.

Taddei, S., Virdis, A., Mattei, P., Ghiadoni, L., Sudano, I., & Salvetti, A. (1996). Defective L-arginine-nitric oxide pathway in offspring of essential hypertensive patients. *Circulation,* 94(6), 1298–1303.

Tepper, D. (1999). Frontiers in congestive heart failure: Effect of Metoprolol CR/XL in chronic heart failure: Metoprolol CR/XL Randomised Intervention Trial in Congestive Heart Failure (MERIT-HF). *Congestive Heart Failure,* 5(4), 184–185.

Tharaux, P. L., Chatziantoniou, C., Fakhouri, F., & Dussaule, J. C. (2000). Angiotensin II activates collagen I gene through a mechanism involving the MAP/ER kinase pathway. *Hypertension,* 36(3), 330–336.

The Joint National Committee on Prevention Detection Evaluation and Treatment of High Blood Pressure and the National High Blood Pressure Education Program Coordinating Committee. (1997). The Sixth Report of the Joint National Committee on Prevention, Detection, Evaluation, and Treatment of High Blood Pressure. *Archives of Internal Medicine,* 157, 2413–2446.

Thun, M. J., Peto, R., Lopez, A. D., Monaco, J. H., Henley, S. J., Heath, C. W., Jr., et al. (1997). Alcohol consumption and mortality among middle-aged and elderly U.S. adults. *New England Journal of Medicine,* 337(24), 1705–1714.

Thurmann, P. A., Kenedi, P., Schmidt, A., Harder, S., & Rietbrock, N. (1998). Influence of the angiotensin II antagonist valsartan on left ventricular hypertrophy in patients with essential hypertension. *Circulation,* 98(19), 2037–2042.

Toto, R. D., Mitchell, H. C., Smith, R. D., Lee, H. C., McIntire, D., & Pettinger, W. A. (1995). "Strict" blood pressure control and progression of renal disease in hypertensive nephrosclerosis. *Kidney International,* 48(3), 851–859.

Touyz, R. M., & Berry, C. (2002). Recent advances in angiotensin II signaling. *Brazilian Journal of Medical and Biological Research,* 35(9), 1001–1015.

Trials of Hypertension Prevention Collaborative Research Group. (1992). The effects of nonpharmacologic interventions on blood pressure of persons with high normal levels. Results of the Trials of Hypertension Prevention, Phase I. *JAMA,* 267, 1213–1220.

Trials of Hypertension Prevention Collaborative Research Group. (1997). Effects of weight loss and sodium reduction intervention on blood pressure and hypertension incidence in overweight people with high-normal blood pressure: the Trials of Hypertension Prevention, phase II. *Archives of Internal Medicine,* 157, 657–667.

Tsao, P. S., Niebauer, J., Buitrago, R., Lin, P. S., Wang, B. Y., Cooke, J. P., et al. (1998). Interaction of diabetes and hypertension on determinants of endothelial adhesiveness. *Arteriosclerosis Thrombosis Vascular Biology,* 18(6), 947–953.

Tu, K., Mamdani, M. M., & Tu, J. V. (2002). Hypertension guidelines in elderly patients: is anybody listening? *American Journal of Medicine,* 113(1), 52–58.

US Department of Health and Human Services. (1996). *Physical activity and health: A Report of the Surgeon General.* Atlanta, Ga: US Department of Health and Human Services, Centers for Disease Control and Prevention, National Center for Chronic Disease Prevention and Health Promotion.

Uzu, T., Ishikawa, K., Fujii, T., Nakamura, S., Inenaga, T., & Kimura, G. (1997). Sodium restriction shifts circadian rhythm of blood pressure from nondipper to dipper in essential hypertension. *Circulation,* 96(6), 1859–1862.

Uzu, T., Nishimura, M., Fujii, T., Takeji, M., Kuroda, S., Nakamura, S., et al. (1998). Changes in the circadian rhythm of blood pressure in primary aldosteronism in response to dietary sodium restriction and adrenalectomy. *Journal of Hypertension,* 16(12 Pt 1), 1745–1748.

Varon, J., & Marik, P. E. (2000). The diagnosis and management of hypertensive crises. *Chest,* 118(1), 214–227.

Vasan, R. S., Beiser, A., Seshadri, S., Larson, M. G., Kannel, W. B., D'Agostino, R. B., et al. (2002). Residual lifetime risk for developing hypertension in middle-aged women and men: The Framingham Heart Study. *JAMA,* 287(8), 1003–1010.

Vasan, R. S., Larson, M. G., Leip, E. P., Kannel, W. B., & Levy, D. (2001). Assessment of frequency of progression to hypertension in non-hypertensive participants in the Framingham Heart Study: a cohort study. *Lancet,* 358(9294), 1682–1686.

Veterans Administration Cooperative Study Group on Antihypertensive Agents. (1967). Effects of treatment on morbidity in hypertension: results in patients with diastolic blood pressures averaging 115 through 129 mm Hg. *JAMA,* 202, 116–122.

Veterans Administration Cooperative Study Group on Antihypertensive Agents. (1970). Effects of treatment on morbidity in hypertension. II. results in aptients with diastolic blood pressure averaging 90 through 114 mm Hg. *JAMA*, 213, 1143–1152.

Vidt, D. G. (1999). Management of hypertensive emergencies and urgencies. In J. L. Izzo Jr & H. R. Black (Eds.), *Hypertension primer* (2nd ed., pp. 437–440). Baltimore: Lippincott, Williams & Wilkins.

Vita, A. J., Terry, R. B., Hubert, H. B., & Fries, J. F. (1998). Aging, health risks, and cumulative disability. *New England Journal of Medicine*, 338, 1035–1041.

Voors, A. W., Webber, L. S., & Berenson, G. S. (1978). Relationship of blood pressure levels to height and weight in children. *Journal of Cardiovascular Medicine*, 3, 911–918.

Wallace, P., Cutler, S., & Haines, A. (1988). Randomised controlled trial of general practitioner intervention in patients with excessive alcohol consumption. *BMJ*, 297(6649), 663–668.

Wang, P. S., Bohn, R. L., Knight, E., Glynn, R. J., Mogun, H., & Avorn, J. (2002). Noncompliance with antihypertensive medications: the impact of depressive symptoms and psychosocial factors. *Journal of General Internal Medicine*, 17(7), 504–511.

Wassertheil-Smoller, S., Oberman, A., Blaufox, M. D., Davis, B., & Langford, H. (1992). The Trial of Antihypertensive Interventions and Management (TAIM) Study. Final results with regard to blood pressure, cardiovascular risk, and quality of life. *AJH*, 5, 37–44.

Weber, M. A. (2002). Clinical implications of aldosterone blockade. *American Heart Journal*, 144(5 Suppl.), S12–18.

Weder, A. B. (1998). Pathogenesis of hypertension: genetic and environmental factors. In N. K. Hollenberg (Ed.), *Hypertension: mechanisms and therapy* (2nd ed., pp. 1.1–1.28). Philadelphia: Current Medicine.

Weinberger, M. H., Cohen, S. J., Miller, J. Z., Luft, F. C., Grim, C. E., & Fineberg, N. S. (1988). Dietary sodium restriction as adjunctive treatment of hypertension. *JAMA*, 259, 2561–2565.

Westheim, A., & Os, I. (1992). Physical activity and the metabolic cardiovascular syndrome. *Journal of Cardiovascular Pharmacology*, 20(Suppl. 8), S49–53.

Whelton, P. K., Appel, L. J., Espeland, M. A., Applegate, W. B., Ettinger, W. H., Kostis, J. B., et al. (1998). Sodium reduction and weight loss in the treatment of hypertension in older persons: a randomized controlled trial of nonpharmacologic interventions in the elderly (TONE). *JAMA*, 279, 839–846.

Whelton, P. K., He, J., Appel, L. J., Cutler, J. A., Havas, S., Kotchen, T. A., et al. (2002). Primary prevention of hypertension: clinical and public health advisory from The National High Blood Pressure Education Program. *JAMA*, 288(15), 1882–1888.

Whelton, S. P., Chin, A., Xin, X., & He, J. (2002). Effect of aerobic exercise on blood pressure: a meta-analysis of randomized, controlled trials. Annals of Internal Medicine, 136(7), 493–503.

Williams, M. V., Baker, D. W., Parker, R. M., & Nurss, J. R. (1998). Relationship of functional health literacy to patients' knowledge of their chronic disease. A study of patients with hypertension and diabetes. Archives of Internal Medicine, 158(2), 166–172.

Wilson, F. H., Disse-Nicodeme, S., Choate, K. A., Ishikawa, K., Nelson-Williams, C., Desitter, I., et al. (2001). Human hypertension caused by mutations in WNK kinases. *Science*, 293(5532), 1107–1112.

Windhauser, M. M., Ernst, D. B., Karanja, N. M., Crawford, S. W., Redican, S. E., Swain, J. F., et al. (1999). Translating the Dietary Approaches to Stop Hypertension diet from research to practice: dietary and behavior change techniques. DASH Collaborative Research Group. *Journal of the American Dietetic Association*, 99(8 Suppl.), S90–95.

Wing, L. M., Reid, C. M., Ryan, P., Beilin, L. J., Brown, M. A., Jennings, G. L., et al. (2003). A comparison of outcomes with angiotensin-converting–enzyme inhibitors and diuretics for hypertension in the elderly. *New England Journal of Medicine*, 348(7), 583–592.

Wolf-Maier, K., Cooper, R. S., Banegas, J. R., Giampaoli, S., Hense, H. W., Joffres, M., et al. (2003). Hypertension prevalence and blood pressure levels in 6 European countries, Canada, and the United States. *JAMA*, 289(18), 2363–2369.

Wong, Z. Y., Stebbing, M., Ellis, J. A., Lamantia, A., & Harrap, S. B. (1999). Genetic linkage of beta and gamma subunits of epithelial sodium channel to systolic blood pressure. *Lancet*, 353(9160), 1222–1225.

Working Group to Define Critical Patient Behaviors in High Blood Pressure Control. (1979). Critical patient behaviors in high blood pressure control: guidelines for professionals. *JAMA*, 241, 2534–2537.

Wright, J. T., Jr., Agodoa, L., Contreras, G., Greene, T., Douglas, J. G., Lash, J., et al. (2002). Successful blood pressure control in the African American

Study of Kidney Disease and Hypertension. *Archives of Internal Medicine*, 162(14), 1636–1643.

Wright, R. R., & Mathews, K. D. (1996). Hypertensive encephalopathy in childhood. *Journal of Childhood Neurology*, 11(3), 193–196.

Xin, X., He, J., Frontini, M. G., Ogden, L. G., Motsamai, O. I., & Whelton, P. K. (2001). Effects of alcohol reduction on blood pressure: a meta-analysis of randomized controlled trials. *Hypertension*, 38(5), 1112–1117.

Young, W. F., Jr. (2003). Minireview: primary aldosteronism–changing concepts in diagnosis and treatment. *Endocrinology*, 144(6), 2208–2213.

Yusuf, S., Sleight, P., Pogue, J., Bosch, J., Davies, R., & Dagenais, G. (2000). Effects of an angiotensin-converting-enzyme inhibitor, ramipril, on cardiovascular events in high-risk patients. The Heart Outcomes Prevention Evaluation Study Investigators. *New England Journal of Medicine*, 342(3), 145–153.

Zhu, X., Chang, Y. P., Yan, D., Weder, A., Cooper, R., Luke, A., et al. (2003). Associations between hypertension and genes in the renin-angiotensin system. *Hypertension*, 41(5), 1027–1034.

Zou, Y., Hu, Y., Metzler, B., & Xu, Q. (1998). Signal transduction in arteriosclerosis: mechanical stress-activated MAP kinases in vascular smooth muscle cells. *International Journal of Molecular Medicine*, 1(5), 827–834.

REFERENCES FOR CLINICAL TRIALS LISTED IN TABLE 39-10

ACC/AHA Heart Failure Guideline (Hunt, Baker et al., 2001)

Merit-HF (Tepper, 1999)

Copernicus (Packer, Coats et al., 2001)

CIBIS ("A randomized trial of beta-blockade in heart failure. The Cardiac Insufficiency Bisoprolol Study (CIBIS). CIBIS Investigators and Committees," 1994)

SOLVD ("Effect of enalapril on survival in patients with reduced left ventricular ejection fractions and congestive heart failure. The SOLVD Investigators," 1991)

AIRE ("Effect of ramipril on mortality and morbidity of survivors of acute myocardial infarction with clinical evidence of heart failure. The Acute Infarction Ramipril Efficacy (AIRE) Study Investigators," 1993)

TRACE (Kober, Torp-Pedersen et al., 1995)

ValHEFT (Cohn & Tognoni, 2001)

RALES (Pitt, Zannad et al., 1999)

ACC/AHA Post-MI Guideline (Braunwald, Antman et al., 2002)

BHAT ("A randomized trial of propranolol in patients with acute myocardial infarction. I. Mortality results," 1982)

SAVE (Hager, Davis et al., 1998)

Capricorn (Dargie, 2001)

EPHESUS (Pitt, Remme et al., 2003)

UKPDS ("Efficacy of atenolol and captopril in reducing risk of macrovascular and microvascular complications in type 2 diabetes: UKPDS 39. UK Prospective Diabetes Study Group," 1998)

ALLHAT ("Major outcomes in high-risk hypertensive patients randomized to angiotensin-converting enzyme inhibitor or calcium-channel blocker vs diuretic: The Antihypertensive and Lipid-Lowering Treatment to Prevent Heart Attack Trial (ALLHAT)," 2002)

HOPE (Yusuf, Sleight et al., 2000)

ANBP2 (Wing, Reid et al., 2003)

LIFE (Dahlof, Devereux et al., 2002)

CONVINCE (Black, Elliott et al., 2003)

NKF-ADA Guideline (Arauz-Pacheco, Parrott et al., 2003; "K/DOQI clinical practice guidelines for chronic kidney disease: evaluation, classification, and stratification. Kidney Disease Outcome Quality Initiative," 2002)

Captopril Trial (Lewis, Hunsicker et al., 1993)

RENAAL (Brenner, Cooper et al., 2001)

IDNT (Lewis, Hunsicker et al., 2001)

REIN ("Randomised placebo-controlled trial of effect of ramipril on decline in glomerular filtration rate and risk of terminal renal failure in proteinuric, non-diabetic nephropathy. The GISEN Group (Gruppo Italiano di Studi Epidemiologici in Nefrologia)," 1997)

AASK (Wright, Jr., Agodoa et al., 2002)

PROGRESS ("Randomised trial of a perindopril-based blood-pressure-lowering regimen among 6,105 individuals with previous stroke or transient ischaemic attack," 2001)

40

Lipid Management and Coronary Heart Disease

JOAN M. FAIR • KATHLEEN A. BERRA

Coronary heart disease (CHD) is the leading cause of death for American women and men and is responsible for 39.4% of all deaths or approximately 1 in every 2.5 deaths (American Heart Association, 2002). Elevated serum cholesterol and, particularly, elevated low-density lipoprotein (LDL) cholesterol are significant and modifiable risk factors associated with the development and progression of CHD. More than 105 million Americans have a total blood cholesterol higher than the desirable level of 200 mg/dL (American Heart Association, 2002). Furthermore, more than 42 million Americans have a blood cholesterol more thane 240 mg/dL, a level at which current treatment guidelines recommend the initiation of dietary or pharmacologic interventions (American Heart Association, 2002; National Cholesterol Education Program, 2001). There is a large body of evidence, including animal studies (Armstrong, 1970), observational studies (Anderson, 1987), and more than 50 clinical trials, that consistently point to a relationship between high blood lipids and CHD.

Table 40-1 summarizes the results of the more recent, large cholesterol-lowering primary and secondary prevention trials (Downs et al., 1988; National Cholesterol Education Program, 2001; Scandinavian Simvastatin Survival Study, 1995; Sacks, 1996; Shepherd et al., 1995; LIPID Study Group, 1998). Meta-analyses of the cholesterol-lowering clinical trials estimated that a 10-mg reduction in total cholesterol results in a 22% reduction in CHD incidence after 2 years of intervention, and a 25% reduction after 5 years (Gould, 1995). There is some evidence that cholesterol lowering begun at an early age (eg, age 40 years) may provide greater risk reduction than if started at a later age (eg, age 70 years) (Law, 1999). It has recently been reported that the total cholesterol levels in American adults have changed little since 1994. In this survey, only 35 % of American adults with total cholesterol levels higher than 200 mg/dL were aware that they had hypercholesterolemia (Ford et al., 2003). This information shows that both the incidence of high blood cholesterol and the benefits of treatment are substantial. Cardiovascular nurses need to understand hyperlipidemia and actively participate in its treatment and management.

In May 2001, the Third Report of the National Cholesterol Education Program (NCEP) Expert Panel on Detection, Evaluation, and Treatment of High Blood Cholesterol in Adults (ATP III) was released. This chapter focuses on new recommendations for evaluation, identification, and treatment based on these new guidelines (National Cholesterol Education Program, 2001).

BLOOD LIPIDS: STRUCTURE AND FUNCTIONS

The complex relationships between genetic and metabolic mechanisms and the molecular interactions within the cell wall help explain the association between lipid abnormalities and CHD. The major lipid particles, cholesterol and triglycerides, both have important functions in the body. Cholesterol is an essential component of cell membranes, functioning to provide stability while permitting membrane transport; it is a precursor to adrenal steroids, sex hormones, and bile and bile acids. Triglycerides are the major source of energy for the body. Both cholesterol and triglycerides are insoluble molecules and must be transported in the circulation as lipoproteins.

Lipoproteins are complexes of nonpolar lipid cores (triglycerides and cholesterol esters) surrounded by a surface coat of polar lipids (phospholipids and free cholesterol) and specific proteins called apoproteins. Total cholesterol, for example, is composed of 18 different lipid and lipoprotein particles (Castelli, 1996). Lipoproteins can be classified according to their density, their migration on an electrophoretic field, or their lipid and apoprotein composition (Schaefer & Levy, 1985).

During the 1980s, significant advances were made in determining the function of the apoproteins, the lipid processing enzymes, and lipoprotein receptors. Apoproteins function as more than transport vehicles; they have variant properties that activate enzyme systems or receptor sites to promote the catabolism or removal of lipoproteins from the circulation (Gotto, 1983). The functions of nine apoproteins in the lipid metabolic cascade have been identified: apo A-I, apo A-II, apo B-100, apo B-48, apo C-I, apo C-II, apo C-III, apo E2, apo E3, apo E4, and lipoprotein(a) [Lp(a)]. In addition, the actions of several lipoprotein-processing enzymes (lipoprotein lipase [LPL], hepatic lipase, lecithin cholesterol acyltransferase [LCAT], and cholesterol ester transfer protein) and the function of cell receptors, including the

Table 40–1 ■ LARGE, RANDOMIZED, CLINICAL TRIALS USING STATIN THERAPY TO LOWER CHOLESTEROL

Trial	Number of Patients	Age (y)	Lipids (mean, mg/dl)	Length of Follow-up	Mean Lipid Reduction	Outcomes
Primary Prevention						
West of Scotland (WOSCOPS)	6,595 men	45–64	TC: 272 LDL: 192	4.9 y	TC: 20% LDL: 26%	Nonfatal MI and CHD death: 31%
AFCAPS/TEXCAPS	5,608 men, 997 women		TC: 221 LDL: 150	5.2 y	TC:18% LDL: 25%	Major coronary events (MI, unstable angina, or sudden cardiac death: 37%)
Secondary Prevention						
Scandinavian Simvastatin Survival Study (4S)	3,617 men, 427 women	35–70	TC LDL: 188	5.4 y	TC: 28% LDL: 38%	CHD deaths: 42% Nonfatal MI and CHD death: 37%
Care	4,159	5	LDL:139		LDL: 27%	Major coronary Events 25%, Coronary Mortality 24%, Total Mortality 9%
Lipid	9,014	5	LDL:150		LDL: 25%	Major Coronary Events 29%, Coronary Mortality 24%, Total Mortality 23%

CHD, coronary heart disease; LDL, low-density lipoprotein; MI, myocardial infarction; TC, total cholesterol.

LDL and chylomicron remnant receptor, are now established. These advances permit an understanding of lipid metabolism, as well as the abnormalities leading to elevated blood cholesterol.

LIPID METABOLISM AND TRANSPORT

The gut and liver are responsible for the production of the six principal lipoproteins. Exogenous lipoproteins are formed in the mucosa of the small intestine after digestion of dietary fats. During the digestive process, hydrolyzed products of ingested fats enter epithelial cells of the small intestine, where they are converted into triglycerides and cholesterol esters. These products are then aggregated into the lipoprotein complexes known as chylomicrons. Chylomicrons pass into small lymph vessels and reach the circulatory system through the thoracic duct. In the peripheral capillaries, chylomicrons are hydrolyzed by the enzyme LPL, located on the capillary endothelium. Free fatty acids and glycerol then enter adipose tissue cells. A cholesterol-rich chylomicron remnant (a second lipoprotein complex) is released into the circulation when lipolysis is nearly complete. Chylomicron remnants are cleared rapidly by the liver (Grundy, 1984; Grundy, 1984) (Fig. 40-1).

In the liver, the endogenous lipoprotein cascade begins with the production of very-low-density lipoproteins (VLDL). Triglycerides are resynthesized from chylomicrons and packaged with specific apoproteins, apo B-100, apo C-I, apo C-II, and apo E, to form VLDL. Once VLDL is released into the circulation, intermediate-density lipoproteins (IDL) and VLDL remnants are formed from VLDL lipolysis. This process takes place in the capillary endothelium and is mediated by LPL, the same enzyme responsible for the hydrolysis of chylomicrons. Apo C-II also acts as a cofactor in these processes (Breslow, 1992).

Low-density lipoprotein receptors in the liver recognize and bind with apo E on the IDL particle and remove approximately half of the IDL from the circulation. The remainder is converted by hepatic lipase into smaller cholesterol-rich lipoproteins known as LDLs. Apo B-100 is the remaining protein left on the surface coat of LDL particles. The LDL receptors on cells of the liver and

EXOGENOUS PATHWAY

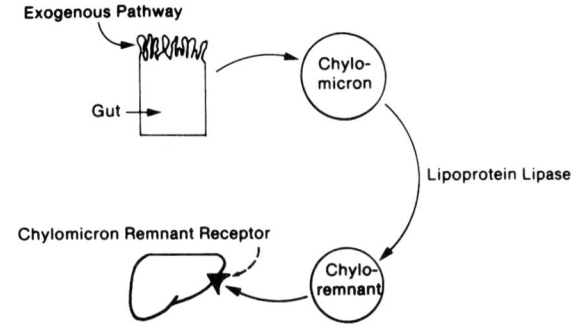

■ **Figure 40–1.** The exogenous metabolism of lipoproteins and the transport of chylomicrons to the tissues and chylomicron remnants to the liver. (From American Heart Association. [1987]. *Professional cholesterol education program.* Dallas: American Heart Association. Reproduced by permission of the American Heart Association, Inc.)

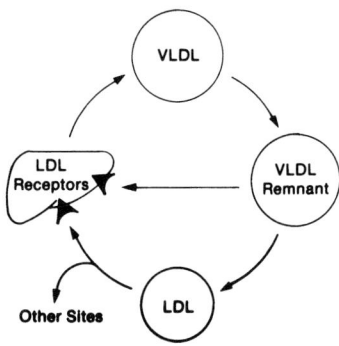

■ **Figure 40–2.** The endogenous lipid transport system originates in the liver. Low-density lipoproteins provide essential cholesterol to the tissue cells. (From American Heart Association. [1987]. *Professional cholesterol education program.* Dallas: American Heart Association. Reproduced by permission of the American Heart Association, Inc.)

other organs that require cholesterol for structural and metabolic functions bind with apo B-100 and facilitate the removal of LDL from the blood. Figure 40-2 illustrates the endogenous pathway. The LDL particle is the major cholesterol-carrying lipoprotein in the blood and, consequently, the most atherogenic lipoprotein Schaefer & Levy, 1985). Under normal conditions, more than 93% of the cholesterol in the body is located in the cells, and only 7% circulates in the blood. Two thirds of the blood cholesterol is carried by LDL. Increased cellular uptake of cholesterol through the LDL receptor pathway suppresses the cell's own synthesis of cholesterol by inhibiting the hydroxymethylglutaryl coenzyme-A (HMG-CoA) reductase enzyme. This enzyme determines the rate of cholesterol synthesis. As cellular cholesterol levels increase, the activity of the LDL receptor is down-regulated, and synthesis of new LDL receptors is inhibited (Goldstein & Brown, 1987). These feedback control mechanisms serve as the rationale for determining the treatment of elevated blood cholesterol.

Several metabolic and genetic disorders can be related to elevated LDL cholesterol levels. Habitually high dietary intakes of saturated fats and cholesterol beyond that needed for cell functions result in blood levels of LDL beyond normal and result in inhibited LDL receptor activity. High LDL levels also can result from a decrease in clearance of LDL because of a deficiency in LDL receptors. This deficiency may be caused by genetic abnormalities in the structure of the receptor binding sites (where apolipoproteins bind) or by a decrease in LDL receptors on the surface of cells. In addition, genetic mutation in apoproteins, particularly apo E and apo B-100, can result in decreased cholesterol clearance. The metabolic consequence is an increased blood level of this atherogenic lipoprotein and the synthesis of cholesterol within cells, a process normally suppressed by LDL uptake.

REVERSE CHOLESTEROL TRANSPORT

The intestine and liver are responsible for synthesizing the precursors for the high-density lipoprotein (HDL). HDL and its major apoproteins facilitate the transport of excess cholesterol from tissues to the liver. The major apolipoprotein components of HDL are apo A-I, A-II, C-II, C-III, and E. The apolipoprotein components, primarily apo A-I and phos-

pholipid constituents, such as lecithin, form incomplete (or nascent) HDL precursors. The precursors are converted to a stable spherical particle through the action of the blood enzyme, LCAT, which converts free cholesterol in the tissues into a cholesteryl ester core (Gotto, 1983; Tall & Small, 1978). Apo A-I has been shown to activate LCAT and may influence the activity of the cholesteryl ester transfer protein (Tall, 1998). Apo C-II is a cofactor for LPL. In the presence of circulating triglycerides, apo C-II moves from HDL to the triglyceride particle, activating LPL and promoting the catabolism of VLDL (Miller, 1990). This mechanism, in part, explains the clinical observation of an inverse association between high triglycerides and low HDL levels. A third apoprotein, apo E, is thought to facilitate direct transfer of cholesterol esters to hepatocyte receptors (Miller, 1990). Cholesterol esters are then excreted in bile or bile acids (Rifkind, 1991). Although the protective effect of HDL has been linked to its role in the reverse transport of cholesterol, it is clear that other factors, particularly genetic factors, determine coenzyme, apoprotein, and receptor activity. In fact, it is estimated that 50% to 70% of the variation in HDL is genetically determined influencing the receptor and enzyme activity involved in the catabolism of HDL (deLemos et al., 2002). Recent studies have found that plasma HDL levels are regulated by a class of enzymes including lipoprotein lipase (LPL), hepatic lipase (HL), and endothelial lipase (EL) (Cohen, 2003). LPL is synthesized by adipose and skeletal muscle cells and acts primarily on hydrolysis of triglycerides. HL is synthesized in the liver cells and acts on triglyceride and phospholipid catabolism. EL is synthesized in endothelial cells and appears to regulate HDL levels by preventing the transfer of triglycerides and remnant particles to HDL. Evidence includes genetically modified animal models that overexpress EL show a marked decrease in HDL levels (Ishida, 2003) and human studies observing genetic variants in the EL gene in persons with high HDL levels (deLemos, 2002). It is still not known if EL alters HDL composition. At present, there are two major subclasses of HDL based on density and apoprotein composition. HDL_3 is richer in apo A-II than HDL_2, which has a higher concentration of apo A-I (Eisenberg, 1984). Production of apo A-I is higher in women than in men and is increased by exercise training, alcohol consumption, and estrogen administration (Schaefer & Levy, 1985). Premenopausal women have more than three-times the concentration of HDL_2 than do men. Studies have also suggested that HDL may act as an antioxidant, preventing the oxidation of LDL (Brown et al., 1998; Tall, 1998).

High-density lipoproteins are not atherogenic; rather, increased circulating levels of HDL may well be antiatherogenic (Grundy, 1984). High HDL has been associated with a reduced risk of CHD (Gordon, et al., 1998; Scandinavian Simvastatin Survival Study, 1995; The Lipid Research Clinic Investigators, 1984). It has been suggested that the protective effect of HDL is greater than the atherogenic effect of LDL cholesterol. For men in the Framingham Heart Study, a 50% reduction in coronary risk was found with every 10-mg/dL increment in HDL (Kannel, 1983). Studies have indicated that increased apo A-I levels may also be inversely related to CHD (Eisenberg, 1984). Clinical trial data demonstrated that pharmacological increases of HDL cholesterol significantly decreased coronary and stroke events among CHD patients (Asztalos & Schaefer, 2003). Given the protective role of HDL, lipid disorders of combined elevated blood LDL and decreased levels of protective HDL present the major risk for CHD (Kannel, 1983).

LOW-DENSITY LIPOPROTEIN VARIANTS

Low-Density Lipoprotein Particle Size

Mounting evidence suggests that the size of the LDL particle plays an important role in its atherogenicity. Particle size is determined by flotation rates after ultracentrifugation procedures. LDL can be separated into a small dense LDL particle (phenotype B) and a larger less dense LDL particle (phenotype A) (Austin, et al., 1994). Clinical trial evidence suggests that people with a predominance of small dense LDL particles have a higher incidence of CHD and more accelerated progression of coronary lesions (Gardner et al., 1996). The exact mechanism of the negative influence of the small dense LDL particle is not completely understood. One possible explanation is that the smaller denser particles have a greater ability to penetrate the endothelial space and participate fully in the subendothelial atherosclerotic process. Small LDL particles also appear to be more susceptible to oxidation than larger LDL particles (deGraaf et al., 1991). In addition, the small dense LDL particle is most commonly found in conjunction with a constellation of other factors, including hypertriglyceridemia, low HDL cholesterol, and insulin resistance (Reaven, 1993).

Research also suggests that it is possible to increase (alter) the size of the LDL particle to the larger (phenotype A) size by reducing triglycerides and normalizing insulin sensitivity. In addition, lipid-lowering drugs such as bile acid-binding resins, niacin, and the fibrates are reported to alter particle size favorably (Austin, et al., 1994).

Oxidized Low-Density Lipoprotein

Ongoing research in lipid metabolism is investigating the issue of oxidation. Molecular biologists have established that modified or oxidized LDL is taken up more rapidly in vitro by monocytes and macrophages than is native LDL (Axelson et al., 1985; Block et al., 1988).

Oxidized LDL has been found to be cytotoxic, and it is postulated that this facilitates endothelial injury, leading to the development of fatty streaks and atherosclerotic lesions. Oxidative inhibitors can block the modification of LDL to an oxidized form. Studies are ongoing in this area.

The Role of Lipoprotein(a)

Genetic researchers investigating variant LDL particles uncovered a lipoprotein, Lp(a), that is similar to LDL except for the addition a large protein linked to apo B-100. Elevated levels of Lp(a) have been shown to be an independent risk factor for CHD, conferring a six-fold increase in risk. Lp(a) has also been detected in atherosclerotic plaques (Lawn, 1992). Gene cloning allowed researchers to determine that the Lp(a) protein is similar in DNA sequence to plasminogen, a substance that breaks up blood clots. It is hypothesized that this variant LDL evolved at a time when our ancestors had markedly lower levels

Table 40–2 ■ LIPID ABNORMALITIES AND ASSOCIATED MECHANISMS

Lipid Abnormality	Mechanisms
Elevated total cholesterol	High dietary intake of saturated fat and cholesterol
	LDL receptor deficiency or down regulation
Elevated LDL-cholesterol	LDL receptor deficiency
	Apoprotein B-100 genetic defect
	High dietary intake of saturated fat and cholesterol
Elevated triglycerides	Deficiency in lipoprotein lipase
	Obesity, physical inactivity, insulin resistance, glucose intolerance
	Excessive alcohol intake
Low HDL	Apoprotein A-1 deficiency
	Reduced VLDL clearance
	Cigarette smoking, physical inactivity
	Insulin resistance
	Elevated triglycerides
	Overweight and obesity
	Very high CHO intake (>60% total calories) Certain drugs (beta-blockers, anabolic steroids, progestational agents)
Increased lipoprotein remnants (VLDL is a surrogate marker for Lipoprotein remnants when Tg is >200 mg/dL)	Defective apolipoprotein E Seen in familial combined hyperlipidemia
Lipoprotein(a)	Level is genetically determined
Small LDL particles	Particle Size is determined by level of Triglycerides; LDL particle is denser and more atherogenic at higher levels of TG
HDL Subspecies	Low levels of HDL 2 and 3 may increase CHD risk ?genetically determined vs lifestyle and other lipid levels
Apoliprotein B	May be potential marker for all atherogenic lipoprotein
Apoliprotein A-1	Increased CHD risk when Apo A-1 is low
Combined dsylipidemias Small, dense LDL, high triglycerides, low HDL Elevated LDL and triglycerides	Defects in VLDL and LDL receptor activities coexisting with environmental influences such as obesity, physical inactivity, diet high in saturated fat, and cigarette smoking

HDL, high-density lipoprotein; LDL, low-density lipoprotein; VLDL, vary-low-density lipoprotein.
National Cholesterol Education Program, 2001; Stone et al., 1997.

of blood cholesterol and that it would assist in wound healing, bringing needed cholesterol to repair cell membranes (Lawn, 1992). More research is needed to provide a full understanding of the role of Lp(a). Like Lp(a), there are a number of emerging lipid risk factors that may further explain the relationship of dyslipidemia to coronary heart disease (Table 40-2).

CHOLESTEROL AND ENDOTHELIAL FUNCTION

Serum cholesterol levels and diets high in fat have been associated with impairments in endothelial functioning. The endothelium acts to regulate vascular tone, platelet adhesion, thrombosis, and growth factors (Fair & Berra, 1996). Studies have demonstrated that elevated cholesterol results in a reduced vasodilation response. Furthermore, when cholesterol is lowered, vasodilation responses improve (Treasure et al., 1995).

Elevated cholesterol also increases platelet aggregation and monocyte adhesion, factors that lead to thrombus formation and plaque rupture (Levine et al., 1995). Continuing research suggests that the lipids influence a variety of endothelial responses that appear to contribute to the atherosclerotic process.

DYSLIPIDEMIC DISORDERS

Although the metabolic processes related to blood lipids are complex and influenced by both genetic and environmental factors, the management of dyslipidemia has been well characterized. National recommendations have been developed based on scientific evidence and taking into account the need for both primary and secondary prevention of CHD (National Cholesterol Education Program, 2001). In general, lipid disorders can be characterized by the specific lipid abnormalities observed (see Table 40-2).

HYPERCHOLESTEROLEMIA

Hypercholesterolemia is the most common dyslipidemia and, in most people, decreased LDL clearance is responsible for the observed abnormality. A high intake of dietary cholesterol and saturated fatty acids down-regulates LDL receptor activity and receptor synthesis, resulting in decreased LDL clearance (Brown et al., 1986).

Familial (Severe) Hypercholesterolemia

Severe hypercholesterolemia is caused most commonly by a genetic disorder and is known as familial hypercholesterolemia (FH). There are two types of FH, heterozygous and homozygous. Plasma LDL cholesterol normally binds to cell membrane receptors and is taken into the cell for several biologic functions. In heterozygous FH, there is one normal gene and one abnormal gene for the LDL receptor.

Because only half the normal number of LDL receptors are synthesized, LDL is removed from the blood at two-thirds the normal rate (Goldstein & Brown, 1987). The result is a two- to three-fold increase in blood LDL levels. One person in 500 is thought to have this genetic disorder, which eventually results in an increased risk for myocardial infarction (MI) (National Cholesterol Education Program, 2001). The homozygous form of FH develops when two abnormal genes are inherited. The 1 in one million people who have this disorder have LDL levels six-times normal and may have an MI as early as age 5 to 15 years (Goldstein & Brown, 1987; National Cholesterol Education Program, 2001). In addition, a genetic defect related to apo B-100 results in marked elevations in LDL cholesterol.

Hypertriglyceridemia

The relationship between triglycerides and CHD is not clear. Elevated serum triglyceride levels have been associated with CHD. However, the strength of the association is diminished when other CHD risks are accounted for, leading some to suggest that elevated triglycerides are a marker for other atherogenic factors (Grundy, 1998). Chylomicrons and VLDL are lipoprotein carriers of triglyceride and, whereas chylomicrons are not considered to be atherogenic, the remnants of VLDL catabolism are smaller particles that are richer in cholesterol esters (Grundy, 1998). These remnant particles, or IDL, are considered more atherogenic (Krauss, 1988). Elevated triglycerides are frequently observed in people who also have low HDL levels and small dense LDL particles. This combination of lipid abnormalities is considered an atherogenic phenotype (Grundy, 1998). In addition, elevated triglycerides (and its associated small dense LDL particle size and low HDL cholesterol) commonly exist with insulin resistance (with or without glucose intolerance), hypertension, obesity (particularly abdominal obesity pattern), and prothrombotic and proinflamatory states. This combination of risk factors is commonly called the metabolic syndrome and is linked to increased CHD risk (National Cholesterol Education Program, 2001). These associations suggest that elevated triglycerides may be a marker for other CHD risk factors. Diabetes also results in increased plasma triglyceride levels because of increased VLDL. HDL is often low in diabetic patients as a result of increased hepatic lipase triglyceride activity. LDL cholesterol is more glycated in diabetic patients compared with nondiabetic subjects. Glycated LDL particles have increased oxidative susceptibility (Grundy, 1998). High triglyceride levels are also related to high carbohydrate and alcohol intake. As a marker for CHD risk, the reduction of plasma triglyceride levels to less than 150 mg/dL is a desirable goal (National Cholesterol Education Program, 2001). Although not designated as an independent risk predictor by ATP III, the importance of elevated triglycerides is recognized in a number of ways. In ATP III, triglyceride level is seen as a marker of elevated atherogenic remnant particle level thought to increase risk of CAD and as an indication of lipid and nonlipid risk factors in the metabolic syndrome (National Cholesterol Education Program, 2001).

In addition, normal triglyceride level has been lowered to 150 mg/dL or less compared to ATP II (Nation Cholesterol Education Program, 2001; National Cholesterol Education Program, 1993). A new target for persons with elevated triglycerides is called "non-HDL cholesterol." Non-HDL cholesterol is the total cholesterol minus the HDL cholesterol. This number represents the sum of the LDL and the VLDL cholesterol in determining a treatment goal for LDL cholesterol. The goal for LDL cholesterol is 30 mg/dL higher in persons with triglycerides of 200mg/dL or more. This is based on a normal VLDL value being 30 mg/dL. (See Display 40-1.)

Hypoalphalipoproteinemia

A familial HDL deficiency state, hypoalphalipoproteinemia, has been linked to premature CHD. Whereas high HDL levels may mobilize cholesterol from arterial luminal surfaces and return it to the liver, low HDL usually reflects an enzymatic or apoprotein abnormality affecting the catabolism of LDL or

DISPLAY **40-1**

ATP III CLASSIFICATION OF TRIGLYCERIDES
(National Cholesterol Education Program, 2001)

Tg Level (mg/dL)	Category
<150	Normal
150–199	Borderline High
200–499	High
≥500	Very High

Risk Category	LDL Goal (mg/dL)	Non-HDL Cholesterol Goal (mg/dL) (National Cholesterol Education Program, 2001)
CHD and CHD Risk Equivalent (10 year risk >10%)	<100	<130
Multiple risk factors and 10 year risk ≤20%	<130	<160
0–1 risk factor	<160	<190

VLDL. Alterations of the human apo A-I gene have been found in those with familial HDL deficiency and premature CHD (Ordovas et al., 1986). This suggests that low HDL may represent a genetic marker for identifying those at risk for CHD. The abnormalities related to VLDL catabolism explain the common coexistence of low HDL with elevated triglycerides. Furthermore, when triglycerides are lowered, increases in HDL are observed. In the absence of a genetic deficiency, lower HDL levels are related to environmental factors such as cigarette smoking and physical inactivity (see Table 40-2 for causes of low HDL cholesterol).

Combined Dyslipidemias

Combined dyslipidemias usually represent a combination of genetic lipoprotein or apoprotein defects and environmental effects. The specific lipid abnormalities observed provide clues to the genetic disorders. Table 40-2 summarizes observed lipid abnormalities and associated mechanisms. An understanding of these mechanisms guides the management of lipid abnormalities.

THE MANAGEMENT OF HIGH BLOOD CHOLESTEROL

Since the late 1980s, a large and convincing body of evidence has associated elevated blood lipids with CHD. Furthermore, clinical trials have demonstrated that reducing blood cholesterol is effective for primary and secondary prevention of CHD. This research has prompted groups such as the National Institutes of Health, American Heart Association, and the American College of Cardiology to establish health policy guidelines for the detection and treatment of lipid disorders (27th Bethesda Conference, 1996; Grundy et al., 1997; National Cholesterol Education Program, 2001; Smith et al., 1995).

Recommendations for Detection of High Blood Cholesterol

Health policy recommendations for detection of high cholesterol include the measurement of total cholesterol and HDL cholesterol in all adults aged 20 years and older, with repeat measurement within 5 years (National Cholesterol Education Program, 2001). Total cholesterol less than 200 mg/dL is considered desirable; levels between 200 mg/dL and 239 mg/dL are classified as borderline-high, and those more than 240 mg/dL are considered high blood cholesterol. Measures of HDL less

Table 40–3 ■ NEW FEATURES OF ATP III

Focus on multiple risk factors

Identifies abdominal aortic aneurysm, peripheral vascular disease, cerebrovascualr disease, and diabetes as a CHD risk equivalent

Uses Framingham projections of 10-year absolute CHD risk (ie, the percent probability of having a CHD event in 10 years) to identify patients with multiple (2+) risk factors for more aggressive LDL-lowering therapy

Identifies persons with the metabolic syndrome as candidates for intensified TLC

Modifications of lipid and lipoprotein classification

Identifies LDL cholesterol level <100 mg/dL as optimal

Raises threshold for low HDL cholesterol from <35 mg/dL (in ATP II) to <40 mg/dL

Lowers triglyceride classification cutpoints

Recommendations for implementation

Recommends a complete lipoprotein profile (total, LDL, and HDL cholesterol and triglycerides) over measurement of total and HDL cholesterol alone

Encourages use of plant stanols/sterols and soluble fiber to enhance LDL-lowering therapy

Offers strategies for promoting adherence to TLC and drug therapies

Recommends treatment beyond LDL lowering for persons with triglycerides ≥200 mg/dL

Adapted from Expert Panel on Detection, Evaluation, and Treatment of High Blood Cholesterol in Adults. (2001). Executive summary of the third report of the National Cholesterol Education Program (NCEP) Expert Panel on Detection, Evaluation, and Treatment of High Blood Cholesterol in Adults (Adult Treatment Panel III). *Journal of the American Medical Association, 285* (19), 2486–2497.

than 40 mg/dL are considered low and constitute a risk factor for CHD. HDL more than 60 mg/dL remains a "negative" risk factor and removes one risk factor from the overall risk profile. Other nonlipid factors that contribute to CHD risk status also should be assessed, including cigarette smoking, hypertension, diabetes mellitus, a family history of premature heart disease, age (men younger than 45 years and women younger than 55 years), and the presence of other CHD "risk equivalents" (abdominal aortic aneurysm, peripheral vascular disease, Framingham risk score of 20% or more in 10 years, presence of multiple risk factors). Table 40-3 provides new features of ATP III: classification of LDL cholesterol, major risk factors for CHD, and goals for LDL cholesterol therapy. Tables 40-4 and 40-5 provide scoring for determination of Framingham risk classification.

If total cholesterol is greater than 200 mg/dL or HDL is less than 40 mg/dL, then a full lipoprotein analysis is required and treatment is based on LDL levels. Risk factor reduction, including weight reduction, dietary therapy, and increased physical activity are major therapies for CHD prevention in patients at low risk and a major component of the therapeutic management of those at high risk or those with established CHD. When dietary interventions fail to achieve desired LDL goal, medical management may be considered (National Cholesterol Education Program, 2001) (Table 40-6).

Recommended Goals for the Treatment of High Blood Cholesterol

The goal for cholesterol management is the achievement of an ideal LDL level (<100mg/dL) in all adults. If a screening cholesterol is greater than 200 mg/dL and the person's risk profile predicts a risk of greater than 20% in 10 years, then a full lipid profile and evaluation is recommended. If CHD, CHD equivalents, and/or multiple risk factors are present, a full lipid profile is also recommended. Health policy guidelines strongly encourage consideration of risk status for both

Table 40–4 ■ ESTIMATE OF 10-YEAR CHD RISK IN MEN (FRAMINGHAM POINT SCORES)

Age (years)	Points	HDL (mg/dL)	Points	Systolic BP (mm/Hg)	Points	
					Untreated	Treated
20–34	−9	≥60	−1	<120	0	0
35–39	−4	50–59	0	120–129	0	1
40–44	0	40–49	1	130–139	1	2
45–49	3	<40	2	140–159	1	2
50–54	6			≥160	2	3
55–59	8					
60–64	10					
65–69	11					
70–74	12					
75–79	13					

Total cholesterol (mg/dL)	Points				
	Age 20–39	Age 40–49	Age 50–59	Age 60–69	Age 70–79
<160	0	0	0	0	0
160–199	4	3	2	1	0
200–239	7	5	3	1	0
240–279	9	6	4	2	1
≥280	11	8	5	3	1
Nonsmoker	0	0	0	0	0
Smoker	8	5	3	1	1

Point total	10-year risk (%)	Point total	10-year risk (%)
<0	<1	9	5
0	1	10	6
1	1	11	8
2	1	12	10
3	1	13	12
4	1	14	16
5	2	15	20
6	2	16	25
7	3	≥17	≥30
8	4		

Adapted from Expert Panel on Detection, Evaluation, and Treatment of High Blood Cholesterol in Adults. (2001). Executive summary of the third report of the National Cholesterol Education Program (NCEP) Expert Panel on Detection, Evaluation, and Treatment of High Blood Cholesterol in Adults (Adult Treatment Panel III). *Journal of the American Medical Association, 285* (19), 2486–2497.

Table 40–5 ■ ESTIMATE OF 10-YEAR CHD RISK FOR WOMEN (FRAMINGHAM POINT SCORES)

Age (*years*)	Points	HDL (*mg/dL*)	Points	Systolic BP (*mm/Hg*)	Points Untreated	Points Treated
20–34	−7	≥60	−1	<120	0	0
35–39	−3	50–59	0	120–129	1	3
40–44	0	40–49	1	130–139	2	4
45–49	3	<40	2	140–159	3	5
50–54	6			≥160	4	6
55–59	8					
60–64	10					
65–69	12					
70–74	14					
75–79	16					

Total cholesterol, (*mg/dL*)	Age 20–39	Age 40–49	Age 50–59	Age 60–69	Age 70–79
<160	0	0	0	0	0
160–199	4	3	2	1	1
200–239	8	6	4	2	1
240–279	11	8	5	3	2
≥280	13	10	7	4	2
Nonsmoker	0	0	0	0	0
Smoker	9	7	4	2	1

Point total	10-year risk (%)	Point total	10-year risk (%)
<9	<1	17	5
9	1	18	6
10	1	19	8
11	1	20	11
12	1	21	14
13	2	22	17
14	2	23	22
15	3	24	27
16	4	≥25	≥30

Adapted from Expert Panel on Detection, Evaluation, and Treatment of High Blood Cholesterol in Adults. (2001). Executive summary of the third report of the National Cholesterol Education Program (NCEP) Expert Panel on Detection, Evaluation, and Treatment of High Blood Cholesterol in Adults (Adult Treatment Panel III). *Journal of the American Medical Association, 285* (19), 2486–2497.

Table 40–6 ■ LDL CHOLESTEROL GOALS, AND CUTPOINTS FOR THERAPEUTIC LIFESTYLE CHANGES (TLC) AND DRUG THERAPY IN DIFFERENT RISK CATEGORIES

Risk Category	LDL Goal	LDL Level at Which to Initiate Therapeutic Lifestyle Changes (TLC)	LDL Level at Which to Consider Drug Therapy
CHD or CHD risk Equivalents (10-year risk >20%)	<100 mg/dL	>100 mg/dL	>130 mg/dL (100–129 mg/dL: drug optional)*
2+ Risk Factors 10 year risk ≤20%	<130 mg/dL	>130 mg/dL	10-year risk 10%–20%: ≥130 mg/dL 10-year risk <10% ≥160 mg/dL
0–1 Risk Factor†	<160 mg/dL	≥160 mg/dL	≥190 mg/dL (160–189 mg/dL: LDL lowering drug optional)

*Some authorities recommend the use of LDL-lowering drugs in this category if an LDL cholesterol <100 mg/dL cannot be achieved by Therapeutic Lifestyle Changes. Others prefer the use of drugs that primarily modify triglycerides and HDL, e.g., nicotinic acid or fibrate.
†Almost all people with 0–1 risk factor have a 10-year risk of <10%, thus 10-year risk assessment **in** people with 0–1 risk factors is not necessary.

the evaluation and the treatment of elevated cholesterol. Table 40-6 provides an overview of LDL goals and treatment considerations.

EVALUATION OF THE PATIENT WITH ELEVATED CHOLESTEROL

It is appropriate that the patient with high blood cholesterol receive a thorough clinical evaluation in addition to a lipoprotein analysis. Several medical diagnoses have been associated with high cholesterol. Abnormal lipid profiles may be the first clue to undiagnosed endocrine disorders such as hypothyroidism or diabetes. A careful family history is also important. Genetic forms of hypercholesterolemia are relatively common in the general population; for example, FH has an estimated frequency of 1 in 500 (Schaefer & Levy, 1985). It is therefore advisable that first-degree relatives be screened for lipid disorders. Hyperlipidemia, like hypertension, is a relatively asymptomatic disorder and is usually first recognized by abnormal laboratory findings. Subcutaneous or tendinous lipid deposits, called xanthoma, are the one physical finding that may be prominent in severe lipid disorders. Xanthelasma palpebrarum are seen in the inner corner of eyelids and are associated with FH in approximately half of patients with this finding. Tendinous xanthomas often are found in extensor tendons of the hands and Achilles tendon. Planar xanthomas are lipid deposits in the webs of the hand and occur in children with FH. Corneal arcus is caused by cholesterol deposition within the corneal rim and can be seen as a white band around the cornea. This finding may be indicative of FH in younger people but may not be meaningful in the older adult (Gotto, 1983).

Certain types of hyperlipoproteinemia are characterized by abdominal pain. Possible causes for the abdominal pain include pancreatitis and hepatosplenomegaly. Abdominal pain of unknown cause also has been documented as a physical finding. This pain may be associated with ischemic bowel and is related to increased blood viscosity, macrophage ingestion of fat particles, or the effect of the size of the lipid particles on abdominal tissue (Gotto, 1983). Patients with chylomicronemia, or markedly elevated triglycerides levels, have a high risk for pancreatitis.

LIPOPROTEIN MEASUREMENT

The measurement of plasma lipids and lipoproteins is essential for the diagnosis of lipid abnormalities and for the identification of those at risk for CHD. These measurements also provide important feedback to the patient modifying his or her risk profile. The most common lipid analysis includes measurement of total cholesterol, total triglycerides, and HDL cholesterol. This allows calculation of LDL using the following equation: LDL = total cholesterol − (triglycerides ÷ 5) − HDL (Friedewald et al., 1972). This indirect assessment of LDL can be used if triglycerides are less than 400 mg/dL. If triglycerides are more than 400 mg/dL, then LDL must be directly

measured using the more complex and costly ultracentrifugation procedure.

To interpret the results of lipid measurements, some knowledge of the accuracy and precision of the measure is useful. One of the common scenarios encountered in lipid management is a laboratory report with values extremely different from previously measured values, and the patient protests, "I have not been doing anything differently." Intraindividual cholesterol measurements have been shown to vary by 4% to 11% over a 1-year period (U.S. Department of Health and Human Services, 1990). Although there are several sources for variability or error in cholesterol measures, the most obvious is analytic variability, or laboratory error, which has been estimated to contribute one third to one half of the intra-individual variability. Laboratories must make their standardization criteria available and should strive to achieve less than 3% measurement variability. Biologic and physiologic factors constitute the other major source for measurement variability. To minimize measurement variability, the National Cholesterol Education Laboratory Standardization Panel recommends the following standards of practice (U.S. Department of Health and Human Services, 1990):

A stable lifestyle, including health status, diet, medication, and activity level, should be followed for at least 2 weeks before measurement.

Cholesterol measures should be made no sooner than 8 weeks after MI, surgical procedure, trauma, or an acute bacterial or viral infection.

Blood collection procedures should include a 12-hour fast (except for water and usual medications) before sampling if lipid measures other than total cholesterol are to be performed.

The patient should sit quietly for 5 minutes before the venipuncture.

The sample should be obtained within 1 minute of tourniquet application.

Standardized procedures for processing and transporting samples should be followed.

DIETARY MANAGEMENT OF HYPERLIPIDEMIA

Evidence of the relationship between dietary intake, plasma cholesterol, and CHD has been steadily accumulating. Population studies have shown that countries with the highest incidence of CHD and elevated blood cholesterol levels also have high dietary intakes of saturated fats (Arntzenius et al., 1985; Keys, 1970; Kushi et al., 1985; McGee et al., 1984). Developing countries with a mean cholesterol level less than 150 mg/dL have a very low incidence of CHD and also have diets low in total fat, saturated fatty acids, and cholesterol (Keys, 1970).

Figure 40-3 illustrates the relationship of CHD mortality to types of fat intake. Animal studies have demonstrated that high-fat diets result in increased total and LDL cholesterol and lead to the development of atherosclerotic vascular lesions (Armstrong et al., 1970). Metabolic ward studies also support the relationship

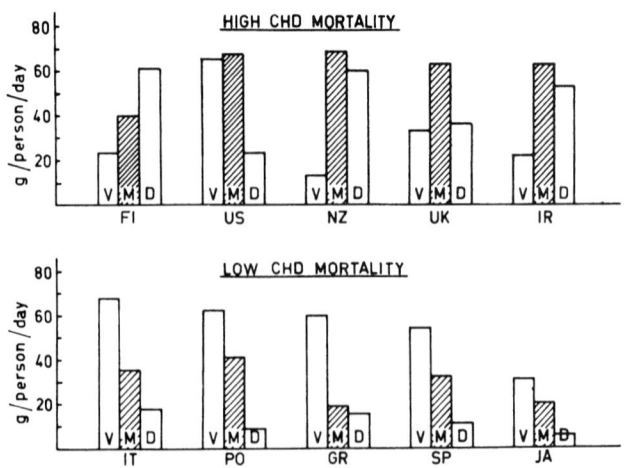

■ **Figure 40–3.** A comparison of the daily intake (in grams) of the major food fats in countries with high and low coronary heart disease (CHD)–related deaths. V, vegetable fats; M, meat fats; D, dairy fats; Fl, Finland; US, United States; NZ, New Zealand; UK, United Kingdom; IR, Ireland; IT, Italy; PO, Portugal; GR, Germany; SP, Spain; JA, Japan. (From Turpienen, O. [1979]. Effect of cholesterol-lowering diet on mortality from coronary heart disease and other causes. *Circulation,* 59, 3. Used with permission of the American Heart Association, Inc.)

Table 40–7 ■ CHARACTERISTICS OF THE METABOLIC SYNDROME

Risk Factor	Comments
Abdominal obesity (waist circumference)	Men: >102 cm (>40 in) Women: >88 cm (>35 in)
Triglycerides	≥150 mg/dL
HDL cholesterol	Men: <40 mg/dL Women: <50 mg/dL
Blood pressure	≥130/≥85 mm Hg
Fasting glucose	≥110–125 mg/dL

Adapted from Expert Panel on Detection, Evaluation, and Treatment of High Blood Cholesterol in Adults. (2001). Executive summary of the third report of the National Cholesterol Education Program (NCEP) Expert Panel on Detection, Evaluation, and Treatment of High Blood Cholesterol in Adults (Adult Treatment Panel III). *Journal of the American Medical Association,* 285 (19), 2486–2497.

between saturated fat consumption and plasma cholesterol (Hegsted et al., 1965; Keys & Parlin, 1966) and have demonstrated that lowering fat intake can achieve as much as a 30% reduction in plasma cholesterol. Clinical trials have used angiography to demonstrate slower rates of CHD progression in subjects adhering to low-fat and low-cholesterol diets (Ornish et al., 1990; Schuler et al., 1992; Watts et al., 1992). Blankenhorn and colleagues examined the relationship of new lesion development and diet in the placebo-plus-diet group of the Cholesterol Lowering Atherosclerosis Study (CLAS). They observed that the dietary fat intake in the subset not acquiring new lesions was 27% of calories, compared with 34% in the subset acquiring new lesions (Blankenhorn et al., 1990). It is the evidence that LDL receptor synthesis and activity are decreased in response to diets high in saturated fat that lends ultimate support to the inclusion of dietary therapy as the cornerstone for lipid management (Brown & Goldstein, 1986; Ornish et al., 1990).

Dietary Recommendations

The goal of diet therapy is to reduce LDL cholesterol to desirable levels predicated by the person's CHD risk status while maintaining a nutritionally sound eating pattern. The dietary intervention recommended by the National Cholesterol Education Program (NCEP III) is called therapeutic lifestyle changes (TLC) (National Cholesterol Education Program, 2001). This diet plan includes reduction in total fat intake to 25% to 35% of total caloric intake. Saturated fats should be no more than 7% of total caloric intake and cholesterol intake should not exceed 200 mg/d. If the LDL goal is not achieved within 6 weeks or if the patient is already adhering to a TLC diet, then it is recommended that the addition of plant stanols/sterols and increasing viscous fiber be considered.

Weight reduction and physical activity should concomitantly be considered for persons following the TLC diet. Many persons are at risk for the metabolic syndrome as a result of obesity and or physical inactivity and a diet high in saturated fats, carbohydrates, and calories (National Cholesterol Education Program, 2001) (Table 40-7).

Before initiating dietary change, an assessment of the patient's current dietary pattern and usual eating habits is necessary. Dietary assessments are based on subjective reports and are predisposed to problems of recall accuracy and reliability. Review articles on dietary assessment issues suggest that food frequency inventories or careful diet history provide the most accurate information on usual eating patterns (Freudenheim, 1993; Friedenreich et al., 1992). Assessment tools are reported in the literature or can be obtained from agencies such as the American Dietetic Association, American Heart Association, the NCEP, or product manufacturers (Connor et al., 1992).

Dietary surveys of Americans between 1976 and 1980 showed that the average American intake of dietary fat was 37% of total calories, saturated fat intake was 13% of total calories, and cholesterol consumption averaged 260 and 430 mg/d for women and men, respectively (Block et al., 1988). When these same data were analyzed by comparing those who reported following a "low-fat diet" with "nondieters," the intake pattern of the dieters averaged 33% of total calories from fat, 11% of calories from saturated fat, and an average cholesterol intake of 287 mg/d.

Extensive professional and public attention has been given to the issue of cholesterol, such that the most recent dietary survey (from 1988 to 1991) in the U.S. population shows a significant 6- to 8-mg/dL decrease in serum cholesterol levels (Johnson et al., 1993). The data from these surveys and from clinical trials on CHD progression suggest that people with established CHD or with CHD risk factors are likely to have adopted a low-fat diet without the intervention and support of health care professionals (Haskell et al., 1994). The new ATP III provides additional saturated fat and cholesterol-lowering recommendations coupled with weight management and physical activity (National Cholesterol Education Program, 2001).

Several aspects related to a lipid-lowering diet remain controversial. Although most experts recommend reducing intake of saturated fats, there is disagreement over what nutrients should replace the reduction in fat. Is the ideal lipid-lowering diet a low-fat, high-carbohydrate diet, or is it a diet that replaces saturated fats with unsaturated fats? Saturated fatty acids, with the exception of stearic acid, raise total and LDL cholesterol, probably through a mechanism decreasing LDL receptor synthesis (Bonanome & Grundy, 1988). Studies suggest that diets high in monounsaturated fat relative to saturated fat convey a desirable plasma lipid profile, with lowering of total and LDL cholesterol and no reduction in HDL (Grundy & Vega, 1983). The major criticism of these studies has been that the addition of only unsaturated fats to the diet is not practical among free-living individuals. For example, food items high in stearic acid usually contain other highly saturated fatty acids as well. Second, studies have yet to determine whether such diets are associated with beneficial outcomes beyond changes to the lipid profile. Low-fat, high-carbohydrate diets produce lower LDL levels than high-fat diets, but such diets may result in higher triglyceride and lower HDL levels. A 1-year study comparing four fat-restricted diets (30%, 26%, 22%, and 18% of calories from fat) found significant reductions in LDL ranging from 5% to 13% (Knopp et al., 1997). Triglycerides increased significantly in the two most fat-restricted diets (18% and 22% of calories from fat). These authors concluded that moderate reduction in fat is beneficial but that more severe restrictions may produce undesirable effects.

The marked increase in obesity of the U.S. population that some attribute to increased carbohydrate consumption has further added to this controversy. In an effort to reduce dietary fat, Americans frequently select low-fat manufactured products containing sugar rather than choosing plant-based carbohydrate foods. This is evident in that the consumption of refined sugar has increased from 120 pounds per person in 1970 to 150 pounds per person in 1995, and fiber intake remains low (Food Surveys Research Group and Agricultural Research Services). Even those researchers who advocated diets high in monounsaturated fats also recommend increased consumption of fruits and vegetables (Connor et al., 1997).

The omega-3 fatty acids, primarily found in fish and fish oils, have also been shown to affect plasma lipids, primarily triglycerides (Connor et al., 1990; Leaf & Weber1988). The response is dose-related and is sufficiently high that it is unlikely to be achieved using food choices only or without supplemental use. The omega-3 fatty acids are postulated to decrease VLDL synthesis and thereby reduce triglycerides. They also exert antithrombotic effects through the thromboxane-prostaglandin pathways, resulting in decreases in platelet aggregation and vasoconstriction. Although the safety of consumption of large amounts of fish oils is an issue, most researchers agree that the inclusion of fish several times each week is a safe and prudent alternative. The response to dietary intervention is variable and appears related not only to the specific fatty acid composition of the diet but to the level of plasma lipids. People with the higher lipid levels usually experience the greatest response to dietary interventions (Kris-Etherton et al., 1988) (see reviews [Gardner & Kraemer, 1995; Kris-Etherton et al., 1988; Mensink & Katan, 1992] for more detailed discussion of the specific effects of fatty acids). The most practical recommendations are to reduce the saturated fat in the diet, change the quality of fat by replacing food items high in saturated fat with foods containing monounsaturated or polyun-

---

DISPLAY 40–2

NUTRIENT COMPOSITION OF THE TLC DIET

• Saturated fat*	Less than 7% of total calories
• Polyunsaturated fat	Up to 10% of total calories
• Monounsaturated fat	Up to 20% of total calories
• Total fat	25–35% of total calories
• Carbohydrate†	50–60% of total calories
• Fiber	20–30% G/day
• Protein	Approximately 15% of total calories
• Cholesterol	Less than 200 mg/day
• Total Calories‡	Balance energy intake and expenditure to maintain desirable weight/prevent weight gain

*Trans fatty acids are another LDL-raising fat that should be kept at a low intake

†Carbohydrates should be derived predominantly from foods rich in complex carbohydrates, including grains, especially whole grains, fruits, and vegetables.

‡Daily energy expenditure should include at least moderate physical activity (contributing approximately 200 Kcal per day (National Cholesterol Education Program, 2001).

Other options found in the new TLC diet are the addition of plant stanols/sterols (2 g/day) and increasing the intake of viscous fiber (10–25 g/day) in order to further reduce LDL cholesterol through dietary means.

---

saturated fatty acids, and increase the quantities of fruits, vegetables, and fiber. The new ATP III approach to lifestyle intervention, TLC, includes nutrition, weight management, and physical activity. The TLC approach applies to all adults for reducing their risk for CHD (Display 40-2).

Dietary Change Strategies

For most patients, recommendations for dietary change are not sufficient to effect dietary change. Substantial knowledge must be acquired and specific behavior skills must be learned and practiced. Required knowledge should include an understanding of the relationship between dietary fat, dietary cholesterol, and blood cholesterol; defining reasonable expectations for dietary change; understanding the differences in the quality of fats; ability to read and interpret food labels; sufficient knowledge about food items to estimate fat content of unlabeled items; and knowledge of food preparation methods that affect fat content. Because eating is a part of our social environment, the behavioral skills must be adapted to a variety of social settings, such as travel, eating out, celebrations, and the work environment. Patients should practice label reading and menu selections and questioning food preparers or servers. Anticipatory responses for avoiding high-fat foods in social situations should be explicitly identified. Adapting recipes and developing grocery-shopping lists that include brand-name selections are also useful skills to learn. Several studies have examined patterns of food and food group changes occurring during adoption of low-fat diets (Buzzard et al., 1990; Gorder et al., 1986;

Kristal et al., 1990; McCann et al., 1990; Schectman et al., 1990; Smith-Schneider et al., 1992).

In general, patients were successful in reducing their consumption of eggs, high-fat meats, and fried food items; substituting lower-fat items for high-fat items, such as skim milk for full-fat milk or low-calorie spreads and salad dressings in place of high-fat dressings; and replacing high-fat items with low-fat items, such as replacing sour cream with yogurt. Although patients were successful at selecting less saturated fats, they were less successful at decreasing their consumption of total and added fats. The most difficult food items to reduce or replace included cheese and snack foods, such as crackers. Until more adequate products become available from food manufacturers, substitution for these areas of difficult change may be a practical strategy.

Computer modeling techniques have been used to examine the effect of dietary fat reduction strategies to determine the most effective strategy for meeting step I dietary goals (Smith-Schneider et al., 1992). The strategies included substitution of low-fat counterparts for high-fat items, reduction in quantity of high-fat foods, replacement of high-fat foods with other types of foods (e.g., beans for meat), and modifying preparation techniques (e.g., broiling instead of frying). For men, the strategy of replacement was the single strategy that met the dietary goals. No single strategy was effective for women. The results suggest that the most significant changes occur using combinations of dietary strategies. Education alone is unlikely to facilitate dietary change. Studies examining educational interventions have found only a small relationship between knowledge, attitudes, and dietary behavior (Axelson et al., 1985).

When behavioral interventions were combined with educational strategies, more positive dietary outcomes were observed (Crouch et al., 1986; Fraser et al., 1988; Gorder et al., 1986). Behavioral strategies are based on the principles of social learning theory (Bandura, 1977). Social learning theory principles include examining the antecedents of the behavior (expectations and values placed on the behavior outcome), the skills and knowledge needed to perform the behavior, and the reinforcement contingencies associated with the behavior (rewards, feedback, and evaluation). Many behavioral techniques, such as self-monitoring, goal setting, defining alternatives and choices, evaluation, rewards, and feedback can be used to assist patients in the change process (Ewart, 1989; McCann et al., 1990).

Daily logs of food patterns, eating habits, environmental setting, and self-efficacy measures provide an opportunity for the patient to evaluate his or her own behavior and to receive feedback on specific successes or assistance in identifying undesirable patterns or trends. The antecedents to the behavior can be examined for positive or negative influences on dietary behavior. Small portable computers are available that can record dietary intake and give an immediate nutrient analysis. This type of device incorporates the techniques of self-monitoring, evaluation, and feedback and, in some cases, can supply alternative choices. Less sophisticated written records that detail the food item, amount, and type of preparation have also been shown to be adequate for the purposes of monitoring and changing behavior. It is not unusual for record-keeping alone to lead to altered behavior. Record analysis can also be useful in determining appropriate goals.

Many behaviorists view goal setting as a key element. The goal should be defined by the patient and should be one that is small, specific, and measurable. Nurses can assist the patient through the process, ensuring that these key goal attributes exist.

A variety of aids have been developed to assist personal monitoring and evaluation of food choices (Buzzard et al., 1990; Connor et al., 1986). Booklets listing the grams of fat for typical portions of commonly consumed foods have been successfully used for this purpose (Pope-Cordle & Katahn, 1991). A daily fat gram goal for both total and saturated fat can be established based on usual daily caloric intake. If daily intake is 2,000 calories, then a diet with less than 20% of calories from fat would restrict fat intake to 44 g (2,000 kcal $\times$ 20% = 400 kcal; 400 kcal $\div$ [9 kcal $\div$ g] = 44 g). Recall that 1 g of fat equals 9 kcal. These booklets usually are pocket-sized and are easily carried while grocery shopping or to restaurants, and they usually include a diary for recording personal daily intake. Behavior can be reinforced using evaluation and feedback techniques.

Feedback can be provided through analysis of food records and by measurement of blood lipids. It is possible to achieve plasma cholesterol reductions of 15% to 20% with adherence to a low-fat and low-cholesterol diet. However, given the individual variability of response, caution should be used in providing feedback based totally on plasma cholesterol measures. Feedback and rewards based on dietary behaviors are likely to provide more positive and long-lasting reinforcement.

WEIGHT CONTROL AND LIPID MANAGEMENT

The prevalence of obesity in the United States has increased since the late 1970s. It is estimated that more than one third (65 million) of adults have a body mass index (weight in kilograms divided by height in meters squared) greater than 31 and would be considered severely obese (Heini & Weinsier, 1997). Because both LDL and the incidence of CHD are reduced in people who maintain a normal body weight, these data are alarming. Studies examining weight loss have reported varying effects on lipid profiles. A meta-analysis of 70 studies examining the effect of weight reduction on lipoproteins found that a 1-kg reduction in weight was associated with a 0.05-mmol/L decrease in total cholesterol (1 mmol/L = 38.67 mg/dL) (Dattilo & Kris-Etherton, 1992). Significant decreases in LDL and triglycerides were also found. The effect of weight loss on HDL varies, decreasing during the active weight loss period and increasing after a period of stable reduced weight. The mechanisms postulated to account for these alterations in lipoproteins include decreased HMG-CoA reductase activity and enhanced cholesterol excretion in bile acids. The release of cholesterol from adipose tissues is also thought to inhibit hepatic synthesis of cholesterol.

For all patients with dyslipidemia, the secondary goal of diet intervention is weight reduction. Patients with dyslipidemia should be counseled to expect an initial reduction in HDL during active weight loss. Increased levels of physical activity may minimize the HDL reduction and facilitate weight loss (Wood et al., 1991).

ALCOHOL AND LIPOPROTEINS

Moderate alcohol intake has been reported to be protective for CHD. France, a country with a low rate of CHD, has a markedly higher per capita consumption of alcohol, particularly of wine (Marmot, 1984). One possible mechanism for this protective effect may be related to the increase in HDL observed with alcohol intake. Researchers have established that moderate alcohol intake increases HDL_3, apo A-I, and apo A-II (Camargo et al., 1985; Haskell et al., 1984).

Alcohol may also alter platelet aggregation and lower fibrinogen levels. Alcohol also increases catabolism of VLDL, the triglyceride-carrying lipoprotein. Patients with elevated triglyceride levels may have dramatic improvements in triglyceride levels with cessation of alcohol. Most researchers agree that the inverse association between alcohol intake and CHD risk is a consistent but weak association (Stampfer et al., 1988). Recommendations to consume alcohol must therefore be considered cautiously, given the potential side effects of impaired judgment, decreased motor coordination, and possible addiction associated with alcohol use. The American Heart Association's recent "scientific advisory" on *Wine and Your Heart* concluded that until randomized clinical trials are undertaken, there is "little justification to recommend alcohol (specifically wine) as a cardioprotective strategy" (Goldberg et al., 2001).

PHYSICAL ACTIVITY AND LIPOPROTEINS

The American Heart Association has added physical inactivity to dyslipidemia, smoking, and hypertension as the fourth major modifiable risk factor for coronary artery and other vascular diseases (Smith et al., 1995). Physical activity works through a variety of mechanisms to lower coronary risk. Regular physical activity aids in weight loss by increasing caloric output. Weight loss decreases serum triglycerides, which can result in increased levels of HDL cholesterol. Exercise improves glycemic control in type II diabetes by lessening insulin resistance and improving insulin sensitivity. In some people, exercise also lowers LDL cholesterol, although LDL reductions usually are modest. Regular physical activity has a positive influence on endothelial function. Research has shown that regular exercise can improve vasodilation responses and reduce platelet adhesion (Fair & Berra, 1996). Given these beneficial effects, regular physical activity should be a part of the multifactorial intervention program used to manage dyslipidemia (Thompson et al, 2003) (see Chapter 41).

HORMONES AND LIPOPROTEINS

Clinical heart disease develops in women almost a decade later in life than in men for reasons not entirely well understood. Several mechanisms have been suggested to account for this beneficial effect. Estrogen decreases LDL and increases HDL and apo A-I levels (Campos et al., 1990). Estrogen use has been associated with lower Lp(a), reduced LDL oxidative susceptibility, and improved endothelial vasodilation responses (Campos et al., 1990; Sullivan, 1996). Large, randomized, placebo-controlled clinical trials are examining the effect of hormone replacement therapy (HRT) for primary and secondary coronary artery disease prevention.

The Heart and Estrogen–Progestin Replacement Study (HERS) evaluated the influence of Premarin plus medroxyprogesterone acetate versus placebo in 2,763 women with CHD at baseline. After an average follow-up of 4.1 years, no differences were detected in acute myocardial infarction and coronary death between the two groups. In addition, there was a pattern of early increased risk of CHD and thrombotic events with a pattern of late benefit in the women randomized to HRT. This increased risk seemed to occur primarily in the first year of treatment and there was a suggestion of potential benefit with long-term treatment (ie, more than 4 years) (Hulley, 1993). Because of this interesting potential late benefit, a follow-up study was undertaken. The investigators found that after 6.8 years of follow-up, use of estrogen–progestin did not significantly decrease the risk of primary or secondary CHD events in postmenopausal women with CHD. The effect of other doses and types of estrogen or estrogen only on CHD was not investigated in this trial; therefore, these conclusions can only be applied to women using this specific estrogen–progestin combination (Grady et al., 2002).

The Women's Health Initiative (WHI) recently received a great deal of media attention as a result of their findings regarding the negative influence of HT on breast cancer and cardiovascular risk in women. The WHI is a double-blind, randomized, placebo-controlled primary prevention trial examining the effects of estrogen and estrogen–progestin combination therapy on various cardiovascular, vascular, breast cancer, and other health outcomes. The Data and Safety Monitoring Board stopped the combined estrogen-plus-MPA arm of the trial because of the fact that the rates of breast cancer in this group were significantly higher compared to placebo. They also found that the overall health risks of the estrogen–progestin combination, including increased risks for acute myocardial infarction, thromboembolism, and stroke, far exceeded the benefits of the combination therapy (Risks and Benefits of Estrogen Plus Progestin in Healthy Postmenopausal Women, 2002). This combined HT was terminated in May 2002, 3 years earlier than its planned completion date of 2006. The increasing risk of breast cancer was the key factor that led the National Heart Lung and Blood Institute (NHLBI) to terminate the combined HT arm of the study (Fletcher & Colditz, 2002). The breast cancer findings along with the negative CVD outcomes discredit short-term or long-term estrogen/progestin use for women with and without CHD (Fletcher & Colditz, 2002; Risks and Benefits of Estrogen Plus Progestin in Healthy Postmenopausal Women, 2002). Women in the WHI with prior hysterectomy were randomized to the Conjugated Equine Estrogen (CEE) only versus placebo group. After 6.8 years of follow-up, the use of CEE was found to increase the risk of stroke and did not affect CHD incidence. As a result, CEE is not recommended for prevention of chronic disease in postmenopausal women (Women's Health Initiative Steering Committee, 2004).

PHARMACOLOGIC MANAGEMENT OF HYPERLIPIDEMIA

The primary rationale for the treatment of hyperlipidemia is the reduction of CHD morbidity and mortality. Studies using hypolipidemic drug therapy to achieve LDL reductions have demonstrated lower CHD morbidity and mortality and lower overall mortality rates (Scandinavian Simvastatin Survival Study, 1995; Shepherd et al., 1995). Angiographic studies using lipid-lowering drugs have demonstrated less progression of angiographically determined CHD with reduction of LDL (Brown et al., 1990; Haskell et al., 1994; Kane et al., Watts et al., 1992). The rate of progression of CHD appears to be a dose-related response, with slower rates of progression associated with greater LDL-lowering. Angiographic studies have been of sufficiently short duration and lack long-term follow-up data such that the effect on total and CHD mortality cannot be determined. Until very long-term studies have been conducted, the safety and efficacy of hypolipidemic drug therapy will be questioned. Meta-analytic techniques have been used to analyze lipid-lowering studies and suggest that the decrease in CHD mortality is offset by increased death rates from other causes, particularly cancer deaths and non—illness-related deaths such as injury deaths and suicides (Hulley et al., 1993; Jacobs et al., 1992; Muldoon et al., 1990). These meta-analyses did not include data from the more recent very large clinical trials investigating lipid-lowering drugs (Downs et al., 1998; Scandinavian Simvastatin Survival Study, 1995; Shepherd et al., 1995). These studies did not observe any increase in cancer or non—illness-related deaths. Although the explanations for these findings remain controversial, the consensus of experts is that hypolipidemic drug therapy should always be instituted with nonpharmacologic interventions, including a low-fat, low-cholesterol diet, regular exercise, weight control, smoking cessation, control of hypertension, and control of blood glucose (in patients with diabetes). Hypolipidemic drug therapy requires careful consideration of individual risks as well as the benefits of such drug therapy. There is mounting evidence that lowering LDL cholesterol, particularly with the use of HMG-COa reductase inhibitors, in persons with known CAD and with CAD equivalents provides substantial benefit to reduced morbidity and mortality.

Lipid Criteria and Goals for Drug Therapy

Consideration of hypolipidemic drug therapy for primary prevention (ie, in people without existing CHD) is indicated in those without CHD risk factors but with LDL levels 190 mg/dL or more, or in people with 0 to 1 CHD risk factors and LDL levels 160 mg/dL or more. The target goals of treatment should be to achieve LDL levels of less than 160 or 130 mg/dL, respectively. In secondary prevention (ie, in patients with established CHD, with CHD equivalents, and/or a CHD risk of >20% in 10 years), drug therapy can be considered if LDL levels are more than 100 mg/dL and should be initiated if LDL levels are more than 130 mg/dL. The goal for all adults, in particular for those with established CHD, is LDL less than

Table 40–8 ■ ATP III CLASSIFICATION OF LDL CHOLESTEROL

LDL Cholesterol Level (mg/dL)	Category
<100	Optimal
100–129	Near or above optimal
130–159	Borderline high
160–189	High
≥190	Very high

Adapted from Expert Panel on Detection, Evaluation, and Treatment of High Blood Cholesterol in Adults. (2001). Executive summary of the third report of the National Cholesterol Education Program (NCEP) Expert Panel on Detection, Evaluation, and Treatment of High Blood Cholesterol in Adults (Adult Treatment Panel III). *Journal of the American Medical Association*, 285 (19), 2486–2497.

100 mg/dL (National Cholesterol Education Program, 2001) (Tables 40-8 and 40-9).

Classes of Hypolipidemic Drugs

The major classes of hypolipidemic drugs include the bile acid-binding resins, nicotinic acid, HMG-CoA reductase inhibitors (statins), fibric acid derivatives, and the intestinal absorption blockers. Individual response to each of these agents is variable, and each of the agents has potential side effects. Nursing can play a major role in the management of patients by assisting the patient to minimize side effects while promoting adherence to the regimen that achieves the desired lipid profile. In this section, the action, indications for use, and specific adherence strategies for each of the classes of hypolipidemic drugs are reviewed (Table 40-10).

Bile Acid-Binding Resins

Actions and Indications for Use. Bile acid-binding resins are insoluble in water and are not absorbed from the intestine. These agents bind with bile acids in the intestine, forming an insoluble complex. The enterohepatic circulation of bile acids is interrupted and fecal excretion of bile acids is increased. This results in increased synthesis of bile acids from hepatic cholesterol stores. Reduced hepatic cholesterol stimulates LDL receptor formation and increases HMG-CoA reductase activity, resulting in increased extraction of LDL from the bloodstream

Table 40–9 ■ GOALS OF LDL CHOLESTEROL THERAPY BY RISK CATEGORY

Risk Category	LDL Cholesterol Goal (mg/dL)
CHD or CHD risk equivalent	<100
Multiple (2+) risk factors	<130*
0–1 Risk factor	<160

Adapted from Expert Panel on Detection, Evaluation, and Treatment of High Blood Cholesterol in Adults. (2001). Executive summary of the third report of the National Cholesterol Education Program (NCEP) Expert Panel on Detection, Evaluation, and Treatment of High Blood Cholesterol in Adults (Adult Treatment Panel III). *Journal of the American Medical Association*, 285 (19), 2486–2497.
*LDL cholesterol goal for multiple risk factor patients with 10-year risk >20% is <100 mg/dL.

Table 40–10 ■ LIPID-LOWERING AGENTS

Drug Class	Average Lipid/Lipoprotein Effects		Side Effects	Contraindications	Clinical Trial Results
HMG-CoA reductase inhibitors (statins)*	LDL-C HDL-C TG	↓18%–60% ↑5%–15% ↓7%–37%	Myopathy Increased liver enzymes	Absolute: 　Active or chronic liver 　　disease Relative: 　Concomitant use with 　　certain drugs†	Reduced major coronary events, CHD deaths, need for coronary procedures, stroke, and total mortality
Bile acid sequestrants‡	LDL-C HDL-C TG	↓15%–30% ↑3%–5% No change or an increase	GI distress Constipation Decreased absorption of 　other drugs	Absolute: 　Dysbetalipoproteinemia 　TG >400 mg/dL Relative: 　TG >200 mg/dL	Reduced major coronary events and CHD deaths
Nicotinic acid§	LDL-C HDL-C TG	↓5%–25% ↑15%–35% ↓20%–50%	Flushing Hyperglycemia Hyperuricemia (or gout) Upper GI distress Hepatotoxicity	Absolute: 　Chronic liver disease 　Severe gout Relative: 　Diabetes 　Hyperuricemia 　Peptic ulcer disease	Reduced major coronary events, and possibly total mortality
Fibric acid derivatives‖	LDL-C (May be increased in patients with high TG) HDL-C TG	↓5%–20% ↑10%–20% ↓20%–50%	Dyspepsia Gallstones Myopathy Unexplained non-CHD 　deaths in WHO study 　with clofibrate	Absolute: 　Severe renal disease 　Severe hepatic disease	Reduced major coronary events
Cholesterol absorption Inhibitors††	LDL HDL TG	↓18% ↑1% ↑8%	Adverse event profile 　similar to placebo	Known hypersensitivity to Ezetimibe	Studies in progress

* Atorvastatin (10–80 mg), fluvastatin (20–80 mg), lovastatin (20–80 mg), pravastatin (20–80 mg), simvastatin (20–80 mg).
† Cyclosporine, macrolide antibiotics, antifungal agents, and cytochrome P-450 inhibitors (fibrates and niacin should be used with appropriate caution).
‡ Cholestyramine (4–16 g), colestipol (5–20 g), colesevelam (2.6–3.8 g).
§ Immediate-release (crystalline) nicotinic acid (1.5–3 g), extended-release nicotinic acid (1–2 g), and sustained-release nicotinic acid (1–2 g).
‖ Gemfibrozil (600 mg BID), fenofibrate (200 mg), clofibrate (1000 mg BID)
†† Not included in ATP III table of medications; approved for use after the guidelines were released.
Adapted from Expert Panel on Detection, Evaluation, and Treatment of High Blood Cholesterol in Adults. (2001). Executive summary of the third report of the National Cholesterol Education Program (NCEP) Expert Panel on Detection, Evaluation, and Treatment of High Blood Cholesterol in Adults (Adult Treatment Panel III). *Journal of the American Medical Association, 285* (19), 2486–2497, and prescribing information for statins.

and a lower plasma concentration of LDL. Hepatic production of VLDL is also enhanced, resulting in increased triglyceride levels. The expected response to resin therapy is seen in 2 to 4 weeks and may result in a 20% to 25% reduction in LDL (Schaefer & Levy, 1985).

Strategies for Increased Efficacy and Adherence. The major side effect of the bile acid-binding resins is constipation; the resins can be unpalatable, which may affect compliance. Resins come in both powder and tablet formulations. In powder form, the resins must be mixed with water. Because they are insoluble, they form a gritty solution. It is helpful to demonstrate the mixing process and allow the patient to taste the drug as part of the prescription process. If constipation develops, instruct the patient in the use of fiber, stool softeners, and other hygienic measures, such as increased fluid intake. Bile acid-binding resins should be taken with meals, particularly with the largest meal of the day, because intestinal bile acids are greatest during that time. Because these drugs are binding agents, they have the potential to bind and interfere with the absorption of other medications. Consequently, the patient should be instructed to take other medications 1 hour before or 4 hours after taking the resin.

Reviewing the mechanism of action with the patient promotes adherence and a better understanding of the rationale for these instructions.

Nicotinic Acid (Niacin)

Actions and Indications for Use. Nicotinic acid, or niacin, is a vitamin B_3 derivative that in large doses blocks the release of free fatty acids from adipose tissues, resulting in less hepatic conversion of free fatty acids into triglycerides (Schectman et al., 1990).

The hepatic production of VLDL is also decreased. Because VLDL is converted to IDL and LDL, decreased VLDL levels lead to favorable reductions in these lipoproteins as well. Contraindications to use include active liver disease and peptic ulcer disease, and caution is needed when it is used in patients with diabetes and atrial arrhythmias.

Strategies for Increased Efficacy and Adherence. The most common side effect of nicotinic acid use is cutaneous flushing caused by a prostaglandin-mediated vasodilation effect on vascular smooth muscle. This effect can be minimized with the use of aspirin taken 30 minutes before the nicotinic acid dose. Other less common side effects include abdominal discomfort; nausea; elevations in glucose, uric acid, and liver enzymes; reversible hepatotoxicity; and potentiation of atrial arrhythmias. Abdominal side effects are reduced if niacin is taken with meals. Niacin use must be monitored by a health professional, with liver enzymes measured before and periodically during therapy. Side effects can be minimized by starting at low doses and increasing the dose gradually. Written instructions, including a suggested dosage schedule, should be provided to the patient. The patient should be informed of the various side effects and instructed to contact a health professional if hepatotoxic side effects, such as flu-like symptoms and malaise, occur (Kashyap et al., 1999).

HMG-CoA Reductase Inhibitors (Statins)

The statins inhibit HMG-CoA reductase, the rate-limiting enzyme in cholesterol synthesis. Reduced cholesterol synthesis in the hepatocytes stimulates increased LDL receptor activity, thereby promoting clearance of VLDL and LDL from the bloodstream (Tobert, 1987).

Strategies for Increased Efficacy and Adherence. The statins are well tolerated. Single daily doses may be sufficient to achieve lipid goals. If single-day dosage is used, lipid response has been shown to be greatest with evening use. Mild gastrointestinal symptoms and headaches are the most common side effects. Liver enzyme elevations occur in 1% to 2% of users and resolve with discontinuation of the drug. Myopathies (muscle aching, soreness, or weakness) associated with elevations in creatine kinase greater than three-times the normal occur in 0.5% of users, but the incidence is increased when statins are used in combination with immunosuppressants, gemfibrozil, and niacin (Gotto, 1992). Patients should be instructed to report muscle aching. If such symptoms are present, liver aminotransferases and creatine kinase should be measured and the drug stopped.

Intestinal Absorption Inhibitors

A new class of medication (intestinal absorption blockers) has recently been released by the FDA. This medication (Ezetimibe) acts by preventing the absorption of cholesterol at the intestinal brush border. The action of Ezetimibe is similar to that of the plant stanols and sterols. This medication appears to be relatively "nonsystemic" in that it works exclusively in the intestine to block the uptake of cholesterol. Through this action, serum cholesterol is lowered, uptake by the liver of LDL is enhanced, and LDL levels decrease. This medication has been shown to lower LDL cholesterol alone or in combination with other cholesterol-lowering medications (Dujovne, 2003; Sudhop, 2002).

Fibric Acid Derivatives

Fibric acid derivatives have been used as hypolipidemic agents. They act primarily to increase LPL activity, which enhances catabolism of VLDL and thereby reduces triglyceride levels (Gotto, 1992). Because of their limited LDL effect, these drugs are not considered first-line therapy for LDL-lowering. They are effective in treating hypertriglyceridemia and low HDL cholesterol states.

General Adherence Strategies

It is estimated that 50% of patients discontinue drug therapy after 1 year and only one-third adhere to dietary interventions beyond 1 year (Houston Miller, 1997; Insull, 1997). Factors related to nonadherence include lack of knowledge, misconceptions, beliefs and attitudes about the therapy, complexity of the regime, side effects, and the strength of the relationship between the patient and the health care provider (Insull, 1997). Patient education should include information about the specific drug regime, how the drug works, when and how to use the drug, and how to minimize potential side effects. Barriers to medication adherence include faulty health perceptions. Beliefs and attitudes may interfere with adherence. Social and environmental barriers may include such problems as difficulty taking medication in social settings or restaurants and lack of equipment for mixing medication. It is appropriate to explore common beliefs, attitudes, and difficulties with the patient and develop strategies together to address these issues. Anticipation of potential side effects should also be explored. Studies indicate that adverse side effects and therapeutic ineffectiveness were the major reasons cited for discontinuing lipid-lowering drugs (Insull, 1997).

Cues to action are important determinants of adherence to medication regimes. Ideal cues are ones that are a part of the patient's habitual routine. Because such cues are habitual, the patient may need assistance in recognizing possible cues. Monitoring and recording medication as it is taken can be useful in identifying potential cues. Feedback is a powerful reinforcer of behavior. Procedures for rapid lipid analysis should be used when possible. Communicating changes in blood lipid response and responding to side effect issues are essential components of lipid management and can often be accomplished by telephone. Consideration should be give to routine telephone contacts to promote adherence and increase the effectiveness of lipid management. Nursing case-managed intervention studies have demonstrated that adherence to lifestyle changes and lipid-lowering drug therapies can be achieved, perhaps caused in part by the strength of the relationship between the nurse and the patient (Haskell et al., 1994).

The nurse is in an excellent position to promote adherence. The focus of the intervention should include the concept of dyslipidemia as a "silent disease," one that is present for life but one for which treatment has been proven effective.

REFERENCES

27th Bethesda Conference. (1996). Matching the intensity of risk factor management with the hazard for coronary disease events. *Journal of the American College of Cardiology, 27,* 957–1047.

American Heart Association. (2002). *Heart and stroke statistics–2003 update.* Dallas, TX: American Heart Association.

Anderson, K. M., Castelli, W. P., & Levy, D. (1987). Cholesterol and mortality: 30 years of follow-up from the Framingham Study. *JAMA, 257,* 2176–2180.

Armstrong, M. L., Warner, E. D., & Connor, W. E. (1970). Regression of coronary atheromatosis in rhesus monkeys. *Circulation Research, 27,* 59–67.

Arntzenius, A. C., et al. (1985). Diets, lipoproteins, and the progression coronary atherosclerosis: The Lieden Intervention Trial. *New England Journal of Medicine, 312,* 805–811.

Asztalos, B. F., & Schaefer, E. (2003). HDL in atherosclerosis: actor or bystander? *Atherosclerosis Supplements,* 4, 21–29.

Austin, M. D., Hokanson, J. E., & Brunzell, J. D. (1994). Characterization of low-density lipoprotein subclasses: Methodologic approaches and clinical relevance. *Current Opinion in Lipidology,* 5, 395–403, 1994

Axelson, M. L., Federline, T. L., & Brinberg, D. (XXXX). AQ1 A meta-analysis of food- and nutrition-related research. *Journal of Nutrition Education,* 17, 51–54.

Bandura, A. (1977). *Social learning theory.* Englewood Cliffs, NJ: Prentice-Hall.

Blankenhorn, D. H., et al. (1990). The influence of diet on the appearance of new lesions in human coronary arteries. *JAMA,* 263, 1646–1652.

Block, G., Rosenberger, W. F., & Patterson, B. H. (1988). Calories, fat and cholesterol: Intake patterns in the US population by race, sex, and age. *American Journal of Public Health,* 78, 1150–1155.

Bonanome, A., & Grundy, S. M. (1988). Effect of stearic acid on plasma cholesterol and lipoprotein levels. *New England Journal of Medicine,* 318, 1244–1248.

Breslow, J. L. (1992). The genetic basis of lipoprotein disorders: Introduction and review. *Journal of Internal Medicine,* 231, 627–631.

Brown, B. G., et al. (1998). Lipid altering or antioxidant vitamins for patients with coronary disease and very low HDL cholesterol? The HDL-Atherosclerosis Treatment Study design. *Canadian Journal of Cardiology,* 14, 6A–13A.

Brown, G., et al. (1990). Regression of coronary artery disease as a result of intensive lipid-lowering therapy in men with high levels of apolipoprotein B. *New England Journal of Medicine,* 323, 1289–1298.

Brown, M. S., Goldstein, J. L. (1986). A receptor-mediated pathway for cholesterol homeostasis. *Science,* 232, 34–47.

Buzzard, I. M., et al. (1990). Diet intervention methods to reduce fat intake: Nutrient and food group composition of self-selected low-fat diets. *Journal of the American Dietetic Association,* 90, 42–50, 53.

Camargo, C. A., et al. (1985). The effect of moderate alcohol intake on serum apolipoproteins A-I and A-II. *JAMA,* 253, 2854–2857.

Campos, H., et al. (1990). Differences in apolipoproteins and lowdensity lipoprotein subfractions in postmenopausal women on and off estrogen therapy: Results from the Framingham Offspring Study. *Metabolism,* 39, 1033–1038.

Castelli, W. P. (1996). Lipids, risk factors and ischaemic heart disease. *Atherosclerosis,* 124(Suppl), S1–S9.

Cohen, J. C. (2003). Endothelial lipase: direct evidence for a role in HDL metabolism. *Journal of Clinical Investigation,* 111, 318–321.

Connor, S. L., Gustafson, J. R., Arthud-Wild, S. M., et al. (1986). The cholesterol/saturated-fat index: An indication of the hypercholesterolemic and atherogenic potential of food. *Lancet* 1(8492), 1229–1232.

Connor, S. L., Gustafson, J. R., Sexton, R., et al. (1992). The diet habit survey: A new method of dietary assessment that relates to plasma cholesterol. *Journal of the American Dietetic Association,* 92, 41–47.

Connor, W. E., Connor, S. L., & Connor, S. L. (1990). Diet, atherosclerosis, and fish oil. *Adv Intern Med,* 35, 135–172.

Connor, W. E., Connor, S. L., Katan, M. B., et al. (1997). Should a low-fat, high-carbohydrate diet be recommended for everyone? A clinical debate. *New England Journal of Medicine,* 337, 562–567.

Crouch, S. J. F., Farquhar, J. W., Haskell, W. L., et al. (1986). Personal and mediated health counseling for sustained dietary reduction of hypercholesterolemia. *Preventive Medicine,* 15, 282–291.

Dattilo, A. M., & Kris-Etherton, P. M. (1992). Effects of weight reduction on blood lipids and lipoproteins: A meta-analysis. *American Journal of Clinical Nutrition,* 56, 320–328.

deGraaf, J., Hak-Lemmers, H., Hector, P. et al. (1991). Enhanced susceptibility to in vitro oxidation of the low-density lipoprotein subfractions in healthy subjects. *Arteriosclerosis and Thrombosis,* 11, 298–306.

deLemos, A. S., Wolfe, M. L., Long, C. J., Sivapackianathan, R., & Rader, D. J. (2002). Identification of genetic variants in endothelial lipase in persons with elevated high-density lipoprotein cholesterol. *Circulation,* 106:1321–1326.

Downs, J. R., Clearfield, M., Weis, S., et al. (1998). Primary prevention of acute coronary events with lovastatin in men and women with average cholesterol levels. *JAMA,* 279, 1615–1622.

Dujovne, CA, et al. (2002). Ezetimibe Study Group. Efficacy and safety of a potent new selective cholesterol absorption inhibitor, ezetimibe, in patients with primary hypercholesterolemia. *American Journal of Cardiology,* 90(10), 1092–7. (Erratum in *American Journal of Cardiology,* 19(11),1399, 2003).

Eisenberg, S. (1984). High-density lipoprotein metabolism. *Journal of Lipid Research,* 25, 1017–1054.

Ewart, C. K. (1989). Changing dietary behavior: A social action theory approach. *Clinical Nutriton,* 8, 9–16.

Fair, J. M., & Berra, K. A. (1996). Endothelial function and coronary risk reduction: Mechanisms and influences of nitric oxide. *Cardiovascular Nursing,* 32, 17–22.

Fletcher, S. W., Colditz, G. A. (2002). Failure of estrogen and progestin therapy for prevention. *JAMA,* 288, 366–368.

Food Surveys Research Group and Agricultural Research Services. (1995). *Data tables: Results from USDA's 1995 Continuing Survey of Food Intakes by Individuals and 1995 Diet and Health Knowledge Survey,* CSFI/DHKS, 1995. Riverdale, MD: Department of Agriculture.

Ford, E. S., Mokdad, A. H., Giles, W. H., & Mensah, G. A. (2003). Serum total cholesterol concentrations and awareness, treatment, and control of hypercholesterolemia among US adults. Findings form the National Health and Nutrition Examination Survey, 1999–2000. *Circulation,* 107, 2185–2189.

Fraser, G. E., Schneider, L. E., Mattison, S., et al. (1988). Behavioral interventions from an office setting in patients with cardiac disease. *Journal of Cardiopulmonary Rehabilitation,* 8, 50–57.

Freudenheim, J. L. (1993). A review of study designs and methods of dietary assessment in nutritional epidemiology of chronic disease. *Journal of Nutrition,* 123, 401–405.

Friedenreich, C. M., Slimani, N., & Riboli, E. (1992). Measurement of past diet: Review of previous and proposed methods. *Epidemiology Review,* 14, 177–196.

Friedewald, W. T., Levy, R. I., & Fredrickson, D. S. (1972). Estimation of the concentration of low-density lipoprotein cholesterol in plasma, with the use of preparative ultracentrifuge. *Clinical Chemistry,* 18, 499–502.

Gardner, C. D., Fortmann, S. P., & Krauss, R. M. (1996). Small low-density lipoprotein particles are associated with the incidence of coronary artery disease in men and women. *JAMA,* 276, 875–881.

Gardner, C. D., Kraemer, H. C. (1995). Monounsaturated versus polyunsaturated dietary fat and serum lipids: A meta-analysis. *Arteriosclerosis Thrombosis Vascular Biology,* 15, 1917–1927.

Goldberg, I. J., Mosca, L., Piano, M. R., & Fisher, E. A. (2001). Wine and Your Heart A science advisory for healthcare professionals from the Nutrition Committee, Council on Epidemiology and Prevention, and Council on Cardiovascular Nursing of the American Heart Association. *Circulation,* 103, 472–475.

Goldstein, J. L., & Brown, M. S. (1987). Regulation of low-density lipoprotein receptors: Implication for pathogenesis and therapy of hypercholesterolemia and atherosclerosis. *Circulation,* 76, 505–507.

Gorder, D., Dolecek, T. A., Coleman, G. G., et al. (1986). Dietary intake in the Multiple Risk Factor Intervention Trial (MRFIT): Nutrient and food group changes over 6 years. *Journal of the American Dietetic Association,* 86, 744–751.

Gordon, D. J., Probstfield, J. L., & Garrison, R. J. (1989). High density lipoprotein cholesterol and cardiovascular disease: Four prospective studies. *Circulation,* 79, 8–15.

Gotto, A. M. (1983). Clinical diagnosis of hyperlipoproteinemia. *American Journal of Medicine,* 74(5A), 5–9.

Gotto, A. M. (1983). High-density lipoproteins: Biochemical and metabolic factors. *American Journal of Cardiology,* 54(4), 2B–8B.

Gotto, A. M., & Pownall, H. J. (1992). *Manual of lipid disorders.* Baltimore: Williams & Wilkins; 1992.

Gould, A. L., et al. (1995). Cholesterol reduction yields clinical benefit: A new look at old data. *Circulation,* 91, 2274–2282.

Grady, et al. (2002). Cardiovascular Disease Outcomes During 6.8 Years of Hormone Therapy. Heart and Estrogen/replacement Study Follow-Up. *JAMA,* 288, 49–57.

Grundy, S. M. (1984). Hyperlipoproteinemia: Metabolic basis and rationale for therapy. *American Journal of Cardiology,* 54, 20C–26C.

Grundy, S. M. (1984). Pathogenesis of hyperlipoproteinemia. *Journal of Lipid Research,* 25, 1611–1618.

Grundy, S. M. (1998). Hypertriglyceridemia, atherogenic dyslipidemia, and the metabolic syndrome. *Am J Cardiol,* 81(4A), 18B–25B.

Grundy, S. M., et al. (1997). Guide to the primary prevention of cardiovascular diseases. *Circulation,* 95, 2329–2331.

Grundy, S. M., & Vega, G.L. (1983). Plasma cholesterol responsiveness to saturated fatty acids. *American Journal of Clinical Nutrition,* 47, 822–824.

Hafner, S. M. (1998). Management of dyslipidemia in adults with diabetes. *Diabetes Care,* 21, 160–178.

Haskell, W. L., et al. (1994). Effects of intensive multiple risk reduction on coronary atherosclerosis and clinical cardiac events in men and women with coronary artery disease. *Circulation,* 89, 975–990.

Haskell, W. L., et al. (1984). The effect of cessation and resumption of moderate alcohol intake on serum high-density-lipoprotein subfractions. *New England Journal of Medicine,* 310, 805–810.

Hegsted, D. M., et al. (1965). Quantitative effects of dietary fat on serum cholesterol in man. *American Journal of Clinical Nutrition, 17,* 281–295.

Heini, A. F., & Weinsier, R. L. (1997). Divergent trends in obesity and fat intake
patterns: The American paradox. *American Journal of Medicine, 102,* 259–264.

Houston Miller, N. (1997). Compliance with treatment regimens in chronic
asymptomatic diseases. *American Journal of Medicine, 102,* 43–49.

Hulley, S. B., Grady, D., Bush, T., et al. (1998). Randomized trial of estrogen
plus progestin for secondary prevention of coronary heart disease in post
menopausal women. *JAMA, 280* (1998), 605–613.

Hulley, S. B., Herman, T. B., Grady, D., et al. (1993). Should we be measuring blood cholesterol levels in young adults? *JAMA, 269,* 1416–1419.

Insull, W. (1997). The problem of compliance to cholesterol altering therapy.
Journal of Internal Medicine, 241, 317–325.

Ishida, T., Choi, S., Kundu, R. K., Hirata, K., Rubin, E. M., Cooper, A. D., &
Quertermous, T. (2003). Endothelial lipase is a major determinant of HDL
level. *Journal of Clinical Investigation, 111,* 347–355.

Jacobs, D., Blackburn, H., Higgins, M., et al. (1992). The Conference on Low
Cholesterol: Mortality associations. *Circulation, 86,* 1046–1060.

Johnson, C. L., Rifkind, B. M., Sempos, C. T., et al. (1993). Declining serum
total cholesterol levels among US adults: The National Health and Nutrition Examination Surveys. *JAMA, 269,* 3002–3008.

Kane, J. P., Malloy, M. J., Ports, T. A., et al. (1990). Regression of coronary atherosclerosis during treatment of familial hypercholesterolemia with combined drug regimes. *JAMA, 264,* 3007–3012.

Kannel, W. B. (1983). High-density lipoproteins: Epidemiologic profile and
risks of coronary artery disease. *American Journal of Cardiology, 52*(4),
9B–12B.

Kashyap, M. L., et al. (1999). Long-term safety and efficacy of a once-daily
niacin/lovastatin formulation for patients with dyslipidemia. *American Journal of Cardiology, 89,* 672–678.

Keys, A. (1970). Coronary heart disease in seven countries. *Circulation,*
41(Suppl I), 1–211.

Keys, A., & Parlin, R.W. (1966). Cholesterol response to changes in dietary
lipids. *American Journal of Clinical Nutrition, 19,* 175–181.

Knopp, R. H., Walden, C. E., Retzlaff, B. M., et al. (1997). Long-term cholesterol-lowering effects of 4 fat-restricted diets in hypercholesterolemic and
combined hyperlipidemic men. *JAMA, 278,* 1509–1515.

Krauss, R. M. (1987). Effects of commonly used sex steroid hormones on
plasma lipoprotein levels in women. In E. D. Eaker, B. Packard, N. K.
Wenger, et al. (Eds.), *Coronary heart disease in women* (pp. 177–180). New
York: Haymarket Doyma.

Krauss, R. M. (1998). Atherogenicity of triglyceride-rich lipoproteins. *American Journal of Cardiology, 26,* 81(4A), 138-178, 81(4A), 13B–17B.

Kris-Etherton, P. et al. (1988). The effect of diet on plasma lipids, lipoproteins,
and coronary heart disease. *Journal of the American Dietetic Association, 88,*
1373–1400.

Kristal, A. R., Shattuck, A. L., & Henry, H. J. (1990). Patterns of dietary
behavior associated with selecting diets low in fat: Reliability and validity of
a behavioral approach to dietary assessment. *Journal of the American Dietetic
Association, 90,* 214–220.

Kushi, L. H., et al. (1985). Diet and 20 year mortality from coronary heart disease. *New England Journal of Medicine, 312,* 811–818.

Law, M. R., Wald, N. J., & Thompson, S. G. (1994). By how much and how
quickly does reduction in serum cholesterol concentration lower risk of
ischaemic heart disease? *BMJ, 308,* 367–373.

Law, M. R. (1999). Lowering heart disease risk with cholesterol reduction:
evidence from observationsl studies and clinical trials. *European Heart Journal Supplement,* Suppl 1, S3–S8.

Lawn, R. M. (1992). Lipoprotein (a) in heart disease. *Scientific American,*
92(6), 54–60.

Leaf, A., & Weber, P. C. (1988). Cardiovascular effects of n-3 fatty acids. *New
England Journal of Medicine, 318,* 549–557.

Levine, G. N., Keaney, J. F., & Vita, J. A. (1995). Cholesterol reduction in cardiovascular disease. *New England Journal of Medicine, 332,* 512–521.

The Lipid Research Clinic Investigators. (1984). The Lipid Research Clinics
Primary Prevention Trials results. *JAMA, 251,* 351–364.

Long-Term Intervention with Pravastatin in Ischaemic Disease (LIPID)
Study Group. (1998). Prevention of cardiovascular events and death
with pravastatin in patients with coronary heart disease and a broad
range of initial cholesterol levels. *New England Journal of Medicine, 339,*
1349–57.

Marmot, M. G. (1984). Alcohol and coronary disease. *International Journal of
Epidemiology, 13,* 160–167.

McCann, B. S., et al. (1990). Promoting adherence to low-fat, low-cholesterol
diets: Review and recommendations. *Journal of the American Dietetic Association, 90,* 1414–1417.

McGee, D. L., Reed, D. M., & Yano, K. A. J. E. (1984). Ten-year incidence of
coronary heart disease in the Honolulu Heart Program: Relationship to
nutrient intake. *American Journal of Epidemiology, 119,* 667–676.

Mensink, R. P., & Katan, M. B. (1992). Effect of dietary fatty acids on serum
lipids and lipoproteins: A meta-analysis of 27 trials. *Arteriosclerosis and
Thrombosis, 12,* 911–919.

Miller, N. E. (1990). HDL metabolism and its role in lipid transport. *European Heart Journal, 11,* H1–H3.

Muldoon, M. F., Manuck, S. B., & Matthews, K. A. (1990). Lowering cholesterol concentrations and mortality: A quantitative review of primary prevention trials. *BMJ, 301,* 309–314.

National Cholesterol Education Program. (2001). *Expert Panel on Detection,
Evaluation, and Treatment of High Blood Cholesterol in Adults.* (Adult Treat-
ment Panel III) National Institutes of Health, Publication no. 01–3670.
Bethesda, MD: U.S. Department of Health and Human Services.

The Expert Panel. (1993). Summary of the second report of the National Cho-
lesterol Education Program Expert Panel on Detection, Evaluation, and
Treatment of High Blood Cholesterol in Adults (Adult Treatment Panel II).
JAMA, 269, 3015–3023.

Ordovas, J. M., et al. (1986). Apoprotein A-I gene polymorphism associated
with premature coronary artery disease and familial hypoalphalipoproteinemia. *New England Journal of Medicine, 314,* 671–677.

Ornish, D., et al. (1990). Can lifestyle changes reverse coronary heart disease?
Lancet, 336, 129–133.

Pope-Cordle, J., & Katahn, M. E. (1991). *The T-factor fat gram counter.* New
York: Norton.

Reaven, G. M., et al. (1993). Insulin resistance and hyperinsulinemia in individuals with small, dense, low-density lipoprotein particles. *Journal of Clinical Investigation, 92,* 141–146.

Rifkind, B. M. (1991). *Drug treatment of hyperlipidemia.* New York: Marcel
Dekker.

Risks and Benefits of Estrogen Plus Progestin in Healthy Postmenopausal
Women. (2002). Principal results for the Women's Health Initiative Randomized Trial. Writing Group for the Women's Health Initiative Investigators. *JAMA, 288,* 321–333.

Sacks, F. M., et al. (1996). for the Cholesterol and Recurrent Events Trial
Investigators. The effect of pravastatin on coronary events after myocardial
infarction in patients with average cholesterol levels. *New England Journal of
Medicine, 335:*1001–9.

Scandinavian Simvastatin Survival Study Group. (1995). Randomised trial of
cholesterol lowering in 4444 patients with coronary heart disease: The Scandinavian Simvastatin Survival Study (4S). *Lancet, 344,* 1383–1389.

Schaefer, E. J., & Levy, R. I. (1985). Pathogenesis and management of lipoprotein disorders. *New England Journal of Medicine, 312,* 1300–1310.

Schectman, G., et al. (1990). Dietary intake of Americans reporting adherence
to low cholesterol diet (NHANES II). *American Journal of Public Health, 80,*
698–703.

Schuler, G., et al. (1992). Regular physical exercise and low fat diet: Effects on
progression of coronary artery disease. *Circulation, 86,* 1–11.

Shepherd, J., et al. (1995). Prevention of coronary heart disease with pravastatin in men with hypercholesterolemia. *New England Journal of Medicine,
333,* 1301–1307.

Smith, S. C., et al. (1995). Preventing heart attack and death in patients with
coronary disease. *Circulation, 92,* 2–4.

Smith-Schneider, L. M., Sigman-Grant, M. J., & Kris-Etherton, P. M. (1992).
Dietary fat reduction strategies. *Journal of the American Dietetic Association,
92,* 34–38.

Stampfer, M. J., et al. (1988). A prospective study of moderate alcohol consumption and the risk of coronary disease and stroke in women. *New
England Journal of Medicine, 319,* 267–273.

Steinberg, D., et al. (1989). Beyond cholesterol: Modification of low-density
lipoprotein that increase its atherogenicity. *New England Journal of Medicine, 320,* 915–924.

Sudhop, T., & von Bergmann, K. (2002). Cholesterol absorption inhibitors for
the treatment of hypercholesterolemia. *Drugs, 62*(16), 2333–47.

Stone, N. J., Blum, C. B., Winslow, E. (1997). *Management of lipids in clinical practice.* Caddo, OK: Professional Communications Inc.

Sullivan, M. J. (1996). Estrogen replacement. *Circulation, 94,* 2699–2702.

Tall, A. R. (1998). Overview of reverse cholesterol transport. *European Heart
Journal, 19,* A31–35.

Tall, A. R., & Small, D. M. (1978). Current concepts: Plasma high-density lipoproteins. *New England Journal of Medicine, 299*, 1232–1236.

Thompson, P. D., et al. (2003). Exercise and physical activity in the prevention and treatment of atherosclerotic cardiovascular disease. A statement from the council on clinical cardiology (Subcommittee on exercise, rehabilitation, and prevention) and the council on nutrition, physical activity, and metabolism (Subcommittee on physical activity). *Circulation, 107*, 3109–3116.

Tobert, J. A. (1987). New developments in lipid-lowering therapy: The role of inhibitors of hydroxymethylglutaryl-coenzyme A reductase. *Circulation, 76*, 534–538.

Treasure, C. B., et al. (1995). Beneficial effects of cholesterol-lowering therapy on the coronary endothelium in patients with coronary artery disease. *New England Journal of Medicine, 332*, 481–487.

U.S. Department of Health and Human Services. (1990). *Recommendations for improving cholesterol measurement: A report from the Laboratory Standardization Panel of the National Cholesterol Education Program.* Bethesda, MD: U.S. Department of Health and Human Services.

Watts, G. F., et al. (1992). Effects on coronary artery disease of lipid lowering diet, or diet plus cholestyramine, in the St. Thomas Arteriosclerosis Regression Study (STARS). *Lancet, 339*, 563–569.

The Women's Health Initiative Steering Committe. (2004). Effects of conjugated equine estrogen in postmenopausal women with hysterecotomy. The Women's Health Initiative Randomized Controlled Trial. *JAMA, 291*, 1701–1712.

Wood, P. D., Stefanick, M.L., & Haskell, W.L. (1991). The effects on plasma lipoproteins of a prudent weight reducing diet with and without exercise in overweight men and women. *New England Journal of Medicine, 325*, 461–466.

Exercise and Activity

JONATHAN MYERS

Since the late 1950s, numerous scientific reports have examined the relationships between physical activity, physical fitness, and cardiovascular health. Expert panels convened by organizations such as the Centers for Disease Control and Prevention (CDC), American College of Sports Medicine (ACSM), American Association of Cardiovascular and Pulmonary Rehabilitation (AACVPR), and the American Heart Association (AHA) (Centers for Disease Control and Prevention, 1993; American College of Sports Medicine Position Stand, 1998; Fletcher et al., 2001; Pate et al., 1995; Leon et al., 1990; American College of Sports Medicine, 2000), along with the 1996 U.S. Surgeon General's report on physical activity and health (U.S. Public Health Service, 1996), have reinforced scientific evidence linking regular physical activity to various measures of cardiovascular health. The prevailing view in these reports is that more active or fit individuals tend to experience less coronary heart disease (CHD) than their sedentary counterparts, and when they do acquire CHD, it occurs at a later age and tends to be less severe (Pate, 1995; American College of Sports Medicine, 2000; Haskell et al., 1992; Paffenbarger, 1986). Cardiac rehabilitation, as an industry, has evolved in large part because of the abundance of scientific evidence indicating that regular exercise improves physical function and reduces the risk of reinfarction and sudden death in patients with known CHD (Leon et al., 1990; O'Conner et al., 1989; Oldridge etl al., 1988; Wenger et al., 1995). Despite this evidence, however, most adults in the United States remain effectively sedentary (Centers for Disease Control and Prevention; 1993; Pate et al., 1995), and more than 80% of patients who sustain a myocardial infarction (MI) are not referred to a cardiac rehabilitation program (Wenger et al., 1995). This is caused in part by the fact that physical activity is not currently integrated into the U.S. health care paradigm, and the majority of physicians fail to prescribe exercise to their patients (Wee et al., 1999; Sherman & Hershman, 1993; Damush et al., 1999; Ribisl, 2001).

It is therefore incumbent on the nurse or other health care provider to encourage patients to become more physically active, to appreciate the role of rehabilitation in cardiac care, and to develop strategies that promote the adoption of physically active lifestyles in all their patients. This chapter describes the scientific evidence linking physical activity and health, summarizes the physiologic changes that occur with a program of regular exercise, and provides an outline for cardiac rehabilitation in the modern treatment era.

ROLE OF EXERCISE IN CARDIOVASCULAR HEALTH

Epidemiologic Evidence Supporting Physical Activity

It has been estimated that as many as 250,000 deaths per year in the United States are attributable to lack of regular physical activity (Hahn et al., 1986; McGinnis & Foege, 1993). Ongoing longitudinal studies have provided consistent evidence of varying strength documenting the protective effects of activity for a number of chronic diseases, including CHD (Fletcher et al., 2001; Pate et al., 1995; Leon et al., 1990; American College of Sports Medicine, 2000; U.S. Public Health Service, 1996; Haskell et al., 1992; Paffenbarger et al., 1986; O'Conner et al., 1989; Oldridge et al., 1988), type II diabetes (Helmrich et al., 1991; Manson et al., 1992; Manson et al., 1991; Myers et al., 2003; Tanasescu et al., 2003), hypertension (Hagberg, 1990), osteoporosis (Marcus et al.,1992;), and site-specific cancers (Thune & Furberg, 2001). In contrast, low levels of physical fitness or activity are consistently associated with higher cardiovascular and all-cause mortality rates (Fletcher et al., 2001; Pate et al., 1995; American College of Sports Medicine, 2000; U.S. Public Health Service, 1996; Haskell et al., 1992; Paffenbarger et al., 1986). Midlife increases in physical activity, through change in occupation or recreational activities, are associated with a decrease in mortality rates (Paffenbarger et al., 1993).

The landmark epidemiologic work of Paffenbarger and associates among Harvard alumni (Paffenbarger et al., 1986, 1993, 1994) has been particularly persuasive in support of physical activity and, thus, the development of the CDC, AHA, and ACSM guidelines. Table 41-1 illustrates the rates and relative risks of death over a 9-year period among 11,864 Harvard alumni by patterns of physical activity. Several findings in Table 41-1 are particularly noteworthy. The largest benefits in terms of mortality appear to occur in engaging in moderate activity levels; *moderate* is generally defined as activity performed at an intensity of 3 to 6 METs (a multiple of the resting metabolic rate), approximately equivalent to brisk walking for most adults (Ainsworth et al., 1993). Note also that regular moderate walking or sports participation is associated with 30% to 40% reductions in mortality (relative risk of

Table 41–1 ■ RATES AND RELATIVE RISKS OF DEATH* AMONG HARVARD ALUMNI, BY PATTERNS OF PHYSICAL ACTIVITY

Physical Activity (weekly)		Person-Years (%)		N of Deaths	Deaths per 10,000 Man-Years	Relative Risk of Death		P-Value of Trend
Walking (km)	<5	26		228	86.2	1.00 ⎤		<0.001
	5–14	42		275	67.4	0.78 ⎬		
	15+	32		194	57.7	0.67 ⎦		
Stair-climbing (floors)	<20	37		341	80.0	1.00 ⎤		
	20–54	48		293	62.9	0.79 ⎬		0.001
	55+	15		80	59.6	0.75 ⎦		
All sports play	None	12		156	88.9	1.00 ⎤		
	Light only	10		152	97.4	1.10 ⎥		<0.001
	Light & moderate	36		208	59.7	0.67 ⎬		
	Moderate only[‡]	42		178	56.4	0.63 ⎦		
Moderate Sportsplay (h)	<1	30		308	92.9	1.00 ⎤		
	1–2	41		126	58.2	0.63 ⎬		<0.001
	3+	29		64	43.6	0.47 ⎦		
Index (kcal)[§]	<500	12 ⎤		197	110.3 ⎤	1.00 ⎤		
	500–999	18 ⎥		135	69.1 ⎥	0.63 ⎥		
	1,000–1,499	15 ⎬ 58		111	68.9 ⎬ 78.9	0.62 ⎬ 1.00		
	1,500–1,999	13 ⎦		73	61.4 ⎦	0.56 ⎦		
	2,000–2,499	10 ⎤		51	52.4 ⎤	0.48 ⎤		<0.001
	2,500–2,999	8 ⎥		44	64.6 ⎥	0.59 ⎥		
	3,000–3,400	6 ⎬ 42		36	74.7 ⎬ 55.4	0.68 ⎬ 0.70		
	3,500+	18 ⎦		82	48.1 ⎦	0.44 ⎦		

METs, metabolic equivalents.
* Age-adjusted.
[†] <4.5 METs intensity.
[‡] 4.5+METs intensity.
[§] Sum of walking, stair climbing, and all sports play.
From Paffenbarger, R. S. Hyde, R. T. Wing A. L., et al. (1994). Some interrelations of physical activity, physical fitness, health, and longevity. In C. Bouchard, R. J. Shephard, T. Stephens (Eds.), *Physical activity, fitness, and health* (pp. 119–133), Champaign, IL: Human Kinetics.

death 0.60 to 0.70). Likewise, the physical activity index, expressed as kilocalories per week (the sum of walking, stair climbing, and sports participation) suggests that a 40% reduction in mortality occurs by engaging in modest levels of activity (1,000 to 2,000 kcal/week, equivalent to three to five 1-hour sessions of activity), whereas only minimal additional benefits are achieved by engaging in greater-intensity activity. These findings agree closely with earlier results among 16,936 Harvard alumni assessed in the early 1960s and followed-up for all-cause mortality for nearly 20 years (Paffenbarger et al., 1984). Similar results have been reported from large studies that have followed-up people for CHD morbidity and mortality in the range of 10 to 20 years among British civil servants (Morris et al., 1966; Morris et al., 1980), U.S. railroad workers (Slattery et al., 1989), San Francisco longshoremen (Paffenbarger et al., 1970), nurses (Rockhill et al., 2001; Hu et al., 2001), physicians (Lee et al., 1999), other health care workers (Albert et al.,2000), and other cohorts (for review, see Kohl [Kohl, 2001] or Lee and Paffenbarger [Lee & Paffenbarger, 1996]). Clearly, the evidence linking a physically active lifestyle and cardiovascular health is substantial.

Physiologic Fitness and Health

A growing number of studies have been published in which physical fitness, determined by standardized exercise testing, was determined among large samples of men and women who have been followed-up for the incidence of CHD morbidity and mortality for up to 10 years (Blair et al., 1989; Ekelund et al., 1988; Paffenbarger et al., 1993; Arraiz et al., 1992; Myers et al., 2002; Roger et al., 1998; Goraya et al., 2000; Snader et al., 1997). Each of these studies demonstrated that higher levels of fitness were associated with lower rates of CHD or all-cause mortality. Importantly, these associations appear to be independent of other CHD risk factors. Moreover, the low levels of fitness in these studies did not appear to be associated with subclinical disease. In general, fitness levels have also been associated with physical activity status assessed by questionnaire (Paffenbarger et al., 1994; Lee & Paffenbarger, 1996; Paffenbarger et al., 1993).

Blair and associates (Blair et al., 1989) assessed fitness by treadmill performance in 10,244 men and 3,120 women and followed them for 110,482 person-years (averaging >8 years) for all-cause mortality. These results are presented in Table 41-2. Mortality rates were lowest (18.6 per 10,000 man-years) among the most fit and highest (64.0) among the least fit men, with the corresponding rates among the women 8.5 and 39.5 per 10,000 man-years, respectively. These findings closely parallel the results from studies relating physical activity levels and mortality (Paffenbarger et al., 1970, 1984, 1993; Morris et al., 1966, 1980; Slattery et al., 1989; Rockhill et al., 2001; Lee & Paffenbarger, 1996). Although physical activity status and physiologic fitness are clearly linked, the latter carries an important genetic component; that is, some people remain comparatively fit without engaging in a great deal of physical activity. The findings of Blair and colleagues (Blair et al., 1989) and others (Williams, 2001) imply that the benefits of physical activity on health and survival are mediated largely through fitness status.

Table 41–2 ■ RATES AND RELATIVE RISKS OF DEATH* AMONG 10, 244 MEN AND 3,120 WOMEN, BY GRADIENTS OF PHYSIC FITNESS

	Men			Women		
Quintiles of Fitness[†]	N of Deaths	Deaths per 10,000 Man-Years	Relative Risk of Death[‡]	No of Deaths	Deaths per 10,000 Woman-Years	Relative Risk of Death[‡]
1(low)	75	64.0	1.00	18	39.5	1.00
2	40	25.5	0.40	11	20.5	0.52
3	47	27.1	0.42	6	12.2	0.31
4	43	21.7	0.34	4	6.5	0.15
5(high)	35	18.6	0.29	4	8.5	0.22

* Age-adjusted.
[†] Quintiles of fitness determined by maximal exercise testing.
[†] P Value for trend 0.05.
From Blair, S. N., Kohl, III H. W., Paffenbarger, Jr. R. S., et al.(1989). Physical fitness and all-cause mortality: A prospective study of healthy men and women. *JAMA*, 262, 2395–2401.

More recently, this issue has been addressed in clinical populations, e.g., patients referred for exercise testing for clinical reasons (Myers et al., 2002; Roger et al., 1998; Goraya et al., 2000; Snader et al., 1997). In a recent study performed among U.S. veterans, 6,213 men underwent maximal exercise testing for clinical reasons and were followed-up for a mean of 6.2 years (Myers et al., 2002). The subjects were classified into five categories by gradients of fitness. After adjustment for age, the researchers observed that the largest gains in terms of mortality were achieved between the lowest fitness group and the next lowest fitness group. Figure 41-1 illustrates the age-adjusted relative risks associated with the different categories of fitness. Among normal subjects and those with cardiovascular disease, the least fit individuals had more than four-times the risk of all-cause

mortality compared with the most fit. Importantly, an individual's fitness level was a stronger predictor of mortality than established risk factors such as smoking, high blood pressure, high cholesterol, and diabetes. Over the past few years, other cohorts, such as those from the Cleveland Clinic (Snader et al., 1997) and the Mayo Clinic (Roger et al., 1998; Goraya et al., 2000), have documented the importance of exercise capacity as a predictor of mortality among clinically referred populations. These clinically based studies confirm the observations of Blair et al. (Blair et al., 1989), Framingham (Kannel et al., 1985), and the Lipid Research Clinics Trial (Ekelund et al., 1988) among asymptomatic populations, underscoring the fact that fitness level has a strong influence on the incidence of cardiovascular and all-cause morbidity and mortality.

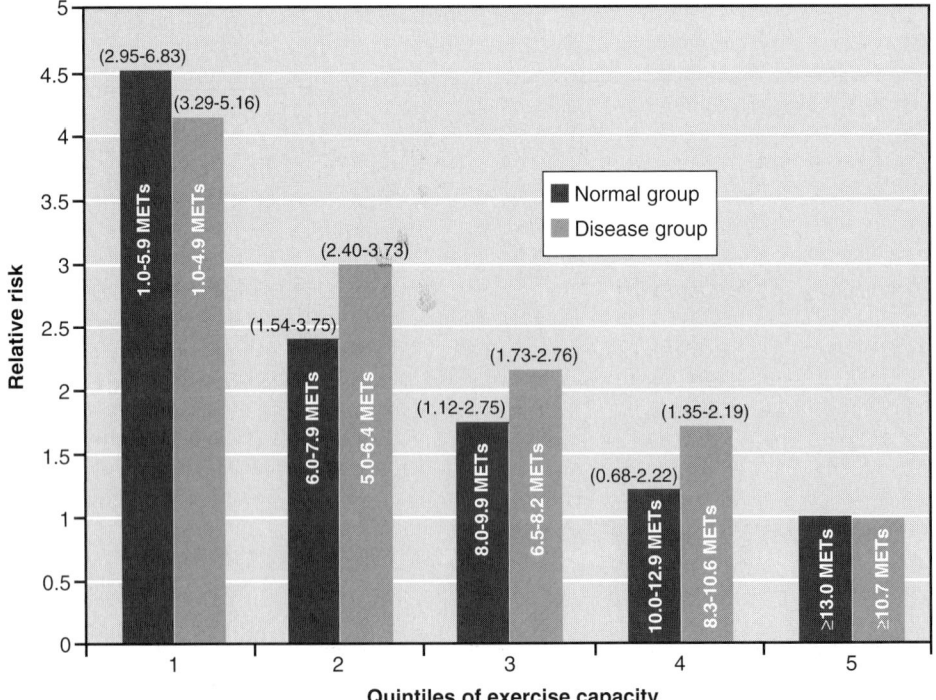

■ **Figure 41–1.** Age-adjusted relative risks of mortality by quintiles of exercise capacity among normal subjects and patients with cardiovascular disease. The subgroup with the highest exercise capacity (group 5) is the reference category. For each quintile, the range of values for exercise capacity represented appears within each bar; 95% confidence intervals for the relative risks appear above each bar. (From Myers, J. N., et al. [2002]. Exercise capacity and mortality among men refered for exercise testing. *New England Journal of Medicine*, 346, 793–853.)

Surgeon General's Report on Physical Activity and Health

Published in 1996, the Surgeon General's Report on Physical Activity and Health represented the strongest policy statement ever made by the U.S. Government concerning physical activity (U.S. Public Health Service, 1996). It represented a historic turning point redefining exercise as a key component to health promotion and disease prevention. The federal government has mounted a multi-year educational campaign based on this report. In this report, the epidemiologic evidence supporting physical activity in the prevention of CHD morbidity and mortality is reviewed in detail. The document also outlines the quantity of exercise necessary to achieve these benefits. It is suggested that each person perform a moderate amount of activity daily, with the amount of activity emphasized rather than the intensity. The concept is that this offers people more opportunities for activities that fit into their daily lives. It is suggested that people perform this moderate amount of activity for 30 minutes or more on most, and preferably all, days of the week. These activities can take the form of brisk walking, yard work or other household chores, jogging, or a wide variety of recreational activities. Within the Surgeon General's report, the National Institutes of Health (NIH) Consensus Conference Statement on Physical Activity and Cardiovascular Health is quoted (NIH Consensus Development Panel on Physical Activity and Cardiovascular Health, 1996).

The latter report more specifically outlines the cardiovascular benefits of exercise and states what is required to achieve these benefits. The NIH document underscores the recommendation that all children and adults should set a long-term goal to accumulate at least 30 minutes or more of moderate-intensity physical activity on most days of the week. Repeated intermittent or shorter bouts of activity (e.g., 10 minutes), including occupational, non-occupational, or tasks of daily living, have similar cardiovascular and health benefits if performed at a level of moderate intensity (e.g., brisk walking, cycling, swimming, home repair, and yard work) with an accumulated duration of at least 30 minutes per day. Individuals who already meet these standards receive additional benefits from increasing this amount to more vigorous activity.

"Health" Versus "Fitness" Benefits of Exercise

A noteworthy theme that is consistent in each of the aforementioned documents is that considerable health benefits are derived from moderate levels of activity; it is generally not necessary to engage in vigorous, sustained activity to derive many of these benefits. Before the release of these reports in the mid 1990s, consensus documents generally promoted the concept that exercise was thought to be effective only if an improvement in some measure of cardiopulmonary function was observed. In recent years, the philosophy on exercise as a means to this end ("fitness" measured by exercise capacity) has changed significantly. It is now appreciated that substantial health benefits can be achieved through more modest amounts of regular exercise, regardless of whether exercise results in a measurable improvement in exercise capacity. Epidemiologic studies have shown that death rates from cardiovascular and all causes are considerably lower even among people who engage in modest amounts of exercise, less than the threshold that was generally thought necessary to increase exercise capacity (American College of Sports Medicine Position Stand, 1998; Fletcher et al., 2001; Pate et al., 1995; Leon et al., 1990; American College of Sports Medicine, 2000; U.S. Public Health Service, 1996; Paffenbarger et al., 1994; Kohl; Lee & Paffenbarger, 1996). It is important for health professionals to be aware of the distinction between "health" and "fitness" when making activity recommendations to patients with cardiovascular disease, those at high risk for its development, and healthy adults. In addition to cardiopulmonary fitness, measures of fat and lean weight, bone density, glucose and insulin metabolism, blood lipid and lipoprotein metabolism, and quality of life should be included under the category of "health." A favorable profile for these variables represents a clear advantage in terms of health outcomes as assessed by morbidity and mortality statistics.

Role of Exercise in Secondary Prevention

During the 1970s and 1980s, numerous controlled trials addressed whether participation in a rehabilitation program influenced morbidity or mortality in patients with CHD. Although the results of these trials independently were inconclusive, most demonstrated a favorable trend for a lower mortality rate among patients who exercised compared with control subjects. For example, the National Exercise and Heart Disease Project was a controlled randomized trial in the United States on the effects of prescribed supervised exercise involving 651 men with acute MI (Shaw, 1981). The cumulative 3-year total mortality rates in this study were 7.3% and 4.6% for the control and exercise groups, respectively, whereas the rates for recurrent MI were 7.0% and 5.4%, respectively. Although this represented 37% and 24% reductions in mortality and reinfarction rates, respectively, for the exercise groups, more than twice as many patients would have been necessary in the study for these differences to be statistically significant. The lack of adequate sample size in this study is typical of the secondary prevention trials that have assessed mortality; although the trends are generally favorable, few have independently demonstrated that patients randomized to an exercise program have a significantly lower mortality compared to control subjects. However, two cardiac rehabilitation trials in Europe were noteworthy for their favorable morbidity and mortality outcomes. Vermuelen and associates (Vermuelen et al., 1983), in a study involving fewer than 100 patients, found that a 6-week rehabilitation program including comprehensive risk factor reduction and exercise resulted in a 50% lower rate of combined CHD morbidity and mortality in the rehabilitation compared to the control patients over a 5-year follow-up period. In the second of these multiple risk factor intervention trials, Kallio and colleagues (Kallio et al., 1979) studied 375 consecutive male and female patients after MI younger than age 65 years in two clinical centers in Finland. After 3 years of follow-up, the cumulative CHD mortality rate was significantly lower in the

Table 41–3 ■ META-ANALYSIS OF CONTROLLED EXERCISE TRIALS IN PATIENTS WITH CORONARY HEART DISEASE

	N of Events (%)		N of Patients (%)	Pooled Odds Ratio (95% CI)	P value
	Treatment		Control		
All-cause death	236/1823 (12.9)		289.1791 (16.1)	0.76 (0.63–0.92)	0.004
Cardiovascular death	204/2051 (9.9)		252/1993 (12.6)	0.75 (0.62–0.93)	0.006

From Oldridge, N. B., Guyatt, G. H., Fischer, M. E., et al. (1988). Cardiac rehabilitation with exercise after myocardial infarction. *JAMA*, 260, 945–950.

intervention group compared to the control group (18.6% vs. 29.4%). This difference primarily reflected a reduction in sudden death in the intervention group during the first 6 months after MI. A favorable trend toward reduction in nonfatal re-infarctions also was observed in the intervention group.

An alternative but less rigorous scientific approach, in the absence of a definitive clinical trial, is to pool data from existing long-term, randomized, secondary prevention trials in which exercise training was a component. A number of such meta-analyses have been published in which data from six to 22 randomized, long-term, clinical trials were pooled using the intention-to-treat principle (O'Conner et al., 1989; Oldridge et al., 1988; May et al., 1982). In the trials included in these meta-analyses, intervention consisted of either a formal exercise program or exercise advice, generally in combination with multiple risk factor management, making it impossible to determine the independent contribution of exercise to subsequent morbidity and mortality. Nevertheless, patients randomized to active cardiac rehabilitation programs after an MI had statistically significant reductions of approximately 25% in 1-year to 3-year rates of fatal cardiovascular events and total mortality compared to control patients (Table 41-3). However, significant differences in general were not found in the rate of nonfatal recurrent re-infarctions in patients undergoing intervention compared with control patients. The reduction in mortality attributed to cardiac rehabilitation by these pooled data is similar in extent to that associated with beta-blocking drugs in clinical trials after MI (May et al., 1982).

Physiologic Benefits of Exercise Training

Regular exercise increases work capacity. Hundreds of studies have been performed cross-sectionally that document higher maximum oxygen consumption (VO$_2$ max) values among active versus sedentary individuals or between groups after a period of training. The magnitude of improvement in VO$_2$ max with training varies widely, usually ranging from 5% to 25%, but increases as large as 50% have been reported. The degree of change in exercise capacity depends primarily on initial state of fitness and intensity of training. Training increases exercise capacity by increasing maximal cardiac output and the ability to extract oxygen from the blood. The physiologic benefits of a training program can be classified as morphologic, hemodynamic, and metabolic (Display 41-1). Many animal studies have demonstrated significant morphologic changes with training, including myocardial hypertrophy with improved myocardial function, increases in coronary artery size, and increases in the myocardial capillary-to-fiber ratio. However, such changes have been difficult to demonstrate in humans (American College of Sports Medicine, 2000; Froelicher & Myers, 2000). The major *morphologic* outcome of a training program in humans is probably an increase in cardiac size; however, this adaptation also appears to occur mainly in younger healthy people and is an unlikely outcome among individuals older than age 40 or in patients with heart disease. However, significant *hemodynamic* changes have been well documented among patients with heart disease after training. These include reductions in heart rate (HR) at rest and any matched submaximal workload, which is beneficial in that it results in a reduction in myocardial oxygen demand during activities of daily living (ADLs). Other hemodynamic changes that have been demonstrated after training include reductions in blood pressure, increases in blood volume, and increases in maximal oxygen uptake. The most important physiologic benefits of training among patients with heart disease occur in the skeletal muscle. The metabolic capacity of the skeletal muscle is

---

DISPLAY 41-1

PHYSIOLOGIC ADAPTATIONS TO PHYSICAL TRAINING IN HUMANS

Morphologic Adaptations
Myocardial hypertrophy

Hemodynamic Adaptations
Increased blood volume
Increased end-diastolic volume
Increased stroke volume
Increased cardiac output
Reduced heart rate for any submaximal workload

Metabolic Adaptations
Increased mitochondrial volume and number
Greater muscle glycogen stores
Enhanced fat utilization
Enhanced lactate removal
Increased enzymes for aerobic metabolism
Increased maximal oxygen uptake

DISPLAY **41-2**

CHANGES IN RISK FACTORS INFLUENCED BY EXERCISE TRAINING

Decrease in blood pressure
Increase in high-density lipoprotein cholesterol level
Augmented weight reduction efforts
Psychological effects
   Less depression
   Reduced anxiety
Improved glucose tolerance
Improved fitness level

DISPLAY **41-3**

PHYSIOLOGIC CONSEQUENCES OF PROLONGED BED REST

1. Loss of muscle mass, strength, and endurance
2. Decreased plasma and blood volume
3. Decreased ventricular volume
4. Increased hematocrit and hemoglobin
5. Diuresis and natriuresis
6. Venous stasis
7. Bone demineralization
8. Increased heart rate at rest and submaximal levels of activity
9. Decreased resting and maximum stroke volume
10. Decreased maximum cardiac output
11. Decreased maximal oxygen uptake
12. Increased venous compliance
13. Increased risk of venous thrombosis and thromboembolism
14. Decreased orthostatic tolerance
15. Incresed risk of atelectasis, pulmonary emboli

From Myers, J. N. (1995). Physiologic adaptations to exercise and immobility. In S. L. Woods, E. S. Sivarajan-Froelicher, C. J. Halpenny, & S. Underhill Motzer (Eds.), *Cardiac nursing* (3rd ed., pp. 147–162.). Philadelphia: JB Lippincott.

enhanced through increases in mitochondrial volume and number, capillary density, and oxidative enzyme content. These adaptations enhance perfusion and the efficiency of oxygen extraction (American College of Sports Medicine, 2000; Froelicher & Myers, 2000). Finally, an important influence of training is a favorable effect on the risk profile in patients recovering from MI (Display 41-2). Although this may include such things as reductions in blood pressure, reduction in body weight, reduction in total cholesterol and LDL, and an increase in HDL, recent studies suggest that the most powerful influence of regular exercise may be an improvement in insulin sensitivity. It is also important to note that although the effect of exercise on any single risk factor may generally be small, the effect of continued regular exercise on overall cardiovascular risk, when combined with other lifestyle modifications such as proper nutrition, smoking cessation, and medication use, can be dramatic.

Cardiovascular Effects of Immobility

The deleterious physiologic effects of prolonged bed rest have been studied extensively. Since the late 1960s, these studies have been an important stimulus for cardiac rehabilitation. Although these effects are commonly attributed to the absence of regular physical activity, an additional important factor underlying the deconditioning of bed rest is the absence of normal hydrostatic pressure caused by orthostatic stress (i.e., caused by gravity). Thus, even short periods of bed rest (2 to 5 days) are accompanied not only by reduced exercise capacity but also by reductions in muscle mass and strength, alterations in body fluid distribution, and orthostatic intolerance (Display 41-3). The importance of the absence of orthostatic stress on the deconditioning response has been documented by studies demonstrating that exercise training during bed rest is only partially effective or fails to maintain VO_2 max (Myers, 1995; Rousseau, 1993).

Through much of the past century, patients were almost completely immobilized in bed for 6 to 8 weeks after MI. As recently as the 1960s, extended periods of bed rest were thought to facilitate myocardial healing for patients recovering from MI. Today, the converse is true. Carefully prescribed and supervised physical activity is recommended as soon as 1 day after the event to counteract the many negative physiologic

effects of bed rest. In addition to their cardiovascular event, patients may be subjected to long periods of immobilization because of severe pain; musculoskeletal or nervous system impairment, including paralysis; generalized weakness; psychosocial problems, such as severe depression; and infectious disease. The extensive literature available on the deleterious effects of immobility has been reviewed elsewhere (Myers, 1995; Rousseau, 1993).

CARDIAC REHABILITATION

Cardiac rehabilitation programs are designed to limit the physiologic and psychological effects of cardiac illness, reduce the risk for sudden death or reinfarction, control cardiac symptoms, stabilize the atherosclerotic process, and enhance the psychosocial and vocational status of selected patients. Cardiac rehabilitation services are typically prescribed for patients who: (1) have had MI; (2) have had coronary revascularization (bypass surgery, PTCA, or stent placement); or (3) have chronic stable angina pectoris. In recent years, cardiac rehabilitation has been expanded to include patients who have chronic heart failure (CHF) and those who have undergone valvular replacement, cardiac transplantation, or pacemaker implantation. Although the spectrum of patients who benefit from rehabilitation has widened, changes in health care economics have drastically altered the way in which cardiac rehabilitation is implemented. Hospital stays are shorter, progression through the program is more rapid, and much of "cardiac rehabilitation" as it was traditionally known has changed. Reimbursement patterns differ considerably from one state to another, and insurance coverage for rehabilitation services differs widely. With shorter periods of time for physicians and nurses to interact with and monitor patients and cover educational materials adequately, there is a greater need for structured outpatient programs in the home or community.

Historically, typical phases that were included in rehabilitation were phase I, which includes the coronary care unit and inpatient care during the first few days after the event; phase II, which involves convalescence, an outpatient program, or a home program; and phase III, which was usually a longer-term community-based or home program. The precise course of each program naturally depends on the individual's needs and clinical status.

In-Hospital Rehabilitation after a Myocardial Event

The purpose of beginning cardiac rehabilitation immediately after a myocardial event is to counteract the negative effects of deconditioning rather than to promote training adaptations. It also provides an ideal time to begin education and psychological support. These first 3 to 5 days after a myocardial infarction or bypass surgery are critical for beginning these processes. The literature is replete with studies documenting the efficacy and safety of beginning activities and education soon after a coronary event in stable patients. Initially, it is worthwhile for the nurse, in concert with the primary physician, to medically evaluate the patient, including assessing the patient's clinical stability and the severity of the myocardial infarction. Details concerning the diagnosis and management of myocardial infarction are presented in Chapter 20. An overview of patient assessment is provided in the context of the patient being considered for cardiac rehabilitation.

History and Physical Examination. The tools for assessment begin with the history and physical examination. The first step in evaluating patients for cardiac rehabilitation is to determine whether the cardiovascular disease is stable. Each patient should be stratified into an appropriate risk category using information usually available from the history and physical examination, as well as diagnostic tests performed as part of the hospital course (Display 41-4). Stability is determined primarily by the presence or absence of myocardial ischemia, CHF, and dysrhythmias.

DISPLAY 41–4

CRITERIA FOR STRATIFYING LOW, INTERMEDIATE, AND HIGH RISK

Low Risk
- No significant LV dysfunction (i.e., EF > 50%).
- Has had successful reperfusion of myocardium (e.g., PTCA, CABG).
- No resting or activity-induced myocardial ischemia manifested as angina or ST segment displacement on the telemetry monitor or from stress test.
- No resting or activity-induced complex arrhythmias.
- No orthostatic BP changes causing patient to become symptomatic.
- Patient followed a regular exercise program or had an "active" lifestyle before hospitalization.
- No other current health problems that would potentially complicate activity regime (e.g., PVD, orthopedic problems, moderate to severe COPD/emphysema, pericarditis).

Intermediate Risk
- Mild to moderately depressed LV function (e.g., EF 31%–49%).
- Has had successful reperfusion of myocardium (e.g., PTCA, CABG).
- No activity-induced myocardial ischemia (1–2 mm ST segment depression on stress test) or reversible ischemic defects (echo or nuclear radiography).
- May have orthostatic BP changes but is not symptomatic.
- Patient did not participate in a regular exercise program before hospitalization but may have had an "active" lifestyle.
- No other current health problems that would potentially complicate activity regime (e.g., PVD, orthopedic problems, moderate to severe COPD/emphysema, pericarditis).

High Risk
- Severely depressed LV function (i.e., EF < 30%).
- Complex ventricular arrhythmias at rest or appearing or increasing with exercise.
- Decrease in systolic blood pressure >20 mm Hg during activity or failure to rise with increasing activity workloads.
- Survivor of sudden cardiac death.
- Myocardial infarction complicated by congestive heart failure, cardiogenic shock, or complex ventricular arrhythmias.
- Severe coronary artery disease and marked activity-induced myocardial ischemia (>2-mm ST segment depression on stress test).
- Orthostatic BP changes and is symptomatic.
- Patient did not participate in a regular exercise program and did not have an "active" lifestyle before hospitalization.

BP, blood pressure; CABG, coronary artery bypass grafting; COPD, chronic obstructive pulmonary disease; EF, ejection fraction; LV, left ventricular; PTCA, percutaneous transluminal angioplasty; PVD, peripheral vascular disease.
From Saint Lake's Shawnee Mission Health System, Kansas City, MO, Mid America Heart Institute 1997. Courtesy of Jan E. Foresman, RN, MS, Cardiac Rehabilitation Specialist.

The hallmark symptom of ischemia is chest pain. Most patients have chest pain of some type, and it is frequently ignored. Once patients are told about heart disease, their routine pains can become frightening. Clinically, it is important to separate non-ischemic from ischemic chest pains. Chest pains that are unrelated to exercise or that are sharp are usually not attributable to ischemia, and not all chest pains should be called angina pectoris. Angina becomes unstable when it changes in pattern (i.e., occurs more frequently, at rest, or at lower workloads). It is important to note that as many as 25% of patients with acute MI have an atypical chest pain pattern, and some will have no chest pain at all. Ischemia can cause transient CHF, and increasing symptoms of CHF should be noted; these include sudden weight gain, edema in the lower extremities, dyspnea on exertion, and paroxysmal nocturnal dyspnea. Combinations of ischemia and CHF are more difficult to manage.

In general, patients can be categorized as those with myocardial damage, those with myocardial ischemia, or those with both. Initially, the ischemic threshold should be determined by the onset of angina pectoris or ST-segment depression at a particular heart rate, double product, or workload. When this threshold is clarified, the amount of mechanical damage should be determined.

Clinical clues that suggest that the patient has myocardial damage include a history of CHF, cardiogenic shock, a previous myocardial infarction, a large anterior myocardial infarction, cardiac enlargement, a large creatine kinase (CK) elevation, multiple Q waves, or underlying problems such as cardiomyopathy or valvular heart disease. These patients must be monitored for signs and symptoms of CHF, whereas patients with ischemia usually do not require such detailed observation. Patients with myocardial damage are limited by reduced maximal cardiac output, which leads to early fatigue and pulmonary symptoms, rather than by chest pain. An effort should be made to explain the symptoms related to CHF in such patients. In the patient with a myocardial infarction, the symptoms could be caused by mitral valve insufficiency secondary to papillary muscle dysfunction, a dilated mitral annulus, or a dysfunctional myocardial segment supporting the mitral apparatus. Secondary processes include cardiomyopathy or a valvular defect. A rare explanation is ventricular septal defect resulting from septal infarction.

In addition to myocardial ischemia and dysfunction, the other key features of heart disease to consider are arrhythmias, valvular function, and exercise capacity. These five features are important because they not only help to determine the patients' prognosis but also help to determine the manifestation of symptoms. Patients should be evaluated for each of these for optimal management, including individualization of the rehabilitation program. The ECG, chest x-ray, and exercise test are next in importance. The exercise test is the key to prescribing exercise (discussed later). Specialized tests, including echocardiography, nuclear scans, and cardiac catheterization, can be used to confirm impressions, clarify incongruous clinical situations, or identify coronary anatomic patterns that necessitate revascularization.

Severity of the Myocardial Infarction. Increases in risk for complications are generally associated with postinfarction ischemia and/or a history of previous myocardial infarction. In addition to ischemia, postinfarction chest pain can be caused by anxiety and pericarditis. These factors can usually be distinguished by a careful history and an electrocardiogram. The ECG pattern predicts the clinical course and outcome surprisingly well. The greater the number of areas with Q waves and the greater the R wave loss, the larger the myocardial infarct. Non-Q wave myocardial infarctions are usually less frequently associated with CHF or shock, but they can also be complicated, particularly when a previous myocardial infarction has occurred.

The concept that an initial subendocardial infarction is incomplete and poses an increased risk has not been substantiated. Inferior infarcts are usually smaller, result in a smaller decline in ejection fraction, and are less likely to be associated with shock or CHF. Anterior infarcts are typically larger, are more often associated with significant wall motion abnormalities, and usually result in a greater decrease in ejection fraction. The perception that exercise may cause further ventricular damage among patients with anterior infarctions and associated left ventricular dysfunction has been refuted by a variety of imaging studies performed over the past 10 years (Fletcher et al., 2001).

The size of a myocardial infarction can be judged by the creatine kinase (CK) level, particularly by the MB fraction released (see Chapter 11). In general, the larger the amount of CK-MB released and the longer the CK level stays elevated, the larger the myocardial infarction. The occurrence of CHF, shock, or pericarditis is also an indicator of a relatively large myocardial infarction.

Complicated Versus Uncomplicated Myocardial Infarctions. Whether an MI is *complicated* is important to consider because it can influence the clinical course and affect when a patient is stable enough to begin rehabilitation. Criteria for classifying an MI as complicated or uncomplicated are presented in Display 41-5. The rates of morbidity and mortality among postinfarction patients who have complicated clinical courses are much higher than among those with uncomplicated myocardial infarctions. The most important clinical predictors of

---

DISPLAY 41-5

CRITERIA FOR CLASSIFICATION OF COMPLICATED* MYOCARDIAL INFARCTION

Continued cardiac ischemia (pain, late enzyme rise)
Left ventricular failure (congestive heart failure, new murmurs, roentgenographic changes)
Shock (blood pressure drop, pallor, oliguria)
Important cardiac dysrhythmias (premature ventricular contractions greater than six per minute, atrial fibrillation)
Conduction disturbances (bundle-branch block, atrioventricular block, hemiblock)
Severe pleurisy of pericarditis
Complicating illnesses
Marked creatinine kinase rise without a noncardiac explanation or after thrombolysis

---

*One or more criteria classify a myocardial infarction as complicated.
From Froelicher, V. F. (1991). Cardiac rehabilitation. In K. Chatterjee, M. D. Cheitlin, J. Karliner, et al. (Eds.), *Cardiology: An illustrated text/reference* (Vol. 2, p. 7,208). Philadelphia: JB Lippincott.

complicated infarctions have been previous MI and the presence of CHF and/or cardiogenic shock. It is possible to assess risk at different temporal points, from presentation in the emergency department through the coronary care unit, as well as before discharge and during later follow-up. This is important because the clinical picture can change over time; a low-risk patient can become a high-risk patient and vice versa. These changes in risk are partially caused by the vicissitudes of the atherosclerosis process, reformation of thrombus, interventions, and disease–host interactions. For instance, a patient may present with premature ventricular contractions that can then disappear or worsen, chest pain may come and go, the ECG may change, or the enzymes may have a late peak. This makes it difficult to classify a patient strictly as high- or low-risk; risk stratification often requires good judgment by the patient's physician, along with that of the nursing staff. In addition, indicators signifying progress or regression of the patient's condition can change quickly during hospitalization. Importantly, any change in clinical status must be considered before initiating physical activity. The pace of rehabilitative steps must often be adjusted for a particular patient.

Psychosocial Considerations. Hospital admission for an acute myocardial infarction is a stressful experience with a powerful impact. However, hospital discharge can be equally stressful after the patient has relied on the highly protective hospital support systems. Discharge into an uncertain future and into a home and work setting in which the patient may be considered a helpless invalid can be as damaging to the patient's self-esteem as the acute event itself. The nurse is faced with the difficult tasks of not only supervising the physical recovery of the patient but also maintaining morale, providing education, helping the family cope, providing support, and facilitating the return to a gratifying lifestyle. Studies have shown that psychosocial intervention, including such things as counseling, group therapy, behavior modification, stress management, and relaxation techniques, are effective in improving psychological well-being, reducing stress, and reducing type A behavior scores (Wenger et al., 1995; American Association of Cardiovascular and Pulmonary Rehabilitation, 1998).

It is also important to consider that a small percentage of patients will have no difficulty exercising on their own and might not need a formal exercise program. However, all patients can benefit from education and secondary risk reduction. Some patients benefit from exercising with a group, whereas others fare better by themselves. The approach to each patient must be individualized because patients' reactions to problems and their needs differ. In addition, nearly all patients will have one or more co-morbidities, and any of these may require different clinical considerations and may also have a different psychosocial impact. For example, an increasing percentage of patients will have obesity, diabetes, or both, and many will have musculoskeletal problems or other metabolic disorders. Triaging or management of these co-morbidities often is within the purview of the cardiac rehabilitation team.

Education of the Patient. Education should be initiated before physical activities are begun; the patient may lack self-confidence and need affirmation that the activities are safe. Patient education during the acute phase usually consists of an explanation of the coronary care unit, the cardiac rehabilitation program, and the delivery of routine diagnostic and therapeutic

---

DISPLAY 41-6

STERNAL PRECAUTIONS AND ACTIVITY GUIDELINES (FOR AT LEAST 6 WEEKS AFTER CARDIAC SURGERY)

Do not lift more than 10 pounds.
Do not push **up** as if getting out of bed or **out** as if pushing a cart.
No pulling.
No arm activities above the level of the heart.

---

modalities. The patient should be educated about the limitations imposed by the disease, the potential for improvement, and precautions to be observed. The program should be individualized for the patient depending on his or her clinical and psychosocial status. The medical status is determined largely by the severity of the myocardial infarction, but the medical history must also be considered.

The activity and exercise component of inpatient education should involve teaching patients about activities they can do, as well as those they should be more cautious in doing, during the first few weeks of their rehabilitation. This differs somewhat between patients having cardiac surgery versus those with MI. The activity limitations after cardiac surgery involve sternal precautions and psychological adjustment to a major surgery. Those activities that put stress on the sternal incision are listed in Display 41-6. It is advisable for cardiac surgery patients to wait at least 4 to 6 weeks before driving a vehicle, partly because the sternal incision would be at risk in an impact. There is also some cognitive adjustment that needs to take place after a major surgery before the patient's reflexes are fully intact. Patients with MI have slightly different reasons for activity limitations. It may be necessary to return to activities gradually because of the added work placed on the healing myocardium. As mentioned, early mobilization of the patient with acute MI is now well accepted; however, there are important reasons to avoid sudden increases in myocardial oxygen demand during the first few weeks of rehabilitation. In addition, those patients who have undergone PTCA and stent placement are often cautioned to refrain from strenuous activity for a somewhat longer period, e.g., approximately 6 weeks. The exercise test is usually postponed until that time as well.

Patients should understand that the conditioning program for patients after MI and surgery should be gradual. Those in a walking program are usually instructed to continue the walking they have been doing in the hospital. In addition, the energy cost of activities in METs should be explained to the patient (Display 41-7) and appropriate household or recreational activities should be recommended accordingly. Patients should also be taught how to take their heart rate and how to use the rating of perceived exertion (RPE) scale. This scale is useful because it is highly correlated with heart rate and, when given a range of RPE, the patient can then objectively judge his or her level of exercise exertion (Table 41-4).

Medications that may have an effect on heart rate or blood pressure should be discussed with the patient (i.e., beta-blockers, calcium-channel blockers). Patients also should be reminded

DISPLAY **41–7**

ENERGY COST IN METs (METABOLIC EQUIVALENTS) OF ACTIVITIES

Very Light Activity

1 MET

Resting
Eating
Writing
Hand sewing
Knitting

2 METs

Light calisthenics
Driving (can be more METs under
    stressful conditions)
Light housework (sweeping, ironing, mopping)
Walking, 2.2 mph

3 METs

Self-care (washing, dressing)

Light Activity

4 METs

Gardening (seeding)
Ballroom dancing
Canoeing, golf (without cart)

5 METs

Mowing lawn, power mower
Washing car
Heavy carpentry (scraping, painting—outdoors)

Moderate to Heavy Activity

6 METs

Shoveling snow
Digging vigorously
Sawing wood
Tennis
Skiing
Walking on level, 5 mph

7 METs

Jogging, moderate pace
Carrying boxes
Skiing, general
Ice skating

8 METs

Cycling, 13 mph
Swimming, 40 yd/min
Level ski touring, 4 mph
Walking upstairs, briskly

Very Heavy Activity

10 METs

Swimming (crawl, 55 yd/min)
Cycle uphill
Walking uphill, 5 mph

---

when and how to take nitroglycerin and when to call for medical assistance. Inpatients' retention of information is low; therefore, it is important to repeat certain guidelines several times and also to provide written information. Patients should have a written walking or cycling program that includes mode,

TABLE 41–4 ■ 6 TO 20 AND 0 TO 10 BORG PERCEIVED EXERTION SCALES

Original Scale		Revised Scale	
6		0	Nothing
7	Very, very light	0.5	Very, very weak
8		1	Very weak
9	Very light	2	Weak
10		3	Moderate
11	Fairly light	4	Somewhat strong
12		5	Strong
13	Somewhat hard	6	
14		7	Very Strong
15	Hard	8	
16		9	
17	Very Hard	10	Very, very strong
18			Maximal
19	Very, very hard		
20			

From Borg, G. A. V. (1999). *Borg's perceived exertion and pain scales.* Champaign: Human Kinetics.

frequency, and duration of exercise. A copy of warm-up and cool-down exercises, preferably the same ones they were taught as an inpatient, can be helpful. A target HR should be provided (usually 20 beats/min above the standing resting HR for the initial phase after discharge); and an RPE scale should be provided, noting the appropriate intensity when exercising (10 to 12 at the beginning). A chart to record HR, RPE, and symptoms can also be useful to track patients' adherence to the exercise prescription and to help determine appropriate progression. It is important that patients are familiar with precautions about exercise (Display 41-8). At the time of discharge, some method of contacting the patient for outpatient cardiac rehabilitation follow-up should be established, and appointments should be made for outpatient cardiac rehabilitation within 1 to 3 weeks after discharge.

Initiation of Inpatient Activity. Once the medical evaluation has been performed and the patient's clinical condition has been stabilized, inpatient activity can be initiated. The objectives for inpatient activity include the following:

To educate the patient and family about the particular cardiac event and diagnostic tests and to prepare them for the stages of cardiac rehabilitation and returning to life at home
To offset the deleterious physiologic and psychological effects of bed rest
To return the patient to activities of daily living
To provide additional medical surveillance for the patient

GENERAL GUIDELINES AND PRECAUTIONS FOR CARDIOVASCULAR EXERCISE

1. Exercise only when feeling well. Wait 2 days until after a cold or flu. Never exercise when you have a fever.
2. Do not exercise vigorously soon after eating. Wait at least 2 hours.
3. Adjust exercise to the weather. Exercise in the cooler time of day on hot days. Exercise at a slower pace and drink more water than usual in hot weather.
4. Slow down for hills. Stay at the same level of exertion for hills.
5. Wear proper clothing and shoes.
6. Understand personal limitations. Find out from your physician what limitations to exercise you have.
7. Select appropriate exercise. Aerobic exercise should be a major component of activities. However, flexibility and strengthening exercises should also be considered for a well rounded program.
8. Be alert for symptoms. If the following occur while exercising of immediately after, contact a physician before continuing exercise:
   a. Discomfort in the upper body
   b. Faintness
   c. Shortness of breath during exercise to the point of uncomfortableness
   d. Discomfort in bones and joints either during or after exercise
9. Watch for the following signs of overexercising:
   a. Inability to finish
   b. Inability to converse during the activity
   c. Faintness or nausea after exercise
   d. Chronic fatigue
   e. Sleeplessness
   f. Aches and pains in the joints
10. Start slowly and progress gradually. Allow time to adapt.

From American Heart Association: Exercise Guidelines.

To introduce the patient to behavior modification with the goal of reducing risk factors

To stratify the patient's risk for future cardiac rehabilitation (Verril et al., 1993) (see Display 41-4)

The patient experiencing MI, CABS, or PTCA is usually transferred from the cardiac or intensive care unit to a telemetry unit and sometimes to a general medicine or surgical unit. However, with decreased length of stays, many are discharged directly from the telemetry or step-down unit. The nurses on each of these units are usually the ones who orient and explain to the patient the processes involved in diagnosis and treatment of the specific cardiovascular event. Education about risk factor reduction and the important aspects of medical observation of the patient are discussed further in Chapters 29 to 33 and 35 to 37. As mentioned, before 1970, patients were generally relegated to strict bed rest after an acute MI. It was thought that any physical activity could lead to complications such as ventricular aneurysm formation, cardiac rupture, CHF, dysrhythmias, re-infarction, or sudden death (Wood, 1968). It has become well established that complications are not increased with early ambulation. One of the important roles of inpatient cardiac rehabilitation is to counteract the detrimental physiologic effects of strict bed rest. There are also data demonstrating that activity during the in-hospital period may help to decrease anxiety and depression, improve self-esteem, and reduce type A behavior characteristics such as hostility and anger (American Association of Cardiovascular and Pulmonary Rehabilitation, 1998).

Traditionally, progressive stepped programs have been used to increase activity levels while the patient was in the hospital, including early mobilization, range-of-motion exercises, and progressive activity. A sample step program is shown in Table 41-5. It should be noted that in the current health care climate, the time available for inpatient rehabilitation is far more limited. Thus, the typical patient must be progressed more rapidly, and a greater emphasis must be placed on education, because exercise progression will often need to be accomplished independently by the patient.

While performing a program of education and increasing activity for the inpatient, measurable objectives should be established that are general and specific to each patient. Some examples of these objectives might include having the patient:

Ambulate 1,000 feet around the unit two to three times per day before discharge

Measure heart rate and relate rating of perceived exertion to activities performed

Climb a flight of stairs without undue symptoms

Relate upper extremity activity guidelines (sternal guidelines) after cardiac surgery

Perform self-care ADLs

Relate plans for resuming other ADLs (i.e., driving, sexual relations, and other strenuous life activities)

Relate plan to perform walking or other exercise program at home

Although the progressive stepped concept has been widely used, approaches to increasing activity can differ considerably between programs and between patients. Inpatient activities should be individualized and can be specific to common activities the patient performs, in addition to walking. Because hospital stays have become shorter (3 to 5 days), it can be important to modify the inpatient program rapidly based on an individual patient's clinical status and needs.

Exercise Testing Before Hospital Discharge

The exercise test after an acute myocardial infarction has been shown to be safe. When performed before discharge, it should be submaximal (e.g., limited to 5 or 6 METs) and should not exceed a Borg Scale level of 16. In many hospitals, a submaximal target heart rate is used (e.g., 110 beats per minute for patients using beta-blockers). The protocol should be modified, given the reduced exercise tolerance of most patients recovering from a myocardial infarction; individualized ramp or Naughton protocols are preferable. An example of a typical submaximal protocol is shown in Table 41-6. Later, when return to full activities is intended, the test can be symptom- and sign-limited.

Table 41–5 ■ SEATTLE VA MEDICAL CENTER CARDIAC REHABILITATION PROTOCOL FOR EARLY PATIENT AMBULATION AFTER MYOCARDIAL INFARCTION

Step	Nursing	Physical Therapy	Occupational Therapy	Dietary
Step 1 (bed rest)* 1 MET	Orient patient to cardiac care unit, use of commode (1.5); arms supported for upper extremity (UE) activities, decrease anxiety, advise patient of activity limitations	Lower extremity (LE), active range of motion (AROM), and evaluation	UE, AROM, and evaluation, intro to sternal precautions and CR progress	
Step 2 survey (in room) 2 METs	Sit in chair for meals, and 20 min at a time, 3–4 times per day, personal activities of daily living (ADLs) at bedside or sink, answer patient questions as they arise	Walking in room, or 50 ft (2.0), warm-ups (WU) and cool-downs (CD) (2.5–3.0)	UE activity with shoulder flexion 45 degrees, 10 reps, education: activity guidelines and risk factor introduction	Diet
Step 3 (short walking) 3 METs	Sitting shower (3.5), continue risk factor education	Walking 100–250 ft with WU and CD, instruction in independent walking	Increasing abduction to 90 degrees and 15 reps, continue energy conservation and showering guidelines	Introduction to heart, healthy eating
Step 4 (long walking) 4 METs	Independent in ADLs and walking on ward, standing shower (3.7); discharge instruction: meds, appts, emergencies, review plans for risk factor reduction efforts	Walking 250–1000 ft 3–4 times per day, one flight of stairs (12 steps) (3.5–4.0) Given and taught home exercise program	Review of ADLs at home work, and leisure (postsurgery and postmyocardial) infarction activity precautions (sex, driving)	Review of dietary follow-up as needed

* All metabolic equivalent (MET) determinations are in parentheses.
From Seattle Veterans Affairs Medical Center, Seattle, Washington.

The pre-discharge test has many benefits, including clarification of the response to exercise, development of an exercise prescription, and recognition of the need for medications or interventions (Sivarajan-Froelicher et al., 1977). It can also have a beneficial psychological impact on recovery and begins the rehabilitation process. The test is considered the first step in the outpatient cardiac rehabilitation exercise program.

The prognostic value of the pre-discharge test has been debated. Meta-analysis has shown that a low exercise capacity or abnormal systolic blood pressure responses are better predictors of increased risk than is ST-segment depression (Froelicher et al., 1987). However, ST-segment depression probably indicates increased risk in men who do not use digoxin and whose resting ECGs do not show extensive damage. The criterion of 2 mm or more ST-segment depression along with symptoms or abnormal hemodynamic responses appears to be useful for identifying higher risk patients who should be considered for cardiac catheterization and revascularization.

Return to Work and Recreational Activities

The economic burden of cardiovascular disability has been enormous, and a great deal of effort has been directed toward vocational rehabilitation. Postdischarge activity recommendations, including determination of disability, are among the biggest challenges facing the health care provider. Historically, the patient's ability to return to work, to drive, and to be sexually active have been based on clinical judgments rather than on physiologic assessments. These decisions should be based on the consequence of the coronary event (e.g., ischemia, symptoms of CHF, or dysrhythmias), the nature of the patient's occupational or recreational activities, and the response to the pre-discharge exercise test.

In general, if patients do not exhibit any untoward responses to submaximal exercise testing and achieve 5 or more METs, it is unlikely that they will encounter difficulties during activities of daily living. More strenuous jobs or recreational pursuits should not be initiated until a symptom-limited exercise test

Table 41–6 ■ EXAMPLE PROTOCOL FOR LOW-LEVEL EXERCISE TESTING

Level	Speed (mph)	Gradient (%)	Time (min)	METs*
I	1.2	0	3	2.1 ± 0.4
II	1.2	3	3	2.4 ± 0.3
III	1.2	6	3	2.7 ± 0.3
IV	1.7	6	3	3.9 ± 0.5

* One MET is defined as the energy equivalent for an individual at rest in sitting position; represents the consumption of 3.5–4.0 mL of oxygen per kilogram of body weight per minute.
From Sivarajan-Froelicher, E. S., & Bruce, R. A. (1981). Early exercise testing after MI. *Cardiovascular Nursing,* 17, 1–5.

can be performed and exercise capacity can be determined and related to the desired physical activities of the patient.

Factors that influence a patient's return to work include age, work history, severity of cardiac damage, financial compensation for illness, employer's ignorance of the patient's capabilities, termination of employment, and, most important, the patient's perception of his or her clinical status. Efforts of the rehabilitation team to help the patient develop a positive attitude, and a sense of well being may facilitate appropriate vocational adjustments. The physician's attitude also greatly affects the patient's return to work; encouragement can be very beneficial.

Contraindications to Exercise Training

Absolute contraindications are the known or suspected conditions that prevent the patient from safely participating in an exercise program. These include unstable angina pectoris, dissecting aortic aneurysm, complete heart block, uncontrolled hypertension, decompensated CHF, uncontrolled dysrhythmias, thrombophlebitis, and other complicating illnesses (American College of Sports Medicine, 2000; American Association of Cardiovascular and Pulmonary Rehabilitation, 1998) (Display 41-9). Relative contraindications, or those that can be superseded by clinical judgment, include frequent premature ventricular contractions, controlled dysrhythmias, intermittent claudication, metabolic disorders, and moderate anemia or pulmonary disease. Studies show that if these contraindications are considered, the incidence of exertion-related cardiac arrest in cardiac rehabilitation programs is extremely low, and because of the availability of rapid defibrillation, serious events rarely occur.

Outpatient Cardiac Rehabilitation

There have been multiple approaches to outpatient rehabilitation, and it has become necessary for programs to be more creative to provide outpatient rehabilitation in the current climate of reduced reimbursement. Traditionally, this phase begins 1 to 2 weeks after discharge from the hospital and may last from 1 to 4 months. Most commonly, patients attend group exercise sessions three times per week; however, frequency of exercise is often modified by the individual patient's overall goals, functional capabilities, reimbursement, proximity to the hospital or clinic, and personal commitment.

The first few exercise sessions after hospital discharge usually emphasize warm-up and cool-down activities, with only a modest aerobic component; some programs use direct electrocardiographic telemetry for the initial sessions to ensure safety. There is less emphasis today than in the past on the need for direct ECG monitoring (see later). A symptom-limited maximal exercise test is usually recommended approximately 6 weeks after the hospitalization to determine an appropriate exercise prescription and activity limitations.

At the beginning of the outpatient program, it is advisable to conduct a patient assessment, discuss the objectives of the program, and develop reasonable goals for the patient based on their needs, capabilities, and clinical condition. Usually the

---

DISPLAY 41-9

CLINICAL INDICATIONS AND CONTRAINDICATIONS FOR INPATIENT AND OUTPATIENT CARDIAC REHABILITATION

Indications

- Medically stable post-myocardial infarction
- Stable angina
- Coronary artery bypass graft surgery
- Percutaneous transluminal coronary angioplasty
- Compensated congestive heart failure
- Cardiomyopathy
- Heart or other organ transplantation
- Other cardiac surgery including valvular and pacemaker insertion (including implantable cardioverter defibrillator)
- Peripheral vascular disease
- High-risk cardiovascular disease ineligible for surgical intervention
- Sudden cardiac death syndrome
- End-stage renal disease
- At risk for coronary artery disease, with diagnoses of diabetes mellitus, hyperlipidemia, hypertension, etc.
- Other patients who may benefit from structured exercise and/or patient education (based on physician referral and consensus of the rehabilitation team)

Contraindications

- Unstable angina
- Resting systolic blood pressure >200 mm Hg or diastolic >110 mm Hg
- Blood pressure drop of >20 mm Hg with symptoms
- Moderate to severe aortic stenosis
- Acute systemic illness or fever
- Uncontrolled atrial or ventricular arrhythmias
- Uncontrolled tachycardia (>100 bpm)
- Uncompensated congestive heart failure
- Third-degree heart block (without pacemaker)
- Active pericarditis or myocarditis
- Recent embolism
- Thrombophlebitis
- Resting ST displacement (>2 mm)
- Uncontrolled diabetes
- Orthopedic problems prohibiting exercise
- Other metabolic problems

From American College of Sports Medicine. (2000). *Guidelines for exercise testing and prescription* (6th ed., pp. 166–167). Philadelphia: Lippincott Williams & Wilkins.

---

patient is scheduled for an initial interview, where baseline data are gathered and information about the program is given to the patient. At this initial interview the nurse should have reviewed the inpatient records so that the patient has been stratified into the appropriate risk category. In general, the objectives of the outpatient program include the following:

Increase activity level and functional capacity

Increase regular exercise participation

Improve the patient's psychosocial status, depression, or anxiety through participation in exercise, education, or counseling when appropriate

Educate and support patients in other risk reduction efforts (i.e., stop smoking, control hypertension, normalize lipid values, and maintain healthy weight)

The exercise prescription for outpatient rehabilitation is based on the exercise test and is described in detail below. A number of fundamental considerations are important when initiating outpatient rehabilitation. Although the typical outpatient session may last approximately 45 minutes, patients should work up to this duration gradually. It is preferable to focus on warm-up, stretching, range of motion, and cool-down exercises for the first 3 to 6 sessions and gradually increase the aerobic portion such that 30 to 45 minutes can be completed. Regardless of the duration of the aerobic portion, all exercise sessions should include warm-up and cool-down periods of 5 to 10 minutes. A variety of exercise modalities should be used, including those that use the upper and lower muscle groups. For example, patients may spend alternating periods using the treadmill, arm ergometer, cycle ergometer, or stair climber. Resistance exercise is also widely recommended today to assist the patient in restoring muscular strength, and complementing aerobic exercise with resistance training has been demonstrated to have favorable effects on cardiovascular endurance, hypertension, hyperlipidemia, and psychosocial well-being (Graves & Franklin, 2001).

Changes in reimbursement patterns have changed outpatient programs more than other components of cardiac rehabilitation. In some circumstances, only a few exercise or educational sessions are reimbursed. The transition from an outpatient to a home-based maintenance program now occurs more rapidly. Randomized trials have demonstrated that patients can return to work quickly and safely during rehabilitation and that participation in rehabilitation facilitates this process. It is also currently appreciated that only a small percentage of patients require continuous ECG monitoring during exercise. Efforts to reduce the cost of rehabilitation in addition to the recognition that most patients can exercise quite safely without continuous telemetry have brought about this change. Although the AHA guidelines suggest ECG monitoring for the first 6 to 12 sessions (Fletcher et al., 1996), recommendations on this issue have varied widely. Patients who should be considered for longer ECG monitoring include those with a history of serious rhythm disorders, ICD implantation, CHF, and abnormal hemodynamic responses to exercise testing (e.g., exercise-induced hypotension).

Exercise Prescription for Outpatient Rehabilitation

The American College of Sports Medicine defines exercise prescription as "the process whereby a person's recommended regimen of physical activity is designed in a systematic and individualized manner" (American College of Sports Medicine, 2000). An "individualized manner" implies specific strategies to optimize return to work or activities of daily living, reduction of risk factors for future cardiac events, and maximization of the patient's capacity to maintain an active lifestyle. The development of an appropriate exercise prescription to meet the individual patient's needs has a sound scientific foundation, but there is also an art to effective exercise programming.

The art of exercise prescription has become increasingly important in this era of cost containment (shorter rehabilitation), surgical and technologic advances (larger numbers of transplantations, pacemaker, or chronic heart failure participants than ever before), and the multitude of new medicines available. There is no single program that is best for all patients or even one patient over time; capabilities, vocational needs, and expectations differ among patients and can change with the passing of time. Thus, the art of exercise prescription relies on the nurse's abilities to synthesize the patient's pathophysiologic, psychosocial, and vocational factors and tailor them to the patient's needs and realistic goals. A final but important consideration is the selection of activities that the individual enjoys, which will provide the best chance that he or she will continue to perform safely after the formal rehabilitation program ends.

Principles of Exercise Prescription. Training implies adaptations of the body to the demands placed on it. A *training* effect is best measured as an increase in maximal ventilatory oxygen uptake, but not all institutions have gas exchange equipment and there are many ways to quantify functional outcomes of rehabilitation. For example, some patients after rehabilitation may be better suited to perform submaximal levels of activity for longer periods, remain independent, continue working, or rejoin their friends on the golf course. All of these can be important goals for a given patient and may occur even with a minimal change in maximal oxygen uptake.

The major ingredients of the exercise prescription are frequency, intensity, duration, mode, and rate of progression. In general, these principles apply for both the patient with heart disease and the healthy adult; however, the ways in which they are applied differ. On the basis of numerous studies performed since the 1950s, it is generally accepted that increases in maximal oxygen uptake are achieved if a person exercises dynamically for a period ranging from 15 to 60 minutes, three to five times per week, at an intensity equivalent to 50% to 80% of the maximum capacity. Dynamic exercises are those that use large muscle groups in a rhythmic manner, such as treadmill walking, cycle ergometry, rowing, stepping, and arm ergometry. As mentioned, short warm-up and cool-down periods are strongly encouraged for participants in cardiac rehabilitation programs. Again, however, an effective exercise prescription must consider the patient's goals, health status, and availability of time in addition to practical considerations such as cost, availability of equipment, and facilities.

Much of the art of exercise prescription clearly involves individualizing the exercise intensity. Typically, exercise intensity is expressed as a percentage of maximal capacity, either in absolute terms (i.e., workload or watts) or in relation to the maximal heart rate, maximal oxygen uptake, or perceived effort. Training benefits have been shown to occur with exercise intensities ranging from 40% to 85% of maximal oxygen uptake, which are generally equivalent to 50% to 90% of the maximal heart rate. However, the intensity that a given individual can maintain for a specified period of time varies widely. In general, the most appropriate intensity for most patients in rehabilitation programs is 50% to 70% of maximal capacity. The actual prescribed exercise intensity for the patient should naturally depend on goals, health status, length of time since infarction or surgery, symptoms, and initial state of fitness.

Training is a general phenomenon; there is no true threshold beyond which patients achieve benefits. Thus, as long as patients exercise safely, setting the exercise intensity is a less rigid practice than it was years ago. In addition, the patient's ability to tolerate activities can change daily. Other factors, such as time of day, environment, and time since medications were taken, can influence the patient's response to exercise, and the exercise prescription must be adjusted accordingly. It is also useful to use a window of intensity that ranges approximately 10% above and 10% below the desired level.

The graded exercise test is the foundation on which a safe and effective exercise prescription is based. To achieve a desired training intensity, oxygen uptake or some estimate of it must be quantified during a maximal or symptom-limited exercise test. Because heart rate is easily measured and is linearly related to oxygen uptake, it has become a standard by which training intensity is estimated during exercise sessions. The most useful method uses a measure known as the heart rate reserve. This method uses a percentage of the difference between maximum heart rate and resting heart rate and adds this value to the resting heart rate. For example, for a patient who achieves a maximum heart rate of 150 beats per minute, has a resting heart rate of 70 beats per minute, and wishes to exercise at intensity equivalent to 60% of maximum:

$$\text{Maximum heart rate} = 150 \text{ bpm}$$
$$- \text{ Resting heart rate} = \underline{70}$$
$$\text{Heart rate range} = 80$$
$$\times \text{ Desired intensity (60\%)}$$
$$= 48$$
$$+ \text{ Resting heart rate} = \underline{70}$$
$$= \text{Training heart rate } 118$$

A reasonable training heart rate range for this individual would be 115 to 125 beats per minute. This is also referred to as the Karvonen formula and is reliable for patients in normal sinus rhythm whose measurements of resting and maximum heart rates are accurate. An estimated target heart rate for exercise should be supplemented by considering the patient's MET level relative to his or her maximum, the perceived exertion, and symptoms.

Patient Education in Outpatient Cardiac Rehabilitation

The education component in an outpatient rehabilitation program usually focuses on modifying risk factors for heart disease. Chapters 29 to 33 and 35 to 37 address risk factor modification in detail. Exercise, as mentioned previously, is usually the main focus of cardiac rehabilitation. However, exercise affects other alterable risk factors such as hypertension, abnormal lipids, obesity, smoking, and diabetes. During exercise, opportunities arise to teach informally about risk factor modification in all these areas. Teaching the patient about exercise is often performed formally through group presentations and informally as each patient progresses with their exercise sessions and as the home program evolves. Other issues can be addressed in formal classroom sessions, in short sessions after the exercise training periods, or by distributing educational materials. The home exercise prescription should be given to the patient soon after starting outpatient cardiac rehabilitation. Patients should be asked to exercise at home on the days they do not come to cardiac rehabilitation. The aim is to gradually have them exercising most days of the week for 30 or more minutes each time, as recommended by the AHA, Surgeon General Report, and ACSM guidelines. If they attempt to exercise every day, they will be most likely to achieve the recommended three to five times per week. When patients walk for exercise, they can be encouraged to gradually increase the duration to 60 minutes. Walking is the most common home exercise, but if the patient has access to other forms of exercise, then prescriptions should be given for these modes. Excellent references for home exercise include the *ACSM Fitness Book* (66), *Take a Load off the Heart* (Piscatella & Franklin, 2003), and numerous other patient education materials that are available on the AHA and ACSM web sites.

Safety of Exercise Training in Outpatient Cardiac Rehabilitation

The safety of outpatient cardiac rehabilitation has been well documented in both the United States and Europe. In 1986, Van Camp and Peterson sent questionnaires to 167 randomly selected cardiac rehabilitation centers (Van Camp & Peterson, 1986). Data were gathered on more than 51,000 patients who exercised more than 2 million hours from January 1980 to December 1984. During this time, there were only 21 cardiac resuscitations (3 of which failed) and eight myocardial infarctions. This amounts to 8.9 cardiac arrests, 3.4 infarctions, and 1.3 fatalities per one million hours of patient exercise. Surprisingly, ECG monitoring had little influence on complications, which suggests that the additional expense of telemetry may not be necessary.

In a 16-year follow-up from William Beaumont Hospital in Michigan, 292,254 patient-exercise-hours were recorded in phase II and III programs (Franklin et al., 1998). During this period, a total of five major cardiovascular complications occurred; the complication rate was 1 per 58,451 patient-exercise-hours. Despite the scarcity of these events, appropriate medical personnel must be available to resuscitate patients should an event occur.

Maintenance Program

Progression to an out-of-hospital maintenance program is desirable after patients have participated in a supervised program for a suitable period. The period of time required before patients move to a maintenance program can vary considerably, depending on reimbursement, the patient's stability, exercise capacity, and the individual patient's needs, but it rarely exceeds 12 weeks. The purpose of this phase is to maintain training adaptations, to prevent recurrence of events or symptoms, and to maintain progress. An important concept to instill in patients at this point in time is that continued maintenance of their exercise capacity and a physically active lifestyle is one of the most important determinants of future health outcomes (Pate et al., 1995; U.S. Public Health Service, 1996; Paffenbarger et al., 1986, 1993; Ribisl, 2001; Tanasescu et al., 2003; Kohl; Lee & Paffenbarger, 1996; Blair et al., 1989; Ekelund et al., 1988; Arraiz et al., 1992; Myers et al., 2002; Roger et al., 1998; Goraya et al., 2000; Snader et al., 1997; Williams, 2001; Kannel et al., 1985; NIH Consensus Development Panel on Physical Activity and Cardiovascular Health, 1996). It is important that patients understand how to monitor their exercise intensity, understand how to recognize symptoms, and have a basic knowledge of their particular disease and medications.

When making occupational activity recommendations for patients, it can be helpful to know the estimated energy requirements of various activities (see Display 41-7). With this knowledge, appropriate recommendations can be made, balancing patients' functional limitations with their need to return to work, desire to continue recreational activities, or both.

It is useful to perform an exercise test before the maintenance program to provide an outgoing exercise prescription, confirm the safety of exercise for a given patient, and assess risk for future cardiac events. Funding for this phase must often be borne by the patient because most types of health insurance do not cover it; however, mechanisms for follow-up should be in place. In recent years, programs have been developed in the YMCA, gyms, and other community facilities that make it less expensive and more accessible for patients in need of maintenance programs.

Rehabilitation in Patients with Chronic Heart Failure

Until the late 1980s, chronic heart failure was considered by many authorities to be a contraindication to participation in an exercise program. Today it is known that most patients with chronic heart failure derive considerable benefits from cardiac rehabilitation (Pina et al., 2003). With improvements in therapy (i.e., thrombolysis, angiotensin-converting enzyme inhibitors, beta-blockers), survival of patients with chronic heart failure has improved considerably, and more of these patients are candidates for rehabilitation. The incidence of chronic heart failure is increasing; it is currently approximately 500,000 per year in the United States. The numerous randomized trials performed during the 1990s in the United States and Europe indicated that the major physiologic benefit from training in chronic heart failure occurs in the skeletal muscle rather than in the heart itself.

The clinical approach to the patient with chronic heart failure who is considered for a rehabilitation program is similar to that for the postmyocardial infarction patient described earlier, although several important differences are worth noting. The risk for sudden cardiac death is higher in patients with chronic heart failure than in patients with normal left ventricular function. This is the population in whom sudden fatal arrhythmias occur most often. There are more medications to be considered that can influence exercise responses, including vasoactive, antiarrhythmic, inotropic, and beta-blocking agents. Exercise capacity tends to be significantly lower than that in the typical patient with coronary disease.

Numerous hemodynamic abnormalities underlie the reduced exercise capacity commonly observed in chronic heart failure, including impaired heart rate responses, inability to distribute cardiac output normally, abnormal arterial vasodilatory capacity, abnormal cellular metabolism in skeletal muscle, higher-than-normal systemic vascular resistance, higher-than-normal pulmonary pressures, and ventilatory abnormalities that increase the work of breathing and cause exertional dyspnea (Pina et al., 2003; Clark et al., 1996; Myers, 2000). Studies performed over the past decade have demonstrated that many of these abnormalities can be improved by exercise training (Pina et al., 2003).

Most patients with reduced left ventricular function who are clinically stable and have reduced exercise tolerance are candidates for exercise programs. It is often necessary to exclude patients with signs and symptoms of right-sided failure or to treat them judiciously before entry into a program. An exercise test is particularly important before initiating the program to ensure safety of participation. Rhythm abnormalities, exertional hypotension, or other signs of instability should be ruled out. Expired gas exchange measurements are particularly informative in this group because they provide an improvement in accuracy and permit an assessment of ventilatory abnormalities that are common in this condition (Myers, 2000) (see Chapter 17). ECG monitoring during exercise is more often indicated in this group. Attention should be paid to daily changes in body weight, rhythm status, and symptoms.

Increasing numbers of patients have undergone cardiac transplantation for end-stage heart failure, and approximately 75% of these patients remain alive after 5 years. These patients are presently considered good candidates for rehabilitation programs. Because the transplantation patient's heart is denervated, some intriguing hemodynamic responses to exercise are observed. The heart is not responsive to the normal actions of the parasympathetic and sympathetic nervous systems. The absence of vagal tone explains the high resting heart rates in these patients (100 to 110 beats per minute) and the relatively slow adaptation of the heart to a given amount of submaximal work. As a result, the delivery of oxygen to the working tissue is slower, contributing to earlier-than-normal metabolic acidosis and hyperventilation during exercise. Maximal heart rate is lower in transplantation patients than in normal subjects, which contributes to a reduction in cardiac output and exercise capacity.

A growing number of reports have addressed the effects of training after cardiac transplantation. These studies have demonstrated increases in peak oxygen uptake, reductions in resting and submaximal heart rates, and improved ventilatory responses to exercise after periods of training. Whether the major physiologic adaptation to exercise is improved cardiac function, changes in skeletal muscle metabolism, or simply an improvement in strength remains to be determined. Psychosocial studies of rehabilitation in transplantation patients are lacking, as are studies of the effects of regular exercise on survival.

New Models of Cardiac Rehabilitation

Changes in reimbursement patterns over the past 15 years, along with the demonstration that clinical outcomes can be improved by multidisciplinary risk factor intervention (Ades et al., 2001; Balady et al., 2000), have led to the development of new models of cardiac rehabilitation. The need for new approaches has also been fueled by the recent observation that a wider spectrum of patients can benefit from cardiac rehabilitation (e.g., valvular surgery, CHF, transplantation, peripheral vascular disease, and the elderly). Moreover, innovative strategies have been proposed to increase the proportion of eligible patients who receive cardiac rehabilitation services despite reductions in reimbursement. In addition, physicians have not been particularly effective in assisting patients in achieving defined risk factor goals (Wee et al., 1999; Sherman & Hershman, 1993; Damush et al., 1999; Sueta et al., 1999; Schrott et al., 1997), and strategies have been suggested to facilitate a greater proportion of patients meeting evidence-based treatment guidelines.

Models that have been developed to meet these needs include the transformation of rehabilitation centers into "secondary prevention centers" (Ades et al., 2001), the "inclusive chronic disease model" (Ribisl, 2002), the implementation of affordable, evidence-based, comprehensive risk reduction in primary and secondary prevention settings (Ades et al., 2001; Gordon et al., 2001), home exercise programs (DeBusk et al., 1985; Ades et al., 2000), and case-management systems (DeBusk et al., 1994; Haskell et al., 1994; Levnecht et al., 1997; Fonarow et al., 2001). The concept that cardiac rehabilitation should be the primary medium to implement comprehensive cardiovascular risk reduction has been embraced by the AHA (Balady, et al., 2000), the AHCPR Clinical Practice Guidelines (Wenger et al., 1995), and the AACVPR (American Association of Cardiovascular and Pulmonary Rehabilitation, 1998). The recent AHA consensus statement on "Core Components of Rehabilitation/Secondary Prevention Programs" (Balady et al., 2000) defines specific evidence-based risk factor goals for management of lipids, blood pressure, weight, smoking cessation, diabetes management, and physical activity (Display 41-10). This model provides an integrated system that includes appropriate triage, education, counseling on lifestyle interventions, and long-term follow-up.

Several studies have demonstrated the efficacy of comprehensive risk factor management using a *case management* approach. In each of these studies, a nurse, as case manager, functions as the coordinator and point of contact who identifies, triages, provides surveillance on safety and efficacy, performs follow-up, and, in many instances, quantifies patient outcomes. Case management has been the cornerstone of recent multidisciplinary efforts to reduce cardiovascular risk. In addition, it has provided a framework for comprehensive management of existing disease, particularly for patients with CHF (DeBusk et al., 1994; Haskell et al., 1994l Levnecht et al., 1997; Fonarow et al., 2001; West et al., 1997). This approach involves the coordination of risk reduction strategies for targeted groups of patients by a single individual, most commonly a nurse or exercise physiologist, with appropriate medical supervision. The case management concept is based on the idea that risk factors are strongly interrelated, and an individualized, integrated approach to management will optimize care such that clinical outcomes will be improved and costs will be saved. The case management approach has been applied in various settings over the past decade and has been successful in reducing risk markers for CAD and improving outcomes in patients with existing disease. Some of the more prominent studies performed during the 1990s using case management approaches are described.

The Butterworth Heath System in Michigan reorganized their cardiac rehabilitation program to focus on improvement in long-term outcomes using a case-management model (Levnecht et al., 1997). The model included the use of referral pathways, education sessions, and intervention by social workers as necessary. In addition, they added regular telephone follow-up to assess the effectiveness of the risk reduction interventions. One year after initiating the program, 77% of patients were on appropriate lipid-lowering therapy, 78% reported exercising at least 3 days per week, and 66% of previous smokers reported smoking cessation.

The MULTIFIT program of DeBusk and colleagues (DeBusk et al., 1994) has been a model for other case management programs, and its success led to it being adopted by the Kaiser Permanente Health Care System. MULTIFIT is a case-managed program for patients hospitalized with acute myocardial infarction in Northern California. Patients were randomized either to special risk reduction intervention by a nurse case manager or to usual care. The intervention patients received education and counseling regarding smoking cessation, regular physical activity, and nutrition. Medical management, such as lipid-lowering therapy, was instituted as indicated for risk factors not controlled by lifestyle change. Much of the intervention was mediated by phone and mail contact. The intervention group showed greater improvement at 6 months and 1 year in functional capacity, rate of smoking cessation, and changes in LDL-C compared to the usual care group, and subsequent analyses have shown MULTIFIT to be cost-effective (West et al., 1997).

The recently completed Cardiac Hospital Atherosclerosis Management Program (CHAMP) (Fonarow et al., 2001) compared outcomes among 302 patients enrolled in a case-managed risk reduction intervention and compared them to 256 control patients. All were discharged from UCLA Medical Center with a diagnosis of CAD or other vascular disease. The case-managed approach emphasized close adherence to appropriate use of aspirin, beta-blockers, ACE inhibitors, and lipid-lowering agents, combined with outpatient exercise, nutrition, and smoking cessation counseling. After the study period, there was greater use of appropriate medications, an increase in the percentage of patients achieving an LDL-C level less than 100 mg/dL, a reduction in recurrent myocardial infarction, and a lower 1-year mortality.

At Stanford, a randomized controlled trial funded by the NIH was performed to evaluate the efficacy of case-managed, physician-directed multi-risk factor intervention (the SCRIP Study) (Haskell et al., 1994). Case managers coordinated care along with a team of nutritionists, psychologists, and physicians to provide clinical and lifestyle interventions, attempting to achieve nationally recognized goals for risk factor reduction. Three hundred subjects were randomized to intervention or usual care groups. After the 4-year study period, the intervention group demonstrated an increase in exercise participation, reductions in dietary fat and cholesterol intake, reductions in systolic blood pressure, body mass index and blood lipids, an improvement in glucose tolerance, and a 27% reduction in Framingham Risk Score. These changes were

DISPLAY **41–10**

CORE COMPONENTS FOR CARDIAC REHABILITATION/SECONDARY PREVENTION PROGRAMS

Lipid Management

- Short-term: Assessment and modification of interventions until LDL < 100 mg/dL.
- Long-term: LDL < 100 mg/dL. Secondary goals include HDL > 40 mg/dL and triglycerides <200 mg/dL.

Hypertension Management

- Short-term: Assessment and modification of interventions until BP < 140 mmHg systolic and <90 mmHg diastolic; in patients with heart failure, diabetes, and renal failure BP < 130 mmHg systolic and <85 mmHg diastolic.
- Long-term: BP < 140 mmHg systolic and <90 mmHg diastolic; in patients with heart failure, diabetes, and renal failure, BP < 130 mmHg systolic and <85 mmHg diastolic.

Smoking Cessation

- Short-term: patient will demonstrate readiness to change by initially expressing decision to quit (contemplation) and selecting a quit date (preparation). Subsequently the patient will quit smoking and use of all tobacco products (action); adhere to pharmacotherapy, if prescribed; practice strategies as recommended; and resume cessation plan as quickly as possible when relapse occurs.
- Long-term: complete abstinence from smoking and use of all tobacco products at 12 months from quit date.

Weight Management

- In patients with BMI > 25 kg/m2 and/or waist >40 inches in men (102 cm) and >35 inches (88 cm) in women:

  -Establish reasonable short-term and long-term weight goals individualized to patient and associated risk factors (eg, reduce body weight by at least 10% at a rate of 1–2 Ibs/wk over a period of time up to 6 months).
- Short-term: Continued assessment and modification of interventions until progressive weight loss is achieved. Have patient participate in on-site weight loss program or provide referral to specialized nutrition weight loss programs such that weight goals are achieved.
- Long-term: adherence to diet and exercise program aimed toward attainment of established weight goal.

Diabetes Management

- In patients with diabetes:

  -Short-term: Develop a regimen of dietary adherence and weight control which includes: exercise, oral hypoglycemic agents, insulin therapy, and optimal control of other risk factors. Drug therapy should be provided and/or monitored in concert with primary healthcare provider.

  -Long-term: Normalization of fasting plasma glucose (80–110 mg/dL or HbA_1c <7.0), minimization of diabetic complications, control of associated obesity, hypertension (<130/85 mmHg) and hyperlipidemia.
- Refer patients without known diabetes whose fasting glucose is ≥110 mg/dL to their primary healthcare provider for further evaluation and treatment.

Physical Activity Counseling

- Increased physical activity, which includes 20–30 minutes per day of moderate physical activity on 5 or more days per week, and increased activity in usual routines; eg, parking farther away from entrances, walking two or more flights of stairs, walking 15 minutes during lunch break.
- Increased participation in domestic, occupational, and recreational activities.
- Improved psychosocial well-being, reduction in stress, facilitation of functional independence, prevention of disability, and enhancement of opportunities for independent self-care to achieve recommended goals.

LDL, low-density lipoprotein; HDL, high-density lipoprotein; BP, blood pressure; BMI, body mass index; HBA1C, glycosylated hemoglobin.
From the AHA and AACVPR. (2000). Scientific statement on core components of cardiac rehabilitation secondary prevention programs. *Circulation*, 102, 1069–1073.

associated with reductions in hospitalizations and coronary events. Angiographic results included less progression of CAD and greater stabilization of plaque in the intervention group.

The home-based model of rehabilitation, validated at Stanford University in the 1980s (DeBusk et al., 1985), has been used in many centers over the past 15 years. This approach uses home exercise that is either unmonitored or monitored via telephone or microprocessor. Some programs feature regular feedback via telephone or home visits, and recent approaches have used exercise monitoring devices such as pedometers, accelerometers, and heart rate recording devices to encourage and document compliance

with prescribed exercise. Safety and efficacy of these home programs have been shown to be similar to those of more conventional programs (DeBusk et al., 1985; Ades et al., 2000).

CLOSING COMMENT

Early and progressive ambulation of patients after a myocardial infarction is now considered routine care. Despite the advent of new therapies in cardiovascular medicine, cardiac rehabilitation maintains an important place in reducing morbidity and mortality. The controlled exercise trials, when combined, demonstrate that the efficacy of rehabilitation in reducing mortality is similar to that of the best medical interventions. Moreover, cardiac rehabilitation has redirected interest to humanistic concerns, providing a balance for the emphasis on complex technology. It also provides an ideal environment for supervision of patients and for ensuring stability after an interventional procedure. Available data suggest that cardiac rehabilitation is economically sound.

Medicine is experiencing an evolution toward technologic efficacy and outcomes assessment. Health economists and legislators are re-examining the value placed on all forms of medical care. Although this movement has changed the way in which cardiac rehabilitation is implemented, studies have confirmed its value. Some of the ways in which the current economic environment has changed cardiac rehabilitation include lessening of direct ECG monitoring, shorter hospital stays, and more rapid progression to home programs. The frequency of interventions has lessened the morbidity associated with myocardial infarction. Modifications in the way cardiac rehabilitation is implemented have encouraged greater referral to and participation in cardiac rehabilitation, and newer models of cardiac rehabilitation have brought a greater focus on secondary risk reduction, case management, and cost efficacy.

Data on efficacy, safety, and technologic advances in the treatment of cardiovascular disease have changed cardiac rehabilitation in such a way that a wider range of patients can benefit from these services than in the past. For example, patients with stable chronic heart failure, once excluded from cardiac rehabilitation programs, are now thought to be among those who benefit the most (Goebbels, 1998). Patients who have had pacemakers, transplantation, bypass or valvular surgery, and claudication now comprise a significant fraction of those in many programs. Despite this fact, most eligible patients (as many as 90%) do not receive these services. It is clear that not all patients need all components of cardiac rehabilitation, but directing these services to patients who need them most remains one of the important challenges for the field.

Lastly, there has been a change in the public health care message toward physical activity as inherently beneficial regardless of objective measurements of fitness. This has caused a shift in focus from morbidity, mortality, and exercise capacity to issues related to maintaining an active lifestyle and optimizing the patient's capacity to perform the physical challenges offered by occupational or recreational activities. Further studies on costs, benefits, and other outcomes should solidify the role of cardiac rehabilitation in the clinical management of patients with cardiovascular disease.

REFERENCES

Ades, P. A., Balady, G. J., & Berra, K. (2001). Transforming exercise-based cardiac rehabilitation programs into secondary prevention centers: A national imperative. *Journal of Cardiopulmonary Rehabilitation*, 21, 263–272.

Ades, P., Pashkow, F., Fletcher, G., et al. (2000). A controlled trial of cardiac rehabilitation in the home setting using electrocardiographic and voice transtelephonic monitoring. *American Heart Journal*, 139, 543–548.

Ainsworth, B. E., Haskell, W. L., Leon, A. S., et al. (1993). Compendium of physical activities: Classification of energy costs of human physical activities. *Medical Science Sports Exercise*, 25, 71–80.

Albert, C. M., Mittleman, M. A., Chae, C. U., et al. (2000). Triggering of sudden death from cardiac causes by vigorous exertion. *New England Journal of Medicine*, 9, 1355–1366.

American Association of Cardiovascular and Pulmonary Rehabilitation. (1998). *Guidelines for cardiac rehabilitation programs*. Champaign, IL: Human Kinetics.

American College of Sports Medicine. (2003). *ACSM fitness book*. Champaign, IL: Human Kinetics.

American College of Sports Medicine. (2000). *Guidelines for exercise testing and prescription* (6th ed.). Baltimore: Lippincott Williams & Wilkins.

American College of Sports Medicine Position Stand. (1998). The recommended quantity and quality of exercise for developing and maintaining cardiorespiratory and muscular fitness, and flexibility in healthy adults. *Medical Science Sports Exercise*, 30, 975–991.

Arraiz, G. A., Wigle, D. T., & Mao, Y. (1992). Risk assessment of physical activity and physical fitness in the Canada health survey mortality follow-up study. *Journal of Clinical Epidemiology*, 45, 419–428.

Balady, G., Ades, P., & Comoss, P., et al. (2000). Core components of cardiac rehabilitation/secondary prevention programs: a statement for healthcare professions from the American Heart Association and the American Association of Cardiovascular and Pulmonary Rehabilitation Writing Group. *Circulation*, 102, 1069–1073.

Blair, S. N., Kohl, H. W. III, Paffenbarger, R. S., et al. (1989). Physical fitness and all-cause mortality: A prospective study of healthy men and women. *JAMA*, 262, 2395–2401.

Centers for Disease Control and Prevention. (1993). Prevalence of sedentary lifestyle-behavioral risk factor surveillance system, United States: 1991. *MMWR Morbidity and Mortality Weekly Report*, 42, 576–579.

Clark, A. L., Poole-Wilson, P. A., & Coats, A. J. (1996). Exercise limitation in chronic heart failure: Central role of the periphery. Department of Cardiac Medicine, National Heart and Lung Institute. *Journal of the American College of Cardiology*, 28, 1092–1102.

Damush, T. M., Stewart, A. L., Mills, K. M., et al. (1999). Prevalence and correlates of physician recommendations to exercise among older adults. *Journal of Gerontology A Biology Science Medicine Science*, 54, M423–M427.

DeBusk, R. F., Haskell, W. L., Miller, N. H., et al. (1985). Medically directed at-home rehabilitation soon after clinically uncomplicated acute myocardial infarction: a new model for patient care. *American Journal of Cardiology*, 55, 25.

DeBusk, R. F., Houston-Miller, N., Superko, H. R., et al. (1994). A case-management system for coronary risk factor modification after acute myocardial infarction. *Annals of Internal Medicine*, 120, 721–729.

Ekelund, L. G., Haskell, W. L., Johnson, J. L., et al. (1988). Physical fitness as a predictor of cardiovascular mortality in asymptomatic North American men: The Lipid Research Clinics Mortality Follow-up Study. *New England Journal of Medicine*, 319, 1379–1384.

Fletcher, G. F., Balady, G., Amsterdam, E. A., et al. (2001). Exercise Standards for Testing and Training: A Statement for Healthcare Professionals from the American Heart Association. *Circulation*, 104, 1694–1740.

Fletcher, G. F., Balady, G., Blair, S. N., et al. (1996). Statement on exercise: benefits and recommendations for physical activity programs for all Americans. A statement for health professionals by the Committee on Exercise and Cardiac Rehabilitation of the Council on Clinical Cardiology, American Heart Association. *Circulation*, 94(4), 857–862.

Fonarow, G., Gawlinski, A., Moughrabi, S., et al. (2001). Improved treatment of coronary heart disease by implementation of a Cardiac Hospitalization Atherosclerosis Management Program (CHAMP). *American Journal of Cardiology*, 87, 819–822.

Franklin, B. A., Bonzheim, K., Gordon, S., et al. (1998). Safety of medically supervised outpatient cardiac rehabilitation exercise therapy: a 16 year follow-up. *Chest*, 114, 902–906.

Froelicher, V. F., & Myers, J. N. (2000). *Exercise and the heart*. Philadelphia: WB Saunders.

Froelicher, V. F., Perdue, S., Pewen, W., et al. (1987). Application of meta-analysis using an electronic spread sheet to exercise testing in patients after myocardial infarction. *American Journal of Medicine*, 83, 1045–1054.

Goebbels, U., Myers, J. N., Dziekan, G., et al. (1998). A randomized comparison of exercise training in patients with normal vs. reduced ventricular function. *Chest*, 113, 1387–1393.

Gordon, N. F., Salmon, R. D., Mitchell, B. S., et al. (2001). Innovative approaches to comprehensive cardiovascular disease risk reduction in clinical and community-based settings. *Current Atherosclerosis Reports*, 3, 498–506.

Goraya, T. Y., Jacobsen, S. J. Pellikka, P. A., et al. (2000). Prognostic value of treadmill exercise testing in elderly persons. *Annals of Internal Medicine*, 132:862–870.

Graves, J. E., & Franklin, B. A. (2001). *Resistance training for health and rehabilitation*. Champaign: Human Kinetics.

Hagberg, J. M. (1990). Exercise, fitness, and hypertension. In C. Bouchard, R. J. Shephard, T. Stephens, et al. (Eds.), *Exercise, fitness, and health* (pp. 455–566). Champaign, IL: Human Kinetics.

Hahn, R. A., Teutsh, S. M., Rothenberg, R. B., et al. (1986). Excess deaths from nine chronic diseases in the United States. *JAMA*, 264:2654–2659.

Haskell, W. L., Alderman, E. L. Fair, J. M., et al. (1994). Effects of intensive multiple risk factor reduction on coronary atherosclerosis and clinical cardiac events in men and women with coronary artery disease; The Stanford Coronary Risk Intervention Project (SCRIP). *Circulation*, 89, 975–990.

Haskell, W. L., Leon, A. S., Caspersen, C. J., et al. (1992). Cardiovascular benefits and assessment of physical activity and physical fitness in adults. *Medical Science Sports Exercise*, 24, S201–S220.

Helmrich, S. P., Ragland, D. R., Leung, R.W., et al. (1991). Physical activity and reduced occurrence of non-insulin-dependent diabetes mellitus. *New England Journal of Medicine*, 325:147–152.

Hu, F. B., Stampfer, M. J., Solomon, C., et al. (2001). Physical activity and risk for cardiovascular events in diabetic women. *Annals of Internal Medicine*, 134, 96–105.

Kallio, V., Lamalainen, H., Hakkila, J., et al. (1979). Reduction of sudden deaths by a multifactorial intervention program after acute myocardial infarction. *Lancet*, 2, 1091–1094.

Kannel, W. B., Wilson, P., & Blair, S. N. (1985). Epidemiological assessment of the role of physical activity and fitness in development of cardiovascular disease. *American Heart Journal*, 109, 876–885.

Kohl, H. W. (2001). Physical activity and cardiovascular disease: Evidence for a dose response. *Medical Science Sports Exercise*, 33 (Suppl), S472–S483.

Lee, I. M., Hennekens, C. H., Berger, K., et al. (1999). Exercise and risk of stroke in male physicians. *Stroke*, 30, 1–6.

Lee, I. M., & Paffenbarger, R. S. (1996). Do physical activity and physical fitness avert premature mortality? *Exercise Sport Science Review*, 24, 5–172

Leon, A. S., Certo, C., Comoss, P., et al. (1990). Position paper of the American Association of Cardiovascular and Pulmonary Rehabilitation: Scientific evidence of the value of cardiac rehabilitation services with emphasis on patients following myocardial infarction. Section 1: Exercise conditioning component. *Journal of Cardiopulmonary Rehabilitation*, 10, 79–87.

Levnecht, L., Schriefer, J., Schriefer, J., et al. (1997). Combining case management, pathways, and report cards for secondary cardiac prevention. *Journal of Quality Improvement*, 23, 162–174.

Levnecht, L., Schriefer, J., Schriefer, J., & Maconis, B. (1997). Combining case management, pathways, and report cards for secondary cardiac prevention. *Journal of Quality Improvement*, 23, 162–174.

Manson, J. E., Nathan, D. M., Kroleski, A. S., et al. (1992). A prospective study of exercise and incidence of diabetes among US male physicians. *JAMA*, 268:63–67.

Manson, J. E., Rimm, E. B., Stampfer, M. J., et al. (1991). Physical activity and incidence of non-insulin-dependent diabetes mellitus in women. *Lancet*, 338:774–775.

Marcus, R., Drinkwater, B., Dalsky, G., et al. (1992). Osteoporosis and exercise in women. *Medical Science Sports Exercise*, 24(Suppl), S301–S307.

May, G. S., Eberlein, K. A., Furberg, C. D., et al. (1982). Secondary prevention after myocardial infarction: A review of long-term trials. *Progress in Cardiovascular Disease*, 24, 331–362.

McGinnis, J. M., & Foege, W. H. (1993). Actual causes of death in the United States. *JAMA*, 270:2207–2212.

Morris, J. N., Everitt, M. G., Pollard, R., et al. (1980). Vigorous exercise in leisure-time: Protection against coronary heart disease. *Lancet*, 2, 1207–1210.

Morris, J. N., Kagan, A., Pattison, D. C., et al. (1966). Incidence and prediction of ischaemic heart disease in London busmen. *Lancet*, 2, 552–559.

Myers, J. N. (1995). Physiologic adaptations to exercise and immobility. In S. L. Woods, E.S. Sivarajan-Froelicher, C. J. Halpenny, & S. Underhill Motzer, (Eds.), *Cardiac nursing* (3rd ed., pp. 147–162). Philadelphia: JB Lippincott.

Myers, J. N. (2000). Effects of exercise training on abnormal ventilatory responses to exercise in patients with chronic heart failure. *CHF*, Sept/Oct, 243–249.

Myers, J. N., Atwood, J. E., & Froelicher, V. F. (2003). Active lifestyle and diabetes. *Circulation*, 107, 2392–2394.

Myers, J. N., Prakash, M., Froelicher, V. F., et al. (2002). Exercise capacity and mortality among men referred for exercise testing. *New England Journal of Medicine*, 346(11), 793–853.

NIH Consensus Development Panel on Physical Activity and Cardiovascular Health. (1996). Physical activity and cardiovascular health. *JAMA*, 27, 241–246.

O'Conner, G. T., Buring, J. E., Yusaf, S., et al. (1989). An overview of randomized trials of rehabilitation with exercise after myocardial infarction. *Circulation*, 80, 234–244.

Oldridge, N. B., Guyatt, G. H., Fischer, M. E., et al. (1988). Cardiac rehabilitation with exercise after myocardial infarction. *JAMA*, 260: 945–950.

Paffenbarger, R. S., Blair, S. N., Lee, I., et al. (1993). Measurement of physical activity to assess health effects in free-living populations. *Medical Science Sports Exercise*, 25:60–70.

Paffenbarger, R. S., Hyde, R. T., Wing, A. L., et al. (1984). Chronic disease in former college students: XXV. A natural history of athleticism and cardiovascular health. *JAMA*, 252, 491–495.

Paffenbarger, R. S., Hyde, R. T., Wing, A.L., et al. (1986). Physical activity, all-cause mortality, and longevity of college alumni. *New England Journal of Medicine*, 314, 605–613.

Paffenbarger, R. S., Hyde, R. T., Wing, A. L., et al. (1993). The association of changes in physical-activity level and other lifestyle characteristics with mortality among men. *New England Journal of Medicine*, 328, 538–545.

Paffenbarger, R. S., Hyde, R. T., & Wing, A. L. (1994). Some interrelations of physical activity, physiological fitness, health, and longevity. In C. Bouchard, R. J. Shephard, & T. Stephens (Eds.), *Physical activity, fitness, and health* (pp. 119–133). Champaign, IL: Human Kinetics.

Paffenbarger, R. S., Laughlin, M. E., Gima, A. S., et al. (1970). Work activity of longshoreman as related to death from coronary heart disease and stroke. *New England Journal of Medicine*, 282, 1109–1114.

Pate, R. R., Pratt, M. P., Blair, S. N., et al. (1995). Physical activity and public health: A recommendation from the Centers for Disease Control and Prevention and the American College of Sports Medicine. *JAMA*, 273, 402–407.

Pina, I. L., Apstein, C. S., Balady, G. J., et al. (2003). Exercise and Heart Failure: A statement from the American Heart Association Committee on Exercise, Rehabilitation, and Prevention. *Circulation*, 107(8), 1210–1225.

Piscatella, J., & Franklin, B. A. (2003). *Take a load off your heart*. New York: Workman Publishing.

Ribisl, P. M. (2001). Exercise: the unfilled prescription. *American Journal of Medicine and Sports*, 3:13–21.

Ribisl, P. M. (2002). The inclusive chronic disease model: Reaching beyond cardiopulmonary patients. In J. Jobin, F. Maltais, P. Poirier, P. Leblanc, & C. Simard (Eds.), *Advancing the frontiers of cardiopulmonary rehabilitation* (pp. 29–36). Champaign: Human Kinetics.

Rockhill, B., Willett, W. C., Manson, J. E., et al. (2001). Physical activity and mortality: a prospective study among women. *American Journal of Public Health*, 91, 578–583.

Roger, V. L., Jacobsen, S. J., Pellikka, P. A., et al. (1998). Prognostic value of treadmill exercise testing: A population-based study in Olmsted County, Minnesota. *Circulation*, 98, 2836–2841.

Rousseau, P. (1993). Immobility in the aged. Department of Geriatrics, Veterans Affairs Medical Center, Phoenix, Arizona. *Archives of Family Medicine*, 2, 169–177.

Schrott, H., Bittner, V., Vittinghoff, E., et al. (1997). Adherence to national cholesterol education program treatment goals in postmenopausal women with heart disease: the heart and estrogen/progestin replacement study (HERS). *JAMA*, 277, 1281–1286.

Shaw, L. (1981). Effects of a prescribed supervised exercise program on mortality and cardiovascular morbidity in patients after myocardial infarction. *American Journal of Cardiology*, 48, 39–44.

Sherman, S. E., & Hershman, W. Y. (1993). Exercise counseling: how do general internists do? *Journal of General Internal Medicine*, 8, 243–248.

Sivarajan-Froelicher, E. S., Snydsman, A., Smith, B., et al. (1977). Low-level treadmill testing of 41 patients with acute myocardial infarction prior to discharge from hospital. *Heart and Lung*, 6, 975–980.

Slattery, M. L., Jacobs, D. R. Jr., & Nichaman, M. Z. (1989). Leisure time physical activity and coronary heart disease death: The U.S. railroad study. *Circulation*, 79, 304–311.

Snader, C. E., Marwick, T. H., Pashkow, F. J., et al. (1997). Importance of estimated functional capacity as a predictor of all-cause mortality among patients referred for exercise thallium single-photon emission computed tomography: report of 3,400 patients from a single center. *Journal of the American College of Cardiology*, 30, 641–648.

Sueta, C., Chowdhury, M., & Boccussi, S. (1999). Analysis of the degree of undertreatment of hyperlipidemia and congestive heart failure secondary to coronary artery disease. *American Journal of Cardiology*, 83, 1303–1307.

Tanasescu, M., Leitzman, M. F., Rimm, E. B., et al. (2003). Physical activity in relation to cardiovascular disease and total mortality among men with type 2 diabetes. *Circulation*, 107, 2435–2439.

Thune, I., & Furberg, A. S. (2001). Physical activity and cancer risk: dose response, all sites, and site-specific. *Medical Science Sports Exercise,* 33 (Suppl), S530–S550.

U.S. Public Health Service, Office of the Surgeon General. (1996). *Physical activity and health: A report of the Surgeon General.* Atlanta, U.S. Department of Health and Human Services, Centers for Disease Control and Prevention, National Center for Chronic Disease Prevention and Health Promotion.

Van Camp, S. P., & Peterson, R. A. (1986). Cardiovascular complications of outpatient cardiac rehabilitation programs. *JAMA,* 256, 1160–1163.

Vermuelen, A., Lie, K., & Durber, D. (1983). Effects of cardiac rehabilitation after myocardial infarction: Changes in coronary risk factors and long term prognosis. *American Heart Journal,* 105, 798–801.

Verril, D., Bergey, D., McElveen, G., et al. (1993). Recommended guidelines for cardiac maintenance (phase IV) programs: A position paper by the North Carolina Cardiopulmonary Rehabilitation Association. *Journal of Cardiopulmonary Rehabilitation,* 13, 87–95.

Wee, C. C., McCarthy, E. P., Davis, et al. (1999). Physician counseling about exercise. *JAMA,* 282, 1583–1588.

Wenger, N. K., Sivarajan-Froelicher, E. S., Smith, L. K., et al. (1995). *Cardiac rehabilitation: Clinical practice guideline No. 17.* AHCOR Publication no. 96–0672. Rockville, MD, U.S. Department of Health and Human Services, Public Health Service, Agency for Health Care Policy and Research and the National Heart, Lung, and Blood Institute.

West, J. A., Miller, N. H., Parker, K., et al. (1997). A comprehensive management system for heart failure improves clinical outcomes and reduces medical resource utilization. *American Journal of Cardiology,* 79(1), 58–63.

Williams, P. T. (2001). Physical fitness and activity as separate heart disease risk factors: a meta-analysis. *Medical Science Sports Exercise,* 33, 754–761.

Wood, P. (1968). *Diseases of the heart and circulation* (3rd ed.). London: Eyre and Spottiswood.

Obesity: An Overview of Assessment and Treatment

LORA E. BURKE • MEGHAN A. CARTWRIGHT*

Obesity is a multifactorial disease involving complex interactions among genetic, metabolic, environmental, cultural, and psychosocial factors. In the United States today, obesity has become a pandemic, the most common nutritional problem, the second most preventable cause of death, a significant contributor to increased health care costs, and a condition that lessens life expectancy and reduces quality of life across the life span (Fontaine, 2003; Manson & Bassuk, 2003; National Heart, Lung, and Blood Institute [NHLBI], 1998; Schwimmer et al., 2003). Around the world, in both developed and less developed countries, the prevalence of obesity is rising to epidemic proportions (Martorell, 2001; WHO, 2003). Data indicate that the countries most affected are Latin America and those in the Caribbean, Central Eastern Europe and the Commonwealth of Independent States, and the Middle East and North Africa (WHO, 2003). The prevalence of obesity in the United States increased from 19.8% in 2000 to 20.9% in 2001, an increase of 1.1% (Mokdad et al., 2003). In 2001, examination of the data from the Behavioral Risk Factor Surveillance System showed that there is a higher prevalence among males (21.0%); blacks (31.1%); those with less than a high school education (27.4%); and those in the 50- to 59-year age group (26.1%) (Mokdad et al., 2003). Recent data from the Centers for Disease Control and Prevention, based on body-mass index, indicate that two thirds of adults in the U.S. are overweight and that over one third are obese (Bonow & Eckel, 2003).

Obesity has been linked to a host of chronic disorders associated with heart disease, including type 2 diabetes, dyslipidemia, and hypertension. It is associated with deleterious effects on the heart and circulatory system, contributing to an increased risk of arrhythmia, sudden death, congestive heart failure, and ischemic heart disease (Saltzman, 1998; Bonow, 2003). Moreover, several physiologic parameters that affect cardiovascular risk factors are associated with obesity, such as lipoprotein oxidizability, arterial blood pressure, hemostatic or fibrinolytic abnormalities, and C-reactive protein, a vascular inflammatory marker (Esposito, 2003; Jialal & Devaraj, 2003; Van Gaal et al., 1997). Obesity was added

to the list of major risk factors for coronary heart disease (CHD) in 1998 (Eckel, 1998).

In the midst of the mounting evidence demonstrating the deleterious effects of obesity on health in general, and the cardiovascular system in particular, research has demonstrated numerous benefits to health by as little as a 10% reduction in initial weight. However, survey data show that approximately one third of men and women are attempting to lose and maintain weight but that only approximately 20% are using a combination of reduced caloric intake and increased physical activity to achieve weight loss (Serdula et al., 1999). Moreover, reports in the literature indicate that those who have been successful in weight loss regain one third of their weight loss during the first year after cessation of active treatment, and that most regain the full amount by the fifth year (Wing, 1998). These facts underscore the importance of identifying the patient at risk and implementing an early treatment course that may prevent the development of obesity.

This major health problem has not gone unnoticed by the scientific community. Several organizations and policymaking groups have joined forces to evaluate the existing obesity treatment programs and to develop guidelines for the identification and treatment of the disorder. More specifically, in 1995, the Institute of Medicine published an extensive report that provided criteria for evaluating three categories of weight-management programs: "do it yourself," nonclinical, and clinical programs (Institute of Medicine, 1995). A year later, the Shape Up America! Organization and the American Obesity Association joined forces to develop and publish *Guidance for Treatment of Adult Obesity* (*Shape Up American & American Obesity Association, 1996*), and in 1998, the National Heart, Lung, and Blood Institute issued the *Evidence Report* (NHLBI, 1998) which provided empirically based guidelines for the identification, evaluation, and treatment of overweight and obesity in adults. On the international level, the World Health Organization (WHO) is addressing the issue through the International Obesity Task Force (IOTF) (Fiore, 1996; Kumanyika et al., 2002; WHO, 2003). However, despite all the attention given to this serious public health problem, this problem is not being addressed by the clinicians or the policymakers to the extent that previous health threats, such as the use of tobacco, have been addressed (Manson & Bassuk, 2003). When patients' visits to their family

*The authors were supported by grant 5RO1 DK58387, National Institute of Health, National Institute of Diabetes, Digestive, and Kidney Disorders.

physicians were observed, only one in four received any nutritional counseling (Eaton et al., 2002). Health care professionals can help slow the trend of excess weight by educating and counseling their patients about maintaining a healthy weight and how to use healthy lifestyle measures to reduce excess weight.

This chapter draws on the rapidly growing volume of empirical literature pertaining to obesity and the evidence-based guidelines to provide an overview of treatment for overweight and obesity. It begins with a review of the process of identification and evaluation of a patient's risk status and the selection of appropriate treatment. The major components of treatment are covered: lifestyle modification, which includes dietary, exercise, and behavioral therapy; drug therapy; and surgical therapy. Finally, maintenance strategies to enhance long-term adherence to the lifestyle changes that facilitated the weight loss are reviewed.

IDENTIFICATION AND ASSESSMENT OF THE OVERWEIGHT OR OBESE PATIENT

Weight Status

In 1988, the United States adopted the cutoff points for the classification of overweight and obese based on body mass index (BMI) developed by the WHO (NHLBI, 1998). These criteria define normal weight as a BMI range of 18.50 to 24.99, overweight as a BMI of 25.00 to 29.99, and obese as a BMI of 30 or more (NHLBI, 1998; WHO, 1997).

BODY MASS INDEX (BMI) MEASUREMENT PROCEDURE

Weight and height measurements, required for the BMI determination, should be taken with the patient wearing undergarments and no shoes. Using the height and weight values, the BMI can be calculated or determined by available nomograms (Gibson, 1990; NHLBI, 1998). The BMI is calculated as follows:

$$BMI = weight\ (kg)/height/squared\ (m^2)$$

The BMI can be estimated from pounds and inches as follows:

$$[weight\ (pounds)/height\ (inches)^2] \times 704.5$$

Waist (Abdominal) Circumference

Visceral obesity is an excess of fat in the abdomen that is out of proportion to total body fat (NHLBI, 1998). Upper body or abdominal obesity is considered more sensitive and specific than BMI as a predictor of obesity-related morbidity and mortality. Visceral obesity can be measured more accurately by computed tomography or magnetic resonance imaging, but these are expensive and impractical for clinical assessment in a practitioner's office (Allison, 1995; Lean et al., 1995). The NHLBI's evidence-based report recommended that waist circumference be included with the BMI in the clinical assessment. An empirical evaluation

of the algorithm found that use of BMI and CVD risk factors alone was sufficient to identify individuals who needed weight-loss treatment, and questioned the clinical utility of this measurement when a clinician is faced with time constraints (Kiernan & Winkleby, 2000). In contrast, Janssen and colleagues have provided substantive evidence that the NIH sex-specific cutoff points for waist circumference help to identify individuals at increased risk within the BMI categories (Janssen et al., 2002). Whether to use these criteria to determine treatment may be a clinical decision made on an individual patient basis. Waist circumference can be a valuable marker to monitor progress and provide feedback to the patient.

The NHLBI guidelines state that measurement of waist circumference is a clinically acceptable method to assess the patient's visceral or abdominal fat content from baseline through weight loss treatment. Sex-specific cutoffs have been established to identify relative risk for development of obesity-associated risks factors. Men with a waistline circumference greater than 40 inches (102 cm) and women with greater than 35 inches (88 cm) are at high risk for development of obesity-related morbidity (e.g., type 2 diabetes, dyslipidemia, and cardiovascular disease) (NHLBI, 1998). Patients of normal weight with increased waist circumference measurements may be at increased cardiovascular risk. Because patients with a BMI in excess of 35 exceed the waist circumference cutoffs, these indicators of relative risk lose their predictive power, making it unnecessary to measure waist circumference in this group (NHLBI, 1998) (Table 42-1) for the classification of overweight and obesity with waist circumference incorporated in the relative risk assessment.

WAIST (ABDOMINAL) CIRCUMFERENCE MEASUREMENT PROCEDURE

The patient should be dressed in undergarments or in an examining gown. Standing to the right of the patient, palpate the upper hip bone to locate the right iliac crest and draw a horizontal mark just above the upper border of the iliac crest. Cross that line with a vertical mark on the mid-axillary line. Place the measuring tape in a horizontal plane (parallel to the floor) around the abdomen at the level of the marked point and hold the tape snug to, but not compressing, the skin. Take the measurement at a normal minimal respiration (U.S. Department of Health and Human Services, 1996).

Assessment of Cardiovascular Disease Risk Factors

Having established the patient's relative risk based on the overweight/obesity and abdominal obesity criteria, the third part of the assessment is determination of the patient's absolute risk status in terms of comorbid conditions or risk factors for cardiovascular disease.

Very High Absolute Risk

Patients who are overweight or obese or have abdominal obesity are considered at very high risk if they have the following disease conditions: established CHD, presence of other atherosclerotic

Table 42–1 ■ CLASSIFICATION OF OVERWEIGHT AND OBESITY BY BMI, WAIST CIRCUMFERENCE AND ASSOCIATED RISK*

| | BMI(kg/m²) | Obesity Class | Disease Risk* Relative to Normal Weight and Waist Circumference | |
			Men≤102 cm (≤40 in) Women≤88 cm (≤35 in)	>102 cm (>40 in) >88 cm (>35 in)
Underweight	<18.5		—	—
Normal†	18.5–24.9		—	—
Overweight	25.0–29.9		Increased	High
Obesity	30.0–34.9	I	High	Very high
	35.0–39.9	II	Very high	Very high
Extreme obesity	≥40	III	Extremely high	Extremely high

* Disease risk for type 2 diabetes, hypertension, and CVD
† Increased waist circumference can also be a marker for increased risk even in persons of normal weight.
Adapted from National Heart, Lung, and Blood Institute. (1998). *Evidence report on detection, evaluation, and treatment of overweight and obesity.* Bethesda, MD. National Institute of Health.

diseases (peripheral arterial disease, abdominal aortic aneurysm, or symptomatic carotid disease), type 2 diabetes, sleep apnea, or target organ damage in the hypertensive patient (NHLBI, 1998). People meeting these profiles require aggressive treatment to reduce their cardiovascular disease risk profiles (e.g., cholesterol-lowering therapy, blood pressure control) (NHLBI, 1998).

High Absolute Risk

Obese patients who have three or more of the following risk factors can be considered at high absolute risk for obesity-related comorbid conditions: cigarette smoking; hypertension; low-density lipoprotein of 160 mg/dL or more, or 130 to 159 mg/dL in the presence of two or more other risk factors; high-density lipoprotein (HDL) less than 35 mg/dL; impaired fasting glucose; family history of premature CHD; and male sex and age 45 years or older, or female sex and age 55 years or older, or postmenopausal status. The provider should follow the established guidelines in estimating absolute risk status and in treating the identified risk factors (Fiore, 1996; NCEP ATP III, 2001; JNC VII, 2003), which are discussed in detail in other chapters.

Additional Factors that Increase Absolute Risk

The presence of additional risk factors (e.g., physical inactivity and elevated triglycerides) can increase a patient's absolute risk to a level higher than that estimated from the preceding categories (NHLBI, 1998; NIH Consensus Conference, 1993; Paffenbarger et al., 1993). A sedentary lifestyle in the presence of obesity heightens the risk for associated disorders. Elevated triglycerides in the obese patient may represent a common manifestation of a lipoprotein phenotype that includes elevated triglycerides, low HDL levels, and small low-density lipoprotein particles, a pattern considered atherogenic (NIH Consensus Conference, 1993).

Conditions Worsened by Obesity

Obese patients who have osteoarthritis, gallstones, gynecologic abnormalities, and stress incontinence are not facing life-threatening consequences, but require appropriate management (NHLBI, 1998). The provider needs to address these conditions and make the patient aware that these conditions are influenced by his or her weight.

Under-Treated Groups

Two groups that providers may be reluctant to treat are patients who are older than 65 years of age and smokers. However, weight reduction improves functional status and reduces concomitant risk factors in the older population in a way similar to that in the younger adult, and therefore this subgroup should at least receive interventions to prevent weight gain, if not achieve weight reduction (NHLBI, 1998; Schwartz, 1998). The overweight or obese smoker carries excess risk from obesity-associated risk factors (NHLBI, 1998). This patient should be advised to quit and prevention of weight gain should be addressed through lifestyle approaches, with the emphasis on smoking abstinence (NHLBI, 1998).

■ CLINICAL EVALUATION

Baseline assessment of the cardiac patient includes the BMI, waist circumference, and cardiovascular risk profile, as well as the noncardiovascular conditions noted previously. These factors need to be evaluated so that obesity is treated in the context of the patient's risk profile and existence of comorbid conditions (NHLBI, 1998). Weight loss frequently ameliorates risks by reducing blood pressure and triglycerides and raising HDL. Therefore, risk factors should be addressed through weight loss treatment (Eckel, 1997; NHLBI, 1998). The NHLBI *Evidence Report* (NHLBI, 1998) includes an algorithm that addresses the treatment decisions based on that assessment (Fig. 42-1). This algorithm is focused on weight-related assessment and treatment and does not include evaluation for other disorders for which the patient may be seeing a health care provider. As noted in Figure 42-1, if the patient's BMI and waist circumference are in the normal range, these parameters should be measured again in 2 years. For the patient who is of normal weight,

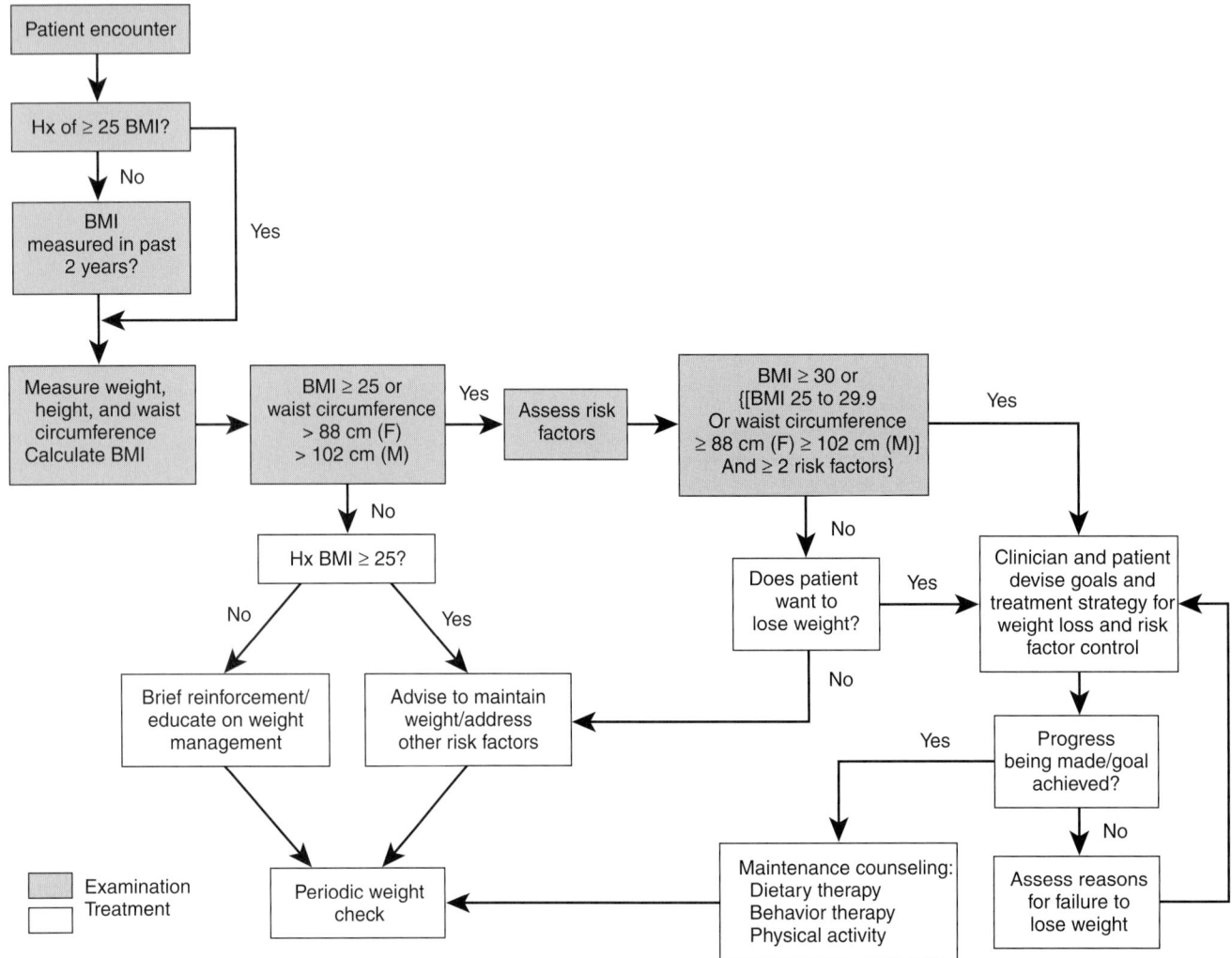

■ **Figure 42–1.** Treatment algorithm. This algorithm applies only to the assessment for overweight and obesity and subsequent decisions based on that assessment. It does not include any initial overall assessment for cardiovascular risk factors or diseases that are indicated. (Adapted from NHLBI. (1998). *Clinical guidelines on the identification, evaluation, and treatment of overweight and obesity in adults. The evidence report.* Bethesda, MD: National Institute of Health.)

brief counseling should be provided about the maintenance of that weight and prevention of future weight gain. Knowing that weight gain can be expected from most, maintenance of weight is a positive outcome (Serdula et al., 2003).

Clinical History. For the patient whose parameters are not normal, assessment needs to include the patient's history, including prior excess weight or weight fluctuations. If not done previously, a physical examination and laboratory measurements to assess lipid profile, glucose level, and related parameters need to be performed. Detection of existing cardiovascular disease and end-organ damage needs to be determined and treated. Serdula and colleagues have adapted the algorithim presented in Figure 42-1 by incorporating other treatment guidelines. However, this tool, while it has practical applications, has not been tested for its effectiveness or ease in clinical use (Serdula et al., 2003).

Eating and Physical Activity Patterns. A nutritional and physical activity assessment provides additional information that can be used in the treatment plan. This can be done by having the patient complete a 3-day food and activity diary,

which should include 2-work and 1-nonwork or leisure-type days. When using a 3-day food and activity diary, the patient needs to be instructed on completion of the diary and the detail that needs to be included (e.g., exact amount of foods eaten and inclusion of recipes or package labels if the food is unusual) (Allison, 1995; Gibson, 1990). Food frequency and activity questionnaires are another means of assessing past year food consumption, or current level of physical activity (Pereira, 1997; Willet, 1990).

Patient Motivation. Before considering treatment options, the patient's motivation for engaging in weight loss treatment needs to be assessed. Embarking on a weight loss and maintenance program requires a commitment to a change in lifestyle and an investment of the patient and provider's resources. Moreover, the change is not for a limited time, but rather lifelong. Factors to consider in the initial assessment include the patient's attitude toward weight loss, prior treatment failures and successes, support system, comprehension of risk posed by weight status, willingness to initiate an exercise program, self-efficacy for achieving weight loss, time commitment, barriers to behavior change, and financial issues if the treatment is not covered by insurance (NHLBI, 1998). Individuals experiencing major life events such as a major move, change in marital status, family illness, or those with significant anxiety, depression, or eating disorders (e.g., binge eating or bulimia) may need to address these issues before initiating a weight loss program, even if health care professionals conduct the program. Patients with the latter clinical problems are best served by a referral to a specialist (Anderson & Wadden, 1999). If the patient is not motivated, the provider needs to review the risks of excess weight and the benefits of initiating treatment and discuss how this treatment may be different and how the patient will be assisted. If the patient remains uninterested in treatment, the provider needs to address coexisting risk factors and initiate management of these, including further weight gain prevention (Eckel, 1997; NHLBI, 1998; Serdula et al., 2003). Having completed the assessment, a treatment plan needs to be considered.

Provider Assessment of Patient's Objectives. The manner and attitude of the health care professional when addressing the patient's obesity and weight management may be an important determinant of the patient's receptivity. The patient needs to define the problem and the clinician needs to be nonjudgmental in discussing the behavior and the weight problem (Stunkard, 1993). Being open and conveying empathetic understanding of the patient when discussing treatment options and the challenges that come with the needed long-term lifestyle changes are important. Finally, eliciting the patient's objective for the treatment and mutually agreeing on a plan of action for the short and long-term will enhance the probability of a positive outcome (Serdula et al., 2003; Burke & Fair, 2003).

TREATMENT OF OVERWEIGHT AND OBESITY

Treatment Approach

Treatment for obesity can be approached through lifestyle modification, which includes dietary and exercise programs, pharmacotherapy, or surgical treatment. The latter two approaches are adjunctive to lifestyle therapy (Table 42-2). The severity of obesity and presence of comorbidities determine the approach to treatment (e.g., the coexistence of non-insulin-dependent diabetes, hypertension, or congestive heart failure) (Eckel, 1997). In the absence of comorbid conditions, patients with a BMI between 25 and 30 can achieve adequate weight reduction through lifestyle approaches. Pharmacotherapy is usually limited to those with a BMI greater than 30 or, in the presence of comorbidities, to those with a BMI between 27 and 30. Surgical therapy is considered for a BMI in excess of 35 with comorbid conditions, or when the BMI exceeds 40. Pharmacologic or surgical therapy is never used in isolation, but rather are adjunctive to lifestyle modification, which needs to be maintained indefinitely after the use of these other treatment modalities.

Table 42–2 ■ APPROACHES TO TREATMENT OF OBESITY BY SEVERITY AND DISEASE RISK

BMI	Comorbid Conditions and/or CVD Risk Factors	Treatment Approaches (Eckel & Krauss, 1998; Wing, 1998)
25–30	Absent	Lifestyle modification* Prevention of wt. gain
27–30	≥2 Present[†]	Lifestyle modification + pharma cotherapy[‡]
>30	Absent	Lifestyle modification + pharma cotherapy[‡]
>35	≥2 Present	Consider surgical therapy
>40	Absent	Surgical therapy[‡]

* Lifestyle modification includes caloric restriction (400 kcal/day defeicit), <30% fat diet, exercise at least 5 days/wk, and behavioral therapy.
[†] Comorbid conditions warranting drug therapy: HBP, CHD, type 2 diabetes, congestive heart failure, and sleep apnea.
[‡] Pharmacotherapy and surgical therapy are adjunctive to lifestyle modification.

Goal of Treatment

The goal of weight loss is not to achieve some cosmetic standard of attractiveness, but rather to reduce morbidity and increase mobility. The recommended initial weight loss goal is 10% of baseline weight, a weight loss that can be maintained for at least a year or longer (Abate et al., 1996; NHLBI, 1998). The rate of loss should be approximately 0.5 to 1 pound per week for the moderately obese and 1 to 2 pounds per week in the severely obese.

It is important to discuss treatment strategies and goals with the patient because these have to be arrived at through mutual decision making, and there could be a discrepancy between the provider's and the patient's goal (Foster et al., 1997; NHLBI, 1998; Stunkard, 1993; Williamson et al., 1992). An example would be a 55-year-old woman who has lower body obesity and no additional risk factors but may wish to lose a certain amount of weight. This patient may achieve the loss and feel better about her appearance, but if she is unable to sustain this loss, she will regain and be frustrated. This person may benefit from guidance for a lower weight loss goal and exercise or a plan for stability of current weight. However, if this same woman had upper body weight or presence of risk factors, she should be counseled for achieving a 10% weight reduction. A 40-year-old woman may wish to achieve a body weight that is significantly below her current weight and one she has not had since she was in her twenties. Not only is achievement of the goal unlikely, but so is maintenance of the weight. This patient may benefit from an initial goal of 10% reduction, and if this is achieved, an additional goal can be established. Other patients may have no desire to reduce and may benefit from a discussion regarding their risk profile and the benefits of weight reduction. If the person is unmotivated to change, a plan of weight gain prevention may be appropriate for the time (NHLBI, 1998; Serdula et al., 2003).

Furthermore, the provider needs to discuss with the patient what other goals she has for weight loss. A patient may think that improved personal relationships or professional opportunities will result from achieving the weight loss goal, but this is rarely the case because more than weight loss usually is necessary for such goals to be realized. The provider needs to emphasize to the patient the health benefits resulting from a 10% loss, and assist the patient in being realistic about weight loss outcomes (Foster et al., 1997; Williamson et al., 1992).

Once the patient and provider have agreed on the treatment approach and the initial goals, it is time to prepare the patient for the course of treatment. Orienting the patient to the active participation required for successful weight loss facilitates cooperation and adherence. Patients need to be oriented to self-monitoring food and caloric intake and expenditure. Conveying to the patient understanding and support during the challenging course and providing reinforcement for behavioral change can go a long way in sustaining the person's motivation (NHLBI, 1998; Stunkard, 1993).

COMPONENTS OF THE TREATMENT

Lifestyle Modification

Lifestyle therapy includes three components: nutritional or dietary therapy, exercise and daily activity, and behavioral therapy. The changes in the patient's dietary and activity habits are facilitated and reinforced through the behavioral strategies used in weight loss treatment. The following sections describe the three components.

Dietary Therapy

During weight loss treatment, the strongest determinant of the rate and amount of weight loss that will occur is the extent of the negative energy balance (Hill et al., 1993). A key component of dietary therapy is a reduction in total caloric intake by 500 to 1,000 kilocalories (kcal)/d, resulting in the patient consuming 800 to 1,500 kcal/d. This is referred to as a low-calorie diet and has been shown to reduce weight by 8% over 6 months. A deficit of 500 kcal/d results in a 1 pound per week weight loss (1 pound is the equivalent of 3,500 kcal). Depending on the patient's baseline weight and the amount of weight loss desired, the patient may follow a diet ranging from 1,000 to 1,200 kcal for women and 1,200 to 1,500 kcal for men (NHLBI, 1998; Wing, 1998).

An important component of dietary therapy is addressing both fat and caloric restriction. Studies have evaluated the restriction of either one alone and have demonstrated less weight loss, especially when fat is restricted in the absence of caloric limitations (Harvey-Berino, 1998). In general, a 20% to 30% fat diet is recommended and the patient is provided a daily fat gram goal along with the calorie goal (Wing, 1998). The recommended diet composition is consistent with the Adult Treatment Panel Step I Diet (Table 42-3), although many programs use a 20% fat eating plan (Wing, 1998; NCEP, ATP III, 2001).

Very-low-calorie diets, which are restricted to less than 800 kcal/d, are no longer recommended for several reasons. They

Table 42–3 ■ LOW-CALORIE STEP I DIET

Nutrient	Recommended Intake
Calories	Approximately 500–1,000 kcal/d reduction from usual intake
Total fat	≤30% of total calories
Saturated fatty acids	8%–10% of total calories
Monounsaturated fatty acids	Up to 15% of total calories
Polyunsaturated fatty acids	Up to 10% of total calories
Cholestrol	<300 mg/d
Protein	Approximately 15% of total calories
Carbohydrate	≥55% of total calories
Sodium chloride	≤100 mmol/d (approximately 2.4 g of sodium or 6 g of sodium chloride)
Calcium	1,000–1,500 mg/d
Fiber	20–30 g/d

From National Heart Lung, and Blood Institute Expert Panel. (1998). *Clinical guidelines on the identification, evaluation, and treatment of overweight and obesity in adults: The evidence report.* Bethesda, MD: National Institute of Health.

provide inadequate nutrition unless supplemented, require medical supervision to monitor the patient's nutritional and electrolyte status, and increase the risk for development of gallstones. Furthermore, studies have shown that the rapid weight loss is followed by a rapid regain, and at 1 year, the percentage of weight loss retained with the very-low-calorie diets is less than with the low calorie diet (Wing, 1998; Paffenbarger et al., 1993).

Low-carbohydrate diets have received considerable attention in recent years by the lay public and the scientific community (Bravata et al., 2003; Foster et al., 2003). One of the biggest concerns about the low-carbohydrate diet, which is accompanied by a high-fat and high-protein intake, is its effects on coronary risk factors. However, the studies that have been conducted to evaluate this dietary approach to weight loss have failed to provide conclusive findings due to uncontrolled assignment to treatment, limited duration of treatment, and, most recently, high attrition with no differences in weight loss between the low-carbohydrate and the standard dietary groups at 12 months (Bravata et al., 2003; Foster et al., 2003).

Programs using the lifestyle approach include nutritional education (Wing, 1998). The focus of the instruction includes the energy value of foods (e.g., fat contains 9 calories per gram compared to protein and carbohydrates, which contain 4 calories per gram), how to read labels, the three types of fat and the recommended distribution of these in the diet, methods to reduce fat and increase fiber and complex carbohydrate intake, and how to prepare foods to reduce the addition of calories. Patients also are instructed on recipe modification and ordering from a restaurant menu (Brownell, 2000; Wing, 1998).

Exercise and Physical Activity

Trials examining weight loss with and without exercise have consistently demonstrated improved weight loss with the combined diet and exercise components (Pavlou et al., 1989; Wing, 1998). Encourage patients to focus on changes in eating patterns during the initial weeks of a program and around the third week, introduce goals for weekly exercise. Increase the goals gradually so that behavior can be shaped to include an exercise routine, eventually achieving a caloric expenditure goal of 1,000 kcal/wk, which can be reached by walking 2 miles per day for 5 of 7 days per week, or by exercising at moderate intensity for 150 minutes per week, as recommended by The American College of Sports Medicine (ACSM). ACSM suggests that there may be advantages to reaching a higher level of exercise duration, e.g., 200 to 300 minutes per week, particularly for the long-term maintenance of weight loss (Jakicic et al., 2001). The single best predictor of weight loss maintenance is exercise (Klem et al., 1997).

Various approaches are available for individuals beginning or expanding their exercise program. Adherence to exercise can be influenced by factors such as environment (e.g., supervised or group exercise classes versus exercising at home) and length of exercise sessions. Having a patient follow an independent exercise program at home may show improved adherence and weight loss (Perri, 1997). Another strategy that may improve exercise adherence as well as weight loss maintenance, includes having the patient use several short bouts (10 minutes) of exercise instead of the conventional long bout (20 to 40 minutes) of exercise (Jakicic et al., 1995; Jakicic et al., 1999).

Daily activity is another way of improving weight loss efforts. Including physically active choices throughout the day (e.g., using the stairs, and walking more through daily activities) can help to increase overall caloric expenditure. Encourage patients to decrease the amount of sedentary activities (i.e., TV viewing or computer use) and replace them with activities such as gardening or recreational sports. Lifestyle activity can result in positive benefits on physical fitness and cardiovascular risk reduction (Dunn, 1999).

Depending on the patient's age, risk factor profile, and concomitant conditions and symptoms, exercise testing to assess cardiopulmonary function and presence of disease may be indicated. This needs to be determined before initiating an exercise program. Patients also require instruction on injury prevention, how to initiate and maintain an exercise program, proper attire, and weather conditions. The kind of activity or exercise and the amount of time spent engaged in it are recorded in the patients' diaries. Lists of activities and their caloric expenditure are provided to patients so they can monitor progress toward their exercise goals.

Behavioral Therapy

Behavioral therapy, based on the earlier work of Stuart (1996), has at its core the functional analysis of behavior (Wing, 1998). Eating and exercise behaviors are analyzed to delineate their association with environmental events, including times, people, places, thoughts, and emotions (Wing, 1998). Patients record their eating and exercise behaviors and use these self-monitoring data to determine specific problem areas. The environment controlling the problem areas is then restructured and the problem behaviors modified (Wing, 1998).

Among the distinguishing features of behavioral therapy is its goal orientation. The objectives of treatment are clearly defined, specific, and measurable. In addition, behavioral therapy attempts to change behavior and, finally, it is a process-oriented approach in that it is a method of learning about one's behavior. Behaviors are broken down into a series of small events, and acquisition of behavior shaped through small steps.

Behavioral treatment programs usually use a multidisciplinary approach and may include a psychologist, nutritionist, exercise physiologist, nurse, or physician (NHLBI, 1998). No studies have been performed evaluating the different health care professionals delivering the intervention, but it is suggested that providers avail themselves of the expertise offered by professionals who have counseled patients in this area (NHLBI, 1998). Duration of treatment is 16 to 24 weeks of either weekly or a combination of weekly and biweekly contacts. More recently, programs are extending treatment to 12 months and use biweekly or monthly meetings during the second 6-month period (Wing, 1998). Behavioral therapy is usually delivered in a closed-group context, that is, the group is formed at the initiation of treatment and no new members are added thereafter. This approach facilitates the development of group cohesiveness and reduces attrition (Wing, 1998). The group approach also offers economic benefits. Behavioral therapy may use numerous strategies to facilitate behavior change. Specific strategies are as follows:

Self-monitoring: often considered the *sine qua non* of behavioral treatment (Wing, 1998). It entails instructing patients to record their food intake, calories, fat grams, and exercise caloric expenditure or time spent in programmed activity. This requires patients to look up these values in books provided and makes them aware not only of their behavior but of the caloric and fat content of foods eaten.

Goal setting: patients are given goals for total calories, fat grams and percent of total calories, and energy expenditure through exercise; goals need to be proximal, specific, and attainable.

Stimulus control: considered the hallmark of behavioral therapy (Stuart, 1996). It is based on the assumption that environmental antecedents control behaviors, and that changing the environment to include positive cues for appropriate eating and exercise behaviors leads to desired behavior-for example, remove high fat foods and replace them with attractive fruits that are ready to eat, store other tempting foods out of sight, restrict places of eating (Wing, 1998).

Problem solving: using the approach described by D'Zurilla and Goldfried (1971), patients are taught four specific steps: identify the problem situation leading to inappropriate eating or exercise behavior, generate solutions, select one solution to test, and evaluate the use of the solution in resolving the problem.

Relapse prevention: patients are taught that lapses are a natural occurrence and should be anticipated and planned for with strategies that can be used in coping with the situation, and thereby prevent relapses (Marlatt & Gordon, 1980).

Cognitive restructuring: entails teaching patients about negative thoughts, rationalizations, comparisons with others, and all-or-none thinking, and how these thoughts serve the patient; patients are taught how to counter these thoughts with more positive thinking and self-statements (Wing, 1998).

Other strategies that can be used include contingency management, reinforcement, dealing with high-risk situations, stress management, and enlisting social support. Patient-centered counseling, an approach that focuses on encouraging patients to set goals, with input from the provider if needed, has been successful in helping patients make dietary behavioral changes and has potential in the treatment of these patients in primary care settings (Ockene, 1999). Another strategy that is showing promise with obese patients when used in clinical settings is motivational interviewing (Simkin-Silverman & Wing, 1997). In summary, the best results for treatment success are attained through a combination of dietary therapy, exercise and physical activity, and use of behavioral therapy (NHLBI, 1998; Wing, 1998). This regimen should be continued for at least 6 months, followed by maintenance strategies.

Acknowledging the chronicity of obesity and the limitations of conventional clinical settings to assist patients to manage their weight, alternative approaches have been evaluated (Heshka et al., 2003; Tate et al., 2003; Tate et al., 2001). Use of the internet to deliver a behavioral weight loss program permits weekly contacts and individualized feedback to participants, and has been successful in achieving weight loss (Tate et al., 2001). However, while the use of technology reduces participant burden by not requiring frequent visits to a study or clinical center, it does not reduce the expense of professional counselors. The widely available structured, commercial weight loss programs that advocate the use of sound, balanced eating plans as well as exercise and behavioral change serve a valuable role in supporting the large number of people who need guidance in weight loss (Heshka et al., 2003). Approaches that address the potential for ongoing contact build on the well-established findings that ongoing contact is essential to promote long-term adherence to lifestyle change (Burke, 1999).

Pharmacotherapy

Drug therapy for the treatment of obesity has had a troubled history (Bray, 1998). This was accentuated by the withdrawal in 1997 of two drugs, fenfluramine and dexfenfluramine, after cardiac valvular abnormalities were noted on echocardiograms in women receiving the popular drugs (Bray, 1998). Subsequently, the approval process of other anti-obesity agents has been slowed. At the same time, these events brought attention to the idea that obesity, like other chronic disorders, needs ongoing treatment, and those who have markedly increased medical risks and who have not been successful with nonpharmacologic therapy, could benefit from adjunctive drug therapy (Yanovski & Yanovski, 2002). However, pharmacologic therapy for treatment of obesity has limited indications, which are treatment of patients with a BMI of 30 or greater in the absence of comorbid conditions, or for patients with a BMI of 27 or greater with concomitant morbidity. Drug therapy needs to be instituted in combination with a program of lifestyle modification.

There are two categories of medications for the treatment of obesity: those that suppress appetite, and those that reduce nutrient absorption; a third category (those that increase energy expenditure) is not currently approved (Yanovski & Yanovski, 2002). Numerous drugs that work through different mechanisms are under study for future treatment (Ettinger, 2003; Gadde et al., 2003; Yanovski & Yanovski, 2002). Other drugs,

originally developed for other indications, are undergoing clinical trial evaluation. These include bupropion, a reuptake inhibitor of norepinephrine, serotonin, and dopamine; topiramate, an antiepileptic agent, and metformin, a drug approved for treatment of type 2 diabetes. Each of these drugs has been associated with small weight losses when used in the treatment of disorders for which they are indicated (Yanovski & Yanovski, 2002). As a greater understanding of the molecular pathophysiology of obesity is achieved, it is likely that new therapeutic agents will be developed (Mertens & Van Gaal, 2000). However, in the interim, the pharmacological agents available are limited.

Two drugs have long-term approval. One agent, sibutramine, blocks the reuptake of serotonin and noradrenaline and thereby reduces food intake and increases thermogenesis (Yanovski & Yanovski, 2002). This drug produces weight loss for approximately one year in clinical trials, but its use is associated with increases in arterial hypertension and heart rate. Thus, it needs to be used with caution in individuals with cardiovascular disease (Haynes & Mark, 2002). A second drug, orlistat, does not act through the central nervous system; it inhibits gastric and pancreatic lipases, which are essential for effective digestion of fats, and thereby decreases fat absorption (G. A. Bray, 1998; Yanovski & Yanovski, 2002; Sharma & Golay, 2002). This agent also has a lowering effect on LDL-cholesterol levels, but it does not affect HDL-cholesterol (Rossner, 2000; Soni, 2000). Orlistat provides the patient with a challenge for adherence because of its thrice-daily dosing schedule within 90 minutes of a meal. Moreover, it requires adherence to a low-fat diet to prevent unpleasant side effects, which include oily or loose stools and fecal leakage. Therefore, patient adherence to diet and medication must be monitored. Since sibutramine and orlistat work through entirely different mechanisms, they may be additive when used in combination (Bray, 1999). Each drug may result in a 10% weight loss, thus used in combination; they may result in a 20% weight loss.

When medications are prescribed for weight loss, it is most likely that long-term use will be needed (National Task Force on the Prevention and Treatment of Obesity, 1996). Numerous studies have shown that weight regain occurs with discontinuation of therapy. Individuals will need to follow a modified eating and exercise program to achieve weight loss even when on drug therapy. Therefore, behavioral or nonpharmacologic therapy should be tried for at least six months prior to the initiation of pharmacological therapy. The limited effectiveness of anti-obesity agents in producing weight loss emphasizes their necessarily adjunctive role (Anonymous, American Society for Hospital Pharmacists, 2001). Several investigators have reported that adding lifestyle modification to the pharmacologic management significantly improved weight loss as well as patients' reported satisfaction with treatment outcome (Berkowitz et al., 2003; Frost et al., 2002; Wadden et al., 2001). Most weight loss occurs within the first 6 months of treatment and averages 5% to 10% of the baseline weight, which translates to 2 to 10 kg (NHLBI, 1998). People who lose weight during the initial 6 months of drug therapy and maintain that loss without side effects may be considered successful and maintained on the drug with periodic follow-up to monitor progress, side effects, weight, blood pressure, and laboratory values, and to provide reinforcement.

Bariatric Surgery

Surgical approaches, which are primarily for the purpose of reducing food intake, are indicated only for patients with severe obesity (BMI ≥ 40) or a BMI of 35 or more and concomitant morbidity, such as sleep apnea, uncontrolled type 2 diabetes, cardiovascular disease, or weight-related problems interfering with daily functioning (Pope, 2002). Selection criteria for patients undergoing bariatric surgery include a BMI of 35 or more with comorbidities or a BMI of 40 or more; failure of at least five to six attempts at weight reduction, and psychological stability, usually established by an evaluation pre-operatively, and an understanding of the surgery and its effects (Brolin, 2002).

There are three surgical procedures: the stapled gastroplasty, the use of which is reduced because of poor maintenance of weight loss; gastric banding; and gastric bypass, which combines restriction of gastric content and intestinal malabsorption (Brolin, 2002). The Roue-en-Y technique is the preferred approach to bypass currently. Substantial weight loss can result from these surgical procedures, e.g., typical weight loss is approximately 65% to 75%, or 35% of the pre-operative weight (Brolin, 2002). However, postoperative outcomes should include improvement of co-morbid conditions, and not just weight loss. Patients undergoing these procedures, including those with overt diabetes, may experience a normalization of glucose. Postoperative weight loss has been associated with improvement in blood pressure, ventricular wall thickness and cardiac chamber size, as well as reductions in total cholesterol and triglycerides, resolution or improvement in sleep apnea, and improvement in several gynecologic disorders, such as menstrual irregularity and amenorrhea, ovulatory infertility and polycystic ovarian syndrome (Brolin, 2002; Deitel, 1988; Foley, 1992). Patients who have undergone bariatric surgery require ongoing medical follow-up and lifestyle adjustments related to diet and exercise.

Maintenance of Weight Loss

Recently, successful long-term weight loss maintenance was defined as intentionally losing at least 10% of initial body weight and maintaining that loss for at least 1 year (Wing & Hill, 2001). Using this definition, successful weight loss maintenance occurs in approximately 20% of overweight or obese individuals. This provides a much brighter picture than the standard reports that 1 year after treatment, patients maintain 60% of their initial weight loss, but return to their baseline weight within 3 to 5 years (Wing, 1998). Still, it remains that the greatest challenge facing health care professionals who treat these patients is identifying the means to assist patients to sustain the initial weight loss (Jeffery et al., 2000). Several strategies have been investigated for their efficacy in improving weight loss maintenance (Perri et al., 1989; Perri et al., 1984a; Perri et al., 1984b; Perri et al., 1987; Perri et al., 1986; Wing, 1996). Those that have most consistently demonstrated improved weight loss maintenance include ongoing contact with the provider (King et al., 1989; Perri et al., 1984), inclusion of aerobic exercise (Perri, 1986), and provision of social support (Wing & Jeffery, 1999). Use of the chronic disease model to treat obesity, an important advance, can facilitate ongoing follow-up and reinforcement beyond the point of

reaching the weight loss goal. Data from the National Weight Control Registry shows that individuals are most vulnerable for regain during the first few years, and those who are able to maintain their loss for 2 to 5 years have a greatly increased likelihood that they will maintain that loss. National Weight Control Registry data reveal that people who are successful in maintaining a weight loss of 13.6 kg (30 lb) or more for at least 1 year report expending 11,830 kJ/wk through physical activity, an amount equivalent to 2,800 kcal/wk, or walking 28 miles (Klem et al., 1997). This finding underscores the importance of exercise as a maintenance strategy. However, adherence to exercise remains a problem (Burke et al., 1997). Maintenance of weight loss is the ultimate form of compliance because it requires long-term adherence to the numerous changes in lifestyle that created the initial weight loss (Burke, 1999). Therefore, the provider needs to implement strategies to enhance adherence throughout the treatment and maintenance phases; these are detailed elsewhere in the text.

▪ SUMMARY

Obesity is a chronic medical condition with numerous adverse effects on the cardiovascular system. The significant increase in its prevalence and the epidemic of type 2 diabetes that is following it demands attention at all levels. The goal of treatment is reduced morbidity and improved health. Current treatment consists of lifestyle interventions and, increasingly, pharmacotherapy. Since 1998, we have evidence-based guidelines for use in the identification, evaluation, and treatment of overweight and obese patients in the clinical setting (NHLBI, 1998). These guidelines emphasize multidisciplinary approaches to the treatment of this chronic disorder. Practitioners can teach patients strategies for self-management by following the precedent established in treating similar conditions (e.g., hypertension, dyslipidemia, and diabetes). Similar to the role nurses play in the treatment of these chronic conditions, nurses need to take the lead in addressing the needs of this ever-growing subgroup of the population. Two important areas to address are prevention of further weight gain and sustaining the weight loss achieved initially.

REFERENCES

Abate, N., Garg, A., Peshock, R. M., Stray-Gundersen, J., Adams-Huet, B., & Grundy, S. M. (1996). Relationship of generalized and regional adiposity to insulin sensitivity in men with NIDDM. *Diabetes, 45*(12), 1684–1693.

Allison, D. B. (1995). *Handbook of assessment methods for eating behaviors and weight related problems: Measures, theory, and research.* Thousand Oaks, CA: Sage.

Anderson, D. A., & Wadden, T. A. (1999). Treating the obese patient. Suggestions for primary care practice. *Archives of Family Medicine, 8*(2), 156–167.

Anonymous. (2001). American Society of Hospital Pharmacists' (ASHP) therapeutic position statement on the safe use of pharmacotherapy for obesity management in adults. Developed by the ASHP Commission on Therapeutics and approved by the ASHP Board of Directors on April 23, 2001. *American Journal of Health-System Pharmacy, 58*(17), 1645–1655.

Berkowitz, R. I., Wadden, T. A., Tershakovec, A. M., & Cronquist, J. L. (2003). Behavior therapy and sibutramine for the treatment of adolescent obesity: a randomized controlled trial. *JAMA, 289*(14), 1805–1812.

Bonow, R. O., & Eckel, R. H. (2003). Diet, obesity, and cardiovascular risk. *New England Journal of Medicine, 348*(21), 2057–2058.

Bravata, D. M., Sanders, L., Huang, J., Krumholz, H. M., Olkin, I., & Gardner, C. D. (2003). Efficacy and safety of low-carbohydrate diets: a systematic review. *JAMA, 289*(14), 1837–1850.

Bray, G. (1998). Drug treatment of obesity: don't throw the baby out with the bath water. *American Journal of Clinical Nutrition, 67*(1), 1–2.

Bray, G. A. (1998). Pharmacological treatment of obesity. In G. A. Bray, C., Bourchard, & W. P. T. James, (Ed.), *Handbook of obesity,* pp. 953–975. New York: Marcel Dekker.

Bray, G. A. (1999). Uses and misuses of the new pharmacotherapy of obesity. *Annals of Medicine, 31*(1), 1–3.

Brolin, R. E. (2002). Bariatric surgery and long-term control of morbid obesity. *JAMA, 288*(22), 2793–2796.

Brownell, K. D. (2000). *The LEARN program for weight control* (8th ed.). Dallas, TX: American Health Publishing Company.

Burke, L., & Fair, J. (2003). Promoting prevention: Skills sets and attributes of health care providers who deliver behavioral intervention. *Journal of Cardiovascular Nursing, 18*(4), 256–266.

Burke, L. E. (1999). Strategies to enhance compliance to weight loss treatment. In G. Fletcher, S. Grundy, & L. Hayman (Ed.), *Obesity: Impact on cardiovascular disease.* Armonk, NY: Futura.

Burke, L. E., Dunbar-Jacob, J. M., & Hill, M. N. (1997). Compliance with cardiovascular disease prevention strategies: a review of the research. *Annals of Behavioral Medicine, 19*(3), 239–263.

Deitel, M., Stone, E., Kassam, H. A., Wilk, E. J., & Sutherland, D. J. (1988). Gynecologic-obstetric changes after loss of massive excess weight following bariatric surgery. *Journal of the American College of Nutrition, 7*(2), 147–153.

Dunn, A. L., Marcus, B. H., Kampert, J. B., Garcia, M. E., Kohl, H. W., 3rd, & Blair, S. N. (1999). Comparison of lifestyle and structured interventions to increase physical activity and cardiorespiratory fitness: a randomized trial. *JAMA, 281*(4), 327–334.

D'Zurilla, T. J., & Goldfried, M. R. (1971). Problem solving and behavior modification. *Journal of Abnormal Psychology, 78*(1), 107–126.

Eaton, C. B., Goodwin, M. A., & Stange, K. C. (2002). Direct observation of nutrition counseling in community family practice. *American Journal of Preventive Medicine, 23*(3), 174–179.

Eckel, R. H. (1997). Obesity and heart disease: a statement for healthcare professionals from the Nutrition Committee, American Heart Association. *Circulation, 96*(9), 3248–3250.

Eckel, R. H., Krauss, R. M. (1998). American Heart Association call to action: obesity as a major risk factor for coronary heart disease. AHA Nutrition Committee. *Circulation, 97*(21), 2099–2100.

Esposito, K., Pontillo, A., Di Palo, C., Giugliano, G., Masella, M., Marfella, R., & Giugliano, D. (2003). Effect of weight loss and lifestyle changes on vascular inflammatory markers in obese women: a randomized trial. *JAMA, 289*(14), 1799–1804.

Ettinger, M. P., Littlejohn, T. W., Schwartz, S. L., Weiss, S. R., McIlwain, H. H., Heymsfield, S. B., Bray, G. A., Roberts, W. G., Heyman, E. R., Stambler, N., Heshka, S., Vicary, C. & Guler, H. P. (2003). Recombinant variant of ciliary neurotrophic factor for weight loss in obese adults: a randomized, dose-ranging study [comment]. *JAMA, 289*(14), 1826–1832.

Fiore, M. C., Bailey, W. C., Cohen, S. J. (1996). *Smoking cessation: Clinical practice guidelines No 18.* Bethesda, MD: Department of Health and Human Services, Public Health Services, Agency for Health Care Policy and Research.

Foley, E. F., Benotti, P. N., Borlase, B. C., Hollingshead, J., & Blackburn, G. L. (1992). Impact of gastric restrictive surgery on hypertension in the morbidly obese. *American Journal of Surgery, 163*(3), 294–297.

Fontaine, K. R., Redden, D. T., Wang, C., Westfall, A. O., & Allison, D. B. (2003). Years of life lost due to obesity. *JAMA, 289*(2), 187–193.

Foster, G. D., Wadden, T. A., Vogt, R. A., & Brewer, G. (1997). What is a reasonable weight loss? Patients' expectations and evaluations of obesity treatment outcomes. *Journal of Consulting & Clinical Psychology, 65*(1), 79–85.

Foster, G. D., Wyatt, H. R., Hill, J. O., McGuckin, B. G., Brill, C., Mohammed, B. S., Szapary, P. O., Rader, D. J., Edman, J. S., & Klein, S. (2003). A randomized trial of a low-carbohydrate diet for obesity. *New England Journal of Medicine, 348*(21), 2082–2090.

Frost, G., Lyons, F., Bovill-Taylor, C., Carter, L., Stuttard, J., & Dornhorst, A. (2002). Intensive lifestyle intervention combined with the choice of pharmacotherapy improves weight loss and cardiac risk factors in the obese. *Journal of Human Nutrition & Dietetics, 15*(4), 287–295; quiz 297–289.

Gadde, K. M., Franciscy, D. M., Wagner, H. R., 2nd, & Krishnan, K. R. (2003). Zonisamide for weight loss in obese adults: a randomized controlled trial. *JAMA, 289*(14), 1820–1825.

Gibson, R. S. (1990). *Principles of nutritional assessment* (pp. 170–195). New York: Oxford University Press.

Harvey-Berino, J. (1998). The efficacy of dietary fat vs. total energy restriction for weight loss. *Obesity Research, 6*(3), 202–207.

Haynes, W. G., & Mark, A. L. (2002). Pharmacotherapy of obesity: lessons from clinical trials in hypertension. *Journal of Hypertension, 20*(9), 1731–1735.

Heshka, S., Anderson, J. W., Atkinson, R. L., Greenway, F. L., Hill, J. O., Phinney, S. D., Kolotkin, R. L., Miller-Kovach, K., & Pi-Sunyer, F. X. (2003). Weight loss with self-help compared with a structured commercial program: a randomized trial. *JAMA, 289*(14), 1792–1798.

Hill, J. O., Drougas, H., & Peters, J. C. (1993). Obesity treatment: can diet composition play a role?[comment]. *Annals of Internal Medicine, 119*(7 Pt 2), 694–697.

Institute of Medicine. (1995). *Weighing the options: Criteria for evaluating weight-management programs.* Washington, DC: National Academy Press.

Jakicic, J. M., Clark, K., Coleman, E., Donnelly, J. E., Foreyt, J., Melanson, E., Volek, J., Volpe, S. L., & American College of Sports, M. (2001). American College of Sports Medicine position stand. Appropriate intervention strategies for weight loss and prevention of weight regain for adults. *Medicine & Science in Sports & Exercise, 33*(12), 2145–2156.

Jakicic, J. M., Wing, R. R., Butler, B. A., & Robertson, R. J. (1995). Prescribing exercise in multiple short bouts versus one continuous bout: effects on adherence, cardiorespiratory fitness, and weight loss in overweight women. *International Journal of Obesity & Related Metabolic Disorders: Journal of the International Association for the Study of Obesity, 19*(12), 893–901.

Jakicic, J. M., Winters, C., Lang, W., & Wing, R. R. (1999). Effects of intermittent exercise and use of home exercise equipment on adherence, weight loss, and fitness in overweight women: a randomized trial. *JAMA, 282*(16), 1554–1560.

Janssen, I., Katzmarzyk, P. T., & Ross, R. (2002). Body mass index, waist circumference, and health risk: evidence in support of current National Institutes of Health guidelines. *Archives of Internal Medicine, 162*(18), 2074–2079.

Jeffery, R. W., Drewnowski, A., Epstein, L. H., Stunkard, A. J., Wilson, G. T., Wing, R. R., & Hill, D. R. (2000). Long-term maintenance of weight loss: current status. *Health Psychology, 19*(1 Suppl), 5–16.

Jialal, I., & Devaraj, S. (2003). Role of C-reactive protein in the assessment of cardiovascular risk. *American Journal of Cardiology, 91*(2), 200–202.

Kiernan, M., & Winkleby, M. A. (2000). Identifying patients for weight-loss treatment: an empirical evaluation of the NHLBI obesity education initiative expert panel treatment recommendations. *Archives of Internal Medicine, 160*(14), 2169–2176.

King, A. C., Frey-Hewitt, B., Dreon, D. M., & Wood, P. D. (1989). Diet vs. exercise in weight maintenance. The effects of minimal intervention strategies on long-term outcomes in men. *Archives of Internal Medicine, 149*(12), 2741–2746.

Klem, M. L., Wing, R. R., McGuire, M. T., Seagle, H. M., & Hill, J. O. (1997). A descriptive study of individuals successful at long-term maintenance of substantial weight loss.[comment]. *American Journal of Clinical Nutrition, 66*(2), 239–246.

Kumanyika, S., Jeffery, R. W., Morabia, A., Ritenbaugh, C., & Antipatis, V. J., (2002). Public Health Approaches to the Prevention of Obesity Working Group of the International. Obesity Task Force: Obesity prevention: the case for action. *International Journal of Obesity & Related Metabolic Disorders: Journal of the International Association for the Study of Obesity, 26*(3), 425–436.

Lean, M. E., Han, T. S., & Morrison, C. E. (1995). Waist circumference as a measure for indicating need for weight management. *British Medical Journal, 311*(6998), 158–161.

Manson, J. E., & Bassuk, S. S. (2003). Obesity in the United States: a fresh look at its high toll.[comment]. *JAMA, 289*(2), 229–230.

Marlatt, G. A., Gordon, J. R. (1980). Determinants of relapse: Implications for the maintenance of behavior change. In P. O. Davidson, & S. M. Davidson (Eds.), *Behavioral medicine: Changing health lifestyles* (pp. 410–452). New York: Bruner/Mazel.

Martorell, R. (2001). *2020 focus 5 (health and nutrition emerging and issues in developing countries, Brief 7 of 11, Feb, 2001): Obesity.* http://www.ifpri.org/. Retrieved June 11, 2003.

Mertens, I. L., & Van Gaal, L. F. (2000). Promising new approaches to the management of obesity. *Drugs, 60*(1), 1–9.

Mokdad, A. H., Ford, E. S., Bowman, B. A., Dietz, W. H., Vinicor, F., Bales, V. S., & Marks, J. S. (2003). Prevalence of obesity, diabetes, and obesity-related health risk factors, 2001. *JAMA, 289*(1), 76–79.

National Heart, Lung, and Blood Institute, Obesity Education Initiative Expert Panel on the Identification, Evaluation, and Treatment of Overweight and Obesity. (1998). *Clinical guidelines on the identification, evaluation, and treatment of overweight and obesity in adults: The evidence report.* Bethesda, MD: National Institute of Health.

National Task Force on the Prevention and Treatment of Obesity. (1996). Long-term pharmacotherapy in the management of obesity. *JAMA*, 276(23), 1907–1915.

NIH Consensus Conference. (1993). Triglyceride, high-density lipoprotein, and coronary heart disease. NIH Consensus Development Panel on Triglyceride, High-Density Lipoprotein, and Coronary Heart Disease. *JAMA*, 269(4), 505–510.

Ockene, I. S., Hebert, J. R., Ockene, J. K., Saperia, G. M., Stanek, E., Nicolosi, R., Merriam, P. A., & Hurley, T. G. (1999). Effect of physician-delivered nutrition counseling training and an office-support program on saturated fat intake, weight, and serum lipid measurements in a hyperlipidemic population: Worcester Area Trial for Counseling in Hyperlipidemia (WATCH). *Archives of Internal Medicine*, 159(7), 725–731.

Paffenbarger, R. S., Jr., Hyde, R. T., Wing, A. L., Lee, I. M., Jung, D. L., & Kampert, J. B. (1993). The association of changes in physical-activity level and other lifestyle characteristics with mortality among men. *New England Journal of Medicine*, 328(8), 538–545.

Pavlou, K. N., Krey, S., & Steffee, W. P. (1989). Exercise as an adjunct to weight loss and maintenance in moderately obese subjects. *American Journal of Clinical Nutrition*, 49(5 Suppl.), 1115–1123.

Pereira, M. A., FitzGerald, S. J., Gregg, E. W., Joswiak, M. L., Ryan, W. J., Suminski, R. R., Utter, A. C., & Zmuda, J. M. (1997). A collection of Physical Activity Questionnaires for health-related research. *Medicine & Science in Sports & Exercise*, 29(6 Suppl.), S1–205.

Perri, M. G., Martin, A. D., Leermakers, E. A., Sears, S. F., & Notelovitz, M. (1997). Effects of group- versus home-based exercise in the treatment of obesity. *Journal of Consulting & Clinical Psychology*, 65(2), 278–285.

Perri, M. G., McAdoo, W. G., McAllister, D. A., Lauer, J. B., Jordan, R. C., Yancey, D. Z., & Nezu, A. M. (1987). Effects of peer support and therapist contact on long-term weight loss. *Journal of Consulting & Clinical Psychology*, 55(4), 615–617.

Perri, M. G., McAdoo, W. G., Spevak, P. A., & Newlin, D. B. (1984). Effect of a multicomponent maintenance program on long-term weight loss. *Journal of Consulting & Clinical Psychology*, 52(3), 480–481.

Perri, M. G., McAdoo, W. G., McAllister, D. A., Lauer, J. B., & Yancey, D. Z. (1986). Enhancing the efficacy of behavior therapy for obesity: effects of aerobic exercise and a multicomponent maintenance program. *Journal of Consulting & Clinical Psychology*, 54(5), 670–675.

Perri, M. G., McAllister, D. A., Gange, J. J., Jordan, R. C., McAdoo, G., & Nezu, A. M. (1988). Effects of four maintenance programs on the long-term management of obesity. *Journal of Consulting & Clinical Psychology*, 56(4), 529–534.

Perri, M. G., Nezu, A. M., Patti, E. T., & McCann, K. L. (1989). Effect of length of treatment on weight loss. *Journal of Consulting & Clinical Psychology*, 57(3), 450–452.

Perri, M. G., Shapiro, R. M., Ludwig, W. W., Twentyman, C. T., & McAdoo, W. G. (1984). Maintenance strategies for the treatment of obesity: an evaluation of relapse prevention training and posttreatment contact by mail and telephone. *Journal of Consulting & Clinical Psychology*, 52(3), 404–413.

Pope, G. D., Birkmeyer, J. D., & Finlayson, S. R. (2002). National trends in utilization and in-hospital outcomes of bariatric surgery. *Journal of Gastrointestinal Surgery*, 6(6), 855–860; discussion 861.

Rossner, S., Sjostrom, L., Noack, R., Meinders, A. E., & Noseda, G. (2000). Weight loss, weight maintenance, and improved cardiovascular risk factors after 2 years treatment with orlistat for obesity. European Orlistat Obesity Study Group. *Obesity Research*, 8(1), 49–61.

Saltzman, E., Benotti, P. N. (1998). The effects of obesity of the cardiovascular system. In G. A. Bray, C. Bourchard, W. P. T. James (Eds.), *Handbook of obesity* (pp. 637–649). New York: Marcel Dekker.

Schwartz, R. S. (1998). Obesity in elderly. In G. A. Bray, C. Bourchard, W. P. T. James (Eds.), *Handbook of obesity* (pp. 103–114). New York: Marcel Dekker.

Schwimmer, J. B., Burwinkle, T. M., & Varni, J. W. (2003). Health-related quality of life of severely obese children and adolescents. *JAMA*, 289(14), 1813–1819.

Serdula, M. K., Khan, L. K., & Dietz, W. H. (2003). Weight loss counseling revisited. *JAMA*, 289(14), 1747–1750.

Serdula, M. K., Mokdad, A. H., Williamson, D. F., Galuska, D. A., Mendlein, J. M., & Heath, G. W. (1999). Prevalence of attempting weight loss and strategies for controlling weight. *JAMA*, 282(14), 1353–1358.

Shape Up America & American Obesity Association. (1996). *Guidance for treatment for adult obesity.* Bethesda, MD: Shape Up America.

Sharma, A. M., & Golay, A. (2002). Effect of orlistat-induced weight loss on blood pressure and heart rate in obese patients with hypertension. *Journal of Hypertension*, 20(9), 1873–1878.

Simkin-Silverman, L. R., & Wing, R. R. (1997). Management of obesity in primary care. *Obesity Research*, 5(6), 603–612.

Soni, S. (2000). What's new in obesity therapy. *Inpharma Weekly*, 1254(9), 3–4.

Stuart, R. B. (1996). Behavioral control of overeating. 1967. *Obesity Research*, 4(4), 411–417.

Stunkard, A. J. (1993). Talking with patients. In A. J. Stunkard & T. A. Wadden (Eds.), *Obesity: Theory and therapy* (pp. 355–363). New York: Raven Press.

Tate, D. F., Jackvony, E. H., & Wing, R. R. (2003). Effects of Internet behavioral counseling on weight loss in adults at risk for type 2 diabetes: a randomized trial. *JAMA*, 289(14), 1833–1836.

Tate, D. F., Wing, R. R., & Winett, R. A. (2001). Using Internet technology to deliver a behavioral weight loss program. *JAMA*, 285(9), 1172–1177.

US Department of Health and Human Services. (1996). *NHANES III anthropometric procedure video.* Washington, DC: US Government Printing Office, Stock Number 017-022-01335-5.

Van Gaal, L. F., Wauters, M. A., & De Leeuw, I. H. (1997). The beneficial effects of modest weight loss on cardiovascular risk factors. *International Journal of Obesity & Related Metabolic Disorders: Journal of the International Association for the Study of Obesity*, 21(Suppl 1), S5–9.

Wadden, T. A., Berkowitz, R. I., Sarwer, D. B., Prus-Wisniewski, R., & Steinberg, C. (2001). Benefits of lifestyle modification in the pharmacologic treatment of obesity: a randomized trial. *Archives of Internal Medicine*, 161(2), 218–227.

WHO International Obesity Task Force. (2003). *About obesity.* International Obesity Task Force: http://www.obesity.chaire.ulaval.ca/iotf.htm. Retrieved June 11, 2003.

Willet, W. (1990). *Nutritional epidemiology* (pp. 52–126). New York: Oxford University Press.

Williamson, D. F., Serdula, M. K., Anda, R. F., Levy, A., & Byers, T. (1992). Weight loss attempts in adults: goals, duration, and rate of weight loss. *American Journal of Public Health*, 82(9), 1251–1257.

Wing, R. R. (1998). Behavioral approaches to the treatment of obesity. In G. A. Bray, C. Bourchard, W. P. T. James (Eds.), *Handbook of obesity* (pp. 855–877). New York: Marcel Dekker.

Wing, R. R., & Hill, J. O. (2001). Successful weight loss maintenance. *Annual Review of Nutrition*, 21, 323–341.

Wing, R. R., Jeffery, R. W., Pronk, N., Hellerstedt, W. L, et al. (1996). Effects of frequent phone contacts and optional food provision on maintenance of weight loss. *Annals of Behavioral Medicine*, 18, 172–176.

World Health Organization. (1997). *Preventing and managing the global epidemic of obesity: Report of the World Health Organization Consultation of Obesity.* Geneva: WHO.

Yanovski, S. Z., & Yanovski, J. A. (2002). Drug therapy: Obesity. *New England Journal of Medicine*, 346(8), 591–602.

43

Diabetes Mellitus

MARGARET I. WALLHAGEN • MARTHA S. NOLTE

Diabetes mellitus is a major risk factor for numerous complications, including cardiovascular disease (American Diabetes Association [ADA], 2003; Centers for Disease Control and Prevention [CDC], 2002; Eberly et al., 2003; Grant & Davies, 2003). However, data increasingly suggest that the incidence of diabetes may be reduced and many of its risks minimized through intensive management (Gaede et al., 2003; United Kingdom Prospective Diabetes Study (UKPDS) Group, 1998; Knowler et al., 2002). In addition, our understanding of the pathophysiologic processes involved in diabetes continues to expand, allowing for the development of more refined and targeted interventions (ADA, 2003; Feldman, 2003). The purposes of this chapter are to discuss: (1) the criteria for diagnosing diabetes; (2) the pathophysiology of type 1 and type 2 diabetes as they relate to complications and therapeutic interventions; and (3) current treatment recommendations. This discussion builds on and emphasizes the importance of understanding and referring to the other topics discussed in this section of the text, i.e., coronary heart disease, hypertension, hyperlipidemia, activity and exercise, obesity, and issues related to adherence, and allows cardiovascular specialists to provide appropriate and comprehensive assessment of people with diabetes and to minimize long-term complications.

DEFINITION AND DIAGNOSIS

Diabetes mellitus describes a heterogeneous group of metabolic disorders characterized by elevated blood glucose levels; disturbances in carbohydrate, protein, and fat metabolism; and relative or absolute deficiencies in insulin secretion or action (ADA, 2003; CDC, 2002). Although two major forms or categorizations of diabetes predominate, type 1 and type 2, the fact that diabetes is a syndrome that incorporates disorders with different causes and clinical presentations is reflected in the classification system (Table 43-1). At the same time, the diagnostic criteria (Table 43-2) recommended by the American Diabetes Association (ADA, 2003) is similar across syndromes and focuses on use of the fasting plasma glucose as the most readily available and easily accomplished test. Choice of a fasting plasma glucose level of 126 mg/dL was based on the view that this is approximately equivalent to a 2-hour glucose tolerance test level of 200 mg/dL. Both findings are associated with

an increased risk of microvascular and macrovascular disease and correlate with a dramatic increase in the prevalence of retinopathy (ADA, 2003). Not everyone agrees with these criteria. Some researchers note that the use of both tests allows identification of several different groups of at-risk individuals: persons with impaired fasting glucose, persons with impaired glucose tolerance, and persons with both (DECODE Group Study, 1999; Schianca, Rossi, Sainaghi, Maduli, & Bartoli, 2003). In addition, researchers suggest that a fasting level lower than 126 may more closely approximate a 2-hour glucose tolerance test of 200 mg/dL and that focusing on the fasting glucose level will underdiagnose diabetes in older adults who frequently have isolated postchallenge hyperglycemia (Elahi et al., 2002; Gabir et al., 2000; Schianca et al., 2003; Shaw, Zimmet, McCarty, & de Courten, 2000). Of most importance, however, is acknowledgement that any increase in blood sugar is associated with negative physiologic processes.

PREVALENCE AND CONSEQUENCES OF DIABETES

Diabetes is an increasingly common problem. The age-adjusted prevalence of diabetes increased 18.4% between 1980 and 1996, and 12% between 1997 and 2000 (CDC, 2003). Approximately 17 million people in the United States are estimated to have diabetes (CDC, 2002). This includes approximately 11.1 million who have diabetes diagnosed and another 5.9 million who have diabetes that remains undiagnosed. Diabetes is more common with increasing age; approximately 20.1% of those age 65 and older in the U.S. have diabetes and account for almost 40% of the total U.S. population with diabetes (CDC, 2003). At the same time, there are growing numbers of children, especially within the African-American and Hispanic/Latino populations, with type 2 diabetes (Dean, 2001; CDC, 2002), a trend that has potentially significant implications for future health care needs.

Diabetes is a global concern (Aschner, 2002; Motala, 2002; Passa, 2002). In 2000, type 2 diabetes affected approximately 141 million adults worldwide, and this may double by 2025 (Green, Hirsch, & Pramming, 2003). The majority of all cases of diabetes (90% to 95%) are classified as type 2, which is especially prominent in African-Americans,

Table 43–1 ■ CLASSIFICATIONS FOR DIABETES MELLITUS

Classification	Description
I. Type 1	Beta cell destruction and absolute insulin deficiency
II. Type 2	A state of insulin resistance with a relative lack of insulin. The primary problem may be either insulin resistance or insufficient insulin secretion. Treatment may include the use of insulin, oral agents, and/or diet and exercise.
III. Other specific types	Includes diabetes related to specific genetic defects and secondary causes such as other endocrinopathies, drugs, or infections.
IV. Gestational (GDM)	Includes any degree of glucose intolerance that is first recognized during pregnancy.
VI. Impaired glucose tolerance (IGT) and impaired fasting glucose (IFG)	While not specifically included in the etiologic classification schema, IGT and IFG are considered a metabolic stage intermediate between normal glucose homeostasis and clinically defined diabetes. These are considered indicators of risk for future diabetes as well as cardiovascular disease.

Adapted from the American Diabetes Association, 2003.

Latinos, and Native Americans (CDC, 2002, 2003). However, the incidence of type 1 diabetes is also increasing, especially in younger children and in regions of the world where the incidence was once low (Atkinson & Eisenbarth, 2001; Gale, 2002; Passa, 2002).

Although the reasons for the increased incidence of type 1 diabetes remain unclear, the steady increase in the overall prevalence of type 2 diabetes since 1958 has been attributed to the aging of the population and a decrease in mortality rates along with an increase in the risk factors for diabetes, including obesity (Mokdad et al., 2003; Skyler & Oddo, 2002). Even over a 1-year time period, from 2000 to 2001, obesity was found to increase in the U.S. from approximately 19.1% to 20.9% (Mokdad et al., 2003).

Both type 1 and type 2 diabetes are associated with negative health outcomes. Persons with diabetes have an increased risk of death that is approximately twice that of persons without diabetes (CDC, 2002). People with type 1 diabetes have a two- to four-fold greater risk of dying in young adulthood and middle age than age-matched peers (Green, Sjolie, & Eshoj,

Table 43–2 ■ DIAGNOSTIC CRITERIA[*]

1. Diabetes: The presence of any one of the following:[†]
   a. The presence of symptoms (such as polyuria, polydipsia, polyphagia, weight loss) along with a casual (random-without regard to meals) blood glucose reading of ≥200 mg/dL (11.1 mmol/L).
   b. A fasting (≥8 hr) glucose level of ≥126 mg/dL (7.0 mmol/L)[‡]
   c. A 2-hour postchallenge plasma glucose reading of ≥200 mg/dL (11.1 mmol/L) during an oral glucose tolerance test.
2. Impaired glucose tolerance: A 2-hour plasma glucose reading of ≥140 mg/dL (7.8 mmol/L) but <200 mg/dL (11.1 mmol/L).
3. Impaired fasting glucose: A fasting plasma glucose of ≥110 mg/dL (6.1 mmol/L) but <126 mg/dL (7.0 mmol/L).

[*] Adapted from the American Diabetes Association, 2003.
[†] It is recommended that a diagnosis of diabetes be confirmed by repeat testing on a subsequent day unless there is unequivocal hyperglycemia with acute metabolic decompensation.
[‡] It is recommended that the FBS be used as the routine screening test.

1997), and people with either type 1 or type 2 diabetes are at significant risk for complications, including retinopathy, neuropathy, amputations, nephropathy, and cardiovascular disease (ADA, 2003; CDC, 2002).

Diabetes also has a significant impact on both the person with diabetes (Bradley & Speight, 2002) and the health care system. The 2002 estimate of the total costs attributed to diabetes was $132 billion (CDC, 2002). Of this amount, $92 billion were related to direct costs, which include medical care and services, and $40 billion were related to indirect costs, which include short-term and permanent disability, lost work, and premature death. Yet even with research supporting the significant impact of diabetes, data suggest that it often remains less than optimally controlled. Analysis of data from the NHANES II study found that as many as 58% of persons with type 2 diabetes had hemoglobin A1c (HbA1c) values of 7 or more and 25% had values of 9 or more (Harris, 2000).

PATHOPHYSIOLOGY OF DIABETES MELLITUS

Glucose Metabolism and Insulin Action

As a heterogeneous group of diseases, the various forms of diabetes mellitus have no single unifying cause (ADA, 2003; Matthaei, Stumvoll, Kellerer, & Haring, 2000). However, knowledge of glucose metabolism and the actions of insulin facilitates an understanding of the multiple sites where alterations may occur. Fuel homeostasis results from the coordination of complex anabolic and catabolic processes involving the interplay of numerous hormones, especially including insulin and the counter-regulatory hormones, glucagon, epinephrine, cortisol and growth hormone (Barrett, 2003; Lingappa & Farey, 2000; Nadel, 2003). These processes keep plasma glucose levels within a very narrow range while maintaining enough substrate (carbohydrate, protein, and fat) to ensure structural integrity as well as central nervous system and enzyme functioning. Insulin plays a central integrating role during the fasting and feeding states of these processes (Barrett, 2003).

Insulin is a protein hormone produced and secreted by the beta cells of the islets of Langerhans in the pancreas through a series of steps; preproinsulin is changed to proinsulin, which is then cleaved to form insulin and a C-peptide fragment. All three substances are stored in granules within the beta cells and released conjointly (Barrett, 2003). Because C-peptide is released in equal amounts with insulin and is not removed from the circulation by the liver, its measurement reflects an individual's ability to secrete insulin (Barrett, 2003).

Small amounts of basal insulin are continuously released (Heinemann, 2003), but these levels are exquisitely sensitive to changes in blood glucose levels. During a meal, increasing blood glucose levels, insulin stimulatory amino acids, and gut hormones trigger a rapid spike of insulin secretion that peaks within 45 minutes and then drifts back toward the baseline (Barrett, 2003; LeRoith, 2002). Investigators have administered nonphysiologic stimuli such as an intravenous bolus or infusion of glucose and two phases of insulin release (Gerich, 2002). A first-phase or acute-phase response causes an initial rapid increase in insulin that lasts approximately 2 to 5 minutes whereas a lower, second-phase release lasts until glucose stimulation ceases. These nonphysiologic studies have been used as a surrogate for beta-cell mass and function. A decrease in the amplitude of the first-phase insulin release correlates with the onset of glucose intolerance and chronic fasting hyperglycemia. Usually, first-phase insulin release is absent with clinically overt diabetes. Under normal conditions, such as consumption of a mixed meal, the increase in glucose is much slower and is accompanied by the presence of other nutrients and enteral hormones, in which case two distinct phases of insulin secretion are no longer distinguishable (Barrett, 2003).

A number of factors other than glucose influence insulin secretion (Barrett, 2003). For example, several amino and keto acids can stimulate insulin secretion. Glucagon stimulates insulin release whereas somatostatin, which is produced in the delta cells of the islets, inhibits insulin and glucagon. In addition, beta-adrenergic stimulation augments insulin secretion whereas alpha-adrenergic stimulation is inhibitory. These latter effects are one reason that beta-blocking agents can influence metabolic control.

Released insulin binds to its receptor on target cells throughout the body, but its actions are especially important within muscle tissue, adipose tissue, and the liver, although glucose uptake is not dependent on insulin in the latter (LeRoith, 2002; Lingappa & Farey, 2000). Binding of insulin to its receptor increases the activity of its tyrosine kinase domain, which initiates a series of phosphorylation reactions that are essential to many of insulin's various actions (Barrett, 2003; Lingappa & Farey, 2000). Insulin's actions are anabolic. It is primarily responsible for activating the transport systems and enzymes that promote the uptake, storage, and use of glucose, amino acids, and fatty acids; and for limiting hepatic glucose production by inhibiting gluconeogenesis and the breakdown of glycogen, protein, and fat.

In the fasting state, insulin levels decrease and the aforementioned processes are reversed. Glucagon, which is released from the alpha cells of the pancreas, promotes the release of glucose from the liver to maintain an adequate supply for neurologic function. Other catabolic counter-regulatory hormones that promote the breakdown of stored supplies for energy use when needed include catecholamines, cortisol, and growth hormone. Data suggest that the kidney may also be important in this homeostatic process, with renal production of glucose accounting for as much as 25% of systemic glucose production (Stumvoll, Meyer, Mitrakou, Nadkarni, & Gerich, 1997).

The various actions of insulin depend on several critical factors: the amount of glucose entering the system from the gut; the ability of the pancreas to respond to glucose stimulation and synthesize and release insulin; and the ability of the target tissues to respond to insulin. Either one or both of the latter two factors are disturbed in diabetes, and all three factors are targets for therapeutic interventions.

Type 1 Diabetes Mellitus

The most common cause of type 1 diabetes mellitus is cell-mediated autoimmune destruction of the beta cells of the pancreas (Akerblom, Vaarala, Hyoty, Ilonen, & Knip, 2002;

ADA, 2003). This may occur rapidly or slowly, but the ultimate outcome is an absolute lack of insulin, necessitating lifelong replacement therapy. The underlying cause of the autoimmune response appears to involve an interplay of a genetic predisposition interacting with environmental factors that promote an immune response. Viral or dietary antigens have been proposed as triggers in susceptible individuals (Akerblom et al., 2002; Laron, 2002). Identifying a specific factor is difficult because the genetic markers and predisposing genes may differ between populations (Akerblom et al., 2002). In addition, although type 1 diabetes most commonly presents during childhood or adolescence, it can occur at any age, and late-onset type 1 diabetes may be more common than previously appreciated (ADA, 1998).

Type 2 Diabetes Mellitus

Type 2 diabetes encompasses conditions characterized by varying degrees of insulin resistance, beta-cell failure, and increased hepatic glucose release (ADA, 2003). Its occurrence requires a genetic susceptibility interacting with environmental factors (LeRoith, 2002). The pathogenesis of all of the various defects found in type 2 diabetes are still not fully understood, and because of the varying causes, one explanation for these defects is unlikely. However, the overt presentation of the disease is usually preceded by a long period of impaired glucose tolerance, a condition associated with increased risk for macrovascular and possibly microvascular complications. Patients often already have long-term complications at the time of diagnosis.

Insulin resistance is a state of decreased responsiveness to the effects of insulin, resulting in a plasma glucose level that is higher than would be expected for a given level of plasma insulin (Evans & Krantz, 2001; Matthaei et al., 2000). The cause of insulin resistance remains unresolved, although many mechanisms are being explored. The response to insulin appears to be especially defective in skeletal muscle and the liver (Matthaei et al., 2000). As noted previously, when insulin binds to its receptor it initiates a series of phosphorylation reactions that are essential to its action. Thus, insulin resistance could be related to alterations in signal transmission or alterations in the intracellular processes involved in initiating a response. Ectopic myocyte lipid deposition also has been proposed as a mechanism of insulin resistance in individuals with diabetes and their nondiabetic but resistant relatives (McGarry, 2002). In addition, a number of genes are being explored as potentially involved in the process (Matthaei et al., 2000). However, attempting to isolate any given cause is complicated by the multiple factors that can influence one or more of the steps noted previously.

Obesity (especially visceral), inactivity, hyperglycemia, hyperinsulinemia, and aging each are associated with altered cellular responsivity and insulin resistance (Chang & Halter, 2003; Goldstein, 2002; LeRoith, 2002). These are risk factors for diabetes as well as factors that influence its management. Thus, on-going tissue exposure to elevated levels of glucose may cause damage to beta cells as well as decrease tissue responsiveness to insulin's actions (Matthaei et al., 2000; Robertson, Harmon, Tran, Tanaka, & Takahashi, 2003), making the achievement of glucose control difficult. In addition, loss of insulin's inhibitory effect on lipolysis and fatty acid oxidation results in elevated levels of free fatty acid, which contribute to tissue insulin resistance, stimulate hepatic gluconeogenesis (increased precursor products), and further diminish beta-cell function (Matthaei et al., 2000). Visceral adiposity may be especially problematic because these adipocytes appear to undergo more lipolysis than those found in subcutaneous tissue (Bloomgarden, 2002).

Another factor that influences the onset of type 2 diabetes is the insulin resistance/metabolic syndrome (Liese, Mayer-Davis, & Haffner, 1998). This condition describes the concurrence of a number of physiologic abnormalities, including hypertension; hyperinsulinemia; a dyslipidemia characterized by elevated triglycerides, decreased high-density lipoproteins, and increased small, dense, low-density lipoprotein (LDL) particles; obesity; and macrovascular disease. Most of these risk factors, including some of the age-related alterations in carbohydrate metabolism, are modifiable through lifestyle interventions such as diet and exercise (Meneilly & Tessier, 2001; Reaven, 2003).

In addition to an altered response to insulin, persons with type 2 diabetes also show altered beta-cell function (LeRoith, 2002). This is supported by the fact that many persons who have insulin resistance do not have progression to overt diabetes. Thus, those who do are unable to increase their insulin secretion enough to compensate (Chang & Halter, 2003; LeRoith, 2002). Under test conditions, data suggest that one of the earliest findings in persons with type 2 diabetes is loss of the first or acute phase of insulin release during an intravenous glucose tolerance test (Matthaei et al., 2000), although not everyone agrees with this finding (Gerich, 2002). However, once started, data suggest that diabetes is a progressive process that leads to worsening glucose homeostasis over time and that requires increasing levels of intervention (UKPDS Group, 1998).

COMPLICATIONS OF DIABETES MELLITUS

The complications of diabetes can be classified as acute or chronic. Acute complications include episodes of hypoglycemia in patients treated with glucose-lowering medications, diabetic ketoacidosis (DKA), and hyperosmolar hyperglycemic nonketotic syndrome (HHNS). Chronic complications are categorized as microvascular or macrovascular. Although chronic complications are the main focus of this chapter, a few points are important in relation to acute events.

Acute Complications

Acute complications are the result of acute changes in glucose levels, are often life threatening, and require immediate intervention. Symptoms of hypoglycemia, generally defined as a blood sugar of less than 50 to 60 mg/dL, occur when insufficient glucose is available for cerebral functioning. This is usually the result of excess insulin (either from injection or from oral hypoglycemic stimulation), decreased or delayed carbohydrate intake, or increased utilization, as through exercise. However, loss of the normal adaptive counter-regulatory hormonal response is also a key factor (Cryer, 2002). As glucose decreases,

persons with long-standing type 1 diabetes are unable to respond with an appropriate increase in glucagon at the same time that their epinephrine response may be attenuated. Although this loss of adaptive capacity is most common in persons with type 1 diabetes, it also occurs in persons with long-standing type 2 (Cryer, 2002). Hypoglycemia is a major limiting factor in the management of diabetes, especially type 1. Because the incidence of hypoglycemia is increased in those undergoing intensive control, it influences the decision-making process regarding diabetes management (ADA, 2003).

Both DKA and HHNS are the result of insufficient insulin and represent the extreme of the diabetic state. DKA is more common in type 1 diabetes, whereas HHNS is most common in older people with type 2 diabetes, although either can occur at any age (MacIssac, Lee, McNeil, Tsalamandris, & Jerums, 2002). Cerebral edema secondary to DKA is a leading cause of death in children with type 1 diabetes (Edge, 2000) whereas the mortality from HHNS is especially high among the elderly (MacIssac et al., 2002). DKA and HHNS are life threatening and can be precipitated by multiple factors, including acute infections (pneumonia, influenza, urinary tract), therapeutic procedures (surgery), alcohol abuse, or acute events (myocardial infarction, trauma). It is therefore always important to look for an underlying co-morbidity.

Microvascular Complications

Classic microvascular complications are retinopathy, neuropathy, and nephropathy. *Retinopathy* is responsible for most new cases of blindness in persons aged 20 to 70, is directly related to the duration of diabetes and blood glucose levels, and can often be prevented by early and intensive management of both glucose levels and blood pressure (ADA, 2003; Knott & Forrester, 2003). The retina has a high metabolic rate and is thus susceptible to damage secondary to changes in the retinal blood supply. Once the process is initiated, retinopathy tends to progress through stages from a mild non-proliferative form to increasingly more severe stages and finally to a proliferative form that is characterized by the growth of new vessels on both the retina and the posterior surface of the vitreous (ADA, 2003; Knott & Forrester, 2003). Unfortunately, progression of later stages in the process is less affected by tight glucose control, emphasizing the importance of early diagnosis and treatment. Macular edema is also associated with duration of diabetes, and cataracts appear earlier and progress more rapidly in people with diabetes than in the general population. Ongoing ophthalmologic evaluations are essential. In general, it is currently recommended that persons with type 1 diabetes have an initial dilated can comprehensive examination by an ophthalmologist or optometrist within 3 to 5 years after onset of the condition and that persons with type 2 diabetes should be evaluated shortly after diagnosis, because they frequently have had the condition for some time (ADA, 2003). Yearly dilated examinations are recommended after this initial evaluation, but more frequent examinations may be necessary if retinopathy is detected and is progressing.

Diabetic *nephropathy* is currently the preeminent cause of end-stage renal disease in the United States and Europe, and treatment of end-stage renal disease cost more than $15.6 billion in the U.S. in 1997 (ADA, 2003; Deferrari, Ravera, &

Berruti, 2003). Although the prevalence of end-stage renal disease is greater in type 1 diabetes, reaching approximately 40%, the numbers of persons with type 2 on dialysis are greater because of their overall numbers. Multiple factors influence the onset and progression of nephropathy, including glucose and blood pressure control, but there also appears to be a genetic susceptibility component that is implicated in the vulnerability of some populations (Gnudi, Gruden, & Viberti, 2003). It is also increasingly recognized that persons with diabetes and any evidence of nephropathy are at significant risk for premature death from cardiovascular disease (Marshall, 2003).

Overt nephropathy is preceded by a phase in which most laboratory values are normal but the excretion of albumin is increased to approximately 30 to 299 mg/24 hours (or 20 to 199 µg/min) (ADA, 2003; Deferrari et al., 2003). This microalbuminuria is not detected on routine dipstick until it reaches approximately 150 mg/L, so more refined tests are needed. These include 24-hour urine collections, which also allow for quantification of glomerular filtration rate; the assessment of urinary albumin-to-creatinine ratio in a random spot collection (although a first-voided morning specimen is recommended); or a timed urinary sample (ADA, 2003). However, because there are day-to-day variations in albumin secretion, two to three separate tests across several months should be performed to confirm a positive finding.

Tight glycemic and blood pressure control minimize the onset of nephropathy. In later stages of the condition when overt proteinuria is present, the impact of glycemic control on further progression is less substantiated (Deferrari et al., 2003). Further, antihypertensives appear to have a differential effect at different times in the course of the progression of nephropathy, and between type 1 and type 2 diabetes; however, angiotensin inhibitors (ACE-I) and angiotensin-receptor blockers (ARB) are currently the most widely supported agents for type 1 and type 2 diabetes, respectively (ADA, 2003; Deferrari et al., 2003).

Neuropathy is another common problem experienced by persons with type 1 and type 2 diabetes and results in significant morbidity and mortality. The major factors involved in the development of neuropathy appear to be the duration of the disease, the age of the patient, and metabolic control. Recent estimates suggest that the annual medical costs of diabetes-related peripheral neuropathy and its complications in the U.S. range between $4.6 to $13.7 billion and account for approximately 27% of the direct medical costs of diabetes (Gordois, Scuffham, Shearer, Oglesby, & Tobian, 2003). However, this does not take into account the personal cost of this condition, because it is often associated with significant and distressing pain (Quattrini & Tesfaye, 2003). Painful sensory neuropathy may even occur in persons with impaired glucose tolerance, before the occurrence of diagnosed diabetes (Singleton & Smith, 2003), emphasizing the role of hyperglycemia in the pathophysiology of the condition.

Diabetic neuropathy encompasses a wide range of clinical patterns and can be either acute and self-limiting or chronic (Quattrini & Tesfaye, 2003; Young, 2003). Hyperglycemia and rapid changes in blood sugar and focal lesions such as carpal tunnel syndrome can cause significant, although generally reversible, pain syndromes. However, the most common chronic problem is distal symmetrical neuropathy, which includes sensory-motor neuropathies and autonomic neuropa-

thy (Quattrini & Tesfaye, 2003; Tomlinson, 2003). The nerve injury that occurs as a result of the underlying pathophysiology can alter the processing of sensory input to the nervous system and lead to ongoing neuropathic pain (Kapur, 2003). Autonomic neuropathies can cause altered sweating patterns, postural hypotension, neuropathic bladders, altered sexual function, and diabetic gastroparesis (Young, R. J., 2003). Altered sweating patterns can increase the risk for decreased thermoregulatory capacity, whereas diabetic gastroparesis can influence metabolic control and cause inconsistencies in the results on various assessments. Gastroparesis may also go unnoticed. Enck and Frieling (1997) note that silent gastroparesis, the occurrence of altered gastrointestinal function without symptoms, may result in the inappropriate assumption that patients are not following their treatment regimen. To detect diabetic autonomic neuropathy, heart rate variability in response to provocative stimuli is noted to be the most sensitive, repeatable, and practical measure (Prendergast, 2001).

Foot complications are strongly associated with diabetic neuropathy; approximately 33% of persons with diabetes are at risk for foot ulcerations secondary to peripheral neuropathy (Young, M. J., 2003), and these ulcerations often lead to future amputations. Neuroarthropathy, or Charcot's joint, is also thought to be related to recurrent trauma to the joints, and surrounding bony structures of the feet that go unnoticed by the person. The resulting deformity contributes to significant morbidity and immobility. Making recognition of the underlying vulnerability more difficult is the fact that the neuropathic foot is often warm, and pulses are often palpable because sympathetic denervation can lead to arteriovenous shunts opening up in the vascular bed (Young, M. J., 2003).

Macrovascular Complications

Steinberg (1997) observed that people with diabetes frequently have microvascular disease but die more commonly from macrovascular (cardiovascular and cerebrovascular) diseases. He also noted that even those with well-controlled diabetes and those who do not have significant lipid abnormalities experience higher risk for premature coronary heart disease, for reasons that are not totally clear. Although macrovascular disease does not correlate strongly with the duration and severity of disease, persons with either type 1 or type 2 diabetes have a two- to four-fold greater cardiovascular risk than those without diabetes (ADA, 2003; Grant & Davies, 2003). The risk for cardiovascular disease in women with type 2 diabetes is three- to four-times greater than in women without the condition; diabetes effectively eliminates the protection afforded to premenopausal women.

PATHOPHYSIOLOGY OF COMPLICATIONS

Hypoglycemic Unawareness

Repeated episodes of hypoglycemia, although not the only cause, are related to hypoglycemic unawareness, a situation in which the normal warning signs of hypoglycemia (neuroglycopenic and neurogenic) do not occur until the blood sugar is so low that the person faints or has a seizure. This may occur because of impaired counter-regulatory neurohormone response or brain adaptation through facilitated uptake at below-normal blood glucose levels. The normal glucagon secretory response to hypoglycemia is lost in people with type 1 diabetes within a few years of disease onset, and the threshold for epinephrine secretion may be altered under conditions of repetitive hypoglycemia, so that lower levels of glucose have to occur for its release (Cryer, 2002). People with hypoglycemic unawareness need to monitor blood sugar levels carefully. Preventing chronic hypoglycemia can often improve awareness of hypoglycemic events.

Chronic Complications

Chronic macrovascular or microvascular complications are the result of long-standing metabolic disturbances created by the underlying pathophysiologic processes that precede and result in increased hyperglycemia as well as the hyperglycemia itself. Microvascular complications appear to be especially related to chronic hyperglycemia. Four major mechanisms are thought to underlie the damage caused by chronic hyperglycemia: increased glucose stimulation of the polyol pathway; increased formation of advanced glycation end products (AGE), activation of protein kinase C; and increased flux through the hexosamine pathway (Brownlee, 2001; Taguchi & Brownlee, 2003; Vlassara & Palace, 2002). It is hypothesized that these pathways may have a common mechanism of action, which is excessive free radical formation. The mitochondrial electron-transport chain is thought to overproduce superoxide, a free radical or reactive oxygen species. A free radical is an atom or molecule that has an unpaired or free electron in an outer orbit, a state that renders it highly reactive and predisposed to interact with almost any biologic substrate. Formed normally during oxidative metabolism and used in many physiological processes (Dröge, 2002), free radicals are counteracted by a complex intrinsic antioxidant defense system. When excessive amounts of free radicals are formed, the biologic antioxidant supply can become depleted and tissue damage can occur. Data suggest that free radicals increase the formation of glycated proteins and contribute to microvascular and macrovascular abnormalities (Feldman, 2003; Ying, 1997).

The cause of the macrovascular complications is multifactorial. There appears to be no qualitative difference in the atheromatous lesions in people with diabetes compared with those without, although they may be more extensive, diffuse, and localized in the distal vessels of the peripheral and coronary circulation (Grant & Davies, 2003). People with type 1 diabetes who are not obese and have good glycemic control also are noted to have near-normal lipid levels (Poirier & Despres, 2003) but have evidence of an accelerated atheromatous process (Nathan et al., 2003). Although the level of glycemia, at least in patients with type 2 diabetes, is less clearly related to macrovascular than to microvascular complications, this may be a consequence of the early occurrence of macrovascular damage with even mild blood glucose elevations (ADA, 2003). There is increasing evidence that glucose intolerance is associated with a significant increase in cardiovascular morbidity and mortality. Increased insulin concentrations, insulin resistance, AGE formation, and defective blood coagulation also are suggested as potential causative factors (Grant & Davies, 2003). There may be interrelationships between the underlying causes of macrovascular and microvascular problems; for example, increased AGE formation has been noted to cause thickening and leakage of the vasculature and decrease vessel elasticity (Brownlee, 2001; Grant & Davies, 2003; Vlassara & Palace, 2002). Interventions aimed at each of these various mechanisms are being explored.

NURSING MANAGEMENT OF DIABETES

Management of diabetes involves a comprehensive multidisciplinary effort that is highly dependent on assisting individuals with diabetes and their families to establish a regimen that will fit their life situations. Types of diabetes differ, occur at different points in the life span, and are associated with varying risk factors. Thus, although the ADA publishes an update of its clinical practice recommendations each year (ADA, 2003), all regimens must be tailored to the individual patient's desires, goals, and concurrent physiologic status. Because type 2 diabetes is especially common in older people, alterations that occur with age are important to consider in discussing treatment options and monitoring response to therapies (Table 43-3).

Because the management of diabetes often involves many lifestyle changes, patients with diabetes not only need to understand their condition and be prepared to make often complex decisions about their care but also need to develop strategies that facilitate self-care (Glasgow & Eakin, 1996). This places the individual in the center of disease management. The role of the health care provider is to facilitate an individual's ability to blend self-management into his or her own life in the best way possible (Anerson & Funnell, 2000). This emphasizes the importance of avoiding blame when clients are unable to attain specific goals and focuses on developing a problem-solving approach to issues that arise.

In general, management of diabetes involves controlling blood sugar, minimizing risk factors, and preventing or treating complications. This includes appropriate screening, monitoring, and intervention. Of major importance is a complete assessment of each person (Table 43-4), with an emphasis on the identification of complications, concurrent physiologic states that alter glucose control, risk factors, and level of knowledge. Data from the other chapters in this section discuss approaches to facilitate behavior change and risk factor reduction. Thus, as much as possible, only aspects of care specific to people with diabetes are included here.

General Goals and Recommendations

Glycemic Control

Maintaining an average hemoglobin A_{1c} of 7.2% was shown to reduce the development of microvascular complications by 50% to 75% in patients with type 1 diabetes (Diabetes Control

Table 43–3 ■ AGE-RELATED FACTORS INFLUENCING CARE OF OLDER ADULTS WITH DIABETES

Change with Age	Implications
Altered renal function:	
Decreased GFR	Decreased renal excretion of many drugs
Decreased capacity to concentrate/dilute urine	Assess renal function, especially before use of Metformin
Altered body composition:	
Decreased LBM	Increased concentration of water soluble drugs
Increased proportion of adipose tissue	Serum creatinine unreliable as measure of renal function; use CrCl
Decreased liver size and blood flow and alerations in phase I metabolism	Deposition and storage of lipid soluble drugs and long T1/2
	Decreased hepatic metabolism and first pass metabolism
Decreased total body fluids	Greater concentration of drug for given dose. Assess/monitor drug response and side effects. Start dose low, go slow with titration.
Altered sensory perception	Altered ability to recognize color, hear instructions (especially high frequencies)
Vision	Use vision and hearing aids; assess perception and need for special aids
Hearing	
Increased prevalence of co-morbidities	Increased potential for drug interactions and use of drugs that alter diabetes control (anti-HTN, anti-lipemics, NSAIDs)
	Consider concurrent CV disease in prescribing exercise
Altered neuromuscular functioning	Possible need for repetition of materials and longer periods of reinforcement; possible need for family member assistance
Slower CNS processing	
Decreased delayed recall	
Possible altered number/sensitivity of receptors	Increased sensitivity to side effects of drugs
Decreased fine motor coordination	Difficulty manipulating syringes, meters
Altered mobility	Decreased ease of access to health care
	Dependence on family/friends for transportation
	Assess social support, community support, safety of setting for exercise
Long-established lifestyle patterns; often highly motivated r/t health	Assess goals, life patterns; assist with strategies to incorporate behavior change

Table 43–4 ■ NURSING ASSESSMENT

Assessment	Comment
History	
Knowledge level and previous education	Many older adults are diagnosed after being admitted for an acute event or HHNS
	Persons with diabetes may need review and updates of new data but also come with extensive personal knowledge of how they respond to treatment
Concurrent chronic conditions	
Recent stressful life events	Stress increases blood sugar
Medications; prescribed/OTC	Many medications influence blood glucose
Physical	
Cardiovascular/peripheral vascular status	CV events such as MI can precipitate DKA or HHNS
Neurological	Autonomic neuropathy can impair the response to hypoxia (Ouellette, 1998)
Signs of infection	High blood glucose levels can impair immune response and wound healing
Skin (cellulitis), feet, oral, urinary tract	Infections can precipitate DKA or HHNS
	Confusion/altered mental status can be the presenting sign of infection in older adults
Renal status	Influences drug dosing, use of Metformin
Laboratory Evaluation	
Blood glucose; lipids; HbA1c	Plasma glucose values are 10%–15% higher than whole blood glucose values
	Some meters still measure whole blood glucose
	Glycosylated hemoglobin assay methods vary; it is important to know laboratory norms and factors that interfere with accurate results

and Complications Trial Research Group, 1993). Subsequently, data from the United Kingdom Prospective Diabetes Study (UKPDS) showed that maintaining a median HbA1c of 7 as compared to 7.9 reduced overall microvascular complications in persons with type 2 diabetes by 25% (ADA, 2003; UKPDS Group, 1998). Given these findings, the goal is to maintain as near euglycemic levels as possible. Current recommendations for blood glucose control in adults are: (1) 90 to 130 mg/dL (5.0–7.2mmol/L) before meals; (2) less than 180 mg/dL (10mmol/L) after meals; and (3) a hemoglobin A_{1c} of less than 7% (ADA, 2003). Treatment modification is considered when these ranges are not established or maintained. However, there are currently no clinical trail data available on how strict glycemic control influences outcomes in persons aged 65 years or older, in children younger than 13, and in those with advanced complications (ADA, 2003). In addition, intensive therapy is associated with higher rates of hypoglycemic events. Thus, certain individuals may not be candidates for strict control; such factors as co-morbid disease, age (very young or very old), and other life circumstances must be considered. For example, older adults with severe cardiovascular or cerebrovascular disease who are at risk for a stroke or myocardial infarction may need different glycemic goals because hypoglycemia can be especially problematic.

To evaluate the effectiveness of an ongoing treatment plan, assessment of glycosylated hemoglobin at 3- to 6-month intervals is recommended to provide data on metabolic control over the past 2 to 3 months. Self-monitoring of glucose is also recommended as an important strategy to facilitate achievement and maintenance of glycemic control because it allows individuals to assess the impact of various foods and life events. After

July, 1998, Medicare started covering the cost of a glucose meter and limited numbers of strips and lancets regardless of whether insulin is being used (Carter, 1998).

Cardiovascular Risk and Lipid Control

Because macrovascular complications are common and significant in type 1 and type 2 diabetes, annual screening and aggressive lipid management is recommended. In persons with type 2 diabetes, elevated triglycerides along with decreased levels of HDL are common (Poirier & Despres, 2003). In addition, although LDL levels are often not very different from those without diabetes, the LDL particles tend to be smaller and denser, characteristics that are associated with increased atherogenicity. HDL, followed by triglyceride levels and total cholesterol, may be most predictive of coronary heart disease in persons with type 2 diabetes, but there are few prospective studies focusing on this issue (ADA, 2003).

In general, goals for the treatment of dyslipidemia, specifically related to LDL, are similar to those established by the National Cholesterol Education Program. Focus is on achieving LDL levels of 100 mg/dL or less, HDL levels of more than 40mg/dL (>50 mg/dL in women), and triglycerides of less than 150mg/dL (ADA, 2003). In those with coronary heart disease, peripheral vascular disease, and cardiovascular disease, drug therapy is initiated if, after diet and blood glucose-lowering interventions, LDL remains more than 100 mg/dL. In those without these concurrent problems, drug therapy is initiated if the LDL level remains more than 130 mg/dL, with a goal of less than 100 mg/dL. When patients have clinical coronary vascular disease or very high LDL levels (≥200 mg/dL), drug therapy may be started concurrent to nutrition and exercise interventions (ADA, 2003).

Blood Pressure Control

Hypertension is discussed in Chapter 39. In diabetes, aggressive treatment of blood pressure is considered of utmost importance to minimize cardiovascular and renal impairment (Onuigbo & Weir, 2003). The goal for blood pressure control in adults with diabetes is less than 130/80 mm Hg, although it is recognized that it is frequently necessary to use three or more drugs to achieve this goal (ADA, 2003). If the blood pressure is 140 or more systolic, or 90 or more diastolic, starting with behavioral and pharmacologic approaches concurrently is recommended. Although data suggest that a number of different agents may successfully reduce blood pressure and have a positive effect on outcomes, ACEI and ARB have been shown to be especially beneficial in reducing cardiovascular events and offering renal protection (ADA, 2003; Onuigbo & Weir, 2003).

Beta-adrenergic blocking agents may mask the symptoms of hypoglycemia, impair insulin release, and have a negative affect on blood lipids (Kaplan, 1997). However, data suggest that they also are shown to reduce the incidence of cardiovascular events after myocardial infarction and are underused in older persons with diabetes (Arnow & Ahn, 2001; Chen, Marciniak, Radford, Wang, & Krumholz, 1999; Di Bari, Marchionni, & Pahor, 2003; Younis, Burnham, Patwala, Weston, & Vora, 2001). Thiazide diuretics are also known to adversely affect blood glucose and lipid levels, but usually at doses higher than 25 mg. If calcium-channel blockers are used, then non-dihydropyridine agents appear to be associated with better outcomes than dihydropyridine agents (Onuigbo & Weir, 2003). However, it is most important to achieve a lower blood pressure, and an individualized approach that takes into account other factors that influence drug choice is still recommended. The importance of lifestyle changes that influence blood pressure should not be overlooked and can be facilitated by input from a health care provider (Egede, 2003).

Foot Care/Neurologic Assessment

Foot ulcers, foot problems, and neurologic dysfunction are major causes of morbidity, mortality, and disability. Minor foot trauma in an insensate foot can initiate a process that ultimately leads to amputation. Performing a foot screen at least annually that includes a vascular, neurologic, musculoskeletal, skin, and soft tissue assessment is essential (ADA, 2003). The neurologic examination should include an assessment of sensation; this can be performed using a 10-g (5.07) Semmes-Weinstein monofilament. Loss of the ability to consistently feel the touch of this monofilament is equated with loss of protective sensation, places the person at risk, and evidences the need for a comprehensive program to prevent foot trauma.

As noted previously, several other neurologic abnormalities can influence the well being of people with diabetes, including orthostatic hypotension, sexual dysfunction, and gastroparesis. Each of these needs careful assessment at ongoing intervals and usually requires a multidisciplinary approach to treatment. Orthostatic hypotension places the person at risk for falls and thus requires assessment of environmental safety features. This symptom is often difficult to manage. Sexual dysfunction may not be openly discussed by many patients but needs to be addressed because there are a number of treatment options. Gastroparesis may need to be considered in those people who have difficulty controlling their blood sugars even when following an active treatment program.

Interventions to Achieve Metabolic Control

Diet and Exercise

Diet and exercise remain the cornerstones of treatment for diabetes. Obesity is discussed in Chapter 35, and exercise and diet for hyperlipidemia are discussed in Chapter 33. In diabetes, approaches to nutritional management have evolved, with increased emphasis on individualizing each regimen and incorporating the expertise of a registered dietitian who is knowledgeable about medical nutrition therapy into any diabetes care team (ADA, 2003). Overall recommendations related to carbohydrates have been liberalized so that simple sugars are no longer proscribed and total grams of carbohydrates consumed are emphasized. Thus, actual amounts of specific foods depend on an assessment of each person's food habits, weight, lipid levels, and management regimen (insulin, oral hypoglycemic, diet). There is debate, however, regarding the most appropriate distribution of carbohydrate versus fat for people with increased levels of triglycerides and very-low-density lipoprotein, especially in those who are obese. Replacing carbohydrates with monounsaturated fats may reduce postprandial blood glucose levels and triglyceridemia but may also promote weight gain (ADA, 2003). Thus an individualized approach is needed and more data are needed on dietary options. Use of a registered dietitian with expertise in diabetes is recommended, and attendance at classes is covered by Medicare.

Exercise remains a key aspect of therapy and can improve glycemic control, decrease cardiovascular risk factors, help with weight maintenance or weight loss, and improve an individual's general sense of well-being (ADA, 2003). Exercise may even prevent the onset of type 2 diabetes. Encouraging activity and exercise is thus a central component of any treatment regimen. At the same time, exercise needs to be adapted to individual condition and lifestyle. In people with type 1 diabetes and in people with type 2 diabetes who are being treated with insulin or glucose-lowering agents, exercise acutely can be associated with either hyperglycemia or hypoglycemia. Hyperglycemia may occur when insulin levels are inadequate because counter-regulatory hormones are produced, elevating glucose and ketone levels–this is generally the case when strenuous exercise is performed when the blood glucose is 250 mg/dL or more. However, if excess insulin is present, it may attenuate counter-regulatory forces and hypoglycemia may occur. Exercise must be adapted to the dietary and medication regimen. In type 2 diabetes, exercise can improve insulin sensitivity and lower the need for medication. Precautions must be taken in people who have been sedentary for many years or who have insensate feet, peripheral vascular insufficiency, proliferative retinopathy, or hypertension (ADA, 2003). People with insensate feet need special shoes and should avoid high-impact sports.

Medications

Therapeutic options for patients with diabetes have expanded dramatically in the 1990s. The newer agents are designed to provide a more physiologic pattern of insulin replacement and restoration of normal or nearly normal glucose levels. Combination oral agent therapy has allowed many individuals with type 2 diabetes to maintain target blood glucose levels and defers the need to initiate insulin therapy.

Insulin. Insulin replacement therapy is necessary for individuals with type 1 diabetes and for 30% to 40% of individuals with type 2 diabetes. Insulin is self-administered as a subcutaneous injection up to multiple times per day or by a continuous subcutaneous infusion (CSII) device (Rassam, Zeise, Burge, & Schade, 1999; Renner et al., 1999).

Insulin formulations can be divided into rapid and short-acting insulins, which are suitable for meal, snack, and high blood glucose correction coverage, and intermediate and long-acting insulins, which are useful for background, between meal, or overnight insulin replacements. Historically, commercially available insulin has been native human insulin produced through recombinant DNA technology, but limitations in the absorption characteristics of the human insulin molecule have resulted in the development of insulin analogs. As of 2003 there are two rapid-acting insulin analogs, insulin lispro

(Humalog®) and insulin aspart (Novolog®), and one very-long-acting insulin analog, insulin glargine (Lantus®). The rapid-acting monomeric insulins, Novolog® and Humalog®, are quickly absorbed with an onset of action in 10 to 15 minutes and time to peak action of approximately 1 hour (Bolli, Di Marchi, Park, Pramming, & Koivisto, 1999; Brange, 1997). Increasing the dose only minimally extends the duration of action. These analogs are preferred for CSII use and for food and glucose correction coverage. In contrast to regular insulin formulations, these analogs may be taken at the time of the meal (rather than 30 minutes before), provide a more physiologic insulin profile, and minimize the risk of late postmeal hypoglycemia.

The long-acting analog Lantus® was developed to provide 24-hour coverage with a minimal peak effect. This is achieved by altering the insulin molecule so that it is soluble under vitalized, acidic conditions but rapidly forms microcrystals after injection into body tissues where the pH is neutral. Insulin begins to appear in the circulation approximately 1.5 to 2 hours after injection, and maximum levels are achieved in approximately 5 to 6 hours. The insulin availability then plateaus over the next 24 hours. In contrast to the traditional intermediate (NPH, Lente) and long-acting (Ultralente) insulin suspensions, the solubility of bottled Lantus® allows more accurate dosing, and the low, steady insulin absorption from the subcutaneous depot minimizes the risk of hypoglycemia (Heinemann et al., 2000; Lepore et al., 2000). Patient quality of life is improved by the convenience of once per day dosing of the background or basal insulin. The different insulin formulations are used alone or in combination, depending on the individual's diurnal insulin sensitivity and overall need for insulin replacement.

Oral Hypoglycemic and Euglycemic Drugs

Insulin Secretagogues

Sulfonylureas. Sulfonylureas are the oldest class of insulin secretagogues and continue to play an important role in the treatment of type 2 diabetes (Buse, 1999; DeFronzo, 1999). They exert their effect by closing adenosine triphosphate (ATP)-sensitive potassium channels in the beta-cell membrane; the resulting depolarization and influx of calcium triggers the release of insulin. Sulfonylureas may bind with potassium channel receptors in extrapancreatic tissues, but the clinical significance of this interaction is uncertain (Gribble, Tucker, Seino, & Ashcroft, 1998). Both first-generation (chlorpropamide, tolazamide, and tolbutamide) and second-generation (glyburide, glipizide, glimepiride) agents have a similar mechanism of action but differ in their pharmacokinetics, pharmacodynamics, metabolism, drug interactions, and side effects. Selection of an agent should be based on its individual profile and the needs of a given patient. Generally, the first-generation agents have limited availability and untoward side effects and drug interactions. Other than tolbutamide, which is a relatively short-acting agent that can be used in older individuals or in mild renal insufficiency, the use of first-generation sulfonylureas is not encouraged. Generic forms of the second-generation agents are becoming available and should become more affordable. Major side effects of sulfonylureas are hypoglycemia and weight gain; the latter may result from retention and subsequent storage of excess calories as the glucose levels come under better control with the medication.

Meglitinides. Repaglinide (Prandin®) is the founding member of a new class of oral insulin secretagogues, the meglitinides (Owens, 1999). Considered a non-sulfonylurea hypoglycemic, repaglinide also stimulates insulin release by attaching to binding sites in the ATP-sensitive potassium channel. It is rapidly absorbed and metabolized, with a peak effect within 1 hour after ingestion but somewhat prolonged duration of action of up to 5 to 8 hours. It is customarily taken before meals in doses of 0.5 to 4 mg. Because it is newly available, there are few data on its long-term effects, although data reported from clinical trials suggest that the adverse events are comparable with those associated with sulfonylureas.

D-Phenylalanine Derivatives. Nateglinide (Starlix®) is the latest insulin secretagogue to be marketed. It also works through closure of the beta-cell membrane ATP-sensitive potassium channels but is distinctive in its rapid onset (approximately 20 minutes), time to peak (approximately 1 hour) action, and limited duration of action (< 4 hr). Nateglinide's hypoglycemic effect is especially blunted during euglycemic and hypoglycemic conditions. Accordingly, nateglinide has a low risk of hypoglycemia and may be especially useful in individuals with milder degrees of glucose intolerance and renal impairment (Dunn & Faulds, 2000; Levien, Baker, Campbell, & White, 2001).

Euglycemics

Biguanides. The only biguanides available for use, metformin (Glucophage®), lowers glucose mainly through its suppression of hepatic and, to a lesser degree, renal glucose production; it is not effective in the absence of insulin (Aviles-Santa, Sinding, & Raskin, 1999; Bailey, 1999; Cusi & De Fronzo, 1998). It also may directly influence gut absorption and metabolism of glucose and secondarily diminish peripheral resistance, but these actions do not appear to be its main benefit. Metformin usually curbs weight gain and promotes a more normal lipid profile; it has become the drug of choice in obese patients. It controls and achieves glycemic control with less hyperinsulinemia than the secretagogues, which is speculated to be a possible cardiovascular benefit. As monotherapy, metformin does not caus hypoglycemia, but this may occur when it is used with other glucose-lowering drugs such as secretagogues or insulin. Side effects of metformin are mainly gastrointestinal.

Of greatest concern is the rare occurrence of lactic acidosis (Chan, Brain, & Feher, 1999; Howlett & Bailey, 1999). This, although infrequent, can be fatal. It usually occurs in people who have contraindications to metformin's use, such as diminished renal or hepatic function, respiratory or cardiac failure, and alcohol abuse. Metformin should not be used in people with serum creatine levels of 1.3 mg/dL in women or 1.5 mg/dL in men or when the glomerular filtration rate is less than 60 mL/min. Metformin should be withheld during most hospitalizations and before any surgery or studies involving the use of iodinated contrast materials. Renal function should be reassessed before metformin is resumed.

Metformin is available in 500- to 850-mg tablets and is usually taken two to four times per day, before meals, and, in some instances, before bedtime. Metformin may have a role in the prevention of diabetes in obese, middle-aged individuals with pre-diabetes (Diabetes Prevention Program Research Group, 2002).

Alpha-Glucosidase Inhibitors. Acarbose (Precose®) and the recently released Miglitol (Glyset®) are alpha-glucosidase inhibitors that delay the digestion and absorption of carbohydrates in the gut by inhibiting enzymes that lead to their breakdown into monosaccharides (Lebovitz 1998). This effectively decreases the postprandial increase in blood sugar levels. Like metformin, these agents would not cause hypoglycemia when used as monotherapy but have less of a glucose-lowering effect by themselves than other agents.

Precose is formulated as 50- and 100-mg and Glyset as 25-, 50-, and 100-mg tablets. The pills need to be taken before each meal and consistent carbohydrate consumption is recommended for the best effect. The major side effects of alpha-glucosidase inhibitors are gastrointestinal and include flatulence and diarrhea. They have limited acceptance in the United States, although they are more popular overseas in regions where there is a relatively high-starch dietary intake. These agents are usually contraindicated in people with inflammatory bowel disease, colonic ulceration, or partial intestinal obstruction. The use of Acarbose by individuals with glucose intolerance has had a modest effect in reducing the progression to overt diabetes and restoring a more normal glucose tolerance (STOP NIDDM trial) (Chiasson et al., 2002).

Thiazolidinediones. Rosiglitazone (Avandia®) and pioglitazone (Actos®) are commercially available thiazolidinedione (TZD) compounds (Day, 1999; Mori et al., 1999; Mudaliar & Henry, 2001; Saleh, Mudaliar, & Henry, 1999). Avandia is available in 4- and 8-mg tablets, and Actos is supplied in 15-, 30-, and 45-mg pills. The dosing is usually once daily, although the 4-mg dose of Avandia may be taken twice daily. These drugs reduce insulin resistance and are euglycemic in that they can restore normal glucose levels without causing hypoglycemia when given as monotherapy or with another euglycemic such as biguanides or alpha-glucosidase inhibitors. As peroxisome proliferator-activator gamma (PPAR-γ) ligands, their primary mechanism of action is the regulation of genes involved with glucose and lipid metabolism and adipocyte differentiation. Chronic TZD therapy is associated with enhanced, new, small, insulin-sensitive, subcutaneous adipocyte differentiation and accelerated, large, visceral, insulin-resistant adipocyte apoptosis. Additional effects are seen in vascular endothelium (protection against atherogenesis), the immune system (decreased inflammatory cytokines), ovaries, and tumor cells.

In a manner reminiscent of synthetic estrogen-receptor modulators, the different thiazolidinediones have varying clinical effects, presumably because their unique side chains confer conformational changes that influence co-activator and co-repressor binding at the nuclear receptor. All the TZDs have common adverse effects, specifically fluid retention that presents as a mild dilutional anemia, peripheral edema, and weight gain. Fluid retention is most common in individuals who are concurrently treated with insulin or insulin secretagogues, and hypoglycemia can also occur in combination therapy with insulin and insulin secretagogues.

The TZDs affect the lipid profile and universally increase HDL and LDL levels. There is a corresponding decrease in triglyceride values, which is greatest in pioglitazone-treated individuals. TZD should not be prescribed for individuals in congestive heart failure, who have significant liver disease, or who are pregnant. As of this writing (2003), because of concern about liver toxicity, the FDA requires bimonthly surveillance of liver function tests during the first year of therapy and periodically thereafter.

There are preliminary reports (TRIPOD Study) suggesting that TZDs may be useful in diabetes prevention and remission (Buchanan, 2001; Buchanan et al., 2002).

HEALTH SCREENING AND MONITORING

Because diabetes is a chronic condition that increases the risk for many complications, ongoing health care maintenance and diabetes monitoring are key elements in therapy. Routine health maintenance activities, including smoking cessation, immunizations, and health screening, should be addressed. In addition to using aspirin therapy as a secondary prevention strategy in people with macrovascular disease, low-dose aspirin therapy is recommended as a primary prevention strategy in men and women with diabetes who have cardiac risk factors (ADA, 2003).

SUMMARY

Diabetes mellitus is a complex, heterogeneous, chronic condition that contributes significantly to individual morbidity and mortality and to health care costs. At the same time, data are continuing to accumulate that support the positive benefits of glycemic control and cardiovascular risk reduction, and new treatment modalities allow a more targeted approach to the underlying pathophysiologic abnormalities. Because diabetes can occur at any time across the life span, may require many lifestyle changes, and involves multiple organ systems, its management necessitates a comprehensive multidisciplinary approach that includes the patient and his or her family.

REFERENCES

Akerblom, H. K., Vaarala, O., Hyoty, H., Ilonen, J., & Knip, M. (2002). Environmental factors in the etiology of type 1 diabetes. *American Journal of Medical Genetics*, 115(1), 18–29.

Anerson, B., & Funnell, M. (2000). *The art of empowerment*. Alexandria, VA: American Diabetes Association.

Arnow, W. S., & Ahn, C. (2001). Effect of beta blockers on incidence of new coronary events in older persons with prior myocardial infarction and diabetes mellitus. *American Journal of Cardiology*, 87, 780–781.

Aschner, P. (2002). Diabetes trends in Latin America. *Diabetes Metabolism Research Review*, 18(Suppl 3), S27–31.

American Diabetes Association. (1998). *Medical management of type 2 diabetes* (4th ed.). Alexandria, VA: American Diabetes Association.

American Diabetes Association. (2003). American Diabetes Association: Clinical Practice Recommendations: 2003. *Diabetes Care*, 26(Supplement 1), S1–S156.

Atkinson, M. A., & Eisenbarth, G. S. (2001). Type 1 diabetes: new perspectives on disease pathogenesis and treatment. *Lancet*, 358(9277), 221–229.

Aviles-Santa, L., Sinding, J., & Raskin, P. (1999). Effects of metformin in patients with poorly controlled, insulin-treated type 2 diabetes mellitus. A

randomized, double-blind, placebo-controlled trial. *Annals of Internal Medicine*, 131(3), 182–188.

Bailey, C. J. (1999). New pharmacological approaches to glycemic control. *Diabetes Review*, 7, 94.

Barrett, E. J. (2003). The endocrine pancreas. In W. F. Boron & E. L. Boulpaep (Eds.), *Medical physiology: A cellular and molecular approach* (pp. 1066–1085). Philadelphia: Saunders.

Bloomgarden, Z. T. (2002). Obesity, hypertension, and insulin resistance. *Diabetes Care*, 25(11), 2088–2097.

Bolli, G. B., Di Marchi, R. D., Park, G. D., Pramming, S., & Koivisto, V. A. (1999). Insulin analogues and their potential in the management of diabetes mellitus. *Diabetologia*, 42(10), 1151–1167.

Bradley, C., & Speight, J. (2002). Patient perceptions of diabetes and diabetes therapy: Assessing quality of life. *Diabetes/Metabolism Research and Reviews*, 18, S64–S69.

Brange, J. (1997). The new era of biotech insulin analogues. *Diabetologia*, 40 Suppl 2, S48–53.

Brownlee, M. (2001). Biochemistry and molecular cell biology of diabetic complications. *Nature*, 414(13 December), 813–820.

Buchanan, T. A. (2001). Protection from type 2 diabetes persists in the TRIPOD cohort eight months after stopping troglitazone. *Diabetes*, 50(Supplement 2), A81.

Buchanan, T. A., Xiang, A. H., Peters, R. K., Kjos, S. L., Marroquin, A., Goico, J., Ochoa, C., Tan, S., Berkowitz, K., Hodis, H. N., & Azen, S. P. (2002). Preservation of pancreatic beta-cell function and prevention of type 2 diabetes by pharmacological treatment of insulin resistance in high-risk hispanic women. *Diabetes*, 51(9), 2796–2803.

Buse, J. B. (1999). Overview of current therapeutic options in type 2 diabetes. Rationale for combining oral agents with insulin therapy. *Diabetes Care*, 22 Suppl 3, C65–70.

Carter, M. (1998). New Medicare law will help seniors pay for supplies and education. *Diabetes Forecast*, 51(8), 43–45.

Centers for Disease Control and Prevention (2002, Last reviewed March 25, 2002). *National diabetes fact sheet: general information and national estimates on diabetes in the United States: 2000*. Department of Health and Human Services, Centers for Disease Control and Prevention. Retrieved June 20, 2003, from the World Wide Web: www.cdc.gov/diabetes/pubs/factsheet.htm

Centers for Disease Control and Prevention (2003, Last reviewed March 17, 2003). *Statistics: Diabetes Surveillance System*. Department of Health and Human Services, Centers for Disease Control and Prevention. Retrieved June 20, 2003, from the World Wide Web: www.cdc.gov/diabetes/statistics/prev/national/notes.htm

Chan, N. N., Brain, H. P., & Feher, M. D. (1999). Metformin-associated lactic acidosis: a rare or very rare clinical entity? *Diabetic Medicine*, 16(4), 273–281.

Chang, A. M., & Halter, J. B. (2003). Aging and insulin secretion. *American Journal of Physiology Endocrinology Metabolism*, 284(1), E7–12.

Chen, J., Marciniak, T. A., Radford, M. J., Wang, Y., & Krumholz, H. M. (1999). Beta-blocker therapy for secondary prevention of myocardial infarction in elderly diabetic patients. *Journal of the American College of Cardiology*, 34(5), 1388–1394.

Chiasson, J. L., Josse, R. G., Gomis, R., Hanefeld, M., Karasik, A., & Laakso, M. (2002). Acarbose for prevention of type 2 diabetes mellitus: the STOP-NIDDM randomised trial. *Lancet*, 359(9323), 2072–2077.

Cryer, P. E. (2002). Hypoglycaemia: the limiting factor in the glycaemic management of Type I and Type II diabetes. *Diabetologia*, 45(7), 937–948.

Cusi, K., & De Fronzo, R. A. (1998). Metformin: A review of its metabolic effects. *Diabetes Review*, 6, 89.

Day, C. (1999). Thiazolidinediones: a new class of antidiabetic drugs. *Diabetic Medicine*, 16(3), 179–192.

Dean, H. (2001). Type 2 diabetes in youth: A new epidemic. In A. Angel, N. Dhalla, G. Pierce, & P. Singal (Eds.), *Diabetes and cardiovascular disease: Etiology, treatment, and outcomes* (pp. 1–5). New York: Kluwer Academic.

DECODE Study Group (1999). Glucose tolerance and mortality: Comparison of WHO and American Diabetes Association diagnostic criteria. *Lancet*, 354, 617–621.

Deferrari, G., Ravera, M., & Berruti, V. (2003). Treatment of diabetic nephropathy in its early stages. *Diabetes/Metabolism Research and Reviews*, 19, 101–114.

DeFronzo, R. A. (1999). Pharmacologic therapy for type 2 diabetes mellitus. *Annals of Internal Medicine*, 131(4), 281–303.

Diabetes Control and Complications Trail Research Group (1993). The effect of intensive treatment of diabetes on the development and progression of long-term complications in insulin-dependent diabetes mellitus. *New England Journal of Medicine*, 329, 977–986.

Diabetes Prevention Program Research Group (2002). Reduction in the incidence of type 2 diabetes with lifestyle intervention or metformin. *New England Journal of Medicine, 346*(6), 393.

Di Bari, M., Marchionni, N., & Pahor, M. (2003). B-Blockers after acute myocardial infarction in elderly patients with diabetes mellitus: Time to reassess. *Drugs and Aging, 20*(1), 13–22.

Droge, W. (2002). Free radicals in the physiological control of cell function. *Physiology Review, 82,* 47–95.

Dunn, C. J., & Faulds, D. (2000). Nateglinide. *Drugs, 60*(3), 607–615; discussion 616–607.

Eberly, L. E., Cohen, J. D., Prineas, R., & Yang, L. (2003). Impact of incident diabetes and incident nonfatal cardiovascular disease on 18-year mortality. *Diabetes Care, 26*(3), 848–854.

Edge, J. A. (2000). Cerebral oedema during treatment of diabetic ketoacidosis: are we any nearer finding a cause? *Diabetes Metabolism Research and Reviews, 16*(5), 316–324.

Egede, L. E. (2003). Lifestyle modification to improve blood pressure control in individuals with diabetes. *Diabetes Care, 26*(3), 602–607.

Elahi, D., Muller, D. C., Egan, J. M., Andres, R., Veldhuist, J., & Meneilly, G. S. (2002). Glucose tolerance, glucose utilization and insulin secretion in ageing. *Novartis Found Symp, 242,* 222–242; discussion 242–226.

Enck, P., & Frieling, T. (1997). Pathophysiology of diabetic gastroparesis. *Diabetes, 46*(Suppl 2), S77–S81.

Evans, A. J., & Krentz, A. J. (2001). Insulin resistance and B-cell dysfunction as therapeutic targets in type 2 diabetes. *Diabetes, Obesity and Metabolism, 3,* 219–229.

Feldman, E. L. (2003). Oxidative stress and diabetic neuropathy: A new understanding of an old problem. *Journal of Clinical Investigation, 111*(4), 431–433.

Gabir, M. M., Hanson, R. L., Dabelea, D., Imperatore, G., Roumain, J., Bennett, P. H., & Knowler, W. C. (2000). The 1997 American Diabetes Association and 1999 World Health Organization criteria for hyperglycemia in he diagnosis and prevention of diabetes. *Diabetes Care, 23,* 1108–1112.

Gaede, P., Vedel, P., Larsen, N., Jensen, G. V. H., Parving, H. -H., & Pedersen, O. (2003). Multifactorial intervention and cardiovascular disease in patients with type 2 diabetes. *New England Journal of Medicine, 348*(5), 383–393.

Gale, E. A. M. (2002). The rise of childhood type 1 diabetes in the 20th century. *Diabetes, 51,* 3353–3361.

Gerich, J. E. (2002). Is reduced first-phase insulin release the earliest detectable abnormality in individuals destined to develop type 2 diabetes? *Diabetes, 51*(Supplement 1), S117–S121.

Glasgow, R. E., & Eakin, E. G. (1996). Dealing with diabetes self-management. In B. J. Anderson & R. R. Rubin (Eds.), *Practical psychology for diabetes clinicians.* Alexandria, VA: American Diabetes Association.

Gnudi, L., Gruden, G., & Viberti, G. F. (2003). Pathogenesis of diabetic nephropathy. In J. C. Pickup & G. Williams (Eds.), *Textbook of diabetes* (3rd ed., Vol. 2, pp. 52.51–52.22). Malden, MA: Blackwell.

Goldstein, B. J. (2002). Insulin resistance as the core defect in type 2 diabetes mellitus. *American Journal of Cardiology, 90*(5A), 3G–10G.

Gordois, A., Scuffham, P., Shearer, A., Oglesby, A., & Tobian, J. A. (2003). The health care costs of diabetic peripheral neuropathy in the U.S. *Diabetes Care, 26,* 1790–1795.

Grant, P. J., & Davies, A. J. (2003). Cardiovascular diseases and diabetes. In J. C. Pickup & G. Williams (Eds.), *Textbook of diabetes* (Vol. 2, pp. 56.51–56.24). Massachusetts: Blackwell Science Ltd.

Green, A., Hirsch, N. C., & Pramming, S. K. (2003). The changing world demography of type 2 diabetes. *Diabetes/Metabolism Research and Reviews, 19,* 3–7.

Green, A., Sjolie, A. K., & Eshoj, O. (1997). Insulin-dependent diabetes mellitus. In J. C. Pickup & G. Williams (Eds.), *Textbook of diabetes* (2nd ed., Vol. 1, pp. 3.1–3.16). Oxford: Blackwell.

Gribble, F. M., Tucker, S. J., Seino, S., & Ashcroft, F. M. (1998). Tissue specificity of sulfonylureas: studies on cloned cardiac and beta-cell K(ATP) channels. *Diabetes, 47*(9), 1412–1418.

United Kingdom Prospective Diabetes Study (UKPDS) Group (1998). Intensive blood glucose control with sulphonylureas or insulin compared with conventional treatment and risk of complications in patients with type 2 diabetes (UKPDS 33). *Lancet, 252,* 854–853.

Harris, M. I. (2000). Health care and health status and outcomes for patients wth type 2 diabetes. *Diabetes Care, 23*(6), 754–758.

Heinemann, L. (2003). Insulin pharmacology. In J. C. Pickup & G. Williams (Eds.), *Textbook of diabetes* (3rd ed., Vol. 2, pp. 42.41–42.15). Malden, MA: Blackwell Science Inc.

Heinemann, L., Linkeschova, R., Rave, K., Hompesch, B., Sedlak, M., & Heise, T. (2000). Time-action profile of the long-acting insulin analog insulin glargine (HOE901) in comparison with those of NPH insulin and placebo. *Diabetes Care, 23*(5), 644–649.

Howlett, H. C., & Bailey, C. J. (1999). A risk-benefit assessment of metformin in type 2 diabetes mellitus. *Drug Safety, 20*(6), 489–503.

Kaplan, N. M. (1997). Hypertension and diabetes. In D. Porte & R. S. Sherwin (Eds.), *Ellenberg and Rifkin's diabetes mellitus* (5th ed., pp. 1097–1104). Stamford, CT: Appleton & Lange.

Kapur, D. (2003). Neuropathic pain and diabetes. *Diabetes/Metabolism Research and Reviews, 19,* S9–S15.

Knott, R. M., & Forrester, J. V. (2003). Pathogenesis of diabetic eye disease. In J. C. Pickup & G. Williams (Eds.), *Textbook of diabetes* (3rd ed., Vol. 2, pp. 48.41–48.17). Malden, MA: Blackwell.

Knowler, W. C., Barrett-Connor, E., Fowler, S. E., Hamman, R. F., Lachin, J. M., Walker, E. A., & Nathan, D. M. (2002). Reduction in the incidence of type 2 diabetes with lifestyle intervention or metformin. *New England Journal of Medicine, 346*(6), 393–403.

Laron, Z. (2002). Interplay between heredity and environment in the recent explosion of type 1 childhood diabetes mellitus. *American Journal of Medical Genetics, 115,* 4–7.

Lebovitz, H. E. (1998). Alpha-glucosidase inhibitors as agents in the treatment of diabetes. *Diabetes Review, 6,* 132.

Lepore, M., Pampanelli, S., Fanelli, C., Porcellati, F., Bartocci, L., Di Vincenzo, A., Cordoni, C., Costa, E., Brunetti, P., & Bolli, G. B. (2000). Pharmacokinetics and pharmacodynamics of subcutaneous injection of long-acting human insulin analog glargine, NPH insulin, and ultralente human insulin and continuous subcutaneous infusion of insulin lispro. *Diabetes, 49*(12), 2142–2148.

LeRoith, D. (2002). Beta-cell dysfunction and insulin resistance in type 2 diabetes: role of metabolic and genetic abnormalities. *American Journal of Medicine, 113*(Suppl. 6A), 3S–11S.

Levien, T. L., Baker, D. E., Campbell, R. K., & White, J. R., Jr. (2001). Nateglinide therapy for type 2 diabetes mellitus. *Annals of Pharmacotherapy, 35*(11), 1426–1434.

Liese, A. D., Mayer-Davis, E. J., & Haffner, S. M. (1998). Development of the multiple metabolic syndrome: An epidemiologic perspective. *Epidemiologic Reviews, 20*(2), 157–172.

Lingappa, V. R., & Farey, K. (2000). *Physiological medicine: A clinical approach to basic medical physiology.* New York: McGraw-Hill.

MacIssac, R. J., Lee, L. Y., McNeil, K. J., Tsalamandris, C., & Jerums, G. (2002). Influence of age on the presentation and outcome of acidotic and hyperosmolar diabetic emergencies. *Internal Medicine Journal, 32,* 379–385.

Marshall, S. M. (2003). Clinical features and management of diabetic nephropathy. In J. C. Pickup & G. Williams (Eds.), *Textbook of diabetes* (3rd ed., Vol. 2, pp. 53.51–53.22). Malden, MA: Blackwell.

Matthaei, S., Stumvoll, M., Kellerer, M., & Haring, H.-U. (2000). Pathophysiology and pharmacological treatment of insulin resistance. *Endocrine Reviews, 21*(6), 585–618.

McGarry, D. (2002). Dysregulation of fatty acid metabolism in the etiology of type 2 diabetes. *Diabetes, 51,* 7.

Meneilly, G. S., & Tessier, D. (2001). Diabetes in elderly adults. *Journal of Gerontology: Medical Sciences, 56A*(1), M5–M13.

Mokdad, A. H., Ford, E. S., Bowman, B. A., Dietz, W. H., Vinicor, F., & Bales, V. S. (2003). Prevalence of obesity, diabetes, and obesity-related health risk factors, 2001. *Journal of the American Medical Association, 289*(1), 76–79.

Mori, Y., Murakawa, Y., Okada, K., Horikoshi, H., Yokoyama, J., Tajima, N., & Ikeda, Y. (1999). Effect of troglitazone on body fat distribution in type 2 diabetic patients. *Diabetes Care, 22*(6), 908–912.

Motala, A. A. (2002). Diabetes trends in Africa. *Diabetes Metabolsim Research and Reviews, 18*(Suppl 3), S14–20.

Mudaliar, S., & Henry, R. R. (2001). New oral therapies for type 2 diabetes mellitus: The glitazones or insulin sensitizers. *Annual Review of Medicine, 52,* 239–257.

Nathan, D. M., Lachin, J., Cleary, P., Orchard, T., Brillon, D. J., Backlund, J. Y., O'Leary, D. H., Genuth, S; Diabetes Control and Complications Trail; Epidemiology of Diabetes Interventions and Complications Research Group (2003). Intensive diabetes therapy and carotid intima-media thickness in type 1 diabetes mellitus. *New England Journal of Medicine, 348,* (23), 2349–2352.

Nadel, E. (2003). Metabolism and nutrition. In W. F. Boron & E. L. Boulpaep (Eds.), *Medical physiology: A cellular and molecular approach* (pp. 1211–1230). Philadelphia: Saunders.

Onuigbo, M., & Weir, M. R. (2003). Evidenced-based treatment of hypertension in patients with diabetes mellitus. *Diabetes, Obesity and Metabolism, 5*, 13–26.

Ouellette, S. M. (1998). AANA Journal course: Update for nurse anesthetists—diabetes mellitus: overview and current concepts in anesthetic management. *American Association of Nurse Anesthetists Journal, 66*(1), 65–76.

Owens, D. R. (1999). Repaglinide: a new short-acting insulinotropic agent for the treatment of type 2 diabetes. *European Journal of Clinical Investtigation, 29* Suppl. 2, 30–37.

Passa, P. (2002). Diabetes trends in Europe. *Diabetes Metabolsim Research and Reviews, 18*(Suppl. 3), S3–8.

Poirier, P., & Despres, J.-P. (2003). Lipid disorders in diabetes. In J. C. Pickup & G. Williams (Eds.), *Textbook of diabetes* (3rd ed., Vol. 2, pp. 54.51–54.21). Malden, MA: Blackwell Science.

Prendergast, J. J. (2001). Diabetic autonomic neuropathy Part 1 - Early detection. *Practical Diabetology, 20*(1), 7–14.

Quattrini, C., & Tesfaye, S. (2003). Understanding the impact of painful diabetic neuropathy. *Diabetes/Metabolism Research and Reviews, 19*, S2–S8.

Rassam, A. G., Zeise, T. M., Burge, M. R., & Schade, D. S. (1999). Optimal administration of lispro insulin in hyperglycemic type 1 diabetes. *Diabetes Care, 22*(1), 133–136.

Reaven, G. M. (2003). Age and glucose intolerance: Effect of fitness and fatness. *Diabetes Care, 26*(2), 540.

Renner, R., Pfutzner, A., Trautmann, M., Harzer, O., Sauter, K., & Landgraf, R. (1999). Use of insulin lispro in continuous subcutaneous insulin infusion treatment. Results of a multicenter trial. German Humalog-CSII Study Group. *Diabetes Care, 22*(5), 784–788.

Robertson, R. P., Harmon, J., Tran, P. O., Tanaka, Y., & Takahashi, H. (2003). Glucose toxicity in beta-cells: type 2 diabetes, good radicals gone bad, and the glutathione connection. *Diabetes, 52*(3), 581–587.

Saleh, Y. M., Mudaliar, S. R., & Henry, R. R. (1999). Metabolic and vascular effects of the thiazoladinedione, troglitazone. *Diabetes Review, 7*, 55.

Schianca, G. P. C., Rossi, A., Sainaghi, P. P., Maduli, E., & Bartoli, E. (2003). The significance of impaired fasting glucose versus impaired glucose tolerance. *Diabetes Care, 26*(5), 1333–1337.

Shaw, J. E., Zimmet, P. Z., McCarty, D., & de Courten, M. (2000). Type 2 diabetes worldwide according to the new classification and criteria. *Diabetes Care, 23*(Suppl. 2), B5–10.

Singleton, J. R., & Smith, A. G. (2003). Painful sensory neuropathy in patients with impaired glucose tolerance: Part 1 - Diagnosis and pathophysiology. *Clinical Geriatrics, 11*(3), 28–34.

Skyler, J. S., & Oddo, C. (2002). Diabetes trends in the USA. *Diabetes Metabolsim Research and Reviews, 18*(Suppl. 3), S21–26.

Steinberg, D. (1997). Diabetes and atherosclerosis. In D. Porte & R. S. Sherwin (Eds.), *Ellengerg and Rifkin's diabetes mellitus* (5th ed., pp. 193–206). Stamford, CT: Appleton & Lange.

Stumvoll, M., Meyer, C., Mitrakou, A., Nadkarni, V., & Gerich, J. E. (1997). Renal glucose production and utilization: New aspects in humans. *Diabetologia, 40*, 749–754.

Taguchi, T., & Brownlee, M. (2003). The biochemical mechanisms of diabetes tissue damage. In J. C. Pickup & G. Williams (Eds.), *Textbook of diabetes* (3rd ed., Vol. 2, pp. 47.41–47.17). Malden: Blackwell Science Inc.

Tomlinson, D. R. (2003). Pathogenesis of diabetic neuropathies. In J. C. Pickup & G. Williams (Eds.), *Textbook of Diabetes* (3rd ed., Vol. 2, pp. 50.51–50.12). Malden, MA: Blackwell Science.

Vlassara, H., & Palace, M. R. (2002). Diabetes and advanced glycation endproducts. *Journal of Internal Medicine, 251*, 87–101.

Ying, W. (1997). Deleterious network hypothesis of aging. *Medical Hypothesis, 48*, 143–148.

Young, M. J. (2003). Foot problems in diabetes. In J. C. Pickup & G. Williams (Eds.), *Textbook of diabetes* (3rd ed., Vol. 2, pp. 57.51–57.19). Malden, MA: Blackwell Science.

Young, R. J. (2003). The clinical features and management of diabetic neuropathy. In J. C. Pickup & G. Williams (Eds.), *Textbook of diabetes* (3rd ed., Vol. 2, pp. 51.51–51.22). Malden, MA: Blackwell Science.

Younis, N., Burnham, P., Patwala, A., Weston, P. J., & Vora, J. P. (2001). Beta blocker prescribing differences in patients with and without diabetes following a first myocardial infarction. *Diabetes Medicine, 18*(2), 159–161.

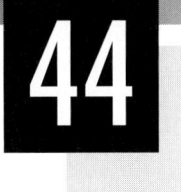

44

Adherence to Cardiovascular Treatment Regimens

LORA E. BURKE • DOROTHY TSCHIRPKE • THERESE A. POLAKOSKI*

The terms *adherence* and *compliance* are used interchangeably in the literature, and are used similarly in this chapter. More than 25 years after it was developed, the definition of compliance given by Sackett and Haynes in 1976 continues to be used, which is "the extent to which patient's behavior (in terms of taking medications, following diets, or exercising other lifestyle changes) coincides with the clinical prescription" (Sackett & Haynes, 1976). More recently, adherence was defined as a partnership between the health care provider and patient, the goal of this relationship being to ensure that the patient is as self-sufficient in managing his or her health as possible (American Hospital Association and the Centers for Disease Control [CDC]). The latter definition emphasizes the mutual responsibility of the patient and provider and reinforces the provider's commitment to enable the patient to implement the recommended treatment. Other terms used in the literature to refer to adherence include *concordance* and *persistence* (McDonald et al., 2002). The terms adherence and compliance are viewed by some as judgmental and suggesting blame of the patient for not following a treatment plan. However, the patient is only one part of the equation when adherence is considered. Adherence, as noted by an expert panel convened by the American Heart Association (AHA), involves the health care professional, the system or organization in which care is delivered, and the patient (Miller et al., 1997). More important than what term is used is recognition that the burden or responsibility is on health care providers to assist patients to follow a treatment plan. Moreover, health care providers need to fulfill their role by adhering to established treatment recommendations and implement evidence-based treatment guidelines (Kottke et al., 2003).

This chapter reviews adherence and the significance of nonadherence in the management of the cardiac patient. Methods used to assess adherence across the behaviors of medication taking, dietary self-management, following an exercise program, and smoking cessation are reviewed. Strategies to enhance adherence are discussed and guidelines for implementing educational and behavioral strategies are provided.

SIGNIFICANCE OF NONADHERENCE

A number of pharmacologic therapies are used in the prevention, as well as the acute and long-term management of cardiovascular disease. However, the extent to which these therapies are effective can be influenced by the patient's adherence to the treatment regimen (Burke et al., 1997; McDonald et al., 2002). The survival benefits of several drugs have been demonstrated in large-scale clinical trials. However, one study showed that at two years, adherence to prescribed statins was 40.1% for those with acute coronary heart disease (CHD), 36.1% among those with chronic CHD, and only 25.4% among those receiving the drug for primary prevention of CHD (Jackevicius et al., 2002). Adherence rates for most pharmacological therapy is similar, e.g., 29% of Americans discontinue their medications prematurely, 22% take less than prescribed, and 12% do not fill their prescription at all (American Heart Association Compliance Action Program, 2003; Haynes et al., 2002). These statistics illustrate how medication nonadherence is a major health problem, the magnitude of which is underscored by a report that 10% of all hospital admissions are the result of medications being taken incorrectly (American Heart Association, 2003).

Although research on ways to improve adherence is ongoing, there remains a huge gap between what is known and beneficial and what is applied in practice (Haynes, 2001). Thus the poor rates of adherence have been relatively static. Nonadherence is observed in regimens affecting lifestyle as well.

Compliance with structured exercise programs has been low. Less than 25% of eligible patients actually participate in cardiac rehabilitation; 25% to 50% of those who enroll discontinue participation within the first 6 months, and 90% by 12 months (Carlson et al., 2000). Among women the rates are lower; only 66% exercise after 1 month in the program, and 50% exercise at 12 weeks (Moore et al., 1998). Smoking cessation rates remain low with the vast majority of those who complete treatment relapsing within 3 months of initial cessation (Ockene et al., 2000). Among those who participate in a formal program, there are fewer relapses compared to self-quitters. However, among program participants, 33% of all relapses

*The authors were supported by grant 5RO1 DK58387, National Institute of Health, National Institute of Diabetes, Digestive, and Kidney Disorders.

occurred during the first month after treatment, and of those who were smoking at 2 years, most had relapsed by 7 months. These early rates of nonadherence are predictive of adherence behavior over the long-term course of treatment (Burke et al., 1997). Adherence to programs that require changing eating habits and physical activity are less than ideal, which is reflected in the current epidemic of overweight, obesity and type 2 diabetes (Manson & Bassuk, 2003). Approximately, 62% of adults in the U.S. are overweight or obese, a trend that is being observed around the world. Moreover, 75% of Americans are sedentary or insufficiently active. These rates of adherence are representative of adherence behavior across cultures, countries, and treatment regimens (Burke et al., 1997).

The duration of treatment is usually a factor influencing compliance, with an initial decline in adherence observed in the first year followed by a gradual decline over time (Haynes, 2001). This pattern is observed repeatedly among those participating in long-term programs, e.g., cardiac rehabilitation and weight loss programs (Burke, 2001; Burke et al., 1997). The prevention and treatment of cardiovascular disease requires ongoing management of lifestyle habits and, increasingly, inclusion of pharmacologic therapy, such as aspirin, hypolipidemic agents, beta blockers or calcium channel blockers. In the absence of sustained adherence, the benefits of prevention or treatment cannot be realized.

In the clinical arena, nonadherence at any point in the treatment continuum poses a threat to satisfactory outcomes. Medication noncompliance has been associated with increased risk of coronary heart disease, precipitated episodes of heart failure, late organ rejection among heart transplant recipients, and mortality (Dew et al., 1995; Evangelista et al., 1999; Irvine et al., 1999; McDermott et al., 1997). These reports emphasize the mediating effects of compliance on clinical outcome, and the impact nonadherence can have on morbidity and mortality associated with cardiovascular disease regardless of when it occurs in the treatment continuum.

In the research arena, noncompliance affects therapy evaluation before its introduction into the clinical setting. Incomplete adherence to the treatment under study underestimates its efficacy, and the diminished effect reduces the study's power to detect a difference between treatment groups, thus preventing the study from meeting the assumptions of the projected sample size. In this situation, when nonadherence to the study protocol results in diminished effect, additional subjects are required. Furthermore, nonadherence to the treatment protocol may mask side effects or result in an overestimation of optimal dosage (Burke et al., 1997). Finally, intermittent or varying adherence to the study protocol may reflect varying adherence to concomitantly prescribed therapeutic modalities, which may affect study outcomes (Urquhart, 1991).

METHODS OF MEASUREMENT

Assessment of adherence needs to be incorporated into each clinical encounter (Dunbar-Jacob et al., 1995). It is important that the clinician separate adherence from therapeutic or clinical outcome, which can be affected by a myriad of variables besides adherence (Dunbar-Jacob & Sereika, 2001). For example,

inadequate control of blood pressure or cholesterol may be due to inadequate drug dosage, individual variation in pharmacokinetic factors of different drugs, day-time or seasonal variations in measurement values, or personal factors (Dunbar-Jacob et al., 1995). Conversely, the absence of symptoms or achievement of goal does not confirm adherence. Clinical outcomes are indirect measures of adherence, whereas patient behaviors (e.g., weight loss, exercise, taking the medication) are direct measures of adherence. Both direct and indirect measures have inherent advantages and disadvantages (Dunbar-Jacob & Sereika, 2001; Urquhart, 2001). Unfortunately, it is difficult to measure behavior directly, and thus there is a great reliance on self-reported behavior. Table 44-1 summarizes the numerous measurement methods and the advantages and disadvantages to their use.

Adherence assessment can be conducted through numerous methods. However, a weakness common to all forms of measurement is a bias toward overestimation of adherence (Dunbar-Jacob & Sereika, 2001). One of the reasons for this measurement error is that the period being measured is usually not representative of the patient's usual behavior. Research has shown that patients' adherence varies in relation to the clinical appointment, with adherence increasing immediately before and after the visit (Cramer et al., 1990). An example of this would be the patient taking medicines very closely to how they were prescribed, or closely following a low-cholesterol eating plan for the 7 days before the clinic appointment. Thus, when the patient is asked to report on his or her behavior, the report may be influenced by the recall of most recent behavior and overestimate adherence for the longer period (Dunbar-Jacob & Sereika, 2001). Cramer's research (1989) also showed that the patient was more adherent in the 7 days after the appointment, and then adherence again tapered off until 1 week before the next appointment. A variety of methods are available to measure adherence in the clinical setting. These include self-report, biologic and electronic measures, pill counts, and records such as pharmacy refills.

Self-Report Measures

Self-report measures consist of interviews, structured questionnaires, and diaries. This form of adherence assessment is used most frequently, which is probably explained by its ease of administration and low cost.

Interviews, often used in the research setting to assess adherence behavior at each contact, can easily be conducted in the clinical setting. Two brief interview scales were developed to assess global medication compliance among hypertensive patients. The four-item scale developed by Morisky and colleagues (1986) pertains to areas of omission, such as forgetting, being careless, and stopping the medication when feeling better or when feeling worse. This scale, for which adequate psychometric properties have been reported, has been used in minority and general populations to assess patient understanding as well as medication adherence. Shea and colleagues (1992) adapted Morisky's scale by making minor modifications in the wording and adding a fifth item, which asked if the blood pressure medication was ever missed for any reason. Again, adequate psychometric properties were demonstrated in a sample predominantly comprised of blacks and Hispanics.

Table 44-1 ■ METHODS OF ADHERENCE MEASUREMENT AND FEATURES OF THEIR USE

Measurement Method	Behavior*	Advantages	Disadvantages
Self-Report			
Interview	All behaviors	Inexpensive, provides details	Tends to over-report adherence
24-hour recall	All behaviors	Increased accuracy due to short recall period	Under representation of time may increase bias if recall day is atypical
Questionnaire	All behaviors	Numerous scales available, does not influence behavior	Requires literacy; may be lengthy, needs to be sensitive & appropriate to age, gender, reading level, & ethnicity
Diaries	All behaviors	Provides detail of circumstances of behavior	May influence the behavior, may under- or over-report adherence, subject to recall bias, requires cooperation of patient, requires patient literacy
Biologic Outcomes (Serum, urine, or saliva level of drug or its metabolite)	All behaviors	May provide a validation of behavior	Are indirect measures of adherence, only measures adherence close to time of measurement
Electronic Monitors (electronic event monitors, heart rate monitors, accelerometers, diaries)	Medication-taking, exercise, smoking cessation, pain control, symptoms, food intake	Provides detailed pattern of adherence, provides data on unsupervised exercise; diaries provide data on adherence to recording protocol, record closer to even so decreased recall bias, record in naturalistic setting	Cost prohibits widespread use, use of the device may influence behavior
Pill Counts	Medication-taking	Inexpensive, easy to conduct	Over estimates, does not provide pattern of adherence
Pharmacy Records	Medication-taking	Provides another source of adherence data	Not available universally, requires use of one pharmacy, does not provide data on adherence pattern

* Medication-taking, eating, exercise, smoking cessation

Adherence can also be ascertained through a 7-day recall interview by asking the patient to report the number of pills and the times at which these were taken for each day of the week before the visit. However, these tend to provide an overestimation of adherence (Dunbar-Jacob et al., 1997). When comparing self-reported interview adherence to electronic measured adherence, Dunbar-Jacob and colleagues (1997) found 97% adherence reported in the interview compared with 84% adherence measured by an unobtrusive electronic event monitor.

Dietary behavior may be assessed through 24-hour recall interviews or through the lengthier diet history interview. Assessing dietary adherence requires a determination of what the person eats and the degree to which the food intake approximates the recommended diet (Burke & Dunbar-Jacob, 1995). The interview allows more exact descriptions of foods (e.g., brands, degree of fat modification). It also requires interviewer skill at eliciting detail and cooperation on the part of the patient. A benefit of the 24-hour recall is that there is increased accuracy because of the shortened recall period, but a disadvantage is that there may be increased bias if the recall is conducted for days on which the eating pattern may vary, such as a weekend or the day before a clinic visit (Block, 1982). To compensate for this weakness, some studies have a 24-hour dietary recall interview performed on three randomly selected days within a certain measurement period, e.g., 2 weeks. The 24-hour recall is usually limited to population-based studies because one day's intake is unlikely to be representative of a person's usual intake (Dolocek et al., 1986). The purpose of the food history is to obtain a detailed description of food consumption over an extended period, including an assessment of normative as well as divergent eating patterns (Wolper, 1995). Validity of this method is threatened by the potential of generalizing recent behavior to long-term behavior, and the person's faulty ability to recall food intake (Burke & Dunbar-Jacob,

1995). Dietary interviews in the Framingham Study, separated by 2 years, showed close agreement across macronutrients (Dawber et al., 1962). A good example of a food history format is the Block Health Habits and History Questionnaire, for which software for analysis purposes is available (Block, 2001; Subar et al., 2001). The most recent version of the Block Questionnaire was based on the National Health and Nutrition Examination Survey (NHANES) III data, and also incorporates additional low-fat food choices and portion-size pictures (Block, 2001).

Adherence to exercise regimens may also be assessed through interviews. Because there are so many dimensions of exercise to assess, e.g., the type of exercise, its frequency, duration, and intensity, as well as the physiological response to exercise, it poses a particular challenge (Dishman et al., 2001). For example, one study reported that sedentary adults overestimate the intensity of their moderate physical activity (Duncan et al., 2001). However, on balance, self-report measures provide the most practical and cost-effective method for assessing adherence. Interviews may be conducted with the use of the questionnaires described below, e.g., the Paffenbarger or the Physical Activity Recall. Questionnaires or diaries are used more often to assess patterns of physical activity or adherence to exercise.

Questionnaires are available to assess adherence across multiple behaviors. Although there are numerous scales available for assessment of eating and exercise behaviors, few exist for medication-taking behavior. The Morisky scale, first published in 1986, has been adapted by several investigators and used as a paper-and-pencil questionnaire in several populations, including those being treated for hypercholesterolemia, rheumatoid arthritis, and HIV. It has also been expanded from a five- to a nine-item scale for its use in a study on HIV (personal communication, J. Erlen, June, 2003). The scale has demonstrated adequate psychometric properties.

Dietary adherence can be measured by several established questionnaires, including the Connor Diet Habit Survey (Connor et al., 1992), the Eating Pattern Questionnaire (Kristal et al., 1990), a Dietary and Risk Factor Questionnaire (Smucker et al., 1989), and the Willet and colleagues (1985) or Block Food Frequency Questionnaires (Block et al., 1986). The first two questionnaires focus on fat intake and have reported psychometric properties when used in cardiac and general populations. Food frequency questionnaires, which typically have precoded forms, are usually used in epidemiologic studies, for which they are extremely practical and inexpensive to score (Willet, 1990). They are best used for averaging long-term diet and for ranking intake of particular food or food groups (Allison, 1995). Their limitation is the number and types of items listed, which reduces their usefulness among ethnic groups (Allison, 1995; Willett et al., 1985). Good reliability and validity of the questionnaires have been established (Allison, 1995). Several of these questionnaires have not been revised to incorporate the numerous low-fat or fat-free food items available today, which may limit their precision. The Block Questionnaire was updated most recently in 1998 (Block, 2001).

Measurement of physical activity, which continues to receive the most attention in the public health field, has relied primarily on the questionnaire (Dishman, 1994; Jakicic et al., 2002; Kriska, 1997). The exercise assessment questionnaires, which are subjective measures, have been validated by objective measures of physical activity, such as measures of total energy expenditure (doubly labeled water), estimates of physical fitness (heart rate), or measures of physical motion by accelerometers (Kriska, 1997). A beneficial trait of the questionnaire is that it does not influence the behavior being measured, and although less precise than the objective measures, it estimates activity relative to others in the population. The questionnaire may range from one item to an array of questions covering a wide range of occupational and leisure activities, and may cover varying time intervals. A compilation of physical activity questionnaires and a review of their psychometric properties was published, providing an excellent resource for anyone wishing to measure exercise adherence (Pereira et al., 1997). In selecting a questionnaire, the investigator must consider characteristics of the population, such as gender, age, culture, and the outcome of interest. Most of the activity questionnaires were developed with men's activities in mind, so they may be less sensitive to differences in physical activity levels in women (Kriska, 1997). Jakicic and colleagues (Jakicic et al., 2002) reported that the Physical Activity Recall and the Paffenbarger Physical Activity Recall were comparable to assess change in activity in a very specific population, sedentary, overweight woman participating in weight loss treatment.

In summary, questionnaires with a shorter time interval are less vulnerable to recall bias and easier to validate with objective measures. However, using a shorter time frame reduces the likelihood of obtaining a picture of usual behavior, because eating and exercise patterns may vary by season. Reliability and validity are affected by the person's ability to store and retrieve information, and by potential influence of the interviewer or respondent bias (Dunbar-Jacob & Sereika, 2001; Kriska, 1997).

Diaries

Daily diaries for food intake or exercise circumvent the bias of recall, but require training and cooperation of the patient or study participant. While diaries may be used as part of an intervention to achieve awareness of one's behavior, the focus here is on assessment of adherence. Food and exercise diaries are often used periodically and cover a 3- or 7-day period, including one non-work or leisure day. Recording for extended periods (i.e., over 3 days) may reduce accuracy, and the recording may begin to influence the recorder's behavior. King et al. (1997), Perri and colleagues (2002) and Jakicic et al. (1999) have used diaries to measure exercise adherence. Using heart rate monitors as a second measure of adherence, King et al. (1991) reported high convergent validity for exercise logs that were corroborated with ambulatory heart rate monitors. However, when comparing self-report to accelerometer data, Jakicic and colleagues demonstrated that nearly half of the overweight women in a behavioral treatment program over-reported their exercise (Jakicic et al., 1998). To summarize, self-report measures are common, easy to use, and inexpensive. Moreover, they provide information on the circumstances surrounding the good or poor adherence. Issues of concern with self-report measures include deliberate and nondeliberate errors in recall or reporting; e.g., one study found that a group of obese subjects underreported their food consumption and over-reported their energy expenditure (Lichtman et al., 1992). Staff should be trained on how to teach participants to record the information, and potential problems with memory and social desirability need to be reduced (Gibson, 1990). For example, recording the behavior immediately reduces forgetting and conveying an expectation of a full range of behaviors may help reduce less than truthful reports.

Biologic Measures

Adherence is often reported in terms of biologic end points, such as serum cholesterol or glycosylated hemoglobin level. Other biologic assays frequently used include serum, urine, or saliva level of a drug or its metabolites. Examples include medication adherence measured by serum digoxin level, dietary adherence measured by urine sodium, smoking cessation by serum or saliva thiocyanate or cotinine, and exercise by direct or indirect calorimetry and maximal oxygen uptake (Burke et al., 1997; Urquhart, 2001). Doubly labeled water ($^2H_2^{18}O$), a procedure that requires the subject to ingest water enriched with ^{18}O and ^2H isotopes, is the most accurate measurement of total energy expenditure available, but is too costly to be used on a widespread basis (Allison, 1995). A limitation of biologic assays is that daily variability in compliance cannot be detected. Instead, they indicate if the person has been adherent close to the time of assessment and may serve as a validation of the behavior. Moreover, biologic assays may be influenced by many other factors such as drug absorption or metabolism (Urquhart, 2001).

Electronic Monitoring

Technology has provided tools for ongoing and detailed assessment of adherence behavior. Electronic methods consist of unobtrusive electronic monitors (Burke, 2001; Cramer, 1989) for medication use, heart rate monitors (King et al., 1997; Perri et al., 2002) and electronic motion detectors for exercise (Jakicic et al., 1998), and electronic diaries for symptom reporting or answering a set of programmed questions on a daily basis (Kamarck et al., 1998; Stone & Shiffman, 2002). The electronic or medication event monitor (Aprex Corp., a division of AARDEX, Ltd., Fremont, CA), which consists of an electronic chip housed inside the medication bottle cap, provides data on the day and time the medication bottle was opened, but does not provide information on the number of pills taken (Bohachick et al., 2002). This method does not guarantee the medication was consumed. Additional applications of the electronic monitor include blister pill packs, eye drop solutions, and aerosol spray nebulizers (Burke, 2001). Several devices can measure exercise adherence. Heart rate monitors can be worn during ambulatory exercises (walking, bicycling), such as the Vitalog (Vitalog Corporation, MountainView, CA) or Polar Beat heart rate monitor (Polar Electro, Inc., Port Washington, NY). These devices include a microprocessor that measures and sequentially stores average heart rate values, providing data on adherence to the exercise prescription (King et al., 1991; King et al., 1997; Perri et al., 2002). Electronic accelerometers are motion sensors that register body accelerations and decelerations, and thus provide a direct and objective measure of movement intensity and frequency during physical activity. Jakicic and colleagues (1999; 1995) reported on the Tri-Trac, an accelerometer that uses three planes of motion (Professional Products, Madison, WI), in a clinical study and suggested there was some discrepancy in the number of exercise bouts reported by the participants and the number recorded by the accelerometer. The newest product available to monitor energy expenditure is BodyMedia's SenseWear Armband (BodyMedia, Pittsburgh, PA). This device, similar to a blood pressure cuff in appearance and worn on the upper arm, includes a 2-axis accelerometer, heat flux sensor, galvanic skin response sensor, skin temperature sensor and a near-body ambient temperature sensor. It is able to measure heat produced by the body as a result of basic metabolism and from all forms of physical activity, detect upper and lower body activity, measure effort created by carrying a heavy load, as well as non-ambulatory physical activity, e.g., upper extremity weight resistance exercise or coitus. It has been shown to reliably determine energy expenditure in both the active and resting state, and thus measure activity adherence in an unsupervised setting (Liden et al., 2002).

Electronic hand-held diaries are available to answer a set of programmed questions, report symptoms or cravings *ad lib*, or when prompted by a sound (Stone & Shiffman, 2002). Because recalling events or symptoms is plagued by biases and inaccuracies, the electronic diaries attempt to avoid this barrier by having individuals record experiences close to the time of their occurrence (Stone et al., 2002). Moreover, these monitoring devices permit objective measurement of adherence to a recording schedule under naturalistic conditions (Kamarck et al., 1998). An added benefit is that the data are directly entered by the person and later downloaded on a computer for analysis. Acceptability of the hand-held computers has been reported as excellent (Hufford & Shiffman, 2003; Stone et al., 2002). Stone and colleagues compared the use of a paper diary equipped with a light sensor to record the day and time of diary openings with an electronic diary (similar to a personal digital assistant). They found that 95% of participants recorded in the electronic diary while 90% reported that they recorded in the paper diary but in reality, only 11% recorded (Stone et al., 2002). Other innovative approaches include the use of web sites for patients to log onto and record diary entries (Baer et al., 2002). In summary, electronic monitors provide a detailed picture of the temporal pattern of adherence, from medication taking to self-reporting of symptoms. With the advancement of technology, more products and software programs are available for assessing adherence in the person's naturalistic environment (Hufford & Shiffman, 2003; Body Media, 2003). However, when evaluating the effectiveness of intervention strategies or therapeutic "failures," consideration needs to be given to the approximation of adherence these devices provide (Urquhart, 2001).

Pill Counts and Pharmacy Refills

Unique to the assessment of medication-taking compliance, these measures provide opportunities for alternative or concurrent measurement methods. The pill count is done by tabulating pills remaining from a previous dispensing for a specific interval, and comparing that number with what should have been remaining. An adherence rate is calculated by dividing the number that should have been taken by the number prescribed and multiplying by 100. These methods tend to overestimate adherence; in one study, the pill count rate of adherence was 94%, compared with 84% for the medication event monitor (Dunbar-Jacob et al., 1997). In the age of managed care and large organizations filling prescriptions, pharmacy refill records are becoming commonplace. The disadvantage with the pill count and pharmacy record is that they do not provide information on the pattern of adherence, which may vary in relation to several factors (Burke et al., 1997). In summary, ongoing assessment of adherence is important, primarily because adherence varies over time. An example is the variability of adherence in relation to the medical appointment, with adherence during the 5 days preceding the appointment averaging 88%, and 5 days after the appointment 86%, with a decline to 67% 1 month later (Cramer, 1990).

Compliance cannot be assumed, nor can the clinician make a clinical judgment that adherence is present. Use of one or more of these various methods provide the clinician or researcher some indication of adherence and possibly some information regarding the circumstances surrounding it. In general, it is recommended that more than one method be used concurrently.

DETERMINANTS OF ADHERENCE

A myriad of factors have been suggested and investigated for their association with adherence, including sociodemographic traits, psychological distress, health beliefs, benefits, and barriers (Dunbar-Jacob et al., 1998; Haynes, 2001). However, many have been inconsistent in their association with adherence, and their predictive power is at best modest (Dunbar-Jacob et al., 1998). Moreover, sociodemographic factors are not remedial. A few exceptions include situational factors, e.g., marital discord or unemployment, and clinical conditions, e.g., mental disorders with paranoid or depressive features may adversely affect adherence (Haynes, 2001; Kozuki & Froelicher, 2003). There are factors that are more consistently identified as related to adherence, and, most important, these factors can be addressed through interventions. They can be divided into categories: patient-related, regimen-related, provider-related, and process-oriented or system-related factors. The salient factors affecting compliance are summarized in Display 44-1. These need to be kept in mind as interventions to improve adherence are reviewed.

MODELS OF BEHAVIOR CHANGE

Improving adherence to treatment regimens is one of the greatest challenges facing health care professionals. The general level of adherence to medication is less than ideal and needs improvement. However, assisting patients with lifestyle changes and, most important, maintaining those changes poses the greatest challenge. Lifestyle modification for the cardiac patient may include adopting a physical activity program, consuming a diet low in fat, cholesterol, and sodium, and possibly adjusting caloric intake to reduce or maintain a healthy weight. In addition, smoking cessation and drug

therapy may be added to an already complex regimen. Various models of behavior change have guided studies investigating determinants of adherence or evaluating strategies to improve adherence. Earlier models included operant learning, which focused on the environment and used stimulus control strategies to restructure the environment. More recently, cognitive-motivational models have focused on beliefs, intentions, and self-efficacy, and most recently, readiness to change. Intervention strategies used today have arisen from research based on these models of behavior change, which have been predominantly based on social cognitive theory (Bandura, 1986b). Social cognitive theory, formerly known as social learning theory, is based on an underlying assumption that behavior, the environment, and cognition function as interacting determinants with a bidirectional influence on each other (Bandura, 1986b).

Using the cognitive-motivational models, studies have examined the role of health beliefs, susceptibility, barriers, and intentions in the explanation of adherence behavior change (Fleury, 1992). However, these constructs explained little variance of behavior change in modifying cardiac risk factors. More recently, the social cognitive models have included self-efficacy. There is evidence that judgments of perceived efficacy predict subsequent performance across a variety of domains, including regaining functional status after an MI or cardiac surgery, smoking cessation, weight loss, and exercise and dietary adherence (Burke et al., 1997).

Self-efficacy is defined as a person's perceived capacity for exerting control over his or her motivation, cognition, behavior, and environmental demands (Bandura, 1986a). It is concerned not with a person's skills, but with the person's judgments of what he or she can do with those skills. Self-efficacy is behavior specific, that is, a person's self-efficacy for exercise may be different from self-efficacy for maintaining a healthy diet. There are four sources of efficacy: (1) mastery experience—the most powerful source comes from achievement of a series of subgoals; (2) modeling or vicarious learning—observing another perform a task; (3) physiologic cues—making inferences from autonomic arousal or other symptoms; and (4) verbal or social persuasion—convincing others they possess the capability to achieve their goal (Bandura, 1986a).

Based on research guided by the models of behavior change, a list of strategies for use in assisting patients to improve adherence to behavior change follows. These strategies are summarized in Display 44-2.

ADHERENCE-ENHANCING STRATEGIES

Self-Monitoring

A key technique in approaches to behavioral change, self-monitoring requires the patient to record behavior (e.g., eating, exercise, or smoking behaviors) and use this information for behavioral analysis (i.e., the patient and provider can identify problem behaviors that could be altered). The provider reviews the self-monitoring record and provides reinforcement for progress.

DISPLAY 44–2

ADHERENCE-ENHANCING STRATEGIES

Self-monitoring—record behavior to increase self-awareness, provider review with patient each visit (e.g., patient can keep track of exercise progression in date book or a separate notebook, same for changes in eating habits).

Stimulus control—arrange environment to be supportive to goals (e.g., remove high-fat foods, have exercise equipment readily available and visible).

Goal-setting—have patient set specific, short-term, attainable goal (e.g., substitute fruit for dessert, begin walking 10 minutes every day), check on progress at each visit or in between.

Reinforcement—commend patient for positive change, for maintaining adherence (e.g., review patient's recording of behavior and attribute success in behavior change to patient's efforts).

Modeling behavior—have credible person demonstrate behavior (e.g., cooking demo, blood glucose testing), watch videotape of similar, successful person exercising.

Self-efficacy enhancement—provide opportunities for success by setting specific, short-term goals, give positive feedback on accomplished changes, convince patient she is capable of doing task or changing behavior, interpret symptoms and meaning (e.g., improved endurance with exercise).

Social support provision—assist patient to enlist support of others (e.g., have an exercise "buddy").

Cueing—set up system of reminders (e.g., beeper on watch for medication-taking, exercise shoes by door).

Habit building—pair a new behavior with an established behavior (e.g., set medicine bottle with toothpaste/take pill with bedtime brushing of teeth).

Contracting—written plan for what, when, how behavior goal will be reached (e.g., plan 5% weight loss through small, specific changes in eating and exercise over specific time).

Problem-solving—assist patient to identify problem, define it in patient's own terms, patient generates solutions, select trial of one solution, evaluate solution strategy; if unsuccessful, select a second solution (e.g., walk through with patient a recurrent problem that interferes with adherence to medication, have patient identify a couple of solutions, test the one the patient thinks will most likely succeed, followup on its effectiveness; if it did not work, do trial of next suggested solution).

Relapse prevention—identify high-risk situation, identify/rehearse coping strategies to deal with situations in advance (e.g., prior to vacation, review how medicines will be remembered, diet maintained).

Tailoring the regimen—develop a regimen plan specific to patient that is realistic and acknowledges cultural preferences and economic limitations (e.g, how, when, where the patient in an inner-city neighborhood will exercise when safety is an issue).

Use of frequent short exercise bouts—have patient develop exercise program in five to six 10-minute bouts per day.

Recommend moderate level of exercise—explain to patient that moderate level of exercise may prevent injury and support his or her following it for the longterm, rather than high-intensity exercise.

Home-based exercise—teach patients how and where to exercise independently; provide guidance in developing plan and progressing from initiation to maintenance phase.

Ongoing contact—continued contact via mail, telephone, or Internet (e.g., have patient send in postcard or diary reports of eating, exercise, medication-taking or smoking-cessation behaviors, call patient with feedback if system capability permits, or use electronic-mail system).

Use of external cognitive aids—use of appointment cards, pill organizer boxes (e.g., demonstrate to patient how a pill organizer can assist when taking multiple medications).

Skill development—provide opportunities for return demonstration and practice by patient, follow up at each visit about how patient is doing; periodically ask for repeat demonstration to check on skills (e.g., glucose monitoring).

Medication adherence enhancement—simplify the regimen to least frequent dosing schedule, use calendar packs when available, provide written instructions regarding medication, discuss adherence and its importance, reinforce and reward adherence, explicitly ask about it at every visit, acknowledge the difficulties of adhering and the patient's efforts, negotiate priorities if nonadherence occurs.

Nurse managed care—serving as case managers, nurses work with patients in initiating behavior change, provide clinic follow-up, ongoing contact, and behavioral change counseling.

Supplementary education and training—teach patient about the regimen to be performed, utilize return demonstration, provide practice opportunities for skill development, provide pertinent reading material as appropriate.

Appointment adherence enhancement—provide reminder of appointment (phone call, post card, electronic mail), immediately follow up on every missed appointment to prevent patient dropping out of system.

Stimulus Control

Using information recorded in the diary on the circumstances of the behavior allows identification of the antecedent or trigger for problem behaviors. The patient is counseled to remove the stimuli and to restructure the environment to minimize the will power needed to overcome strong stimuli.

Goal Setting

Goal setting entails working with the patient in developing realistic and attainable goals that are specific and proximal. The goal should include what will be done, when, and how:

for example, "will walk for 15 minutes three times per week for the next 2 weeks." As each sub-goal is reached, the duration, frequency, or intensity of the next goal is increased (Bandura, 1986a).

Reinforcement

Giving positive feedback to the patient on progress made, supporting self-motivation by highlighting accomplishments, encouraging continued progress, and instilling confidence in the person's capability of meeting a goal all constitute reinforcement. When providing positive feedback, focus on the behavior rather than on the clinical outcome.

Modeling Behavior

The patient can observe a credible model perform a task or have an activity demonstrated, which may be done by watching a video or live action. It is important that the patient find the model credible and the activity feasible, such as observing fellow patients exercising in cardiac rehabilitation programs.

Self-Efficacy Enhancement

Self-efficacy enhancement strategies are based on the sources of self-efficacy and include providing opportunities for successful performance or mastery. Provide feedback and praise for progress and achieving specific behavioral goals, convince the person he or she is capable of performing the activity, and interpret symptoms of physiologic response, such as breathlessness due to inactivity and diminished symptoms after a program of regular exercise.

Social Support

Social support includes enlisting others to assist the patient through the behavior change process, and inclusion of supportive others from various aspects of the patient's life (e.g., family, friends, coworkers, community). The purpose of this strategy is to have supportive allies in place during successes and failures. This may take the form of enlisting a "buddy" for exercise or eating behavior change, or having someone there for reinforcement. Social support has been shown to be important in most behavior change, but particularly in programs of dietary change.

Cueing

Cueing consists of setting up a system of reminders or cues to perform certain activities (e.g., a sticker to remind the person to take a medication, or setting out exercise shoes as a prompt to exercise on a busy day).

Habit Building

Habit building is derived from the stimulus control model and is based on the premise that a large amount of behavior is automatic and responsive to stimuli. It further suggests that behavior can be modified by establishing a relationship between the behavior stimulus and the target behavior, such as pairing a new behavior (medication taking) with an established behavior (brushing teeth). Using cues, as described previously, is a related strategy. These techniques may be particularly helpful when in an unusual environment (e.g., traveling). Pairing the medication bottle with the toothpaste or adding a note to the travel alarm clock may prevent an episode of nonadherence.

Contracting

A form of public commitment, contracting involves the patient in the development of the plan and clearly specifies in writing what is expected, the time frame, and any conditions for a reward if the goal is achieved. The contract needs to specify a behavior rather than the health outcome, and should specify the incremental steps necessary to achieve a goal that is attainable and valued by the patient. A contingency reward may be included for achievement of the goal. This needs to be a reward valued by the person and reinforcing to the healthier behavior, such as a new outfit for someone in a weight reduction program, but not dinner at their favorite restaurant.

Problem Solving

Problem solving involves several steps, beginning with identification or acknowledgment of a problem, defining the problem, generating potential solutions, selecting one solution or set of actions to resolve the problem, and then evaluating the success of the attempt to resolve the problem (D'Zurilla et al., 1971). This technique is integral to maintenance of behavior change and is facilitated by reviewing self-monitoring records and identifying high-risk situations. Anticipatory problem solving can help a patient prepare for an upcoming situation, such as a major social event or vacation.

Relapse Prevention

Based on the work of Marlatt and Gordon (1980), the relapse prevention technique emphasizes that slips or lapses are natural occurrences in the process of behavior change. Patients are taught to anticipate high-risk situations and to identify ways to cope with the situation. When possible, patients should practice problem solving to develop these skills better and rehearse the strategies they would use to resolve the threat to adherence or maintenance.

Tailoring the Regimen

Tailoring the regimen addresses the patient's capability to carry out the plan, that is, what is realistic for the patient to achieve in behavior change. It includes accommodating the patient's schedule for appointments, being sensitive to cultural issues in recommending dietary change or other behavior, and being sensitive to financial constraints in general. It is an important consideration in medication-taking compliance (e.g., considering the costs, memory requirements, and schedule when prescribing a drug that may be available in numerous dosing forms).

Use of Frequent, Short Bouts, Home-Based, or Moderate Intensity Exercise Sessions

Individuals can be reassured that they can be flexible in planning their exercise routine, e.g., exercise for 10-minute bouts four to six times per day and still receive the benefits of exercise, or follow the more standard 30- to 45-minute exercise session (Jakicic et al., 1999). For patients for whom it is safe to exercise in unsupervised settings, assisting the patient in planning a home-based exercise program might facilitate long-term adherence. Patients often do better in terms of long-term adherence and fewer injuries if they are instructed to follow a moderate intensity exercise program (Perri et al., 2002).

Ongoing Contact

Continued contact, through mail, telephone, or the Internet has consistently demonstrated improved adherence in maintaining behavior change (Castro & King, 2002; Martin et al., 2000; Tate et al., 2003). The mail can be used as a method of ongoing contact by having patient's return preprinted postcards or weekly diaries of eating, exercise, or medication-taking behaviors. These may be followed by a brief phone call to provide feedback. This technique adds the accountability factor and encourages ongoing communication with the provider. Similarly, the telephone provides ongoing support and assistance with problem solving. A brief phone call to a patient can provide encouragement that may help the patient sustain the behavior during a challenging period. Regular telephone contacts need to have a structure in terms of purpose, what is to be accomplished, approximate time allowed, and a schedule of when the calls should occur. Scripting or outlining the main steps to follow in the contact can help maintain a focus and ensure that each point is addressed. When considering initiating a telephone or telemedicine follow-up system, the nurse needs to consider the purpose or goal of the system, if these can be met given the frequency and duration of the planned contacts, and the costs in terms of staff time.

Use of External Cognitive AIDS

External cognitive aids include appointment reminder letters, follow-up letters for missed appointments, reminder cards for medication refill, medication calendars or reminder charts, and unit-of-use packaging of pills. Any of these strategies can enhance adherence to appointment keeping and to medication taking (Raynor et al., 1993).

Nurse Case-Managed Care

Serving as case managers, nurses provide clinic and telephone follow-up, initiate therapy for risk reduction, and provide counseling for behavior change (e.g., smoking cessation, dietary change). Use of this treatment model has demonstrated improved clinical outcome in studies of patients with coronary heart disease in which several of the previously described strategies were incorporated into the treatment plan (Allen, 1996; DeBusk et al., 1994; Haskell et al., 1994).

Patient-Centered Counseling

Patient-centered counseling is an intervention developed by Ockene et al. (1999) and is based on provider training in the technique. The counseling approach includes advising the patient about nutrition change, assessing strengths and barriers,

reviewing the patient's food frequency questionnaire that was completed in the waiting room, developing a plan for change, and arranging follow-up. In the trial the intervention took 8 to 10 minutes of the clinic visit time, has been successful in helping patients make dietary behavioral changes, and has potential in primary care settings.

Motivational Interviewing

This is a directive, client-centered counseling style for helping patients examine and resolve ambivalence about behavior change. In settings where time and possibly clinician expertise is limited, an abbreviated version of the technique can be applied. There are four tasks to accomplish in the clinical setting: set an agenda, conduct a quick assessment of motivation and confidence, make a decision and set a target, and exchange information (Emmons & Rollnick, 2001).

EDUCATIONAL STRATEGIES TO IMPROVE ADHERENCE

Didactic, cognitive interventions may be used to transmit information about the disease process or the treatment regimen. Often a behavior change requires educating the patient about the regimen, such as how to follow a low-fat diet or initiate an exercise program. The underlying aim may be to increase the person's knowledge in the expectation that behavior change will follow. However, the association between knowledge and behavior is small (Burke et al., 1998). Educational interventions alone have not yielded positive results (Mullen et al., 1997). Supplementing educational interventions with behavioral strategies increases the effectiveness of the teaching intervention. A list of guidelines for delivering educational interventions is presented in Display 44-3. It is important to incorporate in the intervention the behavioral strategies previously described.

QUESTIONNAIRES RELEVANT TO ADHERENCE-ENHANCING INTERVENTIONS

Most interventions to improve adherence focus on one or more of the constructs of social cognitive theory (i.e., barriers, self-efficacy, or readiness to change). Research has produced several psychometrically sound instruments to measure the constructs that may influence adherence across several behavioral domains, e.g., attitudes and perceived risks and benefits related to blood pressure control and treatment (Hill & Berk, 1995), health behaviors, compliance, and overall satisfaction related to treatment of hypertension (Taneda et al., 2002). Because of their behavioral specificity, self-efficacy scales have been developed for several behavioral domains, including following a general cardiac diet and exercise program (Hickey et al., 1992; Resnick & Jenkins, 2000; Sallis et al., 1988), for adhering to a cholesterol-lowering diet (Burke et al., 1995; McCann et al., 1990), for following a

---

DISPLAY **44–3**

GUIDELINES TO FOLLOW IN DELIVERING EDUCATIONAL INTERVENTIONS

- Keep instructions specific to the activity
- Assess the reading level of material; make sure it is understandable, accurate, and appropriate
- Deliver informational material over time
- Provide verbal instructions in small amounts
- Use printed materials to reinforce verbal instructions
- Provide printed materials in small amounts over time
- Encourage questions of patient and ask patient questions to determine level of comprehension
- Focus on the regimen, not the disease
- Utilize a variety of media formats (videotapes, interactive computer programs, visual illustrations)
- Provide demonstrations to augment verbal instructions
- Provide for return demonstrations and practice opportunities, e.g., mixing medications, taking nitroglycerin, completing diaries, counting pulse
- Utilize community resources, e.g., AHA, local hospital for health classes, cardiac rehabilitation programs
- Provide patients information on additional appropriate resources, e.g., web sites, lay organizations, and lay literature

---

weight-loss diet (Clark et al., 1991; Glynn & Ruderman, 1986), for smoking cessation (Baer et al., 1986), and for medication taking (De Geest et al., 1994). More recently, instruments have been developed that apply the processes of change to risk reduction behavior, including an instrument that measures readiness for change to a low-fat diet (Bowen, 1994) and one to measure future success in smoking cessation (Kristeller et al., 1992). These represent just a few of the self-administered scales that can be used in the clinical or research setting.

■ BUILDING A THERAPEUTIC RELATIONSHIP WITH THE PATIENT

Working with a patient to ensure adequate adherence at the initiation of treatment, and over the long-term either to enhance compliance or to remediate poor adherence, requires good rapport and clear communication lines between the patient and provider. Having a good therapeutic relationship allows ongoing assessment of the patient's adherence and also provides an environment conducive to the patient confiding in the provider when barriers to adherence arise (Burke & Fair, 2003). The patient needs to be queried regularly if he or she has any concerns about the condition or the treatment, and should be commended for seeking and following through on the treatment process.

Listening reflectively to the patient and being supportive can facilitate communication. The provider should try to listen more than talk. Encourage the patient to express problems he or she anticipates having or has encountered in implementing the treatment. Listen with interest. Acknowledge how difficult the new, possibly complex, treatment is and the demands it places on the patient, for example, "I am sure all of this is overwhelming to you. What concerns you the most about your treatment?" Assist the patient to identify barriers to implementing or following the treatment, such as no available time or place where he or she can exercise safely, or, for the patient who needs to quit smoking, a spouse who smokes and has no intentions of quitting. Determine what the patient's view of the treatment is, and clarify what the patient's responsibilities will be in carrying out the treatment. If possible, give priority to the patient's goal in the treatment plan (Burke & Fair, 2003).

When it is time to begin working on the treatment plan, the nurse may begin by acknowledging the challenge, "I know how difficult it is to make changes in long-established eating habits. We are asking you to make changes gradually over time and will work with you in making those changes. What may we do to assist you with this?" and "What would you like to focus on first?" Express confidence in the patient's ability to implement the treatment, and in the treatment having a beneficial effect if it is followed. Assist the patient gradually to assume responsibility for the treatment. Involve the patient in development and implementation of the treatment. Before the close of the session, review with the patient exactly what will be performed: "Now let's go over this plan once more just to make sure I have given you all the information you need. What is the medication you're going to be taking?" Or, to avoid putting the patient in an awkward position: "The name of the drug is . . . Now please tell me how many pills you plan to take and when. Are there any symptoms you should report to us?" In follow-up sessions, acknowledge each time how difficult it is take medications or follow whatever treatment regimen has been recommended (e.g., smoking cessation, dietary change, or regular exercise) and assess how the patient is doing. The nurse may say, "I know it can be difficult to remember to take your pills each time. Do you find that you forget to take your pills sometime?" or "Sometimes when patients feel better, they skip their medications. Do you ever skip taking your pills when you feel good?" A general question may also be asked, such as "Tell me about your medicines and how you are taking them." Ask the patient to go through each medication and describe how many pills are being taken and when. The same general questions can be applied to other behaviors or activities.

An important part of follow-up is providing encouragement and reinforcement. The nurse needs to acknowledge the difficulties the patient faces, but also must be firm regarding the importance of the treatment and continue to instill confidence in the patient. Reinforcement should be given for the behavior change made, not for the clinical outcome. Providing information on clinical outcomes (e.g., blood cholesterol levels) can be an additional reinforcement to the patient, showing the progress he or she has made in changing behavior and its positive effects on health. However, focusing only on the clinical outcomes does not acknowledge the behavioral efforts made by the patient, and moreover, clinical outcomes such as serum cholesterol can be influenced by several intervening variables such as concomitant medications or laboratory changes.

The greatest challenge in compliance is to assist the patient to maintain the behavioral changes for the long-term. As noted previously, there is a decline in adherence during the first year of treatment, with continued erosion over time. This decline is usually accelerated in the absence of any contact with the health care professional. Thus, adherence needs to be addressed at each visit with the previously suggested questions. Slips, lapses, or relapse can be expected and should be prevented when possible. A slip is missing the treatment for a very brief period, e.g., one or two doses of medication missed, a lapse is when the person does not adhere for 3 to 4 days, and a relapse is usually when a person stops following the treatment regimen for at least 1 week. If there is an indication the patient is lapsing, additional attention needs to be provided. It may take the form of periodic telephone contacts and or mail contact. This may include the patient reporting on progress made toward a goal, or the nurse assisting with problem solving in difficult situations, correcting any further problems, providing reinforcement for attempts and progress, and helping the patient set new goals, if appropriate. It may help to have the patient self-monitor behavior for a period and have these records returned before each phone call, or have the patient bring them in at each visit. It is important that these be reviewed and used in pointing out positive behaviors and making suggestions for healthier behaviors (Burke & Fair, 2003; Haynes et al., 2001).

SUMMARY

Inadequate adherence to the recommended treatment plan remains a significant problem facing health care professionals in all settings and populations. Progress has been made in the measurement of adherence and in identifying strategies that may enhance adherence. However, these measurement methods remain limited and often unaffordable (Haynes et al., 2002). Moreover, the intervention strategies are not applied in the clinical setting often enough to significantly affect adherence. Furthermore, the nurse faces additional challenges because of the changing health care environment, including shortened length of hospital stay, increased level of acuity of patients during their hospitalization and at discharge, reduced number of visits after acute events, and increasingly complex treatment regimens that patients need to learn how to implement. However, the nurse is often in the best position to address adherence. As nursing assumes an expanded role in an array of settings, the nurse often assumes responsibility for patient education, ensuring that the patient understands the regimen, and arranging needed follow-up.

Just as the nursing profession has shown leadership in promoting patient education in past decades, and more recently in assuming case-management roles, nursing needs again to take the lead in improving adherence. This requires looking at how health care is provided and determining where in the system interventions need to be directed (i.e., at the level of the provider or system, the treatment regimen, or the patient). Most likely, all three components of the system need to be addressed when making changes to facilitate improved adherence. Moreover, the changes need to be addressed over the continuum of care provision, particularly during the maintenance phase, when nonadherence is most likely to become an issue.

REFERENCES

Allen, J. (1996). Coronary risk factor modification in women after coronary artery bypass surgery. *Nursing Research, 45,* 260–265.

Allison, D. B. (1995). *Handbook of assessment methods for eating behaviors and weight related problems: Measures, theory, and research.* Thousand Oaks, CA: Sage.

American Heart Association. (2003). *Compliance action program.* [Online]. Available: http://www.americanheart.org.

Baer, A., Saroiu, S., & Koutsky, L. A. (2002). Obtaining sensitive data through the Web: an example of design and methods. *Epidemiology, 13*(6), 640–645.

Baer, J. S., Holt, C. S., & Lichtenstein, E. (1986). Self-efficacy and smoking reexamined: Construct validity and clinical utility, *Journal of Consultation and Clinical Psychology, 54,* 846–852.

Bandura, A. (1986a). Self-efficacy. In *Social foundations of thought and action: A social cognitive theory.* Englewood Cliffs, NJ: Prentice-Hall.

Bandura, A. (1986b). *Social foundations of thought and action: A social cognitive theory.* Englewood Cliffs, NJ: Prentice Hall.

Block, G. (1982). A review of validations of dietary assessment methods. *American Journal of Epidemiology, 115,* 492–504.

Block, G. (2001). Invited commentary: another perspective on food frequency questionnaires.[comment]. *American Journal of Epidemiology, 154*(12), 1103–1104; discussion 1105-1106.

Block, G., Hartman, A. M., Dresser, C. M., et al. (1986). A data-based approach to diet questionnaire and testing. *American Journal of Epidemiology, 124,* 453–469.

Bohachick, P., Burke, L. E., Sereika, S., Murali, S., & Dunbar-Jacob, J. (2002). Adherence to angiotensin-converting enzyme inhibitor therapy for heart failure. *Progress in Cardiovascular Nursing, 17*(4), 160–166.

Bowen, D. J., Meischke, H., & Tomoyasu, N. (1994). Preliminary evaluation of the processes of changing to a low-fat diet. *Health Education Research Theory and Practice, 9,* 85–94.

Burke, L., & Fair, J., (in press 2003). Promoting prevention: Skills sets and attributes of health care providers who deliver behavioral interventions. *Journal of Cardiovascular Nursing,.*[AQ1]

Burke, L. E. (2001). Electronic measurement. In L. E. Burke & I. S. Ockene (Eds.), *Compliance in health care and research.* Armonk, NY: Futura Publishing Company, Inc.

Burke, L. E., & Dunbar-Jacob, J. (1995). Adherence to medication, diet, and activity recommendations: From assessment to maintenance. *Journal of Cardiovascular Nursing, 9,* 62–79.

Burke, L. E., Dunbar-Jacob, J., & Hill, M. N. (1997). Compliance with cardiovascular disease prevention strategies: a review of the research. *Annals of Behavioral Medicine, 19*(3), 239–263.

Burke, L. E., Dunbar-Jacob, J., Orchard, T. J. et al. (1998). Is there an association between self-reported dietary adherence and nutrition knowledge? *Annals of Behavioral Medicine, 20*(Suppl), 199.

Burke, L. E., Ewart, C., Thompson P. D. et al. (1995). Psychometric evaluation of the Cholesterol-Lowering Diet Self-Efficacy Scale. *Circulation, 92*(Suppl.), 66.

Carlson, J. J., Johnson, J. A., Franklin, B. A., & VanderLaan, R. L. (2000). Program participation, exercise adherence, cardiovascular outcomes, and program cost of traditional versus modified cardiac rehabilitation. *American Journal of Cardiology, 86*(1), 17–23.

Castro, C. M., King, A. C. (2002). Telephone-assisted counseling for physical activity. *Exercise & Sport Sciences Reviews, 30*(2), 64–68.

Clark, M. M., Abrams, D. B., Niaura, R. S., et al. (1991). Self-efficacy in weight management. *Journal of Consultation and Clinical Psychology, 59,* 739–744.

Connor, S. L., Gustafson, J. R., Sexton, G., et al. (1992). The Diet Habit Survey: A new method of dietary assessment that relates to plasma cholesterol changes. *Journal of the American Dietetic Association, 92,* 41–47.

Cramer, J. A., Mattson, R. H., Prevey, M. L., et al. (1989). How often is medication taken as prescribed? A novel assessment technique. *JAMA, 261,* 3273–3277.

Cramer, J. A., Scheyer, R. D., & Mattson, R. H. (1990). Compliance declines between clinic visits. *Achieve of Internal Medicine, 150,* 1509–1510.

Dawber, T. R., Pearson, G., Anderson, P., et al. (1962). Dietary assessment in the epidemiologic study of coronary heart disease: The Framingham Study. *American Journal of Clinical Nutrition, 11,* 226–234.

De Geest, S., Abraham, I., Gemoets, H., et al. (1994). Development of the long-term medication behaviour self-efficacy scale: Qualitative study for item development. *Journal of Advanced Nursing, 19,* 233–238.

DeBusk, R. F., Miller, N. H., Superko, H. R., et al. (1994). A case management system for coronary risk factor modification after acute myocardial infarction. *Annals of Internal Medicine, 120,* 721–729.

Dew, M. A., Roth, L., Thompson, M. E., et al. (1995). Medical compliance and its predictors in the first year after heart transplantation. *Journal of Heart and Lung Transplantation, 14,* S70.

Dishman, R. K. (1994). *Advances in exercise adherence.* Champaign, IL: Human Kinetics.

Dishman, R. K., Graham, R. E., Buckworth, J., & White-Welkley, J. (2001). Perceived exertion during incremental cycling is not influenced by the Type A behavior pattern. *International Journal of Sports Medicine, 22*(3), 209–214.

Dolocek, T. A., Milas, N. C., Van Horn, L. V., et al. (1986). A long-term nutrition intervention experience: Lipid responses and dietary adherence patterns in the Multiple Risk Factor Intervention Trial. *Journal of the American Dietetic Association, 86,* 752–758.

Dunbar-Jacob, J., Burke, L. E., Rohay, J. M., et al. (1997). How comparable are self-report, pill count, and electronically monitored adherence data? *Circulation, 96*(8 Suppl), I-738.

Dunbar-Jacob, J., & Sereika, S. (2001). Conceptual and methodological problems. In L. A. Burke & I. S. Ockene, (Eds.), *Compliance in health care and research.* Armonk, NY: Futura Publishing Company, Inc.

Dunbar-Jacob, J., Sereika, S., Rohay, J., & Burke, L. (1998). Electronic methods in assessing adherence to medical regimens. In D. S. Krantz (Ed.), *Perspectives in behavioral medicine: Technological and methodological foundation* (pp. 95–113). New Jersey: Erlbaum.

Duncan, G. E., Sydeman, S. J., Perri, M. G., Limacher, M. C., & Martin, A. D. (2001). Can sedentary adults accurately recall the intensity of their physical activity? *Preventive Medicine, 33*(1), 18–26.

D'Zurilla, T. J., & Goldfried, M. R. (1971). Problem solving and behavior modification. *J Abnormal Psychology, 78,* 107–126.

Emmons, K. M., & Rollnick, S. (2001). Motivational interviewing in health care settings. Opportunities and limitations. *American Journal of Preventive Medicine, 20*(1), 68–74.

Evangelista, L., Doering, L., & Dracup, K. (1999). Noncompliance predicts multiple hospital admissions in heart failure patients [abstract]. *Journal of Cardiac Failure, 5*(74).

Fleury, J. (1992). The application of motivational theory to cardiovascular risk reduction. *Image, 24,* 229–239.

Gibson, R. (1990). *Measurement errors in dietary assessment.* New York: Oxford University Press.

Glynn, S. M., & Ruderman, A. J. (1986). The development and validation of an eating self-efficacy scale. *Cognitive Therapeutic Research, 10,* 403–420.

Haskell, W. L., Alderman, E. L., Fair, J. M., et al. (1994). Effects of intensive multiple risk factor reduction on coronary atherosclerosis and clinical cardiac events in men and women with coronary artery disease. *Circulation, 89,* 975–990.

Haynes, R. B. (2001). Improving patient adherence: State of art, with a special focus on medication taking for cardiovascular disorders. In L. E. Burke & I. S. Ockene (Eds.), *Compliance in health care and research.* Armonk, NY: Futura Publishing Company, Inc.

Haynes, R. B., McDonald, H. P., & Garg, A. X. (2002). Helping patients follow prescribed treatment: clinical applications. *JAMA, 288*(22), 2880–2883.

Hickey, M. L., Owen, S. V., & Froman, R. D. (1992). Instrument development: Cardiac diet and exercise self-efficacy. *Nursing Research, 41,* 347–351.

Hill, M. N., Berk, R. A. (1995). Psychological barriers to hypertension therapy adherence: Instrument development and preliminary psychometric evidence. *Cardiovascular Nursing, 31,* 37–43.

Hufford, M. R., & Shiffman, S. (2003). Assessment methods for patient-reported outcomes. *Disease Management and Health Outcomes, 11*(2), 77–86.

Irvine, J., Baker, B., Smith, J., et al. (1999). Poor adherence to placebo or amiodarone therapy predicts mortality: results from the CAMIAT study. Canadian Amiodarone Myocardial Infarction Arrhythmia Trial. *Psychosomatic Medicine, 61*(4), 566–575.

Jackevicius, C. A., Mamdani, M., & Tu, J. V. (2002). Adherence with statin therapy in elderly patients with and without acute coronary syndromes. *JAMA, 288*(4), 462–467.

Jakicic, J. M., Polley, B. A., & Wing, R. R. (1998). Accuracy of self-reported exercise and the relationship with weight loss in overweight women. *Medicine & Science in Sports & Exercise, 30*(4), 634–638.

Jakicic, J. M., Wing, R. R., & Winters-Hart, C. (2002). Relationship of physical activity to eating behaviors and weight loss in women. *Medicine & Science in Sports & Exercise, 34*(10), 1653–1659.

Jakicic, J. M., Winters, C., Lagally, K., et al. (1999). The accuracy of the TriTrac-R3D accelerometer to estimate energy expenditure. *Medicine & Science in Sports & Exercise, 31*(5), 747–754.

Jakicic J. M., W. R., Butler, B. A., et al. (1995). Prescribing exercise in multiple short bouts versus one continuous bout: Effects on adherence, cardiorespiratory fitness, and weight loss in overweight women. *International Journal of Obesity, 19,* 893–901.

Kamarck, T. W., Shiffman, S. M., Smithline, L., et al. (1998). The diary of ambulatory behavioral states: A new approach to the assessment of psychological influences on ambulatory cardiovascular activity. In D. S. Krantz (Ed.), *Perspectives in behavioral medicine: Technological and methodological foundation* (pp. 163–193). New Jersey: Erlbaum.

King, A. C. (1991). Community intervention for promotion of physical activity and fitness. *Exercise & Sport Sciences Reviews, 19,* 211–259.

King, A. C., Oman, R. F., Brassington, G. S., et al. (1997). Moderate-intensity exercise and self-rated quality of sleep in older adults. A randomized controlled trial. *JAMA, 277*(1), 32–37.

Kottke, T. E., Stroebel, R. J., & Hoffman, R. S. (2003). JNC 7- Its more than high blood pressure. *JAMA, 289*(19), 2573–2575.

Kozuki Y., Froelicher E. S. (2003). Lack of awareness and nonadherence in schizophrenia. *Western Journal of Nursing Research, 25*(1), 57–74.

Kriska, A. M., & Caspersen, C. J. (1997). Introduction to a collection of physical activity questionnaires. *Medicine & Science in Sports Exercise, 29,* S5–S9.

Kriska AM, C. C. (1997). Introduction to a collection of physical activity questionnaires. *Medicine & Science in Sports Exercise, 29,* S5–S9.

Kristeller, J. K., Rossi, J. S., Ockene, J. K., et al. (1992). Processes of change in smoking cessation: A cross-validation study in cardiac patients. *Journal of Substance Abuse, 4,* 263–276.

Lichtman, S. W., Pisarska, K., Berman, E. R., et al. (1992). Discrepancy between self-reported and actual caloric intake and exercise in obese subjects.[comment] *New England Journal of Medicine, 327*(27), 1893–1898.

Liden, C. B., Wolowicz, M., Stivoric, J., et al. (2002). Benefits of the SenseWear armband over other physical activity and energy expenditure measurement techniques. White Paper [Online] Available: http://www.bodymedia.com/products/swpro.jsp [Accessed 2003, June 18].

Manson, J. E., & Bassuk, S. S. (2003). Obesity in the United States: a fresh look at its high toll. *JAMA, 289*(2), 229–230.

Marlatt, G. A., & Gordon, J. R. (1980). *Determinants of relapse: Implications for the maintenance of behavior change.* New York: Brunner/Mazel.

Martin, K., Froelicher, E. S., & Miller, N. H. (2000). Women's initiative for nonsmoking (WINS) II: the intervention. *Heart & Lung: Journal of Acute & Critical Care, 29*(6), 438–445.

McCann, B. S., Retzlaff, B. M., Dowdy, A. A., et al. (1990). Promoting adherence to low-fat, low-cholesterol diets: Review and recommendations. *Journal of the American Dietetic Association, 90,* 1408–1414, 1417.

McDermott, M. M., Schmitt, B., & Wallner, E. (1997). Impact of medication nonadherence on coronary heart disease outcomes. A critical review. *Archives of Internal Medicine, 157*(17), 1921–1929.

McDonald, H. P., Garg, A. X., & Haynes, R. B. (2002). Interventions to enhance patient adherence to medication prescriptions: scientific review. *JAMA, 288*(22), 2868–2879.

Miller, N. H., Hill, M., Kottke, T., & Ockene, I. S. (1997). The multilevel compliance challenge: recommendations for a call to action. A statement for health care professionals. *Circulation, 95*(4), 1085–1090.

Moore, S. M., Ruland, C. M., Pashkow, F. J., & Blackburn, G. G. (1998). Women's patterns of exercise following cardiac rehabilitation. *Nursing Research, 47*(6), 318–324.

Morisky, D. E., Green, L. W., Levine, D. M. (1986). Concurrent and predictive validity of a self-reported measure of medication adherence. *Medical Care, 24,* 67–74.

Mullen, P. D., Simons-Morton, D. G., Ramirez, G., et al. (1997). A meta analysis of trials evaluating patient education and counseling for three groups of preventive health behaviors. *Patient Education and Counseling, 32,* 157–173.

Ockene, I., Hayman, L., Pasternak, R., et al. (2002). Task Force 4. Adherence issues and behavioral changes: Achieving a long-term solution. *Journal of the American College of Cardiology, 40*(4), 630–640.

Ockene, I. S., Hebert, J. R., Ockene, J. K., et al. (1996). Effect of training and a structured office practice on physician-delivered nutrition counseling: The Worcester-area trial for counseling in hyperlipidemia (WATCH). *American Journal of Preventive Medicine, 12*(4), 252–258.

Ockene, J. K., Emmons, K. M., Mermelstein, R. J., et al. (2000). Relapse and maintenance issues for smoking cessation. *Health Psychology, 19*(1 Suppl), 17–31.

Pereira, M. A., FitzGerald, S. J., Gregg, E. W., et al. (1997). A collection of physical activity questionnaires for health-related research. *Medicine & Science in Sports Exercise* 29(Suppl.), S1–S205.

Perri, M. G., Anton, S. D., Durning, P. E., et al. (2002). Adherence to exercise prescriptions: effects of prescribing moderate versus higher levels of intensity and frequency. *Health Psychology,* 21(5), 452–458.

Raynor, D. K., Booth, T. G., & Blenkinsopp, A. (1993). Effects of computer generated reminder charts on patients' compliance with drug regimens. *British Medical Journal,* 306, 1158–1161.

Resnick, B., & Jenkins, L. S. (2000). Testing the reliability and validity of the Self-Efficacy for Exercise scale. *Nursing Research,* 49(3), 154–159.

Sallis, J. F., Pinski, R. B., Grossman, R. M., et al. (1988). The development of self-efficacy scales for health-related diet and exercise behaviors. *Health Education Research Theory and Practice,* 3, 283–292.

Shea, S., Misra, D., Ehrlich, M. H., et al. (1992). Correlates of nonadherence to hypertension treatment in an inner-city minority population. *American Journal of Public Health,* 82, 1607–1611.

Smucker, R., Block, G., Coyle, L., et al. (1989). A dietary and risk factor questionnaire and analysis system for personal computers. *American Journal of Epidemiology,* 129, 445–449.

Stone, A. A., & Shiffman, S. (2002). Capturing momentary, self-report data: a proposal for reporting guidelines. *Annals of Behavioral Medicine,* 24(3), 236–243.

Stone, A. A., Shiffman, S., Schwartz, J. E., Broderick, J. E., & Hufford, M. R. (2002). Patient non-compliance with paper diaries. *BMJ,* 324(7347), 1193–1194.

Subar, A. F., Thompson, F. E., Kipnis, V., et al. (2001). Comparative validation of the Block, Willet, and National Institute food frequency questionnaires: the Eating at America's Table Study. *American Journal of Epidemiology,* 154, 1089–1099.

Taneda, K., McDonell, M., & Fihn, S. D. (2002). Evaluation of a questionnaire to monitor patients with hypertension. *Journal of the General Internal Medicine,* 17(Suppl.1), 213–214.

Tate, D. F., Jackvony, E. H., & Wing, R. R. (2003). Effects of Internet behavioral counseling on weight loss in adults at risk for type 2 diabetes: a randomized trial. *JAMA,* 289(14), 1833–1836.

Urquhart, J. (1991). Patient compliance as an explanatory variable in four selected cardiovascular studies. In J. A. Cramer & B. Spilker (Eds.), *Patient compliance in medical practice and clinical trials* (pp. 301–322). New York: Raven Press.

Urquhart, J. (2001). Biological measures. In L. E. Burke & I. S. Ockrene (Eds.), *Compliance in health care and research.* Armonk, NY: Futura Publishing Company, Inc.

Willet, W. (1990). *Nutritional epidemiology.* New York: Oxford University Press.

Willett, W. C., Sampson, L., & Stampfer, M. J. (1985). Reproducibility and validity of a semi-quantitative food frequency questionnaire. *American Journal of Epidemiology,* 122, 51–65.

Wolper, C., Heshka, S., & Heymsfield, S. B. (1995). Measuring food intake: An overview. In D. B. Allison (Ed.), *Handbook of assessment methods for eating behaviors and weight related problems* (pp. 215–240). Thousand Oaks, CA: Sage.

ADDITIONAL READING

Ammerman, A. S., Lindquist, C. H., Lohr, K. N., & Hersey, J. (2002). The efficacy of behavioral interventions to modify dietary fat and fruit and vegetable intake: A review of the evidence. *Preventive Medicine,* 35, 25–41.

Burke, L. E. & Ockene, I. S. (Eds.) (2001). *Compliance in health care and research.* Armonk, NY: Futura Publishing Company

Kahn, E. B., Ramsey, L. T., Brownson, R. C., Health, G. W., Howze, E. H., Powell, K. E., Stone, E. J., Rajab, M. W., Corso, P., & the Task Force on Community Preventive Services. (2002). The effectiveness of interventions to increase physical activity. A systematic review. *American Journal of Preventive Medicine,* 22(4S), 73–107.

Roter, D. L., Hall, J. A., Merisca, R., Nordstrom, B., Cretin, B., & Scarstad, B. (1998). Effectiveness of interventions to improve patient compliance: A meta-analysis. *Medical Care,* 36(8), 1138–1161.

Whitlock, E. P., Orleans, C. T., Pender, N., & Allan, J. (2002). Evaluating primary care behavioral counseling interventions. An evidence-based approach. *American Journal of Preventive Medicine,* 22(4), 267–284.

45

Complementary and Alternative Medicine in Cardiac and Vascular Disease

ELEANOR F. BOND • MARGARET M. HEITKEMPER

People often seek complementary or alternative medicine (CAM) approaches to delay the onset of, slow the progression of, or treat a cardiac or vascular condition, or to promote cardiovascular health. CAM approaches can provide useful adjuncts to health assessment, health promotion, and disease and symptom management. Alternatively, CAM methods can lack specificity or efficacy. In some cases, CAM approaches to cardiovascular health can mask symptoms, alter the efficacy of traditional clinical strategies, evoke unjustified confidence in a course of treatment, or cause new problems. Commonly, the effects of these approaches and the interaction with traditional clinical care have not been well studied and are not fully understood.

It is important that health care providers understand the power and limitations of CAM approaches and integrate this information into their care delivery. It is important that scientists consider CAM issues when they design trials of conventional therapies and that they design studies to clarify the effects of CAM approaches. In the past, conventional health profession schools such as nursing have given insufficient attention to CAM. This pattern is changing as educators, researchers, care providers, and patients become aware of CAM approaches.

In this chapter, CAM therapies are described. Some CAM therapies commonly used in cardiovascular disease are reviewed along with evidence regarding the efficacy, untoward effects, and interaction with conventional treatments. Included are suggestions for assessing a patient's underlying health beliefs and CAM use, and for integrating CAM into clinical nursing management.

CAM DEFINITIONS AND CHARACTERISTICS

CAM refers to healing practices and accompanying theories and belief systems other than those that are part of the local culture's dominant health system (Panel on Definition & Description, 1997). Terms used in discussing such practices include the following:

Allopathic medicine denotes conventional health care approaches as taught in a country's medical and nursing schools.

Alternative medicine approaches are used to replace conventional health practices.

Complementary medicine approaches are those used in conjunction with conventional health practices.

Holistic health care approaches view the patient's physical condition and emotional responses in the context of his environment and support system (family, home, communities). Nursing models are usually holistic.

Integrative medicine combines elements of CAM and allopathic health care.

There is a tendency for treatments to migrate from being considered a complementary or alternative treatment to being classified as a component of allopathic medicine as the approaches are proven effective and gain acceptance. For example, exercise prescriptions, once considered an alternative approach, are now a core element of mainstream clinical management of diabetes mellitus, heart disease, arthritis, cancer-related fatigue, and bone health. In a similar way, cognitive-behavioral therapies, once part of CAM, are now a component of allopathic care, for example, for irritable bowel syndrome.

CAM DOMAINS

The National Institute of Health's National Center for Complementary and Alternative Medicine (NCCAM) describes five major CAM domains. These are listed along with some common examples of therapies within the domain.

1. *Alternative medical systems* include *traditional Chinese medicine* or other types of *Oriental medicine* (involves qi, acupuncture, herbal medicine, oriental massage, qi gong);

Ayurvedic medicine (involves diet, exercise, meditation, herbs, massage, sunlight exposure, controlled breathing to produce inner harmony); *naturopathic medicine* (involves diet/clinical nutrition; homeopathy, acupuncture, herbal medicine, hydrotherapy, spinal and soft-tissue manipulation, therapies using electric currents, ultrasound, and light therapy, therapeutic counseling); and *homeopathic medicine* (involves prescription of minute doses of plant, mineral, or animal materials; based on the notion that "like cures like," i.e., a substance that sickens the well will stimulate innate healing powers to cure a patient presenting a similar disease pattern).

2. *Mind–body interventions* are techniques to facilitate the mind's capacity to affect bodily function and symptoms. Included are *meditation*, some applications of *hypnosis, dance, music, art therapy, prayer and mental healing, biofeedback,* and *yoga.*

3. *Biologically based treatments* include *herbal remedies, special dietary remedies,* and *aromatherapy.*

4. *Manipulative and body-based methods* include *chiropractic manipulation, massage therapy,* and *reflexology.*

5. *Energy therapies* include manipulation of energy fields originating within the body (*biofields*) or those from other sources (*electromagnetic fields*). Included in this category are *acupuncture, Tai Chi, qi gong, Reiki,* and *therapeutic touch.*

PREVALENCE OF CAM

CAM disease prevention and treatment strategies are commonly used. The World Health Organization classifies 65% to 80% of the world's health care services as "alternative medicine" (Kessler et al., 2001; Jonas, 1998). In the United States, it is estimated that 40% of the population uses some form of CAM (Eisenberg et al., 1998; Astin et al., 2000). The number of visits to CAM providers increased by nearly 50% from 425 million visits in 1990 to 629 million visits in 1997. In 1997, approximately 42% of United States health care consumers spent $27 billion on CAM therapies (Kessler et al., 2001; Jonas, 1998).

Many health providers use CAM therapies to manage their own health. Burg and colleagues surveyed conventional health care providers at a major United States health care center regarding their personal use of CAM therapies (1998). Approximately 50% of those responding indicated that they had themselves used one or more CAM therapies. Highest overall use was by allied health professionals, followed by nurses, dentists, pharmacists, and physicians. Fontaine (2000) suggests that nurses' use of CAM therapies is related to the profession's emphasis on self-care.

Several factors have contributed to increased CAM use in the United States and Canada. As the populations age, so increases the incidence of chronic health problems (e.g., arthritis) that are only partially managed by allopathic approaches. Immigration from countries where CAM therapies are common has enhanced North American CAM use. There is a growing trend for United States third-party payers to cover CAM therapies, with state legislatures increasingly mandating this coverage. Patients sometimes express dissatisfaction with what is perceived to be technologically focused allopathic medicine. Patients increasingly value the CAM caregiver approach, which usually involves less emphasis on the issuing of orders and more emphasis on the patient–caregiver relationship. In CAM venues, that relationship is likely to be more like a partnership than a hierarchical association. Thus, CAM approaches may provide the patient with an increased sense of individual responsibility and control over health problems.

Prevalence of CAM Approaches in Cardiovascular Diseases

Several studies describe CAM usage in heart and vascular disease. Foster and colleagues (2000) conducted a randomized household telephone survey in 1997. This revealed that 9% of individuals older than age 65 years used CAM to treat their heart disease; of those with hypertension, 12% used CAM remedies. The study did not specify what types of CAM therapies people used. Wood and colleagues (2003) administered a telephone questionnaire to patents in a Canadian cardiovascular disease registry and found much higher CAM use: 64% of those surveyed used CAM, most commonly herbal remedies and nutritional supplements. Acupuncture was used by 12% of the patients and chiropractic care by 11%. Most cardiac patients were using CAM treatments for cardiac or vascular disease, but some were using the treatments for non-cardiac conditions such as arthritis or psychological symptoms. Patients generally reported they believed that the treatments were safe and proven effective. Most of those surveyed believed that the CAM treatments had improved their health. Another survey revealed that the most commonly used CAM remedies for hypertension were nutritional supplements (coenzyme Q10, vitamin E), the herbal product hawthorn, and relaxation techniques (Eisenberg et al., 1998).

Ai and Bolling (2002) conducted a telephone survey of mixed gender middle-aged and older patients on the day before scheduled cardiac surgery and elicited information about CAM usage. Of 225 patients, more than 80% used CAM. The most common therapies were relaxation techniques, lifestyle/diet modification, megavitamins, spiritual healing, massage, herbal remedies, and imagery. CAM usage was higher in those with more education and in those with better functional status; men and women used CAM equally. Former cigarette smokers, patients with more co-morbidities, and those with heart failure were more likely to use CAM than those with cardiac arrhythmias or co-existing cerebrovascular disease.

ALTERNATIVE MEDICAL SYSTEMS

Alternative systems of medicine, such as traditional Chinese medicine (TCM), ayurvedic medicine (AM), other forms of Oriental medicine, and naturopathic medicine include multiple approaches to maintain or restore cardiovascular health. The following briefly summarizes the general approach taken with some prevalent alternative medicine systems. No studies were found systematically comparing clinical outcomes using an alternative medical system versus an allopathic approach.

However, specific remedies that are part of the alternative medical systems have been studied individually and are discussed in subsequent sections.

Traditional Chinese Medicine (TCM)

TCM has been practiced for thousands of years. TCM relates health to concepts about a person's energy. The practitioner's role is to guide the patient toward restored energy balance and, thus, health. Several types of energy are involved. *Qi* (pronounced *chee*) is the energy of life. In disease, qi is imbalanced. Related to qi are *yin* (associated with cold, moist, internal aspects) and *yang* (associated with heat, dry, external aspects). Yin and yang are constantly interrelated; when imbalanced, illness results (Fig. 45-1). Qi flows along channels called *meridians* (Fig. 45-2). Disease blocks qi flow and upsets the balance between yin and yang. In TCM, *five elements* (water, fire, earth, wood, metal) describe a person's physical and emotional characteristics. TCM assessment involves history taking and physical examination, particularly of the tongue, pulse, and abdomen. Treatments prescribed include *acupuncture,* the inserting of needles at specific points along the meridians to improve qi flow (Fig. 45-3). *Moxibustion* treatments involve holding a burning herb to provide heat along a meridian. *Cupping* treatments involve placing a warmed glass over the skin; as the cup cools, the resulting vacuum pulls blood toward the area. Other TCM treatments include consuming proper foods (*nutrition*), preparing and ingesting Chinese herbs (*herbal medicine*), massaging, and exercising the body through prescribed movements such as qi gong and tai chi. Herbs have energies and are characterized as *yin* or *yang*. Herbs with cold energy treat hot syndromes; herbs with hot energy treat cold syndromes. For example, anemia or weak pulse might be considered a cold syndrome; treatments would warm the blood and strengthen the energy.

Ayurvedic Medicine

Like TCM, AM is thousands of years old. It is commonly practiced in India. In AM, the human body thought to be a replica of the universe and composed of the same basic matter (earth, water, air, fire, ether). Non-material aspects of the person include *Sattva* (consciousness, intelligence), *Rajas* (motion, action), and *Tamas* (inertia resisting motion and action). The goal in AM is to maintain or restore harmony between the individual and cosmic forces. This involves increasing *Sattva* while reducing *Rajas* and *Tamas*. AM involves a holistic approach, with treatments customized to match the individual's characteristics (*Prakruti*). Appropriate food, sleep, and sexual activity are the three pillars of good health in AM. Treatments emphasize mental and physical hygiene and discipline, adherence to moral and spiritual values, massage, exercise, meditation, herbs, sunlight exposure, and controlled breathing to produce inner harmony. Strict adherence to diet (*Yama*) and behavior (*Niyama*) is part of AM. AM treatments sometimes include accessing pressure regions (*Marma*), similar to TCM acupuncture or yoga exercises stressing the ability to bend, flex, extend, and stretch. Physical fitness from the AM viewpoint involves the capacity to withstand heat, cold, hunger, thirst, and fatigue.

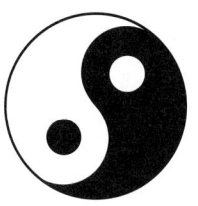

■ **Figure 45–1.** Yin-yang symbol. In traditional Chinese medicine, yin and yang are constantly interrelated forces; disease results when these forces are imbalanced. Yin is associated with cold, moist, internal aspects and yang is associated with heat, dry, external aspects. (From Lewis, S. M., Heitkemper, M. M., & Dirksen, S. R. [2004]. *Medical surgical nursing: Assessment and management of clinical problems* [6th ed.]. St. Louis: Mosby; used with permission.)

Other Oriental Medicine

Other forms of Oriental medicine are practiced in Korea, Japan, and Tibet. Korean medicine includes *Koryo Sooji Chim*, a form of acupuncture in which meridians are mapped on the hand. There is scant information published on the use of this approach in cardiovascular illness.

Naturopathic Medicine

Naturopathy is an alternative medical system developed in the United States. It emphasizes the body's natural healing powers and personal responsibility for prevention and treatment of diseases. Treatments are designed to amplify the natural tendency of the body to heal and eliminate toxins from the body. Therapies involve use of naturally processed foods and herbs; application of heat, water, air, or electricity; physiotherapy, acupuncture, or manipulations; homeopathy; and psychotherapy and counseling. Not included are major surgery, drug prescription, or use of radioactive substances for diagnosis and treatment. Some of the herbal and dietary remedies that a naturopath would prescribe for heart diseases are discussed.

■ MIND–BODY INTERVENTIONS FOR CARDIOVASCULAR DISEASE

Some mind–body interventions are based on a belief that the content of thoughts, beliefs, and emotions can affect physical functioning. Therapies are designed to improve physical functioning by evoking a more positive attitude, for example, using hypnosis or mental healing. Another mind–body approach promotes health by freeing the mind of troubling thoughts or focusing of thought to the exclusion of usual mental patterns. Examples include meditation or yoga, prayer, music, dance, or art therapy. Some mind–body therapies such as biofeedback

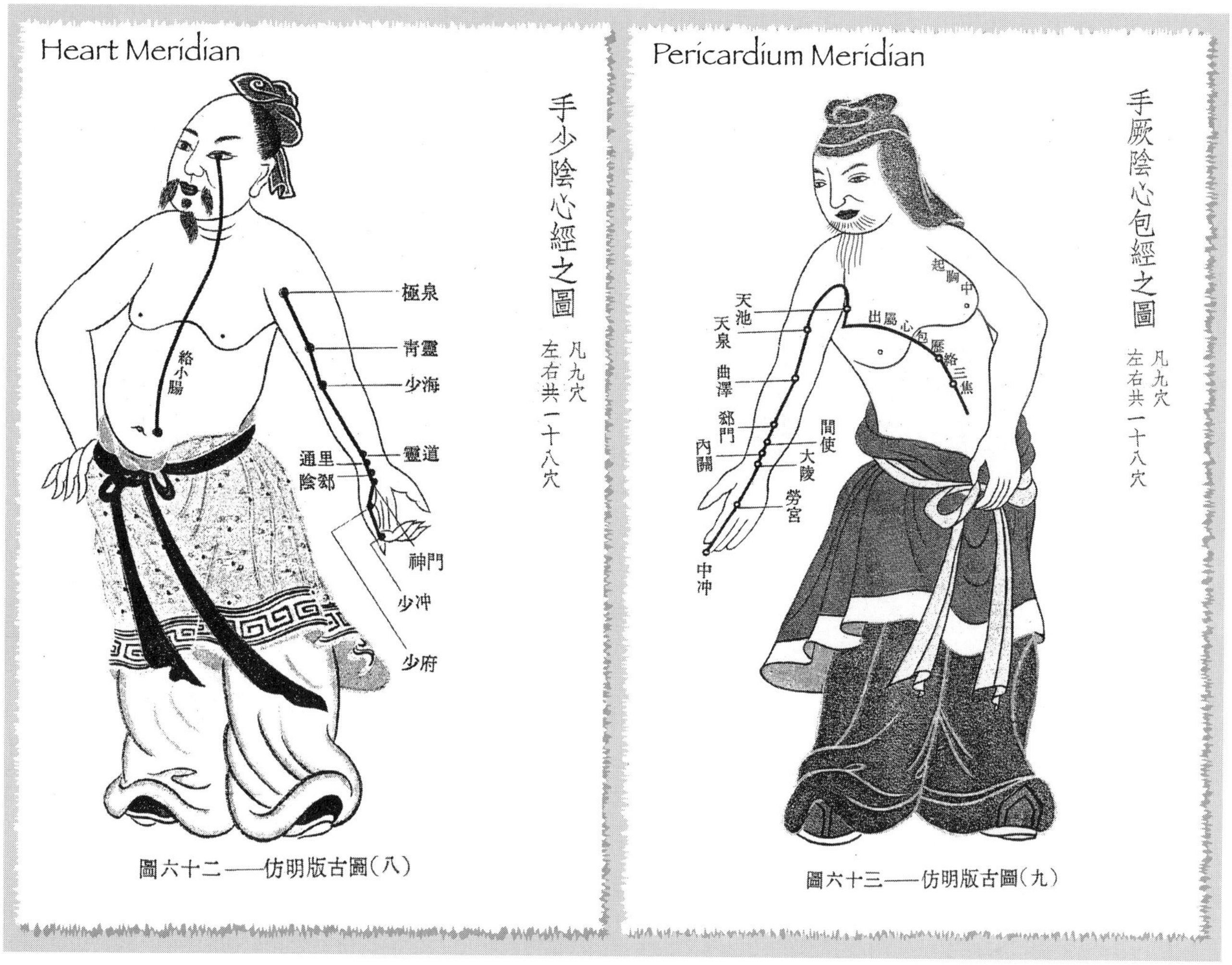

Heart Meridian

手少陰心經之圖

凡九穴
左右共一十八穴

極泉
青靈
少海
靈道
通里
陰郄
神門
少沖
少府

絡小腸

圖六十二——仿明版古圖(八)

Pericardium Meridian

手厥陰心包經之圖

凡九穴
左右共一十八穴

起胸中
出屬心包
歷絡三焦

天池
天泉
曲澤
郄門
內關
間使
大陵
勞宮
中沖

圖六十三——仿明版古圖(九)

■ **Figure 45–2.** Meridian flow chart for the heart and the pericardium. In traditional Chinese medicine, the Oi, or life energy, flows along meridians. Illustrated are meridians associated with the heart (*A*) and pericardium (*B*). (Adapted from Choi, Y. W. [1973]. *The topography of the fourteen meridians.* Pasadena, CA: Cunningham Press; with permission.)

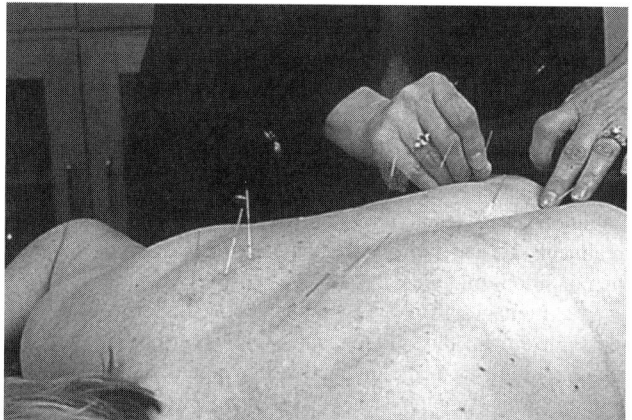

■ **Figure 45–3.** Person receiving acupuncture treatment. (From Lewis, S. M., Heitkemper, M. M., & Dirksen, S. R. [2004]. *Medical surgical nursing: Assessment and management of clinical problems* [6th ed.]. St. Louis: Mosby; used with permission.)

involve teaching the patient to control and regulate physical functioning and reduce stress.

Meditation

There are several types of *meditation*. Generally, meditation involves focusing, centering, and relaxing the mind and body by using techniques such as listening to the breath, repeating a phrase (called a *mantra*), avoiding thought, or focusing thought. Because relaxation reduces the stress response, and because stress is linked with cardiac disease, meditative techniques have sometimes been recommended to reduce heart rate, lower blood pressure, reduce body weight, or improve the lipid profile. However, it is not clear whether meditation has a long-term effect in cardiovascular health. An early meta-analysis by Eisenberg and colleagues (1993) reported that many early meditation studies were poorly controlled and that meditation evoked minimal effects on blood pressure. A study comparing transcendental meditation with an education intervention reported that 3 months of meditation was associated with significant reductions in systolic (women: 10.4 mm Hg; men: 12.7 mm Hg) and diastolic (women: 5.9 mm Hg; men: 8.1 mm Hg) blood pressure (Schneider et al., 1995). However, a nursing study showed that Benson mediation (similar to transcendental mediation) failed to significantly alter blood lipids, weight, or blood pressure in elderly men with hypercholesterolemia when added to a risk reduction program (Carson, 1996). There remains a need for carefully designed studies.

Biofeedback

Biofeedback methods alter acute cardiac parameters such as heart rate, blood pressure, temperature, and health rate variability. However, no comprehensive studies have demonstrated a chronic effect on these parameters on outcomes in cardiovascular patients.

Yoga

The term *yoga* derives from a Sanskrit word meaning to join or unite. Yoga methods include physical and mental disciplines designed to produce unity (e.g., unity of the body with the mind, of the mind with the soul, of the individual with a higher power). This unity is thought to result in a happy, balanced, useful life and possibly improved health. Yoga methods include *Asanas* (yoga postures) (Fig. 45-4), *Pranayamas* (regulated breathing), *Mudras* (hand gestures), and *mantras* (chanted words). Several small studies suggest that that yoga-based techniques can improve cardiac health. Vempati and Telles (2002) studied healthy young adult males and found that yoga activities

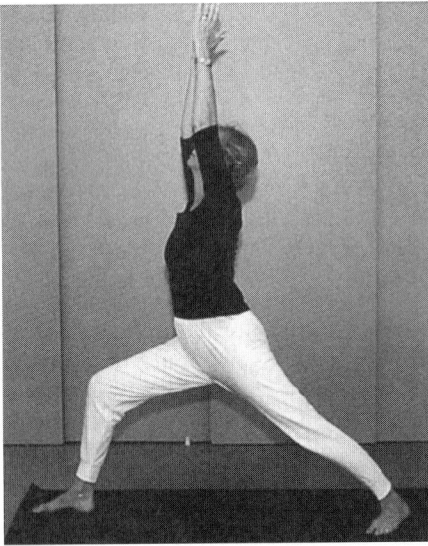

■ **Figure 45–4.** Yoga posture. (From Lewis, S. M., Heitkemper, M. M., & Dirksen, S. R. [2004]. *Medical surgical nursing: Assessment and management of clinical problems* [6th ed.]. St. Louis: Mosby; used with permission.)

were associated with acute reductions in heart rate and sympathetic tone (indicated by changes in heart rate variability). Yoga lifestyle changes have been associated with improved cardiovascular risk factors such as lower body weight, improved lipid profile, and improved blood pressure regulation (Mahajan et al., 1999; Manchanda et al., 2000; Schmidt et al., 97). As with meditation, good experimental studies of yoga are needed but difficult to design.

■ BIOLOGICALLY BASED TREATMENTS

Herbal and special dietary remedies are commonly used for cardiac and vascular disease. Aromatherapy is also considered a biologically based therapy. However, no report was found related to the prevalence or efficacy of aromatherapy for cardiac conditions.

Herbal Remedies

Use of herbal derivatives for heart disease dates to ancient times. Some ancient herbal products such as aspirin, reserpine, digitalis, and caffeine have become mainstays of conventional pharmacotherapy. Two herbal remedies commonly prescribed today include Crataegus oxycantha (hawthorn) and Terminalia arjuna.

Hawthorn. Hawthorn (also known as maybush, maythorn, or may; the formal name is Crataegus oxycantha) is traditionally used as a cardiac tonic. It has been recommended to treat angina, hypertension, hypotension, arrhythmias, heart failure, hyperlipidemia, atherosclerosis, and gastrointestinal symptoms. A poultice of the hawthorn fruit is sometimes used to treat skin lesions. As reviewed in the *Natural Medicines Comprehensive Database*, hawthorn preparations increase myocardial contractile force and lengthen the refractory period. The *Database* notes that hawthorn preparations reduce peripheral vascular resistance (afterload) and thus reduce myocardial oxygen consumption; they may vasodilate coronary vessels, increasing coronary blood flow. Hawthorn's cardiac inotropic properties are possibly caused by phosphodiesterase inhibition or to increasing calcium ion currents into cardiac muscle cells. Hawthorn may reduce lipid levels. It may have antibacterial, spasmolytic, and analgesic effects. Several studies have demonstrated that standardized leaf and flower extract preparations (known as LI 132 or WS 1442) improve ejection fraction, exercise tolerance, and reduce subjective symptoms in patients with New York Heart Association stage II heart failure (Schmidt et al., 1994; Zapfe, 2001). Tauchert (2002) reported that WS 1442, when combined with diuretics, improved exercise tolerance and reduced symptoms in patients with New York Heart Association stage III heart failure. Many of the other alleged uses of hawthorn have not been tested in humans.

Hawthorn should not be taken with drugs and herbs containing cardiac glycosides (i.e., digoxin preparations, black hellebore, Canadian hemp root, digitalis leaf, hedge mustard, figwort, lily of the valley roots, motherwort, oleander leaf, pheasant's eye plant, pleurisy root, squill bulb leaf scales, strophanthus seeds). When taken with digoxin, it increases the chance of digoxin toxicity. It should not be taken with other cardioactive herbs (e.g., calamus, cereus, cola, coltsfoot, devil's claw, European mistletoe, fenugreek, fumitory, ginger, Panax ginseng, white horehound, mate, parsley, quassia, scotch broom flower, shepherd's purse, and wild carrot). If taken with cardioactive drugs, it could amplify or counteract the therapeutic efficacy of those drugs. Side effects reported with hawthorn products include gastrointestinal symptoms, sleep problems, fatigue, rash (particularly on the hands), and palpitations.

Terminalia arjuna Tree Bark. The bark of the terminalia arjuna tree (sometimes called Indian almond) has a long history of use as a cardiac tonic. Two other plants, terminalia chebula and terminalia belerica, are also said to have medicinal properties. Terminalia arjuna has been used in India for more than 3,000 years. Terminalia arjuna is used to treat coronary artery disease, heart failure, and hypercholesterolemia. It has been used for relief of angina pain; also, it is sometimes used as an antibacterial, antimutagen, or aphrodisiac. Related products made from the fruit of terminalia chebula and terminalia belerica are used in AM as a "health harmonizer" or to balance the vital humors. Terminalia chebula is sometimes used to treat veneral disease or is used as a vaginal douche. No large-scale, long-term, well-controlled studies of the efficacy of arjuna in cardiac disease have been published, but there are many small studies. Dwivedi and others conducted small clinical trials in patients with angina, comparing usual care (in this case, nitrates, aspirin, and/or a calcium channel blocker) with and without powdered terminalia arjuna bark for 3 months. Subjects receiving terminalia arjuna bark experienced less angina compared to patients receiving the usual care (Dwivedi & Agarwal, 1994; Dwivedi & Jauhari, 1997). In another small study, patients with severe refractory congestive heart failure (treated with digitalis, diuretics, vasodilators) had reduced symptoms and improved left ventricular function when terminalia arjuna was added to the treatment regimen (Bharani et al., 1995). No studies were found analyzing the efficacy of terminalia arjuna in combination with more recently recommended conventional régimes with demonstrated efficacy in heart failure (i.e., beta-blockers, ACE inhibitors). The mechanism of action for terminalia arjuna is not known. The herb is thought to be relatively safe, but it may increase blood pressure.

Clinical Care Considerations Regarding Herbal Remedies

Patients might use these or any of a large number of other remedies for cardiac and vascular disease. Care providers can refer to the *Natural Medicines Comprehensive Database* web site, http://www.naturaldatabase.com, for up-to-date information about herbal products their patients are using.

It is useful to remember that plant preparations do not have uniform composition of active ingredients. Labeling can be confusing. The concentration of active compounds in a type of plant can vary according to climate, soil conditions, and growing season. Components of the plant such as flowers, leaves, and stems vary in concentration and proportion of active compounds. Extraction methods can produce highly variable concentrations of active ingredients. For example,

hawthorn products are usually described as containing a certain amount (mg) of extract from the plant. The extract can be from flowers or leaves or both. Extractions can be performed using water, ethanol, or methanol; each of these methods results in different quantities and ratios of active ingredients. When Vierling et al. (2003) tested the activity of the various hawthorn extractions on contractility of an aortic strip, the pharmacological effects were remarkably diverse. Thus, it is difficult to standardize a dose of hawthorn. This same problem occurs with many other herbal products. Often herbal products contain multiple ingredients. For example, the *Natural Medicines Comprehensive Database* lists more than 100 patented compounds containing hawthorn, each with variable co-ingredients.

Patients may be consuming herbal products for non-cardiac conditions. These products could have adverse cardiac effects. For example, aconite (sometimes called "chuanwu" or "caowu") is used in TCM to treat neuromuscular and arthritic-related pain conditions. Aconite herb contains diterpenoid alkaloids, which are toxic to neurons and to the heart. Fatal cardiac arrhythmias (bradycardia, hypotension, ventricular tachycardia, supraventricular tachycardia, bi-directional tachycardia, heart block, *torsade de pointes*) have been reported with aconite. There is no known antidote. Atropine may be helpful if there are bradyarrhythmias. Electrical cardioversion tends not to work in aconite poisoning.

Some herbal remedies are associated with drug interactions. For example, several herbs increase the risk of bleeding with anticoagulants. Bleeding has been reported with gingko biloba, garlic, and the Chinese herbs danshen and dong quai. Herbal products can reduce drub absorption. For example, guar gum and psyllium reduce absorption of some pharmaceutical or herbal remedies. Herbs can be contaminated with various active and inactive ingredients. For example, products sometimes contain heavy metals such as lead or chromium, toxins such as fusarium, or microbial elements such as Aspergillus. Because the testing, labeling, and manufacturing regulatory standards are significantly less rigorous with herbal products than with pharmaceutical products, the consumer is not well protected.

The 1994 *Dietary Supplement and Health Act* permits the sale of herbal products that are not toxic as long as they make no claims related to curing conditions. Lacking are regulations that mandate quality control. In 2003, in an attempt to try to improve product purity, potency, and consistency, the United States Food and Drug Administration proposed rules called good manufacturing practices (GMPs) to guide herbal product manufacturing practices. These rules have not been mandated. However, some herbal product manufacturers have adopted voluntary GMPs. US Pharmacopoeia is an independent group that serves as the official standard-setting body for all United States medicines; some herbal manufacturers have sought US Pharmacopoeia certification. Patients can be directed to seek products with the USP logo indicating the product has passed stringent quality-control standards (Fig. 45-5).

Special Dietary Remedies

Fish Oils. Eskimos and some other populations with high dietary intake of omega-3 polyunsaturated fatty acids (O$_3$-PFA)

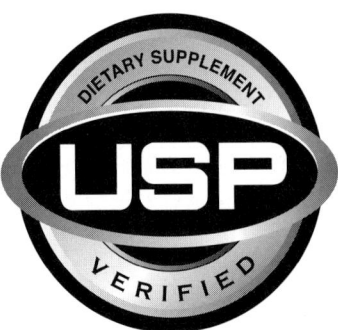

■ **Figure 45–5.** USP logo. This label on a dietary supplement indicates the product in the container has passed the stringent purity, potency, and consistency standards set forth by US Pharmacopeia. (From the US Pharmacopeia website [*http://www.usp-dsvp.org/,* accessed 12 Nov 2003]; used with permission.)

have low rates of heart disease (Rissanen et al., 2000). Dietary sources of O_3-PFAs include fatty fish (especially salmon), flaxseed and flaxseed oil, canola and soybean oil, and certain nuts. Bucher et al. (2002) conducted a meta-analysis of 11 studies comparing dietary or supplemental O_3-PFA to placebo. Subjects in O_3-PFA groups had significantly reduced risk of fatal myocardial infarction (risk ratio 0.7), sudden death (risk ratio 0.7), and all-cause mortality (risk ratio 0.8). A large study known as the *GISSI Trial* was included in the meta-analysis. The GISSI study randomly studied more than 11,000 subjects who had experienced a myocardial infarction within the past 3 months time. Subjects were randomly assigned to one of four groups: fish oil (1 g daily), vitamin E (300 mg daily), both fish oil and vitamin E, or neither. Subjects receiving fish oil had significantly reduced risk of sudden death at 4 months (relative risk 0.47) and at 42 months (Marchioli et al., 2002; GISSI Group, 1999). The fish oil group also had reduced risk of vascular and coronary death beginning at 8 months. Other prospective trials report a similar inverse relationship between fish oil intake and coronary events (Kromhout et al., 1985; Daviglus et al., 1997). In the US Physicians' Health Study of more than 20,000 men, those who consumed more than one fish meal weekly had 52% less risk of sudden death compared with those consuming fish less than once monthly (Albert et al., 2002, 1998).

The mechanism underlying this effect is speculated to be the lowering of serum triglyceride levels; this in turn causes an increase in LDL particle size (Mori et al., 2000; Contacos et al., 1993; Suzukawa et al., 1995). Triglyceride concentration is a determinant of LDL concentration; thus, O_3-PFA is expected to lower LDL as well. In addition to lowering triglycerides, fish oils are reported to have other cardiovascular effects, including reductions in blood pressure, cardiac arrhythmias, and coagulability in patients with hypercholesterolemia (Goodfellow et al., 2000).

Side effects of high levels of fish oil consumption include gastrointestinal effects (nausea, bloating, flatulence, eructation). It has been suggested that fish oil worsens glycemic control in patients with type 2 diabetes mellitus (Vessby &

Boberg, 1990); however, a meta-analysis found that hemoglobin A1C was not adversely affected with fish oil consumption (Farmer et al., 2001). Vitamin E levels decrease with high doses of O_3-PFAs (Schectman et al., 1989; Brown & Wahle, 1990). Some fish oil preparations (e.g., cod liver oil) contain large amounts of fat-soluble vitamins and could cause vitamin A or D toxicity. Fish products may be contaminated with toxins such as mercury or pesticides if the fish were caught in contaminated waters. Mercury is more likely to contaminate fish tissue than fish oil products. Fish oils (as all oils) have a high caloric content and can contribute to weight gain. Because fish oils could possibly lower blood pressure, there is potential for additive effects in patients treated with antihypertensive drugs. Higher-serum fish oil levels were associated with reduced stroke risk in one study (Yamori et al., 1994), but another study suggested that very high dietary fish oil consumption increased the risk of hemorrhagic stroke (Pederson et al., 1999).

Chinese Red Yeast Rice. Chinese red yeast rice, called *Xuezhikang,* is the fermentation product resulting when red yeast (Monascus purpureus) is grown on rice. Ancient documents from the Tang Dynasty (800 AD) describe the product and the ancient Ming Dynasty (1368–1644) pharmacopoeia *Ben Cao Gang Mu* notes that the product evokes mild useful circulatory improvements (Li). The product remains common in the diets of Chinese and Japanese people in Asia and in North America. Animal (Li et al., 1995; Wei et al., 2003) and human studies (Heber et al., 1999) note reductions in serum cholesterol and triacylglycerol concentrations. Heber et al. (1999) conducted a double-blind, repeated measures, random, controlled trial of 46 men and 37 women (ages 34–78 years) with moderate hypercholesterolemia. Half the subjects took 600 mg of red yeast rice in a capsule; the control group took a similar-appearing placebo capsule; all subjects were counseled to consume the American Heart Association Step 1 diet. LDL cholesterol and triacylglycerol were significantly reduced in the test group (by approximately 16% and 7%, respectively) compared with the placebo control group; HLD cholesterol did not change. Improvements were noted at 8 weeks and sustained through the end of the experiment at 12 weeks. Several subjects in the placebo group noted adverse effects (headaches, pneumonia, rash); one test subject noted chest pain. None of the subjects had abnormal liver or renal function studies during the trial (although these complications are reported for Chinese red yeast rice). The menopausal status of the women was not discussed, nor were results separated for men versus women. Because ovarian hormone state is known to affect lipid metabolism, studies are needed explicating the interaction of this dietary component with ovarian hormone status.

Chinese red yeast rice contains various monacolins (including monacolin K, also known as lovastatin, a HMG-CoA reductase inhibitor that is an allopathic drug prescribed to lower serum cholesterol). Also present in Chinese red yeast rice are sterols, isoflavone glycosides, and monounsaturated fatty acids. It is likely that the cholesterol-lowering effects are caused by multiple active ingredients, not just the monacolin K. In the Heber et al. (1999) study, the monacolin K concentration consumed by the test group was lower than in clinical trials of lovastatin alone (Downs et al., 1998), yet the lipid reductions were almost as large. This could suggest that other ingredients in Chinese red yeast rice contribute to its therapeutic effect. More studies are needed to determine the efficacy, mechanism, and safety of the Chinese red yeast rice effects.

Many precautions are needed if the patient is taking Chinese red yeast rice. Side effects associated with oral consumption of Chinese red yeast rice include gastrointestinal symptoms and elevated liver enzymes (Robbers et al., 1999); anaphylaxis has been reported after inhalation (Wigger-Alberti et al., 1999). Because they have a similar chemical composition, Chinese red yeast rice has a potential to cause the same side effects and drug interactions that are associated with HMG-CoA reductase drugs such as lovastatin. Similar to lovastatin, rhabdomyolysis has been reported with Chinese red yeast rice (Prasad et al., 2002). The effects of Chinese red yeast rice and HMG-CoA reductase-inhibiting drugs could be additive. It is well known that grapefruit products can increase the serum levels of lovastatin by inhibiting the cytochrome P450-based drug metabolism (Kantola et al., 1998); the same is likely to be true of Chinese red yeast rice. Incorrect fermentation can result in the presence of citrinin (nephrotoxin) in Chinese red yeast rice products (Heber et al., 2001). The American Heart Association cautions against using Chinese red yeast rice pending the results of long-term studies (American Heart Association, 1999).

Garlic. Garlic is used to treat a various cardiac and vascular conditions, but there is controversy about its effectiveness. Some studies have shown that garlic reduces hyperlipidemia, but other studies have shown no benefit (Isaacsohn et al., 1998; Berthold et al., 1998). In a meta-analysis of 45 randomized clinical trials, Stevinson and colleagues (2000) concluded that when used for 4 to 25 weeks, garlic usually lowers total cholesterol levels by 4% to 12%. However, the six studies judged to be the most rigorous failed to show a significant difference between the garlic and placebo groups. By comparison, "statin" drugs typically decrease cholesterol levels by 17% to 32%. Garlic's antihyperlipidemic effects are possibly caused by a component of garlic (S-allyl cysteine), likely an HMG-CoA reductase inhibitor (Yeh & Liu, 2001; Gebhardt & Beck, 1996). HMG-CoA reductase inhibitors inhibit hepatic cholesterol synthesis; statin-type drugs and Chinese red yeast rice act via a similar mechanism.

Garlic is sometimes used for hypertension. There is some evidence that garlic can modestly reduce blood pressure by 2% to 7% after 4 weeks of treatment (Silagy & Neil, 1998). This effect is thought to be caused by nitric oxide release, which relaxes smooth muscle, causing vasodilatation.

Garlic is sometimes used as an anticoagulant (Rahman & Billington, 2000; Chutani & Bordia, 1981). Other alleged medicinal properties of garlic are as an antifungal, antibacterial, anthelmintic, antiviral, antispasmodic, diaphoretic, expectorant, and immunostimulant. These effects are not proven (*Natural Medicines Comprehensive Database*).

It is difficult to compare studies of garlic and to achieve consistent dosing. There are several active ingredients present; it is not always clear which component might induce a therapeutic effect. Because some components are more labile than others, this issue complicates clinical trials and treatment recommendations. Garlic's pharmacological properties are attributed to organosulfur compounds, particularly allicin and ajoene. Alliin is an odorless compound in the garlic bulb. When the bulb is crushed, the cells release an enzyme called allinase. Allinase converts alliin to the unstable, odiferous compound, allicin, and then to ajoene. The compounds present in a garlic preparation depend on how the products are prepared. Processes that macerate the garlic clove increase allinase activity. Freeze-dried garlic may contain little or no allicin. Gastric acids may degrade products without enteric coating before the active ingredients are absorbed. When heat and steam distillation are used to produce garlic oil from crushed garlic, allicin is converted to less biologically active allyl sulfides. Garlic is sometimes aged to reduce the content of sulfur compounds and the odor commonly associated with garlic. However, the process of producing odorless aged garlic extract reduces the alliin content to only 3% of what is typically contained in fresh garlic. Aged garlic extract is usually standardized to S-allylcysteine, another major organosulfur constituent in garlic, but this is not the compound thought to be the most biologically active. All these factors make it difficult to know what dose of garlic the patient is receiving.

Garlic is associated with noxious breath and body odor; it can burn the skin and irritate the gastrointestinal track. Garlic's effects could be additive with warfarin. Patients taking cyclosporine are advised to avoid garlic because it may activate the liver enzyme (cytochrome P450 3A4), which metabolizes cyclosporine (Piscitelli et al., 2002). Other drugs that are potentially affected by this mechanism include some calcium channel blockers (diltiazem, nicardipine, verapamil), chemotherapeutic agents (etoposide, paclitaxel, vinblastine, vincristine, vindesine), antifungals (ketoconazole, itraconazole), glucocorticoids, alfentanil (Alfenta), cisapride (Propulsid), fentanyl (Sublimaze), lidocaine (Xylocaine), losartan (Cozaar), fexofenadine (Allegra), midazolam (Versed), the protease inhibitor saquinavir, and others.

Flaxseed. Whole flaxseed has been linked with lowered serum cholesterol in subjects without (Cunnane et al., 1993, 1995) and with hypercholesterolemia (Bierenbaum et al., 1993; Jenkins et al., 1999). Flaxseed products can be used for non-cardiac uses, for example, as a laxative for constipation and for arthritis, cancer, anxiety, benign prostatic hyperplasia (BPH), vaginitis, weight loss, and dry eyes. Flaxseed oil contains alpha-linolenic, linoleic, and oleic acids. Linoleic acid and alpha-linolenic acid are required to maintain cell membrane structure. Alpha-linolenic acid raises serum O_3-PFAs, associated with lower incidence of cardiac disease and improved outcomes in cardiac patients (Prasad, 1997). Flaxseed oil might decrease platelet aggregation (Allman et al., 1995; Prasad, 1997). Linoleic acid is an omega-6 fatty acid; it possibly reduces the risk of ischemic stroke (Iso et al., 2002). Flaxseed oil may have antiinflammatory effects; this in turn could slow the progression of coronary vascular disease. Alpha-linolenic acid suppresses production of interleukin-1, tumor necrosis factor, leukotriene B4, and oxygen free radicals by polymorphonuclear leukocytes and monocytes (Prasad, 1997). Alpha-linolenic acid from flaxseed oil might have anti-tumor effects.

Coenzyme Q10. Coenzyme Q10 is a fat-soluble vitamin-like compound occurring naturally in the heart, liver, pancreas, and kidney. Some foods such as soybean oil contain the compound. Commercial preparations are made from fermented beets, sugar cane, and yeast. Coenzyme Q10 has antioxidant properties and serves as a co-factor in some metabolic cycles; it contributes to ATP production. It is used extensively in Japan, Europe, and Russia to treat cardiovascular diseases including heart failure, angina, hypertension, and Adriamycin-induced cardiotoxicity. Several studies suggest that coenzyme Q10 in combination with conventional therapy improves quality of life, improves symptoms such as dyspnea, edema, and insomnia, and decreases the number of hospitalizations in patients with New York Heart Association class II–IV heart failure (Morisco et al., 1993; Hofman-Bang, et al., 1995). Other studies found no effect on exercise tolerance or on ejection fraction (Mortenson, 2000). Coenzyme Q10 may enhance the efficacy of antihypertensives in lowering blood pressure (Singh et al., 1999). Coenzyme Q10 may be most effective when endogenous levels are low, as they are in some types of heart failure. It is also recommended for some non-cardiac diseases including Huntington disease, Parkinson disease, chronic fatigue syndrome, alopecia, and topically for periodontal infection. Coenzyme Q10 is generally thought to be safe; side effects, which include gastrointestinal symptoms, are minimal. It should be used cautiously in combination with pharmaceutical antihypertensives because the effects can be additive.

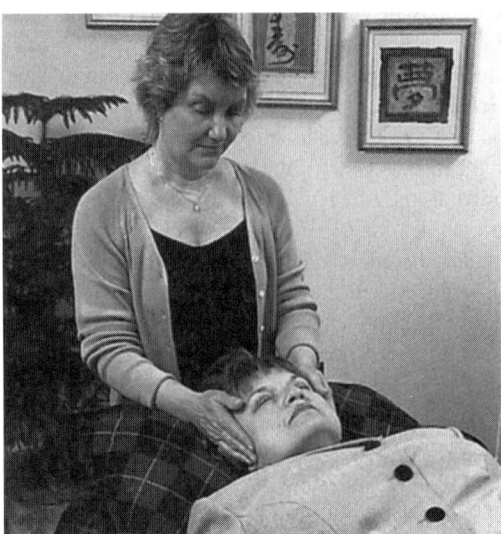

■ **Figure 45–6.** Therapeutic touch. (From Lewis, S. M., Heitkemper, M. M., & Dirksen. S. R. [2004]. *Medical surgical nursing: Assessment and management of clinical problems* [6th ed.]. St. Louis: Mosby; used with permission.)

MANIPULATIVE AND BODY-BASED METHODS AND ENERGY THERAPIES

In theory, manipulative and body-based methods and energy therapies (e.g., chiropractic manipulation, massage therapy, Reiki, qi gong, therapeutic touch) could improve cardiac disease by promoting relaxation and blunting stress responses. There have not been large-scale trials of these approaches, although a recent study probed the feasibility of such a study of chiropractic adjustments and massage (Plaugher et al., 2002). Tai chi–qi gong, a type of energy therapy, has been prescribed as a low-impact exercise in cardiac rehabilitation; it is equivalent to approximately 3 METS (Chao et al., 2002). Acupuncture is another form of energy therapy; it may be helpful in reducing blood pressure in patients with hypertension (Guo & Ni, 2003). Acupuncture is associated with risk of transmission of infectious diseases, including hepatitis, HIV, and AIDS.

Healing touch is a non-verbal communication technique, a mechanism used by care providers to be present in the moment with a patient who is experiencing physical or psychological pain. Nurses with specialized training sometimes practice this form of energy therapy (Fig 45-6). Healing touch could potentially improve the provider–patient relationship, promote relaxation, reduce the stress response, or alter cardiac variables. More studies are needed of the efficacy in cardiac diseases.

LEGAL ASPECTS OF CAM

Most forms of CAM require specialized training and licensure. Naturopathy, traditional Chinese medicine, acupuncture, homeopathy, and chiropractic medicine all require years of training. Other therapies such as massage therapy, Reiki, therapeutic touch, and yoga require some, but less, extensive training. License regulations vary from state to state. Nurses who are making referrals or assisting patients to evaluate various treatment approaches should become familiar with the state regulatory statutes.

INTEGRATION OF CAM INTO NURSING ASSESSMENT AND CLINICAL MANAGEMENT

Structured Approach to Assessing CAM Use and Underlying Health Beliefs

It is important to specifically query patients regarding their CAM usage. Metz et al. (2001) evaluated the intake interviews of 196 cancer patients. Each patient received a standard history and physical including queries about over-the-counter treatments. After completion of the usual interview, patients were asked explicit questions about use of CAM treatments. Although only 13 patients (6.6%) initially disclosed CAM treatments; after directed questioning, an additional 66 patients (36%) disclosed CAM treatments. Thus, CAM usage should be integrated into the health interview rather than relying on the patient to initiate it. The nurse or health care provider should approach the interview with an attitude of being willing to learn from the patient as well as being able to teach. The nurse should proceed in an open, non-judgmental fashion, avoiding terms that suggest disapproval, such as "unproven." The nurse should ask the patient how well the remedy has worked or not worked before stating an opinion. It may be appropriate to ask the patient's permission to coordinate with the other therapists. Some suggested questions are as follows:

1. What are your values and beliefs related to health and illness?
2. Are there health practices that are part of your cultural, spiritual, or religious beliefs?
3. What therapies have you used to maintain or improve your health?
4. Have you consulted with or been treated by a naturopathic, acupuncturist, or homeopathic provider? (Elicit specific details.)
5. Have you consulted with any specialized healers, such as practitioners of Oriental medicine or Native American healing practices?
6. Do you meditate or practice yoga or tai chi?
7. Have you used any herbal treatments?
8. Have you tried any dietary modifications such as increasing your consumption of vitamins or fish oils?
9. Have you consulted with a chiropractor or massage therapist?
10. Do you use magnets or crystals to alter your health status?
11. Why did you select this approach?
12. What is your attitude toward conventional medical care?

Nursing Management Related to CAM

Some CAM approaches are within the scope of nursing practice and can be integrated into the plan of care. Massage, relaxation therapy, or music therapy may be useful adjuncts to the care plan. Nurses conduct most Reiki and therapeutic touch treatments. As with any procedure, the nurse should acquire training in the correct applications of the procedure, review the evidence that the therapy is useful, devise a means to evaluate the efficacy of the treatment, and act in conjunction with the institutional protocols and procedures. There is considerable need for patient education in regard to CAM approaches. Patients often use products or approaches that they learn about from lay people, the World Wide Web, or television advertisements. The nurse can assist the patient with understanding the risks and benefits of a particular treatment approach. Also, the nurse can assist patients to identify licensed and certified providers of therapies.

SUMMARY

It is critical that practitioners understand CAM and the interaction of CAM and conventional medicine and nursing. The widespread and increasing use of CAM by the consuming public amplifies the imperative for health care professionals to become familiar with the range of CAM care options and the roles they play in health promotion, clinical assessment, and management. Unfortunately, nursing curricula have not been inclusive with regard to CAM therapies. The implications of this breach in preparation of direct care providers have obvious

consequences in the care delivered to patients. At the same time, there is a clear need for greater research related to the effectiveness of CAM practices either as sole therapies or as adjuvant therapies in disease prevention and management.

REFERENCES

Ai, A. L., & Bolling, S. F. (2002). The use of complementary and alternative therapies among middle-aged and older cardiac patients. *American Journal of Medical Quality,* 17(1), 21–7.

Albert, C. M., Campos, H., Stampfer, M. J., Ridker, P. M., Manson, J. E., & Willett, W. C., et al. (2002). Blood levels of long-chain n-3 fatty acids and the risk of sudden death. *New England Journal of Medicine,* 346, 1113–8.

Albert, C. M., Hennekens, C. H., O'Donnell, C. J., Ajani, U. A., Carey, V. J., Willett, W. C., et al. (1998). Fish consumption and risk of sudden cardiac death. *JAMA,* 279(1), 23–8.

Allman, M. A., Pena, M. M., & Pang, D. (1995). Supplementation with flaxseed oil versus sunflower seed oil in healthy young men consuming a low fat diet: effects on platelet composition and function. *European Journal of Clinical Nutrition,* 49(3), 169–178.

American Heart Association. Comment: the Am Heart Assn urges caution on cholestin. http://www.americanheart.org/presenter.jhtml?identifier=2925. (Accessed 12 July 2003).

Astin, J. A., Pelletier, K. R., Marie, A., & Haskell, W. L. (2000). Complementary and alternative medicine use among elderly persons: one-year analysis of a Blue Shield Medicare supplement. *Journal of Gerontology A Biological Science and Medical Science,* 55(1), M4–M9.

Berthold, H. K., Sudhop, T., & von Bergmann, K. (1998). Effect of a garlic oil preparation on serum lipoproteins and cholesterol metabolism. *JAMA,* 279(23), 1900–1902.

Bharani, A., Ganguly, A., & Bhargava, K. D. (1995). Salutary effect of Terminalia Arjuna in patients with severe refractory heart failure. *International Journal of Cardiology,* 49(3), 191–9.

Bierenbaum, M. L., Reichstein, R., & Watkins, T. R. (1993). Reducing atherogenic risk in hyperlipemic humans with flaxseed supplementation: a preliminary report. *Journal of the American College of Nutrition,* 12(5), 501–4.

Brown, J. E., & Wahle, K. W. (1990). Effect of fish oil and vitamin E supplementation on lipid peroxidation and whole blood aggregation in man. *Clinial Chim Acta,* 193, 147–56.

Bucher, H. C., Hengstler, P., Schindler, C., & Meier, G. (2002). N-3 polyunsaturated fatty acids in coronary heart disease: A meta-analysis of randomized controlled trials. *American Journal of Medicine,* 112, 298–304.

Burg, M. A., Kosch, S. G., Neims, A. H., & Stoller, E. P. (1998). Personal use of alternative medicine therapies by health science center faculty. *JAMA,* 280(18), 1563.

Carson, M. A. (1996). The impact of a relaxation technique on the lipid profile. *Nursing Research,* 45, 271–6.

Chao, Y. F., Chen, S. Y., Lan, C., & Lai, J. S. (2002). The cardiorespiratory response and energy expenditure of Tai-Chi-Qui-Gong. *American Journal of Chinese Medicine,* 30(4), 451–61.

Chutani, S. K., & Bordia, A. (1981). The effect of fried versus raw garlic on fibrinolytic activity in man. *Atherosclerosis,* 38, 417–421.

Contacos, C., Barter, P. J., & Sullivan, D. R. (1993). Effect of pravastatin and omega-3 fatty acids on plasma lipids and lipoproteins in patients with combined hyperlipidemia. *Arteriosclerosis Thrombosis,* 13, 1755–62.

Cunnane, S. C., Ganguli, S., Menard, C., Liede, A. C., Hamadeh, M. J., & Chen, Z. Y., et al. (1993). High alpha-linolenic acid flaxseed (Linum usitatissimum): some nutritional properties in humans. *British Journal of Nutrition,* 69, 443–53.

Cunnane, S. C., Hamadeh, M. J., Liede, A. C., Thompson, L. U., Wolever, T. M., & Jenkins, D. J. (1995). Nutritional attributes of traditional flaxseed in healthy young adults. *American Journal of Clinical Nutrition,* 61, 62–68.

Daviglus, M. L., Stamler, J., Orencia, A. J., Dyer, A. R., Liu, K,. & Greenland, P., et al. (1997). Fish consumption and the 30-year risk of fatal myocardial infarction. *New England Journal of Medicine,* 336(15), 1046–1053.

Downs, J. R., Clearfield, M., Weis, S., Whitney, E., Shapiro, D. R., & Beere, P. A., et al. (1998). Primary prevention of acute coronary events with lovastatin in men and women with average cholesterol levels: results of AFCAPS/TexCAPS. Air Force/Texas Coronary Atherosclerosis Prevention Study. *JAMA,* 279(20), 1615–1622.

Dwivedi, S., & Agarwal, M. P. (1994). Antianginal and cardioprotective effects of Terminalia arjuna, an indigenous drug, in coronary artery disease. *Journal of the Association of Physicians of India,* 42(4), 287–289.

Dwivedi, S., & Jauhari, R. (1997). Beneficial effects of Terminalia arjuna in coronary artery disease. *Indian Heart Journal,* 49(5), 507–510.

Eisenberg, D. M., Davis, R. B., Ettner, S. L., Appel, S., Wilkey, S., Van Rompay, M., et al. (1998). Trends in alternative medicine use in the United States, 1990-1997. *JAMA,* 280, 1569–1575.

Eisenberg, D. M., Delbanco, T. L., Berkey, C. S., Kaptchuk, T. J., Kupelnick, B., Kuhl, J., et al. (1993). Cognitive behavioral techniques for hypertension: are they effective? *Annals of Internal Medicine,* 118, 964–972.

Farmer, A., Montori, V., Dinneen, S., & Clar, C. 2001. Fish oil in people with type 2 diabetes mellitus. *Cochrane Database Systematic Review,* 3, CD003205.

Fontaine, K. L. (2000). *Healing practices, alternative practices for nursing.* Upper Saddle River, NJ: Prentice Hall.

Foster, D. F., Phillips, R. S., Hamel, M. B., & Eisenberg, D. M. (2000). Alternative medicine use in older Americans. *Journal of the American Geriatric Society,* 48(12), 1560–1565.

Gebhardt, R., & Beck, H. (1996). Differential inhibitory effects of garlic-derived organosulfur compounds on cholesterol biosynthesis in primary rat hepatocyte cultures. *Lipids,* 31, 1269–1276.

GISSI Group (Gruppo Italiano per lo Studio della Sopravvivenza nell'Infarto miocardico). (1999). Dietary supplementation with n-3 polyunsaturated fatty acids and vitamin E after myocardial infarction: results of the GISSI-Prevenzione trial. *Lancet,* 354, 447–455.

Goodfellow, J., Bellamy, M. F., Ramsey, M. W., Jones, C. J., & Lewis, M. J., et al. (2000). Dietary supplementation with marine omega-3 fatty acids improve systemic large artery endothelial function in subjects with hypercholesterolemia. *Journal of the American College of Cardiology,* 35, 265–270.

Guo, W., & Ni, G. (2003). The effects of acupuncture on blood pressure in different patients. *Journal of Traditional Chinese Medicine,* 23(1), 49–50.

Heber, D., Lembertas, A., Lu, Q. Y., Bowerman, S., & Go, V. L. (2001). An analysis of nine proprietary Chinese red yeast rice dietary supplements: implications of variability in chemical profile and contents. *Journal of Alternative and Complement Medicine,* 7, 133–139.

Heber, D., Yip, I., Ashley, J. M., Elashoff, D. A., Elashoff, R. M., & Go, V. L. (1999). Cholesterol-lowering effects of a proprietary Chinese red-yeast-rice dietary supplement. *American Journal of Clinical Nutrition,* 69, 231–236.

Hofman-Bang, C., Rehnqvist, N., Swedberg, K., Wiklund, I., & Astrom, H. (1995). Coenzyme Q10 as an adjunctive treatment of congestive heart failure. *Journal of Cardiac Failure,* 1, 101–107.

Isaacsohn, J. L., Moser, M., Stein, E. A., Dudley, K., Davey, J. A., Liskov, E., et al. (1998). Garlic powder and plasma lipids and lipoproteins, a multicenter, randomized, placebo-controlled trial. *Archives of Internal Medicine,* 158, 1189–1194.

Iso, H., Sato, S., Umemura, U., Kudo, M., Koike, K., & Kitamura, A., et al. (2002). Linoleic acid, other fatty acids, and the risk of stroke. *Stroke,* 33(8), 2086–2093.

Jenkins, D. J., Kendall, C. W. C, Vidgen, E., Agarwal, S., Rao, A. V., & Rosenberg, R. S., et al. (1999). Health aspects of partially defatted flaxseed, including effects on serum lipids, oxidative measures, and ex vivo androgen and progestin activity: a controlled, crossover trial. *American Journal of Clinical Nutrition,* 69, 395–402.

Jonas, W. B. (1998). Alternative medicine–learning from the past, examining the present, advancing to the future. *JAMA,* 280(18), 1616–1618.

Kantola, T., Kivisto, K. T., & Neuvonen, P. J. Grapefruit juice greatly increases serum concentrations of lovastatin and lovastatin acid. *Clinical Pharmacological Therapy,* 1998 63, 397–402.

Kessler, R. C., Davis, R. B., Foster, D. F., Van Rompay, M. I., Walters, E. E., Wilkey, S. A., et al. (2001). Long-term trends in the use of complementary and alternative medical therapies in the United States. *Annals of Internal Medicine,* 135(4), 262–268.

Kromhout, D., Bosschieter, E. B., & de Lezenne Coulander, C. (1985). The inverse relation between fish consumption and 20-year mortality from coronary heart disease. *New England Journal of Medicine,* 312(19), 1205–1209.

Li, C., Zhu, Y., Wang, Y., Jia-Shi, Z., Chang, J., & Kritchevsky, D. (1995). Monascus purpureus-fermented rice (red yeast rice): a natural food product that lowers blood cholesterol in animal models of hypercholesterolemia. *Nutrition Research,* 18, 71–81.

Li, S. (1973). *Ben cao gang mu.* (English: *Chinese medicinal herbs.*) Translated and researched by F. Porter Smith and G. A. Stuart. San Francisco: Georgetown Press.

Mahajan, A. S., Reddy, K. S., & Sachdeva, U. (1999). Lipid profile of coronary risk subjects following yogic lifestyle intervention. *Indian Heart Journal,* 51(1), 37–40.

Manchanda, S. C., Narang, R., Reddy, K. S., Sachdeva, U., Prabhakaran, D., Dharmanand, S., et al. (2000). Retardation of coronary atherosclerosis with yoga lifestyle intervention. *Journal of the Association of Physicians of India,* 48(7), 687–694.

Marchioli, R., Barzi, F., Bomba, E., Chieffo, C., Di Gregorio, D., & Di Mascio, R., et al. (2002). Early protection against sudden death by n-3 polyunsaturated fatty acids after myocardial infarction: time-course analysis of the results of the Gruppo Italiano per lo Studio della Sopravvivenza nell'Infarto Miocardico (GISSI)-Prevenzione. *Circulation,* 105, 1897–1903.

Metz, J. M., Jones, H., Devine, P., Hahn, S., & Glatstein, E. (2001). Cancer patients use unconventional medical therapies far more frequently than standard history and physical examination suggest. *Cancer Journal,* 7(2), 149–154.

Mori, T. A., Burke, V., Puddey, I. B., Watts, G. F., O'Neal, D. N., Best, J. D., et al. (2000). Purified eicosapentaenoic and docosahexaenoic acids have differential effects on serum lipids and lipoproteins, LDL particle size, glucose, and insulin in mildly hyperlipidemic men. *American Journal of Clinical Nutrition,* 71, 1085–1094.

Morisco, C., Trimarco, B., & Condorelli, M. (1993). Effect of coenzyme Q10 therapy in patients with congestive heart failure: A long-term, multicenter, randomized study. *Clinical Investigation,* 71(Suppl 8), S134–S136.

Mortensen, S. A. (2000). Coenzyme Q10 as an adjunctive therapy in patients with congestive heart failure. *Journal of the American College of Cardiology,* 36, 304–305.

National Center for Complementary and Alternative Medicine. Major Domains of Complementary and Alternative Medicine. http://nccam.nih.gov/fcp/classify/ (accessed 6/2003).

Natural Medicines Comprehensive Database. http://www.naturaldatabase.com. Accessed 6/1/2003.

Panel on Definition and Description, CAM Research Methodology Conference. (1997). Defining and describing complementary and alternative medicine. *Alternative Therapy and Health Medicine,* 3, 49–57.

Pedersen, H. S., Mulvad, G., Seidelin, K. N., Malcom, G. T., & Boudreau, D. A. (1999). N-3 fatty acids as a risk factor for haemorrhagic stroke. *Lancet,* 353, 812–813.

Piscitelli, S. C., Burstein, A. H., Welden, N., Gallicano, K. D., & Falloon, J. (2002). The effect of garlic supplements on the pharmacokinetics of saquinavir. *Clinics in Infectious Disease,* 34, 234–238.

Plaugher, G., Long, C. R., Alcantara, J., Silveus, A. D., Wood, H., Lotun, K., et al. (2002). Practice-based randomized controlled-comparison clinical trial of chiropractic adjustments and brief massage treatment at sites of subluxation in subjects with essential hypertension: pilot study. *Journal of Manipulative Physiological Therapy,* 25(4), 221–239.

Prasad, G. V., Wong, T., Meliton, G., & Bhaloo, S. (2001). Rhabdomyolysis due to red yeast rice (Monascus purpureus) in a renal transplant recipient. *Transplantation,* 74, 1200–1201.

Prasad, K. (1997). Dietary flax seed in prevention of hypercholesterolemic atherosclerosis. *Atherosclerosis,* 132, 69–76.

Rahman, K., & Billington, D. (2000). Dietary supplementation with aged garlic extract inhibits ADP-induced platelet aggregation in humans. *Journal of Nutrition,* 130(11), 2662–2265.

Rissanen, T., Voutilainen, S., Nyyssonen, K., Lakka, T. A., & Salonen, J. T. (2000). Fish oil-derived fatty acids, docosahexaenoic acid and docosapentaenoic acid, and the risk of acute coronary events: the Kuopio ischaemic heart disease risk factor study. *Circulation,* 102, 2677–2679.

Robbers, J. E., & Tyler, V. E. (1999). *Tyler's herbs of choice: The therapeutic use of phytomedicinals.* New York: The Haworth Herbal Press.

Schectman, G., Kaul, S., Cherayil, G. D., Lee, M., & Kissebah, A. (1989). Can the hypotriglyceridemic effect of fish oil concentrate be sustained? *Annals of Internal Medicine,* 110, 346–352.

Schmidt, T., Wijga, A., Von Zur Muhlen, A., Brabant, G., & Wagner, T. O. (1997). Changes in cardiovascular risk factors and hormones during a comprehensive residential three month kriya yoga training and vegetarian nutrition. *Acta Physiologica Scandinavia Supplement,* 640, 158–162.

Schmidt, U., Kuhn, U., Ploch, M., & Hubner, W. D. (1994). Efficacy of the Hawthorne (Crataegus) Preparation LI 132 in 78 patients with chronic congestive heart failure defined as NYHA functional class II. *Phytomedicine,* 1, 17–24.

Schneider, R. H., Staggers, F., Alexander, C. N., Sheppard, W., Rainforth, M., Kondwani, K., et al. (1995). A randomised controlled trial of stress reduction for hypertension in older African Americans. *Hypertension,* 26, 820–827.

Silagy, C., & Neil, A. (1994). Garlic as a lipid lowering agent–a meta-analysis. *Journal of the Royal College of Physicians (London),* 28, 39–45.

Singh, R. B., Niaz, M. A., Rastogi, S. S., Shukla, P. K., & Thakur, A. S. (1999). Effect of hydrosoluble coenzyme Q10 on blood pressures and insulin resistance in hypertensive patients with coronary artery disease. *Journal of Human Hypertension,* 13, 203–208.

Stevinson, C., Pittler, M. H., & Ernst, E. (2000). Garlic for treating hypercholesterolemia: a meta-analysis of randomized clinical trials. *Annals of Internal Medicine,* 133, 420–429.

Suzukawa, M., Abbey, M., Howe, P. R., & Nestel, P. J. (1995). Effects of fish oil fatty acids on low density lipoprotein size, oxidizability, and uptake by macrophages. *Journal of Lipid Research,* 36, 473–484.

Tauchert, M. (2002). Efficacy and safety of crataegus extract WS 1442 in comparison with placebo in patients with chronic stable New York Heart Association class-III heart failure. *American Heart Journal,* 143, 910–5.

Vempati, R. P., & Telles, S. (2002). Yoga-based guided relaxation reduces sympathetic activity judged from baseline levels. *Psychology Report,* 90(2), 487–494.

Vessby, B., & Boberg, M. (1990). Dietary supplementation with n-3 fatty acids may impair glucose homeostasis in patients with non-insulin-dependent diabetes mellitus. *Journal of Internal Medicine,* 228, 165–171.

Vierling, W., Brand, N., Gaedcke, F., Sensch, K.H., Schneider, E., & Scholz, M. (2003). Investigation of the pharmaceutical and pharmacological equivalence of different Hawthorn extracts. *Phytomedicine,* 10(1), 8–16.

Wei, W., Li, C., Wang, Y., Su, H., Zhu, J., & Kritchevsky, D. (2003). Hypolipidemic and anti-atherogenic effects of long-term Cholestin (Monascus purpureus-fermented rice, red yeast rice) in cholesterol fed rabbits. *Journal of Nutrition and Biochemistry,* 14(6), 314–318.

Wigger-Alberti, W., Bauer, A., Hipler, U. C., & Elsner, P. (1999). Anaphylaxis due to Monascus purpureus-fermented rice (red yeast rice). *Allergy,* 54, 1330–1331.

Wood, M. J., Stewart, R. L., Merry, H., Johnstone, D. E., & Cox, J. L. (2003). Use of complementary and alternative medical therapies in patients with cardiovascular disease. *American Heart Journal,* 145(5), 806–812.

Yamori, Y., Nara, Y., Mizushima, S., Sawamura, M., & Horie, R. (1994). Nutritional factors for stroke and major cardiovascular diseases: international epidemiological comparison of dietary prevention. *Health Report,* 6, 22–67.

Yeh, Y. Y., & Liu, L. (2001). Cholesterol-lowering effect of garlic extracts and organosulfur compounds: human and animal studies. *Journal of Nutrition,* 131(3s), 989S–93S.

Zapfe, G. (2001). Clinical efficacy of crataegus extract WS 1442 in congestive heart failure NYHA class II. *Phytomedicine,* 8, 262–6.

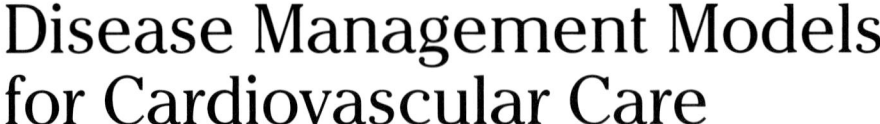

46

Disease Management Models for Cardiovascular Care

NANCY HOUSTON MILLER • ERIKA SIVARAJAN FROELICHER

Disease management is gaining increasing acceptance as an approach to providing evidence-based treatment of cardiovascular conditions. In a health care system faced with an overburden of chronic illnesses, disease management is a concept that will likely enable Americans to live differently in the future. It is necessary to a society whose population is growing older and a health care system focused on managing the acute aspects of illness. Many of the conditions described earlier in this text such as heart failure (Chapter 28) and risk factor management (Chapters 30, 38–43) would benefit from the approaches undertaken in managing individuals with chronic diseases.

By 2030, it is expected that one in five Americans will enter the older than age 65 group (National Center for Health Statistics, 1999). Moreover, average life expectancy has increased by 1 year every 5 years since 1965. In 1997, the average life expectancy was 79 years for women and 74 years for men. Life expectancy at ages 65 and 85 also increased over the past fifty years; women who survive to age 65 can expect to live to age 84, and those who survive to age 85 can anticipate living to 92 (Robert Wood Johnson Foundation [RWJ], 2000). Although the average American then can expect to live much longer, will their quality of life enable them to enjoy independence and function?

More than 100 million Americans now have a chronic condition defined as an illness lasting longer than 3 months (Hoffman et al., 1996). This figure is expected to grow to 134 million by 2020, of whom 29% (or 39 million) will be limited in their activities (RWJ, 2000). Many of these conditions are related to the vascular system, including hypertension, diabetes, obesity, and heart failure. Treatment is complicated by the coexistence of multiple medical conditions and the social and psychological sequelae that accompany them.

The costs associated with caring for an individual with a chronic condition are more than twice as high as those associated with acute conditions (RWJ, 2000). Of the $425 billion spent annually on direct medical costs for persons with chronic diseases, almost two-thirds were for hospital care and physician services, 39% and 25%, respectively (RWJ, 2000). Many of these costs go to treat acute exacerbations of chronic conditions. A major potential exists to prevent these chronic conditions from occurring initially and slow their progression, or to avoid the acute exacerbations leading to hospitalization.

The resources to manage those with an acute illness are quite different from those with a chronic condition. Acute care services are provided primarily by physicians and nurses, often in intensive, hospital-based care requiring the use of expensive technology. In contrast, effective chronic care requires a comprehensive approach that combines social, educational, vocational, and medical services provided in a variety of settings that increasingly focus on the home as the locus of care. The scope of chronic care is broad, encompassing social, community, and personal services as well as medical and rehabilitative care. The management of chronic conditions also requires a network of health care professionals including nurses, social workers, family, and caregivers. Finally, much of chronic care requires education and support of patients and family members to maximize self-management.

In the late 1990s, in a review of the literature, Wagner (Wagner et al., 1996) identified five important elements associated with improved outcomes for those with chronic conditions such as hypertension and diabetes. Successful programs tended to be those that (1) incorporated guidelines and protocols in practice; (2) used a multidisciplinary team with careful allocation of tasks and ongoing patient contact; (3) provided counseling, education, information feedback, and other support to patients; (4) offered access to necessary clinical expertise such as referral to specialists, collaborative care models, and computer-decision support; and (5) used supportive information systems that offer reminders for preventive care and follow-up as well as feedback to providers on patient compliance and service use. Various disease management models have been developed to meet the needs of those with chronic conditions, incorporating many of these elements associated with chronic care delivery. Moreover, a systems approach to care delivery is needed to enhance long-term adherence (see Chapter 44) (Miller et al., 1997). This chapter focuses on various models of disease management, including clinic and nurse case management approaches developed for cardiovascular care. Elements important to care delivery are discussed.

DISEASE MANAGEMENT: DEFINITION AND MODELS

Disease management is a term that has been used for almost a decade to encompass the way in which care is delivered to individuals, but more specifically to groups of patients. Many associate the term with managed care and a way to control health care services (Unger & Warren, 1999). Although numerous definitions for this term exist, Ellrodt (Ellrodt et al., 1997) defines disease management as an approach to patient care that emphasizes coordinated comprehensive care along a continuum of disease and across health care delivery systems. In 1997, because of excessive costs associated with chronic conditions such as heart failure and diabetes, Congress mandated that a better way needed to be found to coordinate care under Medicare. Thus, they requested the Secretary of Health and Human Services to evaluate best practices of coordinated chronic care. The Mathmatica Policy Research Group (Chen et al., 2000) was awarded the contract to review chronic illness care coordination. Of 157 programs reviewed, 67 reported reductions in hospital use or cost, and 24 were selected for further review. And what did they find?

Two prevailing programs existed to deal with the chronically ill: case management and disease management (Table 46-1). Those programs targeting case management included patients at high risk for expensive outcomes, whereas programs for disease management were more narrowly focused on a specific diagnosis. Case management, as defined by the American Nurses Association is a collaborative process that assesses, plans, implements, coordinates, monitors, and evaluates the options and services to meet an individual's health needs using communication and available resources to promote quality cost-effective outcomes (Flarey & Blancett, 1996). The term here is used to define the clinical aspects of case management rather than utilization review. Case management incorporated explicit written plans of care, including referral to community services or organizations, extensive education in symptom identification and self-monitoring of a clinical worsening, compliance with medications, diet, and medical follow-up, and ways of accessing physicians and emergency rooms appropriately. In addition, clear guidelines were delineated with the patient about advanced directives and health care power of attorney. Patients were followed-up either by telephone or by home visits.

In contrast, disease management programs used guidelines for a particular disease, placed less emphasis on coordination of services with community agencies, and provided more standardized patient education. In addition, disease management had more specific guidelines for follow-up, used more technology to monitor services, and some kept patients in their programs continuously, recognizing that conditions such as diabetes and heart failure are not amenable to cure and that patients are likely to lapse into old behaviors.

Both types of programs for chronic care addressed similar needs: (1) assessing and planning a program of care delivery for the patient; (2) implementing and delivering interventions that enable ongoing relationships with patients, families, and primary care providers and foster patient education; and (3) periodically reassessing and adjusting the plan of care (Chen, 2000). These programs also did not require reorganization of practices or new staff and did not threaten the doctor–patient relationship.

It is unclear as yet whether case management or disease management, or the overlap of both models, will significantly decrease health care expenditures. This is now being tested in Medicare demonstration projects. However, it is clear that many of the elements of both case management and disease management are necessary to ensure that patients are cared for appropriately.

VARIOUS MODELS OF DISEASE MANAGEMENT IN CARDIOVASCULAR CARE

Since the early 1970s, unique models for delivering care to individuals with chronic conditions by nurses have evolved. Much of this early work in disease management occurred in hypertension control in the United States and Europe (Runyan, 1975; Aldermann & Shoenbaum, 1973). Most often, attempts were made to deliver high-quality care in various settings that were convenient to the population being studied. In one of the first disease management programs (Runyan, 1975), patients with hypertension, diabetes, or cardiac disease chose to be followed by specially trained nurses in decentralized clinics close to their homes or in a hospital-based outpatient clinic for chronic disease that was staffed by internists. Patients had similar socio-demographic and clinical characteristics. After 2 years, hypertension control rates were superior in those patients cared for by specially trained nurses, and they had 50% fewer hospital admission days. The authors of this study attributed the success of the nurse-run clinics to greater follow-up and time devoted to helping patients manage their chronic conditions.

In another early trial (Alderman & Schoenbaum, 1973), nurses played a key role in the screening and follow-up of individuals within a work site setting in New York City. Nurses screened and enrolled patients over an 11-day period and

Table 46-1 ■ DIFFERENCES IN CHRONIC ILLNESS CARE COORDINATORS

Case management (High risk patient-expensive outcomes)
- Broad assessment of needs (e.g., medical, functional, social, emotional)
- Referral to community resources
- Education on symptom management, compliance with medications, diet, medical follow-up
- Access ways to contact md/emergency rooms
- Guidelines for advanced directives

Disease Management (Patient-Specific Diagnosis)
- Guidelines for a particular disease
- Standardized patient education related to disease
- Specific guidelines for frequency of follow-up
- Technology for monitoring
- Long term participation

Chen, A., Brown, R., et al. (2000). *Best practices in coordinated care.* Princeton, NJ: Mathematica Policy Research.

followed up hypertensive individuals over 1 year. Working closely with a medical director, they performed an initial medical history, obtained preliminary laboratory data, and followed treatment algorithms, initiating and titrating medications for hypertension treatment. Diuretics were chosen as first-line therapy for hypertension treatment, and after controlling blood pressure to goal, patients were seen for review of therapy and were monitored for compliance every 3 months by the nurses. At the end of the year, 84% of the work site had been screened, 97% of those followed up by the nurses remained in therapy, and 81% succeeded with optimal blood pressure lowering. The cost per patient of $100 offset the costs associated with hypertension, including the time lost from work.

These early studies suggested that the convenience of helping individuals manage their health in settings conducive to work and home offered an optimal opportunity for disease management to be brought to the patient. Since the 1970s, disease management by nurses has applied not only to hypertension (Alderman & Shoenbaum, 1973; Hill et al., 1999; Logan et al., 1979; Perry et al., 1982; Pheley et al., 1997; Reighcott et al., 1983; Runyan, 1975) but also to other aspects of cardiovascular management, including dyslipidemia (Allen et al., 2002; Becker et al., 1998; Blair et al., 1998; Schaeffer and Wexler, 1995), tobacco dependence (Hollis et al., 1993; Martin et al., 2000; Miller et al., 1997; Rigotti et al., 1994; Taylor et al., 1990), diabetes (Aubert et al., 1998; Peters et al., 1995; Piette et al., 2001; Taylor et al., 2003; Weinberger et al., 1995), coronary artery disease (Campbell et al., 1998; Cupples & McKnight, 1994; DeBusk et al., 1994; Fonorow et al., 2000; Gordon et al., 2002; Haskell et al., 1994; Murchie , 2003; Naylor et al., 1999; O'Malley et al., 2003, Pozen et al., 1977, Sivarajan et al., 1981, 1982, Sivarajan et al., 1983), and heart failure (Benatar et al., 2003; Cline et al., 1998; Ekman et al., 1998; Fonorow et al., 1997; Jaarsma et al., 1999; Kasper et al., 2002; Koronowski et al., 1995; Laramee et al., 2003; Rich et al., 1995; Riegel et al., 2002; Stewart et al., 1998, 1999, 2003; Weinberger et al., 1996; West et al., 1997). Much of the early work before the term disease management was coined occurred in managing postmyocardial infarction patients using a multidisciplinary approach to managing risk factors, adherence to diet, exercise, medications, and medical regimens to improve functioning and quality of life through the provision of individual and group education, counseling, and behavioral interventions, which included the patient and family as part of rehabilitation (Sivarajan & Newton, 1984).

The largest number of studies related to disease management is in heart failure, in which considerable interest has arisen about how to care for a large and growing population of high-risk patients with the most costly cardiovascular condition (see Chapter 28). The aforementioned body of work and the reviews conducted by investigators in the area of heart failure (Rich, 2001; Philbin, 1999; McAlister et al., 2001; Riegel & LePetri, 2001), diabetes (Renders et al., 2003), and hypertension (Curzio and Beevers, 1997) offer insights and guidance to nurses on the application of disease management systems for care delivery. Disease management systems have now been applied in randomized controlled trials (Allen, 2002; Becker, 1998; Hill, 1999; Taylor, 2003) and clinical practice settings (Unger, 1999), which include younger (Becker, 1998) and older (Rich, 1995; Naylor, 1999) populations, clinics (Fonorow, 1997; Campbell, 1998), hospitals (Miller, 1997; Rigotti, 1994;

Martin, 2000), work sites (Alderman & Shoenbaum, 1973), and home-based (DeBusk et al., 1994; Taylor, 2003) settings, and the use of multidisciplinary (Fonorow, 2000; Haskell, 1994; Riegel, 2002) or physician–nurse teams (West, 1997; Campbell, 1998) to direct care delivery. Moreover, these disease management programs have been shown to effectively reduce multiple risk factors (Haskell, 1994; DeBusk, 1994; Gordon, 2002; Aubert et al., 1998), improve quality of life (Campbell, 1998; Kasper, 2002); and functional status (Fonorow, 1997), increase short-term compliance (Miller, 1997), reduce total admissions, and cardiovascular readmissions (Koronowski, 1995; Naylor, 1999; Riegel, 2002; Stewart, 1998), improve survival (Stewart, 1999), reduce days of hospitalizations (Stewart, 1999; Benatar, 2003), and reduce rehospitalization costs (Naylor, 1999; Stewart, 1999). Further work is still needed to determine the most cost-effective models, how to support long-term adherence including the frequency of interactions to ensure maintenance of health behavior changes, and whether improved outcomes such as a reduction in rehospitalizations are achieved through most disease management programs. In addition, further work must establish the benefit of these systems in ensuring improved outcomes in difficult high-risk populations such as the indigent and those with multiple conditions (Berra et al., 2002).

Approaches to disease management have shown considerable promise and documented the leadership and contribution nurses can make in the care of cardiovascular conditions. Although the names of such models may differ, the specific components, format, and distribution of health care professionals contributing to the multidisciplinary approaches vary by setting and scope of practice according to various health care professional practice acts, geographic region, health care payors, and internationally. Examples of beneficial models have been cited from Europe, Australia, the United States, and Canada.

COMPONENTS OF DISEASE MANAGEMENT SYSTEMS

Identifying a Patient Population

Effective disease management involves a process of identifying at-risk populations, coordinating systems of care delivery, obtaining outcomes, and managing outcomes most appropriately to improve care. The process is shown in Figure 46-1. Most often, disease management programs are developed for chronic conditions that are costly, such as coronary artery disease, diabetes, heart failure, renal failure, and chronic obstructive pulmonary disease. Populations are moderate-risk to high-risk individuals. They may be identified through hospital discharge records as high users of care (Naylor, 1999), through health plan databases for those looking to reduce costs associated with a disease condition (Aubert, 1998), or through a team of individuals such as nurses and physicians attempting to improve the quality of care through a quality-improvement process to meet national guidelines (Fonorow, 2000).

Disease management is most effective when there are incentives tied to outcomes. For example, the goal of managed care organizations may be to reduce re-hospitalizations for heart

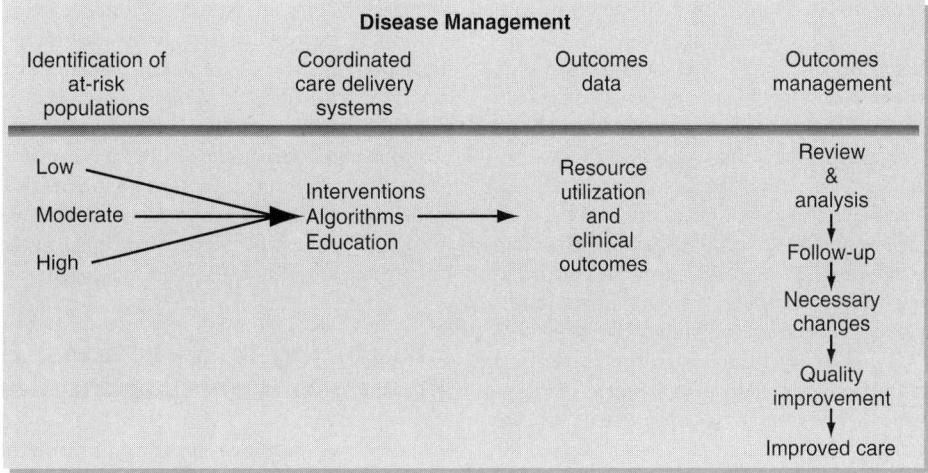

■ **Figure 46–1.** Process of disease management.

failure as reimbursement for patients readmitted within 30 days of hospitalization may be poor. Thus, the goal of a program developed for heart failure must first be to better understand why patients are being admitted so frequently. For a health plan, the goal may be to ensure that all individuals' cardiovascular risk factors are screened and to focus on intensive disease management programs for those individuals with multiple risk factors who assume the greatest risk for future cardiovascular events. Noting that it may be costly to include all patients in disease management programs, organizations, such as Kaiser Permanente of Northern California, have focused their chronic disease efforts by segmenting populations, offering lower-risk individuals educational and supportive services individually or in groups and offering moderate-to-high risk individuals what they term "care management." Their experience is invaluable to those considering the development of disease management efforts.

Once a population in need has been identified, it is critical to learn as much as possible about the population. Knowing the demographic (age, gender, race, socioeconomic, and cultural) characteristics of the population being addressed enables one to structure appropriate and effective interventions. Moreover, being sensitive to the individual educational needs of the population is critical to success.

Coordinating Delivery Systems for Disease Management

Although disease management models have operated in a variety of settings including clinics, hospitals, and work sites, a few systems have also used telephonic care to structure the majority of interactions with the patient to optimize care within the home setting (DeBusk, 1994; West, 1997). Whereas there is much diversity related to structured interventions among programs, the majority have incorporated patient education, multidisciplinary or physician–nurse teams, and specialized follow-up. Furthermore, the development of algorithms and protocols for delivering structured care has been crucial to the success of disease management systems.

Disease management involves a process of care delivery. Because that process of care delivery is different than the typical structure within an office visit or hospital that is well known to most health care professionals, many different models for care delivery in disease management exist today. Although populations differ, interventions have ranged from a single face-to-face visit with telephone follow-up to comprehensive management teams comprising multiple team members (Rich, 2001). Moreover, few have been able to specify which components are most important to overall outcome (Philbin, 1999). Although this is because of the system's approach to care using multiple interventions, specifying primary and secondary goals is key to developing intervention activities. Goals for a disease management program are often to improve patient and caregiver knowledge of the disease, enhance self-management through skill-building, increase medication and treatment adherence, and improve health-related outcomes (Sivarajan, 1981, Ott, 1983; Sivarajan, 1983; Froelicher & Kozuki, 2002).

Education as a Part of Disease Management

Education is a key intervention component of disease management systems. Most often, education surrounds aspects of lifestyle changes including diet, exercise, and smoking cessation, as well as ways to self-monitor a disease condition, including using medication, recognizing important signs and symptoms, and daily monitoring of indicators such as weight, glucose, or blood pressure. The format for education differs from one program to another. Some have used face-to-face individualized education (DeBusk, 1994; Aubert, 1998), whereas others have used a group approach followed by individualized education (Sivarajan, 1982; Sivarajan, 1983; Taylor 2003). In a review of programs offering structured educational interventions for cardiovascular disease, Mullen (Mullen et al., 1992) found that more than two thirds of successful programs, many directed by nurses, were focused on behavioral approaches directed at skill-building. Rather than focusing on providing information, these programs succeeded by offering a range of health behavior skills, such as contracting, goal-setting, self-monitoring, feedback, and problem-solving (Miller & Taylor, 1995). Many used theories of stages of change (Prochaska et al., 1983), social learning (most specifically, self-efficacy) (Bandura, 1977, 1997), and relapse prevention training (Marlatt & Gordon, 1985; Sivarajan Froelicher 2002) to plan successful educational interventions. In addition, offering education materials in multiple formats (e.g., print and video) has also been shown to increase adherence to long-term behaviors as individuals learn in different ways and are given and an opportunity for reinforcement of information (Miller, 1997).

Developing educational interventions based on the critical behaviors to be changed is key to successful disease management efforts. For example, Stewart (1998) formulated a disease management program educating patients in a single face-to-face visit about medication use behaviors to improve heart failure outcomes. The goal of the intervention was to focus on the problems associated with medication adherence for each patient after hospital discharge. With support of a pharmacist and a nurse in a single face-to-face visit in the home, Stewart planned an approach to manage each individual's problems associated with medication use and sought methods for improving adherence. Patients with multiple problems were offered additional support through telephone calls by the pharmacist. At the end of 18 months and 4 years, this disease management intervention resulted in decreased hospitalizations, improved survival, and lower cost associated with heart failure (Stewart, 1999; Stewart et al., 2002). The authors attribute their success to the focused problem solving and tailoring that occurred for each individual patient and the additional efforts applied to more difficult patients through individualization of care (Stewart, 1998).

The success of educational interventions for disease management appears to be related to individualized approaches to education, offering multiple formats, use of behavioral approaches, and a focus on more intensive education in those with the greatest need.

Medical Management of Care Delivery: Protocols and Algorithms

In addition to education, one of the main objectives of disease management programs is to ensure that patients are using prescribed medication regimens that optimize outcomes. Irrespective of disease state, this may be actualized through careful and appropriate dose titration of medications. Strong emphasis has also been placed on the achievement of high adherence rates to prevent exacerbation of symptoms or deterioration of outcomes known to impact future risk (Cline, 1998). Although national guidelines, such as those developed by the National Institutes of Health (NCEP, 2001), the American Heart Association (Smith et al., 2001), and the American Diabetes Association (ADA et al., 2002), are a starting point for key decisions about initiating pharmacotherapy, they are often insufficient in supplying the important aspects of dose titration necessary for disease management, especially in critical populations such as those with heart failure. Thus, protocols or algorithms that delineate appropriate dosing and that are developed based on

formulary decisions of institutions are key to managing medications effectively in disease management programs. Nurses have played a key role in the management of the pharmacological aspects of disease management. Many state practice acts require that nurses follow strict protocols for managing medications in an outpatient setting that must be updated annually (Board of Registered Nursing). Moreover, the development of protocols for medication management is often a shared responsibility of nurses, physicians, and pharmacists within the local institution offering the disease management program.

Structuring Interventions: The Process of Coordinating Care

Interventions that focus on education and medication management as part of any disease management program must be structured in a way to optimize outcomes. As previously mentioned, there is large variation in the frequency of interactions with patients, the use of face-to-face visits versus telephone follow-up, how much follow-up is needed, and the number of health care professionals including the expertise of nurses required for disease management. However, several investigators suggest that there are key factors that must be addressed in making decisions about how to structure the frequency of interactions. These include (1) understanding the needs of the patient population based on problems (e.g., lack of adherence, material support, frequent hospitalizations, inadequate risk factor control); (2) deciding whether face-to-face, group, or individual interventions will enhance overall success, or whether telephone or electronic encounters are sufficient to enhance motivation; (3) determining if a home visit is needed; (4) noting what the time-frame is for problematic behaviors; and (5) considering how much tailoring is needed to support individual patients. Irrespective of whether face-to-face interventions or telephone or electronic encounters are used most often, interactions occur more frequently in the early phases of disease management programs and are designed to taper-off as patients and family members learn how to better self-manage behaviors and pharmacotherapies. Many groups have successfully operationalized disease management in research settings through several studies (Sivarajan, 1981, 1982, 1983; Stewart, 1998,1999, 2003; Miller, 1995, 1997; Naylor, 1994, 1999) and offer their experience, whereas others who have had success in clinical practice settings for more than 10 years (Sivarajan 1984; Miller et al., 1996; Unger, 1999; Von Korff et al., 1997) offer important perspectives on the structuring of interventions and the coordination of care delivery.

Communication With Physicians and Other Personnel

The frequency of interactions with other key personnel involved in disease management efforts is important to overall care. One of the failures of our present system in managing those with chronic conditions has been the frequency of visits to multiple physician providers and the lack of communication among them. In disease management models, nurses most often assume the role of coordinating care among two or more providers. Electronic medical records within large systems have often facilitated that communication. They are still in their infancy, however. In some instances, the disease management program lies outside the normal care delivery system being instituted by a disease management company, or a database for disease management is separate from the existing paper-based or electronic medical record. Thus, to facilitate clear communication about ongoing management, letters updating physicians and documentation of care within the medical record become crucial. These can be facilitated through computer-generated reports highlighting clinical progress to physicians and the development of standard tools for receiving responses from physicians. The frequency of phone-based interactions and the format for receiving information about the care being delivered to patients as part of disease management should be addressed as part of the development of algorithms and protocols. Interactions with physicians most often relate to medication and symptom changes that must be addressed by the team. Key physician champions who can facilitate problem-solving and offer expertise to nurses in the absence of primary care or specialty physicians facilitates success with program implementation.

Anticipating the needs of patients and family members, nurses also play a role in coordinating the care delivered by other health care professionals such as social workers, pharmacists, dietitians, and psychologists. These disciplines offer specialized expertise in defined fields often required for managing long-term chronic conditions. Overseeing the aspects of social isolation and depression, the need for economic and material support, and continued education related to diet and medications, their support is key to improving patient outcomes, such as reduction in utilization.

Collecting Clinical and Resource Utilization Outcomes

Irrespective of a research or clinical initiative in disease management, collecting data on outcomes is crucial to evaluating a program. Many disease management programs collect process and outcome data including resource utilization, quality of life, patient satisfaction (Atkinson 1996), physician satisfaction, and program costs, which is important to substantiate the need for these programs. Health insurance companies and payers of care are most interested in outcomes associated with a reduction in emergency room visits, in hospitalizations or re-hospitalizations, length of hospital stay, and costs of care. This type of information is obtained from financial records or review of medical records and insurance information. Keeping accurate process data in an individual database that is part of the disease management program assists in determining whether adequate pharmacotherapies were delivered, thus ultimately influencing outcomes.

Quality of life is most often measured within the research setting. However, patients and family members place high value on the improvement of quality of life as an outcome of disease management programs. Thus, measurement of this outcome is important in clinically based programs. Although researchers have difficulty agreeing on what constitutes overall quality of life, comprehensive tools exist to measure many of the important components including biologic or physiologic, symptoms, functioning, health perceptions, and overall well being. Some of the most commonly used tools include the Medical-Outcomes Short Form-36 Item Questionnaire (SF-36) (Stewart et al., 1988; Tarlov et al., 1989) and the Sickness Impact Profile. (Bergner et al., 1981; Ott et al., 1983). Shorter tools such as the Short-Form 12 (Jenkinson et al., 1997), which is a modification of the SF-36, are much easier to administer in clinical practice settings but do not provide measurements of changes that are offered through longer instruments.

Whereas general quality-of-life questionnaires can useful, some researchers believe that disease-specific tools are more valuable in defining patient outcomes. For example, the Minnesota Living with Heart Failure tool (Rector et al., 1993), which measures multiple domains of quality of life in heart failure patients and contains 21 items, correlates well with assessments of dyspnea and fatigue, important in this population (Wilson et al., 1993). Measuring functional status of patients, which may be significantly impacted as a result of disease management programs, should also be considered in developing outcome measures for disease management. The Duke Activity Status Instrument (DASI) (Hlatky et al., 1989) is an example of a simple self-administered questionnaire that correlates well with functional activities in heart failure subjects. Other tools that measure symptoms and function include the Canadian Cardiovascular Society Functional Classification (CCS) used for functional disability and angina (Campeau, 1976).

Measuring patient satisfaction is an important way to market your disease management program. Most large organizations are committed to measuring satisfaction as part of quality assurance. However, measuring overall program satisfaction and satisfaction with individual key components of the program may be helpful not only to administrators but also to enhancing program delivery. Assessment of patient satisfaction has also been initiated as part of quality-assurance assessments (Attkinson et al., 1996). Likewise, brief physician satisfaction surveys may help program administrators to monitor and restructure aspects of a disease management program. Because these programs are designed to support the physician's care, physician satisfaction surveys should measure items such as help in improving self-management, a reduction in physician's time for various aspects of care, and support in achieving national guidelines for quality care such as those established by the Joint Committee on the Accreditation of Health Care Organizations (www.jcaho.org) or the National Committee for Quality Assurance (NCQA) (2002).

Finally, many process measures enable disease management personnel to better understand the important aspects of program delivery. Observing the frequency of face-to-face or telephone contacts, length of contacts, and the type of daily tasks performed, completed through time-analysis records, enable one to determine the need for program restructuring. This type of process evaluation is helpful in determining whether nonclinical tasks could be allocated to other personnel so nurses are performing the most important clinical tasks. Process measures also enable one to determine the actual implementation of intervention activities, important to outcomes.

Outcomes Management

Outcomes management includes using evaluation data to make necessary changes in program implementation for continued quality improvement. Although the goal of a disease management model may not be to lower the cost of care, specific outcomes such as reducing the frequency of physician visits for those in a disease management program may be an important outcome of a busy HMO. Moreover, increased patient satisfaction as a result of the program may enable payers to retain patients in their delivery system, thus increasing competition among health industry providers. Finally, looking for more efficient ways to deliver the program to a larger number of patients is often a goal for those actively involved in disease management efforts.

Program Marketing

Whereas the clinical aspects of disease management are critical to success, continual marketing of the program to hospital administrators, payers, physicians, and other health care professionals is key to sustaining a program. Key marketing activities should include (1) a plan for recruiting program participants using brochures, flyers, letters, and other announcements, which is continually maintained; (2) updating key administrators and decision-makers about program implementation through quarterly, bi-annual, or annual reports and presentations; and (3) ensuring that physicians and other health care professionals outside the disease management program are continually informed of program delivery changes, successes, and program volume. Satisfied patients and family members are often willing to write letters to key decision-makers about the value of the program to their overall care.

TRAINING AND JOB QUALIFICATIONS FOR DISEASE MANAGEMENT

Managing a caseload of patients as part of disease management requires sound clinical expertise and a number of other important qualifications. Qualifications for those involved in these programs include strong physical assessment skills, interpersonal skills (warmth, empathy, good listening and problem-solving, an ability to work with families and a multidisciplinary team), the ability to work independently, leadership capability (advocate for patients and families, the disease manager's role, and the program), and good organizational skills (ability to use information systems and time-management skills). Knowledge of and skills in conducting groups is essential when the program is offered in a group format (Sivarajan, 1984). Most often, nurses have bachelor degrees or master degrees and are prepared and have been specially trained for the position. Many are clinical nurse specialists or nurse practitioners specializing in case management or disease management. A strong background in cardiovascular nursing (minimum 3 years) and cardiac rehabilitation are desirable qualifications for disease management.

Core competencies in chronic disease management may be mastered through a curriculum that includes knowledge of the disease process, medical management of risk factors, treatment protocols, lifestyle and psychosocial interventions, information systems, and institutional operations. Strong physical assessment,

patient education, and behavioral counseling skills are also needed. An ability to operationalize treatment protocols surrounding the initiation and titration of medications, symptom management, documentation in medical records, and coordination of care are core competencies that must be mastered. Like those involved in public health and community nursing, disease management nurses must be committed to following patients and families on a long-term basis.

Much of the training for disease management occurs on the job. Best practice programs (Miller, 1996) offer in-depth training to nurses managing multiple risk factors occurring over 2 weeks. Didactic lecture, role-playing, and case study presentation are followed by 1 week of preceptorship training with other experienced disease management nurses in the field. Various nursing organizations, such as the Preventive Cardiovascular Nurses Association (PCNA), are committed to educating nurses to take on expanded roles in preventive cardiology. They offer regional and national training as well as important publications that support those undertaking disease management roles.

THE UNRESOLVED ISSUES FOR DISEASE MANAGEMENT

Although disease management has not yet reached widespread application in clinical practice, it holds promise as a new way of delivering care to those at high-risk for and those with established cardiovascular disease. The success of using nurses to coordinate disease management programs has most often resulted in more frequent medication changes, an increase in the use of combination drug regimens, less expensive medications, and an increase in short-term adherence. These results are in large part because of the use of defined protocols and increased patient contact time for education and behavioral counseling. In addition, a greater achievement of goals such as a reduction in blood pressure, cholesterol, and glucose control has been realized. A byproduct of comprehensive care in these patients has produced a reduction in utilization for all causes (emergency room visits and hospitalizations), something not expected by many in the field (Ades et al., 2002). As noted in Table 46-2, organizations implementing disease management programs for more than 10 years suggest several important lessons for those developing or implementing programs. In addition, Stewart (Stewart & Horowitz, 2003) has highlighted a number of factors that appear to be important in the overall development of those disease management programs that

Table 46–2 ■ IMPORTANT LESSONS FOR PROGRAM IMPLEMENTATION IN DISEASE MANAGEMENT

- Physician leadership/support is key to program viability
- Ongoing marketing is essential
- Program modifications save time and resources
- Protocols require annual updates and alignment with national guidelines
- Defining caseload requirements and re-evaluating is necessary for quality control

Table 46–3 ■ KEY FEATURES OF SUCCESSFUL
PROGRAMS OF CARE IN CHF

- A commitment to individualized health care
- A multidisciplinary approach to managing the patient
- A major role for a specialist nurse to assess patient needs and provide for ongoing management within a supportive multidisciplinary environment
- At least one home visit for a comprehensive assessment of the patients circumstances
- The promotion of self-care behaviors
- Increased levels of monitoring in "high-risk" patients
- The application of optimal, evidence-based pharmacological treatment with flexible protocols for changes in patient status and titration to maximal tolerated doses.

Adapted with permission from Stewart, S., & Horowitz, J. (2003). Specialist nurse management programmes. *Pharmacoeconomics*, 21(4), 22–240.

successfully reduced re-hospitalization rates and costs for heart failure. These are highlighted in Table 46-3.

Many challenges continue to confront those involved in disease management, offering future opportunities for research and for those conducting clinical programs. Disease management programs have typically focused on what is often called a "single disease state" or "carve out." These specialty programs for high-cost patient populations treat only a single chronic condition such as diabetes or heart failure. However, many individuals have predisposing risk factors and co-morbid conditions that determine their functional status and prognosis. For example, more than half of all re-hospitalizations for heart failure are caused by other attributable conditions that impact the disease, such as hypertension and coronary artery disease, or unrelated conditions, such as chronic obstructive pulmonary disease (DeBusk et al., 1999). Moreover, the overlap of cardiovascular risk factors (dyslipidemia, obesity, hypertension, and smoking) is significant. Thus, the need for managing multiple risk factors concurrently is noteworthy and requires further research. As adherence to guidelines by physicians and systems becomes more commonplace, allowing achievement of better patient outcomes, a more central role for nurses in disease management is likely to reside with an elderly and aging population that is burdened by multiple diseases and associated conditions. Certainly, models that have addressed many of the factors associated with the elderly, such as the work by Naylor (Naylor et al., 1994, 1999), hold promise for the future.

A second challenge relates to intervention components and the duration of follow-up. Although disease management models focus on multiple interventions, there is large variation in the frequency of contact, the context for what is provided to patients, and whether patients are followed-up for 1 month, 1 year, or indefinitely. To date, few programs have analyzed the most important components of their programs, and none has compared the effectiveness of different programs or the individual components or combinations of components within programs (Grady et al., 2000). In addition, it is likely that case management and disease management models will be refined over time. Both models offer important components for overall management of chronic conditions. However, those demonstrating high accountability through good patient outcomes at a reasonable cost and that also offset the high costs of acute

exacerbations will most likely prevail. Finally, it is likely that web-based technology will afford the opportunity for health care professionals to follow-up patients over an extended period of time. The use of electronic blood pressure monitors, blood glucose meters, and voice recognition technology offers data that are sometimes difficult to achieve. Real-time data that are linked to patient reminders will enhance management. Whether such technology improves patient outcomes is presently being tested.

Although disease management models have been effectively implemented in research and clinical practice, it is likely that such programs will be delivered to only select groups of patients in the future, because of economic constraints. Peer support models for self-management of chronic conditions have also been tested (Lorig et al., 1999; Lorig et al., 2001). These offer significant promise as an alternative modality supporting individuals with chronic conditions in the self-management of symptoms. The Chronic Disease Management Program is a community-based peer-led program designed to help those individuals with chronic conditions such as cardiovascular disease, arthritis, pulmonary disease, and stroke. Offered to 10 to 15 participants over 7 weeks in 2.5-hour group sessions and led by a trained leader, this program focuses on improving self-management skills based on self-efficacy theory, drawing on peers for support. Weekly sessions focus on action planning and feedback, modeling of behaviors and problem-solving by participants for one another, group problem-solving, and individual decision-making. Supported by a program guide entitled "Living a Healthy Life with Chronic Conditions," weekly content includes the following: adopting exercise programs; use of cognitive symptom management techniques, such as guided relaxation and distraction; fatigue and sleep management; use of medications and community resources; managing the emotions of fear, anger, and depression; training in communication with health care professionals and others; health-related problem-solving; and decision making.

In a study of 831 subjects, Lorig and colleagues (Lorig, 2001) found that compared with baseline, for each of 2 years, emergency room and outpatient visits were reduced ($p = 0.05$) and self-efficacy improved in those attending the sessions ($p = 0.05$). This model, now widely used by health care organizations in the United States and abroad, offers another important alternative for disease management.

A final important challenge facing disease management relates to the transitional aspects of care and the health care delivery system. Acute care that has been linked to the hospital must truly be linked to the delivery of chronic care. A problem confronting some patients has been the perceived loss of control over the health care system (Nelson & Arnold-Powers, 2001). Through qualitative research, Nelson found that impersonal service, health care system navigation, and, for many, feeling discounted by the medical care system are problems many elderly patients face today. Conversely, feeling cared for and enhanced support were frequently cited by those patients participating in nurse case management. Structured appropriately, disease management models must help to support a successful transition from home to hospital and other settings. Ensuring a smooth transition with the disease manager operating in partnership with the patient at the center is likely to reduce the sense of loss of control for patients and families. More opportunities will arise to improve care as communication technologies improve and our capability to monitor patients in the home environment is extended.

In summary, disease management models offer the promise of better care for millions of individuals with multiple risk factors and known cardiovascular diseases. Although much has been studied, the challenge of implementation needs further research and the application of a superior health care delivery system in this century. Much of this challenge rests in the hands of nurses who participate in newly defined disease management roles.

REFERENCES

Ades, P., Kottke T., Houston Miller, N., et al. (2002). 33rd Bethesda Conference: Preventive Cardiology: How can we do better? Task force #3—getting results: who where and how? *JACC,* 40(4), 615–630.

Alderman, M. H., & Shoenbaum, E. F. (1975). Detection and treatment of hypertension at the work site. *New England Journal of Medicine,* 293, 65–68.

Allen, J., Blumenthal, R. S., Margolis, S., Young, D. R., Miller, E. R., & Kelly, K. (2002). Nurse case management of hypercholesterolemia in patients with coronary heart disease: results of a randomized clinical trial. *Am Heart J,* 144, 678–86.

American Diabetes Association. (2002). Clinical practice recommendations. *Diabetes Care,* 25, S5–S21.

Attkinsson, C. C., & Greenfield, T. K. (1996) The client satisfaction questionnaire (CSQ) scales and the services satisfaction scale-30 (SSS-30). In L. I. Sederer & B. Dickey (Eds.), *Outcomes assessment in clinical practice* (pp. 120–128). Baltimore: Williams and Wilkins.

Aubert, R. E., Herman, W. H., Waters, J., Moore, W., Sutton, D., Peterson, B. L., Baley, C. M., & Koplan, J. P. (1998). Nurse case management to improve glycemic control in diabetic patients in a health maintenance organization. *Annals of Internal Medicine,* 129, 605–612.

Bandura, A. (1997). *Self-efficacy: The exercise of control.* New York: W. H. Freeman and Co.

Bandura, A. (1977). *Social learning theory.* Englewood Cliffs, NJ: Prentice Hall.

Becker, D. M., Rqueno, J. V., Yook, R. M., Kral, B. G., Blumenthal, R. S., Moy, T. F., Bezirdjian, P. J., & Becker, L. C. (1998). Nurse mediated cholesterol management compared with enhanced primary care in siblings of individuals with premature coronary disease. *Archives of Internal Medicine,* 158, 1533–1539.

Benatar, D. B., Ghitelman, M., & Avitall, J. Outcomes of chronic heart failure (2003). *Archives of Internal Medicine,* 163, 347–351.

Bergner, M., Bobbitt, R. A., Carter, W. B., & Gilson, B.S. (1981). The sickness impact profile: development and final revision of a health status measure. *Medical Care,* 19, 787–805.

Berra, K., Haskell, W., Clark, A., Klieman, L., Duff, S., Weaver, D., Christopherson, D., & Myle, J (2002). *Multifactorial risk reduction in low income patients: opportunities and changes in implementing a case management model.* National Cardiovascular Health Conference, National Heart Lung and Blood Institute, Washington, DC.

Bessette, L., Sangha, O., & Kuntz, K. M., et al. (1998). Comparative responsiveness of generic versus disease-specific and weighted versus unweighted health status measures in carpal tunnel syndrome. *Medical Care,* 36, 491–502.

Blair, T. P., Bryant, J., & Bocuzzi, S. (1988). Treatment of hypercholesterolemia by a clinical nurse using a stepped-care protocol in a non-volunteer population. *Archives of Internal Medicine,* 148, 1046–1048.

Blue, L. L., McMurray, E., Davie, J. J., McDonagh, A. P., Murdoch, D. R., Petrie, M. C., Connolly, E., Norrie, J., Round, C. E., Ford, I., & Morrison, C. E. (2001). Randomized controlled trial of specialist nurse intervention in heart failure. *BMJ,* 323, 715–718.

Campbell, N. C., Ritchie, L. D., Thain, J., Deans, H. G., Rawles, J. M., & Squair, J. L. (1998). Secondary prevention in coronary heart disease: a randomized trial of nurse led clinics in primary care. *Heart,* 80(5), 447–452.

Campeau, L. (1976). Grading of angina pectoris [letter]. *Circulation,* 54, 522–523.

Chen, A., Brown R., et al. (2000). *Best practices in coordinated care.* Princeton, NJ: Mathematica Policy Research.

Cline, C. M. J., Israelsson, B., Willenheimer, R. B., et al. (1998). Cost effective management programme for heart failure reduces hospitalization. *Heart,* 80, 442–446.

Cupples, M. E., & McKnight, A. (1994). Randomized controlled trial of health promotion in general practice for patients at high cardiovascular risk. *BMJ,* 309(6960), 993–996.

Curzio, J. L., & Beevers, M. (1997). The role of nurses in hypertension care and research. *Journal of Human Hypertension,* 11, 541–550.

DeBusk, R. F., Houston Miller, N., West, J. A., & Taylor, C. B. (1999). Treating the patient with disease(s) vs. treating disease(s) in the patient. *Archives of Internal Medicine,* 159, 2739–2742.

DeBusk, R. F., Miller, N. H., Superko, H. R., Dennis, C. A., Thomas, R. J., Lew, H. T., Berger, III W. E., Heller, R. S., Rompf, J., Gee, D., Kraemer, H. C., Ghandour, G., Clark, M., & Fisherl L. (1994). A case management system for coronary risk factor modification following acute myocardial infarction. *Annals of Internal Medicine,* 120, 721–729.

Ekman, I., Andersson, B., Ehnforst, M., Matejka, G., Persson, B., & Fagerberg, B. (1998). Feasibility of a nurse-monitored, outpatient-care programme for elderly patients with moderate-to-severe, chronic heart failure. *European Heart Journal,* 19, 1254–1260.

Ellrodt, G., Cook, D. J., Lee, J., Cho, M., Hunt, D., & Weingarten, S. (1997). Evidence-based disease management. *JAMA,* 278, 1687–1692.

Executive Summary of the third report of the National Cholesterol Education Program (NCEP). (2001). Expert panel on detection, evaluation, and treatment of high blood cholesterol in adults (Adult Treatment Panel III). *JAMA,* 285, 2486–2497.

Flarey, D. L. & Blancett, S. S. (1996). Case management: delivering care in the age of managed care. In D. L. Flarey & S. S. Blancett (Eds), *Handbook of nurse case management.* Gaithersburg, MD: Aspen Publishing.

Fonarow, G., et al. (1997). Impact of a comprehensive heart failure management program on hospital readmission and functional status of patients with advanced heart failure. *Journal of the American College of Cardiology,* 30, 725–732.

Fonarow, G., Gawlinksi, A., et al. (2001). Improved treatment of cardiovascular disease by implementation of a cardiac hospitalization atherosclerosis management program: CHAMP. *American Journal of Cardiology,* 87, 819–822.

Gordon, N. F., English, C. D., Contractor, A. S., et al. (2002). Effectiveness of three models for comprehensive cardiovascular disease risk reduction. *American Journal of Cardiology,* 89, 1263–1268.

Grady, K. L., Dracup, K., & Kennedy, G., et al. (2000). Team management of patients with heart failure: a statement for healthcare professionals from the cardiovascular nursing council of the American Heart Association. *Circulation,* 102, 2443–2456.

Haskell, W. L., Alderman, E. L., Fair, J. M., et al. (1994). Effects of intensive multiple risk factor reduction on coronary atherosclerosis and clinical cardiac events in men and women with coronary artery disease. The Stanford Coronary Risk Intervention Project (SCRIP). *Circulation,* 89, 975–990.

Hill, M. N., Bone, L. J., Hilton, S. C., Roary, M. C., Kelen, G. D., & Levine, D. M. (1999). A clinical trial to improve high blood pressure care in young urban black men. *American Journal of Hypertension,* 12, 548–554.

Hlatky, M., Boineau, R. E., Higginbotham, M. B., et al. (1989). A brief self-administered questionnaire to determine functional capacity (the Duke Activity Status Index). *American Journal of Cardiology,* 64, 651–654.

Hoffman, C., Rice, D., & Sung, H. Y. (1996). Persons with chronic conditions: their prevalence and costs. *JAMA,* 276 (18), 1473–1479.

Hollis, J. F., Lichtenstein, E., Vogt, T. M., Stevens, V. J., & Biglan, A. (1993). Nurse-assisted counseling for smokers in primary care. *Annals of Internal Medicine,* 118, 521–525.

Jaarsma, T., Halfens, R., Huijer Abu-Saad, H., et al. (1999). Effects of education and support on self-care and resource utilization in patients with heart failure. *European Heart Journal,* 20, 673–682.

Jenkinson, C., Layte R., et al. (1997). A shorter form health survey: can the SF-12 replicate results from the SF-36 in longitudinal studies? *Journal of Public Health,* 19, 179–186.

Joint Commission on Accreditation of Healthcare Organizations. Disease-Specific Care Certification. [On-line] Available at: www.jcaho.org/dscc/index.htm.

Kasper, E., Gerstenblith, G., Hefter, G., VanAnden, E., Brinker, J. A., Thiemann D. R., Terrin, M., Forman, S., & Gottlieb, S. H. (2002). A randomized trial of the efficacy of multidisciplinary care in heart failure outpatients at high risk of hospital readmission. *Journal of the American College of Cardiology,* 39(3), 471–80.

Kornowski, R. Zeeli, D., Averbuch, M., Finkelstein, A., Schwartz, D., Moshkovitz, M., Weinreb, B., Hershkovitz, R., Eyal, D., Miller, M., Levo,

Y., & Pines, A. (1995). Intensive home-care surveillance prevents hospitalization and improves morbidity rates among elderly patients with severe congestive heart failure. *American Heart Journal, 129*, 762–766.

Laramee, A. S., Levinsky, S. K., Sargent ,J., Ross, R., & Callas, P. (2003). Case management in a heterogeneous congestive heart failure population. *Archives of Internal Medicine, 163*, 809–817.

Logan, A. G., Milne, B. J., Achber, C., et al. (1979). Work-site treatment of hypertension by specially trained nurses. A controlled trial. *Lancet, 2*, 1175–1178.

Lorig K., Ritter, P., Stewart, A., Sobel, D., Brown, B. W., Bandura, A., Gonzalez, V. M., Laurent, D. D., & Holman, H. (2001). Chronic disease self-management program. 2-year health status and health care utilization outcomes. *Medical Care, 39*(11), 1217–1223.

Lorig K., Sobel, D. S., Stewart, A. L., Brown, B. W., Bandura, A., Ritter, P., Gonzalez, V. M., Laurent, D. D., Holman, H.R. (1999). Evidence suggesting that a chronic disease self-management program can improve health status while reducing hospitalization: a randomized trial. *Medical Care, 37*(1), 5–14.

Marlatt, G. A., & Gordon, J. R. (1985). *Relapse prevention: Maintenance strategies in the treatment of addiction.* New York: Guilford Press.

Martin, K., Froelicher, E., & Houston Miller, N. (2000). Women's Initiative for Nonsmoking (WINS) II: The intervention. *Heart & Lung: The Journal of Acute and Critical Care, 29*, 438–445.

McAlister, F. A., Lawson, F., Teo, K. K., & Armstrong, P. W. (2001). A systematic review of randomized trials of disease management programs in heart failure. *American Journal of Medicine, 110*(5), 378–384.

Miller, N. H. (1997). Compliance with treatment regimen in chronic asymptomatic diseases. *American Journal of Medicine, 102*, 43–49.

Miller, N. H., Hill, M. N., Kottke, T., & Ockene, I. S. (1997). The multilevel compliance challenge: recommendations for a call to action. A statement for healthcare professionals. *Circulation, 95*, 1085–1990.

Miller, N. H., Smith, P. M., DeBusk, R. F., Sobel, D. S., & Taylor, C. B. (1997). Smoking cessation in hospitalized patients. Results of a randomized trial. *Archives of Internal Medicine, 157*, 409–415.

Miller, N. H., & Taylor, C. B. (1995). Lifestyle management for patients with coronary heart disease. In E. Giles & S. Moore (Eds.), Champaign[AQ1], IL: Human Kinetics.

Miller, N. H., Warren, D., & Myers, D. (1996). Home-based cardiac rehabilitation and lifestyle modification: The MULTIFIT model. *Journal of Cardiovascular Nursing, 11*(1), 76–87.

Mullen, P. D., Mains, D. A., & Velez, R. (1992). A meta-analysis of controlled trials of cardiac patient education. *Patient Education and Counseling, 19*,143–62.

Murchie, P., Campbell, N., et al. (2003). Secondary prevention clinics for coronary heart disease: four year follow up of a randomized controlled trial in primary care. *BMJ, 326*, 84.

National Center for Health Statistics (1999). *Health, United States 1999.* Hyattsville, MD: US Government Printing Office.

National Committee for Quality Assurance. (2002). *The state of health care quality 2002, health plan employer information and data set (HEDIS).* Washington, DC: Author.

Naylor, M., Brooten, D., Campbell, R., Jacobsen, B. S., Mexey, M. D., Pauly, M. V., & Schwartz, J. S. (1999). Comprehensive discharge planning and home follow-up of hospitalized elders. *JAMA, 281*(7), 613–620.

Naylor, M., & Brooten D., et al. (1994). Comprehensive discharge planning for the hospitalized elderly: a randomized clinical trial. *Annals of Internal Medicine, 120*, 999–1006.

Nelson, J., & Arnold-Powers, P. (2001). Community case management for frail, elderly clients: the nurse case managers role. *Journal of Nursing Administration, 31*(9), 444–450.

O'Malley, P. G., Feurstein I. M., & Taylor, A. J. (2003). Impact of electron beam tomography, with or without case management, on motivation, behavioral change, and cardiovascular risk profile. *JAMA, 289*(17), 2215–2223.

Ott, C. R., Sivarajan, E. S., Newton, K. M., Almes, M. J., Bruce, R. A., Bergner, M., & Gilson, B. S. (1983).A randomized study of early cardiac rehabilitation: the sickness impact profile as an assessment tool. *Heart and Lung, 12*(2), 162–170.

Perry, H. M., Schnapner, J. W., Meyer, G., & Swatzell, R. (1982). Clinical program for screening and treatment of hypertension in veterans. *Journal of the National Medical Association, 74*, 433–444.

Board of Registered Nurses State of California. [On-line] Available: www.rn.ca.gov.

Peters, A. L., Davidson, M. B., & Ossorio, R. C. (1995). Management of patients with diabetes by nurses with support of specialists. *HMO Practice, 9*, 8–13.

Pheley, A. M., Terry,P., Peitz, L., et al (1995). Evaluation of a nurse-based hypertension management program: Screening, management, and outcomes. *Journal of Cardiovascular Nursing, 9*, 54–61.

Philbin, E. (1999). Comprehensive multidisciplinary programs for the management of patients with congestive heart failure. *Journal of General Internal Medicine, 14*, 130–137.

Piette, J. D., Weinberger, M., Kraemer, F. B., & McPhee, S. J. (2001). Impact of automated calls with nurse follow-up on diabetes treatment outcomes in a Department of Veterans Affairs Health Care System. *Diabetes Care, 24*, 202–208.

Pozen, M. W., Stechmiller, J., Harris, W., Smith, S., Fried, D. D., & Voigt, G. C. (1977). A nurse rehabilitator's impact on patients with myocardial infarction. *Medical Care, 15*, 830–837.

Preventative Cardiovascular Nurses Association. Madison, WI. Available at: www.pcna.net.

Prochaska, J. O., & DiClemente, C. C. (1983). Stages and process of self-change of smoking: Toward an integrative model of change. *Journal of Consulting and Clinical Psychology, 51*, 390–395.

Rector, T. S., Kubo, S. H., & Cohn, J. N. (1993). Validity of the Minnesota living with heart failure questionnaire as a measure of therapeutic response to enalapril or placebo. *American Journal of Cardiology, 71*, 1106–1107.

Reichgott, M. J., Pearson, S., & Hill, M. N. (1983). The nurse practitioner's role in complex patient management: Hypertension. *Journal of the National Medical Association, 75*, 1197–1204.

Renders, C. M., Valk, G. D., Griffin, S., Wagner, E. H., Eijk, J. T. H. M., & van Assendelft, W. J. J. (2003). *Interventions to improve the management of diabetes mellitus in primary care, outpatient and community settings.* Amsterdam: Institute for Research in Extramural Medicine. Cochrane Review.

Riegel, B. C., Kopp, Z., LePetri, B., Glaser, D., & Unger, A. (2002). Effect of a standardized nurse case-management telephone intervention on resource use in patients with chronic heart failure. *Archives of Internal Medicine, 162*, 705–712.

Reigel, B., & LePetri, B. (2001). *Improving outcomes in heart failure. Heart failure disease management models* (pp. 267–281). Gaithersburg, Maryland: Aspen Publishing.

Rich, M. W. (2001). Heart failure disease management programs: efficacy and limitations. *American Journal of Medicine, 110*(5), 410–2.

Rich, M. W., Beckham V., et al. (1995). A multidisciplinary intervention to prevent the readmission of elderly patients with congestive heart failure. *New England Journal of Medicine, 333*(18), 1190–5.

Rigotti, N. A., McKool, K. M., & Shiffman, S. (1994). Predictors of smoking cessation after coronary artery bypass graft surgery: Results of a randomized trial with 5-year follow-up. *Annals of Internal Medicine, 120*, 287–293.

The Robert Wood Johnson Foundation. Health and healthcare 2010:The forecast, the challenge. Princeton NJ: The Robert Wood Johnson Foundation, 2000. Online. Available at http://www.rwjf.org/publications/publicationsPdfs/iftf/index.htm

Runyan, K. W. Jr. (1975). The Memphis Chronic Disease Program. Comparison in outcome and the nurse's extended role. *JAMA, 231*, 264–267.

Shaffer, J., & Wexler, L. F. (1995). Reducing low-density lipoprotein cholesterol levels in an ambulatory care system. *Archives of Internal Medicine, 155*, 2330–2335.

Sivarajan, E. S., Bruce, R. A., Almes, M. J., Green, B., Belanger, L., Newton, K. M., & Mansfield, L. W. (1981) In-hospital exercise after myocardial infarction does not improve treadmill perfomance. *New England Journal of Medicine, 305*, 357–62.

Sivarajan, E. S., Newton, K. M., Almes, M. J., Kempf, T. M., Mansfield, L. W., & Bruce, R. A. (1983) Limited effects of out-patient teaching and counseling after myocardial infarction: a controlled study. *Heart and Lung, 12*, 65–73.

Sivarajan, E. S., Bruce, R. A., Lindskog, B. D., Almes, M. J., Belanger, L., & Green, B. (1982). Treadmill test responses to an early exercise program after myocardial infarction: a randomized study. *Circulation, 65*, 1420–1428.

Sivarajan, E. S., & Newton, K. M. (1984) Symposium on cardiac rehabilitation: Exercise, education and counseling for patients with coronary artery disease. *Clinics of Sports Medicine, 2*, 349–369.

Sivarajan Froelicher, E., & Kozuki, Y. (2002) Application of theory to smoking cessation intervention. Women's Initiative for Non-smoking IV. *International Journal of Nursing Studies, 39*, 1–15.

Smith, S., Blair, S., et al. (2001). AHA/ACC Scientific Statement: AHA/ACC guidelines for preventing heart attack and death in patients with atherosclerotic cardiovascular disease: 2001 update: a statement for healthcare professionals from the American Heart Association and the American College of Cardiology. *Circulation, 104*, 1577–1579.

Stewart, A. L., Greeenfield, S., Hays, R. D., et al. (1989). Functional status and well being of patients with chronic conditions. Results from the Medical Outcomes Study. *JAMA, 262,* 907–913.

Stewart, A. L.. Hays, R. D., & Ware, J. E. (1988) The MOS short form general health survey: reliability and vailidy in a patient population. *Medical Care,* 724–735.

Stewart, S., & Horowitz, J. (2002). Home-based intervention in congestive heart failure: Long term implications on readmission and survival. *Circulation,* 105, 286–6.

Stewart, S., & Horowitz, J. (2003). Specialist nurse management programmes. *Pharmacoeconomics,* 21(4), 225–240.

Stewart, S., Horowitz J., & Pearson, S. (1998). Effects of a home-based intervention among patients with congestive heart failure discharged from acute hospital care. *Archives of Internal Medicine,* 158, 1067–1072.

Stewart, S., Marley, J. E., & Horowitz, J. D. (1999). Effects of a multidisciplinary, home-based intervention on planned readmissions and survival among patients with chronic congestive heart failure: a randomized controlled study. *Lancet,* 354, 1077–83.

Stewart, S., Vanderbrock, A. J., Pearson, S., & Horowitz, J. D. (1999). Prolonged beneficial effects of a home-based intervention on unplanned readmissions and morality among patients with congestive heart failure. *Archives of Internal Medicine,* 159, 257–261.

Tarlov, A. R., Ware, J., Greenfield, S., Nelson, E., & Zubkoff, M. (1989). The medical outcomes study: an application of methods for monitoring the results of medical care. *JAMA,* 262, 925–930.

Taylor, C. B., Miller, N. H., Killen, J. D., & DeBusk, R. F. (1990). Smoking cessation after acute myocardial infarction: Effects of a nurse-managed intervention. *Annals of Internal Medicine,* 13, 118–123.

Taylor, C. B., Houston Miller, N., Reilly, K. R., Greenwald, G., Cunning, D., Deeter, A., & Abascal, L. (2003). Evaluation of a nurse-care management system to improve outcomes in patients with complicated diabetes. *Diabetes Care,* 26, 1058–1053.

Unger, B. T., & Warren, D. A. (1999). Case management in cardiac rehabilitation. In N. K. Wenger, K. L. Smith, et al. (Eds.), *Cardiac rehabilitation: A guide to practice in the 21st century* (pp. 327–341). New York: Marcel Dekker, Inc.

Von Korff, Michael, S. D., Gruman, J., Schaefer, J., Curry, S. J., & Wagner, E. H. (1997). Collaborative management of chronic illness. *Annals of Internal Medicine,* 127(12), 1097–1102.

Ware, J. E., Jr. (1976). Scales for measuring general health perceptions. *Health Services Research,* 11, 396–415.

Wagner, E. (1998). Chronic disease management: what will it take to improve care for chronic illness? *Effective Clinical Practice,* 1, 2–4.

Wagner, E. H., Austin, B., & Von Korff, M. (1996). Organizing care for patients with chronic illness. *Milbank Quarterly,* 74(4), 511–542.

Weinberger, M., Kirkman, M. S., Samsa, G. P., Shortliffe, E. A., Landsman, P. P. B., Cowpe, P. A., Simel, D., & Fuessner, J. R. (1995). A nurse-coordinated intervention for primary care patients with non-insulin-dependant diabetes mellitus: impact on glycemic control and health-related quality of life. *Journal of General Internal Medicine,* 10, 59–66.

Weinberger, M., Oddone, E., & Henderson, W. G. (1996). Does increased access to primary care reduce hospital readmissions? *New England Journal of Medicine,* 334(22), 1441–1447.

West, J., Miller, N. H., Parker, K. M., et al. (1997). A comprehensive management system for heart failure improves clinical outcomes and reduces medical resource utilization. *American Journal of Cardiology,* 79(1), 58–63.

Wilson, J. R., Rayos, G., Yeoh, T. K., & Gothard, P. (1995). Dissociation between exertional symptoms and circulatory function in patients with heart failure. *Circulation,* 92, 47–53.

Index

Note: Page numbers followed by *f* indicate figures, *t* tables, *d* displays, and *ncp* nursing care plans.

A

Abciximab
for myocardial infarction, 575–576
for percutaneous coronary interventions, 596
Abdomen, physical assessment of, 262–263, 263*f*
Abdominal (waist) circumference, measurement of, 938, 940*f*
Abdominal pain, in hypercholesterolemia, 905
Abdominojugular reflux, 242
Aberrancy, in arrhythmias, 402, 402*f,* 402*t,* 403*f*
Abrupt closure, in percutaneous coronary interventions, 592
Acarbose, for diabetes mellitus, 958
Accelerated idioventricular rhythm, 385–386, 562
Accelerometers, for exercise adherence, 965
Accessory pathways, impulses in, 391–394, 393*f*–396*f*
Acebutolol, for hypertension, 878*t*
ACE inhibitors. *See* Angiotensin-converting enzyme (ACE) inhibitors
Acetylcholine
in blood pressure regulation, 87–88, 88*f*
electrophysiologic effects of, 28, 29*f*
Acetylcysteine, for contrast agent complications, 168
Acid(s)
buffering of, 189–190, 190*t*
definition of, 189
excretion of, 190–191
production of, 189
Acid-base balance, 189–191, 191*t*
acid buffering in, 189–190, 190*t*
acid excretion in, 190–191
acid production in, 189
terminology of, 189
Acid-base imbalances, 191–195
arterial blood gas reports and, 194–195, 195*t*
compensation in, 191
correction of, 191
metabolic acidosis as, 192–193, 192*t,* 193*t,* 195*t*
metabolic alkalosis as, 193*t,* 194, 194*t,* 195*t*
mixed, 195, 195*t*
respiratory acidosis as, 191–192, 192*t,* 193*t,* 195*t*
respiratory alkalosis as, 193–194, 193*t,* 195*t*
Acidemia, definition of, 189
Acidosis
definition of, 189, 191
in diabetes mellitus, 951
electrophysiologic effects of, 19
metabolic, 192–193, 192*t,* 193*t,* 195*t*
respiratory, 191–192, 192*t,* 193*t,* 195*t*
Actigraphy, in sleep measurement, 200
Actin, in vascular smooth muscle, 53
Action potential, 22–27
of atrial cells, 25, 25*f*
of atrioventricular node cells, 25, 25*f*
of bundle of His, 25, 25*f*
definition of, 17
factors modifying, 28–29, 29*f*
hypercalcemia effects on, 183
hyperkalemia effects on, 181
hypocalcemia effects on, 182
of myocardial cells, 22–24, 23*f*

phases of, 23–24, 23*f*
properties of, 22, 22*f,* 22*t*
of Purkinje-type cells, 25
refractory period in, 25–26, 26*f*
of sinus node-type cells, 24–25
Activated clotting time (ACT), 157*t,* 284
Activated partial thromboplastin time (aPTT), 157*t,* 266, 284
Activation gate, of ion channels, 21
Active ion transport, across cell membrane, 21–22
Active vasoconstriction, 96
Active vasodilation, 96
Activity, physical. *See* Exercise
Activity intolerance, after cardiac transplantation, 654*ncp*
Acupuncture, 976, 978*f,* 982
Acute coronary syndromes. *See also* Angina; Myocardial infarction; Myocardial ischemia
definition of, 342
epidemiology of, 550
nursing implications of, 547
phases of, 342
spectrum of, 550, 551*f*
Acute marginal branch, of right coronary artery, 14
Acute rejection, in cardiac transplantation, 19
Acute respiratory distress syndrome, radiography in, 303*t,* 306*f*
Adaptive AV delay, in pacing, 712*d*
Adenosine, for arrhythmias, 367*t,* 373*t*
Adenosine triphosphate (ATP)
formation of, creatine kinase in, 272
in myocardial metabolism, 41
ADH. *See* Antidiuretic hormone (ADH)
Adherence (compliance), 961–973
behavior change for, 966, 967*d*
to cholesterol-lowering therapy, 912
definition of, 961
determinants of, 965–966, 966*d*
measurement of, 962–965, 963*t*
biologic measures in, 963*t,* 964
diaries in, 963*t,* 964
electronic monitoring in, 963*t,* 964–965
pill counts in, 963*t,* 965
self-reporting in, 962–964, 963*t*
vs. nonadherence, 961–962
statistics on, 961–962
strategies for enhancing, 966–971, 966*d*
educational, 969, 970*d*
questionnaires for, 963–964, 969–970
therapeutic relationship for, 970–971
Adhesion molecules, as inflammatory markers, 129
Adrenal gland dysfunction, hypertension in, 862*d,* 863
Adrenal hormones, in shock, 663–664, 664*f*
Adrenergic effects, on electrophysiology, 28, 29*f*
Adrenergic receptors
agonists of, for hypertension, 878*t*
blockers of, for hypertension, 878*t*
in blood pressure regulation, 84, 86, 86*t*
classification of, 84
in skin, 86
stimulation of, 58–59
in venous system, 98

Adrenergic receptors
aging effects on, 223
in blood pressure regulation, 84, 86, 86*t*
classification of, 84
epinephrine stimulation of, 89
stimulation of, 59, 59*f*
in venous system, 98
Adrenomedullin, in heart failure, 608
Adult advanced cardiac life support, 691–695, 693*f*–695*f*
Adult respiratory distress syndrome
postoperative, 640
in shock, 666
Advanced cardiac life support
algorithms for, 695, 695*d,* 696*f,* 697*f,* 698–699, 698*d*
description of, 691–695, 693*f*–695*f*
Advanced glycation end products, in diabetes mellitus, 953
Adventitia, 49, 50*f*
Adventitious breath sounds, 261
Afterdepolarization, triggered activity from, 362–363, 363*f*
Afterload, 36, 36*f*
cardiac output and, 93–94
force-velocity relationship and, 38–39, 38*f*
hemodynamic characteristics of, 507*t*
Aging. *See also* Older adults
physiologic adaptations with, 220–226
cardiovascular system, 222–223
concepts of, 220
general, 221–222
heart rate variability, 532
kidney, 224–225
liver, 225
pharmacokinetics, 225
respiratory system, 223–224, 224*f*
sleep, 201–202, 201*f*
thirst, 174
theories of, 220
AH interval, in electrophysiology studies, 425
AICDs. *See* Implantable cardioverter defibrillators (ICDs)
Air embolism, in pulmonary catheter removal, 497
Akinesis, of myocardium, 312
Alanine aminotransferase, measurement of, 288
Alcohol use and abuse
heart rate variability and, 534
lipoprotein levels and, 909
reduction of, in hypertension, 873–874
smoking cessation and, 850, 850*f*
Aldosterone
antagonists of, for heart failure, 619–620
in blood pressure regulation, 89*f,* 91–92
in kidney regulation, 175*t*
Aldosterone receptor blockers, for hypertension, 879*t*
Aldosteronism, hypertension in, 862*d,* 863
Alert period, in pacing, 712*d*
Alkalemia, definition of, 189
Alkaline phosphatase, measurement of, 288
Alkalosis
contraction, 194
definition of, 189, 193

Alkalosis (continued)
    electrophysiologic effects of, 19
    metabolic, 193t, 194, 194t, 195t
    respiratory, 193–194, 193t, 195t
Allen test, 241
    modified, 484, 484t
Allergy
    to contrast agents, 472, 593–594
    in history taking, 232
Allicin, for cardiovascular disease, 981
Allografts, for prosthetic valves, 764
Allopathic medicine, definition of, 974
Alpha-adrenergic receptors. See Adrenergic
        receptors
Alpha-glucosidase inhibitors, for diabetes
        mellitus, 958
Alternative medicine. See Complementary and
        alternative medicine
Alveolar pressure, in lung zones, 73–74, 73f
Alveoli, aging effects on, 224, 224f
American Association of Cardiovascular and
        Pulmonary Rehabilitation, model of,
        932, 933d
American College of Cardiology
    cardiac catheterization guidelines of,
        459–460, 460t
    coronary artery bypass surgery guidelines
        of, 631
    exercise testing guidelines of, 440
    heart failure classification of, 612–613, 613t,
        616–617, 616t
    implantable cardioverter defibrillator guidelines
        of, 739, 740d
    myocardial infarction criteria of, 545
American College of Physicians, exercise testing
        guidelines of, 440
American College of Sports Medicine, exercise
        prescription definition of, 929
American Heart Association
    advanced cardiac life support procedure of
        algorithms of, 695, 695d, 696f, 697f,
        698–699, 698d
        description of, 691–695, 693f–695f
    cardiac catheterization guidelines of,
        459–460, 460t
    cardiac rehabilitation model of, 932, 933d
    chest pain management algorithm of,
        562, 563f
    coronary artery bypass surgery guidelines
        of, 631
    exercise testing guidelines of, 440
    heart failure classification of, 612–613, 613t,
        616–617, 616t
    implantable cardioverter defibrillator guidelines
        of, 739, 740d
    lesion classification system of, 139–143, 140f
Amiloride, for hypertension, 878t
Amino acids, in myocardial metabolism, 41
Aminocaproic acid, for postoperative
        bleeding, 637
Amiodarone
    for arrhythmias, 367t–368t
    for cardiac arrest, 698d, 706
    for heart failure, 620, 621
    for hypertrophic cardiomyopathy, 785
Amlodipine, for hypertension, 879t
Ammonia, in acid excretion, 190
13N-Ammonia, in positron emission
        tomography, 322
Amplatz catheter, for coronary arteriography,
        467, 468f
Amyl nitrate, heart sounds and, 257t, 258
Amyloid A, as inflammatory marker, 133

Anaphylactic shock, pathophysiology of, 662
Anatomic reentry, 365, 365f
Anemia
    in heart failure, 615
    hemolytic, from prosthetic valves, 766
Anemic hypoxia, 77
Aneroid manometers, for blood pressure
        measurement, 243–244, 244f
Aneurysms
    aortic
        intra-aortic balloon pump contraindicated
            in, 677
        radiography in, 303t, 305f
        repair of, 635–636
    atherosclerotic, 145
    left ventricular, in myocardial infarction, 560
Anger, coronary artery disease and, 827, 834
Angina, 550–556
    in aortic stenosis, 771
    cardiac catheterization in, 459–460, 460t
    chronic stable, atherosclerotic lesion types
        in, 146
    classification of, 553t, 554, 554t
    description of, 231
    in exercise testing, 450, 450d
    heart rate variability in, 531
    in hypertrophic cardiomyopathy, 784
    intra-aortic balloon pump for, 675
    in myocardial infarction, 557
    in myocardial ischemia, 545, 923
    nursing management in, 555–556
    pathophysiology of, 541, 542f
    in percutaneous coronary interventions,
        592, 598
    in sleep, 208
    stable (classic), 545, 550–553
        angiography in, 552–553
        cardiac rehabilitation in. See Cardiac
            rehabilitation
        diagnosis of, 552
        history in, 550–551
        physical assessment in, 551–552
        prognosis for, 553
        risk factors for, 551
        treatment of, 553, 553t
        triggers of, 550–551
    unstable, 545, 553–555, 554t
    variant (Prinzmetal's), 208, 545, 555
Anginal equivalents, 550, 557
Angiogenesis, in myocardial ischemia, 545
Angiography
    computed tomography, 324
    coronary, 467–469, 468f–471f, 552–553
    magnetic resonance, 322–323
        in angina, 552
        in atherosclerosis, 143t
    pulmonary, in pulmonary embolism, 168
Angiojet thrombectomy, 589
Angioplasty, coronary
    creatine kinase after, 273–274, 274f
    laser, 589
    percutaneous transluminal, 587–588, 588f
Angioscopy, in atherosclerosis, 143t
Angiotensin, in blood pressure regulation, 89f,
        91–92
Angiotensin-converting enzyme, gene of,
        polymorphisms of, 7–8
Angiotensin-converting enzyme (ACE) inhibitors
    for dilated cardiomyopathy, 783
    for heart failure, 616–619, 617t, 619t
    for hypertension, 879t, 880t
    for myocardial infarction, 574–575
    for myocardial ischemia, 705

Angiotensin II receptor blockers
    for heart failure, 619, 619t
    for hypertension, 879t, 880t
Anion gap, measurement of, 287
Anisotropic reentry, 365
Anisoylated plasminogen streptokinase activator
        complex, for myocardial infarction, 564
Annuloplasty, in mitral regurgitation, 768
Antegrade cardioplegia, 630
Anterior hemiblock (left anterior fascicular block),
        341, 345f
Antiarrhythmic drugs
    for cardiac arrest prevention, 427–428, 706
    classification of, 366t
    for heart failure, 621
    implantable cardioverter defibrillator and, 749
    for myocardial ischemia, 705
Antibiotics, for endocarditis, 789
Anticoagulants
    for angina, 555
    cardiac catheterization and, 460
    for deep vein thrombosis, 164–165, 165t
    for heart failure, 618
    natural, 156–157
    for percutaneous coronary interventions,
        595–596
    for pulmonary embolism, 168–169
Antidepressants
    for depression, 834–835
    for heart failure, 618
Antidiuretic hormone (ADH)
    in blood pressure control, 89–90, 90f
    excess of, in heart failure, 608, 610f
    in kidney regulation, 175t
    postoperative, 638t
Antidromic atrioventricular reentry tachycardia,
        397, 399f
Antioxidants, coronary artery disease and, 820
Antiplatelet drugs
    for angina, 555
    coagulation studies and, 283–284
Antitachycardia pacing, 734–735, 737f
Antithrombin III, 156
    deficiency of, deep vein thrombosis in, 163
Antithymocyte preparations, for cardiac
        transplantation, 648t, 649–650
Anxiety
    in congenital heart disease, 804ncp
    coronary artery disease in, 827, 833
    with implantable cardioverter
        defibrillator, 750
    in myocardial infarction, 579
    in percutaneous coronary interventions,
        597–598
Aorta
    aneurysms of
        intra-aortic balloon pump contraindicated
            in, 677
        radiography in, 303t, 305f
        repair of, 635–636
    atherosclerosis of, 146
    balloon pump for. See Intra-aortic
        balloon pump
    blood flow velocity in, variation in, 502t
    blood volume in, 61, 62f
    coarctation of, 796f, 797–798, 797t, 863
    cross-clamping of, myocardial protection
        with, 630
    dissection of, repair of, 635–636
    stenosis of. See Aortic stenosis
    structure of, 50f
    thrombosis of, in heparin-induced
        thrombocytopenia, 170

topographic location of, 250
transposition of, 796f, 802–803
vascular resistance in, 61, 62f
Aortic ejection sound, 255, 255f
Aortic impedance, in afterload, 36
Aortic pressure, in cardiac cycle, 44–45, 44f, 64, 64f
Aortic pressure wave, 484–486, 484f–486f
Aortic root
    dilation of, insufficiency in, 772–774, 773t
    echocardiography of, 316
Aortic stenosis, 770–772
    cardiac arrest in, 690
    cause of, 770
    clinical manifestations of, 771
    congenital, 796–797, 796f
    diagnosis of, 771, 772f
    echocardiography in, 315
    exertional syncope in, 82–83
    medical management of, 771
    murmurs of, 762t
    pathology of, 770
    pathophysiology of, 770–771
    physical assessment of, 771
    surgical management of, 771–772
Aortic valve
    anatomy of, 6f, 8–9
    bicuspid, in aortic coarctation, 796f, 797–798
    cardiac cycle and, 44f, 46
    conduction system to, 11, 12f
    echocardiography of, 314–315
    function of, 8–9, 8f
    heart sounds and, 44f, 46
    regurgitation of, 772–774
        cause of, 772–773
        clinical manifestations of, 773
        diagnosis of, 773–774
        echocardiography in, 315
        heart rate variability in, 532
        intra-aortic balloon pump contraindicated in, 677
        medical management of, 774
        murmurs in, 256
        pathology of, 773
        pathophysiology of, 773
        physical assessment of, 773, 773t
        shock in, 661
        surgical management of, 774
    replacement of, 305f, 634–635
        minimally invasive technique for, 764–765
        in regurgitation, 774
        in stenosis, 772
    in Ross procedure, 764, 764f
    stenosis of. See Aortic stenosis
    stentless bioprosthesis for, 764
Apex impulse
    assessment of, 251–252
    in chest wall, 251
Apical branches, of left coronary artery, 15
Apical–radial pulse rate, 239
Apnea, sleep, 209–210, 209f
    hypertension in, 862d, 863
Apolipoproteins
    abnormalities of, 900t
    functions of, 897–899
    as inflammatory markers, 133
    measurement of, 277–278
Apoptosis, of myocardial cells
    in heart failure, 610
    in shock, 665
Appetite suppressants, for obesity, 944
Aprotinin, for postoperative bleeding, 637

Argatroban
    for deep vein thrombosis, 165t
    for heparin-induced thrombocytopenia, 170–171
Arginine vasopressin. See Antidiuretic hormone (ADH)
Arousal state
    definition of, 197
    heart rate variability in, 533
Arrhythmias. See also specific names of arrhythmias and Conduction disorders
    in aortic stenosis, 771
    in atrial septal defect, 798–799
    blood pressure measurement in, 248
    cardiac arrest in, 689, 691
    after cardiac catheterization, 474
    after cardiac transplantation, 646
    complex, 391–421
        atrioventricular dissociation, 417–418, 417f–419f
        concealed conduction, 420–421, 421f, 422f
        differential diagnosis of, 401–408, 402f–410f, 402t
        multilevel atrioventricular block, 413–417, 415f, 416f
        parasystole, 418–420, 419f, 420f
        preexcitation syndromes, 391–394, 393f–396f
        supraventricular tachycardias, 394–398, 397f, 398f
        ventricular tachycardia, 398–401, 399f–401f
        Wenckebach conduction, 408–413, 410f–415f
    in conduction blocks. See Conduction blocks
    in dilated cardiomyopathy, 783
    vs. dysrhythmias, 365–366
    in Ebstein anomaly, 800–801
    electrocardiography in. See Electrocardiography
    electrophysiology studies of. See Electrophysiology procedures
    evaluation of, for cardiac rehabilitation, 923
    in exercise testing, 450
    in heart failure, 601, 618, 621
    heart rate variability in, 531
    in hypercalcemia, 183
    in hyperkalemia, 181
    in hypocalcemia, 182
    in hypokalemia, 180
    in hypomagnesemia, 184
    in hypophosphatemia, 186
    in magnesium deficiency, 287
    mechanisms of, 361–365
        abnormal impulse conduction, 363–365, 364f, 365f
        abnormal impulse initiation, 361–363, 362f, 363f
    in myocardial infarction, 562
    origins of
        in atria, 379–383
        in atrioventricular junction, 383–384
        sinus node, 366, 376–379
        in ventricles, 384–388
    in percutaneous coronary interventions, 593, 598
    postoperative, 638–640, 639f
    in pulmonary artery catheter removal, 497
    sinus, resting, 93
    in sleep, 208–209
    in sleep apnea, 210
    in stress, 827
    treatment of. See Antiarrhythmic drugs; Implantable cardioverter defibrillators; Pacemaker(s) (artificial)

Arterial baroreceptors, in blood pressure regulation, 81, 82f, 102–103, 103f, 104f
Arterial blood gases. See also specific gases, eg, Carbon dioxide; Oxygen
    in acid-base imbalances, 194–195, 195t
    in heart failure, 615
    measurement of, 78, 286
    in shock, 667
    in sleep, 203
Arterial light reflex, in hypertension, 866
Arterial pressure, 63–64, 64f
    in lung zones, 73–74, 73f
    monitoring of, 483–488
        catheter placement for, 484, 484t
        complications of, 488, 488t
        data interpretation in, 486–487
        direct vs. cuff, 487, 487f
        indications for, 483
        pressure wave in, 484–486, 484f–486f
Arterial pressure wave, 484–486, 484f–486f
Arterial pulse, assessment of, 239–241, 240f, 241f
Arterial switch procedure, for transposition of great arteries, 802
Arteriography. See Angiography
Arterioles, 50, 50f
    basal tone of, in blood pressure regulation, 95–96, 95f
    blood volume in, 61, 62f
    vascular resistance in, 61, 62f
Arteriosclerosis, risk factors for, hypertension as, 865
Arteriovenous fistula, in percutaneous coronary interventions, 594–595
Arteriovenous nicking, in retina, 238, 238f
Artery(ies), 49–50, 50f
    aging effects on, 223
    blood volume in, 61, 62f
    catheters in, blood drawing from, 483
    coronary. See Coronary artery(ies)
    dilators for, 621
    pulmonary. See Pulmonary artery(ies)
    thickening or hardening of. See Atherosclerosis
    thrombosis of, in heparin-induced thrombocytopenia, 170, 170t
    vascular resistance in, 61, 62f
Aschoff nodules, in rheumatic fever, 757
Ascites, in heart failure, 612
Ashman's phenomenon, 404–405
Aspartate aminotransferase, 270f, 270t, 288
Aspirin
    for heart failure, 618
    for myocardial infarction, 572–573
    for percutaneous coronary interventions, 595–596
Assessment, physical. See Physical assessment
Asynchronous pacing, 711d, 716
Asystole
    prognosis for, 704
    treatment of, 375t, 697f, 698
    ventricular, 387–388
Atelectasis, postoperative, 640
Atenolol
    for arrhythmias, 368t, 373t
    for hypertension, 878t
Atherectomy, coronary, 588–589, 589f
Atheromas, 141–142, 147t, 542–543
Atherosclerosis, 139–149. See also Atherosclerotic lesions
    with aging, 223
    amyloid in, 133
    aortic, 146
    cardiac arrest in, 690

Atherosclerosis, *(continued)*
  cardiogenic shock in, 659
  cerebrovascular, 146
  coronary. *See* Coronary artery disease
  C-reactive protein in, 131
  definition of, 139
  electron beam computed tomography in, 324
  genetic factors in, 116–118, 116*t*
  high-density lipoprotein protection
        against, 899
  inflammation in, 158
  interleukin 6 in, 132–133
  pathophysiology of, 116, 128, 158,
        542–543
    oxidized LDL in, 900
    triglycerides in, 901
  percutaneous procedures for. *See* Percutaneous
        coronary interventions
  peripheral, 146, 249–250
  polymorphisms in, 119–120, 119*t*
  posttransplantation, 647
  risk factors for, 139, 140*t*, 938–939
    hypertension as, 865
    laboratory tests for, 279–281, 279*f*
    smoking as, 839
  vascular resistance in, 43
Atherosclerotic lesions
  aneurysms in, 145
  angina in, 146
  aortic, 146
  appearance of, 147*t*
  cerebrovascular, 146
  clinical correlations of, 146
  components of, 143–145, 147*t*
    calcium as, 144–145
    collagen as, 144
    elastin as, 144
    fibrinogen as, 144
    lipids and lipoproteins as, 144
    lymphocytes as, 143–144
    macrophages as, 143
    proteoglycans as, 144
    smooth muscle cells as, 143
  coronary. *See* Coronary artery disease
  evaluation of, 142, 143*t*
  formation of, 158
  histology of, 147*t*
  ischemic coronary syndromes in, 146
  in myocardial ischemia and infarction
        development, 542–543
  paradoxical vasoconstriction due to, 541
  percutaneous procedures for. *See* Percutaneous
        coronary interventions
  peripheral, 146
  stenosis caused by, 145–146
  thrombi in, 145
  type I (initial), 139–140, 147*t*
  type II (fatty streaks), 140–141, 147*t*
  type IIa (progressive), 141
  type IIb (progression-resistant), 140–141, 147*t*
  type III (intermediate, transitional,
        preatheroma), 141, 147*t*
  type IV (atheroma), 141–142, 147*t*
  type V (fibroatheroma), 142, 147*t*
  type VI (complicated, disrupted), 142, 147*t*
"Athletes heart," 604*f*
ATP (adenosine triphosphate)
  formation of, creatine kinase in, 272
  in myocardial metabolism, 41
Atrial branches, of right coronary artery, 14
Atrial capture, in pacing, 730
Atrial defibrillators, 744*d*
Atrial escape interval, in pacing, 712*d*, 727

Atrial fibrillation, 382–383
  atrial defibrillators for, 744*d*
  blood pressure measurement in, 248
  electrocardiography in, 405
  in heart failure, 618
  in hypertrophic cardiomyopathy, 785
  in magnesium deficiency, 287
  in mitral stenosis, 759
  in myocardial infarction, 760
  postoperative, 638–639
  radiofrequency catheter ablation for, 432*d*,
        434, 435*f*
  treatment of, 373*t*–374*t*, 393, 618
  in Wolff-Parkinson-White syndrome,
        392–393, 395*f*
Atrial flutter, 381–382
  electrocardiography in, 405, 407*f*
  postoperative, 639, 639*f*
  radiofrequency catheter ablation for, 432*d*,
        434, 435*f*
  treatment of, 373*t*–374*t*
Atrial natriuretic peptide
  in blood pressure regulation, 89*f*, 90–92, 91*f*
  in heart failure, 606–608, 609*f*, 610*f*
  in kidney regulation, 175*t*
  measurement of, 280–281
Atrial overdrive pacing, 733–734, 736*f*
Atrial pacing state, 728, 729*f*
Atrial pressure, in cardiac cycle, 44–45, 44*f*
Atrial refractory period, in pacing, 712*d*, 727
Atrial sensing, in pacing, 730
Atrial septum
  cardiac catheterization through, 465–466, 466*f*
  defects of
    congenital, 796*f*, 798–799
    percutaneous interventions for,
        596–597, 597*f*
Atrial tachycardia, 380–381
  multifocal, 380
  paroxysmal, 380–381
  treatment of, 373*t*–374*t*
Atrial tracking, in pacing, 712*d*, 728, 729*f*
Atriobiventricular pacing, 736
Atriohisian fibers, 391, 394
Atrioventricular block(s), 388–391
  blood pressure measurement in, 248
  first-degree, 388
  high-grade, 390–391
  multilevel, 413–417, 415*f*, 416*f*
  pacemakers for, 710*d*
  in pacing, 730–731, 731*f*
  second-degree, 388–390
    with 2:1 conduction ratio, 389–390,
        414–415, 415*f*, 416*f*
    type I (Wenckebach), 389, 408–410,
        410*f*–412*f*
    type II, 389
    third-degree (complete), 390–391
  treatment of, 375*t*
Atrioventricular dissociation, 417–418,
        417*f*–419*f*
  blood pressure measurement in, 248
Atrioventricular interval/delay, in pacing, 712*d*, 727
Atrioventricular junction, arrhythmias originating
        in, 383–384
Atrioventricular nodal reentrant tachycardia, 396,
        397*f*, 398*f*
  radiofrequency catheter ablation for, 431, 431*f*
  treatment of, 373*t*–374*t*
Atrioventricular node
  action potential of, 25, 25*f*
  aging effects on, 222
  anatomy of, 10–11, 11*f*

blood supply of, 13*t*, 14
  conduction through, 30
  function of, 326
Atrioventricular reentrant tachycardia,
        radiofrequency catheter ablation for,
        432*d*, 433–434, 433*f*, 434*f*
Atrioventricular reentry tachycardia using
        accessory pathway, 373*t*–374*t*,
        397–398, 399*f*
Atrioventricular septum, anatomy of, 8
Atrioventricular sequential pacing state, 728, 729*f*
Atrioventricular valves. *See also* Mitral valve;
        Tricuspid valve
  anatomy of, 8
Atrium (atria). *See also subjects starting with* Atrial
  anatomy of, 3, 4*f*, 5*f*, 6–7, 7*f*
  arrhythmias originating in, 379–383
  blood supply of, 13*t*, 14–15
  conduction in, 30, 30*t*
  contraction of, 44*f*, 45–46
  electrograms in, 405, 409*f*, 425, 427*f*
  enlargement of, 349–351, 354*f*
  function of, 7, 8*f*
  innervation of, 16
  left
    echocardiography of, 314
    enlargement of, 349–350, 354*f*
    myocardial cells of, action potential of, 25, 25*f*
  right
    in Ebstein anomaly, 800–801
    enlargement of, 350, 354*f*
    pressure monitoring in, 488–489,
        490*d*–491*d*, 492*f*
    topographic location of, 250
Atropine
  for arrhythmias, 368*t*
  for asystole, 697*f*
  for bradyarrhythmias, 375*t*, 703
Auscultation
  in abdominal assessment, 262
  in blood pressure measurement, 245–246,
        245*f*, 245*t*, 246*f*
  of bruits, 241
  of heart, 252–258
    dynamic, 257–258, 257*t*
    extra diastolic sounds in, 254, 254*f*, 255*f*
    extra systolic sounds in, 255, 255*f*
    murmurs in, 255–256, 255*f*, 255*t*.
        See also Murmurs
    normal heart sounds in, 253–254, 253*f*
    pericardial friction rubs in, 256–257, 256*f*,
        777–778
    stethoscope for, 252, 252*f*
    technique for, 252–253, 252*t*
  in lung assessment, 259–260, 262, 262*f*
Austin Flint murmur, in aortic regurgitation, 773
Autacoids, 53
Automated external defibrillators, 692–693,
        706, 706*d*
Automatic interval, in pacing, 711*d*
Automaticity
  abnormal, 362
  definition of, 18
  enhanced normal, 361–362, 362*f*
  factors modifying, 28
  normal, 361
Autonomic nervous system
  aging effects on, 223
  in blood pressure regulation, 84–89, 85*f*
    co-transmitters, 88–89, 88*f*
    cutaneous vasculature, 86–87
    neuropeptide Y, 88, 88*f*
    neurotransmitters, 87, 87*f*

parasympathetic branch, 85f, 86t, 87–88
sympathetic branch, 84, 86, 86t
vasoactive intestinal peptide, 89
dysfunction of, hypertension in, 861
of heart, 16
heart rate variability and, 526
aging changes with, 532
in alcohol use, 534
in angina, 531
in arrhythmias, 531
body position and, 533
in brain injury, 534–535
in cardiac surgery, 532
in COPD, 535
in depression, 535
in diabetes mellitus, 535
in heart failure, 531–532
in Huntington disease, 535
in hypertension, 531
in myocardial infarction, 530–531
in pain, 534
in Parkinson disease, 535
in sleep-wake cycle, 533
in smoking, 534
structure of, 84, 85f, 87
Autoregressive method, for heart rate variability
analysis, 529
Autoregulation, of blood flow, 96–98, 97f
cerebral, in hypertension, 866–867
AV node. See Atrioventricular node
a wave, in pulmonary artery wedge pressure,
494, 496f
Axillary artery, catheter placement in, 488
Axis determination, in electrocardiography,
336–337, 337f–340f
Azathioprine, for cardiac transplantation,
648t, 649

B

Background outward current, 27
Backward heart failure, 601–602
Balke treadmill protocol, for exercise testing, 444
Balloon
in coronary angioplasty, 587–588, 588f
in directional coronary atherectomy,
588–589, 589f
intra-aortic. See Intra-aortic balloon
pump (IABP)
on pulmonary artery catheters, 492, 492f, 493
in valvuloplasty
for aortic stenosis, 771–772
for mitral stenosis, 760–761, 761f
Bandura model, for smoking cessation, 840
Bariatric surgery, for obesity, 945
Barlow syndrome. See Mitral valve, prolapse of
Baroreceptors, in blood pressure regulation
arterial, 81, 82f, 102–103, 103f, 104f
cardiopulmonary, 81
Barrel chest, 258, 260f
Basal tone, arteriolar, in blood pressure regulation,
95–96, 95f
Base. See also Acid-base balance; Acid-base
imbalances
definition of, 189
Base rate, in pacing, 711d
Basic interval, in pacing, 711d
Basiliximab, for cardiac transplantation, 650
Basophils, 151f, 152, 153t
count of, 282
Batista procedure
for dilated cardiomyopathy, 783
for heart failure, 618, 635

Bazett's formula, 328
BEARS acronym, for sleep assessment, 211
Beck Depression Inventory, 829
Bed rest, cardiovascular effects of, 921, 921d
Bedside testing, 269
Behavioral assessment, of sleep, 200
Behavioral change
for adherence, models of, 966, 967d
for cholesterol-lowering diet, 907–908
Behavioral therapy, for obesity, 943–944
Beliefs, in history taking, 234
Benazepril, for hypertension, 879t
Beta-adrenergic blockers
for arrhythmias, 373t, 639
for dilated cardiomyopathy, 783
for heart failure, 616–618, 617t, 619t,
620, 620t
hyperkalemia due to, 181
for hypertension, 878t, 880t
for hypertrophic cardiomyopathy, 784–785
for myocardial infarction, 573–574
for myocardial ischemia, 705
Beta-adrenergic receptors. See
Adrenergic receptors
Betaxolol, for hypertension, 878t
Bezold-Jarisch reflex, in blood pressure regulation,
81–83, 83f
Biatrial enlargement, 350–351
Bicarbonate buffer system, 189–190, 190t
Bicarbonate ion
in acid-base imbalances, 195
excess of, in metabolic alkalosis, 194,
194t, 195t
measurement of, 287
Bicycle ergometer, for exercise testing, 442–444
Bifascicular blocks
electrocardiography in, 342, 345f, 346f
pacemakers for, 710d
Bigeminal pulses, 240, 240f
Bigeminal rhythms, blood pressure measurement
in, 248
Biguanides, for diabetes mellitus, 958
Bile-acid binding resins, for hyperlipidemia,
911–912, 911t
Bileaflet prosthetic valves, 763, 763f
Bilirubin, measurement of, 288
Biofeedback, 978
Biologic measures, of adherence, 963t, 964
Biomarkers, for cardiovascular disease.
See Inflammatory marker(s)
Biopsy
endomyocardial, in myocarditis, 786
heart, in transplant rejection, 646–647, 646f
Bipolar leads
in electrocardiography, 331–332, 333f
in pacemaker, 711d, 716, 719f
Bisoprolol
for heart failure, 619t, 620
for hypertension, 878t
Bivalirudin, for percutaneous coronary
interventions, 596
Biventricular pacemakers, 714–715, 715f,
735–737, 737f
Bjork-Shiley valves, 763f
Bladder, distention of, assessment of, 263
Blanking period, in pacing, 712d, 727,
732–733, 734f
Bleeding. See Hemorrhage
Bleeding disorders, 158–162, 159d, 160f, 161t,
162d, 162t
Bleeding time (BT), 157t
Block Food Frequency Questionnaire, 964
Block response, in pacing, 730–731, 731f

Blood
components of, 150
pH of, 189
physiology of, 150
Blood cardioplegia, 630
Blood cells. See also specific type
morphology of, 282
Blood chemistries, 286–291
alanine aminotransferase, 288
alkaline phosphatase, 288
aspartate aminotransferase, 270f, 270t, 288
bilirubin, 288
catecholamines, 289
creatinine, 289
electrolytes, 286–288
glucose, 289
glycated hemoglobin, 289, 289t
glycated serum protein, 289–290
lactate dehydrogenase, 290
nursing considerations after, 291
osmolality, 287
postoperative, 287–288, 290
protein, 290
reference ranges for, 277t
specimen collection for, 291
urea nitrogen, 290
uric acid, 290
Blood culture, in endocarditis, 757–758, 788
Blood flow. See also Circulation
autoregulation of, 96–98, 97f
cerebral, during sleep, 204
coronary
control of, 42–43, 42f
regulation of, 542
definition of, 63
determinants of, 63
in microcirculation, 65
pulmonary, 71, 73–74, 73f
impairment of, in congenital heart disease,
794–798, 796f, 797t
increased, in congenital heart disease,
798–800
Blood gases, arterial. See Arterial blood gases
Blood lipids. See Lipid(s); Lipoprotein(s)
Blood oxygen content, 77
Blood pressure, 63–64, 64f
arterial. See Arterial pressure
as blood flow determinant, 63
components of, 478
decreased. See also Hypotension
arterial baroreceptor response to,
102–103, 103f
in extracellular fluid deficit, 176
definition of, 63
diastolic, 64, 64f
in hypertension, 856, 857t
measurement of, 245–246
distribution of, within vascular system, 62, 62f
in extremities, differences in, in aortic
coarctation, 797
vs. heart rate, 92
increased. See also Hypertension
arterial baroreceptor response to, 103, 104f
Korotkoff sounds in, 245–246, 245t
measurement of, 243–249, 887–888
after cardiac catheterization, 474
cuff vs. direct, 487, 487f
diastolic, 245–246
in exercise testing, 446–447
palpation in, 244
paradoxical, 247–248, 248f
position for, 244, 244f
postural, 247

Blood pressure, measurement of *(continued)*
    pulse pressure, 246–247, 246*f*
    in special conditions, 248–249
    sphygmomanometer in, 243–246, 243*t*,
        244*f*–246*f*, 245*t*
    systolic, 244–245
    in thigh, 248–249
  normal, 243
  regulation of
    antidiuretic hormone in, 89–90, 90*f*
    autonomic nervous system, 84–89, 85*f*, 86*t*,
        87*f*, 88*f*
    baroreceptors in, 81, 82*f*, 102–103,
        103*f*, 104*f*
    Bezold-Jarisch reflex in, 81–83, 83*f*
    cardiopulmonary receptors in, 81
    central nervous system, 83–84
    chemoreceptors in, 83
    epinephrine in, 89
    kallikrein-kinin system in, 89*f*, 92
    long-term, 94–96, 95*f*
    natriuretic peptides in, 89*f*, 90–92, 91*f*
    norepinephrine in, 92
    renin-angiotensin-aldosterone system in, 89*f*,
        91–92
    Valsalva maneuver and, 54, 54*f*
    venous system in, 50–51, 51*f*
  in shock, 662–666, 663*f*–665*f*
  in sleep, 203, 208
  in sleep apnea, 209–210
  systolic, 64, 64*f*
    in hypertension, 856, 857*t*
    measurement of, 244–245, 447
    vs. respiration, 501–502, 502*f*
Blood specimens
  collection of, 265–267
    for blood culture, 283
    for coagulation studies, 285
    for creatine kinase measurement, 272, 276
    guidelines for, 265–267
    labeling of, 267
    patient preparation for, 265
    results influenced by, 267–268
    tubes for, 267
    universal precautions for, 265
  contamination of, 266
  handling of, 267
  types of, 267
Blood urea nitrogen, in heart failure, 615
Blood vessels. *See* Vascular system; *specific*
    blood vessels
Blood volume
  distribution of, 61, 62*f*
  muscle pump and, 101
  pulmonary, 71
  respiratory pump and, 101
B lymphocytes, 151*f*, 152–153, 153*t*
  in atherosclerotic lesions, 143–144
  count of, 282
BMI (body mass index), 235–236
  measurement of, 938, 940*f*
  vs. treatment approach, 941, 941*t*
Body fluids. *See also* Fluid balance;
    Fluid imbalances
  compartments of, 173
  distribution of, 174
  excretion of, 174, 175*t*
  loss of, 174–175
  osmolality of, 173
Body mass index, 235–236
  coronary artery disease and, 817–818, 817*f*
  measurement of, 938, 940*f*
  vs. treatment approach, 941, 941*t*

Body temperature. *See* Temperature, body
Body weight. *See* Weight
Bohr effect, 76–77, 76*f*
Bone marrow, hematopoiesis in, 150
Borg perceived exertion scale
  in cardiac rehabilitation, 924, 925*d*
  in exercise testing, 451, 451*d*
Bowel sounds, 263
Brachial artery
  cardiac catheterization via, 463, 464*f*
  catheter placement in, 484
Brachial plexus injury, in cardiac surgery, 641
Brachial pulse, assessment of, 241, 241*f*
Brachytherapy, percutaneous methods for, 592
Bradyarrhythmias. *See also specific arrhythmias*
  in myocardial infarction, 562
  postoperative, 638
  treatment of, 375*t*
Bradycardia
  after cardiac surgery, 636
  in conduction blocks, treatment of,
    703–704, 703*f*
  implantable cardioverter defibrillators
    for, 748
  junctional, treatment of, 375*t*
  pacemakers for, 709
  sinus. *See* Sinus bradycardia
  in sleep, 208–209
  in sleep apnea, 210
  symptomatic, 709
  treatment of, 703–704, 703*f*
Bradykinin, in heart failure, 608
Bradypnea, 258, 260*f*
Brady-tachy syndrome, 378–379
Brain
  altered perfusion of, in percutaneous coronary
    interventions, 598
  arteries of, atherosclerosis of, 146
  blood flow in, during sleep, 204
  hemorrhage of, in percutaneous coronary
    interventions, 598
  hypertension effects on, 866–867
  injury of, heart rate variability in, 534–535
  metabolism of, in sleep, 204
  resuscitation of, in cardiac arrest,
    704–705, 704*d*
  shock effects on, 666
Brain death, of heart donor, 644
Brain natriuretic peptide
  in blood pressure regulation, 89*f*, 90–92, 91*f*
  in heart failure, 606–607, 609*f*, 610*f*,
    615, 615*f*
  as inflammatory marker, 129
  in kidney regulation, 175*t*
  measurement of, 280–281
  in shock, 667
Breathing, in sleep, 203
  disordered, 209–210, 209*f*
Breath sounds, 260–261, 262*f*
British Pacing and Electrophysiology Group,
    pacemaker nomenclature of,
    715–716, 715*t*
Brokenbrough needle, for cardiac catheterization,
    466, 466*f*
Bronchial sounds, 260
Bronchovesicular sounds, 260
Bruce treadmill protocol, for exercise testing, 444
Brugada syndrome
  cardiac arrest in, 690–691
  electrocardiography in, 357, 360*f*
Bruits, evaluation of, 241
Buffer systems, 189–190, 190*t*
Bumetanide, for hypertension, 878*t*

Bundle branch(es)
  anatomy of, 11–12, 11*f*
  blood supply of, 13*t*
  function of, 326
  Wenckebach conduction in, 412, 413*f*
Bundle-branch blocks, 12, 338–339, 342*f*–344*f*
  wide QRS complex rhythms and, 402*t*,
    403–404, 405*f*, 406*f*
Bundle of His
  action potential of, 25, 25*f*
  anatomy of, 10–11, 11*f*
  blood supply of, 13*t*
  conduction through, 30–31, 30*t*
  electrophysiology studies of, 430
  function of, 326
Bupropion
  for obesity, 944
  for smoking cessation, 847–849
Bursts, in ventricular tachycardia, 386
Butterworth Health System, cardiac rehabilitation
    program of, 932
BX VELOCITY stent, 591, 591*f*

C

CABG surgery. *See* Coronary artery bypass
    surgery
Cachexia, cardiac, in heart failure, 614
CAD. *See* Coronary artery disease
Caffeine
  heart rate variability and, 534
  in myocardial infarction, 571
Caged-ball prosthetic valves, 763, 763*f*
Calcification
  of aortic valve, 770, 796–797, 796*f*
  electron beam computed tomography in, 324
Calcineurin inhibitors, for cardiac transplantation,
    647, 648*t*, 649
Calcium ATPase pumps, 22
Calcium channel(s)
  in action potential
    in late rapid repolarization, 23*f*, 24
    in plateau, 23*f*, 24
  in automaticity, 362
  in excitation-contraction coupling, 31–32, 32*f*
  in pacemaking, 27
  types of, 27
Calcium channel blockers. *See also specific drugs*
  for arrhythmias, 373*t*
  for heart failure, 621
  for hypertension, 879*t*, 880*t*
  for hypertrophic cardiomyopathy, 785
  for myocardial infarction, 575
Calcium currents, 27
Calcium ion
  in atherosclerotic lesions, 144–145
  balance of, 178*t*, 182
  in contraction, 34, 35*f*
  distribution of, in myocardium, 18*t*
  equilibrium potential of, 20
  imbalance of. *See* Hypercalcemia; Hypocalcemia
  ionized, 182
  measurement of, 286–287
  movement of, 21–22
  in relaxation, 34–35, 36*f*
  signaling by, 60–61, 61*f*
  sources of, 60
  in vascular tone regulation, 60–61, 61*f*
Calmodulin
  in excitation-contraction coupling, 31–32, 32*f*
  in vascular tone regulation, 60–61, 61*f*
CAM. *See* Complementary and alternative
    medicine

Canadian Cardiovascular Society, angina
　　classification of, 553*t*
Cancer, pericarditis in, 776
Candesartan
　　for heart failure, 619*t*
　　for hypertension, 879*t*
Cannon a waves
　　in venous pulse, 243
　　in wide QRS complex rhythms, 407
Capillary(ies), 50*f*, 51
　　blood volume in, 61, 62*f*
　　coronary, 15
　　filtration in, 174
　　lymphatic, 52
　　pulmonary, gas exchange in, 74, 75
　　vascular resistance in, 61, 62*f*
Capillary filtration coefficient, 67
Capillary pressure, 66
　　vs. pulmonary artery wedge pressure, 493
Capillary refill time, 249
Capnography, sublingual, for oxygenation
　　monitoring, 517–518
Captopril
　　for heart failure, 619*t*
　　for hypertension, 879*t*
Capture, in pacing, 711*d*, 717–718, 724–725,
　　725*f*, 730
Capture beats, 402*t*, 404
Carbon dioxide
　　carbonic acid produced from, 189
　　excess of, in respiratory acidosis, 191–192,
　　　192*t*, 193*t*, 195*t*
　　exchange of, 74, 75
　　measurement of, 287
　　oxyhemoglobin dissociation and, 76–77, 76*f*
　　partial pressure of, 75
　　　in acid-base imbalances, 195, 195*t*
　　　measurement of, 78
　　　sublingual, 517–518
　　in partial rebreathing system, for cardiac output
　　　measurement, 508*t*, 512
　　sublingual, measurement of, 517–518
　　transcutaneous monitoring of, 519
　　transport of, 75
Carbonic acid
　　in bicarbonate buffer system, 189–190, 190*t*
　　deficit of, in respiratory alkalosis, 193–194,
　　　193*t*, 195*t*
　　production of, 189
Carbon monoxide, in tobacco smoke, harmful
　　effects of, 839
Cardiac allograft vasculopathy, 650
Cardiac arrest
　　creatine kinase-BB in, 273
　　definition of, 689
　　in hyperkalemia, 181
　　incidence of, 689
　　management of, 691–704
　　　adult advanced cardiac life support in,
　　　　691–695, 693*f*–695*f*
　　　algorithms for, 695, 695*d*, 696*f*, 697*f*,
　　　　698–699, 698*d*
　　　impending, 699, 699*d*, 700*f*–703*f*,
　　　　703–704
　　pathophysiology of, 689–691
　　　cardiomyopathy, 690
　　　coronary artery disease, 689–690
　　　structural abnormalities, 689–690
　　　valvular heart disease, 690
　　　without structural heart disease, 690–691,
　　　　691*d*, 692*d*
　　prevention of, 704, 706*d*
　　survival rates in, 689

survivors of
　　electrophysiology studies in, 427–428
　　medical management of, 704–706, 704*d*,
　　　705*f*, 706*d*
　　nursing management of, 706–707
　　prognosis for, 704, 707*d*
Cardiac cachexia, in heart failure, 614
Cardiac care unit
　　esophageal Doppler monitoring in, 509–510,
　　　510*f*, 511*t*
　　myocardial infarction treatment in, 568–572,
　　　568*f*, 570*t*
　　postoperative care in, 636
　　radiography in, 296–297, 297*f*
　　sleep in, 207, 212–213
Cardiac catheterization, 459–477
　　in aortic regurgitation, 773
　　in aortic stenosis, 771
　　approaches to, 463–464, 464*f*, 465*f*
　　in cardiac output determination, 469, 471–472
　　complications of, 472
　　contraindications for, 460–461
　　contrast agents for, 461, 469–471
　　coronary. *See* Coronary artery(ies),
　　　angiography of
　　creatine kinase after, 273
　　data interpretation in, 474–476, 474*t*,
　　　475*f*–476*f*
　　direct brachial approach to, 464
　　discharge instructions for, 473, 473*t*
　　for electrophysiology procedures.
　　　See Electrophysiology procedures
　　history of, 459
　　indications for, 459–460, 460*t*
　　laboratory setting and equipment for, 463
　　left heart, 464–466, 466*f*
　　in mitral regurgitation, 767
　　in mitral stenosis, 760
　　in mitral valve prolapse, 769–770
　　normal values in, 474*t*
　　nursing considerations in, 461–462,
　　　472–474, 473*t*
　　outpatient, 462–463, 4*t*
　　patient education on, 461–462, 473, 473*t*
　　patient preparation for, 461–463, 462*t*
　　percutaneous approach to, 463–464, 464*f*, 465*f*
　　in pericarditis, 779–780
　　postprocedure care in, 472–474, 473*t*
　　right heart, 464, 465*f*, 667–668
　　transseptal left heart, 465–466, 466*f*
　　ventricular, 466–467, 467*f*
Cardiac cycle, 43–47, 44*f*
　　arterial waveform during, 484, 484*f*
　　clinical applications of, 46–47
　　diastole in, 44*f*, 45–47
　　heart sounds in, 44*f*, 46
　　left ventricular events in, 44–46, 44*f*, 45*t*
　　right ventricular events in, 44*f*, 46
　　systole in, 44–46, 44*f*, 45*t*
　　valvular events in, 44*f*, 46
Cardiac enzymes. *See specific enzymes, eg,*
　　Creatine kinase; Lactate dehydrogenase
Cardiac Hospital Atherosclerosis Management
　　Program (CHAMP), on case-managed
　　coronary artery disease, 932
Cardiac index
　　equation for, 513*t*
　　in shock, 668
Cardiac output
　　afterload and, 93–94
　　in blood pressure calculation, 63–64
　　cardiac reserve and, 40, 40*f*
　　central venous pressure and, 99–100, 99*f*, 100*f*

contractility and, 93–94
　　definition of, 35
　　in heart failure, 602, 622–623
　　heart rate and, 93
　　in hypertension, 860
　　in intra-aortic balloon pump use, 681*ncp*
　　in mean arterial pressure calculation, 486
　　measurement of, 503–512
　　　cardiac catheterization in, 469, 471–472
　　　continuous, 506–507
　　　contrast agents for, 469, 471–472
　　　direct Fick method for, 469
　　　Doppler ultrasound in, 508*t*, 509–510,
　　　　510*f*, 511*t*
　　　echocardiography in, 508*t*, 510–511
　　　impedance cardiography in, 508*t*, 511–512
　　　partial carbon dioxide rebreathing system in,
　　　　508*t*, 512
　　　pulse contour analysis in, 508–509, 508*t*,
　　　　509*f*
　　　thermodilution method in, 469, 503–505,
　　　　504*d*, 505*d*
　　　transpulmonary indicator dilution in,
　　　　508, 508*t*
　　　transpulmonary thermodilution in, 480
　　natriuretic peptide effects on, 89*f*, 90–92, 91*f*
　　optimization of, 514*t*
　　oxygen delivery and, 77, 78
　　in oxygen delivery-oxygen consumption
　　　balance, 78
　　in percutaneous coronary interventions, 598
　　pericardial limitation and, 94
　　in pericarditis, 778
　　preload and, 93
　　in pulmonary embolism, 167
　　respiration and, 102, 102*f*
　　in shock, 660*t*, 662–666, 663*f*–665*f*, 670–672,
　　　670*f*, 671*d*, 671*f*, 674
　　in sleep, 202–203
　　after transplantation, 652*ncp*
　　Valsalva maneuver and, 102, 102*f*
　　venous system and, 98–99, 99*f*
Cardiac plexus, 16
Cardiac rehabilitation, 921–933
　　after cardiac transplantation, 650–651,
　　　650*f*, 651*t*
　　contraindications to, 926, 928*d*
　　guidelines for, 925, 926*d*
　　indications for, 921–922
　　in-hospital, 922–926
　　　exercise testing in, 926–927, 927*t*
　　　history in, 922–923, 922*d*
　　　initiation of, 925–926, 927*t*
　　　vs. myocardial infarction severity and
　　　　complications, 923–924, 923*d*
　　　objectives of, 926
　　　patient education for, 924–925,
　　　　924*d*–926*d*, 925*f*
　　　physical examination in, 922–923, 922*d*
　　　psychosocial considerations in, 924
　　　purpose of, 922
　　　risk stratification for, 922, 922*d*
　　new models of, 931–933, 933*d*
　　outpatient
　　　beginning of, 928
　　　exercise prescription for, 929–930
　　　in heart failure, 931
　　　information sources for, 930
　　　maintenance program in, 930–931
　　　objectives of, 928–929
　　　patient education for, 930
　　　reimbursement for, 929
　　　safety of, 930

Cardiac rehabilitation (continued)
  phases of, 922
  precautions for, 925, 926d
  return to work and recreation and, 927–928
Cardiac reserve, 39–40, 40f, 222
Cardiac resynchronization therapy, 618, 735–737, 737f, 743d
Cardiac rhythm. See also Arrhythmias
  in electrocardiography, 330
Cardiac surgery, 628–658. See also specific procedures
  for aortic aneurysm or dissection, 635–636
  for atrial septal defect repair, 799
  blood chemistries after, 290
  cardiopulmonary bypass in, 629
  coagulation studies after, 285
  complete blood count after, 282
  complications of
    cardiovascular, 636–640, 638t, 639f
    gastrointestinal, 640–641
    late, 641, 642f
    neuropsychological, 641
    pulmonary, 640
    renal, 640
  for coronary artery revascularization. See Coronary artery bypass surgery
  creatine kinase after, 275, 275f
  deep hypothermic circulatory arrest in, 631
  electrolytes after, 287–288
  evolving trends in, 628
  fast-track recovery program in, 636
  for heart failure, 618, 635
  heart failure during, intra-aortic balloon pump for, 675
  heart rate variability in, 532
  hypomagnesemia after, 287
  left ventricular assist device after, 683
  minimally invasive techniques for, 629
  myocardial protection in, 630
  preoperative assessment for, 628–629
  preparation for, 628–629
  rehabilitation after, sternal precautions in, 924, 924d
  sleep after, 207
  for tetralogy of Fallot, 800
  transmyocardial laser, 634
  transplantation. See Cardiac transplantation
  for valvular disease. See Valves, cardiac
  for ventricular septal defect, 635
Cardiac tamponade, 781. See also Pericardial tamponade
  paradoxical blood pressure in, 247–248, 248f
  in percutaneous coronary interventions, 593
  postoperative, 637, 641
Cardiac transplantation, 642–651
  activity intolerance after, 654ncp
  age considerations in, 642
  cardiac output maintenance after, 652ncp
  cardiac rehabilitation after, 931
  in children, 642–643
  complications of, 650
  contraindications to, 643–644, 643t
  for dilated cardiomyopathy, 783
  discharge preparation in, 651
  donor characteristics in, 644
  donor heart allocation in, 643
  dyspnea index in, 651, 651t
  exercise testing after, 456
  heart rate variability in, 532
  infection prevention after, 653ncp–654ncp
  intra-aortic balloon pump as bridge to, 675
  knowledge deficit in, 655ncp–656ncp
  left ventricular assist device use before, 683

  medical management of, 644–650
    cardiac function maintenance in, 645–646, 646t
    immunosuppressive drug side effects in, 647–650, 648t
    infection monitoring in, 647
    preoperative status and, 644–645
    rejection monitoring in, 646–647, 646f, 647t
  nursing management of, 651, 652ncp–656ncp
  postoperative care in, 636
  recent developments in, 642–643
  recipient evaluation for, 643–644, 643t
  rehabilitation after, 650–651, 650f, 651t
  self-concept disturbances in, 655ncp
  statistics on, 642–643
  surgical procedure for, 644, 645f
  survival rates in, 642–643
Cardiac veins, 13f, 14f, 15–16, 16f
Cardiogenic shock. See Shock, cardiogenic
Cardiography, impedance, 508t, 511–512
Cardiomyopathy, 782–787
  cardiac arrest in, 690
  concentric, 604f, 605, 607f
  definition of, 782
  dilated, 782–784
    clinical manifestations of, 782–783
    echocardiography in, 312–313
    etiology of, 782, 782d
    heart failure and, 604f
    medical management of, 783
    nursing management of, 783–784
    pacemaker for, 710d
  eccentric, 604f, 605, 607f
  echocardiography in, 312–314
  hypertrophic, 784–785
    assessment of, 784
    cardiac arrest in, 690
    echocardiography in, 313–314
    etiology of, 784
    in heart failure, 607t, 609–610, 611f
    heart failure and, 604, 604f, 607t
    medical management of, 785
    nursing management of, 785
    pacemaker for, 710d
    pathophysiology of, 784
  infiltrative, 314
  restrictive, 785–786
  transplantation for, 643
  types of, 782
Cardiomyoplasty, dynamic
  for dilated cardiomyopathy, 783
  for heart failure, 635
Cardiomyostimulator, for cardiomyoplasty, 635, 783
Cardioplegia, 20, 630
Cardiopulmonary bypass, 629–630, 640
Cardiopulmonary receptors, in blood pressure regulation, 81
Cardiovascular disease. See also specific diseases, eg, Coronary artery disease
  genetic factors in, 115–116
  pathophysiology of, 127–128, 128f
  risk factors for, 140t, 839, 938–939
  sleep in, 205–208
Cardioversion, 699–703
  algorithms for, 700f–703f, 703
  for arrhythmias, 373t
  definition of, 691
  energy requirements of, 699, 699d
  with pacemakers, 722
  procedure for, 699

Carey-Coombs murmur, in mitral regurgitation, 757
Carotid artery(ies), pulse in, 240–241
Carotid baroreceptors, in blood pressure regulation, 81, 82f
Carotid sinus massage
  in syncope diagnosis, 430
  in wide QRS complex rhythms, 407–408, 410f
Carotid sinus syndrome, pacemaker for, 710d
Carpentier-Edwards xenograft valve, 763f, 764
Carvedilol
  for heart failure, 619t, 620
  for hypertension, 878t
Case-managed care, for adherence, 967d, 969
Case management, 987, 987t
  in cardiac rehabilitation, 932
  definition of, 989
Catecholamines
  coronary artery disease and, 828–829, 828f
  electrophysiologic effects of, 28, 29f
  measurement of, 289
  in myocardial infarction, 546
Catheter(s)
  Amplatz, 467, 468f
  for arterial pressure monitoring, 483–488, 484f–486f, 484t, 488t
  blood drawing from
    in hemodynamic monitoring, 483
    for laboratory testing, 266–267
  central venous, 299t, 302f, 483
  complications of, 426–427
  for electrophysiology procedures, 425–426, 426f, 427f
  infection control with, 480, 482t
  of intra-aortic balloon pump, 675, 676f
  in percutaneous coronary interventions. See Percutaneous coronary interventions
  placement of
    arterial, 484, 484t
    central venous, 488–489
  pulmonary artery. See Pulmonary artery catheters
  in radiofrequency ablation. See Radiofrequency catheter ablation
  radiographic appearance of, 299t, 300f–302f
Catheterization, cardiac. See Cardiac catheterization
Caval interruption, for pulmonary embolism, 168
Center for Epidemiological Studies Depression Scale, 829
Central cyanosis, 236
Central nervous system. See also Brain
  in blood pressure regulation, 83–84
Central sleep apnea, 210
Central venous pressure
  vs. cardiac output, 99–101, 99f, 100f
  in cardiac tamponade, 781
  monitoring of, 488–489, 490d–491d, 492f
  in myocardial infarction, 559
  in shock, 660t
Central venous pressure catheter
  blood drawing from, 483
  radiographic appearance of, 299t, 302f
Cerebrovascular atherosclerosis, 146
CHAMP (Cardiac Hospital Atherosclerosis Management Program), on case-managed coronary artery disease, 932
Charcot's joint, in diabetes mellitus, 952
Chemoreceptors
  in blood pressure regulation, 83
  in heart rate control, 92–93
Chest, configuration of, assessment of, 258, 260f

Chest leads, in electrocardiography, 332, 333*f*
Chest pain. *See also* Angina
  differential diagnosis of, 230*t*
  evaluation of, 231
  history of, 231–232
  in myocardial infarction, 557, 576–577, 577*d*
  in pericarditis, 777
Chest radiography, 296–306. *See also specific conditions*
  in acute care, 297, 299*f*–302*f*, 299*t*
  in angina, 552
  in aortic regurgitation, 774
  in aortic stenosis, 771, 772*f*
  in cardiovascular disease, 297, 303*f*–306*f*
  in dilated cardiomyopathy, 783
  in heart failure, 615
  interpretation of, 297, 298*f*
  in mitral regurgitation, 767
  in mitral stenosis, 760
  in mitral valve prolapse, 770, 770*f*
  principles of, 296–297, 297*f*
  in pulmonary embolism, 168
  in shock, 667
  views for, 296, 297*f*, 298*f*
Chest tube, radiographic appearance of, 299*t*
Chest wall, inspection of, 250–251, 251*f*
Cheyne-Stokes respiration, 207, 258, 260*f*
Chief complaint, in history taking, 230–231
Children
  cardiac transplantation in, 642–643
  hypertension in, 857–858, 858*t*, 859*t*, 861
Chinese medicine, 976, 976*f*–978*f*
Chinese red yeast rice, for cardiovascular disease, 980–981
Chiropractic, for cardiovascular disease, 982
Chlamydia pneumoniae infections, atherosclerosis in, 543
Chloride ion
  in action potential, in early repolarization, 23–24, 23*f*
  distribution of, in myocardium, 18*t*
  equilibrium potential of, 20
  measurement of, 286
Chlorthalidone, for hypertension, 878*t*
Cholecystitis, postoperative, 641
Cholesterol
  absorption of, inhibitors of, for hyperlipidemia, 911*t*, 912
  cellular vs. blood distribution of, 899
  endothelial function and, 900–901
  excess of. *See* Hypercholesterolemia
  function of, 897
  lowering of
    for CAD prevention, 120
    clinical trials of, 897, 898*t*
    diet in, 905–908, 906*f*, 906*t*, 907*d*
    exercise in, 909
    goals of, 903, 904*t*, 905
    pharmacologic, 909–912, 910*t*, 911*t*
    weight control in, 908
  measurement of, 276–278, 278*t*, 279*t*
  reverse transport of, 899
Cholinergic effects, on electrophysiology, 28, 29*f*
Cholinergic receptors, in blood pressure regulation, 87–88
Chordae tendinae, anatomy of, 7*f*, 8
Chordoplasty, in mitral regurgitation, 768
Christa supraventricularis, 6
Chromosomes, 112–113, 113*f*
Chronic obstructive pulmonary disease
  heart rate variability in, 535
  sleep in, 208
Chylomicrons, 898, 898*f*

Cigarette smoking. *See* Smoking
Circadian process, in sleep regulation, 202, 202*f*, 203
Circle of Vieussens, 14
Circulation
  arterial, assessment of, 249–250, 249*f*
  assessment of, 249–250, 249*f*
    in shock, 666–667
  collateral
    coronary, 43, 545
    in hand, 484, 484*t*
  coronary. *See also* Coronary artery(ies)
    anatomy of, 12–15, 13*f*, 13*t*, 14*f*
    collateral, 43, 545
    control of, 42–43, 42*f*
    physiology of, 41–43, 42*f*
  lymphatic, 52–53, 52*f*
  microcirculation as, 50–51, 65–67, 66*f*.
    See also Capillary(ies)
  peripheral, assessment of, 241, 241*f*
  pulmonary. *See* Pulmonary circulation
  systemic. *See also* Vascular system;
    components, eg, Vascular resistance
    calcium and, 60–61, 61*f*
    local regulation of, 53–58, 53*t*, 54*f*–58*f*, 54*t*
    neurohumoral stimulation of, 58–60, 59*f*, 60*f*
    structure of, 49–53, 50*f*, 52*f*
  venous, assessment of, 250
Circulatory assist devices, 674–675.
    See also Intra-aortic balloon pump;
    Left ventricular assist devices
Circulatory support, for heart failure, 617
Circumflex artery, anatomy of, 13*f*, 15
Clarithromycin, for rheumatic fever, 757
Click-murmur syndrome. *See* Mitral valve, prolapse of
Clicks, systolic, 255, 255*f*
Clonidine, for hypertension, 878*t*
Clopidogrel
  for heart failure, 618
  for percutaneous coronary interventions, 596
Clostridium difficile infections, postoperative, 641
Clotting. *See* Coagulation; Thrombus(i)
Clubbing, 249, 249*f*
Coagulation
  disorders of, 162–171
    deep vein thrombosis as, 163–166, 163*t*, 165*t*, 166*t*
    heparin-induced thrombocytopenia as, 169–171, 169*f*, 170*t*
    nursing considerations in, 285–286
    pathophysiology of, 162–163, 162*f*
    postoperative, 637
    pulmonary embolism as, 166–169, 167*f*
  inflammation and, 157–158
  laboratory tests for, 157*t*, 283–286
    activated clotting time, 284
    activated partial thromboplastin time, 284
    after cardiac surgery, 285
    fibrinogen, 284
    nursing considerations after, 285–286
    partial thromboplastin time, 284
    platelet count, 283–284
    protein C and protein S, 285
    prothrombin time, 284
    specimen collection for, 266
    thrombin time, 284–285
  regulation of, 156–157
  in shock, 666
Coagulation cascade, 155, 156*f*
Coagulation factors, 153–154, 153*t*

Coarctation, aortic, 796*f*, 797–798, 797*t*, 863
Cockcroft-Gault equation for kidney function, 224
Codes, for pacemakers, 715–716, 715*t*
Codons, 111
Coenzyme Q10, for cardiovascular disease, 982
Cognitive behavioral therapy, for psychosocial risk factors, 831, 831*f*
Cognitive dysfunction, postoperative, 641
Cognitive-motivational models, for behavior change, 966, 967*d*
Cognitive-perceptual status, in history taking, 234
Cognitive restructuring
  for depression, 833
  for weight loss, 943
Collagen, in atherosclerotic lesions, 144
Collateral circulation
  coronary, 43, 545
  in hand, Allen test for, 484, 484*t*
Colony-forming units, in hematopoiesis, 150, 151*f*
Colony-stimulating factors, in hematopoiesis, 150, 151*t*
Color, of skin, assessment of, 236
Color flow Doppler echocardiography, 309
Comfort, for sleep, 213
Common pathway, for coagulation, 155, 156*f*
Communication
  in adherence, 970–971
  in disease management, 990–991
Community, blood pressure screening in, 249
Compensation
  in acid-base imbalances, 191, 195
    metabolic acidosis as, 192–193
    metabolic alkalosis as, 194
    respiratory alkalosis as, 193–194
  in mitral regurgitation, 767
  in shock, 662–666
    clinical manifestations of, 665–666
    in initial stage, 663–664, 663*f*
    in intermediate stage, 664–665, 664*f*
    in irreversible stage, 665, 665*f*
Complementary and alternative medicine, 974–985
  Ayurvedic, 976, 976*f*–978*f*
  biofeedback, 978
  biologically based, 978–982, 980*f*
  characteristics of, 974
  definition of, 974
  dietary remedies in, 980–982
  domains of, 974–975
  herbal remedies in, 978–980, 980*f*
  homeopathic, 975
  legal aspects of, 982
  manipulative methods in, 982, 982*f*
  meditation, 977–978
  mind-body interventions in, 976–978, 978*f*
  naturopathic, 976
  nursing management integrated into, 982–983
  Oriental, 976
  prevalence of, 975
  systems of, 975–976, 976*f*–978*f*
  traditional Chinese, 976, 976*f*–978*f*
  yoga, 978, 978*f*
Complete blood cell count, 281–283
Compliance
  myocardial, 37–38, 38*f*
  with treatment. *See* Adherence (compliance)
  venous, 65
Computed tomography
  in atherosclerosis, 143*t*
  electron beam, 324
  in pericarditis, 779
  in pulmonary embolism, 168

Computed tomography angiography, 324
Concealed conduction, 420–421, 421f, 422f
Concordance. See Adherence (compliance)
Conduction, 29–32
    atrial, 30, 30t
    concealed, 420–421, 421f, 422f
    decremental, 30
    disorders of. See Conduction blocks;
        Conduction disorders
    excitation-contraction coupling in, 31–32, 32f
    junctional, 30
    origin of, 327
    path of, 327
    ventricular, 30–31, 30t, 31f
    Wenckebach, 408–413, 410f–415f
Conduction blocks. See also specific type
    bifascicular, 342, 345f, 346f
    bradycardia in, 703–704, 703f
    bundle-branch, 12, 338–339, 342f–344f
    decremental conduction in, 363–364
    electrocardiography in, 337–342, 341f–346f
    fascicular, 340–341, 345f
    mechanisms of, 363–365, 364f, 365f
    in myocardial infarction, 562
    phase 3 (short-cycle aberrancy), 364, 364f
    phase 4 (long-cycle aberrancy), 364–365, 364f
    postoperative, 638
    as radiofrequency catheter ablation
        complication, 431
Conduction disorders. See also Conduction
        blocks; specific disorders
    concealed conduction, 420–421, 421f, 422f
    in percutaneous coronary interventions, 593
    reentry, 364, 365f
Conduction system
    aging effects on, 222–223
    anatomy of, 10–12, 11f, 12f, 13t,
        326–327, 327f
    disorders of. See Conduction blocks;
        Conduction disorders; specific disorders
    impulse propagation in. See Conduction
    impulse velocity in, factors modifying,
        28–29, 29f
    velocity in, factors modifying, 28
Congenital heart disease, 794–806
    aortic coarctation as, 796f, 797–798, 797t
    aortic stenosis as, 796–797
    atrial septal defects as, 796f, 798–799
    classification of, 794, 795f
    Ebstein anomaly as, 800–801
    Eisenmenger reaction as, 803
    incidence of, 794
    medical management of, 803
    nursing management in, 803, 803ncp–805ncp
    patent ductus arteriosus as, 796f, 798
    pericardial, 776, 777d
    prevalence of, 794
    pulmonic valve stenosis as, 794–796, 796f
    survival in, 794, 795t
    tetralogy of Fallot as, 796f, 800
    transposition of great arteries as, 796f, 802–803
    tricuspid atresia as, 801, 801t
    truncus arteriosus as, 801–802
    ventricular septal defects as, 796f, 799–800
Congestive heart failure. See Heart failure
Connor Diet Habit Survey, 964
Consciousness, assessment of, in shock, 667
Constriction, pericardial, hemodynamic
        characteristics of, 506t
Constrictive pericarditis, 778–780
Consumptive coagulopathy (disseminated
        intravascular coagulation), 158–162,
        159d, 160f, 161t, 162d, 162t

Contact, ongoing, for adherence, 967d, 969
Continuous endothelium, of exchange vessels, 51
Continuous positive airway pressure, for sleep
        apnea, 210
Continuous wave Doppler, 309
Contraceptives, oral
    coronary artery disease and, 818–819
    hypertension due to, 863
Contractility, 39, 39f
    cardiac output and, 94
    hemodynamic characteristics of, 507t
    hypocalcemia effects on, 183
    hypophosphatemia effects on, 186
    metabolic acidosis effects on, 193
    myocardial oxygen consumption and, 42
    postoperative, 637, 638t
Contracting, for adherence, 967d, 968
Contraction
    of heart
        atrial, 44f, 45–46
        calcium ion modulation in, 35
        force of, hemodynamic characteristics
            of, 507t
        isometric, 32–33, 33f
        isotonic, 32–33, 34f
        isovolumic ventricular, 44–45, 44f
        molecular basis for, 33–34, 35f
        overview of, 32–33, 33f, 34f
    of vascular smooth muscle, 53
Contraction alkalosis, 194
Contrast agents
    allergy to, 472
    for cardiac catheterization, 461, 469–471
    for cardiac output measurement, 469, 471–472
    complications of, 593–594
    hemodynamic effects of, 471–472
Contrast echocardiography, 317
Conus arteriosus (infundibulum), anatomy of, 6
Conus branch, of right coronary artery, 14
Cook-Medley Hostility Inventory, 830
Coordination
    of delivery systems, for disease
        management, 989
    in disease management, 990
COPD (chronic obstructive pulmonary disease)
    heart rate variability in, 535
    sleep in, 208
Coping
    in congenital heart disease, 805ncp
    evaluation of, in history taking, 233, 234
Copper wire arteries, in retina, 238, 238f
Corneal arcus, 236, 237f
Cornell index, for left ventricular
        enlargement, 355t
Coronary angioplasty
    creatine kinase after, 273–274, 274f
    laser, 589
    percutaneous transluminal, 587–588, 588f
Coronary artery(ies)
    abrupt closure of, in percutaneous coronary
        interventions, 592
    anatomy of, 12–15, 13f, 13t, 14f, 467,
        469f–471f, 475f–476f
    angiography of, 467–469, 468f–471f
    in angina, 552–553
    atherectomy of, 588–589, 589f
    atherosclerosis of. See Atherosclerosis;
        Atherosclerotic lesions
    blood flow in, regulation of, 42–43, 42f
    dominance of, 12–15
    individual variations in, 12
    innervation of, 43
    left, 12, 13f, 13t, 14–15, 14f

left anterior descending, 13f, 14f, 14–15,
        356, 359f
    magnetic resonance angiography of, 322–323
    percutaneous interventions for.
        See Percutaneous coronary interventions
    perforation of, in percutaneous coronary
        interventions, 593
    reocclusion of, after thrombolytic therapy, 566
    restenosis of, 592, 594
    revascularization of. See Revascularization;
        specific procedures
    right, 13, 13f, 13t, 14, 14f
    silent occlusion of, 146
    spasm of, 543. See also Variant angina
        in hypomagnesemia, 185
        in percutaneous coronary interventions, 593
    stent placement in. See Stents, coronary
    thrombosis of, myocardial infarction locations
        and, 556–557
    wall of, normal, 140f
Coronary artery bypass surgery, 631–633
    for angina, 553
    bypass conduits for, 631–632, 632f
    complications of, 636–641, 638t, 639f, 642f
    contraindications to, 631
    creatine kinase after, 275, 275f
    heart rate variability in, 532
    indications for, 631
    minimally invasive, 629, 633–634, 633f
    postoperative care in, 636
    results of, 632–633
Coronary artery disease
    animal models of, 119
    asymptomatic, cardiac catheterization
        guidelines for, 459, 460t
    cardiac arrest in, 689–690
    cardiac catheterization in, 459–460, 460t
    collateral circulation development in, 43
    in diabetes mellitus, 952
    echocardiography in, 312, 315f
    environmental factors in, 117, 117t
    epidemiology of, 897
    exercise testing in
        ancillary methods for, 453–454
        electrocardiographic response in, 448–449,
            448f, 449f
        in special populations, 455–456
    facial characteristics in, 236
    familial aggregation studies of, 118
    genetic factors in, 116t, 117–120, 117t, 119t
    heart failure in, 614–615
    inflammatory markers of. See Inflammatory
        marker(s)
    laboratory tests for, 279–281, 279f
    lipids and. See Lipid(s); Lipoprotein(s)
    management models for. See Disease
        management
    mortality rates in, 809–810, 810f
    myocardial perfusion imaging in, 320–322,
        320f–322f
    pathophysiology of, 541–543
    posttransplantation, 647
    prevention of, 120–121
    prognosis for. See Psychosocial risk factors, for
        coronary artery disease
    revascularization for. See Revascularization;
        specific procedures
    risk factors for, 118, 543, 809–824. See also
        Psychosocial risk factors, for coronary
        artery disease
        additive effects of, 810, 839
        antioxidant deficiency as, 820
        definition of, 809

demographics of, 810
diabetes mellitus as, 815–817, 816*f*
family history as, 810–811
folate deficiency as, 819–820
homocysteine elevation as, 819–820
hypertension as, 812, 813*f*
lipids and lipoproteins as, 812–813, 813*t*
low physical activity level as, 813–815,
    814*f*, 815*f*
obesity as, 817–818, 817*f*, 938–939
relative risk in, 809, 810*f*
reproductive hormones as, 818–819
smoking as, 811–812, 811*f*, 839
secondary prevention of, exercise for, 919–920,
    920*t*, 932, 933*d*
sleep in, 205–207
smoking cessation in, 840–841
snoring and, 210
treatment of, percutaneous interventions for.
    See Percutaneous coronary interventions
twin studies of, 118
Coronary atherectomy, 588–589, 589*f*
Coronary capillaries, 15
Coronary care unit. *See* Cardiac care unit
Coronary flow reserve, measurement of, in
    percutaneous coronary
    interventions, 595
Coronary laser angioplasty, 589
Coronary precautions, 570–571
Coronary reactive hyperemia, 542, 544
Coronary stents. *See* Stents, coronary
Coronary sulcus, anatomy of, 3, 4*f*, 5, 5*f*
Coronary veins, 13*f*, 14*f*, 15–16, 16*f*
Corpuscular indices, measurement of, 281–282
Correction, of acid-base imbalances, 191
Corrigan's pulse, 240
Corticosteroids
    for cardiac transplantation, 648*t*, 649
    for septic shock, 673–674
Co-transmitters, in blood pressure regulation,
    88–89, 88*f*
Cotton wool patches, in retina, 239, 239*f*, 866
Cough
    assessment of, 258
    in pulmonary embolism, 167
Counseling
    on adherence, 967*d*, 969
    on heart failure, 622, 622*d*
Crackles, 261, 262*f*
Crataegus oxyacantha (hawthorn), for cardiovascular
    disease, 978–979
C-reactive protein
    in atherosclerosis, 131
    as inflammatory marker, 130–131, 131*f*, 546
    measurement of, 279–280, 279*f*
Creatine kinase, 272–276
    action of, 272
    after cardiac surgery, 275, 275*f*
    factors affecting, 273
    isoenzymes of, 272, 272*t*
    isoforms of, 275–276
    measurement of, 276, 276*t*, 277*t*
    after myocardial infarction, 272–275, 274*f*
    during myocardial infarction, 546, 559, 923
    reference values for, 272–273, 276*t*
    specimens for, 272
    tissue distribution of, 272, 272*t*
Creatine kinase-BB, 272, 272*t*, 273, 276
Creatine kinase-MB, 272–275, 272*t*, 274*f*
    after cardiac surgery, 275
    isoforms of, 275–276
    mass concentration of, 275
    measurement of, 276, 276*t*

    in myocardial infarction, 546, 559
    reference values for, 276*t*
Creatine kinase-MM, 272*t*, 273, 275–276
Creatine phosphate, in myocardial
    metabolism, 41
Creatinine, measurement of, 289
Crisis, hypertensive, 881, 882*t*
Cross-bridge theory, of contraction, 33–34, 35*f*,
    37, 37*f*
Crosstalk, in pacing, 712*d*, 732–733, 734*f*
Crown-Crisp Experiential Index, 830
Crystalloid solutions, for hypovolemic shock, 673
C-type natriuretic peptide
    in blood pressure regulation, 89*f*, 90–92, 91*f*
    in heart failure, 606–607, 609*f*, 610*f*
    in kidney regulation, 175*t*
    measurement of, 280–281
Cueing, for adherence, 967*d*, 968
Culture, blood, 283
Cupping, 976
Cushing's syndrome, facial characteristics in, 236
Cutting balloon coronary angioplasty,
    587–588, 588*f*
Cyanosis, 236
    in congenital heart disease
        with decreased pulmonary blood flow,
            800–801, 801*t*
        with increased pulmonary blood flow, 796*f*,
            801–803
    in pulmonary embolism, 167
Cycle length variations, in rhythms, 404–405
Cyclic adenosine monophosphate (cAMP), in
    excitation-contraction coupling,
    32, 32*f*
Cyclic guanosine monophosphate, in vasodilation,
    58–59, 59*f*
Cyclooxygenase-1, in thromboxane synthesis,
    57–58
Cyclosporine
    for cardiac transplantation, 647, 648*t*, 649
    for transplantation, 642
Cytokines. *See also specific cytokines, eg,* Tumor
    necrosis factor alpha
    in atherosclerosis, 158, 543
    in heart failure, 609
    in hematopoiesis, 153
    in myocardial infarction, 546
    in shock, 664–665, 664*f*

D

Daclizumab, for cardiac transplantation, 650
Dalteparin, for deep vein thrombosis, 164, 165*t*
Damping coefficient, in hemodynamic
    monitoring, 480, 483*f*
Danaparoid, for heparin-induced
    thrombocytopenia, 171
DASH (Dietary Approaches to Stop
    Hypertension) diet, 871–872,
    872*t*, 873*t*
Data collection, for disease management, 991
David procedure, for aortic aneurysm, 636
D-dimer assay, 157*t*, 168
Dead space, in lung, 73
Death. *See also* Mortality
    causes of, 221*f*, 810*f*
    in electrophysiology studies, 426–427
    of heart donor, 644
    in older adults, causes of, 221*f*
    smoking contribution to, 838
    sudden. *See* Sudden cardiac death
Deconditioning, cardiovascular effects of,
    921, 921*d*

Decremental conduction, 30
Deep hypothermic circulatory arrest, for cardiac
    surgery, 631
Deep vein thrombosis, 163–166
    assessment for, 166
    clinical manifestations of, 164
    etiology of, 163, 163*t*
    in heparin-induced thrombocytopenia, 170
    medical management of, 164–165, 165*t*
    nursing interventions for, 166
    pathophysiology of, 163
    prophylaxis of, 165–166, 166*t*
    risk factors for, 166*t*
Defibrillation. *See also* Implantable cardioverter
    defibrillators
    atrial, 382–383
    for cardiac arrest, 691–695, 694*f*, 695*f*
    definition of, 691
    electrode position for, 694, 695*f*
    energy requirements for, 694, 694*f*
    equipment for, 692–693
    with pacemakers, 722
    procedure for, 694–695
    for pulseless ventricular tachycardia, 698, 708*d*
    transthoracic impedance in, 693–694
    for ventricular fibrillation, 698, 708*d*
Defibrination syndrome (disseminated
    intravascular coagulation), 158–162,
    159*d*, 160*f*, 161*t*, 162*d*, 162*t*
Delayed afterdepolarizations, 363
Delirium, postcardiotomy, 641
Delta Down, in systolic blood pressure, 502–503,
    502*f*, 502*t*
Delta wave, in Wolff-Parkinson-White syndrome,
    392, 394*f*, 395*f*
Demand, in pacing, 711*d*, 716–717
Demand ischemia, 541
Denial, in acute coronary events, 831
Dental hygiene, in endocarditis prevention, 789
Deoxyribonucleic acid. *See* DNA
    (deoxyribonucleic acid)
Depolarization, 17
    in electrocardiography, 327, 328*f*, 334,
        335*f*, 336
    excitation-contraction coupling and,
        31–32, 32*f*
    hypokalemia effects on, 180
    spontaneous. *See* Automaticity
    in ventricle, 30–31, 31*f*
Depression
    coronary artery disease risk in, 825–826,
        829, 833
    in heart failure, 618
    heart rate variability in, 535
    smoking cessation and, 849–850
Desarginine vasopressin, for coagulation
    promotion, 162*t*
Devices, radiographic appearance of, 297,
    299*f*-302*f*, 299*t*
Diabetes mellitus, 948–960
    age-related factors in, 953, 954*t*
    cardiac transplantation in, 644
    classification of, 948, 949*t*
    complications of, 951–953
    consequences of, 948–949
    as coronary artery disease risk factor,
        815–817, 816*f*
    definition of, 948, 949*t*
    diagnosis of, 948, 949*t*
    economic impact of, 949
    epidemiology of, 815–816, 816*f*
    glycated hemoglobin measurement in,
        289, 289*t*

Diabetes mellitus *(continued)*
  health screening in, 958
  heart rate variability in, 535
  hypertension and, 879–880
  hypertriglyceridemia in, 901
  management of, 953–958
    goals of, 953–955
    interventions for, 955–958
  nephropathy in, 951–952
  neuropathy in, 952
  pathophysiology of, 949–951
  percutaneous coronary interventions in, 586
  prevalence of, 948–949
  prevention of, 816
  retinopathy in, 951
  type 1, pathophysiology of, 950
  type 2, pathophysiology of, 950–951
Diagonal branches, of left coronary artery, 13*f*, 15
Diaphragmatic excursion, in lung percussion, 259, 261*t*
Diaphragmatic surface, of heart, 3, 5*f*
Diaries, for adherence measurement, 963*t*, 964, 965
Diarrhea, postoperative, 641
Diastole
  auscultation of, 252, 253
  coronary blood flow and, 42, 42*f*
  late, 44*f*, 45
  ventricular, 44*f*, 45–47
Diastolic augmentation, by intra-aortic balloon
    pump, 676, 676*f*, 678, 678*f*
Diastolic blood pressure, 64, 64*f*
Diastolic cardiac reserve, 40, 40*f*
Diastolic dysfunction, in heart failure, 602–603, 610–611, 614–615, 617–618, 617*t*
Diastolic filling
  aging effects on, 222
  heart sounds in, 254, 254*f*, 255*f*
Diastolic inward current, transient, 27
Diastolic murmurs, 255, 255*f*
Diastolic potential change, 24
Diastolic run-off period, 484, 485*f*
Diazoxide, for hypertension, 882*t*
Dicumarol, for deep vein thrombosis, 164
Diet. *See* Nutrition
Dietary and Risk Factor Questionnaire, 964
Dietary Approaches to Stop Hypertension
    (DASH) diet, 871–872, 872*t*, 873*t*
Dietary Supplement and Health Act of 1994, 980
Differential AV delay, in pacing, 712*d*
Diffusion
  of charged particles, 19
  in microcirculation, 65
  in respiration, 72–74
Digitalis
  for heart failure, 616–617, 617*t*, 620
  hyperkalemia due to, 181
  in sarcoplasmic calcium ion modulation, 35
  toxicity of, in hypomagnesemia, 184
Digital techniques, in echocardiography, 318
Digoxin
  for arrhythmias, 368*t*
  for heart failure, 620
Dilated cardiomyopathy. *See* Cardiomyopathy, dilated
Dilation, of heart, oxygen supply and, 43
Diltiazem
  for arrhythmias, 368*t*, 373*t*
  for hypertension, 879*t*
Dilution methods, for cardiac
    output measurement
  indicator method as, 508, 508*t*
  thermodilution as, 503–505, 504*d*, 505*d*, 509, 509*f*

Dipyridamole, in myocardial perfusion imaging, 2
Direct Fick method, for cardiac output
    measurement, 469
Directional coronary atherectomy, 588–589, 589*f*
Discontinuous endothelium, 51
Discrete Fourier Transform, for heart rate
    variability analysis, 529
Disease management, 986–996
  acute vs. chronic, 986
  vs. case management, 987, 987*t*
  components of, 988–992
    collecting data, 991
    communication, 990–991
    coordinating delivery systems, 989
    education, 989–990
    medical, 990
    outcomes management, 991–992
    patient population identification,
        988–989, 989*f*
    program marketing, 992
    structuring interventions, 990
  definition of, 987
  demographics and, 986
  duration of, 993
  models for, 987–988, 987*t*
  multiple diseases involved in, 993
  qualifications for, 992
  successful programs for, 986
  training for, 992
  unresolved issues in, 992–994, 992*t*, 993*t*
Disopyramide, for arrhythmias, 368*t*–369*t*
Disruption, of atherosclerotic lesions, 142, 147*t*
Dissection, aortic, repair of, 635–636
Disseminated intravascular coagulation, 158–162
  clinical manifestations of, 160–161
  etiology of, 158–159, 10*d*
  nursing interventions for, 161–162, 161*t*,
      162*d*, 162*t*
  pathophysiology of, 160, 160*f*
  prognosis for, 161
  in shock, 666
  treatment of, 161
Distal protection devices, in percutaneous
    coronary interventions, 595
Distributive shock
  diagnosis of, 669
  pathophysiology of, 660*t*, 662
Diuresis
  extracellular fluid volume deficit in, in
      percutaneous coronary interventions,
      598–599
  at rest, in heart failure, 612
Diuretics
  for heart failure, 616, 619*t*, 620
  for hypertension, 878*t*, 880*t*
  hypokalemia due to, 179
  for mitral regurgitation, 767
  potassium-sparing, 181
Dizziness
  in exercise testing, 450
  in postural hypotension, 247
DNA (deoxyribonucleic acid)
  in chromosomes, 112–113, 113*f*
  diagnostic tests based on, 114, 120
  in genes, 113
  human diversity and, 113
  identification of, in Human Genome
      Project, 114
  satellite, 114
  structure of, 111, 112*f*
  synthesis of, 111
  variations in, 113–114
    drug responses and, 114–115

DO₂. *See* Oxygen delivery (DO₂)
Dobutamine
  for heart failure, 671–672, 672*d*
  for myocardial infarction, 572, 673
  postoperative, 638*t*
  for shock, 669*t*, 671–672, 672*d*
  in stress echocardiography, 311
Dofetilide, for arrhythmias, 369*t*
Dominance, of coronary vasculature, 12–15
Dopamine
  after cardiac transplantation, 646
  electrophysiologic effects of, 28, 29*f*
  for heart failure, 608
  for myocardial infarction, 572
  postoperative, 638*t*
  receptors for, in blood pressure regulation, 84
  for shock, 669*t*
Doppler echocardiography, 309, 314*f*, 614
Doppler ultrasonography
  in blood pressure measurement, 248
  in cardiac output measurement, 509–510,
      510*f*, 511*t*
  in circulation assessment, 241
Dor procedure, for heart failure, 635
Dorsalis pedis artery, catheter placement in, 484
Dorsalis pedis pulse, assessment of, 241, 241*f*
Doxazosin, for hypertension, 878*t*
Drainage tubes, for cardiac surgery, 636–637
Dreams, 201
D receptors, in blood pressure regulation, 84
Dressler's syndrome, 562, 780
Driving, automobile, with implantable
    cardioverter defibrillator, 751
Drugs. *See also specific drugs*
  exercise testing impact of, 441, 441*t*
  in history taking, 232
  hyperkalemia due to, 180–181
  hypertension due to, 862*d*
  injection abuse of, endocarditis in, 788, 790
  metabolism of, genetic variations in, 114–115
  monitoring of, laboratory tests for, 268,
      291, 291*t*
  myocarditis due to, 786, 786*d*
  pharmacokinetics of, aging effects on, 225
  platelet inhibition by, 283
  QT interval prolongation due to, cardiac arrest
      and, 690, 692*d*
  refills of, for adherence measurement, 963*t*, 965
  sleep disorders due to, 212
  for sleep promotion, 213
  in stress exercise testing, 454
  therapeutic reference ranges of, 291, 291*t*
Ductus arteriosus, patent, 796*f*, 798–800
Duke criteria, for endocarditis, 788
Duke Treadmill Score, 321, 322*f*
Dullness, in lung percussion, 259, 261*t*
Dynamic auscultation, 257–258, 257*t*
Dynamic cardiomyoplasty
  for dilated cardiomyopathy, 783
  for heart failure, 635
Dynamic response characteristics, in
    hemodynamic monitoring, 480,
    483, 483*f*
Dyskinesis, of myocardium, 312
Dyslipidemias, 900*t*, 901. *See also*
    Hypercholesterolemia; Hyperlipidemias
  combined, 900*t*, 902
  genetic factors in, 116–117
Dyspnea
  in aortic regurgitation, 773
  in exercise testing, 450, 450*d*
  in heart failure, 610–612
  in hypertrophic cardiomyopathy, 784

in mitral stenosis, 759
in myocarditis, 786
in pulmonary embolism, 167
in restrictive cardiomyopathy, 785
Dyspnea index, in cardiac transplantation,
   651, 651*t*
Dysrhythmias, vs. arrhythmias, 365–366
Dyssomnias, 204, 206*t*
dZ/dt waveform, in impedance cardiography, 512

E

Early afterdepolarizations, 362–363, 363*f*
Early ejection sounds, 255, 255*f*
Early systolic murmurs, 255, 255*f*
Eating Pattern Questionnaire, 964
Ebstein anomaly, 800–801
Echocardiography, 307–318
   in angina, 552
   in aortic insufficiency, 315
   in aortic regurgitation, 773
   of aortic root, 316
   in aortic stenosis, 315, 771
   of aortic valve, 314–315
   in bacterial endocarditis, 317
   in cardiomyopathy, 312–314
   contrast, 317
   in coronary artery disease, 312, 315*f*
   digital techniques in, 318
   in dilated cardiomyopathy, 783
   Doppler, 309, 314*f,* 510–511
   in embolism, 317
   in endocarditis, 758, 758*f,* 788
   in exercise testing, 454
   in heart failure, 614
   of interventricular septum, 314
   in intracardiac masses and foreign objects, 317
   of left atrium, 314
   of left ventricle, 312, 313*f*
   in mitral regurgitation, 316, 767
   in mitral stenosis, 316, 759–760
   of mitral valve, 315–316
   in mitral valve prolapse, 316, 769, 769*f*
   M-mode, 308, 308*f,* 309*f*
   in myocardial infarction, 559
   in pericardial effusion, 780
   in pericarditis, 778
   of pericardium, 316–317
   of prosthetic cardiac valves, 317
   of pulmonic valve, 316
   of right ventricle, 313*f,* 314
   in septal hypertrophy, 314
   in shock, 667
   stress, 309–311
   in syncope, 430
   three-dimensional, 317–318
   transesophageal, 311–312, 510–511, 778
   transthoracic, 308–309, 308*f*–313*f*
   of tricuspid valve, 316
   two-dimensional, 309, 310*f*–313*f,* 552
   in ventricular septal defects, 314
Economic factors, in hypertension, 860
Edema
   assessment of, 250
   in deep vein thrombosis, 164
   in heart failure, 612, 623–624
   optic disc, 238
   pathophysiology of, 174
   peripheral, in heart failure, 614
   pulmonary. *See* Pulmonary edema
Education
   level of, hypertension incidence and, 860
   patient and family. *See* Patient/family education

Effective refractory period, in action potential,
   25–26, 26*f*
Effusion
   pericardial, 780–781
      echocardiography in, 317
      radiography in, 303*t*
   pleural
      postoperative, 641, 642*f*
      radiography in, 303*t,* 304*f,* 306*f*
Eisenmenger reaction, 803
Ejection fraction
   definition of, 46
   in heart failure, 604–605, 605*f*
Ejection murmurs, 255, 255*f*
Elastic arteries, 49
Elastin, in atherosclerotic lesions, 144
Elderly persons. *See* Older adults
Electrical characteristics, of myocardial cells,
   17–22, 18*t,* 19*f*
   modification of, 28–29, 29*f*
Electrical currents, 19–21, 19*f*
   sarcolemmal, 26–28, 26*t*
Electrocardiography, 326–360
   aging effects on, 223
   in angina, 552, 555
   in aortic regurgitation, 773–774
   in aortic stenosis, 771
   in atrial enlargement, 349–351, 354*f*
   axis determination in, 336–337, 337*f*–340*f*
   in bifascicular blocks, 342, 345*f,* 346*f*
   in Brugada syndrome, 357, 360*f*
   in bundle-branch blocks, 12, 338–339,
      342*f*–344*f*
   in cardiac cycle, 44*f*
   vs. central venous pressure, 489, 490*d*–491*d*
   conduction system physiology and, 326–328,
      327*f*–330*f,* 329*t*
   definition of, 326
   in dilated cardiomyopathy, 783
   in electrolyte imbalances, 353–356, 357*f*–359*f*
   in electrophysiology studies, 425–426, 427*f*
   in exercise testing
      preparation for, 441, 442*f*
      responses to, 448–449, 448*f,* 449*f*
   in fascicular blocks, 340–341, 345*f*
   heart rate in, 329–330, 331*f*
   in heart rate variability, 528–529, 528*f*
   in hypercalcemia, 183
   in hyperkalemia, 181
   in hypermagnesemia, 185
   in hypertrophic cardiomyopathy, 784
   in hypokalemia, 180
   in hypomagnesemia, 184–185
   in intra-aortic balloon pump use, 678, 678*f*
   in mitral regurgitation, 767
   in mitral stenosis, 760
   in mitral valve prolapse, 770
   in myocardial ischemia and infarction,
      342–349, 346*f*–350*f,* 347*d,* 350*d,* 545,
      557–559, 558*f,* 559*f,* 568–569, 568*f*
      anterior, 346, 351*f*
      inferior, 346–347, 352*f*
      lateral, 347
      for location of infarct, 346, 350*t,* 351*f*
      non-Q wave, 348–349, 353*f*
      posterior, 347–348, 353*f*
      right ventricular, 348, 352*f*
   in myocarditis, 786
   in pacemaker evaluation, 723–727, 724*f*–726*f*
   in pericarditis, noneffusive, 778, 779*f*
   postoperative, 639, 639*f*
   principles of, 328–330, 330*f,* 331*f*
   rhythm in, 330

vs. right atrial pressure, 489, 490*d*–491*d*
   in shock, 667
   in syncope, 430
   twelve-lead, 330–336, 332*f*
      bipolar leads in, 331–332, 333*f*
      hexaxial reference system for, 334, 334*f*
      normal adult results in, 336, 336*f*
      posterior leads in, 332, 333*f*
      right chest leads in, 332, 333*f*
      twelve views of heart in, 334, 335*f,* 336
      unipolar leads in, 332, 333*f*
   in ventricular enlargement, 351–352, 354*f,*
      355*f,* 355*t,* 356*d,* 356*f*
   waveform configurations in, 329*t*
   in Wellens syndrome, 356, 359*f*
   in wide QRS rhythms, 402–405, 402*t,*
      403*f*–409*f*
Electrodes
   for defibrillation, 694, 695*f*
   for electrocardiography, 331–332, 333*f,*
      336, 336*f*
   in electrophysiology catheters, 425
   of pacemakers, 711*d*
Electroencephalography, in sleep, 197, 198*f,*
   200–201
Electrograms, intra-atrial, in arrhythmias, 405,
   409*f,* 425, 427*f*
Electrolyte(s). *See also specific electrolytes*
   balance of, principles of, 177, 178*t*
   after cardiac surgery, 287–288
   measurement of, 286–287
Electrolyte imbalances
   calcium, 182–183, 182*t,* 183*t*
   electrocardiography in, 353–356, 357*f*–359*f*
   in heart failure, 615
   magnesium, 183–185, 184*t,* 185*t*
   phosphate, 185–186, 186*t*
   potassium, 179–182, 179*t,* 180*t. See also*
      Hyperkalemia; Hypokalemia
Electromagnetic radiation
   implantable cardioverter defibrillator
      interference from, 748–749
   pacemaker interference from, 711*d,* 721–722
Electromechanical dissociation, treatment of,
   698–699
Electromyography, in sleep, 197, 198*f,* 200
Electron beam computed tomography, 324
Electronic monitoring
   of adherence, 963*t,* 964–965
   of blood pressure, 244
Electro-oculography, in sleep, 197, 198*f,* 200
Electrophysiology procedures, 425–438
   diagnostic, 425–430
      in cardiac arrest survivors, 427–428
      complications of, 426–427
      indications for, 428–430, 428*d,* 429*d*
      patient preparation for, 425
      in syncope, 429–430, 429*d*
      techniques for, 425–426, 426*f,* 427*f*
      in wide-complex tachycardias, 428–429, 428*d*
   nursing care in, 435–437
   radiofrequency catheter ablation as.
      See Radiofrequency catheter ablation
Elements, in Chinese medicine, 976
Elimination, in history taking, 234
Embolectomy, pulmonary, 168
Embolism
   air, in pulmonary catheter removal, 497
   definition of, 162
   from endocarditis, 757, 788–789
   intracardiac, echocardiography of, 317
   from prosthetic valves, 765
   pulmonary. *See* Pulmonary embolism

Emergency department, myocardial infarction care in, 567–568
Enalapril
    for heart failure, 619*t*
    for hypertension, 879*t*
Enalaprilat, for hypertension, 882*t*
Encephalopathy, hypertensive, 867
Endarteritis
    in patent ductus arteriosus, 798
    septic, in percutaneous coronary interventions, 595
End diastolic volume, aging effects on, 222
End-diastolic volume, 605
Endless loop tachycardia, 712*d*, 731–732, 733*f*
Endocarditis
    infectious, 787–790
        assessment of, 788–789, 789*t*
        clinical manifestations of, 757, 757*t*
        complications of, 757
        diagnosis of, 757–758, 758*f*
        echocardiography in, 317
        epidemiology of, 787
        medical management of, 789
        native valve, 788
        nosocomial, 788
        nursing management of, 789–790
        pathogenesis and pathology of, 757, 788
        predisposing factors in, 787, 787*d*
        prevention of, 758, 789
        prosthetic valve, 765, 788, 789
        right-side vs. left-side, 789
        risk factors for, 757, 758*d*
        treatment of, 758, 758*d*
        types of, 787–788
        valvular disease in, 757–758, 757*t*, 758*d*, 758*f*
    nonbacterial thrombotic, 788
    in rheumatic fever, 756
Endocardium, anatomy of, 10
Endocrine function, in sleep, 204
Endomyocardial biopsy, in myocarditis, 786
Endothelial lipase, in cholesterol transport, 899
Endothelin-1
    in heart failure, 608
    as vasoconstrictor, 54*f*, 57, 57*f*
Endothelium
    cholesterol levels and, 900–901
    dysfunction of, hypertension in, 861, 864–865
    of exchange vessels, 51
    in hemostasis, 154
    injury of, pathologic events after, 154
    low-density lipoprotein adherence to, 158
    of pulmonary circulation, 72
    vascular smooth muscle cell interaction with, 61*f*
    vasoactive substances derived from, 53–58, 53*t*, 54*f*–58*f*, 54*t*
Endothelium-derived contracting factors, 56–58, 57*f*, 58*f*
Endothelium-derived hyperpolarizing factors, 54*f*, 56, 56*f*
Endothelium-derived relaxing factors, 53–56, 54*f*–56*f*, 54*t*
Endotracheal tube, radiographic appearance of, 299*t*, 300*f*
Enhanced Recovery in Coronary Heart Disease (ENRICHD), 830–834
Enoxaparin, for deep vein thrombosis, 164, 165*t*
ENRICHD (Enhanced Recovery in Coronary Heart Disease), 830–834
ENRICHD Social Support Instrument, 829
Environment, for sleep, 212–213

Enzyme(s), cardiac. *See specific enzymes, eg,* Creatine kinase; Lactate dehydrogenase
Enzyme-linked immunosorbent assay
    for adhesion molecules, 129
    for heparin-associated platelet antibody, 170
    for interleukin 6, 133
Eosinophils, 151*f*, 152, 153*t*
    count of, 282
Epicardial pacemakers, 714, 714*f*, 719, 720*f*, 722
Epicardium, anatomy of, 9
Epigastric artery, inferior, as coronary artery bypass graft, 632
Epinephrine
    for arrhythmias, 369*t*
    for asystole, 697*f*
    in blood pressure control, 89
    for bradyarrhythmias, 375*t*
    electrophysiologic effects of, 28, 29*f*
    measurement of, 289
    postoperative, 638*t*
    in sarcoplasmic calcium ion modulation, 35
    for shock, 669*t*
Epipericardium (visceral pericardium), 776
Eplerenone, for hypertension, 879*t*
Epoch, in polysomnography, 200
Epresartan, for hypertension, 879*t*
Eptifibatide
    for myocardial infarction, 575–576
    for percutaneous coronary interventions, 596
Epworth Sleepiness Scale, 199, 199*t*
Equilibrium potential, calculation of, 19–20
Ergometer, bicycle, for exercise testing, 442–444
Erythema, in deep vein thrombosis, 164
Erythrocyte(s). *See* Red blood cell(s)
Erythrocyte sedimentation rate, 282
Erythrocytosis, in cyanotic heart disease, 803
Erythropoietin, in red blood cell production, 152
Escape interval, in pacing, 711*d*
E-selectin, as inflammatory marker, 129
Esmolol
    for arrhythmias, 369*t*, 373*t*
    for hypertension, 882*t*
Esophageal probe
    in Doppler ultrasonography, for cardiac output measurement, 509–510, 510*f*, 511*t*
    in echocardiography, 510–511
Estes' Scorecard, for left ventricular enlargement, 355*t*
Estrogen
    coronary artery disease and, 818–819
    heart rate variability and, 532
    lipoprotein levels and, 909
Ethical considerations, in genetic disease, 120
Ethnic differences, in hypertension, 859–860
Euglycemics, for diabetes mellitus, 957–958
Everolimus, for cardiac transplantation, 650
Excessive daytime sleepiness, 205
Excitation, myocardial, 18, 18*t*, 19*f*
Excitation-contraction coupling, in conduction, 31–32, 32*f*
Exercise, 916–936. *See also* Exercise testing
    adherence to program schedules and, 961–965
    angina in, 550
    arterial waveform during, 486
    benefits of, 920–921, 920*d*, 921*d*
    in cardiac rehabilitation programs. *See* Cardiac rehabilitation
    after cardiac transplantation, 650–651, 650*f*, 651*f*
    contraindications to, 928, 928*d*
    coronary artery disease risk and, 813–815, 814*f*, 815*f*
    current view of, 916

for decreasing physiological arousal, 832
for deep vein thrombosis prevention, 166
for depression, 825, 833
for diabetes mellitus, 955–956
    diary for, 963*t*, 964, 965
    dynamic, 929
    for heart failure, 622
    heart rate variability and, 534
    in history taking, 234
    for hostility, 834
    for hypertension, 872–873
    vs. immobility, 921, 921*d*
    importance of, evidence supporting, 916–917, 917*t*
    intensity of, 929–930
    isometric, heart sounds in, 257*t*, 258
    lipoprotein levels and, 909
    metabolic equivalents of, 925*d*
    moderate, benefits of, 919
    after myocardial infarction, 570
    in obesity, 942–943
    for outpatient rehabilitation, 929–930
    prescription for, 929–930
    program for enhanced adherence, 968–969
    safety of, 930
    in secondary prevention, 919–920, 920*t*
    in stress echocardiography, 309–311
    Surgeon General's report on, 919
Exercise capacity
    determination of, 447, 448*f*
    vs. mortality risk, 918, 918*f*, 918*t*
Exercise testing, 439–458
    accuracy of, 452–453, 452*d*, 453*d*
    ancillary methods with, 453–454
    in angina, 552
    in aortic regurgitation, 773
    in aortic stenosis, 771
    Balke treadmill protocol for, 444
    benefits of, 439
    Bruce treadmill protocol for, 444
    contraindications to, 440, 440*d*
    creatine kinase after, 273
    cycle ergometer in, 444
    drug impact on, 441, 441*t*
    echocardiography with, 454
    in elderly persons, 455–456
    electrocardiography in, preparation for, 441–442, 442*f*
    for fitness evaluation, 917–918, 918*f*, 918*t*
    gas exchange techniques in, 454–455
    graded, 930
    before hospital discharge, 926–927, 927*t*
    indications for, 439
    low-level, 926, 927*t*
    in mitral valve prolapse, 770
    modalities for, 442–443
    after myocardial infarction, before hospital discharge, 926–927, 927*t*
    myocardial perfusion imaging with, 453–454
    Naughton treadmill protocol for, 444
    objectives of, 439
    personnel for, 439–440
    pharmacologic stress techniques in, 454
    prestest considerations in, 440–441, 441*t*, 442*f*
    prognostic value of, 446*d*, 455
    protocols for, 443–444, 443*f*
    ramp testing in, 444
    recovery period after, 452
    responses in, 445–450, 445*d*–446*d*
        arrhythmias, 450
        blood pressure, 446–447
        electrocardiographic, 448–449, 448*f*
        exercise capacity in, 447, 448*f*

false-positive and false-negative, 452–453, 452*d*, 453*d*
heart rate, 445–446, 447*f*
subjective, 450, 450*d*
safety in, 439–440
submaximal, 444–445
termination of, 450–451, 451*d*
after transplantation, 456
ventricular function studies with, 454
in women, 455
Exit block, Wenckebach, 413, 414*f*, 415*f*
Exons, 111, 113
Expiration, heart sounds in, 253, 253*f*, 257, 257*t*
Expressive hostility, coronary artery disease and, 827
External cognitive aids, for adherence, 967*d*, 969
Extracardiac obstructive shock
pathophysiology of, 660*t*, 662
treatment of, 673
Extracellular fluid
composition of, 173
definition of, 173
distribution of, 173, 174
Extracellular fluid volume, 175–176
deficit of, 175–177, 175*t*
in percutaneous coronary interventions, 598–599
excess of, 176, 176*t*
in heart failure, 623–624
Extrinsic coagulation pathway, 155, 156*f*
Eye
diabetes mellitus manifestations in, 951
hypertension effects on, 866, 866*t*
physical assessment of, 236–239, 236*f*–239*f*
Ezetimibe, for hyperlipidemia, 911*t*, 912

F

Facial characteristics, assessment of, 236
Factor V Leiden, pulmonary embolism with, 166
Fallback response, in pacing, 731, 732*f*
False aneurysms, left ventricular, 560
Familial hypercholesterolemia, 901
Family care and support. *See also* Patient/family education
in cardiac arrest, 707
in endocarditis, 790
in intra-aortic balloon pump use, 682–683*ncp*
in myocarditis, 787
in shock, 674
Family history, 232, 859
Fascicles, anatomy of, 12
Fascicular blocks, electrocardiography in, 340–341, 345*f*
Fast inward current, 27
Fast-response cells, 22, 22*t*
Fat(s), dietary, hyperlipidemia and, 905–908, 906*f*, 907*d*
Fatigue
after cardiac transplantation, 654*ncp*
in heart failure, 207, 611
in mitral stenosis, 759
in myocarditis, 786
Fatty acids
free, in myocardial metabolism, 41
omega-3, hyperlipidemia and, 907
Fatty streaks, 140–141, 147*t*
Fear, in myocardial infarction, nursing management of, 579
Feeding tube, radiographic appearance of, 299*t*, 302*f*
Felodipine, for hypertension, 879*t*

Femoral artery
atherosclerosis of, 146
catheter placement in, 463, 464*f*, 465*f*, 488, 488*t*
for coronary angiography, 467
postprocedure care in, 473–474, 473*t*
injury of, in percutaneous coronary interventions, 594–595
intra-aortic balloon pump insertion through, 675, 676*f*
Femoral pulse, assessment of, 241, 241*f*
Femoral vein, cardiac catheterization through, 466
Fenestrated vascular endothelium, 51
Fenning procedure, for transposition of great arteries, 802
Fenoldopam, for hypertension, 882*t*
Fibric acid derivatives, for hyperlipidemia, 911*t*, 912
Fibrillation. *See* Atrial fibrillation; Defibrillation; Ventricular fibrillation
Fibrin
degradation products of, 155–156, 157*t*
formation of, in coagulation, 155, 156*f*
Fibrinogen
in atherosclerotic lesions, 144
as inflammatory marker, 130
measurement of, 157*t*, 284
Fibrinoid arteriolar necrosis, hypertension and, 865
Fibrinolysis, 155–156, 157*t*
Fibroatheromas, 142, 147*t*
Fibrosa layer, of pericardium, 776
Fibrosis, of skin, in edema, 250
Fibrous skeleton, of heart, 6, 6*f*
Fick equation, 77, 508*t*, 512
Fight-or-flight response, coronary artery disease and, 828–829, 828*f*
Filaments, myosin, in contraction, 33, 34*f*, 35*f*
Filtration
in microcirculation, 65–67, 66*f*
principles of, 174
Finger(s), clubbing of, 249, 249*f*
Fish oils, for cardiovascular disease, 980
Fistula, arteriovenous, in percutaneous coronary interventions, 594–595
Fitness, *vs.* health, 919
FK506 (tacrolimus), for cardiac transplantation, 648*t*, 649
Flaxseed, for cardiovascular disease, 981–982
Flecainide, for arrhythmias, 369*t*–370*t*
Flow-limited diffusion, 65
Fluid(s)
intake of, 173–174
retention of, in heart failure, 606–607, 609*f*
status of, impedance cardiography and, 512
Fluid balance
body compartments and, 173
extracellular volume, 175–176, 175*t*, 176*t*
osmolality and, 173, 176–177, 176*t*, 178*t*
processes involved in, 173–175, 175*t*
Fluid imbalances
extracellular volume, 175–177, 175*t*, 176*t*
in hypernatremia, 177, 177*t*
in hyponatremia, 176–177, 176*t*
mixed, 177
Fluid therapy
after cardiac surgery, 636
in heart donor, 644
hemodynamic indices in, 500, 500*f*
for hypovolemic shock, 673
for myocardial infarction, 572
for septic shock, 673

18F-Fluorodeoxyglucose, in positron emission tomography, 322
Foam cells, in fatty streaks, 140, 143
Folic acid
deficiency of, as coronary artery disease risk factor, 819–820
for homocysteinemia, 132
Fontan procedure, for tricuspid atresia, 801
Food. *See* Nutrition
Foot complications, in diabetes mellitus, 952, 955
Foramen ovale, patent, percutaneous interventions for, 596–597, 597*f*
Force-velocity relation, 38–39, 38*f*, 93–94
Forebrain, in blood pressure regulation, 84
Foreign objects, in heart, echocardiography of, 317
Forrester subsets, of shock, 668, 668*f*
Forward heart failure, 601–602
Fosinopril
for heart failure, 619*t*
for hypertension, 879*t*
Fractional flow reserve, measurement of, in percutaneous coronary interventions, 595
Frank-Starling law of the heart, 36–38, 37*f*, 38*f*, 94
in heart failure, 604–605, 605*f*
Free fatty acids, in myocardial metabolism, 41
Free radicals, in diabetes mellitus, 953
Fremitus, 258
Frequency, natural, in hemodynamic monitoring, 480, 483*f*
Frequency domain analysis, in heart rate variability, 528–529, 529*t*, 530*f*
Friedewald formula, 277, 278*f*
Full recovery time, in action potential, 26, 26*f*
Functional patterns, in history taking, 233–234
Funduscopic examination, examination of, 237–239, 237*f*–239*f*
Furosemide
for heart failure, 619*t*
for hypertension, 878*t*
for pulmonary edema, 671
Fusion beats, 402*t*, 404, 407*f*, 711*d*

G

Gallavardin phenomenon, in aortic stenosis, 771
Gallops, in heart sounds, 254, 254*f*
Gangrene, in heparin-induced thrombocytopenia, 170
Gap junctions, of myocardial cells, 17
Garlic, for cardiovascular disease, 981
Gas exchange, 75
measurement of, in exercise testing, 454–455
ventilation-perfusion matching for, 74
Gas transport, 73, 75–77, 76*f*
Gastric banding, for obesity, 945
Gastric tonometry, for oxygenation monitoring, 79, 517
Gastroepiploic artery, as coronary artery bypass graft, 631–632
Gastrointestinal system
bleeding from, in percutaneous coronary interventions, 599
disorders of, postoperative, 640–641
shock effects on, 666
Gastroplasty, for obesity, 945
Gating, of ion channels, 18, 21
Gender
heart rate variability and, 532
hypertension and, 859
percutaneous coronary interventions and, 585

Gene(s)
  description of, 113
  formation of, 111
  variation in, 113–114
Genetic(s). *See also* Genetic disease(s)
  diagnostic tests based on, 114
  in dilated cardiomyopathy, 782
  DNA in. *See* DNA (deoxyribonucleic acid)
  genetic variation and, 113–114
  in heart rate variability, 532–533
  Human Genome Project, 114
  pharmacogenomics and, 114–115
  terminology of, 112*d*
Genetic disease(s), 115–118, 116*t*, 117*t*, 810–811
  atherosclerosis as, 116, 118
  biochemical basis of, 115
  coronary artery disease as, 118–121, 119*t*
  ethical considerations in, 121
  hypertension as, 859–861, 862*d*
  mutations in, 113–114
  overview of, 115–116
  stroke as, 115–116
  sudden cardiac death as, 116
Genome
  definition of, 112
  Human Genome Project and, 114
  number of genes in, 113
Geographic differences, in hypertension, 859–860
Geriatric Depression Scale, 829
Gianturco-Rubin Flex-Stent, 590, 590*f*
Glomerular filtration rate, aging effects on, 224–225
Glucagon, action of, 950
Glucose
  control of, in diabetes mellitus, 953–955
  infusion of, hypophosphatemia in, 186
  intolerance of, from corticosteroids, 649
  measurement of, 289
  metabolism of, in diabetes mellitus, 949–950
  in myocardial metabolism, 41
Glycated hemoglobin, measurement of, 289, 289*t*
Glycated serum protein, 289–290
Glycolysis, in myocardial metabolism, 544
Glycoprotein IIb/IIIa receptor inhibitors
  for myocardial infarction, 575–576
  for percutaneous coronary interventions, 596
Goal setting
  in adherence, 967, 967*d*
  in weight loss, 943
Gradient-echo magnetic resonance imaging, 322–323
Granulocytes, 151*f*, 152–153, 153*t*
Great vessels. *See also* Aorta
  echocardiography of, 310*f*
  transposition of, 796*f*, 802–803
Greenfield filter, for pulmonary embolism, 168
Groin complications, in percutaneous coronary interventions, 594–595
Guanfacine, for hypertension, 878*t*
Guidewires, for coronary angioplasty, 587–588, 588*f*

H

Habit building, for adherence, 967*d*, 968
Hair, excessive growth of, from cyclosporine, 649
Hancock porcine valve, 763–764
Hard exudates, in retina, 239, 239*f*
HAV (hypotension, acidosis, and vasodilation) syndrome, 193
Hawthorn, for cardiovascular disease, 978–979
HDL. *See* Lipoprotein(s), high-density

Head, physical assessment of, 236–239
  color in, 236
  eye appearance in, 236–239, 236*f*–239*f*
  facial characteristics in, 236
  temperature in, 236
Head-upright tilt test, in syncope, 430
Health care organizations, hypertension control and, 884
Health care providers, sleep in, 213
Health habits, in history taking, 233
Health history. *See* History taking
Health perception, in history taking, 233
Heart
  adrenoreceptors in, 84, 86
  aging effects on, 222–223
  anatomy of, 3–6, 4*f*, 5*f*
    blood vessels, 12–16, 13*f*–14*f*, 16*f*
    chambers, 6–8, 7*f*, 8*f*
    fibrous skeleton, 6, 6*f*
    lymph drainage, 16
    nerves, 16
    tissue, 9–12, 9*f*–12*f*, 13*t*
    topographic, 250, 251*f*
    valves, 8–9
  axis of, 3
  biopsy of, for transplant rejection, 646–647, 646*f*
  dilation of, oxygen supply and, 43
  foreign objects in, 317
  innervation of, 16, 43, 86*t*
  morphology of, exercise effects on, 920, 920*d*
  perforation of
    in electrophysiology studies, 426
    in radiofrequency catheter ablation, 431
  physical assessment of
    auscultation in. *See* Auscultation
    inspection in, 250–251
    palpation in, 251–252
  radiographic appearance of, 296–297, 297*f*
  temperature changes in, electrophysiologic effects of, 29
  transplantation of. *See* Cardiac transplantation
  twelve views of, 334, 335*f*, 336
  weight of, 5–6
Heart blocks. *See* Conduction blocks
Heart failure, 601–627
  acute, 602
    vs. chronic, 661, 661*t*
    diagnosis of, 667–669, 668*f*
    medical management of, 616
    shock in. *See* Shock, cardiogenic
    treatment of, 670–673, 670*f*, 671*d*, 671*t*, 672*d*
  in aortic regurgitation, 773
  assessment in, 621–622
  backward, 601–602
  cardiac rehabilitation in, 921, 931
  in cardiac surgery, intra-aortic balloon pump for, 675
  centers for, 622
  central sleep apnea in, 210
  chronic, 602
    vs. acute, 661, 661*t*
    acute decompensated
      diagnosis of, 668–669
      treatment of, 670–673, 670*f*, 671*d*, 671*t*, 672*d*
    decompensation of, 661
    medical management of, 616–618, 616*t*, 617*t*
  classification of, 612–613, 613*t*
  clinical manifestations of, 610–612, 612*f*, 613*t*
  counseling on, 622, 622*d*

creatine kinase in, 274
definitions of, 601–603, 602*t*
diastolic, 602–603
etiology of, 601–603, 602*t*
forward, 601–602
heart rate variability in, 531
hemodynamic indices of, 500, 500*f*
high cardiac output, 602
in hypocalcemia, 182–183
hyponatremia in, 177
impedance cardiography in, 512
incidence of, 601
inflammatory mediators in. *See* Inflammatory marker(s)
left-sided, 602, 611–612
low cardiac output, 602
management models for. *See* Disease management
medical management of, 613–621
  acute, 616
  adjunctive therapy in, 616–618, 616*t*, 617*t*
  chronic, 616–618, 616*t*, 617*t*
  diagnostic tests in, 614–615
  history in, 613–614
  laboratory tests in, 614–615, 615*f*
  pharmacologic, 618–621, 619*t*, 620*t*
  physical assessment in, 614
in myocarditis, 786
nursing management of, 621–624, 622*d*
pathophysiology and pathogenesis of, 603–610, 603*t*
  hemodynamic abnormalities in, 604–606, 604*f*–607*f*
  neurohormonal response in, 606–610, 607*t*, 608*t*, 609*f*–611*f*
in pulmonic stenosis, 799
radiography in, 303*t*, 304*f*
in restrictive cardiomyopathy, 785–786
right-sided, 602, 612
sleep in, 207
sudden death in, 531–532
surgical management of, 635
systolic, 602–603
transient, in myocardial ischemia, 923
HeartMate ventricular assist device, 686
Heart rate
  aging effects on, 222
  assessment of, 239
  after cardiac catheterization, 474
  cardiac output and, 40, 40*f*, 93
  vs. contraction, 39, 40*f*
  control of, 92–93
  in electrocardiography, 329–330, 331*f*
  in exercise testing, 445–446, 447*f*
  in heart failure, 614
  in myocardial infarction, 557
  myocardial oxygen consumption and, 42, 541–542
  normal, 92
  respiration effects on, 93
  in sleep, 202–203
  target, for exercise training, 930
  variability of. *See* Heart rate variability
Heart rate variability, 527–538
  in angina, 531
  in arrhythmias, 531
  in cardiac surgery, 532
  definition of, 527
  factors influencing, 532–535
    age as, 223, 532
    body position as, 533
    brain injury as, 534–535
    COPD as, 535

Jaundice, 236
Jervell and Lange-Nielsen syndrome, cardiac arrest in, 690
Job stress, coronary artery disease and, 827–828
Joint National Committee of the National High Blood Pressure Education Program, 856–857, 857t
 hypertension algorithm of, 875, 876f, 877t–880t
Judkins technique, for coronary arteriography, 467, 468f
Jugular veins, assessment of, in shock, 667
Jugular venous distention, in heart failure, 612
Jugular venous pressure, assessment of, 241–243, 242f
Jugular venous pulse, assessment of, 241–243, 242f
Junctional bradycardia, treatment of, 375t
Junctional conduction, 30
Junctional rhythm, 384
Junctional tachycardia, 384

K

Kallikrein-kinin system, in blood pressure regulation, 89f, 92
Kent bundles, 11
Ketoacidosis, diabetic, 951
Kidney
 acid excretion from, 190–193, 191t
 aging effects on, 224–225
 assessment of, in shock, 667
 in blood pressure regulation, 94–95
 dysfunction/failure of
  from contrast agents, 593
  in diabetes mellitus, 951–952
  in heart failure, 615
  in hypertension, 865–866, 880
  hypertension in, 861, 862d, 863, 865–866, 880
  pericarditis in, 776–778
  postoperative, 640
  in shock, 664, 664f, 666
 fluid excretion from, 174, 175t
 function of, in sleep, 204
Kinins, in blood pressure regulation, 89f, 92
Knowledge deficit
 after cardiac transplantation, 655ncp–656ncp
 in congenital heart disease, 803ncp–804ncp
 in heart failure, 624
 in hypertension, 886ncp
 in myocardial infarction, 579–580
Korean medicine, 976
Korotkoff sounds, 245–246, 245t
Krogh model, of cardiac output vs. central venous pressure, 100–101, 100f
Krvonen formula, for training heart rate, 930
Kussmaul's sign
 in myocardial infarction, 557
 in pericarditis, 780
Kyphoscoliosis, chest configuration in, 258, 260f

L

Labetalol, for hypertension, 878t, 882t
Laboratory tests. *See also* Echocardiography; Electrocardiography
 for angina, 552
 blood, 265–295
  for alanine aminotransferase, 288
  for alkaline phosphatase, 288
  arterial blood gases. *See* Arterial blood gases
  for aspartate aminotransferase, 288
  for bilirubin, 288
  for catecholamines, 289
  for coagulation, 157t, 283–286
  for C-reactive protein, 279–280, 279f
  for creatine kinase, 272–276, 272t, 274f, 275f, 276t, 277t
  for creatinine, 289
  cultures, 283
  drawing from catheters, 483
  for drug concentrations, 268, 291, 291t
  for electrolytes, 286–288
  for glucose, 289
  for glycated hemoglobin, 289, 289t
  for glycated serum protein, 289–290
  hematologic, 281–283
  for homocysteine, 280
  for hypercholesterolemia, 905
  interpretation of results of, 267–268
  for lactate dehydrogenase, 270f, 270t, 271t, 290
  for lipids, 276–278, 278t, 279t
  for lipoprotein-associated phospholipase A_2, 280
  for myocardial proteins, 269–271, 270f, 270t, 271t
  for natriuretic peptides, 280–281
  for osmolality, 287
  after percutaneous coronary interventions, 586–587
  point-of-care, 269
  postoperative, 287–288, 290
  for protein, 290
  reference ranges for, 268, 277t
  sensitivity and specificity of, 268–269
  specimen collection for, 265–267, 291
  for urea nitrogen, 290
  for uric acid, 290
 for sleep assessment, 213
Lactate, as measure of oxygen supply and demand, 517
Lactate dehydrogenase, 270f, 270t, 271t, 290
Laplace, law of
 afterload and, 94
 intramyocardial tension and, 41–42
Lasers
 in coronary angioplasty, 589
 in transmyocardial revascularization, 634
Latissimus dorsi muscle, in cardiomyoplasty, 635, 783
LDL. *See* Lipoprotein(s), low-density
Leads
 for implantable cardioverter defibrillator, 742, 742f, 743f
 for pacemakers, 711d, 716, 718f, 738
Lecithin cholesterol acyltransferase, in cholesterol transport, 899
Left anterior fascicular block, 341, 345f
Left atrial pressure
 in mitral regurgitation, 766
 vs. pulmonary artery wedge pressure, 493, 494
Left bundle branch, function of, 326
Left bundle-branch block, 339, 344f, 402t, 403–404, 406f
Left heart. *See also* Atrium (atria), left; Ventricle(s), left
 catheterization of, 464–466, 465f, 466f
Left posterior fascicular block, 341, 345f
Left ventricular assist devices, 680, 683–686
 axial flow pumps in, 684
 centrifugal-kinetic energy type, 684, 684f
 continuous-flow, 683, 684, 684f
 for dilated cardiomyopathy, 783
 for heart failure, 617
 indications for, 683
 mechanisms of, 683–684
 pulsatile, 684–686, 685f, 686f
 roller pump in, 684
Left ventricular function curves, in heart failure, 605, 605f
Left ventricular outflow obstruction, in hypertrophic cardiomyopathy, 784
Legal aspects, of CAM, 982
Length-tension relationship, preload and, 36–38, 37f, 38f, 94
Lepirudin
 for deep vein thrombosis, 165t
 for heparin-induced thrombocytopenia, 170–171
Leukocyte(s). *See* White blood cell(s)
Levine's sign, in angina, 550
Lidocaine, for arrhythmias, 370t
Lifestyle modification
 for hypertension, 870–874, 870t, 872t, 873t
 for obesity, 942–944, 942t
Life support, cardiac
 algorithms of, 695, 695d, 696f, 697f, 698–699, 698d
 description of, 691–695, 693f–695f
Lightheadedness, in exercise testing, 450
Limb leads, in electrocardiography, 331–332, 333f
Lines, invasive, radiographic appearance of, 297, 299f–302f, 299t
Lipid(s). *See also* Lipoprotein(s); Triglycerides
 in atherosclerotic lesions, 144
 blood, measurement of, 276–278, 278t, 279t
 functions of, 897–898
 metabolism of, 898–899, 898f, 899f
 reverse transport of, 899
 structures of, 897–898
 transport of, 898–899, 898f, 899f
Lipid bilayer, of myocardial cells, 18, 19f
Lipofuscin accumulation, with aging, 222
Lipoprotein(a), 900
Lipoprotein(s), 900t
 alcohol and, 909
 in atherosclerotic lesions, 144
 excess of. *See* Hypercholesterolemia; Hyperlipidemias
 exercise and, 909
 heart rate variability and, 534
 high-density
  vs. coronary artery disease risk, 903t, 904t
  deficiency of, hypoalphalipoproteinemia in, 901–902
  estrogen effects on, 909
  function of, 899
 hormones and, 909
 intermediate-density, 898
 low-density
  abnormalities of, 900t, 901–902
  adherence of, to endothelium, 158
  classification of, 910, 910t
  as coronary artery disease risk factor, 812–813, 813t
  in diabetes mellitus, 955
  measurement of, 905
  metabolism of, 898–899, 898f, 899f
  oxidation of, 143–144, 900
  particle size of, 900
  receptors for, 898–899, 898f, 899f, 901
 measurement of, 276–278, 278t, 279t, 905
 very-low-density, 898, 899, 899f
Lipoprotein-associated phospholipase A_2, 280
Lipoprotein lipase, in cholesterol transport, 899

 depression as, 535
 diabetes mellitus as, 535
 gender as, 532
 general health as, 533–534
 genetic, 532–533
 Huntington disease as, 535
 pain as, 534
 Parkinson disease as, 535
 sleep-wake status as, 533
 in heart failure, 531–532
 in heart transplantation, 532
 in hypertension, 531
 interventions for, 535
 measurement of, 527–529, 528f, 528t, 529t, 530f
 mechanisms of, 527
 in myocardial infarction, 530–531
 in sudden death, 531
Heart sounds. *See also* Murmurs
 in aortic stenosis, 771
 in atrial septal defect, 798–799
 in cardiac cycle, 44f, 46
 in heart failure, 614
 in mitral stenosis, 759, 760t
 in myocardial infarction, 557
 normal, 253–254, 253f
 in pulmonic stenosis, 795
 in ventricular tachycardia, 406–407
Heat pulses, in continuous cardiac output measurement, 506–507
Height, measurement of, 235–236
Hematocrit, 281
Hematologic studies, 281–283
Hematoma
 in atherosclerotic lesions, 142, 145–146
 groin, in percutaneous coronary interventions, 594
Hematopoietic cells, 150–153
 growth factors for, 150, 151t
 platelets as, 151f, 153
 red blood cells as, 151–152, 151f
 types of, 150, 151f
 white blood cells as, 151f, 152–153, 153t
Hemiblocks (fascicular blocks), 340–341, 345f
Hemodynamic(s)
 of cardiac catheterization, 474–476, 474t, 475f–476f
 exercise effects on, 920, 920d
 of heart failure, 604–608, 604f–607f, 607t, 608t, 609f, 610f
 of hypertension, 860
 of myocardial infarction, 547
 of myocardial ischemia, 544–545
Hemodynamic monitoring, 478–526. *See also specific procedures*
 blood drawing from catheters in, 483
 cardiac output in, 503–505, 504d, 505d, 506t, 507t
  continuous, 506–507
 less invasive methods for, 507–512, 508t, 509f, 510f, 511t
 after cardiac surgery, 636
 in cardiopulmonary bypass, 629
 central venous pressure in, 488–489, 490d–491d, 492f
 direct arterial pressure in, 483–488, 484f–487f, 484t, 488t
 dynamic response characteristics in, 480, 483, 483f
 infection control in, 480, 482t
 in myocardial infarction, 559, 571
 oxygen supply and demand in, 512–519, 513t, 514t, 516f, 518t
 pulmonary artery pressure in. *See* Pulmonary artery pressure
 referencing in, 478–480, 479f, 480f, 480t, 481d–482d
 in shock, 667–668, 668f
 zeroing in, 479–480, 481d–482d
Hemoglobin
 glycated, measurement of, 289, 289t
 measurement of, 281
 optimization of, 514t
 in oxygen transport, 75–76, 76f
 in red blood cells, 151
Hemolysis, in blood specimens, 267
Hemolytic anemia, from prosthetic valves, 766
Hemoptysis, in pulmonary embolism, 167
Hemorrhage
 in atherosclerotic lesions, 142
 in bleeding disorders, 158
 blood pressure regulation in, 90, 90f
 brain, in percutaneous coronary interventions, 598
 in disseminated intravascular coagulation, 160
 eyelid, 236
 at femoral artery catheterization site, 474
 gastrointestinal, 640–641
 hypovolemic shock in, treatment of, 673
 oxygen delivery-oxygen consumption balance in, 78
 in percutaneous coronary interventions, 599
 postoperative, 636–637
 retroperitoneal, in percutaneous coronary interventions, 594
 in thrombolytic therapy, 566
Hemostasis, 154–157
 coagulation cascade in, 155, 156f
 endothelium in, 154
 fibrinolysis in, 155–156, 157t
 natural anticoagulants in, 156–157
 platelet phase of, 154–155
 vascular spasm in, 154
Henderson-Hasselbalch equation, 190
Heparin
 for cardiopulmonary bypass, 629
 for deep vein thrombosis, 164, 165, 165t
 hyperkalemia due to, 181
 low-molecular-weight, for deep vein thrombosis, 164–165, 165t
 for myocardial infarction, 573
 for percutaneous coronary interventions, 586, 596
Heparin cofactor II, 157
Heparin-induced thrombocytopenia, 169–171
 clinical presentation of, 170
 complications of, 170, 170t
 etiology of, 169
 medical management of, 170–171, 170t
 nursing interventions for, 171
 pathophysiology of, 169–170, 169f
Hepatic lipase, in cholesterol transport, 899
Herbal remedies, 978–980, 980f
Hexaxial reference system, 334, 334f
High blood pressure. *See* Hypertension
High cardiac output syndrome, in heart failure, 602
High-density lipoproteins. *See under* Lipoprotein(s)
High-frequency component, of frequency domain analysis, of heart rate variability, 529, 529t, 530f
Hirudin, for heparin-induced thrombocytopenia, 171
His bundle. *See* Bundle of His
History taking, 229–234
 chief complaint in, 230–231
 components of, 229
 family history in, 232
 functional patterns in, 233–234
 identifying information in, 230
 New York Heart Association's Functional and Therapeutic Classification in, 234, 235t
 past history in, 232
 personal history in, 232–233
 present illness history in, 231–232
 presenting problem in, 230–231
 social history in, 232–233
 systems review in, 233
Histotoxic hypoxia, 77
Holistic health care, definition of, 974
Holosystolic murmurs, 255, 255f, 256
Holter monitoring, in heart rate variability, 528, 528f
Homan's sign, in deep vein thrombosis, 164
Homeopathic medicine, 975
Homocysteine
 elevation of, as coronary artery disease risk factor, 819–820
 in heart failure, 615
 as inflammatory marker, 115, 131–132, 132d
 measurement of, 280
Homografts, for prosthetic valves, 763–764
Hook intervention, for hostility, 834
Hormone(s)
 lipoprotein levels and, 909
 reproductive, coronary artery disease and, 818–819
Hormone replacement therapy, postmenopausal, coronary artery disease and, 819
Hospice care, in heart failure, 617
Hostility, coronary artery disease and, 827, 834
Human Genome Project, 114
Human immunodeficiency virus infection, pericardial effusion in, 780
Huntington disease, heart rate variability in, 535
HV interval, in electrophysiology studies, 425–426, 430
Hydralazine
 for heart failure, 619t, 621
 for hypertension, 878t, 882t
Hydraulic conductivity, in microcirculation, 67
Hydrochlorothiazide
 for heart failure, 619t
 for hypertension, 878t
Hydrogen ions, excretion of, 190, 191t
Hydrostatic pressure
 fluid distribution and, 174
 referencing for, 478
Hydroxymethylglutaryl coenzyme-A reductase, 899
 inhibitors of (statins), for hyperlipidemia, 911t, 912
Hyperacute rejection, in cardiac transplantation, 19
Hypercalcemia, 183, 183t, 354, 356, 359f
Hypercapnia, arousal from sleep from, 203
Hypercholesterolemia
 as coronary artery disease risk factor, 812–813, 813t
 detection of, 902–903
 endothelial function and, 901
 epidemiology of, 897
 evaluation of, 905
 familial (severe), 901
 hypertension and, 880–881
 risks of, 902t–904t

depression as, 535
diabetes mellitus as, 535
gender as, 532
general health as, 533–534
genetic, 532–533
Huntington disease as, 535
pain as, 534
Parkinson disease as, 535
sleep-wake status as, 533
in heart failure, 531–532
in heart transplantation, 532
in hypertension, 531
interventions for, 535
measurement of, 527–529, 528f, 528t,
529t, 530f
mechanisms of, 527
in myocardial infarction, 530–531
in sudden death, 531
Heart sounds. See also Murmurs
in aortic stenosis, 771
in atrial septal defect, 798–799
in cardiac cycle, 44f, 46
in heart failure, 614
in mitral stenosis, 759, 760t
in myocardial infarction, 557
normal, 253–254, 253f
in pulmonic stenosis, 795
in ventricular tachycardia, 406–407
Heat pulses, in continuous cardiac output
measurement, 506–507
Height, measurement of, 235–236
Hematocrit, 281
Hematologic studies, 281–283
Hematoma
in atherosclerotic lesions, 142, 145–146
groin, in percutaneous coronary
interventions, 594
Hematopoietic cells, 150–153
growth factors for, 150, 151t
platelets as, 151f, 153
red blood cells as, 151–152, 151f
types of, 150, 151f
white blood cells as, 151f, 152–153, 153t
Hemiblocks (fascicular blocks), 340–341, 345f
Hemodynamic(s)
of cardiac catheterization, 474–476, 474t,
475f–476f
exercise effects on, 920, 920d
of heart failure, 604–608, 604f–607f, 607t,
608t, 609f, 610f
of hypertension, 860
of myocardial infarction, 547
of myocardial ischemia, 544–545
Hemodynamic monitoring, 478–526. See also
specific procedures
blood drawing from catheters in, 483
cardiac output in, 503–505, 504d, 505d,
506t, 507t
continuous, 506–507
less invasive methods for, 507–512, 508t, 509f,
510f, 511t
after cardiac surgery, 636
in cardiopulmonary bypass, 629
central venous pressure in, 488–489,
490d–491d, 492f
direct arterial pressure in, 483–488,
484f–487f, 484t, 488t
dynamic response characteristics in, 480,
483, 483f
infection control in, 480, 482t
in myocardial infarction, 559, 571
oxygen supply and demand in, 512–519, 513t,
514t, 516f, 518t

pulmonary artery pressure in.
See Pulmonary artery pressure
referencing in, 478–480, 479f, 480f, 480t,
481d–482d
in shock, 667–668, 668f
zeroing in, 479–480, 481d–482d
Hemoglobin
glycated, measurement of, 289, 289t
measurement of, 281
optimization of, 514t
in oxygen transport, 75–76, 76f
in red blood cells, 151
Hemolysis, in blood specimens, 267
Hemolytic anemia, from prosthetic valves, 766
Hemoptysis, in pulmonary embolism, 167
Hemorrhage
in atherosclerotic lesions, 142
in bleeding disorders, 158
blood pressure regulation in, 90, 90f
brain, in percutaneous coronary
interventions, 598
in disseminated intravascular
coagulation, 160
eyelid, 236
at femoral artery catheterization site, 474
gastrointestinal, 640–641
hypovolemic shock in, treatment of, 673
oxygen delivery-oxygen consumption balance
in, 78
in percutaneous coronary interventions, 599
postoperative, 636–637
retroperitoneal, in percutaneous coronary
interventions, 594
in thrombolytic therapy, 566
Hemostasis, 154–157
coagulation cascade in, 155, 156f
endothelium in, 154
fibrinolysis in, 155–156, 157t
natural anticoagulants in, 156–157
platelet phase of, 154–155
vascular spasm in, 154
Henderson-Hasselbalch equation, 190
Heparin
for cardiopulmonary bypass, 629
for deep vein thrombosis, 164, 165, 165t
hyperkalemia due to, 181
low-molecular-weight, for deep vein
thrombosis, 164–165, 165t
for myocardial infarction, 573
for percutaneous coronary interventions,
586, 596
Heparin cofactor II, 157
Heparin-induced thrombocytopenia, 169–171
clinical presentation of, 170
complications of, 170, 170t
etiology of, 169
medical management of, 170–171, 170t
nursing interventions for, 171
pathophysiology of, 169–170, 169f
Hepatic lipase, in cholesterol transport, 899
Herbal remedies, 978–980, 980f
Hexaxial reference system, 334, 334f
High blood pressure. See Hypertension
High cardiac output syndrome, in heart
failure, 602
High-density lipoproteins. See under
Lipoprotein(s)
High-frequency component, of frequency domain
analysis, of heart rate variability, 529,
529t, 530f
Hirudin, for heparin-induced
thrombocytopenia, 171
His bundle. See Bundle of His

History taking, 229–234
chief complaint in, 230–231
components of, 229
family history in, 232
functional patterns in, 233–234
identifying information in, 230
New York Heart Association's Functional and
Therapeutic Classification in,
234, 235t
past history in, 232
personal history in, 232–233
present illness history in, 231–232
presenting problem in, 230–231
social history in, 232–233
systems review in, 233
Histotoxic hypoxia, 77
Holistic health care, definition of, 974
Holosystolic murmurs, 255, 255f, 256
Holter monitoring, in heart rate variability,
528, 528f
Homan's sign, in deep vein thrombosis, 164
Homeopathic medicine, 975
Homocysteine
elevation of, as coronary artery disease risk
factor, 819–820
in heart failure, 615
as inflammatory marker, 115, 131–132, 132d
measurement of, 280
Homografts, for prosthetic valves, 763–764
Hook intervention, for hostility, 834
Hormone(s)
lipoprotein levels and, 909
reproductive, coronary artery disease and,
818–819
Hormone replacement therapy, postmenopausal,
coronary artery disease and, 819
Hospice care, in heart failure, 617
Hostility, coronary artery disease and, 827, 834
Human Genome Project, 114
Human immunodeficiency virus infection,
pericardial effusion in, 780
Huntington disease, heart rate variability in, 535
HV interval, in electrophysiology studies,
425–426, 430
Hydralazine
for heart failure, 619t, 621
for hypertension, 878t, 882t
Hydraulic conductivity, in microcirculation, 67
Hydrochlorothiazide
for heart failure, 619t
for hypertension, 878t
Hydrogen ions, excretion of, 190, 191t
Hydrostatic pressure
fluid distribution and, 174
referencing for, 478
Hydroxymethylglutaryl coenzyme-A
reductase, 899
inhibitors of (statins), for hyperlipidemia,
911t, 912
Hyperacute rejection, in cardiac
transplantation, 19
Hypercalcemia, 183, 183t, 354, 356, 359f
Hypercapnia, arousal from sleep from, 203
Hypercholesterolemia
as coronary artery disease risk factor,
812–813, 813t
detection of, 902–903
endothelial function and, 901
epidemiology of, 897
evaluation of, 905
familial (severe), 901
hypertension and, 880–881
risks of, 902t–904t

Hypercholesterolemia (continued)
    treatment of, 902–905
        dietary, 905–908, 906f, 906t, 907d
        goals of, 903, 904t, 905
        pharmacologic, 898t, 909–912, 910t, 911t
        weight control in, 908
Hypercoagulability
    deep vein thrombosis in, 163, 163t
    in Virchow's triad, 162, 162f
Hyperemia, reactive, 58, 542, 544
Hyperglycemia, in diabetes mellitus, 953
Hyperkalemia, 180–182
    cardiac effects of, 181–182
    causes of, 180–181, 180t
    electrocardiography in, 353–354, 358f
    in heart failure, 615
    vascular effects of, 181–182
Hyperlipidemias. See also Hypercholesterolemia
    combined, 900t, 902
    in diabetes mellitus, 955
    hypertension and, 880–881
    treatment of, 898t
        dietary, 905–908, 906f, 906t, 907d
        pharmacologic, 909–912, 910t, 911t
        weight control in, 908
Hypermagnesemia, 185, 185t, 356
Hypernatremia, 177, 177t
Hyperosmolar hyperglycemic nonketotic
        syndrome, 951
Hyperpolarization, 17–18
    endothelium-derived hyperpolarizing factors
        for, 54f, 56, 56f
    in hypokalemia, 180
Hyper-resonance, in lung percussion, 259, 261t
Hypertension
    pulmonary. See Pulmonary hypertension
    renovascular, 863
    systemic, 856–896
        age factors in, 223, 858–859
        in aortic coarctation, 797–798
        after cardiac catheterization, 474
        after cardiac surgery, 636
        after cardiac transplantation, 646, 650
        causes of, 860–863
            primary, 860–861
            secondary, 861–863, 862d
        in children, 857, 858t
        classification of, 856–857, 857t
        clinical manifestations of, 864–867
            cardiac, 865
            neurologic, 866–867
            ocular, 866, 866t
            renal, 865–866
            vascular, 864–865
        as coronary artery disease risk factor, 812, 813f
        crisis in, treatment of, 881, 882t
        definition of, 243, 856–857, 857t
        diagnosis of, 867–869, 867t, 868d, 868t
        disease management programs for, 989–990
        educational level and, 860
        encephalopathy in, 867
        epidemiology of, 812, 813f, 857–860
        ethnic differences in, 859–860
        family history of, 859
        gender differences in, 859
        genetic factors in, 859
        geographic differences in, 859–860
        heart failure in, 601
        heart rate variability in, 531
        hemodynamics of, 860
        from immunosuppressive agents, 649
        incidence of, 857–858
        income and, 860

    vs. normal blood pressure, 856–857, 858t
    nursing diagnosis of, 885
    prevalence of, 857–858
    prevention of, 869–870
    primary, causes of, 860–861
    prognosis for, 869
    vs. pseudohypertension, 249
    secondary, causes of, 861–863, 862d
    signs and symptoms of, 864, 864d
    in sleep apnea, 209–210
    sleep in, 208
    systolic, in older adults, 223, 875–877
    target organ damage in, 864–867, 864d, 866t
    treatment of, 869–888
        adherence to, 884d
        alcohol intake reduction in, 873–874
        algorithm for, 875, 876f, 877t–880t
        benefits of, 874–875
        client role in, 883–884
        community-based programs in, 884–885
        in crisis, 881, 882t
        in diabetes mellitus, 879–880, 955
        dietary, 871–872, 872t, 873t
        evaluation of, 888
        exercise in, 872–873
        goals of, 869, 885
        health care organization role in, 884
        health care professional role in,
            881–883, 884d
        in hyperlipidemia, 880–881
        indications for, 857t
        in kidney disease, 880
        nonpharmacologic, 870–874, 870t, 872t, 873t
        nursing considerations in, 885, 886ncp–888ncp
        in older adults, 875–877
        patient education on, 888
        pharmacologic, 874–875, 876f, 877t–880t
        policy in, 885
        in pregnancy, 877, 879
        preventive, 869–870
        risks of, 874–875
        sodium restriction in, 871
        team approach to, 885
        weight and, 859, 870–871
Hyperthermia, cutaneous vascular changes
        in, 86–87
Hypertriglyceridemia, 900t, 901, 902d, 902t
Hypertrophic cardiomyopathy. See
        Cardiomyopathy, hypertrophic
Hyperventilation, respiratory alkalosis in, 193
Hypoalphalipoproteinemia, 901–902
Hypocalcemia, 182–183
    cardiac effects of, 182–183
    causes of, 182, 182t
    electrocardiography in, 354, 358f
    vascular effects of, 183
Hypoglycemia, in diabetes mellitus, 951,
        952–953
Hypoglycemic drugs, for diabetes mellitus,
        956–958
Hypokalemia
    cardiac effects of, 180
    electrocardiography in, 353, 357f
    etiology of, 179, 179t
    in heart failure, 615
    postural hypotension in, 180
    vascular effects of, 180
Hypokinesis, of myocardium, 312
Hypomagnesemia, 183–185
    cardiac effects of, 184–185, 287
    causes of, 184, 184t
    electrocardiography in, 356
    vascular effects of, 185

Hyponatremia, 176–177, 176t, 615
Hypoperfusion, in myocardial infarction, 561
Hypophosphatemia, severe, 186, 186t
Hypopolarization, in hypokalemia, 180
Hypotension
    after cardiac catheterization, 474
    after cardiac surgery, 636
    in myocardial infarction, 561
    postural, blood pressure measurement in, 247
    in shock, 665
Hypothermia
    for brain protection, in cardiac arrest,
        704–705, 704d
    cutaneous vascular changes in, 86
    deep, with circulatory arrest, for cardiac
        surgery, 631
Hypothermic cardioplegia, 630
Hypothyroidism, facial characteristics in, 236
Hypoventilation
    hypoxemia in, 75
    in sleep, 203
Hypovolemia
    after cardiac surgery, 636
    hemodynamic characteristics of, 506t
    in myocardial infarction, 561
Hypovolemic shock. See Shock, hypovolemic
Hypoxemia
    causes of, 74–75
    in pulmonary embolism, 168
Hypoxia
    classification of, 77
    lactate in, 517
    in shock, 665, 665f
    ventilation-perfusion matching in, 74
Hypoxic hypoxia, 77
Hypoxic spells, in tetralogy of Fallot, 800
Hysteresis, in pacemakers, 711d

IABP. See Intra-aortic balloon pump (IABP)
Ibersartan, for heart failure, 619t
Ibutilide, for arrhythmias, 370t, 373t
ICDs. See Implantable cardioverter defibrillators
Identification, in history taking, 230
Idiopathic hypertrophic subaortic stenosis, 314
Iliac artery, atherosclerosis of, 146
Immobility, cardiovascular effects of, 921, 921d
Immune function
    in endocarditis, 789, 789t
    in shock, 666
    sleep and, 202
Immunoglobulin G, in heparin-induced
        thrombocytopenia, 169–170, 169f
Immunosuppressive drugs
    for cardiac transplantation, 647–650, 648t
    for myocarditis, 786–787
Impedance cardiography, in cardiac output
        measurement, 508t, 511–512
Impedance plethysmography, in deep vein
        thrombosis, 164
Implantable cardioverter defibrillators (ICDs),
        738–754
    atrial, 744d
    for bradycardia, 748
    for cardiac arrest survivors, 427–428, 740–741
    complications of, 748–749, 748d, 749d
    development of, 738–739, 739f
    external defibrillation of, 749, 750f
    follow-up care of, 752–754, 752d, 752f, 753f
    functional characteristics of, 741–745,
        742f–745f, 744d
    for heart failure, 618

implantation of, 748
indications for, 739–741, 740*d*
low-energy mode of, 747
nursing considerations with, 750–751, 751*d*
operation of, 745–748, 746*f*, 747*f*
pacemaker interaction with, 749–750
precautions with, 749–750, 750*f*
prophylactic, for high-risk patients, 741
psychosocial issues with, 751–752
statistics on, 738
for syncope of unknown origin, 741
troubleshooting for, 753–754, 753*f*
for ventricular fibrillation, 746, 746*f*
for ventricular tachycardia, 741, 746–747, 747*f*
Impulse(s)
    abnormal conduction of, 363–365, 364*f*, 365*f*.
        See also Conduction blocks
    concealed conduction and, 420–421,
        421*f*, 422*f*
    generation of
        abnormal, 361–363, 362*f*, 363*f*
        factors modifying, 28–29, 29*f*
    in heart palpation, 251
Inactivation gate, of ion channels, 21
Incompetency, valvular. See *specific valves*,
    regurgitation of
Indapamide, for hypertension, 878*t*
Indeterminate axis, in electrocardiography, 336,
    337*f*, 339*f*
Indian almond tree bark, for cardiovascular
    disease, 979
Indicator dilution method, for cardiac output
    measurement, 469
Infarction, myocardial. See Myocardial infarction
Infection(s)
    after cardiac transplantation, 647,
        653*ncp*–654*ncp*
    endocardial. See Endocarditis, infectious
    myocarditis in, 786, 786*d*
    of pacemaker system, 738
    in percutaneous coronary interventions, 595
    pericarditis in, 776
    wound, postoperative, 641
Infection control
    after cardiac transplantation, 647
    in hemodynamic monitoring, 480, 482*t*
Infective endocarditis. See Endocarditis, infectious
Inferior vena cava filter, for pulmonary
    embolism, 168
Infiltrative cardiomyopathy, echocardiography
    in, 314
Inflammation
    in atherosclerosis, 543
    in cardiopulmonary bypass, 629
    coagulation and, 157–158
    definition of, 127
    in heart failure, 608–609
    myocardial. See Myocarditis
    in myocardial infarction, 546
    pericardial. See Pericarditis
    in shock, 665
Inflammatory marker(s), 127–128
    adhesion molecules as, 129
    amyloid A as, 133
    brain natriuretic peptide as, 129
    C-reactive protein as, 130–131, 131*f*
    fibrinogen as, 130
    homocysteine as, 115, 131–132, 132*d*
    interleukin 6 as, 132–133
    tumor necrosis factor alpha as, 133–134
    von Willebrand factor as, 134
Informed consent, for exercise testing, 441
Infundibulum (conus arteriosus), anatomy of, 6

Inhibited response, in pacing, 711*d*
Inhibited state, in pacing, 728, 729*f*
Initial atherosclerotic lesions, 139–140, 147*t*
Innervation, of heart, 16, 43
Inositol triphosphate, in vasoconstriction, 60, 60*f*
Inotropic agents
    contractility effects of, 39, 39*f*
    for heart failure, 617
    postoperative, 637, 638*t*
    for septic shock, 673
    for shock, 669, 669*t*
Insomnia, 204
Inspiration
    heart sounds in, 253, 253*f*, 257, 257*t*
    paradoxical blood pressure in, 247–248, 248*f*
Insufficiency, valvular. See *specific valves*,
    regurgitation of
Insulin
    action of, in diabetes mellitus, 949–950
    replacement of, in diabetes mellitus, 956
    resistance to, 861, 950–951
Integrative medicine, definition of, 974
Intensive care unit. See Cardiac care unit
Interatrial septum, anatomy of, 6
Intercalated disc, 17, 17*f*
Interleukin 6, as inflammatory marker,
    132–133
Intermediate atherosclerotic lesions, 141, 147*t*
Intermediate-density lipoproteins, 898
Internal mammary artery, as coronary artery
    bypass graft, 631–632, 632*f*
International normalized ratio (INR), 157*t*, 284
International Society of Heart and Lung
    Transplantation, cardiac rejection
    classification of, 647, 647*t*
International Society of Hypertension, guidelines
    of, 856–857, 857*t*
International System of Units, 268
Internodal conduction pathways, anatomy
    of, 10
Interstitial spaces, fluid in, 174
Intervention(s), structuring of, for disease
    management, 990
Interventional cardiology, 585–600
    adjunctive modalities in, 595, 595*f*
    angiojet thrombectomy as, 589
    in aortic stenosis, 771–772
    complications of, 592–596, 595*f*
    coronary atherectomy as, 588–589, 589*f*
    future of, 597
    management during, 586–587
    noncoronary, 596–597, 597*f*
    nursing management in, 597–599
    patient selection for, 585
    patient subgroups in, 585–586
    percutaneous transluminal coronary angioplasty
        as, 587–588, 588*f*
    radiation in, 592
    radiofrequency catheter ablation in. See
        Radiofrequency catheter ablation
    stent placement in, 589–592, 590*f*, 591*f*
    valvuloplasty as. See Valvuloplasty
Interviews, for adherence evaluation, 962–963,
    963*t*, 967*d*, 969
Intestinal absorption blockers, for hyperlipidemia,
    911*t*, 912
Intima, 49, 50*f*
Intra-aortic balloon pump (IABP), 675–679
    for cardiac catheterization complications, 472
    complications of, 21
    contraindications to, 677–678
    description of, 675, 676*f*
    history of, 675

nursing management of, 21, 680*ncp*–683*ncp*
physiologic principles of, 675–676, 676*d*,
    676*f*, 677*f*
purpose of, 675
radiographic appearance of, 299*f*, 299*t*
timing of, 678–679, 678*f*, 679*f*
Intra-atrial electrograms, in arrhythmias, 405,
    409*f*, 425, 427*f*
Intracellular adhesion molecule I, as inflammatory
    marker, 129
Intracellular fluid, 173, 174
Intracranial pressure, in sleep, 204
Intramyocardial tension, 41–42
Intravascular ultrasonography, in percutaneous
    coronary interventions, 595, 595*f*
Intraventricular septum
    blood supply of, 13*t*
    clinical manifestations of, 799
    defects of
        congenital, 796*f*, 799–800
        echocardiography in, 314
        hemodynamic characteristics of, 506*t*
        repair of, 635
        shock in, treatment of, 673
        in tetralogy of Fallot, 800
        in tricuspid atresia, 801
        in truncus arteriosus, 802
    echocardiography of, 314
    hypertrophy of, 314
    management of, 799–800
    pathophysiology of, 799
    rupture of, in myocardial infarction, 561
Intrinsic coagulation pathway, 155, 156*f*
Introns, 113
Inward currents, 26*t*, 27
    rectifier, 24
Ion(s). See also *specific ions*
    distribution and movement of, across
        membrane, 18–22, 19*f*
Ion channels, 18, 19*f*. See also *specific channels, eg,*
    Sodium channels
Ionic activity, in myocardial cells, 21
Ionic currents, sarcolemmal, 26–28, 26*t*
Irbesartan, for hypertension, 879*t*
Ischemia
    in disseminated intravascular coagulation,
        160, 161
    myocardial. See Myocardial ischemia
    in shock, 664–665, 664*f*
Ischemic hypoxia, 77
Isoforms, of myosin, 33
Isometric contraction, 32–33, 33*f*
Isometric exercise, heart sounds in, 257*t*, 258
Isoproterenol, postoperative, 638*t*, 645–646
Isorhythmic dissociation, 418, 419*f*
Isosorbide dinitrate
    for heart failure, 619*t*, 621
    for myocardial infarction, 573
Isosorbide mononitrate, for heart failure, 619*t*
Isotonic contraction, 32–33, 34*f*
Isotonic fluids, 173
Isotonic twitch, myocardial oxygen consumption
    and, 42
Isovolumic ventricular contraction, 44–45, 44*f*
Isovolumic ventricular relaxation, 44*f*, 45
Isradipine, for hypertension, 879*t*

J

James fibers, 391
Janeway lesions, in endocarditis, 789, 789*t*
Jarvik Heart 2000, 684

Jaundice, 236
Jervell and Lange-Nielsen syndrome, cardiac arrest in, 690
Job stress, coronary artery disease and, 827–828
Joint National Committee of the National High Blood Pressure Education Program, 856–857, 857*t*
  hypertension algorithm of, 875, 876*f*, 877*t*–880*t*
Judkins technique, for coronary arteriography, 467, 468*f*
Jugular veins, assessment of, in shock, 667
Jugular venous distention, in heart failure, 612
Jugular venous pressure, assessment of, 241–243, 242*f*
Jugular venous pulse, assessment of, 241–243, 242*f*
Junctional bradycardia, treatment of, 375*t*
Junctional conduction, 30
Junctional rhythm, 384
Junctional tachycardia, 384

K

Kallikrein-kinin system, in blood pressure regulation, 89*f*, 92
Kent bundles, 11
Ketoacidosis, diabetic, 951
Kidney
  acid excretion from, 190–193, 191*t*
  aging effects on, 224–225
  assessment of, in shock, 667
  in blood pressure regulation, 94–95
  dysfunction/failure of
    from contrast agents, 593
    in diabetes mellitus, 951–952
    in heart failure, 615
    in hypertension, 865–866, 880
    hypertension in, 861, 862*d*, 863, 865–866, 880
    pericarditis in, 776–778
    postoperative, 640
    in shock, 664, 664*f*, 666
  fluid excretion from, 174, 175*t*
  function of, in sleep, 204
Kinins, in blood pressure regulation, 89*f*, 92
Knowledge deficit
  after cardiac transplantation, 655*ncp*–656*ncp*
  in congenital heart disease, 803*ncp*–804*ncp*
  in heart failure, 624
  in hypertension, 886*ncp*
  in myocardial infarction, 579–580
Korean medicine, 976
Korotkoff sounds, 245–246, 245*t*
Krogh model, of cardiac output vs. central venous pressure, 100–101, 100*f*
Krvonen formula, for training heart rate, 930
Kussmaul's sign
  in myocardial infarction, 557
  in pericarditis, 780
Kyphoscoliosis, chest configuration in, 258, 260*f*

L

Labetalol, for hypertension, 878*t*, 882*t*
Laboratory tests. *See also* Echocardiography; Electrocardiography
  for angina, 552
  blood, 265–295
    for alanine aminotransferase, 288
    for alkaline phosphatase, 288
    arterial blood gases. *See* Arterial blood gases
    for aspartate aminotransferase, 288

for bilirubin, 288
for catecholamines, 289
for coagulation, 157*t*, 283–286
for C-reactive protein, 279–280, 279*f*
for creatine kinase, 272–276, 272*t*, 274*f*, 275*f*, 276*t*, 277*t*
for creatinine, 289
cultures, 283
drawing from catheters, 483
for drug concentrations, 268, 291, 291*t*
for electrolytes, 286–288
for glucose, 289
for glycated hemoglobin, 289, 289*t*
for glycated serum protein, 289–290
hematologic, 281–283
for homocysteine, 280
for hypercholesterolemia, 905
interpretation of results of, 267–268
for lactate dehydrogenase, 270*f*, 270*t*, 271*t*, 290
for lipids, 276–278, 278*t*, 279*t*
for lipoprotein-associated phospholipase A₂, 280
for myocardial proteins, 269–271, 270*f*, 270*t*, 271*t*
for natriuretic peptides, 280–281
for osmolality, 287
after percutaneous coronary interventions, 586–587
point-of-care, 269
postoperative, 287–288, 290
for protein, 290
reference ranges for, 268, 277*t*
sensitivity and specificity of, 268–269
specimen collection for, 265–267, 291
for urea nitrogen, 290
for uric acid, 290
for sleep assessment, 213
Lactate, as measure of oxygen supply and demand, 517
Lactate dehydrogenase, 270*f*, 270*t*, 271*t*, 290
Laplace, law of
  afterload and, 94
  intramyocardial tension and, 41–42
Lasers
  in coronary angioplasty, 589
  in transmyocardial revascularization, 634
Latissimus dorsi muscle, in cardiomyoplasty, 635, 783
LDL. *See* Lipoprotein(s), low-density
Leads
  for implantable cardioverter defibrillator, 742, 742*f*, 743*f*
  for pacemakers, 711*d*, 716, 718*f*, 738
Lecithin cholesterol acyltransferase, in cholesterol transport, 899
Left anterior fascicular block, 341, 345*f*
Left atrial pressure
  in mitral regurgitation, 766
  vs. pulmonary artery wedge pressure, 493, 494
Left bundle branch, function of, 326
Left bundle-branch block, 339, 344*f*, 402*t*, 403–404, 406*f*
Left heart. *See also* Atrium (atria), left; Ventricle(s), left
  catheterization of, 464–466, 465*f*, 466*f*
Left posterior fascicular block, 341, 345*f*
Left ventricular assist devices, 680, 683–686
  axial flow pumps in, 684
  centrifugal-kinetic energy type, 684, 684*f*
  continuous-flow, 683, 684, 684*f*
  for dilated cardiomyopathy, 783

for heart failure, 617
indications for, 683
mechanisms of, 683–684
pulsatile, 684–686, 685*f*, 686*f*
roller pump in, 684
Left ventricular function curves, in heart failure, 605, 605*f*
Left ventricular outflow obstruction, in hypertrophic cardiomyopathy, 784
Legal aspects, of CAM, 982
Length-tension relationship, preload and, 36–38, 37*f*, 38*f*, 94
Lepirudin
  for deep vein thrombosis, 165*t*
  for heparin-induced thrombocytopenia, 170–171
Leukocyte(s). *See* White blood cell(s)
Levine's sign, in angina, 550
Lidocaine, for arrhythmias, 370*t*
Lifestyle modification
  for hypertension, 870–874, 870*t*, 872*t*, 873*t*
  for obesity, 942–944, 942*t*
Life support, cardiac
  algorithms of, 695, 695*d*, 696*f*, 697*f*, 698–699, 698*d*
  description of, 691–695, 693*f*–695*f*
Lightheadedness, in exercise testing, 450
Limb leads, in electrocardiography, 331–332, 333*f*
Lines, invasive, radiographic appearance of, 297, 299*f*–302*f*, 299*t*
Lipid(s). *See also* Lipoprotein(s); Triglycerides
  in atherosclerotic lesions, 144
  blood, measurement of, 276–278, 278*t*, 279*t*
  functions of, 897–898
  metabolism of, 898–899, 898*f*, 899*f*
  reverse transport of, 899
  structures of, 897–898
  transport of, 898–899, 898*f*, 899*f*
Lipid bilayer, of myocardial cells, 18, 19*f*
Lipofuscin accumulation, with aging, 222
Lipoprotein(a), 900
Lipoprotein(s), 900*t*
  alcohol and, 909
  in atherosclerotic lesions, 144
  excess of. *See* Hypercholesterolemia; Hyperlipidemias
  exercise and, 909
  heart rate variability and, 534
  high-density
    vs. coronary artery disease risk, 903*t*, 904*t*
    deficiency of, hypoalphalipoproteinemia in, 901–902
    estrogen effects on, 909
    function of, 899
    hormones and, 909
  intermediate-density, 898
  low-density
    abnormalities of, 900*t*, 901–902
    adherence of, to endothelium, 158
    classification of, 910, 910*t*
    as coronary artery disease risk factor, 812–813, 813*t*
    in diabetes mellitus, 955
    measurement of, 905
    metabolism of, 898–899, 898*f*, 899*f*
    oxidation of, 143–144, 900
    particle size of, 900
    receptors for, 898–899, 898*f*, 899*f*, 901
  measurement of, 276–278, 278*t*, 279*t*, 905
  very-low-density, 898, 899, 899*f*
Lipoprotein-associated phospholipase A₂, 280
Lipoprotein lipase, in cholesterol transport, 899

Lisinopril
  for heart failure, 619*t*
  for hypertension, 879*t*
Lithium, in transpulmonary thermodilution
    method, 508
Liver
  aging effects on, 225
  dysfunction of, postoperative, 641
  enlargement of, in heart failure, 612
  ischemia of, in shock, 664, 664*f*
  lipid metabolism in, 898–899, 898*f*, 899*f*
  pulsation of, 252
  shock effects on, 666
  size of, assessment of, 262–263, 263*f*
Living circumstances, in history taking, 233
Long QT syndrome, 400
  cardiac arrest in, 690
  genetic factors in, 116, 116*t*
Losartan
  for heart failure, 619*t*
  for hypertension, 879*t*
Loss, sense of, in smoking cessation, 850
Low cardiac output syndrome
  in heart failure, 602
  postoperative, 636
Low-density lipoproteins. *See under* Lipoprotein(s)
Low-frequency component, of frequency domain
    analysis, of heart rate variability, 529,
    529*t*, 530*f*
Lung. *See also* Pulmonary circulation;
    subjects starting with Pulmonary
  acid excretion from, 190, 221*t*
  aging effects on, 223–224, 224*f*
  dead space in, 73
  diffusion in, 74
  examination of, in heart failure, 614
  gas exchange in, 75
  non-gas exchange functions of, 72
  physical assessment of, 258–262, 259*f*
    anterior chest, 261–262, 262*f*
    inspection in, 258, 260*f*
    posterior chest, 258–261, 261*f*, 262*f*, 261*t*
  physiology of, 72–75, 73*f*
  radiographic appearance of, 296, 298*f*
  shock effects on, 666
  ventilation-perfusion matching in, 74
  zones of, 73–74, 73*f*
    pulmonary artery pressure differences in,
    495–496, 497*f*
Lunulae, of valves, 9
Lying down, heart sounds in, 257*t*, 258
Lymphatic system
  of heart, 16
  microvasculature of, 50
  physiology of, 52–53, 52*f*, 67
Lymphocytes, 151*f*, 152–153, 153*t*
  in atherosclerotic lesions, 143–144
  count of, 282
Lymphoid stem cells, 150, 151*f*

M

Macrophages, in atherosclerotic lesions, 143
Magnesium ion
  for arrhythmias, 370*t*
  balance of, 178*t*, 183
  imbalance of, 184–185, 184*t*, 185*t*, 356
  measurement of, 287
  total body depletion of, 185
Magnet(s)
  implantable cardioverter defibrillator and,
    749, 749*d*
  pacemakers and, 711*d*, 721

Magnetic resonance angiography, 322–323
  in angina, 552
  in atherosclerosis, 143*t*
Magnetic resonance imaging, 322–323
  in angina, 552
  functional, in oxygenation monitoring, 79
  in pericarditis, 778
Magnetic resonance spectroscopy, 322–323
Mahaim fibers, 11, 391–392, 394
Mammary artery, internal, as coronary artery
    bypass graft, 631–632, 632*f*
Manipulation, for cardiovascular disease, 982
Manometers, for blood pressure measurement,
    243–244, 244*f*
Marginal branches, of circumflex artery, 15
Marketing, of disease management programs, 992
Mason-Likar limb lead placement, for exercise
    testing, 441, 442*f*
Massage therapy, for cardiovascular disease, 982
Maximal diastolic potential, 24
Maximum tracking rate, in pacing, 712*d*, 727,
    730–731, 731*f*, 732*f*
Maybush (hawthorn), for cardiovascular disease,
    978–979
Mean arterial pressure, calculation of, 486
Mean corpuscular hemoglobin, 281–282
Mean corpuscular hemoglobin concentration,
    281–282
Mean corpuscular volume, 281–282
Mechanical ventilation, pulmonary artery pressure
    in, 496, 500–501, 501*f*, 502*t*
Mechanoreceptors, in blood pressure regulation,
    81, 82*f*
Media layer, of blood vessels, 49, 50*f*
Medical management, of care delivery, in disease
    management, 990
Meditation, 832, 832*d*, 977–978
Medtronic Hall tilting-disk valve, 763
Medtronic Mosaic porcine bioprosthesis, 763–764
Medulla, ventrolateral, in blood pressure
    regulation, 83–84
Megakaryocytes, 151*f*, 153
Megaloblasts, 282
Meglitinides, for diabetes mellitus, 958
Melatonin, sleep and, 204
Membrane resting potential
  calculation of, 20–21
  in myocardial cells, 17
Mendelian disorders, 115
Menopause, hormone replacement therapy after,
    coronary artery disease and, 819
Mercury manometers, for blood pressure
    measurement, 243
Meridians, in Chinese medicine, 976, 977*f*
Messenger RNA, 113
Meta-analysis, of exercise testing, 452
Metabolic acidosis, 192–193, 192*t*, 193*t*, 195*t*
Metabolic alkalosis, 193*t*, 194, 194*t*, 195*t*
Metabolic equivalents
  in cardiac rehabilitation, 924–925, 925*d*
  in exercise testing, 443–444, 443*f*, 447
Metabolic hypothesis, of blood flow
    autoregulation, 97–98
Metabolic syndrome, 861, 901, 906, 906*t*, 951
Metabolism
  acid production in, 189
  in blood flow control, 58, 58*f*
  cerebral, in sleep, 204
  exercise training effects on, 920–921, 920*d*
  in history taking, 233
  myocardial, 41, 544, 544*f*
    in coronary blood flow regulation, 542
    positron emission tomography of, 322

Metformin
  for diabetes mellitus, 958
  for obesity, 944
Methoxamine, heart sounds and, 257*t*, 258
Methyldopa, for hypertension, 878*t*
Metolazone
  for heart failure, 619*t*
  for hypertension, 878*t*
Metoprolol
  for arrhythmias, 370*t*–371*t*, 373*t*
  for heart failure, 619*t*, 620
  for hypertension, 878*t*
METs. *See* Metabolic equivalents
Mexiletine, for arrhythmias, 371*t*
Mibefradil, for hypertension, 879*t*
Microcirculation. *See also* Capillary(ies)
  diabetes mellitus effects on, 951–952
  physiology of, 65–67, 66*f*
  regulation of, 96–98, 97*f*
  structure of, 50–51
Microcytes, 282
Microreentry, 365
Mid-axillary line, as reference point, 478
MIDCAB (minimally invasive direct coronary
    artery bypass), 633–634, 633*f*
Miglitol, for diabetes mellitus, 958
Milrinone
  for dilated cardiomyopathy, 783
  for heart failure, 672*d*
    postoperative, 638*t*
  for shock, 669*t*, 672*d*
Mind-body interventions, 976–978, 978*f*
Minimally invasive techniques, for cardiac
    surgery, 629
  coronary artery bypass as, 633–634, 633*f*
  valve replacement as, 764–765, 765*f*
Minoxidil, for hypertension, 878*t*
Minute ventilation, in sleep, 203
Minute volume (VE), 73
Mitochondria, of myocardial cells, 17, 17*f*
Mitral valve
  anatomy of, 6*f*, 8
  cardiac cycle and, 44*f*, 46
  conduction system to, 11, 12*f*
  displacement of, in hypertrophic
    cardiomyopathy, 784
  echocardiography of, 311*f*, 315–316
  function of, 8, 8*f*
  heart sounds and, 44*f*, 46
  prolapse of, 768–770
    cause of, 768
    clinical manifestations of, 769
    diagnosis of, 769–770, 769*f*, 770*f*
    echocardiography in, 316
    medical management of, 770
    murmurs of, 762*t*
    pathology of, 768–769
    pathophysiology of, 769
    physical assessment of, 769
    prognosis for, 770
    surgical treatment of, 770
  regurgitation of, 766–768
    acute, 673, 766–767, 766*t*
    causes of, 766, 766*t*
    chronic, 766–767, 766*t*
    clinical manifestations of, 766–767
    diagnosis of, 767
    in dilated cardiomyopathy, 783
    echocardiography in, 316
    hemodynamic characteristics of, 506*t*
    medical management of, 767
    murmurs of, 762*t*
    in myocardial infarction, 561–562

Mitral valve, regurgitation of *(continued)*
  pathology of, 766
  pathophysiology of, 766
  physical assessment of, 767
  primary, 766
  in rheumatic fever, 757
  secondary, 766
  shock in, 661
  surgical management of, 767–768, 768*f*
repair of, 634
  for heart failure, 618
  for regurgitation, 767–768, 768*f*
replacement of, 634, 761
  minimally invasive technique for, 764–765, 765*f*
  for regurgitation, 767–768, 768*f*
stenosis of, 759–761
  assessment of, 759, 760*t*
  cause of, 759
  clinical manifestations of, 759
  diagnosis of, 759–760
  echocardiography in, 316
  medical management of, 760
  pathology of, 759
  pathophysiology of, 759
  surgical management of, 760–761, 761*f*
Mixed venous oxygen saturation (SvO$_2$)
  measurement of, 79, 286, 513*t*, 515, 516*f*
  variations in, 513*t*
M-mode echocardiography, 308, 308*f*, 309*f*
Modeling behavior, in adherence, 967*d*, 968
Mode switching, in pacing, 712*d*
Moexipril, for hypertension, 879*t*
Monacolins, in Chinese red yeast rice, 981
Monitoring, hemodynamic. *See* Hemodynamic monitoring
Monoclonal antibodies, for cardiac transplantation, 650
Monocyte(s), 151*f*, 152, 153*t*
  count of, 282
Monocyte chemotactic protein-1, in atherosclerotic lesions, 143
Morphine
  for angina, 555
  for myocardial infarction, 569
Morphologic adaptations, to exercise, 920, 920*d*
Mortality. *See also* Death
  causes of, 810*f*
  in coronary artery disease, 809–810, 810*f*
  vs. exercise capacity, 918, 918*f*, 918*t*
  in myocardial infarction, 809–810, 810*f*
    hemodynamic variables predicting, 668, 668*f*
  in pulmonary embolism, 166
Motivational interviews, for adherence, 967*d*, 969
Moxibustion, 976
MULTIFIT program, for cardiac rehabilitation, 932
Multifocal atrial tachycardia, 380
Multiple gated acquisition study, 319–320, 320*f*
Multiple Sleep Latency Test, 200
Murmurs, 255–256
  in aortic regurgitation, 256, 760*t*, 773, 773*t*
  in aortic stenosis, 771, 797
  classification of, 255, 255*f*, 255*t*
  configuration of, 255, 256*f*
  innocent, 255–256
  in mitral regurgitation, 767
  in mitral stenosis, 759, 760*t*
  in papillary muscle dysfunction, 256
  in pulmonic regurgitation, 760*t*
  in tricuspid regurgitation, 761–762, 762*t*
  in tricuspid stenosis, 760*t*
  in valvular heart disease, 760*t*, 762*t*

Muscarinic receptors, in blood pressure regulation, 88
Muscle(s). *See also* Myocardium
  creatine kinase-MM in, 273
  of respiration, 72
Muscle pump, in cardiac performance maintenance, 101
Mustard procedure, for transposition of great arteries, 802
Mutations, 113–114
MVO$_2$. *See* Oxygen consumption, myocardial
Mycophenolate mofetil, for cardiac transplantation, 648*t*
Mycoplasma pneumoniae infections, atherosclerosis in, 543
Myelocytes, 282
Myeloid stem cells, 150, 151*f*
Myocardial cells
  action potential of, 22–24, 23*f*
  aging effects on, 222
  apoptosis of, in heart failure, 610
  death of, pathophysiology of, 546
  electrical characteristics of, 17–22
    diffusional force as, 19
    electrical force and current as, 19–21, 19*f*
    excitation as, 18, 18*t*, 19*f*
    ion distribution as, 18–21, 19*f*
    ion movement as, 21–22
    modification of, 28–29, 29*f*
  equilibrium potential of, 19–20
  hyperkalemia effects on, 181
  hypertrophy of, in heart failure, 609, 611*f*
  mechanical characteristics of, 32–35, 33*f*–35*f*
  membrane resting potential of, 20–21
  number of, 18
  oxygen deprivation of, 544
  remodeling of, in heart failure, 609, 611*f*
  shock effects on, 666
  structure of, 16–17, 17*f*
  working, function of, 9–10
Myocardial infarction, 556–582
  anterior, 346, 348*f*, 351*f*, 556, 923
  anterolateral, 346, 351*f*
  anxiety in, 827, 833
  arrhythmias in, 562
  atrioventricular block with, pacemaker for, 710, 710*d*
  Bezold-Jarisch reflex in, 82
  bradydysrhythmias in, 562
  cardiac arrest in, 705
  cardiac catheterization in, 460, 460*t*
  cardiac rehabilitation after. *See* Cardiac rehabilitation
  cardiogenic shock in, 659–660, 661*f*
  causes of, 542–543
  cellular mechanisms and events caused by, 545–546
  classification of, 556–557
  clinical manifestations of, 547
  complications of, 560–562, 660, 923–924, 923*d*
  creatine kinase after, 272–275, 274*f*
  critical pathway for, 569, 570*t*
  diagnosis of, 557–560, 558*f*, 558*t*, 559*f*
  discharge planning for, 572
  echocardiography in, 559
  electrocardiography in, 342–349, 346*f*–347*f*, 347*d*, 557–559, 558*f*, 559*f*, 568–569, 568*f*
  evolution of, 346, 546–547
  free wall rupture in, 673
  genetic factors in, 810–811
  heart rate variability in, 530–531

  hemodynamic effects of, 547
  hemodynamic monitoring in, 559
  history in, 557
  hypokalemia in, 179
  hypomagnesemia in, 184
  implantable cardioverter defibrillator for, 741
  incidence of, 545
  infarct expansion in, 560
  inferior, 346–347, 352*f*, 556
  inflammatory markers of
    C-reactive protein as, 4
    tumor necrosis factor alpha as, 8
  lateral, 347, 350*f*, 556
  left ventricular, vs. right ventricular, 557, 558*t*
  left ventricular aneurysms in, 560
  left ventricular failure in, 560–561
  left ventricular remodeling in, 560
  location of, 346, 350*t*, 351*f*
  medical management of, 562–568
    algorithm for, 562, 563*f*
    in cardiac care unit, 568–572, 568*f*, 570*t*
    coronary precautions in, 570–571
    dietary, 571
    in emergency department, 567–568
    goals of, 562
    in hemodynamic disturbances, 571
    infarct size limitation strategies in, 571–572
    pain management in, 569
    percutaneous coronary interventions in. *See* Percutaneous coronary interventions
    pharmacologic, 572–576
    physical activity plan in, 570
    prehospital care in, 567
    right ventricular, 571–572
    thrombolytic therapy for, 562, 564–566, 565*t*
  mitral regurgitation in, 561–562
  mortality in
    hemodynamic variables predicting, 668, 668*f*
    rate of, 809–810, 810*f*
  non–Q-wave (non-transmural), 345, 348–349, 353*f*, 556–557
  non–ST-segment elevation, 553–555, 554*t*, 593
  nursing management of, 576–580
    in anxiety, 579
    in chest discomfort, 576–577, 577*d*
    in decreased myocardial tissue perfusion, 577–578
    in decreased systemic perfusion, 578–579
    in knowledge deficit, 579–580
    plan for, 580, 580*ncp*–582*ncp*
  old, 346
  oral contraceptives and, 818–819
  pathogenesis of, 342, 346*f*, 556
  pathophysiology of, 541–543, 542*f*, 545
  after percutaneous coronary interventions, 592, 593
  pericarditis in, 562, 780
  perioperative, 637–638
  physical assessment in, 557, 558*t*
  posterior, 347–348, 353*f*, 556
  psychosocial considerations in, 924
  Q-wave (transmural), 345, 556–557
  radionuclide studies in, 559–560
  remodeling after, 546–547
  right ventricular, 348, 352*f*, 556, 561
    electrocardiography in, 559, 559*f*
    hemodynamic characteristics of, 506*t*
    vs. left ventricular, 557, 558*t*
    medical management of, 571–572

nursing management in, 580,
580*ncp*–582*ncp*
shock in, 673
treatment of, 673
risk factors for. *See also* Coronary artery disease,
risk factors for
diabetes mellitus, 815–817, 816*f*
exercise training effects on, 921, 921*d*
laboratory tests for, 279–281, 279*f*
low physical activity level as, 813–815,
814*f*, 815*f*
risk stratification in, cardiac catheterization in,
460, 460*f*
serum markers in, 559
severity of, vs. cardiac rehabilitation plans,
923–924, 923*d*
shock in, 659–660, 661*f*, 675
sleep in, 206–207
social support in, 826
ST elevation, after percutaneous coronary
interventions, 593
stiffness after, 38
in stress, 827–828
tachydysrhythmias in, 562
tests for, 270, 270*f*, 270*t*. *See also specific tests*
therapeutic ethanol-induced, for hypertrophic
cardiomyopathy, 785
uncomplicated, 923–924
of undetermined age, 346
ventricular septal rupture in, 561, 635
wall rupture in, 561
white blood cell count after, 282
Myocardial ischemia
atherosclerotic lesion types in, 146
causes of, 542–543
cellular mechanisms and events caused by,
544–545, 544*f*
clinical manifestations of, 545
collateral circulation development in, 43
demand, 541
echocardiography in, 312, 315*f*
electrocardiography in, 342, 346*f*, 347*f*
in hypertrophic cardiomyopathy, 784
incidence of, 543–544
pathophysiology of, 541–543, 542*f*
in percutaneous coronary interventions, 598
postrevascularization, cardiac catheterization
in, 460
reduction of, 705–706
reperfusion after, 544
risk stratification in, 922–923, 922*d*
in shock, 664–665, 664*f*, 670, 670*f*
silent, 543, 550
in sleep, 208
smoking and, 839
supply, 541, 542*f*
transplantation for, 643
Myocardial perfusion imaging, 320–322,
320*f*–322*f*
in exercise testing, 453–454
Myocardial protection, in cardiac surgery, 630
Myocarditis, 786–787
assessment of, 786
dilated cardiomyopathy in, 782, 782*d*
etiology of, 782, 782*d*, 786, 786*d*
medical management of, 786–787
nursing management of, 787
pathophysiology of, 786
in rheumatic fever, 756–757
Myocardium. *See also subjects*
starting with Myocardial
akinesis of, 312
anatomy of, 9–10, 9*f*, 10*f*

blood supply of. *See* Coronary artery(ies)
compliance of, 37–38, 38*f*
contractility of. *See* Contractility
creatine kinase in. *See* Creatine kinase-MB
depression of, postoperative, 637, 638*t*
dyskinesis of, 312
hibernating, 660
hypertrophy of, collateral circulation
development in, 43
hypokinesis of, 312
inflammation of. *See* Myocarditis
injury of, electrocardiography in, 342,
344, 347*f*
ion distribution in, 18*t*
mechanical properties of, 35–41
afterload. *See* Afterload
assessment of, 41
cardiac reserve, 39–40, 40*f*
contractility. *See* Contractility
force-velocity relationship, 38–39, 38*f*
length-tension relationship, 36–38, 37*f*, 38*f*
preload. *See* Preload
treppe, 39, 40*f*
metabolism of, 41, 322, 544, 544*f*
necrosis of, electrocardiography in, 344, 347*f*
oxygen balance in, 541, 542*f*
oxygen consumption of, 41–42
oxygen supply of, 42–43, 42*f*
perfusion of, decreased, 577–578
primary disease of. *See* Cardiomyopathy
stiffness of, 38, 38*f*
stunned, 660
Myocytes. *See* Myocardial cells
Myofibrils, of myocardial cells, 17, 17*f*
Myogenic hypothesis, of blood flow
autoregulation, 96–97
Myoglobin, 270*t*, 271
in myocardial infarction, 559
Myopotential, in pacing, 711*d*
Myosin
in contraction, 33–34, 34*f*, 35*f*
in vascular smooth muscle, 53
Myxedema, facial characteristics in, 236
Myxomatous tissue, in mitral valve prolapse,
768–770

N

Nadolol, for hypertension, 878*t*
Nails, floating, 249, 249*f*
Nateglinide, for diabetes mellitus, 958
National Center for Complementary and
Alternative Medicine, CAM domains
of, 974–975
National Cholesterol Education Program
cholesterol detection recommendations of,
902–903, 902*t*–904*t*
dietary recommendations of, 906–907, 906*t*
Natriuretic peptides
in blood pressure regulation, 89*f*, 90–92, 91*f*
in heart failure, 606–607, 609*f*, 610*f*
in kidney regulation, 175*t*
measurement of, 280–281
in shock, 667
Natural frequency, in hemodynamic monitoring,
480, 483*f*
Natural killer cells, 153
Natural Medicines Comprehensive
Database, 979
Naturopathic medicine, 976
Naughton treadmill protocol, for exercise testing,
444
NBG code, for pacemakers, 715–716, 715*t*

Near-infrared spectroscopy, in tissue perfusion
monitoring, 518–519, 518*t*
Neck veins, pulsation in, in wide QRS complex
rhythms, 407
Necrosis
fibrinoid arteriolar, hypertension and, 865
myocardial, electrocardiography in, 344, 347*f*
in myocarditis, 786
Nephropathy
contrast-induced, 593–594
diabetic, 951–952
Nernst equation, 19–20
Nerves, cardiac, 16
Nesiritide
for heart failure, 671, 671*t*
for shock, 671, 671*t*
Netherlands clues, in wide QRS complex
rhythms, 406*f*
Neuroendocrine response theory, in coronary
artery disease, 828–829, 828*f*
Neurogenic shock, pathophysiology of, 662
Neurohumoral stimulation, of vascular system,
58–60, 59*f*, 60*f*
Neurologic disorders
in diabetes mellitus, 952
in hypertension, 866–867
hypertension in, 862*d*
postoperative, 641
Neuropeptide Y, in blood pressure regulation,
88, 88*f*
Neurotransmitters. *See also*
specific neurotransmitters
in blood pressure regulation, 87, 87*f*
electrophysiologic effects of, 28, 29*f*
Neutrophils, 151*f*, 152, 153*t*
count of, 282
New York Heart Association
Functional and Therapeutic Classification,
234, 235*t*
heart failure classification of, 613,
613*t*, 616*t*
Nicardipine, for hypertension, 879*t*, 882*t*
Nicotine
harmful effects of, 839
replacement of, for smoking cessation,
846–847, 846*f*, 848*d*
Nicotinic acid (niacin), for hyperlipidemia,
911–912, 911*t*
Nicotinic receptors, in blood pressure
regulation, 87
Nifedipine
for aortic regurgitation, 774
for hypertension, 879*t*
Nisoldipine, for hypertension, 879*t*
Nitrates, for myocardial infarction, 573
Nitric oxide
in blood pressure regulation, 95–96
in heart failure, 608
as vasodilator, 53–54, 54*f*–56*f*
Nitric oxide synthase, 55
Nitroglycerin
for angina, 555
arterial pressure wave and, 486, 486*f*
for heart failure, 621, 671*t*
for hypertension, 882*t*
for myocardial infarction, 569, 573
postoperative, 638*t*
for shock, 671*t*, 672*d*
Nitroprusside
for aortic regurgitation, 774
for heart failure, 671*t*, 672, 672*d*
for hypertension, 882*t*
for myocardial infarction, 572

Nitroprusside (continued)
    postoperative, 638t
    for shock, 671t, 672, 672d
NN doublet, in heart rate variability, 528–529,
        528f, 528t
Nodal cells, function of, 10
Nomograms, for exercise capacity, 447, 10f
Nonadherence (noncompliance). See Adherence
        (compliance)
Nonbacterial thrombotic endocarditis, 788
Noncarbonic acids, 189
Non-competitive atrial pace, 712d
Noncompliance. See Adherence (compliance)
Nonrapid eye movement sleep, 200–201, 201f
    cardiovascular function in, 202–203
    cerebral blood flow and metabolism in, 204
    heart rate variability in, 533
    respiratory function in, 203
    snoring in, 210
    thermoregulation in, 203
Norepinephrine
    in blood pressure regulation, 87, 87f, 92
    electrophysiologic effects of, 28, 29f
    in heart failure, 607, 608
    measurement of, 289
    in myocardial infarction, 546
    postoperative, 638t
    for shock, 669t, 673
    in venous system stimulation, 98–99, 99f
Normoblasts, 282
Normothermic cardioplegia, 630
North American Society of Pacing
        and Electrophysiology
    guidelines of, 436–437
    implantable cardioverter defibrillator guidelines
        of, 739, 740d
    pacemaker nomenclature of, 715–716, 715t
Nosocomial endocarditis, 788
Novacor ventricular assist device, 685–686,
        685f, 686f
NREM sleep. See Nonrapid eye movement
        sleep
NTpro-brain natriuretic peptide, as inflammatory
        marker, 129
Nuclear scans. See Radionuclide studies
Nucleus ambiguus, in blood pressure regulation,
        83–84
Nucleus tractus solitarius, in blood pressure
        regulation, 83–84
Nurse case-managed care, for adherence,
        967d, 969
Nursing care plans
    for cardiac transplantation, 652ncp–656ncp
    for coping in congenital heart disease, 805ncp
    for hypertension, 885, 886ncp–888ncp
    for intra-aortic balloon pumps, 21,
        680ncp–683ncp
    for myocardial infarction, right ventricular,
        580ncp–582ncp
Nutrition
    adherence to programs and, 963, 964
    in Ayurvedic medicine, 976
    in complementary and alternative medicine,
        980–982
    in diabetes mellitus, 955–956
    diary for, 963t, 964, 965
    drugs reducing absorption in, 944
    heart rate variability in, 534
    in history taking, 233
    in hypercholesterolemia, 905–908, 906f,
        906t, 907d
    in hypertension, 871–872, 872t, 873t
    in myocardial infarction, 571

in myocarditis, 787
in obesity, 942, 942t
postoperative, 644–645

O

Obesity, 937–947
    assessment of, 938–939, 939t
    blood pressure measurement in, 248
    body mass index and, 235–236
    cardiovascular disease risk factors in,
        938–939
    clinical evaluation of, 939–941, 940f
    as coronary artery disease risk factor,
        817–818, 817f
    definition of, 938
    diabetes mellitus and, 950–951
    disorders associated with, 937
    epidemiology of, 937
    heart rate variability in, 534
    history in, 940
    hyperlipidemia and, 908
    treatment of, 941–945
        algorithm for, 939–940, 940f
        approach to, 941, 941t
        behavioral, 943–944
        dietary, 942, 942t
        exercise in, 942–943
        goal of, 941–942
        lifestyle modification in, 942–944, 942t
        motivation for, 940–941
        pharmacologic, 944
        surgical, 945
        weight loss maintenance after, 945
    under-treatment of, 939
Objective assessment, of sleep, 200
Obstructive sleep apnea, 209–210, 209f
Occlusion, after percutaneous coronary
        interventions, 592, 594
O₂ER. See Oxygen extraction ratio (O₂ER)
Off-pump coronary artery bypass (OPCAB),
        633–634, 633f
Ohm's law, 19
Oimesartan, for hypertension, 879t
OKT3, for cardiac transplantation, 648t, 649
Older adults. See also Aging
    demographics of, 220, 221f
    exercise testing in, 455–456
    heath status of, 220, 221f
    hypertension in, 858–859, 875–877
    percutaneous coronary interventions in, 586
    pharmacokinetics in, 225
    thirst in, 174
Omega-3 fatty acids, in complementary and
        alternative medicine, 980–982
Oncotic pressure, in microcirculation, 66, 66f
OPCAB (off-pump coronary artery bypass),
        633–634, 633f
Opening snaps, in heart sounds, 254, 255f
Ophthalmitis, 236
Optic disc, examination of, 237–238
Oral contraceptives
    coronary artery disease and, 818–819
    hypertension due to, 863
Orlistat, for obesity, 944
Orthocione OKT3, for cardiac transplantation,
        648t, 649
Orthodromic atrioventricular reentry tachycardia,
        397, 399f
Orthostatic (postural) hypotension, blood
        pressure measurement in, 247
Oscillometric blood pressure measurement,
        487, 487f

Osler's nodes, in endocarditis, 789, 789t
Osmolality, 173
    imbalance of, 176–177, 176t, 177t
    measurement of, 287
Osmotic pressure, in fluid distribution, 174
Osteoporosis, after cardiac transplantation, 651
Ostium primum atrial septal defect, 798–799
Ostium secundum atrial septal defect, 798–799
Outcomes, of disease management programs,
        991–992
Outpatient procedures
    cardiac catheterization, 462–463, 462t
    cardiac rehabilitation. See under Cardiac
        rehabilitation
Output
    cardiac. See Cardiac output
    in pacing, 711d
Outward currents, 23–24, 23f, 26t, 27–28
Overdrive suppression, in automaticity, 361
Oversensing, in pacing, 711d, 725, 727
Overweight, definition of, 938, 939t
Oxidized low-density lipoprotein,
        143–144, 900
Oximetry, pulse, 78–79
Oxygen
    exchange of, 74, 75
    partial pressure of, 75, 76
        in acid-base imbalances, 194, 195t
        measurement of, 78
Oxygenation
    in cardiopulmonary bypass, 629
    monitoring of, 78–79, 517
Oxygen consumption (VO₂), 77
    in cardioplegia, 630
    equation for, 513t
    global indicators of, 513–514, 513t
    myocardial, 41–42, 541–542, 542f
    oxygen delivery relationship to, 78
Oxygen consumption index, 513t
Oxygen content, 41, 77
Oxygen delivery (DO₂), 77
    alterations in, 513–514
    equation for, 513t
    global indicators of, 513–514, 513t
    optimization of, 514
    oxygen consumption relationship to, 78
    in septic shock, 674
Oxygen delivery index, 513t
Oxygen extraction ratio (O₂ER), 77–78, 513t,
        516–517
Oxygen saturation (SaO₂), 76
    central venous, 516
    measurement of, 286
    mixed venous (SvO₂), 513t, 515, 516f
    optimization of, 514t
    response to, 513–514
Oxygen supply
    global indicators of, 513–514, 513t
    myocardial, 42–43, 42f, 541–542, 542f
Oxygen supply and demand balance, evaluation
        of, 512–519, 513t
    central venous oxygen saturation in, 516
    global indicators in, 513–514, 513t
    lactate in, 517
    mixed venous oxygen saturation in, 515, 516f
    oxygen extraction ratio in, 516–517
    regional indicators in, 517
    sublingual capnography in, 517–518
    tissue perfusion monitoring in,
        518–519, 518t
Oxygen therapy
    for myocardial infarction, 569, 571
    for pulmonary embolism, 168

Oxygen transport, 75–77, 76f
  equations for, 513t
  goals of, 514t
  in red blood cells, 151–152
Oxyhemoglobin dissociation curve, 76–77, 76f

P

Pacemaker(s) (artificial), 709–738
  asynchronous, 711d, 716
  for asystole, 698
  bipolar, 716, 719f
  biventricular, 714–715, 715f, 735–737, 737f
  for bradycardia, 703–704, 703f
  capture in, 711d, 717–718, 724–725, 725f, 730
  after cardiac transplantation, 646
  for cardiomyoplasty, 635
  cardioversion with, 722
  classification of, 715–716, 715t
  codes for, 715–716, 715t
  complications of, 737–738
  components of, 716, 717f, 718f
  DDD mode, 715–716, 727–728, 727t, 729f, 730
  DDI mode, 727t
  defibrillation with, 722
  demand mode, 711d
  in demand mode, 716–717
  dual-chamber, 714
    antitachycardia pacing in, 734–735, 737f
    atrial overdrive pacing in, 733–734, 736f
    biventricular, 735–737, 737f
    crosstalk in, 711d, 732–733, 734f
    evaluation of, 728, 730
    initiation of, 720, 720f
    modes of, 727, 727t
    pacemaker-mediated tachycardia in, 731–732, 733f
    rate-adaptive pacing in, 733, 735f, 736f
    for resynchronization, 735–737, 737f
    states of, 728, 729f
    temporary, 719–720
    terminology of, 900d–901d
    timing cycles of, 727–728, 728f, 729f
    upper-rate behavior of, 730–731, 731f, 732f
  DVI mode, 727t
  electrical safety with, 722–723
  epicardial, 714, 714f, 719, 720f, 722
  evaluation of, 723–727, 724f–726f, 727t
  for heart failure, 618
  heart rate variability in, 532
  for hypertrophic cardiomyopathy, 785
  implantable cardioverter defibrillator interaction with, 749–750
  indications for, 709–710, 710d
  insertion site care with, 722
  nursing considerations with, 720–723
  permanent, 713, 713f
    electromagnetic radiation and, 711d, 721–722
    indications for, 710d
    magnets and, 711d, 721
    nursing considerations with, 721–722
  postoperative, 638–639, 639f
  principles of, 716–718, 717f–719f
  radiographic appearance of, 299t, 301f
  sensing in, 711d, 718, 725, 726f, 727
  sensitivity threshold testing of, 723
  single-chamber, 711d–712d, 714
  stimulation threshold test for, 723
  stimulus release in, 723–724, 724f

  temporary, 713–714, 713f, 714f
    indications for, 709–710
    initiation of, 718–720, 720f
    nursing considerations with, 722–723
  transcutaneous, 375t, 714, 714f
  transvenous, 375t, 713–714, 713f, 718–719, 720f
  types of, 710, 711d–713d, 713–715, 713f–715f
  unipolar, 716, 719f
  VDD mode, 727t
  VVI mode, 715, 723, 724f, 726f
Pacemaker(s) (physiologic). See also Sinoatrial node
  currents of, 27
  dissociation of, 248, 417–418, 417f–419f
  dominant, 361
  latent, 361
  subsidiary, 361–362, 362f
Pacemaker mediated tachycardia, 712d, 731–732, 733f
Pacemaker syndrome, 711d, 738
Pacer spike, 711d
Pacing interval, 711d, 724f, 727
Pacing lead, 716, 718f
Pain
  chest. See Angina; Chest pain
  in deep vein thrombosis, 164
  heart rate variability in, 534
  in myocardial infarction, 569
  in pulmonary embolism, 167
Pallor, 236
Palmaz-Schatz coronary stent, 590, 590f, 591
Palpation
  in abdominal assessment, 263, 263f
  in blood pressure measurement, 244
  in circulation assessment, 249
  in heart assessment, 251–252
  in lung assessment, 258, 261f, 261
Palpitation, in myocarditis, 786
Pancreatitis, postoperative, 641
Papillary muscles
  anatomy of, 7f, 8
  dysfunction of, murmurs in, 256
  rupture of, in myocardial infarction, 561–562
Papilledema, 238, 238f, 866
Paradoxical blood pressure, measurement of, 247–248, 248f
Paradoxical movement, of chest wall, 251
Paradoxical pulse. See Pulsus paradoxus
Paradoxical splitting, of heart sounds, 253–254, 253f
Parasomnias, 204, 206t
Paraspecific fibers of Mahaim, 11
Parasympathetic nervous system
  in blood pressure regulation, 85f, 86t, 87–88
  of heart, 16
  in heart rate control, 92
  heart rate variability and, 526
Parasystole, 418–420, 419f, 420f
Parkinson disease, heart rate variability in, 535
Paroxysmal atrial tachycardia, 380–381
Partial thromboplastin time, 284
Passive ion movement, across cell membrane, 21
Passive vasoconstriction, 96
Passive vasodilation, 86, 96
Past history, in history taking, 232
Patent ductus arteriosus, 796f, 798–800
Patent foramen ovale, percutaneous interventions for, 596–597, 597f
Patient/family education
  on adherence, 969, 970d
  on cardiac arrest, 707

  on cardiac catheterization, 461–462, 473, 473t
  on cardiac rehabilitation, 924–925, 924d–926d, 925t, 930
  on cholesterol-lowering diet, 907–908
  on dilated cardiomyopathy, 784
  on disease management, 989–990
  on hypertension, 888
  on implantable cardioverter defibrillators, 750, 751d
  on weight loss diet, 942
Pectinate muscles, anatomy of, 6
Pediatric patients
  cardiac transplantation in, 642–643
  hypertension in, 857–858, 858t, 859t, 861
Penbutolol, for hypertension, 878t
Penicillin G, for rheumatic fever, 757
Percussion
  in abdominal assessment, 262–263, 263f
  in lung assessment, 259, 261f, 261t, 262, 262f
Percutaneous coronary interventions, 585–600
  adjunctive modalities with, 595, 595f
  alternatives to, 585
  for angina, 553
  angiojet thrombectomy as, 589
  cardiac rehabilitation after. See Cardiac rehabilitation
  complications of, 592–596, 595f
  coronary angioplasty as, 587–589, 588f
  future of, 597
  management during, 586–587
  for myocardial infarction, 566–567
  nursing management of, 597–599
  patient subgroups in, 585–586
  radiation in, 592
  stent placement in, 589–592, 590f, 591f
Perfusion
  in intra-aortic balloon pump use, 680ncp
  monitoring of, 518–519, 518t
  in myocardial infarction, 578–579
  in respiration, 73
  in shock, 669–674, 669t, 670f, 671d, 671t, 672d
Perfusion pressure, 42
Pericardectomy, for constrictive pericarditis, 780
Pericardial cavity, anatomy of, 4f, 9
Pericardial effusion, 780–781
  echocardiography in, 317
  radiography in, 303t, 304f
Pericardial friction rub
  auscultation of, 256–257, 256f
  in pericarditis, 777–778
Pericardial tamponade, 781
  arterial pressure waveform in, 492f
  hemodynamic characteristics of, 506t
  shock in, 662
Pericardiocentesis
  in cardiac tamponade, 781
  in pericardial effusion, 780–781
Pericarditis, 776–780
  acute clinically noneffusive (dry), 777–778, 779f
  constrictive, 778–780
  etiology of, 776–777
  facial characteristics in, 236
  in myocardial infarction, 562, 780
  in rheumatic fever, 756
  uremic, 777–778
Pericardium
  anatomy of, 9, 776
  congenital abnormalities of, 776, 777d
  constriction of, hemodynamic characteristics of, 506t
  disease of. See also specific types, eg, Pericarditis
    nursing management of, 781–782
    types of, 776, 777t

Pericardium (continued)
    echocardiography of, 316–317
    function of, 776
    restrictive effects of, on cardiac output, 94
Peripheral cyanosis, 236
Peripheral inserted central catheter, radiographic
        appearance of, 299t, 301f, 302f
Peripheral vascular disease, intra-aortic balloon
        pump contraindicated in, 677–678
Persistence. See Adherence (compliance)
Personal history, in history taking, 232–233
Personal information, in history taking, 230
PET (positron emission tomography), 322
Petechiae, of eyelid, 236
pH
    blood
        in acid-base imbalances, 194–195, 195t
        measurement of, 78
    definition of, 189
Phagocytes, 151f, 152–153, 153t
Phantom shocks, with implantable cardioverter
        defibrillator, 751–752
Pharmacogenomics, 114–115
Pharmacokinetics, in older adults, 225
Phasic rapid eye movement sleep, 201
Phasic smooth muscle, 53
Phentolamine, for hypertension, 882t
Phenylalanine derivatives, for diabetes
        mellitus, 958
Phenylephrine
    heart sounds and, 257t, 258
    postoperative, 638t
    for shock, 669t, 673
Pheochromocytoma, facial characteristics in, 236
Phlebostatic axis, 488, 479f, 480f
Phlebostatic level, 488, 479f, 480t
Phlebotomy, for laboratory tests. See Blood
        specimens, collection of
Phonocardiography, 253
Phosphate ion
    balance of, 178t, 185
    as buffer, 190t
Phospholamban, in excitation-contraction
        coupling, 32, 32f
Phospholipase A₂, lipoprotein-associated, 280
Physical activity. See Exercise
Physical assessment, 234–263
    of abdomen, 262–263, 263f
    of blood pressure, 243–249, 243t, 244f–246f,
        245t, 248f
    general appearance in, 235–236
    of head, 236–239, 236f–239f
    of heart, 250–258, 251f
        auscultation in. See Auscultation
        inspection in, 250–251
        palpation in, 251–252
    of jugular venous pulse, 241–243, 242f
    of lungs, 258–262, 259f
        anterior chest, 261–262, 262f
        inspection in, 258, 260f
        posterior chest, 258–261, 261f, 261t, 262f
    order of, 235
    of peripheral vascular system, 249–250, 249f
    of pulse, 239–241, 240f, 241f
    timing of, 234–235
Physiologic cup, in optic disc, 238, 238f
Piezoelectric crystal, in echocardiography, 308
Pigmentation, in edema, 250
Pill counts, for adherence measurement, 963t, 965
Pindolol, for hypertension, 878t
Pioglitazone, for diabetes mellitus, 958
Pitting edema, 250
Plaques, atherosclerotic. See Atherosclerotic lesions

Plasma proteins, as buffers, 190t
Plasmin, in fibrinolysis, 155–156
Plasminogen, in fibrinolysis, 155–156
Plateau phase, of action potential, 23, 23f, 24
Platelet(s), 151f, 153
    aggregation of
        deep vein thrombosis in, 163
        in hemostasis, 154–155
        hypercholesterolemia and, 901
        inhibitors of, for percutaneous coronary
                interventions, 596
    count of, 157t, 283–284
    deficiency of, in heparin-induced
            thrombocytopenia, 169–171,
            169f, 170t
    nitric oxide effects on, 55
Platelet-activating factor acetylhydrolase, 280
Pleural effusion
    postoperative, 641, 642f
    radiography in, 303t, 304f, 306f
Pleural friction rubs, 261, 262f
Pneumonia
    after cardiac transplantation, 647
    radiography in, 303t, 306f
Pneumothorax
    in pacemaker insertion, 738
    radiography in, 303f, 303t, 305f
Point-of-care testing, 269
Point of maximal impulse, 3
Poiseuille's law, blood flow and, 63
Polymorphisms, genetic, 113–114
Polysomnography, 197, 198f, 200
    in cardiac care unit, 207
    in sleep apnea, 209–210, 209f
Popliteal pulse, assessment of, 241, 241f
Population, for disease management,
        988–989, 989f
Porcine valves, 763–764
Position, body
    heart rate variability and, 533
    laboratory results and, 267–268
Positron emission tomography, 322, 552
Postcardiotomy delirium, 641
Posterior hemiblock (left posterior fascicular
        block), 341, 345f
Posterior tibial pulse, assessment of, 241, 241f
Postextrasystolic beats, 257t, 258
Postextrasystolic potentiation, 39, 40f
Postpericardiotomy syndrome, 641, 642f
Postural hypotension
    blood pressure measurement in, 247
    in hypokalemia, 180
Posture, change in, heart sounds in, 257t, 258
Post-ventricular atrial refractory period (PVARP),
        712d, 727
Potassium channels
    in action potential, in plateau, 23f, 24
    ATP-dependent, 27–28
    in automaticity, 362
    in outward currents, 27
    in pacemaking, 27
Potassium ion
    in action potential, in early repolarization,
        23–24, 23f
    balance of, 178t, 179
    distribution of, in myocardium, 18t
    equilibrium potential of, 19–20
    imbalance of. See Hyperkalemia; Hypokalemia
    measurement of, 286
    replacement of, 179
Potential difference, in myocardial cells, 17, 19
Potential for hostility, coronary artery disease
        and, 827

Prazosin, for hypertension, 878t
Preatheromas, 141, 147t
Precordial examination, 250–251, 251f
Precordial leads, in electrocardiography,
        331–332, 333f
Predictive value, of exercise testing, 452, 452d
Preexcitation syndromes, 391–394, 393f–396f
Pregnancy
    aortic coarctation in, 797, 797t
    hypertension in, 877, 879
Prehypertension, definition of, 856, 857t
Preload, 35–36, 36f
    aging effects on, 222
    cardiac output and, 93
    in extracellular fluid deficit, 176
    hemodynamic characteristics of, 507t
    indices of, 500, 500f
    length-tension relationship and, 36–38,
        37f, 38f
    in pulmonary embolism, 167
    in ventricular function curves, 505
Premature atrial complexes, 379
Premature ectopic beats, blood pressure
        measurement in, 248
Premature junctional complexes, 383
Premature ventricular complexes, 384–385, 450
Premature ventricular contractions
    postoperative, 639–640
    in sleep, 208–209
Preoptic nuclei, median, in blood pressure
        regulation, 83–84
Preponderance (dominance), of coronary
        vasculature, 12–15
Prescription, exercise, 929–930
Present illness, in history taking, 231–232
Presenting problem, in history taking, 230–231
Pressure-volume work, myocardial oxygen
        consumption and, 42
PRIME-MD instrument, for psychosocial risk
        factors, 829–830, 830t
PR interval, 328
Prinzmetal's angina, 545, 555
Problem solving
    in adherence, 967d, 968
    in weight loss, 943
Procainamide, for arrhythmias, 371t, 373t
Programmed electrical stimulation, in
        electrophysiology studies, 425
Propafenone, for arrhythmias, 371t
Propranolol
    for arrhythmias, 371t
    for hypertension, 878t
Prostacyclin, as vasodilator, 54f, 55–56, 56f
Prostaglandins
    in heart failure, 608
    as vasoconstrictors, 54f, 57–58
Prostanoids, as vasoconstrictors, 54f, 57–58
Prosthetic valves, 762–766
    for aortic valve. See Aortic valve, replacement of
    cardiac arrest due to, 690
    complications of, 765–766
    degeneration of, 766
    dysfunction of, shock in, 661
    echocardiography of, 317
    endocarditis of, 765, 788, 789
    leakage of, 766
    malfunction of, 765–766
    mechanical, 763, 763f
    minimally invasive placement of,
        764–765, 765f
    for mitral valve, 634
        in regurgitation, 767–768, 768f
        in stenosis, 761

placement of, 634–635
selection of, 762–763, 763*t*
thrombosis of, 765
tissue, 763–764, 763*f*, 764*f*
types of, 763, 763*f*
Protamine
for coagulation promotion, 162*t*
for heparin reversal, in cardiopulmonary
bypass, 629
for postoperative bleeding, 637
Protein(s)
serum, measurement of, 290
synthesis of, 111
Protein C, 157, 157*t*
deficiency of, deep vein thrombosis in, 163
measurement of, 285
Protein S, 157
deficiency of, deep vein thrombosis in, 163
measurement of, 285
Proteoglycans, in atherosclerotic lesions, 144
Prothrombin time (PT), 157*t*, 284
Protodiastole, 44*f*, 45
PSD (power spectral density) plot, in heart rate
variability, 529, 529*t*
Pseudoaneurysm, of femoral artery, in
percutaneous coronary
interventions, 594
Pseudofusion beats, 711*d*
Pseudohypertension, 249
Pseudopseudofusion beat, 712*d*
Psychiatric disorders, sleep disorders in,
204, 206*t*
Psychological assessment, after cardiac
catheterization, 473
Psychosocial issues, in myocardial infarction, 924
Psychosocial risk factors, for coronary artery
disease, 825–837, 826*t*
anger, 827, 834
anxiety, 827, 833
assessment of, 829–830, 830*t*
depression, 825–826, 829, 833
hostility, 827, 834
interventions for, 830–835
anxiety, 833
decreasing arousal, 832, 832*d*
depression, 833
hostility and anger, 834
pharmacological, 834–835
self-monitoring of negative reactions and
responses in, 831–832, 831*f*
social support, 833–834
mechanisms for, 828–829, 828*f*
social support and, 826, 829, 833–834
stress, 827–828
Public health, hypertension control and, 884–885
Pulmonary angiography, in pulmonary
embolism, 168
Pulmonary artery(ies)
anatomy of, 71
topographic location of, 250
transposition in, 796*f*, 802–803
Pulmonary artery catheters
balloon on, for pulmonary artery wedge
pressure, 492, 492*f*, 493
blood drawing from, for laboratory testing, 266
in cardiac output measurement
continuous, 506–507
thermodilution method in, 503–505,
504*d*, 505*d*
description of, 489, 492, 492*f*
insertion of, 492, 493*d*
manipulation of, 496–497, 498*t*, 499*d*
pulmonary effects on, 495–496, 497*f*

radiographic appearance of, 299*t*, 300*f*
removal of, 496–497, 498*t*, 499*d*
in shock, 668, 668*f*
troubleshooting for, 497, 498*t*
Pulmonary artery diastolic pressure,
492–493, 494*f*
Pulmonary artery end-diastolic pressure (PAEDP),
493–495, 494*f*, 497*f*
in pericardial tamponade, 492*f*
Pulmonary artery end-diastolic pressure
(PAEDP)-pulmonary artery wedge
pressure (PAWP) gradient,
495–496, 497*f*
Pulmonary artery pressure
measurement of, protocol for, 481*d*–482*f*
monitoring of, 489–503
catheter for, 489, 492, 492*f*, 493*d*
delta Down in, 502–503
indications for, 489
limitations of, 503
in mechanical ventilation, 500–501,
501*f*, 502*t*
pulse pressure variation in, 503, 503*f*
respiratory variations and, 501–502,
501*f*, 502*f*
right ventricular volumetric measures in,
499–500, 499*t*, 500*f*
in spontaneous ventilation, 500
stroke volume variation in, 503
technical aspects of, 495–496, 497*f*,
498*t*, 499*d*
waveform characteristics in, 492–495,
494*f*–497*f*
in myocardial infarction, 559
waveform of, 492–493, 494*f*
Pulmonary artery systolic pressure,
492–493, 494*f*
Pulmonary artery wedge pressure (PAWP)
in heart failure, 612
measurement of
protocol for, 481*d*–482*f*
troubleshooting for, 498*t*
waveform characteristics in, 493, 494,
494*f*, 495*f*
in myocardial infarction, 559
in shock, 660*t*
Pulmonary capillaries, gas exchange in, 74, 75
Pulmonary circulation, 71–80, 72*t*
anatomy of, 71–72
gas transport in, 75–77, 76*f*
non-gas exchange functions of, 72
oxygen in, 77–79
physiology of, 72–85, 73*f*
Pulmonary congestion
in heart failure, 611
in hypertrophic cardiomyopathy, 784
Pulmonary edema
in endocarditis, 788
in heart failure, 611–612
postoperative, 640
radiography in, 304*f*
in shock, 666, 670–671, 671*d*
Pulmonary embolism, 166–169
clinical manifestations of, 167–168
diagnosis of, 168
in endocarditis, 788–789
etiology of, 166
hemodynamic characteristics of, 506*t*
in heparin-induced thrombocytopenia,
170, 170*t*
incidence of, 166
medical management of, 168
mortality in, 166

nursing interventions for, 168–169
pathophysiology of, 166–167, 167*f*
postoperative, 640
prevention of, 168–169
shock in, 662
Pulmonary hypertension, transplantation
contraindicated in, 643
Pulmonary surface, 3
Pulmonary vascular resistance
in atrial septal defect, 798–799
calculation of, 63
in Eisenmenger reaction, 803
Pulmonary veins, anatomy of, 8, 8*f*
Pulmonic ejection sounds, 255
Pulmonic valve
anatomy of, 6*f*, 8–9
cardiac cycle and, 44*f*, 46
conduction system to, 11, 12*f*
echocardiography of, 316
function of, 8–9, 8*f*
heart sounds and, 44*f*, 46
insufficiency of, echocardiography in, 316
in Ross procedure, 764, 764*f*
stenosis of
congenital, 794–796, 796*f*
murmurs of, 762*t*
in tetralogy of Fallot, 800
Pulsations
in chest wall, 250
in heart palpation, 251–252
Pulse
assessment of, 239–241
amplitude, 240–241, 240*f*, 241*f*
bruits in, 240
contour, 240–241, 240*f*, 241*f*
in dilated cardiomyopathy, 783
in heart failure, 614
jugular venous, 241–243, 242*f*
rate, 239
rhythm, 239–240
in shock, 667
paradoxical. *See* Pulsus paradoxus
Pulse contour analysis, in cardiac output
measurement, 508–509, 508*t*, 509*f*
Pulsed Doppler echocardiography, 309
Pulse generator
of implantable cardioverter defibrillator,
741–742, 742*f*
of pacemaker, 711*d*, 716, 717*f*
Pulseless electrical activity
prognosis for, 704
treatment of, 696*f*, 698–699
Pulse oximetry, 78–79
Pulse pressure
calculation of, 64
diagnostic use of, 246–247, 487
measurement of, 246–247, 246*f*
variation in, 502*t*, 503, 503*f*
Pulse-wave velocity, aging and, 223
Pulsus alternans, 240, 240*f*
blood pressure measurement in, 248
in heart failure, 614
Pulsus bisferiens, 240, 240*f*
Pulsus paradoxus, 240, 240*f*
after cardiac catheterization, 474
in cardiac tamponade, 781
Pulsus parvis et tardus, 240, 240*f*
Pump, heart as, 35, 41
Pump/exchange currents, 26*t*
Purkinje cells
action potential of, 23*f*, 25, 25*f*
conduction through, 30–31, 30*t*
function of, 10

Purkinje fibers
  anatomy of, 11*f,* 12
  function of, 326
Purkinje system, electrophysiology studies of, 430
PVARP (post-ventricular atrial refractory period), 712*d,* 727
P wave, 327, 328*f,* 329*t*
  in atrial enlargement, 349–350, 354*f*
  in wide QRS complex rhythms, 402–403, 402*t,* 403*f*–405*f*

Q

Qi, in Chinese medicine, 976, 977*f*
QRS axis, 336–337, 337*f*–340*f*
QRS complex, 327, 328*f,* 329
  in ventricular enlargement, 351
  wide
    in complex rhythms, 402*t,* 403–404, 405*f,* 406*f*
    differential diagnosis of, 401–408, 402*f*–410*f,* 402*t*
    electrophysiology studies in, 428–429, 428*d*
QT interval, prolonged, 328, 330*f*
  drug-induced, 690, 692*d*
  genetic factors in, 116, 116*t*
Quadruple rhythm, in heart sounds, 254, 254*f*
Quality of life
  evaluation of, for disease management, 991
  with implantable cardioverter defibrillator, 751–752
Questionnaires
  for adherence to treatment, 963–964, 969–970
  for sleep measurement, 199
Quinapril
  for heart failure, 619*t*
  for hypertension, 879*t*
Quinidine, for arrhythmias, 371*t*–372*t*
Q wave, 329*t*
  in myocardial infarction, 556–557
  in myocardial necrosis, 344–346, 348*f*–350*f*

R

Radial artery
  cardiac catheterization via, 463
  catheter placement in, 484, 488, 488*t*
  as coronary artery bypass graft, 632
  pressure wave in, 486*f*
Radial pulse, assessment of, 241, 241*f*
Radiation therapy, percutaneous methods for, 592
Radiofrequency catheter ablation, 430–435
  for arrhythmias, 374*t*
  for atrial arrhythmias, 435, 436*f*
  for atrial fibrillation and flutter, 432*d,* 434, 435*f*
  for atrioventricular nodal reentrant tachycardia, 431, 431*f*
  for atrioventricular reentrant tachycardia, 432*d,* 433–434, 433*f,* 434*f*
  complications of, 431
  indications for, 431–435, 432*d*
  nursing care in, 435–437
  techniques for, 431
  for ventricular tachycardia, 432*d,* 435
Radiography, chest. *See* Chest radiography
Radioimmunoassay, for brain natriuretic peptide, 129
Radionuclide studies, 319–322
  in angina, 552
  in aortic regurgitation, 773
  in aortic stenosis, 771
  in exercise testing, 453–454
  in heart failure, 614

in myocardial infarction, 559–560
  myocardial perfusion imaging as, 320–322, 320*f*–322*f*
  pharmaceuticals for, 319
  positron emission tomography as, 322
  risks of, 322
  ventriculography as, 319–320, 320*f*
Ramipril
  for heart failure, 619*t*
  for hypertension, 879*t*
Ramp exercise testing, 444
Rapammune, for cardiac transplantation, 648*t*
Rapid eye movement sleep, 200–201, 201*f*
  in angina, 208
  after cardiac surgery, 207
  cardiovascular function in, 203
  cerebral blood flow and metabolism in, 204
  heart rate variability in, 533
  kidney function in, 204
  respiratory function in, 203
  snoring in, 210
  thermoregulation in, 203
Rapid ventricular ejection, 44*f,* 45
Rate-adaptive pacing, 733, 735*f,* 736*f*
Rate drop response, in pacing, 712*d*–713*d*
Rate response/modulation/adaptation, in pacing, 711*d,* 713*d*
Rate smoothing, in pacing, 713*d,* 731, 732*f*
Reactive hyperemia, 58
  coronary, 542, 544
Reactive oxygen species, as vasoconstrictors, 58, 58*f,* 542
Rebreathing system, carbon dioxide, in cardiac output measurement, 508*t,* 512
Rectifying currents, outward, 27
Red blood cell(s), 151–152, 151*f*
  abnormal morphology of, 282
Red blood cell count, 281–282
Red reflex, in eye, 237
Red spots, in retina, 239
Reduced ventricular ejection, 44*f,* 45
Red yeast rice, for cardiovascular disease, 980–981
Reentrant pathways, Wenckebach conduction in, 412–413, 414*f*
Reentry, 364, 365*f*
Reference ranges, for laboratory tests, 268, 277*t*
Referencing, in hemodynamic monitoring, 478, 479*f,* 480*f,* 480*t*
Reflection coefficient, in microcirculation, 67
Reflex, Bezold-Jarisch, 81–83, 83*f*
Refractory period
  in action potential, 25–26, 26*f*
  atrial, 712*d,* 727
  hypokalemia effects on, 180
  in pacing, 711*d,* 712*d,* 723
  post-ventricular atrial (PVARP), 712*d,* 727
  total atrial (TARP), 713*d,* 727
  ventricular, 713*d,* 727
Regimen, tailoring of, for adherence, 967*d,* 968
Regulatory proteins, in contraction, 33
Regurgitant murmurs, 255, 255*f*
Regurgitation. *See also specific valves, regurgitation of*
  definition of, 756
Rehabilitation, cardiac. *See* Cardiac rehabilitation
Reiki, for cardiovascular disease, 982
Reimbursement, for cardiac rehabilitation, 929
Reinforcement, in adherence, 967, 967*d*
Rejection, in cardiac transplantation, 646–647, 646*f,* 647*t*
Relapse prevention
  in adherence, 967*d,* 968
  in weight loss, 943

Relationships, in history taking, 234
Relative refractory period, in action potential, 25–26, 26*f*
Relaxation, 832, 832*d*
  endothelium-derived relaxing factors for, 53–56, 54*f*–56*f,* 54*t*
  molecular basis for, 34–35, 36*f*
  for sleep, 213
  ventricular, 44*f,* 45
REM sleep. *See* Rapid eye movement sleep
Renal arteries, atherosclerosis of, 146
Renin-angiotensin-aldosterone system
  in blood pressure regulation, 89*f,* 91–92
  dysfunction of, hypertension in, 861, 863
  in heart failure, 606–607, 609*f*
  inhibitors of, for heart failure, 618–620, 619*t*
  in shock, 663–664, 664*f*
Renovascular hypertension, 863
Repaglinide, for diabetes mellitus, 958
Reperfusion, after myocardial ischemia, 544, 546
Repolarization, 17
  early, 23–24, 23*f*
  in electrocardiography, 327–328, 328*f*
  late rapid, in action potential, 23*f,* 24
  in ventricle, 31
Reproductive hormones, coronary artery disease and, 818–819
Reserpine, for hypertension, 878*t*
Resistance, electrical, 19
Resonance, in lung percussion, 259, 261*t*
Respiration. *See also* Ventilation
  assessment of, 258, 260*f*
    in shock, 667
  vs. blood pressure, 247–248, 248*f*
  Cheyne-Stokes, in heart failure, 207
  events in, 72, 73*f*
  heart rate and, 93
  heart sounds in, 253, 253*f,* 257, 257*t*
  hemodynamic response to, 102, 102*f*
  muscles of, 72
  in red blood cells, 151
  vs. right atrial pressure, 501, 501*f*
  in sleep, 203
  vs. systolic blood pressure, 501–502, 502*f*
Respiratory acidosis, 191–192, 192*t,* 193*t,* 195*t*
Respiratory alkalosis, 193–194, 193*t,* 195*t*
Respiratory excursion, assessment of, 258, 261*f*
Respiratory pump, in cardiac performance maintenance, 101
Respiratory rate, assessment of, 258, 260*f*
Respiratory system
  aging effects on, 223–224, 224*f*
  dysfunction of
    in heart failure, 623
    postoperative, 640
Restenosis
  in aortic stenosis, 772
  of coronary arteries, 592, 594
Resting potential, 19, 19*f,* 20
Rest potentiation, 39, 40*f*
Restrictive cardiomyopathy, 785–786
Resuscitation. *See* Advanced cardiac life support
Resynchronization therapy, 618, 735–737, 737*f,* 743*d*
Reteplase, for myocardial infarction, 564
Reticulocytes, 282
Retina, examination of, 237–239, 237*f*–239*f*
Retinopathy
  in diabetes mellitus, 951
  in hypertension, 866, 866*t*
Retractions, in chest wall, 250
Retrograde cardioplegia, 630

Retroperitoneal hemorrhage, in percutaneous coronary interventions, 594
Revascularization, coronary. *See also* Coronary artery bypass surgery
　for angina, 553, 553*t*
　for cardiac arrest prevention, 705
　complications of, 636–641, 638*t*, 639*f*, 642*f*
　laser angioplasty, 589
　percutaneous transluminal angioplasty, 587–588, 588*f*
　postoperative care in, 636
　for shock, 670
　transmyocardial laser, 634
Reverse cholesterol transport, 899
Rheumatic heart disease, 756–757, 757*f*
　aortic regurgitation in, 773
　facial characteristics in, 236
　mitral stenosis in, 759
Ribosomes, in protein synthesis, 113
Rick method, direct, for cardiac output measurement, 469
Right atrial pressure, vs. respiration, 501, 501*f*
Right atrial pressure (RAP)
　monitoring of, 488–489, 490*d*–491*d*, 492*f*
　in ventilation, 500–501, 501*f*, 502*t*
Right bundle branch, function of, 326
Right bundle-branch block, 339, 343*f*, 364, 364*f*, 402*t*, 403, 405*f*, 406*f*
Right heart. *See also* Atrium (atria), right; Ventricle(s), right
　catheterization of, 464, 465*f*
Right ventricular end-diastolic volume (RVEDV), 499, 499*t*
Right ventricular end-diastolic volume index (RVEDVI), 499, 499*t*
rmsSD (square root of mean squared differences between successive NN intervals), in heart rate variability, 528*t*, 529
RNA (ribonucleic acid), 113
Robotics, in valve replacement, 765
Romano Ward syndrome, cardiac arrest in, 690
Rosiglitazone, for diabetes mellitus, 958
Ross procedure, for valve replacement, 764, 764*f*
Rotational atherectomy, 589, 589*f*
Roth's spots, 239, 789*t*
Roux-en-Y technique, for obesity, 945
RR interval, in heart rate variability, 528–529, 528*f*, 528*t*
R wave, 329*t*
　in heart rate determination, 329, 331*f*
　in ventricular enlargement, 351, 352, 354*f*, 356*f*
Ryanodine receptors, in excitation-contraction coupling, 31, 32*f*

S

Safety
　in cardiac rehabilitation, 930
　in exercise testing, 439–440, 440*d*
　with pacemakers, 722–723
Safety pacing, 713*d*, 733, 734*f*
St. Jude's Medical bileaflet valve, 763, 763*f*
Salvos, in ventricular tachycardia, 386
San Francisco clue, in wide QRS complex rhythms, 406*f*
Saphenous vein, as coronary artery bypass graft, 631–632, 632*f*
Sarcolemma
　ionic currents of, 26–28, 26*t*
　of myocardial cell, 16–18, 17*f*, 18*t*, 19*f*
Sarcomeres, in contraction, 32
Sarcoplasm, of myocardial cell, 16, 17*f*

Sarcoplasmic reticulum
　calcium-ATPase pump of, in heart failure, 605, 606*f*
　of myocardial cells, 17, 17*f*
　of vascular smooth muscle, 53
Satellite DNA, 114
Scar tissue, formation of
　in myocardial infarction, 546–547
　in pericarditis, 778
S7 coronary stent, 591*f*
Scotts criteria, for left ventricular enlargement, 355*t*
SDANN (standard deviation of averages of NN intervals), in heart rate variability, 528*t*, 529, 530
SDNN (standard deviation of all NN intervals), in heart rate variability, 528*t*, 529, 530
SDNN index, in heart rate variability, 528*t*, 529
Seattle Medical Center cardiac rehabilitation protocol, 927*t*
Seldinger technique, for cardiac catheterization, 463, 464*f*, 465*f*
Selectins, as inflammatory markers, 129
Selectivity, of ion channels, 18, 21
Self-care deficit, in shock, nursing management of, 674
Self-concept
　disturbances in, after cardiac transplantation, 655*ncp*
　in history taking, 234
Self-efficacy
　in adherence, 966, 967*d*, 968
　in smoking cessation, 840
Self-monitoring
　of adherence, 966, 967*d*
　of negative reactions and responses, 831–832, 831*f*
　in weight loss, 943
Self-perception, in history taking, 234
Self-report measures, of adherence, 962–964, 963*t*
Semilunar valves. *See also* Aortic valve; Pulmonic valve
　anatomy of, 8–9
Sensing
　in implantable cardioverter defibrillation, 742–745, 745*f*
　in pacing, 711*d*, 718, 725, 726*f*, 727
　atrial, 730
　ventricular, 730
Sensing threshold, in pacing, 711*d*
Sensitivity
　of exercise testing, 452, 452*d*
　of laboratory tests, 268
Sensitivity threshold testing, in pacing, 723
Sensory/perceptual alterations, in intra-aortic balloon pump use, 682*ncp*
Septal branches, of left coronary artery, 15
Septal hypertrophy, echocardiography in, 314
Septic endarteritis, in percutaneous coronary interventions, 595
Septic shock. *See* Shock, septic
Septum (septa). *See specific septa, eg,* Intraventricular septum
Serosa layer, of pericardium, 776
Serum, definition of, 267
Sex chromosomes, 113, 113*f*
Sex hormones
　coronary artery disease and, 818–819
　heart rate variability and, 532
Sexual dysfunction, after cardiac transplantation, 650
Sexuality, in history taking, 234
Shear stress, nitric oxide release in, 55, 55*f*

Sheath removal, after percutaneous coronary interventions, 587
Shock, 659–688
　anaphylactic, pathophysiology of, 662
　blood pressure measurement in, 248
　cardiogenic
　　compensation in, 662–663
　　diagnosis of, 668–669
　　intra-aortic balloon pump for, 675
　　in myocardial infarction, 561
　　pathophysiology of, 659–661, 660*t*, 661*f*, 661*t*
　　prognosis for, 669
　　pulmonary edema in, 666
　　treatment of, 670–673, 670*f*, 671*d*, 671*t*, 672*d*
　classification of, 659
　compensatory mechanisms in, 662–666
　　clinical manifestations of, 665–666
　　in initial stage, 663–664, 663*f*
　　in intermediate stage, 664–665, 664*f*
　　in irreversible stage, 665, 665*f*
　definition of, 659
　diagnosis of, 667–669, 668*f*
　distributive
　　diagnosis of, 669
　　pathophysiology of, 660*t*, 662
　extracardiac obstructive
　　pathophysiology of, 660*t*, 662
　　treatment of, 673
　hypovolemic
　　compensation in, 662
　　diagnosis of, 669
　　pathophysiology of, 660*t*, 662
　　prognosis for, 669
　　treatment of, 673
　medical management of, 667–674
　　diagnosis in, 667–669, 668*t*
　　prognosis in, 669
　　in specific situations, 673–674
　　treatment in, 669–673, 669*t*, 670*f*, 671*d*, 671*t*, 672*d*
　neurogenic, pathophysiology of, 662
　nursing management of, 674–686
　　circulatory assist devices in. *See* Circulatory assist devices; *specific types*
　　in decreased cardiac output, 674
　　in decreased tissue perfusion, 674
　　family care in, 674
　　in self-care deficit, 674
　pathophysiology of, 659–662, 662*t*
　　cardiogenic, 659–661, 660*t*, 661*f*, 661*t*
　　distributive, 662
　　extracardiac obstructive, 662
　　hypovolemic, 662
　physical assessment in, 666–667
　prognosis for, 669
　septic
　　compensation in, 663
　　diagnosis of, 669
　　hemodynamic characteristics of, 506*t*
　　pathophysiology of, 662
　　treatment of, 673–674
　vasogenic, compensation in, 662–663
Shock liver syndrome, 641
Shock lung, 666
Shortening relation
　force-velocity, 38–39, 38*f*
　myocardial oxygen consumption and, 42
Shunting, hypoxemia in, 75
Sibutramine, for obesity, 944
Sick sinus syndrome, 378–379
Silent ischemia, 543, 550

Silver wire arteries, in retina, 238, 238*f*
Single-photon emission computed tomography, 320–321, 321*f*
  in angina, 552
  in exercise testing, 453
Sinoatrial node
  action potential of, 24–25, 25*f*
  anatomy of, 10, 11*f*
  arrhythmias originating in, 366, 376–379
  blood supply of, 13*t*, 14, 14*f*, 15
  dysfunction of
    after cardiac transplantation, 646
    pacemaker for, 710*d*
  electrophysiology studies of, 430
  function of, 326, 327
  impulse initiation in, 361–362
  Wenckebach conduction in, 411, 412*f*
Sinus arrest, 377
Sinus arrhythmia, 239–240, 376–377
  resting, 93
  in sleep, 208–209
Sinus bradycardia, 376
  after cardiac surgery, 636
  in sleep, 208–209
  in sleep apnea, 210
  treatment of, 375*t*
Sinus exit block, 377–378
Sinus node. *See* Sinoatrial node
Sinus pause, 377
Sinus rhythm, normal, 366
Sinus tachycardia, 376
Sinus venosus, in atrial septal defect, 798–799
Sirolimus
  for cardiac transplantation, 650
  in coronary stents, 591, 591*f*
Skin
  assessment of
    in heart failure, 614
    in shock, 666
  color of, assessment of, 236
  edema effects on, 250
  fragility of, from corticosteroids, 649
  temperature of, in circulation assessment, 249
  vasculature of, in blood pressure regulation, 86–87
Sleep, 197–219
  in aging, 201–202
  angina in, 208
  arrhythmias in, 208–209
  assessment of, 211, 211*t*
  in cardiac care unit, 207
  cardiac events in, 208–209
  after cardiac surgery, 207
  in cardiovascular disease, 204–205, 205*f*, 206*t*
    adverse outcomes of, 210–211
    nursing management in, 211–213, 211*t*
  cardiovascular function in, 202–203
  cerebral blood flow and metabolism in, 204
  in chronic obstructive pulmonary disease, 208
  cycle of, 201, 201*f*
  definition of, 197, 198*f*, 199*f*
  deprivation of, 204–205, 205*f*
  disordered breathing related to, 209–210, 209*f*
  disorders of, 204–205, 205*f*, 206*t*, 211–212
  disruption of, 204–205, 205*f*
  endocrine function in, 204
  function of, 202
  in health care providers, 213
  in heart failure, 207
  heart rate variability in, 533
  in history taking, 234
  in hypertension, 208
  kidney function in, 204

  laboratory testing during, 213
  loss of, physiologic effects of, 202
  measurement of, 197, 199–200, 199*t*
  physiology during, 202–204
  regulation of, 202
  respiratory function in, 203
  stages of, 200–201
  thermoregulation in, 203
Sleep apnea, 209–210, 209*f*
  coronary artery disease and, 206
  hypertension in, 862*d*, 863
Sleep hygiene, 212
Sleepiness
  definition of, 197, 198*f*, 199*f*
  excessive daytime, 205
  in heart failure, 207
  measurement of, 197, 199–200, 199*t*
Sleep rate, in pacing, 713*d*
Slow-response cells, 22, 22*f*, 22*t*, 24
Small vein filling time, in extracellular fluid deficit, 176
Smoking
  assessment of, 842, 842*d*
  as coronary artery disease risk factor, 811–812, 811*f*
  economic impact of, 838
  environmental pollution by, 812
  harmful effects of, 839
  heart rate variability and, 534
  statistics on, 811–812, 811*f*, 838
Smoking cessation, 838–855
  alcohol use and, 850, 850*f*
  benefits of, 812, 840
  clinical practice guidelines for, 841–849
    assistance for, 843–849, 845*f*, 846*f*, 848*d*
    follow-up, 849
    identification of users, 842, 842*d*
    identification of users willing to attempt, 843, 843*d*
    strong urging for, 842–843, 843*d*
  in coronary artery disease, 840–841
  depression and, 849–850
  relapse prevention in, 844–846, 845*f*
  sense of loss after, 850
  social support for, 851, 851*f*
  stress and, 849
  theoretical framework for, 840
  trends in, 841
  vulnerable populations in, 851–852
  weight gain after, 850–851
  in women, 852
Smooth muscle, vascular, 53
  adrenergic receptors in, 58–59, 59*f*
  cells of, in atherosclerotic lesions, 143
  endothelium-derived contracting factors action on, 56–58, 57*f*, 58*f*
  endothelium interaction with, 61*f*
  hypocalcemia effects on, 183
  nitric oxide action on, 55, 55*f*, 56*f*
Snoring, coronary artery disease and, 210
Social cognitive theory, adherence and, 966, 967*d*
Social history, in history taking, 232–233
Social support
  for adherence, 967*d*, 968
  in coronary artery disease, 826, 829, 833–834
  for smoking cessation, 851
Socioeconomic status, hypertension and, 860
Sodium-calcium exchange, 21–22
Sodium channels
  in action potential
    in early repolarization, 23–24, 23*f*
    in plateau, 23*f*, 24
    in upstroke, 23, 23*f*

  in automaticity, 362
  fast currents in, 27
  function of, 21
  in pacemaking, 27
Sodium chloride, excretion of, in blood pressure regulation, 95
Sodium ion
  distribution of, in myocardium, 18*t*
  equilibrium potential of, 20
  excretion of, aging effects on, 224–225
  imbalance of, 176–177, 176*t*, 177*t*
  measurement of, 286
  reabsorption of, defects of, hypertension in, 861
  restriction of, in hypertension, 871
Sodium-potassium-adenosine triphosphate pump, 21
Sotalol, for arrhythmias, 372*t*
Spasm
  coronary artery, 543
    in hypomagnesemia, 185
    in percutaneous coronary interventions, 593
    in variant angina, 208, 545, 555
  vascular, in hemostasis, 154
Specificity, of tests
  exercise, 452, 452*d*
  laboratory, 268–269
Specimens, blood. *See* Blood specimens
SPECT (single-photon emission computed tomography), 320–321, 321*f*
  in angina, 552
  in exercise testing, 453
Spectral (frequency domain) analysis, in heart rate variability, 528–529, 529*t*, 530*f*
Spectrophotometry, for oxygenation monitoring, 79
Spectroscopy, near-infrared, in tissue perfusion monitoring, 518–519, 518*t*
Sphygmomanometer, 243–246, 243*t*, 244*f*–246*f*, 245*t*
Spin-echo magnetic resonance imaging, 322–323
Spironolactone
  for heart failure, 619, 619*t*
  for hypertension, 879*t*
Spleen, ischemia of, in shock, 664, 664*f*
Splitting, of heart sounds, 253, 253*f*
Sputum, assessment of, 258
Square root hemodynamic pattern, in restrictive cardiomyopathy, 785
Squatting, heart sounds in, 257*t*, 258
Stable angina. *See* Angina, stable (classic)
Staircase phenomenon (treppe), 39, 40*f*
Standing, sudden, heart sounds in, 257*t*, 258
Stanford classification, of aortic dissection, 635–636
Starling's hypothesis of microvascular fluid exchange, 65–67, 66*f*
Starling's law of the heart. *See* Frank-Starling law of the heart
Starr-Edwards caged-ball valves, 763
Stasis, in Virchow's triad, 162, 162*f*
State-Trait Anxiety Inventory, 830
Statins, for hyperlipidemia, 911*t*, 912
Stem cells, 150, 151*f*
Stenosis. *See also specific valves,* stenosis of
  in atherosclerosis, 145–146
  definition of, 756
Stents, coronary, 589–592
  acute thrombosis of, 592
  clinical trials of, 591
  drug-eluting, 591–592, 591*f*
  history of, 590, 590*f*
  technology for, 591, 591*f*
  types of, 590, 590*f*

Sternal rise, in chest wall, 251
Stethoscope, for heart assessment, 252, 252f
Stiffness, myocardial, 38, 38f
Stimulation threshold, in pacing, 712d, 723
Stimulus control
    in adherence, 967, 967d
    in weight loss, 943
Stimulus release, in pacing, 723–724, 724f
Stomach, surgery on, for obesity, 945
Storage granules, in platelets, 153
Streptococcal infections, rheumatic heart disease
        in, 756–757, 757f
Streptokinase
    for deep vein thrombosis, 165, 165t
    for myocardial infarction, 564–566
Stress
    angina in, 551
    coronary artery disease and, 827–828
    in history taking, 234
    smoking cessation and, 849
Stress echocardiography, 309–311, 454
Stress myocardial perfusion imaging, 320–322,
        320f–322f
Stroke
    creatine kinase-BB in, 273
    genetic factors in, 115–116
    heart rate variability in, 535
    in hypertension, 867
    in percutaneous coronary interventions,
        594, 598
    postoperative, 641
    in shock, 666
Stroke volume
    in cardiac output, 93
    definition of, 35
    variation in, 502t, 503
ST segment, 328, 329t
    in exercise testing, 448–449, 448f, 449f
    in myocardial infarction, 345–346, 348f–350f,
        568–569, 568f
    in myocardial ischemia, 342, 347f
    in ventricular enlargement, 352, 355f
Subjective measurement, of sleep, 199, 199t
Sublingual capnography, for oxygenation
        monitoring, 517–518
Submaximal exercise testing, 444–445
Sudden cardiac death. See also Cardiac arrest
    in aortic stenosis, 82–83
    definition of, 689
    in dilated cardiomyopathy, 783
    genetic factors in, 116
    heart rate variability in, 531
    in hypertrophic cardiomyopathy, 784–785
    implantable cardioverter defibrillator use after,
        740–741
    incidence of, 689
    instantaneous, 689
    in sleep, 209
    in stress, 827
Sudden infant death syndrome, position and, 533
Sulfonylureas, for diabetes mellitus, 956–957
Summation gallop, in heart sounds, 254, 254f
Superoxide anions, as vasoconstrictors, 58, 58f
Supply ischemia, 541, 542f
Support system, in history taking, 233
Supraventricular arrhythmias, in myocardial
        infarction, 562
Supraventricular tachycardia, 383, 394–398,
        397f–399f
    electrophysiology studies in, 428–429, 428d
    treatment of, 699, 699d, 700f–702f, 703
Surgeon General's Report on Physical Activity and
        Health (1996), 919

Surgery
    bariatric, for obesity, 945
    cardiac. See Cardiac surgery; specific procedures
    pacemaker function during, 721–722
Sutter valves, 763
SvO2. See Mixed venous oxygen saturation (SvO2)
S wave, 329t
Sympathetic nervous system
    in blood pressure regulation, 84, 86, 86t,
        102–103, 103f
    of heart, 16
    in heart rate control, 92
    heart rate variability and, 526
    stimulation of, in heart failure, 608
Syncope
    in aortic stenosis, 771–772
    electrophysiology studies in, 429–430, 429d
    in hypertrophic cardiomyopathy, 784
    in postural hypotension, 247
    in pulmonary embolism, 167
    of unknown origin, implantable cardioverter
        defibrillator for, 741
    vasovagal, 81–83, 83f
Systemic inflammatory response syndrome, in
        shock, 666
Systemic lupus erythematosus
    facial characteristics in, 236
    pericarditis in, 777
Systemic vascular resistance
    vs. afterload, 93–94
    in blood pressure calculation, 63–64
    calculation of, 63
    in hypertension, 860
    in mean arterial pressure calculation, 486
    in shock, 660t, 668
Systole
    auscultation of, 252, 253, 255, 255f
    coronary blood flow and, 42, 42f
    heart sounds in, 255, 255f
    ventricular, 44–46, 44f, 45f
Systolic blood pressure, 64, 64f
    vs. respiration, 501–502, 502f, 502t
Systolic cardiac reserve, 40, 40f
Systolic clicks, 255, 255f
Systolic dysfunction, in heart failure, 602–603,
        610, 614
    treatment of, 616–617, 616t, 617t

T

Tachyarrhythmias
    in myocardial infarction, 562
    postoperative, 638–639
Tachycardia(s)
    antidromic atrioventricular reentry, 397, 399f
    atrial. See Atrial tachycardia
    atrioventricular nodal reentrant. See
        Atrioventricular nodal reentrant
        tachycardia
    differential diagnosis of, 401–408,
        402f–410f, 402t
    endless loop, 712d, 731–732, 733f
    junctional, 384
    in myocardial infarction, 557
    pacemaker mediated, 712d, 731–732, 733f
    in pulmonary embolism, 167
    sinus, 376
    supraventricular. See Supraventricular
        tachycardia
    ventricular. See Ventricular tachycardia
Tachypnea, 258, 260f
Tacrolimus, for cardiac transplantation, 648t, 649
Tai chi, for cardiovascular disease, 982

Tamponade. See Cardiac tamponade; Pericardial
        tamponade
TARP (total atrial refractory period), in pacing,
        713d, 727
Technetium 99m compounds, in myocardial
        perfusion imaging, 319, 320
    in exercise testing, 453
    in myocardial infarction, 559–560
Telmisartan, for hypertension, 879t
Temperature
    body, measurement of, 236
    skin, in circulation assessment, 249
Tenecteplase, for myocardial infarction, 564–565
Terazosin, for hypertension, 878t
Terminalia arjuna tree bark, for cardiovascular
        disease, 979
Tetralogy of Fallot, 800
Thallium 201, in myocardial perfusion imaging,
        319–321, 453
Thebesian veins, 15–16, 16f
Therapeutic lifestyle changes, for hyperlipidemia,
        904t, 906–907, 907t
Therapeutic relationship, for adherence, 970–971
Therapeutic touch, for cardiovascular disease,
        982, 982f
Thermodilution method, for cardiac output
        measurement, 469, 503–505,
        504d, 505d
    pulse contour, 509, 509f
    transpulmonary, 508, 508t
Thermoregulation
    cutaneous vasculature and, 86–87
    sleep and, 202, 203
Thiazolidinediones, for diabetes mellitus,
        958–959
Thick filaments, in contraction, 33, 34f, 37, 37f
Thigh, blood pressure measurement in, 248–249
Thin filaments, in contraction, 33, 35f, 37, 37f
Thirst, 173–174
Thoracotomy, for minimally invasive coronary
        artery bypass, 633
Thoratec ventricular assist device, 685, 685f
Three-dimensional echocardiography, 317–318
Thrills, in heart palpation, 251
Thrombectomy, angiojet, 589
Thrombin, formation of, in disseminated
        intravascular coagulation, 160
Thrombin time (TT), 157t, 284–285
Thrombocyte(s). See Platelet(s)
Thrombocytopenia, 283
    heparin-induced, 169–171, 169f, 170t
Thrombolytic therapy
    creatine kinase after, 274
    for deep vein thrombosis, 164–165, 165t
    fibrinogen measurement in, 284
    fibrin selective, 564
    for myocardial infarction, 562, 564–568
        agents for, 564–565
        contraindications to, 565t
        outcome of, 565–566
        patient selection for, 565, 565t
    nonselective, 564
Thrombomodulin, 154
Thrombophlebitis, assessment of, 250
Thromboplastin, in disseminated intravascular
        coagulation, 158–159
Thrombopoietin, 153
Thrombosis
    arterial, in heparin-induced thrombocytopenia,
        170, 170t
    coronary, pathogenesis of, 543
    coronary stent, 592
    deep vein. See Deep vein thrombosis

Thrombosis *(continued)*
  femoral artery, in percutaneous coronary
      interventions, 594
  in heparin-induced thrombocytopenia,
      169–171, 169f, 170t
  after percutaneous coronary interventions, 592
  from prosthetic valves, 765
  risk factors for, 162, 162f
Thromboxane A$_2$, as vasoconstrictor, 54f, 57–58
Thrombus(i)
  in atherosclerotic lesions, 142, 145
  definition of, 162
  formation of, 162–163, 162f
Ticlopidine
  for heart failure, 618
  for percutaneous coronary interventions,
      595–596
Tidal volume (VT), 73
Tight junctions, in endothelium, 51
Tilting-disk prosthetic valves, 763, 763f
Tilt test, in syncope, 430
Time domain analysis, in heart rate variability,
      528–529, 528t
Timolol, for hypertension, 878t
Tirofiban, for myocardial infarction, 575–576
  for percutaneous coronary interventions, 596
Tissue factor, in disseminated intravascular
      coagulation, 158
Tissue perfusion. *See* Perfusion
Tissue plasminogen activator, 155, 165, 165t
Tissue pressure hypothesis, of blood flow
      autoregulation, 98
Tissue prosthetic valves, 763–764, 763f, 764f
Tissue-type plasminogen activator, for myocardial
      infarction, 564–566
T lymphocytes, 151f, 152–153, 153t
  in atherosclerotic lesions, 143–144
  count of, 282
Tobacco smoking. *See* Smoking
Tocainide, for arrhythmias, 372t
Tonic rapid eye movement sleep, 201
Tonic smooth muscle, 53
Tonometry, gastric, for oxygenation monitoring,
      79, 517
Topiramate, for obesity, 944
Torsades de pointes, 399–401, 400f, 401f
Torsemide, for hypertension, 878t
Total atrial refractory period (TARP), in pacing,
      713d, 727
Touch, therapeutic, for cardiovascular disease,
      982, 982f
Tourniquet, in blood specimen collection,
      265–266
Tracheostomy tube, radiographic appearance
      of, 299t
Traditional Chinese medicine, 976, 976f–978f
Training, for disease management, 992
Trandoapril, for hypertension, 879t
Transcellular fluid, 173
Transcendental meditation, 832, 832d
Transcription, of genes, 111
Transcutaneous monitoring
  of blood gases, 79
  of tissue oxygenation, 519
Transcutaneous pacing, 375t, 714, 714f
Transducers, in echocardiography, 308, 308f
Transesophageal Doppler ultrasonography, for
      cardiac output measurement, 509–510,
      510f, 511t
Transesophageal echocardiography, 311–312,
      510–511
  in cardiac output measurement, 510–511
  in endocarditis, 758, 758f

in mitral regurgitation, 767
in mitral valve prolapse, 769
in pericarditis, 778
Transfusions
  after cardiac surgery, 636
  for disseminated intravascular coagulation,
      161–162, 161t
  hyperkalemia due to, 181
  hypocalcemia due to, 182
  for hypovolemic shock, 673
Transient diastolic inward current, 27
Transient outward current, 27
Transitional atherosclerotic lesions, 141, 147t
Translation, of genes, 111
Transluminal coronary angioplasty, percutaneous,
      587–588, 588f
Transmyocardial laser revascularization, 634
Transplantation, cardiac. *See* Cardiac
      transplantation
Transposition of great arteries, 796f, 802–803
Transpulmonary indicator dilution method, for
      cardiac output measurement, 508, 508t
Transseptal approach, to cardiac catheterization,
      465–466, 466f
Transtheoretical Model, for smoking cessation, 840
Transthoracic echocardiography, 308–309,
      308f–313f
Transthoracic impedance, in defibrillation,
      693–694
Transvenous pacing, 375t, 713–714, 713f,
      718–719, 720f
Treadmill, for exercise testing, 442–444
*Treating Tobacco Use and Dependence: Clinical
      Practice Guideline*, 841–849
Treppe, 39, 40f
Triamterene, for hypertension, 878t
Tricuspid valve
  anatomy of, 6, 6f, 8
  atresia of, 801, 801t
  cardiac cycle and, 44f, 46
  conduction system to, 11, 12f
  disease of, facial characteristics in, 236
  displacement of, in Ebstein anomaly, 800–801
  echocardiography of, 316
  function of, 8, 8f
  heart sounds and, 44f, 46
  regurgitation of, 761–762, 762f
  stenosis of, 762
Trifascicular blocks, pacemaker for, 710d
Triggered beats, 363
Triglycerides
  excess of, 900t, 901, 902d, 902t
  functions of, 897
  measurement of, 276–278, 278t
  normal level of, 901, 902d
Tropomyosin, in contraction, 33–34, 35f
Troponins, 269–271, 270f, 270t, 271t
  in contraction, 33–34, 35f
  in myocardial infarction, 546, 559
True aneurysms, left ventricular, 560
Truncus arteriosus, 801–802
T-tubule system, of myocardial cells, 17, 17f
Tube(s)
  chest, radiographic appearance of, 299t
  radiographic appearance of, 297, 299f–302f,
      299t
Tuberculosis, pericarditis in, 778
Tumor, of heart, echocardiography in, 317
Tumor necrosis factor alpha
  in atherosclerotic lesions, 143
  as inflammatory marker, 133–134
Tunica adventitia, 49, 50f
Tunica intima, 49, 50f

Tunica media, of blood vessels, 49, 50f
T wave, 327, 328f, 329t
  in myocardial ischemia, 342, 344, 347f
  in ventricular enlargement, 352
Twiddler syndrome, 738
Two-dimensional echocardiography, 309,
      310f–313f
Two-Process Model of Sleep Regulation,
      202, 202f
Type A behavior, coronary artery disease and,
      827, 834

U

Ulnar nerve injury, in cardiac surgery, 641
Ulnar pulse, assessment of, 241, 241f
Ultrafiltration, in microcirculation, 65–67, 66f
Ultrasonography. *See also* Echocardiography
  in atherosclerosis, 143t
  in deep vein thrombosis, 164
  Doppler, for cardiac output measurement,
      509–510, 510f, 511t
  intravascular, in percutaneous coronary
      interventions, 595, 595f
Undersensing, in pacing, 712d, 725, 726f
Unipolar leads
  in electrocardiography, 332, 332f
  in pacing, 712d, 716, 719f
United States Pharmacopoeia, herbal remedies
      in, 980
Universal precautions, for blood specimen
      collection, 265
Upper airway resistance, coronary artery disease
      and, 210
Upper rate limit, in pacing, 712d, 730–731,
      731f, 732f
Upstroke, of action potential, 23, 23f
Urea nitrogen, measurement of, 290
Uremic pericarditis, 777–778
Uric acid, measurement of, 290
Urinary output, measurement of, after cardiac
      catheterization, 474
Urine, formation of, 174
Urine output, in shock, 667
Urokinase, 155, 165, 165t
U wave, 327–328

V

Vagal stimulation
  in heart rate control, 92
  in wide QRS complex rhythms, 407–408, 410f
Vagus nerve, in heart innervation, 16
Valsalva maneuver
  avoidance of, in myocardial infarction, 571
  heart sounds in, 257–258, 257t
  hemodynamic response to, 102, 102f
  in wide QRS complex rhythms, 407–408, 410f
Valsartan
  for heart failure, 619t
  for hypertension, 879t
Values, in history taking, 234
Valves
  cardiac. *See also specific valves*
    anatomy of, 6f, 8–9
    cardiac cycle and, 44f, 46
    conduction system to, 11, 12f
    disease of. *See* Valvular heart disease; *specific
        disorders*
    prosthetic. *See* Prosthetic valves
    repair of, 634
    replacement of, 634–635
  venous, 51–52

Valvular heart disease, 756–775. *See also specific valves*
  cardiac arrest in, 690
  cardiac catheterization in, 459
  causes of, 756–759
  infectious endocarditis, 757–758, 757*t*, 758*d*, 758*t*
  rheumatic heart disease, 756–757, 757*f*
  classification of, 756
  congenital, 794–797, 796*f*, 800–801, 801*t*
  definition of, 756
  diagnosis of, 759
  epidemiology of, 756
  postoperative care in, 636
  repair in, 634
  replacement in, 634–635. *See also* Prosthetic valves
  in endocarditis, 789
  shock in, 673
Valvuloplasty
  for aortic stenosis, 771–772
  for mitral regurgitation, 768
  for mitral stenosis, 760–761, 761*f*
Variant angina, 208, 555, 545
Varicose veins, 250
Vascular adhesion molecule I, as inflammatory marker, 129
Vascular closure devices, after percutaneous coronary interventions, 587
Vascular resistance. *See also* Systemic vascular resistance
  in afterload, 36
  as blood flow determinant, 63
  in blood pressure regulation, 95–96, 95*f*
  respiratory acidosis effects on, 192
  in venous system, 64
  vs. vessel diameter, 62, 62*f*
Vascular system. *See also components, eg,* Artery(ies); Vein(s)
  acid-base imbalance effects on, 193*t*
  arterial, 49–50, 50*f*, 63–64, 64*f*
  blood flow in. *See* Blood flow
  circulation in. *See* Circulation
  classification of, 49, 50*f*
  cutaneous, in blood pressure regulation, 86–87
  diabetes mellitus effects on, 951–952
  fluid in, 174
  hypercalcemia effects on, 183
  hyperkalemia effects on, 182
  hypermagnesemia effects on, 185
  hypocalcemia effects on, 183
  hypokalemia effects on, 180
  hypomagnesemia effects on, 185
  hypophosphatemia effects on, 186
  injury of
    by intra-aortic balloon pump, 679
    in Virchow's triad, 162, 162*f*
  layers of, 49, 50*f*
  lymphatic drainage in. *See* Lymphatic system
  microcirculation in, 50–51, 65–67, 66*f*
  neurohumoral stimulation of, 58–60, 59*f*, 60*f*
  peripheral, assessment of, 249–250
  resistance in. *See* Systemic vascular resistance; Vascular resistance
  respiratory acidosis effects on, 192
  spasm of, in hemostasis, 154
  structure of, 49–53, 50*f*, 52*f*
    arteries, 49–50, 50*f*
    lymphatics, 52–53, 52*f*
    microvascular bed, 50–51
    smooth muscle, 53
    veins, 51–52
    venules, 51

sympathetic stimulation of, 86
  venous, 51–52, 64–65
  volume distribution of, 61, 62*f*
Vasculitis, pericarditis in, 776–777
Vasculopathy, transplant, 650
Vasoactive intestinal peptide, in blood pressure regulation, 89
Vasoactive substances. *See also* Vasoconstriction; Vasodilation; *specific substances*
  endothelium-derived, 53–58, 53*t*, 54*f*-58*f*, 54*t*
  in oxygen delivery-oxygen consumption balance, 78
Vasoconstriction, 52
  active, 96
  adrenergic receptors in, 58–59
  antidiuretic hormone in, 90, 90*f*
  in atherosclerosis, 541
  baroreflexes in, 87
  in blood pressure regulation, 95–96, 95*f*
  compensatory, 66–67, 66*f*
  in cutaneous vasculature, 86–87
  endothelium-derived contracting factors in, 56–58, 57*f*, 58*f*
  in heart failure, 607–608, 610*f*
  in hemostasis, 154
  intracellular signals for, 60, 60*f*
  passive, 96
  in pulmonary circulation, 72
  in respiratory alkalosis, 194
  in ventilation-perfusion matching, 74
Vasodilation
  active, 96
  adrenergic receptors in, 59, 59*f*
  arterial pressure wave in, 486, 486*f*
  in blood pressure regulation, 95–96, 95*f*
  cerebral, in respiratory acidosis, 192
  in cutaneous vasculature, 86–87
  distributive shock in, 662
  endothelium-derived relaxing factors, 53–56, 54*f*-56*f*, 54*t*
  intracellular signals for, 59–60
  local metabolic factors in, 58, 58*f*
  mechanisms of, 59, 59*f*
  passive, 86, 96
  in pulmonary circulation, 72
  in ventilation-perfusion matching, 74
Vasodilators
  for heart failure, 620–621, 672, 672*d*
  for hypertension, 878*t*, 882*t*
  for shock, 672, 672*d*
Vasopressin. *See* Antidiuretic hormone (ADH)
Vasopressors
  for septic shock, 673
  for shock, 669, 669*t*
Vasovagal reaction, in percutaneous coronary interventions, 593
Vasovagal syncope, 81–83, 83*f*
Vegetations, in endocarditis, 787, 788
Vein(s)
  blood volume in, 61, 62*f*
  catheters in, blood drawing from, 483
  compliance of, 65
  coronary, 13*f*, 14*f*, 15–16, 16*f*
  dilators for, 621
  structure of, 50*f*, 51–52
  varicose, 250
  vascular resistance in, 61, 62*f*
Venography, in deep vein thrombosis, 164
Venous banking, in retina, 238, 238*f*
Venous insufficiency, chronic, 250
Venous pressure, 64
  in lung zones, 73–74, 73*f*
  neurohumoral effects on, 98–99, 99*f*

Venous stasis, in Virchow's triad, 162, 162*f*
Venous system
  circulation in, assessment of, 250
  neurohumoral stimulation of, 98–99, 99*f*
  physiology of, 64–65
Venous thrombosis, deep. *See* Deep vein thrombosis
Ventilation, 72. *See also* Respiration
  acid excretion in, 190, 191*t*
  mechanical. *See* Mechanical ventilation
  pulmonary arterial pressure variation in, 496
Ventilation-perfusion matching, 74
Ventilation-perfusion mismatching, in pulmonary embolism, 167, 168
Ventricle(s)
  anatomy of, 3, 4*f*, 5*f*, 6–8, 7*f*, 8*f*
  arrhythmias originating in, 384–388
  blood supply of, 13*t*, 14–15
  conduction in, 30–31, 30*t*, 31*f*
  contraction of, isovolumic, 44–45, 44*f*
  ejection from, afterload and, 39
  enlargement of, electrocardiography in, 351–352, 354*f*-356*f*, 355*t*, 356*d*
  function of, 7, 7*f*, 8*f*, 454
  hypertrophy of, oxygen supply and, 43
  innervation of, 16
  left
    aneurysms of, in myocardial infarction, 560
    cardiac cycle and, 44–46, 44*f*, 45*t*
    in Ebstein anomaly, 800–801
    echocardiography of, 310*f*, 312, 313*f*
    enlargement of, electrocardiography in, 351–352, 355*f*, 355*t*
    failure of, 602, 611–612
      hemodynamic characteristics of, 506*t*
      in myocardial infarction, 560–561
    filling of, in heart failure, 605–606, 606*f*, 607*f*
    hypertrophy of
      cardiac arrest in, 690
      in hypertension, 865
    outflow obstruction of, in aortic stenosis, 796–797, 796*f*
    topographic location of, 250
    workload of, in shock, 672–673, 672*d*
  muscle fibers of, 9, 9*f*, 10*f*
  remodeling of, after myocardial infarction, 546–547
  right
    cardiac cycle and, 44*f*, 46
    echocardiography of, 313*f*, 314
    enlargement of, electrocardiography in, 352, 356*f*, 356*t*
    failure of, 602, 612
    hypertrophy of, in tetralogy of Fallot, 800
    infarction of. *See* Myocardial infarction, right ventricular
    outflow obstruction in, 794–796, 796*f*
    topographic location of, 250
    volumetric measures of, 499–500, 499*t*, 500*f*
    rupture of, in myocardial infarction, 546, 561
Ventricular arrhythmias
  in cardiac catheterization, 472
  from pacemakers, 738
  in sleep, 209
Ventricular assist devices. *See* Left ventricular assist devices
Ventricular asystole, 387–388
Ventricular branches, of right coronary artery, 14
Ventricular dysynchrony, 735
Ventricular ejection, 44*f*, 45

Ventricular fibrillation, 387
  cardiac arrest in, 691
  defibrillation of, 691–695, 694*f*, 695*f*
  implantable cardioverter defibrillators for,
    746, 746*f*
  postoperative, 639–640
  prognosis for, 704
Ventricular flutter, 387
Ventricular function curves, 505
Ventricular parasystole, 419, 419*f*
Ventricular refractory period, in pacing,
    713*d*, 727
Ventricular relaxation, isovolumic, 44*f*, 45
Ventricular sensing, in pacing, 730
Ventricular septum. *See* Intraventricular septum
Ventricular tachyarrhythmias, in myocardial
    infarction, 562
Ventricular tachycardia, 386–387, 398–401
  bidirectional, 386
  blood pressure measurement in, 248
  classification of, 386
  defibrillation of, 691–695, 694*f*, 695*f*
  electrophysiology studies in, 426
  in exercise testing, 450
  implantable cardioverter defibrillators for, 741,
    746–747, 747*f*
  monomorphic, 386, 398–399, 399*f*
  nonsustained, 386
  polymorphic, 386, 399, 400*f*
  postoperative, 639–640
  prognosis for, 704
  pulseless, treatment of, 698, 698*d*
  radiofrequency catheter ablation for,
    432*d*, 435
  sustained, 386, 741
  torsades de pointes in, 399–401, 400*f*, 401*f*
  treatment of, 373*t*–374*t*, 699, 699*d*,
    700*f*–702*f*, 703
Ventricular tracking limit, in pacing, 712*d*
Ventriculography, 319–320, 320*f*, 466–467 ,
    467*f*
Ventriculoplasty, reduction
  for dilated cardiomyopathy, 783
  for heart failure, 635
Venules, structure of, 50*f*, 51
Verapamil
  for arrhythmias, 372*t*, 373*t*
  for hypertension, 879*t*
Very-low-density lipoproteins. *See under*
    Lipoprotein(s)
Vicious cycle, of overloaded heart, 610, 611*f*
Viral infections
  myocarditis in, 786, 786*d*
  pericarditis in, 777–778, 779*f*

Virchow's triad, 162, 162*f*
Visceral pericardium (epipericardium), 776
Vision, assessment of, 236
Vitamin B$_6$, for homocysteinemia, 132
Vitamin B$_{12}$, for homocysteinemia, 132
Vitamin C, coronary artery disease and, 820
Vitamin E, coronary artery disease and, 820
VLDL. *See* Lipoprotein(s), very-low-density
V$_{max}$ (maximal velocity of depolarization), 23
VO$_2$. *See* Oxygen consumption (VO$_2$)
Voice sounds, transmitted through chest wall, 261
Volume overload, from contrast agents, 594
von Willebrand factor, as inflammatory marker, 134
v wave, in pulmonary artery wedge pressure,
    494, 496*f*

W

Waist (abdominal) circumference, measurement
    of, 938, 940*f*
Waking
  heart rate variability in, 533
  regulation of, 202
Wallstent, 590
Wandering atrial pacemaker, 379
Warfarin
  for deep vein thrombosis, 164, 165*t*
  for heart failure, 618
  monitoring of, 284, 285
  for myocardial infarction, 576
  for percutaneous coronary interventions, 596
Warming, in cardiopulmonary bypass
    discontinuation, 630
Water
  body. *See also* Body fluids; Fluid balance; Fluid
      imbalances
    amount of, 173
    excretion of, in blood pressure regulation, 95
Water-hammer pulse, 487
Wavelet Dynamic Discrimination Criterion, for
    implantable cardioverter
    defibrillators, 745
Weakness, in heart failure, 611
Weight
  control of
    in hyperlipidemia, 908
    in hypertension, 870–871
  excess. *See* Obesity
  gain of, in smoking cessation, 850–851
  measurement of, 235–236
  normal, 938

Wellens syndrome, electrocardiography in,
    356, 359*f*
Wenckebach conduction
  alternating, 414, 415*f*
  atrioventricular, 408–410, 410*f*–412*f*
  in bundle branches, 412, 413*f*
  with exit block from ectopic focus, 413,
    414*f*, 415*f*
  in reentrant pathways, 412–413, 414*f*
  sinoatrial, 411, 412*f*
Wenckebach upper-rate response, in pacing,
    730, 731*f*
West zones, in lung, 73–74, 73*f*
Wheezes, 261, 262*f*
White blood cell(s), 151*f*, 152–153, 153*t*
  count of, 282
Wide-complex tachycardias, electrophysiology
    studies in, 428–429, 428*d*
Windkessel effect, 49, 484
Wolff-Parkinson-White syndrome, 392–393,
    393*f*–395*f*
  cardiac arrest in, 691
  radiofrequency catheter ablation for, 432*d*,
    433–434
Women
  exercise testing in, 455
  hypertension in, 859
  smoking cessation in, 852
World Health Organization, hypertension
    guidelines of, 856–857, 857*t*
Worry, control of, 833
Wound infection, postoperative, 641

X

Xanthelasmas, 236, 237*f*, 905
Xanthomas, in coronary artery disease, 120
X-rays, principles of, 296–297, 297*f*

Y

Yin-yang symbol, in Chinese medicine, 976, 976*f*
Yoga, 978, 978*f*

Z

Zeroing, in hemodynamic monitoring, 479–480,
    481*d*–482*d*

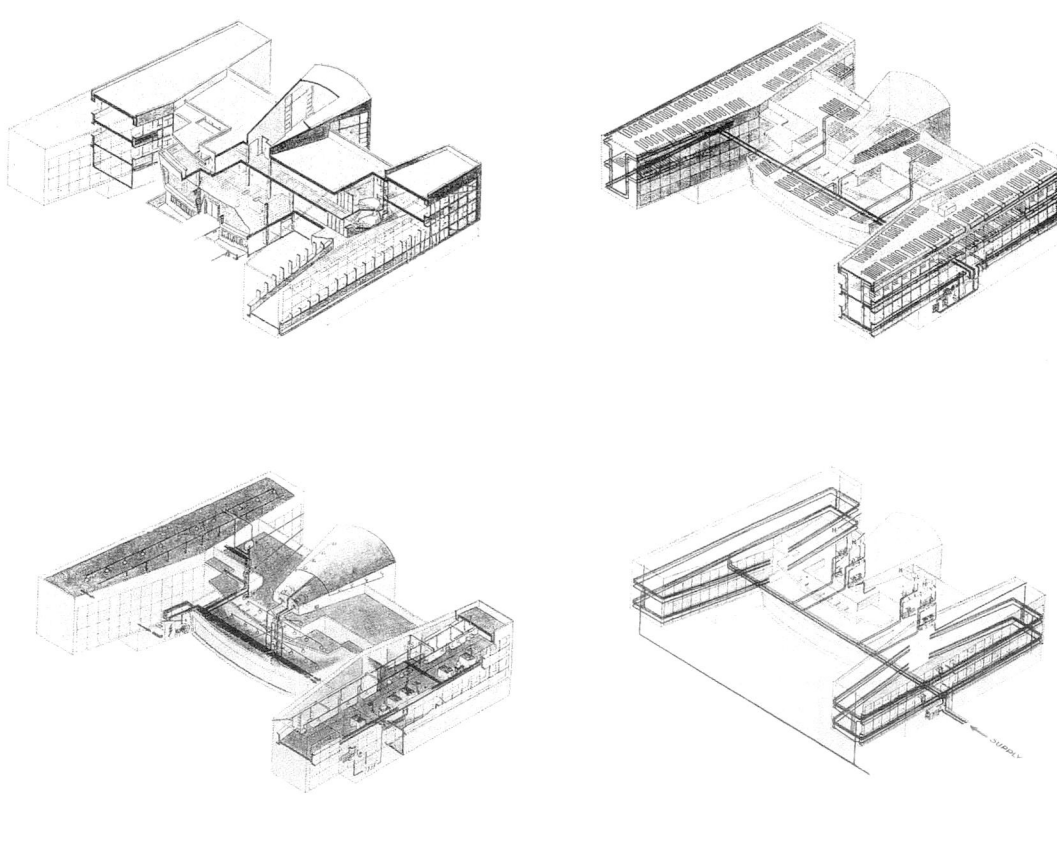

apparatus of heating, ventilation and artificial lighting.

Le Corbusier directly addressed this question in some of his early 'white' villas. In the living room of the Villa Savoye, for example, the purpose-made linear light fitting became a key element of the composition, and no attempt was made to conceal the cast-iron radiators beneath the wide sills of the fenêtre en longueur (fig. 17). At the Cité de Refuge, however, while artificial light fittings were conspicuous in all the main spaces, the elaborate original systems for heating and ventilation were much more discreetly accommodated (fig. 18). Careful provision was made in the plan for the vertical ducts, but these were not visibly expressed as such.

In *The Architecture of the Well-tempered Environment*, Reyner Banham identifies two approaches to the physical incorporation of plant and services into the fabric of a building: 'concealed power' and 'exposed power'. Many important developments occurred in the technologies of environmental control, particularly in the mechanisms of refrigeration and air-conditioning, but Banham suggests that the predominant approach to the physical incorporation of services systems in the buildings of the Modern Movement was their concealment rather than their expression.

A particularly sophisticated relationship between engineering and architectural intention was achieved in the 1930s through the collaboration of Berthold Lubetkin and a group of consultant engineers.[21] At the Highpoint apartment buildings in

fig. 22 Le Corbusier, Unité d'Habitation, Marseilles, 1947-1952, sol artificiel; after Le Corbusier, *Oeuvre Complet.*

fig. 23: Le Corbusier, Unité d'Habitation, Marseilles, 1947-1952, cheminée de ventilation; after Le Corbusier, *Oeuvre Complet.*

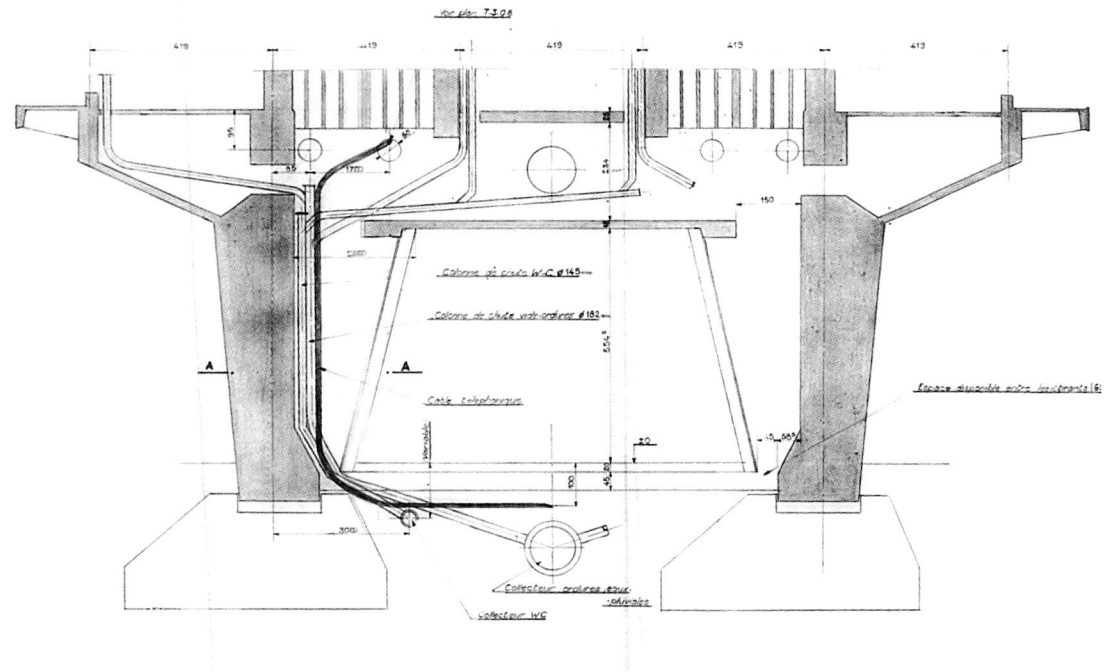

Highgate, north London, and at the Finsbury Health Centre, Lubetkin worked with the structural engineer Ove N. Arup and the services engineers G. N. Haden & Sons. The consultants were involved from the inception of each design, and as a result the architecture, structural design and environmental services achieved a high degree of integration.

The environmental emphasis at Highpoint was on the Modernist virtues of natural light and fresh air, but, in addition to large windows and planning for cross-ventilation, the apartments were equipped with concealed radiant ceiling heating providing, as Lubetkin stated, 'pleasant heat with no draughts. Air not stuffy.' All the plumbing was located in accessible ducts, as were the extensive electrical services (fig. 19). The Finsbury Health Centre had a more demanding environmental programme than Highpoint, and the integration of the services systems within the structure was realized in total accord with the functional and architectural intentions. Four distinct but interconnected technical systems were defined: the construction system, the heating system, the electrical system and the plumbing system (fig. 20). The primary service runs for each system were located within a void formed between the main structural beams and the curtain walling. From this position they were fed into the building (fig. 21).

The development of the independent structural frame, curtain wall and suspended ceiling as the kit from which buildings for many purposes could be made allowed the concealment of extensive plant in

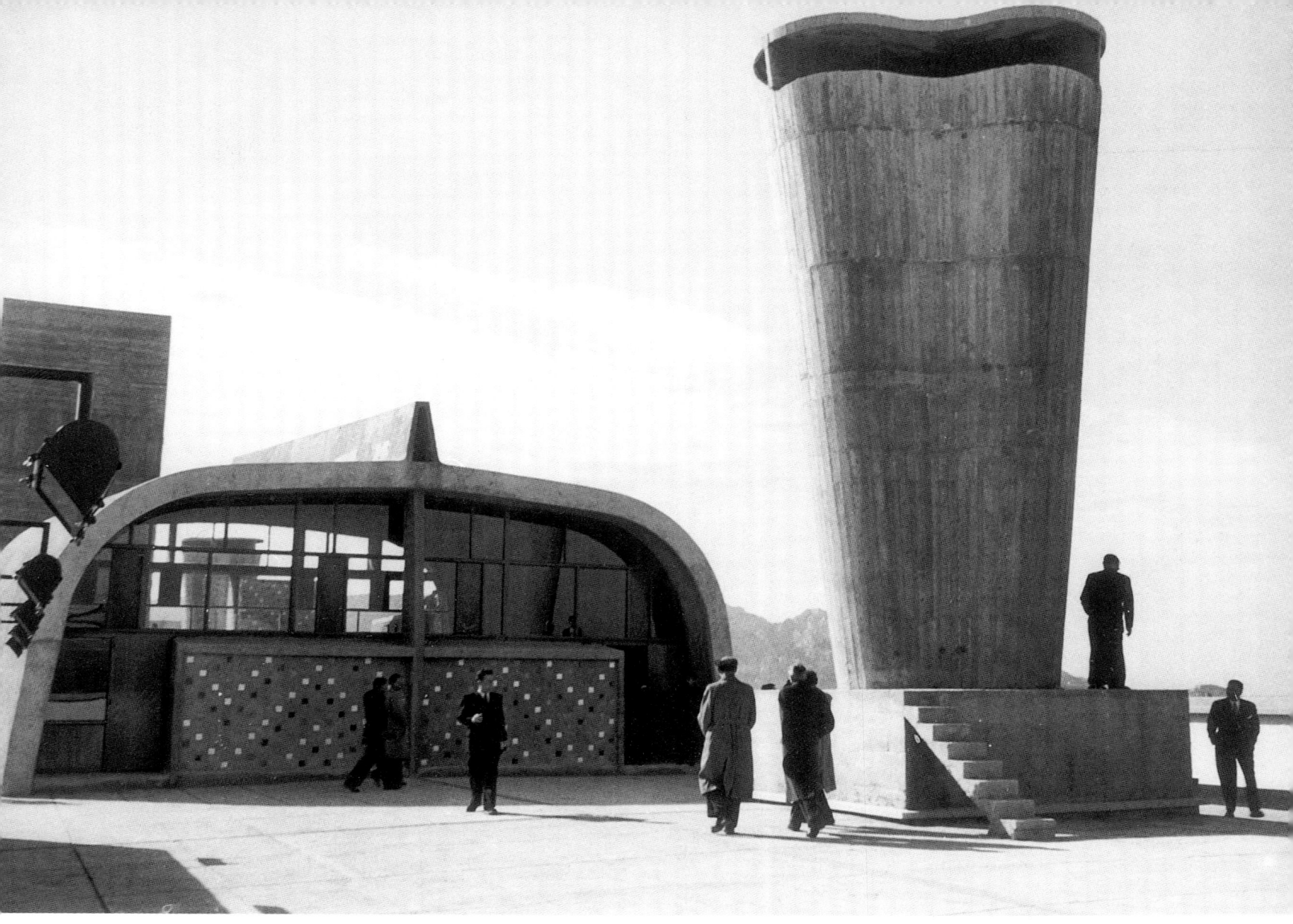

deep ceiling voids. While this kit-of-parts became the 'vernacular architecture' of corporate 20th-century culture, it has its origins in the works of Mies van der Rohe. But, as Kenneth Frampton shows in *Studies in Tectonic Culture*, the tectonic was, for Mies, not an end in itself, but the instrument through which he might seek 'the embodiment of the spirit in the banality of the real'.[22] The suspended ceiling was not merely a convenient covering for the service mechanisms in the void above but became a representation of 'abstract materiality'

in contradiction of the actual materiality of his structures and the natural materials of his floors. This was further sustained by Mies's open embrace of the idea of concealed power. Frampton writes, 'Mies recognised modern technology as a dichotomous destiny that was at once both destroyer and provider. He saw it as the apocalyptic demiurge of the new era and as the inescapable matrix of the modern world.'

If you look at the collage of the interior of the project for a Museum for a Small City (1943), you may deduce

that the shadowless uniformity of the visual field is the product of an even distribution of artificial illumination issuing from a diffusing ceiling. This is intended not as a night-time substitute for natural light but as the primary light source at all times of day or night. The heating also issues, silently and continuously, from concealed outlets in the ceiling and, perhaps, from other elements of the building fabric. Exactly this effect was anticipated in the silk exhibition that Mies designed in colla-boration with Lily Reich at the German section of the Barcelona International

↓

fig. 24: Marco
Zanusso, Olivetti
Factory, Argentina,
1964, cut-away
perspective showing
relation of structure
and mechanical plant;
after Banham.

1 Exposed end of
  hollow concrete
  beam
2 Main roof structure
3 Air conditioner unit
  attached to end of
  hollow-beam duct
4 Monitor lights
  in roof

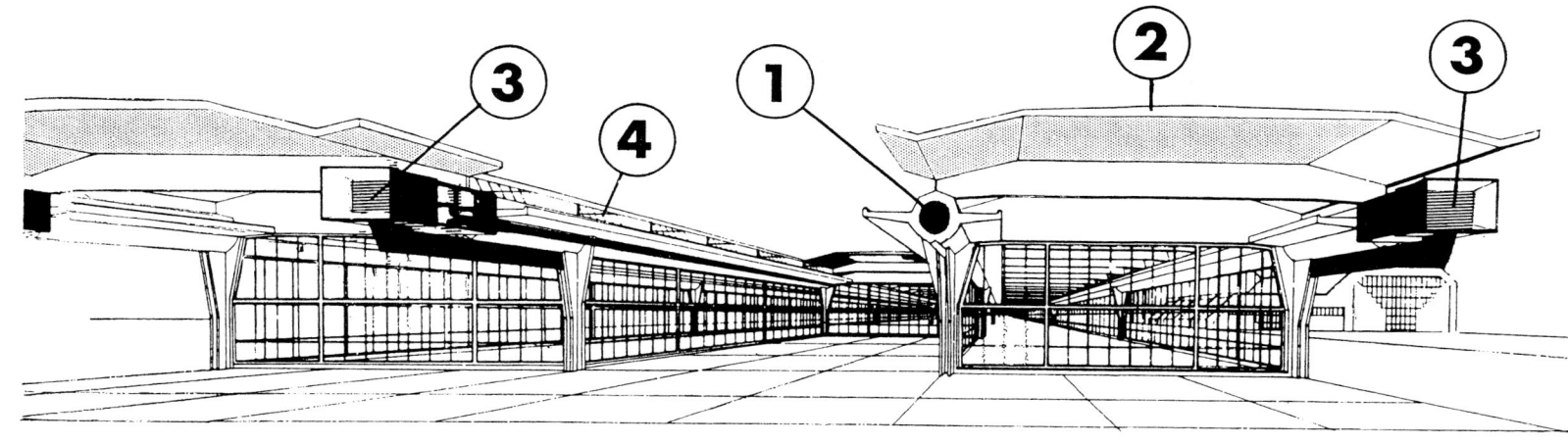

Exposition in 1929. In Mies's built projects during his mature period from the early 1940s, it can be seen how this environmental complement to his tectonic visions was brought to masterly realization. At the IIT campus in Chicago, particularly in the central buildings such as Crown Hall (1956), at the National Gallery in Berlin (1958) and, perhaps most influential of all, at the Seagram Building in New York (1958), this vision of the seamless, imperceptible, but 'ideal' environment, invisibly supplied, is brought to complete realization.

Banham argues that the invisibly serviced glass enclosure satisfied a primary aesthetic objective of the Modern Movement. On the other hand, it contradicted the 'moral imperative' that the functions and elements of a building should be given honest expression. In the years after the Second World War this position was challenged by designs such as Le Corbusier's Unité d'Habitation at Marseilles. There the extensive services networks were gathered and organized sectionally in the sol artificiel, poised over the piloti

(fig. 22), and the air extract ducts were given sculptural form in the playful composition of the roof terrace (fig. 23). Other architects began to explore ways to express the new relationship between structure and services. Banham illustrates Marco Zanusso's Olivetti Factory in Argentina (1964), with its exposed air-conditioning units plugged directly into hollow tubular roof beams (fig. 24). Here the extensive roof of the single-storey building becomes a combined structural and environmental canopy over the production space. In Rome,

fig. 25: Franco Albini,
Rinascente department
store, Rome, 1961, cut-
away axonometric
showing services ducts
integrated into façade;
after Banham.

1 Plant room in roof
2 Vertical distribution duct
3 Precast cladding
4 External steel framing
5 Distribution duct to
  sales space

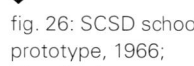

fig. 26: SCSD school
prototype, 1966;
after Banham.

1 Mixing boxes for
  air from conditioner
  on roof
2 Rigid distribution ducts
3 Flexible distribution
  ducts
4 Ceiling outlets
5 Lighting system
6 Roof space acting as
  return air plenum

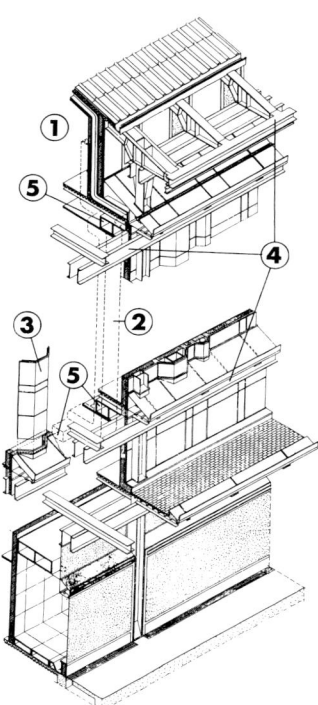

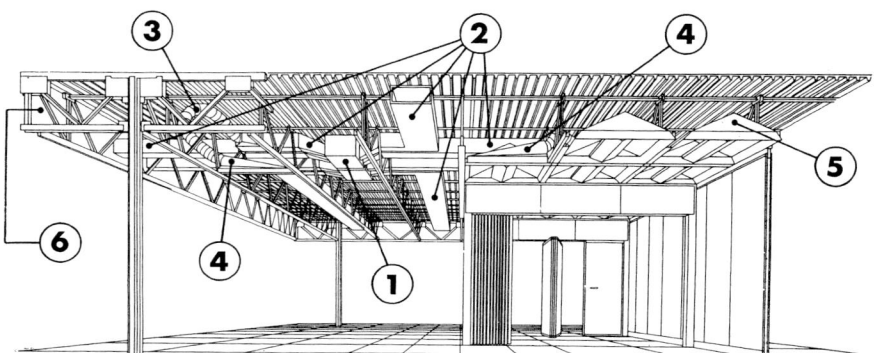

Franco Albini designed a modern palazzo for the department store La Rinascente (1961), in which the service systems are carried in voids formed within the precast concrete cladding, all supported on an exposed steel structure (fig. 25).[23]

In the USA during this period the idea of rationalized construction and the exploitation of mechanical technology in environmental design was given its most utilitarian and in some respects most influential expression in the Schools Construction System Development (SCSD) programme.[24] Evolving from a research project carried out under the direction of Ezra Ehrenkrantz at Stanford University, the idea of the system was to construct a light steel roof structure over a deep-plan space within which internal partitions could be placed to provide many alternative arrangements, all serviced by adjustable artificial lighting and air-conditioning supplies. The image of the rooftop air-conditioning unit being delivered by helicopter (fig. 26) spoke loudly of the triumph of technology over nature, as the fully artificial environment replaced the benign climate of California.

The most influential building of this time was almost certainly Louis Kahn's Richards Memorial Laboratories in Philadelphia, completed in 1961 (fig. 27). 'I do not like ducts, I do not like pipes,' said Kahn. 'I hate them really thoroughly, but because I hate them so thoroughly, I feel that they have to be given their place. If I just hated them and took no care, I think that they would invade the building and completely destroy it. I want to correct

↓
fig. 27: Louis Kahn, Richards Memorial Laboratories, Philadelphia, 1961, axonometric showing service towers; after Hawkes.

(1) Service towers; (2) Stair tower; (3) Air intakes.

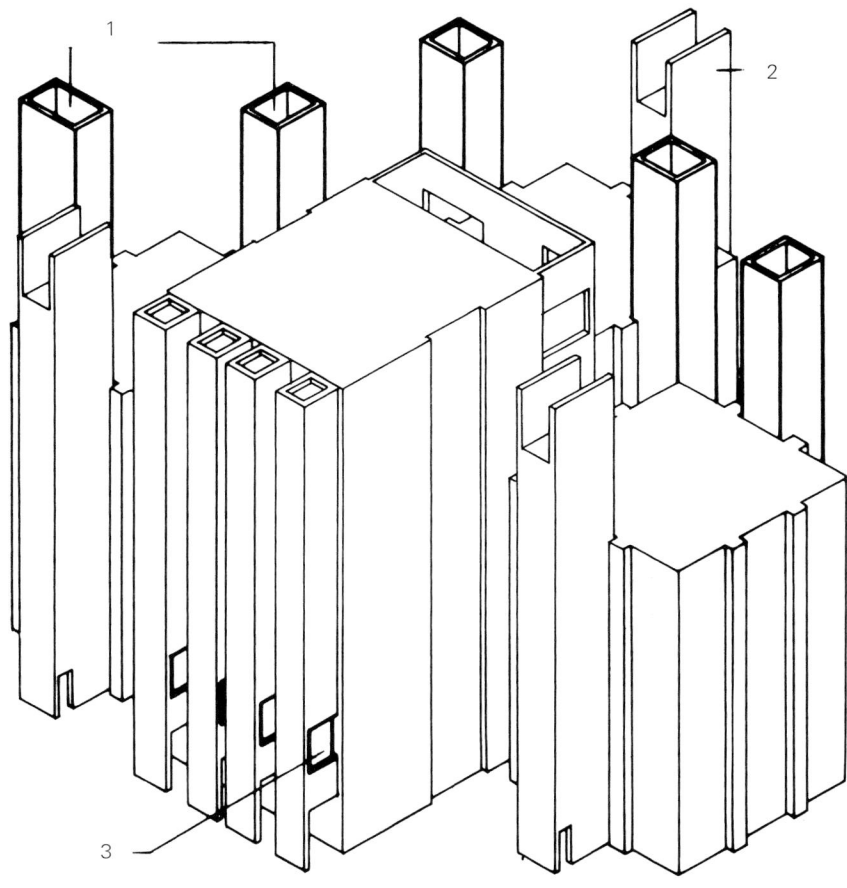

any notion you may have that I am in love with that kind of thing.'[25] Kahn issued this cri de coeur after the completion of the Richards building. Along with his distinction between 'served' and 'servant' spaces, this building provoked a new phase in the approach to the deliberate exposure of service systems, but it was the specific nature of the laboratory building, with service systems far more extensive than those of most other building types, that led Kahn to his particular and, in many ways, radical solution. In all his later designs, whether for art museums or centres of government, however carefully he organized the distribution of services in relation to space and structure, the approach was conceived in strict observance of the implications of the programme. Technical display for its own sake was anathema to Kahn, as attested by the subtle integration and concealment of the services installations at the Kimbell Art Museum at Fort Worth (1972) (fig. 28) and the Mellon Center for British Art at New Haven (1974) (fig. 29).

In a line that continues to the present day, the influence of the Richards building can be traced to many later designs. Perhaps the clearest early example of influence may be seen in the early works of the 'high-tech' school in the 1970s.[26] Although they adopt a completely different approach to questions of materiality and representation from that of Kahn, both the Pompidou Centre (Renzo Piano and Richard Rogers, 1977) (fig. 30) and the Lloyds Building (Richard Rogers, 1984) (fig. 31) owe a clear debt to Kahn in their

fig. 28: Louis Kahn,
Kimbell Art Museum,
Fort Worth, 1972,
sectional perspective
showing relation of
structure and
services – 'served'
and 'servant' spaces.

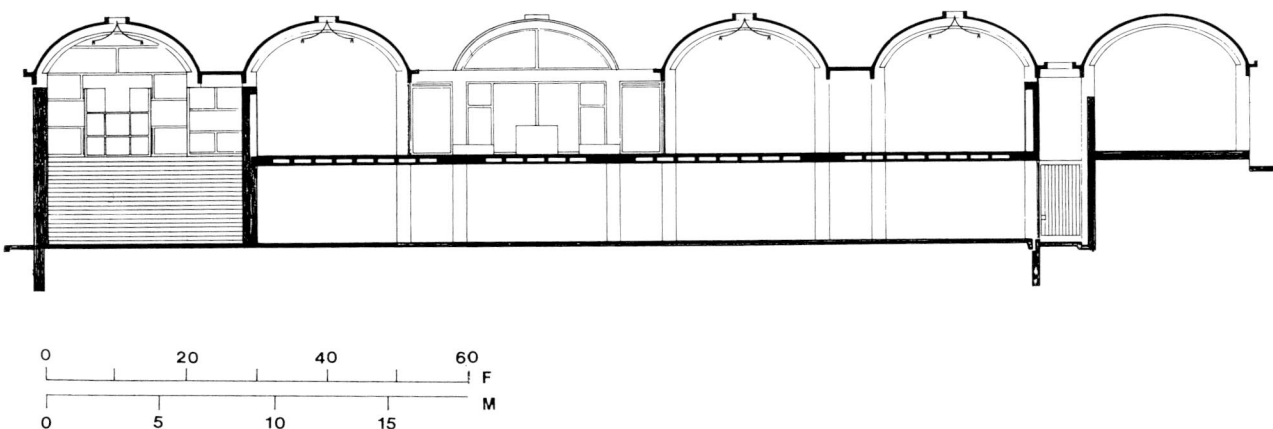

```
0        20        40        60
└──┴──┴──┴──┴──┴──┴──┘ F
└────┴────┴────┴────┘   M
0        5        10       15
```

emphatic location and expression of mechanical plant as 'servant' space relative to the 'served' enclosure.

In the 1980s this lineage was challenged, albeit briefly, by the emergence of architectural Postmodernism.[27] At the heart of this movement, in most of its various and varied manifestations, was the rejection of the kind of 'objectivity' and 'instrumentality' that had informed the development of architecture, in theory and practice, through much of the 20th century. With its preoccupation with new kinds

of interpretation, historicism and, as Frampton put it, the scenographic over the tectonic,[28] questions of environmental control and of the systematic organization of services installations received little attention in Postmodern theory. But, as is so often the case in architecture, buildings are as revealing as theory.

The Postmodern environment can be characterized by Robert Venturi's design for the Sainsbury Wing at the National Gallery in London, completed in 1991 (fig. 32).[29] In the modern picture gallery strict control of

lighting and air quality are crucial for the safe display and conservation of works of art. In addressing this need, Venturi's design began, not with Modernist analysis, but with reference to what he describes as 'the body of traditional practice'. The picture galleries in the Sainsbury Wing were modelled on John Soane's Dulwich Picture Gallery. The two buildings have the same arrangement of clerestorey windows providing even and controlled illumination of the walls and pictures, but in Venturi's building all is not what it seems.

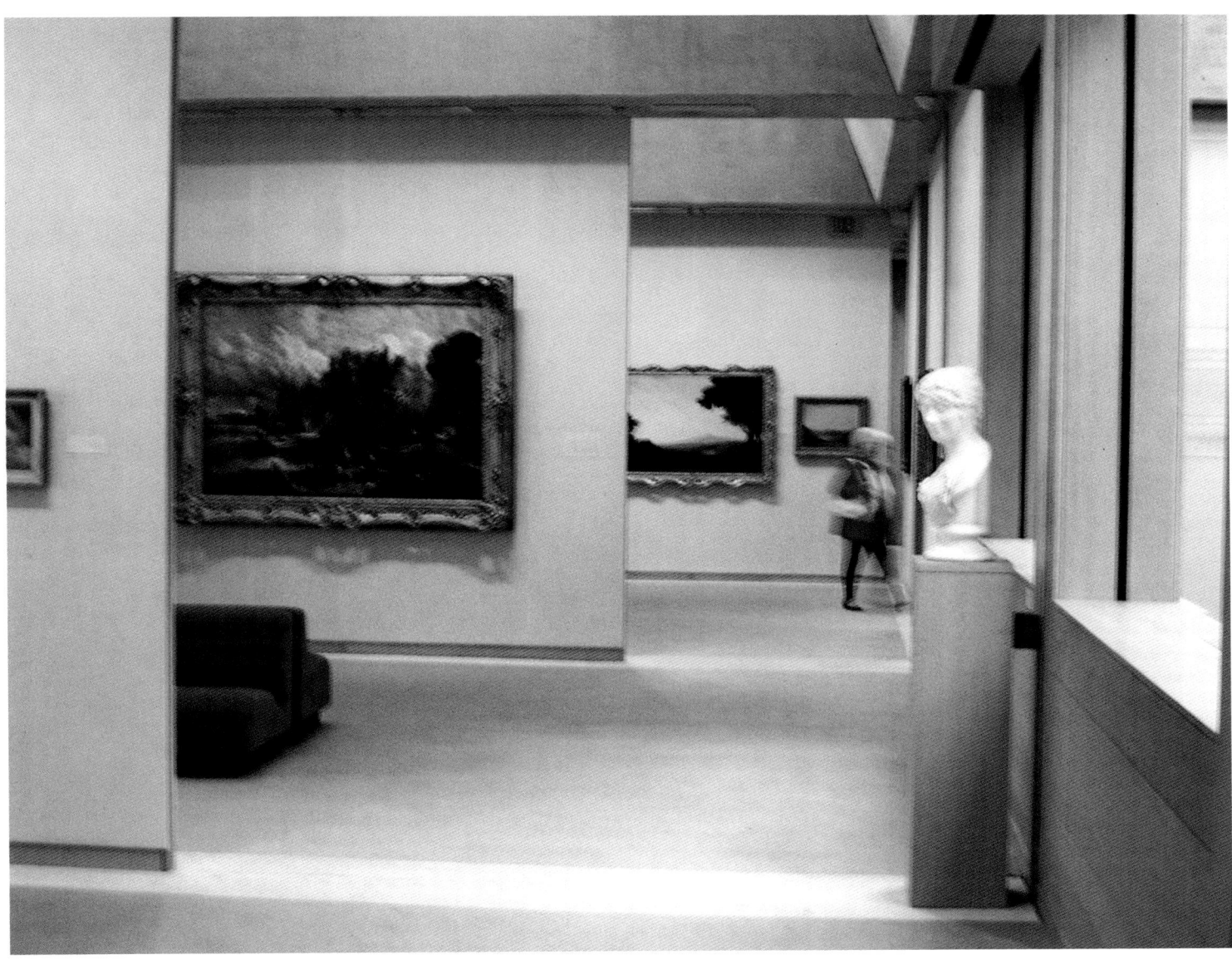

Beyond the clerestorey, which is glazed with etched glass, there is a further layer of rooftop structure and enclosure. This is an elaborate mechanism of environmental control, in which banks of adjustable louvres and fluorescent lamps operate in concert to regulate the amount of light that enters the galleries. This creates an illusion of constant natural light in the galleries, but for much of the time, even in daytime, the light source is artificial. This is pure environmental scenography; the pictures are lit individually and precisely by spotlamps mounted in the ceiling.

The building is fully air-conditioned, a necessary requirement of the modern urban art museum, but artifice rather than expression of the extensive installation is again at work. Its cellular plan gives the impression of massive, load-bearing construction – the openings between rooms are lined with solid stone architraves and this continues as a deep skirting – but the building is actually a steel-framed construction and the thick walls are made of plasterboard supported on a light steel framing system, providing plenty of voids in which the air-conditioning ducts can be concealed.

So, after the Modern Movement had attempted to define clear geometrical and functional relationships between, space, construction and environmental systems, at the end of the 20th century architects demonstrated that all the complexity of the controlled environment could be organized in the service of the picturesque. The delivery of 'concealed power' resumed its subservient position in the architectural hierarchy.

fig. 30: Renzo Piano
and Richard Rogers,
Pompidou Centre,
Paris, 1977, east
'service' façade.

fig. 29: Louis Kahn,
Mellon Center for
British Art, New
Haven, 1974, interior
of picture gallery.

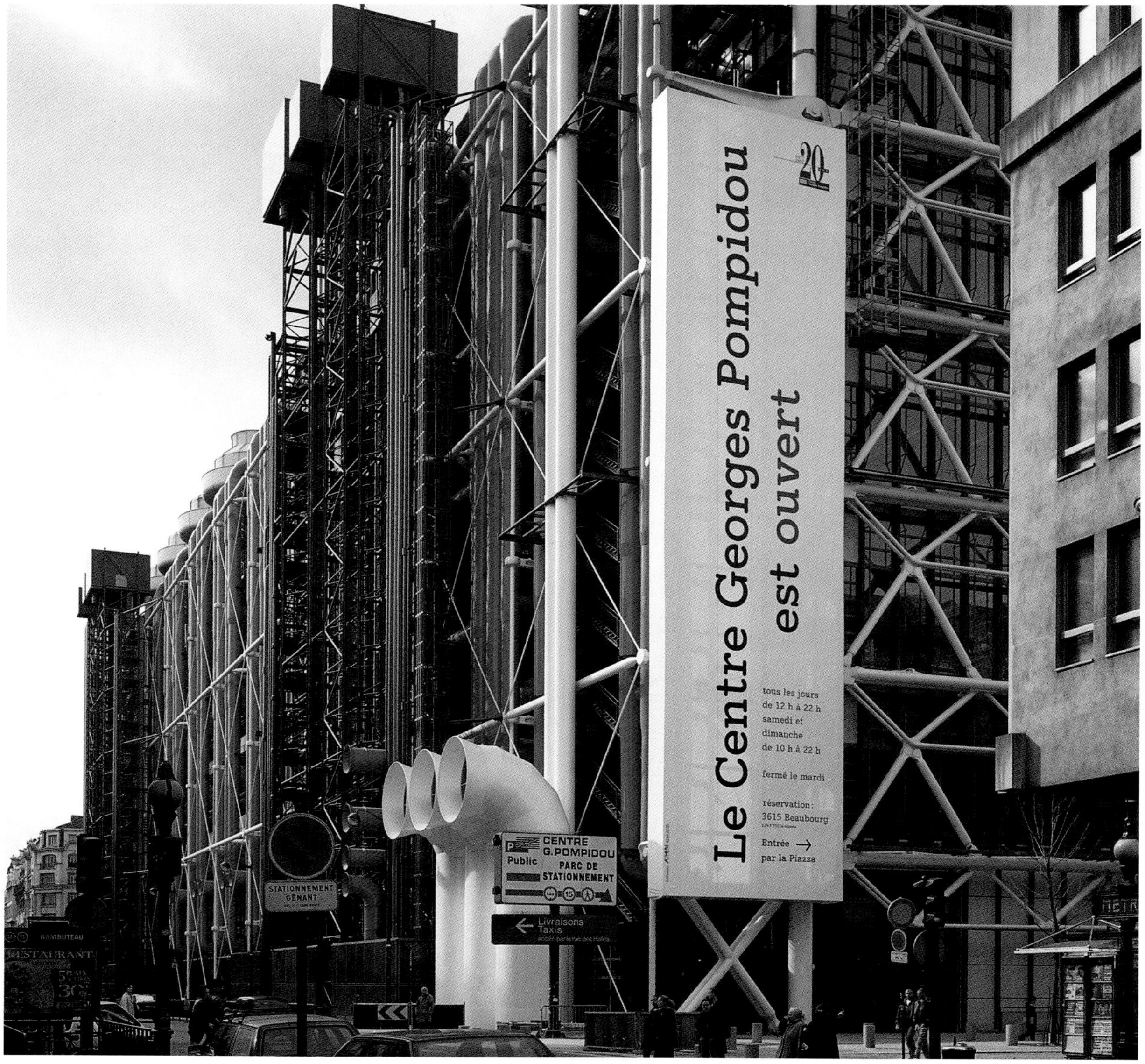

The evolving envelope

In the 1930s Le Corbusier added a new element to the apparatus of modern architecture with his invention of the brise-soleil. It first appeared in his project for an apartment building in Algiers in which the south and west façades were shaded by a concrete 'egg-crate' structure. The most celebrated early installation was in the design of the Ministry of Education building in Rio de Janeiro (1936–45) (fig. 33), a collaboration with Lucio Costa, where the brise-soleil were added to the standard repertoire of the cinque points, 'columns, glass façades, independent framework, roof garden, etc.'[30] This signalled the beginning of a process by which the external envelope of the modern building has become progressively more complex in the service of environmental control.

Writing in 1962, Alan Colquhoun pointed out that, by the mid 20th century, the clarity of the cinque points on the separation of structure and enclosure had been replaced in many buildings by a revival of interest in heavy and traditional methods of construction: 'It is as if the urge to create the world anew by means of structures which had the lightness and tenuousness of pure thought had given way to the desire to create solid hideouts of the human spirit in a world of uncertainty and change, each one a microcosm of an ideal world.'[31]

The late buildings of Louis Kahn exemplify this trend. The Richards Laboratory, the Kimbell Art Museum and the Mellon Center all retain a clearly articulated distinction between frame and envelope, but in every case the envelope combines areas of solid

33

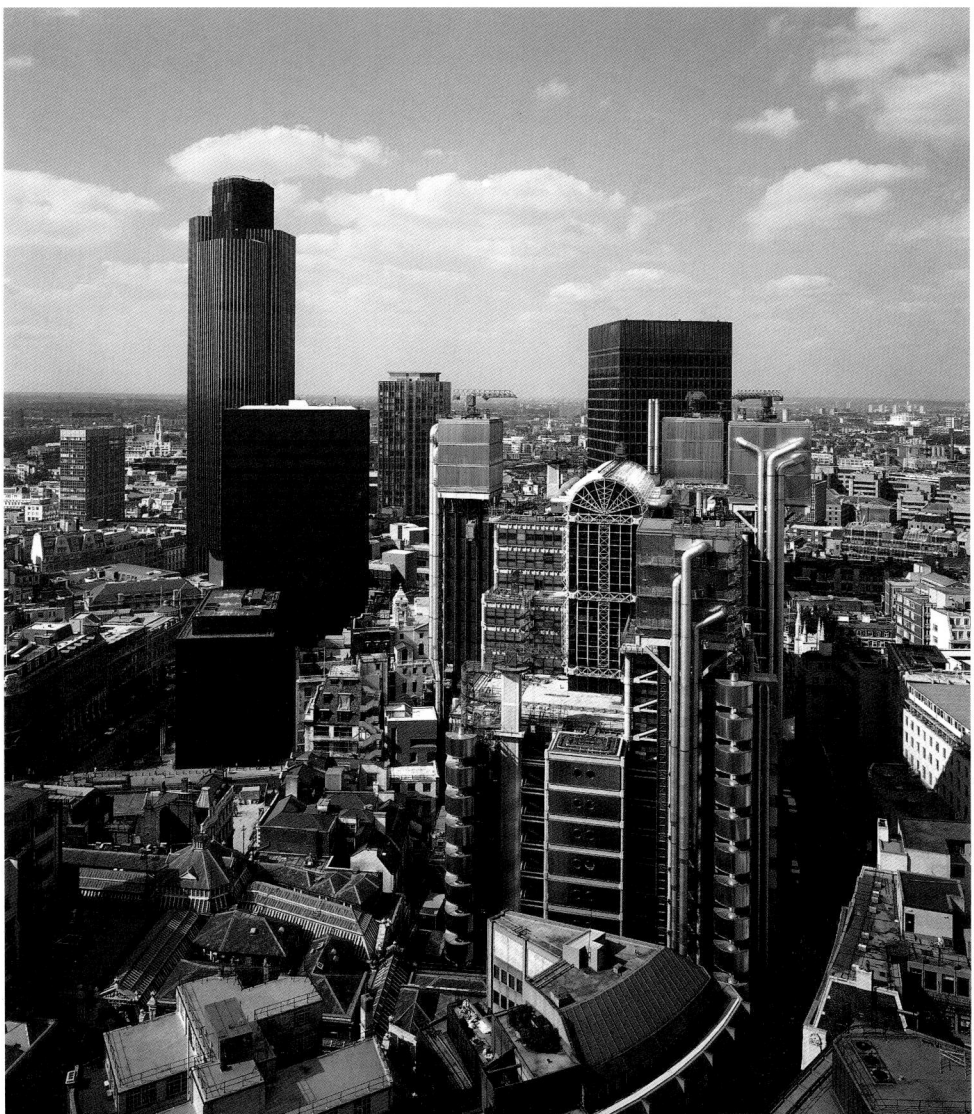

fig. 31: Richard
Rogers, Lloyds
Building, London,
1984.

and void in proportions appropriate to the function of the building. In Kahn's first project outside the USA – the unbuilt design for the US consulate in Luanda, Angola (1959–61) (fig. 34) – he responded to the equatorial climate by constructing a deeply layered envelope with unglazed screens standing in front of deeply recessed windows and by surmounting the 'rain roof' with a structurally independent 'sun roof' to provide shade and promote natural ventilation. In the library at Philips Academy, Exeter, New Hampshire (1965–71) (fig. 35), where climate was less of a challenge, the entire envelope was enclosed, but distinct environmental zones were established within the plan's concentric territories. Readers sit in the brick-built, daylit perimeter, where aedicular desks are located within the oak window frames, and books, which are more environmentally sensitive than readers, are placed in the thermally massive *in-situ* concrete core, where it is easier to maintain a stable environment.

These projects helped to reassert the environmental function of a building's external envelope, whereby it acts as a mediator, a 'filter', between internal and external climates. Although the highly serviced glass box continues to exert its appeal, the potential of the more complex, environmentally considered façade is explored increasingly often in contemporary designs. A discipline has emerged in which arbitrary form-making and stylism have no place but which opens up rich possibilities for the development of architectural language. In asserting the authority of the tectonic in architecture, Kenneth

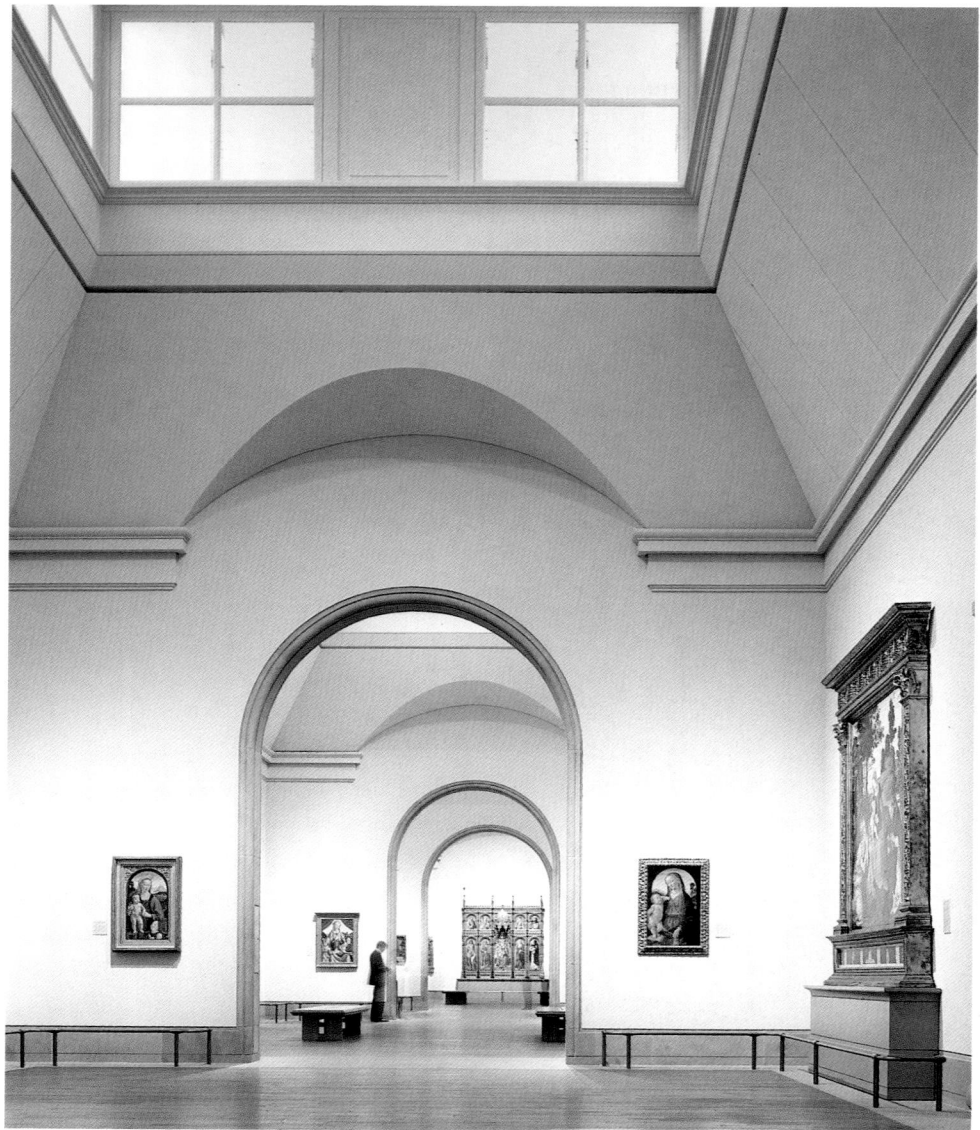

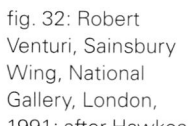

fig. 32: Robert Venturi, Sainsbury Wing, National Gallery, London, 1991; after Hawkes.

Frampton has argued that 'the tectonic does not necessarily favour any particular style'.[32] The same may be said of environmental design principles, which are neither formally nor stylistically determinate; good architects and engineers may adapt them creatively to the programme, context, economy and culture of each project. The buildings described in detail later in this book illustrate the diversity and sophistication of the modern environmental envelope.

Natural versus mechanical energy

Pointing to the ever-accelerating consumption of mineral reserves, as industrialization provided more and more tools for an increasingly urbanized world, Derry and Williams argued that a crucial change had taken place in Western man's relationship with natural resources in the period between 1750 and 1900.[33] In the field of architecture and building, one of the central themes during this period was the conversion of the energy stored in fossil fuels to power consumed in devices for environmental control. This paradigm survived the arrival of architectural Modernism and was given impetus by the emergence of the idea of an 'International Style' in which, as Le Corbusier put it in *Précisions*, 'international scientific techniques [allow us] to propose only one house for all countries'. Building trends throughout the 20th century confirmed the potency of this idea. The air-conditioned glass skyscraper has become that 'one house for all countries', providing international business and recreation interests with

→

fig. 33: Le Corbusier
and Lucio Costa,
Ministry of
Education, Rio de
Janeiro, 1936–45.

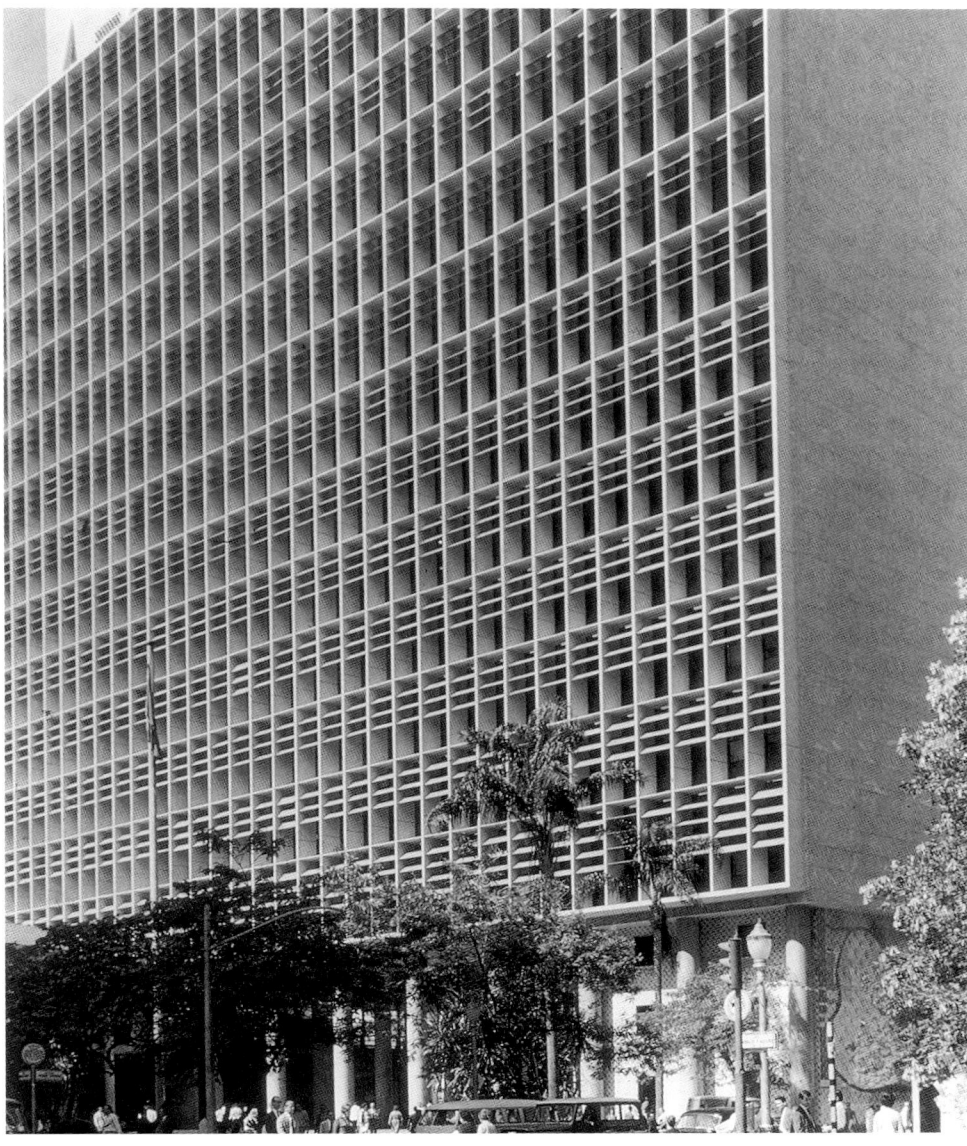

a uniform, controlled internal environment wherever they may be. In the last quarter of the 20th century, however, the assumption that the march of technological progress would, and should, continue indefinitely was seriously questioned – first by a growing awareness of the limits of the earth's fossil-fuel resources, and then by the apprehension that their continued consumption at established rates was having an irreversibly destructive effect on the world's climate. A new perspective on the objectives and

methods of environmental control in buildings emerged, which focuses on ways of reducing demand for non-renewable sources of energy and mechanical power and explores ways in which they might be replaced by renewable natural resources.

The environmental strategy applied in architecture, whether consciously or unconsciously, before the Industrial Revolution may be described in terms of the 'Vitruvian model' (fig. 36).[34] According to this model, 'architecture', as a portmanteau term embracing all elements of building, is represented

as the mediation between the unpredictable climate and the more stable conditions necessary to sustain the functions of human society.

In *Design with Climate*, one of the 20th century's most important books about the relationship between climate and architecture, Victor Olgyay proposed a model of 'interlocking fields of climate balance' (fig. 37) which explicitly extends the Vitruvian model by distinguishing between architecture (the static organization and fabric of a building) and the new element, technology

fig. 34: Louis Kahn,
Project for US Consulate,
Luanda, Angola, 1959–61,
cut-away axonometric
showing environmentally
layered envelope.

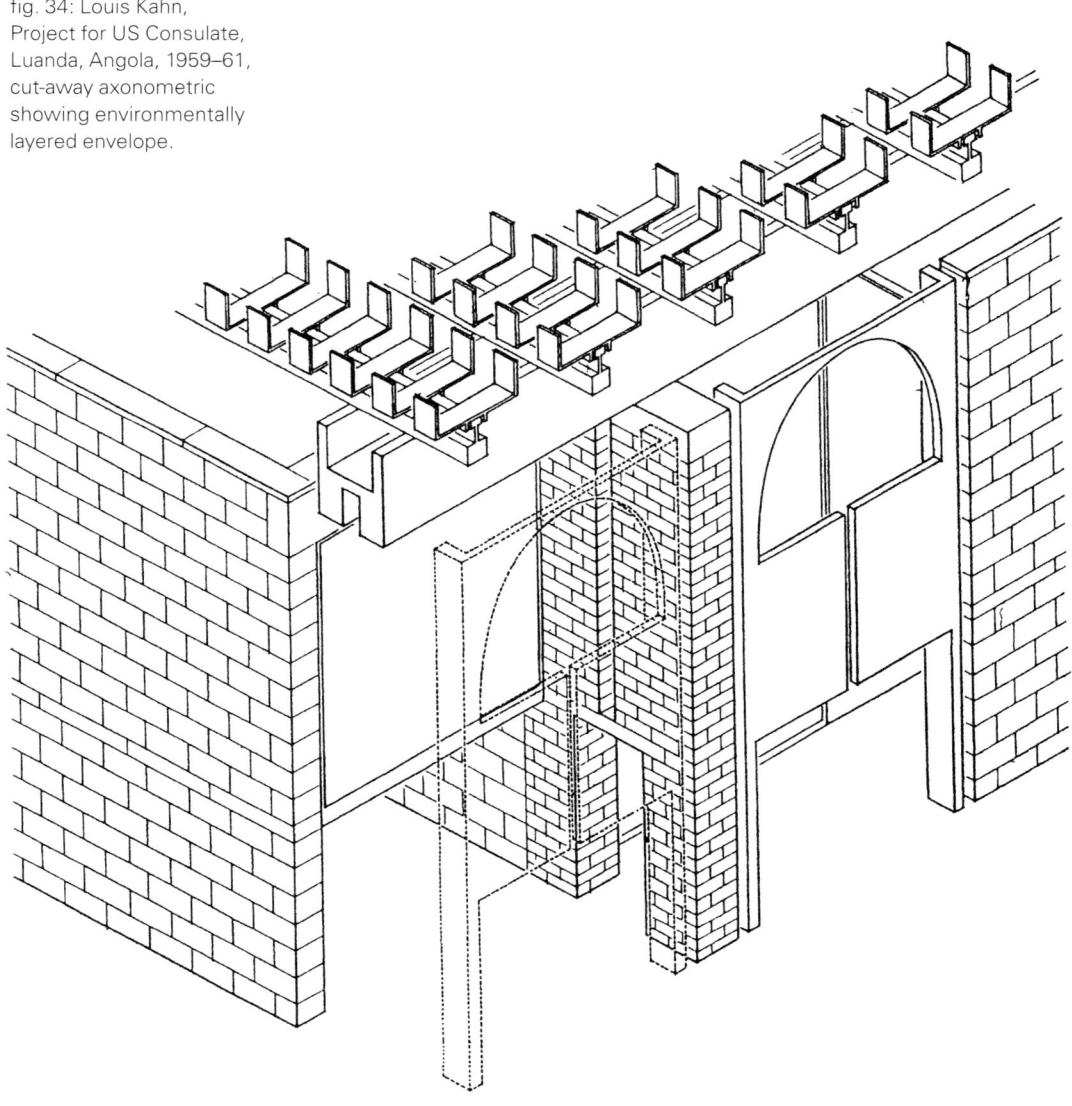

(mechanical services), in the process of environmental control.[35] This distinction describes the basis of almost all contemporary environmental design in architecture and suggests the primacy of the collaboration between architect and engineer. But, writing in 1963, Olgyay was constructing a framework that more precisely represented the balance between the environmental functions of architecture and technology. In an elegantly simple diagram related to the 'interlocking fields' model and called 'flattening the curve' (fig. 38), Olgyay defined the stages by which wide variations of climate – in this instance of temperature – might be progressively modified. In this he distinguishes between the roles of 'microclimatology', 'climate balance of the structure' and, finally, 'mechanical heating or cooling'. The point of the exercise was to show how manipulation of the first two of these variables might significantly reduce the demands placed upon the mechanical plant. In effect this is an argument for the whole building, its architecture and its technology, to be conceived as a system of complementary and interlocking parts.

Olgyay's book is one of the key documents in the development of an environmentally friendly approach to architecture. In it he uses the term 'bioclimatic architecture' to describe designs that set out to work with rather than against nature. Much of the pioneering work in bioclimatic architecture was in designs for small dwellings, in most cases using the techniques of 'passive solar' design to meet some, if not all, the space-

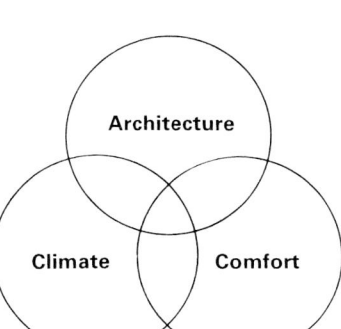

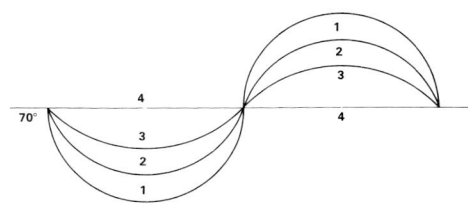

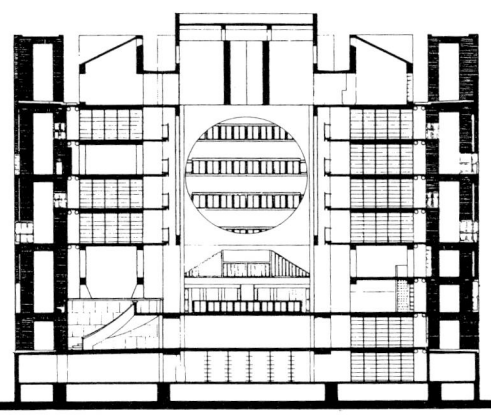

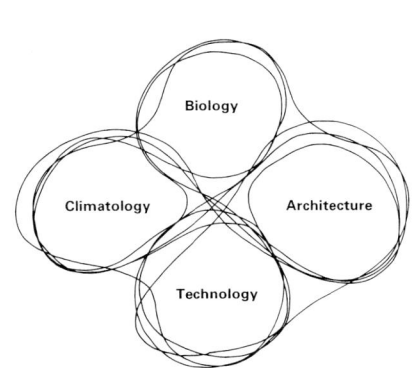

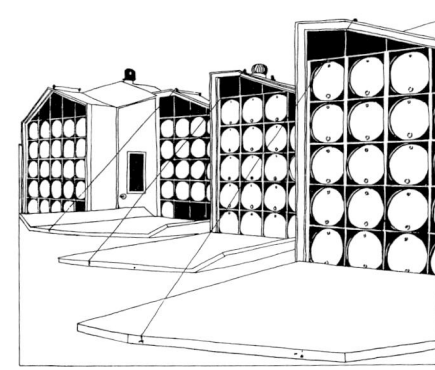

heating requirements (fig. 39).[36] Other projects sought the more ambitious goal of 'autonomy' (fig. 40), in which all a dwelling's servicing needs could be met without dependence on mains services of any kind.[37] Such ventures made it possible to test new ideas before they gradually found their way into the design of larger buildings. By the late 1980s there was an increasing number of designs for various building types in which some of these lessons were being effectively applied.[38] Norman Foster's Lycée Polyvalent at Fréjus in the south of France (1991–93)

(fig. 41) exhibits, in its array of brise-soleil, the respect for orientation that is one of the cornerstones of bioclimatic design. The concrete structure provides thermal mass to moderate extremes of temperature and the cross-section is manipulated to promote controllable natural ventilation. In their design for the Queen's Building at De Montfort University at Leicester in the English Midlands (1989–93) (fig. 42), Short Ford & Associates combined references to the brick tradition of English architecture with a powerful

expression of the terminals of the building's natural ventilation stacks, although the impact of this gesture was compromised by the building's curious appropriation of quasi-Victorian stylism. In Austria, Thomas Herzog reinterpreted the idea of the 'crystal palace' in his design for a congress and exhibition hall at Linz (1986–94) (fig. 43). The complex layering of glazing and louvres achieves a high level of natural light in the hall without the disadvantage of uncontrollable solar-heat gains. The form of the arched roof also promotes

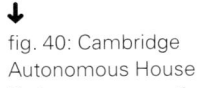

fig. 40: Cambridge
Autonomous House
Project, cross-section.

fig. 41: Norman
Foster, Lycée
Polyvalent, Fréjus,
France, 1991–93.

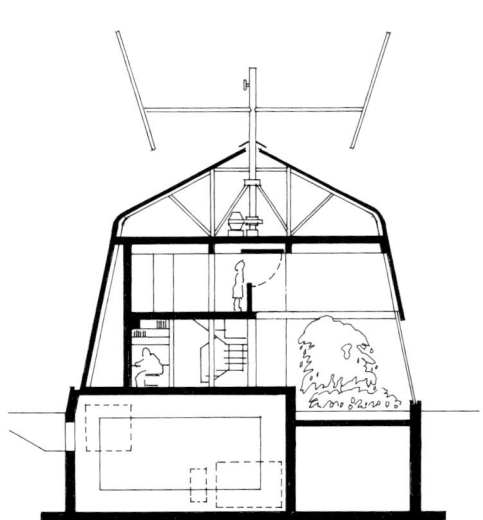

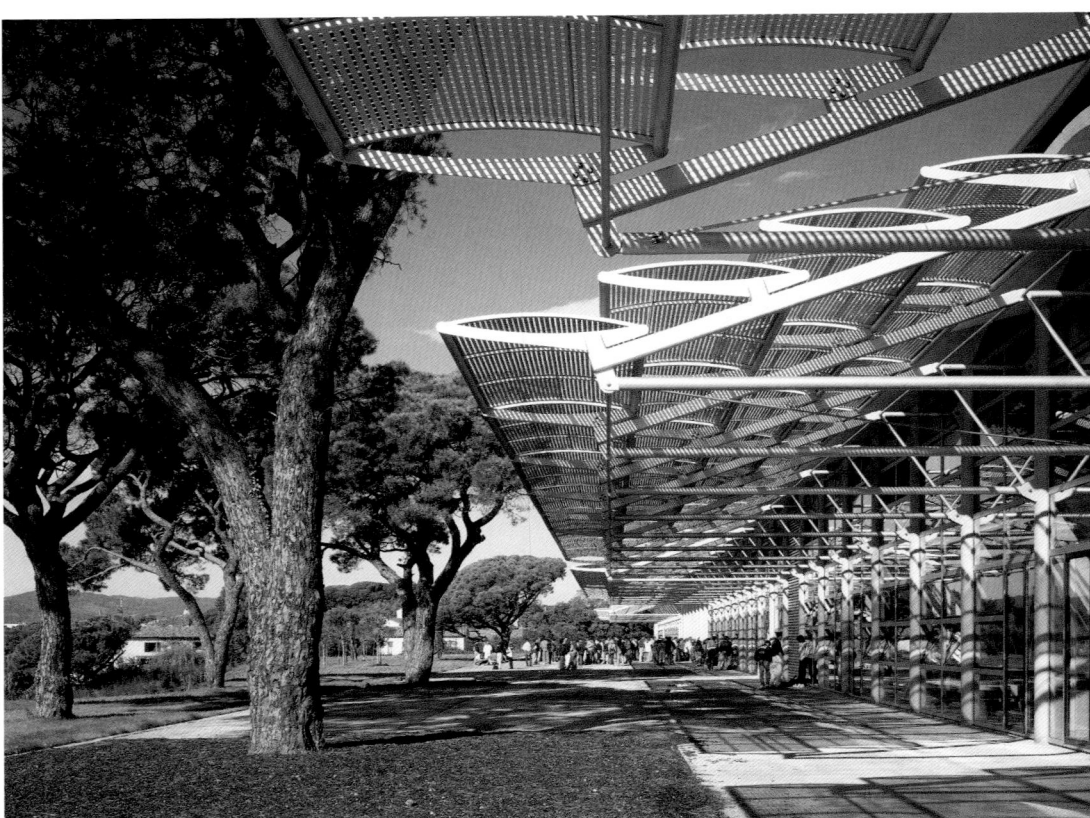

natural ventilation of the vast space.

The Malaysian architect Ken Yeang has developed his own interpretation of bioclimatic design.[39] His bioclimatic skyscraper projects in South-east Asia have brought a systematic approach to the design of the building envelope to bear on the extreme climate of that region. The Menara Mesiniaga office building in Selangor, Malaysia (1989–92) (fig. 44) fuses understanding of environmental principles with late 20th-century structural and material technologies.

A taxonomy of environmental architecture

The recent history of architecture has seen the development of a new and more sophisticated synthesis and collaboration between leading architectural and engineering practices. Numerous developments in the technology of building have greatly expanded the tectonic and environmental repertoire and, as a consequence, the scope of environmental design. Contemporary practice exhibits a greater diversity of approach than ever before.

As we have tried to show in our outline of the environmental history of architecture since the 18th century, the basis of this diversity rests on the relationship between the environmental function of form and fabric of a building and its mechanical service systems. Before the development of mechanical service systems it was form and fabric that, through their configuration and materiality, provided a permeable and, often, highly effective boundary between the external climate and the internal environment – the Vitruvian model.

fig. 42: Short Ford,
Queen's Building, De
Montfort University,
Leicester, UK,
1989–93; after
Hawkes.

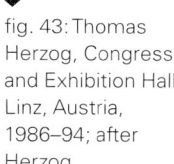

fig. 43: Thomas
Herzog, Congress
and Exhibition Hall,
Linz, Austria,
1986–94; after
Herzog.

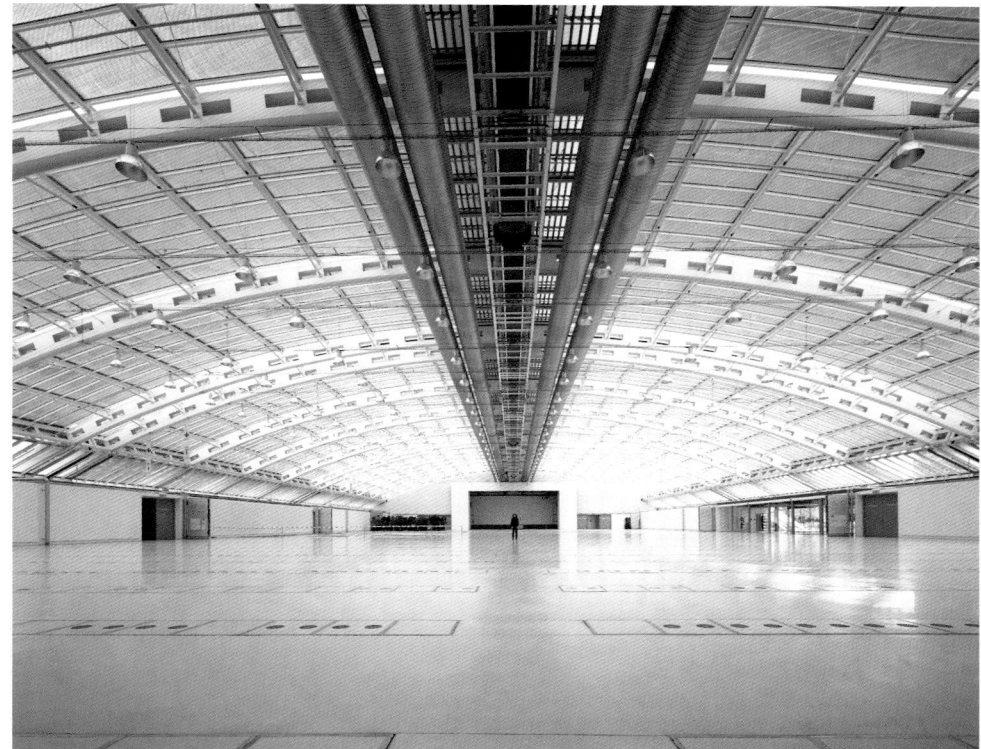

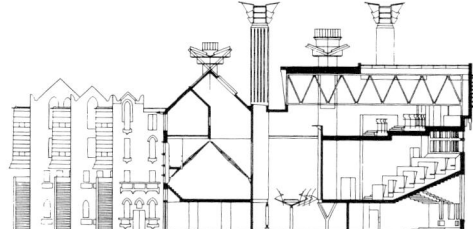

As service systems developed in the 19th and 20th centuries, they added to the environmental scope of form and fabric and, in the process, produced higher and more predictable standards of comfort. With the full apparatus of modern mechanical servicing – plant for heating, cooling, ventilating, lighting – and with the achievement of the sealed envelope, it became possible to deliver a controlled, and by implication 'perfect', artificial environment within a building.

The enormous diversity of present-day environmental design practice is based on alternative interpretations and adaptations of this history. Some designs continue to work with a combination of form and fabric operating in a calculated relationship with mechanical systems. Others separate the external and internal climates with a sealed enclosure and apply mechanical services as the main providers of the internal environment. These two *modes* of environmental control have been defined as, respectively, the *selective* and the *exclusive*.[40]

This classification distinguishes between designs that, in *selective* mode, *selectively* accommodate and filter the ambient environment as their primary strategy and those that, in *exclusive* mode, configure and construct the building enclosure to achieve maximum *exclusion* of the external climate in order to minimize the demands placed on environmental plant. Such a distinction broadly characterizes the predominant environmental options, but the richness and complexity of modern practice demands a more refined taxonomy.

To structure the discussion of the 'critical studies' that follow we

↓
fig. 44: Ken Yeang,
Menara Mesiniaga,
Selangor, Malaysia,
1989–92; after
Powell.

↓
fig. 45: A taxonomy
of environmental
architecture and
engineering.

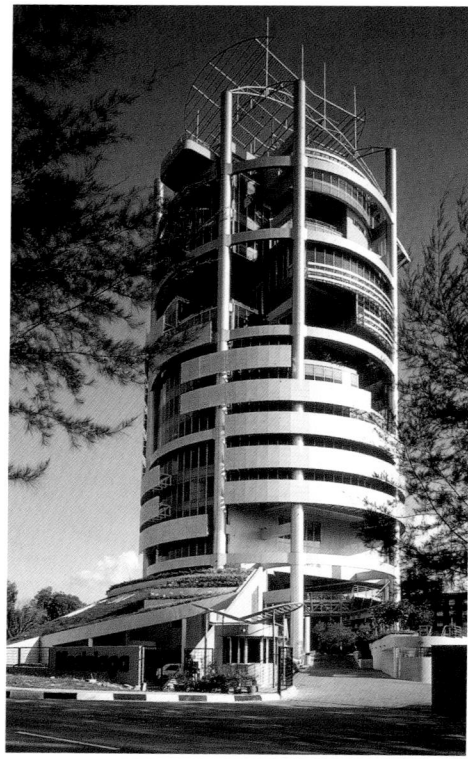

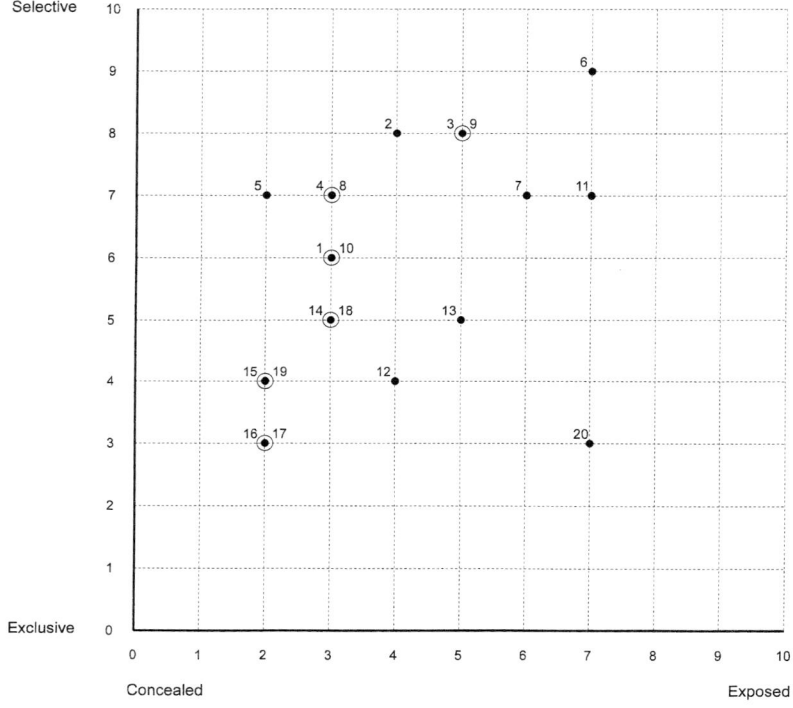

propose a descriptive scheme that extends the distinction between *selective* and *exclusive* by taking note of the way in which the environmental systems of a building are, in a key distinction drawn by Banham, either *concealed* or *exposed*.

In combination, these factors provide a means of characterizing the environmental strategy of a building. A simple graphic representation is given at fig. 45. Each of the buildings has been given a 'score' between 0 and 10 on the two axes, *selective/ exclusive* and *concealed/exposed*

and, on this basis, is located on the 'solution space' of the diagram. The order in which the projects appear in the book has been used to identify the buildings on the graph:

1 Offices for Apicorp
2 Eastgate
3 Arup Campus
4 Howlands Farm Student Housing
5 Marzahn Low-Energy Apartment Building
6 BedZED Sustainable Development
7 Mont Cenis Training Centre
8 Study Centre, Darwin College

9 Jubilee Campus, University of Nottingham
10 Cultural Centre
11 Carmel Mountain Ranch Public Library
12 Helicon Building
13 Villa VPRO Offices
14 Beyeler Foundation Museum
15 Byzantine Fresco Chapel Museum
16 Museum of Contemporary Art
17 Walsall Art Museum
18 Tate Modern
19 Portuguese Pavilion
20 Velodrome

The Selective Mode

Offices for Apicorp
DEGW
Al Khobar, Saudi Arabia
2000

➜
The building envelope
as climatic filter:
model of the Apicorp
project.

Any review of Middle Eastern modern architecture would reveal a body of work that has relied largely on the borrowing of ideas from other, mainly Western cultures. This penchant for cut-and-paste architecture has almost obliterated the best traditions of the regional architecture that had evolved in response to climate and culture. The energy-guzzling glass towers and malls of the temperate Western climates seem even more absurd when transported to hot arid zones.

The Arab Petroleum Investments Corporation (APICORP) is an investment company based at Al Khobar in Saudi Arabia. The company was established in 1975 by the governments of the member states of OPEC. In 1995, when the company needed a new headquarters, an international competition was held to find a suitable design. The brief stipulated that the new building 'should respect the existing context and allude to traditional Arab architecture without resorting to

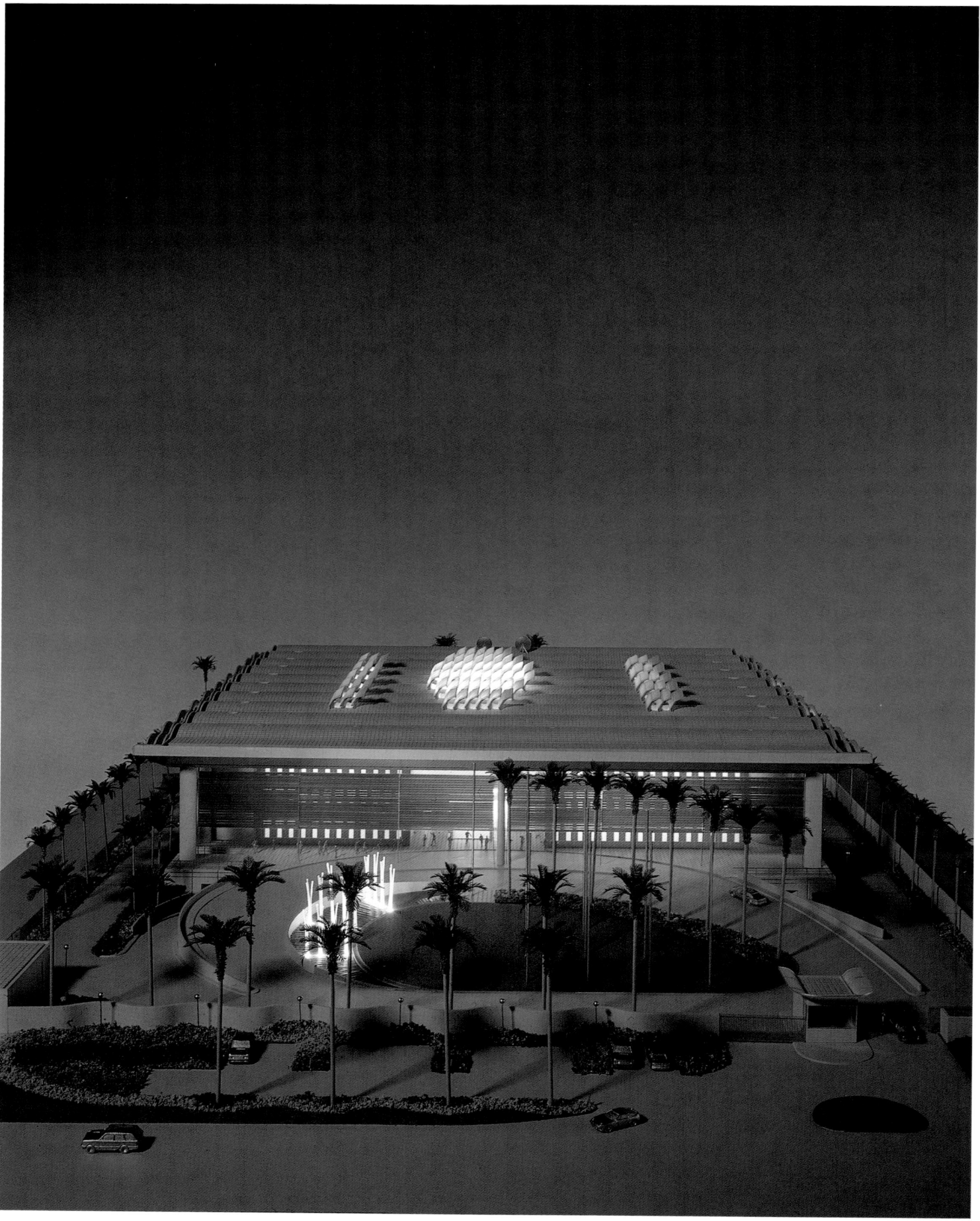

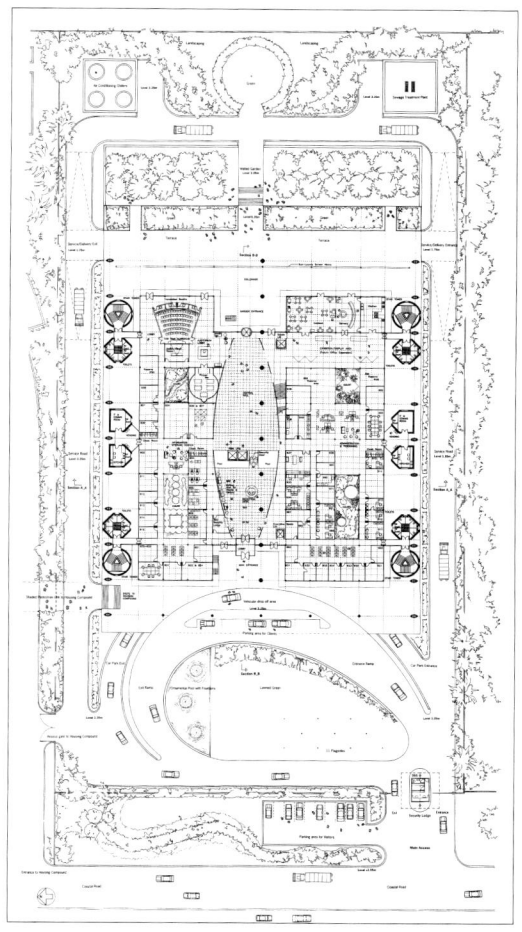

↑
Site plan

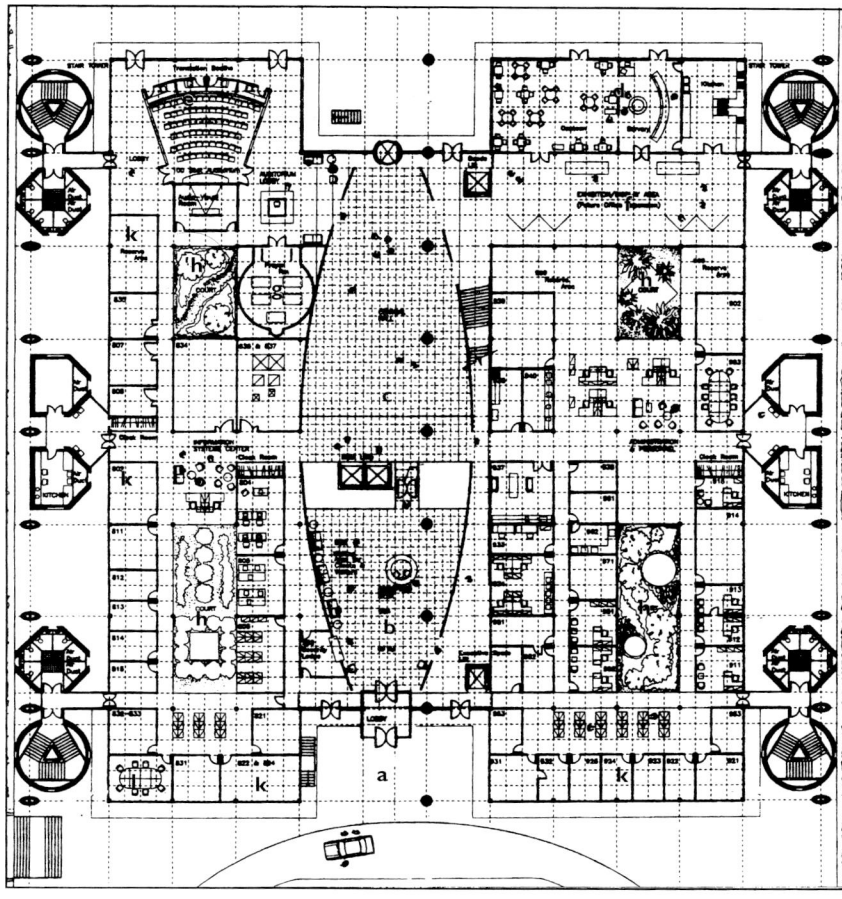

↑
Ground-floor plan.

→
Model at design
stage.

pastiche'.[1] The six ranked
competition entries were designs by
Harry Seidler, Henning Larsen, HOK
International, Fitzroy Robinson, Alberts
& Van Hunt, and DEGW.

Site

The site is next to the company's
existing housing compound, designed
in the late 1970s by Studio Nervi,
which consists of two monumental
curved apartment blocks that lock
together around a central courtyard.
The blocks are stepped back in section
from the courtyard, providing shaded
balconies, but little shelter is provided
in the large central courtyard, and it is
difficult to imagine any architecture
less responsive in form to the location
and local climate.

The competitors' responses to the
brief are worth comparing. They
varied from attempts to harmonize

with the existing formal language of
Nervi (Seidler Associates) to
'grandiose external expression'
(Fitzroy Robinson and HOK
International) and exercises in
singular 'self-contemplation'.[2]

Only two entries seemed to respond
to place and climate, but Henning
Larsen's concept was regarded as
lacking respect for Apicorp's corporate
identity and programming
requirements, while DEGW's
proposals resolved issues of
corporate identity, organizational
needs and response to regional
climate and place, if not to the
immediate context – and the company
emerged as a clear winner.

Located on the Gulf coast of Saudi
Arabia, the site is a challenge for
designers of the modern workplace.
Daytime temperatures rise above 40°C
(104°F) for six to seven months of the

year. Relative humidity is also high –
frequently 70 per cent, and sometimes
as high as 90 per cent. The coastal
location makes for a heavily saline
atmosphere that is potentially
corrosive not only to many metallic
building materials but also to
reinforced-concrete structures unless
they are detailed carefully and
protected. From October to April,
temperatures fall to a mean of
20–30°C (68–86°F). At night,
temperatures can fall to below 10°C
(50°F). Although annual average
rainfall is not high, occasional
rainstorms can be heavy because of
the coastal location.

Building form and organization
The architectural response to the
demands of site, context and
organization is simple and elegant. A
massive sinusoidal roof is employed

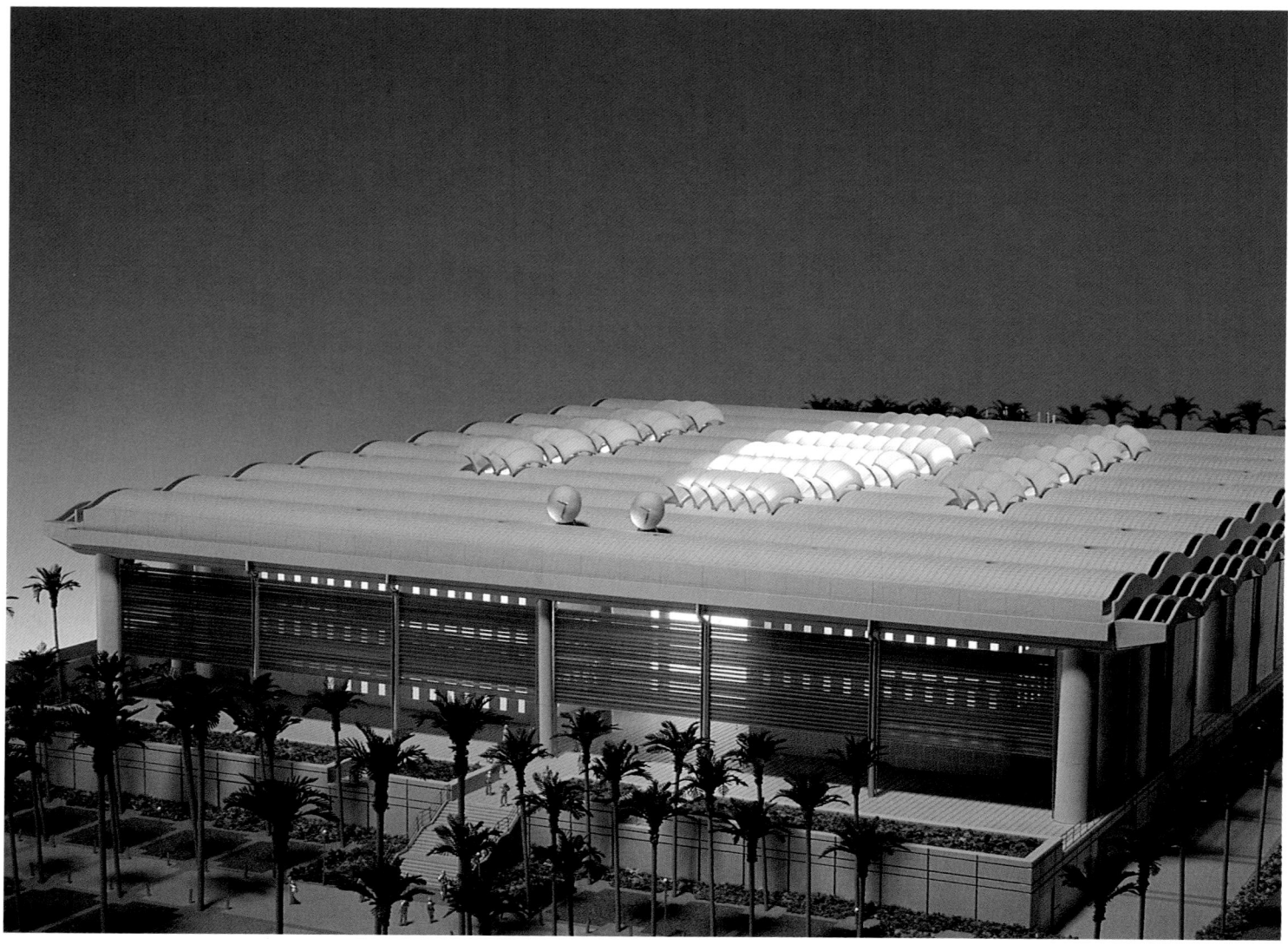

as a sheltering element. It is designed to act as a sunshade and also as an all-embracing form for the concept of 'office as village'. DEGW have a long and notable track record in office-building research and design. Francis Duffy, one of the founders of DEGW, presented a doctoral thesis on office organizations at Princeton in 1974 [3] and in 1976 the DEGW book *Planning Office Space* was published. [4] These publications established DEGW's identity as a practice whose approach to office design was founded on matching building and organizational characteristics, post-occupancy evaluation, space budgeting and participating briefing. Design proposals and built reality are both tested through research.

DEGW drew on this tradition in the design for Apicorp. In recognition that the client needed a building that

would provide the potential for a range of different kinds of workplace, the 'office as village' was organized around a series of courtyards. Essentially, Apicorp is conceived as a conventional shell-and-core building but subtly manipulated to suit programme and place. The large central elliptical courtyard is surrounded by four subsidiary courtyards flanked by perimeter 'outboard' service towers, all sheltering under the great roof canopy. These cores are expressed externally as free-standing silos and they articulate the external wall. Flanked by two three-storey office wings, the toplit central courtyard at the heart of the building contains a public reception area at the front and access to auditorium, prayer room and refectory at the rear. Above ground floor the elliptical courtyard

space is crossed by a bridge connecting the two office wings. The wings are not symmetrical: one floor plate is 24m (79ft) wide and the other is 18m (59ft), and these are effectively narrowed by the penetration of the secondary courtyards. Although such a variety of floor plates offers a high degree of workspace flexibility, the initial need of the client is for mainly cellular spaces.

Organizationally Apicorp is a world away from the current norm of northern European offices, with their 'hot desking', 'romp' anywhere, 'home base' mix of space that is capable of 'overnight' change, but Apicorp's cells can also be transformed when required. The floor-plate depth combines with the planning grid to enable a range of workplace configurations. At occupation the building is 90 per cent cellular but it

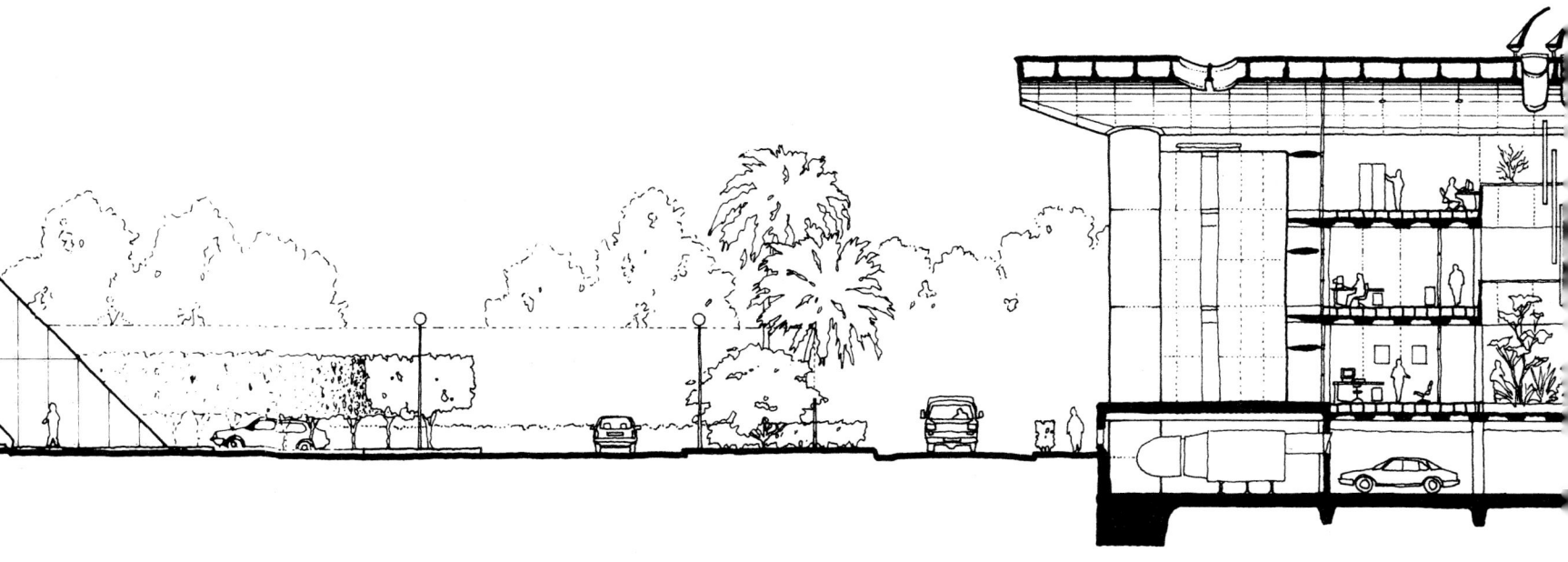

has been designed to promote social interaction. As the social heart of the building, the central courtyard is a key component in this design. The whole building sits on a podium above an underground car park.

Structure and construction

Apicorp's shell, structure, services and scenery are based on DEGW's preferred office-planning module of 1.5m by 1.5m (5ft by 5ft). The structure consists of a primary and secondary structural grid, the primary element of which is the great barrel-vaulted roof supported on gigantic elliptical columns on the north and south perimeters placed at 9m (30ft) centres. The full span of 72m (236ft) from perimeter column to perimeter column is divided by a central column placed asymetrically in the elliptical courtyard. The 36m (118ft) span is

further subdivided by secondary columns at 6m (20ft) centres, and the resulting overall 9m by 6m (30ft by 20ft) structural grid supports the planning and constructional module.

The 9m (30ft) span from column to column is covered at roof level by ribbed precast-concrete vaults supported on primary *in-situ* concrete beams. Profiled metal decking has been laid over these and a layer of in-situ concrete poured over this insulation and placed on top of the concrete. Ceramic tiles have been laid as an external finish. As well as enhancing Apicorp's corporate identity (a primary requirement of the competition brief), the roof also plays a central role in the building's environmental control. In addition to providing solar shading and reflection, layered roof construction, in conjunction with the large hollow

columns, forms part of the distribution system for ventilation to the courtyard. The three floors of office space are supported on a waffle *in-situ* concrete slab. The whole floor zone is 800mm (32in) deep and incorporates a raised floor; clear floor-to-ceiling height in the offices is 3m (10ft) with a structural floor-to-floor height of 3.8m (12ft). This extends to 5.2m (17ft) on the floor where the barrel vault is exposed.

The traditional elements of the international commercial façade – full-height glazing and in-board perimeter columns – have been eschewed in favour of a system that meets local environmental demands. Solid spandrels, clad in local marble and fixed flush with the double-glazed window units, provide thermal mass and privacy. The glazing pattern is designed to reflect Arabic tiling and

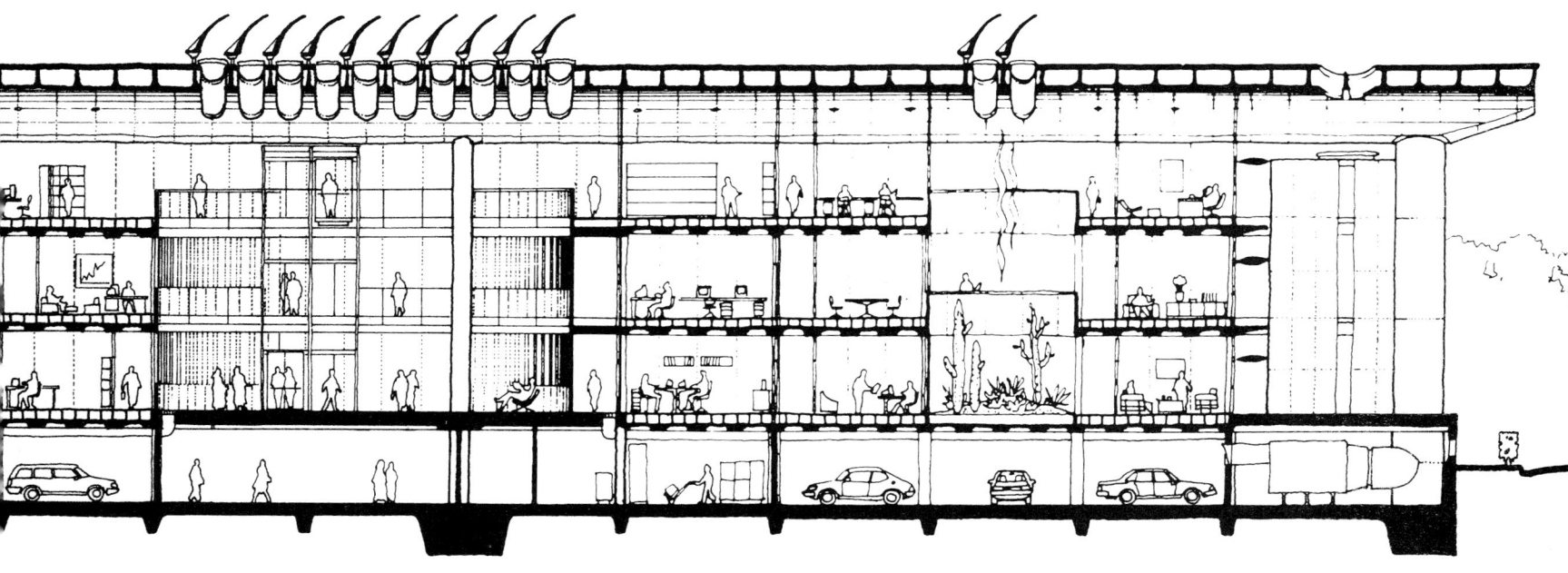

screens. A chequer-plate pattern of smaller windows is placed at eye level, and larger windows are positioned at a higher level to throw light deeper into the plan and add reflected light from the ceilings. The vertical surfaces of walls and windows are protected from direct sun by the over-sailing roof and louvred screens on the east and west façades.

Energy and environment

Thermal mass is traditionally used to modify climate in hot arid zones, but the maritime nature of the site limited the effectiveness of this traditional strategy for Apicorp's new headquarters. Arup calculated that, although there is some potential for free night cooling between October and May (by drawing cool night air through the building), the fan energy needed to push the air through

the filtration and heat-recovery equipment exceeded energy savings through passive cooling because of high air resistance.

The environmental strategy was therefore based on careful integration and balance between building services and structures and fabric. The effects of roof shade and filtered daylight reduce energy demands for heating and cooling. The environmental strategy, even without the benefit of passive cooling, demonstrates a 60 per cent reduction in annual energy consumption compared with a typical North American office.

All the courtyards are daylit through the roof. Rooflights, elliptical on plan, are cut into the barrel vaults over the central and subsidiary courtyards. Direct solar gains are prevented by elegantly designed shades. High sun

angles can make rooflighting design very difficult, and at Al Khobar during the summer the sun reaches an angle of 81 degrees from the horizon – but, even though the sun can be virtually overhead, the depth of the roof construction combined with the external screening admits only first or second reflections.

The deep-plan building is divided into two environmental zones. Its perimeter is subject to the modified effects of the external climate; fluctuations in room loads are dealt with by fan-coil units located in the raised floor. In the more stable zones deeper in the plan, a conventional displacement ventilation system operates. The raised floor acts as a plenum for supply air and low-velocity floor outlets provide delivery. The double-skin roof also forms part of the building's mechanized ventilation

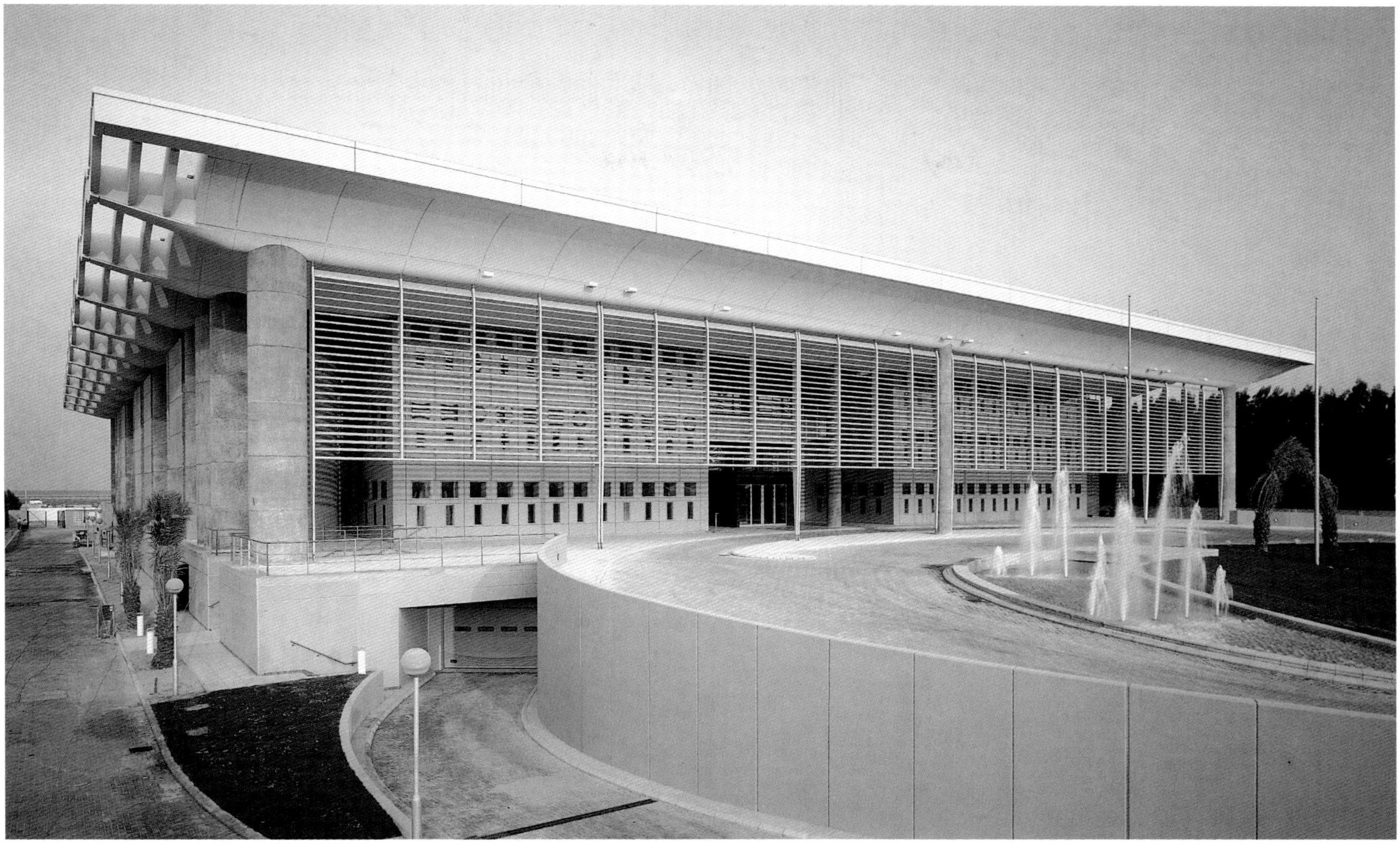

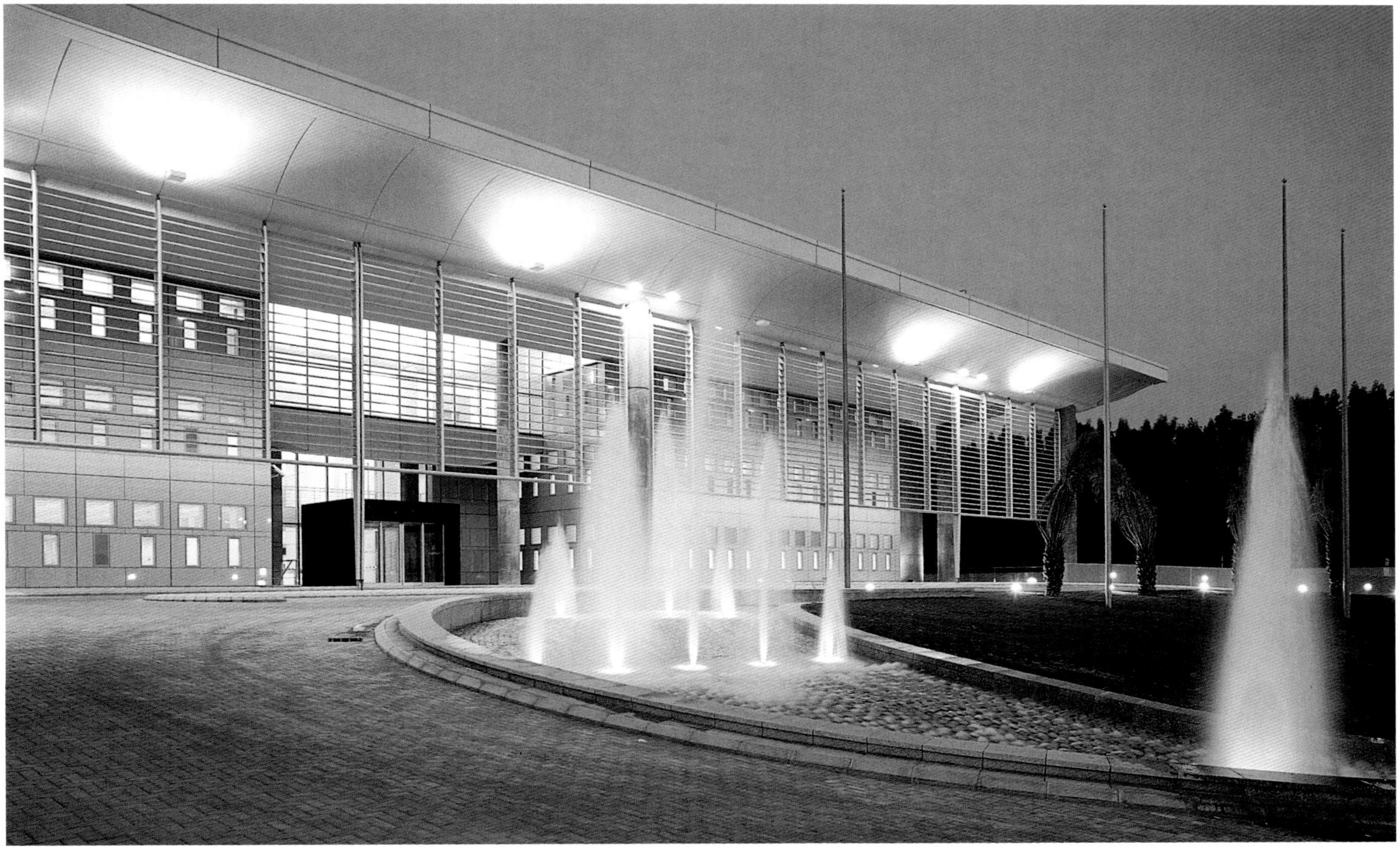

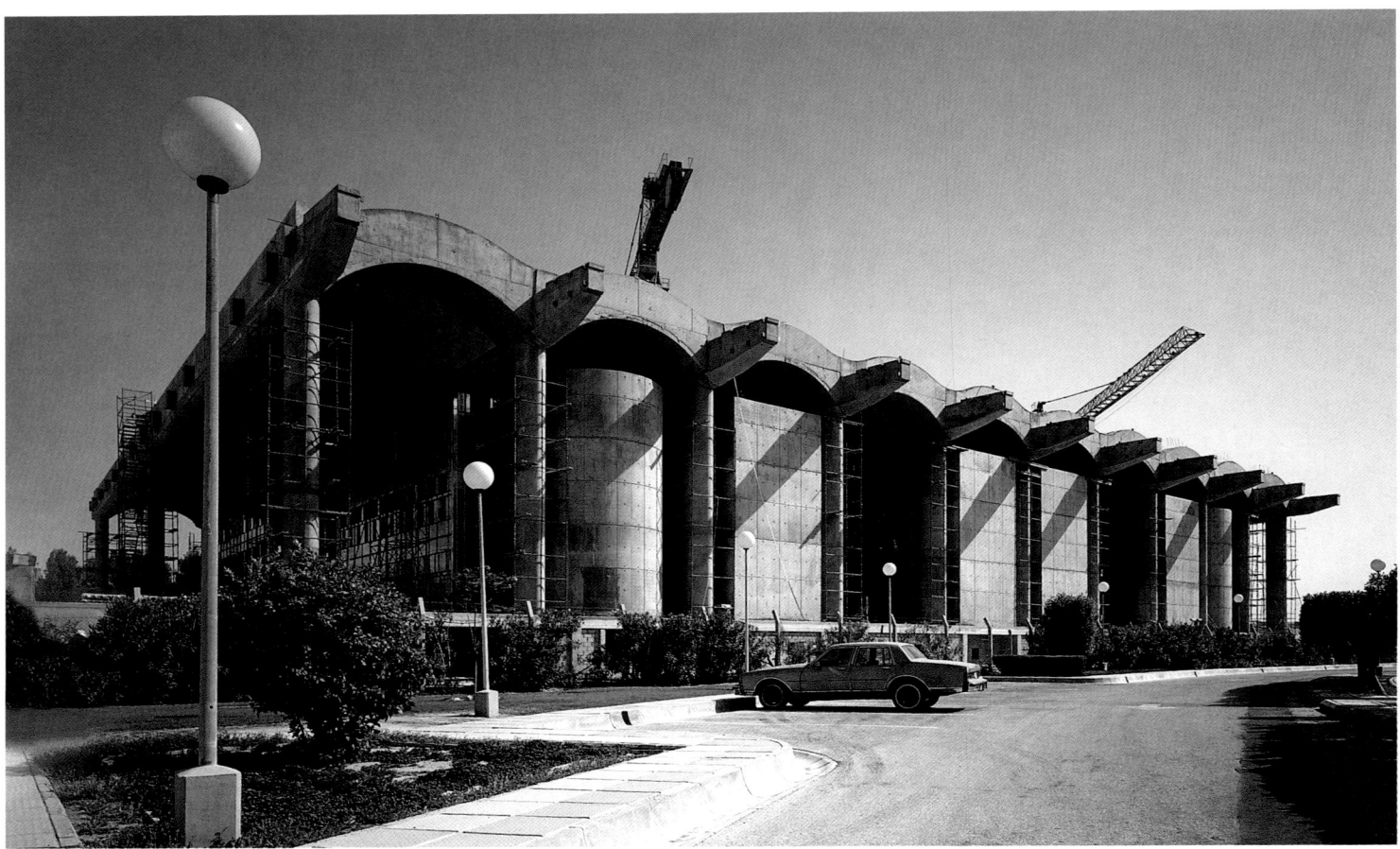

← Building façade at entry: day (top) and night (bottom).

↑ A construction shot, clearly showing the sinusoidal roof.

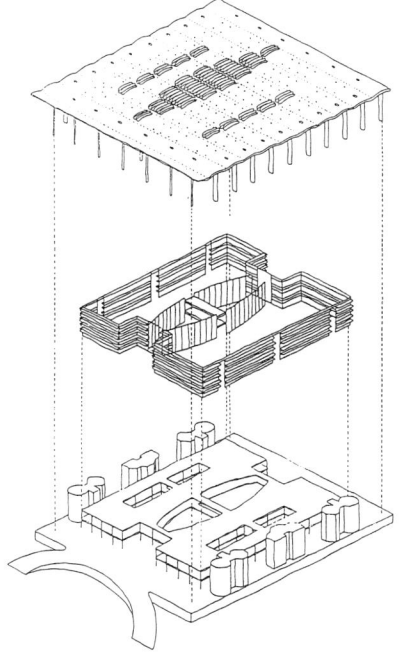

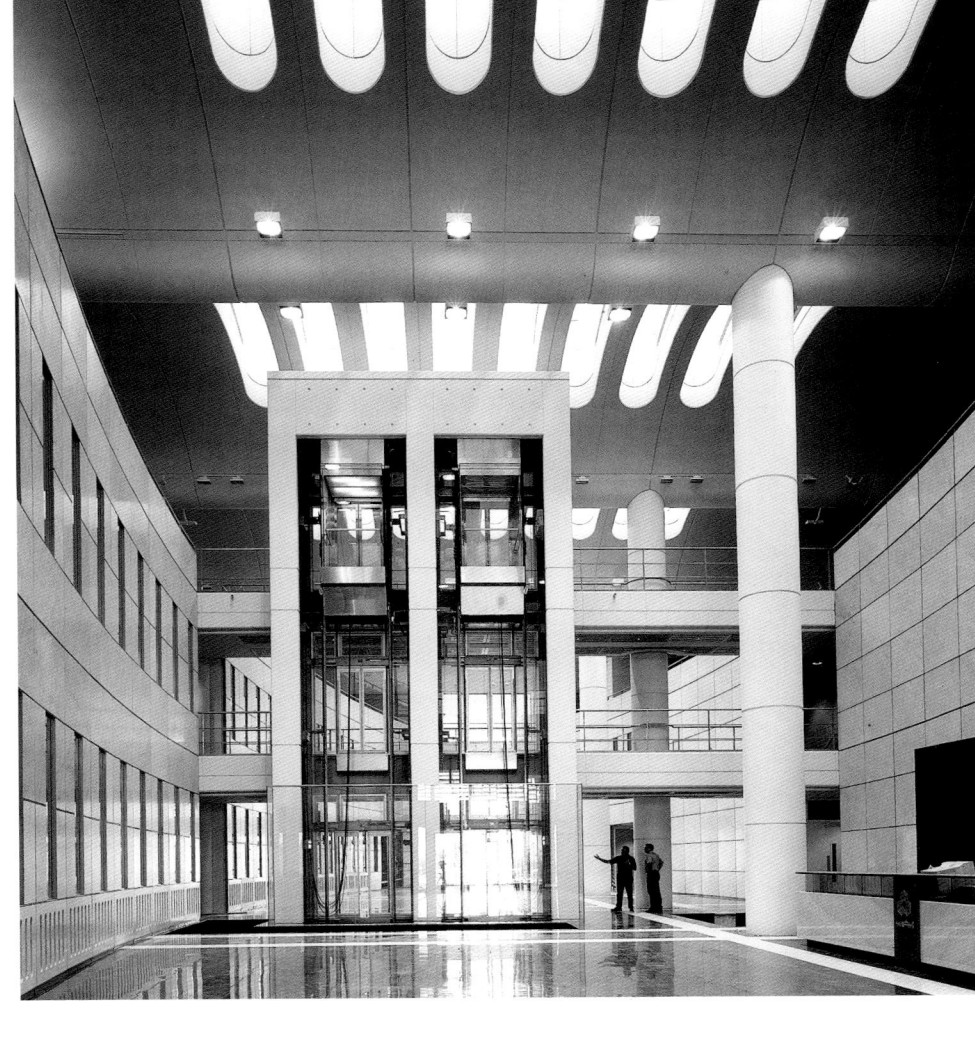

system: air rises from floor level and enters the hollow roof structure; exhaust air is drawn through the void and down vertical ducts in the large hollow columns to the plant rooms in the basement plinth. In summer, exhaust air is dumped into the enclosed car park to aid cooling.

Conclusion

The new Apicorp headquarters exemplifies a new regional architecture that responds to the demands of climate in a traditional way but is also based on selective borrowing from other cultures. In the development of modern architecture in the Middle East, the borrowing of ideas has sometimes been reduced to the cloning of images but, as Khaled Asfour suggests, 'Borrowed ideas do interact with different circumstances on transfer, giving birth to interpretations so particular (and so private) that outcomes become self-sustainable.... Once a tradition is established in this field, borrowing ideas becomes an advantage, not a burden on design quality.' [5]

It may be too soon to see benefits from the combination of borrowing and the exploitation of local energy resources, but Apicorp's design team have suggested how these resources used in conjunction with intelligent architectural form may lead to a new discourse among those who practise architecture in the Middle East.

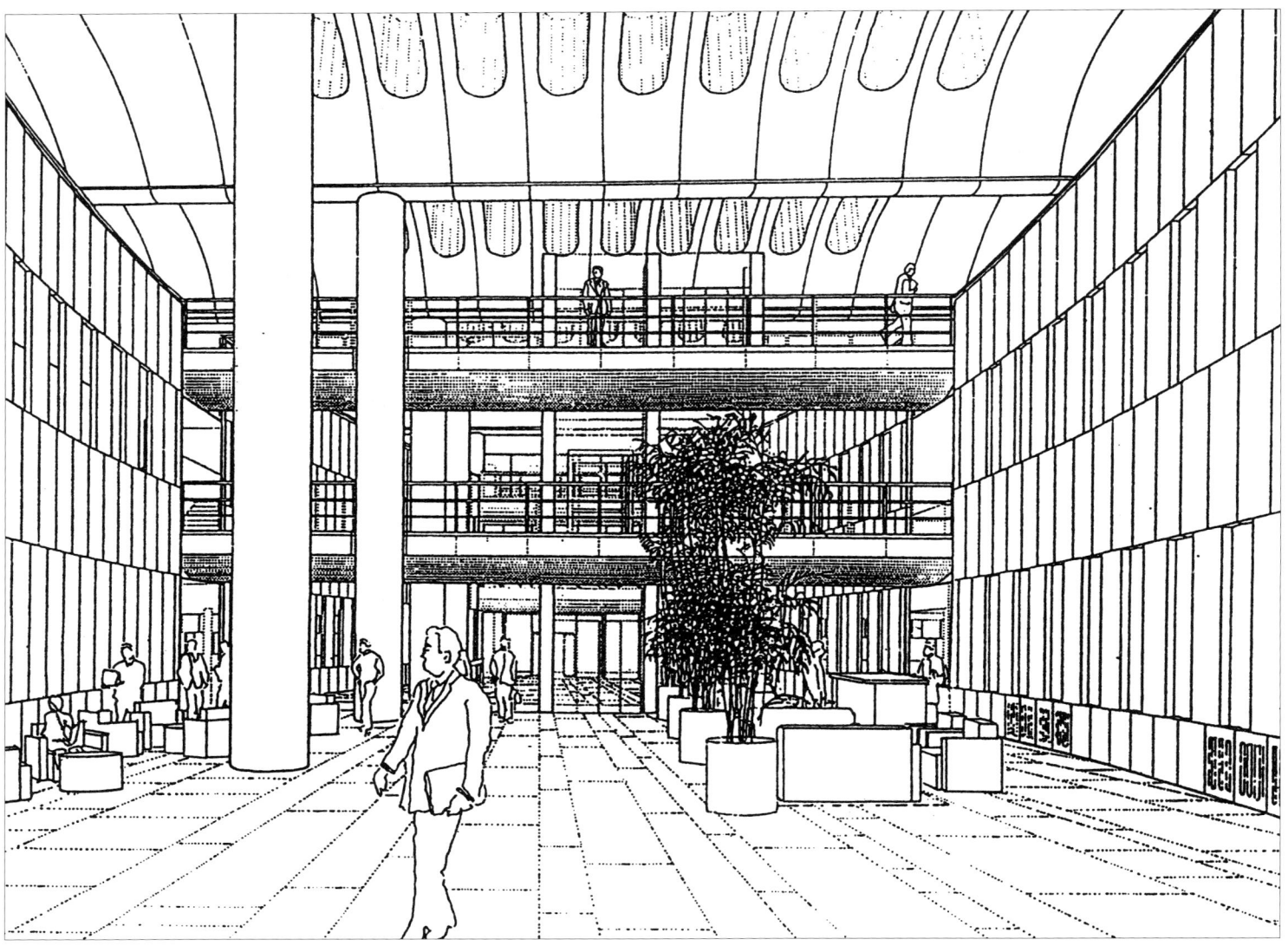

↑
Early design sketches
of central court.

Eastgate
Pearce Partnership
Harare, Zimbabwe
1996

At the beginning of a new millennium the question of globalism versus regionalism has assumed great significance in the political, economic, social and cultural debate. It can be argued that, in some respects, architecture led the way towards global culture. The image of the glass skyscraper was proposed in Mies van der Rohe's Berlin projects of 1919 and 1922. Le Corbusier's declaration –

'I propose only one house for all countries, the house of exact breathing' – made in Buenos Aires in 1929, implied the domination of technology over climate. These and other statements laid the foundations for the high-rise corporate office building that dominates the skylines of cities in all continents and has come to be the ubiquitous visible symbol of globalization.

The skyscraper makes use of a standard technological 'kit' of structural frame, curtain-walled envelope, suspended ceiling and air-conditioning to provide an environment for the processes of administration and commerce. Wherever it is located, this 'technical fix' allows the maintenance of similar conditions of temperature, ventilation, humidity and illumination, whether

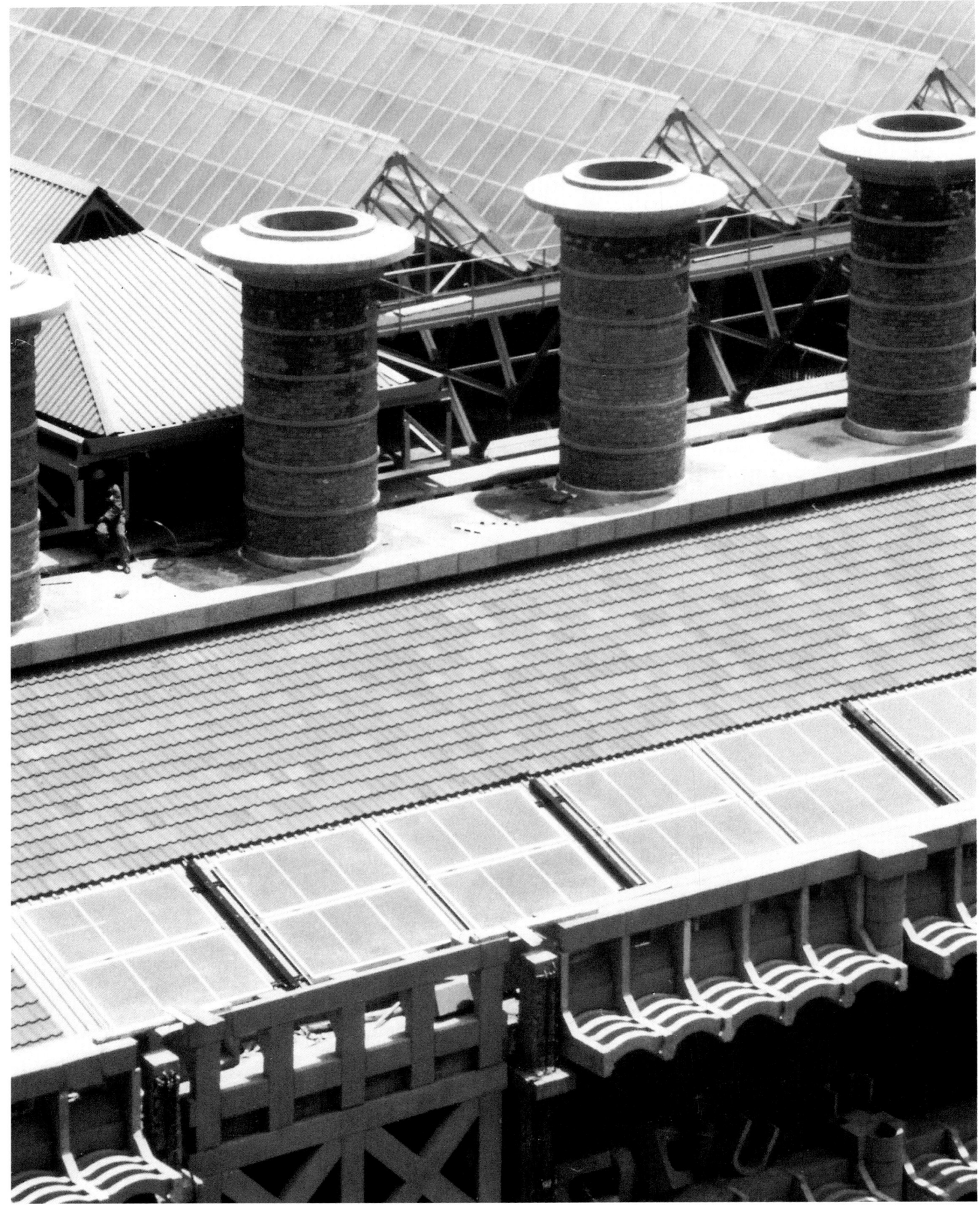

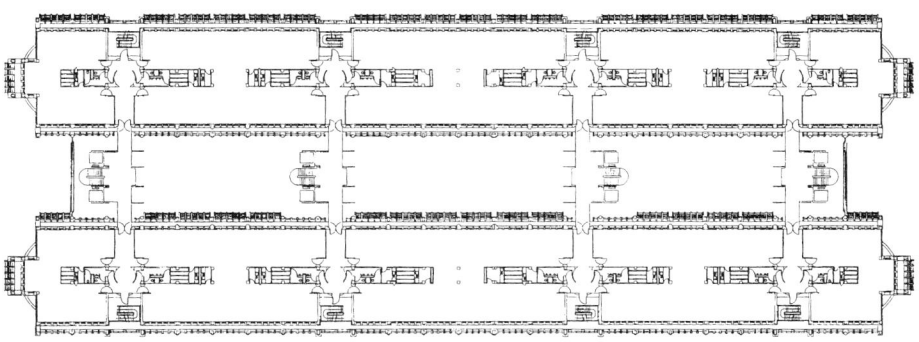

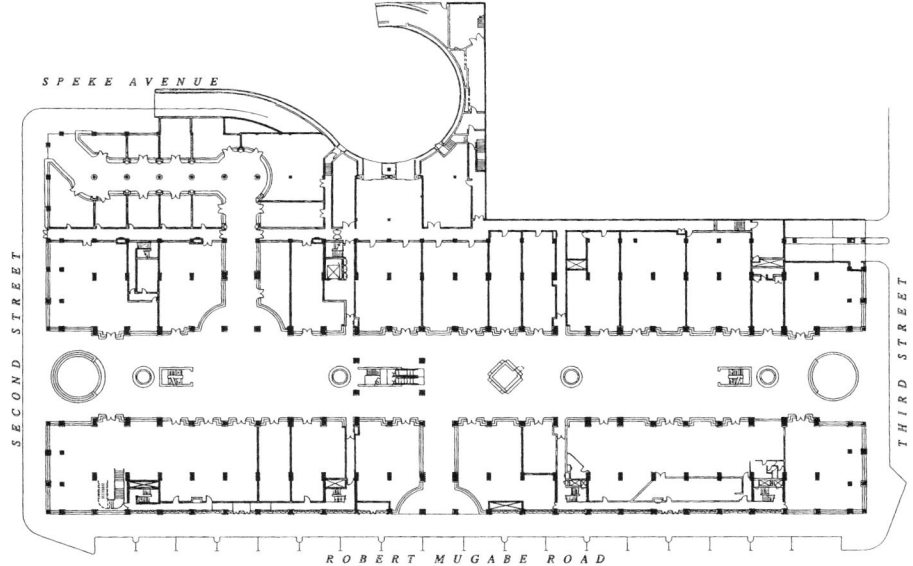

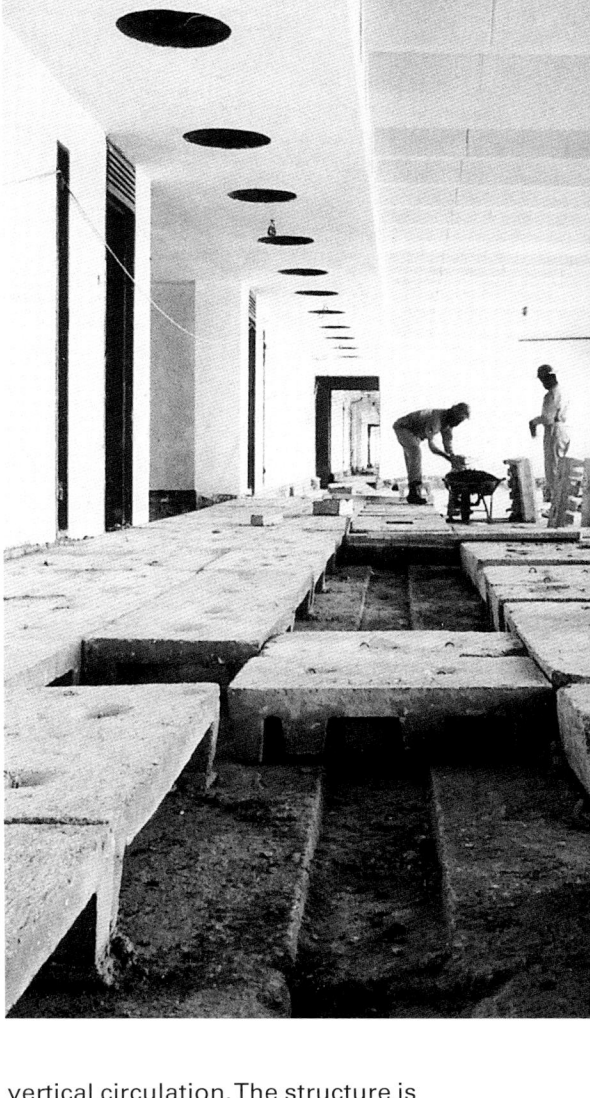

the local climate is hot or cold, dry or humid, temperate, tropical or equatorial.

A 'regional' alternative

The Eastgate Building in Harare offers a powerful challenge to the stereotypical solution. From the beginning the building was designed to provide a good commercial environment without the use of air-conditioning. In the developing economy of Zimbabwe many of the components of environmental plant have to be imported – a process that is expensive and leads to maintenance problems. As an alternative, the designers examined the idea of passive cooling.

The environmental logic of the building makes use of principles widely applied during the 19th century. Eastgate has many

similarities with Barry's and Reid's work at the Palace of Westminster and Jebb's designs for prisons, but there are significant differences, the most obvious of which spring from differences in climate and, to some extent, in function. In addition, computer modelling and, subsequently, quantitative performance modelling invest the design process with a degree of precision that would have been impossible a century and a half ago.

The building occupies an entire city block, 104m by 70m (341ft by 230ft), on the edge of the central business district of Harare. It comprises 26,000m² (279,760ft²) of office space and 5,600m² (60,256ft²) of shops in two, parallel, nine-storey blocks which are oriented with their long axes east–west. Between these is a glass-roofed atrium containing the principal

vertical circulation. The structure is principally reinforced concrete, which plays a crucial role in the environmental strategy. Within the concrete structure the enclosing walls are of brickwork.

The climate of Harare is warm and sunny, with a pattern of warm days and cool nights. Passive cooling works by using this diurnal temperature fluctuation to reduce the temperature of the structure during the night-time hours and, thereby, to reduce the temperature of air delivered to the interior during the day. This is achieved by the complete integration of the building fabric and its environmental processes.

The cross-section illustrates the essentials of the design. The two parallel blocks are 15m (49ft) wide, as is the central atrium. Each block has seven floors of offices above two

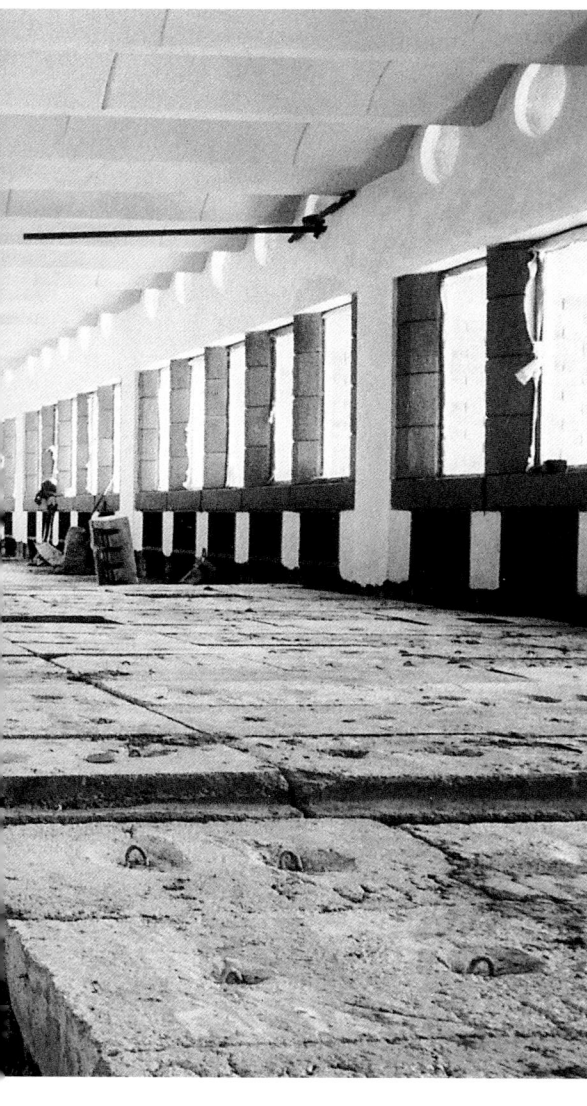

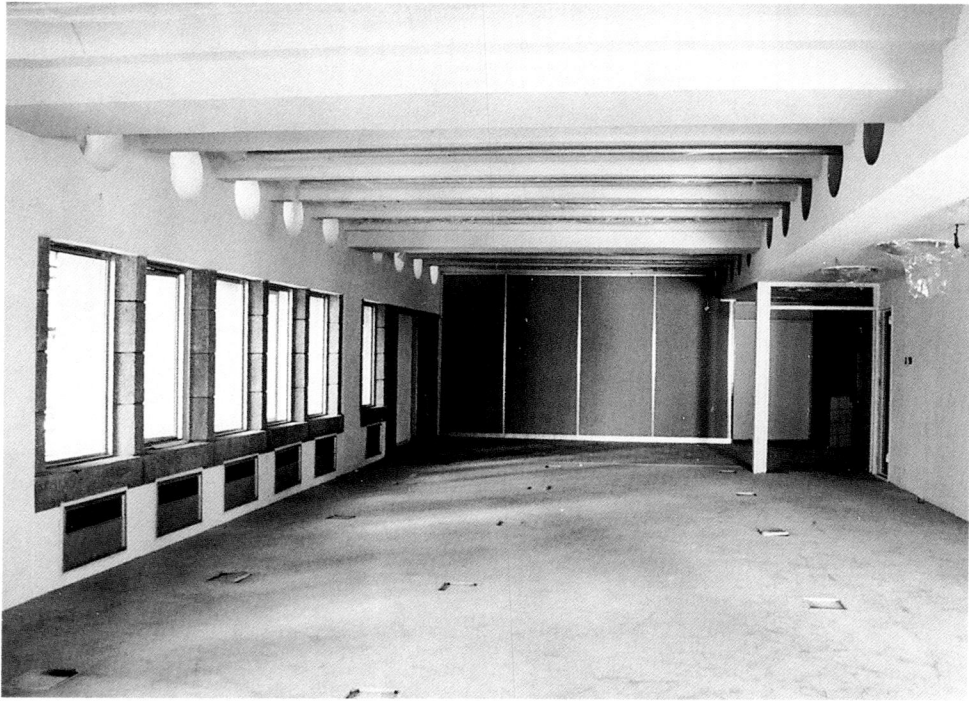

←

Plans at ground level, showing the shopping mall, and at a typical upper floor showing the office layout.

Office space under construction, showing the installation of the precast concrete

raised floor units. The void between these and the structural concrete slab is the supply plenum for the displacement ventilation system. It also houses electrical services.

↑

General view of office space. The exposed concrete mass of the construction is a fundamental element of the environmental system of the building.

lower floors containing shops, a food court and some parking. Between these zones is a service mezzanine. The incoming air for the offices is drawn through this and is then distributed through a network of vertical ducts. Air is extracted through a second system of ducts and is exhausted through brickwork chimneys above the roof.

The incoming air is taken from the atrium, where it is cleaner than that in the surrounding streets. It is then filtered and driven mechanically through the structure by locally manufactured fans. From the main vertical shafts, air is passed through a void in each concrete floor slab and enters the offices through grilles beneath the windows in the perimeter walls. This low-level supply acts to displace the air in the space, which exits through a high-level vent directly

into the vertical extract duct. The extract cycle has no mechanical assistance and is driven entirely by natural stack effect, assisted by the effect of the sun warming the brick chimneys and increasing the velocity of the extracted air. The architect has called these 'solar accelerators'. The building has four principal supply zones that correspond to the four façades – two exposed to the external climate and two to the internal atrium. Cooling is achieved by running the intake fans at a relatively high speed, achieving ten air changes per hour, during the night cycle; this was calculated to provide the best balance between the cooling effect and the amount of power consumed by the fans. During the daytime the fans supply air at only two air changes per hour, which is enough to achieve good ventilation of the offices and to

maintain good comfort temperatures. The central atrium is ventilated by stack effect that vents through a gap between the glazed canopy and the roof of the office wings.

For the few occasions when heating is necessary in Harare, the building has individual electric room heaters, located under the windows. These can be controlled by the occupants, but the system is overridden by a thermostatic control to prevent its use when the ambient temperature is above a certain point.

The orientation of Eastgate, with its long façades facing north and south, makes it relatively easy to protect the building from the high angle of the sun at this latitude. All the long elevations, in and outside the atrium, have deep structural overhangs, in the form of precast concrete hoods, and planting to provide shade to the

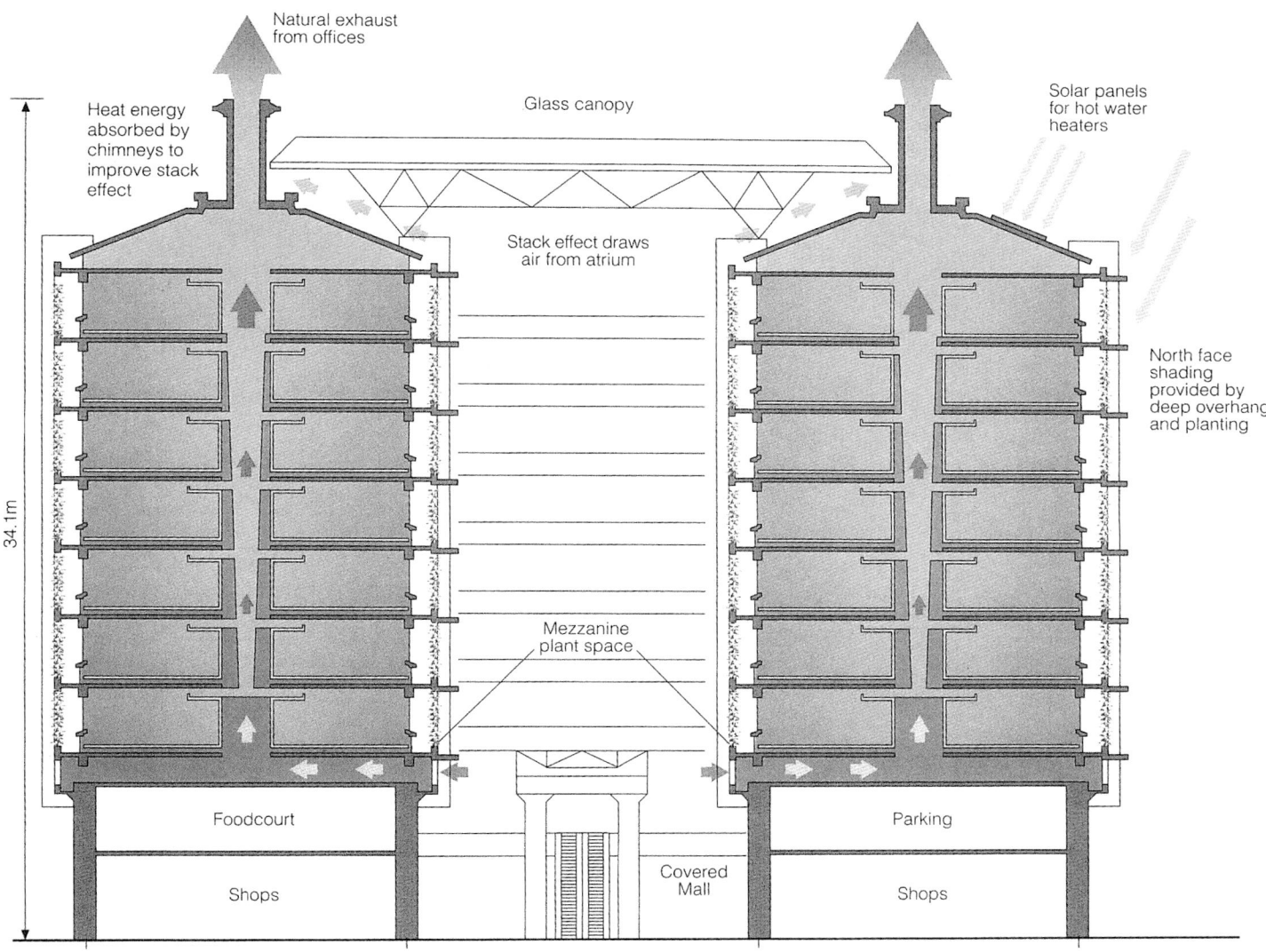

Natural exhaust from offices

Heat energy absorbed by chimneys to improve stack effect

Glass canopy

Solar panels for hot water heaters

Stack effect draws air from atrium

North face shading provided by deep overhang and planting

34.1m

Mezzanine plant space

Foodcourt

Parking

Covered Mall

Shops

Shops

windows. The windows occupy 25 per cent of the façade, and each has an internal blind that can be operated manually to control local solar gains or glare. This ratio was calculated using a computer model which simulated the sun's path and the effect of alternative shading devices, and optimized the balance of lighting and temperature in the offices.

The artificial lighting system is also completely integrated, physically and operationally, into the building. The principal lighting is from fluorescent uplighters suspended from the exposed concrete ceilings, which provide evenly distributed illumination that avoids undesirable reflections on computer screens. The control gear of fluorescent lamps produces heat that would affect the temperature of the offices. To avoid this, they are placed in the exhaust-air

shaft above a lowered ceiling at the rear of the space. This ceiling supports low-energy downlight fittings that supplement the output of the fluorescent lamps.

An array of solar collectors runs along the roof of the northerly block. These are the primary sources for the hot water supplied to the tea kitchens within the offices. They are supplemented by electric heaters, located in the water storage tanks, that can be operated only at night-time.

The performance of the building has been monitored by the consultant engineers, Ove Arup & Partners Zimbabwe, who have established their own offices there. Initial results show that, on days of typical variation in diurnal temperature, 4.5 degrees of cooling of the temperature in the offices can be achieved. When the

diurnal variation is lower, the cooling effect is less marked, but these conditions typically occur when the peak temperature is lower. Initial measurements of total energy consumption indicate that the building performs very well in comparison with recent air-conditioned buildings in Harare. This is in a range of 48 per cent to 83 per cent of the energy demand of these other buildings.

Conclusion

Eastgate stands as a potent symbol of the way in which the standard assumptions and solutions of technological globalism may be challenged by inventive, culturally appropriate and scientifically informed design. The design adapts principles that, as explained in the introduction, have a long and reliable

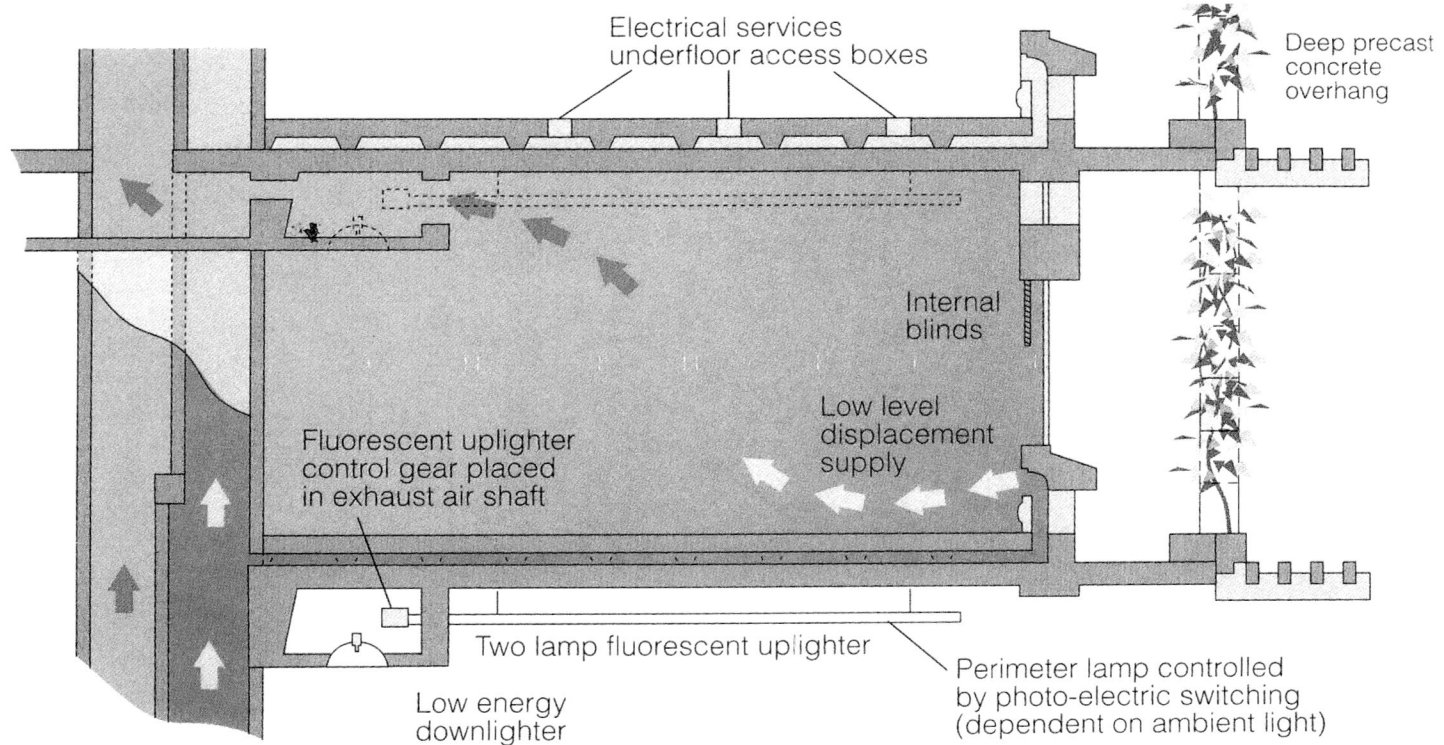

Electrical services
underfloor access boxes

Deep precast
concrete
overhang

Internal
blinds

Fluorescent uplighter
control gear placed
in exhaust air shaft

Low level
displacement
supply

Two lamp fluorescent uplighter

Low energy
downlighter

Perimeter lamp controlled
by photo-electric switching
(dependent on ambient light)

← Operational cross-section that describes the principal features of the building's environmental logic.

↑ Detailed cross-section through a typical office space. This shows the principal air supply and extract routes and the integration of the electrical installation with the structure of the building.

pedigree. With the support of the analytical and predictive tools that have emerged from 20th-century building science, architects and engineers have collaborated in investing these principles with a new precision and reinterpretation. The result is a building that fits precisely into its specific economic and technological and climatological context.

In achieving this, the building embodies aspects of the 19th century's confident synthesis of structure and environmental process. It also shows how the 20th century's engagement with the expression and organization of the machinery of environmental control – Louis Kahn's 'served and servant' – can be reinterpreted in the realization of passive, selective strategies.

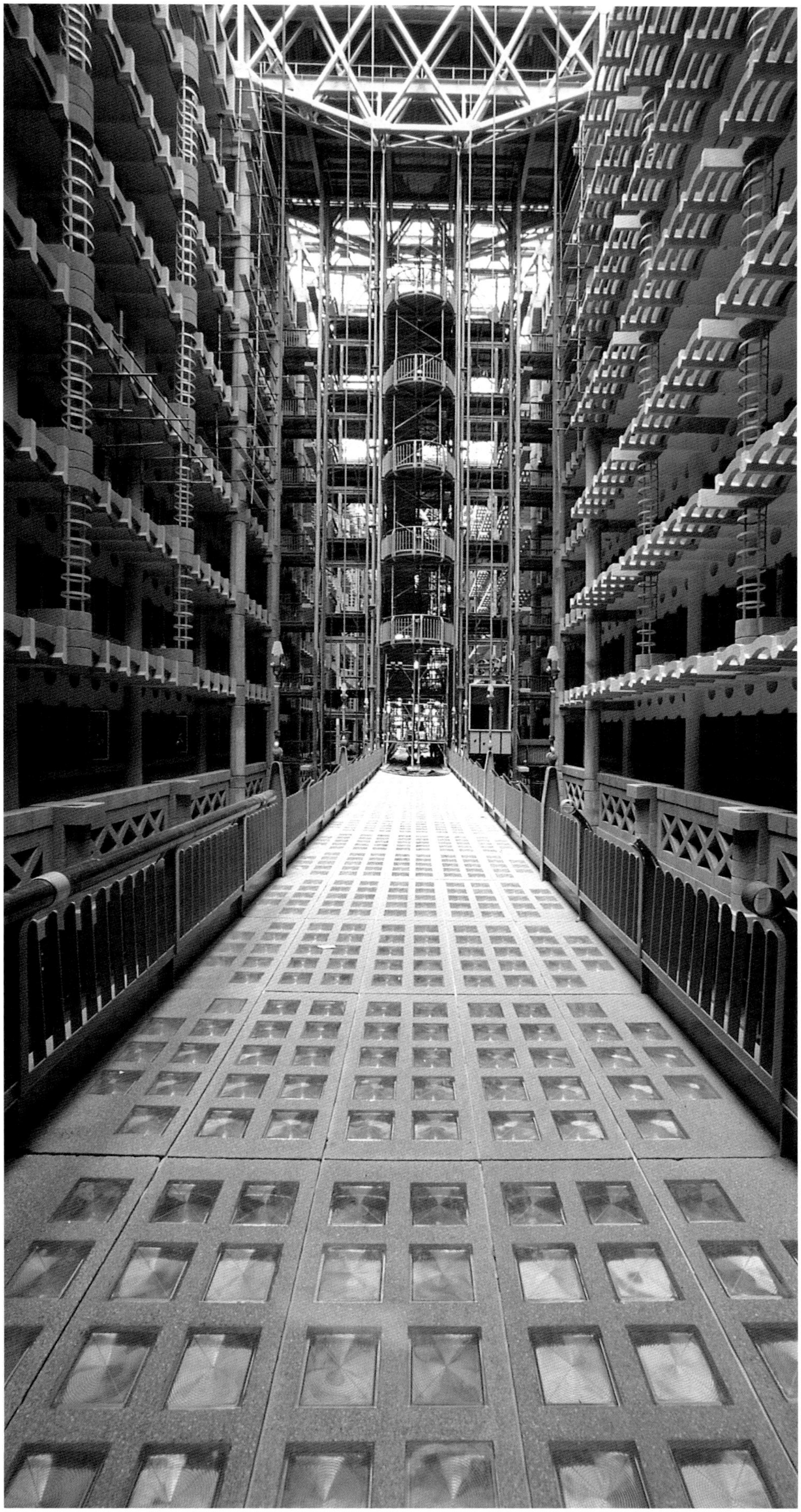

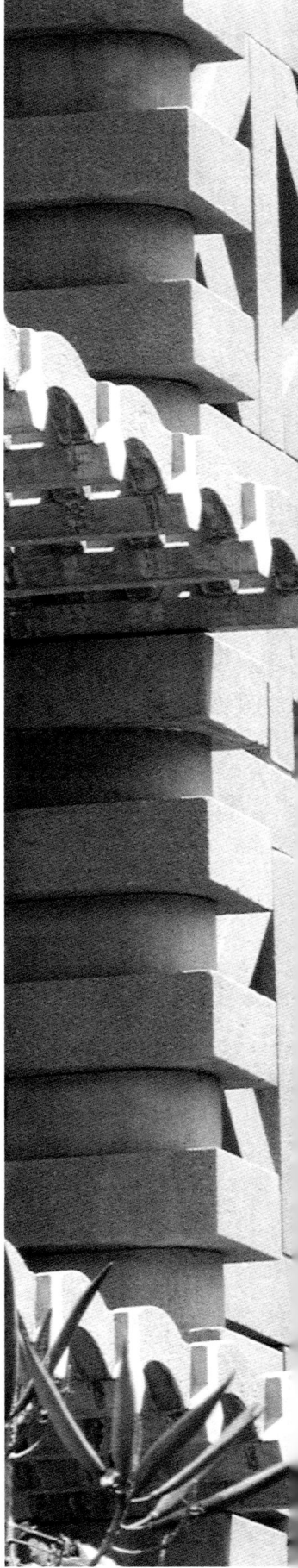

The central atrium, defined by offices rising above the shopping areas.

Detail of the precast concrete shading system that articulates the exterior of the building.

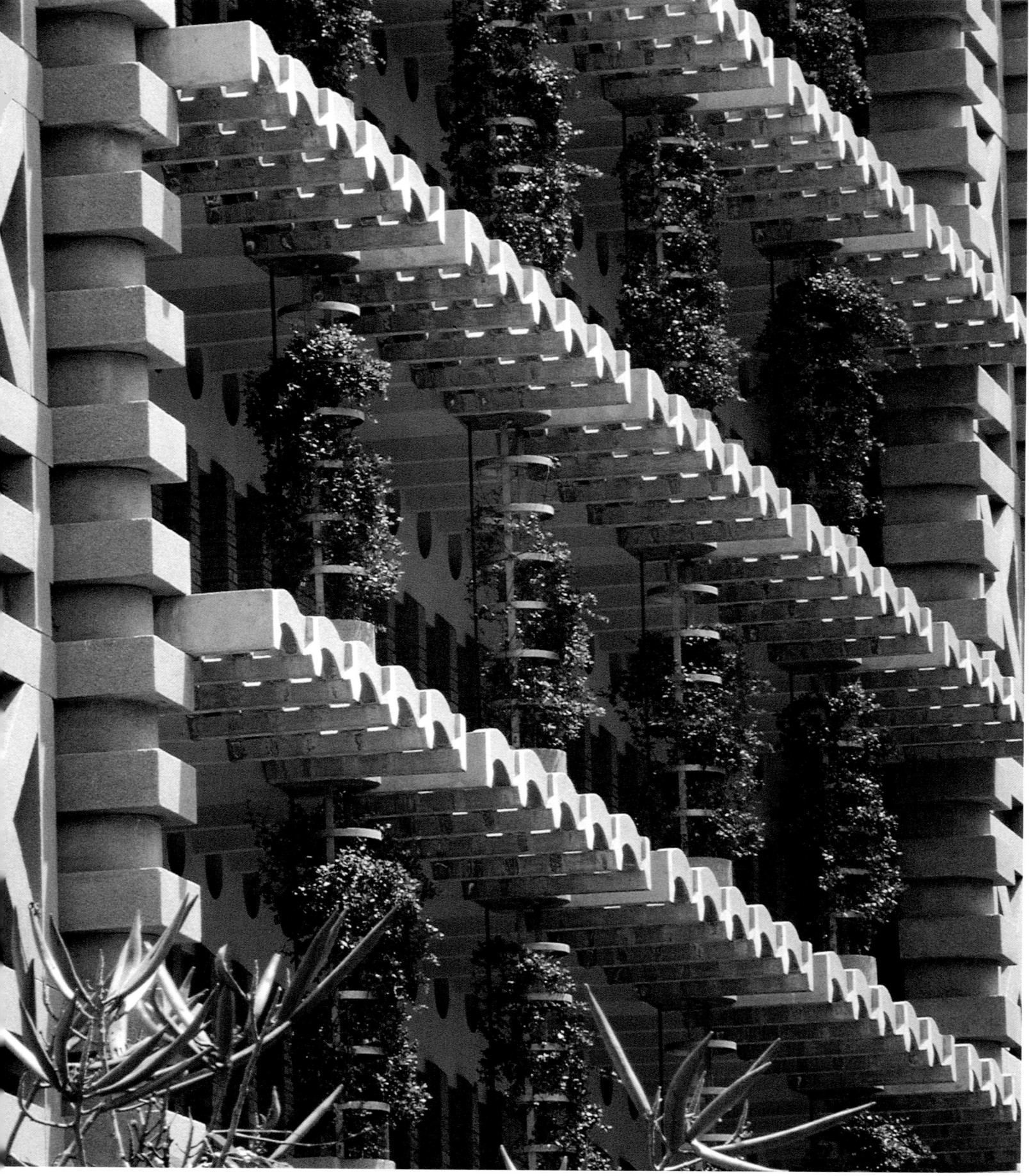

Arup Campus
Arup Associates
Solihull, UK
2001

➜
The Campus building, with its roof-mounted passive design elements and dynamic façade.

A question frequently asked by designers who have strongly held practices, philosophies and beliefs is 'Can these tenets survive when the designers become their own developers?' Arup faced this question in the design and construction of their new £7 million Midland headquarters. Although designed by their sister practice, Arup Associates, a brief was set that not only included aspects of effective commercial development, but also focused on the application of the organisation's core skills in comfortable, low-energy and sustainable design. This had to be more than just wishful thinking and these aspects had to be incorporated into the building in a demonstrable way. The interdisciplinary ethic, for which Arup is famous, also needed to be accommodated spatially.

The brief for the new building specified floor plates that would encourage communication within teams and throughout the company, and provide an appropriate level of flexibility and adaptability. 'We envisaged a new set-up whereby as many diverse Arup skills as possible would be co-located, so that we could co-operate to provide integrated services for the whole range of client requirements. Additionally, we wanted the offices to be stimulating and efficient, and also represent us to the outside world.' [1]

A vast reservoir of experience is, of course, available. A brief scan of Arup Associates' pedigree in the design of business park-type offices reveals a lineage from the CEGB Headquarters and Wiggins Teape, Basingstoke, through to many phases of Stockley Park, each of which provided lessons that were assimilated into the design of the organization's new building.

Site
The sloping site occupies part of some land earmarked for a proposed

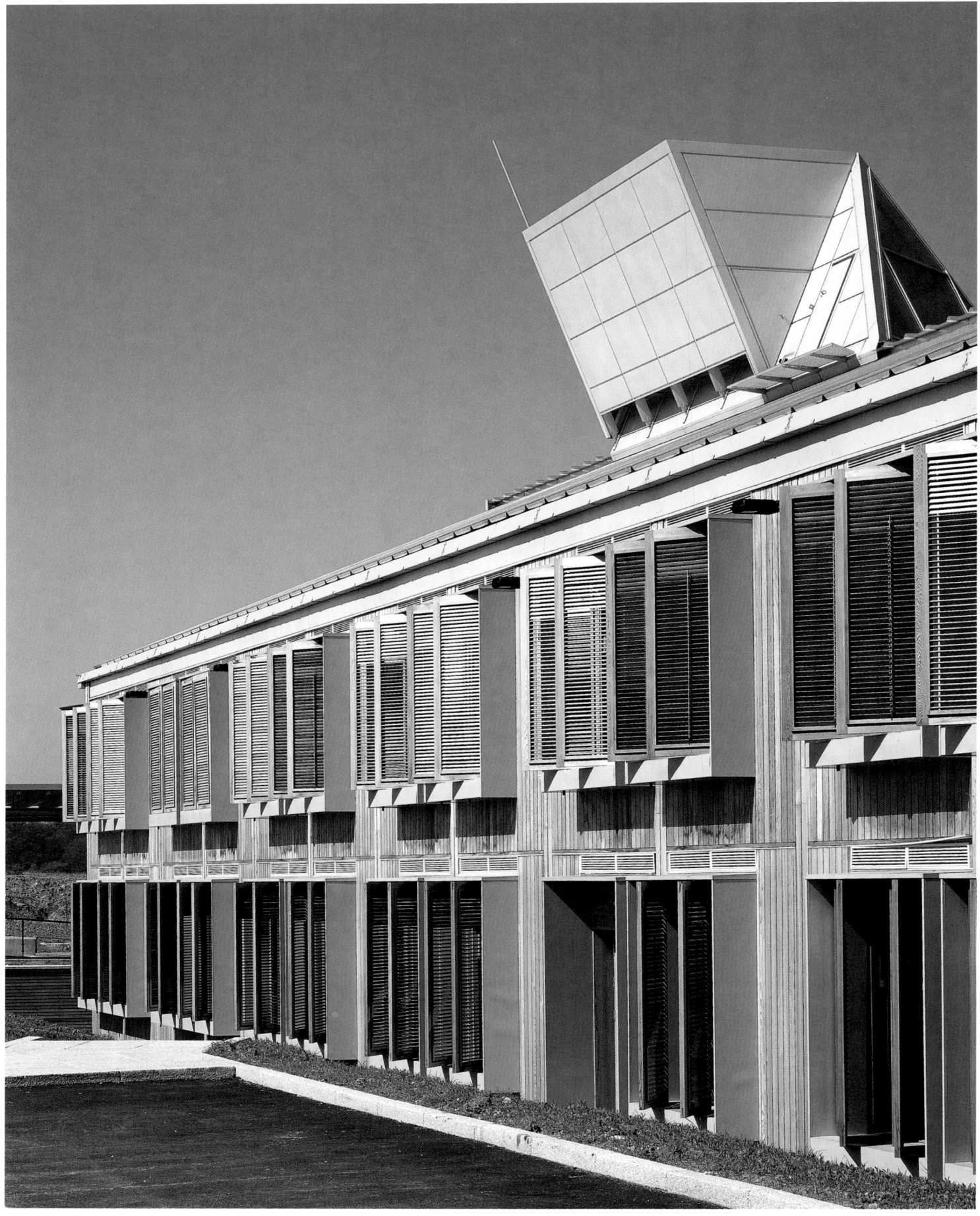

Site plan showing the
relationship of the
pavilions to the
landscape.

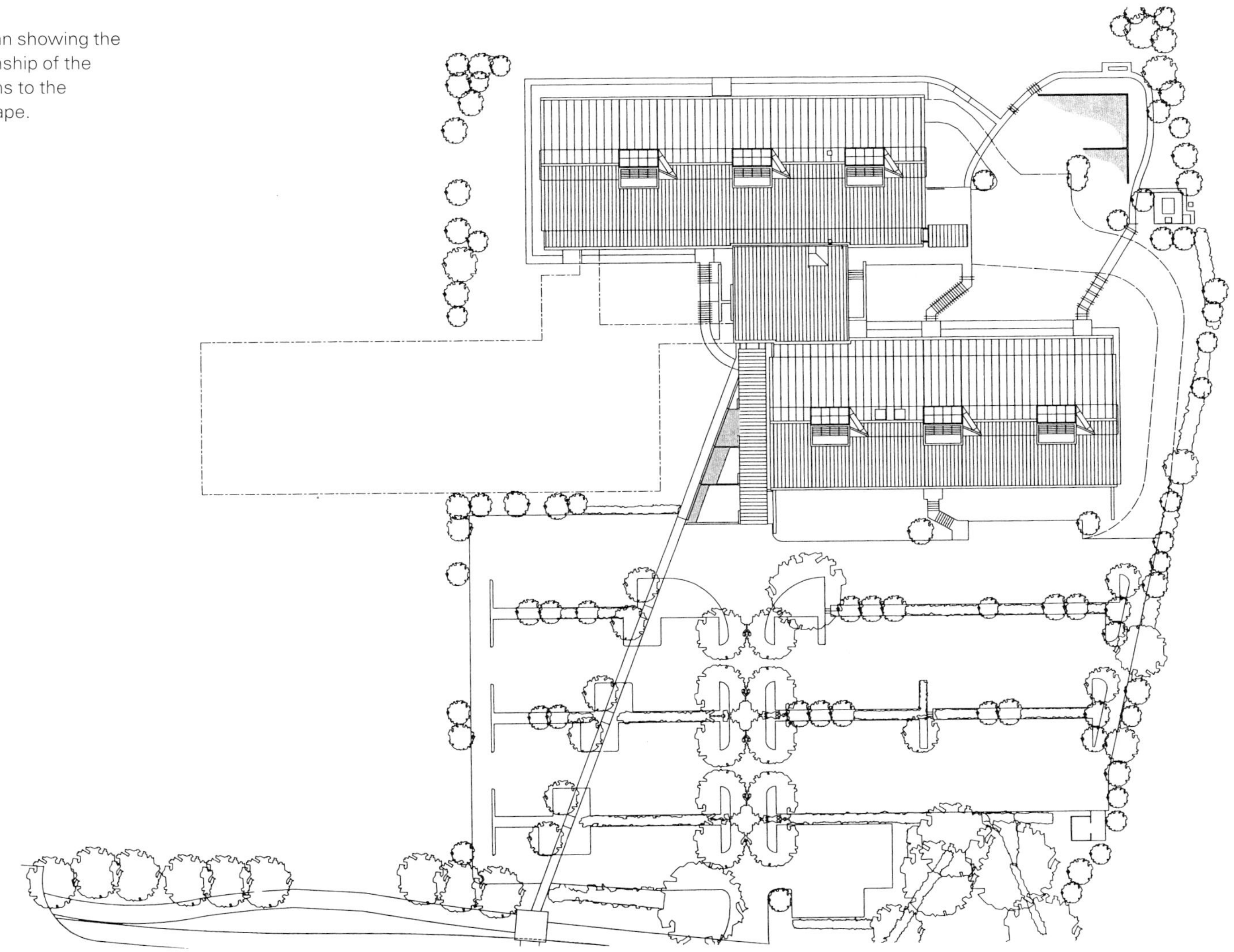

business park in Solihull in the
English Midlands. The decision to
develop on this particular site was
influenced by the need to amalgamate
activities previously located in two
separate Midlands centres –
Birmingham and Coventry.

The positioning of the new
buildings is based on the following
responses to site:

· exploit panoramic views to the
  north-west
· exploit and work with the existing
  site contours
· buildings to address the proposed
  lake
· accommodate entry from the south,
  already fixed by the business park
  distribution road

Furthermore, the development had
to be planned for construction in

stages. The development will
comprise three pavilions (two in
Phase 1, and another in Phase 2) that
step down the slope of the site. The
long dimensions of the pavilions run
along the site's contours and take
advantage of the views over the lake.
At the heart of the plan, an auditorium
and café form the focus of the
complex. Floors are arranged at half
levels and a central link connects the
circulation of the Phase 1 pavilions. A
central, terraced and landscaped
courtyard acts as a potential outdoor
work area and social space.

Building Form
The following priorities of the brief
have determined the building form:

· a comfortable and energy-efficient
  working environment
· flexible space

· minimal vertical spatial separation
· a cohesive campus atmosphere
· allowance for tenancy sub-division

The priority for comfort and energy
efficiency was further defined as:

· naturally ventilated through outside
  air supply
· good levels of daylight, contributing
  to a comfortable visual environment
· a coherent office layout
· visual communication between
  floors
· views and contacts with outside
  landscape
· flexibility and adaptability

The formal development of the
pavilions is based on these
requirements, starting with
aspirations for a single space; a clear-
span, deep-plan box is described,

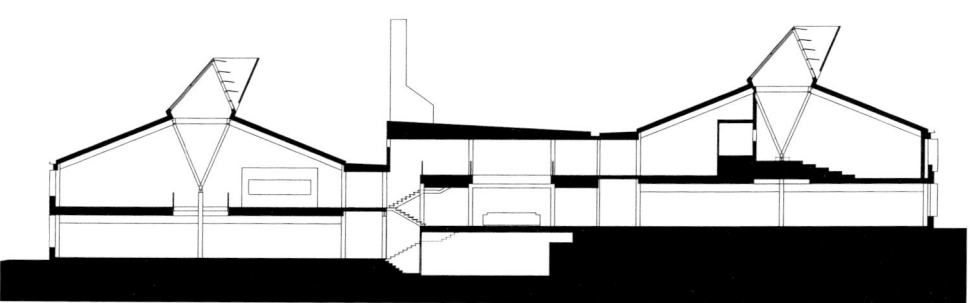

←

Section through
auditorium and office
floor.

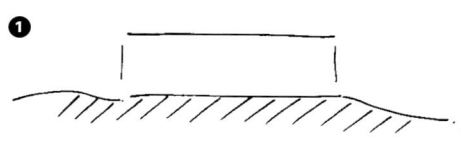

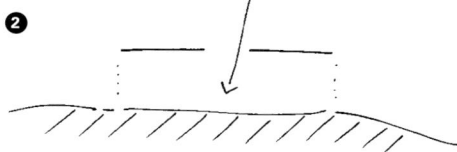

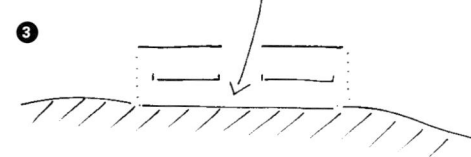

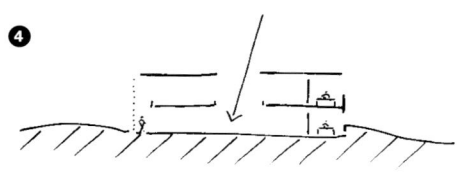

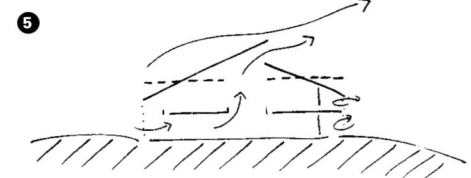

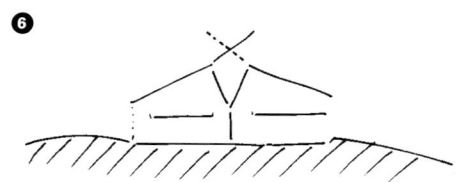

↑

1 A single space...
2 penetrated by light.
3 Cost considerations
   reduce external
   wall: introduction
   of mezzanines...
4 which extend to

walls to ensure
lettable space.
5 Pitch roof upward
   to increase internal
   environment then...
6 open structure to
   light with V-supports.

which is then punctured at mid-span roof level to provide daylight. These first two moves are radical, as they break, or at least recast, the mould for the standard campus office model. The desire for daylight and natural ventilation would ordinarily limit the depth of office space to between 12m (39ft) and 14m (46ft). At Solihull, the window-to-window dimension was set at 24m (79ft) almost reverting to the kind of floor plates that would have to rely on a permanently electrically lit and mechanically ventilated interior, like those of the CEGB Headquarters from over 20 years ago. The deep plan deals effectively with the organization's needs; in particular, it can provide the physical context to accommodate a high degree of flexibility and adaptability. Larger spaces, such as auditorium and cafeteria, can fit

alongside a range of different workplace scenarios.

The dumb, and potentially 'exclusive', box is thus transformed into an intelligent, and potentially 'selective', one. The enclosure is layered and pierced to enable daylight penetration and the openings for this, on the ridgeline of a pitched roof, allow for ventilation through stack effect. The environmental section is further developed to optimize daylight and natural modes of ventilation.

Construction and Materials
The buildings are constructed in a sparse, lean and almost stringent manner, sadly not often seen in the UK construction industry. This may have been driven by budget as much as anything else, but it is refreshing to see buildings dealt with in this straightforward way. The structural

system is designed to meet not only the needs of economic structural support, but also the environmental system – embodied energy and re-use. The 24m (79ft) window-to-window dimension is simply split by placing a column at mid-span. This column supports the intermediate floor, then separates into a 'wish-bone' form to hold the two different leaves of the sloping roof apart, to allow daylight penetration. Columns like these, allowing environmental control, are not new to Arup Associates and may be seen as a classic motif, having been employed as early as 1954 in the Duxford Aero Factory.

The steel frame is made visible and exposed, and supports a precast concrete floor and roof panel, which spans 6m (20ft) from beam to beam. The steelwork is bolted to allow

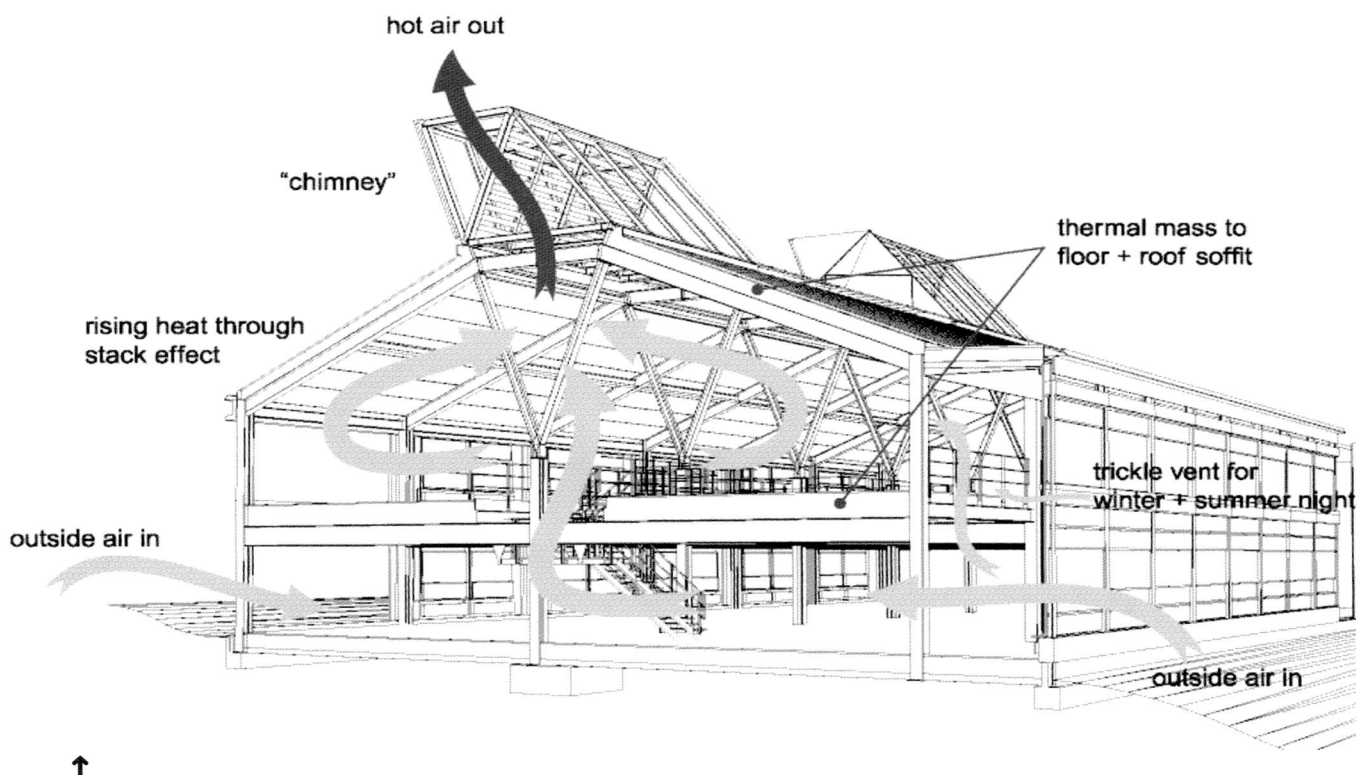

hot air out

"chimney"

rising heat through
stack effect

thermal mass to
floor + roof soffit

outside air in

trickle vent for
winter + summer night

outside air in

↑
Stack-assigned
natural ventilation.

disassembly and re-use at the end of the building's life cycle. The principle of design for re-use runs throughout the building elements, as part of the overall quest for sustainability. Composite construction is eschewed. The soffits of these precast units are left exposed and painted to provide thermal mass.

The external envelope is clad predominantly in untreated western red cedar (from certified, environmentally managed sources) and façades are carefully designed according to orientation. Windows are equipped with moveable, external louvred blinds, again made of cedar, which provide solar control. These windows combine with the opaque façade elements to make refreshingly calm and ordered building façades, which are in stark contrast to the typical call-centre sheds and

speculative office blocks that are its neighbours. The repose of the pavilions is punctuated by aluminium roof 'pods'. These are purpose-designed enclosures that appear at regular intervals and are designed to promote daylight and ventilation. They were designed for ease of assembly and were delivered to site flat-packed, constructed on the ground and erected into position.

Energy and Environment
The design is based on an orthodox approach to the passive design of offices – high levels of daylighting and solar control, with modes of natural ventilation, all within a thermally efficient envelope. The aim of the design team was to achieve a very good rating on the Building Research Establishment Environmental Assessment Method. The building will

probably exceed this standard and achieve an excellent rating, as the combination of passive design (resulting in a reduction in the use of natural resources and CO_2 emissions, and greater recycling) and global factors, such as transport (a Green Transport Plan has been devised for occupiers) add up to an integrated approach to the Campus.

Visual environment
The areas and disposition of glazing were determined in the physical and computer modelling carried out by Arup Associates and in the Artificial Sky at the Bartlett faculty, University College London. In particular, studies were made to ensure that the glare index from perimeter windows and roof-mounted pods was controlled. Daylighting is achieved through the combination of top and sidelight by

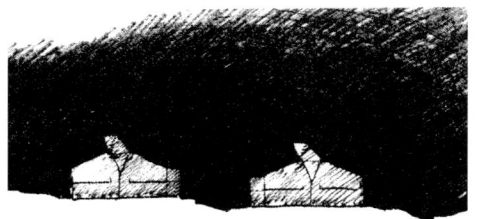

↑
Design sketch
section shows
pavilions sited on
contours.

→
Early design
sketches illustrate
environmental
principles and formal
development.

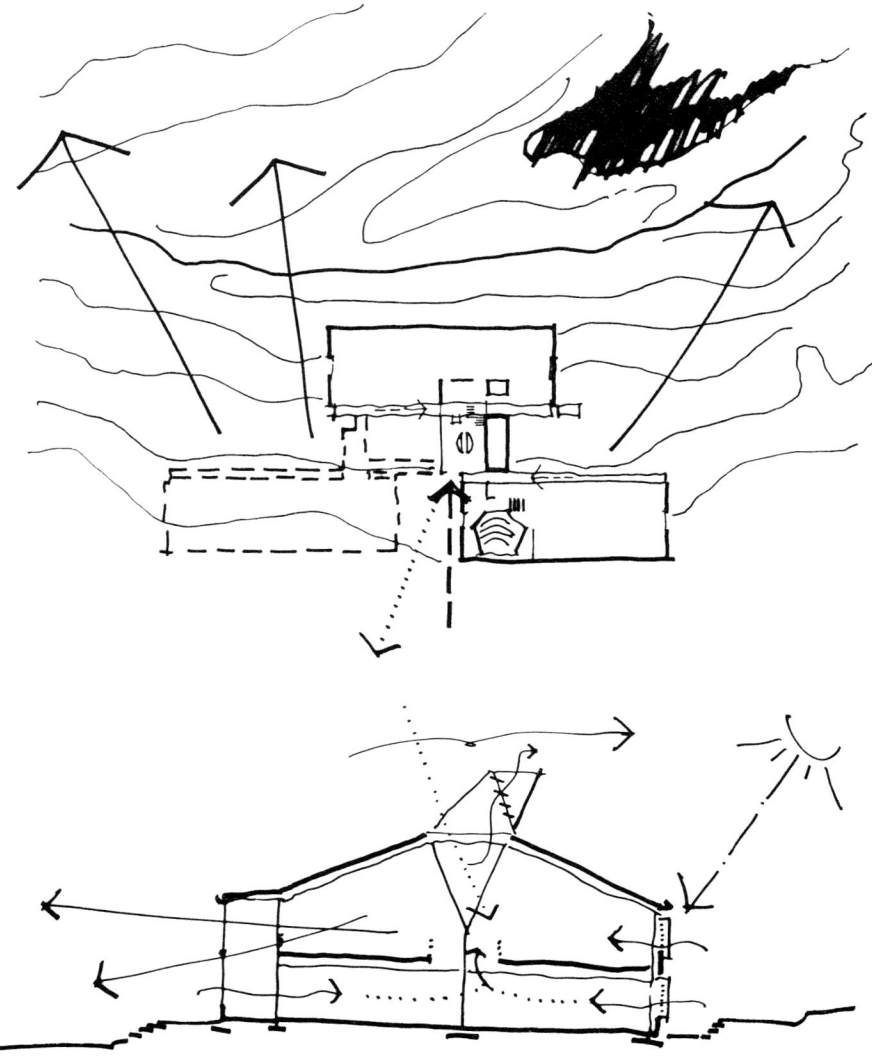

external louvres and manually
operated shutters to south façades,
and manually and electrically
operated internal blinds to other
façades.

The lighting systems have been
designed to achieve a 400 lux level of
illumination over the work surface.
Whilst much of this is through
daylight during normal working
hours, an automatic lighting control
system is linked to, and balances,
lighting conditions.

Ventilation
The office is designed for natural
ventilation under most conditions.
Defying the current orthodoxy of 14m
(46ft) floor plates, window to window,
the Campus floor plate is a ground-
breaking 24m (79ft). The ridgeline
'pods' supplement normal passive
design strategies. The perimeter walls

incorporate windows with openable
vents at high and low levels. Trickle
vents, linked to the building
management system, add to these
openings. In summer conditions,
windows are opened as necessary,
this being linked to stack effect
ventilation via the roof pods. Draught-
free, controlled ventilation is achieved
in the winter by motorized louvres,
designed as integral parts of the
cladding system. The same
mechanisms operate to provide useful
night-time cooling.

Heating is provided by a simple low-
pressure hot-water system, with
perimeter radiators, again linked to
the building management system. A
number of temperature sensors are
located throughout the building and
activate the building management
system, which operates the damper
devices to control ventilation rates.

The auditorium and computer
rooms are air-conditioned, based on a
displacement system, with free
cooling using outside air for the
majority of the year.

Conclusion
For many designers, it seems obvious
that sustainability should be integral
to the development of architectural
practice. However, more often than
not, atypical projects tend to get this
kind of treatment – landmark projects
or, at the other end of the scale,
modest projects designed by
environmentally committed
practitioners. Sustainability is worn
on the sleeve of the completed
buildings. To attempt to transform the
established and well-known typeform,
in order to achieve high performance,
may be a tougher challenge than
making bespoke buildings and, in the

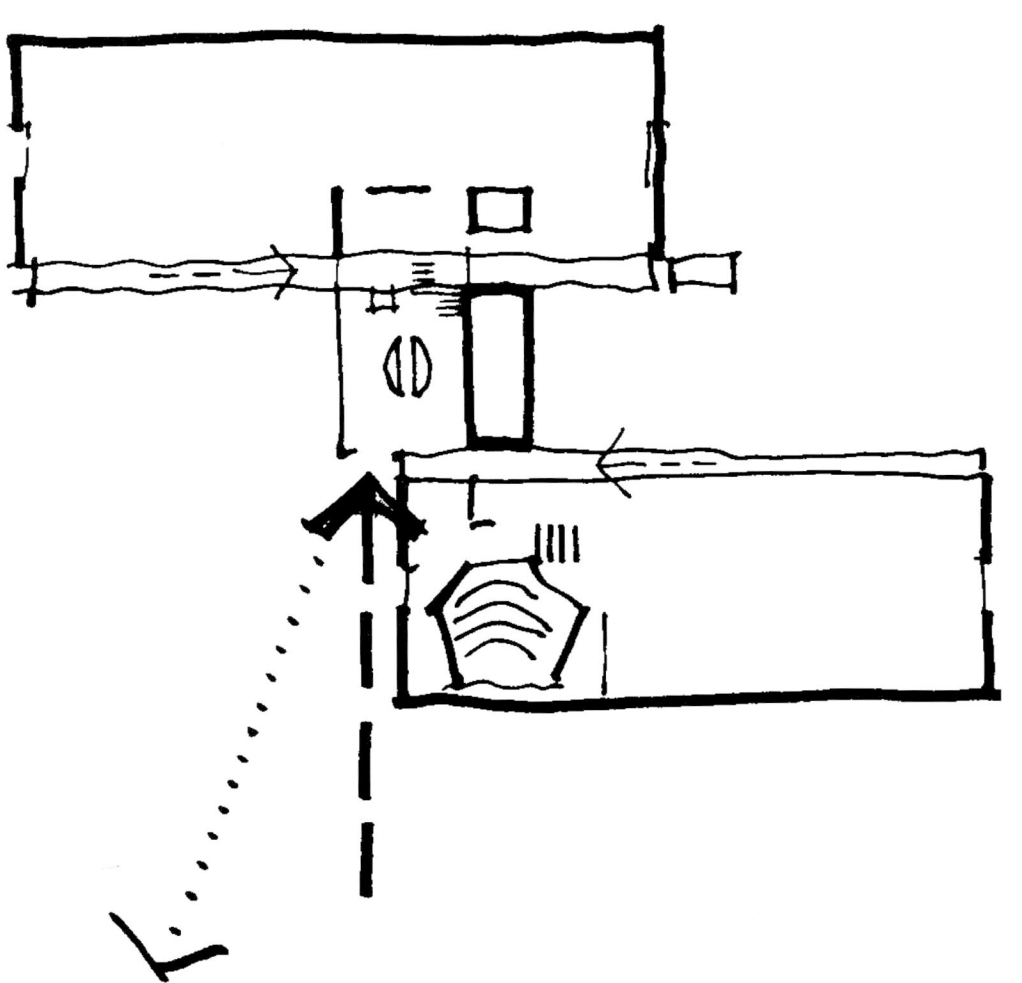

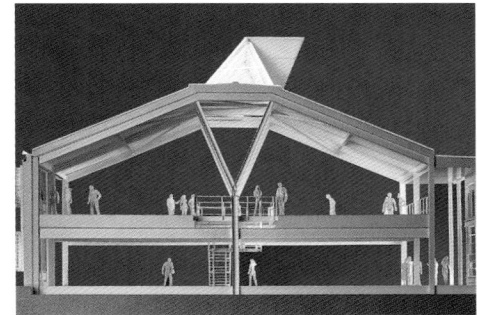

long run, may be more important. At Solihull, a new approach to the design of the office campus building has been adopted and the resulting architecture is relaxed, site-responsive and stringent, but also humanely modern. It also has green credentials. Taking on such challenges places particular demands on the design team who set and pursue these goals. Mindsets have to be changed, research and validation takes place in the midst of fast-track development and the results, although significant, rarely make the pages of the respected architectural journals.

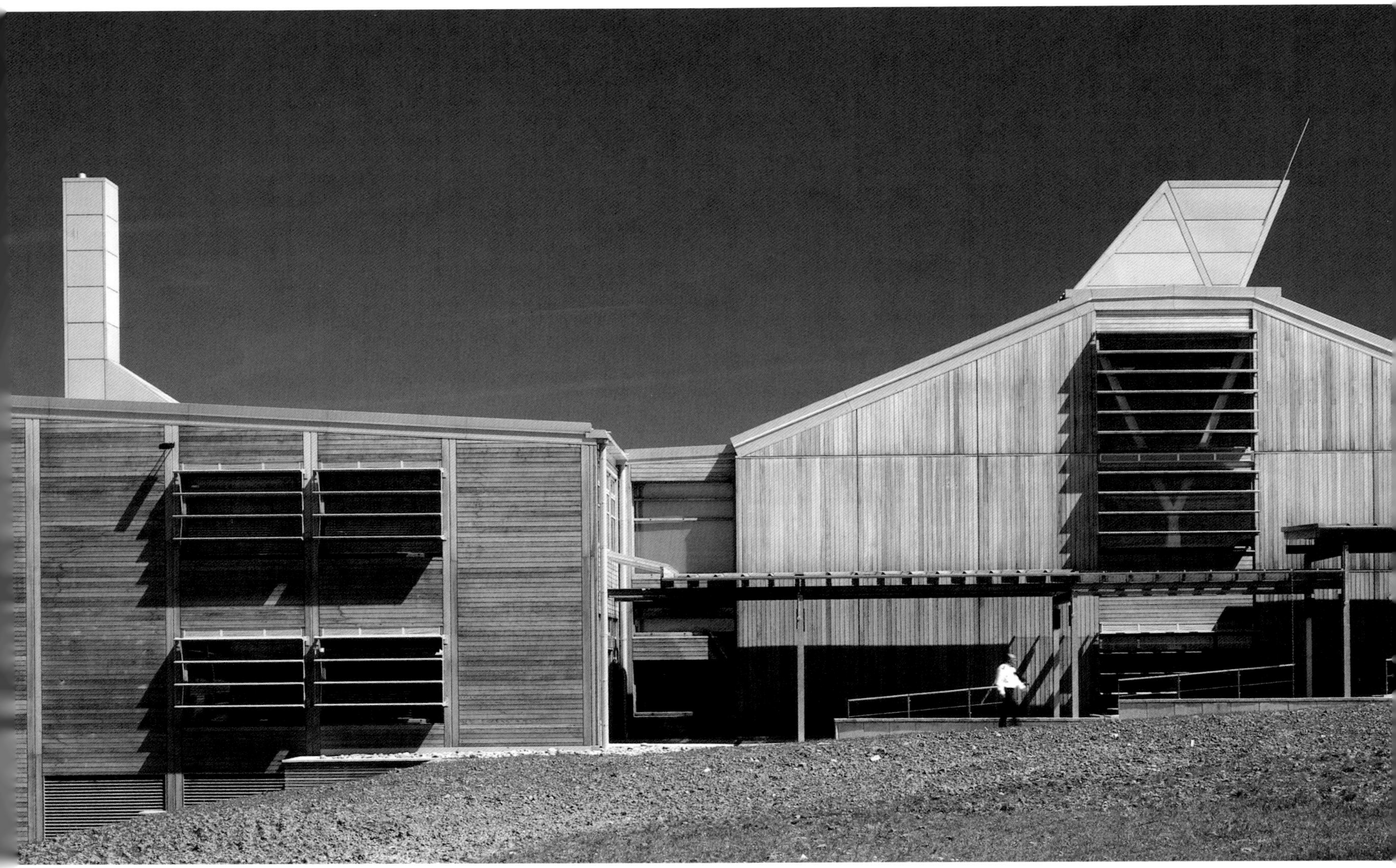

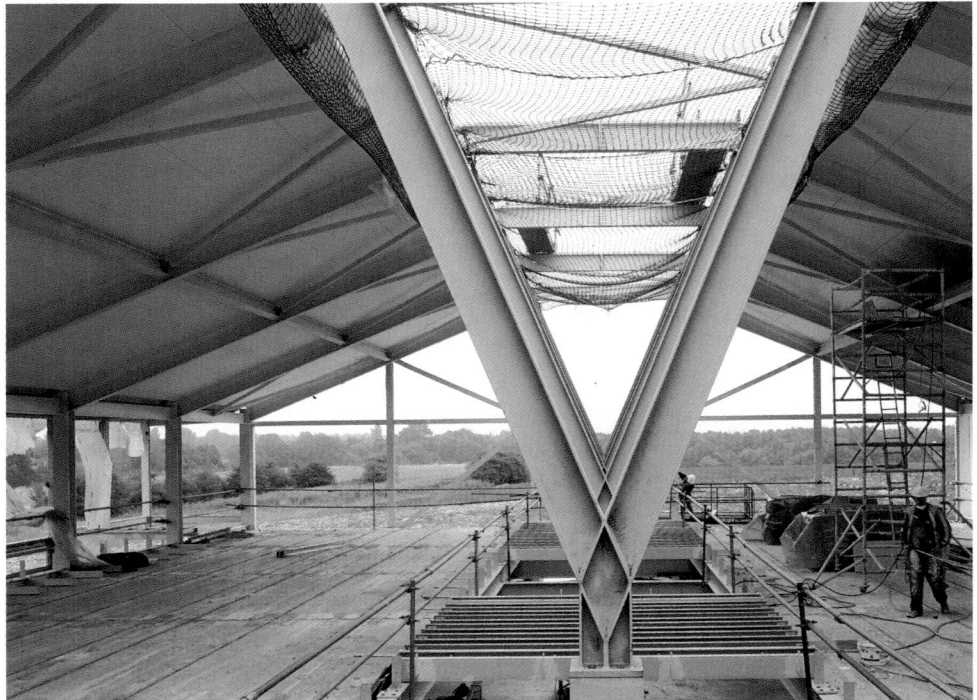

←
Campus under construction: the wishbone atrium at mid-span.

↑
Solar control to the campus pavilion façades.

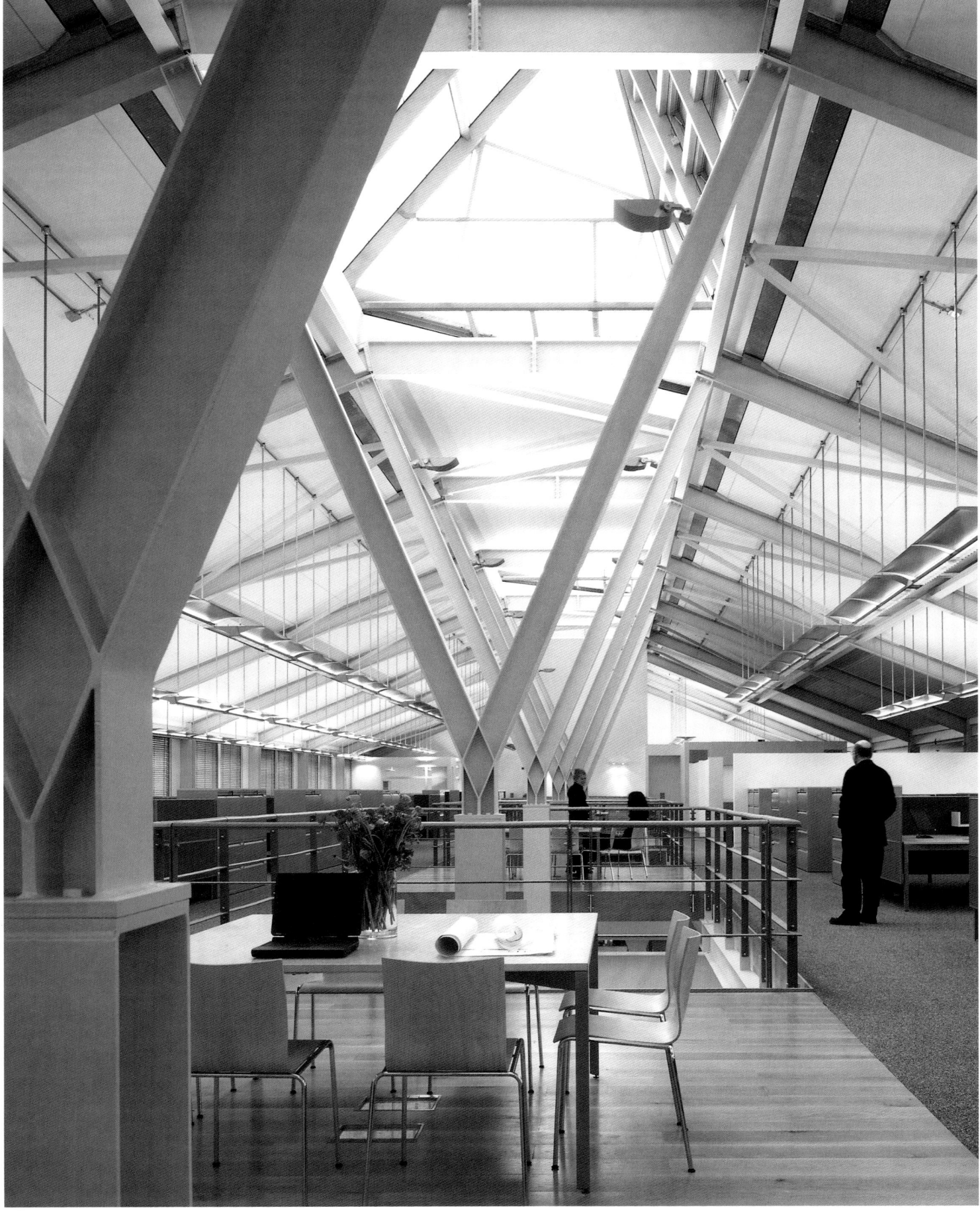

First-floor offices:
daylit interior.

Detail of window.

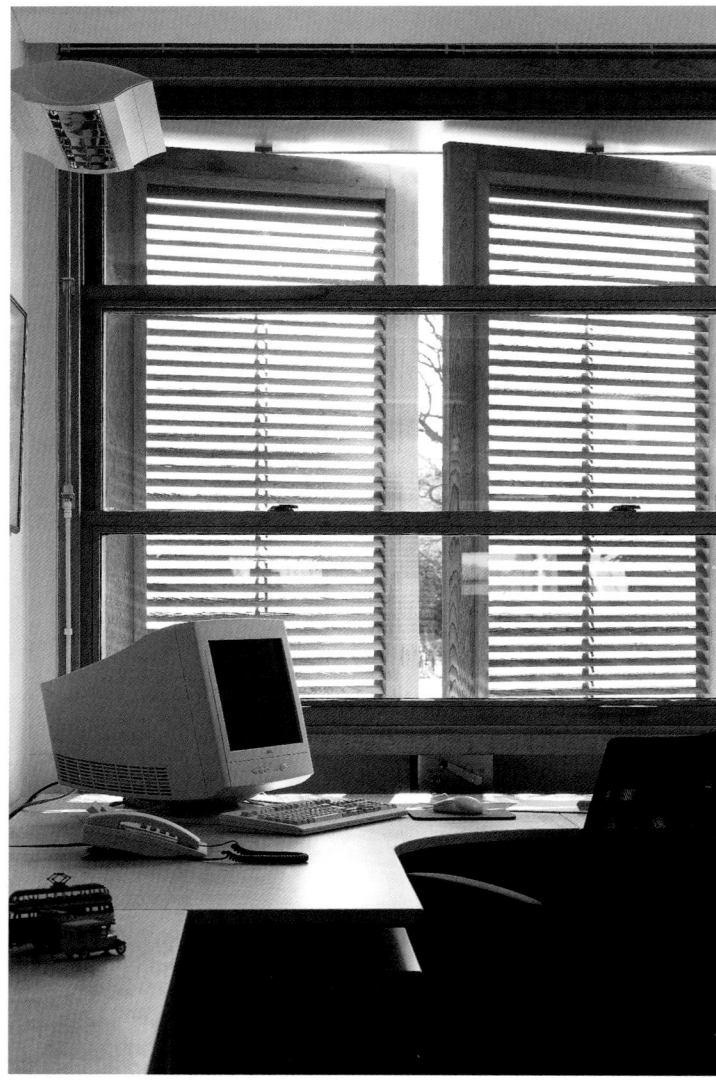

The dynamic façade
provides
environmental
control for the user.

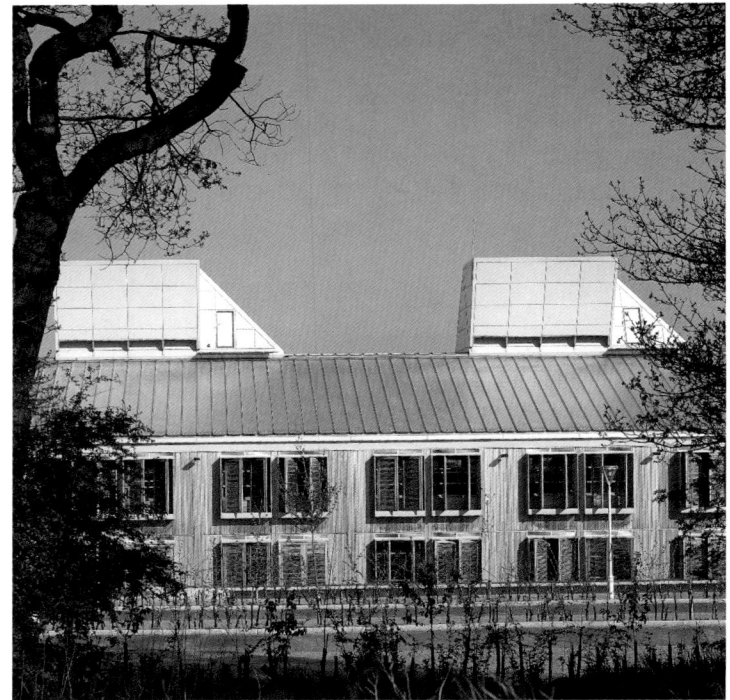

→

Roof-mounted 'pod'
structures for
daylight and natural
ventilation.

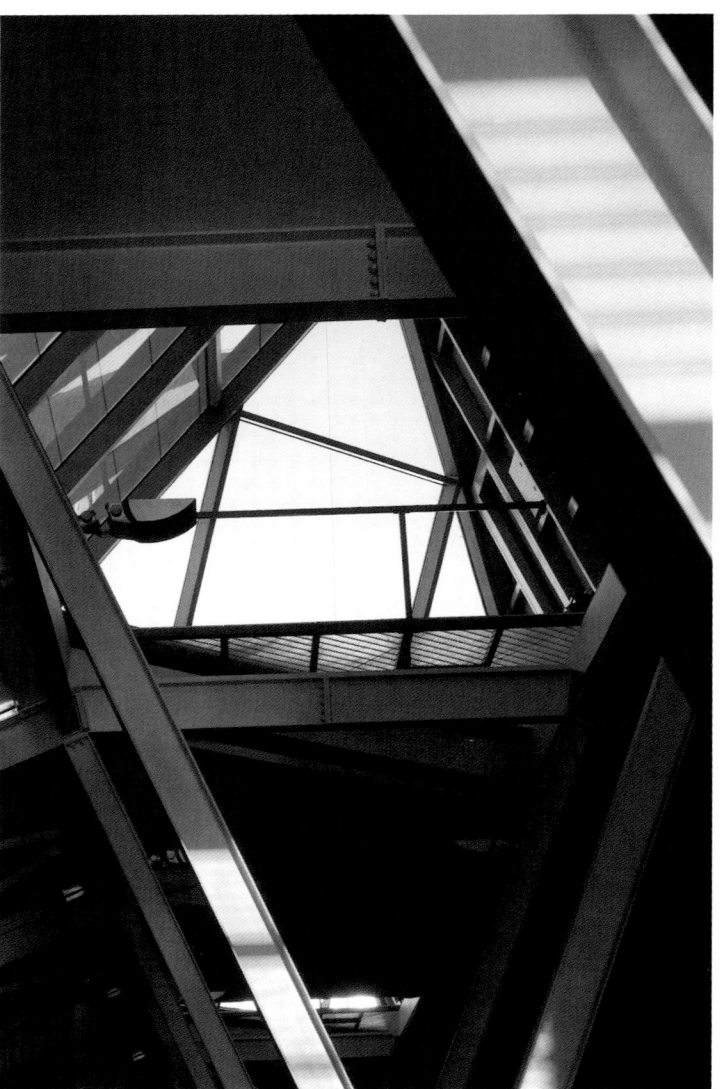

Howlands Farm
Student Housing
Arup Associates
Durham, UK
1999

➔
General view showing
brick pavilions and
timber ventilation
towers.

Nikolaus Pevsner described Durham as 'one of the great experiences of Europe....The group of cathedral, castle and monastery on the rock can only be compared to Avignon and Prague.'[1] The University of Durham was founded in 1832 and received its first students the following year. University College took over the castle, which had been the seat of the prince-bishops of Durham, and during the first century of the university's existence its principal institutions and

buildings were accommodated on the rock, woven into the tissue of the old city. In response to the expansion of British universities that began in the 1960s, new buildings, including teaching departments and student housing, were built in open country to the south of the city.

The expansion continued, and in 1994 the university held an architectural competition, won by Arup Associates, for the design of more student housing on a site at

Howlands Farm on the crest of a south-west-facing slope. The competition brief was for an extensive development, which Arup Associates conceived as a hilltop 'village' of 21 individual 'villas' and a large communal building. The programme for the project explicitly asked for an environmentally responsible approach. Requirements ranged in scale from a request that all excavated construction material should be kept on the site to a prescription that the

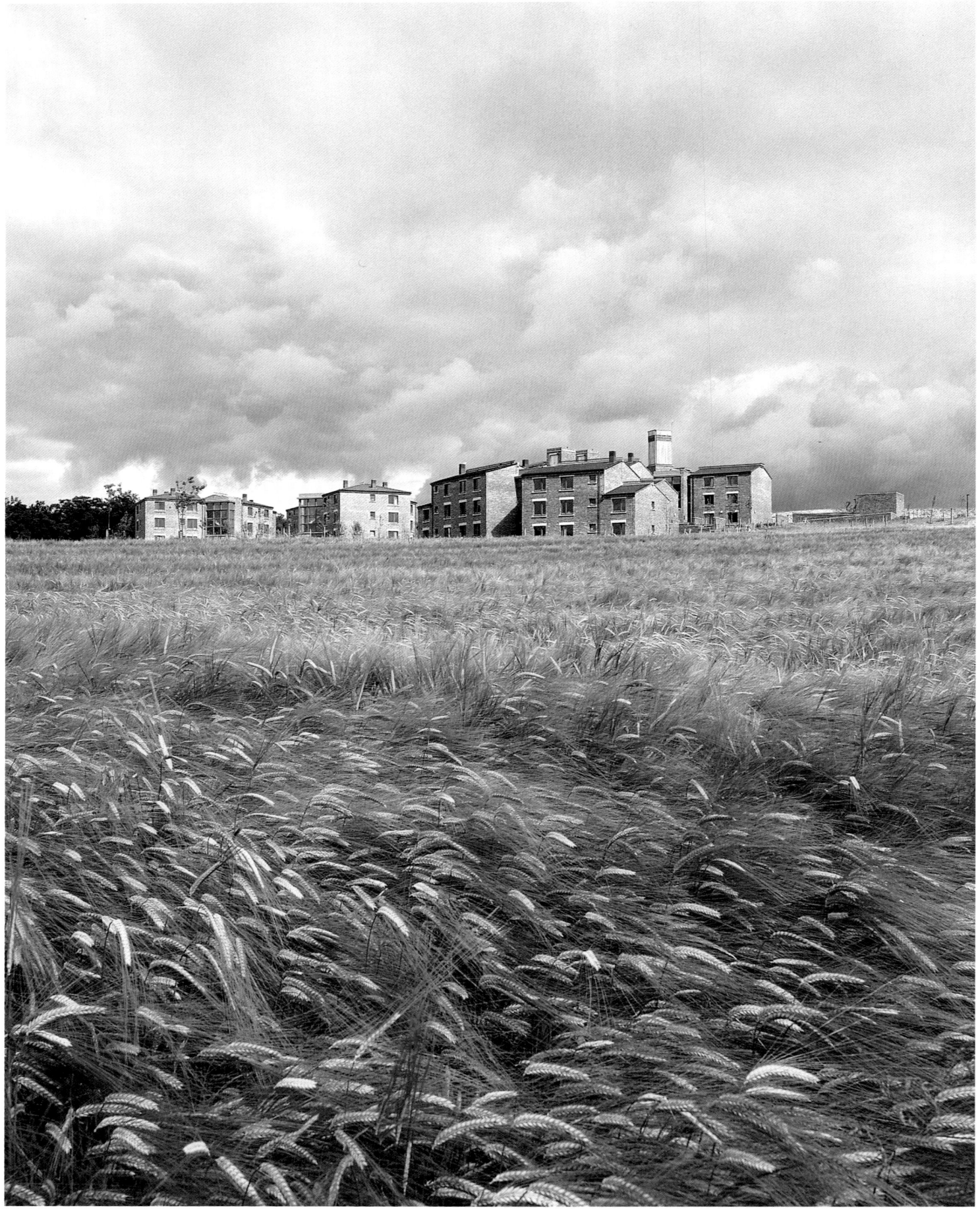

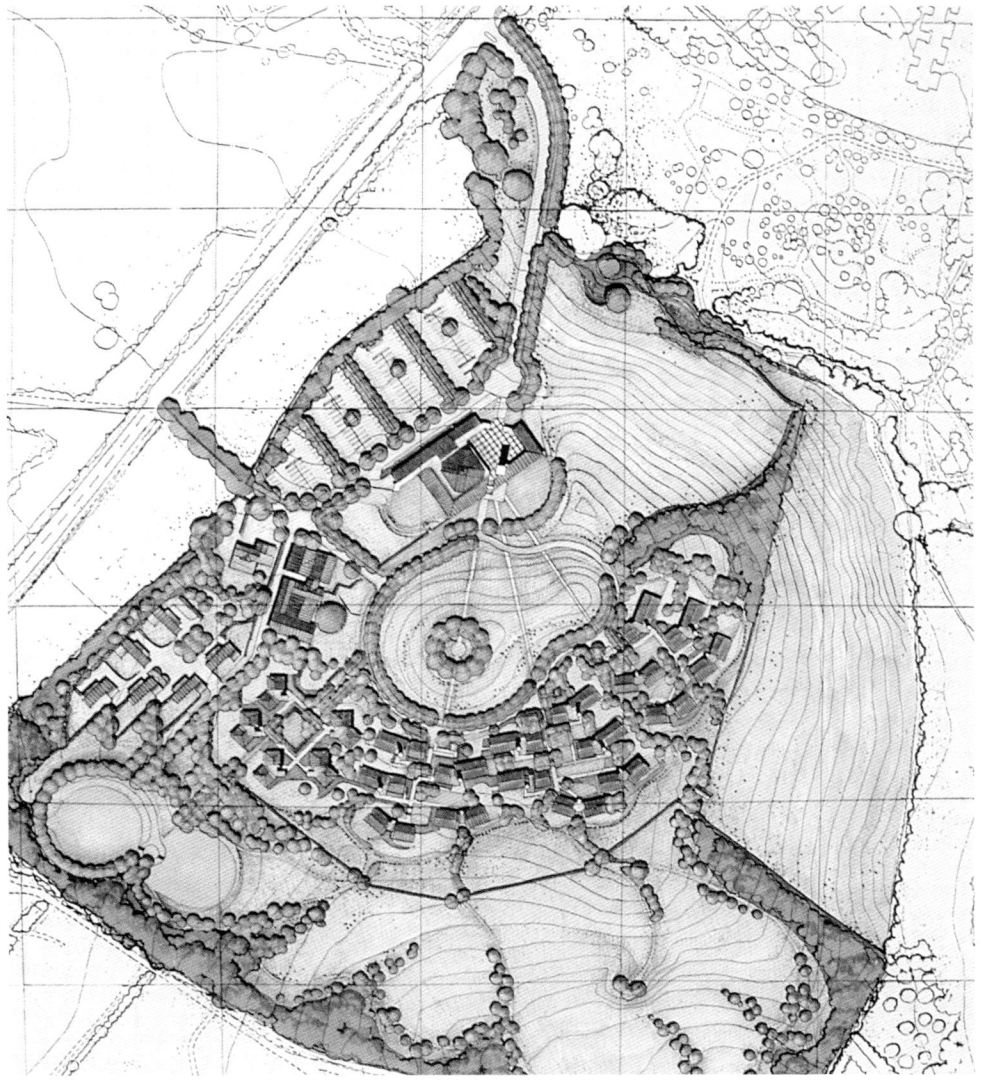

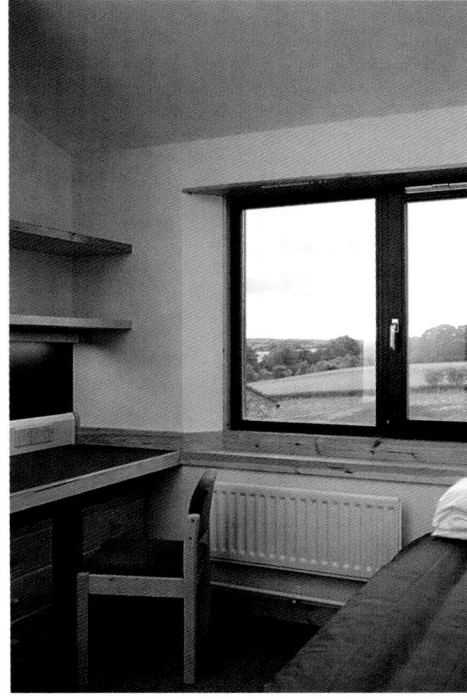

↑
Interior of study-bedroom.

←
Site plan.

individual buildings should achieve low overall energy consumption. The first stage of the project, consisting of eight villas and a small communal building converted from an existing barn, has been completed.

Dwelling form and energy use
Early in the 1970s, immediately after the energy crisis, much of the pioneering research into low-energy design focused on using small houses to test the principles of harnessing solar power – a process that continues to the present day. In many respects, this approach underlies Arup Associates' design at Howlands Farm, which opens up the possibility of a domestic-scale solution to a project that, in other interpretations, could have been larger and more monolithic.

There are, of course, significant differences between the design of a single-family house and a collective dwelling for a community of students. Student accommodation requires a different spatial organization from that of a house. In the Durham development, the plan form of each three-storey villa consists of two blocks containing simple study-bedroom cells. A linking element contains the entrance and the staircase, and the configuration of this in relation to the accommodation blocks is adjusted in response to the building's location and its relation to its neighbours.

Within this general form there are three variations in the accommodation provided. Five of the villas each provide accommodation for 21 students, including one shower room shared between two and a kitchen shared between seven. Two other buildings have a more complex mix, with 29 study-bedrooms, each with its own washbasin, but with the shower rooms each shared between three students, and the kitchens each shared between four or six students. The final block of the nine so far completed has en suite bathrooms for each of its 28 study-bedrooms, and the kitchens are shared between either nine or ten students.

In a single-family house the daytime rooms – the living room, dining room and kitchen – usually account for at least 50 per cent of the total floor area. In most passive solar designs the aim is to maximize the potential solar gains to reduce the requirement for conventional space heating. It is the daytime spaces that benefit most from this, and one of the fundamental principles of passive design applied to house design is to provide the principal rooms with a southerly

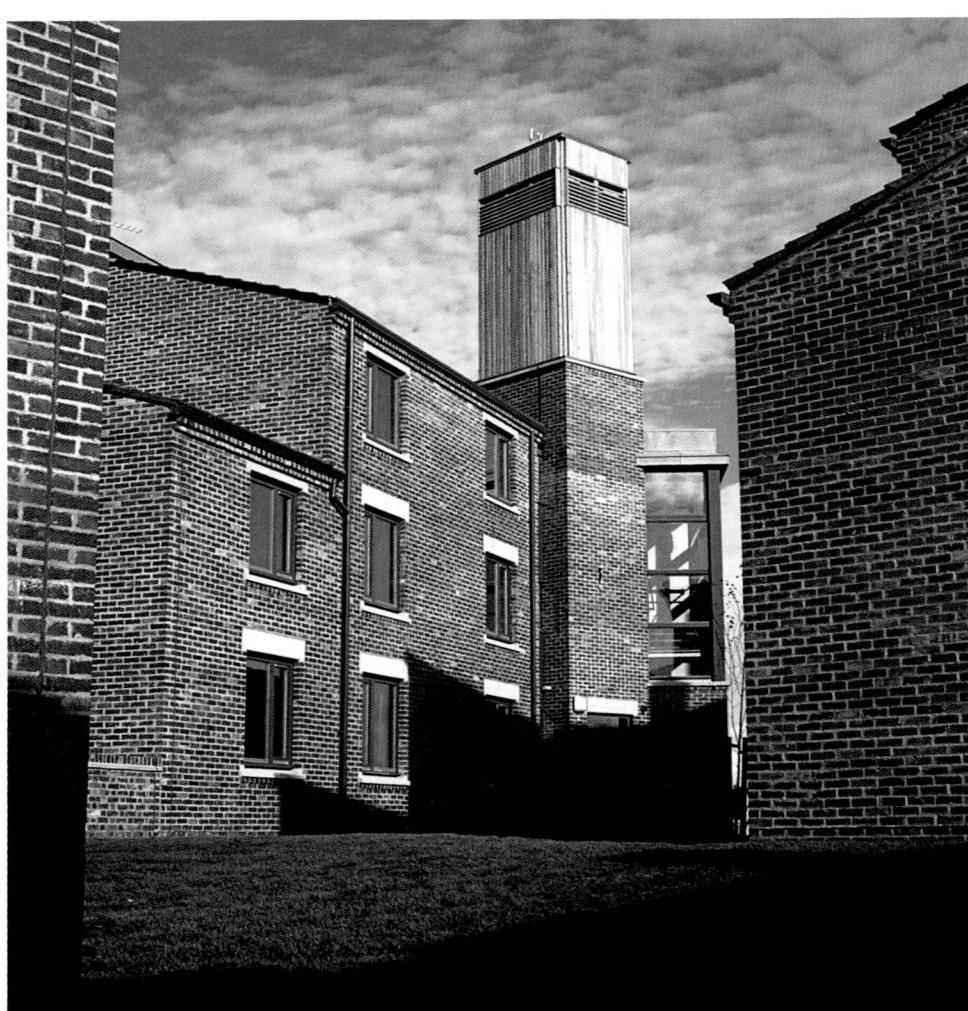

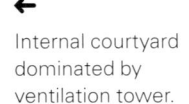
Internal courtyard dominated by ventilation tower.

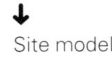
Site model.

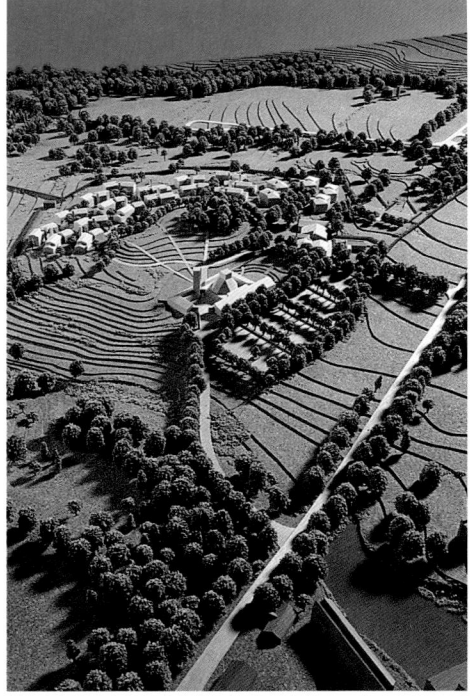

orientation to maximize the capture of solar heat.

At Howlands Farm the predominance of individual study-bedrooms over communal spaces has led to a different interpretation. In their load-bearing brick construction, with small window openings and strongly expressed concrete lintels and sills, the simple forms of the residential blocks allude to the 19th-century industrial vernacular housing of the former coal-mining villages that surround the city of Durham. As with those dwellings, there is no preferential orientation of the individual rooms. A significant difference is that the new buildings are constructed to a very high standard of thermal insulation. With their relative compactness of form, the new buildings suffer a low overall heat loss, thereby reducing energy demand.

It is at the junction of the two blocks that the passive design strategy is brought to bear. The entrance and staircase block becomes both a solar collector and the motive power for a system of natural ventilation that serves all the shower rooms, lavatories, kitchens and communal spaces. The external expression of these facilities is found in the large south-facing windows that enclose the stairwells and, most dramatically, in the brick ventilation shafts, surmounted by tall timber 'wind-catchers', which rise above the entrances.

Passive energy systems

The wind towers are used as inlets and outlets for the natural ventilation system. Each tower is divided vertically to form two stacks. One captures incoming air and delivers this downwards through a duct

network to the spaces below. A parallel network of ducts carries the extracted air back to the tower and away through the other stack. The extract stack is equipped with a heat exchanger that, in winter, removes heat from the warm exhaust air and transfers it to the adjacent stack to preheat the incoming fresh air. A fan has been installed to guarantee that the building is adequately ventilated on the few days when the air is still.

In passive design terminology, the glazed stairwells operate as a 'direct gain' system. In this, the direct insolation raises the temperature of the air, which is circulated by the ventilation system into the communal spaces. Absorbed heat continues to be re-radiated from the heavy masonry construction of the stairwells and partitions at night, after the sun has set and the temperature begins to

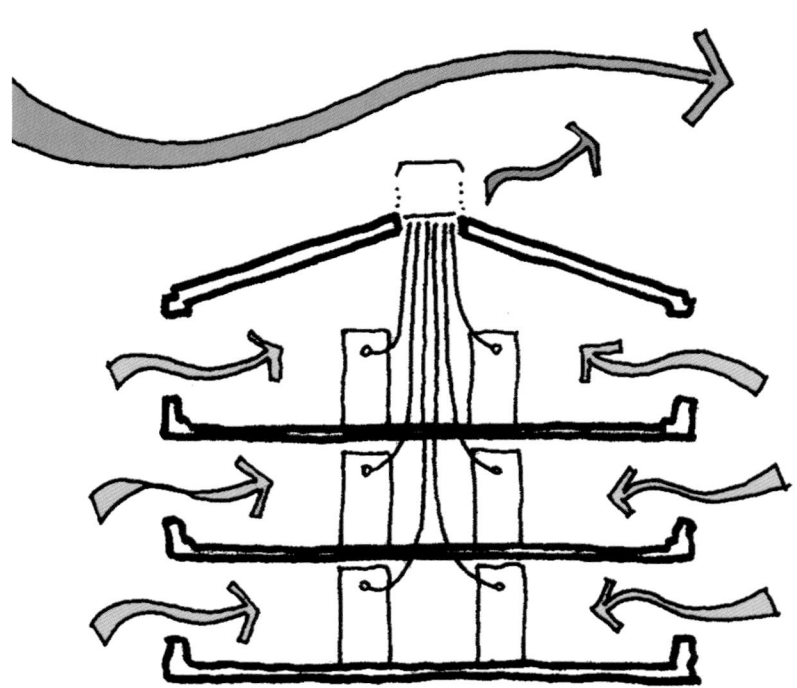

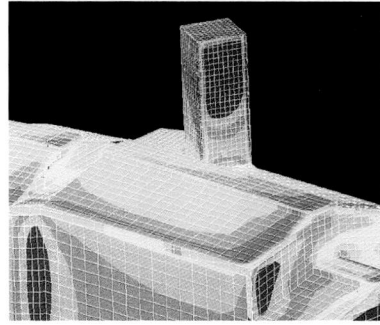

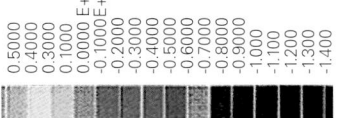

Pressure
Relative PA
Local:
max 0.6320
min 0.9471

↑
CFD model output
showing pressure
distribution over the
building envelope.

←
Cross-section
showing ventilation
processes.

→
View from the south
showing ventilation
tower and glazed
staircase block.

fall, helping to spread the useful heat through the diurnal cycle.

Conclusion

The Durham project is, at first sight, modest in its ambitions and unremarkable in its architectural language. But, as is often the case, appearances are deceptive. There is a deep strand of British architecture, characterized by J. M. Richards as 'the Functional Tradition', that rests on the celebration of the necessary, and it is in this lineage that Howlands Farm takes its place.[2] Its originality comes not from contrived novelty but from the transformation of the conventional. The simple, strong brick volumes and pitched roofs of the villas conceal new standards of construction and performance. It is the juxtaposition of these forms with the glazed expanses of the stairwells and the vertical extension of the ventilation towers that produces something new. Everything is expressive of its purpose.

The apparent simplicity of this project may seem out of place in the wider discourse about the relationship between architect and engineer, but such apparently effortless integration of form and performance requires mutual understanding and unity of purpose within the design team equal to that necessary to produce the more demonstrable synthesis evident in large-scale, technologically complex designs.

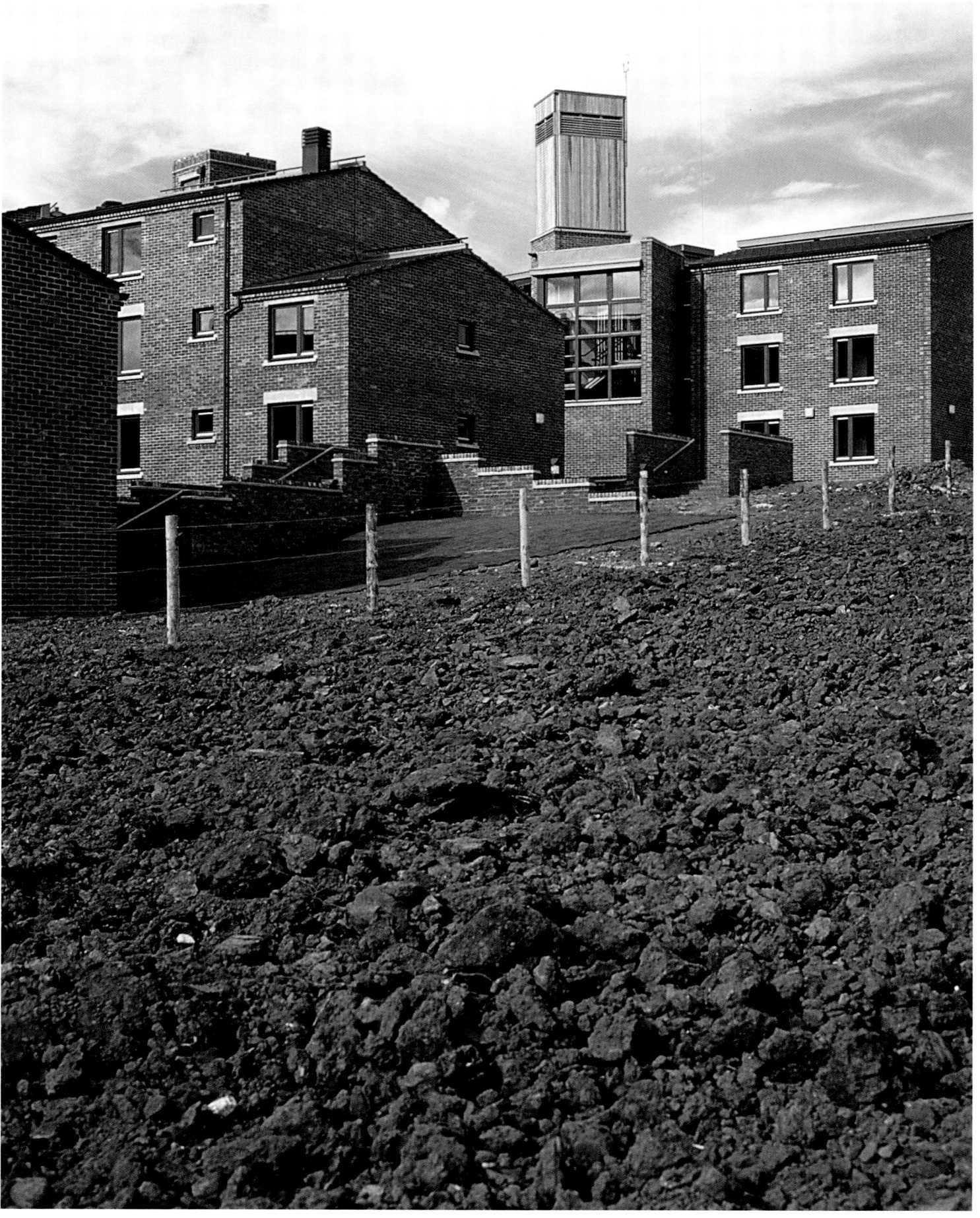

Marzahn Low-Energy Apartment Building, Assmann, Salomon & Scheidt Berlin, Germany 1994–97

→
View from south-east showing glazed façade.

One of the key questions in the design of a building is the selection of its fundamental form. The history of architecture shows how certain forms have been consistently used, adapted or transformed to meet recurrent and changing needs. In *The Classical Language of Architecture*, Summerson shows how building forms that were first established in antiquity have proved to be appropriate models for many subsequent buildings.[1] For example, the cylindrical form of the Pantheon in Rome, with its attached portico, has been adapted to serve as, among many uses, church, dwelling,

academic institution and public library. Reference to past forms was given more formal recognition and structure at the beginning of the 19th century through the development of the idea of type by theoreticians such as J. N. L. Durand.[2]

Our contemporary concern about the design of low-energy buildings means that the question of form, and its relation to typology, has a new and important role to play. 'What shape is a low-energy building?' is an obvious and easy question to ask, but the answer is neither obvious nor necessarily easy. One assumption made in some of the early theoretical

studies of the question was that there is a direct relation between the ratio of the surface area of a form and the volume it encloses; because energy is consumed in compensating for heat loss, it seemed self-evident that an efficient form would be that which minimized the surface area to volume ratio. A quarter of a century ago the literature was scattered with confident statements such as: 'Buildings should be large rather than small and have circular or square plans, heated buildings should be near cubical in shape.'[3] Subsequently, these simple prescriptions were more thoroughly investigated, and the complexity of

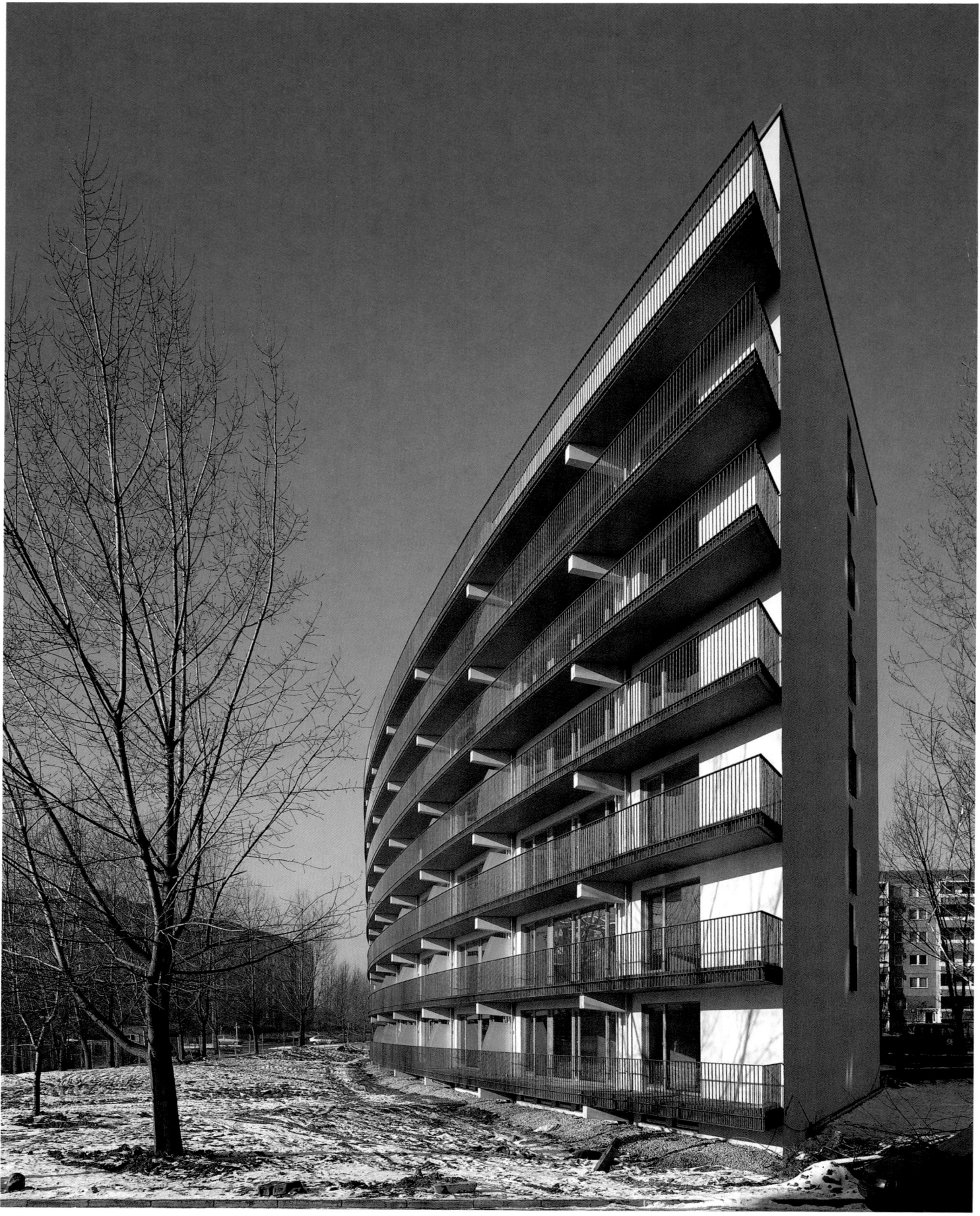

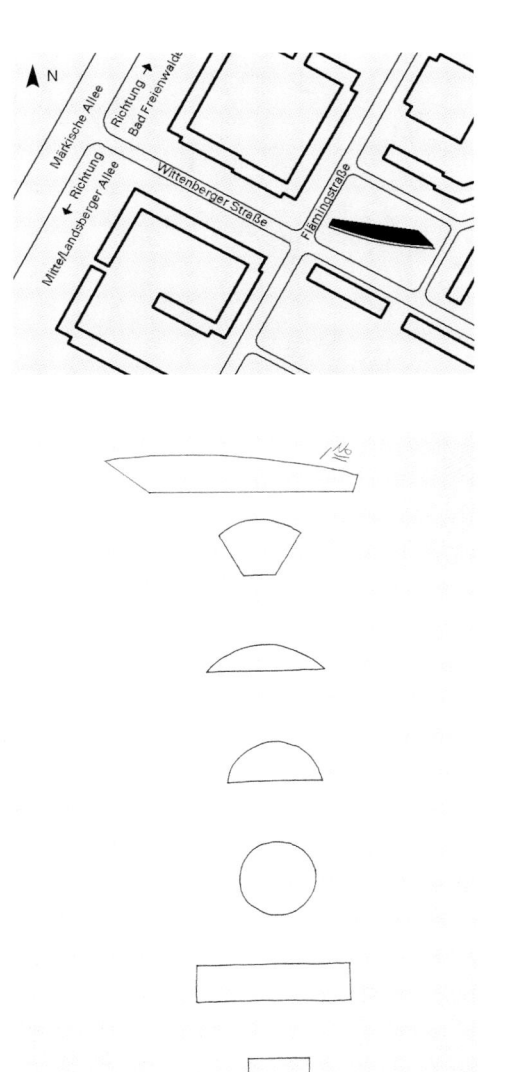

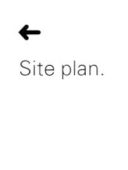

Site plan.

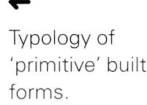

Typology of
'primitive' built
forms.

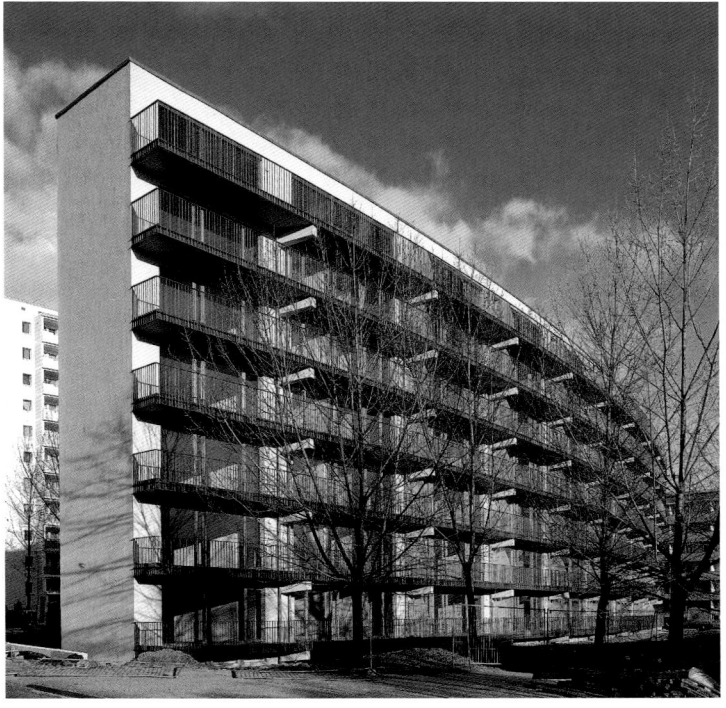

↑
View from south-east
showing projecting
balconies that
provide shade in the
summer months.

→
The minimally glazed
north façade.

the question is now more thoroughly understood, but the question of shape remains at the heart of low-energy design – and it is this that makes the design of the apartment building at Marzahn in Berlin of such great interest.[4]

The development of form
Marzahn is a suburb of eastern Berlin where the client, a housing association, sought to build 56 apartments. The housing association had entered into an agreement with the local government by which they would qualify for additional funding as long as the design achieved a target for energy demand 20 per cent below the newly introduced regulations. The client determined that the design should, from the outset, be subject to a close collaboration between the architects and the

consultant engineers. In addition to their conventional responsibilities for structure and building services, Arup had been appointed as energy consultant.

The design process began with a study of the relationship between form and energy use. During the cold Berlin winters the principal demand for energy would be in space heating, so the researchers looked at the question of surface area to volume. A typology of six 'primitive' built forms was constructed. In plan these were a square, a rectangle, a circle, a semicircle, an arc and a truncated fan-shape. All were assumed to be six storeys high and with a gross floor area of $6,000m^2$ ($64,560ft^2$). Calculations were made to assess the annual heating energy demand for each of the forms to enable comparisons to be made. In making

the calculations, standard assumptions were made about the insulation value of the envelope and, crucially, allowance was made for the contribution to heating requirement that would be made by solar heat gain from the southerly orientation. In the extended forms it was assumed that the long façade would face south, a condition that could be met on the site for the building.

The results of the study showed that a cylindrical building would, at $35kWh/m^2$ ($11.09 BthU/ft^2$), have the lowest winter-heat energy demand of the first five built forms. But the truncated fan shape could, by a process of manipulation of its proportions, be shown to equal this. To achieve this result, the north façade was kept as short as possible and the lengths of the east and west façades were varied systematically until an

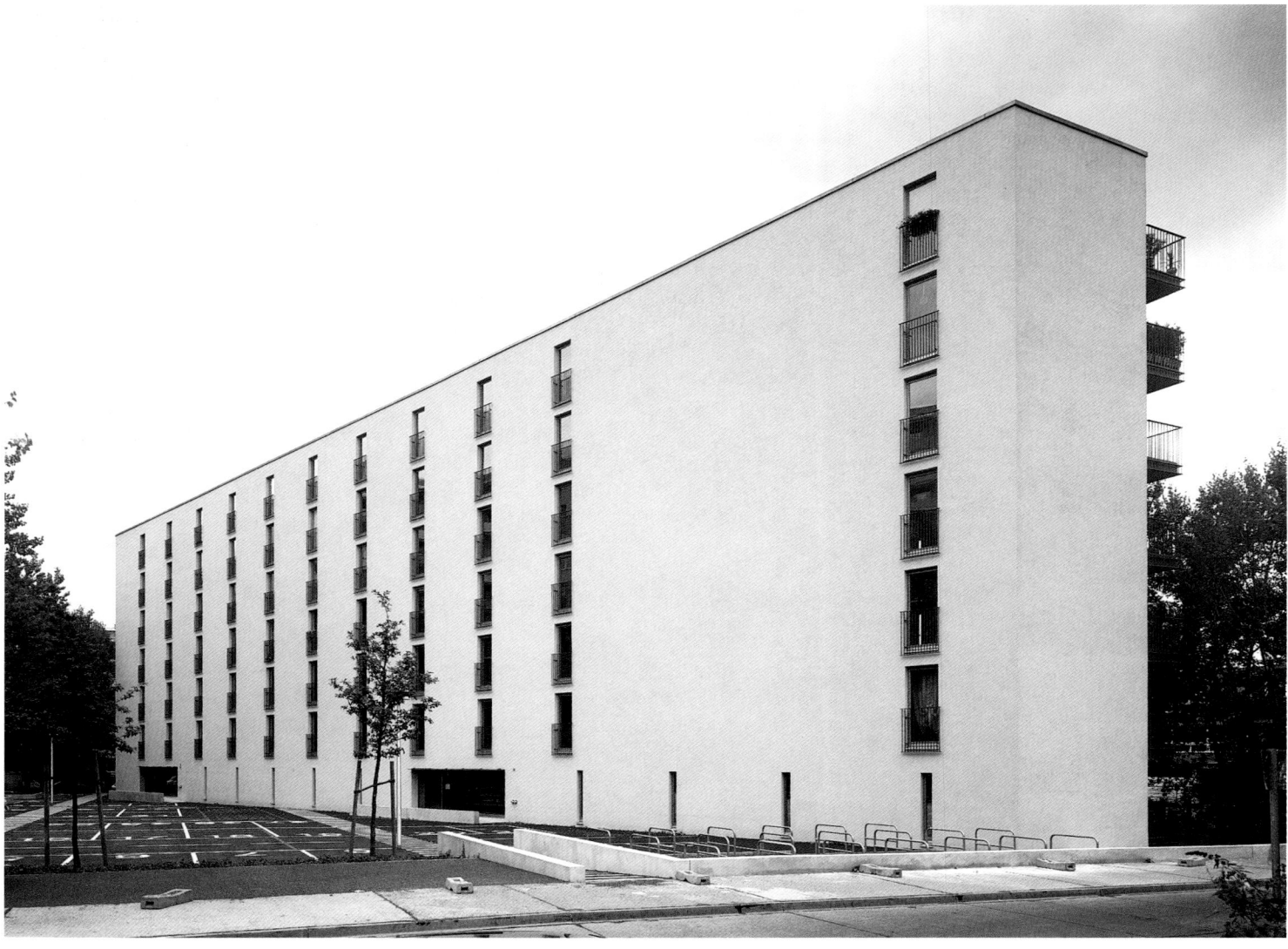

'optimum' was reached. The advantage of this form, in comparison with the cylinder, is that all the apartments could have a southerly aspect.

The determination of the overall built form is only the starting point in the design of any building. The initial studies were followed by more detailed investigations into the arrangement and detailed design of the individual apartments within the block. These led to a particular plan form in which the principal rooms – living room, kitchen and bedrooms – face south, and the entrances, hallways and bathrooms are all located at the north side. Beyond these the circulation areas, containing lifts and stairs, act as an unheated buffer zone. The curved façade means that the precise orientation of the individual apartments varies, so they

do not enjoy equal amounts of solar gain throughout the day. To allow the inhabitants to overcome this to some degree, the partitions between these rooms have sliding doors that allow the entire apartment to be opened up to the sun.

The building is constructed with load-bearing cross-walls of precast concrete that form the divisions between the apartments. The floors are also precast units, prestressed to span 8.6m (28ft). The internal partitions within the apartments are non-loadbearing. The envelope is constructed to a high standard of thermal insulation, typically less than $0.2W/m^2/°C$ (0.035 BthU/ft^2/°C), and the glazing is specified to balance heat loss and the collection of useful solar gain.

Structure and service
In the general terminology of environmental architecture, the design that evolved through this analytical process is described as 'direct-gain, passive-solar'. In some instances, and in certain climates, it may be possible to design a building using the principles of passive-solar design that achieves acceptable levels of thermal comfort without recourse to any auxiliary heating system. In Berlin's relatively extreme winter climate, and in the design of mass-housing, it would be difficult to contemplate such a solution. But the integration of an auxiliary heating system with passive solar elements is not a trivial task. The heating system uses hot water supplied, via a heat exchanger, from a local district heating network. The rooms are heated by conventional radiators.

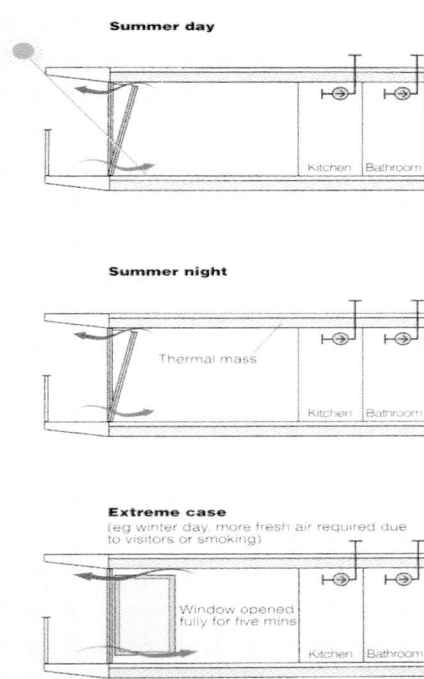

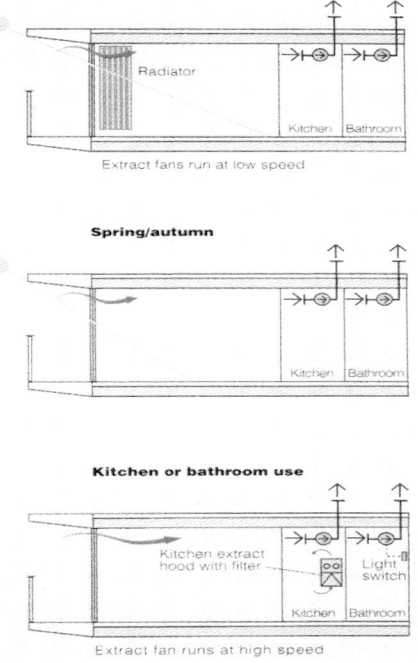

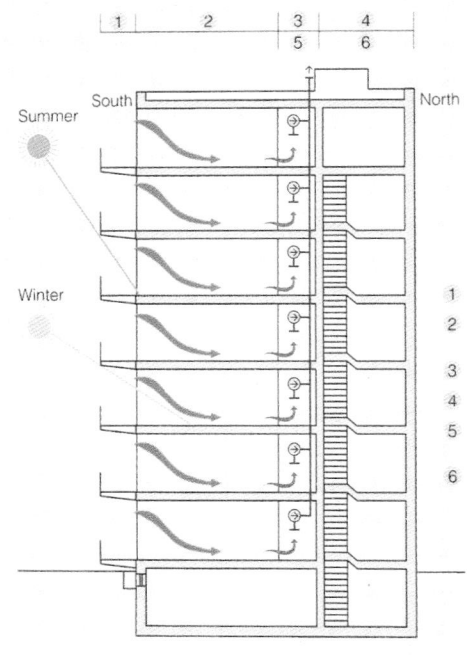

↑
Detailed cross-sections showing seasonal and diurnal operation of the environmental systems.

↑
Cross-section showing assisted ventilation of appartments.

In a highly insulated building there is a risk that heat loss due to uncontrolled ventilation could be extremely wasteful. To avoid this, each apartment at Marzahn has two extract fans, one in the kitchen, the other in the bathroom. These provide most of the ventilation that is needed in winter by drawing fresh air in through controllable vents in the window frames of the south-facing rooms. If there is a need for more ventilation, the large windows can be opened, but when this is done the heating system and the mechanical ventilation are automatically turned off. This quickly lowers the room temperature and implicitly instructs the inhabitants about how to get the best out of their building.

The building has a computer-controlled building management system that, in addition to linking the heating system to the opening windows, allows the users to receive, from a touch screen display in each apartment, information about their energy consumption (expressed in Deutschmarks), room temperatures and so forth. The hope is that these data will further inform the inhabitants about the performance of the building and, thereby, produce greater efficiency of use.

In the summer months the building is naturally ventilated and the overhang of the continuous balconies of the south façade provides solar shading. The depth of the overhang was calculated to balance winter insolation with summer shading, and further shading, if required, is provided by internal blinds. A group of deciduous trees provides more shade but allows the sun to reach the building in winter when they have shed their leaves. The building management system provides a visible warning to the occupant at times when the windows could provide more effective ventilation than the mechanical fans. It is intended that the windows should be left open on summer nights, both to provide ventilation and to cool the thermal mass of the exposed ceilings. This will then assist in maintaining comfort temperatures during the following day.

Conclusion

In architecture the relationship between theory and practice is complex. The design office and the building site frequently play as important a part in the development of theory as the research institute. The lesson of Marzahn is a clear example of this. The design of an apparently

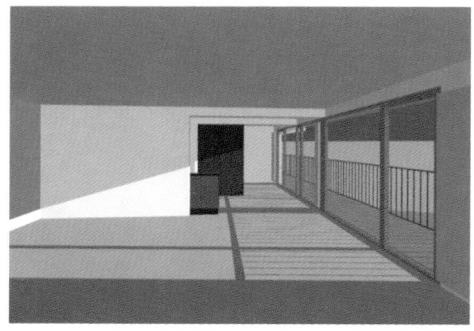 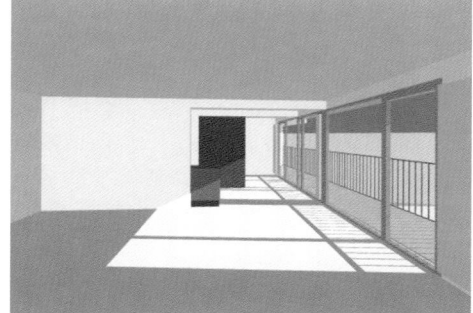 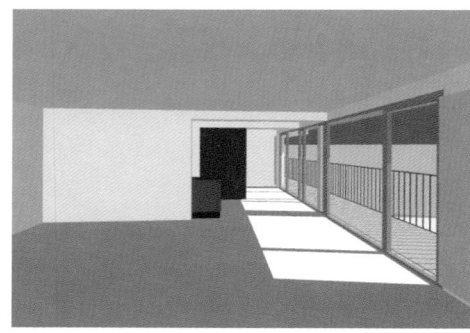

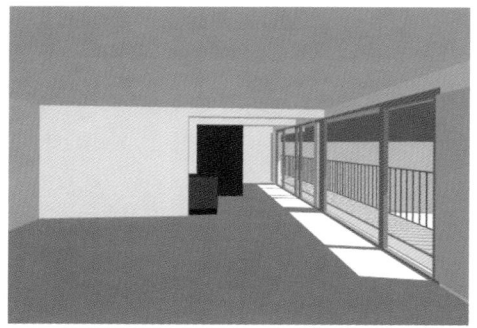 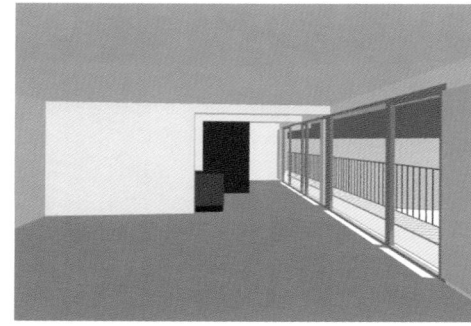 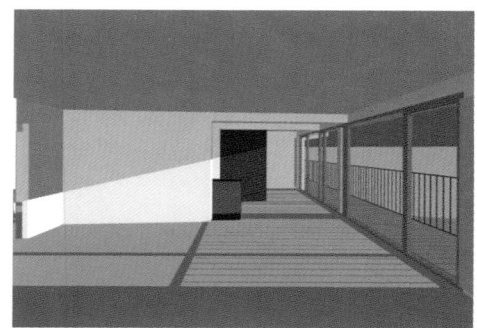

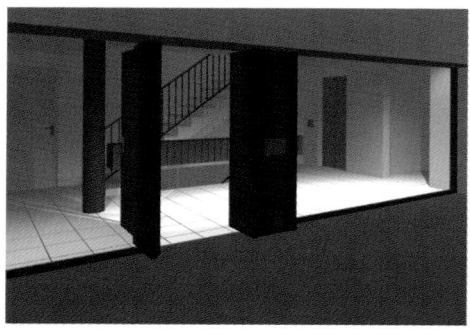 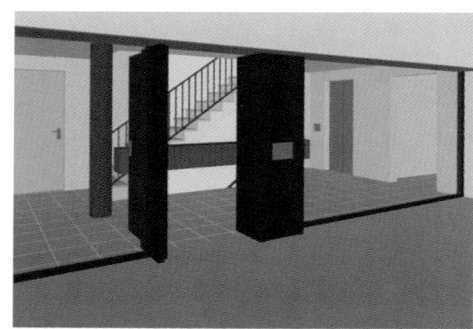

←
Computer simulation
of sunlight
penetration into
appartments and
circulation space.

straightforward building project proves to be a valuable vehicle for research into the relationship between built form and performance. The studies carried out here by the design team show how simple prescriptions may be refined to add to the evolving typology of low-energy architecture. The further development of the design, through its constructional system, detailed planning and its mechanical services and their controls, shows that the technical success of a building depends equally upon its practical realization as upon its initial conception.

To return to broader questions of form, type and architectural method, it is interesting to compare the Marzahn design, the product of an explicitly systematic design procedure, with Alvar Aalto's 'Neue Vahr' apartment building in Bremen, designed in 1958 and completed in 1962.[5] At that date, low-energy design was not acknowledged as part of the main agenda of architecture, but the work of many architects evinced a profound, often intuitive, sense of the interdependence of architecture and nature, and between architecture and environment. Among the major architects of the 20th century, Aalto exhibited this sensibility more than most: 'a truly serious problem is the discovery of form, the basic design for our century'.

The Bremen building logically and eloquently responds to the environmental difference of north and south exposures, closed and orthogonal to the north, open and undulating to the south. It is certain that Marzahn will be superior to Neue Vahr in its energy performance – the explicit energy brief will guarantee that. On the other hand, the similarity between it and the product of Aalto's informed intuition about architecture's place in relation to nature serves to connect the new building, and the research that it embodies, to the significant mainstream. The development of architecture as a comprehensive discipline, embracing the arts and the sciences, will only be properly achieved if we make connections, as Le Corbusier urged in *Vers une architecture*, between the realms of objectivity and intuition.[6]

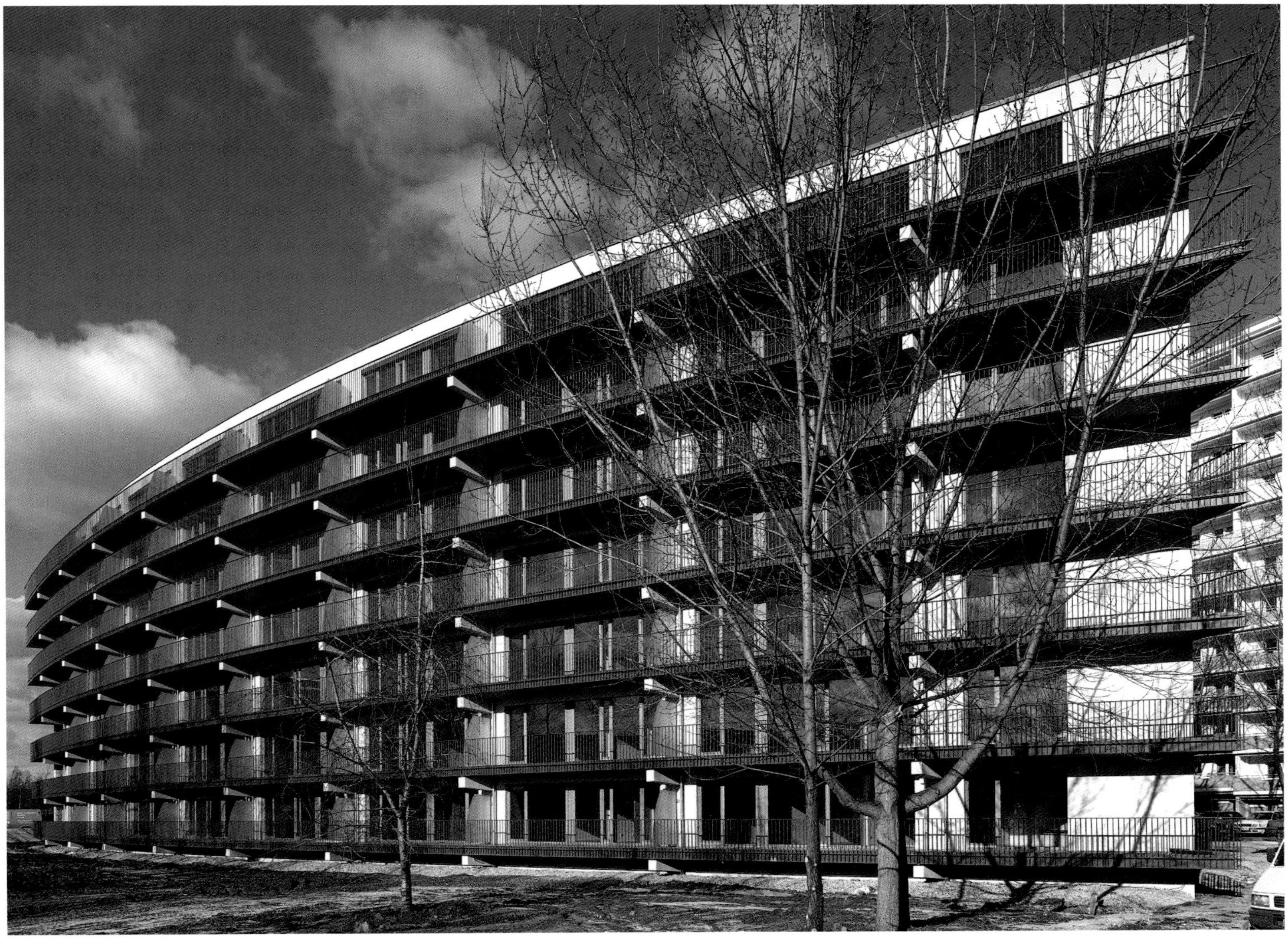

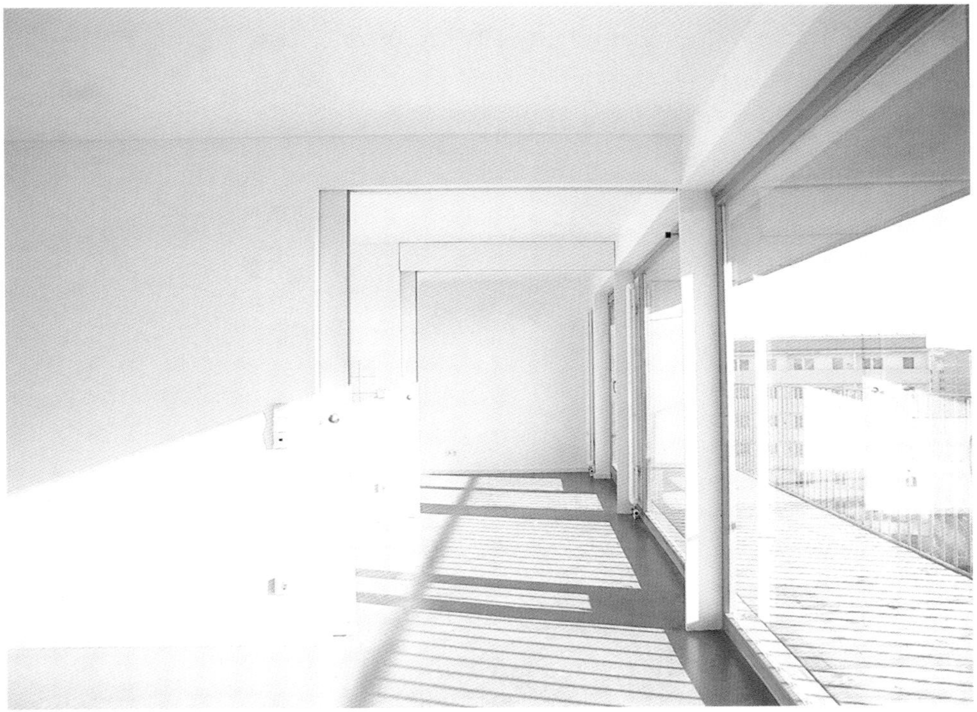

← Appartment interior showing sliding partitions between the principal rooms.

↑ South façade.

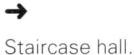

Staircase hall.

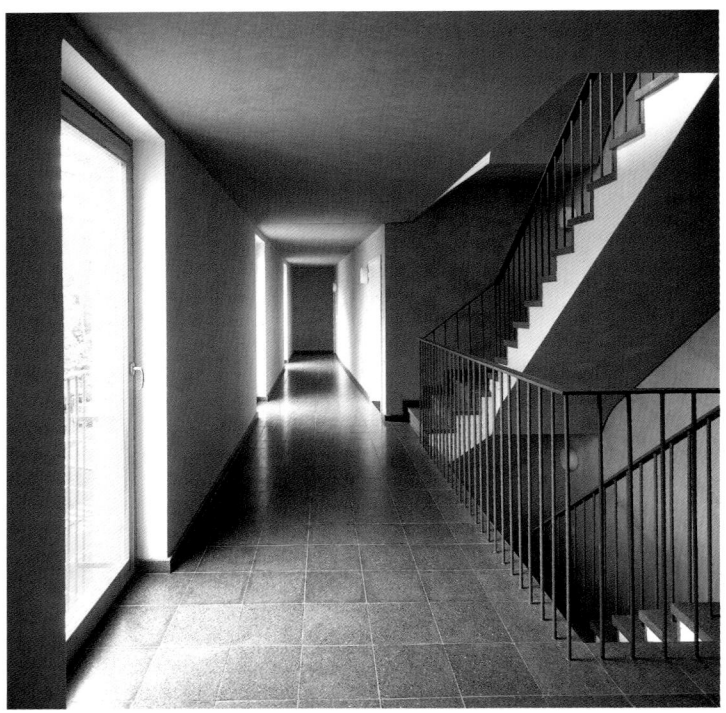

Detail of south-facing glazing.

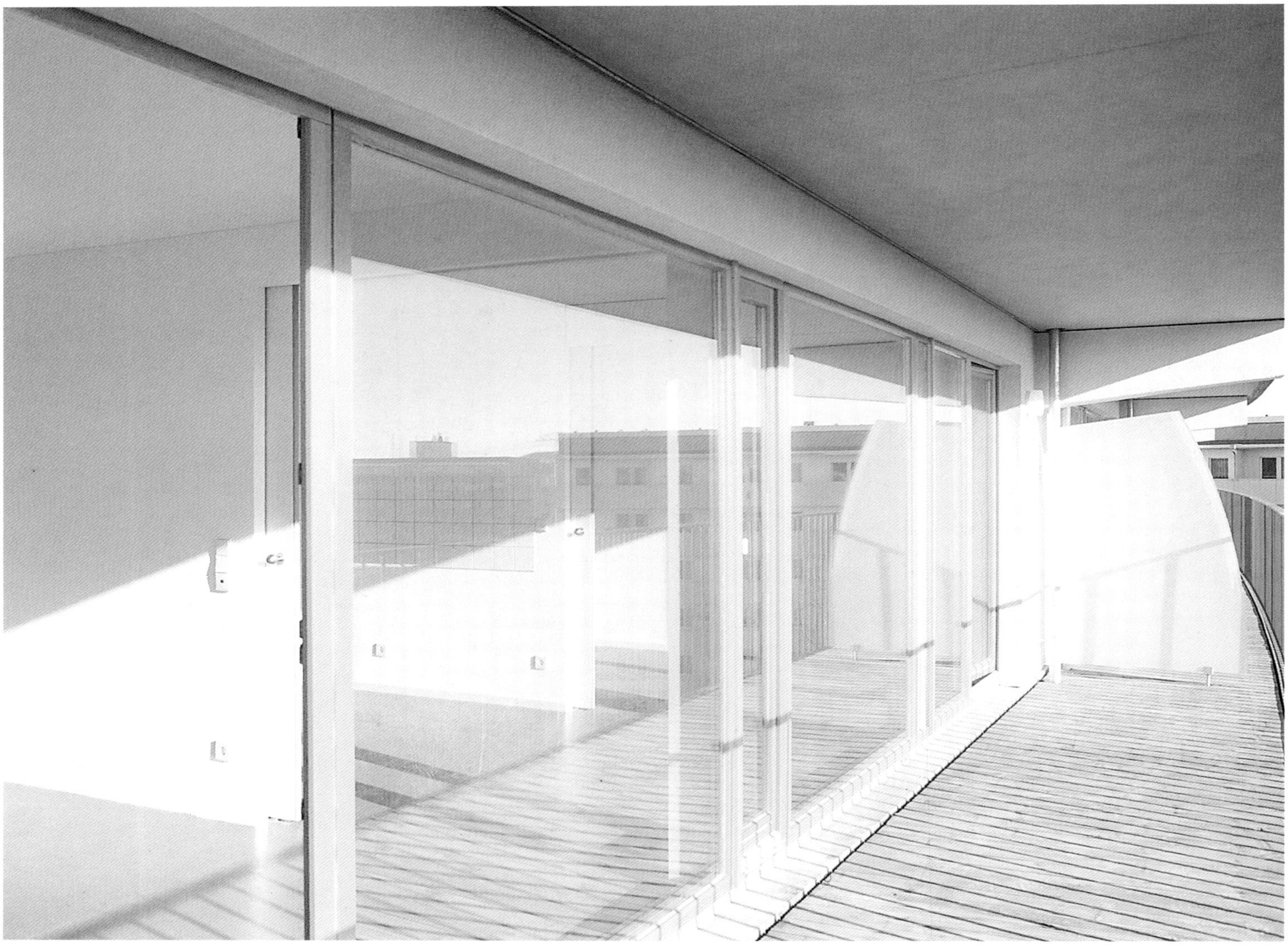

BedZED Sustainable Development

Bill Dunster
London, UK
2002

→
BEDZED is a compact live/work development that exploits the potential for sustainable futures.

In 1999 the UK government published *Towards an Urban Renaissance*, a report that aimed to provide guidelines for practical solutions to the design of cities, towns and urban neighbourhoods. It claimed to establish 'a new vision for urban regeneration founded on the principles of design excellence, social well being and environmental responsibility within a viable economic and legislative framework'. [1]

Counter-urbanization was one of several factors identified to have contributed directly to 20 per cent increases in energy consumption by households in England over the previous 25 years. Underperformance in waste management and increases in motor-vehicle traffic were also contributors to the huge environmental burden. The report's conclusions were that a much greater

mix of building types and tenures in more compact urban forms close to existing and new transport interchanges were needed.

The London borough of Sutton took up the challenge in the form of the Beddington Zero Energy Development, a ground-breaking project that aims to prove that sustainable living is not only economically and technically viable

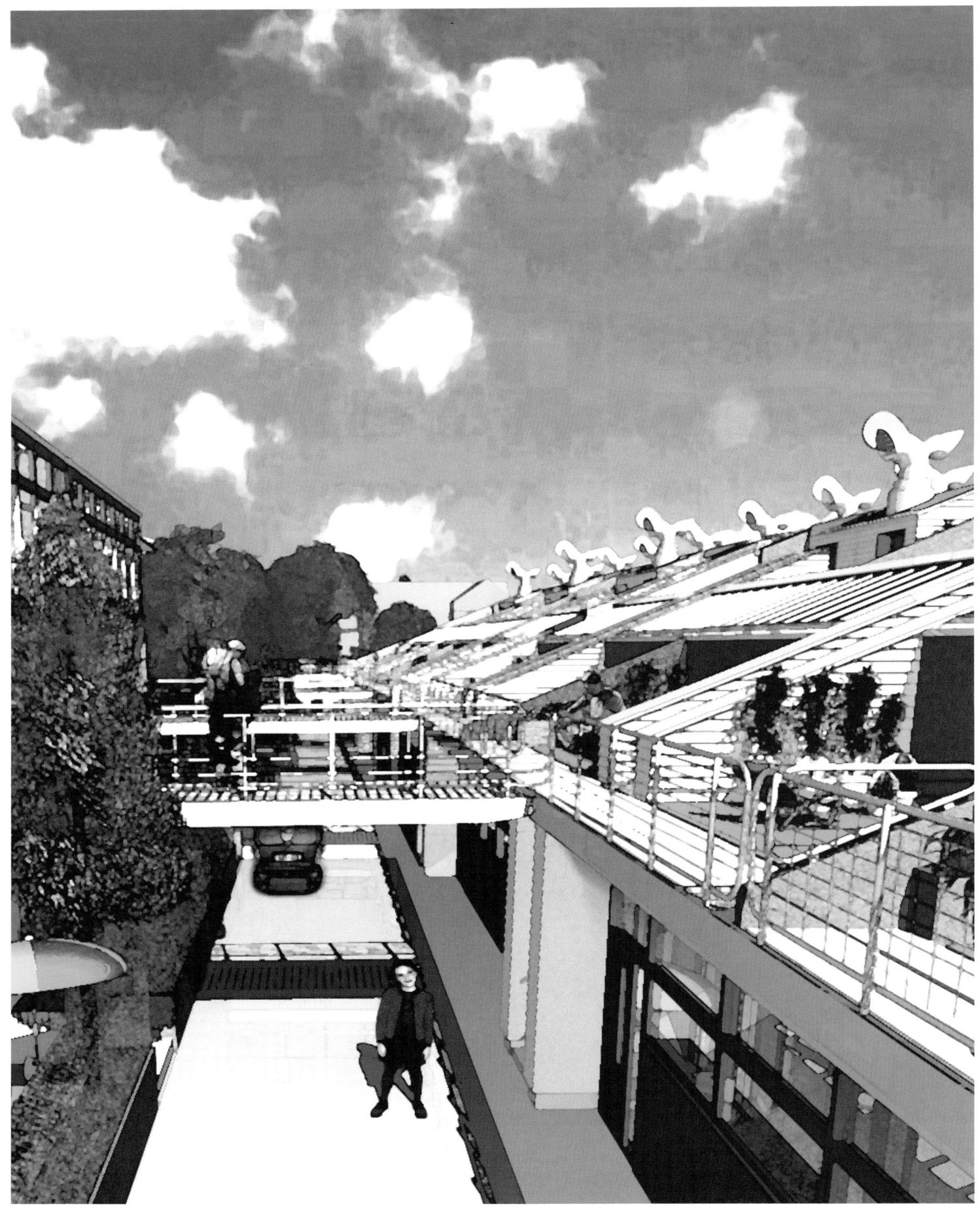

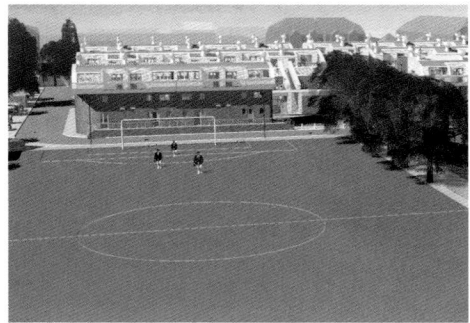

↑
The development
includes a number of
community facilities.

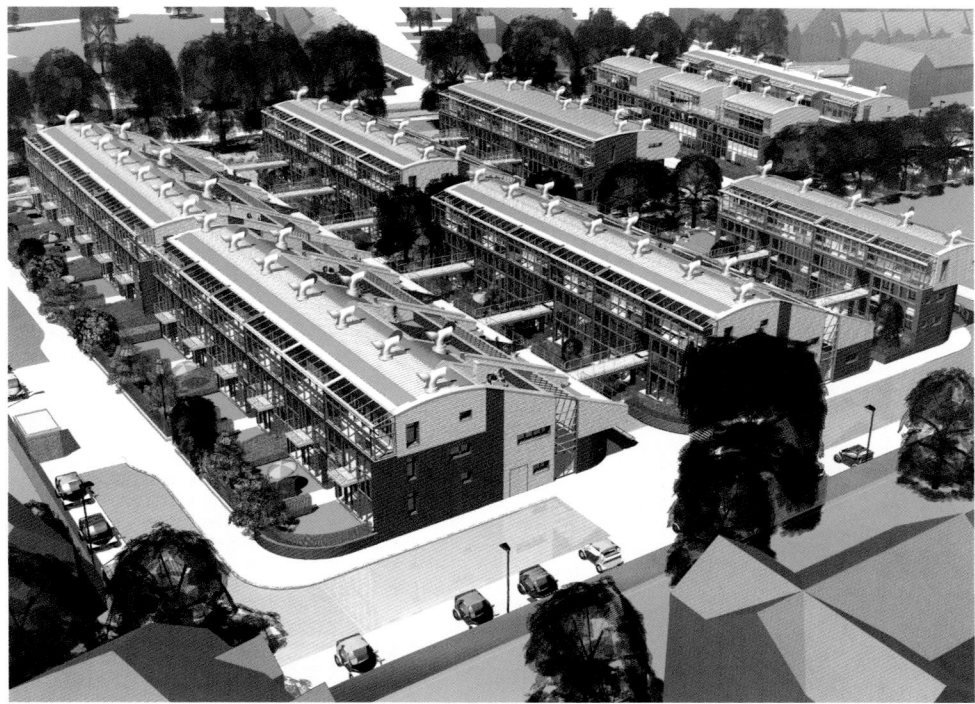

↑
The BedZED layout
consists of five rows
of terraces, running
east–west.

but can also be comfortable and
manageable for ordinary people. The
development has its roots in a
collaboration between Bioregional
Developments, an environmental
charity, and Bill Dunster Architects.
BedZED is designed to provide 82
homes and 1,600m² (17,220ft²) of work
space on a 1.4ha (3¹/₂ acre) site, as well
as a number of other facilities,
including a sports club, a football
pitch, a nursery, an organic-food shop
and a health centre. BedZED is the
largest sustainable development of its
kind in the UK, and it anticipated in
many ways the outcome of recent UK
planning policies.

The BedZED strategy for sustainable
design is holistic, embracing health
and safety, water-use efficiency,
recycling, waste minimization and
green transport as well-known
principles of low-energy design.

Heating requirements in a BedZED
home are expected to be around 10
per cent of those of a typical UK home
of the same size.

Site, location and climate
The site, a former sewage works on
the southern edge of London, was
sold to the client, Peabody Trust, even
though BedZED was not the highest
bidder. For the first time in the UK, a
scheme's sustainability credentials
had been taken into account in the
adjudication of tenders. Peabody,
however, was not sole developer of
the site. The site was found by
environmental advisers Bioregional
Developments, who approached
Peabody for funding. The core of
Bioregional's design team had been
developing the design to a relatively
detailed stage prior to Peabody's
involvement. The site is 15 minutes'

walk from Mitcham station and on the
new Wimbledon to Croydon tramline.
Anticipating many of the principles
discussed in *Towards an Urban
Renaissance* by architect Lord Richard
Rogers, head of Britain's Urban Task
Force, the designers addressed the
question of how to build an urban
community that provides a high-
quality lifestyle without profligate use
of scarce global resources.

The layout is very straightforward:
five rows of terraces run east–west.
This results in an overall density of 50
dwellings and 120 workspaces per
hectare after allowing for the sports
facility, clubhouse and landscaping.
The design team estimates that
approximately 1¹/₂ million dwellings of
this kind could be built on existing
'brownfield' land in the UK –
satisfying almost half the predicted
need by 2016.

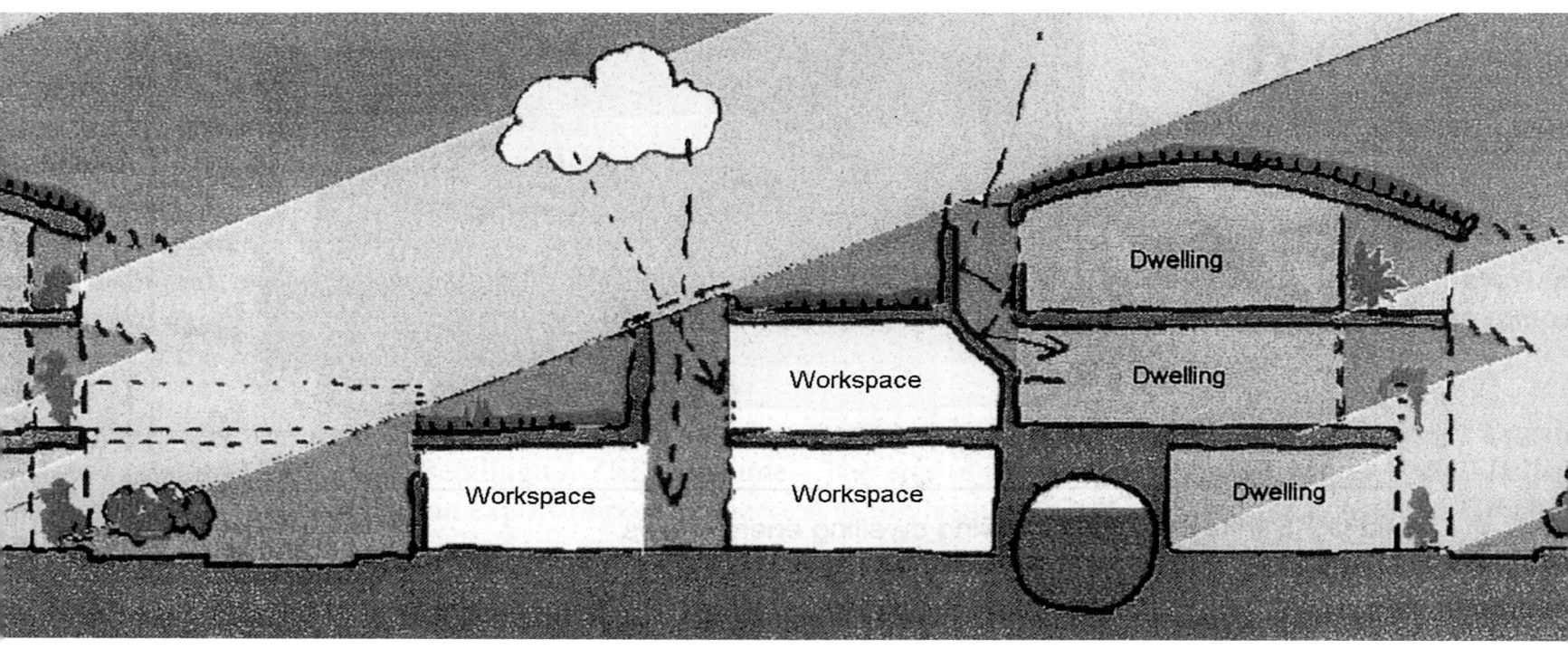

Labels within image: Dwelling, Dwelling, Dwelling, Workspace, Workspace, Workspace

↑
Sketch section depicting solar strategy.

Houses are placed on the south side of the terraces to promote maximum solar potential and workspaces are on the north side, shaded by the dwellings, and may therefore be north-lit and naturally ventilated. Although the layout is compact, green amenity space is made available wherever possible – for example, workspace roofs are used as gardens for adjacent dwellings. In this way, every dwelling has a private garden at densities that would normally only allow for balconies. This relieves the scheme of the monotonous one-dimensional layouts of the early generation of passive solar housing schemes. The integrated nature of the project with its social amenities and shared community spaces is more closely related, in fact, to the garden suburb model.

Construction and materials
The thermal performance of the building envelope at BedZED is three times more efficient than the current UK regulations require and will also outstrip projected performance standards for 2003; 300mm (12in) thickness of insulation provides U values that still justify description of 'super-insulated dwelling'. The building form is clearly based on Hope House, Bill Dunster's own house built four years earlier.[2] Although built as a 'one-off', the house has always been considered a prototype for a high-density form of urban dwelling. The original house can be defined as a classic solar design, with a south-facing conservatory backed up by a well-insulated fabric with high thermal mass. As at Hope House, thermal mass – provided by intermediate concrete floors – is an

integral part of the strategy of the BedZED dwellings.

BedZED is built from natural recycled materials. New wood is sourced from FSC (Forest Stewardship Council) sources and all other materials have been sourced within a 35 mile (56km) radius of the site, often using salvaged materials especially for timber studwork. Energy and pollution generated from transport is thereby kept to a minimum and the local economy benefits. Local contractors are preferred. The BedZED philosophy of employing local resources to deal with global concerns is one of the first examples of 'glocal' architecture in the UK.

Building form
The typical modern dwelling in the UK has a relatively low occupancy, low intermittent heat gains and a wide

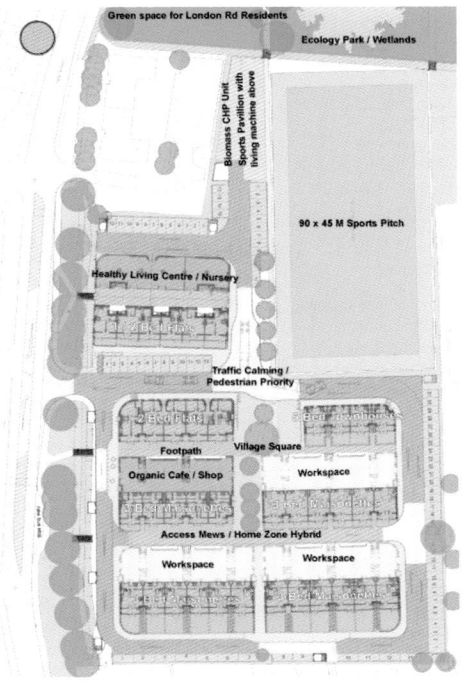

↑
Site layout.

BedZED U VALUES OUTSTRIP PROJECTED UK STANDARDS				
Element	Fabric U values W/m²/°K (Btu/h/ft²/°F) *Current value*	Proposed value *for 2001*	Proposed value *for 2003*	Bedzed value
roof	0.25 (0.044)	0.2 (0.035)	0.16 (0.028)	0.1 (0.018)
ground floor	0.45 (0.079)	0.3 (0.053)	0.25 (0.044)	0.1 (0.018)
exposed floor	0.45 (0.079)	0.3 (0.053)	0.25 (0.044)	0.1 (0.018)
exposed walls	0.45 (0.079)	0.35 (0.062)	0.3 (0.053)	0.11 (0.019)
windows, doors and rooflights	3.3 (0.581)	2.2 (0.387)	2 (0.352)	1.2 (0.211)

↑
Table showing how U
values at BedZED
exceed projected UK
standards.

→
Ventilation strategy
for both dwelling and
work spaces.

range of summer comfort conditions. There are huge potential benefits in energy and comfort terms from south-facing passive solar heating. On the other hand, the workplace has high internal heat gains and a more precisely defined comfort range. The consequence is often installation of expensive solar-shading devices, high lighting use and uneven daylighting provision across the workspace. These features combined to provide the design team with straightforward solutions in terms of building form:

· dwellings are orientated south in terraces
· workspaces are orientated north in terraces
· terraces are positioned to avoid overshadowing, wherever possible
· heat loss through exposed surface area is minimized

· south-facing glazed sun spaces are included in all dwellings.

Design for sustainability
Sustainable design aims not only to reduce our dependence on non-renewable resources but also addresses issues of environmental impact, social progress and economic prosperity. The design team at BedZED have taken a step towards a holistic approach to the design of new housing schemes, aiming to make sustainable living 'easy, attractive and affordable'. They have put the following issues at the forefront of the project:

· reduction in energy demand and renewable sourcing
· land reuse, higher than normal urban density and biodiversity through landscape design

· integration with existing communities
· innovative home/work arrangements
· reduced travel for material miles, food miles, home/work miles
· promotion of walking, cycling and use of public transport
· material environmental impact, embodied energy, durability and recycling
· reduced water consumption
· consumable waste and recycling
· buildings as energy producers for transport.

Energy demand
The objective is to match energy demand with available renewable energy sources so that the buildings at BedZED do not add to carbon dioxide emissions in the atmosphere. Renewable energy sources in the UK

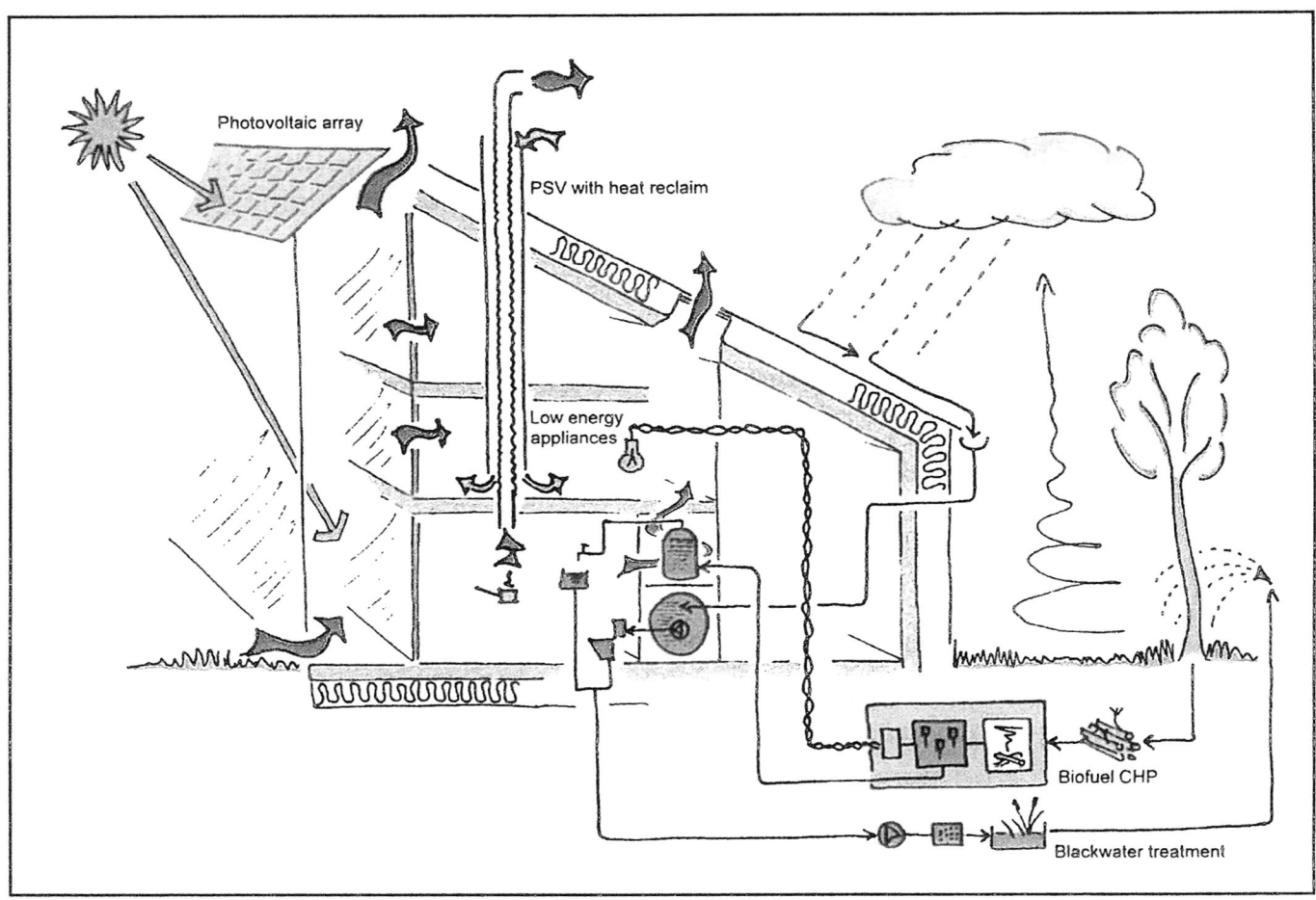

Photovoltaic array

PSV with heat reclaim

Low energy appliances

Biofuel CHP

Blackwater treatment

are difficult to match and balance with demand as well as being expensive in terms of capital costs. It is therefore vital to reduce energy demand through other design strategies, for example, high-performance building fabric.

As BedZED consists of a mixture of dwellings, office shops and community accommodation, Arup initially carried out a review of typical energy consumption for the various building types and established target consumption figures. The grade of energy being consumed was also considered. In the UK, in general terms, electricity is the highest-grade energy and is the most difficult to replace through renewable sources. The production of hot water is the next most difficult, and space heating is the easiest. As a result of this early analysis the following design principles were adopted:

· super-insulation to match fabric heat loss to internal and passive solar gain
· room surface has high thermal capacity to store internal heat until needed
· passive cooling using thermal mass to avoid mechanical cooling
· reduction of uncontrolled ventilation and air infiltration
· avoidance of parasitic energy by mechanical means (high grade energy...by fans, pumps, etc.)
· installing systems that are easy to understand and operate manually
· ventilation heat recovery
· good natural daylight
· high-efficiency initiatives
· low-energy domestic appliances

Energy sources
The following renewable sources of energy were identified by the design team as useful for BedZED:

· passive solar heating
· heat from occupants
· heat from lighting and appliances
· heat from cooking and domestic hot water
· daylight
· bio-fuelled combined heat and power unit (CHP)

It was proposed that BedZED would become a nett producer of energy through the use of renewable resources. The building of integrated photovoltaics was also proposed to provide power for electric cars. Low-grade energy for space heating will be provided by passive solar means combined with internal heat gains. For the system to operate successfully, an efficient means of storing low-grade heat is essential. At BedZED extensive exposed high-thermal-capacity room surfaces will absorb heat when room

BIO-FUELLED COMBINED HEAT & POWER
CHP

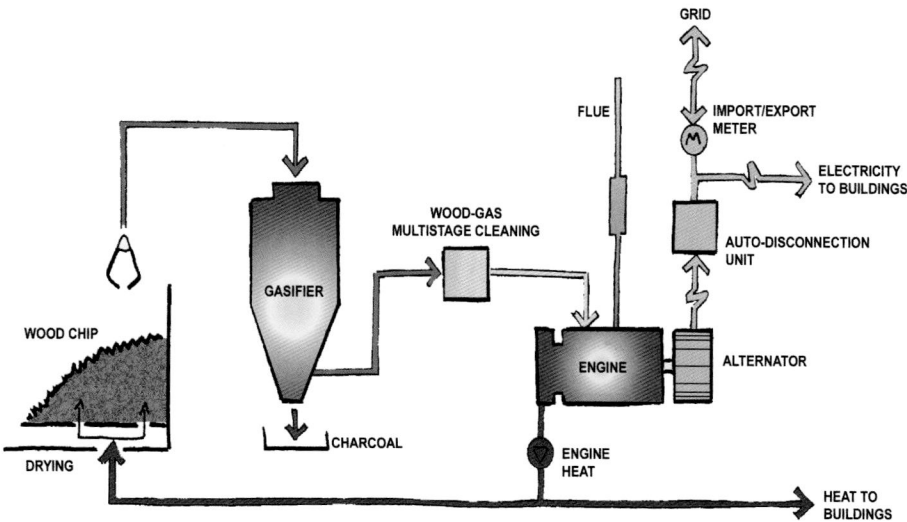

Bio-fuel system for
the development.

temperatures start to rise and release heat back into the atmosphere when temperatures fall.

A combined heat and power unit (CHP) fuelled by chipped and dried tree waste will generate BedZED's electricity. The nominal 130KW capacity CHP is equipped with an export/import connection to the national grid, allowing constant electrical output of the CHP to balance demand changes. By eliminating space-heating loads which fluctuate through seasonal demand, a more constant heat output can be designed for the CHP. For example, the CHP supplies domestic hot water whose daily total demand is relatively constant all year round. Some heat storage is needed to deal with daily fluctuations, however, and this is provided by large domestic hot-water cylinders in each dwelling and

workplace. The CHP 'trickle' charges them and the peak hot-water demand is designed to match the peak CHP output, thereby avoiding the cost of peak-load boiler plant. Cylinder immersion heaters provide a hot-water standby. Energy meters are located in prominent positions so that users can monitor their own energy consumption.

Daylighting

A primary goal of the BedZED team is to provide good daylighting in offices and dwellings in order to save energy through reduced use of electric light and also to improve the overall visual environment. Daylighting in offices is considered especially important because offices are used predominantly during the day and have higher illumination requirements. Particular attention was paid to the

sectional development of the terraces and window design. The performance characteristics of the windows in dwellings were defined as follows:

· low emissivity
· clear triple-glazing to all windows
· clear double glazing on room side and exterior of solar spaces
· daylight obstruction through frame to be no greater than 30 per cent
· windows to have larger panes due to both internal and external framing obstruction
· average room surface to be reflective

Ventilation

The strategy at BedZED is 'build tight and ventilate right' to limit ventilation heat loss and eliminate the need for a conventional heating system. It is based on using natural ventilation to minimize capital costs and energy

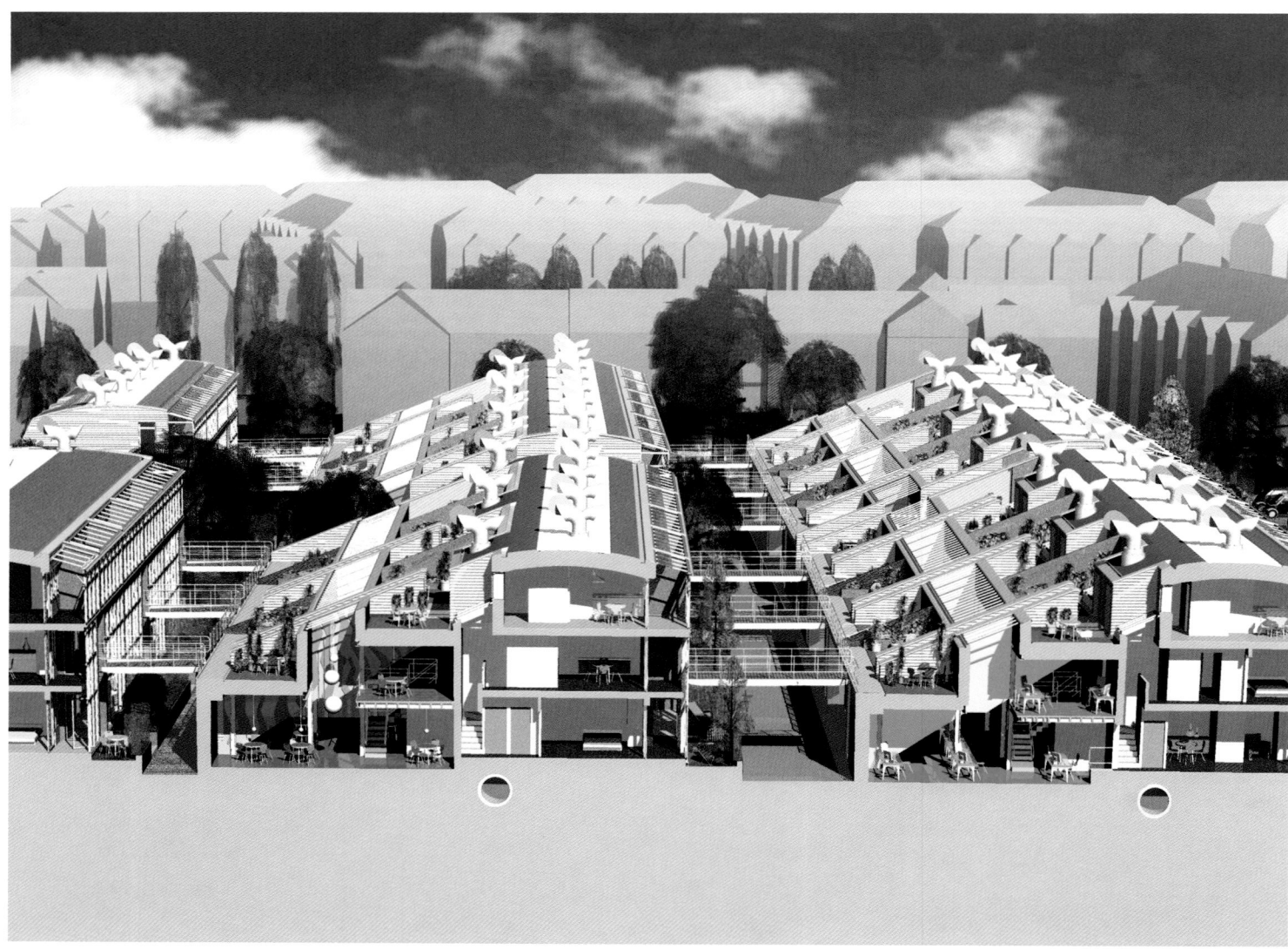

consumption. Ventilation is needed for fresh air, periodic purging (of pollutants), cooling during occupancy, night-time cooling, removal of local moisture gains and removal of smells.

The BedZED design is founded on the provision of occupant-controlled opening windows of an area equal to at least 5 per cent of the floor area in all habitable rooms. For night-time cooling, secure locking allows windows to be held with a minimum clear 50mm (2in) opening. Wind- and winter buoyancy-driven roof cowls supply fresh air and extract moisture and pollutants.

In naturally ventilated domestic and non-domestic buildings a minimum supply of fresh air is normally provided by window trickle ventilators. However, in a low-energy building without room-heat emitters, such ventilators become a significant

energy drain, particularly on a cold windy day. Ventilation design for BedZED seeks to provide preheated fresh air by using passive stack ventilation with heat recovery. This takes advantage of the sealed building envelope to create a balanced air supply and exhaust using a combination of internal heat buoyancy and wind pressure through a both positive and negative heat exchanger fitted with a roof wind cowl. The air supply enters the living rooms and bedrooms, and the exhaust comes from the kitchens, bathrooms and toilets.

Mechanical systems
The low-energy strategy is based on exploiting the use of low-tech building fabric form and materials and avoiding heavy dependence on sophisticated electrical and

mechanical systems in the individual buildings. Large capital investments have been made in providing the long-life passive building fabric components, while savings have been made by not supplying conventional heating systems. Over the long design life of the building this strategy will result in the lowest 'cradle-to-grave', embodied and consumed energy needs. The mechanical services systems consist of:

· potable water supply from mains
· rainwater greywater system
· domestic hot water cylinder assembly in each dwelling/workspace
· site-wide bio-fuelled mini-CHP serving each domestic hot-water cylinder
· wind and passive stack drum ventilation with heat recovery

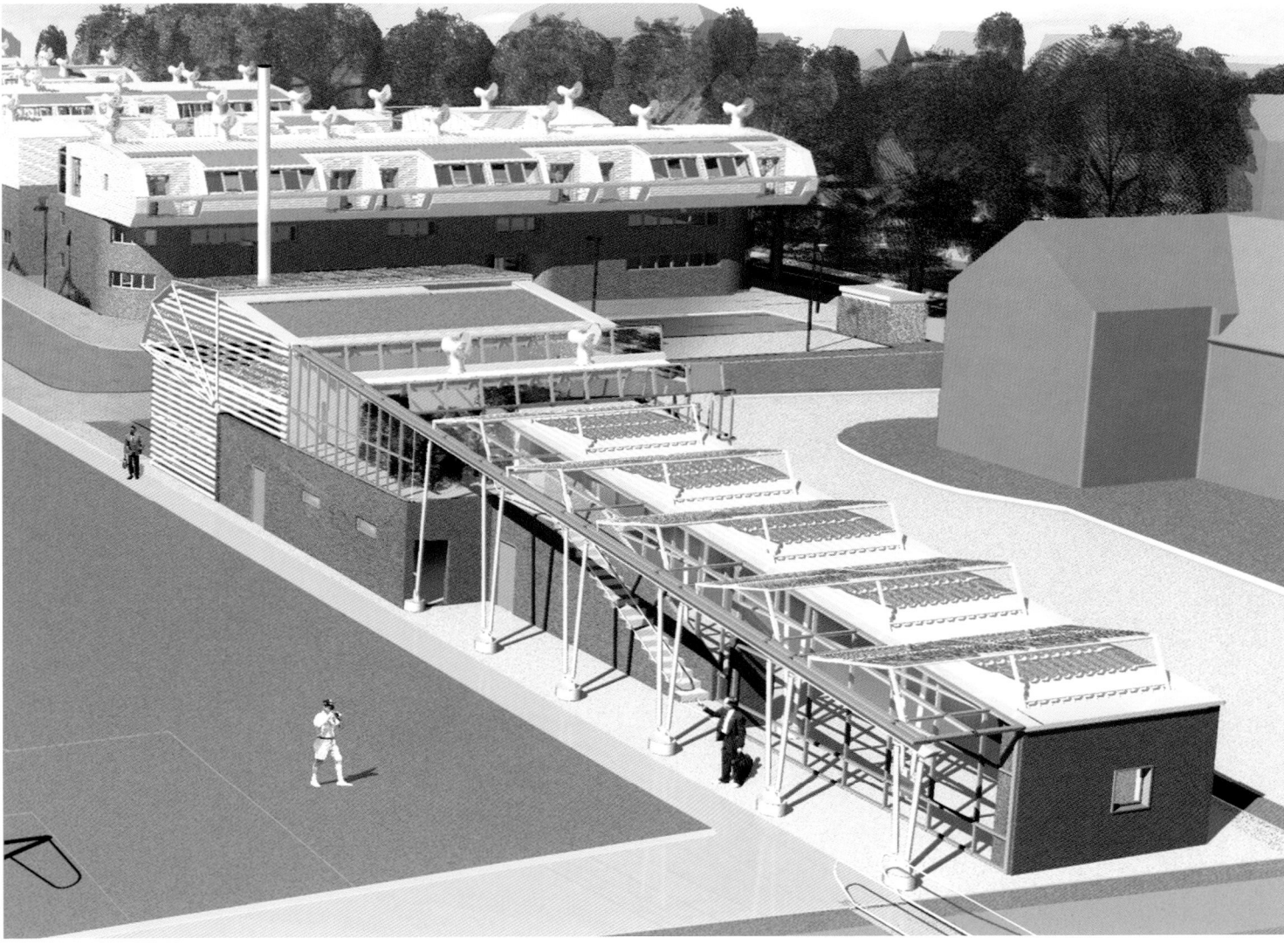

Heating

The strategy is to avoid the need for a conventional mechanical system by designing the building fabric so that the natural heat gains are more than adequate to cope with the heat losses. This is achieved by using:

· heat gains from people
· heat gains from lighting and appliances
· heat gains from cooking and domestic hot water
· solar heat gain
· super-insulation
· very high envelope air-tightness
· ventilation heat recovery
· high thermal inertia room surfaces to store excess heat until it is needed

The goal is to achieve room temperatures almost constantly above 19°C (66°F) if occupants wish. Alternatively, rooms can be vented by opening windows manually. During longer periods when the building is unoccupied, and therefore experiencing minimum heat gains, the aim is to maintain a background temperature using a thermostatically controlled vent from the domestic hot-water cylinder cupboard. The piped CHP primary hot-water mains serve the domestic hot-water needs of the buildings through a coil inside the hot-water cylinders of each dwelling and workspace. The CHP main return pipe goes via a bathroom towel rail in each dwelling.

Water consumption

One of the aims of the project is to reduce potable water consumption by avoiding power showers and installing outlet-flow limiters and low-water-consuming appliances. A range of water-recycling methods has been investigated, with the recovery of rainwater to serve low-water flush toilets being identified as most suitable. Design aims are as follows:

· potable water demand could be reduced by about 50 per cent
· water system has low mechanical plant requirement
· proven component availability
· self-cleaning filtration
· almost no maintenance
· standard drainage components, eg. rainwater store is a large drainage pipe
· main roof as impermeable collection surface, as it should be noted that garden and street run-off unsuitable due to fouling by animals, cars and garden chemicals

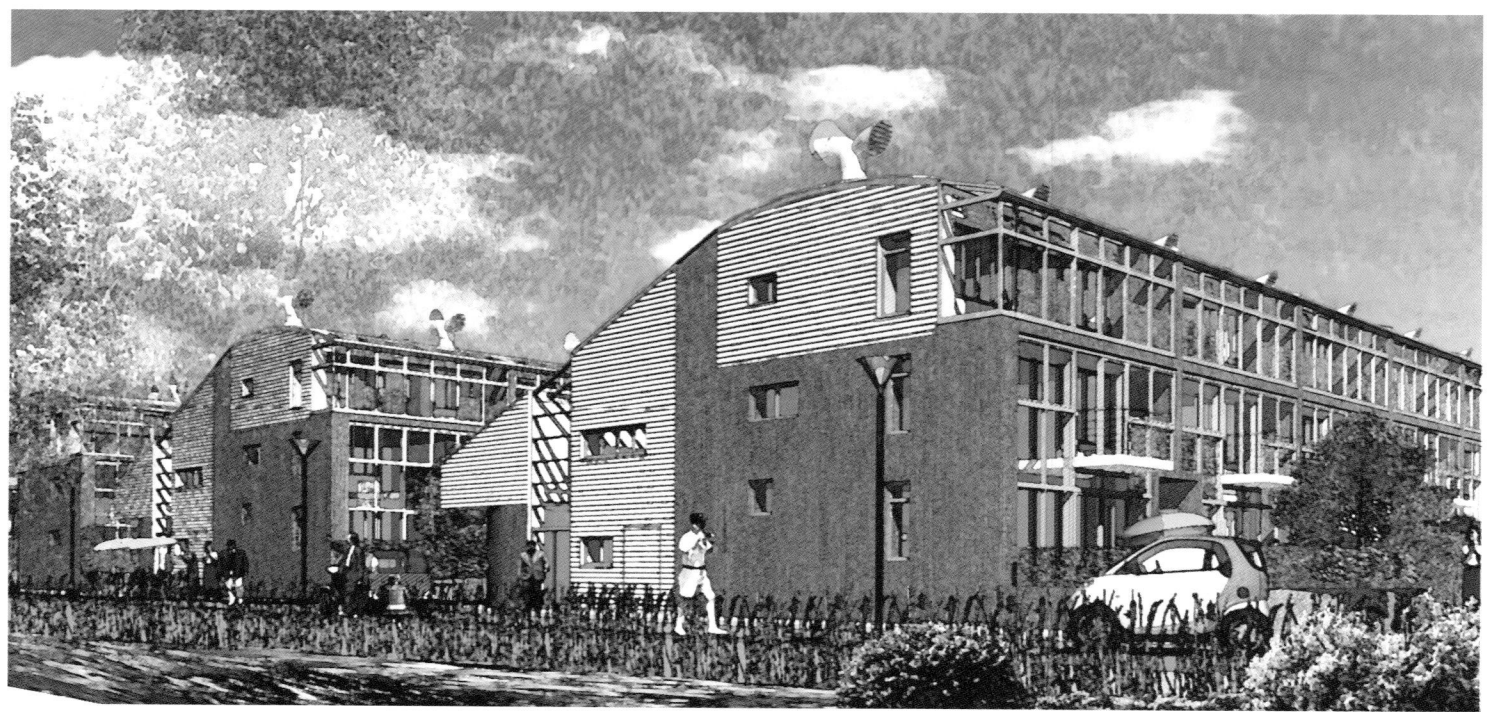

← Community building flanking the recreation area.

↑ The integrated sustainable community.

Conclusion

BedZED is the most ambitious sustainable development in the UK. Designed to be energy-efficient, it is based on well-known and orthodox technologies, but it goes way beyond the previous generations of 'low-energy' housing. It is based on a new way of integrated communal living. This is not as new or radical in other mainland European countries as it is in England, where the general quality of housing is poor. Much of the housing in the Netherlands and Germany, for example, has higher space standards. This can be partly attributed to the culture of research and development that exists in these countries. The lessons from BedZED should be absorbed and transferred to new UK developments.

Mont Cenis
Training Centre
Jourda & Perraudin
Herne-Sodingen
Germany
1997

➜

The dynamic skin of
Mont Cenis acts as a
climatic filter.

In 1991 a competition was organized jointly by IBA Emscher Park and Land Nordrhein–Westphalia in Herne-Sodingen, Germany, for a government training centre including seminar facilities, meeting rooms, hotel-type accommodation, a restaurant, a gymnasium, a library and leisure facilities including sports fields. The two-stage competition was won by architects Jourda & Perraudin from Lyons, France.

As far back as 1980, Jourda & Perraudin had been exploring the idea of an architecture in which different climatic zones in a building would provide different comfort conditions to match particular activities.[1] The idea of a house within a house – similar in concept to a Russian doll – has been a constantly recurring theme in their work, and the competition entry for the German academy was rooted in this tradition.

In 1993 Jourda & Perraudin with consulting engineers Arup Partners and Agibat MTI completed a research project under the Joule II programme of the European Union Directorate General XII based on the design strategy of 'a microclimatic envelope'. Their conclusions were that real environmental benefits might accrue from an envelope of this kind. Further proposals were added to incorporate approximately 10,000m^2 (107,600ft^2) of photovoltaic cells to act as a solar-power generator integrated with the roof of the envelope. The original competition brief was modified to include a public library, a multi-purpose hall and local authority offices.

A new company, EMC (Entwicklungsgesellschaft Mont Cenis), was founded to represent the various client bodies, and construction began in 1997. That year, the design was exhibited in the German pavilion at the Architecture Biennial in Venice and at the world conference for

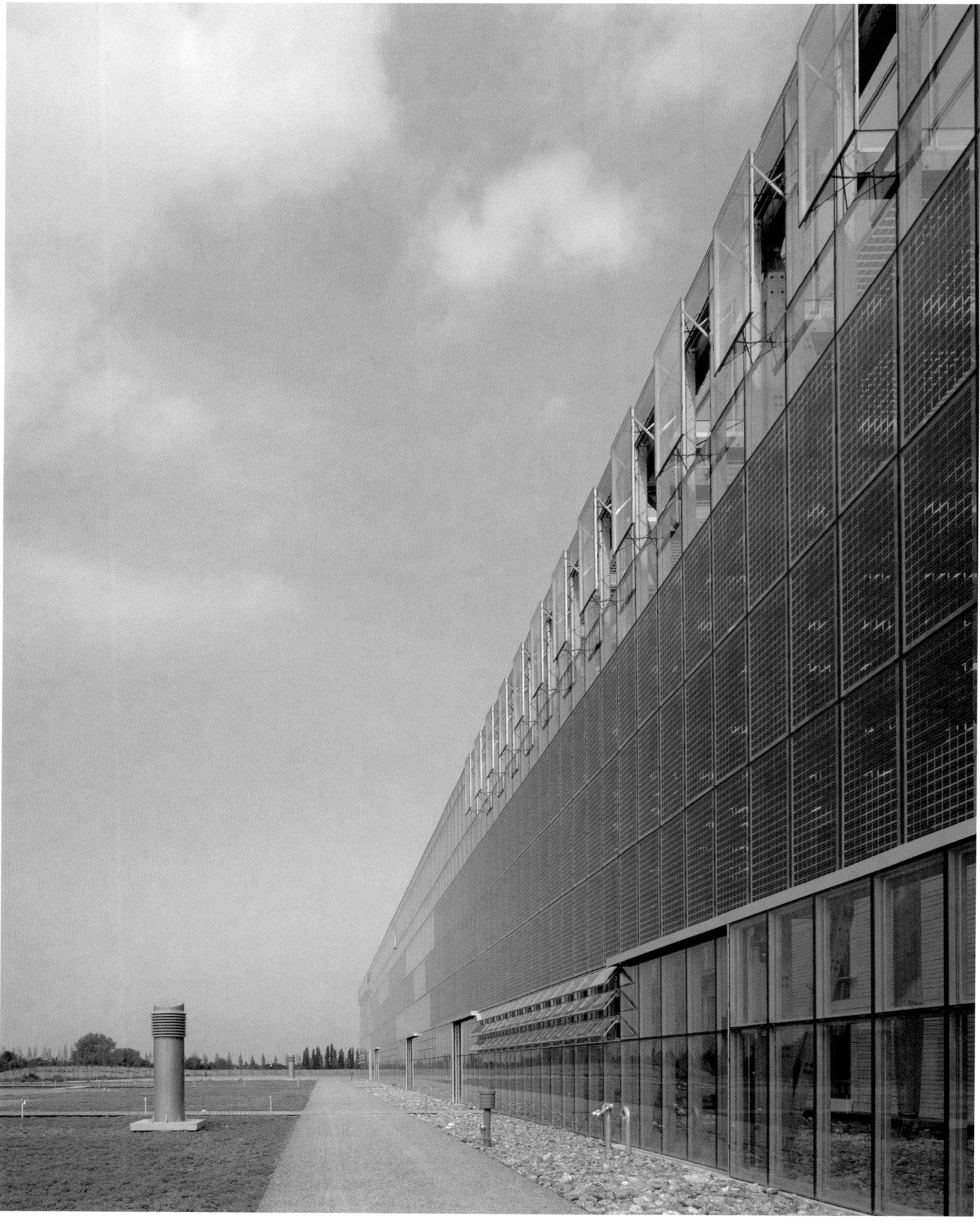

CFD study of chilled ceiling displacement (typical internal office).

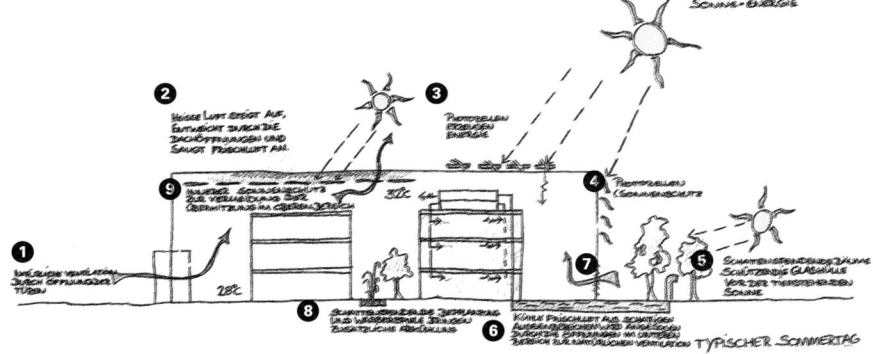

Typical summer's day

1 Doors open for views and natural ventilation
2 Hot air rises and escapes through open rooflights, drawing fresh air in at low level
3 Solar water heater
4 Photovoltaic cells (solar shades)
5 Trees shade glasshouse from low-angle sun
6 Cool fresh air drawn in from shade areas outside glasshouse
7 Low-level openings from natural ventilation
8 Vegetation and water features shade and evaporatively cool glasshouse
9 Internal shades trap solar heat at high level

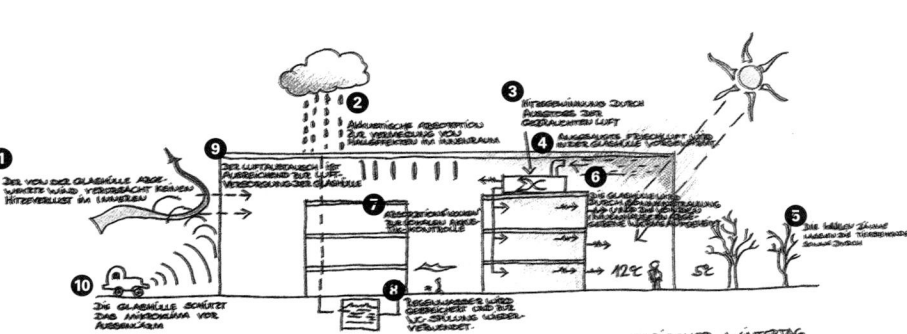

Typical winter's day

1 Wind, deflected by glasshouse, minimizes wind heat losses from the inner building
2 Acoustic absorption to limit glasshouse reverberation
3 Heat reclaimed from exhausted air
4 Fresh air drawn in and preheated by glasshouse
5 Trees shed leaves, allowing in low-angle sun
6 Glasshouse heated by sun and heat loss from buildings
7 Absorption 'cloud' for local acoustic control
8 Rainwater stored and reused to flush toilets
9 Infiltration rate sufficient to keep glasshouse fresh
10 Glasshouse protects microclimate from outside noise

environmental protection in Kyoto, and the building was completed in 1999. It is ground-breaking in its use of the microclimatic envelope to provide environmental comfort with large-scale energy savings.

Location

Herne is situated in the heart of the Ruhr, an area traditionally dominated by heavy industry, which has become a focus for urban and economic regeneration. The town of Sodingen – once dominated by the coal mine at Mont Cenis, now closed and demolished – is the site for the new development, which is part of the International Bauausstellung Emscher Park (International Architecture Exhibition).

The project aims to be a beacon for regeneration in the area, not only socio-economically but also environmentally – by developing a redundant and contaminated mine site and using new clean-energy sources and bioclimatic building. The development has five main elements:

· an education centre for the minister of the interior of Nordrhein-Westphalia
· municipal buildings including a multi-purpose meeting hall, a civic administration building and a library
· new shops, public services and offices connected to an existing shopping centre
· 250 units of housing extended from the neighbouring area
· a landscaped park

Urban context

The strategy was to convert the former mine site into parkland, which would be linked in the south to the existing town centre and in the north to the open green space of Vosshacken. Also to the north is a square bordered by an extension to an existing shopping centre.

A set of steps lined on both sides by buildings leads up to the park from the town centre. At the head of the steps is the academy, planned as a conspicuous landmark, with the education centre – the heart of the project – located in an oval clearing. To the east is a car park accessible from Kirchstrasse. The housing can be reached by the same route, and at the end of the main axis lies the Belvedere, a geometric form created from demolition waste. The contaminated land to the north has been drained by a network of trenches and embankments, and planted. Raised wooden walkways will form

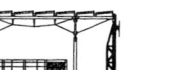

← Cross-section.

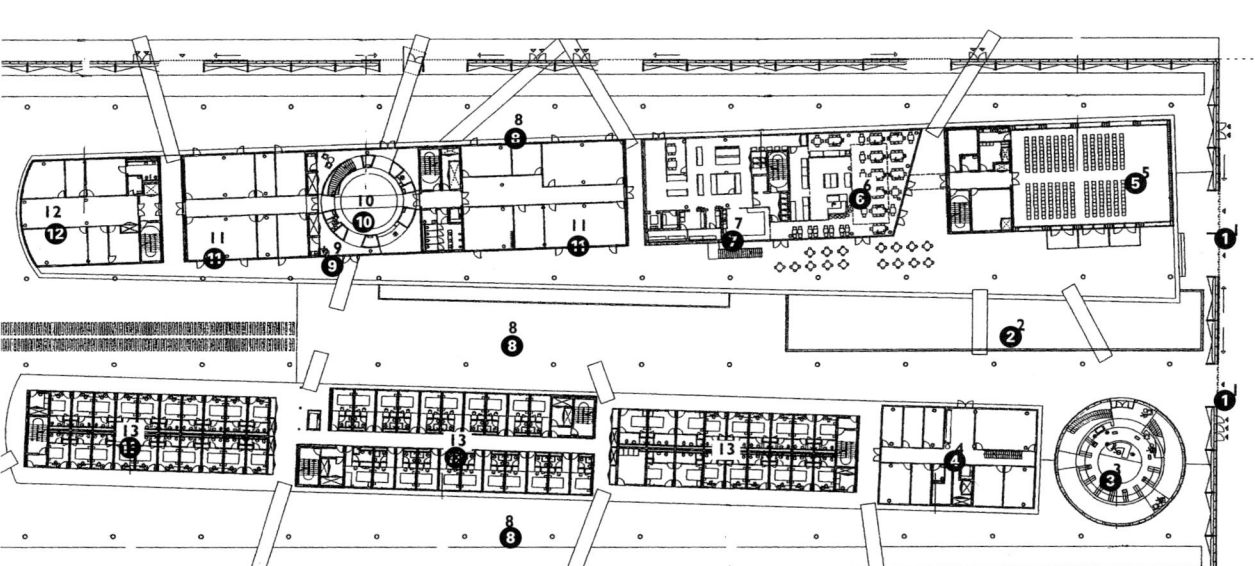

← Site plan.

1   Main public entrance
2   Pool
3   Library
4   Municipal offices
5   Multi-purpose hall
6   Café
7   Recreational facilities
8   Winter garden
9   Training Centre
10 Reception
11 Classrooms
12 Training Centre offices
13 Residential
     accommodation

part of a new public square on previously inaccessible land.

Form

The concept of the microclimatic envelope consists of a glazed 'blanket' thrown over a group of buildings to create a controlled environment between the buildings. The interior of the envelope is characterized by a temperate climate protected from rain and wind, making it a more attractive setting for social activities. In Herne-Sodingen the buildings are grouped in two blocks around a communal space. The zone between the microclimatic envelope and the buildings links occupied spaces with the landscape and surrounding park, making it a spatial as well as a climatic buffer between inside and outside.

The glass envelope is therefore the scene of a climatic shift – the buffer space is climatically Mediterranean rather than northern European. This has had a 'knock-on' effect in the design of the buildings contained by the envelope, which have been effectively re-sited to a more temperate climate. In summer, parts of the façade can be opened to improve ventilation. The vegetation and the water basin contribute to summer cooling in the buffer zone, while the interiors of the buildings are cooled and ventilated by air drawn through tunnels.

Layout

Within the microclimatic envelope lies a new urban village offering community, educational and leisure amenities. The buildings are a collection of rational, cool, almost neutral timber boxes placed within the envelope; they are arranged in two long blocks tilted towards one another to force a long perspective to the park to the north. At the centre of the complex is the academy, a three-storey lineal block dominated by a glazed entrance in the form of a three-storey toplit conical column containing reception, stairs and meeting rooms. Beyond this area is a series of flexible classrooms arranged in six zones on either side of a central circulation spine. Opposite the academy is a hotel consisting of three blocks, each of three levels arranged lineally on a deck. The two end blocks can be accessed directly from this galleried deck, made possible by the climatic modification of the envelope. The central block is more traditionally served by a central corridor, with hotel rooms each side.

The civic accommodation is placed close to the main entrance at the

The timber structure is reminiscent of Victorian boat building sheds.

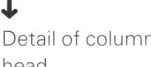
Detail of column head.

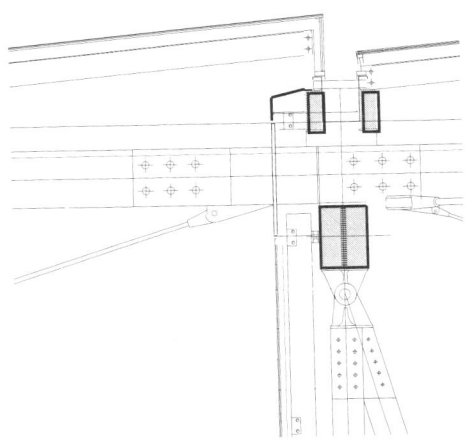

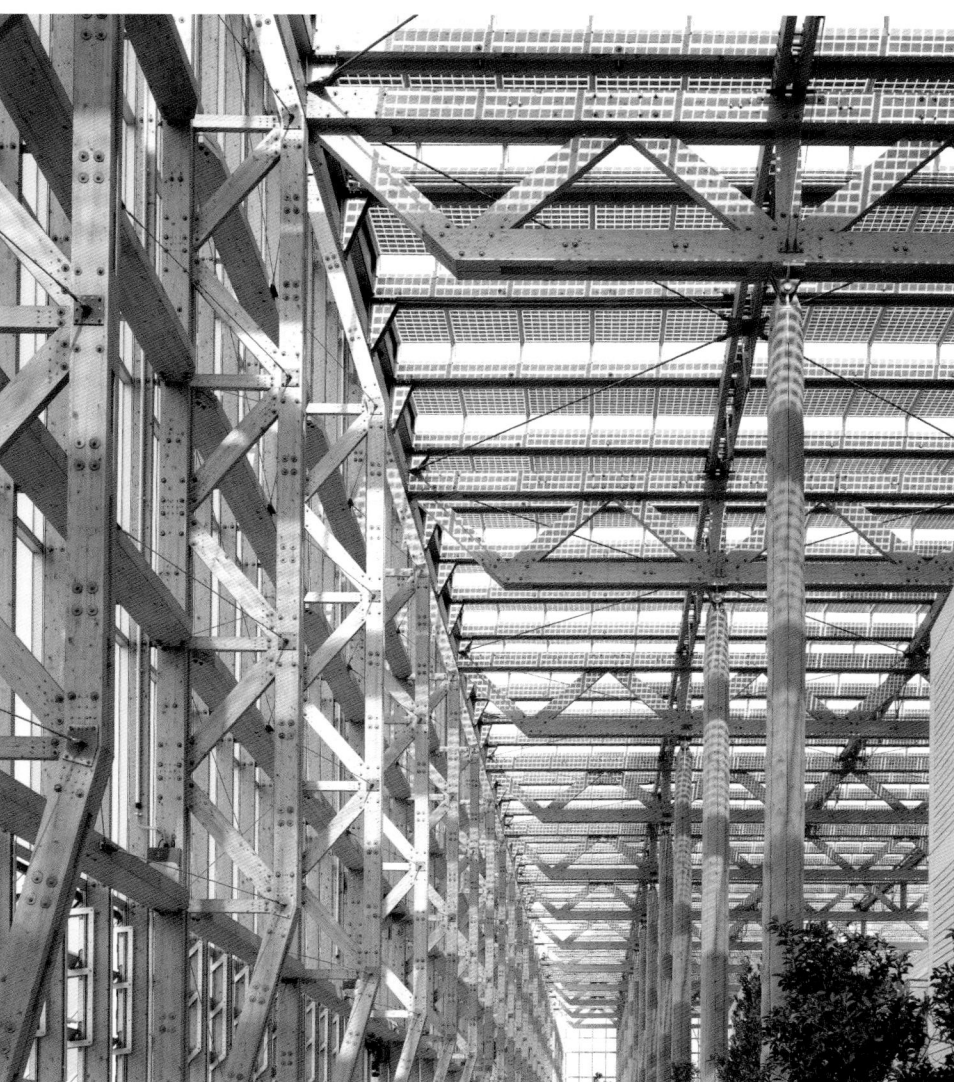

southern end of the hotel wing. This also consists of a three-storey block of mainly cellular rooms served by a central corridor. Also at the southern end of the academy wing is the public meeting room, a large versatile space used for receptions, meetings, shows and banquets; the southern elevation is fully glazed to provide visual contact with the town. The restaurant opens onto a landscaped deck on the ground floor sandwiched between the public meeting room and the academy. Located above the restaurant are a gymnasium, a sauna and a terrace. In the same way that the meeting hall punctuates the academy wing, the library – accessible from the public entrance in the south façade – punctuates the hotel wing. The library's conical shape makes it stand out when seen through the glazed envelope. It contains library

documentation for the education centre and the town and is intended to be a more enclosed and meditative space.

Structure and construction

The structure of the microclimatic envelope is a striking timber-column and lattice-beam hall reminiscent of great Victorian structures such as boat-building sheds and exhibition halls. As at the Crystal Palace, the principles of repetition have been applied for ease of construction. Primary and secondary structural grids are constant and allow for economical construction with an emphasis on prefabrication. The primary columns are made of trunks of pinewood from local renewable sources and their trunk-like shape has been maintained. Some of the buildings are made of reinforced

concrete, and the thermal mass acts as a balancing factor between differences in daytime and night-time temperatures. The repetitive 1.2/2.4m (4/8 ft), 12m and 24m (40ft and 80ft) module contribute to waste minimization.

Energy use and the microclimatic envelope

As well as providing shelter from the wind and rain, the envelope reduces overall energy consumption. In comparison with other similar buildings of the same insulation, a 23 per cent energy saving is predicted. There will also be a 28 per cent reduction in carbon dioxide emissions. The heating system will use less than 50KWh/m^2/year (15,850 Btu/f^2/annum) and the total energy consumption is predicted to be approximately 32KWh/m^2/year (10,144

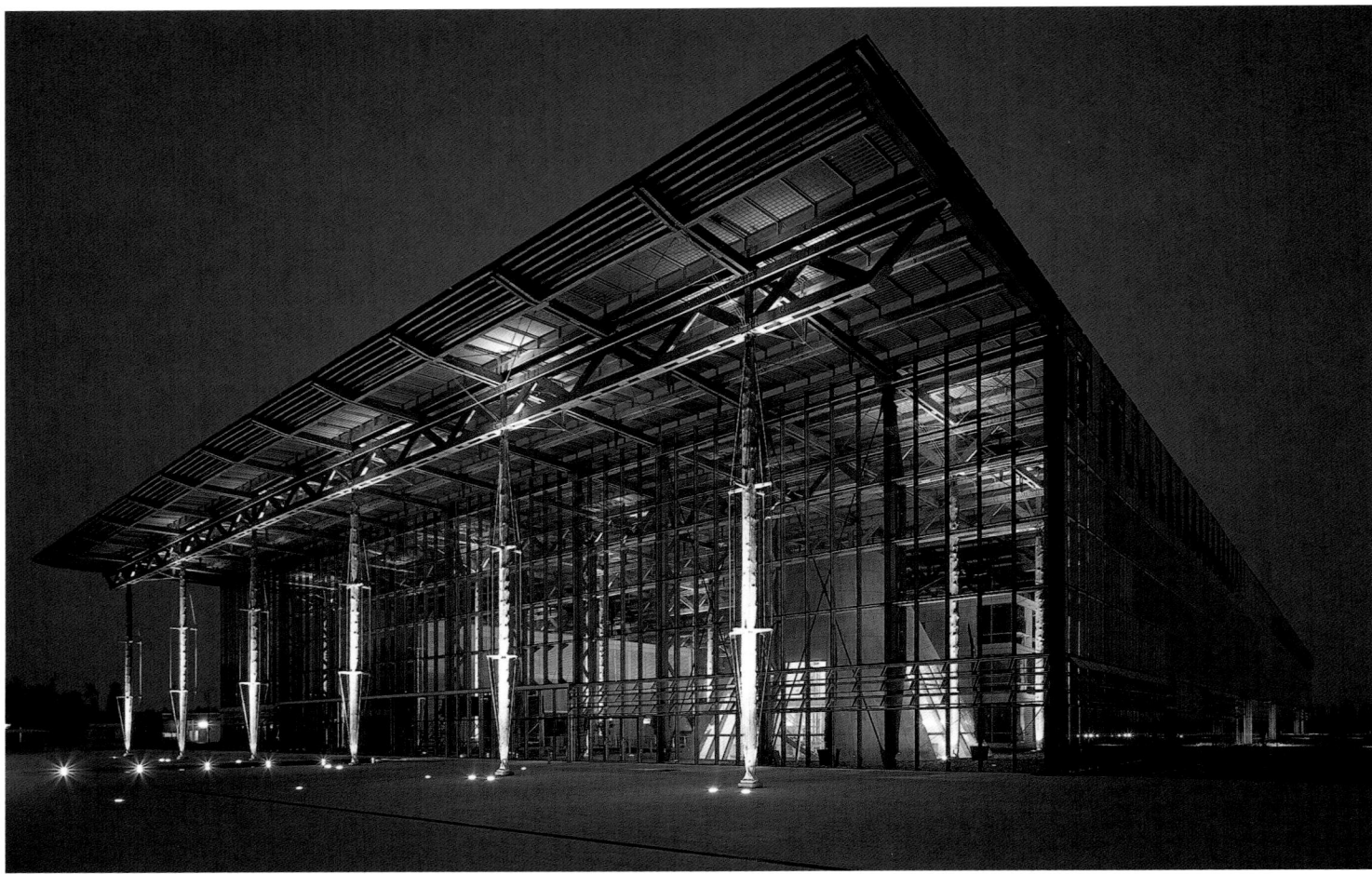

↑
The building complex
makes a dramatic
landmark at night-time.

Btu/f^2/annum) when the system is at maximum use.[2]

Ventilation and thermal insulation
In winter, wind is deflected by the envelope and heat loss from the buildings is minimized. Fresh air is preheated by solar gain in the glasshouse and drawn into the buildings. The infiltration rate is controlled to keep the 'buffer zone' fresh. An air-handling unit with a heat exchanger has been installed to reclaim and redistribute heat from exhaust air. In summer, the doors of the envelope can be opened to promote natural ventilation; warm air rises and is vented through open roof vents, and cooler fresh air is drawn in at low level. The great glass roof is predominantly shaded by photovoltaic cells, while the walls are protected by trees, thereby avoiding

excessive solar gains even on the warmest days.

Daylight
The envelope has been carefully designed to provide appropriate levels of daylight throughout the buffer zone and in the interiors of the buildings. The roof was designed as a cloud canopy simulating optimal sky conditions. Photovoltaic cells were arranged in varying density over the roof to provide shade in the appropriate spaces. Light shelves are incorporated into certain façades of the buildings to enable daylight penetration to deep spaces, and the two truncated cones of the library have a holographic film incorporated into the roof glazing to direct daylight by means of heliostat effects. A rainbow effect is created in the entrance hall.

Energy sources
The glazed roof of the building incorporates 8,400m^2 (90,380ft^2) of photovoltaic cells within the 12,600m^2 (135,580ft^2) total roof area. This generates a 1MW solar-power generation station. Arranged in cloud patterns, the modules provide optimal shading and protection from glare and direct solar gains. The density of the photovoltaic cells per panel varies from 58 per cent to 86 per cent, and energy production varies accordingly. Solar panels are also incorporated as shading into the west façade of the envelope. The total installation generates far in excess of the 750,000 KWh that the building demands; 600 inverters transform the DC current to AC current, and surplus energy can be fed back to the general grid. As well as the solar power, a number of other energy sources are integrated into the

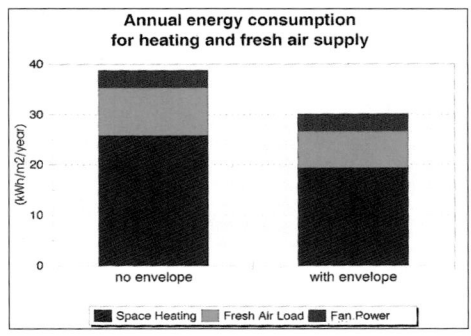

Annual energy consumption for heating and fresh air supply

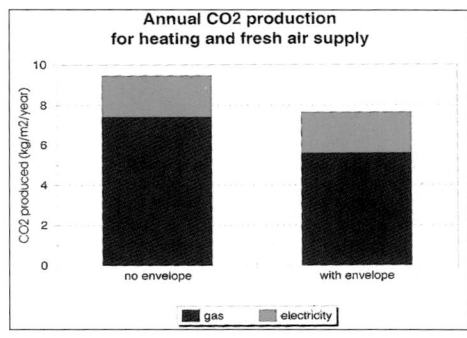

Annual CO2 production for heating and fresh air supply

←

Comparative studies of energy use and CO₂ production.

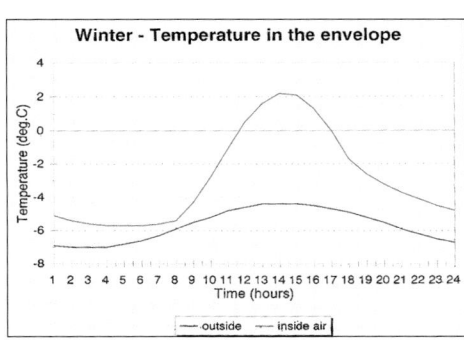

Winter - Temperature in the envelope

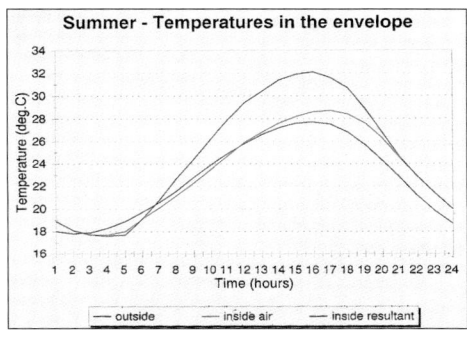

Summer - Temperatures in the envelope

←

Modelling the effect of temperatures in the envelope.

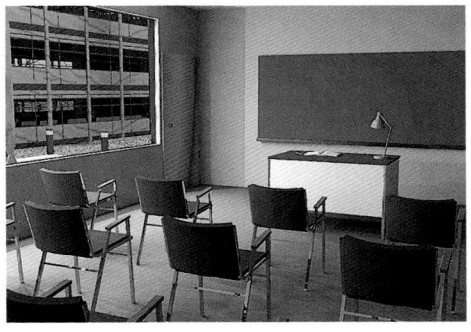

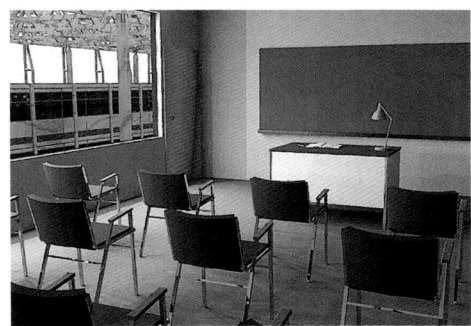

←

Daylight studies to ensure the daylight penetration of training spaces.

complex. The colliery pits release more than 1 million m³ (1,308,000yd³) of gas per year, 60 per cent of which is methane; the gas is used to fuel two co-generation units, producing both electricity and heat. The heat is used not only for the academy but also for the houses and a nearby hospital. Harnessing the excess gas from the disused colliery means that carbon dioxide emissions into the atmosphere are reduced by 12,000 tonnes (11,800 tons).

Conclusion

The development of the microclimatic envelope in the work of Jourda & Perraudin has reached its logical conclusion at Herne. Achieving a climatic shift by sheltering a collection of buildings – almost a civic precinct with a diverse range of occupancies – huge energy savings have been

achieved. However, apart from the energy issues, the complex at Herne suggests a new kind of communal living – all under one roof. The notion of an 'in-between' hybrid space is not new, but has been neglected, if not forgotten. At Herne the roof admits daylight but also provides solar shading and is a solar collector; the walls supply the inhabitants with air, light and shade, making the envelope more of a climatic filter than an umbrella.

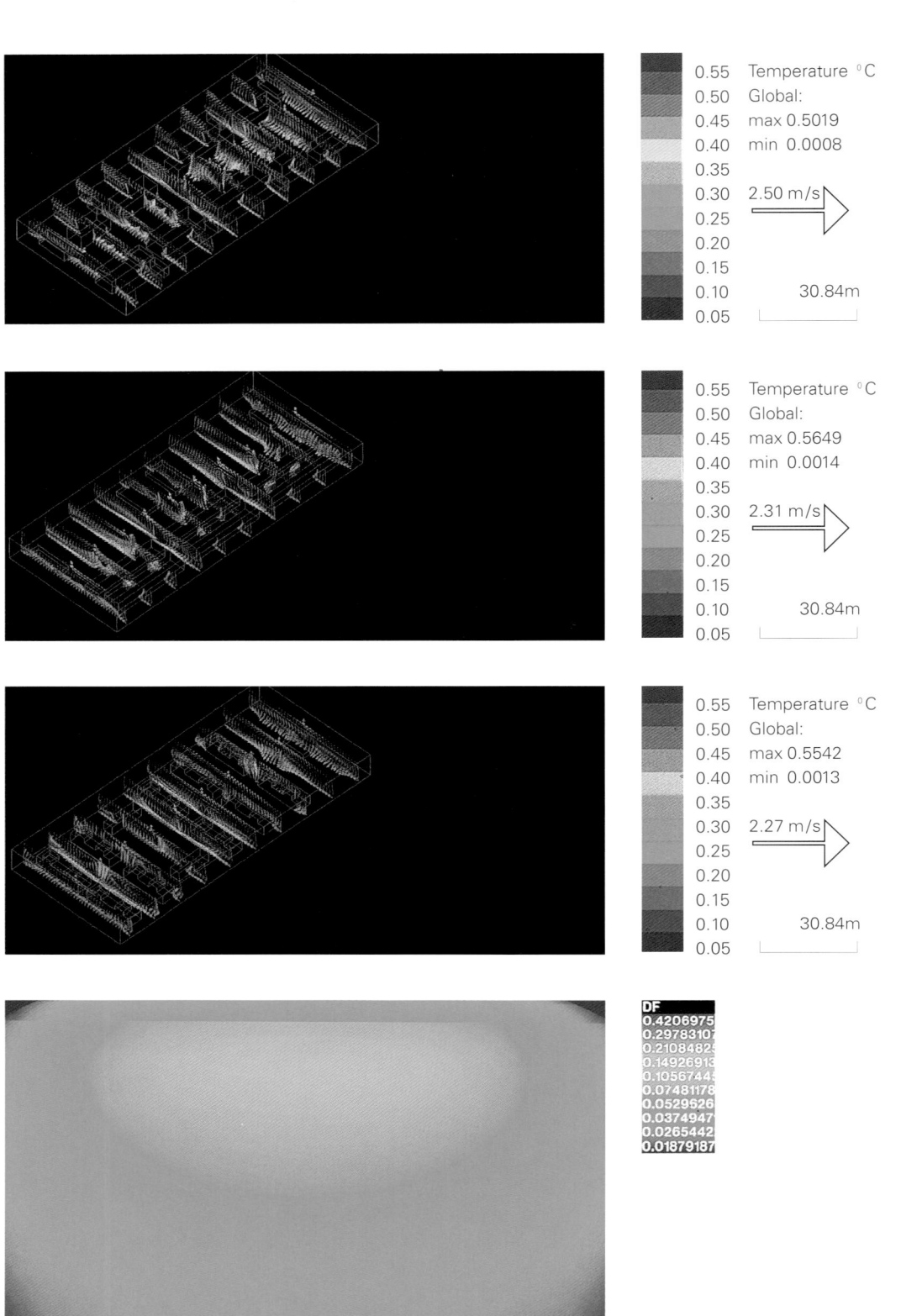

	Temperature °C
0.55	Global:
0.50	max 0.5019
0.45	min 0.0008
0.40	
0.35	
0.30	2.50 m/s
0.25	
0.20	
0.15	
0.10	30.84m
0.05	

	Temperature °C
0.55	Global:
0.50	max 0.5649
0.45	min 0.0014
0.40	
0.35	
0.30	2.31 m/s
0.25	
0.20	
0.15	
0.10	30.84m
0.05	

	Temperature °C
0.55	Global:
0.50	max 0.5542
0.45	min 0.0013
0.40	
0.35	
0.30	2.27 m/s
0.25	
0.20	
0.15	
0.10	30.84m
0.05	

DF
0.4206975
0.29783107
0.21084825
0.14926913
0.10567445
0.07481178
0.0529626
0.0374947
0.0265442
0.01879187

←

CFD studies were used to analyze an internal environment under different external conditions.

←

Daylight studies of the glazed roof.

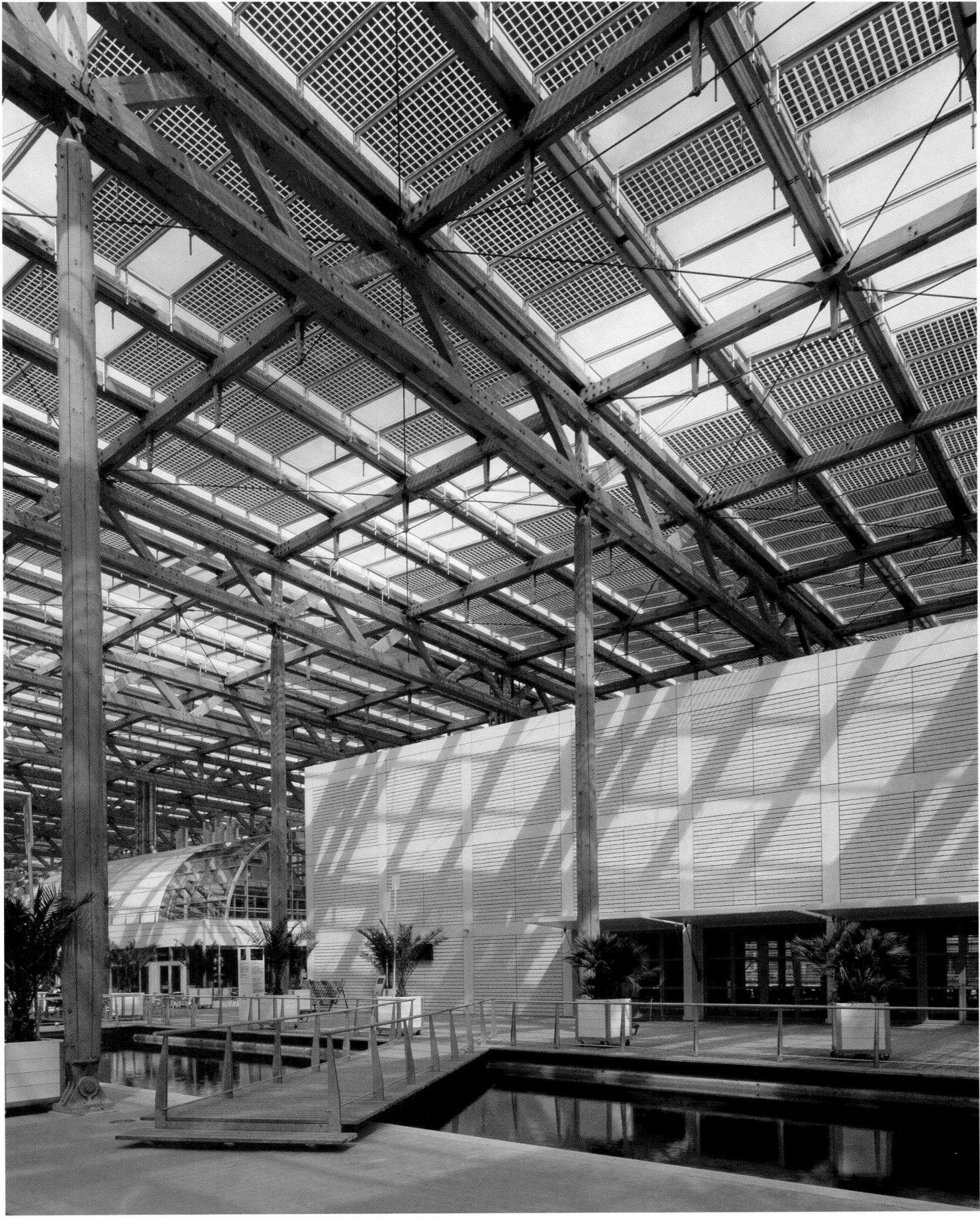

Interior showing photovoltaic shading of roof.

Varying density of photovoltaics to simulate cloud canopy.

↓

The envelope creates a 'climatic' shift.

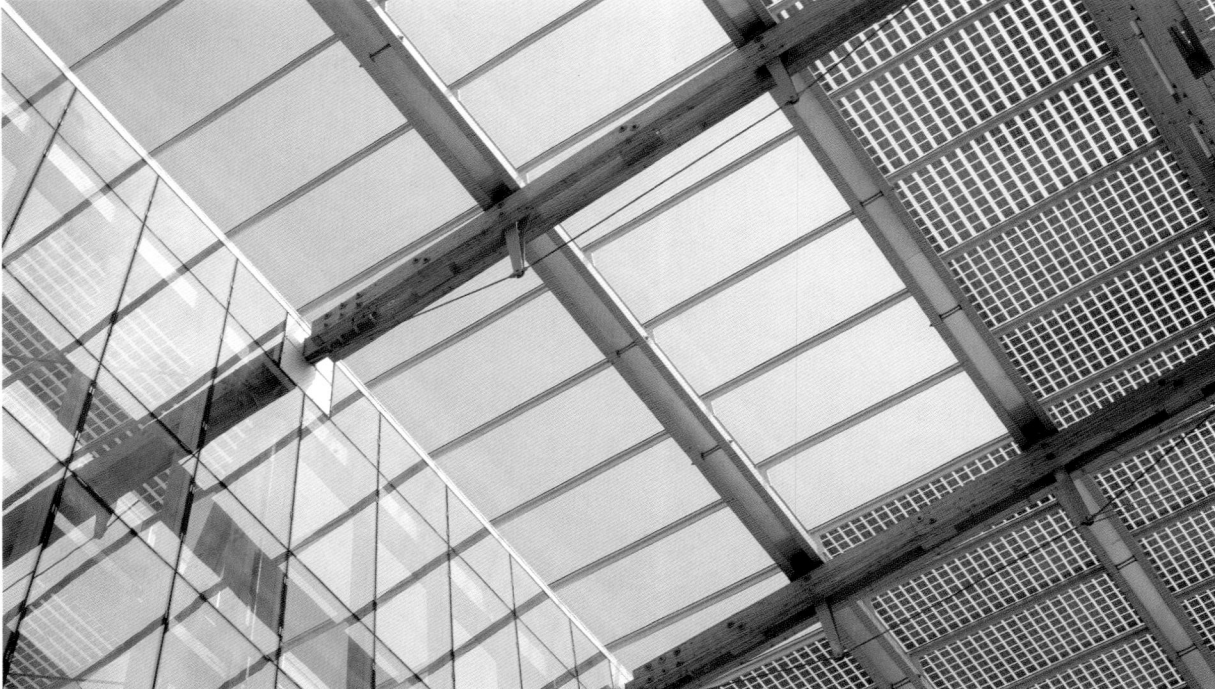

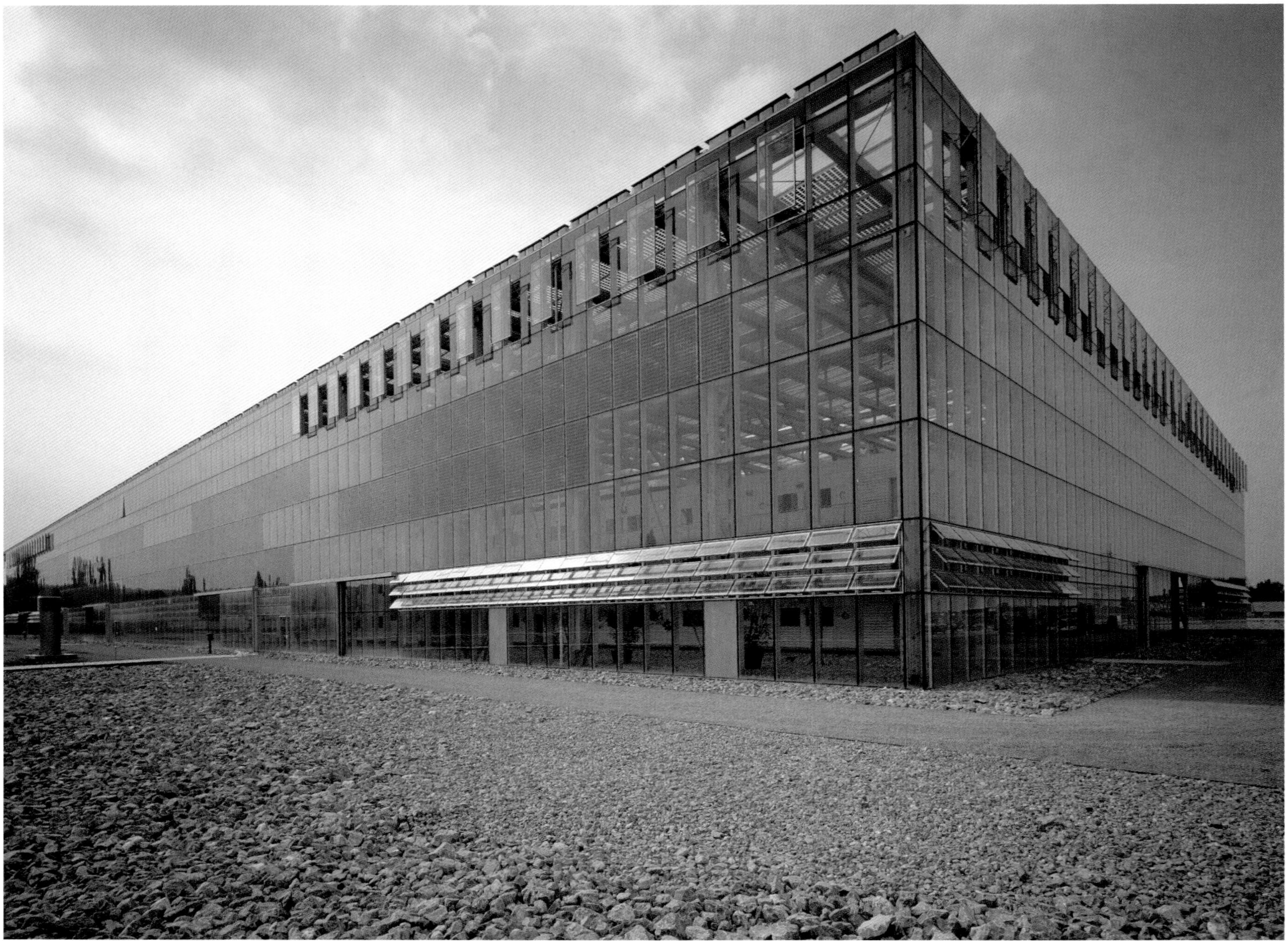

Study Centre Darwin College

Jeremy Dixon and Edward Jones Cambridge, UK 1994

The collegiate system of education practised in the ancient universities of Oxford and Cambridge enjoys a particular relationship with its architecture. In the historic colleges a particular morphology has evolved in which the principal elements of the college are organized around open courtyards – referred to as 'quads' at Oxford and 'courts' at Cambridge. In one way or another each college adopts and adapts this form to organize both the general spaces of students' living accommodation and the highly specific spaces of chapel, dining hall, master's lodging and, as

perhaps the most significant expression of the institution's scholarship, the library.

Darwin College, the first college in Cambridge exclusively for post-graduate students, was founded as recently as 1965. Its very modernity and its particular constitution make it distinctive within the long history and traditions of the university, and this is inevitably reflected in its architecture. At its foundation Darwin was expected to be a small college, with some 20 fellows and 40 or 50 students. Its chosen site was a beautiful but small area close to the

city centre, set between two busy roads and the river. Three existing houses, two of which had been in the ownership of the Darwin family, were joined together and enlarged by the construction of new buildings. This resulted in a linear arrangement in which the buildings acted as a buffer between the roads and the tranquillity of the garden and its river frontage. Within this plan the college put priority on providing residential accommodation for students, and it was decided to do without a chapel and a master's lodging, but a new dining hall was constructed and a

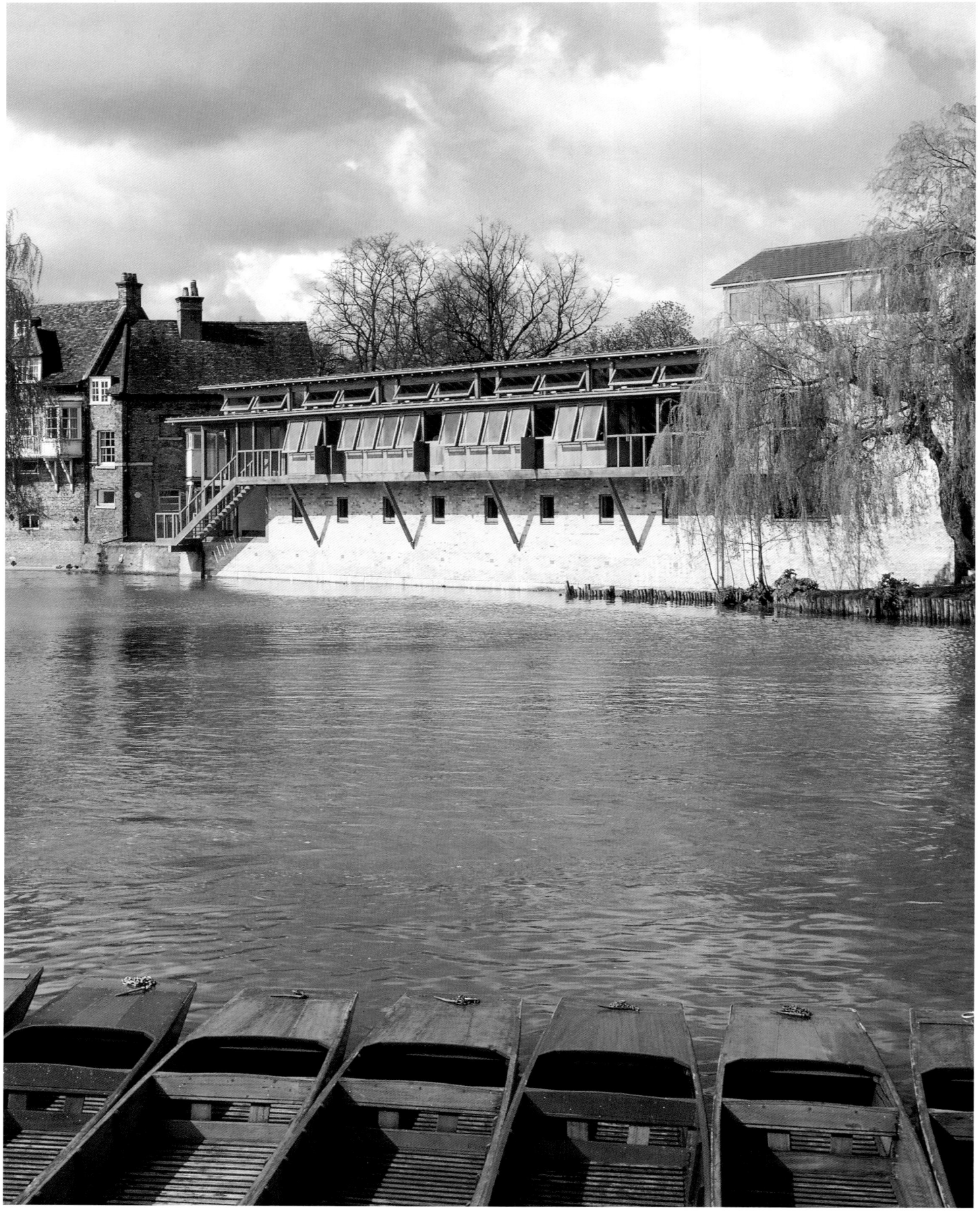

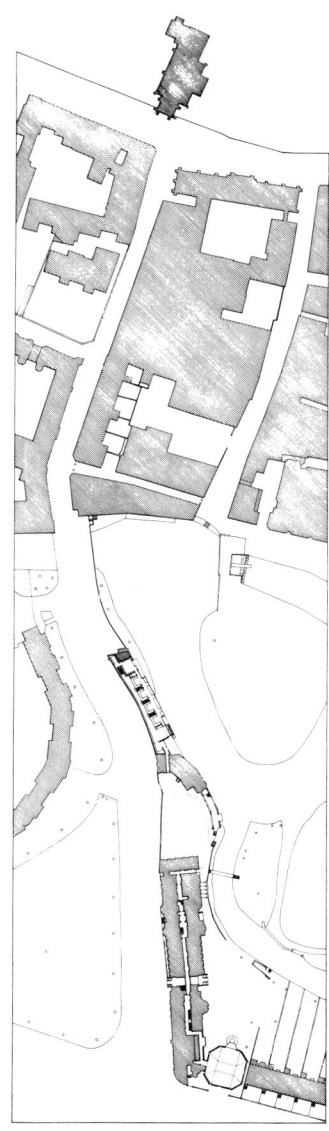

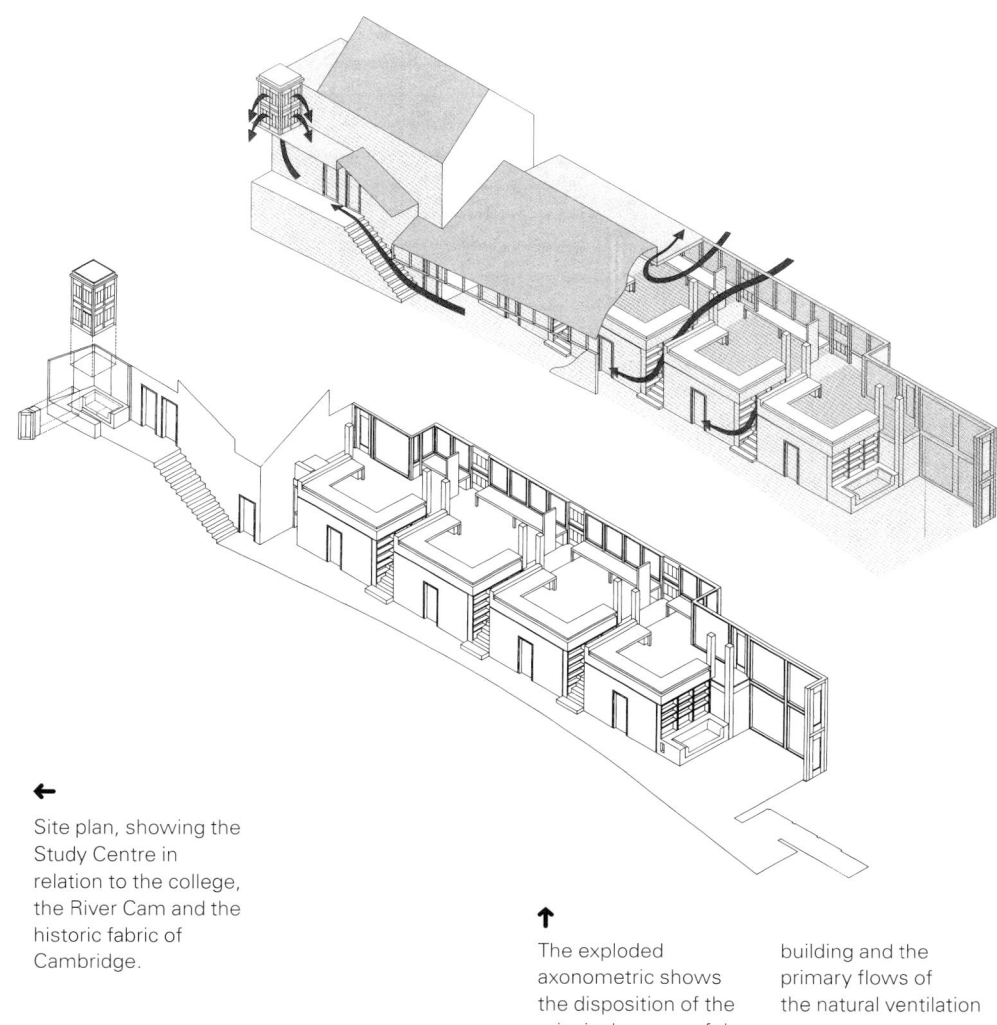

← Site plan, showing the Study Centre in relation to the college, the River Cam and the historic fabric of Cambridge.

↑ The exploded axonometric shows the disposition of the principal spaces of the building and the primary flows of the natural ventilation system.

small library was created by adapting two rooms in one of the existing houses.

In the last decades of the 20th century post-graduate study grew exponentially in British universities. By the late 1980s Darwin had more than 300 students from over 50 countries researching the entire range of academic disciplines. This put pressure on the central facilities and, in particular, on the small library, leading the college to explore the prospect of building a larger library to meet the demand for space and of providing students with access to IT facilities. Within the limitations of the small site there was only one possible location for the new building – a long, narrow piece of land wedged between a boundary wall and the river that had been the Darwin family's kitchen garden. This was the challenge that faced the architects Jeremy Dixon and Edward Jones when they won a competition for the design of the building.

Site and programme

The site is 45m (148ft) long and varies in width between 6m (20ft) and 8m (26ft). Silver Street to the north is one of the few routes into the city centre over the River Cam, which it crosses by means of a bridge designed by Edwin Lutyens. Next to the site for the new building is the set-down point for the fleets of tourist buses that descend on Cambridge throughout the year. The river frontage, orientated slightly east of due south, looks across a wide millpond to Laundress Green, an open space much used in the summer by picnickers, that leads on to an area of open common lining the river.

The brief acknowledged that it would be impossible for an ordinary college library to satisfy the specialized needs of postgraduate students working in many different subject areas. At Darwin the aim is to provide a wide range of standard works of reference, guides, maps, critical and cultural works, particularly of an interdisciplinary nature, and major works of fiction. A tradition has been established for members of the college to donate copies of any books they write. One major element of the collection is the entire library of a former master, Sir Moses Finley, who bequeathed his unique collection of works – principally, but not exclusively, on ancient history – to the college. The college wanted to create a building that was more a place for private study than a store for books. In some cases the medium would be the

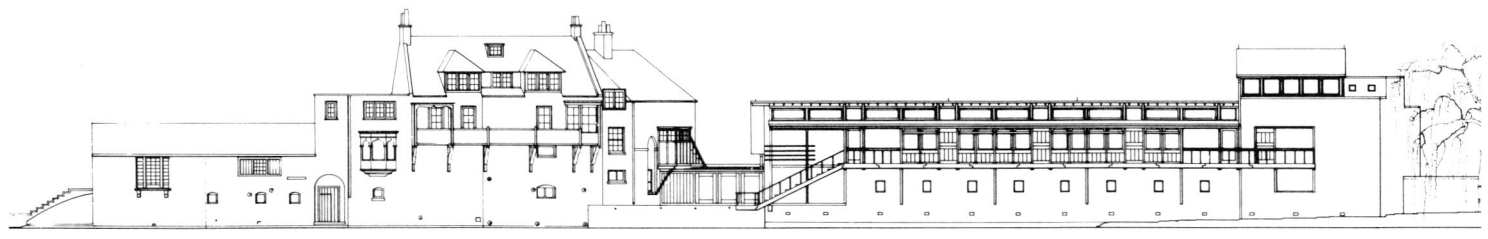

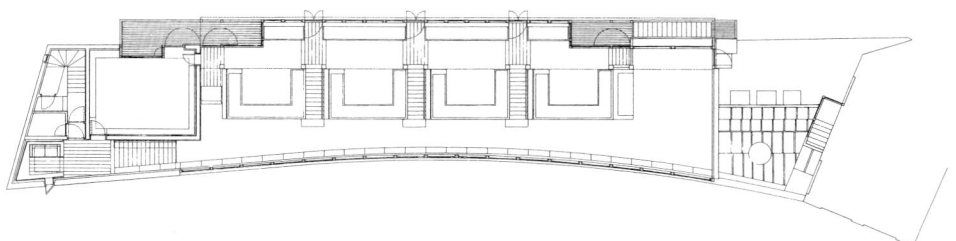

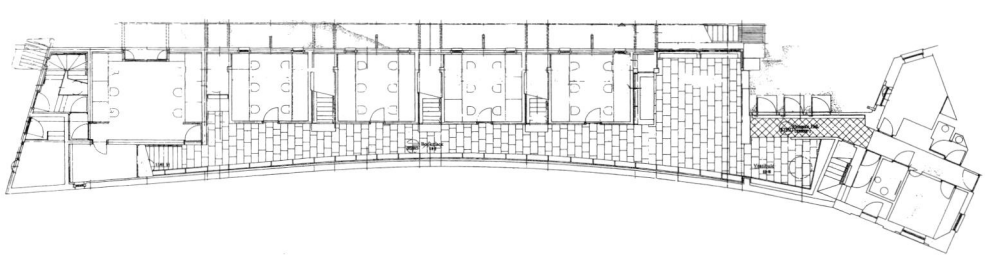

← Upper floor plan, showing the open-plan, principal study area.

↑ The river elevation of the new building extends and transforms the language of the 19th-century Old Granary by J.J. Stevenson.

← The ground plan shows the cellular arrangement of the computer rooms.

book and the notepad; in more and more cases it would involve IT. A final element of the brief was to provide a flat for a research fellow.

Environmental synthesis

Any new building in the core of a historic city such as Cambridge carries obligations to its setting, so the form and language of the building are very specific to its site and programme. The site is at a major point of entry to the city, both by road over Lutyens' bridge and by river, where the bridge acts as a portal to the lyrical reach of the Cam known as 'the backs'. Within Darwin College grounds the site is immediately adjacent to a building known as 'the old granary', a former granary building converted in the 19th century into a dwelling for the Darwin family by J. J. Stevenson, a leading light of the so-called Queen Anne

Movement in architecture.

These facts, along with the dimensional constraints of the site, clearly influenced the arrangement of the building. But architectural invention is not purely a matter of mechanical response to constraint. What matters is the interpretation that is placed upon the facts. In this case a long, sloping roof rises from the northern boundary along the street towards the warmth of the southerly prospect across the river; this keeps the hostile street at bay and offers the possibility of creating a rich and diverse environment in which to study.

The cross-section places an expressed and expressive oak-framed structure above a solid brick-built base. A gently curved former garden wall has been reconstructed as a barrier to the street and to act within

the building as the principal location for book stacks. At the lower level, four enclosed rooms contain the fixed computer terminals. Above these and projecting above the river is a continuous but subtly differentiated study space which is covered in part by the bowed form of the sloping roof and, at its edge above the river, by a low flat ceiling.

The building is lit from a range of windows looking across the river and two clerestories, one to the south below the apex of the roof, the other sitting above the boundary wall to the north. A dynamic natural light suffuses the interior, its quality varying from room to room and changing with the seasons and the time of day. Rippling reflections from the river play across the ceiling of the study space. At the point of entry into the building, the full dimension and

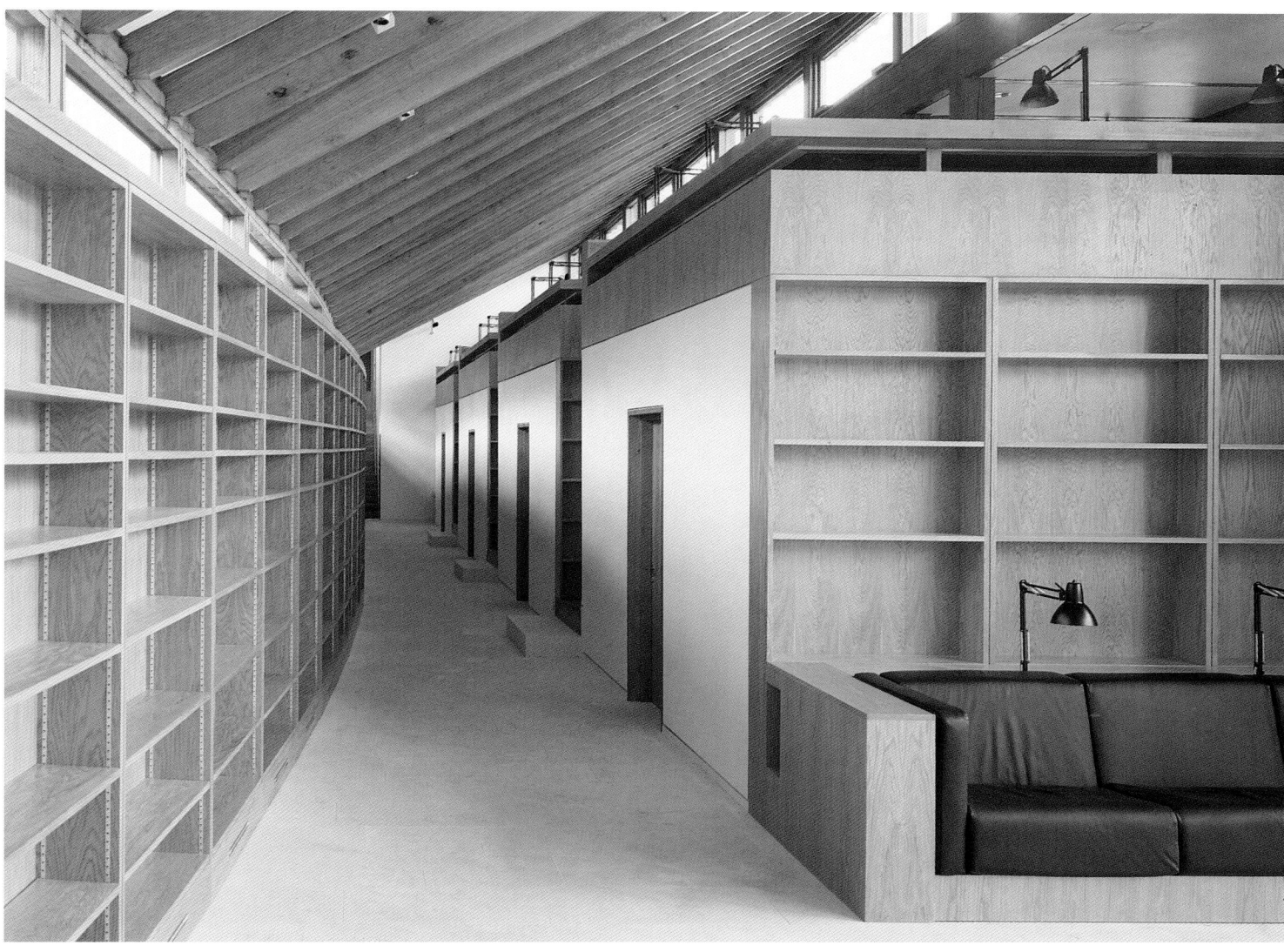

anatomy of the cross-section is revealed in a tall space filled with light from an enormous floor-to-ceiling window flanked by a large reading table. At the eastern end of the slender plan there is a three-storey brick block that at ground level has another computer room; above is a seminar room lined with bookcases containing Sir Moses Finley's library. The top floor houses the fellow's flat.

The sweeping range of bookcases that lines the wall to the street leads to a flight of stairs ascending to the seminar room on the first floor. At the head of the flight is a small private study space with an elegant leather seat. There is a rooflight at the top of an oak-lined lantern and a small window gives a view of the street outside – but neither of these is quite what it appears. Upon close examination, the window reveal is

found to house an inclined mirror showing a view, not of the buildings of Queens' College directly across the street, but along the flank of the building towards the city centre. The rooflight lantern is similarly complex, embodying an essential element of the building's environmental control systems. The lantern's solid walls are in fact a series of mechanically operated flaps that can provide summer ventilation to the entire open volume of the study space.

Arup's environmental control strategy is based on a set of precise relationships between the form and materials of the building and relatively simple mechanical systems. The building is sealed from the noise and fumes of the coach stop in the street. The clerestory window that runs above the bookcases is triple-glazed with no opening lights. People

using the library can open the south-facing windows above the continuous desk in the main study space to provide local ventilation. The south-facing clerestory opens automatically, in tandem with the vents of the timber lantern. This promotes cross and linear ventilation through the building, drawing fresh air from over the river. The mechanisms respond to temperature, wind speed and rain. A computer simulation model was used to test the effectiveness of this passive system at the design stage. Heating for the main body of the building is supplied by radiators located under the windows and underfloor heating beneath the limestone floor of the book-lined gallery on the ground floor. The computer rooms have different environmental requirements from those of the open study space. These are lit by relatively small

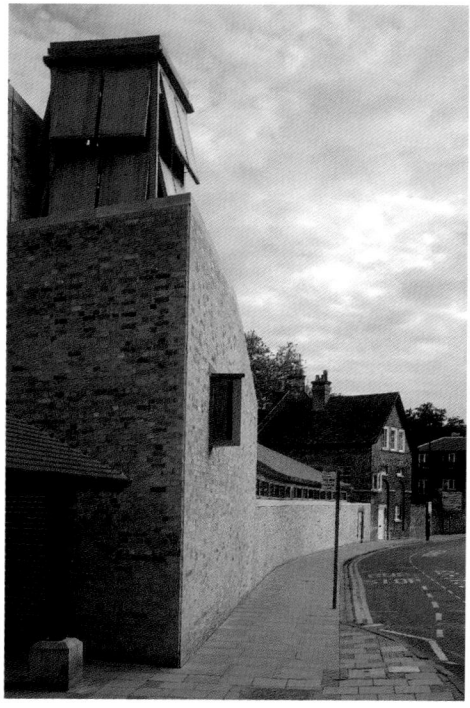

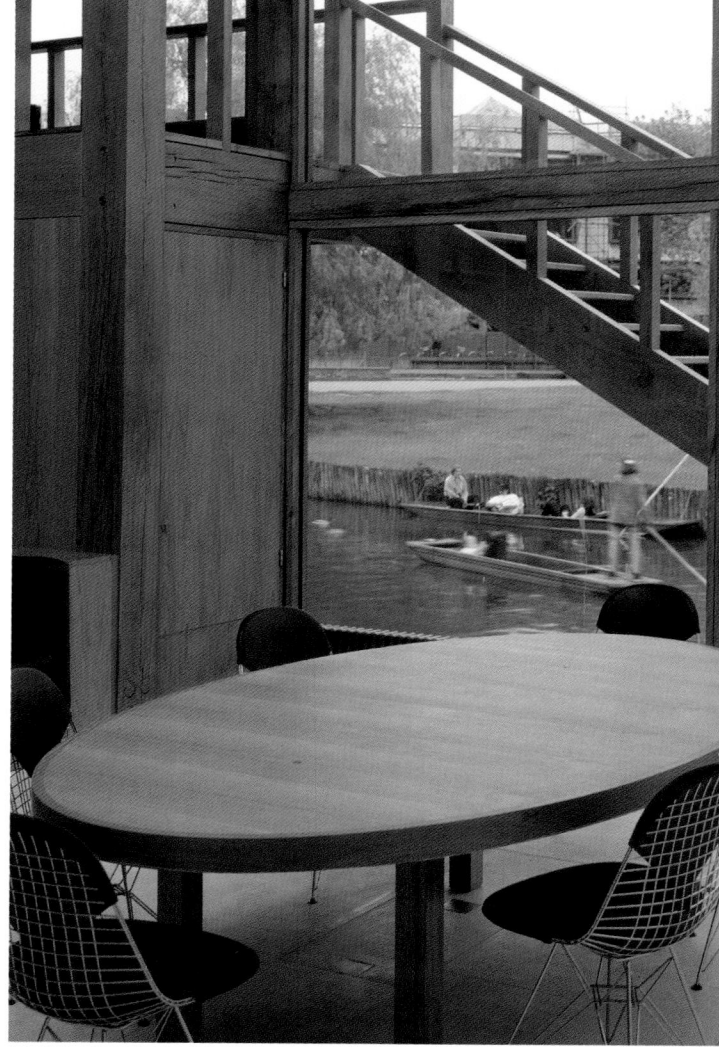

←
The structural and environmental logic of the building are expressed in the cross-sectional view from the entrance.

↑
The reconstructed garden wall becomes the northern face of the building. The oak ventilation box is a major element of the composition.

→
Readers enjoy visual contact with activity on the river.

windows giving views of the river, so the architects had to provide adequate background lighting while avoiding reflections in computer screens. The rooms have local fan-coil heating and cooling devices, which means they can be closed off from the general space to contain noise from keyboards and printers.

The building's artificial lighting is a subtle combination of low-level background illumination and focused pools of light emanating from the individual desk lamps that punctuate the work surfaces and establish individual territories within the collective space. This arrangement is another example – one of many found throughout the building – of the thoughtful analysis that has been made of users' needs.

Conclusion

In addition to producing an enjoyable environment for study, the building unobtrusively demonstrates an understanding of the principles of low-energy design. Its well-insulated envelope minimizes heat loss and the asymmetry of the cross-section differentiates between the conditions to north (relatively hostile) and south (relatively benign). The structural form is precisely related to the environmental strategy.

The principles that inform the environmental design of Darwin college library are very simple. They are not far removed from those that might be found in a house designed by one of the leading architects of the Arts and Crafts Movement. Indeed, the observance of the difference between a northerly and a southerly aspect is one of the defining characteristics of houses by C. F. A.

Voysey, M. H. Baillie Scott and their contemporaries. But, compared with what may be appropriate in a house, a late 20th-century academic library, or 'study centre', demands a more predictable and controllable environmental system.

The achievement of the designers, architects and engineers of the Darwin building is that its synthesis – achieved with apparent effortlessness – is based on quite sophisticated architectural science. The building is quite small, no bigger than many Arts and Crafts houses, and is the product of a unique set of circumstances. It nonetheless stands as a potent example of how architecture and engineering can collaborate in responding to the challenges of the new environmental agenda.

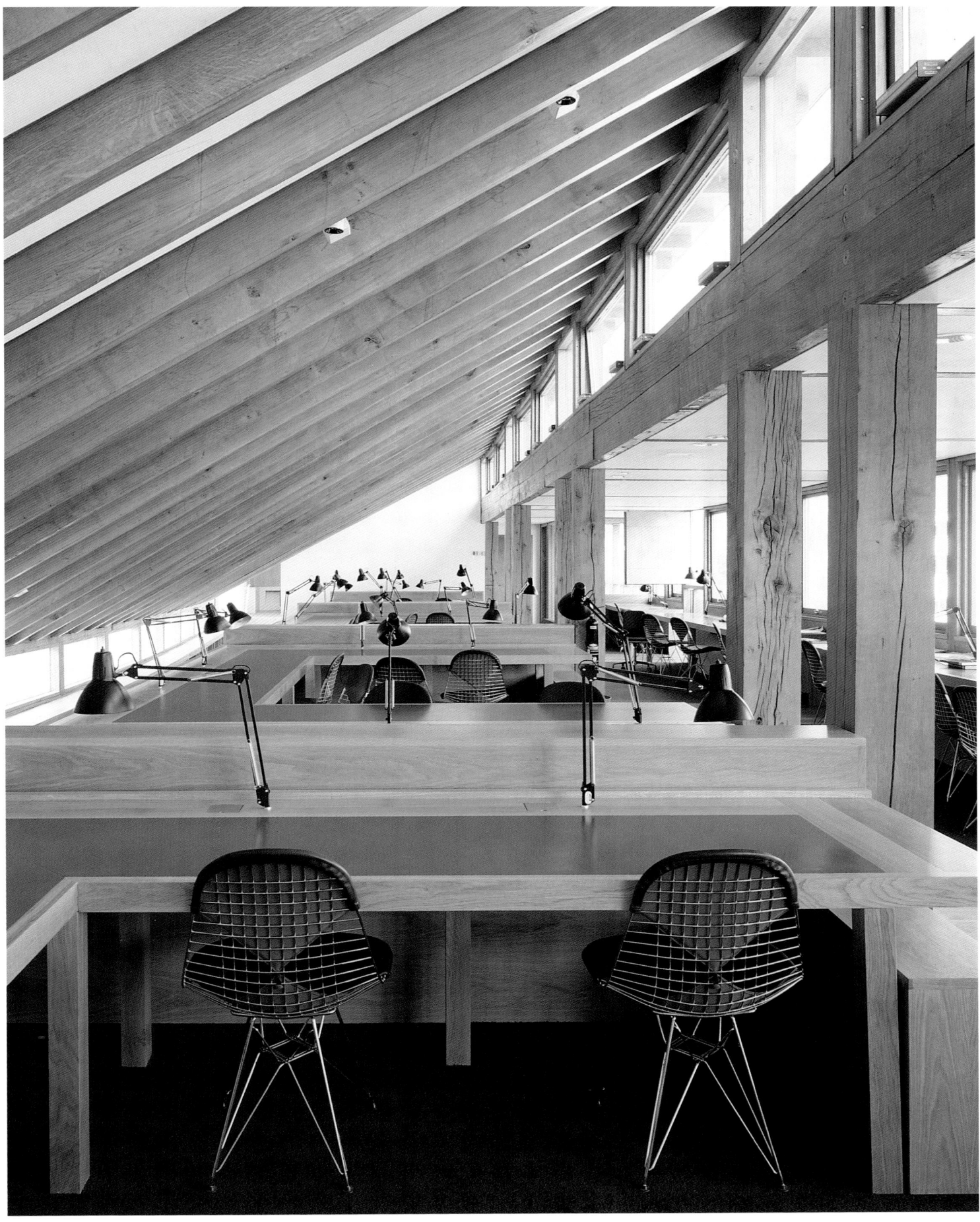

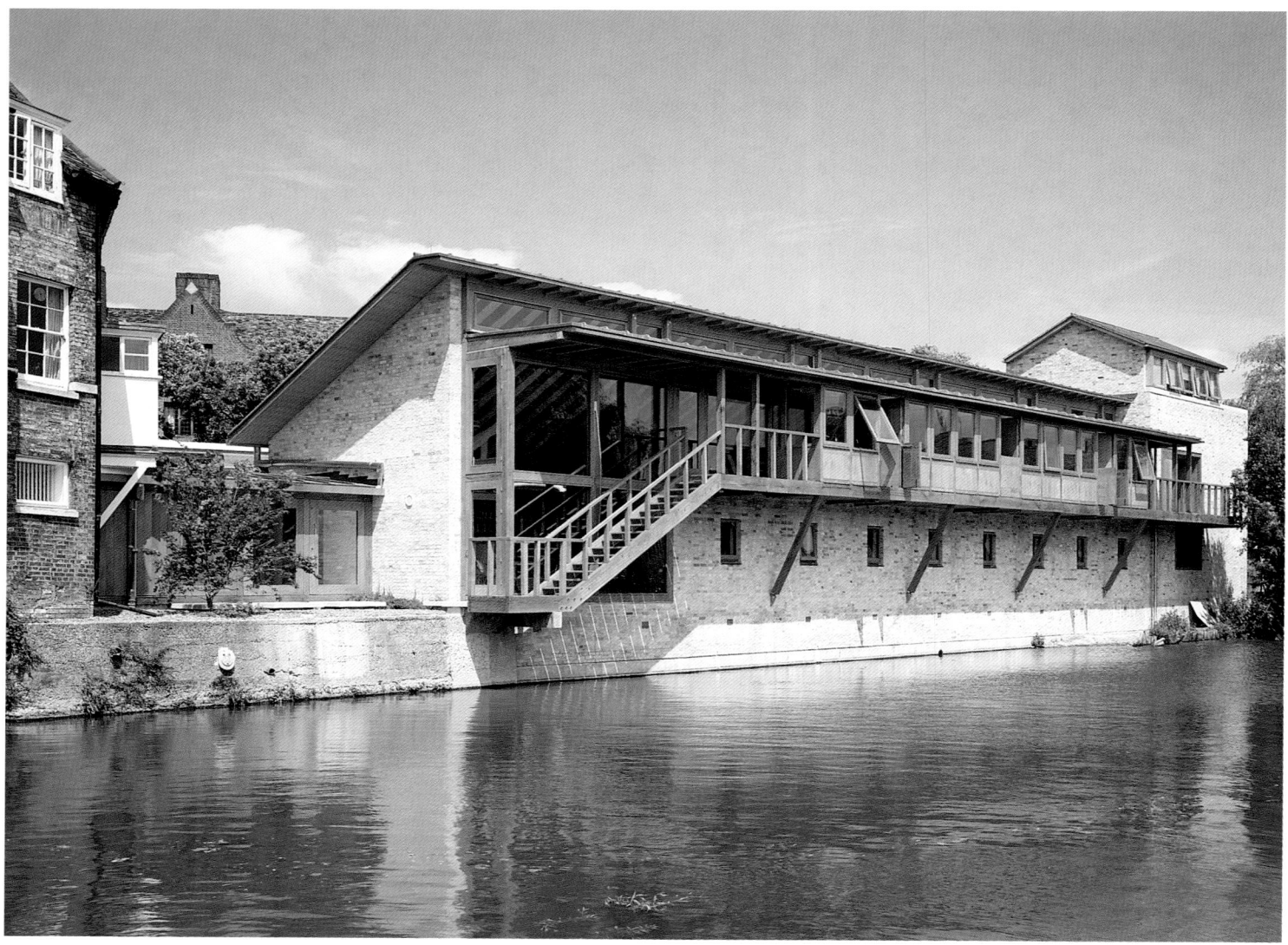

← The principal study space inhabits the oak roof structure and is illuminated and ventilated by the continuous clerestory.

↑ From the south-west, the glazed, timber-framed reading areas wrap around and overhang the masonry base.

Jubilee Campus
University of Nottingham
Michael Hopkins
& Partners
Nottingham, UK
2000

➜

The learning resources
centre at Nottingham
University's Jubilee
Campus is a free-
standing inverted
cone.

In 1996 the University of Nottingham held a design competition for a proposed Jubilee Campus to commemorate the university's 50th anniversary. The campus was envisaged as a model for sustainable development in the East Midlands and as an example of the affordable and sustainable regeneration of a former industrial site. The limited competition involved top UK architects in the field of design for higher education and sustainability (including Feilden Clegg and Macormac Jamieson & Pritchard). The architects Michael Hopkins & Partners were appointed with Ove Arup & Partners as services and structural engineer and Battle McCarthy as landscape architect.

The brief for the campus consisted of 41,000m² (441,160ft²) of buildings including undergraduate and postgraduate accommodation, three faculty buildings, a central teaching building and a learning resources centre. Nottingham University is among a group of postwar institutions that grew from previous university college status and expanded again in the 1960s. It has been described as a place where 'Basil Spence's progressive, but eclectic Modernism co-existed with the Banker's Georgian

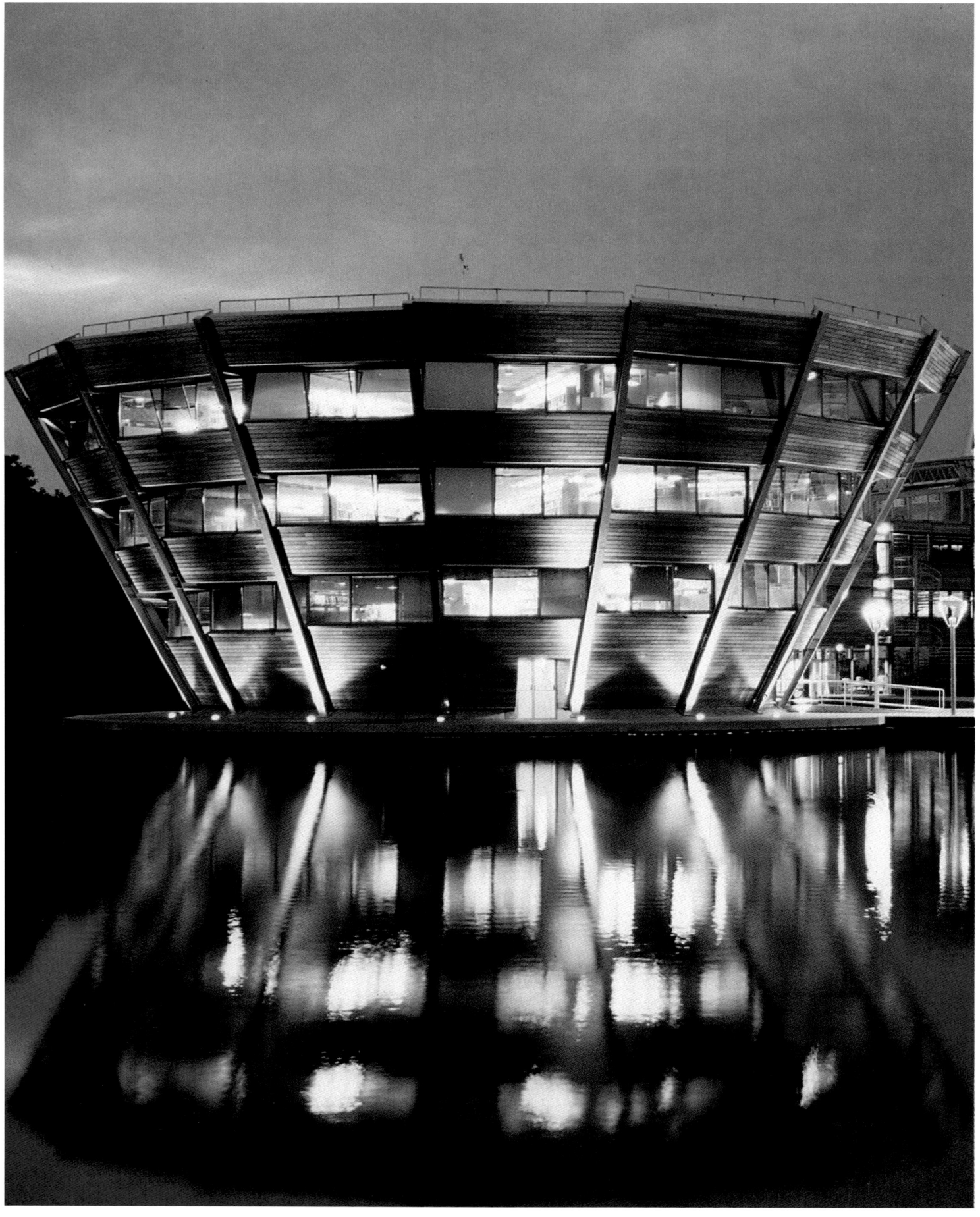

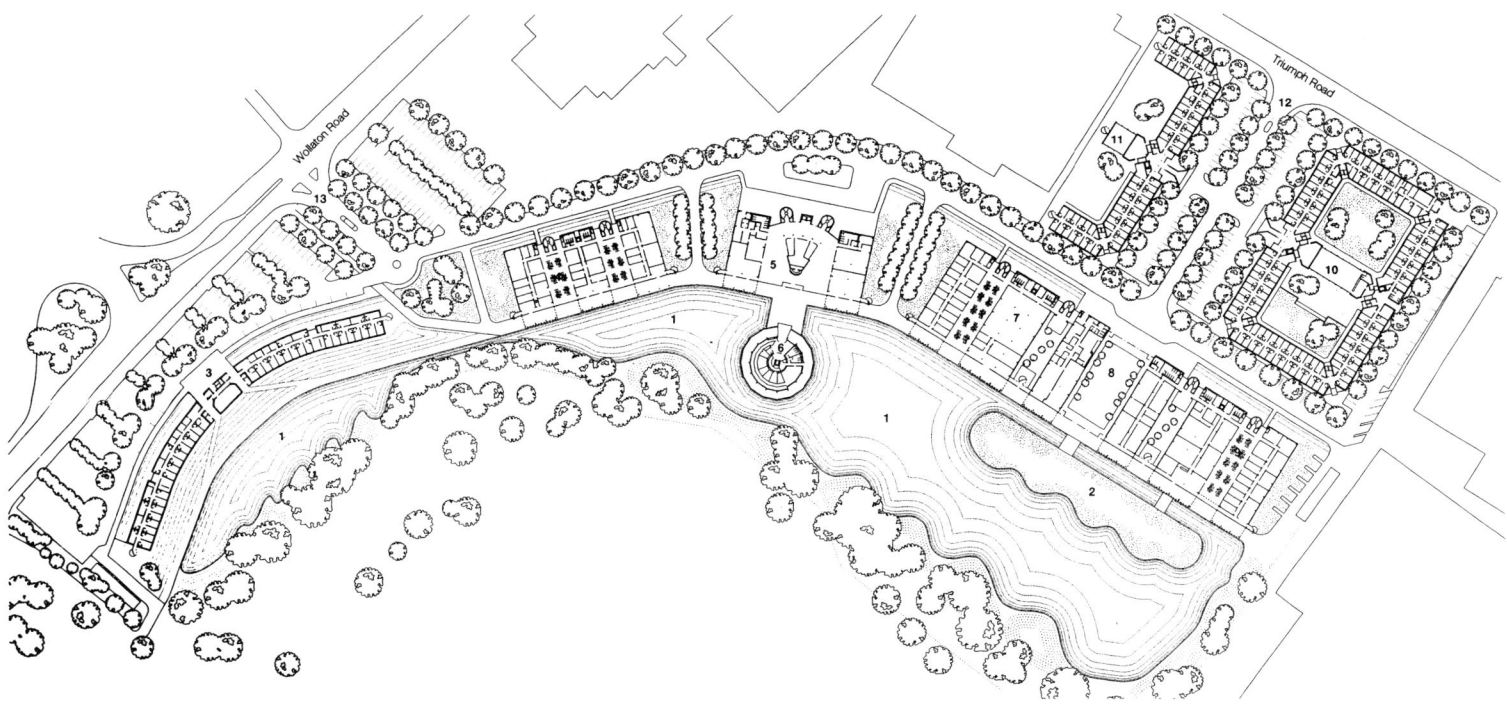

Site layout.

1 Lake	6 Learning Resource	9 Departments of	11 Undergraduate
2 Grassed island	Centre	Education / Higher	Halls
3 Postgraduate Hall	7 Department of	Education	12 Entrance
4 Business School	Computer Science	10 Undergraduate	13 Main entrance
5 Central Teaching	8 Central Catering	Halls	
Facility	Facility		

of Morley Horder and Cecil Howitt'. [1]

The building type developed at Nottingham over the period since its Royal Charter and before can be called pavilions set within a romantic landscape. Hopkins's competition entry responds to and builds on this typology of pavilions in a parkland; it also builds on the Inland Revenue buildings by the same architects and engineers less than a mile from the proposed new campus.

Site location and layout

About 1.6km (1 mile) away from its existing Beeston Campus, the university secured a 7.5ha (18½ acre) 'brownfield' site, where a Raleigh bicycle factory once stood, set between an industrial zone and interwar suburban housing. The centre point of the proposal is a 13,000m² (139,880ft²) linear lake that

forms a buffer between the new campus and the housing. As well as providing waterside promenades and reintroducing wildlife to the area, the lake echoes the use of water on the main campus.

Pedestrian movement is given priority over cars by containing parking and traffic to the north. Buildings are sited to exploit views over the lake and to benefit from the possibilities of passive design. Teaching and social spaces face west and south-west. Student residences are treated differently, with undergraduate halls taking the more familiar quadrangle form (although, unlike Oxford and Cambridge, they are served by corridors rather than stairs), whereas the postgraduate accommodation snakes along the side of the lake, recalling Alvar Aalto's halls of residence at MIT.

The entrance to the site is flanked by the undergraduate halls of residence and trees, making a formal avenue, again echoing the city of Nottingham. At the end of the avenue is the transparent three-storey refectory, allowing glimpses through to the lake beyond, which is flanked by teaching pavilions lining the banks of the lake. These pavilions effectively contain the park to the west of the lake and are also based on a typology. Rational corridor-served blocks contain either closed or open atria. Views from the teaching pavilions are therefore varied – either into the atria or across the lake and into the park. The pavilions are interspersed with places of high-intensity student activity, including the refectory and the central teaching facility, which contains a number of lecture theatres stacked vertically within an atrium flanked by facilities such as a bank, a

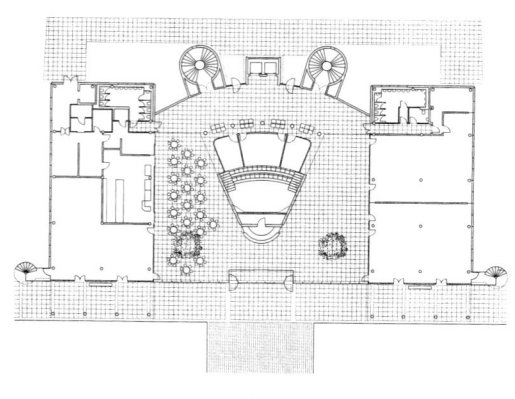

← Plan of lecture theatre, ground floor.

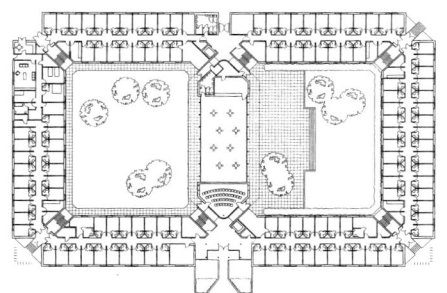

← Undergraduate rooms, ground floor.

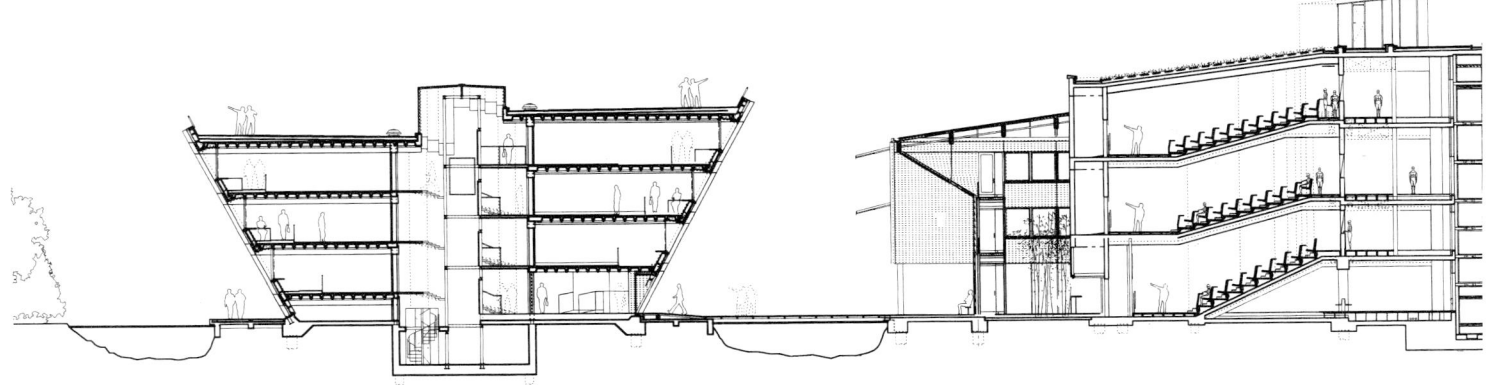

↑ Section through learning resources centre and lecture theatres.

shop and students' union meeting rooms.

Sited opposite the learning resources centre, the central teaching facility is the only element in the whole composition that has been allowed to break free from the banks of the lake and occupy a peninsula jutting out into it. The functional dialogue between the two elements of the campus seems more appropriate than the formal one. The learning resources centre takes the form of an inverted polygonal cone intended to provide panoramas over the lake. Whereas the largest lecture theatre in the central teaching facility is placed at the top of the stack and the smallest at ground level in order minimize the footprint in the public atrium, the form of the learning resources centre is less rooted in the rationale of the campus and appears

to be perched rather uncomfortably on its promontory.

Structure and materials

The structure for the teaching pavilions is simple and straightforward. In-situ concrete floors are supported by columns on a 6m by 6m grid, exposed to provide thermal mass. External envelopes are designed to be thermally efficient and made of materials from sustainable sources. Roofs, for example, are green and are planted with tundra species, giving a U value of $0.22\,\mathrm{W/m^2/^\circ C}$ ($0.04\,\mathrm{Btu/h/ft^2/^\circ F}$). Faculty buildings are clad predominantly in western red cedar from a Canadian source chosen because it holds WWF/FSC certification. These prefabricated timber panels cloak a layer of cellulose Warmcell insulation incorporated into a breathing wall construction with a U

value of $0.287\,\mathrm{W/m^2/^\circ C}$ ($0.05\,\mathrm{Btu/h/ft^2/^\circ F}$). The overall performance of the walls and the low maintenance costs of the cladding helped to persuade the initially sceptical client of the suitability of the timber as a cladding. Cedar is also used in the interior of the atria, where panels incorporate a layer of hessian-covered quilt to ensure acceptable acoustic qualities. The timber will weather to a silver colour over time – the exterior long before the interior.

Prefabricated cladding panels and windows are framed in hot-dipped galvanized steel, a material that is also used for the glazed elements of atria and walkways. As well as being a cheaper alternative to stainless steel, the galvanized steel was considered by the architects to be more eco-friendly. Motorized retractable fabric blinds – which animate and enliven

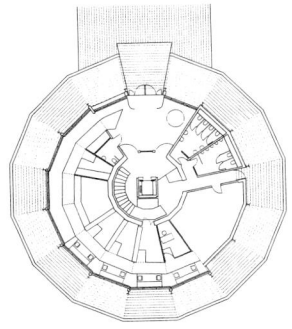

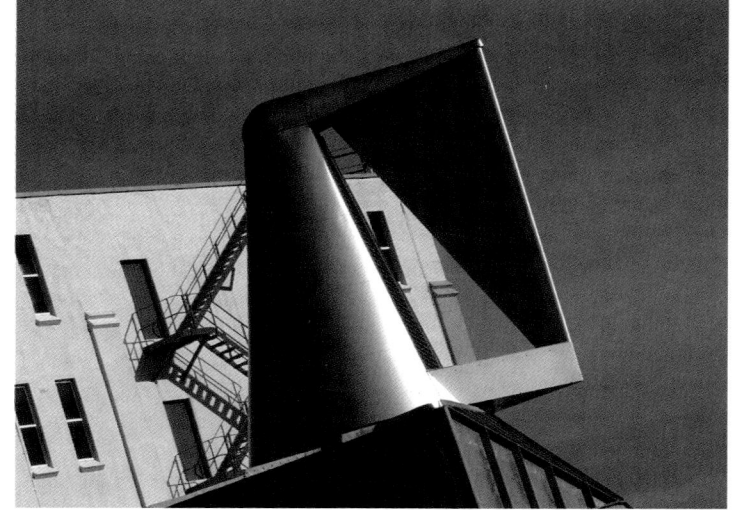

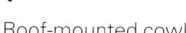
Roof-mounted cowl.

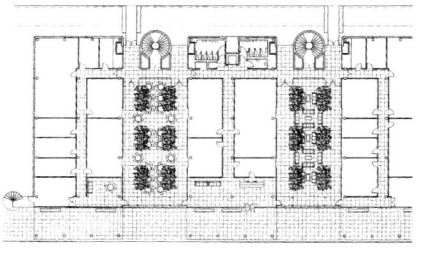

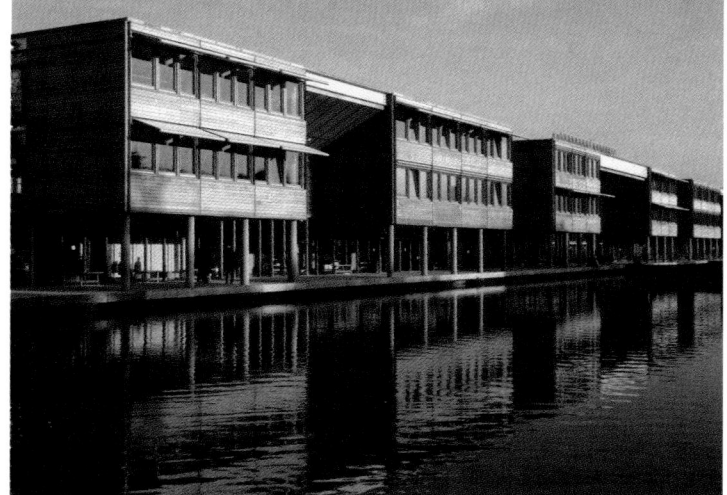

The central teaching facility.

the building forms and help to reduce fabric temperatures and shade windows – relieve this spare and perhaps austere palette of materials.

Energy and environment
Although the original competition brief specified that buildings should be low-energy and naturally ventilated 'wherever possible', the design team did not find it too prescriptive. The three faculty buildings – dedicated to education, computer science, and management and finance – appeared to offer the main opportunities for low-energy services. Arup's previous collaborations with the Hopkins office at the Inland Revenue building in Nottingham, the Saga Headquarters in Folkestone and Portcullis House, Westminster, provided models for an elementary low-pressure ventilation

system. This was augmented by Arup's own European Union-funded research into solar and wind energy and wind-tunnel testing of alternative chimney terminals.

Ventilation
Background data suggested that low-pressure mechanical ventilation geared to heat recovery would provide a more energy-efficient system than natural ventilation. The system is predicted to operate in this mode for the majority of the year but windows can be controlled to enable the building to be entirely naturally ventilated by stack effect.

In the mixed mode, air is drawn into air-handling units mounted at roof level, where it is filtered electrostatically and blown through vertical air ducts into floor voids, where it is delivered into teaching

rooms through low-pressure floor diffusers at a rate of 2.5 l/s (0.089 ft³/s) for each square metre (11ft²) of room space. Exhaust air is returned using the corridor as the extract path. Acoustic separation is maintained through the use of a low-pressure attenuated floor path between teaching rooms and the corridor. From the corridor the air is drawn into the stairwell and returned to the atria for heat recovery or evaporative cooling – or extracted through the roof cowls.

A key feature of the low-energy mechanical system is that fan power is minimized through pressure drops. Ducts, which must be as large as possible to reduce air pressure, lead into floor voids and carry air with velocities as low as 1.5 m/s (4.92 ft/s). Floor voids are also larger than standard, with a 350mm (14in) deep void. The plant is equipped with a

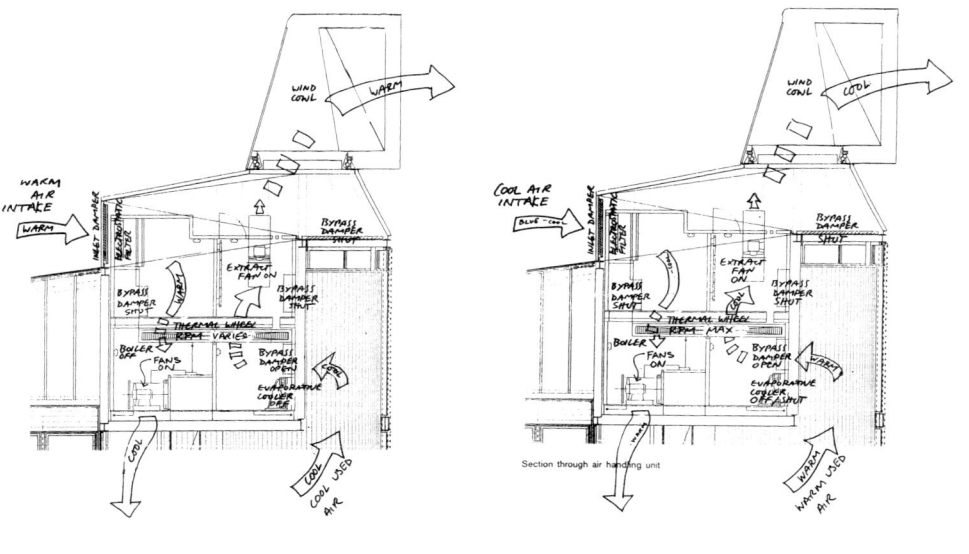

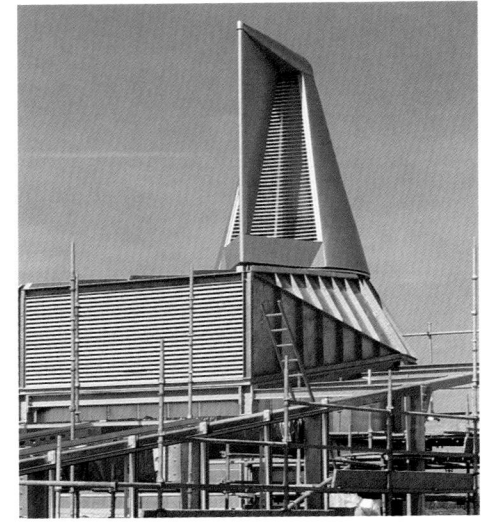

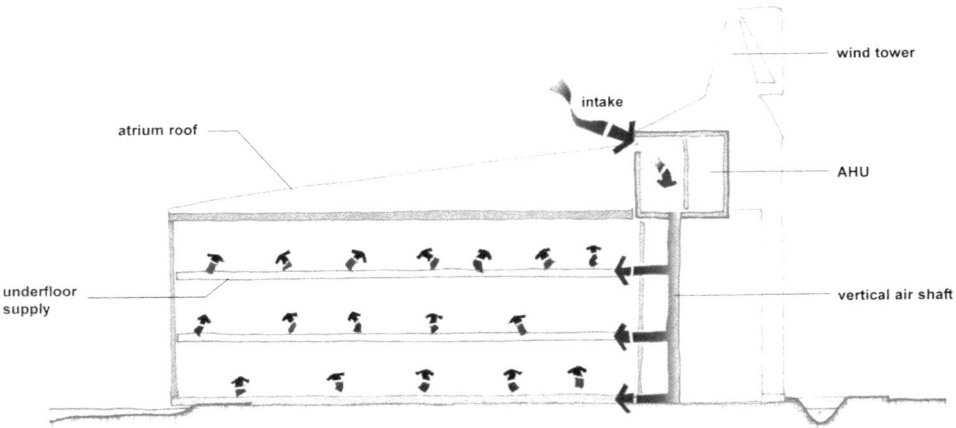

← Supply air and extract air routes. Air intake is through the roof-mounted AHHs via a thermal wheel. It is then blown through vertical ducts into the floor void. Exhaust air returns through the stairwell to the AHU for heat recovery or evaporative cooling and is expelled via the cowl.

↑ The roof-mounted cowls.

sophisticated bypass system so that components that create pressure drops, such as the evaporative humidifier, can be eliminated when not in use. Arup designed a balanced flue boiler for the system, instead of a heating coil that would again create a pressure drop.

Efforts to reduce pressure drop have paid off in that the fans now deal with pressures from 28 to 34 Pa depending on season (a conventional system deals with 1200 Pa to 1600 Pa). Mechanical ventilation will probably be used for much of the year, but natural ventilation is possible by opening windows to admit fresh air and stack effect for exhaust though the stairwell chimney.

The steel cowls that punctuate the roof forms, located above the modular air-handling units, are designed to revolve and turn in the wind so that the exhaust vents always face downwards, thereby maintaining extraction of exhaust air. They also reflect a desire to add a finishing touch, in the form of a bonnet, to the rather self-consciously 'green' uniform that the buildings wear. Indeed, this display of 'exposed power' is hardly merited – as the designers acknowledge, 'the reality of wind in suction mode provides only a very small force indeed'.[2] This mode of passive ventilation may operate when external temperatures are between 18°C (64°F) and 25°C (77°F).

The central teaching facility operates on the same principles as the main teaching blocks. There, however, air is cooled and delivered below lecture theatre seating. While the buildings will not be tested for air tightness ducts and floor voids have been pressure-tested to ensure that infiltration rates are as predicted. The campus atria are single-glazed and unheated, and ventilation is independent and non-powered. Atria are designed with profiled nose-shaped south facades to promote natural ventilation.

Wind-tunnel tests demonstrated that the cowls would turn in wind speeds of as little as 2m/s (6.56ft/s) and were stable in winds in excess of 40m/s (131.23ft/s), but design figures indicate that the fan energy saved by using the cowl is less than 1 per cent of total fan power.

Ventilation fans are powered by a total area of 450m² (4,840ft²) of photovoltaic solar cells integrated into the atrium roofs. As well as providing 51,240 Wh of annual energy output, the four arrays of monocrystalline cells effectively shade the atrium roofs.

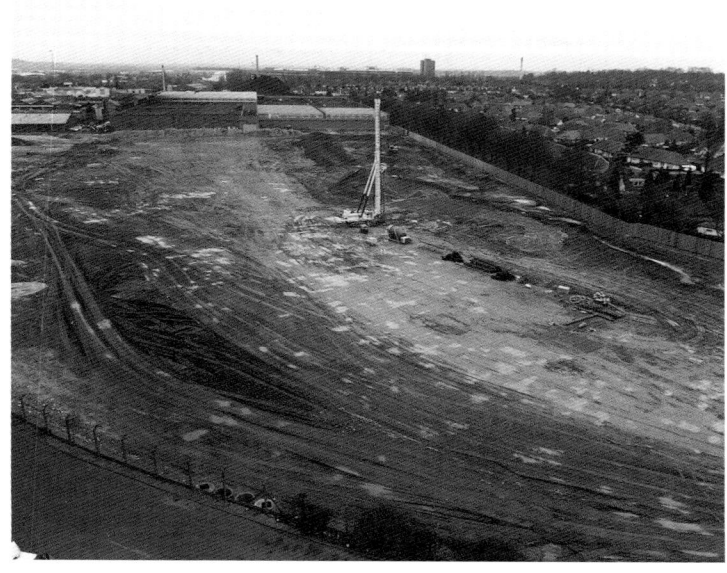
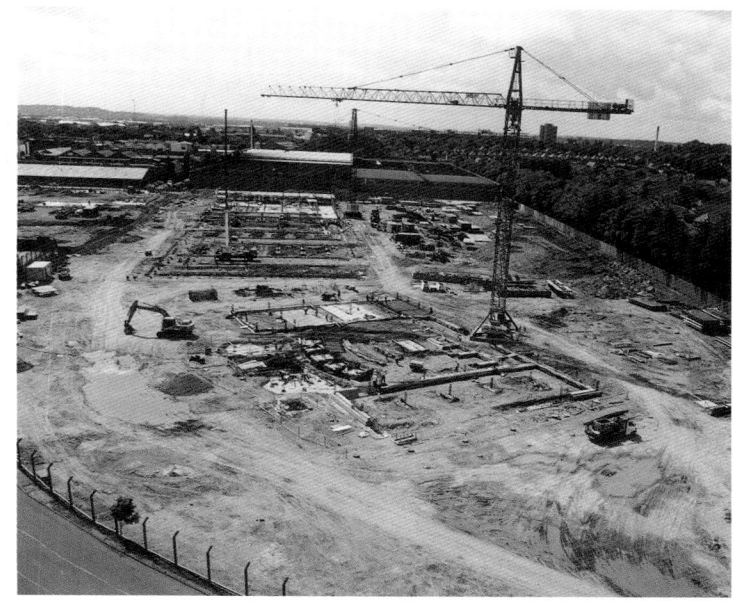
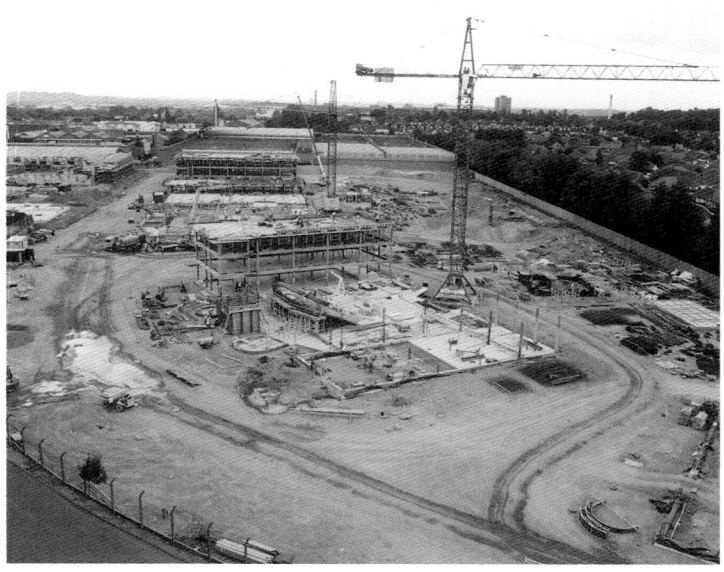
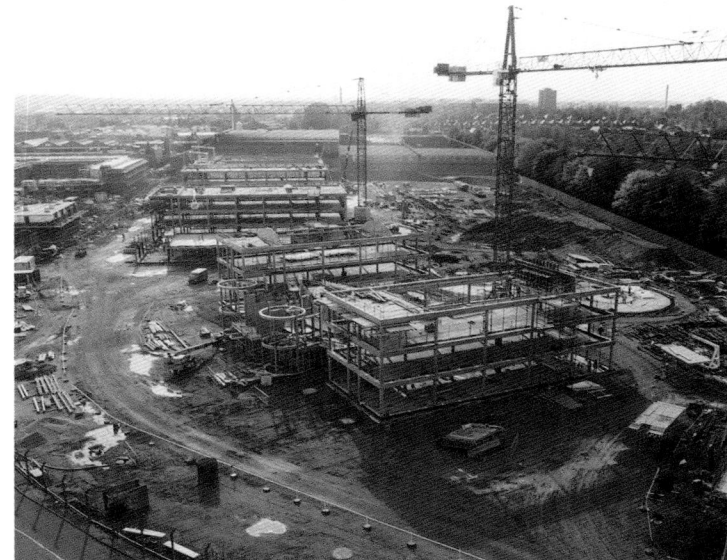
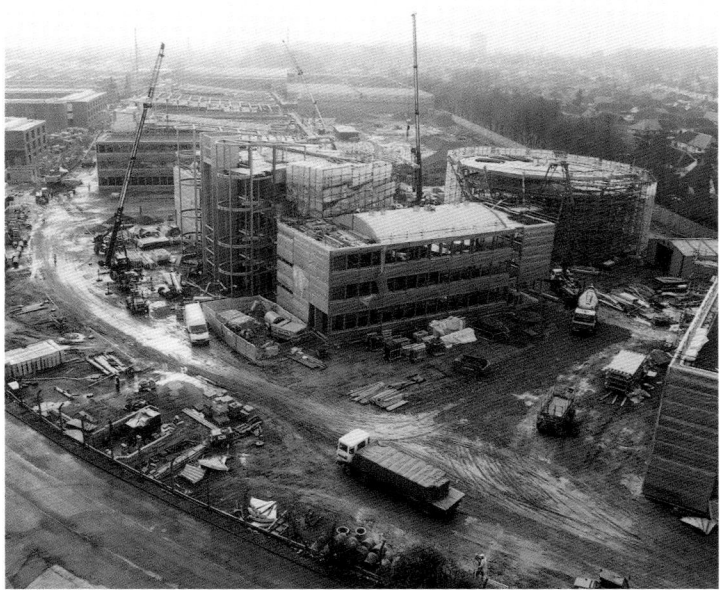
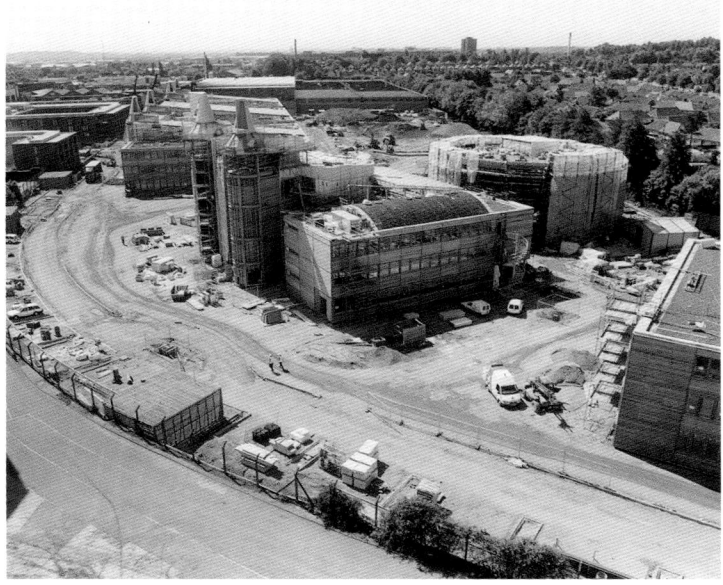

Construction process
from the brownfield
site of the campus.

450m² (4,840ft²) of
pv cells are designed
to match annual fan
power.

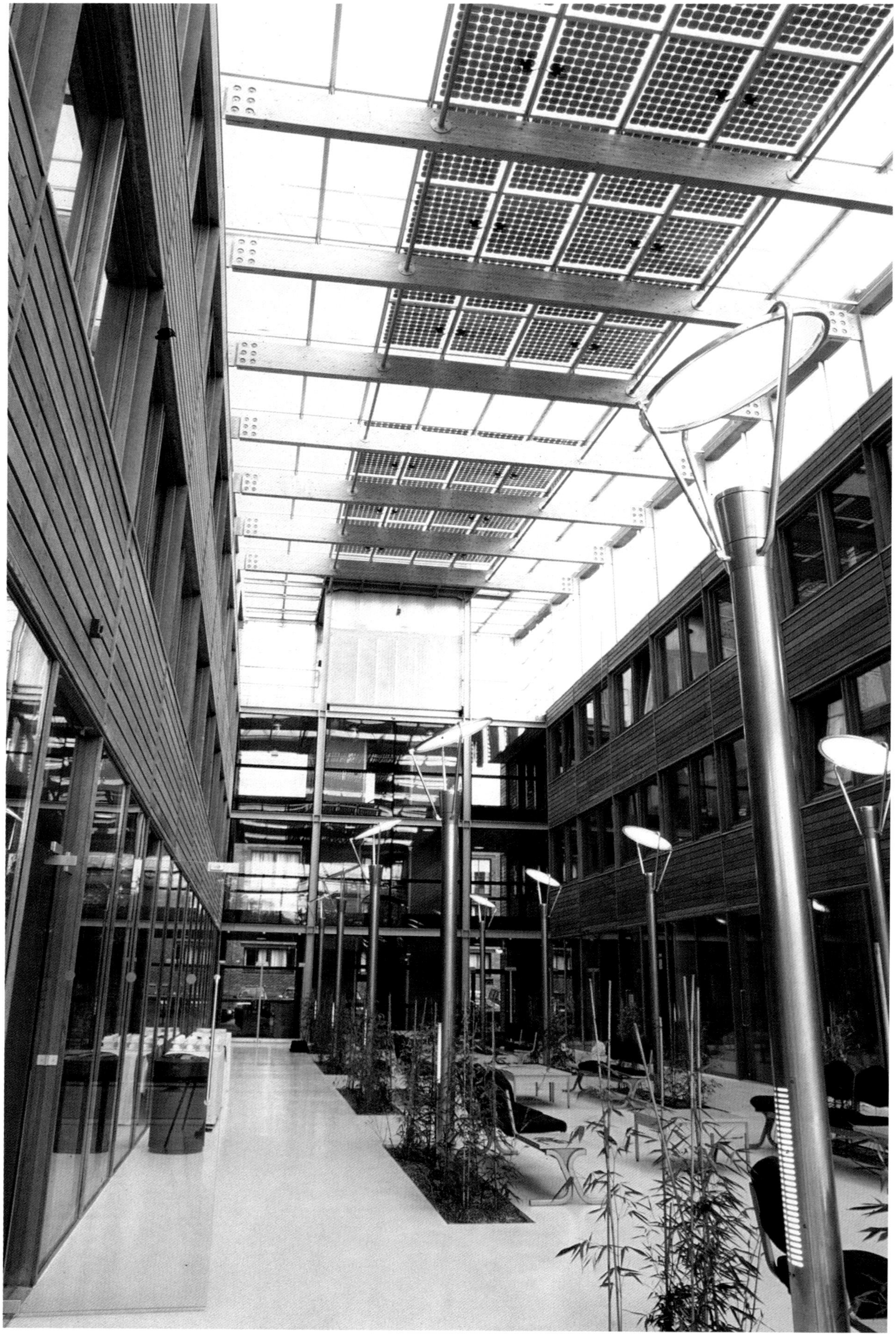

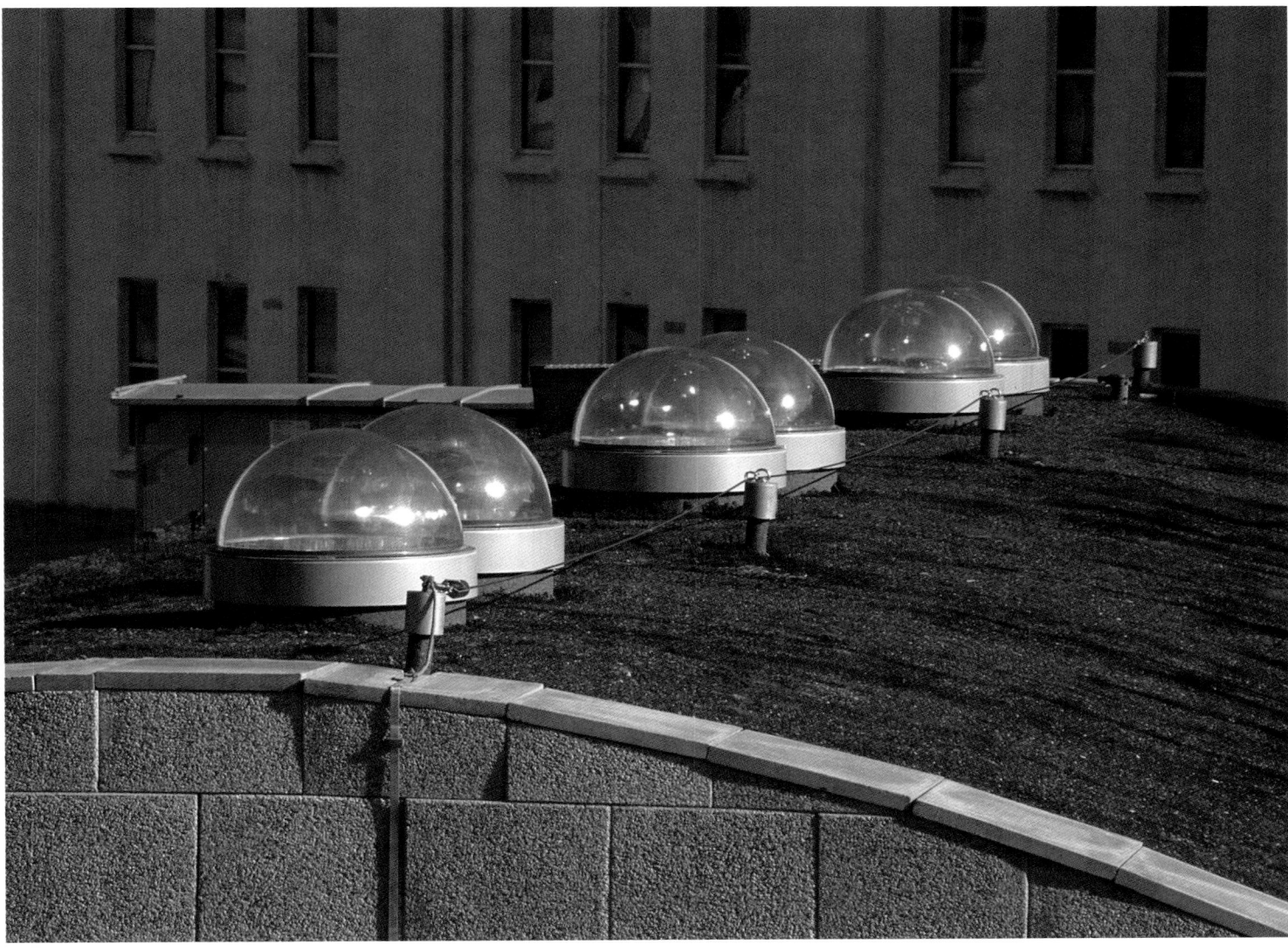

Heating
Condensing gas boilers on the roof of each building deliver heat through standard radiators fitted with thermostatic valves. The heating system is sized to integrate with the cooling system and to take account of the beneficial effect of energy stored in thermal mass. Incoming fresh air is heated to 18°C (64°F) by being passed through thermal wheels. When external temperatures fall below 2.3°C (36°F) heating is supplemented by a 30KW gas-fired boiler mounted on the air-handling unit. Predictions, based on weather data for Nottingham, show that the boiler will be used for only 10 per cent of hours when the buildings are occupied.

Lighting
Daylight is used as the primary light source wherever possible. The teaching spaces are lit through ribbon windows; this is controlled by fixed horizontal louvres that cover the top halves of east- and west-facing windows. The white-coloured louvres and internal light shelves combine to reduce glare and produce even distribution of daylight across the room depths.

Toplighting is supplied in top-floor seminar rooms through light tubes. The electric lighting is controlled by a stand-alone intelligent lighting management system linked to passive infrared detectors in every room, and custom-made luminaires at the perimeter of rooms have daylight sensors, which switch and dim them depending on daylight levels.

Conclusion
Overall energy use is predicted to be two-thirds that of naturally ventilated cellular offices – but the Jubilee Campus displays its environmental credentials in other ways. Its palette of recognizably eco-friendly features includes green space, water and wildlife, plenty of timber, and green roofs topped with the almost mandatory chimneys. The buildings lean slightly away from the more neutral but highly crafted creations of Hopkins's traditional work. The overall result is interesting in the light of the current drive for efficiency, prefabrication and value for money in the UK construction industry. Mass customization meets William Morris at the Jubilee Campus. As Peter Fawcett comments, 'It generates a quintessentially English campus, free from the empty formal posturing, or equally techno-fetishism of his competitors.'[3]

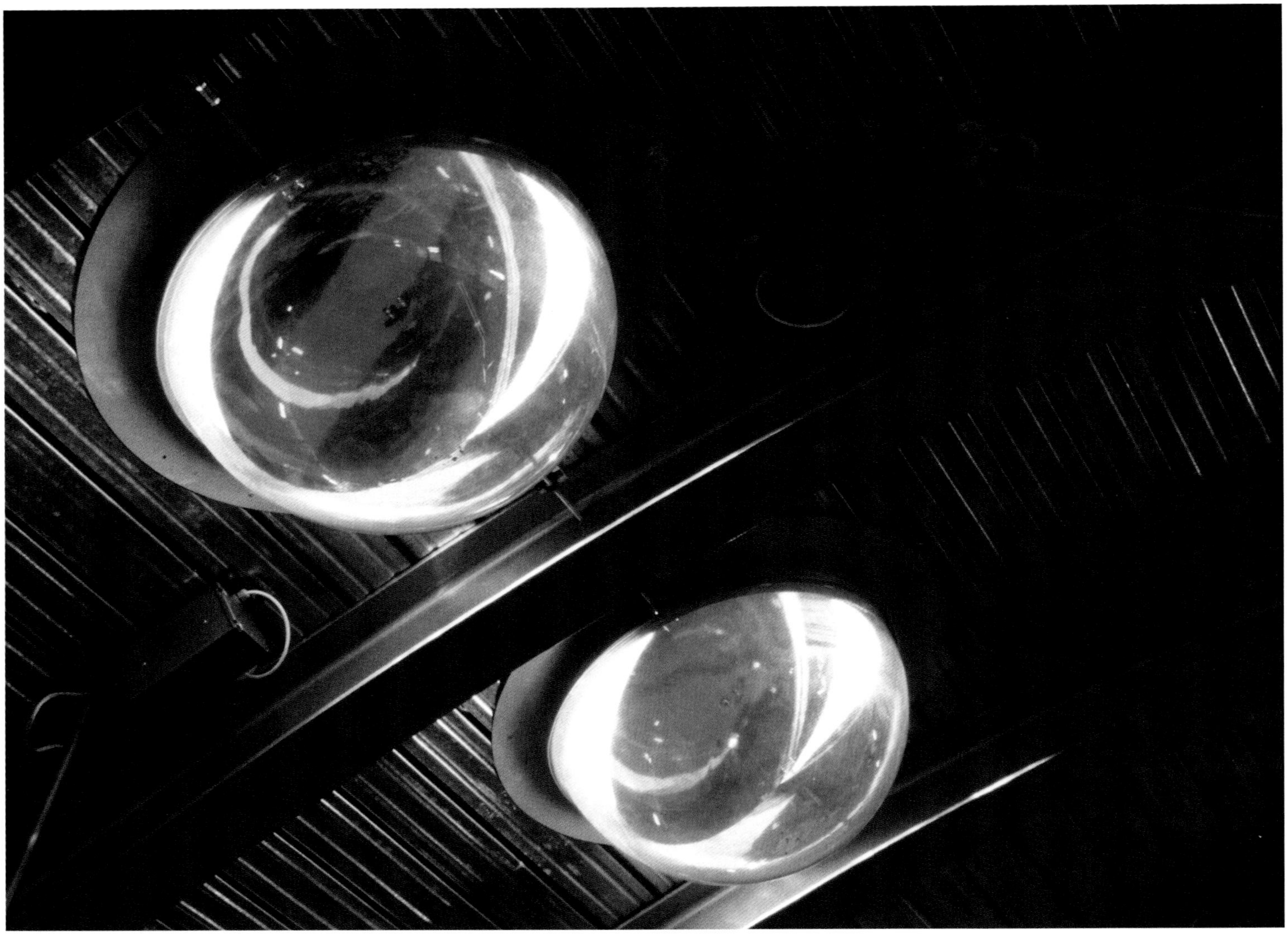

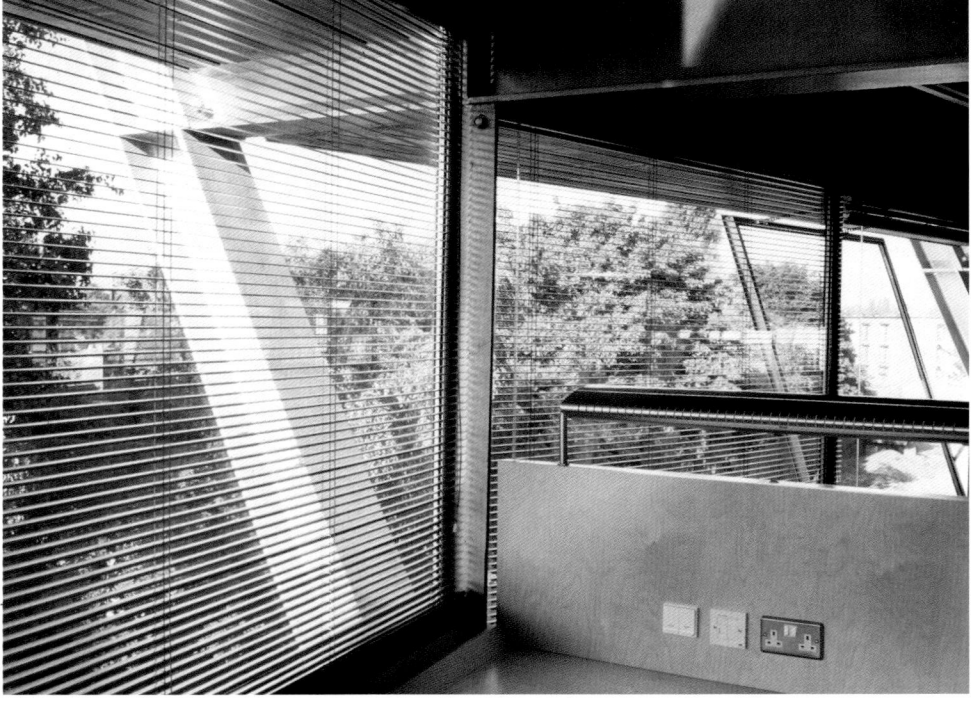

← Toplighting is used to daylight top-floor seminar rooms.

↑ Roof lighting.

→ Solar control to the learning resources centre.

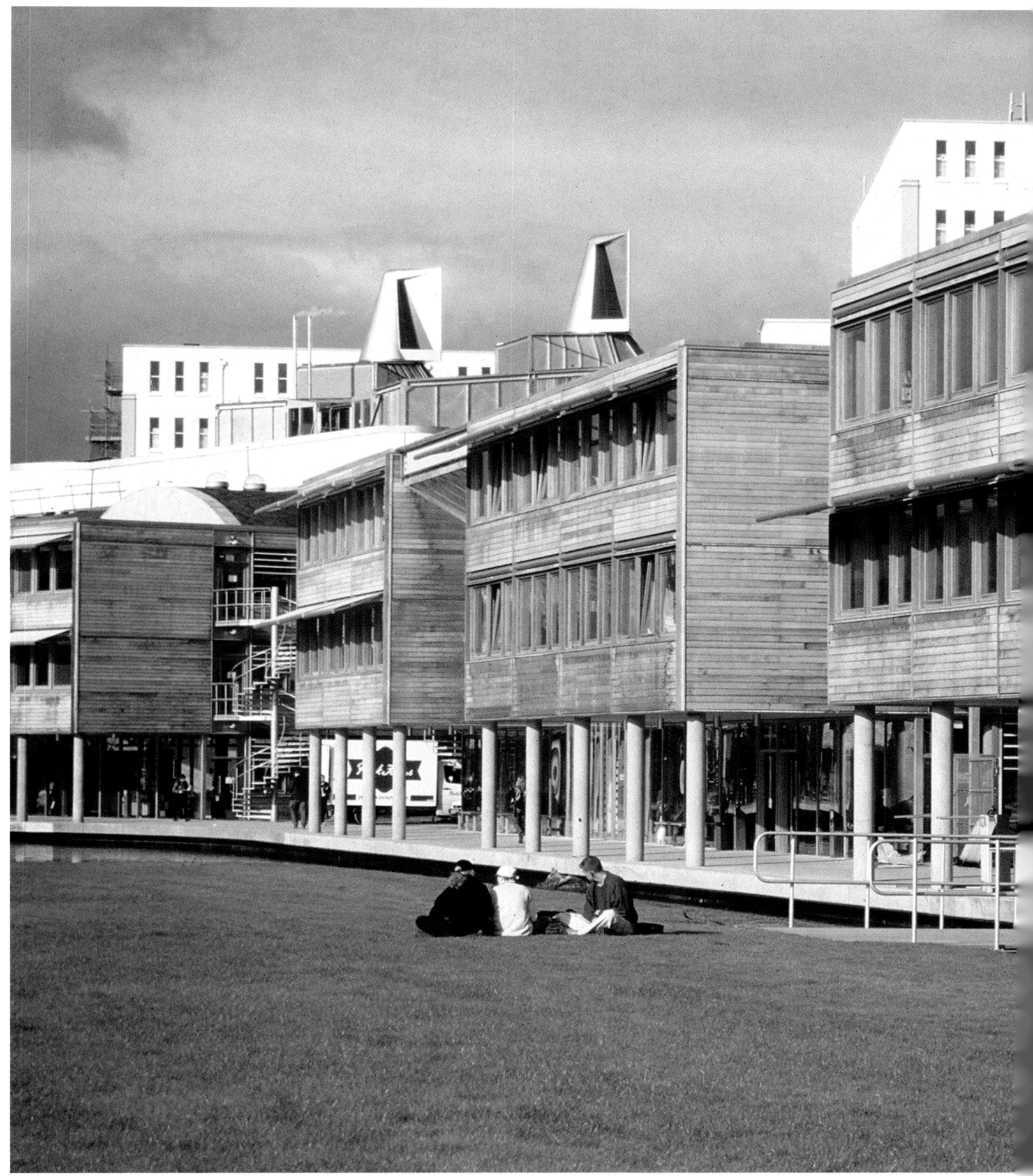

←

Campus in use: the lakeside arcade has an appropriate scale and form.

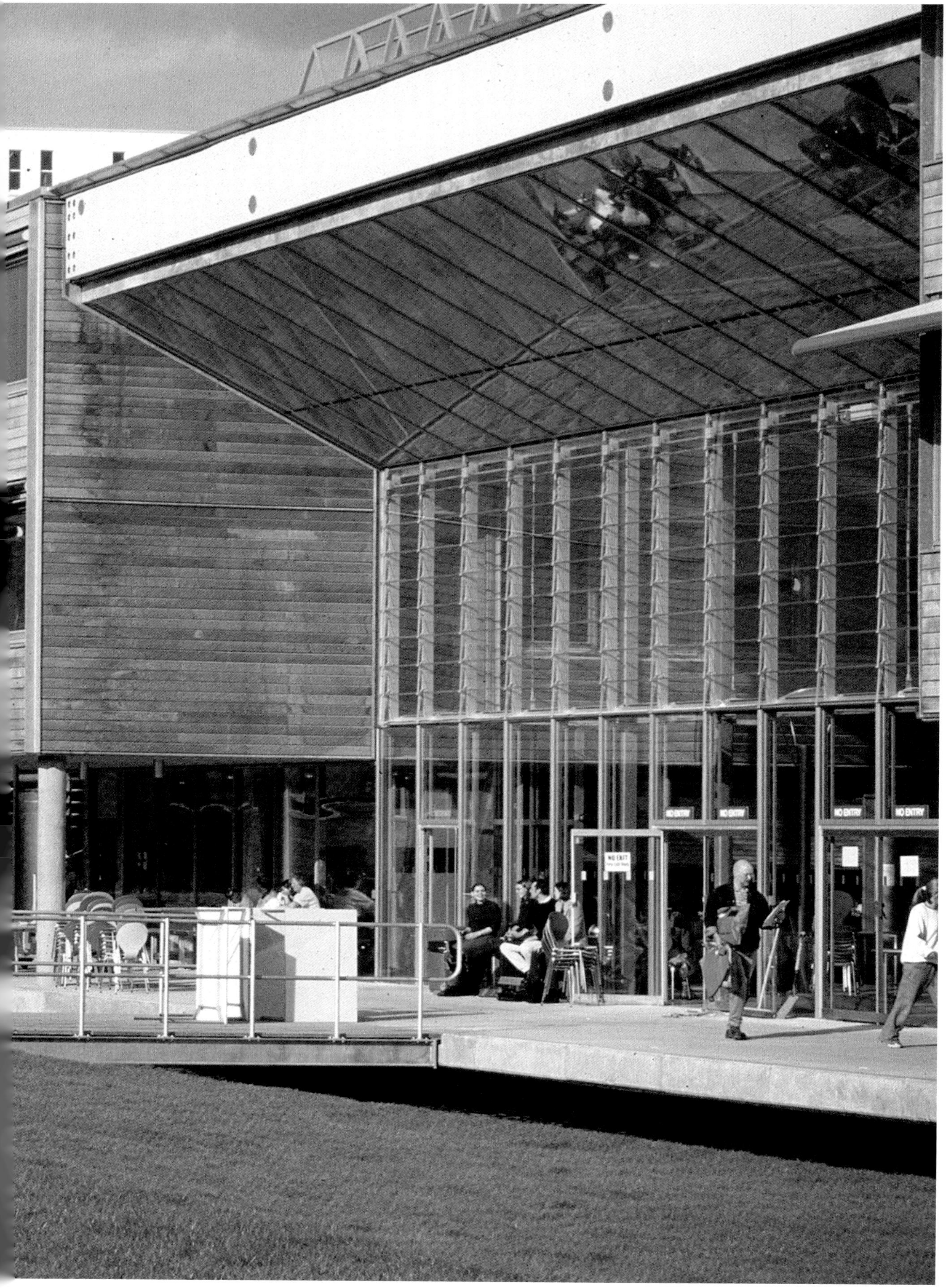

Cultural Centre
Renzo Piano
Nouméa
New Caledonia
1997

➔

The 'cases' of the
Nouméa complex.

'The return to tradition is a myth.... No people has ever achieved that. The search for identity, for a model, I believe it lies before us...our identity is before us.'[1] These words provide the inspiration for the design of a new cultural centre at Nouméa in New Caledonia. They belong to Jean-Marie Tjibaou, who was the leader of the New Caledonian independence movement. His vision for the people of New Caledonia to achieve a balance of their tradition with the modern world is paralleled in Renzo Piano's creation.

Piano appears to be one of a few living architects who can successfully face up to the challenge of cultural devaluation brought on by the 'all pervasive thrust of the media and the market'.[2] The work of the Renzo Piano Building Workshop is based on rigorously investigating the needs of people who use buildings and interpreting these through constructional discipline. This method, however, is always inflected by a contextual and cultural sensibility and the collaborative approach of the 'workshop'. The Nouméa design passed through a number of stages as the workshop studied, researched and reinterpreted the scheme. The result is a building which, though completely original,

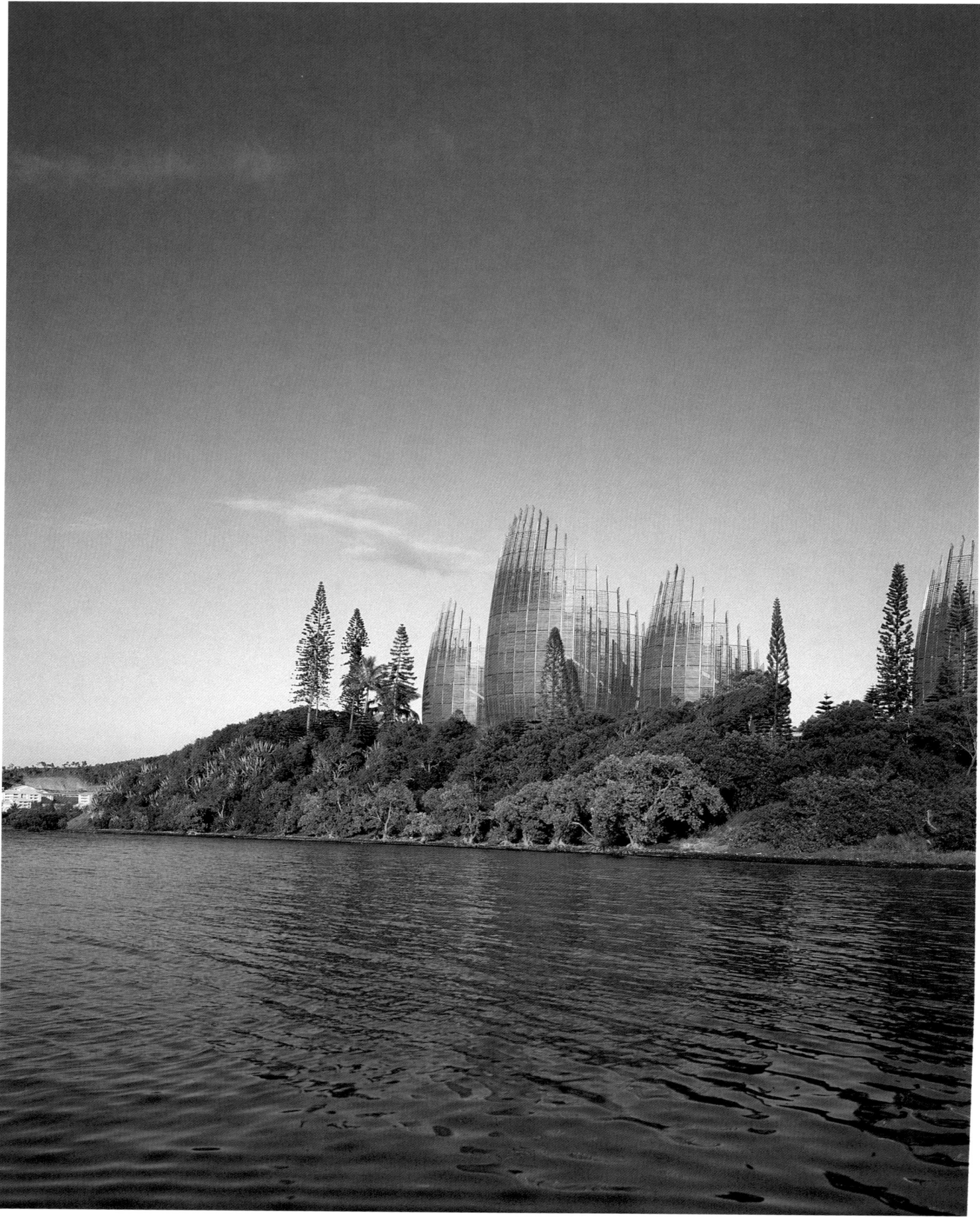

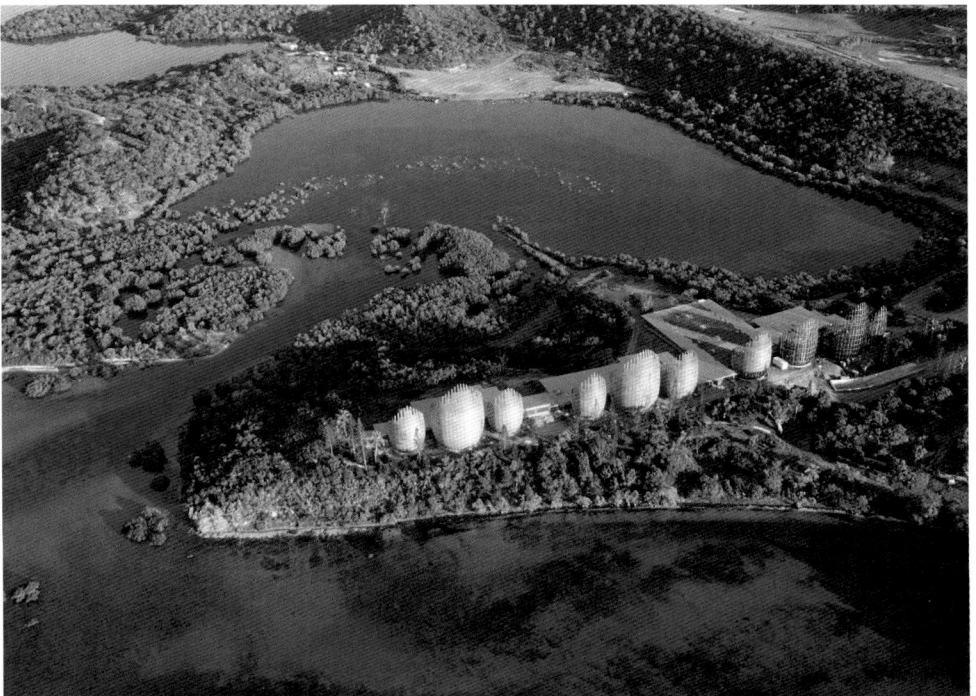

↑
The buildings in the
'oceanic tropical'
setting.

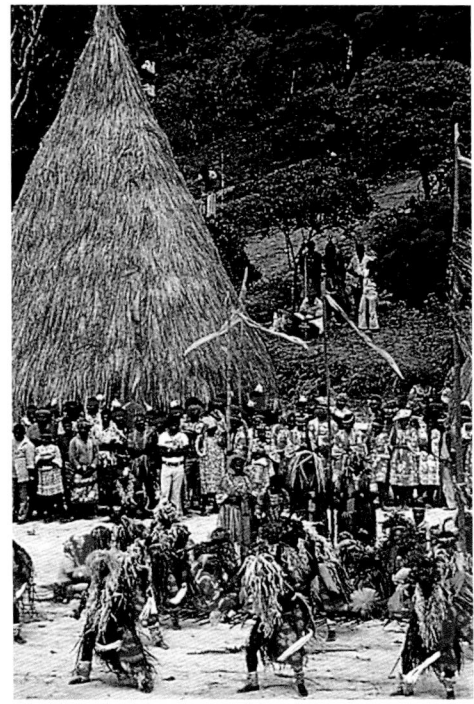

↑
Typical Kanak huts –
inspiration for the
case forms.

evokes elements of traditional indigenous settlements and plant forms.

Before Tjibaou's death in 1989, at the hands of Kanak extremists who opposed the referendum on independence agreed with the French, it had already been decided to build a centre dedicated to Kanak culture. An international design competition, held in 1991 on behalf of the Agence de Développement de la Culture Kanak (ADCK), was won by the Renzo Piano Building Workshop, working with Arup. Given to ADCK by the municipality of Nouméa, the site was the place where Tjibaou had held the Melanesia 2000 festival in 1975 – one of the milestones in the struggle for political and cultural recognition.

Location and site
New Caledonia is an island in the Pacific Ocean approximately 1,600km (1,000 miles) east of Australia. The site is set on a promontory covered in palm and pine trees which separates the Bay of Magenta from a small lagoon on the eastern edge of Nouméa, the capital. The climate is 'oceanic tropical', meaning that it is generally humid throughout the year with only moderate variations in temperature.

A full annual weather record was recorded at Nouméa airport and analysed for temperature, humidity and wind speed and direction. The average winter minimum is 18°C (64°F) and the average summer minimum is 28°C (82°F). The relative humidity is very high at about 75 per cent, with average monthly maximums of 90 per cent and lows of 60 per cent. It is no easy task to provide comfort conditions using passive design in such a climate.

Design development
The competition design of April 1991 sought to establish the centre as part of the landscape and culture of New Caledonia by evoking vegetal analogies and formal echoes with traditional settlements both in plan and section.[3]

A covered promenade, curved like a stalk, was laid out on the crest of the promontory to link the various departments. The major spaces, circular in plan, were held inside shell-like elements made predominantly of timber. Tall, layered and curved, these were known as 'cases' and – in addition to their evocative connections to programme and place – were intended as primary means of shelter and climate modification. The cases relate formally and visually to, but do not mimic, the indigenous bush and Norfolk Island pine trees

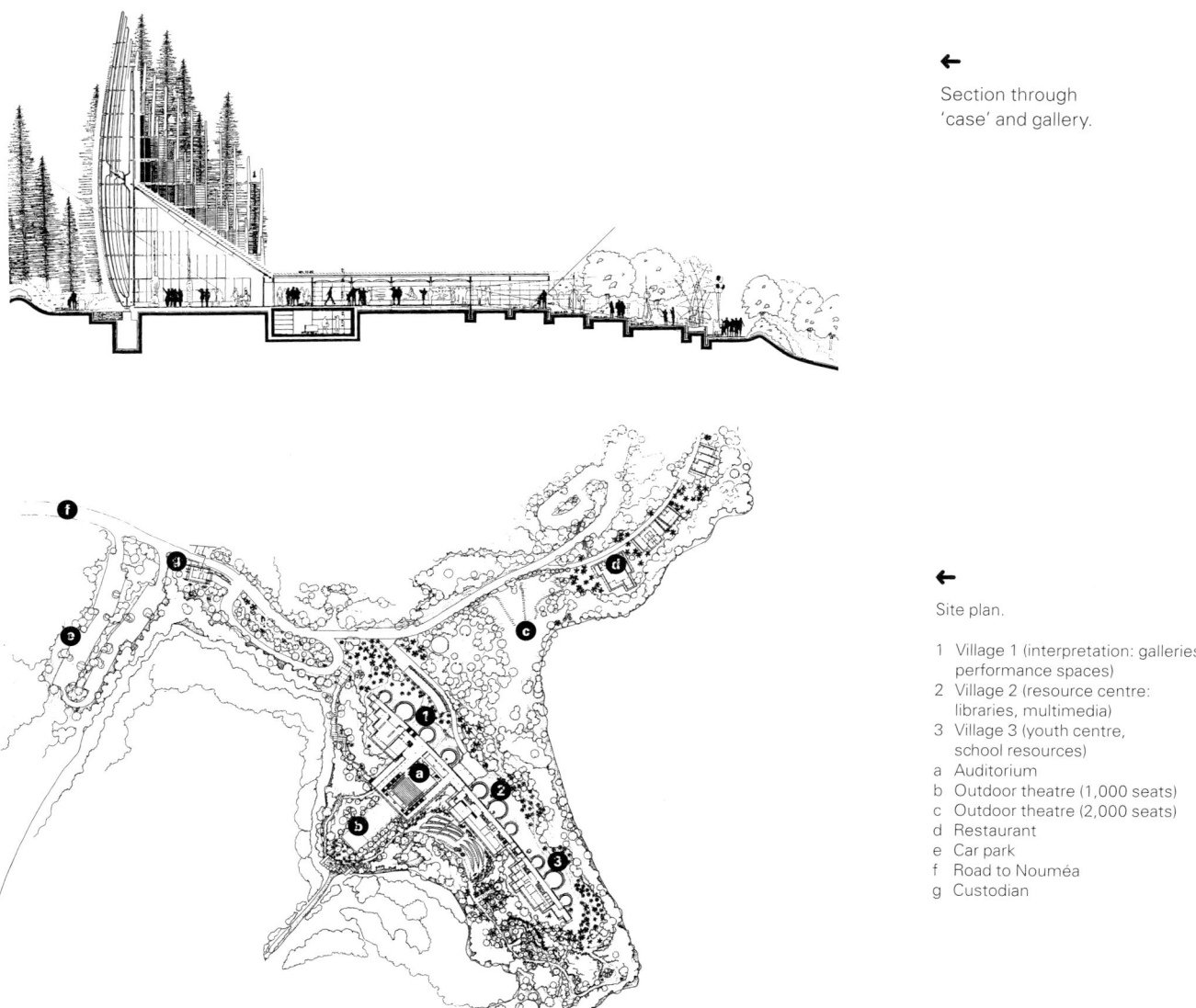

←

Section through
'case' and gallery.

←

Site plan.

1 Village 1 (interpretation: galleries,
  performance spaces)
2 Village 2 (resource centre:
  libraries, multimedia)
3 Village 3 (youth centre,
  school resources)
a Auditorium
b Outdoor theatre (1,000 seats)
c Outdoor theatre (2,000 seats)
d Restaurant
e Car park
f Road to Nouméa
g Custodian

and the traditional Kanak huts and settlements. They were also designed to promote natural wind-driven ventilation by directing and accelerating breezes into internal spaces and by setting up convective stack ventilation within the buildings. In the original competition design, the cases were placed on both sides of the curved promenade.

Access to the site is from the north and the access road skirts the lagoon to reach the promenade through a shaded car park before turning east towards a residential quarter for visiting artists. The area between the residential quarter and the cultural centre was planned to contain an arc of traditional huts with spaces between each – a showcase for traditional Kanak life and Kanak ceremonies. The constituent parts of the centre were located at appropriate places along the promenade: public facilities close to the entrance, an auditorium and media theatre on the quiet lagoon side, a multi-purpose hall on the lagoon side, with a bar/cafeteria and lounge on the opposite side. This original zoning survived the development of the design but has been changed as the brief was modified.

Piano's cases are the most striking feature of the scheme. They are as tall as the surrounding pine trees (nearly 30m (98ft)) and were designed originally from a mixture of specially adapted local materials. Although reminiscent of the ribbed construction of Kanak huts, the cages are not a literal reinterpretation of the vernacular. They are much larger than the huts and are constructed of laminated iroko tied with stainless-steel tubes and rods. Therefore, while the overall forms are traditional, the construction of the cases relies on innovation. Equivalent in height to ten-storey structures, they must be built to resist cyclonic and earthquake conditions. Not an indigenous timber, iroko was chosen on account of its strength and durability; it needs no decorative protection and weathers to a silver grey similar to that of the surrounding pines.

The layout of the scheme developed from the original competition entry. In the feasibility study of January 1992 the cases are grouped to resemble three separate village clusters and they are more sculptural than in their finally developed form. By January 1993 the flat roof had been swept up to become an integral part of the case, and the cases themselves had evolved into a double layer of laminated timber ribs.

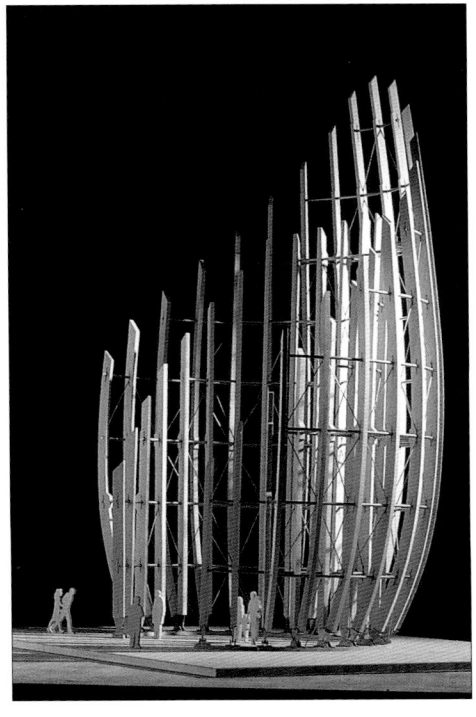

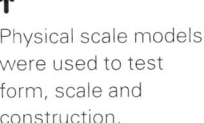
Physical scale models
were used to test
form, scale and
construction.

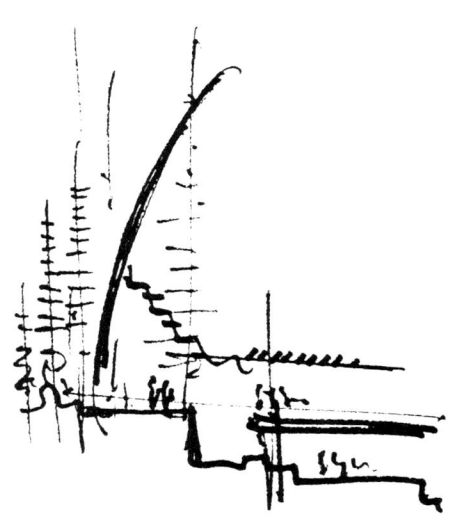
Sketch of a 'case'.

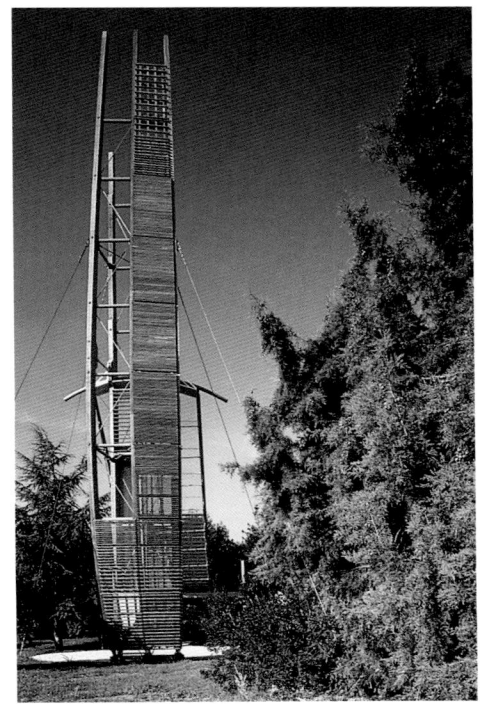
Part of a full-scale
'case' mock-up in
France.

The varying dimensions of the
horizontal slatted cladding – widely
spaced at the top and bottom, more
narrowly spaced in the middle – were
determined by the ventilation studies.
The cases eventually detailed in April
1993 defined only about two-thirds of
a circle on plan. They had also
acquired straight sloping roofs of
glass or metal. The cases had also
been evenly spaced, and the original
concept of the three villages becomes
difficult to read.

The layout of the complex also
changed from the original
competition entry and early feasibility
study, although the original zoning
survives. Three groups of cases, or
villages, are set along the southern
side of a curved promenade. Village 1
contains interpretation galleries and
performance spaces. Village 2 has a
resources centre and libraries. Village

3 accommodates the youth centre and
educational resources.

Structure and construction

Arup was responsible for the concept
design and analysis up to tender
stage, while the French company
Agibat MTI took charge of formal
design completion.

There are three sizes of cases all
sharing a similar structure designed
to resist cyclonic winds that can gust
up to approximately 65m/s (213.25
ft/s) from any direction. The tallest
case is 28m (92ft) high with an internal
diameter of 14m (46ft). Structural and
formal development was determined
by wind conditions and passive
ventilation mechanisms. In the final
form, two concentric walls are set out
from a common centre point. The
structural elements of both skins
consist of glue-laminated columns –

arched in the outer ring and straight in
the internal ring. They are tied
together and braced to provide overall
wind resistance.

The timbers are braced with steel
tubes placed at 2.25m (7ft) vertical
centres with single diagonal ties in
each bay, apart from the lower
internal ring where opening windows
are placed. To prevent distortions, the
inner and outer walls are tied together
with up to three levels of belt trusses;
the sloping roof is designed to lie
inside the inner walls, allowing the
roof to be free from stresses from wall
movements and also to be relatively
lightweight. Connections were
carefully considered to enable the
cases to be externally skinned with
horizontal slats; a steel casting is
inserted into the timber columns
accommodating compact fixings for
diagonal steel rods.

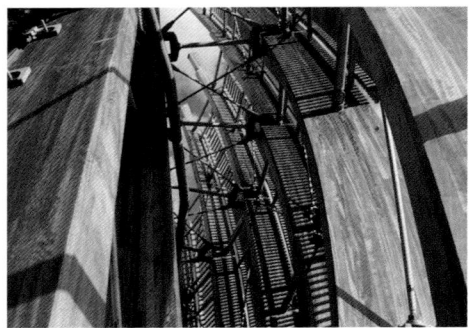

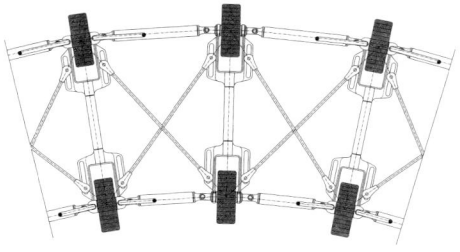

↑
Detail of paired ribs to 'case'.

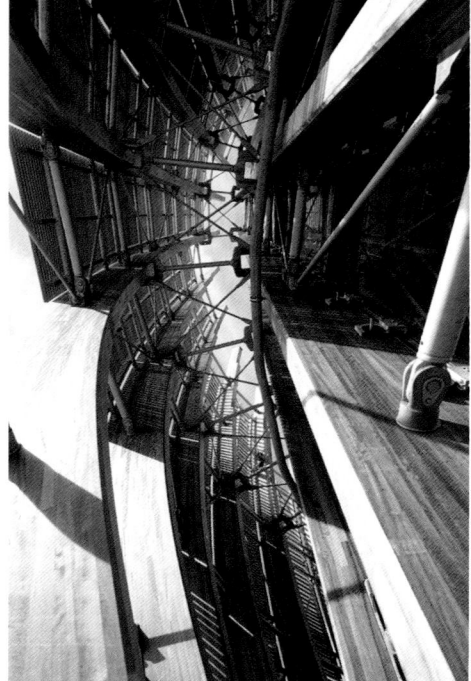

↑
Void between two skins.

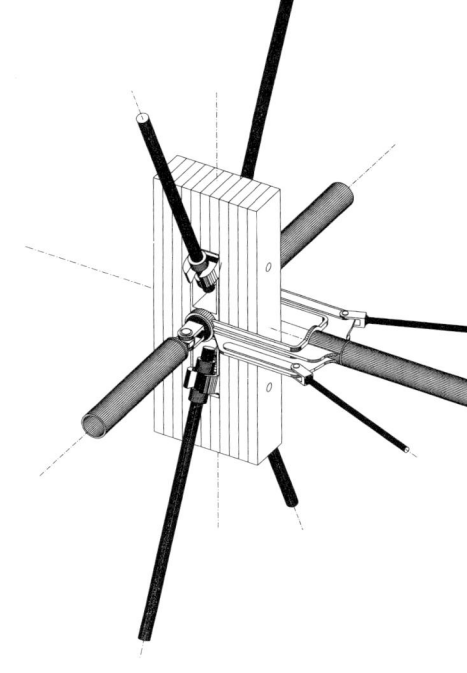

↑
Timber construction to bracing tubes and diagonals.

The connection of the feet of the timber columns to concrete foundations is equally carefully and elegantly resolved. The choice of iroko for the structure was determined by a number of performance factors but durability was critical: humidity, maritime conditions, termite resistance and gluing characteristics were all taken into account.

The structure and construction, while unique, are products of the developmental and constructional discipline of the Renzo Piano Building Workshop. Material development stems from the timber technology developed by the architects on previous projects, eg. the IBM travelling exhibition. Similarly, structural relationships can be identified in a number of other projects, including the workshop's own offices and the envelope,

particularly the modular double roof, is another identifiable motif.

Energy and environment
The principal spaces are cocooned in circular cases connected along one edge by a circulation spine. Environmental conditions inside the spaces are protected and modified by the cases. The other side of the spine consists of pavilions with stainless-steel flat roofs supported on laminated iroko posts and beams. The cases are clad in horizontal iroko slats and the pavilions in glass and iroko louvres positioned and regulated to promote a passive ventilation system. In order to achieve natural wind-driven ventilation for a wide variety of wind speeds and directions, a five-stage control strategy was devised by Arup.

Louvres in the case of the building are opened and closed in response to

wind conditions. Several openings allow ventilation. Two face towards the prevailing winds; one opening is set 2m (6½ft) above ground, another 0.5m (1½ft) above ground. On the other side of the case, a series of openable windows allow for cross ventilation. The windows have three positions – open, closed or half closed – and are controlled automatically. The opening position is dependent on external wind speed and is open only enough to achieve internal air speeds to a maximum of 1.5m/s (4.92 ft/s).

Each case has a double-louvred opening at a high level; when this is open, the case can operate as a chimney, providing ventilation (through stack effect or natural ventilation) on days when wind-driven cross ventilation is impossible. On windy days, the curved form of the case directs the wind up and over the

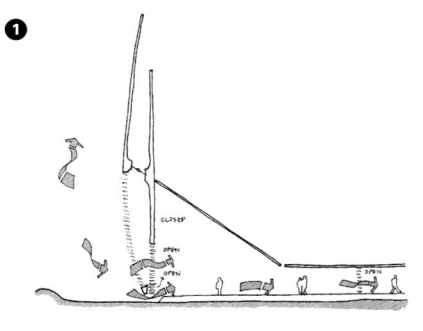

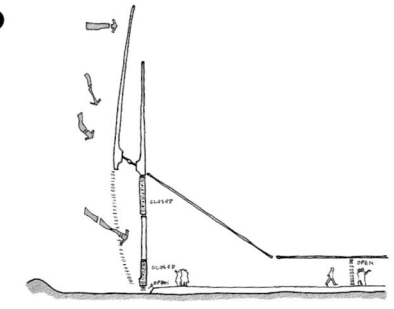

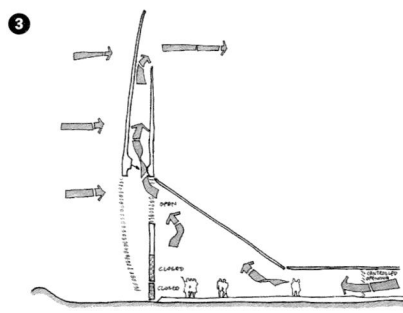

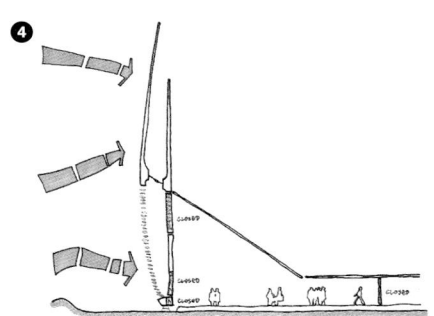

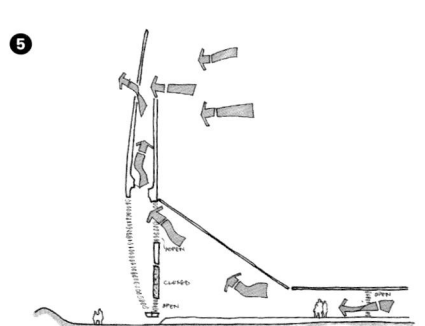

← Various modes of operation for openings in the case.

1 Light winds
2 Moderate winds
3 Strong winds
4 Cyclonic conditions
5 Reverse winds

chimney, setting up a negative pressure that draws air up and over the chimney and pushes it through the internal space from the louvred openings on the opposite side of the case. When the prevailing winds are from an opposite direction, the chimney acts in reverse. If a cyclone occurs, the envelope is closed, 'battened and hatched'.

Prediction of comfort conditions
Comfort conditions were analysed by means of the Arup Room program, using weather data for the peninsula. Air temperature, radiant temperature and humidity were calculated for each hour every day of the year at a number of points in occupied spaces for each of the control modes. This information was supplemented with information on how outside wind conditions would generate air

movement in spaces. To accomplish this, a 1:50 scale model was constructed and wind-tunnel tested by Arup and CTSB in Nantes. Internal air velocity was predicted for each mode of operation based on coefficients for each location and wind direction applied to the wind speed data.

This data was combined with temperature and humidity calculations to arrive at a comfort index at each position and for each hour during the critical months of the year. The results were compared against indices of comfort for people living in naturally ventilated conditions in a tropical climate. The predictions showed that in February, the hottest month, comfort criteria were met for all but 5.8 per cent of the time the building was occupied.

Conclusion
In 1992 Piano made a forthright statement about the role of the architect: 'Unless an architect is able to listen to people and understand them, he may simply become someone who creates architecture for his own fame and self-glorification instead of doing the real work he has to do...an architect must be a craftsman. Of course any tools will do. These days, the tools might include a computer, an experimental model, and mathematics. However, it is still craftsmanship – the work of someone who does not separate the work of the mind from the work of the hand. It involves a circular process that draws you from an idea to a drawing, from a drawing to an experiment, from an experiment to a construction, and from construction back to an idea again. For me, this cycle is

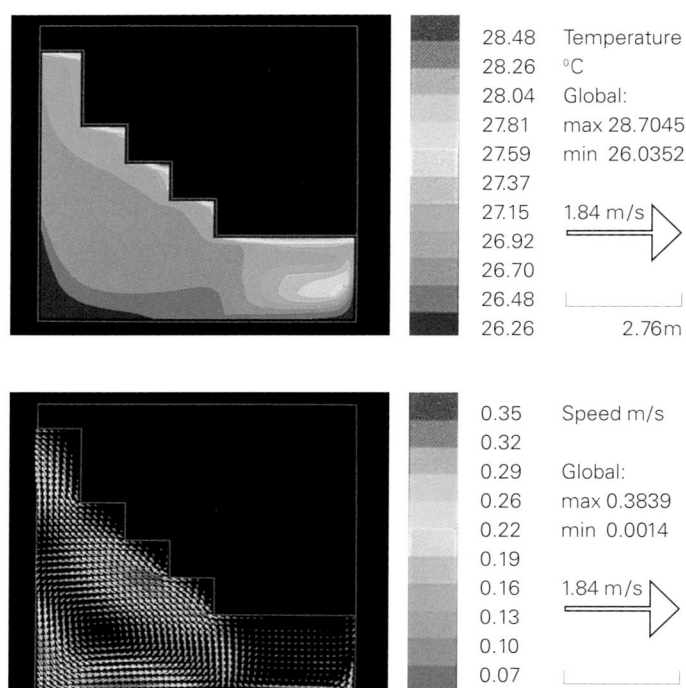

28.48	Temperature
28.26	°C
28.04	Global:
27.81	max 28.7045
27.59	min 26.0352
27.37	
27.15	1.84 m/s
26.92	
26.70	
26.48	
26.26	2.76m

1.51	Speed m/s
1.37	
1.23	Global:
1.10	max 1.6423
0.96	min 0.0046
0.82	
0.69	8.40 m/s
0.55	
0.41	
0.28	
0.14	2.76m

0.35	Speed m/s
0.32	
0.29	Global:
0.26	max 0.3839
0.22	min 0.0014
0.19	
0.16	1.84 m/s
0.13	
0.10	
0.07	
0.03	2.76m

↑

CFD analyses of air speed and temperature through the case, in varying conditions.

fundamental to creative work. Unfortunately, many have come to accept each of these steps as independent.... Teamwork is essential if creative projects are to come about. Teamwork requires an ability to listen and engage in a dialogue.'[4]

This analysis describes precisely the process of creating the Nouméa cultural centre – a building that makes a powerful contribution to Tjibaou's ambition to tell the work 'that we are neither escapees from prehistory nor archaeological remains, but men of flesh and blood'.[5]

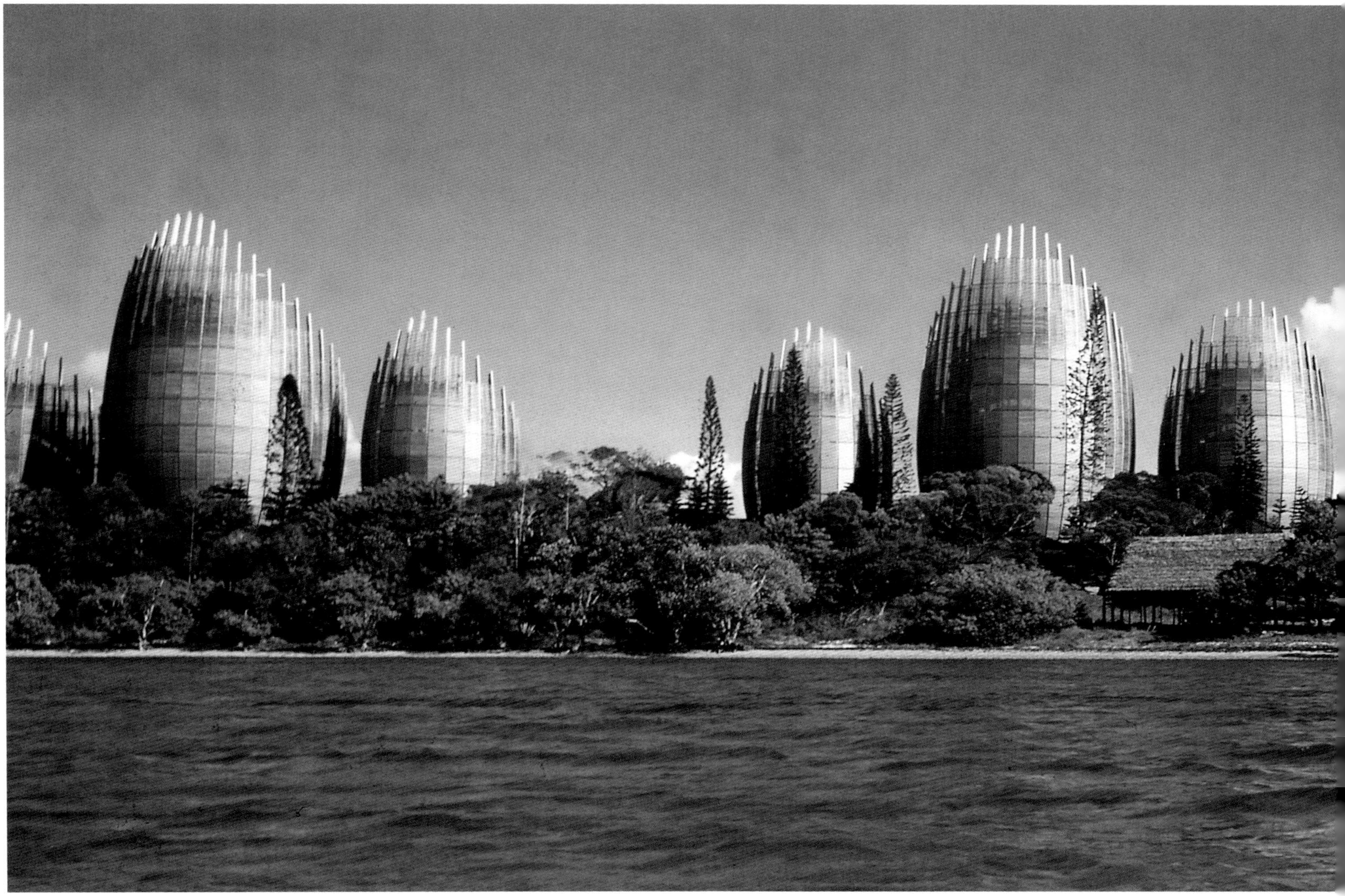

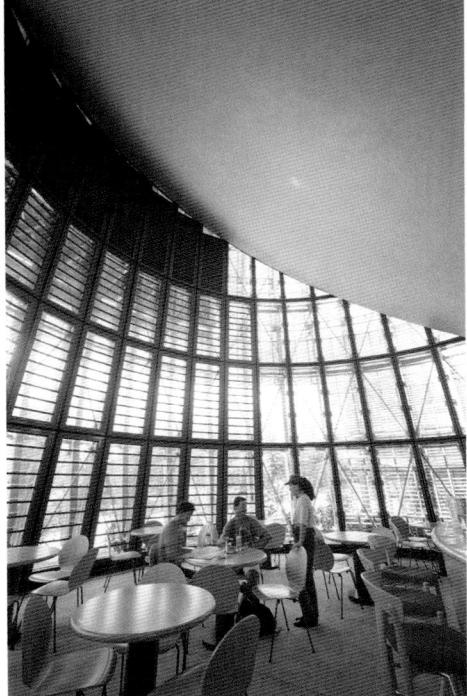

↑
Cultural and
contextual
sensitivity: the
complex from off-
shore.

→
Dining and library
facilities.

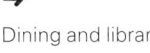
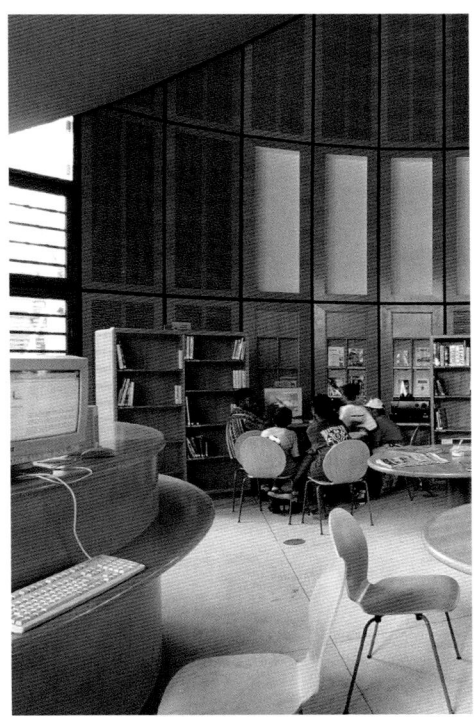

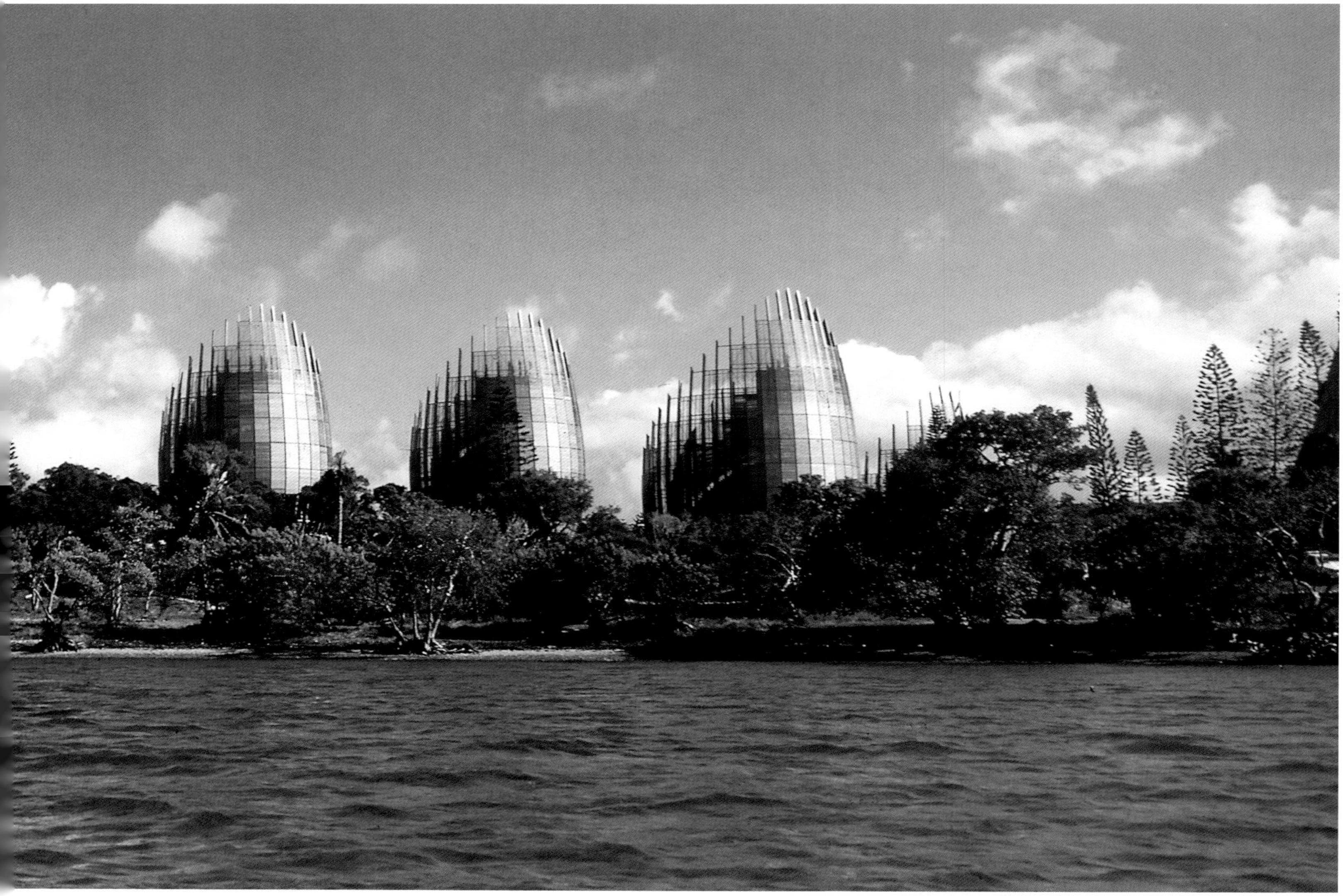

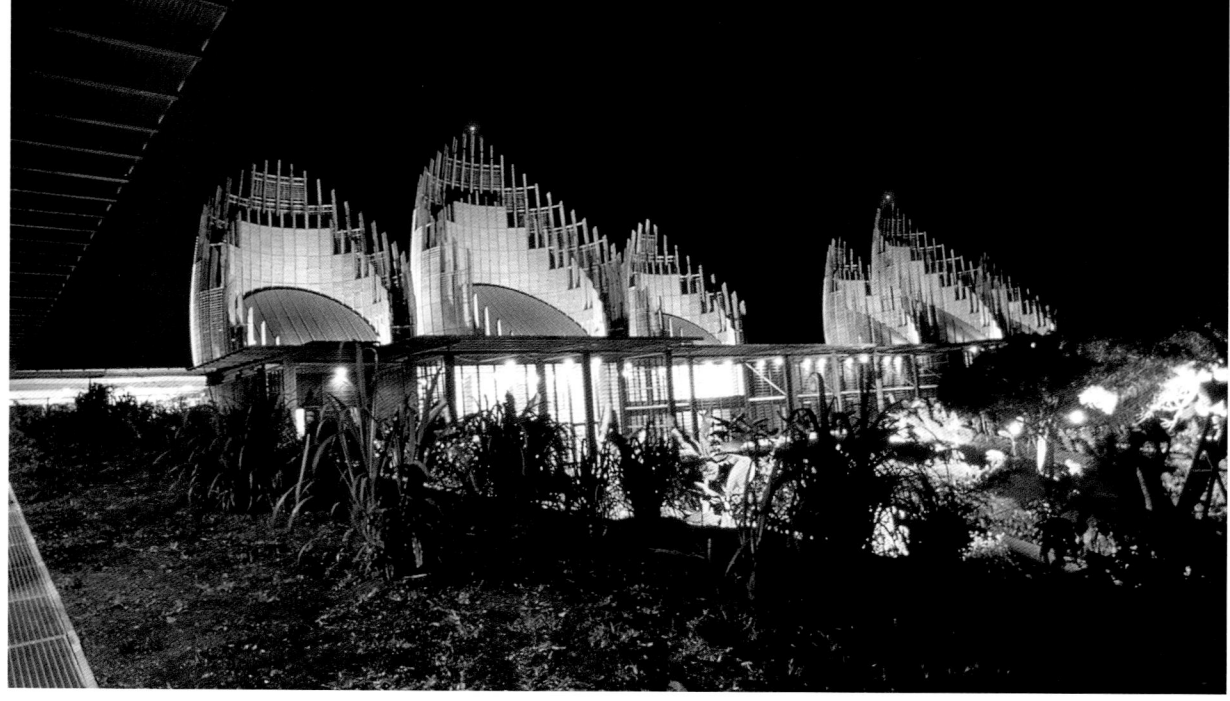

→
The complex at night:
the profile of the
cases is accentuated
by silhouetting.

Carmel Mountain Ranch Public Library

M.W. Steele Group Inc.
San Diego
California, USA
1996

→
Detail of the structural
overhang.

With its mild winters and abundant sunshine, the climate of Southern California is most agreeable, in spite of atmospheric pollution in downtown areas – and the odd Hollywood downpour like the one Gene Kelly danced through at the highpoint of *Singing in the Rain*. The sequence of wonderful Californian houses that began with Greene and Greene – and continued through the work of Frank Lloyd Wright, Rudolf Schindler, Marcel Breuer and Richard Neutra up to the mid-20th century 'Case Study' houses by Craig Ellwood and Charles Eames – amply demonstrates how a happy synthesis of architecture and climate can be achieved there.[1] In all these buildings, form and fabric are organized to filter and moderate the ambient environment. Wide roof overhangs, widely opening doors and windows, shades and blinds, shaded terraces and patios are all part of the architectural and environmental language. Identical elements were found in other building types, for example, in a number of schools Neutra designed in the 1930s.

It was predictable that California should have been one of the first regions of the world where mechanical environmental control was adopted as the norm for buildings of all types. The influence of the aerospace industry and, more recently, of 'Silicon Glen', led to a predisposition for a technically based architecture. As explained in the

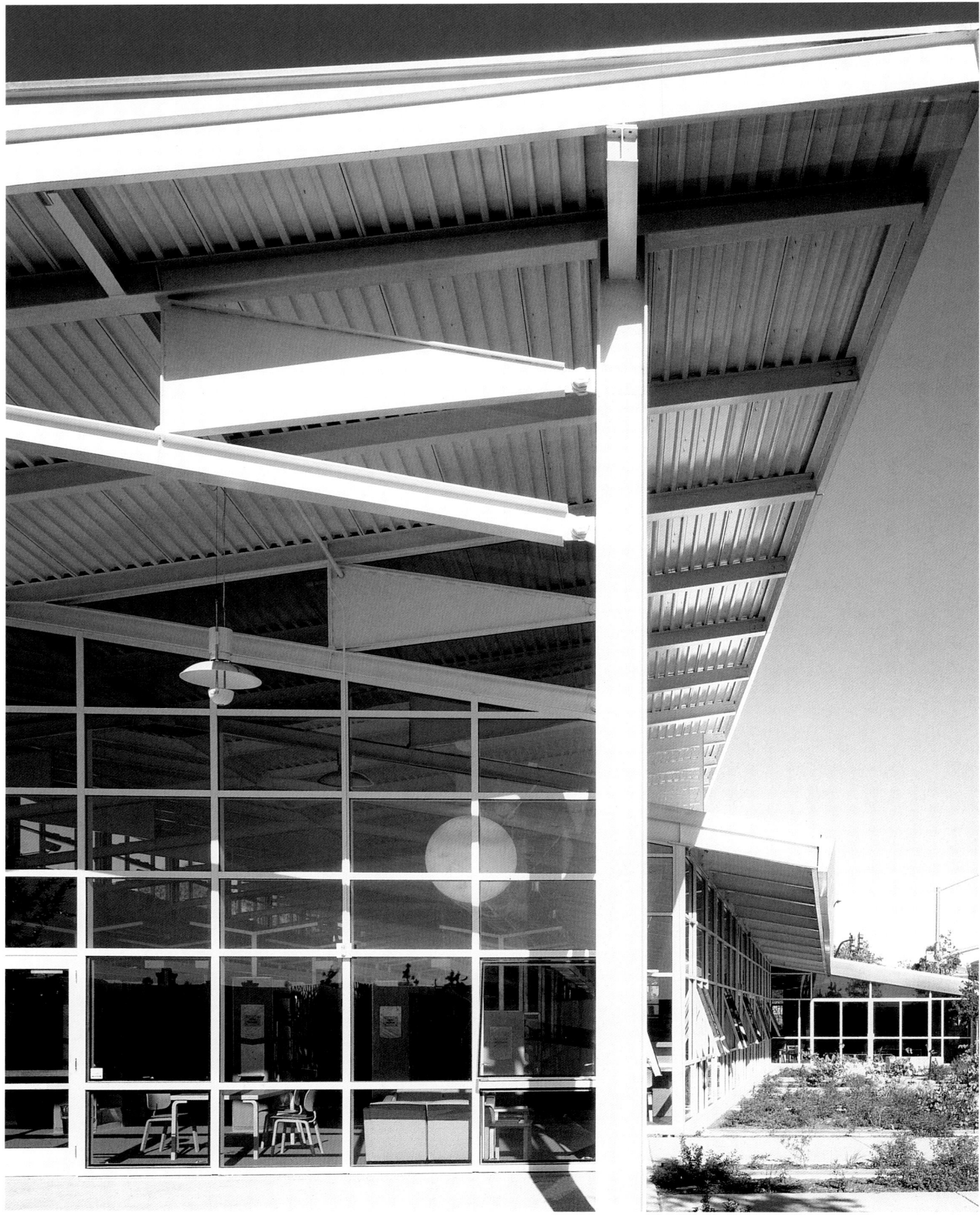

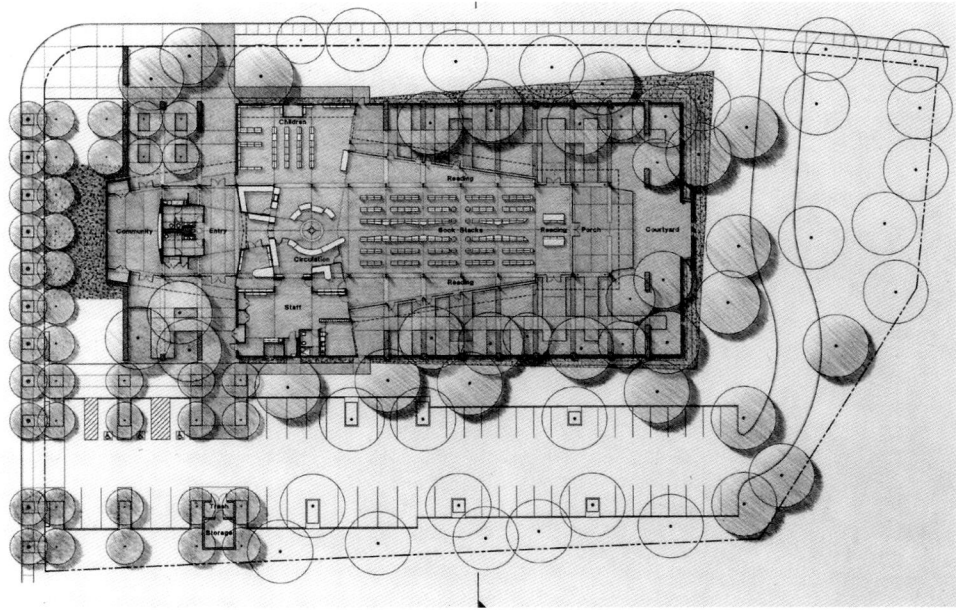

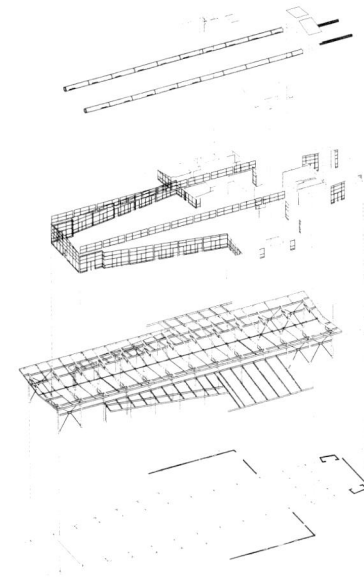

introduction, the 1960s SCSD schools programme, under the direction of Ezra Ehrenkrantz, was a symbol of this, bringing as it did the benefits of a fully air-conditioned, sealed environment to California's classrooms, in contrast with Neutra's earlier climate-filtering designs.

The design for Carmel Mountain Ranch Public Library by the M.W. Steele Group represents a return to California's environmental tradition in architecture. Working closely with Ove Arup & Partners California, M.W. Steele have produced a building that brings together that tradition with engineering systems in a functional relationship that seeks to combine the best of both worlds.

The library environment
The design of a public library, however small, is a rich architectural challenge. In addition to its traditional function as a lending and reference source, a library is a place for private study by people of all ages and has also become an important point of access to digital information. Many people visit a library simply to borrow or return books and spend a relatively short time in the building. Others may spend many hours there working on projects, using books and/or digital sources of reference. There is often a separate children's section and many libraries provide a room, or rooms, for community use. Library staff, who spend all their working days in the building, have their own particular needs.

It would be possible to deal with these complex requirements in a simple environmental brief in which uniform and standardized levels of heat, light and sound are delivered constantly throughout the building. Such a proposition was at the heart of the SCSD schools programme. Its advantage is precise environmental control regardless of the seasonal and diurnal variations in the natural world. But it is equally plausible to argue that the richness and diversity of a library's uses should be reflected in the provision of a diverse environment. This approach has been followed at Carmel Mountain Ranch and the whole character of the building flows from it.

Form and environment
The environment of the building ranges from the relatively stable conditions at the heart of the plan to the widely dynamic conditions of the tree-shaded courtyard that surrounds the main library space. The scissor-form roof structure and the newly

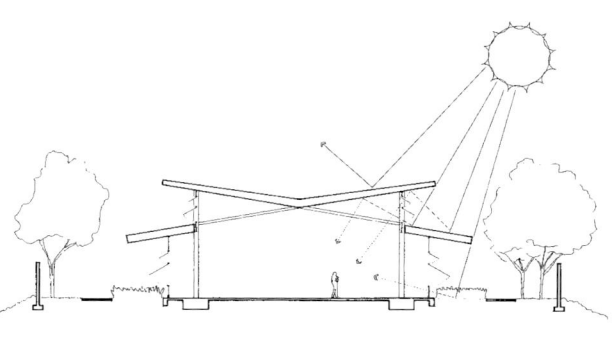

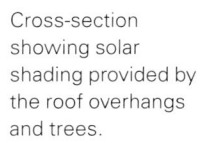

Cross-section showing solar shading provided by the roof overhangs and trees.

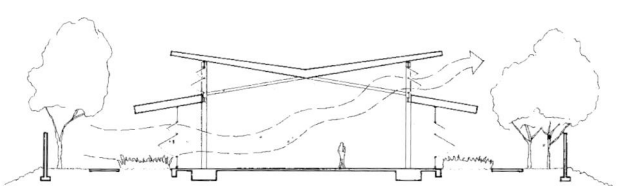

Cross-section showing natural cross-ventilation through the building.

Detailed cross-section showing the distinct environmental zones of garden and interior.

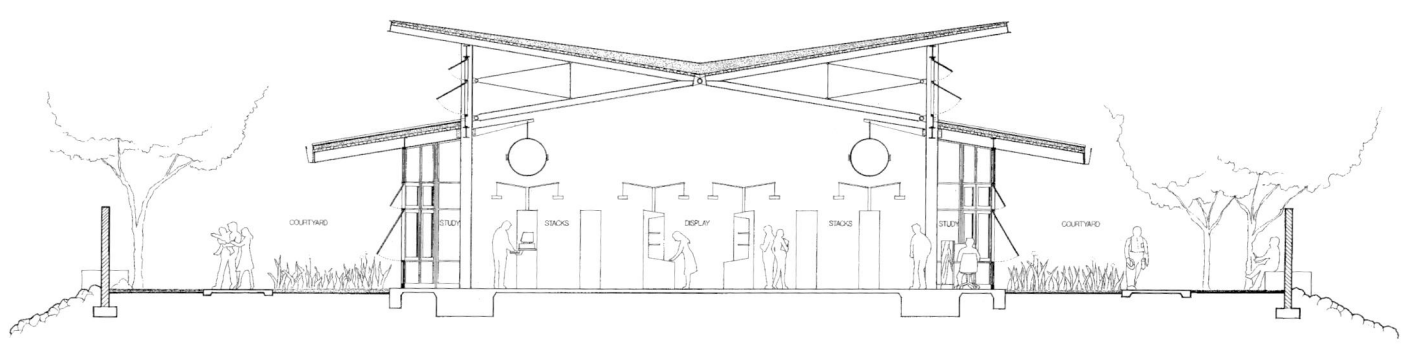

planted trees create an almost continuous canopy, making the steel structure into a natural metaphor. In the 19th century Henri Labrouste adopted the same metaphor in his design for the reading room at the Bibliothèque Nationale in Paris, where the array of top-lit domes, supported on branching cast-iron columns, is a clear allusion to the luminous qualities of a forest glade – a point reinforced by the painted frieze of tree-tops around the perimeter of the room.

At Carmel Mountain Ranch the roof form is a direct expression of the environmental strategy. The primary mode of ventilation and cooling for the building is 'passive' or, in our terminology, 'selective'. Natural ventilation occurs through clerestory windows above the central 'nave' of the plan, and the wide eaves, which

overhang the main structure by 2.1m (7ft) provide shade for the windows in the heat of summer. At the perimeter, under the lower eaves of the aisle-like spaces, library visitors can open and close windows at will, but a small air-conditioning plant has been installed to provide 'peak trimming' of the temperature, either cooling or heating, in extreme conditions. The intention is to minimize energy consumption and running costs. The highly insulated roof deck reduces heat gain and the mass of exposed concrete floor slabs and dense masonry walls moderate internal temperature variations. Glazing provides a further degree of solar control. Plenty of daylight penetrates the building – the central bookstacks are lit from the clerestories and the reading areas from the windows that look out onto the courtyard. Energy-

efficient lamps, with automatic controls, supply artificial lighting at night.

The courtyard garden was laid out by the landscape artist Marty Poirier as an extension of the library environment. Within the high enclosing wall, which provides security, readers may, on most days of the year, find places to read beneath the trees, and the trees to the south give extra shade to the building. Scented plants such jasmine and sage add a sensory dimension both to the garden and, when the windows are open, to the interior of the building.

In its architectural language the building reflects the Modernist type that flourished in Southern California in the mid-20th century. The repetitive steel frame calls to mind the 'Case Study' houses. This lineage is clearly revealed in the architects' exploded

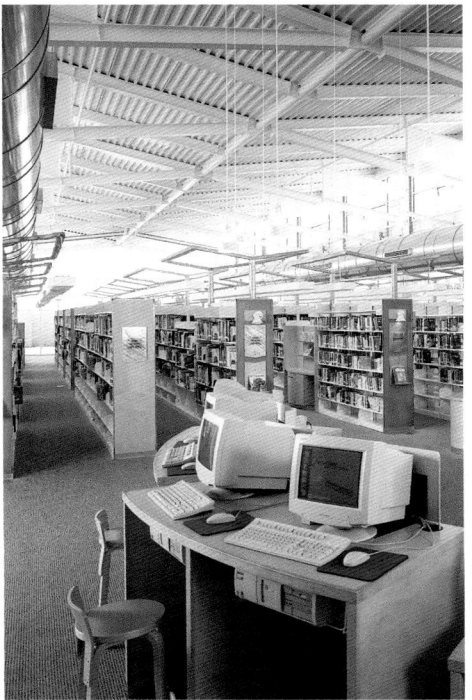

↑
General view of the interior. This shows the clear differentiation and expression of structure and services.

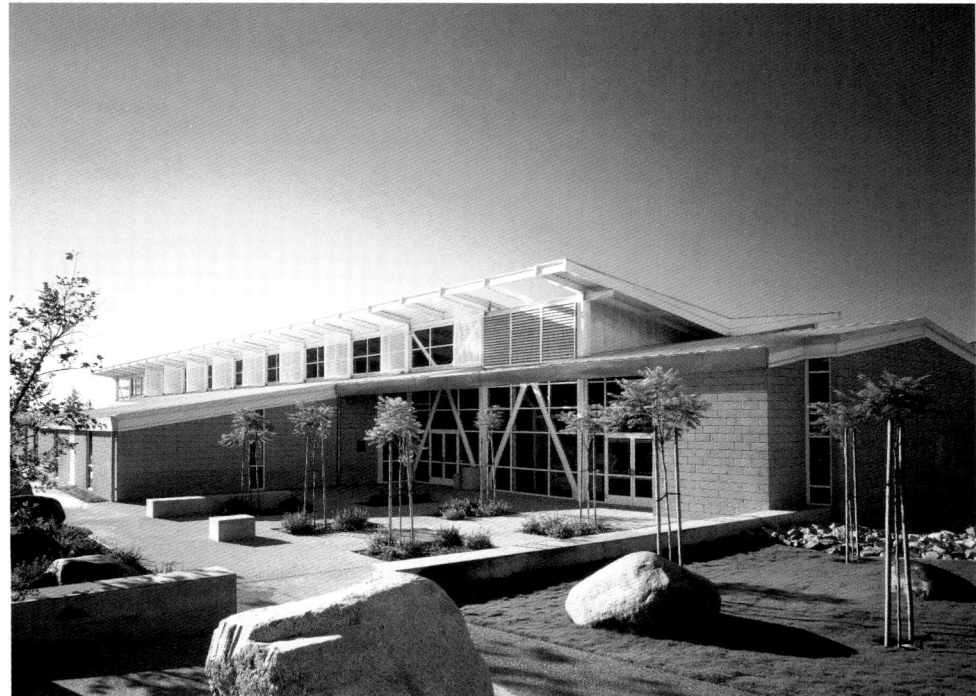

↑
View of the main entrance from within the garden courtyard.

axonometric drawing that shows the building as three distinct tectonic systems located above the foundation plan: the structural system, the enclosure system and the mechanical system. These distinct systems are clearly expressed in the execution of the building, where the artificial light fittings and the air-conditioning ducts are seen suspended below the unadorned roof structure. All the other elements – bookcases, book-check desk, study carrels – stand in a coherent relationship within this ordered space.

Environmental quality
The result is an internal environment that captures and responds to the variations of temperature and light that occur outside. Only when those variations compromise comfort – when it is too hot or cold or too dark –

is it necessary to resort to mechanical services. For much of its life the building will gently moderate the Californian climate to sustain the life of the library in all its rich diversity. Visitors are invited to make their own contribution to this process by choosing where to work, in the sun or in the shade, inside the building or in the garden. They can open or close windows at will. It is predicted that the building will consume only about half the energy of a typical modern library elsewhere in San Diego.

In a state where energy consumption often exceeds supply, a building like this clearly indicates a solution to the crisis. It suggests that it is not necessary to abandon the Kyoto resolutions on the global environment in favour of ever-higher consumption of fossil fuels or to expand our reliance on nuclear energy.

Conclusion
At face value the Carmel Mountain Ranch library is a modest building. It occupies an unambiguous position in our taxonomy of environmental architecture, being emphatically 'selective' in its strategy and adopting a tectonic of 'exposed power'. It is clear-cut and lucid and, as such, is a good example of the successful collaboration between architect and environmental engineer. A reinterpretation of the spirit of the 'Case Study' houses, which played such an important part in adapting the original propositions of the Modern Movement to the culture and climate of Southern California, it illustrates that these principles continue to be relevant as a response to the more specific and urgent environmental agenda of the 21st century.

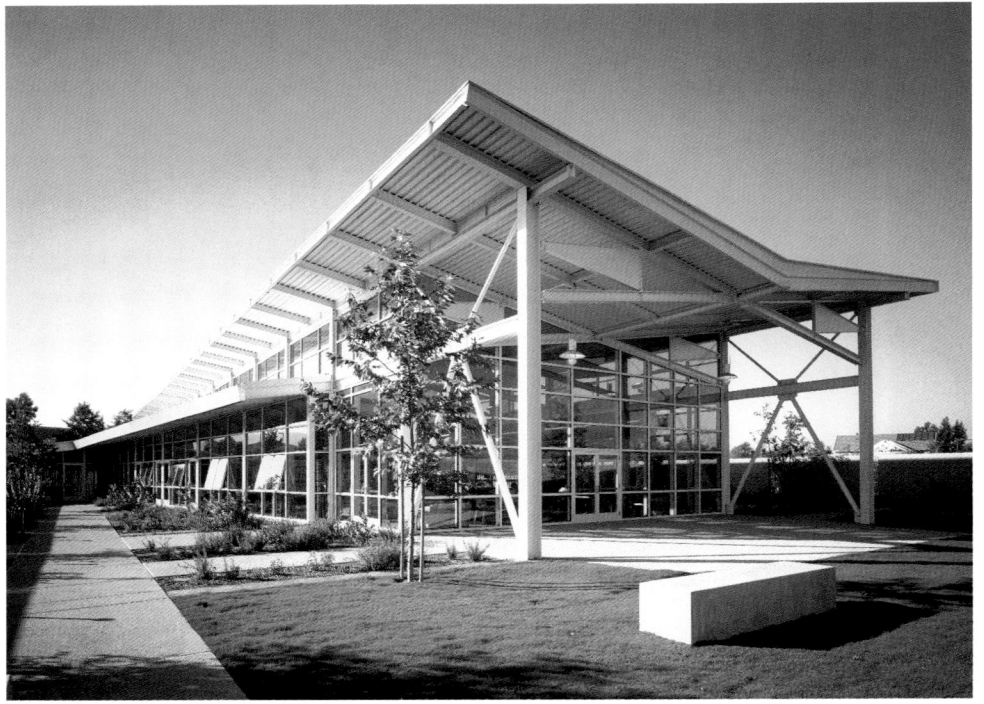

↑
The over-sailing roof creates a sheltered outdoor reading space.

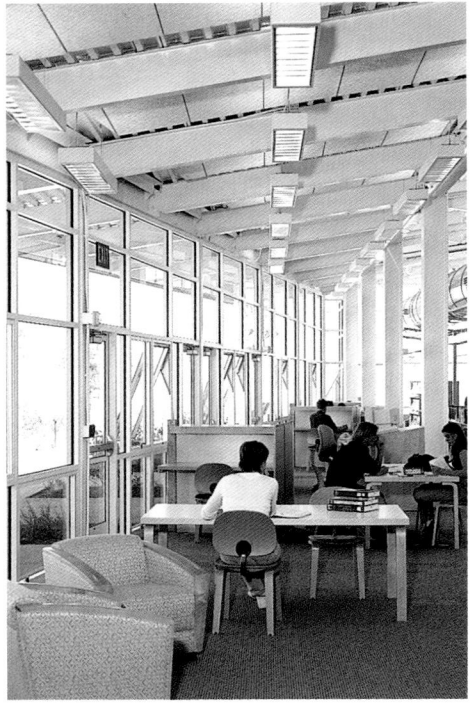

↑
Interior showing study area with individually openable windows.

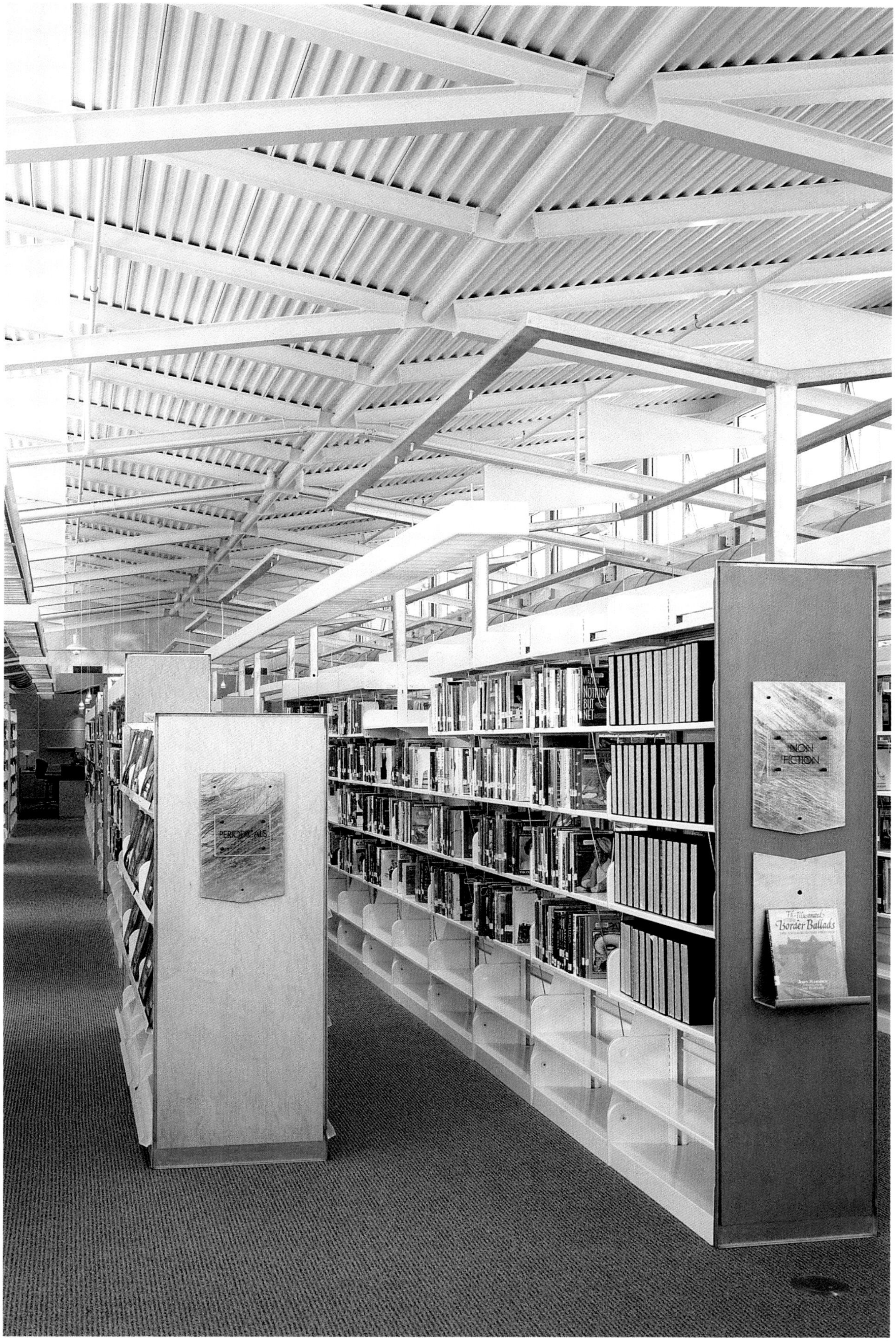

Bookstacks at the environmentally stable core of the building.

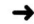

An individual study place, with its open window and view into the garden.

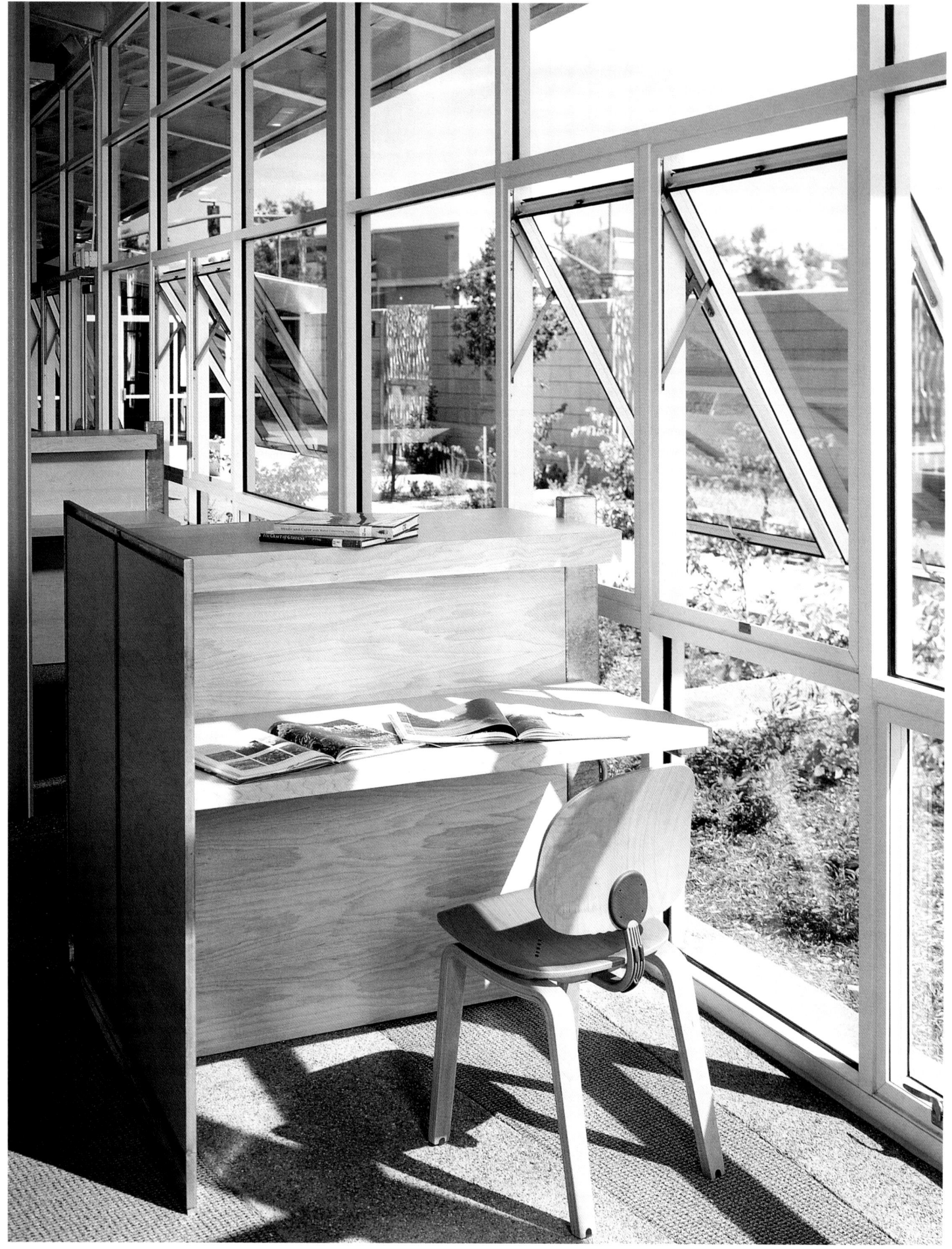

The Exclusive Mode

Helicon Building

Sheppard Robson
London, UK
1996

→
The envelope of the
Helicon Building is an
integral part of the
environmental
system.

Modern developments in urban office design can be traced back to a seminal paper by Leslie Martin and Lionel March, 'Land Use and Built Forms'.[1] Published in 1966, it demonstrated that, on large urban sites, court forms, through their inherent geometrical properties, achieve more efficient land use than isolated pavilions, and that court forms offer environmental advantages, particularly in respect of daylighting. A later study by Dean Hawkes and Richard MacCormac,

published in 1978, examined the environmental and energy-demand implications of glazing over the central courtyards of urban buildings.[2] This showed that such forms could, if carefully designed, achieve significant energy savings, up to 50 per cent, compared with typical air-conditioned buildings of that date.

The Helicon office project draws on these classic studies in that it involves the specific environmental and energy concerns embraced by the notion of

'sustainability'. The studies investigated a transformation of the urban courtyard form in which the central space has the potential to become a 'sustainable island' within the established urban fabric. Designed in the early 1990s, the Helicon project continues this line of thought by proposing a way in which the existing unsustainable city might be progressively transformed through adaptive design. For example, the layered wall conceived as a protective

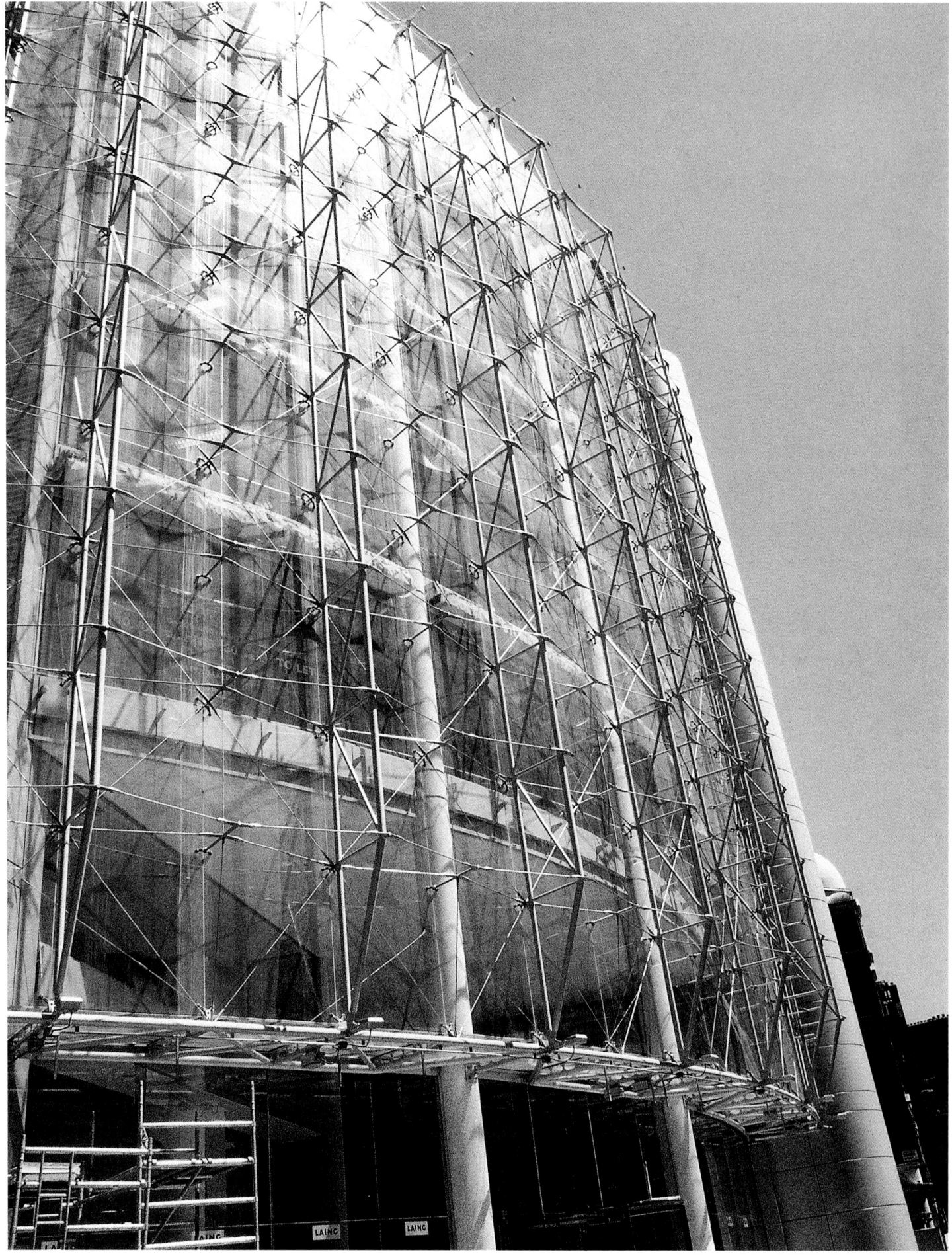

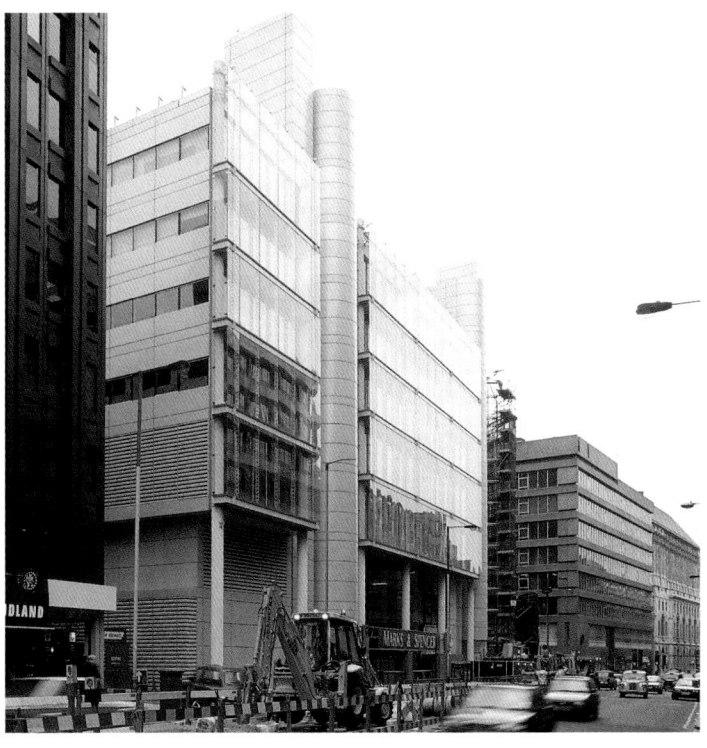

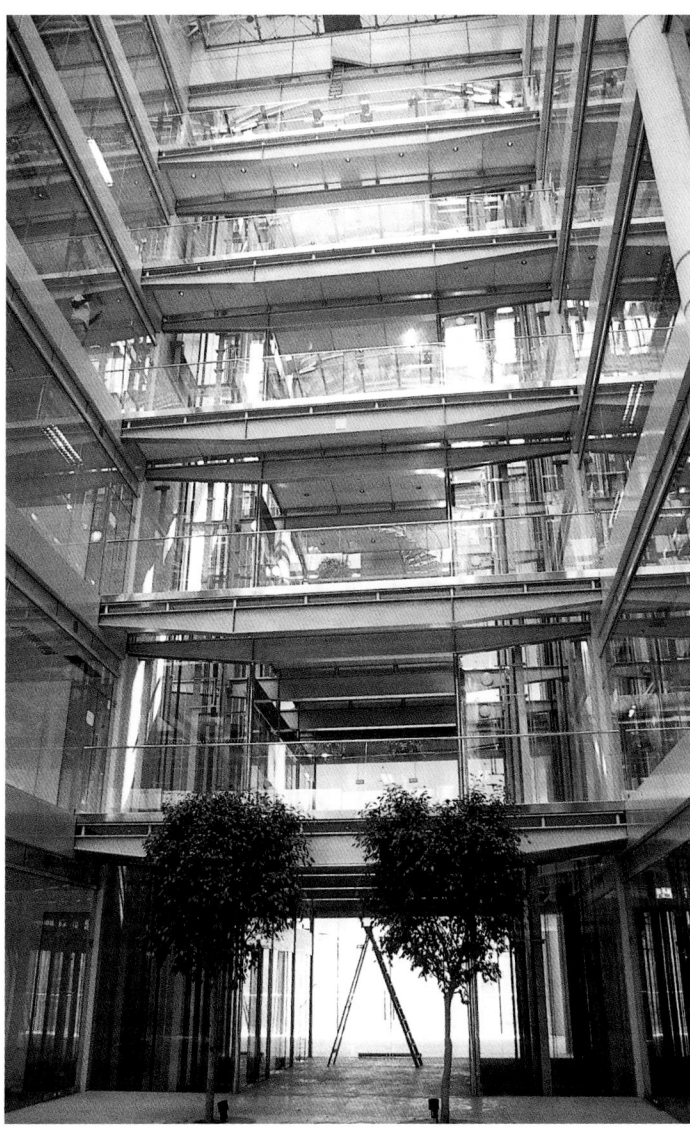

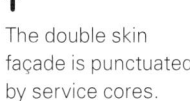
The double skin façade is punctuated by service cores.

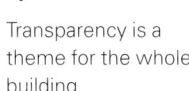
Transparency is a theme for the whole building.

and adaptable skin designed to lessen the energy load is carefully integrated with the environmental system.

In the early 1990s the retailer Marks & Spencer opened a takeaway food store in Moorgate, London. The store was so successful that it struggled to cope with demand and facilities on the site were found wanting. In particular, unloading facilities were inadequate to cope with store turnover and articulated trucks were forced to drive around the narrow city streets waiting for gaps in the loading and unloading sequence. The city block on the other side of Moorgate bounded by Finsbury Pavement, South Place, Dominion Street and Lackington Street had been acquired by London and Manchester Assurance in the recession of the early 1990s. Although at the time the acquisition may have appeared unpromising,

Marks & Spencer, who were prepared to take a 125-year lease, and another potential anchor tenant, Midland Bank, suggested that the development of the site might be commercially viable. The developer decided to combine offices with retail, and the eventual achievement of almost 50 per cent potential pre-let space allowed a start to be made on the development of the Helicon.

Site and climate

The building occupies a full city block in London's financial district. Bounded by busy city streets on all four sides, the block is virtually an island. Office developments in the heart of cities – where high levels of atmospheric pollution, noise and unwanted solar gain combine to make an unattractive cocktail – are generally confined to hermetically sealed boxes that can

keep out the worst of the city's environmental effects.

Form

Recent city building design has been typified by bland, blind boxes or overblown exercises in 'look-at-me' architecture. In the few developments where contextual design has been on the agenda, the result has been confused and confusing stylistic gestures. The Helicon combines retail accommodation, offices and a bank, which gave the designers the opportunity not only to respond to the complexity of the site's former uses but also to tackle the issue of the deep-plan high-energy city-office building. Six floors of speculatively developed office floors sit on top of three floors of retail. The six floors wrap around the ubiquitous atrium, but in this case the floors are terraced

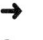
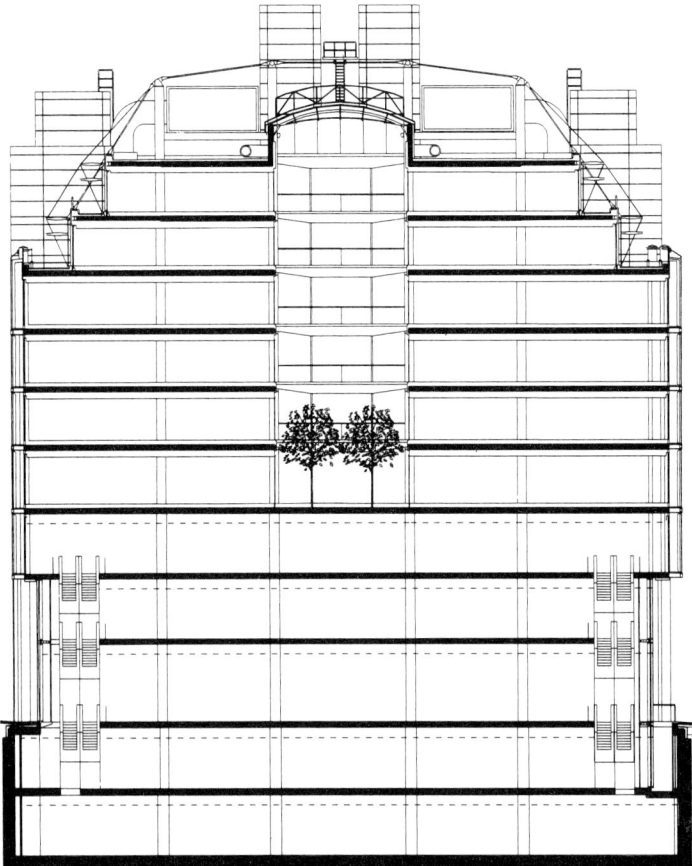

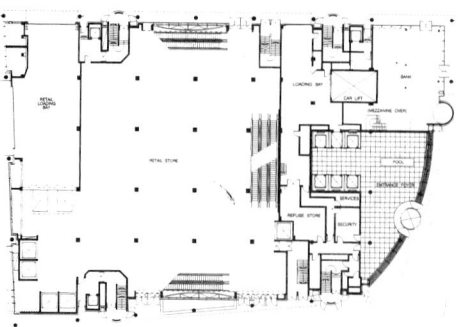

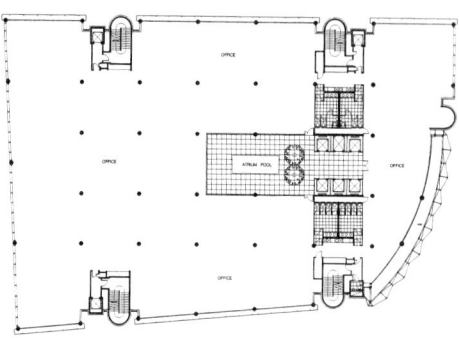

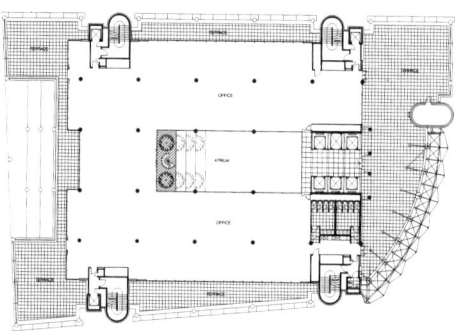

in the manner of a vineyard. Upper floors are set back like attic storeys from the pavement edge to diminish the overall bulk of the building mass. Punctuating the block is a stair and lift tower; these elements are 'inset' so that they appear to be 'outboard' of the main floor plates in the manner of the Lloyds Building. Graham Anthony of Sheppard Robson had been responsible for the design of the services towers for Richard Rogers in the Lloyds Building, and the same clear articulation, if not total separation, of served and servant spaces is also evident at the Helicon.

The stairs are bull-nosed and the lifts are rectangular. Their twin shafts are clad in silver metal panels (also reminiscent of Lloyds), making solid elements that provide a counterpoint to the glazed transparent elements of the remainder of the building

envelope. The main entrance to the offices is signalled by a curved suspended glass screen over double-height doors on the corner of Moorgate. The quadrant-shaped entrance, with entry on the diagonal, is simply shifted back to the orthogonal grid so that the main core including toilets and lift shafts runs the entire width of the block at the head of the atrium.

Layout
The width and depth of the office floors vary from level to level, but the floor plates reflect a traditional modular approach to office planning. The floors are based on a 1.5m (5ft) planning grid to provide maximum flexibility for the wide-ranging needs of potential tenants. The width of the floor plate is generally 16.5m (54ft) – made up of 9m (30ft) and 7.5m (25ft)

structural bays – from external window to atrium window. Exceptions to this occur in the section of floor that steps with the atrium. At the widest point the floor is more than 20m (66ft), but this reduces to approximately 10m (33ft) for the top two office floors. The atrium is roofed with a glazed barrel vault and sits above the Marks & Spencer store linked to the double-height entrance by an all-glass lift core. The atrium consists of a 9m (30ft) wide slot scooped out of the middle of the building form. The floors are sealed to the atrium with clear glazing to optimize daylighting to this edge of the office floor.

Structure and construction
The structure consists of a post-tensioned *in-situ* concrete-floor structure supporting raised floor offices above headroom. Walls are

149

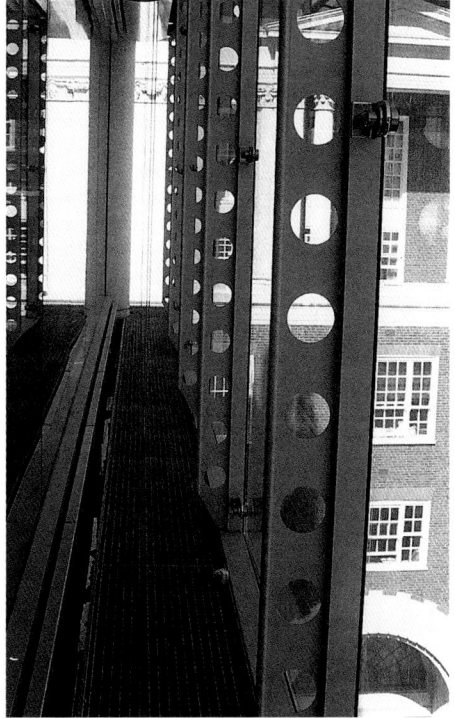

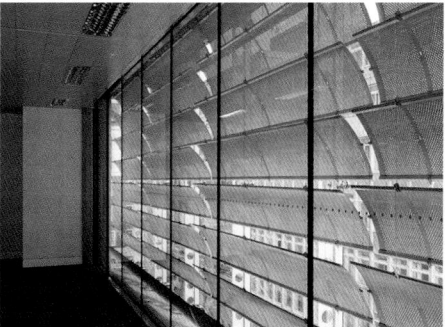

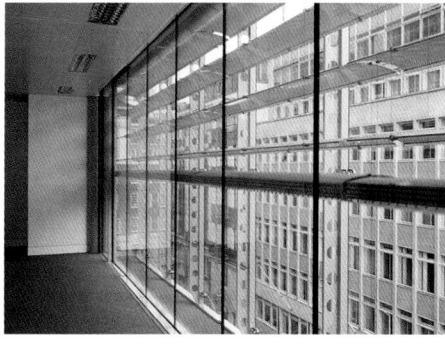

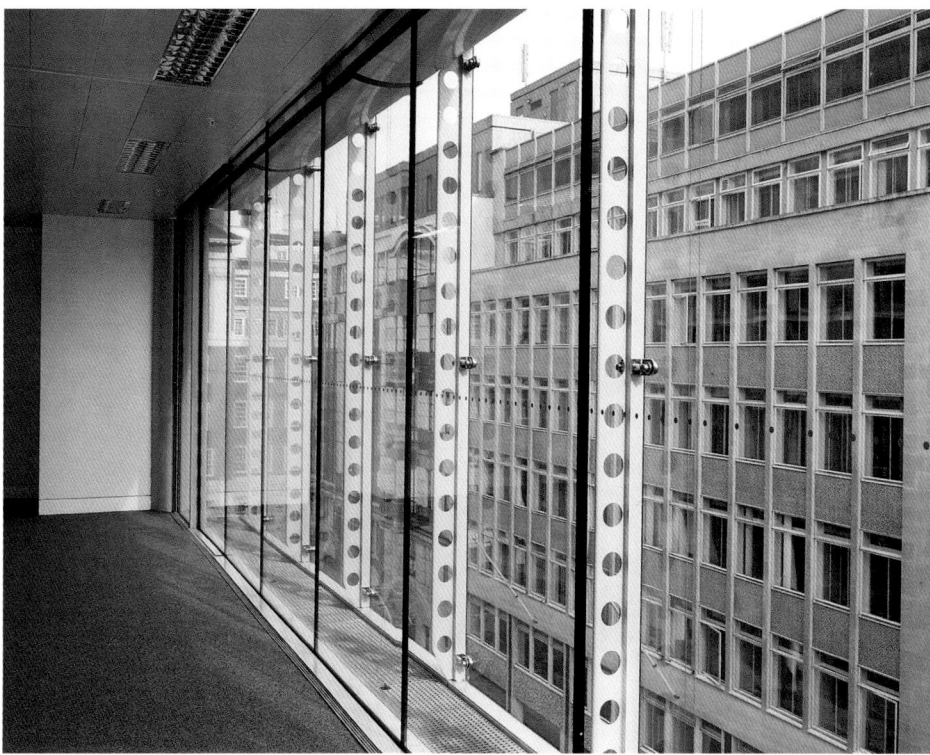

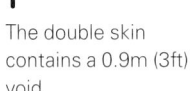
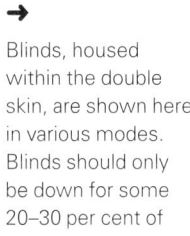

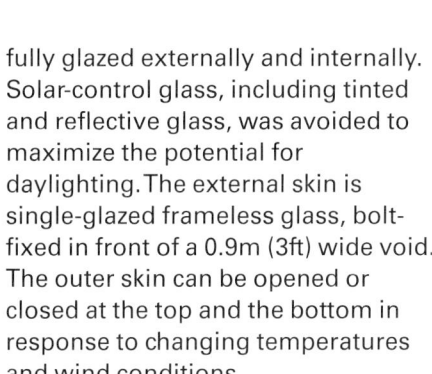

↑
The double skin
contains a 0.9m (3ft)
void.

→
Blinds, housed
within the double
skin, are shown here
in various modes.
Blinds should only
be down for some
20–30 per cent of
the year.

fully glazed externally and internally. Solar-control glass, including tinted and reflective glass, was avoided to maximize the potential for daylighting. The external skin is single-glazed frameless glass, bolt-fixed in front of a 0.9m (3ft) wide void. The outer skin can be opened or closed at the top and the bottom in response to changing temperatures and wind conditions.

While the inner skin remains sealed, the outer skin acts as a buffer to noise and temperature. Inside the void, large horizontal louvres are fitted between skins. Like giant Venetian blinds, these may be raised or lowered, tilted or turned, depending on solar conditions. The louvres are carefully spaced to avoid visual obstruction and they are perforated so that some daylight penetration is possible even when they are fully

tilted. The gap between the two skins makes a 0.9m (3ft) void – wide enough to allow access for full maintenance of the external envelope. Detailing of the external envelope and the skin inside the atrium is crisp and spare, heightening the whole building's sense of transparency.

Energy and environment
The standard solution for providing comfortable and healthy office environments in dense urban contexts in the 1980s and 1990s was variable-air-valve air-conditioning. At Helicon the objective was to find a low-energy alternative which would integrate with the external envelope and overall form of the building.

The ventilated façade
While a fully glazed façade is useful in maximizing daylight penetration,

problems of solar gain and glare have to be solved in order to provide a comfortable visual environment and also to limit cooling loads. In the design of the Helicon, Sheppard Robson worked with Arup to maximize transparency of the envelope while including a low-energy heating and ventilation system. A range of commonly used techniques including tinted and mirrored types of glass and external sun-shading were considered, but all were found to have a number of disadvantages. None of the coated glasses met the need for transparency, while external sun-shading added to maintenance and cleaning difficulties. The best option proved to be the glazed double-skin façade.

The double skin is an environmental buffer that moderates the effects of

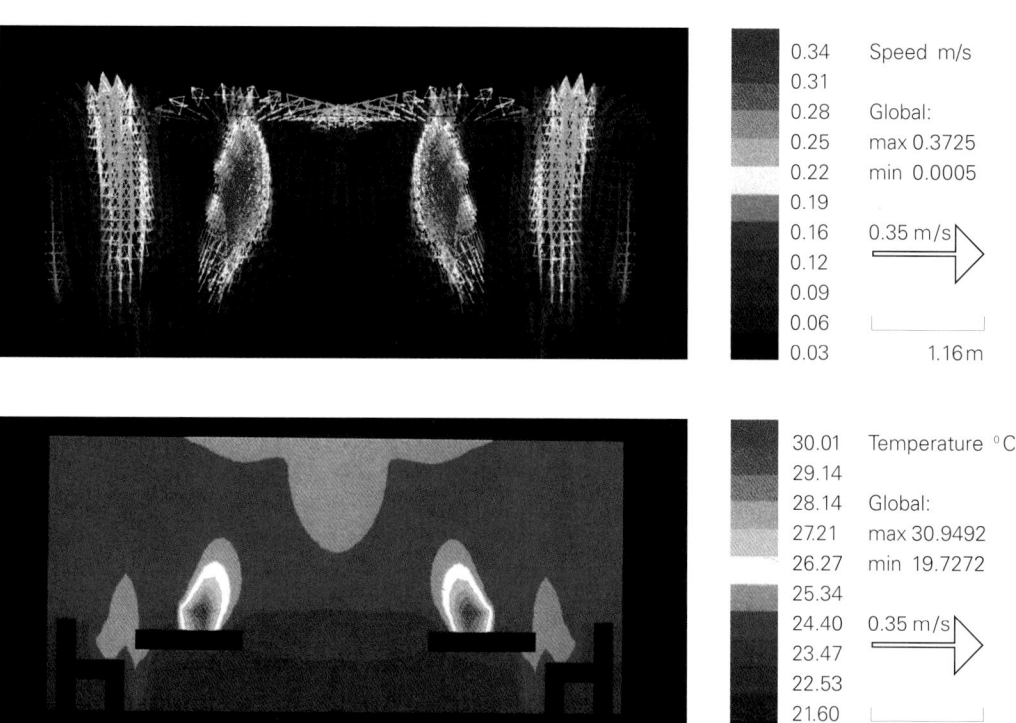

0.34	Speed m/s
0.31	
0.28	Global:
0.25	max 0.3725
0.22	min 0.0005
0.19	
0.16	0.35 m/s
0.12	
0.09	
0.06	
0.03	1.16 m

30.01	Temperature °C
29.14	
28.14	Global:
27.21	max 30.9492
26.27	min 19.7272
25.34	
24.40	0.35 m/s
23.47	
22.53	
21.60	
20.66	1.16 m

← CDF studies of the office environment.

climate on the internal environment. When the air temperature is below 20°C (68°F), the void of the double skin is closed so that the whole wall can provide a warm layer of air next to the inner glazed wall. In summer the void is ventilated at the top and bottom. Acting as a thermal flue, a flow of air is created to promote a cooler layer of air. This is supplemented by carefully designed solar control.

Within the 0.9m (3ft) wide zone are perforated maintenance walkways and binds with 4.5m (15ft) wide perforated blinds that can be lowered and tilted. The mechanism for raising and lowering the blinds is automatically controlled by a solarimeter that measures the intensity of solar radiation and a light sensor on the façade. A light sensor and thermostat are positioned inside the offices to control the inclination of the louvre blades. The louvres on either side of each given floor are controlled as a group. A full-size mock-up of the system was made and tested by the design team in collaboration with Technical Blinds and carefully integrated with the design of the building services. The shading and ventilation of the void was predicted to reduce peak summertime solar gain by two-thirds, in turn reducing peak cooling requirements. The floor-to-ceiling glazing on both external and atrium skins optimizes potential for day-lighting across the office floor plate. Electric lighting is designed to supple-ment the daylighting and provide a general lighting level of 400 lux.

Chilled ceilings

Reductions in solar gain permitted the use of chilled ceilings to deal with the office cooling loads. This is fairly standard practice today, but in the early 1990s, when Helicon was in the design phase, the integration of an intelligent skin with this kind of system was a design innovation. In 1992 Arup made comparative studies of heating and ventilation systems, highlighting the fact that, while the combination of chilled ceilings and underfloor heating was not the lowest cost alternative, other benefits would accrue from this system. Although fan-coil units were about 15 per cent cheaper, plant space required by chilled ceilings was about 50 per cent that of a conventional variable-air-volume system. Fan-coil units appeared to be higher maintenance than chilled ceilings, and the comparison also indicated that chilled ceilings could allow a 16 per cent saving in energy costs.

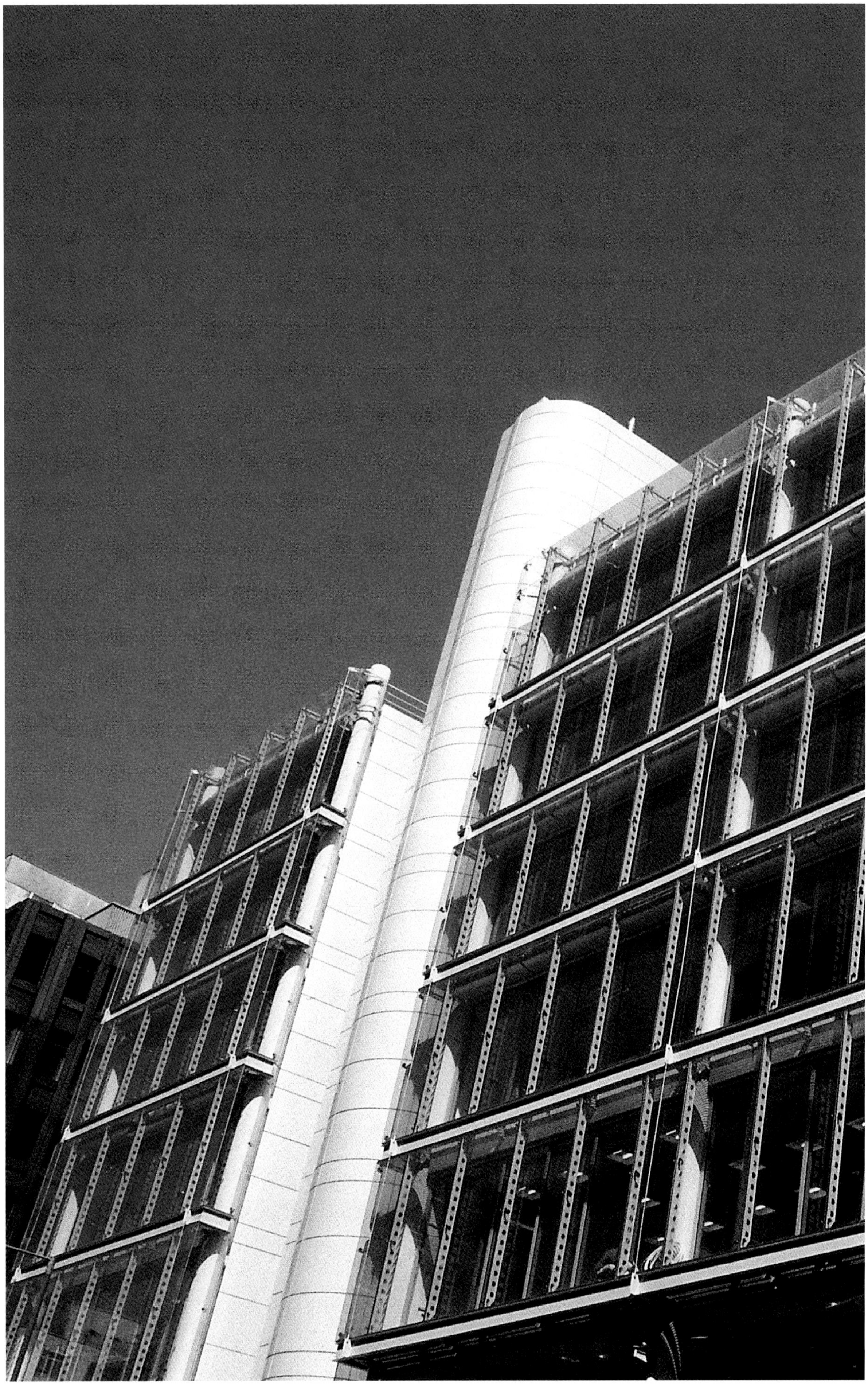

The ventilated façade means that solar gain is managed, despite maximizing glazing for daylight.

Delicate detailing of the envelope articulates the office entrance at the south-west corner.

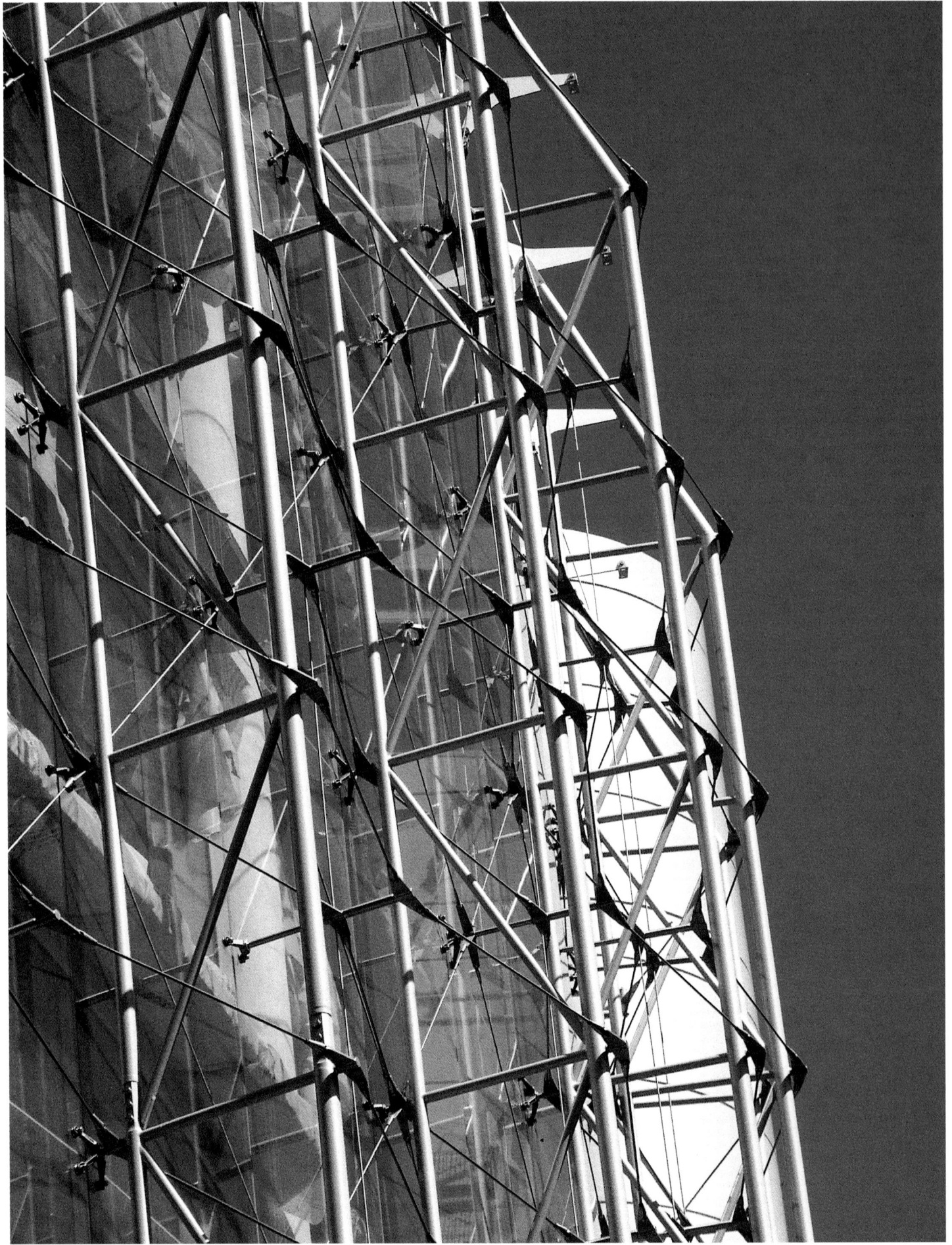

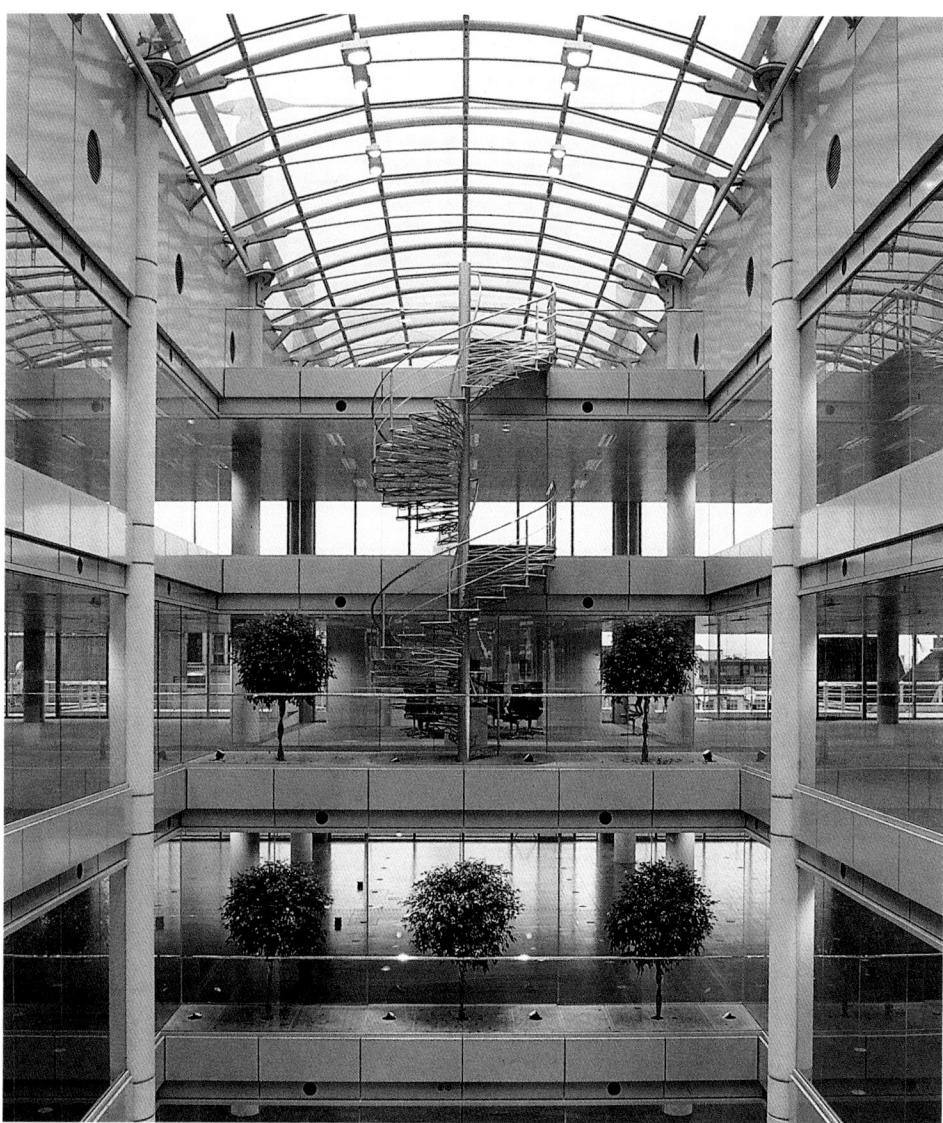

←
View across the
atrium to office
floors.

→
The building at night.
The articulation and
layering of the
external envelope
deals effectively with
the mass and bulk of
the block.

As chilled beams were considered by the design team to be visually intrusive, other options for chilled ceilings were investigated. Arup was not keen to use chilled ceiling panels that had to be clipped to the ceiling tiles, but just at that time a system was launched that incorporated demountable perforated metal ceiling tiles concealing flattened copper tubes with braided steel flexible connections to the chilled water supply. This is the system adopted in the building.

Air is supplied at 18°C (64°F) from under the floor at 2.5l/s/m² (0.0082ft³/s/ft) – approximately three air changes per hour– while the flow temperature to the chilled ceiling is 15°C (59°F). Computational flow design studies showed that the combination was enough to maintain the temperature at a summer maximum of 23°C (73°F), while the radiant effect of the ceiling would make the space more comfortable.

Plant and distribution

Although it would have been possible to tap into the heating and cooling network of the City of London – allowing what would have otherwise been plant-room space to be replaced by office space – this appeared to have little economic benefit, and the need for reliability persuaded the design team to opt for on-site plant. Chillers, boilers, switch rooms and tank rooms are located in the basement, while the landlord's generator, air-handling units and cooling towers are at roof level. Four vertical cores distribute services to the floors, and air is ducted from the risers to the pressurized floor plenum. The system demands that the building skin is tight and a strict leakage specification of 0.35l/sm² (0.0011ft³/s/ft²) at 50 Pa was set. Extract is via a similar plenum at high level as exhaust air through the luminaries. Air supplied is not 100 per cent fresh; up to 40 per cent is recirculated depending on the enthalpy of the outside air.

Conclusion

Helicon represents a milestone in the development of the sustainable urban office. The combination of intelligent skin and covered atrium allows the installation of efficient low-energy servicing systems and improved comfort for office workers. This marks a step function change in the design of the office building and represents a new stage towards the development of urban offices as producers, rather than consumers, of energy.

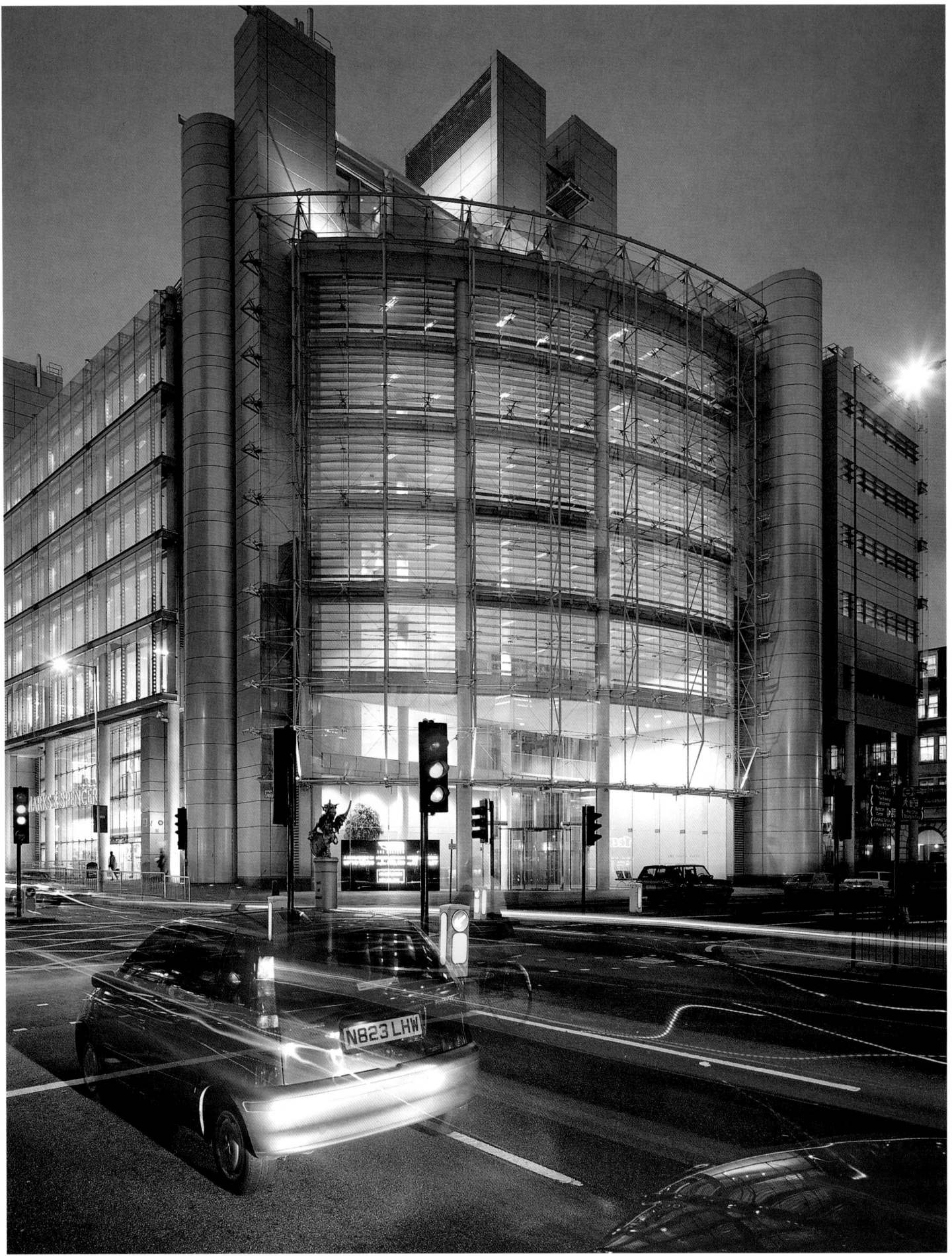

Villa VPRO Offices
MVRDV
Rotterdam, Netherlands
1997

The design of the workplace, particularly of the late 20th-century office, has been virtually reduced to a system based on 'shell, core and fit out'. Efficient in its use of space and with built-in ease of construction and servicing, the system is loved equally by developers and facilities managers – but all too often the result is neutral space that can be occupied by anyone but belongs to no one. Individuality is crushed and privacy is eroded. As Peter Davey has commented, 'the acres of hot-desking are as spiritually uplifting as a visit to the Gobi Desert, where grey sand is blown in your teeth and stuffs your nose'.[1]

Have architects done anything to improve the workplace? Only one or two examples spring to mind, among them Centraal Beheer at Apeldoorn by Herman Hertzberger (1973), where spaces in which individuals can work in isolation or as part of a community are arranged around communal pedestrian streets. The Dutch architectural tradition attaches more importance to real life than to theory. As might be expected, therefore, when a young firm of Dutch architects was commissioned to design a new workplace for a Dutch broadcaster, the traditional 'shell, core and fit out' system was not top of the agenda.

VPRO is an independent broadcasting company based in Hilversum which enjoys a reputation for high-quality television and radio programmes and is funded by voluntary subscriptions. Its popularity – reflected in increasing subscriber numbers – led VPRO in 1993 to decide to move to a purpose-built headquarters on a greenfield site in the grounds of the National Broadcasting Centre in Hilversum. The company originally operated from villa-type properties that, as a result of expansion, had become scattered across the city, with staff increasingly working in a variety of rooms, ranging from first-floor

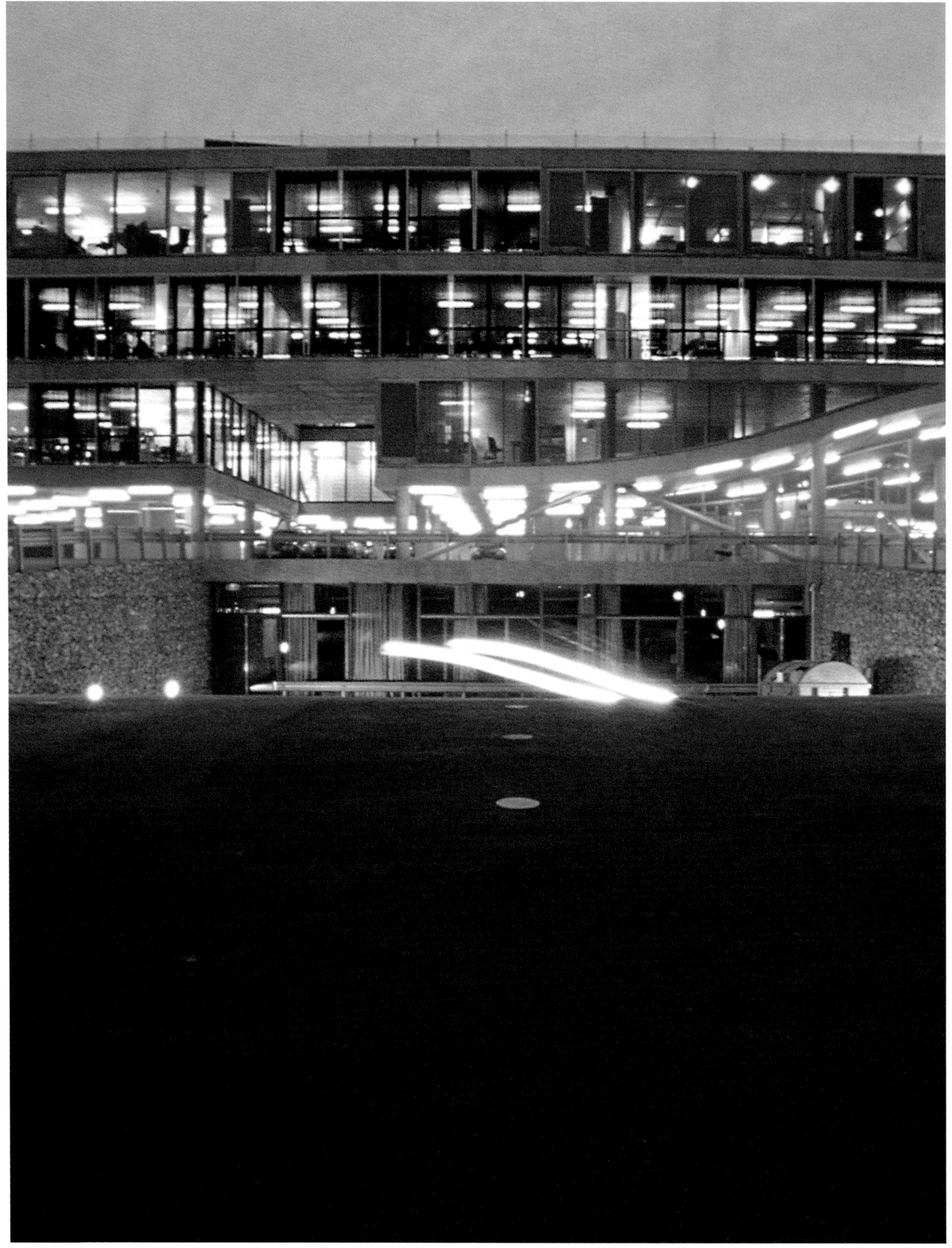

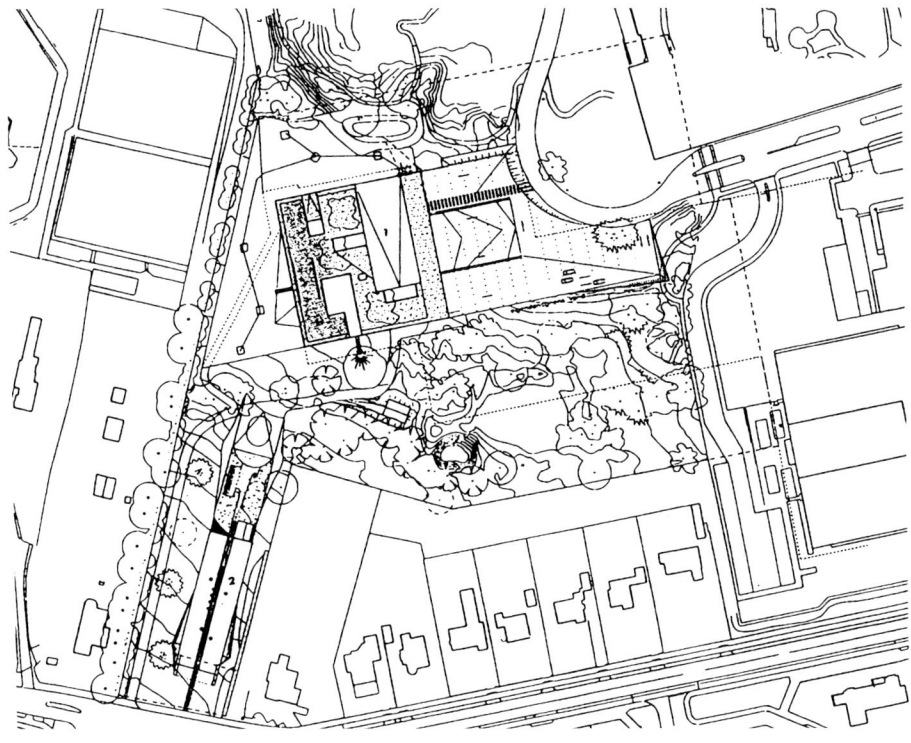

↑
Site plan showing the
56m by 56m (184ft by
184ft) building
amongst its
neighbours.

piani nobili to attics and sun lounges.
The villas had played a vital role in
establishing VPRO's identity.

Having decided to rationalize
operations in a single building on a
campus shared with other television
and broadcasting companies, VPRO
wondered how it could preserve its
accustomed workplace informality in
a modern office building. The brief
was that the new building should
evoke the spirit and atmosphere of the
villas without replicating them, and
allow informal and vital connections
between people inside and outside
the organization to be re-created.
The main activities at VPRO are
programme research and design,
radio broadcasting, programme
editing, central archiving and
customer services. Through research
by MVRDV and extensive discussion
with the company and individual staff,

the original standard headquarters
building brief was revised, and the
concept of the 'big villa' emerged
from a holistic approach.

Site and context
The idea of the 'big villa' was
compromised by a number of site
constraints. Zoning and height
restrictions meant that the building
had to be developed in very compact
form. The result is a five-storey
building, 9,000m² (96,840ft²) in area
with a footprint of 56m by 56m (184ft
by 184ft) – thought to be the deepest
office plan in the Netherlands. It is
hard to determine the relationship
between the new VPRO building and
the surrounding villas. The site
constraints and strict building codes
forced MVRDV to develop informal
and intimate interconnecting spaces
by subtracting from the deep plan,

rather than by the more obvious step
of additive pavilion-type structures.
The building is partly recessed into its
hilly site to stay within height
restrictions.

Building form and organization
Differences between the inside and
outside of the building have been
blurred by what is called 'precision
bombing', which has produced a
number of deep shafts and slits in the
plan, enabling spaces to flow into
each other and connect.[2] The
distinction between different levels is
also unusual in that the conventional
orthogonal floor plates are stepped
and ramped. The building is entered at
first-floor level via a sloping
landscaped car park that continues as
the first-floor slab into the building
and then folds back on itself to form
the second floor. These folding floor

↓

Sections of the
building: south–north
(top) and east–west.

→

Floor plans: (from
bottom to top, left
to right) basement;
ground; second;
third; fourth; and
fifth.

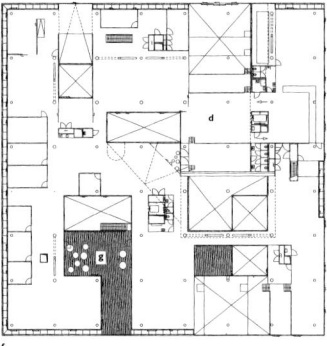
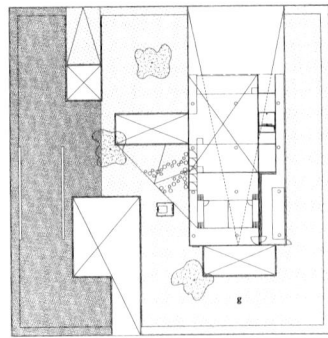
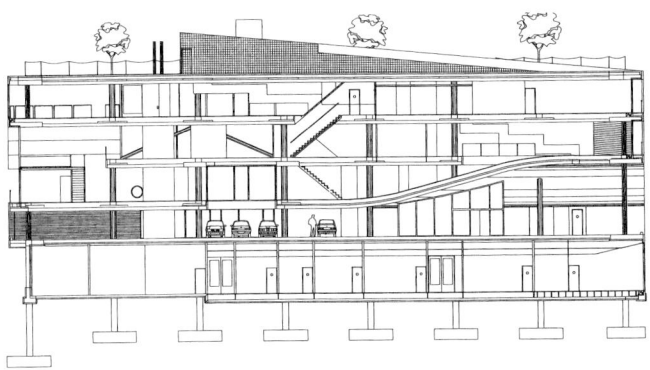
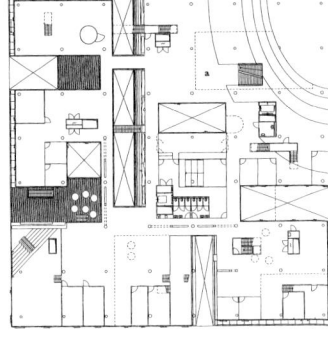
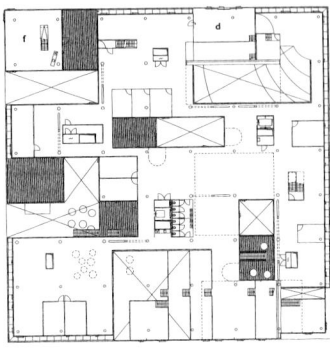
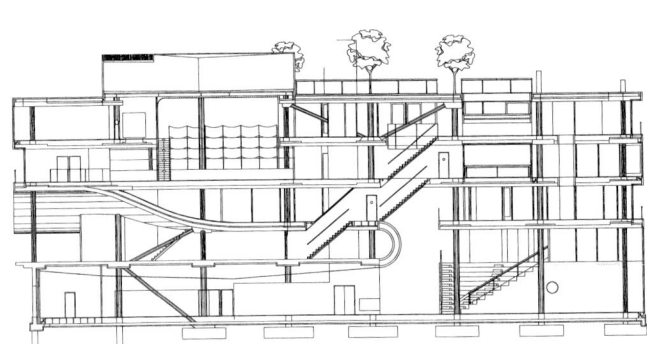
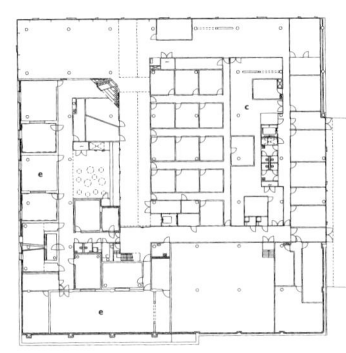
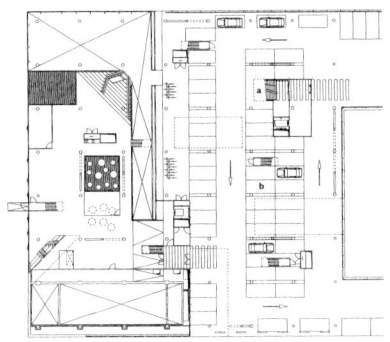

plates form a relatively continuous interior space incorporating hills, ramps, stairs and small faults negotiated by small flights of steps, offering as wide (if not wider) a range of spaces as that enjoyed in the original villas.

The car park runs under the porch framed by the canopy of the folded slab, and the main entrance to the building is through a glass box that sits in the car park occupying most of the plan at that level. The entrance 'is neither welcoming nor even immediately obvious. It's just that there can be nowhere else to go.'[3] From here visitors have to negotiate either Dutch 'stepladder' stairs or lift to reach the double-height reception area.

Structure and materials

Arup's VPRO structure is principally a reinforced-concrete floor slab supported on an orthogonal grid of circular columns. The grid is 7.5m by 7.5m (25ft by 25ft); while this integrates with the car park, the wide variety of workspaces is not determined by a regular planning grid. The system was chosen because it offered maximum flexibility in terms of the deformation and stopping of floor plates and the creation of voids. The fact that the two-way spanning slab could be cantilevered, cut, slotted and folded without using beam elements was put to maximum use. The floor-slab profile is expressed externally and the twists, turns and steps in the building can be read on all four elevations. Beams were confined to spaces such as the stepping restaurant. The vertical part of the folded plate acts as a beam as well as a wall in this condition. Steel cruciform shear heads are embedded

in the slabs at each column/floor junction and column up-stand shear heads are also used to enable slab thickness to be minimized. As well as limiting overall floor-to-floor heights, the spatial compression of the folded slab is accentuated. Columns are not permitted through voids. In the situation where the void is a double-grid width the two deep-transfer beams are employed at roof level and these become part of the urban landscape at this level.

The building form at Villa VPRO eliminated the traditional cores and the structural stability they provide in skeletal office buildings, so stability was added through the development of structural steel tube stability braces; these appear to be distributed randomly around the building but they transfer wind loads from one floor to the next. The floor plate then

159

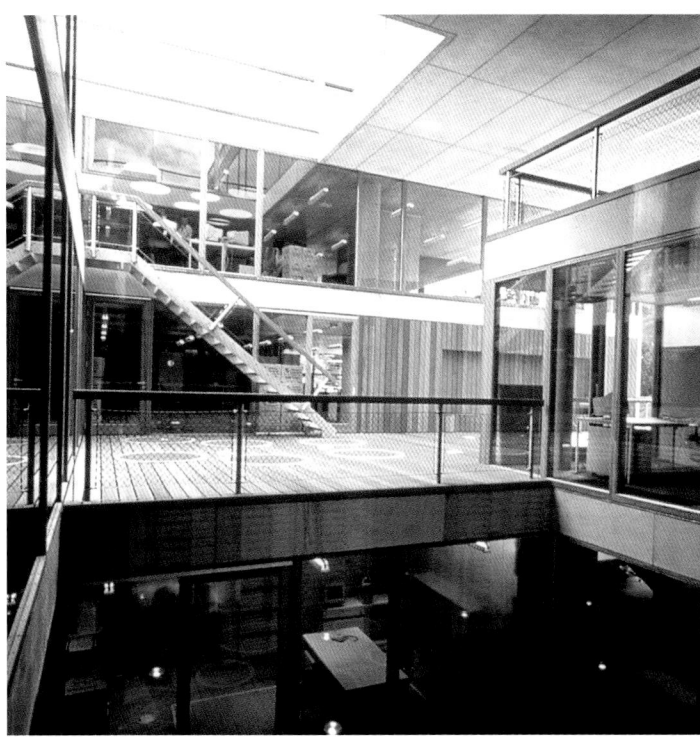

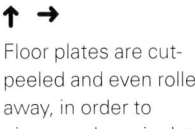

Floor plates are cut-peeled and even rolled away, in order to pierce and manipulate what would otherwise be a very deep plan.

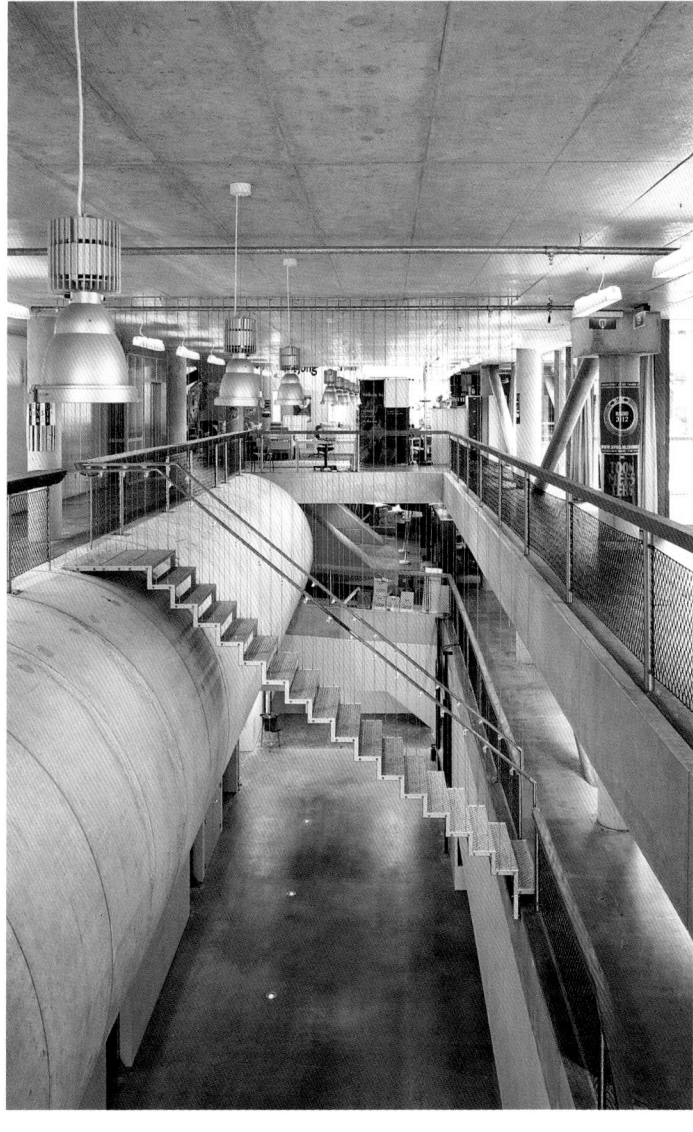

distributes these forces to the next layer of braces on the level below. Such a system provides a high degree of flexibility when it comes to where to position bracing; visible bracing is placed around floor plates in order to open or close vistas, or to create visual elements that are severe or dynamic and dissonant.

To enable the structural topography to be expressed externally, façades are almost entirely glazed. Thirty-five types and colours of glass are used to deal with solar gain and thermal performance. Each particular type of glass is matched to its place and orientation, and supplemented with fixed and dynamic shading, balcony overhangs, blinds and plants. The result is a vivid geometry (especially when seen at night) that creates an exciting mosaic matching the dynamic of the building's interior.

Environment and services

Villa VPRO meets the Dutch regulations for office spaces regarding natural lighting and the requirement for all work stations to be within 5m (16ft) of a view. The building mass is cut, slotted, scooped and 'kebab'd' to provide slots for air and light. Nearly every office has access though a door to a patio, garden, terrace or balcony, and the distinction between inside and outside is constantly subdued even in the middle of the building. The primary aim of providing a wide variety of spatial settings for work is met by these formal moves but this strategy sets new challenges for the environmental designer.

Studies using both physical and computational models were carried out by Arup and DGMR to establish daylight conditions, façade heat gains

and losses, internal and external shading, and acoustics. These studies were part of an interactive process and helped to establish the final form, position and geometry of voids. Arup adopted a number of servicing approaches to support the multitude of different spaces and workplace configurations, and at the same time to minimize the visual impact of services. Given that the folded concrete slab leading people through the interior was a key concept of the design, it was not an option to adopt the conventional discreet distribution of services through suspended ceilings. Exposed concrete surfaces to floor and ceilings could not be cluttered with service ducts. Maximum use was therefore made of natural ventilation in spaces close to the envelope edge.

In most parts of the plan a raised floor plenum delivers conditioned air

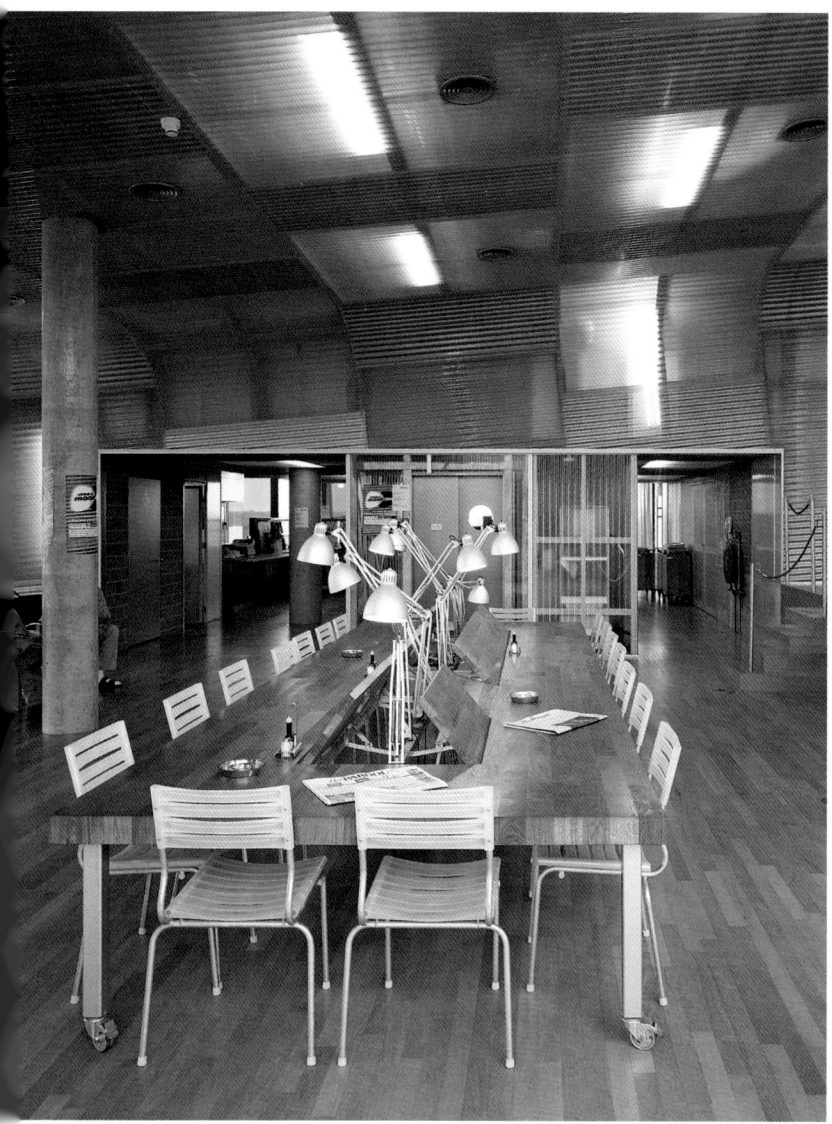

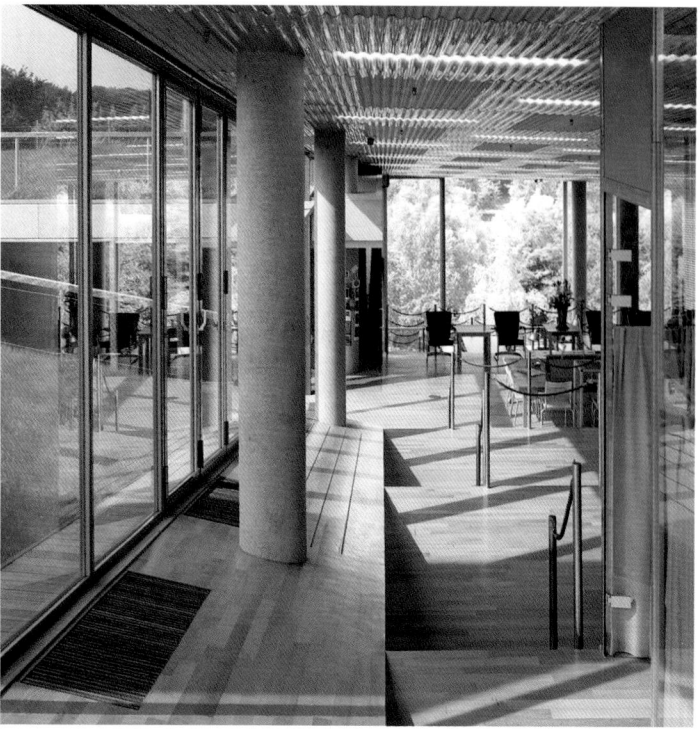

←↑
A wide range of
working contexts and
environments are
available for the
building users.

to the spaces, while in areas such as the restaurants and studio dedicated air-handling units deal with the higher loads demanded by increased ventilation rates. Editing suites incorporate chilled beams to complement the optimized fresh air delivered from the main air-handling units. The pedestal-type raised floor has a solid screed finish, and the void was used for power and communications distribution as well as a plenum.

The irregular floor plates, each with their particular and peculiar floor voids, present challenges for the integration of services. Discontinuity and remote spaces were a special problem. The building is designed with six principal risers carefully situated to deliver services to all areas of the building. Service runs are therefore minimized and the floor void

is optimized. The complexity of form over the deep plan means that the challenge of service rationalization and distribution is extended to the design of drainage above ground.

Conclusion
In the work of MVDRV the demands of programme, once defined, are cast in stone through their method of 'systematic realization'.[4] These programmatic constraints and the strict Dutch regulations have been applied to the letter at Villa VPRO to generate a bewildering variety of spaces. In the hands of an engineer and environmental designer not in tune with each space, this complex situation could result in chaos. At VPRO the system of 'shell, core and fit out' has not been abandoned entirely but intelligently modified to accommodate the spatial complexity

while providing an appropriate system of structural and environmental support. Villa VPRO may be regarded as characteristic of the architecture of the emerging global age and christened by some as 'Supermodernism'.[5] In the Dutch tradition of the nondescript box with a spatially complex inner world, the building challenges preconceived ideas about the workplace but is not as cold and scenographic as, say, the work of Rem Koolhaas.

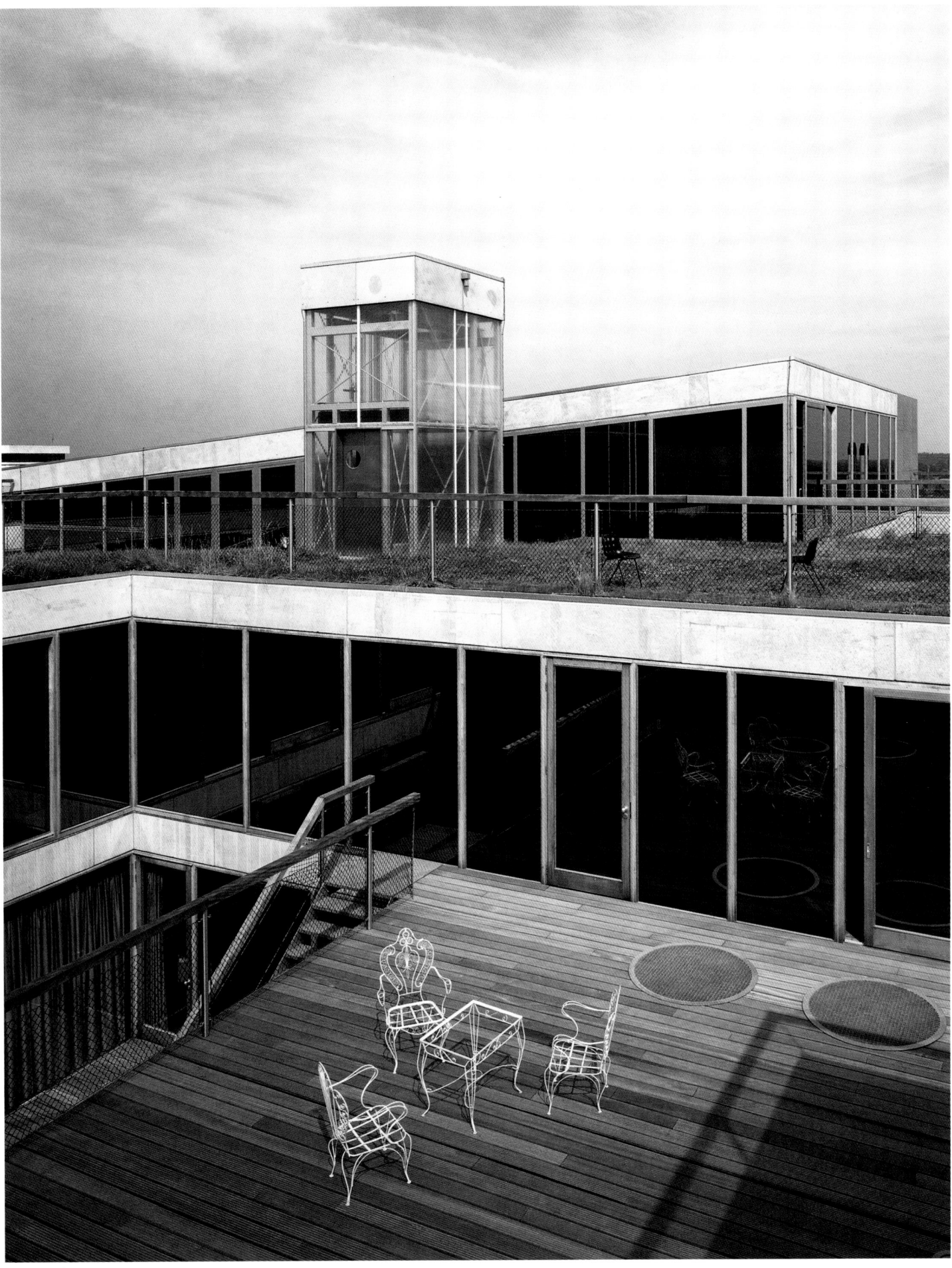

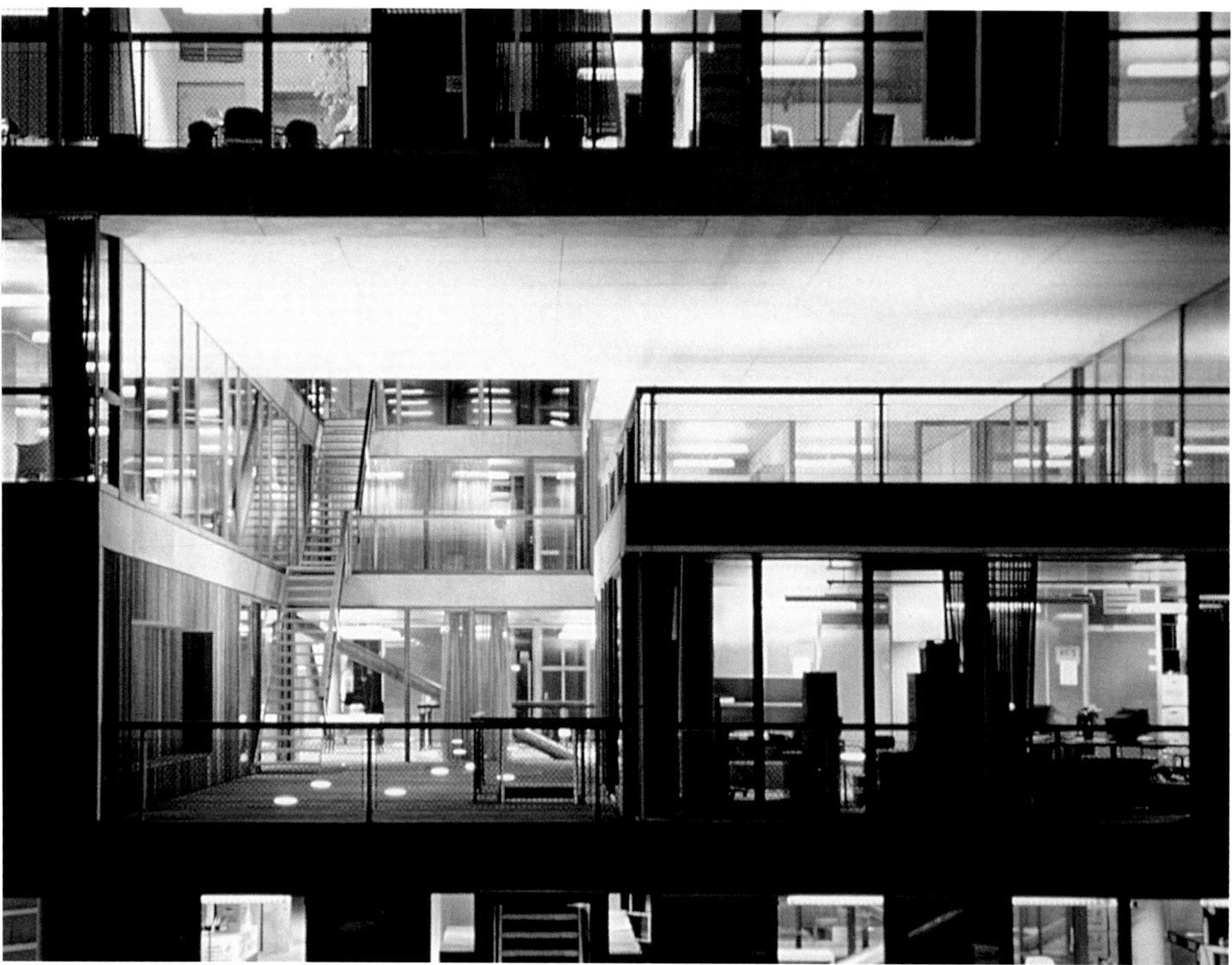

←

The roof is an integral part of the promenade.

↑

Façade detail showing how the building form has been manipulated to ensure inhabitants have access to daylight and views.

Beyeler Foundation Museum

Renzo Piano
Riehen, Basel
Switzerland
1997

➜

The 'intelligent' roof
of the Beyeler
Foundation Museum,
at the southern
approach to the
building.

The first art galleries were private affairs. Pictures collected by wealthy men were displayed in private salons for personal pleasure and enjoyment and to impress a close circle of friends and acquaintances. The first buildings providing public access often resembled what Tom Markus has described as 'a safe well-lit warehouse'.[1] Since then the art gallery has evolved, often to meet the environmental conditions demanded by the conservation of fragile but valuable artefacts. The gallery has incrementally been reduced to more of a safe warehouse and the designer's role is now often confined

to exercises in formal excess in order to signify that here lies culture accompanied by some new image of civitas. To challenge the technical migration of the gallery towards the scenographic and exclusive mode of environmental control and head back towards a selective functional tradition requires the marriage of a particular client with a particular collection and a design team with the technical wherewithal.

The Beyeler Foundation Museum was designed and constructed to house the private collection of modern art belonging to Ernst Beyeler. The collection was built up

over a long period and consists of about 180 paintings, ranging from works by Monet to recent East German art. It includes works by Cézanne, Matisse, Picasso, Klee, Kandinsky, Rauschenberg and Lichtenstein, as well as sculptures by Giacometti and pieces from Easter Island and Oceania. International awareness of the collection was sparked by exhibitions in Madrid's Centro Reina Sofia, and a purpose-built gallery in Switzerland to house the collection was proposed. Ernst Beyeler wanted a naturally lit environment of calm and repose. In 1981 Dominique de Menil had

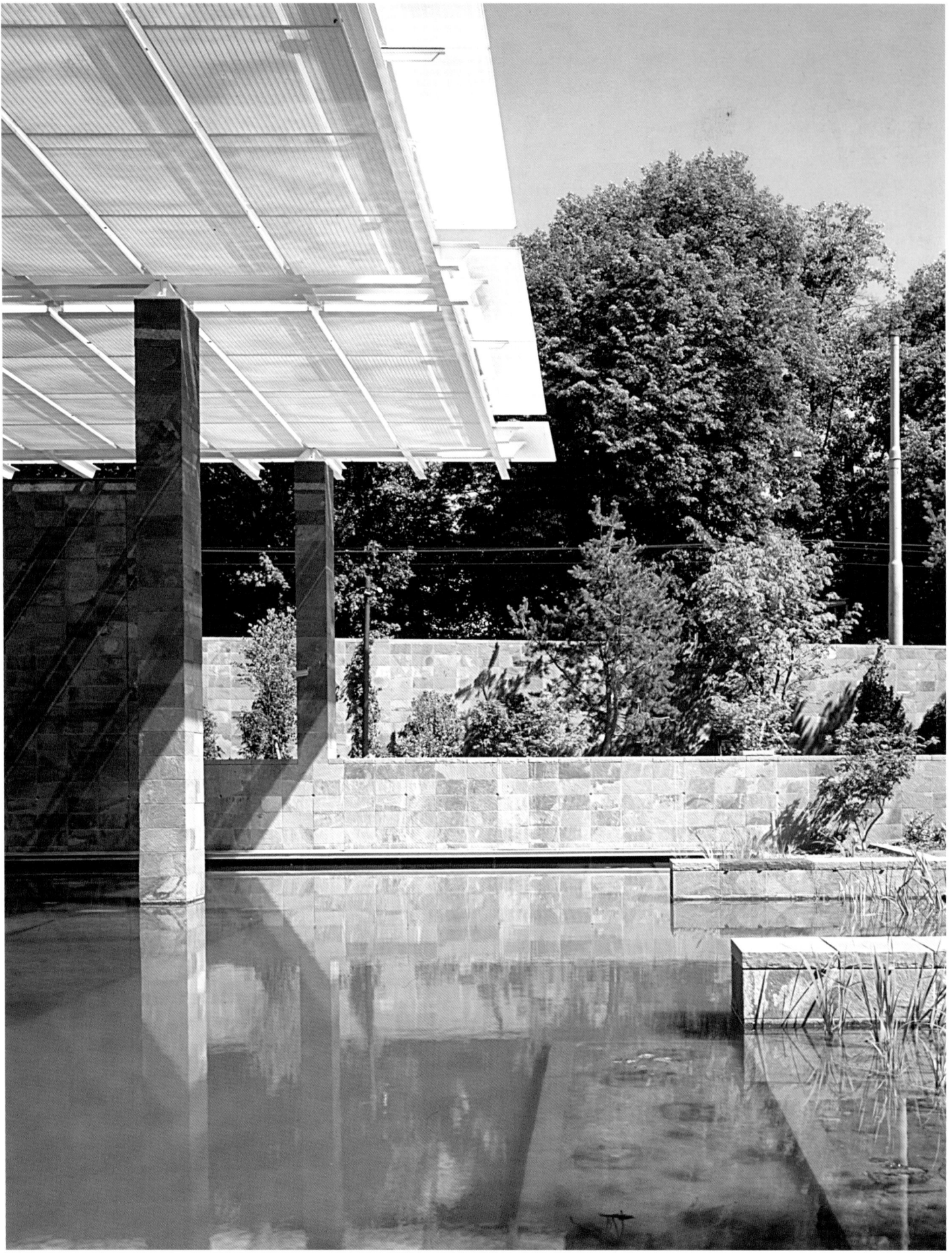

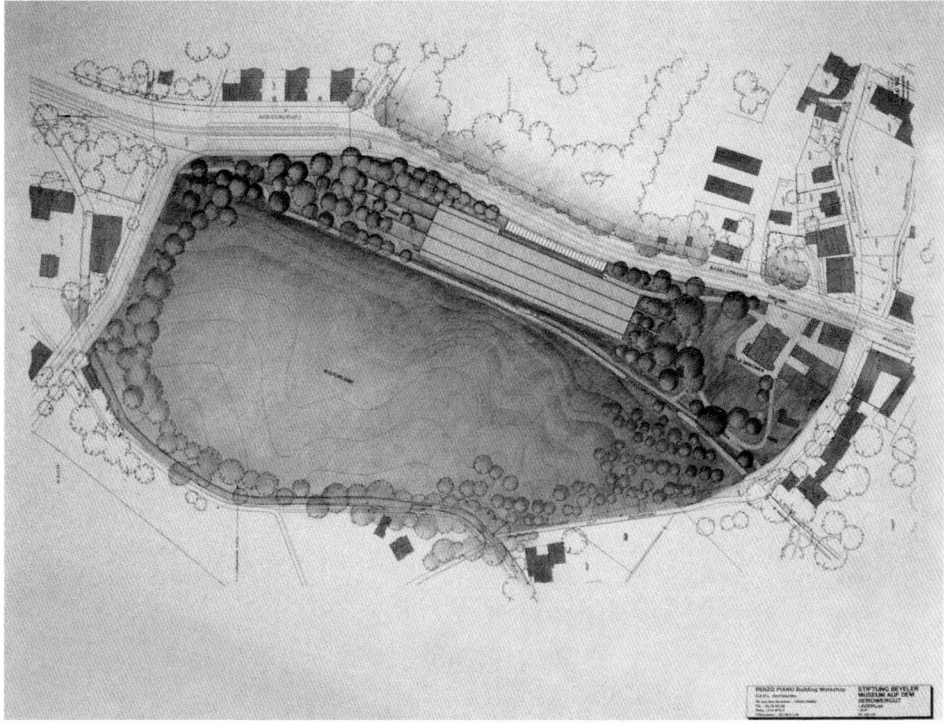

↑
Site plan: the gallery
runs parallel to the
north–south road.

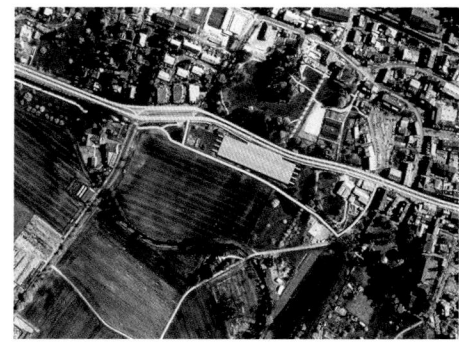

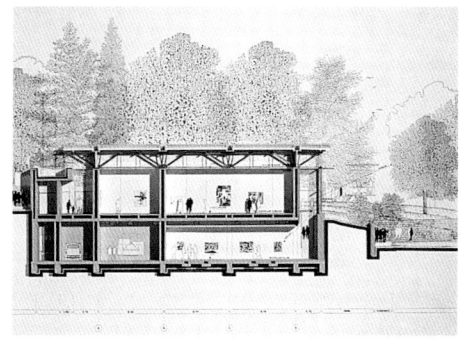

↑
Aerial photography
and sectional model
show buffering and
containment of site.

entrusted Renzo Piano with the design of a new museum in Houston for the Menil Collection (see pages 174–181), one of the most important corpuses of surrealist and primitive African art. The idea was to create a non-monumental space open to contact with nature, facilitating a direct and relaxed relationship between visitor and artefact. Piano's solution – based on the design of daylit spaces under a sheltering roof that filtered the sky – was the inspiration for Beyeler. Impressed by the tranquil spaces of the Menil and determined to display his collection in natural light wherever possible, Beyeler asked his design team to create a protective lightweight canopy for the galleries which would modulate the effects of the sky and hover over the walls that the art is exhibited on.

Site

Riehen is an affluent suburb of Basel near the German border. The museum site is in parklike grounds that extend northwards along a road leading from the 18th-century Villa Berower. The entrance to both is marked by gates that stand opposite a tram terminus. Once inside the gates, visitors may enter the villa, which now houses the museum bookshop, cafeteria and offices, or walk on to the museum.

The new museum is designed as a pavilion running 120m (395ft) south–north from the villa and parallel to the road. The narrow rectangular plan is contained between a new boundary wall to the road and an existing stone retaining wall that runs alongside a path on the eastern edge of the park. The building offers a calm haven in which to study art and enjoy the views of the countryside to the west.

Form and layout

The form of the gallery is determined by long parallel walls running north–south which are expressed externally but disintegrate and break down internally. The 7.5m (25ft) wide space between the walls accommodates gallery spaces. Entry through the existing garden is along a path between boundary walls on the southern edge of the building. Here the ends of the 700mm (27½in) wide parallel walls are expressed below a great oversailing roof as they run beyond glazed openings to the galleries. This striated layering has been described as providing a 'view inwards...like an X-ray, cutting through this southerly elevation deep into the gallery space and the precious works of art'.[2] An angled boundary on the northern side of the building channels visitors towards the

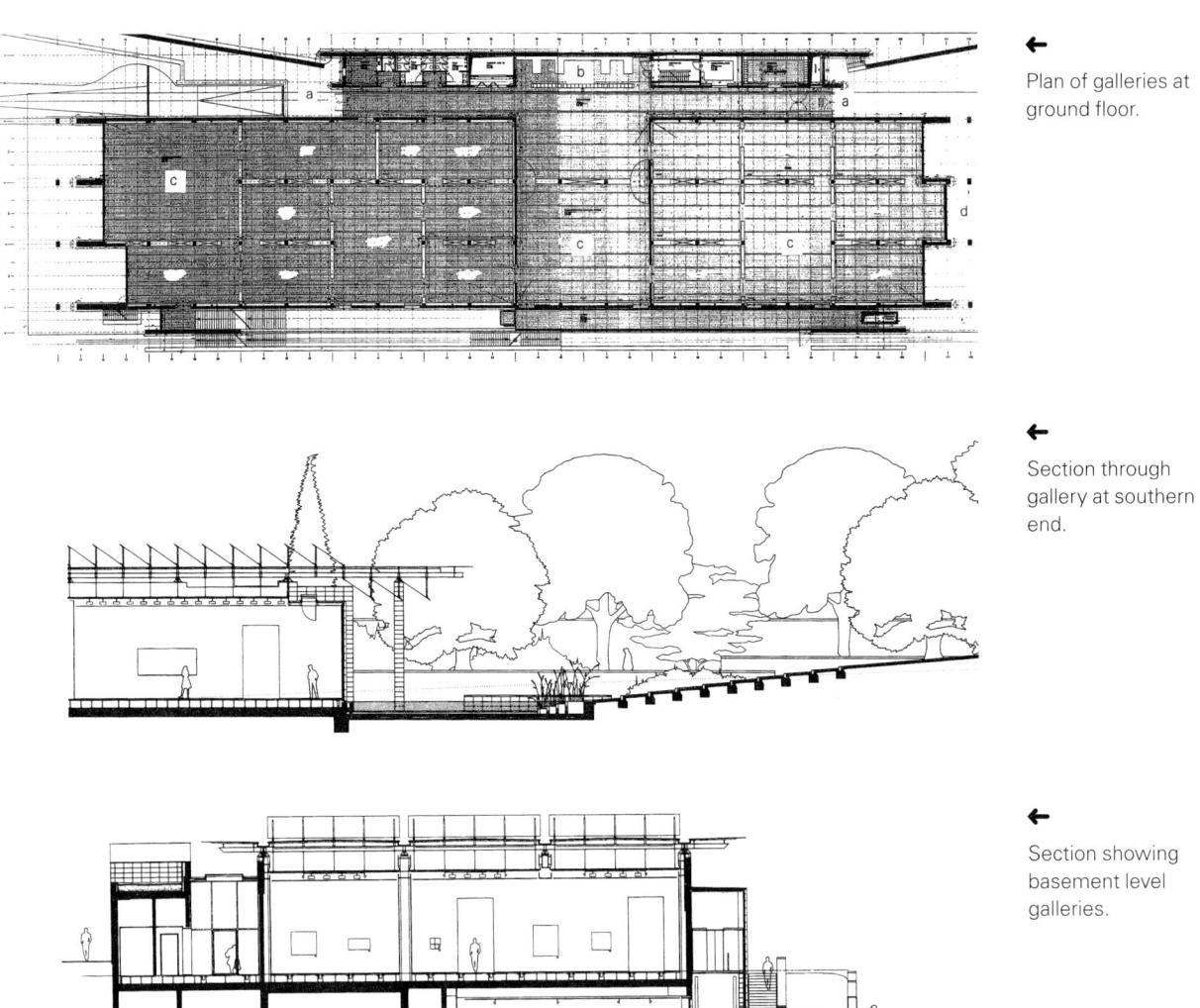

←

Plan of galleries at
ground floor.

←

Section through
gallery at southern
end.

←

Section showing
basement level
galleries.

entrance. On this side there is a
secondary set of doors and a
vehicular ramp that leads to the
basement storey, which provides
accommodation for staff car parking,
loading, storage space, workshops,
plant rooms and an artificially lit
gallery for light-sensitive works.

The lightweight oversailing roof
canopy contrasts with the apparent
heavyweight archaic walls,
emphasizing the distinction between
'tectonic' and 'stereotomic' elements.
The walls are interrupted and broken
in order to provide a range of gallery
spaces, typically 12m by 7.2m (39ft by
24ft) punctuated with larger exhibition
spaces of 7.2m by 18m (24ft by 59ft)
and 15.1m by 18m (50ft by 59ft).

Structure and construction
The lineal pavilion is constructed over
a 4.3m (14ft) deep reinforced-concrete

basement. The walls of the galleries
are not structural but they contain
reinforced-concrete columns at 6m
(20ft) centres to support the roof. Roof
overhangs are supported by steel
columns also encased in stone. The
four long walls, spaced at 7.8m (26ft)
centres, each 108m (354ft) long and
6.1m (20ft) high, sit under a
lightweight crystalline roof canopy
28.3m by 127m (93ft by 417ft) on plan.

The steel roof structure gives
continuous support for the various
glass layers, comprising glass ceiling
and internal louvres, double-glazing,
and the posts that carry the external
inclined glass shading. Primary
beams span continuously from east to
west, while the secondary beams are
arranged in pairs on either side of the
columns, spanning 6m (20ft) in the
north–south direction. Additional
primary beams spanning north–south

on the main column lines create
longer exhibition spaces. The 250mm
(10in) deep beams, formed from steel
plates, are carefully detailed. Primary
beams have a box section with the
flanges projecting outside the webs,
so that their appearance is similar to
that of the fabricated 'I' sections used
for the secondary beams. The beam
and column connections are also
carefully configured. Using steel
castings and bolts, the continuity of
construction is broken on the centre
line of the column. Forces and
moments are transferred from inside
to outside structural elements but
cold-bridging is eliminated by the
physical separation of the elements.

The complex roof construction is
completed by white glass *brise-soleil*,
supported on vertical steel tubular
posts bolted to the top of beams on
site with steel castings. Steel castings

167

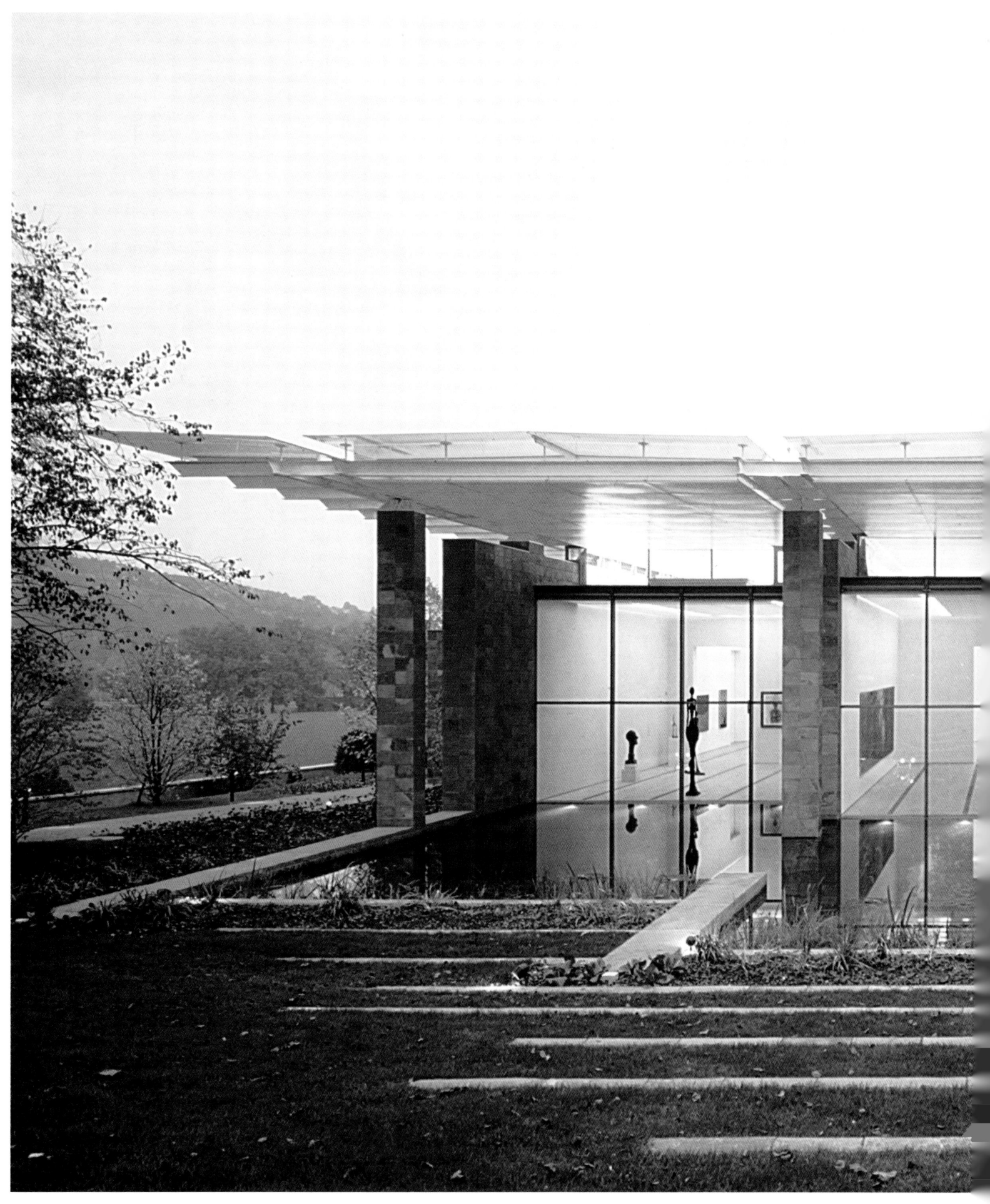

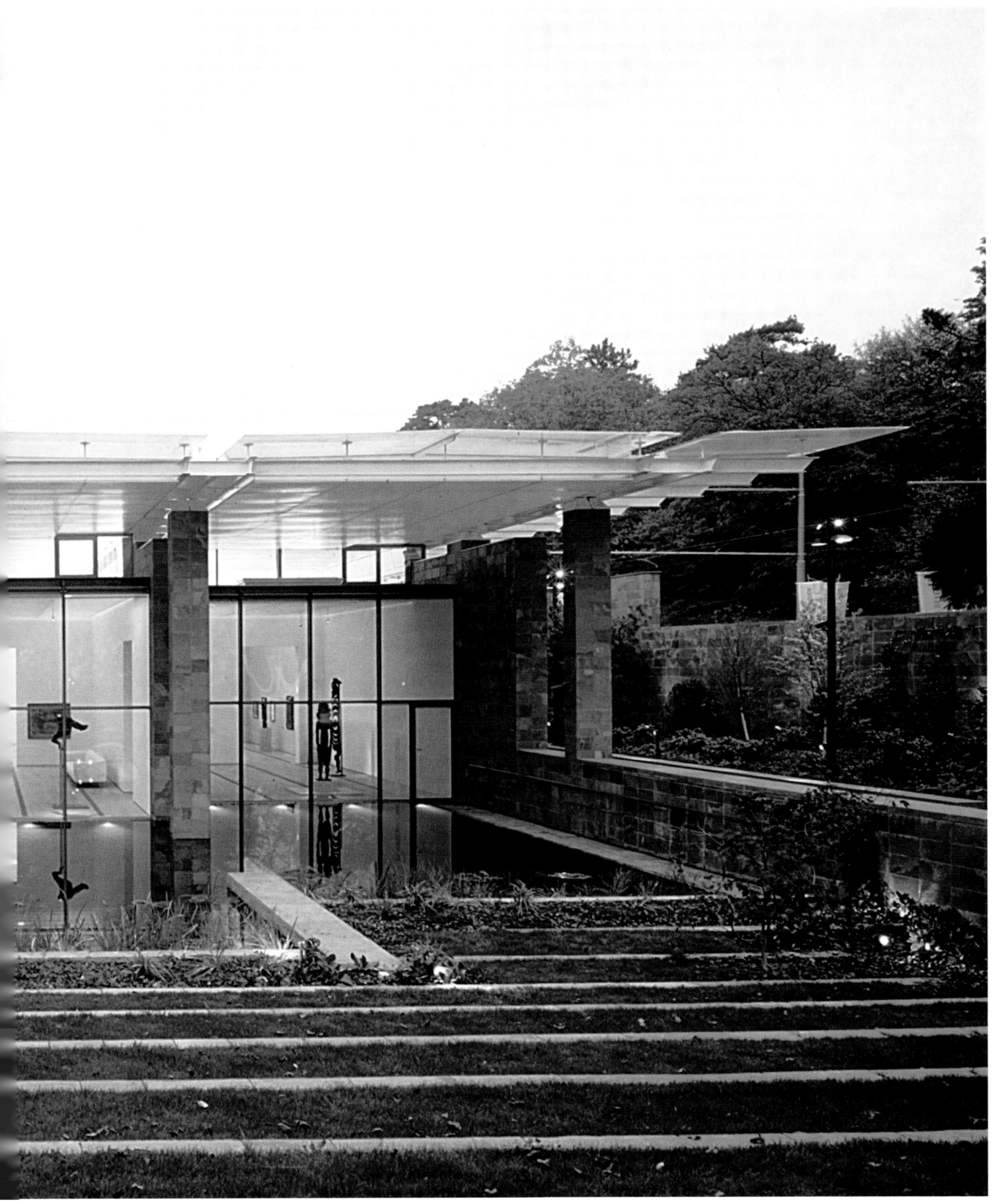

The approach to the building from the south, exposing the clear tectonic of the structure.

→ Looking south, out to the lily pond.

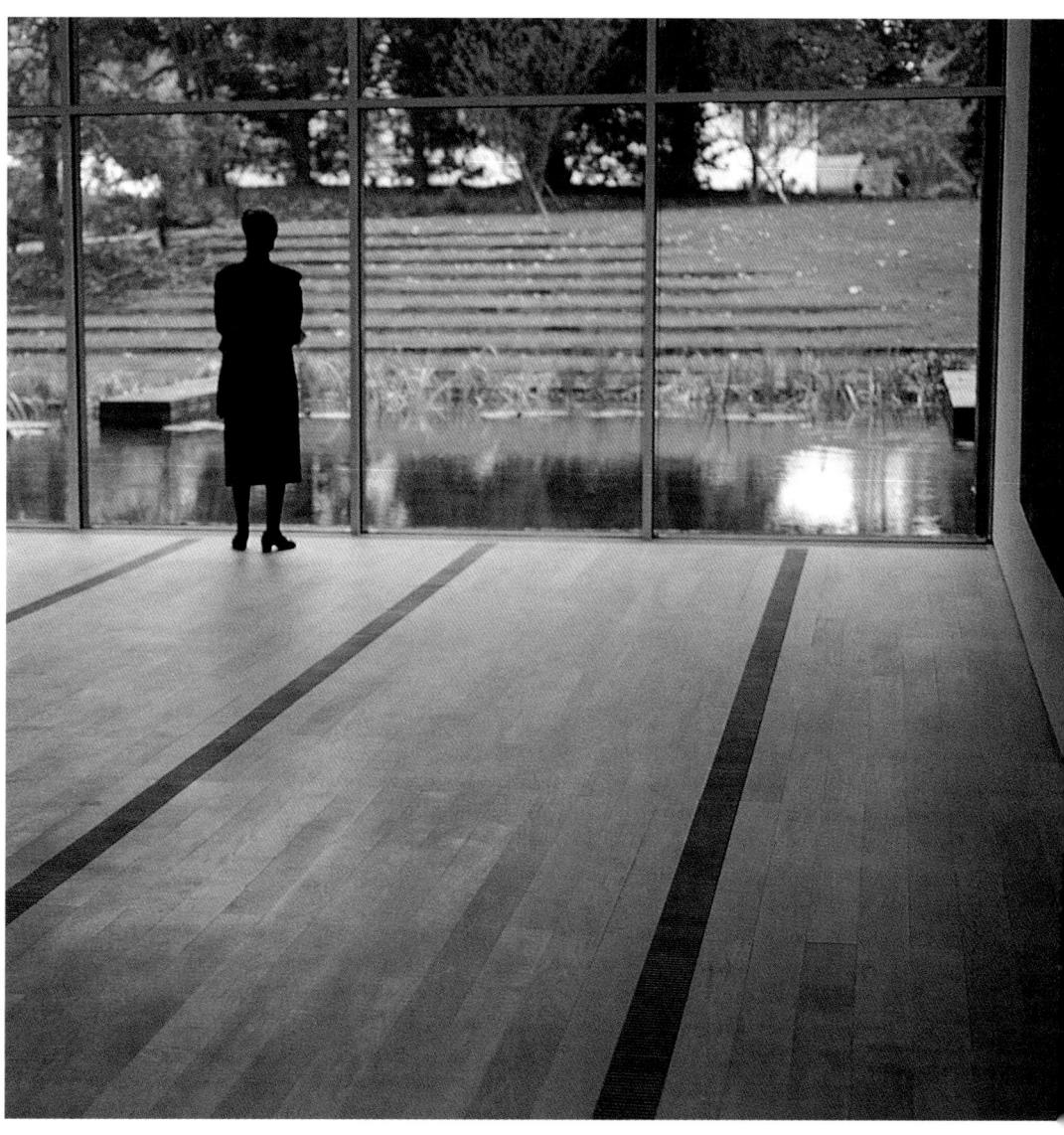

are also used at the top of the posts to fix the *brise-soleil*. These top-bolted connections allow glass to slide parallel to glass, but also to take wind loads perpendicular to the glass so that differential deflections of the beams supporting the top and bottom of the plane of glass do not induce high stresses into it. The structure was designed to Swiss building codes to accommodate relatively high snow loading; as the building also lies within a seismic zone, horizontal forces are limited to around 7 per cent of the total vertical loads.

Visual environment

Ernst Beyeler had seen the Menil building in Houston designed by Piano and Arup and was committed to securing the same qualities of daylight in his museum as those at the Menil. It was agreed that daylight should be used as the light source across the whole ground floor, and that the design of the building should seek to maximize the number of hours during which the collection could be viewed by daylight. However, best-practice standards for exposure of works of art to daylight in terms of time, levels and spectral content could not be compromised by the desire to provide a daylit environment.

Following studies of lighting conditions in Basel, Arup recommended a target daylight factor of 4 per cent, which is around double that in most European galleries. An active shading system to control internal light levels within predetermined limits, particularly on bright summer days, was also prescribed as an essential part of the lighting strategy. These performance requirements were met by the development of a universal multi-layered roof. The outermost element is the layer of fitted glass brise-soleil inclined and positioned to prevent direct sun penetration during all museum opening times but also to maintain optimum admittance of diffused light. Below this lies the weatherproof layer consisting of a double-glazed skin with an ultraviolet filter that removes those parts of the electromagnetic spectrum most likely to damage the paintings to be displayed on the ground floor of the museum. Immediately below this layer are computer-motorized aluminium louvre blades that control light levels in each room of the museum. These levels can be arranged to suit the management of the building and the conservation of the collection. When the museum is closed, for example, the louvres are

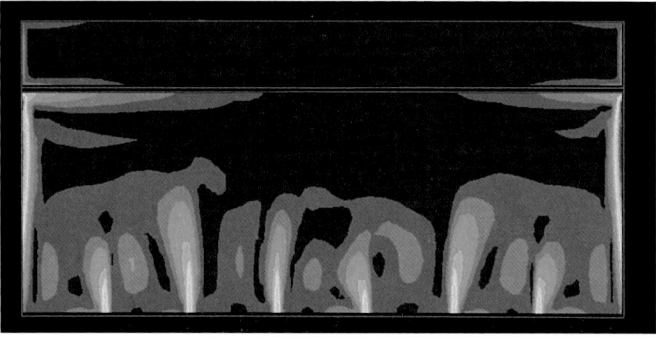

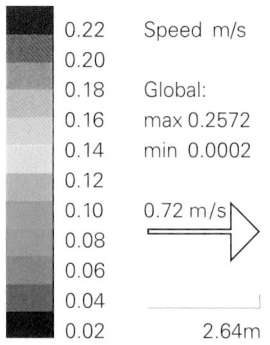

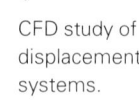

CFD study of displacement systems.

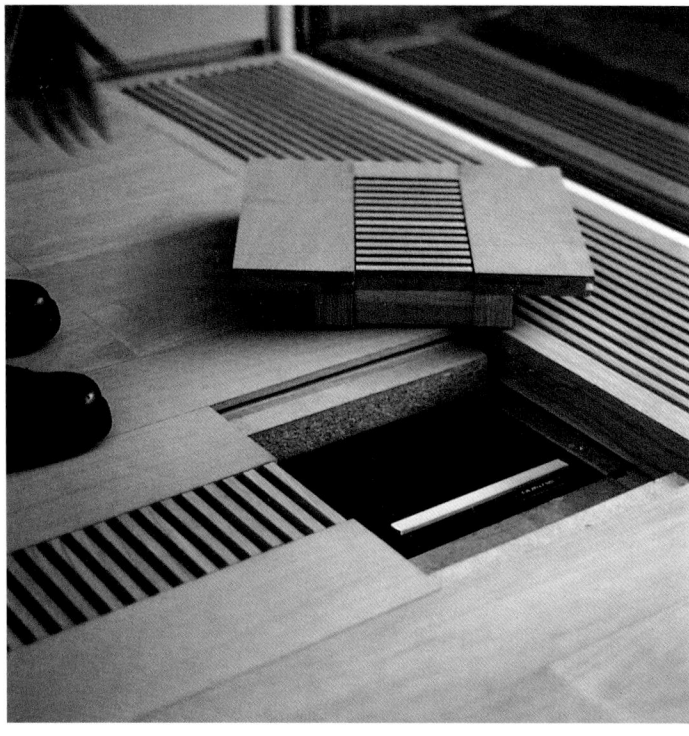

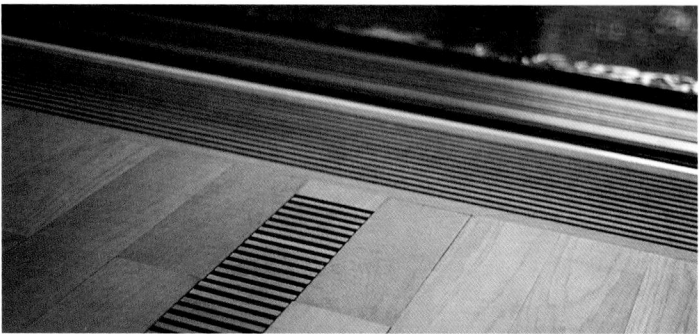

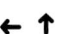

Air is delivered at low velocity through carefully integrated floor grilles.

closed to prevent exposure of artworks to daylight.

The louvre system lies in the zone between ceiling and roof, which is designed as a 'loft thermal buffer zone'[3] and combines with the external *brise-soleil* to prevent 98 per cent of incident solar radiation from reaching the gallery spaces below. The lower boundary of the loft is formed by a laminated-glass ceiling designed to support maintenance access to the louvre-blind motors and electric illumination in the loft. The electric illumination is designed to complement the daylighting strategy: as daylight fades, triphosphor linear fluorescent fittings gradually compensate for the loss, contributing to the maintenance of ideal lighting levels. The lowest layer in the system forms the visible ceiling of the ground-floor galleries: a grid of perforated-

metal panels incorporates a paper that diffuses light once more and adds a layer of opacity to the contents of the 'loft thermal buffer zone'. The uniform lighting system is augmented by small low-voltage spotlights positioned on stems at the junctions of each ceiling panel. These can add high-lighting and directional light essential for modelling effects of sculpture.

Energy and environment

Thermal buffer spaces extend from the roof to the east and west sides of the façade, helping to limit the effects of climatic extremes on the building (-11°C (12°F) in winter, 33°C (91°F) in summer). The heated and ventilated loft means that, despite the 100 per cent glazed roof, perimeter heating is needed only in the north and southernmost galleries. The east façade is climatically buffered by the

service and ancillary rooms, and to the west the 'winter garden' performs the same task, as well as providing a resting place with views across the countryside.

These buffer zones help to reduce reliance on mechanical systems – particularly important in Switzerland, where air conditioning is strongly discouraged in line with the national policy to abandon development of nuclear power and to reduce the country's reliance on predominantly nuclear-generated power from France. Regulatory frameworks therefore focus on the reduction of energy demand. In the case of this particular building type, a 'statement of need' must be submitted to the local authority that justifies the requirement for mechanical systems. The case for the Beyeler – based on the intention to display, conserve and

171

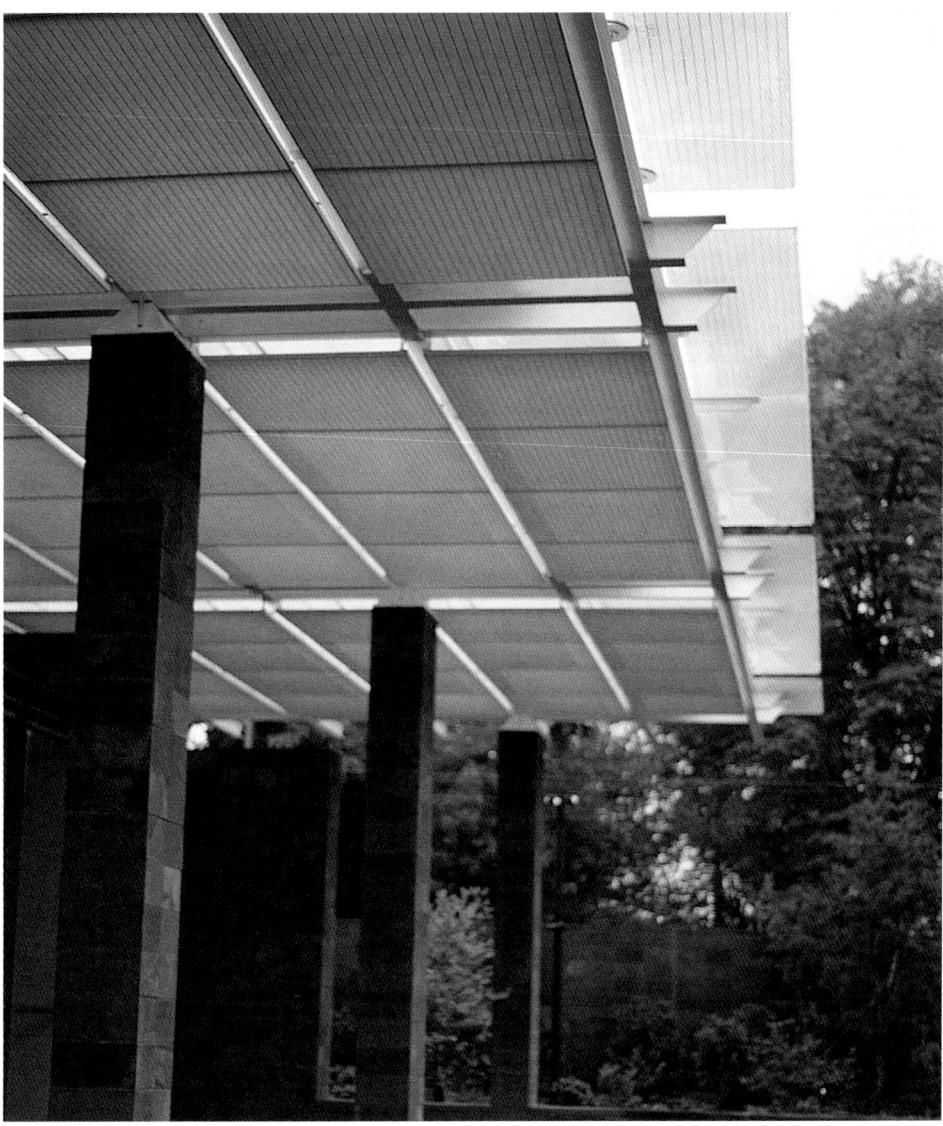

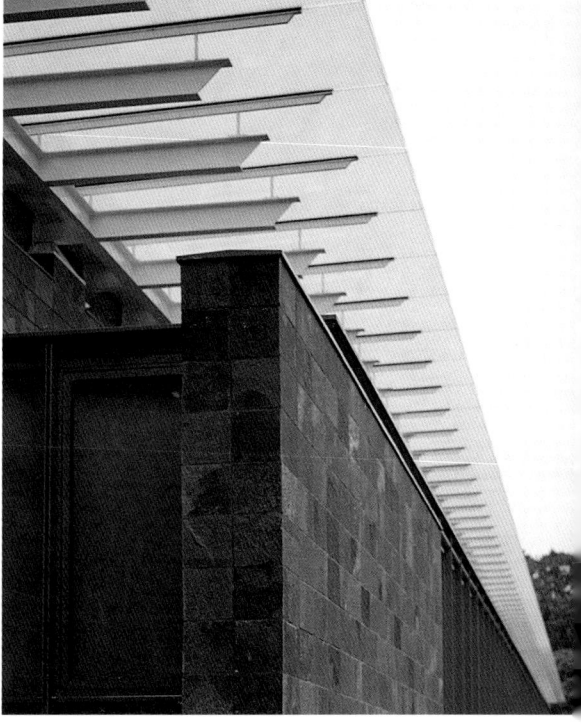

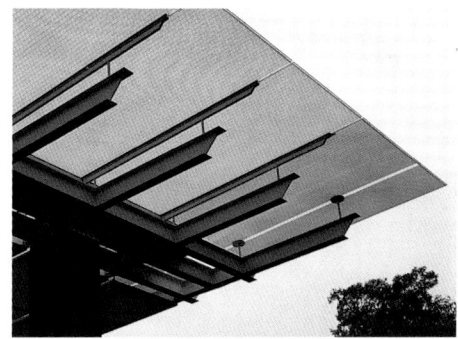

store valuable works of art – was supplemented by a dynamic analysis of annual energy use, as required by the local authority.

Heating and ventilation system

A true displacement system of ventilation was chosen for the Beyeler. This was designed to minimize air velocities in proximity to artwork. The air is delivered at very low velocities from linear floor grilles, which are made from wood to integrate both visually and functionally with the oak strip floor. Floorboards on either side of the grills can be removed to enable access to the ductwork plenum below (for cleaning) and to electrical sockets (for flexible display). Heating is limited to perimeter heating through trench connectors installed below the same wooden grilles under perimeter windows. The air supply to each

gallery module is controlled by variable-air-volume boxes installed in the services corridor at basement level. This 1.8m (6ft) wide space runs for most of the building length and contains supply and extract ducts, which are fed by two air-handling units, each able to provide up to 50 per cent fresh air in favourable external conditions. Additionally, the primary air-handling units each incorporate thermal wheels to recover heat from exhaust air in winter and also obtain further heat following dehumidification by transferring heat from the extract air.

Energy analysis

Using their own computer model, 'Energy 2', Arup carried out energy analysis. This model makes use of the thermal and radiation algorithm of the program 'Room' to analyze

dynamically the major spaces of the museum. Energy required by the building was calculated for every hour of the year based on real weather data from Basel.

The glass roof

The glass roof consists of approximately 4,000m² (43,060ft²) of conventionally supported, double-glazed insulating units. As structural glazed roofs have become more in demand, codes of practice and design guidelines have been developed, but at Beyeler the roof included elements not covered by design guidance. In particular, the cantilevered glazed overhangs at the edge of the roof canopy presented a new challenge. The overhangs are outside the envelope of the building volume and therefore do not need to be double-glazed insulating units.

Carefully detailed roof overhangs at the south and west façades.

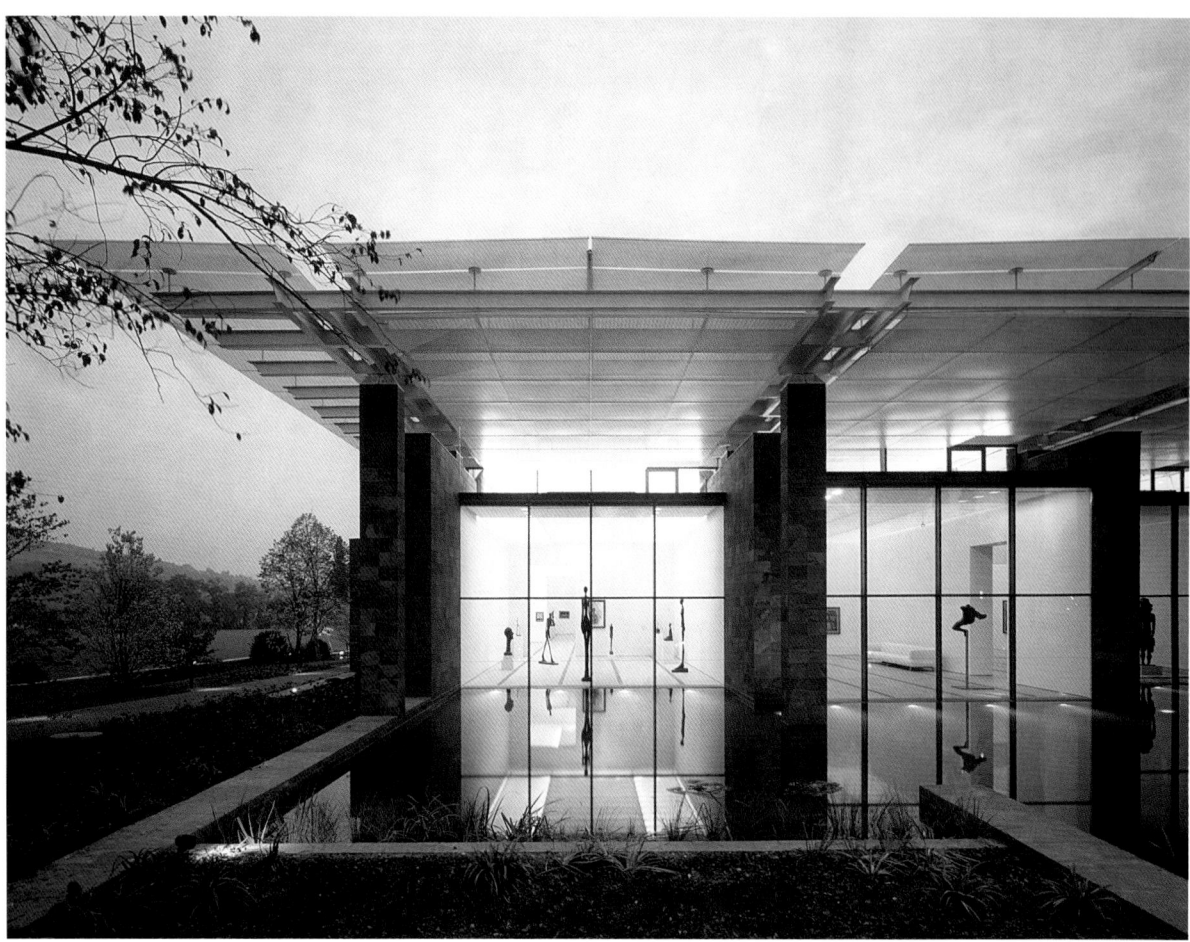

Laminated single-glazed panels were chosen, but the design of the four cantilevering corner panels required special attention. These panels are subject to loading conditions not covered by any codes because of their unique asymmetric configuration. Glass has a low tensile strength (compared with steel and reinforced concrete), which cannot be appreciably increased by variations in chemical composition. However, glass can effectively be pre-stressed by heat-treating; this produces different levels of residual compressive stress, which must be overcome before tensile failure can occur.

The corner panels therefore comprise a single pane 3.2m by 2.4m (10ft by 8ft) of heat-strengthened glass 8mm ($^1/_3$in) thick laminated on top of a 12mm ($^1/_2$in) thick toughened glass pane using four layers of 0.38mm ($^1/_{100}$in) thick polyvinyl butryl. The single pane is supported 0.9m (3ft) in from the short edge and 1.2m (4ft) in from the long edge, creating a 1.5m (5ft) cantilever to the free corner. If the toughened layer were placed on top in the conventional manner and were to break, collapse would be possible. Therefore, in this case, by placing the strengthened glass on top and employing the building layer if the toughened glass fractures, collapse is prevented as the upper layer works compositely with the broken layer.

Conclusion

Ernst Beyeler's collection had originally been installed in his home, where the works were daylit and came alive in naturally changing conditions. He wanted to re-create these conditions in the new gallery, and his desire has been largely fulfilled by means of the distillation of architecture and engineering in the art of the environment. The spaces for display are tranquil and undisturbed by the intrusive visual noise of engineering and constructional technique.

Byzantine Fresco Chapel Museum

François de Menil Houston, Texas USA, 1997

➔
The concrete-clad
exterior from the
garden court.

The Menil Foundation in Houston has a distinguished record as a patron of the fine arts and of the work of contemporary architects. It has twice commissioned buildings from Renzo Piano: the Menil Collection museum, completed in 1986,[1] and the Cy Twombly Gallery, completed in 1995.[2] In 1990 it asked François de Menil to design a chapel museum to house two important Byzantine frescoes that had

been stolen, during the late 1970s, from a small chapel at Lysi in Cyprus. Following their recovery and restoration, the frescoes were acquired by the Menil Foundation and returned to the Church of Cyprus, which handed them back to the foundation to be kept in safe custody on extended loan.

The frescoes, depicting Christ and the Virgin Mary, were taken from the

dome and apse of the original chapel. In their restored form they are supported on back-up shells designed with the help of Peter Rice at Arup.[3] They are installed in the new building as two geometrical figures, of hemisphere and demi-hemisphere, dome and apse.

François de Menil's intention was to create a building that was simultaneously a museum and a

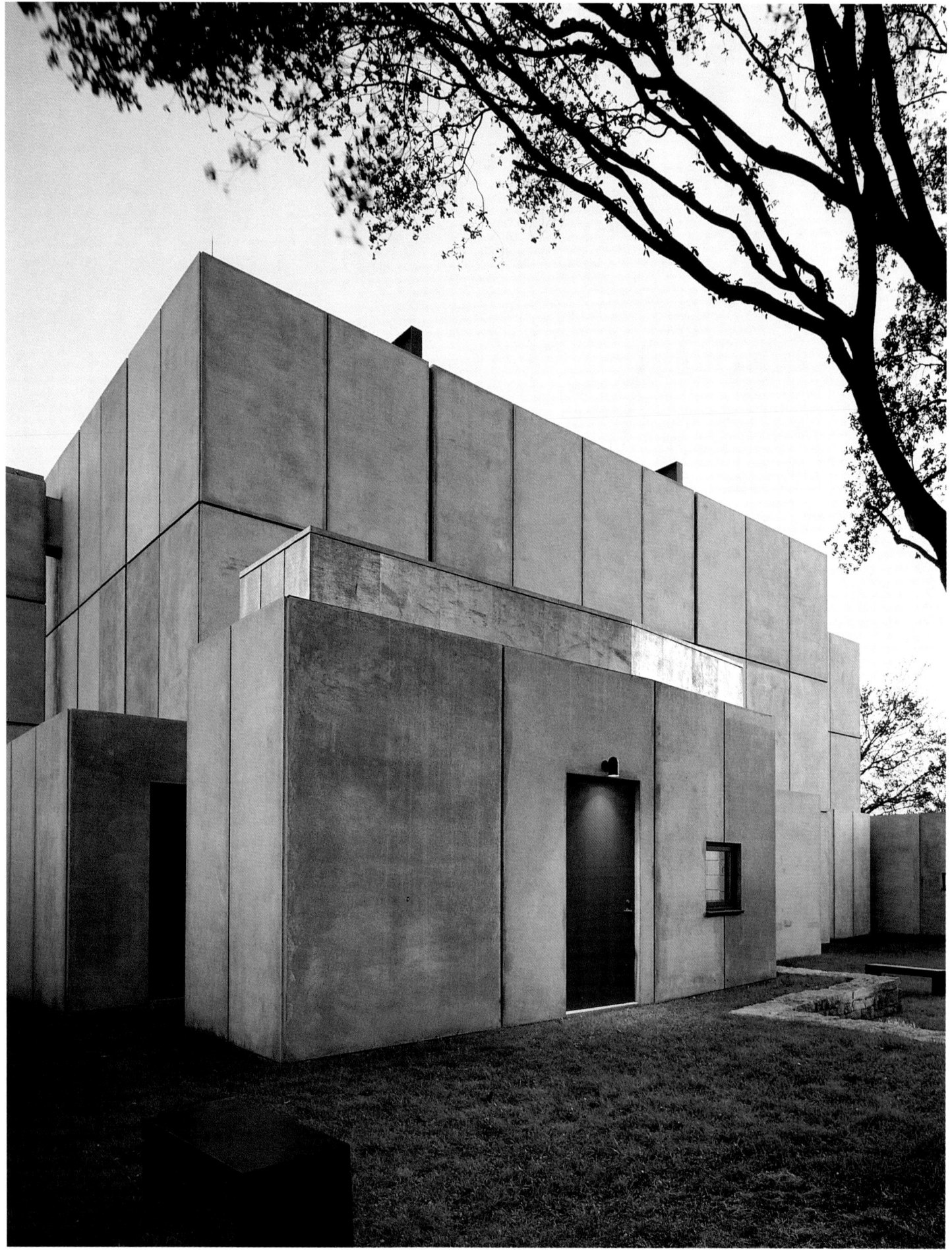

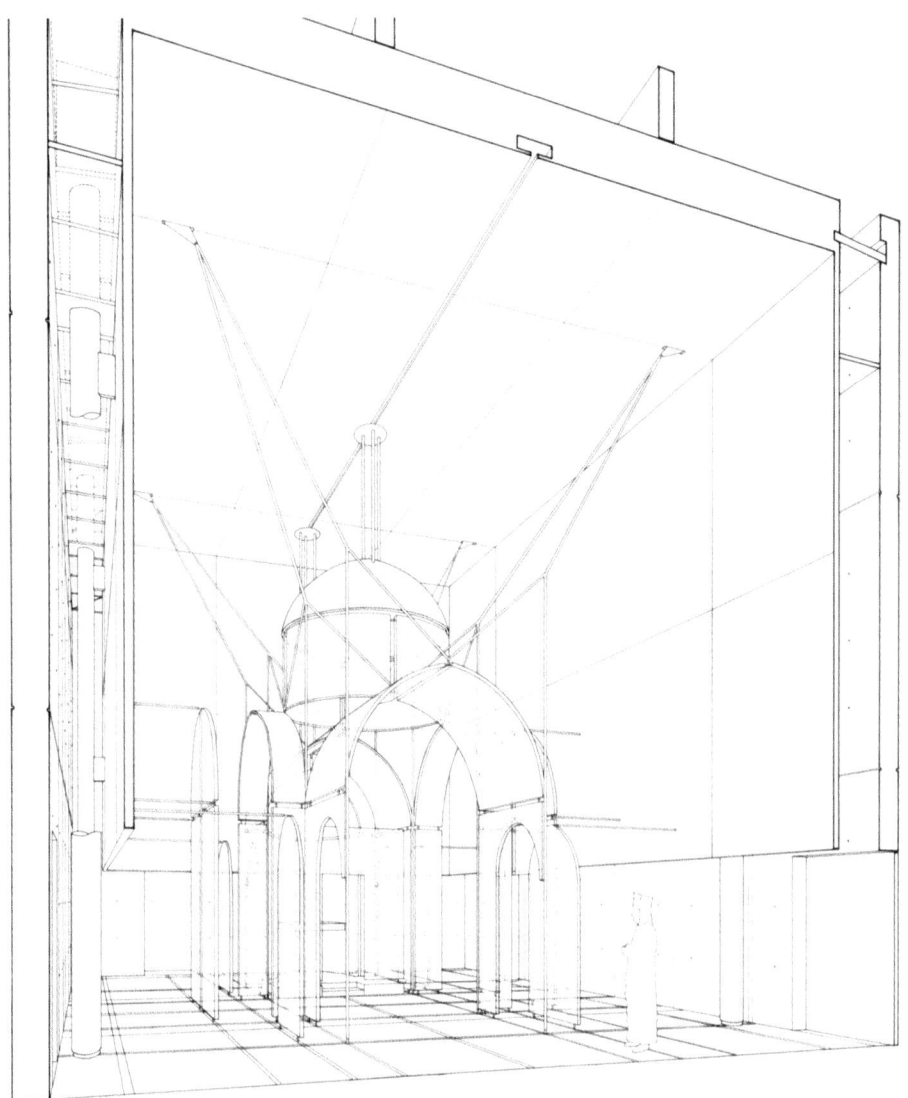

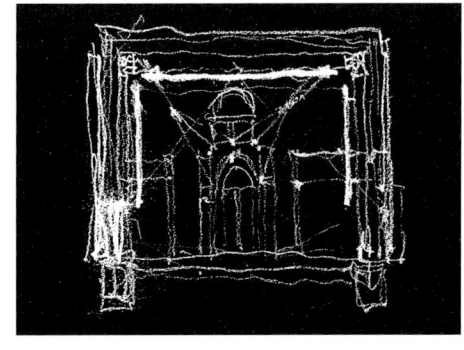

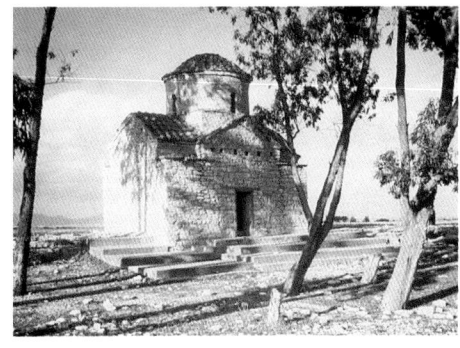

← The sectional perspective reveals the cross-sectional hierarchy of the concrete enclosure, the secondary steel lining and the skeletal steel and glass of the chapel.

↑ An early sketch by François de Menil.

↑ The Byzantine chapel at Lysi, Cyprus, where the frescoes were originally painted.

consecrated Greek Orthodox chapel. The solution is a layered composition in which a skeletal 'reliquary box', which evokes the form of the historic chapel in Cyprus, is placed within a massive enclosing structure. The development of the design is a vivid demonstration of intensive collaboration between architect and engineer. Arup undertook all aspects of the engineering design.

Quantity and quality

It is a paradox that, in their dislocation from their original setting in a historic chapel, the frescoes have become subject to a set of environmental requirements that could not possibly have been met there. The technical brief demanded that, in their new home, they must be kept in an environment that met the most stringent curatorial standards for an art museum, including precise control of temperature, humidity, air quality and illumination exposure, but an overriding aim was to make a place in which the frescoes would resume their original status as objects of contemplation – to address the technical needs in a manner that, however elaborate the engineering, would sustain respect for the sacred.

Layers of environmental space

The site in the suburbs of Houston is enclosed by a rough-hewn perimeter wall of limestone, a reference to the materiality of the chapel in Cyprus. Within this, the box-like volume of the chapel has been constructed from load-bearing *in-situ* concrete, clad with precisely formed and finished precast concrete panels. The space is 9.1m (30ft) wide, 14m (46ft) long and 8.8m (29ft) high. Smaller concrete and lead-clad volumes, containing ancillary spaces, including the sacristy, cluster around this. Entrance is through a narthex-like space that slips between the perimeter wall and the chapel enclosure.

The strategy of layering continues in the interior, where a steel-framed structure supports a further enclosure of dark, sheet-steel walls and the roof slab. This internal volume is suspended from eight tubular steel columns and terminates 2.4m (8ft) above the floor. It is separated from the concrete box by a 600mm (23½in) wide toplit space. Within this, the form of the chapel is delineated by a delicate and precise framework of steel tubes which, in their turn, carry panels and arches of 38mm (1½in) thick laminated, annealed, white water glass. In a precise recreation of the form and dimensions of the original building, the frescoes of dome and

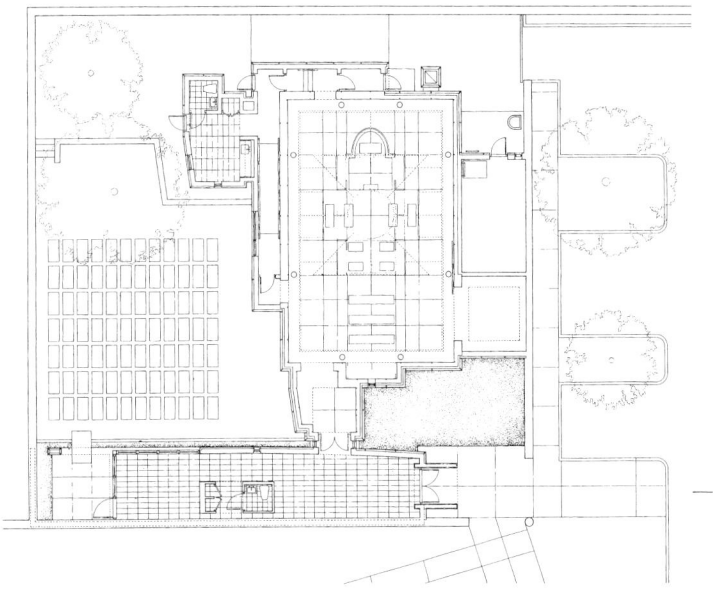

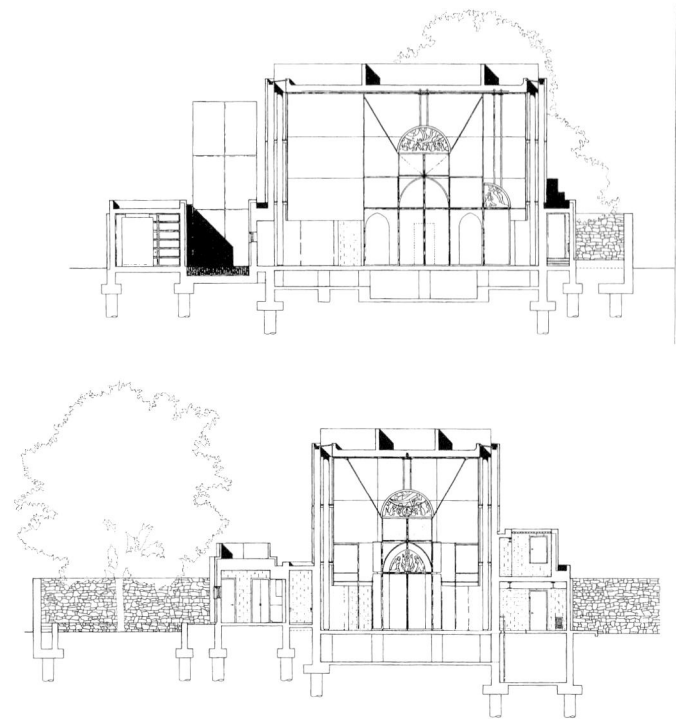

↑
The plan of the
building shows the
chapel within the
perimeter enclosure
of the courtyard.

→
The cross-sections
show how the glass
chapel is enclosed and
sustained by the
surrounding
structures. The
underfloor plenum
space plays an

essential role in the
environmental
strategy of the
building.

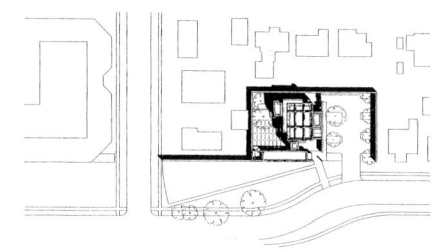

apse float in their new space. The overlapping of the external and internal enclosures ensures that direct daylight and sunlight are excluded from the centre of the space. Natural light cascades down the finely finished grey concrete and is reflected upwards by a perimeter strip of limestone paving. Within the inner space all surfaces are dark – black-painted steel and a dark slate floor. These absorb the daylight and create the setting in which the fictional recreation of the chapel may establish its presence.

The chapel structure is a welded tubular-steel plane frame that, almost imperceptibly, supports the laminated glass elements that define its overall form. Concealed artificial light sources reflect and refract from and within the thick sheets of glass and the structure appears to float weightlessly in the

space. These gently glowing surfaces bathe the frescoes in an even and controlled light. Artificial light comes from two sources. First, an array of fluorescent lamps is positioned in narrow slots cut into the floor directly beneath each vertical glass panel to uplight them delicately. The second source is a series of small tungsten halogen luminaires attached to the steel structure. Wiring concealed within the structural frame carries the low voltage supply to these. At night fluorescent lighting between the steel and concrete enclosures replaces daylight and maintains the calculated balance of illumination.

Thermal control

Environmental layers are key to the thermal strategy of the design. The almost unpunctured, sealed envelope acts to exclude the heat of the

Houston summer and its thermal mass stabilizes the internal environment. The reflectant surface of the precast concrete cladding helps to reduce the transmittance of direct solar radiation. The process of exclusion is further supported by the function of the entrance and sacristy, which act as buffer zones and are air-conditioned independently by heat-pump units mounted on their rooftops. The chapel is positively pressurized further to reduce the infiltration of outside air.

The function of the building as a place of worship created the need to make an environment fit for human habitation. Computer models were used extensively in the design process to analyse thermal performance and to reduce the loads and operation of the mechanical plant. The chapel is air-conditioned as a

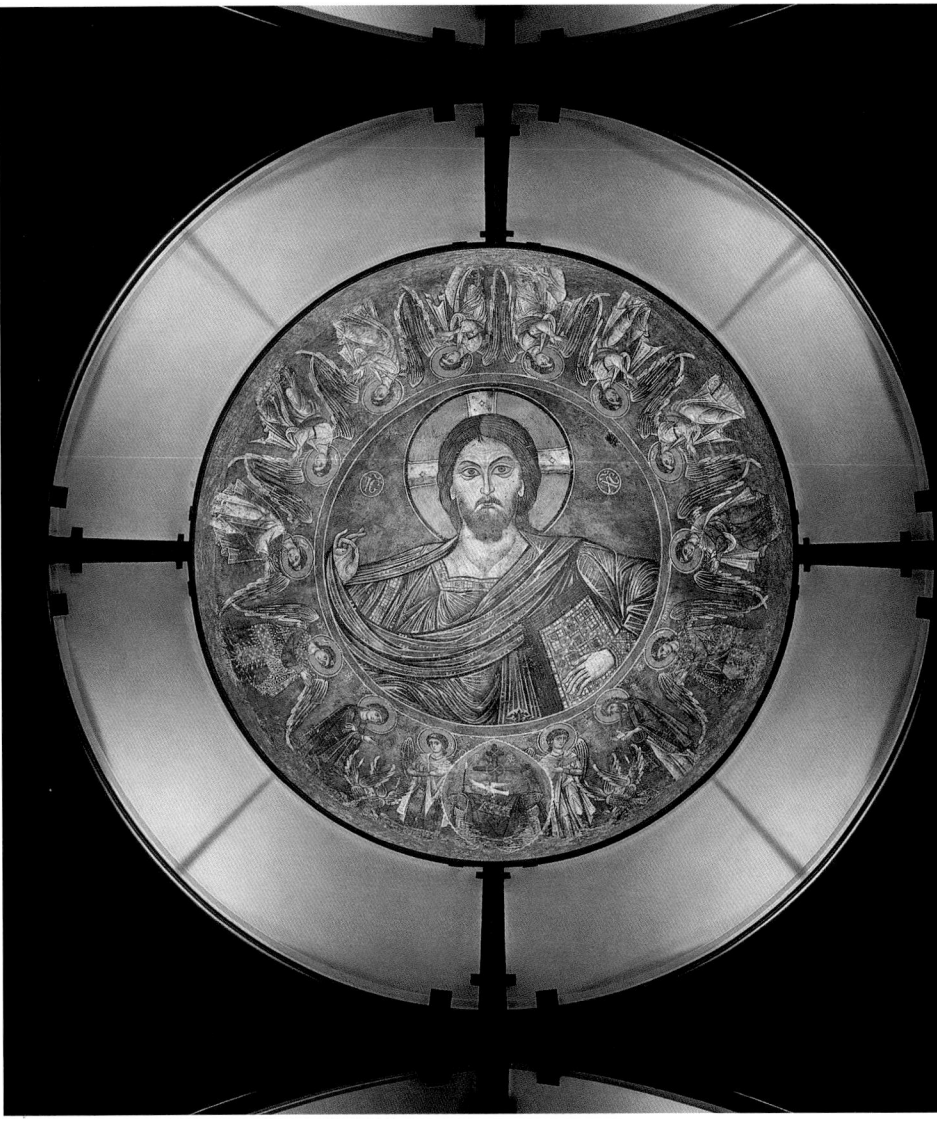

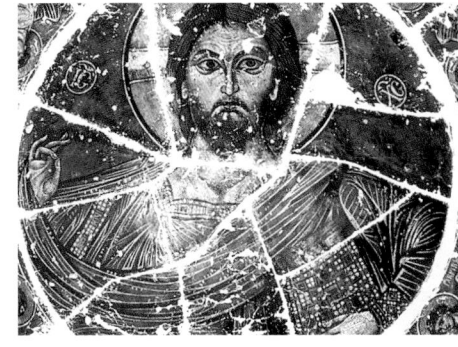

← The restored fresco as it 'floats' above its new enclosure.

↑ The fresco before restoration.

→ Detail of the softly illuminated glass structure.

single zone with a dedicated air-handling unit located in the basement, which delivers conditioned air to a sealed basement plenum below the chapel floor and, from there, into the space through a continuous grille at the perimeter, between the limestone and slate floors. This delivers air precisely to control the effects of any solar gains or heat losses that result from the perimeter rooflight directly above. A second series of inlets is positioned directly beneath the vertical glass panels, where they mark the outline of the enclosure in the floor. These inlets are also occupied by the concealed fluorescent lamps that light the panels, elegantly combining both systems.

The installation uses the principle of displacement air distribution within the chapel, which ensures that the conditions are uniform throughout the space, meeting the needs of both the frescoes and the human visitors. Extraction is through an opening in the ceiling above the frescoes, and the condition of the returned air is monitored to control the condition of the supply air. The system uses a relatively high air-change rate so that effective filtration of the supply can be achieved; this required thorough acoustic analysis and the design of noise-control measures to ensure that the plant is appropriately quiet. Before the frescoes were installed, the entire system was tested *in-situ*.

Conclusion

In comparison with most of the other works in this book, the chapel museum is a small and specialized building but, as we suggest above, its significance in this context lies in the fact that re-housing the frescoes demanded such precise and complex collaboration of architecture and engineering to ensure their survival.

In our modern culture we have assumed a new sense of responsibility for and custodianship of the past, so that such contrivance has become a necessity. In his essay *Travels in Hyperreality*, Umberto Eco proposed that this is a particularly American phenomenon, in which the authentic and the ersatz may be confused by the perfection with which they are executed.[4] But the demand for the long-term conservation of works of art is now universal and this small building in Houston stands as a demonstration of the capability of contemporary architectural and engineering practice to reconcile the needs of the qualitative and the quantitative.

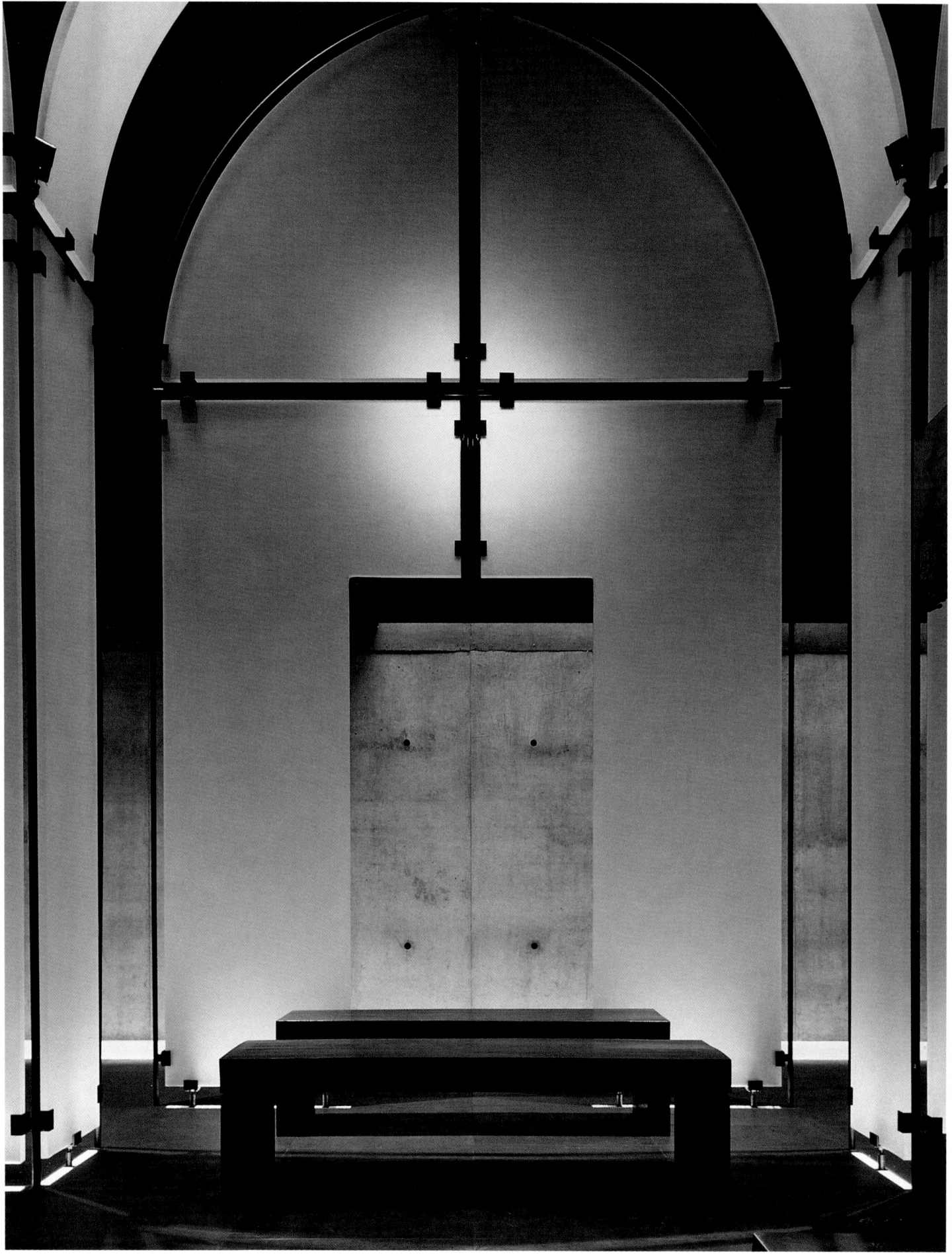

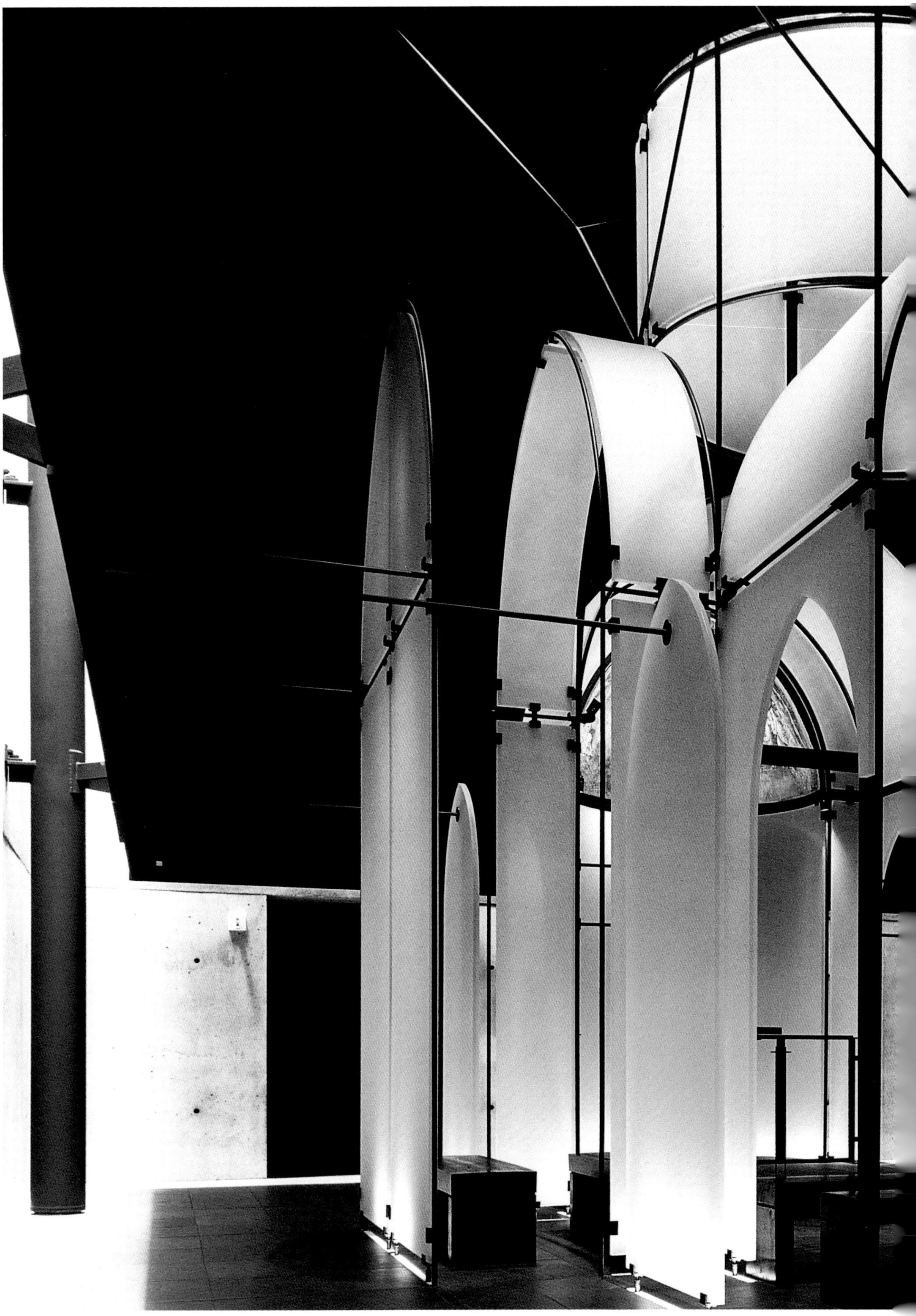

In the completed building, the chapel is suspended in its layers of natural and artificial illumination.

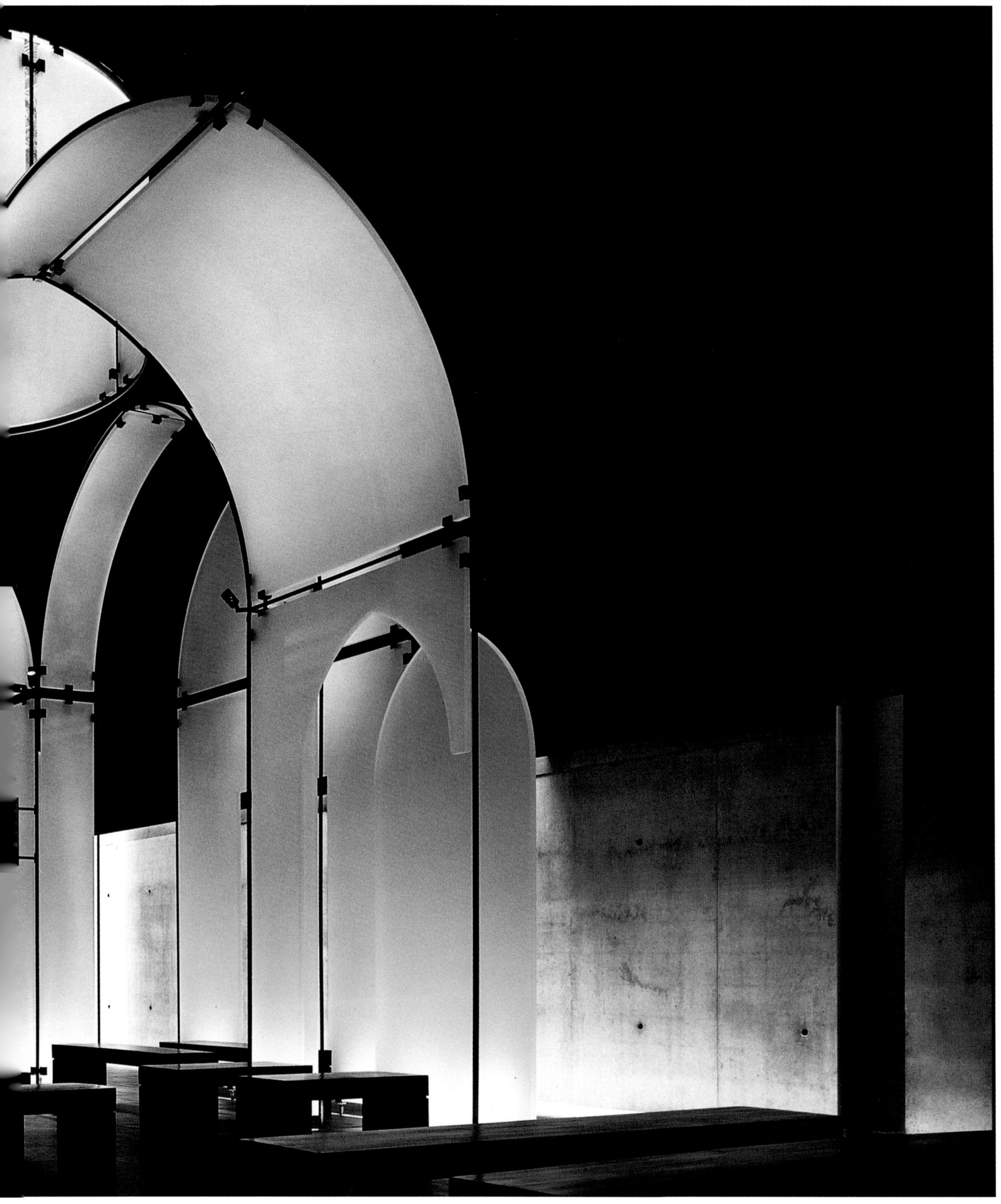

Museum of Contemporary Art
Josef Paul Kleihues
Chicago, USA
1996

When Chicago's Museum of Contemporary Art was founded in 1967, it was housed in a building that a decade later was no longer able to meet the needs of either the growing permanent collection or the expanding programme of temporary exhibitions. In 1990 the site of the National Guard Armory building, on a well-preserved strip of parkland between Michigan Avenue and Lake Michigan, was chosen as the location for a new museum. One year later, the Berlin-based architect Josef Paul Kleihues was chosen to design the building, which was completed and opened to the public in 1996.

According to Andrea Mesecke and Thorsten Scheer, the authors of *Museum of Contemporary Art Chicago*, Kleihues, in formulating his approach, was influenced by 'a combination of European classicism, which of course was the origin of what was called rationalism in architecture since the late 1920s and something that is typical of Chicago...and the pragmatism that characterises Chicago's best architecture, its naked concentration on the task at hand'.[1]

In elaborating this analysis, Mesecke and Scheer referred explicitly to the work of the great 19th-century

German classicist Karl Friedrich Schinkel.[2] Schinkel's designs for public buildings in Berlin, the Schauspielhaus (1818–21) and the Altes Museum (1822–28), provide strong authority for the representation of the cultural institution as an austere pavilion set axially in relation to a major public open space in the city. In addition, the Altes Museum serves as a powerful precedent for an art museum organized according to strict symmetrical principles. Both of these features are reflected in Kleihues's design for the Chicago museum.

The Chicago School of Architecture had its origins in the rapid

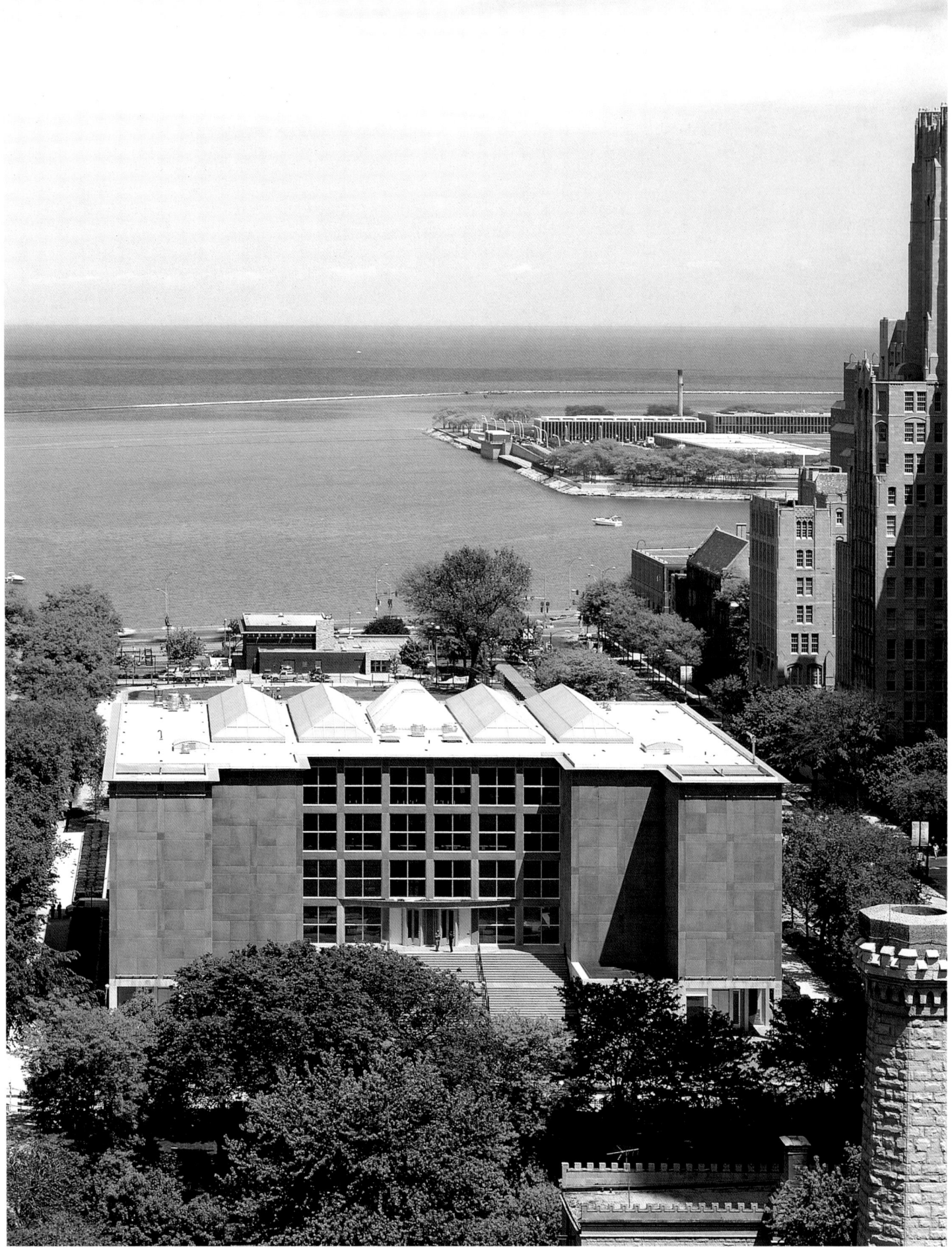

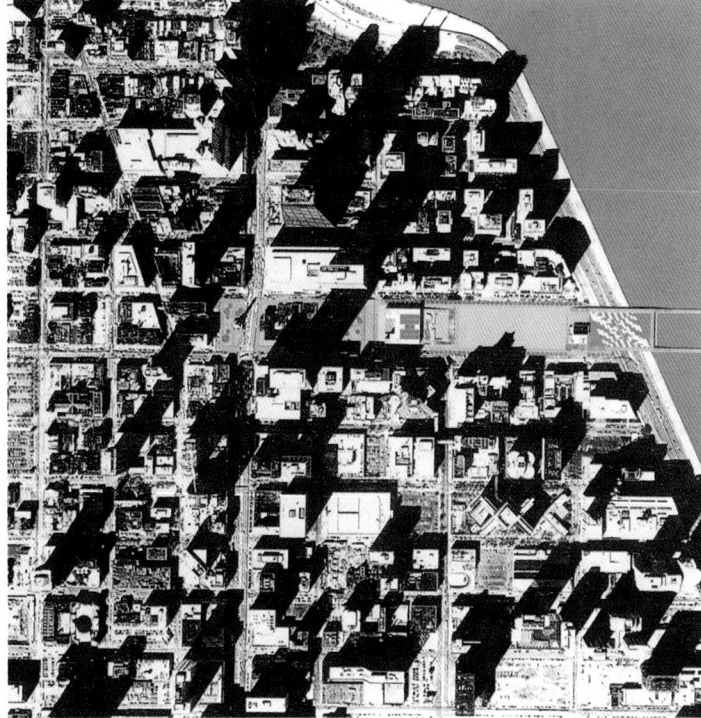

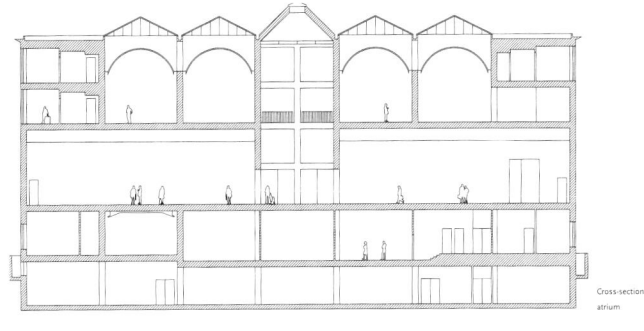

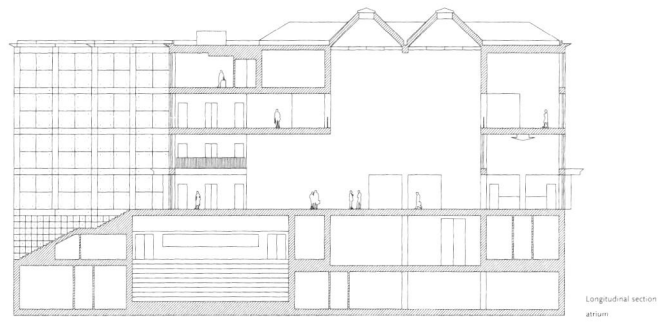

↑

The site plan showing
the Museum of
Contemporary Art in
a green canyon in the
central business
district of Chicago.

↑

The north–south
section (top) shows
the top-lit permanent
exhibition galleries
above the artificially-lit
spaces for temporary

exhibitions. In the
east–west section
(above) the spatial
significance of the
central atrium
is shown.

reconstruction and expansion of the
city in the decades after 1871, when a
fire destroyed much of the downtown
area. During that period, architects
such as William leBaron Jenney, H. H.
Richardson, Burnham & Root,
Holabird & Roche and Adler &
Sullivan created a confident
architectural language for the
realization of the building
programmes of the new metropolis.[3]
In doing so, they rapidly assimilated
and applied the developments in
building technology that were taking
place at the time. The result was an
architecture that directly expressed its
purpose and construction – the 'naked
concentration of the task at hand' that
was so admired by Kleihues. As
regards the wider cultural background
to the design for the Museum of
Contemporary Art, it is worth noting
that Chicago was the city in which

Mies van der Rohe settled in 1938,
after his departure from Germany.

Site and programme

The site of the Museum of
Contemporary Art has been described
as a 'green canyon' within the dense
urban fabric of Chicago's business
district.[4] It is a 66.8m by 126.8m (219ft
by 416ft) rectangle, with its long axis
running east to west. To the west is the
water tower and pumping station that
has been a landmark in the city since
the 19th century, and to the east an
open park extends to the shores of
Lake Michigan. Tall office blocks rise to
the north and south.

The new building includes galleries
for the museum's collection of
contemporary art and for its rich
programme of temporary exhibitions.
There is also an outdoor sculpture
garden, as well as the Mayer

Education Center, which incorporates
a 300-seat auditorium, studio-
classrooms and areas for live
performances and symposia. Other
amenities include a shop, a 15,000-
volume art library and a café, as well
as extensive storage and service
spaces.

The design of a museum
environment is governed by the need
to maintain precise control over both
the condition of the internal air and
the illumination levels. In this case,
the fact that Chicago suffers from
severe atmospheric pollution –
caused by gaseous and particulate
pollutants carried into the city by the
prevailing westerly winds – made
particularly stringent demands on
Arup's design of the mechanical
services. From the start Kleihues was
emphatic that the principal exhibition
rooms should be naturally lit. He was

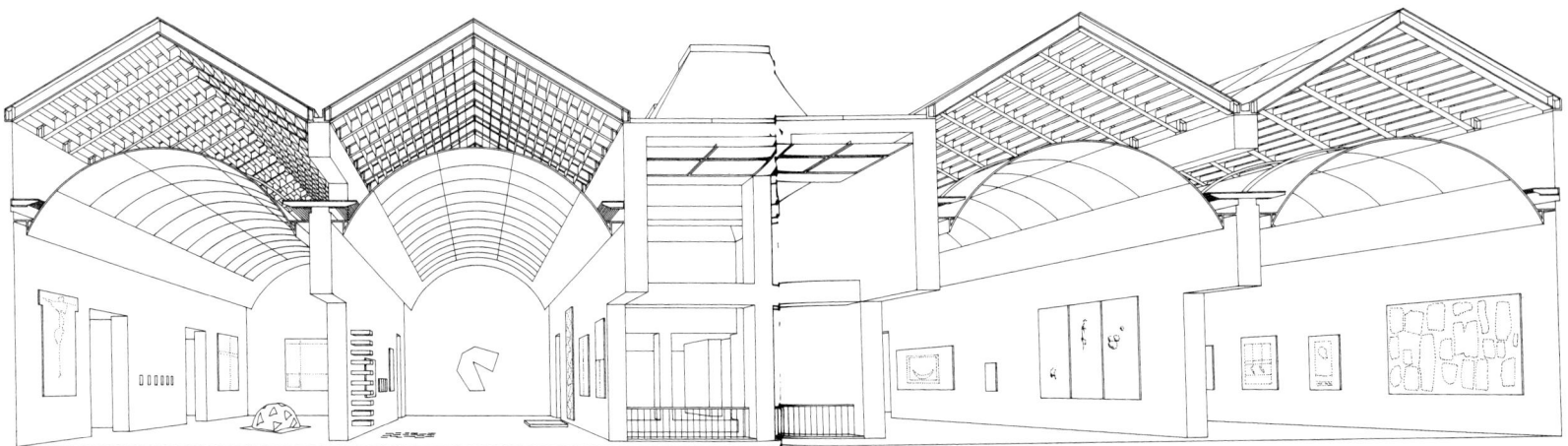

 The permanent exhibition galleries achieve controlled daylighting through their layered system of translucent laylights, above which further control is provided by automatically operated louvres.

equally insistent that, rather than a 'cold', 'grey' northern light, there should be 'a wealth of light with all spectral colours'.

The classical tradition

Among the most apparent classical influences in the design of the museum are the symmetry of its plan and the adoption of the conventional horizontal organization into base, wall and cornice. The main entrance is reached by a sweeping flight of steps cut into a limestone-clad base reminiscent of Schinkel's Altes Museum. The entire building adheres to a geometrical order based on a repeated square of 7.8m by 7.8m (26ft by 26ft) and its subdivision into a secondary system of 3.9m (13ft). The overall plan of the building is contained within a seven by seven grid of these 7.8m (26ft) squares,

giving 54.6m (182ft), plus 0.3m (1ft) either side to allow for structural thickness – a total of 55.2m by 55.2m (184ft by 184ft). This geometrical discipline also applies to the cross-section. A module of 0.6m (2ft) is used to regulate all the minor dimensions and details of the building.

During the classical revival of the 19th century, complex environmental installations were incorporated into buildings. Eminent architects such as Adam, Soane, Barry and Elmes in England, Labrouste in France and Semper in Germany achieved a discreet synthesis of new technology and conventional architectural language. By declaring the influence of the European classical tradition, and in particular its revival in the 19th century, Kleihues implies a similar discretion in his environmental approach at the Chicago museum.

Structure and planning

The building consists of a reinforced-concrete structure based on the 7.8m (26ft) grid. At its heart is an atrium rising four storeys from first to fourth floors and topped by two truncated pyramidal rooflights, which establishes a sense of spatial continuity and orientation throughout the museum. The first-floor entrance on the west side of the building opens directly into a double-height vestibule that evokes the great entrance loggia of the Altes Museum. A broad passage leads ahead to the atrium and beyond to the double-height café, which overlooks the sculpture garden to the east. The temporary exhibition galleries are located on either side of the atrium.

As an alternative to the grand approach to the *piano nobile*, the building may be entered at ground

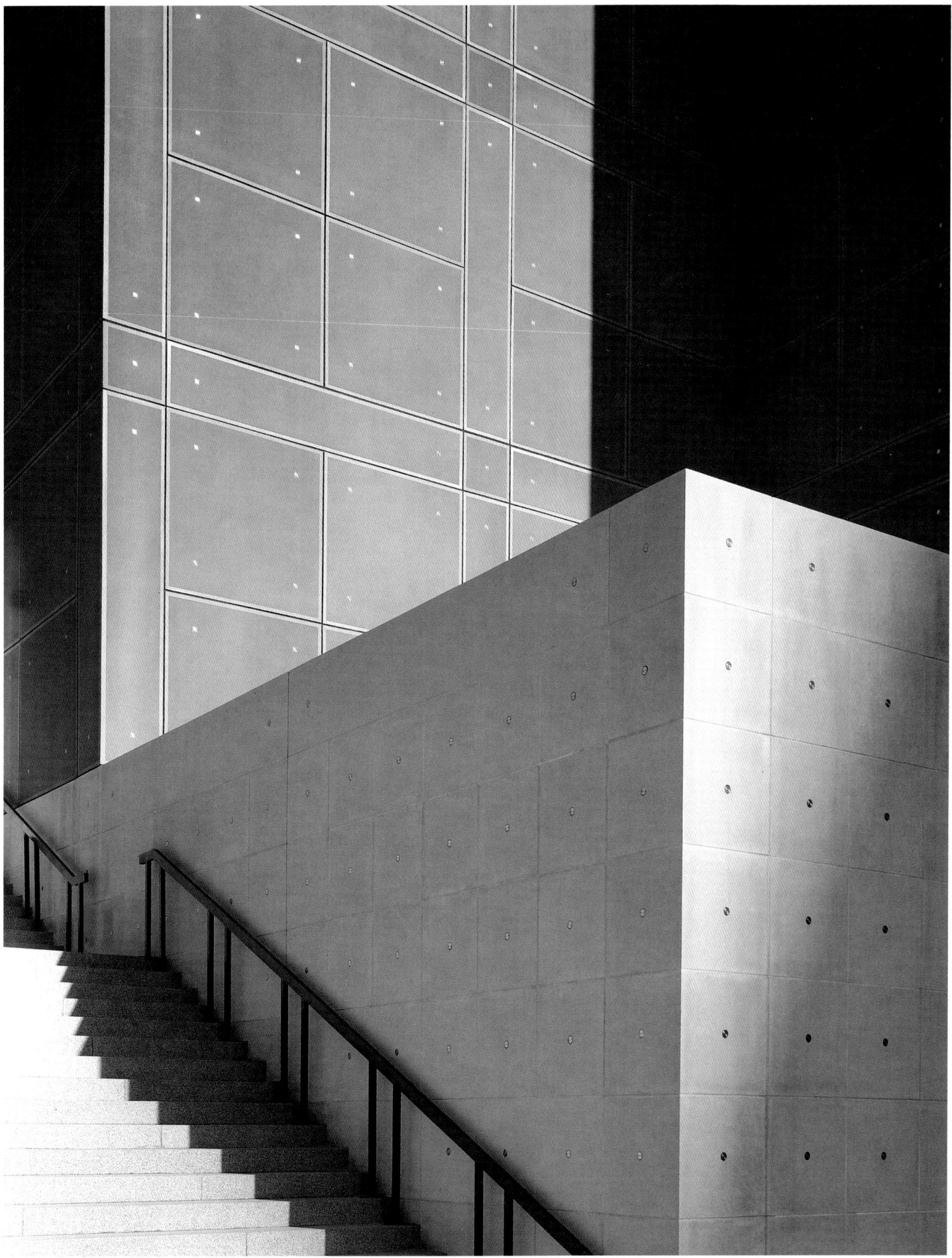

←

The stairs to the main entrance, cut into the limestone-clad base, above which rises the cast-aluminium cladding of the body of the building.

→

Looking up the steel and stone main staircase.

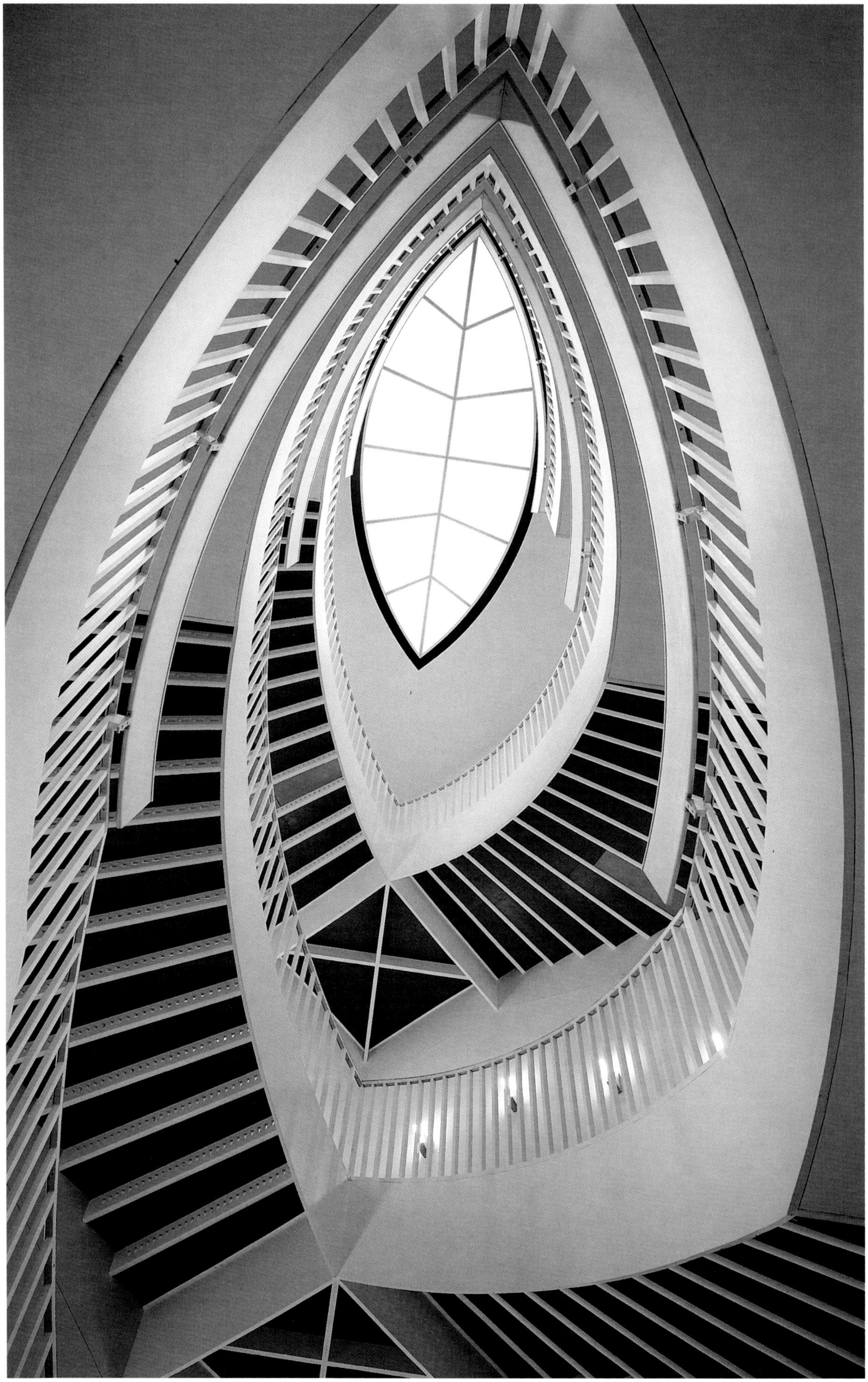

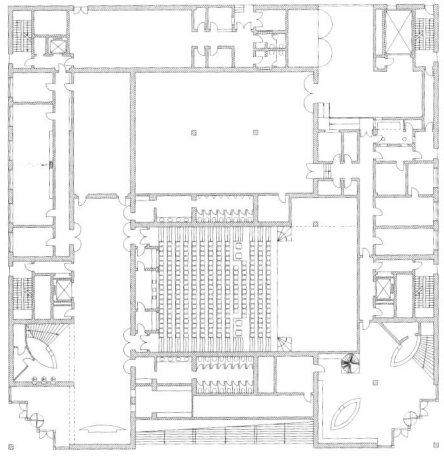

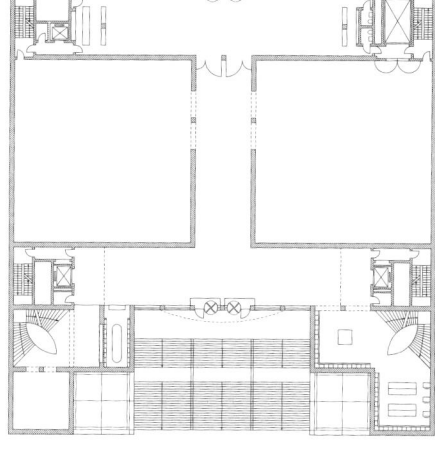

→

At the plinth level, in addition to the Meyer Education Center, the plan accommodates the principal service and plant rooms.

At the level of the main entrance, and of the temporary exhibition spaces, the dominant symmetry of the plan is established. The position of the four vertical service cores is clearly legible.

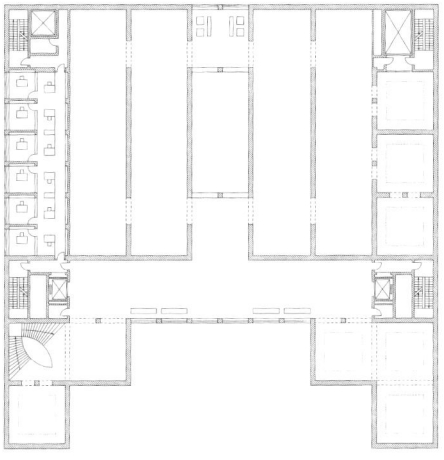

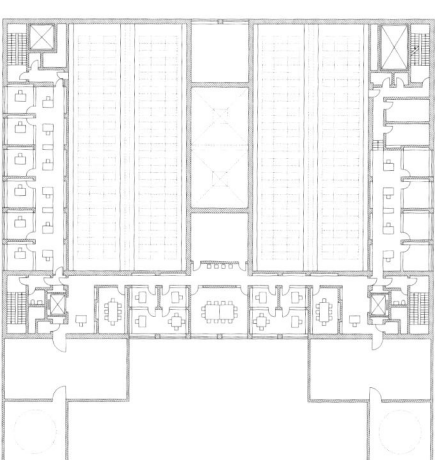

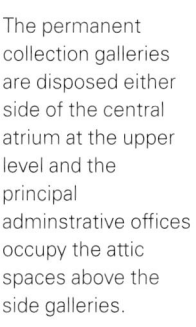

← →

The permanent collection galleries are disposed either side of the central atrium at the upper level and the principal adminstrative offices occupy the attic spaces above the side galleries.

Looking west across the atrium at the upper level. The geometrical regulation of the entire building is expressed in the coordination of the grids of structure, fenestration and illuminated ceiling.

level through openings recessed into the stone base either side of the west façade. The northern entrance leads into the foyer of the Mayer Education Center, from which the main staircase rises through the full height of the building. The southern entrance gives access to the museum shop, whose two levels are connected by a smaller version of the principal staircase, which is itself linked to the main entrance vestibule.

On the fourth floor are the galleries for the permanent collection, which take the form of four rooflit, barrel-vaulted rooms placed two on either side of the atrium. Works that need protection from natural light are displayed in three small, artificially lit rooms opening off the southernmost gallery. The museum administration is located in a U-shaped mezzanine on the fifth floor.

The simple clarity and order of its materiality and detail reinforce the geometric logic of the building. Externally, above the limestone base, the structure is clad in cast-aluminium panels that delineate the underlying regulating dimensions. Window openings, where they occur, also conform to this order. Reminders of the geometry, evident throughout the interior, are most clearly identifiable in the atrium, in the pyramids of the rooflights and in the expressed structural frame. Elsewhere the gridded ceilings follow precisely the same system and organize the relationship of artificial light sources and outlets for the air-conditioning. The structural frame and walls are finished in unadorned white paint.

This quiet austerity is continued in the galleries for the permanent collection. Kleihues's desire to use

natural light as the principal light source in these rooms has led to a multi-layered roof construction in which translucent glass vaults are suspended beneath four continuous rooflights. A system of automatically controlled louvres in the ceiling void precisely regulates the light levels to which the pictures are exposed. Artificial lighting is integrated into this system. The temporary exhibition galleries on the lower floor are permanently artificially lit, providing the flexibility needed for the diverse exhibitions shown there.

Environmental response
The basis of the building's lighting design was the 'lux-hours' principle, which establishes maximum exposure levels for the various kinds of art work, defined as the product of light levels and hours of exposure per

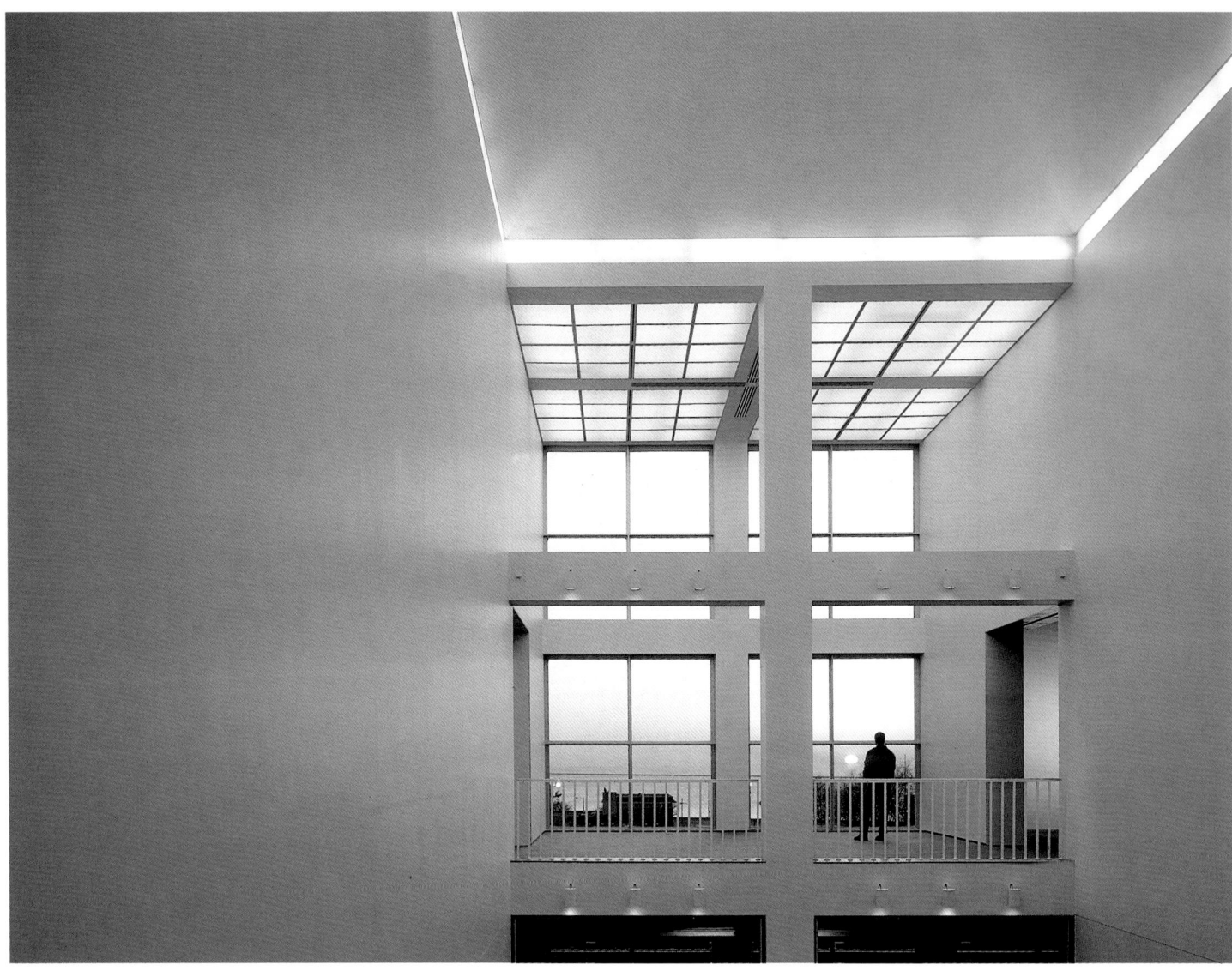

annum. It proved necessary to prevent direct penetration of sunlight into the building. To ensure that exposure does not exceed the permitted levels, the illumination in the galleries is continuously monitored by photocells, which adjust the louvres above the ceiling vaults to reflect and filter the daylight without eliminating the full spectrum, in accordance with the architect's intentions. A filtering laminate incorporated in the external layer of the roof glazing excludes ultraviolet light, which is damaging to coloured pigments. The effect within the galleries of shadows cast by the surrounding tall buildings on the museum's glazed roof was reduced, but not eliminated, by using the adjustable louvre system.

Excluding atmospheric pollution was the greatest challenge in the design of the mechanical installations.

The Illinois Environmental Protection Agency confirmed that Chicago's atmosphere contained high levels of sulphur dioxide, nitrous oxides, ozone and chlorides, all of which are potentially damaging to works of art. The galleries are served by an air-handling unit that incorporates layers of filtration to eliminate particulate and chemical contaminants before the temperature and moisture content of the air is adjusted to the required levels. The system uses a network of sensors spread throughout the galleries to maintain the internal environment within the necessary narrow limits. It includes a heat recovery unit that helps to reduce the building's total energy demand.

Such precise control is unnecessary in the offices and social spaces. In the offices there is a fan-coil system that allows recirculation of air and

provides the occupants with local control over their environment. The volume of air delivered to the restaurant and auditorium varies in response to the number of people in those areas at different times.

Integration and concealment
A combination of the classical tradition and the pragmatism of the Chicago School has demonstrably influenced the overall form and tectonic method of the building, but architectural theory and culture had to be reconciled with a technically demanding environmental brief. Provision for services is made in four vertical risers at the four corners of the gallery spaces. Horizontal service distribution, concealed in the floor and ceiling construction, is carried from these. Such a simple, rational arrangement is strikingly similar to that of a modern office building.

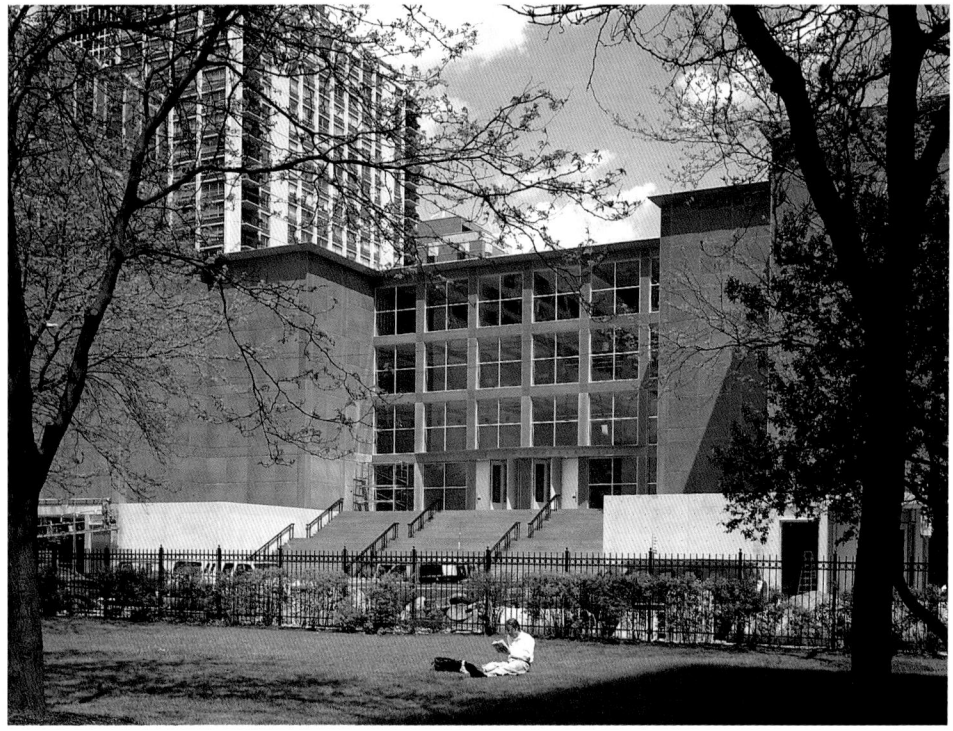

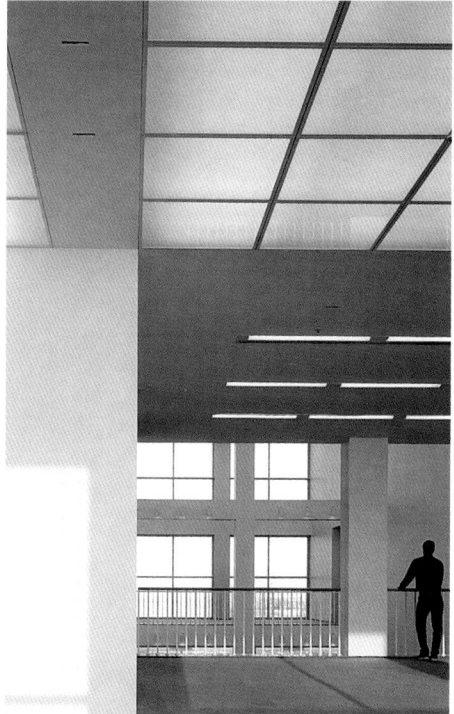

↑
The main entrance
stair from the east.

↑
Upper-level
vestibule.

→
The clarity of form
and detail in the
permanent exhibition
galleries conceals the
complexity of the
services installation
that sustains them.

Within the public areas of the building, vestibules and galleries, the suspended ceiling serves as the principal, discreet expression of environmental services. In the temporary exhibition galleries and the foyers, the gridded ceilings, whose dimensions are derived from the building's geometric order, allow for precise organization of the apparatus of artificial lighting, air grilles and fire safety systems. The permanent exhibition galleries, with their translucent glass vaults, make reference to the lengthy tradition of the rooflit art museum, from Sir John Soane through Schinkel to Louis Kahn – and even to Robert Venturi's reinterpretation of Soane's Dulwich Picture Gallery at the National Gallery in London.

In their calm uniformity, the temporary and permanent exhibition spaces also call to mind the image of Mies van der Rohe's Museum for a Small City project. In the central atrium Kleihues creates a delicate illusion by installing a strip of diffused artificial light around the bases of each of the two roof pyramids. This visually detaches the roof from the orthogonal structure below.

Since the roof of the building is overlooked from the adjacent skyscrapers, the nature and location of the rooftop elements of the environmental plant needed careful thought. All the major elements have been placed beneath the roof surface, with only the essential terminals being visible from above. These are organized symmetrically in relation to the gallery rooflights and the pyramids of the atrium.

Conclusion

The Chicago museum is a highly serviced building with a demanding environmental programme. Its compact form, sealed envelope, controlled areas of glazing and comprehensive mechanical systems define it, according to our taxonomy, as environmentally exclusive. From the environmental standpoint, the design has comprehensively integrated a coherent architectural philosophy with the technical demands of the brief. It is in this respect that the architect has most demonstrably reconciled the conventions and discipline of the classical tradition with the pragmatism of the Chicago School.

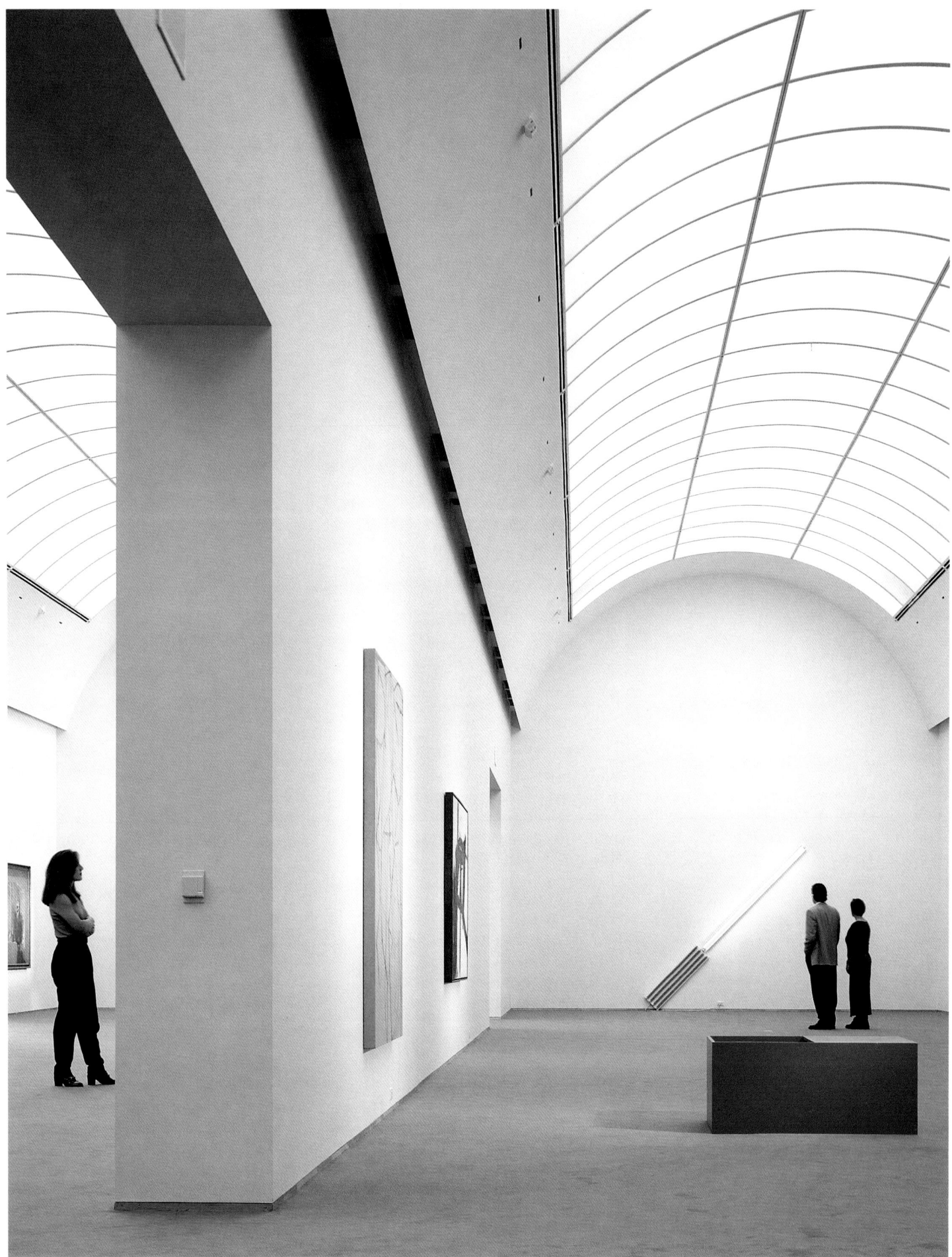

Walsall Art Gallery

Caruso St John
Walsall, UK
2000

→
The new Walsall Art
Gallery, viewed across
the canal basin. The
fenestration differentiates
between the cellular
spaces of the Garman
Ryan Collection – small
rectangles – and the
larger volumes of the
temporary exhibition
galleries – horizontal
clerestory.

The art museum has played a significant role in the history of environmental design. For example, as noted in the introduction to this book, John Soane's Dulwich Picture Gallery (1811–14) was an example of the architect's deep interest in applying early methods of central heating, and the building is equally important in establishing a strategy for the controlled illumination of paintings by natural light. The manipulation of the cross-section in order to establish a precise relationship between work of art, viewer and light source has become a paradigm for the design of the art museum that has survived to the present day. Louis Kahn's Kimbell Museum (1972) and Renzo Piano's designs for the Menil Collection at Houston (1987) and the Beyeler Museum in Basel (1997) represent a continuation of the tradition.

This model was challenged, however, by Mies van der Rohe's project for the Museum for a Small City (1943), where a 'universal' and uniform environment for art is proposed, exploiting the potential of totally controlled artificial lighting. The vision of a new kind of gallery space was realized in Mies's National Gallery in Berlin (1958), where the major artificially lit galleries are located in the windowless crypt beneath the transparent entrance pavilion.

Since the 1960s a new demand has been placed upon the designers of art museums, following the discovery of the extent to which paintings can be physically damaged by exposure to light. Research has shown how works in all media are affected by both the intensity of the illumination to which they are exposed and the duration of exposure. Paintings can also be damaged by the quality of air in a gallery. These findings have brought about a major review of gallery design, with the result that the

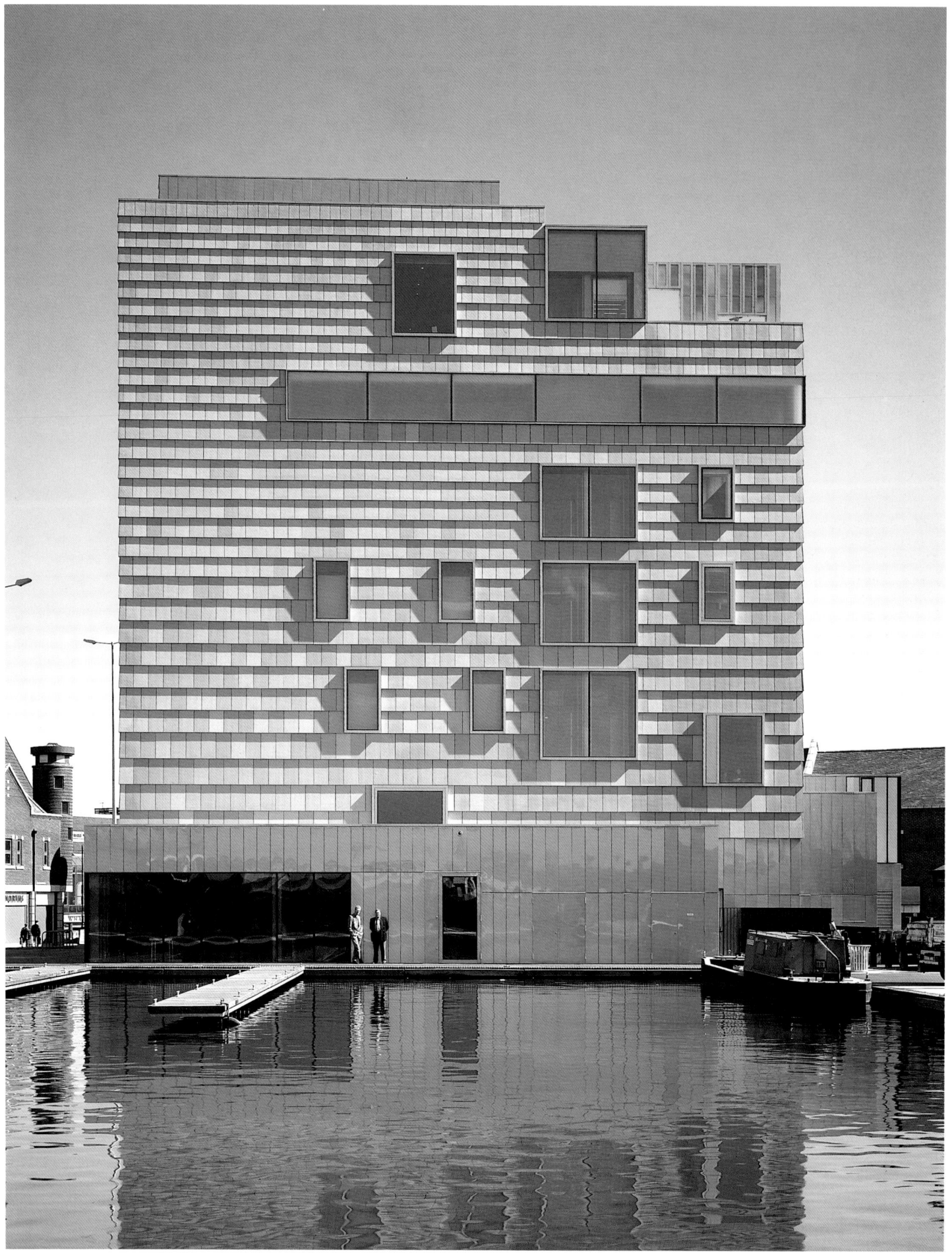

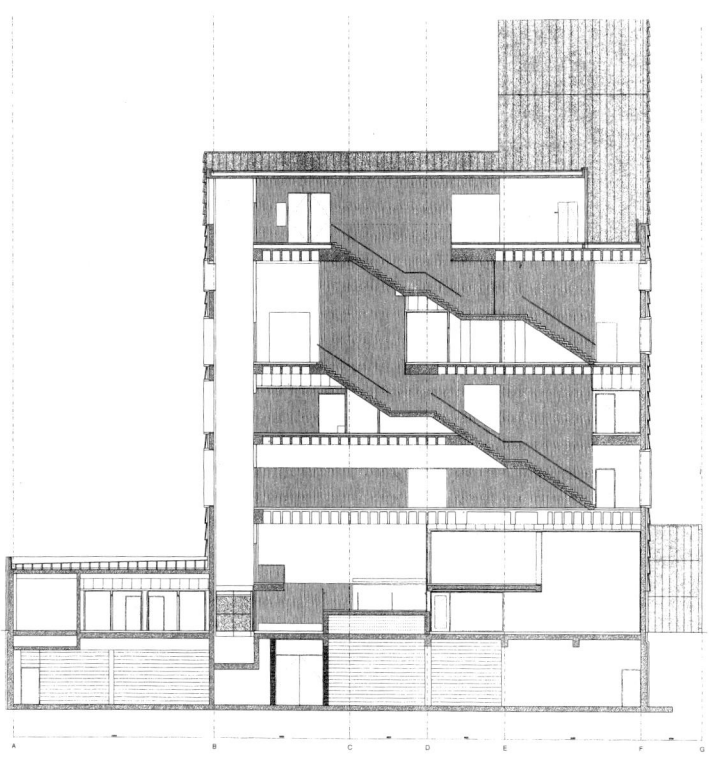

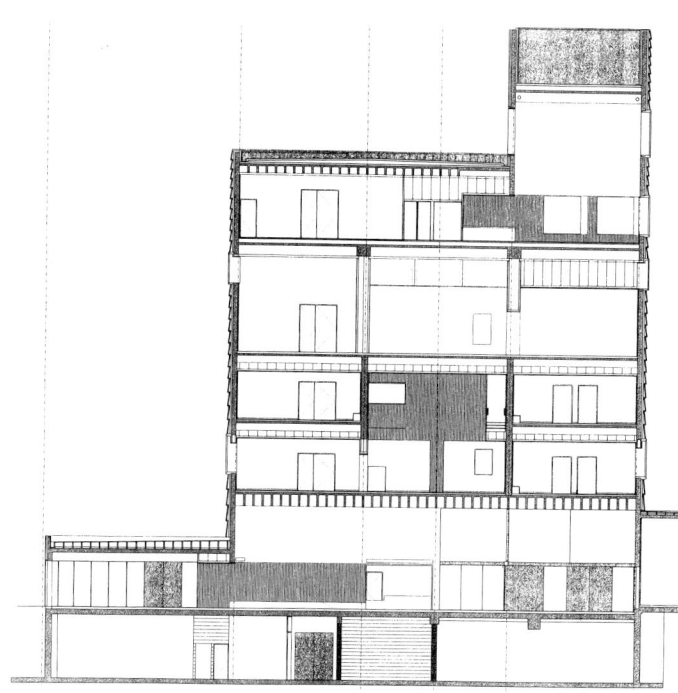

↑
The complex cross-sections, with their exposed structure and construction, suggest little of the conventions of structure-service relationships.

→
The plans show the clear distinction between the cellular structure of the Garman Ryan Collection and the less specific arrangement of the temporary exhibition galleries. They also show the vital vertical service cores.

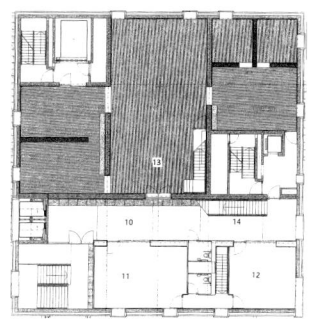

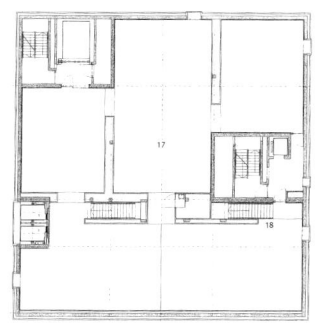

modern urban art museum has, in almost all instances, become an exercise in the exclusive mode of environmental design.

Robert Venturi developed a critique of gallery design in which he argued that the articulation of the cross-section as the principal element of daylight control has, over time, become as much a symbol of the art museum as it is necessarily functional.[1] In his design for the Sainsbury Wing in London's National Gallery (1990), Venturi paid homage to Soane by constructing a sequence of Dulwich-like galleries. But, in response to the central urban location and the environmental demands of art conservation, the form derived from historical precedent is enclosed within an envelope that renders the form more scenographic than functional.

The Walsall environment
In 1996 Caruso St John won a competition for the design of the Walsall Art Gallery. The programme required specific gallery spaces for the permanent display of the Garman Ryan collection of paintings and sculpture, as well as galleries for temporary exhibitions. The site is in the centre of this industrial town, adjacent to a canal basin and close to the main shopping centre and the bus and train stations. It is also close to a number of still-functioning factories, and there is a relatively high level of atmospheric pollution. It was part of the brief that the air delivered to the exhibition rooms had be filtered to reduce the levels of acidic gases to 20 times less than those found outside.

It is impossible to design an art gallery without defining the nature of the exhibition spaces, but there are many other factors to take into account. In the Walsall Art Gallery there were requirements for education rooms, artists' studios, a library, a café, a shop and administrative offices. Environmentally, this has been acknowledged in the adoption of a *mixed mode* strategy, that is part *exclusive* and part *selective*. The galleries and art store are air-conditioned, with close control of temperature and humidity. The conference room is comfort cooled. The lavatories are mechanically ventilated. All other areas are naturally ventilated. In the galleries the difference between displaying a specific collection such as the Garman Ryan and providing for the inevitable diversity of temporary exhibitions is emphatically registered in the arrangement, materiality and

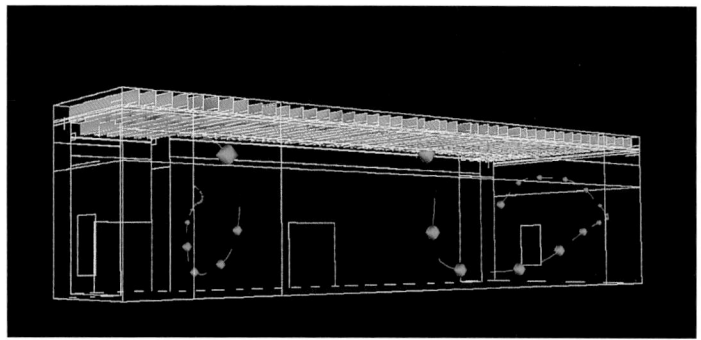
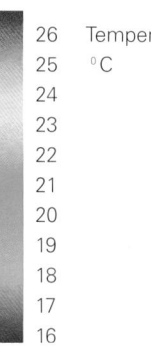

26 Temperature
25 °C
24
23
22
21
20
19
18
17
16

←

Computer-generated representation of summer air movements.

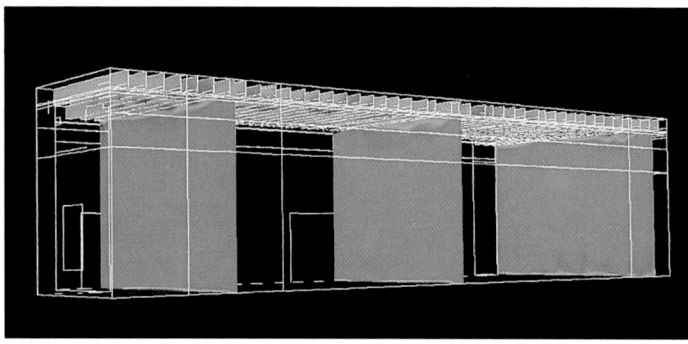
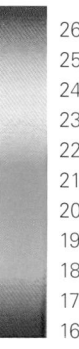

26 Temperature
25 °C
24
23
22
21
20
19
18
17
16

←

Computer-generated representation of vertical sections, showing summer air temperature distribution.

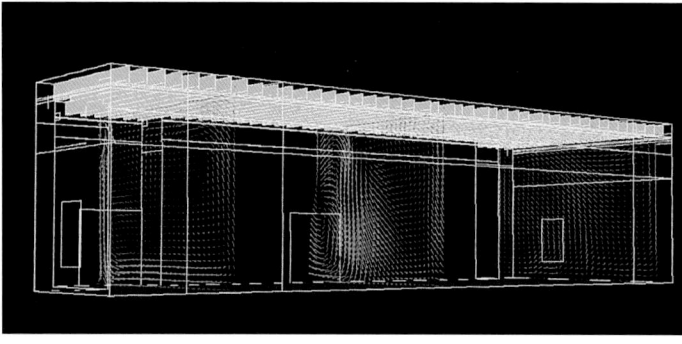
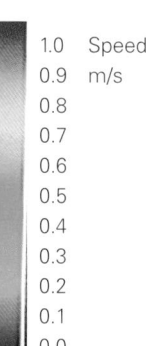

1.0 Speed
0.9 m/s
0.8
0.7
0.6
0.5
0.4
0.3
0.2
0.1
0.0

←

Computer-generated representation of vertical sections, showing summer air velocity distribution.

fenestration of the respective parts of the building.

The Garman Ryan collection consists of pictures in all media – oils, watercolours, engravings and drawings – and sculpture, again in a range of materials and techniques. Most of the works are relatively small and a condition of their donation to the town was that they should be displayed in defined thematic groupings. The architects' response to this was to create a two-storey 'house' in which a series of quite small galleries was planned around a double-height space located on the first and second floors of the five-storey building. The height of the rooms – 3m (10ft) from floor to ceiling – is relatively modest, and each room has at least one window. The floors and suspended ceilings are made of Douglas fir and the walls are white-painted plaster. In both scale and material, these rooms allude to a domestic setting.

Arup's lighting design in these rooms achieves the illusion of domestic space through the careful design and positioning of the windows, but the stainless-steel and etched-glass 'laylights' are the principal source of illumination. The conservation lighting design is based on the 'kilolux hour per year' principle. This is a calculation of the cumulative exposure of the art works over a year and, in this installation, allows the diverse media to co-exist in the same room without risk to the more delicate works. The artificial lighting operates in response to the level of daylight entering the windows: levels are automatically adjusted, and white blinds are raised or lowered to control the amount of daylight that enters. Individual works can be highlighted by spotlights fixed to the laylights.

Externally, an almost continuous band of glazing is the most obvious symbol of the building's purpose. This is the clerestorey window, which is the primary source of light in the temporary galleries. Located on the third floor, these are essentially neutral spaces, waiting to receive whatever works might constitute a travelling exhibition. But, as in the Garman Ryan galleries, first appearances are deceptive. The clerestorey is a complex mechanism of environmental control. Between its outer double skin and its inner single skin of etched glass, there are artificial light fittings and motorized blinds that allow the control of light levels to meet the requirements of a particular exhibition. Blinds are adjusted

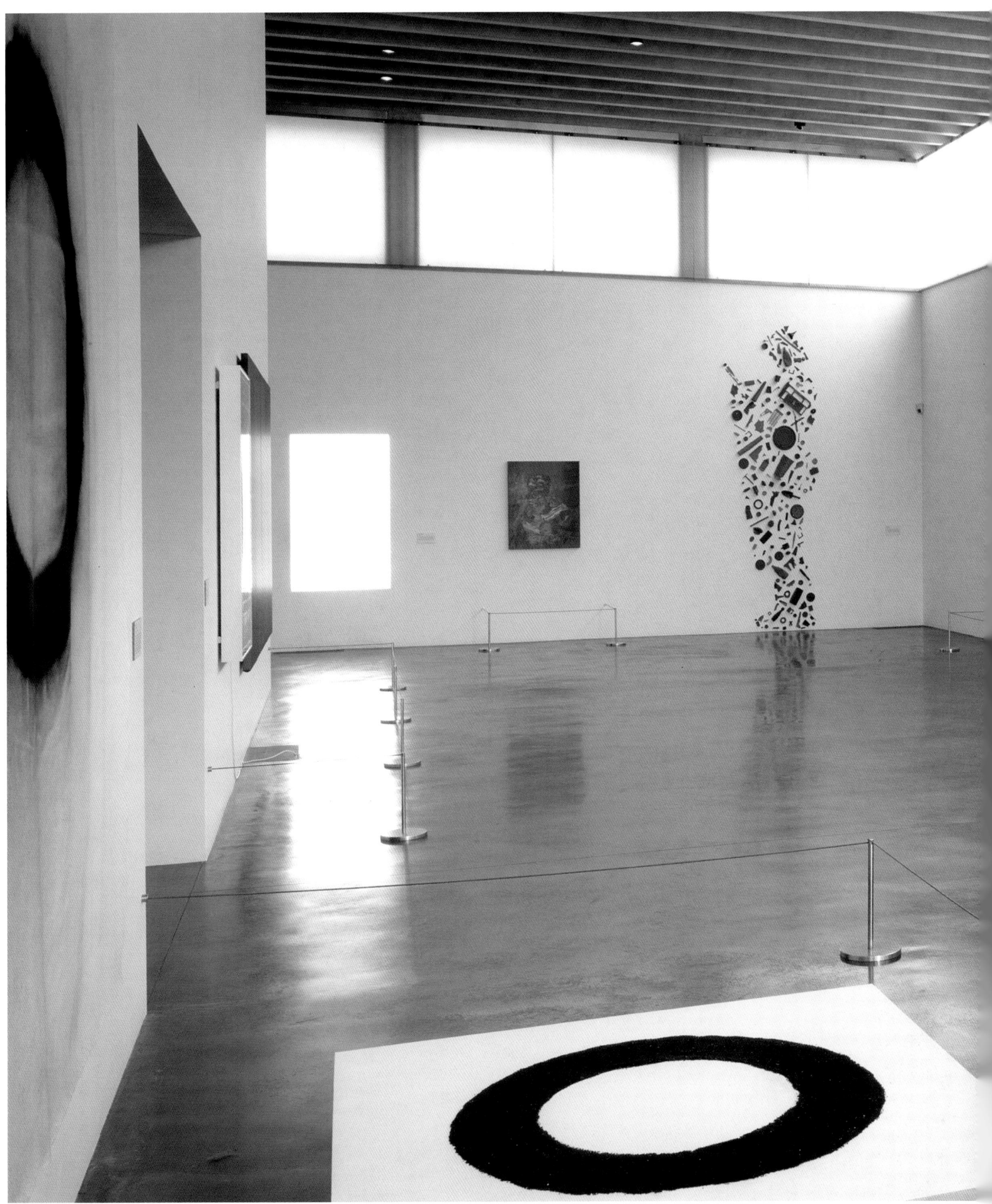

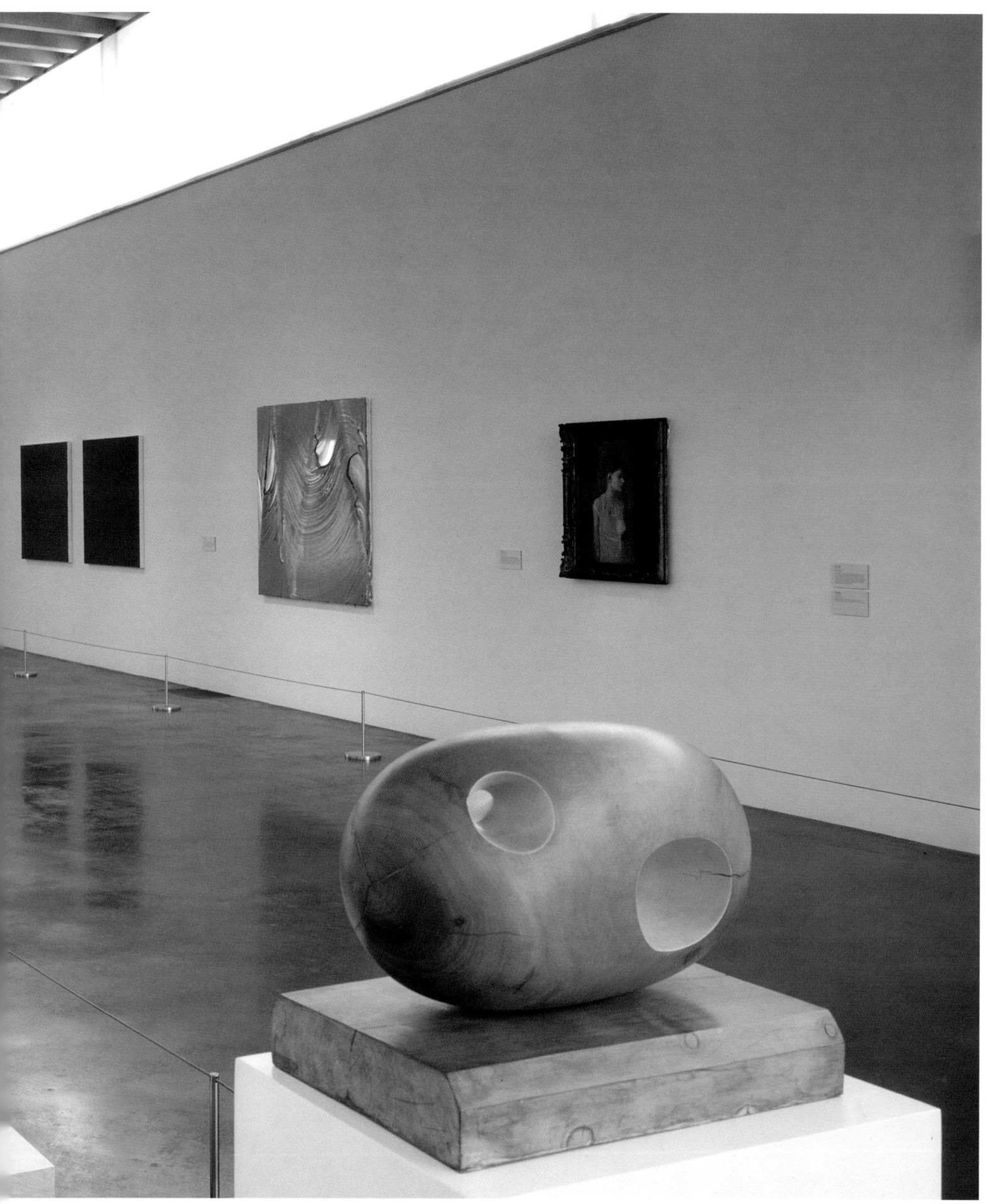

← Temporary exhibition gallery, with the exposed concrete structure above the translucent clerestory lighting.

→ The temporary exhibition galleries under construction. The framed structure at the centre of the plan provides essential flexibility for the installation of the mechanical systems.

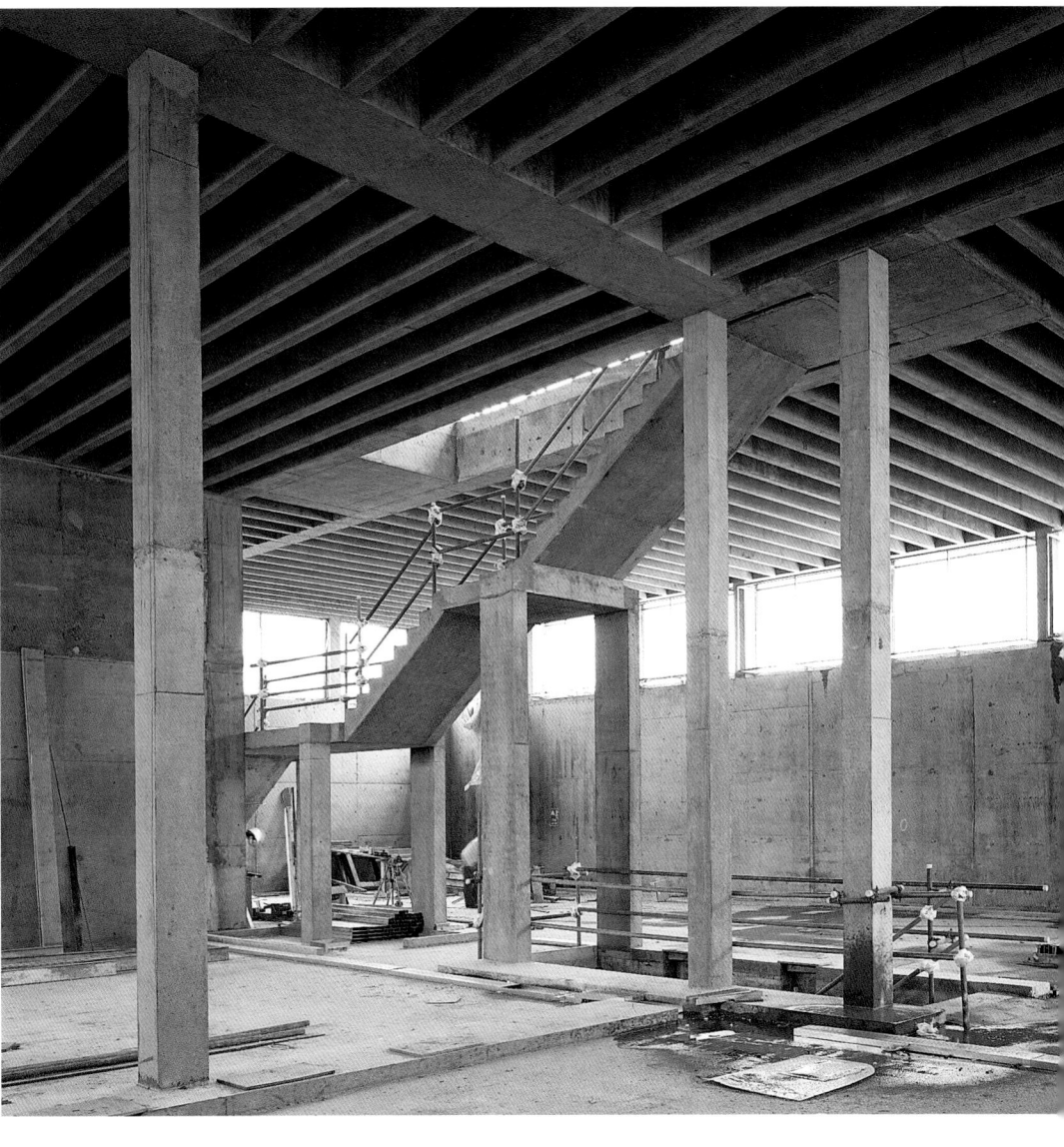

constantly to maintain the required levels, and the artificial lighting responds to daylight levels. At night the clerestorey becomes a giant luminaire, lighting up the galleries and shining out above the town. Spotlighting for individual works is provided from points within the ribbed concrete ceiling. In the second largest gallery, the clerestorey occupies the space above the two shorter walls – but this is another illusion, since only one of these is an outer wall: the clerestorey in the other wall is an artificial light source.

In the tradition of the rooflit gallery, the golden rule is to locate the light source outside the field of vision of the viewer when he or she is looking at a work of art. The clerestorey window almost always contradicts the rule, thereby producing an unacceptable glare. The Walsall design

seeks to overcome this through a singular clerestorey design, in which the glazing acts to diffuse light, and the internal blinds act to reduce the contrast between the window and the wall below, and the narrow proportions of the spaces produce a relatively uniform distribution of the light. This is not technological determinism. In terms of Venturi's critique, the balance of symbol and function has been redefined.

Thermal conditions in the gallery spaces and the meeting rooms are maintained by the use of full air-conditioning, which keeps the internal air within strict limits of temperature, humidity and filtration. The background noise level of gallery spaces is, conventionally, kept low and this was a further factor in the design of the plant. Computational fluid dynamic (CFD) modelling was

used to evaluate the design.

The architects held strong views on preserving the carefully crafted construction and materiality of the building and sought to conceal all the principal service systems. Two main service risers run vertically through the full height of the building, but, because of the complexity of the planning, the secondary distribution is more pragmatic. There are, however, absolutely lucid strategies for the distribution of air in the gallery spaces. In the rooms of the Garman Ryan collection, the Douglas-fir-clad suspended ceilings conceal the supply ductwork. Extract air is returned to the risers using the ceiling void. Incoming air is delivered around the long sides of the laylights and is extracted through slots cut into the ceiling. The temporary exhibition galleries have exposed ribbed-

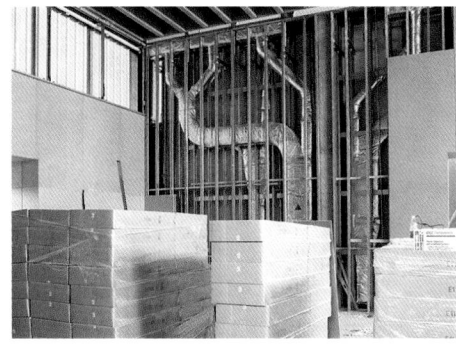

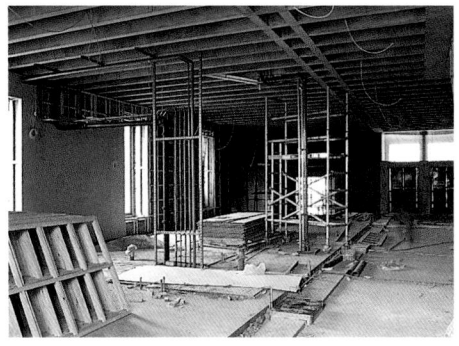

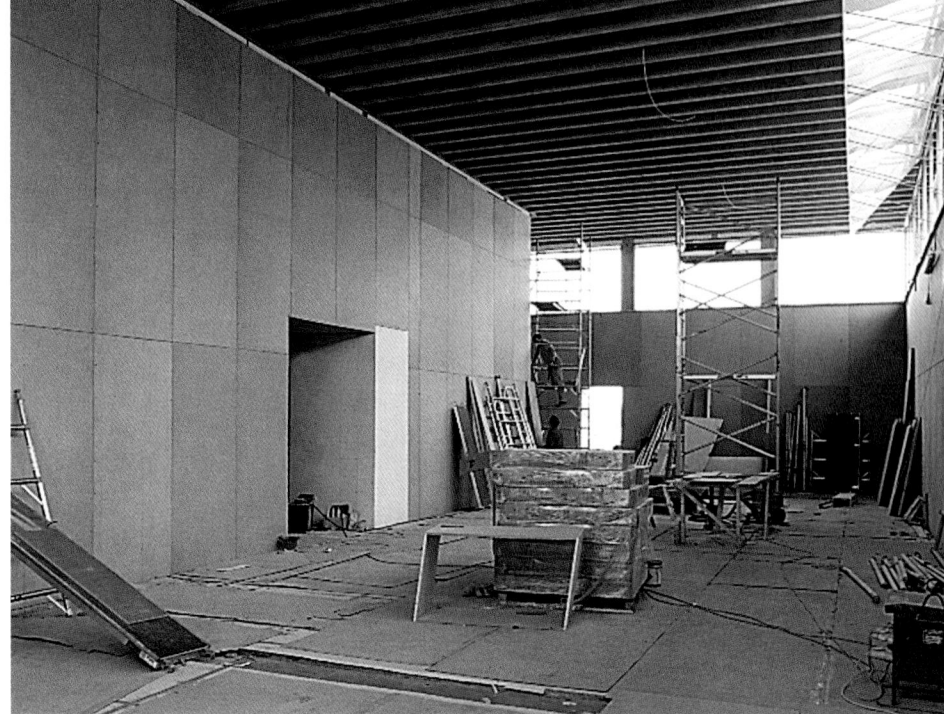

↑
Temporary exhibition gallery with major services installations, before fixing of cladding to steel studwork.

Garman Ryan Gallery showing services installations during construction.

↑
Temporary exhibition gallery after enclosure of structural frame with steel stud-frame construction.

concrete ceilings that prohibit any technical installation at high level. The ductwork is accommodated by a concrete frame structure at the core of the plan at this level, which allows the walls between the galleries to be constructed from steel stud frames and become, in effect, large service voids. Air is supplied through long slots at the top of the walls and extracted through the clerestorey windows.

In the *selective* mode areas of the building, such as the circulation spaces, the shop and the café, underfloor heating is installed under the powerfloat concrete floors. In other areas, a relatively conventional central heating system, with radiators or floor trench heaters, has been installed. Natural ventilation is provided, where appropriate, by openable windows. Elsewhere there

are high-level motorized windows, in keeping with the architects' desire to maintain the clarity of their tectonic language.

Conclusion

This building occupies an interesting position in the annals of environmental architecture. The overriding concerns of the architects belong to a world of subtle allusion and metaphor. As Brian Carter has observed, the abstract language of its form, spatiality and materiality carry references to the particularly English strand in Renaissance architecture that reached its height in Robert Smythson's Hardwick Hall (1597).[2] That building is amenable to an explicit environmental interpretation, but here at Walsall it is not that which is important.[3] We are far removed from the tradition of environmental

determinism.

In a building such as this, the job of the environmental consultant is to engineer solutions to an extremely complex programme in ways that support the poetic intentions of the architects and, crucially, are consistent with their tectonic objectives. Perhaps the closest analogy is with the collaborations between the architects and engineers of the 19th century, Soane with Perkins and Barry with Reid. As they sought to define the concept of the environmental function of buildings, these men achieved a remarkable synthesis of art and technology that was as inventive and undogmatic as the Walsall environment.

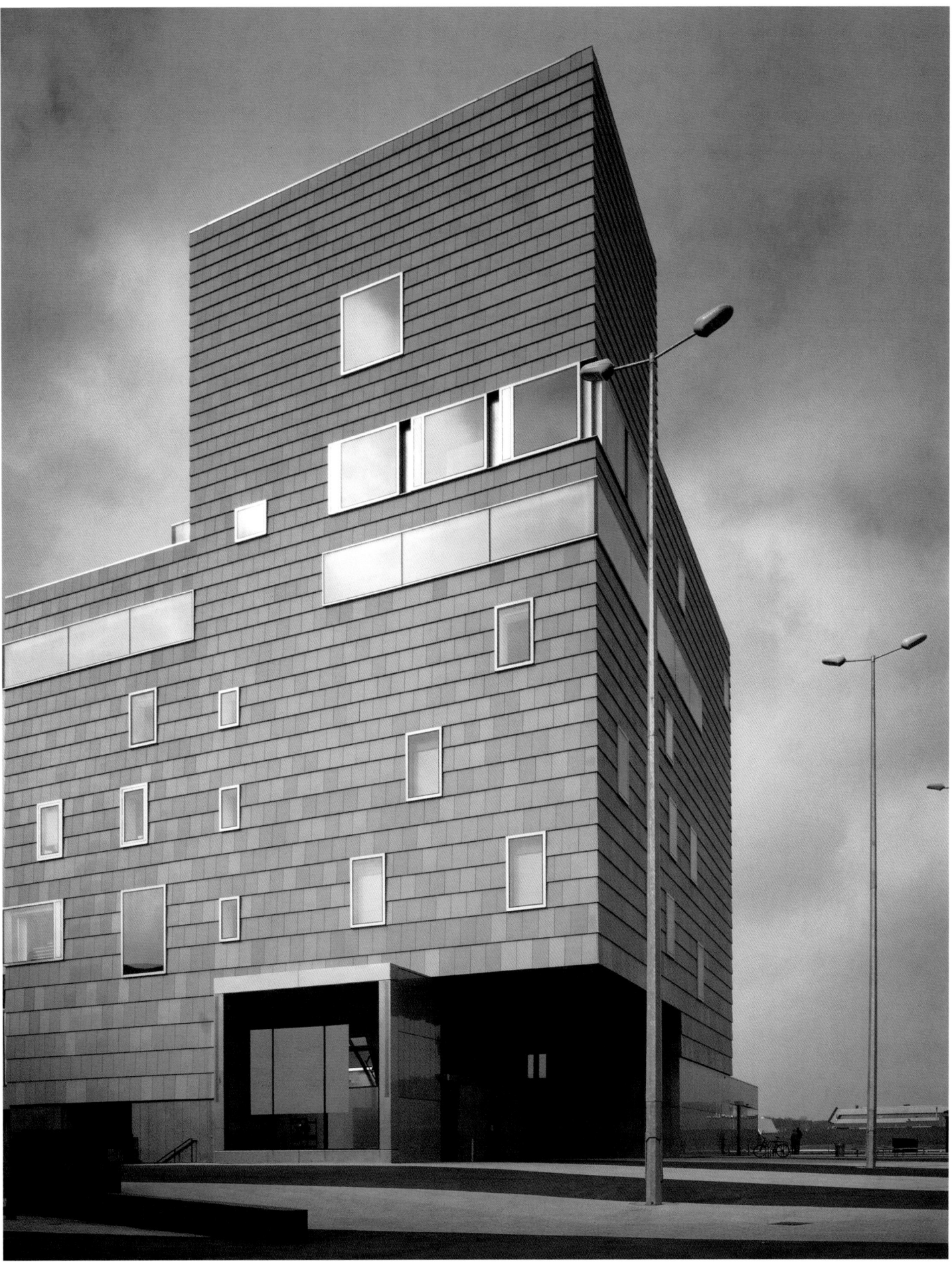

←

The entrance to the
building is set
beneath a
spectacular two-way
cantilever.

→

A computer-
generated
representation of
the illumination
of a temporary
exhibition gallery.

The central space
of the Garman Ryan
Gallery. The timber
ceilings conceal the
principal services
installations.

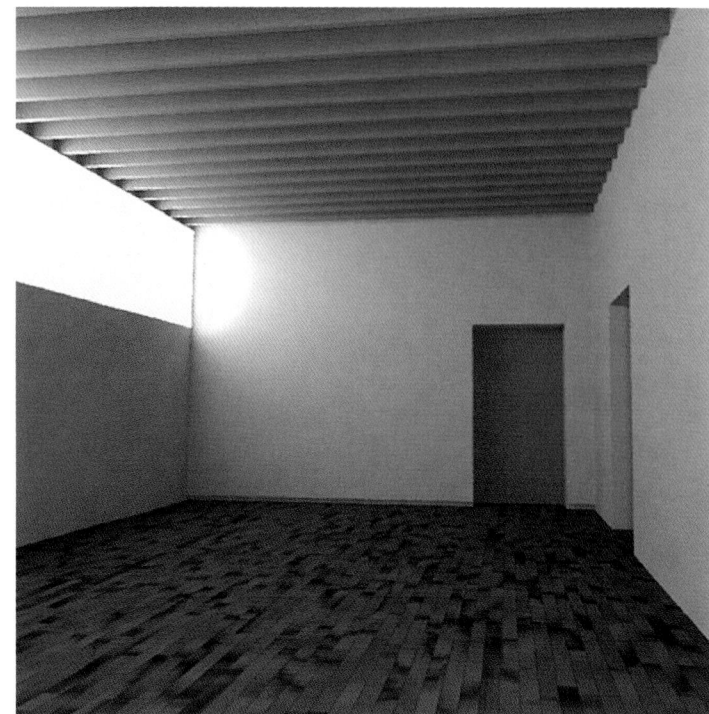

↓

Distant view along
the canal.

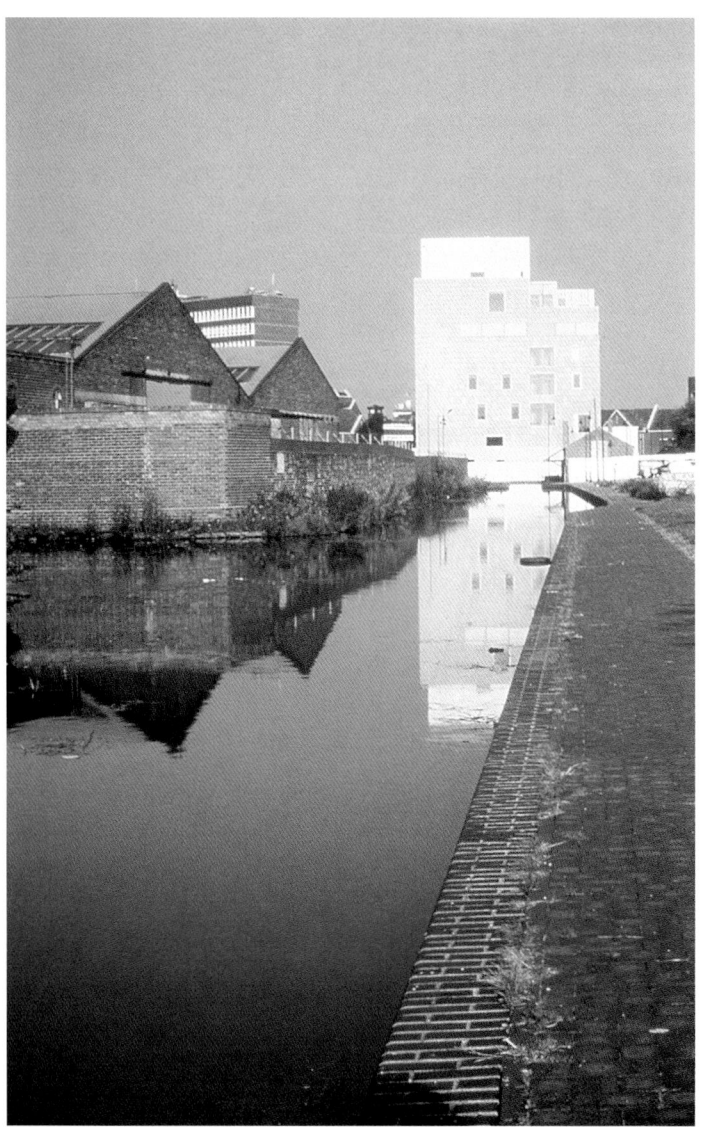

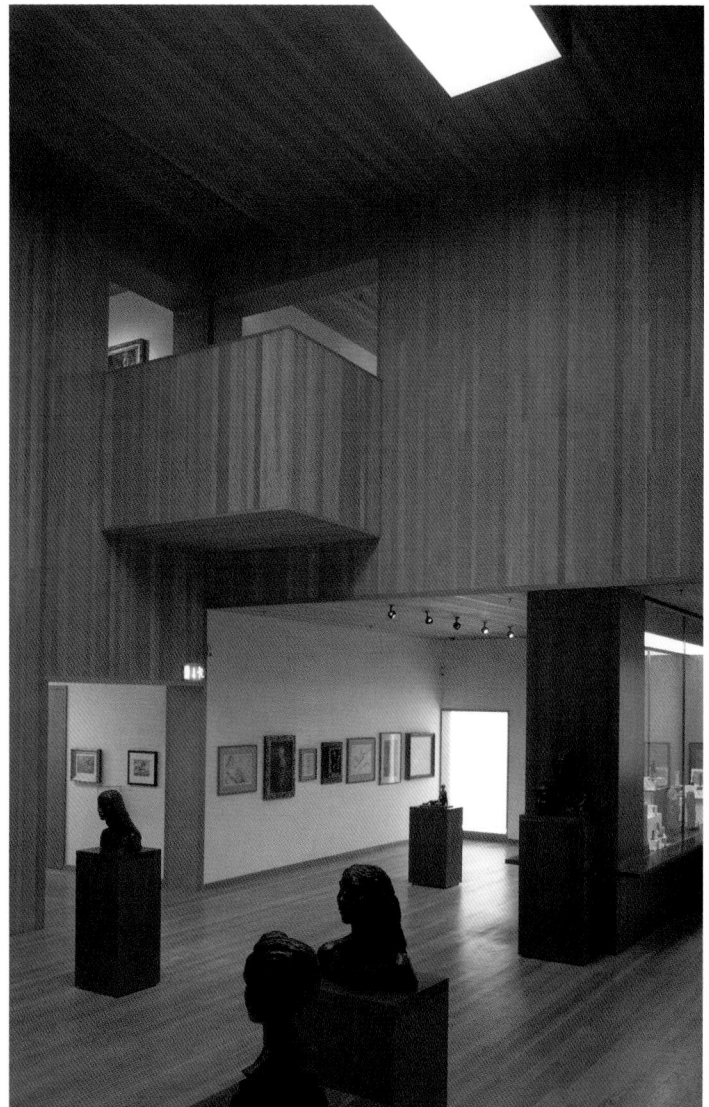

Tate Modern

Herzog & de Meuron
London, UK
2000

→
Night view across the
River Thames.

'Those wishing to grasp the full compass of the arts must, in addition to notions, also possess a perceptiveness trained to understand their various creative spheres. The Tate Modern is divided into two parts: a "vast void" and a space containing the art collection. The eye is led along a path through a succession of perfectly laid out spaces in which vanishing points, atmosphere and colour vary as required. All the technology is invisible. Without being an expressive force, the technology is what it ought to be: simply a service. The interdisciplinary approach creates a constant dialogue between architecture and art, and a harmonious synthesis within a historical monument regained to inject life into an area through the dynamics of culture.'

In this statement about their design for Tate Modern, the Swiss architects Herzog & de Meuron establish the essential continuity of art, architecture and context that defines the essence of their interpretation of the programme for the building.[1] They stress their 'interdisciplinary' approach and make clear their position on technology, emphatically declaring that it should be 'simply a

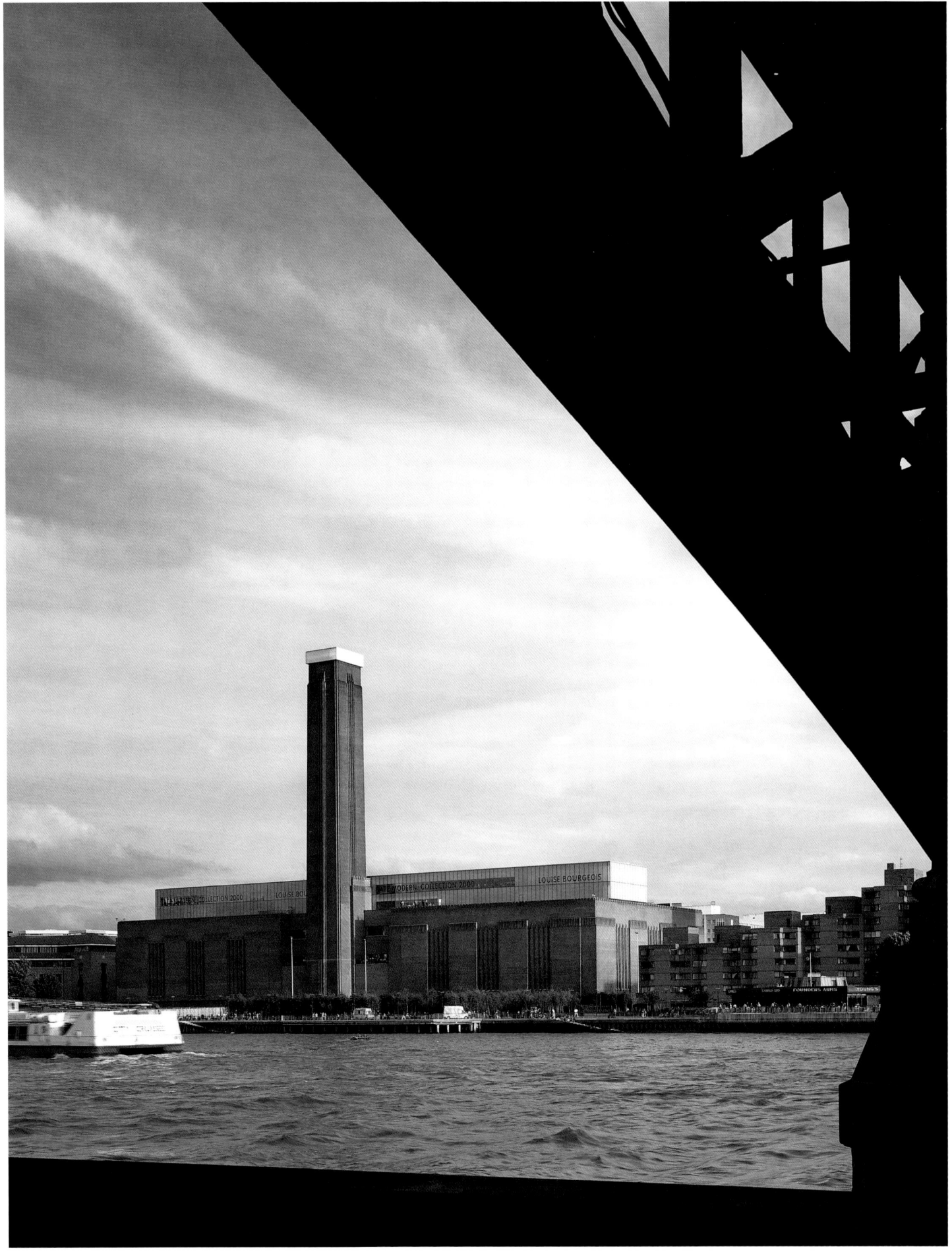

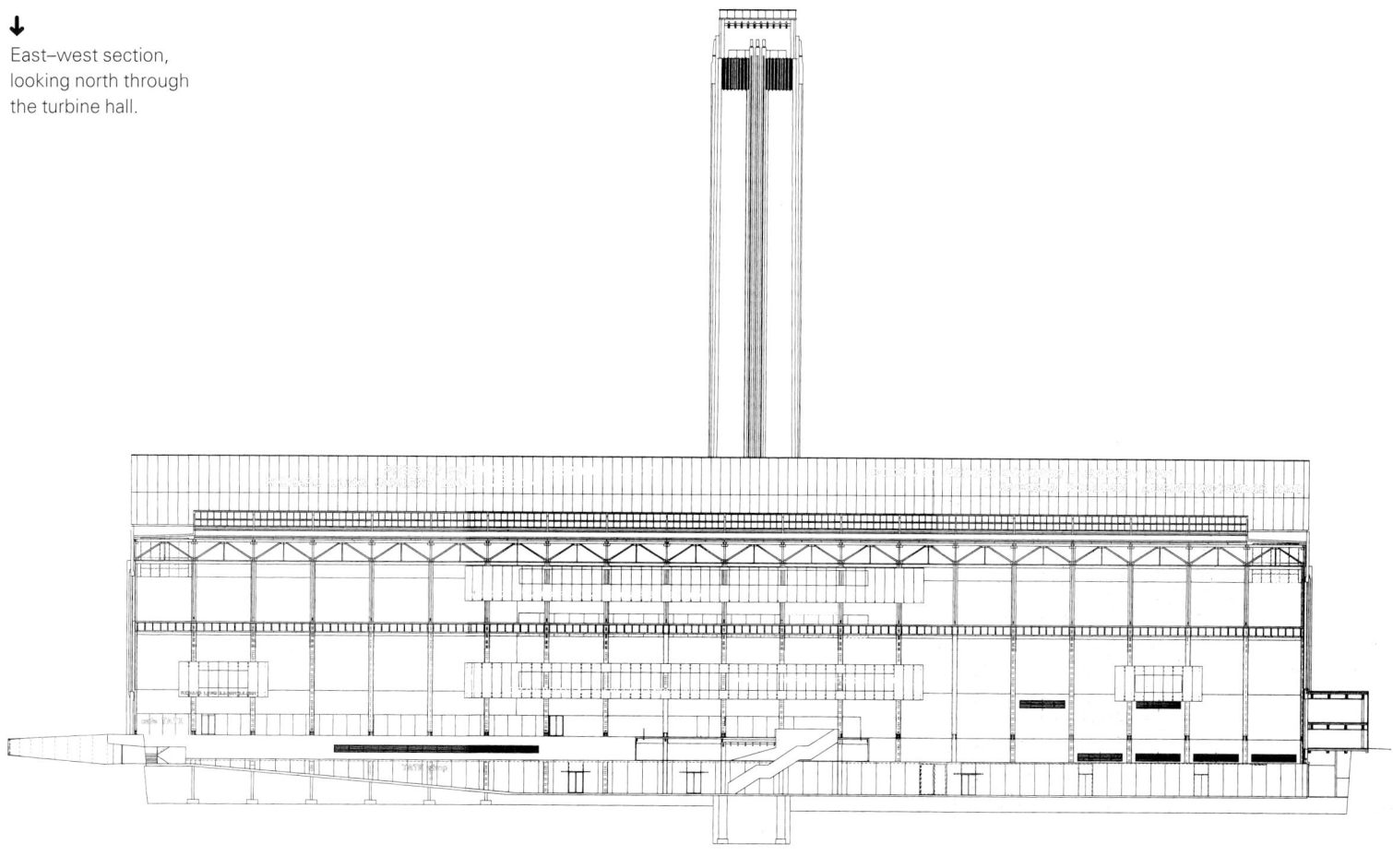

service'. In the same discussion the architects made some forthright comments about contemporary British architecture, describing it as 'all straightforward in the Gothic tradition. Architecture, they think here, always has to give expression to the technical side. We found that out time and time again in the form of a cultural confrontation during the building phase.'

Power to art
The London Borough of Southwark has a rich history.[2] By the 19th century it was a major industrial area packed with factories, wharves and dense slum housing. This contrasted with the wealth and grandeur of the City of London on the opposite bank of the River Thames – a state of affairs that persisted through much of the 20th century. In 1947 Bankside power

station was designed by Sir Giles Gilbert Scott to provide electricity supplies for much of the City. It opened in 1963 and was decommissioned in 1981. In 1994, the disused building was chosen as the site of Tate Modern – a location for the display of the Tate Gallery's collection of international modern art as well as for temporary exhibitions. The development of Tate Modern helped to transform this area of the south bank of the Thames into a major cultural centre close to the City.

Scott's vast brick-clad structure has become one of London's major landmarks. His design gave powerful expression to the building's utilitarian function through its symmetrical composition, with a single chimney gathering the flues from an array of boilers placed at the centre of the river frontage – where it acts as

counterpoint to the dome of St Paul's Cathedral on the opposite bank. Inside the building were two full-height volumes, the boiler house and the turbine hall, both of which ran the full length of the northern part of the building. A third major element, the switch house, offers space to accommodate the expected expansion of the museum.

Plan and section
The volume of the boiler house and turbine hall together was 160m (525ft) long, 54m (177ft) wide, and 34m (112ft) from basement to roof. After the surviving generating plant had been removed, the differentiation between the two major spaces was retained. The turbine hall was opened up to its full height and becomes an enormous covered public space, entered by a sweeping ramp leading

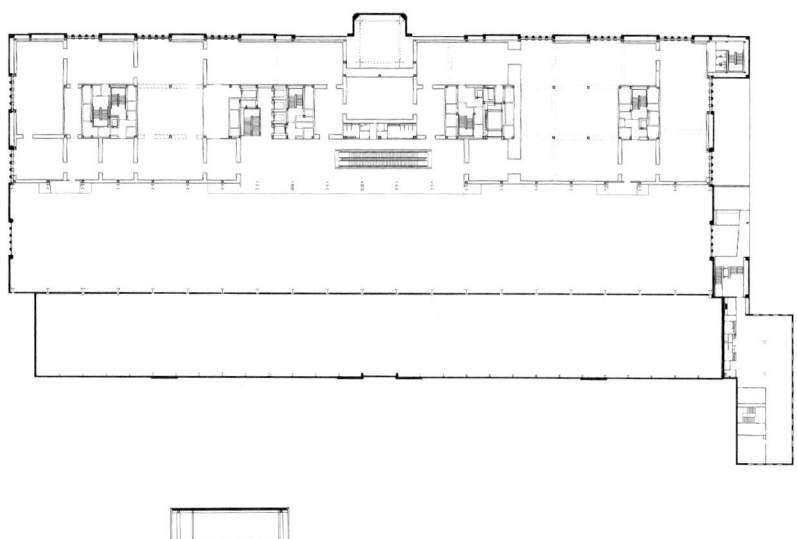

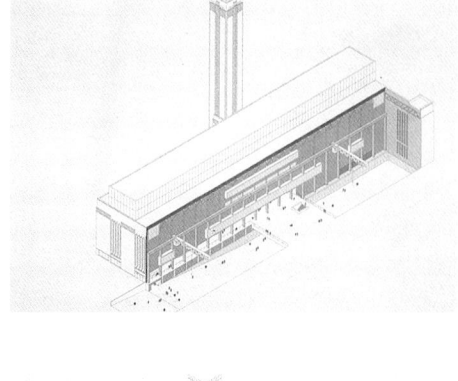

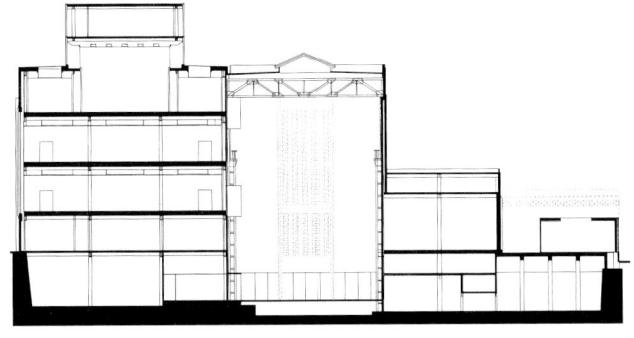

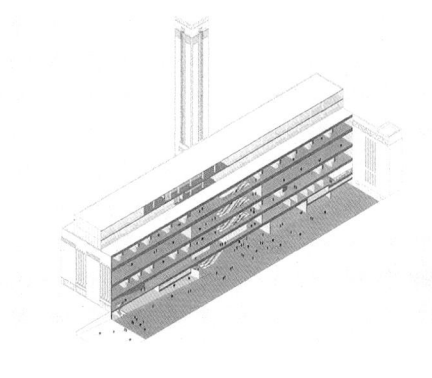

↑
Cut-away
axonometrics

↑
Gallery floor plan,
showing the relation
of gallery spaces to
service cores and
circulation.

Cross-section, looking
east, showing the
turbine hall (centre)
with the gallery
spaces inserted within
the former boiler
house.

down from the western entrance. To
the north, at the foot of the chimney, is
a second entrance approached from
the river frontage. A seven-storey
steel structure has been inserted into
the boiler house to form the art
museum itself. This rises above the
brick mass of the power station to
emerge as a translucent 'light beam',
signalling the building's new function
across the London skyline. The
internal façade between the gallery
and concourse holds a composition of
similarly translucent 'light boxes'.

Within the seven-storey section the
galleries are at levels 3, 4 and 5, and
the other elements of the museum –
shop, lecture theatre, administrative
offices, cafés and restaurant – are
below, at levels 1 and 2, or above, at
levels 6 and 7. The galleries at levels 3
and 5 contain works from the Tate's
permanent collection and level 4 is

designated for temporary exhibitions.
Within the gallery areas, the internal
subdivision is formed by wide hollow
partitions faced in medium-density
fibreboard. The principal circulation
and service spaces rise through the
central part of the plan and open out
into concourses that overlook the
turbine hall at each level.

Form and environment

Arup's environmental design strategy
is based on the architects' decree that
the technology of the building should
be 'simply a service'. In developing
this position further, they pointed to
the power exerted over them by the
existing building: 'whenever we
departed – in the dialectically
anticipatory sense – from what was
there, that became in a sense quite
ridiculous, because the existing fabric
was always stronger'.

The gallery spaces have a precisely
calculated set of relationships with the
existing fabric. Levels 3 and 4 occupy
the volume defined by Scott's huge
windows to north, east and west. At
level 5 the perimeter galleries sit
beneath the parapet of the former
boiler house, from where they are lit
by concealed rooflights, and the
central spaces penetrate up into the
lower part of the 'light beam'. This
defines two strips of continuous
clerestory window, facing north and
south.

The lighting design of the spaces
follows directly from these
relationships between old and new.
The aim was to bring daylight into the
galleries wherever possible and to
balance this with the needs for control
and conservation and the need to
provide supplementary artificial
lighting. At level 5 the rooflights of the

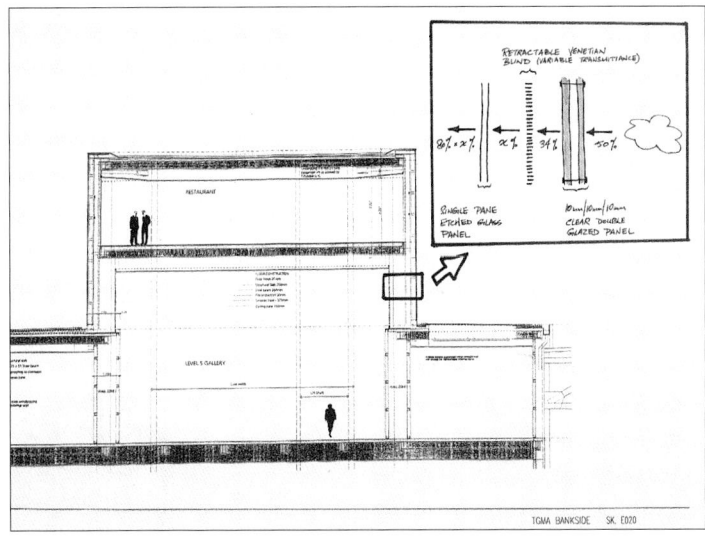

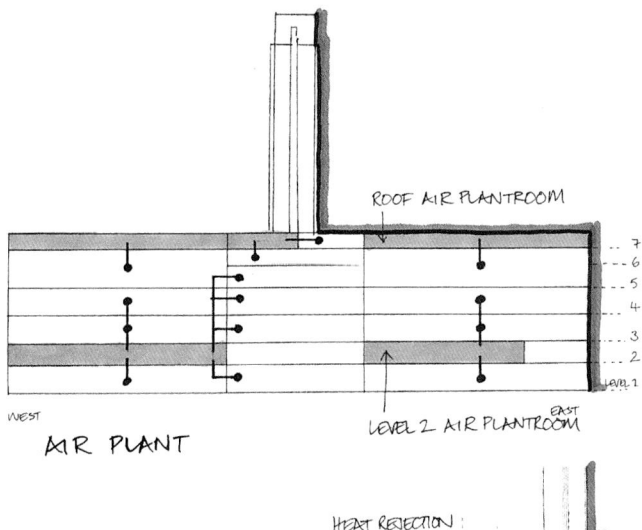

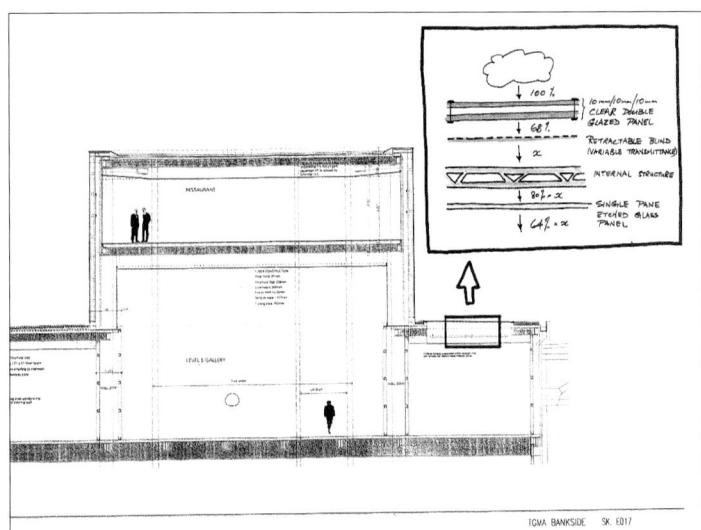

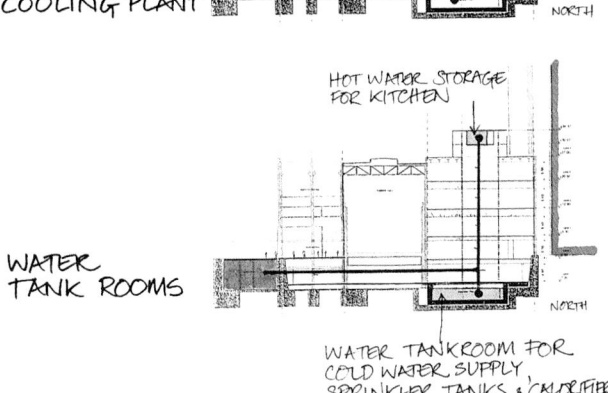

perimeter galleries have diffusing 'laylights' of translucent glass. Concealed blinds control levels when there is an excess of daylight and there is artificial lighting for use on dull days and at night. The clerestories in the central double-height galleries have a double layer of translucent glazing. In the void between the layers, adjustable louvred blinds control the level of daylight that is admitted and artificial lighting provides night-time illumination. Artificial lighting also illuminates the 'light beam' as it glows above the museum's rooftop at night. At levels 3 and 4, daylight enters through Scott's windows – 'cathedral' windows, as Herzog & de Meuron describe them – supplemented by artificially lit laylights that simulate the effect of the rooflights on level 5. In all the galleries further artificial lighting can be

installed, in the form of spotlights, to illuminate individual works. Opaque roller blinds allow all the windows and rooflights to be completely blacked out.

This strategy makes it possible to bring varying levels and qualities of light into each of the galleries, allowing visitors to experience a sense of the progression of the seasons and changes in the local weather. In their architectural development these spaces are elaborately unassertive. All junctions of floor and wall, wall and ceiling, clerestory or laylight and ceiling, are unadorned and flush. Sawn oak boards bring warmth and texture to the lower galleries; on the upper floor, wood is replaced by a polished concrete finish.

The turbine hall – used for temporary exhibitions of large-scale

works – retains its original roof structure. The continuous central rooflight has been reconstructed and provides copious daylight. Banks of fluorescent lamps running along the blind south wall supplement this at night – but the dramatic light in this space is provided by the 'light boxes' that project from the opposite wall. By their use of translucent glass, these bring the principal material theme of the new intervention, expressed on the exterior by the light beam, into the heart of the building. The light beam plays a consciously ambiguous part in the life of the building, acting as a bringer of light during the day and as a beacon at night. The light boxes also have dual functions – as inhabited space, extending the galleries and concourses into the turbine hall, and as enormous luminaires.

← Engineer's design drawings, showing detailed explorations of specific conditions of the enclosure in the exhibition galleries (far left, top and bottom) and schematic layouts of the air plant, heating and cooling plant and water services (left).

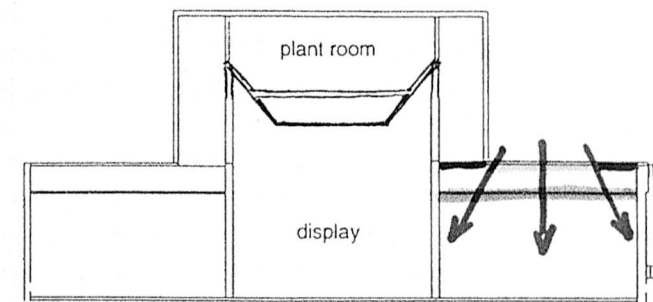

↓ Computer-generated studies of relative humidity in exhibition spaces

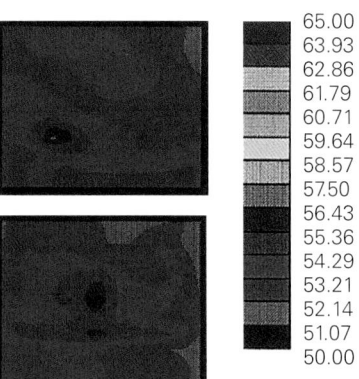

65.00
63.93
62.86
61.79
60.71
59.64
58.57
57.50
56.43
55.36
54.29
53.21
52.14
51.07
50.00

Relative humidity in percentages.

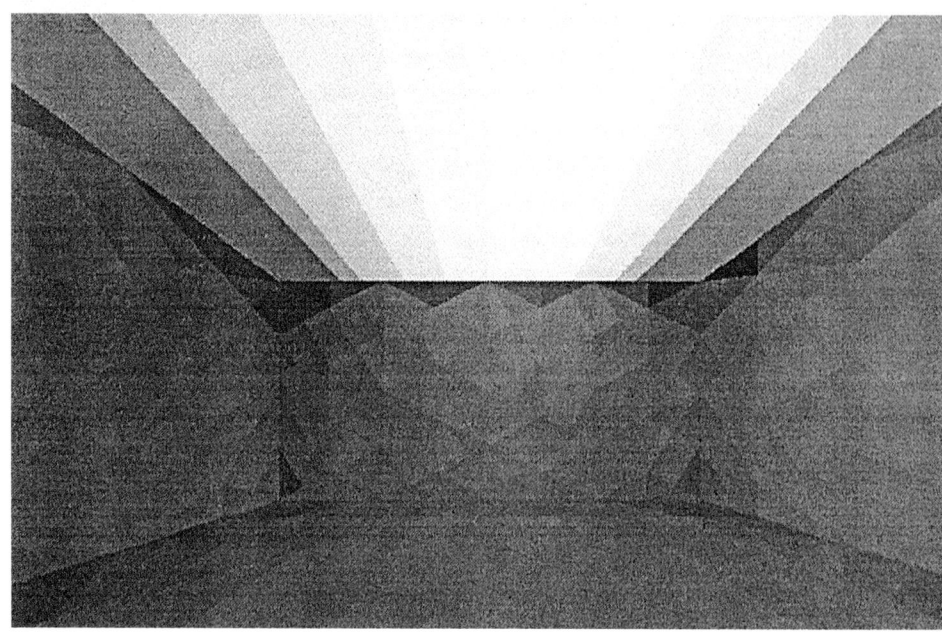

↑ Daylighting studies of roof-lit gallery.

Invisible service

Designing the environment of an art museum is not solely a question of controlled lighting. Modern standards of conservation demand that, almost without exception, works of art must be displayed in spaces where every measurable element of the environment is controlled. The envelope of the modern gallery is a sealed box – exclusive, in our terminology – within which mechanical systems operate to admit, filter, temper, supply and extract air at precisely calculated levels of temperature, humidity and cleanliness. To achieve this, a building must incorporate extensive networks of ducts and voids connecting every conditioned space to centrally located plant rooms.

The architectural philosophy of Herzog & de Meuron eschews what they identify as a particularly British preoccupation: 'to give expression to the technical side'. For them, 'All the technology is invisible.' In Tate Modern, the air-conditioning to the galleries is a low-velocity displacement system. The supply air is carried from the plant room through the vertical service cores and is then distributed horizontally at each floor at high level. From there it travels downwards, in ducts located within the hollow walls that define the sequence of galleries. A plenum space extends beneath the floors, and air is finally delivered from this to the galleries through cast-iron grilles. Return air is extracted through the ceiling void. To achieve efficient distribution and to limit the depth of the structural and servicing zone, a double slab section was devised: a second slab was placed 460mm (18in) above the main concrete floor slab, creating the supply plenum.

The cast-iron grilles, set into floors of either sawn oak or polished concrete, are a carefully thought-out element of the iconography of the building and, in particular, of the architects' position on the visual status of the services installations. 'The building has, first of all, this roughness. That's why we took these grilles. Without creating industrial architecture in the strict sense. There's more at issue here than just moods...but architecture does have to do with atmospheres and images. If I have smooth aluminium grilles, for example, then I want to demonstrate that we have a ventilation system which contrasts with the stuffy old industrial building. And with these cast-iron grilles, I blur this question of old and new, I don't even ask it.'[3]

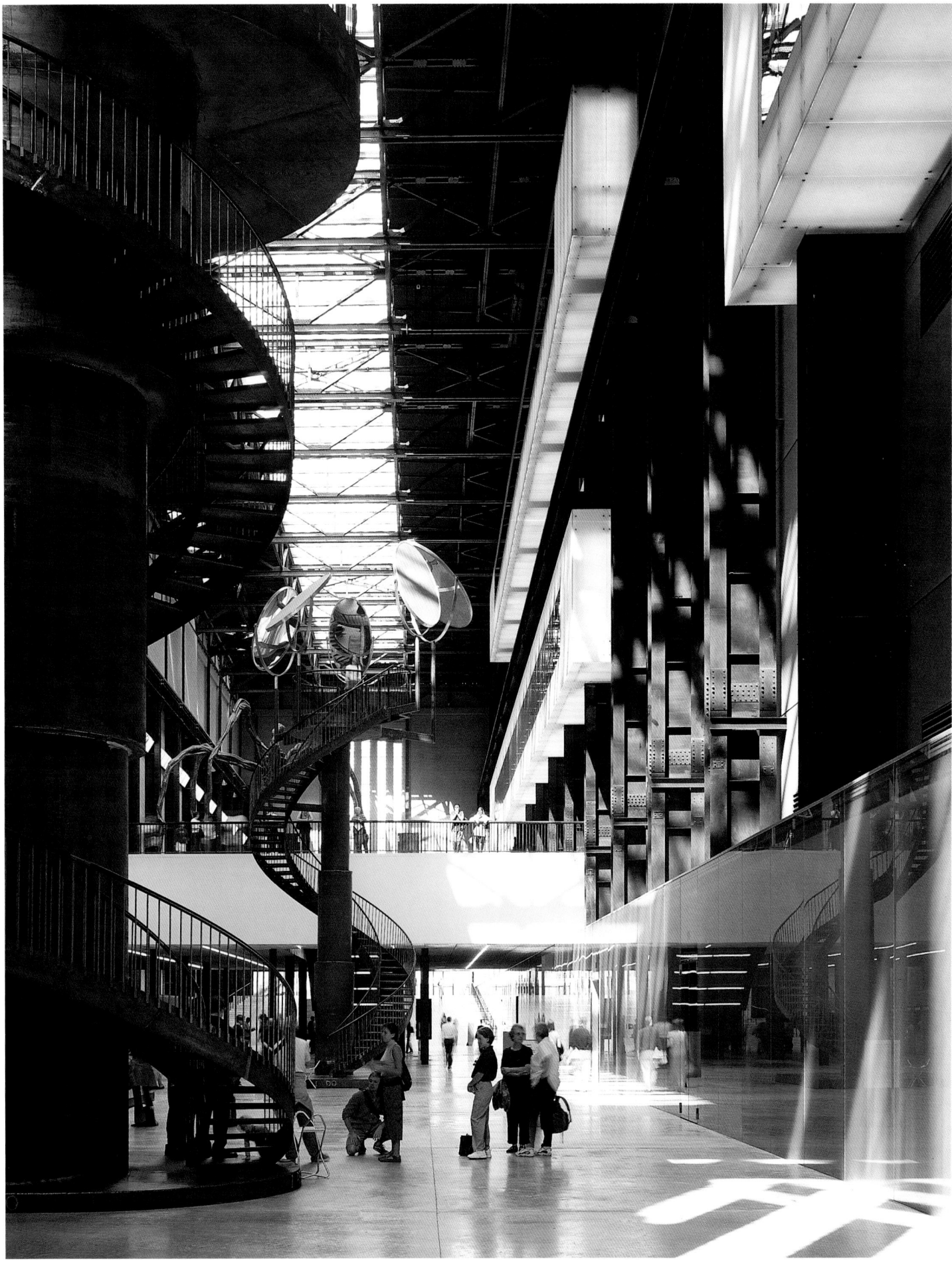

The turbine hall, with sculpture installation by Louise Bourgeois.

Detail of cast-iron air conditioning grille set in sawn oak floor.

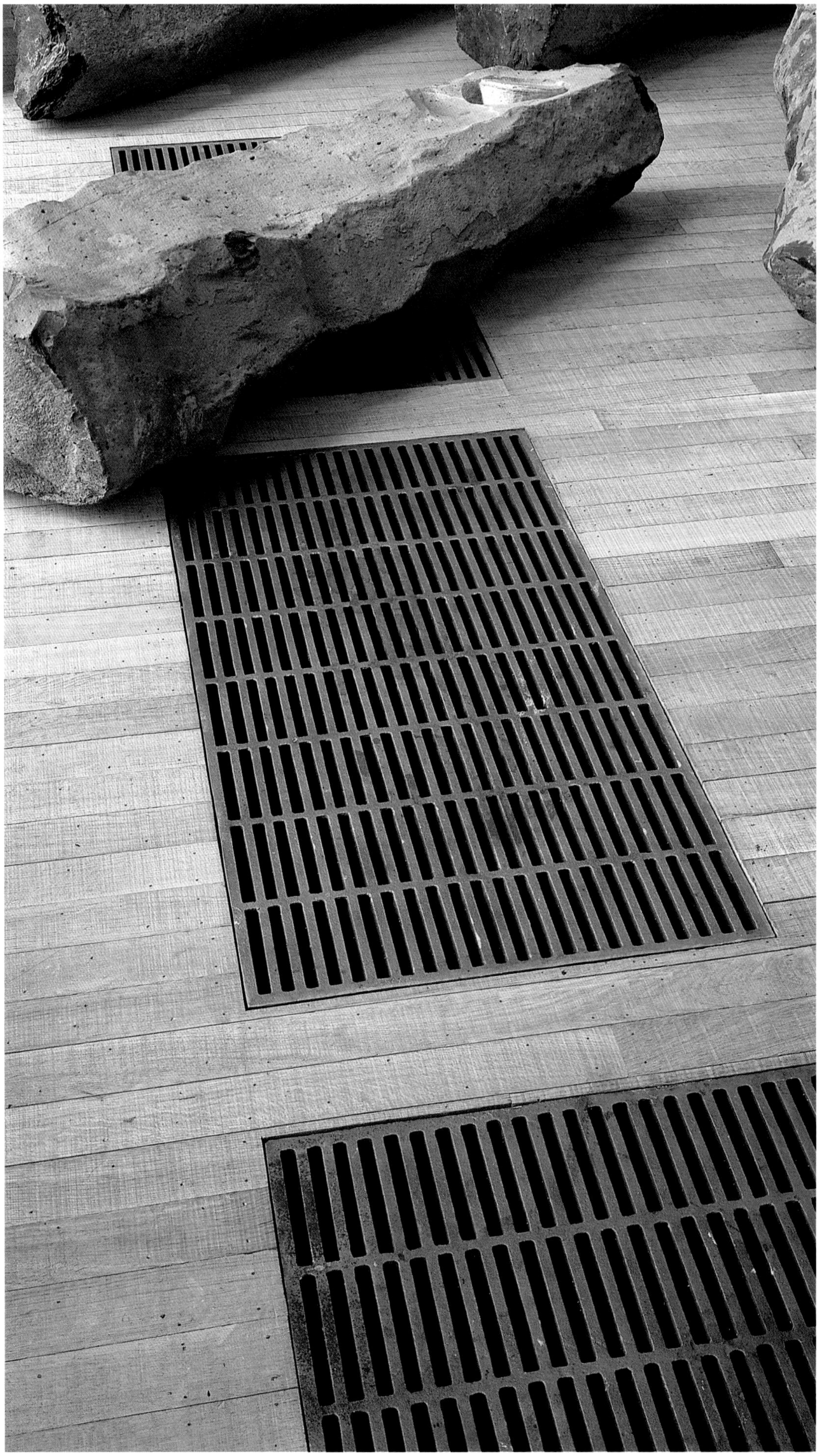

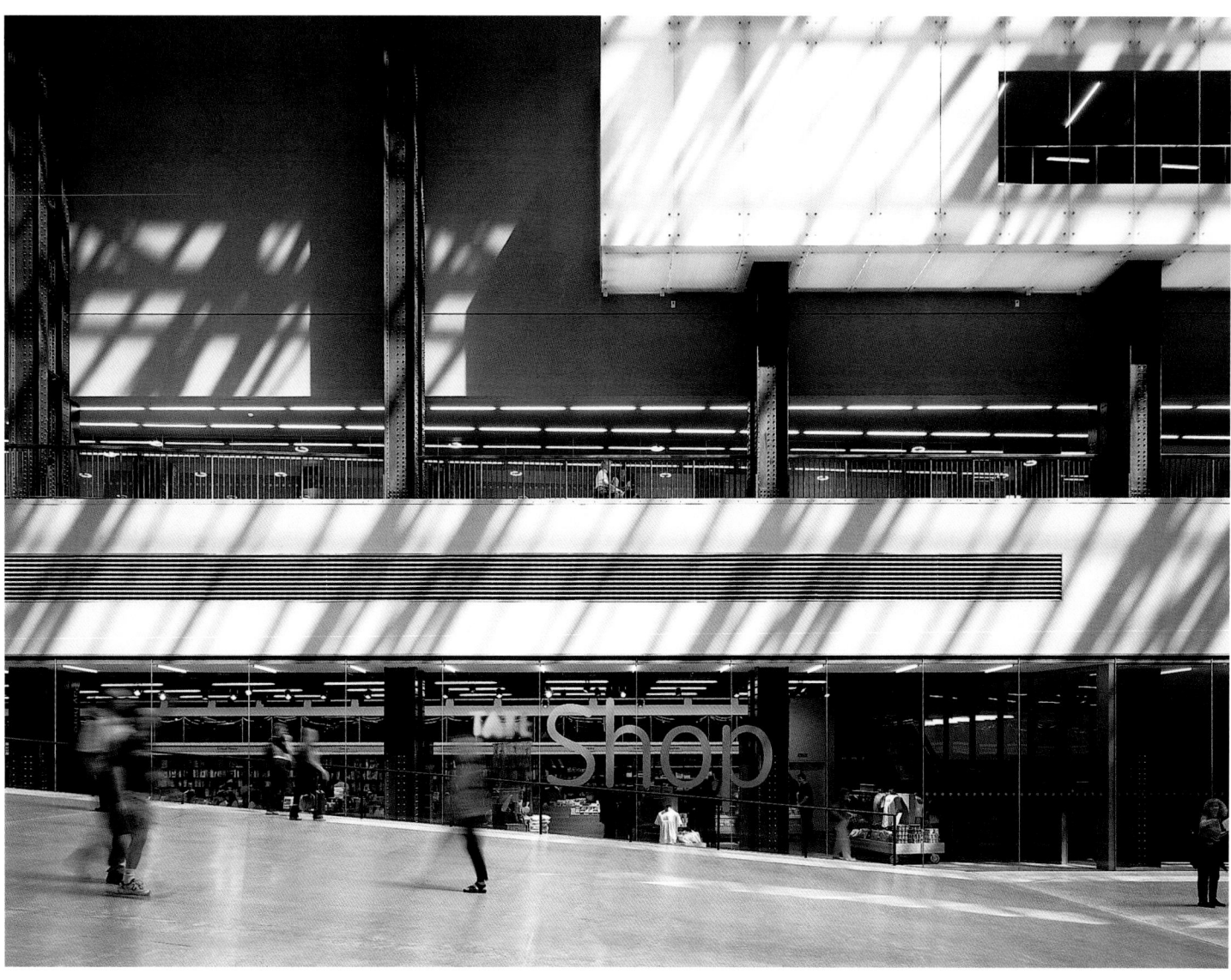

At certain critical points in the building the doctrine of 'invisible technology' has been abandoned. The most notable of these is in the circulation concourses, where the suspended ceiling has been omitted to reveal the network of black-painted air ducts and electrical conduits beneath the exposed concrete slab. A similar, but perhaps more self-consciously ironic installation is to be found in the café, where haloes of fluorescent light are suspended beneath an array of exposed machinery, this time finished in metallic silver paint.

Conclusion

In transforming Bankside power station into Tate Modern, Herzog & de Meuron challenged the specifically British interpretation of the relationship between architecture and technology, the approach that they characterize as 'all straightforward in the Gothic tradition', where architecture, 'give[s] expression to the technical side'. Although the roots of this tradition may be traced back to the material theories of John Ruskin and Augustus Pugin, in the lineage proposed by Nikolaus Pevsner in *Pioneers of Modern Design*, equal authority for a kind of technological display may be found in the European traditions of Henri Labrouste and Gottfried Semper.[4] More recently, Franco Albini's works and Louis Kahn's strictures about 'ducts and pipes' indicate its universal diffusion.

The wider perspective offered by our historical review of the relationship between the architecture and engineering of environment may more specifically locate Herzog & de Meuron's position in the tradition of,

in Banham's terminology, 'concealed power'. That interpretation, as explained in the introduction, runs through the unfolding of this history over the last two centuries, alongside the alternative of 'exposed power', in the work of architects as different as Karl Friedrich Schinkel, Mies van der Rohe and Robert Venturi. It is in this context that the subtle clarity of the engineering of this design makes its greatest contribution.

← Detail of internal façade of turbine hall.

→ Concourse at Level 5. The omission of a suspended ceiling in the circulation areas provides one of the few occasions in the building where services are exposed to public view.

↓ Exhibition gallery at Level 5, with clerestory lighting flowing from the externally expressed light beam.

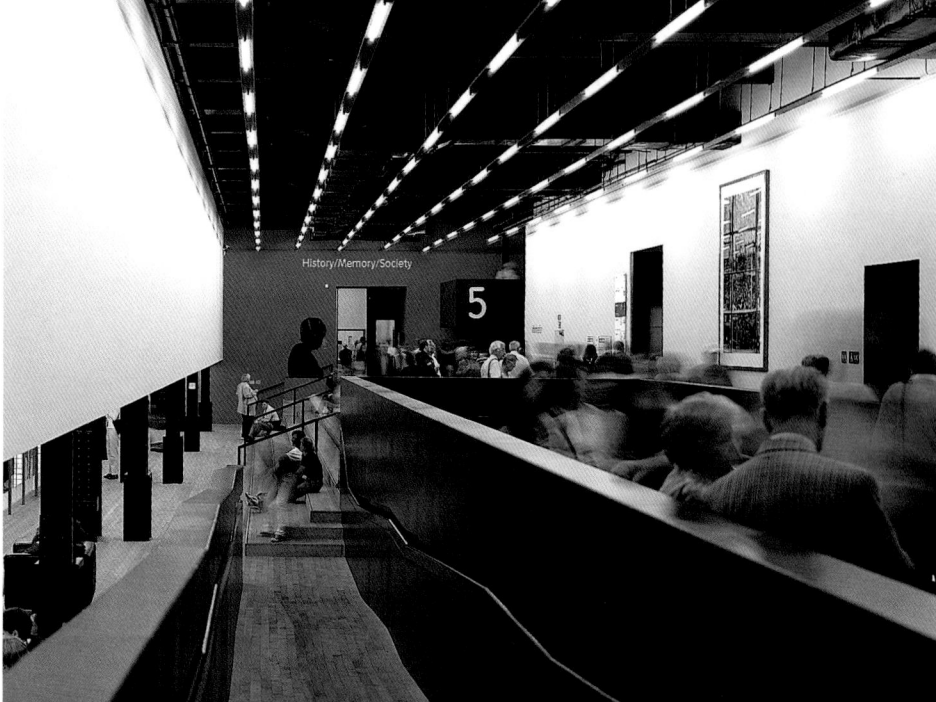

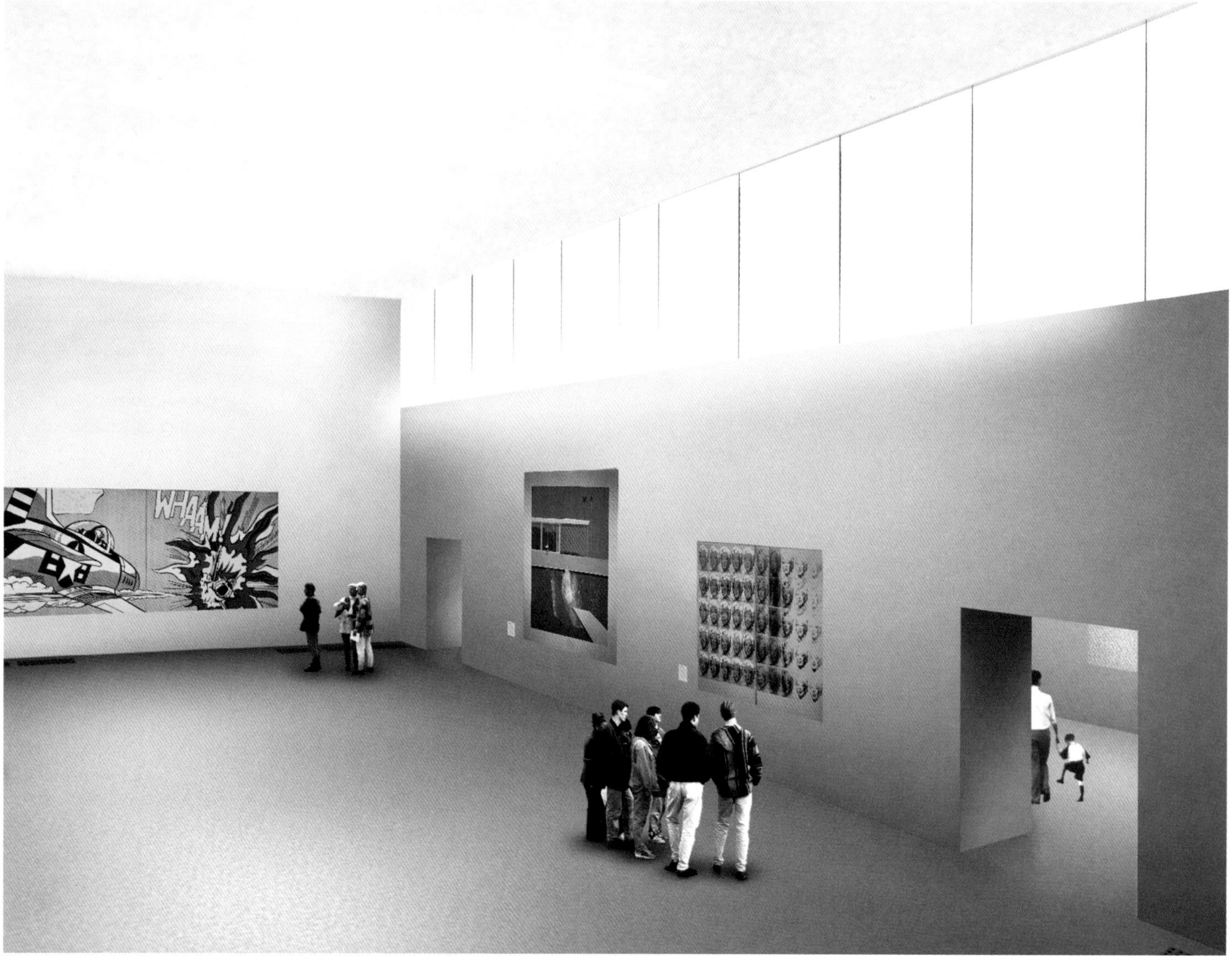

Portuguese Pavilion Expo 98
Álvaro Siza
Lisbon, Portugal
1998

→

The entrance canopy provides a protected microclimate before entering the building.

'Working in a team is like working alone, but with a capacity for analysis and invention multiplied by X,' writes the architect Álvaro Siza.[1] 'Each person's discoveries, each hypothesis launched into the flow, generate further hypotheses and further discoveries on their part and other's – as happens with my ideas when I work alone – but here at a giddy rate.... It is therefore urgent, not least for the work of these agents, that we extend information early on and to everyone, to bring to an end the myths of specialisation, of the incommunicable complexity of all the different specialisms.'

Admiration for the work of Álvaro Siza focuses on the way in which his buildings appear to transform the tenets of international Modernism into a decorous and culturally grounded vocabulary that is responsive to the issues of globalization. As Kenneth Frampton writes, 'Siza pursues an architecture of resistance. The global has always to be offset by the local at every level, not in terms of some categoric rejection of universal technology, but rather in recognition of the need to mediate technique through culture.'[2] In view of his pronounced sensitivity to context, it is surprising that little

critical attention has been given to Siza as an environmentalist. He regards teamwork as crucial to the success of contemporary architecture, and his design for the Portuguese Pavilion at Expo 98 makes an important contribution to the developing relationship between architecture and environmental engineering.

Site and programme
In addition to its function as an international showground, Expo 98 played a role in the planned expansion of Lisbon. The site on derelict land to the north of the

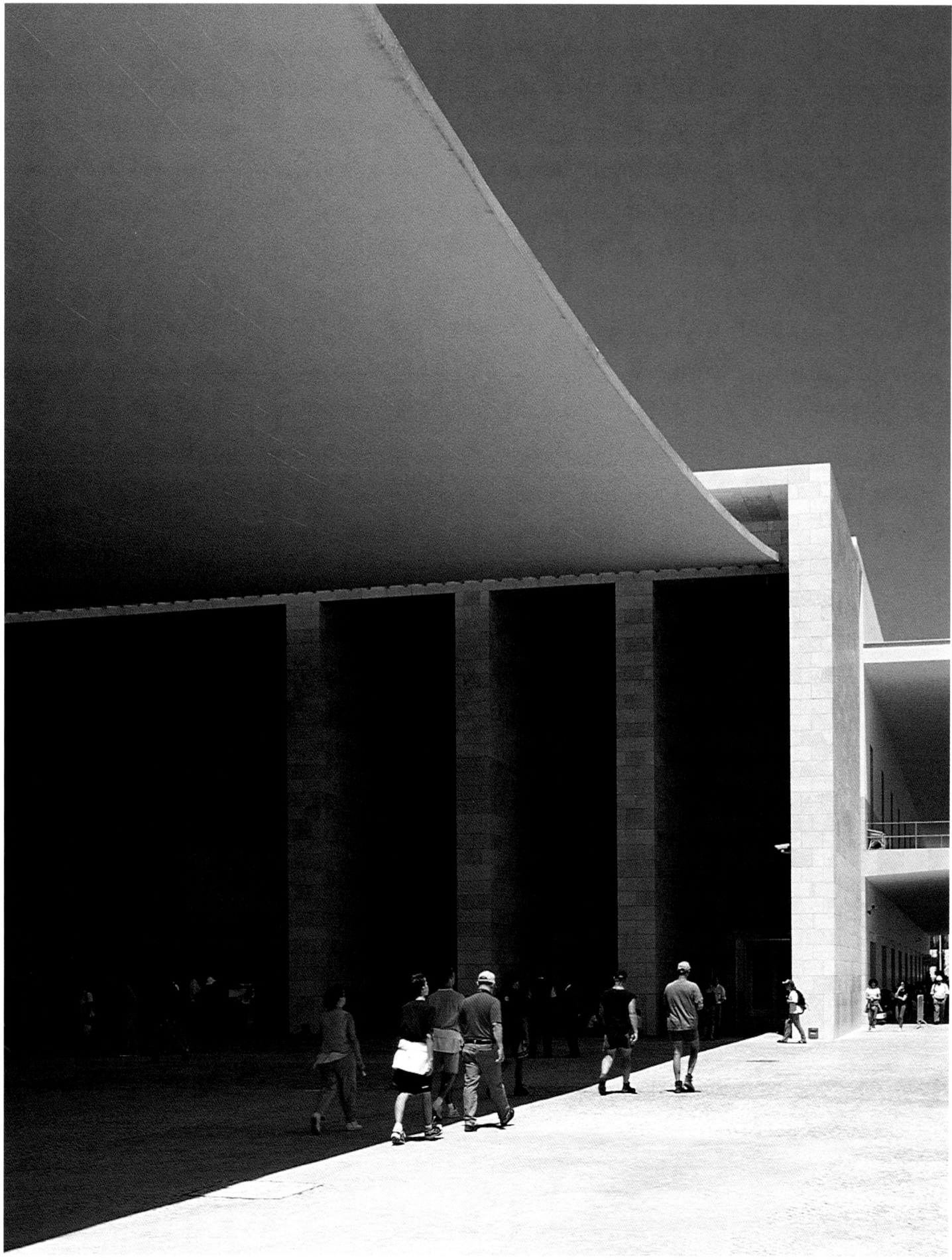

213

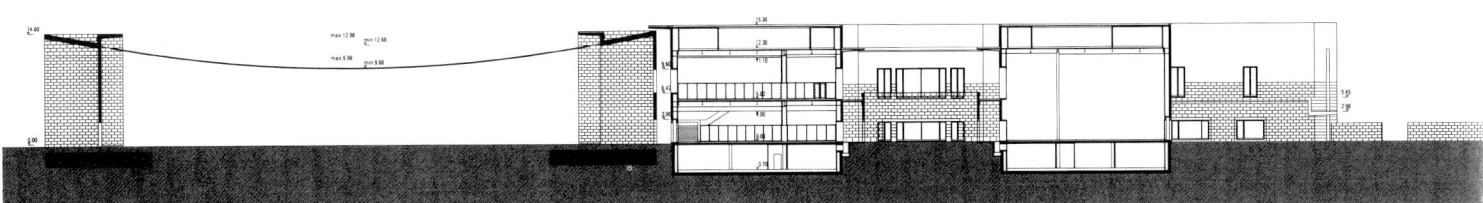

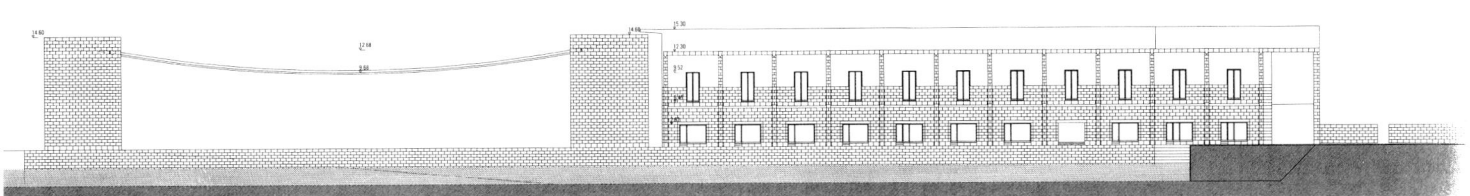

historic centre, on the banks of the Tagus, is close to the international airport and on the main railway route to Coimbra and Porto. As part of the preparations for Expo 98, the metro system, which in recent years has transformed the city's transport infrastructure, was extended to the site. Santiago Calatrava's remarkable Oriente Station – which marks a meeting point of metro, main railway and local bus network – links the Expo site directly to local, regional, national and international transport networks, laying the foundations for major expansion. At the time of Expo 98 a major retail and commercial centre had already been completed and a start had been made on a residential development programme.

The Portuguese Pavilion was designed symbolically and functionally to represent the host nation and to provide a venue for all the important ceremonies that took place during Expo 98. It was also the location of a major multimedia installation designed by Eduardo Souto de Moura. The pavilion occupies a spectacular position overlooking the lagoon of Doca dos Olivais at the centre of the Expo site. Its form is both simple and remarkable. A two-storey pavilion faced in stone and stucco stands to the north of an independently supported entrance canopy whose scale and construction are awe-inspiring. A shallow concrete catenary hangs on steel cables between two stone- and tile-clad supporting structures, spanning 67.5m (221ft). The space defined becomes, simultaneously, piazza, providing a microclimate sheltered from the summer sun, and porte cochère,

signalling the entrance to a important public building.

Indeterminacy and environmental design
Uncertainty about the long-term use of the building was a major factor in its design, which might have led towards an architecture of overt 'adaptability'. The apparatus of 'free space' and its concomitant of 'flexible services' have played a major part in recent architectural methodology. The arguments that underpinned the design of a building such as the Centre Pompidou might have been brought to bear on the Portuguese Pavilion. As *The Architectural Review* wrote of Pompidou, 'nothing is rigid, immutable, the container is flexible, adaptable through the use of "soft" mechanisms, articulated so that it can be adapted'.[3]

Conceptual sketch showing the relationship between the sweeping canopy and the body of the building.

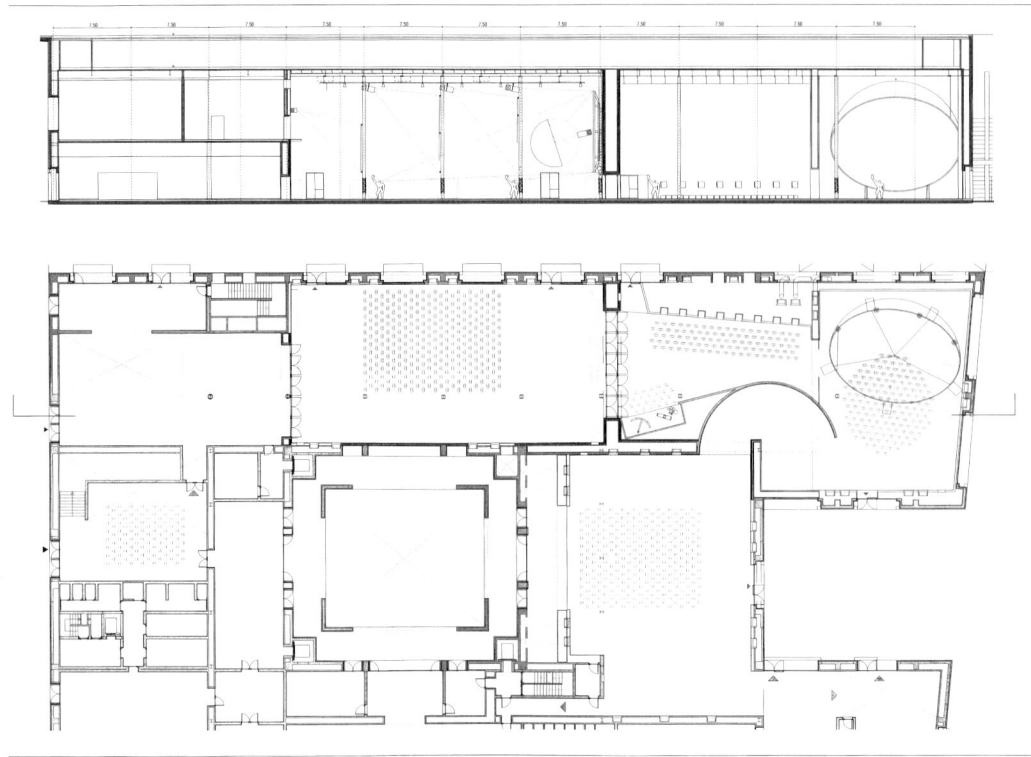

Longitudinal section through the building showing the internal courtyard.

Ground floor plan.

South elevation.

With two comprehensive internal refits since its completion, the Centre Pompidou appears to have been well served by such an approach to its design. But Siza's architecture is not concerned with the kind of functional openness and technological display represented by the Centre Pompidou; in his eyes, if the future role of a building is uncertain, a less demonstrative solution has to found.

The pavilion is organized around an open atrium. To the west and north are the main double-height exhibition spaces, with the more cellular ceremonial spaces and services occupying the two-storeyed south and east wings. The structure of the building is a hybrid of reinforced-concrete external envelope with a steel frame within supporting lightweight concrete on profiled steel decking to form the slabs. This

solution was devised by the engineers in response to the seismic risk in the Lisbon region and also to allow removal of floors and partitions if that became part of a replanning strategy in the future.

To meet the demands for comfort during summer ceremonies, the building is air-conditioned, but the envelope and mechanical systems are integrated to make its operation both efficient and adaptable. The inhabited spaces are sandwiched between an extensive basement and an array of rooftop plant enclosures concealed behind a continuous high parapet. The perimeter walls and the walls around the atrium are double-skinned and become, from a services point of view, continuous voids containing all the service systems, including the air supply and extract ducts. These walls also provide the structural stability of

the building, allowing flexibility of internal planning. The complete integration of architectural, structural and environmental needs is testimony to the relationship between the architect and Arup.

The body of the building is punctured with small window openings that are deeply recessed into the double-skin construction, giving some protection against solar gains, while adjustable external shutters give complete solar exclusion if this becomes necessary. To the east the façade is further sheltered by an oversailing arcade that forms a grand walkway alongside the Doca dos Olivais. The proportion and disposition of the fenestration set in the thermally massive enclosure is a clear response to the climate and architectural traditions of Lisbon and its region and, also, a demonstration

215

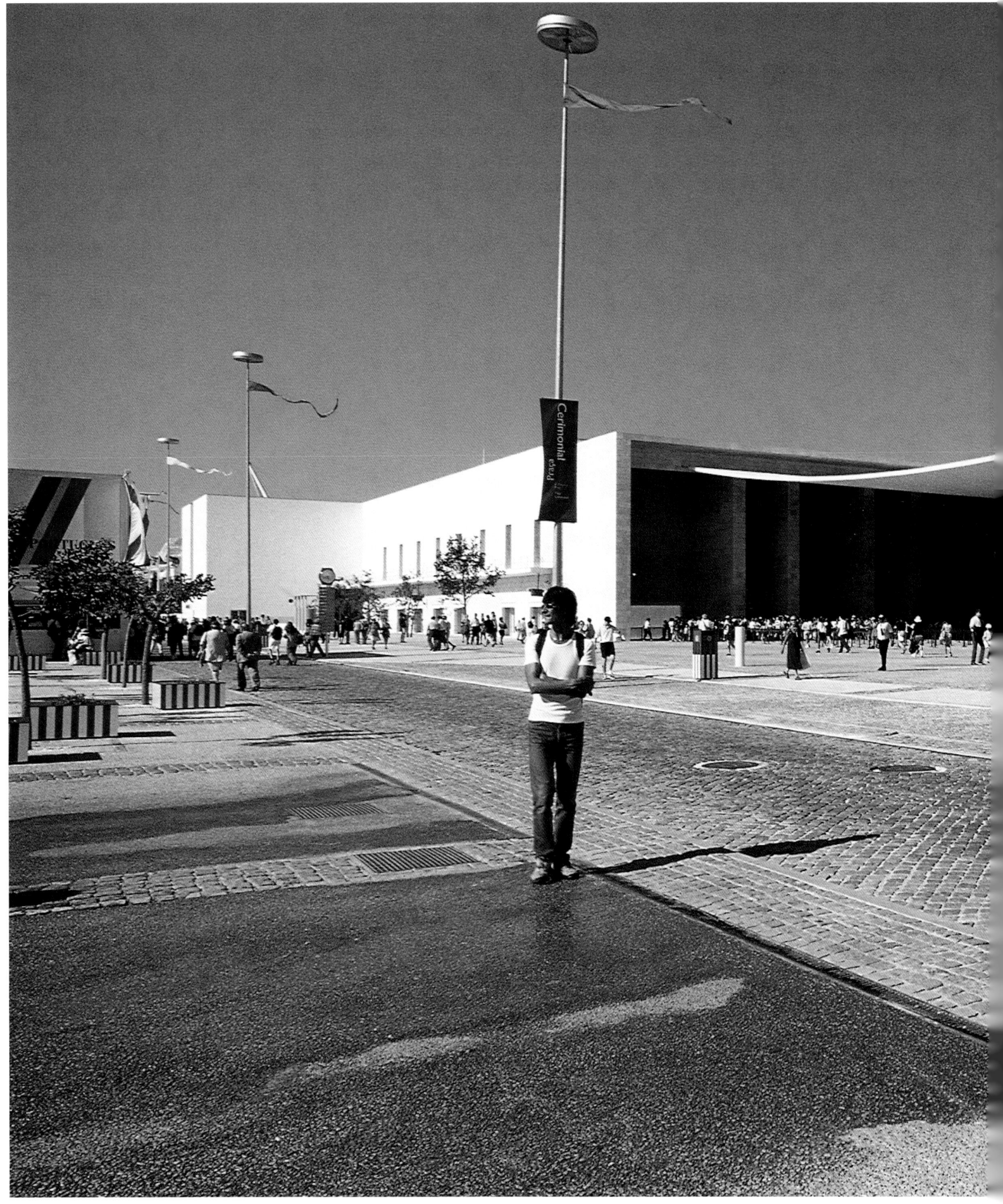

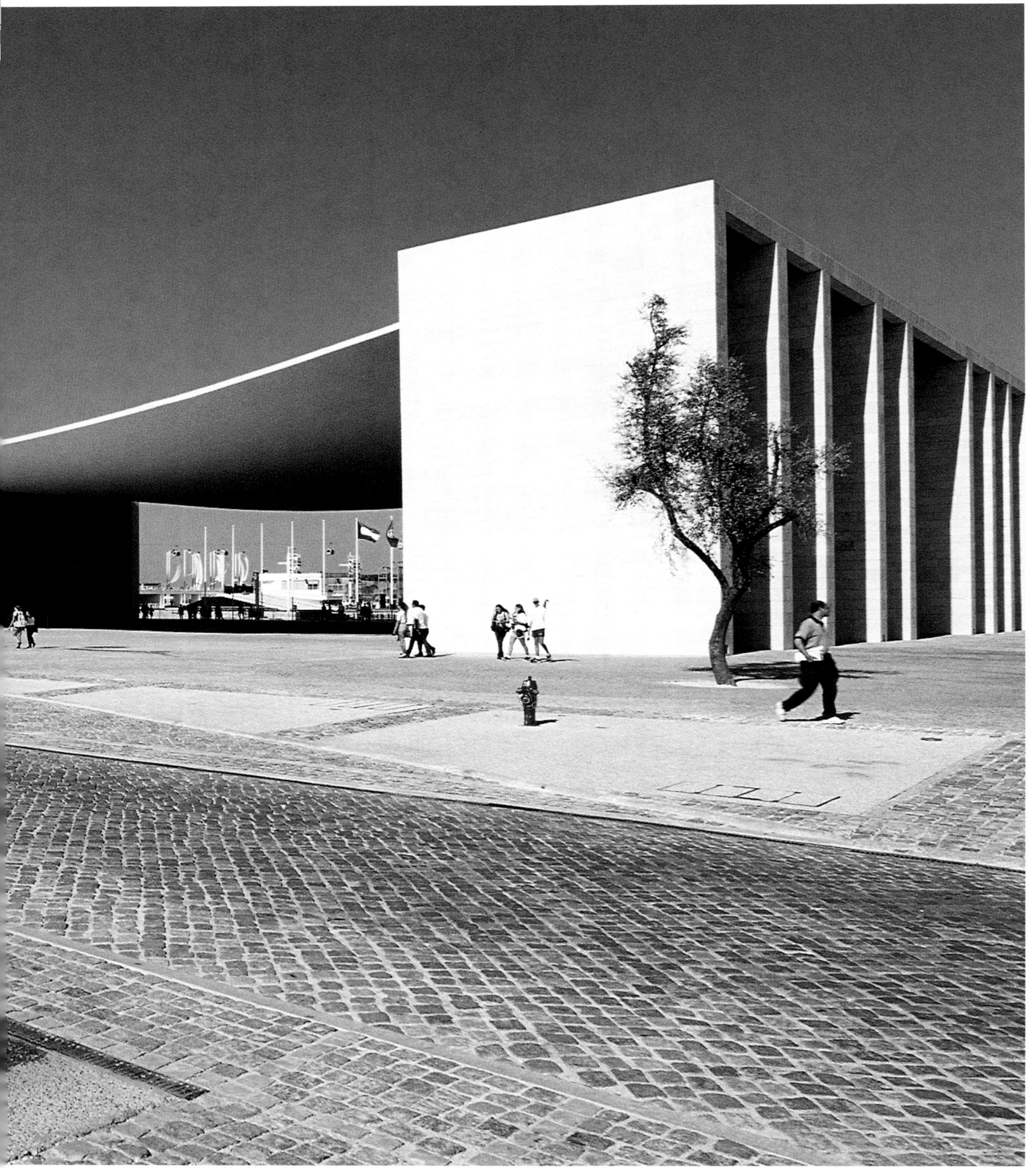

← The canopy forms at once a piazza and a porte cochère, signalling the entrance to an important building.

→ Schematic elevation showing the relative position and dimension of the fenestration of the south façade and the mechanical systems.

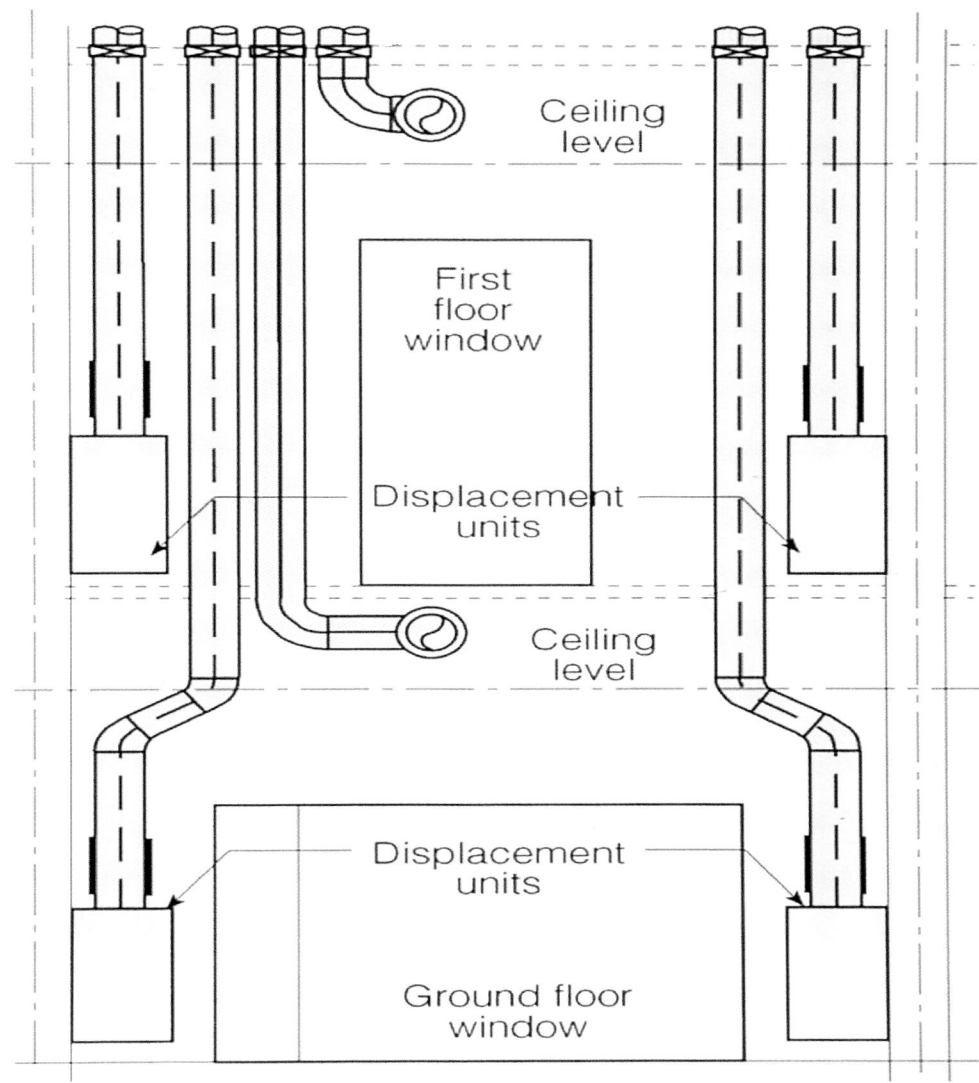

of Frampton's proposition of Siza's mediation of 'technique through culture'.

A combined heat and power (CHP) system delivers heated and chilled water and electricity to all the main buildings at the Expo site. Within the Portuguese Pavilion heat exchangers are used to transfer the energy delivered to the building's own water circuits. These supply heating and cooling to seven separate air-handling units housed in the rooftop plant spaces. Each of these units controls a distinct vertical zone of the building through ductwork concealed in the double skin.

Supply ducts are carried down to low-level displacement units concealed within the wall at each floor. These deliver conditioned air to each space, which is extracted by displacement at high level, from where it is returned to the plant room by a system of ducts, again hidden in the wall voids. All these systems are discreetly incorporated in the refined layering and restrained detail of Siza's interiors.

Conclusion

In terms of our 'environmental taxonomy', this building is located towards, respectively, the exclusive and concealed ends of the two principal axes, exclusive/selective mode and concealed/exposed power. It is a highly serviced structure in which the external enclosure acts to hold at bay the effects of extremes of climate, in particular the heat of the summer, in order to minimize demands on the mechanical plant. Equally, it succeeds in subtly integrating an extensive array of plant into its structure and fabric.

One of the themes in Álvaro Siza's

work throughout his career has been a concern with the expression of consistency rather than that which is conspicuously new. 'After years of passionate invention, of separation from History...after the Modernist movement, a reading, albeit transitory, of the huge amount we have received from the previous generation seems fairly clear to me,' he writes. 'In spite of new materials and new techniques...the essence of Architecture has not changed.' [4] The achievement of the Portuguese Pavilion has two sides to it. A collaboration of architect and consultants has led to a synthesis and organization of structure and services that is as coherent as Louis Kahn's distinction between 'served' and 'servant', but which is subsumed into form and language that are subtly related to context and culture.

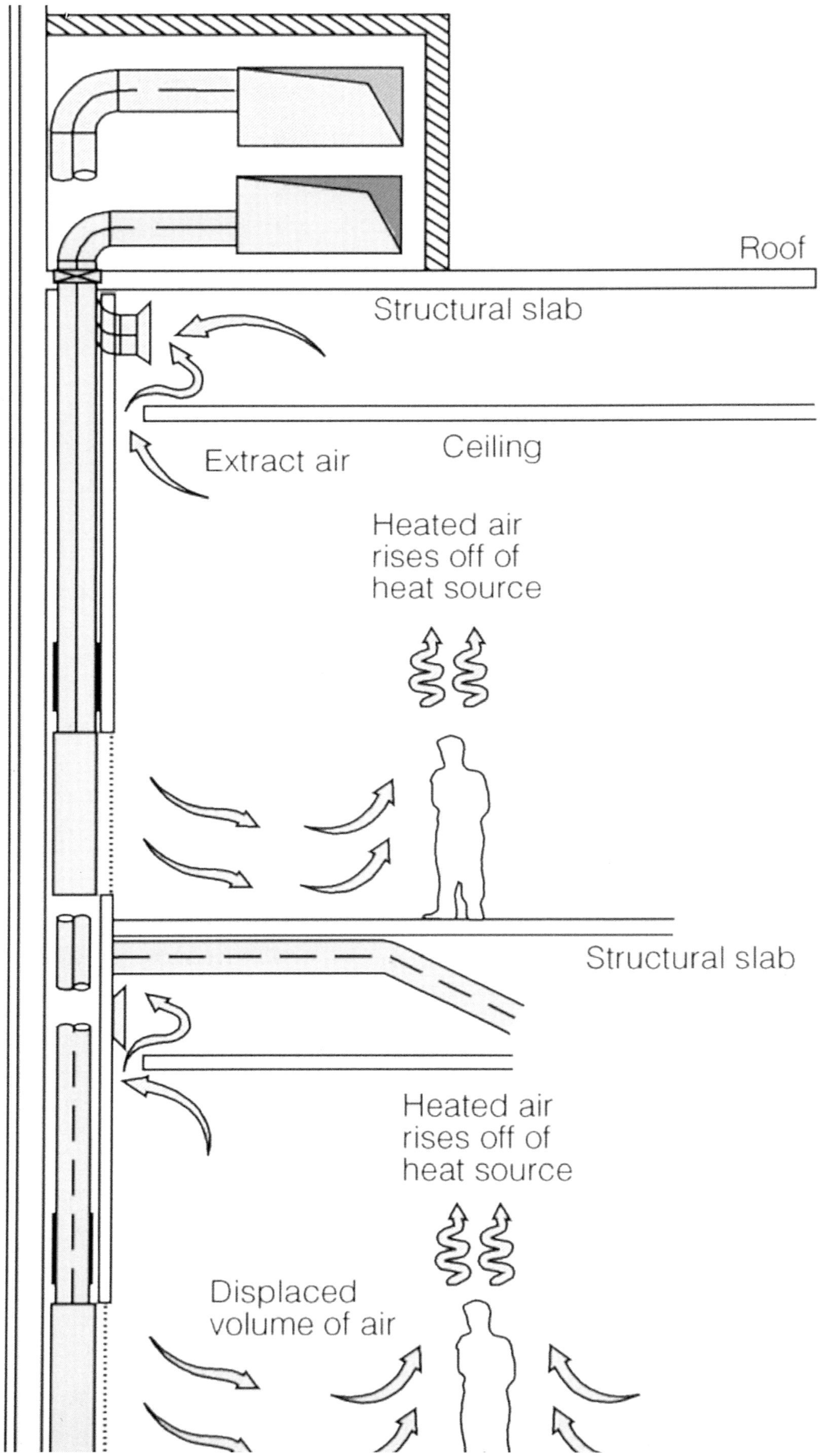

Roof

Structural slab

Ceiling

Extract air

Heated air
rises off of
heat source

Structural slab

Heated air
rises off of
heat source

Displaced
volume of air

Technical cross-
section showing the
relationship of
structure and
servicing
installations. The
intention is to achieve
maximum efficiency
with concealed
power systems.

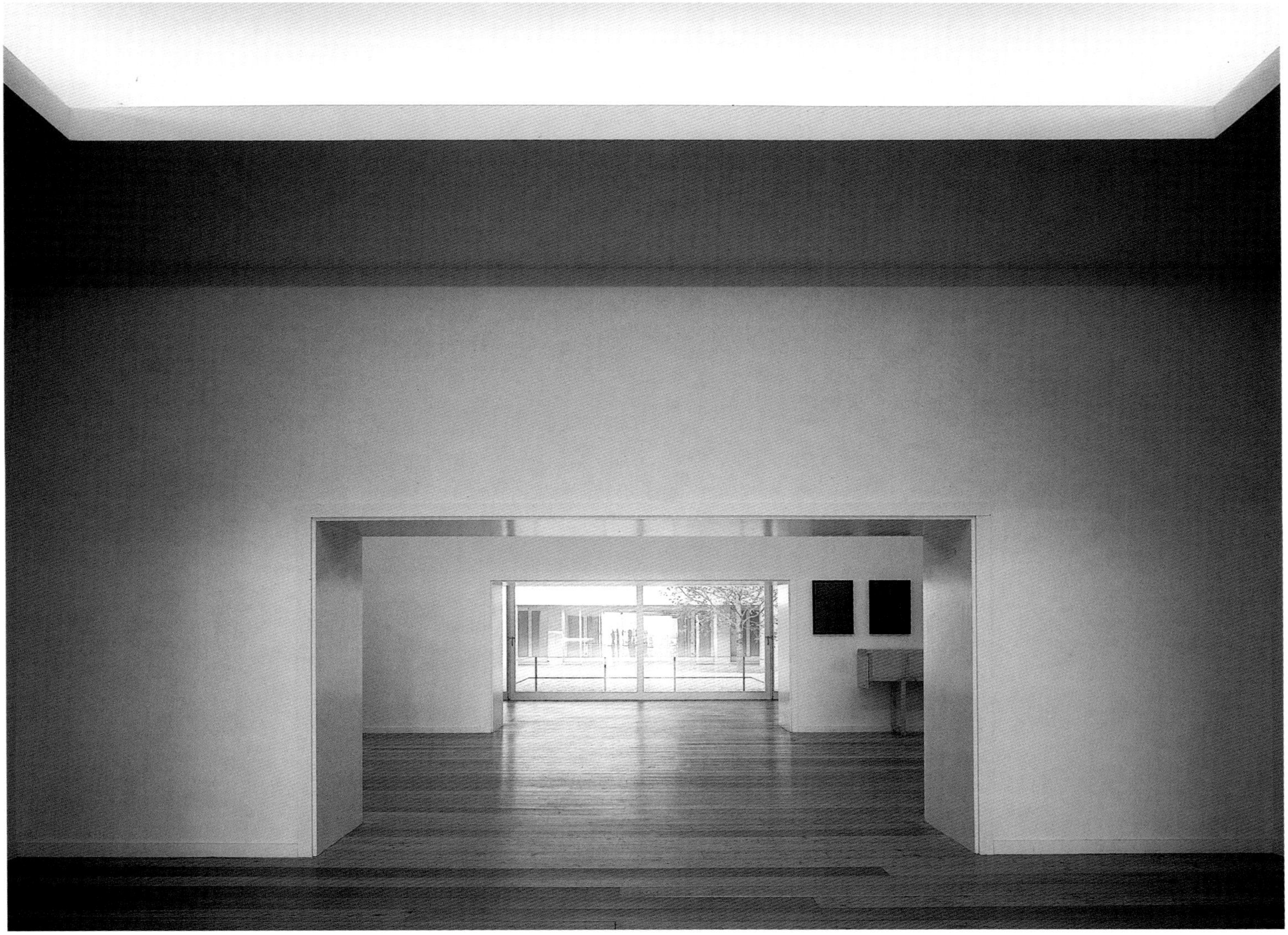

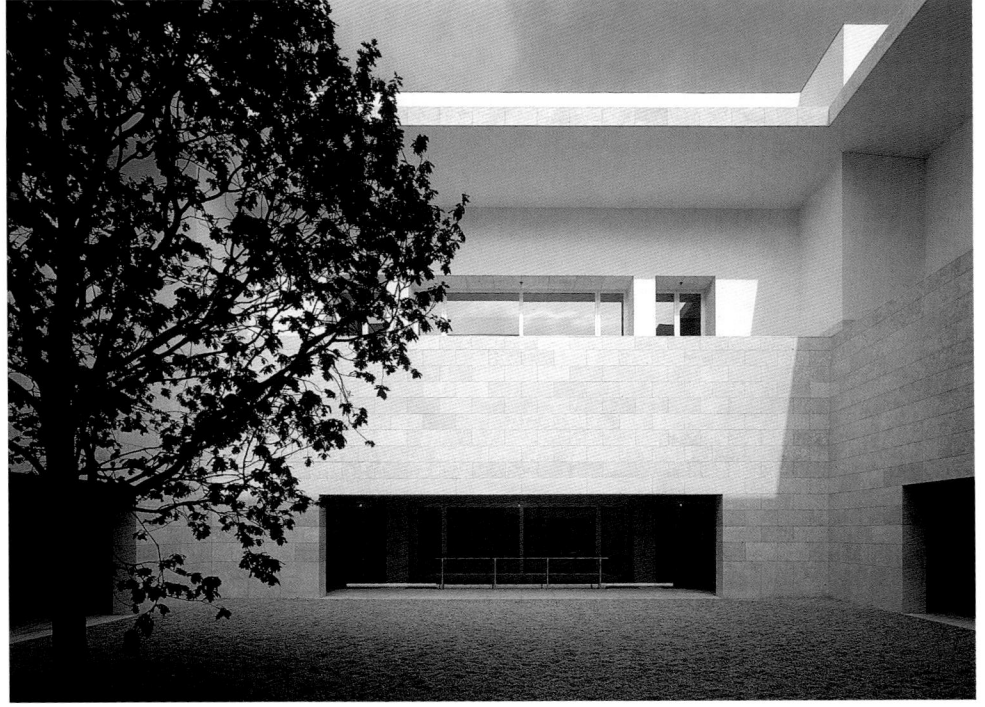

↑
Gallery space.

→
Internal courtyard.

←

First-floor reception room, showing relationship with the internal courtyard.

↑

Furniture and murals by Álvaro Siza.

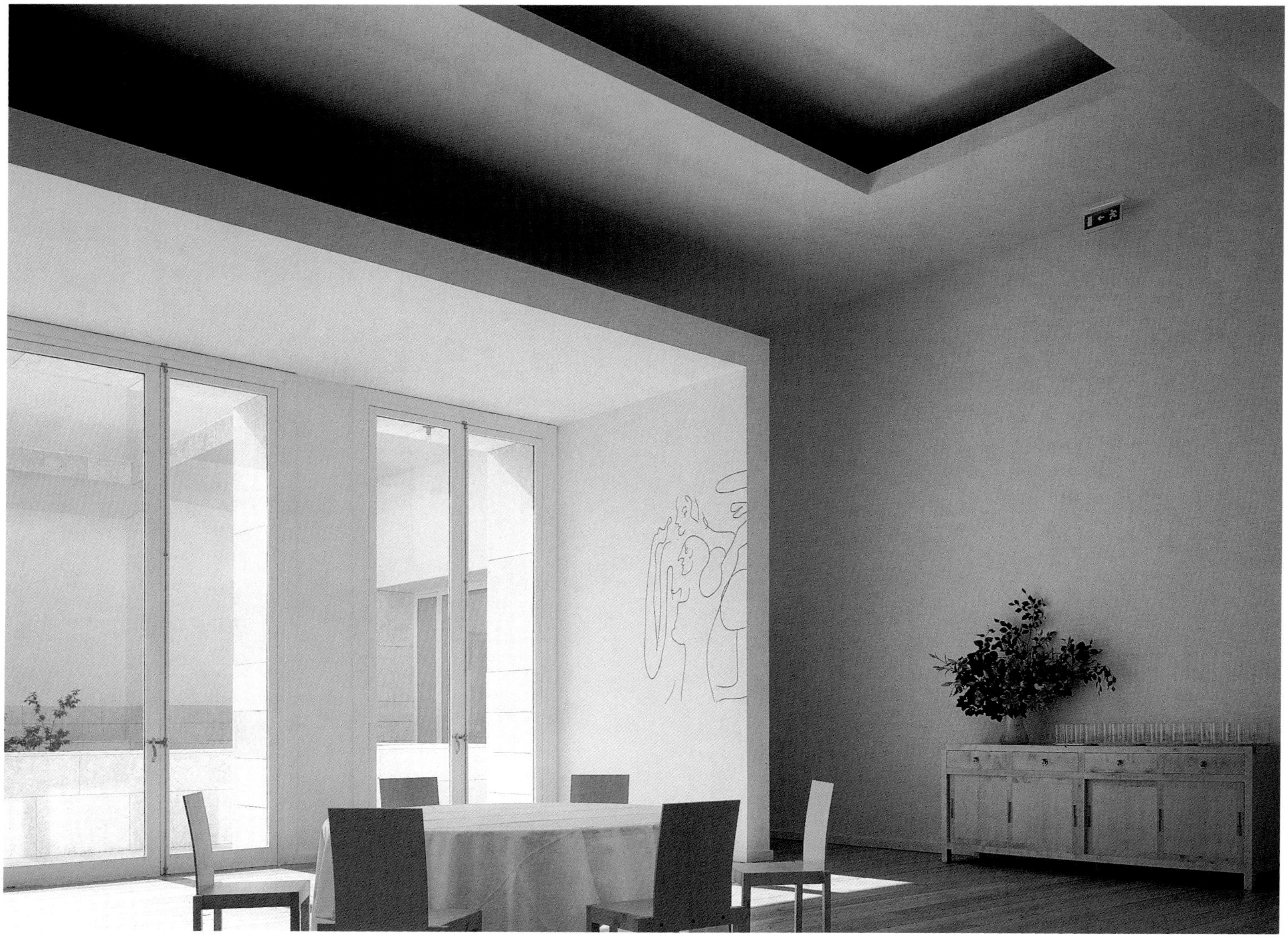

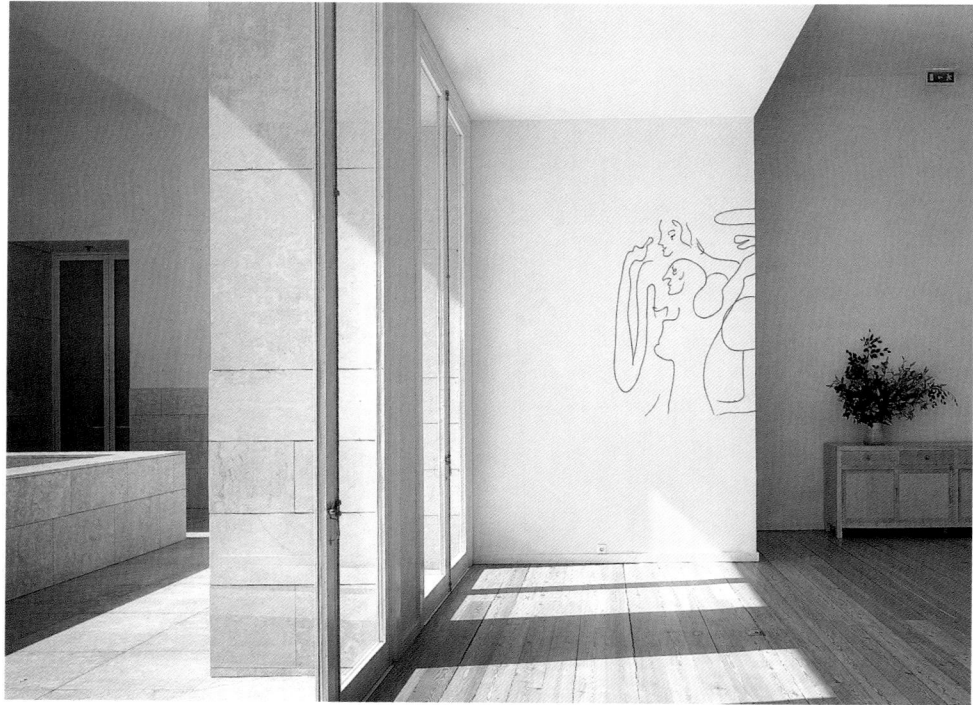

Velodrome

Dominique Perrault
Berlin, Germany
1997

➜

Plan view of model,
showing velodrome
and swimming pool,
set in the raised
plinth with its orchard
of Normandy
apple trees.

Track cycling is both an outdoor and an indoor sport. In its early days, when cycling was a predominantly European passion, there was a clear distinction between the summer and winter versions. Summer events, which often included the sprint finish of a road race, were usually staged in large outdoor arenas such as the Parc de Princes in Paris, and the short-track winter meetings, which often took the form of six-day team races, were indoors. There were a few permanent indoor tracks – the best known was probably Vel d'Hiv in Paris, now demolished – but in many cases these events took place on temporarily erected circuits within large exhibition halls, for example. As a consequence, the tracks varied enormously in size and quality. In recent years the sport has become much more popular and there have been moves to standardize tracks. New tracks have been built around the world, the majority of which are indoor, allowing year-round use.

In 1991, Berlin city council made a bid for their city, the capital of a reunited Germany, to be the venue of the 2000 Olympic Games. Work began on the development of a number of new sports installations, including a

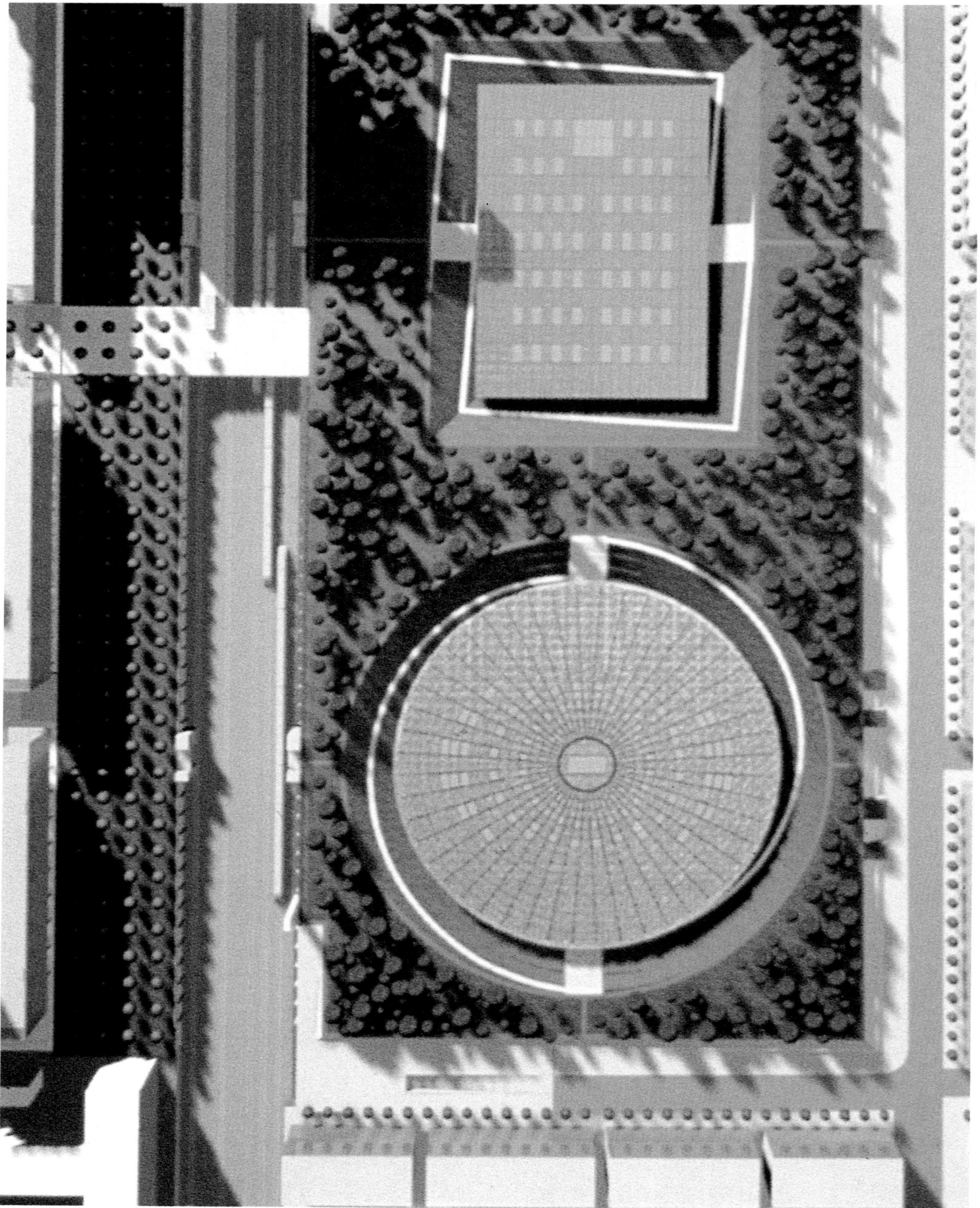

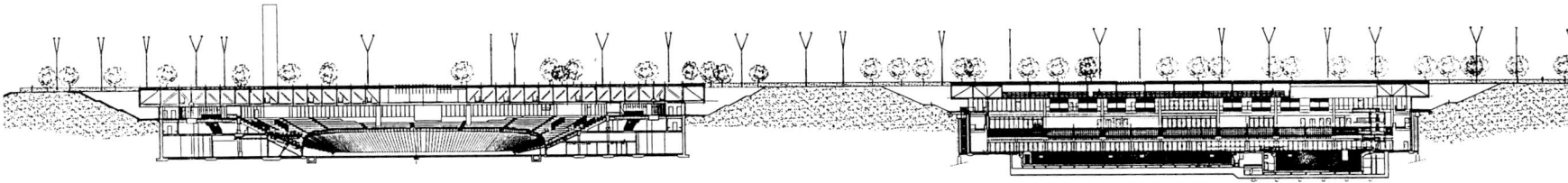

↑

Long-section, with velodrome (left) and swimming pool (right).

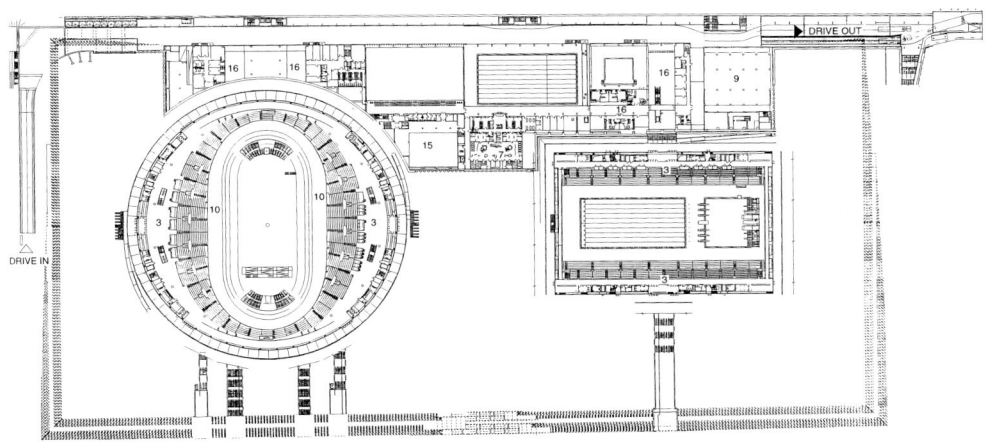

←

The plan shows the connection between the two primary arenas and the shared service zones beneath the plinth.

velodrome and swimming pool complex on a site in the Prenzlauerberg district in Berlin's former eastern zone. The Paris-based architect Dominique Perrault won an international competition for the project, held in 1992. As concrete evidence of Berlin's commitment to the Olympics, the project moved quickly to site. The Berlin Olympic bid was ultimately unsuccessful, but the project continued to completion of the velodrome in 1997 and completion of the swimming pool a year later.

Perrault's design puts the entire building below ground level. In the open, Modernist structure of Prenzlauerberg, with its ranks of high-rise apartments and commercial buildings, he has created an 'orchard' of Normandy apple trees in which the roof planes of the two sports halls resemble glistening lakes, one

circular, the other rectangular. Each consists of a concrete-lined excavation covered by a large-span steel roof. The entire roof plane and the edges of each enclosure are covered in a fine steel mesh whose appearance constantly changes with the light.

The sporting environment

A sports building has to provide comfortable conditions for both athletes and spectators. Regulating temperature, ventilation, lighting and acoustics is more complex in such a place than in many other building types. The Berlin Six-Day cycle race, held each year in January, has sessions each day from six o'clock in the evening until three o'clock in the morning. As the two-man teams race around the track, a crowd of up to 13,000 fills the perimeter seating and

the central piste, and a carnival takes place as the cyclists circle around. The demands this places on the environmental systems of the building are easy to imagine. In addition to its primary function as the venue for cycling, the velodrome is also used for other sports, such as tennis, concerts, both classical and pop, trade shows, political rallies – all of which add to the environmental brief. The continental climate of Berlin has long cold winters, with temperatures often down to -15°C (5°F), and hot summers, when temperatures as high as 35°C (95°F) may be experienced.

In Perrault's design, the circular roof structure hovers over an elliptical enclosure within which is the oval cycle track. The main body of the building is below natural ground level. Above this rises the plateau of

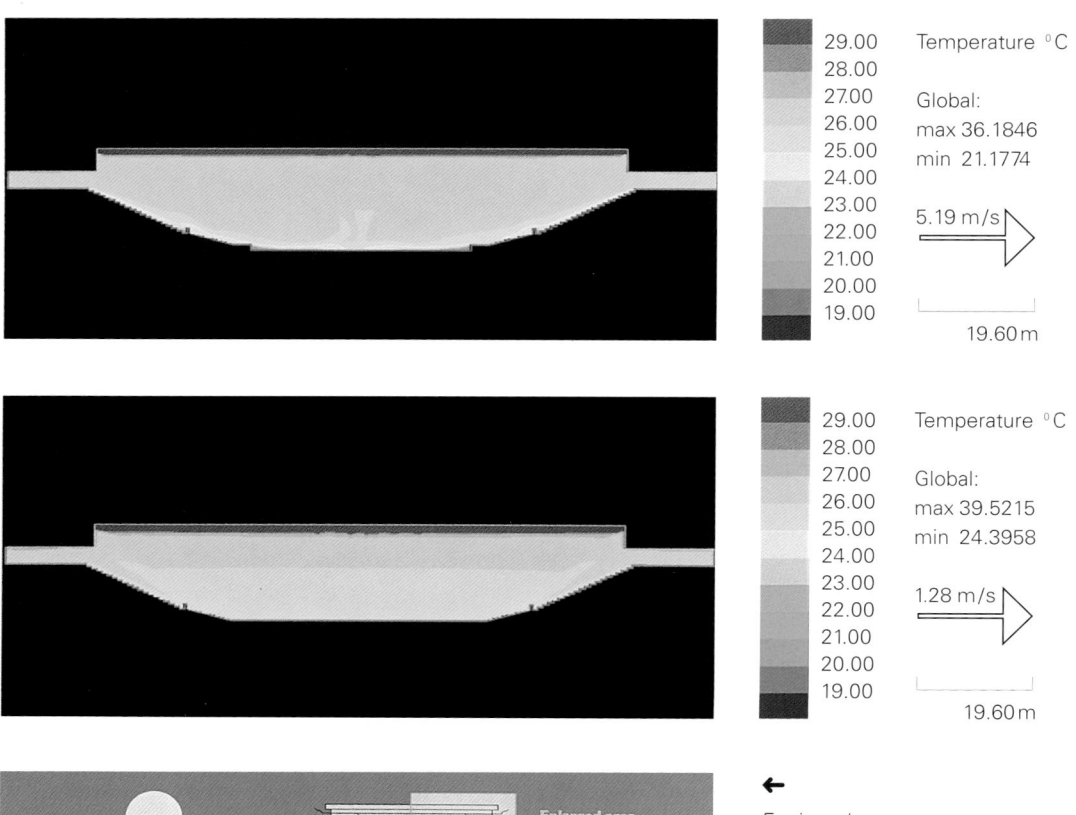

Temperature °C

Global:
max 36.1846
min 21.1774

5.19 m/s

19.60 m

Temperature °C

Global:
max 39.5215
min 24.3958

1.28 m/s

19.60 m

←
Computer models, showing predicted temperature distributions in the velodrome for alternative cycling and concert configurations.

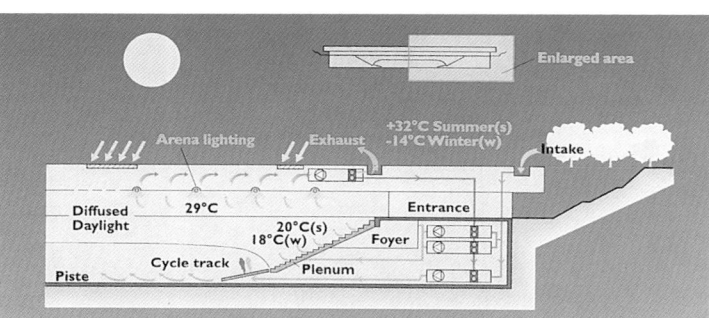

Enlarged area

Arena lighting   Exhaust   +32°C Summer(s)   Intake
                           -14°C Winter(w)

Diffused Daylight   29°C   Entrance
              20°C(s)
              18°C(w)   Foyer
Piste   Cycle track   Plenum

←
Engineer's schematic section, showing principles of the environmental strategy.

the 'orchard', and the steel-mesh cladding of the roof floats 1m (3ft) above this. The cross-section defines and articulates the essential elements of the environmental strategy. The roof disc is 140m (459ft) in diameter. It consists of 48 steel radial trusses that span from a circumferential ring of 16 concrete columns with linking trusses, and a 14.4m (47ft) radius ring truss at the centre. Each radial truss is restrained by tie-down elements at a radius of 65.2m (214ft). Secondary beams connect the trusses in both their top and bottom planes. A major feature of the design is the circular rooflight that spans the central opening, bringing a pool of natural light into the heart of the arena.

Heat

The air supply to this huge enclosure is delivered at low level, through the vertical surface of the precast-concrete steps that form the seating terraces, and at the inner rim of the cycle track. Extract is by mechanical exhaust close to the perimeter of the disc, where it does not obstruct the rooflight and is relatively unobtrusive visually. The natural buoyancy of the air assists the extraction process. This configuration is an economical means of creating a microclimate at the lower, inhabited level of the arena. Supply to the seating and the piste is from separate units. Arup's design was validated using a computational fluid dynamics (CFD) model, which allowed a series of occupancy patterns related to the potential uses of the building to be simulated for a range of climatic conditions. A centralized plant serves both the velodrome and the swimming pool. This incorporates a combined heat and power plant (CHP)

which delivers both heat and electricity. Additional heat is drawn from the district heating system that serves much of Berlin. The system is configured so that the CHP plant is used to heat the water in the swimming pool and to run the pool ventilation. It also provides emergency power.

Light

The velodrome has an extensive artificial lighting installation to allow events to be held there after dark. Illumination for the major sporting events is provided by an array of floodlights, concentrically arranged to follow the geometry of the roof structure. To achieve uniform lighting within the geometrical constraints of the architecture, the lamps were designed with asymmetric reflectors. This installation is supplemented by a

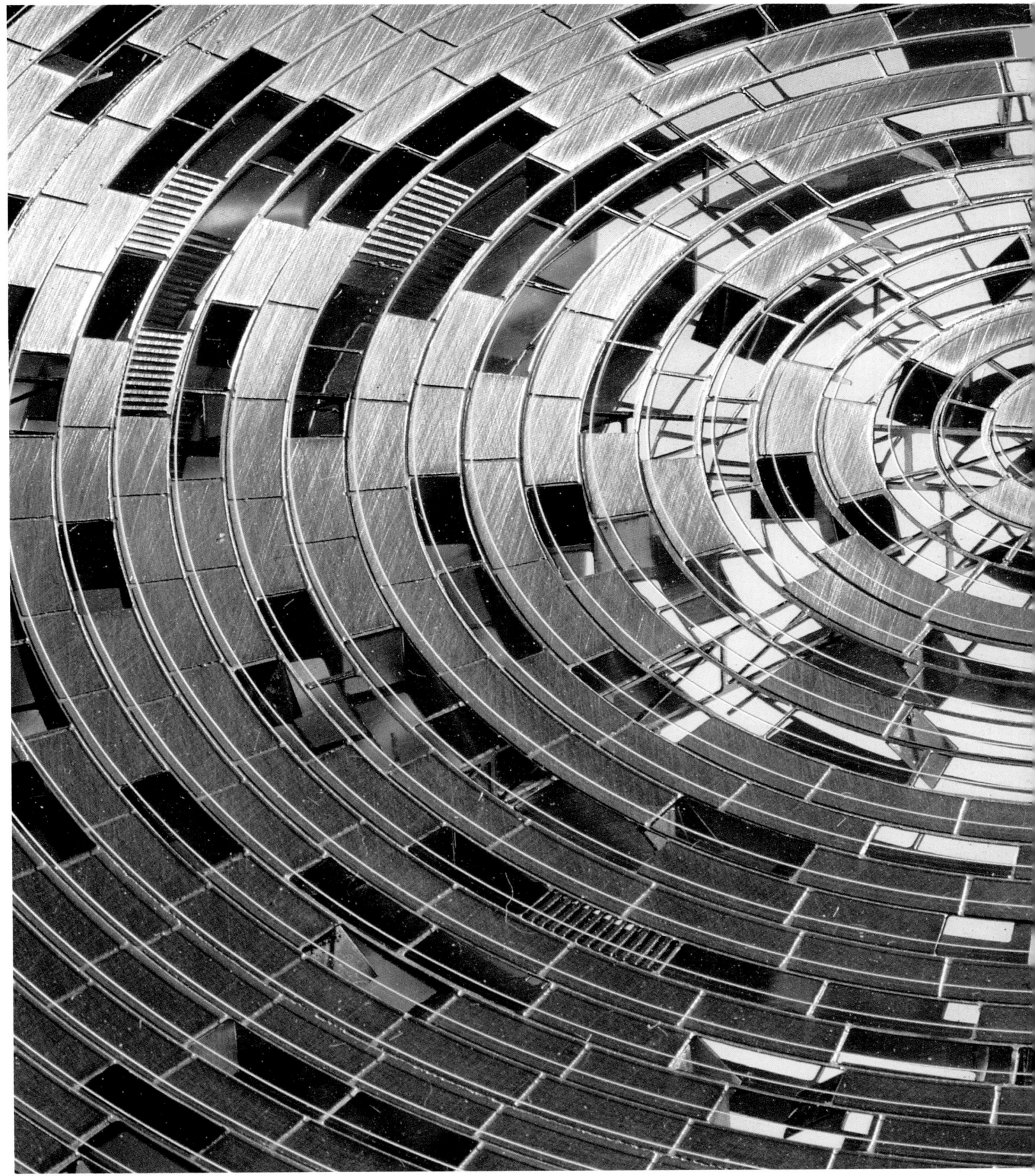

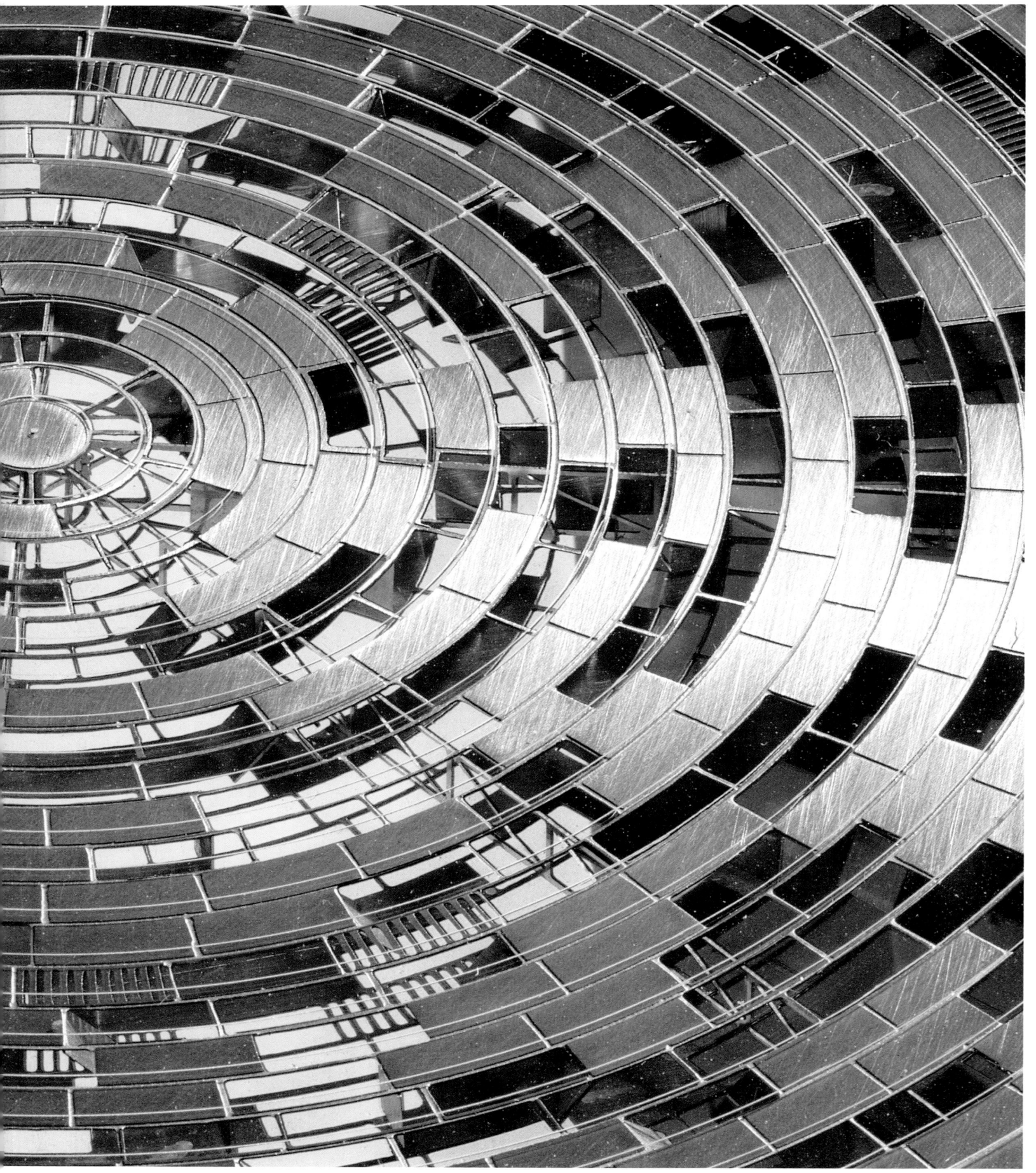

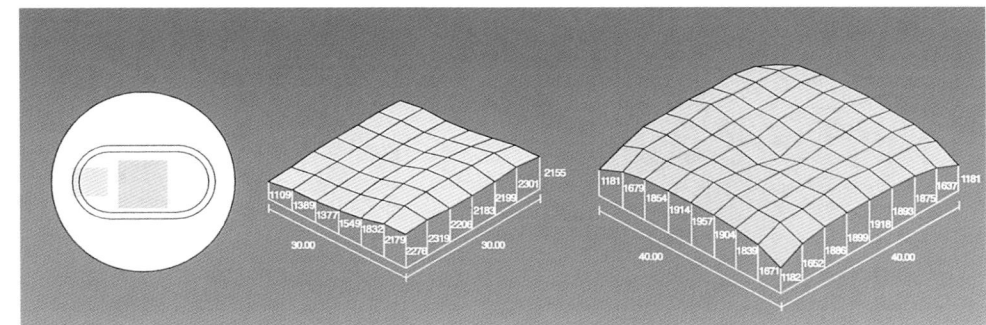

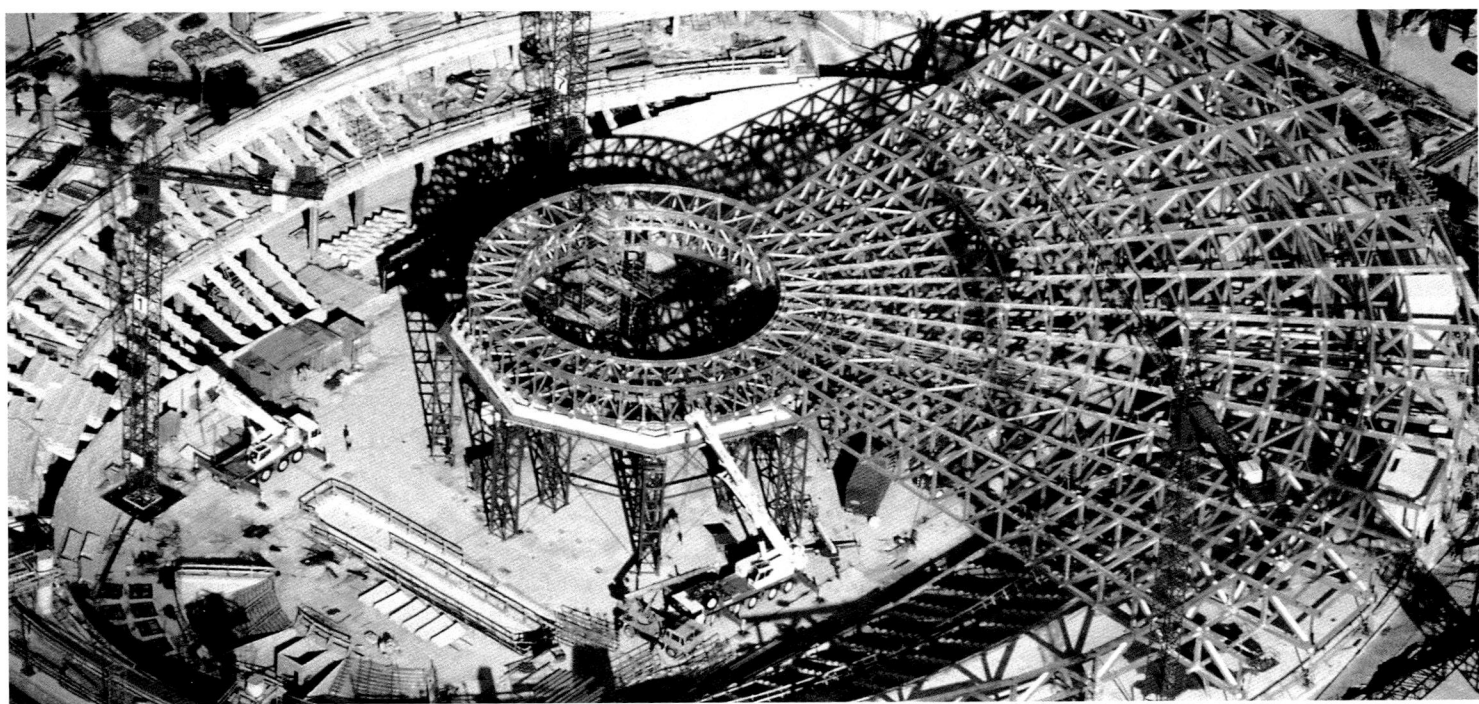

secondary set of powerful lamps to provide the higher level of light needed for televised events. Each lamp can be individually addressed by the computer control system. This makes it possible to provide appropriate lighting for all the other, non-sports events that take place in the building. Once again, computer modelling played an essential role in the design of the installation.

Sound

Acoustics may seem of secondary importance in the design of a sports building, but the noise of an enthusiastic crowd contained within an enclosure must be properly controlled. First, the response of the enclosure has to be analysed to make sure that an atmospheric but comfortable acoustic is achieved. Second, particularly in a residential district such as Prenzlauerberg, it is important to limit the noise that is transmitted through the enclosure to the surroundings. In this case it was also necessary to achieve an acoustic that would support other uses of the space, particularly musical performances.

The form and materiality of the velodrome are determined by the needs of the sport. Perrault's elegant geometrical system of superimposed figures – circle, ellipse and oval – invests the space with a clear order. The materials of the arena, mainly concrete, are acoustically reflective. In a space such this, the roof is the main source of acoustic control. A liner tray system was suspended below the roof deck, whose construction was optimized to provide both sound insulation and low-frequency absorption. Together the deck and the hanging system control the high- and mid-frequency reverberations, and the hanging trays optimize the low frequencies. The design achieves a reverberation time of 2.1 seconds across the frequency range, thereby avoiding the exaggeration of low frequencies often suffered in large volumes. Within the arena itself, the design was detailed to avoid focused reflection from the curved forms. Sound-absorbent materials were used wherever possible, and the continuous glazed strip above the upper seating was angled to reflect sound up onto the absorbent panels in the roof.

The acoustic needs of most kinds of performance are met by an extensive electro-acoustic installation. Three types of loudspeaker are arranged in a concentric configuration, directed respectively towards the upper

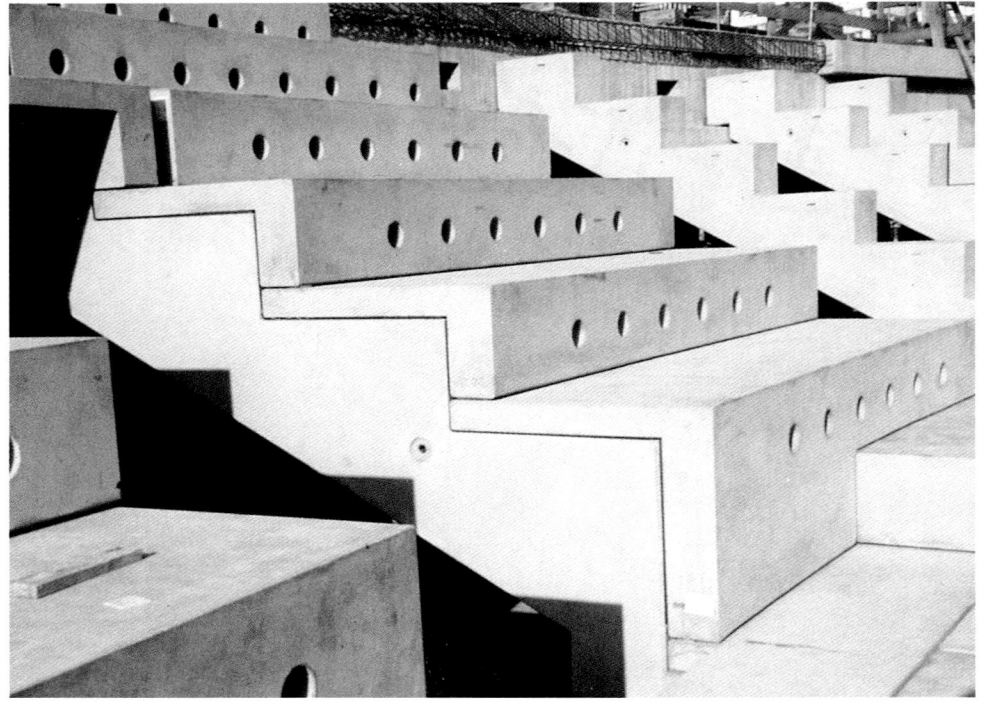

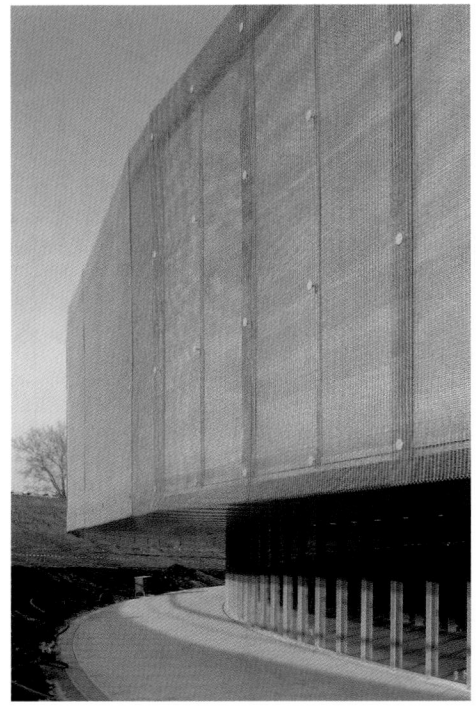

↑
Precast concrete
seating tiers of the
velodrome. The
circular holes in the
risers are the supply
inlets from the air
system.

↑
The perimeter of the
roof disc, clad in
steel mesh, floats
above the perimeter
concourse.

seating, lower seating and the piste
area; the whole system is computer-
controlled to allow it to be configured
to suit each individual event. It is
compatible with the powerful sound
systems used by rock bands.

Conclusion

The Berlin Velodrome is one of the few
modern sports arenas that transcend
the pragmatics of the geometry of the
playing area, the provision of
acceptable sight lines for the
spectators and muscular structural
expression. Perrault's formal play of
circle and rectangle, set into the
manmade landscape of the
Normandy 'orchard', is a poetic
addition to the arid urban fringe of
Prenzlauerberg.

The building is a wonderfully
explicit demonstration of creative
collaboration between architect and
engineer. Central to this is the cross-
sectional order that elegantly resolves
the complex environmental
requirements of the modern indoor
sports arena. Within the sealed,
exclusive envelope, the mechanical
systems are physically and
functionally integrated with the
structure so that they deliver heat,
light and sound in correct measure
where and when they are needed.

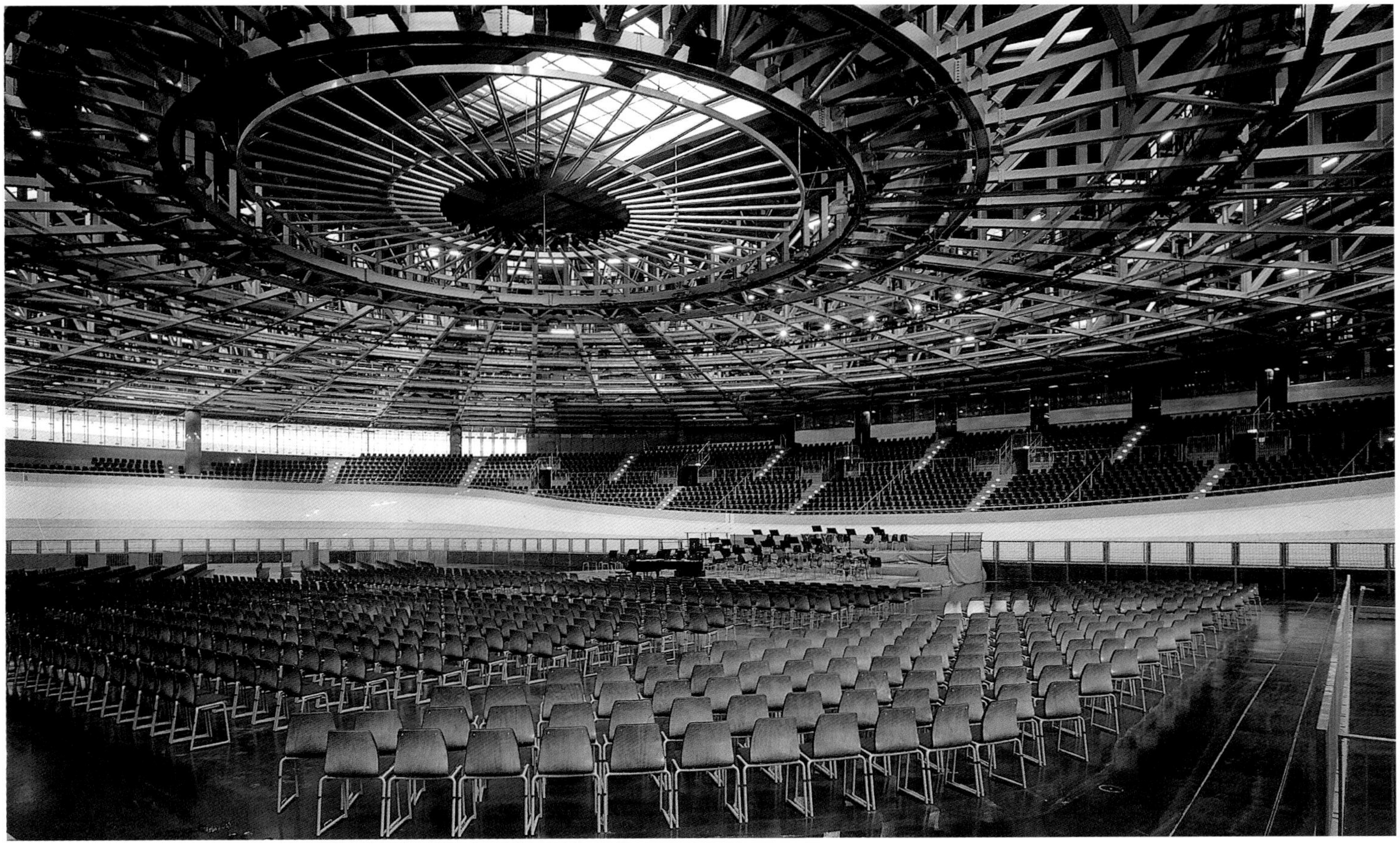

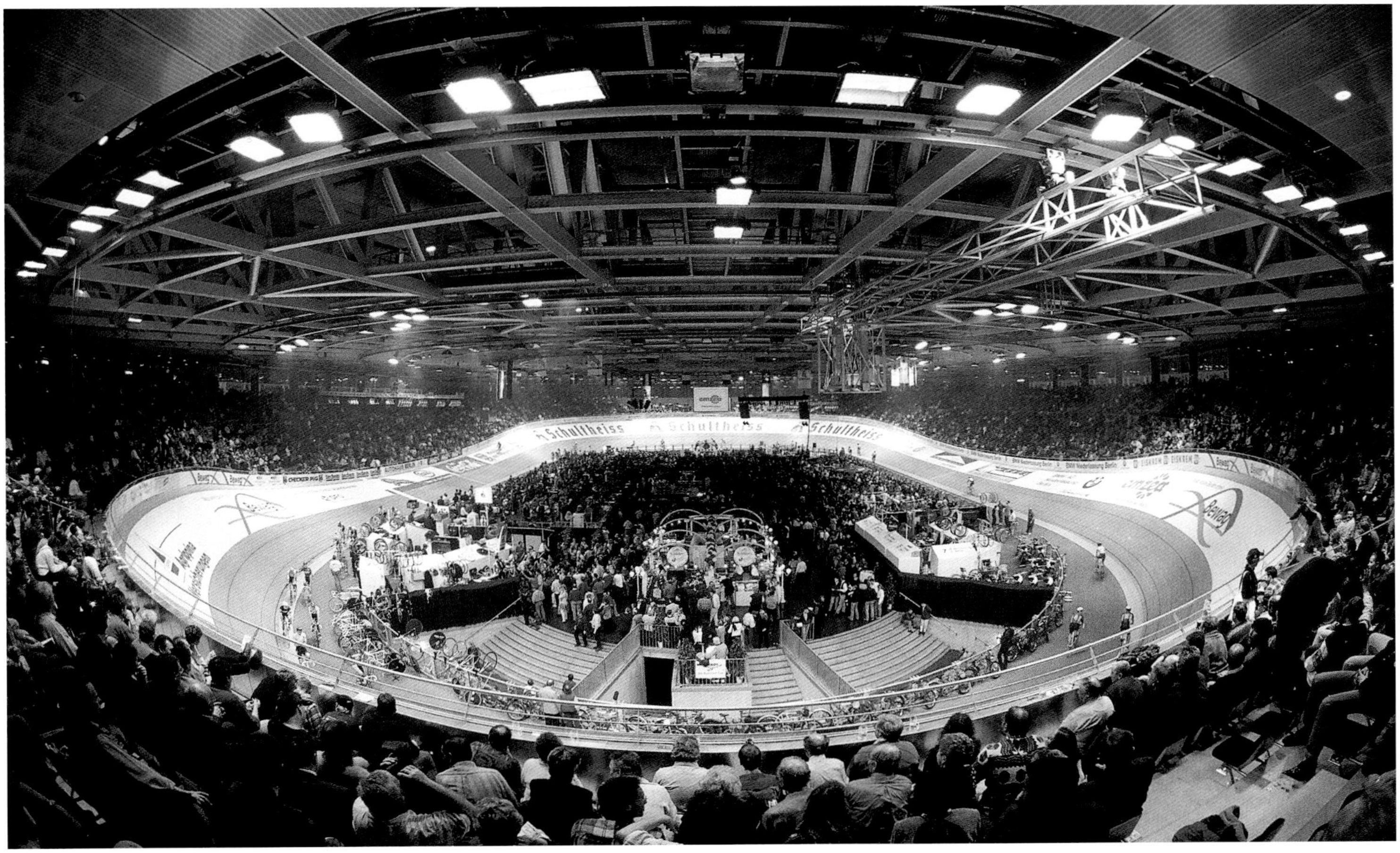
Schultheiss
Schultheiss
Schultheiss

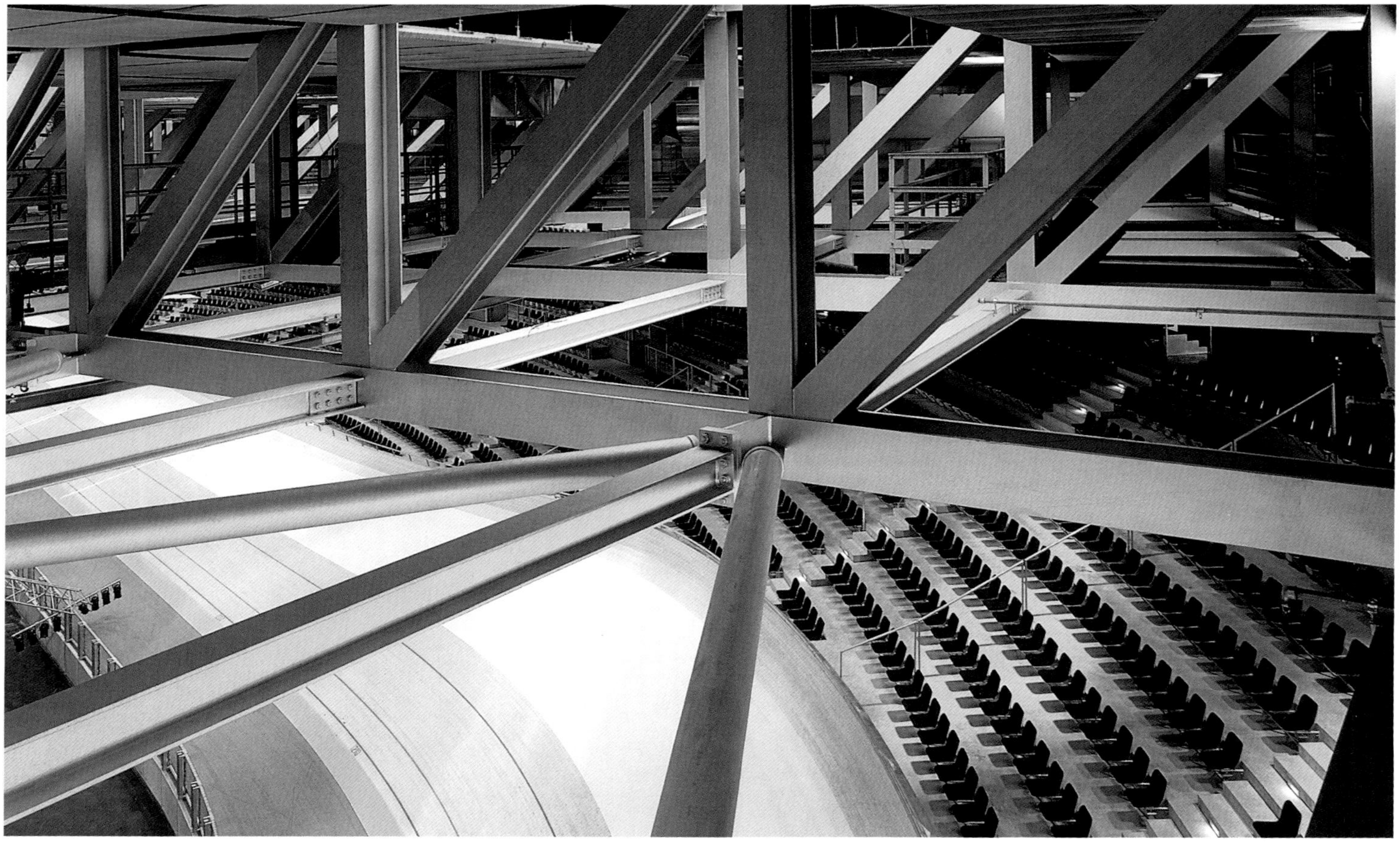

The velodrome set out for its secondary use as a concert hall. The roof structure is seen to perform its additional function of integrating elements of the environmental services.

A major cycle race in progress. The computer-controlled artificial lighting concentrates attention on the oval of the track within the circular arena.

The roof structure in detail.

Appendix

INTRODUCTION

1. Le Corbusier, *Vers une architecture*, Paris, 1923. English translation by Frederick Etchells, *Towards a New Architecture*, London, 1926.
2. Nikolaus Pevsner, *Pioneers of Modern Design*, revised edition, Penguin Books, Harmondsworth, 1960. First published as *Pioneers of the Modern Movement*, Faber & Faber, London, 1936.
3. Sigfried Giedion, *Space, Time and Architecture*, Harvard University Press, Cambridge, Mass., 1941. Fourth revised edition 1962.
4. Reyner Banham, *The Architecture of the Well-tempered Environment*, The Architectural Press, London, 1969.
5. T. K. Derry and Trevor I. Williams, *A Short History of Technology: from the earliest times to AD 1900*, Oxford University Press, Oxford, 1960.
6. Robert Bruegmann, 'Central Heating and Forced Ventilation: Origins and Effects on Architectural Design', *Journal of the Society of Architectural Historians*, XXXVII, 1978, pages 143–60.
7. Todd Willmert, 'Heating Methods and Their Impact on Soane's Work: Lincoln's Inn Fields and Dulwich Picture Gallery', J*ournal of the Society of Architectural Historians*, LII, 1993, pages 26–58.
8. M. H. Port (ed.), *The Houses of Parliament*, Yale University Press, New Haven, 1976.
9. John Olley, 'The Reform Club', in Dan Cruickshank (ed.), *Timeless Architecture*, The Architectural Press, London, 1985.
10. John Olley, 'St George's Hall, Liverpool, Parts One and Two, *The Architects' Journal*, 18 and 25 June 1986.
11. See Pevsner, op. cit.
12. See Giedion, op. cit.
13. See E. O. Sachs, *Modern Opera House and Theatres*, 3 vols. London, 1896–98, for a full description of this building and its installations. Sachs's work is a key reference for theatre design in the 19th century.
14. D. B. Reid, *Illustrations*, cited in Bruegmann, op. cit.
15. Fernand Léger, 'The origins of painting and its representational value', Montjoie, Paris, 1913. Reprinted in E. F. Fry, *Cubism*, Thames and Hudson, London 1966.
16. Le Corbusier, programme of *L'Esprit Nouveau* no. 1, October 1920.
17 Le Corbusier and Pierre Jeanneret, *Cinque points d'une architecture nouvelle*, 1925.
18. Brian Brace Taylor, *Le Corbusier: the City of Refuge, Paris, 1929/33*, University of Chicago Press, Chicago and London, 1987. First published as *La Cité de Refuge di Le Corbusier 1929/33*, Officina Edizione, Rome, 1978.
19. Le Corbusier, *Precisions: On the Present State of Architecture and City Planning*, English translation, MIT Press, Cambridge, Mass., 1991. First published as *Précisions sur un état de l'architecture et de l'urbanism*, Cres et Cie., Paris, 1930.

20. For a detailed account of the controversy over the performance of the executed design, see Brian Brace Taylor, op. cit.
21. See John Allen, *Berthold Lubetkin: Architecture and the Tradition of Progress*, RIBA Publications, London, 1992, for a detailed account of Lubetkin's life and work.
22. Kenneth Frampton, *Studies in Tectonic Culture: The Poetics of Construction in Nineteenth and Twentieth Century Architecture*, MIT Press, Cambridge, Mass., 1995.
23. Pierre van Meiss, 'The aesthtics of gravity: La Rinascente Department Store, Rome' in *arq*, vol. 4, no. 3, 2000, pp. 237–45.
24. See Rayner Banham, *The Architecture of the Well-tempered Environment*, The Architectural Press, London, 1969, for an outline of the environmental aspects of SCSD.
25. Louis I. Kahn, quoted in *World Architecture 1*, Studio Books, London, 1964.
26. See 'Space for services: the architectural dimension', in Dean Hawkes, *The Environmental Tradition: Studies in the Architecture of Environment*, E. & F. N. Spon, London, 1996.
27. Charles Jencks, *The Language of Post-Modern Architecture*, 4th edition, Academy Editions, London, 1984.
28. Kenneth Frampton, 'Towards a critical regionalism: six points for an architecture of resistance', in Hal Foster (ed.), *Postmodern Culture*, Pluto Press, London & Concord, Mass., 1985.
29. Dean Hawkes, 'The Sainsbury Wing, National Gallery, London', in *The Environmental Tradition: Studies in the Architecture of Environment*, E. & F. N. Spon, London, 1996.
30. W. Boesiger and H. Girsberger, *Le Corbusier 1910–1965*, Les Editions d'Architecture, Zurich, 1967.
31. Alan Colquhoun, 'Symbolic and literal aspects of technology', *Architectural Design*, November 1962, reprinted in *Essays in Architectural Criticism: Modern Architecture and Historical Change*, Oppositions Books, MIT Press, Cambridge, Mass., 1981.
32. Kenneth Frampton, *Studies in Tectonic Culture: The Poetics of Construction in Nineteenth and Twentieth Century Architecture*, MIT Press, Cambridge, Mass., 1995.
33. T. K. Derry and Trevor I. Williams, op. cit.
34. See Introduction to Dean Hawkes, *The Environmental Tradition: Studies in the Architecture of Environment*, E. & F. N. Spon, London, 1996, for a detailed account of the derivation of this proposition.
35. Victor Olgyay, *Design with Climate*, Princeton University Press, Princeton, 1963.
36. See Philip Steadman, *Energy, Environment and Building*, Cambridge University Press, Cambridge, for a comprehensive summary of these early designs.
37. A pioneering autonomous project was the Cambridge Autonomous House Project. See *Architectural Design*, November 1974. The work of Brenda and Robert Vale, *The New Autonomous

House: Design and Planning for Sustainability, Thames and Hudson, London, 2000, has carried these principles into built reality.
38. Thomas Herzog (ed.), *Solar Energy in Architecture and Urban Planning*, Prestel, Munich and New York, 1996, brings together an extensive and representative sample of these designs.
39. See Robert Powell, *Ken Yeang: Rethinking the Environmental Filter*, foreword by Kisho Kurokawa, Landmark Press, Singapore, 1989; and Ken Yeang, *The Green Skyscraper: The Basis for Designing Sustainable Intensive Buildings*, Prestel, New York, 1999.
40. See Dean Hawkes, 'Building shape and energy use', an essay first published in 1980 and reprinted in revised form in *The Environmental Tradition: Studies in the Architecture of Environment*, E. & F. N. Spon, London, 1996. The potential of the selective mode in contemporary design is developed further in Dean Hawkes, Koen Steemers and Jane MacDonald, *The Selective Environment*, E. & F. N. Spon, London, 2001.

SELECTIVE MODE

Offices for Apicorp
notes
1. C. Slessor, 'Sheltering Sky', *The Architectural Review*, March 1998, vol. CCIII, no. 1213, p. 34.
2. *RIBA Journal*, April 1995, 102/4.
3. F. Duffy, 'Office Interiors and Organisations – A comparative study of the relation between organisational structure and the use of interior space in sixteen office organisations', Princeton University PhD, 1974.
4. DEGW, *Planning Office Space*, Architectural Press, London, 1976.
5. K. Asfour, 'Cultural Crisis', *Architectural Review*, March 1998, vol. CCIII, no. 1213, pp. 52–60.
sources
Architectural Review, March 1998, vol. CCIII, no. 1213.
Building Design, 26 May 1995, no. 1222.

Eastgate
sources
1. Robert de Jager, et al, Special Issue: 'Sustainable Architecture', *Architecture SA*, no. 7/8, July/ August, 1997, pp. 23–29.
2. Fred Smith, 'Eastgate, Harare, Zimbabwe', *The Arup Journal*, vol. 32, no. 1, 1/1997, pp. 3–8.
3. Marian Giesen, 'Eastgate office and shopping complex, Harare, Zimbabwe', *Planning (Johannes burg)*, no. 154, November, 1997, pp. 42–45.
4. Bram Posthumus, 'Het gebouw als organism (The Building as Organism): Eastgate in Harare', *Archis*, no. 5, May, 1999, pp. 77–80.
5. Marc Gosse, et al, Special Issue: 'Villes en développement', *A plus*, no. 161, Dec/Jan, 1999/2000, pp. 64–65.

6. Liane Lefaivre, 'Making a midrise out of a termite hill', *Architecture (New York)*, vol. 89, no. 11, November, 2000, pp. 89–90.

Arup Campus

notes

1. John Harvey, quoted in *Arup Bulletin*, No. 165, May 1999, p. 1.

Howlands Farm Student Housing

notes

1. Nikolaus Pevsner, *The Buildings of England: County Durham*, second edition, revised by Elizabeth Williamson, Penguin Books, Harmondsworth, 1983.
2. J. M. Richards, *The Functional Tradition*, The Architectural Press, London, 1958.

sources

Martin Spring, 'Nature studies: Howlands Farm student accommodation, Durham', *Building*, 9 June 2000.

Marzahn Low-energy Apartment Building

notes

1 John Summerson, *The Classical Language of Architecture*, revised edition, Thames and Hudson, London, 1980.
2. J. N. L. Durand, *Recueil et parallèle edifices de tous genres, anciens et modernes*, Paris, 1801.
3. W. P. Jones, 'Built form and energy needs' in A. F. C. Sherratt (ed.), *Energy Conservation and Energy Management in Buildings*, Applied Science, London, 1976.
4. Dean Hawkes, 'Building shape and energy use' in D. Hawkes and J. Owers (eds.), *The Architecture of Energy*, Longmans, Harlow, 1980. Reprinted in Dean Hawkes, *The Environmental Tradition*, E. & F. N. Spon, London, 1996.
5. Karl Fleig (ed.), *Alvar Aalto: the complete works*, 3 vols., Birkhauser Verlag, Basel, Boston, Berlin, 1971.
6. Le Corbusier, *Vers une Architecture*, Paris, 1923, English Translation *Towards a New Architecture*, by Frederick Etchells, London, 1926.

sources

Brian Cody, 'Low energy apartment building in Berlin', *The Arup Journal*, vol. 33, no. 3, 3/1998.

BedZED Sustainable Development

notes

1. Department of the Environment, Transport and the Regions, *Towards an Urban Renaissance: Final Report of the Urban Task Force*, E. & F. Spon, 1999.
2. D. Turrent, 'Hope for the Future', *RIBA Journal*, vol. 103, no. 1, January 1996, pp. 24–9.

sources

K. Long, 'Health Resort', *Building Design*, no. 1453, 25 August 2000, pp. 15–7.
K. Long, 'Green and Pleasant Land', *Building Design*, no. 1473, 9 February 2001, pp. 12–3.
A. Pearson, 'Clean Living', *Building*, vol. 265, no. 8143 (26), 30 June 2000, pp. 44–7.
Ove Arup and Partners, 'A practical solution for

sustainable living in Sutton', Concept Stage Report, July 1999.

Mont Cenis Training Centre

notes

1. R. M. Lebens (ed.), *Passive Solar Architecture in Europe: The Results of the First European Passive Solar Competition*, 1980, Architectural Press, London, pp. 92–5.
2. 'Entwicklungsgesellschaft Mont-Cenis, Fortbildungsakademie Herne', a special report on the project, published by Stadt Herne, Montan Grundstückgesellschaft, 1998.

sources

Architectural Review, vol. 206, no. 1232, October 1999, pp. 30–1 and 46–71.
Detail 'Special Issue', vol. 39, no. 3, April/May 1999, pp. 358–60.
Techniques and Architecture, no. 443, June/July 1999.
World Architecture, no. 80, October 1999, pp. 44–9.

Study Centre, Darwin College

sources

Peter Davey, 'Heart of Oak', *The Architectural Review*, October 1994, pp. 50–3.
Simon Hancock, Roger Hyde and Mick White, 'Darwin College Study Centre, Cambridge', *The Arup Journal*, vol. 33, no. 1, 1/1996, pp. 16–8.
Sabine Schnieder, 'Bibliothek in Cambridge', *Baumeister*, June 1995, pp. 33–9.

Jubilee Campus, University of Nottingham

notes

1. P. Fawcett, 'Campus Arcadia', *Architectural Review*, no. 1236, February 2000, pp. 42–7.
2. J. Palmer, 'Under Pressure', *Building Services Journal*, August 1999, pp. 24–9.
3. P. Fawcett, op. cit.

sources

J. Berry, 'Super-Efficient Mechanical Ventilation', *Indoor and Built Environment*, March–April 2000, pp. 87–96.
P. Fawcett, 'Campus Arcadia', *Architectural Review*, no. 1236, February 2000, pp. 42–7.
J. Palmer, 'Under Pressure', *Building Services Journal*, August 1999, pp. 24–9.
'Green Agenda: Hopkins & Partners at Nottingham', EcoTech 1, issue 1, *Architecture Today*, March 2000, pp. 32–36.

Cultural Centre

notes

1 S. McInstry: Tjibaou quoted in 'Sea and Sky', *Architectural Review*, no. 1222, December 1998, p. 30.
2. K. Frampton, *Studies in Tectonic Form and Culture: The Poetics of Construction in Nineteenth and Twentieth Century Architecture*, MIT Press, 1995, p. 382.
3. P. Buchanan, *Renzo Piano Building Workshop*, vol. 2, Phaidon Press, 1995, p. 192.

4. K. Frampton, op. cit., p. 382.
5. S. McInstry, op. cit. p. 36.

sources

M. Banfi and A. Guthrie, 'Kanak Cultural Centre, Nouméa, New Caledonia', *The Arup Journal*, no. 2, 1999, pp. 26–9.
M. Chown and A. Guthrie, 'The Design of a Naturally Ventilated Cultural Centre in French New Caledonia', *Proceedings of CIBSE National Conference, Brighton, 2–4 October 1994*, vol. 2, pp. 121–133.

Carmel Mountain Ranch Public Library

notes

1. Esther McCoy, Case Study Houses 1945–1962, Hennessey & Ingalls, second edition 1977.

EXCLUSIVE MODE

Helicon Building

notes

1. L. Martin and L. March, 'Land Use and Built Form', *Cambridge Research*, April 1996.
2. D. Hawkes and R. MacCormac, 'Office Form, Energy and Land Use', *RIBA Journal*, 1978.

sources

Building Services Journal, September 1996.
Building Services Journal, October 1996.
Architecture Today, no. 73, November 1996.
T. Herzog, *Solar Energy in Architecture and Urban Planning*, Prestel, Munich, 1996.

Villa VPRO Offices

notes

1. P. Davey, 'Work Ethics', *Architectural Review*, no. 1232, October 1999, p. 30.
2. Peter Buchanan, *A&U*, no. 9 (336), September 1998, p. 48.
3. P. Stam, 'Villa VPRO', *Architectural Review*, no. 1225, March 1999, p. 42.
4. B. Lootsma, '*Pays Bas Prospective*', L'Architecture d'Aujourd'hui, September, 1996.
5. H. Ibelings, 'Supermodernism: Architecture in the Age of Globalisation', *NAI*, Amsterdam, 1998.

sources

P. Stam, 'Villa VPRO', *Architectural Review*, no. 1225, March 1999.

Beyeler Foundation Museum

notes

1. T. Markus, *Buildings and Power*, Routledge, London, 1993, p. 171.
2. R. Ryan, 'Pastoral Pavilion', *Architectural Review*, December 1997.
3. A. McDowell, A. Sedgwick, A. Smith and J. Wernick, 'Beyeler Foundation Museum, Riehen, Switzerland', *Arup Journal*, 2/1999, p. 19.

sources

P. Buchanan, *Renzo Piano Building Workshop*, vol. 2, Phaidon Press, 1995.
A. McDowell, A. Sedgwick, A. Smith and

J. Wernick, 'Beyeler Foundation Museum, Riehen, Switzerland', *Arup Journal*, 2/1999, pp. 18–21.
R. Ryan, 'Pastoral Pavilion', *Architectural Review*, December 1997, pp. 59–62.
A. Tichhauser, 'Silent Light: Piano in Basel', *Architecture Today*, no. 86, March 1998, pp. 14–20.

Byzantine Fresco Chapel Museum
notes
1. Renzo Piano, Menil Art Museum, Houston, Texas, 1986.
2. Renzo Piano, Cy Twombly Gallery, Houston, Texas, 1993.
3. Peter Rice, *An engineer imagines*, Artemis Press, London, 1993; and Andy Brown, *Peter Rice*, Thomas Telford, London, 2000.
4. Umberto Eco, *Travels in Hyperreality*, translated by William Weaver, Harcourt Brace Jovanovitch, San Diego, 1990.
sources
Catherine Slessor, 'Out of this world', *The Architectural Review*, May 1998, pp. 82–85.
Ignacio Barandiaran, Varughese Cherian, Ray Quinn, Andy Sedgwick, 'Byzantine Fresco Chapel Museum, Houston, Texas', *The Arup Journal*, vol. 33, no. 1, 1/1998.

Museum of Contemporary Art
notes
1. Josef Paul Kleihues, quoted in Andrea Mesecke and Thorsten Scheer, *Museum of Contemporary Art Chicago*, Gebr. Mann Verlag, Berlin, 1996.
2. Andrea Mesecke and Thorsten Scheer, op. cit.
3. Carl W. Conduit, *The Chicago School of Architecture*, University of Chicago Press, Chicago and London, 1964.
4. Andrea Mesecke and Thorsten Scheer, op. cit.
sources
Nicola Martin and Andrew Sedgwick, 'Chicago Museum of Contemporary Art', *The Arup Journal*, vol. 31, no. 3, 3/1996, pp. 3–5.

Walsall Art Gallery
notes
1. Robert Venturi, 'From Invention to Convention in Architecture', in I*conography and Electronics upon a Generic Architecture: A View from the Drafting Room,* MIT Press, Cambridge, Mass., 1996.
2. Brian Carter, *The Architectural Review*, May 2000, pp.62-66.
3. Mark Girouard, *Robert Smythson and the Elizabethan Country House,* Yale University Press, New Haven, 1983.

Tate Modern
notes
1. Dietmar Steiner, 'Tate Modern, London', interview with Jacques Herzog, *Domus*, 828, July/August 2000, pp. 32–43.
2. Doreen Massey, 'Bankside: International Local', in, Iwona Blazwick and Simon Wilson (eds.), *Tate Modern: the handbook,* Tate Publishing, London, 2000, pp. 24–7.

3. Dietmar Steiner, op. cit.
4. Nikolaus Pevsner, *Pioneers of Modern Design*, revised edition, Penguin Books, Harmondsworth, 1960.
sources
1. Dietmar Steiner, op. cit.
2. Tony Fretton, 'Into the void: Herzog & de Meuron's Tate Modern', *Architecture Today*, No. 109, June 2000, pp. 34–57.

Portuguese Pavilion
notes
1. Alvaro Siza, *Siza: Architectural Writings*, Antonio Angellillo (ed.), Skira, Milan, 1997.
2. Kenneth Frampton, *Alvaro Siza: Complete Works*, Electra, Milan, 1999. English edition, Phaidon Press, London, 2000.
3. *The Architectural Review*, November, 1985
4. Alvaro Siza, op. cit.
sources
Philip Jodidio, *Alvaro Siza*, Benedikt Taschen Verlag GmbH, Cologne, 1999.
Kenneth Frampton, *Alvaro Siza: Complete Works*, Electra, Milan, 1999. English edition, Phaidon Press, London, 2000.
Mike Gilroy, Fred Ilidio, Andrew Minson, Martin Walton, 'The Portuguese National Pavilion', *The Arup Journal*, vol. 34, no. 2, 2/1999.

Velodrome
sources
Mike Banfi, David Deighton, Paul Nuttall, Raj Patel, Alan Tweedie and Mohsen Zikri, 'Radsporthalle, Berlin', *Arup Journal*, vol. 32, no. 4, 4/1997, pp. 3–10.
Andy Cook, 'Buried leisure', *Building*, 16 May 1997, pp. 50–2.
Sebastian Redeke, 'Velodromo, Berlino', *Domus*, 812, February 1999, pp. 12–21.

Offices for Apicorp
Client: Apicorp
Architect: DEGW Ltd
Arup role: Structural, mechanical, electrical, public health, infrastructure, and communications engineer
Quantity surveyor: Davis Langdon & Everest

Eastgate
Project manager and building developer: Old Mutual Properties, Zimbabwe
Architect: Pearce Partnership
Arup role: Structural, mechanical, electrical, public health and civil engineer
Quantity surveyor: Hawkins Leshnick & Bath

Arup Campus
Client: Ove Arup Partnership
Architect, structural, mechanical, electrical, and public health engineer, quantity surveyor: Arup Associates
Other Arup role: Acoustic, communications, fire, and transportation engineer

Howlands Farm Student Housing
Client: Durham University Developments Ltd
Architect, structural, mechanical, electrical, and public health engineer, quantity surveyor: Arup Associates
Other Arup role: Geotechnical, acoustic, and infrastructure engineer

Marzahn Low-Energy Apartment Building
Client: Wohnungsbaugesellschaft Marzahn mbH
Architect: Assmann Salomon und Scheidt
Arup role: Structural, mechanical, electrical, public health engineer and energy consultant

BedZED Sustainable Development
Client: The Peabody Trust
Architect: Bill Dunster Architects
Arup role: Building services and building physics engineer, and energy consultant
Structural engineer: Ellis & Moore Consulting Engineers
Quantity surveyor: Gardiner & Theobald

Mont Cenis Training Centre
Client: Innenminister des Landes Nordrhein-Westfalen
Architect: Jourda & Perraudin
Associate architect: HHS Planer & Architekten
Arup role: Concept and scheme structural, mechanical, electrical, public health lighting engineer
Quantity surveyor: BDM Development

Study Centre, Darwin College
Client: Darwin College, Cambridge
Architect: Jeremy Dixon & Edward Jones
Arup role: Structural, mechanical, electrical, public health engineer
Quantity surveyor: David Langdon & Everest

Jubilee Campus, University of Nottingham
Client: University of Nottingham
Architect: Michael Hopkins and Partners
Arup role: Structural, mechanical, electrical, public
health, building physics, and civil engineer
Quantity surveyor: Gardiner and Theobald
Construction manager: Bovis Midlands

Cultural Centre
Architect: Renzo Piano Structural, mechanical,
electrical, public health Workshop
Arup role: Structural concept and mechanical,
electrical, and public health engineer
Climate control feasibility: CSTB

Carmel Mountain Ranch Public Library
Client: Carmel Mountain Ranch Library
Architect: MW Steele Group Inc
Arup role: Structural, mechanical, electrical, and
public health engineer

Helicon Building
Client: London & Manchester Assurance Co Ltd
Building user: Marks & Spencer plc
Architect: Sheppard Robson
Arup role: Structural, mechanical, electrical, public
health, fire, and acoustic engineer
Quantity surveyor: Silk & Frazier

Villa VPRO Offices
Client: VPRO Broadcasting Company, Hilversum
Client representative: Heidemij Advies BV, Arnhem
Architect: MVRDV, Rotterdam
Arup role: Scheme structural, mechanical, electrical,
public health engineer and site supervision
Building physics consultant: DGMR, Arnhem

Beyeler Foundation Museum
Client: Beyeler Foundation
Architect: Renzo Piano Structural, mechanical,
electrical, public health Workshop
Arup role: Structural concept, scheme roof design
(including glazing), mechanical, electrical, public
health and lighting engineer, and energy consultant

Byzantine Fresco Chapel Museum
Client: The Menil Foundation
Architect: François de Menil
Arup role: Structural, mechanical, electrical, public
health, acoustic, and communications engineer,
and lighting concept

Museum of Contemporary Art
Client: Board of Trustees, Chicago Museum of
Contemporary Art
Architect: Josef Paul Kleihues
Arup role: Structural, mechanical, electrical, public
health, lighting, and acoustic engineer to scheme and
detail design

Walsall Art Gallery
Client: Walsall Metropolitan Borough Council
Architect: Caruso St John Architects

Arup role: Structural, mechanical, electrical, public
health, lighting, fire, acoustics, and communications
engineer, planning supervision
Quantity surveyor: Hanscomb
Project managers: The London Group and Bucknall
Austin

Tate Modern
Client: The Tate Gallery
Project manager: Stanhope Properties Ltd
Architect: Herzog & De Meuron Architekten
Associate architect: Sheppard Robson
Arup role: Structural, mechanical, electrical, public
health, civil, lighting, fire, traffic/transportation,
acoustic, and communications engineer, planning
advice

Portuguese Pavilion
Client: Parque Expo '98
Architect: Alvaro Siza Vieira
Arup role: Scheme structural, mechanical, electrical,
public health, lighting, fire, and acoustic engineer

Velodrome
Client: OSB Sportstättenbauten GmbH, Berlin
Architect: Dominique Perrault, Paris
Arup role: Structural, mechanical, electrical, public
health, geotechnical, specialist lighting,
communications, and acoustic engineer, quantity
surveying, cost control, construction management

Many people have provided assistance in the
production of this book. We are particularly grateful
to Arup, who have made available the considerable
resource of their archive relating to the buildings
discussed in the Critical Studies. Bob Emmerson,
the Chairman, has guided the project throughout
and David J Brown, Editor of The Arup Journal, and
Arup's Archivist, Pauline Shirley, have given day-to-
day support in gaining access to material. In Cardiff
we have made much use of the Architecture Library
at the Welsh School of Architecture and wish to
thank Sylvia Harris and her staff for their tolerance
and help. As always in a project of this kind, many of
the ideas and arguments derive from the
conversations that we conduct daily with colleagues
and students. We wish to thank them for this.

Wayne Forster
Dean Hawkes
Cardiff 2001

All pictures reproduced with kind permission
from Arup, except for the following:

2   Christian Gahl
17   Fondation Le Corbusier / © DACS, London, 2002
18   V G Bild Kunst Bonn / © DACS, London, 2002
19   Fondation Le Corbusier / © DACS, London, 2002
20   Fondation Le Corbusier / © DACS, London, 2002
21   RIBA / © DACS, London, 2002
22   Fondation Le Corbusier / © DACS, London, 2002
26   Fondation Le Corbusier / © DACS, London, 2002
27   Fondation Le Corbusier / © DACS, London, 2002
33   Dennis Gilbert / VIEW
34   Alastair Hunter
35   Matt Wargo
36   Fondation Le Corbusier / © DACS, London, 2002
39   right Dennis Gilbert / VIEW
40   right John Edward Linden / Arcaid
41   courtesy of T R Hamzah & Yeang
45, 50 top, 51 courtesy of DEGW
47, 50 bottom, 52 Samir Sadir
55, 60–1 Wideangle Inc., Harare
63   Peter Cook / View
68   centre Andrew Putter
69   top Peter Cook / View
69   bottom Grant Smith
70–1 Peter Cook / View
74 right, 75 left, 77 Grant Smith
79, 80, 81, 84 top, 85 top Christian Gahl
84 bottom, 85 bottom ASS Archive
87, 88, 94, 95 Bill Dunster Architects
97, 100, 101, 104–5 H.G. Esch Fotographie
107,110–1 Dennis Gilbert / VIEW
120   University of Nottingham
115, 121, 122, 123–5 Paul McMullin
127, 128 left, 131, 134 bottom, 135 bottom
        John Gollings
130 left Renzo Piano
130 right Gerard Martron
134–5 P.A. Pantz
137, 140–3 David Hewitt/Ann Garrison
157 Hans Werlemann
160 left, 163 MVRDV
165, 168–9, 173 Christian Richters
166 Renzo Piano
175, 178 left, 179, 180–1 Paul Warchol
176, 178 right François de Menil
183, 186, 187, 190 left, 191 Hedrich Blessing
193, 198 Peter MacKinven / VIEW
196–7, 200, 201 bottom right Paul McMullin
201 Hélène Binet
203, 208–10, 211 top Dennis Gilbert / VIEW
211 bottom Hayes Davidson
220–1 Christian Richters
223 Perrault Projets
226–7 Michel Denance
229 right Ulrich Schwarz
230–1 Gerhard Zwickert
230 bottom Willebrand Photographie

a
Aalto, Alvar 83, 116
Adam, Robert 185
        Edinburgh Register Office *10*, 15
ADCK *see* Agence de Développement
        de la Culture Kanak
Adler and Sullivan 184
Agence de Développement de la Culture
        Kanak (ADCK) 128
Agibat MTI 96
Alberts & Van Hunt 46
Albini, Franco 210
        Rinascente department store, Rome 29, *29*
Al Khobar, Saudi Arabia: Apicorp office building
(DEGW)
        44–53
Anthony, Graham 149; *see* Sheppard Robson
Apeldoorn, Netherlands: Centraal Beheer
(Hertzberger)
        156
Apicorp (Arab Petroleum Investments Corporation)
        offices, Al Khobar, Saudi Arabia (DEGW) 44–53
Architectural Review 214
Arts and Crafts Movement 111
Arup, Ove/Arup Group/Arup Associates:
        Apicorp offices, Al Khobar 49
        Arup Campus, Solihull 62–71
        Beyeler Museum 170, 172
        Byzantine Fresco Chapel Museum, Houston 174
        Carmel Mountain Ranch Public Library,
          San Diego 138
        CEGB Headquarters 62, 65
        Duxford Aero Factory 65
        Finsbury Health Centre, London 26
        Helicon Building, London 150, 151, 154
        Highpoint apartment buildings, Highgate 25–6
        Howlands Farm Student Housing, Durham 72–7
        Inland Revenue building, Nottingham 118
        Menil Collection museum, Houston 170
        Nottingham University Jubilee Campus 114, 118
        Portcullis House, Westminster 118
        research projects 96, 118
        Asfour, Khaled 52
Assmann, Salomon & Scheidt: Marzahn Low-energy
        Apartment Building, Berlin 78–85

b
Banham, Reyner: *The Architecture of the Well-
        tempered Environment* 12, 25, 28, 41, 210
Bank of England, London (Soane) 15
Barry, Charles 185, 199
        Houses of Parliament *12*, 16–17, 24
        Reform Club *12*, 17
Basel: Beyeler Foundation Museum, Riehen (Piano)
        164–73, 192
Battle McCarthy 114
BedZED Sustainable Development, London (Dunster)
        86–95
Berlin:
        Altes Museum (Schinkel) 182, 185
        glass skyscraper projects (Mies van der Rohe)
        18, 22, 54
        Marzahn Low-energy Apartment Building

        (Assmann, Salomon & Scheidt) 78–85
        National Gallery (Mies van der Rohe) 28, 192
        Schauspielhaus (Schinkel) 182
        Velodrome (Perrault) 222–31
Beyeler, Ernst 164, 165, 170, 173
Beyeler Foundation Museum, Basel (Piano)
        164–73, 192
bioclimatic architecture 37–9
Bioregional Developments 88
Boulton, Matthew, and Watt, James: cotton mill
        8, 10, 14–15
Brighton: Royal Pavilion (Nash) *8*, 10
Bruegmann, Robert 14, 16–17, 19–20
Buchanan, R.: *Essays on the Economy of Fuel* 19
Burnham & Root 184
Byzantine Fresco Chapel Museum, Houston,
        Texas (de Menil) 174–81

c
Calatrava, Santiago: Oriente Station, Lisbon 214
Cambridge: Darwin College Study Centre
        (Dixon and Jones) 106–13
Cambridge Autonomous House Project 38, *39*
Carter, Brian 199
'Case Study' houses 136, 140
CEGB Headquarters (Arup) 62, 65
ceilings, suspended 26–7
central-heating systems, early 13–18, 19–20
Chabannes, Marquis de: *On Conducting Air
        by Forced Ventilation* 19
Chicago:
        IIT campus (Mies van der Rohe) 28
        Museum of Contemporary Art (Kleihues) 182–91
Cité de Refuge (Le Corbusier) *18*, 22–4, *23*, 25
cockle-stove heating system *9*
Colquhoun, Alan 33
Cook, William: steam heating system *9*, 14
Costa, Lucio: Ministry of Education,
        Rio de Janeiro 33, *36*

d
Darwin College Study Centre, Cambridge
        (Dixon and Jones) 106–13
Davey, Peter 156
Davy, Sir Humphry 16
DEGW: Apicorp offices, Al Khobar,
        Saudi Arabia 44–53
Derby Infirmary 14
Derry and Williams 13, 35
Dixon, Jeremy, and Jones, Edward:
        Darwin College Study Centre, Cambridge 106–13
Dresden, Germany: Opera House (Semper) 19
Duffy, Francis 47; *see* DEGW
Dulwich Picture Gallery, London (Soane)
        15, 31, 190, 192, 194
Dunster, Bill:
        BedZED Sustainable Development, London 86–95
        Hope House 89
Durand, J. N. L. 78
Durham 72
        Howlands Farm Student Housing (Arup) 72–7
Duxford Aero Factory (Arup) 65

e

Eastgate Building, Harare (Pearce Partnership) 54–61
Eco, Umberto: *Travels in Hyperreality* 178
Ecole des Beaux-Arts, L' 11, 18
Ecole Polytechnique, L' 10–11
Edinburgh Register Office (Adam) *10*, 15
Ehrenkrantz, Ezra 29, 138
Elmes, H. L. 185
    St George's Hall, Liverpool *13*, 17
Exeter, New Hampshire: Philips Academy (Kahn) 34, *38*

f

Fawcett, Peter 122
Feilden Clegg 114
Finley, Sir Moses: library 108, 110
Fitzroy Robinson 46
Folkestone, Kent: Saga Headquarters (Hopkins & Partners) 118
Fort Worth: Kimbell Art Museum (Kahn) 30, *31*, 33–4, 192
Foster, Norman: Lycée Polyvalent, Fréjus, France 38, *39*
Frampton, Kenneth: *Studies in Tectonic Culture* 27, 34–5, 212
Fréjus, France: Lycée Polyvalent (Foster) 38, *39*

g

Giedion, Sigfried: *Space, Time and Architecture* 10, 11, 14–15, 18

h

Haden (G. N.) & Sons 26
Harare, Zimbabwe: Eastgate Building (Pearce Partnership) 54–61
Hardwick Hall (Smythson) 199
Hawkes, Dean, and MacCormac, Richard: study 146
Helicon Building, London (Sheppard Robson) 146–55
Herne-Sodingen, Germany: Mont Cenis Training Centre (Jourda & Perraudin) 96–105
Hertzberger, Herman: Centraal Beheer, Apeldoorn, Netherlands 156
Herzog, Thomas: Congress and Exhibition Hall, Linz 38–9, *40*
Herzog & de Meuron: Tate Modern, London 202–11
Hofburg Theatre, Vienna (Semper) *16*, 19
HOK International 46
Holabird & Roche 184
Hopkins (Michael) & Partners:
    Inland Revenue building, Nottingham 118
    Nottingham University Jubilee Campus 114–25
    Portcullis House, Westminster 118
Houses of Parliament, London (Barry) *12*, 16–17, 24
Houston, Texas:
    Byzantine Fresco Chapel Museum (de Menil) 174–81
    Menil Collection museum (Piano) 166, 170, 174, 192
    Twombly Gallery (Piano) 174
Howlands Farm Student Housing, Durham (Arup) 72–7

i

Institution of Civil Engineers 13
International Style 35

j

Jeanneret, Charles-Edouard *see* Le Corbusier
Jeanneret, Pierre 22
Jenney, William LeBaron 184
Jones, Edward *see* Dixon, Jeremy
Jourda & Perraudin: Mont Cenis Training Centre, Herne-Sodingen 96–105

k

Kahn, Louis 29–30, 59, 210
    Kimbell Art Museum, Fort Worth 30, *31*, 33–4, 192
    Mellon Center for British Art, New Haven 30, *33*, 33–4
    Philips Academy, Exeter, New Hampshire 34, *38*
    Richards Memorial Laboratories, Philadelphia 29–31, *30*, 33–4
    US Consulate, Luanda (unbuilt) 34, *37*
Kanak culture 128; huts *128*, 129
Kimbell Art Museum, Fort Worth (Kahn) 30, *31*, 33–4, 192
Kleihues, Josef Paul: Museum of Contemporary Art, Chicago 182–91

l

Labrouste, Henri 18, 185, 210
    Bibliothèque Ste-Geneviève *14*, 18–19, 139
Larsen, Henning 46
Le Corbusier 8, 21, 33, 54
    air-conditioning diagram *20*
    Cinque points d'une architecture nouvelle 16, 22
    Cité de Refuge, Paris *18*, 22–4, *23*, 25
    Ministry of Education, Rio de Janeiro 33, *36*
    Précisions 23, 35
    Unité d'Habitation, Marseilles *26*, 28
    Vers une Architecture 83
    Villa Savoye, Poissy *20*, 25
Léger, Fernand 21
Leicester: Queen's Building, De Montfort University (Short Ford & Associates) 38, *40*
Lincoln's Inn Fields, London (Soane) *11*, 15–16
Linz, Austria: Congress and Exhibition Hall (Herzog) 38–9, *40*
Lisbon: Portuguese Pavilion, Expo 98 (Siza) 212–21
Liverpool: St George's Hall (Elmes) *13*, 17
Lloyds Building, London (Rogers) 30–1, *34*, 149
London:
    Bank of England (Soane) 15
    BedZED Sustainable Development (Dunster) 86–95
    Dulwich Picture Gallery (Soane) 15, 31, 190, 192, 194
    Finsbury Health Centre (Lubetkin) *24*, 26
    Helicon Building (Sheppard Robson) 146–55
    Highgate flats, Highgate (Lubetkin) *23*, 25–6
    Houses of Parliament (Barry) *12*, 16–17, 24
    Lincoln's Inn Fields, London (Soane) *11*, 15–16
    Lloyds Building (Rogers) 30–1, *34*, 149
    Portcullis House, Westminster (Hopkins & Partners) 118

Reform Club (Barry) *12*, 17
Sainsbury Wing, National Gallery (Venturi) 31–2, *35*, 190, 194
Tate Modern (Herzog & de Meuron) 202–11
Lubetkin, Berthold:
    Finsbury Health Centre, London *24*, 26
    Highgate flats, Highgate *23*, 25–6
Lutyens, Edwin: bridge, Cambridge 108
Lycée Polyvalent, Fréjus, France (Foster) 38, *39*

m

MacCormac, Richard *see* Hawkes, Dean
Macormac Jamieson & Pritchard 114
March, Lionel *see* Martin, Leslie
Marks & Spencer, Moorgate 148, 149
Markus, Tom 164
Marseilles, France: Unité d'Habitation (Le Corbusier) *26*, 28
Martin, Leslie, and March, Lionel: 'Land Use and Built Forms' 146
Marzahn Low-energy Apartment Building, Berlin (Assmann, Salomon & Scheidt) 78–85
mechanics institutes, 19th-century 13
Mellon Center for British Art, New Haven (Kahn) 30, *33*, 33–4
Menara Mesiniaga office building, Selangor (Yeang) 39, *41*
Menil, Dominique de 164
Menil, François de: Byzantine Fresco Chapel Museum, Houston 174–81
Menil Collection museum, Houston (Piano) 166, 170, 174, 192
Mesecke, Andrea, and Scheer, Thorsten: *Museum of Contemporary Art, Chicago* 182
Mies van der Rohe, Ludwig 27, 28, 184, 210
    glass skyscrapers, Berlin *18*, 22, 54
    IIT campus, Chicago 28
    Museum for a Small City 27, 190, 192
    National Gallery, Berlin 28, 192
    Seagram Building, New York 28
    silk exhibition, Barcelona Exposition 27–8
Modern Movement 8, 9, 11, 23, 25, 26, 28, 32, 140
Mont Cenis Training Centre, Herne-Sodingen (Jourda & Perraudin) 96–105
Museum for a Small City (Mies van der Rohe) 27, 190, 192
MVRDV: Villa VPRO Offices, Rotterdam 156–63

n

Napoleon Bonaparte 11
Nash, John: Royal Pavilion, Brighton 8, 10
National Gallery, London: Sainsbury Wing (Venturi) 31–2, *35*, 190, 194
Neutra, Richard 136
New Caledonia: Cultural Centre, Nouméa (Piano) 126–35
New Hampshire: Philips Academy, Exeter (Kahn) 34, *38*
New Haven: Mellon Center for British Art (Kahn) 30, *33*, 33–4
New York: Seagram Building (Mies van der Rohe) 28
Nottingham:
    Inland Revenue building (Hopkins & Partners) 118

Jubilee Campus, Nottingham University
(Hopkins & Partners) 114–25
Nouméa, New Caledonia: Cultural Centre (Piano)
126–35

o

Olgyay, Victor: *Design with Climate* 36–7, *38*
Olivetti Factory, Argentina (Zanusso) 28, *28*
Olley, John 17

p

Paris:
Bibliothèque Ste-Geneviève (Labrouste)
14, 18–19, 139
Cité de Refuge (Le Corbusier) *18,* 22–4, *23*, 25
Pompidou Centre (Piano and Rogers)
30–1, *33*, 214–15
Peabody Trust 88
Pearce Partnership: Eastgate Building, Harare 54–61
Peclet, Eugène: *Etude sur la Chaleur* 20
Perkins, Jacob 15, 199
Perrault, Dominique: Velodrome, Berlin 222–31
Pevsner, Nikolaus: *Pioneers of Modern Design*
10, 11, 18, 72, 210
Philadelphia, PA: Richards Memorial Laboratories
(Kahn) 29–31, *30*, 33–4
Philips Academy, Exeter, New Hampshire (Kahn)
34, *38*
Piano, Renzo:
Beyeler Foundation Museum, Basel 164–73, 192
Menil Collection museum, Houston
166, 170, 174, 192
Nouméa, New Caledonia: Cultural Centre 126–35
Pompidou Centre, Paris 30–1, *33*, 214–15
Twombly Gallery, Houston 174
Poirier, Marty 139
Poissy, France: Villa Savoye (Le Corbusier) *20*, 25
Pompidou Centre, Paris (Piano and Rogers)
30–1, *33*, 214–15
Portcullis House, Westminster (Hopkins & Partners)
118
Postmodernism 31

q

Queen Anne Movement 109
Queen's Building, De Montfort University,
Leicester (Short Ford & Associates) 38, *40*

r

Reform Club, London (Barry) *12*, 17
Reich, Lily 27
Reid, David Boswell 199
Houses of Parliament *12*, 16–17, 24
*Illustrations of the Theory and Practice
of Ventilation* 20
St George's Hall, Liverpool *13*
Rice, Peter 174
Richards, J. M. 76
Richards Memorial Laboratories, Philadelphia
(Kahn) 29–31, *30*, 33–4
Richardson, H. H. 184
Rio de Janeiro: Ministry of Education (Le Corbusier
and Costa) 33, *36*

Rogers, Lord Richard 88
Lloyds Building, London 30–1, *34*, 149
Pompidou Centre, Paris 30–1, *33*, 214–15
Rome: Rinascente department store (Albini) 29, *29*
Rotterdam: Villa VPRO Offices (MVRDV) 156–63

s

Sainsbury Wing, National Gallery, London (Venturi)
31–2, *35*, 190, 194
St John, Caruso: Walsall Art Gallery 192–201
Salford: cotton mill (Boulton and Watt) *8*, 10, 14–15
San Diego, California: Carmel Mountain Ranch
Public Library (Steele Group) 136–43
Scheer, Thorsten *see* Mesecke, Andrea
Schinkel, Karl Friedrich 182, 210
Altes Museum, Berlin 182, 185
Schauspielhaus, Berlin 182
Schools Construction System Development (SCSD)
programme 29, *29*, 138
Scott, M. H. Baillie 111
SCSD *see* Schools Construction System
Development
Seagram Building, New York (Mies van der Rohe) 28
Seidler, Harry 46
Selangor, Malaysia: Menara Mesiniaga office
building (Yeang) 39, *41*
Semper, Gottfried 185, 210
Dresden Opera House 19
Hofburg Theatre, Vienna *16*, 19
Sheppard Robson: Helicon Building, London 146–55
Short Ford & Associates: Queen's Building,
De Montfort University, Leicester 38, *40*
Siza, Alvaro: Portuguese Pavilion, Expo 98,
Lisbon 212–21
Smeatonian Club 13
Smythson, Robert: Hardwick Hall 199
Soane, Sir John 19, 185, 199
Bank of England 15
Dulwich Picture Gallery 15, 31, 190, 192, 194
Lincoln's Inn Fields, London *11*, 15–16
Tyringham Hall, Buckinghamshire 15
Solihull: Arup Campus (Arup) 62–71
Souto de Moura, Eduardo: multimedia installation
214
Steele (M.W.) Group Inc.: Carmel Mountain Ranch
Public Library, San Diego 136–43
Stevenson, J. J.: Old Granary, Cambridge 109, *109*
Strutt, William 14
Summerson: *The Classical Language of
Architecture* 78
Sylvester, Charles: *The Philosophy of Domestic
Economy* 20

t

Tate Modern, London (Herzog & de Meuron) 202–11
Tjibaou, Jean-Marie 126, 128
Towards an Urban Renaissance (Government
report) 86, 88
Tredgold, Thomas: *Principles of Warming and
Ventilation* 20
Twombly Gallery, Houston (Piano) 174
Tyringham Hall, Buckinghamshire (Soane) 15

u

Unité d'Habitation, Marseilles (Le Corbusier) *26*, 28

v

Velodrome, Berlin (Perrault) 222–31
ventilation systems, early 14, 16–18, 19–20
Venturi, Robert 210
ainsbury Wing, National Gallery, London
31–2, *35*, 190, 194
Vienna: Hofburg Theatre (Semper) *16*, 19
Villa Savoye, Poissy, France (Le Corbusier) *20*, 25
Villa VPRO Offices, Rotterdam (MVRDV) 156–63
Viollet-le-Duc, Eugène: *Entretiens* 18
'Vitruvian' model of environmental design 36–7, *38*
Voysey, C. F. A. 111

w

Walsall Art Gallery (St John) 192–201
Watt, James *see* Boulton, Matthew
Willmert, Todd 15, 19
Wren, Sir Christopher 16

y

Yeang, Ken 39
Menara Mesiniaga office building, Selangor *39*, *41*

z

Zanusso, Marco: Olivetti Factory, Argentina 28, *28*

Tuesday, December 15, 1992
New York

Mornings were always a bad time for Nick Angel. He lay in bed, eyes closed, unwilling to surrender the peaceful darkness, fighting the fact that he had to get up and face another day. Especially this day. His birthday.

Thirty-five.

Nick Angel was thirty-five.

Jesus! The newspapers would have an orgasmic overdose on this one. He was no longer the boy wonder. Age was creeping up on him.

He lay very still. It was probably past noon, but the longer he delayed getting up the better, for he knew that once he stirred they'd be all over him. Honey – his live-in girlfriend. Harlan – his so-called valet. And Teresa, his faithful karate champion assistant.

He heard a sudden movement in the room. A subtle rustle of silk and the faint aroma of White Diamonds – Honey was a big Liz Taylor fan. In fact Honey was a fan. Period.

So . . . why was he with her?

Good question. The problem was there were too many questions in his life and not enough answers.

Honey was on the prowl. Pretty blonde Honey with the lethal body and vacant mind. He sensed her standing by the bed staring down at him, willing him to wake up.

Too bad, sweetheart. Get lost. Not in the mood.

As soon as he was sure she'd left, he quickly rolled out of bed and made it to the safety of his steel and glass high-tech bathroom where he immediately locked the door.

Ah . . . Nick Angel in the morning. Not the man he once was, although still handsome in spite of ten pounds of excess flesh, bloodshot eyes, and an altogether dissipated demeanour.

He hated the way he looked. The extra weight he'd put on disgusted him. Had to stop drinking. Had to get his life together.

Nick Angel. Longish black hair. Indian green eyes. A pale skin, stubbled chin. At five feet ten inches he was tall without being overpowering. His handsomeness was not perfect. More brooding . . . mesmerizing. And in spite of being bloodshot his green eyes were hypnotic and watchful. His nose – once broken – gave him the dangerous edge he needed.

And now he was thirty-five.

Old.

Older than he'd ever thought he'd be.

But the world still loved him. His fans would continue to worship because he was Nick Angel and he belonged to them. They'd elevated him to a rare and crazy place where nobody could expect to remain sane.

It's too much, he thought bitterly, splashing cold water on his face. *The adulation, the never-ending attention. Crushing . . . stifling . . . suffocating . . . Too fucking much.*

He smiled grimly.

Welcome to the insane asylum.

Welcome to my life.

Reaching for the phone he buzzed the underground garage, connecting with one of his team of driver/bodyguards.

"I'm on my way down," he said, keeping his gravelly voice low. "Get out the Ferrari. No driver. And call the airport, tell them to have my plane ready, I'm taking it up."

"Right, Nick. Oh, an' happy birthday, man."

Screw this birthday crap. He knew he'd hear nothing else all day.

Finishing in the bathroom he dressed quickly in the trademark black he always wore. Pants, shirt, leather jacket and black tennis shoes. All he had to do now was make it out of the apartment before he was forced to endure more congratulations.

As soon as he hit the hall they came at him. Honey, all pearly teeth and rounded breasts encased in a pink angora sweater, her short skirt swishing sexily around her thighs.

Harlan – a crazed black man with wild hair extensions and subdued make-up.

2

And Teresa – who was six feet tall with a face like a man.

What a mismatched trio! But they were his. He owned them. He paid for every move they made.

"Gotta go," he said, edgily.

"Where?" Honey asked, thrusting angora clad tits in his direction.

"Where?" echoed Teresa, staring at him accusingly. "I should come with you."

"Yeah, where ya goin', man?" added Harlan, joining the chorus.

"I'll be back soon."

Maybe.

Maybe not.

Cleverly, he timed his words to coincide with the arrival of the elevator, and before they could nail him further he was out of there, downstairs, in his Ferrari, driving out of Manhattan as fast as he could.

It took him forty-five minutes to reach the private airstrip where he kept his two-engine Cessna plane. Several mechanics greeted him with birthday wishes.

Surprise, surprise. He'd known today was going to be a bummer.

He climbed aboard his plane, settled in the cockpit and guided the small aircraft down the runway until he was given clearance to take off into the unseasonably blue sky.

He sighed, a long heavy sigh. When did it all begin to get out of control?

Nick Angel.

Free at last.

But he had a solution. A plan he was about to put into action.

Colour me dead.

BOOK ONE

Chapter 1

Louisville, Kentucky 1969

"Do it!" the young girl gasped urgently, her breath coming in short frantic gasps. "Do it, *do* it!"

"I'm tryin'," Nick Angelo replied, heatedly. And indeed he was, but to his dismay the girl was so wet he kept slipping out.

Her voice was shrill and commanding. "Do it!" she insisted, wriggling back into position. "C'mon, Nicky. C'mon, c'mon, c'*monnnn!*"

Beginning to panic he jammed the point of entry yet again, and thank goodness managed to stay in place.

"*Uuuuuummm* . . ." The desperate shrillness faded from her voice and she began to sound pleased. "*Ooooooh* . . ." She continued to sigh sweetly as he pumped away.

Nick hung on, even though he was sweating and uncomfortable, but he hung on anyway because jamming himself inside this girl was the most important act in the entire world.

Vaguely he remembered one of his friends telling him sex was like riding a horse – mount up – get in the saddle – and take the trip.

Nobody had warned him it would be such a dangerous, hot, sticky journey.

And then it hit him. The most exciting, throbbing, out-of-control feeling he'd ever experienced. Holy cow! He was coming! And he was inside a real female – his hand and some dirty magazine had nothing to do with it.

The girl screamed out her satisfaction.

7

He felt like doing the same thing. But he was cool, a guy had to stay cool – even if it *was* his first time.

Nick Angelo was finally making out – and he couldn't think of a more mind-blowing way of celebrating his thirteenth birthday.

Evanston, Illinois 1973

"Please, Nick, *pleeease* . . . I can't take any more."

Maybe. Maybe not. But he'd been giving it to her for twenty minutes and she'd only now started to complain – although it was hardly a complaint, more an agonized cry of ecstasy.

"Ooh, Nicky, you're the best!"

Yeah? So he'd been told. Now if he could only teach them not to call him Nicky . . .

Making out was his specialty. It sure beat homework or any of that learning crap. And it certainly beat spending time at home watching his old man drink himself unconscious while his mother was out busting her ass working two jobs to keep the lazy slob in beer.

Family life. You could shove it. Just like he was shoving it up Susie or Jenny or whatever her name was.

One of these days he planned on taking off, getting out of this dump, and bringing his mother with him. But first he needed a job so he could score some bucks, then there'd be no holding him back.

Right now he was stuck in school because his mother thought education was important. Mary Angelo had this crazy fantasy that one day he'd get a scholarship to college.

Yeah, sure – a make-out college was the only place *he'd* get in.

Mary wasn't into reality – she was into dreams. At thirty-seven she looked ten years older. A bird-like woman – slight and nervous, with faded prettiness and wispy hair. She'd met Nick's father, Primo, on a blind date when she was sixteen and he was thirty. They'd gotten married exactly one week before Nick was born and Primo had hardly worked a day since. A carpenter by trade, he'd soon realized that picking up unemployment while

8

sending his wife out to work was a far better deal than actually doing anything himself.

The Angelo family moved often, trudging from state to state, living in rented accommodations, always ready to be on the move whenever Primo felt that restless urge. And he felt it often.

Growing up, Nick couldn't remember being in the same town for longer than a few months at a time. As soon as he began to settle in they were on their way again. Eventually he gave up on any permanent relationships. New town. New girls to conquer. And on to the next. Now he'd gotten used to it.

"Can we go see a movie tomorrow?" Susie or Jenny or whatever her name was asked. "It'll be my treat."

"Nah." He shook his head as he got up, pulling on his pants. They were in the back office of a small car showroom – a venue he used often on account of the fact he sometimes ran errands for one of the salesmen, and in return he got to borrow the keys.

"Why not?" the girl asked. At eighteen she was two years older than him. She had short hair, freckles, and a well-developed chest. He'd picked her up the day before behind the counter of a Kentucky Fried Chicken outlet.

He tried to come up with a quick excuse. He excelled at sex. Hated to stick around. Past experience told him she wouldn't appreciate the truth. A screw is a screw – who needs it to be anything else?

"Gotta work," he said, brushing a hand through his unruly black hair.

"What do you do?" she asked, curiously.

"I'm an undertaker's assistant," he lied, straight-faced.

That shut her up.

He waited for her to adjust her clothing, even helped her up. Then he took her to the bus stop, left her there and walked the mile home.

Currently they were living in a run-down house with Mary's sister – his aunt Franny – a big woman with dyed yellow hair and a bleached moustache. It was only a small house, but as long as Primo had a television to watch and a plentiful supply of beer, he was satisfied.

Nick hoped Mary was home from work. If she was, there'd be a chance of something to eat. Franny never bothered to cook. She was on a diet of Reese's peanut-butter cups and diet soda – screw fixing meals.

Sure. Franny got fatter and everyone else starved to death.

9

Sex always made him hungry. Right now he'd kill for a hamburger, but he was broke as usual, so the only chance he had was working on Mary with his charm. Not that he'd have to do much work, his mother adored him, she put him before everyone, including Primo when she could get away with it, which wasn't often, for Primo demanded most of her attention when she wasn't working.

Nick's goal in life was to have as little to do with his father as possible. He hated the way Primo treated Mary. He couldn't stand listening to him bitch and complain about everything. And most of all he despised the way Primo sat on his big, fat can doing nothing.

The truth was that Primo scared him. He was a huge, over-powering man, and whenever he was in a bad mood Nick felt the back of his hand or the sting of his rough leather belt across his backside. Mary always tried to stop the beatings – protecting him as best she could – even if it meant getting beat herself. Primo didn't care who got in his way – he lashed out good.

Sometimes Nick wanted to kill him. Other times he accepted the beatings as a fact of life. The rage he felt was muted, buried. There was nothing he could do – not until he was older, then he'd get him and his mother out.

Halfway home it started to rain. Pulling up the collar of his old denim jacket he bent his head down and began jogging along the kerb, thinking about how great it would be to have wheels, imagining that one of these days he'd get himself a car – a gleaming red Cadillac with chrome wheels and a real fine radio.

Yeah . . . one of these days.

Primo was sitting on the steps outside Franny's house. Nick could see him as he approached. He tensed up, something was wrong. Why else would his old man have deserted his precious television and be sitting outside in the rain?

He approached warily. "What's up?" he asked, stopping and jogging in place.

Primo wiped the back of his hand across his nose and glared up at him, bloodshot eyes bulging. "Where've ya bin?" he demanded, slurring his words.

Nick felt the cold rain trickling down the back of his collar and he shivered – anticipating bad news. "Out with friends," he mumbled.

Primo heaved a mournful, beer-soaked sigh and hauled himself to his feet. His shirt was stuck to his body. His thick greying hair fell in greasy clumps on his prominent forehead. Raindrops continued to drip from the end of his nose.

"She's gone," he said, glumly. "Your goddamn mother went an' died on us."

Chapter 2

Bosewell, Kansas 1973

Lauren Roberts was sixteen when a man stopped her in the street and asked if she'd ever considered a modelling career. Lauren had laughed in his face. Who was this stranger? And why was he picking on her?

It turned out there was a film crew passing through town, an odd bunch of people. Lauren had been warned – along with everyone else in school – to have nothing to do with them.

When she got home she told her father.

Phil Roberts nodded sagely and said, "A pretty girl will always be bothered, but a wise girl soon learns to take no notice."

Lauren agreed. Pretty was one thing, but wise was better. Her father was smart. He'd always taught her that relying on her exceptional good looks to get by was a mistake. Being an A student was better. Getting good grades. Excelling at sports. Helping out with community service. And even though Bosewell was only a small town – population no more than six thousand people – there was always plenty of community service.

Lauren was certainly pretty. At five foot seven she was taller than most of the other girls in her class. She had long legs, a slender body, and her hair was thick and chestnut, falling beneath her shoulders, framing an oval-shaped face with expressive, long-lashed, tortoiseshell eyes, a straight nose and a wide mouth concealing a dazzling, heart-warming smile.

Lauren Roberts was one of the most popular girls in school, everyone liked her – even the teachers.

She was standing in the school yard with her best friend,

Meg, when Meg nudged her conspiratorially and whispered, "Here he comes. You'd better watch out!"

"He" was Stock Browning – Bosewell High's very own football star. Lately he'd been noticing Lauren in a big way.

Lauren frowned. "Shut up," she muttered, "he'll hear you."

"So what?" replied Meg, tossing her blonde curls. "I bet he's going to ask you out."

"No he's *not*."

"Bet he is."

Stock walked like a cowboy with a wide-legged rolling gait. His hair was white-blond and crew cut, and his eyes a teutonic blue. Big and tanned, he was well aware he could get anything or anyone he wanted. It helped that his father owned Brownings, the only department store in town.

"Hiya, Lauren," he drawled, stifling a strong desire to pat his crotch – snug in track suit pants.

It was the first time he'd called her by her name, even though they'd attended the same school for years.

I guess sixteen must be the magic number, she thought, skittishly.

"Hello, Stock," she responded, wondering, as she had many times before, where his parents had come up with his name.

"How 'bout you an' me taking in a movie?" he suggested, getting straight to the point.

Lauren considered his invitation. In a way she was flattered, after all, Stock Browning was looked on as the catch of the year. But then again she didn't – unlike most of the other girls in school – feel "that way" about him. He wasn't her type.

"Hmm . . ." she said, caught off guard and stalling.

He couldn't believe she was actually hesitating. "Is that a yes?" he asked.

"It's a when," she replied, carefully.

His blue eyes narrowed. "When what?"

"When did you have in mind?" she asked, trying to keep it light.

Goddamn it! Was she being difficult? Any other girl would be singing at the chance of a date with him. "Tonight. Tomorrow night. Whenever you like."

I'd like you to leave me alone, she decided. Even though she didn't have a boyfriend she was not interested in dating him. Absolutely not. He was too full of himself by far.

"Well?" He towered over her, and she couldn't help thinking of his big, sweaty body pressing down on hers if they ever did it. Not that she had any intention of doing it. Not until

13

she was married to the man she loved – whoever he might be.

She continued to stall as she hated hurting anyone's feelings – even his. "I don't know, I've got a busy week," she demurred.

Now it was his turn to frown. A busy week! Was little Lauren Roberts actually turning down a date with him? Surely it wasn't possible?

"Call me when you make up your mind," he said brusquely, and stalked off.

Meg, hovering on the sidelines, giggled nervously. "You didn't say no, did you?"

Lauren nodded. "I said no."

"You *didn't*!" Meg clapped a hand over her mouth.

"I did."

They both burst out laughing and hugged each other.

"Holy cow!" exclaimed Meg. "I bet that's the first no *he's* ever had."

"Serves him right for ignoring us all these years," Lauren said, crisply.

"You're right," Meg agreed, although if Stock Browning had invited *her* out she would be boogeying down Main Street handing out flyers. "What are you going to do if he asks you again?" she asked, curiously.

Lauren shrugged. "I'll worry about it when it happens, and quite honestly, I don't think it will."

"It will," Meg said wisely.

"So I'll deal with it." Lauren felt that Stock Browning had occupied enough of their time. "Let's go get a malt."

Later that night she told her parents about the encounter, expecting them to agree that Stock was rich and spoilt and even though he was the son of the most affluent man in town she'd done the right thing in turning him down.

Jane and Phil Roberts had been married twenty-five years – the first ten childless. Just when they'd given up hope, along came Lauren. She had received nothing but their love and devotion – it would be hard to find a more united family. So it came as a shock to discover that no – her parents did not agree with her. It seemed they considered Stock a very nice boy with a bright future, and certainly a suitable candidate for their only daughter to go out with.

Lauren was crushed they felt that way. "I'm *not* dating him," she said stubbornly, before rushing up to her room.

14

Twenty minutes later her father knocked on her bedroom door. Phil Roberts was a pleasant looking man with sandy hair parted in the middle, a small moustache and a weak chin. "Lauren, dear," he said, soothingly. "We want the best for you, surely you know that?"

The best, don't you mean the richest?

"Yes, Daddy, I know."

Phil paced around her room, uncomfortable and ill at ease. "Spend an evening with the boy, give him a chance."

A chance at what? Her virginity?

"Okay, Daddy – maybe," she mumbled, noticing that tonight her father looked tired, and she didn't want to upset him.

"Good girl," Phil said, looking relieved.

Meg was right, it didn't take Stock long to ask again. A few days later he invited her to his cousin's twenty-first birthday party. "Black tie," he announced, grandly.

"I don't have a black tie," she dead-panned.

He didn't laugh. Bad sign.

"I'll pick you up at six-thirty," he said, patting his crotch – obviously a favourite habit.

Her parents were suitably pleased.

"We'll go to Brownings and I'll buy you a new dress," her mother said.

Lauren nodded. *Do we get a discount if I let him jump me?*

On the appointed evening Stock turned up washed and brushed – bristly blond crew cut, reddish tan, well-fitting white dinner jacket. Her parents were impressed. In fact she'd never seen her mother so giggly and girlish as she lined them up for a series of quick snapshots.

Lauren's new dress was sludge green. She hated it. "Made in New York," the saleslady had pronounced in hushed tones. After that her mother had refused to look at anything else.

Stock put his arm around her for the photographs. She felt the heat of his hand through the thin material of her dress and held her breath. The rumour was that Ellen-Sue Mathison had been forced to leave town because he'd gotten her pregnant. And Melissa Thomlinson swore he'd tried to rape her.

She shuddered.

"Are you cold?" Stock asked, solicitously.

"Oh, no, I'm just fine, thank you, Stock," replied her mother, twinkling gaily.

"Try this." Phil Roberts thrust a glass of champagne drowned

15

in orange juice into his beefy hand. "One for the road. No harm, eh?"

Lauren was seeing her parents in a new light and she wasn't sure she liked it.

Stock drove a sleek Ford Thunderbird. He opened the door for her and helped her in, trying for a surreptitious peek up her skirt.

"Nice parents," he said, settling behind the wheel.

"Nice car," she responded, dully.

"It gets me there."

Not with me it doesn't.

Now that he had her he didn't know what to say, and she wasn't about to make it easy. She was here by default, and if he made one wrong move he'd find himself very, very sorry indeed.

Chapter 3

Evanston, Illinois 1973

Friday morning dawned bleak and icy. The rain beat down relentlessly, forming a muddy sludge on the ground.

Crammed into the back of a cab between Aunt Franny and his father, Nick felt the bile rise in his throat. They both smelt strongly of mothballs – due to the fact that they'd borrowed black clothes from the neighbours, one of whom, Mrs Rifkin, had magnanimously decided to accompany them to the funeral.

Mrs Rifkin sat in the front of the cab, chewing Chiclets and attempting to make conversation with the black driver who was more interested in breaking the speed limit and dumping them fast. He sensed a small tip, and nothing pissed him off more.

Franny extracted a half-melted peanut-butter cup from her worn purse, popped it into her mouth and said to Primo, "Well now . . . when do you think you'll be moving on?"

Great, Nick thought sourly, his mother wasn't even cold and this old bag was trying to get rid of them. So much for family attachments.

Primo opened his mouth to reply, and the foul aroma of bad teeth and stale beer wafted in the air jockeying with the mothballs for attention.

"What's your hurry, Fran?" Primo asked, letting out a not so discreet burp.

"Without Mary's pay-cheque I can't be lettin' you stay. Can't afford it," Franny stated, munching away.

"So you're throwin' us out? Is that it?" Primo said, nastily.

Franny smoothed down the folds of her skirt, rubbing a

17

newly discovered spot on the cheap material. She was damned if she was going to let her sister's lazy slob husband live off her. She hated the sight of his ugly face. "I plan on renting out your rooms," she announced. "The sooner the better. I – "

"Not to darkies I hope," interrupted a panicked Mrs Rifkin, forgetting who she was sitting next to.

The cab careered around a corner, throwing Nick up against his aunt's ample bosom. He wished he could throw up all over her, the old cow deserved it.

"An' how about Nick?" Primo asked, as if he wasn't sitting right there beside them.

"You'll take him with you," Franny replied, not even considering the idea of inviting him to stay on.

"He'll be better off with you," Primo insisted.

Franny rummaged for another chocolate. "What am I expected to do with a sixteen-year-old boy?" she said, in an exasperated voice.

Primo wasn't about to drop it. "At least he'll have a home."

Was his father actually thinking of him, or was it the thought of being free that urged him on?

"Yes. An' extra food t'buy. An' clothes, and all that other stuff young boys need," Franny said, indignantly. "No thank you. He's *your* son. He goes with *you*."

Case settled.

Nick leaned forward, trying to stop the despair that was rising up within him, a despair so great he could barely manage to breathe. One day his mother was there. The next – gone – just like that. Heart failure they said.

Heart failure at thirty-seven years of age? Desertion more like. She'd left him alone with Primo because she simply couldn't take any more.

When they got out of the taxi outside the cemetery Primo stood there fidgeting, until Franny realized he expected her to pay for the ride. She threw him a filthy look.

"Must've left my wallet home," Primo mumbled, sheepishly.

"Cheap monkey," she said sourly, counting out the exact fare. "You always were and you always will be."

The cab driver snatched the money and zoomed off, the wheels of his vehicle splashing them all with mud.

Mrs Rifkin was not pleased. She sprung open a faded umbrella, all the while muttering under her breath, "They shouldn't let 'em drive, that's what *I* say."

Nick shivered. How could his mother leave him alone with Primo?

Despair was replaced with anger. He wanted to shout and scream. If he could have gotten hold of her he would have shaken the life out of her.

Only it was too late wasn't it? She was already dead.

A thin man in a shiny grey slicker with a sinister hood announced he would be escorting them graveside. "Is this all of you?" he sniffed, sounding disappointed.

"Yeah," said Primo, belligerently. "Wanna make somethin' of it?"

The man ignored him.

"We haven't lived here long," Nick felt compelled to explain, as they trudged past endless rows of neatly lined up graves. "My mother didn't have time to make friends."

"Oh, dear," said the man, with about as much interest as a fish. He was into getting rid of this motley group as fast as possible.

"She was a wonderful woman though, really wonderful," Nick added, speaking too quickly, his words tripping over each other.

"I'm sure she was," said the man in the slicker.

Finally they arrived at a freshly dug plot of land where a cheap wooden coffin waited to be lowered into the ground.

My mother's in that box, Nick thought, suddenly losing it. *Oh, Jeez! My mother's in that box.*

And so the short ceremony began. And the rain pounded down. And Nick didn't know whether he was crying or not because his face was wet, so very, very wet . . .

Three days later they left. Franny was relieved to see them go. Just to make sure she packed them stale cheese sandwiches and a flask of lukewarm instant coffee. She stood outside her house waving them on their way, even though it was still raining and bitterly cold.

"Fat bitch!" mumbled Primo, as they drove away in the shabby old van he'd had for ten years.

"Where we goin', Dad?" Nick ventured.

"Don't ask no questions an' you won't hear no lies," Primo said grimly.

"I just thought – "

"*Don't* think," Primo interrupted, harshly. "Sit there an' keep

19

your big ugly mouth shut. Ain't it enough I gotta be responsible for you?"

There was a thickness in Nick's throat. Oh sure, he was used to leaving town, abandoning his friends and starting afresh every few months. But he was not used to being without his mother's protection. She'd always been the buffer between him and Primo, and now there was no one who cared.

"Soon as we get where we're goin' I'll look for a job," he said, staring at the windscreen wipers as they worked on the relentless rain, scratching against the windscreen with a dull scraping sound.

"Nah. Ya gotta stay in school," Primo said.

"I don't," he objected.

"That's where ya wrong. I made ya mother a promise."

"*What* promise?"

"Mind your business."

It was *his* life they were discussing, surely he was entitled to know? And since when did Primo care about keeping promises?

Primo slumped into silence, his bloodshot eyes fixed on the road ahead, his big hands clutching the steering wheel.

Nick's mind kept on drifting back to his mother being lowered into the ground, the rain soaking through the cheap wooden coffin. He was overcome with an unbearable sense of suffocation and loneliness.

Was she cold?

Was her body slowly beginning to rot?

Some kind of horrible wail began to beat and pound inside his head.

Why couldn't it have been Primo?

Why couldn't it have been his goddamn father?

They stopped for gas a couple of hours later. Nick got out and stretched his legs while Primo vanished into the men's room and didn't come out for twenty minutes. When he finally emerged he ignored his son and headed straight for the convenience store, where he purchased a pack of Camels and a six-pack of beer. Then he stationed himself by the pay phone and began making calls.

Nick knew better than to ask who he was phoning. He didn't care. It didn't matter what his father said, as soon as possible he would find a job, save his money and get the hell out.

He wandered outside and got back in the van. It stunk of

gas. Idly he rolled down the window and watched a blonde in a miniskirt and boots make a dash from her car to the ladies room, somewhat futilely holding a soggy magazine over her black roots.

Girls. They were all the same. He'd made out with enough of them to know exactly what they were like. In all his travels there hadn't been one girl he'd wanted that he hadn't had. It was hard to understand how some poor jerks agonized over getting laid because it was so easy – kind of like fishing. Put out the bait. Reel 'em in easy. Go for the kill. And then take off. Fast.

Nick Angelo could score with anyone. And he did – as frequently as possible – it gave him his only real sense of identity.

Primo lumbered out to the van, threw the six-pack – depleted by one can – into the middle of the seat, and started the engine.

"Uh . . . it's illegal to drive with alcohol in the vehicle," Nick muttered.

Primo wiped his nose with the back of his hand. "What're you, a cop?"

"Just pointing it out."

"Well, don't."

Yeah. Shut up. Sit still. Butt out. The story of his life.

Leaning back he closed his eyes, drifting into a sort of half sleep – until he was jolted awake when they almost skidded into the back of a massive truck parked on the side of the highway.

"Fuckin' drivers!" screamed Primo. "They don't give a crap where they dump it."

"Why don't *I* drive?" Nick suggested. It was beginning to get dark and Primo was already gulping down his third beer.

"Since when did *you* drive?" Primo sneered.

"I got taught driver's ed. in school. Took a test, got my licence."

"Don' remember that."

No, he wouldn't, would he? And even if he did he'd never have allowed him to use the van, but he'd taken it out on more than one occasion when Primo was slumped in a drunken stupor and he'd had no fear of getting caught.

The van skidded again. Primo grunted, finally deciding he'd had enough. Pulling over, he slid across to the passenger side, shoving Nick out into the icy rain.

Nick ran around the back and quickly jumped in the driver's seat. "Where we headin'?" he asked, gripping the steering wheel, anxious to get wherever they were going.

Primo finished his beer, crushing the can in his big hand and flinging it out the window. "Kansas," he said, burping loudly. "Some piss-assed town called Bosewell."

"Why there?"

"'Cause I got a wife there, that's why."

This was big news to Nick.

Chapter 4

Bosewell, Kansas 1973

What started out as a simple date seemed to be turning into a relationship, and everyone was pleased except Lauren. She'd fallen into some kind of dumb routine with Stock. Dinner and a movie on Friday night. Dancing and a party every Saturday. And two family brunches. This had been going on for six weeks.

"What's happening?" she wailed to Meg. "I used to be a free person, how did I get myself into this?"

"Has he tried anything yet?" Meg asked, lighting up a forbidden cigarette.

"No," she shook her head. "And stop pumping me all the time, you're like a district attorney!"

"No I'm not. I'm dying to find out the dirty details."

"Why?"

"C'*mon*, Laurie," Meg pleaded. "You *know* we share everything. He must've kissed you at least."

"Maybe," she said, mysteriously.

"Has he?" Meg pressed.

"Maybe," she repeated.

They were in Lauren's bedroom, and Meg began to bounce up and down on the bed, her face red with the frustration of not being able to get any good scoop out of her best friend. "Tell me, you rotten little B-word!"

She didn't particularly wish to confide in Meg – after all it wasn't that exciting – but now there seemed to be no choice. "Okay, so he's kissed me. Big deal. End of subject."

Meg's eyes gleamed. "Is he a good kisser?"

"He's got big teeth."

"What does *that* mean?"

"They get in the way. And besides," she sighed, "I *told* you, I don't feel anything for him."

Meg jumped off the bed. "Perhaps *I* should take him over. How's that for an idea?"

"Yes!"

"You don't mean it."

"I do! I do!"

Meg was exasperated. "You've got the hottest hunk in town panting all over you, and you're acting like it's no biggie."

"It's not."

"Then why don't you stop seeing him?"

She sighed again. "Because I can't. My parents like him. They like *his* parents. In fact, if you want to know the truth – my father's selling his dad some kind of big insurance thing."

Meg dragged on her cigarette like a veteran. "Oh, that's not so good."

"Don't I know it," she said glumly, trying to figure out exactly how it had happened. Their first date had been uneventful, Stock had behaved himself perfectly – he didn't even get drunk, while all around his football buddies were staggering zombies.

She'd had no reason to turn down his second invitation, especially with her parents urging her on. And then suddenly *her* father was selling *his* father insurance, and there was no way she could mess that up.

Before she knew it, everyone considered that she and Stock were a couple.

Now she was stuck. And she wasn't happy.

Mr Lucas, Bosewell High's history teacher droned on. Lauren attempted to concentrate but it was difficult – the man was dull – and getting anything out of his class was almost impossible, he had no idea how to fire his students' imaginations. They sat in front of him – twenty-four bored teenagers engaged in a variety of activities. Joey Pearson – the class clown – was busy writing dirty limericks and passing them around. Dawn Kovak – the school tramp – negotiated with one of the boys about what she might do to him during lunch hour. Meg sketched fashion designs beneath the cover of *World History*. And Lauren day-dreamed.

Her biggest day-dream was always about New York. When she was little her parents had taken her to see Audrey Hepburn in

24

Breakfast at Tiffany's and she'd never forgotten the thrill of seeing the big city on the movie screen.

New York . . . she'd definitely decided that one of these days she was going there just like Audrey Hepburn. And she'd have her own apartment, a fulfilling job and a cat. Oh, yes, she'd *definitely* have a cat. And of course a boyfriend. A *real* boyfriend. Not Stock Browning with his white crew cut and macho walk. A man more along the lines of Robert Redford or Paul Newman – she was quite partial to the dirty-blond look.

"Lauren!" Mr Lucas's waspish voice interrupted her reverie. "Kindly answer the question."

Question. What question? She quickly glanced at the blackboard and figured out what he'd been teaching, coming up with the correct answer just in time.

"You're amazing!" Meg whispered, stifling a giggle. "Even *I* could see you were somewhere in China!"

"New York," Lauren whispered back, "although I wouldn't mind visiting China one day."

"Fat chance!"

Meg and she viewed their futures differently. Meg saw herself married with kids living happily in Bosewell. Lauren knew there was a whole other world out there and she planned to explore it before settling down.

The bell sounded, signifying the end of class.

Stock was leaning on the lunch counter waiting for her. "I'll pick you up at six-thirty tonight," he said.

"You will?"

"Don't tell me you've forgotten."

"Forgotten what?"

"Dinner with my parents."

"Oh, yes," she said, listlessly.

"Don't go crazy with excitement."

What did he want from her? She was going wasn't she? Surely that was enough?

Bending down he pecked her on the cheek. He smelt of sweat and camphor. The sweat she could take, but the camphor almost made her gag. It was definitely time she had a chat with her father about the insurance he was selling Mr Browning. Was it a done deal? And if she stopped seeing Stock would it upset everything? She was sure that any moment he was going to make the big move, and she had no desire to star as the struggling victim trapped beneath his bulk in the cramped interior of his Ford Thunderbird.

On the way home she stopped at her father's small office – located on Main Street above the Blakely Brothers hardware store. The door was locked, the shade pulled down covering the glass. *Philip M. Roberts, Insurance*, was printed on the door. One day he'd hinted it would read *Philip M. Roberts and Daughter*. Lauren hadn't summoned up the courage to inform him she had no intention of going into the insurance business.

Disappointed he wasn't there, she carried on home.

Her mother was in the kitchen making a cake.

"Where's Dad?" she asked, sticking her finger in the mixing bowl and scooping out a taste of the creamy mixture.

"Stop that!" Jane Roberts scolded. She was a dark-haired woman with fine features and high cheekbones. It was easy to see where Lauren had inherited her good looks.

"Umm! Delicious!" Lauren stuck her finger in again.

"I said stop it," Jane repeated, sternly. "There'll be nothing left. This cake is for you to take to the Brownings tonight."

"No way!" she said, horrified. "I'm *not* taking them a cake, Mother."

"Then I'll have to ask Stock."

"No, mother, *no!* You can't embarrass me this way."

Jane stopped what she was doing and wiped her hands on her apron. "What's embarrassing about baking the Brownings a cake?"

Lauren hesitated. "Well, you know, it's sort of like . . . uh . . . sucking up."

Jane narrowed her eyes. "Sucking up?"

"You *know* what I mean."

"No. I'm afraid I don't." Jane glared at her only child with a *how dare you talk to me like that – wait until your father gets home* expression.

Uh oh. Mother was p.o.'d. Maybe she'd gone too far. "Okay, okay, I'll take the dumb cake," she mumbled, and rushed upstairs to her room.

It was quite obvious suck up was the name of the game, and right now there was nothing she could do about it.

Daphne Browning was a big woman with multiple chins and bright scarlet lips. She greeted Lauren graciously. "Your mother's *so* thoughtful. What a perfectly *lovely* gesture," she gushed.

"Of course my doctor forbids that *I* eat chocolate, but Benjamin simply adores it, don't you, darling?"

Benjamin Browning barely glanced up from his newspaper. He was a tall man, thick around the middle – with terse features, iron grey hair and matching bushy eyebrows. "Trying to diet," he grunted.

Stock prowled around the room, while Lauren settled herself stiffly on a damask chair in the very formal living room. A hovering maid whisked the cake away never to be seen again.

"When are we eating?" demanded Stock.

Daphne ignored him. "Tell me, dear," she said, scarlet lips quivering as she turned towards Lauren. "Is Stock your first boyfriend?"

Lauren could not believe she was being asked such a personal question. If she wasn't so polite she would have replied, "None of your business." Instead she began furiously petting Mrs Browning's Pekinese – a ferocious little dog who bared its teeth and growled viciously.

"What a cute puppy!" she exclaimed, trying to sound sincere. "How old is he?"

"She," corrected Mrs Browning.

"And her name is?"

"Princess Pink Pontoon."

"How unusual." She patted the dog again and the little rat snapped at her with its lethal teeth.

Stock guffawed. "It'll take your hand off if it can."

"Stock!" admonished Daphne. "Princess would *never* do that."

"Dinner is served," announced a black maid, appearing at the door.

Mr Browning put down his paper. "About bloody time," he said, irritably.

Dinner was a drag. This was one evening Lauren had no wish to repeat. Mrs Browning was a snob. Mr Browning was plain rude. And Stock was . . . well he was Stock.

On the drive home he got straight to the point. "They like you," he said.

"That's nice."

"Even though you're young."

What was *he* – all of eighteen? "I'm thrilled," she said, dryly.

He missed her sarcasm. "They gave us permission."

"For what?" she asked, stifling a yawn.

"To get engaged."

Chapter 5

Aretha Mae Angelo opened the door of her trailer home and glared at Primo as if she'd seen him the day before. Actually it was seventeen years since he'd walked out on her, but she certainly wasn't about to let seventeen years stand in the way of a vigorous tongue-lashing.

Hunched in the van, Nick could hear every word as she tore into his father.

"What *you* want? Cheatin' slime. How come you sniffin' round here again? Y'ain't nothin' but a bum, so get outta here. Y'hear me? *Out.*"

She might be telling him to get lost, but Primo whined some kind of weak excuse, and before Nick could make out exactly what was happening the woman yelled more insults, dragged Primo inside the trailer and slammed the door shut.

Nick sat in the van and contemplated the last week. He was sixteen years old – nearly seventeen – and his life was over. Who cared about anything? He certainly didn't. His whole existence had been a lie.

Mary and Primo. His loving parents. Now Primo had informed him they weren't even legally married, because he'd still been married to this woman when he and Mary had exchanged their wedding vows.

Primo Angelo was a bigamist.

And if that was so, what did it make him?

He didn't care to think about it.

The rain had slowed to a drizzle but it was still icy cold. Nick huddled in the van, hungry and tired – empty of any emotion.

Some time later Primo emerged from the trailer followed by the woman. Yanking open the door of the van he thrust a

28

dirty blanket at Nick. "You'll sleep out here," he said, gruffly. "No room inside."

The woman pressed forward trying to get a look at him.

Nick noticed she was dark-skinned, very dark-skinned. With a sudden jolt he realized she was black.

In the morning the rain had stopped. Asleep across the two front seats Nick was awakened by a faint scratching sound. For a moment he couldn't figure out where he was. He sat up, banging his head on the roof. His gut ached with hunger, and he felt an urgent need to pee.

Staring at him through the side window were two small black boys. One of them was scraping his fingernails against the window. As soon as they saw he was awake they ran away.

In the light of day he took in his surroundings. The van was parked in the middle of a sparsely populated trailer park. A few skinny dogs loped around a cluster of dilapidated looking trailers, while all around was mud, weeds and over to one side a massive garbage dump.

This place made Aunt Franny's run-down house in Evanston seem like a palace.

He got out of the van. Crouching on the ground a few feet away lurked the two black kids, still staring at him.

"Hey –" he said. "What's up?"

They didn't respond.

"Gotta take a piss."

One of the boys pointed to a ramshackle hut next to the garbage pile.

He made it to the hut and wished he hadn't, the stench was unbearable.

After doing what he had to do he hurried back to the van, his stomach rumbling uncontrollably. In his pocket he had exactly thirty-five cents. Not enough to do shit.

Leaning against the van he thought about his future and decided that things certainly couldn't get any worse. He was stuck in a strange town, waiting around in some crummy trailer park while his father re-acquainted himself with the woman he'd been married to for seventeen years and never told anyone.

One of the boys edged towards him, a handsome kid with bright eyes and dark chocolate skin. "What's your name, mister?" the boy asked, curiously.

"Nick. What's yours?"

"Harlan. I'se ten. How olds you?"

"Sixteen."

"What you doin' here?"

He shrugged. "Beats me."

After a while Primo emerged from the trailer clad only in his grubby underwear, scratching his bulging belly, a rare smile lighting up his unshaven face. Nick knew the look. It was his father's *I just got laid, aren't I a fine stud* look.

"Howdja sleep?" Primo asked, as if they'd spent the night in a fancy hotel.

"I didn't. I was too hungry," he muttered, angry with his father, and yet not sure how to express himself. What he'd really like to do was beat his stupid lying brains out.

"Doncha worry 'bout that," Primo said jovially, as if nothing was amiss. "Aretha Mae's one fine little cook." He clapped his hand on his son's shoulder. "C'mon, I wancha t'meet her."

Reluctantly he followed Primo into the trailer while the two boys hovered close behind.

Inside it was a crowded mess with clutter everywhere – clothes, magazines, old newspapers and junk piled high on every surface. In one corner was an unmade bed, and on the floor rested two mouldy sleeping bags.

Aretha Mae busied herself at a kerosene stove frying ham and potatoes in greasy bacon fat. She was a sinewy black woman with frizzy, dyed red hair and a wary look in her eyes.

"Sit yourself down, boy," she said to Nick over her shoulder. "You must be real hungry."

He squeezed on to a torn plastic covered bench next to a rickety table stacked with dirty dishes.

Aretha Mae dumped a plate of food in front of him, sweeping the used dishes to one side. "Eat," she commanded.

Primo chuckled, he saw a home in his future. "I knew you two would get along."

"Shut your mouth," Aretha Mae said. "We be talkin' 'bout who gets along later. Don't go thinkin' you're movin' in."

Nick was impressed by her nerve, although he half expected his father to smack her across the mouth.

Primo didn't. Primo laughed, a big-bellied laugh. "Still a feisty bitch," he said. "I like that in a woman. You haven't changed."

Aretha Mae threw him a stern look. "Don' use no bad language in front of my kids," she said, indicating the two silent boys by the door.

"Listen who's talkin'," Primo said, scratching his stomach. "I can remember when that's *all* you used."

"Things was different then," Aretha Mae said, primly. "Those was different times."

Primo continued to laugh and grabbed her ass. "They sure was."

She slapped his hand away and turned to Nick, busy wolfing down the greasy but delicious meal. "What your old man tell you 'bout me?" she demanded. "He tell you we was married? He tell you he ran out on me when I got pregnant? He tell you 'bout your half-sister he ain't never seen – let alone supported?"

Nick stopped eating. Sister? What kind of crap was coming his way now?

"I didn't know . . ." Primo whined. "You threw me out. I didn't know you was pregnant."

"Liar!" she snapped. "The baby in my belly was *why* you ran." She glared at him balefully. "An' then whaddaya do? Fix another woman so youse trapped anyhow. Dumb chickenshit!"

Primo wrapped his arms around her from behind, caressing her bony body. "C'mon, hon, I'm back," he crooned. "You always *knew* I'd be back, didn't'ja?"

Aretha Mae made a cross sound in the back of her throat. Not that cross. In fact it was becoming quite obvious she didn't mind having Primo's lumbering arms around her one little bit.

Nick thought of his hard-working mother lying in her grave and the greasy food turned in his stomach. He hated his father. He hated the whole stinking set-up.

Abruptly he stood up. "What sister?"

"She be away right now," Aretha Mae said, quickly. "She be visiting relatives in Kansas City."

"I got me a daughter," Primo marvelled. "I always wanted a girl."

"You got one all right," Aretha Mae said. "Oh, yessir me, you *really* got one."

Several days later they moved in after spending a few nights in Bosewell's only motel. Since there wasn't room for all of them in one trailer, Primo made a deal with the couple next door to take over their rat-infested storage dump – a place with no wheels and cardboard covering the window spaces. "It'll do for the kids t'sleep in," he convinced Aretha Mae. "Should clean up nice."

Nick spent three days hauling out junk, dodging rats, cockroaches and spiders while Harlan and his younger brother, Luke, helped out. They were jumpy little kids, petrified of their mother who ruled them with an acid tongue.

The two boys attended school every day. They walked the several miles, leaving the trailer park at six in the morning. Aretha Mae left shortly after that to go to her job as a maid to a rich family in Bosewell. This gave Primo plenty of time to himself, and although he promised Aretha Mae he'd start looking for a job he had no intention of doing so. The moment she left he settled in front of her small black-and-white portable television – a six-pack nearby. Nothing had changed for Primo. He knew his priorities and he stuck to them.

Nick hung around, he had nowhere to go.

After a couple of days Primo said, "Gotta get you back in school."

"I'd sooner get a job," he said, feeling restless and trapped. "Maybe –"

"I promised your ma," Primo interrupted, staring at the television. "Thought I told y'that."

"So what?"

Whack! Right across the mouth. It caught him by surprise cutting the side of his lip. He tasted blood and was filled with fury. There was no Mary to protect him now. School was in his future and there was nothing he could do about it, at least for now. As soon as he could he'd find a job, save his money and get out.

Nick Angelo planned to run, and nobody was going to stop him.

Chapter 6

"How exciting!" screamed Meg.

"Darling, I couldn't be more pleased for you," said her mother.

"This is great news," announced her father, like she'd just concluded a complicated insurance deal.

Idiot! She should have kept her mouth shut. All she'd done was tell them Stock had mentioned they should get engaged, and the next thing it was the town gossip. Now she was more trapped than ever in a relationship that totally confused her.

She was sixteen. She was too young. Oh sure, her mother had gotten married at seventeen – but that was a love match between two people who were crazy about each other, they'd told her the story enough times.

Her situation was different – she hardly even *knew* Stock – and what she *did* know she didn't much like.

"I'm not getting engaged," she informed her parents, panic-stricken at the thought.

Jane Roberts smiled and patted her daughter like she was an excitable puppy that needed calming. "Nerves, darling," she said. "Marriage is a big step. You'll have a long engagement, get to know each other. Stock's a nice boy from a fine family. Your father and I are very happy."

Oh, good, *they* were happy. What about her? Wasn't *she* the one supposed to be grinning uncontrollably and walking ten feet above the ground?

Love. From everything she'd seen and read it was a magical feeling and all *she* felt was sick.

In second grade she'd had a crush on Sammy Pilsner. She'd been eight years old and ecstatic. He'd made her shiver and shake whenever she saw him.

At twelve she'd fallen in love with one of her cousins –

Brad – a bony looking boy three years older than her. He and his family only visited at Christmas so she'd soon grown out of that.

At thirteen she'd had her first date. Disaster.

At fourteen her first kiss. Even worse.

And at fifteen she went steady for a satisfying six months with Sammy Pilsner.

Sammy didn't make her shiver and shake as much as he had when she was eight, but he was a good kisser and they got into many long lustful nights of heavy petting, although she never let him go all the way – she was too frightened of getting pregnant – even though he drove over fifty miles to a neighbouring town to buy rubbers, and tried to convince her they should do it.

Eventually Sammy's father got promoted at his job, and they moved to Chicago. She was a little bit heartbroken. She and Sammy corresponded for a few months, then his letters tapered off, and she realized she was free to see whoever she wanted. She dated several different boys. They all wanted one thing. If she hadn't given it to Sammy, why would she surrender it to a casual date?

One thing about Stock, he hadn't jumped her. Yet.

"I don't want to get engaged," she confided to Meg.

"Everyone's *soooo* jealous!" Meg squealed. "Has he given you a ring? When are you going to *do* it? You'll *have* to do it now you're engaged."

"But I'm not," Lauren protested.

Meg squinted at her. "Not what? Not engaged? Or not going to do it?"

"Not engaged, asshole."

"Nice talk from a virgin!"

"Asshole," Lauren repeated.

If her father ever heard her say that he'd kill her. Neither of her parents swore, at least not in front of her, although she'd once heard her father loudly groaning, "Christ! Christ!" when she was eleven and listening outside their bedroom door.

At least she knew what men said when they had sex. Although Sammy didn't. In the throes of passion, when she was doing something to him nice girls weren't supposed to do, Sammy Pilsner used to yell out, "Cowboys and Indians! This is an attack! Go for it! Go for it!"

Thinking of Sammy made her grin. His was the first and only penis she'd ever seen – she didn't count the time she'd walked in on her father getting out of the shower. He'd gone red in the face and screamed at her to leave the room immediately. She was ten at the time. Shortly after, her mother had taken her to one side and told her to please knock when entering their bathroom.

Knock knock.

Who's there?

Daddy's penis.

I promise I won't look.

Sammy Pilsner was very proud of his penis, he wanted her to look all the time. In fact he wanted her to do a lot more than look.

She'd obliged, because at the time she thought she loved him, and at least you couldn't get pregnant that way.

She knew all about oral sex having read about it in *Playboy*. Her father kept copies of the magazine locked in a storage closet in the basement. She'd discovered his stash one day and over the course of the next few weeks had read them all. Each magazine was full of naked women, sexist cartoons and articles about all kinds of sexual activities. She didn't enjoy looking at it, but it certainly taught her a lot. Sammy Pilsner couldn't believe his luck!

But that was the past – now she had Stock to deal with.

A few days later he sidled up to her in lunch break and informed her that his parents had decided to throw a big engagement party for them.

She wanted to say, "But I never said we'd get engaged." Instead she found herself nodding and listlessly agreeing.

Maybe that's what Stock liked about her – her total lack of enthusiasm. As the football hero and son of the town's richest man, he'd had girls fawning all over him since sixth grade. Perhaps he found her cool attitude a refreshing change.

"Saturday night," he said, sliding his arm around her shoulders. "My mother's talking to yours."

Oh, great! She should put a stop to this now. Somehow it just seemed easier to go along with it. Like that girl in *The Graduate* she could take it all the way to church – and then some handsome hero would rush in to save her and she'd run off with him leaving Stock with his mouth open – probably patting his crotch to make sure she hadn't taken it with her!

One question. Who would the rescuing hero be? Sammy Pilsner? She didn't think so. Sammy was probably getting his penis licked by a cute little Chicago girl with long legs and a big mouth.

Idly she wondered if her mother ever did *that* to her father. The very thought made her shudder. No way. He probably didn't even let her *look* at it.

"I've got a big surprise for you," Stock said, surreptitiously checking out her bra strap through her sweater.

"What?" she asked, impatiently.

"Never you mind, you'll see."

Asshole.

On the way home from school she stopped by her father's office. Once more he'd closed up early. She rattled the handle just to make sure. Nobody home.

Downstairs she popped into the Blakely Brothers hardware store. The Blakely brothers were identical twins, both fat and fifty with jovial smiles and drooping bushy eyebrows. She had no idea how to tell them apart.

"Hi'ya, Mr Blakely," she said, cheerily. "How's your wife?"

He beamed. "If I had one she'd be fine."

Foiled again! One was married. One single. The rumour around town was that the single one was a homosexual.

She grinned. "Just testing. I knew it was you!"

"No, you didn't." He winked. "I hear you're engaged. That's very nice, Lauren."

Her father the blabbermouth. This was obviously no secret.

"Have you seen my dad? He seems to have left early again."

"Didn't notice him go."

She had a ton of homework. Perhaps it was just as well her father wasn't around, they would have started talking, she'd get home late, and then she'd have to work all through dinner.

She'd never told her father she knew about his secret stash of *Playboys*. She'd never told her mother either.

"Your mom ordered lightbulbs," Mr Blakely said. "Since your dad has left . . ." he trailed off.

"I'll take them," she volunteered.

He handed her a large brown supermarket bag piled high. When her mother ordered she did it in bulk imagining it saved her money.

The package wasn't heavy – merely cumbersome. Lauren slung her school bag over her shoulder and grasped the bag with both hands. "Bye, Mr Blakely."

"Goodbye, Lauren. You're marrying into a fine family. One of the best."

I'm not marrying into anything, Mr Blakely. I am merely getting engaged. Temporarily. Because I can't stand the fuss of wriggling out of it. Because I'm always trying to please people. Because I hate to hurt anyone's feelings.

Because I'm an idiot!

Crash! Some jerk ran right into her at the swing door, and her package fell to the ground, followed by the sound of breaking glass.

"Shit!" the jerk said. No "Sorry." No "Excuse me." Just a short, terse "Shit!"

She waited.

"You should look where you're goin'," he said, rudely.

She was outraged. "*I* should?"

"Yeah. *You* walked into *me*."

"I did no such thing."

"Sure you did."

"No. I didn't."

They stared at each other, two furious strangers.

He was skinny and not very tall, with jet black curly hair, a pale complexion, a slight indentation in the centre of his chin and intense green eyes. He wore a grubby white T-shirt under a battered denim jacket, indescribably filthy torn jeans and battered sneakers.

Against her better judgment she felt a shiver of excitement. "Aren't you going to help me pick everything up?" she asked, wondering who he was.

Nick returned her stare. Not bad. A bit square looking. Hardly his usual type. But he was horny, God, he was horny!

"Okay," he mumbled, bending to help her.

"What about the broken bulbs?" she asked, finding two smashed ones.

"Get the store to replace 'em, you're on their property," he said, trying to decide how long it would take to screw her. Small-town girl. Possibly a virgin. Definitely more than one date.

He leaned closer catching a whiff of her scent. She smelt like lemon soap, no cheap dime store perfume. And her hair – long and shiny – was some sort of chestnut colour. He checked out her body. Slim but definitely acceptable.

"I can't do that," she said, primly. "You'll have to pay for them."

He laughed. Not a very nice laugh. A sarcastic *who do you think you're talking to* laugh.

37

"Sweetheart, I got enough to buy one pack of smokes an' that's *it*."

"Am *I* supposed to pay for them?" she countered.

"No," he nodded over to the counter where Mr Blakely was busy with another customer. "I told you – go talk to old fatso. He'll give you back your money."

"Don't call Mr Blakely that," she whispered, furiously.

"He can't hear me."

"Maybe he can."

"What's he got – X-ray ears?"

Just as she was about to reply her father appeared, hurrying down the stairs that led from his office.

"Daddy!" she exclaimed, forgetting about the green-eyed stranger for a moment.

As soon as Nick heard the word "daddy" he was out of there. He'd learned at an early age to stay as far away from fathers as possible.

"Where have you been?" Lauren asked, grabbing her father's arm.

"Upstairs, working."

"But I went upstairs. The shade was down, the door locked."

"Nonsense. What's all this?" he indicated the mess on the floor.

Flustered, she looked around. The boy who'd so rudely crashed into her was gone. "Oh, I dropped Mom's lightbulbs."

Phil chuckled. "What's the woman doing – stocking up for the next three years?"

Lauren giggled, they were conspirators in her mother's excesses. "You know Mom," she said.

"Indeed I do," he replied. "By the way, Lauren, I haven't had a private moment to tell you how happy I am about your engagement. Stock is an upstanding boy with traditional values, his family is first class." A pause. "Your mother and I are very proud of you."

Shit! If a stranger could say it she could certainly think it.

I guess I'm engaged, she thought gloomily. *No way out. For now*.

Chapter 7

Aretha Mae arranged to get him into Bosewell High mid-term. "Cyndra goes there," she informed him.

"Who's Cyndra?"

"She be your sister, boy, an' don' go forgettin' it. Good-lookin' girl, that's her problem. An' I don' wan' it bein' yours, seein' as you all be sleepin' in together."

Wasn't it bad enough he had to squeeze in with Harlan and Luke?

He cadged a couple of bucks off his father and made his way into town. They'd stayed in some one-gas-station towns in their time, but Bosewell scored the prize. He explored Main Street, wandering into the hardware store where he bumped – literally – into a girl he considered making out with for a moment, but then her father appeared and he was out of there fast. She wasn't his type anyway, too clean-cut.

The waitress in the drugstore was more like it. Mid-twenties, big knockers and a slight squint.

He slid up to the counter and ordered coffee.

"Black?" she asked, hardly taking any notice of him.

He winked to get her attention. "With cream, sweetheart. Lots of it."

"You new in town?"

"How'd'ja guess?"

"'Cause if you wasn't you wouldn't be tryin' to hit on me. You'd know Dave was my husband." She jerked her thumb at the short-order cook, a burly man about ten years older than her with muscles to spare.

Nick refused to give up. "He keep you happy?"

She raised a sarcastic eyebrow. "Does Mommy know you're out?"

39

They both burst out laughing at the same time.

"Louise," she said. "Welcome to Bosewell."

"Dave's a lucky guy."

"And you're a fresh kid. What you doin' here anyway? Passin' through on your way to reform school?"

"My old man moved us here."

She poured him a cup of coffee, adding a generous amount of cream. "An' what does *he* do?"

"Fucks up a lot."

Louise sighed, "Don't we all, dear. Don't we all."

"I gotta go to school," he said, gulping his coffee. "But I wanna work nights an' weekends, score some bucks. Got any ideas?"

"What do you think I am? An employment agency?" she said, smoothing down her gingham apron.

"Just askin'."

She softened. "Maybe Dave'll know of somethin'."

Her attention was taken by a group of High school kids who came crowding in making a lot of noise. She moved over to take their orders.

Nick checked them out. He was used to joining new schools halfway through the semester, it was always the same deal. The other kids regarded him with suspicion – usually there was some jerk who tried to start a fight, while most of the girls pretended they didn't notice him – although they did.

Every time he had to prove himself, every fuckin' time. It meant pounding the shit out of the school bully and screwing the prettiest girl. Somehow he always managed to do both.

He had one golden rule. Don't play fair. It worked good.

One of these days he'd be out of school once and for all, the routine was getting him down. Exactly how many times did he have to prove himself?

The group was asking Louise about him and staring over. A couple of the girls nudged each other. A big guy with a blond crew cut made a smart remark and they all laughed.

Instinctively he knew that this was the guy he'd have to deal with.

Tough shit, big guy. I'll give you a shot in the balls that'll take you all the way to Miami and back.

Louise returned and filled his cup.

He nodded towards Mister Crew Cut.

"Don' mess with him, honey," Louise warned. "His daddy owns most of this town."

"Yeah?"

"You'd better believe it." She brushed a strand of lank brown hair out of her squinty eyes. "Lemme go talk to Dave, his brother George runs the gas station. You know anythin' 'bout cars?"

"If it stops I can fix it. That good enough?"

"We'll see, hon, we'll see."

Back at the trailer it was the same old scene. Primo sat glued to the television, burping, swigging beer and picking at a bag of pretzels.

Aretha Mae stood in front of the kerosene stove, her shoulders slumped as she heated up two-day-old meatloaf – a gift from her employer, who allowed her the choice of throwing old food away or taking it home.

Harlan and Luke played outside, kicking around old tin cans and jumping in and out of the skeleton of what was once a car.

Nick strolled outside and joined them. "One of these days I'm gonna get me a Cadillac," he confided. "A goddamn red Cadillac with chrome bumpers an' leather seats."

"Can we ride in it?" Harlan asked, believing every word.

"Sure. Every day if you like."

The next morning he rode the bus to school with Aretha Mae. She told him where to get off and handed him a dollar.

"What's this for?" he asked, not wanting her charity.

"In case y'need it," she replied stoically, staring straight ahead.

He wondered what the going rate was for maids in Bosewell? Or maybe her employer piled her up with old food and clothes and considered that payment enough.

Bosewell High was a pale grey concrete building surrounded by green lawns on one side and an enormous parking lot on the other.

Clusters of students headed towards the imposing front entrance, most of them coming from the parking lot.

Nick felt the usual hollow feeling in the pit of his stomach. He tried to ignore it. Stay cool. No nerves.

Don't let the fuckers get you down.

Without having to ask he found registration and made himself official. The school secretary ran a disapproving eye over his grubby uniform of jeans, T-shirt and jacket.

"While we have no dress code here at Bosewell High, we do expect our students to look clean and well-groomed," she said.

"That means washed and pressed clothes at all times. And no torn jeans."

"Yes, ma'am." Hopefully he'd never have to see her again.

"Classroom number three, Mr Angelo. Your teacher will tell you what books you need."

"Thank you, ma'am."

Old cow. He could charm her if he wanted to.

Who wanted to?

Chapter 8

"Ohh . . . feast your eyes on *him*!" Meg nudged Lauren excitedly. "Now he's what I call *gorgeous*!"

Lauren glanced up from her desk, her mind elsewhere. "Who?" she asked, vaguely.

"*Him*. Standing by the door. He must be the new student. Dawn spotted him yesterday at the drugstore and she's in *love*."

"Dawn's in love every day."

"I know. But this one is – oh – I dunno – so sort of moody looking." Meg jumped up. "I'm going over to welcome him."

Lauren looked over at the door. And then she looked again. Meg was talking about the boy she'd run into at Blakely's hardware store. The one with the green eyes and smart mouth.

"Who is he?" she asked.

Too late. Meg was halfway across the classroom, while Dawn was fast approaching from the other direction.

Lauren sat tight. Let them make fools of themselves if they wanted to. He wasn't *that* great. Just different . . .

Meg was speaking to him now, eyes sparkling, cheeks flushed. Lauren watched her go for it. They were best friends, had been since elementary school, but sometimes Meg was too impulsive. She should have waited, let him come after her. Well-known fact. Boys liked to chase after girls, not the other way around.

Meg was pretty, with fluffy yellow hair and blue eyes. She was ten pounds overweight and on a permanent diet. Her two front teeth were crooked which sometimes gave her a rabbity look.

Dawn Kovak on the other hand was a tramp. She had dyed black hair, a prominent bosom, and wore too much make-up. She didn't look sixteen, she looked thirty.

Lauren observed them both in action, her best friend and the school dump – as Dawn was nicknamed.

He'd probably go for Dawn with her black hair and big bosom – they always did. Meg had virgin written all over her.

Surprisingly he chose Meg, allowing her to lead him to the only vacant desk, listening as she chattered on, giving her all his attention.

Lauren felt the smallest shiver of jealousy. Which was ridiculous really, because she certainly wanted nothing to do with him. She was engaged to Stock Browning. She was *very*, *very* busy thank you very much.

Hmm . . . maybe she should go over and greet him?

No need. Meg seemed to be doing a perfectly wonderful job of making him feel more than welcome.

She stopped watching and opened up her English Lit. book. Concentrating was not easy. She couldn't help glancing up to see what Meg was doing. Meg was heading back to her desk with a triumphant expression.

Just as she got back, their teacher entered the classroom.

"He's *fantastic*!" Meg whispered, sitting down, a silly smile lighting up her face. "*And* he's asked me out."

"He has?"

"Yep. Tonight."

"Where?"

"Who knows? I'm meeting him in front of the drugstore at eight."

"Your parents'll never let you out on a school night."

"I'll say I'm over at your place studying."

"Meg, you don't know anything about him, how can you go out with him?"

"Holy cow, Lauren, you sound like my mother."

"I do not!"

"Yes you do."

"Girls!" The high-pitched tones of Miss Potter – their English Lit. teacher – interrupted them. "Will you be joining us today?" she continued, sarcastically. "Or shall we set up a table for you two outside so that you may carry on your conversation uninterrupted?"

"Sorry, Miss Potter," they chorused, sounding like a couple of good little students.

Lauren couldn't resist one more quick glance over at the new boy. He caught her look and returned it.

Meg picked up her book trying to choke down a giggle. "I'm so excited!" she whispered. "He's really gorgeous!"

"You're crazy," Lauren muttered, and for one brief moment wished that *she* was the crazy one.

The chubby little blonde came on to him like gangbusters. He chose her over the dark one because he had a strong suspicion the dark one had nailed every guy in school, and while he was interested in getting laid, he was not interested in catching a dose of the clap – or even worse – crabs.

It was easy. As usual. Had something to do with his green eyes. He could fix them on a girl – just for a moment – and they had this sort of crazy, hypnotic effect.

Jeez! He was allowed to have *something* wasn't he? And God had given him the eyes.

He caught the girl he'd bumped into yesterday watching him from across the room. She didn't mean to, but he could see she couldn't help herself. Maybe after he was finished with the blonde he'd go for her, give her a cheap thrill. Maybe . . .

Bosewell High was going to be easy compared to some of the inner city dumps he'd been forced to attend. This school was strictly small-town, he could take his pick.

So far he hadn't spotted the beefy guy with the crew cut. The schlump was probably in a different grade, and that was good. If he played it smart perhaps he could avoid him altogether.

Deep down he knew this wasn't possible. Deep down he knew there was always one dumb asshole who'd go for his throat.

When school got out for the day he planned to return to the drugstore, find out if Louise had come up with a job for him, and then, if he was lucky, cadge a meal and hang around until it was time to meet Blondie.

The teacher noticed him and made him stand up and introduce himself to the class. *Jeez! What a drag!* He hated the way they all looked him over. Why didn't they ask for his rank and serial number while they were at it?

At lunch break he fell in behind the crowd and drifted down to the school cafeteria where he bought a cheese sandwich and a Coke, found a corner table and sat down.

Before long, Crew Cut made his entrance – trailed by an admiring group busy hanging on to his every word.

Nick munched his sandwich and surveyed the scene. Blondie waved at him from across the room. She was probably dying to

45

talk to him again, but had decided to play it cool. Ha! He could even figure out how they thought.

And then the girl from the hardware store made her entrance, pausing in the doorway.

He knew she noticed him and half-hoped she'd come over, but she didn't.

And what was this? Crew Cut was on his feet, racing across the room, putting his arm around her and leading her over to a table. Shit! She was his girlfriend!

Immediately Nick wondered if she was gettable.

Yeah. Why not? He was always up for a challenge.

"The party's all set," Stock said.

"I know," Lauren replied. "My mother and your mother are like this." She held up two fingers to show exactly what they were like.

Stock smirked. "My mother likes bossing your mother around."

Lauren took offence. "What do you mean?"

He shrugged. "My mother likes bossing everyone, including me."

Just for a second Lauren felt sorry for him. It must be awful having a mother like Daphne, a huge, commanding woman with scarlet lips telling everyone what to do.

"Meg's got a date tonight," she found herself saying, anything to make conversation.

"Really?" He couldn't care less.

"With that new guy," she added.

"What new guy?"

"You know, the one that started school today."

"Yeah?" His lack of interest was quite apparent.

She gave up, there was only so much she could do.

Meg arrived at her house an hour before her date, barely able to conceal her excitement. She rushed up to Lauren's room making a mad dash for the mirror. "How do I look?" she demanded, fluffing out her newly-washed hair.

"Horrible," Lauren teased.

"*Whaaat?*"

"Only kidding."

"Don't do that," Meg wailed. "This is the first decent date I've had in months."

Lauren sat cross-legged on her bed. "How do you know he's decent?"

Meg was exasperated. "What's the *matter* with you?"

"What's the matter with *me*?" she retorted, sharply. "Take another look in the mirror. You're all excited over a guy you don't even know. He could be a sex maniac, a rapist, anything . . ."

"You're really weird," Meg said, shaking her head. "I mean, *really*."

"Thanks. All compliments gratefully accepted."

"Anybody would think *you* liked him."

She flushed, and jumped off the bed. "Don't be ridiculous."

"Forget it. *I* saw him first and he's mine. Anyway, you're engaged, or had you conveniently forgotten?"

Lauren pulled a face. "Would that I could."

"Nice talk," Meg said, adjusting the waistband of her new black skirt to make it shorter. "How do my legs look?"

"Like legs. What'll I tell your mother if she calls?"

"Tell her I'm in the bathroom. Anyway, she's not likely to."

"It could happen."

"You're a big help."

"Call me as soon as you get home. I want a full report."

Meg gave a jaunty wink. "You bet!"

"Hi." Meg felt suddenly shy as she approached Nick. He was leaning against the wall outside the drugstore, smoking a cigarette.

When he saw her coming he flicked the butt towards the kerb with an elaborate flourish. "Hi," he replied, taking her arm as if they'd been dating for months. "You look nice."

"Thanks," she giggled, nervously.

"I mean it," he replied "very nice." He'd scored a free hamburger off Louise, and a promise from Dave he could work at his brother's gas station Saturday nights. Things were looking up. Now all he had to do was get laid and perhaps he could get a good night's sleep, although it wasn't easy with Harlan and Luke coughing and farting the night away.

"Where are we going?" Meg asked, as he guided her along Main Street.

"Thought we'd catch a movie."

She'd already seen *The Poseidon Adventure* playing at The Bosewell, but so what? "Super," she said, eager to please.

Super. Hmm . . . Maybe he should have picked the sure thing with the black hair; this one was a baby.

When they reached the theatre he steered her away from the box office. "Buy your ticket, go inside, an' then let me in through the fire-escape door. Like I'm busted, y'know?" He gave her arm an encouraging squeeze. "Okay?"

Buy her own ticket? Usually on a date the boy paid. Lauren would *love* this. Still . . . it made life exciting. "Okay," she agreed.

He gave her a little shove. "It's easy, you'll see."

She purchased her ticket and entered the almost empty theatre. Then, when she was sure she wasn't being observed, she raced down the side aisle to the fire exit, opened the heavy door and let Nick in.

"Yeah!" he said, guiding her to the back row, which was conveniently empty.

The movie had already started. Putting his arm around her he settled back to watch. After a few minutes he moved closer. "I knew you and me would get along soon as I saw you," he said in a low voice. "It was like . . . y'know . . . uh . . . special."

"I know," she whispered back, thrilled they were thinking along the same lines.

"Sometimes these things happen," he said, massaging her back through her sweater.

"Right," she agreed, beginning to feel rather warm.

"Like it's meant t'be or somethin'," he added, his hand creeping around to the front, dangerously close to her left breast.

She opened her mouth to agree again and without warning his lips were on her, kissing insistently, his tongue probing.

She gasped for breath. This was all happening so fast. The last boy she'd dated had waited three whole weeks before trying anything. Now Nick's hand was definitely on her breast and she knew she should push him away, but at least she could enjoy it for a minute, couldn't she?

Nick circled her nipple through her sweater, his thumb and forefinger moving in circles.

She let out an involuntary groan as he slowly began to push her sweater up, fumbling in the dark for her bra clip.

"Don't," she managed, realizing she'd better put a stop to this now.

He didn't listen. He was too busy unhooking her bra.

Cupping her left breast he bent his head, licking her nipple with practised ease.

She tried to push his head away. "No!" she whispered, urgently.

"Yes!" he whispered back.

48

"Someone will see."

"It's empty in here."

"I don't want you to do this."

"Yes you do."

And it was true. She did. For a moment she relaxed, giving herself up to this glorious feeling sweeping over her. Was it so bad to feel so good?

He began to suck her nipple, at the same time reaching for her hand and jamming it on his penis – which somehow or other he'd managed to release.

Oh God! She'd never touched one before. Oh, dear! There was no way she should be doing this. Nice girls didn't do this – unless, of course, they wanted to be labelled easy or a tramp – like Dawn Kovak.

With a sudden burst of resolve she attempted to pull her hand away.

He was having none of it. "Hold it," he commanded. "It ain't gonna bite!"

"I can't," she said, desperately.

"Yes, you can." He groaned, helping her hand move up and down – faster . . . faster . . .

And then it happened. He spurted all over her. Hot, sticky, wet.

"Jeez!" he groaned again. "Ohhh . . . jeez!"

"My skirt!" Meg wailed, horrified. "You've done it all over my new skirt!"

He leaned his head back, closed his eyes and took a deep, satisfied breath.

Welcome to Bosewell. It had been one helluva day.

Chapter 9

Nick made the long trudge home thinking about Blondie. Nice tits. Too shy. Not for him. Jerk-off action was for boys Harlan's age.

Who was he kidding? Once in a while a jerk-off was better than nothing, and he knew if he'd tried to screw her she'd have bolted. As it was she was hysterical about her stupid skirt. What was it with girls and clothes?

Best not to see *that* one again, he thought. Better off to invest in a packet of rubbers and give the dark haired one a chance.

Girls, they were all the same. Easy. And he never cared if he saw any of them again. Once the sex was over he felt an emptiness, a void.

When he got back to the trailer the two boys were sitting on their pile of blankets flicking through well thumbed comic books.

"What's up?" he asked cheerfully, taking off his jacket.

"What's up with you?" Harlan retorted.

"Nothin' much." He nodded over at Luke. "How come he never speaks?"

"He jest don't," Harlan replied, suddenly sullen.

"Somethin' happen to him?" Nick asked, stripping off the rest of his clothes.

"Not your business."

"I'm only askin' 'cause I thought I might help."

"Not your business," Harlan repeated, fiercely.

Nick shrugged and settled himself down on his lumpy mattress, trying to find a comfortable spot. "No farting tonight," he said sternly, staring menacingly at the two boys.

Harlan stood up, pulled down his shorts, bent his rear end in Nick's direction and let one rip.

"Aw, god*damnit!*" Nick wrinkled his nose in disgust. "If I wasn't so beat I'd slap your skinny butt halfway across this trailer park."

Harlan burped. Luke laughed. At least he could do that.

Nick closed his eyes, and for some unknown reason began thinking about the other girl, old Crew Cut's girlfriend. No, he told himself sternly, mustn't look for trouble. The truth is they're all the same in the dark, and he'd never met a girl who could give him anything more than a hard-on.

In the morning he followed the two boys into the main trailer hoping to cadge breakfast. Aretha Mae handed out stale slices of bread smeared with congealed bacon fat. He grabbed one.

Primo snored loudly, sprawled across the rumpled bed.

Aretha Mae looked tired, her eyes sunken, her mouth pinched into a thin line. She clapped her hands together. "Out," she told the two younger boys. "Get movin' or you be late." She turned to Nick. "How 'bout I pay y'bus fare the rest a the week. After that you be on your own."

"Don't worry, I got a part-time job," he said quickly. "I'm workin' down at the gas station Saturday nights."

She was impressed that he didn't take after his idle father. "That's good," she said, wiping her hands on an old cloth. "That's real good."

He nodded. "Yeah."

Meg was late for class. She slipped into her seat and shuffled a few books around, attempting to look industrious.

"You didn't call," Lauren hissed. "I don't appreciate that kind of behaviour when I'm supposed to be your alibi."

"I had more important things to worry about," Meg hissed back.

"Like what?"

"Like a ruined skirt."

Mr Lucas coughed meaningfully and glared across the room at them.

Lauren returned her attention to her books. She'd had a miserable morning listening to her parents carry on about her engagement party. They were turning into a couple of social-climbing phonies right before her eyes – discussing what to wear, who would be there, how they should act.

"Today I'm going shopping for a new outfit," Jane had declared, enthusiastically. "And Lauren, dear – we'll buy you a pretty new dress too."

Lauren hated the word "pretty": it conjured up visions of pale pink ruffles. "I don't need a new dress," she'd said.

"What nonsense! We'll go shopping after school today. Bring Meg."

She'd been unable to wriggle out of it. This engagement thing was getting out of hand.

As soon as Mr Lucas signalled freedom she grabbed Meg. "Well?" she asked, breathlessly.

Meg shook her curls. "You were right. He's a sex maniac."

"He *is*?"

"Oh, yes."

"*Really*?"

"I'm not lying."

"What happened?"

"He's crazy about me."

"I'm sure. But what did you *do*?"

Meg sighed, ready to tell her story. Before she could, Nick put in his first appearance of the day, strolling by on his way to Math. Clinging on to his arm as if she owned him was Dawn Kovak.

He winked at Meg, greeting her with a cavalier, "Hey – How're ya doin'?"

"Fine," she managed, her cheeks burning with rage and humiliation.

"They're tenting the garden," Stock said, flexing his muscles.

"Isn't it too cold?" Lauren asked.

He smirked. "They've got those heater things."

"*Why* are they tenting the garden? Your house is so large, they could have everyone inside."

He proceeded to do a series of knee bends. "Beats me."

"Stock . . ." she began, tentatively.

"Yes?"

"Maybe we don't need a big party."

He continued doing knee bends. "Sure we do. Once we get rid of the old farts it'll be a blast."

"But everyone's making such a fuss. I'm not certain it's what I want. I –"

"Listen, hon," he interrupted, standing up straight. "We're talkin' a good time here. Relax, you'll love it."

"I will?" she said, unsurely.

"Course you will."

"Okay," she said, still not convinced, watching her mother pull into the driveway in the family station wagon. "I have to go. We're going shopping."

"Buy something sexy," he leered, unexpectedly pinching her on the ass.

She swatted his hand away. "Don't *do* that!"

He chuckled. "Why not? We're engaged. I'll soon be doin' a lot more than pinchin' your butt!"

Oh, no you won't, she thought, angrily. *I'm putting a stop to this as soon as I summon up the courage to tell my parents.*

"Okay, babe, see ya. I got football practice anyway." He swiped a kiss on her cheek and loped off.

"Lucky thing!" sighed Suzi Harden, coming up behind her.

Lucky thing indeed! Lauren didn't feel lucky. She felt like a cornered fieldmouse waiting for the trap to snap shut.

Sex with Stock was unthinkable. His big sweaty hands all over her. Crushed beneath his enormous bulk. No way!

"Where's Meg?" Suzi asked. "You two are usually always together."

"She didn't feel well – went home early."

And who could blame her? She was broken up over Nick's appearance with Dawn Kovak. One moment he was all over her, and the next he was consorting with "Anything Goes Kovak". Boys! Who could understand them? Who wanted to?

Her mother swerved the station wagon over to the kerb and she got in.

"Where is Meg?" Jane asked, adjusting her rear-view mirror. "I thought she was coming with us."

Maybe she should have a little card printed:

Meg is not coming.

Meg is humiliated and heartbroken.

All humans of the male species are sex-crazed animals.

Lauren shrugged. "She didn't feel up to it."

Jane looked concerned. "Is she sick? I hope not. We don't want *you* catching anything."

"She's sick of boys."

Jane laughed. "You girls!"

Ha Ha! Lauren thought sourly, catching a glimpse of Nick

Angelo – she knew his name – sauntering out of school with Dawn Kovak clinging to his arm. Obviously Dawn was now a permanent fixture.

He was real moody looking, a regular bad boy. She'd warned Meg, told her not to get involved, she should have listened.

Nick Angelo. Hmm . . . Meg had said he was a great kisser . . .

So what?

One thing he'd learnt in life – if you're going to dump a girl, do it quickly. No excuses. No hanging around. One sharp cut and it's over.

Blondie was a mistake. Dawn was definitely more his speed.

"How come it took you so long to get here?" she'd asked, approaching him on the way into school.

"What's *that* supposed to mean?" he'd replied, checking her out.

She'd touched his cheek with a long red fingernail. "I've been waiting for a guy like you all my life."

Soul mates. She was even using his lines!

"So," he'd said, "here I am."

"So," she'd said, with a provocative wink, "I'm ready."

Dawn Kovak lived with her alcoholic mother on the wrong side of town. Not quite as bad as the trailer park, but getting there. She didn't have much going for her except her curvaceous figure and sultry looks, so she used them to full advantage. She might be the school screw, but at least her assets made her popular. During the day she filled him in about Bosewell. Small town. Small thinkers. No fun. No action. The nearest place where anything happened was fifty miles away – a town called Ripley – where there were bars and places to dance and a cool bikers' hang-out.

"You got a car?" was one of the first questions she asked.

"I can get hold of one," he'd replied, thinking of taking the van one night when Primo was out cold.

"You an' me – we'll make our own good times," she'd promised, seductively.

For now, Nick had thought, *while it suits me. Don't get too close, I'm only passing through.*

Chapter 10

When the Brownings did something they did it big. The garden was tented. A three-piece group played what was supposed to be dance music. The food was catered. And the tables set with fancy pink linen and fine silverware. After all, the Brownings were the richest family in town and once in a while they liked to show it.

Stock collected Lauren early and drove her straight to his house, proudly showing off the party preparations.

"When the old folks hit the sack we've got a disco all set up," he boasted. "And plenty of beer. I mean we're talking *plenty*."

He was telling her like she was a big beer drinker or something. "Great," she managed, tugging at the bodice of the pale yellow dress her mother had talked her into buying. She hated the dress: it made her look like a flower girl at somebody's wedding.

"Right now I have something *just* for you," he said, grabbing her hand and pulling her over to the corner of the garden.

Oh no! Was this the big moment? Was this the great attack?

"What?" she mumbled, praying he wasn't going to jump her – although it was highly unlikely in his parents' tented garden with sixty guests due any minute.

"This," he said, proudly pushing a small leather box into her reluctant hand.

She held it gingerly.

"Go on, open it," he said, encouraging her.

Easy for *him* to say. But when she opened it the net would tighten, for any fool knew it was an engagement ring.

"I always dreamt of going to New York," she blurted out, postponing the inevitable.

"We will," he assured her. "On our honeymoon if you like."

When was *that* going to be? Next week? Things were moving so fast she almost couldn't breathe.

"I figure we'll get married after I finish college," he said, as if reading her thoughts. "I know that sounds a long time – but when we're officially engaged it'll almost be like being married, won't it?"

Reprieve! Reprieve!

"Course, if you get pregnant we can do it earlier," he added.

Pregnant! Was he kidding? You had to have *sex* to get pregnant, and there was no way she was doing anything with him. *No way.*

With a feeling of relief she realized this was the answer to all her problems. No sex. No engagement. When she refused to put out he'd break the engagement. *He'd* break it off. *She'd* be the injured party, and her parents couldn't be mad at her. Whew!!! What an escape.

With renewed vigour she sprung the box open and stared at a heart-shaped sapphire surrounded by more than a dozen small baguettes. "Wow!" she exclaimed. "This is beautiful."

"I knew you'd like it," he said, smirking proudly. "My mother picked it out."

"How romantic," she said, dryly. As usual, her sarcasm was lost on him.

"Put it on," he urged. "See if it fits."

She did so – imagining the day she would give it back.

He took her hand, pressing it on his tuxedo-clad crotch. "Feel this," he said, with another proud smirk. "This is what you do to me."

She jerked her hand away. Their engagement was going to be shorter than anyone could possibly imagine.

Dawn Kovak was the girl of his wet dreams – ready, willing and always able. He knew her reputation – not that it came as any surprise because Joey Pearson had already filled him in. Joey was a good guy – funny, clever, a touch off-beat. They'd palled up instantly when it turned out they were both doing Saturday night shifts at the gas station.

"Look," he'd explained to Joey, "I won't be stayin' long. What do I care if she's screwed every guy in town? She's just the way I like 'em – experienced."

Joey had laughed. "Yeah, there's nothin' like a girl who knows what she's doin'."

Both of them had been recruited to park cars at the Brownings' party – anything to earn a few extra bucks.

A maroon Cadillac made its way up the circular driveway. Nick ran around to the driver's side and opened the door. A man got out. His wife was in the passenger seat. Meg emerged from the back and made a quick dash into the house.

"What happened with you an' her?" Joey asked. "Didn't you take her to the movies or somethin'?"

"Nothin' happened," Nick lied, easily. He wasn't about to tell tales. "My mistake. Picked the wrong girl. It was my first week in town, y'know how it is."

Yes. Joey knew how it was. His mother and he had arrived in Bosewell from Chicago a year ago. His father – a cop – had been killed in a bank hold-up, and his mother immediately decided they should move to the safety of a small town.

"When we first came here my ma said it was for my protection," Joey grimaced. "Like the minute I'm eighteen I'm outta here. It's back to Chicago for me. I'm gonna do stand-up."

Nick looked vague. "Stand-up?"

"Y'know, like tell jokes 'n stuff. Make people laugh."

"Sounds good t'me."

Joey searched through his pockets and produced a battered cigarette. He snapped it in two and handed Nick half. They shared a match.

"So . . ." Joey said, taking a deep drag. "I know what *I'm* doin' here. What brings *you* to this pisshole?"

Nick sucked on his half of the cigarette. "My old man," he said.

"What does *he* do?"

Nick laughed bitterly. "Fuck all."

"That's nice."

"Very nice. Like he was married to this woman . . . this black woman . . ." He paused, Joey didn't need to know this, nobody did. "Aw, shit. It's a bummer, it doesn't matter."

"Tell me about it," Joey urged.

Nick wasn't in the mood to reveal himself. "Some other time," he said, dropping the subject.

Joey shrugged. "I'm not goin' anywhere."

More cars arrived and they got busy.

"Y'know Stock Browning is the asshole of the world," Joey said, running back from parking a Buick. "The schmuck tried to beat me up once – I kicked him in the nuts an' got myself a knife."

Nick laughed. "I knew we'd get along."

"The funny thing is," Joey continued, "when I was goin' to school in Chicago I never got beat up once."

57

"Maybe 'cause your dad was a cop."

"Bullshit. There weren't any jerks like Stock Browning around."

"You really love the guy, doncha?"

"He's a prick. I'd sure like to know why Lauren's gettin' engaged to him. Dumb move."

"You ever take her out?"

"No way, man. She and Meg – it's virgin city."

"Maybe she's changed."

"Yeah," Joey said, disgustedly. "That can happen. Girls! Show 'em a wad of money an' it's legs in the air an' let's party!"

Another car entered the driveway and pulled up in front of the house.

"I'll toss ya for it," Nick said.

"What's the difference?" Joey replied. "We're splittin' all the tips anyway."

Nick nodded. "Right."

Meg was furious. "He's outside!" she complained to Lauren.

"Who?"

"Don't ask me who!" Meg snapped. "You *know* who. It's him. Nick. Isn't it enough that I have to see him at school? Now he's here, parking cars. I'm so humiliated. I arrived with my *parents*! How could you do this to me?"

"Calm down, Meg. I had no idea he'd be here."

"Oh, no, *sure*. You're too busy getting engaged to notice *any*thing or anybody. How do you think I *feel*?"

"Meg," Lauren said, patiently. "Your date with him was three weeks ago. Forget it."

"Easy for you to say. Try putting yourself in my place." Her voice rose hysterically. "He practically *raped* me!"

Lauren looked concerned. "You didn't tell me that. You said he got your bra off and ruined your skirt. You certainly didn't tell me he tried to rape you. If he did, you should report him to the police."

"It's too late."

"If that's what happened, it's never too late."

Meg's face crumpled. "I hate him!" she cried out.

"So do I," agreed Lauren, ever the supportive friend. Although truthfully she couldn't say that she hated him, because she didn't even know him.

Of course, she knew he had green eyes; and black curly hair; and a great chin; and a James Dean slouch.

58

She also knew he was working part-time at the gas station, and that he and Joey Pearson were friends, and that most nights he saw Dawn Kovak.

She certainly found him intriguing, although she couldn't tell Meg, had to keep a tightly buttoned lip on *that* little piece of info.

"Are you enjoying the party?" she asked, moving the conversation along.

Meg narrowed her blue eyes and reached for a glass of watered-down punch. "Will you have to call your first-born Stock Junior?" she asked, in a mean voice.

"Not if it's a girl." Lauren smiled sweetly and moved over to join her parents who seemed to be having a perfectly fine time sucking up to the entire Browning clan.

Dawn was the uninvited guest – at least her name wasn't on the official list.

"Suprise!" she greeted Nick, arriving just before midnight in a car full of leather-clad friends who looked like they'd strayed out of *West Side Story*. "Stock told me to get here late."

This was not the rich kids' group. These were the tougher, older kids who smoked pot, drank alcohol, and blasted Joplin and Hendrix day and night.

Nick hadn't exactly fallen in with them – but thanks to Dawn he knew most of them, and they'd accepted him as a cool guy.

Behind the car were six or seven motorcycles. Dawn had recruited more friends from Ripley.

"Hiya, Nicky," she licked his ear, suggestively sticking her tongue deep. "Now the party can *really* get goin'. Dump this gig an' let's go inside."

"Yeah, go on, man," Joey encouraged. "There's only a few more cars. I'll take care of 'em."

"I don't wanna stick you –" Nick began.

"Go. We'll split the tips tomorrow."

Why not? If Dawn was invited he was entitled to tag along. He was certainly as good as any of these other creeps.

They blasted in noisy and out for a good time.

Stock greeted them surrounded by several of his football buddies all well on the road to oblivion.

"Hi'ya, sexy," Dawn said, provocative in an off-the-shoulder sweater and short tight skirt. She nuzzled in for a deep French kiss. "Takin' *you* outta circulation is a crime!"

Stock guffawed, winked and burped. "Let's get the disco goin' – you take care of it, Dawn."

"Sure thing, handsome – anything you want. An' I *mean* anything."

He stuck his tongue out, flipping it obscenely from side to side. "I've had *that.*"

His friends roared. Dawn did too.

Nick headed for the bar. So Stock had screwed her. Big surprise.

He helped himself to a cold beer, swigging from the bottle and checking everything out. This was some set up, it must have cost big bucks – what with the tent, a full bar, dozens of tables and chairs – flowers and all that crap. There was even a dance floor, which Dawn was now dragging Stock on to as the disc jockey took over from the sedate three piece group, blasting everybody out of their seats with the Stones' raunchy rendition of "Satisfaction".

The last of the adults scurried towards the exit. Daphne and Benjamin Browning were long gone.

Nick helped himself to another beer.

"Oh, no!" Meg yelped. "He's here. What's he *doing* in here?"

Lauren was truly fed up with her friend; she'd done nothing but complain all night.

"I've got to go," Meg said, frantically.

Lauren was in no mood to stop her. "I'll see you tomorrow," she said, coolly.

"Are you staying?" Meg asked, surprised.

"It's my engagement party. Or had it slipped your mind?"

"I suppose *you* have to stay until the end. You don't mind if I go, do you?"

As a matter of fact she did mind, but there was no way she was begging Meg to stay. "No, that's okay."

"Thanks." Meg took off without a second thought.

Lauren sighed – so much for best friends. She wished she could say to Meg, "Stay. I need you." And she wished she could say to Stock, "Goodbye. I don't need you."

Her parents had enjoyed the evening. Phil Roberts had turned on the charm and talked up more prospective insurance to more clients than he could remember. Jane Roberts had declared herself belle of Bosewell, dancing with every old man in town.

Lauren had danced with Stock and all his buddies. She'd even had to dance with Benjamin Browning who'd held her too close and breathed whisky breath in her face. Now she was ready to call it quits, but Stock had other ideas. He was all set to let the good times begin.

He reeled off the dance floor fresh from Dawn, and grabbed Lauren. "C'mon, sugar, let's rock 'n roll," he said, leering drunkenly.

"I'm really tired," she said. "It's been a long night."

"Are you kidding?" he rolled his eyes. "The evening's just beginning."

"Do your parents know you've invited all these other people?" she asked, gesturing at the crowd.

"What do *you* think? I told them I was havin' a few more friends come by, they don't care. This is my party, I can do whatever I want."

"*Our* party," she corrected. "And *I* want to go home."

He shook his head, perplexed. "Sometimes you're a real pain. Have a glass of punch. Relax. Get with it."

"I had a glass of punch, thank you."

"So have another one. One of the guys spiked it. Now the party'll *really* swing." He attempted a kiss. She pulled away.

He laughed bitterly. "You're a helluva fiancée."

The Stones gave way to a raucous Rod Stewart. Lauren gave him a little shove towards the dance floor where all his cronies seemed to be having a great time. "Go dance with Dawn again. She loves it, I don't."

"If you're with me you'd better learn to love it," he slurred, beckoning Dawn.

What did he think this was, school? She'd learn to do exactly what she pleased and that was it.

Over by the door Nick caught the action. He didn't care about Dawn taking off – it didn't matter. Lauren was the girl that interested him, may as well admit it. And now was as good a time as any to do something about it.

Just as he was about to head towards her, a familiar voice said, "What in hell *you* doin' here, boy?"

It was Aretha Mae, a different looking Aretha Mae with her

frizzy red hair pinned back and a starched white maid's uniform covering her skinny body.

"I could ask you the same," he said, smartly.

She glared at him. "*I* work here," she said. "An' you better be gettin' your ass outta here." She balanced a tray of dirty glasses and marched back into the house.

Screw her. She wasn't his mother. He didn't have to listen to anything she said.

Lauren was still by herself. Seizing the opportunity he sauntered over, sitting down beside her. "How ya doin'?" he asked, casually.

She turned to look at him. They'd never been formally introduced, but what did that matter?

Oh, God! Meg would be furious if she talked to him.

"Uh, hi," she replied, trying to sound equally casual.

He nodded at Dawn and Stock on the dance floor. "They make quite a couple, huh?"

"Hmm," she said, non-committally.

"Isn't it supposed to be you up there with him?" he asked, helping himself to a cigarette from a box on the table.

He had a nerve. He knew perfectly well it was supposed to be her.

"How come *you're* not dancing with him?" he persisted. "Don't you like to dance?"

"Don't you?" she countered.

He gave her the benefit of his green-eyed stare. "Only if it's with somebody special."

She met his eyes for a moment, found them too dangerous and quickly broke the look. "I . . . I have to go," she said, getting up.

"Mr Football Hero's in no state to take you home," he said, also standing.

She wondered why her heart was beating so fast. "That's not your concern, is it?"

He kept on staring at her. "Maybe it could be."

"I beg your pardon?"

This girl wasn't reacting the way they usually reacted. A little warmth would be nice. "How come you're so uptight?" he asked, trying to throw her off balance.

"I'm not uptight," she answered defensively. "You're rude."

"Yeah?" he challenged. "What've I done?"

"Nothing – to me," she said, quickly.

62

"What's that mean?"

"You know."

"No, I don't. What?"

She wished she hadn't brought the subject up, but there was no stopping now. The words tumbled out. "The way you treated Meg. You took her out, jumped all over her, and then dropped her. How do you think she feels?"

Shit! That was the trouble with girls, they always confided in each other. "She told you about it, huh?"

"Meg's my best friend."

The truth, he decided, was the way to play it with this one. "And she's nice," he explained. "But not for me, so I . . . uh . . . didn't see her again. I thought I did her a favour."

Lauren faced up to him, fighting Meg's battle. "*That's* a favour?" she asked incredulously. "You don't lead someone on then dump them."

Time to change the subject. "Why are you getting engaged to this jerk anyway?"

Two bright red spots stung her cheeks. "You're the jerk. You don't even know him."

"C'*mon*, you know he's a jerk." He paused for a moment. "I suppose you're gonna tell me you're the happiest girl in the world."

"Just exactly who do you think you are?" she asked, angrily.

"Me? I'm just passing through, honey."

"And *don't* call me honey."

"Why?" he teased. "Does it turn you on?"

Their eyes met for a moment. He held the stare. Once more she broke it by walking away.

For some unknown reason her heart was still pounding as she hurried outside. Nick Angelo was dangerous and she knew it.

Chapter 11

Cyndra Angelo had been travelling on the bus for hours. She was tired and dirty. Her clothes were rumpled and uncomfortable. Her feet hurt and she was hungry. She peered out the window. It was raining. It was always raining.

She'd had to move seats three times. Every time the bus stopped and new passengers got on there was always some guy who chose to sit next to her. After a few minutes he moved too close, started to talk, and she was forced to shift seats again.

It wasn't as if she did anything to encourage them, they came on to her whether she wanted them to or not. Pigs!

Kansas City had been a nightmare. Staying with distant relatives of her mother's, she'd found the men in the family only too eager to put their hands all over her. It seemed that every male she met wanted to lure her into bed. What was it about her? What did she do to encourage them?

Nothing that she knew about.

She opened up her old tote bag, took out a compact with a broken mirror and studied her face. She wasn't white. She wasn't black. She was nothing.

It never occurred to her that she had the best of both worlds. That her skin was the most glorious olive – smooth and blemish-free. Her jet black hair was long and thick. Her eyes a deep rich brown. Her jawline strong and her cheekbones etched. She looked different from everybody else. The truth was that she was a very beautiful young girl indeed.

The bus stopped and two men got on. It didn't take long before one of them came sidling up the aisle and sat down beside her. "Hi'ya, sweetie," he drawled. "Where you headin'?"

"None of your business," she replied, turning her back to face the window.

"No need to be unfriendly," he complained.

She ignored him until he finally got the hint and moved away.

Maybe she was crazy for going home when she could've stayed in Kansas City and gotten herself a job.

Oh yeah . . . sure . . . some sensational job. Hooker, Call Girl, Stripper, Go-Go Dancer . . . There were a million and one opportunities for a girl like her. But Cyndra had bigger ideas. Somehow she was going to make something out of her life, and nobody was going to stop her.

She'd gone to Kansas City for an abortion. Paid for, she suspected, by the man who'd raped her. Of course, nobody would admit he'd raped her. Her mother had said it was her own fault, that she'd encouraged him.

She'd never done any such thing. She hated him, always had.

Mr Benjamin Browning. Big business man. Happily married family man. Big phoney son-of-a-bitch.

The Brownings. Her mother's employers. The fine, upstanding Brownings.

Oh yeah, she could tell the town a thing or two about the fine, upstanding Browning family. She'd had the unfortunate distinction of knowing them all her life.

When she was a little girl her mother used to take her to the house all the time and leave her in a back room while she worked. Sometimes Benjamin Browning would come to that back room and touch her. She was too young to understand what he was doing, but as she got older she began to dread going there.

When she was five she'd tried to tell her mother. Aretha Mae had slapped her sharply and said, "Don't you dare talk 'bout Mr Browning like that. I work for these people. Don't you *never* make up no bad things again."

So Cyndra had learned to shut up. At least her mother stopped taking her there – she put her into Kindergarten instead, dropping her off on the way to work.

School was another bad experience. She was jeered at because of her dark skin, and ostracized because her mother worked as a maid. Several times she was beaten up by the older kids. Eventually she'd learned to look after herself. Not quite well enough, it seemed.

Damn Benjamin Browning. Mister fine upstanding pillar of the community. Damn him and his money and everything about him.

She'd been away for a month. The abortion had turned out to be a frightening experience. It had taken place in the run-down house of a hatchet-faced woman and a grey-haired man with bony white hands, who'd called her Girlie and treated her as though she was a prostitute. For hours after she'd bled uncontrollably, until they'd had to rush her to the nearest hospital, dumping her on the front steps and abandoning her like a delivery of prime beef.

"What happened to you?" the doctor at the hospital had demanded. "We need names. You have to tell us who did this to you."

But she couldn't do that, so she kept quiet, just as she'd kept quiet her whole life.

Now she was on a bus coming home, and she didn't know if she was happy or sad.

"How old are you?" the doctor in Kansas City had asked.

"Twenty-one," she'd lied.

"I don't think so," he'd replied.

And he was right. She was sixteen. Sweet sixteen.

With a deep sigh she began day-dreaming. One of these days she was going to get out of Bosewell. One of these days the name Cyndra Angelo was going to mean something.

By the time the bus dropped her off the rain had almost stopped. The driver waved goodbye and she grabbed her bag and began the long trek to the trailer park. In a way she was pleased to be coming home. At least she had Harlan and Luke to look forward to. They were good kids and she genuinely loved them. She did not love Aretha Mae, although she grudgingly respected her for managing to survive on her own with three children to raise.

When Cyndra was six she'd asked who her father was.

"Never you mind," Aretha Mae had replied. "That be my business, not yours."

She knew he was white and that's all she knew. Harlan and Luke were the offspring of a black man called Jed who'd lived in the trailer for two years, then moved out one day when Aretha Mae was at work. Jed had never been seen or heard from again – which was just as well, for his interest in little Cyndra had been more than stepfatherly.

As she walked along the deserted pathway she started thinking about Benjamin Browning and what she would like to do to him. Kill him for starters. Maim him if that didn't work. String him up by his grungy old balls.

The truth was that she knew in her heart there was nothing she *could* do. It was her dirty secret and she was stuck with it.

She thought about how it had happened, and if there was anything she could have done to stop it.

No. Impossible. The man was an animal. Besides, he was over six feet tall and weighed at least two hundred pounds. Whereas she was only five feet five inches and one hundred and fifteen pounds. No contest.

It had happened on a Tuesday. Aretha Mae was sick with flu, so at her request Cyndra had taken time off from school to help out. The Brownings had another maid, but she was out sick too, so Cyndra found herself alone in the house. Mrs Browning was shopping, Stock was at school, and Mr Browning was at his office.

He came home early coughing and spluttering. "I feel lousy. There's this damn flu going around," he complained, loosening his tie. "Be a good girl and fix me a hot tea with lemon. I'll be upstairs."

She didn't like him, but she had no reason to be frightened of him. She was a big girl now, and he hadn't touched her since she was five.

She made the tea in the spacious kitchen, putting the china cup on a tray with a matching saucer next to it containing several slices of lemon. Then she carried the tray upstairs to the master bedroom.

He was in his bathroom. "Leave it on the bedside table and turn the bed down," he called out.

She did as he asked, touching the fine quality linen sheets, wondering what it must feel like to sleep between such luxury.

Mr Browning emerged from the bathroom clad in a terry cloth robe. It was a warm day and the window was open. Outside the gardener worked on the lawn.

"Close the window," Mr Browning said, clearing his throat.

She went over to the window and pulled it closed. Before she could turn around he grabbed her from behind and wrestled her on to the bed, pushing up her skirt and ripping off her cotton panties.

She was so startled she hardly had time to put up a struggle. "Stop!" she managed, trying to get away.

"Cunt, gimme that black cunt," he mumbled excitedly, thrusting himself roughly inside her.

She was too shocked to scream, it all seemed to happen so fast.

Mr Browning was enjoying himself. "C'mon, black bitch. Give it to me. Give it to me *good*," he grunted.

Frantically she struggled, still trying to push him off.

"That's what I like!" he crowed. "Keep on moving – I like it! I like it when you fight me."

He ripped into her, tearing at her insides, hurting her terribly. She thought she screamed but she wasn't sure. Whatever she did he had no intention of stopping, he was beyond control – until, with a long drawn out cry, he was finally finished.

He collapsed on top of her for a few moments – almost suffocating her. Then he got off, and she heard him go into the bathroom.

Drawing her legs up to her stomach she began to sob.

After a few minutes he came out of the bathroom fully clothed as if nothing had happened. "I'm not going to shower," he said in a conversational tone. "I want your smell on me all day." He walked to the door and stopped. "Oh, and by the way, Mrs Browning will be home soon, so you'd better stop that snivelling and get those sheets changed – they're covered in blood."

Six weeks later she'd realized she was pregnant. She had nowhere to turn except her mother, so she'd told her everything.

Aretha Mae had listened silently, her face clouding over with anger.

When she was finished her mother said harshly, "You're never done makin' up stories 'bout these people, are you?"

"It's the truth –" she began.

Aretha Mae slapped her across the face. "Shut up, you hear me, girl? I'll take care of it – but you must *never* talk 'bout this again. *Never*."

Somehow Aretha Mae had come up with the extra money to send her to Kansas City for the abortion.

Now she was back, and she hoped Aretha Mae wasn't going to force her to continue school. It would be far better if she dropped out and got a job, they could certainly do with the extra money.

The rain had stopped, but the ground was still muddy. She wasn't frightened walking through the dark. There were no streetlights but she knew every inch of the trailer park – it was the only home she'd ever known.

When she arrived outside their trailer she was surprised to see lights on and hear the television blaring. It wasn't like her mother to stay up so late.

She opened the door and walked in.

A man was sprawled on the bed watching television. He had a can of beer in one hand and a stupid smile on his face. He was laughing at something Johnny Carson had just said.

Cyndra stopped abruptly. "Who're you?" she asked, alarmed.

Groggily he sat up. "Who am *I*? Who in hell're *you*?"

"Where's my mother?" she demanded. "Where's Aretha Mae?"

Primo's eyes focused on this beautiful slip of a girl. "Shee . . .it!" he exclaimed. "You must be my daughter. Come on over here an' say a big hello to your daddy."

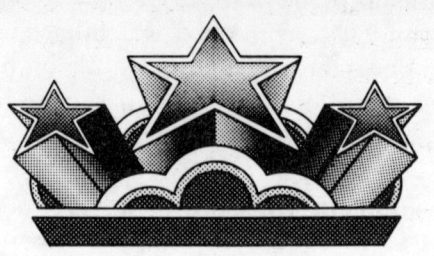

Chapter 12

Since their engagement party Stock had been suitably deflated. He'd caught hell from his parents for inviting too many people, and allowing the party to get totally out of control. When Lauren left he'd been drunkenly reeling around the place with his so-called friends – who'd proceeded to wreck the place, smashing glasses and bottles, pulling down half the tent, generally causing chaos. Mr Browning was not amused.

"It wasn't my fault," Stock whined to Lauren. "You were there, why didn't you stop me from letting them all in?"

"Because I'm not your keeper," she said, crossly. "It's your own fault." And it *was* his fault. Who did he think she was – his mother?

They bickered on and off. Lauren was miserable and yet she didn't know what to do. Should she give him back his ring? She knew that's what she *should* do, but she didn't want to do it while he was having trouble with his parents. His father had cut his allowance. His mother was barely speaking to him. How could she turn against him too?

Stock did nothing but complain. She decided that as soon as his complaints stopped she would make her move. Meanwhile, she threw herself into a student production of *Cat on a Hot Tin Roof*. She'd landed the plum role of Maggie the Cat, which was exciting, and her husband, Brick, was played by one of the older boys, Dennis Rivers. Apart from being very good-looking, Dennis was a terrific actor. The rumour was that he liked boys instead of girls. Lauren couldn't care less who or what he liked, she felt privileged to be working with him.

Betty Harris was in charge of the drama group. They met after school at the old church hall once a week.

Betty was unlike the other teachers. A large, billowy woman

in her fifties, she had flushed cheeks and straw-coloured hair that never looked combed. She favoured loose, gypsy clothes and spoke in a breathy, excited voice encouraging her students to excel.

As far as Lauren was concerned drama group was the high point of her week.

"I hear you got engaged Lauren, dear," Betty Harris greeted her. She nodded.

"Too young," Betty said, shaking her head knowledgeably. "Much too young."

Lauren nodded again. At least *someone* understood.

When all of her students were assembled, Betty made an announcement. "I have a big surprise for everyone," she said, fluttering her hands. "You've often heard me mention my brother, Harrington Harris, the famous New York stage actor. Well, next week he's actually coming to visit us here in Bosewell."

An appreciative hum went around the room.

"So you will see that I am not actually making him up," Betty continued, her rosy cheeks glowing. "He will be with us very soon.' She paused, her protruding eyes darting around until they settled on someone at the back. "And on another note, before we start rehearsals today, I'd like to welcome a new student into our group. Will all of you please say hello to Nick Angelo."

Lauren turned around, startled. Lounging at the back of the room in his familiar outfit of jeans and dirty denim jacket was Nick.

Meg nudged her. "I just died!" she whispered. "If I can only keep him away from Dawn maybe I've got another chance."

"Do you still want one? I thought you hated him."

"I know," Meg agreed, "but who else *is* there? I mean, you've got to admit, he *is* gorgeous."

Yes, reluctantly Lauren had to admit it – in his own intense way, he certainly was.

Cyndra was shocked and angry to discover that while she'd been away her mother had allowed her long-time missing husband and his scummy son to move in. A husband Cyndra hadn't even known existed. And what's more, the man claimed he was her father. Her father for God's sake! A white trash piece of shit who made her sick just looking at him.

"I'm getting out of here," she threatened.

71

"Where you goin', girl?" Aretha Mae asked, her lip curling.

Cyndra was close to tears. "I'll get a job – find something, but I'm *not* stayin' here."

They argued back and forth until finally Cyndra realized it was useless. She had no money and nowhere to go. Once again she was trapped.

"You be sharin' the other trailer with your brothers," Aretha Mae said, glad to see her daughter, but sorry about the trouble she was bound to cause.

Reluctantly Cyndra moved into the battered old trailer next door. She put up a sheet dividing the already crowded trailer in two, and refused to speak to Nick. "Stay on your side," she warned him, "an' we won't have no trouble. Got it?"

He'd just looked at her, still trying to reconcile himself to the fact that he actually had a half-sister, and a black one at that.

"What've I done to you?" he asked one day. "It ain't my fault we're stuck here."

"You and your goddamn daddy," she replied, her brown eyes flashing. "He's nothing to me."

"Oh yeah – nothin' 'cept your dad."

"My dad your dumb ass," she fired back. "I hate both of you."

She was pretty but a real pain. He made no further attempt to speak to her.

Meanwhile he was doing okay at the gas station. Apart from Saturday nights he now came in on Saturday mornings too. He stashed away most of the money he made, handing a few bucks to Aretha Mae each week. When Primo found out he had a part-time job he soon had his hand out.

"Nothin' left," Nick said.

"What'n t'hell am *I* supposed t'do?" Primo complained.

"Whyn't you try getting a job?" Nick replied, standing up to his father for once.

Whack! Primo lashed out, his heavy hand swinging through the air. Nick was old enough and wise enough to know when it was coming and duck out of range.

Cyndra refused to walk with him in the mornings or even sit next to him on the bus. At school he noticed she was even more of a loner than he was, although on Saturday nights she hung out with the biker crowd from nearby Ripley.

Primo seemed to think they were living the great American

dream. Now that Cyndra had returned he tried to play the concerned father. "Don't want that girl runnin' around all times of night," he informed Aretha Mae.

"You've left it too late to be givin' her no orders," she said. "She ain't gonna take nothin' from you."

"She's my daughter," Primo roared. "An' *I* make the rules 'round here."

Aretha Mae shook her head wearily. She had Primo back after seventeen years, but the question was – did she really want him?

The scene from *Cat on a Hot Tin Roof* went extremely well. Lauren was glowing, she loved playing Maggie the Cat, especially with Dennis as Brick.

After class Betty Harris praised her. "Excellent, Lauren, dear. You really have talent."

She was delighted. "I do? You know one day I'd like to go to New York. Would I have a chance?"

"Acting is a tough business," Betty replied. She was wearing a voluminous caftan with multiple hanging gold necklaces, and every time she spoke the chains rattled against each other. "Too many actors chasing too few parts."

"But I'd love to give it a try," Lauren said, earnestly.

"A try would be good, dear, but don't depend on acting to make a living, it's far too treacherous a profession."

Stock met her after class, took her arm possessively, noticed Nick and said, "What's that creep doing here?"

Lauren jumped to his defence. "He's not a creep."

"Says who? Take a look at him – always in that stupid get up. Who does he think he is – James Dean?"

"Not everyone has to look like you," Lauren said, coolly.

"Not everyone *can* look like me," he boasted.

They went to the drugstore for a soda. *The Way We Were* was playing at the local cinema. Lauren wanted to see it, but Stock wasn't interested.

"I hate that sentimental crap," he jeered. "Give me Clint Eastwood any day."

She sighed. "You *promised* we could see it tonight."

"I got other ideas."

"Like what?"

"Going for a drive, talking about our future. It's about time."

"I guess so," she said hesitantly, taking a long deep breath. A drive was good; it would give her an opportunity to tell him she didn't think they had a future.

Stock drove like a rich kid showing off. His father had weakened and promised him a new car for Christmas, so he really let the Ford Thunderbird rip, zooming down Main Street as though he was competing in a drag race.

"Not so fast," she said, clutching the dashboard.

"Calm down."

She hated being told to "calm down" – like she was hysterical or something. "Where are we going?" she asked.

"Over to the old athletic field," he replied, taking one arm from the steering wheel and placing it around her shoulders.

The deserted field just outside town was a notorious necking spot. "No," she said quickly.

"Why not?"

"You know why."

"We're engaged. We can go anywhere."

"That's what I want to talk to you about."

"I thought *I* was the one wanted to talk."

"We should both talk," she said, seriously.

Against her better judgment she allowed him to drive to the edge of the old field, where he parked the car, dipped the headlights and immediately swooped.

"What are you *doing*?" she said, pushing him off.

"What I should've done a couple of months ago," he replied, his big hands roaming all over her.

She slapped his hands away. "C'mon, Stock, don't start this."

"What are you, Lauren? Some kind of ice queen?" he said, managing to clamp his lips down on hers.

She struggled free. "Will you stop it!"

He drew away from her clenching his fists. "Christ! When do I get to first base with you?"

"Never," she replied, heatedly. "This engagement thing's a big mistake. We weren't meant to be together."

He sat up straight. "What the hell do you mean by *that*?"

"I never should have said yes. I don't know why I did. My parents encouraged me . . . they like you . . . they like your family . . . they think we make a great match." She knew she was speaking too fast, but now she was on a roll and couldn't stop. "I'm not ready to be involved."

"You were involved with Sammy Pilsner," he said, slyly.

74

"What do you know about me and Sammy?" she snapped, her cheeks reddening.

"Nothing much. Just that he used to tell all the guys he was getting a blow-job from you."

She couldn't believe Sammy would have betrayed her. "I don't believe you," she said, fiercely.

"It's true isn't it? And if you did it to him – I want the same." And with that he launched himself upon her again.

She wasn't Meg about to let some oaf have his way with her. "If you don't stop I'm getting out of the car," she threatened, once more slapping his hands away.

"Go ahead," he replied, confidently. "It's a long walk home."

"You think that's going to stop me?"

"Aw, shit, you're behaving just like a dumb girl," he whined. "Anybody else would love being here with me."

He was nothing but a braggart and a bully. She glared at him furiously. "I'm *not* anybody else, it's about time you realized that."

Sensing her anger he rapidly changed tactics. "C'mon, Lauren," he wheedled. "I only wanna love you up a little." And it was hands all over her again.

Every time he launched an attack she felt incredibly vulnerable. He was so big and strong, it would be easy for him to overpower her. Right now she knew she had to make a move and make it fast. Hurriedly she groped for the door handle, sprung it open and bolted. "I'm out of here," she yelled. "You're nothing but a sex maniac!"

"And you're nothin' but a prick tease!" he yelled back.

"Get lost Stock Browning!" Burning with fury she set off down the road.

Stock suddenly realized she was serious. He started the engine, turned the car around and drove after her. Winding down the window he leaned out. "Get back in. Stop being stupid."

"I don't need this," she replied, marching along the bumpy country road.

He was contrite. "I won't touch you again. I swear I won't."

She stopped walking and whirled around to face him. "What do you swear on?" she demanded, not relishing the thought of a five-mile walk home.

"My father's life."

"Big deal."

"Okay, okay, I'll swear on my *own* life. Does that make

you happy? Now get back in the car." He threw open the passenger door and she climbed in. "I'll behave myself," he said, backing down all the way. "I'll wait until we're married. That's a promise."

You'll have a long wait, she thought. *A real long wait.*

Chapter 13

The school play was due to take place in December a few days before the Christmas break. Lauren was so immersed in her role that she decided to put the incident with Stock behind her and deal with him after Christmas. Her New Year resolution was to get rid of him once and for all.

Her parents were driving her crazy – all they wanted to talk about were wedding dates.

"I was married to your father when I was barely eighteen," her mother said.

"I'm only sixteen," she pointed out. "And I'm *not* getting married."

"Why not?" Jane and Phil chorused.

What was it with them? Were they trying to get rid of her? Or couldn't they wait to share in all the perks that being related to the Brownings would bring them?

Rehearsals became the most important thing in her life. The only interruption was the arrival of Betty's brother. Harrington Harris looked like a famous actor. Tall, in his early forties, he had a receding hairline, long sideburns to compensate, lecherous eyes and a disarming manner. Every girl in the class immediately fell in love, including Meg.

"Harrington's the most exciting man I've ever met," she confided to Lauren.

"Too old for me."

Meg winked. "Certainly *not* too old for me. *And* he's asked me out."

Here we go again, thought Lauren. "Maybe he's married," she said.

Meg was silent.

"Well, *is* he?"

"How do I know?"

Are you going out with him?"

"Of *course* I am. It's an adventure."

"And I suppose I'm your excuse?"

"Of *course* you're my excuse."

At least Meg finally seemed to have gotten over Nick, which meant that maybe she could talk to him now. It wasn't easy pretending she didn't notice him – even though they kept on exchanging long looks, and she was painfully aware of everything he did.

Meg set off for her date with Harrington Harris full of her usual enthusiasm. The following day her enthusiasm had turned to outrage. "He jumped me," she complained.

Lauren shook her head in wonderment. "What did you expect? A cup of coffee and an intellectual chat? Naturally he jumped you. Sex. That's all men want. Didn't your mother teach you that?"

Meg giggled, "As a matter of fact she did."

"So what did you do this time?"

"I told him I was a virgin. That frightened him off."

"At least you're learning."

A few days later Meg came down with the mumps. Twenty-four hours later so did Harrington Harris. Unfortunately, several other members of the cast caught the dreaded disease, including Dennis, much to Lauren's disappointment.

"What will we do about the play?" she asked Miss Harris.

Betty was as upset as she was. She surveyed her class of high school students searching their eager young faces for someone to replace Dennis, her eyes finally falling on Nick. He was such a handsome boy in an intense kind of way, and he certainly looked as if he might be able to handle it. Not that she had any idea if he could act or not, but she waved a script at him, and told him to get on stage and read with Lauren.

Sitting at the back of the class he jumped to attention. "I . . . I can't do this," he mumbled.

"Come along, dear," Betty said crisply. "You joined this group, I'm sure you're perfectly capable of giving it a try."

Reluctantly he got up and made his way to the stage where Lauren sat at a makeshift dressing table brushing her hair.

"This is the scene at the beginning of the play where Maggie and Brick have a confrontation," Betty explained. "You've watched the scene, Nick, you can do it."

He clutched the script tightly. Christ! He'd joined the group to get closer to Lauren, but he hadn't expected to get this close. What if he made a fool of himself?

He opened the script and stared blankly at the written words. It wasn't like he hadn't watched Dennis say them enough times, and if Dennis could do it so could he. Angry at himself for getting trapped he began to read.

Lauren turned around and responded to his lines, her eyes flashing.

Soon he relaxed and started to get into it. Hey – it wasn't as bad as he'd imagined. Suddenly he wasn't Nick any more, he was just an actor playing a role, and, jeez, it was a kick!

When the scene was finished he dropped the script to the floor and reality came flooding back.

Lauren was staring at him. She had the most beautiful eyes he'd ever seen. He turned to Betty Harris, anxious for her reaction.

"That was very good, dear," Betty said, beaming happily. "I'm impressed. Now all you have to do is learn the words."

Learn the words. Was she kidding? "Ah . . . yeah, yeah, sure," he assured her, sounding a lot more confident than he felt.

"Then there's no panic," Betty said, relieved. "Class, you can relax – we have our Brick."

Outside the old church hall it was cold and dark. Tiny white snowflakes were beginning to fall, silently hitting the ground. Nick emerged and leaned against the old bike Dave's brother had lent him. It certainly beat taking the bus. He waited patiently for Lauren. According to Aretha Mae, Stock and his parents were in Kansas City attending a family funeral, so there'd be no boyfriend lurking about.

She came out a few minutes later.

He stepped forward. "Hey . . . uh . . . I just wanted to say thanks," he said, kicking a pebble on the ground.

She stopped. "For what?"

"Y'know, for not letting me look like a jerk."

She held out her hand to catch a snowflake. "You handled it really well, you must have acted before."

He laughed. "Who, me? No way."

"Then you're a natural."

Now he was embarrassed. "Well, like I've seen a lotta movies, stuff like that."

"It's not easy the first time you have to get up in front of people. But honestly – you knew what you were doing."

He stamped his feet on the ground, warming up. "Thanks. That's a nice present."

"Present?"

"Yeah, it's my . . . uh . . . birthday today."

"Really?"

"Yep."

"How come you didn't tell anyone?"

"Hey . . . seventeen . . . s'no big deal."

"My parents always make sure *my* birthday's a big deal. I have a huge cake and friends over to the house and lots of presents. What did you get?"

"My family don't give presents."

She wondered about his family; there'd certainly been enough gossip about them in school. "Aren't you going to celebrate at all?" she asked, half-expecting Dawn to put in an appearance and drag him off.

He pulled up the collar of his denim jacket and stamped his feet again. "Nah, guess not."

"You *have* to do *something*," she said, prolonging the moment. "At least let me buy you a cup of coffee and a piece of cake."

He wasn't about to turn *this* invitation down. "Great," he said quickly, "let's go."

"I've got a car," she said. "Leave your bike here and we'll pick it up later."

"Do I get to drive?"

"It's the family station wagon," she said, apologetically. "Only I'm allowed to drive it."

He grinned. "What they gonna do, shoot you?"

"I guess they'll let me live," she said, smiling back.

Oh, God! Why was she doing this? She tried to tell herself she felt sorry for him, that nobody should be alone on their birthday. But it was more than that and she knew it. Nick Angelo was exciting, and she wanted some of that excitement.

They walked over to the car.

"Like one of these days I'm getting me a bright red Cadillac," he said. "Yeah, a Cadillac – that's the car for me."

"Why a Cadillac?"

"I dunno. It's just kinda . . . a cool car. An' it's made pretty good. It's American."

She smiled again. "You're very patriotic."

"You gotta be something, right?"

Their eyes met. "Right," she said.

80

The snow kept everyone home, and by the time they reached the drugstore it was almost empty. Nick guided her into a booth and slid across the other side. "What'll you have?"

"*I'm* buying," she reminded him.

"I'm driving so *I'm* buying," he countered.

She laughed. "No way. It's your birthday."

Louise came over, tapped her order pad and threw Nick a disapproving look. "What'll it be?" she asked, pen poised.

"I'm starving," Lauren said. "How about two cheeseburgers?"

"Yeah, an' let's go for a couple of chocolate malts along with that," Nick added, winking at Louise.

"And fries –" Lauren said.

"With ketchup –" he interrupted.

"And fried onions –"

"Yeah! Right!"

They both burst out laughing as Louise walked briskly to the kitchen.

"I like a girl who eats," he said, grinning.

"From what I hear you like all girls," she replied, immediately thinking – *Oh, no! Why did I say that? It makes me sound like a jealous idiot!*

"That's 'cause *I'm* not engaged," he said, staring pointedly at her ring.

She caught him looking and hurriedly slid her hands under the table. "Stock's very nice," she said, defensively.

"Very nice my ass."

"I don't know . . . maybe it's not going to work out the way everybody thinks." Why was she revealing herself to him?

He leant across the table. "Are you telling me you're *not* engaged?"

She hesitated for a moment, then plunged right in. "I'm just saying certain people have expectations. My parents think we make a great couple. But what I really want is to go to New York and give acting a try. When I'm older, of course."

"Sounds cool to me. You told him?"

"No," she said defensively. "I don't have to tell him. My future doesn't necessarily lie with Stock Browning."

He nailed her with an intense stare. "So take his ring off."

"I didn't *say* I was getting disengaged. I just said my future might not lie with him."

Louise marched over, slammed their order on the table and

threw Nick another sharp look as if to say, *What the hell you doing with her?*

Lauren took a bite of her cheeseburger. "Where's Dawn tonight?" Damn! She'd said it again. Why couldn't she keep quiet about Dawn?

He shrugged. "Who knows? I only see her when I feel like it."

She wanted to know more about him, but she didn't dare ask.

He wanted to know more about her, but he figured he shouldn't push it.

They ate in silence.

"I guess this turned out to be a pretty good birthday after all," he said at last.

She wondered why she felt so light-headed. "It did?"

"Yeah – like y'know – bein' with you, getting the part in the play, it kinda makes today special."

"That's if Dennis doesn't recover and come back," she reminded him.

"Whatever," he said casually, pretending it didn't matter, although by this time he was hooked and it did matter a great deal. "Y'know, this is my first birthday since my mother died. She never made me a cake or any of that birthday stuff – she was always too busy working. But sometimes she would like – y'know – slide me ten bucks."

"When did she die?" Lauren asked, softly.

"A few months ago, that's why we came here. Turns out my father married Aretha Mae seventeen years ago, then skipped town. He never got a divorce – so he an' my mother weren't legally married. She didn't know – nobody did. When she died, my aunt threw us out so we came here. We live over in the trailer park."

"What's it like?"

"Believe me, you never wanna know. I got this half-sister who refuses to speak to me, an' a couple of half-brothers – Harlan and Luke – they're okay. I share a trailer with 'em. My old man sits on his ass all day while Aretha Mae goes out to work. I'm stuck here until I get enough money to split."

"Where will you go?" she asked, widening her eyes.

"I dunno. New York. Maybe." He paused and grinned. "Wanna come?"

"My parents would *love* that."

He was suddenly serious. "They wouldn't have to know. We'd just take off . . . Ever thought of doing something like that?"

Why was she feeling so dizzy? "You're crazy, Nick. I don't even know you."

He looked at her very gravely. "One of these days you will. That's a promise."

Chapter 14

"Uh . . . the Christmas play is coming up," Nick mumbled, not quite sure whether to mention it or not.

Primo was lounging on the unmade bed, scratching his beer belly. "What?" he said, dragging his eyes away from *All In the Family* for a brief moment.

"I said it's the school play coming up," Nick repeated. "And . . . uh . . . one of the actors got the mumps, so I'm playing the lead." He hesitated for a moment. "I dunno . . . thought you might wanna come."

"*I* wanna come," piped up Harlan. "Me and Luke."

"No, you don't," said Aretha Mae, busy at the stove.

"Sure they do," Nick said. "I'll get 'em seats."

"Wanna go. Wanna take Luke," Harlan chanted.

"No," Aretha Mae said, sharply.

"Why not?" Nick asked.

"Because we don't belong with those people. We ain't gonna sit in no fancy theatre watchin' you make a damn fool of yourself."

"I don't make a fool of myself," he objected. "I'm good."

"Good?" Aretha Mae arched her eyebrows and curled her lip. "You be good for nothin', boy."

What was *she* bitching about? He gave her money every week, which was more than anybody else in the family did. How come she didn't pick on Primo? The lazy slob hadn't even attempted to get a job.

"I'm going into town," he said, like anybody cared.

He left the trailer, got on his bike and started the long ride. God, it was freezing. He didn't know why he was going into town anyway considering it was Sunday, and there was never anything to do. Everyone went to church in the morning and then retired into their houses never to be seen again. The drugstore was

84

closed. The gas station was closed. The movie house was closed. What was he planning? A fast ride up and down Main Street? Very exciting.

He decided that maybe he'd pay Dawn a visit seeing as they hadn't been together lately, and he was feeling decidedly horny. Since he'd been rehearsing for the play he hadn't seen much of anybody except Lauren. And there was no way he could make a move on her.

Ah, Lauren . . . He couldn't figure her out. One moment she was his best friend – the next cool and businesslike – as if the play was the only important thing. They met at rehearsal and went through their scenes. The moment they finished she hurried off to meet Stock who was always outside waiting to take her home.

He'd imagined things would be different after their one night together sharing hamburgers and a few home truths. But no. Everything was back to the way it was before.

He was mad that he'd opened up and told her about Aretha Mae and his father. It wasn't her business. She was just some rich girl, stuck up like all the rest.

When he reached Dawn's house, her mother told him she was away for the weekend. Great, now he didn't even have Dawn to take his mind off things.

"When's she comin' back?" he asked.

"Tomorrow," Mrs Novak replied, clutching a scarlet cardigan across her scraggy breasts. She was one of those rail-thin women with bulging eyes and a nervous tongue that kept on darting in and out, licking her dry thin lips. She smelt of whisky and stale cigarette smoke.

"Why don't you come in anyway and have a lemonade," she suggested.

Jeez, Nick thought, if she and Primo ever met they'd make the perfect couple. Fat and thin and both zonked out of their minds.

He declined Mrs Novak's invitation and got out of there fast.

"How are you feeling, Dennis?" Lauren asked over the phone.

Dennis told her he was depressed about not being able to appear in the play with her.

"Don't worry," she said, comfortingly. "We'll manage without you, but it won't be the same."

85

Liar, she thought to herself as soon as she hung up, *it'll be even better because Nick Angelo is playing your part.*

She felt disloyal and confused, and yet she was savvy enough to know that Nick meant trouble. She also knew she couldn't stop watching him at every opportunity, and she loved acting with him. But there was such a thing as self-preservation, and she was aware that it was essential to stay away from him, which wasn't easy, because every time they did the opening scene between Maggie and Brick she sensed a great surge of electricity between them.

Now it was almost time to perform the play on the stage with half the town watching. She shivered. Would everyone be able to spot the chemistry between them?

Stock was back in her life with a vengeance. Big and bossy and full of himself because he'd taken delivery of his new car — a super-fast Corvette. She stuck by his side whenever she could. It was safer than allowing Nick to get close.

"You don't have to come to the play if you don't want to," she told Stock.

"I'll be there," he said, confidently. "You're my girl – wouldn't miss it. I'm sittin' with my parents in the front row."

Oh great, that's all I need.

"I'm just saying you shouldn't feel obligated, I'm perfectly okay with the fact that you . . . you might be bored." She was almost stammering.

He didn't get it. "Is Dennis back yet?"

"Uh . . . no. That new guy's playing the role."

"That jerk, you mean," he said, sourly.

It seemed that both Stock and Nick were programmed to insult each other whenever they could.

Sometimes she felt as if she was going to explode. There was nobody she could confide in. Not her parents, and certainly not Meg who'd kill her if she knew she had these feelings for Nick.

Bury them, she told herself. *And Nick Angelo will go away. He's the kind of boy who comes to town, causes trouble and then takes off.*

There was plenty of activity in Bosewell at Christmas. First there was the play, followed by the school dance on New Year's Eve. Naturally, Stock had plans. "After the dance," he informed her, "Some of the guys have booked rooms over at the motel. We'll have a party."

"What kind of party?"

86

"Oh, you know, music, good times an' a few strong blasts . . . Relax, Lauren, you're such a square sometimes."

She hated being told to relax – it was so patronizing. "Remember what happened last time," she said, to her horror sounding just like her mother. "Your allowance was cut off and you told me I should've warned you about inviting all those extra people."

"This'll be different," he promised. "Oh – and ask your girl-friend, Meg, if she wants to go with Mack Ryan."

Mack was Stock's best friend. Bigger than Stock. Blonder than Stock. But not as rich.

"Why doesn't he ask her himself?"

"Maybe he doesn't want to, guys don't dig the idea of getting rejected."

Meg was delighted, she said yes immediately. *At least we'll be a foursome*, Lauren thought. Anything was better than being alone with Stock.

As the play drew nearer Betty insisted on more rehearsals. Lauren didn't mind, in fact she loved it.

Nick grabbed her arm one day on her way out. "Hey," he said. "Do I have to wait until my next birthday for you to talk to me like a human being?"

"I'm talking to you now," she said, trying to remain calm.

"Ha!" he laughed, bitterly. "You're back in the same old groove. You've got your rich boyfriend, your nice organized life, an' no time for me."

"We're working together," she said. "What gave you the impression it was more than that?"

He stared at her so intently she thought she might dissolve.

"You *know* it's more than that," he said.

"I . . . I have no idea what you're talking about."

"Yes, you do," he said. "Only you won't admit it."

She pulled free and rushed outside. To her relief Stock was waiting. Stock was always waiting.

The night of the play there was a blizzard. Betty Harris was in a bad mood because Harrington, whom she'd planned to show off, was still sequestered away with a bad case of the mumps.

Lauren was shaking. Why had she agreed to play the lead? Did she really want to stand up in front of the whole town in a skimpy silk slip and play Maggie the Cat, a sexual older woman? God, everybody would laugh her off stage.

Nick was nervous too – he couldn't figure out how he'd got conned into this.

Before going on they wished each other luck. "Break a leg," Lauren said.

He looked at her incredulously. "Break a leg?"

"That's what they say in the theatre for good luck."

"I always figured actors were a crazy bunch," he said, shaking his head.

She grinned. "I guess they are."

His throat was dry and he had a strong desire to run. "Well, anyway – we're gonna kill 'em. Right?"

"Right!"

Lauren made her entrance first. Nick waited in the wings, his heart thumping. When he made it to the stage he lost all fear and became the character.

Shit, he thought, *I can do this – I can really do this*. And he was right, because the play was a smash. Shocking and *risqué* for a small town like Bosewell, Betty had taken a risk putting it on – but the audience loved it anyway.

As they were taking their bows, Lauren spotted a scowling Stock sitting in the front row with his parents. She couldn't care less, she was too busy enjoying the applause.

After five curtain calls the elated cast mingled backstage. She looked around for Nick, found him and hurried over. "You were great," she said, warmly.

"So were you." He broke into a grin. "Hey – we both were."

Betty Harris approached them, beads and gold chains jangling. "We're a hit!" she gushed. "You were *all* wonderful. If only my brother were here to enjoy our triumph."

"I'm sorry he's still sick," Lauren said.

"His balls probably look like an elephant on a bad day," Nick muttered in her ear.

"What?" She couldn't believe what he'd just said.

"It's the mumps," he replied straight-faced. "Gets 'em every time!"

She choked back a giggle as a vivid picture of Harrington Harris with swollen elephant balls flashed before her eyes. Fortunately her parents appeared before she burst out laughing. She tried to introduce them to Nick, but he'd taken off.

A glowering Stock hovered behind them. "You never told me you were going to be up on stage half-naked for everyone to get an eyeful," he complained.

Wasn't he supposed to be congratulating her?

"You never asked," she replied.

"We'll see you later, dear," her mother said, wandering off with Phil in tow.

"How does it make *me* look?" Stock demanded. "You up there with that creep playing opposite you. You made a fool of me tonight, Lauren."

"I did not," she said, heatedly.

"Yes, you did," he argued.

She sighed. "Don't spoil it, Stock. This is a special night for me."

"It isn't for me."

"Then maybe you should go home."

"And what will *you* do?"

"I'll stay here and celebrate with the rest of the cast."

"Without me?"

"Yes, without you."

"You do that." He said, storming off.

Too bad. She wasn't exactly heartbroken.

Betty Harris had arranged dinner in one of the adjoining rooms for the cast. They were high with excitement, milling around congratulating each other. When they sat down Lauren found herself next to Nick.

"So . . . I guess that's it," he said, picking at a bread roll. "I won't get to see you until school starts next year."

She sipped a glass of water. "Next year sounds like forever. Vacation's only a few weeks, and we'll see each other at the New Year's dance. You are going, aren't you?"

"Nah . . . don't think so."

"Why not?"

"I can't get into all that organized crap where everybody's supposed to have a good time."

She bit her lip and tried not to say it, but out it came anyway. "Surely Dawn will want you to take her?"

He gave her a quizzical look. "I thought I told you, me and Dawn, we're not a couple."

"That's not what she says." *Oh God, Roberts. Shut up!*

"How come you're so concerned anyway? You've hardly talked to me lately."

"I'm talking to you now."

He stared at her. "Maybe I'd like t'do more than talk."

She looked away. She should have known he'd want to jump her, just like he'd done to Meg. Why were boys so interested in sex? Didn't feelings or getting to know someone ever come into it?

89

"Excuse me," she said, pushing her chair away from the table and getting up.

"Where are you going?"

"I've got a present for Betty in my car."

Leave me alone, Nick Angelo. I am not interested.

Oh yes you are, Roberts. Oh yes you are.

She hurried outside to the station wagon, opened the door and reached inside for the brightly wrapped gift.

"Hey –" He was right behind her.

She turned around, feeling weak and vulnerable.

Without saying a word he moved very close and kissed her.

It was not like any kiss she'd ever felt before. His lips were insistent and yet soft. His tongue was exploring, and yet not in a conquering way. Without thinking she began kissing him back.

"I've wanted to do this ever since I first saw you," he mumbled, pulling her in close.

She took a deep breath. "Blakely's hardware store. I was scrambling around on the floor –"

"Yeah, an' you looked pretty good that day."

She was about to say, "So did you," but before she could he kissed her again, and the second time was so incredible that she let herself fall into it and get lost. She'd kissed boys before – Sammy Pilsner, Stock, several boys she'd dated, but it had never been like this. Never.

He pushed his hands through her long hair. "You're so . . . I dunno . . . beautiful."

Nobody had ever called her beautiful before. Pretty – yes. Nice – naturally. Beautiful was something else. But even so . . . she mustn't get carried away. "We can't do this," she murmured, softly.

"I'm not forcin' you," he replied, pressing close.

She took another deep breath willing herself to make a move. "I have to go." Without waiting for a reply she turned around and rushed back inside.

For the rest of the evening she tried not to look in his direction or even think about him.

Betty Harris made a speech praising all her students, and when it was time to leave Nick was right behind her. "Can I drive you home?" he asked.

"No, I'm the one with the car, remember?" Lauren replied.

He grinned. "You're right."

"Good night, Nick," she said, politely.

"Good night, beautiful."

All the way back to the trailer park he thought about her. Then his mind started racing in different directions. The play had been such a triumph. He'd really got off on the feel of an audience watching him, studying his every move. On stage he wasn't some nothing kid, he was Brick, he was someone they responded to in a positive way.

And then his thoughts returned to Lauren. When he'd kissed her it had been like nothing he'd ever known. Oh sure, he'd had enough girls, but none of them had been like her – he'd never had that feeling of wanting to look after a girl, protect her, be with her all the time. This had nothing to do with scoring. This was different.

Was he in love?

Don't even think about it.

Maybe he could be an actor. The thought sneaked into his head unexpectedly.

Nah. He didn't stand a chance.

Or did he?

Chapter 15

Once Nick decided what he wanted to do he went all out. His first move was to visit Betty Harris and ask if she'd consider giving him private coaching.

"I can't pay you," he explained, "But one of these days I'll make it, an' then I'll pay you big."

Betty laughed. "If only I had a dime for every boy that thought he could be the next Marlon Brando or Montgomery Clift. You're no different, Nick. You're good, but you're no different."

"Hey – you don't understand," he said. "I'm not gonna be a nuclear scientist. I ain't got a chance of runnin' for President. I gotta go for *something*, an' I've decided this is it."

"Ah yes, but I *do* understand," Betty said, pacing around her small living room. "When I was young I had the same ambition. In fact I even went to New York."

He was surprised. "You did?"

"Yes. I made the rounds of auditions only to be told I was too tall, too short, too fat, too thin, too ugly, too pretty. Believe me, Nick, nobody knows what they want. They only know they want a carbon copy of somebody who's made it."

"So what did you do?"

"I got married," she said. "I married a man who liked to dress up in my clothes. He left me for another woman." She laughed, dryly. "Thank God it wasn't for another man!"

"Go on," he encouraged.

"I suppose I got older and certainly wiser. Every so often I landed bit parts here and there, until eventually I came back to Bosewell," she sighed, "and here I am, teaching the High school acting class. Teaching you all to do something you're never going to have a chance at."

"Everybody's got a chance, Betty."

She smiled, wryly. "Full of optimism. How old are you? Sixteen?"

"Seventeen."

"Well, Nick, I went to New York when I was twenty, came back when I was thirty. I'm now fifty. The last twenty years . . ." She trailed off, shaking her head, wondering where the time had gone.

"But your brother made it," he pointed out.

"It depends what you call making it," she said matter-of-factly. "In a town like Bosewell he's a star. But the truth is he's played three butlers on Broadway in the last six years, and that's the extent of his stardom. The last time he worked was advertising a cure for haemorrhoids on television."

"Harrington Harris?"

"Yes, the great Harrington Harris. But it makes everybody feel good when he comes back here. They *think* he's a star, and that's all that matters."

"Betty," he said earnestly, fixing her with his green eyes. "You gotta help me. I need to study, an' I have to do it with somebody who'll teach me things."

There was something about him that was so intensely sincere. Betty knew she shouldn't encourage the boy, but what did she have to lose? The winter was cold and lonely, and there were five weeks before school and acting class resumed. What else was she going to do with her time?

"Very well," she said. "You'll come over here three times a week at noon and we'll work from twelve until four. Be prepared to work hard and *never* call to tell me you have something else to do."

"I swear it," he said, excitedly. "I'll be here."

She smiled. "Good. It's a start."

Life at the trailer park was hard during the winter. The roofs of both trailers leaked, causing a rancid damp smell and numerous little puddles. It was almost like living outside.

Primo refused to do anything about it. "My arm hurts," he whined. "I ain't fixin' nothin'."

"You musta hurt it lifting a can of beer," Nick muttered, disgustedly.

"You're gettin' a real smart mouth," Primo slurred. "I could throw you out any time."

"I thought you promised my mother I had to graduate High school?"

"Don't be so sure," Primo grumbled.

Out of school, Luke and Harlan were bored. They ran into town every day and Aretha Mae couldn't stop them. One day Harlan came home beaten up.

"What happened to you?" Nick demanded.

"Nothin'," Harlan said, sulkily.

Nick turned to Luke. "What happened to him?"

Luke stared blankly.

"Jeez!" Nick exclaimed. "Open your mouth and talk, god-damnit!"

Luke ran out of the trailer, crying.

Aretha Mae stood in front of the sink stoically washing dishes. Primo snored in his usual position.

"Don't either of you give a shit?" Nick demanded.

"He better learn to defend hisself. This won't be the last time," Aretha Mae said.

Cyndra had gotten herself a job working down at the canning plant. She left early in the morning and arrived home late at night, barely acknowledging Nick's existence.

"You're a freakin' pain," he exploded one day. "When you gonna lighten up?"

"When you leave," she replied, brusquely.

"Don't hold your breath. I'm outta here on *my* time – not yours."

"Good," she said. "Make sure it's soon."

He kept himself busy. What with the work at the garage, and visiting Betty Harris three times a week, and trying to do a few repairs around the trailers, he never had a moment to himself.

Working with Betty was a kick. She chose plays she knew would interest him. He particularly loved *A Streetcar Named Desire*. Reading Stanley to her Blanche was a real blast. The good thing was that he'd finally found something he could absorb himself in and it was pretty exciting.

The honeymoon was over for Aretha Mae and Primo. Whenever she was home they'd taken to having long, vicious yelling matches. Primo beat up on her pretty good. Smack! That's all the bastard seemed to know.

Nick wished he could apologize for his father. He wanted to say, *Look it's not my fault. Throw us out. We'll go somewhere. Anywhere. We don't have to screw your life up, too.*

94

But now that she had him back, Aretha Mae had no intention of letting Primo go.

Christmas came and went. It was a dismal holiday. Aretha Mae brought home the remains of the Brownings' turkey and made a thick soup – that was the extent of their festivities. No tree. No presents. No nothing.

Nick didn't mind, he was more or less used to it, but he felt sorry for the kids – especially Harlan – it was useless trying to get through to Luke.

Occasionally he hung out with Joey who wanted to know if he was going to the New Year's dance.

"Haven't thought about it," he said.

"There's nothin' else to do," Joey said. "We gotta make plans."

"How do we get in?" Nick asked. "Don't we have to buy tickets?"

"Nah, it's a High school thing. Whyn't you take Dawn?"

He hadn't really thought about Dawn lately. He'd been so busy that the need to get laid hadn't arisen. "Yeah, I'll give her a call. Who'll you bring?"

Joey dragged on his cigarette and attempted to sound casual. "Maybe I'll ask your sister."

Nick looked surprised. "My sister?"

"Cyndra," Joey said. "I mean, it's not like I think she'd say yes or anything, but she always seems so . . . kinda – y'know – all by herself."

Nick made a face "Hey, if you wanna get your balls crushed, go ahead."

He had no feelings for Cyndra. Maybe as a brother he was supposed to feel protective, but what the hell – she was a bitch, he didn't care who she went out with.

"What do we wear to this thing?" he asked.

"Tux," Joey replied. "We'll take a ride to Ripley an' hire a couple of monkey suits."

They set off for Ripley the next afternoon. Joey had a second-hand motorcycle and they made it in a couple of hours. The rental place was crowded with manic people struggling to get themselves an outfit for New Year's Eve. Joey pushed his way to the front, grabbed a salesman and picked out two tuxedos.

"I feel like a jerk," Nick said, trying his on.

"You look like one," Joey guffawed. "But that's okay, so does everyone on New Year's."

He paraded in front of the mirror. The pants were too long, the jacket too big. "Have I really gotta wear it?"

95

Joey slapped him on the back. "Only for a night. You'll live."

They paid their money and left.

"I know a bar where they got naked girls," Joey said with a wink. "Bare tits an' ass."

They'd both acquired fake I.D.s so they swaggered into the bar full of confidence. Nobody stopped them. Nobody cared.

The place was jammed with construction workers busy watching the parade of half naked waitresses – girls who wore nothing but black stockings, garter belts, frilly aprons and phoney smiles.

Nick couldn't believe what he was seeing. He nudged Joey. "Ain't there some law against this?"

Joey sniggered. "Don't tell me you've never been in a topless bar before. They're the coming thing."

"Hey, hey, talkin' of comin'," Nick joked.

Joey laughed. "Let's have a little control here. You can look, not touch."

"Do they put out?"

"If you've got the bread."

He patted the top pocket of his denim jacket. "I got it," he said. "Yesterday was pay-day." He already had his eye on one girl – a pretty brunette with a sweet face who reminded him of Lauren. He hadn't seen her since the play, and sometimes he thought about her. But he tried not to – she wasn't exactly available. When the girl took their order he came on to her. "What're you doing later?" he asked.

She peeked at her watch. "I get off at three."

"I'm about ready to get off now," he joked. "How much?"

She tried to look insulted. "You think I'm a hooker?"

"Course not," he said. "How much?"

"Twenty."

"Twenty," he repeated. "What is it, mink lined?"

"Ten for you because you're cute."

"You got a room?"

"If you wanna go to my place it'll be an extra five."

He weighed up the possibilities. He'd never had to pay for it before, but somehow it seemed fitting, a New Year's present to himself, a girl he didn't have to sweet talk. "Okay," he agreed.

Her name was Candy and she lived in one room with two smelly cats roaming around, and a hamster in a cage.

"I don't usually bring people back here," Candy announced, shrugging off her coat. "But you seem like a nice guy. How old are you anyway?"

"Twenty-one," he lied. "How about you?"

"Twenty."

More like thirty, he thought. "You bin doin' this long?"

"Doing what?" she said, scrambling in her purse for a joint.

"A little action on the side."

"Oh. I don't really do this," she said vaguely, lighting up. "I needed extra money this week . . . and like I said, you're kinda cute."

Sure, he thought to himself.

She offered him a drag and began to undo the buttons on her blouse.

He drew deeply on the joint – it wasn't the first time he'd had marijuana – and watched her as she took her time removing her blouse. He'd already seen the goods on display in the bar, but it was more of a kick watching them revealed slowly just for him.

Underneath the blouse her small breasts were covered by a skimpy black bra. With a theatrical flourish she threw the blouse on the floor and unzipped her skirt, daintily stepping out of it. Quite obviously she hadn't bothered to wear panties. He felt that good old familiar stirring.

"What shall I leave on?" she asked.

He noticed she was chewing gum. "Your ear-rings," he replied.

She laughed, casually fingering her nipples. "Never heard *that* one before."

He stripped off his clothes. This girl was a challenge. She was a professional, and he wanted to see if he could make her feel as good as all his other conquests.

Candy plumped herself down on the bed and beckoned him over.

He made the trip across the room in record time and climbed aboard.

She took another drag of her joint and placed it in a chipped glass ashtray next to the bed.

"You're not really twenty-one," she said slyly. "Tell me the truth?"

No way was he admitting to seventeen. "Nah. Twenty-two," he lied, pumping away.

Candy had obviously expended all her energy down at the bar. She lay there like a corpse, chewing gum and looking blank as he gave her a little of the Angelo magic.

As soon as he was finished he couldn't wait to get away. Forget about pleasing her – this was the first and last time he'd ever pay for it. He left the money on the table and beat a hasty retreat.

Later Joey met him at the bar and they got on the bike and headed for home.

"What happened, man?" Joey wanted to know. "Gimme all the filthy details."

"You want details, pay for it yourself," he replied, shortly.

"What's the matter? You fall in love?" Joey teased.

He groaned. "Don't even mention the word."

Love. Was *that* the feeling he had for Lauren? He missed her and yet he was nervous about seeing her when school started because he didn't know what would happen. He was so used to being in control with girls. He got beat up enough at home, at least there was one part of his life where he had the upper hand.

Now he had this dumb feeling and it wouldn't go away.

Lauren Roberts. She was the only special girl he'd ever met and she belonged to somebody else.

The truth was it was about time he did something about it.

Chapter 16

Lauren spent a miserable Christmas. Over the holidays her mother's brother, Will, and his wife, Margo, came to visit from Philadelphia. This time they did not bring Brad – their nineteen-year-old son. Lauren's crush on him had been a long time ago and she didn't miss his presence.

The day after Christmas they spent at the Brownings' house. Stock gave her a cashmere sweater and two cookbooks – obviously chosen by his mother. She gave him a simple pewter money clip and a photo frame. And all day long she wondered what Nick Angelo was doing.

At night she lay in bed and thought about her future.

Only another two years and she'd be out of school. She was already campaigning for enrolment in an Eastern college. Her parents said Kansas City was as far as they'd let her go, but she had her mind set on New York.

Meg came by the house to find out about the New Year's dance. "What are you wearing?" As usual she was obsessed with clothes.

"I haven't thought about it," Lauren replied, vaguely. "Maybe that dress I wore to my engagement party."

Meg frowned. "You *can't* wear the same thing again."

"Yes I can," she said, stubbornly.

"What's the *matter* with you? You're so . . . sort of . . . different, lately."

Lauren wondered if she was different. All she ever thought about was Nick. On his birthday he'd seemed so sensitive and understanding, and the night of the play, when he'd kissed her, it was definitely something special. She couldn't believe he'd practically attacked Meg. The truth was that Meg had probably encouraged him and then backed off at the last moment, always a dangerous practice.

"I'm wearing black," Meg announced, dramatically.

"That's exciting," Lauren murmured. Frankly she couldn't care less.

The night of the New Year's dance there was thick snow on the ground. Lauren stared out of her window watching the snowflakes falling. She wondered if she could get out of going altogether.

No such luck. Stock called to announce he would be picking her up at seven. "Be ready," he said.

God, he was so overbearing. When had she ever kept him waiting? New Year resolution. Get out of this engagement once and for all. Stop thinking about it and do it.

For a Christmas present the Brownings had insisted she visit their store and pick out an outfit. She'd done so reluctantly, and only at her mother's insistence. She'd chosen a short, black off-the-shoulder dress. When her mother saw it she had a fit. "You can't possibly wear that, it's quite unsuitable."

"Why?"

Jane was perplexed. "It's too sophisticated. Besides, young girls don't wear black."

"This young girl kind of likes the idea."

Jane sighed. "I don't know what's the matter with you lately, you're so argumentative."

Hmmm. Had she and Meg been talking?

Stock arrived with a corsage of white orchids and an appreciative, "Wow! You look –" He was about to say sexy, but since Mr and Mrs Roberts were hovering in the front hall he changed it to "– sensational."

She smiled. For once he'd said the right thing.

Jane produced her camera. "Photo time!" she exclaimed, gaily.

Dutifully she posed for a picture with Stock, then kissed her parents, said, "See you later," and left the house. Usually there was a discussion about what time her curfew was, but since it was New Year's Eve and she was with Stock, it didn't seem to matter. All they were interested in was cementing the deal.

Mack Ryan was waiting in the car, and they set off to pick up Meg. When they arrived at her house she gave Lauren a filthy look. "You didn't tell me you bought a black dress. How *could* you? *I'm* wearing black," she muttered, furiously. "And you *knew* I was."

Lauren shrugged. Quite truthfully she'd forgotten. "It doesn't make any difference. We don't look alike."

"I wanted to stand out," Meg said, shaking her head petulantly. "Now we look like twins!"

"You do stand out," Lauren replied, thinking that her friend had put on a pound or two.

"No. *You* do," Meg said. "It's *always* you."

They got to the dance late, having stopped for champagne in the car. Lauren wasn't used to drinking – she hated the taste, but she'd decided this New Year was going to be different from any other. It was time she grew up.

When they arrived the dance was in full progress. Stock grabbed her by the arm cutting a swath through his cronies as he led her on to the dance floor. "You're looking hot tonight," he said. "I didn't want to say it in front of your parents, but boy – have you got a body!"

Was this the first time he'd noticed? She decided to respond in kind. "Boy, have you got a body, too!"

He wasn't sure quite how to take this, so he pretended he hadn't heard, and began to gyrate his hips to the strains of "Honky Tonk Woman' played by the local band. Not quite Mick Jagger – as a matter of fact not even close.

Lauren felt a little dizzy as she started to dance, her eyes continually searching the room.

What are you looking for, Roberts?

I'm looking for Nick Angelo. Want to make something out of it?

To Nick's surprise, Cyndra said yes when Joey asked her to the dance. "I hear you're going with Joey," he said.

She glared at him.

"One of these days you're gonna realize you're taking it out on the wrong person," he said, trying to fix his stupid bow tie.

"When that day comes I'll let you know," she replied, brushing back her long, dark hair.

"Gee, I'm holding my breath," he said, irritated by her pissy attitude.

They were interrupted by the sound of banging and screaming coming from the trailer next door. It was nothing new – ever since Christmas, Primo and Aretha Mae had been at each other's throats.

Cyndra glared at him with a spiteful expression as if it was his fault. "Maybe you won't be around here much longer."

"How many times I gotta tell you? This wasn't my choice."

"You belong to him, an' he ain't nothin' but dirt," she said, vengefully.

"Yeah . . . well, let me tell you this – you belong to him too."

Her eyes were full of fury. "I don't believe it."

"Are you telling me your ma lied to you, is that it?"

Her dark eyes continued to blaze brightly. "I don't believe that dumb ox is my father."

"He is. Get used to it."

Joey arrived to pick her up on his motorcycle.

Cyndra stood at the door of the trailer peering out with an angry expression. "It's snowing," she said. "How we gonna get anywhere on that dumb bike?"

Joey produced a rolled-up plastic raincoat, unrolled it with a flourish and threw it over her. "There you go. How's that for service?"

"Oh, this is classy," she grumbled. "A real classy date."

"What did you expect? A Kennedy?"

"Nothing," she said, curling her lip sourly. "Absolutely nothing."

Nick had been planning to ask Primo if he could borrow the van, but what with all that screaming coming from the trailer he decided to ride his bike over to Dawn's and see if they could borrow her mother's car.

He hated the rented tux: it was too big for him, and what the hell was he supposed to wear on his feet?

Fuck 'em. He'd wear his sneakers, and if anybody had anything to say about it he'd smash 'em in the mouth.

Harlan told him he looked nice. Luke stared at him like a zombie. It occurred to Nick that the kid should be getting some kind of professional help. Fat chance.

"What are you two doin' tonight?" he asked.

Silly question. What *could* they do? They had no way of getting into town unless they walked and the snow was pretty deep on the ground. They couldn't even slide into the other trailer and watch television on account of the fact that Aretha Mae and Primo were busy killing each other.

"Tell you what," he said, trying to cheer them up, "tomorrow I'll treat you both to the movies."

Harlan nodded, his face lighting up.

He set off for Dawn's on the bike. It was a long ride and by the time he got there he was soaked through.

Dawn greeted him wearing the tightest dress he'd ever seen. She did not believe in leaving anything to the imagination.

"Great date you are!" she said, shaking her head. "We've gotta get you dry before we can go anywhere."

"Can we borrow your mom's car?"

"It's all ours, handsome. She *was* gonna use it, but then she passed out. C'mon, get your clothes off, I'll try to dry 'em."

He followed her upstairs to her room and stripped off. Two large posters of Elvis Presley sneered down at him.

She ran an appreciative eye up and down his body. "Hmm . . . sure you wanna go to the dance? My mom won't surface until tomorrow."

"Hey, I didn't ride all the way into Ripley to hire a freakin' tux to sit at home."

She winked, suggestively. "Sitting wasn't what I had in mind."

"We can do that later, okay?"

"Whatever you want, big boy."

That was the thing about Dawn, she was much too obliging.

Lauren spotted him the moment he came in. In a way she hadn't expected him to turn up. In another way she'd hoped he would. And now here he was with Dawn hanging on to his arm like a leech.

She tried not to stare – she certainly didn't want him catching her. He looked great in his tuxedo – even if it was a little big. He'd obviously made an effort. Was it because of Dawn? *Bitch!*

Lauren immediately felt guilty. The trouble was that Dawn wasn't a bitch at all, she was a perfectly pleasant girl who just happened to be the school tramp. Lauren suspected Stock had slept with her. Not that he admitted it. Not that she cared.

Stock was having a fine time twirling her around the dance floor, full of himself as usual.

"Let's get a drink," she said breathlessly, breaking away.

He beamed, "That's more like it. How about going for the rest of the champagne out in my car?"

"I meant a soft drink."

"Excuse *me*."

She hated it when he tried to be sarcastic.

Over by the bar Nick handed Dawn a glass of watered-down punch. "Try this poison."

Her eyes scanned the room and she shook her head. "I dunno what *we're* doing here. We shoulda gone to Ripley." She threw him a sly look. "Or stayed home."

He had to agree with her, they didn't belong.

She swallowed a fake yawn. "We came, we saw, we got bored. Let's get the hell outta here, we can have more fun at my house. I'll show you mine if you show me yours!"

He wasn't prepared to leave until he'd seen Lauren, after all, she was the reason he'd hired a tuxedo and shown up.

"Hey – you told me you were such a hotshot dancer. How about showing 'em what a *real* dancer can do?"

Dawn was always up for a challenge. "Honey, I can beat any of 'em. Any time. Any way."

"What are we waitin' for?" He pulled her on to the crowded floor. Not that he was into dancing, but he could make the moves if he had to.

Dawn enjoyed showing off. She had her assets and she knew how to shake them – especially in her favourite tight dress.

A small crowd gathered as they put on a show.

And then he spotted Lauren. She was sitting at a table with Stock and a group of his friends, and naturally she looked sensational.

He knew he had to make a move. He didn't know what he was going to do or when he was going to do it, but he wasn't leaving until he did.

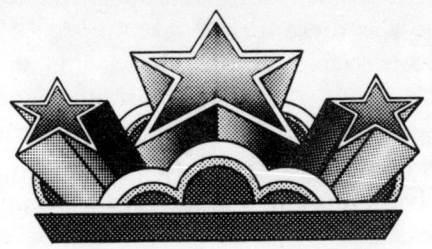

Chapter 17

"So?" Joey asked, leaning across the small table. "Do you like to dance?"

"No," Cyndra said, checking out the room with her dark moody eyes, wondering why Joey had invited her.

"How come?"

"How come what?" she snapped. "Just because I'm half-black I'm supposed to have rhythm?"

"I didn't say that."

"No, but you sure thought it. Is *that* why you asked me tonight? Black chick ain't got no morals – she'll be easy."

"Huh?"

"You heard me."

"I heard someone with a big hang-up."

"What?"

"A hang-up – like in chip on the shoulder shit."

She smoothed down the skirt of her green velvet dress – purchased at a second-hand shop – and tried to compose herself. She certainly hadn't dressed up and come out to get involved in a slanging match. "I don't have no chip," she said, controlling her temper.

"Maybe you should," he remarked. "It's a lousy deal – black mother, white dad, you can't figure out *what* colour you are."

Unexpectedly tears stung her eyes. He was right on, she wasn't one thing or the other and it hurt.

"*My* dad was Jewish," Joey continued. "A Jewish cop in Chicago married to a nice Irish Catholic girl. I never tell anyone I'm half-Jewish, s'not worth the aggravation."

"What aggravation?" she ventured.

"Y'know – the name calling, the dirty words. You know."

Yes. She knew all right. Mr Browning crying out in the

105

throes of his lust – "black cunt." Every man she ever met looking her over like she was there for the taking.

"You gotta learn to live with it," Joey said, wisely. "*I* did."

She sneaked a quick glance at him. He was kind of funny looking, tall and lanky with a shock of brown hair, a lopsided grin and crooked teeth. She didn't know why she'd accepted his invitation. Maybe because it was the first time anyone had asked her anywhere formal.

"Wanna dance?" He jerked his thumb towards the crowded floor.

She saw Nick out there breaking his butt with Dawn Kovak to the strains of "Sugar Sugar". "I . . . I don't think so."

He noticed her watching. "What've you got against him?" he asked.

She shifted uncomfortably. "Who?"

"Nick. What's he done to you?"

"He came here, that's what," she said, fiercely.

"It wasn't his choice." Joey said, taking a pack of Camels from his pocket and offering her one. "He's a cool guy. You should give him a chance."

She waved the package of cigarettes away. "You don't understand."

"Maybe one day you'll explain it to me. Sometimes it's good to talk – get it out in the open." He paused, realizing he was dealing with a touchy subject. "Whenever you like – I'm here. Okay?"

She narrowed her eyes and regarded him suspiciously. "What do you want from me?"

He shrugged. "Nothin', if that's all right with you."

"What time is it?" Meg asked, clinging on to Mack Ryan as if *they* were the engaged couple.

Stock consulted his expensive waterproof watch – a present from his parents. "Twenty-five minutes before midnight. Come five past an' we're on our way."

"You got it," said Mack, placing his hand on the back of Meg's neck and giving her a rub and a tickle. "This little lady an' I – we want some privacy."

Meg giggled. "We do?" she said, coquettishly.

Sure, Lauren thought. *And tomorrow this little lady is going to be complaining about how you nearly raped her.*

"Are we gonna *party* tonight!" Stock proclaimed.

Lauren took a hearty gulp of punch and immediately regretted it – the stuff tasted disgusting.

"C'mon," Stock urged, pulling her out of her chair. "They're playing my favourite."

His favourite turned out to be a soapy rendition of "Rocket Man". She hated it, especially when he began to get romantic, pulling her close, rubbing his crotch up against her leg and singing off key in her ear.

Tonight's the night, she thought gloomily. *He's going to make a move and when he does I'm giving him back his ring.*

About time too.

Across the dance floor Nick edged his way nearer to Lauren, guiding Dawn until she finally realized something was up and said, quite testily, "Where are we *going*? You're pushin' me around like I'm a vacuum cleaner!"

"We're gonna play excuse me."

"Huh?"

"Like I'll ask Lauren t'dance – an' you'll take care of Stock."

"I will?"

"Yeah. We gotta liven things up."

"That'll liven things up all right,' she said, getting the picture and not particularly liking it. If Nick thought he was about to score with Miss Thighs Together Roberts he had another think coming. Sweet little Lauren wouldn't give him a second glance. And Stock would punch his brains out if he made a move on his precious fiancée.

As soon as he'd manoeuvred them next to Lauren and Stock, he gave Dawn a little shove and an encouraging, "Go for it!"

Dawn smiled provocatively at Stock – after all she knew him well enough – they'd been secretly sleeping together on and off since eighth grade; his engagement had certainly made no difference to his sex life. "My turn," she said gaily, pulling him away from Lauren, throwing a perfunctory, "You don't mind, do you?" over her shoulder.

"Go ahead," Lauren said, one eye on Nick – who winked as if to say *how did you like the way I arranged this?*

Stock was easily led. Could he help it if girls found him irresistible? Dawn played her part, dragging him off to the middle of the dance floor, clinging on to him tightly.

"Hey –" Nick said, staring intently into Lauren's eyes. "Looks like you need someone to dance with."

She felt her heart begin to beat erratically. All of a sudden she could hardly breathe. "I guess so."

He took her in his arms pulling her in real close. "Tonight you're breakin' your engagement," he said, very quietly.

"I know," she found herself replying.

He held her even closer. "Just so long as you know."

"There's gonna be trouble," Joey said.

"What kind of trouble?' Cyndra asked.

"Big trouble," Joey replied, nodding towards the dance floor.

Cyndra had no idea what he was talking about, as far as she could see everybody seemed to be having a good time.

"You don't get it, do you?" he said.

She wondered what she was supposed to get.

"Stock Browning."

Browning. The very sound of that name made her shudder. Damn the whole disgusting Browning family, they were the worst kind of people.

"What about Stock?" she asked, trying to stay cool.

"Your brother's makin' a move on his girl."

She frowned. "How many times do I have to tell you? Nick's *not* my brother."

"Don't make no difference, he's gonna get his ass kicked."

"Good."

"You want him gettin' beat up?"

"I don't care."

"Yeah, well . . . I'll hav'ta get into it."

"Why?"

"'Cause he's my friend."

She studied the dance floor. Stock was gyrating with Dawn. Nick was way over the other side slow dancing with Lauren. "Nothing's going to happen," she said.

"I hope you're right."

"I usually am."

"What's Lauren doing with *him*?" Meg said, staring furiously across the dance floor.

"Y'know," Mack was not listening to a word she said, "I

always had eyes for you – even when I was going steady."

Meg was distracted. She was enjoying all the attention, but at the same time she didn't appreciate her best friend cosying up to Nick Angelo. "Where's Stock?" she demanded. "He should put a stop to this."

"You got the cutest little butt I've ever seen."

A compliment was a compliment. She forgot about Lauren for a minute. "I do?"

"Yeah. Cute butt. Cute face. I really dig you, Meg. Always did."

"Yes?"

"Let's go outside an' sit in the car for a minute."

"It's cold out there."

"We'll put on the heater, play the radio, finish up the champagne. C'mon . . . say yes . . . I wanna tell you about when I first noticed you."

How could she resist? "You won't . . . try anything?"

He looked suitably hurt. Girls were the most stupid creatures on Earth; did she really imagine it was conversation he was after?

"Who – *me*? I have too much respect for you, Meg. I surely do."

She allowed herself to be persuaded, after all he was pretty damn cute himself.

"Well . . . all right."

Ten minutes to touch down! With a great deal of effort he tried to keep his eyes off her plump, ripe breasts as he steered her outside.

As midnight approached a sense of anticipation hung over everyone. Excitement was definitely in the air.

The band blasted out a Beatles medley while Nick held Lauren very tight.

"This is a special night," he said, his voice low and warm. "The start of somethin' new."

"I know," she said, softly.

"This time in ten years we'll be old."

"Sort of."

"Very."

"I guess."

"But we'll be together."

He sounded so sure, and yet she knew this wasn't going to be easy. Stock she could deal with – but her parents would go crazy if she ever started dating Nick Angelo.

Don't be negative, Roberts.
Okay, okay. Take it easy. I'll try to be as positive as I can.

The Beatles medley ended, and the band blasted into their own noisy version of "Born To Be Wild".

Dawn grabbed Stock's hand as soon as he began backing off. "Where *you* goin' big boy? We was just getting into it." She licked her lips suggestively and wriggled her hips. "Don't flake on me now."

Stock felt altogether foggy. "Gotta find Lauren, it's almost midnight."

"Oh, yeah, midnight," Dawn sneered. "Big deal. I can show you a better time than little Miss Goody – *an'* you know it."

"Gotta find her," Stock repeated, slurring his words, his face red from too much Scotch surreptitiously sipped from his father's silver flask hidden deep in his pocket.

Dawn felt she'd done her part, she wasn't going to beg. Screw Nick Angelo – this wasn't how she'd planned on spending her New Year's.

Over by the edge of the dance floor Nick and Lauren were locked in each other's arms, oblivious to everyone around them. Stock spotted them and started over.

Joey stood up. "Here we go," he groaned, stubbing out his cigarette.

Cyndra toyed with her glass of watered-down punch. "Nothing's gonna happen."

The leader of the band grabbed his microphone. "Five minutes to midnight!" he roared, excitedly. "Five minutes to blast off! Are we ready?"

"Yeah," the crowd roared back, "we're ready!"

The band switched to "Crocodile Rock" – they were in an Elton John mood.

"Lauren –" Stock placed his hand on her shoulder and whined a plaintive "I didn't mean to dance with Dawn for so long. C'mon . . . it's time to go."

Lauren was startled, for a moment she'd forgotten about everyone and everything except Nick; Stock had ceased to exist. She turned to face him. "I . . . I don't want to go," she said quietly, her heart pounding.

"Why not?" he demanded, belligerently.

"Because I don't."

Stock began to get angry. Was she giving him a hard time on account of his dancing with Dawn? For a moment he stood there swaying, suddenly realizing that while he'd been busy, Lauren had been cosying up to Nick Angelo.

"What the hell you dancin' with *this* dumb prick for?" he demanded. "Take a look at him – he's wearing sneakers for crissake, can't even afford shoes."

She felt Nick stiffen, ready for battle. Quickly she touched his arm hoping to restrain him.

"Three minutes to midnight!' yelled the bandleader.

"You come with me where you belong," Stock said.

"No," she replied.

"You're my fiancée. Cut the shit an' do like I tell you."

Without saying a word she removed her engagement ring and handed it to him.

He was stunned. "What's this?" he said blankly, staring at the sparkling diamonds.

"It's over, Stock," she said, finally feeling in control.

"Over?" he said, incredulously. "It can't be over."

"It is," she replied calmly, experiencing an overwhelming sense of relief.

He raised his voice, his face becoming even redder. "Nothin's over until *I* say it is."

She stifled a hysterical giggle. Was it her imagination or did he look like a boiled lobster? "Don't yell at me," she managed, without breaking up.

"Two minutes!" from the bandstand.

"Shit!" from Stock.

Now people were beginning to notice something was going on and couldn't help watching.

Nick decided the time had come to join in. He put his arm around her waist. "Let's go," he said.

"*You* – fuckin' butt out," Stock shouted, enraged. "This has *nothing* t'do with you."

"You've got it wrong there," Nick replied, evenly. "It has *everything* to do with me."

"Fuck you!" Stock screamed.

"We're rollin' into countdown," the leader of the band yelled, his microphone outshouting everyone. "So let's all do it together. Countin' back from sixty. Fifty-nine. Fifty-eight. Fifty-seven –"

"Jesus!" Stock smacked his forehead with the palm of his hand and glared at Lauren. "Now I know why I couldn't get into your friggin' pants. This nigger-lovin' prick got there first!"

"How *dare* you talk to me like that," she said.

"I'll talk to you any way I want. You're nothing but a cheap tramp – I should've listened to my mother."

Nick stepped forward. "This asshole is askin' for it."

"No!" She tried to block him from getting to Stock.

"Nineteen. Eighteen. Seventeen –"

"Yeah, out the goddamn way," slurred Stock. "I'm teachin' this white trash punk a lesson."

"Don't!" She tried to stop them, she hadn't wanted it to come to this.

"– Eleven. Ten. Okay – Everybody together. Let's hear you all!"

The crowd launched into a raucous chant.

Joey fought his way through, hoping to stop the inevitable. Cyndra trailed behind him.

"– Five. Four. Three –"

Stock shoved Lauren roughly aside. Nick went to protect her, and before he realized it was coming, Stock hauled back and let one rip, taking him by surprise.

"– Two. One. HAPPY NEW YEARRR!!"

Nick didn't have a chance. He fell like a slab of concrete. Just before he lost consciousness he saw balloons. Hundreds and hundreds of pretty pink balloons floating through the air.

Chapter 18

He came to gradually, gasping for breath, his head aching like it was going to bust right open. Groaning he raised his hand to his face and touched sticky blood. Slowly he opened his eyes.

Lauren was sitting on the floor – his head cradled in her lap. They were in the corridor outside the gym. A few people stood around watching – waiting to see if he was dead, no doubt.

Mr Lucas, one of the school chaperones for the night, glared down at him. "That was disgusting behaviour, Angelo," he said sharply. "We don't condone fighting in this school."

"*He* didn't do anything, Mr Lucas," Lauren protested. "Stock hit *him.*"

Mr Lucas ignored her. "Somebody better get him home," he said impatiently, puffed up with his own importance. "I have to go back inside."

Now the excitement was over the few onlookers drifted away. Only Joey remained, Cyndra hovering close behind him.

"Jesus, man, you all right?" Joey asked. "I was on my way over when that moron laid one on you."

Nick tried to think straight. He felt like shit. Gingerly he touched his throbbing nose. "I . . . I think it's broken."

"Then we'd better get you over to the Emergency Room," Joey said, taking charge.

"What Emergency Room?" Cyndra joined in. "This isn't Chicago, y'know. We've got two doctors in town and they're probably both out celebrating."

"Are you sure it's broken?" Lauren asked, filled with guilt.

He touched his nose again. "Yeah, I'm sure."

His face was covered in blood, some of it had dripped on to the skirt of Lauren's dress, leaving big wet stains.

"I didn't mean this to happen," she whispered, softly. "I'm really sorry."

He tried to make light of it. "Hey, a broken nose is worth it if it gets that asshole out of your life."

She considered his words. Yes. Stock was certainly gone, there was no doubt about *that*. "He is out of my life," she said, quietly. "Forever."

"Well," Joey said, "this is all very cosy, but what're we gonna do?"

"We could take him over to the hospital in Ripley," Cyndra suggested. "They've got an Emergency Room."

"How'll we get him there?" Joey said, scratching his chin. "It's snowing, freezing cold, an' it's New Year's Eve. How'll we do it? On the back of my bike?"

"I guess not," Cyndra said.

"He can't go to the trailer park," Lauren said, firmly. "It's too far. I'll call my father and ask him to pick us up. He can stay at my house tonight."

"Are you nuts?" Joey exclaimed. "Your parents will freak when you tell 'em you've finished with Stock."

"You're right," she said glumly, "but it's my fault he's hurt and I'll take responsibility."

Nick groaned, "I'd like t'kick that asshole in the balls."

"What makes you think he's got any?" Cyndra said, coolly.

He attempted a weak laugh. "So, it takes something like this for you to talk to me, huh?"

She shrugged. "Don't get carried away."

Lauren hurried off to call her parents. She stood at the pay phone, impatiently waiting for someone to answer. Then she remembered they'd gone to a party and probably weren't back, which was all the better to smuggle Nick into the house before they could object. She called the local taxi service and was lucky enough to get a cab.

By the time she got back Nick was on his feet.

"Listen – I can walk. Don't let's make a big deal out of this," he said, feeling embarrassed.

"Are you sure?"

"Yeah, I'm sure." He looked at Cyndra. "Tell 'em I won't be back tonight. Not that they give a shit."

"Like I'll be talking to them when I get home," she said, sarcastically.

Back at her house Lauren led Nick straight up to her room. "How are you feeling?" she asked, anxiously.

"Like a jerk. Your boyfriend took me by surprise. We should've taken it outside and I could've given as good as I got."

"Ex-boyfriend," she said matter-of-factly, pulling down the cover on her bed. "You'll sleep here."

He managed a weak grin. "With you?"

She smiled back. "Let's get serious."

He sat down on the side of her bed. "Okay okay, just asking."

She soaked a washcloth and gently cleaned the blood off his face. "Ouch!"

"Don't be a baby."

When she was finished he said, "Now what? Am I gonna roll between the sheets with all my clothes on?"

"I'll take care of everything," she assured him.

He grinned again. "Including undressing me?"

She shook her head, smiling. "One of these days . . . maybe. But right now you can do it yourself. You should get some sleep, we'll talk in the morning."

"Your dress is messed up. Hadn't you better change before your parents see it?"

He was right, her new black dress was stained with dark patches of blood. "I hated this dress anyway," she said, wryly. "Let's call it my farewell present from the Brownings."

"Hey, Lauren," he said, reaching for her hand. "It was worth it."

"Say that in the morning when you look in the mirror."

By the time her parents arrived home she'd made up a bed for herself on the couch, changed into her robe, and was waiting to greet them.

As they came through the front door she heard her father's angry voice. "Don't threaten me, Jane. Don't *ever* threaten me."

"I'm not threatening you," Jane replied in a strained voice. "But I can tell you this –" She spotted her daughter and abruptly stopped. "Lauren, what are you doing home so early?"

This was a new one. Home so early? It was one o'clock in the morning. "Uh . . . somebody got hurt at the dance."

"Not you?" Phil said, quickly.

"No, I'm fine," she replied.

"Who then?" Jane asked.

"It . . . it's, uh, Nick Angelo. Remember? He was in the school play with me."

"What happened to him?" Jane asked, totally uninterested.

"He was . . . he was in a fight. He didn't start the fight – but he got a broken nose and there was no way he could get home tonight what with the snow and everything, so I brought him here." She knew she was speaking too fast, but she couldn't stop. "Actually, he's asleep in my bed. It's all perfectly respectable, Mother. I'm sleeping on the couch."

Her father looked furious. "That boy is here – in your bed?"

"Yes, Daddy," she said, patiently. "But *I'm* not. I'm downstairs with you. Right?"

Phil and Jane exchanged horrified glances.

"I do wish you hadn't done this without asking us," Jane fretted. "I don't like strangers sleeping over. Who is he anyway?"

"I told you, Mother," she replied, patiently. "Nick Angelo. He was Brick in the play."

"Oh, him. Strange looking boy," Jane said. "Somebody told me he lives over in the trailer park. Is that true?"

"Does it make any difference?" Lauren challenged.

Jane frowned. Her daughter could be very stubborn, and she could see that this was one of those times. "Well, if you wish to sleep on the couch, I suppose there's nothing we can do about it. We'll see you in the morning."

Lauren gave them half an hour. She waited until they'd both used the bathroom and she heard their bedroom door close. After that there was the faint murmur of conversation, and eventually silence.

When the house was absolutely quiet she crept upstairs and looked in at Nick. He lay on his back, arms outstretched, eyes closed.

She stared down at him for a long moment.

Nick Angelo, you've changed my life, she thought. *And I am so very, very grateful!*

In the morning Lauren was up at six. She'd decided it was better to get Nick out of the house before he had to face her parents. If she moved quickly and quietly she could borrow the family station wagon and drive him over to the hospital in Ripley before they were awake.

She'd hardly slept at all. Everything was changing and so was she. She knew she had to be strong, ready to stand up to all the opposition she was bound to face. For so many years she'd been good little Lauren – hard-working little Lauren. Now she'd be labelled naughty little Lauren because she didn't wish to remain engaged to the richest boy in town.

Too bad. She could deal with it – the problem was, could they?

Upstairs in her room Nick sat on the side of her bed clad in his ruined tux. She entered the room, put a finger to her lips and whispered, "Shhh . . . We're leaving."

He nodded, relieved to be getting out of there.

She hurried into her closet and pulled on jeans, sweatshirt and a heavy duffle jacket. "Follow me," she whispered. He did as she asked and they crept downstairs.

In the kitchen she scribbled a note explaining why she'd taken the car and taped it to the refrigerator door.

Within minutes they were outside. "Whew!" she sighed, unlocking the car. "It's not easy acting like a criminal."

"I'll drive," he said.

"No," she replied, firmly. "Not this time."

"Did you get any sleep?" he asked, getting into the passenger side without a fight.

"No. Did you?"

Ruefully he touched his swollen nose. "What do *you* think?"

She eased the car away from the kerb. It had stopped snowing, and although the roads were wet and slushy they were driveable.

"I think we're both insane!" she exclaimed, perfectly happy.

"And you like it."

"I love it!" she replied recklessly. "I feel free for the first time in ages."

He looked at her intently. "Yeah?"

"Oh, yes. Stock was like a big dark cloud hovering over me."

"So why did you stay with him?"

"It seemed the easiest thing to do."

"Easy ain't always easy," he remarked, sagely.

She snuck a quick glance at him. "You look awful."

"Thanks!"

"How do you feel?"

"Like a tractor ran over my face. Apart from that – great."

"The doctor'll fix your nose."

"What doctor?"

"We're driving to Ripley."

"We are?"

"I owe you a new nose. It was my fault you got hit."

"Hey – any time, if it means sleeping in your bed." He grinned. "Loved the Snoopy sheets!"

"Don't make fun of me. My mother never throws anything out."

His nose continued to throb and he was in serious pain. So why did he feel like singing? After all, Lauren was only another girl – yeah – only the most beautiful girl in the world!

He studied her perfect profile. "What're your parents gonna say about everything?"

She grimaced. "I'll let you know."

He reached for the radio, tuning it to a rock station. If only they could stay in the car and keep on going. Was it too much to ask her to give up everything and run away with him?

They made it to Ripley in an hour and a half and drove straight to the Emergency Room. New Year's Eve had taken its toll – the place was crowded with survivors of various battles. There were bloody knife wounds, a shooting or two, a couple of beaten women and a large black man screaming obscenities. Lauren clung to Nick's arm as they took a seat.

"Hey – take it easy," he said, feeling somewhat queasy himself.

They waited nearly five hours before getting any attention, and then a harassed young doctor rushed him into an examining room and confirmed that yes his nose was indeed broken. He set it and covered it with bandages.

"I feel like I was in a war," Nick joked, as they left the hospital. Deep down he was wondering what he'd look like when the bandages came off. Hell, he'd always been happy with his appearance – now what? Another stroke against him?

"Don't worry," Lauren said, reading his mind. "You'll look fine."

Outside the snow had started up again with a vengeance. "Big cities," she said, shivering. "They frighten me."

He laughed. "This ain't no big city. This is Disneyland compared with New York or Chicago." He clapped his hands together. "Jeez! I'm freezing!"

"So am I. And starving!"

"Me too."

She glanced at her watch. "It's nearly three. My parents will murder me! We'd better start back."

"Not until we get something to eat."

Her parents were going to kill her anyway, what difference did another half hour make? "Okay," she said, wondering if she should phone them. No, she decided, save the big confrontation for later.

They left the station wagon in hospital parking and ran, slipping and sliding on the wet sidewalk, to a nearby hamburger joint.

A waitress approached their table. She had a cigarette hanging from the corner of her mouth and a jaded expression. "Yeah? What'll it be?"

"Double burger with everything on, a Coke and fries," Lauren ordered breathlessly. "Twice." She smiled at Nick. "Okay?"

He had twenty dollars in his pocket. "I'm buyin'," he said.

"No. *I* am," she insisted. "It's my fault we're here."

"Can't let you do that."

"Yes, you can."

"Two burgers or *what*?" The waitress was bored, she couldn't care less who was paying as long as the check got settled. Lauren nodded, and the waitress left.

Nick leaned across the table and kissed her.

"What's that for?" she asked, wide-eyed.

"Uh . . . I guess for bein' you."

She smiled. He decided she had the most beautiful smile in the world.

"Hey –" he blurted, unable to stop himself. "I think I . . ."

"Yes?" she asked, eagerly.

"Aw – Forget it."

Her eyes shone brightly, urging him to continue. "What?"

"Uh . . . like I think . . . uh . . . y'know – like I think I love you."

"Me too," she whispered softly, feeling as if she was going to melt with happiness. "Me too."

Chapter 19

At first Jane Roberts was pleased when she awoke and found that Lauren had left with Nick Angelo, she hadn't relished dealing with a stranger in the morning. Besides, she had other things on her mind, there was no time to worry about her stubborn daughter right now.

She frowned when she reached the kitchen and discovered Lauren's note. Phil was not going to be pleased to find that Lauren had taken the car without his permission, it was so unlike her.

She re-read her daughter's note.

> BORROWED CAR
> BACK SOON
> LOVE
> LAUREN

When Phil came downstairs he was furious. "We give that girl too much freedom," he grumbled. "How dare she presume she can drive out of here in my car."

"What'll Stock say?" Jane fretted. "I hope she's back in time for the New Year's lunch with the Brownings. We're expected there at one."

"She'll be back," Phil said, gruffly. "She's probably taken that boy home."

"I wonder who he was in a fight with."

"Who knows? Who cares?" replied Phil, opening the kitchen cupboard and reaching for a packet of cornflakes. "Whoever it was he was probably bigger. Lauren always protects the underdog."

"Yes," Jane said, "but it wasn't very nice of Stock to leave her alone."

Phil tipped the cornflakes into a dish and added milk. "We have to talk about us, Jane," he said.

Her face reddened. "We talked last night."

"Not enough."

"It was enough for me," she replied, her lips tightening into a thin line.

The phone interrupted what was about to be another fight. Phil picked up. "Yes?"

"Sorry, Mr Roberts, did I wake you?"

"No," he said tersely.

"It's Meg. Can I speak to Lauren?"

"She went out early."

"Where did she go?"

He ignored her question. "She'll call you when she gets back."

"Uh . . . thank you, Mr Roberts."

Shortly before noon Jane Roberts sat at her dressing table adding a touch of powder here, a dab of rouge there. She had a new cinnamon outfit with matching pumps. Over the top she'd decided to wear her fur coat. It was five years old, but perhaps when Lauren married into the Browning family and Phil's business started improving he would be able to buy her a new one.

Phil walked into the room and stood behind her tapping impatiently on his watch. "She's not back."

"Oh, dear," Jane said. "How can she do this to us?"

"It's snowing again," Phil said, moving over to the window and staring out. "I hope she hasn't had an accident."

"Lauren's an excellent driver."

"I know," Phil said, pacing up and down. "I don't understand where she can be."

"Nor do I," said Jane, more than slightly irritated that her daughter would choose today to mess things up.

The phone rang. "That'll be her," Phil said, grabbing the receiver.

It was not Lauren, it was Daphne Browning. "Phil," she said, in her commanding and slightly imperious voice, "let me speak to Jane."

"Certainly, Daphne." He covered the mouthpiece with his hand. "She wants to talk to you – don't mention Lauren."

Jane rushed to pick up. "Happy New Year, Daphne," she

gushed. "You left the Lawsons' party awfully early last night, but it was fun, wasn't it?"

Daphne was not into pleasantries. "I simply cannot believe your daughter's behaviour," she said, flatly.

Jane was startled. "I beg your pardon?"

"Lauren's behaviour," Daphne repeated, as if she was talking to an extremely backward child.

"What happened?"

"Surely you know?"

Jane took a stab in the dark. "About the fight?"

"Disgusting!" Daphne exclaimed. "You might think Lauren would have the decency to stay with her fiancé rather than go running off with that no-account boy from the wrong side of town."

Jane took a deep breath; she had known Lauren's engagement to Stock was too good to be true. "Are you still expecting us for lunch?" she said tentatively, knowing the answer before she asked.

"I don't believe there's any point, do you?" Daphne replied. A long, cold pause. "I'm extremely disappointed in Lauren. You should be, too."

"Lauren's always done the right thing," Jane said, finally coming to her daughter's defence.

"Certainly not this time."

"Well," Jane hesitated. "I'm sure whatever happened between them, Stock and Lauren will work it out."

"You're making very light of this," Daphne said, disapprovingly. "You *do* know she gave him back his ring?"

"Oh," said Jane, blankly.

"He doesn't care," said Daphne, her tone snappy and spiteful. "Not after the way she treated him."

"I have to go," Jane said, not wishing to prolong the conversation.

"Fine," sniffed Daphne, hanging up.

Phil walked back into the room, adjusting his tie. "We should leave," he said. "You'd better write Lauren a note telling her we've gone ahead."

"Too late," Jane said. "The engagement is off. We are no longer invited to lunch."

By noon the news was all over town that Lauren Roberts had broken off her engagement to Stock Browning. It was

122

also common knowledge that Stock had smashed Nick Angelo in the face, and nobody seemed to know where Nick and Lauren were.

Joey was alarmed; he'd seen the electricity between the two of them and knew it meant trouble. Shortly before noon he rode over to pick up Cyndra.

"Did you hear anything from Nick?" she asked.

"No. Did you?"

"We don't have a phone in case you hadn't noticed."

Harlan was hanging around outside. "Nick was gonna take us to a movie," he said, sounding mournful.

"He got hurt," Cyndra explained. "He was in a fight."

"When's he coming back?"

"Later."

"He promised," Harlan said sadly. "Luke was lookin' forward to it."

"He'll take you another day," Cyndra said.

"Whyn't *you* take us?" Harlan asked, his eyes big.

"Some other time," she answered quickly. "Come on, Joey, let's go."

Cyndra didn't care to admit it, but she was pleased to see Joey. When he'd taken her home the night before he hadn't even tried for a kiss good-night. She felt safe with him. It made a welcome change to feel safe with a member of the opposite sex.

They rode into town on his bike and stopped by the drugstore. Joey settled her in a corner booth and went off to talk to some of his friends. When he came back he said, "Okay, so this is the story goin' around. Nick took a slug at Stock an' the big guy creamed him."

"But that's not true," Cyndra said, heatedly. "Nick didn't have a chance. Stock hit him when he wasn't looking."

"Yeah, *we* know it," Joey agreed. "But since he's on the missing list it's difficult to defend him. Oh, an' Meg says Lauren's not around either. She's been tryin' to call her all day."

They both thought about it for a minute.

"Hey –" Joey said at last, as if he'd had some kind of big revelation. "You don't think they ran off and did it, do you?"

Cyndra smiled, a sly smile. "Did *what*, Joey?"

He grinned back. "*You* know. What *we're* gonna do one of these days."

Oh, yeah? That's what *he* thought. "Don't bet on it," she said, sipping her Coke.

He threw up his hands. "Okay, okay. Only jokin'."

By late afternoon the light smattering of snow flakes had turned into a fierce storm.

"I'm calling the police," Phil Roberts said. "I'll give them the licence number and they'll track them down."

Jane looked dismayed. "How can she do this to us?" she asked. "Doesn't she know we're worried out of our minds?"

Phil shook his head as he marched across the room to the phone. "I'm calling the police," he repeated.

Jane nodded. There seemed to be no other answer.

Chapter 20

They sat in the hamburger place for two hours. They talked. They got to know each other. They gazed into each other's eyes. They held hands. They giggled. Neither of them had any idea of the time.

The two of them made a strange couple. Lauren all bundled up in her winter clothes, and Nick in his battered tuxedo, his nose bandaged, his dark hair falling on his forehead, his green eyes as intense as ever.

Eventually the waitress approached their table. "You can't sit here nursing a Coke forever," she said, sharply. "Either order somethin' else or leave."

Nick stood up. "We're outta here."

"Old bitch!" Lauren whispered.

"No bad language," he said, laughing.

"I'm not the little goody-goody everybody thinks I am."

"Yeah – like I've noticed."

He grabbed her hand and they ran outside. Now the snow was really coming down in icy blasts.

"I'd better phone home," Lauren said, feeling guilty.

"They'll only yell at you," he said. "Let's hit the road an' get back."

When they reached the station wagon it was piled high with snow. It was so cold that some of it had already turned to slabs of ice. Lauren got a shovel out of the trunk, and handed it to Nick who began trying to crack the ice.

"I'm gonna end up with no hands," he complained. "My fingers are frozen!"

"Can I help?"

"Yeah, get in the car an' start the engine. We'd better get goin' before it's dark."

The car didn't want to start. Lauren tried to no avail. She moved across the seat while Nick got behind the wheel. He gave it a couple of shots until the engine finally turned over and they set off.

The car began to skid and slide on the slippery roads. He tuned the radio to a news station. A weather warning announced blizzards, heavy snow falls and impassable roads.

"What now?" Lauren asked, helplessly.

"We can try an' make it."

"And if we get stuck?"

"I dunno."

"Maybe we should stay here," she said, tentatively.

"Then you're *really* gonna have to call home. You can't let 'em think you're never comin' back."

"Okay."

"There's a motel over by the gas station at the edge of town," he said. "Let's see if we can make it."

"Fine," she replied, thinking about how she would explain this to her parents.

By the time they reached the motel she was shivering with nerves. While Nick booked them in she hurried to a pay phone. Her father answered with a sharp, "Yes?"

"Daddy?" she ventured.

"Lauren," he replied, his voice harsh. "Where are you? Your mother and I are worried sick."

"I know. I'm sorry."

"You're *sorry*? We imagined you dead and buried under a snow drift, and you're calling to say you're sorry. Get home *right* now! Do you understand me? Right now!"

"Daddy, I can't, I'm in Ripley. The roads are closed."

There was an ominous silence. "Who are you with?"

"I . . . I'm with Nick. I took him to the hospital. You see it's my fault his nose is broken. I know I shouldn't have borrowed the car without asking you, but I didn't want to wake you. The Emergency Room was filled with people, we had to wait . . . I . . . I didn't realize it would take so long."

"Are you telling me you can't get home?"

"We thought we'd stay in a motel and drive back tomorrow."

"My daughter – in a motel? With that scum?"

"Nick's not scum," she said, defiantly. "He's a very nice person. It wasn't his fault Stock smashed him in the face, it was mine."

"You'd better speak to your mother."

Jane grabbed the phone. "Your behaviour is absolutely disgraceful," she said, in a low, tight voice.

"I'm sorry –" Lauren began.

"I don't wish to hear your excuses. If the roads are closed it's quite obvious you can't get home tonight. Since you are forced to stay in Ripley, promise me you'll stay in separate rooms and have nothing to do with that boy whatsoever. Can you promise me that, Lauren?"

There was no point in arguing. She crossed the fingers of her left hand and just to make sure her right hand too. "I promise, Mother."

"We'll deal with this tomorrow, young lady," Jane said, "and don't expect us to be lenient."

The motel room had fringed orange lampshades with scorch marks on. The faded yellow bedspread had seen better days. The blue rug was threadbare. But there was a television, and Nick found out there were soft drinks and a candy machine in the manager's office.

"It cost too much to get two rooms," he'd explained when she'd come back from the phone. "You don't mind sharin', do you?"

She didn't mind. She knew that when she got home it would all be over anyway – so why not make this a night to remember?

Once they were settled they both decided they were having a wonderful time. They'd stocked up with candy and potato chips, Cokes and 7-Ups, and now they sat cross-legged on the bed munching and watching an *I Love Lucy* re-run on television.

"This is great," Nick said, swigging Coke from the can.

"I can't believe we're here together," Lauren smiled, happily.

"Y'know," he said, "I always had you figured as a timid little small-town girl – frightened to make a move."

"Then why did you come after me?"

"'Cause I figured you were worth savin'."

"Thanks a *lot!*"

"You're welcome."

She began to laugh. "You look so silly with your nose all bandaged."

"Maybe I should rip 'em off. That doctor didn't seem to know what he was doin'."

"You were too handsome before."

"You thought I was handsome, huh?"

"Very."

"Not your type though?"

"Yes."

"Nope. You like 'em big an' beefy."

She reached for a pillow and threw it at him. "Will you *stop*."

"Only if you make me."

"I'll make you all right," she giggled, rolling on top of him, attempting to pin his arms to the bed.

With one swift move he reversed the situation and had her trapped beneath him. "Now you're my prisoner," he joked. "I can do anything I like."

"Go ahead," she whispered, suddenly serious. In her heart she knew that when they returned to the real world she would be forbidden to see him, and while she could she wanted to be as close to him as possible.

He was filled with mixed emotions. His body was urging him to go for it – but his head kept insisting he'd better hold back. Lauren Roberts wasn't just another one night conquest. She was pretty and sweet and talented and most of all special.

And yet he had a hard-on that could crack ice.

She gazed up at him, her eyes dreamy and inviting.

"Uh, y'know, maybe we shouldn't –" he began.

"Yes – we should," she said earnestly, reaching up to touch his face. "I'm ready, Nick. It's what I want. It's what we both want, isn't it?"

"Hey – only if you're sure –" he said, uncertainly.

"I'm *very* sure."

He started to kiss her, slowly at first, but as things began to heat up it was all he could do to control himself. For a girl who hadn't been around she could certainly kiss.

He reached under her sweatshirt, touching her breasts, groping for the clasp on her bra.

She helped him pull the sweatshirt over her head and went for the buttons on his shirt, tearing the material in her haste to get it off him.

He traced her breasts with the tips of his fingers – touching her softly, stroking her nipples until she began to make small gasping sounds.

Jeez! Her skin was like smooth satin, her hair long and silky fanning out over the sheets. And she smelt so clean and fresh. Most girls he'd slept with favoured heavy perfume and had cigarette breath. Dawn Kovak wore musk, he had to scrub to get her scent off him.

"Come on, Nick." Now she was leading *him*, reaching for his zipper, wriggling out of her jeans.

She had the longest legs he'd ever seen.

He peeled down her panties and tossed them on the floor, dipping his fingers, feeling her urgent need, and finally getting on top of her and carefully easing into the trip of a lifetime.

She opened up to him with no inhibitions. It was her first time but it didn't matter.

He broke through as gently as he could and took her all the way.

When they were both finished he held her in his arms – cradling her until she fell asleep, a smile on her face.

He'd made love a hundred times since the first time when he was thirteen – but never like this – never had feelings been part of it.

Lauren Roberts.

Lauren Angelo.

It sounded good.

He'd finally found a soul mate, and as far as he was concerned their lives were forever entwined.

Chapter 21

"You will *never* see him again," Phil Roberts thundered. "Do you understand me, Lauren? Do you?"

She understood him all right, and his harsh words came as no surprise – so why was her heart breaking into a thousand tiny pieces? Why was there a feeling of dread in the pit of her stomach? Why did she want to die?

She glanced over at her mother. Jane's mouth was set in a tightly compressed line. Lauren knew the expression – it meant *I'm not getting involved – don't ask me.*

"Daddy –" she began.

He held up his hand. "No! I do not wish to hear your excuses. What you did was unforgivable. Taking the car. Staying out all night."

"I called," she said, defiantly. "I explained the roads were closed. I *couldn't* get home."

"And as for the way you've treated Stock, it's beyond my comprehension."

"He's a jerk, Daddy. He called me a prick tease."

"Lauren!" gasped Jane.

"How dare you speak like that in front of your mother," Phil roared.

Lauren imagined herself as a stranger watching this dramatic family scene. Phil Roberts – red in the face, puffed up with self-righteous anger.

Jane Roberts – a faded beauty in a small town, her shoulders tense – standing by while her husband took charge.

And then there was Lauren. Sixteen years old and no longer a virgin. Sixteen years old and desperately, wildly, incredibly in love.

They couldn't stop her from seeing Nick. What were they

going to do – lock her in the house?

The moment she'd walked through the door they'd started on her.

Why did you break your engagement?

Nick Angelo is nothing but trash.

How can you do this to us?

What will people think?

Who cared what people thought? *She* certainly didn't. For once in her life she felt absolutely totally alive.

"Go to your room," her father said, harshly. "And stay there until we give you permission to come out."

Good. All she wanted was to be alone so she could think about Nick, re-live every wonderful, magical moment. The touch of him, the taste of him, the sheer thrill of being in his arms. She turned to go upstairs.

"We're very disappointed in you, Lauren." This from her mother.

Oh, go bake a cake! You have no idea who I am any more.

Her room was a mess, just the way she'd left it – her bed unmade, the sheets rumpled from Nick's overnight stay. She bent to sniff them, maybe catch his odour. Oh God! She had to see him again soon, she missed him already.

Her rock heroes – John Lennon and Emerson Burn – gazed down at her from above her bed. Once her idols, it now seemed silly to worship from afar. She unpinned the posters, rolled them up and put them in her closet. Then she stared at herself in the mirror, deciding that she looked exactly the same – no real change, except maybe the expression in her eyes. There was something new there – something intangible.

After making love she and Nick had slept in each other's arms all night as close as two people could be. And in the morning they'd made love again, and this time she'd enjoyed it even more. She'd cried out for him to fill her up, and then she'd cried out from sheer pleasure as her body jerked in response to his loving and she'd experienced a feeling so sensational, so amazing that she'd wanted to burst into happy tears.

"What was *that*?" she'd gasped.

"What?"

"That feeling I just had."

"You came," he'd told her.

"Came where?"

And he'd explained that making love wasn't only for the man's satisfaction.

"How do you know so much?" she'd asked, feeling a strong twinge of jealousy.

"'Cause I got taught by a whole bunch of older women. Now I can teach you."

She'd reached for him. "How about teaching me more?"

They didn't leave the motel until eleven in the morning. He drove slowly along the treacherous icy roads, while she snuggled next to him. By the time they reached Bosewell it was almost two thirty.

"I'll get off at the gas station," he'd said. "Unless you'd like me to come in an' face your parents with you. I don't mind."

"*I* do. It's better I handle them alone."

He'd pulled the car up across the street and jumped out. "I'll call you later."

She'd laughed and slid behind the wheel.

He'd come around and kissed her through the open window. "I . . . uh . . ."

She had a right to be demanding. "What? *Say* it?"

He'd attempted to make light of it. "I love ya."

"You too."

And she'd watched him run across the street – her hero in a blood-stained tux with a battered nose.

Now she was back to reality.

As soon as she reached the safety of her room she picked up the phone to call Meg and find out what had been going on in her absence. Before she'd finished dialling her father appeared at the door. "No phone privileges," he said, his face long and dour.

"But, Daddy –" she started to object.

"I said you will *not* use the phone," he repeated sternly, entering her room, pulling the phone from its jack and carrying it off under his arm.

They were angrier than she'd thought, probably because she'd broken up with Stock. It wasn't that they resented Nick, she rationalized, they didn't even know him. Maybe after a few weeks she could introduce him into their lives and they'd soon realize what a terrific guy he was.

The real truth was there was no way they could stop her from seeing him. School resumed in a couple of weeks and then she'd be with him every day whether her parents liked it or not.

Right now it was quite obvious they weren't going to let her out of the house. No car. No phone. No contact with friends. She was a prisoner. A prisoner with her thoughts.

Ah . . . but her thoughts were going to keep her very happy until she saw Nick again. Very happy indeed.

"You dumped on us," Harlan said accusingly, sitting on the steps outside the trailer, zinging pebbles at an empty can.

"Hey – couldn't help it. I had an accident. Take a look at my face," Nick said.

"You promised us a movie," Harlan said, glumly.

"I wasn't here," he explained, edging past him into the trailer. "I told you why."

Luke lay listlessly on top of the mattress he shared with Harlan.

"What's the matter with *him*?" Nick asked.

"I dunno," Harlan followed him in, shrugging. "He got sick."

"What's your ma say?"

"She ain't here."

He went over to Luke and placed his hand on his forehead. The kid was burning up.

"When did he get like this?"

"Dunno," Harlan said, sighing.

Nick stripped off his clothes realizing there was no way he could ever return the tuxedo. It was good that when Joey had checked out the clothes from the rental place he'd given a phoney address. "Where's Cyndra?" he asked, pulling on his jeans.

"Out with Joey." Harlan leaned against the door looking miserable.

"Tell you what," Nick said, cheerfully, "soon as Luke's better we'll go to that movie."

"You said that before."

"Yeah – but this time I ain't gonna be stuck in Ripley with a broken nose."

"You look funny," Harlan said, staring at him, his head on one side.

"Yeah, yeah, I know."

He wondered what Lauren was doing. After she'd dropped him at the gas station he'd worked for a couple of hours, but it was so quiet he'd finally made the trek home, picking up his bike from outside Dawn's without ringing her doorbell. Joey hadn't been at work, so he had no idea what the buzz around town was. He'd been planning on going back to the drugstore to see Louise and Dave, but now he didn't feel he should leave Luke.

"Anybody got a thermometer around here?" he asked.

Harlan gazed at him solemnly. "What that?"

"Forget it," he said, quickly. "Hang on, I'll ask Primo."

His father was in his usual position – stretched out like a sleeping rhino, snoring heavily. The television played loudly, and there were three cans of beer stacked in a row on the floor next to the bed. He wore a torn undershirt and dirty underpants. A half-eaten packet of potato chips spilled out on his chest.

Roughly Nick shook him until Primo came to, bleary-eyed and puce-faced. "Whassamatter? Wass goin' on?" he griped, burping loudly as he hoisted himself into a sitting position. His rheumy eyes focused on his son. "Wadda *you* wan'?"

"It's Luke," Nick said, trying to get through to him. "He's burnin' hot an' just lyin' there."

"Ain't my problem," Primo yawned, automatically reaching for a beer.

"It could be if anythin' happens to him," Nick said, hating his father even more if that was possible.

"Whyn't ya tell Aretha," Primo's attention was now taken by a bikini-clad blonde with jiggling tits cavorting across the television screen.

"She's at work," he said, shortly.

"Quit botherin' me. Throw a bucket a water over him – that'll cool him down 'til she gets back." Primo reached into his underpants and had a vigorous scratch. "An' don't tell her 'bout Luke 'til she done fixin' my supper."

For a moment Nick stood there trying to figure out what to do. Then he spotted the keys to the van on the table and swiped them on his way out. Fuck Primo. Fuck the fat pig.

By the time he got back to the other trailer Luke was breathing funnily.

He made a fast decision. "We're takin' him into town," he told Harlan. "Wrap him in a couple of blankets an' let's get movin'."

"Sit down, Aretha Mae," Benjamin Browning said.

Aretha Mae hovered in the doorway of his study, her expression wary and suspicious. "Why?"

Benjamin picked up a silver pen from his desk top and twirled it between his thick fingers. He did not relish the job Daphne had landed him with; the sooner it was done the better. "Because I say so," he said, irritably. "Come in. Close the door behind you and *sit down goddamnit*."

She did as he requested, albeit reluctantly. Once she was seated he swivelled his leather desk chair at an angle so that he didn't have to look her in the eye.

"Yes?" Her voice betrayed her impatience.

"I am terminating your employment," he said, coldly.

She was startled. "What you sayin'?"

"I'm firing you. Your services are no longer required."

A nerve twitched beneath her left eye. "Oh, they ain't, huh?"

"Mrs Browning and I have decided you deserve six weeks severance pay on account of your years of service with us." He passed a signed cheque across the desk. "Mrs Browning has requested that you do not return to work after today. Is that clear?"

"Clear . . ." she muttered.

He thought she was accepting her termination without argument. Thank God for that.

"Well . . ." he said, willing her to go quietly. "That's all."

"That's all," she repeated his words, not moving.

"You may go," he said, dismissing her with a cursory wave.

Aretha Mae stood up, placed both hands on his desk and glared at him. "I ain't goin' nowhere y' son-of-a-bitch," she said, forcing him to make eye contact.

He'd known she would try to cause trouble. It was too much to expect for her to go quietly. Once . . . many years ago when she'd first come to work for them she'd been lovely. Young and vibrant with long legs, big breasts and a sassy smile – just like Cyndra – a juicy little piece – hot and sexy. Now – seventeen years later – she was a dried-up bitter old woman. Skinny and wild-eyed with sunken cheeks and dyed red hair. Even Daphne had aged better than her, and Daphne was ten years older. Not that he fucked his wife any more, but once a year on their anniversary he made her get down on her knees and give him a suck. He knew how much she hated it, and it gave him immense pleasure to watch his penis vanish into that scarlet slash of a mouth. Daphne didn't dare refuse him. Daphne would never give up the grand title of Mrs Browning.

"I'm firing you," he repeated. "Don't you understand English? You *have* to go."

"No such thing as Aretha Mae havin' t'do nothin'," she snapped, sitting back down. "No such thing, an' you know it."

He threw his silver pen down on the desk, full of exasperation. "I'll double your severance pay if that's what you're after. Three months' money and out of here today."

"Ain't goin'," she said, stubbornly.

Now he was getting really angry. "Why not?"

"'Cause three months down the line I ain't got no job, no money, no nothin'."

"You can find another job."

"In Bosewell? No shit? What other family got themselves a full-time maid?"

"There's always work in the paper factory or the canning plant."

She jumped up again. "No!" she said, forcefully. "I work here – an' this'n where I stay."

He was silent for a moment before saying, "What do you want?"

"Same money I'se gettin' now for the rest a my natural life. An' five thousand dollars in the bank for my Cyndra. Oh, yeah, an' a lawyer's letter t'say I gets it regular."

"That's blackmail."

"*Your* word – ain't mine."

"And if I refuse?"

"Then the whole town gets t'know who Cyndra's daddy is, an' the filthy things y'done t'her."

"What are you saying?"

"You *know* what I'se sayin'. Cyndra's *your* child."

Benjamin paled. "It's . . . it's not possible."

"That it is."

"How?"

"Remember when I first came t'work here?"

His throat was restricted. "Yes."

"You was chasin' me day an' night – soon as your wife left the house you was after me – an' I was sleepin' in that room down in the basement. Well, one night you came there, held your hand over my mouth, an' shoved your thing inside me even though I didn't want it."

"You wanted it," he said, angrily. "After the first time you were begging for it."

"You got me pregnant an' I didn't know what t'do. So I ended up marryin' the first man who'd have me – an' we moved t' the trailer park. Thing is – when I told him I was pregnant he ran out on me – an' all these years I bin alone. But I kept on workin'

136

for you – an you kept on pokin' me 'till I wasn't young 'nuff for you no more."

"My wife and I supported you, and this is how you pay us back – by lying?"

She gave a hollow laugh. "Supported me – *sheeit*! I worked my black ass off for you an' your family, an' don' you forget it. Washin' your dirty underdrawers, cleanin' the shit in your johns, wipin' up all the mess."

"And now you're going to blackmail me with this far-fetched story?"

"I'm gonna get what's right for me an' that child a yours."

"She's not my child," he said, vehemently.

"Want me t'tell the town 'bout how you was screwin' me all those years? Want me to tell them how you raped your own daughter?"

"You wouldn't do that."

"Honey," she said, bitterly, "*I* ain't got nuttin' t'lose. How 'bout you?"

Chapter 22

Nick drove the van to the drugstore, parked in back, and entered through the kitchen, grabbing Louise as she passed by carrying an order of ham and eggs.

She stopped and let out a whistle. "Lookit you! Your damn face is one big mess."

"I need a doctor," he said, urgently.

"Seems like you should'a thought of that before."

"Not for me. Luke's sick – my kid brother. I got him in the van. Who can I take him to?"

"Gee . . ." She hesitated. "Doc Marshall's away, an' Doc Sheppard don't like bein' bothered at home."

"Where does he live?"

She placed her order on the counter and gave him her full attention. "What's wrong with the kid?"

"I dunno. He's hot, can't breathe good."

"Maybe I should take a look before you go waking up Doc Sheppard – he's an ornery old bastard." She untied her apron. "Hey – Dave –" she yelled, "I'm takin' a break; have Cheryl fill in."

Out in the van Luke was shivering uncontrollably. Harlan sat beside him looking miserable.

"Thought you said he was hot," Louise said accusingly, placing a hand on the child's forehead. "Oh, shit, yeah – he's hot all right."

"What do you think it is?" Nick asked.

"Dunno. But it ain't good." She climbed into the van. "Let's go – we'll wake up old Doc Sheppard. Hang a left, then take the second street on the right. An' Nick – put your foot down."

The bus ride took longer than ever. Aretha Mae sat by the

window gazing out. Usually she let her mind go blank – ridding herself of the cares of the day. But today she was filled with pent-up emotions – feelings she hadn't allowed to surface for seventeen years.

Benjamin Browning was Cyndra's father and she was glad she'd finally told him. Yes – glad to see the expression on his pompous white face when the full impact struck and he'd realized what he'd done.

Filthy pig. He was no good – only his money saved him from wallowing in the gutter.

With a deep sigh she recalled the day she'd started work at the Brownings. Her mother had answered an ad in the newspaper, and Mr Browning had agreed to pay her bus fare from Kansas City if she could start immediately. "My girl be there," her mother had assured him, delighted to be rid of one of seven daughters. Her mother had lied and said she was eighteen. The truth was she was barely fifteen and just out of school. "Work hard. Stay quiet. Don't get in no trouble." Those had been her mother's parting words.

Six months after she left home her mother was killed by a drunken driver. She had no father.

At first Aretha Mae liked working in a house with running water, indoor toilets, and unheard of luxuries like a refrigerator and TV. But Daphne Browning was not pleasant to work for. She'd recently given birth to Stock, and she had no intention of caring for the child unless he was clean and fresh at all times and never crying. Although she had all the housework to do, Aretha Mae soon found herself caring for the baby as well as attending to her other duties.

Benjamin Browning watched her like a tiger stalking its prey. She was aware of his lecherous eyes and roaming hands, but she managed to stay clear. He was in his early thirties then and quite good-looking. A self-made man with an abundance of energy and a canny mind. Daphne had pale skin, yellow hair and large breasts. They made love every night. Aretha Mae knew because she got to change the messy sheets.

The first night Benjamin came to her room he'd been out at a bachelor party. It was late, he was drunk, and she was asleep. He'd ripped the covers off her bed, placed a firm hand over her mouth, lifted her nightdress and thrust himself inside. She hadn't dared to complain. What good would it do? She had nowhere to run to.

139

When he was sure of her silence it became a weekly habit – sometimes twice or three times a week, depending on his mood.

After a while he stopped putting his hand over her mouth.

After a while – to her shame – she began looking forward to his nocturnal visits.

And then she got pregnant.

Aretha Mae was no fool – she knew if she mentioned it they'd throw her out, so she said nothing, merely bided her time, desperately taking hot baths, swigging gin when they were out, and hoping the baby growing in her belly would quietly go away.

Primo Angelo arrived in town at exactly the right time. He was a big handsome man with a cocksure swagger and a glint in his green eyes. A carpenter by trade he was doing work on the new school building. Aretha Mae did everything in her power to seduce him. She flattered him, babied him, told him he was the most handsome man she'd ever seen, and refused to sleep with him.

What was a man to do? He married her and they moved to the trailer park – although she did not give up her job at the Brownings.

Primo stopped working immediately. "I need my strength to make love to you," he told her. The man with the silver tongue and the lazy ass.

When she informed him she was pregnant he took off without so much as a fast goodbye. She was miserable for five minutes. Men – what could you expect? They were never faithful – never true.

When she had her baby everyone believed her vanished husband was the father. But she knew the truth, and she hugged it to herself like precious gold. One day the information would pay off.

Now – finally – that day had come.

The bus reached her stop and she climbed off, weary but triumphant. Benjamin Browning had agreed to her terms. He'd promised to arrange the papers with his lawyer, and soon – for the first time in her life – she'd be secure.

Doctor Sheppard lived in a large comfortable house with a big garden and a sign hanging over the front door that read: *COME*

ALL YE LITTLE SHEPHERDS AND GATHER HERE FOR SUSTENANCE AND COMFORT. Nick pounded on the door while Louise and Harlan stayed in the van with a steadily worsening Luke.

Nobody answered, so he pounded some more.

An upstairs window shot open and a white-haired old man in bright red pyjamas leaned out. "What's all that din?" he shouted in a crotchety voice.

"Somebody's sick. Can we come in?" Nick shouted back.

"Now?" replied Doctor Sheppard, his surprise evident.

"No, tomorrow morning, jerk," Nick muttered under his breath.

By this time Louise was beside him. "Doctor Sheppard," she yelled. "It's me. Louise. From the drugstore. Remember? You gave me that internal examination a couple of months ago. Said I had a lovely pelvis."

She'd succeeded in getting his attention. "I'll be right down," he croaked.

"Dirty old geezer," Louise said, disgustedly. "Stuck his finger up me like he was flippin' a pearl! Never again."

"You get the door open, I'll carry Luke inside," Nick said.

By the time he got back to the van Harlan was crying. "What's the matter, kid?" he asked.

"Is Luke gonna die?" Harlan worried, seeking assurance, tears rolling freely down his cheeks.

"No, he ain't gonna die," Nick assured him, gathering Luke up into his arms. "Don't think nothin' like that. You stay out here – he'll be fine."

He carried the small boy up to the house, not sure what was going to happen – he only knew it didn't look good.

Louise had the door open and was proceeding to charm Doctor Sheppard – a short man with hairy hands, a halo of white hair and big pop eyes. He was old and crusty and took a lot of charming.

"What's this?" he said, when Nick appeared with Luke in his arms.

"This child is sick," Louise said quickly. "Can you take a look at him, Doc? *Please.*"

"I'm off-duty," the miserable old man said.

"I know." Louise kept her voice soft and persuasive. "But I figured you'd do us this one favour – what with Doc Marshall bein' away an' all, an' you bein' the only doctor left in town."

She paused, giving him a seductive look. "I'm coming in to see you next week. I had those stomach cramps again, thought you could look me over."

Doctor Sheppard cheered up.

Louise continued to pour it on. "I guess I need another of those . . . uh . . . exams you're so good at giving. I felt so much better after the last time."

"Yes, yes," the old man said. "Bring the boy into the examining room."

She winked at Nick. He carried Luke into the examining room and laid him on the cold table.

The doctor bent down and peered at Luke. "This boy is black," he said, indignantly.

So? Nick wanted to say. *What the fuck does that matter?*

"We thought he was too sick to drive to Ripley," Louise said, quickly.

"That's where *black* people are supposed to go," Doctor Sheppard muttered bad-temperedly, rubbing his bulbous nose with the tip of his thumb. "I'm not supposed to look after coloureds."

"Hey –" Nick couldn't help himself. "It's nineteen seventy-four for God's sake, an' we ain't even in the South."

Doctor Sheppard turned to glare at him. "Who are you, young man? I've never seen you before."

"Thank God for that," Nick muttered, and then loud enough for the Doctor to hear, "I'm his brother."

Doctor Sheppard's bushy eyebrows shot up. "His brother?"

"Just take a look at the kid, will you?"

Ten minutes later they were out of there. "Nothing wrong with the boy," Doctor Sheppard had said. "All he needs is a good night's sleep and an aspirin."

Nick didn't believe him, but what could he do? "How about that other doctor he was talking about – the one in Ripley?" he asked Louise.

She shrugged. "I dunno. Never heard of him. I'm sorry, I gotta get back to work. Dave's gonna be pissed, y'know what he's like."

He dropped Louise off and began the drive to the trailer park. Maybe the old doctor was right – maybe all Luke needed was rest and an aspirin.

On the way home he spotted Aretha Mae trudging along the side of the road. He swerved over to the side.

142

"What you doin' with your father's van, boy?" Aretha Mae asked, sharply.

Quickly he explained about Luke. She jumped in the back, took one look at Luke and was as panicked as he was.

"I told him not to play out in the snow," she fretted, "I told him he was gonna catch cold. He's got somethin' bad, I know it."

"Yeah," Nick agreed. "That's why I took him to see Doctor Sheppard."

"That dumb old fool – he's no good," she said, shaking her head in disgust. "He won't treat us – whatever the law says. We gotta take him to Ripley."

"The roads ain't clear yet. It took hours to get back earlier."

"We have t'go," Aretha Mae said, obstinately.

"What about Primo? He don't know I've taken the van."

"Too bad," she said.

"Okay," he shrugged. "Ripley it is."

He drove as fast as he could considering the conditions of the roads – even so, it was midnight by the time they reached Ripley.

Aretha Mae directed him to a house in a run-down neighbourhood, and when he got there she jumped out of the van and rang the bell.

An Indian woman in a sari answered the door. She didn't seem at all surprised to have patients arriving in the middle of the night.

"It's my child," Aretha Mae said. "He be real bad."

"Bring him in," the woman said, graciously. "I'll fetch my husband."

Doctor Singh Amroc was a slightly built Indian man, totally bald with a thin black moustache. After a cursory examination of Luke he said, "This boy has pneumonia. It's essential he's admitted to a hospital at once."

They all set off, crowding into the van, the doctor too.

On the way to the hospital Nick began thinking about Lauren. He hadn't called her, would she be mad? Girls were funny about things like phoning when you said you would – and yet he was sure that when he explained everything she'd understand.

He wondered if her parents had given her a hard time. He missed her already and couldn't wait to see her again.

At the hospital he sat in the waiting room with Harlan while the Doctor and Aretha Mae filled out the forms to get Luke admitted.

Harlan stared at his half-brother. "Thanks, Nick," he said, solemnly. "You're my best friend."

"Hey –" he shrugged, embarrassed, "it was nothing."

Primo's rumbling stomach awoke him. Bleary-eyed he groped for the large clock ticking away on the floor. It was late, very late, and where the hell was Aretha Mae?

He staggered to his feet, brushed a scurrying cockroach off the side of the bed and rolled outside, taking a piss in the nearby brush.

Then he lurched back inside, grabbed a can of beer and sat and brooded. After ten minutes he went outside again and kicked open the door of the kids' trailer. Nobody was around.

"Where *the fuck* is everybody?" he yelled. "Where *the fuck* is my dinner?"

Outside he noticed his van was missing. "Goddamn it!" he muttered, making his way back to the main trailer. The bitch had taken his van and the kids. The bitch would pay for being home late. *Nobody* treated him this way. *Nobody* kept Primo Angelo waiting and got away with it.

Luke had to stay in hospital.

"There ain't no way I'm leavin'," Aretha Mae said, her mouth set in a stubborn line. "No way at all."

"Hey – if you're stayin', we're stayin'," Nick said.

She shook her head. "No – you'd best get back. When Primo finds his van's missin' he'll be mad."

"I'm not goin' back without you and Luke."

"Yeah, me too, Ma," Harlan joined in.

"Suit yourself." She was too tired to argue.

"I know a cheap motel," Nick said. "We can all spend the night there."

"What'll we do about Primo?" Aretha Mae worried.

"I'll call Joey in the morning. He'll stop by the trailer an' tell him what's goin' on."

She nodded. "Good. Now you take Harlan to this motel while I stay here."

"Why don't we stay with you?"

"No," she shook her head. "Don't want Harlan comin' down sick, too. You go rest up."

Reluctantly he got up. "We'll be back first thing tomorrow."

"You got money, boy?"

"Well . . . dunno if I've got enough."

"Here." She rummaged in her purse and counted out fifteen dollars in worn bills.

"Thanks," he said, pocketing the money. "We'll get back here early."

They left the hospital and drove straight to the motel. The man in the manager's office recognized him. "You here again?" he said, winking lewdly. "Must've been a good one."

Nick ignored the comment. "We'll be stayin' one night," he said, paying in advance.

He took Harlan into the room, settled him in front of the television and hurried to the pay phone. For a moment he stood in the ice-cold booth wondering if he could phone Lauren at this late hour. No way. It was even too late to contact Joey – his mother would be seriously pissed. Shit! There was nothing left to do except go to bed. He'd call everyone in the morning.

Harlan awoke at six a.m. "I gotta bad feeling, my gut hurts," he whined.

"Hey –" Nick got out of bed and stretched. "Don't worry about it. Everything's gonna be fine."

Harlan shook his head. "No, it ain't, Nick. It ain't."

"Quit worryin' an' get dressed. We'll get to the hospital early."

Outside the wind was howling. Shivering, Nick pulled up the collar of his jacket, stuffed his hands in his pockets and ran over to the van. Harlan followed him and jumped in the passenger seat.

Five minutes later they were standing at the hospital reception. "Luke Angelo," Nick said.

The nurse consulted her admittance book. "Ward Five, fifth floor."

They took the elevator. At reception on the fifth floor Nick asked again, "We're here to see Luke Angelo."

The nurse glanced up. "Relative?" she enquired.

"Yeah – I'm like . . . uh . . . his brother."

"The doctor is with Mrs Angelo right now," the nurse said, all business. "Please take a seat."

"Uh, Luke . . . he's okay, right?"

"Take a seat."

They waited over ten minutes before Aretha Mae appeared, clutching her thin winter coat – a Brownings cast-off – around her.

Harlan ran down the corridor and clung to his mother's legs.

Nick knew it before she said a word. He got up and walked slowly towards her. His throat was dry and his stomach churning.

Aretha Mae shook her head, hopelessly. "He's gone," she said, her voice no more than a hoarse whisper. "My baby is dead."

Harlan let out a wail that could be heard from one side of the hospital to the other. It was a sound Nick would never forget.

Chapter 23

"Did Nick call?" Every morning Lauren asked the same question, and every morning her parents gave her the same stupid answer. "It doesn't matter whether he did or not. You are *never* seeing him again."

"I don't care," she replied, her heart beating fast. "I just need to know."

"It makes no difference," her father said, harshly.

"It makes a difference to me," she replied, wondering how she had ever imagined her father to be a kind and sensitive man.

"Then in that case he has *not* called you."

She didn't know whether they were telling the truth or not. She sat in her room and brooded. Did Nick consider her easy? Is sex all he'd wanted? *Oh, God, no! Please God, no!*

They'd been so close and now they seemed so far apart. She knew he didn't have a phone, so she couldn't call him. Not that her parents would let her get within ten feet of a telephone. They had her trapped in the house, guarding her as if she was a maximum security prisoner.

"What have I done that's so terrible?" she asked one day.

"You were engaged to one of the finest boys in town," her father replied, his face stony. "You should have taken into consideration that I was doing business with Stock's father before recklessly breaking off your engagement."

"I didn't realize it was a business arrangement," she muttered.

"You owed us the information," her father said.

She couldn't believe they were being so mean. "I've never done anything to upset you in my life," she said. "No alcohol, drugs or any of the things some of the kids at school get into. All I did was borrow the family car, and you're punishing me like I'm a criminal."

Together – the perfect team. "You have to learn the hard way, Lauren, or you won't learn at all."

"What will happen when school starts?" she asked. "You can't watch over me every day then."

"When the new semester commences we hope you'll have learnt your lesson," Phil said.

And what if I haven't? she wanted to reply. *What if the first time I see Nick we run off together?*

As if reading her mind her mother chimed in with, "If you see Nick Angelo at school, I want your solemn promise you'll have nothing to do with him."

She crossed her fingers behind her back, a habit she was getting used to. "Okay, Mother, if that makes you happy."

Yeah. Good little Lauren was learning to play the game their way – and it was their fault.

On her first day back she bumped into Meg on the way to history class.

"OhmiGod! OhmiGod!" Meg exclaimed excitedly. "I've been *desperate* to see you. I've called you *dozens* of times. I even came by your house and begged your mom. She wouldn't let me in. What *is* going *on?*"

"*You* tell *me*," Lauren said. "I've been held prisoner, cut off from everything."

Meg lowered her voice. "There's been rumours you were *pregnant* and had to have an abortion."

"Are you serious? Surely *you* know what happened?"

"You mean at the New Year's dance?"

"Right – when Stock hit Nick, broke his nose, and I drove him to the hospital in Ripley. I'm sure you heard we got stuck there overnight, the roads were closed and we couldn't get back. My parents were furious."

"Oh," Meg said, sounding disappointed, "is that all?"

"Isn't that enough?"

Meg wanted to know more. "What happened with you and Nick?"

"Nothing," Lauren lied. "I was punished for absolutely nothing."

"Nick Angelo is the worst. How come you drove him to the hospital? Stock's been so upset. Mack and I have tried to look after him, but he's like – heartbroken." Meg shook her head. "You treated him badly."

Lauren was incensed. "*I* treated *him* badly? How about the way *he* carried on?"

148

Meg continued as if she hadn't heard a word. "Throwing his ring at him and everything. *I* heard it was Nick tried to attack *him* and *that's* why Stock broke his nose – he was only defending himself."

"That's not true."

"Yes, it is. Nick Angelo is a real deadbeat. Look what he did to me."

Lauren attempted to remain calm. "What *did* he do to you, Meg?"

"Practically raped me."

She had a strong desire to smack her friend's smug face. "Oh, and I suppose you didn't provoke it?"

"What do you mean?"

"It seems to me that every time you go out with a boy the same thing happens."

Meg flushed. "It certainly doesn't."

"I thought you were my friend," Lauren said, sadly.

"And I thought you were a friend worth having," Meg replied, with a spiteful toss of her blonde curls.

Miserably Lauren sat in class, her eyes searching the room for Nick. He failed to appear.

Shortly before lunch break she spotted Joey in the corridor and hurried over. "Hi. Can we talk?"

He gave her a dirty look. "Oh, *you* resurfaced, huh?"

"What does *that* mean?"

"It would've been nice if you'd called Nick after all that happened."

"After *what* happened?"

"His little brother dying and all."

She was genuinely shocked. "*What?*"

He could see she wasn't acting. "You didn't hear?"

"I've been grounded since New Year's."

Joey felt uncomfortable. "I'm sorry. Nick told me you wouldn't talk to him."

She wondered how much Joey knew. "Why would I avoid him?" she asked, carefully.

"He called your house enough times. Your parents said you didn't want to speak to him."

"That was them talking – not me. Please, Joey, tell me what happened?"

"His half-brother got sick with pneumonia. Doc Sheppard refused to treat him, so they had to take him to another doctor in Ripley. The kid died in hospital there."

149

"Oh, God! That's so awful."

"Yeah."

"Where is Nick? I have to see him."

"He won't be back in school."

"Why not?"

"He was thrown out on account of your boyfriend."

"You mean expelled?"

"Yeah – the Browning family didn't want him around – they put on the pressure. Course it didn't help that he smashed up the sign in front of Doc Sheppard's house, and threatened to beat the shit outta the old fart."

"He did?"

"Yeah, Cyndra went with him. The old fuck called the Sheriff. Nick spent the night in the can. Cyndra wanted to join him – but I managed to persuade her it wasn't the coolest move in the world."

"Where is he now?" she asked, thinking about what he must have gone through.

"Workin' down at the garage full-time. Old man Browning tried to stop that too – but George wouldn't listen. If the Brownings had their way they'd run him out of town."

"Can you take me there?"

"Sure, but if we get caught there'll be big trouble."

"Don't tell *me* about trouble."

"Okay. Meet me in the parking lot in five minutes."

"I'll be there."

"An' don't mention it to your big-mouthed girlfriend either. She's real tight with Stock an' all his buddies."

"I understand."

She hurried to her locker and grabbed her purse and jacket. On her way downstairs she ran straight into Stock and a group of his ever-present cronies. Their eyes met. The group went silent.

"Uh . . . hi," she said, trying to make the most of an awkward situation.

Stock's jaw tightened, his right eye twitched, his hand strayed toward his crotch and he totally ignored her – pushing by as if she didn't exist.

Okay with me, she thought. *If that's the way you want it, Stock Browning, I can handle it.*

Joey was waiting out in the parking lot revving up the engine of his motorcycle. "Climb aboard," he instructed. "We'd better split before we get ourselves busted."

150

She jumped on the back of his bike and they took off. Whatever the consequences she didn't care. She was on her way to see Nick, and that's all that mattered.

Chapter 24

"Thanks, sweetie." The woman in the maroon Cadillac had enormous breasts stretching the confines of a tight pink sweater. She'd been in twice this week to gas up her car – not that she needed to, the second time he'd almost had an overflow at three gallons.

Nick strolled casually around the car. "Want me to check your oil an' water?" he asked.

"Why not, sweetie?"

While he was checking under the hood he noticed she was checking out her face in a flashy silver compact. The woman scrutinized. First the eyes – heavily mascaraed and outlined in black. Next the nose – powder, powder. And lastly the lips – full, sexy lips glossed and ready for action. She had long reddish hair and wore a fur coat which did not succeed in covering her outstanding sweater-clad breasts. She was old, at least thirty. Nick was an expert at figuring women's ages.

"Who is she?" he'd asked George, the first time she'd come in.

"Never seen her before," George had said, chewing tobacco. "Illinois plates – must be visiting."

"You got a johnnie here?" the woman asked, snapping shut her compact.

"A what?"

"Little girl's room."

He pointed.

She got out of the car.

She was tall – which was fortunate Nick thought, because with the pair she was carrying falling flat on her face was a distinct possibility. Her fur coat ended at the hip. Under it she wore a short skirt and thigh-high black patent leather boots.

"You from around here?" he asked, knowing she wasn't.

She ran her tongue across her front teeth. "Passing through on my way to civilization. Staying a week with my sister."

"Having fun?" He could have kicked himself. What kind of a dumb question was that. How could anyone have fun in Bosewell?

She looked him over slowly – seductive eyes raking him from top to bottom. "Nope," she said, sauntering off to the rest room.

George winked conspiratorially. "She's got the hots for you, boy. Better watch it! Didja get an eye-full of those gazumbas? Wouldn't mind a mouthful myself." George began to chuckle and wheeze.

A few weeks ago, Nick thought, this woman might have been a challenge. But now . . . who cared? All he was interested in was making money – plenty of money – and as soon as he'd saved five hundred bucks he was on his way out of this pisshole.

The woman had left her open purse on the front seat. He noticed her wallet poking out – crammed with bills. When she came back he pointed it out to her. "You shouldn't leave your purse open like that – it's askin' for trouble."

"Story of my life," she said, smiling laconically. "How was my oil?"

"Fine."

"I don't need anything?"

"You're perfect."

She handed him a credit card and he put it through the machine. Genevieve Rose. He'd already noticed the wedding ring – a fat band of diamonds.

"Where you from?" he asked, as she signed with a flourish.

"Chicago. Ever been there?"

"My friend has. His dad was a cop."

Another dumb remark. Jeez! What was the matter with him today?

"A cop, huh? The worst kind." She slipped him a five-buck tip and drove off without another word.

"Hey – she gave me a five," he told George.

"Frame it," George said. "It's the first an' last time you'll see a tip like that."

"Yeah." He went into the rest room and sniffed – her perfume lingered. He rinsed his face with cold water and noticed the mirror above the sink was still cracked, George said it wasn't worth having fixed. Peering at himself he gingerly touched his nose. It wasn't the same – it would never be the same – but it didn't look too bad. Not straight like before, slightly bent and rough looking. But somehow it gave his face more character and certainly made him appear older than seventeen. Betty Harris said his broken nose gave his face a strength it hadn't had before.

He wasn't sure.

"When you're famous you can always have it fixed," she'd said.

Famous! Holy shit! For her to say a thing like that was a compliment indeed.

Betty Harris had turned out to be the one constant presence he could trust. Now that he no longer had school to contend with he divided his time between work for money and work for pleasure. The long sessions with Betty Harris were pure pain mixed with intense pleasure. Acting satisfied him in a way nothing else had. Since he was thirteen he'd always had sex to get lost in, but after Lauren, mindless sex did not hold the same appeal, so now he took all of his pent-up energy and channelled it into the roles Betty allowed him to play. Hamlet was a particular favourite, and Stanley in *Streetcar*. Oh yeah, he could really let rip – pouring every emotion into the highly charged complex characters.

Betty was impressed. She praised him constantly, and her encouragement really helped. When he'd got himself thrown into jail for messing up the outside of Doctor Sheppard's house, Betty had put up his bail. He'd been charged with defacing property. If he'd had his way he'd have defaced the old white-haired gnome of a doctor from here to eternity. But for the old man Luke might still be alive.

After the initial shock Aretha Mae had reverted to her usual stoic self. Primo was unaffected – Luke hadn't meant anything to him. Cyndra was sad. And Harlan inconsolable. Night after night Nick listened to the kid sob himself to sleep. A few times Cyndra took Harlan into her bed and comforted him with stories and songs. Sometimes Nick joined in. The three of them formed a bond. For the first time since his mother died he really felt he had a family.

Primo had tried to cause trouble over him borrowing the van. For once Aretha Mae shut him up with an acid tongue-lashing he wouldn't forget in a hurry. Primo had slunk off like a beaten dog.

When they'd thrown him out of school he hadn't bothered telling his father. What was the point? George gave him a permanent job at the garage, and every buck he made he put away – stashing it under his mattress – watching the pile of bills grow larger every week.

As for Lauren – he'd shut her out of his mind. When he didn't hear from her . . . when there was never any message, he'd felt a deep sense of betrayal. He'd opened himself up to another human being and look where it had gotten him – exactly nowhere. Never again. Love – you could shove it.

Emerging from the rest room he bumped into George, who said, "You got a visitor. Use the office."

"Who?" he asked, but George was off doing something else.

He entered the small, crowded office and there she was – Lauren – perched on the edge of the old warped desk, looking as beautiful as ever.

"Hi," her soft voice was almost a whisper.

Jeez! Who needed this? "What're *you* doin' here?" he asked, roughly.

She got off the desk and came towards him. "I made Joey bring me."

"Good for him."

"I came as soon as I could."

"A few weeks late," he said coldly, "but I s'pose you were busy."

"My parents wouldn't let me out. I had no idea what happened." She moved closer. "Nick, I'm so sorry to hear about your brother. I didn't know. I thought I'd see you in school today and when I didn't . . ." She trailed off, shrugging helplessly. "You've got to forgive me – it wasn't my fault."

It sounded logical. Only why had both her parents sounded so sincere when they'd informed him she had no wish to speak to him and would he kindly stop bothering her? Still . . . parents . . . those fuckers could lie better than anyone.

He made one last effort to back away. "Hey – I'm cool, you don't havta feel sorry for me."

Her eyes filled with tears. "Sorry for you? Is that what you think?"

"Listen, it's –"

"I *love* you," she interrupted, her voice breaking. "I honestly love you."

Her words melted the ice, and suddenly she was in his arms, soft and sweet-smelling. There was no way he could resist her. There was no way he wanted to.

They talked for over an hour, clearing everything up, and by the time she left, they'd worked things out. Joey would be their liaison – he'd deliver notes and set up meetings.

"One of these days I'll talk my parents into you," Lauren

promised, "and then we can be together as much as we want."

Yeah, he thought, *don't bet on it*. Parents and him – not a good mix.

She kissed him before leaving. She wasn't even gone and he couldn't wait to see her again.

"Soon," she promised.

He wasn't so sure it would be as easy as she thought.

Chapter 25

And that's how they handled it – as carefully and secretly as possible. Of course, there's no such thing as a secret once more than two people know. Joey knew, and Cyndra. Harlan, of course, and George – who confided in Louise and Dave.

As the months passed and they grabbed furtive meetings here and there, Lauren began to show the strain of lying to her parents. She'd become an expert at inventing elaborate excuses that wouldn't rouse their suspicions, but still it was tough.

Nick felt it too. He didn't want to pressure her, but being with her in short sharp bursts was doing him no good. He wasn't a kid, and he was beginning to think he couldn't take one more evening of groping and fumbling – he needed more. He needed to be as close to her as two people can get.

As the weather improved and Spring took root he came up with the idea of bringing her to the trailer. Harlan was at school, Cyndra at work, and Primo never stirred.

The trailer was hardly the ideal place – but it was a lot better than the old abandoned car in the back of the gas station where they'd been forced to spend most of their time together.

He set it up, arranging for Joey to bring her to meet him at the gas station.

She was excited when he told her of his plans, and on the appointed day she warned her parents she was doing community service after school and would be home later than usual.

The day of their meeting dawned crisp and sunny. Lauren had settled into a stilted polite relationship with her parents. They thought she'd forgotten all about Nick Angelo – the bad boy who'd come to town and disrupted her life. Little did they know.

She left for school at the usual time, entered through the

front, avoided roll call and exited through the back. She knew she was living dangerously; skipping school was full of risks – the wrong word in the wrong place and she could be busted; then what?

The risk was worth it.

Fortunately she didn't run into anyone likely to question her. The close friendship she'd had with Meg was long over. Meg was part of Stock's group now, and Stock refused to speak to her.

How her life had changed over the last few months – and yet she was happier than she'd ever been.

Joey was revving up his bike in the parking lot ready to go. "Come on," he said. "Jump aboard an' let's get the fuck outta here."

At first it was awkward – the trailer being such a dump and all. Nick had tried to clean it up – shoving all the clothes into a corner, smoothing out the worn blanket on his mattress, but there wasn't much he could do to improve twelve square feet of space shared by three untidy people.

He could see Lauren was shocked by the shabby conditions, but she covered it well.

"Okay, so it's a pisshole," he said with a cocky grin. "But who promised you The White House?"

She pretended to look solemn. "I'll have to leave then."

"Yeah?"

"Maybe."

"Oh, really?"

"I think so."

"Come here."

"Why?"

"You know why."

He fell on the mattress, pulling her down beside him. They started to kiss, slowly at first – savouring each other's lips – and then faster until they both wanted it to be more.

He moved his hands under her sweater feeling her breasts. "I've missed you so much," he mumbled, working his way under her bra, trying to concentrate on something other than the feeling he was experiencing.

"You too," she managed.

He pulled her sweater over her head and unclipped her bra,

bending to kiss her breasts – his tongue moving slowly from nipple to nipple.

She sighed – a long drawn out sound.

It was too much. The moment of no return was upon them before either of them had time to stop and think, and even though she'd planned to ask him to wear a rubber – who cared? It didn't matter. Nothing mattered except the fusing of their two bodies.

He was more aggressive than the time before – entering her with a burst of energy – riding her like his life depended on it. And now that she knew what to expect she responded with a wildness and abandon she had not known she possessed.

Together they rocked the world – riding the roller-coaster until it peaked on the highest point of all – pausing for several mind-blowing seconds – before cruising smoothly all the way to stop.

"Oh . . . jeez!" he exclaimed. "That was the best ever."

"It was?"

"It was."

"Me too."

"C'mere, me too."

And she curled into his arms, wet and sticky, and fell into a blissful sleep.

When she awoke it was afternoon and he was lying on his back beside her, hands behind his neck. Slowly she traced the contours of his chest with her tongue – tentatively at first because she wasn't sure if he'd like it. He obviously loved it – so she really got into it – licking and sucking – teasing him with little love bites.

"Where'd you learn t'do this?" he asked, groaning.

"Hmm . . . wouldn't *you* like to know?"

"Yeah," he reached for her breasts but she brushed his hand away. "I think I would."

"Lie back and enjoy it," she said, leisurely travelling down his body until she reached his hard penis.

"Lauren –" he began. "You don't havta –"

"Yes I do," she whispered, teasing him with her tongue. "Because I want to."

By late afternoon they both knew they had to make a move. "You'd better get dressed," he said, wishing they could stay in bed forever.

"Uh . . . where's the bathroom?"

"I don't know how t'break this to you, but we ain't got one."

She thought he was joking and laughed.

159

"No, seriously – we don't."

"No bathroom?"

"Sorry."

"Where do you shower?"

"Down at the gas station. It's not exactly a shower – but I don't think you want the details."

She felt bad that she'd asked, she didn't want to embarrass him.

"Maybe we can come here every week," he said, getting up and pulling on his jeans. "Just you an' me – shut out the world."

"I can't take too many days off school."

"Yeah. An' I suppose George wouldn't be too happy if I ducked work on a regular basis."

"Nick," she stared at him, her face composed and serious, "What if I got –"

"Whoa – *no way*! I pulled out in time."

She was relieved. "You did?"

"Course I did. Wouldn't risk it."

"Thank goodness."

"Hey – you gotta learn to trust me – y'know that I . . . uh . . ."

"Say it!"

He grinned – "Love ya."

She smiled and softly touched his face. "Yes, I know."

"How was school today?"

"Huh?" Lauren tried to squeeze past her mother – who was standing in the front hall blocking the stairs.

"School?" Jane Roberts repeated.

If Lauren wasn't so intent on getting upstairs she would have noticed a tenseness in her mother's voice.

"Oh, the usual – boring math – dull history. And P.E. I *hate* P.E. In fact the showers were out of order – I feel all sweaty – maybe I'll take a shower now."

Jane did not budge. "Anything unusual happen?"

Warning bells rang in Lauren's head. Something had gone on at school that she didn't know about.

Gotta play it smart, Roberts. Wouldn't do to get busted.

"The thing is, Mother," she said quickly, "I wasn't going to worry you – but after P.E. I didn't feel so good. The nurse suggested I lay down for a while."

"Really?" Jane's tone did not warm up. Usually she would have been full of concern.

160

There was a short, uncomfortable silence. Since her mother didn't seem inclined to move, she decided to head for the kitchen. Jane followed her in – there was no escape.

Opening the ice-box she grabbed a carton of milk and turned around to find her mother staring at her with cold, accusing eyes.

She couldn't take it any more. "Is something wrong?"

"Why do you ask?"

She shrugged, reaching for a glass. "I don't know. You seem kind of . . . funny."

She wondered if she could make a dash past Jane and get upstairs without further questioning.

"Lauren," her mother said, in slow measured tones. "We've always brought you up to be a good girl. Truthful at all times."

Oh God, something was definitely up.

She tried to look innocent. "Yes, Mother?"

"You weren't at school today, were you?"

Now she had a choice. Did she continue to lie and take a chance? Or did she tell the truth?

Dear Mother, I spent the day in bed having sex with Nick Angelo.

Did you, dear? How nice.

Gee, thanks, Mom, you're so understanding.

She bit her bottom lip – there was only one way to go. "I told you, I *was* at school, but I didn't feel good."

"The school secretary phoned to inform me you have probably been playing truant on and off for the last few months."

She managed to look amazed. "What?"

"Apparently you've been absent on several occasions with various excuses. A sore throat, a cold, a visit to the dentist. And all your excuse notes were supposedly signed by me. Miss Adams is no fool. Eventually she became suspicious – especially as this morning you were seen leaving on the back of a motor-cycle."

Oh God, here it came. She was in deep trouble.

"We've always trusted you, Lauren, and now this. Your father is on his way home."

Naturally.

"It's *your* fault," she blurted out, her cheeks reddening. "You can't stop me from seeing Nick. We're in love."

"In love?" Jane laughed, derisively. "You're sixteen years old, what do *you* know about love?"

More than you think, she wanted to yell out. *More than you'll ever know.*

161

Words came tumbling out. "Don't you understand? Nick doesn't have anybody except me. I can't turn my back on him like everyone else. I can't do it."

"You'll do exactly what your father and I say you will."

Dread swept over her. This was no idle threat. Somehow she was going to have to deal with it.

Chapter 26

"We're outta here," Joey said.

"Huh?" Nick slid from under the Lincoln he was servicing. "Whatcha talkin' about?"

"I mean we're leavin' town, me and Cyndra."

"You don't have enough money," Nick said, wiping oil off his hands.

"Sure we do," Joey replied. "I bin workin' two jobs, remember? And Cyndra's bin doin' time at the factory. We've had it here."

Joey and Cyndra – the two people he was closest to were taking off. Wasn't it bad enough that he couldn't see Lauren any more?

"Anyway," Joey said, lighting up a butt, "we did some talkin' – an' we figured if you wanted to come with us it's okay."

"Where you plannin' on goin'?"

Joey shrugged. "Chicago. I got relatives there, friends, people who'd put us up until we find a place."

"You told your mother?"

Joey dragged on the butt, inhaling every last bit of smoke into his lungs. "Are you shittin' me? I'll leave her a note. She'll freak whatever I say."

"How about Cyndra?"

"She ain't tellin' nobody, only you." He dropped the butt on the ground crushing it underfoot. "We're goin' tomorrow."

Nick shook his head. "Jeez! Tomorrow! Like how about givin' me notice?"

"I know it's kinda sudden, but if we don't do it now we'll never make the move. You comin' with us or not?"

He was torn. Sure he wanted to go, but how could he leave Lauren? Even though he hadn't seen her for six weeks he still loved her. It wasn't her fault she'd gotten busted – it was his – he should have made certain they were more careful.

Things were a mess. They'd really blown it. Her parents had gone crazy. Phil Roberts had even turned up at the trailer. He'd listened when Phil had attempted to confront Primo – like the fat slob gave a shit. Some fucking joke.

"I want your assurance your son will have nothing more to do with my daughter," Phil Roberts had said, standing stiffly at the door.

"What in hell ya talkin' about? Get the fuck outta here," Primo had replied, a true gentleman.

Phil Roberts had retreated fast.

Nick unbuttoned his greasy overalls. "I dunno what t'say, Joey. I'm real tempted."

"Look . . . I understand it ain't easy."

"I can't run out on Lauren without seein' her."

"Whyn't you write her a letter? Tell her you'll be back for her when you got the bucks."

"Like when?"

"What am I? A fortune teller? Who knows? But you're sure not securin' any future for the two of you hangin' 'round here."

Joey was right. If he took off he could do anything he wanted – start a new life – anything – and when Lauren was eighteen she could tell her parents to screw off and they'd be together.

"Let me think about it," he said, peeling off his overalls.

"Don't think – do," Joey encouraged. "'Cause I ain't plannin' on endin' up here – an' neither is Cyndra. We're on our way, Nick – an' if you're smart you'll come with us."

He thought about it all day, and the more he thought, the more appealing the prospect became. Take off. Say goodbye to Primo, Bosewell, all the negative shit that plagued his life. Jeez – it was tempting.

Then he began thinking about Harlan. How could he dump the kid? Especially with Cyndra leaving too.

Hey man, what are you, a babysitter? Think about yourself for a change.

He needed to see Lauren but that wasn't possible. Writing her a letter seemed like a good idea. He could explain everything so she'd understand. That way she wouldn't think he'd run off without her.

After work he stopped by the drugstore. Louise greeted him, her usual cheery self. "What's up, Nick?"

"I need a big favour."

"What else is new?"

"Can you see Lauren gets a letter if I leave it with you?"

"You mean hand it to her when she comes in?"

"Yeah. Only not if she's with her mother."

"No problem."

"Lend me a pen an' paper, I gotta write it."

Louise was obliging as ever; she set him up with paper and pen and he hunched in a corner booth trying to figure out what to write.

Dear Lauren, I'm going, but I'll be back for you. It's dumb for me to hang around since we can't see each other anyway, so I'll keep in touch and you'll always know where I am.

It didn't exactly cut it. He tried again.

Dearest Lauren.

Too formal. And once more . . .

Lauren – I miss you so much that every night when I go to sleep all I can think about is you. I see your face. I feel your body. I smell you.

Nah, that sounded rude. He started again, and finally got the words right. Then he sealed it in an envelope, marked her name on it, adding a large PRIVATE! and URGENT! on the front. Now all he had to do was tell Joey he was going with them.

As he left the drugstore, Stock Browning drove up and got out of his car with a couple of his cronies. He swaggered past Nick, seeing this as a perfect opportunity to show off – his favourite sport. "Smell something, guys?" Stock said with a rude snigger. "Like an open trash can?"

His friends guffawed.

Nick had been waiting for this ever since his broken nose. "Hey, man," he countered. "How come y'always travel with bodyguards? Scared shitless you might run into me, huh?"

"Into *you*?" Stock smirked, showing off for his pals. "I squash white trash like you under my feet."

"Yeah – well they're sure big enough."

"What did you say, *jerk*?"

"You heard me, *asshole*."

Stock thought he'd be a big man in front of his friends. Since he'd creamed Nick once he figured it was easy. He turned towards him, his hefty right arm raised, ready to throw a punch.

This time Nick was ready – "Fuck you," he spat out, kneeing

Stock in the balls, following up with a sharp kick below his knee.

Stock let out a roar of pain.

Nick chopped him across the neck, and before anyone knew what was happening Stock was sprawled on the ground.

"Hey –" Nick said, prodding him with the tip of his sneaker. "I guess I owed you that." Turning his back he walked away.

Cyndra was in the trailer when he got home, busy cramming everything she owned into a small backpack.

"Joey told you, huh?" she said, rolling up her favourite sweater and squeezing it in.

"Yeah."

"What have you decided?"

"I'm gonna come."

She jumped up, threw her arms around his neck and kissed him. "I'm real happy, Nick."

"So am I."

They grinned at each other. It had taken time but they'd finally formed an alliance.

When Harlan came home he immediately knew something was up. "Where're you goin'?" he asked Cyndra, his big eyes accusing.

"Nowhere," she said, unable to look at him.

"We gotta tell him," Nick warned her in a low voice.

"Look – I love him as much as you do, but there's no way we can drag a kid along. I know my mom – she'll get used to me splittin' – but if we take Harlan, she'll send the cops after us."

"We can't just dump on him."

She stared at Nick, sour-faced. "If we tell him, he'll run straight to Aretha Mae."

"Not if he makes us a promise."

"What's goin' on?" Harlan asked, edging nearer.

"C'mere, kid," Nick said, patting the end of his mattress. "Howdja like to have this trailer all to yourself? You're gettin' older now, you can bring girls here, throw wild parties, huh?"

Harlan's eyes filled with tears. He'd known it was bad news. "You an' Cyndra goin' away, ain'tcha?"

"Yeah – we gotta go," Nick said, wrinkling his forehead. "But it ain't that bad."

Cyndra joined in. "Look – one of these days I'll come back for you. That's a promise."

Harlan shook his head. "No, you won't."

"Yes I *will*," she insisted. "Wanna bet?"

"I'll take the bet," Nick said. "An' if she don't – I will. How's that?"

Harlan was unconvinced. He wiped away his tears with the back of his hand and tried to pretend it didn't matter.

Nick felt bad – but what could he do? He'd made a decision and he intended to stick to it.

The next morning dawned exceptionally bright and clear. Since it was pay-day the plan was for everybody to go to work, pick up their pay-cheque and meet around six. Joey told his mother he would be away for the weekend. Cyndra told Aretha Mae the same thing. Unfortunately Primo overheard and launched himself into a sitting position. "Where you goin'?" he demanded, as if he had a right to know.

"None of your business," Cyndra replied sharply, hating the sight of him.

Aretha Mae sensed something going on. She pulled her daughter to one side and said in a hoarse whisper. "You got money comin'. Real money."

Cyndra was surprised. "I have?"

"Mr Browning – he came through."

"Why?" Cyndra asked, suspiciously.

"'Cause I told him he hadda do what's right."

"I thought you didn't believe me."

"Maybe I did – maybe I didn't. It don't matter – he owes you."

"How much money?" Cyndra asked, quickly.

"We'll talk about it next week," Aretha Mae said.

"Why not now?"

"Now's not the time."

On their way to work Cyndra told Nick about the conversation. "She knows," she said, nervously biting her thumb-nail. "That's why she's telling me 'bout this money now. Whyn't she tell me before?"

He shrugged. "Dunno. Why is old man Browning givin' you money anyway?"

"It's a long story," she said, clamming up.

He didn't push it; she'd tell him when she was ready.

Now that he'd made the decision to leave he was impatient, although he did want to take the time to say goodbye to Betty Harris, she'd been good to him and he owed her that.

★

167

Since leaving the Brownings, Aretha Mae had been working over at the canning plant. It was a tougher job than private service, but at least it was a job. She hadn't told Primo she'd quit the Brownings, it was none of his damn business. Taking Primo back had been a mistake. She'd thought she might enjoy having a man around again, but what did he give her? Pure nothing.

Benjamin Browning had kept his word – he'd had no choice really – he couldn't risk Aretha Mae revealing him for the pervert he was. She'd banked the five thousand dollars he'd handed over in cash. What a fine day that had been!

At first she hadn't planned on telling Cyndra about the money – it was there for an emergency. But that morning she'd had a funny feeling when Cyndra said goodbye. The girl was up to something – and that's why she'd mentioned the money. She didn't want her daughter doing anything foolish – like running off with Joey Pearson. A girl with Cyndra's looks could do far better than him.

On Fridays Aretha Mae worked a half-day. Lately she'd been meeting Harlan from school, taking him down Main Street and treating him to an ice-cream. They were both lonesome since Luke's death.

She thought of Luke often, and her heart was filled with sadness. Poor Luke . . . poor baby . . . he'd never had a chance.

Harlan was standing outside school when she arrived. She tried to take his hand but he pulled away from her.

"How ya doin', baby," she asked, thinking what a fine looking boy he was.

"Don' call me that, Mama." Harlan glanced around, making sure none of his school-mates had heard.

"Gonna buy you ice-cream," Aretha Mae promised.

Harlan's heart was heavy. He didn't want ice-cream – he wanted God to bring Luke back. And maybe at the same time God could persuade Cyndra and Nick to stay.

Betty Harris wasn't surprised. "I knew you'd be on your way one of these days," she said, inviting Nick into her living room. "I didn't realize it would be so soon."

"There's nothing for me to hang around here for," he explained, flopping down on her over-stuffed couch. "I gotta get away from my old man before I end up like him."

"What makes you think that would happen?" Betty asked.

"'Cause if I stay anywhere near him I ain't got no chance."

"And you imagine you'll have a chance in Chicago?"

"Why not? It's a big city."

"Big cities can sometimes be cruel places," she said, quietly. "You're young and good-looking. I'm sure you'll get plenty of offers – perhaps not always the ones you expect."

"I can take care of myself," he said, edgily.

"I know that." She sighed, thinking how vulnerable he was – in spite of his tough exterior. "I'll miss you, Nick. Teaching you has been a wonderful experience, you're really a talented boy. You have a natural ability to become whatever character you're portraying." She hesitated before giving him what she considered the ultimate compliment. "Sometimes you remind me of a young James Dean."

He laughed, slightly embarrassed. "Hey – let's not get carried away or maybe I won't go."

Betty Harris watched him, her expression serious. "If people see you, if you get the right opportunities . . . I shouldn't encourage you because acting is the most difficult profession in the world." She sighed again. "You *do* know that most actors are out of work most of their lives, don't you?"

"I gotta take the chance," he said, wishing she'd cut out the negative shit.

She nodded wisely. "Yes, that's the right attitude. Positive thinking. Wait here a minute."

She left the room and he got up and paced around. He loved being in Betty's living room, it was so warm and comfortable, a real home. There were photographs in silver frames and stacks of interesting books. God, how he wished he'd been encouraged to read as a child. He hadn't even known what a book was until his first day of school.

He picked up a picture of Betty in a white lace gown, her hair tumbling in soft curls around her youthful face.

"I was pretty, wasn't I?" she said, coming back into the room and startling him.

"You still are," he replied, gallantly.

"So young and so smart. There'll always be a woman to look after you."

"That's not what I want."

"I know." She smiled and handed him a padded envelope.

"What's in it?" he asked, weighing it from hand to hand.

"Something I want you to have," she said, earnestly.

"If it's money I can't take it."

"It's not."

"Can I open it?"

"Go ahead."

He tore the envelope open. It was Betty's precious signed copy of *A Streetcar Named Desire*.

"Betty – jeez – this is great."

"Good. I want you to have it."

He tucked the book under his arm. "Betty, I gotta tell you . . . you've been so good t'me, I'll always remember you."

"I'll remember you, too, Nick. Take care of yourself." Impulsively she stepped forward and hugged him. He hugged her back – tightly. Betty represented his last vestige of security and he was going to miss her and their intense sessions.

When he left her house he did so without a backward glance. It was time to move on. His new life was just beginning.

They met at six o'clock on Friday night – excited – maybe a little bit frightened – but none of them showed it.

Joey had the trip all planned. The last bus to Ripley – and then they'd hop a freight train all the way to Kansas City, and from there – Chicago.

The three of them stared at each other.

"This is it!" Joey said.

"Goodbye Bosewell," Cyndra said.

"I ain't comin' back 'til I've made it," Nick said confidently. "And I *will* make it. Then I'll come back for Lauren. Bet on it."

Chapter 27

Every morning Lauren awoke with the same blank feeling. As soon as she opened her eyes she felt a dull ache of despair, and there was nothing she could do about it.

She'd begun to hate her parents. Walking into the kitchen and having breakfast with them was an effort. Sitting at the table and listening to their inane conversation. Didn't they realize they were killing her inside? Didn't they realize they were mean-spirited and unrelenting and above all – wrong?

She thought about Nick all the time and in her heart she knew she had to see him. But how? That was the big question – how?

Every day her father took her to school, later on her mother met her, driving up in the family station wagon, giving her no chance to escape. This had been going on for six weeks – ever since she'd been caught.

"When are you going to trust me?" she asked one day.

"When your father and I feel that we can," her mother replied, with a pious expression.

There was no point in pursuing it. Trying to change their opinion of Nick was useless.

Today it was Monday, and Nick was on her mind more than ever. She walked over to her bedroom window and gazed out. The sun blazed hot and steady – unseasonably so. Downstairs she could hear her mother calling out, "Lauren! Breakfast is ready."

Soon she would have to sit in the car next to her father as he dropped her off at school. Delivered and collected. And she knew they checked with the school secretary every day to make sure she hadn't taken off.

Listlessly she wandered downstairs, ate the breakfast her mother had prepared – picking at the food with absolutely no appetite at all, and collected her books.

Phil Roberts appeared five minutes later. Was it her imagination or did the atmosphere between her parents seem tense? They hardly seemed to talk any more. She was sure she was responsible. It had to do with the fact that her father had not concluded the insurance deal with Benjamin Browning, therefore her mother had not received the social and financial boost she'd expected, and this had obviously put a strain on their relationship.

Too bad. It was nothing compared to what she was going through.

"It's hot today," Phil grumbled, struggling into his jacket and grabbing a slice of toast on his way through the kitchen.

"The weather report says it will be hotter than yesterday," Jane remarked.

Phil did not look in her direction. He walked into the hall and examined himself in the mirror, reaching up to pull out a strand of grey hair. "I'll be home late tonight," he called out, picking up his briefcase.

Jane did not respond. She slammed dishes into the sink and ran the water.

On the way to school Lauren decided to open up a conversation. "Daddy, can we talk?" she began, determined to get through to him.

"Not today, Lauren," he said, his eyes fixed on the road ahead. "I'm not in the mood."

"When *will* you be in the mood?"

"Stop bothering me."

Her life was breaking into little pieces and all her father could say was "Stop bothering me". Once she'd felt she could go to him with any problem, now there was a cold war between them. Didn't he care that he was driving her away?

When he dropped her off she didn't even bother saying goodbye.

Dawn Kovak lingered near the lockers. She and Dawn were not exactly close friends, but Dawn greeted her as if they were. "Did you hear what Nick did to Stock?" Dawn asked.

Lauren was immediately alert. "What?"

Dawn was determined to draw it out. "You mean you haven't heard?"

"No. Are you going to tell me or not?"

Dawn smoothed down her tight skirt. "No need to get edgy."

"I'm not edgy. If you have something to tell me, go ahead."

"Well, from what I hear, Nick knocked Stock on his ass." Dawn couldn't help giggling.

Lauren waited to hear more. "Are you sure?"

"It happened outside the drugstore. Stock was on his way in with a couple of guys, and Nick was on his way out. They got into some kinda beef and Nick creamed him. Funny, huh?"

Even though she was dying to hear all the details Lauren attempted to stay cool. "Is . . . is Nick all right?"

"To tell you the truth," Dawn replied matter-of-factly, "me and Nick — we don't see each other any more."

Lauren nodded. "Oh."

"Look," Dawn said, suddenly sympathetic, "I got the message about how he feels about you. I wouldn't interfere with that."

Lauren felt tears sting her eyelids. Nobody had spoken to her about Nick before, there wasn't anyone she could confide in. "My parents won't allow me to see him," she said, miserably. "I don't know what to do."

Dawn looked suitably concerned. "Yeah, Joey told me. Listen," she added jauntily, "parents are a pain — maybe they'll change their minds."

Lauren shook her head. "Not my parents." She paused for a moment. "I feel so bad about everything. It's my fault Nick got kicked out of school, I mean if it wasn't for me . . ." she trailed off.

"Don't sweat it — he's happy working down at the gas station, beats school any day. And it's *not* your fault. Stock's the one that had his parents do the dirty."

"I know you're right, but sometimes I wake up in the morning and all I want to do is run away."

Dawn nodded understandingly. "We all get that feeling."

"Really?"

"Sure — it's natural."

A couple of girls rushed past on their way to class. "C'mon, Lauren, you'll be late," one of them called out.

She hesitated for a moment. "What are you doing for lunch today?"

Dawn was surprised. "Who? Me?"

"I don't see anybody else standing here."

"What I normally do. Hang out. Why? You wanna eat with me?"

"I'd like it if we could talk some more," Lauren said.

Dawn seemed pleased. "So would I."

173

After dropping Lauren off, Phil drove straight to his office. Before going upstairs he stopped in at the hardware store and picked up the new kitchen scissors Jane had ordered.

Kitchen scissors, he thought grimly, *she's probably going to stab me to death.*

He collected them in the morning because he knew by the time he was ready to go home the last thing he'd be thinking about was picking up something for his wife.

Upstairs he unlocked his office door and entered. Eloise, his secretary, had not yet arrived. The place smelt stuffy and humid. He threw open the windows and settled behind his desk, thinking that perhaps he should have allowed Lauren to talk to him in the car. It wasn't right – this distance between them. If things were different at home maybe it would be easier for him to communicate with his daughter, but there was so much tension between him and Jane that he didn't seem to have the time to deal with anything else.

He considered calling Benjamin Browning. They'd been almost ready to conclude a business deal when Lauren had broken her engagement; after that he'd been unable to reach him.

The hell with it! Picking up the phone he dialled Benjamin's office before he changed his mind.

A secretary answered, cool and efficient. "Who may I say is calling?"

"Phil Roberts."

"Just one moment, Mr Roberts, I'll see if he's available." A beat of ten. "I'm sorry, Mr Roberts, Mr Browning is tied up in a meeting. May I take a message?"

"Yes, I've called several times. I need to speak to him as soon as possible. Can he return my call."

"I'll see Mr Browning receives the message. I'm sure he'll get back to you."

Yes, I'm sure he will, Phil thought, sourly.

Harlan told Aretha Mae he had a sore throat.

"Is it bad?" she asked.

"It feels real bad," Harlan lied.

"Where's your sister?" Her see-all eyes searched the empty trailer.

"She ain't back yet," Harlan said.

Aretha Mae fixed him with a steely stare, daring him to tell a fib. "Is she comin' back?"

He refused to meet her stare. "I dunno."

Aretha Mae screwed up her face, knowing perfectly well Cyndra wasn't coming back. She'd known it on Friday when the girl had come to her with some story about staying away for the weekend.

She started to poke around the trailer – all of Cyndra's favourite things were gone and Nick's too. So he'd run off as well. She wondered if she should tell Primo. No. She'd wait and see if he noticed his only son was missing – it would probably take him weeks – that's how much he cared.

In a way she didn't mind now she knew Nick was with Cyndra – at least he'd keep a watchful eye on her, and maybe the two of them together could forge a better life for themselves.

"It's okay," she told Harlan. "You can stay home."

He was delighted. He hadn't thought he'd get away with it. Harlan never told anybody about how bad school was, the names they called him – nigger and dirt poor and stinking bastard. He'd gotten used to it – he'd even gotten used to defending himself when they beat him up.

As soon as Aretha Mae left for work he sneaked into her trailer to see if he could scrounge some food. Primo was in his usual position, fast asleep with the television blaring. Harlan noticed his mouth was wide open and he couldn't help wondering if anything ever crawled in. Stifling a chuckle he crept inside the trailer, edged over to the small ice-box and peered inside. He spotted a leg of chicken – and without considering the consequences grabbed it and hurriedly slid out of the trailer before he was discovered.

Primo heard the door bang shut and woke up. He sat up, scratching his stomach. Even though it was early it was goddamn hot – he could feel the sticky sweat trickling down his body.

He got up, went to the door and stepped outside. A skinny mutt growled at him. Primo picked up a beer can and hurled it at the mangy animal.

Lately Primo found himself getting restless. He'd never liked staying in one place for long. Aretha Mae might be a good woman, but he was bored. After a while being with one woman always bored him. Maybe the time had come to move on – after all there was a whole country out there – and plenty of other women who'd be only too happy to take him in. He was still a fine-looking man. Yeah – fine looking *and* a stud. What more could any woman ask?

Continuing to scratch his belly he headed for the outhouse and relieved himself.

When he emerged he caught Harlan sitting on the steps of his trailer chewing a chicken leg. "What'ya starin' at, boy?"

Harlan lowered his eyes. "Nothin'."

"Don't give me that nothin' crap. How come ya ain't in school?"

Harlan didn't look up. "I ain't feelin' good," he muttered.

Aretha Mae and her chickenshit kids – they were always getting sick. Except Cyndra. His daughter. Now she was a real nice-looking girl. If she wasn't his own flesh and blood he would certainly consider bedding her down. She needed an experienced older man who could teach her a thing or two.

"Wanna take a ride?" he asked Harlan.

The boy's eyes widened. Primo had never spoken to him before, let alone offered him a ride. "Where to?" he asked, suspiciously.

"Into town, unless you gotta better idea."

"Nope."

"Okay – hop in the truck."

Primo wondered why he was being so generous allowing the kid to tag along.

Because there was nothing to do in Bosewell, that's why. It was a one-horse, hicksville town. No decent bar, no dancing girls, no nothing.

A new thought began nagging inside his head. If he decided to leave Bosewell, would he have to take Nick with him?

Nah, why should he? The boy was old enough and ugly enough to manage on his own. Besides, Aretha Mae seemed to have taken a shine to him – let *her* have the responsibility for a while.

Not that he was taking off today. Right now he was riding into town and stocking up with beer and pretzels. He'd leave the following weekend – right after Aretha Mae came home with her pay-cheque. There was nothing to stop him from borrowing it.

He'd leave in the middle of the night, that way he'd be a couple of hundred miles away before they realized he was gone.

Primo Angelo deserved a life too, and the sweet thing was – if there was nothing out there for him he could come back. Aretha Mae would always be waiting.

Eloise Hanson arrived at Phil Roberts' office at twelve noon exactly. She worked for him three afternoons a week – typing and filing – those were her duties. Not that there was much to file lately – business was grim.

Eloise was a small plump woman in her mid-thirties, with pink cheeks, a scrubbed complexion and gentle brown eyes. Widowed a year previously – her husband was killed in a freak accident at the canning plant – she'd needed extra money to support herself and her elderly mother.

At first the relationship between herself and Phil Roberts had been strictly businesslike, but as the months passed they'd formed a close bond that eventually turned into a love affair.

Both of them felt guilty.

Both of them hated the duplicity involved.

Both of them could not keep their hands off each other.

As soon as Eloise walked into the office, fanning herself and murmuring about the heat, Phil realized that work was over for the day. He took her hand and led her into his office. "No work today,' he said, squeezing her moist palm.

She blushed a little, knowing full well what he had in mind. "But there's letters to get out."

"Too bad."

She accepted his desire without question and slowly began unbuttoning her blouse.

Phil went to the outer door, pulled the shade down and locked it – hanging out the "Closed" sign.

Jane suspected the affair was still going on, even though he'd assured her it was absolutely over. He wasn't certain she believed him, but somehow he couldn't stop. Eloise was such a caring woman, so giving and kind. Most of all she was a tiger in bed – a woman without inhibitions. She made Phil feel like a real man in her arms.

Not that sex with his wife hadn't always been good – over the years they'd enjoyed a satisfactory relationship – satisfactory bordering on dull. Eloise was different – she brought out a passion in him he'd thought was extinguished. Eloise allowed him to re-live the excitement of his youth. After all, he was not even fifty, surely he was allowed this final fling?

Recently Jane had given him an ultimatum. "Fire her," she'd said, her tone allowing no argument.

"Why should I?" he'd replied, struggling to maintain control of his marriage. "She's an excellent secretary. And you know there's nothing between us any more."

"I couldn't care less," Jane had replied. "I do not want that bitch anywhere near you."

Jane never swore. To hear her say "bitch" was quite shocking.

Phil knew that firing Eloise was inevitable, but he kept on delaying the moment. Eloise was his escape, and without her – what exactly did he have?

Lauren and Dawn sat on the grass together sharing a tuna-fish sandwich.

"I know you went out with Nick," Lauren said, not anxious for the details, but unable to stop herself from finding out how serious it had been.

"It was before he started seeing you," Dawn explained. "As soon as you came into the picture it was over." She shrugged. "Look, I understand. I've met plenty of boys like Nick. I'm like a stop gap, you know? I'm there when they need me and then they move on. He loves you – he never loved me."

"Can I tell you something?" Lauren said, hesitantly.

"Go ahead," Dawn replied, biting into her sandwich.

"It's . . . it's embarrassing."

"Ha!" said Dawn. "Trust me. I've heard it all. *Nothin'* embarrasses me."

Lauren sighed – a long weary sigh. "It's just that my parents are very strict, and I haven't been allowed to see Nick in nearly two months, and the fact is – I don't know what to do."

"What is it?" Dawn asked. "You can tell me."

The words were difficult to say, but Lauren managed to get them out. "I . . . I think I'm pregnant."

Until she'd actually said it out loud she hadn't been prepared to believe it. Now that she'd voiced her suspicions she felt a great wave of relief.

"Damnit!" Dawn said. "How late are you?"

Lauren studied the grass. "Almost six weeks," she mumbled. "I daren't tell my parents. I . . . I have to see Nick. I have to tell him."

"Sounds like a good idea to me."

"How can I?"

"How *can't* you is more like it. If I was you I'd head straight over to the gas station and tell him. You shouldn't have to handle this alone."

"What if they find out?"

"You can't be any worse off than you are now, can you?"

Dawn had a point.

"I'll do it," she decided.

"Maybe the two of you can run off and get married," Dawn said, getting carried away. "*Very* romantic."

"That'll *really* thrill my parents."

"Stop worrying about them. Talk it over with Nick. The way I see it you've got two choices — marry him and have the baby, or get an abortion."

The word abortion petrified her. If there was a baby growing inside her she would never consider doing it any harm.

"Has this ever happened to you?" she asked.

"To tell you the truth, no. But I always take precautions. Didn't Nick wear a rubber?"

Lauren couldn't believe she was discussing anything as intimate as this with Dawn. "No . . . I, uh . . . he told me he . . . uh . . . pulled out."

"Oh, Jesus!" Dawn looked disgusted. "*Never* let 'em tell you that, it's the oldest line in the book. That and — let me just lay down next to you, I swear I won't put it in." She stood up and held out her hand. "Come on, get up, we gotta make plans. If you skip out of school now an' make it over to the gas station you can hear what he's got to say an' decide what you'll do. If you're lucky you'll be back before your mother gets here."

"You're right," Lauren said, drawing a deep breath. "It's the only answer, isn't it?"

"Sure — it's just as much *his* responsibility as yours. He's the asshole supposed to take precautions. An' don't worry, whatever you decide — I'm your friend, an' I'll help you if I can."

Lauren nodded gratefully, and felt sorry for all the bitchy things she and Meg had said about Dawn in the past. "Thanks," she said, squeezing her hand. "You've been great. I owe you one."

Chapter 28

Early Monday morning they made it into Chicago. Dirty, tired and hungry but totally elated.

"This is my kinda town, Chicago is," Joey sung, happily.

"Enough with the singin' – where we goin'?" Nick asked.

"Yeah, where?" Cyndra joined in. "I'm beat."

"Hey –" Joey said, "I got it all under control."

"I wish you'd get my stomach under control," Cyndra complained. "Travelling on that stinkin' freight train all night has made me starvin'."

"Okay, okay – I get the message. Let's go in here."

They entered a dingy looking café. Cyndra pulled a face while Joey ordered bacon and eggs, hot coffee and orange juice.

"Can we afford it?" she whispered. "Maybe we shouldn't be blowing our money like this."

"It's okay," Nick said. "We deserve a decent breakfast."

"This is the plan," Joey said, taking charge. "After we eat I'll make a few calls. Don't worry, we'll be sleeping in beds tonight."

"I hope so," Cyndra said, wearily. "'Cause I can't take another night sleeping rough." She went off to the rest room to wash up.

A rag-clad old tramp approached their table. "Gotta dime?" he wheezed.

"Buzz off!" Joey said, sharply.

Nick reached in his pocket and fumbled for loose change, handing the old man a quarter.

"What in hell're you doing? We might need that," Joey said, indignantly.

"It's like a superstition," Nick replied. "Never turn a beggar down."

"Oh – some superstition. They'll be following you like the freakin' Pied Piper!"

Cyndra returned from the ladies room having brushed her long dark hair and washed her face. "I feel better now," she said, ravenously attacking the runny eggs and greasy bacon.

"This'll havta last us until dinner," Joey warned, grabbing a piece of toast and mopping up his eggs. "Think I'll go make those calls now."

Fifteen minutes later he was back. "Friends," he said, sourly. "You can shove 'em."

"What happened?" Nick asked.

"Well, like, y'know, I had this best friend at school. He told me there's no way we can go to his house on account of he's havin' trouble with his dad – so strike him off."

Cyndra pressed forward. "Who else did you call?"

"This girl I used to go with, but when I told her there were three of us she cried off, so then I called my cousin."

"I thought we were forgetting about relatives."

"Don't sweat it. He changed his number – no new one."

"Is that it?" Nick asked. "These are the friends and relatives that were gonna put us up?"

"Hey – things change," Joey said. "We've got enough money for a hotel."

"Not for long." Nick said. "We've only got enough for three or four days – then we're out on the street."

"We'll get jobs," Joey argued.

"What jobs?" Cyndra asked.

"I'm gonna try out at a few comedy clubs," Joey said, cheerfully. "Face it – I'm young, I'm hot, I'm theirs!"

"I suppose I could do some waitressing," she said thoughtfully.

"And you can get a gig at a gas station, Nick." Joey said.

"Hey – if I wanted a job at a gas station I'd have stayed in Bosewell," Nick retorted, sharply.

"Stop bitchin'," Joey said. "We're here. We're outta Bosewell. Something good'll come along. Right now the most important thing is finding a cheap hotel for the night."

"I'm not sleeping on any park benches," Cyndra said, flatly.

"Nobody's askin' you to, sweetheart," Joey replied.

After an hour of traipsing the streets they checked into a fleabag hotel with flashing neon signs, vibrating beds and in-house porno movies. Joey and Cyndra registered as Mr and Mrs Pearson while Nick slipped around to the back alley. As soon as they reached their room they let him in through the fire escape.

"Some dump!" Cyndra complained, trying out the lumpy bed.

"You were expecting the Plaza?" Joey countered.

"Quit it," Nick said. "I'm not listenin' to you two fight all night long."

They began studying the newspaper, circling job opportunities. Joey found what he was looking for and got ready for action. He combed his hair, slicked it down with oil, put on his best jacket and said, "I'm visiting the Comedy Club. How old do I look?"

Cyndra leaned back, narrowing her eyes. "'Bout seventeen."

"You're full of it." He turned to Nick. "Whaddaya think?"

"Y'could pass for twenty."

"I'm growin' a beard, that'll do it."

Cyndra wrinkled her nose. "Ugh . . . I hate beards."

"You hate everything," Joey said.

"No, I don't," she argued.

Nick was getting edgy. "C'mon you two," he said.

"Listen to this." Cyndra pounced triumphantly, reading aloud from the paper. "'Beautiful young girls wanted for modelling jobs. Ability to travel abroad essential.' Sounds great," she jumped off the bed and paraded around the room. "I could be a model, couldn't I?"

"Sounds great," Joey mimicked. "They'll have you on a slow boat to China with a needle in your arm."

"Huh?"

"That's what they do to girls once they get hold of 'em. Ship 'em off to whorehouses in Bangkok."

"You and your imagination."

"I'm not kiddin'."

"I'm gonna take a walk," Nick said. "See you two later."

"Yeah, yeah," Joey said. "I'm doin' the same. Cyndra, you're on your own, so don't go signing with no modelling agency unless you check it with me first."

"Sure, Mr Bigshot," she said, sarcastically.

Joey grinned, he liked her sassiness. "You'd better believe it. We'll meet back here in a coupla hours."

Trudging around the streets of Chicago Nick felt his adrenalin begin to pump. Walking the streets was a kick – people-watching, getting the feel of the city. He passed a couple of Help Wanted signs and went inside only to find both positions filled. Who wanted to work in a hamburger joint or a barber shop anyway?

After a while he passed a restaurant/bar with the same old sign in the window. What the hell – he'd make a pretty good bartender. He ventured inside the dim interior and checked it out. The place was dingy – with low lights and a tired stripper gyrating to a gloomy sounding Glen Campbell on the jukebox. There were few customers.

He headed towards the bar where a gnarled old man with a Marine crew cut and bloodshot eyes stood guard.

"Yeah?" the man rasped. "What kin I getcha?"

"I'm interested in the job," he said.

The man snorted and turned away. "Round the back."

"What job is it?"

"Washin' dishes."

"That's not exactly what I had in mind."

"What *didja* have in mind?" the man said, picking up a glass and giving it a cursory polish with a grubby cloth.

"Your job."

"Ha ha, the kid's a comedian. Get your skinny ass around the back."

Nick decided he was better off repairing cars than washing dishes, but he was here anyway, so he made his way into the alley coming face to face with a large rat balanced on top of an overflowing garbage can. He dodged past it and entered through the back door into a filthy kitchen.

A very thin man in what once might have been a white apron sat on a stool, his legs propped on a counter top near the sink. He was smoking a cigarette, blowing lazy smoke rings towards the ceiling. On the stove a huge pan of fries sizzled in a sea of greasy black oil.

"Yeah?" the man said, looking down his long thin nose.

"I was wondering 'bout the job," Nick said.

"You wanna do some washin', jump right in," the man said, gesturing toward a chipped sink piled high with dirty dishes.

"How much?"

"Two fifty an hour – cash."

"That ain't enough."

"Whaddaya think I am – Rockefeller? You want the job or not?"

"How many hours a day?"

"A coupla hours lunchtime, two or three in the evenings."

Thirteen bucks a day if he was lucky, and he'd still have mornings and afternoons free to go on auditions. "Make it a straight three bucks an hour an' I'm yours."

183

"Don't go bargaining with me, kid. I can get a Mexi t'do it for half the price."

"Why don't you?"

The man blew smoke in his face. "Oh, you gotta smart mouth too, huh? Fuckin' Mexis break everything."

"Two seventy-five," Nick said.

"Jesus!" the man slapped his forehead. "Start now and you got the job – or shift your ass outta here. Take it or leave it."

He took it. It sure beat walking the streets.

Chapter 29

By the time Lauren reached the gas station she was hot and tired. The forecourt was deserted so she made her way to the office and tapped on the door.

George sat behind his desk going over some outstanding accounts. "Yes?" he called out.

"Excuse me," she said, putting her head around the door. "I'm looking for Nick Angelo."

"Nick don't work here no more," George said, gruffly.

"He doesn't?"

"Nah – he quit."

She was stunned. How could he quit his job just like that? She was about to ask more questions when the phone rang and George settled himself into a conversation.

She left the gas station, trying to decide what to do.

You've gone this far, Roberts. May as well go all the way. Take a bus over to his trailer and find out what's going on.

She was more nervous about telling Nick than facing up to her parents, but it had to be done. What would he say when she told him she was pregnant? Oh, God! Would he hate her? She couldn't stand it.

She hurried to the bus stop and waited ten minutes before the bus arrived. It was stiflingly hot and stuffy, and she was beginning to feel nauseous.

"Bad weather up ahead," the driver said, accepting her fare.

What was he talking about? It was a beautiful day, much too hot, but it certainly didn't look like rain.

"Thunderstorms," the driver said, nodding his head knowingly. "I can hear 'em miles away."

Settling into a window seat she looked outside – there wasn't a cloud in the sky.

As soon as the bus began to move she started thinking about her father. Phil Roberts had always taught her to be honest and true, so why couldn't she be honest with him? Because that's what she really wanted to do.

On impulse she jumped off at Main Street, deciding to visit him at work and make one last attempt to communicate.

By the time she reached the stairs leading to his office she'd made up her mind exactly what she would say. She'd tell him her life was over if she wasn't allowed to see Nick Angelo. And then she'd tell him about the baby.

The shade was down on his office door, and the "Closed" sign was displayed. Disappointed, she went downstairs to the hardware store and spoke to one of the Blakely brothers.

"When will my father be back?"

"He's upstairs, Lauren."

"He's not, the office is closed."

"I'm almost sure he's up there. Here – take the spare key, you can wait for him."

She took the key and went back upstairs. Her father was probably out having lunch. This break was good, it would give her time to compose herself. When he came back she'd be ready with a perfectly reasonable speech that he couldn't fail to understand and respond to.

She put the key in the lock and let herself into the small reception area. As soon as she stepped inside she knew she wasn't alone – there were strange muffled sounds coming from the inner office.

He's being robbed, was her immediate thought. Without thinking she opened the door and stood on the threshold.

Eloise, her father's secretary, was spread-eagled naked across the couch. Crouched above her, also naked, was her father.

Lauren's hand flew to her mouth and she gasped. Eloise let out a little screech of horror, and Phil Roberts turned his head around to meet his daughter's shocked stare.

"Lauren!" he said, rolling off Eloise and frantically grabbing for his pants. "Oh my God! This is not what you think. Lauren, what are you *doing* here?"

She turned around and ran from the room, stumbling down the stairs, trying not to cry. *This* was her father? *This* was upstanding Phil Roberts – the man she'd looked up to all her life?

He was a phoney. He was a nothing. And she'd never, ever forgive him.

Primo Angelo lumbered into the liquor store and bought four six-packs of beer. Harlan trailed behind him.

When he was finished in the store and the van was loaded he said, "I'm starvin', wanna grab a bite?"

Harlan could hardly believe his luck. "*Yessir*," he said, quickly. "I'se always hungry."

"Where can we find us a good 'burger?" Primo asked.

Harlan pointed down Main Street. "The drugstore."

Primo set off with Harlan loping behind.

Louise greeted them with a smile, a menu, and a crisp, "Hi there, folks," as they sat down at the counter.

Primo nodded. Nice looking piece of ass. Good tits too. "Coupla 'burgers," he said. "Make 'em plump an' juicy an' fast." He winked suggestively. "Just like you, honey."

The smile vanished from her face. "Cheeseburger, chilliburger, or plain?" she asked, curtly.

"Make it two cheeseburgers – well done," Primo said, undressing her with his eyes. He could see little slivers of sweat between her breasts and it began to excite him. He'd had it with Aretha Mae, she was old and dried up, he needed somebody younger, juicier – somebody like this hot-looking waitress with the big tits and sassy ass.

Louise stopped by the kitchen, gave the order to Dave, and went in the back room grumbling to herself. Some men had no manners. All they thought about was sex.

She removed her purse from the shelf and took out her lipstick and a hairbrush. Then she fluffed out her hair and teased her bangs, before applying more lipstick. Louise always liked to look her best, especially when dealing with sexist jerks. Just as she was putting everything away she noticed the letter Nick had left for her to give to Lauren lying on the bottom shelf.

Can't give it to her if she ain't been in, she thought.

Nick had marked it URGENT! and IMPORTANT! If Lauren didn't show up soon maybe she'd hand it to her friend Meg to pass on.

Louise propped the letter up so she wouldn't forget, and returned to the kitchen.

The school secretary phoned Jane Roberts at one o'clock. "Mrs

Roberts, I'm sorry to have to tell you this – but it seems Lauren is missing again. She was here this morning and now she appears to have left."

Jane's lips tightened. "You mean she's not in school?"

"I'm sorry, Mrs Roberts, but I must warn you if this behaviour continues . . . Well, I don't have to tell you the consequences."

"Thank you." Jane put down the phone and immediately dialled her husband's number. Nobody answered.

Why did Lauren have to put her through this? Wasn't it enough that Phil had been sleeping with his secretary? Wasn't it enough that she'd been humiliated by the Brownings' rejection?

Jane's perfect life was falling to pieces around her and she couldn't stand it.

She snatched up her car keys and rushed from the house.

Lauren ran down Main Street until she was away from her father's office and the whole sordid scene. She didn't stop running until she reached the bus stop.

Pictures of her father, bare-assed, pumping away on top of Eloise kept playing before her eyes.

Now it all became clear why her parents were always fighting. Her father was having an affair, and her mother probably suspected.

Oh, God! Was this the man who'd told her how to live her life? The man she'd respected and looked up to?

She wanted to cry, but tears wouldn't come. *Poor Mommy,* she thought miserably. *Poor me.*

There were so many thoughts crowding her head she thought it might crack wide open.

The bus trundled up and she leapt on. There was no doubt about where she was going now. She had to see Nick, he was the only person she could talk to. The only person in the world she could trust.

Two women got on the bus and sat across from her.

"I spoke to my sister this morning," said the first woman, a straggly blonde. "She told me they're having a big thunderstorm over in Ripley."

"Yes?" the other woman did not seem particularly interested. She was several months pregnant and looked exhausted.

"Heard a rumour we might be expecting a twister around these parts," said the straggly blonde.

"Not a chance." The pregnant woman shook her head. "It's beautiful here today – we're lucky."

Lauren tuned out. Her life was destroyed and these women were discussing the weather.

What was she going to do, that was the big question – *what was she going to do?*

Primo took a five-dollar bill from his pocket, rolled it into a tight cone and attempted to poke it down Louise's cleavage.

Forcefully she slapped his hand away, glaring at him. "What the hell you think *you're* doing?"

"Giving you one helluva tip."

"Hey, mister – you can take your tip and stick it up your –" She caught Harlan watching them. "Ah, forget it."

Primo got up and lumbered to the door. Harlan grabbed a few stray french fries from the basket on the counter and followed him out to the truck.

"You saw that bitch in there," Primo said sourly. "Women – mark what I say – they're all whores. You don't want nothin' t'do with any of 'em. Remember that." He sprung open a can of beer and took a couple of hearty swigs, then passed the can to the boy. "Try it," he commanded.

"Don't wanna," Harlan replied, kicking the asphalt.

"Try it!" Primo repeated. "Be a goddamn man."

Gingerly Harlan took the can and managed a few sips, almost choking.

Primo laughed, grabbing the can back.

He felt like action.

He felt like doing something.

He felt like getting laid.

"It's not your fault, Eloise," Phil Roberts kept on assuring her.

Eloise, dressed and pink-cheeked, sat on the office couch sobbing into a dainty lace handkerchief. "She'll tell your wife, I know she will."

"Not if I get to her first," Phil said, attempting to calm her. "I can explain what happened. Lauren's a good girl – she'll understand."

"What is there to understand?" Eloise raised her voice. "What we had together was special and now it's . . . it's dirty."

"It's not dirty," Phil objected.

"Yes, it is," Eloise insisted, continuing to sob. "Everything's ruined."

He didn't know how to cope with her. "Go home," he urged. "Let me take care of this. By tomorrow it'll all be forgotten."

Eloise shook her head. "Your wife will destroy my reputation."

Prudently, Phil had not told her that Jane already knew about their affair. "Go home, Eloise," he repeated, firmly. "I have to find Lauren."

I have to find her before she gets to Jane and opens up her mouth.

By the time the bus reached the stop nearest the trailer site it had started to rain – huge wet droplets. And yet the sun was still shining and the temperature remained muggy.

Lauren had visited Nick's trailer only once, but she was certain she could find her way from the bus stop. She walked quickly down the country lane trying not to think about her father any more. Nick would solve all her problems. Nick would make everything all right.

It was a strange day what with the heat and the rain – there seemed to be a stillness in the air, everything was so quiet. A van roared past her. She kept her head down and continued walking.

Eventually she spotted the trailer site up ahead and quickened her pace. A pack of dogs foraged by the overflowing piles of garbage. How could Nick live here? How could he put up with such a slum?

She recognized his trailer and hurried towards it. A big man was getting out of the van parked outside, a small black boy by his side.

The man noticed her. "Lookin' for someone?"

"Yes . . . Nick Angelo. Do you know if he's home?"

"Nick's my boy."

"I beg your pardon?"

"My boy, my son. Who're you?"

"Are you Mr Angelo?"

"Yeah – that's me all right. I'm the good-lookin' one in the family." He roared at his own humour, and patted her on the arm.

So this was Nick's father, this big untidy lout with a can of beer clutched in his right hand and a smarmy gap-toothed smile. Perhaps this wasn't the right time to be visiting.

190

"I . . . I don't want to disturb anyone," she said, unsurely. "Maybe I should come back another time."

"Disturb? What's to disturb? Come on in," Primo said, flinging open the door of the trailer.

Harlan attempted to attract her attention. "If you're lookin' for Nick –" he began.

Primo pushed him roughly aside. "Come in," he insisted. "Nick'll be here soon. You can wait, I'll enjoy the company."

Reluctantly she entered the cramped trailer and almost gagged – the stench of stale beer and sweat was overwhelming.

Harlan tried to follow them, but Primo shoved him out kicking the door shut. He gestured expansively, "Take a seat, anywhere'll do. Wanna beer?"

"No . . . no, thank you. Is Nick here?"

"The kid'll find him."

Primo checked her out. She was a pretty girl, a very pretty girl. More than likely Nick had been slipping her a slice of the old Angelo magic. Like father, like son. Yeah – the Angelo men – real studs.

Lauren felt extremely uncomfortable as she hovered nervously near the door wishing Nick would appear.

"Will'ya sit down," Primo insisted. "He'll be here soon. So –" he leered at her, "you two old friends, is that it?"

"We go to school together. That is we did – until Nick . . . uh . . . left."

Primo snapped to attention. "Whaddaya mean, left?"

She hesitated, it was more than likely Nick hadn't told his father about getting expelled. She corrected herself quickly. "Oh . . . I mean *when* he leaves . . . to go to his job, you know?"

"Yeah, yeah – his weekend job down at the gas station." Primo ran his tongue across his teeth. "Didja try there?"

"They told me he'd . . . quit." She knew as soon as she said it that she shouldn't have.

He squinted at her. "Whaddaya mean, quit?"

"Uh, for the day. He quit for the day."

"Oh." Primo sprang open another can of beer. "Wanna swig?"

"I really have to be going, Mr Angelo, my parents are expecting me."

He moved over to her, so close she could smell his foul breath. "Pretty girl like you, bet there's someone always waitin'."

Now she felt more than uneasy. His huge physical presence was threatening. Very carefully she began to edge towards the door.

With one fast move he blocked her. "Where ya goin'?"

"I . . . I told you, I must get home."

His voice turned to a lewd whisper. "You an' Nick doin' it? You an' my boy gettin' it on?"

Her stomach turned, and she tried to move. He lunged forward, grabbing her breast.

"Don't touch me! Don't you dare touch me!" she yelled, shrinking away from him.

Primo chuckled, "Hey – feisty little chickie, huh? If'n Nick's doin' it to ya, why can't I?"

Her eyes flashed angrily. "You'd better let me out of here or I'll scream," she said, trying not to panic.

"Who's gonna hear ya, girlie? Ya think there's anyone 'round here cares?"

Out of the corner of her eye she noticed a kitchen knife lying on the side of the sink. Slowly she backed towards it.

Primo was enjoying himself. "C'mon, chickie, loosen up. Ya fucked the boy, doncha wanna fuck the man?" he said, leering lecherously as he moved closer.

Her back was up against the sink. Carefully she manoeuvred one hand behind her groping for the knife. "I said let me out of here," she repeated in a low angry voice, managing to get a firm grip on the handle.

"When I'm ready," Primo replied, fiddling with his belt buckle. "When I'm *good* an' ready."

Outside the sky suddenly darkened and lightning flashed across the window followed by heavy peals of thunder.

She clutched the knife tightly. "You'd better let me go or –"

He guffawed. "Or *what*, Princess?"

The lightning flashed again, once more followed by huge cracked rumbles of thunder. Outside the sky turned even darker, and the light rain swelled to a heavy downpour.

Primo took no notice, so intent was he on getting what he wanted.

She decided that if this man touched her one more time she would stab him.

Outside Harlan started hammering on the door. "Lemme in," he shouted. "Lemme *in*!"

"Get lost," Primo shouted back, unzipping his fly. "Get the fuck outta here."

Harlan continued to yell and hammer on the door. He sounded desperate.

A strong wind howled eerily outside the trailer and the rain turned into pelting hailstones.

"C'mere, girlie," Primo said, pulling at her as she tried once again to dodge past him.

"Don't!" she warned.

He was in no mood to listen to her objections. He grabbed her – forcing his fleshy lips down on hers.

At school she'd learned self-defence and she put it to good use – bringing her knee up hard and sharp, catching him in the groin.

He let out a grunt of pain, but managed to hold on to her – bending her backwards until she could feel his disgusting hardness pressing up against her, and she knew she had to do something drastic. Gripping the knife behind her back she readied herself for action.

Primo pulled at her skirt, pushing it up and ripping at her panties. "C'mon, y'hot little bitch, you're gonna love this," he muttered, dropping his pants.

She lunged with the knife, blindly striking out as the trailer began to rock in the wind and there was a frighteningly loud roaring sound.

Tornado – the thought flashed through her mind. *Oh God, it's a tornado!*

Chapter 30

Jane Roberts was driving towards Main Street when the sky suddenly turned ominously black and from out of nowhere giant hailstones began pounding the windscreen of her car.

She pulled over to the side of the street, petrified, and waited for the ferocious rain to stop, prayed for it to subside – for Jane had lived in the Midwest all her life and she knew what this kind of weather could bring.

Louise peered out the wide front window of the drugstore and yelled to Dave, "Honey, you'd better c'mon out here right now an' get a load of this weather. It's raining hailstones bigger than golf balls."

Dave had hardly taken one step forward when in the distance they heard a thunderous roar – getting louder by the second.

"Shit!" Dave said, running to the window.

"What?" Louise asked, catching his note of alarm.

"Sounds like a twister to me. Jesus! Can you see it out there?"

Indeed she could. A writhing grey funnel of death and destruction. And it was heading in their direction.

Eloise was at the door of Phil's office, ready to leave when the sudden loud howling wind forced her to stand still. She turned to Phil. "What's that?" she asked, her voice quavering with fear.

He looked concerned. "I . . . I don't know. Put on the radio."

Eloise ran to the portable radio on her desk and switched it on. A country and western singer twanged about her man doing her wrong.

The howling wind was getting louder by the second, and

outside the sunshine vanished and the sky turned black.

"Find the news," Phil snapped.

"I'm trying," Eloise said, frantically searching for the right station.

"Try harder, I think we're in trouble."

Stock and Mack were in the middle of football practice on an open field, while Meg was nearby rehearsing a new routine with the cheerleading squad, when the physical ed. teacher spotted the tornado in the distance and began yelling – "Everybody inside! Everybody into the gym! Hurry! Go now! Hurry!"

Stock and Mack looked at each other. The sky was darkening, but they hadn't thought a little bit of rain would interfere with football practice.

Stock started to say, "What's his problem –" when Mack spotted the powerful cone bearing down on them.

"Holy shit!" he said, hoarsely. "We'd better move."

Mr Lucas ran out of the main building. "Inside!" he yelled. "Everyone get under cover. Do it!"

Mack dashed over and grabbed Meg by the hand. She wished it was Stock. "What's the matter?" she asked. "What's all the panic?"

"We gotta get inside," Mack said. "Can't you see? There's a tornado on the way."

Aretha Mae hurried to the side exit of the factory, looked outside and shuddered. There, only miles away and moving fast – she saw it – an enormous, howling, writhing funnel of grey dust bearing down in their direction, destroying everything it passed.

Aretha Mae had never been a religious woman, but now she crossed herself and fell to her knees. "Save Harlan, God," she whispered. "Please, God – save my little boy."

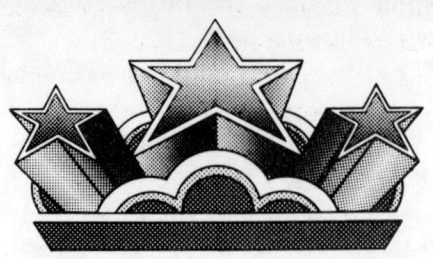

Chapter 31

"Mop the floor."

"I wasn't hired to mop the floor."

"Fuckin' *do* it. I got health inspectors up my ass."

Q.J. was the boss. Rat-faced, with long greasy hair, an aquiline nose and slit eyes. He wore a grubby white suit, cheap black shirt and bright green tie. He wasn't very tall and he walked with a limp and smoked thin cheroots. He hadn't reached forty yet, but was well on the way if he didn't get knocked off first. Q.J. had plenty of enemies.

Reluctantly Nick grabbed a mop and went to work. He'd only been there a few hours and was already thinking of quitting.

"Where'd ya find this bozo?" Q.J. demanded of Len, the so-called chef.

Len looked down his long thin nose. "He walked in off the street. I hired him on a temporary basis."

"Tell him I don' expect no lip."

"Yeah, yeah, I'll tell him."

They spoke about him as if he didn't exist. Surely they realized they were fortunate to get anyone to work in such a crummy place.

The tired-looking stripper he'd caught a glimpse of earlier strolled into the kitchen wearing nothing but a short kimono and a bright yellow hairband.

"Hi'ya, Q.J."

"Hi'ya, doll."

"Lousy business."

"It's that time of year."

She opened the big industrial ice-box, reached for the milk, drank from the carton and put it back.

"That's a filthy habit, Erna," Q.J. grumbled. "Some poor schnook's gonna get your spit in his coffee."

"They should be so lucky." Erna yawned, reaching inside her kimono for a vigorous scratch. "Who's the kid, Len?"

"We're tryin' him out," Len replied. "If he can break less than zero he's got himself a job."

"He's cute," Erna remarked, with a little wink in Nick's direction. "Put him out front – make him a busboy."

"Excuse *me*," Q.J. interjected. "*I'm* runnin' this place."

"Just a suggestion," Erna said, throwing Nick another wink. "Maybe the ladies wanna look at somethin' for a change."

"Shit," Q.J. said, shaking his head at Len. "Now I gotta listen to hirin' crap from your wife."

Len ignored him, he was busy pulling the innards from a dead chicken.

Nick wondered how Joey and Cyndra were doing. Before the night shift began he wanted to get back to the hotel and check in. He took a quick peek at his watch – it was almost six which meant he'd been cleaning up for three hours.

"What time you want me back?" he said, addressing himself to Len.

"Whaddaya mean – back?" demanded Q.J., stepping over a box of wilted lettuce stashed on the floor. "We're comin' up to busy. You'll stick around 'til we close."

"He told me a coupla hours lunchtime, an' two or three in the evenings," Nick said, nodding at Len.

Q.J. couldn't care less. "What can I tell ya? He lied."

"Do I still get paid by the hour?"

"Yeah, yeah," Q.J. said impatiently, shooting his cuffs, revealing over-size pearl and gold cufflinks.

Nick wondered if they were real. "When's pay-day?" he asked.

"Friday. Jesus! That's all I need – a fuckin' dishwasher with a mouth!"

"Leave him alone, Q.J. He's workin' hard." So spoke Erna – his new guardian angel. "This place looks almost clean – for once."

By the time he got out of there it was past one in the morning. If his figures held up he'd made himself over twenty bucks. But jeez he was tired – ready to drop, and now he couldn't remember where the dumb hotel was.

He walked the streets for an hour before giving up, diving into the subway and curling up on a bench outside the men's room.

He'd find the hotel in the morning, right now all he could think about was sleep.

Just before oblivion hit he thought about Lauren and he fell asleep with a smile on his face.

Hands awoke him. Frantic hands, insistent hands. He opened his eyes to find an elderly well-dressed man bending over him struggling with the zipper on his jeans.

"What the hell –" he began, shoving the man's hands away.

"I'll pay you," the man interrupted, a feverish gleam in his eyes. "I'll pay you good. Ten dollars to blow you – or if you'd sooner the other way round I'll –"

Nick leapt up, startling the man who cowered against the wall.

"I . . . I . . . can go to fifteen," the man offered, licking dry lips. "Even twenty . . ."

"Fuck you!" Nick snarled, running down the platform towards the stairs. "*Fuck you, pervert!*"

"No need to get –"

Nick made it up to the street and fresh air. He took a deep gulp. Shit! If this was the big city he'd better learn to watch out.

He glanced at his watch; it was past seven and the streets were already busy. Now that it was light it didn't take him long to find the hotel, sneak past the front desk and make his way upstairs to their room.

Cyndra and Joey were asleep. Nice. Like they'd really been worried about him. He gave Joey a hefty shove.

"Wassup?" Joey mumbled, opening one eye.

"I'm back, that's what's up."

Joey struggled to sit up. "Where were you, man?"

"Workin'. Where were *you*?"

Joey was impressed. "You got a job?"

"No big deal. Washin' dishes. I'll do it 'til I score somethin' else."

"Washin' dishes," Cyndra mumbled, surfacing from under the covers. "I didn't leave home t'do that."

"Yeah, well, *you're* not doin' it, are you? I am," Nick replied. "An' it's only 'til we connect."

"That'll be soon," Joey said confidently, leaping out of bed. "Real soon."

Unfortunately Nick discovered he was the only one who'd found work. Neither Cyndra nor Joey had been so lucky. Secretly he was proud of himself; he'd proved he could manage on his own and that was a big achievement – maybe he should have run from his father a long time ago.

Later, when he reported for work he felt more at home. The foraging rat by the garbage cans seemed like an old friend, and Len in his soiled apron even threw him a friendly wave, cigarette ash scattering everywhere.

Nick Angelo. Dishwasher. Some beginning.

But it was better than nothing.

Cyndra might be only seventeen but she knew the look – it was in most men's eyes as soon as they saw her.

This man was no different. This skinny little jerk with a bald spot, glasses and a nervous tic.

"How oldja?" he asked, picking his nose.

She was interviewing for a job as an usher in a movie theatre. How old did you have to be to direct people to their seats? She took a wild guess. "Twenty."

"Got references?"

"Nope."

He stopped digging for treasure and peered at her through his thick glasses. "No references, huh?"

Big deal. Try a smile. "This would be my first job," she said, politely.

The man stared at her breasts. "I'd hire ya – but the management needs references."

"How can I have references if I've never had a job?" she said reasonably, wishing she'd worn a heavier sweater.

The man pushed at his glasses. "Can't risk it."

This was her fifth interview of the day – probably her fiftieth for the week. She'd been out looking every day, and so had Joey. How come Nick walked in off the street and scored an immediate job? It wasn't fair.

She wondered if she wrote to the canning plant back in Bosewell if they'd mail her a reference.

To whom it may concern:

Cyndra Angelo worked her black ass off for several months making sure an extra peach didn't fall into the wrong can. She stood on an assembly line for ten hours

*a day and we paid her minimum wage. Oh yes, and every
man in the place tried to fuck her.*

No way. She'd left without giving notice. Gallagher – the
foreman of her section – was probably still pissed off.

She left the cinema and hit the streets again. It was hot and
her feet hurt. She sat down on a bench by the bus-stop and tried
to figure out her next move.

Use your looks, a little voice whispered in her head. *Make
'em work for you.*

She remembered an interview a couple of days back. DANC-
ING GIRLS NEEDED the ad had stated. She'd gone to a loft
in the city and lined up with about twenty other girls while a
shirtless man with a video camera had filmed the line. When he
was finished he'd said, "Okay – now the nude shots. Anyone who
don't wanna strip get out now."

She and three other girls had beat a hasty retreat. The
rest had started to disrobe.

What would have happened if she'd stayed?

She shuddered, not wanting to know. No way was she
parading around naked, it wasn't her style. And she did have
style. Whatever happened to her, whatever the future held, she
always had to believe in herself – otherwise she was finished.

"I gotta coupla friends – they both need jobs," Nick blurted
out.

Tonight Q.J. was in a maroon velvet smoking jacket well worn
at the elbows. As far as he was concerned Cary Grant better watch
out. "Whatcha think this is? A fuckin' charity set up?" Q.J. said,
pulling a face at Len as if to say *Who is this schmuck? And why is
he workin' for me?*

Len pounded on a slab of rabbit shortly to be served up as
Chicken Surprise. "Ya don't want conversation don' come in the
kitchen. This kid never stops. He thinks he's an actor."

"An actor?" Q.J. managed to look amazed. "Only *I* would
hire a fuckin' dishwasher who thinks he's a fuckin' actor."

As usual they were talking about him as if he didn't exist.
That was okay. He was used to it by now. Two weeks working
at Q.J.'s and he was used to anything. The place was a dump –
but it had turned out to be a popular dump. It hadn't taken Nick
long to find out that Q.J. was a reformed house burglar who'd
spent so much time in jail that a couple of years previously he'd

decided to give up his life of crime and open a restaurant/bar with his brother-in-law, Len – a former waiter at one of Chicago's more fashionable hotels. Erna – Q.J.'s sister, had declared herself in as head stripper. Every time she wasn't around Q.J. complained. "Ya gotta retire her, Len. When she takes 'em off half my customers get up an' leave!"

"*You* tell her," was Len's standard reply. "*I* havta sleep with her."

Q.J.'s clientele consisted of ex-cons, present cons and the more colourful element of Chicago's criminal population. Strictly small-time, but they all had money to spend, and Q.J. made sure everyone had a good time – in spite of Erna and her dance of the seven veils.

Q.J. was a genial host who did a touch of fencing on the side, and in spite of his tough talk he was a real easy touch. Which is why Nick decided to repeat his words.

"I gotta coupla friends – they both need jobs."

"Do I look like an employment agency?" Q.J. demanded, throwing his arms wide. "I gotta pay nine people a week – ten if ya wanna include the cleaner who don't clean shit. I am not –" he raised his voice for effect "– a fuckin' refuge for fuckin' teenage schmucks from the East."

"West," Nick corrected.

Q.J. threw him a filthy look. "Now I gotta stay outta my own kitchen on account of your mouth. What I do to deserve this?"

Len reached for his cigarette smouldering on the counter top. He took a puff, causing thick ash to drop on the pounded rabbit flesh. Neither Q.J. nor Len seemed bothered.

"Can I bring 'em in?" Nick asked, expertly stacking clean glasses ready to return to the bar.

"No," said Q.J.

"No," said Len.

"You'll like 'em both," said Nick.

Two nights later he arrived at six with Cyndra and Joey lurking behind him.

Q.J. took one look at Cyndra and rolled his eyes. "Too pretty," he said. "The broads'll hate her. Can't have a stripper better lookin' than the customers – they don't like it."

"I'm not a stripper," Cyndra said hotly, glaring at Nick.

Q.J. squinted in her direction. "What are ya, doll? A brain surgeon with tits?"

"A singer."

"A what?"

"You heard me."

Q.J. adjusted the collar of his striped shirt and loosened his cerise tie. The girl was a beauty – a little dark for his taste and dangerously young, but she had class. Maybe his customers would go for her if he had Erna dress her up in a tight red dress with plenty of cleavage. Yeah – maybe he'd be Mister Nice Guy and give her a chance.

"I gotta be crazy," he said, shaking his head. "One night. Ten bucks. If they don' like you, you're out."

"What about me?" Joey asked. "I'm a –"

"Save it, sonny. I did my good deed for the day."

Joey knew when to shut up.

Cyndra's singing debut was inauspicious. Dressed up by Erna in a tight revealing gown she hated, with teased hair and too much make-up, she stood in front of a boozy crowd and attempted to warble her version of Aretha Franklin's "Respect". A mistake. The only singing Cyndra had ever done was in private, and although her voice was pleasantly husky she had no idea how to use it.

After a few minutes the crowd became restless. "Get 'em off, sweetie," yelled one man, and others soon took up the chant.

Standing at the back of the room Q.J. chewed on a toothpick and scowled. He'd thought he might have made a discovery – but as usual he was wrong. The girl had faked him out – convincing him she could do something she wasn't capable of.

"You fuckin' her or what?" asked Petey the Frog, one of his regulars, his bug-eyes bulging.

"Nah – just givin' her a chance." Q.J. replied, smoothing down his velvet smoking jacket.

"C'mon, ya gotta be fuckin' her," Petey the Frog said, slurping his drink.

"Too young," Q.J. said shortly, walking away.

Cyndra finished to desultory applause and a few more raucous cries of "Get 'em off!" She ran from the small stage.

"I quit!" she told an amazed Q.J.

"You quit?" he managed. "You fuckin' quit? I'm firin' ya, doll."

She glared at him. "You can't fire someone who already quit."

"And I ain't payin' ya, either," Q.J. added, red in the face.

"Oh yes you are," she said, fiercely. "I performed. You'll pay. It's not my fault your customers are a bunch of stupid apes."

Q.J. had never come across a girl like Cyndra before. She was a young one – but she had guts and he couldn't help admiring her. It was a shame she had no talent.

His first wife had been like that – Sassy Sarah everyone had called her. She'd run off with their electrician while he'd been languishing in jail. His second wife had chosen the plumber. He'd been single now for eight years and that's the way he planned to stay.

He paid Cyndra her ten bucks. She didn't seem particularly grateful. "I don't havta do this," he informed her.

"Yes you do," she replied, walking out into the night.

Q.J. did not appreciate her attitude, a little ass kissing would have been nice.

"Don't bring in no more of your friends," he warned Nick.

"You shoulda let her practise or somethin'," Nick said.

Q.J. shook his head at Len. "What the fuck's goin' on here? I gotta dishwasher lippin' off, an' a broad that can't sing shit givin' me a hard time. Do I deserve this?"

"That's life," Len said, dipping his finger into a bowl of cream.

"Shit!" said Q.J. "*Shit!*"

"Listen –" Nick began.

"One more word outta you an' you're fired," Q.J. said, gruffly.

Erna entered the kitchen beaming. "Big hit, huh?"

"With all due respect," Q.J. said to his sister, "You wouldn't know a big hit if it landed on ya ass an' bit you!"

By the time Nick finished work and got back to the hotel Cyndra and Joey were waiting outside with their bags packed. It was two in the morning.

"What's up?" he asked, dreading the answer.

"We got thrown out," Joey said, stamping his feet against the cold night air.

"How come?"

"'Cause we owe 'em."

"But I gave you the money to pay."

Joey looked sheepish. "I kinda lost it in a street hustle."

"Jerk!" muttered Cyndra.

"Hey – this place cost too much anyway," Joey said, quickly. "Tomorrow we'll get us a one-room apartment – it'll be cheaper."

Nick was angry. He was still the only one working – and now Joey was taking his hard-earned money and blowing it on street con games for dumb tourists. Maybe it was time to split up.

"I'm cold," Cyndra said, sounding like a little girl. "Where'll we sleep?"

She was his sister, he couldn't desert her.

"C'mon," he said, "we'll find you a nice comfortable park bench, cover you with newspapers an' you'll sleep like a baby."

She recovered her edge. "Gee, I can't wait."

Joey snapped his fingers. "Whaddaya want? The penthouse at the Ritz Carlton?"

She looked at him as if he was a lowly worm. "Yes," she said. "And one of these days that's exactly what I'll get."

"Sure," Nick agreed. "But tonight it's the park, so let's hit it."

They picked up their belongings and set off.

As they trudged towards the park he began thinking about Lauren and how much he missed her. By this time she'd have read his letter, and maybe if he got a post office box and wrote again, care of Louise, she'd reply.

The first thing they had to do was find somewhere to live. Joey was right: the hotel – cheap as it was – had been too expensive – they should have moved weeks ago.

An icy wind blasted them as they turned the corner. Joey stopped to gather a stack of old newspapers sticking out of a garbage can – disturbing a mangey cat. It ran off down the street screeching. Two drunken old tramps staggered by. A couple of junkies huddled in a doorway busy shooting up.

Cyndra clung to Nick's arm, shivering. "I'm frightened," she whispered.

"Don't worry," he said, trying to reassure her, "we'll be all right."

She clung tighter. "Promise?"

"Hey listen, kiddo – as long as y'hang out with me I'll never let you down. Okay?"

"Yes, Nick."

He may have sounded full of confidence, but it was a cold hard world out there and sometimes he was frightened, too.

Chapter 32

It all seemed to happen at once – one moment she was fighting off Primo, and then everything became a horrifying deadly blur. First the howling wind, followed by a thunderous roar as the tornado bore down on them, catching the trailer in its path, scooping it into the air and carrying it along for several hundred yards as if it were made of papier mâché.

Lauren could hardly remember anything as she was hurled from the door to the ground outside and knocked unconscious. When she came to, the tornado was off in the distance, sweeping a path of destruction, ripping up everything as it headed for the centre of town.

Lying on the ground, she groaned, lifted her hand and felt blood on her cheek. She tried to sit up, overcome with an overwhelming sense of despair as she attempted to remember exactly what had happened.

Primo . . . grabbing her . . . tearing at her clothes . . . the knife.

Oh, God, the knife! Had she killed him?

Panic stricken she staggered to her feet forcing herself to think clearly. All she could remember was the power of the tornado descending, and being propelled from the door as if by some magic hand as the trailer was lifted up and swept away.

Somehow she'd been saved. Why?

She looked around the trailer site – it was more or less obliterated, everything gone. Even the trees had been plucked from their roots.

Living in the Midwest she'd heard about tornadoes all her life, but she'd never experienced one. Now the reality was upon her and she saw for herself the devastation it could cause.

In the distance she could still see the wreathing grey funnel twisting on its way, its awesome destructive power demolishing everything it encountered.

There was no more rain, just an eerie stillness, and a deathly silence.

She tried to force herself to move, but her legs felt weak and could hardly hold her weight. Somewhere a dog barked mournfully.

I've got to get home, she thought. *They'll be so worried about me.*

She began to walk. Back towards town. Back to the house she hoped was still standing.

The tornado swept down Main Street like a lethal weapon, cutting its deadly path with incredible strength. Everything in its way was sucked up into its white-grey funnel. Trees, people, animals, cars – it was not selective.

Picking up strength as it travelled on its way it hit Main Street at its peak, propelled by winds of up to two hundred and fifty miles an hour.

The plate glass windows of the drugstore caved in, sending great shards of glass smashing to the ground.

Louise held tightly on to Dave, fervently praying.

He dragged her out into the street as the ceiling collapsed and falling debris crashed around them. Protecting her as best he could he threw her to the ground and lay on top of her – both of them trembling with fear. A sheet of glass sliced through his leg, cutting it off below the knee.

Louise let out a long, anguished scream as the blood from Dave's injury pumped all over her.

The tornado continued on its way, demolishing the Blakely Brothers hardware store, above which Phil Roberts and Eloise clung together in his office. They hardly knew what hit them. The very last words Phil Roberts heard was Eloise screaming, "I never meant to do it, God. Forgive me for my sins. Please forgive me!"

And then there was nothing.

Jane Roberts' car with her inside was swept up into the wind funnel and carried along for almost a mile. She died of shock.

The car, containing her body, was recovered twenty-four hours later – miraculously, it was still perfectly intact.

Bosewell High School suffered a direct hit. As the students raced into the gym, the tornado sucked the roof off the building, pelting everyone with flying glass and jagged chunks of concrete. Crashing debris hit a gas main causing a major fire.

Meg managed to grab hold of Stock as he hung on to the climbing rails, the only part of the gym that remained. She held on for dear life, trying to ignore his hysterical sobs and keep a clear head.

Mack had vanished – sucked away in the awesome cone of dust.

"Help me!" Stock sobbed, hysterically. "Somebody help me!"

"I'm here," Meg cried, soothingly. "Don't worry, I'll look after you, I'm here."

Aretha Mae watched the factory vanish before her very eyes. She stood in the middle of the destruction completely unharmed and continued to pray.

By the time the tornado left Bosewell fourteen people were dead, over a hundred and fifty injured. More than sixty buildings were damaged or destroyed and the small town declared a disaster area.

In the big story nobody bothered to mention Bosewell – for the killer tornado cut a path of death and destruction throughout the Midwest, making the small town of Bosewell only a minor victim.

By the time the story hit the major news services, Bosewell was hardly mentioned.

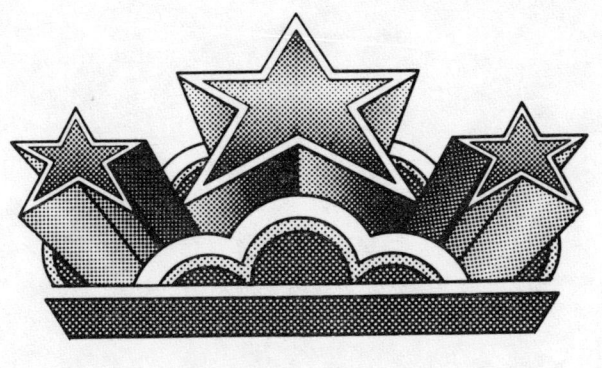

BOOK TWO

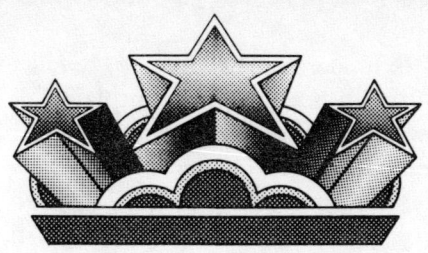

Chapter 33

Chicago, 1979

Nick lay back in bed his eyes following the naked redhead prowling around his tiny one-room apartment. Her name was DeVille and she was a natural redhead.

He liked watching her in his home, it sure beat observing her gyrate on stage while dozens of horny old men got off ogling her considerable charms. She was, at twenty-six, an older woman, but only by four years, which fazed neither of them.

DeVille had a sweep of long hair, pale aquamarine eyes, pouty lips, voluptuous breasts and a sunny disposition. She'd been living with him for almost six months.

"Can I fetch you anything, sweet thing?" she asked, prancing around his apartment, all curves.

"Yeah." He leaned back in bed putting one arm behind his head. "Get over here."

DeVille did not argue, she never argued. Sometimes he wished she would. He'd heard of easy, but she was ridiculous.

She approached the bed and stood beside him. He reached up and touched one perfect size thirty-six tit – no silicone – DeVille was all natural, the only phoney thing about her was her name.

Rolling her extended nipple between his fingers he made a suggestion she was not about to turn down.

DeVille was pleased. Her last lover had been twenty years older than her and a grouch. Nick was a real treat.

"My, oh my!" she exclaimed, pulling the sheet off him and widening her eyes. "What big . . . *thighs* you have."

"All the better to grab your ass!" He pulled her on top of him and they both laughed as she straddled him with her long white

211

legs. DeVille liked being on top. He didn't mind, he knew it was her one power play.

They started to make frantic love – DeVille was a screamer – their neighbours did nothing but complain.

When they were finished he rolled out of bed and strolled into the cramped bathroom.

"How about I make pancakes?" DeVille called out.

"I ain't hungry," he said, quickly. The one thing she couldn't do was cook.

He noticed a spider crawling along the side of the tub. Picking it up by one of its legs he carefully placed it on the window-sill and watched it dart to safety across the fire-escape.

"I'll make coffee then," she sang out.

At least she could do that. He stepped into the rusty tub and turned the knob to activate the wall shower – as usual, getting nothing but a trickle of lukewarm water.

He had a hangover. The night before had been a long one, plenty of action and he hadn't gotten home until three in the morning.

Who'd have thought Q.J.'s would become *the* place? And who'd have thought he'd become the manager?

Yeah, some success story. From dishwasher to manager. And all it had taken was five years. Wow!

"What shall we do today?" DeVille asked, popping her head around the bathroom door.

"I'm easy."

"Maybe we could catch a movie – there's a new Paul Newman."

Yeah – Paul Newman. That meant he'd definitely get laid again. "Sure," he said, easily.

By the time he emerged from the bathroom, DeVille was dressed. On Sundays she liked to play at being ordinary. She'd put on jeans, a sweater, and braided her long red hair. Looking at her today nobody would guess she performed one of the horniest acts in town.

"Oh – I forgot to tell you. This letter came for you yesterday," she said, handing him an envelope.

He studied the writing on the front – it was from Cyndra. "How many times I gotta tell you? When I get mail I want it right away," he said, irritated.

"I told you – I forgot."

The envelope looked in bad shape. "What did you do, steam it open?"

"As if I would!"

"As if you wouldn't."

DeVille had a jealous streak he didn't appreciate.

"Is it from your sister?" she said, peering over his shoulder.

"You *did* open it," he accused.

"No, I did not. Her name's on the back, big deal."

It was a stupid thought, but one of these days he still hoped he might receive a letter from Lauren. Yeah – a real stupid thought. Lauren was his past, long gone. He'd written her many times and never gotten a reply. After a while he'd given up, it was obvious she didn't care about him.

But that didn't mean he couldn't think about her once in a while, did it? He imagined her still in Bosewell, married with kids, happy, never giving him a second thought – she probably didn't even remember his name.

He opened Cyndra's letter. She'd left Chicago with Joey over four years ago. The two of them had taken off when the winter got too cold and neither of them could keep a job. They'd tried to persuade him to go with them, but by that time he was settled at Q.J.'s doing everything from taking over the bar to running errands for Q.J.

Cyndra had stayed in New York with Joey for a couple of years, until eventually she'd met some sharp-shooter called Reece Webster, who'd lured her out to California with a few phoney promises. She was still with him. From what Nick could gather the guy was married, but on the brink of leaving his wife. He'd been on the brink for the last two years.

He scanned her letter.

Dear Nick:

Well, things are good in Los Angeles, you'd really love it here. It's hot all the time and there's these great palm trees everywhere – but I guess I've told you that enough times – right?

Why don't you come visit me? I've got plenty of room if you don't mind sleeping on a sofa-bed. Reece is never here at weekends so we could have fun and you know how much I miss you.

As far as my career . . . well, I'm taking singing lessons – ha ha! Aren't you glad? I'm also meeting lots of people Reece says can help me.

I haven't heard from Joey in a while. I think he's driving a cab. You know Joey, always waiting for the big break. Aren't we all – ha ha!

I'm serious, Nick – please think about coming out here even if it's only for a long weekend.

I love you and I miss you lots.

As always,
Your sister,
Cyndra

She wasn't the world's greatest letter writer, but at least she bothered to write.

"You ever been to California?" he asked DeVille, folding the letter and putting it in his pocket.

"Once," she replied. "When I was eighteen. There was this rich guy with his own private plane. He flew me and three other girls to a party in Vegas. We put on a show *they* didn't forget in a hurry!"

"What kind of show?"

"Stripping, parading the goods, what else?"

"Did you ever do any hooking?"

Her mouth tightened. "Why are you asking me that?"

"I'm throwing it into the conversation."

"Throw it out again, Nick," she said, glaring at him. "I take my clothes off, and that's *all* I do."

"Yeah, yeah, I'm sorry. I don't know why I said that."

"Nor do I." She marched into the bathroom slamming the door behind her.

She'd sulk for five minutes and then come out. DeVille never stayed angry for long.

Q.J. had this theory about women. He considered them all hookers under the skin. Sometimes he'd give Nick the benefit of his wisdom. "You gotta look at it like this – when they marry a guy, what the hell ya think they're doin'? They're havin' sex for money, right? So the husband screws her one night, an' buys her a dress the next day. The poor schmuck pays for everything. Why don't he leave a hundred buckerooneys on the bedside table an' call it quits?"

Q.J. was a true cynic. Maybe that was the way to be. Nick had no intention of ever getting married. Every time DeVille so much as hinted he'd laughed, not taking her seriously.

Once again his thoughts drifted back to Lauren. He couldn't help thinking about her – she hovered at the back of his mind – a distant memory he couldn't forget. He'd hoped that over the

214

years Joey or Cyndra would go back to Bosewell for a visit – but neither of them seemed inclined. As far as he knew Joey had never contacted his mother, and Cyndra had no urge to get in touch with Aretha Mae, although she occasionally mentioned Harlan. They both felt guilty about leaving the kid. "When I make it I'll go get him," Cyndra said.

Yeah. Sure.

Once in a while he thought of calling Louise at the drugstore – just to find out what was going on in town. But something always stopped him. The truth was he really didn't want to know.

Over the years he'd worked hard, helping to make Q.J.'s the successful place it was today. Five years ago it was a hang-out for petty con artists and their one-night stands, offering nothing but bad food and a couple of tired strippers. When disco got really big he'd started badgering Q.J. about dumping the strippers and bringing in a disc jockey.

"Are you outta your fuckin' skull?" Q.J. had said. "My customers get off on the girls – anyhow, we ain't got no space for dancin'."

"Make it," he'd urged. "You gotta get into this disco thing before it's over."

"I hire a fuckin' dishwasher an' all of a sudden he's tellin' me what to do."

"I ain't a dishwasher no more."

"What are you then?"

"Your assistant."

"If you say so."

Q.J. was too cheap to hire a disc jockey, and too nervous to risk losing customers by firing the strippers, so he'd compromised by making Nick the disc jockey, and persuading Erna to stop stripping – putting her in charge of two new girls he hired. Business had picked up immediately.

Nick was triumphant. "I told ya," he'd said.

"Yeah, yeah, you told me," Q.J. had replied. "Like I didn't already know."

Nick really got into the music. It was a kick hanging out at the record stores listening to all the new sounds and picking out the latest hits.

The sound system Q.J. elected to put in was shit, but he quickly learned how to work the room – mixing the old with the new – a little bit of Elvis, followed by Al Green, throw in some

Bobby Womack, then calm them down with Dionne Warwick and Smokey Robinson.

When he wasn't working the turntables he was behind the bar.

The resident bartender didn't like it. "Get that ratty kid away from me," he'd complained, "or I'm outta here."

There was nothing Q.J. liked better than a threat. Plus he could get away with paying Nick half the money he was paying the old man. "So quit," he'd said.

The bartender did, and Nick had found himself in charge of the bar, too.

"We gotta hire somebody else," he'd complained. "I can't play records *and* run the bar."

"Jesus Christ, you're gonna break me," Q.J. complained.

"No," he'd corrected. "I'm gonna make you."

Erna was his biggest supporter. Even Len got into the spirit of things by hiring an assistant chef who could actually cook. Q.J.'s really took off.

Not that anybody had ever thanked him. He didn't need thanks – a steady job was enough.

He considered the situation. He'd walked in off the street five years ago with exactly nothing, and now he was the son Q.J. never had. Not bad. Not good. He'd come to Chicago hoping to be an actor and done nothing about it. He was twenty-two years old – if he didn't start soon he never would. While he stayed at Q.J.'s there was no time for anything else – not even acting class. He'd managed to save a couple of thousand dollars over the years, and now California beckoned. The letter from Cyndra was a sign. If he didn't make a move he'd be stuck at Q.J.'s forever, wearing cerise shirts and shooting his cufflinks just like Q.J. himself. A frightening thought!

DeVille bounced out of the bathroom. She was pretty, sexy and amiable.

It was over. Six months was his limit. Besides, he couldn't take her with him; excess baggage was never a good idea.

"Are we going to the movie?" she asked.

"Sure."

God, she had a great mouth.

It would be tough kissing it goodbye.

Chapter 34

Philadelphia, 1979

"Excuse me, Miss Roberts."

"Yes, Mr Larden?"

"I notice that it's raining outside, and I wondered if I might offer you a lift home."

"That's very nice of you, Mr Larden, but my cousin is meeting me."

"Oh." Mr Larden stared at her. He was a man of medium height in his thirties with thinning hair and a drooping mouth. He was also a married man with two children, one dog and several hamsters. He was her boss.

"Are you sure, Miss Roberts?" he asked, hopefully.

"Yes, I'm sure, Mr Larden."

They played this game all the time. He pretended to be the concerned boss always looking out for his secretary's welfare. She pretended that he really did want to give her a lift out of the kindness of his heart because it was raining outside. They both knew this was a lie. He wanted to get her into bed any way he could.

Lauren had worked for him as his personal secretary for two years now, and she knew she had to leave or go completely crazy.

"Well," he said, collecting his briefcase. "I'll see you tomorrow, then."

"Yes, Mr Larden."

She waited until he'd left before picking up the phone. "Brad," she said, in a low voice. "I can't see you tonight."

"What do you mean you can't see me?" he spluttered.

"It's difficult to explain now. Let's talk tomorrow." She put the phone down quickly before he could argue.

Bradford Deene, her cousin. Good old Brad. Without him she probably couldn't have gotten through the last five years. But their relationship was sick, it had to stop, and she was the one who was going to end it.

Five years ago she'd arrived in Philadelphia a shivering wreck. Her mother's brother, Will, along with his wife, Margo, had met her at the airport.

"We're so sorry, dear, so very, very sorry," Margo had said, but she hadn't shed a tear.

Will seemed more sincere. "Your mother was a wonderful woman – always a good sister to me. We shall miss her."

The Deenes had taken her to their house on Roosevelt Boulevard. It was a nice house, but it certainly wasn't home. Brad, her nineteen-year-old cousin, was away at college and they allowed her to stay in his room. At night she overheard them whispering. Margo first – "What are we going to do with her? We can't keep her here."

Then Will. "Lauren is my sister's daughter, Margo. She has no other relatives. We *have* to take her in, after all, she's only sixteen."

"I know, I know. But for how long?"

Jane and Phil Roberts had both perished in the deadly tornado that had practically totalled Bosewell. Lauren remembered very little of the nightmare. She'd arrived in Philadelphia still numb with shock. And shortly after arriving she'd had to tell Margo she was pregnant.

Her aunt had gone completely crazy. "How did this happen? Were you raped?" she'd demanded.

"It just . . . happened . . ."

"Was it that boy you were engaged to? Stock? Because if it was we can force him to marry you."

"No, it wasn't Stock."

"Who was it then?"

"It doesn't matter."

"Your poor parents . . . they'd be so . . . so . . . disappointed in you."

"I want to have the baby," Lauren had said, quietly.

Margo had shaken her head. "Absolutely out of the question. It's enough that *you're* here – we cannot look after a baby, too."

"There *is* no choice in this matter," her uncle had said. "You'll have to have an abortion."

She remembered the termination as if it were yesterday. Margo had taken her to a male gynaecologist – a bald man with sleepy eyes and rubber-gloved hands.

"What have you been up to, young lady?" he'd said with a jovial wink as she lay on the cold hard examining table, feeling naked and vulnerable beneath the paper garment the nurse instructed her to wear.

"Come along, put your legs in the stirrups, dear."

He'd probed and poked until she could stand it no more.

"I don't want to lose my baby," she'd whispered.

"It's nothing," he'd said. "Don't worry about it. Next time you open your legs be a little more careful, that's all."

Then they'd given her an injection, and she remembered nothing much at all except the harsh feel of cold steel between her legs.

After that there was no more baby, no more Nick.

At the time she'd thought about him every second of the day, but now she'd forced herself to stop. Nick Angelo had left her, run out of town without so much as a goodbye, and she'd never heard from him again – not even after the tragedy.

In a way she hated him. He'd used her for his own selfish reasons and then dumped her – leaving her pregnant and alone. She was shocked that he'd left. No note, no word, no nothing. She hardened her heart towards him, but for some inexplicable reason she still didn't want to lose his baby.

Margo and Will insisted she go back to school. She did so reluctantly because she'd had no choice.

One night Margo and Will had called her into their living room and given her the bad news. "Your father's estate left nothing. Death taxes took what little there was. He was heavily in debt."

"I'm sorry, Lauren," Margo added. "There's no money to send you to college. You must understand that we can't afford it. We've worked hard all our lives to allow Bradford all the advantages he's had, and now we're entitled to enjoy what's left."

"I don't want to go to college," she'd said. "As soon as I graduate High school I'll find a job."

"You could always try for a scholarship," Will ventured, feeling guilty. "After all, you're a smart girl."

They didn't understand that she meant it when she said she had no wish to attend college.

For several years she'd had nightmares about the tornado. In her mind she could see it sweeping down on the trailer – and sometimes in her dreams the tornado would turn into Primo. He would be part of it – leering at her . . . touching her . . . saying lewd things – until he forced her to raise the knife and strike out.

She'd killed Primo.

Or had she?

The uncertainty drove her crazy.

As soon as she graduated High school she'd taken a job at the local bank and started saving money. The moment she had enough she planned to move out of the Deene household.

Since coming home from college Brad was always around. He was good-looking with curly brown hair and a ready smile. He was taller than Nick, more muscular. She still compared every man she met to Nick, it was a habit she couldn't break.

By the time she was nineteen she'd saved enough money to move out. She had good secretarial skills and immediately got a job at Larden and Scopers, Attorneys at Law. Mr Larden himself had interviewed her and informed her she was perfect – exactly what he was looking for.

Her life was simple until Brad complicated it. He'd dropped by her small apartment one night, stayed too long and drunk too much. Then he'd confessed he thought he loved her, and somehow or other they'd ended up in bed even though they'd both known it was wrong. She'd tried to make it one time only but he wouldn't let her. He'd talked her into it, and once in she couldn't get out. Besides, it felt good to be with someone who cared.

Their affair had been going on for several months and she was suffocated with guilt. She wanted out. All she had to do was tell him.

She left the office and took the bus to her small apartment, running the last few hundred yards to her building, getting soaked.

Brad was inside, sitting on *her* couch, his feet up on *her* table watching *her* television.

"I told you I couldn't see you," she said, removing her raincoat.

"You didn't mean it," he replied.

"I want my key back," she said, clicking off the TV.

He frowned. "What's with you lately?"

"Brad, you know this isn't right. It has to end."

"No way, baby," he settled back, totally at ease.

The way he said "baby" made her stomach turn. She knew for sure she wasn't the only girl he was sleeping with.

"Please," she said. "I want it to be over."

He held out his arms. "Come over here."

"No, Brad."

"Are we playing hard to get?"

He wouldn't leave and she couldn't make him.

"What if I told your parents," she threatened.

"You wouldn't do that."

"I might."

"They'd blame you."

"Do you think I care? They never wanted me to come and live with them anyway."

He considered her threat. He wouldn't put it past her. "What is it, the wrong time of the month?" he asked, clicking the television back on.

She had a plan. If he wouldn't go, she would.

A week later at the office Christmas party, a drunken Mr Larden grabbed her in his office, trapping her up against his desk.

She knew exactly how to deal with men who tried to force her to do something she didn't want to do. She grabbed a letter opener and stabbed him in the arm.

Mr Larden yelled out his surprise and pain. "Are you *insane*?" he shouted.

"Try taking no for an answer," she said, making it to the door.

"You're fired," he said.

"Good."

By the time Christmas arrived she had every detail of her departure planned. On Christmas Day she went to Margo and Will's for lunch – they'd been a lot nicer to her since she'd moved out and they weren't obliged to support her. Brad was there with a girl called Jennie. The two of them spent the entire day giggling and necking.

"I think they might get engaged," Margo confided in the kitchen.

"That's nice," Lauren said. If he'd brought his girlfriend to make her jealous it wasn't working.

Sitting at the dining table she noticed Brad's hand creep under the table and up Jennie's thigh.

"You know," Margo said, turning to Lauren, obviously unaware of her son's furtive adventure, "you're perfectly welcome to bring a date here. Are you seeing anyone?"

Lauren shook her head. "No."

"A pretty girl like you," Will said, cheerfully. "You should have dozens of boyfriends."

"She's probably hiding them from us," Brad said, laughing confidently as his fingers played with the elastic on the brief panties guarding his girlfriend's moist crotch.

Lauren sighed. He was good in bed and he knew it. He played her like an expert, touching everything in just the right way.

Later that night when he'd gotten rid of Jennie, he arrived unannounced at her apartment. She allowed him to make love to her for the last time, only he didn't know it was the last time – he was under the misguided impression she was going to be available for him whenever he felt like it.

As soon as he left she hurried to the shower, washing him away forever. Then she packed, and early the next morning she took a cab to the bus station and boarded a Greyhound bus bound for New York.

She left no forwarding address. As far as she was concerned she'd been in mourning long enough.

Lauren Roberts was about to start a new life.

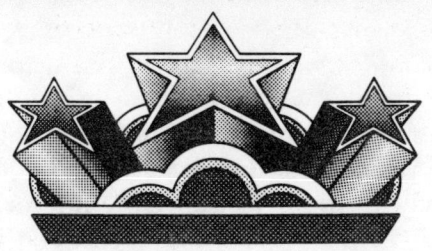

Chapter 35

Several things convinced Nick it was time to move on, not the least being the Carmello Rose incident. Carmello was a short grizzly man in his fifties with a beak nose, dark skin and a raspy, menacing voice. He was a rumoured Chicago hit man who visited Q.J.'s from time to time, always with several nubile young girls in tow, always with an eye to pick up more.

This particular night he arrived with only one woman – a tall redhead in her late thirties with large breasts and a sour expression.

"Fuck!" Q.J. said, agitatedly. "That broad's his wife."

"So," Nick asked "what's the big deal?"

"You'd better make sure nobody says nothin' 'bout none of the other skirts he's bin hangin' out with – 'cause if his wife finds out she'll blow his shrivelled ass to Cuba an' back. She's a wild woman."

"You worry too much," Nick said, calmly. "I'll take care of Mr Rose myself."

And why not? Carmello Rose was known for leaving hundred-dollar tips.

When he got near the table and took a closer look he had a feeling he'd seen this woman somewhere before. She was wearing a dangerously low-cut black cocktail dress, and he couldn't help his eyes from straying down her generous cleavage.

Carmello caught him catching a peek and fixed him with a frog-eyed stare that said all right to look, but no touching.

"What can I get you, Mr Rose?" Nick asked.

Carmello ordered a bottle of champagne.

"I just found out it's his wife's birthday," Q.J. said, agitatedly, stalking Nick behind the bar. "Get Len to arrange a cake."

"What does his wife do?" Nick asked.

"What does she *do*? What the fuck you *think* she does – looks after him."

"Then how come he's always hangin' out with other women?"

Q.J. looked testy. "We don't know nothin' 'bout that, do we? Take him a bottle of the best – my compliments."

"How come *you're* not going over?"

"'Cause Carmello frightens the crap outta me. Is that a good enough reason? Ya just gotta look sideways at his old lady an' he has a freakin' fit."

"Y'know, I got a feeling I've seen her somewhere before."

"Jesus, Nick, ain'tcha got enough broads of your own? This one's too old for you, anyway."

"Who's interested? I just wanna recall where I seen her."

Q.J. shook his head. "Forget it."

He took the champagne to the table informing them it was from Q.J. "On account of it bein' Mrs Rose's birthday an' all," he said, with a smile.

Carmello grunted.

"Thanks, sweetie," Mrs Rose said.

Was it his imagination or did she throw him a wink? He took another peek at her impressive breasts and it suddenly came to him. She was the woman whose car he'd gassed up in Bosewell a few years ago. The one in the sweater with the attitude. Who could ever forget those tits!

"How's your sister?" he asked, pouring her a glass of champagne.

She ran her tongue across her front teeth and darted a nervous glance at Carmello. "Huh?" she said, blankly.

Carmello snapped to attention. "Whadda *you* know about her sister?"

"She lives in Bosewell, right? I used to live there too."

Obviously he'd made no impression on her. She had no idea what he was talking about.

"Hey – I gassed your car a coupla times. You were visiting your sister, remember?"

Carmello threw her a filthy look. "You know this guy?"

"No, I certainly don't," she snapped, three large, diamond rings flashing on her fingers.

"He sure seems to remember you."

"Everyone remembers me," she said, defiantly.

"Hey, listen, no big deal," Nick said quickly, sensing trouble. "I musta made a mistake," he added, pouring more champagne into Carmello's glass before walking away.

Five minutes later he was in the stockroom when Carmello entered, kicking the door shut behind him. Before he could say a word Carmello took out a gun and shoved it in his stomach.

He lost his legs, it was like they weren't even there. "*Jesus*! What the hell you *doin'*?" he mumbled, panic-stricken as his life flashed before his eyes.

"Ya wanna know what *I'm* doin'," Carmello snarled gruffly, jabbing him with the gun. "What the fuck was *you* doin' with my wife?"

His throat was so dry he could barely speak. "I gassed her car, nothin' else."

"You gassed her car, huh? That it?"

He was breaking out in a cold sweat. "I swear. I was a kid – I promise you." Jesus! He needed to pee in the worst way.

Carmello shoved the gun into his stomach even harder. "Swear a little louder, ya dumb punk. Get down on your knees and fuckin' swear."

"It's the truth – God help me it's the truth."

"Turn around an' get down on your knees, fuckhead."

Maybe Carmello was going to shoot him, maybe he wasn't. He'd never know, because at that moment Q.J. opened the door and walked in on them. "Everything all right?" he asked calmly, like he didn't know anything was going on, although of course he did.

Reluctantly Carmello put his gun away. "Sure, sure. The kid an' me – we was talkin'."

And that was that. Crisis over. But Nick knew the time had come to get out.

Two days later he visited Q.J. in his office.

"I quit," he said.

"You *what*?"

"You heard me."

"Sure I heard you, but I don't believe what I'm hearin'."

"I've been in Chicago long enough."

Q.J. glared at him. "Yeah. Long enough to learn everythin' I know, is that the deal? You're gonna open your own place. I shoulda known it." He got up, marching angrily around the room. "I took you in, treated you good, now you're gonna stab me in the heart."

"That's not it," Nick said. "I'm plannin' on takin' a trip to California."

Q.J. rubbed together nicotine stained fingers. "What for?"

225

"For a chance."

"*I* gave you a chance. Ain't that enough?"

"I always had this thing 'bout gettin' into acting. If I don't try it now I never will."

Q.J. snorted his disgust. "Act. Schmact. You're in the bar business, that's where you belong."

"When I get settled I'll call, let you know how I'm doing."

"Who gives a shit? All I care about is you stayin' here. You're my manager, you take care of things. How about showin' some appreciation?"

"When I came to work here I never said it was a lifetime thing," he explained, hoping Q.J. would understand.

"Jesus!" Q.J. rolled his eyes. "You can't trust nobody no more."

"I'll stay 'til you find a replacement."

Q.J. was steaming. "I don't need nobody else. Don't worry 'bout a thing – you ungrateful little prick. Shift your ass outta here, see if I give a shit."

He knew Q.J. didn't mean it. "How about I stay around for two weeks?" he suggested.

"Do what you want," snapped Q.J.

Later Erna grabbed hold of him. "There's a rumour you're going to Hollywood," she said, thrilled at the thought.

"Yeah, I'm gonna give it a shot."

She nudged him slyly. "Like me to come with you?"

"Uh – I don't think Len would appreciate it."

She giggled. "Perhaps you're right," she said, tugging at an escaping bra strap. "I had a chance to go there once. I coulda been a famous starlet." She winked, knowingly. "Course, it meant sleeping with a fat old producer, so I stayed here, married Len, and now look at me."

"You're happy, aren't you?"

"I'm married to Len, that doesn't make me ecstatic."

"He seems like a nice guy."

"He's no Q.J."

Erna had confirmed his suspicions – she definitely had a crush on her brother.

When DeVille heard the news of his imminent departure she flew into a fury because he hadn't told her himself. Usually she left the club before him, but this particular night she stayed, joining the table of a customer – something she never did.

Nick realized this meant trouble. If he was smart he'd have taken off without telling anybody.

At closing time, DeVille dumped the customer and left with him, hanging on to his arm. She was drunk and angry – not a happy combination.

"Y'know something, Nicky," she slurred in his ear, well aware that he hated being called Nicky.

"What?" he said, steering her unsteady body into a cab.

"You're a son-of-a-bitch, that's what you are." She nodded, reassuring herself. "Yeah, a son-of-a-bitch."

"Hey, listen, I *was* gonna tell you," he said, defending himself. "But I had to tell Q.J. first. I owed him that."

"You owed him that," she mimicked. "And what do you owe me?"

He raised an eyebrow. "Y" think I owe you somethin"?"

"Bastard," she spat.

The cab driver – a weary veteran – glanced warily in his rear-view mirror.

"Goddamn bastard," DeVille said, hauling back in an attempt to slap him. "We live together – doesn't that mean *anything* to you?"

The cab swerved over to the side of the street and the driver turned around. "I don't want no trouble," he said. "Out. Both of you."

"It's all right, man," Nick said, gripping DeVille firmly by the wrist. "There ain't gonna be no trouble. Keep driving."

"The last couple hadda fight in my cab wrecked it," the driver muttered, sourly.

"I said keep driving," Nick repeated. "I'll take care of you good."

Still muttering under his breath the driver set off.

DeVille began to cry. Her anger he could take, but crying always got to him.

"Hey," he said, trying to comfort her. "I'm only going for a month or two."

"You're lying," she cried, leaning all over him, getting mascara on his one and only jacket.

"Maybe I'll send for you."

"Now you're *really* lying," she sobbed.

DeVille was no fool; they both knew it was over.

As soon as they reached his apartment she began to pack, hurling her things into a suitcase, well recovered from her crying jag. "I thought you were different," she yelled. "But no way – you're just like every other guy – selfish, self-centred, all you care about is your precious dick."

227

She looked good when she was angry and somehow or other they ended up in bed. DeVille thought if she was the best she'd ever been he might take her with him. It was quite an experience. At four o'clock in the morning their neighbours couldn't take the moaning and groaning any longer and called the police. They ended up hysterical with laughter.

In the morning they parted company. DeVille was sober and tense and, in a funny sort of way, dignified.

When she left he almost missed her – only almost.

"You're a scumbag, you know that? No loyalty." Q.J. was on a kick and he didn't intend to stop.

"Leave the kid alone," Erna said, coming to Nick's defence.

Q.J. glared angrily at his sister. "Did I ask for your input?"

"No, but –"

"I treat him like a son," Q.J. interrupted. "Grooming him, y'know what I mean?"

"Grooming him for what?" Erna asked, sharply. "To be in the bar business all his life like us? Who wants that?"

They were at it again, talking about him as if he didn't exist.

Len entered into the conversation. "He'll be back," he said, nodding wisely. "It's too hot in California."

Q.J. didn't seem so sure. "Ya think?" he said.

"No," said Erna, spitefully. "He won't be back. Why would he?"

On his last night Q.J. relented and threw him a big farewell party after the bar closed. For the first time he wondered if he was making the right move. Everybody was so warm and friendly. The waitresses, strippers, Erna, Len – even Q.J. In a way, this was his family now – the family he'd never had.

DeVille put on a show – and what a show it was! Enough bumping and grinding to turn on a priest! Maybe she wanted him to know exactly what he was leaving behind. He knew all right, but he still couldn't help himself.

Q.J. clapped him around the shoulders. "Ya know somethin', Nick, if y'ever wanna come back, y'got your job waitin'. I ain't never said that to nobody who worked for me before. Consider yourself honoured."

"I consider myself honoured," he said, grinning.

"In the meantime," Q.J. continued, "when ya get to LA I want ya t'look up my ex-partner."

"Who's your ex-partner?"

"Some guy used to be known as Manny the Menace, now he's strictly legit. Call him Mr Manfred and don't go mentioning his nickname – it drives him beserko."

"What does he do?"

"Runs a car service. Respectable. Just like me."

Nick burst out laughing. "Whoever said *you* were respectable?"

"Very funny." Q.J. smoothed an imaginary crease in his pin-stripe pants which did not go with his bright red jacket and green polka-dot tie.

"You're sure this guy is straight?" Nick asked, thinking that tonight Q.J. looked like a waiter in a whorehouse.

"Would I lie to you?"

"Yes."

"Go see him, Nick. He'll give you a job. All ya gotta say is I'm callin' in the favour he owes me. Q.J.'s collectin' – that's what ya tell him. He'll know what you mean."

"Shouldn't you contact him first?"

"We don't speak."

"So why would he want to –"

"Trust me." Q.J. scribbled on a piece of paper and handed it over. "Here's his number. Do like I say and phone him soon as y'get there."

"Thanks," he said, shoving the paper in his pocket. It was certainly better than arriving in LA cold.

Erna hugged him, covering him in her cloying scent. "Don't forget about us now, you hear me?"

"How –" he grinned, "could I ever forget *you*?"

'Not much chance of that," she giggled, coyly.

Len was his usual stoic self. They shook hands. "You'll be back," Len said, knowingly.

"Maybe – one of these days."

Now he was really beginning to regret his decision to leave. He had no idea what Los Angeles was like. He had no friends there, no job, just Cyndra, and he hadn't even warned her he was coming, figuring a surprise would be good.

In the morning Q.J. was on the missing list. "He don't like goodbyes," Erna explained, as she and Len drove him to the airport. "Gotta see you off in style," she added, with a saucy wink.

They couldn't park so they dropped him off kerbside. He grabbed his carry-on bag from the trunk and stood on the sidewalk waving to them as they drove away in Len's two-toned gold Chevrolet with the dented front fender.

As soon as they were gone he felt alone, but only for a moment. Then he picked up his bag, turned and strode purposefully towards the airline desk.

Chapter 36

The Greyhound bus delivered Lauren into New York at noon. She waved goodbye to the driver, collected her suitcase and stood alone in the middle of the busy bus station.

Before she could take two steps a scruffy looking man stinking of cheap aftershave approached her. His long greasy hair hung in strands around his face, and a cigarette dangled from the corner of his chapped lips.

"Hi'ya, lovely. Lookin' for a place t' stay?"

She was no naïve little country bumpkin getting off the bus in New York ready to be picked off by some lurking pimp.

"I have somewhere, thank you," she said, giving him a withering look.

"Just askin'. Can't do more than that, pretty chick like you."

She hurried away, only to be accosted a few yards later by a dark-skinned man in a filthy white suit who sidled up behind her.

"Wanna be a model?" he offered, speaking out of the corner of his mouth.

She kept walking.

"Wanna be a model an' make a lotta bucks?" he said, keeping pace with her.

She ignored him.

"Wanna fuck me?"

She stopped, turned to look at him, and said in a very loud voice, "Leave me alone or I'll call a cop. Got it, pervert?"

He slunk off.

Outside the bus station she found a cab, got in and gave the driver the address of the Barbizon Hotel for Girls.

"How many times you get hit on in there?" the driver asked, shoving his foot on the gas and zooming away from the kerb – missing another cab by mere inches.

231

"Enough," she replied, gazing out of the window at the dirty sidewalks, scurrying crowds and snarled traffic.

It was like a dream. Here she was, finally in New York, and she was free, she had nobody to answer to except herself.

She'd booked a room at the Barbizon before leaving Philadelphia. She'd also been buying the New York papers and circling job opportunities, setting up several appointments by phone.

After she'd unpacked and settled in, she took a walk over to Fifth Avenue. Oh yes, it was just like *Breakfast at Tiffany's*. The same wide street, the same expensive stores. She found herself outside Tiffany's staring into the windows like a tourist. She stifled a giggle – all she needed now was a cat and she was all set!

The next day she awoke early. It was autumn and the weather was brisk. She dressed carefully in a simple dark blue dress, adding low-heeled shoes and her mother's pearls. Over the top she belted a navy trench coat. She pulled her thick chestnut hair back securing it with a barrette, and wore very little make-up. The plainer the better, she thought. But there was no disguising the fact that at twenty-one Lauren was a natural beauty with her perfect oval face, unusual tortoiseshell colour eyes and dazzling smile.

Before doing anything else she opened a bank account and deposited her four-thousand-dollar savings. Then she set off on the first of three interviews.

The first one was with a law firm housed in a tall chrome and glass building on Park Avenue. There she was interrogated by an attractive black woman, who asked her a series of probing questions, and made her fill out a personality analysis form. After that she had to sit in a room and produce a sample of her typing.

The woman timed her. "Excellent!" she exclaimed. "Where can we reach you?"

Her next interview was with a firm of accountants on Lexington Avenue. The building was not so nice, although it was near Bloomingdale's and she'd certainly heard plenty about Bloomingdale's. The man who interviewed her was a junior partner. He was friendly and didn't seem on the make. He read through her references twice and asked if she could start the following week. She told him she'd have to let him know.

Her third interview was with a modelling agency on Madison Avenue called Samm's. They'd advertised for a booker. Lauren had no idea what a booker did – but working at a modelling agency might be fun, and she could certainly do with a little fun in her life.

A harassed girl in a purple jumpsuit told her that she'd made a mistake and better come back the next day because there was nobody to see her.

"I can't come back tomorrow," she said. "My appointment was for today. I have two other jobs under consideration and I have to make a decision."

The girl looked at her like she was nuts. "So don't come back," she said. "Take one of the other jobs, I should care."

"I'd like to make a choice," Lauren said, reasonably. "Why can't somebody see me today?"

"They're all over at the big photo shoot for Flash Cosmetics. Is that a good enough reason for you?"

She nodded, went downstairs, found a phone booth, and looked up Flash Cosmetics. Then she called their main office. "Can you tell me where the ad. photo session is taking place?" she asked. "This is Lauren from Samm's."

"Sure, just a moment," said a voice on the other end of the phone. Two minutes later she had the information – and the address of a photographer's studio on Sixty-fourth Street.

She walked to the studio. It only took her fifteen minutes and when she arrived she informed the girl at reception that she had something to deliver from Samm's. The girl told her to go to the studio in back.

She made her way down a narrow corridor which led into a large, brightly-lit studio jammed with people.

The first person she noticed was a short, flamboyant man hovering behind a camera set-up, while several other people stood around watching. In front of the camera languished the most startling looking girl Lauren had ever seen. She was an exceptionally tall blonde with masses of curly hair, huge blue eyes, pouty lips and a low-cut, slinky, silver sequin gown. Lauren recognized her as Nature, the current darling of the fashion magazines.

"Get yer finger out, Antonio," Nature screamed. She had a voice like a fishwife and a cockney accent that could sharpen knives. "I'm freezing me balls off."

"Close your legs, darling, maybe that will help," murmured a thin, fortyish, redhead standing to one side.

Lauren hovered on the periphery.

Nature struck a pose.

Antonio started shooting. "*Bellissima,* darling, *bellissima!* You are the most fantastic woman in the world!"

The more he flattered her the more Nature loved it. She postured and preened, making intimate contact with the camera, her glossy lips quivering with emotion. Her big blue eyes mesmerizing.

Antonio shot several rolls of film before calling for a break.

Everybody clapped. Nature threw her head back and laughed, sounding like a demented parrot. "Me bleedin' feet are killin' me," she roared, collapsing into a chair while make-up and hair rushed forward to attend to her every need.

"Excuse me," Lauren tapped one of the camera assistants on the arm. "Can you tell me who the executives from Samm's are?"

"Over there." He jerked his thumb in the direction of the redheaded woman.

Tentatively Lauren approached her. The woman was in the process of lighting up a long, thin cigarillo.

"Uh . . . excuse me," she said. "My name's Lauren Roberts. I had an appointment today with someone at Samm's, but the girl told me everyone was here."

The woman dragged on her cigarette and stared at her. "Too short, too heavy, too eager."

Lauren frowned – at five feet seven she'd never been called short – and as for heavy . . . no way. This woman was definitely peculiar. "I beg your pardon?" she said, hotly.

"You'll never make it, darling. You don't have the attitude."

"I'll never make what?"

"A model. Isn't that what you want to be? Isn't that what they all want to be? Although, I must say, it's *très* original, following me to the studio."

She stood her ground. "I didn't follow you anywhere. And nobody's ever called me heavy before."

"For a real person you're not the least bit heavy. For a would-be model you're grossly overweight."

"We had an appointment," Lauren said. "Someone was supposed to interview me about the booker's job. I went to your office and the girl said there was nobody to see me."

"So you decided to come here?"

She couldn't stop herself from staring at the woman's blood-red, inch-long nails – talons her mother would've called them. "Yes."

"In that case you get full marks for using your head. Can you type?"

"I sent in my résumé."

"Can you type?" the woman repeated, impatiently.

Don't get aggravated, Roberts, stay cool. "Yes, I can type."

"Can you answer phones?"

She couldn't keep the sarcasm out of her voice. "It sounds like a really challenging job."

The woman was unfazed. "Oh, don't worry, dear, it's challenging all right. I'll try you out. Be at the office at nine o'clock tomorrow."

"*If* I decide to take the job, I can start Monday."

The woman looked at her like she wasn't quite sure she'd heard correctly. "If you *decide* to take the job? My God, little Miss Independent, aren't we?"

"I have two other job offers I'm looking into."

"And what would you do if I said this offer was only open now, this very moment, and if you turn it down, don't bother coming back."

There was a brief silence, broken by Nature screaming, "Get yer bleedin' arses in gear – I'm ready ter shoot."

Lauren took a moment to consider the possibilities. She could accept the job with the law firm, but she already knew what that would be like – boring, boring, boring. Or she could say yes to the position with the accountancy firm – another laugh a minute. Her third alternative was to take the job with this bossy, redheaded woman. It could prove to be interesting.

"Well?" the woman said, abruptly. "Are you joining us or not?"

"What's the salary?"

"Not enough," the woman replied, brusquely.

"I need to make a decent salary. I have to get an apartment and afford to eat."

"You can share an apartment and starve. Builds character. Let me know when you make up your mind. You have exactly five minutes to think about it. After that, my dear girl, this job opportunity is over."

Chapter 37

Reece Webster had her exactly where he wanted her – pinned beneath him – waiting for the big moment – almost begging. He knew he gave her good loving, the best she'd ever had, so he could afford to keep her hanging.

He paused mid-thrust. "What's your name, little lady?" he demanded.

"Cyndra," she gasped.

He prolonged the moment. "Cyndra what?"

"Don't torture me, Reece."

"Cyndra *what*?"

"Cyndra Webster."

He laughed, and let her feel him move inside her. "Who owns you now?"

She moaned, almost there. "You do."

"An' who's gonna love you 'til you drop?"

"You are."

Now he heated up the action, giving her his best shot. "And who am I?"

"You're . . . my . . . husband."

"Damn right, baby. Damn right!" He let rip and she came on cue. What a stud! Nobody did it like he did.

Cyndra shuddered and rolled away from him, curling her beautiful body into a tight little ball. Some guys might be offended by her immediate withdrawal, but not Reece Webster – he was a man – a real man – and he could take it. In fact, it was a relief – women who wanted to cuddle and talk after sex gave him that *let's get outta here* feeling.

The good news was he'd finally had the smarts to shed his first wife, a going nowhere blonde, and two days later he'd turned around and married his little darkie songbird –

236

Cyndra. Now *this* was a girl destined to go places, and *he*, Reece Webster, was going right along with her. Cyndra Angelo was an investment – his. He'd married her to protect himself.

Reece Webster was five feet ten inches tall, with sandy hair, a thin blond moustache, slit eyes and a penchant for wearing flashy cowboy clothes, even though he'd been born in Brooklyn thirty-eight years ago. He was sixteen years older than Cyndra, but as far as he was concerned this was a good thing. It meant she didn't know as much as he did. He could mould her any way he wanted, and that's exactly what he was doing.

They'd met in New York at a club where her boyfriend was working as a temporary bouncer. Joey hadn't stood a chance once Reece Webster moved in.

After introducing himself as a personal manager he'd asked her what she did.

"I'm plannin' to be a professional singer," she'd said, very full of herself.

"Then you just met the man who's gonna make you a star," he'd replied, equally confident.

Corniest line in the world, but it worked every time.

At first his interest had been purely sexual. A quick lay and on to the next. But she wasn't interested in accompanying him to his apartment. She had no desire for a quickie – not even when he'd told her he produced records and had something to do with the rise of John Travolta's career. Both lies of course – but who was listening?

Usually he didn't like them so young – but there was something special about Cyndra, so he'd continued the pursuit, reeling her in carefully. The key word was career. He'd hired a studio for a couple of hours and paid for her to cut a demo. She'd had no idea what she was doing – but there was a voice there somewhere – and he'd decided that if he could bring it out they'd be rolling in dollar bills.

"I'm goin' back to Hollywood," he'd told her casually one day. "Yeah . . . Hollywood's the place a girl like you could really score."

"Well –" she'd hesitated. "One of these days Joey and I –"

"Forget about Joey. He's a loser. Hang out with him an' you'll end up like him. On the other hand – come with me an' I'll do somethin' 'bout that singin' career of yours."

And so it came to pass that she finally dumped Joey, and drove with Reece across country in his shocking pink 1969 Cadillac, consummating their relationship in a Holiday Inn somewhere near Galveston.

Once they'd settled in LA Reece had arranged singing lessons for her. He wasn't disappointed, she was a natural.

Now, two years later, all his hard work and well invested money was hopefully beginning to pay dividends. He'd managed to interest a couple of record companies in her – and they were both considering meeting with her and maybe cutting a demo.

In the meantime he'd married her. Reece knew a lifetime meal ticket when it stared him in the face.

Curled up in a ball, knees hugging her chest – Cyndra couldn't figure out why she didn't feel any different. She was married for God's sake. Married! And yet she still felt the same.

Well, I've only been married one day, she reasoned, maybe I'll feel different tomorrow.

She thought about Aretha Mae and wondered what she'd have to say about this. For the first time since leaving Bosewell, she almost considered going home. Just for a visit of course – a very short visit. She'd ride up in Reece's big old Cadillac and Harlan would come running to greet them. God, he must be a big boy now – sixteen. Aretha Mae would cook up some of her special fried chicken and greasy fries. What a treat!

The only problem was she'd never told Reece about her poor beginnings. He thought she came from a nice middle-class family. As far as he knew, her mother was a housewife and her father made his living as a car salesman. She didn't have the nerve to tell him the truth. The fact was she was ashamed of where she came from.

Reece Webster had entered her life at exactly the right time – just when she and Joey were beginning to fight non-stop. New York was tough; she'd had seven different jobs and it was getting her down. If she'd had to serve one more plate of beans and hash she knew she'd go nuts.

When Reece Webster first came on to her she'd thought he was just another on-the-make hustler. "You haven't even heard me sing," she'd said scornfully, when he announced he'd make her a star.

"I don't have to," he'd replied. "With your looks all you gotta do is open your mouth an' every guy in the place will do the fandango. Get it?"

Yes, she got it. He didn't have to tell her about men and their reaction to her.

Joey had been furious when she'd informed him she was leaving; they'd argued non-stop. "What do you know about this guy?" he'd said.

"Enough," she'd replied.

"You're making a big mistake."

Maybe she was and maybe she wasn't, but she had to take the chance. It was time to leave, so she'd packed up and taken off in spite of Joey's objections.

In Los Angeles Reece had set her up in what she considered total luxury. A nice apartment on Fountain Avenue, no roaches or rats, and a palm tree outside her window. A palm tree! She thought she was in heaven.

Reece vacillated between staying with her, or spending time with his wife who lived in Tarzana. For two years he'd threatened to get a divorce, now he'd done it, and they'd jumped in his Cadillac, driven to Vegas and gotten married.

"Just you wait," Reece had said. "When you're rich an' famous we'll do it again. An' this time the world will come. You'll see, honey, you'll see."

The first thing that hit Nick when he stepped off the plane in Los Angeles was the sunshine – dazzling, blinding sunshine. And his next impression was one of a laid-back, casual friendliness, the like of which was not evident on the streets of Chicago.

Out on the sidewalk, with the sun beating down, he hailed a cab and gave the driver Cyndra's address.

On the ride in he took in the scenery. Wide streets, tall, dusty palm trees, and a proliferation of gas stations, fast food chains and used car lots. Pedestrians were sparse on the street, but cars were everywhere.

As they got closer into town the greenery overwhelmed him. Every garden seemed to be filled with exotic plants, and every street lined with trees.

He couldn't help feeling excited. After all, this was the real thing, he was in Los Angeles for crissake. Hollywood. Land of the movies. Jeez! If he was lucky he might even bump into Dustin Hoffman or Al Pacino walking down the fucking street!

The cab pulled up in front of Cyndra's apartment house – a three-storey pink stucco building. He jumped out and checked the row of buzzers by the main door. Sure enough one of them was marked with her name, so he pressed and waited.

Five minutes later when she still hadn't replied he realized he should have called.

A well-preserved woman in tennis whites and running shoes walked up to the door balancing two bags of groceries.

"Hi," he said.

"Hi," she replied, groping for her key.

He went to help her with the grocery bags. "Can I give you a hand?"

She flashed a row of perfect white teeth. "Why not?"

Hmm . . . in Chicago she'd have told him to get lost. People were obviously more trusting in LA.

He balanced her grocery bags in one arm, picked up his bag with the other, and followed her in as she opened the gate.

The first thing he saw was a swimming pool. Holy shit! Cyndra must be rolling in it.

Around the swimming pool there were several apartments.

"You wouldn't happen to know where Cyndra Angelo lives?" he asked.

"Are you a friend of hers?"

"I'm her brother."

"Apartment three, across the other side."

He handed her groceries over. "Thanks."

She smiled again. "You're welcome. Have a nice day."

"I plan to, but thanks anyway."

He went over to Cyndra's apartment – knocked just to make sure, and when nobody answered, placed his bag against her front door and tried to decide what to do. Since this was his first day in LA and there was nobody out by the pool he decided to take a swim. Stripping down to his shorts he leaped in, splashing around like a fish. Goddamn it! This was luxury!

He spent the afternoon on a lounger catching some rays and waiting for his sister. By six o'clock it was obvious she was going to be late. Other people were arriving home from work and entering their apartments. A couple of them gave him strange looks.

He knew he'd better make a move before someone became suspicious. With a few deft strokes he used his credit card to spring her lock. Nobody was around to notice as he slid inside. Mental note – make sure Cyndra got herself a decent lock.

Once inside he looked around. Little sis was living pretty good. He opened the refrigerator and uncovered a dish of cold spaghetti. It looked inviting so he ate it, then he drank from a carton of milk and began roaming around the small apartment. He didn't mean to be nosy, but he couldn't help checking out the bathroom cabinets and opening up the closet. There was definitely a man in residence – some asshole who favoured cowboy boots and ten gallon hats.

On top of the Sony stereo in the living room was a framed picture of Cyndra with an older guy. He picked it up and studied it.

So this was the notorious Reece Webster. The man looked old enough to be her father – skinny and blondish with a thin mouth, droopy moustache and shifty eyes. Cyndra looked sensational in a sexy tank top and shorts. Little Cyndra was all grown up.

He lit a cigarette and settled in front of the television. After a few minutes he dozed off.

When he awoke it was way past midnight and the cigarette had burnt a hole in the arm of the couch. There was still no sign of Cyndra, so he grabbed a blanket from the bedroom, curled up on the couch and went back to sleep.

Cyndra didn't want to go home. She'd fallen in love with Las Vegas.

"This place is the best," she told a dumbfounded Reece.

"This place is a pisshole, honey," he replied, amazed that anyone could actually like Vegas.

"Then why did you bring me here?"

"Because this damn pisshole is gonna make us a whole lotta money."

"How come?"

"You're gonna be a star here, baby. I feel it."

She wanted to believe him. She basked in his enthusiasm. "I am?"

"Sure you are. Tomorrow I've set up appointments for you to meet the talent scouts from a couple of the big hotels. You're gonna impress the custom-made pants off 'em."

"How'll I do that?"

"By lookin' sexy an' singin' for 'em, sugar."

"Why? When we've got those record companies waiting to cut demos with me back in LA?"

"Good business," Reece said, very sure of himself. "Never put it all in one place. When we go in an' see these guys, you listen – don't talk."

That night he took her around all the best hotels. The Sands.

Desert Inn. Tropicana. Cyndra was thrilled; she'd never seen anything like the lavish hotels with their multi-coloured fountains, oversize sculptures and enormous colourful casinos filled with middle America losing their hard-earned money.

"Consider this little tour an educational trip,' Reece said, as he swaggered from hotel to hotel in his cowboy boots and ten gallon hat masquerading as a Texas millionaire. He jerked his thumb at a girl singer in the lounge of The Golden Nugget. "You see her? She can't sing for shit, but she sure puts in a pretty appearance."

"Why are you telling *me*?" Cyndra asked.

"'Cause, Mrs Webster, not only do you look good, but you can sing too. An' we're gonna use everything we got to make you bigger and better than anyone else."

Reece made her feel she could achieve anything. "Can we stay a couple of extra days?" she begged, "Can we? *Please*. After all, it *is* our honeymoon."

He tilted his hat. "What'll you give me if I say yes?"

She smiled. "I'll make it simple. Anything you want, Reece. Anything at all."

Nick awoke in the morning uncomfortable and hot. There was no Cyndra around – she must have taken off somewhere. He should've called to let her know he was coming. Shit! Too late now.

He helped himself to a banana, made a cup of instant coffee and then sauntered outside to the pool.

An athletic looking girl in a one-piece swimsuit swam lengths, her brown arms and legs flashing through the inviting blue water.

"Hey," he called out. "Any chance you know where Cyndra Angelo is?"

The girl took no notice of him as she pounded the water, hardly coming up for breath. He squatted down beside the pool waiting for her to surface.

After a few minutes she swam to the shallow end and climbed out, shaking herself like a shaggy dog. The girl wasn't pretty in a conventional way, more interesting looking – with a pert face, snub nose and bright blue eyes. She was five feet three with a sensational compact body and very short red hair.

"Excuse me," he said. "I'm trying to find Cyndra Angelo."

"Who're you?"

"Her brother."

"*You're* her brother?" she said disbelievingly, grabbing a towel and drying herself. "Cyndra never mentioned she had a brother."

"I flew in from Chicago – figured I'd surprise her – I guess it wasn't such a good idea."

"What did you do, break into her apartment?" she said knowingly, towelling a bronzed thigh.

"Technically, yeah, but I know she'd want me to make myself at home."

"Tell *that* to the Super."

"Is he around?"

"I wouldn't dig him up if I were you, he'll throw you out."

"So you can't help me?"

"Come to think of it – I did see Cyndra walking out of here carrying a bag on . . . let's see – maybe it was Thursday. She's probably away for a long weekend."

"Today's Tuesday, I'll wait."

The girl threw him a suspicious look. "Are you sure her boyfriend's going to like that?"

"Who is this boyfriend?"

She laughed. "He's okay – if you like watered down cowboys." She finished drying herself and walked towards her apartment across the other side of the pool. "See ya," she called over her shoulder.

She certainly had a body.

"Yeah – see ya. Uh . . . what's your name?"

She turned around at her apartment door. "Annie Broderick. Oh, and by the way, if you rip her off, I *can* identify you to the police. And I will."

He stared at her quizzically. "Do I look like I'd do a thing like that?"

"No. You look like an actor. Worst kind." She entered her apartment slamming the door behind her.

She couldn't have said anything nicer if she'd tried. An actor, huh? Some compliment. He hadn't performed in so long he wondered if he still remembered how.

By noon he was bored; sitting around waiting was not his style. Out of curiosity he picked up the phone and called the number Q.J. had given him.

"Manfred Glamour Limousines," a woman's voice said.

Glamour Limousines – was she kidding? "Let me speak to Mr Manfred," he said quickly, before he changed his mind.

"Who's calling?"

"Tell him . . . uh . . . tell him it's a friend of Q.J.'s."

Her voice rose. "Q.J.'s?"

"Yeah – he'll know who you mean."

There was a long wait. A very long wait. So long that he almost hung up. Then a gruff voice snapped, "Who's this?"

"You don't know me," he explained, speaking fast. "But your ex-partner said I should give you a call when I got to LA. Q.J. mentioned you might have a job for me."

"Who the fuck are ya?"

"Nick Angelo. I ran Q.J.'s bar in Chicago."

"And what ya got in mind t'do for me?"

"Anything you want if it's legit."

"I don't fuckin' believe this," Manny grumbled. "You pick up a phone, mention that putz to whom I don't speak no more, and ya really think I'll give ya a job?"

"Hey – listen, if it's a problem, forget it. Q.J. insisted I call. He told me to say Q.J.'s collecting – for that favour you owe him. But if it means nothing to you . . ."

A weary sigh. "Come in and see me."

"When?"

"Be here in an hour."

"Where's here?"

"Sunset past La Brea. You can't miss it." Manny hung up without so much as a goodbye.

Nick decided to go for it. After all, he had nothing to lose.

Chapter 38

"Don't you ever date?" Nature asked, studying her face in a large magnifying mirror she'd extracted from her enormous purse.

"Not if I can help it," Lauren replied.

"Not if you can 'elp it," Nature shrieked, in her sharp cockney tones. "Cor blimey – that's a funny one. Me – I can't get through the day if I don't 'ave a fella waitin' for me at the end of it."

"You're you and I'm me," Lauren said, sensibly.

"Bleedin' right," Nature agreed, searching for imagined blemishes on her perfect peaches-and-cream skin.

Lauren had been working at Samm's for three months. It was certainly different. Definitely not boring. In fact she was so busy she never had time to think about anything except work. A booker, she'd soon found out, did everything for the band of models who trudged in and out of the place like a constant parade of dazzling beauty. They were all gorgeous, but every one, it seemed, had a screwed-up personal life.

Nature, Samm's most famous client, was the most screwed-up of all. She'd taken to dropping by and sitting on Lauren's desk so they could chat. Nature had confided she was fed up with people who brown-nosed her to death.

"You're like a real person," she'd told Lauren. "I can talk to you, you're so sort of normal."

That's nice, Lauren wanted to say, *but I have work to do.*

The phone at Samm's never stopped. Along with Nature, the agency handled three of the other top models in New York – Selina, Gypsy and Bett Smith. At the agency they were known as the Big Four. Selina was a willowy blonde with cat eyes. Gypsy was Eurasian, exotically beautiful. And Bett Smith was an all-American blonde with a cute snub nose and just enough freckles.

Samm herself had turned out to be the woman Lauren had encountered at the first photo session she'd crashed. Samm Mason, former top model – now a very successful agent.

In the late fifties Samm had been one of the top models in the country. When she retired she'd opened her own agency, and over the years built it into a formidable rival to Eileen Ford and the Casablanca Agency. Samm was tough, but it worked for her. She ran a tight operation, protected her girls and expected everybody in her employ to do the same. "I know how easy it is to get treated like a piece of shit in this business," she'd often tell her employees. "That's not going to happen to any of my girls. Not while they work for me."

Lauren palled up with an American-born Chinese girl called Pia who'd worked at the agency for several years as Samm's personal assistant. Without Pia to help her through the early days she might have given up. It was certainly nothing like working in a law office – the modelling world was chaos. People on the phone day and night screaming for this girl or that girl. The models yelling that they didn't want to go to Alaska, they would prefer to do the shoot in the Bahamas. Boyfriends calling up, men trying to track them down, clients complaining. In fact, the phones never stopped for one reason or another. Lauren's job was to see that everybody arrived in the right place at the right time. She was also expected to keep everyone happy. She soon became adept.

After a few weeks Pia had said, "You're doing okay, Samm's really pleased. Are you having fun?"

Fun was not exactly the best way to describe her first couple of months in New York. She'd hardly had time to think, let alone have fun, there was always something going on. Early on Samm had asked if she minded working weekends. Like an idiot she'd said she didn't mind. But still, she had nothing else to occupy her time, and it meant making extra money.

She'd moved from the hotel to a one-room apartment in the Village. It wasn't the perfect location. Upstairs an angry woman practised the piano at all hours. And downstairs a young boy who claimed he was a performance artist turned tricks.

The good thing about being in New York was there was never time to feel lonely, she was always busy doing something.

"So," Nature said, leaning across her desk. "Last night I met this tall geezer, sort of a Euro-trash type. He was 'anging out at one of the discos. Bleedin' hell, he came on so strong even

I couldn't fight him off – an' that's sayin' something!" Nature snorted with laughter. "Bloody Italians – they've got their hands all over you before you so much as find out their name. Good job I know 'ow to fight back. Kick 'em in the cobblers an' run. Me mum taught me that."

"Did you go out with him?" Lauren enquired, thinking that a kick in the balls from Nature was enough to kill any normal man. Nature was over six feet tall and extremely well-built – not skinny like her main rival, Selina.

"Out with 'im? *In* with 'im is more likely," Nature chortled. "He dragged me back to 'is hotel and we 'ad a party."

"What kind of party?"

"What kind of party do you think? Some grass, plenty of rock 'n roll – although 'e wanted to play Julio Iglesias. I put a stop to that *dead* quick, I can tell you."

Lauren finished typing a sheet of paper and handed it over. "Here's your instructions for the Acapulco shoot. You leave on Thursday. I've arranged a car and driver to pick you up at your apartment and you'll be back the following Tuesday in time to be in the studio Wednesday morning for the *Cosmopolitan* cover session."

Nature grabbed the piece of paper barely looking at it. "Acapulco," she snorted. "It's so bleedin' hot."

"Have you been there before?"

"About ten times."

Lauren sighed – sometimes she envied the models and the exotic trips they all seemed to take for granted. "It must be absolutely marvellous," she said, wistfully.

Nature made a face. "If you like sunshine and a bunch of dark geezers runnin' about all over the place. Personally, if I 'ad me choice, I'd be back in London with me mum 'aving a nice cuppa tea."

"How long is it since you've been home?"

"Must be a year now. Samm promised I can take a few weeks off at Christmas."

"Do you need her permission?"

Nature chortled. "Don't knock it when it's all happenin'. Samm got me where I am today. I listen to what she 'as to say, she's a smart old bird. Which reminds me, I gotta see 'er. Is she by 'erself?"

"Let me buzz her."

"Thanks, darlin'. You're such a sweetie."

Samm was available. Nature marched into her office leaving Lauren with the ever-ringing phones. There were two other bookers, but neither of them paid as much attention as she did. She hadn't intended on making herself indispensable, but deep down she knew everyone depended on her. It was a big responsibility – but at least she felt needed.

The rest of the day passed quickly – everything happening at the usual breakneck speed. By the time she was ready to leave she was wiped out.

Pia caught her by the door. "It's Samm's birthday next week; the girls want to throw her a surprise party. She'll hate it. What'll I do?"

"If she'll hate it, tell them no."

Pip tapped long red fingernails on the side of her fake Chanel purse. "Have you ever tried telling those spoilt bitches no?"

"You can do it."

"It's Samm's big one," Pia worried. "I suppose we *should* have a party. Can you make arrangements for food and music, flowers and whatever else you think we need? Selina's offered the use of her boyfriend's apartment."

"Which boyfriend?"

"Haven't you heard? She's in love again."

It was a well-known fact that the models changed boyfriends as often as they changed their panties. Men were one of the perks of the business.

"Who's she in love with now?" Lauren asked.

"That English rock star, Emerson Burn," Pia giggled. "When Nature finds out she'll kill her – she thinks anything British is automatically hers."

Lauren tried to remain cool. In a way it was all too much – one minute she was sitting in Philadelphia slogging away at a job she hated with a boss who was always chasing her – not to mention her affair with Brad. Now she was in New York mixing with models and rock stars. Emerson Burn was famous. And she was going to meet him. Emerson Burn! It wasn't so long ago that she'd had his poster on her wall hanging next to John Lennon.

Calm down, Roberts, he's only a person. And from the sound of his publicity not a very nice one.

"Can I depend on you to handle it?" Pia asked, already on her way out. "I'd do it myself but you're so good at everything – so organized."

I'm not so organized, she wanted to scream. *I'm twenty-one years old and I'd like to have a life too.*

"Sure," she said. "Leave the numbers on my desk and I'll get started tomorrow."

"Gee!" Pia peered at her watch. "It's past seven, my guy's gonna kill me. We're seeing *Manhattan*. I'm crazy about Woody Allen. Can you check all the lights are off and lock up?"

Thanks a lot, Pia. Why don't I collect your pay-cheque too?

She took the subway home, ignoring an elderly flasher in the requisite grubby raincoat.

Two giggly girls sitting opposite her screamed with laughter when the flasher turned his attention on them. "Get it blown up an' frame it!" one of them yelled, making a rude gesture.

The flasher slunk off down the train searching for more docile victims.

Lauren stopped at the corner market near her apartment and bought a can of beans and a loaf of fresh bread. *Another gourmet dinner coming up*, she thought, wryly.

Since arriving in New York she hadn't been out once. Her routine was work and home – it didn't deviate. A couple of guys had asked her for a date – one a photographer who'd dropped by the office to see Samm, and the other an assistant to Samm's accountant. She'd declined both offers. Who needed the hassle of a man? She certainly didn't.

Nick Angelo.

Every so often his name popped into her head for no reason at all, and she found herself wondering where he was and what he was doing, and most of all – was he happy?

Who cared? Nick Angelo was her past. She didn't give a damn if she never saw him again.

Chapter 39

Manny Manfred was without doubt the fattest man Nick had ever seen. Manny wasn't just fat, he was gargantuan – with beady eyes, layers of jowls and chins and dyed yellow hair sporting inch-long black roots. He sat in a specially made naugahyde chair behind a cluttered desk, sucking 7-Up through a straw and tossing handfuls of cashew nuts into his greedy little mouth. He was not what Nick had expected. Q.J. and Manny together must have been the sight of the century!

"I'm Nick."

"So what?"

"You told me to come by."

"Oh, yeah, Q.J. sent ya."

"That's right."

"Whaddaya want?"

"A job. Part-time. I need to be free to go on auditions if they come up."

"What auditions?"

"I'm an actor."

"Says who?"

"Says me."

Manny shifted his enormous bulk and sighed. "Can ya drive?"

"Yes."

"Can ya drive good?"

"Yes."

"Ya gotta clean licence?"

"You bet."

"See Luigi. Tell him I said t'put you on the airport run."

"Is that it?"

"Whaddaya want – a kiss an' a cuddle? Scram."

He scrammed. Saw Luigi – a bullet-headed man with a broken

250

front tooth and a sour expression – got a short lecture on the dos and don'ts of driving a limo, and was told to report back at eight p.m. It was as easy as that.

It wasn't so easy getting back into Cyndra's apartment. The Super pounced on him just as he was using his credit card on her door. The Super was a ferocious looking man with shoulder length dreadlocks, two gold teeth and a take-no-prisoners attitude. He clamped his burly hand on Nick's shoulder. "What you up to, mon?"

He attempted to explain.

The Super was having none of it. He threw him out.

Nick realized he was lucky to get away without the Dreadlock King calling the police.

He hung around outside the building until Annie Broderick emerged. She looked different in clothes. A track suit covered her curvy body, and a baseball cap hid her short red hair.

"Remember me?" he said.

"No," she said.

"Sure you do," he said, laying on the irresistible green-eyed stare.

"What do you want?" she asked, unimpressed.

"Your help."

She walked over to an old brown Packard and opened the door. "Why?"

He spread the charm waiting for the usual reaction. "'Cause you know me. We're friends."

She seemed surprised. "We are?"

"Sure we are," he said, persuasively.

Annie had wasted enough time. "Now, listen," she said, sharply. "Cyndra's brother – or whoever you are – stop bugging me. I may look like an easy touch – but trust me – no way."

"I'm not after your money," he said, quite affronted.

"That's good, 'cause I don't have any."

"All I want to do is leave a note for Cyndra. Tell her where she can reach me."

"Who's stopping you?"

"The Super's on my case. I can't even get my bag outta her apartment – I need to explain."

"Explain to me. I'll pass it on," she said, waiting expectantly.

He didn't say a word.

"Well?" she was getting impatient. "Where shall I say you'll be?"

"I don't have a place."

251

Now this is where she was supposed to feel sorry for him and offer the use of her couch.

"You don't have a place," she repeated, blankly. "Too bad."

So much for the old Angelo charm. This female had a cold heart.

"No – but I got a job," he said quickly, as if that might change her mind.

"Good for you." She glanced meaningfully at her watch. "I'm late for class."

Maybe she was a dyke – anything was possible. "Just tell her I was here and I'll be calling her. Okay?"

Annie nodded and took off.

He spent the rest of the day wandering around Hollywood – checking out the star's names embedded in the sidewalk, mooching through a small shop filled with stills and photos from movies, and finally ending up at Farmer's Market on Fairfax where he ordered corn-beef and cabbage from one of the many open-air counters offering all different kinds of traditional fare.

He thought about what he was going to do next. Money was no problem: he'd left Chicago with twelve hundred bucks in his pocket – not bad considering he spent as he earnt. If he wanted he could rent an apartment and get himself settled – although it made more sense to wait for Cyndra to get back and camp out on her couch for a few weeks until he got the feel of the city and decided whether he wanted to stay or not.

Renting a car was definitely a priority. He'd soon realized that in LA the buses ran slow and did not cover the city. There was no subway – so a car was a necessity. He looked up rentals in the yellow pages and arranged himself a month-long deal on an old Buick.

Behind the wheel of the car he felt a lot more secure. At least he had a place he belonged – somewhere to call home.

"Ya ain't plannin' on wearin' what ya got on?" Luigi demanded, squinting at Nick with a disgusted expression.

"What's wrong with what I got on?"

"Ya gotta be fuckin' kiddin'." Luigi ran his hand over his bullet-head. "Ya look like a bum."

They glared at each other. This was not an auspicious start.

"I don't have anything else," Nick said. "I lost my bag."

"There's a closet in there." Luigi indicated the back room.

"Find somethin' that fits you. And for crissakes move, you're on the airport run."

"Who am I meeting?"

"Mr Evans. He's a businessman. Ya hold up the card with his name on, ya escort him out to the limo, ya shut the privacy glass, an' you drive him anywhere he wants to go. Oh, an' remember t' drive nice an' smooth. Mr Evans don't like no sudden stops."

"Sure."

"An' another thing – no talkin' unless he speaks first. Them's the rules of the game. These people pay good money for a limo, they don't want no conversation."

Ha! Like he was looking for a meaningful communication with a total stranger. What kind of schmuck did Luigi take him for?

He searched through the closet in the back room and found a pair of black pants, a dark jacket and a none-too-clean white shirt. The clothes didn't fit properly but what the hell – he'd be sitting behind the wheel of a car, anyway.

There were a couple of other drivers back there smoking and playing cards. Neither of them took any notice of him.

Luigi thrust a form at him. "Fill it out," he ordered.

He put down Cyndra's address and lied about his driving experience, writing that he'd driven for a limo company in Chicago. That information took the edge off Luigi's scowl.

Idly, he wondered what favour Manny owed Q.J. One of these days he intended to find out.

Luigi gave him a silver limousine to drive. It was shined and polished pretty good, but once he got in he realized the limo had seen better days. The back, where the passengers sat, was all spruced up with a single rose in a glass vase, a fresh bowl of fruit and side compartments stocked with booze. But in front the leather covering the seat was cracked, and there were plastic strips peeling off the side windows. So much for Glamour Limousines. The car reminded him of a gorgeous girl with the clap.

"You know the way to the airport?" Luigi scowled.

He had no idea how to get there but he nodded anyway. As soon as he left the garage he parked the limo on a side street and studied a map he'd found in the glove compartment. No big deal. LA was all straight roads going in different directions like one big board-game. He clicked the radio on and zoomed out to the airport listening to Jimi Hendrix at full volume.

He reached L.A.X. twenty minutes early and had no idea

where to park. Traffic cops were everywhere – yelling and shouting – making sure all the vehicles kept moving.

Rolling down his window, he waved ten bucks at a porter and asked where he could put the car.

The porter grabbed the money and obligingly told him where to leave it so he wouldn't get a ticket.

His passenger arrived on a flight from Switzerland. Mr Evans was a swarthy man with patent-leather hair and wrap-around black shades. Kind of strange at ten o'clock at night, but Nick was getting used to the foibles of people who lived in Los Angeles.

Mr Evans had no luggage except a snake-skin briefcase that he clutched firmly to his side, snarling ungratefully when Nick attempted to take it.

"Only trying to help," Nick said with a shrug, accompanying the man to the limo.

Mr Evans lived in a high-rise on Wilshire. Nick dropped him off and waited for a tip, a word of thanks – anything.

Mr Evans was not into pleasantries. He walked into his building without a backward glance.

"Screw you, too, buddy," Nick muttered, deciding that maybe the life of a limo driver was not for him.

Back at Glamour Limousines, Luigi sat in his office picking his nose while speaking on the phone. "I'm gonna hump your juicy ass off, sweetie. I'm gonna –" He stopped abruptly when Nick entered. "What the fuck *you* want?" he asked, covering the mouthpiece.

"I brought the car back. Thought you'd like to know I delivered your passenger safely."

"Whaddaya want – a medal?" Luigi was like a lesser version of Manny – they'd obviously both graduated from the same charm school.

"Same time tomorrow?" Nick asked, wondering what kind of woman Luigi had panting on the other end of the phone.

"Yeah," Luigi snapped, anxious to get back to his sweetie.

"I'll be here."

Maybe.

If nothing better comes along.

He got in his rented Buick and cruised down Hollywood Boulevard, finally stopping at a motel where he booked a room for the night.

"Wanna hooker?" the desk clerk enquired, reluctantly shifting his attention from a well-thumbed porno magazine.

254

"Not tonight."

The clerk regarded him suspiciously. "Why doncha?"

He didn't bother replying.

Lying on a lumpy bed watching Johnny Carson do his monologue he wondered if he'd made the right move leaving Chicago. He'd left a good job at Q.J.'s, a great-looking woman – and for what? A fleabag motel and a shit job servicing other people.

He'd give it a couple of weeks and if things didn't improve he was on a plane out of there.

Chapter 40

Emerson Burn had a mane of hair better than any girl. Lauren couldn't help staring. She'd been a fan for so many years, loved his music, and now she was in his presence. It didn't seem possible. His thick, shaggy, honey-coloured hair fell way below his shoulders. His eyes were a dreamy grey shadowed by long curling lashes. His nose aquiline and his lips surprisingly full for a man.

You're staring, Roberts.

I can't help it!

Lauren wasn't alone with him. Also present were his manager, his publicist, his personal assistant and Selina, who – clad in a leopard-skin catsuit – prowled his apartment as if she owned it. Selina was incredibly thin and almost as tall as Nature. She had straight white-blonde hair that hung to her waist and incredible cat eyes set in a classically beautiful face. She kept fixing her eyes on Emerson as if to say *This is mine and I don't want anybody touching it.*

"So," said Emerson, standing up and stretching. "I guess that's it."

Even though he was in his late thirties he was still in great shape. He wore skin-tight black leather pants on his long skinny legs, scuffed boots and a white shirt with some kind of ridiculous frill down the front. Ridiculous or not, on him it worked.

Lauren, busy making notes on an oversized pad, realized he hadn't looked at her once. And why should he? She was only the hired help.

Selina floated over to Emerson and kissed him full on the mouth, making sure everyone noticed the little bit of tongue play she indulged in. "You're such a sport, letting us use your apartment," she sighed. "Samm's going to be absolutely amazed."

"S'long as we 'ave fun, darlin'," he replied, putting his arm around her, pressing her in the small of her back and guiding her in for another kiss.

They kissed as if nobody else was in the room – in fact their smooching session went on for so long that Lauren thought they were going to leave the meeting and rush off into the bedroom. Nobody else seemed to take any notice. She imagined they'd seen it all before.

When the kiss was finished so was Emerson. "Bye, everyone," he called, striding to the door.

His entourage leapt to their feet and followed him.

"Later, strong man," Selina whispered, blowing him more kisses.

As soon as he was gone Selina stopped being the ethereal little flower and turned into the tough balls-breaker she really was. "Are we all organized, Laura? I don't expect any fuck-ups."

"Yes, Serina," Lauren replied, sarcastically. "Everything's under control."

"It better be," Selina said threateningly, as if Lauren was her personal slave. "And," she spun around, "if Samm finds out about the party before it happens I'm holding you personally responsible."

Lauren decided that out of all of the girls Selina was the worst bitch.

Back at the office Samm gave her a blast. "And exactly where have you been all morning?"

"I had to go to the dentist," she lied.

"Not good enough," Samm said, curtly. "Make dental appointments on your own time, not when you're supposed to be working."

"I don't have any personal time," Lauren explained. "You've got me working weekends and I'm here late every night. I had a toothache – what was I supposed to do?"

"Hmm . . . I suppose you had no choice," Samm said, giving in. She frowned. "I hate to say it, but this place is chaos without you."

"You managed very well before I came along," Lauren pointed out.

"Yes, well, that was then and this is now. Let's get back to work." Samm tapped her painted nails on her desk top. The polish looked like the high gloss finish on a car.

Lauren sat down and prepared to take notes.

"First I want you to send a bottle of champagne to Antonio,"

Samm said. "He had a vile time on the Selina shoot. I'm really going to have to talk to that girl before she trips over her own ego. Oh – and then call Flash Cosmetics, they need Nature in the studio on the same day she has that big *Vogue* shoot. Contact Nature and tell her she'll have to start earlier. Ignore her screaming. After that talk to *Swimwear Magazine*, they need all the girls on the tenth. I've told them it's impossible to get anybody out to the Virgin Islands before the twelfth – but they're insisting. You deal with it, Lauren, you're so good with people."

"Consider it all taken care of," she said, getting up.

As soon as she reached her desk Pia was beside her whispering, "Everything okay?"

"All systems go."

Pia looked relieved. "You're so good at this!"

Yes, Pia. I should be doing your job and making your salary.

At lunchtime several of the girls stopped by the office with a cake and faked Samm out.

"God, I hate birthdays," Samm said, reluctantly blowing out the candles. "Who told you all?"

Nobody owned up.

"At least she thinks it's over and done with now," Pia murmured. "Boy, will she be surprised!"

"How are you getting her up to Emerson's apartment?" Lauren asked. It was the one detail she hadn't been in charge of.

"Selina's taking her. She's told Samm that she and Emerson have a surprise they want to tell her personally."

"Did Samm fall for it?"

"Absolutely. She thinks they're planning marriage, and she's all set to talk them out of it."

Later, Nature managed to corner her at her desk. She was all blonde hair, blue eyes and glowing Acapulco tan. "I can't believe Selina "as bagged Emerson Burn," she complained. "She's not "is type, too bloody skinny. He likes a bird with a bit of meat on "er bones – me fer instance!"

"Do you know him?" Lauren asked.

Nature licked her lips. "No, but I intend to."

Lauren sensed trouble ahead.

As soon as she could she left the office and raced over to Emerson Burn's apartment to check on all the arrangements. She was wearing a pleated skirt and plain blue sweater, her hair pulled back in a thick braid. There was obviously not going to be time for her to get back to her apartment and change into something more festive. So what? Nobody cared how she looked, as long as she stayed in the background and did her job.

Selina was already there, floating around the apartment issuing orders. Emerson's four servants hovered in the background with surly expressions. They did not appreciate every single one of his girlfriends coming in and trying to take over.

"Thank God you're here," exclaimed Selina. "Do go and talk to the caterers. Check that they know what they're doing. Oh, and Laura, you did make sure everyone was told to be here promptly at eight o'clock?"

"All taken care of." She paused. "By the way, my name is Lauren not Laura."

"Whatever." Selina waved a beautifully manicured hand in the air.

Bitch! Lauren thought as she hurried into the kitchen to confer with the caterers.

Various members of Emerson's entourage skulked around unhappy because he'd thrown open his apartment for Samm's surprise party.

After she was done with the caterers she viewed the flower arrangements, checked out the guest list with a burly guard at the door, and finally found a moment to spend alone.

Locking herself in the guest bathroom she gazed at her reflection in the mirror. Was this how she planned to spend her life? Arranging parties for other people to have a good time? She'd wanted to become a famous New York stage actress. Now she was this unimportant little gofer doing things for other people. Lauren Roberts – invisible.

Somebody tried the door of the bathroom. She ignored them, they could wait.

Whoever it was hammered on the door again.

Angrily she flung it open and came face-to-face with Emerson Burn.

"Who're you?" he demanded.

"Lauren," she replied, curbing a strong desire to reach out and touch his shaggy mane of honey-coloured curls. "From Samm's Agency. I'm organizing the party – remember? We did meet."

He shook his golden hair and took her arm. "Follow me, I want you to "ear something."

"Pardon?"

"Don't argue," he said, grabbing her arm and leading her down a plushly carpeted corridor into the back part of the apartment where he'd built a state of the art recording studio. "Sit down an' "ave a listen to this."

Exactly who did he think he was bossing around?

"Mr Burn," she said, "I have no time to listen. I'm trying to organize a party for you – I have to see everything runs the way it's supposed to."

"This is *my* bloody apartment. *I'm* paying for the bleedin' party, so sit down an' shut up."

He sounded like Nature. Maybe the two of them *did* belong together, after all they shared the same accent.

She sat stiffly on a chair while he marched over to a control panel and pressed a couple of buttons. Suddenly the room was flooded with sound.

She recognized his voice immediately – that sexy, cocksure rasp. She'd been thirteen when he'd burst on to the scene and taken America by storm with his most famous single "Dog Days and Wild Women".

The song playing was a love song, not the romantic kind, but a driving, hard love song called "Viper Woman".

"Listen to this and tell me what you think," Emerson said, pacing up and down his studio.

She studied his leather-clad legs. "Does it matter what *I* think?"

"Yeah, you're the public," he said, speaking quite slowly as if she was an idiot. "You're the girl in the street. You won't kiss my ass – you'll tell me the truth." He turned up the volume, almost blasting her out of the room.

The lyrics hammered her senses.

She loves me for my money
She loves me for my power
She even goddamn loves me for my big fat car
She's a Viper Woman
Loves to rock 'n roll
She's a Viper Woman
She only got one goal
Oh yeah!
Money money
Sex and honey
She got her eye on it all
Money money
Sex and honey
This bitch is pretty damn cool!

The record certainly wasn't vintage Emerson Burn.

He turned the volume down and stared at her. "Well?"

"It's . . . it's okay," she said, standing up and smoothing down her skirt.

"Okay." He repeated okay like it was a dirty word. "What are you – deaf?" Then he raised his voice. "It's my new single for crissake. It's a fuckin' *hit*!"

Hmm . . . obviously he didn't care to hear the truth. Maybe she should lie and say it was the best thing she'd ever heard.

Oh, the hell with it, why should she?

"I don't like it," she said. "I don't appreciate you calling women bitches. If it's a love song why isn't it more loving?"

"Who *the fuck* do you think you are?" he exploded. "'Viper Woman's' one of the best things I've ever recorded."

"Who the hell do you think *you* are?" she blazed back. "I'm not some burned-out groupie who's going to tell you it's wonderful if I don't think so. You asked for my opinion and you got it."

"Get the fuck outta my sight," he snarled. "You don't know shit."

She was furious, but there was nothing she could do. A party was about to take place and she had to make sure everything ran smoothly.

With as much dignity as she could muster she left the room.

"I knew this was going to be a good day."

Lauren turned around and faced Jimmy Cassady, the photographer who'd asked her out a few weeks earlier.

"Hi," she said, glad to encounter a friendly face.

"Hi," he replied, with a smile.

She groped for conversation. "Do you think Samm was surprised?"

"Surprised?" he laughed. "More like pissed."

"I guess it's not much fun being forty."

"Forty?" He laughed even louder. "You think Samm's forty? The woman is fifty."

"What?" Lauren was amazed. "She doesn't look it."

"She doesn't even look forty," Jimmy said. "Samm's a phenomenon. Have you seen pictures of her when she was modelling?"

"No."

"Dynamite!"

Lauren's eyes darted around the crowded party. Most of the guests had arrived on time and when Samm put in an appearance with Selina on one side and Emerson on the other they'd all screamed "**SURPRISE**!" right on cue. And now everything was going so well she thought she might sneak out.

"What's *your* story?" Jimmy asked, lighting a cigarette.

She turned to look at him. He was in his early thirties, short and wiry with a pointed face and hair that was thinning on top and long in the back. He wore it in a pony-tail. He also wore John Lennon eye glasses and tight blue jeans. The jeans immediately reminded her of Nick.

Sternly she put Nick Angelo out of her head.

"I don't have a story," she said, deciding she could exit through the kitchen without anyone noticing.

"Everyone has a story," he replied, confidently. "And I'm interested in finding out yours."

She shrugged. "Small-town girl, came to New York, got a job. That's it."

"There's a lot more to you than that. I could tell the moment I asked you out."

"Not used to getting turned down, huh?"

He drew on his cigarette and regarded her with a contemplative expression. "You're not married, are you?" He looked pointedly at her left hand, bereft of rings.

"No, I'm not married," she said, defensively.

"Going steady? I don't notice a guy with you."

"I'm not seeing anyone."

"Then why can't we go out?"

Good question, but she owed him no explanation. "Has it occurred to you that I might not want to?" she said, hoping to put an end to the conversation.

He refused to be put off. "Is it just me or does everyone get the big no?"

"I'm leaving," she said, and then added, "Everything's going nicely, they don't need me any more."

He took the hint. "You organized this event?"

"Right," she began a slow edge towards the kitchen.

He followed her. "You did a pretty fine job, but you'd better not leave."

"Why?"

He gestured over to the corner. "Because Selina is just about to kill Nature. Take a look."

Lauren looked. Nature was all over Emerson Burn, who lounged on a couch, his leather-clad legs stretched out before him.

Her shrieking laugh could be heard all the way across the room.

Selina hovered behind him clad in a floating chiffon dress, her cat eyes signalling immediate danger.

"It's not my problem," Lauren said.

"How come?" Jimmy asked. "You're known around the office as the solver of all problems."

"I am?"

He grinned. "Yeah – have you any idea what they call you behind your back?"

She wished he'd leave her alone. "I'm sure you can't wait to tell me."

He seemed amused. "Miss E."

Now she was really irritated. "Miss E? What's that supposed to mean?"

He laughed. "Miss Efficiency."

"Oh, thanks a lot," she said, not exactly thrilled with the title.

He pressed on. "It's true isn't it? You do everything for everybody. You've made yourself indispensable. How long have you been there – three months? The other bookers must love you. I bet even Pia's getting nervous about her job."

How come he knew so much about her? "What are you talking about?"

He stubbed his cigarette in a nearby ashtray. "I'm talking about you. You're the ideal personal assistant – and don't think it's escaped Samm's notice, because nothing escapes Madam."

"I'm not after anyone's job," Lauren said. "I'm perfectly happy doing what I'm doing."

He stared at her from behind his John Lennon specs. "Yes?"

"Yes," she replied defiantly, preparing to take off.

"Oh, shit!" he exclaimed.

"What?"

"Take a look at them now."

She glanced over at Selina, Nature and Emerson in time to observe Selina slowly and deliberately pour a full glass of champagne over Emerson's head.

"Leave 'em to it," Jimmy said, putting a restraining hand on her arm just in case she was about to take care of that problem too. "They'll work it out between 'em."

Emerson Burn was now on his feet, stoned and swaying, champagne dripping down his face. "Yer stupid bleedin' cow," he shouted. "You've ruined me bleedin' hair."

"Yeah," Nature joined in. "Look what you've done."

"Stay out of it, bimbo," yelled Selina.

"What'd you call me?" Nature yelled back.

And before anyone could stop them they were at each other like a couple of wildcats, tearing at hair, chiffon, ear-rings – anything they could get their hands on.

Emerson prevented anyone from getting near them. "Let 'em at it," he shouted, happily. "This is the best part of the bleedin' party."

"Come on," said Jimmy, taking Lauren's arm. "I'm escorting you out of here."

Before she could argue he steered her to the door and they slipped away into the night.

Chapter 41

Cyndra stormed around her apartment raging in disbelief. "Some-one's been in here. I don't believe it! Look, Reece, *look*, there's cigarette butts in the ashtrays and a burn hole on the arm of the couch."

"Even better," Reece shouted from the bedroom, where he was investigating further. "Instead of taking *our* stuff they've left a bag here."

"What?" she said, marching into the bedroom to see what he was talking about. Sure enough, there was somebody's bag full of clothes. She began searching through it.

"I don't understand," Reece said, scratching his chin.

"*I* do," Cyndra said, pulling out a pair of worn jeans. "This is Nick's stuff."

"Who's Nick?"

"I told you about him – he's my brother."

Screw it! Reece thought. *Relatives! That's all I need.* "How'd he get in? An' where is he?" Reece demanded.

"Knowing Nick, he broke in. Is there a note or something?"

"That's a helluva thing, breakin' into a person's apartment," Reece grumbled.

"Oh, like *you* wouldn't."

He chewed on his lip. "How long is it since you've seen this brother of yours?"

"Going on four years."

Reece's imagination began running wild. Cyndra, his little darkie beauty, probably had a brother who was over six feet tall and black as his patent-leather shoes. What's more, it was likely that he'd want to beat the shit out of him. "You gotta be careful of relatives," he cautioned.

She turned on him angrily. "Nick's my brother. I love him."

265

"Well," Reece said, hoping the brother would not put in a return appearance, "There's nothing we can do about it. I'll store his bag in the closet and we'll see if he contacts you. One thing, honey – if he does – I've had experience – don't get too cosy with relatives, 'cause they come to stay and then you can never get rid of 'em."

"Thanks, I'll take your advice," she said, sarcastically. "I'll throw my own brother out on the street and hope he doesn't bug me again."

If they'd been married longer Reece might have smacked her – he didn't appreciate sassy women. But he knew that the moment you hit a woman you had to have her in a position where she couldn't leave, and since they'd only just gotten married, she might take off on him, and then where would he be, what with the money he'd laid out on singing lessons, clothes and all the rest.

"I'm going to a meeting,' he said, adjusting the tilt of his stetson.

She didn't reply. She was too busy thinking about where Nick might be.

The second night of working for Glamour Limousines Nick landed the airport run again. This time his passenger was an anorexic woman producer with cropped hair and a bad-tempered attitude. Julia something or other. She sat in the back of his limo snorting coke and talking non-stop on a portable phone.

When they reached Bel Air he got lost in the winding hills, and she screamed at him, calling him a dumb fuck and a stupid prick. He almost stopped the car and threw her out, but wisdom prevailed.

When they reached her house she changed moods and invited him in.

"What for?" he asked.

She had desperate eyes and bad breath. "A fuck."

"Sorry – got another job."

Sweet revenge. Not that he'd have fucked her with somebody else's dick.

So far he was not having a wonderful time in LA.

That night he stayed at the motel again, and in the morning he called Cyndra.

"Nick!" she exclaimed, excitedly. "I've been waiting for your call, I *knew* you were here. I went through your bag and unpacked it. Naturally I had to wash all your clothes, you filthy hog. Nothing's changed, huh?"

"Where've you been?" he demanded. "I came all this way and you weren't even home."

"Where are you?"

"In some crappy motel on Hollywood Boulevard."

"Get over here fast! You'll stay with me and Reece. Hurry up, I'll make you breakfast."

"Since when did you cook?"

"This is California. I take it from the freezer, put it in the toaster and call it waffles. You'll *love* my cooking!"

He made it over to her apartment as fast as possible, parking his car on the street.

She greeted him at the door, almost jumping up and down with excitement. Throwing her arms around him she hugged him tightly and dragged him inside.

"It *was* you, wasn't it? You broke into my apartment."

He grinned. "What could I do? You weren't around, so I spent the night here, an' when I came back the next day the Super wouldn't let me in."

"Don't mess with Rasta," she giggled. "He's a wild man."

They went into the tiny kitchen where she poured him coffee and toasted her famous frozen waffles.

"So where were you?" he asked again.

"Guess?" she said, grinning happily.

He hated playing games. "I can't guess."

She took a deep breath. "I got married."

Oh great. "You did?"

"Yes – me and Reece got married in Las Vegas." She looked at him with a half-guilty, half-delighted expression – seeking his approval. "Oh, Nick, I hope you like him. He's helping me with my career – he really cares about me."

"Good. 'Cause if he didn't I'd have to kill him," Nick said, making it sound like a joke.

"He does, you'll see. I mean, when you first meet him you might think he's a tiny bit older than me, and y'know, like maybe his cowboy clothes are kinda silly, but he's gonna help me make it big."

"If you say so."

Her marriage had taken him by surprise. He'd imagined them sharing an apartment and hanging out together just like Chicago. Now she had a husband and there was no way he could stay.

He tried to find out more. "What does this character do?"

"Personal manager," she said, proudly.

"Who does he manage?"

"Who do you think? *Me*, of course!"

Of course. "So how does he make money?"

She waved her hands vaguely in the air. "I don't know, he has an office he goes to. We don't discuss money. He always has enough."

Sometimes his sister was extremely naïve, how could she not know what her husband did?

"You'll stay here," she said. "The couch turns into a bed – you'll be very comfortable."

It was different now, he was certainly glad to see her, but he didn't plan on moving in. "No, it won't work out – not with you bein' newly married an' all."

She couldn't hide her disappointment. "You've *got* to stay here, Nick."

How could he resist her big brown eyes? "Maybe just for tonight, but then I'll find my own place."

"You can listen to my tapes," she said, proudly. "They're professional. I'm a real singer now."

"Yeah?" He remembered her singing debut at Q.J.'s – a total disaster.

"I've been taking lessons," she said. "Reece has a record company interested in cutting a demo with me. Oh yes, and when we were in Vegas I met a couple of the talent bookers at the big hotels, and they might hire me to sing in one of the lounges."

"Sounds great."

"And it's all because of Reece."

"I'm glad you're happy."

"So what made you come to LA? I thought everything was going so well in Chicago."

Yeah – going so well – all the way to nowhere.

"I finally decided I hadda give acting a shot. You know it's what I've always wanted to do."

"This is the right place. Maybe Reece can be your manager, too."

Sure. Bring him in on a family package.

When Reece arrived home he and Nick sized each other up, circling warily.

Nick thought Reece looked like a dumb asshole with his fringed suede jacket, stupid cowboy hat and droopy moustache. Not good enough for Cyndra by a long way. And too old.

Reece was relieved to discover that Nick was white. All day long his imagination had been running riot – Cyndra's brother had been getting bigger and blacker as the day progressed. Now here was this skinny white kid, and he didn't feel threatened at all.

"What do you do, Nick?" he asked, going for the friendly brother-in-law approach.

"I was running a bar in Chicago, but I came out here to get into acting."

Reece couldn't help himself. "Yeah – you and every other schmuck in town."

"Excuse me?" Nick said, holding his temper in check because he didn't want to upset his sister.

"Oh . . . no offence. I mean kids come to Hollywood all the time tryin' to make it. Everyone wants to be a star."

"Oh, I'll make it," Nick said, confidently.

"That's nice," Reece replied. "Y'see, with me behind her, your sister's gonna be a big star."

"Is that why you married her?" he asked, hitting pay dirt.

Reece glared at him. "I married her 'cause I love her."

"That's nice," Nick replied, giving him a long hard stare. "Because if anyone ever hurts my sister, they're dead."

Reece couldn't wait to corner Cyndra in the kitchen. "How long is he gonna stay?" he asked, agitatedly.

"Only for the night," she said, not catching his concern. "I'm trying to persuade him to hang around longer. Why don't *you* talk to him?"

"Sure," he said, although he had no intention of doing so. The sooner the brother was out of their way the better.

The next morning Nick sat at the kitchen table studying the newspaper, circling apartment possibilities. "I fancy gettin' a place at the beach," he said.

"That's easy," Cyndra replied. "I've heard the rent is lower in Venice, we could look around later today."

"Good idea," he said, folding the newspaper.

Later, when they were driving along Santa Monica, he asked her if she ever heard from Joey.

She brushed back her long black hair. "I wish I did – I wrote him several times, he never bothered to reply. The last time I called, someone said he'd moved and left no forwarding address."

"Sounds like Joey."

She nodded, wistfully. "Sometimes I miss him. We shared so much together."

Nick felt the same way. "Yeah, we did, didn't we?" he said, thinking of the good old days when the three of them had faced the world alone – hitching rides, sleeping on park benches, sharing a motel room.

The first apartment they looked at was a rat-hole with broken windows, stained carpets and barely hidden roach motels. As soon as they got outside, Cyndra said, "Ugh, if that's the kind of places available I still say you should stay with us. Reece wouldn't mind. He likes you."

Sure, Nick thought. *Like a rat loves a cobra.*

"Will you think about it? Please?"

He promised he would, but of course he wouldn't. One night with Reece Webster was one night too many.

The second apartment they saw was better. Unfortunately, the rent was too high so they moved on. The next three were hopeless. On their sixth try they found a pleasant if somewhat run-down house on the beach in Venice divided into one room apartments.

The landlady – a slovenly woman in a grubby orange robe and fluffy carpet slippers – showed them the front-room apartment overlooking the beach. It was a large, sunny room with a small kitchenette.

"No bathroom?" Nick asked.

"You share with the other apartment in front," the landlady said, a cigarette dangling from the corner of her mouth.

"I dunno –"

"The tenant is never here – she travels all the time, so you more or less got it all to yourself."

He looked at Cyndra. "What d'you think?"

"It certainly beats anything else we've seen."

"You superstitious?" the landlady asked, picking tobacco from her teeth.

Nick noticed a hole in one of her slippers. "Why?" he asked, trying not to stare.

"'Cause a guy died in here last week. Hung himself." She hoisted an escaping bra strap. "I'm up-front about it – don't wanna fool you. If you're into that karma thing, you may not wanna live here."

He shook his head. "Karma thing? Shit, the rent is right an' it's on the beach – I'll take it."

270

Cyndra squeezed his hand. "Reece and I will help you fix it up. If we all come here next weekend with a bucketful of paint we can make it look terrific."

"You got yourself a job. And you –" he said, turning to the landlady, "got yourself a tenant."

After leaving a deposit he drove Cyndra back to Hollywood. She talked all the way about old times and the future and her career. Finally she just threw it into the conversation. "Did you ever hear from Lauren? Remember – that girl you liked in High school?"

As if he was going to forget. Was she crazy? He would *never* forget Lauren.

"Nope. I guess she dumped me," he replied, making it sound casual. "I wrote her a lot – she never replied."

"She probably married that big jerk she was engaged to," Cyndra said, rolling down the window. "Strick – wasn't that his name?"

"Stock," he corrected.

"Oh, yeah, Stock." She giggled. "Dumb oaf! Hey – remember that New Year's Eve when he broke your nose?"

"What a prick!"

"And then a few weeks later you beat *him* up."

"Those were the good times," he said, dryly.

"Would you ever go back?" she asked, wide-eyed.

"Would you?" he countered.

She hesitated. "Only if I was a star. A real big star. I'd be driven into town for a visit in a fancy limo – and I'd show 'em *all* who I was – every damn one of them." Now she was warming to her subject. "I'd be wearin' one of those big fox fur coats like Diana Ross, an' some kinda slinky sequinned dress. And I'd have a car load of presents for Aretha Mae and Harlan."

"Do you miss him?" Nick asked, pulling up at a stop light.

Her expression was wistful. "Sometimes I feel bad about leavin' him behind – kinda guilty."

"Yeah, I know what you mean. But we couldn't have taken him."

"I know."

"Hey – maybe we'll *both* make it big an' we can go back together. How's that?"

She nodded enthusiastically. "Yeah! We'll show that damn town a thing or two."

As he was dropping her off at her apartment they bumped into Annie Broderick getting into her car.

"I see you two found each other," Annie said. "Is he really your brother?"

Cyndra nodded happily, clinging to his arm. "Absolutely. Didn't you believe him?"

"You aren't exactly the same colour," Annie said, bluntly.

"We share the same father, not the same mother," Cyndra explained matter-of-factly.

"I was only looking out for your interests," Annie said, pushing her hand through her short red hair. "Didn't want some stranger breaking into your apartment."

"You looked after her interests all right," Nick said. "I almost had to sleep in my car."

"At least you've got a car. Think yourself lucky."

"Thanks, Annie," Cyndra said quickly – defusing the situation.

"What's *her* problem?" Nick asked, as soon as she left.

"It's tough being a single girl alone in LA."

"No boyfriend?"

"She's into her career."

"What does she do anyway? She said something about going to class the other night."

Cyndra looked amused. "What do you *think* she does? What do you think *everyone* does in LA? She's an actress of course."

"So – how do you get into this class of hers? Do you have to pay?"

"Dunno – never been. Talk to Annie about it."

"Maybe I will."

A few weeks later Nick had settled into the LA routine. He had his job at Glamour Limousines. He had his apartment at the beach. He'd even started to work out a little and eat healthier foods, and he spoke to Cyndra on the phone every couple of days.

All she could talk about was the deals Reece was about to make on her behalf. He didn't trust Reece. The guy had con artist written all over him – he'd seen enough cheap hustlers in Q.J.'s to recognize that combination of smarmy charm and bullshit a mile away. Still . . . it wasn't his business, Cyndra seemed happy enough.

One day he asked her for Annie Broderick's number.

"Why? Are you plannin' on taking her out?" Cyndra asked.

He hadn't considered it, but it wasn't such a bad idea if he wanted to find out more about her acting class. Plus he was feeling horny, oh was he feeling horny! Of course, Annie Broderick was not his usual type, too gamine looking and short – but he had to admit she did have a sensational body – and it had been too long between pit stops. He was even starting to miss DeVille.

Cyndra gave him Annie's number. He waited a day and called. "I'd like to buy you lunch," he said, expecting an immediate yes.

"Why?" she asked, suspiciously.

Oh, shit, he was going to have to work for it. "'Cause I kinda think we got off on a downer, an' I don't have many friends here."

She was silent.

He was prepared to work – but not that hard. "Hey – big deal – you wanna have lunch or not?"

She was not exactly filled with enthusiasm. "Maybe."

Didn't she realize this was Nick Angelo calling? "Maybe. What's that supposed to mean?"

"Well . . . can you come to where I work?"

"Tell me where –"

"The Body Beautiful on Santa Monica."

"Are you kidding me? What's the Body Beautiful?"

"It's a health club."

Glamour Limousines. The Body Beautiful. They sure loved to foster illusions in LA. "Okay," he said.

"I get a break at noon."

"I'll be there."

The Body Beautiful was a big white building on Santa Monica. The place was alive with people hurrying in and out, all wearing shorts, tank tops, cut-outs, tights, every kind of variation on work-out gear.

"Can I help you?" asked a California blonde, perched behind the reception desk, her perky breasts covered by a white Body Beautiful T-shirt.

"I'm looking for Annie Broderick," he said, checking out her attributes.

She caught him looking, fluttered long fake lashes and smiled. "Oh . . . you must be Nick."

He was surprised Annie had mentioned him – maybe she liked him better than she'd let on.

"Is she around?"

"She's getting changed. She'll be with you in a minute." The girl's smile brightened. "I understand you're new in town."

"Sort of."

"How did you meet Annie?"

"She lives in the same building as my sister," he said, noticing that she wasn't wearing a bra.

"Hmm . . ." she eyed him hungrily. "I wish *I* did."

He knew a come-on when it hit him in the face. "What's *your* name?" he asked, going along for the ride.

Annie cut him off at the pass by appearing at the reception desk. "Let's go," she said briskly, taking his arm and leading him out of the building.

"Where are we going?" he asked, thinking she looked healthy and glowing and really quite attractive – even if she wasn't his type.

"There's a health food place across the street. Have you ever tried a turkey burger?"

"Is that like a hamburger without the taste?"

She smiled. "Come on – you'll love it."

"I will?"

"Yes, you will," she said, firmly.

They crossed the street, entered the restaurant and sat at a window table. Annie immediately ordered two health burgers. "Turkey, soya and seasonings. It's the most delicious thing you've ever tasted," she assured him.

"I'm drooling!"

"You're funny."

They exchanged smiles.

"So," he said. "You work at a health club, eat healthy foods and exercise in the pool. What are you in training for – the Olympics?"

She tapped her fingers on the table. "I don't know if I told you or not, but I'm really an actress. That's why I have to stay in great shape."

"Isn't being a good actress enough?"

"Producers expect you to have a Raquel Welch body."

"In case you have to do a nude scene, huh?"

"Maybe."

"Would you?"

"If it was an integral part of the story."

He burst out laughing. "Come *on* – that's like me saying I read *Playboy* for the articles."

274

She couldn't help laughing too. The waitress delivered their turkey burgers to the table. Nick looked at his suspiciously.

"Go ahead, taste it," Annie encouraged.

"Can I have ketchup?"

"You can have anything you like."

"Anything?" he teased.

"Within reason," she replied, beckoning the waitress. "Susie, bring us a couple of glasses of the big A, oh, and a bottle of ketchup."

"You come here all the time, huh?"

"It's convenient." She paused for a moment. "Uh, Nick, I'm sorry I might have seemed a little tense with you when we first met, but I had no idea who you were. And it seemed kind of strange – you know, Cyndra being, well . . ." She hesitated, then blurted it out. "Black."

"Yeah – I see your point."

The waitress brought the ketchup and two large glasses of deep brown liquid.

He picked up his glass. "What's this?"

"Pure apple juice," she explained. "No preservatives. Drink up – you'll enjoy it."

"Jeez! I've *really* gotta get used to you."

"Maybe you'll have a chance," she said, casually.

Was he finally getting through? "Cyndra told me you go to acting class," he said, smothering his burger in ketchup.

"That's right."

He took a bite – it wasn't half bad. "Howdja get into that?"

She sipped her apple juice. "If you're not working you have to study, it's important to keep on learning."

"What kind of class is it?"

Her eyes shone with enthusiasm. "It's an actors' workshop. We do all kinds of interesting things. Scenes from plays and movies. Improvisation. A lot of working actors go there."

"Yeah?" he said, taking a gulp of apple juice. "Sounds interesting."

"It is."

He studied her pertly pretty face. "Have you ever had a professional job? Like in a movie or on television?"

She looked pleased that he'd asked. "As a matter of fact I've been in three commercials."

He was impressed. "I guess you've got an agent then?"

"How come all these questions, Nick?"

He decided to confide in her. "Why do you think? Listen, I had a great job in Chicago running a bar – I was the king of my own little kingdom. But ever since High school I've had a thing about acting."

"You can't just do it. You have to be good."

"Oh, I'm good," he boasted.

"Glad to hear it, because one thing you need is plenty of confidence." She sighed. "It helps when you get rejected twenty times a day."

He had no intention of getting rejected. Once he got through the door – whoever's door it was – he was going to make such an impression they'd never let him go.

"I'd like to come to class with you – I could sit in back and watch."

"I don't see why not. You're allowed to observe two sessions, after that you have to pay – that's if Miss Byron accepts you."

"Who's Miss Byron?"

"Joy Byron – the best acting coach in town."

If she was the best he wanted her. "When can I come?"

"How about tonight?"

"No, nights are out. I got this gig driving for a limo company."

"I had a friend who sold a script to a producer while he was driving him to Santa Barbara."

"Really?"

"It can happen. You have to find out exactly who you've got in the car and go for the pitch. That's what my friend says. It certainly worked for him. His point is if they can afford to hire a limousine they must be someone."

He remembered Luigi and his ferocious scowl. "I got strict orders not to talk to the paying customers."

"You don't look like a man who follows orders."

She was right, it was about time he found out who he was driving and did something about it.

"I'll let you in on a little secret about this town," Annie confided, her bright eyes meeting his. "I've been here three years, and if there's any way you can make a connection, go for it. Don't let anything stand in your way."

He leaned across the table and took her hand which was surprisingly small and soft. "Thanks, I like good advice."

They finished lunch, and as they were parting company she suggested he might want to come to class with her on the following Saturday.

"Sounds good," he said. "I'll pick you up."

"Okay. I'll see you at four."

That night, when Luigi assigned him Mr Evans again, he was not exactly thrilled. This Evans guy was a deadbeat, no connections to be had there.

It turned out to be the same routine as before. The same bad-tempered face, the same briefcase clutched to his side, the same non-tip. Nick had a good mind to tell Luigi he didn't want to drive him again. He'd talked to the other drivers and found out that most customers handed out cash tips on top of the percentage added to the bill. No chance with this tight-wad.

"That Evans guy is a real cheapo," he complained to Luigi when he dropped the limo back. "Do me a favour an' stop assigning me to him."

"Am I hearin' right?" Luigi demanded, eyes bulging. "Mr Manfred gives ya a job outta the kindness of his fuckin' heart – an' now you're mouthin' off an' tellin' me who ya will an' who ya won't drive."

"I'm entitled to an opinion," he said, stubbornly.

"You're entitled t'suck my nuts if I tell ya to," Luigi steamed.

"I guess I'll pass on that tempting offer."

Luigi made a rude gesture. "In your eyes, punk."

The next night when he reported for work Luigi greeted him with a knowing sneer. "Mr Manfred wants ta see ya."

"What about?"

"Do I strike ya as a fuckin' information centre?"

Manny Manfred greeted him looking fatter than ever. It didn't seem possible, but could he have gained another twenty pounds?

"How's it goin', Nick?"

Surprise. The fat man remembered his name.

"Okay," he said, carefully.

"An' the actin' thing? Any auditions yet?"

"I'm lookin' into it."

"That's the way ta do it," Manny said, reaching into a bowl of jelly beans, grabbing a handful, and promptly stuffing them into his surprisingly small pink mouth.

Nick noticed he was wearing a Rolex – the heavy gold watch gleamed as it caught the light.

"I talked to Q.J.," Manny said, munching away.

"You did?"

"He likes ya."

"I know."

"He trusts ya."

"I should hope so. I worked for him nearly four years."

Manny spat out a red jelly bean. It landed with a disgusting blob of spit on his huge knee. He brushed it to the floor.

"Loyalty an' trust – them's the things ya can't buy."

"Right." Nick waited for the pitch he knew was on its way.

"So . . ." Manny said, not disappointing him, "I gotta proposition."

"Yeah?"

"Ya look like a smart kid."

Jeez! Compliments! From the fat man himself.

Big fucking deal.

"I can handle myself," he said, carefully.

"That's what I like t'hear," Manny said, beaming. "Soon as Luigi told me ya was complainin' I knew ya wasn't satisfied sittin' behind the wheel of a car – drivin' some rich motherfucker ya knows you're better than."

"It's a job."

"An' so's what I got in mind for ya."

"Is it legal?"

"Are you bothered?"

"Whyn't you tell me about it?"

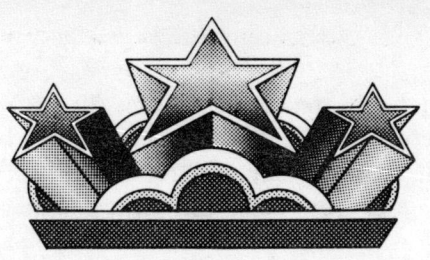

Chapter 42

Lauren had been out with Jimmy Cassady several times – four dates exactly – the last two ending with a chaste kiss on her front doorstep. Now they were on their fifth date and she knew that tonight he expected more. Not that he actually came out and said so – he wasn't that obvious – but she picked up little signs here and there, and after a quiet dinner in a romantic Italian restaurant he hailed a cab, and instead of giving the driver her address he gave him his.

"I want you to hear the new Joni Mitchell album," he said, putting his arm around her.

"I'd love to," she replied.

Well, Roberts, she thought. *What are you going to do?*

I don't know.

You'd better decide.

I can't.

Why?

Good question. Why couldn't she decide?

The answer came out of nowhere.

Because I still love Nick Angelo.

"You're quiet tonight," Jimmy said, taking her hand in his. "Something I said?"

She shivered, trying to block the memory of Nick from her mind. "No, I'm tired. I had a tough day."

"Too tired to listen to Joni Mitchell?"

He was asking one question with his mouth and another with his eyes.

"I can't think of anything I'd rather do," she replied, while voices continued to scream inside her head.

All he wants is a quick lay – that's what they all want.

You sound like your mother.

I'll sound like her if I want!

"We're here," he said, paying the driver and helping her from the cab.

She followed him into the elevator – filled with trepidation. Jimmy Cassady seemed like a genuinely nice guy.

Sure, they all do until they get what they want, and then they dump you, run out on you, leave you alone and pregnant. Leave you . . . leave you . . . leave you . . .

"What are you thinking?" he asked, squeezing her hand.

"Nothing," she said, banishing Nick from her thoughts and concentrating on Jimmy. What did she know about him? Not that much. He'd told her he'd come to New York from Missouri seven years ago and started out as a photographer's assistant – moving out on his own four years later. For the past three years he'd been building his reputation as one of the most innovative photographers around with his stark black and white images.

In the course of talking to some of the girls she'd discovered nothing about his personal life. Usually the models gave chapter and verse on every photographer they'd worked with – including graphic details of size, sexual preferences and how many times they liked to do it a night. There were no reports on Jimmy – except from Nature, who'd worked with him once and then announced, wide-eyed with surprise, "Well, 'e's gotter be gay, ain't 'e? 'Cause 'e 'din't even hit on me once!"

After their fourth date, when he'd dropped her outside her apartment with only a kiss, she'd thought that maybe Nature was right. But tonight she knew it wasn't so; he had that look in his eyes and she was well aware he was all set to make the big move.

His apartment wasn't an apartment at all – it was loft space, divided into compartments by six-foot stucco walls that ended long before the soaring ceilings. His furniture was minimal modern – everything either black, white or stainless steel. Stark, like his photographs.

"This place is amazing," she exclaimed, wandering around taking in every detail. "Did you design it yourself?"

He laughed. "No professional decorator could come up with this. Besides, I happen to like it."

"So do I," she said, exploring further. "But you have to admit – it *is* different."

"That's *why* I like it," he said, following her into the compact stainless steel kitchen. He moved closer. "That's why I like you,"

280

he added, unexpectedly pinning her up against the cold steel of the refrigerator door and kissing her on the mouth. No, *Would you like a drink? Can I give you a tour?* He didn't even bother putting on the Joni Mitchell album he'd been talking about all night.

Just the kiss.

Hard and sensual. Not like his usual goodnight peck. This was definitely the real thing.

She gasped for breath, but he didn't stop.

For a moment she resisted, her body rigid – not allowing him to get too close.

He persevered, and slowly she felt herself begin to respond – a warmth sweeping up her body – a tidal wave of desire so long repressed that it took her by surprise – rendering her helpless to resist.

After a few minutes his hands moved down to her breasts – touching – feeling – stroking.

She began a half-hearted objection. "Jimmy . . . I don't know –"

"I do," he said surely, hands creeping down the neckline of her dress, moving around to the back and unsnapping her bra.

And all the while his lips remained on hers, his insistent tongue exploring her mouth, his warm breath all over her.

She threw her head back and surrendered as he exposed her breasts and his lips travelled slowly down to the tips of her nipples.

Gently he pushed both her breasts together, tongueing her nipples simultaneously as his hands worked the zipper on her dress and it fell to the floor.

She closed her eyes trying not to think of Nick, trying to forget him once and for all. This was all happening so fast, and yet she felt powerless to stop him.

"You smell so good," he whispered.

It didn't matter any more, nothing mattered. She'd reached the point of no return, he could do whatever he liked.

He picked her up and carried her to the bedroom, placing her gently in the middle of his large water-bed.

She lay back and opened up her soul to him. There was no choice any more, she'd been lonely too long.

And Nick Angelo was never coming back.

"I'm getting married," Lauren said, nervously clenching her fists.

Samm glanced up from a contract she was studying and

raised her oversized horn-rimmed glasses. "What did you say?"

"Married," she replied, as if this wasn't a major announcement.

Now she had Samm's full attention.

"I don't believe it!" the older woman said, placing her glasses on the desk.

"It's true," she managed, sounding a lot calmer than she felt.

Samm reached for one of her long thin cigarillos, her blood red nails lethal weapons. "And may I ask to whom?"

"Jimmy Cassady."

"*My* Jimmy Cassady?" Samm was very possessive of all the photographers who worked with her girls – she considered every one of them belonged to her.

Lauren nodded. "I guess so."

Samm was silent for a moment while she digested this unexpected information. Then she said, "Isn't this rather . . . sudden?"

Lauren felt like a school kid standing in front of the principal. Why was she putting herself through this? She didn't owe Samm an explanation. "We've been seeing each other for six weeks," she said. *And sleeping together for three* – she wanted to add, but didn't. Her sex life was her business.

Samm picked up a thin gold pen and tapped it on her lacquered desk top. "Six weeks is not a long time to get to know someone."

"Long enough for me," she replied, thinking that she certainly didn't need a lecture from Samm.

"Don't you think –" Samm began.

"Congratulations would be nice," Lauren snapped, shattering her "good little Lauren" image once and for all. "Oh, and I'm giving you two weeks notice – Jimmy wants me to work with him."

Samm was too wise to say another word – Lauren was obviously under Jimmy Cassady's influence and nothing she said would make any difference. Men! They'd caused her more problems over the years than she cared to think about. Usually it was the models who got hooked by a glamorous playboy or some fast-talking would-be manager. She certainly hadn't expected Lauren to get swept away.

Samm might be sceptical, but the girls in the office thought it was sensational news. Pia seemed especially pleased for her. And when Nature heard, she made a special trip to the office, shrieking, "This is bleedin' smashing! So, 'e's not a fag after all!"

Trust Nature to come right out with it.

From the moment they'd slept together Jimmy had started talking about marriage. He wanted to do it immediately. "What's the point of waiting?" he'd demanded.

The point of waiting, she'd thought, *is to decide whether we're making a mistake.* Samm was right – six weeks was not a lot of time to get to know somebody. But the more she got to know Jimmy, the more special she decided he was, and certainly different from the other men she'd come across in New York.

Even so, at first she'd said no.

"Why not?" Jimmy persisted.

She could think of no good reason.

He'd pressed until she'd finally changed her mind. Jimmy was attractive, serious about his work, a good lover, and he genuinely seemed to care for her. Besides, she was swept up in the excitement of his desire. And the thought of belonging to someone and being safe was too tempting to resist.

She didn't love him – whatever love was. But maybe that would come in time.

Once she'd said yes, they both agreed they should do it as soon as possible. For one rash moment she'd considered calling her aunt and uncle in Philadelphia, but then she'd changed her mind. Who needed Brad knowing? Besides, both she and Jimmy wanted the ceremony to be as simple as possible.

"What about your family?" she'd asked.

"We lost touch," he'd said, vaguely.

"How come?"

He'd raised an eyebrow. "Am *I* questioning *you*?"

Soul mates.

Pia announced she wanted to throw her a wedding shower, but she was soon overruled by Nature, who decided a proper bachelor-girl bash was more in order. "You deserve it," Nature announced cheerfully. "You work ever so hard lookin' after us all, now it's our turn to do something for you."

In a way Lauren wished she hadn't told anybody. Maybe it would have been better if they'd just done it quietly with no fuss.

Too late now, Nature had plans.

Lauren protested, but Nature – as usual – refused to listen. "Be at me apartment next Saturday at six o'clock. And don't expect to get home until three in the morning – that's if you're lucky!"

There was no point in fighting Nature, she was like a great

283

big Mack truck – the safest thing to do was climb aboard and enjoy the ride.

As the days passed Lauren realized leaving Samm's was going to be a wrench – she'd made so many good friends there. But Jimmy assured her it would be fun for her to help him out at his studio, and it didn't seem like such a bad idea.

Meanwhile there was so much to do. They had to take blood tests, get a wedding licence – and finally she went shopping with Pia, searching for the perfect outfit which Samm insisted on paying for.

By the night of the wedding shower she was a wreck. Nature herself was in top form – screaming and yelling all over the place. She'd ordered a convoy of limos for the night, and following behind the limos she surprised everyone with six leather-jacketed bikers sitting astride their Harleys.

"Ain't it nice 'aving an escort," Nature joked, winking conspiratorially at the convoy of guys. "Muscles an' black leather – me favourite combination!"

First they went to an Italian restaurant where everyone presented Lauren with their gifts. She managed to put a good face on it, opening the presents one by one and dutifully exclaiming that each gift was exactly what she wanted.

Nature presented her with a huge black vibrator, which elicited much mirth around the table.

When she was finished with her gifts, one of the better-looking bikers swaggered into the restaurant, hit a button on a tape machine, and proceeded to do a raunchy strip to the Stones "Satisfaction". He was merely the appetizer, because from there they all piled back into the limos and headed for a male strip club.

Lauren watched in fascinated amazement as the guys at the club proudly presented their assets – thrusting them into the eager audience's faces.

"Too many dicks," Pia said, solemnly.

"Don't you mean assholes," Lauren murmured, longing to get out of there.

Nature was in her element – hooting and hollering at the guys to take it off. Sticking ten dollar bills down their skimpy G-strings – loving every minute.

At last it was over, and they dropped her back at her apartment. She fell thankfully into bed. As far as she was concerned the evening had been a nightmare. Still . . . they'd meant well, and she was lucky to have people who cared about her.

The next day she gave up her apartment and moved all her things over to Jimmy's place. That night they ate dinner by candle-light and made love. For the first time since leaving Bosewell Lauren felt she finally belonged somewhere, and she knew that her decision to marry Jimmy was the right one. She fell asleep in his arms, happy and content.

The day before the wedding Pia picked her up and took her over to her place. "You can't stay with your future husband the night before the wedding," she scolded. "It's big bad luck."

In the morning Nature arrived, breezing through Pia's apartment, bossily taking over. "'Ere," she said, removing a large sapphire ring from her finger. "You'll wear this. It covers borrowed, blue *and* new. Now all we've got to worry about is getting you something old."

Pia produced a pair of exquisite filigree ear-rings. "These were my great-grandmother's," she said, handing them over. "I'd be honoured if you wore them."

Lauren put on the oyster satin suit Samm had bought her, Pia's ear-rings and the sapphire ring.

Nature peered at her critically. "I wish you'd let *me* fix your 'air."

"I like it just the way it is."

"Yeah, all neat and understated," Nature replied. "Unlike me," she added, fluffing out her blonde curls.

"You look beautiful, Lauren," Pia whispered.

They set off in a stretch white limousine – Nature's choice. "Shut your eyes and pretend you're a rock star," she giggled.

By the time they arrived at City Hall Lauren's stomach was doing somersaults. The driver helped her out of the car and she entered the building, flanked by her friends.

They bumped into Samm by the elevator. "How are you feeling?" Samm asked, chic as ever in a scarlet Chanel suit.

"Nervous," she replied.

"It doesn't show. You look lovely."

"Thanks." Her throat felt dry as she clutched her corsage of white orchids and wished that everything was over and done with.

Pia and Nature ushered her into a side room to await the arrival of the bridegroom. Jimmy was coming alone. When she'd asked him who his best man was, he'd replied he didn't want one. "I travel alone," he'd said.

Fine with her. Maybe that's why they got along so well.

She couldn't sit still. She got up, pacing nervously up and

285

down the small room, her mind racing this way and that. A few minutes seemed like an eternity.

Nature kept checking her watch. "'E's bleedin' late, ain't 'e," she finally said in an exasperated voice.

"Maybe it's the traffic," Pia said, giving her a warning look.

"Yeah, well, bleedin' traffic or not, 'e's late. S'not nice to be late for your own wedding."

After fifteen minutes, Pia slipped out of the room, found a pay phone and called Jimmy's apartment. There was no reply.

Nature cornered her in the corridor. "What the 'ell's going on? Where *is* the scummy bastard?"

Pia shook her head. "I have no idea."

"You wait downstairs," Nature said, "while I keep 'er busy here."

Another twenty minutes passed and Jimmy still hadn't shown up. Pia called Samm out of the main room and Nature joined them in the corridor for a conference.

"Looks like 'e's dumped her," Nature said. "What a low-life!"

"Has somebody called his apartment?" Samm asked.

"Yes, I did," Pia said. "There's no answer."

Samm shook her head, she'd had a feeling about Jimmy Cassady.

"What shall we do?" Pia asked.

"Fuck 'im!" Nature said, cavalier as usual. "Men! They're all no bleedin' good."

By the time an hour had elapsed it was obvious Jimmy wasn't coming. Lauren took the news stoically, although she was breaking up inside.

Pia, Nature and Samm accompanied her back to his apartment. There was a note pinned to the refrigerator door.

Sorry! he'd scrawled. *Gone on assignment to Africa. Be back in a few months. You can stay at the apartment until you find somewhere.*

Lauren read the note twice before handing it to the others.

"Bastard!" exclaimed Nature, scanning it quickly.

"Oh, dear," said Pia.

Samm was more eloquent. "That lousy son-of-a-bitch!" she said, forcefully. "I never trusted him."

Lauren felt totally blank. Another rejection. It didn't matter. Nothing mattered. One thing she knew. She would never trust another man again. Never. Of that she was sure.

Chapter 43

The proposition was this – Manny wanted him to take the limo across the border into Tijuana, pick up a passenger at the Tijuana Sunset Hotel and then drive back into the US. It sounded simple enough.

"That's it?" Nick asked, warily.

"Easy, huh?" Manny leaned back in his oversized chair, double chins wobbling.

"Sure," he replied. "Depending on what the passenger's carrying."

"Let's make it none of your business," Manny said, rubbing his chin. "That way you don't know from nothin'."

Nick decided he wouldn't trust Manny with a nun, but he sensed an opportunity to make money, and since his stash from Chicago was fast running out he investigated further. "How much?"

Manny shot him a knowing wink. "More than you're making now."

"Listen," he said, "I don't know what I'm bringing in, but I ain't crossin' the border for less than two grand."

"That's a lotta money."

"The way I'm hearin', it's a lotta risk."

"Okay, okay," Manny said, grudgingly.

The fat man had agreed too readily. Nick immediately wished he'd asked for more. "When's this supposed to take place?" he asked.

"Sometime next week. Things are bein' set up now."

"Who's the passenger?"

"A school kid."

"A school kid?"

"Yeah – wanna make something outta it?"

Nick knew he was stepping on to dangerous territory. There was no way Manny's activities were legal. He took a beat. Did he really want to get involved?

Yeah – for two grand he *really* wanted to get involved.

"I got somebody for ya t'meet," Manny said.

"Who?"

"A special broad, so keep her outta your dirty mind."

Oh. Like he was going to hit on a girl that had anything to do with Manny. Big chance.

Manny hit a buzzer and the door opened.

"Say hello to Suga," Manny said, presenting her as if she was the Queen of England. "Suga an' me – we bin together five years. Married for two," he added, proudly. "Happy as a coupla sandbugs."

Suga was twenty-three, looked sixteen, and acted as if she was twelve. Her choice of dress was black rubber, barely making it to the top of her chubby thighs, worn with lace-up white boots and as much fake gold jewellery as she could manage without falling down. She was top heavy, short, her flesh was rosy and her hair shoulder-length spikes of dyed blonde with inch-long black roots. She smoked non-stop, chewed gum, and bit her nails.

Stationing herself next to her husband she stared balefully at Nick. She had small beady eyes surrounded by too much make-up and mean little lips curved in a perpetual sneer.

"Suga's a classy broad," Manny said. "Helps me with a lotta things."

Yeah, Nick thought. *I bet she does.*

"I figured you two should meet," Manny continued, touching his wife on the thigh, "on account a it's Suga you'll be collectin' in Tijuana."

Jesus Christ, what was he getting into? "You said it was a school kid."

"Don't worry – she'll be dressed like one."

"You're putting me on?"

Suga spoke up, her voice a shrill squeak. "Screw you," she said, chewing gum like an angry cow.

This was going to be some trip.

Joy Byron's acting class was held in a disused warehouse on the wrong side of Wilshire. Joy Byron herself was an elderly English woman with a voice like a hack-saw. She wore a long flowered dress on her bony body and carried a parasol, giving her a somewhat eccentric Mad Woman of Chaillot look.

Nick would never admit it to anyone, but he was dead nervous. "So, uh, like what do I do?" he asked, trying to sound cool.

"Nothing," Annie said. "You're merely an observer. Will you relax?"

"Okay, okay," he said, wondering why he was putting himself through this.

She grabbed his hand. "Come on, I'll take you over to meet her."

Reluctantly he allowed himself to be led across the room.

"Miss Byron," Annie said. "This is a friend of mine. Is it okay for him to sit in?"

Joy Byron turned around and studied him. "And what is your name, young man?" she asked, in imperious tones.

"Nick," he mumbled.

"Do we have a surname?"

"Nick Angelo."

"Lose the 'O'." She gestured theatrically. "Nick Angel, I can see it on marquees now."

"Yeah?"

"But of course." She turned to speak to another student and Annie pulled him away. "She likes you."

"How do you know?"

"I can tell."

He grinned. "Yeah, well, I'm not just anybody."

"That's what I like about you, Nick – no ego. Come on, we'll grab a seat over here."

His eyes darted around the large musty room. There were a bunch of guys in T-shirts and jeans doing their best Brando imitations, and lots of pretty girls who seemed to take themselves much too seriously. Actors. Just like him.

When everybody was settled Joy Byron stood at the front and addressed her class. "Today we shall speak about motivation," she said. Long dramatic pause. "When I worked with Olivier, Gielgud, in fact *all* the English greats, one of their first thoughts before going on stage was motivation, motivation, what exactly *is* my motivation."

Nick could see this was going to be different from drama classes with Betty Harris way back in Bosewell. And he was right. Joy Byron revelled in lecturing her students on what she thought they should know, talking a great deal about her fabulously successful career in England.

"Was she some kind of big star over there?" he whispered to Annie.

Annie nodded, eyes shining. "She's a great teacher."

"How come she gave it up?"

"I don't know."

Halfway through the class Joy summoned two of her students to the front and instructed them to improvise a scene about anger. Nick watched carefully as the two young actors went to work.

They were good.

He was better.

After they were finished Joy stood up again, gave a long harsh critique and then invited the class to comment. Some of the students couldn't wait to pick the two actors to pieces, while a few of them were quite flattering.

"You have to take the good with the bad," Annie murmured. "Everybody has their say. Believe me – it can be brutal up there."

He couldn't make up his mind whether to get involved in this shit. Acting in Bosewell was one thing, but this was Hollywood and who needed criticism?

On his way out Joy Byron stopped him, laying a dainty blue-veined hand on his arm.

"You've got the look, dear boy," she said, in her gravelly English voice.

"I have?" he replied, carefully.

"Oh, yes. I always recognize it," Joy said. "You've got the look."

He took a deep breath, inhaling her scent of musty roses mixed with mothballs. "Yeah, well, uh . . . glad to hear it."

She fixed him with watery eyes. "On your next visit you'll perform something for me."

"I haven't joined the class yet."

"Ah, yes, but sometimes I accept students without fees. We'll see. Next time come prepared."

"What did she say?" Annie wanted to know as soon as they were outside. When he told her she got really excited. "My God, you never even did anything and you made an impression on her."

"Maybe she's horny," he joked.

Annie was unamused. "That's not funny," she said, sternly. "Joy Byron is a true professional."

He took her arm. "Hey – there's something I've been meaning to ask – do you have a permanent guy in your life?"

"Why?" she asked, suspiciously.

"I thought you'd help me out. Like if you don't have a boyfriend you'd come by my place on Saturday night."

There was a long pause before she answered. "Nick," she said hesitantly, "I'm not looking to get involved with anybody."

"Hey – who's asking? All I want you to do is read with me. I have to prepare something, don't I?"

"Oh," she was embarrassed at having gotten the wrong impression, "I'd be happy to."

Saturday night his landlady was having her usual weekend party. He ignored the hangers-on lingering outside and steered Annie straight through to his apartment. The smell of marijuana was overwhelming. "Don't breathe too deeply," he joked. "One lungful and you're stoned for the rest of the week!"

She walked over to the large windows overlooking the beach. "How did you find this place?"

"Cyndra helped me."

"Nice view."

"Yeah, I was lucky."

The landlady's stereo blasting reggae almost blew them out of the room.

"This is the down side," he explained. "She throws a party every Saturday. You gotta be in the mood." He opened his refrigerator and inspected the contents. "How about a drink? I got rootbeer or Coke. Take your choice."

"Both bad for you," Annie said. "I'll have plain water."

"Don't you do *anything* that's bad for you?" he teased, reaching for a glass.

"Not if I can help it," she said, primly.

He found his precious signed copy of *Streetcar*, and flipped it open to a scene he particularly liked, handing it to Annie. "How about I read Joy a scene from this?"

"Hmm," she flicked through the pages. "You want to do it with me?" she asked, settling on the couch.

"Do I want to do *what* with you?" he replied, still teasing.

Her cheeks were flushed. "Nick, get serious."

He moved in on her knowing he shouldn't. "I *am* serious," he said, sliding his arm around her shoulders and pulling her close.

She was vulnerable and jumpy as he began to kiss her. Feebly she tried to push him away.

"Relax," he coaxed, well aware he had her nailed. "You gotta have *some* fun in life," he added, pressing his lips down on hers.

Just as he was getting somewhere they were interrupted by a loud knock on the door. Annie seized the moment to wriggle out of his grasp and jump guiltily to her feet.

"Ignore it," he said. "It's probably someone looking for the john."

"You'd better see who it is," she said, glad of the distraction.

"Jeez, just when we were gettin' comfortable, huh?" he said, walking over to the door and flinging it open.

Standing there was DeVille carrying a suitcase.

"Hi, honey," she said. "I'm here."

Chapter 44

Pia wanted Lauren to stay with her, but Nature insisted she'd be more comfortable at her place. Frankly, Lauren couldn't care less where she went – Jimmy's behaviour had left her without any feelings. It didn't matter, nothing mattered. She packed up her things and moved into Nature's huge white apartment without an argument.

Nature was delighted. She led Lauren into the guest bedroom announcing proudly, "This is where me Mum stays. You'll like it. It's ever so cosy."

Lauren decided it was a good place to hide. Maybe she'd stay forever – who needed the real world?

Nature yelled at her assistant to cancel all her appointments for the rest of the week.

"You can't do that," Lauren protested. "You have the *Vogue* shoot, and the Antonio session for *Harper's*. You're booked solid."

"I can bleedin' do what I want," Nature replied, tartly. "I'm not a bloody work machine. I understand what you're goin' through – the truth is it 'appened to me once."

"What happened to you?"

"Course, it was when I was young an' innocent – ha ha!" Nature threw herself down on the bed, ready to talk. "There was this geezer I was seeing before I was a model – a right layabout. I worked in a 'airdressing salon, and this bloke used to come in all the time. He seemed ever so nice. And sexy – wow! Anyway, the truth is 'e dumped me – just like that. Ran off with me best friend an' married her. I bet 'e's sorry now – she's a fat old cow an' I'm a big star – well sort of. I never forgave 'im."

"I had no idea," Lauren murmured, sympathetically.

"I'm not gonna bloody advertise it, am I? After that I got meself discovered an' flown to New York. Never looked back.

Course me Mum's not thrilled – but *I* am. It's great gettin' away from the family. Where's your family anyway?"

"I don't have anybody," Lauren said, admitting it for the first time. "My mother and father are both dead."

"Oh, sorry, luv."

"That's all right."

Nature jumped up. "Well, listen, you're welcome to stay as long as you want."

And that's exactly what she did. For two weeks she hid away in the guest room, huddled under blankets watching television day and night, until Pia visited one day, marched into the room and said, "Okay, enough. Time to get back to work. Samm says your job is waiting."

"No." She shook her head. "Too many bad memories."

"You can't force her," Nature said, entering the room.

"Staying here doing nothing certainly won't help her," Pia said sharply, not appreciating Nature's interference.

Lauren spoke up, after all it was her they were discussing. "Pia's right. It's time I found an apartment and another job."

"Jobs aren't so easy to find," Pia warned. "If you're smart you'll come back to Samm's."

"I've got it!" Nature shrieked, joining in as usual. "I've bleedin' got it!"

"What?" Lauren asked.

"You'll work for *me!* You can be my new assistant. It'll be a lot more fun than sitting in an office picking up the bleedin' phone all day."

"I don't know," she said, unsurely.

Nature was on a roll. "So now you don't 'ave to move out. It'll be nice 'aving you 'ere permanently – someone to talk to when I get 'ome."

"Yes, very nice," Pia interjected. "Don't do it, Lauren. You'll be on call twenty-four hours a day."

"Well?" Nature questioned, flashing her big blue eyes.

Lauren shrugged; she had nothing else in mind. "Why not?"

Pia sighed, "You'll regret it."

"No, she bleedin' won't," snapped Nature.

And that was that.

Sometimes Lauren thought it was the best decision she'd ever made and sometimes she thought it was the worst. Working for

Nature filled her days, and living in the same apartment filled her nights. If she'd thought she had no life working at Samm's, she certainly had none at all working for Nature, although it was never boring.

Nature did not lead a dull life. As her personal assistant she was expected to do everything from collecting the dry cleaning to watering the plants. She soon delegated the duties she had no wish to do to the maid, and concentrated on getting Nature's life as organized as possible – which was not easy, because Nature was a true gypsy and had thrived on chaos for years.

"You're fantastic!" Nature said one day. "'Ow did I ever manage without you?"

"Beats me," she replied dryly, thinking was this her lot in life – to be the girl nobody could manage without?

Nature had aspirations to act. "Can't be a model forever," she confided. "I gotta grab all the opportunities I can."

"You're twenty-two," Lauren pointed out. "What's your hurry?"

"I won't look like this for long. Once the lines start 'appening, an' I get a bit of sag here and there, it'll be over."

"You're crazy," Lauren said. "You've got another twenty years of looking great."

Nature shook her head. "Twenty years? You must be jokin'! All those little sixteen-year-olds sneakin' up behind, sniffing at me heels – wanting what *I* got. This modelling lark ain't easy."

Lauren realized it was true – modelling was not easy, and the most successful girls worked hard to keep themselves at the top. Nature never allowed herself to gain an extra pound – every day – no matter how early she had to get up – she worked out for a solid hour, pushing her strength to the limit.

Emerson Burn arrived back in town from a world tour. Nature read about it in the *New York Post* and immediately hatched a plot. She had Lauren call his apartment.

"Tell 'im I wanna 'ave a dinner party for him."

"When?"

"Any night he likes. Now that 'e's dumped that stupid Selina cow I'm in with a chance."

Lauren called and spoke to his personal assistant who rudely informed her Mr Burn's social calendar was full.

She waited a day and phoned again saying it was Candice Bergen. This time she was put right through.

Emerson Burn sounded like a male version of Nature. "'Allo?"

"Emerson Burn?" Lauren asked, just to make sure.

"Candy Bergen?" he countered.

"No, this is Lauren Roberts – Nature's assistant. She'd like to invite you to dinner next week."

He sounded disappointed. "I thought you was Candy Bergen."

"Your secretary must have gotten your calls mixed up."

"Okay . . . dinner with Nature. She's on."

"What night?"

"Tuesday – eight o'clock. But only if she'll cook."

Lauren choked back laughter. Nature in the kitchen – that was a good one. "Do you have any special requests?"

"Yeah – tell 'er I want roast beef, Yorkshire pud and roast potatoes."

When Lauren informed Nature of his request she panicked. "Oh Gawd! I can't bleedin' cook. Can you?"

"Don't worry, we'll hire a caterer."

"I don't *want* a bleedin' caterer," Nature wailed. "This has gotta taste like a 'ome-cooked meal. Look – find a cooking school and learn – then I'll pretend I made it. 'Ow's that?"

Lauren laughed. "It's different."

And that's how she found herself attending a cooking class learning how to make roast beef and Yorkshire pudding. She learned fast.

The night of Nature's date with Emerson she prepared the meal, gave strict instructions how to serve it, and retreated to her bedroom in the back of the apartment.

At three a.m. she awoke, walked quietly out of her room preparing to turn the lights off in the living room, and discovered Nature and Emerson asleep on the white bear skin rug, naked and wrapped in each other's arms.

For a moment she stood quite still staring at them. Then she felt too much like an intruder and hurried back to her room, closed the door and attempted to sleep.

It was impossible. She knew the time had come to move on. No more hiding behind Nature. She had to resume living.

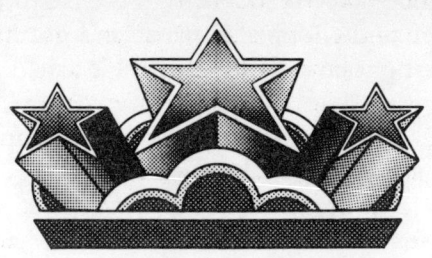

Chapter 45

On the morning of the Tijuana run Nick awoke at seven. He wasn't into getting up early, but today he was on edge and found it impossible to sleep.

DeVille lay quietly beside him. DeVille with her pale red hair and glorious white body. He hadn't sent for her, but she'd arrived anyway, and since she was standing on his doorstep he'd taken her in. He'd tried to explain to Annie, who'd pretended it didn't matter, grabbed her purse and run out of his apartment like she'd had a rocket up her ass.

He couldn't make up his mind whether she was angry with him or not. Probably she was. Women were like that – overly sensitive.

For a couple of days he'd lost himself in sex. It was so good it should be illegal – especially with DeVille, who knew everything he liked and made sure he was the happiest man on the block.

"I can get my own apartment if you want," she'd offered, not really meaning it.

"That's a good idea," he'd replied, not really meaning it either, and they'd fallen back into bed.

Now she'd been at his place for five days and he knew it was time for her to go – only he hadn't gotten around to mentioning it.

Tomorrow I'll do it, he thought. Give her fifty bucks and ease her out gently by telling her that living together was not a good idea on account of his career.

What career?

The career he was going to have after Joy Byron saw him perform and found him an agent – who in turn would secure him his first professional acting job.

Confidence, you had to have confidence – and he was brimming with it.

By eight o'clock he'd taken a run on the beach, eaten a healthy breakfast of bran and chopped bananas and got himself mentally ready for his first phone call of the day. He called Annie. She was suitably cold.

"Hey, listen," he said. "Remember I was supposed to work on some kinda scene for Joy Byron?"

"Yes?" she said in her *who gives a damn* voice.

"You promised to help me out. I haven't had a lot of time this week –"

"I can imagine," she interrupted.

"I've found the scene I want to do. I thought that I'd drop by tomorrow and read through it with you."

"I'm working tomorrow," she said, coolly.

"I'd really like to rehearse before I do it for Joy," he said, hoping to persuade her.

"Miss Byron," she corrected. "Nobody calls her Joy."

"You *will* read with me, won't you, Annie?"

"Did I say I would?"

Time to turn on the charm, not so easy over the phone – he did better in person. "Are you pissed at me?"

"Should I be?"

He shrugged, "I dunno." A short pause. "Hey – about DeVille arriving on my doorstep – she's an old girlfriend from Chicago who blew into town with nowhere to stay. She'll be moving on soon." He glanced over at DeVille – still asleep on his bed. DeVille wasn't moving anywhere.

There was a long awkward silence, finally broken by Annie. "I bumped into Cyndra yesterday," she said. "She'd like to hear from you."

"I've been meaning to call her."

"What are you waiting for? She *is* your sister."

"I'll call her tomorrow. I'm driving to Mexico today."

"Mexico?"

"Yeah, I'm picking up a passenger. Somebody's kid's getting out of boarding school."

"Boarding school – in Mexico?"

"You think I'm making it up?"

"I'm never sure what you make up and what's the truth."

He got off the subject. "So . . . can I see you tomorrow?"

There was another long pause before she finally said, "Okay, I guess so. Come by at five, we'll go to class together."

"I'll be there," he said, hanging up and deciding that after scoring the two grand he was going to tell Manny goodbye. One trip was enough. Soon he'd have an acting job and wouldn't need this crap.

Manny had told him to go out and buy a chauffeur's uniform. He'd done so reluctantly. Jeez! There was nothing worse than dressing up in a uniform, feeling like somebody's lackey.

The uniform hung in his closet. He took it out, looked at it, put it away and went back to bed.

DeVille groaned in her sleep as he snuggled up behind her, letting her know he was awake. Tomorrow he really would tell her to leave. May as well make the best of this last opportunity.

"I finally heard from your brother," Annie remarked, rubbing suntan oil on her legs.

"What's he up to?" Cyndra asked, turning on her lounger beside the pool. "I call him all the time – he's never home."

"That's because his girlfriend came in from Chicago."

Cyndra sat up. "*What* girlfriend?"

"Some tall showgirl type with long red hair."

"Jealous?"

"Who, *me?*"

"Come *on,* Annie. I *know* you like him."

"Well . . . I must admit I thought there might be something between us, but that was before I found out he was the Don Juan of the out-of-work actors."

Cyndra nodded knowingly. "Nick's always been like that. Back in High school he could have any girl he wanted."

"You should have warned me."

"I didn't think you were planning on getting involved."

"*You're* the one who gave him my phone number."

"I had a feeling you two might be good together."

"Listen, the *last* thing I need in my life is a guy who can't keep it in his pants."

Cyndra laughed. "Okay, okay, I get the message." She glanced up as Reece emerged from their apartment wearing a pair of striped madras shorts with several heavy gold chains swinging around his neck.

"Hi, Reece." Annie greeted him with a desultory wave. "Another hard day's work?"

"Don't look like *you're* exactly bustin' *your* ass," he said, throwing her a dirty look before settling down on the lounger next to Cyndra.

"Reece likes to work on his tan," Cyndra said, quickly.

"You don't have to explain nothin' to her," Reece snapped.

"I wasn't explaining."

Annie jumped up before they got into a fight. Lately she'd heard a lot of yelling coming from their apartment. "What's happening with that demo record you were supposed to do?" she asked.

"These things take time," Cyndra said.

Annie nodded. "I guess they do. See you guys later."

Luigi managed to ignore Nick when he arrived to collect the car. Nick ignored him back as he made his way through to Manny's office.

"The uniform suits ya," Manny wheezed, looking him up and down. "Now, make sure ya got this right. Ya drive across the border, pick up Suga from the hotel, an' drive straight back to LA. If they stop ya at the border ya don't know from nothing. Ya was hired to pick up a school kid." He sucked on his cigar. "Who was ya hired by?"

"Prince Limos," Nick said, reciting his part.

"Yeah – no mention of Glamour. Ya got the address I gave you?"

"All set."

"Did Luigi put new plates on the car?"

"They're on."

"Okay, you're ready."

Yeah, Nick thought. *As long as I don't get busted.*

What was he bringing back? He hoped it wasn't drugs.

Who was he kidding? Sure, it was drugs. What else could it be?

On the drive to San Diego he played Rolling Stones tapes non-stop, making the trip in record time. He was ahead of schedule, so he parked the car in an underground garage and sat in a Burt Reynolds movie killing time. After that it was all the way to Tijuana.

Once there he parked outside the hotel, slid inside and searched the lobby looking for Suga.

He couldn't see her. *Shit!* Manny had said she'd be standing right in front.

Yeah, sure.

Just as he was about to approach the desk an apparition snuck up behind him and tapped him on the arm. It was Suga, looking twelve. Scrubbed of make-up, her hair in braids, a school cap on her head and in full uniform she resembled a truculent tomboy.

"Are you blind?" she hissed from the corner of her sulky mouth. "I bin standin' here forever."

He did a double take – the transformation was quite remarkable.

"Pick up my goddamn suitcase," she commanded, marching outside.

He followed her, carrying the case which weighed a ton. Maybe he should spring it open before they crossed the border and check out the contents. For all he knew he could be carrying a goddamn body, it was heavy enough.

Suga stood next to the limo stamping her feet impatiently.

He sprung the trunk open, loaded the suitcase, then got into the driver's seat.

"Bust your ass outta here," Suga squeaked, jumping in the back. "I hate these runs – they make me wet my pants."

"How many times you made this trip?" he asked, sliding the car away from the kerb.

"Too many," she replied, popping bubble gum.

They drove in silence for a while until he couldn't contain himself any longer. "What's in the suitcase?"

"Did Manny say you could ask questions?" she snapped. "Whyn't ya just drive. You're making your money – what do you care?"

He eased the limousine along the crowded streets. Now he was getting nervous. Two grand was one thing, but it wasn't worth getting busted.

Yeah, well two thousand dollars is a lot of bucks, he reasoned. It would take months of real work at Glamour Limousines to score that kind of money – especially with clients like cheapskate Evans. Although right now, as he headed towards the border, Mr Evans seemed like a dream passenger.

Suga didn't care for his Rolling Stones tapes. "Turn that crap off," she whined. "I hate Mick Jagger."

He saw no reason to take her crap. "Anybody ever told you to shut up?"

"Oh," she said, sarcastically. "*You're* gonna tell me. Big fat chance."

"How much older than you is Manny?"

"Mind your fuckin' business."

"Why'd you marry him?"

"Get fucked."

So much for conversation with little Miss Charm.

There was a long line of cars at the border. It was getting dark and he was more nervous by the minute.

Suga sat in the back, chewing gum, perfectly calm.

By this time he imagined the suitcase was filled with cocaine. They'd throw him in jail for fifty years if he was caught. Never again. This was *it*.

By the time they reached the guard, he was sweating through his clothes.

The guard leaned down and looked through the window. "Do you have any fruits, vegetables or plants?" he asked, peering into the back of the car.

"No, just one juvenile delinquent I'm delivering to her parents," Nick said, pleasantly. Jeez, he actually sounded cool!

"Okay," the Guard said, walking away.

Okay? Did that mean they could go?

Apparently it did. He put his window up and drove the car out of there.

"Faster!' Suga urged from the back.

"I gotta stop an' take a piss."

"No!" she yelled. "Get away from the fuckin' border."

By the time they reached San Diego he was high. It was so easy, like nothing. Christ, he could make this trip twice a day if he had to. He checked out the rear-view mirror. Suga was busy wriggling out of her schoolgirl clothes and struggling into a short skirt and tight sweater.

"Hey –" he said. "Now you can tell me. What's in the case?"

"Two hundred and fifty thousand buckeroonies in cash," she said, casually. "Wanna take it an' run off together, Nick?"

"Are you shittin' me?"

She hitched her skirt down. "Would I do that?"

"No drugs?"

"You think I'd have anything to do with drugs?" she sniffed, indignantly. "What *I* need is to find me a guy with enough balls to split. Manny would track us, but we'd have the money, wouldn't we? We could vanish good."

Two hundred and fifty thousand dollars! Holy shit! What if he dumped *her* and took off by himself?

For a moment he thought about it. But only for a moment.

He had no desire to spend the rest of his life running from Manny Manfred.

"Well?" Suga challenged. "You got the balls or not?"

The little bitch was testing him so she could report back to Manny. "Whyn't you shut up," he said.

"Dumb prick," she muttered. "I meant it, you know."

He never found out if she was putting him on or not, because as soon as they got back to the garage she jumped out of the car and vanished.

Luigi opened the trunk, removed the suitcase and brought it to Manny's office.

"When do I get paid?" Nick asked, following him.

"Don't sweat it. Nobody's leaving town," Luigi said.

I made a mistake, he thought. *I should have gotten the money up front. Now they're gonna screw me.*

"I made the run, I took the risk. I want my money."

"Later," Luigi threw over his shoulder.

He followed him all the way into Manny's office where Luigi put the suitcase down. "I want my money," he repeated.

"Yeah, Nick, sure," Manny said, producing a thick bankroll and peeling off several hundred dollar bills. "Here ya go, ya did a nice job."

He didn't trust the fat man. Standing in front of his desk he counted the bills. "There's only one thousand here,' he said, when he was through.

"That's right," Manny answered, reaching for a handful of cashews. "A thousand for the first run, two grand for the second."

"No – we had a deal – two grand for this run."

"Tell ya what I'll do," Manny said magnanimously, crunching on the nuts. "I'll split the difference. Ya get fifteen hundred for this run, an' two an' a half for the next. How's that?"

Nick was angry. "Who the fuck d'you think you're dealing with?"

Manny's voice hardened. "Some punk kid who's lucky to have a job."

"I want my two thousand, Manny, or you'll regret it."

Manny's beady little eyes froze. "*I'll* regret it? You're *threatening* me?"

"I know what's in the suitcase."

"Howdja know that?"

Suga might be a pain in the ass but he wasn't about to put her away. "Do I get my two grand?"

303

Manny wheezed with laughter. "You're okay, kid. Q.J. said ya was." He peeled off several more bills and handed them over. "Ya can work for me any time."

Yeah, like he wanted to. Snatching the money he walked out.

"See ya tomorrow," Luigi called after him. "Mr Evans is comin' back t' town. Nine p.m. L.A.X. Don't be late."

Fuck Mr Evans.

Fuck Glamour Limousines.

He had his two grand – this was the last they'd see of him.

Chapter 46

"You can't leave," Nature shrieked.

"I have to," Lauren said.

"But why?" Nature demanded, petulantly. She was so used to getting her own way that she didn't understand the word no.

Nature was involved in a full-fledged affair with Emerson Burn. It was not peaceful – another reason why Lauren had decided to move on. Their screaming fights were legendary. Even worse, their passionate reconciliations.

Valiantly she tried to explain. "I feel like I'm living in your shadow. It's time I got my life back on track."

Nature pouted. "We're having fun, ain't we?"

"Yes, but it's not enough for me."

Reluctantly Nature accepted defeat. "What will you do? Work for Samm again?"

She shook her head. "I was thinking of starting my own business – kind of a . . . you know, like a Girl Friday."

"Girl Friday, what's that?" Nature asked, hooting with laughter.

"Someone who does everything. I'll put myself out for hire and people will pay me by the hour. I can even work for you occasionally."

"That's nice."

"Actually, I've been speaking to Pia and she's going to be leaving Samm's."

Nature raised a sceptical eyebrow. "Pia's quitting? Samm'll have a freaking fit."

Lauren hadn't planned on confiding in Nature, but now she couldn't stop herself. "We've already talked about going into business together. We'd call ourselves Help Unlimited."

Nature nodded. "Sounds good to me – but only if I can get you back any time."

Lauren grinned. "Pay my hourly rate and I'm all yours!"

Help Unlimited was an instant hit. Word travelled fast, and before they knew it Lauren and Pia were inundated with clients. In fact, so many, that after the first three months they had to hire two helpers. It was a hectic existence. One day Lauren found herself watering house plants in a Park Avenue duplex and the next organizing a fantastic midnight dinner for thirty on top of the Empire State building!

Pia had met a man she was crazy about. His name was Howard Liberty, and he was an executive with Liberty & Charles – one of the most prestigious advertising agencies in New York. Howard was short and sandy-haired with a pleasing personality. Lauren liked him immediately.

"Good, because we're talking marriage," Pia admitted, excitedly.

Nature's affair with Emerson Burn continued on its erratic course. Once in a while he used their services, but Lauren always made sure Pia dealt with him; somehow she never felt comfortable in his presence.

Every so often someone tried to fix her up even though they knew she wasn't open to a new relationship. She'd erected a wall around her emotional life and it was there to stay. All her energy was directed towards creating a successful business.

"What are you gonna do – stay celibate?" Nature demanded.

"I don't have to jump in and out of bed to be happy," she replied, calmly. "I'm building a business."

"You're *really* strange," Nature said, shaking her head. "No way *I* could go without sex."

Big surprise!

Pia and Howard fixed a wedding date.

"I hope this doesn't mean you'll be leaving the business," Lauren worried.

"No way!" Pia replied, adamantly. "I certainly don't plan on sitting home having babies."

"Good!" Lauren said, relieved.

One Monday morning Nature called at six a.m. Lauren groped for the phone in her sleep.

"It's me!" Nature screeched. "I'm in Vegas. I bleedin' got hitched, didn't I?"

"Hitched?"

"Married, of course! Me an' Emerson finally did it."

306

"Oh, no," Lauren mumbled.

"What do you mean, *oh no*? 'Ang out the flags. I'm bleedin' Mrs Emerson Burn, ain't I?!"

Lauren couldn't think of a worse combination. The two of them together were much too volatile – they'd kill each other. She struggled to sit up. "Why did you do it?"

"Oh, this is nice," Nature said. "You're the first person I call, an' all I get is negative shit. We're in *love*, Lauren. In love!"

"Do the press know?"

"Not yet."

"When they find out they'll be all over you."

"Emerson's calling 'is manager. I expect he'll arrange a press conference. Can you fly out here to be with me? I'll pay."

"You don't have to pay. If you want me, I'm there."

"We're flying back to LA this afternoon. Emerson's a bleedin' maniac at the tables – there's no controlling 'im. Gotta get 'im outta 'ere quick. Tell you what, why don't you meet us at 'is LA house tomorrow? Oh, an' do me a big favour."

"Name it."

"Call Samm, an' tell her. If I call 'er, she'll only scream at me."

Samm took the news stoically. It wasn't the first time one of her girls had run off and married a rock star, and it wouldn't be the last.

Pia wasn't thrilled when Lauren informed her she was flying to LA. "You know I'm getting married next week. I need you here," she said.

"I'll be back," Lauren assured her. "All the arrangements are in place – everything will go smoothly – and I promise you I'll be here."

"*Why* do you have to go?" Pia complained.

"Because Nature is my friend," Lauren said.

"Ha!" Pia exclaimed. "Nature likes you because you do things for her."

Trust Pia to be cynical.

"Thanks a lot."

Pia sighed. "What will you do? Sit by the pool watching them fight while I run the business all by myself?"

"Come on, Pia", she said, persuasively. "I've never been to LA. I'll only stay a few days."

By the time she'd organized her departure, Nature and Emerson's marriage had hit the airwaves in a big way. Even though Nature had said there were no press present,

307

photographs of them began appearing everywhere – Nature in a short white mini dress lovingly feeding Emerson wedding cake. Emerson in black leather, his mane of shaggy hair falling way below his shoulders. Nature grinning. Emerson scowling.

They looked happy.

They looked stoned.

Lauren sat on the American flight studying the *New York Post*. A picture of Nature and Emerson dominated the front page.

"Rock stars," sniffed a blue-haired woman in the next seat. "They're all degenerates, you know."

Lauren ignored the woman and closed her eyes. She was *en route* to LA. It was a long way from Bosewell.

Disembarking from the plane she felt like a movie star. A uniformed driver greeted her at the gate and accompanied her to the luggage carousel where she pointed out her one small suitcase.

He looked surprised. "That it?"

"That's it," she replied, sure it must be a disappointment for him having to meet a nobody like her. But he seemed quite cheerful as she followed him outside to the limo.

Everything in Los Angeles seemed bigger and better. The sky was bluer, the trees greener, and the limousine she climbed into was longer and more luxurious than any limo she'd ever seen. It was white with black windows, and inside there were little fairy lights dotted all around the sides.

"Ever been to LA before?" the driver asked, as they cruised along the freeway.

"Never," she replied, settling back into the luxurious leather upholstery.

"It's a trip," he said, peering at her through the rear-view mirror. "I've been out here ten years now. Came from Chicago. Name's Tucker."

"And you like it better here?" she asked, politely.

"LA life is easy."

"How long have you worked for Emerson Burn?"

"Six months. He's a good guy. Sometimes I get to travel with him."

"I guess his marriage surprised you."

Tucker laughed. "When it comes to rock 'n rollers, *nothing* surprises me."

Emerson lived in a mansion high in the hills of Bel Air. A guard waved Tucker through, and the huge gates closed behind them as the limo snaked its way up a long, winding driveway. At the top of the hill was the largest house Lauren had ever seen.

As soon as the limousine drew up to the front door Nature came running out, wearing a red polka-dot bikini and little else. "You're here!" she screamed, happily. "About bleedin' time." They hugged, warmly. "Come on in," Nature said, pulling her through the massive front door. "Welcome to me ever so humble home."

The house was a palace. High vaulted ceilings, old masters on the wall and heavy over-stuffed furniture. "Course," Nature said matter-of-factly, dragging Lauren through a domed ceiling hallway towards the pool in the back. "S'not exactly my taste, but I'll soon get 'im to change everything."

"It doesn't look like his taste, either," Lauren remarked, taking it all in.

"Some queen decorator did it," Nature said offhandedly. "Probably wanted to give 'im one." She laughed at the thought. "C'mon outside an' congratulate the bridegroom."

Emerson Burn rested on a lounger beside an enormous blue pool wearing nothing but a brief black Speedo bikini.

Lauren's eyes travelled to the bulge. Either he used padding, or everything you saw up on stage was the real thing.

His shaggy mane was bunched into a pony-tail emerging from a black baseball cap. Ominous black shades covered his eyes. On either side of him were small tables. One held a phone, a tall jug of apple juice, two bottles of Stolichnaya vodka and several glasses. The other table was piled high with scripts.

Nature bounced over. "You remember Lauren, don't you, darling?"

Emerson removed his shades and stared at her with his dreamy grey eyes.

Lauren stared back, wondering if he used mascara on his long curling lashes. "Uh . . . congratulations,' she mumbled.

"Thanks," he said, putting his shades back on and lifting his chin to catch more sun.

"Come back inside," Nature giggled. "I'll give you the grand tour."

By the time Nature had dragged her all around the huge mansion she was exhausted. "Can I take a shower?" she asked hopefully.

"Yeah, 'ave a sleep, too, 'cause tonight we're gonna party!"

"I didn't come here to party," she objected. "I came to help you out."

"Don't need any help, luv – Emerson's got sixty thousand people working for 'im. I'm entitled to 'ave a friend visit, ain't I? I just got married, for God's sake." She paused by a mirror in the hallway attracted by her own reflection. "Hmm . . . I'm gettin' fat," she remarked, pinching her curvaceous waistline.

"No, you're not," Lauren said, firmly. "How can you say that?"

"It creeps up on you, luv," Nature replied, frowning as she turned this way and that – inspecting her body. "Oh, by the way, what did Samm say?"

"She wasn't exactly ecstatic."

"I *bet* the old bag wasn't. Did you tell 'er to cancel all me bookings for the next month?"

"No, I thought we'd discuss it first."

"There's nothing to discuss."

"Just because you're married doesn't mean you should give up your career."

"Who's giving it up? But I ain't workin' me bleedin' arse off when I can stick with Em." She lowered her voice to a confidential whisper. "'E can't be trusted, y'know. 'Ave you any idea what happens on these tours? Rock stars got dumb little groupies crawlin' all over 'em like bleedin' fungus. I'm gonna travel with 'im, protect me interests."

"You won't be very popular if you cancel your bookings."

"This ain't a popularity contest," Nature retorted, flinging open a door and leading Lauren into a large sunny room overlooking the pool. "'Ere's your room."

"Oh my God! It's bigger than my apartment!"

"Everything's bigger and better in California," Nature announced. "You'll soon get used to it. How long can you stay?"

"Three days."

"You 'ave t' stay at least a week."

"I can't run out on Pia."

"She'll manage."

"Three days, Nature."

"Four days."

"Okay, deal."

Nature smiled, knowingly. "By that time you'll be beggin' to stay longer. 'Ave a lie down – someone will wake you at six."

Lauren took a shower in the marble bathroom and then lay in the middle of the king-size bed. Within minutes she was asleep.

When she awoke it was late in the afternoon. She wandered over to the window and observed Emerson Burn in the pool. He was swimming lengths as if his life depended on it. Anything to keep in shape.

Her first Hollywood party and everyone was dressed to overkill. The mansion, owned by a record tycoon, was bigger and better than Emerson Burn's. Servants abounded.

"'Ave a gander over there," Nature said, nudging Lauren sharply in the ribs. "It's Jack bleedin' Nicholson, ain't it? Wanna meet him?"

"No," Lauren said, horrified at the thought.

Nature giggled. "When you're out with me you can meet anyone you want – who do you fancy?"

"I fancy sitting in a corner by myself."

"You're 'aving fun, ain'tcha?"

"You know my idea of fun. I prefer to watch."

"Very kinky!"

"Do me a favour – go off with your husband and enjoy yourself. I'm perfectly happy."

Nature didn't need much encouragement. "Okey-doke – I'll check you later."

Looking around, Lauren couldn't get over the fact that there were more waiters than guests. She requested a club soda from one with a blond crew cut, and found a corner for herself, trying to remember everything she saw to tell Pia.

Not only was Jack Nicholson present, but she recognized a whole slew of other famous faces. A smiling Burt Reynolds, a gorgeous Angie Dickinson, a strutting Rod Stewart and a dignified looking Gregory Peck.

The little girl in her said, *Why didn't I bring my autograph book?* The big girl said, *I don't want to be here. Let me out!*

Everybody kissed each other, only their lips never touched. Conversation seemed transient. The women wore jewels the like of which she'd never seen.

Nature revelled in it. Lauren watched her as she fluttered from person to person – blonde, big and luscious. Emerson didn't follow her around, he sat at the bar and everybody came over to pay homage. He was a rock star. It was his due.

Lauren found it easy to blend into the background. Although at one time she'd been the prettiest girl in Bosewell, she certainly didn't impress anybody in Hollywood. Not that she was trying. In fact, as usual she'd played her looks down – her hair was neatly drawn back, and she wore no make-up and her simple outfit blended into the background. Nature often screamed at her about the way she dressed, and Pia was into giving lectures claiming she didn't make the most of herself. "I'm perfectly happy the way I am," she'd told them both.

By midnight she was ready to leave, but Nature was still going strong and Emerson showed no signs of moving. The house had its own discotheque – a mirrored room with flashing strobe lights, black granite floors and a disc jockey stand complete with a wasted looking disc jockey.

Lauren managed to grab hold of Nature as she fluttered by on her way to dance. "I'm falling asleep," she whispered. "Do you mind if I go?"

"Don't worry," Nature screeched. "We'll be out of 'ere soon."

"Maybe I can take the car and send it back for you?"

"Do what you want," Nature replied vaguely, continuing on her way.

Tucker was outside talking to a group of drivers.

"They're not ready," Lauren said, "but I am."

Tucker nodded. "I'll bring the car around."

Sitting in the back of the luxurious limo she closed her eyes all the way back to Emerson's mansion. When she arrived she couldn't wait to fall into bed.

Sometime before dawn she was awakened by a screaming fight between Nature and Emerson.

What else was new?

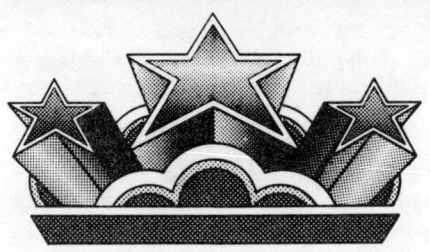

Chapter 47

The next few months passed quickly. Nick had his apartment, a stash of money from the Tijuana job, and Joy Byron's class to keep him busy. Joy Byron had turned out to be the teacher of his dreams. She didn't criticize, she nurtured – carefully watching every move he made. The other students in the class couldn't wait to pick everyone's performance to pieces. Fuck 'em. As long as Joy thought he was good, that's all that mattered.

"I've decided to give you extra coaching," Joy announced one day, her watery eyes darting around the room.

"Can I afford it?" he asked, half-jokingly.

"Probably not," she replied, crisply. "But you'll pay me back . . . one day."

He began visiting her run-down house way up in the Hollywood Hills on a regular basis, and in her dusty living room he got to do anything he wanted. Joy Byron had bookshelves piled high with every play ever written – it was better than a trip to the library. She allowed him to indulge himself – reading with him, giving pertinent advice and teaching him about diction, posture, timing, make-up and the best lighting and camera angles.

"This information is invaluable," she said. "You, my dear boy, are going to be big."

He wasn't intimidated by her. "Hey – *I* know that," he replied, cockily.

"Good," she said, unfazed by his sureness. "Confidence is everything."

When she came on to him he was taken aback, the woman had to be at least sixty-five. He quickly made up a fiancée, a true love, waiting patiently for him in his home town.

Joy did not believe him, but she backed off anyway, remarking that she had plenty of lovers and certainly didn't need the likes of him.

He wondered if it would make any difference to their student/teacher relationship. It didn't.

Annie was not pleased. The only time he ever saw her was in class and she'd taken to ignoring him.

"What's the matter?" he asked one day. "You're treatin' me like I got a bad case of BO."

"You used me," she said, turning on him full of pent-up anger. "All you wanted was an introduction to Joy, and now you're her pet project nobody hears from you. I don't appreciate being used, Nick."

"Hey – what's wrong with me gettin' everything I can out of this?"

Annie refused to be placated. "You're kissing her ass."

It didn't take long to realize most of the other students felt the same way. Well fuck 'em – if they didn't like it that was their problem; he fully intended to learn everything he needed to know.

Joy announced she was putting on a student production of *On the Waterfront*. Naturally she gave Nick the coveted Marlon Brando role. This did not go down well with the rest of the class who resented him even more.

So far Joy had advised him not to seek out an agent or manager. "Many important people come to my shows," she informed him. "I'll find you the right agent. Follow my guidance, dear boy, and we can't fail."

That was okay with him; he had no desire to traipse around agents' offices getting a series of turn-downs.

DeVille was still living in his apartment – somehow she'd never gotten around to moving out. He didn't mind. It meant he didn't have to go looking for sex – she was always ready and available. Occasionally he asked her to read with him. She wasn't half bad and soon started dropping hints about maybe accompanying him to class.

That, he didn't need. He was having trouble enough – he could just imagine what would happen if he showed up with DeVille on his arm.

As for Manny Manfred and Glamour Limousines, he'd never gone back. As long as he had enough money who needed to work for a living?

Cyndra called to complain she never saw him. "I'm going

to be playing Vegas," she said, full of enthusiasm. "Reece has me booked to sing at one of the best hotels. Will you fly out?"

He assured her he would, but he still hadn't gotten around to it, he was too busy putting all his energy into preparing for his upcoming role.

In between rehearsals he continued to spend most of his time at Joy's house. The night before the big event she came on to him stronger than ever.

"I bring people luck, Nick," she announced grandly, her bony hand hovering dangerously near the top of his thigh.

"Yeah?" he said warily, backing off as usual.

Her watery eyes bored into his. "If I told you about some of the men I've slept with, famous men . . . powerful men. They all claim I bring something . . . *special* into their lives."

By this time her hands were all over him.

He knew there was no way he could get it up and yet he couldn't risk disappointing her. "Hey – listen, Joy, you're a very attractive woman," he lied, speaking fast while desperately removing her hand from his leg. "But like I said – I got this fiancée, an' we promised we'd never cheat on each other."

Joy muttered something lethal under her breath and threw him out.

He drove back to his apartment hoping he hadn't made a mistake.

Hell, no – gotta have some principles.

When he arrived home DeVille was sitting in a chair facing the door dressed for business. Next to her were two packed suitcases.

"Going somewhere?" he asked, throwing off his jacket.

She smiled, a trifle sheepishly. "I'm finally moving out. Remember, we discussed it a couple of months ago?"

He threw open the fridge and surveyed the meagre contents. DeVille was a lousy housekeeper. "Hey, I didn't ask you to go," he said, reaching for a can of beer.

She pushed back her pale red hair. "I know, Nick, but I've stayed long enough."

"Where's your next stop?"

She lowered her eyes, almost afraid to tell him. "I met this guy."

Funny, but he wasn't at all jealous. "Yeah? What guy?"

"A producer."

He snapped the can open. "A *real* producer? Or some Hollywood phoney?"

"He's asked me to live with him."

"How come you never mentioned him before?"

"It didn't seem necessary."

Nick wasn't used to being walked out on, but so what – there was no way he was begging her to stay. If she wanted to get conned by some would-be producer it was her problem.

That night he slept restlessly. He had a hunch that starting tomorrow everything was going to be different.

"Come over here, darlin'," Reece said, patting the empty seat beside him.

Cyndra hesitated. She had no intention of sitting with Reece at the small round table in the cocktail lounge of the busy downtown casino. The night before she'd joined him and two of his so-called "friends". As soon as she'd sat down he'd got up and vanished for over an hour. The men had started making suggestive remarks and trying to grope her. She'd soon put them straight. When Reece had returned he'd been furious.

"Those were important guys," he'd told her. "*Real* important. What's the *matter*? You dumber than you look?"

His words had stung like a slap. How dare he talk to her in such a way – he never had before. But since they'd been in Vegas he'd changed, and it wasn't for the better. First of all there was the matter of the hotel where she was to perform. Reece had assured her it was going to be one of the big ones.

"Which one?" she'd asked, imagining her debut was to be at The Sands or Desert Inn.

"It's a surprise," he'd said mysteriously, not looking her in the eye.

Some surprise. A downtown dump full of hookers and hustlers with only a pianist to back her – a surly Puerto Rican who could barely talk English and was usually half-drunk.

"What happened?" she'd asked, furiously.

"We gotta get you more experience before we hit the big time," Reece explained. "This is a fine start, honey."

Reece talked a good game. First the demo recordings which failed to take place. Now Vegas and this crummy place.

Cyndra told herself she shouldn't blame him – at least he was trying. But he'd made such big promises and look where they'd got her.

When they'd returned to their motel room she'd refused to

speak to him. Now he was sitting in the audience like nothing had happened, expecting her to join him.

Well screw him, he could think again.

She narrowed her eyes and checked out the table. At least he was alone.

Hmm . . . he probably wanted to apologize.

Hmm . . . maybe she'd give him a second chance.

There was a buzz about performing for an audience – a buzz he'd never felt before. Better than sex – almost orgasmic in a way. Jeez! This was it. Give him a steady diet of applause and he'd be a happy man.

Joy hovered at the side of the stage encouraging, criticizing, whispering in his ear every time he came off. Do this. Do that. More gestures. Use your voice.

Fuck you, lady, I'm flying! I don't need your help.

And the audience loved him. They fucking loved him! Marlon move over – Nick Angelo is here to stay!

By the end of the show he was on fire – adrenalin pumping through his veins like pure heroin.

Joy was pleased. She had a big smirk on her face, especially when half the audience came piling backstage to congratulate her.

He wished he knew who was important and who wasn't – it wouldn't do to waste his charm on the wrong person. He looked to Joy for guidance. She was deluged by people.

"Not bad," Annie said grudgingly, passing by with a group. "We're going to the Hamlet on Sunset. Want to join us?"

Hamburger Hamlet was not exactly what he had in mind to celebrate his triumph. Plus Annie was really beginning to piss him off. Why couldn't she tell him he was fantastic; what was with this "not bad" shit? She was such a downer.

"Maybe," he mumbled. *If nothing better comes along.*

Joy beckoned him. "Nick, come over here – I want you to meet someone."

The someone turned out to be Ardmore Castle – a small-time agent well-known for his penchant for good-looking young actors.

"Hello . . . Nick." Ardmore had anxious eyes, plump jowls and a hungry expression. He was chasing fifty.

Joy moved away. Nick nodded, scanning the room. Ardmore Castle's reputation preceded him. Maybe Joy figured if *she* couldn't have him then Ardmore was in with a chance.

The agent fixed him with a lecherous stare. "I enjoyed your performance."

"Uh . . . thanks."

"Very macho."

"Yeah, well, it's written that way."

"You brought something special to it."

Major eye contact. Jeez! Where was Joy when he needed her?

Ardmore cleared his throat. "Perhaps you'd care to join me at my house later. I'm having a few friends drop by."

"Gee . . . sounds great, but I got a date."

"Bring him," Ardmore said, boldly.

"It's a her," he responded, quickly.

Ardmore realized he was getting a brush. He pursed his lips. "Suit yourself."

"I intend to."

"*Very* bold. For an unknown."

Joy descended, accompanied by a hatchet-faced middle-aged woman in a man's pin-stripe jacket and black pants. The woman brushed past Ardmore as if he didn't exist.

"Hello, Frances dear," Ardmore said, determined to be acknowledged.

She blew cigarette smoke in his face, barely nodding in his direction.

Joy grabbed Nick's arm in a proprietary way. "Nick, dear – meet Frances Cavendish, the casting director." She said casting director in meaningful tones. He got the message.

Frances didn't bother with pleasantries. She was a strong-jawed woman with a stern demeanour. She was also fast-talking and to the point. "My office. Tomorrow. Noon," she said, flicking a business card at him. "Might have something for you."

Deftly Joy plucked the card from his hand. "We'll be there, Frances dear," she said, smiling sweetly.

"Don't need you, Joy. I'm sure Nick can walk and talk on his own."

What was this little scene? He felt uncomfortably like a piece of meat lying on a slab while the dogs sniffed around deciding who'd get lucky.

Ardmore expressed his disapproval. "You need an agent," he said. "Someone who'll protect your interests."

"Yes," Frances said, dryly. "Someone who'll allow you to keep your pants on."

Nick took a deep breath, snatched Frances Cavendish's card back from Joy and mumbled, "I'm outta here."

"Where are you going?" Joy asked, hands fluttering.

"Gotta get some fresh air. See ya."

And he was gone before any of them could object.

Chapter 48

Nature took on the role of tour guide, deciding that Lauren had to see everything there was to see in Los Angeles.

"Can we take a break?" Lauren begged, after they'd been to Disneyland, Universal City and Magic Mountain all in one day.

Nature looked surprised – "What for? You're only here a few days – we gotta do everything we can – besides, I've never been to any of these places myself. It's a kick!"

While they were exploring, Emerson lay out by the pool working on his suntan and reading scripts.

"He's looking for a movie for us to do together," Nature confided.

Sure, Lauren thought.

Every day around noon his entourage arrived at the house and stayed until he threw them out – usually not until two or three in the morning. They laughed at his jokes, assured him he was the best thing since Elvis and freebied all over the house.

The pack was led by his manager, Sidney Fishbourne – a lanky man in his forties with shoulder-length frizzy black hair. Sidney was usually accompanied by April – a thirty-year-old married redhead he referred to as his executive assistant, although everyone knew she was his mistress.

The rest of the entourage consisted of Emerson's clothes designer, his make-up artist, his hair-stylist and his personal publicist.

The group spent most of their time discussing Emerson's image for his upcoming world tour.

"You gotta get wilder," Sidney insisted. "Break a few guitars, throw stuff around the stage, get the girls screaming."

"No fuckin' way," Emerson said adamantly. "I'm not doin' all that sixties shit again."

"He should be involved in a cause," his publicist said, twirling her worry-beads. "Perhaps something to do with nuclear power – or the environment."

"It's all in the clothes," his designer insisted. "No more black leather. I think suits."

"Suits are old," Sidney snapped. "We gotta start appealing to a younger audience."

His designer persevered. "Sophistication is very in."

"Who gives a shit," Emerson said flatly, and that was the end of the suit discussion.

Nature complained to Lauren that she felt left out. "All we ever talk about is 'im – what about *me*?" she demanded. "I'm famous, too."

"You married a rock star," Lauren pointed out. "His first interest is obviously going to be himself, especially with a world tour coming up."

"It's not that I'm jealous or anything," Nature continued, "but I'm hardly the bleedin' girl next door. I *should* get more attention, don't you think?"

"It depends," Lauren said, carefully. "Do you really *want* attention from that bunch of ass kissers?"

Nature giggled. "You're right as usual. Who cares about them?"

"What you *should* do is get back to work. You're not the type to sit at Emerson's feet. Show him you're independent – that's why he married you, isn't it?"

"Hmm . . ." Nature wasn't entirely convinced. "I dunno."

"Well *I* do," Lauren said, forcefully. "*Never* give everything up for a man."

It didn't take long before Nature and Emerson were embroiled in another of their famous fights. This one was triggered off by April, who innocently remarked she'd seen Selina, Nature's arch rival, on television discussing her first movie role.

"Ha!" Nature said, spitefully. "What's *she* playing – dumb cunt of the year?"

They were all sitting in the breakfast room picking at an array of salads and fruit plates. Emerson was into losing a few pounds which meant no real food allowed.

"C'mon, luv," Emerson said, mildly. "Selina's never done anything to you."

That was all Nature had to hear. She exploded in a jealous rage, lashing out at everyone.

"Got the rag on, 'ave we?" sneered Emerson, furious with her display of temper in front of everyone.

"Fuck you!" Nature screamed, picking up her plate of Caesar salad and flinging it in his face. "Go back to Selina if that's who you really want!" And with that she stormed from the room.

Lauren was embarrassed for both of them – Emerson with small pieces of oil-covered lettuce stuck to his face and hair – and Nature, who'd made a jealous fool of herself in front of everyone.

Emerson glared at his entourage. "Get the fuck out," he commanded. "Show's over for today."

Obediently they all filed out. Lauren started to follow. "*You* don't 'ave t'go," Emerson called after her.

She pretended not to hear and hurried upstairs to her room where she called the airline and booked a flight back to New York the following morning. She'd kept her promise and stayed four days. It was more than enough.

Later that afternoon she ventured down to the pool. She'd seen Emerson leave in the limo, and Nature had not returned from her lunchtime exit.

Lying out in the sun with nobody around was wonderfully peaceful. No rock music blaring. No Nature shrieking. No entourage clinking glasses and making inane conversation.

She closed her eyes and allowed her mind to drift – thinking about Bosewell and her parents. Meg, Stock – all the old crowd. And finally Nick.

Oh, God, she didn't want to think about Nick. She tried to keep him out of her thoughts as much as possible – it wasn't worth re-living memories so bitter-sweet and painful.

Nick Angelo with his black hair, green eyes and killer smile.

Nick – whom she'd given herself to totally.

Nick – who'd taken off without so much as a goodbye, leaving her pregnant and alone.

She opened her eyes forcing him from her thoughts. Standing over her, straddling the end of her lounger, was Emerson.

"What are you doing?" she asked, startled.

"Watching you," he replied, and she smelt the liquor on his breath.

She attempted to move her legs so she could get into a sitting position, but moving meant touching his crotch – and, oh no, she could see his hard-on – the brief bikini bottom he wore did nothing to hide it.

Stay calm, she warned herself. *Stay in control and nothing will happen.*

"Is Nature back?" she asked, trying to sound casual as she quickly pulled up the top of her swimsuit.

"I want you t'suck my cock," Emerson announced, swaying drunkenly.

Voices screamed inside her head. *Don't react! Don't panic! Stay cool!*

There was a long moment of silence. Neither of them moved. She noticed the small, spiky, black hairs on the insides of his thighs and the tiny spot of moisture staining his bikini briefs.

"Emerson, don't do anything you'll regret later," she said, trying to keep her voice even.

"Who says I'll regret it?" he slurred.

Where were the servants and Tucker? If she screamed would they hear? Would they care?

Damn Nature for putting her in this position.

She remembered Bosewell and Primo and that fateful day five years ago.

I think I killed a man.

No. The tornado killed him.

She'd never know the truth.

Her mind began to race, formulating a plan of action. If she raised one knee sharply and unexpectedly she'd catch him right on target, probably giving her enough time to run. But where would she run to? Surely if there was no one in the house she'd be putting herself in an even more vulnerable position?

Emerson stuck his fingers in the top of his briefs and began pulling them down.

Perfect! As soon as they were down far enough he'd immobilize himself and she'd make her move.

She made one more attempt to warn him off. "Don't do this, Emerson. Please don't. You're drunk. You're not thinking straight."

He looked surprised. "C'mon, Lauren, y'know you've been dyin' t'suck my dick ever since you got here."

They moved together like clumsy ballet partners. He pulled his pants down. She brought her knee up. He fell to one side, cursing. She struggled to her feet and started running towards the house. A count of three and he was behind her, kicking his bikini away from his ankles, running naked.

She sprinted swiftly across the marble terrace, hardly daring to glance behind because she knew he was close.

323

He caught her by the steps to the house, slammed her from behind, and they both fell to the ground.

"Gotcha!" he yelled triumphantly, like they were in the middle of a fun game. Then he pinioned her arms behind her head and rolled on top of her. "Now I'm gonna fuck you like you never bin fucked before," he rasped, gripping both her arms with one hand, while attempting to roll the top of her swimsuit down with the other.

"Don't you have enough girls," she gasped, turning her head. "Girls who want to be with you. Understand me, Emerson – *I* don't."

"Try to believe it, baby," he said, ripping at her swimsuit, rolling it down around her waist and grabbing her breasts. "You'll want me so much you'll be beggin' for it. You hear me? *Beggin'* for it."

He tore at the crotch of her swimsuit, pushing it to one side, doing his best to enter her.

"You son-of-a-bitch!" she screamed, suddenly losing all control. "LEAVE ME THE FUCK ALONE!" If she'd had a knife she would have stabbed him, just like she'd stabbed Primo.

Now he was really enjoying himself. He had her where he wanted and there was no way she could escape. "Temper, temper!" he mocked. "Mustn't use dirty words. Mummy wouldn't like it."

She felt the tip of his penis about to force an entry and she was filled with despair.

Suddenly a new voice filled the air. "You dirty low-life, scumbag *rat!*" It was Nature's unmistakable shriek. "You lying, cheating, mother-fuckin' *pig!*"

Emerson's hard-on deflated.

Lauren seized the moment and rolled out from under him, pulling up her swimsuit, fighting back angry tears.

"And as for you," Nature turned on her, blue eyes blazing. "I thought you was me bleedin' friend – but you're just like all the rest of the slags – couldn't wait t'get your hands on me old man."

"Now wait a minute –"

"Get outta me house," Nature shouted, her cheeks red with anger. "I *never* want to speak to you again."

Emerson began to rock with laughter. He had no intention of coming to her defence.

What a couple. The truth was they deserved each other.

She ran into the house without looking back.

Chapter 49

"Are you straight?" Frances Cavendish asked as if it was the most normal question in the world.

"Want me to pull down my pants an' prove it?" Nick replied, damned if she was going to embarrass him.

Frances leaned back behind her desk and adjusted the *diamanté* studded glasses covering her flinty eyes. "Go ahead," she drawled, challenging him.

"Don't bet me, lady," he warned, still trying to figure her out.

Frances laughed – a big bawdy laugh. "The kid's got attitude. I like it."

He didn't appreciate her talking down to him. "The *kid* is a hell of an actor. What I need from you, lady, is a job."

Coolly Frances appraised him, dragging on her cigarette. "What's your professional experience?"

"I done a lot of stuff," he mumbled.

Frances' expression said she didn't believe him. "Do you have a résumé? A tape? Photographs?"

"Uh . . ." He trailed off. She wasn't going to do anything for him. He'd made the trip to her fancy office for nothing. Frances Cavendish, casting agent. She must have known he had no experience. The old broad probably got off on humiliating people.

Frances continued to drag on her cigarette and squinted at him. "Are you fucking Joy Byron?"

"Now wait a minute –"

"No. *You* wait a minute," she said, sharply. "You slouch in here in your tight jeans with your bad-ass scowl expecting exactly what?"

"You asked me to come," he fired back.

"Did I?" She took off her glasses and studied him further.

He felt her gaze penetrating beneath his clothes. She wanted a fuck. That's what they all wanted. And if he wasn't giving it to Joy – who at least treated him like a human being – he certainly wasn't giving it to this one. He turned, making his way towards the door; there was no point in hanging around.

Frances stopped him at the threshold, her voice strong and commanding. "I'm sending you on an audition."

He threw her a look. "Yeah?"

"It's a small role – but juicy."

"I got all the juice y'want."

"I'm sure you have," she said coolly, putting her glasses back on. "Conditions."

"What?" he asked, suspiciously.

"Take my advice and get rid of Joy – she'll hang around your neck like a cement block. Oh yes, and stay away from agents like Ardmore Castle. If you get the part I'll recommend a legitimate agent to take care of you."

He felt obliged to defend Joy, after all she'd been good to him. "Joy's a great teacher," he said, quickly.

Frances was having none of it. "Joy's an old hack living in the past. Drop her now, Nick, before it's too late."

"You're a hard lady."

"I'm honest – an almost impossible attribute to come by in this town."

He wondered what she wanted. Then decided he had nothing to lose by asking. "So . . . uh . . . what am I gonna owe you?"

"Occasional escort services. When I need you. Get yourself a tuxedo – you already have the attitude." She paused, inhaling deeply, heavy smoke drifting from her nostrils. "Escort duties end at the door. Which is more than you can say for Joy or Ardmore. Do we have a deal?"

This was some straight-talking old broad. "What's the part?"

"Small-time hood with a heart of mush. It's a minor role – but showy. I'm sending you over to meet the director and producers. If they ask about experience – lie. Tell them you've done stock, off-Broadway and commercials. If they ask for photos refer them back to me. I'll make an appointment for you to have photographs taken later this week. You'll pay me back when you get your first cheque."

He couldn't figure her out. "Why are you doin' all this?"

"Because when you make it you'll owe me. I like that. Write

down your number. I'll call you tomorrow and give you their reaction."

He was apprehensive. "You mean I'm goin' on an audition *now?*"

She stubbed her cigarette out in a full ashtray, immediately reaching for a fresh package. "Unless you'd prefer to wait a day or two."

He didn't hesitate. "Lady – I'm ready."

"That's *exactly* what I thought."

"You'll do things my way, or you're gonna find yourself doing nothin' at all." So spoke Reece.

Cyndra felt a shiver of fear. This was not the man she'd married – the laid-back cowboy with the big promises. This was someone else – a stranger. "You'd better stop getting on my case or I'm likely to walk," she said sharply, challenging him.

He caught her with a slap around the face, taking her by surprise. "Get it into your head – you're my wife," he said, harshly. "*My wife,* do you understand me? I fucking married you – that means you belong to me, and you'll do anything I tell you to do."

Her hand flew to her face stinging from his slap. "I don't belong to *anybody!*" she yelled.

"That's where you're wrong," he yelled back. "And if you don't believe me, maybe you'll believe this."

To her horror he pulled a gun from his belt and waved it in her direction.

She backed into a corner of their motel room, her eyes wide with fear. "Reece . . . Reece, what are you doing?"

"What the hell you think?" he replied.

"Where did you get a gun?"

He strutted around the room. "I always had it. Never know when it might come in useful. Man's gotta protect himself."

She took a deep breath and tried to stay in control.

"Put it away . . . put it away now."

"I got your attention, huh?" he smiled slyly, pleased with himself. "So maybe you'd care to give some of that attention to my friends 'stead of making me look like a jerk."

Her mouth was dry; she couldn't believe what was happening. Within the last few minutes her life had crumbled around her. Wasn't it enough that she'd had to escape from Bosewell? Did she have to escape from this man, too?

327

"Listen to me *good*, bitch," Reece said, enjoying her attention. "I found you bumming around New York – now you're singin' in Vegas, so don't ever forget it's *me* got you here. An' if I expect you to be nice to my friends, then you'll do it. Understand?" As he spoke he waved his gun in the air.

"Yes, Reece," she whispered.

"Say it louder," he commanded.

"*Yes!*"

"*That's* what I like to hear." He stuck the gun back in his belt. "Tomorrow night mebbe I'll have a coupla guys join us after the show, an' you'll be nice to 'em, honey. You'll do whatever I tells you t'do."

She nodded blankly.

Later, when he was asleep, she thought about creeping from the room and running. But where could she run to? If she took off she knew Reece would come after her.

With a feeling of deep despair she realized there was no escape. Once more she was trapped. It was a bad feeling.

Nick did exactly what Frances had told him to do. He lied. When they asked him about his experience, he made up a travelling stock company he'd performed in, then mentioned a few commercials and several original off-Broadway plays. In fact, he lied pretty good.

There were two producers in the room. A tall, nervy man who sat in the background, staring. And a middle-aged woman with great legs that she kept on crossing and uncrossing. The director was Italian/American, short, with swarthy features and a shock of greasy brown hair.

Nick checked them out. Three assholes all in a row. Fuck it. He wasn't nervous – although the casting assistant was really pissing him off – when they read together she didn't know acting from shit. But still, the three assholes seemed to like him – in fact they made him read through the scene twice.

When he'd arrived the girl in reception had handed him several pages of dialogue. He'd had half an hour to study them. He'd also had half an hour to study the other actors waiting to go in. Talk about a cattle call – you could feel and smell the competition.

He remembered Frances' words – "small-time hood with a heart of mush" – and that's who he became. Not Nick Angelo

– an actor chasing a role – just a small-time hood with a heart of mush. Some fucking description!

He finished reading the second time and waited for their reaction.

"Good seeing ya, Nick," said the director, dismissing him as though they were old friends.

"Thank you," said the woman producer, crossing her legs again, while eyeing him contemplatively.

The tall man said nothing.

Before he could think about it he was out of there.

He stopped at the reception desk and spoke to the girl. "How long before I get to hear?" he asked.

She looked amused. "New at this?"

"Nah . . . well, yeah, I guess. I'm new in town. I was, uh . . . workin' in Chicago an' New York."

"Oh, you're a New York actor," she said, a little bit impressed. "Don't worry, you'll soon get to know the routine. Sometimes these auditions go on for months. They see you, like you, then they see fifty other guys. After that maybe they'll call you back. You never know."

"So it's like a long wait?"

She shrugged. "Face it. This town is a crap shoot."

She was using his dialogue! He wondered if she ever got to listen in on the producers' conversation after the actors left the room.

"Hey, what's your name?" he asked, going for the friendly approach. "And when do you wanna have dinner?"

"Marilyn," she replied, still smiling. "*Married* Marilyn," she added, holding up her hand to display a wedding ring. "But thanks for asking anyway."

Outside in the parking lot he contemplated driving back to Frances' office and giving her a report.

Nah. Instinct told him he should wait until he heard from her. But now he was high from the audition and there was no way he could sit around waiting for the phone to ring. He decided to pay Annie a visit.

She was vacuuming when he arrived and didn't look thrilled to see him. "Oh, the big star is here," she said, continuing to vacuum.

He pulled the plug from the outlet. "What is this crap with you?"

She sighed. "How many times have we had this conversation?

329

Like last night – why didn't you join us at Hamburger Hamlet? What *did* you do, take off with Ardmore Castle?"

"You calling me a fag, Annie?" he said, feigning indignation.

"I'm not calling you anything, but you . . ." She shook her head. "Oh – I don't know, Nick, you confuse me."

"I went home – alone."

"That's nice."

"I met this casting director – Frances Cavendish. I dropped by and saw her today and she sent me on an audition."

"What audition?"

"Small part in a movie."

"Did you get it?"

"Dunno."

"Did you read?"

He grinned. "I was great!"

"Mister Modest."

"Listen – if *I* don't sing 'em – who will?"

She pushed the vacuum over to a corner closet and stored it. "Are you coming to Joy's class tomorrow night?"

He wandered around her small apartment. "I kinda figured I might drive to Vegas, see Cyndra. Beats sitting around waiting for the call to tell me I didn't get the part. This is like difficult shit."

"Nobody ever said it was easy."

"Whaddaya think? Should I go to Vegas?"

"Cyndra would love to see you."

"How long's the drive?"

"Five, six hours, I'm not sure."

"Wanna come?"

She shook her head but he could tell she was tempted.

"C'mon – live dangerously – throw a few things in a bag, it'll be fun," he said, encouragingly.

Annie began to relate a list of excuses.

Nick shot them all down.

An hour later they were on their way.

Chapter 50

Back in New York Lauren refused to talk about her LA trip.

"What happened?" Pia was anxious to know.

"Nothing," she replied, quickly. "Exactly nothing."

"Why aren't you telling me anything?" Pia complained. "And how come if Nature calls you don't want to speak to her? *Something* must have gone on."

Lauren's only desire was to forget about LA, and with that in mind she threw herself back to work. In her spare time – of which there was little – she began attending a self-defence class, studying French, and also taking a gourmet cooking class. These activities left her no time for a social life, and if anyone tried to fix her up they got a blank "No thanks".

Shortly after getting back, Lauren attended Pia and Howard's wedding in the garden of his uncle Oliver's house in the Hamptons. Oliver Liberty was one of the founders of Liberty & Charles. He was a distinguished looking man in his late fifties, with a dry sense of humour – the complete opposite of his wife, Opal, a vacuous blonde he'd married on the rebound after an expensive divorce from his first wife of thirty-one years.

It was a beautiful wedding. Lauren sat back and day-dreamed about how it might have been if things had been different with Jimmy. She even allowed her mind to drift back to Nick. So many years ago . . . but when she thought about him it still hurt and she shut off the thoughts abruptly.

Oliver Liberty strolled over and sat down beside her after dinner. "I hear you and Pia are building quite a business," he said, one eye on his flashy wife who was cavorting on the dance floor in a too-tight red dress.

"We're doing okay," she replied, adding with a smile, "I'm sure you can't wait to steer all your clients in our direction."

331

He nodded. "Always thinking ahead. That's what I like – a smart woman."

If that's what he liked how come he'd married the blonde – who, according to Pia, had an IQ of zero?

"So . . . will we be getting your clients?"

He smiled. "I'm sure, Lauren, you always get exactly what you want."

Shortly after Pia moved out the calls started. The first one came at two o'clock in the morning. Lauren groped for the phone in her sleep mumbling a groggy, "Hello."

"I wanna talk to you," a familiar voice said.

She knew immediately it was Emerson Burn. For a moment she held her breath before quietly replacing the receiver.

He called back within seconds. "Don't 'ang up on me," he complained. "That's not nice."

"What do you want?" she asked, amazed at his nerve.

"It's about time we got together," he said, confidently.

"Are you crazy?" she said, struggling to sit up.

"Seems like a normal request to me."

"Have you forgotten what happened in LA?"

"Nothin' happened."

"That was because Nature came back."

"What are you gettin' so uptight about? So I came on to you. Big deal. Most girls would give their left tit to 'ave me come on t'them."

"I don't *believe* this. You tried to rape me, and the only reason you didn't get away with it was because your wife came home. *Your wife* – remember her? She used to be my best friend – now she no longer talks to me thanks to you. You're an asshole, you know that?" She slammed the phone down.

It rang again immediately.

She took the receiver off the hook and buried it under her pillow.

The next day three dozen red roses arrived at the apartment with a note. The note read, *Sorry! E.* She dropped the flowers off at a nearby hospital.

A few days later while lunching with Samm she casually enquired about Nature.

"Did you two fall out?" Samm asked, raising an elegant eyebrow as she picked at her tomato and lettuce salad.

"You know what Nature's like better than anyone," she replied cagily, sipping a glass of water.

"That's true," Samm replied, with a weary sigh. "The girl can be absolutely impossible. I don't know what she sees in that mangy rock star, he looks like he's in desperate need of a shower – several in fact. Those leather pants stick to his body like tacky tape – and I *do* mean tacky."

"So they're still very much together?"

"About as close as two enormous egos *can* be," Samm said dryly, before adding, "You *do* know she's been bad-mouthing you all over town."

Lauren sighed – this was all she needed to hear. "She has?"

"I wouldn't worry – nobody takes her seriously."

Emerson called again the following week. "Changed your mind?" he asked casually, like they chatted every day.

"About what?"

"Gettin' together."

The man was in ego overdrive. "I have a news flash," she replied, sharply. "You've finally met the one person who doesn't want to go out with you."

He was not to be put off. "If you're worried about Nature she's in LA."

"I thought she came with you on every trip to hold your hand."

"Nah, can't 'ave her trailin' me, can I? S'not good for the image. Come on, we'll hit a few clubs, 'ave us a time."

"You know what, Emerson?"

"*What*, babe?"

"Stop calling me."

It seemed inconceivable that Emerson Burn had decided to pursue her. Did he honestly think that a near-rape was prelude to a romantic relationship?

Three months after getting married Pia announced she was pregnant. "Howard and I talked it over, and we want you to be godmother."

"I'd be honoured," Lauren replied, thinking how lucky Pia was to be married to the man she loved *and* pregnant.

Help Unlimited was doing so well that they'd finally rented proper office space. Pia decided to keep working until a month before the baby was due. "I'm not the sitting-at-home type," she explained. They now employed six people which gave Lauren the luxury of choosing the jobs she wished to do. Since she'd taken the cooking course, small dinner parties were her forte. She enjoyed organizing incredible meals, and it also kept her busy most nights – which suited her fine.

Sometimes, late at night, lying in bed, a wave of unbearable loneliness swept over her. But she'd decided it was better to be lonely than to suffer another broken heart.

Now that Pia had moved out of the apartment they'd shared, she decided to re-decorate. It wasn't the most luxurious place in the world, but it was comfortable and cosy and she was happy there. Weekends she liked nothing better than strolling along Eighth Avenue exploring the antique shops and picking out special things.

One Saturday afternoon she was walking across Park and turning on Madison when she noticed a long white limousine crawling along the kerb behind her.

She quickened her step, but the limousine kept pace, and when she stopped at a street corner the door of the car was flung open and Emerson Burn leaped out.

Emerson – the leather-clad rock star with the mane of golden hair – grabbed her arm and spun her around to face him. "You bin avoiding me," he said, accusingly.

Was he so dumb he really thought she was ever going to talk to him again?

"What now?" she said, attempting to shake his arm off.

His grip tightened. "Get in the car an' I'll tell you."

"Forget it."

"I ain't forgettin' it, darlin'," he said, loudly. "*That's* the friggin' point."

Two girls spotted him and froze as if they'd just seen Jesus.

Emerson's bodyguard jumped out of the car. "Time ta split, Em," he said, watchful eyes raking the street.

Emerson ignored him.

The girls clutched on to each other and braced themselves for the rush.

"You ain't bein' fair t'me," Emerson complained, holding tight. "I wanna explain. I was drunk. I had a problem."

"Now look –" she began.

The girls sprung into action – sprinting towards him with purposeful looks in their eyes. The bodyguard saw them coming. So did Emerson. "Oh, shit!" he exclaimed. "Here comes trouble."

Lauren felt a thump in the small of her back and was rudely shoved aside as one of the girls moved in on him.

"I'm insane about everything you do!" the girl yelled hysterically, pulling at his jacket. "I love you! I *really, really* love you!"

Before Lauren could think about what to do the bodyguard bundled Emerson into the limo – somehow pushing her in behind him. The car immediately took off.

"Well,' Emerson said. "That settles it. You're trapped, darlin', an' there ain't nothin' you can do about it."

Chapter 51

"I've never done anything like this before," Annie said, throwing Nick a sideways glance.

He laughed. "Anybody would think we were planning on robbing a freakin' bank!"

"You know what I mean, taking off like this – it's . . ." she looked at him questioningly, "I guess it's fun."

"*Now* you're beginning to learn."

They'd been driving for several hours. The freeway ride was long and boring, but the thought of seeing Las Vegas for the first time excited both of them.

"Hey, how much money you got on you?" he asked, realizing he hadn't come prepared.

"About fifty dollars. Why?"

"'Cause we're gonna blow it, that's why."

"Oh no, not with my money," she said, indignantly.

Grinning, he steered the old Chevrolet on to an off ramp. "C'mon, Annie, you gotta take *some* chances in life."

"It's my rent money," she objected.

"So we'll double it. How's that?"

She glanced over at him. "You know, Nick, you're really strange."

"Oh, so now I'm strange. What's *this* leading up to?"

"Can I be honest with you?" she asked, earnestly.

"You can be whatever you like," he replied, pulling into a Chevron station.

"It's just that sometimes it seems you're coming on to me, and then other times you act as if you're my brother."

Oh, shit – the last thing he needed was Annie developing a crush on him. But then again, why not? DeVille was long gone and he was bored with the endless stream of one-night stands he could have any time he wanted.

"Are you interested in me or not?" she asked, putting it firmly on the line.

He stalled for time. "Is this a proposition?" he said lightly, winding down his window.

"I . . . I need to know."

"Hey, I'm here with you, we're driving to Vegas."

"Is that your idea of a commitment?"

Commitment! The very word gave him nightmares. What was it with women and commitments? Why couldn't they take it day by day?

The gas station attendant leaned into his window – saving him a reply. "What'll it be?" the old man asked, scratching his grizzled beard.

"Fill her up," Nick said. "An' check the oil an' water while you're at it."

"Well?" Annie demanded, not letting him off the hook.

He took his time before replying. "We're goin' on a trip," he said, carefully. "Whyn't we take it nice an' easy and maybe we'll find out."

Reece Webster sat back in the smoky atmosphere of the small casino bar and watched Cyndra sing. She was good. She was *really* good. So how come she wasn't getting anywhere? The record labels hadn't liked the deal he'd proposed, and the bigger hotels had said she needed experience. Experience goddamn it! He was giving her experience, and what kind of thanks was he getting? Exactly nothing. Cyndra had no appreciation of the things he did for her.

Well, what did he expect? Women were all takers and Cyndra was no exception.

He hoped he hadn't wasted his time marrying her – he'd been so sure she was going to be his ride to the big time – now all he did was pay the bills. The money she made at the casino didn't even cover his expenses. Some dud investment. He'd put two years into singing lessons and grooming and it simply wasn't paying off.

His narrow eyes raked the room. Several men were watching Cyndra with that look on their faces. Reece knew the look well. It was the *I wanna fuck your brains out* look.

He studied her dress. Not sexy enough. She needed more

cleavage and maybe a deep slit in the skirt. She had great tits and long legs. He'd have to deal with that. He'd have to pay for it, too.

Cyndra was beginning to remind him of his first wife. That bitch had dragged him down like a lead weight; all she'd been capable of was grabbing everything he had. Now Cyndra was falling into the same category, and it was about time he did something about collecting on his investment.

The other night he'd overheard a couple of guys talking while Cyndra was on stage. "I wouldn't mind a piece of that," one of them had said.

"Yeah, with gravy all over it!" the other one replied.

Reece had sidled over. "Wanna meet the little lady?" he'd offered. "'Cause if you do, I'm the man can arrange it."

Both men had nodded eagerly, so Reece had negotiated a deal. The problem was he'd forgotten to tell Cyndra, and when he'd sat her down with the two guys and they'd come on to her she'd insulted them both. The men were real riled up – and who could blame them? Much to his chagrin he'd had to return their money.

So what the hell was wrong with a little light hooking on the side? The truth was, convincing Cyndra was a bitch. Except that today he'd asserted himself – put the fear of God into her. *That's* what women expected – a little fear in their lives. They had to know who the boss was; they *needed* to know.

Sipping his malt whisky he scoped out likely prospects, focusing on a stocky man sitting alone at a corner table watching Cyndra like he'd just discovered candy for the first time. The man was middle-aged with a florid complexion. A brightly-coloured Hawaiian shirt and open sandals on his feet announced tourist.

Casually Reece wandered over. "Howdy," he said, tipping his cowboy hat.

The man looked up. "Do I know you?"

"No," Reece said, "but I got a strong suspicion you'd like to."

"Get your homo ass away from me," the man said, his florid face reddening even more.

"You got it wrong," Reece replied, scowling. "I ain't that way. I came over here t'do you a favour."

"What favour?" the man asked, suspiciously.

Reece gestured towards Cyndra. "Y'see that little lady standing up there? She's what I got in mind for you, but if insults is what I get – then we got no more conversation." He turned to go.

"Wait a minute," the man said.

Reece stopped. "You interested or not?"

The man glanced around furtively. "I'm interested," he said, lowering his voice. "How much will it cost me?"

"Did you win or did you lose? 'Cause if you lost you can't afford this baby."

"I won at craps."

"Then you're a lucky son of a gun, 'cause she's gonna cost you two hundred and fifty big ones."

The man licked his lips and thought quickly. His flabby wife was upstairs sleeping off the effects of winning at the slots. His snotty teenage son was out chasing girls. This was the opportunity of a lifetime and he didn't want to blow it. But two hundred and fifty bucks was an awful lot of money – he could buy a second television for that much money. "I . . . I don't know," he said, hesitantly.

"You don't know," Reece repeated, as if he couldn't believe what he was hearing. "You got a chance for a piece a that and *you don't know?*"

Sweat beaded the man's thick neck. "Is she good?" he asked, hoarsely. "Is she worth it?"

Reece tilted his cowboy hat even further back on his head. "Are you shittin' me? Does Kentucky give fried chicken? Does Cadillac give the smoothest ride goin'? Man, this little lady is the best *you* ever had."

They came upon Las Vegas like a shimmering jewel sitting in the middle of the desert. It was dark and they'd been driving for hours without any light at all. Now, in the distance they saw the flat city spread out before them and it was a startling sight.

"It's incredible!" Annie gasped.

Nick grinned. "I told you – you gotta get out an' do things. No good sittin' on your ass all day expecting . . . I dunno –" he looked at her quizzically. "What *do* you expect, Annie?"

She shrugged. "I work hard, go to class . . . one of these days I'll get a break."

"Yeah, I guess that's what we all think." He pulled the car over to the side of the road, sliding his arm around her shoulders. "I'm glad you came."

"So am I."

They were silent for a while staring at the mirage ahead – at least that's what it looked like in the middle of the barren desert. Finally he broke the silence. "I never asked you before – where's your family?"

"They're in Florida where I grew up. I left three years ago and took the bus out to LA." She snuggled closer. "What about you? Cyndra's never talked about your family. Where are your parents? Do you have any other brothers or sisters?"

He drew away from her on the pretext of reaching for a cigarette. "No sad stories," he said, shaking loose a Camel. "Cyndra and me – we got a father in common, a real charmer. Neither of us has seen him in years."

"You don't speak to him?"

"Nope."

"That's a shame. Family is all we really have."

"Yeah, well, you ain't met mine," he said flippantly.

"What about your mother?"

He struck a match and lit up. "She died when I was sixteen. Left me."

"She didn't leave you, Nick," Annie said, softly. "Dying is not exactly making a choice."

He didn't need to dredge up any more memories, it was painful enough without having to talk about it.

"Hey, can we quit this conversation? Let's appreciate what we got in front of us. Take a look at that view!"

"It's beautiful," she murmured.

"Yeah," he said, starting the car. "Let's go get us a piece of it."

"This is my friend," Reece said.

Cyndra nodded, not looking anywhere near the man in the Hawaiian shirt.

"My *good* friend," Reece added, in case she hadn't quite gotten the message.

"Uh huh," she said, dully.

The man nudged Reece. "When we gettin' out of here?" he asked, perspiration beading his forehead. "It's not good for me to be seen with you people. Where we going anyway?"

"Close by," Reece replied, reassuringly.

"You're not like those con people I seen on TV," the man said, anxiously. "They lure you to a room with a girl, take your money and beat up on you."

Reece tipped his cowboy hat. "Do I look like a con man?"

340

he said, his lip curling. "Does she look like a con woman? Don't worry, partner – *you* are about to have the dream trip of your life."

Cyndra caught snatches of the conversation. She knew what Reece expected, he'd made that very clear, but she still couldn't believe it.

"Okay, hon," Reece said, all nice and friendly. "Let's go so you an' this fine gentleman can get to know each other better."

"I'm warning you," she hissed under her breath, just loud enough for him to hear. "I'm not doing this."

His hand strayed towards his belt. "Co-operate, hon. I told you this mornin' – I bin carryin' you too long; it's about time you gave something back."

The three of them walked out of the casino into the parking lot where the humid night-time air enveloped them like a heavy cloud. She wondered what Reece would do when she refused to go through with this. He'd probably blow her head off – he was crazy enough. But still, he wouldn't be in the room watching them, and once he left she'd tell the guy the position she was in – appeal to his better nature. He looked like a family man, although he sure didn't smell like one. He stunk of beer and pretzels. She shuddered – his smell reminded her of Primo.

They rode to the motel room in Reece's shocking pink Cadillac. By the time they got there the man was sweating even more profusely.

"Take my licence number," Reece suggested, sensing that this dude could back off at any moment. "It'll make you feel more secure."

"No, no, I trust you," the man said, although he didn't. "How'm I gonna get back?"

"I'll stay around," Reece said. "Whistle when you're done an' I'll drive you."

Cyndra got out of the car and stood stiffly beside it.

"Get your cute little butt to the room, honey," Reece said, coaxingly. "An' don't forget t'leave the door open for our friend." He waited until she was out of sight and then snapped his fingers; it was time for business. "Gotta have cash," he said. "No cash, no pussy."

The word pussy turned the man on. Feverishly he counted out several large bills.

Reece checked it through twice. When he was satisfied he said, "Room eight, near the pool." Then he winked. "Do the double loop for me, partner, compliments of the house."

When Cyndra reached their room she thought about locking the door and keeping everyone out. Unfortunately she knew it wouldn't work – if she didn't let the man in Reece would only kick the door down.

She was pretty, she was young, she had talent – why hadn't her career taken off? If it had, everything would be all right. Reece was doing this to punish her. *How about divorcing him?* a little voice whispered in her ear. *How about getting out while I still can?* But she knew it was hopeless, he'd never let her go unless she paid back every cent he'd spent on her.

There was a knock on the door. Swallowing hard, she smoothed down her dress, walked over and threw it open.

The man barged past her into the room, his Hawaiian shirt sticking to his chest. "Let's do this quick," he blurted. "I'm about ready – so hurry it up."

"I'll fix you a drink," she said, stalling for time. "There's a Coke machine down the hall and we got a bottle of Scotch or vodka. What'll it be?"

"Nothing," he said, already fumbling with the buttons on his fly.

She noticed the gleam of a wedding ring on his finger. "Does your wife know you're doing this?" she asked, sharply.

He stopped short. "What's my wife got to do with anything?"

"I . . . I just wondered, that's all."

His eyes darted around the room, settling on the bed. "I do it the conventional way," he announced. "Whyn't you lie back and take your clothes off?"

"I'm not a conventional girl," she replied quickly, continuing to stall.

"I don't got all night," he said, glancing at his watch.

"If you'd sooner forget it . . ." she ventured.

He jumped to attention at that. "I paid good money for you."

"How much?"

"What's it to you?"

His words infuriated her. "It's *me* you're supposed to fuck, isn't it?"

He reached over, pinching her left nipple through her dress. "I'm not used to women talkin' dirty."

She shrunk away. She was no hooker and she wasn't about to act like one. If Reece wanted to blow her head off, then so be it. "There's been a mistake," she said, her voice a dull monotone.

His eyes began to bug. "What mistake?"

342

Still with the flat voice. "I don't do this sort of thing."

"But I was told –"

"I don't care *what* you were told. Zip up your pants and get out of here. Go home to your wife."

Without any warning he burst into tears. "I knew I shouldn't a come here," he sobbed. "I knew it was a bad thing to do."

Cyndra was taken aback, she'd expected a violent reaction, not this. "Look," she said, showing some compassion. "I'll get Reece to drive you back to the casino. He doesn't have to know nothing happened."

The man continued to sob.

"We'll tell him it was the greatest. That way we'll both come out of this okay – you'll look like a real stud and I won't get my head bashed in." Gently she began steering him to the door. "This'll work out, you'll see. We'll –"

With a sudden spurt of anger he threw her arm off and choked out a frustrated, "What about my money?"

"I can't help you with that."

"I paid good money for you. I want it back."

"You'll have to ask Reece, and if you ask him he's gonna know."

The man seemed to have recovered from his crying jag. Now he was red-faced and angry. "I want my money," he said, stubbornly.

"I told you – I don't have it."

"Then you'd better get it, you cheap little hooker."

"He's got a gun," she said, in a flat voice. "He could blow both our heads off. Whyn't you do us both a favour an' go quietly?"

"This was a set-up all along," the man said, bitterly. "I seen you people on television, you had no intention of putting out."

"Listen, mister, you're the one started to whine like a baby."

"You black bitch – if I'm not getting my money, I'll sure get my money's worth." Unexpectedly he grabbed her, his wet lips slobbering all over her neck.

She shoved him off, but he came at her again.

Suddenly she was back in the Browning house in Bosewell and he was Mr Browning – grabbing her – forcing her to do things. Every bad memory flooded over her.

"I . . . won't . . . do . . . this,' she screamed, kicking out.

"You'll do it unless I get my money back," he said, roughly squeezing her breasts.

Was money all anybody cared about? Mr Browning's words

343

hung in the air – *black cunt . . . black bitch . . .* She could hear his voice, his insults. It was like it had all happened yesterday.

They fell back on the bed and her screams became louder. Somebody knocked on the dividing wall yelling a terse, "Shut up!"

The door flew open and Reece marched in. "What in hell-fire's goin' on here?" he demanded, narrow eyes pinning Cyndra accusingly.

"He . . . he . . . tried to attack me," she gasped.

"Damn whore," the man muttered. "The bitch wouldn't give me nothin'."

"I left you two to have a good time," Reece said patiently, tapping one of his pointy-toed cowboy boots on the frayed carpet. "An' all you're doin' is fighting. "*Course* she's gonna give you any sweet thing you want." He threw her a warning look. "Get it together, hon, or you *know* what'll happen."

"Screw you, Reece," she spat. "You can't treat me like this."

His hand hovered near his belt. "Oh, I can't, huh?"

The man decided the time had come to get back to his hotel room and his flabby wife. "I want my money," he said, making one last attempt to claim what was his.

"No refunds," Reece snapped.

"You had no right to pull this on me," Cyndra said, tears stinging her eyes. "I'll divorce you, that's what I'll do."

Reece stood dangerously still. "Honey, you'll *do* what *I say* you'll do."

"Why don't I take my money and leave," the man suggested, not liking the way this was going.

"Shut your mouth an' stay out of this," Reece said, not even looking in his direction. This was between him and Cyndra, and she had to learn a lesson.

"Maybe what I *should* do is call the cops," the man threatened. "You stole from me."

Reece jumped to attention, pulling back his jacket and revealing his gun stuck casually into his belt. "You ain't going nowhere, partner."

"Aw, Jesus!" the man groaned, the colour draining from his face. "Aw, sweet Jesus!"

Reece turned his attention back to Cyndra. "You – get your clothes off. I hear one more scream outta this room an' you *know* what'll happen."

The man began a slow edge towards the door.

Cyndra stared at Reece, a deep rage burning inside her. "You know what, Reece – you're nothing but a dumb pimp," she said, the words spilling out. "In fact, that's all you're capable of – pimping. How does it feel to be pimp of the year? Pimp of the fucking century?' Her voice rose. "How does it feel to know you CAN'T DO ANYTHING ELSE?"

The person next door hammered on the wall again.

"You callin' *me* a pimp?" Reece yelled. "Well, what does that make you? A whore, honey. A drippin' bloodsuckin' whore."

"Oh, I ain't no whore, mister. Don't you get it? *I ain't no whore!*" She leaped off the bed furious.

Removing the gun from his belt Reece waved it in her face.

"Don't threaten me," she yelled, hysterically. "You can't control my life. You can't control *me.*" She lunged at him grabbing for the gun.

The man reached the door, sweat coursing down his face. These two were crazy. And he was equally crazy to have been tempted.

His hand clutched the door-knob as Cyndra and Reece struggled for possession of the gun. His hand was so slick with sweat he couldn't get it open.

And then a shot rang out. One lone shot.

The bullet ricocheted against the wall and hit the man in the back of his head. He fell to the ground without a sound. There was a long moment of frozen silence.

"Oh, *shit*," Reece said, panic-stricken. "Look what you done, you crazy bitch – you shot the dumb motherfucker. You killed him, you stupid cunt. You gone and goddamn killed him!"

Chapter 52

"I'm not as bad as you think," Emerson said.

"How do you know *what* I think?" Lauren replied, sliding along the leather seat as far away from him as she could get.

"It's not exactly difficult figuring you out."

"Figure this out, Emerson. I'd like to get out of this car, and I'd like to get out now."

He shrugged. "Okay, I'll admit it – I was bombed outta my skull – I gave you a hard time – so I'm sorry – I'll make it up to you."

She shook her head. "What does it take to get you to understand that I don't want anything to do with you?"

He began to laugh. "That's what I like about you. You're different from the rest of 'em. You can even string two words together."

"So can Nature," she snapped.

"*You* try living with Nature," he said, gloomily. "It's a bloody nightmare. Anyway – we split – didn't she tell you?"

Lauren leaned forward and tapped on the smoky black glass separating them from the driver.

"Whattaya doin'," he asked, lounging back and stretching out his long, leather-clad legs.

"Telling your driver to stop the car."

He looked amused. "I thought I told you – you're my prisoner."

"This is kidnapping."

He shrugged. "So arrest me."

She sat back trying to decide what to do. In spite of everything there was no denying that he was a very charismatic figure, and if she really wanted to face up to it she *was* attracted to him in spite of what had happened. Besides, what did she have to lose? Exactly nothing. Nature wasn't talking to her anyway.

"Okay," she said, with a weary sigh.

"Okay what?"

"I'll have lunch with you. Impress me. Dazzle me with your charm. Show me that you're really just like the boy next door."

He chortled with laughter. "Babe, I 'aven't been like the boy next door in twenty years."

"Make an effort."

"For you – anything."

He took her to a small Italian restaurant on Third Street. The jovial owner ushered them to a table in the back, treating Emerson like a king, while his bodyguard stayed at the front of the restaurant scanning the sidewalk for trouble.

"Champagne, caviar, what'll it be?" Emerson asked, tossing back his mane of hair.

She glanced at her watch. "It's three o'clock in the afternoon."

He couldn't have cared less. "So?"

"So I'll have a small green salad and some pasta. Then I have to go. Besides, this place doesn't have champagne and caviar."

"Wanna bet? I can get anything I want any time I want," he boasted.

"And if you don't get it you take it. Story of your life, right, Mr Burn?"

"What's with this Mr Burn crap?"

"I'm giving you a little respect, you should try it some time."

He leaned across the table staring directly into her eyes. "You're beautiful, y'know that? You got somethin' I really get off on."

She hit him with a little light sarcasm. "Gee, you certainly have a way with words."

He didn't seem to mind. "It's me upbringin'," he said, cheerfully.

"Where was that?"

"Elephant an' Castle – or asshole as we liked to call it back in the good old days. Sorta Brooklyn with a cockney accent."

"You and Nature have a lot in common – including a country."

He laughed, derisively. "Me and Nature 'ave exactly nothing in common."

"You married her."

"Big friggin' deal. I 'ad a hangover at the time."

"Is that your excuse for everything?"

"Oh – now you're gonna give me the "you drink too much" speech."

"I really don't care what you do."

"You're wrong."

"About what?"

"About not caring. From the first time I saw you I knew we had something goin'. You were like this little mouse runnin' around organizing that party for Samm up at my apartment – remember? I noticed you immediately 'cause you seemed different – you still are – that's what I like about you."

"I'll tell you what you like about me," she said, crisply. "You like the fact you can't have me, because you're so used to having every girl that breathes, and now finally somebody says no. *That's* the only thing you like about me."

"Wrong."

"I don't think so."

"Whyn't we put it to the test?"

"How?"

"Sleep with me an' see if I'm still around tomorrow."

"Very funny."

"Glad I got you laughin'."

After lunch he decided he had to buy some books so they stopped at Doubleday's on Fifth Avenue. Two minutes after leaving the limo word was on the street and he was mobbed. He grabbed her hand and ran her back to the limo. As soon as they were inside, the car took off.

"Home. Mine," she said, breathlessly.

"Deal," he replied. "I'll pick you up at ten."

"I'm asleep at ten."

"Tonight's different. Be dressed and ready to hit the town."

"I didn't say I'd go out with you."

"You didn't say you wouldn't. Just remember, I could have kept you prisoner for the rest of the day, but I'm letting you go. Now you owe me."

"Exactly nothing."

"Do you always 'ave to 'ave the last word?"

"Yes."

Upstairs in her apartment she found herself unable to settle down. This was crazy. Emerson Burn was a dilettante rock star. She wanted nothing to do with him. Or did she?

How come you had lunch with him, Roberts?

Why shouldn't I?

Do you find him attractive?

Yes, as a matter of fact I do.

The phone rang and she grabbed it, ready to tell Emerson

she was definitely not going out with him that night or any other night for that matter.

"Hi," Pia said, brightly. "What are you doing?"

"I just walked in. Why?"

"Howard and I want to take you to dinner."

"I don't like the sound of your voice."

"What's wrong with my voice?"

"Whenever you use that tone there's always some single guy you think is perfect for me."

"I resent that," Pia said, indignantly. "As a matter of fact, we're dining with Howard's uncle, and we thought it would be nice if you made up the foursome."

"Where's his wife?"

"At their house in the Hamptons."

"Hmm . . ."

"Lauren. We're talking about Howard's *old married* uncle – he's hardly likely to jump all over you."

"He's a man, isn't he?"

"Oh, *please!*"

"Okay, I'll come."

Pia was so used to getting a no that this was a surprise. "We'll pick you up at eight," she said quickly, before Lauren changed her mind.

Hmm . . . dinner with Howard's uncle. At least it got her out of the house, and when Emerson arrived and found nobody home maybe he'd take the hint and leave her alone.

Or then again – maybe not.

Chapter 53

She didn't know how long she'd been sitting there, she only knew that Reece had gone and left her. Left her with a dead man lying on the floor.

She crouched on the bed, hugging her knees to her chest, her eyes wide with fear, while the man's body lay in a huddle behind the door.

"*I* didn't shoot him, *you* did it," she'd screamed at Reece when it had happened, breaking away from him, her body trembling.

"Oh no no *no* – *baby*, I don't take the rap on this one," Reece had said, frantically stuffing his clothes in a suitcase and running for the door.

"You . . . can't . . . leave . . . me," she'd said, the words sticking in her throat.

"Just watch me, honey," he'd said, throwing the gun at her.

And then he was gone.

At first she'd thought about calling the police. In fact, she wouldn't have been surprised if they'd turned up, because the people next door must have heard the gun shot. But nothing happened. Absolutely nothing. So she stayed on the bed too frightened to move, knowing she should have followed Reece and taken off. But how could she? He had the car and all their money – she was left with nothing.

So she sat in the middle of the bed, tears rolling down her cheeks, clutching on to the gun – her only protection.

Her life was over and there was nothing she could do about it.

"This is just like I've seen it on television!" Annie exclaimed. "Look at all these lights!"

"Yeah, this is really something," Nick agreed, pulling into

the parking lot of a downtown hotel.

"Where are we going?" she asked. "Shouldn't we find Cyndra?"

"First we're gonna gamble. That's what you're supposed t'do in Vegas."

"Nick –"

"Try an' enjoy yourself, Annie," he said, teasingly. "Today's your day for takin' chances. Bring it t'the edge – you never know – you might enjoy it." He got out of the car, grabbed her by the hand and they ran across the parking lot into the hotel lobby.

"Holy shit!" Nick exclaimed, taking in the banks of slot machines all in constant use. A grin spread over his face. "Y'know, I always wanted to do this." He groped in his pocket for change, coming up with several quarters. "C'mon, pick a machine – we're gonna win big time!"

"We are?" she asked, unsurely.

"You bet your ass we are!"

They played the slots for two hours straight, ending up ten dollars ahead. By this time Nick had the fever – he was all set to carry on, but Annie was ready to quit. "We'd better go find Cyndra," she worried. "It's one o'clock. What will they say when we turn up in the middle of the night?"

"They won't care. Tomorrow night we'll catch Cyndra sing, then we'll drive back to LA."

"I can't take off work again tomorrow," Annie objected.

"You'll call in sick. Big deal."

She sighed. "You're making me as bad as you are."

"Hey – that can only be an improvement, right?"

"Thanks a lot!"

Armed with directions they drove to the motel where Cyndra and Reece were staying. It was not the most glamorous place in the world – just a few rooms located around a small pool.

"I bet they're asleep," Annie said, accusingly. "I told you we should have come earlier."

"I bet they're not," he retorted, confidently. "Nobody sleeps in Vegas."

They parked the car, found the room and knocked a few times getting no answer.

"I gotta stop making a habit of this," he grumbled. "I'll spring the lock – no problem."

"You can't do that," Annie said, alarmed.

"Yeah, *right*," he said, working his magic on the lock and pushing the door open.

351

The first thing they saw was Cyndra sitting in the middle of the bed holding a gun. The second was the body slumped on the floor behind the door.

"Oh my God!" Annie gasped.

Cyndra stared at them blankly while Nick edged his way towards her. "Take it easy," he said, speaking fast. "Take it real easy." Gently he removed the gun from her hands. "What happened?"

She covered her face with her hands and began to sob. "Oh, Nick . . . Nick . . ."

He put his arms around her, cradling her to him.

"C'mon, baby, you can tell me."

Slowly she began to choke out her story. "Reece wanted me to sleep with this . . . man. He brought him to our room . . . and then . . . then the guy wanted his money back because I wouldn't do it, and . . . and . . . Reece took out his gun . . . we were fighting . . . and . . . it went off. It was an accident, Nick, it really was."

"Where's Reece?"

"He ran."

"And left you like this?"

"What's going to happen, Nick? Nobody's gonna believe me. The cops won't understand."

Cyndra was right, she wouldn't stand a chance.

He went over to the man, staring down at his immobile body, hoping this was all a big mistake and that the guy would breathe – move – *something*.

No such luck.

"I'll phone the police," Annie said, pale and shaken.

"No," he said, quickly. "This don't look so good." He turned back to his sister. "You're *sure* you didn't know him?"

She shook her head. "Reece picked him up in the casino; I never saw him before."

"So there's no connection between the two of you?"

"Not unless we were seen leaving together."

He bent down, gingerly groping inside the man's jacket for his wallet. It was imitation leather and contained five hundred dollars cash, a couple of credit cards and a driver's licence made out to George Baer.

"We gotta get him out of here – an' fast," he muttered, thinking aloud. "Yeah, that's what we gotta do."

Annie asserted herself. "No. What we must do is call the police."

352

"Will you shut up about the cops," he said, glaring at her. "Cyndra's in trouble, we gotta help her."

"I can't be an accessory," Annie said, stiffly.

"I'm asking you a favour."

"It's too big a favour."

He pinned her with his green eyes. "I'm worth it, aren't I?"

She hesitated. "I . . . I don't know."

"Do it for me, Annie," he said, persuasively. "Nobody has to know what happened here tonight."

"*I'll* know," she said, vehemently. "And I can't live with it."

She was getting on his nerves. Fuck her if she didn't want to co-operate. "If that's the way you feel you'd better take a walk."

"Don't you understand," she said, her eyes filling with tears. "This is wrong."

"Cyndra's my sister – she needs me, so get off my fuckin' case."

"I'm not leaving," Annie said, stubbornly.

"If you're staying you're helping, an' that makes you part of it."

"What are you going to do?"

"I'll deal with it, okay?" he replied, tired of her questions.

He coaxed Cyndra off the bed and told her to pack her things. Then he stripped the blanket from the bed and began the arduous task of trying to roll the man's body into it. No easy job. There was blood everywhere and Annie's accusing eyes nailed him every move he made. Sweat enveloped him. His mouth was dry and his heart pounding. Shit! He didn't even know if he was doing the right thing, but if he was to get Cyndra out of this mess there seemed to be no other alternative.

Finally he had the body wrapped in the blanket. The next move was to get it out of the stinking motel room and into the trunk of the car. He stood back and took a beat.

"Nick, I'm really frightened," Cyndra said, clinging to his arm.

"Don't be," he said, sounding more confident than he felt. "It's almost taken care of. I'm gonna drive the body out to the desert and bury it. You two'll stay here until I get back."

"No," she said, sharply. "I can't let you do this alone. I'm coming with you."

"If you're going so am I," Annie said, quickly joining in.

The two of them were beginning to drive him crazy, but it was probably safer to take them with him. "Okay, okay," he said, reluctantly. He went outside and took a look around. When he was sure it was all clear, he backed his car up as close as he could get. Then, still keeping a wary eye out, he dragged the body out of the room and somehow or other bundled it into the trunk.

By the time they set off everyone was tense and on edge.

"We're taking this nice and easy," he said, trying to keep them both calm. "If we get pulled over for anything – anything at all – stay cool, right?"

He drove carefully out of town through the gaudy neon-lit streets until they reached the quieter outskirts, and then eventually the desert. Then he drove another half hour before pulling over to the side of the road, lugging the man's body from the trunk, dragging him across the sand for what seemed like an eternity – and then digging a makeshift shallow grave using his hands.

When he was finished he rolled up the blood-soaked blanket and carried it back to the car. "We'll bury this somewhere else," he said, throwing it in the trunk. "Don't want any connection between the body and the hotel room."

"What about the gun?" Cyndra asked, anxiously.

"I'll get rid of it on the way back to LA."

"This is a nightmare," Annie said, shaking her head. "I wish I'd never met either of you."

"Well, sweetheart – you did, an' now you're part of it, so shut up," he said roughly, not in the mood to listen to any more of her complaints.

Within minutes they were on their way back to LA.

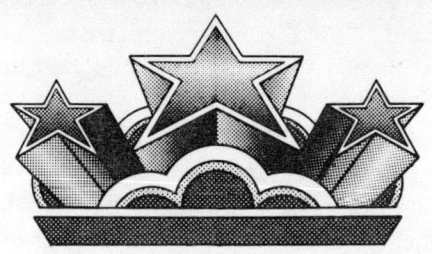

Chapter 54

"I made a mistake," Oliver Liberty said.

"Excuse me?" Lauren replied.

They were sitting in an exclusive New York club, sipping brandies while Pia and Howard clung together on the small dance floor. The sound of Frank Sinatra singing "In the Wee Small Hours of the Morning' flooded the darkly panelled room.

Oliver puffed on a long thin cigar – it suited his aquiline features. "I said I made a mistake," he repeated.

"About what?" she asked, politely.

"When my wife left me I was very angry. We'd been together for over thirty years until one day she decided she'd had enough. She became an overnight feminist, and suddenly I was the enemy."

"That's not good."

"An understatement, my dear."

"So you met Opal –"

"And foolishly married her."

Lauren wasn't sure she wanted to hear this. Sitting in a nightclub listening to Howard's uncle tell her all about his failing marriage was not her idea of heaven. But then again she'd had a nice enough time. They'd been to an expensive French restaurant, talked about everything from politics to the latest fashions and although he might not be the youngest man in the world, he certainly had an abundance of charm.

"Are you sure you should be telling me this?" she asked.

"I can talk to you," he said, nodding as if to reassure himself. "You have a certain quality."

"What quality is that?" she asked, lightly.

"Something in your eyes. An understanding. And let us not forget, you're also a very beautiful woman."

This certainly seemed to be her week for compliments. "I'm flattered," she said, "but I'm no psychiatrist."

"I didn't say you were," he replied, nodding towards the dance floor. "Shall we?"

"Okay," she said, getting up.

He stubbed out his cigar, took her hand and led her on to the crowded floor. For a moment he held her at a discreet distance, and then without warning pulled her into his embrace. "I've already spoken to my lawyers," he said.

"About what?" she asked, inhaling his expensive aftershave.

"A divorce."

"Why are you telling me?"

"Because you're easy to talk to, and I want to see you again. That's if you don't mind being in the company of an older man." He smiled when he said it, taking the curse off his words.

She thought about saying *I have no intention of getting involved*, but it seemed presumptuous to assume anything at this early stage, so instead she murmured, "I'd like that."

"So would I," he replied. "How about tomorrow night?"

Outside the club Oliver's Japanese chauffeur and sleek black Rolls waited patiently.

"Not bad, huh?" Pia whispered, climbing in the back while Oliver and Howard discussed business on the sidewalk. "Do you like him?"

"He's married," Lauren whispered back. "Stop trying to fix me up."

"Ah, but he's getting a divorce."

"Pia, he's old enough to be my father, maybe even my grandfather."

"So what?"

"Do me a favour – quit trying to match-make."

They dropped Howard and Pia off first, and then the Rolls proceeded to Lauren's apartment. On the street she spotted Emerson's limousine parked outside her building. The last thing she was in the mood for was another confrontation. Turning to Oliver she said, "Do you have a guest room?"

He looked at her, quizzically. "A guest room?"

"There's somebody I want to avoid, and uh . . . it seems to me if I went home with you it would save me a problem."

"Certainly," he said, only too happy to oblige.

Oliver's apartment was sumptuous by anybody's standards. Located in a stately old building overlooking Central Park the

356

ceilings were high, the rooms large, and the view incredible. He led her into the living room and offered her a drink.

She shook her head. "I have to work tomorrow. Would you mind if I went straight to my room?"

"Not at all," he said, leading her down a spacious corridor into a guest bedroom. "Can I get you something to sleep in?"

"Maybe an old shirt?"

"I'll be right back."

She explored the tastefully decorated room obviously designed by a woman – certainly not his current wife – perhaps a decorator?

Picking up a silver frame she studied the photograph of a younger Oliver and a woman who was obviously his previous wife. They made a handsome couple.

Oliver returned and handed her a plastic wrapped toothbrush, a tube of toothpaste, a silk shirt and a hairbrush. "All settled?" he asked, smiling.

She smiled back. "Thank you, I've got everything I need – you must have done this before."

"No, Lauren," he replied, seriously. "I can assure you I haven't." He hesitated at the door. "Tell me, my dear, exactly *who* are you avoiding?"

She shook her head. "Nobody important."

The next morning she was dressed and ready to leave by eight thirty. A housekeeper greeted her in the hallway.

"Mr Liberty has already left. He asked me to tell you that his driver is downstairs waiting to take you wherever you wish to go."

She felt a tinge of disappointment – she'd hoped to see him, but apparently he was an earlier riser than she.

Taking advantage of his car she had the driver drop her at her apartment where she quickly changed clothes. No messages from Emerson. She felt relieved – or did she? Too confusing, she couldn't make up her mind.

At the office Pia bombarded her with questions. "What do you think of him? I told you he's getting a divorce, didn't I? Hmm . . . he *is* attractive, isn't he?"

Lauren shook her head. "*Stop* fixing me up."

"I'm not fixing you up – I'm trying to marry you off! One day you'll be old and shrivelled – what then?"

"I'm sure I'll be very happy, thank you."

Pia pulled a face. "You know what, Lauren – you're a hopeless case. Oh, and by the way – Emerson Burn called you three times this morning. What does *he* want?"

"If I knew I'd tell you."

"*Sure* you would."

"I would."

"Oh yes, and pigs will wear tutus and fly down Fifth Avenue!"

"Very funny."

"You don't need a rock star, Lauren. You need Oliver. He's stable, rich and crazy about you."

"I'll tell his wife."

"Ex-wife."

"Not yet."

"Sooner than you think."

"Yeah?"

"Yeah."

Chapter 55

Back in LA Nick found two messages from Frances Cavendish. Good sign? Bad sign? He didn't know. He'd brought Cyndra and Annie back to his place because he'd figured it wasn't safe for either of them to go to their own apartments, but now they were getting on his nerves. Cyndra wandered around in a daze, and Annie complained hotly because he hadn't dropped her home.

"We gotta get our stories straight before anybody goes anywhere," he said. "I'll call Frances Cavendish back – then we'll talk."

Annie glared at him. He ignored her.

"Where have you been?" Frances said, testily.

"Out of town."

"In future leave a number where I can reach you."

Who the fuck did she think she was talking to? "Yes, *ma'am*," he said, biting back a sharper retort.

"They like you, sonny," she drawled, calming down. "They like you a lot."

"What does that mean?" he asked, suspiciously.

"They want to see you again. In fact they might even test you."

"Is that good or bad?"

She made an exasperated sound in the back of her throat. "How long have you been in this business, Nick? A test costs them money – if they're paying of course it's good."

He wound the phone cord around his wrist, snapping it back and forth. "When do I get to do this?"

"Today, be at my office at ten." She hung up before he could reply.

Well, why not? She knew he'd be there. He was an actor after all, and when a casting agent says jump it's all systems go.

Annie had stationed herself by the door. "I want to go home," she said, daring him to say no. "I want to go home now."

"Okay, okay. But Cyndra stays here. And listen carefully, if Reece shows up, you know nothin'. You never went to Vegas, you've been with a girlfriend for the last twenty-four hours. Got it?"

She continued to glare at him. "Yes."

"And don't go making any phone calls you might regret. Whatever happened in Vegas – it's history."

"If you say so," she said, tightly.

"What's that mean?"

"I've never had to bury a body before."

"I said forget about it, Annie, it never happened."

"Maybe *you* can pretend it never happened. I can't."

"Okay – I'll take you home." He glanced over at his sister. She sat by the window staring out. "Cyndra, you stay here. Don't answer the door or phone. I'll get back soon as I can."

She nodded, dully.

Annie gave him the silent treatment on the drive to her apartment. Her attitude was shit, but there was nothing he could do about it.

"Call you later," he promised, dropping her off on the street.

She didn't say a word as she marched inside. He had a strong suspicion she was going to cause trouble.

Regrettably there was nothing he could do about it.

The woman producer had eyes for him. No mistaking that hungry look.

The tall man hated him. Probably a closet queen with a yen he didn't want to let loose.

The director was into pleasing everyone.

"I don't think we need to test him," the woman said. "Do you, Joel?"

The tall man shrugged. "Whatever."

"I'm happy," the director said.

Nick sat in the room listening to them talk about him as if he wasn't there.

"Shall we have him read again?" asked one of the casting people.

"Not necessary," said the woman, tapping her foot impatiently.

"The camera'll love him," said the director, running a hand through his greasy brown hair. "He's got the eyes."

"I'd like to see his body," the woman said, crossing her legs, silk stockings crackling.

He wasn't sure but he thought he caught a glimpse of suspenders.

"Would you mind removing your shirt?" said one of the casting people.

Where was Frances when he needed her? Nobody had warned him he'd have to strip off.

"There's a scene in the movie where he's in bed with the hero's girlfriend," explained the director. "Can't have you looking better than the star."

They all laughed.

He stood up and awkwardly removed his shirt.

"Fine," said the woman.

"No competition," said the director.

"We'll get back to you," said the tall man.

Getting out of there was a pleasure.

Outside he sat in his car trying to re-live the events of the last twenty-four hours. He'd buried a body for crissakes. He'd buried a fucking body in the Nevada desert, and that made him an accessory to murder. Jesus. Maybe Annie was right. Maybe they should have called the police and let Cyndra explain.

No way. She wouldn't have stood a chance.

The woman producer strode out of the building and got into a cream coloured sports Mercedes. She wore large mirrored sunglasses and a knowing smile.

Nick wondered who she was fucking. The tall man for sure. The director – maybe.

He hadn't liked removing his shirt in there, it was demeaning. He was an actor, not a stripper.

The woman drove off and he followed her for a while. Her Mercedes sped down Sunset. He drew alongside her at a stop light and said, "Hi." She looked at him as if she'd never seen him before in her life.

"Nick Angel," he said, dropping the O, just as Joy had advised.

"Do I know you?" she said, adjusting her huge mirrored shades.

Bitch!

He gunned the light and drove straight home. Cyndra was gone. This wasn't his day.

His landlady was sunning herself outside. "You're two days late on the rent," she reminded, as he rushed past.

"You'll get it."

"I'd better or you're out."

Money was a problem. He'd almost blown the Tijuana stash and there was nothing coming in. If he paid his rent there'd be hardly anything left.

"Did you see my sister leave?"

"Your sister," his landlady sneered. "No, I didn't see your *sister*."

He jumped back in his car and headed for Annie's.

"We're going to the police," Annie said. She was dressed and ready for action, a silent Cyndra by her side.

He'd arrived just in time, they were almost out the door.

"You can't do that," he said.

"Oh, yes, we can."

He appealed to Cyndra. "I helped you out – you go to the cops now an' it'll be me who gets it. Don't kid yourself – we'll all be in deep shit. Is that what you want?"

"I don't know . . ." she said, unsurely. "Annie says it's the right thing to do, otherwise this'll always be hanging over us."

"Fuck!" he muttered angrily, turning on Annie.

She backed away.

"Don't you understand?" he said, angrily. "It's *too goddamn late*. We're in this together an' we'd better learn to trust one another, so stop this runnin' to the cops shit. I can't take it every time I leave the house."

"But –" Annie began.

"But nothing – you do this again an' so help me I'll –"

"You'll what?" she asked, defiantly.

He'd almost raised his arm to her. He'd wanted to strike out – just like Primo, just like his father. Oh, God! There was no way he'd ever allow himself to become like that fucking loser. He slumped into a chair. "Don't do this to us, Annie. You gotta let it go."

Her eyes filled with tears. "I'm trying."

"Try harder."

She nodded, acquiescing.

They were safe – for now – but who knew how long it would be before she spilled it all? Annie was dangerous. But he had a solution, and the sooner he put it into action the better.

Chapter 56

Emerson dropped out of sight and Oliver moved in. Lauren had never been courted before and it was strangely seductive. Oliver sent her flowers every day, called at noon without fail, always checked out his plans with her, and never so much as attempted a good-night kiss.

After three weeks of this courtly treatment she was beginning to wonder what was wrong with her.

"He adores you!" Pia confided, perching on the side of her desk. "He told Howard."

"That's nice," Lauren replied, busily organizing a pile of papers.

"Stop being so cool and in control," Pia said, hardly able to hide her exasperation. "What do *you* think of *him*?"

"He's a very charming man."

"You're so non-committal."

"What do you *want* me to say?"

"Have you slept with him?"

"Pia – if I had, you'd be the last to know."

"Why?"

"Because since you've become a married woman you do nothing but gossip."

Pia's eyes gleamed. "Is he sensational in bed? Older men are supposed to have fantastic technique," she giggled, slyly. "I hear they give great head."

"I wouldn't know."

"What are you waiting for?"

Good question. What *was* she waiting for?

Actually she was waiting for Oliver to make a move. The fact that he hadn't intrigued her. Was there something wrong with her? Did she turn him off? It was about time she found out.

363

Later that week they went to the opening of a Broadway show and the following party. Oliver seemed to know everyone. The musical comedy actress who starred in the show; a slew of New York socialites whom he jokingly called night runners; a famous senator and his equally famous model girlfriend. Lauren guessed that he probably even knew Emerson Burn – crazy Emerson who'd flashed into her life and vanished just as quickly. A good thing – because he was definitely trouble. She'd read that he'd left on a world tour.

On the ride home they discussed the evening. Oliver enjoyed filling her in on everyone – he had interesting stories and was not shy about telling them. According to him the musical comedy actress liked other women; the senator wore red sequinned stockings to bed; and the model only slept with men worth over ten million dollars.

"How do you know all this?" she asked, studying his distinguished profile.

"I'm in advertising. It's my business to know everything."

"Then who's going to be the new Marcella girl? I hear they want Nature and she's holding out for too much money."

Oliver frowned; he hated it when somebody knew something before he was prepared to tell them. "Who told you that?"

"Samm."

"If she was worth it, I'd recommend they pay her."

"You don't think she is?"

"Too many covers in too short a time," he said, brusquely. "Her face is overly familiar."

"Is it your account?"

"Between us?"

"No. I'm taking an announcement in *Ad Weekly*."

"Very amusing, Lauren."

"Well?" she pressed. "*Is* it your account?"

"It wasn't, but it will be."

"Really?"

"They're coming in to see what we have to offer tomorrow."

"And what *do* you have to offer?"

"A surprise."

She grinned. "I love surprises."

"Good."

The car drew up outside her building. She'd never asked him before, but the time seemed right. "Would you like to come up for a drink, Oliver?"

364

He shook his head. "I didn't want to bother you with this before, but my charming wife has detectives following me. Apparently she feels she'll get even more of my money if she can prove I'm sleeping around."

"I asked you up for a drink, nothing else."

"My dear, *I* know that. But I would never put you in a compromising position."

Thoughtful as well. He was turning out to be the perfect man.

"Tomorrow night – I'll pick you up at eight," he said.

"Not possible, I'm catering a dinner."

"Have someone else do it."

"No."

"Why not?"

She hated it when he tried to tell her what to do. "Because I want to do it myself."

He went to say something, then changed his mind. Lauren had that determined look, he knew better than to argue.

Chapter 57

Things happened fast. "You've got the part," Frances told him over the phone. "Shooting begins in two weeks. I've made an appointment for you to see an agent friend – she'll handle the deal. And I've booked you a photo session with another friend of mine. The session's gratis – all you have to pay for are the prints."

"Hey, Frances – this is great. I –"

Frances was a fast talker. "Saturday night. Escort duties. You're taking me to an industry party – wear a suit."

He started to say something but she cut him off again.

"I'm putting you on to my assistant, she'll give you the details. Oh, and Nick, don't forget who got you started."

"Frances, I –" She was gone.

He had a role in a fucking movie. He was about to get an agent. He was going to be a star! Things were definitely moving in the right direction.

His new agent was a short, middle-aged woman called Meena Caron. She had dark, bobbed hair and thick "no nonsense" glasses. She was with a large important agency, which was reassuring.

"It's two days work," she said, all business. "You'll be shooting in New York. They'll fly you in the day before – tourist – only above the title gets first."

"What does that mean?"

"Above the title?"

"Yeah."

She looked at him quizzically. "You *are* new to the business, aren't you."

"Gotta learn sometime," he said, cheerfully.

Meena tapped a silver Cartier pen on her desk top. "*Stars* get their name above the title. The star of your movie is Charlie

Geary. He's young, red-hot and a real-life pain. Stay away from him – he'll do his best to get you fired. And don't try to screw the leading lady – that's Charlie's privilege."

Oh, yeah?

"Who's the girl?"

"Carlysle Mann. Very pretty. Very crazy."

"I never went for crazy."

Meena didn't crack a smile. "As soon as you get your photos bring them in. There's a pilot at NBC you could be right for. You *can* act, can't you?"

"Frances wouldn't've sent me to you if I couldn't."

Meena stood up – she was finished with him. "Frances has her own reasons for doing things. You look good. I'm sure she's taking you on the party circuit."

He didn't answer. It was none of her goddamn business. Maybe he should have opted to go with Ardmore Castle instead of this storm trooper.

The photographer Frances set him up with was a tall gawky woman who worked fast, shrieking directions at her harassed assistant. Didn't Frances ever deal with men?

She circled him like a predatory animal. "Stop trying so hard," she kept on telling him. "For God's sake attempt to look natural. Dump the put-on scowl, it's so phoney."

He hated her too. He was used to women falling all over him. The agent and the photographer didn't appear to give a fast fuck.

After the session he figured he should go home – check up on Cyndra. But then again Joy was probably wondering where he'd vanished to, and he didn't want her mad at him. Christ, this was like walking a tightrope without a net. Surrounded by women and he wasn't even getting laid.

Joy greeted him frostily.

He told her about the movie.

"Bit part," she said, screwing up her nose in disgust. "You should have held out for better."

"At least it's a job. My first professional one."

"Crap movie. Crap director."

Why couldn't she be pleased for him instead of criticizing everything? "Gotta start somewhere," he said easily, refusing to let her get to him.

"Ha!" she sniffed.

He told her about Meena Caron.

367

"Second rate."

"She's with a big agency," he pointed out.

"You'll get lost. You should have signed with Ardmore."

"I don't like Ardmore."

She narrowed her eyes. "Who said you have to like people? It's what they can do for you that counts."

Maybe. Maybe not. But right now Joy was bringing him down, so he got out of there fast and stopped by to see Annie at the health club. She was suitably cool.

"My movie's shooting in New York," he said. "Maybe Cyndra can stay with you while I'm away."

"*Your* movie," she sneered.

He'd had it with her attitude. "Yeah. *My* fuckin' movie. Two days work – it's more than you're doin'."

She looked hurt. "Thanks, Nick. Remind me that I can't get a job. Remind me that every time I go on an interview all they want is a six foot blonde with big tits."

He did his best to soften her up. "Two days, Annie. I can't leave her alone."

"Why not?" she said, bitterly. "I'm here to do anything you want. Right?"

Slowly Cyndra recovered and tried to think positively. After all it wasn't her fault, *she* hadn't shot the man, Reece had. It was *his* gun, *his* responsibility.

Damn Reece Webster. He'd gone. Vanished. Good riddance.

"I'm moving back to my apartment," she told Nick.

"You can't do that,' he said, trying to reason with her.

Cyndra had a strong stubborn streak. "Why not?" she asked, tilting her chin, preparing for a fight.

"'Cause you're not ready."

She sighed, brushing a hand through her long dark hair. "Stop worrying about me, Nick. I won't go to the cops, and nor will Annie."

"An' what'll you do if Reece comes back?"

"He won't."

"You don't know for sure."

"Look – if he does, I'll tell him the guy got up an' walked away."

Was she stupid or what? "The man was dead, Cyndra, fuckin' *dead.*"

"Reece doesn't know that. He ran out of there so fast he

doesn't know anything. Go off and do your movie, it's a great break for you. It'd be nice if *one* of us made it."

He couldn't argue with that.

Frances worked a room good. She knew everyone and everyone knew her. Nick trailed behind, feeling out of place and inadequate in his rented suit. He was in a freakin' mansion for crissake – the like of which he'd never seen. It made the Browning house back in Bosewell resemble a shack.

Frances ordered a drink and made him carry it. She didn't bother introducing him to anyone – not that anyone seemed interested in meeting him – they looked right through him as if he didn't exist. As the evening progressed so did his sense of aggravation. He felt invisible, unimportant – it wasn't a feeling he enjoyed.

Dinner was seated, and he was not seated next to Frances. He found himself between a fat woman in a maroon cocktail dress and an older man in an ill-fitting tuxedo. He didn't have to be a genius to figure out it was the worst table in the room.

The fat woman talked to a vivacious blonde on her other side. The older man morosely sipped his drink.

Frances was across the room at a table filled with familiar faces. Everyone at her table was laughing and talking. Shit! How did he get stuck in these situations?

He gave conversation a shot, asking the man what he did.

"Banking," was the cold reply.

"You work in a bank or you own it?" he said, going for the flippant approach.

The man was unamused.

After a while he got up and made his way outside to the bar. Two waiters were sneaking a smoke. "Anybody know who's giving this party?" he asked.

"Some studio exec," said one of the waiters.

"That's his daughter," said the other waiter, gesturing across the well-kept gardens, where a young blonde was entwined around a guy with long hair. They were making their own entertainment.

"At least someone's having a good time," he mumbled.

It took forever before Frances was ready to be escorted home. He got behind the wheel of her old Mercedes and gunned the engine.

"Did you enjoy yourself?" she asked, puffing on a cigarette.

Was she kidding?

He stared unseeingly at the road ahead. "I had a lousy time."

She couldn't have cared less. "Really?"

"Those people don't wanna know you unless you're important."

"That's Hollywood, dear," she said, matter-of-factly. "Make the most of it – when you're famous they'll be crawling all over you."

He liked the sound of her words. Glancing at her quizzically he said, "You really think I'm gonna be famous, Frances?"

She blew smoke in his face and regarded him with her flinty grey eyes. "Yes, Nick, as a matter of fact I think you're going to be very famous indeed."

Chapter 58

"I'm finally divorced," Oliver announced over the phone. "Tonight we're celebrating."

Lauren was at work. Cradling the receiver under her chin she doodled on a yellow legal pad. "How did it happen so fast?" she asked.

"We made a deal. My ex-wife loves deals."

She drew a circle enclosing it with a square. "Congratulations, Oliver."

"Thank you, my dear."

"Where are we going?"

"We're staying home. My chauffeur will pick you up at seven." A slight pause. "Oh, and Lauren . . . bring a toothbrush."

Was this his way of telling her they were finally going to consummate their relationship? Hardly romantic, but Oliver was nothing if not to the point.

She went home early, washed her hair, took a leisurely bath, rubbed perfumed cream into her skin and thought about the evening ahead. She liked Oliver – he was entertaining. He had panache and style, wore great suits, always got the best table in restaurants. He was a good dancer, charming and witty.

But I don't love him.

So what? Who do you think's going to come rushing into your life? There are no Prince Charmings left.

But I don't love him.

Get real. He's the man for you.

He's old enough to be my grandfather.

It doesn't matter.

She dressed carefully, still thinking about what lay ahead. She'd slept with three men. Nick – who'd gotten her pregnant and dumped her. Brad – her bad seed cousin. And Jimmy – who'd taken off the day of their supposed wedding.

Some trio.

Except Nick is special.

Bullshit. Nick Angelo is nothing but a loser.

I loved him.

No you didn't.

I still love him.

For God's sake!

Oliver's apartment was filled with white orchids; his favourite jazz pianist – Erroll Garner – played background music on the stereo – the lights were low and Oliver was in a very good mood indeed. He greeted her with compliments and a glass of champagne, while the butler served small wedges of toast loaded with caviar from a silver tray.

"I don't like caviar," she said, wrinkling her nose.

Oliver looked amused. "It's an acquired taste. Acquire it, my dear, you'll soon grow to adore it."

They ate in the dining room with candles lighting the table and Erroll Garner giving way to the smooth sound of Ella Fitzgerald.

Lauren picked at her food and gulped two glasses of wine, wondering if she should encourage him.

A little late, Roberts. You've encouraged him for three months. Why stop now?

After dinner he dismissed his servants and led her into the darkly panelled library where they sat in front of a burning wood fire sipping brandies.

"I don't usually drink –" she began.

"I know," he interrupted, removing the glass from her hand and leaning over to kiss her.

This was not the first time they'd kissed, but it was certainly the most intense. She was glad she'd had the champagne and the wine at dinner and now the brandy.

God! She was nervous.

He moved slowly, kissing her for a long time before suggesting they go into the bedroom.

Her affair with Jimmy had taken place over a year ago – she hadn't been with anyone since, and yet she did not feel that incredible rush of excitement. Instead she felt apprehensive – as if she was about to embark on a trip she might regret.

The bedroom was alive with red roses, the seductive scent of them filling the air. Oliver touched her lightly on the cheek. "Do you want to undress in the bathroom? There's a robe in there for you."

She hadn't planned on undressing herself, but that was apparently what he expected.

Shutting the bathroom door she stared at herself in the mirror. Little Lauren Roberts. High school prude. About to embark on a sexual adventure with a man who was older than her father. Oh, God!

For a moment she flashed on to the memory of Phil Roberts that fateful day in Bosewell. Her father and his . . . woman. Her father and that cheap tramp.

And then she saw Primo, leering at her with his wild eyes. She could almost feel his beer gut pushing up against her, and his filthy laugh began ringing in her head.

You killed him, Lauren.

I'm not sure . . .

Oh yes, Lauren, you killed him all right.

She removed her clothes and put on the silk robe Oliver had so thoughtfully provided. The material was soft and sensuous. She pulled it around her protectively.

He was waiting under the covers with the lights off. A single candle lit the room. The scent of the roses was overwhelming.

Standing next to the bed she slipped the robe from her shoulders, allowing it to fall to the floor.

"You're so beautiful," Oliver murmured, holding the covers open.

She dived for safety.

Slowly he began stroking her naked body – apparently in no hurry – content to touch and caress her, until she felt herself longing for more.

Tentatively she stretched her hand beneath the sheet, reaching for him. To her surprise and disappointment he was not hard.

"Don't worry, it'll happen," he murmured, unconcernedly. "Lie back, my darling, before anything else I plan to make you feel wonderful."

His head began to move down her body, his tongue tracing little patterns on her breasts and stomach as he descended, until finally his head was between her legs and his fingers started prying her apart – all the better for his tongue to gain entry.

She gasped. This was a first and she was unprepared and wary of what to expect.

373

"Relax, my sweet, relax and enjoy," he said soothingly, his tongue flicking in and out with practised ease.

"Oh . . . my . . . God," she whispered. This was so intimate, so private, and yet – she had to admit – so breathtakingly enjoyable.

She threw her head and arms back and did as he requested, allowing herself to fall into the beauty of the moment.

He held her open with his thumbs – all the better to penetrate as far as he could.

Was this what Pia had been talking about when she'd said older men gave great head? Was this it? – because if it was Oliver certainly knew what he was doing.

Before long she began to feel little shock waves of pleasure. They started in her toes and travelled up her entire body – causing her to moan softly. Shivering uncontrollably she threw her legs wide.

He devoured her with a passion until she climaxed with a long drawn out cry of ecstasy.

Oliver surfaced, a smile on his face. "I can't think of a better time to ask you." He paused for a moment. "My beautiful Lauren, will you do me the honour of becoming my wife?"

"Let me see the ring," Pia said for the hundredth time – at least it seemed to Lauren it was the hundredth time.

She held out her hand while Pia admired the four-carat emerald surrounded with baguette diamonds.

"Gorgeous!" Pia sighed.

Lauren patted her friend's evergrowing stomach. "Gorgeous!" she said, enviously.

"Seriously, Lauren, I'm so happy for you."

When I'm thirty he'll be almost seventy, Lauren thought. *When I'm fifty he'll be dead.*

"Is he okay about you continuing to work?" Pia asked.

"About as okay as Howard is with you."

"That's encouraging. Howard begs me daily to give it up."

Lauren looked perplexed. "Why is it that men are always so threatened by working women?"

"Because it means we have our own money," Pia said, wisely. "And with our own money comes independence. Samm is my shining example."

"Samm is a lonely old spinster."

"But a beautiful one. *And* she doesn't have to wash anyone's socks."

"Pia, you have a maid."

Pia giggled. "I'm only joking. I *love* washing Howard's socks!"

Lauren knew that was something she'd never have to do. It was quite obvious Oliver had no plans to change his lifestyle. He was very comfortable, a man of habit. He had his live-in housekeeper, two daily maids, a butler when he entertained, and his trusty Japanese chauffeur. At the office he had a slew of assistants who obviously adored him.

They planned on getting married in the Bahamas where Oliver kept a bank account and a house. "You'll love it there," he'd assured her. "It's very peaceful and the people are delightful."

Their target date was six weeks.

Since that night nothing much had changed. Oliver was totally into pleasuring her, and when she tried to reverse the situation he always had the same answer. "Give me the joy of making you happy now – when we're married it'll be different."

She didn't fight it, there was no hurry – after all she was marrying the man – she had the rest of her life to make him the happiest man alive.

Chapter 59

Working on a movie was a new experience and Nick immediately knew he was going to love it. He'd arrived in New York to be met at the airport by a car and driver – not a limo, only a sedan, but it sure beat taking the subway. They had him staying at a small hotel near Times Square where most of the crew were, and upon arrival he found a typed call sheet giving him instructions for the next day.

In the meantime, he had to meet with Waldo, the men's costumer. They spent the afternoon shopping in the Village for a suitable outfit. Actually he could have used his own clothes, because they ended up purchasing tight jeans, black shirt and leather jacket.

"Do I get to keep the clothes?" he joked. "They'll blend right into my closet!"

"Only if it's in your contract," Waldo replied, fussing with the leather jacket.

"My agent's got the contract."

"Then it's probably too late." Waldo stood back and surveyed him. "Steal 'em," he said, archly. "They'll never notice."

Nick laughed. "*Now* you're talkin'!"

"I'm surprised you got this role," Waldo remarked, pursing his lips.

"How's that?"

"Our macho young *star* is hardly going to be thrilled when he sees you."

"Oh, you mean Charlie?"

"Do you know him?"

"Nah, never met him, but we'll get along."

"Don't be so sure."

"C'mon, Waldo, believe me – I get along with everyone."

How wrong he was. Charlie Geary was the jerk everybody said he was. A former television star, Charlie had hit the movies in a big way with two box office bonanzas. He was shorter than Nick with a baby face, a shock of reddish hair and a bad cocaine habit. The moment he saw Nick he was on the director's case.

"What the fuck you hire him for? *I'm* supposed to be the star of this movie."

"We gotta have someone who looks halfway decent," the director replied. "In the movie he's in bed with your girlfriend – why else would she hop in the sack with him?"

Charlie's baby face creased into a sour expression. "Do I give a fuck? Do I care? Fire him."

"Too late," the director said.

"Don't fucking tell *me* it's too late," Charlie replied, his eyes popping. "Because I'll tell you it's never too late for me to walk."

The director conferred with his producers. The producers, who'd had enough of Charlie Geary and his enormous ego said they weren't firing anyone.

Their first scene together took place in a bar. Charlie Geary was at a table with his cronies and Nick had to enter the shot, exchange insults with Charlie, and walk off camera.

Although Charlie only had a few lines, he managed to blow them every time. The director kept calling "Cut" and going for another take.

Nick had his lines down pat. He loved the feeling on the set, the family atmosphere, the way everybody fussed around him. Plus it was a real blast being in front of a camera.

Make the most of it, he told himself. *You're only here for two days.*

Because of Charlie the scene took all day, continuing into overtime. The director was pissed, the producers more so as they worked into the night.

Waldo took Nick to one side. "You'd better plan on being here an extra day," he said. "They'll never get to your scene with Carlysle by tomorrow."

"Hey – I'm here for as long as they want me," Nick replied. "I could really get used to this."

Back at his hotel he tried calling the number he had for Joey.

"Joey moved outta here a year ago," a female voice said. "I took over the apartment from him."

"You got any idea where he went?"

"Yeah, there's a number somewhere."

"Can you find it?"

She did not sound enthusiastic. "I dunno."

He went into persuasive overdrive. "I'd really appreciate it if you could."

"You visiting or what?"

"I'm shooting a movie here."

Her voice perked up. "Oh, you're an actor?"

"You got it."

"Well, um . . . you here alone?"

"Find me the number an' we'll talk."

Her voice heated up considerably. "Whyn't you come over and I'll give it to you personally."

"Because I need to call him now."

"I like actors."

Oh, shit! Why did he always get lumbered with the maniacs? "So I'll send you an autographed picture. Be a sweetheart an' get me the number."

She finally delivered and he called Joey. A stoned woman answered.

"Joey around?" he asked.

"Who wants him?"

"An old friend."

"He owe you?"

"No, I told you – I'm an old friend."

She snorted, derisively. "Sure, same old story. It's always an old friend, an' he always ends up gettin' his brains beat out. I told you, mister, he ain't here."

"Tell him it's Nick – Nick Angelo. Okay?"

"Wait a minute." She kept him on hold for a while, then she got back on the phone and gave him the address of a club. "You'll find Joey there."

This was like playing tag. Find Joey in the big city. Christ!

The club she sent him to was a dump. Nude photos displayed outside proclaimed, "*SEVEN BEAUTIFUL GIRLS – TOTALLY NAKED.*" An Indian bouncer slumped wearily on a canvas folding chair picking his nose. It cost ten bucks to get inside, and once there he was immediately pounced on by a topless waitress with droopy tits who offered him a complimentary glass of champagne and the choice of a hostess to sit with him.

He declined both offers. "I'm lookin' for Joey."

She lost interest in him and jerked a finger towards the bar.

He walked over. It was not difficult finding Joey – he was the only customer. Nick tapped him on the shoulder. "Joey?"

Joey spun around. "What the fu – Jesus! *Nick?*"

"Yeah, it's me."

Joey almost fell off the bar stool. They hugged awkwardly and grinned at each other.

"How're you doing, man?" Nick asked, thinking that Joey did not look good at all. He was skinny and pale, with dark circles under his sunken eyes and a nervous facial tic. "Don't even tell me – you look like shit."

Joey managed a weak grin. "Thanks. S'good to see you, too." He dragged on his cigarette. "How come you're here? I heard you were livin' in LA."

"Can you believe it – I'm in a movie."

"A movie, huh? You're finally doin' that acting thing."

"Yeah, well, I stayed in Chicago for a while – then moved to LA, found myself an agent, went on this audition and got lucky. It's only a small role, but at least I'm workin'."

Joey snapped his fingers at the girl behind the bar. She bounced over wearing nothing but a short sequinned miniskirt and long fake eyelashes. "Get my movie star friend a beer – an' don't water it down."

"Anything you want, Joey," she said, squinting at Nick. "Movie star, huh? What you bin in?"

"Never mind," Joey said, waving her away.

The girl moved off and Joey gestured around the dingy club. "Classy joint, huh? My place of work. I come on between strippers – the crowd really gets off on me. I'm doing stand-up like I always wanted."

Yeah, and from the looks of you that's not all you're doing.

"That's great, Joey."

"Don't give me polite crap. This gig is about as great as a rattlesnake up your ass. I'm doin' a shit job in a shit place, but it's all I got right now." He stubbed out his cigarette, immediately reaching for another. "So," he added, rubbing his bloodshot eyes. "What's happening with Cyndra? You seen her?"

"She married that Reece Webster guy – who incidentally turned out to be creep of the century. He's not around any more."

"What's she doing?"

"She was singing in a Vegas hotel. Small stuff, she'll do okay."

"We kinda lost touch."

"Looks like you lost touch with everyone."

Joey laughed, ruefully. "It's always that way, huh?"

"Did you ever make it back to Bosewell?" Nick asked.

"No. Did you?"

"Nope."

"I guess once we got outta there – that was it."

The topless bar-girl delivered his beer in a cracked glass. "Enjoy," she said, holding out her hand for money.

"Put it on my tab," said Joey, irritated.

"Your tab's overd –"

"I said put it on my fuckin' tab," he snarled.

She flounced off.

"You look like you could do with a break," Nick said. "How about flyin' to LA an' staying with me for a while?"

"Oh, yeah – an' give up my job?"

"There's plenty of comedy clubs in LA."

"I can't afford to take the chance."

"Why? You got such a wonderful life here?"

"Nah, I'm living with this girl."

"Somebody special?"

"If I told you, you wouldn't believe me."

"Try it."

"She's a hooker."

"Okay, so I believe you."

They both laughed.

"Seriously. She's the proverbial hooker with a heart of gold. I met her at a party. She likes having me around. I like being around. She pays the rent an' I give her what I can. It works out okay."

"Hey, Joey," shrieked a blowsy blonde. "Get your ass up on stage. *Now.*"

Joey shrugged, stubbed out his cigarette. "My boss. Charming lady. Hang around, Nick, catch the act."

"I'd love to, but I got an early call tomorrow. Whyn't you come by the set? Here, I'll give you the address." He scribbled on a piece of paper and handed it over. "Drop by tomorrow an' we'll talk about you coming to LA."

"Yeah, maybe."

When he got back to the hotel he called Cyndra. "Everything okay?"

"Everything's fine."

"No sign of Reece?"

"No."

"Is Annie behaving herself?"

"I told you, Nick, everything's fine. Stop worrying."

He cleared his throat, ready to give her the big news. "Guess who I saw tonight?"

"Who?"

"Joey."

There was a long silence. "How is he?" she finally asked.

"Not in great shape. I'm trying to talk him into flying back to LA with me."

"Not on my account. I've had it with men."

"Listen – the three of us went through some hard times together. Be nice to hang out, huh?"

She answered a touch too fast. "I told you, Nick, don't drag him back because of me. I'm not interested."

"I get the message."

She changed moods. "How did the filming go today?"

"It's a trip."

"What's Charlie Geary like?"

"A stoned prick."

"Really?"

"Wouldn't kid you."

"Y'know, Nick, I've been thinking. Tomorrow I'm going to contact the record company Reece was dealing with and see if they're still interested in me."

"Sounds like a good idea."

"You think so?"

"What's to lose?"

"That's how I feel," she said, glad to have his confirmation.

"I'll call you tomorrow," he said. "Take care, little sis."

"'Bye, Nick."

Running into Charlie Geary early in the morning in the make-up room was not a pleasant sight. The famous actor was wasted; he looked worse than Joey.

"Boy, did I have a night last night!" Charlie boasted. "Even though I say it myself I gotta cock that never quits. I had this little pussy creamin' herself all over me – I mean she was comin' an' com –"

"Shut up, Charlie," the make-up girl said, wearily.

"Don't tell *me* to shut up, sweetheart. You wanna stay on this film you'll suck my dick if I tell you to."

Nick sat down in the second chair. Charlie stretched and burped in his direction. "So – where'd they dig you up from?"

"I been around," Nick said.

"Yeah?" Charlie yawned, throwing his arms up and back, almost hitting the make-up girl in the face. "Couldn't tell it from your performance. You really fucked up yesterday – I hate working with amateurs."

He was not about to take this little asshole's shit. "You got a short memory – it wasn't me that fucked up, it was you."

"Don't bother with him," the make-up girl murmured, moving past. "He's not worth it."

"What didja say, cunt?" Charlie demanded, almost falling off his chair.

"Why don't you leave the girl alone?" Nick said.

"Why don't you get fucked."

Fortunately an assistant entered, summoning Charlie to the set. He got out of the chair unsteady on his feet and lurched to the door.

"He's stoned," the make-up girl said.

"No kiddin'?" Nick replied.

Later, on the set, Charlie played the same game – screwing up his lines, forgetting cues, generally messing up.

Nick noticed the two producers conferring in a corner. The woman wore a bright scarlet suit, her long legs in matching tights and very high heels. The tall man had assumed a permanently grim expression, while the director ran around looking frantic.

After the lunch break Charlie failed to appear at all. The A.D. said she couldn't get him out of his trailer. Forming a group, the two producers and the director stormed off to personally escort him to the set. They returned with no Charlie.

"Tell you what, Nick," the director said. "We'll shoot your close-ups. Charlie's not feeling good – he may not be able to do the rest of the scene this afternoon."

As little as Nick knew about production, he realized this did not bode well for the shoot. But screw it – he wasn't complaining – close-ups sounded good to him.

Joey did not show, so at the end of the day he called him again. This time Joey picked up the phone himself.

"Where were you?" Nick asked.

"Hadda meetin'."

"You couldn't've come by after?"

"Hey, man, what's the problem?" Joey said, belligerently. "We don't see each other for a few years – you come back inta my life an' I'm supposed t'jump?"

"Forget it. I'll see ya."

"C'mon, Nick, don't go gettin' pissed. I'll be there tomorrow. Right now I got a lot on my mind."

"Anythin' I can help out with?"

"Nah. Just small problems."

"See you tomorrow."

"Bet on it."

Nick settled back to study his script. Tomorrow he had his big scene with Carlysle Mann – and he didn't want to blow it. This filming shit was seductive.

He fell asleep with the script clutched tightly in his hands.

The next morning he was sitting in make-up at seven a.m. calm as can be, when the A.D. entered looking flustered.

"They need to see you at once," she said.

"Who needs to see me?" he asked, patiently.

"The producers."

"Yeah?"

Oh, shit. This is it. Charlie Geary's getting his way and I'm about to be canned.

"He's nearly through," the make-up girl said, blending dark pancake on his neck.

Yeah, sweetheart, you can say that again.

"There's a crisis," the A.D. said. "They need him immediately."

"Better let you go," the make-up girl said.

He got out of the chair and followed the A.D., silently rehearsing his objections.

It didn't matter what he said, he was out and he knew it.

Chapter 60

Lauren was frantic, suddenly there seemed so much to do before she left for the Bahamas. Pia was not much help – seven months pregnant, she waddled around with a smile on her face, arriving late and leaving early. Lauren didn't blame her, but still it left most of the responsibilities of the business to her.

"I wish Howard and I were coming with you," Pia said with a wistful sigh, obviously expecting Lauren to say, "Why don't you?" But she'd decided it was going be her and Oliver – nobody else. She'd experienced one wedding where everybody stood around waiting and the bridegroom didn't show up, and she did not plan on doing it again.

"Who'll run the business while I'm away?" she worried.

"*I* will," said Pia.

"You're hardly here any more."

"Don't obsess. I'll be around all the time while you're away."

Lauren knew that the business only survived because of her personal touch. She'd gained such a good reputation, especially with her dinner parties. Lately, all Pia took care of was the financial side.

She had one more dinner to organize before leaving for the Bahamas. This was at the house of Quentin and Jessie George. Quentin was the managing editor of *Satisfaction*, the avant garde magazine of the moment, and Jessie was a social whirlwind. She'd catered dinner parties for them before and it was always an enjoyable experience. The Georges put together an eclectic group of guests, mixing politics and fashion, rock 'n roll and movies. Jessie was a delightful character – a woman of indeterminate age, not conventionally pretty, but loaded with style.

The night before the dinner Lauren visited their brownstone

to go over the final details. Jessie had heard about her upcoming marriage and couldn't wait to complain.

"I suppose we'll be losing you," she lamented. "You won't want to do this any more."

"I didn't say that," Lauren objected.

"Ah, but Oliver will never let you."

"Oliver's not going to control what I do and what I don't do."

Jessie nodded, knowingly. "Darling, when you're married you'll see."

"Jessie, when I'm married I'll see nothing. I'll carry on exactly the way I please."

"Hmm," Jessie said. "That's what *I* thought when I married Quentin, and look at me now."

"It seems to me you have a fantastic life."

"Some would say so." Jessie waved her bracelet-adorned arms in the air. "Now, let's get down to business. I have a brilliant idea for hors-d'œuvres – imagine scooped out melon balls filled with golden caviar – doesn't it sound divine?"

Oliver was very much involved with the Marcella girl campaign. Marcella was a very successful, large make-up manufacturing corporation in Italy who were all set to take a large chunk out of the American market. They planned to rival Revlon and Estée Lauder. Now that Oliver's firm had landed the account, the search was on for the perfect girl. So far they'd tested and photographed at least thirty candidates.

Lauren viewed the photos and watched the video tapes with Oliver. He was extremely critical – as far as he was concerned this one was too glamorous, this one too old, this one too young and so on.

"Your expectations are too high," she said. "I can see at least seven or eight of them who'd be great."

"No," he said, shaking his head. "None of them have it. The Marcella girl has to have a special quality that appeals to the public, something that makes women say, "I want to look exactly like her – and if I wear Marcella make-up I can." She has to have a certain ordinariness, combined with that magical something else."

"I've no idea what you're getting at."

"It's a quality. Grace Kelly had it. Marilyn didn't. Ingrid Bergman had it."

385

"Who's Ingrid Bergman?"

"Never mind." He stared at her closely. "You have it."

"I have what?"

"The quality I'm talking about."

"Is that good or bad?"

"If you were in the running for the Marcella girl it would be good."

She walked over to his desk and helped herself to an apple from a bowl of fruit. "Fortunately, Oliver, I'm not."

He frowned, looking at her intently. "But you could be."

"You *are* joking."

"No," he said, very seriously, "I'm not."

She laughed. "Oliver, I am *not* a model, I do not want to be a model, I am perfectly happy doing what I'm doing, so kindly forget it."

"Will you do something for me before we leave?"

She sighed. "What?"

"Will you let my people organize a photo session with you?"

She crunched her apple. "Now why would I do a thing like that?"

"Because it would be very helpful if I could show them exactly who I'm looking for."

She flopped into an armchair. "You're so funny."

"Then humour me."

"I don't have time."

"Do I ask for much, Lauren? Wouldn't you enjoy having your hair done and your make-up and wearing beautiful clothes? It could be fun."

"It might be your idea of fun, but believe me, I have better things to do."

"Please, Lauren – for me? As a wedding present. Think of the money you'll save."

"Oliver –"

"Yes?"

She weakened. "Well, as long as you promise not to take it seriously."

"You have my solemn promise."

Humouring Oliver turned out to be more enjoyable than she'd thought. To go into a studio and be totally made over by professionals was an interesting experience. Pia thought it was a hoot and insisted on accompanying her. They giggled like a couple of schoolgirls as the make-up artist and hairdresser went to work.

386

"At least you'll have some incredible photographs to show your grandchildren," Pia said, perching behind her on a high stool.

"*What* grandchildren?" Lauren exclaimed. "I haven't even got any children yet – let's not get carried away."

"You *are* going to have some, aren't you?" Pia asked, anxiously. "I need a playmate for mine," she added, patting her huge belly.

"I guess so," Lauren agreed. "But give me time to enjoy my marriage first."

"You got fab 'air, darlin'," said the English hairdresser, his cockney accent reminding her of Emerson. "The colour needs livening up a bit, an' you're in desperate need of a cut – apart from that you're perfect!"

"I've always had long hair," she said, alarmed.

"Yeah, but it's just 'angin' there, ain't it? Let me work it over – leave it to me."

"Don't take off too much," she said, when he started wielding his scissors.

"Trust me, darlin', you'll be thankin' me."

She shut her eyes and hoped he knew what he was doing. The make-up artist was next. He came at her with a pair of tweezers, plucking at her eyebrows, squinting at the shape of her face.

"I don't like to wear much make-up," she ventured.

"Nor do I," he said, tartly. "What we have to do here is the illusion of no make-up at all while I create *the* most incredible face."

And so they transformed her. Lauren Roberts – small-town beauty – was turned into Lauren, face of the moment. The hair-dresser had added ever so subtle light streaks into her chestnut hair, and the cut had given it more body and shape, so that although it still fell below her shoulders, it was fuller and more flattering.

The make-up artist had worked on her face with a palette of natural colours – playing with browns and beiges, bringing out her eyes in a way they had not been emphasized before.

"My God!" Pia said, genuinely amazed. "You look fantastic!"

"Oh, thanks a lot," Lauren said, pretending to frown. "Was I such a dog before?"

"You know what I mean. You've always been pretty, but my God, now you're absolutely stunning!"

Next it was the photographer's turn. Antonio worked fast

with a minimum of fuss and the maximum of assistants. He knew exactly what he wanted, and even though Lauren had never been in front of a camera before, she fell into the poses easily, having watched Nature so many times. It was a kick. There was great music playing, she was clad in beautiful designer clothes. When it was all over she confided to Pia that she'd actually enjoyed it.

"Who wouldn't?" Pia said, shaking her head in amazement. "You really *do* look incredible."

"I wish you'd stop saying that. God knows what I must have looked like before."

"I can't wait to see the photos," Pia said.

"And I can't wait to wash this make-up off."

Later, Oliver asked her how she'd enjoyed the session.

"It was okay," she said, laughing. "Never again, though. You can only talk me into it once."

The next morning was a different kind of frantic. She left early for the market accompanied by a couple of her young, college student assistants. They picked out fresh fruit and vegetables, and then stopped to buy flowers. Jessie and Quentin were very particular and that's exactly the way she liked it.

"Have Oliver come to the dinner," Jessie urged, when she arrived at their house.

"No way," she objected. "I don't want him sitting there while I'm working."

"But I adore Oliver – he's so droll," Jessie said. "At least have him drop by to pick you up."

She called Oliver at his office. "Do you want to come by later and pick me up from the Georges' dinner party?"

"I'd like that," he said.

"Jessie particularly requested you. How well do you know her?"

"We had a hot and steamy affair once."

She almost believed him. "Oliver – *did* you?"

He laughed. "No, my dear. I am not the hot and steamy affair type."

"You could have fooled me."

"Ah," he promised. "Wait until our honeymoon."

From four o'clock on she commandeered the Georges' kitchen. It was the kind of kitchen she liked, large and spacious, with all modern conveniences. The menu she'd planned was one of Jessie's favourites. Cold vichyssoise followed by rib-sticking chicken casserole with creamy mashed potatoes, lightly sautéd carrots and creamed spinach, all accompanied by a healthful chopped salad.

"I love it when you serve those kind of meals,' Jessie confided. "It makes people feel comfortable and relaxed, and when they're in that kind of mood the conversation *really* sparkles. Oh dear, Lauren, what am I going to do when Oliver takes you away from all this?"

"I'll still keep the business," she said. "I'll cook occasionally."

"Shall we bet on this?" Jessie suggested.

Lauren grinned. "Only if it's cash."

Later Oliver called her at the Georges'. "Remember how you said the other day you loved surprises?"

"Did I say that?"

"Yes. Well, I have a surprise for you."

"What is it?"

"If I told you it wouldn't be a surprise. When I come by later I'll bring it."

"Does it have four legs?" she asked, remembering her recent request for a puppy.

"Be patient, my dear. I'll show you later."

Chapter 61

Carlysle Mann was pretty beyond belief. She had one of those etched faces with alabaster skin, huge blue eyes, a snub nose and a beguiling overbite. She was petite, with baby-fine blonde hair curling around her face, and a perfect figure.

For the first time in his life Nick felt intimidated meeting somebody. He'd seen her in a couple of movies, but actually meeting her was something else.

"Hi," he said, almost shyly.

"Congrats," she replied, pretty blue eyes gazing into his. "This is some great break for you."

Yeah, congratulations were definitely in order. He had not been canned. Instead he had gotten the chance of a lifetime. While Charlie Geary was being rushed off to a drug rehab centre, he, Nick Angelo – excuse me, Nick Angel – had been presented with the big break. He'd been given the lead in the movie, and it was a career-making role – that of a young hood who reforms, finds true love, and ends up as the hero.

"You've got the look," the woman producer had said, crossing and uncrossing her elegant legs.

Yeah, I've got the look all right, he'd wanted to say. *A look you didn't even recognize when I pulled alongside you in my car in LA.*

"We're giving you this chance," the director had said, "in the hope you'll deliver."

"We've spoken to your agent," the tall man had added. "You'll probably want to give her a call."

Want to give her a call? Holy shit! He couldn't believe this was happening. Charlie was dumped and he was in.

"I can do it," he'd blurted. "I've studied the script – I can do this good."

"That's exactly why you're getting this opportunity," the woman had said.

The truth was they didn't have much choice. Charlie Geary was out of action and they couldn't afford to shut down production while they waited to negotiate for another star. They were prepared to take a chance on Nick.

The next few days were crazy time. His main worry was Cyndra and Annie. Could he trust them alone in LA? Would they be all right without him? Or would Annie go running to the cops, ruining everything. It was a chance he had to take.

He called them both. Annie sounded sulky as usual. She didn't even rustle up any enthusiasm when he told her about his lucky break.

"Tell you what," he suggested. "Give me a few days, then maybe you'll fly to New York for a weekend. I'll spring for your ticket and room. I talked to my agent, I'm making okay money."

"I don't think so," she said coolly.

"C'mon," he persuaded. "You want to see New York, don't you? You've never been here."

"I'll let you know."

Cyndra was genuinely thrilled. "You'll be sensational Nick," she assured him.

"I'll do my best. Can't do more than that."

His agent had been suitably businesslike. "It's an excellent opportunity for you to show them how good you are. Of course, you're still very inexperienced. It may not work out – don't get your hopes up."

"How come they went with me?" he asked.

She told him the truth. "This is not a big budget movie. If they wait for a replacement for Charlie it'll hold them up and cost them money they can't afford. You're there, and as far as they're concerned you seem capable of doing the job. Carlysle's name will carry the film. Oh, and Nick – remember what I told you – don't screw her – it'll get in the way of your performance."

"You told me not to screw her before because it would get in the way of Charlie Geary. Now he ain't around."

"Nick, you're new to this business – *don't* screw her."

Frances expressed the same sentiments. "Save everything you've got. Getting laid takes time and energy. Put all that sexual juice into your performance."

Once he met Carlysle he knew exactly where all his sexual

391

juice was going. They'd hit it off immediately. He asked around and found out her story. She'd been a child star since the age of eight, now she was twenty-two, recently divorced from a rock and roll drummer, and very career orientated. She had a mother who usually accompanied her on shoots, but so far had not arrived in New York.

"Watch out for the mother," Waldo warned. "The woman is a complete nightmare."

"Why are you telling *me*?" he asked.

"Because we all know what's about to happen between you two," Waldo replied, with an evil chuckle.

Nick laughed. "How about fillin' *me* in?"

Their second day on the set Carlysle invited him out. "I have to go to this dinner party tomorrow night," she said. "My mother was coming with me, but since she's not here . . . Will you take me?"

She gazed up at him with her big blue eyes and he wasn't about to say no.

"Yeah, sure. Should we go from the set?"

"No, I'll have to go home and change first. Pick me up at my apartment."

"I thought you lived in LA."

"I do. I've got a house in LA and an apartment here."

Wow! This girl really had it all together. "What time?" he asked.

"The dinner starts at seven-thirty, but they probably won't sit down to eat until nine. Get me at eight-thirty and we'll make a late entrance."

"Uh, what do I wear?"

She smiled. "Whatever you like. I'm sure you look fine in anything."

Cyndra was determined the incident in Vegas was not going to drag her down. She'd come so far and she was not allowing it to pull her under. It was unfortunate, but it was her past – just like Mr Browning, her abortion, and all the other bad things she'd gone through.

Annie, on the other hand, kept on insisting they had to do something about it. If Nick knew he'd throw a fit.

"You'd better shut up about this," Cyndra warned her. "'Cause the only thing you can do is get us all into big trouble."

"You agreed with me at first," Annie reminded her.

392

"I was upset then. I wasn't thinking clearly. Understand, Annie, Nick is right, it's *our* secret, and if none of us blow it we'll keep it that way."

"How can you forget what happened?" Annie demanded. "That poor man – what about his family? Don't you *care?*"

"Stop giving me that poor man crap," Cyndra said, angrily. "He was in a motel room with me, wasn't he? He thought I was a hooker. You should have heard the names he called me."

"He didn't deserve to die for it."

"It was an *accident*, Annie. Reece didn't shoot him purposely, it was just one of those things. Like when you get on a plane you don't expect it to crash. When you go for a ride in a car you don't expect it to be totalled. These things happen."

"I still think –" Annie began.

"Will you shut up," Cyndra said, finally losing her temper, her dark eyes blazing. "Shut up about it, Annie."

She went through her apartment and packed all of Reece's clothes into two suitcases, stacking them in a closet by the front door. Nick had suggested that as he was going to be in New York for at least six weeks she should give up her apartment and move into his. Since she didn't have any money it struck her as an excellent idea. He'd also left her his rented car to drive, so at least she was mobile.

Searching through Reece's papers she found the name of the producer he'd been dealing with at Reno Records. Marik Lee. She called him on the phone and asked if she could drop by.

"Where's your manager?" Marik asked, sounding guarded.

"You mean Reece Webster?"

"That's the guy."

"He's no longer my manager."

"Good," he said.

"Good?" she questioned. "How come?"

"Drop by and we'll discuss it."

She didn't need a second invitation. Within the hour she was at his office – dressed to make an impression in a tight red dress which showed off her figure and flattered her glowing skin. Her hair, dark and lustrous, fell almost to her waist.

Marik Lee did a double take when she walked in. "*You're* Cyndra?" he said, standing up.

She nodded, checking him out. He was black, a little over-weight, and kind of homely looking, but he had nice eyes and a big friendly smile. "Why do you sound so surprised?" she asked, sitting in a chair across from his desk and crossing her legs.

His eyes wandered. "I had no idea you were so . . . so . . . pretty."

"Thank you," she said demurely, accepting the compliment.

"Now tell me," he continued. "That guy you were hitched up with – that uh – Reece Webster. He definitely out the picture?"

"Yes," she replied. "Very definitely."

"Between you and me he was a bad case. We don't like to get involved in those situations."

"What situations?"

"Y'know what I'm saying. He talked about you like you were a slab of meat, like you'd do anything he wanted. We expect our talent to be able to talk for themselves."

She sat up very straight. "Oh, I can talk for myself all right."

He looked at her appreciatively. "Yeah, I can see that."

She thought about Nick in New York about to get his big chance. She wasn't planning on playing the little sister role – dragging along behind. She had every intention of making it just as big as he.

"Mr Lee," she said, boldly.

"Call me Marik."

"Marik. Tell me the truth – do Reno Records and I have a future together, or am I wasting my time?"

Nick was in the wardrobe trailer trying on different clothes.

"They're very happy with the dailies," Waldo confided, *sotto voce*.

"Dailies?" he said, zipping up a pair of tight black jeans.

"Oh, Nick, *please*. Surely you know what I'm talking about? The dailies are the scenes from the previous day. My friend is the projectionist – I get a full report."

He was pleased. "So they like me?"

"Yes, they certainly do. Why do you think they hired you in place of Charlie? They took one look at your close-ups and realized they had something with you. According to my friend the camera simply loves you." He reached for a pair of cowboy boots. "Try these, please."

Nick sat down grabbing the boots. "Yeah, well – I always knew I could do this," he said, pulling on the left boot.

"You can do it all right, although of course, there's no such

394

thing as a sure thing. You might have what it takes and the audience can still hate you."

"No way they'll hate me," he said, confidently. "I'm putting everything I've got into this performance. They're gonna respond. You'll see – they're gonna respond big time."

"I'm sure they will," Waldo said, selecting a denim jacket from the rack. "And what are we wearing tonight when we take little Miss Madam out?"

He pulled on the other boot and stood up. "How come my date with Carlysle is public knowledge?"

"This is a film set, Nick. If you fart in the privacy of your dressing room everyone knows about it."

"Great!"

"Just be careful with little Madam. She appears to be angelic, but watch out."

He grinned. "Hey – Waldo – this may come as a big shock to you, but when it comes to women I know my way around the block an' back again."

"Actresses are not women," Waldo murmured. "Oh dear me, no."

Nick burst out laughing. "You're a character, you know that?"

"You have been warned," Waldo said, primly. "Nobody can say you haven't been warned."

"Thanks, but I guess I'll take a chance."

Waldo rolled his eyes.

"Hi," Carlysle said, greeting him at her apartment door wearing nothing but a welcoming smile and a skimpy bath towel wrapped sarong style around her body.

"Uh . . . hi," he said, standing on the threshold.

"Come on in," she said. "As you can see, I'm not quite ready."

Oh, he could see all right!

She led him into a comfortable living room and waved him in the direction of a small bar. "Fix yourself a drink. I'll be quick – I promise."

"Take your time," he said, checking the place out.

"Ooops!" Her towel slipped and she quickly hitched it up, but not before he caught a glimpse of her large, rosy, disturbingly erect nipples.

She noticed him looking and giggled, her blue eyes widening. "Isn't it stupid the way we all try to hide ourselves? Wouldn't it be better to walk around without anything on? After all, we weren't born fully dressed, were we?"

"Works for me," he said, opening the ice-box behind the bar and extracting a beer.

"Good," said Carlysle, dropping the towel.

Instant erection. He didn't even have time to think about it.

"Why don't you take your clothes off, too?" she said, with an innocent little smile.

"Hey –" he began.

"You're not shy, are you?" she teased.

No, baby, I'm not shy, but I am used to being the instigator and this is a different trip.

He shrugged off his jacket and began unbuttoning his shirt.

Carlysle was not a patient girl. She ran towards him and went right for his zipper, pulling down his pants and underwear. Before he knew what was happening she had him in her mouth giving him one of the finest blow jobs known to man! He came in record time because it was so unexpected and so good, and the truth was he hadn't gotten laid in a while and he was beyond horny.

"Ah . . . Jesus!" he groaned. "That was . . ."

"Yes?" she asked breathlessly, still on her knees.

"Pretty . . . damn . . . good."

"Good? Surely you mean sensational?"

"That, too. C'mere," he said, reaching for her breasts.

She jumped to her feet, skipping out of his range. "Later," she said, in a little girl voice. "Gotta get dressed. It wouldn't do to be late for the party, would it now?"

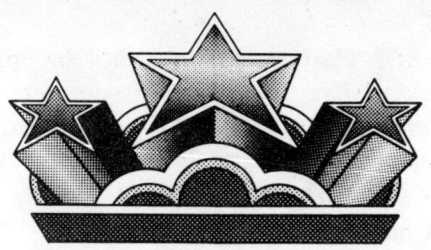

Chapter 62

The guests had all arrived, the hors-d'œuvres had been served and Lauren began her own private countdown to dinner. Her two assistants, Hilary and Karen, knew her well, anticipating her every request. Actually, the truth was she'd trained them so efficiently they could probably do it without her. Which was good, because when she and Oliver were married she'd have to delegate a lot more. Oliver had already told her he wanted her to travel with him, and why not – she was dying to see Europe. He took six weeks' vacation every year, travelling through Italy, France and England. Help Unlimited would just have to manage without her for a few weeks.

Jessie popped into the kitchen. "Almost ready," she said, beaming in her severe, man's-style velvet suit. "The melon and caviar was a riot!"

"We're all set when you are," Lauren said, adjusting the flame under her sautéd carrots.

"Spectacular!" exclaimed Jessie.

One of the things Lauren liked about catering dinners for the Georges was their unbridled enthusiasm. Quentin – whenever he appeared – was exactly like his wife. The two of them enjoyed life and it was infectious.

"Who's out there tonight?" Lauren asked Hilary, who'd been busy serving hors-d'œuvres.

Hilary recited a list of celebrities – including a controversial black politician, an avant-garde dress designer, a famous ball player and two movie stars. Jessie sure loved to mix people up.

Lauren decided Oliver would be happy when he dropped by. He enjoyed hanging out with celebrities. She didn't. If she was lucky she wouldn't have to emerge from the kitchen all night long.

"Did you like it?" Carlysle giggled, holding tightly on to his arm in the back of her limo. "Was it the best – the very *very* best you've ever had?"

He grinned, lazily. "The best."

She squeezed his arm. "Don't lie to me, or I'll have to do it again – right now – in the car."

He laughed. "Sure."

Her blue eyes sparkled. "You think I wouldn't?"

"I'm positive you would."

"Want me to?" she asked, stroking his thigh.

He felt himself getting hard again. "What about the driver?" he said.

She pressed a button and the black privacy glass slid up. "Oh, he's not getting any – he's *definitely* not on my list."

Before he could question her about what list that might be, she was on him again – going for his zipper with practised hands – springing him free – and bending her blonde curls.

He gave himself up to the moment, pressing the top of her head, forcing himself into her mouth as deep as she could take him.

This time he lasted longer, and when he came it was an explosion. "*Shit!*" he exclaimed, falling back on the leather seat. "Holy *shit!*"

She laughed, triumphantly. "I'm good, huh?"

"You're great."

"The greatest?"

What was it with this girl? All she wanted to hear was how great she was. "Yes," he said.

"The greatest you've ever had?"

He reached for her breasts again, but she slapped his hands away. "We're here," she said. "Didn't you notice the car stop?"

"Sweetheart," he sighed, "I didn't notice anything but you."

He'd said the right thing. Carlysle beamed like a cat who'd just devoured a saucer full of cream – and in a way she had.

"Later I'm gonna fuck you," he said.

"Later I'm going to let you," she replied.

Grinning, they alighted from the limo and entered the house.

The vichyssoise was served. The guests were happy. In the

kitchen Lauren concentrated on the mashed potatoes, making sure they had just the right combination of cream, butter and milk. Cooking was therapeutic. She really enjoyed creating a meal and watching as all the empty plates came back into the kitchen.

"Carlysle Mann just arrived," Hilary said. "She's *sooo* pretty."

"You're pretty, too," Lauren said, crisply. "You're equally as pretty as any movie star."

"No way!"

"Yes, you are."

"She's got fantastic skin," Hilary said, enviously.

"Talking of skin – did you see the guy she's with?" Karen said, joining in.

"Cute," they both said in unison. "Very *veree* cute." They burst out giggling.

Oh, to be young again, Lauren thought. Hilary and Karen were so bright-eyed and full of life. She was only six years older than them, but sometimes she felt like a staid old lady. "Come on, girls, concentrate," she said. "Let's get this meal on the road."

Carlysle's hand began creeping up his leg again. Shit! She was actually doing it in front of all these people. And important people, too. He glanced around the table and couldn't believe he was sitting amongst them.

"Hey – stop that," he whispered.

"Why?" she whispered back.

"'Cause somebody's gonna see."

"So what?" she replied.

"So what? You're crazy – you know that?"

She leaned very close and nibbled on his earlobe. "If I had my way I'd give you a blow job right under the table now."

This girl was not bluffing. "You would too, wouldn't you?"

"Ooops! I dropped my napkin – excuse me." She started to dive under the table.

He grabbed her arm, stopping her. "Don't you dare!" he warned.

"So, Carlysle sweetie," said Jessie, turning in their direction. "How's your new film going?"

"We only just started," said Carlysle, abandoning her under-the-table plan. "I guess you heard about Charlie? He had a kind of . . . uh, virus."

"I'm so sorry. Is he in the hospital?"

"Not exactly. Well, sort of – yeah, I guess you could say he is."

"I always thought you two made such an adorable couple," Jessie said.

"Uh . . . thanks."

Jessie turned away to talk to the politician on her other side.

Nick nudged Carlysle. "I didn't know you and Charlie were a couple."

"We weren't," she said, shortly.

"Then why'd she say that?"

"We went on a few dates – that's not exactly being a couple."

He imagined her on her knees in front of Charlie and he wasn't too thrilled. But still, he hardly knew her, he couldn't start acting possessive at this stage.

Soon she began trying to unzip his jeans again, her hands working feverishly.

"Give me a break!" he objected, catching a look from the dress designer on his other side who had orange hair and an attitude.

Carlysle giggled. "Stop acting like a prude."

This girl was a wild one.

Oliver arrived at the dessert stage.

"The dinner was simply divine," Jessie informed him. "You're marrying the best cook in the world."

Oliver was amused. "I'm not marrying Lauren for her cooking, Jessie, dear."

"I'm sure you're not."

He put his head around the kitchen door. Lauren was busy organizing desserts. She'd baked two *tartes tatins*, and a batch of double chocolate brownies.

"You're busy," he said.

"Very astute," she said.

"Jessie wants you to come out and join the party."

"I can't do that. Anyway, I'm not dressed."

"You're more beautiful than any of the guests."

"You're such a smooth talker, Oliver."

"Which is *exactly* why I'm where I am today."

She ladled whipped cream into a cut glass dish. "Oliver, please – I'm trying to get this together."

He nodded, understandingly. "Very well, I'll go and sit down and wait patiently. When you're ready I'll take you home."

What about my surprise? she wanted to say. She'd been looking forward to a puppy all night, but then again he couldn't have brought it to the Georges' house. Maybe he had it waiting at home.

Everybody carried on about the delicious desserts. Jessie had squeezed Oliver in between Quentin and a vivacious book editor with teased black hair. Suddenly she stood up, tapping the side of her champagne glass. "Listen, everyone, I have an announcement," she said, beaming around the table.

Nick felt Carlysle's hand slide inside his zipper. This was wild, but he couldn't help being aroused.

"I know you've all enjoyed the excellent food tonight, and I'm bringing our chef out to allow you to thank her personally. You may also congratulate her, because she and Oliver Liberty are engaged. You all know Oliver, but I don't think you've met his lovely fiancée." Jessie beckoned a waiter. "Have Lauren come out," she said.

In the kitchen Lauren was mortified. "I'm not going out there," she said, backing into a corner. "What does she think this is – a show?"

Karen gave her a little shove. "You have to, she's waiting."

"Oh, no!" Lauren groaned.

"Oh, yes!" Karen and Hilary chorused, enjoying every minute. They loved working for Lauren, and they were delighted to see her get the kind of attention she deserved.

Reluctantly she allowed herself to be propelled to the dining-room doorway. If there was one thing she hated it was being the centre of attention.

"Ah, Lauren, dear, there you are." Jessie raised her champagne glass. "Here's to you."

There was an enthusiastic round of applause from the guests.

She felt like a total fool. Her eyes scanned the dinner table, checking out the guests. She looked once, twice and couldn't believe her eyes. Nick Angelo was there. *Her* Nick was actually at this dinner.

No, it couldn't be.

Yes, it was.

She looked again. He was older, more handsome than ever, skinnier. His eyes were still deep green and intense. His hair

401

that incredible jet black. Oh, God! She wanted to die. The only good thing was the fact that he hadn't seen her. He was all over the girl sitting beside him, who happened to be Carlysle Mann, the movie star.

Desperately Lauren tried to breathe, to recover her composure. *Move slowly. Get out before he spots me. Get the hell out!*

As she turned to bolt from the room he looked up and their eyes met. He was as startled as she was. They gazed at each other in disbelief before she broke the stare and rushed back into the kitchen. She didn't hesitate, grabbing her coat and purse she ran for the back door.

"Where are you going?" Hilary asked, startled.

"I don't feel good. I have to get out of here," she mumbled. "Tell Oliver I had to go."

"One of us should come with you," Hilary insisted.

"No – I have to get out now," she said, flinging open the door and racing out of the apartment before anyone could stop her.

"What's the matter?" Carlysle said. "What happened?"

His hard-on had deflated. "Nothing," he said, brushing her hand away as he surreptitiously tried to zip up his pants.

"What do you mean, nothing?" she said, her chin tilting belligerently.

He got up from the table. "'Scuse me, I gotta take a piss."

"I'll come with you," she volunteered. "You'd be surprised what we can get up to in the john."

"Hey – Carlysle, I'm not surprised at anything you do. Stay here. I'll be back."

Outside the dining room he grabbed a hovering waiter. "Where's the kitchen?"

"Through there, sir. Can I get you something?"

"Nah, it's okay," he said, hurrying into the kitchen.

She wasn't there. He stopped a pretty girl in a striped apron. "Where's Lauren?"

"She left," Hilary said, quite intrigued by this intense looking guy. "She didn't feel good."

"Where can I contact her?"

"Do you need to have a party catered? We have a very comprehensive service. Here – let me give you one of our cards."

402

She handed him a card and he stared at it. Help Unlimited was printed in the middle with an address and phone number. In neat script on either side were two names – Lauren Roberts and Pia Liberty.

"You can contact us any time," Hilary said, wishing he'd flirt with her. "During business hours, of course."

"Oh, I will," Nick said, pocketing the card. "Bet on it."

Chapter 63

The couple entwined on the bed made love fast and furiously until they climaxed with a series of grunts and moans.

"Oh, baby, baby, that was freakin' sensational!" said Marik.

Cyndra rolled away from him, flushed and surprised at her own boldness, yet at the same time strangely exhilarated. Marik had only been in her life a week, and she already had him in her power.

"Was it good for you too, baby?" he asked, sitting up and reaching for a cigarette.

"You *know* it was good for me," she replied, coming out with all the right words. "You're an amazing lover, Marik. The best."

They'd been to dinner at a cosy Italian restaurant, following an afternoon in the studio where she'd finally cut a demo record. Marik had liked what he'd heard. When they were finished in the studio he'd said, "We're goin' out to celebrate, 'cause when the big boss hears your sound – you're gonna be signin' your life away!"

She'd glowed with delight. "Really?"

"Yeah, babe. Really."

Cyndra liked Marik, he seemed nice enough. But more than that, she wanted something from him, and she was beginning to learn that if you wanted something you had to offer a prize in return. Her way of doing this was to get him into bed where she knew she had the power.

"Do you really like my voice?" she asked again, anxious to hear him repeat the compliment.

"Hey, baby, how many times I gotta tell you? You sound *good!* A little raw in places – nothing I can't fix when we record your first single."

She'd been waiting to hear those words from somebody legitimate all her life. She moved closer to him, brushing her breasts against his chest. "What happens next?"

"Anything you want," he said, puffing on his cigarette with a blissful smile.

"I want a contract."

"Baby, as far as I'm concerned – you got it."

"I want to start making money."

"I'm the man to do it for you."

"And I need somewhere to live. I moved out of my apartment. Right now I'm staying at my brother's."

"Oh, wow, you're in a bad way, huh?"

"I had to get away from Reece. Now I plan to start fresh."

"You will, baby. When the big boss hears your voice and takes a look at you, we're goin' all the way."

"That's exactly what I needed to hear."

He laughed. "Come back here, and I'll show you *exactly* what *I* need."

Marik was true to his word. Within a week she was installed in a new apartment, she'd signed a contract with Reno Records, and finally met the big boss. His name was Gordon D. Hayworth, and he was a powerful looking black man in his forties.

Gordon D. Hayworth was handsome – he was also married. As soon as Cyndra stepped into his office she'd noticed the family pictures on his desk. One wife – very beautiful. And two young children. The perfect American family.

"You've got some voice," he told her. "It's not strong – more soulful and sexy – but I like that."

"You do?" she asked, widening her eyes.

"Yes, I do," he replied. "We'll find the right single for you to record and see what happens."

"Really?"

He looked at her very seriously. "It's what you want, Cyndra, isn't it?"

"It's what I've always wanted, ever since I was a little girl."

"You must've been a cute little girl," he said, smiling.

She wondered how cute he would've thought she was when Mr Browning was raping her, when she was having the abortion, and all the other bad things that had happened to her.

"Yes, I was very cute," she said, smiling back.

"We're happy to have you with us, Cyndra," he said, standing up and walking around his desk to pat her on the shoulder in a fatherly fashion.

"I'm happy, too," she said.

"We'll be seeing lots of each other."

I hope so, she thought.

He continued to smile as he escorted her to the door.

She walked out of his office and realized for the first time in her life she'd met a man she knew she could fall in love with.

"I'm flying to New York to see Nick," Annie said.

"That's nice," Cyndra replied. "It'll be a break for you."

Annie frowned. "I have to be honest with you. I'm going there to tell him I can't keep quiet any longer."

Cyndra turned on her, her eyes flashing angrily. "*No,* Annie. How many times must I tell you? It's not just Nick you'll hurt – it's me. And now my career is about to take off, you mustn't do this."

"I have to," Annie said, stubbornly. "I can't live with myself and keep this secret."

"Screw you!" Cyndra exploded. "I'll deny it ever happened. Let them go out and search for the body. You'll look like a fool 'cause I'll deny everything. You're not dragging me down, girl, so don't you try it. I'll tell them you're crazy, I'll tell them you've always been crazy."

"You can say what you like," Annie said, refusing to look her in the eye. "But I'm going to the police when I get back."

As soon as she was alone Cyndra called Nick. "Annie's gonna blow it," she said. "You'd better be prepared to do something about her."

"I know what I have to do," he said.

"Good, 'cause otherwise we've both had it."

Chapter 64

"What happened?" Oliver said, standing on her doorstep trying to conceal his anger.

"I didn't feel well. I had to get out of there."

He tapped his foot impatiently. "May I come in?"

She wasn't in the mood to deal with him. "I still don't feel good, Oliver."

He walked past her into the living room. "Why didn't you tell me? I could have driven you, my car was downstairs."

She trailed behind him. "I needed some air. I walked halfway home."

He looked at her as if he didn't quite believe what he was hearing. "You left me there and walked home? You left me looking like a fool, Lauren."

"No, I didn't," she said, refusing to admit she might be wrong. "Nobody knew I'd gone."

"I'm sure they did."

"Please, Oliver, I'm not in the mood for a fight. I told you, I don't feel well."

"Do you need a doctor?"

"No, I'll be all right. It was just the pressure of cooking dinner, and their kitchen was so hot, and I just . . ." She trailed off and sighed. "Oliver, don't you ever feel that you're about to explode?"

"No," he said, in an irritated voice. "And if I did I would tell you."

"Thanks," she said, listlessly.

"Sometimes, Lauren, I don't understand you."

He could say that again. Perhaps she should enlighten him before it was too late.

"There's a lot about me you don't know. Maybe we should think about this marriage thing."

Now he was really aggravated. "I don't have to think about it, and nor do you."

"If I told you about my past you might change your mind."

"Oh, now you're going to tell me you have a hidden past, is that it?"

"It hasn't all been exactly *Little House on the Prairie*."

"Listen, my dear, everyone has secrets. I have no need to hear yours. I love you, that's enough for me."

She was determined to be heard whether he liked it or not. "When my parents were killed I went to live in Philadelphia with my aunt and uncle. I had an affair with my cousin."

"Am I supposed to be upset about that?"

"Then I came to New York, met Jimmy and slept with him."

Oliver frowned; he was not enjoying this. "Lauren, how old are you?"

"Twenty-four."

"You're twenty-four years old and you've had affairs with two men. You wouldn't be normal if you hadn't." His tone softened. "You know, darling, I hardly imagined you were a virgin."

"There was somebody else – somebody I knew when I was very young."

"Who was that?" he asked, patiently.

"A boy in High school."

"What about him?"

"Oh, nothing . . ." She trailed off. There was no point in telling him about Nick. "Please, Oliver, I really need to be alone. We'll talk tomorrow. Go home."

"I was going to give you your surprise," he said, refusing to budge.

"Give it to me tomorrow."

His lips formed a thin tight line. "Very well," he said, obviously not at all pleased. "Get a good night's rest." He pecked her on the cheek and left.

As soon as he was gone she paced around her apartment a nervous wreck. God! She was so confused. She didn't know what to do or what to think. She'd never imagined running into Nick. As far as she was concerned he was out of her life forever. And yet there he was, sitting at the dinner party with that Carlysle person, and every feeling she'd ever had for him came flooding back over her. She'd loved him so very much, she would have given her life for him.

Seeing him again had unnerved her. Her memories of him were so vivid. And he'd looked so good, so great, so fantastic.

Get real. Nick Angelo is your past.

It doesn't have to be that way.

Yes, it does.

Had he seen her? Had he recognized her? Their eyes had met for an instant and yes – she knew without a doubt he'd recognized her.

If only she could tell somebody, but there was nobody to confide in. Who would understand about her and Nick? They'd say it was a teenage crush, a stupid little affair. But it wasn't. She'd lived for him and he'd crushed her.

Nick Angelo – why was she getting in such a state? He was a son-of-a-bitch. He'd dumped her like all the others. He'd set the pattern.

Well, she'd show him. She was marrying Oliver Liberty, a man of substance. And when she was Mrs Liberty he couldn't touch her ever again.

The next morning she woke up and fervently wished it had all been a dream. She showered, brushed her teeth, put on her make-up, dressed and went into the office.

As soon as she walked in Pia was on her case. "Nick Angelo called," she said. "He sounded anxious to reach you. Who is he?"

Her stomach did a somersault. "Nobody important – tear the message up."

On her desk there were a dozen red roses from Oliver and a note asking her to meet him for lunch. She knew he must be feeling anxious; they were supposed to leave for the Bahamas in two days and her behaviour had obviously unsettled him.

"Uh, Pia . . . do me a favour," she said, staring at the roses.

"Yes?"

"If Nick Angelo calls again, say I've left town. In fact, you can tell him I'm about to be married and don't give him any other information."

"Who is he?" Pia asked, curiously.

"Oh . . . just somebody I knew a long time ago in High school."

"He's got a great voice," Pia said. "Kind of sexy."

"That's nice," she replied, wishing Pia would get off the subject.

Oliver was waiting when she arrived at the restaurant. "Feeling better today?" he asked, solicitous as ever.

"Much better, thank you," she said, sliding in beside him.

"Good. Because I have your surprise."

"Does it bark and eat plenty of food?"

"No, my dear, it is not a puppy, you know how I feel about puppies. I refuse to have them peeing all over my Persian rugs."

"Then I'm very disappointed, Oliver."

"You won't be," he said, groping for a large envelope on the banquette seating. "Take a look," he said, handing it to her.

"What is it?"

"Open it and you'll see."

She opened the envelope and pulled out a large poster. Staring at her was her own image. Above the photograph in bold lettering were the words: THE NEW MARCELLA GIRL!

"What's this?" she asked.

"You can see what it is. It's your photograph from the session."

"I know, but why does it say The New Marcella Girl?"

"Because, my darling, that's exactly who you're going to be."

Carlysle tried every way she knew how, but she could not get any further action out of Nick that night. Unbeknown to her he was in a state of shock because he couldn't believe he'd run into Lauren after all those years. It was all he could do to escort Carlysle home.

"Aren't you coming up?" she asked, as he helped her from the limo.

"Nah, early call," he explained.

"So've I," she pointed out. "We could go in to the studio together."

"I got a headache," he said.

"*You've* got a headache?" she laughed, hysterically. "Isn't that supposed to be *my* line?"

She went for his zipper again. He slapped her hand away.

"What happened?" she demanded. "I thought we were having a good time."

"We were. It's nothing personal."

"God, you're behaving really strangely."

He was behaving strangely? Had she ever thought about her own behaviour?

"Look, I'll see you on the set tomorrow," he said.

She marched into her apartment building without a backward glance. Her driver took him back to his hotel.

He couldn't get over seeing Lauren. What exactly was she doing in New York? And who was the old guy she was engaged to?

How could she be engaged to a man old enough to be her grandfather? And how come she hadn't acknowledged him? She must have busted her ass to get out of there so fast.

He had so many questions and he needed answers. It wasn't that he was going to forgive her for not answering his letters, but it would be nice to find out why.

At the hotel there was a message from Annie. He returned her call.

"I'm coming in," she announced.

"Oh . . . that's great," he said, thinking it wasn't so great. The last thing he needed was Annie.

"I'll be arriving tomorrow at four. Will you meet me?"

"I'm on the set," he said. "But I'll arrange to have someone there."

"We have to talk," she said.

Oh, Christ! Cyndra was right, this didn't sound good.

First thing in the morning he called Help Unlimited.

A female voice said, "Pia Liberty. Can I help you?"

"Yeah, let me talk to Lauren."

"She's not in yet."

"I need to get in touch with her like immediately."

"I'll see she gets the message."

"Maybe you can give me her home number."

"No, I'm sorry."

"We're friends from way back."

"I'm sure you are, but we never divulge personal numbers. Why don't you call again at ten?"

He took off for the studio. Carlysle greeted him with a scowl; she was obviously unused to not getting her own way.

He studied his script, conferred with the director and tried to throw himself into character, but it was difficult holding his concentration. As soon as he got a break he rushed to the phone. "Is Lauren in yet?"

"I'm sorry, you've missed her. She's left town. She's getting married, you know."

"Is this Pia?"

"Good memory."

"Listen, Pia, I *have* to talk to her. It's very important."

"I gave her your message. Maybe she'll call you."

"You don't understand. We really go back a long way."

"She said she'd contact you."

"She did?"

"Yes."

He hung up the phone feeling depressed. What was he chasing her for anyway? She'd dumped him. What more could he have done than written her a hundred times without receiving one single reply.

The truth was – if he wanted to face up to it – Lauren Roberts had never wanted him. It had all been a game for her. Nick Angelo – the jerk from the wrong side of the tracks – and pretty little Lauren Roberts, who'd amused herself at his expense.

Well screw her. Let her go off and marry some rich old man. What did he care?

But deep down he did care. And although he'd never admit it, seeing her again had stirred up every painful memory of the love he'd once had for her.

He wanted Lauren to be his past. Somehow he knew it wasn't possible.

Chapter 65

Annie had her own agenda – he knew it as soon as she arrived direct from the airport and came straight to the set. In New York she looked very Californian with her deep suntan, athletic body and brightly coloured clothes.

"Who's she?" Carlysle demanded, the moment Annie hit the set.

"A friend," Nick replied.

Carlysle smiled a secret smile. "I bet she doesn't give head like I do."

Waldo, hovering on the sidelines, raised his eyebrows and tut tutted.

"She's not my girlfriend," Nick explained to Carlysle.

"You haven't fucked her?" Carlysle questioned.

"No."

"But she wants you to."

"Why do you say that?"

"Take a look at her, Nick, she's mooning after you like a baby who wants to suck mama's tit," Carlysle giggled, wickedly. "Only it's not your tit she wants to suck."

"Has anybody ever told you you've got sex on the mind?"

"Something wrong with that?"

One thing about Carlysle, she wasn't a clinger. She didn't give a damn who he was sleeping with – which was just as well because he didn't plan on answering to anyone.

He introduced Annie to the director, which pleased her. Later she sat in his chair and watched while they shot a restaurant scene. When it was done she reluctantly admitted he was good.

"Thanks," he said.

"Joy would be proud of you. Aren't you glad I took you to her class?"

Was this her subtle way of telling him that if she hadn't taken him to Joy Byron's class none of this would have happened?

Filming finished shortly before seven, and they rode back to his hotel in a cab.

"I booked you a room," he said. "It's one floor up from me. Oh, and they need to know how long you're staying."

"That depends on you," she said, in an edgy voice.

Shit! Why did it depend on him?

"What d'you mean?" he asked.

She stared straight at him. "How long do *you* want me to stay?"

Carlysle was right. Annie was waiting for him to make a move, and unfortunately the only way he could stop her from opening up her mouth to the cops was to make her his girlfriend.

They ate Chinese food in a nearby restaurant, talked about the movie and LA and Cyndra's record deal. Then they got down to the real reason she'd come to New York.

"I suppose Cyndra warned you," she said, sipping Chinese tea. "I'm sorry to do this to you, Nick – but it's too big a burden for me to carry any longer."

"Yeah," he said, thinking about how to handle her. "I understand."

She was surprised. "You do?"

"I know how difficult it must be for you, Annie. You're all alone – you've got nobody to talk to – you're trying to get connected and acting jobs aren't easy. Yeah, I understand." He moved right along, talking about Joy and the class and her job at the health club.

She was confused. She'd expected him to try and talk her out of going to the police and she'd had all her arguments ready. But no, he'd gone completely in the opposite direction and it wasn't what she'd expected.

On the walk back to the hotel he put his arm around her, held her hand and told her how pretty she looked. By the time he got her to his room on the pretext of rehearsing the next day's scene, she was all his. But still he proceeded carefully, and when he started to undress her she was more than ready.

He took it slowly – pacing himself – going at her speed, which was slow. She did have a terrific body – compact and muscled, not really his type – he liked his women on the more voluptuous side.

When they finally made it he was shocked to discover she

was a virgin. "You must be the only virgin left in Hollywood," he joked, trying not to hurt her as he went for the final thrust.

"Don't joke about it, Nick," she gasped. "I believe in waiting."

He broke through and felt her gush. Then he proceeded to make her very happy indeed.

By the time he was finished he knew the cops would be the last place she'd go.

Annie stayed a week. The moment she left he resumed service with Carlysle, whose only comment was why hadn't the three of them got it on.

"You're somethin' else," he said, shaking his head.

With Annie safely back in LA they proceeded to have sex whenever and wherever they could. It became a standing joke that if either of them were needed on the set they had to be prised apart first. Their on screen love scenes were sizzling, especially when Carlysle did things to him under the sheets that nobody knew about except the two of them.

He got to see the dailies and knew it was working for him. Carlysle and he had great chemistry.

Most nights they went out. Carlysle was invited everywhere, and there was always a party or opening. She really got off on public sex – the more dangerous the better. They'd done some form of sexual activity everywhere from the first night of a Broadway show to the toniest restaurant. And he never made a limo trip without Carlysle giving him one of her famous blow jobs.

"Don't you ever get tired?" he asked, only half-jokingly.

"I've got the rest of my life to get tired. Live for the moment, Nick – we won't be around forever."

If she carried on at this pace she'd wear out his dick! And then where would he be?

The female producer started paying more attention to him. He figured her to be in her early forties, but extremely well-preserved. One day she informed him she had a script she'd like him to read and invited him up to her hotel suite.

"Can *I* come, too?" Carlysle begged.

"No," he said firmly.

"She wants to fuck you," Carlysle said.

"According to you everyone wants to fuck me."

"When this movie comes out they will. You can take odds on it."

Carlysle, as usual, was right. The producer poured him a vodka on the rocks and sat opposite him, crossing and uncrossing her long elegant legs while he attempted to read the script. She'd already informed him it was under wraps and could not leave her hands.

Twenty pages in and she dropped her skirt, revealing a black lace garter belt, stockings and a black bush. She obviously did not believe in panties.

He remembered the stop light where she'd ignored him and he fucked her good.

Afterwards she asked him what he thought of the script.

"Not bad," he said, confidently. "But the fuck was great."

Carlysle wanted details. She savoured every juicy one, and it so turned her on that they made out in an alley behind the latest hot disco where they were attending a party.

Meanwhile he called Annie every other day. She sounded fine. He was relieved; at least he had her under control.

One day he received a distraught call from Joey's hooker girlfriend.

"Those bastards beat Joey up good," she said. "He's in the hospital."

As soon as he finished work he rushed over to visit. Joey lay in a public ward with bandaged limbs and a pulped face. His eyes were mere slits and his lips swollen to twice their size.

"This is really nice," Nick said, cheerfully. "Can't leave you alone for a minute. How'd it happen?"

"Got inna fight," Joey mumbled.

"What with – a meat truck?"

Joey tried to raise his arm. "Don' make me laugh."

Later he talked to Joey's girlfriend again and found out the true story. According to her Joey owed big drug money on account of a heroin habit he wasn't about to quit.

"I'll take care of it," Nick promised, and he went to Carlysle and asked to borrow money so he could help Joey out. "I wanna put him into some kinda clinic – get him straight," he explained. "It costs, an' I don't have that kinda bucks. This'll be a loan – I'll even pay interest."

Carlysle was unconcerned. "My mother handles all my money," she said, blithely dismissing his problem. "I can't touch it."

You could if you wanted to, bitch.

He went to his producer. She asked questions. Satisfied with his answers she agreed to the loan in exchange for an option agreement making him available for her next film.

In Los Angeles Meena Caron objected bitterly. "I'm hearing excellent reports, Nick. It would be suicide to tie you up now."

"Gotta help a friend," he explained, and signed the agreement.

Before the movie was over the word was out. There was a new hot property on the horizon. And his name was Nick Angel.

Chapter 66

"Do you, Lauren Roberts, take this man, Oliver Liberty, to be your lawfully wedded husband?"

She hesitated for only a second. "I do," she said, breathlessly.

"Do you, Oliver Liberty, take this woman, Lauren Roberts, to be your lawfully wedded wife?"

He turned to look at her, his eyes full of pride. "I do."

They stood on the terrace of his house in the Bahamas over-looking a glorious never-ending white beach and a bluer-than-blue ocean. The setting was idyllic. Lauren wore a simple white dress and flowers in her hair. Their witnesses were Oliver's housekeeper and her husband – a friendly black couple who did nothing but beam happily.

When she said, "I do," Lauren felt a shudder of apprehension. She was giving her life to another human being. She was joining with Oliver and things would never be quite the same.

It's what you want, isn't it, Roberts?

No.

Don't think that way.

What I want is Nick Angelo.

Oh, for God's sake.

Oliver bent to kiss her and she quickly shut out the images of her past.

Later that night they dined quietly, just the two of them on the terrace overlooking the sea.

"So, my darling," he said, clasping her hand. "How do you feel?"

She wasn't sure how she felt. "Light-headed, I guess."

"That's good, because I feel I'm the luckiest man in the world," he said, clinking his champagne glass with hers.

She sipped her champagne, and listened to the soothing sound of the surf.

I'm Mrs Oliver Liberty.
He's forty years older than you.
I don't care.
You've married a father figure.
That's not true.

After dinner Oliver retired to his study to make a few phone calls. "It'll give you time to relax," he said.

Why would she require time to relax on her wedding night?

She wandered around the house, finally settling in the master bedroom. It was a light and airy room with another picturesque view. Decorated in earth tones, there was an intricate white lace cover on the bed and piles of luxurious cushions. She wondered who'd decorated it. Wife number one or wife number two? She decided it was wife number one – far too tasteful for wife number two.

In the pale beige limestone bathroom she took a shower and slipped into the sheer white nightgown she'd purchased especially for her wedding night. By the time she returned to the bedroom Oliver was lying on the bed in silk pyjamas perusing a stack of mail.

"Don't you ever stop?" she asked, standing silhouetted in the doorway.

"I believe in taking advantage of every moment. This is correspondence I didn't have time to deal with before I left."

She moved over to the bed. "Was it absolutely necessary to bring it on our honeymoon?"

He must have noticed her tone of annoyance, because he pushed the mail to one side. "I'm sorry," he said, reaching for her hand. "You, my darling," he continued, looking at her for the first time, "are absolutely ravishing."

Will you ravish me tonight, Oliver?
Will you ravish me until I can't breathe?

"Thank you," she murmured.

"Come over here," he said, pulling her down on to the bed.

This was the first night of their married life and she wanted it to be memorable. So far their sex life had not progressed very far. Oliver kept on telling her that when they were married things would be different, and she was ready for the change. She needed a man to take her on a passionate trip. Only Nick had managed to satisfy her every need, and she craved that same satisfaction.

Oliver began to kiss and caress her. She responded with a passion she'd kept hidden from him before.

419

"Oliver, tonight should be memorable . . ." she murmured, voicing her thoughts.

"Isn't our lovemaking always memorable?" he asked, smoothly.

No, it's not, she wanted to reply. *We've never made love properly. All you've done is make love to me with your tongue.*

She demonstrated with actions what she wanted to do to him. As she began to bend her head, he stopped her abruptly.

"What are you doing?"

"I'm going to make you very happy."

"No, Lauren, I don't like you to do that."

"But you do it to me all the time. In fact, that's all you do."

"Because you deserve it."

Deserve it? What kind of comment is that?

"Oliver, let me do this to you. You know you'll love it."

"No, Lauren, I will not love it. I refuse to see you in that position."

"I only want to please you," she said.

"I know, my darling, but that doesn't please me. It's an act I associate with sex for sale. It's demeaning and I don't expect you to do it."

She was shocked by his words. Surely, when two people were married, nothing was demeaning if it was something they both desired? But if that's the way he wanted it, so be it.

They kissed and caressed some more. His hands fondled her breasts, stroking her gently. Then his head began travelling down her body, heading for what he considered to be his proper destination.

Some women might be wild with joy at the thought of a man who gave them non-stop oral sex, but she'd had enough. Especially as he wouldn't allow her to do it to him.

"No, Oliver," she said, moving. "I want you to make love to me properly."

"But, my darling, you enjoy every second of what I do to you."

"Tonight it should be different," she said, reaching to feel his hardness – disappointed to discover he was only semi-erect.

"Lauren, my darling," he said, drawing away.

"Yes?"

"I have no desire to disappoint you."

"Why would you disappoint me?"

"Because I'm not twenty-five."

She couldn't help being sarcastic. "Oh, really? And I thought you were."

"Don't be flippant. When I was a young man I made love all night long. When I got to be older I realized there were other pleasures that could give a woman more joy than anything else."

"What are you saying?"

"I'm not sure I can satisfy you in the way you expect."

"Why can't we try?"

"It's simply that . . ." He hesitated. "Well . . . since I had my pacemaker –"

"Pacemaker?" she said, alarmed.

"Surely I mentioned it? About two years ago I had a heart irregularity, nothing serious. My doctors decided a pacemaker would solve the problem."

"You never told me, Oliver."

"I probably didn't think it was that important."

"Of course it's important. We're married. I should know everything about you."

"Why – would it have made a difference?"

"No . . ." Her mind was racing. A pacemaker. Did that mean he was sick? If they made love could he suddenly die? Oh God, what had she gotten herself into?

He stepped off the bed and walked over to the window. "I'm sorry, my dear. You're right, I should have told you."

She tried to make it better for him. "Well, you didn't and now I know. But we can still make love, can't we?"

"Yes."

"Then come back to bed. I'm not demanding. All I want is to be close to you."

They stayed in the Bahamas for ten days, during which time Lauren realized she'd married a man who was not prepared to consummate their marriage in the normal way. The truth was he wanted to make love to her his way or not at all. And although his way was very pleasant, it was hardly the same as being joined together with another person.

Oliver was also obsessed with business. She'd thought that once he was away from the office he'd be able to relax.

She'd imagined long walks on the beach, swimming, snorkelling, maybe taking a boat out. She did all of those things by herself, because Oliver spent most of his time on the phone.

Occasionally the subject of the Marcella girl came up. When he'd first suggested the idea she'd said a very resounding no. However, he wasn't prepared to take no for an answer. Every other day he asked if she'd changed her mind.

"I told you, Oliver, I'm not a model, nor do I want to be."

"I understand," he replied. "But this is hardly a modelling assignment. You'll be spokesperson for Marcella. You'll also make a lot of money, become well-known and enjoy every minute of it."

She disagreed. The idea of making money was appealing, but she had no wish to become well-known.

Pia called from New York. "Well? Are you going to do it or not?"

"Not," she said, firmly.

"You're blowing an opportunity if you don't," Pia said. "What have you got to lose? Oh, and by the way, take a look in yesterday's *New York News*. There's a photo of that Nick Angel guy – the one who called you. You didn't tell me he was an actor. And you certainly didn't tell me he was gorgeous."

When Lauren hung up she immediately searched for yesterday's New York papers. Sure enough, on page five of the *News* there was a picture of Nick with Carlysle Mann. She studied the picture, then read the copy:

Carlysle Mann, out on the town with her new co-star, Nick Angel. Carlysle and Nick are shooting Night City *on location in New York. Word has it that Nick lights up the screen – especially in the sex scenes – of which there are many. Ladies look out . . . he could be your new Saturday night rave . . .*

Nick was actually in a movie! She could hardly believe it. Nick Angel – whatever happened to Angelo? God! He was a professional actor. He'd done what they'd both talked and dreamed about.

She stared at his picture again, and hated Carlysle – which was stupid, because she didn't even know her. Then she read the copy through three times, folded the paper and put it in a drawer.

Later that day she approached Oliver. As usual, he was on the phone.

"Hang up," she said, standing in front of him.

He covered the mouthpiece. "What's the matter?"

"Hang up. I have to talk to you."

422

He excused himself and put the phone down. "I hope this is important," he said, irritably.

"It is."

"Well?"

"I'm accepting."

"You're accepting what?"

"I'll be the Marcella girl."

He perked up. "Really?"

"Yes, Oliver. And I want Samm to be my agent. She'll negotiate my price."

He laughed. "*She'll* negotiate your price?"

"I'm expensive," Lauren said. "But if you want me you'll pay."

Back in New York Pia waddled around looking like she was going to drop the kid any moment. Lauren realized that if she was going to embark on this Marcella girl campaign, then it was time to think seriously about Help Unlimited.

"What do you want to do?" she asked Pia. "You're having a baby, you've got the responsibility of Howard. Maybe we should dissolve the business."

"I *like* having the business," Pia said. "Although I suppose you're right. I won't have the time to spend there. And if you get the Marcella job, nor will you."

It was sad, but they decided the best thing to do was to close it down.

Lauren met with Samm, who was quite amused by the turn of events. "Do you realize how many of my models will want to scratch your eyes out, darling?" she said. "They'll say you used your influence with the boss."

"No, Samm – he used *his* influence with *me*. But I want a killer deal, otherwise I'm not doing it."

Samm nodded. "I like killer deals. Are you giving me permission to walk in and make the deal of the century?"

Lauren smiled. "That's *exactly* what I'm doing."

"And can I stroll casually away if they don't care to accept it?"

"I wouldn't expect you to do anything else."

"Lauren – you're my kind of girl."

Oliver came home that night with raised eyebrows. "Are you insane? You're asking for more money than a top model."

"Sweetheart, this was your idea, not mine. If Marcella would like me to represent them, then this is what they'll have to pay."

He shook his head. "I didn't realize I'd married a tough business woman."

"It wasn't my idea to be the Marcella girl, kindly remember that."

"I've talked with the client," Oliver said. "They have my recommendation. I've also given them several other suggestions. The final decision is theirs."

"Good," Lauren said. "Because I don't care either way."

Although deep down she did. Deep down she knew that she wanted to be somebody. Just like Nick Angel was going to be somebody. She didn't want to be left behind. She wanted to be just as important as he.

Chapter 67

"You need a publicist," Frances said.

"What for? I'm getting plenty of publicity. Carlysle and I are all over the columns."

"You need somebody to shape an image for you. Give you a profile – a very high profile."

"Forget it. I don't have the money."

"What did you do with the money you got for the option agreement you so foolishly signed against Meena's advice?"

He shrugged. "I had a friend in trouble. That was the deal."

"How sweet," Frances said, dragging deeply on her cigarette. "He has a kind heart."

"I always thought it was cool to help out friends," he said, throwing himself on her couch. "Isn't that the way it's supposed to work?"

"You really are a genuinely nice person," said Frances, sounding surprised.

"So I guess you've got a publicist you want to recommend," he said, reaching for a cigarette, deciding it was his turn to blow smoke in her face.

"You have to admit," Frances replied, "you *do* like my recommendations. Your new photographs are excellent and Meena is doing well for you. Of course, she could do better if you hadn't tied yourself up to that ridiculous option deal."

"Hey," he shrugged. "What's so ridiculous about signing for another movie? A couple of months ago I couldn't have gotten arrested. Why the big fuss?"

"Learn to understand this business," Frances said, sternly. "From all reports, when *Night City* comes out you're going to be hot. When you're hot is the time to act. But since you've tied yourself up for another film, Meena cannot do anything for you."

"Yeah, Frances, but I'm not a total jerk. I don't have to do the film immediately. There's a clause in there that says I can do something else if they're not ready by a certain date. It's cool."

"So now you've decided to be your own lawyer?"

"Hey, I've been meaning to talk to you about that. Can you recommend a good lawyer?"

"There's a cocktail party tomorrow night," Frances said. "You'll take me. There'll be several top lawyers there. You can quietly audition them."

"I don't know if I can make tomorrow night."

She looked at him sharply. "Nick, I don't expect you to forget our deal so early on in our relationship."

"Okay – I'll make it," he said.

He'd only gotten back to Los Angeles the day before after nearly two months shooting in New York, and although he'd spoken to Annie on the phone he hadn't seen her. He'd promised to take her out the next night for a welcome home dinner. Now that Frances required his company he'd just have to switch nights on her.

Frances wrote down the name and phone number of a publicist and handed him the paper. "Go see her," she said.

"Another woman?"

Frances narrowed her flinty eyes. "What's the matter? Don't you like dealing with women? Believe me, dear, they'll look after you much better than men."

Like she was telling him something new.

Marik, Cyndra had decided, was too nice for his own good. He treated her like a princess. Initially she'd lured him into bed – although he didn't take much luring – to get him under her power. Now she had him where she wanted him and more besides, because not only was he producing her single, but he was also her attentive and caring companion. The trouble was she didn't want a companion. She was perfectly happy making it on her own. Being married to Reece was enough companionship to last her a lifetime.

Marik was a California boy. He wanted her to meet his mother and sisters. She said no until she ran out of excuses and then she accompanied him one sunny Sunday afternoon. His family lived in the valley and they were all equally as nice as Marik.

Unfortunately, he was in love with her. She liked him, but she certainly didn't love him.

Gordon Hayworth was another matter. Every time she saw him she experienced exquisite little chills running up and down her spine, and a nervous stomach that drove her crazy. He dropped by the recording studio when she was making the demo and she spied him talking to Marik through the glass. She wanted to stop everything and go over just to be near him.

Casually she asked around. Usually the secretaries had the scam on everyone, but Gordon had no scandal attached. He was married to a beautiful ex-model and never came on to anyone else.

Gordon Hayworth had a presence and dignity she'd never observed in a man before. And she wanted him almost as much as she wanted a big career.

Marik was excited. The song he'd found for her was called "Child Baby", and it was written by a couple of up-and-coming songwriters. He'd put together a backing ensemble that really complimented her voice, and the arrangement was killer.

"Reno Records is behind you all the way, baby," he told her. "When this little old record hits the airwaves people gonna find out about you big time!"

The next weekend Marik wanted to take her to Palm Springs. He was so anxious to please that she didn't want to disappoint him, even though she'd sooner not have gone.

They drove down on a Friday night in his white Corvette and stayed at a small hotel surrounded by a backdrop of magnificent mountains.

"What was the story with you and that Reece guy?" Marik asked as he unpacked his overnight bag.

"Why?" she said carefully, unfolding her clothes.

"'Cause I'm interested. He said you were married. True or false?"

"No, we weren't married," she said, quickly. "We lived together for a while. I was young and stupid – I didn't know any better."

She didn't care to tell him the truth. If he'd known she was married to Reece it may have affected their business relationship, not to mention their personal one.

Later that night they sat outside in the bubbling Jacuzzi gazing up at the stars.

"This is oh so very, very nice," Marik said, stretching his legs.

"Yes, it's really pretty," she replied.

"No, baby – *you're* really pretty."

She threw her head back, her long hair trailing in the bubbling water. "So, tell me, Marik, how long have you been with Reno Records?"

"I've kinda been around Reno for five years."

"Where were you before that?"

"I put in time at a couple of the big companies. Produced some damn good artists. Then Gordon came along and offered me this job. It was a chance to do bigger and better." He laughed. "Gordon kinda stole me away."

"I expect he's good at that," she said.

His hand touched her leg. "Yeah, Gordon's a powerful personality. He's sure heavy on charisma."

"Why don't you tell me about him, he seems like an interesting guy."

"He had a small record company in New York, sold it for mucho bucks and moved out to LA about ten years ago. Then he started Reno, and the rest is a big success story."

"Is he married?" she asked, knowing full well that he was.

"Yeah."

"Who's his wife?"

"She was a top model – gave it all up when they married – Gordon didn't want his wife working."

"Are they happy?"

"Very happy." His hand snaked up her leg. "Hey, baby – what's with all the questions?"

"I should know who I'm working for."

"Stick with me, girl, and you don't have to know nothin'!"

He held open his arms and she moved into his bubbly softness. California was so health conscious, she wondered if Marik had ever thought about attending a gym. He should firm up his pecs, work on those stomach muscles. She didn't want to hurt his feelings by asking.

He was a good kisser so she leaned back and let him do his business. Marik was taking her all the way to stardom – why fight it?

Bridget Hale, Nick's new publicist, reminded him of a thinner, less cheerful Meena – what did these women have – a club? At least she seemed to know what she was doing; she'd already set him two interviews for later in the week – one with a news service for a piece that would run throughout the country, and one with a popular entertainment weekly magazine. He'd done a few interviews on the set and found it to be kind of a kick talking about himself.

Bridget trained him in the ways of the world. "We have to make up an interesting background for you," she said. "I don't know where you're from and I don't particularly care. We'll start from zero."

"I'm from the Midwest," he said.

"No, I don't think so. Something foreign will do. Your father was in the CIA – you were raised in China. Let me work on it."

"You gotta be kidding."

"Another point to remember – never tell them your age – let them guess. The more mysterious you are the better. Hollywood loves a loner."

"How come?"

"Because when you're on the cover of *Time* we don't want some nosy journalist visiting your home town and checking with all your old friends. If we can maintain it, mystery is the best, remember that."

"So what *do* I say when they ask me?"

"That you don't believe in pasts, only futures."

He laughed. "Sounds good to me."

"Frances and Meena are very high on you," she said. "And their praise does not come easily."

"They haven't seen me on film yet."

"Frances and Meena hear everything first. If you're good in this movie then they're aware of it."

He knew he should visit Joy, but he also knew she'd do nothing but bitterly criticize everything he'd done, and he wasn't in the mood for that. While he was prepared to acknowledge her help for introducing him to Frances, he was not prepared to listen to her negative comments. He wanted to feel good about himself. He was finally on the road and the main thing was to enjoy it.

He'd gotten Joey out of the hospital in New York and now he was safely stashed in a drug rehab clinic somewhere in the middle of the country. As soon as Joey was through with his treatment he'd arranged for him to come straight to LA.

In the meantime there was Annie to deal with.

They had dinner at a little restaurant near the Santa Monica Pier, and talked about what they'd both been doing. Towards the end of dinner she leaned across the table and fixed him with a penetrating stare. "Nick, am I going to move in with you?" she asked. "Is that what we're planning?"

He hadn't been planning anything of the sort, but it was obviously what she expected. He stalled for time, finally saying, "Uh, you mean you'd give up your apartment?"

She nodded. "If we're going to be together it seems only sensible. Why waste money paying rent on two places?"

The last person he'd lived with had been DeVille. Towards the end he'd felt beyond claustrophobic. "Are you sure it's what you want?" he asked, hoping she'd say no, but knowing she'd say yes.

"Very sure," she said firmly, just as he'd predicted.

He knew if he backed away she was going to start with the *I'm going to the cops* crap again. He couldn't afford to take the risk.

"If that's what you want, you should move in."

"Are you sure, Nick?"

He took her hand and squeezed it. "Yeah, course I'm sure."

What a lie. He liked Annie as a friend. He didn't love her, and the last thing he wanted was to live with her.

Trailing Frances around another industry party was the same old story. However, he felt a little more secure. He'd starred in a movie and a couple of people seemed to know who he was even though the movie hadn't come out yet.

He felt even more secure when he bumped into Carlysle. He'd missed the on-the-edge excitement of being with her. This was a different Carlysle from the girl he'd known in New York. She wore a neat little dress with a Peter Pan collar and a sweet angelic smile.

"This is my mother," she said, introducing him to an untidy looking woman who practically ignored him. "Mommy, this is Nick Angel – he starred in *Night City* with me. Remember? I told you about him."

"Oh," Mommy said. "So you're Nick. I hear you've done a good job."

"I'm hoping," he said.

Carlysle did not make a pass at him. Carlysle was a different person when she was with Mommy.

After the cocktail party Frances took him to dinner. "So, you did fuck her," she said, studying the menu.

"Who?"

"Carlysle. It was all over New York."

He grinned. "I had no choice."

"A word of advice," Frances said, sipping a J&B on the rocks. "Never let your cock interfere with your career."

"I'll remember that, Frances," he said, trying to keep a straight face.

A week later Annie moved in. He hated having to share his closet. She hated the fact that the bathroom was down the hall. "I'll look for something better," he promised, although he was fond of his little place by the beach.

Six weeks later he was invited to view a rough cut of the movie. Annie and Cyndra accompanied him. He sat in the theatre sweating, wondering what it was going to be like seeing himself on the screen. He'd attended a couple of day's rushes, but that was it. Meena, Frances and Bridget were in the audience. Having them there made him extra nervous. He nodded at his two producers – the woman didn't even crack a smile. Carlysle was there with her mother, looking demure.

Cyndra squeezed his hand. "This is so exciting!" she whispered.

"Yeah, almost as exciting as your record debut. When's it coming out?"

She grinned. "Two weeks. I can hardly stand it!"

"We'll celebrate," he said.

"You *bet* we will."

He wished something would come along for Annie; he knew she must be feeling left out, working at the health club watching their careers take off while she never got a break. It couldn't be much fun.

When the lights dimmed, he slid down in his seat barely able to watch the screen. Carlysle got star billing. He got an, *INTRODUCING NICK ANGEL AS PETE.*

Jesus! That was his name up on the screen. He'd actually made it – he was in a fucking movie!

The film was fast paced, gritty and surprisingly good. At the end of the screening there was a burst of spontaneous applause. Bridget was smiling – unusual for her.

Frances came up to him. "I like the film, I like you in it."

"Lunch, tomorrow," Meena said on her way out. "It's about time you met the head of the agency."

Cyndra was more excited than anybody. "Oh God, Nick, this is so great! You're fantastic, you really are!"

431

Annie was more controlled. Naturally. It wasn't in her nature to get excited about anything.

The three of them went to a restaurant on the Strip where they celebrated with double Margueritas and huge steaks.

Later, at home alone with Annie, he felt like making love, but not with her – she failed to turn him on. He was only with her because he had to be – it was a sad thought.

But tomorrow was another day and he'd figure out something – maybe.

He lay awake for a long while thinking about the movie, wondering what would happen next.

Eventually he fell asleep with a smile on his face.

Chapter 68

Lorenzo Marcella was the quintessential Italian man. Tall, exquisitely dressed in the finest Armani had to offer, proudly handsome in an aristocratic way. His dirty-blond hair was longish and lightly touched with silver at the temples. His jewellery was discreet and solid gold. His car was a black Masarati – not exactly ideal for Manhattan – but he would not dream of letting down the image. He was forty-two years old and the only heir to the family fortune. While he waited to inherit he'd been sent to America to spearhead the Marcella girl launch.

Lorenzo had no idea Lauren was married to the head of the powerful advertising agency Liberty & Charles – the very agency who were handling the Marcella account. And even if he had it wouldn't have made any difference. "This is the girl we use," he announced, picking out Lauren's photo from a select group.

"She's expensive," Oliver said, trying to curb his amusement, for he'd known there was no contest.

"How expensive?" Lorenzo demanded.

"Very," Oliver replied, straight-faced.

"Does she represent any other product?"

"No," said Howard, sitting in on the meeting with several other Liberty & Charles executives.

Lorenzo studied Lauren's photographs one more time. "Then we sign her to an exclusive Marcella contract. I don't mind what she costs. She is the girl."

"Good," said Oliver. "I think you've made the perfect choice."

Lorenzo flashed a movie star smile. "But of course!"

"Well, my dear," Samm said, her cat eyes gleaming. "You *are* the new Marcella girl – it's a done deal."

433

"You got my price?" Lauren asked.

"Yes, this was a record breaker and I am very happy indeed. Of course, as I mentioned before, most of my models will want to kill me. They'll blame me for not getting *them* the job. You're going to be a star."

Lauren laughed. It didn't seem possible. "I'll be in a lot of magazines, and my face will be around, but that hardly makes me a star, Samm."

"Just you wait," Samm said, nodding wisely. "Hollywood will come chasing after you. Didn't you once tell me you wanted to be an actress?"

"That was a long time ago."

"Well, sweetie, you're hardly ancient. How old are you now?"

"I'll soon be twenty-five."

"An old hag," Samm laughed. "I'd like to see Jimmy Cassady's face when he picks up the first magazine with you on the cover."

"Being the Marcella girl does not mean I'll be on any covers."

"Oh," Samm said, acidly. "If they want you in *Vogue* you'll turn them down?"

"Yes, I told you – I'm doing this for the money."

"I'm sure Oliver can look after you very nicely indeed."

"Yes, he can – but I prefer to be independent."

"You *do* know that Nature was up for this job, don't you?"

"How is she?"

"Living in LA with a producer."

"What happened to Emerson?" Lauren asked, trying to sound casual.

"According to Nature, he sent her a telegram from Japan announcing he was ending the marriage. By that time she'd moved in with her producer so she didn't much care. Don't you read the gossip columns?"

"Actually, I don't."

"Smart girl. Who needs to fill one's mind with trivia."

Oliver, who'd been so enthusiastic at the idea of her being the Marcella girl, was now not so pleased. "Perhaps I've created a monster," he said.

"Don't be silly, Oliver."

"I know what's going to happen. I'll never see you."

"Representing Marcella will not take all my time. I've read the contract carefully. Two photo sessions a year, six public appearances and one commercial."

434

He shook his head. "You have no idea how much of your time they'll require."

"You were the one that got me into this in the first place."

She was confused. She hadn't wanted a career in the public eye, but now it seemed that's exactly what she was about to have. All she'd really wanted was to marry Oliver and live a happy, fulfilled life. Only this was not to be; her husband could never fulfill her. Oliver could not make love the way she expected, and whenever she raised the subject he dismissed it as though it wasn't important.

Did he really think she was going to want nothing but oral sex from him their entire married life? If the truth were known, he'd tricked her into marriage. He should have told her about the pacemaker.

Meeting Lorenzo Marcella was an experience. The only Italian man she'd ever come in contact with before was Antonio the photographer, and he was gay. Lorenzo was the complete opposite. He kissed her hand, gazed into her eyes, inundated her with white orchids and told her she was the most beautiful woman who'd ever breathed.

"You *are* my Marcella girl," he said. "You will make every woman in the world want to be you. And every man want to be with you."

She backed off; his avid attention made her edgy. "I'll do my best," she said.

"Ah, but your best is going to make me a very happy man," Lorenzo crooned, continuing to gaze into her eyes.

They were at a luncheon in her honour – arranged so she could meet the other executives from Marcella.

"Did you tell them we're married?" she whispered to Oliver.

"No," he shook his head. "I imagine they'll find out soon enough."

"But he's coming on to me."

"Take no notice, my dear. Italian men come on to every woman. Whether they be six or sixty – it doesn't make any difference to them."

Obviously, Lorenzo's outrageous flirting did not bother Oliver, so she went along with it.

Lorenzo had many plans and he was not shy about revealing them. "I will have a wonderful party to present you to the press. It will not be another boring press conference. It will be a fantasy ball – and you will make a divine entrance in the middle of the party."

"I will?"

"Yes, *bellissima*! You shall introduce Marcella Cosmetics to the world as only you can. Everyone will fall in love with you – just as I have."

"You have?"

Lorenzo flashed his dazzling smile. "But of course!"

Chapter 69

The next few months proved challenging and exciting for both Cyndra and Nick. Neither of them could really comprehend what was happening to them.

"It's like a dream come true," Cyndra said. "Can you believe it, Nick – you and me? My record's taking off and your movie's like a big hit. It's incredible."

It was incredible. If he wasn't stuck with Annie he might have enjoyed it a lot more. He was so tired of faking his emotions – pretending to be someone he wasn't.

And Annie smothered him. Because her own career had failed to go anywhere, she leeched on to his – voicing her opinion on everything. This was exactly what he didn't need. It was enough he had Frances giving him advice, Meena handling his career, and Bridget guiding him through the maze of hungry press.

He also had his producer friend anxious for him to start her next movie. He'd read the script. It was not exactly what he wanted to do. Meena said they'd try to get him out of the contract.

"How?" he'd asked.

"With the right lawyer we can do anything," she'd replied, confidently.

Night City had launched his career. It was one of those low budget films the critics loved and the public flocked to. His reviews were excellent and suddenly he was an actor people were talking about. He'd followed Bridget's advice and made up a past for himself, not revealing too much.

"Try not to smile in interviews," she'd told him. "Cultivate that moody look. Women love it."

He did as she asked. Especially with the reporter from *Satisfaction*. They ran a cover story on him that blew his mind. He was on the cover of a fucking magazine and everybody in the world was going to see it!

In the meantime, Cyndra's record was getting plenty of air play. Gordon Hayworth had financed a trip for her and Marik to visit some of the most influential disc jockeys in the country. Marik loved the idea of travelling with her, but she wasn't so thrilled. She would have preferred that it was Gordon accompanying her.

Shortly after she got back Nick took her for a long drive. It had been a while since they'd been alone and had a chance to talk privately. He drove his rented car to Paradise Cove and parked. It was a beautiful September day and they got out and strolled along the beach.

"So," he said, stopping to flip pebbles in the sea. "How you feelin', kid?"

"Sensational! What about you?"

"The agency is trying to get me out of that contract. They have another film for me to do. This time it's a big movie with an important director."

"Is it what you want, Nick?"

"Yeah, I'm doing all the things I always dreamt of."

"So am I," she said. "Thanks to you."

"Why me?"

"Because you're stuck with Annie. You've saved us both."

He shrugged. "Annie's a nice girl."

Cyndra pinned him with her eyes. "But she's not the girl for you, is she?"

"You can talk. Marik's not the guy for you – but sometimes we do stuff to make things work."

"How do you know Marik's not for me?"

"I see it in your eyes."

"Oh, thanks a lot, Nick. Am I that obvious?"

"Hey – I'm your brother. I should be able to read you, huh?"

She stopped walking and flopped down on the sand, hugging her knees to her chest. "Wait until *that* little item hits the press."

He zoomed another pebble and watched it skim across the smooth ocean. "What, that I'm your brother?"

"Somebody's bound to find out."

"Y'know, I've been thinking," he said, squatting on the sand beside her.

"What?"

"Now that we're both getting all this publicity, maybe it's time to go back to Bosewell."

"Really, Nick? Y'know, sometimes I wake up in the middle of the night and I get all these guilty feelings about leaving Harlan."

He nodded. "I know what you mean."

She rushed on. "I always thought I'd send for him, but it was never the right time. It would be nice to go back and let them see how well we're doing – although I'll catch hell from Aretha Mae."

He frowned. "God knows why I'd want to see Primo."

"'Cause you wouldn't let me go by myself."

"You really think we should do it?"

"Definitely."

"Okay – so this is the plan," he said, jumping up.

"What?"

He reached out his hands and pulled her to her feet. "Now that I'm in a position to buy a car, I'm gonna get me the biggest, reddest Cadillac you've ever seen. And I'll take delivery in Kansas, then we'll drive to Bosewell. How'd'ja like *that* image?"

She began to laugh. "With fifty copies of *Satisfaction* on the back seat so you can hand them out. Right?"

He grinned. "Hey – Bosewell's a small town – maybe they haven't heard."

"But we'll tell 'em, huh?"

"If we're goin' back we gotta do it big time."

"Right on, Nick. When shall we do this?"

"How about next weekend."

"Just the two of us?"

He nodded. "Just the two of us."

They flew to Kansas and took a cab directly to the car showroom. When Nick saw his gleaming red Cadillac it was one of the happiest moments of his life. He'd always dreamt about it, but he'd never actually thought the day would come.

The car dealer in Kansas handed him the keys with a shit-eating grin. "Enjoy. This little baby's gonna give you plenty of pleasure."

Nick tried to stay cool – had to keep his image – he was getting good at it.

"Uh . . . thanks."

"Finest car on the market."

439

"I know."

"Liked you in *Night City*."

"Thanks."

He finally got rid of the salesman. Then he sat behind the wheel of the Cadillac with Cyndra beside him and let out a whoop of joy. "Holy shit! I got it! It's all mine! It's all fuckin' mine!"

"I know," Cyndra said, bouncing up and down on the seat. "It's so fantastic."

"Hey – get a load of the radio, look at the chrome, feel the leather. I *love* this freakin' car. I goddamn *love* it!"

She leant across the seat and hugged him. He started the engine and switched on the radio.

"It's my record!" Cyndra screamed. "They're playing my record!"

"Shit!" he said, grinning. "This day belongs to us!"

Their plan was to drive to Bosewell, visit Aretha Mae and Harlan, take a walk around town and then drive back to LA. Nick had estimated it would take them a couple of days, but they'd both decided they needed the break.

When he and Cyndra had first talked about visiting Bosewell he'd hoped that Joey might come with them. He'd called him up and asked. Joey had said no.

He wasn't about to argue and Cyndra was hardly disappointed.

"Joey's a loser," she'd said. "He always was and he always will be."

When Joey had gotten out of the drug rehab clinic he'd run straight back to New York. Nick had decided he'd done all he could.

Later that day they arrived in Ripley. Nick had booked them the biggest suite in the best hotel. They ordered room service and recalled old times. Then they drove around the city, and Nick detoured past the spot where the motel he'd spent his first night with Lauren was situated. The motel had been replaced with a gas station. So much for memories.

Cyndra stared out at the grimy streets. Maybe it wasn't such a good idea coming back. She was starting to remember all the bad things. What if she came face to face with Mr Browning? Would she talk to him?

Hell, yes! She had nothing to be scared of now.

Early Saturday morning they set off for Bosewell. In the back seat of the car were stacks of Cyndra's single and piles of *Satisfaction* with Nick on the cover.

440

"We should've found out if *Night City* played there yet," Cyndra said, snapping open a can of 7-Up.

"Don't worry, I already did," he said, laughing. "I had somebody call – it was on a month ago."

"Where's our first stop?" she asked, sipping from the can.

"The trailer park, where else? Then we'll go to the drugstore and drive up and down Main Street."

She giggled. "Handing out records and magazines!"

"Right on!"

Suddenly she felt anxious. "Oh, Nick, I hope we've made the right move. It feels so strange being back, doesn't it?"

He glanced out of the window. "It sure does. Small-town people stuck in a one-gas-station town. I bet nothing's changed."

"You're probably right."

He'd gone to the bank before he'd left and withdrawn a thousand dollars in cash. He planned on making an extravagant gesture and handing it to Primo. Let the asshole see what a big man his son had become.

Here, Dad, thought you might need some money.

Fuck you, Dad. Make the most of it because I'm never coming back.

He drove straight to the trailer park. They were both startled to discover it no longer existed. In its place there was now only wild brush, overgrown grass and huge mountains of abandoned garbage.

They looked at each other in surprise. "Probably moved them somewhere," Nick said. "We'd better drive into town – see what we can find out."

She squeezed his arm. "Nervous?"

"Yeah. How about you?"

She nodded.

They started the drive towards town. When they reached Main Street they both realized it did not look the same. The buildings were different. Everything was different. It was almost as if they were visiting an alien place.

"What the hell happened around here?" Nick said. "I don't recognize anything."

"I guess they've done a lot of improvements," Cyndra said. "Look how built-up everything is."

He drove slowly down the street. "Christ! Where's the freakin' drugstore?"

"Look over there," she said, pointing. "Isn't that where Blakely's hardware store used to be – now it's like one of those mini shopping malls."

He pulled the car into a parking space and they got out in front of a book store and a fast food place – both new stores.

"Do you see anybody you know?" he asked.

She shook her head.

"Some triumphant return, huh?"

"How are we going to find anybody?"

"We'll ask."

They walked into the book store and up to the counter.

"Can I help you?" said a woman with frizzy grey hair.

"Yeah, as a matter of fact, you can," Nick said.

Standing on a ladder behind the woman was a girl stacking books on a shelf. She took one look and did a double take. "Oh, my goodness!" she said, almost falling off the ladder. "Aren't you . . . aren't you Nick Angel?"

"Uh . . . yeah."

"I saw *Night City*," she said, excitedly. "I saw it three times!"

"I guess you enjoyed it."

She could hardly speak. "Oh, I did! I did!"

The woman was looking at him with a new respect.

"How long's this store been here?" he asked.

"Five years," she said. "Although I've only been working here for two. Can I find you a particular book? We have a very large selection."

"There was a hardware store here before. Uh . . . Blakely's hardware. Have the Blakely brothers still got a place in town?"

The woman shrugged. "I don't know – never heard of them."

The girl stepped forward, clutching a raggedy piece of paper. Her hand was shaking. "Can I have your autograph?" she asked, staring at him as if he was Clint Eastwood.

He and Cyndra exchanged glances. "Yeah, sure," he said, self-consciously scribbling his name.

She took the scrap of paper and gazed at it in awe.

They walked out of the book store and stood on the sidewalk. "This is what I think we should do," he said.

"What?"

"Go see George at the gas station. He'll know everything."

"You're right."

They got back in the Cadillac and drove to the gas station – a familiar sight at last. There didn't seem to be anybody around, so

Nick got out of the car and walked into the office. Sitting behind the desk, speaking on the phone, was Dave.

"Hey," Nick said, in a loud voice. "I got a red Cadillac outside needs a lot of attention. Anyone around here care?"

Dave didn't look up – he waved his hand as if to say *Don't bother me, can't you see I'm on the phone?*

"Where's George?" Nick said, speaking even louder. "Tell the old bastard to haul his lazy butt out here."

Dave covered the mouthpiece of the phone and glanced up. "'Scuse me?"

Nick burst out laughing. "You fuckin' old fart."

Dave's mouth dropped open. "Holy cow! Nick! It's you, ain't it?"

"You bet your ass it is." He beckoned Cyndra into the office. "You remember my sister, Cyndra. You've probably heard her record on the radio."

"Sure have," Dave said, beaming widely. "Everyone's heard it. You two are famous around here."

"We are?" Nick said, getting off at the thought.

"I saw your movie. Haven't gotten so lucky with Louise in a long time."

Nick walked around the familiar office remembering old times. "Oh, Jesus, it's good to see your ugly face," he said. "We went to the trailer park – it's gone. We drove down Main Street – everything's different. Where's the drugstore? Where's Blakely's? We come back and nothing's the same."

Dave nodded. "Since the tornado there's been a lot of changes."

"What tornado?" Cyndra asked.

Dave rubbed his chin. "You weren't here when it happened?"

Cyndra looked concerned. "When what happened?"

"The big tornado of 1974. The whole town was darn near wiped out."

Cyndra stepped forward. "What are you talking about?"

"Gone. Everything gone. People killed, devastation. You must've read about it."

"Oh, Jesus," Nick said. "We didn't read anything. We didn't know – we were in Chicago."

Dave shook his head. "I'm sorry I had to be the one to tell you."

"What about my mother?" Cyndra asked, clasping her hands tightly together. "Do you know where Aretha Mae is?"

"Plenty of people left town," Dave said. "There weren't any jobs here – not until we started to rebuild."

"How about Louise?" Nick asked. "Is she okay?"

"She's doing good," Dave said. "Fact is, we've managed to have us a few kids. They keep her busy."

"Hey, at least there's some good news," Nick said.

"You can say that again," Dave said, reaching for his crutches behind the rickety old desk.

Nick glanced down and saw that half of Dave's leg was missing. "Oh, jeez – what happened?"

"The tornado," Dave said, matter-of-factly. "Cut my damn leg in half. One of these days I'm gonna get myself a false limb. Can't afford it now – what with the kids an' all. But I manage – doesn't bother me that much."

"How am I going to find my mother and Harlan?" Cyndra worried. "I have to find them."

Dave propelled himself around the table. "I don't know what to tell you. Maybe Louise knows – she's always in on everybody's business."

"Where is she?" Nick asked.

"Stop by the house," Dave suggested. "She's at home with the kids. It'll give her a thrill to see you. We watched your movie together. Couldn't darn believe it was you up on the screen."

"Are the Brownings still in town?" Cyndra asked.

"Yep. You know what they say – when the poor get poorer the rich get richer. He built another store; he's got two places now. They're still living in that big house. The tornado never touched them."

"Give Louise a call and tell her we're coming," Nick said.

Dave shrugged. "I would if we had a phone. Things been tough around here these last few years. Ring the doorbell and say hello – she'll be real glad to set eyes on you."

"Where's George? I'd like to say hello before we go."

"George fell victim to the big C. Died last year."

"I'm sorry, Dave. That's too bad."

"Yes, we were all sorry to see him go. He left me this piece of property, makes life a little easier."

"I'm sure it does."

Outside the gas station they sat in the Cadillac and stared at each other.

"Shit!" Nick said. "Nothing but bad news. I don't fucking believe it."

"We have to find Aretha Mae and Harlan," Cyndra said,

444

clasping her hands together. "They must think we deserted them."

"We didn't desert them. We had no idea what happened."

"I only hope they're all right."

"Primo would've taken care of them."

"Get serious, Nick. Your old man probably ran the moment it happened."

"Yeah, you're right. But don't worry, we won't leave until we find 'em."

Louise was not the same sharp-tongued woman they'd once known. She looked twenty years older and thirty pounds heavier. She stared at Nick with saucer eyes, as if she was a fan. "OhmiGod! OhmiGod!" she kept repeating, wiping her hands on a grubby apron. A couple of whining toddlers crawled on the floor of the untidy living room and a baby cried lustily in its crib. The place was run-down and a mess. So was Louise.

"Let me make you a cup of coffee," she said, after she'd gotten over her initial shock. "I can still do that."

"I'm sorry about Dave," Nick said, shaking his head. "I never knew. We took off to Chicago – and that was the last we heard of Bosewell."

"You're lucky to have missed it. A lot of people lost everything. Fortunately, there weren't too many died, but it was an unbelievable scene, like someone dropped a big fat bomb on us."

"Who got killed?" he asked.

"Remember that girl you liked – Lauren Roberts?"

"Lauren's okay," he said, quickly. "I just saw her in New York."

"No – not her, but both her parents. Her mother was carried away in her car – literally swept up into the air. It was terrible. And her father was in his office when the entire block got wiped out. He was killed instantly. So was his secretary."

Nick suddenly realized that Lauren had probably never received any of his letters. "Uh . . . Louise – do you remember if you handed Lauren that note I gave you the night I left town? I know it's dumb to ask after all that's gone on, but did she ever get it?"

Louise shook her head. "You've got to be joking. The drugstore was completely destroyed – nothing left except rubble. Me an' Dave – we're lucky to be alive."

"It must've been tough for you."

"It was tough for everyone," she said. "Especially Lauren. We all felt so bad for her, she took such a big loss."

445

"I'm trying to find my mother and brother," Cyndra said. "They lived at the trailer park."

"That was all gone, too," Louise said. "But I heard Aretha Mae went back to work for the Brownings." She shrugged. "Look, I wish I could tell you more. It was one big nightmare for everyone."

"What about Betty Harris – is she still in town?" Nick asked.

"You mean that acting teacher?"

"Yeah."

"If I recall she moved to New York – even though the houses on that side of town weren't touched. People got nervous it could happen again. Trouble is, with three kids I don't get around much any more. I used to know everything. Now I'm trapped in the house all day."

"Mommy! Mommy!" One of the toddlers dragged on her apron strings, his chocolate covered face crinkling into tears. "I'm hungry!"

"I gotta feed 'em," she said, apologetically. "It's been a treat to see you both. You here for long?"

"Just long enough to find Aretha Mae and Harlan."

"Try the Brownings. I'm sure they can tell you where she is."

"Thanks, Louise." He leaned forward and kissed her warmly on the cheek.

She blushed. "You were always a nice kid, Nick. You deserve every bit of your success."

The Browning mansion looked the same as ever, although after living in LA it was not the palace they'd both once thought it was.

"Is it okay to walk up to the front door and ring the bell?" Cyndra asked, unsurely.

"What do you wanna do – go around the back?"

"I don't know, Nick . . . this is so strange . . ."

"What is it with you and the Browning family? Just because your mother worked for them –"

"It's more than that."

"Wanna tell me about it?"

"Not now. Maybe on the drive back to LA."

They rang the bell and waited.

The door was opened by a plump blonde in tennis shorts with heavy thighs and a dissatisfied twist to her mouth. She stared at

446

them, they stared at her, and then her mouth fell open and she said, "Nick Angelo," in reverent tones.

He didn't recognize her. "Do I know you?" he said, politely.

"Do you know me?" she laughed, gaily. "I was your first girlfriend in Bosewell. I'm Meg."

"Meg?"

"Remember *The Poseidon Adventure*? When you made me sneak you in the back without paying?"

He recognized her. It was Lauren's ex best girlfriend, Meg.

"What are you *doing* here?" she asked, looking flushed.

"What are *you* doing here?" he countered.

She sucked in her cheeks and stood up straighter. "I'm Mrs Browning. Stock and I got married five years ago."

"You did?"

She nodded. "Nick, we're all so excited by your success. The whole town is talking about it ever since your movie played here. And Cyndra dear, nobody can believe you're doing so well. Oh, I'm so rude leaving you standing on the doorstep. Do come in."

"We're trying to find out what happened to Cyndra's mother,' he said, following her inside the house. "We heard she was working for the Brownings again."

Meg looked blank. "Cyndra's mother?"

"Aretha Mae," Cyndra said.

"Oh, yes, of course, she's your mother. Well, as far as I know, Aretha Mae went to live in Ripley – it must have been a year or so ago."

"Do you have an address for her?" Cyndra asked.

"No," Meg said. "I have no idea where she went." She turned to Nick again – far more interested in speaking to him. "You look wonderful," she gushed. "We saw *Night City* twice. Stock loved it. He's such a fan of Carlysle Mann. Is she nice? What's Hollywood like? We're both so *proud* to be your friends – we always knew you'd do it."

He couldn't believe the crap that was coming out of her mouth. Stock had hated his guts. And so had she. What a couple of major phonies.

"Is Benjamin Browning here?" Cyndra asked.

"He's in the breakfast room. Do you wish to see him?"

"Yes, maybe he can help me with the information we need."

"This is so exciting," Meg said, leading them through the hall, tugging at the back of her shorts, failing to hide ripples of cellulite.

447

"So you married Stock?" Nick said, thinking to himself, *So you married the asshole. Well, somebody had to get stuck with him – it may as well be you.*

"We have two adorable children," Meg announced, proudly. "Miffy and JoJo."

"We only just heard about the tornado," Nick said. "Must've been a tough time here."

"It was terrible. You have no idea – the destruction was tragic."

"I heard about Lauren's parents."

"Yes, it was a terrible tragedy. She was devastated. Went to live with her aunt and uncle in Philadelphia. We lost touch a long time ago. I have no idea where she is now."

"You two were such good friends."

"We were children," Meg said. "Babies."

They all trouped into the breakfast room. Benjamin was sitting at the table drinking coffee and reading a newspaper. He looked up, startled. Cyndra was satisfied to see that he was older, greyer and fatter.

"Remember me, Mr Browning," she said, standing in front of him, hands on her hips. "Or should I call you Benjamin?"

He stumbled to his feet. She noticed he'd grown a thin Hitler-like moustache.

He stared at her, his mouth twitching. "What are *you* doing here?" he said.

"Looking for my mother. I thought you might be able to help me."

His shifty eyes darted this way and that, searching for an escape.

"You were always very close to my mother, weren't you?" Cyndra continued, watching him squirm.

He cleared his throat and shot a filthy look at Meg for letting them into his house. "Aretha Mae moved to Ripley," he said.

"Do you have an address for her?"

"I'll get it," he said.

"I recall coming to this house so many times," Cyndra called after him, as he left the room. "I have so many fine memories, Mr Browning . . . Benjamin, don't you?"

Meg, oblivious to the tension, said, "Stock is playing tennis, but I know he'd adore to see you both. Can you come back later? We could all go out and have a drink – wouldn't that be nice?"

"We gotta get back to LA," Nick said. "We only came to see Cyndra's mother and my dad."

"Oh yes, your father," Meg said.

"What about him?"

She looked embarrassed. "I really don't want to be the one to tell you."

"Tell me what?"

"He's . . . he's dead."

Nick felt absolutely nothing. He knew he should be upset, but the news didn't affect him. "How did it happen?" he asked, blankly.

"The tornado," Meg replied. "I'm so sorry."

Mr Browning returned with Aretha Mae's address written on a piece of paper.

"Why did she leave?" Cyndra wanted to know.

"I have no idea," he replied, his face an impassive mask.

"She wasn't hurt in the tornado?"

"No. Her trailer was destroyed, which is why Mrs Browning and I took her in out of the kindness of our hearts."

"What a prince you are," Cyndra said, sarcastically. "And did you take Harlan, my brother, in too?"

"He came here for a while and then went to Ripley. Your mother followed him."

"Thank you so much . . . Benjamin. C'mon, Nick, let's go."

They sat in the Cadillac and contemplated the latest information.

"Are you upset about Primo?" she asked, squeezing his hand.

"I guess I'm supposed to be . . ."

"It doesn't matter if you're not. You don't have to feel guilty."

She was right. Primo had never given a shit about him – why should he care?

But still . . . Primo *was* his father . . .

"So many changes here," Cyndra murmured. "And we knew nothing."

"You know what this means," Nick said, starting the car. "Lauren never got my letters. She must've thought I ran out on her."

"It was a long time ago."

"You don't understand. *I* was mad at *her*. I thought *she* didn't care. A few months ago I saw her in New York."

"You never told me."

"I was at a dinner party with Carlysle. Lauren was catering it. She was engaged to this old rich guy – one of the guests. I tried to contact her the next day, but I was told she'd gone off to get married."

"Did you speak?"

"No, we made eye contact, an' you know what? It was like time stood still."

"Really?"

"I always loved her, and I guess I always will."

"Don't go getting romantic on me, Nick. I can't stand it."

"There'll never be another girl like Lauren."

"Listen to you – it's pure soap opera."

"Fuck you, Cyndra. I've got to find Lauren and explain what happened."

"Didn't you tell me she got married?"

"It doesn't matter – I have to see her."

"I wouldn't mention this to Annie if I were you. She might not appreciate it."

"Annie has nothing to do with this."

"I know, but be careful. Annie could rock our future."

"Don't worry, Cyndra, I'm more aware of it than you."

"I'm sorry, Nick."

"About what?"

"Vegas. What happened there."

"It's nothing. Everything's gonna work out just fine. Now let's go find Aretha Mae and Harlan."

Chapter 70

Apparently it did not concern Oliver one little bit that Lorenzo Marcella was launching a kamikaze attack on his wife.

"I'm going to tell him we're married," she informed Oliver.

"Do whatever you wish, my dear, but I can assure you – it won't make any difference to the attention he pays you. Italian men are incorrigible."

"Don't you care?"

"Naturally I care. However, I trust you. You know how to handle yourself."

She didn't understand him. He refused to make love to her, and now a much younger, attractive Italian was all over her and it didn't appear to bother him. As a matter of fact, the more time she spent with Lorenzo the more she enjoyed his company. He was outrageously phoney, but his charm was addictive. His latest plan was for her to come to Italy and visit the big Marcella factory.

"This will be important," he announced.

"Can my husband come, too?" she asked.

They were in his office on Park Avenue, only it looked more like a luxurious apartment. Sheepskin rugs on the floor, an enormous white desk, oversized couches and leopard skin throws.

"You mention this husband all the time," Lorenzo said. "And yet I have never seen him. Who is he? Tell me and I will have him killed." He smiled.

She smiled back. "You know my husband, Lorenzo."

"I do?"

"I thought somebody would have told you by now."

"Told me what?"

"My husband is Oliver Liberty."

Lorenzo looked at her with a quizzical expression. "You are not serious?"

"Yes."

"I do not believe you."

"Why would I lie?"

"He's too old for you."

"That's rather a presumptuous thing to say."

"You are young, beautiful, vital. Oliver is – how do you say in English? Ah yes, he is over the mountain."

"You don't have to be young in years to be vital. Oliver has a tremendous amount of energy – probably more than you and me put together."

"Ah, well," Lorenzo said, sighing. "I will simply have to steal you away from him."

She laughed. "You're incorrigible."

"But you like it."

She had to admit that she did. Lorenzo made her smile. He made her feel young and light-hearted. Living with Oliver had turned into all business.

Pia gave birth to a baby girl, a golden child they named Rosemarie. Lauren was appointed godmother. She loved going over to Pia's apartment and cradling the baby in her arms; all her maternal instincts sprung to life. The thought occurred to her – if Oliver never made love to her, how was she going to get pregnant?

As the months passed she found herself drawing away from him. If he didn't want to make love to her properly, she didn't want him to touch her at all. Whenever she tried to discuss it he walked away as if it didn't matter.

You made a mistake, Roberts.

I'm getting good at that.

One Saturday afternoon she went by herself to see *Night City.* She sat in the dark movie theatre and watched Nick up on the screen. He was so good. His intensity worked for the camera. When he was in bed with Carlysle Mann she closed her eyes – she couldn't bear to watch.

Their affair was long ago and far away – and yet it seemed like yesterday. Maybe she should have taken his call the day after the Georges' dinner party. Instead of speaking to him she'd run off to the Bahamas and married Oliver. Foolish girl. She should have listened to what he had to say.

Too late now. Nick Angelo was a movie star, and she was about to be launched upon an unsuspecting public.

"Lorenzo wants us to go to Italy," she told Oliver.

"I can't go anywhere," he replied. "I'm in the middle of landing an important client."

"What client?"

"Riviera Champagne."

"Surely you can get away for a few days?"

"No," he said, abruptly. "The owner is coming to town. It's a personal thing. Only *I* can talk him into switching his account to Liberty & Charles."

"Can't Howard handle it?"

"Howard is *not* me, Lauren. I'm training him, but it will take time and experience before he can pull an account from another agency the way I do."

"Do you mind if I go with Lorenzo?"

"What is this trip for?"

"He wants me to meet the other Marcella executives and visit the factory. He feels that if the campaign works in America they'll want me to spearhead the whole European campaign. I've spoken to Samm, she likes the idea and so do I. Of course, it will mean more money."

"Are you asking me what I think?"

"Yes."

"Then you should go – it's important."

"You wouldn't mind?"

"Of course not."

Screw Oliver. He honestly didn't care. He was sending her to Europe with an eligible, devastatingly attractive Italian lech.

"It's settled then," she said.

The next morning she had coffee with Pia in her apartment.

"You're going to Rome with Lorenzo?" Pia said, almost spilling her coffee.

"Oliver seems to think there's nothing wrong with it."

Pia leapt up. "Ha! Howard wouldn't let me exchange a hand-shake with Lorenzo Marcella! Those Italian men are lethal – especially when they look like him."

"Why?" Lauren asked, casually. "Do you think he's attractive?"

"What a ridiculous question. The guy is devastating – he looks like a movie star."

It wasn't his looks that attracted Lauren, it was his attitude.

"When do your ads start appearing?" Pia asked.

"They'll be in the Christmas magazines, which means they'll hit the stands at the end of November."

"Wow, that's exciting."

"Can I see the baby?" Lauren asked.

"She's sleeping."

"Why don't we wake her?"

Pia grinned. "Why not?"

The private jet was the most luxurious form of travel Lauren had ever imagined.

"It's nothing," Lorenzo said, with a sweeping wave of his hand.

His idea of nothing was a state of the art cabin fitted out with full stereo equipment, a kitchen, a marble bathroom and a bedroom in the back. The interior of the plane was decorated as though it was a penthouse apartment. It was the company plane, but Lorenzo had full use of it whenever he wanted.

"I'm sorry your husband was unable to accompany us," he said, strapping himself into the seat next to her, not meaning a word he said.

"I'm sure you are."

"No, really, *bellissima*. I would never pay attention to another man's wife."

He could have fooled her. "Have you ever been married?" she asked.

"No, my princess, I have yet to meet the woman of my dreams. Besides, we have one life to live – why confine oneself to the same meal every day?"

She wrinkled her nose. "You're beginning to sound like a chauvinist."

"What is a chauvinist?" he asked, innocently.

"You know what I mean – comparing a woman to a meal. That's hardly very nice."

Watching her closely he said, "You are the most beautiful woman in the universe. I love it when you speak. The way your mouth moves, the way your lips quiver. Everything about you is so . . . so tempting."

"You're full of it, Lorenzo."

It was her first trip to Europe and she couldn't help being excited.

Lorenzo was amused. "I have crossed the Atlantic so many times that I have lost count," he boasted.

"Lucky you," she replied, fastening her seatbelt and tensing for take-off. Every time she flew it made her nervous.

Lorenzo seemed totally at ease. He took her hand and turned it palm up.

"Ah . . . you, too, will be very lucky," he said, studying her palm. "I see it here."

"What, Lorenzo?"

"Did I not tell you that my grandmother was a gypsy? I read palms, I can foresee the future."

"And what do you see in my future?"

"You will be very famous, and very rich. Ah – you notice this broken line here – it means you will have a divorce."

"Lorenzo," she scolded, pulling her hand away.

"No, no, my princess, I am not joking." He took her hand again. "Maybe lots of little bambinos – two, three, ah yes, four." He frowned. "I see something else," he said, peering closely.

"What?" she asked, alarmed.

"I see they are not American babies – they are half-Italian."

She began to laugh. "You're bad, you know that?"

"Ah, yes, I've been told many times. But I am not bad where it matters."

"And where's that?"

"In the bedroom."

He had seductive eyes, a thin nose and carved cheekbones. She liked looking at him, and so did the two stewardesses who paid him avid attention.

After take-off they sipped champagne, ate a delicious meal, and then Lorenzo watched a movie while she fell asleep.

He woke her gently when they were preparing to land. "Ah, *bellissima,* you were exhausted. Twenty minutes and we will be in my home country."

She struggled awake and went into the bathroom to repair her make-up and brush her hair. What had her life become? Here she was on a plane with a very attractive Italian while her husband had elected to stay behind in America. She knew she was going to be tempted. It was inevitable.

Let's see how you handle this one, Roberts.

I can do what I want.

There was a welcoming committee waiting to greet them. A small child in a long white dress rushed to present her with a

455

bouquet of roses. She accepted it gracefully, although several of the thorns stuck into her flesh. A television crew captured every moment.

Lorenzo introduced her to several people at once. They shook her hand and kissed her on both cheeks. She was overwhelmed by all the attention.

Lorenzo rushed her out of the airport into a limo which sped through the streets of Rome as if it was competing in a race. She hardly had a chance to view the sights. The limo deposited her at the Villa Marcella, where the guest suite was bigger than the apartment she'd lived in when she was single in New York.

"Tonight you will rest," Lorenzo said. "And tomorrow there will be a big reception gala in your honour." He put both hands on her shoulders and placed a tender kiss on each cheek. "I have things to do now. Anything you want, just ring. Tomorrow, *bellissima*."

The next few days were magical. Rome was the most beautiful city she'd ever seen. Lorenzo arranged a tour for her and she saw everything from the incredible ruins of the Coliseum to the Appian Way and all the fine buildings and monuments in between. She particularly loved the narrow cobblestone streets and colourful kerbside cafés.

She met Lorenzo's family. His father was an older version of him and his mother was a frighteningly chic blonde woman. Everybody treated her like a queen. She visited the factory and met many of the employees. Her picture was everywhere.

"They love you," Lorenzo smiled. "They have named you the innocent American girl."

"I'm not so innocent," she said.

"You have that special quality Grace Kelly possessed. It's very appealing to Europeans."

She'd expected him to make a pass, but Oliver was obviously right – Italian men flirted a lot, but took it no further.

On their last night in Rome he invited her to dinner at an open-air restaurant located near the bottom of the Spanish Steps. She'd expected it to be the usual group of people, but it turned out to be just the two of them.

"Tonight we enjoy the typical Italian meal," he said. "No champagne, no caviar. We have pasta, a little fish, plenty of vino – we relax."

He amused her with stories about his past and she found herself having a wonderful time. Later he invited her back to his apartment. "You will see the best view in Rome," he boasted. "Or maybe you'd prefer to go to a disco?"

"No, I'd like to see your apartment."

She knew she was treading on dangerous territory. She'd drunk too much wine and the city was a seductive siren, luring her to misbehave.

He held her captive with his eyes. "Are you sure, Lauren? I don't want to force you to do anything you do not wish."

"All I'm doing is coming back to your apartment."

He smiled. "Yes, *bellissima,* that is all." Although they both knew this was not the case.

His apartment did indeed have the best views in Rome and was furnished most luxuriously.

"Now is the time for champagne," he said. "To finish the evening."

He poured them both a glass, put Billie Holiday on the stereo and held open his arms. "Good Morning Heartache" serenaded her and for a moment she thought about Nick. Then she closed her eyes and allowed Lorenzo to sweep her into his arms. They danced together slowly, their bodies pressed closely against each other.

I wonder what Oliver is doing now?

Ha! Working. What else.

You never loved him, Roberts, why did you marry him?

That's my business.

Lorenzo's fingers pressed through the thin material of her dress. When he started to lower her zipper she didn't stop him. He peeled the dress from her shoulders and expertly unclipped her bra.

She knew she was about to be unfaithful to her husband, but somehow she couldn't stop herself.

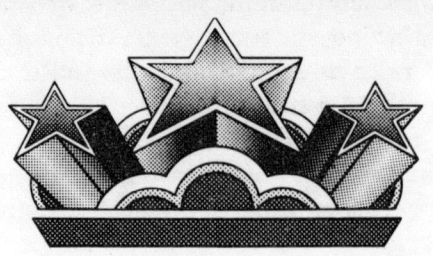

Chapter 71

Aretha Mae stared at Cyndra as if she'd seen a ghost.

"Mama?" Cyndra said softly, shocked at how thin and wasted her mother looked. "Mama, it's me, Cyndra."

Aretha Mae shook her head in disbelief.

"Can we come in?" Cyndra asked, standing at the door.

"Oh, girl, lookit you," Aretha Mae said, speaking in a low shaky voice. "You so pretty."

Cyndra's face lit up. "Yes, Mama, you think so? You really think so?"

"I should be spanking your ass," Aretha Mae said, recovering her composure. She peered at Nick. "And what you have to say for yourself?"

Christ! This was just like being a kid again. "It took us a while to find you," he mumbled.

"I would've left you an address if I'd known where you run off to," she said, tartly – the same old Aretha Mae.

They followed her into the small room she called home. The place was cluttered with stacks of newspapers and magazines. On the mantel were two old photos of Luke, surrounded by several burnt-out candle stumps.

"What are you doing now, Mama?" Cyndra asked, running her finger along the mantel and finding thick dust.

"Don't work no more," Aretha Mae said, fiddling with the glasses hanging on a string around her neck. "Don't have to. Got me some money, 'nough to manage on."

"Is Harlan here?" Nick said, anxious to see him and get the hell out.

"What you wanna know 'bout him for?" Aretha Mae said, suspiciously.

"Is he okay, Mama?" Cyndra asked. "The tornado happened

after we left. We knew nothing about it – we only heard today. Were you all right?"

"'Bout as all right as a person can be when their home gets destroyed," Aretha Mae snapped.

Cyndra sat down on the worn old couch. "If I'd known I would've come back."

Aretha Mae pursed her lips. "You did right, girl, gettin' out."

"I'm a singer now," Cyndra said, proudly. "I got a record; they're playing it on the radio. And Nick's in a movie."

Aretha Mae shook her head from side to side, her expression blank. "Don't get out much," she muttered, her voice weak again.

"Maybe Harlan knows?" Cyndra said, hopefully. "Where is he?"

"I don't see your brother no more," Aretha Mae said, sharply.

"Isn't that why you moved to Ripley – to be close to him?"

Aretha Mae stared accusingly at them both. "Who told you those lies?" she demanded.

"Mr Browning," Cyndra said, frightened by her mother's strange behaviour.

"You saw that cracker?" Aretha Mae sneered. "Why'd you see him?"

"We had to track you somehow."

"Why'd you go near him?" Aretha Mae asked, narrowing her eyes. "You shouldn't've done that."

"'Cause I had to find you."

"You found me, girl. Here I am."

"We heard about Primo," Nick said.

Aretha Mae began to cough, the harsh sounds racking her thin body.

Cyndra jumped to her feet. "Are you all right? Mama? You sound terrible."

"I feel fine."

"Have you seen a doctor about your cough?"

"Doctors! Ha!" Aretha Mae shrieked with crazy laughter.

"You should see one. You're too thin."

Aretha Mae frowned. "Don't go tellin' *me* what to do, girl."

Cyndra tried to put her arms around her mother. "I'm sorry I left you. I always meant to write. I know I didn't, but that doesn't mean we can't be close now, does it?"

Aretha Mae darted across the room to escape her daughter's embrace. "You always saw things your way, Cyndra. It always had to be your way or nothin'."

"That's not true," Cyndra objected.

"Oh yes it is."

"No, it's not."

"Where're you living?"

"We live in California. Los Angeles."

"That Hollywood place – fulla sex an' drugs an' all those bad things I read 'bout," Aretha Mae said, churlishly.

Cyndra laughed. "It's not full of sex and drugs. Maybe you'll visit me one day. I'd like that."

"*I* wouldn't."

"So tell us about Harlan. Is he working?"

"You don' want nothin' t'do with him."

"Why not?"

"He got himself in trouble."

"Maybe we can help," Nick suggested.

"You don' wanna help him, oh dear me, no."

"That's our choice."

Aretha Mae glared at him. "You don' wanna help no pansy boy."

"What?"

"Pansy boy. Sells himself down on Oakley Street. Gets in a car with anybody he does. He ain't my son no more. Luke's my son – the only one I care about – him and Jesus."

"Jesus?" Cyndra said, glancing quickly at Nick.

"Yes, girl, Jesus. An' you better learn to repent your ways. Otherwise, Jesus gonna shut you out, an' your fancy black ass gonna burn in hell."

"Mama, I never did anything wrong."

"Oh, yes, you did wrong, girl," Aretha Mae said, her eyes burning feverishly. "Oh, yes, you led Mr Browning on. You led him into Satan's bedroom."

"I didn't," Cyndra said, her eyes filling with tears. "You know I didn't."

Aretha Mae sat down in an old chair, wrapped her arms across her chest, and rocked back and forth. "Deny all you want, but Jesus knows, Jesus sees."

Nick took Cyndra's arm. "We gotta get goin'."

"Don't *say* that, Mama," Cyndra said, pushing his hand off. "Don't say that to me."

Aretha Mae cackled. "An' the guilty shall burn in hell. An' the fire'll take out their eyes. An' a girl like you – a temptress – will be the devil's playmate. You done things no decent person can forgive."

Cyndra was frantic. "What are you *talking* about? I didn't

do anything. Benjamin Browning *raped* me – you know it."

A strange smile snaked around the corners of Aretha Mae's downturned mouth. "You sinned, girl. Mr Browning – he be your daddy. And you let him sin with you." Her voice rose. "You gonna burn in hell. Oh, yes you are."

"He's not my father," Cyndra screamed, angrily.

"He be your daddy for sure, girl. When you got rid of that baby – you murdered your own brother. You killed Luke, didn't you?" She leapt up. "You killed Luke, you little whore!"

Nick grabbed Cyndra's arm again and physically dragged her out of the room. She was sobbing hysterically. He pulled her down the stairs and into the street.

"What's she talking about?" Cyndra yelled. "Nick, help me, tell me what she's saying? What's she trying to do to me?"

"Can't you see she's crazy. God knows what happened here."

"I have to see Harlan."

"Okay, okay – we'll find him."

"When?" she demanded.

"Now," he replied, pushing her into the car.

They drove to Oakley Street, parked the Cadillac and sat in it and waited. After a while Nick left her in the car and went into a nearby bar to find out what the action was.

"You can get anything you want on Oakley Street," the barman told him. "Only ya gotta watch out – it can look like a girl, it can talk like a girl, but you're likely to find a big old surprise swingin' between their legs."

"Transvestites, sweetie," crooned a fat woman sitting at the bar downing a vodka surprise. "This street is crawling with them. Now, why don't you sit down with me, buy me a drink and I'll tell you everything you ever wanted to know."

"Thanks, another time," he said, hurrying back to the car. Cyndra had been crying.

"You don't wanna take any notice of Aretha Mae," he said, trying to comfort her.

Her voice was shaky. "She said Benjamin Browning was my father. Do you know what that means?"

"She doesn't know what she's talking about."

"Oh, yes, she does. She's telling the truth. I'm sure of it."

"Hey," he said, flippantly. "Look on the bright side – Benjamin's your father you can claim half his money when he drops."

"Be serious, Nick. You don't seem to understand. When I was sixteen Benjamin raped me, and my mother did nothing. He made me pregnant, and I had to have an abortion. You remember when you came to live at the trailer? I was in Kansas – getting rid of my own father's baby."

Nick decided this trip was a horrible mistake. They'd have been better off leaving Bosewell in their past where it belonged. Now all of this bad stuff was happening and he didn't like it.

By dusk the transvestites began to hit the street in full drag. Several of them cruised past the car in pairs, bending down to peer in the window.

"We're looking for Harlan," Cyndra said, talking to them in a friendly voice. "Do you know him?"

"What's wrong with me?" lisped a beefy six footer in a long blonde wig and transparent white mini dress.

"You're lovely," Nick said. "But we want Harlan."

"If the bitch puts in an appearance I'll send her over," the man said, patting his wig.

"I've got a big feeling we're not gonna like this," Nick said.

"Whatever – he's still my brother," Cyndra said, fiercely. "If Aretha Mae's telling the truth – you're not."

He was hurt. "Hey, Cyndra, we'll always be brother and sister. It doesn't matter who your father is."

"I know, I know," she said, sorry for what she'd said.

They sat in the car for a long while, watching the parade from the window.

"How will we recognize him?" she asked. "What if he's all dressed up? We left a little boy behind – now he's a man."

"I hate to point this out," Nick said, "But black faces aren't exactly heavy on the street."

"You're right."

Around nine o'clock Cyndra thought she spotted him.

"Are you sure?" Nick said, peering into the darkness.

"I don't know, but like you said, black faces aren't exactly common."

"Okay, whyn't I go see." He got out of the car and approached what appeared to be a black woman in a scarlet dress, feather boa and long black wig. "Harlan?" he questioned, edging close so as to get a better look.

"Don't you mean Harletta?" the creature shrieked.

"Harlan, it's me – it's Nick."

The creature put a finger to its chin. "Do I know you? Have I *had* you?"

"Harlan, for Christ's sake, it's Nick. Cyndra's in the car. Come talk to us."

The creature backed further into the shadows. "Harletta never goes anywhere unless she's paid handsomely."

He fumbled in his pocket and produced several bills which he shoved at the creature. "Get in the goddamn car!"

"Oooh!" Harlan shrieked. "I love it when you talk rough."

And so that's how they found Harlan. A drugged-out street hustler. An embittered young man who'd had no chance to be anything else. They'd taken him back to their hotel and counselled him for hours, but he apparently had no desire to change his lifestyle. He laughed at them.

"Come back to LA with us," Cyndra pleaded.

"My friends are here," Harlan replied, roaming restlessly around the hotel suite.

"Your friends are street people," Nick pointed out. "Hookers and hustlers. What kind of friends are those?"

"At least they're here when I need them," Harlan sniffed, suddenly pulling off his wig and throwing it petulantly across the room. "You two ran off an' left me. You don't know what it was like after you'd gone. There was no money, no place to live. Aretha Mae had to take charity from that Benjamin Browning pig."

"Did he touch you? Did he do anything to you?" Cyndra asked.

"What do you think?" Harlan replied, his grotesquely painted lips twisting contemptuously.

"I'll kill that bastard one of these days,' Cyndra said, staring blankly ahead. "I'll blow his fucking head off."

"Calm down," Nick said.

"He deserves it."

"Oh yes," Harlan agreed. "An' I'll watch. Front row seats, please," he added, archly.

They couldn't persuade Harlan to leave with them. But he did accept their money and after hours of discussion he reluctantly promised to keep in touch. Not that either of them believed him. "We'll be lucky if we ever see him again," Nick said.

Finally they got in the red Cadillac and made the long drive home to Los Angeles.

The moment he arrived back Nick sold the car.

"I don't understand you," Annie complained. "Why would you do that? You've dreamt about owning a Cadillac all your life."

463

"There's a lot of things you don't understand about me, Annie," he said.

"Maybe we should try spending more time together," she suggested.

Wasn't it enough they were living in the same apartment? What did she want from him?

He went out that night by himself and called Carlysle from a phone booth. "Are you with your mother?" he asked.

"She's out of town," Carlysle replied. "Why? Want to party?"

"Yes."

"Come on over."

When he arrived at her house he found she was not alone. There was another girl there, an exotic Indonesian model. The three of them ended up in the jacuzzi playing games he'd never played in school.

He lost himself in a round of hedonistic pleasures. He needed the release. By the time he left Carlysle's house he felt better.

The next day Meena informed him they'd gotten him out of his contract for the movie with the woman producer and arranged a deal for him to star in *Life* – a big budget movie about a young killer and his father.

"This is an excellent break, Nick," Meena said, briskly. "Top director, first-class production – and here's the best news – I've doubled your money."

He wasn't as elated as he should have been. He had Lauren on his mind and somehow or other he knew he had to see her.

He went home and told Annie that he had to go to New York for a couple of days.

"Can I come with you?" she asked, hopefully.

"No. It's business." He kissed her on the cheek. "See you in a couple of days."

At the airport he made out a cheque for six thousand dollars and sent it to Dave. It was all the money he had in his account. But he was lucky, there was more coming in.

He made the evening flight. Soon he would get to see Lauren, one way or another. He didn't know what he'd say to her. He only knew that he had to resolve the situation. And the sooner the better.

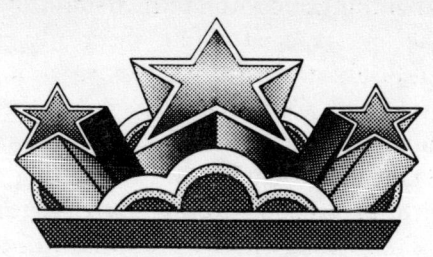

Chapter 72

Lauren was filled with guilt because she'd slept with Lorenzo and hadn't meant to. It had only happened once – the last night she was in Rome – and she had no excuse. The experience was memorable – which didn't please her because she would have preferred to have forgotten it.

Maybe I take after my father, she thought, miserably. *Why should I feel guilty – he obviously never did.*

Upon their return to America, Lorenzo behaved like a perfect gentleman. She told him she regretted it had happened, it would never happen again, and would he please never refer to it.

"I respect your wishes," he'd said. "But when you get rid of your husband, I will be waiting."

Oliver suspected nothing. "How was your trip?" he'd asked.

"I wish you'd been with me," she'd said.

"Next time," he'd promised. "In fact, I was thinking that in the summer we might cruise the Riviera on a yacht."

"That would be nice, Oliver. Can you get the time away?"

"I'll make time."

She'd already done the photographs for the Marcella girl campaign, and now it was time to shoot the commercial. Digging down into her past she drew on her acting experience, relaxed and had fun in front of the camera. It was quite an elaborate commercial and took a week to shoot.

Lorenzo visited the set every day, still behaving like a perfect gentleman. He did nothing more than flirt with his eyes – but, oh, those Italian eyes! She remembered their one night together in Rome and her body screamed out for more. It was only her mind that kept her from doing anything about it.

You're a married woman, Lauren.

You don't have to keep on reminding me.

She enjoyed making the commercial, being the centre of attention. It made her feel special – like she really mattered in the scheme of things.

It seemed that now Oliver possessed her he paid less and less attention to her. Work, as usual, came first.

She decided that if he could put work first, so could she. Over lunch with Samm she told her that if any other good modelling jobs came along she was prepared to do them.

"I thought you weren't interested in modelling," Samm remarked, sipping a glass of white wine.

She picked at a salad. "I've changed my mind."

"You won't be able to represent other products, but you can certainly do photographic work," Samm said, thoughtfully. "I'll see what I can get you."

"Get me the cover of *Vogue*," Lauren said, with a persuasive smile. "You know you can do anything."

Samm waved at a fashion editor, leant back and also smiled. "My, my – aren't *we* getting ambitious."

"Why not? It's about time."

"By the way," Samm said. "Did you hear about Jimmy Cassady?"

"What about him?" Lauren asked, coolly. As far as she was concerned he was ancient history – even hearing his name failed to bother her.

"He emerged from the closet."

"Huh?"

"Gay, my sweet. Positively festive in fact!"

So there was the answer to that little mystery.

Most weekends she spent with Pia, Howard and the baby. Sometimes they stayed in town – other times they drove to Oliver's large estate in the Hamptons where he spent most of his time in his study on the phone – relaxing was not for him.

Sunbathing on the beach one day, Pia said, "Do you realize you have three homes now? The apartment in New York, the house in the Bahamas and this place."

"They're Oliver's homes," Lauren said, enjoying the hot sun. "I never chose any of them."

"If you feel that way you should sell them and buy something else. Be nice to start fresh, wouldn't it?"

Lauren reached for the suntan oil. "I'm sure Oliver would let me do exactly what I like. He probably wouldn't even notice."

"Hmm," Pia said. "Do I detect a note of dissatisfaction?"

She rubbed the greasy oil over her legs. "You detect a note

of 'I've married a man who never stops working'."

"Ah," Pia said, wisely. "That's *why* you have three houses."

"Very quick."

Pia looked thoughtful. "I think Howard's following in Oliver's footsteps," she said, pensively. "He didn't come home last night until nine o'clock. Maybe he's got a mistress."

"Howard?" Lauren started to laugh. "I can't imagine Howard with a mistress."

"Why?" Pia said, quite affronted. "Don't you think he's sexy?"

"To you he's sexy – to other women he's your husband."

"Sometimes I wish we'd kept the business," Pia said, wistfully. "I love Rosemarie and looking after her, but playing mommy is not my life."

"Get a job," Lauren suggested, lying back.

"I don't want to go that far. Being my own boss is one thing, but working for somebody else – no, that's not for me. Unless you'd like me as your personal assistant – I'd be very efficient."

"I'm not busy enough for an assistant," Lauren murmured, closing her eyes.

"You will be. Wait until the ads start appearing. And Samm tells me you want to start doing other work."

"I wouldn't mind."

"Nature's turned to acting, you know."

"Really?"

"Yes, she's living with this producer guy and he's put her in his movie. She's the new discovery on the block."

"That'll make her happy."

"And I read in one of the columns that Emerson Burn gets back from his world tour this week."

"You're a regular little gossip monger."

Pia sighed, enviously. "You certainly have some interesting exes. And when you came to work at Samm's we all thought you were so quiet."

"Emerson's not an ex."

"Is Nick Angel?" Pia asked, curiously. "You never speak about him. He sure was anxious to talk to you, though."

"I went out with Nick in High school," she said casually, like it really meant nothing.

"Wow! High school – was he gorgeous then?"

"Yes," she said, very quietly. "He was."

As soon as Nick arrived in New York he called Help Unlimited. The operator told him the number was no longer in service.

"Shit!" he said, slamming down the phone. He thought for a moment, then called Carlysle in LA.

"Oh, boy!" she exclaimed. "That was *some* good time! I didn't realize you were so adventurous."

"Yeah, well, that makes two of us."

"Can you come over now? My friend's still here."

"I'm in New York."

"Shame."

"I need a favour."

"What?"

"You remember that dinner party you took me to when we were shooting *Night City*?"

"We went to so many places."

"The hostess had on all those crazy bracelets."

"You mean Jessie George."

"That's the one. What's her number?"

Carlysle giggled. "Oooh, Nick, isn't she a little old for you?"

"I need to ask her something."

"Wait a sec, I'll get my book."

She gave him the number and he hung up and dialled. All he had to say was, "Nick Angel," and Jessie knew exactly who he was.

"Nick, how nice to speak to you," she said. "I so enjoyed *Night City*. Memorable performance."

"Thanks."

"What can I do for you?"

"Do you have the number of Help Unlimited?"

"Unfortunately they're not in business any more."

"They're not?"

"No. I'm sad myself. But I do have another caterer I can recommend."

"Remember that girl . . . the one who did all the cooking?"

"Do you mean Lauren?"

"Who was that guy she was about to marry?"

"Oliver Liberty. They got married in the Bahamas."

"What does he do?"

"Oliver owns the biggest ad agency in New York – Liberty & Charles."

"Can you give me his home number?"

"Certainly. By the way, I'm having a dinner party tomorrow night. I'd love you to come."

"Well, uh, I don't know . . . I'm only here for a few hours. Gotta get back to LA."

"What a shame – Oliver and Lauren will be here."

"Maybe I don't have to get back so fast," he said, quickly.

"Eight o'clock. Casual. I'm putting you on my list."

So, Lauren had actually gone ahead and married the guy. This wasn't good news. But then again all he wanted to do was apologize; it wasn't like they were going to fall into each other's arms. A long time had passed. They were both different people now.

Yeah, sure. And what else was new?

Odile Hayworth was the most exquisite woman Cyndra had ever seen and she hated her on sight. Gordon belonged to Odile. Odile belonged to Gordon. It was patently obvious.

Marik had arranged a cosy dinner for four at a French restaurant and Cyndra was loathing every minute of it. Odile was uncommonly pretty, with amber eyes, fashionably short black hair and a wide smile. She was also at least thirty-five.

Old, Cyndra thought. *Surely he needs someone younger?*

"Marik tells me you used to be a model," Cyndra said politely, not that she cared.

"I was a model all right – until Gordon came along and rescued me," Odile replied, squeezing her husband's hand. He squeezed hers back.

How sweet, Cyndra thought.

"I saw her across the room at a crowded party," Gordon said. "Took one look and knew my life was over."

They all laughed.

"Hmm," Odile said, pretending to sound cross. "Your life was only just beginning, *and* you know it."

He smiled. "She's right. Before Odile I was a womanizer. After I met her I repented."

"Oh, yes, did you repent," smiled Odile. "Before you met me you were a *dog*!"

Marik took Cyndra's hand in his. "I kind of feel the same way myself."

This was news to her. She knew he liked her a lot, but he'd never expressed any serious intentions.

"It looks like you two are pretty cosy already," Odile said. "Do I hear moving in together noises?"

Gordon sipped a glass of brandy. "We like to see our artists happy. And I have some news, Cyndra, that should make you very happy indeed."

"Yes?"

"Your record broke the top forty."

She was wild with excitement. "It *did*?"

"True."

"Oh, this is so great!" She turned to Marik. "Did you know about this?"

He grinned, sheepishly. "Yeah, I knew, but Gordon's the boss – he wanted to tell you himself."

"I needed some good news in my life."

"Baby, you're gonna get all the good news you can handle," Marik said.

Later they made love. She thought about Gordon at home with his pretty wife and his two little children. He'd never so much as second glanced her. She was a recording artist – *his* recording artist – and that was all she meant to him. One of these days he'd look at her in a different fashion. One of these days he'd want her as much as she wanted him.

Cyndra knew there was no such thing as an ungettable man.

Later that night Nick dropped by to catch Joey's act. The club had not improved in his absence, nor had the lack-lustre hostesses.

Joey was funny – he had genuine talent – a talent he was pissing away in this joint.

"You promised you were comin' out to stay with me," Nick said.

"Hey, man, you're like a nursemaid," Joey complained. "Stop checkin' up on me."

"Tell you what – you come to LA an' I'll try to get you a role in my new movie."

Joey's lip curled. "Oh, big star now. You can get me a role, huh?"

"Maybe. But not if you're sitting on your ass in New York."

"I ain't sitting on my ass, man. I'm workin' for a living."

Nick took a good look at Joey. He wasn't an expert, but he could've sworn his friend was back on drugs.

"I'm sending you a ticket,' he said.

"I can buy my own ticket."

"Hey, listen – I got more money than you. Take advantage of it while you can."

"Fuck you," said Joey, grinning.

"Likewise," Nick replied.

He called Meena when he got back to the hotel. "I need a favour."

"Just tell me one thing," she said, sounding annoyed.

"What?"

"Who said you could fly to New York without telling me?"

"Am I supposed to check in?"

"No, but you *are* supposed to be in costume fittings tomorrow morning at nine a.m. sharp."

"I'll be back in forty-eight hours."

"In future, tell me."

"Yes, Mommy."

"Hilarious, Nick," Meena said, dryly. "What's the favour?"

"I got this talented friend. I'd like him to have a part in the movie."

She couldn't control her amusement. "Who do you think you are – Burt Reynolds?"

"At least get him in for a reading."

"What part did you have in mind?"

"He'd be good as the jail snitch."

"They've got someone they like."

"Make 'em see him, Meena, he's good."

"Very well, Nick, I'll try and arrange it. By the way, what *are* you doing in New York?"

"My publicist taught me one thing."

"What's that?"

"Always keep 'em guessing!"

In the morning he took a brisk walk through Central Park. A couple of girls recognized him, clutched on to each other and fell into fits of hysterical giggles.

Back at the hotel he called Jessie and told her he was definitely coming to her dinner.

"I'm delighted," she said. "Will you be bringing a date?"

"No, I'll be alone." He paused for a moment. "Uh, Jessie?"

"Yes?"

"Put Lauren next to me."

"You mean Oliver's wife?"

"Yeah, yeah. You see, Lauren and I . . . we, uh . . . we knew each other a long time ago."

"I wasn't aware of that."

471

"We lost touch, so it would be nice to catch up on old times. No big thing – but if you can seat her next to me I'd appreciate it."

"Of course, Nick. I look forward to seeing you."

Jessie put the phone down thoughtfully. Far be it from her to read anything into it, but it did seem rather odd that at first Nick had called to get Oliver's number and now he was requesting that Oliver's wife be seated beside him.

Oh well, it wasn't for Jessie to question, it was just for her to do. She had an interesting group planned, and Nick Angel would make it even more so.

If her instincts were correct it was going to be quite an evening.

Chapter 73

Lauren had been back from her trip to Rome for five weeks when she realized something was wrong. She'd been feeling queasy for a few days, and when she checked her calendar she realized she was late. This was unusual because she was never late.

One big thought loomed at the centre of her mind – was she pregnant?

Once she'd started to think about it she couldn't stop. She went to the gym and vigorously worked out. Then she came home and sat in a hot bath for an hour. She wanted a baby, and yet it wasn't possible because Oliver had never made love to her. So, if she *was* pregnant, how was she going to explain it?

I will not have an abortion, she thought. *I will not kill another baby.*

What are you going to do now, Roberts?

I don't know.

See where your little jaunt in Rome got you?

Shut up! Shut the fuck up!

There was only one answer: she had to get Oliver to make love to her properly.

He arrived home from the office early for a change.

"Can we talk?" she asked, handing him a martini.

He seemed distracted. "If we're going to the Georges' tonight, I have several calls to make before we leave."

"Oliver," she said, evenly. "I'm requesting a conversation. Is that too much to ask?"

"Of course not. I am merely pointing out I must make these calls before we go. Can our talk wait until later?"

"You're always tired when we come home."

"I won't be tired," he promised. "I'll make time for you."

473

Oh, how generous! The truth was he was beginning to get on her nerves.

She wondered if she could cancel the Georges. If they didn't go she'd have Oliver to herself and then who knew what could happen.

You have to get it up before you can get it in, Roberts.

I told you – shut the fuck up!

The thought of calling Jessie and cancelling out at this late hour was not one she relished. Jessie would throw a fit, especially as they hadn't seen her in a while.

With a sigh she realized they'd have to go.

She put on a simple black dress, brushed her hair and applied a careful make-up. Then she stood back and surveyed her image. Since she'd been doing the Marcella girl campaign there was a certain glow about her. Oliver called it the glow of success.

She wondered if it was the glow of having great sex with Lorenzo.

Once.

Once was not enough.

She was too guilty to do it twice.

Walking into the Georges' apartment she felt as if she should head straight for the kitchen and start cooking.

Jessie had gathered together her usual interesting mix, it would not be a dull evening.

She lifted a drink from a passing waiter, and spoke briefly to one of Oliver's competitors from a rival agency.

"Congratulations," the man said, standing too close. "I've seen the Marcella ads – they're very sleek. Trust Oliver to find the face of the year and marry it."

"I'm glad you like them," she said, surreptitiously backing off. "You have excellent taste."

He chortled. "So does Oliver."

She had her back to the door, but she sensed somebody important entering. Turning around she was startled to see Emerson Burn. His mane of hair was longer and wilder and he had acquired an even deeper suntan. Pale beige leather pants emphasized his long legs and he wore a stylish fringed jacket. The girl with him looked about twelve.

It didn't take long before he made his way over to her. "How you doin', luv?" he said, like they'd spoken the day before. "I 'ear you got married."

"I hear *you* got divorced," she responded, coolly.

He didn't seem too concerned. "It was bound to 'appen. Nature drove me bleedin' bonkers. Crazy bird."

Lauren indicated the young girl hovering by the door. "Is that your daughter you're with – or a date?"

"Ha, ha, still a comedian."

"You always bring out my sense of humour, Emerson."

"That's not exactly what you bring out in me." He pointed at Oliver across the room. "Is that the old geezer?"

"Don't call Oliver an old geezer."

"He ain't exactly in the first flush of youth." he said, scrutinizing her. "You're lookin' pretty good. Marriage must agree with you."

"You should know. *How* many times have you done it now?"

"Enough to know better."

Lorenzo swept down on them. Lorenzo in his impeccably tailored suit with his charming accent. He kissed her on both cheeks. "Ah, *bellissima*, every other woman in the room pales beside you."

"Cor, blimey," Emerson said. "I've 'eard a load of cobblers in me time, but this takes the cake."

"Emerson, meet Lorenzo Marcella."

"It is my pleasure," Lorenzo said, proffering a manicured hand. "I listen to your music – it brings me much delight."

"What do you do, Lorenzo?" Emerson asked.

"He owns Marcella Cosmetics," Lauren said, quickly. "It's an Italian firm whose products are just about to hit the American market."

"Em," Emerson's petite young girlfriend marched determinedly over with a frown on her face and a plaintive whine in her voice. "You left me standing over there by the door. I don't know anybody here. How can you do that to me?"

"Shush, love, there's grown-ups present."

"Yes," Lorenzo said, ignoring the interruption. "Lauren is the Marcella girl. Starting next month you will see her face everywhere."

"Well," Emerson said cheerfully, "it's a pretty enough face."

Shortly before dinner she began to feel queasy. She hurried into the bathroom, soaked a towel with cold water and held it to her forehead.

I'm pregnant.

How do you know?

Because I do.

Then it's your own fault.

475

Oh God! How was she going to explain it to Oliver?

Sweetheart, I know we've never had proper sex, but something miraculous has happened. We've had an immaculate conception.

It didn't sound too convincing.

When she emerged from the bathroom everyone was seated. She entered the dining room and slid into her empty seat. Lorenzo was on her left. "Are you feeling all right?" he asked, solicitously.

"Fine, thank you."

She turned to see who was seated on her other side and could not believe it.

"Hi, Lauren," said a familiar voice. "It's been a long time."

Nick.

Nick Angelo.

Her past swept over her rendering her speechless.

Their eyes met and locked together. For a moment she couldn't catch her breath. She felt her heart pounding in her chest and she didn't know what to do. There was no escape. She had to face up to him – it was inevitable.

"Hello, Nick," she said, weakly. "This is a surprise."

"I guess we're destined to meet at Jessie's parties, huh?" he said.

"It seems that way," she replied, trying to sound as casual as him.

Oh, God! His eyes were the same piercing green. His hair jet black and curly. He still had the indentation in the middle of his chin which drove her totally crazy.

"It's good to see you," he said, thinking that she looked more beautiful than ever.

"You too," she murmured.

They talked all the way through dinner. She never turned to her other side and Lorenzo was not pleased.

They started off with surface talk, gradually getting more personal, until eventually he mentioned his trip back to Bosewell and that he'd heard about her parents and how sorry he was.

She nodded. "It was a frightening time."

"You do know I wrote you," he said, staring at her intently.

"No, I didn't know that."

"Yeah, many times. I guess there was nowhere for the letters to go. I also wrote you a long letter when I left town explaining why I had to leave."

"Where did you send it?"

"I left it with Louise at the drugstore. She said she never had a chance to give it to you, but I didn't know that until I went back." He continued staring into her eyes. "How're you doing?"

476

"Fine," she said, not knowing how she was managing to talk at all.

"So you got married," he said.

"Yes. That's my husband at the other table," she said, pointing Oliver out.

He took a good look. "I don't mean to be rude or anything, but isn't he too old for you?"

"You *are* being rude," she said, trying to breathe evenly.

He grinned. "Yeah, well, remember me? I was never Mister Polite."

She couldn't help smiling back. Yes, she remembered him, she remembered him only too well. For a moment she got lost in his green eyes and it was all over. "I thought you didn't care," she murmured, softly.

"I thought the same about you."

She broke the stare and grabbed her glass of wine. Her hand was shaking and she wished it wasn't, but there was nothing she could do about it. "It was a long time ago – we were both very young."

"Yeah," he agreed. "Little kids."

"Not that little."

He leaned closer. "You're so . . . goddamn . . . beautiful."

She gulped more wine. "Nick . . . I . . ."

"Yes?"

"Oh . . . nothing." Desperately she tried to change the subject. "Who else did you see in Bosewell?" She held her breath, waiting for him to tell her his father was dead.

How did he die, Lauren?

You killed him.

"Saw your old friend, Meg. Guess what?"

"What?" she asked, breathlessly.

"She married that asshole Stock Browning."

"No! Really?"

"Are you surprised?"

"Well . . . I guess they do make a perfect couple."

"Jeez! What a pompous prick he was. And you were engaged to him."

"Only by default," she said, quickly.

"Don't use big words on me."

She picked up her wine glass again. "Remember the night he broke your nose?"

"Oh, yeah," he said, ruefully. "Like I'm gonna forget that.

477

You took me home with you and your parents were really thrilled."

"And in the morning we drove to Ripley."

He fixed her with another long stare. "Now *that* was memorable."

"Very," she said, returning his look.

He shook his head. "Jesus, Lauren – it seems like such a long time ago."

She turned the stem of the wine glass in her hands. "I thought about you a lot, Nick. Where did you go?"

"Chicago. Got a job in a club, ended up doing everything – barman, disc jockey, you name it I did it. Then I moved to LA."

"It must have been exciting."

"Hey, anything was exciting after Bosewell." He hesitated for a moment, then added, "Missing you wasn't."

"Did you think about me?" she asked, softly.

"Every single day."

"Me, too."

"There's something I need to say –" he began.

"Lauren." Lorenzo had had enough. He jabbed her sharply in the ribs. "Introduce me to your friend."

She was shaken back to reality. "Oh, uh, this is Nick . . . Nick Angelo."

He cleared his throat. "It's Angel now."

"Of course. How could I forget." She began to giggle hysterically. "Angel. What kind of name is that?"

He grinned. "Hey – it's my professional name, don't make fun of it."

"Oh, well," she said, still giggling, "in that case – Lorenzo, meet Nick Angel, we used to go to High school together."

"We used to do a lot of things together," Nick said, catching her with his eyes.

They exchanged intimate smiles.

I love you, Nick. Nothing's changed.

Get real, Roberts. You're a married woman carrying another man's baby.

Lorenzo did not appreciate this situation one little bit. He sensed competition and reacted fiercely. The husband was one thing – easy to deal with. But this man was a threat, and Lorenzo did not like threats.

"Recently Lauren and I were in Rome together," he said,

478

snaking a possessive arm across her shoulders. "Ah, such a romantic city! Have you been there . . . Rick?"

"It's Nick," Lauren said quickly, moving so that she dislodged his arm.

"Whatever," Lorenzo said, disdainfully.

"No," Nick said. "But I may make a movie there next year." He was lying – but screw this Italian prick who quite obviously had big eyes for Lauren.

"Gina Lollabrigida is a very good friend of mine," Lorenzo said, adjusting a perfect silk cuff.

Nick looked at him blankly. "Gina who?"

"Gina is one of the biggest movie stars in Italy. And a great beauty."

"This'll be a contemporary film," Nick said, winking at Lauren.

She pushed her chair away from the table and stood up. She was feeling queasy again.

"You look pale, *bellissima*," Lorenzo said, leaping to his feet.

"No . . . no, I'm fine. I'll be right back," she said, glancing over at the other table. Oliver was making conversation with Emerson Burn. Good. She had enough to handle with Nick and Lorenzo surrounding her, she didn't need any more complications.

The guest bathroom was occupied, so she made her way down the corridor to Jessie's bedroom where she sat on the edge of the bed and attempted to think straight. It was all too much. Oliver, Emerson, Lorenzo . . . and Nick.

The only person she really cared about was Nick. In fact, she loved him just as much as she always had. He was in her heart and in her soul, but she was trapped in an impossible situation, and there was nothing she could do about it.

"What's going on, Lauren?" Nick walked in, startling her.

"Uh . . . nothing."

"Can I see you?" he asked, urgently.

"You are seeing me."

His green eyes captured her attention. "You know what I mean."

She knew exactly what he meant.

He walked over and stood very close, pulling her to her feet.

She was melting inside. Falling . . . falling . . . And when he began to kiss her it was like time stood perfectly still and nothing else mattered. They kissed feverishly.

His hands touched her face. "Oh God, Lauren, I missed you so much."

She managed to push him away, fighting for her life, desperately trying to gain control of the situation. "Nick, you're forgetting something. I'm married. *Very* married."

"Get a divorce."

"It's not that easy."

"We'll make it easy."

"No . . . I . . . I can't."

He kissed her again, forcing her to be silent.

She closed her eyes and she was sixteen again, and there was no more pain. She was safe with Nick; she'd always been safe with him.

He held her tightly and she felt his urgent desire pressing against her. She knew she should break their embrace, but she didn't have the strength nor the inclination.

"I love you, Lauren." He whispered the words she was waiting to hear. "I've always loved you."

She wasn't sixteen any more. She was a grown woman and she could do what she liked.

How do you know he's not lying to you? It's easy for him to say he wrote you. But remember – he left you pregnant, and now you're pregnant again.

"Nick . . . I . . ."

It was too late to protest. She was just as caught up in the passion of the moment as he was.

They fell back on the bed locked in a dangerous embrace.

His hands began exploring her body beneath her clothes and she lost all sense of time and place.

"I love you, Lauren," he kept on repeating like a mantra. "I love you – love you –"

"Excuse *me*," a woman's voice interrupted them.

Guiltily they broke apart.

Jessie hurried over to her dressing table pretending she hadn't noticed what they were up to. "Lauren, Oliver is looking for you," she said casually, picking up her silver hairbrush. "Oh, and Nick, why don't you stay here for a few moments?"

Lauren felt her cheeks burning. She adjusted her dress and fluffed her hair. Real life was back with a vengeance.

"Call me, I'm at the Plaza," Nick said in a low voice. "I'll wait for your call."

She nodded, knowing she wouldn't call.

It was too late to go back.

Nick Angelo was her past. It had to stay that way.

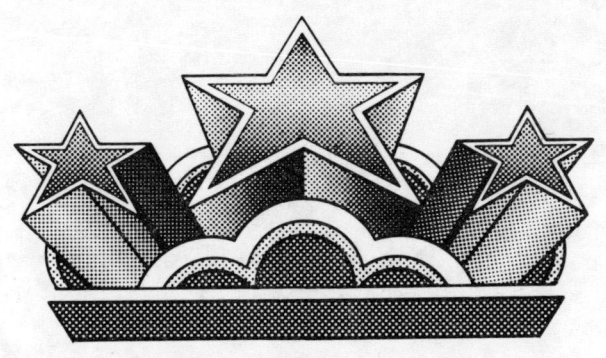

BOOK THREE
1988

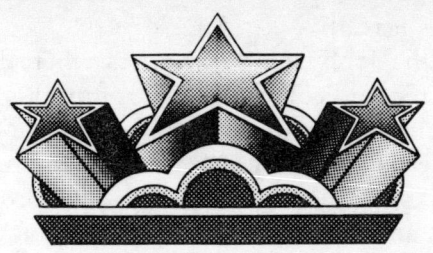

Chapter 74

The crowds went crazy. Totally berserk. Nick could hear them before he left the safety of his limo, screaming his name, yelling hysterically. Annie sat beside him, impassive as usual. He took another swig of Scotch from the leaded glass in his hands, put it on the carpet of the limo and said to his bodyguard, "Okay, let's go."

Igor, an enormous bald black man, said, "Yes, boss," in a feathery little voice that did not quite match his looks.

They had a routine. Igor left the limousine first and met up with his other two bodyguards who followed in a back-up car. Then the three of them formed a shield around Nick, and Annie trailed behind as they made a rush for the entrance of the theatre.

It was the première of Nick's new movie, *Hoodlum*. On each side of the red carpet press and paparazzi lined up, thrusting cameras at him, screaming his name. They were almost as bad as the fans.

He'd learnt how to handle it. Stare straight ahead – don't look to the left or right – just keep walking, never stop.

Stardom.

It was a pisser.

The crowds tonight were unruly. They began trying to break through the barriers, struggling with the police holding them back.

He quickened his step, holding on to Annie's hand, dragging her along behind him. After all, she was his wife, it wouldn't do to lose her.

The crowd began to chant. "NICK! NICK! WE LOVE YOU! WE LOVE YOU!"

Yeah, it was all very nice, but sometimes he felt like such a phoney. Who was this person they'd created? This icon. Was it really him? Was it really Nick Angelo?

They made the lobby of the theatre, where he was greeted by his agent, Freddie Leon. Meena Caron no longer handled his career, he was now looked after by Freddie, the head of a rival company to Meena's – I.A.A. – International Artists Agents.

Freddie was a poker-faced man in his early forties, with cordial features and a quick bland smile. His nickname was The Snake, because he could slither in and out of any deal. Nobody ever called him The Snake to his face.

Since Nick had been with him – which was over four years, now – Freddie had guided his career to superstardom status.

Freddie gave Annie a quick peck on the cheek and then ignored her. She was Mrs Angel. She deserved an acknowledgement, but that was about it. Stars' wives had to know how to stay in the background, look attractive and keep quiet.

Annie was not good at it. Her anger bubbled beneath the surface like a volcano about to erupt.

Freddie put his arm around Nick's shoulders and they walked into the theatre together – the superagent and the superstar. The celebrity-filled audience turned to look. These two men were Hollywood royalty.

Mrs Freddie Leon waved to Annie and they exchanged empty kisses on the cheek.

Everybody was smiling except Nick. Bridget, his original publicist had taught him well. Moody was best. Moody worked every time.

Bridget was no longer his publicist. He was now represented by Ian Gem, a wiry PR dynamo with flat red hair that looked like a wig, although it was all his own.

Nick sat down in his reserved seat with Freddie on one side and Annie on the other. He wished he'd brought his drink in with him, but that would have caused Ian to throw a fit. It wouldn't do to be seen drinking in public.

Why the hell not? He could do what the fuck he liked.

Carlysle Mann walked down the aisle and waved at him. She was with her new husband – a studio head with a tired expression and crinkle-cut hair. Christ! Living with Carlysle was enough to make anybody exhausted.

He and Annie rarely exchanged words any more. Nearly seven years of a loveless marriage and they were growing more apart every day. The more famous he became the more hostile Annie was. She would never forgive him for the career she'd never had.

He'd married Annie for two reasons: One – the anonymous body buried somewhere in the Las Vegas desert; Two – the fact that she was pregnant. He had a daughter now – the one light of his life. She was called Lissa.

The audience settled into their seats, twisting and turning, greeting him if they could, waving, blowing air kisses, generally brown-nosing. These were the same people who'd once ignored him. Fuck 'em. He could play the Hollywood game as well as anyone.

He'd seen the movie at least fifty times. One of the enjoyable things about making movies was the editing process. He'd gotten into that on his third movie, and now with every film he made, he liked to sit in with the editors – viewing the film frame by frame, shaping it to make it exactly what he wanted.

He knew he was only allowed to do this because he had the power. Last week he'd told Freddie that he wanted to direct.

"Whatever you want," Freddie had replied, totally unfazed.

Being a superstar meant never having aspirations you couldn't achieve.

The lights began to dim. Nick hunched his shoulders and slid down in his seat. It was all so unreal, this movie stardom shit. He'd done nothing to deserve it, and yet he was now at a place where the atmosphere was so heady he could hardly breathe.

Nick Angel – superstar. How had it all happened?

He tried to think – clear his mind. Every day there was so much going on – so many demands on his time. He never had a moment alone. Sitting in the darkened theatre was a pleasure – no one to bother him – no fucking leeches clinging on to his every word.

Annie fidgeted beside him. Annie who'd turned into the definitive Hollywood wife. She gave great charity – yes, Annie was extremely generous with his money.

This was the first time she'd seen *Hoodlum*. She hadn't gone to any of the previews or special sneak screenings that gauged early audience reaction. No. Annie had told him she didn't care to sit through his latest movie more than once. Bitch! If she could find an opportunity to put him down she did.

According to Annie he'd sold out, become a movie star instead of the fine actor he could have been. *Bullshit*. What was wrong with making six million bucks a movie? He noticed she had no trouble spending it.

They'd moved three times in the past seven years. First the modest little house above Sunset with a breathtaking view of the city. Then the larger house in fashionable Pacific Palisades. And finally the Bel Air mansion.

Who needed a fucking mansion? He certainly didn't.

Annie was into decorating. She'd surrounded herself with a bunch of gay interior designers and they all had a high old time spending, spending, spending.

His name appeared on the screen and there was a ripple of applause. Hey – he didn't have to turn in a performance, they loved him anyway.

He wasn't quite sure how it had happened – he only knew it had happened fast. From modest success to cult superstardom. Three easy steps. Meena Caron had taken him the first two levels – Freddie Leon had whisked him into the stratosphere.

The movie started and his image filled the screen. His co-star was a moody blonde with downturned lips and smoky eyes. They'd had an affair. It was one of the perks of being a superstar – you got to fuck whoever you wanted – and leading ladies were up for grabs.

Freddie could get to do the same thing if he wanted, but Freddie never availed himself. He'd once told Nick that the high he got from a great deal was far more satisfying than any transient fuck.

Lucky Freddie. He had his power base agency, an attractive intelligent wife who'd been his college sweetheart, and a couple of well-behaved teenage kids. He had it all.

Nick did not consider himself so lucky – although some might say he was the luckiest man in the world. How many red-blooded males would love to be in his position? He was a star. He could have any woman he wanted. People laughed at his jokes. He got the best tables in restaurants. He was fêted wherever he went. He was adored, worshipped and loved.

But it wasn't enough. He didn't have Lauren.

He often thought about the last time he'd seen her. It was in New York at Jessie George's dinner party. When they were together it was like no time had passed. They'd ended up in the bedroom, about to renew their relationship when Jessie had interrupted them.

Lauren had promised to call. He'd never heard from her again. Five long gut-wrenching days he'd sat in his hotel room waiting before he was forced to fly back to LA to start the new movie.

When he'd got back he'd tried to contact her, but she'd refused to take his calls.

Soon after their meeting in New York, photographs of her had started appearing in all the magazines. He'd been prepared to forget her, but it wasn't possible. There she was staring out at him – that beautiful, incredible face. The Marcella Girl.

Over the years she hadn't gone away. As his star had risen so had hers. She was probably the most famous model in America now. And he was probably the most famous movie star.

But it wasn't enough. Not by a long way.

When he'd returned to LA after the New York trip Annie had been waiting as usual. He'd been considering having a talk with her, saying it wasn't working out. But he was sure if he did, she'd run straight to the police. She had him where she wanted him – and she knew it.

Annie had greeted him with unexpected news. "We're having a baby."

What did he have to lose? Lauren was married, and obviously didn't want anything to do with him, so he'd married Annie because he didn't like the idea of his baby growing up with no father.

Bridget and Meena had thrown a fit. According to them marriage was a career killer. They'd made him keep it secret for two months, until one day Annie had blurted it out to a reporter – by accident, she'd said, but nobody believed her.

After that she'd started getting the attention she thought she deserved. Mrs Nick Angel got a lot more kudos than plain Annie Broderick.

Joey had finally made his way out to the coast and Nick kept his promise and got him a part in his movie. Joey had taken to California immediately, and Nick was so pleased that he'd made it a habit to put Joey in every movie he made. Eventually Joey had overdosed on his minor success. Three years after coming to live in LA he was found dead in his girlfriend's apartment with an empty vial of crack beside him.

Nick had not blamed himself. He'd done everything he could for his friend – but drugs won. Joey's death was inevitable.

Sitting in his seat Nick began getting that old restless feeling. Watching his face on the screen drove him crazy. Sometimes he wished it had never happened. Hadn't he been happier in Chicago running the bar for Q.J. and living with DeVille? No pressure

487

then. Now there was so much fucking pressure he sometimes thought he'd explode.

He got up.

"Where are you going?" Annie hissed.

"Gotta take a leak."

He walked outside, grabbed an usher and handed him a hundred-dollar bill. "Do me a favour, run to the liquor store and buy me a quart of Scotch. Keep the change."

"Yes, *sir*," said the young guy, fully impressed.

He paced around the lobby until the usher returned, then he took the bottle into the john and took a few solid swigs. The strong liquor burned a hole in his stomach. He hadn't eaten all day, had to keep the gaunt look, had to keep the Nick Angel image.

Peering in the mirror he wondered why it had happened to him. Oh yeah, sure he looked okay, but he was certainly no Redford or Newman.

Shit! The trouble was he had everything, and yet he knew for a fact it could all vanish tomorrow.

Why wasn't he happy?

Because he was living with a woman he didn't love, and it made him feel empty inside.

He swigged enough Scotch to give him the strength to go back to his seat.

As soon as he sat down Annie smelt the liquor on his breath. "Couldn't you wait?" she said, in an angry whisper.

Screw you, he wanted to say. *Get out of my life. Go to the police if you want. I've paid for burying that body a million times.*

And yet at the back of his mind he knew she could ruin everything if she exposed him.

Cyndra was unconcerned, but Cyndra lived in her own world; she thought nobody could touch them.

After the movie there was the obligatory party. He didn't mingle – he didn't have to. He sat at a table with Freddie, while people trouped over to pay their respects.

"Sometimes I feel like the Godfather," Freddie joked, loving every minute of his silent authority.

"You've got the power," Nick said, gulping a glass of Scotch.

"So've you," Freddie replied, sticking to Perrier.

Nick got along with Freddie because Freddie didn't give a damn about anything except the deal. There was something likeable about his steely single-mindedness.

Freddie's wife, Diana, engaged Annie in light conversation. They weren't exactly bosom buddies, but Annie was about as friendly with Diana as she was with anybody.

Annie was no social butterfly. Women didn't warm to her because she was too critical and outspoken. She was also bitter and a bitch. She and Cyndra had stopped speaking long ago. Cyndra knew that Annie had forced him into marriage, even though he tried to deny it. "Listen, I made her pregnant," he'd explained. "I wanted to be a father to my baby." Cyndra wasn't having it.

He had to admit that he loved his little girl; Lissa was quite a character. The only time he was really at peace were the afternoons he spent with her – teaching her to swim in the pool, running around the garden with her, watching her play with her toys.

Annie always managed to spoil their times together. She'd appear at just the wrong moment and summon Lissa in for a piano lesson or a dancing class.

"Leave the kid alone," he'd say.

"I want her to have all the advantages I never had. Don't try and stop her progress."

"Fuck you, Annie."

It had become his lament. *Fuck you, Annie.*

Hoodlum was well-received. The critics loved it. Right now he could do no wrong. Each movie he did received more and more praise.

The brooding intensity of Angel's performance propels this movie to new heights read one glowing review.

Angel scores again! A dark performance filled with pain and bitterness as only Angel can portray it, read another.

He'd thought about taking a break, maybe visiting Hawaii with Lissa and the nanny.

Annie soon put a stop to that. "She has to go to summer school," she said. "I want her to learn Spanish."

"She's six years old," he objected. "Give her a chance to have some fun."

Annie glared at him. "You control your career. At least let me control what happens to our child."

Over the next few months he met with the writer and director of his upcoming movie, *Miami Connection*. It was the

489

kind of role he hadn't tackled before and he liked it a lot. A young cop who gets caught up in a drug scam, is coerced by the villains, and eventually turns the tables.

The search was on for a suitable co-star. The director wanted a star. Freddie, who had very good instincts, suggested they go with somebody new.

"Let's discover somebody," Freddie said, enthusiastically. "I'm in the mood to make a new star!"

Carlysle Mann phoned Nick and told him she wanted the part.

"It's not up to me," he said.

"You're full of shit," she said.

Ah, Carlysle . . . still as sweet as ever.

A few days later he was having lunch in the private dining room at the I.A.A. offices when Freddie picked up a magazine and threw it across the table.

"Take a look at this girl," he said. "She's the top model in the country. I've been asked to represent her. What do you think? Should we bring her out for a screen test?"

Before Nick looked at the magazine he knew who it was.

Lauren.

"Yeah," he said. "I'll test with her myself. Fly her out."

Chapter 75

Lauren sat behind the desk in her Park Avenue office. The room was light and bright, furnished with sleek bird's-eye maple furniture and comfortable beige couches. On the walls were framed covers of all the top fashion and women's magazines featuring her. The Lauren Roberts image dominated. Sexy. Sweet. Thoughtful. Provocative. She could be anything the photographer required – hence her enormous success. A block of *Vogue* covers took pride of place. She'd asked Samm for one cover. She'd got it and gone on to be their favourite cover girl for the last seven years.

Concluding a meeting she stood up, walked around her desk and shook hands with the two men and one woman she'd been meeting with. "I like your ideas," she said. "Put everything in writing and I'll give you my decision."

"As soon as possible I hope," said one of the men, his bull neck flushed with the thought of success.

"It's your move," Lauren replied, smiling.

"I think we can lay out a deal that'll please you."

"Good. I'll look forward to it." She ushered them from her office and closed the door. "No way," she said, turning to Pia, who sat unobtrusively in the corner.

"How come?"

"'Cause they're a nickel-and-dime operation. I knew it was a waste of time meeting with them."

"They're offering you a lot of money for one simple exercise video."

"What do you want to bet it's all deferred payments? I'd sooner deal with legitimate people and make less money."

"In that case why did you agree to see them?"

Lauren grinned. "To test out my gut instinct. Trust me, it's still working."

Her secretary buzzed. "Mr Liberty on line two."

"I'll take it." She picked up the phone. "Oliver, what can I do for you?"

It struck Pia that she talked to her husband as if they were working colleagues rather than man and wife.

"Okay," Lauren said, rather irritably. "I know. I'll be there." She put down the phone and glanced at the Art Deco Cartier clock on her desk. "Oliver's getting panicky. I promised I'd go to the Raleigh cocktail party. Damn! I'm late, aren't I? Do you think I have time to go home and change?"

"You look great," Pia said, and marvelled at exactly how great Lauren looked. She was staggeringly beautiful, although it was no longer the innocent somewhat naïve beauty she'd once possessed. Lauren was sleek, almost feline with her long thick chestnut hair streaked with blonde, unusual tortoiseshell eyes and full sensuous lips.

At thirty she was more stunning than she'd ever been. Glossy, slick – but still with that faint vulnerability – Lauren was the face of the decade.

Sometimes Pia thought she envied her. Other times she knew she didn't. Lauren had everything, and yet she had nothing. She had an empty marriage, no children, a business empire and great fame, but she was always chasing more. She wanted to be tops at everything she did. It wasn't enough that she was one of the most sought after models in the world. That she had lent her name to a very successful clothing line, and co-authored a beauty book. Now she was looking into an acting career.

"Why don't you take some time off and enjoy your success?" Pia said to her one day. "You're always in such a hurry to conquer new mountains."

"I love working," Lauren had replied. "Working is my life!"

No wonder she and Oliver got along. Twin personalities.

Outside her Park Avenue office Lauren got into her car. She had her own limo and driver – preferring not to share Oliver's. Their schedules were never in sync so they needed separate cars.

She told her driver where to go, and reached for the day's newspapers stacked neatly on the seat opposite her. Lauren did not believe in wasting time; car journeys allowed her the perfect opportunity to scan the newspapers.

She went through the *New York Post* in record time, perused the *Wall Street Journal*, glanced at *Newsday* and stopped at a column piece in *The News*. It was a short gossip item about Nick. He'd been spotted out and about with his latest leading lady. Nothing new about that.

Hmm, she thought – *if Nick Angel had screwed every woman he was linked with he'd be dead.*

She put the paper down and frowned. She wished she could stop thinking about him. She wished that he would vanish. But this was not to be. Nick Angel was a superstar. He was everywhere she went.

She thought about the last time she'd seen him in Jessie George's New York apartment and shivered. Every so often she re-lived that night in her head. Being in the same room with Emerson, Lorenzo and Oliver was unnerving enough – but when she'd seen Nick everything had changed. At first it had been so good to see him, so wonderful – and she'd gotten carried away with the moment. But it was only for a moment, because reality soon reminded her that she was a married woman. And not only that, she was pregnant – or at least she'd thought so at the time.

A week later she'd gotten her period. It had all been a false alarm.

"Probably the European trip threw you off schedule," her gynaecologist had told her. "It often happens."

If there wasn't Oliver to consider she would have been a free person. She'd thought about calling Nick and seeing him again, but she didn't have his number in LA, although it would have been easy enough to find if she'd really wanted to. But did she?

She woke up one morning a few months later and realized that yes, she did. Maybe if she divorced Oliver there'd be a chance for her and Nick to be together after all.

She'd decided to use her connections, find out where he was and call him.

Before she had a chance, the papers were full of the news. Nick Angel had gotten secretly married.

With a dull feeling of hopelessness she'd known it was too late for her to do anything.

Lauren arrived at the cocktail party late. Oliver glowered at her. "It was important for me that you were here earlier," he snapped.

"I'm sorry," she replied coolly, not really sorry at all. "I was in a meeting. Surely you understand better than anyone that business comes first?"

493

She knew why he wanted her there. People were impressed when they found out she was his wife.

After the cocktail party there was a boring dinner with business people. She excused herself and left early, much to Oliver's chagrin.

Back at the apartment there were several messages on her private answering machine. Two were from Lorenzo.

Ah, sweet faithful Lorenzo. He'd never given up hope, even though he was now a married man. He'd wed a beautiful eighteen-year-old Italian girl, but he still lusted after Lauren.

She called him first. "What can I do for you, Lorenzo?"

He laughed. "You know what I would like you to do for me, *bellissima*."

"Cut it out, Lorenzo. It's late, I'm tired and I'm not in the mood for your phoney Italian bullshit."

"Ah, such a lady. Whatever happened to the sweet innocent girl I used to know?"

"She grew up."

"I was thinking," he said. "Would you entertain the idea of adding a line of cosmetics to your fragrance line?"

Lorenzo sure knew how to make a girl interested.

"It's a great idea – when did you come up with it?"

"Your fragrance has been so successful the other directors and I thought it might be a good idea if we started a limited line. We would call it The Lauren Roberts Collection. You like that?"

"I like it," she said, enthusiastically. "Can you stop by my office, say at noon tomorrow, and we'll discuss it?"

"But of course," he replied, pleased because he had her full attention.

She hung up the phone and smiled. The more she achieved the better she liked it. Three years ago Marcella had financed her with her own scent collection. It had been an enormous success. To branch into make-up would be an interesting challenge.

Being a model had never been enough for Lauren. She felt that her beauty was a gift and that taking advantage of it and forging a good professional career was an excellent way to handle her gift. Her business acumen she'd developed. In a way it was much more important to her than merely looking good. She wasn't going to be a model forever. She was thirty now and she had to protect her future.

There were several more messages on her answering machine.

The only call she decided to return was the one from Samm. It was past eleven, but Samm was a night person.

"I'm not waking you, am I?" she asked.

"Not at all," Samm replied. "I was hoping you'd get back to me tonight."

"What's up?"

"Can you fly to Los Angeles tomorrow?"

She laughed incredulously. "No, Samm, I cannot fly to Los Angeles tomorrow. What are you talking about?"

"I'm talking about that big chance you've been waiting for."

"I've had plenty of big chances," Lauren replied. "And I'm not waiting for anything."

"Short memory," Samm said, crisply. "For the last eighteen months you've been badgering me about a film career."

"And you've told me it's not something I should pursue. You said models do not make good actresses – all they make is fools of themselves."

"Yes, Lauren, but when you talk I listen. You're very smart."

"Thanks, Samm. Coming from you I guess that's a compliment."

"Without your knowledge I've been speaking to Freddie Leon. Do you know who he is?"

"Oh, come on, I took the straw out of my hair a long time ago."

"Anyway, I thought if you were going to have representation in LA it should be the best. As you know, Freddie handles only a very few select clients, and they're all top stars."

"So?"

"So, he's interested in representing *you*. He wants you to fly to LA tomorrow to test for the new Nick Angel movie." There was a long silence. "Lauren – are you there?"

"Yes, I'm here."

"Will you do it?"

She took a deep breath. "Yes, I'll do it."

Chapter 76

"How many times must I tell you, Marik? I have no desire to get married."

"But, baby, baby, we're so good together."

"I know," Cyndra relented – but only a little. Marik was the sweetest man she'd ever met and she didn't want to hurt his feelings. "I don't see us married," she said.

Actually she did see them married, but it was impossible. Somewhere out there was a man called Reece Webster, and she had no idea where. All she knew was that she was legally married to him, and there was nothing she could do about it.

Or maybe there was. Lately she'd been considering confiding in Gordon. He was an important and powerful man and now she was his important and powerful recording star. If she went to him in strict confidence maybe he could help her.

Of course, she wouldn't tell him anything about the shooting, that was privileged information. She would just tell him she was once married to this guy who'd run out on her, and how could she get a divorce.

Over the years Gordon and she had forged a good friendship. There'd been one little glitch three years ago when she'd come right out and confessed her feelings for him. He'd sat her down and talked to her like a father.

"Cyndra," he'd said. "When you find what *I* have, you never want to risk losing it. You're a beautiful and fine woman, and I love you in my own way. But Odile is my life, and nothing will ever change that."

Strangely enough she'd understood exactly what he was saying and accepted it. Since that time they'd been best friends.

Marik and she were still an item. It was better to be with

one guy than fight off the lines of men that came sniffing around after she became a star.

Stardom. Nick hated it. She loved it. What a trip! She'd had eight hit singles, three mega albums and was even now contemplating the offer of her own television series.

One night she and Nick had started laughing about it.

"Maybe there was something in the water at Bosewell High," he'd joked. "It's crazy that we've all made it so big. You, me and Lauren."

"What about the rest of them?" she'd asked.

"Yeah, well, you had to drink the water and *then* get out fast," he'd explained, laughing. "That's the way it works."

A year ago she'd persuaded Aretha Mae to come and live with her. The old woman was very sickly and stayed in her room all day muttering to herself.

"Are you out of your mind?" Nick had said. "What do you want her around for?"

"Because she brought me up. Because she busted her ass so I could go to school and have food on the table. And I couldn't live with myself if I didn't care for her now."

Marik also thought she was nuts. "I hate the way that batty old lady looks at me," he complained.

"What do you mean, looks at you? She never comes out of her room."

"She spies on me from her window."

"Big deal. It shouldn't bother you."

"She's loco – and you know it."

"Yeah, but she's also my mother."

Neither she nor Nick had achieved any success with Harlan. He'd never contacted them. They weren't even sure if they had the right address any more, but they both regularly sent money.

"One of these days," Cyndra said, "I'm gonna ride into town in a big old limo with an entourage and a couple of strong bodyguards. Then I'm gonna find Harlan, throw him in the back of my car, and bring him back here."

Nick had no doubt that one day Cyndra would do it. She was strong-willed enough.

Every couple of weeks she and Nick spoke on the phone.

"Why don't you ever come by the house?" he asked.

"You know why. I try to avoid that wife of yours – she's such a bad-tempered witch."

"Lissa misses you."

"Really?"

"You know she likes seeing you."

"So bring her over to my house one day. Maybe she'll lure Aretha Mae out of her room."

He changed the subject. "Lauren's coming to town."

"How do you know?"

"Because she's testing for my new movie."

"I'm proud of you, Nick. How did you fix that?"

"Freddie's thinking of representing her. He suggested it."

"Oh, and you didn't exactly fight it?"

He laughed. "Nope. I guess not."

"You'd better not let Annie find out," Cyndra warned. "She'll slice your balls up and lay 'em out for the fans."

"You got a graphic way with words."

"How long is it since you've seen Lauren?"

"I look at her every day. All I have to do is pick up a magazine."

"You're not exactly out of the limelight yourself, Nick. Anyway, she's still married, isn't she?"

"Yeah."

"Then you're both perfectly safe."

"Gee, thanks. That's just what I wanted to hear."

Freddie was totally unaware that Nick and Lauren were already acquainted. He sent one of his minions to meet her at the airport, and then visited her when she was installed in a bungalow at the Beverly Hills Hotel.

He called Nick later. "I'm not usually impressed," he said, "but I have just met the most beautiful woman I've ever seen. And sweet, too. And sharp. And intelligent."

"You met Lauren, huh?"

"What's with the Lauren bit?"

"Neither of us advertise the fact, but we went to High school together."

"You're kidding?"

"No, I'm not kidding."

"Then how come you didn't nail her? She's gorgeous. And you know me, Nick, I do not get enthusiastic about anybody."

This was true. Freddie rarely noticed or commented on women. Sexual chemistry was not his thing.

"Uh . . . do me a favour," Nick added. "Keep this information to yourself. I'm not sure Lauren wants people knowing. And I certainly don't think it's a good idea to spread it around."

"Why? What's the big secret about going to High school with someone?"

Nick sighed. "We did more than go to High school."

"You *did* nail her?"

It was so unlike Freddie to talk like one of the guys that he was quite shocked.

"Hey, Freddie," he said, edgily. "Maybe she nailed me. What's the difference? I don't answer questions like that."

Freddie didn't seem to notice his aggravation. "She's *really* beautiful, Nick."

"I know."

After he hung up he was unreasonably pissed off. What the fuck was Freddie getting interested for? Before he had a chance to think about it further, Annie buzzed him on the intercom.

"Dinner's ready," she said.

They had a cook who usually attended to such menial tasks as cooking, but recently Annie had been attending a gourmet cooking class, and now, three nights a week, they were treated to her culinary concoctions.

He went downstairs, sat at the dining-room table and toyed with a plateful of pumpkin ravioli.

"Don't you like it?" she asked, accusingly.

"It's bitter," he replied, pushing it around the plate.

"God, I can never do anything right, can I?"

"You asked for my opinion."

"You're at home now, Nick," she said, angrily. "You're not on show for the fans. You don't have to make a fuss about everything – I'm not waiting on you hand and foot, so don't expect me to."

"Annie, you know what?"

She turned on him, eyes blazing. "What?"

"Aw, shit . . . forget it."

That night he couldn't sleep. He lay in bed imagining Lauren ensconced in the Beverly Hills Hotel. What was she thinking? Was she looking forward to seeing him as much as he was looking forward to seeing her?

Annie came to bed wearing her peach peignoir. It signalled sex.

Christ! Occasionally he did it with his wife. He had to, didn't he? He never would have thought that sex would become a chore, but it was.

The next morning he was up early and out of the house

before Annie awoke. Lauren was going to be testing with him. He didn't want to keep her waiting.

The studio limo picked her up at seven. She wore jeans, sweat-shirt, a baseball cap, no make-up and huge shades.

"Morning, Ms Roberts," her driver greeted her, checking her out in the rear-view mirror. He was young and good-looking, standard Hollywood fare. "It's a clear day today. No smog."

"That's nice," she said.

"Unusual," he said.

Damn, he wanted conversation and she wasn't in the mood. Once she would have humoured him, been polite, chatted all the way to the studio even though she didn't want to. Now she was a different Lauren, no longer into pleasing everyone. She pressed the privacy glass cutting him off mid-sentence.

Pia had wanted to come with her, but she'd said no, this was one trip she had to make by herself. This trip was a test. She was all grown up and she wasn't about to turn to mush when she saw Nick again.

Arriving at the studio she was hustled straight through to make-up. "I have my own ideas," she said to the make-up artist.

"Fine with me," the girl said. "I'll do whatever you want."

"I see this character as tough looking – yet with a vulnerable streak. Smoky eyes, natural eyebrows, not much lipstick."

"Sounds good," the girl said.

Lauren had studied the script on the plane. As usual, the female role was somewhat passive, but if she got the part she had lots of ideas.

"I heard a rumour that Nick Angel is coming in to test with you himself," the girl said, in reverent tones.

Lauren wasn't surprised. She'd known he'd be around. Well, she was prepared. They were both married now – they were even.

"He's a nice guy," the make-up girl volunteered. "His wife's a real pain, though. She doesn't visit the set often, but when she does – oh boy, run for the hills. You'd think she was royalty."

"Is she an actress?" Lauren asked.

"From what I hear she tried to be and never made it."

"Oh," Lauren said. She'd seen pictures of Nick with his wife. She wasn't the woman she'd imagined he'd marry.

I am not tingling with anticipation, she told herself, sternly.

500

When I see him I will not fall to pieces like I did last time. I'm a different person now. I've finally grown up. It's been a long time.

Yes, Roberts?

Yes.

They met on the set, so there was no time to get personal as they were surrounded by people.

"Hey, congratulations on all your success," Nick said, a polite but friendly stranger. "It's really great to see you again."

"You, too, Nick. You're amazing. I can't believe your career."

He smiled. "I know – it's good, huh?"

She smiled back. "Very good."

He peered at her closely. "Now – let me see – there's something different about you."

She grimaced. "Yeah, wrinkles – I'm older."

"You – *never*."

"Thank you."

The director came over to introduce himself, and ask her if she was comfortable with the scene. She assured him she was.

"I've studied the script. I understand this character."

"Good," said the director, moving off to confer with his lighting cameraman.

"Freddie Leon's very high on you," Nick said, impressed with the way she handled herself. "He thinks you could be big."

"I'm glad I have the opportunity to test for this movie. You know I always loved acting."

He nodded, remembering Betty and their acting class in Bosewell. "This sure takes me back. Remember *Cat on a Hot Tin Roof*?"

She smiled. "How could I ever forget it?"

"You were the actress then," he admitted. "I was the amateur."

"And now it's the other way around."

"Hey, don't knock it – you're just as famous as I am."

She nodded. "It's funny, isn't it?"

"Yeah – Cyndra and I were talking the other night. We decided there must have been something in the water at Bosewell High."

"In that case . . ."

"I know what you're gonna say –" he interrupted, laughing. "So what happened with Stock an' Meg and all the rest of 'em?

The scam is this – you had to drink the water, *then* get out of town."

They were both quiet for a moment before she continued the conversation. "Congratulations, Nick," she said. "I haven't seen you since you got married. I understand you have a child."

"Yeah, Lissa – she's a little beauty."

For one painful moment Lauren thought about the baby she'd aborted. Nick's baby. She'd never told him. She'd never told him about what happened between her and his father, either. It was better that way.

The director returned and asked if they were ready.

"Let's do it," Nick said. "Let's make it as good as old times." He looked at her. "Right, Lauren?"

She took a deep breath. "Right, Nick."

He made sure the scene went smoothly, filling her in on camera angles, lighting and the best way to play to the camera. "It's different than working in the theatre," he explained. "You play it down instead of up. The camera catches everything."

He obviously hadn't seen her commercials; she knew exactly what she was doing.

When they played the scene, he gave it to her – wanting her to get the role. They were finished before lunch. "Okay," he said, "I'm buying."

"No, Freddie Leon is," she replied, quickly. "He's sending a car for me."

Nick felt a stab of uncontrollable jealousy. What the fuck was Freddie up to? "Am I invited?" he asked lightly, walking her back to her dressing room.

She shrugged. "I don't know – you'd better ask Freddie."

"Hey – I don't have to ask, he's my agent." He paused for a moment. "You don't *mind* if I come, do you?"

She stopped at the door to her dressing room. "Not at all."

"I'll have someone call Freddie – tell him I'll bring you to the restaurant. Why don't I meet you here in fifteen minutes?"

As soon as he left she rushed to the mirror, staring at her reflection.

Nothing had changed. Absolutely nothing. She was still as hooked as she'd ever been.

Tough luck, Roberts.

Screw you.

★

Freddie dominated lunch. He was charming, funny and completely unlike himself. They ate at Le Dôme on Sunset, sitting at a round table in the back room. Nick settled back and watched Lauren in action. She was different, he decided. More sophisticated, stylish, and definitely more worldly. But underneath the gloss he knew there was still the same sweet Lauren he'd fallen in love with.

"You know," Freddie said, with his new charming smile. "This lunch was for me to persuade Lauren to become an I.A.A. client. I guess I can't do that with you sitting in on the meeting, Nick."

"You're doing a pretty good job," he replied, determined to stick around.

Lauren sipped a glass of Perrier, well aware of the interaction between the two men. "It's so good to see you again, Nick," she said, as if they were nothing more than polite strangers. "And meeting you, Freddie, is a pleasure."

He wanted to touch her so badly he didn't know how he controlled himself. And he wanted to smash his best friend, Freddie Leon, in the face.

Eventually Freddie left the table to go to the john.

He waited until he was out of sight and leaned across the table. "Can we have dinner tonight?"

She kept her voice even. "I'm planning on taking the late flight back to New York."

"You just got here," he pointed out.

"I know, but I have an important meeting tomorrow morning. Marcella has offered me a deal to start my own cosmetic line."

"Oh, like you're not busy enough?"

She was immediately defensive. "How do you know how busy I am?"

"I read the papers. You're always in the New York columns doing this and that."

"I read the papers, too, Nick," she replied, staring straight at him. "You're always in the paper, screwing this and that."

He laughed. "Nice talk."

"How's your marriage?" she couldn't help asking.

"How's yours?" he countered.

Their eyes met and there was a long moment of silent intimacy.

Freddie bounced back to the table. "Lauren," he said. "I know you're not making any decisions today, but I'll be in New York next week, so why don't we have dinner and talk about it then?"

Why don't we have dinner and talk about it then? Nick couldn't believe what he was hearing. This was Freddie – faithful Freddie. Freddie Leon with a definite hard-on.

"I'd like that," Lauren said. "Do you get to New York often?"

"Only when it's important," Freddie replied, homing in on her.

"Are you taking Diana?" Nick interjected.

Freddie shot him an annoyed look. "No."

"Who's Diana?" Lauren asked.

"Freddie's wife," Nick replied. "Terrific woman. They've got a couple of great kids. You should meet the family."

Freddie continued to glare at him. Lauren looked from one to the other. She knew exactly what was going on and it amused her.

Freddie signed the cheque, and they got up to leave.

"I'll drop Lauren back at her hotel," Freddie said.

"That's okay," Nick said. "I'll take care of her."

"As a matter of fact," Lauren said, "I'm not going to my hotel. I thought I'd stop by Neiman's and do some shopping – I never get time in New York."

"My offices are right there," Freddie said. "Maybe you'd like to come up and meet some of the other agents."

"Not today. Perhaps next time."

"Yeah, stop hustling her, Freddie," Nick said. "She hasn't signed with you yet."

"She will. Won't you, Lauren?"

She smiled her dazzling smile. "I'll have to see."

Lauren walked around Neiman Marcus in a daze. She hadn't seen Nick in seven years, and yet he had this incredible effect on her. She was still the same stupid wreck.

What kind of hold did he have over her?

What kind of a hold did she want him to have?

She sighed. They were both married. It was an impossible situation.

She wandered around the store – tried on a Donna Karan jacket, picked out a couple of Armanis, and charged it all to her American Express. Shopping was not her thing, but it was better than going back to her hotel and sitting there until she had to leave for the airport.

"Hey –"

She turned around, startled. It was Nick. "What are you doing here?" she asked, her heart immediately starting to pound uncontrollably.

"I'm taking my fucking life in my hands," he said.

"What do you mean?"

"I don't travel anywhere without bodyguards. I'll get mobbed in here."

She laughed. "Oh, come on, nobody's taking any notice of you. This is Beverly Hills, they're used to movie stars."

A saleswoman rushed up to him. "Can I have your autograph for my daughter," she gushed. "She loves you. She sees everything you do."

He shot Lauren a triumphant look.

"And you're the Marcella Girl, aren't you?" the woman continued, turning to Lauren. "My daughter loves you, too. Oh, this is so thrilling!"

They both signed the piece of paper she proffered, and then Nick took Lauren's shopping bags and said, "Let's go, we're getting out of here. Walk swiftly and don't make eye contact."

She giggled. "You sound like the CIA."

He took her hand and she found herself beginning to melt.

The valet had his car waiting outside. Nick slid him a twenty.

"Get in, fasten your seatbelt – we're gonna talk whether you like it or not."

"I told you," she protested, knowing it was useless. "I have a plane to catch."

"I'll see that you do."

She got into the passenger seat of his red Ferrari. "I thought a Cadillac was the car of your dreams," she said, remembering how he used to talk about it all the time.

"It was – the dream turned into a nightmare."

"Oh, not so patriotic any more?"

"You could say that." He revved the engine and zoomed off down the street.

"Where are we going?" she asked.

"To the beach. I have a house there."

"Of course you do," she said, dryly.

They didn't talk in the car. He pushed in a Van Morrison tape and concentrated on his driving. She stared straight ahead as they sped down Wilshire on their way to the Pacific Coast Highway.

It took twenty minutes before he made a dangerous left turn

505

into a winding driveway, pulling up outside a shuttered house. "This is my retreat," he said. "The only place I get any privacy."

"How do you know your wife's not here?"

"'Cause she doesn't know about this house. I bought it without her. I needed somewhere that's all mine. A place that's not filled with servants, ringing telephones and people driving me crazy."

"You don't sound too happy," she said, as he helped her from the car.

"Hey – I got a lotta demands in my life, don't you?"

"Yes, but I love every one of them."

He walked her to the front door. "That's because you've turned into a workaholic. Can't pick up a magazine without seeing you."

"Can't go to the movies without seeing you."

They both began to laugh, breaking the tension.

He pulled out a key, opened the massive door and she entered paradise. The house was located on top of a bluff with full-length glass windows overlooking the ocean. Perched on the edge of the grounds was an infinity swimming pool – creating the optical illusion of disappearing into the sea, even though it was hundreds of feet above it.

"This is absolutely breathtaking," she said, as they strolled outside.

He turned her towards him, placing his hands on her shoulders. "You never called me in New York. I sat in that fucking hotel room for five days waiting."

"I would have, if I'd thought we could be together," she found herself saying.

"Why *can't* we be together?" he said, urgently. "Let's cut out the shit. You know as well as I do it's what we both want."

"Nick, be serious. I'm still married, and now you're married too."

"Are you happy, Lauren?" he asked, staring at her.

"No," she replied, getting lost in his green eyes. "But what's that got to do with anything?"

"How about this for a plan," he said. "We could both get divorced."

She shook her head. "You make it sound so simple. Life isn't like that."

"Life's what you make it, Lauren. We've both worked hard, why *can't* we be together?"

"Are you suggesting I go home, say, 'Hey, Oliver, I went

to LA, met this old friend of mine and I've decided to divorce you.' You think he'll accept that? And what about you? What'll you say to your wife? 'Hey – Lauren's back – goodbye.' She's the mother of your child, Nick. You have responsibilities."

He refused to take no for an answer. "If we really wanted to we could work it out."

She shook her head again, trying desperately to stay cool. "I don't know if I want to, Nick. What kind of a life would we have together? You're this big movie star, and I work all the time. We'd never see each other."

"Hey – why are you making it so difficult?"

"I'm not. We're two different people. This isn't Bosewell; we're not kids."

He kissed her, taking her by surprise.

She didn't fight it. They stood quietly on the terrace entwined in each other's arms, their lips pressed closely together.

"I love you," he said very quietly, drawing back. "I always have and I always will. Nothing's gonna change that."

She felt weak. "Don't say it, Nick."

"I have to, because it's the truth."

They began to kiss again. Feebly she attempted to pull away. "I must get back, my plane . . ."

"I don't give a shit about your plane. You're staying here tonight. We'll have a night together neither of us will ever forget."

Oh, yes, that's what I want. That's what I really want. "Nick . . . you don't understand. I can't . . ."

"Hey, Lauren – this is the way it's gonna be," he said, forcefully.

She continued to fight it. "I don't know . . ."

He still wasn't taking no for an answer. "Yeah . . . well . . . I do."

His lips were on hers again and all was lost.

She'd promised herself that after the pregnancy scare with Lorenzo she'd never cheat on Oliver again. But this was her life and she had to live it. Damn the consequences. Nick was right. They deserved one magical night together.

Chapter 77

Nick awoke first. Rolling over he stared at Lauren asleep beside him. Jesus! She was the most perfect, beautiful woman in the world – everything he remembered and more.

He got out of bed, moving quietly so as not to disturb her. He'd known when he'd purchased this house it would come in useful one day. The only person who knew about it was Freddie – he'd arranged the deal and paid for it with money Annie was unaware of.

Christ! Annie. He hadn't phoned her – she'd be freaking out. She'd probably called the police by now and reported him as a missing person. He could just imagine the headlines. *Nick Angel vanishes. Wife inherits everything.* Oh, yes, Annie would love that. She'd finally be the centre of attention. Maybe it would even kick-start her acting career.

He knew he wasn't being fair; it wasn't Annie's fault that she was a pain in the ass. It was just that the guilt of what they'd done in Vegas weighed heavily on all of them.

He padded barefoot and naked into the kitchen. There was nothing in the fridge except champagne and 7-Up. He opened the cupboard and found a can of orange juice. Then he picked up the phone and called home.

Annie answered with a terse, "Yes?"

"It's me."

"Where are you?"

"I'm at a friend's."

Icily, "And what friend is that?"

"Don't question me, Annie," he warned.

"Then don't treat me like a fool. You're with a woman, aren't you?"

"Hey – wherever I am and whoever I'm with, I'm letting

you know I'm okay and I'll be home later."

"Maybe you shouldn't bother coming home."

"Is that a threat, Annie?"

"I don't appreciate being treated like nothing."

"We gotta talk," he said.

"Maybe *I* should have talked a few years ago."

He knew exactly what she meant and it was time they got it out in the open, but not now, not on the telephone. "I'll be home later," he said.

She slammed the phone down.

He took a deep breath. There was no way she was going to ruin his day. Swigging orange juice from the can he realized it was the first morning in a long time he hadn't wanted to add vodka to it.

Back in the bedroom Lauren was still asleep. He sat on the bed and stared at her. She was naked, covered only by a thin silk sheet. Her skin was smooth and white and very soft. He ran his fingers across the tips of her breasts. She sighed and made little groaning noises. Slowly she opened her eyes. "I thought this was all a dream," she murmured, stretching luxuriously.

"We actually got to spend the night together," he said. "First time we did that."

She sat up, hugging the sheet to her bosom, "Oh, God! I missed my plane."

"I love you," he said, stroking her arm.

She tried to sound firm. "Nick, this is hopeless."

"What's hopeless? I'll speak to Annie, you'll talk to Oliver. We'll work this out, Lauren, after all we've waited long enough."

She sighed. "You make it all sound so easy."

"It *can* be easy, if it's what we both want."

"I'm not so sure."

"You're wrong."

"It's more complicated than you think, Nick. We're not two unknown people. The press will be after us, watching our every move. Everything we do will be public knowledge."

"Hey – so what else is new?"

"It's not just you – now you have a child to consider. What about her?"

"Believe me, Lauren, we'll work it out."

She sighed again, completely hooked – he had some kind of hypnotic power over her. She was too weak to resist, and what's more, she didn't want to. His love embraced her and she wanted more.

"If you say so," she murmured.

"I say so," he said, cradling her in his arms and kissing her very, very slowly. "I want you to know that last night was the most incredible night of my life. And you are the most incredible woman."

"Last night I should have been on a plane," she said, ruefully.

"But you weren't. You were in bed with me where you belong – and you have to admit it was the greatest."

Why was it that every time she was with him her heart started to race and her body tingled? Yes, he was right, it was the greatest and she couldn't deny it. Together they had something very special.

They continued to kiss, slowly at first, but more heatedly as his hands began to explore her body.

She craved his touch. He electrified her. Sex with Lorenzo had been pleasurable. Sex with Nick was beyond anything she'd ever known. He took her to new heights and then back again.

Eventually they made love fast and passionately. He teased her – taking her almost there and then making her wait until she begged for more.

"Tell me what I want to hear," he said, urgently. "Tell me – I want to hear you say it."

She couldn't stop herself. "I love you, Nick – I always have."

It was noon before they even thought about getting dressed.

"I've got to go," she said, reaching for her clothes.

"Why?"

"Because I have to get back."

"Do you want to?"

She touched his chin. "Silly question."

Before he could convince her not to she called the airline and booked another flight.

"We'll stop by your hotel, pick up your bags and I'll drive you to the airport," he said. "Maybe I should come with you."

"Oh – you'll sit there while I tell Oliver? That'll be very helpful."

"You're right," he agreed. "I'll take care of things here, and we'll talk tomorrow. It won't be like last time."

"No?"

"We're going to be together."

"Do you think so?"

He bent to kiss her again. "I *know* so."

510

She flew back to New York filled with confusion. The last forty-eight hours seemed like a dream. She'd come out to California so full of confidence, knowing she could handle any situation, especially Nick Angel.

But no, it was not to be. Once she was with him all her resolve failed, and having spent the night in his arms she knew there was no going back. It was time to tell Oliver their marriage was over. And when she was free, if Nick was able to extract himself from his marriage, they would be together. It was truly their destiny.

Halfway to New York she realized she hadn't called anyone to tell them she was arriving a day late. Knowing Oliver he was too busy to notice, but Lorenzo was probably furious she'd missed their meeting. She'd called her driver from L.A.X. and told him to be at the airport. Her plan was to go straight to the office, reschedule her meeting with Lorenzo and then tell Oliver they had to talk.

It was raining in New York, the skies were black and heavy with thunder.

"Pia Liberty would like you to phone her as soon as you arrive," her driver informed her.

She picked up the car phone. "Hi, Pia, I'm back."

Pia sounded distraught. "Oh, Lauren, thank God! I've been trying to reach you."

"What's the matter?" she asked, anxiously.

"It's Oliver. Last night he had a massive heart attack."

"Oh, no!"

"Come straight to the hospital, Lauren. Come quickly."

"As far as I'm concerned," Freddie Leon said, "she's got the part. You want her, don't you?"

"Ask a stupid question," said Nick.

"The studio people ran her test early this morning – they love her. In fact they're ready to make an offer." He paused. "And guess what?"

"What?"

Freddie looked pleased with himself. "I'll negotiate her deal."

Nick reached for a cigarette. "I've never seen you so interested in a woman."

"Me? Interested?" Freddie said casually. "I'm a happily married man."

"Yeah, yeah, just like all the rest of 'em."

"What is it between you and her, Nick?" Freddie asked, curiously. "I sense there's more to this."

"I told you," Nick replied, speaking slowly. "We're old friends."

"So if I *was* interested . . ."

"Forget it," he said, sharply.

Freddie nodded knowingly. "That's what I thought."

Nick had stopped by to see Freddie on his way home because he wasn't that anxious to face Annie. He had a feeling he should talk to his lawyer first, fill him in on all the facts. But no, surely Annie wasn't going to come up with the same old threat? And if she did – would they ever find the body in the desert? It must have decomposed by now, nobody would be able to identify the man. And how could they pin it on him anyway?

When he finally got back to the house the housekeeper handed him a note from Annie.

"Mrs Angel and Lissa have gone away for a few days," the woman informed him.

"Where to?" he asked, aggravated.

"Mrs Angel didn't say," the housekeeper replied.

He was pissed. Annie had known he wanted to talk to her, she'd done this purposely. And how dare she take Lissa without telling him where they were going.

Angrily he walked into his study, threw himself into the leather chair behind his desk and ripped open her letter.

Dear Nick,

I refuse to be humiliated in this fashion. It is common knowledge in Hollywood that you sleep with whores. I do not intend to be made a laughing stock. If your behaviour continues, I will take Lissa and you will never see your child again.

You should also remember the information I have. Information that has been a burden for me to keep all these years and would be a great relief for me to reveal to the authorities.

I like being Mrs Angel and I plan to remain Mrs Angel, so I suggest that if you continue to whore around you are more discreet. Remember what is at stake.

Your loving wife,
Annie

He read the letter twice and couldn't believe it. Bitch! Black-mailing bitch! She wasn't going to quit until they were both dead.

He picked up the phone and called his lawyer. "Kirk, I need to see you. Can you drop by the house this afternoon?"

Kirk Hillson – along with Freddie Leon – was one of the Hollywood power elite. As a top lawyer he had plenty of clout and knew all of the right people in all the right places. Nick had a feeling Annie was not going to be easy to get rid of – and he needed Kirk's full support – which meant there could be no secrets. It was about time he got the Vegas thing off his mind – all he'd done was bury a body – he hadn't murdered anyone for Christ's sake. The way Annie carried on you'd have thought he'd pulled the fucking trigger.

He didn't mind paying Annie a bundle – after all, he could certainly afford it. But there was no way he was allowing her to give him a hard time when it came to seeing Lissa. His daughter, along with Lauren, was one of the most precious things in his life; he'd fight for her all the way.

When Kirk arrived he told him the whole story – omitting Cyndra's name. It wasn't fair to involve her until he checked it with her first.

Kirk, a sleek, well-preserved man with startling horse teeth, was non-committal. "It makes you an accessory," he remarked, sipping a glass of unchilled Evian.

"I know," Nick agreed. "Why do you think I've stuck with Annie all these years?"

"On the other hand, maybe she imagined the whole thing," Kirk said, getting up and walking to the window.

"What do you mean?"

"Well – what's she going to prove? Does she know where you buried the body? Do *you* know?"

"I kinda remember," Nick said, hesitantly. "I think I know where I drove to – I'm not sure."

"By this time the evidence will be gone, believe me."

"Yeah, but is it worth taking a risk?"

Kirk glanced at his Rolex – he was late for a golf game. "It's one of those things. You're Nick Angel – they won't dare touch you."

"Then I want out," Nick said, firmly.

"Have you met someone else?" Kirk enquired.

"There is someone else," Nick explained. "She's been in my

life a long time – it's just that we've never gotten together before now."

"Is she worth it?"

"She's worth anything it'll cost me."

"It would be better if there wasn't somebody else," Kirk said, admiring his manicure. "You know what they say about a woman scorned?"

"Annie won't be scorned. She doesn't give a shit about me, anyway. All she cares about is the money and status. She's pissed my career took off the way it did and she never made it."

"I've heard that story a hundred times," said Kirk. "But whatever you say she'll try to hurt you."

"I want out," Nick repeated. "It's time."

"Does she have a lawyer?" Kirk asked.

"You're her lawyer."

"I can't represent both of you. Perhaps I should recommend someone. By the way, have you told Freddie?"

"Not yet."

"You should bring him in on this."

"You mean tell him about Vegas?"

"Not at this stage. But he should know you're planning to divorce Annie."

"I'll tell him."

"Excellent." Kirk headed for the door. "I don't foresee any problems. If you're prepared to give her ninety-nine per cent of your money we'll be fine."

Nick laughed. "Jeez, lawyer's humour – just what I need."

Kirk smiled. "It'll cost you, so I hope your freedom's worth it."

"You know something, Kirk? I'd pay her every dime I had if I could be free tomorrow."

And he meant it. Being with Lauren was the most important thing in his life. He couldn't wait.

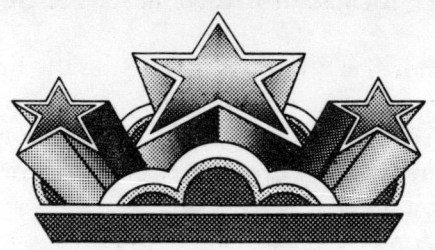

Chapter 78

Aretha Mae had been bedridden for several weeks. Cyndra had nurses there day and night to look after her. The doctor had recently informed her that Aretha Mae was suffering from bronchial pneumonia and should really be in the hospital.

"No hospitals," she said, firmly. "I want her at home where I can watch her."

"She'd get better care in the hospital," the doctor pointed out.

"No," Cyndra replied, remembering what had happened to Luke. "My mother stays here."

Marik tried to persuade her. "C'mon, baby, let them take her to the hospital."

"No," Cyndra said, flatly. "Those places kill people."

"She's dying anyway," Marik said.

"Oh, that's encouraging."

But she knew he spoke the truth. Aretha Mae did not have long to go.

Every evening at six o'clock she went into her mother's room and sat with her. She held her hand, the frail little hand that had once cooked greasy fries and bacon, slapped her kids, brought them up and allowed them to survive.

"How you doin', Mama?" she whispered, leaning in close.

Aretha Mae stared at her. "I soon be with Luke," she said. "Soon be happy."

"Mama – I have something to ask you," Cyndra said, speaking softly.

"Yes?"

"You have to be very truthful with me. You must promise."

"Tell me, girl, what is it?"

"Who's my real father?"

Aretha Mae looked up at her with sunken eyes and was silent

for a long while. "Benjamin Browning – he be your father," she said at last.

Cyndra nodded. She'd known it was true the first time Aretha Mae had told her, but she'd needed to hear it again. "Is there any proof?" she asked.

Aretha Mae nodded, weakly. "There's a letter in the bank in Bosewell. You'll get it when I die."

"You're not gonna die, Mama."

"I don't mind dying, girl. I be with Jesus, an' my sweet baby Luke."

"No, Mama, you are *not* going to die," Cyndra repeated fiercely.

Aretha Mae smiled mysteriously. "I always knew you'd survive, girl. I was always sure."

Later that night Cyndra sat with Marik and talked about her past in a way she never had before. He listened quietly while she told him about Benjamin Browning, the rape, the abortion, and all the other bad things that had happened to her.

"Oh, baby, baby, I had no idea," he said, holding her tight.

"Why should you?" she replied. "It's my pain – I can handle it."

"That Benjamin Browning must be one bad son-of-a-bitch,' Marik said. "We could have somebody sent down there who'd fix him good."

"No," she said, sharply. "Benjamin will pay for his sins, just like Mama would want him to. But it'll be my way."

The next day she signed a contract to star in her own television show. She took the contract home and proudly waved it in front of Aretha Mae. "You see, Mama, you see? I'm gonna be on television all over the country. Everybody will watch me. Everybody in Bosewell. What do you think of that?"

Aretha Mae smiled a sad little smile and managed to nod her head. "You be a star, girl, you did real good."

And then she shut her eyes and died peacefully.

Cyndra threw herself on her mother's body and started sobbing. The nurse called for Marik. He rushed to the room, took Cyndra in his arms and comforted her.

"I want you to be my wife, baby," he crooned. "It's time you had somebody looking after you."

"We'll see," she said, between sobs. "We'll see."

Nick couldn't believe she was doing it to him again. Lauren had been gone for two days, and although he'd left countless messages on her private answering machine she still had not returned his calls. What was it with her? She'd done the same thing to him in New York when he'd sat in his hotel room waiting for five days. This time he wasn't going to stand for it.

He contacted a girl who worked at I.A.A. in New York and told her to go to Lauren's office.

"Make sure she calls me immediately," he said. "And don't leave until you see her. I'll be waiting by the phone."

The girl did as he asked and then called him in Los Angeles. "I'm sorry, Mr Angel, Ms Roberts is at the hospital."

"What's wrong?" he asked, panicking.

"Her husband had a heart attack."

"A heart attack?" he repeated, blankly.

"Yes, I spoke to her personal assistant and she said she'd try to get a message to Ms Roberts that you're trying to reach her."

He put the phone down and shook his head. Had Lauren told her husband and then he'd promptly had a heart attack? Was it Oliver's way of hanging on? Jesus, this was not good.

Freddie called and said, "You're not going to believe this."

"What?"

"Lauren Roberts turned us down. According to Samm, her New York agent, she doesn't want to do the part."

"Why not?"

"Her husband's in hospital."

"He's going to be all right, isn't he?" Nick asked, flatly.

"Nobody knows. Apparently she's at his bedside day and night."

It was bizarre. Fate brought them together every so often, and fate split them apart. If he knew anything about Lauren at all, he was certain she would not leave Oliver while he was sick.

"Any suggestions?" Freddie asked.

"About what?"

"Your leading lady."

"Give it to Carlysle. She wants it."

"I don't think the studio'll go for Carlysle Mann – she's old news."

"She's not even thirty for crissakes – she's right for the part. Tell 'em I want her, that should do it."

"Are you sure?"

"Very sure."

And he was. Carlysle Mann was exactly what he needed to

get him through the next few months. Because Lauren was not going to be around. Of that he was sure.

Oliver smiled, weakly. "Somebody should have told me I was overdoing it."

"They did. Constantly," Lauren replied, fussing around his hospital bed.

"They did?" Oliver asked, innocently.

"Yes. *I* told you, Howard, Pia. We all did. Non-stop work and no play makes Oliver a candidate for a very big heart attack."

"It wasn't that big."

"With a pacemaker anything's big."

A nurse entered the room carrying more flowers. The room already resembled a flower shop.

"I'll slow down. I promise."

Lauren nodded. "If you wish to stay around I suggest you do."

He held out his hand. "Come over here, my beautiful neglected wife."

Inexplicably her eyes filled with tears. She was so relieved he was alive. According to Pia, if their butler hadn't been working late when Oliver collapsed, he would not have survived.

While your husband was almost dying, Roberts, you were in LA in bed with Nick Angel. Proud of yourself?

I didn't want this to happen.

Well, it did, and you're lucky he's still here.

Every time she cheated on him something bad happened. First the false pregnancy – now this. It was a sign. She and Nick were not meant to be.

He squeezed her hand and gazed helplessly into her eyes. "I'm making plans," he said. "We'll go to Rome and Venice. We'll travel together. I don't know what I'd do without you, my darling. I'd be lost."

He was her husband and she was fond of him, but if she were to tell the truth he was more like a father figure than a husband. He'd never made love to her. In fact, for the last four years they'd had no physical contact at all.

Oliver was almost seventy. She was thirty. Oh God! She was totally and absolutely trapped.

"Don't worry, Oliver," she said. "I'm here. I always will be."

Later that night she called Nick.

"I heard," he said.

"I don't know what to say."

"You don't have to say anything, I understand."

"I can't tell him now – not while he's sick. Maybe in a few months when he gets better."

"Lauren, you don't have to explain to me."

"But I do. This time I didn't want to leave you hanging."

"I'll always be hanging."

"Don't make me cry, Nick."

"Look, you must do what you have to do. I'm divorcing Annie whatever happens. I don't intend to stay in a meaningless relationship."

"Yes, well, your wife's not lying in a hospital bed."

"Can we at least speak?"

"It's not a good idea."

"You're killing me, Lauren, you really are. You come into my life every so often, screw me up, and vanish. You're fucking killing me."

"Nick, if it means anything at all, I love you. I truly love you, but I can't leave this man, not now."

"When you're free, call me," he said. "I hope I'll still be waiting."

Nick attended Aretha Mae's funeral with Cyndra. She was buried at Forest Lawn, and there was a good turn-out of people showing their respect for Cyndra.

"Actually, Nick," she told him, "they're showing their respect for my stardom, but what do I care?"

"Are you sure she wants to be buried here?" he asked. "Wouldn't you be better off sending her body back to Bosewell?"

"I thought about it," she said. "But then I remembered she had nothing but bad times there. She'll rest in peace here."

A few weeks later she informed him she was going to visit Bosewell.

"What do you want to do that for?" he argued.

"Marik's coming with me," she said. "I have people to confront before I can be at peace with myself."

"Are you crazy?" he said, trying to talk her out of it. "You're a big star now. If the tabloids get hold of your story you'll be sorry."

"I don't care," she said, stubbornly. "It's something I have to do."

He realized her intentions. "You're after Browning, aren't you?"

She nodded.

"How does Marik feel about this?"

"He'll go along with me."

"And Gordon? Have you told him?"

"No," she said, irritably. "I don't have to tell him. He's not my father confessor."

"Maybe you should listen to his advice."

"I know what his advice will be. He'll tell me not to go, just like you. But some things are unavoidable."

"Well, lots of luck, Cyndra. You know I mean it."

"Want to come with me, Nick?"

"You've *gotta* be kidding. I wouldn't go back there for all the money in the world."

That afternoon Annie arrived home. Lissa rushed into the house first, raced up to him and threw herself into his arms.

"Daddy! Daddy! I missed you *sooo* much!"

"I missed you, too, little kid," he said, hugging her tightly.

"Gotta go pee!" she giggled, wriggling out of his arms and running off.

Annie marched in with a sour face.

"Where the fuck have you been?" he demanded.

"With friends," she said coldly, going to the bar and pouring herself a drink.

He followed her. "What friends?"

"The same friends you were with. How do you like it when *I* vanish?"

"Don't ever take off with my kid," he said, sharply. "Don't ever do that to me, Annie, because you'll regret it."

She arched her eyebrows. "*I'll* regret it?"

"I want a divorce," he said.

"No," she replied, sipping straight gin.

"It's too late. I've already talked to my lawyer. I want out of this marriage. Neither of us are happy. It's not good for Lissa – all she ever sees us do is fight."

"Didn't you read my note, Nick? I *like* being Mrs Angel. There's no way I'm letting you go."

"You have no choice, Annie."

"Oh, but I do. You seem to forget what I know."

"I'm not forgetting anything. Kirk will recommend a lawyer for you. I'll be fair with you, but it's over."

"Oh, yes," she said, spitefully. "It'll *really* be over when I tell everything I know."

"You know something, Annie?" he said, wearily. "You've held

this over me for too many years now – I don't give a shit what you do or who you tell. I'm through – get it into your fucking head. I'm through."

"You'll regret it. I'll take Lissa and you'll never see her again," she said, playing her trump card.

"Oh no, that's where you're wrong," he said, curtly.

"Your career will be over, Nick."

"You can't touch me, Annie."

She smiled, contemptuously. "We'll see who's right."

Chapter 79

Oliver's recovery was slow, but true to his word he began to take it much easier. This affected Lauren because she was used to getting on with her own career and not worrying about Oliver being lonely or wondering where she was. Now he demanded her attention.

She informed Lorenzo she did not wish to proceed with the cosmetic line at this particular time.

Lorenzo was upset. "What will you do? Stay at home and look after an old man?"

"I don't think it's any of your business."

"You cannot waste your life like this, Lauren," he said, genuinely concerned. "You are at the peak of your career, you can achieve anything."

"I'm taking some time," she said, quietly. "I have to look after Oliver. He needs me."

Samm was equally outraged. "You fly to Hollywood, test for a role in a Nick Angel movie, get the part – and then tell me you can't do it. I don't believe this!"

"Samm, sometimes life comes before fantasy. Making a movie is fantasy, being with my husband is real life. I'm looking after him until he's better."

Samm shook her head, too perplexed to argue.

"And another thing," Lauren added. "No more modelling assignments until I feel Oliver is back on his feet."

"You have your commitment to Marcella," Samm pointed out.

"I'll keep that commitment. Right now put everything else on hold."

As soon as Oliver was out of the hospital she accompanied him to their house in the Hamptons where they spent several weeks sitting around doing nothing. She bought him piles of magazines and books, classical tapes and videos.

"You know, I rather like doing nothing," Oliver confessed. "Especially with you beside me."

She smiled, wanly. "I thought you might."

"We've spent so little time together over the last few years. I'm going to make it up to you, Lauren, you'll see."

She tried not to think about Nick. It was quite obvious their relationship was not to be, and Oliver's heart attack was God's way of warning her. She'd been very blessed. Having Nick was not part of the deal.

When Oliver was feeling better she booked them on a long cruise and they took off for several months.

She'd thought about phoning Nick before she left, but then decided against it. They both had their lives to lead. They had to do it separately.

"C'mon, stud – fuck me!" Carlysle urged, in a feverish voice. "C'mon, Nick, fuck me good."

She was unbelievable. What the hell did she *think* he was doing?

"Hey – we're already rocking the trailer back and forth," he pointed out.

She laughed hysterically. "What do you care? You think the crew don't know what we do in here all the time? You and me, Nick Angel, we're a pair – right?"

"Yeah, right," he said, giving it to her just the way she liked.

She caught her breath. "Mmm . . . that's nice. We should've gotten together a long time ago."

"We did get together a long time ago," he panted.

"No, I mean permanently. Like married."

He started to laugh, only Carlysle managed to fuck and carry on a conversation at the same time. "You want to get married?"

"I've tried it twice," she gasped. "You could be third time lucky."

Oh God, he was almost there. "Did you say lucky?"

"Hmm . . ." She let out a deep groan. "Don't forget I knew you when, and I *screwed* you when. All these little girls running after you now – they want you because you're Nick Angel. I had you when you were nothing. Remember?"

"Yeah, I remember," he said, thinking about the apartment in New York and the way she'd greeted him in nothing but a bath towel.

"Think about it, Nick," she said, speaking very fast. "You're getting divorced – we'd be good together. And we wouldn't have to worry about that whole boring faithful thing. I could bring girls home for you whenever you wanted. You know how you love threesomes."

He groped for a nearby bottle of vodka taking a healthy swig.

"Shouldn't drink when you're working," Carlysle admonished. "Especially when you're fucking."

She was right and he knew it.

One final thrust and he climaxed.

Carlysle joined him, letting out a blood-curdling scream.

Someone hammered on the trailer door.

"God!" exclaimed Carlysle, struggling into a sitting position. "You'd think they'd be used to us by now." Giggling, she yelled out, "Who is it?"

"You're wanted on the set, Ms Mann. Is Mr Angel there?"

"Haven't seen him," she yelled back, pulling on her panties. "Try his trailer."

He got up and zipped up his pants. Carlysle made him feel like a teenager. Dirty sex on the floor. Getting it on anywhere they could. Getting it on anywhere that would make him forget Lauren.

He took another swig of vodka from the bottle. Carlysle wagged a finger at him.

"Don't sweat it," he said. "It works for the part."

"Okay, okay."

He left her trailer and returned to his.

"Your lawyer called," said his personal assistant.

"Anything interesting?" he asked.

"Yes, he left a message for you to call him. Something about Las Vegas."

Las Vegas. So Annie was finally making her play. They'd been separated for a couple of months. He'd become a weekend father, seeing Lissa on Saturdays and Sundays, taking her on jaunts to Universal, Disneyland and the movies – always accompanied by his bodyguards. He didn't like it.

At least Annie hadn't gone through with her threat to keep Lissa from him. But still . . . being a weekend father did not cut it.

Grabbing the portable phone, he waved his assistant out of the trailer and called Kirk. "What's going on?" he asked.

"I don't want to discuss it on the phone," Kirk replied. "How about a drink later?"

"Come by the set. I don't know what time we'll be through tonight. Could be shooting late."

Kirk sighed. "I don't do sets, Nick."

"For me you'll do it," he said, persuasively.

"All right, have your secretary call my secretary with the address. And I hope the location is in Beverly Hills because my Rolls doesn't leave the vicinity."

"C'mon, Kirk, you're such an old pussy. We're shooting downtown – risk it."

"No, Nick, call me when you get back to your house. I don't do downtown."

"I'll be tired when I get home."

"Do you want to hear what Annie is planning or don't you?"

"Okay, okay, I'll call you."

He didn't need to hear what she had planned. He already knew. She was going to screw him, and she was going to screw him good.

Cyndra arrived in Bosewell in a blaze of glory. She did it the way she'd always wanted to – in a huge limo, followed by two back-up limos containing her entourage. She wore a red fox coat, wild extensions in her long dark hair, and a glamorous gown. The town of Bosewell wished to present her with the keys to the city at a special luncheon ceremony. The prodigal daughter was returning a huge star.

A TV crew followed her, recording her visit to be made into a television special. Small-town girl made good. Big, big star. What could be better?

Returning with Nick seven years earlier had been a small happening. Now she was coming back as a mega-star.

Marik was by her side – along with two publicity people from the record company, a producer from her new television show, her personal make-up artist, her hairdresser, and her clothes co-ordinator. Plus the television crew.

They all stayed in the big Hilton in Ripley and made the cavalcade limousine journey to Bosewell on Saturday morning.

They were escorted into town by the Bosewell police and taken straight to the Town Hall for a reception in her honour.

The town turned out in force. Cyndra looked around as she was led inside and recognized many of the faces. Nobody had given two cents about her welfare when she'd lived in Bosewell. Now they were fawning all over her – touching and grabbing – telling her how wonderful she was and how they were so proud of her and how they'd always known she could do it. Well, fuck 'em. Let 'em weep.

A dark woman wearing too much eye make-up and a tight orange dress grabbed her arm. "Hi, Cyndra, remember me?"

"Dawn," she said, remembering immediately.

Dawn Kovak beamed. "What a memory! We were at school together."

"We sure were," Cyndra said, recalling that Dawn had been one of the few people who'd talked to her. "Still here, huh? I thought you'd have gotten out long ago."

Dawn waved her hand, flashing a sizeable diamond ring. "I stayed," she said. "And last year I married Benjamin Browning." She beamed, triumphantly. "His wife died a few years ago, so now *I'm* Mrs Browning. Ain't that a kick? Now everyone really has to kiss my ass."

"*You're* Mrs Browning?" Cyndra said, barely concealing her surprise. "*You* married Benjamin?"

"Yeah," Dawn nodded, happily. "You can imagine the scandal. Not much goes on here, but when I bagged him, boy, was there an uproar! Stock went nuts – couldn't accept it. Ben and me – we hadda throw him an' his wife outta the house. She's such a pain anyway."

The crowds were pushing and shoving. Marik attempted to hustle her along.

"I'm sorry, Dawn, I can't talk now," she said.

"I'll see you later," Dawn said, moving off into the crowd.

There were so many people and they all wanted a piece of her. One by one they came up to her saying things like – "You remember me?" "What fun we had in school." "It's *so* good to see you again!"

Some phoney group. If she wasn't Cyndra, big singing star, they wouldn't even remember her name.

So Dawn Kovak, the school tramp, had bagged the richest man in town. In fact, Dawn had bagged her daddy. Well, they were all in for a big shock.

She saw Stock fighting his way through the crowds to get near her. Stock, once the handsome football hero, was now thirty pounds overweight with heavy jowls and a puffy red face. An overweight Meg clung to his side.

526

The TV crew captured every moment as they finally fought their way over to her.

"I always knew you'd be a star," Meg breathed, excitedly. "When you visited a few years back I said to Stock – 'She's going to be such a big star.' I love your records. You know, we were planning on coming out to Los Angeles with the children for a vacation. What do you think? We'd adore to see your house."

Stock eyeballed her with lecherous eyes. He'd been one of the worst offenders at school, calling her dark meat and other offensive names. She wondered how he was going to take the fact that she was his half-sister.

"Is your daddy around?" she asked him.

"You heard the news?" Stock said, scowling. "He married Dawn. He's damn senile."

"It's shocking," Meg added, in a hoarse whisper. "She only married him for his money. But we're seeing a lawyer. We're not going to let him change his Will. Stock's entitled to everything."

Cyndra smiled. *That's what you think.*

"How long we gotta stay here, baby?" Marik asked. "I'm getting depressed."

"Just long enough for me to attend the lunch," she assured him. "Then they'll hand me the keys to the city, an' we're on our way."

"I still don't understand why you wanted to do this," he grumbled. "This town treated you badly. Why *did* you want to come back?"

"You'll see," she said, smiling sweetly.

She had not revealed her plans to Marik, but they were all in place. She knew exactly what she was going to do.

They were finally seated. The lunch was long and boring. People got up and made little speeches about what an excellent student she'd been, how they'd all known she would do so well, even the school principal spoke glowingly of her.

Eventually it was time for the presentation. The Chief of Police stood up, made a short speech and handed her the keys to Bosewell. A round of applause rippled around the room.

She smiled and got to her feet.

"A long time ago this town was my home," she said, speaking clearly. "I lived in the trailer park. Nobody took much notice of any of us then, but we just about survived. My mother worked as a maid. In fact she worked for the illustrious Browning family

527

who I'm sure you all know." She shot a vindictive glance at Benjamin, sitting with his new wife. "Oh, the Browning family was very good to my mother. They used to give her their cast off clothes and stale food."

A buzz echoed around the room.

"And when I was a little girl," Cyndra continued, "my mother took me with her to their house. It was always fun at their house. Well, let me put it this way – I was too little to understand what fun was all about – but I think Mr Browning had a good time. He used to come into that back room when I was a little girl and pat me on my cute ass, and run his hand up my panties, and sometimes he even lifted my dress so he could *really* get a good feel."

A murmur of consternation from the crowd.

Cyndra checked to see that the TV cameras were recording everything. They were.

"Yes," she continued. "That filthy bastard abused me good when I was a child. And then when I was a young girl, he raped me." She paused for effect. "I was sixteen and a virgin. His wife was out shopping at the time, and his spoilt bigoted son was at school, screwing all the girls. Mr Browning raped me, and called me every foul name he could think of. I had to go to Kansas to get an abortion. Before my mother died she told me the truth. When she first went to work for the Brownings she was a young, innocent girl. Benjamin Browning raped her too. And you want to hear the twist to this lovely American folk story? I'm his daughter. *I'm* Benjamin Browning's daughter. And I have a letter to prove it."

The room erupted.

"Oh, baby, baby, when you do it, you really do it," muttered Marik. "Let's get the hell outta here, and fast."

Cyndra refused to be stopped; she kept right on going. "I've come back to town," she said, in a loud clear voice, "because I know there's nothing you all love better than a good old American success story. And I thought you'd enjoy hearing the truth."

Cyndra's story made every TV news programme in America, and she was thrilled. "I *had* to bring it out into the open," she explained to Marik. "I needed to. It was my life and he tried to ruin it. Now I've ruined his. I'm a survivor, but there's lots of kids out there who'll never survive – because their fathers or uncles or somebody else is abusing them every day. This is something we shouldn't hide. I refuse to be ashamed any more."

"Right on, baby," Marik said. "I'm with you all the way."

Marik had supported her royally. On the way back to LA she'd made him stop in Ripley and, with her two security guards, they'd searched for Harlan and kidnapped him just as she'd sworn to do. They'd found him in a bar dressed in tattered clothes and drugged out of his mind. He hadn't recognized her at first, but when he had he'd broken down in tears and allowed himself to be taken without a fight. He was such a pathetic sight. She'd vowed there and then that she'd look after him and help him make a decent life for himself. He was her brother and she loved him.

Back in LA, she'd put him into a private clinic to break him of his habit, visiting him every few days.

Three weeks after getting back she and Marik were married in a lavish ceremony in Beverly Hills.

She'd long forgotten about Reece Webster. As far as she was concerned he was dead.

Chapter 80

"She wants five million dollars in a bank in Switzerland. This demand is separate from the divorce settlement."

"Shit!" Nick exclaimed.

"I know," Kirk agreed. "Apparently it's the price of her silence." He paused. "Is it worth it or do you wish to take a risk?"

"I don't know," Nick said, pacing up and down. "You tell me."

"You're a big star. You'll make a lot more movies. In the long run five million dollars won't mean that much to you. My advice is to pay it."

"Jesus – she's getting half my money as it is, and she wants another five million bucks on top of it. How greedy can you get?"

"I've seen worse," Kirk said. "In Hollywood it's often this way. When the husband is famous and the wife isn't, there's always resentment. Usually the wife came to Hollywood to be an actress. Instead she marries a famous man, and has the compensation of being a wife with clout. When that clout is taken away she wants revenge – usually the revenge is financial."

"And what about Lissa?" Nick said. "Can I spend as much time as I like with her? I don't want to have to ask permission to see her. I refuse to be a weekend father. Oh, yeah – and when I'm not working I'd like her to be able to come and live with me."

"If you're amicable to the agreement I'm sure we can work it out."

"Do I have the money?"

"I've spoken to your business manager; right now it's tied up in bonds, but he can make arrangements. Yes, you have it, Nick. You're doing pretty damn good."

"Okay," he said. "If this is what it takes to get my freedom."

"Good," Kirk said. "I'll have the papers drawn up."

"Fast, Kirk, fast."

As soon as Kirk left he called Carlysle. "I'm lonely," he said.

"Naughty boy, I just left you. We did it three times today in the trailer – what more do you want?"

"Come over. Bring a friend."

She pretended to be insulted. "I'm not a hooker, you know."

"What's the matter, Carlysle, you getting old?"

These were the dreaded words for any actress. "I'll be there," she said. "Who do you fancy?"

"Remember that Indonesian friend of yours? Is she still around?"

"No, she's in New York. But there's this girl I met on the set the other day – she's an extra. Great bod. I'll see if I can contact her."

She turned up an hour later with Honey, a seventeen-year-old nymphet. Honey had huge eyes, a delectable mouth, an unbelievable body and she was a fan.

"I can't believe I'm here with Nick Angel," she sighed, gazing around his house in awe.

"You won't be unless you shut up," Carlysle said, sharply. "Don't talk, enjoy. That's the way he likes it."

He got through half a bottle of Scotch and still managed to make love to them both. Honey was one of the most obliging girls he'd ever come across. Anything he wanted she did.

In the end Carlysle got jealous; she could see he was really getting off on Honey and she didn't like it.

"Don't forget your promise," she whispered, as they left.

"What promise?" he slurred, squinting at her.

"After your divorce – you and me – we'll be together."

He might be drunk, but he wasn't that far gone. "I never said that."

"Oh, yes, you did."

"Oh, no, I didn't."

When they finally left he staggered up to bed and got two hours sleep before his early call.

He got through the week, and on Friday night he stayed sober, preparing for his Saturday visit with Lissa.

He picked her up early in the morning.

"Where are we going today, Daddy?" she asked.

"Wherever you want, sweetheart."

He took her to the toy store and out to lunch. But even with his ever watchful bodyguards it was impossible. Everywhere he went people stopped him, requesting autographs, wanting to take his photograph, telling him how much they loved him. There was no privacy.

Lissa was upset. "I don't like it, Daddy," she said, beginning to cry. "Why can't people leave you alone?"

"Hey, kid – my sentiments exactly."

Eventually they went back to his house and Lissa settled in front of the television watching a video of *The Sound of Music* for the hundredth time. "I like this movie, Daddy," she said, cheering up. "It's nice."

He didn't take Lissa home when he was supposed to.

A furious Annie called up. "Where is she?"

"She wants to stay here tonight," he said.

"She can't," Annie replied.

"What are you going to do about it?"

"I'll get a court order."

"You won't get a court order until Monday."

"You'd better send her home, Nick. I'm warning you."

"Stop threatening me, Annie. It's over."

He went into the kitchen and told the cook to make Lissa a hamburger and a milkshake. Then he sat beside her and watched the film.

An hour later a furious Annie was at his door. She barged into the house. "Lissa, come with me," she said, her tone brooking no argument.

"No, my Daddy says I can stay here tonight," Lissa said defiantly, curling up on the couch.

"You see," Nick shrugged. "She *wants* to stay here. There's nothing you can do."

Annie turned on him. "You son-of-a-bitch."

He stood up. "Don't use language like that in front of Lissa. And don't let's fight in front her either."

Annie's lip curled. "I can't imagine why I ever married you. You're nothing but a piece of shit."

"Oh, and I suppose you're Mother Theresa."

Annie went up to Lissa and grabbed her by the arm, yanking her off the couch. "You're coming home with me."

Lissa's eyes filled with tears. "Daddy! Daddy! You said I could stay."

Annie was in a rage. "You're coming with me, you little bitch!"

Nick tried to stop her. "Don't talk to her like that, Annie."

"I'll do what the fuck I want. I don't have to listen to you, I *hate* you." She pulled the reluctant child towards the door.

Lissa began screaming and crying.

532

"Don't do this, Annie," he said, going after them. "Can't you see she doesn't want to go?"

"I'll do what I damn well please."

He wanted to slap her down, but he couldn't do it in front of his daughter – this scene was traumatic enough for Lissa to deal with.

He followed them outside. Christ! Money, fame, none of it mattered when it came to Lissa.

Annie shoved the child into her car. "Don't you ever pull this stunt again, Nick, or you won't see her at all."

"Quit threatening me, Annie, 'cause I'm through taking your crap. I'm talking to Kirk about this."

She jumped into the car. "Your high-priced Beverly Hills lawyers can't help you get Lissa," she sneered. "I'm her mother; she'll always stay with me." She started the car and roared off down the driveway.

"Don't bet on it," he yelled after her, filled with an impotent fury.

It was the last he saw of either of them. Their car was in a head-on collision. Neither Lissa nor Annie survived.

BOOK FOUR
December 1992

Chapter 81

Two over-ripe teenagers in short, black knit dresses with black hose and "fuck me" shoes boogeyed the night away beneath the midnight tent, where lights sparkled like mini stars and an assortment of predatory deadbeats circled the dance floor on the lookout for a score of some kind or the other.

Honey Virginia, bleached blonde hair pulled demurely back, finely tuned body clad in strapless lace, sat on Nick's knee, purring sweet sexual promises into his ear.

Diana Leon, sitting across the table next to her husband, watched from the corner of a jaundiced eye. Nick Angel never failed to amaze her. His capacity for everything was overwhelming. Honey entered his life on and off, and in between Nick covered the waterfront.

Diana often urged Freddie to talk to him. "Does he practise safe sex? Does he understand about AIDS?"

Freddie always placated her. "I'm his agent, not his sex therapist."

"But he's so . . . irresponsible. You *should* talk to him. You're his friend."

Freddie knew better than to discuss women with Nick Angel. Nick was a legend, having steadily laid every fuckable woman in Hollywood since he'd first arrived in town. It was surprising he could still get it up. But then little Honey could raise the dead if the mood took her, and Nick was by no means dead – just a touch jaded. And at age thirty-four showing definite signs of wear and tear. Freddie decided that maybe he *would* have a talk with him. Nick was getting out of control – it was becoming increasingly obvious. It had been a steady build-up since Lissa's death in the car crash with Annie. At first Nick had been inconsolable, he'd gone off to a retreat and stayed there for several months. When he'd returned it was like nothing had ever happened. He refused to discuss the accident. But Freddie knew he was breaking up inside. Nick had always been a drinker, and as the months turned into years his habit escalated.

"You should get into one of those twelve step programmes," Freddie had suggested one day. "I think you've got a problem."

Nick had turned on him, green eyes full of a deep hidden anger. "You think it's time I started looking for a new agent, Freddie?" he'd asked.

Freddie knew when to back off. It was one of his strengths.

"Can we go?" Diana whispered in his ear. She hated parties and had only attended this one because the woman for whom the party was being given was Freddie's latest client – a blonde video superstar called Venus Maria.

"Five minutes," Freddie promised, "and we're out of here."

Honey removed herself from Nick's knee, stood up and stretched. Every man at the party craned his neck to get a better look at her spectacular body.

Nick had been with her for four years on and off. In between he screwed all his leading ladies and anybody else he fancied. He was playing a dangerous game – AIDS was not selective.

Diana was getting restless. She rose from the table. "Good night, Nick. Good night, Honey, dear," she said, politely.

Nick leant back. "Are you two going?"

"Past my bedtime," Diana said, with a stretched smile.

"See ya," Nick said. He'd always considered Diana Leon a tight-assed broad. The older she got the more tight-assed she became.

Honey decided to join the two over-ripe teenagers on the dance floor. She put them to shame with moves even strippers hadn't thought of.

Nick watched her. The next morning they were leaving for New York. He had a birthday coming up and he didn't care to celebrate it in Los Angeles. Not that there was any cause for celebration; getting older was a pisser.

Two years ago he'd purchased a New York apartment. He liked having a place in the same city as Lauren, although they hadn't seen each other in four years. She'd called him when the news of the accident hit the headlines.

"Is there anything I can do?" she'd asked, full of concern.

Yes, be here with me, he'd wanted to say. But he knew she wasn't going to leave Oliver.

538

He decided it was time to get the hell out. Honey was still busy on the dance floor. He walked over and pulled her by the arm. "C'mon, we're going."

"I don't wanna . . ."

"I *said* we're going."

She followed him dutifully. Twenty-one years old and an idiot with the best body in town. That was all right – he wasn't interested in conversation. Meaningless sex. His life.

"Why did we have to leave so early?" Honey complained in the car on the way home.

"'Cause I might feel like flying the plane tomorrow. If I do I want to be able to see where I'm going."

He'd been taking flying lessons for a couple of years; it was the one thing he did where he tried to remain sober.

Back at the mansion Honey did a slow striptease for his benefit.

She was undeniably luscious.

He watched her for a few minutes, then passed out.

She might be luscious but he'd seen it all before.

"You look tired, *bellissima*," Lorenzo said, full of concern.

"Thank you," Lauren replied, crisply. "That's just what I want to hear when I'm about to go before the camera."

"The camera loves you. You will always look beautiful. Me – I know you too well, and you do look tired."

"I *am* tired," she confessed. "I had so much more energy when I was working all the time. Every morning was a challenge – I'd get up and there was always something new to do. Now that Oliver's retired I do nothing but sit around at home."

"Why?"

"Because he likes me there. It makes him feel secure."

"You don't have to do this, Lauren."

"Yes, I do," she said, defensively. "I'm his wife."

"You don't love him."

"What's love got to do with it?"

"When I married my wife I loved her. When I fell out of love we got a divorce."

"Well, Lorenzo, you do things in a much more simple fashion than I do. I believe in loyalty and sticking with somebody through bad times."

"Oliver is perfectly healthy now."

"I know, but he got used to not working. He liked it so much he decided to retire."

"That doesn't mean *you* have to waste your life."

"I'm doing the new Marcella campaign," she said. "What more do you want?"

"Yes, but that's all you're doing. Before you were so vital – everything excited you."

"I guess I'm not excited any more, Lorenzo. This is the last year I'll do the Marcella campaign. As you know, we're moving to the south of France."

"Lauren, you're making a mistake – shutting yourself away from the world."

"It's not a world I particularly want to be in any more. Anyway, the south of France is beautiful. And Oliver's found this wonderful old farmhouse way up in the hills – miles from anywhere."

Lorenzo shook his head. He simply didn't understand her.

It was Sunday afternoon and Cyndra was entertaining. She paused at the top of the stone stairs leading to her patio. She paused just long enough for people to notice she was making an entrance.

Smiling at her guests she watched Marik leap to his feet. He was always so attentive and concerned about her welfare. He was also a consistently good lover. It was a shame he wasn't more attractive.

Don't think that way, she scolded herself. *Marik is the best thing that ever happened to me. He's kind and caring, and he genuinely loves me. Apart from that he's a wonderful producer, and he made me a star.*

Behind her, Patsy, their plump English nanny, carried their little girl, Topaz. Topaz was the pride of her life. Three years old and adorable. Cyndra would do anything for her child – so would Marik; he worshipped their daughter.

"Hi," Cyndra greeted her guests graciously, going from table to table, smiling and chatting warmly.

Marik crept up behind her hugging her tightly. "You look fantastic, woman," he said, nibbling her ear. "Every year you get better looking."

"Thank you, dear."

Out of the corner of her eye she noticed Gordon and Odile

arriving. Gordon was still her best friend. She confided in him, went to him for advice, discussed most things with him – including the incident in Vegas – which he'd told her to forget about.

She went over to greet them. "Hi, Gordon."

"Hi, beautiful." Gordon said, kissing her on both cheeks.

"Hello, Odile," she said, with a smile.

"You're looking hot, Cyndra."

"Thank you. From you that's a compliment."

Over the years she'd actually gotten to like Odile. Yes, she was beautiful and, yes, she was Gordon's wife. But she was also an extremely nice woman.

Gordon and Odile were Topaz's godparents, along with Nick, who was godfather number one. She was upset Nick hadn't been able to come. He'd flown off to New York complaining he was depressed.

"Why don't you stay here for your birthday?" she'd asked.

"I don't feel like it," he'd said.

She wished he'd dump Honey. The girl made dumb look intelligent. But Nick was on some sort of self-destruct course; he didn't seem to care about the company he kept. Ever since the accident he hadn't been the same man. Unfortunately he blamed himself.

"It wasn't your fault," Cyndra repeatedly assured him.

"If I hadn't been fighting with Annie, it would never have happened."

"No, Nick, you mustn't think that way."

But he did, and she knew there was nothing she could do about it.

Maybe Nick would have a good time in New York. At least he'd be away from the pressures of Hollywood, and there was always Harlan to keep him company.

Ah, Harlan . . . What a character he'd turned out to be. After kidnapping him and getting him off drugs she'd moved him in with her. He'd quite taken to Hollywood, and met an older man whom he'd decided to go work for as his valet. When the man died of AIDS two years later Harlan had not wanted to stay around. Cyndra had arranged for him to work for Nick in New York. He loved it.

Marik took her arm and led her over to sit down. She was surrounded by friends and loving family. Little Topaz created a furore wherever she went, running from table to table, giggling and cute.

541

Cyndra surveyed her guests, her family and her beautiful home. *I'm so lucky*, she thought to herself. *I have everything*.

Only sometimes, late at night, the thought occurred to her that maybe she was too lucky. Then she shuddered and hugged herself and prayed to God that her good luck would last. For family meant everything to her and she didn't want to lose it.

Chapter 82

Reece Webster had not had a good time in prison. For once in his life his looks had not worked in his favour. In jail they were particularly fond of snake-hipped white guys with blond hair and nice looks, and he'd had two choices – give it up or get the crap beaten out of him.

Reece soon learnt which way to turn. Not that he was a faggot. No way. But taking it up the butt from one big black brother, as opposed to watching his ass every move he made, seemed to be the better deal.

Eleven years. Eleven fucking years of his life and now he was out.

He lingered outside the jail in North Carolina trying to decide what to do first. He wanted a woman bad, but he also wanted a fat juicy steak. An inmate had given him the name of a whorehouse that served up the best women, and food, too. What more could he ask for?

He tilted his rather beat-up stetson and took the bus into town. He didn't have much money. Fuck! He didn't have much of anything. But he sure as hell knew how he was going to get plenty. He'd studied up on that. In eleven years a man could do a lot of studying.

The whorehouse served him a dried-up steak and a dried-up hooker who'd seen better days. It was not a first-class operation. But any woman was better than none at all.

He wore a condom supplied by the house. He didn't argue because he'd heard it was pretty dangerous out on the streets now. Sex was not the carefree pastime it once was.

He fucked the whore three times.

"You bin in jail, dear?" she asked, not particularly impressed by his stellar performance.

"Howdja know?"

"I can tell. You convicts are always the horniest."

Yeah. He'd been in jail all right. Sixteen years was the sentence he'd been handed, and he was out in eleven for good behaviour. Sixteen lousy years for something he'd never done.

When he'd split Vegas he'd travelled all the way to Florida, where he'd met a nightclub hostess who took a shine to him and let him move in with her. He hadn't been living with the bitch two weeks when Max, her old boyfriend, returned. She'd omitted to tell him that Max was a convicted felon who specialized in robbing banks. Since Max was with his latest girlfriend – a ditsy redhead – there seemed no need for him to move on, so the four of them had palled up.

"People who work legitimate make me sick," Max told him one day. "Me – I kin take any bank I fancy. I jest walk in, show 'em my gun, scoop out the money an' I'm on easy street."

"What if you get caught?" Reece enquired, thinking it sounded simple enough, but there was always a downside.

Max chortled. "You realize how many people git busted? Outta a hundred hits mebbe five people git themselves caught. I bin doin' this goin' on twenny years."

"But you were in jail once."

"Only short time – it weren't nothin'."

They went on a car ride through several states, and Max showed Reece exactly how easy it was. On their ninth job Max blew away the security guard.

They were caught, arrested and charged with armed robbery and murder. The sentence was not light.

Screw it. He hadn't pulled the trigger, but nobody took that into account – he was sentenced along with the rest of them.

Now he was out and he was bitter as hell. If Cyndra hadn't gotten him into that mess in Vegas, he'd never have met the nightclub hostess in Florida, and he'd never have spent eleven years of his precious life in jail.

Fuck little Cyndra. While he was away she'd become a big star and so had Nick Angel. He'd watched their rise carefully – oh yeah, he was no fool.

Now he was out and he knew exactly where to go and what to do. Little Cyndra must be worth millions, and he was going to get himself some of that great big score.

Yes. Reece Webster had a plan.

California, here I come . . .

544

Chapter 83

The new Marcella photos were done and Lauren had nothing left to keep her in New York. Oliver was anxious to leave. For some time he'd been severing his ties in America, selling the East Hampton house, putting the New York apartment on the market and preparing for their move to France. At first Lauren had been unsure. It was a radical move, but, on the other hand, what was the point in sitting around New York when Oliver wasn't working. In France he would have his garden, the view, the tranquil surroundings.

Christ! You're beginning to sound like an old lady, Roberts.

It's my life – I have to accept it.

Pia came by with Rosemarie, a particularly bright little girl, and watched her pack. "Are you sure you're making the right move?" Pia asked, wandering around the room.

"Yes, I'm sure," Lauren said, although she wasn't sure at all.

"It's just that everything's so different for you now," Pia remarked. "I mean, you went through a period where you really loved your life, it showed on your face. Now you're kind of like . . ."

"Are you calling me a zombie, Pia?" Lauren asked, gathering together a pile of sweaters.

"You said it, not me."

Lauren placed the sweaters in a suitcase. "I'll do things in the south of France. Maybe even start an interior design business."

"Oh, that sounds very challenging. Decorate houses for senile old millionaires who've moved there to retire."

"Can I come visit, Auntie Lauren?" Rosemarie asked, a polite little girl with a sweet smile.

"Of course you can, darling, any time you want."

She packed several pairs of Charles Jourdan shoes and wondered why she was taking them anyway. Where was she going to wear them? Even in New York they never went out any more.

"How's Howard?" she asked.

"Howard has turned into Oliver," Pia said. "He works day and night, never gets back from the office before nine, then goes straight to his study where he spends the rest of the evening on the phone. I told him the other day if this goes on I'm not standing for it."

Lauren laughed. "You know you love it."

"Love what?"

"Being Mrs Howard Liberty. It's a lot of fun when your husband's the head of a big important company."

"I'm not so sure I do," Pia said, thoughtfully. "It was all right for you when you had your high-powered career – but I don't enjoy being the little wife. Half of the parties we go to I'm ignored. He's the big gorilla."

"Pia, I'm sure you're never ignored."

"You'd be surprised."

Lauren shut the suitcase. "Why don't you and Rosemarie stay for dinner tonight?"

"We'd like that. I'll call Howard and tell him if he gets through early enough he can join us."

At dinner Oliver was particularly animated. He was looking forward to the move and it showed.

In the middle of dinner Lauren had a phone call from Lorenzo.

"I have unfortunate news," he said, sounding upset.

"What is it, Lorenzo?" she asked.

"There was an accident in the lab – the negatives of the new photographs are ruined."

"You're kidding me?"

"No, this is a freak thing. It's never happened before. You must stay and shoot again."

"I can't do that. You know we're leaving tomorrow."

"Oliver will have to leave without you. You'll join him a few days later. I'll organize everything as quickly as possible."

"Lorenzo," she said, crossly. "This is most inconvenient."

He was more than apologetic. "I know, my darling, for me too."

"What's the matter?" Pia asked, when she hung up.

Lauren sighed. "The Marcella photographs are ruined. Lorenzo wants me to do the shoot again."

"But you're leaving tomorrow."

"That's exactly what I told him."

"Don't worry, my dear," Oliver said, perfectly calm. "I'll go ahead without you."

"You can't fly all that way by yourself."

"I'm not an invalid, Lauren," he said, rather snappily. "Our travel agent has perfectly good people on both ends to meet me and take care of the luggage. I'll settle in and you'll be there when you can. No problem."

"Are you sure?"

"Yes, I'm very sure."

She went into the bedroom and called Lorenzo back. "This better not be one of your crazy scams."

"Lauren, I can assure you."

"Okay, I'll stay. Tell me tomorrow what time we're going to do the photos."

"My darling," he said happily, "you are a princess."

"And you are a prince – the prince of bullshit."

"I'm so glad our relationship gets closer every year."

The next morning she was up early helping Oliver with last minute packing.

"How about if you postpone the trip?" she said. "Then I can come with you."

"It's all arranged, my dear. You worry too much."

"I'm coming to the airport," she said.

"You don't have to – the traffic . . ."

"I'm coming to the airport."

She sat next to him in the limo and saw him safely on the plane. Then she rode back to New York, alone and thoughtful. Soon she would be leaving the city and her life would change. She'd come a long way from Bosewell and the little girl she once was.

Nick . . . Every so often he lingered in her thoughts. She wondered how he was, how he was doing. She missed him. She always missed him.

"What do you want for your birthday?" Honey demanded.

Peace. "No celebrations," he said, sternly.

"Why not? I get off on birthdays," she said, toying with a strand of her long hair.

He hoped she wasn't planning anything – at twenty-one it was easy to love birthdays, but he was not in the mood.

"I'm telling you, I don't want anything. No surprises," he repeated, hoping she'd get the message.

She pouted. "I'll think of something."

"Don't," he said.

Had he made a mistake bringing Honey with him? He wasn't sure. Sometimes it was nice to have a warm body lying next to him in the middle of the night when he woke up and thought about Lauren. And he thought about her often. Over the years he'd grown to accept the fact that she was an obsession. Only the drinking made her go away.

In the New York apartment there was a stack of scripts waiting for him to read. Word was out that he wanted to make his next movie in New York, and every producer in town seemed to know it. There was a pile of faxes, a ton of mail and a list of phone calls waiting for him.

"Teresa, you deal with this shit," he said, calling upon his assistant.

Teresa had worked with him for a year now. She was the best assistant he'd ever had. He figured she was gay because she'd never come on to him, and that suited him just fine. Before her he'd had a series of assistants who'd looked at him with mournful eyes day and night, and eventually confessed undying love. Who needed that?

Teresa was all business. A black belt karate champion who could also type. The perfect combination.

"I'm taking the week off," he told her. "Don't bother me with anything – you deal with whatever comes up, okay?"

Teresa nodded. She looked like a man. He wondered if she had a girlfriend; he hadn't noticed any lurking about.

Tomorrow he was going to be thirty-five. It was a milestone. Ever since he'd started acting it had always been young Nick Angel. He'd always played the rebel, the kid without a cause. Now he was moving into a different age group. He was going to have to start playing responsible roles, and he wasn't sure if he was ready for it. He still felt like a kid at heart, sometimes a very weary kid, but always young.

He shut himself in his den and put his favourite Van Morrison on the CD player. Honey tried to come in and annoy him, but he waved her away.

Closing his eyes he let the music sweep over him.

He wasn't happy, but he hadn't quite figured out what he could do about it.

548

Chapter 84

It wasn't difficult finding out where Cyndra lived. Reece purchased a map to the stars' homes from a street vendor and thumbed through it. Sure enough, there was Cyndra's address printed clearly for all to see.

He chuckled to himself. Sweet little Cyndra. Sweet little bigamist.

Who did she think she was fooling? He reached for the latest copy of *People Magazine*. There was a big story on her and he read it for the sixth time. Sitting in his rented car he studied the pictures. Cyndra in her fancy bathroom. Cyndra by her fancy pool. And Cyndra with her cute little girl, Topaz, sitting on her daddy's lap.

Cyndra had gone and married one of her own kind. A producer they called him. Marik Lee – he was no Billy Dee Williams. But the two of them together seemed like they had it all their own way – and nobody was worried about Reece Webster.

He'd spent eleven years in jail and they didn't give a damn. Motherfuckers! They'd soon find out he was back.

He pulled the car up to a hot-dog stand and bought himself a greasy dog with plenty of relish and onions. Life's small pleasures, how he'd missed them in jail.

Later he drove down Melrose, stopped at a store and bought himself a new stetson, and some sharp looking leather boots. He handed the sales clerk a cheque that would bounce, but he'd be long gone by the time they discovered it was no good.

He admired himself in a full-length mirror. Still looked good. Still had that lean body and handsome face. Nobody would guess where he'd been for the last eleven years. He could do with a suntan. Didn't have time to wait to get one. Shame.

By three o'clock in the afternoon he was ready to start the

action. He knew exactly where Cyndra's house was. He drove up into the hills, through the winding streets, until he reached her security gates. Then he leaned out of his car window and pressed the entry buzzer.

A man's voice said, "Yes?"

"Cyndra?"

"No, she's not here. Who is this?"

"I'm here to see Cyndra," he said.

"I just told you, mister, she's not home."

"Then I'll wait."

"Who are you?"

Should he spoil the surprise? Tell this moron that he was her husband?

No, it was better to confront her face to face.

"I'm a relative," he said. "What time will she be back?"

"I can't reveal that information. Leave a note in the mailbox and I'll see she gets it."

What kind of garbage was this? He was leaving no note. He drove the car half a block away, turned it around and sat in it waiting and watching.

After a while a fancy white limousine drove down the street and turned into the gates.

Reece started his car, and as soon as the gates opened he followed the limo in, thinking to himself how stupid these people in Hollywood were if they actually thought a pair of fancy gates were enough to keep anybody out.

He followed the limousine up a long driveway until they reached the grand entrance to an imposing mansion.

A driver got out of the limo, noticed Reece's car behind him and rushed over.

"Can I help you?" the driver said.

The back door to the limo opened and a man that Reece recognized as Cyndra's supposed husband got out. "Hey, Clyde, what's going on?" the man called.

"I'm looking into it," Clyde replied, embarrassed because he was at fault for not noticing the car before.

Reece got out of his rented car. "I'm here to see Cyndra," he said.

"I'm sure you are," Clyde replied, very hostile. "A lot of people would like to see her. If it's an autograph you want, leave your address and we'll see you get one."

"You don't understand," Reece said. "I'm a relative."

Marik walked over. "What's going on here?" he said.

550

"I want to see Cyndra," Reece said.

"You shouldn't follow people into private property. We're going to have to call the police."

"I don't think you'll want to do that," Reece said.

"Look, man," Marik said, patiently. "I know you're a fan – and you love her. A lot of people love Cyndra – but you cannot follow her into her private home. Get it? Now I suggest you get back in your car, turn around, go away and we'll forget about this."

"You don't recognize me, do you?" Reece said.

"No," Marik said. "I don't."

"Think back," Reece said. "And fuckin' weep. I'm Cyndra's husband."

Cyndra had been crying on and off for hours. In the back of her mind she'd known the good life would not last. One moment she had everything she'd ever wanted, and the next Reece Webster came back like a ghost from the past to ruin it all.

At first she'd tried to deny she knew him. She'd gotten out of the limo, stared him in the face and said, "I don't know this man. I've never seen him before."

"Hey, bitch," Reece had taunted. "Would you sooner I went to the newspapers with this? I'm giving you the courtesy of coming here first."

They went into the house and the story began to unfold. How she'd married him. How he'd used her. And then Vegas. "She shot a guy," Reece said. "Shot him stone cold dead."

"I didn't do it – you did it," she said, accusingly.

Marik looked from one to the other and shook his head. Then he stared at Cyndra with hurt eyes. "Why didn't you tell me, baby?"

Her world was crumbling. "'Cause I never thought Reece would come back."

"Here I am," said Reece. "Would've been here sooner – but I got myself put in jail on a false charge. That's where I've been."

"What do you want?" Marik asked.

"Why, I would imagine that's pretty obvious," Reece said, taking in the luxurious surroundings. "I want my wife back."

"Let's talk straight here," Marik said, grimly. "What do you *really* want?"

"Well," Reece said, tilting his stetson at a rakish angle. "If I can't have the little lady, then I guess I'll have to be compensated for my loss."

"Yes," Marik said. "I understand you want money. And Cyndra wants her freedom. We'll pay. And the money will buy a quiet divorce."

One thing about this Marik guy – he certainly wasn't stupid. "How much you got in mind?" Reece said.

Marik glanced at Cyndra. She was too upset to look at him. "We have to discuss it," he said. "In private. I'll talk to my lawyer and we'll come back to you with an offer."

"It better be a big offer," Reece said. "Oh, and by the way, I thought I might pay me a visit to Nick Angel."

"What's Nick got to do with this?" Cyndra snapped.

"He helped you out, didn't he, sweetheart?" Reece said, slyly. "I saw what happened that night. You thought I left, but I didn't – I stuck around, followed you. So y'see, I know exactly what went on. You took that good old boy out into the desert and buried him. You're all as guilty as hell. I think Nick Angel will want to contribute to my future well-being, don't you?"

"Leave him out of this, Reece. We'll make a deal, but leave Nick out."

"Now, now, don't go getting upset."

Cyndra's mouth twitched dangerously. If she had a gun she'd blow his head off. All her life she'd been a victim, and now, just when she'd thought she was through with being victimized, this creep had to come back to haunt her with his threats.

"Calm down, Cyndra, we'll settle this," Marik said, taking charge.

"We're not talking pennies here," Reece said, warningly.

"I understand," Marik replied.

"When will I hear from you people?" Reece asked.

"Tomorrow," Marik said. "Where are you staying?"

"Give me a thousand bucks cash for now, an' I'll contact you tomorrow."

"I don't have that much cash."

"What *do* you have?"

"Five hundred."

"It'll do."

As Marik was escorting Reece to the front door, Topaz came running out of her room. "Mommy! Mommy! Look at my new dress. Isn't it pretty?"

Reece stopped. "Yeah, sugar, that's *real* pretty. You're the image of your mama."

"Stay away from her," Cyndra turned on him, her dark eyes stormy. "Get out of my house and stay away from my family."

He shrugged. "Trouble with you, Cyndra, is you got no appreciation. Who gave you singing lessons, taught you how to dress an' fix your hair? You were nothing when I found you hanging out in New York. Now you're a big star. I expect plenty of compensation for all I did."

"You'll get it. I told you that," said Marik, leading him to the front door.

Cyndra rushed over to Topaz and picked her up. "Come here, sweetie."

"Bye, little girl," said Reece, waving. "See you around."

She ran upstairs with Topaz and tried to call Nick in New York. He was out. She left a message with Harlan for him to call her back. Then she went to her closet and searched behind her clothes for the secret compartment where she kept her most valuable possessions. There, alongside her diamond necklace and ear-rings, was a small pearl-handled gun. One of her security guards had given it to her as a gift. He'd told her how to use it, too.

"Never hurts for a lady to have a gun," he'd said. "Especially a famous lady like yourself."

She'd never told anybody about the present, otherwise the guard would have gotten fired. But she'd always appreciated it.

Soon she had a feeling she might be forced to use it.

Chapter 85

Lauren called Oliver in the south of France to make sure he'd arrived safely and was settled in.

"I'm perfectly fine," he said. "In fact, last night Peggy invited me over for dinner."

Vaguely Lauren remembered Peggy – a titled English widow who'd sold Oliver the farmhouse.

"That's nice," she said. "I'll be there soon."

"You don't have to rush," he said. "It's beautiful here, so peaceful and quiet. I'm very content."

Oh, God! Should she bring her knitting?

Oliver seemed perfectly satisfied with the tranquil life, but she wasn't so sure it was for her. Maybe she was making a mistake after all. She wished she had the courage to tell him. No. It was impossible. This was her life.

Lorenzo called bright and early to inform her that the photo session was on for the next day.

"No more fuck-ups, Lorenzo," she said, sternly. "I have to get out of here."

He was hurt. "Please, Lauren, do not insult me."

She got dressed and wandered around the apartment she'd grown to love. It was on the market and every day people came to see it. She hated showing them around and tried to stay out of the way, leaving the tour in the hands of their realtor. It had been her home for almost twelve years and she was certainly going to miss it.

She sipped her morning coffee sitting at a table on the outside terrace overlooking Manhattan. It was a chilly December day, but clear. She loved looking out at the bustling city laid out below her.

The maid brought her the newspapers. She glanced through

them quickly, stopping at an item in *USA Today*. She scanned it once, then read it more slowly a second time.

> *Today millions of fans across the world celebrate the*
> *thirty-fifth birthday of cult superstar, Nick Angel, and*
> *the opening of his latest movie,* Killer Blue. *A statement*
> *issued by Panther Studios disclosed that Nick will not*
> *be present at the Los Angeles premier of* Killer Blue *as*
> *expected.*
>   *A personal spokesman for Angel reported that the*
> *actor will spend his birthday in New York.*

Nick Angel . . . he was in New York and it was his birthday . . . Was she ever going to forget him?
I can call him if it's his birthday.
No, you can't.
Why not?
Because he'll want to see you and you're leaving for a new life with Oliver in France.
She shut her eyes for a moment, saw his face, and wanted to be with him more than anything else in the world.
So why are you punishing yourself, Roberts?
I'm not punishing myself.
Yes, you are. If you want to be with him you should.
I murdered his father.
Maybe. Maybe not.
I murdered his baby.
You had no choice.
She reached for the phone. Her hand hovered over the receiver for a few minutes. Then she shook her head. No, it wasn't right. She'd be tempting fate again – just forget it.

Honey took the second phone call from Cyndra. "He left here early," she said. "I think he's taken his plane up."
"But I need to speak to him," Cyndra said.
"He'll be back later. I'm having a surprise party for him."
"Nick doesn't like surprises."
Honey giggled. "He'll like this one."
"Let me talk to Harlan," Cyndra said.
Harlan got on the phone sounding swishier than usual. Since his move to New York he'd become extremely caustic. "Sister,

dearest – and *what* can I do for you?"

"I need to talk to Nick. Is there any way I can reach him?"

"He's *not* in the best of moods," Harlan said. "Raced outta here like he had a ferret playing tag up his ass."

"Tell him to call me as soon as he gets back."

"Will do."

He'd got out of his apartment, left them all standing there, and now he was completely alone.

Behind the wheel of his small plane Nick felt a glorious freedom. There was something about being alone, totally un-surrounded by people – a rarity for him. Oh, sure, he had his retreats, but one by one they got discovered. The *National Enquirer* had the number of his beach house. Every fan in town knew where he lived. Most of his business acquaintances had somehow or other gotten hold of his private phone number.

Now he was totally cut off from everything and everyone, and it was a wonderful feeling.

Flying was something he'd never imagined himself doing. He'd taken it up because of some macho bet with an old actor who'd appeared in one of his movies. Now he enjoyed it better than anything.

Colour me dead.

It was a tempting thought. He could fly this little mother right into the fucking ocean and vanish forever. The ultimate thrill. No more hassles. No more fame. Because the fame was suffocating the life out of him. And there was nothing that made him happy any more . . . except Lauren . . .

And what had he done about that situation?

He'd let her get away again. Hadn't even bothered to pursue her.

"Call me when you're free," he'd said. And four years had passed.

She was never going to leave Oliver. She'd stay with him until he dropped.

Well, shit, he couldn't take it any more.

On a sudden impulse he turned his plane around and headed back to base.

Reece thought about Cyndra, he thought about her a lot. Damn, she looked hot – a real juicy piece. He'd been right about her

556

all along. Cyndra was a star – and only because he'd had the foresight to pay for her singing lessons and the rest. The truth was that he'd discovered her before anyone. He was the one that deserved all the credit. Goddamn it! He'd even introduced her to Reno Records. They owed him plenty, too. They should all be sucking his dick.

He was bored in his hotel room, there was no way he was sitting there waiting to hear from Marik. He had five hundred dollars. The idea was to go out and spend it.

He got in his car and drove down Sunset, cutting up La Brea to Hollywood Boulevard. A sign caught his eye. *Naked Live Beauties. Topless, Bottomless, Big Bare Babes.*

He parked his car, went inside and got himself a seat at the bar where he watched a long-legged dyed blonde bump and grind as she removed strips of black leather from her sinewy person.

He beckoned her over with a twenty dollar bill.

"Come here, doll. Get that sexy ass over here."

She edged closer to the side of the bar – which doubled as the stage.

He folded the bill into a thin strip.

She squatted down, and he inserted the money into her G-string, grabbing a quick feel at the same time.

"Later," she hissed. "It'll cost you more than twenty."

He was insulted. He'd only ever paid for it once, and that was the day he got out of jail. But still, paying for it wasn't such a bad thing. At least you knew where you were.

He winked at her. She winked back. As far as he was concerned they had an agreement.

After coffee on her terrace Lauren went inside and finished off packing. Lorenzo had wanted to come round, but she'd put him off.

"What are you doing tonight?" he'd asked.

"Staying home."

He'd sighed. "Lauren, Lauren – one more night on the town before you fade into retirement, please, I beg you."

"Well . . . maybe."

Going to dinner with Lorenzo was a temptation she didn't need. She'd accustomed herself to the life she had now. No sex.

What are you, a nun, Roberts?

No, but I have the strength of character not to play around on my husband.

Oh, get off your soapbox.

At two o'clock her phone rang again. If it was Lorenzo she decided to tell him that she wouldn't have dinner with him after all. Why tempt fate?

"Hey, Lauren."

She held her breath for a moment. "Who's this?" she asked, although of course she knew immediately who it was.

"Nick."

"Nick," she repeated, dumbly.

"It's been a long time. How are you?"

"I'm leaving in a couple of days," she said, quickly. "Oliver and I are moving to France."

"I want to see you."

"It's not possible."

"Lauren, it's my birthday. Remember old times? You always looked after me on my birthday."

"You know what happens every time we see each other, Nick," she said, weakly.

"Five minutes of your time, that's all I need."

"For what?"

"You can't spare me five minutes on my birthday?"

"Oh, Nick, come on, this is ridiculous."

"Be downstairs in half an hour; I'm on my way."

Before she could say anything he hung up.

She paced around the apartment undecided about what to do. Then she realized that since there was obviously no stopping him she'd better see him.

You don't have to.

Oh yes I do!

She felt totally wired as she ran into her bedroom, stripping off the boring silk shirt and skirt she had on, and reaching for her favourite faded jeans and a familiar sweatshirt – it wouldn't do to look like she'd tried. Then she brushed her hair, added soft shadow around her eyes and a blusher to her cheeks. She stared quickly at her reflection. Talk about glowing. She looked alive for the first time in a long while.

Here we go again.

She put on tennis shoes, grabbed her Oliver Peoples shades and ran downstairs.

"Do you need a cab, Mrs Liberty?" the doorman asked.

"No, no, that's okay," she said.

"It's cold out," he said.

"It's not that cold. The sun's shining."

"If you're going for a walk you'll need a coat."

"I'm not walking, Dave, somebody's picking me up. I'll only be out for five minutes."

What was she explaining herself to the doorman for?

"Oh, by the way, Mrs Liberty," he said, handing her an envelope. "I was supposed to give you this letter today. Mr Liberty left it for you. I was about to bring it up to your apartment when you came down. Saved me a trip."

She glanced at the envelope and recognized Oliver's handwriting. Quickly she opened the letter and read it.

My dear Lauren,

I have known for some time now that you are not completely happy. The truth is – neither am I. I feel that both of us are compromising our true feelings, and that we would be better off apart. I have never wished to be treated as a burden, and whether you know it or not, that's what our relationship has become. Over the last few months I have become quite close to Peggy during the course of our negotiations on the farmhouse. She is a wonderful woman – nearer to me in age, and quite ready for a settled life. You, my dear, are not. So I arranged with Lorenzo to keep you in New York. It's where you belong.

I am releasing you, Lauren, because I love you, and we will have better lives apart.

Of course, I quite understand –

The letter continued on in the same vein, and she read it filled with mixed emotions. Oliver wanted out! *He* was releasing her!

Oh God!

Free at last!

Free to do whatever she wanted!

The timing was unbelievable. And the best thing was, she didn't have to feel guilty, because he'd found someone else. Pocketing the letter she peered through the glass doors, impatiently waiting, pacing up and down until eventually she saw the Ferrari approaching – red of course.

She rushed outside. It had been four years since she'd seen him, and her heart was in overdrive. He looked a little ragged, but it was still her Nick.

He leapt out of the car. "Hey –"

"You're crazy, you know that?" she said, speaking too fast.

He took her hand. "Get in the car."

"Five minutes," she said, her heart beating wildly.

"Yeah, yeah."

Dave was standing at the entrance staring. He'd suddenly realized it was Nick Angel she was with. Before he could recover she jumped in the car and Nick took off.

"Happy birthday," she said, looking at him sideways.

"You're my present," he said.

"I am, huh?"

"I need to tell you something."

"What?"

"I've waited for you ever since I left Bosewell, and I'm not waiting any longer."

She sighed. "Nick, don't do this to us again."

"Why?"

"Because . . ."

"Listen, Lauren – I love you and you love me. You can't fight it any longer."

For a moment she thought how simple it would be to agree with him, because that's what she really wanted to do. But there was too much he didn't know about her. He didn't know she'd killed his father. He didn't know she'd killed his baby. And if he knew those things he wouldn't want to be with her anyway.

She glanced at her watch. "Your five minutes is up."

"What five minutes?" he said, steering the Ferrari on to the freeway.

"You said five minutes."

"I lied."

"Oh, God, Nick, don't start."

"I'm taking you for a ride in my plane."

"I'm not going in your plane."

"Oh yes you are."

"No way."

"Will you shut up? Just shut up for once."

Why did I let him talk me into this?

Because you wanted him to.

So do like he says – shut up and enjoy it.

She leaned back in her seat and didn't say another word.

Forty-five minutes later they were at the private airstrip. "Come on," he said. "Out."

"I told you, I'm not going in a plane with you."

"Maybe I should knock you out and carry you over my shoulder. What do you think?"

"You're crazy, Nick Angel."

He grinned, so happy to see her. "Yeah, yeah, you told me that before. Shouldn't come as a shock to you."

She knew she should back out, but she was already drawn into the game. She got out of the car and walked with him over to the plane.

"Five minutes," she said, sternly.

"Sure," he said.

She shook her head. "This is the last time I'm going anywhere with you, Nick."

"Hey – never say never."

"Why not?"

"'Cause you could live to regret it."

He took her hand and helped her aboard.

"Five minutes," she repeated.

"Hey – whatever you say."

Chapter 86

"How much do you think he wants?" Cyndra asked.

"It's not the money," Marik responded. "It's what he can do to us."

"What do you mean?" she said, fearfully.

"Think about it," Marik said, sounding calmer than he felt. "Over the last few years you've had massive national publicity. You've been on all the shows talking about pride and strength and women not allowing themselves to be abused. How do you think it'll look if Reece spills his guts?"

"Where's he staying?" she said, thinking about how she could put a stop to Reece Webster once and for all.

"Our driver followed him. He's at the Hyatt on Sunset." Marik peered at her, suspiciously. "Why'd you want to know?"

"Why not?" she said, flatly.

"You're not to try and talk to him," Marik said, warningly. "You're to leave this to me and Gordon."

"What's Gordon got to do with it?"

"We'll need his help," Marik said. "I've already called him, he's coming right over."

"Damn!" she said.

"What?"

"I don't want him involved."

"Cyndra, baby," Marik said, patiently. "This is big-time stuff. We gotta work it out carefully. A pay-off has gotta mean just that. A one time score – no coming back for more. We need Gordon's brain in on this."

"All right," she said, reluctantly. "But I don't want to see him – it's too humiliating. I'm going to bed."

He came over and kissed her. "Don't worry, baby, it'll all be taken care of."

You bet it will, she thought to herself. *By tomorrow morning Reece Webster will be history.*

The sinewy blonde took him back to her apartment, fucked him, then demanded three hundred dollars.

He laughed in her face.

"Pay up, bastard," she said, "or I'll set my boyfriend on you."

"I'm Reece Webster," he said, disdainfully. "That's who I am. Not some dumb john off the street."

"I don't give a cocksucking crap *who* you are," the blonde replied, showing her true vulgarity. "You're payin' an' ain't that the truth."

Reece zipped up his pants, pulled on his boots and reached for his stetson. He'd been threatened by bigger and better than this dumb cooze. "You ain't worth three bucks, let alone three hundred," he sneered.

"I hate cheap cocksuckers," she said.

"And I hate cheap whores," he responded, walking through her front door.

She picked up a heavy glass ashtray and hurled it after him. The jagged edge of the ashtray hit him on the side of the head, making a deep gash in his temple and knocking his stetson to the ground.

"Bitch!" he started to say, reaching up and feeling sticky blood pumping from the cut.

She ran over and slammed the door shut, leaving him out in the hallway.

At least he hadn't paid the whore.

He stooped to pick up his hat and felt dizzy. For a moment he slumped against the wall, his hand holding the wound. Soon his hand was covered with slippery blood.

Better get out before her boyfriend arrives, he thought, feeling quite unsteady on his feet. The goddamn bitch had hurt him. She'd pay for this.

He staggered downstairs, blood dripping on to his jacket, soaking through the material.

Out on the street a woman walking past took one look at him and quickly shrank away.

Christ! What was going on? He hardly had the strength to walk.

He blinked once, twice, tried to clear his head and remember where he'd parked his car.

The street light reflected an eerie shadow. He sat down on the kerb, putting his head in his blood-soaked hands. Nausea overcame him and he threw up.

563

Goddamn it, better get to his car and get out of here.

Cyndra crept into Topaz's room and watched her baby sleeping. The little girl was so cute. She had a snub nose, wide eyes and Marik's tight curly hair.

Carefully Cyndra extracted her thumb from her mouth. "No buck teeth, Topaz," she whispered, softly. "Gotta think beautiful."

Back in her own bedroom she went to her closet and changed into a black track suit. Then she pulled her hair severely back, covering it with a squashy Garbo type hat. Large sunglasses completed her disguise. Unrecognizable, she thought. As Cyndra, her public image was cascades of long dark hair, shimmering gowns and provocative make-up.

Reece Webster was threatening her future. Marik thought money would solve the problem. Cyndra knew it wouldn't.

She reached for her purse, checked that the small pearl handled revolver was loaded and in place, and slipped quietly down the back stairway into the garage.

Reece slumped behind the wheel of his car. He was lucky to have made it. He had a headache from hell and blood was still pumping from his wound. Ripping off his jacket he held it to his head and started the engine.

One hand on the wheel and one hand holding his head, he set off towards his hotel.

Cyndra took the nanny's station wagon – best not to call attention to herself with her Rolls or Marik's Jaguar. She locked the doors – second nature for a woman driving alone in LA – and drove down the hill.

The car was weaving. Reece felt it swaying this way and that – he couldn't seem to control it. All he had to do was get back to the hotel, put a dressing on his head and lie down. He'd be fine after a rest.

It occurred to him that maybe he needed to go to the Emergency Room – but those places were always filled with the lowest of the low – gunshot wounds, stabbings, heart attacks and worse. Who needed it? Besides, he should be at the hotel in case Marik phoned. Didn't want to miss the deal of the century.

Three million bucks. That's what he'd decided to ask for. And cheap at the price.

The sound of a blaring horn almost made him swerve off the road. Bastards! Why didn't people concentrate on their driving instead of hassling him?

He saw the hotel in the distance and slowed down.

More blaring horns.

Goddamn it, people didn't know how to behave any more.

Cyndra decided against valet parking. She found a space on the street and left the station wagon, locking the doors with a remote control.

Bump! Big bump!

Fuck, someone hit him. What did he care, it wasn't his car, only a rental.

Christ, his head was getting ready to explode. Was he at the hotel yet? Must be. He could hear noise, confusion. Leaning on the steering wheel he closed his eyes while blood dripped steadily on to his new cowboy boots.

There was something going on outside the hotel. Cyndra hurried along the street glancing over as she approached the entrance. A car had crossed over to the wrong lane and smashed into two other cars. The hotel doorman was running over to investigate.

A figure in the offending car was slumped over the driving wheel, his weight on the horn which let out an incessant noise.

She covered her ears and was just about to detour by when she realized the yellow car – a Chevrolet – looked awfully familiar. In fact it was the same car Reece Webster had been driving when he'd followed her limo up her driveway.

She stopped, watching – while the doorman – assisted by two other people – opened up the door and extracted the driver.

"He's dead," she heard one of them say. "Looks like he bled to death."

She edged closer for a better look as they laid the figure on the ground. No mistaking those cowboy boots. Reece Webster was certainly dead.

"Thank you, God," she whispered, and quietly made her way back to her car.

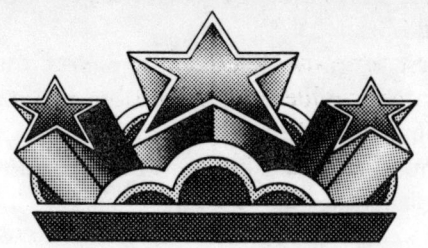

Chapter 87

"I didn't know you could fly a plane."

He put it on auto pilot and raised his arms. "Look, Ma, no hands!"

"Very funny," she said, sternly.

"Hey –" he caught her with a green-eyed stare. "Have I told you lately that I love you?"

"Nick –"

"Yeah?"

"Please stop," she begged.

"What? Stop loving you? I'm sorry, but I can't seem to do that."

"I think you can."

"How's that?"

She lowered her eyes. "There's things I've never told you."

"What things?" he asked.

She turned away from him, staring out of the window at the clear blue sky, determined to be truthful so there could finally be an end to this.

"Nick," she said, hesitantly. "When you left Bosewell, I was . . . I was pregnant with our baby."

"Oh Jesus, Lauren, I had no idea –"

"I know you didn't." She hesitated before carrying on. "I went to the trailer park to tell you – I guess it was the day after you left. Your father was there –"

"Yes?" He had a feeling he wasn't going to like what he was about to hear.

"He . . . he tried to attack me," she continued. "I stabbed him – then the tornado came and I don't remember anything else. When I woke up I was on the grass and the trailer was gone. The town was in chaos – my parents were both victims. I was sent to live in Philadelphia with relatives. Shortly after I arrived they made me have an abortion." Her eyes filled with tears. "Nick – they made me kill our child."

It was the first time she'd spoken of any of this and the relief was overwhelming. Suddenly it wasn't her secret any more – the burden was not hers alone.

"I didn't know," he said. "If I'd known I'd never have left. We would have worked it out somehow – Jesus, Lauren – I don't know what to say except that I love you. I always have and I always will. I'm sorry for what happened. I'm sorry I wasn't there with you, and for everything you had to go through without me."

All these years she'd expected him to be angry, to blame her for what had happened. Now he was the one that was sorry.

"I murdered our baby, Nick," she cried out, in case he hadn't understood.

"Come here, sweetheart," he said, taking her in his arms. "You had no choice. You were a kid – we both were. You did what you had to do – so stop blaming yourself."

It felt so good in his arms. She was at peace. It was as if she belonged there.

"As for Primo," he said, holding her tight. "You didn't kill him – he died of head injuries. It's public record".

"It is?"

"Yup. I had it checked out."

"All these years I thought I'd killed him."

"Why didn't you tell me this before?"

"Because . . ."

"Because what?"

"I don't know."

"You're crazy. And I love you."

"Nick," she said hesitantly, feeling like a kid again.

"Yes?"

"I love you, too."

He grinned. "So what are we going to do about it?"

"We're going to be together."

"We are?"

"Yes," she said, filled with a sudden strength and determination. "Forever."

"Fasten your seatbelt," he said, relinquishing his hold and concentrating on piloting the plane. "We're preparing to land."

"Where are we?" she asked.

"Canada."

"*Canada?*"

"I figured I had to take you somewhere remote – where nobody can bother us – not unless we want them to. There's this little log cabin –"

"How did you arrange it? And how did you know I'd come with you?"

"Hey – it's my birthday."

She smiled, softly. "Happy birthday, Nick."

"Thank you, Lauren."

They stared into each other's eyes and smiled.

The dream was finally coming true.

They were together and they both knew without a doubt that this time nothing would ever split them apart again.